Saunders Comprehensive Veterinary Dictionary

2nd Edition

Saunders Comprehensive Veterinary Dictionary

2nd Edition

D. C. Blood OBE

BVSc HonDVSc FACVSc HonLLD HonAssRCVS
Emeritus Professor, School of Veterinary Science,
University of Melbourne, Victoria, Australia

& V. P. Studdert

BS DVM
Professor of Veterinary Clinical Sciences, School of Veterinary Science,
University of Melbourne, Victoria, Australia

Anatomical Tables by

John Grandage

B VetMed MRCVS DVR

WB Saunders

EDINBURGH LONDON NEW YORK OXFORD
ST LOUIS SYDNEY TORONTO 19

WB SAUNDERS
An imprint of Elsevier Limited

First Edition 1988
Second Edition 1999

Paperback ISBN 0 7020 2034 6
Reprinted 1999, 2000 (twice), 2001, 2003 (twice), 2004, 2005
Hardback ISBN 0 7020 2442 2
Reprinted 2000, 2002 (twice), 2003, 2004, 2005

British Library Cataloguing in Publication Data
A catalogue record for this book is available from the British Library

Library of Congress Cataloging in Publication Data
A catalog record for this book is available from the Library of Congress

Medical knowledge is constantly changing. As new information becomes available, changes in treatment, procedures, equipment and the use of drugs become necessary. The editor, advisers and the publishers have taken care to ensure that the information given in this text is accurate and up to date. However, readers are strongly advised to confirm that the information, especially with regard to drug usage, complies with the latest legislation and standards of practice.

Commissioning Editor: Catriona Byres
Development Editor and Project Supervisor: Tim Kimber

The Publishers and authors have made every effort to trace the copyright holders for borrowed material. If they have inadvertently overlooked any, they will be pleased to rectify the matter at the first opportunity.

ta system by Compulexis Ltd, Oxford
hotosetting, Charham, Kent

The Publisher's policy is to use **paper manufactured from sustainable forests**

Contents

Contents

Consultants

Douglas C Blood OBE BVSc FACVSc HonLLD HonAssRCVS. Emeritus Professor, School of Veterinary Science, University of Melbourne, Victoria, Australia

Virginia P Studdert BS DVM. Professor of Veterinary Clinical Sciences, School of Veterinary Science, University of Melbourne, Victoria, Australia

Ian Beveridge DVSc PhD. Reader in Parasitology, School of Veterinary Science, University of Melbourne, Victoria, Australia

Pauline Brightling MVSc BAnimSci BVSc. Senior Lecturer in Veterinary Medicine, School of Veterinary Science, University of Melbourne, Victoria, Australia

Kathleen Brock BVSc MS DipACVA MACVSc. Previously Lecturer in Veterinary Anesthesiology, School of Veterinary Science, University of Melbourne, Victoria, Australia

Glenn F Browning BVSc DipVetClinStud PhD. Reader in Veterinary Microbiology School of Veterinary Science, University of Melbourne, Victoria, Australia

Robert M Cannon MSc. Biometrician, Bureau of Rural Science, Department of Primary Industries and Energy, Canberra ACT, Australia

Colin B Chapman, BPharm BVSc PhD. Professor of Pharmacology, Victorian College of Pharmacy, Monash University, Victoria Australia

Bruce Christie BVSc MVSc MACVSc DiplomatACVS. Senior Associate in Veterinary Surgery, School of Veterinary Science, University of Melbourne, Victoria, Australia

Nick Costa BAgSci PhD. Associate Professor, Biochemistry and Nutrition, School of Veterinary Studies, Murdoch University, West Australia, Australia

David B Galloway BVSc VMD FRCVS MACVSc. Previously Associate Professor in Animal Reproduction, School of Veterinary Science, University of Melbourne, Victoria, Australia

Robin Gasser BVSc Drmedvet PhD. Reader in Veterinary Parasitology, School of Veterinary Science, University of Melbourne, Victoria, Australia

John Grandage BVetMed MA MRCVS DVR. Fellow, St Catharine's College, Cambridge, Clinical Veterinary Anatomist, Department of Anatomy, Cambridge University UK

Trevor Heath BVSc MA PhD FACVSc FAIBiol. Professor of Veterinary Anatomy School of Veterinary Science, University of Queensland, Queensland, Australia

Ross A Mckenzie BVSc MVSc DVSc. Principal Veterinary Pathol… Department of Primary Industries, Animal Research Institute… Senior Lecturer Veterinary Toxicology, University of Quee… Australia

Deborah Joan Middleton MVSc PhD DipVetClinStud. Senior L… Pathology, School of Veterinary Science, University of Melbourn…

Consultants

Russell W Mitten BVSc DVR DipACVR. Senior Lecturer in Veterinary Medicine, School of Veterinary Science, University of Melbourne, Victoria, Australia

Barry Munday DVSc MACVSc. Reader in Aquaculture, Department of Aquaculture, University of Tasmania, Tasmania, Australia

Michael J. Studdert BVSc MVSc PhD DVSc MACVSc FASM. Professor of Veterinary Virology, Director, Center for Equine Virology, School of Veterinary Science, University of Melbourne, Victoria, Australia

Andrew L Vizard BVSc MPVM. Associate Professor in Veterinary Epidemiology, School of Veterinary Science, University of Melbourne, Victoria, Australia

Preface to the Second Edition

After ten years of the first edition there were enough new words, especially in biochemistry, molecular biology and immunology, to justify a new edition of the dictionary. The challenge was to include all the new material which fitted our criteria and to delete the words which no longer had currency in modern veterinary medicine, without increasing the number of entries unnecessarily. The number of entries has been increased from 55,000 to 65,000 and the number of tables is now increased by five to 23.

The objective of the dictionary is unchanged—to include all the veterinary technical and scientific words and phrases which veterinary undergraduates might encounter in their university courses. This has been its most successful function, to provide a professional vocabulary for veterinary students on their first day at university and for their entire stay. Part of this success is due to the composition of the individual entries. For the most part they go beyond just defining the word or phrase, and give a supplementary description of the structure or function of the pathogen or the disease.

Our sources have again been the standard textbooks for the various subjects, but the selection of words to be included has been made more difficult because of the enormous expansion of the textbook list during the past few years; there were many more books to consult. That disadvantage was offset by the generally great improvement in the quality and coverage of the books.

For the definition of entries outside the competence of the authors we depended again on the assistance of consultants, eighteen for this edition, compared to eight for the first edition. To a large extent the need for this expansion of the contributor list has been the increased complexity and sophistication of the veterinary knowledge base. There has also been a determination on the part of the authors to increase the depth of the information provided in such subjects as histology, embryology, genetics, molecular biology and immunology. No fields of veterinary endeavor have been deleted from the list but fish health, in response to the dramatic increase in fish culture for human food production, acupuncture, ultrasound imagery, endoscopy and mycology are now specified items. We owe a great deal to the consultants for their assistance, in most cases as an added burden to an already overburdened university teacher.

We commented in the first edition on the difficulty of devising a policy which would best establish the alphabetical location of each word or expression in the text, a problem greatly magnified by the large number of expressions which contain more than one word; the problem being to alphabetize on the first or second, or even the third word. To alphabetize on both words, with a cross-reference between them would greatly increase the size of the book. Because the problem has not been resolved we have retreated to the compromise of the first edition. 'When there is a c
at the point where common use will dictate that the reader will lo
add the admonition 'If the phrase is not found at the location of yo
sure you search at the alternate location.'

In our continuing effort to keep apace with the veterinary vocab
be expected to emails addressed to doug@melbpc.org.au contai

relevant to the scope of the dictionary but are not included in it. Please set the words in the context in which they are observed.

Our sincere thanks are due to Tim Kimber and Catriona Byres of the WB Saunders editorial staff for advice and support, and to Robert Branton and the staff at Compulexis Ltd for indefatigable computer back-up at any hour and on any day.

Douglas Blood

Virginia Studdert

Notes on the Use of this Dictionary

This book is a compilation of terms, alphabetically arranged, together with their definitions. In order to economize on space, and to facilitate word searches, a number of conventions have been adopted. These are summarized below.

Terms within this Dictionary are located either as main entries, which are printed in **bold type** (see Section 1 below) or as sub-entries printed in smaller **bold type**, which occur after the main entry and its definition (see Section 2 below).

1 MAIN ENTRIES

The main entries of this Dictionary occur as single words, hyphenated words or two or more words separated by spaces. They are alphabetized as follows:

1.1 Single words: single words, acronyms and abbreviations are alphabetized letter by letter, with capital letters coming *before* lower-case letters. For example:

PT
Pt
pt
PTA
ptarmic

REM
rem
remedy

1.2 Multiple words: main entries of more than one word which are separated by spaces, hyphens or dashes are alphabetized according to the first word and then (if needed) according to the second word (or other subsequent words). For example:

heart
heart-base tumour
heart block
heart failure
heart-lung unit
heart sounds
heartbeat

thin
thin ewe syndrome
thin-shelled egg
thin sow syndrome
thinness

(see also Section 1.3 below.)

However, where the hyphen simply separates two identical vowels, the word is treated as though it were a single word without a hyphen. For example:

intra-
intra vitam
intra-abdominal
intra-aortic
intra-arterial
intra-articular
intracanalicular

cricoarytenoid
cricoid
cricoidectomy
cricolaryngotomy
crico-esophageal
cricopharyngeal

1.3 Compound terms: when a term is composed of two or more words, it will usually be found under more than one of the words, although discretion has been used to avoid unnecessary repetition of the definition. For example, benign prostatic hyperplasia is found under both **benign** and **prostatic**, but the main definition is found under **prostatic** (with appropriate cross-referencing). Similarly, feline sarcoma virus is found under both **feline** and **sarcoma**, but the main definition is found under **feline**, with appropriate cross-referencing (see Section 3 for an outline of cross-referer

1.4 Combining forms (word elements): prefixes and suffixes are listed alphabetically, including any characters in parentheses. For example:

cheilitis
cheil(o)-
cheilognathopalatoschisis
cheilognathoschisis

macrencephalia
macro
macr(o)-
macroamylase

1.5 Terms with unusual characters: certain characters of the main entry are ignored in the alphabetization, i.e. Greek letters, numbers, small capital characters and subscript/superscript characters. For example:

aminophylline
β-aminopropionitrile
aminopterin
4-aminopyridine
aminopyrine
4-aminoquinoline
aminosalicylic acid
ρ-aminosalicylic acid
aminosidine

glutamine
β-(γ-L-glutamyl) aminopropionitrile
L-glutamyl-β-cyanoalanine
γ-glutamyl cycle
γ-glutamyl transferase
γ-glutamyl transpeptidase
glutaral

1.6 Eponyms/possessive terms: where the suffix *'s* occurs, it is ignored in the alphabetization. For example:

Crustaceae
Cushing's disease
Cushing-like disease
Cushing suture pattern
Cushing's syndrome
cushingoid

sal
Sala's cells
salamander

1.7 Mc/Mac and St./Saint terms: entries beginning with Mc- are listed as if they were spelled Mac-. Similarly, those beginning St. (for Saint) are listed as if they were spelled Saint.

1.8 Homographs, i.e. words that have the same spelling but have different *etymological derivations* are designated as separate main entries with superscript bold numbers. For example:

lead[1] a chemical element, atomic number 82, ...
lead[2] 1. ... electrodes. 2. ... to facilitate walking a dog.

Not to be confused with different *definitions* of the same word! For example, in the second of the two examples above, there are two different (numbered) definitions. Another example is:

film 1. a thin layer or coating. 2. a thin sheet of material (e.g. gelatin, cellulose acetate) specially treated for use in photography or radiography; ...

2 SUB-ENTRIES

The term being sought may be a main entry or a sub-entry under the main entry. In general, the word will be a sub-entry if it has a common area of interest with the main entry. The sub-entries are listed alphabetically under the main entry, with the initial letter(s) of the main entry repeated. For example:

chylous
  c. ascites
  c. hydrothorax
  c. peritonitis

skim milk
  s. m. extender
  s. m. powder

enterocolitis
  antibiotic-associated e.
  hemorrhagic e.
  pseudomembranous e.

The alphabetization of sub-entries *ignores* the repeated main entry (and such words as *a, and, in, of, on, the, to,* etc.). For example:

organ
o. of Corti
effector o.
enamel o.
genital o.
Golgi tendon o.
gustus o.
o. of Jacobson
ocular o.

tendon
bowed t.
calcaneal t.
congenital t. contracture
contracted t's
t. contracture
cunean t.

Occasionally, the repeated main entry is spelt out in full when needed. For example, when the irregular plural form is referred to:

linea
l. aspera
lineae atrophicae

macula
maculae acusticae
m. atrophica

3 CROSS-REFERENCING

Throughout the Dictionary, cross-references are given within the text as SMALL CAPITALS.

When two or several entries have the same meaning (synonyms), we have placed the definition under the most commonly used and best understood term in our judgment. At the alternative entry(ies), a cross-reference is given. They appear as 'see'. For example:

sand rat see GERBIL.

rat-tail syndrome see SARCOCYSTOSIS.

auricular ...
a. mange infestation with ear mites. See OTODECTIC MANGE.

gerbil mouse or rat-like, nocturnal creature, sand-coloured on top, ...

sarcocystosis a rare clinical disease in all food animal species caused by the intermediate stage of the protozoan parasite *Sarcocystis* spp.

otodectic mange the ear and the skin disease caused by infestation with *Otodectes cynotis*.

There are also situations where it is simply more convenient to define the word in a different location, to which the reader is then referred.

In some instances it is appropriate to direct the reader to definitions other than that specifically sought. These cross-references are supportive in that they provide ancillary information to the basic definition and act as a cue to consult the related entry. For example:

REM rapid eye movement. See also SLEEP.

Thea chinensis one of the few plants that absorbs fluorine ... See also CAMELLIA, which is much more toxic.

uncinariasis the disease caused by UNCINARIA in cats and dogs. Similar to, but less severe than ANCYCLOSTOMIASIS, with only mild bloodloss and enteritis.

Cross-references are either to main entries (see the examples above) or to sub-entries. In the latter case, only the main entry word(s) appears as small capitals. For example:

wall ...
abdominal w. see ABDOMINAL wall.

abdominal ...
a. tunic see TUNICA flava abdominis.

galactocerebrosidosis see globoid cell LEUKODYSTROPHY.

tympanic ...
t. plexus see tympanic PLEXUS.

abdominal ...
a. wall consists of the parietal peritoneum, ...

tunica ...
t. flava abdominis an extensive sheet of elastic tissue that helps to support the abdomen.

leukodystrophy ...
globoid cell l. an inherited lysosomal storage disease of polled Dorset sheep, cats and dogs, ...

plexus ...
tympanic p. a network of nerve fibres supplying the mucous lining of the tympanum and auditory tube.

4 ALTERNATIVE FORMS

In many entries, alternative spellings or terms are given as part of the definition. (These variant terms may or may not be entries elsewhere in the dictionary.) They are indicated by 'called also'. For example:

paraffin ... Called also alkane, kerosene, lamp oil.

shell rot softening and ulceration of the carapace and plastron of softshell turtles ... Called also rust, ulcerative shell disease.

5 ADJECTIVAL FORMS

Adjectives are indicated in **bold type** immediately following the abbreviation adj. For example:

fetus [L.] the developing young in the uterus, ... adj. **fetal.**

rectum the distal portion of the large intestine ... adj. **rectal.**

6 IRREGULAR PLURALS

Where a noun takes an irregular plural, this is indicated in *italic type* immediately following the abbreviation pl. For example:

fistula pl. *fistulae, fistulas;* any abnormal, tubelike passage ...

imago pl. *imagoes, imagines* [L.] the adult or definitive form of an insect.

7 TRANSLATIONS

Where a translation of a foreign term occurs, it is indicated in *italic type* immediately following the abbreviation for the language (which is in square brackets). For example:

hydrargyrum [L.] *mercury* (symbol Hg).

-iasis word element. [Gr.] *condition, state.*

8 ABBREVIATIONS USED IN THIS DICTIONARY

adj.	adjective	pl.	plural
Af.	Afrikaans	Scand.	Scandinavian
Ar.	Arabic	Span.	Spanish
Fr.	French	spp.	species
Ger.	German	St.	Saint
Gr.	Greek	syn.	synonym
L.	Latin		

9 TABLES

All tabular material is presented as an Appendix at the end of the Dictionary.

10 DRUG NAMES

Where possible, only generic names are used.

A

A accommodation; adenine; ampere; anode (anodal); anterior; axial; mass number.

A_2 aortic second sound (see HEART SOUNDS).

A_w water activity. Relative to food for human consumption it is an indication of the amount of water available in the food as a substrate for bacterial growth. An A_w of 1 means pure water and no chance of bacterial growth.

Å angstrom.

a- word element. [L.] *without, not.*

(A-a) *Po_2* alveolar–arterial oxygen tension difference.

A fibers nerve fibers in nerve trunks and peripheral nerves which have the fastest rate of transmission of nervous impulses.

A-mode amplitude mode. See A-mode ULTRASONOGRAPHY.

A–R–F sequence remodeling sequence of bone cell activity; means activation–resorption–formation.

A site see aminoacyl-TRNA binding site.

āā [Gr.] *ana* (of each), in prescriptions.

aa. pl. *arteriae* [L.] arteries.

AA protein a product of α-globulin and the major protein component of reactive amyloid.

AAFCO American Association of Feed Control Officials.

aalveld poisoning by the plant *Narthecium ossifragum* characterized by a crystal-associated cholangiohepatopathy.

Aanes' method surgical reconstruction after a third-degree perineal laceration in the mare. There are two stages: the first operation constructs a shelf between the rectum and the vagina, the second reconstructs the perineal body.

aardvark the only living member of the order Tubulidentata. It is a 100 to 150 lb, 5 to 7 ft long animal with a long snout, a massive body, spadelike claws and a short, sparse haircoat. They are gray-brown in color, nocturnal in habit, live in burrows and exist mainly on a diet of ants. Called also earth pig, *Orycteropus afer.*

aardwolf member of the family Hyaenidae. Resembles a striped hyena; lives in an earth and feeds on termites, carrion and small wildlife. Called also *Proteles cristatus.*

AAUAAA sequence see POLYADENYLATION.

Ab antibody. Called also gamma globulin (γ). See IMMUNOGLOBULIN.

ab [L.] preposition, *from.*

ab- word element. [L.] *from, off, away from.*

abalone HALIOTIS.

abamectin a mixture of avermectins derived from STREPTOMYCES *avermitilis.*

abandoned patient a hospital patient whose owner cannot be located or is unwilling to take the patient away.

abarthrosis abarticulation.

abarticular not affecting a joint; away from a joint.

abarticulation 1. synovial joint. 2. a dislocation.

abasia inability to walk.
a.–astasia astasia–abasia.
a. atactica abasia with uncertain movements, due to a defect of coordination.
choreic a. abasia due to chorea of the limbs.
paralytic a. abasia due to paralysis.
paroxysmal trepidant a. abasia due to spastic stiffening of the limbs on attempting to stand. Called also spastic abasia.
spastic a. see paroxysmal trepidant abasia (above).
trembling a., a. trepidans abasia due to trembling of the limbs.

abattoir a building for the slaughter of animals for human food. It may vary in size and sophistication depending on location and local government ordinance but it should contain the following facilities or have them close by: a slaughter area, an area for emergency slaughter, refrigeration area, condemned meat area and space for holding suspect meat, offal, gut and tripe area, hide and skin area, cutting room, despatch area, amenities for personnel, a veterinary officer's room, preferably including a laboratory, and accommodation for animals awaiting slaughter, called lairage. Called also slaughterhouse, meat packing plant.
a. fever see Q FEVER.

abaxial situated away from the axis of the body, limb or part.

abbokinase see UROKINASE.

Abbreviata a genus of nematodes in the subfamily Physalopterinae, parasites of reptiles (especially saurians) or more rarely in amphibians and primates.

ABC aspiration biopsy cytology.

abdomen the portion of the body between the thorax and the pelvis containing the abdominal cavity. See also ABDOMINAL.
acute a. an acute intra-abdominal condition of abrupt onset, usually associated with pain due to inflammation, perforation, obstruction, infarction or rupture of abdominal organs, and usually requiring emergency intervention. Called also surgical abdomen.
gaunt a. decreased abdominal size.
surgical a. see acute abdomen (above).

abdominal pertaining to, affecting or originating in the abdomen. See also abdominal PARACENTESIS, ABDOMINAL SOUNDS.
a. binding a wide bandage applied to the abdomen to raise intra-abdominal pressure. Its primary purposes are (1) to limit the displacement of the diaphragm during thoracic compression of cardiopulmonary resuscitation, thereby raising intrathoracic pressures achieved and improving forward blood flow, and (2) to maintain blood volume in the central circulation during hemorrhagic shock.
a. breathing an abnormal form of respiratory movement in which the thorax is fixed and the inspiratory and expiratory movement of the lungs are carried out by the diaphragm and the abdominal muscles so that there are exaggerated movements of the abdominal wall.
a. cavity the body cavity between the
the pelvis; contains the a
a. enlargement may
(transudate, exudate or
cera (neoplasia, dilatatio
logical phenomena, e.g. p
masses or fat. Weakness
ally results in a pendu
abdomen.
a. lavage see abdominal

a. muscle ischemia an unexplained ischemic necrosis of the internal oblique muscle of ewes in late pregnancy which are carrying twins or triplets. Results in ventral hernia but often with little apparent effect on the ease of lambing.

a. muscles the paired muscles of the flank and belly that surround and support the abdominal viscera.

a. pad see abdominal PAD.

a. pain may arise from an abdominal organ, the peritoneum or be referred as from spinal nerves.

a. regions arbitrary, descriptive subdivisions of the abdomen made up of three groups of three (like a noughts-and-crosses grid), three along the middle—xiphoid, umbilical and pubic, and three lateral pairs—hypochondriac, lateral abdominal and inguinal.

a. silhouette the shape of the abdomen viewed from behind.

a. trier see TRIER.

a. tunic see TUNICA flava abdominis.

a. viscera the organs contained within the abdominal cavity; they include the stomach, intestines, liver, spleen, pancreas, and parts of the urinary and reproductive tracts.

a. wall consists of the parietal peritoneum, the deep and superficial layers of fascia, the transverse abdominal, internal and external abdominal oblique muscles, the subcutaneous tissue and the skin. It contains the umbilicus, the cicatrix marking the entry point of the umbilical cord, and is traversed by the inguinal canal, and at its caudal extremity carries the prepubic tendon, the ventral attachment of the wall to the pubic bones.

a. wall rigidity reflex response to pain of peritonitis, accompanied by pain on palpation or percussion.

abdominal sounds sounds heard on auscultation of the abdomen. In horses gastric and small intestinal sounds are not sufficiently identifiable to be of clinical value. Absence of ileocecal valve, cecal and colonic sounds indicates paralytic ileus, increased sounds indicate enteritis or spasmodic colic. In ruminants only reticuloruminal sounds are of value as diagnostic aids; their absence suggests atony, hyperactivity indicates chronic distension. Muffling of normal sounds suggests the presence of obstructing material especially fluid. See also abdominal AUSCULTATION.

abdomin(o)- word element, *abdomen*.

abdominocentesis paracentesis of the abdomen. See also abdominal PARACENTESIS.

abdominocystic pertaining to the abdomen and gallbladder.

abdominohysterotomy hysterotomy through an abdominal incision.

abdominoparacentesis abdominocentesis.

abdominopelvic pertaining to the abdominal and pelvic cavities.

abdominoperineal pertaining to the abdomen and the perineum.

abdominoscopy examination of the abdomen with an endoscopic instrument inserted through the abdominal wall.

abdominovaginal pertaining to the abdomen and vagina.

abduce to abduct, or draw away.

[illegible]ducens [L.] *drawing away*.

[illegible] nerve see ABDUCENT nerve, and Table 14.

[illegible]ent abducting.

[illegible]**e** the sixth cranial nerve; it arises from the [illegible] supplies the lateral rectus and retractor [illegible]les of the eyeball, allowing for motion. Paralysis of the nerve causes a medial strabismus and absence of third eyelid protrusion when the corneal reflex is tested. See also Table 14.

abduct to draw away from an axis or the median plane.

abduction the act of abducting; the state of being abducted. For a digit, the drawing away from the axis of the limb.

abductor that which abducts.

Aberdeen Angus a black, polled breed of beef cattle. Known inherited defects in the breed include MANNOSIDOSIS, DWARFISM and inherited spastic PARESIS.

aberrant pigment metabolism see inherited PORPHYRIA.

aberratio [L.] *aberration*.

aberration 1. deviation from the normal or usual. 2. imperfect refraction or focalization of a lens, e.g. the lens of the eye.

chromatic a. inability to focus a pencil of light through a lens because of the different refrangibilities of the colored constituents of white light. In an optical instrument such as a microscope this represents an error in the lens system.

spherical a. that due to failure of a spherical mirror to focus all the light rays at one point; a fault of construction in an optical instrument.

Abildgaard method named after P.C. Abildgaard, a Danish veterinarian; a method of casting horses and cattle. The horse method is a combination of sidelines and hobbles in which all four feet are included in a rope and harness system which brings all four hooves up to the belly. The cattle method is also one in which all four hooves are trapped and pulled together, but they are not brought up to the midline. The harness is made entirely of rope.

abiosis absence or deficiency of life.

abiotrophic disease see ABIOTROPHY.

abiotrophy premature progressive loss of vitality of certain tissues or organs, usually of the nervous system, leading to disorders or loss of function; applied especially to degenerative hereditary nervous system diseases of postnatal onset.

cochlear a. an inherited degeneration of the cochlear duct of dogs causing deafness which becomes evident after several weeks of age.

hereditary neuronal a. of Swedish Lapland dogs an autosomal recessive trait with lower motor neuron abiotrophy causing arthrogryposis, tetraplegia and muscle atrophy from 5 weeks of age.

spinal cord a. see hereditary neuronal abiotrophy of Swedish Lapland dogs (above).

abirritant 1. diminishing irritation; soothing. 2. an agent that relieves irritation.

abirritation diminished irritability; atony.

ablactation weaning.

ablastin serum antibodies that inhibit protozoan replication.

ablate to remove, especially by cutting.

ablatio [L.] *detachment*.

a. retinae detachment of the retina.

ablation 1. separation or detachment; extirpation; eradication. 2. removal, especially by cutting.

ear canal a. a surgical procedure in which the cartilaginous external ear canal is removed. Indicated in neoplasia of the canal or chronic otitis externa in dogs which are unresponsive to all other forms of treatment.

subconjunctival a. a method of removal or enucleation in which the globe is removed leaving the conjunctiva.

ablepharia congenital reduction or absence of the eyelids.

ablepharon see ABLEPHARIA.
ablepsia blindness.
abluent 1. detergent; cleansing. 2. a cleansing agent.
abnormality 1. the state of being unlike the usual condition. 2. a malformation.
inherited a. a defect of anatomy or function acquired by the patient from its parents by way of inherited material passed through the germ cells from which the patient originated. See also INHERITANCE.
abnutzen pigment see LIPOFUSCIN.
abomasal pertaining to, affecting or originating from the abomasum.
a. anterior displacement syndrome in cattle in which the abomasum is displaced anteriorly to a position between the reticulum and the diaphragm; characterized clinically by anorexia, ketonuria, and absence of abomasal sounds in the right or left flanks as in right or left displacement.
a. atony lack of tone of abomasal wall, thought to be basic cause of displacements and torsion. Possibly due to prolonged feeding on finely ground concentrates.
a. bloat distension of abomasum with gas produced by fermentation of milk in abomasum of young ruminants, especially artificially reared lambs fed large volumes of warm milk infrequently.
a. dilatation see right abomasal displacement (below).
a. displacement see left abomasal displacement, right abomasal displacement (below).
a. emptying defects cause weight loss, anorexia, abdominal distension and grossly enlarged abomasums in sheep.
a. fundus the cranial blind end of the abomasum, lying over the xiphoid process of the sternum and to the right of the reticulum.
a. gastrocentesis cannulation of a distended abomasum, usually through the right flank, to allow evacuation of the distending gas. The technique may be used for diagnostic reasons, but is more commonly used therapeutically to gain temporary relief for the animal before surgery is undertaken.
a. groove the third and last part of the gastric groove of ruminants that occupies the lesser curvature of the abomasum and which is free from mucosal folds. See also gastric GROOVE.
a. impaction a disease of beef cows with large energy requirements, e.g. during very cold weather or when fed poor quality roughage with low energy content and poor digestibility. The abomasum impacts with dry roughage and the abdomen distends on the right; clinical signs are scant feces and emaciation.
left a. displacement chronic disease of recently calved cows characterized by a distended abomasum trapped under the rumen, detectable on the left side, anorexia, acetonemia and abdominal gauntness.
a. perforation may be perforation by erosion through a pre-existing ulcer, or by rupture along the greater curvature due to dilatation. Perforation results in acute or peracute peritonitis; rupture is followed by sudden death. See also abomasal ulcer (below).
a. phytobezoar see PHYTOBEZOAR.
a. reflux the reflux of fluid from the abomasum into the rumen. When flow to the intestine is obstructed, the abdomen distends, serious changes in acid–base balance occur, and there may be regurgitation of fluid from nostrils. See also INTESTINAL obstruction, PYLORIC obstruction.
right a. displacement a disease of recently calved cows characterized by lack of feed intake, persistent acetonemia, distension in the right abdomen and fluid sounds in right flank. May terminate as abomasal torsion.
a. rupture see abomasal perforation (above).
a. torsion a disease of sudden onset in dairy cows, often following a subacute illness due to abomasal dilatation. There is shock, acute abdominal pain, distension of the right abdomen with sounds of fluid present, blood-stained feces and a fatal outcome in 24–48 hours.
a. trichobezoar see TRICHOBEZOAR.
a. tympany see abomasal bloat (above).
a. ulcer many calves have clinically silent ulcers during the period of change from a milk diet to one of fiber. In adult animals the ulcer may be hemorrhagic, with a sudden onset of subacute abdominal pain with alimentary tract stasis and heavily blood-tinged feces, or perforating. See abomasal perforation (above).
a. volvulus the same condition as abomasal torsion (see above) and probably the more accurate name.
abomasitis inflammation of abomasum; occurs as part of many gastroenteritides but seldom diagnosed as a separate condition. The organ's location aboral to the forestomachs provides some protection against dietary insults. See also ABOMASUM.
abomasopexy fixation of the replaced abomasum, after correction of a displacement, by suturing the abomasal wall or its attached omentum to the abdominal wall. See also OMENTOFIXATION.
abomasotomy surgical opening of the abomasum, usually to remove impacted food or foreign material, especially phytobezoars.
abomasum the fourth compartment of the ruminant stomach. It is an elongated sac, comparable in structure and function to the stomach of nonruminants. It lies in the right half of the abdominal cavity, largely on the abdominal floor, except in late pregnancy when it is pushed cranially by the enlarging uterus and may also be lifted from the abdominal floor. See also ABOMASAL.
Abondance cattle French breed of dual-purpose cattle, mostly red, some red on belly and extremities.
aborad away from the mouth; aborally.
aboral away from the mouth.
abort 1. to arrest prematurely a disease or developmental process. 2. to expel the products of conception before the fetus is viable.
abortifacient 1. causing abortion. 2. an agent that induces abortion.
abortion premature expulsion from the uterus of the products of conception; termination of pregnancy before the fetus is viable.
complete a. complete expulsion of all the products of conception.
early a. abortion within the first third of pregnancy.
epizootic bovine a. characterized by serious fetal disease followed by abortion. Occurs only in California, USA. Necropsy findings in the fetus are diagnostic; they include profuse petechiation and severe granulomatous hepatitis. Cause not identified but probably *Chlamydia* spp. Transmitted by the tick, *Ornithodoros coriaceus*.
habitual a. spontaneous abortion occurring in three or more successive pregnancies.
incomplete a. abortion in which parts of the products of conception are retained in the uterus.
induced a. abortion procured by the veterinarian to eliminate a misalliance, to reduce wastage in animals in a feedlot, to encourage commencement of lactation earlier than would otherwise occur. In cattle manipulation through the rectal wall is a possible way

of destroying the viability of the fetus. Induction by the administration of prostaglandins or corticosteroids is more usual. See also PREGNANCY termination.

infectious a. the common causes in the various species are:

CATTLE *Brucella abortus* (brucellosis); *Campylobacter fetus* var. *venerealis* (vibriosis); *Campylobacter fetus* var. *intestinalis*; *Leptospira pomona*, *L. hardjo* (leptospirosis); *Listeria monocytogenes* (listeriosis); *Aspergillus*, *Absidia* and *Mucor* spp. (fungal abortion); bovine virus diarrhea virus; infectious bovine rhinotracheitis herpesvirus; *Chlamydia psittaci*; an unidentified agent (epizootic bovine abortion); *Coxiella burnetii* (Q fever), *Neospora caninum*.

SHEEP *Campylobacter fetus* (vibriosis); *Chlamydia* spp. (enzootic ovine abortion); *Listeria monocytogenes* (listeriosis); *Salmonella abortus-ovis*; *Toxoplasma gondii* (toxoplasmosis); *Brucella ovis* (limited occurrence).

GOAT Listeriosis, salmonellosis and toxoplasmosis are listed.

HORSE Equine herpesvirus (EHV1), equine viral arteritis (EVA).

PIG *Leptospira pomona*, *L. grippotyphosa*, *L. canicola*, *L. icterohaemorrhagiae* (leptospirosis).

DOG AND CAT *Brucella canis*, feline leukemia virus, feline herpesvirus.

missed a. retention of a dead embryo or fetus for more than 1 to 2 weeks.

a. rate number of abortions as a percentage of the cows in the herd which were diagnosed pregnant in early pregnancy; the target is <2%.

septic a. abortion associated with serious infection of the uterus leading to generalized infection.

spontaneous a. abortion occurring naturally. See also SPONTANEOUS abortion.

a. storm a cluster of abortions occurring at about the same time or in rapid sequence within a group of pregnant females. See also equine VIRAL abortion.

therapeutic a. abortion induced by a veterinarian for medical or other health reasons.

abortive 1. incompletely developed. 2. abortifacient.

abortus a dead or nonviable fetus.

ABP see ANDROGEN binding protein.

ABPEE acronym for acute bovine pulmonary emphysema–edema. See ATYPICAL INTERSTITIAL PNEUMONIA.

ABR test abortus-bang-ring test. See also BRUCELLOSIS testing, MILK ring test.

abrachia congenital absence of the forelimbs.

abrachiocephalia a developmental anomaly with absence of the head and forelimbs.

abrasion a wound caused by rubbing or scraping the skin or mucous membrane. A 'skinned knee' and a 'rope burn' are common examples.

dental a. abnormal wearing away of tooth substance caused by mechanical process such as chewing of rocks or metal cages.

abrasive 1. causing abrasion. 2. an agent that produces abrasion.

abrin toxalbumin in the seeds of *Abrus precatorius*. Causes purging and paralysis.

Abrus pantropical plant genus of the legume family Fabaceae.

A. precatorius seeds contain a toxin, abrin, which causes severe diarrhea and paralysis. Called also jequirity, love precatory, lucky or paternoster bean, rosary or coral pea, crab's eye, minnie-minnie, Indian liquorice.

abscess a localized collection of pus in a cavity formed by the disintegration of tissue. Most abscesses are formed by invasion of tissues by bacteria, but some are caused by fungi or protozoa or even helminths, and some are sterile. Their effects are determined by their location and the pressure that they exert on nearby organs, and the degree of toxemia that they create from their bacterial content and the amount of tissue destroyed. So that for a reasonably active abscess the syndrome presented will be one of local pain, anorexia and fever, and a leukocytosis. For specific abscesses see under anatomical sites, e.g. brain abscess.

Brodie's a. a circumscribed abscess in bone, caused by hematogenous infection, that becomes a chronic nidus of infection.

cervical a. see VERTEBRAL abscess.

cold a. one of slow development and with little inflammation, e.g. caseous lymphadenitis of sheep and goat.

cornea stromal a. small ulcers or puncture wounds of the corneal epithelium may permit entry of bacteria then heal, creating an abscess. Particularly important in horses.

diffuse a. a collection of pus not enclosed by a capsule.

facial subcutaneous a. a disease of cattle eating hay or pasture containing mature grass awns.

gas a. one containing gas, caused by gas-forming bacteria such as *Clostridium perfringens*.

grass seed a. in cattle occurs as a cold, subcutaneous abscess at the throat or on the mandible and is often diagnosed but rarely confirmed. In dogs it occurs in many sites, but most commonly between the toes. The causative grass awn(s) may be recovered by forceps or, in more extensive lesions, surgical exploration.

infraorbital a. occurs in birds as a sequel to chronic upper respiratory infection with sinusitis.

injection site a. an iatrogenic lesion resulting from incomplete skin disinfection before injection; usually contains *Actinomyces pyogenes*.

intra-abdominal a. include diaphragmatic, mesenteric, retroperitoneal; many are subclinical; clinical signs include those of chronic peritonitis. Called also omental bursitis.

maxillary a. see MALAR abscess.

mediastinal a. a very large abscess in this site may cause signs of congestive heart failure due to compression of pericardium and venae cavae.

miliary a. one of a set of small abscesses.

milk a. abscess of the mammary gland occurring during lactation.

pectoral a. a disease of horses in which abscesses occur in the pectoral muscles and ventral midline, and in some cases in internal organs, causing local pain and swelling and eventually rupturing and draining to the exterior.

periapical a. inflammation and destruction of dental pulp and surrounding tissues, including the periodontal membrane and alveolar bone. The radiographic appearance is a translucency of the tooth apex and adjacent alveolar bone. Most common in dogs.

periorbital a. firm masses above or below the eyes occur in birds as a sequel to chronic respiratory disease and sinusitis.

phlegmonous a. one associated with acute inflammation of the subcutaneous connective tissue.

primary a. one formed at the seat of the infection.

rete mirabile a. see PITUITARY abscess.

retroarticular a. one located between the intermediate phalanx and the deep flexor tendon in the hoov of cattle. It may be caused by extension of infection from the navicular bursa or from suppurative arthritis of the distal interphalangeal joint.

retrobulbar a. behind the orbit of the eye; cause pain on opening of the mouth, chemosis and exophthalmos, protrusion of the nictitating membrane, and systemic signs of infection. Most common in dogs and cats.

stitch a., suture a. one developed about a stitch or suture.

vertebral body/epidural a. usually of cervical or lumbar vertebrae; causes compression of cord manifested by incoordination, paresis, paralysis.

wandering a. one that burrows into tissues and finally points at a distance from the site of origin.

abscessation formation of an abscess.

abscise to cut off or remove.

abscissa the horizontal line in a graph along which are plotted the units of one of the factors considered in the study, as time in a time–temperature study. The other line is called the ordinate.

abscission removal of a part or growth by cutting.

abscopal pertaining to the effect on nonirradiated tissue resulting from irradiation of other tissues of the body.

absence from practice a convention in the veterinary profession recognizing that clients who are accustomed to obtain professional services at a particular premises are entitled to expect that those services will always be available, either directly or by being referred to another, comparable service with which suitable arrangements have been made beforehand.

Absidia a genus of nonseptate fungi in the class Zygomycetes. *A. ramosa* and *A. corymbifera* cause bovine abortion resulting from a severe placentitis. *Absidia* spp. are also associated with ZYGOMYCOSIS, causing disease of the gastrointestinal tract, and less commonly oral cavity, larynx and subcutaneous tissue.

absolute in mathematical terms, the magnitude of a number regardless of sign.

a. refractory period extends from the onset of the action potential as the nerve impulse is generated to the stage where the fiber is repolarized and susceptible to the transmission of another impulse.

absorb 1. to take in or assimilate, as to take up substances into or across tissues, e.g. the skin or intestine. 2. to stop particles of radiation so that their energy is totally transferred to the absorbing material.

absorbable gelatin sponge see GELATIN.

absorbance in radiology, a measure of the ability of a medium to absorb radiation, expressed as the logarithm of the quotient of the intensity of the radiation entering the medium divided by that leaving it.

absorbefacient 1. causing absorption. 2. an agent that promotes absorption.

absorbent 1. able to take in, or suck up and incorporate. 2. a tissue structure, lymphatic or other vessel, involved in absorption. 3. a substance that absorbs or promotes absorption.

Absorbents used pharmaceutically are usually finely ground inert substances applied locally to prevent friction and reduce tissue irritation, e.g. talc, zinc stearate, a mixture of boric acid and calcium oxide. Similar substances, e.g. finely ground charcoal, kaolin, are administered orally for the same purposes and also to absorb toxins.

absorption 1. the act of taking up or in by specific chemical or molecular action; especially the passage of liquids or other substances through a surface of the body into body fluids and tissues, as in the absorption of the end products of DIGESTION into the villi that line the intestine. 2. in radiology, uptake of energy by matter with which the radiation interacts.

chemical a. any process by which one substance in liquid or solid form penetrates the surface of another substance.

Compton a. effect see COMPTON EFFECT.

differential a. the difference in the absorption of x-rays by different tissues.

digestive a. the passage of the end products of DIGESTION from the gastrointestinal tract into the blood and lymphatic vessels and the cells of tissues. Absorption of this kind can take place either by diffusion or by active transport.

percutaneous a. a passive process in which noxious or therapeutic substances pass through the skin into the body.

radiation a. the dissipation of radiant energy as it passes through matter. This phenomenon is of particular importance in diagnostic and therapeutic radiology, which depends on the interaction between ionizing radiations and matter. As radiation passes through matter, it is absorbed by an amount dependent on the atomic and molecular structure and thickness of the substance, and the energy of the primary photons. If radiations pass through a medium of living or nonliving material without absorption (loss of energy), no biological or photographic effects can occur. In true absorption the photons of radiation waves give up or transfer all of their energy to electrons within the atoms of the matter through which they are passing.

a. tests are used to assess absorptive function of the small intestine. Glucose, D-xylose and fats are substances administered orally and at timed intervals later measured in the blood. See also digestive absorption (above), FAT absorption test.

absorptive having the power of absorption; involving absorption.

abu nini [Sudanese] see CONTAGIOUS caprine/ovine pleuropneumonia.

abuse misuse, maltreatment or excessive use.

animal a. a modern day concept by which the trust that animals should have in humans, in return for the benefits that they bestow, is betrayed when humans abuse animals physically or psychologically. The abuses often stop short of cruelty in a legal sense but can be classified as harassment. The term has a variable but generally wide scope and includes physical cruelty by assault, by deprivation of adequate food, water, transport and shelter, and proper care during illness, pregnancy and parturition, and participation in sporting events at a level beyond the animal's capacity to perform. This form of abuse covers such misuses as riding horses in rodeos, excessively arduous endurance rides, ignominious performances and exhibits, oppressive displays of obedience. Mental or psychological abuse is less readily defined but in today's culture is usually taken to include undue confinement, demeaning performance as entertainment and harassment by teasing.

ABVP American Board of Veterinary Practitioners.

ABVT American Board of Veterinary Toxicology.

Abyssinian cat a shorthaired breed of domestic cat with yellow or green eyes and a characteristic coat that results from the double or triple bars of pigmentation (agouti ticking) on individual hairs giving an appearance similar to that of a hare. The breed is affected by amyloidosis and retinal atrophy.

Ac chemical symbol, *actinium*.

a.c. [L.] *ante cibum* (before meals).

Acacia a large genus of trees and shrubs of warm, dry regions, belonging to the legume family Mimosaceae, which provides valuable browse for grazing ruminants but also contains some poisonous plants.

Acacia spp. capable of causing cyanide poisoning: *A. binerva* (*A. glaucescens*), *A. burrowii*, *A. caffra*, *A. cheelii* (*motherumbah*), *A. concurrens* (*A. cunninghamii*), *A. crassa* (*A. cunninghamii*), *A. cunninghamii* (black wattle), *A. erioloba* (camel thorn), *A. glaucescens* (sally wattle), *A. gregii* (catclaw), *A. lasiopetala* (*A. sieberana*), *A. leiocalyx* (*A. melanoxylon*), *A. longifolia*, *A. longispicata* (*A. cunninghamii*), *A. osswaldii*, *A. sieberana*.

A. aneura see LIPOFUSCINOSIS. Called also mulga.

A. berlandieri contains tyramine which causes ataxia in sheep and goats. Called also guajillo.

A. cana can accumulate selenium if the soil selenium content is unusually large.

A. catechu cyanogenic plant. See CATECHU.

A. erioloba host plant of *Gonometa* spp. (molopo moth); the moth larva produces indigestible silk in its cocoon; causes rumen impaction; a South African phenomenon.

A. georginae has a high concentration of fluoroacetate and can cause sudden death. Called also Georgina gidgee or Georgina gidyea.

A. melanoxylon contains toxic tannins; rarely causes ataxia, recumbency, alimentary tract irritation.

A. mellifera host plant for *Gonometa* spp. (molopo moth), the larva of which produces indigestible silk in its cocoon; causes ruminal impaction.

A. nilotica* subsp. *kraussiana pods contain toxins which cause hemolysis, methemoglobinemia and diarrhea.

A. salicina contains toxic tannins; raraly causes incoordination, recumbency.

acacia the dried exudate from *Acacia senegal* and other *Acacia* species of African origin, used as an emulsifier, stabilizer and suspending agent. Called also gum arabic.

academic associates extramural instructors appointed by universities who have much experience in the vocational aspects of veterinary science. Undergraduate and postgraduate students are sent to the practices of these veterinarians to acquire practical experience which may not be available over the whole scope of the profession's interests at the university. See also SEEING PRACTICE.

academic education education in the principles of the subject or course. In veterinary science this includes anatomy, physiology, biochemistry, pharmacology, nutrition, genetics, general pathology, microbiology and parasitology. Complemented by vocational education aimed at the more practical aspects of the profession.

acampsia rigidity of a part or limb.

acantha 1. a spine. 2. a spinous process of a vertebra.

acanthamebiasis infection by amebae of the genus *Acanthamoeba*; has been observed rarely in dogs.

Acanthamoeba small amebae, found in soil and water; they have been found in tissue cultures and in sporadic cases of pneumonia, general systemic infection and have produced meningoencephalitis after experimental administration. Possibly associated with granulomatous encephalitis in greyhounds. Includes *A. castellani*, *A. culbertsoni*.

acanth(o)- word element. [Gr.] *sharp spine, thorn.*

Acanthocephala a phylum of elongate, mostly cylindrical organisms (thorny-headed worms) parasitic in the intestines of all classes of vertebrates.

acanthocephalans members of the phylum Acanthocephala.

acanthocephaliasis infection with worms of the phylum Acanthocephala.

acanthocephalid see ACANTHOCEPHALANS.

Acanthocephalus a genus of thorny-headed worms of the family Echinorhynchinae. Includes *A. jacksoni* (in trout).

Acanthocheilonema see DIPETALONEMA.

acanthocyte an erythrocyte with protoplasmic projections giving it a thorny appearance; may be seen in dogs with liver disease and related disturbances of lipid metabolism and in dogs with hemangiosarcoma. Morphologically similar to spur cells, but biochemically distinct. See also spur-cell ANEMIA.

acanthocytosis the presence in the blood of acanthocytes.

acantholysis loss of cohesion between the epidermal cells, resulting in intraepidermal clefts, vesicles and bullae. Seen in inflammatory, viral and autoimmune skin diseases, particularly the pemphigus complex.

a. bullosa see EPIDERMOLYSIS bullosa.

familial a. a congenital disease of Aberdeen Angus calves characterized by ulceration of the oral mucosa and the skin over the distal limb joints and the coronet.

acanthoma a tumor in the prickle cell layer of the skin. See intracutaneous cornifying EPITHELIOMA.

infundibular keratinizing a. see intracutaneous cornifying EPITHELIOMA.

Acanthophis antarcticus see death ADDER.

A. a. pyrrhus see desert death ADDER.

acanthor larva contained within the mature eggs of Acanthocephalans: the egg is thick-shelled and the larva carries an anterior circlet of hooks and spines.

acanthosis an increased thickness of the stratum spinosum, due to either an increased number or hypertrophy of cells.

frictional a. see acanthosis nigricans (below).

a. nigricans a skin disease of dogs characterized by hyperpigmentation, lichenification, seborrhea, and alopecia commencing in the axillae and often spreading to involve flexural surfaces of all limbs, and the ventral body. Dachshunds are particularly predisposed to primary acanthosis, often developing the first changes at a young age. Sporadic cases are secondary to systemic disease, endocrinopathies, hypersensitivity reactions and friction in body folds.

Acanthospermum plant genus of the Asteraceae family; originated in tropical America.

A. hispidum contains a hepatotoxin and causes hepatic insufficiency. Called also star burr.

Acanthospiculum see ONCHOCERCA.

acapnia decrease of carbon dioxide in the blood.

acarbia decrease of bicarbonate in the blood.

acardia a developmental anomaly with absence of the heart.

acardiacus [L.] *having no heart.*

acardius an imperfectly formed twin fetus without a heart and invariably lacking other body parts.

acariasis infestation with arthropod parasites of the order Acarina including the ticks and mites. See also tick INFESTATION.

cutaneous a. see MANGE.

nasal a. see NASAL acariasis.

oto-a. see OTODECTES *cynotis*.

otodectic a. see OTODECTES *cynotis*.

pulmonary a. see PNEUMONYSSUS.

acaricide an agent that destroys ticks and mites. The common ones are the organophosphorus compounds, the synthetic pyrethroids, and the carba mates. The chlorinated hydrocarbons are no longer much used on farm animals because of the problems with tissue residue that result.

acarid a tick or a mite of the order Acarina.

Acarina an order of arthropods (class Arachnida), including mites and ticks.

acarine pertaining to or of the nature of members of the order Acarina including the ticks and mites.

acarinosis any disease caused by mites. Called also acariasis.

acarodermatitis skin inflammation due to bites of parasitic mites (acarids).

Acaroidea a superfamily of the order Acarina.

Acarus includes *A. farinae*, *A. longion*, *A. siro*, *A. tawinae*; see TYROGLYPHUS.

acaryote 1. non-nucleated. 2. a non-nucleated cell.

ACAT acyl CoA : cholesterol acyltransferase; an important enzyme that removes the inhibitory influence of free cholesterol on activity of HMG CoA reductase and the synthesis of LDL receptors.

acathexia inability to retain bodily secretions.

accelerated conduction syndrome see accessory tract atrioventricular CONDUCTION.

accelerator [L.] an agent or apparatus that increases the rate at which something occurs or progresses.

developing a. alkaline constituent of an x-ray developer which controls the rate of development. Called also activator.

a. factor, a. globulin factor V, one of the blood CLOTTING factors. Called also proaccelerin.

serum prothrombin conversion a. (SPCA) clotting factor VII; see PROCONVERTIN.

acceptability of food the measure of whether an animal will consume enough of a food to meet its caloric needs.

acceptable daily intake the amount of a drug or chemical residue to which an animal can be exposed daily for a lifetime without suffering a deleterious or injurious effect, on the basis of all of the facts known at the time.

acceptor a substance that unites with another substance.

hydrogen a. the molecule accepting hydrogen in an oxidation–reduction reaction.

access 1. surgical term for the ease of reaching the target organ or site in an operation. 2. computer term for getting access to a file or other collection of data.

a. time the time required for a program to locate data from its storage on a disk and load it into the memory of the processor.

accessibility ease of gaining access.

data a. when large amounts of data are accumulated into banks and accessed by computer it is desirable to create systems that limit access to the data at a variety of levels, usually by the use of identification codes. In this way the confidentiality of the data can be protected. One of the great challenges of the age is the cracking of these entry codes.

government document a. as part of the open government policy adopted in some Western countries there are statutes entitled Freedom of Information Acts that entitle members of the public to have access to government files concerning their daily lives. This may affect the performance of some animal disease control enactments.

test result a. the results of laboratory tests and radiographic examinations are often sought by owners of the subject animals. Veterinarians usually believe that the results are their property and that the owner is entitled only to an interpretation of them. The question is not resolved.

accessory supplementary or affording aid to anoth similar and generally more important thing.

a. nerve see Table 14.

a. sex glands any gland, other than the gonad, associated with the genital tract, such as the ampulla of the ductus deferens and the bulbourethral, prostate and vesicular glands of the male.

accident prone specially susceptible to accidents.

Accipiter gentilis see GOSHAWK.

acclimation the process of becoming accustomed to a new environment.

acclimatization the adaptation of an animal to the climatic conditions in an area. The ability to adapt in this way is an important characteristic of livestock.

accommodation adjustment, especially adjustment of the eye for seeing objects at various distances. This is accomplished by the ciliary muscle, which controls the LENS of the eye, allowing it to flatten or thicken as is needed for distant or near vision.

amplitude of a. the total amount of accommodative power of the eye.

histological a. changes in morphology and function of cells following changed conditions.

accountancy trail the sequence of actions taken in the completion of a financial transaction which an auditor can follow in an examination of the adequacy of the system used.

accounts the bill provided to the client by the veterinarian setting out the sums owing for services rendered.

itemized a. the provision of accounts for professional services in which all of the medicines, materials and services supplied are itemized. The disadvantage of the procedure is the opportunity that it provides to vexatious clients to argue with the charges. It is standard procedure to provide an itemized account if the client asks for one.

a. payable the monies owed to other accounts by the practice and to be paid during the month.

a. receivable the accounts that owe the practice money and which can be expected to pay during the month.

accreditation given a stamp of dependability by an authorized agency.

accredited recognition by an appropriate authority that the performance of a particular institution has satisfied a prestated set of criteria.

a. herds cattle herds which have achieved a low level of reactors to, e.g., the tuberculin or brucellosis agglutination tests; chicken flocks proven to be free of pullorum disease.

a. inspectors veterinarians who have attended appropriate continuing education courses and performed well enough through a probationary period to be accredited as part-time veterinary inspectors; employed by governments or more local authorities.

a. schools in some countries a governmental or professional body conducts periodic examinations of the country's veterinary schools to determine their efficacy as teaching schools. Schools which lose their accreditation usually lose their status as providers of veterinary graduates who are adequate to the needs of the country's animals.

accretion 1. growth by addition of material. 2. accumulation. 3. adherence of parts normally separated.

accumulator plants plants which accumulate unusually large amounts of particular elements; includes facultative accumulators, e.g. *Aster*, *Atriplex* spp. which accumulate a particular element, e.g. selenium, but can grow quite well without it, and obligate accumulators which only grow in soils where high concentrations of the elements exist, e.g. *Oonopsis*, *Xylorrhiza* and some *Astragalus* spp.

accumulator plates battery components made of lead and a frequent cause of poisoning when chewed or licked.

accuracy the closeness with which an observation or a measurement of a variable approximates its true value. An important component of diagnostic tests. An accurate test implies freedom from both random and systematic error. See also PRECISION.

ACD acid citrate dextrose.

ACD solution an anticoagulant solution used for the collection of blood for purposes of storage and transfusion. The active principle is sodium citrate with citric acid and dextrose.

ACE angiotensin-converting enzyme.

ACE inhibitors a group of drugs used as vasodilators in the management of heart failure. They act to decrease circulating levels of angiotensin II and aldosterone. See CAPTOPRIL, ENALAPRIL, LISINOPRIL.

ace acepromazine.

acedapsone a sulfone, related to dapsone, used in the treatment of leprosy in humans and atypical mycobacterial infections in animals.

acellular not cellular in structure.

acelomate having no celom or body cavity.

acemannan a complex polysaccharide derived from the plant ALOE *barbadensis* (ALOE *vera*) and used as an immunomodulator.

acenocoumarol, acenocoumarin a warfarin derivative used as an anticoagulant. Called also nicoumalone.

acentric 1. not central; not located in the center. 2. a chromatid or chromosome which which lacks a centromere.

acephalobrachia congenital absence of the head and forelimbs.

acephalocardia congenital absence of the head and heart.

acephalocardius a monster without a head or heart.

acephalochiria congenital absence of the head and forefeet.

acephalogaster a fetus without a head or stomach.

acephalogastria congenital absence of the head, chest and stomach.

acephalopodia congenital absence of the head and hindfeet.

acephalopodius a fetus without a head or hindfeet.

acephalorachia congenital absence of the head and vertebral column.

acephalostomia congenital absence of the head, with the mouth aperture on the upper aspect of the body.

acephalothoracia congenital absence of the head and thorax.

acephalous headless.

acephalus a headless fetus.

acepromazine, acetylpromazine one of the phenothiazine derivative psychotropic drugs, used in animals as a means of chemical restraint. Its principal value is in quietening and calming frightened and aggressive animals. The standard pharmaceutical preparation, acepromazine maleate, is used extensively in horses, cats and dogs, especially as a preanesthetic agent.

Acer trees of the family Aceraceae.

A. rubrum ingestion of wilted or dries leaves of this tree causes acute hemolytic anemia characterized by red urine, jaundice, anemia and methemoglobinemia in horses. Called also red maple, swamp maple.

acervuli calcified granules sometimes found in the pineal body and choroid plexus, especially in horses; structure similar to hydroxyapatite crystals; appear to have glial or stromal origin. Called also brain sand, corpora arenacea, psammoma bodies.

acervuline aggregated; heaped up; said of certain glands.

acervulus pl. *acervuli* [L.] sandy calcifications in or about the pineal body and choroid plexus.

acetabular pertaining to the acetabulum.

a. dysplasia see HIP dysplasia.

a. sourcil thickening of subchondral acetabular bone. Used as an indicator of biomechanics in the canine hip joint and in radiographic assessment for HIP dysplasia.

acetabulectomy excision of the acetabulum.

acetabuloplasty plastic repair of the acetabulum.

acetabulum the cup-shaped socket of the hip joint that receives the head of the femur. See also ACETABULAR.

inherited a. defect in Dole horses; clinically normal at birth, osteoarthritis and round ligament disruption develop later.

acetal an organic compound formed by a combination of an aldehyde with an alcohol.

acetaldehyde a colorless volatile liquid, CH_3CHO, found in freshly distilled spirits, which is irritating to mucous membranes and has a general narcotic action. It is also an intermediate in the metabolism of alcohol.

acetaminophen, paracetamol an analgesic and antipyretic drug in dogs. It is contraindicated for cats because of serious side-effects which include intravascular hemolysis, methemoglobinemia and hepatic necrosis.

acetanilid an analgesic and antipyretic. Like the other para-aminophenol derivatives, its toxicity is greater than that of salicylates and other analgesics so that it is not much used.

acetarsol, acetarsone an organic arsenical used as an antiprotozoal agent, especially in turkeys and geese. See also organic ARSENIC poisoning.

acetate a salt of acetic acid.

a. base cellulose acetate sheet used as support or base for x-ray film.

a. tape slide a method of collecting ectoparasites such as mites, lice or fleas, and their eggs, for diagnostic purposes by pressing the sticky side of the tape against the skin and haircoat and applying the tape to a glass slide which is then examined microscopically.

acetazolamide a carbonic anhydrase inhibitor used as a diuretic, most commonly to reduce intraocular pressure in the treatment of glaucoma.

Acetest trademark for reagent tablets containing sodium nitroprusside, aminoacetic acid, disodium phosphate and lactose. A drop of urine is placed on a tablet on a sheet of white paper; if significant quantities of acetone are present the tablet changes from a purple tint (1+), to lavender (2+), to moderate purple (3+) or to deep purple (4+). Extensively used for field testing of cows for acetonemia and ewes and cows for pregnancy toxemia.

acetic pertaining to vinegar or its acid; sour.

a. acid CH_3COOH, a short-chain, saturated fatty acid, the characteristic component of vinegar and one of the principal acids formed in the rumen by fermentation. It has the odor of vinegar and a sharp acid taste. A 36.5% solution of acetic acid is used topically as a caustic and rubefacient. A dilute acetic acid solution (6%) may be used as an antidote to alkali, e.g. in urea poisoning in cattle where the urea is converted to ammonia in the rumen. Glacial acetic acid is a 99.4% solution.

acetoacetate see ACETOACETIC ACID.

acetoacetic acid CH_3COCH_2COOH, one of the KETONE bodies formed in the body in metabolism of certain substances, particularly in the liver in the oxidation of fats. It is present in the body in increased amounts in abnormal conditions such as uncontrolled DIABETES mellitus and starvation, and in bovine ACETONEMIA and PREGNANCY toxemia of cows and ewes. Occurs in the body as acetoacetate.

acetoacetyl CoA intermediate in ketogenesis and utilization of the ketones, beta-hydroxybutyrate and acetoacetate. Penultimate intermediate in the beta-oxidation of fatty acids.

acetohexamide a first generation sulfonylurea derivative, used as an oral hypoglycemic agent in the treatment of diabetes mellitus.

acetohydroxamic acid a hydroxamic acid that specifically inhibits urease; it retards alkalinization of the urine caused by urease-producing bacteria and may inhibit bacterial growth. Used in the prevention and dissolution of uroliths, but in dogs causes a dose-related, reversible hemolytic anemia and blood dyscrasia. Abbreviated AHA.

acetokinase enzyme catalyzing the phosphorylation of acetate using ATP.

acetonaemia see ACETONEMIA.

acetone a compound, CH_3COCH_3, with solvent properties and characteristic odor, obtained by fermentation or produced synthetically; it is a by-product of acetoacetic acid. Acetone is one of the KETONE bodies produced in abnormal amounts in uncontrolled DIABETES mellitus, metabolic ACIDOSIS, PREGNANCY toxemia and ACETONEMIA of ruminants.

a. bodies acetone, acetoacetic acid and beta-oxybutyric acid, being intermediates in fat metabolism. Called also KETONE bodies.

a. poisoning in companion animals causes narcosis, gastritis and renal and hepatic damage.

acetonemia 1. ketonemia. 2. wasting acetonemia, a disease of recently calved cows characterized by rapid weight loss, indifferent appetite and severe ketonuria which responds well to treatment with parenteral glucose or glucocorticoids. Rarely there are nervous signs of circling, constant licking and chewing, somnolence and frequent, hoarse bellowing. Called also ketosis. See also NERVOUS acetonemia, KETONEMIA.

acetonuria see KETONURIA.

acetophenazine a phenothiazine, similar to chlorpromazine, used as a tranquilizer.

acetophenetidin a para-aminophenol-derivative analgesic, similar to acetanilide. Its toxicity is much higher than that of the salicylates and other analgesics, especially for cats, so that it is not much used. Called also phenacetin.

Acetosella vulgaris RUMEX *acetosella*.

acetrizoate sodium the sodium salt of acetrizoic acid, used as a contrast medium in radiography.

acetyl the monovalent radical, CH_3CO, a combining form of acetic acid.

acetyl CoA key intermediate in aerobic intermediary metabolism of carbohydrates, lipids and some amino acids. Allosteric regulator of the activity of the pyruvate dehydrogenase complex and pyruvate carboxylase. Present in low concentrations but with high turnover. Dependent on B-group vitamin, pantothenic acid for structure of coenzyme A.

acetyl CoA carboxylase a biotin-containing enzyme which participates in the synthesis of fatty acids by catalyzing the carboxylation reaction in which acetyl-CoA is converted to malonyl-CoA. It has the important effect of regulating the rate of fatty acid synthesis and is itself influenced in its activity by the local concentration of magnesium, citrate, palmitylcarnitine and ATP and is stimulated by the action of insulin.

5-acetyl-deoxynivalenol see DEOXYNIVALENOL.

2-acetylaminofluorine a thyroid initiator credited with direct stimulation of the thyroid resulting in a higher incidence than normal of neoplasms in the gland.

acetylandromedol andromedotoxin.

acetylation one of the synthetic biotransformations which operate in the metabolism of drugs in which metabolites are produced that are more readily excreted than the parent drug. Dogs are exceptional amongst the domesticated species in that acetylation does not occur in their tissues. Acetylation is one of the principal metabolic pathways of the sulfonamides.

acetylator an organism capable of metabolic acetylation. Those animals that differ in their inherited ability to metabolize certain drugs, e.g. isoniazid, are termed fast or slow acetylators.

acetylcarnitine a substance which can act as a carrier for acetyl groups across the inner mitochondrial membrane in mammalian liver.

acetylcholine the acetic acid ester of choline, normally present in many parts of the body and having important physiological functions. It is a neurotransmitter at cholinergic synapses in the central, sympathetic and parasympathetic nervous systems. It is not used clinically but it is the classical cholinergic agonist. Abbreviated ACh.

a. receptors structures located at the endorgans, e.g. at the skeletal muscle fibers. The myofibers are stimulated to contract by the interaction of acetylcholine with acetylcholine receptors which are located on the motor end plate or postsynaptic sarcolemma. See also NEUROMUSCULAR junction.

acetylcholinesterase an enzyme present in nervous tissue, muscle and red cells that catalyzes the hydrolysis of acetylcholine to choline and acetic acid; called also true CHOLINESTERASE. Abbreviated AChE.

a. antagonists organophosphorus compounds and carbamates that act by inactivating acetylcholinesterase; hence poisoning by these compounds has parasympatheticomimetic manifestations.

acetylcoenzyme A acetyl-CoA, the carrier of acetyl groups into the tricarboxylic acid (Krebs) cycle and the chief precursor of lipids; it is formed by the attachment to coenzyme A of an acetyl group during the oxidation of pyruvate, fatty acids or amino acids.

***N*-acetylcysteine** a mucolytic agent used to reduce the viscosity of secretions of the respiratory tract. The principal method of administration is by aerosol, which in animals requires the use of a face mask or aerosol chamber. Also used parenterally in the treatment of acetaminophen poisoning in cats where it aids in detoxification of the drug and enhances its elimination, and topically in the treatment of collagenase-associated corneal ulcers.

acetylene a colorless, combustible, explosive gas, the simplest triple-bonded hydrocarbon.

acetylethylenimine one of a group of related alkylating agents used in the preparation of inactivated vaccines.

***N*-acetylgalactosamine** one of the repeating disaccharide units in glycosaminoglycans.

***N*-acetyl-glucosamine-6-sulfatase** an enzyme which when deficient in Nubian goats causes a condition similar to Sanfilippo's III-D syndrome in humans; the clinical syndrome includes delay in rising and walking in neonates, ataxia, bowing of front limbs, clouding of the cornea, dwarfism, and cartilaginous and bony deformities; histological examination reveals lysosomal overload.

***N*-acetylglutamate** compound produced from acetyl CoA and glutamate that provides the regulator stimulus to the activity of carbamoyl synthetase II of the urea cycle.

***N*-acetyl loline alkaloid** a compound thought to contribute to fescue poisoning.

acetyl-β-methylcholine see METHACHOLINE.

acetylsalicylic acid see ASPIRIN.

acetylstrophanthidin a semisynthetic cardiac glycoside, similar to STROPHANTHIN.

AcG accelerator globulin (clotting factor V).

ACh acetylcholine.

acha see DIGITARIA *exilis*.

achalasia failure to relax of the smooth muscle fibers of the gastrointestinal tract at any junction of one part with another; especially failure of the lower esophagus to relax with swallowing, due to an abnormality of innervation. Called also cardiospasm. See also MEGAESOPHAGUS.

cricoesophageal a. failure of the cranial esophageal sphincter to relax during swallowing to accommodate the approaching bolus. Gagging, nasal regurgitation and aspiration result. Called also cricoesophageal incoordination.

cricopharyngeal a. is motor dysfunction of the cricopharyngeal sphincter in which a failure of relaxation prevents the bolus from entering the esophagus during swallowing. Called also cricopharyngeal dysphagia.

esophageal a. see MEGAESOPHAGUS.

pyloric a. failure of the pylorus to open in neonates so that distension of the stomach occurs and causes continuous vomiting. This may be reflex in response to local ulceration, e.g. in young calves, or be a congenital defect.

reticulo-omasal sphincter a. is probably a factor in the development of the gut stasis in bovine vagal indigestion with onward passage of ingesta obstructed at the exit from the rumenoreticulum. Results in rumen distension and frothiness of contents.

AChE see ACETYLCHOLINESTERASE.

ache 1. continuous pain, as opposed to sharp pangs or twinges. An ache can be either dull and constant, as in some types of backache, or throbbing, as in some types of headache and toothache. An ache is a subjective sensation and its occurrence in animals is only assumed. 2. to suffer such pain.

acheilia a developmental anomaly with absence of the lips.

acheiria a developmental anomaly with absence of the forefeet.

acheiropodia a developmental anomaly characterized by absence of all feet, both fore and hind.

Achilles tendon the group of tendons that insert on the calcaneus near the point of the hock made up of the tendons of the gastrocnemius, soleus, superficial digital flexor, semitendinosus and biceps femoris muscles. Called also common calcaneal tendon. See also GASTROCNEMIUS MUSCLE tendon.

achillobursitis inflammation of the bursae about the gastrocnemius tendon.

achillodynia pain in the Achilles tendon or its bursa.

achillorrhaphy suturing of the gastrocnemius tendon.

achillotenotomy surgical division of the gastrocnemius tendon.

achlorhydria absence of hydrochloric acid from gastric juice.

Achly fungus which causes white, cotton-wool like growths on cutaneous trauma sites of fish and their newly spawned eggs; most common at colder water temperatures.

Achnatherium inebrians STIPA *inebrians*.

Acholeplasma a genus of the class Mollicutes and very closely related to the genus *Mycoplasma*.

A. laidlawii a common isolate in the lungs of calves with enzootic pneumonia but of doubtful significance.

A. oculi is a common finding in the conjunctivae of sheep with contagious ophthalmia but the bacteria have not been proven to be pathogenic in this situation.

acholia lack or absence of bile secretion.

acholic feces gray, putty-colored feces resulting from an absence of oxidized bile pigments in the intestinal tract; usually indicative of complete bile duct obstruction, but pale color can also be caused by dietary factors or reduced bacterial activity in the intestine, e.g. decreased transit time, or by antibacterial therapy.

acholuria absence of bile pigments from the urine.

achondrogenesis a hereditary disorder characterized by hypoplasia of bone, resulting in markedly shortened limbs; the head and trunk are normal.

achondroplasia a failure of growth of cartilage in the young, leading to a type of DWARFISM. Several breeds of dogs display this in their standard conformation, e.g. Dachshund, Basset. See also CHONDRODYSPLASIA.

inherited congenital a. see achondroplastic DWARFISM.

inherited a. dwarfism see achondroplastic DWARFISM.

inherited a. with hydrocephalus see BULLDOG CALVES.

Achorion see TRICHOPHYTON.

achromasia 1. lack of normal skin pigmentation. 2. the inability of tissues or cells to be stained.

achromat an achromatic objective.

achromatic 1. producing no discoloration, or staining with difficulty. 2. refracting light without decomposing it into its component colors.

achromatism the quality or the condition of being achromatic; staining with difficulty.

achromatophil 1. not easily stainable. 2. an organism or tissue that does not stain easily.

achromatosis 1. deficiency of pigmentation in the tissues. 2. lack of staining power in a cell or tissue.

achromatous colorless.

achromaturia colorless state of the urine.

achromia the lack or absence of normal color or pigmentation, as of the skin.

achromocyte a red cell artefact that stains more faintly than intact red cells.

achromoderma amelanosis; lack of pigment in the skin.

achromophil see ACHROMATOPHIL.

achromotrichia loss or absence of pigment in hair. It may be complete or patchy, affect the length of the fiber or be in well-defined bands or speckled. Can be caused by nutritional deficiency, selective freezing, radiation or pressure. See also VITILIGO, COPPER nutritional deficiency, SNOWFLAKES.

achropachia ossea see pulmonary hypertrophic OSTEOPATHY.

Achtheres a genus of the class Crustacea which parasitize freshwater fish.

Achyla a genus of fungi which cause disease in fish reared by fish culturists and aquarists.

achylia absence of hydrochloric acid and enzymes in the gastric secretions.
achylous deficient in chyle.
achymia deficiency of chyme.
acicular needle-shaped.
acid 1. sour. 2. a molecule or ion with a tendency to give up a proton to the solvent according to Bronsted and Lowry theory.

All acids react with bases to form salts and water (neutralization). Other properties of acids include a sour taste and the ability to cause certain dyes to undergo a color change. A common example of this is the ability of acids to change litmus paper from blue to red.

Acids play a vital role in the chemical processes that are a normal part of the functions of the cells and tissues of the body. A stable balance between acids and bases in the body is essential to life. See also ACIDIC, ACID–BASE BALANCE, and individual acids.

amino a. any one of a class of organic compounds containing the amino and the carboxyl group, occurring naturally in plant and animal tissues and forming the chief constituents of protein. See also AMINO ACID.

bile a's steroid acids derived from cholesterol. See also BILE acids.

a. excretion blood buffers prevent a sudden change in pH of body fluids when they receive excess acid or alkali from absorption or metabolic processes. This temporary measure is supplemented by a mechanism for the excretion of hydrogen ions via the kidney in the form of dihydrogen phosphate and ammonium ions.

fatty a. any monobasic aliphatic acid containing only carbon, hydrogen and oxygen. See also FATTY acids.

a. hydrolases major group of enzymes present in lysosomes.

inorganic a. an acid containing no carbon atoms.

keto a's compounds containing the groups CO (carbonyl) and COOH (carboxyl).

a. methyl green stain stains protozoal nuclei a bright green and is recommended for the detection of *Balantidium coli* in fecal smears.

nucleic a's substances that constitute the prosthetic groups of the nucleoproteins and contain phosphoric acid, sugars, and purine and pyrimidine bases. See also NUCLEIC ACIDS.

a. phosphatase see acid PHOSPHATASE.

a. retention retention of metabolic acids, including sulfates and phosphates, as a result of acute and chronic renal disease.

acid–antigen plate test see ROSE BENGAL test.
acid–base balance a state of equilibrium between acidity and alkalinity of the body fluids; called also hydrogen ion (H+) balance because, by definition, an acid is a substance capable of giving up a hydrogen ion during a chemical exchange, and a base is a substance that can accept it. The positively charged hydrogen ion (H+) is the active constituent of all acids.

Most of the body's metabolic processes produce acids as their end products, but a somewhat alkaline body fluid (pH 7.4) is required as a medium for vital cellular activities. Therefore chemical exchanges of hydrogen ions must take place continuously in order to maintain a state of equilibrium. An optimal pH (hydrogen ion concentration) between 7.35 and 7.45 must be maintained; otherwise, the enzyme systems and other biochemical and metabolic activities will not function normally.

Although the body can tolerate and compensate for slight deviations in acidity and alkalinity, if the pH drops below 7.30, the potentially serious condition of ACIDOSIS exists. If the pH goes higher than 7.50, the patient is in a state of ALKALOSIS. In either case the disturbance of the acid–base balance is considered serious, even though there are control mechanisms by which the body can compensate for an upward or downward change in the pH. Shifts in the pH of body fluids are controlled by three major regulatory systems which may be classified as *chemical* (the buffer systems), *biological* (blood and cellular activity), and *physiological* (the lungs and kidneys).

Imbalances of the acid–base ratio are discussed under ACIDOSIS and ALKALOSIS. Diagnosis and monitoring of either of these conditions are greatly enhanced by periodic determination of the plasma pH and by BLOOD GAS ANALYSIS.

acid citrate dextrose see ACD.
acid-detergent fiber see FIBER.
acid etch technique the use of dilute acid, commonly phosphoric acid, on teeth to improve their ability to retain restorative materials.
acid-fast 1. not readily decolorized by acids after staining; said of bacteria, especially *Mycobacterium* spp. 2. stain demonstrating this characteristic. See also Ziehl–Neelsen STAIN.

modified a.-f. bacteria resist decolorization by mild acid solutions; includes *Brucella*, *Nocardia* and *Chlamydia* spp.

acid phosphatase see acid PHOSPHATASE.
acid-proof acid-fast.
acid rain rain which contains materials, sulfates and oxidation products of nitrogen and sulfur particularly, produced by combustion of coal and oil in industrial processes and by motor vehicles; lowers the pH of water bodies; see ACID WATERS; credited with local decline of fish culture.
acid waters waters with a low pH occurring naturally and where water contaminated by ACID RAIN and run-off from mine sites; acid waters often contain higher concentrations than normal of cadmium, copper, zinc and lead. Water affected by heavy leaching from soil may contain high levels of aluminum, copper, manganese and iron. These waters adversely affect production in fish cultures. See also water ACIDITY.
acidaminuria see AMINOACIDURIA.
acidemia abnormal acidity of the blood.
acidic of or pertaining to an acid; acid-forming.

a. urine is usual in carnivores, that of herbivores is usually neutral or slightly alkaline. Urine increases in acidity when a large load of acid is passed into the extracellular fluid and is excreted by the kidneys. If the kidneys can cope with the excretion load the pH of the blood will return to normal. If the acid load is too great or the kidney function inadequate, acidemia results.

acidified milk replacer liquid milk substitute acidified to pH 5.2 to preserve it and to reduce the intake so that the calf takes more frequent but smaller meals during the day.
acidifier an agent that causes acidity; a substance used to increase gastric or urine acidity.
acidifying solution a solution used in fluid therapy for alkalosis.
acidity 1. the quality of being acid; the power to unite with positively charged ions or with basic substances. 2. excess acid quality, as of the gastric juice.

gastric a. is maintained by the secretion of hydrochloric acid by the oxyntic or parietal cells located in the mucosa of stomach or abomasum.

water a. fish can tolerate only a narrow range of pH

in the water in which they swim. Naturally occurring acidification, such as occurs in waters draining from acid soils, can cause fish deaths.

acidophil 1. a histological structure, cell, or other element staining readily with acid dyes. 2. an alpha cell of the anterior lobe of the pituitary gland or the pancreatic islets. 3. an organism that grows well in highly acid media. 4. acidophilic.

a. neoplasms adenomas and adenocarcinomas of the pars distalis of the pituitary gland are recorded in cats, dogs, sheep and rats. These are infrequently functional but may have space-occupying effects on the pituitary and hypothalamus. They have been associated with diabetes mellitus in cats, galactorrhea in ewes, and metahypophyseal diabetes in dogs.

acidophile see ACIDOPHIL.

acidophilic 1. easily stained with acid dyes. 2. growing best on acid media.

hepatocellular a. bodies see CYTOSEGRESOME FORMATIONS.

acidosis a pathological condition resulting from accumulation of acid or depletion of the alkaline reserve (bicarbonate content) in the blood and body tissues, and characterized by increase in hydrogen ion concentration (decrease in pH).

The optimal ACID–BASE BALANCE is maintained by chemical buffers, biological activities of the cells, and effective functioning of the lungs and kidneys. The opposite of acidosis is ALKALOSIS.

It is rare that acidosis occurs in the absence of some underlying disease process. The more obvious signs of severe acidosis are muscle twitching, involuntary movement, cardiac arrhythmias, disorientation and coma.

compensated a. a condition in which the compensatory mechanisms have returned the pH toward normal.

diabetic a. a metabolic ACIDOSIS produced by accumulation of ketones in uncontrolled DIABETES mellitus.

hypercapnic a. respiratory acidosis.

iatrogenic a. may result from administration of drugs, such as urinary acidifiers, or anesthetic agents which depress respiration.

lactic a. the accumulation of lactate in the rumen in ruminants and the stomach of horses, and hence in the blood, as a result of overfeeding with readily fermentable carbohydrate. See also CARBOHYDRATE ENGORGEMENT.

metabolic a. acidosis resulting from accumulation in the blood of keto acids (derived from fat metabolism) at the expense of bicarbonate, thus diminishing the body's ability to neutralize acids. This type of acidosis can occur when there is an acid gain, as in diabetic ketoacidosis, lactic acidosis, poisoning and failure of the renal tubules to reabsorb bicarbonate. It can also result from bicarbonate loss due to diarrhea or a gastrointestinal fistula.

mixed alkalosis and a. characterized by low serum chloride, normal or slightly elevated plasma bicarbonate and a very high anion gap.

organic a. accumulation of organic anions occurs in uremia, diabetic acidosis and lactic acidosis, and ingestion of salicylates, ethylene glycol or methanol.

renal tubular a. renal tubular malfunction leads to faulty resorption of bicarbonate or excretion of acid and the production of alkaline urine; types I (distal tubular acidosis) and II (proximal tubular acidosis) are identified.

respiratory a. acidosis resulting from ventilatory impairment and subsequent retention of carbon dioxide.

ruminal a. acidosis caused by an altered metabolic state, usually lactic acidosis, in the rumen.

starvation a. a metabolic acidosis due to accumulation of ketones following a severe caloric deficit.

uncompensated a. a condition in which the compensatory mechanisms have not been applied sufficiently to return the pH of the blood to normal.

uremic a. see metabolic acidosis (above).

acidum [L.] *acid.*

aciduria the excretion of acid in the urine. See also specific forms, such as aminoaciduria, orotic aciduria.

orotic a. appearance of orotic acid, an intermediate of pyrimidine synthesis, in the urine due to a lack of orotate phosphoribosyltransferase activity.

paradoxical a. occurs when a metabolic alkalosis caused by severe vomiting or pooling of gastric secretions in the abomasum leads to renal bicarbonate reabsorption and sodium–hydrogen exchange with the inappropriate production of acid urine.

aciduric capable of growing in extremely acid media.

acinar pertaining to or affecting an acinus or acini.

acinetic see AKINETIC.

Acinetobacter gram-negative bacteria commonly found in the environment and often normal flora in animals and humans, but has been associated with nosocomial infections and with bronchopneumonia in mink.

aciniform grapelike.

acinitis inflammation of the acini of a gland.

acinitrazole used as a treatment and prophylactic for blackhead in turkeys; low toxicity but excessive dosing causes infertility and liver and kidney damage.

acinonodular aciniform.

Acinonyx jubatus spotted, long-legged, nonclimbing, big cat. Easily trained and used for hunting. Called also cheetah, hunting leopard.

acinose, acinous made up of acini.

acinus pl. *acini* [L.] any of the smallest lobules of a compound gland.

liver a. the smallest functional unit of the liver made up of two wedge-shaped masses of liver parenchyma that are supplied by two neighboring branches of the portal vein and hepatic artery and drained by two central veins and by terminal branches of the bile duct.

acitretin an active metabolite of ETRETINATE, with similar actions and also used in dermatology.

ACLAM American College of Laboratory Animal Medicine.

aclasia, aclasis pathological continuity of structure, as in chondrodystrophy.

acleistocardia an open state of the foramen ovale of the fetal heart.

acme the critical stage or crisis of a disease.

acne a disorder of the skin characterized by comedones that arise from papules and pustules. Secondary bacterial infection of hair follicles often occurs.

canine a. a skin disease of young, shorthaired dogs affecting the chin and lips.

contagious equine a. see CANADIAN HORSEPOX.

feline a. occurs in cats of any age, involving the skin on the point of the chin and the lips. Also known as fat chin.

interdigital a. see interdigital PYODERMA.

mammary a. see MAMMARY pustular dermatitis.

acnegenic producing acne.

acneiform resembling acne.

Acokanthera a genus of the plant family Apocynaceae used in Africa in the preparation of arrow poisons. Poisoned livestock show diarrhea, irregular heartbeat and sudden death. Contain cardiac glycosides. Includes *A. longiflora*, *A. oblongifolia*, *A. oppositifolia*, *A. schimperi*, *A. spectabilis* (*A. oblongifolia*), *A. venenata* (*A. oppositifolia*). Some species were formerly classified in *Carissa* spp.

acokantherosis the state of being poisoned by *Acokanthera* spp.

Acomatacarus a trombidiform mite of the family Trombiculidae. The larvae are parasitic. Called also chiggers, scrub itch-mite. Includes *A. australiensis* (humans, dogs), *A. galli* (chickens, mice, rats, rabbits).

acomia see ALOPECIA.

Acomys hirinus the spiny mouse, a desert rodent subject to the development of diabetes when fed large quantities of laboratory chow.

aconite see ACONITUM.

aconitine a mixture of alkaloids in ACONITUM *napellus*. Causes abdominal pain, dyspnea, vomiting, diarrhea, cardiac irregularity.

Aconitum a genus of the Ranunculaceae family from northern temperate areas. Includes *A. chasmanthum*, *A. columbianum*, *A. ferox*, *A. vaccarum*, *A. vulpari*.

A. napellus one of the most poisonous of British plants. All parts of the plant contain aconitine, one of the plant's toxic alkaloids. The dried tuberous root was used pharmaceutically as a counterirritant and local anesthetic. The plant is not usually eaten and field poisoning with it is uncommon. Signs of poisoning include vomiting, colic, slow heart rate, paralysis, pupillary dilatation and death due to asphyxia. Called also monkshood, wolf's bane, aconite.

acoprosis absence or paucity of feces in the intestines.

acorea absence of the pupil.

acoria insatiable appetite.

acorn the fruit of the oak—*Quercus* spp. Called also oak buds. In many countries the acorns are ground and used as a carbohydrate-rich food but there is some danger of causing renal damage. See also QUERCUS.

acorn calves congenital defect of calves characterized by an abnormally short or long head, shortened limb bones and bent joints, difficulty in standing, deformity of the back, incoordination and bloating. See also achondroplastic DWARFISM.

acoustic relating to sound or hearing.

a. coupler used in the low speed transmission of data over a telephone line.

a. enhancement an artifact seen in ultrasound examination. There is an area of increased brightness underneath fluid resulting from the lack of impedance when sound waves pass through fluid and increased echoes from underlying structures.

a. gel see COUPLING.

a. nerve see VESTIBULOCOCHLEAR. See also Table 14.

a. reflex test used primarily in humans to differentiate between sensorineural and conductive hearing loss.

a. shadowing an artifact seen in ultrasound imaging in which an intensely echogenic line appears at the surface of structures which block the passage of sound waves.

a. window the body surface area selected for application of the ultrasound transducer, through which sound waves will be transmitted. Consideration must be given to underlying bone or gas-filled structures which would impair image quality.

acoustics the science of sound and hearing.

acoust(o) combining form meaning sound.

ACP acronym for acepromazine; acyl carrier protein.

ACPV American College of Poultry Veterinarians.

acquired incurred as a result of factors acting from or originating outside the organism; not inherited.

a. bleeding a tendency to bleed caused by factors other than inherited and congenital ones. Includes dicoumarol and warfarin poisonings, nutritional deficiency of vitamin K, liver disease and autoimmune thrombocytopenias.

feline a. immunodeficiency syndrome see FELINE immunodeficiency virus.

acral affecting the extremities.

a. lick dermatitis a skin disorder in dogs caused by their licking of a localized area of skin, usually on the lower limbs and particularly over the carpus or metatarsal region. The initiating cause is believed to be psychological but the area quickly becomes traumatized, often secondarily infected, and apparently pruritic which serves to intensify the licking and worsening of the lesion. Called also neurodermatitis, acral pruritic nodule, acropruritic nodule or granuloma, acral lick granuloma.

a. mutilation syndrome see hereditary sensory NEUROPATHY.

a. pruritic nodule see ACRAL lick dermatitis.

acrania partial or complete absence of the cranium.

acranius a monster in which the cranium is absent or rudimentary.

Acremonium a genus of endophytic fungi with species symbiotic in *Lolium perenne*, *festuca arundinacea*; produce toxic lolitrems and ergot alkaloids respectively. Unspecified species have been reported as a cause of eumycotic mycetoma in dogs.

A. coenophialum a clavicipitaceous endophytic fungus that parasitizes tall fescue grass and causes tall fescue poisoning. See FESCUE foot.

A. loliae an endophytic fungus that grows in *Lolium perenne* and produces a tremorgenic mycotoxin which is the cause of RYEGRASS staggers in sheep and cattle.

acridine a dibenzopyridine compound used in the synthesis of dyes and drugs. Derivatives of acridine are successful as antibacterial agents, finding their principal use as local antiseptics. They were popular at one time as antibabesial and trypanocidal agents. See also ACRIFLAVINE, PROFLAVINE.

a. orange stain binds nonspecifically to nucleic acids, proteins, polysaccharides and glycosaminoglycans. Together with fluorescent microscopy, it is reportedly more sensitive than conventional staining methods for demonstrating *Haemobartonella felis* in blood smears.

acriflavine an antiseptic dye used for topical application; average strength is 1 : 1000 to 1 : 8000 solution.

a. hydrochloride used as a solution for local antiseptics. Acid in reaction and slightly irritant.

acritical having no crisis.

acro- word element. [Gr.] *extreme, top, extremity.*

acroanesthesia anesthesia of the extremities.

acrobrachycephaly abnormal height of the skull, with shortness of its anteroposterior dimension.

acrocentric having the centromere toward one end of the chromosome or chromatid; see TELOCENTRIC CHROMOSOME.

acrocephalia see OXYCEPHALY.

acrocephalic see OXYCEPHALY.

acrocephaly see OXYCEPHALY.

Acrochordineae a subfamily of the major family

Colubridae of snakes. They have no fangs and are not venomous. Called also aglypha.
acrochordon see fibrovascular PAPILLOMA.
acrocinesis see ACROKINESIA.
acrocyanosis a human condition characterized by symmetrical cyanosis of the extremities; seen in calves recovering from septicemia, often accompanied by gangrene.
acrodermatitis inflammation of the skin of the extremities, particularly the paws or feet. See also ACRAL lick dermatitis.
enteropathic a., a. enteropathica a hereditary disorder of humans associated with a defect of zinc uptake. Gastrointestinal disturbances accompany the dermatological signs. Inherited PARAKERATOSIS in calves (lethal trait 46) resembles this disorder.
lethal a. an inherited, autosomal recessive abnormality of zinc metabolism in Bull terriers. Clinical signs include stunted growth, severe hyperkeratosis of foot pads and pressure points, and secondary infections, particularly in the skin.
acrodermatosis any disease of the skin of the extremities, particularly the paws or hooves.
acroesthesia 1. exaggerated sensitiveness. 2. pain in the extremities.
acrokinesia abnormal motility or movement of the extremities.
acrolein aldehyde of allyl, formed by the destructive distillation of glycerin and during the burning of fat; has a pungent odor.
a. poisoning exposure to fumes causes conjunctivitis, rhinitis, pulmonary edema.
acromegaly abnormal enlargement of the extremities of the skeleton due to overgrowth of connective tissue and increased appositional growth of bone caused by hypersecretion of growth hormone (GH) from the PITUITARY gland in adults. The condition has been reported in cats and dogs. Called also hypersomatotropism.
iatrogenic a. may be caused by the administration of drugs that stimulate growth hormone-secreting acidophils. Progestational agents, usually administered for estrus control, have been responsible for this disorder in dogs. Affected dogs show coarsening of facial features, widening of interdental spaces, enlargement of the abdomen, thickening of skin with excessive hair growth, and inspiratory stridor.
acromelanism genetically determined, temperature-dependent pigmentation pattern, with full expression only occurring on legs, ears, tail and face. Seen in Siamese and Himalayan cats, and rabbits.
acromelic pertaining to the end of a limb.
a. dysplasia dysplasia of the extremities of limbs.
acromicria abnormal smallness of the extremities of the skeleton—nose, jaws and feet.
acromio- word element. [Gr.] *acromion*.
acromiohumeral pertaining to the acromion and humerus.
acromion the prominence at the distal end of the spine of the scapula.
acromionectomy resection of the acromion.
acromiothoracic pertaining to the acromion and thorax.
acromotrichia see LEUKOTRICHIA.
acromphalus 1. bulging of the navel; sometimes a sign of umbilical hernia. 2. the center of the navel.
acroneurosis any neuropathy of the extremities.
acropachia see hypertrophic OSTEOPATHY.
acroparalysis paralysis of the extremities.
acropathy any disease of the extremities.
acropodium the part of the limb made up of digits.
acroposthitis inflammation of the prepuce.
Acroptilon repens CENTAUREA *repens*.
acrosin one of the enzymes in the acrosome on the head of a mammalian spermatozoon. Involved in the penetration of the zona pellucida of the ovum by the spermatozoon.
acrosomal vesicles a structure participating in the conversion of the spermatid to the spermatozoon. Proacrosomal granules coalesce to form a single large vesicle which contains the acrosome. The vesicle collapses on the nucleus forming the head cap of the spermatozoon.
acrosome the caplike, membrane-bounded structure that covers the anterior portion of the head of the mammalian spermatozoon; it is bounded by an inner and an outer membrane and contains enzymes involved in penetration of the ovum.
a. reaction fusion of the outer acrosomal membrane with the sperm plasma membrane, and the breakdown of the fused complex, after the attachment of the spermatozoon to the zona pellucida. It is induced by substances from the egg investments and releases enzymes involved in penetration of the ovum.
acrosoxacin see ROSAXOACIN.
acroteriasis congenital absence or part absence of limbs. Called also amputates.
bovine a. an inherited defect involving amputation of limbs, defects of facial bones, cleft palate and mandibular shortness.
acrotism absence or imperceptibility of the pulse.
acrylic glue a glue used to repair damaged beaks of birds; care must be taken to avoid inhalation of vapors.
ACT[1] activated clotting time.
ACT[2] American College of Theriogenologists.
Actaea a genus of the Ranunculaceae family.
A. spicata contains a gastrointestinal and buccal irritant. Called also baneberry, herb Christopher, dolls' eyes, black cohosh.
ACTH adrenocorticotropic hormone; produced by the anterior lobe of the PITUITARY gland that stimulates the cortex of the ADRENAL gland to secrete its hormones, including corticosterone. If production of ACTH falls below normal, the adrenal cortex decreases in size, and production of the cortical hormones declines. Called also adrenocorticotropin and corticotropin.

Its principal use is as a diagnostic agent: e.g. in the differentiation of primary adrenocortical neoplasia and adrenocortical hyperplasia.
ACTH assay determination of plasma levels of ACTH may be used to identify pituitary-dependent hypo- or hyperadrenocorticism.
ACTH cells see CHROMOPHOBE.
ACTH gel a commercially available form of ACTH in gelatin with prolonged action.
ACTH response test, ACTH stimulation test measures the secretory capacity of the adrenal cortex in response to a supraphysiological dose of exogenous ACTH. This test is commonly used in the diagnosis of hyperadrenocorticism in dogs. An increased response is consistent with adrenocortical hyperplasia.
ACTH-secreting adenoma see CORTICOTROPH ADENOMA.
actin a muscle protein localized in the I band of myofibrils; acting along with myosin particles, it is responsible for the contraction and relaxation of muscle.
a. F assembly of actin G monomers into filaments.
a. filaments smallest filamentous proteins involved in a static role in cell structure and a dynamic role in cell movement.

a. G monomeric globular protein which assembles into actin filaments.

Actinea see HYMENOXYS.

actinic producing chemical action.

a. dermatitis that produced by exposure to actinic radiation, such as that from the sun, ultraviolet waves, or x- or gamma radiation. Called also dermatitis actinica.

a. radiation said of rays of light beyond the violet end of the spectrum.

actinium a chemical element, atomic number 89, atomic weight 227, symbol Ac. See Table 6.

actino- word element. [Gr.] *ray, radiation.*

actinobacillary caused by infection with *Actinobacillus* spp.

equine a. peritonitis see PERITONITIS.

a. glossitis see ACTINOBACILLOSIS.

a. mastitis an occasional occurrence in ewes.

ovine a. epididymitis see EPIDIDYMITIS.

a. seminal vesiculitis see SEMINAL vesiculitis.

actinobacillosis an infectious disease characterized by inflammation of the soft tissues of the head, especially the tongue, pharyngeal lymph nodes and esophageal groove in cattle and the subcutaneous tissues of the head and neck in sheep by *Actinobacillus lignieresi.* The acute disease in cattle is characterized by a swollen, painful tongue and hypersalivation. Called also wooden tongue.

cutaneous a. of sheep and cattle there are ulcers and nodules in the subcutaneous tissue, often on lymphatics, which contain yellow to green pus. Local lymph nodes are often involved. The lesions are mostly about the head, often in the mouth, but do not affect the tongue.

nasal a. in sheep is characterized by nasal obstruction and stertor and a nasal discharge. See also NASAL actinobacillosis.

perinatal a. of foals is a septicemia caused by *Actinobacillus equuli.* The disease is usually endemic on individual farms and can cause many deaths. The clinical syndrome is one of collapse and coma. Surviving foals show signs related to localization of infection in specific organs. Called also shigellosis, sleepy foal disease.

a. of rumenoreticulum causes interference with normal motility and development of a vagus indigestion.

Actinobacillus a genus of bacteria which are gram-negative, pleomorphic rods.

A. actinoides a secondary agent in seminal vesiculitis in bulls and enzootic pneumonia in calves.

A. actinomycetemcomitans associated with epididymitis in rams and periodontal disease and endocarditis in humans.

A. capsulatus the cause of arthritis and septicemia in rabbits.

A. equuli the cause of septicemia and subsequent focal lesions in young foals. Previously called *Shigella equirulis.*

A. lignieresi the cause of ACTINOBACILLOSIS of cattle and sheep, and occasionally in pigs, dogs and humans.

A. mallei see BURKHOLDERIA *mallei.*

A. pleuropneumoniae causes severe pleuropneumonia and pleuritis in pigs. Previously *Haemophilus pleuropneumoniae.*

A. salpingitidis the proposed name for a bacteria which is isolatable from cases of salpingitis, peritonitis, airsacculitis and pneumonia in birds. Called also *Pasteurella salpingitis.*

A. seminis the cause of epididymitis and periorchitis in rams.

A. suis the cause of septicemia and subsequent focal lesions in young pigs.

A. ureae may be a cause of abortion in sows.

Actinocleidus a genus of flukes parasitic in fish.

actinodermatitis dermatitis from exposure to x-rays.

actinolyte an apparatus for concentrating the rays of electric light in phototherapy.

Actinomadura a dubious genus of the Nocardiaceae family; credited with causing cutaneous granulomata in horses.

Actinomyces a genus of non-acid-fast, gram-positive organisms that form a mycelium of branching filaments that fragment into irregular-sized fragments.

A. bovis the cause of ACTINOMYCOSIS of cattle and sheep.

A. congolensis, A. dermatonomus see DERMATOPHILUS *congolensis.*

A. hordeovulneris a cause of abscesses, pleuritis and systemic infections in dogs where it is often associated with penetration by grass awns (foxtails) of *Hordeum* spp.

A. israelii an uncommon cause of actinomycosis in cattle and pigs.

A. necrophorus see FUSOBACTERIUM *necrophorum.*

A. pyogenes capable of producing suppurative lesions in any organ or tissue in animals. In farm animals, especially ruminants, it is much the most common bacteria found in infected wounds and abscesses. An important cause of MASTITIS in cattle. Previously called *Corynebacterium pyogenes.*

A. suis the cause of actinomycosis of the swine mammary gland.

A. viscosus the cause of periodontal disease in hamsters, and opportunistic infections of dogs.

actinomyces an organism of the genus *Actinomyces.*

actinomycete a mold-like bacterium (order Actinomycetales) occurring as elongated, frequently filamentous cells, with a branching tendency.

actinomycetoma see actinomycotic MYCETOMA.

actinomycin a family of antibiotics from various species of *Streptomyces,* which are active against bacteria and fungi; it includes the antineoplastic agents actinomycin C (CACTINOMYCIN) and actinomycin D (DACTINOMYCIN).

actinomycoma a tumorlike reactive lesion due to *Actinomyces* spp.

actinomycosis in cattle, caused by *Actinomyces bovis,* commonly a rarefying osteomyelitis of the bones of the head particularly the maxilla and mandible. There is obvious swelling of the bone which is painful and causes interference with eating, and sinuses onto the cheek which discharge sticky, honey-like material containing granules. Rare occurrences are granulomatous lesions of the skin about the head, soft tissue lesions in the testicles and sow mammary gland, and infection of the esophageal groove causing a vagus indigestion. Called also lumpy jaw. See also ACTINOBACILLOSIS, ACTINOMYCOTIC.

In dogs and cats, actinomycosis usually consists of localized pyogranulomatous infections, most often in subcutaneous tissues around the head and neck, bone, and thoracic or abdominal cavities. Disseminated infections are uncommon. See also NOCARDIOSIS.

cutaneous a. see MYCOTIC dermatitis.

actinomycotic caused by infection with *Actinomyces* spp.

a. fistulous withers see FISTULOUS withers.

a. lesion 'actinomycotic' lesions resemble those caused by *Actinomyces* spp. and may contain small particulate granules, such as occur in actinomycosis.

These granules also have an asteroid appearance under the microscope. The lesions are slow growing and often caused by *Aspergillus* spp. or *Coccidioides immitis*.

a. mandibular osteomyelitis see ACTINOMYCOSIS.

a. mycetoma see MYCETOMA.

a. poll evil see POLL evil.

action 1. the accomplishment of an effect, whether mechanical or chemical, or the effect so produced. 2. the gait or type of movement of an animal.

cumulative a. the sudden and markedly increased action of a drug after administration of several doses.

a. lists are produced by a computerized herd health program from the analysis of reproduction data, which set out which cows are to be examined for a variety of reproductive reasons, such as pregnancy, failure to conceive and postnatal clearance for resumption of breeding.

action potential the nerve impulse, the sign of activity and the basis of activity in individual neurons in the nervous system. The measure of the activity of an individual nerve cell is indicated by the frequency of its discharge.

compound a. p. the sum of the activity in a number of nerve fibers. It applies to the degree of activity in a nerve trunk in which a variable proportion of nerve fibers are discharging.

activated a state of being more than usually active. In biological systems this is usually brought about by chemical or electrical means. Commonly said of pharmaceutical and chemical products.

a. clotting time (ACT) a simplified version of the activated partial thromboplastin time which measures the intrinsic clotting activity of the whole blood. See also activated COAGULATION time, CLOTTING time.

a. partial thromboplastin time (APTT) a test of intrinsic clotting activity of whole blood. Partial prothrombin, usually rabbit or human brain prothrombins, is added to plasma activated with kaolin or ellagic acid. The time required for the test is short and the results are dependable.

a. sludge a method of dealing with sewage and abattoir effluent. Consists of an aeration tank in which biologically active, previously sedimented sludge is mixed with incoming effluent and agitated in the presence of an ample supply of air.

activation the process of activating.

a. analysis a method of analyzing the content of elements in samples of biological material. The sample is bombarded with nuclear particles and the elements in it measured by the radiation emitted by their radioactive daughter products. Called also radioactivation analysis.

a. energy the difference in energy between the ground state of the reactants in a reaction and the point of maximum energy or transition state of the reactions. Usually lowered by enzyme catalysts.

a. factor see HAGEMAN FACTOR.

a. unit the combination of complement (C4, C2 and C3) that binds to the antigen–antibody complex in the initial reaction step in the classical pathway of complement activation. See also COMPLEMENT.

activator a substance that makes another substance active or that renders an inactive enzyme capable of exerting its proper effect.

developing a. see developing ACCELERATOR.

plasminogen a. a substance that activates plasminogen and converts it into plasmin.

active not passive.

a. principle the drugs or chemicals in a pharmaceutical preparation that exert an effect pharmacologically; as distinct from the inert fillers, wetting agents and other excipients also often included.

a. site that region of a protein, usually an enzyme, that binds to another molecule such as the substrate of the enzyme.

a. transport the movement of ions or molecules assisted by a carrier protein across the cell membranes and epithelial layers, usually against a concentration gradient, resulting directly from the expenditure of metabolic energy. For example, under normal circumstances more potassium ions are present within the cell and more sodium ions extracellularly. The process of maintaining these normal differences in electrolytic composition between the intracellular fluids is active transport. The process differs from simple diffusion or osmosis in that it requires the expenditure of metabolic energy.

activin a gonadal peptide hormone isolated from follicular fluid; has an unidentified role in stimulating FSH secretion.

activity the quality or process of releasing energy or of accomplishing an effect.

displacement a. an instinctive behavior pattern, exhibited out of context and believed to be a means of relieving tension in the animal. Usually performed when the animal is in a state of high arousal or when it is frustrated in the performance of some instinctive activity. Seen as sexual mounting, digging, tail chasing, or excessive grooming in cats.

economic a. a method of producing a specific product, e.g. fine wool, white veal.

enzyme a. the catalytic effect exerted by an enzyme, expressed as units per milligram of enzyme (*specific* activity) or molecules of substrate transformed per minute per molecule of enzyme (*molecular* activity).

a. gross income the total value of production, rather than the income, for a particular activity.

a. gross margin the gross income of an activity less its variable costs.

intermediate a. production of a commodity which is not sold but is used as an input to some other enterprise, e.g. crop used on the farm as stock feed.

optical a. the ability of a chemical compound to rotate the plane of polarization of plane-polarized light.

actomyosin the complex of actin and myosin constituting muscle fibers and responsible for the contraction and relaxation of muscle.

acts of veterinary science those acts, such as making diagnoses, performing surgical operations, anesthetizing, performing embryo transfers, carrying out radiographic examinations which are considered, in law, to be the prerogative of registered, professional veterinarians. Persons who are not veterinarians and who perform these acts are liable to prosecution under the registration legislation.

actual focal spot the actual area of the focal spot on the radiographic target as viewed at right angles to the plane of the target.

actuarial methods statistical techniques relating to preparation of mortality and other analytical tables.

Acuaria a genus of nematode parasites. Includes *A. hamulosa* (see CHEILOSPIRURA *hamulosa*), *A. spiralis* (see SYNHIMANTUS *spiralis*), *A. uncinata* (see ECHINURIA *uncinata*).

acuchi see MYOPROCTA.

acuity acuteness or clearness.

acuminate sharp-pointed.

acupoint specific locations at which treatment by acupuncture is delivered; called also acupuncture point.

acupressure compression of a blood vessel by inserted acupuncture needles.

acupuncture the Chinese practice of inserting needles into specific points (acupoints) along the 'meridians' of the body to relieve the discomfort associated with painful disorders, to induce surgical anesthesia, and for preventive and therapeutic purposes. In recent years, the techniques have been adapted for use in veterinary medicine.

a. instruments includes cups for vacuum creation, needles, hot needles, moxibustion, electronic heating devices, coolant spray, ultrasound, electroacupuncture machines, laser equipment.

a. points areas of skin specified in animal 'maps' as being related to certain internal organs; the practical basis of Chinese acupuncture.

special action a. points acupoints used only to influence specific organs or tissues.

acus a needle or needle-like process.

acute 1. brief. 2. common usage is 'having severe signs and a short course of 12 to 24 hours'. See also under organ (e.g. pancreatitis), system (e.g. respiratory), causative agent (e.g. arsenic) or lesion (e.g. myonecrosis).

a. bovine pulmonary emphysema-edema see ATYPICAL INTERSTITIAL PNEUMONIA.

a. care see SECONDARY health care.

a. death syndrome of chickens sudden death, for no apparent reason, in 2 to 3 week old broiler chicks; clinical signs of falling, wing flapping and convulsions may occur for about a minute before death.

a. phase response the rapid change in composition of certain plasma proteins, largely due to alteration in hepatic synthesis, in response to infection or inflammation. Although the purpose is not well understood, these changes are believed to assist in immune response. Erythrocyte sedimentation rate (ESR) is a laboratory indicator of the acute phase response. See also C-REACTIVE PROTEIN and TUMOR necrosis factor.

a. physiology and chronic health evaluation (APACHE) see APACHE SYSTEM.

a. respiratory distress syndrome (ARDS) see acute RESPIRATORY distress syndrome.

acute equine respiratory syndrome (Morbillivirus) a fatal disease of horses recorded only in Queensland, Australia in 1994. A virus of the *Paramyxoviridae* family, possibly a morbillivirus, has been isolated and is considered to be the cause of the disease in horses and of a fatal disease in humans working with them. Clinical signs in horses include fever, dyspnea, copious, clear or blood-tinged, frothy nasal discharge, death in 1 to 3 days, with a case fatality rate of 60–70%. Necropsy lesions include pulmonary congestion and edema and acute interstitial pneumonia. The virus is considered to have originated from fruit-eating macrobats (*Pteropus* spp.) present in Eastern Australia. See EQUINE morbillivirus.

In one fatal human case the clinical syndrome resembled in general that observed in horses while in a second case death occurred after a prolonged clinical course including central nervous system signs one year after infection.

acute-phase proteins see ACUTE phase response.

ACVA American College of Veterinary Anesthetists.

ACVB American College of Veterinary Behaviorists.

ACVCP American College of Veterinary Clinical Pharmacology.

ACVD American College of Veterinary Dermatology.

ACVECC American College of Veterinary Emergency and Critical Care.

ACVIM American College of Veterinary Internal Medicine.

ACVM American College of Veterinary Microbiologists.

ACVN American College of Veterinary Nutrition.

ACVO American College of Veterinary Ophthalmology.

ACVP American College of Veterinary Pathologists.

ACVPM American College of Veterinary Preventive Medicine.

ACVR American College of Veterinary Radiology.

ACVS American College of Veterinary Surgeons.

ACVSc Australian College of Veterinary Scientists.

acyanotic not characterized or accompanied by cyanosis.

a. heart malformations congenital cardiac malformations which permit life-sustaining levels of activity; includes pulmonary STENOSIS, aortic STENOSIS, INTERATRIAL septal defect, small VENTRICULAR septal defect, DEXTROCARDIA and some cases of ECTOPIA cordis.

acycloguanosine acyclovir.

acyclovir, aciclovir a synthetic analog of guanosine which selectively interferes with viral DNA synthesis. Used parenterally and topically as an antiviral agent in herpesvirus infections in humans and to a limited extent in animals.

acyesis 1. sterility in a female animal. 2. absence of pregnancy.

acyl 1. an organic radical derived from a fatty acid by removal of the hydroxyl group. 2. generic term for fatty acid groups.

a. carrier protein ACP; a carrier protein molecule which is part of the fatty acid synthesizing enzyme complex in non-mammalian systems and which carries acyl groups.

a. CoA thioester of coenzyme A and a fatty acid of unspecified, but usually more than 14 carbon length.

a. CoA dehydrogenase deficiency lack of the first enzyme of beta-oxidation, acyl CoA dehydrogenase, a flavoprotein which catalyzes the removal of two hydrogens from the acyl chain.

acylaminopenicillins see UREIDOPENICILLINS.

acylation introduction of an acyl radical into the molecules of a compound.

1-acyl-sn-glycerol-3-phosphate acyltransferase enzyme catalyzing the preferential transfer of unsaturated fatty acids to the 2-position of the glycerol backbone of phospholipids and triacylglycerols.

acystia congenital absence of the urinary bladder.

acystinervia paralysis of the urinary bladder.

ACZM American College of Zoological Medicine.

AD see ALEUTIAN MINK DISEASE.

ad [L.] preposition, *to*.

-ad suffix meaning toward.

ad- prefix meaning towards.

ad. lib. ad libitum.

ad libitum without restraint.

a. l. feeding food available at all times with the quantity and frequency of consumption being the free choice of the animal.

ada-a see MORINDA RETICULATA.

adactylia, adactyly congenital absence of the digits.

adamantine pertaining to the enamel of the teeth.

adamantinoma see AMELOBLASTOMA, acanth... EPULIS.

adamantoblast see AMELOBLAST.

adamantoblastoma, adamant... BLASTOMA.

Adams Autocrit a centrifuge use...

of the packed (red blood) cell volume in capillary tubes.

Adams–Stokes disease see STOKES–ADAMS DISEASE.

adamsite an arsenical smoke which causes sneezing, malaise and vomiting, and is used in crowd control and riot control. Called also DM. See also STERNUTATOR.

Adamson's fringe in growing hairs, the margin between the mitotically active hair bulb and the inactive hair shaft.

adaptation 1. adjustment of the pupil to light, constricting with increased light intensity, dilating with decreased intensity. 2. any anatomical, physiological, developmental or behavioral adjustment to the environment of an organism which enhances its chances of leaving descendants. The ability of animals to adapt to a limited supply of drinking water and to high or low environmental temperatures is an important aspect of animal husbandry. The selection of animals which are capable of a high level of such adaptation has made it possible to improve the productivity of herds and flocks in some countries. See also GENERAL ADAPTATION SYNDROME. 3. the process by which organisms are modified so as to improve their chances of survival in an environment.

dark a. adaptation of the eye to vision in the dark or in reduced illumination.

light a. adaptation of the eye to vision in sunlight or in bright illumination (photopia), with reduction in the concentration of the photosensitive pigments of the eye.

negative a. see HABITUATION.

a. rate the rate at which afferent sensory receptors discharge into their afferent axons. The rates differ between different types of receptors. For example, there are slow adaptors which signal the more persistent changes such as steady pressure. See also receptor adaptation (below).

receptor a. sensory receptors vary in their individual response to stimuli, the response declining after an initial period of rapid response. The rate at which different kinds of receptors change these responses is the adaptation rate (see above).

adaption see ADAPTATION.

adaptive nephron hypothesis see INTACT-NEPHRON HYPOTHESIS.

ADCC antibody-dependent cell-mediated cytotoxicity.

addax a North African antelope with long, ribbed, spiral horns. Called also *Addax nasomaculatus*.

added filtration sheets of metal placed in the path of the primary x-ray beam to make it a more penetrating beam.

adder a loose nomenclature of snakes which cuts across scientific classification. Includes puff adder, common English adder which are VIPERINE snakes, and the Australian adder which is an ELAPINE snake.

death a. gray-brown, dark, banded, 30 inch Australian elapid snake which is aggressive and a rapid striker. The venom is a potent toxin. The bite often leaves no mark but is usually fatal. Called also *Acanthophis antarcticus*.

desert death a. a specially adapted, smaller desert form of the death adder. Called also *Acanthophis antarcticus pyrrhus*.

puff a. *Bitis arietans*, an unaggressive but highly poisonous African snake, 3 to 5 ft long with a thick body.

addiction physiological dependence on some agent, usually a plant, with a tendency to increase its use. Whether true addiction ever occurs in animals is doubtful. Field evidence does point to preferential grazing of some known toxic plants, e.g. *Astragalus*, *Swainsona* spp.

drug a. abuse of narcotic drugs is a hazard of veterinary practice because of the availability of addictive agents to registered veterinarians. The same laws apply to members of the veterinary profession as to the medical profession and are designed to protect them against becoming dependent upon any drug. Deregistration and a consequent isolation from the prohibited substances is the usual penalty.

Addis count the determination of the number of red blood cells, white blood cells, epithelial cells, casts, and the protein content in an aliquot of a 12-hour urine specimen. Used in the diagnosis and management of kidney disease. Not commonly used in veterinary medicine.

Addison's disease see primary HYPOADRENOCORTICISM.

addisonian crisis signs of weakness, vomiting, diarrhea and sometimes collapse accompanying an acute adrenocortical insufficiency. See also HYPOADRENOCORTICISM.

additive 1. characterized by addition. 2. a substance added to another to improve its appearance, increase its nutritive value, etc. See FEED additive.

food a. material added to food; includes preservatives, emulsifiers, stabilizers, acids, nonstick agents, humectants, firming agents, antifoaming agents, colorings and flavorings, solvents, and even nutritive materials such as minerals and vitamins.

a. gene action 1. total contribution made by all loci to a polygenic trait. 2. when the heterozygote is intermediate in phenotype between the two homozygotes, i.e. a lack of dominance.

a. genetic relationship the degree of relationship (number of genes held in common) between two individuals neither of which is inbred; the minimum relationship is 0 and the maximum is 1.0.

a. genetic variance variance attributed to the mean effect of substituting one allele for another at any given loci.

intramammary infusion a. agents, e.g. anti-inflammatories, added to improve pharmacological efficacy.

a. relationship see additive genetic relationship (above).

address the specific location of a piece of information in the storage media of a computer.

addressins tissue-specific molecules in vascular endothelium which are involved in directing extravasation of recirculating lymphocytes.

adduct to draw toward a center or median line.

adduction the act of adducting; the state of being adducted.

adductor that which adducts.

thigh a. muscles include the pectineus, gracilis and the adductor itself. These and the external obturator muscle can be affected by obturator paralysis which allows the legs to spread. Section of the pectineus and adductor has been suggested as a palliative treatment for canine hip dysplasia.

adeciduate placenta see epitheliochorial PLACENTA.

Adema disease see inherited PARAKERATOSIS of cattle.

adenalgia pain in a gland.

adenasthenia deficient glandular activity.

adendritic without dendrites.

adenectomy excision of a gland.

adenectopia displacement of a gland.

Adenia digitata plant genus in family Passifloraceae; contains cyanogenetic glycosides and a potent toxal-

bumin—modeccin. *A. volkensi* may be similarly toxic.
adeniform gland-shaped.
adenine a purine base present in nucleoproteins of cells of plants and animals. Adenine and guanine are essential components of NUCLEIC ACIDS.
a. arabinoside see VIDARABINE.
a. nucleotide translocator protein in the inner mitochondrial membrane; exchanges ADP produced by reactions in the cytosol for ATP produced in the mitochondrion by oxidative phosphorylation.
adenitis inflammation of a gland.
granulomatous cervical a. granulomatous inflammation of the lymph nodes of the neck in pigs; asymptomatic and found only at slaughter; caused by *Rhodococcus equi* or atypical mycobacteria, rarely by *Mycobacterium tuberculosis*, *M. avium*, *M. bovis*.
granulomatous sebaceous a. see SEBACEOUS adenitis.
lacrimal gland a. see DACRYOADENITIS.
adenization assumption by other tissue of an abnormal glandlike appearance.
adeno- word element. [Gr.] *gland*.
adeno-associated virus a replication-defective, single-stranded DNA virus classifed in the genus *Dependovirus* of the family *Parvoviridae*. They depend on help provided by coinfection with adenoviruses for their replication. Not known to cause disease.
adenoameloblastoma an odontogenic tumor with formation of ductlike structures in place of, or in addition to, a typical ameloblastic pattern.
adenoblast an embryonic cell capable of forming gland tissue.
adenoCa an abbreviation used in medical records for adenocarcinoma.
adenocarcinoid see goblet-cell CARCINOID.
adenocarcinoma carcinoma derived from glandular tissue or in which the tumor cells form recognizable glandular structures. Some are listed under the tissues or organs they invade.
a. of the ileum a higher than usual prevalence is described in sheep and cattle in some very localized geographical areas, and a relationship to a high intake of bracken hypothesized. The lesions may be symptomless or cause intestinal obstruction. See also PTERIDIUM.
nasal a. see enzootic NASAL adenocarcinoma.
renal a. causes little clinical abnormality in large animals but may be detectable as kidney enlargement during physical examination.
adenocele a cystic adenomatous tumor.
adenocellulitis inflammation of a gland and the cellular tissue around it.
adenochondroma a tumor containing both glandular and cartilaginous elements.
adenocystoma adenoma in which there is cyst formation.
adenodynia pain in a gland.
adenoepithelioma a tumor composed of glandular and epithelial elements.
adenogenous originating from glandular tissue.
adenohypophyseal pertaining to the adenohypophysis.
a. aplasia see PITUITARY hypoplasia.
a. corticotrophs cells which secrete ACTH, beta lipotropin.
a. gonadotrophs cells which secrete follicle-stimulating and luteinizing hormones.
a. hypoplasia see PITUITARY hypoplasia.
a. mammotrophs cells which secrete prolactin.
a. neoplasms include ACIDOPHIL and BASOPHIL adenomas, normally inactive CHROMOPHOBE adenoma and an ACTH-secreting corticotroph adenoma.
a. pouch see RATHKE'S POUCH.
a. somatotrophs cells which secrete growth hormone.
a. system includes the hypothalamus, the pituitary gland and the interconnecting blood supply.
a. thyrotrophs cells which secrete thyroid-stimulating hormone.
adenohypophysis the so-called anterior lobe of the hypophysis cerebri (see also PITUITARY), which in domestic animals mostly surrounds the posterior lobe. It develops from the roof of the embryonic mouth and is divided into a large pars distalis, a smaller pars tuberalis and a pars intermedia. It secretes hormones under the control of releasing agents which arrive from the hypothalamus via a hypothalamohypophyseal portal system. The hormones include growth hormone, ACTH, beta-lipotropin, prolactin, thyrotropic hormone, follicle-stimulating hormone and luteinizing hormone.
See also ADENOHYPOPHYSEAL.
adenoid 1. resembling a gland. 2. enlarged pharyngeal tonsils.
adenolipoma a tumor composed of both glandular and fatty tissue elements.
adenology the sum of knowledge regarding glands.
adenolymphitis lymphadenitis; inflammation of lymph nodes.
adenolymphoma a cystic salivary-gland tumor containing epithelial and lymphoid tissue.
adenoma a benign epithelial tumor in which the cells form recognizable glandular structures or in which the cells are derived from glandular epithelium. Called also PITUITARY tumor (acidophil), ADRENAL GLAND tumor, APOCRINE tumor, ceruminous gland tumor, ECCRINE tumor.
adenomalacia undue softness of a gland.
adenomatoid resembling adenoma.
congenital a. malformation see BRONCHIAL hypoplasia.
adenomatosis the formation of numerous adenomatous growths.
enzootic bovine a. see ATYPICAL INTERSTITIAL PNEUMONIA.
porcine intestinal a. a disease of recently weaned pigs characterized by a sudden appearance of anorexia and weight loss, a short course of a few weeks and recovery in most cases. The diagnostic feature is the adenomatous thickening of the intestinal wall. *Campylobacter hyointestinalis* has been suggested as a possible etiological agent. See also ovine PULMONARY adenomatosis, PROLIFERATIVE hemorrhagic enteropathy, NECROTIC enteritis, terminal ILEITIS.
adenomatous pertaining to adenoma or to nodular hyperplasia of a gland.
a. polyps see POLYP.
a. intestinal hyperplasia see porcine intestinal ADENOMATOSIS.
adenomere the blind terminal portion of a developing gland that will become the functional portion of the organ. Used also as a title for a mature secretory endpiece. Depending on the type of gland the adenomere may be mucous or serous. It may also be tubular, alveolar, acinar or tubuloalveolar.
adenomyoma a tumor made up of endometrium and muscle tissue, found in the uterus, or more frequently, in the uterine ligaments.
adenomyometritis adenomyosis of the uterus.

adenomyosarcoma adenosarcoma containing striated muscle.

adenomyosis invasion of the muscular wall of an organ (e.g. uterus) by glandular tissue.

epididymal a. occurs in aged dogs and bulls, probably due to chronic estrogenic stimulation, such as occurs in dogs with Sertoli cell tumors. Spermatic granulomas are a common sequel.

uterine a. a rare lesion seen occasionally in cows and bitches.

adenopathy enlargement of glands, especially of the lymph nodes.

adenosarcoma adenoma blended with sarcoma.

adenosclerosis hardening of a gland.

adenosine one of the four bases that make up RNA and DNA containing the pentose sugar, 2-deoxy-D-ribose. Adenosine nucleotides are involved in the energy metabolism of all cells. Adenosine can be linked to a chain of one, two or three phosphate groups to form *adenosine monophosphate* (AMP), *adenosine diphosphate* (ADP) or *adenosine triphosphate* (ATP). The bond between the phosphate groups in ADP or the two bonds between the phosphate groups in ATP are called *high-energy bonds* because hydrolysis of a high-energy bond provides a large amount of free energy that can be used to drive other processes that would not otherwise occur spontaneously. The energy that is derived from the oxidation of carbohydrates, fats or proteins is used to synthesize ATP. The energy stored in ATP is then used directly or indirectly to drive all other cellular processes that require energy, of which there are four major types: (1) the transport of molecules and ions across cell membranes against concentration gradients, which maintains the internal environment of the cell and produces the membrane potential for the conduction of nerve impulses; (2) the contraction of muscle fibers and other fibers producing the motion of cells; (3) the synthesis of chemical compounds; (4) the synthesis of other high-energy compounds.

cyclic a. monophosphate (cyclic AMP, cAMP, 3′,5′-cAMP) a cyclic nucleotide, adenosine 3′,5′-cyclic monophosphate, involved in the action of many hormones, including catecholamines, ACTH and vasopressin. The hormone (first message) binds to a specific β-receptor on the cell membrane of target cells. This activates an enzyme, adenylate cyclase, which produces cyclic AMP from ATP. Cyclic AMP acts as a second messenger activating other enzymes via covalent modulation within the cell.

a. deaminase key enzyme in degradation pathway of adenosine; catalyzes the deamination of adenosine to inosine. Many cases of severe combined immunodeficiency syndrome in humans result from a heritable lack of adenosine deaminase.

a. diphosphate (ADP) a nucleotide, adenosine 5′-pyrophosphate, produced by the hydrolysis of adenosine triphosphate (ATP). It is then converted back to ATP by oxidative, substrate or photosynthetic phosphorylation. See also ADP.

a. monophosphate (AMP) a nucleotide, adenosine 5′-phosphate, involved in energy metabolism and nucleotide synthesis. Called also adenylic acid.

a. triphosphatase a term used to refer to the enzymatic activity of certain intercellular processes that split ATP to form ADP and inorganic phosphate, when the energy released is not used for the synthesis of chemical compounds. Examples are the splitting of ATP in muscle contraction in myosin head-groups and the transport of ions across cell membranes. Called also ATPase.

a. triphosphatase test used as a quantitative assay of the amount of avian leukosis virus in chicken tissues or tissue cultures. It depends on the virus's characteristic of carrying on its surface a phosphatase enzyme that dephosphorylates adenosine triphosphate.

a. triphosphate (ATP) a nucleotide, adenosine 5′-triphosphate, occurring in all cells, where it stores energy in the form of high-energy phosphate bonds. Free energy of hydrolysis is supplied to drive metabolic reactions or to transport molecules against concentration gradients, when ATP is hydrolyzed to ADP and inorganic phosphate or to AMP and inorganic pyrophosphate. ATP is also used to produce high-energy phosphorylated intermediary metabolites, such as glucose-6-phosphate.

adenosis 1. any disease of a gland. 2. abnormal development of a gland.

adenosquamous carcinoma a primary epithelial bronchogenic tumor.

adenotomy anatomy, incision or dissection of glands.

Adenoviridae the family of viruses containing two genera, *Mastadenovirus*, which are the mammalian adenoviruses, and *Aviadenovirus*, which contain the bird adenoviruses. Virons are nonenveloped, 70 nm diameter and contain a double-stranded DNA molecule of about 30 to 35 kilobase pairs. They grow in cell cultures producing cytopathology and each species has a relatively narrow host range. Adenoviruses are common causes of relatively mild upper respiratory disease and of enteric infections. The type species is human adenovirus h1.

adenovirus a member of the family ADENOVIRIDAE.

avian a. types 1–11 cause respiratory or enteric disease, aplastic anemia, atrophy of bursa of Fabricius, egg-drop syndrome.

bovine a. types 1–9 cause conjunctivitis, pneumonia, diarrhea, pneumoenteritis.

canine a. type 1 (CAV-1) causes infectious canine HEPATITIS.

canine a. type 2 (CAV-2) is a cause of KENNEL COUGH (tracheobronchitis).

equine a. type 1 causes pneumonia, the most severe form being primary, severe combined immunodeficiency disease of Arab foals.

equine a. type 2 associated with enteric infections.

ovine a. types 1–5 cause mild respiratory and enteric diseases.

porcine a. types 1–4 cause respiratory disease; type 4 causes diarrhea and/or meningitis.

turkey a. causes respiratory or enteric disease, marble spleen disease.

adenyl cyclase see ADENYLATE cyclase.

adenylate a salt, anion or ester of adenylic acid.

a. cyclase an enzyme that catalyzes the conversion of adenosine triphosphate (ATP) to cyclic adenosine monophosphate (cAMP) and inorganic pyrophosphate. It is activated by the attachment of a hormone or neurotransmitter to a specific membrane-bound receptor.

a. kinase enzyme catalyzing the conversion of two moles of ADP to ATP and AMP, thereby equilibrating ADP with ATP and AMP. Controls the adenylate energy charge of a cell, particularly muscle cells. Called also myokinase.

adenylic acid adenosine monophosphate; a component of nucleic acid, consisting of adenine, ribose and phosphoric acid.

adermia congenital defect or absence of the skin.

adermin see PYRIDOXINE.

ADF acid-detergent fiber.

ADH antidiuretic hormone.

ADH response test see ANTIDIURETIC hormone.

adhesins substances which confer virulence on bacteria by enabling them to adhere to epithelial surfaces. See also PILUS, FIMBRIA.

adhesion union of two surfaces that are normally separate; also, any fibrous band that connects them. Surgery within the abdomen sometimes results in adhesions. As an organ heals, fibrous scar tissue forms around the incision. Fibrinous exudate and scar tissue may cling to the surface of adjoining organs, causing them to kink. Adhesions are usually painless and cause no difficulties, although occasionally they produce obstruction or malfunction by distorting the organ. They can also occur following peritonitis and other inflammatory conditions. They may also occur in the pleura, in the pericardium, and around the pelvic organs. Surgery is sometimes recommended to relieve adhesions.

bowel a. see peritoneal adhesion (below).

cervical a's adhesions in the uterine cervix; they usually result from infection and in mares encourage the development of PYOMETRA.

interthalamic a. the midline union of the two halves of the thalamus; during development of the brain the two thalami encroach into the primitive disk-shaped third ventricle transforming it into a ring.

intestinal a. takes the form of nonelastic bands between loops of intestine or between the intestine and other organs, or of constricting bands around the intestine. They often cause no clinical signs. Long bands may cause intermittent colic due to obstruction of the intestinal lumen which is relieved spontaneously. When they are not relieved they are life-threatening. Cicatricial bands within the wall of the intestine are more likely to cause persistent, subacute abdominal pain. See also equine COLIC.

pericardial a's fibrous adhesions that restrict the action of the heart and that follow late stages of pericarditis. This may cause cardiac inefficiency that leads to congestive heart failure.

peritoneal a. part of the healing process in peritonitis, and disruption by surgical means or by violent activity may result in recrudescence of peritonitis. In the late cicatrization stage, adhesions may, by contraction, cause partial obstruction of the intestine and chronic or intermittent pain; a common cause of chronic colic in horses.

pleural a. develops in the healing stages of pleurisy but is soon attenuated by constant thoracic movement and causes little respiratory insufficiency.

reticular a. if extensive, can restrict the movements of the reticulum so much that the reticular groove cannot open to allow emptying of the rumen through the reticulo-omasal orifice. Chronic distension and frothy bloat result.

vaginal a's common only in mares. Interfere with mating by preventing penetration of the penis, or with fertilization by blocking the movement of spermatozoa. Vaginal and rectal examination reveal bands of adhesion across the passage, or transverse partitions that completely block it. In the latter there may be an accumulation of exudate or secretion cranial to it. Three-dimensional adhesions convert the vagina into a solid mass with a similar obstructive effect. See also VAGINAL.

adhesiotomy surgical division of adhesions.

adhesive 1. pertaining to, characterized by, or causing close adherence of adjoining surfaces. 2. a substance that causes close adherence of adjoining surfaces.

tissue a's materials, mainly cyanoacrylates, used for control of hemorrhage from cut surfaces, oral surgery, intestinal anastomosis and corneal ulcerations.

ADI acceptable daily intake.

adiaphoria nonresponse to stimuli as a result of previous exposure to similar stimuli.

adiaspiromycosis a respiratory disease of humans and many animal species caused by the fungus *Chrysosporium* spp. and characterized by large, thick-walled spherules (adiaspores).

adipectomy excision of adipose tissue.

adipic pertaining to fat.

adip(o)- word element. [L.] *fat.*

adipocele a hernia containing fat.

adipocellular composed of fat and connective tissue.

adipocyte a cell specialized for the storage of fat; the fat is stored in a large cytoplasmic vesicle.

embryonic a. develop in the subcutis during the second half of pregnancy.

adipofibroma a fibrous tumor with fatty elements.

adipogenic, adipogenous producing fat.

adipokinesis the mobilization of fat in the body.

adipokinin a factor from the anterior pituitary that accelerates mobilization of stored fat.

adipolysis the digestion of fats.

adiponecrosis necrosis of fatty tissue.

a. neonatorum induration of subcutaneous fat, thought to be caused by obstetric trauma, in the newborn. Called also adiposis subcutanea.

adipopexis the fixation or storing of fat.

adipose fatty.

brown a. tissue a connective tissue that contains multilocular fat cells whose color results from cytochrome pigments and a high density of mitochondria; it functions primarily in heat production and control of body weight. Is especially notable in young and hibernating animals for non-shivering thermogenesis.

white a. tissue a connective tissue that contains large spherical or polyhedral fat cells each storing a single fat droplet; it is the form in which a majority of the body's available energy is stored as triacylglycerols.

adiposis a condition marked by deposits or degeneration of fatty tissue.

a. cerebralis fatness from cerebral pituitary disease.

a. dolorosa a painful condition due to pressure on nerves caused by fatty deposits.

a. hepatica fatty degeneration of liver.

a. neonatorum see ADIPONECROSIS neonatorum.

adiposity obesity.

adiposogenital dystrophy, adiposogenital syndrome a disease characterized by abnormal distribution of fat (obesity) accompanied by underdevelopment of the genitalia. The condition is caused by damage to certain parts of the HYPOTHALAMUS, with a decrease in the secretion of gonadotropic hormones from the anterior lobe of the PITUITARY gland. Treatment depends on the primary cause of the condition, usually a tumor or infection involving the hypothalamus. Called also Fröhlich's syndrome.

adiposuria the occurrence of fat in the urine.

adipsia absence of thirst; abnormal avoidance of drinking.

aditoprim an antibacterial agent that inhibits dihydrofolate reductase; similar to TRIMETHOPRIM.

aditus pl. *aditus* [L.] an entrance or opening.

a. laryngis the entrance to the larynx.

a. pharyngis the aperture between the palatoglossal arches through which the mouth communicates with the oropharynx.

adjustment summarization of statistical measures in which the effects of differences in composition of the populations being compared have been minimized by statistical methods.

adjuvant 1. assisting or aiding. 2. a substance that aids another, such as an auxiliary remedy. Commonly used in reference to substances, commonly mineral oil or alum, added to vaccines to enhance antigenicity. See also FREUND'S COMPLETE ADJUVANT.

adlay *Coix lachryma-jobi*. Called also Job's tears.

adluminal connected to the lumen.

admission criteria the rules for the establishment of comparable groups in any comparison of differences in the performance or responses of the group. The criteria may be permissible age group, the previous productivity, the freedom from disease and so on.

adnerval, adneural toward a nerve.

adnexa [L.] *appendages;* accessory organs, as of the eye (*adnexa oculi*), uterus (*adnexa uteri*) or epidermal appendages, e.g. hair, sweat glands, sebaceous glands and claws or nails.

adnexal pertaining to, or emanating from, the adnexa.

a. tumors see under names of individual structures such as sebaceous gland adenoma.

adonidin cardiac glycoside present in weeds of the *Adonis* genus.

Adonis a genus of the plant family Ranunculaceae; contain adonitoxin, adonidin, cardiac glycosides which cause diarrhea. Includes *A. autumnalis* (*A. microcarpa*), *A. aestivalis*, *A. annua* (*A. microcarpa*), *A. microcarpa*, *A. vernalis*.

adonitoxin cardiac glycoside in plants of genus ADONIS.

adontia absence of teeth.

adoption 1. of alien young. Individual dams of all species may adopt strange neonates, and some ewes will even attempt to poach from others, but special measures have to be taken in most cases to foster alien young. Sows are probably the easiest to deceive. Queens will accept foster kittens if they are within about 2 weeks of the age of their own kittens. Reluctant ewes may accept strange lambs only if they are rubbed with secretions from their own. 2. also used in reference to the placing of stray or otherwise unwanted dogs and cats into ownership, as stray animals obtained from an animal shelter.

adoptive transfer the transfer of cells, commonly lymphocytes from an immunized individual, to a non-immune recipient.

adoral 1. situated near the mouth. 2. directed toward the mouth.

ADP 1. ADENOSINE diphosphate. 2. automatic data processing.

ADP-ribosylation the attachment of ADP-ribose to elongation factor 2 that blocks the translocation of the nascent polypeptide. The mode of action of diphtheria toxin.

ADR adverse drug reaction; abbreviation for colloquial expression 'ain't doing right'.

adrenal 1. near the kidney. 2. of or produced by the adrenal glands. 3. an ADRENAL GLAND.

a. cortex the outer part of the adrenal gland made up of an external zona glomerulosa, a deeper zona fasciculata and a zona reticularis. It produces three main groups of hormones, the glucocorticoids which are concerned with increasing blood glucose levels, the mineralocorticoids concerned with the maintenance of electrolyte levels in the extracellular fluid, and androgens which have the same masculinizing effect as the hormone testosterone produced by the testis. Called also adrenal gland cortex. See GLUCOCORTICOID, MINERALOCORTICOID, ANDROGEN.

a. cortex inhibitors see ADRENOLYTIC.

a.-cortical see ADRENOCORTICAL.

a. cortical dysfunction see HYPERADRENOCORTICISM, HYPOADRENOCORTICISM.

a. corticoids see MINERALOCORTICOID, GLUCOCORTICOID, CORTICOSTEROID.

a. function tests see ACTH response test, DEXAMETHASONE suppression test, V-TEST.

a. hyperplasia-like syndrome a congenital abnormality of adrenal steroidogenesis reported in dogs which results in hyperprogestinism and hyperandrogenism. Clinical signs include bilaterally symmetrical alopecia resembling that seen with other endocrinopathies.

a. insufficiency hypofunction of the adrenal gland, particularly the cortex, leading to signs of weakness and loss of sodium, chloride and water. See also primary HYPOADRENOCORTICISM.

a. medulla a glandular extension of the effector fibers of the sympathetic nervous system that releases into the bloodstream the hormones EPINEPHRINE (adrenaline) and NOREPINEPHRINE (noradrenaline). When the sympathetic nervous system is stimulated the adrenal medulla responds also and its hormones are carried via the bloodstream to cause increases in cardiac output and metabolic rate, vasoconstriction and reduction of gastrointestinal peristalsis. The hormones have similar functions but epinephrine is removed from the bloodstream more slowly and has a more prolonged effect. Called also adrenal gland medulla.

Adrenal medullary hormones are not essential to life. Hypersecretion, such as occurs in some functional pheochromocytomas, causes tachycardia, edema and cardiac hypertrophy.

a. steroids cortisol, corticosterone, cortisone, 11-dehydroxycortisone, deoxycorticosterone, 17-hydroxy-11-deoxycorticosterone, aldosterone, the adrenal corticoids from the adrenal cortex. Called also corticosteroids.

adrenal gland one of the pair of endocrine organs located near the cranial pole of the kidneys. Each is composed of two parts, an outer cortex and an inner medulla, that are anatomically, embryologically and functionally distinct. See also ADRENAL cortex, ADRENAL medulla.

a. g. fetal cortex the first adrenal cortex in the fetus; it is subsequently surrounded by a permanent cortex and has disappeared by the time of birth; the function is unknown.

a. g. hormones includes epinephrine, norepinephrine from the adrenal medulla and cortisol, corticosterone, cortisone, 11-dehydroxycortisone, deoxycorticosterone, 17-hydroxy-11-deoxycorticosterone, aldosterone, the adrenal corticoids from the adrenal cortex.

a. g. medulla see ADRENAL medulla.

a. g. tumors includes myelolipoma and cortical adenomas and carcinomas. Cause local tissue compression and the adenomas and carcinomas can cause hypersecretion of cortisol. Tumors specific to the medulla include neuroblasoma and ganglioneuroma, both of which may cause local tissue compression.

adrenalectomy surgical excision of an adrenal gland. This procedure is indicated when a disorder of the adrenal gland, such as CUSHING'S SYNDROME or PHEOCHROMOCYTOMA, causes an overproduction of adrenal hormones.

adrenaline see EPINEPHRINE.

adrenergic 1. activated by, characteristic of, or

secreting epinephrine or substances with activities similar to those of epinephrine. The term is applied to those nerve fibers of the sympathetic nervous system that release norepinephrine (and possibly small amounts of epinephrine) at a synapse when a nerve impulse passes. 2. an agent that acts like epinephrine. Called also sympathomimetic.

a. agents sympathomimetic amines which exert their effects on adrenergic receptors of effector cells innervated by the sympathetic nervous system. The administration of these adrenergic agonists mimics the physiological effects of sympathoadrenal discharge.

a. alpha-blockers, beta-blockers see ADRENERGIC blockade.

a. amines these are the sympathomimetic amines. They have similar but not identical structures and actions. Epinephrine, norepinephrine and isoproterenol are catecholamines but differ in their effects. Norepinephrine is primarily an activator of alpha-receptors whereas isoproterenol is a selective beta-receptor agonist. Epinephrine is an active agonist for both alpha- and beta-receptors. Ephedrine is the classical noncatecholamine sympathetic agonist.

a. blockade adrenergic blocking agents prevent the activation of adrenergic receptors. They may be alpha-blockers, e.g. ergot, or beta-blockers such as propranolol.

a. blocking agent a drug that blocks the secretion of epinephrine and norepinephrine at the postganglionic nerve endings of the sympathetic nervous system. By blocking these adrenergic substances, which cause constriction of blood vessels and increased cardiac output, adrenergic blocking agents produce a dilatation of the blood vessels and a decrease in cardiac output.

a. nerves see adrenergic (1) (above).

a. nervous system see SYMPATHETIC nervous system.

a. receptors class of receptors named after the action of adrenalin(e), the alternative name for epinephrine. Alpha receptors, which are stimulated by norepinephrine and blocked by agents such as phenoxybenzamine, are categorized into two classes, α_1 and α_2, which have different actions. α_1 adrenergic actions include contraction of the iris, decreased motility in the intestine, and potassium and water secretions from the salivary glands. α_2 adrenergic receptors inhibit adenylate cyclase, rather than activating it. Beta receptors, which are stimulated by epinephrine and blocked by agents such as propranolol, are also categorized into two types; β_1 adrenergic receptors, which produce lipolysis and cardiostimulation, and β_2 adrenergic receptors, which produce bronchodilatation and vasodilatation.

α-adrenergic blocking agent see ADRENERGIC blocking agent.

β-adrenergic blockade the blockade of beta-adrenergic receptors by beta-blockers, e.g. propranolol.

adren(o)- word element. [L.] *adrenal glands.*

adrenochromes pigments produced by chromaffin-positive granules contained in the glandular cells of the adrenal medulla.

adrenocortical pertaining to or arising from the cortex of the adrenal gland.

a. hormones any of the corticosteroids elaborated by the ADRENAL cortex, the major ones being the glucocorticoids and mineralocorticoids, and including some androgens, progesterone and perhaps estrogens. See also CORTICOSTEROID.

a. hyperplasia may be bilateral, resulting from stimulation by a functional corticotropic adenoma of the pars distalis or the pars intermedia of the pituitary gland. See HYPERADRENOCORTICISM.

a. neoplasms adenomas usually do not cause clinical signs and are incidental findings at autopsy. Carcinomas are highly invasive of surrounding tissues and into the caudal vena cava. Rarely, adrenal neoplasms are functional and may cause signs of HYPERADRENOCORTICISM.

adrenocorticoid a compound produced by the adrenal cortex.

adrenocorticomimetic having effects similar to those of hormones of the adrenal cortex.

adrenocorticosteroid one of the steroid compounds produced by the adrenal cortex.

adrenocorticotrophic adrenocorticotropic; corticotropic.

a. hormone a hormone elaborated by the anterior lobe of the PITUITARY gland that stimulates the action of the ADRENAL cortex. See also ACTH.

a. hormone secreting tumor adenoma of either posterior or intermediate lobe; causes a syndrome of cortical excess (Cushing's syndrome).

adrenocorticotrophin adrenocorticotropic hormone, or corticotropin.

adrenocorticotropic having a stimulating effect on the adrenal cortex; corticotropic.

a. hormone ACTH, a hormone secreted by the anterior PITUITARY gland which has a stimulating effect on the ADRENAL cortex. Called also corticotropin.

adrenocorticotropin adrenocorticotropic hormone (ACTH) or corticotropin.

adrenocorticotropin-releasing factor thought to be released from the fetal hypothalamus late in gestation in normal pregnancy. Stimulates release of adrenocorticotropin from the anterior pituitary.

adrenodoxin a nonheme iron protein.

adrenolytic 1. antagonizing the action of adrenaline (epinephrine). See also ANTIADRENERGIC; ADRENERGIC blocking agent. 2. inhibits secretions of the adrenal gland. See MITOTANE.

adrenomedullary pertaining to or arising from the medulla of the adrenal gland.

adrenomegaly abnormal enlargement of the adrenal gland.

adrenomimetic having actions similar to those of adrenergic compounds; sympathomimetic.

adrenopathy any disease of the adrenal glands.

adrenoreceptor a receptor essential to neurohumoral transmission, situated on or within the surface membranes of cells innervated by adrenergic neurons and in some cells which are not so innervated.

adria cell myocytic vacuolar degeneration; one of the manifestations of microscopic myocardial changes in dogs poisoned with the antineoplastic ANTHRACYCLINE antibiotics. The clinical picture is one of congestive heart failure.

adriamycin doxorubicin.

Adson tissue forceps standard thumb-operated, wishbone type forceps for grasping tissue but distinguished by having rows of very fine teeth at the edges of the tips.

adsorb to attract and retain other material on the surface.

adsorbent 1. pertaining to or characterized by adsorption. 2. a substance that attracts other materials or particles to its surface.

gastrointestinal a. a substance, usually a powder, administered to adsorb gases, toxins and bacteria in the stomach and intestines. Examples include activated charcoal and kaolin.

adsorption the action of a substance in attracting and holding other materials or particles on its surface.
adtorsion a turning inward of both eyes.
adult having attained full growth or maturity, or an organism that has done so.
adulteration addition of an impure, cheap or unnecessary ingredient to cheat, cheapen or falsify a preparation. Adulteration of ox beef with horsemeat is an example. See also SUBSTITUTION.
adulticide the medication used to kill adult heartworms (*Dirofilaria immitis*) as distinct from that used to kill the microfilaria. Some drugs are capable of both effects.
advancement detachment of a portion of tissue, especially muscle, and reattachment at an advanced point.
adventitia the outer, connective tissue coat of an organ or structure, especially the outer coat of an artery or vein.
adventitious 1. accidental or acquired. 2. not in the usual place.
a. breath sounds see BREATH sounds.
a. movements purposeless movements; as seen in distemper MYOCLONUS in dogs.
adversarial law a legal system which depends on contests between or confrontations by contesting parties, one of which is often the state, with judgments made by judges, magistrates or juries who observe the adversaries in action. The opposite of the inquisitorial LAW system.
adverse opposing the interests of the patient.
a. drug reaction (ADR) an undesirable and unintentional effect caused by a drug administered at the normal therapeutic dose.
a. food reaction an abnormal response to ingested food components. It may be immunologic or non-immunologic. See also FOOD.
a. syndrome lesions of the rostral thalamus causing head turning, circling or deviation of the eyes toward the side of the lesion.
advertising the making of public statements about services offered and facilities available in a professional practice. Personal advertisement in this way is frowned upon because of the risk that there will be misrepresentation and that it will unfairly attract business to the detriment of the client. The contrary view is that the public is disadvantaged because they will not be aware of the range of services offered and the fees attached to them. In most countries now, in which it used to be controlled by the registering authority, the scope of personal advertising is left to the discretion of the individual. Corporate advertising which advertises the profession as a whole is encouraged.
advisory services advisory services provided to the public, in their capacity as owners and managers of animals, are an important part of veterinary science. They may be provided by government bureaux, by commercial companies who deal in pharmaceuticals or animals or animal products, or by veterinary species specialists practicing privately or in incorporated institutions.
adynamia lack of normal or vital powers.
adynamic ileus see ILEUS.
Aedes a genus of the family Culicidae, the mosquitoes, and known to transmit the *Plasmodium* spp. of bird malaria, and the viruses of Rift Valley fever and Japanese B encephalitis. Some species are vectors of equine encephalomyelitis virus. *Dirofilaria immitis* uses *Aedes* spp. as intermediate hosts for the development of microfilariae. Also cause insect worry in animals and vicious species, e.g. *A. vigilex*, may cause fatalities amongst puppies and piglets.
AEEC attaching–effacing *Escherichia coli.*
aegobronchophony see EGOBRONCHOPHONY.
aegophony see EGOBRONCHOPHONY.
Aegypius monachus see VULTURE.
Aegyptianella a genus of the family of rickettsia-like organisms called Anaplasmataceae.
A. pullorum the bacterial cause of AEGYPTIANELLOSIS in birds.
aegyptianellosis the disease of birds caused by *Aegyptianella pullorum*, and possibly other organisms of the same genus. It is characterized by fever, anorexia, diarrhea and paralysis.
Aelurostrongylus a genus of lungworms of the family Angiostrongylidae; cause chronic cough and weight loss. Includes *A. abstrusus* (cat), *A. falciformis* (badger), *A. pridhami* (wild mink).
-aemia word element; for words ending thus see words ending -emia. [Gr.] *condition of the blood.*
Aepyceros melampus see IMPALA.
aeration 1. the exchange of carbon dioxide for oxygen by the blood in the lungs. 2. the charging of a liquid with air or gas.
aerial part the part of the plant above the ground.
aerial surveys an epidemiological technique for surveying animal populations and their habitat, especially the latter, over a very wide area. Requires special techniques adapted to sensing of electronically marked animals from a distance, and infrared scanning of vegetation.
aeriform resembling air; gaseous.
aero- word element. [Gr.] *air, gas.*
Aerobacter aerogenes a name formerly used to describe some strains of KLEBSIELLA *pneumoniae.*
aerobe a microorganism that grows in the presence of free oxygen and utilizes oxygen for oxidative phosphorylation.
facultative a. one that can live in the presence of oxygen.
obligate a. one that cannot live without oxygen.
aerobic a microbe or microbiological process that functions fully only in the presence of free oxygen.
a. effluent treatment the ACTIVATED sludge method of handling sewage and abattoir effluent.
a. exercise moderate exercise performed in the circumstance where the blood supply is able to maintain an adequate supply of oxygen to the tissues during the exercise.
aerocele a tumor formed by air filling an adventitious pouch, such as laryngocele and tracheocele.
aerodermectasia subcutaneous or surgical emphysema.
aeroembolism obstruction of a blood vessel by air or gas.
aerogen a gas-producing bacillus.
aerogenesis formation or production of gas.
aerohydrotherapy therapeutic use of air and water.
Aeromonas a genus of facultatively anaerobic, gram-negative rod-shaped bacteria in the family Pseudomonadaceae, usually resident in richly organic water and soil, and on fish species.
atypical *A. salmonicida* miscellaneous infections of fish, not the identified *A. salmonicida salmonicida,* the cause of goldfish furunculosis, but may cause goldfish ulcer disease.
A. hydrophilia causes ulcerative stomatitis (mouthrot, canker) of captive reptiles. Ulcerative lesions in the mouth may extend to cause osteomyelitis of the jaw bone, inflammation of the harderian gland and invasion of the corneospectacu-

lar area causing severe swelling. This bacterium may also cause septicemia, especially in aquatic snakes with access to infected water; causes fin, tail and snout erosions (RED SORE DISEASE) in captive fish. May also cause diarrhea in foals.

A. liquefaciens a group of closely related, motile aeromonads which cause hemorrhagic septicemia in many cultured pond-fish, aquarium fish and salmonids.

A. salmonicida salmonicida causes GOLDFISH ulcer disease, FURUNCULOSIS in salmonids and ERYTHRODERMATITIS in carp.

aerophagia habitual swallowing of air. See CRIB-biting.

aerophilic, aerophilous requiring air for proper growth.

aeroplethysmograph an apparatus for graphically recording respiratory volumes.

aerosinusitis barosinusitis.

aerosol a colloid system in which solid or liquid particles are suspended in a gas, especially a suspension of a drug or other substance to be dispensed in a cloud or mist.

a. clearance removal of particles that have been deposited in the respiratory tissues. Clearance may occur by ciliary transport, by phagocytosis, by encapsulation and immobilization in a deposit of fibrous tissue (in which case the particles remain in the body), and by dissolving in tissue fluid and subsequently diffusing into the general circulation where the particles are metabolized.

a. deposition the depositing of aerosol particles onto a nearby surface, especially deposition or retention of the particles within the respiratory system. Closely related to aerosol penetration and affected by the same factors.

a. penetration the maximum distance aerosol particles can be carried into the respiratory tract by inhaled air. Depth of penetration increases as particle size decreases. Factors affecting where aerosol particles will be deposited and how deeply they can penetrate are: gravity, kinetic activity of gas molecules, inertial impaction, physical nature of the particle, and the ventilatory pattern.

a. therapy nebulization; delivery of a therapeutic agent as a fine mist or spray to the mucociliary layer of the respiratory tract.

aerotolerant surviving and growing in air; said of anaerobic microorganisms.

aerotropism growth of aerobic organisms towards or around a source of oxygen.

Aeschynomene a genus of shrubs in the family Leguminosae used as browse by grazing animals.

aesculin esculin.

Aesculus a genus of the family Hippocastanaceae of shrubs and trees. Called also horsechestnut, buckeye. Contains a toxic hydroxycoumarin glycoside esculin in seed pods and shoots; causes depression, tremor, incoordination, paralysis. Includes *A. californica* (California buckeye), *A. glabra* (Ohio buckeye), *A. hippocastanum* (horsechestnut), *A. pavia* (red buckeye), *A. octandra* (sweet buckeye).

aestivation see ESTIVATION.

aethimizol a xanthine derivative; a stimulant to respiration at the brainstem level and to adrenocorticotropic function of the hypophysis.

Aethusa a member of the plant family Umbelliferae; contains a piperidine alkaloid cynapine capable of causing posterior paralysis which may be fatal. Includes *A. cynapium* (fool's parsley, lesser hemlock).

aetiology see ETIOLOGY.

af- prefix meaning towards.

afebrile without fever.

Affenpinscher a very small (6–9 lb), lively dog with a prominent chin, small erect ears and docked tail. The coat, usually black, is shaggy and in general short, but longer around the eyes, nose and chin, giving a typical monkey-like appearance. Called also monkey dog.

afferent conducting toward a center or specific site of reference; incoming.

a. arterioles branches of the interlobular arteries of the kidney that supply the glomerular capillaries of the renal corpuscle.

a. loop syndrome chronic partial obstruction of the proximal loop (duodenum and jejunum) after gastrojejunostomy, resulting in duodenal distension, pain and nausea following ingestion of food.

a. nerve any nerve that transmits impulses from the periphery toward the central nervous system. See also NEURON, afferent nerve fibers (below).

a. nerve fibers nerve fibers in the peripheral nervous system carrying information to the brain and spinal cord. Their cell bodies are in ganglia and their telodendria in the central nervous system.

a. nervous activity the number of afferent nerve fibers that are activated by the stimulus. This depends on the number of receptive fields that are included in the zone being stimulated.

a. system the collective sensory fibers from all parts of the body.

affinity 1. attraction; a tendency to seek out or unite with another object or substance. 2. in chemistry, the tendency of two substances to form strong or weak chemical bonds forming molecules or complexes. 3. in immunology, the thermodynamic bond strength of an antigen–antibody complex.

antibody a. the strength of the binding interaction between antigen and antibody.

drug a. the attraction of a particular class of receptor to a drug, at a level sufficient to give an observable reaction. Such a drug is an AGONIST.

a. maturation the increased affinity of antibody for an antigen which occurs during the course of an immune response.

Afghan hound a tall, long silky-coated dog with pendulous ears, high tail carriage and a very elegant appearance. The breed originated on the Sinai peninsula and was later used as a sight hunter in northern Afghanistan. Called also Tazi. The breed suffers from inherited cataracts and a hereditary MYELOPATHY.

Afghan melon CITRULLUS *lanatus*.

afibrinogenemia absence or deficiency of fibrinogen in the circulating blood. The defect is inherited in goats, causing a severe hemorrhagic diathesis. See also HYPOFIBRINOGENEMIA, DYSFIBRINOGENEMIA.

AFIP (United States) Armed Forces Institute of Pathology.

aflatoxicosis the disease caused by the toxin aflatoxin. It is a toxin of major importance being hepatotoxic, carcinogenic, teratogenic and immune suppressant. The common syndrome in animals is of hepatic insufficiency including jaundice, blindness, circling, falling and convulsions. Called also groundnut poisoning.

aflatoxin a mycotoxin produced by growth of the fungus *Aspergillus flavus*, usually on groundnuts or stored grain. See also AFLATOXICOSIS.

AFP alpha-fetoprotein.

African buffalo includes black Cape buffalo, red Congo buffalo and red-brown varieties from Abyssinia to Niger. See also BUFFALO.

African clawed toad see XENOPUS LAEVIS.
African daisy see SENECIO *pterophorus*.
African elephant *Loxodonta africana*. See ELEPHANT.
African farcy epizootic lymphangitis.
African glanders see EPIZOOTIC lymphangitis.
African green monkey CERCOPITHECUS *aethiops*.
African horse sickness a highly infectious, fatal disease of horses, donkeys and mules. It is caused by an orbivirus transmitted by mosquitoes and possibly *Culicoides* sp. The clinical picture includes an acute pulmonary form manifested by dyspnea, cough and profuse nasal discharge, and a subacute, cardiac form in which the principal signs are edema of the head and internally, oral petechiation and esophageal paralysis. The mortality rate is very high.
African lion hound see RHODESIAN RIDGEBACK.
African milk bush SYNADENIUM ARBORESCENS.
African mouth breeder African freshwater tropical fish distinguished by their behavior of carrying the fertilized eggs in their mouths. Called also *Tilapia macrocephala*.
African pig disease see AFRICAN SWINE FEVER.
African pygmy pig see miniature PIG.
African redwood see MANSONIA ALTISSIMA.
African rue see PEGANUM *harmala*.
African star grass CYNODON *nlemfuensis*.
African swine fever a peracute, highly contagious, highly fatal disease of pigs caused by African swine fever virus, previously a member of the family *Iridoviridae*, now an unclassified virus. The virus is carried by wart hogs in which it produces no disease and is transmitted to European pigs via the tick *Ornithodoros moubata porcinus*. The disease was originally confined to southern Africa, but has spread to North Africa, to Europe, including Spain, Portugal and Belgium, and also to Cuba and the Dominican Republic.

The disease resembles classical swine fever (hog cholera). Clinically there is high fever, severe depression, purple skin discoloration, incoordination and posterior paresis. Death occurs about 2 days after the first signs of illness. In recent times the proportion of outbreaks which have been mild in severity has increased markedly.
African trypanosomiasis nagana. See TRYPANOSOMIASIS.
Africander an African breed of cattle derived from British breeds (about 25%) and Brahmans (about 75%). A Sanga type with long lateral horns, used usually for red meat and draft. Africa's answer to the Santa Gertrudis. See also SANGA, BONSMARA, DRAKENSBERGER, AFRIKANER.
Afrikander a common misspelling for AFRICANDER.
Afrikaner Afrikaans name for *Bos indicus* cattle. Called also Africander.
afterbirth the special tissues associated with the development of a fetus in the uterus that are expelled after the birth of a neonate. These are the PLACENTA, or the structure attached to the wall of the uterus through which nourishment passes from the mother to the fetus, and the umbilical CORD, which attaches the fetus to the placenta. See also FETAL membranes.
afterbrain metencephalon.
aftercare the care and treatment of a convalescent patient, especially one that has undergone surgery.
aftercongestion a chronic reactive hyperemia of nasal mucosa that may follow prolonged use of topical decongestants.
afterdepolarization in myocardial activity a polarization, sufficient to trigger a cardiac cycle, which results from a preceding impulse or series of impulses.
afterdrop a decrease in body temperature observed as a complication during rewarming of a hypothermic patient. It is believed to be the result of redistribution of cooler blood.
afterfeather a small feather underneath the large main feather produced by most plumaceous and pennaceous feather follicles. It varies from a simple tuft to a structure identical to the main feather. It is missing in some birds including the ostrich and some passerines.
afterglow small amounts of light emitted by a phosphor after the stimulating radiation has ceased. Seen in x-ray intensifying screens and fluoroscopic screens.
afterhyperdepolarization similar to AFTERDEPOLARIZATION but does not trigger conducted impulses.
afterload see CARDIAC afterload.
aftermath the exuberant autumn regrowth of pasture which has been harvested for meadow hay in the late summer. Grazing cattle on it is a common history preceding an outbreak of atypical interstitial pneumonia. Called also fog, foggage, feg.
a. disease see ATYPICAL INTERSTITIAL PNEUMONIA.
a. emphysema see ATYPICAL INTERSTITIAL PNEUMONIA.
aftosa the Mexican name for foot-and-mouth disease. Called also aphthous fever.
Ag 1. chemical symbol, *silver* (L. *argentum*). 2. abbreviation for antigen.
A–G ratio the ratio of albumin to globulin in blood serum, plasma or urine.
agalactia partial or complete absence of milk flow in the absence of disease of the mammary gland. It may be due to the presence of other disease, to emotional disturbances or to lack of let-down hormones or hormonal stimulation for the development of the mammary glands. See also MASTITIS–METRITIS–AGALACTIA, FARROWING hysteria.
contagious ovine/caprine a. see CONTAGIOUS agalactia.
primary a. reduced milk flow is the only abnormality.
agammaglobulinemia severe or complete deficiency of immunoglobulins (antibodies) in the blood. Most domestic animals are agammaglobulinemic at birth, prior to suckling. An inherited defect is not commonly recorded in animals, but does occur as a primary inherited condition and as part of a combined immune deficiency, both of them in horses. The deficiency or absence of antibodies results in severe and recurrent infections. See also HYPOGAMMAGLOBULINEMIA, COMBINED IMMUNE DEFICIENCY SYNDROME (DISEASE).
Bruton's a. an inherited, X-linked recessive condition in humans involving a deficiency of B lymphocytes and plasma cells. A similar condition, though less well characterized, has been recognized in horses.
aganglionic lacking ganglion cells.
a. colon see colonic AGANGLIONOSIS.
a. intestine see colonic AGANGLIONOSIS.
aganglionosis, agangliosis congenital absence of parasympathetic ganglion cells.
colonic a. congenital defect manifested by stenosis, but patency, of the colon, an absence of ganglia of the myenteric plexus and an almost complete absence of skin pigment in white foals resulting from matings between OVERO horses. The foal develops colic at birth and dies after about 48 hours. See also ATRESIA. Occurs also in some spotted mutant strains of mice. Called also congenital megacolon, aganglionic megacolon.

Agapornis see LOVEBIRD.

agar a dried hydrophilic, colloidal substance extracted from various species of red algae. When suspended in a liquid medium and heated to 212°F (100°C), the agar dissolves. When it is allowed to cool to 110°F (43°C) the medium becomes a solid gel. It is used in culture media for bacteria and other microorganisms, in making emulsions, and as a supporting medium for immunodiffusion and immunoelectrophoresis. Because of its bulk it is also used in medicines to promote peristalsis and relieve constipation.

birdseed a. one containing *Guizotia abyssinicia* (Niger) seed and creatinine, used for growing *Cryptococcus neoformans*. Called also Niger agar.

bismuth sulfite a. a special preparation used for isolation of salmonellae from food.

blood a. a culture medium used for the growth of bacteria. Consists of agar and intact erythrocytes.

brain heart infusion a. used for cultivating the yeast phase of dimorphic fungi.

brilliant green a. used to cultivate salmonellae.

chocolate a. an enriched agar for the growth of *Hemophilus*, some *Actinobacillus*, and *Taylorella* spp. A molten agar and blood mixture is held at 122°F (50°C) prior to pouring plates. The additional nutrients supplied are hemin and NAD.

a. diffusion test see ANTIMICROBIAL sensitivity test.

eosin-methylene blue (EMB) a. used for the identification of *Eschericha coli*.

a. gel immunodiffusion test see IMMUNODIFFUSION tests.

MacConkey a. contains bile salts, lactose and neutral red indicator for isolation of enterobacteria.

mannitol salt a. selective for staphylococci.

milk a. contains skim milk and used to demonstrate casein digestion.

Niger seed a. see birdseed agar (above).

nutrient a. the basic growth medium for bacteria, composed of beef extract and peptone.

potato dextrose a. used in cultivating fungi; promotes sporulation and pigmentation.

Sabouraud's dextrose a. one used for isolation of fungi. See also DERMATOPHYTE test medium.

a. sausage see MEDIUM sausage.

xylose lysine (XLD) a. used to differentiate Enterbacteriaceae.

agarose more highly purified form of agar with similar uses to agar and widely used in the separation of nucleic acid fragments.

agastric having no stomach.

Agauria salifolia a poisonous shrub, in the family Ericaceae; contains andromedotoxin. Ingestion by ruminants causes salivation, vomiting, colic, staggering, collapse and death.

Agavaceae plant family containing the toxic genera *Agave* and *Nolina*.

Agave a genus of the plant family Agavaceae.

A. americana contains an unknown toxin; causes lameness, recumbency and muscle damage. Called also century plant, American aloe.

A. lecheguilla contains a steroidal or lithogenic saponin; causes photosensitive dermatitis. Called also lecheguilla, tula ixtle.

AGD amebic gill disease.

age 1. the duration, or the measure of time of the existence of an animal or object. 2. to undergo change as a result of passage of time.

a. adjustment see DATA adjustment.

a. associated disease diseases which occur at particular ages, either because of changes in the animal's biochemistry or immunity or because of variations in exposure of the animals because of a change in management.

a. descriptor terms other than years used to indicate the age of animals, e.g. two-tooth, first-lactation.

a. determination in the absence of explicit records about birth dates the estimation of age is a frequent task for veterinarians. The eruption, then the growth of teeth to apposition and then the wear of the teeth are the best guide to age in horses, cattle, sheep and goat, but not in the pig. In the pig and the dog some assistance can be obtained from examination of the teeth, but the general appearance of the animal and the history are the best means. See also RULE OF SIX.

a. distribution the proportion of the total population which is in each of the specified age groups.

first joining a. a critical point in the economy of a herd or flock. In seasonal animal production systems unnecessary delay may cause loss of a year's productivity for each female. Starting too early may cause losses due to difficult parturition in small dams and a poor conception rate.

a. groups cattle and sheep being grazed extensively are commonly segregated into age groups because they are dealt with as groups for purposes of mating, vaccination, prophylactic treatment and eventually culling for old age.

a.-matched control in a comparison of performance between groups it is desirable to create the groups by pairing a series of treatment animals and control animals for all significant variables, of which age would be one of the most important.

a. pigment lipofuscin.

slaughter a. the age at which the animals in a group are to be slaughtered. Varies with the meat objective, the price in the market, opportunities for replacement and the capacity to carry additional animals on the feed available.

a.-specific death rate the death rate for a specified age group as a proportion of a total number of specified animal × time period, such as cow × years.

weaning a. see WEANING age.

age classes the classification of animals according to age is an important part of animal farming but is difficult to carry out and has limited value because of varying interpretations of the terms used. Some of the classifications, based on average farming practices, are:

Calf, birth to 1 year, yearling 1 to 2 years, heifer to first calf born. Calf and yearling may be classified as bull or heifer. Cow is female after first calf: bull is entire male over 2 years old. Castrated males: steer calf to 1 year, steer or bullock—over 1 year, stag—adult, castrated when mature.

Lamb, birth to weaning (average 4 months), weaner—4 months to 2-tooth. 2-tooth to 15 months. 4-tooth to 2 years. 6-tooth to 3 years. Full mouth to 4 years. All groups may be subdivided into ram and ewe groups. Females are ewe lambs, 2-tooth ewes, etc. Ewes at first lambing. Gimmer is ewe that has not borne a lamb. Adult entire males are rams or tups. Castrated males are wethers or hoggets or hoggs; these may also be subdivided into age groups, e.g. 2-tooth hoggets.

Piglet—birth to undetermined period, probably synonymous with suckler. Suckler—birth to weaning. Weaner—after weaning to attainment of 30 kg bodyweight. Boar—entire male over 6 months old, usually for breeding but not necessarily so. Maiden gilt—female in the breeding herd, over 6 months old but not yet mated. Gilt—female in breeding herd but not yet farrowed for first time. Sow—female that has farrowed. First litter sow—from first fertile mating to second. Barrow—castrated male in fattening herd.

Foal—birth to one year, filly or colt foal. Yearling—1 to 2 years, filly or colt. Then, 2 year old, 3 year old and so on. Filly—under 4 years. Mare—4 years and over. Then, classified on a use basis—e.g. brood mare. Colt 2 to 4 years. Stallion—entire male 4 years and over. Gelding—castrated male any age.

Show classes for pups have different age limits in different places. Males and females graduate from puppydom at sexual maturity when about 6 months old.

Kittens until sexual maturity at 5 to 6 months for females, slightly older for males.

Chicken, hatching to 4 weeks. Pullet—4 weeks to 5 months. Cockerel—4 weeks to 5 months. Rooster and hen—over 5 months. Turkeys—as for fowls except that young birds are poults and adult males are toms. Ducks similarly, with young birds called ducklings, the adult females are ducks and the males are drakes. In all species the dividing line between adult and young birds is not age but sexual maturity as evidenced by commencing egg laying or, in the case of males, mating females.

age-specific rate a rate which specifies the age parameter for the rate.

aged animals of advanced age; in horses, more than 8 years old.

agene process bleaching of flour with nitrogen chloride, a process no longer in use. The denatured protein in the treated flour is toxic and causes a condition of hysteria in dogs eating biscuits made from the flour.

agenesis absence of an organ due to nonappearance of its primordium in the embryo.

agenitalism a condition due to lack of secretion of the testes or ovaries.

agenized flour see AGENE PROCESS.

agenosomia imperfect development of reproductive organs.

agent 1. any power, principle or substance by which something is accomplished, or which is capable of producing a chemical, physical or biological effect such as a disease. 2. of disease; any factor whose excessive presence or relative absence is essential for the occurrence of a disease.

adrenergic neuron blocking a. one that inhibits the release of norepinephrine from postganglionic adrenergic nerve endings.

alkylating a. a cytotoxic agent, e.g. a nitrogen mustard, which is highly reactive and can donate an alkyl group to another compound. Alkylating agents inhibit cell division by reacting with DNA and are used as ANTINEOPLASTIC agents.

anesthetic a. substance capable of producing reversible general or local anesthesia.

anticholinergic a. cholinergic blocking agent.

a. change change in an animal's chemical or antigenic configuration can alter its pathogenicity. For example, a case of nitrate–nitrite poisoning in a cow can become a case of nitrite poisoning after conversion of the nitrate in the rumen. Mutation and antigenic drift are other types of change that vary agent pathogenicity.

chelating a. a compound that combines with metals to form weakly dissociated complexes in which the metal is part of a ring, and is used to extract certain elements from a system.

chemical a. substance that produces change by virtue of its chemical composition and its effects on living tissues and organisms.

cholinergic blocking a. one that blocks the action of acetylcholine at nicotinic or muscarinic receptors of nerves or effector organs.

determinant a. only some agents are determinants of diseases in that they always cause disease, and the same disease, and the disease does not occur without the agent. Many agents require the intervention of other factors, such as anaerobicity of tissue, hepatic insufficiency or physiological stress before they can establish their pathogenicity.

ganglionic blocking a. one that blocks cholinergic transmission at autonomic ganglionic synapses.

immobilizing a. see NEUROMUSCULAR blockade.

infectious a. an organism able to live in or on the tissue of a living animal; may not necessarily cause disease.

a. interaction is the interaction between precipitating and predisposing causes of disease.

oxidizing a. a substance that acts as an electron acceptor in a chemical oxidation–reduction reaction.

a. properties are the properties which determine the pathogenicity of the agent, the solubility and acidity or biodegradability of a chemical, the virulence, adhesiveness, resistance to antibacterial agents of bacteria and viruses and so on.

reducing a. a substance that acts as an electron donor in a chemical oxidation–reduction reaction.

surface-active a. a substance that exerts a change on the surface properties of a liquid, especially one, such as a detergent, that reduces its surface tension. Called also surfactant.

therapeutic a. a substance capable of producing a curative effect in a disease state.

a. without disease exemplified by the orphan viruses. The agent is of a type that causes disease, but none is associated with the presence of the particular agent.

Ageratina a genus in family Asteraceae; contains unidentified toxins. Includes *A. altissima* (causes syndrome of trembles or milk sickness), *A. riparia*, *A. adenophora* (Crofton weed).

agger an elevation or eminence.

agglomerated of particles, compacted together into a mass.

a. feeds particulated feeds compacted or extruded into pellets and similar forms.

agglutinable capable of agglutination.

agglutinant 1. acting like glue. 2. a substance that promotes union of parts.

agglutinate to stick together and form clumps.

agglutination aggregation of separate particles into clumps or masses; especially the clumping of bacteria or blood cells by antibody specific to, or directed against, surface antigenic determinants. See also AGGLUTININ.

bacterial a. test a diagnostic procedure that employs serum or other body fluid of unknown antibody titer, titrated with standard suspension of bacteria as antigen. These may be performed quantitatively in 96-well microtitration plates or qualitatively on slides.

cross a. the agglutination of particulate antigen by an antibody raised against a different but related antigen; see also group agglutination (below).

group a. agglutination—usually to a lower titer—of various members of a group of biologically related organisms by an agglutinating antibody made to one of that group.

intravascular a. clumping of particulate elements within the blood vessels; used conventionally to denote red blood cell agglutination.

latex a. test see passive agglutination test (below).
microscopic a. test one in which the test mixtures are examined microscopically to detect the agglutination.
mucus a. test see MUCUS agglutination test.
passive a. test an agglutination reaction in which a soluble antigen, such as gonadotropin, is linked to inert particles such as latex beads or tanned erythrocytes.
platelet a. the clumping together of platelets owing to the action of platelet agglutinins. Such agglutinins are important in platelet typing.
slide a. test a rapid screening or semiquantitative test in which antibody and antigen are mixed on a glass slide and observed for agglutination.
a. test see bacterial agglutination test (above).
tube a. test an agglutination test for the identification of bacteria carried out in a test tube, a positive reaction consisting of a clearing of a prior opalescence.

agglutinin any substance causing agglutination (clumping together) of cells, particularly a specific antibody formed in the blood in response to an invading agent. Such agglutinating antibodies (see IMMUNOGLOBULIN) function as part of the immune mechanism of the body. When the invading agents that bring about the production of agglutinins are bacteria, the agglutinins produced bring about agglutination of the bacterial cells both in vivo and in vitro.

Erythrocytes also may be agglutinated by agglutinins that are naturally present in the blood, such as the presence of anti A antibody in humans with the blood group B erythrocytes, or such agglutinins may also be formed in response to the entrance of noncompatible blood cells into the bloodstream. A transfusion reaction is an example of the result of agglutination of blood cells brought about by agglutinins present in the recipient's blood.
cold a. antibody that acts only at low temperature.
cold a. disease an autoimmune disease in which erythrocyte autoantibodies, usually IgM, are most active at temperatures below 98.6°F (37°C). Agglutination occurs in capillaries of the extremities (tail, ears, nose and feet), particularly on exposure to cold, resulting in tissue necrosis in those areas. Hemolytic anemia is a variable feature.
group a. antibody made against a particular organism. One that has a specific action on certain organisms, but will agglutinate other, usually related species as well.
H a. one that is specific for flagellar antigens of bacteria.
immune a. a specific antibody found in the blood after recovery from the disease or injection of the microorganism.
incomplete a. antibody that at appropriate concentrations fails to agglutinate the homologous antigen for steric reasons.
normal a. a specific antibody found in the blood of an animal or of humans that has had no known exposure to the antigen with which it combines; these may be natural antibodies such as those directed against A and B blood group antigens in humans or cross-reacting antibodies produced after infection with a related microorganism.
O a. antibody specific for somatic or cell wall antigens of a bacterium.
partial a. antibody which agglutinates organisms closely related to the specific antigen, but at a lower dilution.
warm a. an incomplete antibody that sensitizes and reacts optimally with erythrocytes at 98.6°F (37°C).

agglutinogen a substance (antigen) that stimulates the animal body to form agglutinating antibody.

aggregate selection criteria the sum of all of the criteria to be used in a selection program with each criterion multipled by its relative importance to the other criteria.

aggregated lymphatic nodules see PEYER'S PATCHES.

aggregation 1. massing or clumping of materials together. 2. a clumped mass of material.
familial a. the occurrence of more cases of a given disorder in close relatives of an animal with the disorder than in control families.
platelet a. platelet agglutination.

aggressin substance or substances formed in the body by bacteria which enhance the bacteria's virulence. Include capsular material, enzymes and toxins. Called also virulin.

aggression behavior that is angry and destructive and intended to be injurious, physically or emotionally, and aimed at domination of one animal by another. It may be manifested by overt attacking and destructive behavior or by covert attitudes of hostility and obstructionism.
fear-induced a. accompanied by fear and usually when escape is not possible; may be associated with previous unpleasant experiences.
interfemale a. dominance aggression between females.
intermale a. fighting between males, most commonly tomcats; includes elements of competitive, territorial and sexual aggression.
maternal a. the dam's protection of her young; a variant of dominance aggression.
pain-induced a. defensive aggression triggered by pain.
play a. biting, nipping and growling at people or other animals during play.
possessive a. a form of DOMINANCE aggression; the animal is reacting against someone or another animal trying to remove something, usually food.
predatory a. directed towards any kind of animal, including dogs and humans, or even inanimate objects. Typically, it is elicited by something that is moving quickly.
protective a. the animal is protecting its territory. See territorial aggression (below).
redirected a. occurs when the animal is touched or restrained by a human or another animal, while it is fighting or threatening.
territorial a. behavior directed toward the defense of an area by an individual or a group against entry by others, usually members of the same species but the trait is developed in guard dogs that protect property from human intruders.

aggressiveness see AGGRESSION.

aging, ageing 1. the process of growing older. It includes a reduction in strength, endurance, speed of reaction, agility, basal metabolism, sexual activity and hearing acuity. The bones are more brittle, the skin drier and less elastic and the teeth are shed. 2. assessing the age of an animal.
a. of fetuses based largely on crown–rump length plus hair follicles and other external features.
a. by teeth often the most convenient means of assessing an animal patient's age; errors occur because of the effect of nutrition and varying rates of dental attrition.

agist to provide grazing for another farmer's livestock on a rental basis.

agistment see AGIST.

Agkistrodon contortrix see COPPERHEAD SNAKES.
aglossia congenital absence of the tongue.
aglossostomia congenital absence of the tongue and the mouth opening.
aglutition inability to swallow.
aglycemia absence of sugar from the blood. See also HYPOGLYCEMIA.
aglycone the noncarbohydrate portion of a glycoside molecule.
aglycosuric free from glycosuria.
aglypha snakes without fangs, hence aglypha, species of the family Colubridae.
aglyphous without venomous fangs.
agnathia congenital absence of the lower jaw.
inherited a. a lethal recessive in sheep which are unable to graze; ventral displacement of the ears is a common accompaniment.
agnogenic of unknown origin.
a. myeloid metaplasia see MYELOID metaplasia.
-agogue word element. [Gr.] *something that leads or induces.*
agonad an animal having no sex glands (gonads).
agonadal having no sex glands; due to absence of sex glands.
agonal pertaining to death or extreme suffering.
a. gasp the spasmodic open mouth with contraction of the diaphragm and retraction of the hyoid apparatus which occurs at death.
agonist 1. in physiology a muscle which in contracting to move a part is opposed by another muscle (the antagonist). 2. in pharmacology, a drug which has affinity for the cellular receptors of another drug or natural substance and which produces a physiological effect.
adrenergic a. (2) see ADRENERGIC agents.
cholinergic a. (2) see CHOLINERGIC.
partial a. (2) a drug that combines with the relevant receptors but not with the efficiency of the agonist.
agonist/antagonist analgesia see SEQUENTIAL analgesia.
agony 1. death struggle. 2. extreme suffering.
agoraphobia in animals, a reluctance to go outside. Includes companion animals and especially horses that have been kept in stables for long periods. See also BARN rat.
agouti 1. speedy, stout-bodied, nocturnal, South American rodent that bounds like a hare. Called also *Dasyprocta aguti*. 2. a pattern of pigmentation in which individual hairs have several bands of light and dark pigment with black tips. Seen in hares, Abyssinian cats, guinea pigs, and the agouti, after which it is named.
-agra word element. [Gr.] *attack, seizure.*
agranular reticulum smooth-surfaced endoplasmic reticulum (SER).
agranulocyte white blood cells such as lymphocytes and monocytes which are without obvious cytoplasmic granules when viewed under a light microscope.
agranulocytopoiesis the absence of granulocyte production.
agranulocytosis a disease state characterized by a marked reduction in the granulocyte count in the blood and in the body's defenses against bacterial invasion. Called also granulocytopenia. See also FELINE panleukopenia.
agranuloplastic forming nongranular cells only.
agranulosis agranulocytosis.
agreement similar results obtained, e.g. by two tests.
chance a. the agreement between results which would be expected by chance.
a. by more than chance similarity of results obtained in excess of that expected by chance, i.e. estimated by statistical tests such as Kappa.
agretope the amino acid residues of a processed antigenic peptide that bind to an MHC molecule.
agricultural advisers agricultural engineers, agronomists, agrostologists, nutritionists, geneticists, accountants, veterinarians and the like.
agricultural chemical industry suppliers and manufacturers of fertilizers, insecticides, anthelmintics, mineral and vitamin supplements, pharmaceuticals, growth promotants, feed additives, sanitation materials. The industry produces much of agriculture's applied research and maintains the data base of agricultural technical and scientific knowledge.
Agriolimax meticulatus the common garden slug, intermediate host of the sheep lungworm, *Cystocaulus ocreatus*.
Agriostomum a genus of the subfamily Chabertinae of nematode worms. Includes *A. vryburgi* (*Bos indicus* cattle).
Agrostemma a genus of the plant family Caryophyllaceae; seeds contain githagin, a toxic saponin which causes diarrhea and nervous signs. Includes *A. githago* (corn cockles).
Agrostis grass in the plant family Poaceae. Includes *A. avenacea* (blowaway, blown, fairy or oat grass).
A. avenacea* + *Anguina agrostis* (*A. funesta*) + *Clavibacter toxicus those grass seed heads which are infested with a nematode produce galls containing the bacteria which produces a toxin tunicamyluracil (corynetoxin), the cause of FLOOD plain staggers.
agrostology the scientific study of grasses.
Aguirre syndrome unilateral periocular loss of pigmentation seen in Siamese cats, usually associated with Horner's syndrome, upper respiratory infection or ocular disease.
agyria see LISSENCEPHALY.
AHF antihemophilic factor (clotting factor VIII).
AHG antihemophilic globulin (clotting factor VIII).
AHV-1 alcelaphine herpesvirus-1.
AI 1. aortic incompetence. 2. aortic insufficiency. 3. apical impulse. 4. artificial insemination.
AI (4) center an establishment for the housing of males, usually bulls, the collection and storage of semen, the despatch of preserved semen, the keeping of records of performance and usually the provision of a problem-solving veterinary service.
AI (4) technician a person qualified to inseminate animals with stored semen. The 'bull in the bowler hat' of modern antiquity.
ai shi in acupuncture, a sensitive, nonspecific acupoint which reflects pain or abnormality in some part of the body.
AIDS *a*cquired *i*mmune *d*eficiency *s*yndrome of humans, caused by the lentivirus, human immunodeficiency virus 1 (HIV1), less commonly HIV2. The virus initially infects macrophages and then attacks and destroys T helper CD4 lymphocytes, thereby producing immunodeficiency and resulting in death, usually after a very prolonged incubation period followed by a very prolonged clinical course. A very similar virus SIV1 causes simian AIDS in captive macaque monkeys. A further similar virus SIV2 has been isolated from healthy green monkeys.
feline AIDS see FELINE immunodeficiency virus.
AIHA autoimmune hemolytic anemia.
ailurophobia morbid fear of cats.
Ailuropoda melanoleuca giant panda. See PANDA.
Ailurus fulgens lesser or red panda. See PANDA.
Aino virus a bunyavirus transmitted by insects.
A. v. disease a disease that causes congenital arthro-

gryposis and hydranencephaly in calves. See also AKABANE VIRUS disease.

air the gaseous mixture that makes up the atmosphere. See also AIR SACS.

a. capillaries the minuscule vessels that connect the parabronchi in avian lungs, in which there are no blind-ended tubules.

a. cell the air-filled space between the internal and external shell membranes of a bird's egg.

a. changes per hour the standard measurements used to indicate the level of ventilation in a building especially with respect to removal of humidity, noxious gases and carbon dioxide.

a. dried said of feed that is dried in the open with only natural movement of air, e.g. conventional hay. Contains about 10% water.

a. filtration used as a means of reducing contamination inside a building, the efficiency depending on the pore size of the filter. A technique of some value when combined with temperature control in reducing the prevalence of pneumonia in calves in intensive veal producing units.

a. flow rates are important in assessing the suitability of a ventilating system in animal accommodation. Standards for suitable flow rates for different species and age groups for heating and cooling are available.

a. hunger a distressing dyspnea affecting both inspiration and expiration which occurs in paroxysms; characteristic of diabetic acidosis and coma. Called also Kussmaul's respiration.

a. movement includes air changes voiding humidity and gases to the exterior plus movements within the space which facilitate cooling.

a. passages the combined air delivery system of the upper and lower respiratory tracts including nasal cavities, pharynx, laryngeal cavity, trachea, bronchi and bronchioles.

a. pollution contamination of the air with deleterious or esthetically unattractive chemical, physical or biological material. Usually reserved for pollutants generated by humans.

a. pump a small electrically driven appliance used to provide a constant stream of air bubbles to aquaria. The bubbles themselves add little oxygen to the water but the constant disturbance of the surface of the water does.

a. quality the determination of air flow rate, temperature, humidity, freedom from bacteria, solid particles, obnoxious effluvia and poisonous gases—especially hydrogen sulfide and methane from sullage pits under the animal accommodation.

a. trapping dilatation of alveoli without destruction of their walls.

a. vesicles extend radially from parabronchi in the lungs of birds and connect with air capillaries, in which gaseous exchange occurs with vascular capillaries.

air plant see BRYOPHYLLUM *pinnatum*.

air sac disease see AIRSACCULITIS.

air sacs sacs that communicate with the respiratory, air-filled membranous system in birds and primates.

avian a. s. there are eight air sacs in the chicken: an unpaired cervical, an unpaired clavicular, a pair of cranial thoracic, a pair of caudal thoracic and a pair of abdominal sacs. They connect with the lungs through ostia along the ventrolateral borders of the lungs. The connections are to large and small bronchi. The sacs are also connected to and aerate the bones of the thoracic cage, including the vertebrae, the pelvis and the upper limb bones. Ducks have a similar pattern of air sacs to that of chickens. Turkeys have seven sacs: an unpaired cervicoclavicular sac, a pair of medial clavicular, a pair of cranial thoracic and a pair of abdominal sacs.

a. s. disease includes AIRSACCULITIS and air sac mite infestation (CYTODITES *nudus*).

a. s. inflammation see AIRSACCULITIS.

a. s. mite CYTODITES *nudus*.

primate a. s. laryngeal diverticula of variable size that reach extreme development in the gibbons.

airborne see airborne TRANSMISSION.

Airedale terrier a large black and tan terrier with a wiry coat, originating in the Aire River valley in the Yorkshire district of England for hunting small game. The breed is subject to cerebellar hypoplasia and an increased risk of certain types of neoplasms. Called also Working terrier, Waterside terrier.

airsacculitis inflammation of the air sacs.

avian a. occurs as part of a respiratory tract infection by *Mycoplasma gallisepticum* infections usually referred to as CHRONIC respiratory disease. Airsacculitis as such is notable for the high rate of carcass condemnations that it causes. Postmortem lesions include the presence of caseous exudate, or a beaded appearance of the lining. There are usually accompanying lesions in the bronchi and lungs.

primate a. a large variety of bacterial species participate in the disease. Clinical signs include cough, dyspnea and swelling of the submandibular area.

airway 1. the passage by which air enters and leaves the lungs. 2. a mechanical device used for securing unobstructed respiration during general anesthesia or other occasions in which the patient is not ventilating or exchanging gases properly. Includes an endotracheal tube and a tracheostomy tube.

artificial a. endotracheal or tracheostomy tubes.

a. obstruction in the unanesthetized animal is usually caused by vomitus or laryngeal spasm due to foreign material in the larynx. In the nonintubated anesthetized animal, it is caused by caudal displacement of the tongue and epiglottis, accumulation of mucus, saliva and blood in the pharynx or laryngeal spasm resulting from that accumulation. In the intubated animal, faulty placement or functioning of the endotracheal tube or kinking of it can cause obstruction of the airway. The signs of obstruction are deep, asphyxial respirations, struggling and great agitation in the conscious animal. Deeply anesthetized animals simply show a decline in respiratory efficiency.

a. reflexes aid in the removal of secretions and foreign material. See also COUGH, SNEEZE.

a. resistance the resistance to airflow through the respiratory tree and any addition to the airway, such as the endotracheal tube and connectors in a closed circuit anesthetic machine.

AIS see ILLAWARRA CATTLE.

aitchbone butcher's term for the hip bone in a carcass.

AIV silage silage to which acid is added during preparation to ensure adequate acidification for preservation. Not a common procedure.

Aix galericulata brightly colored mandarin duck with a white front and red, green, yellow, brown patches; pairs show great mutual affection; the Chinese symbol of conjugal fidelity!

Ajellomyces see BLASTOMYCES *dermatitidis*.

Akabane virus a bunyavirus transmitted by insects, including *Culicoides brevitarsis*, and the cause of arthrogryposis and hydranencephaly, recognized in newborn calves and lambs following in utero infection in the early months of gestation.

A. v. disease the causative bunyavirus is carried by insects, e.g. *Culicoides brevitarsis*, and affects only young fetuses in pregnant ruminants. At birth the calves are either without intelligence (imbecile calves) or have joint fixation, in flexion or extension, and create a dystocia (curly calves). See also AINO VIRUS disease, HYDRANENCEPHALY. Called also enzootic bovine arthrogryposis.

akaryocyte, akaryote a non-nucleated cell, e.g. an erythrocyte.

Akbash dog a Turkish flock-guarding dog; it is very large (80–140 lb) with a thick, smooth or long, double coat in solid white.

AKC American Kennel Club.

akinesia 1. abnormal absence or poverty of movements. 2. the temporary paralysis of a muscle by the injection of a local anesthetic agent.

eyelid a. produced by performing an auriculopalpebral nerve block.

akinetic affected with akinesia.

Akita a large, robust dog with a dense coat, a tail that curls over the back, small eyes and erect ears. Called also Japanese Akita, the name taken from Akita Prefecture on the island of Honshu, and Akita Inu. See also NIPPON INU.

Al chemical symbol, *aluminum*.

-al suffix meaning pertaining to.

Al-Dhabh see MUSLIM SLAUGHTER.

AL protein a proteolytic digestion product of immunoglobulin light chains found in immunogenic amyloid.

ALA δ-AMINOLEVULINIC ACID.

Ala alanine.

ala pl. *alae* [L.] a winglike process, e.g. the cervical and caudal alae of nematodes; the wing-like structures at the esophageal and tail regions of the worm.

a. cinerea an area on the floor of the 4th ventricle; the trigonum nervus vagi of the medulla oblongata.

a. lobuli centralis a lobule of the rostral part of the cerebellar hemispheres that extends from the vermis.

a. nasi the wing of the nose; the cartilaginous flap on the outer side of either nostril.

a. ossis illium wing of the ilium.

sacral a. the lateral parts of the base of the sacrum which carry the articular surfaces for the ilium and the transverse processes of the last lumbar vertebra.

a. spuria the alula.

Alabama rot see idiopathic CUTANEOUS and renal glomerular disease.

alacrima a deficiency or absence of secretion of tears.

congenital a. a rare condition occurring mainly in toy breeds of dogs.

ALAD δ-aminolevulinic acid dehydratase.

Alaeuris brachylophi oxyurid worms found in the intestines of lizards and turtles.

alafosfalin a phosphonic acid compound with antibacterial activity.

Alagar virus a Brazilian subtype of the VESICULAR stomatitis virus.

alanine a naturally occurring, nonessential amino acid.

a. cycle cycle of alanine produced in muscle from transamination of pyruvate produced from glycolysis of glucose during exercise, transported in the plasma to the liver where the alanine amino-nitrogen is converted to urea for excretion and the carbon from the keto-acid of alanine, pyruvate, is recycled via gluconeogenesis to glucose, which is finally transported back to the muscle.

alanine aminotransferase an enzyme that catalyzes the reversible transfer of an amino group in the reaction:

$$\text{alanine} + \text{2-oxoglutarate} \rightleftharpoons \text{pyruvate} + \text{glutamate}$$

requiring the coenzyme pyridoxal phosphate. Abbreviated ALT. It is present in high concentrations in hepatocytes of dogs, cats and humans. The serum concentration is elevated, especially when there is acute damage to liver cells, as in viral or toxic hepatitis, and obstructive jaundice. Significant elevation of the serum levels of ALT is a specific indicator of liver damage only in small animals and primates. Called also glutamic–pyruvic transaminase (GPT).

alar 1. pertaining to or like a wing. 2. pertaining to the axilla.

a. cartilage a nasal cartilage which supports the rim of the nostril of some animals such as the horse.

a. fold extends from the nostril to the ventral nasal concha. It forms the medial and ventral walls of the false nostril in the horse.

a. foramen a third foramen which perforates the wing of the atlas in some animal species.

a. plate dorsal bulge of the embryonic neural tube, destined to develop into the dorsal horn of the spinal cord.

rostral a. fold one of a group of foramina in the caudal part of the orbit.

Alaria a genus of the family Diplostomatidae of digenetic trematodes. Includes *A. alata* (largely nonpathogenic, found in intestines of wild and domestic carnivores).

alariasis infestation with the intestinal fluke *Alaria* spp. Many affected animals are clinically normal. Very heavy infestations may cause an increase in fecal mucus and occasionally hemorrhagic enteritis.

alarm points in acupuncture, points located on the ventral abdomen, one for each of the *Zang-fu* organs. Called also *MU* points.

alarm reaction the response of the sympathetic nervous system either to physical stress or to a strong emotional state. Called also stress reaction and fight or flight reaction. It is an automatic and instantaneous response that increases the body's capability to cope with a sudden emergency.

The physiological changes occurring during this reaction increase physical strength and mental activity. The blood pressure is elevated, the blood glucose level is raised for additional energy, the blood coagulates more readily, and the flow of blood to muscles needed for activity is increased, while those organs not needed for fight or flight receive a diminished blood supply. One of the most striking manifestations of this reaction is the involution of lymphoid tissues due to the action of adrenal hormones.

Alaskan malamute a heavy boned, powerfully built, gray or black and white, thick-coated dog with great strength and endurance, used originally for pulling sleds in Alaska. The breed is subject to an inherited chondrodysplasia with hemolytic anemia, factor VII deficiency and hemeralopia.

alba [L.] *white*.

albamycin see NOVOBIOCIN.

Albanian cattle yellow to red-black dual-purpose Albanian cattle; similar brachyceros-type cattle breeds in Yugoslavia and Greece.

albatross a large, 25 lb, ocean flying bird with a very wide wingspan, 10 ft, which enables it to glide for long distances at a height of about 50 ft above the sea. There are several genera, the commonest being *Diomedea* and *Phoebetria*. The commonest species is the Wandering Albatross, *Diomedea exulans*.

albendazole a benzimidazole anthelmintic with high efficiency in sheep and cattle against all intestinal nematodes, except *Trichuris* spp., and intestinal tapeworms and lungworms and, with increased dose rates, will kill adult liver fluke.

Albers–Schönberg disease a rare inherited disorder of humans characterized by severe generalized osteosclerosis. OSTEOPETROSIS of cattle and rabbits resembles this disease.

Alberta Certified Preconditioned Feeder Program a government backed certification program for PRECONDITIONING calves going into feedlots for fattening in Canada.

albicans [L.] *white*.

albiduria the discharge of white or pale urine.

Albini's nodules gray nodules of the size of small grains, sometimes seen on the free edges of the atrioventricular valves of the newborn; they are fetal remnants.

albinism congenital absence of normal pigmentation in the body (hair, skin, eyes).

inherited equine a. true albinism is very rare in animals. A true white can be produced by mating two Overo horses, but the foals have congenital atresia of the colon. There is a true albino Icelandic sheep with no other apparent defects. There are a number of pseudoalbinos, one in horses being a lethal trait because of early fetal death.

albino an animal affected with albinism.

true a. true albinos have pink eyes without pigment, impaired vision and white skin; so-called albino horses are usually pseudo-albinos because they have pigmented eyes.

albino muscle a condition in which all muscle, except cardiac, diaphragmatic and coccygeal, are lighter in color than normal in cattle that appear normal in other respects.

albinuria albiduria.

Albizia a genus of legumes in the plant family Mimosaceae; seed pods of the toxic species contain 4-methoxy-pyridone a pyridoxine analog which causes cardiomyopathy, pulmonary edema and polioencephalomalacia. Includes *A. chinensis* (*A. stipulata*), *A. versicolor* and *A. tanganyicensis* (*A. lebbeck* var. *australis*, *A rhodesia*, fever tree, red paperbark).

albuginea 1. a tough, whitish layer of fibrous tissue investing a part or organ. 2. the tunica albuginea.

albugo a translucent corneal opacity.

albumen the white of the egg; typically comprising 60% of a bird egg. It consists of a middle dense layer surrounded by an inner liquid layer and an outer liquid layer. It surrounds the yolk and is surrounded by the egg membrane and shell.

albumin 1. any protein that is soluble in water and moderately concentrated salt solutions and is coagulable by heat. 2. serum albumin; a plasma protein, formed principally in the liver and constituting about four-sevenths of the 6 to 8% protein concentration in the plasma. Albumin is responsible for much of the colloidal osmotic pressure of the blood, and thus is a very important factor in regulating the exchange of water between the plasma and the interstitial compartment (space between the cells).

The presence of albumin in the urine (see ALBUMINURIA) indicates malfunction of the kidney, and may accompany kidney disease or heart failure.

A decrease in the serum albumin level may occur with severe disease of the kidney. Other conditions such as liver disease, malnutrition and extensive burns may result in serious decrease of plasma proteins.

aggregated a. heat-denatured human albumin, which is labeled with radioisotopes for pulmonary perfusion scanning. Called also macroaggregated albumin. See also TECHNETIUM.

^{51}Cr-labeled a. excretion a method of determining gastrointestinal protein loss. After intravenous administration of ^{51}Cr-labeled albumin, radioactivity in the feces is measured.

a.–globulin (A/G) ratio the ratio of albumin to globulin in blood serum, plasma or urine.

iodinated ^{125}I a. a radiopharmaceutical used in plasma volume determinations, consisting of albumin human labeled with iodine-125.

iodinated ^{131}I a. a radiopharmaceutical used in blood pool imaging and plasma volume determinations, consisting of albumin human labeled with iodine-131.

macroaggregated a. (MAA) aggregated albumin.

serum a. albumin of the blood.

albuminocytologic dissociation increase in the level of albumin in cerebrospinal fluid without an accompanying increase in the number of cells.

albuminoid, albuminous 1. resembling albumin. 2. an albumin-like substance; the term is sometimes applied to scleroproteins.

albuminuria the presence in the urine of serum albumin. It indicates RENAL dysfunction and occurs in primary RENAL failure (glomerular) and congestive HEART FAILURE. There may be a sufficient loss to cause HYPOALBUMINEMIA.

albuterol a relatively selective β_2-adrenergic bronchodilator used for relief of bronchospasm in patients with reversible obstructive airway disease. Called also salbutamol.

Alca torda erect, short-legged ungainly black and white arctic bird, called also razorbill, razor-billed Auk.

Alcaligenes a genus of saprophytic obligately aerobic bacilli occasionally found in the intestines of vertebrates or in dairy products and sometimes in nosocomial infections. *A. fecalis* is now called *Bordetella avium*.

alcapton, alkapton a class of substances with an affinity for alkali, found in the urine and causing the condition known as alkaptonuria. The compound commonly found, and most commonly referred to by the term, is homogentisic acid.

alcaptonuria, alkaptonuria excretion in the urine of homogentisic acid and its oxidation products as a result of a genetic disorder of phenylalanine–tyrosine metabolism in humans and orang-utans.

Alcataenia cerorhincae a cestode found in the bird, the rhinoceros auklet (*Cerorhinca monocerata*).

Alcataenia fraterculae a cestode found in horned puffin (*Fratercula coniculata*).

alcelaphine pertaining to the members of the family Alcelaphinae of antelopes of which the hartebeest and wildebeest are members.

a. herpesvirus-1 the cause of wildebeest-related bovine malignant catarrh in European cattle; abbreviated AHV-1.

Alcelaphus caama Called also *A. buselaphus*, *A. buselaphus cokei* (Coke's hartebeest). See HARTEBEEST.

Alces americana see AMERICAN MOOSE.

alcian blue a basic phthalocyanin dye that stains mucopolysaccharides blue.

alcid members of the bird family Alcidae, the northern counterpart of the southern hemisphere penguin; includes auks, guillemots, puffins.

alcohol 1. any organic compound containing the hydroxy (–OH) functional group except those in which the OH group is attached to an aromatic ring, which are called *phenols*. Alcohols are classified as *primary*, *secondary* or *tertiary* according to whether the carbon atom to which the OH group is attached is bonded to one, two or three other carbon atoms and as *monohydric*, *dihydric* or *trihydric* according to whether they contain one, two or three –OH groups; the latter two are called *diols* and *triols*, respectively. 2. common name for ethyl alcohol (ethanol). See also ALCOHOLIC.

absolute a. ethyl alcohol free from water and impurities.

complex plant a. includes cicutoxin, oenanthotoxin, tremetol, all toxic, causing heavy mortalities and signs including incoordination, tremor, convulsions, vomiting.

denatured a. ethyl alcohol made unfit for consumption by the addition of substances known as denaturants. Although it should never be taken internally, denatured alcohol is widely used on the skin as a cooling agent and skin disinfectant.

ethoxylate a. detergents alcohols containing an ethyl radical with an attached oxygen group; used in the treatment and prevention of ruminal bloat.

ethyl a. a transparent, colorless, mobile, volatile liquid miscible with water, ether or chloroform, and obtained by the fermentation of carbohydrate with yeast. It is the major ingredient of alcoholic beverages consumed by humans. Called also ethanol and grain alcohol. It is used in veterinary medicine in the preparation of mixtures for topical application and for skin disinfection.

grain a. see ethyl alcohol (above).

isopropyl a. a transparent, volatile colorless liquid used as a rubbing compound. Called also isopropanol.

methyl a. a mobile, colorless liquid used as a solvent. Called also wood alcohol or methanol. It is a useful fuel, but is poisonous if taken internally. Consumption may lead to blindness or death.

a. nerve block permanent anesthesia to a part can be produced by blocking the relevant nerve with isopropyl alcohol. Adverse effects are likely due to continued loss of sensation and motor power.

a. poisoning in animals this does not present the social problems that it does in humans even in cattle and sheep fed on brewer's grains and distiller's solubles. Ethyl alcohol is produced in some feeds which are fermented accidentally, but overt alcohol poisoning is not recorded. Carbohydrate engorgement is a more likely occurrence. Isopropyl alcohol is an end product of ketone body degradation in the rumen in cattle and does cause signs of inebriation in cows with nervous acetonemia.

Small companion animals are sometimes exposed to toxic levels of ethyl alcohol by owners and it may be readily consumed. Excessive amounts can lead to vomiting, various levels of central nervous system depression, including excitement, seizures and respiratory depression.

wood a. methyl alcohol.

alcuronium chloride a muscle relaxant, a derivative of toxiferene obtained from curare. It is an antidepolarizing agent with a medium duration of action.

ALD aldolase.

aldehyde an organic compound containing the aldehyde functional group (–CHO); that is, one with a carbonyl group (C=O) located at one end of the carbon chain. Aldehydes are formed in meat during the rancidification of fat and in the degradation of alcohols in biological materials. They have an acrid unpleasant taste and are toxic if taken in sufficient quantities. Some aldehydes (formaldehyde and glutaraldehyde) are used as disinfectants and fixatives.

alder buckthorn RHAMNUS *cathartica*, RHAMNUS *frangula*.

aldicarb a carbamate pesticide.

aldolase an enzyme involved in the Embden–Meyerhof or glycolytic pathway which reversibly catalyzes the reaction fructose-1,6-bisphosphate to glyceraldehyde-3-phosphate and dihydroxyacetone phosphate. Present in all cells and may be measured in the serum as an indicator of muscle, heart or liver disease. Called also ALS and ALD.

aldopentose any one of a class of sugars that contain five carbon atoms and an aldehyde group (–CHO).

aldose a sugar containing an aldehyde group (–CHO).

aldosterone the main MINERALOCORTICOID hormone secreted by the adrenal cortex, the principal biological activity of which is the regulation of electrolyte and water balance by promoting the retention of sodium (and, therefore, of water) and the excretion of potassium; the retention of water induces an increase in plasma volume and an increase in blood pressure. Its secretion is stimulated by angiotensin II. Deficiency is HYPOADRENOCORTICISM (Addison's disease).

aldosteronism an abnormality of electrolyte balance caused by excessive secretion of aldosterone; hyperaldosteronism.

primary a. that arising from oversecretion of aldosterone by an adrenal adenoma, characterized typically by hypokalemia, alkalosis, muscular weakness, polyuria, polydipsia and hypertension. Called also Conn's syndrome.

pseudoprimary a. that caused by bilateral adrenal hyperplasia and having the same signs and symptoms as primary aldosteronism.

secondary a. that due to extra-adrenal stimulation of aldosterone secretion; it is associated with edematous states, as in nephrotic syndrome, hepatic cirrhosis and heart failure.

aldoxycarb a carbamate pesticide.

aldrin an insecticide. See CHLORINATED HYDROCARBONS.

alecithal having no distinct yolk.

alecrim see HOLOCALYX GLAZIOVII.

Alectryon genus in the plant family Sapindaceae; plants capable of causing cyanide poisoning. Includes *A. excelcus* (titoki), *A. oleifolius* (boonaree, rosewood, *Heterodendron oleifolium*).

Aleppo button, Aleppo boil see LEISHMANIASIS. Called also Aleppo boil.

alertness the mental state of aroused awareness. Inferred in animals.

aleukemia 1. absence or deficiency of leukocytes in the blood. 2. aleukemic LEUKEMIA.

aleukemic leukemia see LEUKEMIA.

aleukia leukopenia; absence of leukocytes in the blood.

aleukocytosis diminished proportion of leukocytes in the blood.

aleurioconidia the single cell conidia produced by extrusion from the conidiophores of fungi such as *Microsporum* and *Trichophyton*.

aleuriospore a terminal or lateral spore that separates by breaking the wall of the hypha.

Aleurites a genus of the plant family Euphorbiaceae. Plants may contain toxic albumins, saponins, diterpenes; cause hemorrhagic enteritis and profuse diarrhea. Includes *A. fordii* (tung oil tree), *A. moluccana* (candlenut tree), *A. montana* (mu tree), *A. triloba* (*A. moluccana*), *A. trisperma*.

Aleutian mink disease a slowly progressive disease of certain mink (e.g. Aleutian mink which are mutants for a pale colored pelt) caused by persistent parvovirus infection and associated with polyclonal, virus specific hypergammaglobulinemia and immune complex-mediated lesions, especially arteritis and glomerulonephritis. It is manifested by emaciation, reproductive inefficiency and death from renal failure. The characteristic laboratory findings are hypergammaglobulinemia and a massive proliferation and infiltration of plasma cells into the swollen kidneys and into the spleen, liver, lymph nodes and bone marrow.

alevin advanced FRY.

Alexander gouge a heavy duty bone gouge with a fluted blade, a sharp chisel point and a rounded end to the shaft adapted to hitting with a hammer.

Alexander's disease a congenital, fibrinoid encephalomyelopathy of humans and described in dogs.

alexin see COMPLEMENT.

aleydigism absence of secretion of the interstitial cells of the testis (Leydig cells).

alfalfa see MEDICAGO.

alfentanil an opioid analgesic; a derivative of fentanyl with lower potency but more rapid action.

alfombrilla DRYMARIA *arenarioides*.

Alfortia edentatus see STRONGYLUS *edentatus*.

ALG antilymphocyte globulin.

algae a group of plants living in the water, including all seaweeds, and ranging in size from microscopic cells to fronds many meters long. A group of unicellular algae, the *Cyanobacter*, growing on dams, ponds and lakes can cause severe mortalities in animals drinking the water. See also ALGAL, MICROCYSTIS, PROTOTHECA. Artificial culture of algae as a source of livestock feed is being tried in some arid countries.

algal pertaining to or caused by algae.

a. infection is very rare but systemic and udder infections are recorded. See PROTOTHECOSIS.

a. mastitis the algae *Prototheca trispora* and *P. zopfii* cause chronic bovine mastitis.

a. poisoning toxic *Cyanobacteria* grow in stagnant water and, in the correct circumstances for massive growth and with certain species of bacteria, the top layer of water can be very poisonous. There are two syndromes: sudden death caused by neurotoxins, and severe liver damage with jaundice and photosensitization caused by hepatotoxins. Called also water bloom. See also ALGAE, ANATOXIN, CYANOBACTERIA, MICROCYSTIN.

algarroba see PROSOPIS JULIFLORIA.

Algerian Arab sheep meat and carpetwool sheep, both horned and polled.

algesia sensitiveness to pain; hyperesthesia.

algesic, algetic pertaining to or emanating from algesia.

a. substances endogenous substances involved in the production of the pain that is associated with inflammation. Includes serotonin, bradykinin and prostaglandins.

algesimetry measurement of sensitivity of pain.

algesthesis a painful sensation.

-algia word element. [Gr.] *pain*.

algicide 1. destructive to algae. 2. an agent that destroys algae.

algid chilly; cold.

alginate a salt of alginic acid, a colloidal substance from brown seaweed; used, in the form of calcium, sodium or ammonium alginate, as foam, clot or gauze for absorbable surgical dressings. Also used as an irreversible hydrocolloid impression material in dentistry for making impressions of jaws in the preparation of orthodontic appliances.

algo- word element. [Gr.] *pain, cold*.

algodystrophy a combination of pain and dystrophic changes in bone.

algogenic 1. causing pain. 2. lowering temperature.

algology 1. the scientific study of pain. 2. phycology.

algometer a device used in testing the sensitiveness of a part.

algometry estimation of the sensitivity to painful stimuli.

algor chill or rigor; coldness.

a. mortis the cooling of the body after death, which proceeds at a definite rate, influenced by the environmental temperature and protection of the body.

algorithm a set of rules designed to solve a specific problem by proceeding through a series of prearranged, logical steps. Originally referred to purely mathematical problems, now used in a wider sphere, e.g. to solve diagnostic problems. Often depicted in the form of a box and line diagram which sets out the logic of the procedure or program.

diagnostic a. mapping of the logical steps to be taken in eliminating potential diagnoses which do not match clinical signs or pathological findings and arranging possible diagnoses in order of probability.

aliasing an imaging artefact in Doppler ultrasound, governed by the Nyquist limit, in which the blood flow direction appears to be reversed. An experienced operator can readily distinguish the aliased image from the true image.

alienation isolation or separation from the standard.

alienia absence of the spleen.

aliflurane a halogenated inhalant anesthetic agent.

aliform shaped like a wing.

aliment food; nutritive material.

alimentary pertaining to or caused by food, or nutritive material.

a. canal all the organs making up the route taken by food as it passes through the body from mouth to anus; it comprises the esophagus, stomach, and small and large intestines. Called also digestive tract. See also DIGESTIVE system.

a. ketosis see ACETONEMIA.

a. system see DIGESTIVE system.

a. toxic aleukia leukopenia due to ingested toxin, e.g. *Fusarium* spp. poisoning, stachybotrytoxicosis.

alimentary tract see ALIMENTARY canal, DIGESTIVE system.

a. t. abnormal motility includes hypermotility, hypermotility, stasis.

a. t. congenital defects includes agenesis, aplasia, achalasia.

a. t. dysfunction inability of the alimentary tract to carry out properly the functions of prehension, swallowing, digestion and absorption of food. The mode of the dysfunction may be one of abnormal motor function, expressed by errors in motility, or of chemical function relating to secretion of digestive juices, including hypersecretion and fluid loss, and absorption of the products of digestion.

a. t. functional movement arrests see ILEUS.

a. t. motility the movements of the stomach and intestines which are the means of propelling food through the tract. They include peristalsis, segmenting movements and sphincter relaxation. Abnormality may take the form of hyper- or hypomotility.

a. t. mycosis see PHYCOMYCOSIS, CANDIDIASIS, ASPERGILLOSIS, HISTOPLASMOSIS.

a. t. pain see COLIC.

a. t. secretory function includes gastric and pancreatic secretion, and secretion of intestinal glands.

a. t. stimulant a traditional pharmaceutical maneuver of increasing gut motility by the oral administration of medicines which cause physical irritation of the mucosa, e.g. aloin, castor oil, croton oil.

alimentation giving or receiving of nourishment.

intravenous a. the administration by intravenous injection of a solution containing sufficient nutrients in appropriate concentration to maintain life.

oral a. feeding by mouth.

total parenteral a. see HYPERALIMENTATION.

alinasal pertaining to the sides or wings of the nostril.

aliphatic 1. fatty or oily. 2. pertaining to a hydrocarbon that does not contain an aromatic ring.

a. organic arsenicals include the pharmaceuticals—cacodylic, phenarsonic acids and the herbicides—monosodium and disodium methanearsontes. See also organic ARSENICAL.

aliquot 1. a sample that is representative of the whole. 2. a number that will divide another without a remainder; e.g. 2 is an aliquot of 6.

alkalemia abnormal alkalinity, or increased pH, of the blood. See also ALKALOSIS.

alkali any one of a class of compounds such as sodium hydroxide that form salts with acids and soaps with fats; a base, or substance capable of neutralizing acids. Other properties include a bitter taste and the ability to turn litmus paper from red to blue. Alkalis play a vital role in maintaining the normal functioning of the body chemistry. See also ACID–BASE BALANCE, ALKALINE, BASE.

a. disease see SELENIUM poisoning.

a. reserve the ability of the combined buffer systems of the blood to neutralize acid. The pH of the blood normally is slightly on the alkaline side, between 7.35 and 7.45. Since the principal buffer in the blood is bicarbonate, the alkali reserve is essentially represented by the plasma bicarbonate concentration. However, hemoglobin, phosphates and other bases also act as buffers. A lowered alkali reserve means a state of acidosis; increased reserve indicates alkalosis. Alkali reserve is measured by the combining power of carbon dioxide, which is the amount of carbon dioxide that can be bound as bicarbonate by the blood.

alkali disease see SELENIUM poisoning.

alkali milk vetch ASTRAGALUS *racemosus*.

alkaline having the reactions of an alkali.

a. incompatibilities a basic chemical fact that acids and alkalis react together so that the mixing of them in medications is likely to render the medicine ineffective. The phenomenon is utilized in the treatment of poisoning when the objective is to combat the effects of an ingested substance.

a. phosphatase a nonspecific enzyme localized on cell membranes that hydrolyzes phosphate esters liberating inorganic phosphate and has an optimal pH of about 9.5. Serum alkaline phosphatase activity is elevated in hepatobiliary disease, especially in obstructive jaundice, and in bone diseases with increased osteoblastic activity such as HYPERPARATHYROIDISM, OSTEITIS deformans and bone cancer. The liver and bone tissue each produce a distinct isoenzyme. Called also AP, alkaline phosphomonoesterase, glycerophosphatase.

a. picrate test a technique for estimating urine creatinine levels.

a. tide see postprandial alkaline TIDE.

a. urine the urine of carnivores is acidic, that of herbivores is alkaline. The presence of an alkaline urine in a carnivore, provided the sample is fresh and uncontaminated, is an indication that the patient is alkalotic, but urine findings must always be interpreted with caution.

alkalinity 1. the quality of being alkaline. 2. the combining power of a base, expressed as the maximum number of equivalents of acid with which it reacts to form a salt.

alkalinizing the capacity to alkalinize, or confer alkalinity.

a. agent sodium bicarbonate, potassium citrate, calcium carbonate or calcium acetate may be added to food in the management of acidosis associated with renal failure.

a. solution one used in fluid therapy of acidosis to raise blood pH, e.g. sodium bicarbonate or sodium lactate.

alkalinuria an alkaline condition of the urine.

alkalization the act of making alkaline.

alkalizer an agent that causes alkalization.

alkaloid one of a large group of small organic compounds, mainly derived from amino acids, and containing nitrogen, found in plants. They are water-soluble, usually bitter in taste and are characterized by powerful physiological activity. Examples are morphine, cocaine, atropine, quinine, nicotine and caffeine. The term is also applied to synthetic substances that have structures similar to plant alkaloids, such as procaine. When treated with acids they are converted to water-soluble salts. In cases of poisoning by alkaloids the recommended antidote is tannic acid, but heavy metal salts and iodine also precipitate them. Includes PYRROLIZIDINE and solanaceous alkaloids.

alkaloidosis alkaloid poisoning.

alkalosis a pathological condition resulting from accumulation of base, or from loss of acid without comparable loss of base in the body fluids, and characterized by decrease in hydrogen ion concentration (increase in pH). Alkalosis is the opposite of ACIDOSIS. See also ACID–BASE BALANCE.

compensated a. a condition in which compensatory mechanisms have returned the pH toward normal.

concentration a. associated with deficit in free body water, hypotonic fluid losses or increased sodium levels.

gastric a. alkalosis due to loss of gastric fluid because of persistent vomiting. See also hypochloremic alkalosis (below).

hypochloremic a. a metabolic alkalosis in which gastric losses of chloride are disproportionately greater than sodium loss because of corresponding increase in potassium loss.

hypokalemic a. a metabolic alkalosis associated with a low serum potassium level; retention of alkali or loss of acid occurs in the extracellular (but not intracellular) fluid compartment; although the pH of the intracellular fluid may be below normal.

metabolic a. a disturbance in which the acid–base status shifts toward the alkaline because of uncompensated loss of acids, ingestion or retention of excess base, or potassium depletion. The condition can occur with vomiting or accompany treatment with diuretics.

respiratory a. reduced carbon dioxide tension in the extracellular fluid caused by excessive excretion of carbon dioxide through the lungs (HYPERVENTILATION). Conditions commonly associated with respiratory alkalosis include pain, hypoxia, fever, high environmental temperature, poisoning, early pulmonary edema, pulmonary embolism and central nervous system disease.

alkalotic pertaining to or characterized by alkalosis.

alkane a saturated hydrocarbon, i.e. one that has no carbon–carbon multiple bonds; formerly called paraffin.

alkavervir a standardized mixture of alkaloids extracted from VERATRUM *viride*, used as a rumenatoric. Called also *Veratrum viride*.

alkene an aliphatic hydrocarbon containing a double bond.

alkyl the radical that results when an aliphatic hydrocarbon loses one hydrogen atom.

a. lead may be in effluent from petrochemical plants and cause poisoning in local wildfowl.

alkylate to treat with an alkylating agent.

alkylating agent a compound containing alkyl groups that combine readily with other molecules. Their action seems to be chiefly on the deoxyribonucleic acid (DNA) in the nucleus of the cell. They are used in chemotherapy of cancer although they do not damage malignant cells selectively, but also have a toxic action on normal cells. Locally they cause blistering of the skin and damage to the eyes and respiratory tract. Systemic toxic effects are nausea and vomiting, reduction in both leukocytes and erythrocytes, and hemorrhagic tendencies. Among the agents of this group used in therapy are the NITROGEN mustards, including mechlorethamine hydrochloride and chlorambucil, and busulfan and cyclophosphamide.

Also used for the inactivation of organisms in the preparation of vaccines as it does not significantly interfere with antigenicity. β-propiolactone is an example.

alkylmethyl-benzyl ammonium chloride used as a disinfectant; accidental contamination of poultry water supplies has caused poisoning.

alkylsulfonates a group of compounds with the carcinotherapeutic activity of the ALKYLATING AGENT.

alkyne an aliphatic hydrocarbon containing a triple bond.

all-in–all-out housing a strategy directed at the control of infectious disease, especially enzootic pneumonia of pigs and viral pneumonia of calves. The barn is emptied of all animals on a particular day, the accommodation is cleaned and disinfected and then refilled, all on the one day.

all-meat syndrome a nutritional secondary hyperparathyroidism with osteodystrophia fibrosa in dogs and cats, resulting from the high phosphorus and low calcium content of a diet consisting mainly of meat.

all-or-none trait patients either have all of the clinical signs of a disease or are clinically normal without any of the signs.

all-or-nothing law the phenomenon, characteristic of individual axons and nerve fibers, of responding only to a stimulus above a specific threshold and then responding with the maximum discharge or contraction of which the unit is capable under the particular conditions operating at the time.

allantochorion the fused or juxtaposed parts of the allantois and chorion as one structure. See also VITELLOCHORION.

allantoic pertaining to the allantois.

a. fluid see FETAL fluids.

a. vesicle the saclike hollow portion of the allantois.

allantoid 1. sausage-shaped. 2. pertaining to the allantois.

allantoidoangiopagous twin fetuses joined by the umbilical blood vessels.

allantoin a crystalline substance, the product of purine metabolism and present in urine of most mammals except primates and Dalmation dogs, and in plants. At one time used topically to promote wound healing.

allantoinuria allantoin in the urine.

allantois a ventral outgrowth of the hindgut of the early embryo, which expands to form a large sac, filled with urine-like fluid, that fuses with the chorion to make up a major part of the placenta; vestigial in humans and some other species.

a. adenomatous dysplasia adenomatous nodules and plaques on the allantois of mares; usually associated with fetal disease.

allele one of two or more alternative forms of a gene at the same site or locus in each of a pair of chromosomes, which determine alternative characters in inheritance. Called also allelomorph.

blank a. an allele which produces an antigen which cannot be detected.

null a. see silent allele (below).

silent a. one that produces no detectable effect.

allelic exclusion the process in which B and T lymphocytes express the rearranged antigen specific heavy and light chains of immunoglobulins in B cells and T-cell receptors in T cells from only one chromosome.

allelomorph see ALLELE.

allelotaxis development of an organ from several embryonic structures.

allergen 1. a substance, protein or nonprotein, capable of inducing allergy or specific hypersensitivity. 2. an extract of any substance known to cause allergy.

Allergens are used to test a patient for hypersensitivity to specific substances (see SKIN test). They are also used to densensitize or hyposensitize allergic individuals. See IMMUNOTHERAPY.

Almost any substance in the environment can be an allergen. The list of known allergens includes plant pollens, spores of mold, food preservatives, dyes, drugs, inorganic chemicals and vaccines. Allergens can enter the body by being inhaled, swallowed, touched or injected. Following primary exposure to an allergen, subsequent exposures result in hypersensitivity (allergic) reactions which may be immediate or delayed, local or systemic and include anaphylaxis and contact dermatitis.

alum-precipated a. an allergen extract used in intradermal and scratch allergy skin testing; the allergen is adsorbed onto alum to slow antigen release and provide a slower, more persistent immune stimulation. Local tissue reactions and skin nodules may follow their use.

aqueous a. a form of allergen extract used in intradermal and scratch allergy skin testing. In hyposensitization regimes, it is rapidly absorbed, but requires more frequent administration.

emulsion a. allergen extracts prepared in propylene glycol glycerin, or mineral oil. They give the most sustained effect when used in hyposensitization regimes.

allergic pertaining to or caused by ALLERGY.

a. alveolitis see ATYPICAL INTERSTITIAL PNEUMONIA.

a. breakthrough a theory which attributes temporary increases in clinical severity of atopy to influences, such as concurrent disease or hormonal variations, acting to inhibit the mechanisms which normally regulate production of IgE at low levels following sensitization.

a. bronchitis see BRONCHITIS, feline BRONCHIAL asthma, PIE SYNDROME.

a. contact dermatitis results from percutaneous sensitization to allergens, usually haptens, that form covalent bonds with epidermal proteins, and the development of a delayed (type IV) hypersensitivity. Lesions typically correspond in location to the area of contact between allergen and skin which in animals is often in relatively hairless areas unless the allergen is presented in liquid form.

a. dermatitis inflammation of the skin resulting from exposure to antigens to which the animal is hypersensitive. Usually involving immediate (type I) hypersensitivity but also commonly applied to reactions involving delayed (type IV) hypersensitivity. The specific skin reaction, lesions and pattern of disease produced depend on many factors including the type of allergen and immune mechanism, route of exposure and species differences. See also ATOPY, SWEET itch, allergic contact dermatitis (above).

a. encephalitis see experimental allergic ENCEPHALOMYELITIS.

equine a. dermatitis an intensely itchy dermatitis along the back of horses caused by sensitivity to the bites of the sandfly *Culicoides brevitarsus* and possibly other insects. Called also sweet itch, Queensland itch.

a. inhalant dermatitis see ATOPY.

a. reaction an immune-mediated, adverse clinical response, following the inhalation, ingestion or injection of an antigen by a sensitized animal. Manifestations include URTICARIA OR ANAPHYLAXIS.

a. rhinitis see ENZOOTIC nasal granuloma, SUMMER snuffles.

a. urticaria see URTICARIA.

allergid a papular or nodular allergic skin reaction.

allergization active sensitization by introduction of allergens into the body.

allergy an altered reactivity following second or subsequent exposure to antigen (allergen). See also HYPERSENSITIVITY, ALLERGIC.

atopic a. hereditary predisposition to develop certain allergies. See ATOPY.

bacterial a. a specific hypersensitivity to a particular bacterial antigen, e.g. *Mycobacterium tuberculosis*; it is dependent on previous infection with the specific organism.

bronchial a. asthma.

cold a. a condition manifested by local and systemic reactions, mediated by histamine, which is released from mast cells and basophils as a result of exposure to cold.

delayed a. see delayed HYPERSENSITIVITY.

drug a. see DRUG allergy.

drying-off a. see milk allergy (below).

food a. called also gastrointestinal allergy; see food HYPERSENSITIVITY.

gastrointestinal a. see food allergy (above).

hereditary a. an allergy with a hereditary predisposition. The tendency to develop some forms of allergy is inherited, but the specific clinical form is not. IgE, formerly called reagin or reaginic antibody, may be involved. See also ATOPY.

induced a. allergy resulting from the injection of an antigen, contact with an antigen, or infection with a microorganism, as contrasted with hereditary allergy.

inhaled a. see ATOPY.

milk a. a hypersensitivity to the milk protein, α-casein. Signs, varying from urticaria to anaphylaxis, have occurred in Jersey cows when milk escapes from the udder into the bloodstream during the drying off period.

physical a. a condition in which physical agents, such as heat, cold or light, trigger an allergic response.

Allerton virus the herpesvirus (bovine herpesvirus 2) which causes a form of lumpy skin disease. Originally named for a region in South Africa. See also LUMPY skin disease.

Allescheria boydii see PETRIELLIDIUM BOYDII.

allescheriosis eumycotic mycetoma caused by the fungus *Petriellidium* (*Allescheria*) spp.

allethrin a first-generation pyrethroid; used to control ectoparasites on dogs.

allidochlor, α-chloro-*N*,*N*-diallylacetamide an amide herbicide, poisonous if given in large amounts but not if used according to instructions. Causes anorexia, salivation, depression and prostration. Called also CDAA.

alligator amphibious reptiles of the order Crocodylia. The closely related crocodile, caiman and gavials are also members.

a. clips spring-loaded, slightly-toothed clamps with long jaws; used particularly as electrodes on an electrocardiograph because they can be easily attached to the animal's skin.

Allis tissue forceps forceps with inward-curving toothed blades and a ratcheted handle. Designed for grasping fascia and tendons.

Allium a genus of plants belonging to the Liliaceae family; contain *N*-propyl-disulfide. A constant heavy diet of many species causes severe hemolytic anemia. Includes *A. ameloprasm* (wild onion), *A. canadense* (wild onion), *A. cepa* (cultivated onion), *A. sativum* (garlic), *A. schoenprasm* (chives), *A. triquetrum* (three-cornered garlic), *A. ursinum* (wild garlic), *A. validum* (wild onion), *A. vineale* (false garlic).

all(o)- word element. [Gr.] *other, deviating from normal.*

alloantibody an antibody produced by one individual that reacts with alloantigens of another individual of the same species.

alloantigen an antigen existing in alternative (allelic) forms in a species, thus inducing an immune response when one form is transferred to members of the species who lack it; typical alloantigens are the blood group antigens.

canine secretory a. system (CSA) a minor histocompatibility system in dogs.

alloantiserum antiserum produced by injecting antigens into another member of the same species.

allobarbital diallylbarbituric acid, an intermediate- to long-acting sedative and hypnotic. Called also allobarbitone.

allobarbitone see ALLOBARBITAL.

allocation the technique of forming groups in a population for the purpose of carrying out comparisons between them. The objective is to create comparable groups and to avoid bias. Techniques used include random allocation, self-selection or clinical judgment.

allochromasia change in color of hair or skin.

allocortex the phylogenetically older part of the cerebral cortex and includes the cortex of the paleopallium and the archipallium. The newer part of the cortex is the neocortex or isocortex.

Allodermanyssus a genus of mites, members of the Dermanyssidae family. Includes *A. sanguineus* (blood-sucker in rodents).

allodynia pain produced by a non-noxious stimulus.

allogen allergen.

allogeneic denoting individuals of the same species but of different genetic constitution (antigenically distinct).

allograft a graft between individuals of the same species, but of a different genotype. Formerly called homograft.

a. rejection see REJECTION.

alloimmune immunity to an alloantigen.
a. hemolytic anemia of the newborn occurs in humans, where it is also called Rh disease, in foals as a naturally occurring disease, and in pigs and cattle receiving vaccines containing allotypic red blood cell antigens. In naturally occurring Rh-like syndrome, there are usually no untoward consequences for the first pregnancy, but at parturition red blood cells from the offspring enter the maternal circulation and, if the red blood cell antigens differ from the dam, result in the production of antibodies. A subsequent pregnancy from the same mating in which an offspring of the same blood type is produced will result in a hemolytic anemia in the offspring when maternal antibodies are acquired in the colostrum.

alloimmunization development of antibodies in response to alloantigens; antigens derived from a genetically dissimilar animal of the same species. See also ALLOANTIGEN.
a. of pregnancy sensitization of the dam against fetal red blood cell antigens that leak into the maternal circulation across the placenta or during parturition is uncommon except in the mare and sow where it gives rise to ALLOIMMUNE hemolytic anemia of the newborn.

allometric scaling scaling of dose rates of drugs, diet rations to relative growth and size of each part of the animal, or each animal relative to the others.

allometry measurement of the changes in shape of an animal relative to increases in its size.

allophenic pertaining to individual animals that have cells of different phenotypes in various tissues of the body.

alloploid the state of having any number of chromosome sets derived from different ancestral species. Called also allopolyploid.

allopolyploidy see ALLOPLOID.

allopurinol a drug that inhibits uric acid production and reduces serum and urinary uric acid levels; used in the treatment of urate uroliths in dogs.

alloreactivity the reaction of lymphocytes or antibodies with alloantigens.

allorhythmia irregularity of the pulse.

allosensitization sensitization to alloantigens (isoantigens) during pregnancy.

allosteric pertaining to an effect on the biological function of a protein, produced by a compound not directly involved in that function (an allosteric effector) or to regulation of an enzyme involving cooperativity between multiple binding sites (allosteric sites).
a. enzymes any enzymes containing an allosteric site, where effector molecules can bind to increase or decrease the rate of reaction, in addition to an active site for substrate binding. Allosteric enzymes exhibit sigmoidal rather than Michaelis–Menten kinetics.
a. site that site on an enzyme molecule which binds with a nonsubstrate molecule, inducing a conformational change that results in an alteration of the affinity of the enzyme for its substrate.

allotherm an organism whose body temperature changes with its environment. Called also poikilotherm.

allotriophagia see PICA.

allotropic exhibiting allotropism.

allotropism existence of an element in two or more distinct forms.

allotropy allotropism.

allotype a genetically determined variation in plasma proteins which may be recognized as antigenic by other members of the same species. Commonly applied to subclasses of immunoglobulins.

alloxan an oxidized product of uric acid which destroys β cells of the islets of Langerhans in the pancreas. It has been used in experimental studies of diabetes mellitus and in the treatment of insulinomas in dogs.

alloxuremia the presence of purine bases in the blood.

alloxuria the presence of purine bases in the urine.

allyl a univalent organic group previously used in the manufacture of pharmaceuticals.
a. alcohol a potent cause of hepatic necrosis. Metabolized in the liver by alcohol dehydrogenase to acrolein, the hepatoxin.
a. formate has the same effect as ALLYL alcohol.
a. isothiocyanate used as a counterirritant and in the manufacture of war gases. Called also volatile oil of mustard. Occurs naturally in members of the plant family Cruciferae which cause acute indigestion in cattle.

***N*-allylnormorphine** see NALORPHINE.

almond PRUNUS *amygdalus*.
a. shells causes abomasal impaction in stall-fed cattle where the shells are added to the ration as a roughage supplement.

Alocasia plant genus in the Araceae family. Contain raphide calcium oxalate crystals which cause severe stomatitis if eaten. Includes *A. brisbanensis* (*A. macrorrhizos*). Called also elephant ear, cunjevoi, giant taro.

aloe the dried juice of plants of the genus *Aloe* of the Liliaceae family. It is an anthraquinone cathartic and was at one time the favored purgative for horses. Called also aloes. The name aloe is also used to refer to the fragrant wood of the tree *Aquilaria agallocha*.
a. vera a mucinous substance obtained from the leaves of the plant, *Aloe vera*. Various therapeutic properties are claimed, including antibacterial, antifungal and anti-inflammatory activity. It is often used on burns.

aloe-emodin the cathartic principle in aloes. Also present in senna and rhubarb.

aloes see ALOE.

aloin the active constituent in aloes; used at one time as a purgative for horses.

alopecia deficiency of the hair or wool coat; may be caused by failure to grow or by loss after growth. There is a significant difference amongst those in which grown fibers are lost, between those in which stumps of fibers remain, and those in which the hair root has been shed from the follicle. See also HYPOTRICHOSIS, ALOPECIC.
a. areata noninflammatory hair loss in sharply defined areas. A rare condition seen in dogs, cats, horses and primates; the cause is unknown, but immune-mediated mechanisms are suspected.
bilaterally symmetric a. a clinical feature associated with endocrine and metabolic causes of hair loss in dogs and cats, although other causes including self-trauma are sometimes responsible.
cicatricial a., a. cicatrisata irreversible loss of hair associated with scarring.
collar frictional a. loss of hair around the neck occurs in some cats wearing collars. It is reversible when the collar is removed.
color dilution a. color mutant alopecia (below).
color mutant a. a clinical syndrome seen in dogs with blue or fawn coat color caused by the dilution gene at the D locus. Clinical signs include bacterial folliculitis, scaling and hair loss, mainly over the back and commencing within the first year or two of life. Hairs contain clumped melanin (macrome-

lanosomes) with distortion and fracture of the shaft. Seen most often in Doberman pinschers but reported in a number of other breeds. Called also blue Doberman syndrome, fawn Irish setter syndrome. Seen also in many breeds of cattle, especially Simmental, Angus. Characterized by short, sparse, curly haircoats and wispy tail switch. Called also color dilution alopecia.

a. congenitalis complete or partial absence of the hair at birth.

endocrine a. hair loss caused by an endocrine abnormality that adversely affects hair growth. Usually characterized by symmetrical distribution and noninflammatory changes in the skin.

feline acquired symmetric a. a bilaterally symmetric hair loss on the posterior abdomen, inner thighs, perineum and, less consistently, ventral thorax, flanks and forelegs of cats, most commonly neutered males. The skin is usually normal and nonpruritic. The cause is unknown; sex hormone deficiency was previously believed to be responsible, but abnormal thyroid function is also suspected. Some cases are in reality self-inflicted by excessive grooming or the cat's response to unrecognized pruritus. Called also feline endocrine alopecia.

inherited symmetrical a. calves born with a normal haircoat lose their hair over bilaterally distributed specific areas of the skin. See also inherited congenital HYPOTRICHOSIS.

a. medicamentosa hair loss due to ingestion of a drug.

a. mucinosa hair loss associated with mucinosis of the epidermis and hair follicles.

pattern a. see pattern BALDNESS.

periodic a. a pinnal alopecia observed in miniature poodles. Regrowth usually occurs in 3 to 4 months.

pinnal a. gradual loss of hair on the pinnae until there is total alopecia. Occurs mainly in Dachshunds and may have an hereditary basis.

pituitary a. see GROWTH HORMONE-responsive dermatitis.

post-clipping a. a failure of hair to regrow, usually for a long period, after clipping. Seen particularly in Chow Chows, Samoyeds and Siberian huskies. The cause is unknown.

postvaccination a. and panniculitis a focal area of hair loss occurring at the site of rabies vaccination; miniature poodles are predisposed.

progressive a., congenital anemia and dyskeratosis a condition seen in Hereford cattle; affected calves are born with sparse, short kinky or curly hair which is gradually lost. They are also anemic.

psychogenic a. hair loss resulting from intensive self-trauma such as licking or biting and for which no cause can be found. Boredom is often considered a factor. See also ACRAL lick dermatitis, idiopathic HYPERESTHESIA syndrome.

seasonal flank a. a cyclic follicular dysplasia which tends to occur seasonally, mainly in spring or fall. There is a nonpruritic hair loss and often hyperpigmentation of the skin in irregular, defined areas on the flanks and lateral thorax. Many cases regrow hair after 3 to 6 months, but recurrences at the corresponding time in following years is common. Boxers, Airedale terriers, English bulldogs, and Miniature schnauzers are predisposed breeds, but it has been reported in others. Called also cyclic follicular dysplasia.

symptomatic a., a. symptomatica loss of hair due to systemic or psychogenic causes, such as general ill health, infections of the skin, nervousness, a specific disease, or to stress. The hair may fall out in patches, or there may be diffuse loss of hair instead of complete baldness in one area.

traction a. loss of hair due to traction, as occurs in dogs of breeds in which hair on the head is held by rubber bands or barrettes.

traumatic a. that caused by self-trauma (licking, scratching, chewing or pulling); possible in any pruritic skin disease in any species, but particularly severe in cats. The area of hair loss corresponds to those areas most accessible to the form of self-trauma.

a. universalis congenital absence of hair from the entire body. A characteristic of the Canadian hairless cat and Sphinx cat.

alopecic affected by alopecia.

a. breeds the Mexican hairless and Chinese crested dogs and Sphinx cat have partial or near total absence of hair as a characteristic of their breed.

Alopex lagopus see arctic FOX.

Alouatta see HOWLER MONKEY.

Alouattamyia parasitic fly of which the larval grub causes cutaneous cysts in *Alouatta* spp., the howling monkeys of New World primates.

Aloysia plant genus in the family Verbenaceae. Cointain a toxin, possibly a toxic indole alkaloid. Includes *A. lycioides* (*Lippia ligustrina*).

ALP alkaline phosphatase.

alpaca a ruminant of the animal family of Camelidae. It is similar to but smaller than the llama and the vicuña and guanaco. It is raised commercially in South America for its wool.

alpestrine clover TRIFOLIUM *alpestre*.

alpha the first letter of the Greek alphabet, A or α; used to denote the first position in a classification system; as, in names of chemical compounds, to distinguish the first in a series of isomers, or to indicate the position of substituent atoms or groups; also used to distinguish types of radioactive decay, brain waves or rhythms, adrenergic receptors, and secretory cells that stain with acid dyes, such as the alpha cells of the pancreas.

a.-adrenergic antagonist see alpha-blocking agents (below).

a.-blocking agents a group of drugs that selectively inhibit the activities of alpha receptors in the sympathetic nervous system. As with beta-blocking agents, alpha-adrenergic blocking agents compete with the catecholamines at peripheral autonomic receptor sites. This group includes ergot and its derivatives, and phenotolamine.

a. brain waves human brain-wave currents during electroencephalography having a frequency of approximately 8 to 13 hertz (pulsations per second), best seen when patient's eyes are closed and the patient is physically relaxed. See also ELECTROENCEPHALOGRAPHY.

a. cells glucagon-producing cells of the PANCREAS.

a.-hemolysin see alpha HEMOLYSIS.

a. hemolysis see alpha HEMOLYSIS.

a. particles a type of emission produced by the disintegration of a radioactive substance. The atoms of radioactive elements such as uranium and radium are very unstable; they are continuously breaking apart with explosive violence and emitting particulate and nonparticulate types of radiation. The alpha particles, consisting of two protons and two neutrons, have an electrical charge and form streams of tremendous energy when they are released from the disintegrating atoms. These streams of energy (alpha rays) are used to advantage in the treatment of various malignancies. See also RADIATION and RADIOTHERAPY.

a.-responsive sympathomimetic drugs drugs which cause vasoconstriction and maintain correct vascular permeability.

a.-sheet, α-sheet a common structural feature of many proteins in which a single polypeptide chain turns regularly about itself to make a rigid cylinder in which each peptide bond is regularly hydrogen-bonded to other peptide bonds elsewhere in the chain.

a. toxin the toxins of many bacteria are classified as alpha, beta, etc.

alpha-adrenergic receptor receptors in effector organs which respond to epinephrine and norepinephrine; includes receptors in heart muscle which are responsible for increasing rate and force of cardiac contractions.

alpha-amylase a salivary enzyme which hydrolyzes starch to dextrins, maltose, maltotriose.

alpha$_1$-antitrypsin a plasma protein (α_1-globulin) produced in the liver, which inhibits the activity of trypsin and other proteolytic enzymes. Deficiency of this protein is associated with ROUND HEART DISEASE in turkeys. Called also α_1-protease inhibitor.

a. mastitis test after the first month of lactation, it is an indication of leakage through damaged endothelium.

alpha carbon atom carbon-2 of a molecule or the carbon atom next to the function group of a molecule, the carbon(s) of which are not included in the lettering.

alpha-fetoprotein a plasma protein produced by the fetal liver, yolk sac and gastrointestinal tract and also by some cancers in humans. In animals it binds testosterone and estrogens in the blood and provides a reservoir for these hormones. Called also AFP. In humans the serum AFP level is used to monitor the effectiveness of cancer treatment, and the amniotic fluid AFP level is used in the prenatal diagnosis of neural tube defects.

alpha-globulin glycoprotein found in saliva, tears, colostrum; present in blood plasma but does not cross placental barrier of animals, collecting instead in the maternal colostrum. Called also IgA.

alpha helix conformation most commonly occurring helical type of ordered molecular structure characterized by a crystallographic repeat, pitch and rise; the repeats occur after exactly 18 residues, and 5 turns which equates to 3.6 residues per turn.

1-alpha-hydroxylase the renal enzyme which participates in the conversion of 1,25-hydroxycholecalciferol into 1,25-dihydroxycholecalciferol and 24,25-dihydroxycholecalciferol.

alpha-naphthylisothiocyanate a compound used experimentally to produce bile duct hyperplasia.

alpha receptors tissue receptors which respond well to epinephrine and norepinephrine but less so to isoprotenerol.

alpha rigidity rigidity which remains after transection of the spinal cord and is due to the hyperactivity of the alpha motor neurons.

alpha subunit first-named chain (or subunit) occurring in the functional organization of macromolecules, usually proteins, containing two or more chains.

alpha$_2$-antiplasmin the most important inhibitor of plasmin mediated fibrinolysis.

alphadolone one of the two pregnanediones in Saffan, the steroidal anesthetic. Called also steroid II. See also SAFFAN.

Alphaherpesvirinae one of the three subfamilies within the family HERPESVIRIDAE.

1-alphahydroxycholecalciferol synthetic analog of 1,25-dihydroxycholecalciferol.

alphanumeric pertaining to letters and numbers.

a. sort the rearrangement of a list of words into a combined alphabetical and numerical order.

alphaprodine an opioid related to meperidine, used as an analgesic and narcotic.

2-4-alphathiazolyl-5 -benzimidazole the carbamate is marketed as fenbendazole.

Alphavirus one of the four genera of the family *Togaviridae*; includes eastern, western and Venezuelan equine encephalomyelitis viruses and Getah virus. All of them replicate in arthropod vectors including mosquitoes.

alphaxalone one of the two pregnanediones in SAFFAN, the steroidal anesthetic used widely in cats. Called also steroid I.

Alphitobius diaperinus a beetle common to the litter in most poultry houses. Suspected of involvement in transmission of Marek's disease. Larval stages called the lesser mealworm.

alpine pasture deaths sudden deaths due to poisoning of drinking water in Swiss alpine lakes during summer months. There is no visible bloom on the water, the causative cyanobacteria growing on submerged rocks. See also BENTHOS.

Alpine sheep see LOP-EARED ALPINE.

alprazolam a benzodiazepine tranquilizer used as an anxiolytic.

alprenolol a β-adrenoreceptor blocking agent used as a cardiac antiarrhythmic drug.

ALS 1. antilymphocyte serum. 2. the serum enzyme, aldolase.

Alsatian see GERMAN SHEPHERD DOG.

Alsike clover TRIFOLIUM *hybridum*.

Alstonia a genus of the Apocynaceae family of creepers and shrubs, many of them toxic. Includes *A. scolaris* (cheesewood, milky pine).

A. constricta contains the indole alkaloids alstonine, alstonidine and reserpine and causes hyperesthesia, tetany and convulsions. Called also quinine tree, bitter bark.

alstonidine one of the toxic group of alstonine alkaloids in bark or root of *Alstonia* spp.

alstonine a group of toxic indole alkaloids in *Alstonia constricta*.

ALT alanine aminotransferase.

alter euphemism for castration of a male animal; sometimes used as a synonym for spay of a female. Called also cut, geld.

alterative a medicine given to a horse with the objective of improving its general condition without purging it. Called also tonic.

Alternanthera denticulata plant in the Ameranthaceae family. Capable of causing nitrate–nitrite poisoning.

Alternaria a saprophytic fungus commonly found on the skin; also has been associated with subcutaneous infections (PHAEOHYPHOMYCOSIS) and reputed to be one of the causes of the indeterminate syndrome of forage poisoning in farm animals. Tenuazonic acid is a toxic metabolite.

alternariosis infection by *Alternaria* spp.

Althaea officinalis non-toxic plant known in UK as marshmallow; not to be confused with *Malva parviflora*.

altitude sickness, altitude disease a disease of animals kept at high altitudes. Those with even a minor impairment of the circulatory or respiratory systems may not be able to find sufficient cardiac reserve to compensate for the extra dynamic load created by the altitudinal anoxia, so that congestive heart failure develops. Called also brisket disease, mountain sickness.

altrenogest a progestogen used in the synchronization of estrus.

altretamine an antineoplastic agent, similar to TRETAMINE.

altricial said of birds which are hatched with their eyes closed.

Alu family interspersed repetitive DNA sequences that occur nearly a million times in the human genome. So called because they are cleaved by the restriction enzyme AluI.

alula, alula spuria the freely articulated first digit of the avian hand. Called also bastard wing.

a. remiges see REMEX.

alum any of several substances, including potassium alum, aluminum alum, ammonium alum, potash alum and aluminum potassium sulfate, with strong astringent properties. May be used as a styptic or hemostatic and as a topical antimycotic agent. It also may be given by mouth to induce vomiting. Large doses may cause gastrointestinal disturbances.

alumina aluminum oxide.

aluminum a chemical element, atomic number 13, atomic weight 26.982, symbol Al. See Table 6.

a. acetate a preparation of aluminum subacetate and glacial acetic acid, used for its antiseptic and astringent action on the skin. Called also Burow's solution.

a. binding agents usually includes aluminum carbonate and hydroxide. See PHOSPHATE binders.

a. chloride a deliquescent, crystalline powder used topically as an astringent solution and antiperspirant.

a. equivalent a radiological measurement expressing the thickness of aluminum that produces the same attenuation of the x-ray beam as the thickness of the material being examined.

a. factory prime source of fluorine pollution of pasture.

a. filter inserted in the window of x-ray tubes to filter out x-rays of long wavelength; reduces potentially harmful and unnecessary radiation.

a. hydroxide, a. phosphate aluminum preparations, available in suspension, as a gel, or in dried form, used as an antacid in the treatment of peptic ulcer in humans and gastric hyperacidity and in PHOSPHATE binders.

a. poisoning pollution of pasture occurs from dust from factories handling aluminum products and in acid rain near such industrial works; contributes to nutritional deficiency of phosphorus by interfering with phosphorus absorption. Bodies of water which receive drainage from soils rich in aluminum may experience fish kills in circumstances in which the amount of aluminum is increased.

a. sulfate see ALUM.

alveld a disease of lambs in Scandinavia caused by poisoning with NARTHECIUM *ossifragum*.

Alveococcus multilocularis see ECHINOCOCCUS *multilocularis*.

alveolar[1] pertaining to or arising from the alveolus of a tooth.

a. abscess a localized, suppurative inflammation of tissues about the apex of the root of the tooth. Causes local pain and swelling and may discharge onto the face or into the maxillary sinus, and thence the nasal cavity.

a. bone the lamellar bone around the roots of a tooth.

a. periostitis new bone growth about the tooth root usually the result of infection. Chronic periostitis causes local swelling and difficulty in extraction of the tooth. Acute periostitis of the posterior upper molars may cause maxillary sinusitis; acute periostitis of the front upper and lower molars causes osteomyelitis, and sometimes a draining sinus.

a. process see alveolar PROCESS.

alveolar[2] pertaining to or arising from the lung alveolar epithelium.

a. capillary comprise the alveolar capillary bed, in immediate contact with the lung alveoli.

a.–capillary membrane the membranous partition between the alveolar space and the venous blood, consisting of an alveolar epithelium and capillary endothelium.

a. cell cover the alveolar surface. *Type 1* cells are flattened and extended, offering maximum opportunity for oxygen diffusion, but vulnerable to damage and slow to repair. They cover the bulk of the healthy alveolar wall. Called also membranous pneumocytes. *Type 2* cells are cuboidal and cover much less of the alveolar surface than do type 1 cells. Their function is to secrete surfactant in response to injury and the renewal and repair of the alveolar wall. Called also granular or secretory pneumocytes. See also alveolar epithelialization (below).

a. collapse the microscopic basis of acquired ATELECTASIS.

congenital a. dysplasia a disease of the newborn in which the alveoli are uneven in distribution and shape and there is too much interstitial tissue. The lungs are poorly aerated and retain their fetal appearance.

a. cyst dilatations of pulmonary alveoli, which may fuse by breakdown of their septa to form large air cysts (pneumatoceles).

a. dead space that part of the dead space located in the alveoli. The space in the alveoli where gaseous exchange does not occur.

a. duct extensions from respiratory bronchioles that terminate in a number of alveoli-lined saccules through a common atrium.

a. dysplasia see congenital alveolar dysplasia (above).

a. echinococcosis see alveolar hydatid cyst (below).

a. emphysema abnormal enlargement of the alveoli, the air spaces at the end of the bronchioles, with some destruction of the alveolar walls. Alveolar emphysema is rarely a problem except in the horse. See also CHRONIC obstructive pulmonary disease.

a. epithelial cells cover the alveolar surface. *Type 1* cells are flattened and extended, offering maximum opportunity for oxygen diffusion, but vulnerable to damage and slow to repair. They cover the bulk of the healthy alveolar wall. Called also membranous pneumocytes. *Type 2* cells are cuboidal and cover much less of the alveolar surface than do type 1 cells. Their function is the secretion of surfactant in response to injury and the renewal and repair of the alveolar wall. Called also granular or secretory pneumocytes. See also alveolar epithelialization (below).

a. epithelialization after severe damage to the alveolar lining there is a significant loss of type 1 membranous pneumocytes which are physiologically effective in gaseous transport but susceptible to injury. Their place may be taken by type 2 cells, the secretory pneumocytes, which are more cuboidal and active as producers of surfactant. The alveolar wall is thickened and is described as being in a stage of epithelialization.

a. fibroblast connective tissue cells in the lungs with contractile functions, cell and matrix interactions, and secrete substances important to the mechanical properties of lung.

a. filling disorders a group of incidental conditions characterized by the filling of alveoli by lipid-filled macrophages with minimal inflammation.

a. gas exchange the diffusion of CO_2 and O_2 across the alveolar–capillary membrane.

a. histiocytosis a pulmonary condition characterized by large, focal accumulations of foamy macrophages.

a. hydatid cyst multivesicular, infiltrative form of hydatid cyst found in rodents, e.g. ground squirrel, field mouse.

a. lipoproteinosis an accumulation of acidophilic, acellular material within pulmonary alveoli. The condition can be experimentally reproduced but has been associated with chronic interstitial pneumonia of goats. See also CAPRINE arthritis–encephalitis.

a. macrophage derived from monocytes in the bone marrow, contains many lysosomes and phagosomes, and forms a major element in the pulmonary defense mechanism.

a. metaplasia a characteristic of pulmonary epithelial cells is their capacity to undergo metaplasia from one cell type to another. Called also transdifferentiation.

a. microlithiasis see MICROLITHIASIS.

a. oxygen tension the measure of oxygen level within the alveoli and a factor influencing diffusion of gases across the alveolar–capillary membrane; increased with oxygen administration to the patient.

a. pattern see ALVEOLOGRAM.

a. phospholipidosis characterized by the accumulation of acidophilic, acellular material in pulmonary alveoli.

a. pore pore of Kohn.

a. saccules the intervening structures between pulmonary alveolar ducts and alveoli.

a. transport system refers to the clearance mechanisms within the lower respiratory system, including alveolar macrophages, mucociliary escalator and peribronchial lymphatics.

a. ventilation the volume of air entering and leaving the alveoli per unit of time.

a. volume the volume of the alveolar space. The dead space volume and the alveolar volume make up the total volume of the respiratory tract.

alveolectomy surgical excision of part of the alveolar process.

alveolitis inflammation of the walls of the alveoli; definition of pulmonary, dental, mammary preferred.

diffuse a. see interstitial PNEUMONIA.

diffuse fibrosing a. see ATYPICAL INTERSTITIAL PNEUMONIA, interstitial PNEUMONIA.

alveolodental pertaining to teeth and the alveolar process.

a. membrane periodontium.

alveologram on radiographs, the irregular, mottled appearance of lung tissue, caused by the contrast in density between some alveoli being filled with fluid or cellular material and others filled with air.

alveolotomy incision of the alveolar process.

alveolus pl. *alveoli.* 1. a small cavity. 2. one of the thousands of tiny sacs borne on the terminal parts of the bronchial tree. 3. a tooth socket. 4. the dilated saclike part of the secretory unit of an alveolar gland such as a lactating mammary gland.

See also ALVEOLAR.

mammary a. because its epithelia produce milk the alveolus is the basic functioning unit of the lactating mammary gland.

alveus pl. *alvei* [L.] a canal or trough.

a. hippocampi the white fibers covering the ventricular surface of the hippocampus that contribute to the fornix.

alymphia absence or lack of lymph.

alymphocytosis deficiency of lymphocytes in the blood.

alymphoplasia failure of development of lymphoid tissue.

thymic a. congenital agammaglobulinemia in which there is thymic hypoplasia.

Am chemical symbol, *americium.*

amacrine without long processes.

a. cell a branched retinal nerve cell without an axon.

amalgam a silver–tin–copper alloy in combination with mercury, commonly used in dental restoration.

a. burnisher an instrument used to smooth the surface of an amalgam filling.

a. condenser, a. plugger an instrument used to pack amalgam into a filling.

a. well a small bowl used to hold amalgam until it is used in the restoration.

amalgamator a piece of equipment used in dentistry for the mixing of restorative materials such as amalgam or glass-ionomer.

Amanita a genus of macro fungi many of which can be poisonous to humans, less frequently to animals unless eaten in large quantities. Called also mushrooms. Include *A. mappa, A. muscaria, A. pantherina, A. phalloides, A. verna, A. virosa.* Contain hepatoxic peptides and hallucinogens.

amanitin one of the toxins in *Amanita* spp. See also PHALLOIDIN.

amantadine hydrochloride an antiviral agent which prevents penetration and uncoating of several RNA viruses.

Amaranthus a genus of the plant family Amaranthaceae, many of them succulent weeds of cultivated fields. Contain high levels of nitrate or oxalate or both. Includes *A. blitum, A. cruentus, A. deflexus, A. hybridus, A. mitchellii, A. palmeri, A. paniculatus, A. powellii, A. retroflexus, A. spinosus, A. thunbergii, A. viridis.*

A. retroflexus if eaten in large quantities is capable of causing non-oxalate-induced nephrosis and fatal uremia in cattle and pigs. Called also Prince of Wales feather, redleg, red amaranth, pigweed.

Amaryllis a genus of the plant family Amaryllidaceae, all with bulbs or tuberous roots. Garden plants reputed to be poisonous. Called also *Hippeastrum.*

amastia congenital absence of one or more mammary glands.

amastigote an early stage in the life cycle of trypanosomes, found in invertebrates. The body is rounded and the flagellum is absent or represented by a short fibril. The kinetoplast is present.

amaurosis loss of sight without apparent lesion of the eye, as from disease of the optic nerve, spine or brain.

amaurotic pertaining to, or of the nature of, amaurosis.

a. familial idiocy a group of hereditary disorders in humans characterized by cerebromacular degeneration, blindness, progressive dementia, and progressive and unremitting paralysis. The term has been applied to ceroid LIPOFUSCINOSIS in English setters and Chihuahuas which have very similar clinical features.

Amazon parrots see AMAZONA.

Amazona a large genus of gaudy parrots in the family Psittacidae.

A. farina the best known of the very large number of species of this parrot genus.

ambenonium chloride a moderately long-acting cholinesterase inhibitor used to increase muscular strength in myasthenia gravis.

amber HYPERICUM *perforatum*.

ambergris a solid, gray intestinal concretion of sperm whales. It has an unpleasant odor but is very valuable in the formulation of expensive perfumes. Is found floating free after evacuation.

ambilateral pertaining to or affecting both sides.

Ambiphyra a ciliate protozoan, a genus of the phylum Ciliophora. Causes heavy mortality in young fish.

ambisexual denoting sexual characteristics common to both sexes.

amble a slower, non-racing version of PACE gait in horses.

broken a. has many characteristics of the amble but there are four beats to the gait with each foot contacting the ground independently. Called also single-foot.

Amblyomma a genus of ticks of the family Ixodidae.

A. americanum a three-host tick which causes painful bites and tick paralysis and transmits Q fever, tularemia and Rocky Mountain spotted fever of humans. Called also the lone star tick.

A. cajennense a three-host tick that transmits spotted fever of human and leptospirosis due to *L. pomona*. Called also cayenne tick.

A. hebraeum a three-host tick that transmits *Rickettsia ruminantium*, the cause of heartwater. It also causes severe bite wounds. Called also bont tick.

A. maculatum a three-host tick which causes paralysis but does not transmit disease. Called also Gulf coast tick.

A. pomposum a three-host tick, a vector for the heartwater rickettsia.

A. variegatum a three-host tick which transmits *Rickettsia ruminantium* (heartwater), *Coxiella burnetii* (Q fever) and Nairobi sheep disease. Called also variegated or tropical bont tick.

amblyopia dimness of vision not due to organic defect or refractive errors.

hereditary a. with quadriplegia a severe cerebellar cortical degeneration with quadriplegia at an early age has been observed in Irish setters. It is believed to be an autosomal recessive trait.

ambo-, ambi- a prefix meaning round, all, both.

amboceptor an old term for hemolysin, which is an antibody that binds to the surface of erythrocytes in such a way that they are lysed in the presence of complement.

ambon the fibrocartilaginous edge of the socket in which the head of a long bone is lodged.

Ambrosia elatir a plant in the family Asteraceae (Compositae). An annual weed producing a highly irritant pollen commonly associated with hay fever in humans. Called also ragweed.

ambulant, ambulatory walking or able to walk.

Ambystoma a genus of amphibians of the class Amphibia; syn. *Seridon*.

A. mexicanum a four-legged, gilled amphibian, a neotenous newt that breeds in the larval stage. Is related to the salamanders but unlike them rarely metamorphoses to the adult stage. Called also axolotl, Mexican axolotl, Mexican walking fish.

amcinonide a glucocorticoid used for topical application in the treatment of corticosteroid-responsive dermatoses.

amdinocillin, mecillinam a semisynthetic penicillin, active mainly against gram-negative bacteria.

amdinopenicillins semisynthetic derivatives of amidinopenicillanic acid. See AMDINOCILLIN, PIVAMDINOCILLIN.

ameba pl. *amobae, amobas* [L.] a minute, one-celled protozoan. The common laboratory example is *Amoeba proteus*.

amebiasis infection with amebae, especially in the intestine with *Entamoeba histolytica*. Saprophytic amebae also occasionally cause disease. See also AMEBIC dysentery, AMEBIC meningoencephalitis, ACANTHAMEBIASIS.

amebic pertaining to, caused by, or of the nature of, an ameba.

a. dysentery an acute amebic dysentery of humans caused by *Entamoeba histolytica* which rarely occurs spontaneously in dogs and cats. A similar disease of reptiles and amphibians is caused by *E. invadens* and *E. ranarum*.

a. gill disease caused by *Paramoeba* spp.; important disease in sea-caged salmonids; manifested by lethargy, flared opercula, rapid death; encouraged by high temperatures.

a. granulomatosis world-wide disease of goldfish; cause not definitely known; characterized by white nodules on the skin, visceral granulomata and ascites.

a. meningoencephalitis caused by *Naegleria fowleri* and is restricted in occurrence to humans.

amebic dysentery dysentery caused by *Entamoeba histolytica* in humans and nonhuman primates; a mild to severe necroulcerative enterocolitis.

amebicide destructive to amebas.

amebocyte a cell showing ameboid movement.

ameboid resembling an ameba.

Amelanchier alnifolia a plant in the family Rosaceae; its foliage is sufficiently cyanogenetic to cause poisoning of animals. Called also Saskatoon serviceberry, juneberry.

amelanosis lack of pigment; see also ACHROMOTRICHIA, ACHROMODERMA.

amelia a developmental anomaly with absence of the limbs; an inherited defect in cattle.

amelification the process of enamel formation by ameloblasts.

ameloblast a cell which takes part in forming dental enamel.

ameloblastic pertaining to the formation of dental enamel.

a. fibro-odontoma see ameloblastic odontoma (below).

a. layer the inner layer of cells of the enamel organ, which forms the enamel prisms of the teeth.

a. odontoma resembles ameloblastic fibroma but the tumor contains enamel and dentine rather than only enamel.

ameloblastoma a locally invasive, highly destructive tumor of the jaw consisting of proliferating odontogenic epithelium in a fibrous stroma.

pituitary a. see CRANIOPHARYNGIOMA.

amelodentinal pertaining to dental enamel and dentine.

amelogenesis formation of dental enamel.

a. imperfecta imperfect formation of enamel, resulting in brownish coloration and friability of the teeth.

amelogenic capable of forming enamel.

amelus an animal exhibiting amelia.

amensalism interaction between coexisting populations of different species, one of which is adversely affected and the other unaffected.

American aloe see AGAVE *americana*.

American Association of Feed Control Officials an association of state officials concerned with the regulation of commercially prepared animal diets; abbreviated AAFCO.

American bison see BISON *bison*.

American blackbird see GRACKLE.

American blue Gascon hound a large hound-type dog with a short, dense coat of white with tan points and heavy black ticking. Called also Big'n blue.

American Board of Veterinary Practitioners see AMERICAN VETERINARY SPECIALTY BOARDS.

American bronze, Australian bronze domestic turkey. See BRONZEWING.

American brown Swiss an American variety of Swiss brown or Brown mountain cattle. A gray-brown breed of dairy cattle, of heavy build, which are used in Europe for beef, draft and milk.

American cherry laurel PRUNUS *caroliniana*.

American cocker spaniel see COCKER SPANIEL.

American College of Veterinary Surgeons a voluntary, professional organization dedicated to the advancement of the art and science of veterinary surgery. It is concerned only with graduate veterinarians and constitutes a certifying agency to qualify members as specialists. It also encourages postgraduate study and research.

American cupped oyster CRASSOSTREA *virginicus*. See Table 23.

American curl a medium-sized cat with short coat. Their distinguishing feature is a smooth curl of the ear cartilage with the tips pointing toward the middle of the head. This is inherited as a dominant trait; kittens develop the curl in the first week of life.

American dog tick see DERMACENTOR *variabilis*.

American dogweed see VERBESINA ENCELIOIDES.

American elk see WAPITI.

American encephalitis see equine viral ENCEPHALOMYELITIS.

American-English spelling the American version of English spelling as distinct from British-English.

American equine encephalomyelitis see equine viral ENCEPHALOMYELITIS.

American foxhound see FOXHOUND.

American hellebore see VERATRUM *viride*.

American Kennel Club a non-profit organization, made up of a large number of individual clubs, devoted to the advancement of purebred dogs. It serves as the official body for maintaining the stud book and registration of purebred dogs, and it conducts competitions.

American mandrake see PODOPHYLLUM PELTATUM.

American miniature horse Shetland ponies 34 inches or less high at maturity; the foals are more susceptible to colonic impaction and development of fecaliths than foals of other breeds.

American moose a large, 6 ft high, 1800 lb, dark brown, wild ruminant with white legs; males are bearded and roman-nosed with a thick, overhanging upper lip. Called also *Alces americana*.

American opossum see OPOSSUM.

American pit bull terrier a powerful, muscular dog with short, smooth hair, broad head and ears which naturally fold over but in some countries are cropped. It has earned a reputation as a fighting dog.

American quarter horse see QUARTER HORSE.

American Rambouillet sheep American adaptation of French Rambouillet; fine-wool, polled or horned.

American rattlesnake see RATTLESNAKE.

American Saddle horse a bay, brown, black or chestnut horse, preferably with white markings, 15 to 16 hands high. A show-ring horse performing as a harness horse or as a three- or five-gaited saddle horse. Very showy in appearance and action. Originated from Thoroughbred, Morgan horse, American Trotter and Canadian Trotter.

American shorthair a medium- to large-sized cat, longer than it is tall, with a large head, large eyes, and a thick, short coat in many different colors.

American singer a song-type canary, bred in the United States by crossing the Roller to the Border Fancy.

American sneezeweed HELENIUM *amarum*.

American Staffordshire terrier a medium-size, muscular dog, similar to the STAFFORDSHIRE BULL TERRIER, but larger. It has a powerful head, well-muscled body, short tail and a short, colored haircoat.

American tiger cat see MARGAY.

American Trotter American horse used in trotting races. Short legs, long body, plain head, about 15.2 hands high. Any solid color. Races as a pacer or diagonal trotter. Originated from Thoroughbred, Hackney and Morgan horse. Called also Standardbred.

American trypanosomiasis a disease of humans caused by *Trypanosoma cruzi* in which many animal species act as carriers. The disease in dogs includes anemia, debility and splenomegaly; in cats there are posterior paralysis and convulsions. The disease is transmitted by reduviid bugs. Called also Chagas' disease.

American Veterinary Boards bodies such as the American Board of Veterinary Practitioners (ABVP), American Board of Veterinary Toxicology.

American Veterinary Colleges[1] need to be differentiated from American veterinary colleges, the educational institutions which provide educational programs leading to the basic, registrable degree of DVM, and the associated postgraduate degrees. See also AMERICAN VETERINARY SPECIALTY BOARDS.

Includes American College of Laboratory Animal Medicine, American College of Poultry Veterinarians, American College of Theriogenologists, American College of Veterinary Behaviorists, American College of Veterinary Anesthetists, American College of Veterinary Clinical Pharmacology, American College of Veterinary Dermatology, American College of Veterinary Emergency and Critical Care, American College of Veterinary Internal Medicine, American College of Veterinary Microbiologists, American College of Veterinary Nutrition, American College of Veterinary Ophthalmology, American College of Veterinary Pathologists, American College of Veterinary Preventive Medicine, American College of Veterinary Radiology, American College of Veterinary Surgeons, American College of Zoological Medicine, American Veterinary Dental College.

American veterinary colleges[2] the state and private educational institutions which provide undergraduate teaching programs leading to the basic, registrable degree of DVM, and the associated postgraduate degrees. Need to be differentiated from AMERICAN VETERINARY COLLEGES[1], which provide professional postgraduate qualifications which earn the recipients recognition as specialists.

American Veterinary Medical Association a non-profit, professional organization of veterinarians in the USA, whose stated objective is to advance the science and art of veterinary medicine, including its relationship to public health and agriculture.

American veterinary specialty boards the American Veterinary Boards and American

Veterinary Colleges which conduct examinations and award diplomas of competence in veterinary professional specialties to graduate veterinarians. Passing the examinations is known colloquially as 'getting your boards' and is one of the most highly prized qualifications in the veterinary world. See also AMERICAN VETERINARY COLLEGES.

American water hemlock CICUTA *maculata*.

American water spaniel a medium-sized (25–45 lb) dog with liver- or chocolate-colored curly coat on the body and ears. The legs and tail have feathering. Similar in appearance to the Irish water spaniel, but smaller and lacking the topknot and rattail of that breed.

American wirehair similar to the American shorthair cat, but with coarse, crimped hair.

American wormseed see CHENOPODIUM *ambrosioides*.

americium a chemical element, atomic number 95, atomic weight 243, symbol Am. See Table 6.

AmerToy see FOX TERRIER.

Ames test a test for mutagenic substances, in which a strain of *Salmonella typhimurium* that lacks the enzyme necessary for histidine synthesis is cultured in the absence of histidine and in the presence of the suspected mutagen treated with liver extract. If the substance causes DNA damage resulting in mutations, an increased number of the bacteria will regain the ability to synthesize histidine and will proliferate to form colonies. An important test for detecting potentially carcinogenic agents such as agricultural chemical and food additives.

ametazole see BETAZOLE.

amethocaine see TETRACAINE.

ametria congenital absence of the uterus.

ametropia the state when the image of a distant object is not in focus on the retina; due usually to some defect in the refraction of the optic system of the eye.

Amianthium muscaetoxicum a plant species belonging to the family Liliaceae. A small onion-like plant; causes salivation, dyspnea, weakness. Called also fly poison, crow poison, staggergrass, *Chrosperma muscaetoxicum*.

amicarbalide an aromatic diamidine used as an antiprotozoal in the treatment of babesiosis, particularly in cattle, and has also been used in ehrlichia infections.

amicrobic not produced by microorganisms.

amiculum a dense surrounding coat of white fibers, as the sheath of the inferior olive and of the dentate nucleus.

amide any compound derived from ammonia by substitution of an acid radical for hydrogen, or from an acid by replacing the –OH group by $-NH_2$.

a. compound herbicides diphenamid and CDAA may cause poisoning if given in large doses. Signs include depression, weight loss and muscular weakness of the hindquarters.

amido the monovalent radical $-NH_2$ united with an acid radical.

amidopyrine see AMINOPHENAZONE.

Amidostomum a genus of the helminth family of Amidostomatidae.

A. anseris parasitic in the gizzard of ducks and geese. Lethal to young birds because of blood-sucking and mucosal damage.

amifloxacin a fluoroquinolone antibiotic, similar in activity to ciprofloxacin.

amikacin sulfate a semisynthetic aminoglycoside antibiotic derived from kanamycin, used parenterally in the treatment of bacterial infections, particularly those caused by gram-negative organisms.

amiloride a potassium-sparing diuretic.

aminacrine, aminoacridine a quinoline antimicrobial dye, similar to acridine, used externally as the hydrochloride salt.

amine an organic compound containing nitrogen.

biogenic a's amine neurotransmitters, e.g. norepinephrine, serotonin and dopamine.

direct-acting sympathomimetic a's activate adrenergic effector cells, e.g. CATECHOLAMINE, directly and do not need adrenergic nerves to exert their effects.

a. hormones enteroendocrine cells, distributed widely in the gastric, intestinal and pancreatic tissue, synthesize peptide and amine hormones that control the secretion of digestive juices. See also APUD CELLS.

a. precursor uptake and decarboxylation cells see APUD CELLS.

toxic a's occur in plants, e.g. cyclopamine, tyramine.

vasoactive a. amine that causes vasodilatation and increases small vessel permeability, e.g. histamine and serotonin.

aminergic hormone hormones classified as being derived from amino acids, e.g. epinephrine or thyroid hormone.

amino the monovalent radical $-NH_2$, when not united with an acid radical.

amino acid any one of a class of organic compounds containing the amino (NH_2) and the carboxyl (COOH) group, occurring naturally in plant and animal tissues and forming the chief constituents of protein.

In certain inherited or acquired disorders of metabolism, specific amino acids accumulate in the blood (*aminoacidemia*) or are excreted in excess in the urine (*aminoaciduria*). Urinary amino acid levels are increased in liver disease, muscular dystrophies, phenylketonuria (PKU), lead poisoning and folic acid deficiency.

acidic a. a's those containing carboxylic acids in their side chains, e.g. aspartate and glutamate.

basic a. a's amino acids containing side chains that accept protons at physiological pH, e.g. lysine, arginine, and histidine.

branched-chain a. a's methyl branched amino acids.

a. a. dehydratase an enzyme which contributes significantly to the total production of ammonia in the body.

essential a. a's the amino acids which animals must ingest with their diets and which vary between species and physiological status. The commonly accepted list of essential amino acids includes arginine, histidine, isoleucine, leucine, lysine, methionine, phenylalanine, threonine, tryptophan and valine. Birds also require glycine and cats require taurine in their diets.

free a. a's amino acids free in the blood, providing an available source for all tissues for catabolism.

glucogenic a. a. an amino acid which yields either pyruvate or oxaloacetate and glucose synthesis can occur.

ketogenic a. a. an amino acid whose carbon skeleton yields ketone bodies; leucine is an example.

a. a. nutritional deficiency the effects may be the same as a deficiency of total protein, reduced growth and production, reduced food intake, loss of body weight, but deficiencies of individual amino acids may have specific effects, e.g. TAURINE in cats. See also METHIONINE, LYSINE, ARGININE.

a. a. poisoning methionine has caused growth retardation and cervical paralysis in turkey poults.
a. a. ratio a decreased ratio of branched chain to aromatic amino acids in plasma can be used to detect chronic liver disease or portacaval shunts in dogs.
a. a. sequencer automatic machine for determining the amino acid sequence of a protein.
sulfur a. a's essential amino acids containing sulfur, CYSTEINE, CYSTINE and METHIONINE.
a. a. transamidation see TRANSAMIDATION.
a. a. transamination see TRANSAMINATION.
urinary a. a's analysis may be used to detect inherited disorders of metabolism, such as cystinuria, tyrosinemia and citrullinemia.

L-amino acid oxidase a group of specialized enzymes which are capable of oxidative deamination of amino acids; they contain flavin mononucleotide as the coenzyme.

aminoacetic acid glycine.

aminoacetonitrile a lathyrogen capable of inducing limb deformities in fetal calves when it is fed to their dams. See also ARTHROGRYPOSIS.

aminoacidemia an excess of amino acids in the blood.

aminoacidopathy any inborn error of amino acid metabolism producing a metabolic block that results in accumulation of one or more amino acids in the blood (aminoacidemia) or excess excretion in the urine (aminoaciduria) or both.

aminoaciduria an excess in the urine of amino acids. Occurs in FANCONI'S SYNDROME, a familial renal disease of Norwegian elkhounds and Basenji dogs, and as a predisposing factor in the development of cystine UROLITHS.

aminoacylation a two stage process whereby amino acids are 'activated' in order to be incorporated into proteins; energy in the form of ATP is required and one of a family of 20 aminoacyl-tRNA synthetases, one specific for each amino acid, links the carboxyl group of the amino acid to either the 2′- or 3′-hydroxyl group of the ribose unit at the 3′-end of tRNA.

***p*-aminobenzoic acid** see PARA-AMINOBENZOIC ACID. Called also PABA.

γ-aminobutyric acid an amino acid that is one of the principal inhibitory neurotransmitters in the central nervous system. Abbreviated GABA.

aminocaproic acid an inhibitor of plasminogen activation, used as an antifibrinolytic agent.

aminocarb a carbamate pesticide.

aminocyclitol see AMINOGLYCOSIDE.

2-aminoethanesulfonic acid see TAURINE.

aminoglutethimide a compound that inhibits the adrenal cortex and peripheral aromatase, thereby blocking production of adrenal steroids. Used in the treatment of hyperadrenocorticism.

aminoglycoside any of a group of bacterial antibiotics derived from various species of *Streptomyces* that interfere with the function of bacterial ribosomes. These compounds contain an inositol moiety substituted with two amino or guanidino groups and with one or more sugars or aminosugars.

The aminoglycosides include gentamicin, streptomycin, tobramycin, amikacin, kanamycin and neomycin. They are used to treat infections caused by gram-negative organisms and are classified as bactericidal agents because of their interference with bacterial replication. All of the aminoglycoside antibiotics are highly toxic, requiring monitoring of blood serum levels at frequent intervals and careful observation of the patient for early signs of toxicity, particularly ototoxicity and nephrotoxicity.

aminogram the pattern of amino acids present in a substance.

aminohippuric acid an acid used in renal function tests. See also PARA-AMINOHIPPURIC ACID.

aminolevulinate the conjugate isomer of aminolevulinic acid.

aminolevulinate dehydratase an enzyme involved in the synthesis of heme; abbreviated ALAD. The enzyme is inhibited by lead. In cases of lead poisoning blood levels of the enzyme fall, protoporphyrins and δ-AMINOLEVULINIC ACID accumulate in the blood. The acid spills over into the urine thus forming the basis of the tests for lead poisoning. Called also porphobilinogen synthase.

aminolevulinic acid see δ-AMINOLEVULINIC ACID.

δ-aminolevulinic acid a precursor of porphyrins and hemoglobin. Serum levels of the acid are elevated in lead poisoning. See also AMINOLEVULINATE DEHYDRATASE.

aminolevulinic acid dehydratase the erythrocytic enzyme which is lowered in lead poisoning in most species.

aminolevulinic acid synthetase the enzyme catalyzing the first step in the synthesis of porphyrins, glycine + succinyl-CoA to delta-aminolevulinic acid (ALA).

aminonitrazole a hormonal weedkiller which can poison animals allowed to graze on sprayed pasture. Signs include colic in horses and incoordination in sheep.

aminonitrile one of the two toxic substances in plants of the *Lathyrus* genus, causing skeletal deformity by virtue of its effect on bone matrix formation. Called also β-aminopropionitrile.

aminonitrothiazole a nitrothiazole derivative used in the treatment of histoplasmosis in turkeys. Excessive dose rates cause infertility and renal and hepatic disease.

aminopenicillins antibiotics which are chemically similar to penicillin G, have some activity against gram-negative bacteria and are not susceptible to acid hydrolysis. The group includes ampicillin, amoxycillin, epicillin and bacampicillin.

aminopentamide an anticholinergic and antispasmodic used in the treatment of vomiting and diarrhea in dogs and cats.

aminopeptidase an enzyme produced by the intestinal mucosa which completes the process of protein digestion by hydrolyzing the amino-terminal amino acids of peptides and some proteins, after the initial breakdown of protein to peptides has already taken place, e.g. the enzyme that removes the methionine coded by the initiation codon AUG.

aminophenazone an analgesic and antipyretic. Called also amidopyrine and aminopyrine.

aminophylline a mixture of theophylline and ethylenediamine; used as a respiratory stimulant, smooth muscle relaxant, myocardial stimulant and diuretic. Administration of the drug may be by mouth, intramuscularly, intravenously or rectally.

aminopromazine a phenothiazine derivative with antispasmodic effects; the fumarate is used as a smooth muscle relaxant.

β-aminopropionitrile see AMINONITRILE. Called also BAPN.

4-aminopyridine 1. a central nervous system stimulant and a pharmacological antagonist to *d*-tubocurarine and ketamine-diazepam. Used experimentally as a neuromuscular potentiator in the treatment of botulism. 2. a bird repellent which will poison animals that eat the treated grain accidentally. Horses show fright, sweating, convulsions and sudden death.

aminopyrine see AMINOPHENAZONE.
***p*-aminosalicylic acid** a derivative of benzoic acid used in the treatment of tuberculosis. It enhances the potency of streptomycin and delays development of bacilli resistant to streptomycin. Also used to treat mycobacterial infections in fish. Abbreviated PAS, PASA.
aminosidine see PAROMOMYCIN.
aminotransferase an enzyme that catalyzes the reversible transfer of an amino group from an α-amino acid to an α-keto acid using the coenzyme pyridoxal phosphate. Called also transaminase.
alanine a. an enzyme that has high serum levels after acute damage to liver cells. Called also ALT. See also ALANINE AMINOTRANSFERASE.
aspartate a. an enzyme that has high serum levels after skeletal muscle damage or acute damage to liver cells. Called also AST. See also ASPARTATE AMINOTRANSFERASE.
aminotriazole a herbicide with relatively low toxicity. Poisoning causes a syndrome of pulmonary edema and alimentary tract hemorrhage.
aminouracils a group of synthetic heterocyclic compounds with diuretic activity due to their direct action on renal tubules.
aminuria an excess of amines in the urine.
amiodarone a drug that lengthens action potential duration and acts as a coronary vasodilator. Used in the treatment of ventricular and supraventricular arrhythmias.
amisometradine an aminouracil diuretic.
amitosis direct cell division; simple cleavage of the nucleus without the formation of a spireme spindle figure or chromosomes.
amitraz a formamidine used as a topical acaricide on cattle, sheep, pigs and fruit crops and miticide in the treatment of generalized demodectic mange in dogs. In horses it causes fatal impaction of the intestine. See also colon impaction COLIC.
amitriptyline a tricyclic antidepressant in humans; used in dogs and cats to treat psychodermatosis and as an antipruritic.
amitrole, aminotrazole a nitrothiazole derivative used in the treatment and prevention of histomoniasis of turkeys. Excessive dosage causes infertility and renal and hepatic disease.
amlodipine besylate a long-acting dihydropyridine calcium channel blocking agent, used in the treatment of hypertension.
ammate see AMMONIUM sulfamate.
Ammi a genus of the plant family Apiaceae; these plants contain furocoumarins which are direct photosensitizing compounds and cause light-sensitive dermatitis. Includes bishop's weed, meadow sweet (*A. majus*), visnaga (*A. visnaga*).
ammodendrine a pyrrolizidine alkaloid found in lupins; possibly a teratogen.
ammonia a colorless alkaline gas, NH_3, with a pungent odor and acrid taste, and highly soluble in water. See also AMMONIUM.
blood a. ammonia is a cerebrointoxicant and a high blood level causes a degenerative brain lesion. High blood levels of ammonia can occur in a number of diseases of the liver, in portacaval shunts, urea poisoning and liver dysfunction.
a. clearance see ammonia tolerance test (below).
a. poisoning ammonia gas may be released from artificial fertilizers or from decomposing manure and urine in slurry pits and silos and cause chronic poisoning manifested by conjunctivitis and coughing, sneezing and dyspnea. May cause dermatitis in animals bedded for long periods on deep litter. Acute poisoning causes heavy mortalities, as in UREA poisoning. A secondary effect of chronic poisoning is hepatic ENCEPHALOPATHY. High ammonia content in water can cause deaths of fish, although additional factors such as high levels of suspended organic matter may be contributory.
a. pollution of barn gases by production from fermentation of urine.
a. tolerance test assesses liver function and is particularly useful in detecting abnormalities of the hepatic portal vascular system. Blood ammonia levels are measured before and after the oral administration of ammonium chloride. See also PORTACAVAL shunt.
ammoniate to combine with ammonia.
ammoniated forage poisoning changes in treated hay cause poisoning manifested in cattle and sheep by restlessness, blinking, pupillary dilation, ear flicking, frequent urination and defecation, dyspnea, frothing at the mouth, bellowing, charging, circling and convulsions.
ammoniated mercury a compound used as an antiseptic skin and ophthalmic ointment.
ammoniemia hyperammonemia.
ammonium a hypothetical radical, NH_4, forming salts analogous to those of the alkaline metals. See also AMMONIA.
a. acetate a weak diuretic and feed supplement.
a. bifluoride wood preservative; causes diarrhea and fall in milk yield in cattle.
a. carbonate, a. chloride saline expectorants used for the purpose of liquefying pulmonary secretions. Effectiveness has not been proven. They are sometimes used as a reflex stimulant because of the strong ammonia given off. The chloride salt is used mainly as a urinary acidifier. Excessive dosage may produce ACIDOSIS.
a. magnesium phosphate see MAGNESIUM ammonium phosphate.
a. metavanadate experimentally causes VANADIUM poisoning.
a. nitrate causes NITRATE poisoning.
a. oxalate causes OXALATE poisoning.
a. phosphate a feed additive for cattle. The monobasic salt provides 27% phosphorus and 13% nitrogen, while the dibasic salt provides 23% phosphorus and 21% nitrogen.
a. sulfamate used as a herbicide; cattle and deer eating treated plants may be poisoned.
a. sulfate causes AMMONIA poisoning.
ammoniuria excess of ammonia in the urine.
Ammotragus lervia an animal that resembles a goat in appearance and habit. Has a great capacity to survive without water. Called also arni, aoudad, Barbary sheep.
Amnicola limosa porosa a snail, the intermediate host of *Metorchis conjunctus*, a liver fluke of cats and dogs.
amniocentesis transabdominal perforation of the amniotic sac for the purpose of obtaining a sample of amniotic fluid, which contains cells shed from the skin of the fetus as well as biochemical substances.
amniochorial pertaining to amnion and chorion.
amniogenesis the development of the amnion.
amniography radiography of the gravid uterus.
amnion the innermost membrane enclosing the developing fetus and which is filled with amniotic fluid; characteristic of reptiles, birds and mammals. See also AMNIOTIC.
a. nodosum a nodular condition of the fetal surface

of the amnion, observed in oligohydramnios associated with absence of the kidneys in the fetus.
amnionitis inflammation of the amnion.
amniorrhea escape of the amniotic fluid.
amniorrhexis rupture of the amnion.
amnioscope an endoscope that, by passage through the abdominal wall into the amniotic cavity, permits direct visualization of the fetus and amniotic fluid.
amniote any animal with amnion.
amniotic pertaining to the amnion.
a. fluid the albuminous fluid contained in the amniotic sac.
a. plaque small, 2 to 4 mm diameter, poxlike lesion on the inside of the amnion. Constant on the bovine amnion during the middle trimester and causes no problems nor has any known function.
a. sac the amnion; the sac enclosing the fetus suspended in the amniotic fluid.
a. vesicle see amniotic sac (above). Palpation of the vesicle per rectum in the cow is a common test for pregnancy between the 35th and 65th day of pregnancy.
amniotome an instrument for cutting the fetal membranes.
amniotomy surgical rupture of the fetal membranes.
amobarbital sodium an intermediate-acting barbiturate used as a sedative and hypnotic. It has been used as an anesthetic agent in fish.
Amoeba a genus of the subphylum Sarcodina. It is a single-celled mass of protoplasm which changes shape by extending cytoplasmic processes called pseudopodia by which it moves about and absorbs nourishment. The majority of amebae are free-living in soil and water. See also AMEBIC.
Amoebotaenia a genus of tapeworms of the family Dilepididae.
A. cuneata a tapeworm of poultry. Heavy infestations cause a hemorrhagic enteritis. Chronic infections cause wasting and reduced growth rate.
A. sphenoides see *Amoebotaenia cuneata* (above).
Amoracia rusticans toxic plant in family Brassicaceae. Causes stomatitis, diarrhea and sudden death. Called also *A. lapathifolia*, *Cochlearia armoracia*, horseradish.
amorph an inactive mutant gene, i.e. one that produces no detectable effect.
amorphia, amorphism state of being amorphous.
amorphous having no definite form; shapeless.
amorphus globosus a rounded structure of normal tissues covered with normal, pigmented skin typical of the breed, which occurs in the uterus of cattle. May cause dystocia. Called also fetal mole.
amotio [L.] *a removing.*
a. retinae detachment of the retina.
amoxapine a tricyclic antidepressant, similar to amitriptyline, used in the treatment of psychogenic dermatoses in dogs and cats.
amoxicillin, amoxycillin an aminopenicillin, similar in action to ampicillin and susceptible to β-lactamase, but more efficiently absorbed from the gastrointestinal tract and with a longer duration of action.
a.-clavulanic acid addition of clavulanic acid widens the spectrum of activity and renders amoxicillin resistant to β-lactamase. A widely used antibiotic in dogs and cats.
AMP adenosine monophosphate.
cyclic AMP, 3′,5′-cAMP cyclic adenosine monophosphate.
amp. ampere, ampoule.
amperage strength of an electric current in amperes or milliamperes.
ampere a unit of electric current strength, the current yielded by one volt of electromotive force against one ohm of resistance.
amphenone an aniline derivative capable of inhibiting the organification of thyroglobulin.
amphetamine a central nervous system stimulant with marked α and β adrenoreceptor activity. Its use is strictly controlled and there are few applications in veterinary medicine. Called also benzedrine.
amphi- word element. [Gr.] *both, on both sides.*
amphiarthrosis a joint in which the surfaces are connected by fibrocartilage, as between vertebrae. Called also cartilaginous JOINT. See also SYMPHYSIS, SYNCHONDROSIS.
Amphibia a class of animals containing the AMPHIBIANS.
amphibians members of the animal class Amphibia. Includes frogs, toads, newts, salamanders and cecilians all capable of living on land or in water.
Amphibolurus barbatus an Australian, desert-dwelling lizard whose neck collar of scales bristles when it opens its mouth. Called also bearded dragon.
amphicelous concave on either side or end as in some vertebrae.
amphicentric beginning and ending in the same vessel, like the branches of the rete mirabile.
amphicytes the neuroglial cells that surround the neurons of ganglia. They are closely related to oligodendrogliocytes.
amphidiarthrosis a joint having the nature of both ginglymus and arthrodia, as that of the lower jaw.
Amphimerus avian digenetic trematodes of the family Opisthorchiidae. Includes *A. elongatus* (blocks biliary, pancreatic ducts in poultry, ducks, pigeons), *A. pseudofelineus* (liver fluke in cats, coyotes).
amphinomids members of the family Amphinomidae, a group of browsing marine worms with bristles that cause skin irritation.
amphipathic molecules containing both polar and non-polar regions in their structure.
amphistomes see PARAMPHISTOMES.
amphistomiasis see PARAMPHISTOMIASIS. Called also stomach fluke infestation.
amphitrichous having flagella at each end.
amphixozes diseases that affect humans and other animals with equal facility, e.g. salmonellosis.
ampholytes see AMPHOTERIC sanitizing agents.
amphophil an amphophilic cell or element. See also HETEROPHIL.
amphophilic staining with either acid or basic dyes.
amphoric pertaining to a bottle; resembling the sound made by blowing across the neck of a bottle.
amphoteric capable of acting as both an acid and a base; capable of neutralizing either bases or acids.
a. sanitizing agents long chain substituted amino acids or betaines, compatible with other detergents, sanitizers and hard water. Called also ampholytes.
amphotericin B an antifungal antibiotic produced by *Streptomyces nodosus*, used to treat deep mycotic infections and also to treat cutaneous and mucocutaneous candidiasis. Potential nephrotoxicity limits its use.
amphotony hypertonia of the entire autonomic nervous system.
ampicillin an aminopenicillin of synthetic origin, susceptible to β-latamase, with activity similar to amoxicillin but shorter duration of activity. It can be administered orally or parenterally.
amplexus in amphibians, the period during which fertilization of eggs by the male occurs as they are passed by the female.

amplification 1. the process of making larger, as the increase of an auditory or visual stimulus, as a means of improving its perception. 2. said of a virus means multiplication; replication. 3. in polymerase chain reaction, the synthesis of multiple copies of a particular nucleic acid template sequence.
amplifier see IMAGE amplifier system.
amplitude largeness, fullness; wideness or breadth of range or extent.
a. mode see A-mode ULTRASONOGRAPHY.
ampoule ampule.
amprolium a widely used coccidiostat that is stable in chicken rations and compatible with most ration ingredients. Needs to be combined with other compounds to achieve all-round protection and treatment.
a. poisoning causes encephalopathy in cattle and sheep, possibly by causing brain swelling because of its antithiamin action. See also POLIOENCEPHALOMALACIA.
ampule a small, hermetically sealed glass or plastic container, e.g. one containing medication for parenteral administration or semen for insemination. Called also ampoule.
ampulla pl. *ampullae* [L.] a flasklike dilatation of a tubular structure, especially of the expanded ends of the semicircular canals of the ear. See also AMPULLAR.
a. chyli cisterna chyli.
a. coli the enormously dilated part of the right dorsal colon of the horse.
a. ductus deferentis the enlarged glandular urethral end of the ductus deferens.
Henle's a. ampulla ductus deferentis.
hepatopancreatic a. ampulla of Vater; in humans, a flasklike cavity in the major duodenal papilla into which the common bile duct and pancreatic duct open.
Lieberkühn's a. the blind termination of the lacteals in the villi of the intestines.
ampullae membranaceae the dilatations at one end of each of the three semicircular ducts.
ampullae osseae the dilatations at one of the ends of the semicircular canals.
phrenic a. the dilatation at the diaphragmatic end of the esophagus in some species.
rectal a. the dilated portion of the rectum just proximal to the anal canal, prominent in the horse.
a. of Thoma one of the small terminal expansions of an interlobar artery in the pulp of the spleen.
uterine tube a. the longest and widest portion of the uterine tube, between the infundibulum and the isthmus of the tube.
vas deferens a. dilatation of the terminal part of the vas deferens caused by glandular thickening of the wall.
a. of Vater hepatopancreatic ampulla.
ampullar pertaining to or originating from an AMPULLA.
a. anomalies unilateral aplasia, fusion of, and appendages to the ampullae of the ductus deferens occur in bulls and unilateral aplasia in stallions.
ampullitis inflammation of the ampulla of the vas deferens. Clinical signs are not usually observed.
amputates see AMELIA, ACROTERIASIS.
amputation the removal of a limb or other appendage or outgrowth of the body. The most common indication for amputation of an upper limb is severe trauma. Other indications may include malignancy, infection and gangrene.
closed a. flap amputation; one in which flaps are made from skin and subcutaneous tissue and sutured over the bone end of the stump.
congenital a. absence of a limb at birth, attributed to constriction of the part by an encircling band during intrauterine development.
a. in contiguity amputation at a joint.
a. in continuity amputation of a limb elsewhere than at a joint.
diaclastic a. amputation in which the bone is broken by an osteoclast and the soft tissues divided by an écraseur.
flap a. closed amputation.
guillotine a. open amputation; one in which the entire cross-section is left open (flapless) for dressing.
interpelviabdominal a. amputation of the thigh with excision of the lateral portion of the pelvic girdle.
interscapulothoracic a. amputation of the forelimb with excision of the lateral portion of the shoulder girdle.
open a. guillotine amputation.
spontaneous a. loss of a part without surgical intervention, as in leprosy, etc.
amrinone a synthetic phosphodiesterase inhibitor compound, used to provide inotropic support to the failing myocardium.
AMS α-amylase. See AMYLASE.
Amsinckia plant genus of the Boraginaceae family. Many of them contain PYRROLIZIDINE alkaloids. Includes *A. calycina*, *A. gloriosa*, *A. hispida*, *A. intermedia*, *A. lycopsoides*, *A. menziesii*; seeds contaminate feed grain. Called also tarweed, ironweed, yellow burrweed.
amyelia congenital absence of the spinal cord.
amyelinic without myelin.
amyelonic 1. having no spinal cord. 2. having no marrow.
amyelus a fetus with no spinal cord.
amygdala 1. the corpus amygdaloideum. 2. (rare) a tonsil.
amygdalin the cyanogenetic glycoside in bitter almonds.
amygdaline 1. like an almond. 2. pertaining to tonsils.
amygdaloid body a complex of nuclei of the telencephalon located in the pyriform lobe deep within the olfactory cortex.
amygdalolith a calculus in a tonsil.
Amygdalus communis tree in the plant family Rosaceae; can cause cyanide poisoning. Called also *Prunus amygdalus*, almond.
amylaceous composed of or resembling starch.
amylase an enzyme that catalyzes the hydrolysis of starch into simpler compounds. The α-amylases occur in animals and include pancreatic and salivary amylase; the β-amylases occur in higher plants. Measurement of serum α-amylase activity is an important diagnostic test for acute pancreatitis and acute attacks of chronic pancreatitis.
a. isoenzymes serum amylase is composed of a number of isoenzymes, isoamylases, probably originating from different tissues. Elevation of an isoenzyme of hepatic origin is found in HYPERADRENOCORTICISM.
a. reaction an identification test, based on an extracellular product of group A β-hemolytic streptococci.
serum a. the most significant laboratory aid in the diagnosis of acute pancreatitis or exacerbations of a chronic pancreatitis. Other organs may also produce the enzyme, or its isoenzymes, but the amounts are normally limited.
urine a. dogs excrete very little amylase in the urine in contrast to humans where urine levels of the enzyme may be valuable in assessing the progress of a case of pancreatitis.

amylin see AMYLOID.
amyl(o)- word element. [Gr.] *starch.*
amylo-1,6-glucosidase deficiency see GLYCOGENOSIS type III.
amylobarbitone see AMOBARBITAL SODIUM.
amylogenesis the formation of starch.
amyloid 1. starchlike; amylaceous. 2. an eosinophilic homogeneous hyaline material deposited extracellularly in glomeruli in particular. Because of its characteristic β-pleated pattern it is resistant to proteolysis and is insoluble.
a. AA derived from serum amyloid A protein in reactive systemic (secondary) amyloidosis.
a. AL derived from immunoglobulin light chains in immunocytic or primary amyloidosis; usually associated with myeloma.
islet a. polypeptide a polypeptide produced in the pancreatic β-cells and co-released with insulin; inhibits insulin release and may counteract insulin action in peripheral tissues. Deposits are found in the pancreas of cats with diabetes mellitus.
amyloidosis the deposition in various tissues of amyloid. This protein is almost insoluble and once it infiltrates the tissues they become waxy and nonfunctioning. Systemic amyloidosis may be immunocytic or reactive (see below).
cutaneous a. multiple cutaneous, hard, painless, chronic plaques occur over the head, neck and shoulders of horses. There may be involvement of the nasal mucosa and resulting dyspnea.
immunocytic a., immunogenic a., primary a. amyloid produced from light chains of immunoglobulins as in plasma-cell dyscrasias. See also AL PROTEIN.
reactive a. is derived from excess serum protein SAA produced as a result of chronic antigenic stimulation. The kidney is most often affected and the amyloid is most often deposited in glomeruli but medullary deposits are seen in cats and cattle. Idiopathic amyloidosis is common in the dog and less common in cats. It is associated with chronic suppurative disease processes in cattle, antiserum production in horses, and it occurs rarely in pigs. Called also secondary alopecia.
renal a. characterized by severe proteinuria and uremia. There is chronic diarrhea, polydipsia and anasarca. Seen particularly in dogs and cats.
secondary a. reactive amyloidosis (above).
Amyloodinium a protozoan, a member of the Sarcomastigophora, the cause of velvet disease of aquarium fish. The gills are the primary site of inflammation, but the lesions may spread to the skin. See also OODINIUM.
amylopectin the insoluble constituent of starch; the soluble constituent is amylose.
amyloplast a starch-forming leuko-plastid in a plant.
amylopsin see AMYLASE.
amylorrhea the presence of an abnormal amount of starch in the stools.
amylose 1. polysaccharide of D-glucose containing α-1→4 glycosidic bonds. 2. the soluble constituent of starch, as opposed to amylopectin.
amyocardia weakness of the heart muscle.
amyoplasia lack of muscle formation or development.
a. congenita generalized lack in the newborn of muscular development and growth, with contracture and deformity of most joints.
amyostasia a tremor of the muscles.
amyosthenia failure of muscular strength.
amyosthenic 1. characterized by amyosthenia. 2. an agent that diminishes muscular power.
amyotonia atonic condition of the muscles.
congenital a. any congenital disease marked by general hypotonia of the muscles.
amyotrophia amyotrophy.
amyotrophic lateral sclerosis a type of motor disorder of the nervous system in humans in which there is destruction of the anterior horn cells and pyramidal tract. The cause is unknown. It is characterized by weakness, spasticity and muscle atrophy and is fatal in most cases. One form of hereditary canine spinal MUSCULAR atrophy is similar to this disease.
amyotrophy atrophy of muscles.
neurogenic a. see MUSCULAR atrophy.
Amyrsidea dedonsai louse of guinea fowl.
amyxia absence of mucus.
amyxorrhea absence of mucous secretion.
AMZ see AUSTRALIAN Milking Zebu.
An chemical symbol, *actinon.*
An. anisometropia; anode.
an hua acupuncture terminology for saddle wound.
an shen acupuncture term meaning sedation.
ANA antinuclear antibody.
ana [Gr.] *of each;* used in prescription writing; abbreviated āā.
ana- word element. [Gr.] *upward, again, backward, excessively.*
Anabaena a genus of planktonic Cyanobacteria which frequents still, fresh water. Important because of its capacity to produce potent toxins including ANATOXIN, SAXITOXIN and MICROCYSTIN. Causes nervous syndrome, highly fatal within a few hours, and hepatic necrosis with photosensitization. Called also water bloom. Includes *A. circinalis*, *A. flos-aquae*, *A. spiroides.*
anabasine teratogenic piperidine alkaloid in *Nicotiana* spp. Called also neonicotine.
anabasis the stage of increase in a disease.
anabiosis restoration of life processes after their apparent cessation.
anabolic pertaining to or arising from anabolism.
a. steroid steroids with a tissue-building effect. Testosterone is an example of a natural anabolic steroid with the, sometimes undesirable, effect of causing masculinization. Synthetic steroids are designed to avoid this problem as much as possible. The purpose of their use includes improvement in body weight in old animals and in the young after debilitating disease or major surgery.
anabolism the constructive phase of metabolism, in which the body cells synthesize protoplasm for growth and repair.

The manner in which this synthesis takes place is directed by the genetic code carried by the molecules of deoxyribonucleic acid (DNA). The 'building blocks' for this synthesis of protoplasm are obtained from amino acids and other nutritive elements in the diet.
anachoresis preferential collection or deposit of particles at a site, as of bacteria or metals that have localized out of the bloodstream in areas of inflammation.
anacidity abnormal lack or deficiency of acid.
gastric a. achlorhydria.
anacrotism a pulse anomaly evidenced by the presence of a prominent notch on the ascending limb of the pulse tracing.
anaculture vaccine containing toxoid and killed bacteria; used to immunize against some clostridial diseases.
Anacystis cyanea MICROCYSTIS *aeruginosa.*
anadipsia intense thirst.

anadrenalism absence or failure of adrenal function.
anadromous said of fish; those living most of their lives in the sea but entering rivers to spawn.
anadromy migration of fish, as adults or subadults, from salt water to fresh.
anaemia see ANEMIA.
anaerobe an organism that lives and grows in the absence of molecular oxygen.
facultative a. a microorganism that can grow with or without molecular oxygen.
obligate a. an organism that can grow only in the complete absence of molecular oxygen.
anaerobic the absence of air.
a. bacteria see ANAEROBE.
a. effluent treatment is usually conducted in deep ponds where air does not penetrate. A fully contained system is also available.
a. exercise exercise at high work intensity during which the needs of muscle metabolism for oxygen exceeds the capacity of the circulation to supply it and an oxygen debt is incurred.
a. infection one caused by aerobic organisms.
anaerobiosis life in the absence of oxygen; a term applied most commonly to microbes.
Anaeroplasma anaerobic commensal found in the rumen.
anaerosis interruption of the respiratory function.
Anaerovibrio lipolytica one of the many ruminal bacteria.
Anafilaroides a subgenus of *Oslerus*. Includes *A. rostratus* (cause of tracheobronchitis in cats).
Anagallis a genus of the Primulaceae family of plants; contains an unidentified nephrotoxin and causes diarrhea. Includes *A. arvensis* (scarlet pimpernel), *A. arvensis* var. *caerulea* (blue pimpernel).
anagen in the cycle of hair growth, the period of active production by the hair follicle.
a. defluxion, a. effluvium loss and abnormal formation of hair that is in the anagen stage of growth; occurs with antimitotic drugs, endocrinopathies, metabolic disorders.
a.-telogen ratio a comparison of the numbers of anagen and telogen hair bulbs, which is an indication of the percentage of active hair follicles. Normally, the majority should be in anagen.
anagyrine an alkaloid in lupins thought to be responsible for the limb deformities of newborn calves following ingestion of lupins by pregnant cows.
anakatadidymus a twin monster, separate above and below, but united in the trunk.
anakusis total deafness.
anal relating to the ANUS.
a. abscess acute, purulent infections in the area of the anus, usually caused by gram-negative organisms. In dogs, these most often arise from the ANAL SACS.
a. atresia, atresia ani congenital absence or stenosis of the anus manifested by an absence of feces and a gradual development of abdominal distension. Fistulae may develop between the rectum and urogenital tract. The anomalous development can occur in several forms and may be accompanied by similar atresia at higher levels of the intestine. There is usually normal development of sphincters. A dimple is usually evident at the point at which surgical intervention is required.
a. canal the short, terminal, retroperitoneal segment of the intestinal tract between the rectum and anus.
a. constriction a congenital constriction combined with vulvar constriction occurs in Jersey cattle.
a. fibroma occurs in cattle and excision effected for esthetic reasons.
a. fistula see PERIANAL fistula.
a. fold see anal FOLD.
a. furunculosis see PERIANAL fistula.
a. membrane the dorsal part of the cloacal membrane in the embryo; when it eventually breaks down the dorsal passage becomes the rectoanal passage.
a.-perineal laceration see RECTOVAGINAL fistula.
a. prolapse the protrusion of a small amount of mucosa through the anus.
a. reflex the pursing of the anal orifice when the perineum is stimulated; indicative of an animal with intact sacral segments of the spinal cord.
a. sac see ANAL SACS.
a. sacculitis inflammation of the anal sacs.
a. sphincter the internal anal sphincter is formed from smooth muscle of the anal canal while the external anal sphincter, which is larger and of greater importance in fecal continence, consists of striated muscle.
a. sphincter hypertrophy occurs in aged dogs and may give rise to difficult and painful defecation.
a. stenosis scar formation after perianal fistulae, trauma, severe anal sac disease, or treatment for neoplasia may result in a reduced lumen and particularly a loss of the capacity to dilate with passage of feces. Straining, passage of ribbon-like feces and constipation result.
a. ulceration inflammation and ulceration of the perianal skin which may be associated with anal sac disease. Seen most commonly in German shepherd dogs.
anal sacs a pair of sacs between the internal and external anal sphincter on either side at the mucocutaneous junction of the anus in carnivores. The walls are lined with large sebaceous glands and in dogs also apocrine glands. The combined secretions are malodorous, gray-brown, granular material that is expelled in small quantities with each defecation, as a form of territorial marking, or in larger amounts from vigorous struggling or due to fear and may occur during treatment by a veterinarian. These sacs are subject to hypersecretion, ductal blockage, impaction and abscess formation which may necessitate surgical removal. Discomfort associated with disease may give rise to 'scooting', rubbing or licking of the anal area in dogs.
a. s. abscess infection, aided by impaction of secretions, of anal sacs can lead to abscess formation which may rupture and drain to perianal skin or into deep tissues surrounding the rectum. See also PERIANAL fistula.
a. s. tumor the most common tumors of the anal sacs are apocrine adenocarcinomas, occurring most often in aged bitches. These tumors are sometimes associated with the paraneoplastic syndrome of PSEUDOHYPERPARATHYROIDISM.
analbuminemia absence or deficiency of serum albumins.
analeptic 1. a drug that acts as a stimulant to the central nervous system, such as caffeine and amphetamine. 2. a restorative medicine.
Analges a genus of the Analgesidae family of mites. Includes *A. passerinus* (in the plumage of passerine birds).
analgesia absence of sensibility to pain, particularly the relief of pain without loss of consciousness; absence of pain or noxious stimulation. See also ANALGESIC.
continuous caudal a. continuous injection of an anesthetic solution into the sacral and lumbar plexuses within the epidural space to relieve the pain

of parturition; also used in general surgery to block the pain pathways caudal to the umbilicus (see also CAUDAL anesthesia).
epidural a. analgesia induced by introduction of the analgesic agent into the epidural space of the vertebral canal. See also EPIDURAL.
infiltration a. paralysis of the nerve endings at the site of operation by subcutaneous injection of an anesthetic.
intrasynovial a. surface analgesia, produced by the introduction of a local analgesic agent into the synovial cavity and massaged into tendon sheaths.
intravenous regional a. the local anesthetic agent is injected intravenously caudal to a tourniquet. The tissues below the tourniquet become anesthetized. The tourniquet and the anesthesia can be maintained for up to 15 minutes. Called also Bier block (technique).
local a. injection of an anesthetic agent to create local analgesia. Includes infiltration, nerve block, epidural, intrathecal, intrasynovial, subarachnoid. See ANESTHESIA.
regional a. see regional ANESTHESIA.
segmental a. see segmental dorsolumbar EPIDURAL block.
spinal a. injection of an analgesic agent into the spinal canal, generally either into the subarachnoid or epidural space. See also spinal ANESTHESIA.
surface a. local analgesia produced by an anesthetic applied to the surface of mucous membranes, e.g. those of the eye, nose, throat and urethra.

analgesic 1. relieving pain. 2. pertaining to analgesia. 3. a drug that relieves pain. See also OPIUM, MORPHINE, METHADONE, MEPERIDINE, PENTAZOCINE LACTATE, PROPOXYPHENE, DIETHYLTHIAMBUTENE HYDROCHLORIDE.
a. antagonist used for the control of excessive reaction to or overdosing with the narcotic analgesics. See also NALORPHINE, NALOXONE.
a. nephropathy papillary necrosis due to local ischemia resulting from the antiprostaglandin effect of aspirin, phenylbutazone and phenacetin.
non-narcotic a. includes SALICYLATE, ACETANILID, ACETOPHENETIDIN, PHENYLBUTAZONE, DIPYRONE, MECLOFENAMIC ACID, INDOMETHACIN, NAPROXEN, FLUNIXIN MEGLUMINE, XYLAZINE.

analgia painlessness.

analog, analogue 1. a part or organ having the same function as another, but of different evolutionary origin. 2. a chemical compound having a structure similar to that of another but differing from it in respect of a certain component; it may have similar or opposite action metabolically.
a. computer see COMPUTER.

analysis separation into component parts.
cohort a. the separation of each of two cohorts into component parts and comparing the results.
current a. analysis performed on contemporary data.
discriminant a. a form of multivariate analysis in which the objective is to establish a discriminate function. The function (typically a mathematical formula) discriminates between individuals in the population and allocates each of them to a group within the population. The function is established on the basis of a series of measurements or observations made on the individuals.
economic a. evaluation of the costs and benefits of a commercial enterprise that takes into account additional returns, returns no longer obtained, additional costs and costs no longer incurred, discounting of gains back to the time when the project began, and opportunity costs relating to potential profitability from alternative use of the investment.
factor a. a multivariate technique which analyzes the underlying structure of a set of data. It is useful in explaining observed relationships amongst a large number of variables in terms of simpler relations.
guaranteed a. declares the range within which nutrients occur in a manufactured animal food.
multivariate a. techniques for the study of simultaneous variation in a number of variables. Includes linear discriminant functions, cluster analysis and factor and principal component analysis.
path a. a statistical technique for testing a limited number of causal hypotheses, the causal relationships between variables, by manipulation of one or more of the variables and predicting the outcome.
qualitative a. determination of the nature of the constituents of a compound or mixture.
quantitative a. determination of the proportionate quantities of the constituents of a compound or mixture.
regression a. a general statistical technique that analyzes the relationship between a dependent (criterion) variable and a set of independent (predictor) variables.
systems a. analysis of the interaction of a system, e.g. a biological system, often for the purpose of analyzing the differences between systems. See also SYSTEM.
a. of variance a statistical method for comparing variables by partitioning the variance of the observations between the effects of the different variables and comparing it with the underlying random variation.
vector a. analysis of a moving force to determine both its magnitude and its direction, e.g. analysis of the scalar electrocardiogram to determine the magnitude and direction of the electromotive force for one complete cycle of the heart.

analyte a substance or material determined by a chemical analysis.

analytical, analytic pertaining to or emanating from analysis.
a. control control of confounding by analysis of the results of a trial or test.
a. epidemiology draws statistical inferences, mostly about causes, about disease in populations based on available samples of it.
a. methods techniques used to draw statistical inferences including multiple regression, path analysis, discriminate analysis and logistic analysis.
a. study a method for testing a hypothesis as part of an investigation of the association between a disease and possible causes of the disease.

Aname one of the three genera of trapdoor spiders.

anamnesis 1. the faculty of memory. 2. the history of a patient and its relatives.

anamnestic 1. pertaining to anamnesis. 2. aiding the memory.
a. response a secondary immune response; occurs with a second or subsequent exposure to an antigen. The antibody or cell-mediated response is more rapid and greater than occurred following the primary exposure.

anamniotic having no amnion.

anamorph the asexual form of a fungus.

anamu see PETIVERIA ALLIACEA.

anaphase the third stage of division of the nucleus of a cell in either meiosis or mitosis.

anaphoresis diminished activity of the sweat glands.

anaphrodisia absence or loss of sexual desire.

anaphrodisiac 1. repressing sexual desire. 2. a drug that represses sexual desire.

anaphylactic pertaining to anaphylaxis.

a. reaction see ANAPHYLAXIS.

a. shock a serious and generalized state of shock brought about by hypersensitivity (ANAPHYLAXIS) to an ALLERGEN, such as a drug, foreign protein or toxin.

anaphylactogen a substance that produces anaphylaxis.

anaphylactogenesis the production of anaphylaxis.

anaphylactoid resembling anaphylaxis, but not involving an immunological mechanism.

a. purpura see anaphylactoid PURPURA.

anaphylatoxin a substance produced in blood serum when complement is activated; serves as a mediator of inflammation by inducing mast cell degranulation, histamine release and increased vascular permeability, and on injection into animals, it causes anaphylactic shock.

a. inhibitor a specific serum carboxypeptidase, one of the complement proteins.

anaphylaxis an unusual or exaggerated allergic reaction of an animal to foreign protein or other substances. Anaphylaxis is an immediate or antibody-mediated hypersensitivity reaction (type I) produced by the release of vasoactive agents such as histamine and serotonin. Release is a consequence of the binding of IgE antibodies to Fc receptors on the surface of particularly mast cells and basophils. Antigen binding to two adjacent IgE molecules causes perturbation of the cell membrane leading to the release of vasoactive substances. Anaphylaxis may be localized, usually cutaneous, or generalized. Called also anaphylactic shock.

Substances most likely to produce anaphylaxis include drugs, particularly antibiotics and local anesthetics; drugs prepared from animals, such as insulin, adrenocorticotropic hormone and enzymes; diagnostic agents, such as iodinated x-ray contrast media; biologicals used to provide immunity, such as vaccines, antitoxins and gamma globulin; protein foods; the venom of bees, wasps and hornets; and pollens and molds. See also HYPERSENSITIVITY, ANAPHYLACTIC.

acquired a. that in which sensitization is known to have been produced by administration of a foreign antigen.

active a. see acquired anaphylaxis (above).

aggregate a. caused by large amounts of antibody–antigen complexes that activate complement and resulting in degranulation of mast cells.

antiserum a. passive anaphylaxis.

cutaneous a. a localized form of anaphylaxis, which follows the injection of antigen into the skin.

cytotoxic a. a form of anaphylaxis triggered by antibodies against self antigens. Blood transfusion reactions and Rh reactions are examples.

cytotropic a. refers to binding of IgE to Fc receptors.

heterologous a. passive anaphylaxis induced by transfer of serum from an animal of a different species.

homologous a. passive anaphylaxis induced by transfer of serum from an animal of the same species.

indirect a. that induced by an animal's own protein modified in some way.

passive a. that resulting in a normal animal from injection of serum of a sensitized animal.

passive cutaneous a. (PCA) localized anaphylaxis passively transferred by intradermal injection of an antibody and, after a latent period (about 24 to 72 hours), intravenous injection of the homologous antigen and Evans blue dye; blueing of the skin at the site of the intradermal injection is evidence of PCA.

reverse passive cutaneous a. antigen is injected first, succeeded by the injection of antiserum.

systemic a. a generalized anaphylactic reaction most often observed when the antigen is injected intravenously but may also be produced after local administration of antigen. The main shock organs in cattle and sheep are the lungs, in the horse, cat and pig the lungs and intestines, and in dogs the liver, specifically the hepatic veins.

anaplasia loss of differentiation of cells, an irreversible alteration in adult cells toward more primitive (embryonic) cell types; a characteristic of tumor cells.

Anaplasma a genus of organisms in the family Anaplasmataceae. They are gram-negative rod-shaped, spherical, coccoid or ring-shaped bodies that multiply only in the erythrocytes of ruminants. They are transmitted by arthropods and are susceptible to tetracyclines.

A. centrale causes a mild form of ANAPLASMOSIS in cattle and has been used as a vaccine against *A. marginale*.

A. marginale a significant pathogen, the cause of ANAPLASMOSIS in ruminants. The infection is transmitted mechanically by many biting insects. *Boophilus* spp. and *Dermacentor* spp. are biological vectors.

A. ovis the cause of ANAPLASMOSIS of sheep.

Anaplasmataceae the family of organisms containing the genera *Anaplasma*, *Paranaplasma*, *Aegyptianella*, *Haemobartonella*, *Eperythozoon*.

anaplasmosis a disease caused by *Anaplasma* spp. In cattle it is a chronic, often remitting disease characterized by fever, jaundice, emaciation and anemia, but never hemoglobinuria. It is transmitted by a number of insect vectors, especially ticks. In sheep and goats the disease is subclinical. See also BABESIOSIS.

anaplastic 1. restoring a lost or absent part. 2. characterized by anaplasia.

anaplerotic reaction a reaction that replenishes the concentration of an intermediate in a metabolic pathway.

anapophysis the accessory vertebral process.

Anas platyrhynchos the mallard, a monogamous, broad-billed dabbling duck. One of the original ducks from which the domestic ducks have originated.

anasarca extensive subcutaneous edema; an expression of a generalized edema such as occurs in congestive heart failure. There is diffuse subcutaneous swelling which is cool to the touch and retains the imprint of a fingertip after pressure is released—hence 'pitting edema'. The principal locations are the intermandibular space and the ventral aspects of the neck and trunk. In horses the limbs are also commonly involved.

anastalsis 1. an upward-moving wave of contraction without a preceding wave of inhibition, occurring in the alimentary canal in addition to the peristaltic wave. 2. styptic action.

anastaltic styptic; highly astringent.

anastole retraction, as of the lips of a wound.

anastomosis 1. communication between two tubular organs. 2. surgical, traumatic or pathological formation of a connection between two normally distinct structures.

arteriovenous a. anastomosis between an artery and a vein.

cobra-head a. a technique used in joining grafts to blood vessels. Ends of grafts are trimmed to form an enlarged lumen.
esophageal a. uniting the free ends after complete resection of a part of the esophagus.
heterocladic a. one between branches of different arteries.
intercarotid a. a naturally occurring communication between the internal and external carotid arteries in birds. It provides a collateral pathway for blood to the brain, the counterpart of the cerebral arterial circle of Willis in mammals.
intestinal a. establishment of a communication between two formerly distinct portions of the intestine.
skin arteriovenous a. frequent natural occurrence; capable of diverting large volumes of blood to splanchnic circulation during cardiovascular stress.
tracheal a. end-to-end anastomosis of the trachea after resection of a part.
ureterocolonic a. see URETEROCOLOSTOMY.
anat. anatomy.
Anaticola a genus of bird lice in the superfamily Ischnocera. Includes *A. anseris, A. crassicornis* (duck lice).
anatid said of birds; members of the family ANATIDAE, ducks, geese and swans.
Anatidae family of aquatic birds, including the ducks, geese and swans.
anatine a bird of the family Anatidae, the ducks, geese and swans.
anatipestifer syndrome see PASTEURELLA *anatipestifer.*
Anatoecus a genus of lice in the suborder Mallophaga. Includes *A. dentatus, A. icterodes* (duck lice).
Anatolian black cattle black dual-purpose brachyceros type Turkish cattle.
Anatolian buffalo dairy and draft Turkish buffalo, dark gray to black often with white on head and tail, sickle or crescentic horns.
Anatolian shepherd dog, Anatolian Karabash a large, tall (28–32 in) dog with a short, dense coat, broad head, and long tail carried over the back. It is usually fawn with a black mask, but other colors also occur. A Turkish breed used for guarding sheep, goats and other livestock.
anatomic, anatomical pertaining to anatomy, or to the structure of the body.
a. dead space (respiratory) the space in the air passages, oral to the parenchymatous lung tissue, where no respiratory exchange takes place.
anatomist one skilled in anatomy.
anatomy the science dealing with the form and structure of living organisms.
comparative a. description and comparison of the form and structure of different animals.
developmental a. the changes in form from fertilization to adulthood, including embryology, fetology and postnatal development.
gross a. that dealing with structures visible with the unaided eye. Called also macroscopic anatomy.
macroscopic a. see gross anatomy (above).
microscopic a. anatomy revealed by microscopy; includes histology and cytology.
morbid a. anatomy of diseased tissues. Called also pathological anatomy.
pathological a. see morbid anatomy (above).
radiological a. anatomy revealed by the techniques of radiography and fluoroscopy.
special a. anatomy devoted to study of particular organs or parts.
topographic a. that devoted to determination of relative positions of various body parts; regional anatomy.
x-ray a. see radiological anatomy (above).
anatoxin neurotoxin produced by some cyanobacteria including species of *Anabaena, Oscillatoria, Aphanizoomenon.* Includes anatoxin-a, a potent nicotinic toxin, which is toxic to a wide range of species, and the cholinesterase inhibitor anatoxin-a(s), which is highly toxic to pigs, dogs and some waterfowl but seems to be unable to reach the brain or the retina in many species. Called also sudden death factor.
Anatrichosoma a genus of the nematode subfamily Capillariinae.
A. cutaneum, A. cuteum parasitizes most Old World nonhuman primates. See also ANATRICHOSOMIASIS.
anatrichosomiasis a creeping eruption of captive Old World nonhuman primates. Cause is ANATRICHOSOMA *cutaneum.*
anatriptic a medicine applied by rubbing.
anchor worm LERNAEA *elegans.*
anchorage fixation, e.g. surgical fixation of a displaced viscus.
anchoring fibers collagenous attachments between bone and ligaments, tendons and fibrous capsules.
anchoring filaments collagenous and reticular fibers connecting endothelial cells of lymphatics to surrounding connective tissue space.
anchoring plaques structures on the plasma membrane of smooth muscle fibers; points of contact between muscle fibers.
anchovies a cause of diarrhea, vomiting, salivation, lacrimation, depression, miosis, polypnea, tachycardia, hypothermia in cats.
anchovy paste as a supplement in poultry diets causes severe hepatitis and nephrosis characterized by low egg production, diarrhea, cyanosis, thirst, paralysis.
anchylo- for words beginning thus, see those beginning *ankylo-.*
ancipital two-edged; two-headed.
Ançon a mutant, achondroplastic sheep that appeared in Massachusetts, USA, in 1791 and became extinct in 1876. A similar mutant appeared in Norway in 1919. Called also Otter.
anconad toward the elbow or olecranon.
anconeal, anconal pertaining to the elbow.
a. process the projection of the ulna that occupies the olecranon fossa of the humerus when the elbow is extended and which develops as a separate ossification center in some dogs.
ununited a. process a failure of the anconeal process to unite with the ulna, resulting in fracture through the growth plate. Seen mainly in young dogs of large breeds, causing varying degrees of weight-bearing lameness and arthritis. Demonstrated radiographically after 5 months of age and usually treated surgically by removal of the fragment. Called also elbow dysplasia.
anconitis inflammation of the elbow joint.
ancoria absence of a pupil.
Ancryocephalus a fluke genus of monogenetic trematodes in the family Dactylogyridae. A parasite of fish.
ancylo- for words beginning thus, see also those beginning *ankylo-.*
Ancylostoma a genus of nematode parasites (HOOKWORM) belonging to the family Ancylostomatidae.
A. brasiliense a species parasitic in dogs and cats in tropical and subtropical regions; its larvae may cause creeping eruption in humans.

A. caninum the common hookworm of dogs and cats.
A. ceylanicum a hookworm of dogs and cats in Asia; resembles *A. braziliense*.
A. tubaeforme the hookworm of cats.

Ancylostomatidae a family of nematode parasites having teeth or two ventrolateral cutting plates at the entrance to a large buccal capsule, and small teeth at its base; the hookworms.

ancylostomiasis infection by worms of the genus *Ancylostoma* or by other hookworms (*Necator americanus*). See also HOOKWORM.

ancylostomosis the syndrome caused by hookworm infestation. It includes melena, pallor of mucosae, hyperpnea, poor exercise tolerance, anasarca, and anemia. Called also hookworm disease.

Ancystropus zeleborii a parasitic mite found under the eyelids and in plugged meibomian glands of Chiroptera bats.

Andalusian, Andalucian breeds of animals named after the Spanish province of Andalusia.
A. ass gray donkey, origin of American and other ass breeds.
A. cattle three varieties, a dark, black-brown, a yellow, and gray, of meat and draft cattle, with open lyre horns, bred in southern Spain.
A. horse Spanish breed of light horse originating from Arab and Barb. Brown, gray or black, about 15.2 hands high. Origin of many breeds of horses and of CRIOLLO and MUSTANG.

Anderson's lupine LUPINUS *andersonii*.

Andersonstrongylus milksi a metastrongyloid nematode found in the respiratory tract of dogs.

Andrachne decaisnei See LEPTOPUS DECAISNEI.

andr(o)- word element. [Gr.] *male, masculine*.

androblastoma 1. a rare benign tumor of the testis histologically resembling the fetal testis; there are three varieties: diffuse stromal, mixed (stromal and epithelial) and tubular (epithelial). The epithelial elements contain Sertoli cells, which may produce estrogen and thus cause feminization. 2. arrhenoblastoma.

Androctonus see SCORPION.

androgen any steroid hormone which promotes male characteristics. The two main androgens are androstenedione and testosterone.
a. binding protein generated by Sertoli cells; binds androgens within the adluminal compartment of the testis.
a. insensitivity see testicular FEMINIZATION.

androgenic steroids the androgens produced in small amounts in the adrenal cortex.

android resembling a human being.

Andromeda japonica PIERIS *japonica*.

andromedotoxin the toxin found in members of the plant family Ericaceae, including azaleas, rhododendron. Ingestion by ruminants causes salivation, colic, vomiting, staggering, collapse, death. Called also grayanotoxin.

Andropogon a large genus of grasses in the family Poaceae. A volunteer in native pasture in many countries. Palatable when young. Makes good meadow hay. Called also bluestem, bluesedge, turkeyfoot.

androstane the hydrocarbon nucleus, $C_{19}H_{32}$, from which androgens are derived.

androstanediol an androgen, $C_{19}H_{32}O_2$, prepared by reducing androsterone.

androstene an unsaturated cyclic hydrocarbon, $C_{19}H_{30}$, forming the nucleus of testosterone and certain other androgens.

androstenediol a crystalline androgenic steroid, $C_{19}H_{30}O_2$.

androstenedione an androgenic steroid produced by the testis, adrenal cortex and ovary. Immunization against it gives excellent results in promoting fertility in ewes by increasing the twinning rate.

androsterone an androgenic hormone, $C_{19}H_{30}O_2$, excreted in the urine. When injected intramuscularly, it counteracts the effects of castration.

anechoic in ultrasonography, an absence of internal echoes.

anectasis congenital atelectasis due to developmental immaturity.

Aneilema accuminatum African plant in the family Commelinaceae; known to cause nitrite poisoning.

anemia a reduction below normal in the number or volume of erythrocytes or in the quantity of hemoglobin in the blood. Clinically it is manifested by weakness, exercise intolerance, hyperpnea which is only moderate, pallor of mucosae, tachycardia and a large increase in the intensity of the heart sounds. There are often accompanying signs related to the site of blood or hemoglobin loss.
aplastic a. a form of anemia generally unresponsive to specific antianemia therapy. It is often chronic, accompanied by granulocytopenia and thrombocytopenia, in which the bone marrow is usually acellular or hypoplastic. It may, however, be rapidly fatal. The term is actually all-inclusive and most probably encompasses several clinical syndromes. See pure red cell APLASIA.
autoimmune hemolytic a. immune-mediated hemolytic anemia, which occurs in many species, particularly dogs, in which autoantibodies directed against red blood cells are produced. Different classes of immunoglobulins may be involved giving rise to differing clinical syndromes. Signs include pallor, lethargy, splenomegaly, and sometimes icterus, bilirubinuria and hemoglobinuria. There may also be an accompanying thrombocytopenia with bleeding tendencies. Diagnosis is based on a positive Coombs test.
avian infectious a. see infectious CHICKEN anemia.
blood loss a. see hemorrhagic anemia (below).
a. of chronic disease see ANEMIA of inflammatory disease (below).
cold antibody a. an immune-mediated hemolytic anemia in which the antibody is maximally active at temperatures below 98.6°F (37°C). See also cold AGGLUTININ disease.
cold (or cold water) a. a disease of cattle, especially calves, housed in warm barns and given near freezing water to drink. Dyspnea and the passage of red urine occur several hours after a large drink.
Coombs-positive a. immunoglobulin-mediated anemia that gives a positive reaction to COOMBS TESTS, indicating the presence of immunoglobulins on the red cell surface. See also autoimmune hemolytic anemia (above), ALLOIMMUNE hemolytic anemia of the newborn.
deficiency a. nutritional anemia.
drug-induced hemolytic a. some drugs such as quinine, quinidine, para-aminosalicylic acid, phenacetin, penicillin, insecticides, chlorpromazine, sulfonamides and dipyrone may be directly injurious to red cells or act to initiate an immune response in which red cells are destroyed.
familial nonspherocytic a. of Basenji dogs an inherited pyruvate kinase deficiency causes a hemolytic anemia with shortened red cell life span. In early stages, the disease is characterized by very active erythropoiesis but eventually, usually by the second or third year of life, a terminal myelofibrosis

and osteosclerosis develops. The disease is inherited as an autosomal recessive trait.

feline infectious a. see FELINE infectious anemia.

fragmentation a. see microangiopathic anemia (below).

Heinz body a. hemolytic anemia resulting from oxidation of globin and formation of Heinz bodies, which are seen in blood smears as dark refractile intracytoplasmic bodies and stain with new methylene blue. Some common causes are ingestion of onions and plants in the Brassicaeae family, phenazopyridine, methylene blue and ACETAMINOPHEN (paracetamol). Cats are particularly susceptible to Heinz BODY formation.

hemolytic a. see HEMOLYTIC anemia.

hemorrhagic a. is caused by loss of whole blood. If this is very rapid hypovolemic shock develops. At a slower rate there is anemic anoxia and the animal is suffering from anemia. Called also blood loss anemia.

hypochromic a. anemia in which the decrease in hemoglobin is proportionately much greater than the decrease in number of erythrocytes.

hypoplastic a. anemia due to incapacity of blood-forming organs, i.e. inactivity of the bone marrow. See also aplastic anemia (above).

idiopathic immune a. see autoimmune hemolytic anemia (above).

infectious equine a. see EQUINE infectious anemia.

a. of inflammatory disease a nonregenerative, usually mild, anemia that occurs in association with malignancy or chronic infection. Although other causes of anemia such as hemolysis and blood loss may also occur with these conditions, there is altered iron metabolism with decreased serum iron and iron-binding capacity but with increased iron storage that results in decreased erythropoiesis.

iron-deficiency a. a form characterized by low or absent iron stores, low serum iron concentration, low transferrin saturation, elevated transferrin (iron-binding capacity), low hemoglobin concentration or hematocrit, and hypochromic, microcytic red blood corpuscles, and thrombocytosis. See also IRON.

isoimmune hemolytic a. see ALLOIMMUNE hemolytic anemia of the newborn.

lizard viral a. produces inclusion bodies in erythrocytes, commonly mistaken for protozoan parasites.

macrocytic a. anemia in which the erythrocytes are much larger than normal. The MCV (mean corpuscular volume) and MCH (mean corpuscular hemoglobin) are increased and the MCHC (mean corpuscular hemoglobin concentration) is normal.

megaloblastic a. anemia characterized by the presence of megaloblasts in the bone marrow and macrocytic erythrocytes. It occurs in vitamin B_{12}, cobalt and folic acid deficiencies and in some myeloproliferative disorders in cats.

microangiopathic a. anemia due to fragmentation of erythrocytes in blood vessels whose endothelium has been badly damaged, usually by an infectious disease such as septicemias, disseminated intravascular coagulation and salmonellosis. Called also fragmentation anemia.

microcytic a. anemia characterized by decrease in size of the erythrocytes.

myelopathic a., myelophthisic a. anemia due to destruction or crowding out of hematopoietic tissues by space-occupying lesions, neoplasms and fibrosis.

nonregenerative a. one occurring without an appropriate erythropoietic response by the bone marrow.

normochromic a. that in which the hemoglobin content of the red cells as measured by the MCHC and MCH is within the normal range.

normocytic a. the anemia in which the red blood cells are normal in size.

nutritional a. anemia due to a deficiency of an essential substance in the diet, which may be caused by poor dietary intake or by malabsorption; called also deficiency anemia. See also PYRIDOXINE, VITAMIN B_{12}, FOLIC ACID, COPPER, IRON.

parasitic a. hemorrhagic anemia due to blood loss caused by blood-sucking parasites such as fleas, hookworms and *Haemonchus contortus*.

pernicious a. see PERNICIOUS anemia.

physiological a. the anemia which occurs as part of a natural event, e.g. in neonates.

piglet a. see IRON nutritional deficiency.

primary immune a. see autoimmune hemolytic anemia (above).

regenerative a., responsive a. associated with active erythropoiesis with increased numbers of reticulocytes, nucleated red blood cells, anisocytosis and polychromasia in the peripheral blood.

spur-cell a. anemia in which the red cells have a bizarre spiculated shape and are destroyed prematurely, primarily in the spleen; it is an acquired form occurring in severe liver disease, and represents an abnormality in the cholesterol content of the red cell membrane.

unresponsive a. see nonregenerative anemia (above).

anemic pertaining to anemia.

Anemone a genus of the plant family Ranunculaceae. Contains the toxic glycoside protoanemonin which causes abdominal pain, oral mucosal erosions, salivation, diarrhea. Includes *A. hortensis* (*A. stellata*), *A. nemorosa* (wood anemone), *A. patens* (*A. pavonina*), *A. pulsatilla* (pasque flower).

anemonin a pharmacologically inert substance which results from detoxication in the animal of PROTOANEMONIN, a toxin in plants of the Ranunculaceae family.

anencephaly congenital absence of the cranial vault, with the cerebral hemispheres completely missing or reduced to small masses.

anephric being without kidneys.

anergy diminished reactivity to specific antigen(s).

anesthekinesia, anesthecinesia combined sensory and motor paralysis.

anesthesia loss of feeling or sensation. Artificial anesthesia may be produced by a number of agents capable of bringing about partial or complete loss of sensation. It is induced to permit the performance of surgery or other painful procedures. See also ANESTHETIC.

balanced a. anesthesia that balances the depressing effects on the motor, sensory, reflex and mental aspects of nervous system function by the anesthetic agents. The philosophy encourages the use of several agents, each designed to affect one of the functions.

basal a. narcosis produced by preliminary medication so that the inhalation of anesthetic necessary to produce surgical anesthesia is greatly reduced.

block a. regional anesthesia. See also BLOCK.

caudal a. injection of an anesthetic into the sacral canal. See also CAUDAL anesthesia.

central a. lack of sensation caused by disease of the nerve centers.

closed a. that produced by continuous rebreathing of a small amount of anesthetic gas in a closed system with an apparatus for removing carbon dioxide.

crossed a. loss of sensation on one side of the face and loss of pain and temperature sense on the opposite side of the body.
dissociated a., dissociation a. loss of perception of certain stimuli while that of others remains intact.
electric a. anesthesia induced by passage of an electric current.
endotracheal a. anesthesia produced by introduction of a gaseous mixture through a tube inserted into the trachea.
epidural a. see EPIDURAL anesthesia.
field block a. the anesthetic agent is injected around the boundaries of the area to be anesthetized, with no attempt to locate specific nerves.
frost a. abolition of feeling or sensation as a result of topical refrigeration produced by a jet of a highly volatile liquid.
general a. a state of unconsciousness produced by anesthestic agents, with absence of pain sensation over the entire body and a greater or lesser degree of muscular relaxation; the drugs producing this state can be administered by inhalation, intravenously, intramuscularly, or rectally, or via the gastrointestinal tract.
infiltration a. local anesthesia produced by injection of the anesthetic solution directly into the area of terminal nerve endings.
inhalation a. anesthesia produced by the respiration of a volatile liquid or gaseous anesthetic agent. Halothane, methoxyflurane, isoflurane, and a combination of nitrous oxide and oxygen are the common agents in veterinary use.
insufflation a. anesthesia produced by introduction of a gaseous mixture into the trachea through a slender tube.
intrasynovial a. injection of a local anesthetic agent into a joint or tendon sheath.
intrathecal a. introduction of local anesthetic agent into the spinal fluid by penetration of the spinal dura. Causes anesthesia in the tissues supplied by the nerves in the spinal cord zone that has been anesthetized. There is danger of injury to the cord and the technique is litte used in veterinary surgery. Called also subarachnoid, subdural or intradural anesthesia/analgesia.
intravenous a. the anesthetic agent, e.g. a barbiturate, is administered intravenously to effect. If an intravenous catheter is used, 'topping-up' amounts can also be administered as required.
intravenous regional a. see BIER TECHNIQUE.
irreversible a. the loss of sensory and motor function of the part is permanent. The local injection of isopropyl alcohol has this effect.
local a. that produced in a limited area, as by injection of a local anesthetic or by freezing with ethyl chloride. Includes infiltration, nerve block, field block, surface, regional, retrograde regional, spinal, epidural.
mixed a. that produced by use of more than one anesthetic agent.
nerve block a. the anesthetic agent is deposited from a syringe and needle as close to the target nerve as possible. Several injections are often made if the landmarks for the location of the nerve are not outstanding.
obstetrical a. see OBSTETRICAL anesthesia.
open a. general inhalation anesthesia in which there is no rebreathing of the expired gases.
parasacral a. regional anesthesia produced by injection of a local anesthetic around the sacral nerves as they emerge from the sacral foramina.
paravertebral a. regional anesthesia produced by the injection of a local anesthetic around the spinal nerves at their exit from the spinal column, and outside the spinal dura.
parenteral a. anesthesia induced by the injection of the agent, either intravenously, intraperitoneally, subcutaneously or intramuscularly.
peripheral a. lack of sensation due to changes in the peripheral nerves.
permeation a. analgesia of a body surface produced by application of a local anesthetic, most commonly to the mucous membranes. Called also surface anesthesia.
rectal a. anesthesia produced by introduction of the anesthetic agent into the rectum.
refrigeration a. local anesthesia produced by applying a tourniquet and chilling the part to near freezing temperature. Called also cryoanesthesia.
regional a. insensibility caused by interrupting the sensory nerve conductivity of any region of the body: produced by (1) field block, encircling the operative field by means of injections of a local anesthetic; or (2) nerve block, making injections in close proximity to the nerves supplying the area.
saddle block a. the production of anesthesia in the region of the body corresponding roughly with the areas of the buttocks, perineum and inner aspects of the thighs, by introducing the anesthetic agent low in the dural sac.
segmental a. loss of sensation in a segment of the body due to a lesion of a nerve root.
spinal a. 1. anesthesia due to a spinal lesion. 2. anesthesia produced by injection of the agent beneath the membrane of the spinal cord.
splanchnic a. block anesthesia for visceral operation by injection of the anesthetic agent into the region of the celiac ganglia.
subarachnoid a. see intrathecal anesthesia (above).
surface a. the application of a local anesthetic agent in solution, as in eye drops, or as a jelly, cream or ointment. The use of cold materials which freeze the superficial layers of skin is not much used in veterinary surgery. See also permeation anesthesia (above).
surgical a. that degree of anesthesia at which operation may safely be performed. There is muscular relaxation, and coordinated movements, consciousness and pain sensations disappear; many of the spinal neuromuscular reflexes are abolished.
topical a. that produced by application of a local anesthetic directly to the area involved.

anesthesiologist a veterinarian or physician who specializes in anesthesiology.

anesthesiology that branch of veterinary medicine or medicine concerned with administration of anesthetics and the condition of the patient while under anesthesia.

anesthetic 1. pertaining to, characterized by, or producing anesthesia. 2. a drug or agent used to abolish the sensation of pain, to achieve adequate muscle relaxation during surgery, to calm fear and allay anxiety. See also ANESTHESIA.
dissociative a. an anesthetic causing interruption of cerebral association pathways between the limbic system and cortical system. It produces a catalepsy-like state, in which the patient feels dissociated from its environment, and marked analgesia. Ketamine, phencyclidine and tiletamine hydrochloride are examples.
gaseous a. inhalation anesthesia. Halothane and isoflurane are commonly used agents.
general a. see general ANESTHESIA.

a.-induced rhabdomyolysis see PORCINE stress syndrome.
inhalation a. gas or volatile liquid that produces general anesthesia when inhaled. The older agents, ether and cyclopropane, have been replaced by halothane, enflurane and isoflurane.
injectable a. sedative-hypnotic drugs produce anesthesia when administered in large doses. It can be administered intraperitoneally, but intravenous injection is much the most common route. Short-acting drugs, such as thiopentone, are used alone for very rapid procedures or for instrument examinations, or as induction for a longer term inhalation anesthetic. See also BARBITURATE. One anesthetic agent that is administered intramuscularly is ketamine.
irreversible a. the injection of a substance that destroys the peripheral nerve, e.g. ethyl or propyl alcohol.
local a. a drug that blocks nerve transmission in the nerves affected by the local presence of the drug. It may be applied topically, e.g. into the conjunctival sac, or by injection into tissues near the target nerve. Most local anesthetics are in the -caine series.
a. machine apparatus or equipment used to administer gaseous anesthetic agents; functions of the apparatus should include, 1. delivery of oxygen, 2. removal of carbon dioxide, 3. quantifiable delivery of anesthetic vapor or gas, and 4. capability of providing artificial respiration to the patient.
a. scavenging the use of any device to reduce the pollution of the air in surgeries caused by exhaled anesthetic gases. May be canisters of filtering material attached to the machine or suction lines at stragetic positions in the theater.
volatile a. see inhalation anesthetic (above).

anesthetist a person trained in administering anesthetics.

anesthetization production of anesthesia.

anestrum see ANESTRUS.

anestrus, anoestrus nonoccurrence of estrus so that the female is not sexually receptive at any time. See also no visible ESTRUS, silent ESTRUS.

anethole trithione a direct-acting salivary stimulant.

anetoderma looseness and atrophy of the skin.

aneuploidy the state of having chromosomes in a number that is not an exact multiple of the haploid number; seen in karyotypes which have a small number of extra chromosomes or have a small number less than normal.

aneurin, aneurine see THIAMIN.

aneurysm a sac formed by the localized dilatation of the wall of an artery, vein or the heart.
aortic a. see AORTIC aneurysm.
arteriovenous a. an abnormal communication between an artery and a vein in which the blood flows directly into a neighboring vein or is carried into the vein by a connecting sac.
atherosclerotic a. one arising as a result of weakening of the tunica media in severe atherosclerosis.
bacterial a. an infected aneurysm caused by bacteria.
berry a. a small saccular aneurysm of a cerebral artery, usually at the junction of vessels in the circle of Willis; such aneurysms frequently rupture, causing subarachnoid hemorrhage. Called also BRAIN aneurysm.
cardiac a. thinning and dilatation of a portion of the wall of the left ventricle, usually a consequence of myocardial infarction.
cirsoid a. dilatation and tortuous lengthening of part of an artery.
compound a. one in which some of the layers of the wall of the vessel are ruptured and some merely dilated. Called also mixed aneurysm.
congenital a. observed sporadically in the aorta and pulmonary artery.
dissecting a. one resulting from hemorrhage that causes lengthwise splitting of the arterial wall, producing a tear in the inner wall (intima) and establishing communication with the lumen of the vessel; it usually affects the thoracic aorta. Seen most commonly in horses and caused by larvae of *Strongylus vulgaris*. See STRONGYLOSIS. A specific disease of turkeys.
fusiform a. a spindle-shaped aneurysm.
infected a. one produced by growth of microorganisms (bacteria or fungi) in the vessel wall, or infection arising within a pre-existing arteriosclerotic aneurysm.
inherited aortic a. causes a high mortality rate in the affected cattle breed. The defect is in the abdominal aorta.
lung a. may result from the lodgement of pulmonary emboli; rupture and pulmonary hemorrhage are potential sequelae.
mixed a. compound aneurysm.
mycotic a. an infected aneurysm caused by fungi.
pseudoaneurysm false aneurysm.
racemose a. cirsoid aneurysm.
sacculated a. a saclike aneurysm.
varicose a. one formed by rupture of an aneurysm into a vein. See also aneurysmal VARIX.
venous a. see VENOUS dilatation.
verminous a. see STRONGYLOSIS.

aneurysmal pertaining to or arising from an aneurysm.
a. bone cyst see BONE cyst.

aneurysmectomy excision of an aneurysm.

aneurysmoplasty plastic repair of an artery for aneurysm.

aneurysmorrhaphy suture of an aneurysm; an intravascular graft insertion used to treat aneurysm.

ANF ATRIAL natriuretic factor.

anfractuous convoluted; sinuous.

angel-fish see SQUATINA SQUATINA.

angel wings a deformity of the scapulae seen with osteodystrophia fibrosa, particularly in kittens. The pull of the scapular muscles causes an outward bowing, hence the name.

angelfish see PTEROPHYLLUM, SQUATINA SQUATINA and Table 23.

angel's trumpet DATURA *candida brugmansia*.

angiectasis dilatation of a vessel.

angiectomy excision of part of a blood or lymph vessel.

angiitis inflammation of the coats of a vessel, chiefly blood or lymph vessels. Called also vasculitis. Local or generalized, the latter e.g. in hypersensitivity states.

angi(o)- word element. [Gr.] *vessel (channel)*.

angioblast 1. the earliest formative tissue from which blood cells and blood vessels arise. 2. an individual vessel-forming cell.

angioblastoma a term applied to certain blood-vessel tumors of the brain.

angiocardiogram the film produced by angiocardiography.

angiocardiography radiography of the heart and great vessels after introduction of an opaque contrast medium into a blood vessel or one of the cardiac chambers.

angiocardiokinetic pertaining to movements of the heart and blood vessels.

angiocardiopathy disease of the heart and blood vessels.
angiocarditis inflammation of the heart and blood vessels.
angiocentric see PERIVASCULAR.
angiodysplasia small vascular abnormalities, especially of the intestinal tract.
angioedema a condition characterized by the sudden and temporary appearance of large areas of painless swelling in the subcutaneous tissue or submucosa, with or without pruritus. Caused by immunological reactions, usually immediate type hypersensitivities. Sometimes referred to as angioneurotic edema.
hereditary a. in humans, the periodic occurrence of angioedema caused by a deficiency of the complement regulatory protein.
angioendothelioma see HEMANGIOENDOTHELIOMA.
angioendotheliomatosis a state marked by the development of multiple endotheliomas; the clinical syndrome which results varies with the location of the major lesions.
angiofibroma angioma containing fibrous tissue.
nasopharyngeal a. a relatively benign tumor of the nasopharynx composed of fibrous connective tissue with abundant endothelium-lined vascular spaces.
angiofollicular pertaining to a lymphoid follicle and its blood vessels.
angiogenesis the development of blood vessels.
tumor a. the induction of the growth of blood vessels from surrounding tissue into a solid tumor by a diffusible chemical factor released by the tumor cells.
angiogenic cord see angiogenic CORD.
angioglioma a form of vascular glioma.
angiogram a radiograph of a blood vessel.
angiograph a radiological demonstration of a blood vessel using a contrast medium. See ANGIOGRAPHY.
angiography radiological demonstration of certain areas of the vascular system by the injection of a radiopaque solution (arteriography, lymphangiography or phlebography).
brain a. radiography of the cranium after the intravenous injection of a radiopaque substance. An area of poor vascularity indicates the presence of a space-occupying lesion in the brain.
fluorescein a. intravenous fluorescein can be visualized in retinal and iris vasculature with the use of blue filters and direct or indirect ophthalmoscopy or photography. See also vitreous FLUOROPHOTOMETRY.
nonselective a. injection of contrast material into a regional vessel or the general circulation.
orbital a. contrast study of the arteries of the orbit, particularly the malar, infraorbital, maxillary and dorsal orbital, using the infraorbital artery for injection of a suitable medium.
pulmonary a. demonstration of pulmonary veins and arteries by introduction of contrast material into the jugular or cephalic vein or via a catheter positioned in the pulmonary artery.
renal a. outlines renal blood flow, usually via a catheter introduced into the femoral artery and passed retrograde into the aorta to the vicinity of the renal arteries.
selective a. placement of the catheter in the vessel or heart chamber being studied in order to provide the best possible contrast study of the suspected lesion.
angiohemophilia see VON WILLEBRAND'S DISEASE.
angiohyalinosis hyaline degeneration of the muscular coat of blood vessels.
angioid resembling blood vessels.
angiokeratoma a benign neoplasm of endothelial origin accompanied by epithelial hyperplasia. Rare in animals.
angiokinetic see VASOMOTOR.
angiolipoma angioma containing fatty tissue.
angiolith a calcareous deposit in the wall of a blood vessel.
angiology scientific study or description of the blood and lymph vessels.
systematic a. angiology of a single body system.
angiolysis retrogression or obliteration of blood vessels, as in embryological development.
angioma a benign tumor made up of blood (hemangioma) or lymph vessels (lymphangioma), e.g. hemangioma, lymphangioma, glomangioma.
a. cavernosum, cavernous a. disseminated cavernous HEMANGIOMA.
telangiectatic a. an angioma made up of dilated blood vessels.
angiomatosis the presence of multiple angiomas.
bovine cutaneous a. nodular vascular lesions in the skin, particularly along the back, occur in cattle. They may be inflamed and can bleed profusely.
juvenile bovine a. a condition in young calves characterized by multiple angioma in all tissues, sometimes by a single lesion.
retinal a. diseased retinal blood vessels with subretinal hemorrhages.
angiomegaly enlargement of blood vessels.
angiomyolipoma a benign tumor containing vascular, adipose and muscle elements, occurring most often in the kidney with smooth muscle elements.
angiomyoma a hamartoma composed of blood vessels and smooth muscle.
angiomyoneuroma see GLOMANGIOMA.
angiomyosarcoma angioma blended with myoma and sarcoma.
angioneurectomy excision of vessels and nerves.
angioneuroma see GLOMANGIOMA.
angioneuromyoma see GLOMANGIOMA.
angioneurosis any neurosis affecting primarily the blood vessels; a disorder of the vasomotor system, as angioparalysis, angiospasm.
angioneurotic edema see ANGIOEDEMA.
angiopathy any disease of the vessels.
angioplasty surgical repair of blood vessels or lymphatic channels.
percutaneous transluminal a. dilatation of a blood vessel by means of a balloon catheter inserted through the skin and into the chosen vessel and then passed through the lumen of the vessel to the site of the lesion, where the balloon is inflated to flatten plaque against the artery wall. Called also PCTA.
angiopoiesis the formation of blood vessels.
angiorrhaphy suture of a blood vessel.
angiosarcoma a malignant tumor of vascular tissue. Called also hemangiosarcoma, lymphangiosarcoma.
angiosclerosis hardening of the walls of blood vessels.
angiospasm spasmodic contraction of the walls of a blood vessel.
angiostrongyliasis infection by nematodes of the genus *Angiostrongylus*.
angiostrongylosis see ANGIOSTRONGYLIASIS.
Angiostrongylus a genus of worms of the family Angiostrongylidae.
A. cantonensis the rat lungworm which may cause eosinophilic meningitis in humans and other species including dogs.
A. costaricensis parasitizes the blood vessels of the alimentary tract of wild rodents and may infect humans causing eosinophilic granulomas in the intestine.
A. mackerrasae a rat lungworm which may also cause eosinophilic meningitis in humans.

A. vasorum the 'lungworm' of dogs; occurs in the pulmonary artery and right ventricle of dogs and foxes. Pulmonary emphysema and fibrosis may be accompanied by congestive heart failure.

angiotelectasis dilatation of blood vessels.

angiotensin a vasoconstrictive principle formed in the blood when RENIN is released from the juxtaglomerular apparatus in the kidney. The enzymatic action of renin cleaves a serum alpha$_2$-globulin, angiotensinogen, forming the decapeptide angiotensin I, which is relatively inactive. It in turn is acted upon by peptidases (converting enzymes), chiefly in the lungs, to form the octapeptide angiotensin II, a powerful vasopressor and a stimulator of aldosterone secretion by the adrenal cortex. By its vasopressor action, it raises blood pressure and diminishes fluid loss in the kidney by restricting blood flow. Angiotensin II is hydrolyzed in various tissues to form heptapeptide angiotensin III, which has less vasopressor activity but more effect on the adrenal cortex.

a. amide an amide derivative of angiotensin II which is a powerful vasoconstrictor and vasopressor, and is used in the treatment of certain hypotensive states; usually administered by slow intravenous infusion, and sometimes intramuscularly or subcutaneously.

a.-converting enzyme (ACE) a peptidase which catalyzes the formation of angiotensin II from angiotensin I. See also ACE.

angiotensinase any of a group of peptidases in plasma and tissues that inactivate angiotensin.

angiotensinogen a serum α_2-globulin secreted in the liver which, on hydrolysis by renin, gives rise to angiotensin.

angiotomy incision of a blood vessel or lymphatic channel.

angiotonic increasing vascular tension.

angiotribe a strong forceps for crushing tissue containing an artery, for the purpose of checking hemorrhage. See also FERGUSSON ANGIOTRIBE.

angiotripsy hemostasis by means of an angiotribe.

angiotrophic pertaining to the nutrition of vessels.

angitis see ANGIITIS.

angle the space or figure formed by two diverging lines, measured as the number of degrees one would have to be moved to coincide with the other.

cardiodiaphragmatic a. that formed by the junction of the shadows of the heart and diaphragm in radiographs.

costovertebral a. the angle formed on either side of the vertebral column between the last rib and the lumbar vertebrae.

filtration a. the angle between the iris and cornea at the periphery of the anterior chamber of the eye, through which the aqueous humor readily permeates. Called also angle of the iris.

glenoid a. the angle of the scapula at the glenoid cavity, or ventral end, of the bone. The cranial and caudal angles are at the dorsal border of the scapula.

a. of inclination see CERVICOFEMORAL ANGLE.

a. of jaw the junction of the ventral and caudal borders of the lower jaw.

nasofrontal a. see STOP.

oral lip a. angle of union of the oral lips. Called also commissura labiorum.

sole a. the angle formed by the inflection of the wall of the hoof to form the bars on the sole of the horse's foot. Called also angulus soleae medialis, lateralis.

angleberry see PAPILLOMA.

Anglo-Arab light horse produced by Arab-Thoroughbred first cross. Also later crosses and breeds derived from such crossbreeding.

Anglo-Nubian English breed of dairy goat. Mostly all black, but may be any color. Characterized by prominent roman nose and large drooped ears. Called also Nubian (USA).

Angora the ancient name of Ankara, Turkey, which has been given to particular breeds in several animal species probably originally to a longhaired cat that was believed to originate in Turkey, and later to the other species because of their long coat.

A. cat a fine-boned, longhaired breed, originally found in Turkey. The build is generally slimmer and longer than other longhaired types. The silky coat is usually white, but other colors have been developed. Called also Turkish Angora.

A. goat a horned, white variety of *Capra hircus,* the domestic and wild goats. Has a long silky haircoat of great commercial value as mohair.

A. rabbit a breed of meat- and fur-producing rabbit in two varieties, English and French. A striking-looking animal like a fluffy snowball with long, silky wool with tufts on the ears and feet. Color usually white but can be fawn, gray-blue or sable and with ruby-colored eyes.

angry cat posture a description sometimes used in reference to cats suffering from HYPERVITAMINOSIS A that crouch with low, rigid extension of the head and neck, arched back and tail sweeping the ground.

angstrom a nonsystematic unit of length equal to 10^{-10} meter or 0.1 nanometer; symbol Å.

Anguilla genus of farmed eels in the family Anguillidae; includes *A. anguilla* (European eel), *A. japonica* (Japanese eel). See also Table 23.

Anguillicola flukes of the swim bladder of eels; cause devastating losses in eels in Europe. Includes *A. australiensis, A. crassus, A. novaezeelandiae.*

Anguina lolii grass nematode that parasitizes grass seedheads and converts the seed into a gall. A toxin is produced when *Clavibacter toxicus* (*Corynebacterium raythi*) is present. The clinical effects are principally nervous ones especially incoordination, convulsions and death. The grasses susceptible to the worm are annual or Wimmera rye (*Lolium rigidum*) and Chewing's fescue (*Festuca rubra commutata*). Called also *Anguina agrostis, A. funesta.*

angular deformity deformity of limbs by angulation at joints or in the bones themselves. See also DIAPHYSEAL, METAPHYSEAL, EPIPHYSEAL dysplasia.

angular pea LATHYRUS *angulatus.*

angular zieria ZIERIA *laevigata.*

angulation 1. the formation of a sharp obstructive angle as in the intestine, the ureter or similar tubes. 2. in conformation, used to describe angles between long bones at joints, especially shoulder, stifle and hock.

angulus pl. *anguli* [L.] angle; used in names of anatomical structures or landmarks.

a. soleae see sole ANGLE.

Angus see ABERDEEN ANGUS, a breed of beef cattle.

anhidrosis absence of sweating. In horses the disease is common in tropical climates and seriously interferes with the racing calendar. Affected animals show respiratory distress even at rest, absence of sweating at times when all of the others in the group are sweating heavily; they are quite unable to race. Disease is akin to anhidrotic asthenia of humans. Called also puff disease, dry coat syndrome.

anhidrotic 1. checking the flow of sweat. 2. an agent that suppresses perspiration.

a. asthenia weight loss, dehydration and lassitude in animals introduced to tropical climates from a temperate area.

anhydrase an enzyme that catalyzes the removal of water from a compound.

carbonic a. a zinc-containing enzyme that catalyzes the decomposition of carbonic acid into carbon dioxide and water, facilitating transfer of carbon dioxide from tissues to blood and from blood to alveolar air. See also CARBONIC ANHYDRASE.

anhydration the condition of not being hydrated.

anhydremia diminution of the fluid content of the blood. See also DEHYDRATION.

anhydride a compound derived from an acid by removal of a molecule of water.

anhydrosis see ANHIDROSIS.

anhydrous containing no water.

a. lanolin the principal animal fat used in the preparation of ointments for animals. Now competes with synthetic materials such as polyethylene glycols.

Anichkov cell see ANITSCHKOW cell.

anideus a parasitic fetus consisting of a shapeless mass of flesh.

anidrosis see ANHIDROSIS.

anileridine an opioid used as an analgesic or sedative.

animal 1. a living organism having sensation and the power of voluntary movement and requiring for its existence oxygen and organic food. 2. of or pertaining to such an organism.

a. behavior any movement made by an animal, as a result of neurological reflexes, inherited traits, conditioned responses, physiological influences such as hormone levels, and psychological state. It is also influenced by the physical status of the animal.

a. bite a wound caused by the bite of an animal. See also animal BITE.

a. boarding establishments commercial places at which food and accommodation are provided for temporary animal residents at a daily or weekly tariff. They are usually required to be registered by a local government authority so that the premises can be inspected to ensure that the services provided avoid misconduct in terms of animal abuse or cruelty. See also BOARDING KENNELS.

a. breeds see under species and names of individual breeds.

a. capture may be by physical means using trap cages or corrals, nets or other devices, or by the use of chemical restraint. Immobilizing agents are injected into the animal by the use of syringes on long poles, or fired as projectiles from guns using compressed gases or explosive devices as propellants, or from crossbows. The constant problem is the avoidance of fatal capture MYOPATHY or exhaustion.

a. clinics conduct of an animal clinic per se by nonveterinarians would not be an offense under most veterinary statutes but conduct of veterinary practice in the premises by unregistered persons would be.

control a. an untreated animal otherwise identical in all respects to one that is used for purposes of experiment; used for checking results of treatment.

a. facilitated therapy the utilization of animals, usually companion pets, in the treatment or management of human problems, usually physical handicaps or psychiatric disorders. Acceptance of this form of therapy has widened in recent years and there are many examples of recent and current programs based on placement of animals in private homes or institutions such as prisons, nursing homes and hospitals. Although the benefits derived are difficult to assess, there is general agreement that morale and motivation of patients or inmates is improved as a result of these programs. Guide dogs for the blind, hearing dogs and horseback riding for the disabled are also sometimes included in this category.

a. feed food materials for animal consumption.

a. fight injuries encompass the wide variety of damage that can be done by teeth, horns, claws and hooves, usually complicated by infection.

a. food food for humans of animal origin or containing materials of animal origin. See also animal feed (above).

a. health insurance comparable to medical insurance in humans. The owner pays a premium in return for disease prevention and health maintenance services at reduced rates. Sometimes used to provide these services to an animal population in a country or state, e.g. Israel, Quebec.

a. health technician person other than a veterinarian trained in animal health techniques and bearing accredited qualifications.

a. housing see HOUSING.

a. identification see IDENTIFICATION.

a. improvement improvement in production efficiency by genetic means, principally by selection and cross-breeding, to a less extent by inbreeding, all facilitated by artificial insemination and embryo transfer.

a. insurance includes insurance against loss by death as a financial asset or against loss of function, especially with respect to reproduction in the case of a male animal. See also animal health insurance (above).

a. liberation a group of animal lovers with activist proclivities who oppose domination of animals by humans. In particular, the movement opposes animal experimentation and close confinement.

a. medicines must be labeled as being for animal use only. Their manufacture and sale is controlled by legislation in most countries. The objective is to protect the human population and the subject animals also.

a. models of human disease diseases of animals which are suitable models for diseases which occur in humans; often used for experimental studies.

a. nurses training programs lasting usually for two years of full-time study are available in most countries for aspiring animal nurses. The term veterinary nurse is used in some countries but avoided in others because of the confusion that it might cause in the minds of the public about who is qualified to do what. Animal nurses are qualified to assist veterinarians to perform ACTS OF VETERINARY SCIENCE.

a. nursing auxiliaries see animal nurses (above).

a. oil lard, whale oil, wool fat.

performing a. see PERFORMING ANIMALS.

a. pound see animal shelter (below).

a. protein protein for animal feed derived from abattoirs, meat-packing plants, fish processors, dairy manufacturers.

a. protein factor a term previously used for an unknown factor present in feeds of animal origin and necessary for growth in swine and poultry. Now known to be vitamin B_{12}. Called also APF.

a. rights a commonly held view is that animals have rights in much the same way as people do. There is no legal support for that view, other than that embodied in legislation dealing with matters of abuse.

a. shelter accommodation provided for and to maintain custody of discarded and unwanted pets, usually provided by animal welfare societies or local government authorities. An unpleasant corollary of this system is the euthanizing of large numbers of dogs and cats because the amount of accommodation is limited. Called also animal pound.

a. technician a person trained in the care of animals including feeding, breeding, housing, training, use, health maintenance. Oriented towards healthy animals in groups or institutions with a particular involvement with laboratory animals. See also animal nurses (above) who are oriented more towards sick animals.

a. use comparable to occupation in humans. Classifications include beef cattle, dairy cattle, dairy or milk goats, fiber goats, wool sheep, mutton or meat sheep, pleasure horse, draft horse, event horse, cattle dogs, companion dogs and so on.

a. welfare the avoidance of abuse and exploitation of animals by humans by maintaining appropriate standards of accommodation, feeding and general care, the prevention and treatment of disease and the assurance of freedom from harassment, and unnecessary discomfort and pain. A code of practice, aimed at owners and custodians, is necessary for each animal species. A more complex problem, which is still to be resolved, is that of infringement of animal rights in law.

Proper application of the principles of animal welfare includes the continuous surveillance of the environment that human beings provide for animals that are in their care, and the promotion of what are considered by the community to be adequate rewards to the animals for the contribution that they make to the physical and psychological well-being of humans.

a. welfare codes of practice rules for the care of animals which set out what is expected by the local community of persons who have animals in their care. Not a legal document but likely to be used as a guide by the courts. They specify feeding, housing, surgical alteration, transport and so on. See also CODE of practice/conduct.

animal husbandry the methods employed in keeping domestic animals in such a way as to avoid their abuse but so as to provide food, fiber, entertainment and company at levels described as love, companionship, physical guidance, protection, shepherding. In many instances the overriding constraint is that the maintenance system must be cost-effective so as to provide an occupation for the owner. In other circumstances the rewards are less tangible and come within the ambit of emotional gratification or psychological dependence. In more pragmatic terms the discipline includes nutrition, genetics and breeding, housing, handling facilities and techniques, hygiene, sanitation, health maintenance and disease prevention, marketing, preparation for contests, physical and psychological training, culling, management in times of drought or other civil disaster, use of animal experiments and codes of practice for the management and transport of various classes of animals.

a. h. advisors a profession which supplies advice to animal owners on matters of husbandry.

animal production the technology applied to the keeping of animals for profit. Includes feeding, breeding, housing and marketing. Of great importance is the making of the financial arrangements necessary to the successful carrying out of each enterprise in the light of the market conditions for the sale of the end products.

a. p. data include milk production, race times for distances, annual egg production weighted for age, clean wool yield, pig litter size, annual pigs weaned per sow. Includes raw data and analyzes of indexes used as measures of performance and as targets in production systems.

a. p. systems include the categories of extensive, ranch, irrigation, dryfarming, intensive, factory farming, pastoral, feedlot, permanent housing, breeding establishments, fattening farms, flying herds.

animal starch see GLYCOGEN.

anion an ion carrying a negative charge. In an electrolytic cell anions are attracted to the positive electrode (anode).

a.-exchange resin see ION-EXCHANGE RESIN.

anion gap method used to evaluate a patient's acid–base status; based on the observation that the sum of blood cations (sodium, potassium, chloride and bicarbonate ions) usually exceeds the sum of the anions (sulfates, phosphates, proteinates, organic acid ions); the difference between the two is the anion gap. Significant departure from the normal level of difference indicates acid–base disturbance.

aniridia congenital complete or partial absence of the iris. Occurs in Jersey calves as an autosomal recessive trait and causes visual impairment, ranging to blindness. May be associated with multiple anomalies such as microphakia and ectopiac lentis.

equine neonatal a. believed to be inherited as an autosomal recessive trait in Belgian horses; sometimes occurs in association with cataracts.

anisakiasis the disease in humans caused by infestation with one of the worms of the genus *Anisakis*. See also PHOCANEMA, TERRANOVA and CONTRACAECUM.

Anisakidae a family of nematode parasites of marine mammals, fish, birds, reptiles and, by accidental infestation, humans. See PHOCANEMA, TERRANOVA and CONTRACAECUM.

Anisakis a genus of nematodes that parasitize the stomachs of marine mammals; found most commonly in wild fish, rarely in cultured fish. Larval stages can cause disease in humans.

anise dried seeds of the plant *Pimpinella anisum* of the family Umbelliferae. Anise oil is extracted and used as a flavoring, as a carminative and in broiler feeding as an appetizer. Has an attraction for animals and sometimes used as a decoy in traps. See also ANISEED.

aniseed aromatic seed sometimes observed as a taint in meat. The taste is due to essential oils in the aniseed plant. See also ANISE.

aniseikonia retinal images in each eye are different sizes.

anis(o)- word element. [Gr.] *unequal.*

anisochromatic not of the same color throughout.

anisocoria unequal or asymmetric pupils.

prechiasmal a. mydriasis caused by disorders of the retina or optic nerve.

anisocytosis the presence in the blood of erythrocytes showing abnormal variations in size. Normal in some species, especially cattle.

anisogamy sexual conjugation in which the gametes differ in structure and size.

anisognathism a form of malocclusion in which the mandible is too narrow. See also narrow BASE.

anisokaryosis inequality in the size of the nuclei of cells.

anisomastia inequality in the size of the mammary glands.

anisopiesis difference in blood pressure recorded in corresponding arteries on the right and left sides of the body.

anisosthenic not having equal power; said of muscles.

anisotonic 1. varying in tonicity or tension. 2. having different osmotic pressure; not isotonic.

anisotropic 1. having unlike properties in different directions. 2. doubly refracting, or having a double polarizing power.

anisotropine an anticholinergic drug which produces relaxation of visceral smooth muscle, and is used as a spasmolytic in various gastrointestinal disorders. Called also octatropine.

anisotropy the quality of being anisotropic.

anisuria alternating oliguria and polyuria.

Anitschkow cell large mononuclear cells with an undulating, ribbon-like formation of nuclear chromatin. These 'caterpillar cells' are found in myocardium and thought to be macrophages or attempts at myofiber regeneration. Called also Anitschkow myocytes.

ankle a human anatomical term often applied to dogs when referring to the hock joint.

ankyl(o)- word element. [Gr.] *bent, crooked, in the form of a loop, adhesion, fixed.*

ankyloblepharon fusion of the eyelids to each other along the lid margins. Normal in the newborn of some species, lasting about 10 days in puppies and kittens. Delayed separation may occur.

ankylocheilia adhesion of the lips to each other.

ankyloglossia tongue-tie; abnormal shortness of the frenulum of the tongue, resulting in limitation of its motion.

a. superior extensive adhesion of the tongue to the palate.

ankylopoietic producing ankylosis.

ankylosed affected with ankylosis.

ankylosing caused by or emanating from fixation of the joint.

a. spondylitis see SPONDYLITIS.

a. spondylosis see SPONDYLOSIS.

ankylosis abnormal immobility and consolidation of a joint.

Ankylosis may be caused by destruction of the membranes that line the joint or by faulty bone structure. It is most often a result of chronic arthritis, in which the affected joint tends to assume the least painful position and may become more or less permanently fixed in it.

Artificial ankylosis (arthrodesis), locking of a joint by surgical operation, is sometimes done in treatment of a severe joint condition.

bony a. union of the bones of a joint by proliferation of bone cells, resulting in complete immobility.

extracapsular a. that caused by rigidity of surrounding parts.

false a., fibrous a. reduced joint mobility due to proliferation of fibrous tissue.

inherited multiple a. calves are affected at birth and cause fetal dystocia. The legs are bent and fixed in flexion, and there is some deformity of the spine. In one breed of cattle there is a combination of ankylosis and cleft palate.

intracapsular a. that caused by rigidity of structures within the joint.

spontaneous a. occurs in the intertarsal and tarsometatarsal joints of horses. Called also bone spavin.

spurious a. extracapsular ankylosis.

stapedial a. fixation of the footplate of the stapes in otosclerosis, causing a conductive hearing loss.

surgical a. performed to immobilize a painful joint or to correct excessive mobility, e.g. carpal ankylosis carried out on large birds as a deflighting procedure.

true a. bony ankylosis.

ankylosis–cleft palate combined defect suspected inherited defect in Charolais cattle.

ankylotia closure of the external meatus of the ear.

ankyroid hooklike; like the fluke of an anchor.

anlage pl. *anlagen* [Ger.] primordium.

annectent connecting; joining together.

annelid a member of the phylum ANNELIDA.

Annelida a phylum of metazoan invertebrates, the segmented worms, including leeches.

annelloconidium conidia that develop from extruded end of a conidiophore as by the fungi *Scopulariopsis* spp.

annual conducted once each year.

a. annuity the present value of a series of equal payments paid annually.

a. beard grass POLYPOGON MONSPELIENSIS.

a. cumulative stress the accumulated stresses for the year from all sources including geographic, climatic, predation, pollution and the like.

a. goldeneye VIGUIERA ANNUA.

a. livestock calendar a calendar setting out the cardinal events and tasks for the year for the relevant farming enterprise, e.g. a beef breeding calendar.

a. mercury MERCURIALIS *annua*.

a. ryegrass see LOLIUM *rigidum*.

a. saltbush ATRIPLEX *muelleri*.

annular ring-shaped.

a. dermatitis inflammation and crusting in an annular pattern is characteristic of dermatophytosis (ringworm), particularly in pigs.

a. vessel of eye a loop of the hyaloid artery which encircles the margin of the optic cup during development of the eye.

annulate lamellae structures identical to cell membranes, occurring singly or stacked in groups, in the cellular cytoplasm. Their function is unknown.

annuloplasty plastic repair of a cardiac valve.

annulorrhaphy suture of a hernial ring.

annulospiral endings afferent nerve endings innervating the equators of muscle fibers.

annulus, anulus pl. *annuli, anuli* [L.] a small ring or encircling structure.

atrioventricular a. a ring of Purkinje cells around the right A-V orifice that serves the myocardium and valves locally and also serves as an alternative connection between the atria and the ventricles.

fibrocartilaginous a. the circular pad which connects the tympanic membrane to the external acoustic meatus.

annuli fibrosi 1. four fibrous rings at the base of the heart to which the myocardium is attached, one around each A-V orifice and one each around the aorta and the pulmonary artery. 2. the intervertebral disks consist of a soft central pulpy nucleus and a peripheral annulus fibrosus.

a. iridis the iris consists of two rings, an inner smooth annulus iridus minoris, and an outer plicated part, the annulus iridis major.

a. preputialis the ring of skin marking the entrance to the cavity of the prepuce.

a. sclerae a roll of connective tissue on the inside of the sclera at the corneoscleral junction.

spermatic a. a small ring condenses around the proximal centriole of the spermatid.

a. vaginalis the ring through which the peritoneal cavity connects with the cavity of the vaginal tunic.

Anoa a small, 3 ft high buffalo of the Celebes. Called also *Anoa depressicornis*, dwarf buffalo.

Anocentor see DERMACENTOR.

anococcygeal pertaining to the anus and coccyx.

anode the positive electrode or pole to which negative ions are attracted.

The stationary anode in an x-ray tube is a solid bar

of copper with an inset of tungsten on the face of the bar opposite the cathode filament. The tungsten target has a high melting point to withstand the intense heat of the x-ray beam—the copper conducts the heat away.

a.-film distance see focal-film DISTANCE.

rotating a. an x-ray tube in which the anode rotates when x-rays are being produced. This means that there is a larger effective target surface of the anode which can be available to generate x-rays.

stationary a. a non-rotating anode in an x-ray tube so that the target surface is comparatively small.

anodontia congenital absence of some or all of the teeth. See also PSEUDOANODONTIA.

anodyne 1. relieving pain. 2. a medicine that eases pain.

anodynia freedom from pain.

anoestrus see ANESTRUS.

anogenital relating to the region of the anus and the genitalia, especially the external genitalia.

a. cleft congenital anomaly in which there is a common opening for anus and genital tract, as in a cloaca.

a. distance physical distance between anus and the genitalia (base of the genital tubercle in the fetus); used to discriminate between the sexes in the neonates in some species, especially cats and guinea pigs.

a. papilloma see anogenital warts (below).

a. raphe line of union between the two halves of the perineum.

a. warts papillomas transmitted venereally. Caused by the papilloma virus. Esthetically unattractive but generally cause little inconvenience.

anomalad a term proposed to designate a single, localized anomaly occurring during morphogenesis, together with the pattern of subsequent morphological defects that stem from it.

anomalous atrioventricular excitation Wolff–Parkinson–White syndrome.

anomaly marked deviation from normal. For specific anomalies see under anatomical location.

developmental a. absence, deformity or excess of body parts as the result of faulty development of the embryo.

lethal a. a defect which is incompatible with life and leads to the natural death or euthanasia on humane grounds of the neonate concerned.

sex-limited a. limited in its occurrence by the sex of the neonate, e.g. cryptorchidism.

sex-linked a. the gene responsible for the defect is located on the X or the Y chromosome, the sex determinative ones.

anomer one of two stereoisomers (designated α or β) of the furanose or pyranose form of a sugar, e.g. α-D-glucose. α-forms have –OH group of the anomeric carbon below the plane of the furanose or pyranose ring.

anonychia absence of the nails.

anophagia see APHAGIA.

Anopheles a genus of the Culicidae family of mosquitoes which may carry filarioid worm microfilariae.

anopheline pertaining to the ANOPHELES genus of mosquitoes.

Anophryocephalus ochotensis a tapeworm of the Californian sealion.

anophthalmia, anophthalmos a developmental anomaly marked by complete absence of one or both eyes or the presence of rudimentary eyes. Occurs most commonly in pigs and sheep.

anoplasty plastic repair of the anus.

Anoplocephala a genus of the tapeworm family of Anoplocephalidae. Includes *A. magna* (horses, donkeys), *A. perfoliata* (horses).

Anoplocephaloides a genus of the tapeworm family Anoplocephalidae. Includes *A. mammillana* found in the small intestine of the horse. Heavy infestations may cause unthriftiness.

Anoplotaenia dasyuri a metacestode found in heart, lungs and skeletal muscles of the Australian marsupials, wallabies and pademelons.

Anoplura lice suborder of sucking lice; includes *Haematopinus*, *Linognathus*, *Solenoptes* spp.

anorchid an uncastrated male animal without testes.

unilateral a. an animal with one testis missing.

anorchidism, anorchism the state of being an anorchid.

anorectal pertaining to, emanating from or affecting the ANORECTUM.

a. abscess see PERIANAL fistula.

a. anastomosis surgical resection of rectal neoplasms may require removal of a bowel segment and subsequent union of rectum to skin.

anorectic 1. pertaining to anorexia. 2. an agent that diminishes the appetite for food.

anorectum the distal portion of the digestive tract, including the entire anal canal and the distal few centimeters of the rectum.

anorexia lack or loss of appetite for food. Appetite is psychological, dependent on memory and associations, as compared with hunger, which is physiologically aroused by the body's need for food. Anorexia can be brought about by unattractive food, surroundings, or the presence of other animals. The existence of appetite in animals is assumed. For strictest accuracy the words aphagia, anophagia, etc. should be used but common usage includes anorexia, hyperorexia, etc. Called also inappetence.

anorexia–cachexia complex seen in association with advanced neoplasia; caused by reduced caloric intake, hypermetabolism and altered metabolism of glucose and protein synthesis.

anorexic anorectic.

anorexigenic 1. producing anorexia. 2. an agent that diminishes or controls the appetite.

anorthosis absence of penile erectility.

anoscope a speculum or endoscope used in direct visual examination of the anal canal.

anoscopy examination of the anal canal with an anoscope.

anosigmoidoscopy endoscopic examination of the anus and distal colon.

anosmatic having no sense of smell.

anosmia absence of the sense of smell; characteristic of lesions of the olfactory lobe, peduncle or mucosa. Such deficiencies are difficult to assess in animals.

anospinal pertaining to the anus and spinal cord.

anostosis defective formation of bone.

anotia congenital absence of the external ears.

anova see analysis of VARIANCE.

anovaginal pertaining to or communicating with the anus and vagina.

anovarism absence of the ovaries.

anovesical pertaining to the anus and bladder.

anovular not associated with ovulation.

anovulation failure to ovulate. The animal may show signs of estrus but the ovum is not shed and fertilization does not take place. This sequence of events can be observed by rectal examination in the cow and mare and by peritoneoscopy in smaller species.

anovulatory pertaining to anovulation.

a. follicular cyst see cystic FOLLICLE.

a. luteinized cyst the theca undergoes luteinization when the follicle fails to ovulate.
a. ovarian cysts see cystic OVARIAN disease.
anovulvar cleft see ANOGENITAL cleft.
anovulvitis see ULCERATIVE dermatosis.
anoxemia lack of sufficient oxygen in the blood.
anoxia absence of oxygen in the tissues; often used interchangeably with *hypoxia* to mean a reduction of oxygen in body tissues below physiological levels. The condition is accompanied by deep respirations, cyanosis, increased pulse rate and impairment of coordination.
anemic a. reduction of oxygen in body tissues because of diminished oxygen-carrying capacity of the blood.
anoxic a. reduction of oxygen in body tissues due to interference with the oxygen supply.
histotoxic a. condition resulting from diminished ability of cells to utilize available oxygen.
stagnant a. condition due to interference with the flow of blood and its transport of oxygen.
ANP atrial natruretic peptide.
Anredera cordifolia a poisonous plant of the family Basellaceae; causes diarrhea. Called also *Boussingaultia* spp., lamb's tail, Madeira vine.
Anrep phenomenon the increase in ventricular volume that results when aortic resistance is increased.
ansa pl. *ansae* [L.] a looplike structure.
a. axillaris a loop between the musculocutaneous nerve and the median nerve.
a. cardiaca a loop of muscle that passes around the dorsal margin of the cardia and forms the margins of the reticular groove in ruminants. It is an essential part of the closing of the cardia.
a. cervicalis a nerve loop attached to the hypoglossal nerve and to the first two or three cervical spinal nerves.
a. coli the loops of the colon including the distal, proximal and spiral loops.
a. distalis a loop of the colon of ruminants that succeeds the spiral colon.
a. of Henle Henle's loop.
a. hypoglossi ansa cervicalis.
a. lenticularis a loop of nerve fibers that connects the globus pallidus with parts of the thalamus and midbrain.
a. nervorum spinalium loops of spinal nerves joining the ventral spinal nerves.
a. peduncularis a complex grouping of nerve fibers connecting the amygdaloid nucleus, piriform area, and anterior hypothalamus, and various thalamic nuclei.
a. proximalis a loop of the colon of ruminants that precedes the spiral colon.
a. sigmoidea the s-shaped curve of the proximal duodenum as it passes over the visceral surface of the liver of the horse, ruminants and pig.
a. spiralis the double loop of colon made up of centripetal and centrifugal coils and a central flexure that run in a vertical plane in ruminants and in a snail-like coil in pigs.
a. subclavia the loop made by the cervical sympathetic trunk as it divides to pass on either side of the subclavian artery at the thoracic inlet.
Anser a genus of birds in the family Anseriformes.
A. anser domestic geese and wild geese.
anseriform, anserine said of birds; refers to ducks, geese, swans, members of the order Anseriformes.
anserine see ANSERIFORM.
anserini see ANSERIFORM.
ant ubiquitous insects, which, among other things, act as intermediate hosts for the trematode *Dicrocoelium dendriticum* and cestodes *Raillietina* spp.
a. bite conjunctivitis recorded in calves and recumbent animals attacked by fire ants (*Solenopsis invicta*).
ant bush SENNA *occidentalis*.
antacid 1. counteracting acidity. 2. an agent that counteracts acidity. Substances that act as antacids include sodium bicarbonate, aluminum hydroxide gel, magnesium hydroxide, magnesium trisilicate, magnesium oxide and calcium carbonate. They are often used in humans in the treatment of PEPTIC ulcer.
antagonism 1. opposition or contrariety between similar things, as between muscles, medicines or organisms, cf. ANTIBIOSIS; the characteristic displayed by an ANTAGONIST. 2. epidemiologically speaking, the opposite of synergism. When the combined effects of two factors is smaller than the effect of any one of them.
antibiotic a. is said to occur when the antibiotic effect of a dual administration is less than the antibiotic efficiency of the most effective of the individual drugs. Chloramphenicol and tetracyclines are considered to be antagonists to penicillins and aminoglycosides but particular combinations do not necessarily have the same effect on all bacteria.
competitive a. the antagonism which blocks or reverses the effects of an agonist, provided that the antagonist is given at an appropriate dosage. The antagonism is completely reversible, and an increase in the biophasic concentration of the agonist will overcome the effect of the antagonist.
drug a. drug antagonists are drugs that compete for the available receptors. They may be noncompetitive and have no pharmacological effect of their own, or competitive in that they are capable of reversing or altering an effect already achieved.
noncompetitive a. is when the antagonist removes the receptor or its response potential from the system; this may be by preventing the agonist from producing its effect at a receptor site by irreversible change to the receptor or its capacity to respond. The antagonism is not reversible by increasing the concentration of the agonist.
antagonist 1. a muscle that counteracts the action of another muscle, its agonist. 2. a drug that binds to a cellular receptor for a hormone, neurotransmitter, or another drug blocking the action of that substance without producing any physiological effect itself. 3. a tooth in one jaw that articulates with one in the other jaw. See also ANTAGONISM.
antalgic 1. counteracting or avoiding pain, as a posture or gait assumed so as to lessen pain. 2. analgesic.
Antarctophthirus a genus of the insect family Echinophthiriidae, lice which infest pinnipeds, e.g. sealions. Includes *A. microchir*.
antarthritic 1. alleviating arthritis. 2. an agent that alleviates arthritis.
antazoline a histamine H_1-receptor antagonist, commonly used topically in eye and nose drops.
ante [L.] preposition, *before*.
ante- word element. [L.] *before* (in time or space).
ante cibum [L.] *before meals;* usually abbreviated a.c. in prescriptions, etc.
ante mortem [L.] *before death*. See ANTEMORTEM.
anteater 1. giant anteater, see EDENTATE. 2. spiny anteater, see ECHIDNA.
antebrachial pertaining to the forearm.
a. growth abnormalities premature closure of a physeal plate, usually caused by trauma, in one bone of the forearm, while growth continues in the other may result in uneven growth and often angular or rotational deformities.

antebrachiocarpal see Table 11; pertaining to the joint between the forearm and carpus. Called also proximal carpal or radiocarpal joint.

antebrachium the forearm. Although the terms arm and forearm do not have common clinical usage relating to animals they are accepted anatomical terms.

antecedent a precursor.

plasma thromboplastin a. PTA; clotting factor XI. See plasma THROMBOPLASTIN antecedent.

Antechinus stuartii free-living macropod in which all males die at the end of the mating season each year.

antecubital situated in front of the cubitus, or elbow.

antecurvature a slight anteflexion.

antefebrile preceding fever.

anteflexion the bending of an organ so that its top is thrust forward.

antegrade performed in the normal direction of flow.

antelope member of the family Bovidae, including the genus *Tragelaphus*, which contains many genera of African antelopes. Includes a large variety of hollow-horned ruminants from dog to cow size. Many types of horns but all simple and persistent.

antelope grass ECHINOCHLOA *pyramidalis*.

antemetic antiemetic.

antemortem performed or occurring before death.

a. handling the management of animals about to be slaughtered for the period immediately prior to slaughter; includes transport, unloading, feeding, watering, housing. Animal welfare considerations are paramount.

a. inspection inspection of live animals prior to slaughter to ensure adherence to rules about cruelty, and to avoid putting sick or harassed animals into the abattoir buildings and the slaughter chain, The objective is to avoid contamination of premises and meat by infective material.

antenatal before parturition. Called also prenatal, antepartal.

antenna one of the appendages on the head of arthropods.

antepartal occurring before the young is born.

a. paralysis see antepartum PARALYSIS.

a. recumbency inability to rise, without other signs, during the last one or two weeks of pregnancy is observed in cows and rarely other species. Thought to be due to pressure of fetus on peripheral nerve supply to hindlimbs. Cesarean section is the preferred and satisfactory treatment.

antepartum performed or occurring before parturition.

antephase the portion of interphase immediately preceding mitosis (or meiosis) when energy is being produced and stored for mitosis (or meiosis) and chromosome reproduction is taking place.

antepubic see PREPUBIC.

antepyretic occurring before the stage of fever.

anterioposterior a term describing the entry of the x-ray beam anteriorly and its exit posteriorly on the patient. Used to describe the view taken in an x-ray. Now referred to as CRANIOCAUDAL.

anterior situated at or directed toward the front; opposite of posterior. In quadrupeds the use of the term is limited to parts of the head but is often used to mean cranially. In bipeds such as humans it is synonymous with ventral.

a. abdomen pain elicited pain in the anterior abdomen caused, in cattle, by reticulitis, hepatic or splenic abscess, abomasal ulcer and intestinal obstruction.

a. chamber the part of the eyeball between the cornea and the iris, filled with aqueous humor.

a. chamber angle see IRIDOCORNEAL angle.

a. compartment chamber of the eye bounded by the iris and cornea; contains the aqueous humor as it moves to the filtration angle; called also anterior chamber.

a. cruciate ligament see cranial (anterior) CRUCIATE ligament.

a. (cranial) drawer sign cranial, nonrotary movement of the proximal tibia in relation to the distal femur. Normally restricted by the cranial (anterior) cruciate ligament and used as a diagnostic test for rupture of that structure.

a. epithelial layer of the cornea is a non-cornified, stratified, squamous epithelium, continuous with the bulbar conjunctival epithelium.

a. functional stenosis achalasia of the reticulo-omasal sphincter causing ingesta to accumulate in the reticulorumen.

a. limiting membrane of the cornea is a combination of the basement membrane, a felted layer of fine collagen fibers; substantial only in primates.

a. pituitary see ADENOHYPOPHYSIS.

a. pituitary hormones see ADENOHYPOPHYSIS.

a. station trypanosomes a section of the genus *Trypanosoma* in which the infectious stages accumulate in the mouthparts and salivary glands of the intermediate host so that the parasite is transmitted when the insect vector takes a blood meal. Called also *Salivaria*. See also POSTERIOR station trypanosomes.

a. vena cava see VENA cava.

anterior-posterior anterioposterior.

antero- word element. [L.] *anterior, in front of.*

anterograde extending or moving forward.

anteroinferior situated in front and below.

anterolateral situated in front and to one side.

anteromedian situated in front and on the midline.

anteroposterior see CRANIOCAUDAL.

anterosuperior situated in front and above.

anteverted tipped or bent forward.

anthelix a low transverse ridge across the medial wall of the first part of the ear canal. The bend in the pinna of lop-eared dogs occurs distal to the anthelix.

anthelminthic anthelmintic.

anthelmintic 1. destructive to worms. 2. an agent destructive to worms. They are classified as antinematicidal, antitrematicidal, anticesticidal.

a. poisoning see under individual anthelmintics.

a. resistance frequent dosing of animals, especially ruminants running at pasture, selectively retains worms with innate resistance to a particular anthelmintic. A population of resistant worms may result. The resistant worm population may be transmitted to other farms. Side resistance to other compounds in the same chemical group may occur. This is observed in the benzimidazole group of compounds and in the levamisole-morantel group.

anthelone E see ENTEROGASTRONE.

Anthemis cotula plant of the Asteraceae (Compositae) family of plants; reported to cause (1) hydrocyanic acid poisoning; (2) irritation to mucosae because of the presence of an acrid substance; (3) milk taint. Called also mayweed.

Anthericum erraticum TRACHYANDRA *laxa*.

Anthochaera carunculata large Australian honeyeater susceptible to thiamine deficiency in urban environments; signs include convulsions, opisthotonos. Called also red wattle bird.

anthocyanin red-colored agent in fruit.

Anthoxanthum odoratum a temperate zone grass which contains coumarin. Called also sweet vernal grass. Moldy hay made from the grass is likely to cause DICOUMAROL poisoning.

Anthozoa a class of predatory marine creatures in the phylum Cnidaria (previously Coelenterata). Includes sea anemones, corals and sea pens.

anthracene a crystalline hydrocarbon, $C_{14}H_{10}$, from coal tar.

anthracic pertaining to or resembling anthrax.

anthracoid resembling anthrax.

anthracosis heavy black deposits of carbon; a common necropsy finding in dogs which have passed a busy working life in a heavily industrialized city.

anthracycline a class of antibiotics isolated from cultures of *Streptomyces peucetius*; it includes the antineoplastic agents daunomycin and doxorubicin. See also anthracycline ANTIBIOTIC.

anthraquinone a derivative of anthracene, a dyestuff. Its derivatives, found in aloes, cascara sagrada, senna and rhubarb, act as cathartics. See also DANTHRON.

anthrax a peracute disease of all animal species, caused by *Bacillus anthracis*, and characterized by septicemia and sudden death. The causative bacteria form long-living spores which maintain the disease on a farm for many years. Significant necropsy findings include exudation of dark, tarry blood from the body orifices, failure of the blood to clot, absence of rigor mortis and splenomegaly. A dangerous zoonosis. Easily controlled by vaccination of livestock.

a. belt regions where anthrax is enzootic, where soil and climate favor persistence of the organism in soil and where routine efforts to control the disease are not sufficient.

cutaneous a. anthrax due to lodgment of the causative organisms in wounds or abrasions of the skin, producing a black crusted pustule on a broad zone of edema. A common form of the disease in humans.

pulmonary a. infection of the respiratory tract resulting from inhalation of dust or animal hair containing spores of *Bacillus anthracis;* an occupational disease of humans usually affecting those who handle and sort wools and fleeces (woolsorters' disease).

anthropo- word element. [Gr.] *human being.*

anthropobiology the biological study of humans and the anthropoid apes.

anthropocentric with a human bias; considering humans to be the center of the universe.

anthropoid resembling humans; the anthropoid apes are tailless apes, including the chimpanzee, gibbon, gorilla and orang-utan; members of the family Pongidae.

Anthropoidea a suborder of primates, including monkeys, apes and humans, characterized by a larger and more complicated brain than the other suborders. They are members of the ape family Pongidae. Closest to humans in development having a well-developed brain, no tail and an upright stance. Includes gibbons, orang-utans, gorillas and chimpanzees.

Anthropoides virgo demoiselle crane.

anthroponoses diseases of humans, transmissible from humans to lower animals.

anthropophilic preferring human beings to animals; said of certain mosquitoes and fungi.

anthropozoonosis a disease of either animals or humans that may be transmitted from one species to the other.

anthropozoophilic attracted to both human beings and animals; said of certain mosquitoes.

anti- word element. [Gr.] *counteracting, effective against.*

anti-invasion factor chondroplasts and chondrocytes secrete an anti-invasion factor.

antiabortifacient an agent that prevents abortion or promotes successful gestation.

antiadrenergic 1. sympatholytic: opposing the effects of impulses conveyed by adrenergic postganglionic fibers of the sympathetic nervous system. 2. an antiadrenergic agent.

a. drugs include ADRENERGIC blocking agents, both alpha- and beta-blockers, and adrenergic neuron-blocking drugs and catecholamine depleting agents.

antiagglutinin a substance that opposes the action of an agglutinin.

antiamebic 1. destroying or suppressing the growth of amebae. 2. an agent that destroys or suppresses the growth of amebae.

antianaphylaxis a condition in which the anaphylaxis reaction does not occur because of free antigens or an excess of circulating antibodies, particularly IgG to the sensitizing antigen in the blood; the state of desensitization to antigens.

antiandrogen any substance capable of inhibiting the biological effects of androgenic hormones.

antianemic counteracting anemia.

a. drugs includes iron preparations, androgenic–anabolic steroids and vitamin–mineral mixtures.

antiantibody a substance that counteracts the effect of an antibody.

antianxiety dispelling anxiety. The term *antianxiety agent* (called also an anxiolytic or minor tranquilizer) refers to a mild sedative, such as diazepam (Valium).

antiarrhythmic 1. preventing or alleviating cardiac arrhythmias. 2. an agent that prevents or alleviates cardiac arrhythmias.

a. drugs include quinidine, procainamide, lidocaine, beta-adrenergic blockers such as propranolol, autonomic drugs including atropine and epinephrine, and digitalis.

antiarthritic 1. effective in treatment of arthritis. 2. an agent used in treatment of arthritis.

antibabesials drugs which are effective against red blood cell parasites of the genus *Babesia*. Older drugs are trypan blue and quinuronium. Modern treatments are aromatic diamidines and carbanilides such as imidocarb, amicarbalide, Berenil (Ganaseg) and phenamidine.

antibacterial 1. destroying or suppressing the growth or reproduction of bacteria. 2. an agent having such properties.

a. agents drugs that destroy or inhibit the growth of bacteria in concentrations that are safe for the host and can be used as chemotherapeutic agents to prevent or treat bacterial infections.

a. resistance consists of genetic factors, hormone levels, nutritional status, tissue enzymes, complement, interferon and immune mechanisms.

a. sensitivity test see ANTIMICROBIAL sensitivity test.

a. withdrawal time the period that must elapse after treatment with an antibacterial agent ceases before the animal or its products can be marketed. Veterinarians who practice food animal medicine have a great responsibility to ensure that food of animal origin complies with pure food laws relating to their acceptable levels of drug residues. Drugs not registered for animal use should not be used and, for those that are, the legal withdrawal times must be observed.

antibechic 1. relieving cough. 2. an agent that relieves cough.

antibiogram antibiotic sensitivity report.

antibiosis an association between two populations of organisms that is detrimental to one of them, or between one organism and an antibiotic produced by another.

antibiotic 1. destructive of life. 2. a chemical substance produced by a microorganism that has the capacity, in dilute solutions, to kill (biocidal activity) or inhibit the growth (biostatic activity) of other microorganisms. Antibiotics that are sufficiently nontoxic to the host are used as chemotherapeutic agents in the treatment of infectious diseases. See also ANTIMICROBIAL. 3. used as feed additives to animals as GROWTH promotants.

anthracycline a's a group of antibiotics which have a tetracycline ring structure substituted with the sugar daunosamine. Includes the antineoplastic drugs doxorubicin and daunorubicin.

antineoplastic a. see ANTINEOPLASTIC.

bactericidal a. one that kills bacteria.

bacteriostatic a. one that suppresses the growth of bacteria.

broad-spectrum a. one that is effective against a wide range of bacteria.

a. detection on-farm and prepackaged laboratory tests available for testing farm products and animal tissues and fluids for antibiotic residues.

a. drugs the range includes the following groups: PENICILLIN, AMINOGLYCOSIDE, TETRACYCLINE, CHLORAMPHENICOL, MACROLIDE, NITROFURAN, CEPHALOSPORINS, and a miscellaneous group including BACITRACIN, TYROTHRICIN, POLYMYXIN, COLISTIN.

a. feed additives see FEED additives.

first generation a. one produced as a natural product, e.g. penicillin G. See second generation antibiotic (below).

a. food preservation is a satisfactory technique but very strictly controlled because of the problem of residues in the food. Used mostly for the preservation of fish.

a.-induced diarrhea see pseudomembranous COLITIS, acute undifferentiated DIARRHEA of the horse.

a. residue in food in human food of animal origin is a seriously regarded pollution in public health surveillance. The residues may arise from systemic administration, or even after absorption from a local site such as the uterus, but the most serious contamination arises from milk from quarters that have been treated for mastitis. It is essential for the safety of the human population, the financial well-being of the farmer and the professional reputation of the veterinarian that ANTIBACTERIAL withdrawal times are observed.

a. resistance see ANTIMICROBIAL resistance.

second generation a. produced by manipulation of the molecular structure of a first generation antibiotic (see above) so that the metabolism and pharmacodynamics of the original compound are significantly altered.

a. sensitivity test see ANTIMICROBIAL sensitivity test.

a. therapy antibiotics vary in their absorption from the alimentary tract, requiring some, e.g. streptomycin, to be given parenterally for systemic effect, freedom from toxicity, the range of bacteria against which they are effective, their capacity to stimulate resistance and whether they are bacteriostatic or bactericidal in their effects. Selection of the most suitable antibiotic to suit a particular circumstance may be guided by an ANTIMICROBIAL sensitivity test, knowledge of the infection present and the price of the drug. In many instances, because of lack of knowledge of the infection present it is necessary to choose an agent with a broad antibacterial spectrum.

a. withdrawal see ANTIBACTERIAL withdrawal time.

antibody specialized serum proteins produced by B lymphocytes in response to an immense number of different antigens (>10^7) to which an animal may be exposed. Antibody produced by a particular antigen combines with that antigen only. The exquisite specificity of Ab for the antigen that stimulated its production is the basis for all antibody–antigen reactions both in vivo and in vitro. Antibodies are heterodimers composed of two light (L) and two heavy (H) chain polypeptide molecules. The amino termini of the L and H chains have a variable amino acid sequence V_L and V_H. The specificity of Ab for Ag is conferred by the V_L and V_H domains. There are five major classes of antibody, designated IgG, IgM, IgA, IgD and IgE. Abbreviated Ab or Ig. Called also IMMUNOGLUBULIN or gamma globulin. See also IMMUNITY.

affinity purification of a. see IMMUNOFILTRATION.

anaphylactic a. antibody, usually IgE, formed after the first injection of certain allergens and responsible for the signs of anaphylaxis following subsequent exposures to the same allergen.

a.–antigen reaction the specific combination of antigen with homologous antibody resulting in the reversible formation of antibody–antigen complexes that differ in composition according to the antibody–antigen ratio. See also ANTIGEN.

antinuclear a. (ANA) autoantibodies directed against components of the cell nucleus, e.g. DNA, RNA and histones; they may be detected by immunofluorescence. A positive ANA test is characteristic of systemic lupus erythematosus, Sjögren's syndrome and rheumatoid arthritis.

anti-idiotype a. antibodies against the antibody variable region.

anti-immunoglobulin a. those produced against an immunoglobulin, often used as reagents to study immunoglobulin molecules.

antiplatelet a. see ANTIPLATELET antibody.

antispermatozoal a. produced following entry of sperm into the bloodstream, e.g. following rupture of the epididymis as in *Brucella ovis* infections.

blocking a. circulating antibody (usually IgG) that reacts preferentially with an antigen, preventing it from reacting with a cell-bound antibody (IgE) and blocking the induction of anaphylaxis.

a. classes see IMMUNOGLOBULIN.

clonotypic a. clone specific antibody.

cold-reacting a. see cold AGGLUTININ.

complement-fixing a. immunoglobulins of the IgG or IgM class which bind complement.

cross-reacting a. one that combines with an antigen other than, but structurally related to, the one that induced its production.

cytophilic a. cytotropic antibody (below).

cytotoxic a. that which binds antigens expressed on the cell surface, which may (a) activate the complement pathway or (b) activate killer cells, resulting in cell lysis.

cytotropic a. those that attach to tissue cells (such as IgE to mast cells and basophils) that have an Fc receptor.

a.-dependent cell-mediated cytotoxicity (ADCC) a cytotoxic reaction in which nonsensitized cells bearing Fc receptors recognize target cells that have antibody bound to antigen exposed in the cell membrane of the target cell.

fluorescent a. see FLUORESCENCE microscopy.
heteroclitic a. one with greater affinity for an antigen other than the one that stimulated its formation.
hormonal a. has been investigated mostly as a means of controlling fertility in animals. See also CONTRACEPTION.
humoral a. see humoral IMMUNITY.
immune a. one induced by immunization or by transfusion incompatibility, in contrast to natural antibodies.
incomplete a. an antibody which combines with antigen without producing an observable reaction such as agglutination; originally used to describe Rh antibodies.
maternal a's those passively transferred from dam to fetus or neonate, transplacentally or via colostrum or yolk sac. See also passive IMMUNITY.
a.-mediated cytotoxicity damage to cells, especially erythrocytes, caused by the reaction of antibodies (IgG, IgM or IgA) with cell surface antigens.
a.-mediated immunity humoral immunity.
monoclonal a. see MONOCLONAL antibodies.
natural a's ones that react with antigens to which the individual has had no known exposure. The best examples are anti a and b antibodies present in serum of humans of blood group B and A, respectively.
neutralizing a. one that reduces, destroys or blocks infectivity of an infectious agent, particularly virus, by partial or complete destruction of the agent.
nonagglutinating a. see incomplete antibody (above).
polyclonal a. a collection of immunoglobulins that react against the same or different antigenic determinants of the one antigen molecule.
protective a. one responsible for immunity to an infectious agent.
reaginic a. see REAGIN and IMMUNOGLOBULIN E.
a. repertoire all the antibody specificities that can be produced by an individual.
saline a. complete antibody.
skin-sensitizing a. see REAGIN.
univalent a. see incomplete antibody (above).

antibrachium see ANTEBRACHIUM.

anticancer drug see ANTINEOPLASTIC.

anticestodal 1. destructive to cestodes. 2. an agent destructive to tapeworms.
a. drugs include the natural organic compound ARECOLINE and the synthetic compounds BUNAMIDINE, NICLOSAMIDE, DICHLOROPHEN, PRAZIQUANTEL, UREDOFOS and RESORANTEL.

anticholagogue an agent that inhibits secretion of bile.

anticholelithogenic 1. preventing the formation of gallstones. 2. an agent that so acts.

anticholinergic blockade of acetylcholine receptors, resulting in the inhibition of the transmission of parasympathetic nerve impulses; parasympatholytic. Used most commonly in the nonspecific treatment of vomiting or diarrhea; includes ATROPINE, PROPANTHELINE, SCOPOLAMINE, ISOPROPAMIDE.

anticholinesterase a drug that inhibits the enzyme acetylcholinesterase, thereby potentiating the action of acetylcholine at postsynaptic membrane receptors in the parasympathetic nervous system.

anticipated calving list the list of dates of expected calvings in a herd provided by a herd health program.

anticipatory care health maintenance programs which check apparently healthy animals for the presence of disease, e.g. tuberculosis and brucellosis testing of cattle, hip dysplasia schemes in dogs.

anticoagulant 1. serving to prevent the coagulation of blood. 2. any substance that, in vivo or in vitro, suppresses, delays or nullifies coagulation of the blood.

There is limited therapeutic use for anticoagulants in animals; their importance is in the collection of blood for testing and for transfusion and in toxicology.
a. drugs see CITRIC ACID, EDTA or EDETATE and HEPARIN, all of which are used for blood collection.
a. poisoning see DICOUMAROL, WARFARIN.
a. rodenticide includes warfarin, pindone, diphacinone, phentolacin, Valone.
snake venom a. see RUSSELL'S VIPER VENOM.

anticoccidials chemicals effective in the treatment and control of coccidiosis in birds and animals. Include CLOPIDOL, QUINOLONES, MONENSIN, LASALOCID, ROBENIDINE, AMPROLIUM, DINITOLMIDE, NICARBAZIN and SULFONAMIDE. Called also coccidiostatic drugs.

anticodon a triplet of nucleotides in transfer RNA that is complementary to the codon in messenger RNA which specifies the amino acid.

anticodon–codon interactions base pairing between the 3 base codon of mRNA and the complementary 3 base anticodon sequence of tRNA.

anticomplement a substance that counteracts complement.

anticomplementary capable of reducing or destroying the power of complement.

anticonvulsant 1. inhibiting convulsions. Any drug that depresses the central nervous system may be used for its anticonvulsant effect. This includes narcotics and sedatives. They have the undesirable effect of depressing all CNS functions. 2. a specific motor depressant, such as anticonvulsant or antiepileptic, which depresses specifically the motor centers and suppresses spontaneous motor activity; examples are PHENOBARBITAL, PHENYTOIN, PRIMIDONE and DIAZEPAM.

anticus anterior.

antidepressants drug used to counteract depression in humans, but sometimes used in the treatment of compulsive behavioral disorders and psychodermatosis in dogs and cats.

antidiarrheal 1. counteracting diarrhea. 2. an agent that counteracts diarrhea.
a. agents medicines used as antidiarrheals in animals. Includes parasympatholytic drugs, e.g. ATROPINE, which act as a SPASMOLYTIC or ANTISPASMODIC, opiates, protectants and absorbents, e.g. activated CHARCOAL, KAOLIN, and astringents, e.g. CATECHU, TANNIC ACID. The classification does not include the treatments that are specific for the diseases that cause diarrhea, e.g. antibiotics.

antidipsetic pertaining to or causing the suppression of thirst.

antidiuresis the suppression of secretion of urine by the kidneys.

antidiuretic 1. pertaining to or causing suppression of urine production. 2. an agent that causes suppression of urine production.
a. hormone vasopressin; a polypeptide hormine from the posterior lobe of the pituitary that suppresses the production of urine; it has a specific effect on the epithelial cells of the renal tubules, stimulating the reabsorption of water independently of solids, and resulting in concentration of urine. Stored and released by the posterior lobe of the PITUITARY gland, it also has vasopressor activity. Called also ADH.
a. hormone response test measures urine specific gravity or osmolality before and after the administra-

tion of vasopressin to determine whether a polyuric condition is caused by a deficiency or reduced responsiveness to antidiuretic hormone. Called also Pitressin tannate test, Pitressin concentration test.

syndrome of inappropriate secretion of a. hormone (SIADH) one in which there is abnormal production of ADH leading to hyponatremia (see also SYNDROME OF INAPPROPRIATE SECRETION OF ANTIDIURETIC HORMONE).

antidotal having the properties of an antidote.

a. therapy treatment specifically directed towards reversing the effects of a poison.

antidote an agent that counteracts a poison.

chemical a. one that neutralizes the poison by changing its chemical nature.

mechanical a. one that prevents absorption of the poison.

physiological a. one that counteracts the effects of the poison by producing opposing effects.

universal a. a mixture formerly recommended as an antidote when the exact poison is not known. There is, in fact, no known universal antidote. Activated charcoal is now being used for many poisons.

antidromic conducting impulses in a direction opposite to the normal.

a. vasodilator impulses produced artificially by electrical stimulation of the peripheral end of a cut dorsal nerve root.

antidysenteric counteracting dysentery.

antiemetic 1. useful in the treatment of vomiting. 2. an agent that relieves vomiting.

antiendotoxic counteracting the effect of endotoxins.

antiendotoxin an antibody that counteracts the effect of endotoxin.

antienzyme agent see *N*-ACETYLCYSTEINE, an anticollagenase drug.

antiepileptic 1. combating epilepsy. 2. a remedy for epilepsy.

a. agent see ANTICONVULSANT.

antiestrogen 1. blocking the action of estrogens. 2. an agent that so acts.

antifebrile counteracting fever.

antifebrin see ACETANILID.

antifibrinolysin see ANTIPLASMIN.

antifibrinolytic inhibiting fibrinolysis.

antifoaming having the capacity to reduce or prevent the formation of foam: (1) for the reduction of foam in pulmonary edema, e.g. by the inhalation of nebulized ethyl alcohol; (2) for the reduction or prevention of formation of foam in the rumen, e.g. oils, alcohol ethoxylate detergents, and poloxalenes.

antifolate drug see FOLIC ACID antagonist.

antifoulant substances used to coat marine netting in fish cages; some may cause unacceptable chemical residues in the farmed fish.

antifreeze see ETHYLENE glycol.

antifungal 1. destructive to or checking the growth of fungi. 2. an agent that destroys or checks the growth of fungi, such as amphotericin B or flucytosine (5-FC). Includes: (1) topical drugs, e.g. UNDECYLENIC ACID, BENZOIC ACID, SALICYLIC ACID, TOLNAFTATE, CANDICIDIN, HALOPROGIN, IODOCHLORHYDROXYQUIN, CUPRIMYXIN, CLOTRIMAZOLE, THIABENDAZOLE and MICONAZOLE; (2) systemic drugs, e.g. GRISEOFULVIN, AMPHOTERICIN B, 5-FLUCYTOSINE and KETOCONAZOLE.

antigalactic 1. diminishing the secretion of milk. 2. an agent that so acts, e.g. mibolerone.

antigen any substance which is capable, under appropriate conditions, of inducing a specific immune response and of reacting with the products of that response; that is, with specific ANTIBODY or specifically sensitized T lymphocytes, or both. Antigens may be soluble substances, such as toxins and foreign proteins, or particulate, such as bacteria and tissue cells; however, only a small portion of the protein or polysaccharide molecule known as the antigenic determinant or epitope is recognized by the specific receptor on a lymphocyte. Similarly the antibody or effector lymphocyte produced by the response combines only with the one antigenic determinant. A bacterial cell or large protein will have many hundreds of antigenic determinants, some of which are more important than others in protective immunity. Abbreviated Ag.

See also IMMUNITY, ANTIGENIC.

allogenic a. one occurring in some but not all individuals of the same species, e.g. histocompatibility antigens and blood group antigens; formerly called isoantigen.

antibody–a. reaction see ANTIBODY–antigen reaction.

blood group a's present on the surface of erythrocytes which vary between individuals of the same species and are used as the basis for blood typing.

a. bridge a link between antigen-specific receptors of two antibodies.

capsular a's K, L and V antigens (below).

carcinoembryonic a. (CEA) see oncofetal antigen (below).

common a. an antigenic determinant present in two or more different antigen molecules and the basis for cross-reactions among them.

complete a. an antigen which both stimulates the immune response and reacts with the products, e.g. antibody, of that response, cf. HAPTEN.

conjugated a. see HAPTEN.

cross-reacting a. 1. one that combines with antibody produced in response to a different but related antigen, owing to similarity of antigenic determinants. 2. identical antigens in two bacterial strains, so that antibody produced against one strain will react with the other.

dog erythrocyte a. (DEA) the antigens found on dog erythrocytes and used to distinguish different blood groups in the species. See Table 7.

environmental a's those found in pollens, fungi, house dust, foods and animal dander.

a. epitope see antigenic DETERMINANT.

feline oncornavirus cell membrane a. (FOCMA) tumor-specific antigen present on the membrane of cells in cats infected with FELINE leukemia virus.

flagellar a. H antigen (below).

flea a. 1. some components of flea saliva, as well as whole flea extracts, are antigenic and certain individuals may become hypersensitive to flea bites; the most common hypersensitivity in dogs. 2. extracts, usually of whole fleas, but sometimes of flea saliva, are used for intradermal skin testing and desensitization procedures.

Forssman a. heterophil antigen occurring in various unrelated species, mainly in the organs but not in the erythrocytes (guinea pig, horse), but sometimes only in the erythrocytes (sheep), and occasionally in both (chicken). Antibody to Forssman antigen is usually recognized by agglutination of sheep red blood cells.

group specific (gs) a. common to a certain group of organisms, e.g. streptococci, oncornaviruses.

H a. [Ger.] *Hauch* (film) the antigen that occurs in the bacterial flagella.

heterogeneic a. see xenogeneic antigen (below).

heterophil a., heterogenetic a. one capable of stimulating the production of antibodies that react with tissues from other animals or even plants.

hidden a. one not normally exposed to circulating lymphocytes, e.g. within central nervous tissue, testicular tissue and certain intracellular components, so they do not normally evoke an immune response.
histocompatibility a's see HISTOCOMPATIBILITY antigen.
H-Y a. a histocompatibility antigen of the cell membrane, determined by a locus on the Y chromosome; it is a mediator of testicular organization (hence, sexual differentiation) in the male.
Ia a's histocompatibility antigens governed by the I region of the major histocompatibility complex (MHC), located principally on B lymphocytes, although T lymphocytes, skin and certain macrophages may also contain Ia antigens.
isogenic a. an antigen carried by an individual, or members of the same inbred strain, which is capable of eliciting an immune response in genetically different individuals of the same species, but not in individuals bearing it.
K a's bacterial capsular antigens.
L a. a capsular antigen of *Escherichia coli.*
Ly a's antigenic cell-surface markers of subpopulations of T lymphocytes, classified as Ly 1, 2 and 3; they are associated with helper and suppressor activities of T lymphocytes.
lymphocyte-defined (LD) a's class II antigens found in lymphocytes, macrophages, epidermal cells and sperm. Important in graft rejection.
M a. a type-specific antigen that appears to be located primarily in the cell wall and is associated with virulence of *Streptococcus pyogenes*.
Marek's tumor-specific a. (MATSA) found on the surface of cells infected by Marek's disease herpesvirus.
Nègre a. an antigen prepared from dead, dried and triturated tubercle bacilli by means of acetone and methyl alcohol; used in serum tests for tuberculosis in humans.
nuclear a's the components of cell nuclei with which antinuclear antibodies react.
O a. [Ger.] *ohne Hauch* (without film) the antigen that occurs in the cell wall of bacteria.
oncofetal a. a gene product that is expressed during fetal development, but repressed in specialized tissues of the adult and that is also produced by certain cancers. In the neoplastic transformation, the cells dedifferentiate and these genes can be derepressed so that the embryonic antigens reappear. Examples are alpha-fetoprotein and carcinoembryonic antigen.
organ-specific a. any antigen that occurs exclusively in a particular organ and serves to distinguish it from other organs. Two types of organ specificity have been proposed: (1) first-order or tissue specificity is attributed to the presence of an antigen characteristic of a particular organ in a single species; (2) second-order organ specificity is attributed to an antigen characteristic of the same organ in many, even unrelated species.
partial a. see HAPTEN.
pollen a. the essential polypeptides of the pollen of plants extracted with a suitable menstruum, used in diagnosis, prophylaxis and desensitization in hay fever.
a. presentation the presentation of peptide derivatives of antigens on the surface of antigen presenting cells (APCs), which include macrophages, dendritic cells and B lymphocytes, in association with class II major histocompatibility complex (MHC) antigens as required for recognition by T lymphocytes. Also includes antigen presentation in association with MHC class I by cells that are targets for lysis by cytotoxic T lymphocytes.
a.-presenting cells cells (macrophages, Langerhans cells, dendritic cells, and B lymphocytes) that process and present antigen to T lymphocytes.
private a's antigens of the low-frequency blood groups, so-called because they are found only in members of a single kindred.
recall a. an antigen to which an individual has previously been sensitized and which is subsequently administered as a challenging dose to elicit a hypersensitivity reaction.
a. receptors immunoglobulin molecules on the cell membranes of B lymphocytes and a structurally related, but quite distinct molecule on the surface of T lymphocytes which recognize particular antigenic determinants of an antigen.
a. recognition see RECOGNITION (2).
sequestered a's certain antigens, e.g. the lens of the eye and thyroid proteins, that are sequestered anatomically from the immune system during embryonic development and thus thought not to be recognized as 'self'. Should such antigens be exposed to the immune system during adult life, an autoimmune response would be elicited.
serologically defined (SD) a. class I antigen of the major histocompatibility complex, identifiable by the use of specific antisera.
synthetic a. chemically synthesized or produced by recombinant DNA technology, the synthesis of polymers, based on sequences found in microbial antigens, has been used in the production of vaccines.
T-dependent a. the immune response of most antigens requires T helper (Th) lymphocytes; lymphokines produced by T lymphocytes determine the characteristics of antibodies produced, which may change during the immune response.
thymus-dependent a. an antigen that requires T lymphocyte participation before an immune response can occur. Most antigens are of this type.
thymus-independent a. an antigen that elicits an antibody response without the participation of T lymphocytes. Usually large carbohydrate molecules with repeating epitopes are of this type.
tolerogenic a. see TOLEROGEN.
tumor-specific a. (TSA) antigens found only in tumor cells.
V a., Vi a. an antigen contained in the capsule of a bacterium and thought to contribute to its virulence.
xenogeneic a. an antigen common to members of one species but not to members of other species; called also heterogeneic antigen.

antigen–antibody glomerulonephritis see immune-mediated GLOMERULONEPHRITIS.

antigenemia the presence of antigen in the blood.

antigenic having the properties of an antigen.
a. competition the immune response to an antigen may be reduced if an unrelated antigen is administered simultaneously or shortly before. These may be between different molecules (intermolecular) or different determinants on the same molecule (intramolecular).
a. drift point mutations in genes resulting in antigenic change. See also ORTHOMYXOVIRIDAE.
a. mimicry similarities between sequences found in microbial proteins and host proteins which may result in cross-reacting immune responses and autoimmune disease.
a. shift genetic reassortment between two subtypes of a viral species resulting in a new subtype with

completely different antigenicity. See also ORTHOMYXOVIRIDAE.

antigenicity the capacity to stimulate the production of antibodies or cell-mediated immune responses.

antiglobulin an antibody to a heterologous antibody, such as goat antihorse IgG antibody, as used in the Coombs test, ELISA, immunofluorescence or other assays.

a. test see COOMBS TESTS.

antiglomerular basement membrane nephritis see immune-mediated GLOMERULONEPHRITIS.

antihelix see ANTHELIX.

antihelmintic see ANTHELMINTIC.

antihemophilic 1. effective against the bleeding tendency in hemophilia. 2. an agent that counteracts the bleeding tendency in hemophilia.

a. factor (AHF) A one of the clotting factors, deficiency of which causes VON WILLEBRAND'S DISEASE and HEMOPHILIA A. Called also factor VIII and antihemophilic GLOBULIN.

a. factor B CLOTTING factor IX.

a. factor C CLOTTING factor XI.

antihemorrhagic 1. exerting a hemostatic effect and counteracting hemorrhage. 2. an agent that prevents or checks hemorrhage.

antihistamine a drug that counteracts the effects of histamine by acting on histamine receptors without activating them but preventing their accessibility to histamine. A competitive and reversible reaction. There are two types:

Those that block H_1 receptors are commonly referred to as the antihistamines and are widely used to relieve the symptoms of allergic reactions, especially urticaria. Some have an antinauseant action that is useful in the prevention of motion sickness and others have a sedative and hypnotic action.

H_2 receptor blocking agents inhibit the stimulation of gastric secretions.

See also HISTAMINE antagonists, H_2-receptor BLOCKER.

antihistaminic 1. counteracting the pharmacological effects of histamine. 2. an antihistamine.

antihormone a substance, usually antibody, that counteracts a hormone. It is produced in animals after repeated injections of a hormone or hormone-bearing protein. Further doses of the hormone may result in the neutralization of the hormone, in neutralization of the patient's own hormone, or in stimulation of an attack of allergy or anaphylaxis.

antihyperlipoproteinemic 1. promoting a reduction of lipoprotein levels in the blood. 2. an agent that so acts.

antihypertensive acting to reduce tension; in medical terms, usually referring to elevated blood pressure. Drugs used for this purpose include diuretics, β-adrenergic antagonists, and vasodilators.

anti-immune preventing immunity.

anti-infective 1. counteracting infection. 2. a substance that counteracts infection. Includes ANTISEPTICS, DISINFECTANTS, ANTIBIOTICS, and ANTIFUNGAL and VIRUCIDAL agents.

anti-inflammatory 1. counteracting or suppressing inflammation. 2. an agent that so acts.

a. drugs those used to reduce the inflammatory response to infectious agents, trauma, surgical procedures or in musculoskeletal disease.

nonsteroidal a. drug see NONSTEROIDAL ANTI-INFLAMMATORY DRUGS.

antiketogenesis inhibition of the formation of ketone bodies.

antiketogenic preventing or suppressing the development of ketones (ketone bodies) and thus preventing development of ketosis.

antilewisite See DIMERCAPROL.

antilithic 1. preventing calculus formation. 2. an agent that prevents calculus formation.

Antilocapra americana see ANTILOCAPRIDAE.

Antilocapridae a family of antelopes containing only one species, *Antilocapra americana*, the pronghorn antelope.

antilogarithm the number whose logarithm is the number in question.

Antilope cervicapra see INDIAN ANTELOPE.

antilymphocyte serum antiserum containing antibodies specific for lymphocyte surface antigens that may be used to suppress delayed type hypersensitivity, particularly graft rejection, responses without affecting humoral immune response; abbreviated ALS. Used in organ transplantation, usually in combination with immunosuppressive drugs. Prepared by hyperimmunizing an animal, e.g. horse, with foreign, e.g. human, lymphocytes. See also antilymphocyte GLOBULIN.

antimere one of the halves of a bilaterally symmetrical part or organism.

antimetabolite a substance bearing a close structural resemblance to one required for normal physiological functioning, and exerting its effect by interfering with the utilization of the essential metabolite.

antimethemoglobinemic 1. promoting reduction of methemoglobin levels in the blood. 2. an agent that so acts.

antimetropia hyperopia of one eye, with myopia in the other.

antimicrobial 1. killing microorganisms, or suppressing their multiplication or growth. 2. an agent that kills microorganisms or suppresses their multiplication or growth.

Antimicrobial agents are classified functionally according to the manner in which they adversely affect a microorganism. Some interfere with the synthesis of the bacterial cell wall. This results in cell lysis because the contents of the bacterial cell are hypertonic and therefore under high osmotic pressure. A weakening of the cell wall causes the cell to rupture, spill its contents, and be destroyed. The penicillins, cephalosporins and bacitracin are examples of this group of antimicrobials.

A second group of antimicrobial agents interfere with the synthesis of nucleic acids. Without DNA and RNA synthesis a microorganism cannot replicate or translate genetic information. Examples of antimicrobials that exert this kind of action are griseofulvin, fluoroquinolones and rifampicin.

A third group of antimicrobial agents change the permeability of the cell membrane, causing a leakage of metabolic substrates essential to the life of the microorganism. Their action can be either bacteriostatic or bactericidal. Examples include amphotericin B and polymyxin B.

A fourth group of antimicrobial agents interfere with metabolic processes within the microorganism. They are structurally similar to natural metabolic substrates, but since they do not function normally, they interrupt metabolic processes. Most of these agents are bacteriostatic. Examples include the sulfonamides, aminosalicylic acid (PAS) and isoniazid (INH).

A fifth group interfere with translation of proteins by the ribosome. This action may be bacteriocidal, if errors in translation are induced (aminoglycosides) or bacteriostatic, if translation is inhibited (macrolides, tetracyclines, chloramphenicol).

a. resistance ability of a microorganism to resist the effects of an antimicrobial agent. May be an intrinsic characteristic or acquired by selection for mutation or by acquisition of a resistance gene from other microorganisms.

a. sensitivity test an in vitro test of the effectiveness of selected antibacterial agents against bacteria recovered from a patient. Paper disks impregnated with various agents are placed on an inoculated agar plate (disk diffusion) or the agent is added to broth cultures. Inhibition of growth is interpreted as an indication of bacterial sensitivity to the antibacterial.

subtherapeutic a. therapy used mainly in mass medication programs as preventive measures against unspecified infectious diseases. Carries the risks of creating resistant strains of organisms, and of resulting in unacceptable residues in human food.

a. therapy antimicrobial agents may be administered topically, orally, or injected. There are special needs for special circumstances. Aquarial fish, for example, may be treated by incorporating the agent in the feed or by injection. Immersing the fish in a tank containing a solution of the agent is satisfactory only for superficial infections because the drug is not absorbed directly through the skin and the intake is very slow.

antimony a chemical element, atomic number 51, atomic weight 121.75, symbol Sb. See Table 6. Trivalent and pentavalent antimony compounds are used in medicine as anti-infective agents in the treatment of tropical diseases, especially those of protozoan origin. All antimony compounds are potentially poisonous and must be used with caution. See also STIBOGLUCONATE, MEGLUMINE.

a. poisoning resembles arsenic poisoning. Signs include vomiting and diarrhea. Postmortem lesions are those of gastroenteritis.

a. potassium tartrate a nauseant expectorant and ruminatoric. Also used as an antiparasitic agent in schistosomiasis, trypanosomiasis and leishmaniasis. Called also tarter emetic.

antimorph a mutant allele which acts in the opposite direction to the normal allele.

antimotility drugs drugs used to inhibit peristaltic activity of the gastrointestinal tract in the treatment of diarrhea; usually parasympatholytics. Called also spasmolytics.

anti-müllerian hormone the factor secreted by the Sertoli cells of the embryonic, developing testis that causes regression of the müllerian ducts, the primordia for the accessory sex glands of the female.

antimuscarinic drugs see MUSCARINIC blocking agents.

antimycin A a respiratory inhibitor isolated from *Streptomyces*. Blocks electron transfer from cytochrome b to cytochrome c_1.

antimycotic destructive to fungi.

antinarcotic relieving narcotic depression.

antinematodal see NEMATOCIDE.

a. drugs includes PIPERAZINE, IMIDAZOTHIAZOLES and TETRAHYDROPYRIMIDINES (e.g. tetramizole, LEVAMISOLE, MORANTEL, PYRANTEL), BENZIMIDAZOLE and pro-benzimidazoles (e.g. THIABENDAZOLE, MEBENDAZOLE, PARBENDAZOLE, FENBENDAZOLE, OXFENDAZOLE, CAMBENDAZOLE, flubendazole, FEBANTEL, THIOPHANATE, NETOBIMIN), macrocyclic lactones (IVERMECTIN, MOXIDECTIN, doramectin), ORGANOPHOSPHORUS COMPOUNDS (DICHLORVOS, HALOXON, TRICHLORFON), SALICYLANILIDES (CLOSANTEL, NITROSCANATE).

antineoplastic 1. inhibiting the maturation and proliferation of malignant cells. 2. an agent having such properties.

a. therapy a regimen of treatment aimed at destruction of malignant cells and utilizing a variety of chemical agents that directly affect cellular growth and development.

The chemicals and drugs used in the treatment of cancer may be divided into three groups. The first group, the *alkylating* agents, are capable of damaging the DNA of cells, thereby interfering with the process of replication. Among these drugs are CHLORAMBUCIL, CYCLOPHOSPHAMIDE, MUSTINE HYDROCHLORIDE and triethylene thiophosphamide (THIOTEPA). The antibiotic actinomycin D (DACTINOMYCIN) is also included in this group.

The second type of drugs used in cancer chemotherapy are the *antimetabolites*. As the name suggests, these drugs interfere with the cancer cell's metabolism. Some replace essential metabolites without performing their function, while others compete with essential components by mimicking their functions and thereby inhibiting the manufacture of protein in the cell. Included in this group are CYTOSINE arabinoside, FLOXURIDINE (FUDR), 5-FLUOROURACIL (5-FU), MERCAPTOPURINE (6-MP), METHOTREXATE and THIOGUANINE.

The third group of chemicals employed in the treatment of cancer are '*natural products*' that directly affect the mechanism of cell division. The plant alkaloids, e.g. VINCRISTINE and VINBLASTINE, stop cell division at metaphase (a subphase in cell mitosis). The enzymes, e.g. L-ASPARAGINASE, starve tumor cells by catabolizing substances (e.g. asparagine) which they need for survival. Hormones change cell metabolism by making the cellular environment unfavorable for growth of certain tumors.

antinephritic effective against nephritis.

antineuritic relieving neuritis.

antinidatory agent one preventing implantation of a fertilized ovum. Used in the treatment of misalliance.

antinuclear antibody see antinuclear ANTIBODY.

antiovulatory suppressing ovulation. In dogs and cats, pharmacological suppression of ovulation with progestins and androgens is common. See also CONTRACEPTION.

antioxidant a substance that in small amount will inhibit the oxidation of other compounds. Used in feeds and foods to prevent rancidification of polyunsaturated fats.

antiparallel orientation two strands of DNA arranged in opposite directions.

antiparallelism in DNA structure, the two strands are aligned in opposite directions.

antiparasitic 1. destroying parasites. 2. an agent that destroys parasites.

a. agent includes insecticides, acaricides and anthelmintics. Their suitability depends on their efficiency in reducing parasite loads, especially of the immature forms, the breadth of their therapeutic spectrum, safety, their ease of administration, cost and freedom from tissue residue problems and the development of resistance.

systemic a. the medication is administered orally or by injection and exerts its effect when the target parasite sucks blood or other body fluids or is in contact with the agent in the gut lumen.

topical a. medication applied directly to the skin.

antipediculotic 1. effective against lice and in treatment of pediculosis. 2. an agent that is effective against lice.

antipepsin an antienzyme that counteracts pepsin.

antiperistalsis reverse PERISTALSIS.
antiphlogistic 1. countering inflammation and fever. 2. an agent that counteracts inflammation and fever, e.g. poultice, hot pack, hot fomentation.
antiphlogistine a proprietary poultice but the name is also used to include other poultices with a kaolin base. Used as a remedy for muscle and joint sprains.
antiplasmin a principle in the blood that inhibits plasmin.
antiplastic unfavorable to healing.
antiplatelet directed against or destructive to blood platelets; inhibiting platelet function.
a. antibody autoantibody against platelets, the cause of immune-mediated THROMBOCYTOPENIA. Detected by the PLATELET factor 3 release test.
a. drugs the prevention of thromboembolic disorders in animals is limited mainly to the treatment of cats with arterial thromboembolism and dogs with heartworms. Platelet aggregation may be impeded by treatment with aspirin, dipyrimadole, sulfinpyrazone or propranolol.
antipolycythemic 1. effective against polycythemia. 2. an agent effective against polycythemia.
antiport a cell membrane structure that transports two molecules at once through the membrane in opposite directions.
antiprostaglandin 1. acting against the formation, release or activity of prostaglandins. 2. a class of drugs with these activities; the nonsteroidal anti-inflammatory drugs. Include ASPIRIN, FLUNIXIN MEGLUMINE, DIPYRONE, PHENYLBUTAZONE.
alpha-1-antiprotease see ALPHA$_1$-ANTITRYPSIN.
antiprothrombin a substance that retards the conversion of prothrombin into thrombin.
antiprotozoal 1. destroying protozoa, or checking their growth or reproduction. 2. an agent with that effect.
a. agent see COCCIDIOSTATIC DRUGS, TRYPANOCIDAL.
antipruritic 1. preventing or relieving itching. 2. an agent that counteracts itching; of special importance in the treatment of animals because of the self-trauma that results from their responses to pruritus.
antipsychotic effective in the management of manifestations of psychotic disorders; also, an agent that so acts. There are several classes of antipsychotic drugs (phenothiazines, thioxanthenes, dibenzazepines and butyrophenones), all of which may act by the same mechanism, i.e. blockade of dopaminergic receptors in the central nervous system. Called also NEUROLEPTIC and major tranquilizer.
antipyretic 1. effective against fever. 2. an agent that relieves fever. Cold packs, aspirin and quinine are all antipyretics. Antipyretic drugs dilate the blood vessels near the surface of the skin, thereby allowing more blood to flow through the skin with increased heat loss by radiation and convection. Also, an antipyretic can increase perspiration, the evaporation of which cools the body.
antipyrine see PHENAZONE.
antipyrotic 1. effective in the treatment of burns. 2. an agent used in the treatment of burns.
antirachitic therapeutically effective against rickets.
antireflux acting to prevent reflux. In gastroesophageal REFLUX disease antireflux surgery restores the abdominal segment of the esophagus and increases pressure at the gastric inlet.
antirickettsial 1. effective against rickettsiae. 2. an agent effective against rickettsiae.
antirotation wiring in the application of wires to stabilize bone fracture fragments, use of a figure-eight pattern reduces the rotational forces.
antiseborrheic 1. effective against seborrhea. 2. an agent with that effect. This includes keratolytics and keratoplastics such as SALICYLIC ACID, TAR preparations, SULFUR and BENZOYL peroxide.
antisecretory 1. inhibiting or diminishing secretion; secretoinhibitory. 2. an agent that so acts, as certain drugs that inhibit or diminish gastric secretions.
antisense nucleic acids natural or synthetic oligonucleotides that are complementary to mRNAs that hybridize to and inactivate mRNA. Proposed as a form of antiviral therapy.
antisense RNA an RNA sequence which is complementary to a functional RNA.
antisense strand one of the two strands in a DNA molecule that is not transcribed.
antisepsis prevention of sepsis by destruction of microorganisms and infective matter. Usually refers to cleansing the skin or mucous membranes of pathogenic organisms, but with resident flora remaining.
antiseptic 1. preventing sepsis. 2. any substance that inhibits the growth of bacteria, in contrast to a germicide, which kills bacteria outright. Antiseptics are not considered to include antibiotics, which are usually taken internally. The term antiseptic includes disinfectants, although most disinfectants are too strong to be applied to body tissue and are generally used to clean inanimate objects such as floors and equipment. Includes physical antiseptics, chemical antiseptics, halogens, alcohols and surfactants.
urinary a. a drug that is excreted mainly in the urine and performs its antiseptic action in the bladder. These drugs may be given before examination of or operation on the urinary tract, and they are sometimes used to treat urinary tract infections.
antiserum a serum containing antibodies. Obtained from an animal that has been exposed to antigen. Used in the prevention, treatment or diagnosis of infectious disease. See also IMMUNITY and IMMUNIZATION.
antishock pneumatic garment a specially designed covering used to apply external pressure to the pelvis, abdomen and hindlegs with inflatable balloons in the treatment of shock.
antisialagogue, antisialogogue an agent that inhibits the flow of saliva.
antisialic checking the flow of saliva.
antispasmodic 1. preventing or relieving spasms. 2. an agent that prevents or relieves spasms. Said of parasympatholytic drugs used in the treatment of gastrointestinal or urinary tract disorders. Called also spasmolytics.
antistreptococcic counteracting streptococcal infection.
antisucking operation a procedure to prevent young cattle from sucking themselves or other cattle. Nose rings may be used or surgical amputation of part of the tongue can be performed. See also CRIB-biting operation.
antisudorific 1. inhibiting sweating. 2. an agent that inhibits sweating.
antitetanic counters tetanus or tetany.
a. serum see tetanus ANTITOXIN.
antithenar placed opposite to the palm or the sole.
antithrombin any naturally occurring or therapeutically administered substance that neutralizes the action of thrombin and thus limits or restricts blood coagulation.
a. III (AT III) an alpha$_2$-globulin synthesized in the liver which is a natural inhibitor of clotting.

antithrombocytic 1. preventing the aggregation of blood platelets (thrombocytes). 2. an antithrombocytic agent. See also ANTIPLATELET.

antithromboplastin any agent or substance that prevents or interferes with the interaction of blood clotting factors as they generate prothrombinase (thromboplastin).

antithrombotic 1. preventing or interfering with the formation of thrombi. 2. an agent that interferes with thrombus formation. See also ANTIPLATELET drugs.

antithyroid suppressing thyroid activity.

a. drugs these include THIOURACIL, METHYLURACIL COMPOUNDS.

antitick serum hyperimmune serum produced in dogs by exposing naturally resistant animals to a continuous and heavy infestation with the tick *Ixodes holocyclus.* Used in treatment and temporary protection of dogs against tick paralysis.

antitoxic effective against a poison; pertaining to ANTITOXIN.

antitoxin a particular kind of ANTIBODY produced in the body in response to the presence of a toxin or toxoid. Most commonly used in the treatment of diseases caused by clostridial toxins, e.g. botulinum and tetanus. See also IMMUNITY.

gas gangrene a. serum containing antitoxic antibodies; prepared from the blood of healthy animals immunized against gas-producing organisms of the genus *Clostridium.*

tetanus a. preparation from the blood serum or plasma of healthy animals immunized against tetanus toxin. Used for prophylaxis after injury because of its immediate effect. Active immunization is preferred for long-term protection, particularly for many clostridial diseases such as tetanus.

antitragus the part of the auricular cartilage that lies caudal to the tragus and with it completes the caudal boundary of the opening into the ear canal.

antitrematodal having efficiency in the treatment of trematodes. Because of the lower susceptibility to injury of immature flukes the measure of efficiency of antitrematodal drugs is measured by their efficiency against immature flukes. Includes ALBENDAZOLE, BITHIONOL sulfoxide, BROMSALANS, CARBON TETRACHLORIDE, CLIOXANIDE, DIAMFENETIDE, TETRACHLORODIFLUORETHANE, HEXACHLOROETHANE, HEXACHLOROPARAXYLENE, HEXACHLOROPHENE, NICLOFOLAN, NITROXYNIL, OXYCLOZANIDE, RAFOXANIDE, TRICLABENDAZOLE.

antitrochanter on the avian pelvic skeleton, a blunt process which articulates with the femoral trochanter so as to limit abduction.

antitrope one of two structures that are similar but oppositely oriented, like a right and a left glove.

antituberculous therapeutically effective against tuberculosis.

a. drugs agents used in the treatment of mycobacterial infections, which in animals is limited to dogs and cats, include isoniazid, rifampicin and ethambutol. Several other drugs may be used in combination therapy to increase effectiveness. In addition, dapsone is effective against *Mycobacterium leprae.* See also FELINE leprosy.

antitussive 1. effective against cough. 2. an agent that suppresses coughing. The narcotics codeine and hydrocodone, and several opioids or opioid-like drugs, including dextromethorphan and butorphanol, are commonly used in small animals.

a.-bronchodilator combination a common therapeutic combination used in the treatment of respiratory diseases in dogs and cats.

antiulcerative 1. preventing the formation or promoting the healing of ulcers. 2. an agent that so acts.

antivenin, antivenene a material used to neutralize the venom of a poisonous animal. Prepared by immunization of serum-producing animals, usually horses. Antivenins against the venoms of most poisonous snakes, spiders and stinging fish and other aquatic species are available, but only in those areas in which the poisonous species occurs.

antiviral 1. effective against viruses. 2. an agent effective against viruses.

a. drugs may be useful in early stages of some virus infections or to prevent recurrences or reactivation in chronic infections. Most drugs exert their effects only during certain stages of viral replication and many are relatively toxic for the host when used systemically. In general, chemotherapy of virus infections in animals is uncommon with limited applications, mainly in topical treatment of ophthalmic infections. Examples are IDOXURIDINE, VIDARABINE, AMANTADINE HYDROCHLORIDE, ACYCLOVIR, RIBAVIRIN.

antivitamin a substance that inactivates or inhibits the normal functioning of a vitamin.

antixerotic preventing dryness.

antizymotic unfavorable to fermentation.

antler single-tined or branched horny outgrowths from the frontal bones of male deer. Reindeer and caribou females also have horns. Antlers grow and are shed each year, becoming more complicated in structure as the buck ages. At the beginning of the season the horns are covered with velvet, the soft, hairy skin which produces the horn and is then shed to expose the horn which is itself shed the next spring.

a. amputation a dehorning technique requiring considerable skill and experience to avoid losing the deer and to ensure regrowth of the antler.

a. farming deer farming conducted for the sole purpose of annual harvesting of the antlers for quasi-pharmaceutical use.

velvet a. the whole of the antler, including the velvet and the outgrowth of the frontal bone, before calcification.

Anton test a test used in the identification of *Listeria monocytogenes*; instillation of a culture into the conjunctival sac of a rabbit or guinea pig causes severe keratoconjunctivitis within 24 hours.

Antoni patterns the characteristic patterns in which nerve cells are arranged in non-anaplastic Schwann cell tumors of the nervous system.

antral pertaining to the antrum; usually the reference is to the pyloric antrum of the stomach. See also PYLORUS.

a. peristalsis responsible for the onward movement of ingesta through the pylorus; when the pylorus is closed the movements assist in the mixing and maceration of the stomach contents.

antritis inflammation of the gastric antrum, the expanded portion of the pyloric part of the stomach.

antr(o)- word element. [L.] *chamber, cavity;* often used with specific reference to the maxillary antrum or sinus.

antrum pl. *antra* [L.] a cavity or chamber.

mastoid a. an air space in the human mastoid portion of the temporal bone communicating with the middle ear and the mastoid cells.

maxillary a., a. maxillare maxillary sinus, especially of humans.

pyloric a., a. pyloricum the lumen of the pyloric part of the stomach; the pump of the stomach, regulating the propulsion of food through the pylorus into the duodenum.

tympanic a., a. tympanicum mastoid antrum.

ANTU see α-NAPHTHYLTHIOUREA.
anuclear having no nucleus.
anulus see ANNULUS.
anuresis 1. retention of urine in the bladder. 2. anuria.
anuria complete suppression of urine formation by the kidney.
anuric failure renal failure in which anuria or oliguria is a prominent sign, as distinct from polyuric failure.
anury absence of the tail.
anus the terminal opening of the alimentary canal. See also ANAL.
imperforate a. congenital absence of the normal opening of the rectum. Called also anal atresia, atresia ani.
a. of Rusconi see BLASTOPORE.
anusitis anal ulceration. See also PERIANAL fistula.
anvil 1. incus; the middle of the three bones of the middle ear. 2. a block of iron, 250–350 lb, with a tapering beak at one end used by farriers to make and shape shoes. There are two holes in the top of the anvil, a square one to hold cutting equipment, and a round one over which holes can be punched in the shoe.
anxiety a demonstration of a feeling of uneasiness, apprehension or dread.
separation a. the display of destructive behavior, vocalization, urination and defecation by some dogs when left alone or separated from their owners.
anxiolytic a mild sedative, such as diazepam, used for relief of anxiety. Called also antianxiety agent and minor tranquilizer.
anxious expression posture and facial expression suggesting apprehension. See also ANXIETY.
Aonyx see OTTER.
aorta pl. *aortae, aortas* [L.] the great artery arising from the left ventricle, being the main trunk from which the systemic arterial system proceeds. See Table 9. See also AORTIC.
abdominal a. the part of the descending aorta within the abdomen.
ascending a. the first part of the aorta which passes dorsally and cranially.
descending a. the aorta after it turns caudally at the aortic arch.
overriding a. see OVERRIDING aorta.
supravalvular a. the portion of aorta immediately above the aortic valve.
terminal a. the segment of the aorta immediately before it divides into the iliac arteries.
thoracic a. the part of the descending aorta within the thorax.
aortic pertaining to or emanating from the AORTA. See also AORTIC ARCH.
a. aneurysm occurs most often in dogs, where it is caused by *Spirocerca lupi* larvae, turkeys and primates, causing dyspnea, cyanosis and coughing. May be congenital affecting the aortic trunk and the arch sometimes associated with aneurysm of an aortic sinus. See also COPPER nutritional deficiency.
a. aneurysm, inherited see inherited aortic ANEURYSM.
a. annulus fibrosus the fibrous ring in the wall of the root of the aorta. In the bovine heart the ring carries the ossa cordis (see OS^2).
a. base rupture rupture of the vessel just above the semilunar valves.
a. bodies small neurovascular structures on either side of the aorta in the region of the aortic arch. The left body is located at the angle between the left subclavian artery and the aorta, and the right at the junction of the right subclavian and right common carotid arteries. They contain chemical receptors which send impulses through the afferent branches of the vagus nerve and are involved in regulating respiration so as to ensure an appropriate partial pressure of oxygen in the arterial blood.
a. body tumors single or multiple nodules within the pericardial sac near the base of the heart. Malignant tumors may invade the anterior mediastinum. Called also heart base tumor.
a. bulb the dilated part of the aorta at its origin, caused by the swellings of the aortic sinuses.
a. coarctation constriction of the aorta at the site of entry of the ductus arteriosus causing a syndrome similar to that of stenosis of the aortic valve.
a. cystic medionecrosis pools of ground substance within the elastic media of the aorta. May predispose to arterial aneurysm but this material is present in the aortas of normal horses.
a. depressor nerve pressure receptors in the aortic arch and thoracic aorta which assist in maintaining circulatory equilibrium by communicating pressure changes through the aortic depressor nerve, an afferent branch of the vagus nerve; stimulation causes heart slowing and vasodilation.
a. dextraposition the aorta receives blood from the right ventricle. There are a number of variations of the basic defect. The common one is the aorta overriding the septum, which is defective, so that the aorta receives blood from both ventricles. The clinical syndrome includes dyspnea and cyanosis from birth, usually with a loud systolic murmur. Affected animals are not viable.
a. embolism occurs in cats in association with feline CARDIOMYOPATHY and rarely in dogs. Acute pain with paresis to paralysis in the hindlegs, cold, cyanotic feet and no femoral pulse are signs of the condition.
a. hiatus an opening in the diaphragm through which the aorta, thoracic duct, the right and/or left azygos veins pass.
a.-ilial embolism see ILIAC artery thrombosis.
a. mineralization is one of the early lesions in poisoning by plants that induce mineralization of tissues, e.g. SOLANUM *malacoxylon*. In combination with lesions in the myocardium causes a syndrome of congestive heart failure.
a. nerve see CARDIAC depressor nerve.
a. palpation the aorta is easily palpable per rectum in cattle and horses; valuable as a clinical sign only in cases of thrombosis at the bifurcation; incision at this point has been used as a means of euthanasia in an emergency.
a.-pulmonary window an anomaly of the aorta in which there is an opening between the the ascending portion of the aorta and the pulmonary artery; clinical signs are similar to those of PATENT ductus arteriosus, but surgical correction is much more difficult.
a. regurgitation see valvular REGURGITATION.
a. root the part of the aorta attached to the atrioventricular fibrous rings and myocardium.
a. rupture 1. in horses is caused by weakening of the wall of the aorta by migrating strongyle larvae. In cattle the cause may be onchocerciasis, in pigs experimental diets deficient in copper. Sudden death results from cardiac tamponade or dissecting aneurysm into the ventricular muscle. 2. sudden death in growing turkeys due to dissecting aneurysmal rupture of the aorta and death due to internal hemorrhage; the cause is unknown.

a. sac the merged ventral aortae of the embryo which supplies blood to the aortic arches.

a. septal defect a congenital anomaly in which there is abnormal communication between the ascending aorta and the pulmonary artery just above the semilunar valves.

a. sinus the three pouch-like dilatations of the aortic bulb which carry the cusps of the aortic valve. The coronary arteries arise from the left caudal and the cranial sinuses.

a. subvalvular stenosis in dogs and pigs is possibly an inherited defect. Characterized by stenosis of the aorta just below the semilunar valves. In pigs, it causes congestive heart failure in the newborn, but in affected dogs severity increases with age so that clinical effects may not be apparent until the patients are older.

a. thromboembolism thrombosis is the usual forerunner of embolism, pieces of the thrombus breaking off the main mass and lodging in more distal parts of the vascular system. See also aortic embolism (above), VERMINOUS mesenteric arteritis, ILIAC artery thrombosis.

a. valve the valve at the entrance to the aorta from the left ventricle made up of three semilunar leaflets or valvulae.

a. valve rupture rupture of the medial cusp is recorded as a cause of sudden death in horses usually as a sequel to endocarditis.

a. valvular disease stenosis is rarely an acquired disorder, but may be an inherited defect in several species. In cats and rarely dogs, restrictive CARDIOMYOPATHY may be a cause of subvalvular aortic obstruction. Valvular incompetence may be congenital or acquired and results in diastolic overloading of the left ventricle with a characteristic water-hammer PULSE and diastolic murmur. See also aortic STENOSIS, aortic subvalvular stenosis (above).

a. vestibule the cranial part of the left ventricular cavity leading to the root of the aorta in the avian heart.

aortic arch the curvature of the aorta where it turns from its cranial path to a caudal one and becomes the thoracic aorta. See also AORTIC.

a. a. anomalies include persistent right aortic arch, double aortic arch, and anomalous arch arteries, which cause compression of areas of the respiratory or digestive tracts.

a. a. branching patterns differ between species; e.g. cat, dog, rabbit are the same; horses and cattle are the same; pigs have one pattern, chickens another.

double a. a. persistence of both right and left embryonic aortic arches creating a vascular ring anomaly that causes esophageal entrapment.

persistent right a. a. persistence of the fourth right aortic arch causes constriction of the esophagus with regurgitation, aspiration pneumonia and dysphagia, and bloat in ruminants. The signs are present at birth.

a. a.-pulmonary artery fistula recorded rarely in horses; a fistula develops after simultaneous perforations occur in the pulmonary artery and the aorta resulting in the development of a fistula and the acute onset of heart failure which is usually fatal within a few days. Possibly results from an inherited defect in the vasa vasorum of the vessels.

a. a. rupture rare occurrence in horses resulting in acute cardiac tamponade or dissecting aneurysm into the myocardium and sudden death; is part of MARFAN'S SYNDROME in calves; rarely a result of onchocerciasis in cattle.

a. a. syndrome any of a group of disorders leading to occlusion of the arteries arising from the aortic arch; such occlusion may be caused by atherosclerosis, arterial embolism, etc.

a. a. transformation the change in the original pattern of aortic arches of the fetus as a result of degeneration of some vessels and differential enlargement of others (see Table 9).

aortic-iliac thrombosis see ILIAC artery thrombosis.

aorticopulmonary septum part of the embryonic development of separating the cardiac chambers from the primordial single sac.

aortitis inflammation of the aorta.

aortocoronary pertaining to or communicating with the aorta and coronary arteries.

aortogram the film produced by aortography.

aortography radiography of the aorta after introduction into it of a contrast material.

aortopathy any disease of the aorta.

aortorrhaphy suture of the aorta.

aortosclerosis sclerosis of the aorta.

aortostenosis narrowing of the aorta.

aortotomy incision of the aorta.

Aotiella aotophilus biting lice found on New World primates.

Aotus trivergatus see OWL MONKEY.

aoudad see AMMOTRAGUS LERVIA.

aoutat see TROMBICULA *autumnalis*.

AP 1. anterior-posterior. 2. alkaline phosphatase.

AP component a basement membrane protein present in reactive amyloid.

AP endonuclease see APURINIC-APYRIMIDINIC (AP) ENDONUCLEASE.

4-AP 4-aminopyridine.

APACHE system Acute Physiology and Chronic Health Evaluation system; a scoring system for assessing severity of disease, used in humans and adapted for use in dogs.

apamine one of the peptides, assumed to be toxic, in bee venom.

apancreatic due to absence of the pancreas.

aparalytic characterized by absence of paralysis.

apathic without sensation or feeling.

apathism slowness of response to stimuli.

apathy failure to respond emotionally to external stimuli.

apatite 1. calcium phosphate; one of the two mineral constituents of bones and teeth. 2. fluorapatite; a naturally occurring rock mineral containing fluorine.

a. calculi see apatite UROLITH.

APC 1. antigen-presenting cells. 2. abbreviation for the combination of aspirin, phenacetin and caffeine, which has been used as an analgesic or antipyretic. 3. atrial premature contraction.

APE anterior pituitary extract.

ape general name for the group of animals which includes the anthropoid apes of the family Pongidae (gibbons, orang-utans, gorillas and chimpanzees) and some other species including the night ape (*Aotus trivirgatus*) and the black Celebes ape (*Cynopithecus niger*).

aperient 1. mildly cathartic. 2. a gentle purgative.

aperistalsis absence of peristaltic action.

apertura pl. *aperturae* [L.] aperture.

aperture an opening.

nasal a. the opening on the skull bounded by the nasal and incisive bones.

nasomaxillary a. the connecting aperture between the middle nasal meatus and the maxillary sinuses.

numerical a. measure of efficiency of a microscope objective proportional to the square root of the amount of light entering the instrument.

apex pl. *apices* [L.] the pointed end of a cone-shaped part.
See also APICAL.
a. beat see cardiac IMPULSE.
cardiac a. lies above the last sternebra and close to the sternal part of the diaphragm.
constricted a. an apical foramen of a tooth is smaller than the adjacent root canal.
dilated a. an apical foramen of a tooth is wider than the adjacent root canal.
nasal a. the dorsal crescent of the snout of the pig.
tooth a. end of a tooth root.
apexification stimulation to form a closed apex in a tooth with necrotic pulp.
apexogenesis stimulation to make the end of a tooth root close in a traumatized tooth with healthy pulp.
aphagia abstention from eating. In the case of animals a suitable translation would seem to be not to take food when it was available.
aphakia absence of the lens of an eye, occurring congenitally or as a result of trauma or surgery. Rare in animals.
aphakic pertaining to aphakia.
a. crescent the crescent-shaped tapetal reflex seen between the iris margin and a subluxated lens.
aphalangia absence of digits.
Aphanizomenon flos-aquae toxic cyanobacterium (algae) contains ANATOXIN; causes sudden death.
Aphanomyces astaci fungal cause of CRAYFISH plague.
apheresis any procedure in which blood is withdrawn from a donor, a portion (plasma, leukocytes, platelets, etc.) is separated and retained, and the remainder is retransfused into the donor. It includes leukapheresis, thrombocytapheresis, etc. Called also pheresis.
aphid an insect of the order Hemiptera. They parasitize many plants during the warm seasons. Of interest in animal health are the black aphids, *Aphis craccivora*, which can exist in very large numbers on burr trefoil, *Medicago polymorpha*, and may stimulate the production of phytoallexins in the plant which then photosensitize animals grazing the infested pasture.
apholate a chemical sterilant for insects; causes congenital ocular defects in sheep.
aphonia loss of the voice; inability to produce vocal sounds.
a. clericorum loss of the voice from overuse, as in dogs barking excessively during kenneling.
aphonic 1. pertaining to aphonia. 2. without audible sound.
aphosphorosis see PHOSPHORUS nutritional deficiency.
aphrodisiac 1. arousing sexual desire. 2. a drug that arouses sexual instinct.
aphtha pl. *aphthae* [L.] see FOOT-AND-MOUTH DISEASE.
aphthosis a condition marked by presence of aphthae.
aphthous characterized by the presence of aphthae.
a. fever see FOOT-AND-MOUTH DISEASE.
Aphthovirus a genus in the family *Picornaviridae*. The seven serotypes of foot-and-mouth disease are the only members of the genus.
aphylaxis absence of phylaxis or immunity.
API 20E a commerically available kit used for the identification of Enterobacteriaceae and some other gram-negative bacteria.
apical pertaining to an APEX.
a. abscess a localized suppurative inflammation of tissues about the apex of a tooth root.
a. delta a foramen made up of multiple fine channels found at the apex of a tooth root through which the blood supply and nerves pass.
a. ectodermal ridge an ectodermal thickening at the end of each limb bud in the developing embryo; of critical importance in the initiation of limb segments.
a. halo a radiological feature of apical abscesses in which the surrounding alveolar bone becomes radiolucent.
a. lung lobe the cranial lobe of the lung.
penile a. ligament a fibrous band along the dorsal surface of the distal part of the penis of the bull which helps to produce a slight twist in the erect state. Abnormality may contribute to the development of deviation of the penis during erection.
apicectomy excision of the apical portion of the root of a tooth through an opening in overlying tissues of the jaw.
apicitis inflammation of the apex of the lung or of the root of a tooth.
apicoectomy see apicectomy.
apicolysis surgical collapse of the apex of the lung.
Apicomplexa a phylum of protozoa, including the coccidia.
Apium graveolens celery; when infected with fungi it may produce phytoallexins including furanocoumarin, and cause photosensitization; can also contain toxic amounts of nitrate.
aplacental having no placenta.
aplasia defective development or complete absence of an organ or tissue due to failure of development.
a. cutis see EPITHELIOGENESIS imperfecta.
pure red cell a. selective depression of erythropoiesis with anemia resulting.
segmental a. aplasia of a segment of an organ, e.g. uterus.
aplastic pertaining to or characterized by aplasia; having no tendency to develop into new tissue.
a. anemia see aplastic ANEMIA.
a. crisis temporary bone marrow failure associated with any disease causing a chronic hemolysis.
Aplopappus heterophyllus HAPLOPAPPUS *heterophyllus*.
apnea 1. temporary cessation of breathing. 2. asphyxia.
sleep a. transient attacks of failure of autonomic control of respiration, becoming more pronounced during sleep and resulting in acidosis and pulmonary arteriolar vasoconstriction and hypertension.
apneic pertaining or relating to apnea or affected with apnea.
a. index a measure of an anesthetic's toxicity with respect to the concentration of the anesthetic necessary to induce respiratory arrest. It compares the concentration of the anesthetic necessary to cause respiratory arrest for one minute to the potency of that particular agent.
apneumia congenital absence of the lungs.
apneusis sustained, gasping inspiration followed by short, inefficient expiration, which can continue to the point of asphyxia. Often associated with lesions in the respiratory center in the brain.
apneustic pertaining to or characterized by apneusis.
a. center a poorly understood part of the respiratory center located in the caudal part of the pons; associated with the taking of deep breaths and in controlling normal respiration.
apo- word element. [Gr.] *away from, separated.*
apocrine denoting that type of glandular mechanism in which the secretory products become concentrat- at the free end of the secreting cell and are throw-

along with a portion of the cytoplasm, as in the mammary gland; cf. holocrine and merocrine.

a. cystic calcinosis see CALCINOSIS circumscripta.

a. cystic dilatation a relatively common finding in dog skin; may be associated with hyperplasia of glandular epithelium or secondary to duct obstruction.

a. cystomatosis see apocrine gland cyst (below).

a. gland cyst cystic hyperplasia of apocrine sweat glands; common in dogs. Often multiple and called apocrine cystomatosis.

a. sweat gland the most abundant type of sweat gland in domestic animals and part of the hair follicle complex; found in haired skin and specialized regions such as the anal sacs. Under sympathetic nervous control and produce sweat by a merocrine mechanism (despite the name) which, in normal quantities, contributes to a protective film on the skin. Specialized apocrine sweat glands are located in the external ear canal and eyelids. Inflammation is called HIDRADENITIS.

a. tumors cystic or papillary adenomas and papillary or tubular carcinomas occur, particularly in dogs and cats. See also ANAL SACS tumor.

apocynin plant toxin found in *Apocynum* spp.; causes gastroenteritis.

Apocynum a plant genus of the family Apocynaceae.

A. cannabinum*, *A. androsaemifolium poisoning by these plants, which probably contain cardiac glycosides, is characterized by a syndrome of gastroenteritis with diarrhea, abdominal pain, teeth grinding with nervous signs of tremor, incoordination and convulsions. Called also dogbane.

Apodemus a genus of the subfamily Murinae of Old World mice and rats.

A. flavicollis the yellow-necked field mouse. See also field MOUSE.

A. sylvaticus the European long-tailed field mouse. See also field MOUSE.

apodia congenital absence of the feet.

apoenzyme the protein component of an enzyme that requires the presence of the prosthetic group (cofactor) to form the functioning enzyme.

apoferritin an apoprotein that can bind many atoms of iron per molecule to form ferritin, the form in which iron is stored in the liver and other tissues.

apogee the state of greatest severity of a disease.

apolar having neither poles nor processes; without polarity.

apolipoprotein a protein moiety occurring in plasma lipoproteins; there are five families of apolipoproteins, designated A–E.

apomorphine an alkaloid from morphine. Used as the hydrochloride; administered parenterally it causes vomiting within 3 to 10 minutes but can also be administered orally. Stimulates receptors in the chemoreceptor trigger zone of the medulla oblongata.

aponeurectomy excision of an aponeurosis.

aponeurorrhaphy suture of an aponeurosis.

aponeurosis pl. *aponeuroses* [Gr.] a broad, sheetlike tendon.

abdominal a. the broad tendinous portion of the oblique and transverse abdominal muscles that attaches to the linea alba.

pharyngeal a. a fascial sheet within the pharyngeal wall, lined with mucous membrane and covered by the pharyngeal constrictors.

aponeurositis inflammation of an aponeurosis.

aponeurotomy incision of an aponeurosis.

Aponomma a genus of ticks occurring almost entirely on reptiles. Resembles *Amblyomma* spp. except that they have no eyes. Includes *A. aruginans* (wombats), *A. concolor* (echidnas).

Apophallus a genus of intestinal flukes (digenetic trematodes) of the family Heterophyidae. Includes *A. muhlingi*, *A. donicum* (dogs, cats).

apophyseal pertaining to an apophysis.

apophysis pl. *apophyses* [Gr.] a bony outgrowth or swelling such as a tuberosity or process, especially one that has no secondary center.

apophysitis inflammation of an apophysis.

apopilosebaceous complex the hair follicle unit consisting of the hair follicle and its associated arrector pili muscle, and apocrine and sebaceous glands. Called also the hair follicle unit.

apoprotein the protein moiety of a molecule or complex, as of a lipoprotein.

apoptosis a process including coagulative necrosis and shrinkage.

apoptotic body degenerate basal epidermal cells, e.g. colloid, hyaline, filamentous, Civatte bodies; round, shrunken, homogeneous, eosinophilic bodies in the stratum basale; are features in lichenoid dermatoses.

aporepressor a repressor that is inactive until it combines with a corepressor.

apostasis 1. an abscess. 2. the end or crisis of an attack or disease.

aposthia congenital absence of the prepuce.

apostome member of the order Apostomatida of ciliated protozoa.

apothecaries' weights and measures a generally superseded system used for measuring and weighing drugs and solutions. It is gradually being replaced by the metric system.

In the apothecaries' system fractions are used to designate portions of a unit of measure: e.g. one-fourth grain is written gr. 1/4. The fraction 1/2 is written ss.

There are two symbols in this system which are sometimes confused and must always be written clearly. These are the symbols for drams (ʒ) and ounces (℥). Small Roman numerals are used after the symbols. For example, ʒiss reads drams one and one-half; ℥iii reads ounces three. See also Tables 4.2 and 4.3.

apothecary a pharmacist; a person who compounds and dispenses drugs.

apotripsis removal of a corneal opacity.

Appaloosa a breed of small riding horses, native to the northwest of the USA, characterized by an irregularly mottled skin and hooves that are vertically striped in black and white. The color patterns vary greatly, but in general there is spotting, speckling or roaning, which can be over the entire body or confined to certain areas, usually the loin and hindquarters. This can be black or brown on a white background or white on a colored background. The breed is known to carry an inherited night blindness.

apparatus 1. an arrangement of a number of parts acting together to perform a special function. 2. certain organ systems such as respiratory or digestive apparatus.

a. digestorius see DIGESTIVE system.

fetlock joint suspensory a. see SUSPENSORY ligament.

forelimb stay a. an apparatus of ligaments and tendons which prevents the forelimb from buckling while the horse is standing for long periods of time; includes mechanisms to prevent flexion of the shoulder and elbow joints, and to prevent overextension or flexion of the carpal joint.

hindlimb stay a. an apparatus of ligaments and tendons which prevents the hindlimb from buckling while the horse is standing for long periods of time; includes mechanisms to lock the stifle and hock joints including the presence of a 'reciprocal apparatus', which ensures that the two joints perform in unison.

lacrimal a. the structures associated with the production, flow and drainage of tears; it includes the lacrimal and accessory glands and their excretory ducts, the lacrimal canals, the lacrimal sac and the nasolacrimal duct.

reciprocal a. consists of two tendinous cords in the hindlimb of the horse, the peroneus tertius and the superficial flexor, which connect the distal end of the femur to the hock, one on the cranial face of the tibia, the other on the caudal face; they ensure that the two joints always move in unison.

Wangensteen's a. a nasal suction apparatus connected with a duodenal tube for aspirating gas and fluid from the stomach and intestine.

append to add to the end of something. In computer terms, adding a character to the end of an existing string of characters or writing data after the end of existing data in a file.

appendage 1. a protuberant outgrowth, such as a tail, a limb or limblike structure. 2. a thing or part appended.

appendicitis inflammation of the vermiform appendix. Occurs in humans and the great apes. The syndrome includes abdominal pain, fever and leukocytosis.

appendicular 1. pertaining to an appendix or appendage. 2. pertaining to the limbs.

a. joint a limb joint.

a. skeleton the skeleton of the limbs.

appendix pl. *appendices* [L.] 1. a slender outgrowth or appendage. 2. the vermiform appendix, a slender diverticulum present in only a few mammals such as the rabbit, humans and the great apes. A structure of doubtful function, rich in lymphoid tissue.

a. epididymis a small, piriform body attached to the head of the epididymis that is a remnant of the blind cranial segment of the mesonephric duct.

a. testis a small cyst adjacent to the head of the epididymis that is a remnant of the paramesonephric (müllerian) duct. Called also Morgagni's hydatid.

Appenzeller a medium-sized, Swiss mountain dog used for herding goats; it has a short, smooth coat in black, tan and white. The tail is curled over the back.

appestat a brain center (probably in the hypothalamus) concerned in controlling the appetite.

appetite the desire for food. It is stimulated by the sight, smell or thought of food and accompanied by the flow of saliva in the mouth and gastric juice in the stomach. Appetite is psychological, dependent on memory and associations, as compared with hunger, which is physiologically aroused by the body's need for food. Its existence in animals can only be conjectured on the response in the form of food intake. Chronic loss of appetite is known as anorexia.

decreased a. see ANOREXIA.

depraved a. see PICA. Called also allotriophagia.

increased a. see HYPEROREXIA, POLYPHAGIA.

salt a. the appetite for salt displayed by animals, especially ruminants, at pasture. Used in the management of cattle on extensive range. See also SALTING.

a. stimulants there are several methods available. Bitters such as gentian and pulv. nux. vomica exert some effect in ruminants, probably by stimulating alimentary tract mucosa. Anabolic steroids are sometimes used for this purpose in dogs and cats. A nutritional deficiency of zinc or the B vitamin complex depresses acuity of appetite and dietary supplementation with it can be effective as an appetite stimulant. Suppression of the medullary satiety center by barbiturates and benzodiazepines is also recommended. There are no well-regarded stimulants of the hunger center of the lateral hypothalamus.

applanometer a mechanical or electronic instrument for determining intraocular pressure in the detection of glaucoma.

apple see MALUS SYLVESTRIS.

a. pulp ingestion of large amounts can cause lactic acidosis, or manganese deficiency resulting in congenital chondrodystrophy.

apple-of-peru see NICANDRA *physalodes*.

apple of Sodom SOLANUM *linneanum*.

application see application PROGRAM.

applicator a device, e.g. a flat wooden stick, used to apply medicaments to a small area of exposed tissue.

apposable capable of being apposed, e.g. edges of a wound.

apposition the placement or position of adjacent structures or parts so that they can come into contact.

apprehension 1. perception and understanding. 2. anticipatory fear or anxiety. See also ANXIETY.

approved veterinary schools schools recognized by the country's registering authority as having educational standards equivalent to the indigenous ones. Graduates of these schools are then accepted for registration to practice in the host country. It may be necessary for applicants to sit an examination to establish that their present proficiency status is adequate. Graduates of schools that are not approved are usually required to undertake further training.

approximal 1. close together. 2. in dentistry the surface of a tooth which faces the adjacent tooth.

approximation 1. the act or process of bringing into proximity or apposition. 2. a numerical value of limited accuracy.

normal a. approximation of the actual distribution of a variable by a normal distribution.

apramycin an aminoglycoside antibiotic, active against gram-negative and gram-positive bacteria. It is water soluble, easily administered in drinking water and has been used largely in treating intestinal infections in pigs and calves.

apricot see PRUNUS.

aprindine an antiarrhythmic drug that acts as a local anesthetic for the myocardial cell membrane; used in the treatment of ventricular arrhythmias.

aprinocid a nucleoside analog used as an anticoccidial agent in chickens and other animals.

aprobarbital, aprobarbitone a crystalline powder, an intermediate-acting sedative and hypnotic.

Aproctella *A. stoddardi* (syn. *Microfilaria fallisi*) a tissue nematode in turkeys, doves, quail, grouse. Necropsy lesions include granulomatous pericarditis.

aproctia imperforate anus.

apron 1. the long hair under the neck and front of the chest seen in rough collie dogs. 2. large skin folds carried on the ventral neck of some strains of merino sheep. 3. a piece of leather suspended under the belly of a ram in front of the prepuce to prevent mating when the ram is used as a teaser. 4. the concrete slab placed in front of feeders in feedlots to reduce muddiness.

aprons outer garments made of lead rubber of a thickness of 0.25–0.5 mm lead equivalent which are worn to prevent x-irradiation of the operator.

aprosopia a developmental anomaly with partial or complete absence of the face.
aprotinin a polyvalent kallikrein-trypsin inhibitor extracted from bovine mast cells; used therapeutically to inhibit fibrinolysis and in the laboratory as a preservative in plasma samples.
Aptenodytes see PENGUIN.
apterium a zone of a bird's skin carrying no feathers or down. The tracts of feathers, carry contour feathers and semiplumes. There are 47 named apteria, e.g. the caudal ventral, the caudal, the postauricular. Called also pterylae.
Apteryx see KIWI.
APTT activated partial thromboplastin time.
aptyalism deficiency or absence of saliva.
APUD cells (*a*mine *p*recursor *u*ptake and *d*ecarboxylation) a group of cells of common embryonic origin that secrete most of the body's hormones, with the exception of steroids. APUD cells comprise both specialized neurons and other endocrine cells. These cells synthesize structurally related polypeptides and biogenic amines. The acronym APUD derives from the fact that polypeptide production is linked to the uptake of a precursor amino acid and its decarboxylation in the cell to produce an amine. Examples of the peptide hormones are insulin, ACTH, glucagon and antidiuretic hormone. Examples of the amine hormones are dopamine, norepinephrine, serotonin and histamine.
APUD tumor see APUDOMA.
apudoma a tumor derived from APUD cells, many of which secrete hormones, e.g. insulinoma and gastrinoma.
Apulian Podolian cattle gray, Italian, meat and draft cattle.
apurinic-apyrimidinic (AP) endonuclease enzyme involved in the excision repair mechanism of DNA. The enzyme nicks the phosphodiester backbone at the depurinized site and excises the sugar phosphate residue, prior to restoration of the damaged strand by the action of DNA polymerase I and ligase.
apus an animal without feet.
apyogenous not caused by pus.
apyretic without fever.
apyrexia absence of fever.
apyrogenic not producing fever.
aq. [L.] *aqua* (water).
aq. dest. *aqua destillata* (distilled water).
AQIS Australian Quarantine Inspection Service.
aqua [L.] 1. water, H_2O. 2. a saturated solution of a volatile oil or other aromatic or volatile substance in purified water.
aquaculture cultivation and harvesting of plants and animals in water. Called also mariculture.
aquapuncture acupuncture terminology for injection therapy; includes injection of any nonirritant therapeutic agent.
Aquareovirus a genus of viruses in the family *Reoviridae*. They cause disease in fish and shellfish.
aquarist student of marine life; curator of an aquarium.
aquarium unit for storage and display of aquatic species; may be fresh water or saline for marine specimens.
aquatic snakes a term which includes some members of the Colubridae family, of very low or nil venomicity, and true sea-snakes of the family Hydrophiidae, which have very powerful venom but keep mostly to the open sea. They can be a hazard if blown to shore in rough weather. They have a capability of staying under water for as long as 8 hours.
aqueduct canal or passage.
cerebral a. a narrow channel in the midbrain connecting the third and fourth ventricles and containing cerebrospinal fluid. Called also aqueduct of Sylvius.
a. of cochlea a narrow canal that unites the perilymphatic space near the base of the cochlea with the subarachnoid space beneath the temporal bone. Called also perilymphatic duct.
a. of Cotunnius vestibular aqueduct.
a. of Fallopius the canal for the facial nerve in the temporal bone. Called also facial canal.
sylvian a., a. of Sylvius cerebral aqueduct. Called also ventricular aqueduct.
ventricular a. see cerebral aqueduct (above).
vestibular a. bony canal that opens onto the medial surface of the temporal bone and passes to the vestibule of the inner ear; houses the endolymphatic duct. Called also aqueduct of Cotunnius.
aqueocentesis surgical puncture of the anterior chamber of the eye for the removal of aqueous humor.
aqueous watery; prepared with water.
a.–blood barrier see blood–aqueous BARRIER.
a. flare turbidity of the aqueous humor caused by increased protein levels and cells.
a. humor the fluid produced by the ciliary process in the eye and occupying the anterior and posterior chambers. It provides nourishment for the lens and cornea and maintains the ocular pressure, and hence the optical integrity of the eyeball. Disturbance of its drainage through the corneoiridial angle can induce glaucoma and other disorders.
a. paracentesis see AQUEOCENTESIS.
plasmoid a. aqueous humor with a protein concentration approaching that of plasma; seen in inflammation or other disruption of the blood–aqueous barrier.
a. suspension a mixture of insoluble particles in water.
Aquila chrysaetos majestic predator bird of Europe, Asia, North America. Called also golden eagle.
Aquilaria agallocha see ALOE.
Aquilegia vulgaris a European member of the plant family Ranunculaceae; it is reputed to be poisonous because of its high content of cyanogenetic glycosides. Called also columbine, granny bonnets.
aquilide A a carcinogen in PTERIDIUM AQUILINUM (bracken).
Aquitaine blond a yellow or yellow-brown breed of meat and draft cattle bred in southern France and Spain. Called also Blond D'Aquitaine.
Ar chemical symbol, *argon*.
-ar suffix meaning pertaining to.
AR5189 virus a flavivirus associated with abortion and stillbirths in cattle in Africa.
ara-A adenine arabinoside; see VIDARABINE.
ara-C cytosine arabinoside; see CYTARABINE.
Ara macao see MACAW.
Arab the purest bred breed of horses and one of great antiquity. A small (14 to 15 hands high, or 55–60 inches at the wither) riding horse, usually bay, chestnut, white or fleabitten gray in color. It has been extensively used in the production of other breeds and crossbreds. It and its crossbreds are noted for the presence amongst them of cerebellar dysplasia, combined immunodeficiency and leukoderma. Called also the Arabian horse.
Arabi black, pied or white fat-tailed, meat or carpet-wool sheep with black head. The males are horned, the females polled. See also NEAR EAST FAT-TAILED.
Arabian having some relationship to Arabia, most conspicuously Arabian horses.

Darley A. the original Arab sire, the founder of the thoroughbred breed, imported into England in 1704.
A. fading syndrome see Arabian FADING syndrome.
A. foal pneumonia see PNEUMONIA.
arabinosyl cytosine see CYTARABINE.
Araceae the plant family of aroids (arums) which can be highly irritant when chewed because of a high content of oxalate as raphide crystals. Genera include *Arum*, *Dieffenbachia*, *Philodendron*, *Monstera*, *Zantedeschia*, *Arisaema*, *Xanthosma*, *Lysichiton*.
arachidonic acid twenty carbon fatty acid containing four double bonds of the n-6 family essential fatty acids from which prostaglandins, thromboxane and leukotrienes are derived. Deficiency, which is characterized by hair loss, fatty liver degeneration, anemia and reduced fertility, occurs most commonly in cats because of their inability to synthesize arachidonic acid from linoleic acid.
Arachis hypogaea see PEANUT.
arachnid a member of the class Arachnida of animals.
Arachnida a class of animals of the phylum Arthropoda, including 12 orders, comprising such forms as spiders, scorpions, ticks and mites.
arachnidism poisoning from a spider bite.
arachnitis see ARACHNOIDITIS.
arachnoid 1. resembling a spider's web. 2. the delicate membrane interposed between the dura mater and the pia mater, and with them constituting the meninges. Called also arachnoidea.
cerebral a., arachnoidea cerebri the arachnoid investing the brain.
a. cyst cysts of the pia and arachnoid containing cerebrospinal fluid; may cause gradually increasing pressure on nervous tissue, especially spinal cord, causing ataxia, paresis.
a. fibroblastoma see MENINGIOMA.
a. granulations villous enlargements of the arachnoid that protrude into dural sinuses or diploic veins and serve to drain cerebrospinal fluid. They are conspicuous in the dorsal sagittal sinus of the horse.
a. membrane arachnoid; middle layer of the meninges.
spinal a. the arachnoid investing the spinal cord.
arachnoidea see ARACHNOID.
arachnoiditis inflammation of the arachnoid.
arachnomelia a congenital anomaly in which the distal extremities of the limbs are excessively long and thin, giving the animal a spidery look.
inherited a. the bones of the elongated limbs are very fragile and there are additional skeletal and cardiovascular defects in affected calves.
aran TRIFOLIUM *repens*.
Aranaeomorpha a suborder of spiders with horizontal fangs; includes the red-backed spider.
Araneida an order of the class Arachnida which contains the spiders.
araphia failure of closure of the embryonic neural tube, the spinal cord developing as a flat plate.
ARAS ascending reticular activating system. See RETICULAR activating system.
arasan a cause of poisoning in poultry due to its content of TETRAMETHYLTHIURAM DISULFIDE.
Araujia hortorum a vine in the family Asclepiadaceae. Its seeds are poisonous to fowl. Probably contains cardiac glycosides. Called also white moth plant, cruel vine.
arbocell purified cellulose; used as a fiber supplement.
arbor pl. *arbores* [L.] a tree.
a. vitae treelike outlines of white substance seen on median section of the cerebellum.
a. vitae cerebelli see arbor vitae (above).
arboreal pertaining to trees, treelike, tree-dwelling.
arborescent branching like a tree.
arborization a collection of branches, as the branching terminal processes of a nerve cell.
a. diagnosis method see DECISION tree, ALGORITHM.
arbovirus (*ar*thropod-*bo*rne) one that replicates in an arthropod, which acts as a vector in transmission of the virus to a susceptible vertebrate host in which replication also occurs. See also TOGAVIRIDAE, BUNYAVIRIDAE, REOVIRIDAE, RHABDOVIRIDAE, ARENAVIRIDAE.
ARC Agricultural Research Council (UK).
arc a part of the circumference of a circle, or a regularly curved line.
binauricular a. the arc across the top of the head from one auricular point to the other.
reflex a. the circuit traveled by impulses producing a reflex action: from the receptor organ, through the afferent nerve, nerve center, efferent nerve, to the effector organ.
arcade see DENTAL arcade.
arcate arcuate.
arch a structure of bowlike or curved outline.
a. of aorta the curving portion between the ascending and descending aorta, giving rise to the brachiocephalic trunk and, in some species, the left common carotid and the left subclavian artery.
aortic a's paired vessels that run from the ventral to the dorsal aortae through the branchial arches of fishes and amniote embryos. In mammalian development, arches 1 and 2 disappear; 3 joins the common to become the internal carotid artery; 4 becomes the arch of the aorta and joins the aorta and subclavian artery; 5 disappears; 6 forms the pulmonary arteries and, until birth, the ductus arteriosus.
arterial a. one or more arteries that form an anastomotic connection between two more or less parallel tributaries; found commonly around joints and other moveable parts.
a. arteriosus, arcus arteriosus a large communicating branch between two arteries.
branchial a's four pairs of mesenchymal and later cartilaginous columns in the pharyngeal wall which in fish develop into gills and in mammals become modified into structures of the ear and neck.
branchial a. derivatives derivatives of the arches are first arch (mandible, ossicles), second arch (hyoid apparatus, ear ossicles), third arch (hyoid apparatus), fourth arch (laryngeal cartilages).
costal a. the rim to the bony thorax formed by the conjoined asternal ribs and their connecting elastic tissue.
cricoid a. the slender ventral half of the cricoid cartilage of the larynx. The most caudal of the palpable landmarks of the larynx.
dental a. the curving structure formed by the crowns of the teeth in their normal position, or by the residual ridge after loss of the teeth.
hemal a. the v- or y-shaped bone borne on the ventral surface of the tail vertebrae of some animals and which protects blood vessels. Called also chevron bone.
hyoid a. the second branchial arch.
ischial a., ischiatic a. the caudal rim of the pelvis formed by the conjunction of the two ischiae. Called also sciatic arch.
lumbocostal a. of the diaphragm the dorsal part of the diaphragm where it crosses the ventral surface of the psoas muscles. Here it is without any attachment and only serous membranes separate the thoracic and peritoneal cavities.

mandibular a. the first branchial arch, being the rudiment of the maxillary and mandibular regions.
neural a. the dorsal vertebral arch.
palatal a. the arch formed by the roof of the mouth from the teeth on one side to those on the other.
palatoglossal a. the thick fold of tissue passing from the soft palate to the lateral border of the tongue.
palatopharyngeal a. a horizontal fold of pharyngeal mucosa that passes from the soft palate and joins with its opposite fold over the entrance to the esophagus.
palmar a. a superficial and a deep vascular arch behind the carpus formed by the conjunction of several arteries of the forearm.
pulmonary a's the most caudal of the embryonic aortic arches, which become the pulmonary arteries.
sciatic a. ischial arch.
subcarpal a. the deep palmar arch, especially of horses.
superficial dorsal a. one of the arterial arches in the foot of carnivores.
supracarpal a. the superficial palmar arch, especially of horses.
tendinous a. a linear arched thickening of fascia that provides attachment for some muscles.
terminal a. the union between the medial and lateral palmar digital arteries, which in horses runs through the solar canal within the distal phalanx.
vertebral a. the dorsal bony arch of a vertebra, composed of paired laminae and pedicles.
zygomatic a. the arch formed by the processes of the zygomatic and temporal bones that is the principal origin of the masseter muscle and is particularly broad and prominent in carnivores.

archaebacteria prokaryotic organisms, distinct from eubacteria, which are found in association with high temperatures or salinity, or are methanogenic. None are pathogens.

archencephalon the embryonic primitive brain from which the midbrain and forebrain develop.

archenteron the central cavity that is the provisional gut in the gastrula; the primitive digestive cavity of the embryo.

archeokinetic relating to the primitive type of motor nerve mechanism as seen in the peripheral nervous system.

arch(i)- word element. [Gr.] *ancient, beginning, first, original.*

archicerebellum the phylogenetically older part of the cerebellum that includes the flocculonodular lobe. Called also vestibular cerebellum.

archicortex see ARCHIPALLIUM.

archinephron the pronephros.

arching back postural abnormality usually accompanied by stiff gait, anxious expression; caused by pain in peritoneum, caused usually by peritonitis.
a. b. downward fleeting postural abnormality occurring during spasms of pain; the back is depressed, often accompanied by crouching.

archipallium that portion of the pallium, or cerebral cortex, which phylogenetically is older and composed of the hippocampus and dentate gyrus.

archistome see BLASTOPORE.

Architeuthidae the family of the giant squids. See SQUID.

archiving removal of infrequently needed data from a computer to a less accessible storage.

arciform see ARCUATE.

Arcobacter a genus of gram-negative, aerotolerant, spiral-shaped bacteria, associated with abortion in pigs and horses.

arctation narrowing of an opening or canal.

Arctic husky see SIBERIAN HUSKY.

Arctictis a genus of one (Viverridae) of the seven families in the order Carnivora. Members have anal scent glands.
A. binturong a cat-sized animal with a long mandible and a prehensile tail. Called also binturong, bear cat.

Arctium lappa a temperate zone plant with burrs which causes granular stomatitis in the dog. Called also burdock.

Arctonyx collaris see hog BADGER.

Arctotheca calendula a plant of the family Asteracea. Good forage plant but may contain toxic amounts of nitrate when it grows profusely after the breaking of a long drought. See also NITRITE poisoning. Called also *Cryptostemma calendula*, capeweed.

Arctotis glutinosa OSTEOSPERMUM *cuneata.*

arcuate bent like a bow.
a. line part of the terminal line that marks the boundary of the pelvic inlet and which extends from the sacrum to the pubic brim.
a. vessels the radicles of the interlobar arteries of the kidney found at the corticomedullary junction that give off the interlobular arteries.

arcuation a bending or curvature.

Arcyophora a genus of moths in the order Lepidoptera.
A. longivalvis, A. patricula nocturnal moths that feed on the secretions of cows' eyes and physically transmit infections of the conjunctival sac between cattle.

Ardea see HERON.

Ardeola see EGRET.

ARDS acute respiratory distress syndrome.

area pl. *areae, areas* [L.] a limited space or plane surface.
association a's areas of the cerebral cortex (excluding primary areas) connected with each other and with the neothalamus; they are responsible for higher mental and emotional processes, including memory, learning, etc.
Brodmann's a's specific occipital and preoccipital areas of the cerebral cortex, distinguished by differences in the arrangement of their six cellular layers, and identified by numbering each area.
cardiogenic a. in the embryo includes heart and pericardial rudiments.
central retinal a. the area of the retina, dorsal to the optic papilla, along the optical axis. Here the retinal vessels are missing.
In cattle the area is poorly defined as two areas; a rounded area concerned with binocular vision and a horizontal strip concerned wuth monocular vision.
a. cerebrovasculosa in anencephaly the cerebral hemispheres are replaced by a sheet of tissue composed largely of blood vessels called the area cerebrovasculosa.
a. cribrosa that part of the renal crest or renal papilla at which the papillary ducts open into the pelvis.
germinal a., a. germinativa embryonic disk.
a. medullovasculosa the central part of a spinal meningomyelocele. It is a raised, reddish protuberance devoid of skin and consists of spinal cord with a surrounding vascular network.
motor a. that area of the cerebral cortex which, on brief electrical stimulation, shows the lowest threshold and shortest latency for the production of muscle movement.
a. nuda an the area on the surface of a viscus that has no serosal covering.

olfactory a. 1. the part of the piriform lobe of the brain associated with olfaction. 2. a more general area including the olfactory bulb, tract and trigone.

a. opaca the opaque area of the embryonic disk of the fertilized avian egg surrounding the area pellucida; it forms some extraembryonic structures.

a. pellucida the clear central part of the developing embryonic disk in a fertilized avian egg. Produces the embryo's tissues.

a. piriformis temporalis the cortical area of the piriform lobe of the brain.

primary a. areas of the cerebral cortex comprising the motor and sensory regions.

psychomotor a. motor area.

a. sampling see area SAMPLING.

silent a. an area of the brain in which pathological conditions may occur without producing clinical signs.

vocal a. the part of the glottis between the vocal cords.

areca nut the fruit of the betel nut tree (*Areca catechu*). Originally used as a cathartic and vermifuge. Its principal ingredient is ARECOLINE.

arecoline an alkaloid obtained from the nut of the tree *Areca catechu*. Previously, a preferred treatment for cestodes in dogs. The acetarsol, hydrobromide and carboxyphenylstilbonate salts have been used for this purpose. Oral administration causes paralysis of the worms and catharsis, so the worms are expelled alive and intact. Lower doses are used as a laxative.

a. challenge test used in the diagnosis of narcolepsy in dogs; pretreatment with atropine reduces the number of cataleptic attacks with exposure to food.

areflexia absence of the reflexes.

detrusor a. a cause of automatic URINARY BLADDER.

Arenaria serpyllifolia a temperate zone plant plant genus of the family Caryophyllaceae. Ingestion causes profuse salivation in horses. Called also thyme-leaved sandwort.

Arenaviridae a family of spherical or pleomorphic, enveloped, single-stranded RNA viruses containing host cell-derived ribosomes, e.g. Lassa fever virus, lymphocytic choriomeningitis (LCM) virus and Tacaribe viruses. The natural hosts are rodents.

arenavirus a virus in the family ARENAVIRIDAE.

areola pl. *areolae* [L.] 1. a narrow zone surrounding a central area, e.g. the darkened area surrounding the NIPPLE of the human mammary gland. 2. any minute space or interstice in a tissue.

placental a. in the epitheliochorial placenta of the sow areolae develop in the placentation zone. They are shallow cups in the chorion opposite the openings of the endometrial glands in the uterine wall.

areolar 1. containing minute spaces. 2. pertaining to an areola.

a. connective tissue loose, spongy connective tissue.

ARF see A–R–F SEQUENCE.

Arg arginase.

argali a wild sheep *Ovis ammon*.

Argas a genus of ticks parasitic on poultry and other birds and sometimes humans.

A. miniatus, A. radiatus, A. robertsi, A. sanchezi similar to *A. persicus* and originally classified with that species.

A. persicus causes tick worry of birds and paralysis of poultry; transmits *Aegyptianella pullorum* and *Borrelia anserina*.

A. reflexus infests pigeons and may transmit *Borrelia anserina* to poultry.

argasid tick tick belonging to the family Argasidae.

Argasidae a family of arthropods made up of the soft-bodied ticks.

Arge pullata larvae of this Scandinavian birch SAWFLY causes severe liver necrosis in sheep which eat them. Contains LOPHYROTOMIN.

Argemone a genus of the plant family Papaveraceae, the poppy family. Includes *A. mexicana*, *A. ochroleuca*, *A. subfusiformis*; contains isoquinoline alkaloids including sanguinarine, which causes mucosal irritation and also interference with pyruvate oxidation in brain tissue. The sanguinarine is excreted in cows' milk and may be linked to the occurrence of endemic primary glaucoma of humans. The seeds of *A. mexicana* and *A. ochroleuca* are frequent contaminants of grain fed to chicken, causing low egg production, edema, ataxia, comb cyanosis and gastroenteritis. Dried plants in hay may cause chronic heart failure in cattle. Called also Mexican poppy.

argentaffin staining readily with silver salts; see also argentaffin CELL.

a. tumor see CARCINOID.

argentaffinoma a tumor arising from argentaffin cells, most frequently in the duodenum, colon and rectum of dogs. Called also carcinoid. Such tumors produce CARCINOID syndrome.

Argenté large, silver-colored, fur rabbits, in several color varieties with different tonings in the fur. Champagne is the largest, with a dark, slate blue coat; Bleu is lavender blue; Brun, silvered-brown; and Creme, silvered yellow.

Argentine having some relationship with the country Argentina.

A. tick MARGAROPUS *winthemi*.

A. tortoise GEOCHELONE *chilensis*.

Argentipallium blandowskianum HELICHRYSUM *blandowskianum*.

argentum [L.] *silver* (symbol Ag).

arginase an enzyme of the urea cycle in the liver that splits arginine into urea and ornithine; abbreviated ARG. Significant amounts occur only in ureotelic mammals such as dogs, cats, sheep, pigs, rats and humans. Elevated blood levels are associated with acute hepatic necrosis and determination of arginase levels in plasma or serum is a good liver-specific test in these species. Called also arginine amidinase, canavanase.

arginine a basic amino acid occurring in proteins and essential for many species, particularly the cat.

a. amidinase see ARGINASE.

a. deaminase test see arginine dihydrolase test (below).

a. dihydrolase test a test for the identification of bacteria, based on the conversion of L-arginine to putrescine. In a positive result, the alkaline product is indicated by bromocresol purple. Called also arginine deaminase test.

a. esterase an androgen-dependent enzyme derived from the prostate which occurs in high concentrations in seminal plasma.

a. nutritional deficiency results in elevated blood ammonia concentration. Cats are particularly sensitive and within hours of eating an arginine-free diet, severe neurological signs develop, leading to death. In other species, cataracts have been reported in dogs and feather abnormalities occur in chickens on deficient diets.

a. vasopressin a potent vasoconstrictor in mammals.

a. vasotocin the normal antidiuretic hormone in birds; released from the avian posterior pituitary.

L-arginine–nitrous oxide pathway a metabolic pathway in which nitrous oxide is liberated from arginine by such factors as acetylcholine or shear stress; the nitrous oxide causes vasodilation and inhibits aggregation of platelets and the development of adhesions.

argininosuccinic acid a compound normally formed as an intermediate in urea metabolism in the liver, but not normally present in urine.

arginosuccinate synthetase a urea cycle enzyme in the liver. A deficiency of the enzyme results in very high blood levels of ammonia. See also CITRULLINEMIA.

argon a chemical element, atomic number 18, atomic weight 39.948, symbol Ar. See Table 6.

ARGT annual ryegrass toxicity.

Argulus a genus in the class Crustacea. Freshwater fish lice which cause cutaneous ulceration leading to secondary infection. They also transmit spring viremia of carp. Heavy infestations cause poor growth and erratic swimming. Includes *A. brachiuran*.

argyria poisoning by silver or its salts; chronic argyria is marked by a permanent ashen-gray discoloration of the skin, conjunctiva and internal organs.

argyric pertaining to silver.

argyrism see ARGYRIA.

argyrophil easily impregnated with silver.

argyrophilia affinity for silver stains.

argyrosis see ARGYRIA.

arhinencephaly congenital absence of the olfactory bulbs, tract or nerves. May be accompanied by prolonged pregnancy. Recorded in Guernsey, Simmental and Aberdeen Angus cattle.

arhinia congenital absence of the nose.

ariboflavinosis deficiency of RIBOFLAVIN (vitamin B_2) in the diet, a condition marked by lesions in the corners of the mouth, on the lips, and around the nose and eyes, malaise, weakness, weight loss and, in severe cases, corneal or other eye changes and seborrheic dermatitis.

Arisaema toxic plant genus in family Araceae. Contains raphide oxalate crystals; causes oral mucosal erosions and stomatitis if ingested. Called also Indian turnip, jack-in-the-pulpit.

Aristida member of grass family Poaceae; seeds cause subcutaneous abscesses. Includes *A. arenaria* (*A. contorta*), *A. ciliata*, *A. obtusa* (*Stipagrostis* spp.).

Aristolochia a plant genus of the family Aristolochiaceae. Contains toxic alkaloid aristolochine which causes purgation; effect resembles that of aloin. Includes *A. bracteata*, *A. clematitis* (birthwort), *A. densivenia*, *A. elegans* (Dutchman's pipe). *A. elegans* is toxic to the larvae of Australian butterflies.

aristolochine the toxic alkaloid in the plants *Aristolochia* spp.

arithmetic mean see MEAN.

Arizona a subgroup of the genus *Salmonella* bacteria. See avian ARIZONOSIS.

arizonosis infection with *Arizona* spp.

avian a. a disease of birds caused by infection with *Salmonella arizonae* (*Arizona hinshawi*). Manifested by diarrhea, leg paralysis, twisted neck and pasted vent. Affected birds squat on their hocks and huddle together.

Arles Merino sheep French finewool sheep originated from local breed plus Spanish merino, horned or polled.

Arlt technique surgical technique for SYMBLEPHARON repair.

arm 1. the limb segment between the shoulder and elbow joints; sometimes called the upper arm as distinct from the lower arm which is the section from elbow to carpus. 2. loosely, the free part of the thoracic limb, especially of bipeds.

armadillo see DASYPUS NOVEMCINCTUS.

Westy a. syndrome see EPIDERMAL dysplasia.

armamentarium the entire equipment of a practitioner, such as medicines, instruments, books.

Armigeres mosquito species thought to be capable of carrying Japanese encephalitis virus.

Armillifer a genus of the class Pentastomida consisting of organisms of uncertain taxonomy. Usually considered to be aberrant crustaceans.

A. armillatus occupies respiratory tract of snakes.

army a group of hippopotami; for full appreciation of this irregular collective noun a lyrical pronunciation of *hippopotarmy* is needed.

Army-Navy retractors a handheld retractor with broad blades used for large muscles.

armyworm the larvae of the owlet moth (*Laphygma exempta*) which migrates in large groups ravaging crops.

Arnebia hispidissima poisonous plant in the family Boraginaceae containing the pyrrolizidine alkaloids monocrotaline and echimidine.

arni see AMMOTRAGUS LERVIA.

Arnoczky procedure an over-the-top technique for intra-articular reconstruction of the cranial cruciate ligament, using a medial patellar tendon graft.

Arnold–Chiari malformation a congenital anomaly in which the cerebellum and medulla oblongata protrude down into the cervical spinal canal through the foramen magnum; it is almost always associated with meningomyelocele, spina bifida and hydrocephalus. Recorded in calves, sheep and dogs.

aromatic 1. having a spicy fragrance. 2. a stimulant, spicy medicine. 3. denoting a compound containing a resonance-stabilized ring, e.g. benzene or naphthalene.

a. diamidines some are useful babesiocides, e.g. imidocarb, amicarbalide, phenamidine.

a. organic arsenicals includes thiacetarsamide, arsphencomplexamine, arsanilic acid, roxarsone, nitarsone.

arousal a readiness response; a state of readiness to make behavioral responses.

arprinocid a nucleoside analog used as a coccidiostat.

Arrabidea toxic South American plant genus in family Bignoniaceae; contains unknown toxins capable of causing sudden death in cattle. Includes *A. bilabiata* (gibata), *A. japurensis*.

arrector pl. *arrectores* [L.] raising, or that which raises; an erector muscle.

a. pili muscle smooth muscle that extends from the papillary zone of the dermis to the base of a hair follicle. Involuntary contraction causes hair erection which, in some species, is most noticeable on the neck and along the back (see HACKLES).

arrest sudden cessation or stoppage.

cardiac a. sudden and often unexpected stoppage of effective heart action. Either the periodic impulses which trigger the coordinated heart muscle contractions cease or ventricular fibrillation or flutter occurs in which the individual muscle fibers have a rapid irregular twitching.

epiphyseal a. premature arrest of the longitudinal growth of bone due to fusion of the epiphysis and diaphysis.

maturation a. interruption of the process of development, as of blood cells, before the final stage is reached.

sinoatrial a. a disturbance in cardiac conduction in which the sinoatrial node intermittently fails to generate an impulse. There are no P waves or PQRS-T complexes for at least twice the normal R-R interval. If the pauses are long enough, junctional or ventricular escape complexes may occur. Occurs most commonly in brachycephalic dogs, causing only minor clinical signs.

arrested larval development see HYPOBIOSIS.

Arrhenatherum elatius hardy, perennial bunchgrass suitable for hay or pasture. Called also tall oatgrass.

Arrhenius' plot a graph which displays calculations from Arrhenius' equation which deals with the temperature dependence of a reaction rate constant. Used in studies of biological effects of heat.

arrheno- word element. [Gr.] *male, masculine.*

arrhenoblastoma a rare ovarian stromal tumor that sometimes causes virilization.

arrhinia see ARHINIA.

arrhythmia variation from the normal rhythm, especially of the heartbeat. See also BRADYCARDIA, TACHYCARDIA.

atrial a. see atrial FLUTTER, atrial FIBRILLATION.

bradycardic a. see BRADYARRHYTHMIA.

benign a. one which is clinically insignificant.

cardiac a. irregularity of the normal heart rhythm, either in frequency or amplitude, or almost always both.

exercise-induced a. a cause of poor racing performance or sudden death while racing; detectable only by telemetered electrocardiography.

sinus a. the physiological cyclic variation in heart rate related to vagal impulses to the sinoatrial node.

supraventricular a's see sinoatrial ARREST, atrial TACHYCARDIA, supraventricular TACHYCARDIA, atrial FIBRILLATION.

ventricular a's see PREMATURE heartbeats, VENTRICULAR tachycardia, ventricular FIBRILLATION.

arrhythmic tachycardia the heart rate is faster than normal, the rhythm is irregular; due usually to myocarditis.

arrhythmogenic producing or promoting arrhythmia.

arrow keys see MOVEMENT keys.

arrow poisons include curare and its active component *d*-tubocurarine.

arrowgrass see TRIGLOCHIN. Called also seaside or marsh arrowgrass.

Arruga forceps capsule forceps with fine, downcurving points tipped with an expanded, hollowed out enlargement designed for handling delicate ocular tissues.

arsanilic acid Called also para-aminophenylarsonic acid. See also organic ARSENIC poisoning.

arsenate an uncommon garden pesticide, as lead arsenate, or as antifungal spray on fruit trees or cattle tick dip as sodium arsenate. Relatively insoluble but will cause arsenic poisoning but less toxic than arsenite.

arseniasis arsenical poisoning.

arsenic a chemical element, atomic number 33, atomic weight 74.92, symbol As. See Table 6. Arsenic compounds have been widely used in veterinary medicine, but they have been replaced for the most part by antibiotics, which are less toxic and equally effective. Some of the arsenicals are used for infectious diseases, especially those caused by protozoa, and some skin disorders and blood dyscrasias also are still treated with arsenic compounds. Since arsenic is highly toxic it must be administered with caution. The antidote for arsenic poisoning is DIMERCAPROL (BAL). See also ARSENICAL.

a. bush *Senna floribunda, S. occidentalis.*

copper–chrome–a. wood preservative see WOOD PRESERVATIVE.

a. deficiency evidence on the response to arsenic supplementation of the diet suggests that it may exert a beneficial effect on patients by controlling deleterious intestinal organisms.

inorganic a. poisoning can occur after ingestion or cutaneous absorption. Acute poisoning is manifested by abdominal pain, diarrhea and dehydration. Chronic poisoning shows a syndrome of emaciation, chronic diarrhea, poor haircoat and greatly reduced productivity.

organic a. poisoning arsanilate poisoning in pigs is characterized by blindness and incoordination and a high recovery rate; poisoning by 4-hydroxyphenyl arsenic acid also in pigs causes a syndrome of tremor and incoordination but only if the affected animals are exercising at the time.

a. poisoning see inorganic arsenic poisoning, organic arsenic poisoning (above).

a. trioxide AsO_3, pollutant on pasture from roasting of arsenical and some iron ores.

arsenical 1. pertaining to arsenic. 2. a compound containing arsenic.

a. herbicide includes monosodium or disodium methanearsonates. See also organic arsenical (below).

organic a. includes **aliphatic** organic arsenicals, e.g. the pharmaceuticals cacodylic and phenarsonic acids, the herbicides monosodium and disodium methanearsonates, **aromatic** organic arsenicals, e.g. trivalent phenylorganic arsenicals like thiacetarsamide, arsphencomplexamine, and pentavalent **phenylorganic** arsenicals like arsanilic acid, roxarsone, nitarsone. Poisoning by organic arsenicals causes blindness and incoordination or restlessness, convulsions, incoordination, screaming. Recovery is spontaneous if the toxin is discontinued but some piglets may remain blind.

a. pyrites an arsenic-rich ore.

a. sheepdip, cattledip usually contains arsenic and sulfur with 20% soluble arsenic and 3% insoluble arsenious sulfide.

a. smoke factory smoke effluent from processes using arsenic-rich ores may pollute local pasture with arsenic trioxide.

a. weedkiller contains sodium or potassium arsenite or thioarsenites. They may contain up to 40% arsenic trioxide.

arsenites soluble arsenic compounds, e.g. sodium arsenite. The most toxic of forms of arsenic. Used as insecticides, herbicides. See also inorganic and organic ARSENIC poisoning.

arsenoblast the male element of a zygote; a male pronucleus.

arsphencomplexamine an organic aromatic arsenical therapeutic agent; a trivalent phenylorganic compound.

Artemia shrimp grown and used extensively as a food source for ornamental and food fish culture. Called also brine shrimp.

Artemisia a genus of the plant family Asteraceae. Includes *A. filifolia, A. canescens, A. spinescens, A. vulgaris* (mugwort) and more than 200 other plants comprising a large part of the sagebrush of the western range of the USA. Under exceptional circumstances and with very heavy grazing they may cause unspecified poisonings. *A. canescens* causes selenium poisoning of sheep.

A. absinthium contains oil of absinthe and may be irritant. Called also wormwood.

arteria pl. *arteriae* [L.] artery.
a. lusoria an abnormally situated vessel dorsal to the esophagus derived from the aortic arch which may cause compression of the esophagus or trachea.
arterial pertaining to an ARTERY or to the arteries.
a. anomaly see ARTERIOVENOUS fistula, PORTACAVAL shunt.
a. baroreceptors pressure-sensitive receptors in the blood vessels which initiate changes in blood volume; include low-pressure receptors in great veins and high-pressure receptors in carotid and aortic bodies.
a. blood pressure see BLOOD PRESSURE.
cerebral a. circle arterial circle created by the conjunction of the caudal communicating artery and the rostral cerebral artery. It encircles the optic chiasma and the hypophysis. Called also the circle of Willis.
cilial a. circle the circle of arteries in the ciliary muscle of the eye of birds.
a. degeneration includes ARTERIOSCLEROSIS, ATHEROSCLEROSIS.
direct a. blood pressure direct measurement via a manometer inserted into the artery; procedure suited only to experimental procedures.
a. embolism see EMBOLISM.
a. hypertrophy hypertrophy of any or all layers of the arterial wall. Usually a response to an increased work load, e.g. in collateral arteries after occlusion of a main supply artery; may be associated with regional, e.g. pulmonary, hypertension.
indirect a. blood pressure see arterial BLOOD PRESSURE.
a. inflammation see ARTERITIS.
iridial a. circle the arterial circle at the periphery of the iris.
a. mineralization see MINERALIZATION, INTIMAL bodies.
a. pulse see PULSE.
a. rupture traumatic rupture is more common than spontaneous rupture; the latter occurs in uterine arteries of hypocuprotic old mares at parturition, in dogs infested with *Spirocerca lupi*, in internal or maxillary arteries ulcerated by fungal infection in horses causing fatal hemorrhage into the guttural pouch.
a. thromboembolism see EMBOLISM, THROMBOSIS, VERMINOUS mesenteric arteritis, saddle THROMBUS.
a. thrombosis the presence of a thrombus in an artery. See also THROMBOSIS.
arterialization the conversion of venous into arterial blood by the absorption of oxygen.
arteriectasis dilatation of an artery.
arteriectomy excision of an artery.
arterio- word element. [L., Gr.] *artery*.
arterio-ureteral fistula aneurysm of the terminal aorta which establishes a fistula into a ureter recorded in horses.
arteriogram a radiograph of an artery.
arteriography radiography of an artery or arterial system after injection of a contrast medium in the bloodstream. See also ANGIOGRAPHY.
cerebral a. a radiographic procedure designed to visualize the blood supply to the brain in order to demonstrate the presence of a space-occupying lesion.
arteriola pl. *arteriolae* [L.] arteriole.
a. rectae renis branches of the efferent juxtamedullary glomerular arterioles of the kidney that supply the renal medulla. Called also straight arterioles.
arteriolar emanating from or pertaining to arteriole.
arteriole a minute arterial branch.
afferent a. enters the glomerulus at the vascular pole and divides into capillaries which subsequently merge to form efferent arterioles.
efferent a. derived from the glomerular capillaries in the renal glomeruli, these arterioles exit from the glomerulus at its vascular pole.
straight a. see ARTERIOLA rectae renis.
arteriolith a chalky concretion in an artery.
arteriolitis inflammation of arterioles.
arteriol(o)- word element. [L.] *arteriole*.
arteriology sum of knowledge regarding the arteries.
arteriolonecrosis necrosis or destruction of arterioles.
arteriolosclerosis sclerosis and thickening of the walls of arterioles. The hyaline form may be associated with nephrosclerosis, the hyperplastic with malignant hypertension, nephrosclerosis and scleroderma.
arteriomotor involving or causing dilatation or constriction of arteries.
arteriomyomatosis growth of muscular fibers in the walls of an artery, causing thickening.
arterionecrosis necrosis of arteries.
arteriopathy any disease of an artery.
arterioplasty plastic repair of an artery.
arteriopressor increasing arterial blood pressure.
arteriorrhaphy suture of an artery.
arteriorrhexis rupture of an artery.
arteriosclerosis a group of diseases of humans characterized by thickening and loss of elasticity of the arterial walls. Of no importance in animals.
Monckeberg's a. medial calcific sclerosis of humans.
arteriospasm spasm of an artery.
arteriostenosis constriction of an artery.
arteriosympathectomy periarterial sympathectomy.
arteriotomy incision of an artery.
pulmonary a. a surgical approach used in the correction of pulmonary stenosis.
arteriotony see BLOOD PRESSURE.
arteriovenous both arterial and venous; pertaining to both artery and vein.
a. anastomosis a direct connection between an artery and a vein that acts as a shunt to bypass the capillary bed. These occur in areas where a high volume blood supply is needed only intermittently, e.g. the intestine.
a. fistula an abnormal communication between an artery and a vein; includes cardiac defects such as VENTRICULAR septal defects and PATENT ductus arteriosus. Peripheral fistulae, especially in the extremities, may be localized, usually acquired and the result of trauma, while congenital defects tend to be more diffuse, involving a network of anastomosing vessels.

The effects of arteriovenous fistulae are variable, depending on their location and the amount of blood carried. Within the liver they usually connect the hepatic artery and portal vein, causing portal hypertension and ascites. Small peripheral fistulae may be noticeable only as warm, reducible swellings, often with an audible thrill, or give rise to edema distal to the site. More severe effects are also possible.
pulmonary a. fistula a congenital anomalous communication between the pulmonary arterial and venous systems, allowing unoxygenated blood to enter the systemic circulation.
arteritis inflammation of an artery. See also ENDARTERITIS, PERIARTERITIS nodosa.
elaeophoral a. see ELAEOPHORA.
equine viral a. see EQUINE viral arteritis.
giant cell a. temporal arteritis.
mycotic a. usually results from extension of an infection by *Mucor* spp. which produce a necrotizing, thrombotic arteritis.

a. obliterans endarteritis obliterans.
uremic a. occurs in acute renal failure in the dog. Often accompanied by an endocarditis.
verminous a. see VERMINOUS mesenteric arteritis.

Arterivirus a genus of viruses in the family *Arteriviridae*, in the order *Nidovirales*, which also includes *Coronaviridae*.

artery a vessel through which the blood passes away from the heart to the various parts of the body. The wall of an artery consists typically of an outer coat (tunica adventitia), a middle coat (tunica media), and an inner coat (tunica intima). For named arteries of the body, see Table 9. See also ARTERIAL.
collateral a. see collateral VESSEL. Horses have collateral radial and ulnar arteries (Table 9).
end a. one that undergoes progressive branching without development of channels connecting with other arteries.
vitelline a. artery to the yolk sac or the ovum of the hen egg.

arthralgia pain in a joint.

arthrectomy excision of a joint.

arthritis inflammation of a joint. See also ARTHROPATHY, POLYARTHRITIS.
bacterial a. arises from penetrating wounds, extension from adjacent tissues or by hematogenous spread, especially umbilical infection in the newborn. More common in farm animals than dogs and cats. Some specific causes are erysipelas in pigs and sheep, *Streptococcus* spp. in pigs, calves and lambs, coliforms in calves, *Haemophilus* spp. in pigs (Glasser's disease) and lambs, *Corynebacterium* spp. in lambs, and *Chlamydia* spp. in calves and lambs.
corynebacterial a. a nonsuppurative arthritis and bursitis of lambs caused by *Corynebacterium pseudotuberculosis*.
crystal-induced a. see GOUT, PSEUDOGOUT.
deforming a. see erosive arthritis (below).
degenerative a. see degenerative JOINT disease.
drug-induced a. a number of antibiotics, particularly sulfonamide-trimethoprin, may cause an immune-mediated arthritis and other clinical signs, including glomerulonephritis, polymyositis and thrombocytopenia.
enteropathic a. arthritis of unknown etiology, but associated with bowel disease such as ulcerative colitis and regional enteritis in humans. A similar condition has been recognized in dogs.
erosive a. characterized by the erosion of articular cartilage and destruction of subchondral bone which is dramatically demonstrated radiographically. Generally are the immune-mediated joint diseases and include canine rheumatoid arthritis (below), POLYARTHRITIS in Greyhounds, feline chronic progressive POLYARTHRITIS. Called also deforming arthritis.
erysipelas a. occurs sporadically in calves, lambs and as a major disease in pigs. In all species it is an acute or chronic, nonsuppurative arthritis.
fibrinous a. the acute inflammatory stage of most infectious arthritides. The joint fluid is increased in volume and is turbid and mucinous, the fibrin appearing as a particulate deposit on the serous surface.
idiopathic nondeforming a. occurs in dogs and uncommonly in cats in the absence of systemic lupus erythematosus or chronic infectious systemic disease. It may involve one or several joints with fever, lameness and muscle atrophy. The disease may be chronic and cyclic with spontaneous remissions and recurrences. Presumed to be immune-mediated.
immune-mediated a. noninfectious joint disease involving immune mechanisms. Seen mainly in dogs and cats. See also nonerosive arthritis (below).
infectious a. may be caused by bacteria, mycoplasma, virus, fungus, rickettsiae, or protozoa in the joint only or as part of systemic infection.
lymphocytic–plasmacytic a. see lymphocytic–plasmacytic SYNOVITIS.
mycoplasma a. *Mycoplasma hyosynoviae* and *M. hyorhinis* cause arthritis in pigs, the former with an accompanying polyserositis.
neonatal a. localization from a systemic infection in the joints causing septic arthritis, often in several joints, and infection in other vulnerable organs. Neonatal susceptibility is due to availability of the umbilical vessels as a port of entry and an inadequate defense until maternal antibodies provide passive immunity. Called also navel ill, OMPHALITIS.
nonerosive a. includes those without significant radiographic changes. Includes the arthritis that occurs in association with canine systemic lupus erythematosus and chronic systemic infections, enteropathic arthritis and idiopathic nondeforming arthritis.
persistent proliferative a. see periosteal proliferative POLYARTHRITIS.
retroviral a. the arthritis of goats caused by a retrovirus. The syndrome also includes encephalitis and pneumonia. Called also big-knee. See also CAPRINE arthritis–encephalitis.
rheumatoid a. (RA) a chronic, autoimmune disease of dogs that causes swelling and lameness in joints, often accompanied by systemic signs of fever, malaise and lymphadenopathy. The erosive, destructive changes in joints can be demonstrated on x-rays. The disease is similar to that described in humans and the diagnosis is usually based on satisfying criteria used for humans.
septic a. acute arthritis due to infection of a kind likely to establish a bacteremia or septicemia.
traumatic a. may be caused by trauma that penetrates the joint capsule, introducing infectious agents and resulting in an infectious arthritis, or injures articular cartilage or soft tissues supporting the joint.

arthritis–encephalitis see CAPRINE arthritis–encephalitis.

arthr(o)- word element. [Gr.] *joint, articulation*.

arthrocele a joint swelling.

arthrocentesis surgical puncture of a joint cavity for aspiration of fluid, usually for diagnostic purposes.

arthrochondritis inflammation of the cartilage of a joint.

arthroclasia surgical breaking down of an ankylosis to permit a joint to move freely.

arthroconidium an asexual spore which is the product of separation and fragmentation of true fungal hyphae. Seen in *Geotrichum* spp.

Arthroderma the perfect state of the fungus *Trichophyton*.

arthrodesis surgical fusion of a joint.

arthrodia a type of synovial joint in which the joint surfaces are flat and allow only a gliding motion; called also gliding joint, articulatio plana.

arthrodynia see ARTHRALGIA.

arthrodysplasia any abnormality of joint development.

arthroempyesis suppuration within a joint.

arthroendoscopy inspection of the interior of a joint with an endoscope.

arthrography contrast radiography of a joint.
air a. pneumoarthrography.

arthrogryposis 1. persistent flexion of a joint. 2. tetanoid spasm.
congenital a. with dysraphism arthrogryposis with delayed or arrested closure of the neural tube. Called also arthrogryposis multiplex congenita.
a. and hydranencephaly see AKABANE VIRUS disease.
inherited a. occurs in catle, pigs and sheep. In cattle it is commonly associated with cleft palate, sometimes with other skeletal defects and also prolonged gestation.
a. multiplex congenita see congenital arthrogryposis with dysraphism (above).
arthrolith a calculous deposit within a joint.
arthrology scientific study or description of the joints.
arthrolysis operative loosening of adhesions in an ankylosed joint.
arthrometer an instrument for measuring the angles of movements of joints.
arthropathy any joint disease.
Charcot's a., neuropathic a. chronic progressive degeneration of the stress-bearing portion of a joint, with hypertrophic changes at the periphery; it is associated with neurological disorders involving loss of sensation in the joint.
degenerative a. a degenerative disease of the joints, e.g. degenerative disease of the stifle or hip joint in the ox. The disease may be primary when there appears to be a metabolic defect in the articular cartilage. Secondary arthropathy occurs consequentially to a disease of the supporting bone.
degenerative coxofemoral a. see degenerative arthropathy (above).
developmental a. results from abnormalities in development or growth that cause structural injury or abnormal function in a joint, e.g. conformational abnormalities, CHONDRODYSTROPHY, OSTEOCHONDROSIS, GROWTH disorders, LEGG–CALVÉ–PERTHES DISEASE and PATELLAR luxation.
dietary a. caused by HYPERVITAMINOSIS A in cats and secondary HYPERPARATHYROIDISM.
metabolic a. is secondary to some systemic diseases such as HEMOPHILIA A and MUCOPOLYSACCHARIDOSIS.
neoplastic a. primary neoplasms of the joint, e.g. synovioma or synovial sarcoma, or metastatic tumors, may cause an arthropathy.
neuropathic a. joint disease secondary to diminished pain and proprioceptive reflexes that cause loss of sensation in the joint, loss of support and instability. Usually the result of trauma. See also Charcot's arthropathy (above).
osteopulmonary a. clubbing of digits and enlargement of ends of the long bones, in cardiac or pulmonary disease. See also hypertrophic OSTEOPATHY.
arthrophyma a joint swelling.
arthrophyte an abnormal growth in a joint cavity.
arthroplasty plastic repair of a joint.
excision a. one that involves removal of some component of the joint, e.g. femoral head or patella.
total hip a. total HIP replacement.
arthropod an individual of the phylum ARTHROPODA.
Arthropoda a phylum of the animal kingdom including bilaterally symmetrical animals with hard, segmented bodies bearing jointed appendages; embracing the largest number of known animals, with at least 740,000 species, divided into 12 classes. It includes the arachnids, crustaceans and insects.
arthropodal pertaining to or emanating from arthropods.
a. allergy see ALLERGY.
a. ectoparasites insects that parasitize the skin of animals.
arthropodic disease disease caused by infestation with arthropod parasites, e.g. tick worry, tick paralysis, lousy.
arthroscintigram a scintigram of a joint.
arthroscintigraphy scintigraphy of a joint.
arthrosclerosis stiffening or hardening of the joints.
arthroscope an endoscope, usually a fiberoptiscope, for examining the interior of a joint.
arthroscopic surgery a surgical procedure carried out through an arthroscope.
arthroscopy examination of the interior of a joint with an arthroscope, usually for diagnostic purposes.
arthrosis 1. a joint or articulation. 2. disease of a joint.
Arthrosolon polycephalus GNIDIA *polycephala*.
arthrospore see ARTHROCONIDIUM.
arthrostomy surgical creation of an opening in a joint, as for drainage.
arthrosynovitis inflammation of the synovial membrane of a joint.
arthrotomy incision of a joint.
arthroxesis scraping of an articular surface.
Arthus reaction a local antibody-mediated hypersensitivity reaction in which antibody–antigen complexes which fix complement are deposited in the walls of small vessels causing acute inflammation with an infiltration of neutrophils. Characteristic of type III hypersensitivity reactions. See also SERUM sickness.
passive cutaneous A. r. antiserum is injected intravenously and the corresponding antigen is injected into the skin.
reverse passive A. r. antiserum is injected into the skin and the antigen is injected into the same site or intravenously.
articular pertaining to a JOINT.
a. capsule see articular CAPSULE.
a. cartilage see CARTILAGE.
a. cartilage disease see ARTHRITIS, degenerative JOINT disease.
congenital a. rigidity caused by inherited defects, intrauterine viral infections, ingestion of poisons including plants and anthelmintics. See also CONTRACTED, contracted FOAL, LUPINUS.
a. meniscus similar to an articular disk but is semicircular or C-shaped.
a. plate the cartilaginous covering at the epiphysis of bones in arthrodial joints. Together with the growth cartilage comprises the joint CARTILAGE.
a. rigidity fixation of a joint, including ARTHROGRYPOSIS and ANKYLOSIS. May be caused by contracture of tendons, ligaments or muscles, by deformity of joint surfaces or by fusion of them.
articulare the point of intersection of the dorsal contours of the articular process of the mandible and the temporal bone.
articulate 1. to unite by joints; to join. 2. united by joints.
articulatio pl. *articulationes* [L.] an articulation or joint.
a. plana see ARTHRODIA.
articulation a joint; the place of union or junction between two or more bones of the skeleton.
articulator a device for effecting a jointlike union.
articulo mortis at the point or moment of death.
artifact a structure or appearance that is not natural, but is due to manipulation (man-made).
dermatohistopathological a. may be due to sampling errors (selection, preparation or technique) or processing of specimens.
radiological a. defects in the x-ray film image due to

faults in the cassette (screen artifact) or in the film (film artifact).

static a. a mark on x-ray film caused by discharge of static electricity.

ultrasound a. irregularities produced in the image display. See ACOUSTIC shadowing, ACOUSTIC enhancement, COMET-TAIL, REVERBERATION.

artifacts see SPECIMEN artifacts.

artificial made by art; not natural or pathological.

a. abortion see PARTURITION induction.

a. bone see skeletal PROSTHESIS.

a. breeding includes diagnosis of estrus, semen collection and handling, and artificial insemination (see below).

a. breeding organization a proprietary or cooperative organization dealing in the selection, purchase and maintenance of selected sires, mass collection, storage and sale of semen, employment of artificial inseminators, and often veterinarians skilled in the diseases of the reproductive tract, and the provision of artificial insemination services to individual cows and to herds, flocks or bands of animals. The responsibility is usually assumed for the keeping of complete records and the provision of these to clients and in the form of a periodic report. It is inherent in the animal industries that artificial breeding has as its objectives the genetic improvement and the prevention of sexually transmitted diseases of the species that it serves. Embryo transplantation and its attendant technologies could become part of an artificial breeding service.

a. digestion for trichinosis a sample of the meat to be examined is incubated with a mixture of pepsin and hydrochloric acid and the digesta examined under a microscope for specimens of *Trichinella spiralis*.

a. drying drying or dehydrating of feed by other than natural means of sun and air movement; usually by fossil fuel.

a. kidney a popular name for an extracorporeal hemodialyser.

a. limb a replacement for a natural limb. See also PROSTHESIS.

a. milk see MILK replacer.

a. organ a mechanical device that can substitute temporarily or permanently for a body organ. Not usually used in veterinary medicine.

a. parturition induction see PARTURITION induction.

a. rearing the rearing of newborn animals by the use of milk replacer as an artificial diet, and often the provision of an artificial environment with a cloth-lined box and a heat lamp or other heating device. The provision of an appropriate amount of relevant antibodies or a prolonged course of antibiotics is an essential part of the program. The need may be a permanent one because of the death or complete agalactia of the dam, or because management insists on early weaning. It may be temporary if the dam is agalactic for a brief period because of illness.

a. vagina a device used in the collection of semen from male animals. The usual construction is of a rigid external tube lined by a flexible, thin rubber sleeve. Water at body temperature is introduced between the tube and the sleeve so as to achieve a spongy warm cavity which is lubricated with inert material. A rubber cone, terminating in a graduated plastic or glass collecting tube, is placed over the distal end of the device which is then ready to use.

artificial insemination the implanting of live spermatozoa into the genital tract of the female. The diluted or otherwise treated semen is usually deposited in the body of the uterus because of the higher fertility rate obtained, but insemination into the uterine cervix or even the vagina may be practiced. Although insemination is usually carried out via the vagina transperitoneal insemination may be the technique used in animals whose anatomy precludes a satisfactory vaginal approach. See also AI.

avian a. i. is practiced extensively; it is used in turkeys where selection for heavy breast muscle has bred male turkeys unable to impregnate large numbers of females. The procedure is approximately the same as in other species with the exception that the semen must be fresh; a technique for freezing is not available.

Artiodactyla the animal order of artiodactylids. Contains the families Antilocapridae (proghorn antelope), Bovidae (antelope, wild cattle, bison, buffalo, wild goats, wild sheep), Camelidae (camels, guanacos, llamas, alpacas, vicuñas), Cervidae (moose, elk), Giraffidae (giraffe, okapi) and Tragulidae (mouse deer).

artiodactylid a member of the order ARTIODACTYLA of animals.

Artionema see SETARIA[1].

Arum a genus of the family Araceae which contains many ornamental plants. Includes *A. italicum*, *A. maculatum*. Causes intense irritation to the oral mucosa, thought to be due to oxalate raphide crystals in the plant. Called also arum lily, cuckoopint, lords-and-ladies.

arum lily see ARUM.

Arvicola see VOLE.

-ary suffix meaning pertaining to.

aryepiglottic fold the mucosal fold connecting the lateral border of the epiglottic cartilage to the mucosa covering the arytenoid and corniculate cartilages.

aryl- in organic chemistry, a prefix denoting any radical having the free valence on a carbon atom in an aromatic ring.

aryl phosphates see TRIARYL PHOSPHATES.

arylamine any of a group of amines in which one or more of the hydrogen atoms are replaced by aromatic groups.

a. acetyltransferase see metachromatic LEUKODYSTROPHY.

arylsulfatase a group of enzymes active in the hydrolysis of sulfates and the metabolism of mucopolysaccharides; found in liver, pancreas, kidneys and immature monocytes. Several species of molluscs and *Aerobacter* spp. serve as commercial sources of the enzyme which is used in analytic endocrinology.

a. A deficiency see metachromatic LEUKODYSTROPHY.

a. B deficiency is the cause of MUCOPOLYSACCHARIDOSIS VI which occurs in humans and cats. Called also Maroteaux–Lamy syndrome.

arytenoepiglottic of or pertaining to the arytenoid and epiglottic cartilages.

arytenoid shaped like a jug or pitcher, as the arytenoid cartilage.

a. abscess see LARYNGEAL chondritis.

a. cartilage one of the paired laryngeal cartilages in the dorsal part of the larynx that provides attachment for the muscles that adduct and abduct the vocal cords. The cartilages form the dorsal boundary of the rima glottis, the vocal cords the ventral boundary.

a. chondritis inflammation of the arytenoid cartilage that causes a syndrome similar to that caused by recurrent laryngeal nerve paralysis.

a. lateralization a surgical technique used to treat laryngeal paralysis in dogs. One or both arytenoid cartilages are fixed in a lateral position with sutures, thereby enlarging the diameter of the laryngeal lumen.

arytenoidectomy excision of an arytenoid cartilage; treatment for laryngeal paralysis in dogs.

arytenoiditis inflammation of the arytenoid muscle or cartilage.

arytenoidopexy surgical fixation of arytenoid cartilage or muscle.

As chemical symbol, *arsenic*.

ASA acetylsalicylic acid (aspirin).

Asaemia axillaris Southern African plant in the family Asteraceae (Compositae); an unidentified toxin causes hepatogenous photosensitization. Called also *Tanacetum axillare*, *Pteronia geigerioides*, voorsiektebossie.

asafetida gum-resin from the rhizome of the plant *Ferula asafoetida*. Has an atrocious smell. Used as a carminative and expectorant and to prevent bandage chewing and as a repellent to dogs and cats.

asbestos a naturally occurring amphibole mineral in fibrous form with the fibers lying in parallel in plates; causes asbestosis in humans. Called also horneblende.

asbestosis a disease of humans consistently exposed to asbestos fibers in the environment. Minimal pneumoconiosis found in ponies in coal mines. The human disease is marked by pulmonary fibrosis, pleural mesothelioma and pneumoconiosis.

asbos, asbosvygie see PSILOCAULON.

ascariasis infection with *Ascaris* spp. The disease affects pigs, principally the young. Signs include poor growth, poor coat and diarrhea due to enteritis. Migration by the larvae results in the development of hepatitis and pneumonia. Other less common sequelae include biliary duct obstruction and a severe interstitial pneumonia when atypical larvae, e.g. *Ascaris suis*, infect cattle.

ascaricide an agent destructive to ascarids.

ascarid any of the phasmid nematodes of the Ascaridoidea, which includes the genera *Ascaris*, *Parascaris*, *Toxocara* and *Toxascaris*.

a. infection see ASCARIASIS.

ascaridata ascarids.

Ascaridia a genus of nematode worms of the family Heterakidae. Includes *A. columbae*, *A. dissimilis*, *A. compar*, *A. numidae* and *A. razia*.

A. galli a parasite of domesticated and wild birds which causes enteritis with diarrhea, and unthriftiness with poor feed conversion especially in birds up to 3 months of age.

ascaridol a terpene, the active principle of OIL of chenopodium. Poisoning with the oil is manifested by enteritis and nervous signs including convulsions, paralysis, coma and death.

Ascaris a nematode parasite found in the intestine of many animal species. The genus is a member of the family Ascarididae. Includes *A. columnaris* (wild animals—see BAYLISASCARIS *columnaris*), *A. equorum* (horse—see PARASCARIS *equorum*), *A. lumbricoides* (humans), *A. schroederi*, *A. suum* (pigs), *A. vitulorum* (see TOXOCARA *vitulorum*).

Ascarops a genus of nematode worms of the family Spirocercidae. Includes *A. strongylina*, *A. dentata* (pig's stomach).

ascending progressing to higher levels, usually used in reference to the nervous system.

a. colon dilation dilation of the spiral or coiled colon in cattle, usually a part of torsion of the mesentery of the colon; characterized by acute abdominal pain and distended loops of intestine in the right flank.

a. hemorrhagic myelomalacia see progressive hemorrhagic MYELOMALACIA.

a. hematomyelia see progressive hemorrhagic MYELOMALACIA.

a. reticular activating system see RETICULAR activating system.

a. syndrome see MYELOMALACIA.

ascensus medullae the shortening of the spinal cord relative to the vertebral column caused by the unequal growth of the two organs.

Aschheim–Zondek test an outdated test which used to be used to diagnose pregnancy in mares. Serum from the mare was injected into the peritoneum of rats. A positive result was edema and enlargement of the rats' uteri. Accurate if performed in the 50 to 80 day period of pregnancy.

ASCII file acronym for American Standard Code for Information Interchange; a standard format for representing characters on a computer.

ascites abnormal accumulation of serous (edematous) fluid within the peritoneal cavity. Characterized by distension of the abdomen, a fluid thrill on percussion, a typical ground glass appearance on radiography and a positive result on paracentesis.

cardiogenic a. that caused by cardiac insufficiency.

chylous a. see CHYLOUS ascites.

fetal a. affected fetuses are usually dropsical and cause dystocia, even the aborting ones; usually accompanies another defect, e.g. achondroplasia.

Asclepiadora decumbens ASCLEPIAS *asperula*.

Asclepias widespread genus of the plant family Asclepiadaceae which contains many poisonous plants, most of them with copious white sap. Contain cardiac glycosides. Cause diarrhea and heart failure syndrome. Includes *A. asperula*, *A. brachystephana*, *A. curassavica* (red cotton bush), *A. eriocarpa* (*A. galioides*), *A. incarnata*, *A. labriformis*, *A. latifolia*, *A. mexicana*, *A. pumila*, *A. physocarpus* (*Gomphrena physocarpus*), *A. speciosa*, *A. subverticillata* (*A. verticillata*), *A. syriaca*. Called also milkweeds, wild cotton.

Ascoli test an agar gel precipitation test used for the detection of anthrax infected hides.

Ascomycetes a class of fungi which contains *Neurospora*, *Penicillium*, *Aspergillus*, true yeasts and the dermatophytes.

Ascomycota a phylum of the fungi kingdom characterized by septate hyphae, asexual reproduction by conidia and sexual reproduction in an ascus containing eight ascospores. Genera of veterinary importance in the phylum are *Aspergillus, Penicillium, Sporothrix*, *Microsporum* and *Trichophyton*.

ascorbate a compound or derivative of ascorbic acid. See also SODIUM ascorbate.

ascorbic acid, L-ascorbic acid VITAMIN C, called also cevitamic acid; a substance found in many fruits and vegetables, especially citrus fruits, such as oranges and lemons, and tomatoes. It is synthesized by most animal species, except primates, guinea pigs, fruit bats and some birds and fish, and so is not a dietary requirement in ordinary circumstances except for the species named.

a. a. nutritional deficiency occurs in primates and guinea pigs with inadequate dietary intake; affected animals are weak, depressed, anorectic, and have enlarged joints. In farm animals the only example of a possible secondary deficiency is a dermatosis of young calves which occurs at a time at which ascorbic acid levels might be expected to be at their lowest. The syndrome includes heavy dandruff, alopecia and a waxy crust on the skin.

ascospore the sexual spore of Ascomycetes.

ascus pl. *asci*; the spore case of Ascomycetes.
-ase suffix used in forming the name of enzymes, affixed to a stem indicating the substrate (luciferase), the general nature of the substrate (proteinase) or the type of reaction effected (hydrolase).
asepsis absence of septic matter; freedom from infection or infectious material.
surgical a. refers to destruction of organisms before they enter the body. It is used in caring for open wounds and in surgical procedures.
aseptic free from infection or septic material; sterile.
a. fever fever in the absence of infection, e.g. due to trauma, surgical manipulation of tissue, tissue necrosis, injection of certain chemicals, e.g. dinitrophenols.
a. necrosis of the femoral head see LEGG–CALVÉ–PERTHES DISEASE.
a. technique required for modern day veterinary surgery, especially orthopedic surgery. Includes a dust-free environment, complete immobilization of the patient, intensive skin preparation, capping, gowning, masking and gloving of the surgeon and assistants, draping and packing of the patient, proper equipment for removal of blood and other liquids and avoidance of the introduction of nonsterile items such as x-rays, stomach tubes, restraint gear into the sterile field.
asexual without sex; not pertaining to or involving sex.
asexualization sterilization, as by castration or vasectomy.
ASF African swine fever.
ash the incombustible, inorganic residue remaining after any process of incineration. See also BONE ash.
dietary a. generally the mineral content.
ash tree see FRAXINUS EXCELSIOR.
asialia aptyalism.
Asian elephant *Elaphus maximus*.
asiderosis deficiency of iron reserve of the body.
ASIF Association for the Study of Internal Fixation.
ASIF system a complete set of instruments for compression bone plating. Includes hand or power drills with detachable bits for boring holes in the bone, bit directors to ensure accurate placement of holes, a tapping instrument to create the thread in the bored hole, screws and plates of various shapes and weights with round holes or slots, a screwdriver and many other ancillary items.
-asis suffix meaning process or condition.
ASLO *Actinobacillus suis* like organism.
Asn asparagine.
***Asn*-X-thr/ser sequence** sequence of amino acids in a polypeptide chain associated with position of attachment of *N*-linked oligosaccharides through the asparagine moiety to form glycoproteins.
Asp aspartate.
asparaginase an enzyme that catalyzes the deamination of asparagine; used as an antineoplastic agent against cancers, e.g. acute lymphocytic leukemia, in which the malignant cells require exogenous asparagine for protein synthesis.
asparagine Asn; the β-amide of aspartic acid, a nonessential amino acid occurring in proteins.
aspartame a synthetic compound of two amino acids (L-aspartyl-L-phenylalanine *o*-methyl ester) used as sweetener in low-calorie drinks. It is 180 times as sweet as sucrose (table sugar); the amount equal in sweetness to a teaspoon of sugar contains 0.1 calorie.
aspartate Asp; any salt of aspartic acid; aspartic acid in dissociated form.
a. carbamoyl transferase enzyme catalyzing the condensation of carbamoyl phosphate and L-aspartate to *N*-carbamoyl-L-aspartate. A regulatory, allosteric enzyme in the synthesis of pyrimidine nucleotides.
a. transaminase see ASPARTATE AMINOTRANSFERASE.
aspartate aminotransferase an enzyme that catalyzes the reversible transfer of an amino group:

$$\text{aspartic acid} + \alpha\text{-ketoglutaric acid} \rightleftharpoons \text{oxaloacetic acid} + \text{glutamic acid}$$

requiring the coenzyme pyridoxal phosphate; abbreviated AST. It is present in many tissues and body fluids. The serum concentration is elevated when damage to tissue cells, especially of the heart and liver, causes a release of the enzyme. AST values are also increased in some muscle diseases, such as enzootic muscular dystrophy. The test has limitations because of its lack of organ specificity. Called also (serum) glutamic–oxaloacetic aminotransferase (GOT or SGOT).
aspartic acid a nonessential dicarboxylic amino acid, widely distributed in proteins.
aspecific not specific; not caused by a specific organism.
aspect 1. that part of a surface viewed from a particular direction. 2. the look or appearance.
dorsal a. a view from the back (bipeds), or from above (quadrupeds).
ventral a. a view from the front (bipeds) or from below (quadrupeds).
aspergilloma a tumorlike granulomatous mass formed by colonization of *Aspergillus* in a bronchus, pulmonary spaces, or pulmonary cavity; the organism may disseminate through the bloodstream to the brain, heart and kidneys.
aspergillosis a disease caused by species of *Aspergillus*, marked by inflammatory granulomatous lesions in the skin, ear, orbit, nasal sinuses, lungs, and sometimes bones and meninges. Abortion due to fungal placentitis is common in cows and occurs also in mares and sows. Subacute pulmonary involvement may be accompanied by lesions at all levels in the respiratory tract. Congenital infection of the fetus, especially manifested by dermatitis, is a rare accompaniment. A gastroenteritis with ulceration in the esophagus and forestomachs occurs in calves. Rarely osteomyelitis, intestinal and central nervous system involvement have been recorded in dogs, the most frequent site of infection being the nasal cavity. See also BROODER pneumonia.
avian a. principal manifestation is as pneumonia but systemic invasion, dermatitis, osteomyelitis, ophthalmitis, encephalitis also occur. Species involved are *A. fumigatus*, *A. flavus*.
disseminated a. in dogs, a disseminated disease characterized by signs of generalized infection, lymphadenopathy, diskospondylitis, and lameness, paresis or paraplegia. *A. terreus* is the most common etiologic agent and German shepherd dogs are predisposed. Cats with disseminated aspergillosis usually have concurrent immunosuppressive disease.
nasal a. a localized form of aspergillosis, involving the nose, ears and paranasal sinuses. In dogs, there is usually a unilateral or bilateral serosanguinous nasal discharge and a characteristic depigmentation and ulceration of skin adjacent to the external nares.
aspergillotoxicosis poisoning caused by *Aspergillus* spp. growing in animal feed. A variety of poisonings may be caused including those due to AFLATOXIN, OCHRATOXIN, CITRININ, OXALATE, FUMITOXIN, STERIGMATOCYSTIN. There are still other poisonings in which the effective agent has not been identified.

Aspergillus a genus of fungi (molds), several species of which are parasitic and opportunistic pathogens. Others produce toxins and when they contaminate animal feeds they can cause heavy losses. Includes *A. amstelodami*, *A. chevalieri*, *A. clavatus*, *A. flavus oryzae*, *A. fumigatus*, *A. maydis*, *A. niger*, *A. ochraceus*, *A. parasiticus*, *A. taumanii*, *A. wentii*.

A. fumigatus a cause of respiratory tract disease in many species. See AIRSACCULITIS, ASPERGILLOSIS.

A. nidulans, A. versicolor produce known carcinogenic toxin, sterigmatocystin.

A. terreus a cause of FESCUE foot and the most common cause of canine disseminated ASPERGILLOSIS.

aspermatogenesis failure to produce spermatozoa.

autoallergic a. caused by an immune response to the animal's own spermatozoa when they are introduced into its tissues experimentally or naturally by trauma.

aspermia failure of formation or emission of semen.

asphalt a suspect but appears not to be poisonous.

asphyxia a condition due to lack of oxygen in inspired air, resulting in actual or impending cessation of apparent life. It includes lack of air to respire. See also SUFFOCATION.

neonatal a. the fetus is deprived of air while on the birth canal and appears to have died during birth. Stimulation of respiratory movements and artificial respiration may cause respiration to resume.

asphyxial pertaining to or emanating from asphyxia.

a. respiratory failure respiratory failure manifested by dyspnea with alternating apnea and gasping respiration before death.

asphyxiant any substance capable of producing asphyxia.

asphyxiate to suffocate; to deprive of oxygen for utilization by the tissues.

Aspiculuris a nematode genus of the oxyurid family *Heteroxynematidae*. Includes *A. tetraptera* (rodents).

Aspidium DRYOPTERIS *filix-mas*.

aspidium the dried products of a genus of plants known as male fern (*Dryopteris filix-mas*). Contains an oleoresin capable of causing liver damage. Used at one time as an anthelmintic.

Aspidogastrea a subclass of trematodes that parasitize fish, turtles, Mollusca, Crustacea.

aspirate 1. to withdraw fluid by negative pressure, or suction. 2. the fluid obtained by aspiration.

aspiration 1. the act of inhaling. Pathological aspiration of vomitus or mucus into the respiratory tract may occur when a patient is unconscious or under the effects of a general anesthetic. 2. removal of fluids or gases from a cavity by the aid of suction.

a. biopsy see BIOPSY.

a. pneumonia is the result of inhalation or aspiration of infected solid or liquid material into the lungs. Large volumes of aspirate cause asphyxia, smaller amounts cause a necrotic or gangrenous pneumonia, in anterior and ventral parts of the lung. There is profound toxemia, cough, gurgling or squeaky rales, and usually an attendant pleurisy producing a friction rub. Called also inhalation pneumonia.

aspirator an instrument for evacuating fluid or tissue by suction.

ultrasonic a. see PHACOEMULSIFICATION.

aspirin acetylsalicylic acid, a common drug generally used to relieve pain and reduce fever.

a. poisoning occurs in dogs and cats, either from accidental ingestion or inappropriate therapeutic doses. The cat is particularly susceptible because of its limited ability to form glucaronide conjugates. Clinical signs are of a hemorrhagic gastritis, hyperexcitability and metabolic acidosis.

asplenia absence of the spleen.

Asplenium flabellifolium fern in the family Aspleniaceae; can cause cyanide poisoning. Called also necklace fern.

asporogenic not producing spores; not reproduced by spores.

asporous having no true spores.

ass see DONKEY.

assassin bug see TRIATOMA.

assay determination of the purity of a substance or the amount or activity of any particular constituent of a mixture.

biological a. bioassay; determination of the potency of a drug or other substance by comparing the effects it has in a biological system with those of a reference standard.

assembly language see COMPUTER language.

assessment the critical analysis and evaluation or judgment of the status or quality of a particular condition, situation, or other subject of appraisal. For example—clinical assessment of a patient's condition as a prerequisite to making a prognosis.

assimilation conversion of nutritive material into living tissue; anabolism.

assist list a list setting out cow identities and the various things that would happen to them; supplied as part of the service by good herd health programs.

assistant one who aids or helps another; an auxiliary; e.g. nursing assistant, technical assistant, laboratory assistant.

association 1. close relation in time or space. In neurology, correlation involving a high degree of modifiability and also consciousness. In genetics, the occurrence together of two characteristics (e.g. blood group O and peptic ulcers) at a frequency greater than would be predicted on the basis of chance. 2. in statistics an association is present if the probability of an event, or the quantity of a variable, depends on the occurrence of other events or the quantity of other variables. If the weight of evidence suggests that the changes in one of the variables causes the alteration in the other the association is said to be causal. In the reverse situation, where no such causal relationship exists, the association is said to be a non-causal one.

a. areas areas of the cerebral cortex (excluding primary areas) connected with each other and with the neothalamus; they are responsible for higher mental and emotional processes, including memory, learning, etc.

epidemiological a. the association between a disease and a cause.

a. points in acupuncture terms all are located on the bladder meridian, along the back 1 to 1.5 inches from the midline. Called also *shu* points.

a. strength (degree) the strength of association between a disease and a cause. Is usually indicated by the relative risk.

association of practices a loose association of practices in which there is a sharing of common resources such as accommodation, equipment and staff.

assortative mating sexual reproduction in which the pairing of male and female is not random.

ass's parsley CHAEROPHYLLUM *sylvestre*.

AST aspartate aminotransferase.

Astacus astacus European crayfish. See Table 23.

astasia motor incoordination with inability to stand.

a.–abasia inability or refusal to stand or walk although the legs are otherwise under control.

astatine a chemical element, atomic number 85, atomic weight 210, symbol At. See Table 6.

asteatosis any disease in which persistent dry scaling of the skin suggests scantiness or absence of sebum.

astemizole a long-acting, non-sedating H_1-blocking antihistamine used in the treatment of pruritus in dogs and cats.

Aster genus of selenium indicator plants in the family Asteraceae; preferentially accumulates selenium from the soil. Includes *A. adscendens*, *A. coerulescens*, *A. commutatus*, *A. ericoides*, *A. glaucoides*, *A. laevis* var. *geyeri*. See also XYLORRHIZA.

aster a structure occurring in dividing cells, composed of microtubules radiating from a centrosome. The two asters are the poles of the mitotic SPINDLE.

asternal 1. not joined to the sternum. 2. pertaining to asternia.

asternia congenital absence of the sternum.

asteroid star-shaped.

a. body 1. found in fungal pulmonary lesions. Small remnants of hyphae are surrounded by radiating acidophilic clubs similar to those of the granules of actinomycosis. 2. an irregularly star-shaped inclusion body found in the giant cells in sarcoidosis and other diseases.

asthenia debility; loss of strength and energy; weakness.

anhidrotic a. see ANHIDROTIC asthenia.

cutaneous a. a group of inherited disorders of collagen synthesis that result in fragility and hyperextensibility of skin, and in some forms, hypermobility of joints. There are many clinical similarities to the group of human conditions known as EHLERS–DANLOS SYNDROME. This disorder has been reported in cattle, sheep, horses, dogs, cats, pigs and mink; within and between species there are clinical, biochemical and ultrastructural variations. Examples of diseases which include cutaneous asthenia as a lesion include hereditary collagen dysplasia, DERMATOSPARAXIS in cattle and sheep, rubber-puppy syndrome in dogs, cutis hyperelastica in pigs.

asthenic pertaining to asthenia.

asthen(o)- word element. [Gr.] *weak, weakness*.

asthenocoria sluggishness of the pupillary light reflex.

asthenometer a device used in measuring the degree of muscular asthenia or of asthenopia.

asthenospermia reduced motility of spermatozoa in the semen.

asthenozoospermia reduction in the vitality of spermatozoa; a high percentage of spermatozoa in the sample have less than normal motility.

asthma a condition marked by recurrent attacks of dyspnea, with wheezing due to spasmodic constriction of the bronchi.

It is also known as *bronchial asthma*. Attacks vary greatly from occasional periods of wheezing and slight dyspnea to severe attacks that almost cause suffocation.

acute equine a. sudden attacks of respiratory distress in horses at pasture; the dyspnea responds dramatically to treatment with corticosteroids combined with antihistamines.

allergic a. extrinsic asthma; bronchial asthma due to allergy. Called also atopic asthma.

atopic a. see allergic asthma (above).

bronchial a. asthma.

cardiac a. a term applied to breathing difficulties due to pulmonary edema in heart disease, such as left ventricular failure.

feline a. see feline BRONCHIAL asthma.

astigmatism an error of refraction in which a ray of light is not sharply focused on the retina, but is spread over a more or less diffuse area; it is due to differences in curvature in various meridians of the refractive surfaces (cornea and lens) of the eye.

astigmometer an apparatus used in measuring astigmatism.

astomia congenital atresia of the mouth.

astragalectomy excision of the astragalus.

Astragalus a genus of the legume family Fabaceae in the Americas, Europe and Asia. Many of the *Astragalus* spp. are poisonous with several forms of poisoning.

A number of species of the genus grow preferentially in selenium-rich soils and accumulate much more selenium than other plants, enhancing the probability of producing selenium poisoning. Included are *A. bisulcatus*, *A. pattersonii*, *A. pectinatus*, *A. praelongus*, *A. preussi*, *A. racemosus*.

Many species of the genus contain toxic aliphatic nitro compounds. Poisoning is manifested by nitrite ('nitro') poisoning or by acute respiratory distress or chronic incoordination, blindness and respiratory stertor. Includes *A. arequipensis*, *A. atropubescens*, *A. bergii*, *A. campestris*, *A. canadensis*, *A. chamissonis*, *A. cryptobotrys*, *A. distinens*, *A. emoryanus* var. *emoryanus*, *A. falcatus*, *A. garbancillo*, *A. hamosus*, *A. hylophylus*, *A. miser*, *A. miser* var. *hylophylus* (locoweed, timber milk vetch), *A. miser* var. *oblongifolus*, *A. miser* var. *serotinus*, *A. oblongifolus*, *A. palenae*, *A. pehuenches*, *A. pterocarpus*, *A. serotinus*, *A. tetrapterus*, *A. toanus*, *A. vesiculosus*.

Long-term ingestion of any one of a series of species of the plant causes 'loco' or locoweed poisoning, an acquired lysosomal storage disease caused by swainsonine, which is manifested by incoordination, extreme hypersensitivity and excitability. Includes *A. allochrous*, *A. argillophilus*, *A. bisulcatus*, *A. diphysus*, *A. earlei*, *A. lentiginosus*, *A. lonchocarpus*, *A. lusitanicus* (*Erophaca baetica*), *A. missouriensis*, *A. mollisimus*, *A. nothoxys*, *A. nuttallianus*, *A. pubentissimus*, *A. strictus*, *A. tephrodes*, *A. thurberi*, *A. wootonii*, *A. variabilis*. Chronic heart failure due to swainsonine is caused by *A. lentiginosus* at high altitudes.

Abortion is a common manifestation and is accompanied by a great variety of skeletal defects including arthrogryposis and hypermobility. Called also locoweed, milk vetch.

astragalus see TALUS.

Astrakhan see KARAKUL.

Astrebla Mitchell grasses, Australian members of the family Poaceae (Graminae), hosts a fungus (*Corallocytostroma*) in the form of 'coral' sclerotia (galls) which produce an unidentified toxin causing fatal BLACK SOIL BLINDNESS in cattle.

astringent 1. causing contraction or arresting discharges. 2. an agent that causes contraction or arrests discharges. Astringents act as protein precipitants; they arrest discharge by causing shrinkage of tissue.

Some astringents, such as tannic acid, have been used in treating diarrhea; others, such as boric acid and sodium borate, help relieve the symptoms of inflammation of the mucous membranes of the throat or conjunctiva of the eye. Skin lotions often contain astringents such as aluminum acetate that help to reduce oiliness and excessive perspiration. Witch hazel is a common household astringent used to reduce swelling. Styptic pencils, used to stop bleeding from small cuts, contain astringents. Zinc oxide and calamine are astringents used in lotions, powders and ointments to relieve itching and chafing in various forms of dermatitis. Astringents have some bacteriostatic properties, though they are not generally used as antiseptics.

astroblast a cell that develops into an astrocyte.

astroblastoma an astrocytoma, composed of cells with abundant cytoplasm and two or three nuclei.

astrocyte a neuroglial cell of ectodermal origin, characterized by fibrous or protoplasmic processes; collectively called astroglia or macroglia.

gemistocytic a. a plump astrocyte which results from injury to nervous tissue. Usually an extensive area is involved.

astrocytin an antigen present on the cell membrane of astrocytes, found in the serum of patients with malignant glial tumors.

astrocytoma a common intracranial tumor composed of astrocytes; classified in order of malignancy as differentiated or undifferentiated groups.

gemistocytic a. comprises gemistocytic astrocytes, plump or swollen astrocytes or gemistocytes.

astroglia the astrocytes considered as tissue; neuroglial tissue made up of astrocytes.

astrogliosis inflammation of the astroglia; proliferation of astrocytes and their processes.

astrosphere 1. the central mass of an aster, excluding the rays. 2. aster.

astrovirus a small, nonenveloped, unclassified, single-stranded RNA virus with characteristic starlike staining pattern that gives it the name. Associated with enteric infections in several species including cattle, sheep and dogs.

Asturian cattle red with pale extremities, dual-purpose, Spanish cattle.

asymmetric hind quarter syndrome a condition of pigs in which there is a suboptimal growth of muscle probably conditioned by an inherited factor. There is no defect of gait. See also IRON poisoning.

asymmetry 1. lack or absence of symmetry; dissimilarity in corresponding parts or organs on opposite sides of the body which are normally alike. 2. in chemistry, lack of symmetry in the special arrangements of the atoms and radicals within the molecule or crystal.

asymphytous separate or distinct; not grown together.

asymptomatic showing no symptoms.

asymptote a mathematical term used for the straight line which is a tangent to a curve at infinity.

asynchronism occurrence at different times; disturbance of coordination.

asynechia absence of continuity of structure.

asynergia lack of coordination among parts or organs normally acting in unison.

asynovia absence or insufficiency of synovial secretion.

asyntaxia lack of proper and orderly embryonic development.

asystole cardiac standstill or arrest; absence of heartbeat.

At chemical symbol, *astatine.*

at. atomic.

at. no. atomic number.

at. wt. atomic weight.

atactic pertaining to or characterized by ataxia; marked by incoordination or irregularity.

Atalaya hemiglauca a small Australian tree in the family Sapindaceae. Poisonous to horses by causing heart failure. Called also whitewood.

ataractic 1. pertaining to or characterized by ataraxia. 2. an agent that induces ataraxia; a tranquilizer.

ataraxia a state of detached serenity without depression of mental faculties or impairment of consciousness.

atavism apparent inheritance of characters from remote ancestors, caused by recessive genes. Called also 'throwback'.

ataxia failure of muscular coordination; irregularity of muscular action.

cerebellar a. ataxia characterized by defects in rate, range, force and direction of movement of limbs. There is a broad based stance, inability to maintain the head in the proper position so that it oscillates, there is hypermetria or hypometria, direction cannot be maintained and the animal falls easily, often in an exaggerated way.

congenital a. cerebellar ataxia due to viral infection of the fetus, e.g. bovine virus diarrhea and feline panleukopenia, or to inheritance, e.g. in cattle. See also CEREBELLAR atrophy.

copper-related a. see COPPER nutritional deficiency.

enzootic a. see ENZOOTIC ataxia.

equine sensory a. see ENZOOTIC equine incoordination.

familial convulsions and a. of cattle see FAMILIAL convulsions and ataxia of cattle.

feline a. see FELINE panleukopenia.

foal a. see ENZOOTIC equine incoordination.

frontal a. disturbance of equilibrium occurring in cases of tumor of the frontal lobe.

hereditary a. see HEREDITARY ataxia.

locomotor a. tabes dorsalis.

otarid a. a syndrome in pinnipeds caused by nutritional deficiency of thiamin or enterotoxemia or hypoglycemia. Signs include heelwalking (elevation and curling of the rear toes) followed by running staggers, ataxia and violent falling.

progressive sensory a. of Charolais see PROGRESSIVE ataxia.

sensorimotor a. caused by moderate spinal cord lesions, manifested by weakness of movement, scuffing of toes, incomplete limb extension, knuckling, wobbly gait, easy falling, difficult rising.

sensory a. ataxia due to loss of proprioception (joint position sense), resulting in poorly judged movements and becoming aggravated when the eyes are blindfolded.

spinal a. see equine protozoal ENCEPHALOMYELITIS.

vestibular a. a loss of balance with preservation of strength. If unilateral, the abnormality is asymmetrical; if bilateral, it is symmetrical.

atelectasis a collapsed or airless state of the lung, which may be acute or chronic, and may involve all or part of the lung. See also MICROATELECTASIS.

The primary cause of atelectasis is obstruction of the bronchus serving the affected area. In fetal atelectasis the lungs fail to expand normally at birth.

congenital a. that present at (primary atelectasis) or immediately after (secondary atelectasis) birth.

lobar a. that affecting only a lobe of the lung.

lobular a. that affecting only a lobule of the lung.

primary a. congenital atelectasis in which the alveoli have never been expanded with air.

secondary a. congenital atelectasis in which resorption of the contained air has led to collapse of the alveoli.

Ateleia glazioviana poisonous South American plant in the order Fabaceae; causes abortion in cattle. The toxin has not been identified. Called also TIMBO DE PALMEIRA.

Ateles see SPIDER MONKEY.

atelia imperfect or incomplete development.

ateliocardia imperfect development of the heart.

ateliosis 1. a condition characterized by failure to develop completely. 2. hypophyseal infantalism.
atelo-, atelio- prefix meaning imperfect, incomplete.
atelocephaly imperfect development of the skull.
atel(o)(io)- word element. [Gr.] *incomplete, imperfectly developed.*
atelomyelia imperfect development of the spinal cord.
ateloprosopia congenital incomplete development of the face.
atenolol a cardioselective BETA-blocker having a greater effect on β_1-adrenergic receptors of the heart than on the β_2-adrenergic receptors of the bronchi and blood vessels.
Athanasia trifurcata a South African plant in the family Asteraceae (Compositae) that causes severe liver damage manifested principally by photosensitization; the toxin is unidentified.
athelia congenital absence of the teats.
athermic without rise of temperature.
athermosystaltic not contracting under the action of cold or heat.
atheroembolism embolism due to blockage of a blood vessel by an atheroembolus.
atheroembolus pl. *atheroemboli*; an embolus composed of cholesterol or its esters (typically lodging in small arteries) or of fragments of atheromatous plaques.
atherogenesis formation of atheromas in arterial walls.
atheroma an abnormal mass of fatty or lipid material with a fibrous covering, existing as a discrete, raised plaque within the intima of an artery.
atheromatosis the presence of multiple atheromas.
atherosclerosis a common form of ARTERIOSCLEROSIS in humans in which deposits of yellowing plaques (atheromas) containing cholesterol, other lipoid material, and lipophages are formed within the intima of large and medium-sized arteries. It is a common finding in cetaceans and sirenians and also in aoudads.
atherosclerotic pertaining to ATHEROSCLEROSIS.
Athesmia a genus of trematode parasites of the family Dicrocoeliidae. Includes *A. foxi* (South American monkeys).
athetoid 1. resembling athetosis. 2. affected with athetosis.
athetosis repetitive involuntary, slow, sinuous, writhing movements. Seen in primates, but not a feature of neurological disorders in domestic animals.
athletic animals domestic animals selectively bred and trained for athletic prowess including sprint and distance running, jumping, agility, steeplechase, weight-pulling, rodeo wrestling, bull fighting, cock fighting, coursing, dog fighting.
athrepsia see MARASMUS.
athymia absence of functioning thymus tissue. See also NUDE MOUSE.
athymism the condition induced by removal of the thymus.
athyreosis hypothyroidism.
athyria 1. absence of functioning thyroid tissue. 2. hypothyroidism.
ATIII antithrombin III, a natural α-globulin coagulation inhibitor.
atipamezole used to antagonize (reverse) the action of the α_2 adrenoceptor agonists medetomidine, xylazine and detomidine.
atlantal pertaining to the atlas.
Atlantic puffin *Fratercula arctica.*
Atlantic salmon SALMO *salar.*
atlantoaxial pertaining to the atlas and axis.
a. joint the articulation between the first two cervical vertebrae.
a. membrane the fibrous sheet which closes the interarcual space between the atlas and the axis.
a. subluxation degeneration or malformation of the dens is seen mainly in toy breeds of dogs predisposing to displacement of the axis. Fracture of the dens can occur in any animal. Compression of the cervical cord is a common sequel that causes neck pain and varying degrees of spastic tetraparesis. Treatment is surgical stabilization. Also reported in Holstein cattle.
atlanto-occipital pertaining to the atlas and occiput, e.g. atlanto-occipital joint.
a. fusion a congenital defect observed in calves; causes tetraplegia at birth or by two months of age.
a. malformation includes hypoplasia of the odontoid process, atlanto-occipital fusion.
a. malformation of Arab horses includes occipitalization of the atlas and atlantalization of the axis. It causes incoordination with a characterisitic extension of the head at birth or soon afterwards.
a. membrane there are two, the dorsal and ventral, each of which connects the cranial edge of the atlas to the margin of the foramen magnum.
atlas the first cervical vertebra, the uppermost segment of the backbone which supports the skull, characterized by the absence of a body and a wide vertebral canal.
atloaxoid pertaining to the atlas and axis.
atm atmosphere.
atmospheric of or pertaining to the atmosphere.
a. pressure see atmospheric PRESSURE.
atocia sterility in the female.
atom the smallest particle of an element that has all the properties of the element.

There are two main parts of an atom: the nucleus and the electron cloud. The nucleus is made up of protons, which carry a positive electrical charge, and (except in hydrogen) neutrons, which contain one proton and one electron and carry no electrical charge. The electron cloud is made up of particles called electrons, which carry a negative electrical charge and move in orbits or 'shells' around the nucleus. Different atoms have different numbers of protons, neutrons and electrons in their makeup.

The atomic number of an element is the number of free protons (those not in neutrons) in the nucleus; it is equal to the net positive charge of the nucleus.

The atomic weight is the weight of an atom of a substance as compared with the weight of an atom of carbon-12, which is taken as 12.
atomic bomb explosion of a nuclear device.
a. b. injury see RADIATION injury.
a. b. fallout subsequent to the explosion of an atomic device is the gradual return to earth of radioactive dust.
a. b. irradiation irradiation of animal tissues by any means, therapeutic, accidental, atomic bomb blast.
atomization the act or process of breaking up a liquid into a fine spray.
atomizer an instrument for dispensing liquid in a fine spray.
atonia, atony absence or lack of normal tone.
atonic lacking in tone.
a. constipation constipation caused by atony of the colon.
atony see ATONIA.
atopen the antigen responsible for atopy.
atopic 1. displaced; ectopic. 2. pertaining to atopy.

a. asthma see allergic ASTHMA.
a. dermatitis called also atopic disease, allergic inhalant dermatitis. See canine ATOPY.
a. disease see atopic dermatitis (above).
a. rhinitis see ENZOOTIC nasal granuloma, ATOPY.
atopy a clinical syndrome involving type I hypersensitivity (allergy) with a hereditary predisposition. Immunoglobulin E (IgE) is involved.
canine a. characterized by pruritus, often seasonal, mainly of feet, face and ventral body, with self-trauma. Secondary pyoderma, hyperhidrosis and otitis externa are often present. Rhinitis, conjunctivitis or gastrointestinal disorders may also occur.
atoxic not poisonous; not due to a poison.
ATP see ADENOSINE triphosphate.
ATPase see ADENOSINE triphosphatase.
ATPS ambient temperature and pressure, saturated; denoting a volume of gas saturated with water vapor at ambient temperature and barometric pressure.
Atractylis gummifera European poisonous plant in the family Asteraceae containing atractyloside, a potent hepatoxin.
atracurium besylate a short-acting, nondepolarizing neuromuscular blocking agent.
atraumatic not producing injury or damage.
Atrax a genus of the suborder of Mygalomorpha spiders with vertical fangs.
A. robustus, A. formidabalis the very poisonous funnel web spider.
atrazine a triazine herbicide; it is not poisonous at levels of intake likely to be encountered in agriculture.
atresia congenital absence or closure of a normal body opening or tubular structure.
anal a., a. ani see ANAL atresia.
aortic a. absence of the opening from the left ventricle of the heart into the aorta.
aural a. absence of closure of the auditory canal.
biliary a. congenital obliteration or hypoplasia of one or more components of the bile ducts, resulting in persistent jaundice and liver damage.
choanal a. see imperforate BUCCOPHARYNGEAL membrane.
follicular a., a. folliculi premature degeneration and resorption of a graafian follicle of the ovary. It may be postovulatory or preovulatory atresia. It is a normal occurrence when several ova mature together. Abnormal atresia may be a cause of anestrus.
ileal a., a. ilei the congenital obstruction in calves may cause sufficient abdominal distension to result in dystocia.
inherited alimentary tract segmental a. occurs in cattle and horses. A variety of segments are involved, including ileum, colon, rectum and anus.
jejunal a., a. jejuni resembles ileal atresia clinically.
lacrimal puncta a. atresia of the lacrimal puncta causing tearing from birth.
mesonephric duct a. causes stenosis or aplasia of epididymis or ductus deferens.
nasolacrimal duct a. atresia of the nasolacrimal duct causing tearing from birth.
paramesonephric duct a. causes uterus unicornis or duplex uterus or segmental aplasia of a uterine horn or tube.
rectal a., a. recti congenital absence of luminal development leading to abdominal distension after birth. There is obvious absence of feces and staining and inability to pass a sound.
salivary duct a. congenital atresia causes distension of the gland followed by atrophy.
tracheal a. common in English bulldogs; may be segmental or affect the entire length of the tube.
tricuspid a. absence of the opening between the right atrium and right ventricle, circulation being made possible by an atrial septal defect.
atretic being in a state of atresia; without an opening.
a. follicle an ovarian follicle in an undeveloped state due to immaturity, poor nutrition or systemic disease; manifested by prolonged anestrus.
atria [L.] plural of *atrium*.
silent a. see ATRIAL standstill.
atrial pertaining to an atrium.
a. contraction contraction of the atrial muscle; plays a part in ventricular filling and opening and closing of the A-V valves.
a. filling return of blood via the venae cavae and the pulmonary veins to the atria. Too slow a return means inadequate cardiac output, too slow emptying means an increase in central venous pressure and possibly the development of congestive heart failure. The rate varies normally with the cardiac cycle, being fastest during atrial diastole and slowest during atrial systole.
a. natriuretic factor (ANF) a peptide hormone found in cardiocytes of the right and left atria and released in response to increases in plasma volume. Plays a role in the regulation of blood pressure and volume, and in the excretion of water, sodium and potassium. Closely related or possibly identical substances include auriculin, atriopeptin, cardionatrin.
a. rupture most often is a complication of endocardiosis and valvular insufficiency in dogs. The resulting acute pericardial hemorrhage may cause death from cardiac TAMPONADE.
a. septal defect a congenital heart defect in which there is persistent patency of the atrial septum, owing to failure of closure of the ostium primum or ostium secundum.
a. standstill complete lack of atrial contraction; ventricular function remains normal. Caused by hyperkalemia, extreme sinus bradycardia, digitalis toxicity and a congenital muscle disorder of dogs and cats.
a. systole see atrial contraction (above).
atrichia absence of hair or of flagella or cilia.
atrichial gland tumor eccrine sweat gland neoplasms occur rarely in cats and dogs.
atrichous 1. having no hair. 2. having no flagella.
atriomegaly abnormal enlargement of an atrium of the heart.
atriopeptin see ATRIAL natriuretic factor.
atrioseptopexy surgical correction of a defect in the interatrial septum.
atrioseptoplasty plastic repair of the interatrial septum.
Atriotaenia a genus of tapeworms of the family Linstowiidae. Includes *Atriotaenia megastoma, A. procyonis* (mustelids and procyonids, e.g. skunk, badger, marten, ermine, mink).
atrioventricular pertaining to an atrium and ventricle of the heart.
accessory tract a. conduction see accessory tract atrioventricular CONDUCTION.
a. block see atrioventricular HEART BLOCK.
a. bundle BUNDLE of His.
common a. canal a congenital cardiac defect in which both sides of the heart share the same atrioventricular orifice. Called also persistent atrioventricular canal, ATRIOVENTRICULARIS COMMUNIS.
a. node a mass of cardiac muscle fibers (Purkinje fibers) lying on the right lower part of the interatrial septum of the heart. Its function is the transmission of the cardiac impulse from the sinoatrial node to the muscular walls of the ventricles. The conductive sys-

tem is organized so that transmission is slightly delayed at the atrioventricular node, thus allowing time for the atria to empty their contents into the ventricles before the ventricles begin to contract.

partitioning a. canal during embryological development partitioning of the cardiac chambers and their orifices may be incomplete, leading to fatal cardiac defects, e.g. persistent atrioventricular chamber.

persistent common a. canal see ATRIOVENTRICULARIS COMMUNIS.

a. stenosis left and right atrioventricular stenosis are recorded; the former is an acyanotic defect, the latter is more serious and a cyanotic defect.

a. trunk see BUNDLE of His.

a. valvular disease may be identifiable on finding of systolic murmur (incompetent valve) or diastolic murmur (stenotic valve) over the apex of the heart with maximum audibility over the left or right sides, depending on the side involved.

Wenckebach a. block see Mobitz atrioventricular HEART BLOCK.

atrioventricularis communis a congenital cardiac anomaly in which the endocardial cushions fail to fuse, the ostium primum persists, the atrioventricular canal is undivided, a single atrioventricular valve has anterior and posterior cusps, and there is a defect of the membranous interventricular septum. Most commonly seen in pigs and cats. Called also persistent common atrioventricular canal.

Atriplex 1. a genus of the plant family Chenopodiaceae; saltbushes. They are an excellent source of feed but are facultative indicator plants and may lead to selenium poisoning when growing on selenium-rich soils. Includes North American species *A. canescens*, *A. nuttalii*, *A. patula*, *A. rosea*. 2. Australian species may be toxic by virtue of a high nitrate or oxalate content, e.g. *A. muelleri*, *A. semibaccata*.

atrium pl. *atria* [L.] a chamber affording entrance, especially the chamber (atrium cordis) on either side of the heart, transmitting to the ventricle of the same side blood received (left atrium) from the pulmonary veins and (right atrium) from the venae cavae. See also ATRIAL.

parabronchi a. extensions of the parabronchial lumen giving rise to the air capillaries.

a. partitioning partitioning of the atrium by the septum primum during embryological development may be defective leading to a congenital malformation, e.g. patent foramen ovale.

ruminal a. the first part of the rumen, and the cranial chamber of its dorsal sac, just caudal to the reticuloruminal fold. Called also *atrium ruminis*.

ventricular a. the shallow vault between the reticulum and the rumen into which the esophagus in the ruminant opens.

Atropa belladonna a plant in the Solanaceae family. Contains L-hyoscyamine and causes tremor, excitement, tachycardia, pupillary dilatation and recumbency. Poisoning is rare and most such diagnoses are based on incorrect identification of the plant; it is confused with *Solanum nigrum* among others. Called also deadly nightshade.

atrophia [L.] see ATROPHY.

a. bulbi a shrunken end-stage eye that contains recognizable ocular structures. See also PHTHISIS bulbi.

atrophic characterized by atrophy.

a. dermatosis characterized by epithelial and connective tissue atrophy; a common accompaniment of endocrine disorders and nutritional deficiencies.

ovarian a. cyst anovulatory cystic follicles causing failure of estrus in most cases; a common cause of infertility in cows.

a. rhinitis a disease primarily of young pigs causing deformities of the facial and turbinate bones which persist for life. Clinically there is an initial attack of acute rhinitis manifested by sneezing and snout rubbing, followed by crumpling of the face often with a distortion to one side.

atrophoderma atrophy of the skin.

atrophy 1. decrease in size of a normally developed organ or tissue; wasting. 2. to undergo or cause atrophy.

disuse a. atrophy of local musculature due to failure to use a part of the body, due usually to pain. Is separate from neurogenic atrophy when nerve damage causes atrophy from both disuse and denervation.

iris a. occurs with aging, particularly in Siamese cats and miniature schnauzers and poodles; may be secondary to trauma, recurrent uveitis and chronic glaucoma.

mammary a. the terminal stage of chronic mastitis; palpation establishes that little mammary tissue remains and inflammatory fibrous tissue has subsided.

optic a. atrophy of the optic nerve; may occur with trauma, prolonged inflammatory diseases of the eye, and retinal degeneration.

retinal a. see progressive RETINAL atrophy.

serous a. in cachexia there is mobilization of depot fat and lipid vacuoles are progressively reduced in size and replaced by proteinaceous fluid which converts the fat depots to gelatinous masses of serous atrophy.

villous a. a common finding in a variety of intestinal diseases of animals, including viral, bacterial and protozoal infections, parasitism, hypersensitivity reactions in the bowel and alimentary lymphosarcoma. Malabsorption and diarrhea result. An idiopathic, possibly immune-mediated, villous atrophy occurs in dogs.

atropine an anticholinergic alkaloid occurring in belladonna, hyoscyamus and stramonium. It acts as a competitive antagonist of acetylcholine at muscarinic receptors, blocking stimulation of muscles and glands by parasympathetic and cholinergic sympathetic nerves; used as a smooth muscle relaxant, as a preanesthetic to reduce secretions, and as an antidote to organophosphate poisoning. Has been used as a spasmolytic in many cases of gut hypermotility, e.g. equine spasmodic colic. Has the disadvantage of causing prolonged pupillary dilatation.

a. challenge test used in the diagnosis of narcolepsy in dogs; pretreatment with atropine reduces the number of cataleptic attacks with exposure to food.

a. methobromide a synthetic muscarinic blocking agent used as a smooth muscle relaxant but less effective against poisoning with organophosphorus insecticides than atropine. Called also methylatropine.

a. poisoning severe toxic reaction due to overdosage of atropine. Signs include dilated pupils, absent pupillary light reflex, dry mouth, high heart rate, excitement, muscle tremor. In animals usually results from atropine overdose.

a. sulfate the pharmaceutical preparation in common use.

atropinic muscarinic.

attachment 1. state of being attached. 2. a connection which achieves attachment.

a. plaque an electron-dense coating of cell membranes in which intermediate filaments are embedded participating in the mechanism of holding cells together.

attack an episode or onset of illness.

a. rate the proportion of a population affected by the disease during a prescribed, usually short, period of time.

attenuated having undergone a process of ATTENUATION.

a. breath sounds normal breath sounds audible via a stethoscope over the lungs.

attenuation 1. the act of thinning or weakening. 2. reduction in the virulence of a pathogenic microorganism induced by passage through another host species, decreasing its virulence for the native host and increasing it for the new host. Some attenuated strains of microorganisms may occur naturally. The possibility now exists of using genetic engineering to attenuate microorganisms in defined ways. Attenuated organisms are used as live vaccines. See also attenuated VACCINE. 3. the change in a beam of radiation or sound beam as it passes through matter. The intensity of the electromagnetic radiation decreases as its depth of penetration increases. A sound beam becomes weaker as it travels through tissue.

attic a small upper space of the middle ear, containing the head of the malleus and the body of the incus. Called also epitympanic recess.

atticotomy incision into the attic or epitympanic recess, the dorsal part of the tympanic cavity which contains the upper half of the malleus and most of the incus.

attitude a posture or position of the body; in obstetrics, the relation of the various parts of the fetal body to one another. See also POSTURE.

attitudinal pertaining to or arising from an attitude or posture.

a. reflexes see POSTURAL reflexes.

atto- a prefix signifying one million-million-millionth, or 10^{-18}; symbol a.

attractant a material used to attract animals for capture purposes.

attraction the force or influence by which one object is drawn toward another.

attributable emanating from or pertaining to attribute.

a. proportion see attributable risk (below).

a. risk a measure of the proportion of the total risk which can be attributed to the risk factor which is under consideration. Called also attributable proportion.

attribute 1. in statistics a qualitative variable which cannot be expressed in numerical terms, e.g. insectivorous as a behavioral attribute. 2. in computer terms an element which determines the appearance of a character, e.g. italics, bold.

attrition the physiological wearing away of a substance or structure in the course of normal use.

dental a. see DENTAL attrition.

atypia deviation from the normal or typical state.

atypical irregular; not conformable to the type.

a. disease a form of a disease which differs significantly in clinical signs or pathological lesions from classical or textbook forms of the disease, e.g. bovine atypical interstitial pneumonia.

a. fever a fever in which temperature variations are irregular.

a. mycobacterial granuloma see opportunist MYCOBACTERIAL granuloma.

atypical interstitial pneumonia the name given to a number of diseases which are closely related clinically but whose etiology is incompletely understood. Clinically there is acute or chronic respiratory distress, gross abnormality of lung sounds, and a complete absence of toxemia and other systemic signs that are characteristic of most other pneumonias of adult cattle. All forms of the disease are unresponsive to treatment. The disease appears to have a number of causes. See also TRYPTOPHAN, 3-METHYLINDOLE. Called also acute respiratory distress syndrome, bovine pulmonary emphysema, enzootic bovine adenomatosis, pulmonary adenomatosis, mold hypersensitivity, fog fever, panters.

AU both (left and right) ears.

Au chemical symbol, *gold* (L. *aurum*).

aubergine SOLANUM *melongena*.

Auchmeromyia a genus of flies of the family Calliphoridae.

A. luteola the larva of this African fly is a bloodsucker and parasitizes pigs and people. Called also Congo floor maggot.

audi(o)- word element. [L.] *hearing*.

audiogenic produced by sound.

audiometer instrument used to measure the quality of a patient's hearing.

audiometry measurement of the acuity of hearing for the various frequencies of sound waves. Not widely used in animals except under laboratory conditions. See also brainstem auditory EVOKED RESPONSE, DEAFNESS.

audiosurgery surgery of the ear.

audit systematic review and evaluation of records and other data to determine the quality of the services or products provided in a given situation.

retrospective a. conducted after the patient's discharge. Methods include the study of closed patients' charts and nursing care plans, questionnaires, interviews, and surveys of patients and other animals in the household.

audition perception of sound; hearing.

auditor trail see ACCOUNTANCY TRAIL.

auditory pertaining to the EAR or the sense of hearing.

a. apparatus comprises the tympanic membrane, the auditory ossicles that connect the membrane to the oval window to the internal ear, the membranous labyrinth and its contained endolymph, the labyrinth's cochlear duct, the organ of Corti, a specialized sensory epithelium lining the duct, the sensory hair cells of the organ of Corti and the sensory receptors of the auditory nerve that terminate at the base of the hair cells.

a. bulb the membranous labyrinth and cochlea.

a. conditioning signals sounds used to condition animals to certain procedures or events, such as gathering at the sound of a bell or trumpet, milking to the sound of a radio, whistle signals to a sheep dog.

external a. meatus air-filled tubular extension of the auricle leading to the eardrum.

internal a. meatus a canal in the petrous temporal bone that accommodates the VIIth and VIIIth cranial nerves.

a. nerve the eighth cranial nerve; called also VESTIBULOCOCHLEAR nerve and acoustic nerve. See Table 14.

a. ossicles the malleus, incus and stapes, the three small bones of the tympanic cavity of the ear. They form a connecting bony system from the tympanic membrane to the oval window that is the opening to the internal ear.

a. tube the narrow channel connecting the nasopharynx to the middle ear. See also PHARYNGOTYMPANIC TUBE.

Auer reaction type III hypersensitivity-induced inflammation.

Auerbach plexus a peripheral plexus of fine autonomic nerve fibers lying between the muscle layers of the intestine. Called also myenteric plexus.
AUG codon codon for methionine; usually, but not always the first AUG sequence encountered as the mRNA is read 5′→3′ is the translational start signal; the methionine encoded is cleaved from the polypeptide.
augnathus a fetus with a double lower jaw.
Aujeszky's disease a disease primarily of pigs but can occur in other secondary host species; caused by porcine herpesvirus 1 and characterized by respiratory, reproductive and nervous signs. In piglets there is incoordination followed by recumbency and convulsions and most piglets die. In older pigs the predominant signs are dyspnea, coughing, sneezing and nasal discharge. Nervous signs follow in some pigs. The mortality rate is low. Infection of sows in late pregnancy causes abortion and stillbirths or mummified fetuses. In secondary hosts infection is acquired from pigs and nervous signs predominate. In cattle the disease is characterized by frenzied scratching, intense excitement, paralysis, convulsions and death of all affected animals. Called also pseudorabies, 'mad itch'.
Aulonocephalus lindquisti a cecal and colonic nematode of uncertain pathogenicity in quail.
aunt a mare that develops maternal behavior and cares for foals belonging to other mares in a herd.
aura a peculiar sensation preceding the appearance of more definite symptoms. It is a well-known phenomenon in humans and, on good clinical grounds, assumed to occur in animals, appearing as behavioral abnormalities.
aural pertaining to the ear.
a. plaque see AURICULAR plaque.
auramine a fluorescent dye used in staining tisues for fluorescence microscopy.
auranofin a compound containing 29% gold; used orally in CHRYSOTHERAPY in dogs and cats.
Aureobasidium pullulans a cause of chromomycosis in animals.
auri- prefix meaning ear.
auric pertaining to gold.
auricle 1. the flap of the ear in the form of a funnel-like organ which collects the sound waves. Called also pinna. 2. the ear-shaped appendage of either atrium of the heart; formerly used to designate the entire atrium.
auricula pl. *auriculae* [L.] auricle.
auricular pertaining to or emanating from the ear.
a. cartilages comprise the auricular, the main funnel-shaped cartilage, the annular, a C-shaped cartilage surrounding the external meatus, and the scutiform cartilage that lies on the surface of the temporal muscle.
a. hematoma bleeding of branches of the great auricular artery, usually caused by head shaking or trauma, result in hematoma formation between the skin on the inner side of the ear and auricular cartilage or in a cleavage within the cartilage. Common in dogs with otitis externa and foreign bodies of the ear canal. Surgical drainage and fixation of tissues is the usual treatment.
a. hillocks small swellings on the embryonic visceral arches; the beginnings of the external ears.
a. mange infestation with ear mites. See OTODECTIC MANGE.
a. muscles see Table 13.1G.
a. plaque hyperkeratotic, depigmented plaques of tissue on the inner aspect of the pinna of a horse's ears. They are verrucae plana or flat warts.
a. veins see Table 15.
auricularis [L.] pertaining to the ear.
auriculin see ATRIAL natriuretic factor.
auriculopalpebral pertaining to the ear and eyelid.
a. nerve block block anesthesia of the auriculopalpebral nerve as it proceeds from the base of the ear over the zygomatic arch. Used to immobilize the eyelids (it does not anesthetize them) for examination of the conjunctival sac. Needs to be complemented with topical anesthetic for removal of foreign bodies.
auriculotemporal pertaining to the ear and the temporal region.
auriculotherapy the most highly developed regional acupuncture therapy in humans but an undeveloped field in animals.
auripuncture myringotomy; surgical puncture of the tympanic membrane.
auris pl. *aures* [L.] ear.
auriscope otoscope; an instrument for examining the ear.
auro- prefix meaning gold or golden.
aurothioglucose a gold preparation used in treating immune-mediated diseases such as pemphigus complex and rheumatoid arthritis. See also CHRYSOTHERAPY.
aurotrichia gold coloring of the hair; gilding. A syndrome seen in young adult Miniature schnauzers in which there is patchy or diffuse distribution of the color change with a decrease in numbers of secondary hairs.
aurum [L.] *gold* (symbol Au).
auscultate to examine by auscultation.
auscultation listening for sounds produced within the body, chiefly to ascertain the condition of the thoracic or abdominal viscera; it may be performed with the unaided ear (direct or immediate auscultation) or with a stethoscope (mediate auscultation).
abdominal a. for the purpose of listening to the sounds created by the movement of gas and fluid in the intestines, and in the forestomachs in ruminants. The presence or absence of sounds is valuable in assessing the motility of the gut.
cardiac a. auscultation of the cardiac area with special attention to location and size of the heart, the rhythm and intensity of the heart sounds, the presence of abnormal sounds and the relationship of the heart sounds to the occurrence of the pulse waves.
a. with percussion auscultation of one part of the region while percussing elsewhere. Used in examining the chest for areas of consolidation, or the bovine abdomen when searching for the displaced abomasum or the distended colon or duodenum.
pulmonary a. auscultation of both sides of the chest with the objective of ascertaining the state of the lungs and air passages. Points observed are the rhythm and depth of breathing, quality of the breath sounds and the size and disposition of the area over which they can be heard.
thoracic a. includes auscultation of the lungs and air passages, the pleural cavity including the presence of extraneous organs such as intestines, and the heart and pericardial sac. The principal rule in the examination is the absolute necessity of auscultating both sides of the chest.
tuning fork a. the tip of a tuning fork is placed over the area to be auscultated and the stethoscope applied nearby. Consolidated lung transmits the sound, normal lung muffles it. See also COIN TEST.
auscultatory pertaining to auscultation.
Australian pertaining to or originating in Australia.

A. cattle dog a medium-sized, compact working dog used for control of cattle. The coat is medium length and dense, but longer and thicker on the neck. It is a characteristic blue or red speckled color with erect ears and a bushy tail. The breed is affected by congenital deafness.

A. College of Veterinary Scientists has the objective of encouraging veterinarians, principally those in practice, to undertake postgraduate study in professional subjects. Awards Membership and Fellowship qualifications, in part to establish credentials as specialists.

A. feedlots are designed to fit Australian grain farming conditions in which grain is available for cattle fattening in only a limited number of years. This restricts expenditure on capital improvements to post and wire fences of limited restraining power. Called also backup feedlots.

A. fireweed SENECIO *bipinattisectus*.

A. heeler see Australian cattle dog (above).

A. Illawarra cattle see ILLAWARRA CATTLE.

A. indigo INDIGOFERA *australis*.

A. itch see PSORERGATES *ovis*.

A. kelpie a medium-sized, moderately short-coated, active dog used for working sheep. It is very alert, active and intelligent. Comes in black (sometimes called a BARB), blue or red.

A. Merino sheep finewool, horned or polled, originated from Spanish merino; comes in superfine, finewool, medium and strongwool strains. See also BOOROOLA MERINO.

A. milking shorthorn see ILLAWARRA CATTLE.

A. Milking Zebu a zeboid breed of dairy cattle produced in Australia by crossbreeding Jersey, Red Sindhi and Sahiwal cattle with later infusions of Guernsey, AIS and Holstein–Friesian breeding. Resembles a Jersey, with drooped ears and dewlap of zebu. Called also AMZ.

A. native dog see DINGO.

A. phalaris PHALARIS *aquatica*.

A. Pony bred in Australia by crossing Arab with ponies of various breeds, usually Welsh. Used as riding ponies for children. Known to carry the inherited cerebellar defect of the Arab. Assorted colors, mostly grays, no broken colors; 12 to 14 hands high.

A. shepherd dog a working sheep dog developed in the United States; it is little known in Australia. A medium-sized, tailless, medium-haired, black, red, red merle, blue merle and white dog, It suffers from an inherited RETINAL dysplasia, ocular colobomas.

A. Shorthorn a horned red or red roan with white patches breed of dairy cattle, bred in Australia from Shorthorn and other dairy breeds. Called also AIS, Australian Illawarra Shorthorn.

A. silky terrier see SILKY TERRIER.

A. Stock horse a class of horses rather than a breed. See CUTTING HORSE, POLO PONY.

A. terrier a small lively dog with a straight, harsh coat of medium length, relatively short legs, erect ears, and a docked tail which is carried erect.

A. umbrella tree see SCHEFFLERA ACTINOPHYLLA.

A. Veterinary Association a voluntary professional organization with the objective of maintaining the highest possible status of the Australian veterinary profession.

A. Waler see WALER.

A. white see WHITE HOLLAND.

Australorp black, dual-purpose poultry breed, descended from Black Orpington. Wattles, comb and earlobes are red, legs and beak black, and body and wing plumage have a characteristic green sheen.

Austrelaps superba see COPPERHEAD SNAKES.

Austrian brown cattle brown, dual purpose, mountain type, Austrian cattle.

Austrian pea PISUM *sativum* var. *arvense*.

Austrian yellow see GELBVIEH.

Austrobilharzia a genus of digenetic trematodes of the family Schistosomatidae.

A. variglandis principally a parasite of waterfowl but can also cause dermatitis in mammals that frequent shallow aquatic environments.

Austrosimulium includes *A. ornatum*; see BLACK FLY.

autacoid a term once proposed to replace the term *hormone* and recently suggested as a general term for various physiologically active, endogenous substances (histamine, serotonin, angiotensin, prostaglandins, etc.) that do not yet fit into existing functional classifications.

aut(o)- word element. [Gr.] *self*.

autoagglutination 1. clumping or agglutination of an individual's cells by its own serum, usually because of the presence of autoantibodies, as in autohemagglutination. Autoagglutination occurring at low temperatures is called *cold agglutination*. 2. agglutination of particulate antigens, e.g. bacteria, in the absence of specific antibodies.

autoagglutinin a factor, usually antibody, in serum capable of causing clumping of the subject's own cellular elements.

autoamputation spontaneous detachment from the body and elimination of an appendage or an abnormal growth, such as a polyp.

autoantibody an antibody formed in response to, and reacting against, an antigenic constituent of the animal's own cells or tissues.

autoantigen a tissue constituent that stimulates production of autoantibodies or self-reactive T lymphocytes in the animal in which it occurs.

autocatalysis catalysis in which a product of the reaction hastens or intensifies the catalysis.

autochthonous 1. originating in the same area in which it is found. 2. denoting a tissue graft to a new site on the same individual.

autoclasis destruction of a tissue by an autoimmune response. See AUTOIMMUNE disease.

autoclave a self-locking apparatus for the sterilization of materials by steam under pressure. The autoclave allows steam to flow around each article placed in the chamber. The vapor penetrates cloth or paper used to package the articles being sterilized. Autoclaving is one of the most effective methods for destruction of all types of microorganisms. The amount of time and degree of temperature necessary for sterilization depend on the articles to be sterilized and whether they are wrapped or left directly exposed to the steam.

a. tape special masking tape used to close packages of surgical materials to be autoclaved. Includes a heat sensitive dye in diagonal stripes. The appearance of the dye can be misunderstood; it does not indicate that the package has been sterilized only that it has been exposed to some heat.

autocoid see AUTACOID.

autocrines chemicals secreted by cells which are themselves affected.

autocytolysin see AUTOLYSIN.

autocytolysis see AUTOLYSIS.

autodigestion dissolution of tissue by its own secretions.

autoeczematization the spread, at first locally and later more generally, of lesions from an originally circumscribed focus of eczema.

autogeneic arising from self; pertaining to an autograft.

autogenesis self-generation; origination within the organism.

autogenous self-generated, originating within the patient's own body.

a. tissue graft a graft comprising tissue from the patient's own body.

a. vaccine see autogenous VACCINE.

autograft a graft transferred from one part of the patient's body to another part.

autohemagglutination agglutination of erythrocytes by an autoantibody.

autohemagglutinin a substance, usually antibody, produced in an animal's body that causes agglutination of its own erythrocytes.

autohemolysin a hemolytic antibody produced in the body of an animal which causes destruction of its own erythrocytes.

autohemolysis hemolysis of the blood cells of an animal by its own autoantibody.

a. test determination of spontaneous hemolysis in a blood specimen maintained under certain conditions, to detect the presence of certain hemolytic states.

autohemotherapy treatment by reinjection of the animal's own blood.

autohistory one completed in written form by an owner in response to a series of questions on a history sheet.

autoimmune the state conferred by AUTOIMMUNITY.

a. disease a disease state characterized by a specific antibody or cell-mediated immune response against the body's own tissues (autoantigens).

The immunological mechanism of the body is dependent on two major factors: (1) the inactivation and rejection of foreign substances and (2) the ability to differentiate between the body's own antigens ('self') and foreign ('nonself'). It is not yet known exactly what causes the body to fail to recognize proteins as its own and to react to them as if they were foreign. Autoimmune reactions are rare in large animal diseases. THROMBOCYTOPENIA, milk ALLERGY and SPERMATIC granuloma are known examples. In dogs and cats there are a number of autoimmune diseases recognized and they occur with some frequency. These include autoimmune hemolytic ANEMIA and THROMBOCYTOPENIA, systemic LUPUS ERYTHEMATOSUS, rheumatoid ARTHRITIS, GLOMERULONEPHRITIS, lymphocytic THYROIDITIS and a variety of dermatological disorders in the PEMPHIGUS group of diseases.

a. reaction includes, most importantly, the acute syndromes of anaphylaxia and pulmonary and cutaneous diseases.

autoimmunity an condition which may result in AUTOIMMUNE disease.

autoimmunization immunization of an animal with its own tissues.

autoinfection spread of an infection from part of the body to another.

autoinoculation inoculation of one's own body.

autointoxication poisoning by toxins formed within the body. In dogs it has been associated with changes and indiscretion in diet.

autoisolysin a substance that lyses cells (e.g., blood cells) of the individual in which it is formed and also those of other individuals of the same species.

autokeratoplasty grafting of corneal tissue from one eye to the other.

autokinesis voluntary motion.

autolesion a self-inflicted injury.

autologous related to self; belonging to the same organism.

autolysate a substance produced by autolysis.

autolysin a lysin originating in an organism and capable of destroying its own cells and tissues.

autolysis the disintegration of cells or tissues by endogenous enzymes. See also POSTMORTEM decomposition.

autolysosome a vacuolar element of the lysosome system of cells to which hydrolases have been added by fusion with lysosomes.

hepatocellular a's participate in the formation of CYTOSEGRESOME FORMATIONS in the liver when damaged hepatocytes are surrounded by an isolating membrane.

automated cell counting systems mechanized procedures for carrying out the various cell counting procedures performed in a clinical pathology laboratory, particularly red and white blood cells, platelets and cytological assessment of fluids. They have revolutionized the diagnosis of subclinical bovine mastitis because of the speed and automaticity with which they perform individual cow MILK CELL COUNTS.

automatic spontaneous; done involuntarily; self-regulating.

a. film processors radiographs can be processed by machine at higher temperatures to give shorter processing times and requiring less labor.

a. sexing circumstances in which identification or separation of the sexes occurs automatically, e.g. by the occurrence of breeds of fowl that indicate their sex by the color pattern of their feathers, or by a genetically engineered lethal gene in a sex chromosome. Called also autosexing.

a. ventilator a small, simple machine used for small animal anesthesia; fits any continuous flow anesthetic apparatus.

automaticity the ability of cells, after activity, to depolarise spontaneously, and then initiate a propagated, transmembranous, action potential; in healthy hearts only the sinus node cells reach threshold potential without an external stimulus.

automatism mechanical, often repetitive motor behavior performed without conscious control.

automobile oil see SUMP OIL.

autonomic not subject to voluntary control.

a. craniosacral outflow the parasympathetic nervous system includes nerve fibers in the oculomotor, facial and glossopharyngeal and vagal cranial nerves. The sacral outflow includes autonomic fibers in the ventral nerve roots of the sacral nerves.

a. drug drugs that have effects similar to those of the effector agents in the two systems are called SYMPATHOMIMETIC and PARASYMPATHOMIMETIC drugs.

a. ganglionic blocking agent nicotine and some synthetic compounds such as hexamethonium, pentamethonium and others specifically paralyze the nerve cells in autonomic ganglia thus neutralizing the sympathetic and parasympathic postganglionic fibers that emanate from that particular ganglion.

a. nervous system see autonomic NERVOUS system.

a. parasympathetic effects include constriction of the pupil and the bronchioles, increased secretory activity of glands, increased tone and motility of the gut, relaxation of the spincters.

a. reflex arc comprises the afferent fibers from sensory end organs which pass into the spinal cord via the dorsal roots, ascend though the sensory columns in the spinal cord to the hypothalamus. Efferent fibers pass from there to subhypothalamic motor levels.

a. sympathetic effects include the fight-or-flight reactions of dilatation of blood vessels to muscles, constriction of others, dilatation of pupils and bronchioles, and inhibition of glandular and plain muscle activity.

a. thoracolumbar outflow the sympathetic nervous system consists of neurons in the intermediolateral gray column of the thoracic and lumbar segments of the spinal cord which leave the cord in the ventral branches of thoracic and lumbar nerves. Once outside the vertebral column the neurons leave the spinal nerve and join the paravertebral sympathetic trunk to enter ganglia from which postganglionic fibers go their separate ways to effector organs.

autonomotropic having an affinity for the autonomic nervous system.

autonomous skin zones skin zones used for testing the integrity of individual nerves.

auto-oxidation see AUTOXIDATION.

autopathy idiopathic disease; one without apparent external causation.

autophagia 1. eating or biting of one's own flesh. 2. nutrition of the body by consumption of its own tissues. 3. autophagy.

autophagic vacuoles cytoplasmic degenerative debris engulfed by primary lysozymes; on completion of digestion form residual bodies later extruded from the cell. Called also cytolysosomes.

autophagocytosis a process similar to but not identical with phagocytosis. Foci of cytoplasmic degeneration within cells are engulfed by primary lysosomes to form cytolysosomes.

autophagosome a secondary lysosome in which elements of a cell's own cytoplasm are digested.

autophagy 1. lysosomal digestion of a cell's own cytoplasmic material. 2. autophagia.

autopharmacological pertaining to substances (e.g. hormones) produced in the body that have pharmacological activities.

autoplasmotherapy therapeutic reinjection of one's own plasma.

autoplasty replacement or reconstruction of diseased or injured parts with tissues taken from another region of the patient's own body.

autopodium distal segment of a limb, comprising the hand or foot.

autopolyploidy the state of having more than two chromosome sets as a result of redoubling of the chromosomes of a haploid individual or cell.

autoprothrombin II see plasma THROMBOPLASTIN component.

autopsy examination of a body after death to determine the actual cause of death; called also postmortem examination and necropsy. Autopsies are also valuable sources of medical knowledge.

a. data data from autopsies used to illustrate the natural history of diseases and changes in their frequency are often flawed by the non-random way in which cases are selected for autopsy.

a. record includes data identifying the corpse including name, address of owner, species of subject, age, sex, breed, use (as occupation in man), identifying marks, plus observations on the gross postmortem examination, the histopathological or other examinations conducted and finally an opinion about the cause of death. Useful additional documents are permission from the owner to conduct the autopsy and details of any insurance or legal interest in the examination.

autoradiograph the film produced by autoradiography.

autoradiography the making of a radiograph of an object or tissue by recording on an x-ray plate the radiation emitted by radioactive material within the object. An immunologic technique used to visualize radioactive molecules in tissue sections or electrophoretic gels. Called also radioautography.

autoreactive pertaining to an immune response directed against the body's own tissues.

autoregulation control of certain phenomena by factors inherent in a situation; specifically, (1) maintenance by an organ or tissue of a constant blood flow despite changes in arterial pressure, and (2) adjustment of blood flow through an organ in accordance with its metabolic needs.

heterometric a. those intrinsic mechanisms controlling the strength of ventricular contractions that depend on the length of myocardial fibers at the end of diastole.

homeometric a. those intrinsic mechanisms controlling the strength of ventricular contractions that are independent of the length of myocardial fibers at the end of diastole.

autosensitization development of sensitivity to one's own serum or tissues.

autosepticemia septicemia from poisons developed within the body.

autoserum serum administered to the patient from whom it was derived.

autosexing see AUTOMATIC sexing.

autosite the larger, more normal member of asymmetrical conjoined twin fetuses, to which the other twin (the parasite) is attached.

autosomal gene a gene located on a chromosome other than the sex chromosomes. Categories are autosomal dominant and autosomal recessive.

autosome any chromosome other than the sex chromosomes.

autosplenectomy almost complete disappearance of the spleen due to progressive fibrosis and shrinkage.

autotomography a method of body-section radiography involving movement of the patient instead of the x-ray tube.

autotopagnosia inability to orient correctly different parts of the body.

autotoxin a toxin developed within the body.

autotransformer a supplementary transformer with insulated primary and secondary windings on one core in a radiographical unit. It corrects fluctuations in the mains input voltage.

autotransfusion reinfusion of a patient's own blood.

autotransplantation transfer of tissue from one part of the body to another part.

renal a. surgical repositioning of a kidney in the same animal, usually to the iliac fossa.

autotroph an autotrophic organism.

autotrophic capable of synthesizing necessary nutrients if water, carbon dioxide, inorganic salts and a source of energy are available.

autovaccination treatment with autovaccine.

autovaccine a vaccine prepared from cultures of organisms from the patient's own tissues or secretions.

autoxidation, auto-oxidation the spontaneous reaction of a compound with molecular oxygen at room temperature.

autumn crocus see COLCHICUM AUTUMNALE. Called also meadow saffron.

autumn fly see MUSCA *autumnalis*. Called also face fly.

autumn saving of pasture. See deferred GRAZING.

auxesis increase in size of an organism, especially that due to growth of its individual cells rather than increase in their number.

auxin plant hormone.

auxochrome a chemical group which added to a chromogen converts it into a dye.

auxotroph an auxotrophic organism.

auxotrophic 1. requiring a growth factor not required by the parental or prototype strain; said of microbial mutants. 2. requiring specific organic growth factors in addition to the carbon source present in a minimal medium.

A-V, AV 1. arteriovenous. 2. atrioventricular.

av. avoirdupois.

AVA see AUSTRALIAN Veterinary Association.

Avahi a lemur-like animal of the suborder Prosimii of mammals.

A. laniger a nocturnal, 10 inch long squirrel-like animal with a very long tail. Called also avahi.

availability the proportion of a specific nutrient or chemical in soil or in animal feed that is available for absorption by plants or by animals that eat the plants. The overall availability of each chemical may vary from time to time in a plant depending on its chemical composition. Represented most simply as the amount of the ingested material not recoverable in the feces. In soil it is the proportion of the content that is eluted by a weak acid.

avascular not vascular; bloodless.

a. necrosis of the femoral head see LEGG–CALVÉ–PERTHES DISEASE.

a. chorion the normally avascular and villous tips of the chorioallantoic membranes in pig, sheep and cattle placentas; colored white to brown, wrinkled; called also the necrotic tips.

avascularization diversion of blood from tissues, as by bandaging.

AVDC American Veterinary Dental College.

Avelina-black Iberian cattle black, meat and draft Spanish cattle.

Avena a genus of cereal plants of the grass family Poaceae (Graminae).

A. pubescens OATGRASS may cause ergotism (see rye ERGOT[1]) when infested with *Claviceps purpurea*.

A. sativa cereal oats, a major feed for animals as grain hay or grazing crop. May cause poisoning by NITRITE, a nutritional deficiency of magnesium leading to HYPOMAGNESEMIA, or MYCOTOXICOSIS when the crop is infested with unspecified fungi. See also OAT grain.

average the sum of the values divided by the number of values. Called also arithmetic MEAN.

a. daily gain average daily increase in liveweight of an animal or group of animals. Measured by weighing on two dates and dividing the difference by the number of days between.

moving a. a series of averages over time, based on a constant number of values, by including the next installment of data, and excluding the oldest data. Used to reduce the variability of a series by calculating a new series based on the average of a constant number of values of the original series. Called also rolling average.

avermectins a group of chemically related anthelmintics belonging to the macracytic lactones, and produced by fermenting *Streptomyces avermitilis*. A number of compounds with anthelmintic activity are produced by this process. The combination of two dehydrogenated avermectins is called IVERMECTIN.

aversion avoidance, as when an animal will not enter a room or yards associated with pain or discomfort.

feed a. when a particular feed is rejected, e.g. feed contaminated by fungal toxin.

Aves a class comprising all of the birds. Any vertebrate, in fact any living organism, that has feathers is a bird. All birds have feathers. Besides the diseases that afflict them as birds, they are also of importance as vectors of disease for other species; known ones include erysipelas, salmonellosis, listeriosis, equine encephalomyelitis.

Aveyron disease French ovine leukopenic enterocolitis caused possibly by the BDV virus.

Aviadenovirus one of the two genera in the family ADENOVIRIDAE, the members of which infect avian species. See also ADENOVIRUS.

avian pertaining to or emanating from members of the class Aves. See also BIRD.

a. air sacs see AIR SACS.

a. broodiness the desire to sit on eggs and hatch them is very strong in birds after they have laid a few eggs at the beginning of a new egg laying season. The procedure is a disaster for the commercial egg producer because egg laying ceases. Temporary measures are available to discourage hens from going broody but the long-term practice has been to select against it so that modern egg laying strains of birds do not show broodiness.

a. diseases diseases affecting birds. For individual diseases see under etiological or pathoanatomic keyword, e.g. avian ARIZONOSIS, MYELOBLASTOSIS (2).

a. hepatitis B-like virus see AVIHEPADNAVIRUS.

a. incubation periods quail hatch in 16–18 days, chickens in 21, ducks in 28 days (Muscovies are an exception—33–35 days) and turkeys in 28 days. In some wild species hatching is synchronized by communication between the eggs.

infectious a. nephrosis see infectious avian NEPHROSIS.

a. influenza a highly contagious disease caused by influenza A virus, affecting fowl, turkeys, pheasants and some wild birds, but rarely waterbirds or pigeons. Clinically there is a short course and very heavy mortality; birds that survive have a nasal discharge, white necrotic spots on the comb and wattles, and edema of the head and neck. Called also fowl plague.

a. leukosis see avian LEUKOSIS.

a. lymphoid leukosis see LYMPHOID leukosis.

a. malaria a disease affecting most species of birds and caused by *Plasmodium* spp. (*P. gallinaceum* in fowl, *P. juxtanucleare* in fowl and turkeys, *P. durae* and *P. griffithsi* in turkeys). The disease is characterized by anemia which may be fatal. Transmission is by mosquitoes. See also PLASMODIUM.

a. molt see MOLTING.

a. nesting a strong biological urge to prepare a nest and lay eggs in it occurs in only some domestic birds. The building of a nest is stimulated by the previous laying of an egg.

a. oogenesis the process from the time that the oocyte leaves the ovary until is produced with the typical avian flourish as a finished egg takes 25–26 hours. The yolk is added to the oocyte in the ovary and over a period of 60–70 days before the ovum is released. The oocyte is enveloped with albumen in the albumen-secreting section or magnum of the oviduct. The two shell membranes are added to the egg as it passes through the isthmus of the oviduct. The shell is added during a stay of about 15–20 hours in the shell gland, the last stop before the vagina. See also EGG (4).

a. pox see FOWLPOX.

a. reticuloendotheliosis virus pathogenic avian retroviruses that are antigenically and genetically unrelated to avian leukosis/sarcoma retroviruses.
a. tuberculosis see *Mycobacterium avium* TUBERCULOSIS.
a. type C retroviruses includes avian leukosis viruses and avian sarcoma viruses.
a. vibrionic hepatitis see avian vibrionic HEPATITIS.

avianized said of an infective agent, usually a virus, which has been attenuated by serial passage through hen eggs, e.g. avianized Flury vaccine for rabies, canine distemper and bluetongue vaccines.

aviary an enclosure for the keeping of birds.

avicide agents, e.g. avitrol (4-aminopyridine), used to poison bird pests.

aviculture the rearing of birds, usually caged birds.

avidin a constituent of normal eggs which inhibits the absorption of biotin. The feeding of large quantities of raw egg whites causes dermatitis, alopecia and cracked hooves in pigs and heavy mortality in mink.

avidity in immunology, an imprecise measure of the strength of antibody–antigen binding based on the rate at which the complex is formed.

Avihepadnavirus a genus of viruses in the family *Hepadnaviridae*. They cause a persistent infection which leads to primary hepatocellular carcinoma in Pekin duck. Called also avian hepatitis B-like viruses.

Avioserpens a genus of nematodes of the family Dracunculidae. Includes *A. taiwana*, *A. mosgovoyi* (ducks, other waterfowl).

Avipoxvirus a genus of viruses in the family *Poxviridae*. Includes the viruses of fowlpox, pigeonpox, turkeypox and others; all poxviruses of birds are related.

avirulence lack of virulence; lack of competence of an infectious agent to produce pathological effects.

avitaminosis disease due to deficiency of vitamins in the diet. See also nutritional deficiency under each vitamin.

Avitellina a nonpathogenic tapeworm genus of the family Thysanosomatidae. Includes *A. centripunctata* (sheep, goats).

avitrol poisoning an avicide; leads to disorientation and vocalization in pigeons which may then be molested by normal birds. Chemical needs to be differentiated from Avitrol, a proprietary name for the anthelmintic levamisole hydrochloride and Avitrol plus (levamisole plus praziquantel).

AVMA see AMERICAN VETERINARY MEDICAL ASSOCIATION.

avocado PERSEA AMERICANA.

Avogadro named after Amedeo Avogadro, an Italian physicist 1776–1856.
A's law equal volumes of perfect gases at the same temperature and pressure contain the same number of molecules.
A's number, A's constant the number of particles of the type specified by the chemical formula of a certain substance in 1 gram-molecule of the substance.

avoidance a conscious or unconscious defensive reaction intended to escape anxiety, conflict, danger, fear or pain.

avoir. avoirdupois.

avoirdupois a system of weight used in English-speaking countries for all commodities except drugs, precious stones and precious metals. See also Table 4.1. Now largely superseded by the metric system.

avoparcin a glycopeptide antibiotic, produced by *Streptomyces candidus*, used as a feed additive.

AVP arginine vasopressin.

AVT avian arginine vasotocin. See VASOTOCIN.

avulsion the tearing away of a structure or part.
brachial plexus a. a common injury in dogs and less often cats, usually resulting from trauma that causes extreme abduction of the forelimb and avulsion of some or all nerve roots from C6 to T1. Depending on the extent of injury, the leg may be completely paralyzed with extensive loss of sensation, or if less severe may be carried with only signs of a radial paralysis.
labial a. stripping of the lip from its underlying attachments. Lower lip avulsion from the mandible is particularly common in cats. Called also stripped chin.
phrenic a. extraction of a portion of the phrenic nerve, producing one-sided paralysis of the diaphragm and partial collapse of the corresponding lung.

Awassi Near East fat-tailed type of sheep, used for milk, mutton and carpetwool. Mostly white, with brown head and legs. Sometimes black, white, gray or spotted face; males are horned, females polled. Used extensively in the Middle East.

awn a long, sharp spine projecting from the coverings about a seed. They assist the seedhead in penetration of the skin and then migration through very large distances into all tissues, including even the canine intervertebral disk. They are common subcutaneous foreign bodies in sheep, where they appear to do no harm, and dogs where they commonly cause abscesses and some chronic, discharging fistulae. They are particularly troublesome in the nasal cavity, ears and eyes of dogs.

axenic [Gr.] *xenos* (stranger); totally free of infection with microorganisms. Axenic mammals are usually produced in the first generation following cesarean section under absolutely sterile conditions and the young are delivered into plastic, sterile isolators where they remain under germ-free conditions; axenic avian species are produced by placing fertile eggs into plastic isolators after carefully sterilizing the egg shell. Called also germ-free animal. See also GNOTOBIOTIC and SPECIFIC PATHOGEN FREE.

axes [L., Gr.] plural of *axis*. The straight lines which intersect at right angles and on which graphs are drawn. Usually the horizontal axis is the x-axis and the vertical one the y-axis. Called also axes of reference.
a. of reference see axes (above).

axial 1. pertaining to or deriving from an axis. 2. pertaining to or deriving from the axis bone of the vertebral column. See also AXIS.
a. skeleton the skeleton of the head and trunk.

axilla pl. *axillae* [L.] the armpit.

axillary of or pertaining to the armpit.
a. lymph node buried deeply between the shoulder muscles and the chest wall; palpable in the living animal only when significantly enlarged and hard.
a. nerve see Table 14.
a. nerve lesion characterized by atrophy of the deltoid muscle.
a. nodular necrosis small, round, hard nodules at the girth or near the axilla in horses.

axio- word element. [L., Gr.] denoting relation to an axis; in dentistry, used in special reference to the long axis of a tooth.

Axis genus of deer in family Cervidae.
A. axis see AXIS DEER.
A. porcinus see HOG DEER.

axis pl. *axes* [L., Gr.] 1. a line through a center of a body, or about which a structure revolves. 2. the second cervical vertebra.

celiac a. celiac trunk.
a. cylinder axon.
dorsoventral a. one passing from the back to the belly surface of the body.
electrical a. of heart the resultant of the electromotive forces within the heart at any instant. See also MEAN electrical axis.
external bulbar a. the optical axis that connects the anterior and posterior poles of the eyeball. Called also optic axis.
frontal a. an imaginary line running from right to left through the center of the eyeball.
a. of heart. a line passing through the center of the base of the heart and the apex.
optic a. see external bulbar axis (above).
orbital a. a line passing through the apex of the bony orbit and the center of the opening of the orbit.
sagittal a. an imaginary line extending through the anterior and posterior poles of the eye.
visual a. an imaginary line passing from the midpoint of the visual field to the fovea centralis.

axis deer a native of India and Sri Lanka; has three-tined antlers. Called also *Axis axis*, chital.

axoaxonic referring to a synapse between the axon of one neuron and the axon of another.

axodentritic referring to a synapse between the axon of one neuron and dentrites of another.

axolemma the surface membrane of an axon.

axolotl see AMBYSTOMA.

axolysis degeneration of an axon.

axon the process of a nerve cell along which impulses travel away from the cell body. It branches at its termination, forming synapses at other nerve cells or effector organs. Many axons are covered by a myelin sheath formed from the cell membrane of a glial or Schwann cell.
a. hillock the elevation on the perikaryon from which the axon emerges.
a. reflex a nerve impulse conducted through nerve pathways limited to the single axon, without the participation of a nerve cell or synapse. Not a true reflex.
a. telodendrion extensive terminal branches of the axon before terminating on the effector organ.
a. terminals the axonal structure capable of forming a synapse with another axon.

axonal pertaining to or arising from an axon.
a. degeneration an axon dies and cannot be replaced if its cell body is destroyed. A damaged axon in the central nervous system similarly cannot undergo regeneration, but a peripheral nerve with an intact nerve cell can regenerate. See also WALLERIAN DEGENERATION.
a. dystrophy specific diseases characterized by nutritional abnormalities of axons include in **sheep**, Suffolk, Coopworth, Merino axonal dystrophies, in **dogs**, Rottweiler, Chiahuahua dystrophies, in **horses** Haflinger, Morgan, in **cats** a dystrophy in lilac coat color domestic shorthaired.
giant a. neuropathy see giant axonal NEUROPATHY.
a. migration the movement of axoplasm from the proximal segment of a severed nerve fiber to the distal portion, following Schwann cell extensions, in the process of peripheral nerve regeneration.
a. reaction central chromatolysis of the axon characterized by eccentric relocation of the nucleus, greater prominence of the nucleolus and a basophilic cap of RNA on its cytoplasmic aspect, dispersal of the Nissl substance to the periphery of the cell, and an increase in the number of neurofilaments.

axonapraxia see NEURAPRAXIA.

axoneme 1. the central core of a cilium or flagellum, consisting of two central microtubules surrounded by nine peripheral microtubule pairs. 2. the gene-string or filament forming the basis of a chromosome.

axonic zone the all-or-none conducting zone of the three functionally significant zones of the neuron; includes axis cylinder and part of the arborizing axonal terminal.

axonopathy a disease of axons.
Boxer progressive a. an inherited, degenerative disorder of the peripheral and central nervous system in Boxer dogs. By 6 months of age, dogs homozygous for the trait show ataxia and weakness in the hindlimbs and an absence of the patellar reflex.
congenital a. Holstein–Friesian calves are recumbent from birth; the necropsy lesion is degeneration in spinal cord and midbrain nerve tracts; considered to be inherited as an autosomal recessive trait.
inherited ovine degenerative a. inherited in several forms in some sheep breeds (Suffolk, Merino, Coopworth); may be congenital or develop at up to 6 months old; signs include ataxia, recumbency, invariable death. Probably the same disease as that called Murrurrundi disease.
peripheral and central distal a. of Birman cats see distal POLYNEUROPATHY of Birman cats.
segmental a. axonopathy affecting a segment of the axons.

axonotmesis nerve injury characterized by disruption of the axon and myelin sheath but with preservation of the connective tissue fragments, resulting in degeneration of the axon distal to the injury site; regeneration of the axon is spontaneous and of good quality.

axoplasm the cytoplasm of an axon; called also hyaloplasm.

axoplasmic pertaining to or emanating from axoplasm.
a. flow the flow of proteins, hormones, enzymes and neurotransmitters along nerve fibers.
a. transport the mechanism by which viruses make their way along the axons.

axosomatic referring to a synapse between the axon of one neuron and the cell body of another.

aye-aye a lemur-like monkey. Called also *Daubentonia madagascariensis*.

Aylesbury an English meat duck, with white plumage and bright yellow legs.

Ayre's T-piece see T-piece CIRCUIT.

Ayrshire a hardy breed of Scottish dairy cattle with a white haircoat splashed with large patches of bay (red-brown) to brown coloring, and long, upward pointing (lyre) horns. Their temperament is inclined to be irascible. Known to carry an inherited predisposition to congenital LYMPHATIC vessel obstruction.

Azadirachta indica toxic Indian plant, known for its insecticidal properties, in the family Meliaceae; an unidentified toxin causes stomatitis, diarrhea, nephrosis; called also neem.

azalea see RHODODENDRON *indica*.
A. indica RHODODENDRON *indica*.
A. occidentale RHODODENDRON *occidentale*.

azaperone a butyrophenone tranquilizer widely used as a tranquilizer or as a premedication for pigs.

azathioprine a mercaptopurine derivative used as a cytotoxic and immunosuppressive agent in the treatment of leukemia and autoimmune diseases and in transplantation therapy.

azeotrope a mixture of two substances that has a constant boiling point and cannot be separated by fractional distillation.

2-azetidinecarboxylic acid toxin found in CONVALLARIA MAJALIS—lily-of-the-valley.

azide inhibitor of cytochrome *c* oxidase (or complex IV) of the respiratory electron-transfer chain.

azidothymidine a thymidine analog with antiviral activity used in the treatment of AIDS in humans and feline leukemia virus infection in cats. Called also AZT, zidovudine.

azinphos-methyl an organophosphorus, nonsystemic insecticide and acaricide. Poisoning with the compound causes typical signs for organophosphates.

azithromycin a macrolide antibiotic used in the treatment of toxoplasmosis.

azlocillin a ureidopenicillin with a broad spectrum of activity, but inactivated by β-lactamase.

azo dyes a group of synthetic dyes with weak antimicrobial properties. Examples are phenazopyridine and scarlet red.

azocarmine a red basic dye.

azole antifungals imidazoles and triazoles which are broad-spectrum antifungal agents and are active against gram-positive bacteria. Includes miconazole, ketoconazole, itraconazole, fluconazole and enilconazole.

azoospermia absence of spermatozoa in the semen, or failure of formation of spermatozoa.

azot- prefix meaning nitrogen.

azote nitrogen.

azotemia the presence of nitrogen-containing compounds in the blood. See also UREMIA.

postrenal a. is caused by reduced renal blood flow caused by increased pressure within the renal collecting system, e.g. hydronephrosis and urine retention from a variety of causes.

prerenal a. is due to extrarenal causes that reduce renal blood flow and glomerular filtration, e.g. dehydration, shock, reduced cardiac output, decreased plasma albumin osmotic pressure.

primary renal a. results from loss of renal functional parenchyma.

azotemic pertaining to or emanating from azotemia.

a. pseudodiabetes the glucose intolerance that occurs with primary renal failure, probably due to peripheral resistance to glucose utilization.

azotenesis any disease due to excess nitrogen in system.

azotorrhea discharge of excessive quantities of nitrogenous matter in the stools.

azoturia excess of urea in the urine (specifically in horses, see PARALYTIC myoglobinuria). Called also sacral paralysis, black water.

azoturia-like syndrome a syndrome similar to that in horses recorded in draft oxen and Greyhounds. See also capture MYOPATHY.

azovan blue see EVANS BLUE.

AZT azidothymidine.

aztreonam a monobactam, β-lactam antibiotic, very resistant to β-lactamase, but with a narrow range of activity. It is used parenterally against infections with gram-negative organisms, particularly *Pseudomonas aeruginosa*.

azure one of three metachromatic basic dyes (azures A, B and C).

azuresin a complex combination of azure A dye and carbacrylic cation-exchange resin used as a diagnostic aid in detection of gastric secretion.

azurophil a tissue constituent staining with azure or a similar metachromatic thiazine dye.

azurophilia a condition in which the blood contains cells having azurophilic granules.

azurophilic staining with azure or similar metachromatic thiazine dyes; pertaining to azurophilia.

a. granules the large, homogeneous, dense, peroxidase-positive granules of progranulocytes and early myelocytes that stain blue with Romanowsky stains because of their acid mucopolysaccharide content. Called also primary granules.

azygogram the film obtained by azygography.

azygography radiography of the azygous venous system.

azygos 1. any unpaired part, as the azygos vein. 2. unpaired. Called also azygous.

a. vein a vein beginning in the abdomen and coursing in the dorsal mediastinum which returns blood from the thorax to the heart. The right azygos is found in most domestic animals (rarely the pig) while the left azygos is found in pigs and ruminants.

azygous see AZYGOS.

azymic not giving rise to fermentation.

B

B chemical symbol, *boron*; Baumé scale; boils at; buccal.

B blood group system the major histocompatibility complex first identified in chicken red cells; responsible for most of the variation in graft survival time in that species.

B cell see B LYMPHOCYTE.

B fibers preganglionic, autonomic efferent nerve fibers with much slower conduction speeds than A cells.

β-galactosidase see GALACTOCEREBROSIDASE.

B immunoplasts cells which gain access to Peyer's patches, and establish populations of B lymphocytes, via permeable, postcapillary venules.

B lymphocyte see B LYMPHOCYTE.

B-mode brightness mode. See B-mode ULTRASONOGRAPHY.

B-virus a herpesvirus of monkeys that shares a common antigen with the pseudorabies and herpes simplex viruses. The infection is common in Old World monkeys especially in rhesus, cynomolgus and vervet monkeys. Clinical signs in the monkeys include fever blisters on the lips, and ulcerative and papillary lesions on the anterior dorsum of the tongue. The infection is transmissible to humans causing a highly fatal ascending encephalitis.

Ba chemical symbol, *barium*.

Baastrup's disease a bony proliferation between the dorsal spinous processes in the lumbar spine of humans. A similar condition has been noted radiographically in dogs, particularly large breeds and especially in Boxers. The clinical significance is unknown.

Babcock forceps forceps with loop blades which are also semicircular in sagittal cross-section. Designed to hold a short length of intestine without compressing it.

Babcock's test a test for determination of the fat content of milk. Based on the centrifugation of a heated sample of milk which has been treated with strong acid to carbonize the milk protein.

Babès–Ernst granules metachromatic granules, characteristic of corynebacteria.

Babès' nodules very small glial nodules found in the brain of animals, especially ruminants, which have died of rabies.

Babesia a genus of large, round to pyriform protozoa, of the family Babesiidae. Includes piroplasms. These protozoa pass part of their life cycle in erythrocytes. Transmission between animals is by ticks.

B. bigemina causes BABESIOSIS of cattle and some wild ruminants.

B. bovis causes BABESIOSIS of cattle and some wild ruminants. Includes *B. argentina, B. berberi, B. colchica.*

B. caballi causes a mild form of BABESIOSIS in horses.

B. canis causes BABESIOSIS in dogs.

B. cati found in cats.

B. colchica see *B. bovis* (above).

B. divergens causes a mild form of BABESIOSIS of cattle and some wild ruminants.

B. equi causes BABESIOSIS in horses.

B. felis causes BABESIOSIS of cats.

B. gibsoni causes BABESIOSIS in dogs.

B. herpaiuri found in cats.

B. hylomysci found in red deer.

B. major causes a mild form of BABESIOSIS of cattle.

B. motasi causes acute BABESIOSIS in sheep and goats.

B. ovis causes a mild form of BABESIOSIS in sheep and goats.

B. pantherae found in cats, leopard.

B. rodhaini found in red deer.

B. vogeli found in dogs.

babesiasis see BABESIOSIS.

babesicide destructive to babesia.

babesiosis a group of diseases caused by the protozoan *Babesia* spp. and transmitted by blood-sucking ticks. Clinically they are all characterized by fever and intravascular hemolysis manifested by a syndrome of anemia, hemoglobinuria and jaundice. Called also tick fever, Texas fever, redwater fever.

Babinski reflex a reflex action of the toes, indicative of abnormalities in the motor control pathways leading from the cerebral cortex. It is elicited in dogs and cats by an upward stroking of the metacarpal or metatarsal bones. A normal reaction is slight flexion of the toes. In a positive sign, the toes extend; seen with upper motor neuron lesions. Called also Babinski sign.

baboon Old World monkeys mostly in the family Cercopithecidae. They are big, with a strong facial resemblance to dogs. They are omnivorous, terrestrial, walk on all fours, and show a great variety of coloring in their distinctive ischial callosities and anogenital skin. Called also *Papio.*

baby pig disease see NEONATAL hypoglycemia.

Babyrousa babyrussa, Babirussa babyrussa a species of the family Suidae of the order Artiodactyla. A nonruminant pig-like animal.

bacampicillin an ester of ampicillin that in vivo becomes ampicillin and has the actions and uses of the parent drug.

Baccharis a genus of plants from the Americas in the Asteraceae (Compositae) family. Sesquiterpenes have been identified in some species, but the toxin originates from *Myrothecium* spp., fungi associated with the roots. Signs include stiffness, trembling, convulsions; lesions include rumenitis, enteritis. Toxic species include *B. cordifolia, B. dranunculifolia, glomeruliflora, B. halimifolia, B. megapotamica, B. pteronioides, B. ramulosa.*

bacillary pertaining to bacilli or to rodlike structures.

b. hemoglobinuria an acute, highly fatal toxemia of cattle and sheep caused by *Clostridium haemolyticum* (*Cl. novyi* type D). It is characterized by fever, hemoglobinuria and jaundice, and at postmortem examination by the presence of necrotic infarcts in the liver.

b. layer layer of rods and cones in the retina.

b. necrosis see NECROBACILLOSIS.

b. pyelonephritis see CONTAGIOUS bovine pyelonephritis.

b. typhlitis see TYZZER'S DISEASE.

b. white diarrhea see PULLORUM DISEASE.

bacille Calmette–Guérin see BCG.

bacillemia the presence of bacilli in the blood.

bacilli see BACILLUS.

bacilliform having the appearance of a bacillus.

bacillin an antibiotic substance isolated from strains of *Bacillus subtilis,* highly active on both gram-positive and gram-negative bacteria.

bacillosis infection with bacilli.

bacilluria bacilli in the urine.

Bacillus a genus of bacteria that are gram-positive, aerobic, spore-forming rods. With the exception of *B. anthracis* and the occasional wound contamination and bovine mastitis caused by *B. cereus,* the organisms are largely saprophytic and do not cause disease. However, they may invade devitalized tissue. They do have importance in the area of food preservation.

B. actinoides STREPTOBACILLUS *moniliformis.*

B. aneurinolyticus, B. thiaminolyticus are thiaminase-producing bacteria which may proliferate in the rumen and contribute to the cerebral lesions in carbohydrate engorgement and polioencephalomalacia in cattle.

B. anthracis characterized by its capacity to form spores when exposed to the air and to survive for long periods in soil and other inert materials. Has a characteristic appearance with McFadyean's stain. Causes ANTHRAX in all species.

B. brevis the source of TYROTHRICIN.

B. cereus a species causing food poisoning, occasional cases of septicemia and bovine mastitis and abortion.

B. circulans, B. coagulans, B. stearothermophilus very heat-resistant bacteria which cause fermentation of cereals in canned meat foods. They cause souring but no gas production so that the can does not bulge. Called also flat sour. *B. stearothermophilus* spores are used to test efficacy of autoclaves.

B. larvae the cause of American foulbrood in honeybees.

B. licheniformis reported as a cause of abortion in cattle, sheep and pigs, and also isolated from suppurative lesions of horses and cattle.

B. piliformis the previous name of CLOSTRIDIUM *piliforme,* the cause of TYZZER'S DISEASE.

B. polymyxa (B. aerosporus) strains of this organism are the source of the antibiotic POLYMYXIN.

B. subtilis a common saprophytic soil and water form, often occurring as a laboratory contaminant, and rarely, in apparently causal relation to pathological processes, such as conjunctivitis.

bacillus pl. *bacilli* [L.] 1. an organism of the genus *Bacillus.* 2. any rod-shaped bacterium.

Battey b. MYCOBACTERIUM *intracellulare.*

Calmette–Guérin b. MYCOBACTERIUM *bovis,* rendered completely avirulent by cultivation over a long period on bile–glycerol–potato medium. See also BCG vaccine.

Friedländer's b. KLEBSIELLA *pneumoniae.*

glanders b. BURKHOLDERIA *mallei* (previously *Pseudomonas mallei*).

Hansen's b. MYCOBACTERIUM *leprae.*

tubercle b. MYCOBACTERIUM *tuberculosis.*

typhoid b. SALMONELLA *typhi.*

bacitracin an antibacterial substance elaborated by the licheniformis group of *Bacillus subtilis*, found in a contaminated wound, and named after the patient, Margaret Tracy; useful in a wide range of infections and usually applied topically.

back see also DORSUM.

b. arched upwards humped back posture as in subacute abdominal pain.

cold b. horse resents the saddle being placed in position and the girth tightened. May be due to pain in back or to disinclination to wear the saddle.

hollow b. the natural concave line of the backbone is exaggerated.

b. muscle necrosis is characterized by pain and swelling over the backs of pigs. The pigs are reluctant to move and there is arching or lateral flexion of the spine. Subsequently there is atrophy of the muscles. See also PORCINE stress syndrome.

b. pain pain expressed when pressure is applied to the back. Spondylosis, injury to dorsal spinous processes and muscle sprain are amongst the common causes. A special area of interest in the horse, because of its importance in restricting movement and causing abnormalities of gait.

b. raking manual removal of the feces from the rectum. Performed often in the preliminaries to pregnancy diagnosis in mares and cows. Carried out cosmetically in horses and especially elephants just before a circus or other performing act.

b. *Shu* points acupuncturese for association points along the back.

back bleeding a slaughtering error in which the pleural sac is punctured during bleeding-out. Blood is aspirated into the sac causing staining. Called also over-sticking.

back-cross a mating between a heterozygote and a homozygote.

double b.-c. the mating between a double heterozygote and a homozygote.

back-fence the fence used to prevent cattle grazing back over already eaten out pasture which is being strip-grazed. As the front fence is moved forwards the back-fence is also moved up.

back-swept said of horns which sweep out, usually horizontally, from the patient's head and point backwards towards the tail.

backband an essential part of most horse harnesses. A strap that goes over the back, sometimes through a backpad, and supports the shafts or the traces.

backbone the vertebral column.

backcross mating the crossbred offspring of a two-way cross back to one of the parent breeds.

backfat a segment of the well-developed panniculus adiposus along the back of the pig; at this location the fat is especially well-formed and firm. The thickness of the layer is used as an index of the fatness of the entire carcass.

b. probe a sharp instrument used to measure backfat thickness without incising the carcass. Electronic probes are available for use in the live pig.

backflow abnormal backward flow of fluids; regurgitation. See also REFLUX.

pyelovenous b. drainage from the renal pelvis into the venous system occurring under certain conditions of back pressure.

background radiation the inescapable radiation received by the entire population due mostly to cosmic radiation, but also due to naturally occurring radioactive materials in the terrestrial environment and to internal isotopes.

background rate the rate, often low, at which some event or agent occurs, at a particular time or in a particular place, in the absence of a specific hazard.

backgrounding the practice of putting yearling cattle onto high energy but nonfattening rations in a special backgrounding feedlot before they go into the terminal fattening lot and are fed the finishing ration.

Backhaus towel clamp a clamp used for fixing drapes to the skin of anesthetized patients. A scissor action with ratchet fixation at the finger loops and sharp, incurving, needle-like blades.

backline the upper outline of the body's silhouette viewed from the side.

backs wool taken from the back section of a fleece of wool.

backscatter in radiology, radiation deflected by scattering processes at angles greater than 90 degrees to the original direction of the beam of radiation. Important in radiotherapy when estimating surface exposure dose.

backstrap see BACKBAND.

backtag a tag of special tough paper, bearing identification codes relating to origin of animals, which are stuck to the back of animals with a very strong glue. Designed for easy reading in saleyards, short life and to help with traceback during investigation of the origin of disease outbreaks. See also TAIL tag.

backtrace see TRACEBACK.

backup the act of saving computer files to ensure that a copy survives a major problem in the computer. Achieved by periodic copying of data in one computer to another unit of the same medium or to a different medium so that the data may be recovered in the event of its loss.

backward tone see OPISTHOTONOS.

baclofen an analog of gamma-aminobutyric acid (GABA) used as a muscle relaxant.

bacon curing preserving of pig meat by dry pickling with salt and saltpetre or by immersion in a brine tank, followed by a period of maturation in a cool place to allow an even distribution of the pickle. Injection of pickling brine into large muscle masses is much used to hasten the curing process.

bacon weight the desirable weight for a pig that is to be used for bacon production—200–220 lb liveweight.

bacteraemia see BACTEREMIA.

bacteremia the temporary presence of bacteria in the blood. The condition is not manifested by any clinical signs but is commonly followed by the development of embolic infections such as arthritis, meningitis, endocarditis, and liver and lung abscesses.

bacteria plural of BACTERIUM.

anaerobic b. derive energy from fermentative processes in the absence of oxygen. Are found in necrotic or abscessed tissues.

cell-wall deficient b. see L-form bacteria (below).

facultatively anaerobic b. are able to derive energy from aerobic or anaerobic metabolism. Includes most intestinal pathogens.

glucose-non-fermenting, gram-negative b. includes *Bordetella*, *Moraxella* and *Pseudomonas* species.

L-form b. abnormal growth forms that can replicate in the form of small filterable elements with defective or absent cell walls. Spontaneously formed by some bacteria, e.g. *Streptococcus* spp., *Bacterioides* spp., and by others when synthesis is impaired. L-forms have been associated with infections in dogs and cats.

marker b. those added to provide a means of identifying the bacteria being studied. See SERRATIA *rubidaea*.

obligate aerobic b. require oxygen as a source of energy and therefore for growth.
putrefactive b. see DECOMPOSITION.
resistant b. see ANTIMICROBIAL resistance.
ruminal b. the ruminal fluid of the normal cow contains 10 to 50 million million organisms per gram. Bacteria outnumber the protozoan population many times over. The genera and species of bacteria present vary between times in the same cow. The function of the ruminal bacteria is to digest the food taken in and thus allow its absorption. This includes the lysis of cellulose, xylanol, starch, dextrin, pectin, protein, lipids, the utilization of glycerol and lactate, and the fermentation of soluble sugars. The end products of the digestive process include methane, formate, acetate, ethanol, propionate, lactate, butyrate, succinate, valerate, caproate, hydrogen and carbon dioxide.
spoilage b. see DECOMPOSITION.

bacterial pertaining to or caused by bacteria.
b. adhesiveness see ADHESINS.
b. allergy see bacterial HYPERSENSITIVITY.
cutaneous b. granuloma see BOTRYOMYCOSIS.
b. diseases diseases in which bacteria play a significant but not necessarily exclusive role.
b. fermentation fermentation is more commonly a function of yeasts but is performed by some bacteria, e.g. those in the rumen. See also FERMENTATION.
b. food poisoning see FOOD poisoning.
b. gill disease see GILL disease.
b. kidney disease of fish a serious disease of salmonid cultures characterized by granuloma in the kidney and spleen, and extensive caseation of muscles. The disease is chronic and causes heavy losses. The cause appears to be a minute gram-positive coccobacillus *Renibacterium salmoninarum*.
b. overgrowth a syndrome of malabsorption causing chronic or recurrent diarrhea in dogs. Believed to be due to the presence in the small intestine of an abnormally large population of *Clostridium* spp. and other enteric bacteria normally found in the colon.

bactericidal destructive to bacteria.

bactericide an agent that destroys bacteria.

bacterid a skin eruption due to bacterial infection elsewhere in the body.

bacterin vaccine consisting of killed bacteria.
oral b. prepared from killed cultures of *Aeromonas* spp. has been used successfully in fish in which individual parenteral prophylaxis is prohibitively expensive.

bacter(io)- word element. [Gr.] *bacteria*.

bacteriocidin a bactericidal antibody.

bacteriocin a peptide produced by some strains of bacteria which inhibits the growth of, or kills, other bacteria. Examples are staphylococcin, produced by *Staphylococcus aureus*, and colicins, produced by *Escherichia coli*.

bacteriologist an expert in the study of bacteria and the diseases they cause.

bacteriology the scientific study of bacteria and the diseases they cause.

bacteriolysin an antibody that lyses bacterial cells.

bacteriolysis destruction or dissolution of bacteria.

bacteriophage or simply phage; a virus that infects bacteria often killing them by lysis; many varieties exist, and usually each attacks only one kind of bacteria. Some bacteriophage are widely used as cloning vectors and for determining DNA sequence. Virulent DNA bacteriophages in the T series adsorb to specific receptor sites on the bacterial cell wall and inject their DNA content into the bacterium. The viral DNA usurps the machinery of the cell for the replication of viral DNA and protein which is assembled into a crop of progeny phage which are released by lysis from the cell. Called also bacterial virus.
M13 b. small rod-shaped, nonlytic, single-stranded DNA phage; used as a template in the Sangar dideoxy method for DNA sequence determination.
ΦX174 b. prototype of a class of phage that are small, icosahedral single-stranded DNA viruses that code for only 10 to 12 proteins and are highly dependent on the host cell for their replicaiton.
RNA b. the genome is RNA instead of DNA; smallest known viruses, encode for only four proteins; they have contributed to basic studies of RNA.
temperate b's typified by λ phage; have a similar lytic life cycle but in addition have an alternate life cycle whereby the injected DNA becomes integrated into the cell DNA where it remains stable, behaving as a cell gene. The integrated DNA is called prophage and the bacterial cell is said to be lysogenic. The phage DNA may be induced whereby it becomes disassociated from the cell DNA and enters the lytic life cycle. Temperate phage may transfer bacterial cell DNA from one cell to another to produce a recombinant.

bacteriopsonin an opsonin that acts on bacteria.

bacteriosis a bacterial disease.

bacteriospermia the presence of bacteria in the semen.

bacteriostasis a state in which the growth or multiplication of bacteria is inhibited without the bacteria being killed.

bacteriostat an agent capable of inhibiting the growth of bacteria.

bacteriostatic arresting the growth or multiplication of bacteria; also, an agent that so acts.

bacterium pl. *bacteria* [L.] any prokaryotic microorganism. Bacteria are single-celled microorganisms that differ from all other organisms (the eukaryotes) in lacking a true nucleus and organelles such as mitochondria, chloroplasts and lysosomes. Their genetic material consists of a single double-stranded DNA molecule, whereas the genetic material of eukaryotes consists of multiple chromosomes, which are complex structures of DNA and protein.

Bacteria reproduce by binary fission and generally have a very high rate of population growth and mutation. Genetic material can be transferred between bacteria by three processes: *transformation* (absorption of naked DNA), *transduction* (transfer by a temperate bacteriophage), and *conjugation* (transfer by independently replicating DNA molecules, called *plasmids*). Some bacteria can also form *spores*, dehydrated forms that are relatively resistant to heat, cold, lack of water, toxic chemicals and radiation.

Most bacteria have a rigid cell wall outside of the cell membrane primarily composed of a dense layer of peptidoglycan, a network of polysaccharide chains with polypeptide cross-links. Some antimicrobial agents, the penicillins and cephalosporins, act by interfering with peptidoglycan synthesis.

Bacteria can have any of three types of external structures: *flagella*, which are rotating locomotor organelles; *pili* or fimbriae, which are minute filamentous appendages; and a *capsule*, which is a layer of gelatinous material around the cell. Large pili called sex pili are involved in conjugation while other pili are involved in adherence of bacteria to mucosal surfaces. The capsule is associated with virulent strains of bacteria and protects the bacterium from phagocytosis. See also BACTERIA.

acid-fast b. one that, because of wax-like composition of the cell wall, is not readily decolorized by acids after staining, especially *Mycobacterium* spp.
coliform b. particularly found in the gut (colon) of animals. See AEROBACTER AEROGENES, ESCHERICHIA and PARACOLOBACTRUM.
hemophilic b. microorganisms of the genera *Haemophilus* and *Bordetella*, which have a nutritional requirement for fresh blood or whose growth is significantly stimulated on blood-containing media.
lactic acid b. bacteria that, in suitable media, ferment carbohydrates to form lactic acid.
lysogenic b. any bacterial cell harboring in its genome the genetic material (prophage) of a temperate BACTERIOPHAGE and thus reproducing the bacteriophage DNA in each cell division; occasionally the prophage becomes nonintegrated (induced), replicates, lyses the bacterial cell, and is free to infect other cells.

Bacterium viscosum-equi see ACTINOBACILLUS *equuli*.

bacteriuria bacteria in the urine.

bacteroid 1. resembling a bacterium. 2. a structurally modified bacterium.

Bacteroidaceae the family of obligately anaerobic, gram-negative, rod-shaped bacteria containing 13 genera, including *Fusobacterium*, *Bacteroides* and *Leptotrichia*.

Bacteroides a genus of the family Bacteroidaceae, a family of gram-negative, non-spore-forming, obligate anaerobes. Common inhabitants of the alimentary tract and necrotic tissue, probably as secondary invaders.
B. amylophilus, B. ruminicola, B. succinogenes the predominant gram-negative bacteria in ruminal contents.
B. asaccharolyticus associated with gingivitis and osteomyelitis.
B. fragilis occasionally infects foals, pigs, lambs and calves, causing diarrhea, mastitis and abscesses.
B. gingivalis associated with dental plaque and periodontal disease in sheep.
B. heparinolyticus associated with oral disease in horses and cats.
B. levii associated with summer mastitis in cattle.
B. melaninogenicus a common finding in FOOTROT of cattle, bite wounds of dogs and cats, and pleurisy and peritonitis in dogs, cats and cattle.
B. nodosus see DICHELOBACTER NODOSUS.
B. salivosus causes subcutaneous abscesses in cats.
B. ureolyticus gram-negative, microaerophilic bacterial species isolated from the genital tract of mares with endometritis.

bacteroides 1. any highly pleomorphic rod-shaped bacteria. 2. an organism of the genus *Bacteroides*.

bacteruria see BACTERIURIA.

baculoviral midgut gland necrosis virus baculovirus causing heavy mortalities in larval and post-larval *Penaeus japonicus* and *P. monodon* prawns.

baculovirus group of rod-shaped, double-stranded, DNA viruses which infect and kill a large number of different invertebrate species especially insects, including Lepidoptera, Hymenoptera, Diptera, Neuroplera, Trichoptera, Coleoptera and Homoptera, and also prawns; used as biocontrol agents, sometimes following genetic engineering of the virus.

Baculovirus pennaei a virus which causes infection with high mortality in larval, postlarval and juvenile prawns, especially *Penaeus vannamei* and other American species of prawns.

bad debt a professional fee that is owed but is not recoverable by the normal procedure of submitting three accounts at one month intervals and rendered from the veterinarian's office. A bad debt must be written off as a loss or placed in the hands of a professional debt collector or a solicitor to collect. If bad debts exceed 2% of the gross income the management of the practice should be investigated.

badger 1. a coat color in dogs that consists of a mixture of white, gray, brown and black. May occur in patches. Seen in a variety of hound breeds and the Great Pyrenees dog. 2. a burrowing carnivore in the family Mustelidae.
American b. *Taxidea taxus*; found in western North America. Called also taxel.
b. dog literal translation of dachshund.
Eurasian b. MELES *meles*.
ferret b. MELOGALE MOSCHATA.
hog b. *Arctonyx collaris*; found in Southeast Asia; called also hog-nosed badger, sand badger.
hog-nosed b. see hog badger (above).
Japanese b. MELES *anakuma*.
sand b. see hog badger (above).

BAER brainstem auditory evoked response.

Baermann technique a laboratory method for separating parasite larvae from feces, soil or herbage for counting or identification.

baffle boards large pieces of rigid material, usually plywood, carried vertically by an attendant between him/her and a large pig or other uncontrollable animal. They are used to shepherd the animal from place to place without the use of force. A useful device in zoos, but no protection against an aggressive animal.

bag a sac or pouch.
b.-in-a-bottle a basic form of ventilator used in gaseous anesthesia in which an expandable bag is enclosed in a bottle. Injection or extraction of air in the bottle causes expansion and contraction of the bag and controls ventilation.
Douglas b. a receptacle for the collection of expired air, permitting measurement of respiratory gases.
fecal b. strapped to an animal in such a way as to catch the fecal output. Used in experimental work or clinical investigation in ambulatory animals especially sheep.
sterilizing b. any of several types of paper or plastic bags used to package individual instruments in the autoclaving process.
urine b. a bag strapped to the animal, usually an ambulatory sheep, in such a way as to collect the total urinary output.
b. of waters the membranes enclosing the AMNIOTIC fluid and the developing fetus in utero.

bagasse the fibrous residue of sugar cane after the extraction of the sugar juice. Used as a fibrous diluent for heavy grain and molasses diets.

bagassosis a hypersensitivity pneumonitis of humans caused by inhalation of thermophilic actinomycetes in moldy bagasse.

bagging nostrils enclosing muzzle in a plastic bag to promote deep breathing in a patient for better auscultation result over lung fields.

bagging up a term which refers to an increase in the size of the udder due to physiological causes. Said of a cow coming close to parturition. It is also not unusual to stop milking a cow for 24 hours before sale or show in order to give the cow a better appearance.

Baghdad boil leishmaniasis.

bagpod SESBANIA *vesicaria*.

Bahia grass PASPALUM *notatum*.
Bahia oppositifolia a North American plant in the family Asteraceae; contains cyanogenetic glycosides and can cause poisoning.
Bailey rib contractor two inward-facing, curved, clawed hands mounted on a ratcheted bar designed for bringing ribs closer together during thoracic surgery.
Baileya multiradiata flowers and fruit of this plant cause nephrosis and hepatitis when eaten.
Bain system see Bain coaxial CIRCUIT.
Bainbridge clamp an instrument similar to intestinal forceps. Used to clamp large blood vessels.
Bainbridge forceps standard intestinal forceps.
Bainbridge reflex a reflex of uncertain validity that states that the intravenous injection of fluid or blood, or the experimental dilatation of the right atrium, causes tachycardia. An alternative statement says that these manipulations cause bradycardia. Called also McDowall reflex.
bait a preparation containing a palatable food substance such as raw meat, carrot or bran and a pharmaceutical or poisonous substance. The purpose is to introduce the medicament or poison into the unsuspecting animal.
baiting the laying of a BAIT. May be done for purposes of medication or control, or for malicious reasons. In urban areas baiting is controlled by law which forbids baiting except, in some countries, on one's own property. Most of the poisonous substances used are controlled by legislation so that the identity of the baiter is recorded.
bajra PENNISETUM *glaucum*.
bakery waste may be overflow bread or dough or be moldy, or contain substances other than farinaceous ones. Normal dough or bread or flour can cause CARBOHYDRATE ENGORGEMENT in horses and ruminants. If the fungi on moldy bread are toxic, poisoning may also result. Bread or pastry containing meat may cause the spread of diseases carried in meat scraps, e.g. foot-and-mouth disease, swine fever.
BAL British antilewisite. See DIMERCAPROL.
balance 1. an instrument for weighing. 2. harmonious adjustment of different elements or parts; harmonious performance of functions. Used to describe symmetry and proportion of conformation.
  acid–base b. the proportion of acid and base required to keep the blood and body fluids neutral. See also ACID–BASE BALANCE.
  analytical b. a laboratory balance sensitive to very small variations of the order of 0.001 mg.
  b. examination simultaneous palpation of muscles on both sides of the body of Greyhounds attempting to locate areas of soreness or spasm.
  fluid b. the state of the body in relation to ingestion and excretion of water and electrolytes (see also FLUID balance).
  nitrogen b. the state of the body in regard to ingestion and excretion of nitrogen. In negative nitrogen balance the amount of nitrogen excreted is greater than the quantity ingested. In positive nitrogen balance the amount excreted is smaller than the amount ingested. See also NITROGEN balance.
  posture b. disturbances of balance, including falling to one side, rotation of the head, walking in circles. These are usually indications of disturbances of the organs of balance in the semicircular canals.
  water b. FLUID balance.
balanced ration see balanced RATION.
balanic pertaining to the glans penis or glans clitoridis.
Balanites aegyptica African member of plant family Zygophyllaceae; fruits may contain steroidal saponins; cause nephrosis, hepatitis, muscle wasting in ruminants.
balanitis inflammation of the glans penis.
balanoposthectomy surgical removal of the penis and prepuce.
balanoposthitis inflammation of penis and prepuce.
  enzootic b. see ENZOOTIC balanoposthitis.
  infectious b. see ENZOOTIC balanoposthitis.
  infectious pustular b. the male manifestation of infectious pustular VULVOVAGINITIS caused by bovine herpesvirus 1. It is manifested by the development of pustules and inflammation of the skin of the penis and prepuce, a mucopurulent preputial discharge, and pain of the organ causing the bull to refuse to serve.
balanopreputial pertaining to the glans penis and prepuce.
balanorrhagia balanitis with free discharge of pus.
Balansia epichloe fungal pathogen of pasture plant seedheads; contains ergot alkaloids and causes gangrene of extremities.
balantidiasis infection by protozoa of the genus *Balantidium*. SWINE dysentery was thought at one time to be a form of balantidiasis caused by *B. coli*. Nowadays, the infection is known to be universal and occasionally to cause a severe enteritis in pigs and dogs. A zoonosis and the infection in humans causes colitis.
Balantidium a genus of ciliated protozoa, including many species found in the intestine in vertebrates and invertebrates, predominantly in primates, pigs and humans. See also BALANTIDIASIS.
  B. coli see BALANTIDIASIS.
bald 1. loss of hair, see ALOPECIA. 2. in cattle and horses used to describe an animal with a white face. Called also BALDY.
  b. faced a horse with a blaze and a snip into a nostril conjoined.
  b. thighs syndrome a condition of unknown cause occurring in racing Greyhounds about four weeks after commencing a training program. There is complete alopecia with no other abnormality of the skin on the caudolateral aspects of the thighs and sometimes also in the axilla and on the ventrolateral aspects of the chest.
baldness absence of hair; alopecia.
  pattern b. occurs in dogs as hair loss of the ears in Dachshunds, predominantly males; hair loss on the ventral neck, caudomedial thighs and tail in American water spaniels and Portuguese water dogs; and hair loss on the postauricular areas, ventral and neck and ventral body in dogs of several small breeds.
baldy, baldy-faced said of cattle to mean a white face and usually indicating a Hereford influence in the animal's breeding.
baldy calves see INHERITED EPIDERMAL DYSPLASIA.
bale 1. a package of wool in a wool pack weighing 150–250 lb depending largely on whether it is greasy or scoured. 2. a compressed bundle of hay, either about 100 lb tied with wire or twine, or large, round, untied bales, as big as a small hay stack and referred to as 'big bales'.
Balfour retractor three individually operable, outward-looking curved loops mounted on a bar. By inserting the blades into an incision and spreading them all the incision is opened to give maximum access to tissues below. Available in standard and pediatric sizes, the latter being suitable for a ventral approach to the vocal cords of the horse.

Bali cattle red to red-black meat cattle from Indonesia, originated from Banteng cattle.
Balinese a breed of cat with the body build, temperament and light-colored body and darker ears, face, tail and legs seen in Siamese, but with semi-long hair. The name is derived from the graceful tail movements that are compared to the sinuous movements of Balinese dancers.
baling wire wire used for baling hay which can cause injury to animals. A constant hazard on farms which use hay baled with wire. The most serious injuries are to the lower limbs of horses when they are accidentally entangled in the wire, and TRAUMATIC reticuloperitonitis when the wire is chopped into small lengths by being passed through a chaffcutter.
balk the action of a horse when it refuses to obey a command to which it usually responds. See also JIBBING.
Balkan grippe see Q FEVER.
Balkan nephropathy an endemic disease of humans in south-western Europe. It has a strong resemblance to ochratoxin A induced porcine nephropathy caused by intoxication by FUSARIUM.
balking, baulking see JIBBING.
ball a more or less spherical mass. See also BOLUS.
fungus b. aspergilloma.
Ballearica pavonina Eastern crowned crane.
balling the act of administering a bolus or a ball to a horse for medicinal purposes.
b. gun a device for administering a BOLUS to an animal. Consists of a short cylinder sufficiently large to contain the average bolus, a hollow stem containing the rod that connects the handle with the plunger in the cylinder, and the handle. The handle needs to be long enough to position the cylinder in the pharynx before the bolus is discharged by pushing the handle. Sophisticated models have a spring-loaded handle. Suitable for use in horses, cattle, sheep, goats and pigs but a mouth speculum is essential in many uncooperative animals, especially pigs.
b. gun trauma cellulitis in the pharynx or the cheek opposite the posterior molar teeth caused by too vigorous attempts to push the nozzle of the gun into the pharyngeal orifice.
ballismus, ballism violent flinging movements of the limbs, sometimes affecting only one side of the body (hemiballismus).
ballistiVet see BIOBULLET.
balloon cotton GOMPHOCARPUS *physocarpus*.
balloon dilatation a technique that uses a catheter with an inflatable balloon to increase the diameter of the lumen of a structure such as the urethra or a heart valve. See balloon VALVULOPLASTY.
balloon kidneys an abattoir expression meaning normal kidneys surrounded by an excessive amount of fat.
ballottement [Fr.] a palpatory maneuver to test for a floating object, especially for detecting pregnancy by pushing the fist, in the case of cows, the fingertips in the case of ewes, into the abdominal wall, causing the fetus to move from and quickly return to the fist or fingers.
balm 1. a balsam. 2. a soothing or healing medicine.
balneotherapy use of baths in the treatment of disease.
balsa a very lightweight timber, easy to carve to fit limbs, used for making individual splints.
balsam a semifluid, fragrant, resinous, vegetable juice. Balsams are resins combined with oils, used in various preparations to treat irritated or denuded areas of the skin and mucous membranes. Stains from these preparations are extremely difficult to remove. Friar's balsam, called also compound benzoin TINCTURE, is used as a topical protectant. Balsam of Peru, or Peruvian balsam, is used as a local protectant and rubefacient. Tolu balsam is used as an ingredient in compound benzoin and as an expectorant.
b. traumatic see FRIAR'S BALSAM.
BALT bronchus-associated lymphoid tissue.
bambatsi panic grass PANICUM *coloratum* var. *nakarikariense*.
Bamberger–Marie disease see hypertrophic OSTEOPATHY.
bambermycin an antibiotic feed additive for poultry, pigs and calves.
ban QUERCUS *incana*.
banana disease see BACK muscle necrosis.
band 1. a part, structure or appliance that binds. 2. in histology, a zone of a myofibril of striated muscle. 3. in cytogenetics, a segment of a chromosome stained brighter or darker than the adjacent bands; used in identifying the chromosomes and in determining the exact extent of chromosomal abnormalities. Called *Q-bands*, *G-bands*, *C-bands*, *T-bands*, etc., according to the staining method used.
b. form an immature polymorphonuclear leukocyte. See also SHIFT to the left.
bandage 1. a strip or roll of gauze or other material for wrapping or binding any part of the body. See also SLING. 2. to cover by wrapping with such material. Bandages may be used to stop the flow of blood, to provide a safeguard against contamination, or to hold a medicated dressing in place. They may also be used to hold a splint in position or otherwise immobilize an injured part of the body to prevent further injury and to facilitate healing. In horses it is standard practice to bandage the cannons while the horse is being transported, and in some animals while they are exercising or working. The objective is to prevent fluid accumulation and to protect against injury while making rapid foot movements.
acrylic b. useful for their strength and in some cases slight flexibility.
carpal flexion b. used in dogs to maintain the carpus in flexion, thereby relaxing flexor tendons, while permitting use of the elbow and shoulder.
compression b. one used to apply pressure, usually to control hemorrhage.
figure-of-8 b. one in which the turns cross each other like the figure 8.
flannel b. used to give warmth, support and protection of the lower limbs of horses; should be 4 in × 10 ft.
many-tailed b. see tailed bandage (below).
occlusive b. see OCCLUSIVE dressing.
plaster b. a bandage stiffened with a paste of plaster of Paris.
pressure b. one for applying pressure, for the purpose of arresting hemorrhage; pressure is applied directly over the wound.
rigid b. used for local immobilization, usually for purposes of allowing soft tissue healing.
Robert–Jones b. a heavily padded bandage consisting of cotton batting or cotton wool in a wrapping material, sometimes with added stiffening devices such as plastic piping or parallel strips of thin metal. It is applied as a pressure bandage to provide temporary support for a fractured limb prior to plaster immobilization or immediately afterwards.
roller b. a tightly rolled, circular bandage of varying widths and materials, often prepared commercially. In an emergency, strips may be torn from a sheet or

piece of yard goods and rolled. When more than a few inches of length is needed, rolling is essential for quick and clean bandaging.

soft padded b. consists of cotton padding, gauze and tape. Provides support and protection of soft tissues.

spider b. see tailed bandage (below).

tailed b. a square piece of cloth cut or torn into strips from the ends toward the center, with as large a center left as necessary. The bandage is centered over a compress on the wound and the ends are then tied separately. Called also many-tailed or spider bandage.

tie-over b. a dressing held in place by suture material anchored in surrounding skin and tied over the dressing. Used for postoperative care of skin grafts.

bandicoot small, 1 ft, fawn, sometimes barred marsupial with a pointed nose, prick ears and long back legs. It is nocturnal, burrowing, insectivorous and a host for *Ixodes holocyclus*. Called also *Perameles* spp.

banding 1. the act of encircling and binding with a thin strip of material. 2. in genetics, any of several techniques of staining chromosomes so that a characteristic pattern of transverse dark and light bands becomes visible, permitting identification of individual chromosome pairs.

bandjibos [Af.] TYLECODON *wallichii*.

Bandl's rings tonic, cuff-like contractions of the uterus about the fetus.

bandy knees outward bowing of the forelimbs. See also VALGUS.

baneberry see ACTAEA *spicata*.

Bang's bacillus see BRUCELLA *abortus*.

Bang's disease BRUCELLOSIS caused by *Brucella abortus*.

bangtail the name given to a horse or cow in which the long hairs on the tail are sheared off horizontally, in the horse level with the hocks. Done partly for show, in cattle mainly as a mark that the cattle have been handled and the usual operations of castration or spaying have been performed. Called also banged tail.

bank a stored supply of animal material or tissues for future use by other individuals, as blood bank, serum bank, bone bank, skin bank, eye bank, etc. See also DATABASE.

bantam a group of miniature poultry breeds, some of them true bantams which have developed naturally, others have been developed from standard breeds. Includes Cochin-China, Silkies, Ancona and Andalusian.

Banteng see BOS *banteng*.

Banzai virus a flavivirus associated with abortion and stillbirths in cattle in Africa.

BAPN β-aminopropionitrile. See AMINONITRILE.

Baptisia leucantha toxic North American plant in the Fabaceae family; may contain quinolizidine alkaloids; causes diarrhea. Called also wild indigo.

BAR abbreviation for bright, alert, responsive; used in medical records.

bar 1. a cgs unit of pressure, being the pressure exerted by 10^5 Newtons per square cm (10^6 dynes per square cm). 2. a metal strip that is attached to the metal arch on each side of a saddle and constitutes its skeleton. The attachments for the stirrup leathers are anchored to the bars. 3. a term for describing the humerus.

hoof b. the reflection of the wall of the horse's hoof at the heel, with one bar on each side of the frog. They contribute to the spreadability of the heels but give them protection against excessive contact with the ground surface. May be erroneously cut back by an overzealous blacksmith.

b. pad a pad, usually of leather, fitted between the shoe and the hoof of a horse so as to protect the sole and bars of the foot.

b. shoe a special horseshoe with a bar connecting the two heels of the shoe so as to make a full circle. Designed for use in horses whose heels are likely to be injured by too frequent contact of the heel with the ground surface.

walking b. a reinforcement placed at the bottom of a cast which allows weight to be transferred from the foot to the upper part of the cast. Used most often in casts for large animals.

bar diagram a method of presenting data in which frequencies are displayed along one axis and categories of the variable along the other, the frequencies being represented by the bar lengths.

baralime, baralyme calcium hydroxide and barium hydroxide mixture in granules, used to absorb carbon dioxide from exhaled air in a closed circuit anesthetic system. See also SODA lime.

Barb 1. originally a distinct line of black Australian kelpies, but now the term is generally applied to any black kelpie. 2. a riding horse of great antiquity native to North Africa; bay, brown, chestnut, black, gray and 14 to 15 hands high. The foundation of the ANDALUSIAN breed.

barba [L.] *beard*.

Barbados Blackbelly sheep tan with black belly, polled, haired meat sheep with mane in rams.

Barbados nut JATROPHA *curcas*.

barban an organic substance used as a weedkiller. Poisoning manifested in cattle by ruminal stasis, recumbency, salivation and tachycardia. In pigs the syndrome comprises incoordination, vomiting and diarrhea.

Barbarea vulgaris toxic North American plant in family Brassicaceae; contains irritant oil, causing enteritis and diarrhea; called also winter cress, yellow rocket.

Barbary sheep see AMMOTRAGUS LERVIA.

barbed wire strong wire with sharp barbs at close intervals, used in fencing to deter livestock. Consists commonly of two strands twisted together and bearing sharp spines every 4 inches (10 cm) or so. Animals accidentally caught in a fence made of the wire can be badly lacerated.

barber scissors sharp-pointed scissors with a finger lever on one of the finger grips. Designed for hand cutting a limited area of hair.

barbering hair-chewing; observed in cats, rodents, rabbits and ferrets.

Barberry see BERBERIS.

barber's pole worm see HAEMONCHUS.

barbicel the hooks borne on the barbules of a bird's contour feather that serve to interlock adjacent barbs to make a stable vane.

barbital, barbitone a long-acting barbiturate, used as a hypnotic and sedative. Largely replaced by PHENOBARBITAL.

barbitine see DITERPENOID ALKALOID.

barbiturate any of a group of organic compounds derived from barbituric acid. There are a number of barbiturates. They all depress the nervous system and are used to induce apathy and sleep, and in high doses, as anesthetics. They vary in their sedative effects, in the duration of their effectiveness and in their toxicity. Those that are used in veterinary medicine are: (1) pentobarbital sodium (Nembutal); largely superseded, but still sometimes used for intravenous anesthesia in companion animals; (2) thiopental sodium, which has a short period of effectiveness, an advantage in many veterinary situations, e.g. examination of a pharynx; (3) thialbarbital sodium, a medium length compound; (4) thiamylal sodium, a compound with ultrashort action.

b. slough skin slough over a vein where a solution of barbiturate intended for injection into the vein leaks into subcutaneous tissue.

barbituric acid a compound, $C_4H_4N_2O_3$, the parent substance of BARBITURATE.

barbone [Fr.] see HEMORRHAGIC septicemia.

barbotage [Fr.] repeated alternate injection and withdrawal of fluid with a syringe, as in gastric lavage or administration of an anesthetic agent into the subarachnoid space by alternate injection of part of the anesthetic and withdrawal of cerebrospinal fluid into the syringe.

barbs the primary, delicate filaments that are given off the shaft of a bird's contour feather. They project from the rachis and bear the barbules.

barbules the hooked processes that fringe adjacent barbs of a bird's feather.

Bard–Parker a proprietary group of surgical equipment.

B.–P. instrument tray Pyrex dish with a rubber-gasketed metal cover, designed to contain a chemical sterilant with instruments permanently in situ in a metal tray that can be raised and locked into a position above the liquid. Suitable for minor procedures in the practice office.

B.–P. scalpel a metal or disposable plastic handle with a patent form of attachment for blades that are available in a wide range of sizes and shapes with specific tasks in view.

B.–P. transfer forceps multipurpose, springloaded tongs for picking up sterilized surgical materials. They are permanently housed in a glass or stainless steel canister of instrument disinfectant with the handles protruding so that they can be picked up without opening the container.

Barden sign a means of demonstrating hip laxity in the diagnosis of hip dysplasia. With the dog in dorsal recumbency, the femur is perpendicular to the surface and the stifle is adducted.

bariatrics a field of medicine encompassing the study of obesity, its causes, prevention and treatment.

barilla see HALOGETON GLOMERATUS.

barium a chemical element, atomic number 56, atomic weight 137.34, symbol Ba. See Table 6. Soluble salts, e.g. the chloride and the carbonate, are toxic.

b. burger, barium meal a mixture of barium and solid food, used as a contrast medium in radiographic studies of the esophagus, instead of liquid barium mixtures.

b. chloride used as a rodenticide. The baits are attractive to dogs. Clinical signs include salivation, convulsions and paralysis.

b. deficiency preliminary experiments showing that diets deficient in barium fed to rats and guinea pigs depress growth have been neither invalidated nor confirmed.

b. enema a dilute (5 to 20%) suspension of barium is introduced into a colon that has been emptied by starvation and previous enema.

b.-impregnated polyethylene spheres radioopaque markers used to demonstrate intestinal obstruction and motility disorders; the spheres are given orally and their movement can be tracked radiographically.

b. meal a strong (usually 100%) suspension of barium sulfate is administered to an animal which has been starved for at least 12 hours.

b. study x-ray examination using a barium mixture to help locate disorders in the esophagus, stomach, duodenum, and the small and large intestines. Called also barium test.

b. sulfate a water-insoluble salt used as an opaque contrast medium for x-ray examination of the digestive tract.

b. swallow a small amount of barium paste or liquid administered orally and observed radiographically or by fluoroscopy for examination of swallowing and esophageal function.

b. test barium study.

bark 1. the voice of the dog. 2. the outer covering of a tree.

b. eating a form of pica often indicative of boredom, nutritional deficiency of fiber or behavioral problem.

b. suppression see DEBARKING, DEVOCALIZATION.

Bark lion sentinel dog see LHASA APSO.

barker a term for an animal that does not usually bark which makes a violent respiratory effort, often during a convulsion, accompanied by a sound which roughly resembles a dog's bark.

b. foals see NEONATAL maladjustment syndrome.

b. pig see barker syndrome (below).

b. syndrome newborn piglets show respiratory distress, and 'bark' and walk aimlessly. They appear to be blind. Death follows in 24 hours.

b. and wanderer see NEONATAL maladjustment syndrome.

barley a genus of cereals and grasses. See HORDEUM.

b. beef a British system of introducing calves into pens at 3 months of age, feeding them intensively on high grain diets and marketing them before 12 months of age.

b. beef rumenitis lesions of rumenitis found at necropsy in calves fed heavy barley diets.

b. grass HORDEUM *jubatum*.

b. scab fungus FUSARIUM *roseum*.

Barlow's disease see hypertrophic OSTEODYSTROPHY.

barn a building usually intended to house animals for long periods during the winter season. Marked by an infinite variety of designs and internal fittings, they usually contain a feed storage area, often as a haymow or loft in a top storey, and animal stalls and handling facilities such as a milking parlor on the ground floor.

b. itch see SARCOPTIC MANGE.

b. rat a horse that shows eagerness or determination to return to the stable. See also AGORAPHOBIA.

b. sheet a sketchy method of recording events, especially reproductive ones, in the lives of the inmates of the barn. Fixed to the barn wall it does provide an opportunity to record events as they happen, but suffers the obvious disadvantage of exposure to disfiguring and obscuring materials, especially fly droppings and cow manure. Its design, aimed at encouraging maximum data storage in minimal space, is a test for farmer ingenuity. Called also SHED sheet.

barnacle an adult cirripede that lives attached to fixed objects; an aquatic member of the subclass Cirrepedia of the class Crustacea.

barnyard fowl those avian species commonly kept on general purpose farms, e.g. ducks, geese, chickens.

barnyard grass ECHINOCHLOA *crus-galli*.

barophilic growing best under high atmospheric pressure; said of bacteria.

baroreceptor a sensory nerve terminal that is stimulated by changes in pressure, as those in blood vessel walls.

b. reflex reflexes triggered by changes in pressure,

usually refers to blood pressure, e.g. carotid sinus reflex.

baroreflex see BARORECEPTOR.

barosinusitis a symptom complex in humans caused by differences in environmental atmospheric pressure and the air pressure in the paranasal sinuses.

barotaxis stimulation of living matter by change of atmospheric pressure.

Barr body a small mass of densely staining chromatin seen during interphase of female cells produced by condensation of one of the two X chromosomes. See also DRUMSTICK.

barramundi see LATES CALCARIFER.

barrel a horseman's expression for the horse's trunk; determined largely by the capacity of the chest.

b. chest enlarged, round cross-section of chest with the ribs appearing to be permanently in an inflated position.

barrel medic MEDICAGO *truncatula*.

barren see INFERTILITY.

barrenness see INFERTILITY.

barrier an obstruction; a partition between two fluid compartments in the body.

blood–air b. alveolocapillary membrane.

blood–aqueous b. the physiological mechanism that prevents exchange of materials between the chambers of the eye and the blood.

blood–brain b. (BBB) the barrier separating the blood from the brain parenchyma. See also BLOOD–BRAIN BARRIER.

blood–CSF b. differs from the blood–brain barrier anatomically, in that it consists of the epithelium of the choroid plexuses, but has similar permeabilities.

blood–gas b. alveolocapillary membrane.

b.–retina barrier endothelium of the retinal capillaries and cells of the retinal pigment epithelium form a nonfenestrated barrier between choroidal tissue fluid and retinal tissue fluid.

blood–synovial b. suggested by the presence of plasma proteins of small molecular size and catabolic products of articular cartilage in synovial fluid.

blood–testis b. a barrier separating the blood from the seminiferous tubules, consisting of special junctional complexes between adjacent Sertoli cells near the base of the seminiferous epithelium. It provides an extravascular environment which is also adluminal and permits selective nourishment of spermatozoa.

b. boot a rubber boot worn by horses to protect the hoof against trauma.

b. cream a nonwettable cream used on the skin of the hands and arms to protect against staining and odor absorption when handling offensive materials, e.g. delivery of an emphysematous fetus.

gastric mucosal b. the poorly defined mechanism that prevents back diffusion of hydrochloric acid from the stomach into the tissues of the stomach wall.

skin b. the protective properties of skin and its relative impenetrability by noxious substances as well as medicaments; usually considered a function of keratinized epithelial cells aided by surface lipids.

b. teat dip material which leaves a physical protective coat on the teat between milkings, used mostly to protect against infection for long periods, e.g. during the dry period. Most contain acrylic, latex or collodion.

barrier saltbush see ENCHYLAENA TOMENTOSA.

Barron ligation see RUBBER-BAND LIGATION.

barrow a castrated male pig.

bartholinitis inflammation of the Bartholin glands.

Bartholin's duct the major sublingual duct. It drains the monostomatic sublingual gland which opens on the sublingual caruncle. It is absent in the horse.

Bartholin's glands the major vestibular glands; two small glands, one in each wall of the vaginal vestibule of the cow, cat and occasionally the sheep that secrete mucus; their ducts open on either side of the urethral orifice. They secrete mucus, providing lubrication for coitus and for the passage of the fetus at birth. When cystic in the cow they are visible through the mucosa and are about 1 inch long and 0.5 inch wide. They are homologs of the bulbourethral glands in the male. Called also Tiedmann's or Duverney's gland, vulvovaginal gland.

Barton tether a leather harness used to tether pigs at pasture. One strap around the neck and one around the chest behind the elbows are tied together at the withers by a third strap, and a fourth one ties them together between the front limbs. A tethering chain is attached at any point.

Bartonella a genus of gram-negative, coccoid or rod-shaped bacteria in the family Bartonellaceae. *B. bacilliformis* is the cause of Oroya fever or Carrión's disease in humans and occasionally dogs, in South America.

B. henselae causes cat-scratch disease, bacillary angiomatosis, and endocarditis in humans.

Bartonellaceae a family of the order Rickettsiales, occurring as pathogenic parasites in or on the erythrocytes of humans and other animals. See BARTONELLA.

bartonellemia the presence in the blood of organisms of the genus *Bartonella.*

Bartter's syndrome chronic potassium depletion leading to hypokalemia; caused by renal potassium wasting, elevated plasma renin activity and aldosterone secretion.

baruria see HYPERSTHENURIA.

Barwon lucerne LOTUS *australis.*

Barychelidae a family of spiders in the Myagalomorph suborder which includes the funnel-web spider. They are characterized by having vertical rather than horizontal fangs.

Bas rouge see BERGER DE BEAUCE.

basal pertaining to or situated near a BASE; in physiology, pertaining to the lowest possible level.

b. body the structure that acts as a template for the characteristic 9 + 2 arrangement of the microtubules of eukaryotic cilia and flagella.

b. cell tumors neoplasms of the multipotential cells within the stratum germinativum of the skin. They are common in dogs and cats, are locally expansive and do not metastasize.

b. energy requirements (BER) see ENERGY requirements.

b. ganglia a collection of masses of gray matter at the base of the cerebral hemispheres, subthalamus and midbrain which are responsible for much of the organization of the activity of somatic muscles. The individual nuclei are the caudate nucleus, putamen, globus pallidus, endopeduncular nucleus, subthalamic nucleus and the substantia nigra. Other nuclei which have a similar function but are usually not included in the group are the amygdaloid nuclei and the red nucleus.

b. layer see STRATUM basale.

b. membrane the deepest layer of the epidermis in the avian skin. Called also dermoepidermal junction.

b. metabolic rate see METABOLIC rate.

b. metabolism the minimal energy expended for the maintenance of respiration, circulation, peristalsis, muscle tonus, body temperature, glandular activity and the other vegetative functions of the body. See also METABOLIC rate.

b. metabolism test a method of measuring the body's expenditure of energy by recording its rate of oxygen intake and consumption. Once a major test of THYROID gland function, it is being replaced by diagnostic tests requiring less extensive preparation and capable of producing more accurate test results, e.g. the determination of the levels of thyroid hormones in the blood and the RADIOIODINE uptake test.

b. nuclei see basal GANGLION.

b. plate the ventral plate of the developing neural tube of the embryo; associated with motor output from the CNS.

b. tone degree of contractile tension remaining in blood vessels after complete elimination of all external excitatory influences.

basalioma a BASAL cell tumor.

base 1. the lowest part or foundation of anything. See also BASIS. 2. the main ingredient of a compound. 3. a molecule or ion with a tendency to take up a proton according to Bronsted and Lowry theory; a substance that combines with acids to form salts. In the chemical processes of the body, bases are essential to the maintenance of a normal ACID–BASE BALANCE. Excessive concentration of bases in the body fluids leads to ALKALOSIS. See also BASAL. 4. the primary entity against which all other entities are compared. 5. the non-sugar components of nucleotides in DNA and RNA.

acid–b. pairs the two molecules forming the matching acid and conjugate base.

b. composition refers to the relative components of a nucleic acid.

conjugate b. the anion or uncharged molecule of an acid once it has given up its proton, e.g. Cl^- is the conjugate base of the acid, HCl.

b. deficit see base excess (below).

b. excess the amount of acid or base required to titrate a sample of whole arterial blood to the normal pH of 7.4. The base excess is determined mathematically by calculations that include measurement of the blood $P\text{CO}_2$ and pH and take into account the hemoglobin level. It is negative (base deficit) in acidosis and positive in alkalosis.

heart b. the wide dorsal part of the heart carrying the atria and the large blood vessels and the attachment to the pericardial sac.

horn b. the widest part of the horn, at its attachment to the skin. In the adult horned animal the horn is hollow at this point, encloses the horn process of the frontal bone and merges with the skin. This is covered with a thin layer of horn similar to the periople of the hoof, called the epiceras.

narrow b. a mandible which is narrow relative to the maxilla; often causes the lower canine teeth to strike the hard palate. See also ANISOGNATHISM.

nitrogenous b. an aromatic, nitrogen-containing molecule that serves as a proton acceptor, e.g. purine or pyrimidine.

omasal b. faces cranially and to the left where it is attached to the reticulum and the abomasum at the reticulo-omasal and omasoabomasal orifices.

b. pair two hydrogen bonded nucleotides in a DNA or RNA molecule.

purine b's a group of compounds of which purine is the base, including uric acid, adenine, guanine, xanthine and theobromine.

pyrimidine b's a group of chemical compounds of which pyrimidine is the base, including uracil, thymine and cytosine, which are common constituents of nucleic acids.

stapedal b. the footplate of the STAPES in the middle ear from which the two legs originate. The stapes lies horizontally with the base facing medially and attached to the vestibular window by the annular ligament.

baseline a known value or quantity used to measure or assess an unknown, as a baseline urine sample.

b. data a set of data collected at the beginning of a study or before intervention has occurred.

basement membrane the delicate extracellular supporting layer of mucopolysaccharides and proteins underlying all epithelia.

b. m. dystrophy see refractory ULCER.

b. m. zone the area corresponding to the dermoepithelial junction, which stains with periodic acid–Schiff. It consists of the basal cell plasma membrane, the lamina lucida, the basal lamina and the sub-basal lamina fibrous components.

Basenji a small (20–25 lb) red or black, with white, shorthaired dog, with prick ears, a furrowed, wrinkled forehead and a tail that coils over its back. Although known as the 'barkless' dog, it does have a characteristic vocal sound. The breed originated in North Africa as a hunting dog. Called also Congo dog. Some inherited and congenital disorders that occur in the breed are familial nonspherocytic ANEMIA, CYSTINURIA, FANCONI'S SYNDROME, giant hypertrophic GASTRITIS and persistent PUPILLARY membrane.

BASIC a computer language; acronym for Beginners All-purpose Symbolic Instruction Code.

basic 1. pertaining to or having properties of a base. 2. capable of neutralizing acids.

b. multicell unit the packet of cells involved in remodeling of bone at a remodeling site.

basicity 1. the quality of being a base, or basic. 2. the combining power of an acid.

basidiobolomycosis infection by fungi in the genus *Basidiobolus*.

Basidiobolus a genus of fungi of the group Phycomycetes.

B. haptosporus, B. ranarum see SWAMP CANCER.

Basidiomycetes a class of fungi.

basidiospore the sexual spore of the class Basidiomycetes.

basidium pl. *basidia* [L.] the clublike fungal organ bearing basidiospores.

basihyoid the body of the hyoid bone.

basil finished dressed leather made from sheepskin.

basilad toward the base.

basilar pertaining to a base or basal part.

b. artery one of the main blood supplies to the brain. It originates from the junction of the two vertebral arteries, runs in a median groove, beneath the medulla and pons, and terminates rostrally at the cerebral circle (of Willis). See also Table 9.

b. fracture at the base of the skull, usually involving the occipital and BASISPHENOID bones.

b. impression see PLATYBASIA.

basilateral both basilar and lateral.

basilemma basement membrane.

basiloma a BASAL cell carcinoma.

basioccipital bone see Table 10.

basion the midpoint of the anterior (ventral) border of the foramen magnum.

basipetal descending toward the base; developing in the direction of the base.

basipodium carpus or tarsus; equivalent of wrist or ankle in the human limbs.

basis the lower, basic or fundamental part of an object, organ or substance, or the part opposite to or distinguished from the apex. See also BASE.

basisphenoid one of the bones of the floor of the skull which, with the presphenoid, constitutes the sphenoid bone.
b. fracture occurs in horses that rear over backwards. Characterized by unilateral facial paralysis, circling gait. Called also occipital fracture.
basket cell see basket CELL.
baso- prefix meaning blue or basic.
basocytophilia see BASOPHILIA.
basoerythrocyte an erythrocyte containing basophil granules.
basophil 1. any structure, cell or histological element staining readily with basic dyes. 2. a granular leukocyte with an irregularly shaped, relatively pale-staining nucleus that is partially constricted into two lobes, and with cytoplasm containing coarse bluish-black granules of variable size. 3. a beta cell of the adenohypophysis. 4. BASOPHILIC.
b. cell a beta cell of the adenohypophysis which produces luteinizing and follicle stimulating hormones.
b. degranulation test an in vitro cellular test for immediate hypersensitivity; it detects degranulation of basophils, by their loss of affinity for staining, when blood from a hypersensitive dog is incubated with allergen extracts.
basophilia 1. the reaction of relatively immature erythrocytes to basic dyes whereby the stained cells appear blue, gray or grayish-blue, or bluish granules appear. 2. abnormal increase of basophilic leukocytes in the blood. 3. basophilic leukocytosis.
basophilic staining readily with basic dyes.
b. bone matrix vitamin D poisoning causes the appearance of intensely basophilic bone matrix of a distincitive pattern.
b. cell see BASOPHIL cell.
b. enterocolitis one of the several types of enterocolitis causing chronic diarrhea in horses characterized by fibrinous and ulcerative typhlocolitis and basophilic infiltrates in the regional mucosa and submucosa.
b. leukemia see LEUKEMIA.
b. rubricyte a stage in cellular maturation of erythrocytes, between the prorubricyte and polychromatophilic rubricyte. Characterized by a narrow rim of dark blue cytoplasm and condensed nuclear chromatin in a 'cartwheel' pattern.
b. stippling distinct or diffuse, fine to coarse, dark granular pattern in erythrocytes, representing aggregated ribosomes and caused by ineffective heme formation. Seen in lead poisoning, mainly in dogs and a characteristic of active erythropoiesis in sheep and cattle.
basophilism abnormal increase of basophilic cells.
basoplasm cytoplasm that stains with basic dyes.
bass tapeworm see PROTEOCEPHALUS AMBLOPLITIS.
Bassaricyon gabbii see OLINGO.
Basset Fauve de Bretagne a wire-coated hunting dog, similar to the BASSET HOUND. Called also Brittany bassett.
Basset hound a medium-sized, shorthaired dog with very short, bowed legs, long ears and a long body. The head is large with loose skin and large, pendulous lips. One of the achondroplastic breeds. It is subject to familial disorders of the platelets and primary glaucoma.
Bassia plants of the Chenopodiaceae family; can cause oxalate poisoning. Includes *B. anisacanthoides*, *B. calcarata*, *B. hyssopifolia* (red burr), *B. quinquecuspis*. Called also *Sclerolaena* spp.
basso macello an Italian system of treating meat which is unsuitable for unconditional release for sale for human consumption. The meat is treated by boiling or by other means of decontamination.
bastard atypical, or unusual form of, a disease or plant.
b. lentil ERVUM *ervilia*.
b. strangles see STRANGLES.
b. wing see ALULA.
bastard toad flax see COMANDRA PALLIDA.
bastard wing see ALULA.
bat see CHIROPTERA.
b. ear an erect, broad-based ear in dogs; seen in the French bulldog and Welsh corgi.
b. rabies caused by rabies-like viruses which are antigenically similar to the classical rabies rhabdovirus. Bats also are common carriers of rabies virus transmitting it to other species and between themselves both by bite and by aerosol inhalation of urine. See also LAGOS and MOKOLA viruses.
batch file a file which contains a number of commands which are carried out sequentially when the file is executed. Called also script file.
batch processing a method of processing in which all of the input transactions of a given type which are to be processed on a computer are collected together and processed at one time. Is much more economical of time than processing each item as it appears chronologically but leads to delays while banks of data are being accumulated. Is undesirable for a practice where instant entry of a debit is critical in maintaining consumer goodwill and cash flow.
bath 1. a medium, e.g. water, vapor, sand or mud, with which the body is washed or in which the body is wholly or partially immersed for therapeutic or cleansing purposes; application of such a medium to the body. 2. the equipment or apparatus in which a body or object may be immersed.
colloid b. a bath prepared by adding soothing agents, such as gelatin, starch, bran or similar substances, to the bath water, for the purpose of relieving skin irritation and pruritus. The patient is dried by patting rather than rubbing the skin. Care must be taken to avoid chilling.
contrast b. alternate immersion of a part in hot water and cold water.
cool b. one in water from 60 to 75°F (15 to 24°C).
emollient b. a bath in a soothing and softening liquid, used in various skin disorders.
fish b. treatment a separate tank prepared for this purpose is best. Is most effective as a means of treating skin conditions. There is insufficient absorption of most drugs from aquarium water.
hot b. one in water from 98 to 112°F (36 to 44°C).
b. oil a dispersible surfactant oil used in the treatment of dry skin disease, particularly seborrhea sicca.
tepid b. one in water 85 to 92°F (30 to 33°C).
warm b. one in water 90 to 104°F (32 to 40°C).
whirlpool b. one in which the water is kept in constant motion by mechanical means. It has a gentle massaging action that promotes relaxation and is used in the treatment of skin diseases.
bath medication medication of fish by immersing them in a dilute solution of the medicament for 15 minutes to 3 hours.
Bathmostomum a genus of the Ancylostomatidae family of blood-sucking nematodes. Includes *B. sangeri* (Indian elephant, cecum).
bathmotropy any influence on excitability or irritability (i.e. the stimulation threshold) of heart muscle.
bathrocephaly a developmental anomaly marked by a steplike posterior projection of the skull, caused by excessive growth of the lambdoid suture.

Bathurst burr XANTHIUM *spinosum*.
bathy- word element. [Gr.] *deep*.
bathyanesthesia loss of deep sensibility.
bathypnea deep breathing.
Batten disease see ceroid LIPOFUSCINOSIS.
battery housing the housing of animals or birds in confined spaces, either singly or in twos or threes, with the compartments packed very closely together and often stacked a number of layers deep. Has economic advantages in the provision of automatic feeding, watering, egg-collecting and dung-removal services. The same system has been used for dairy cattle with the cows in mobile cubicles which travel past a milking point at the appointed times. The system is a point of contention between farmers and animal liberationists.
battlement blood smears a method of counting blood cells in which the edge of the smear, where the counting is done, is traversed in a track similar to the silhouette of a castle battlement. It is thought to avoid a biased count due to the greater adhesiveness of some leukocytes and their preponderance at the very edge of the smear.
baud a unit of speed in telecommunication. One baud = 1 bit per second.
bay 1. a tan or red-brown coat color of horses. Light bay is light tan; mealy bay is a redder but lighter, rust color; blood bay is a much deeper, redder color; golden bay has a tinge of yellow in a deep red-brown color. 2. prolonged bark or howl of a hunting hound.
Bayer gag used in the examination of a cow's mouth. A metal block with opposite faces shaped as grooves into which molar teeth slide, on a long steel rod. The block is pushed up between the molar teeth on the opposite side. The retaining rod has a loop and is tied to the headstall to prevent the block from moving. The Swale and Young gags are similar. See also mouth WEDGE.
Bayes theorem a statistical means of including local general information, intuitive judgment, clinical skill as learned over a long period, and similar subjective influences, in the assessment of probability, e.g. in making a diagnosis. The formula relates, for example, the CONDITIONAL PROBABILITY P(D/S), of a disease (D) being present when a particular sign (S) is observed, to three other probabilities: the prevalence of the disease P(D), the frequency of the sign P(S), and the probability of the sign occurring for the disease P(S | D).

$$\Pr(D \mid S) = \frac{\Pr(S \mid D) \times \Pr(D)}{\Pr(S)}$$

Baylisascaris a genus in the Ascarididae family of nematodes which cause cerebrospinal nematodiasis. Includes *B. columnaris* (dogs), *B. transfuga* (captive and zoo bears), *B. procyonis* (rodents).
Bayliss mechanism the myogenic response to stretch in blood vessels.
BBB see BLOOD–BRAIN BARRIER.
BCAA : AAA ratio of branched chain amino acids to aromatic amino acids; used in the assessment of abnormalities in nitrogen metabolism, particularly those associated with hepatic insufficiency, hepatic encephalopathy and chronic renal failure. Low levels of branched chain amino acids are found and supplementation to restore a normal ratio has been used in treatment.
BCG bacille Calmette–Guérin, an avirulent strain of *Mycobacterium bovis*.
BCG test is sometimes used in the diagnosis of tuberculosis in dogs as being more reliable and sensitive than tuberculin testing.
BCG vaccination has been used in the control of tuberculosis in cattle but has many disadvantages, especially interference with tuberculin testing, and is not recommended for use unless the prevalence of the disease is very high.
BCG vaccine contains living BCG organisms. It was developed for use in the control of tuberculosis in humans. Contains living BCG organisms. Is used as a nonspecific stimulant to antibody production in chronic diseases, e.g. equine sarcoid and neoplasia in dogs.
BCNU see CARMUSTINE.
b.d. [L.] *bis die* (twice a day). Called also b.i.d.
Bdellonyssus see ORNITHONYSSUS.
BDV border disease virus.
Be chemical symbol, *beryllium*.
be-still tree THEVETIA *peruviana*.
beach disease LANTANA *camara*.
Beagle a medium-sized, shorthaired hound, bred originally for hunting but much used now as a genetically stable experimental animal. Some congenital and inherited disorders seen in the breed are epilepsy, factor VII deficiency, hemophilia A, lymphocytic thyroiditis, and a number of ophthalmic abnormalities.
B. pain syndrome severe meningitis and polyarthritis of unknown etiology with fever and severe cervical pain; seen in mature Beagles.
beak the hard keratinization (or rhamphotheca) which provides the horny covering of the beak bones, plus the beak bones, of birds. The dorsal ridge of the upper beak is the culmen, the similar keel of the lower beak is the gonys. The cutting edges of the beak are the tomia. Called also bill.
b. avulsion traumatic separation of the upper and lower beak at the base requires hand feeding for survival of the bird. Some attempts at devising an artificial beak have been made, but attachment is a major problem.
b. fracture occurs with trauma and requires immobilization, often with innovative procedures (see ACRYLIC GLUE), without restricting food intake by the bird during recovery. Severe trauma may result in avulsion of upper or lower beak.
b. necrosis can occur as a flock problem possibly associated with a keratolytic bacteria.
b. overgrowth can result from malocclusion, liver disease, lack of wear, ageing, nutritional deficiency, and most commonly infestation by the mite, *Cnemidocoptes pilae*.
psittacine b. and feather disease see PSITTACINE beak and feather disease.
b. sign the radiographic feature of contrast material extending through an elongated, concentrically narrowed pylorus indicative of hypertrophy of the sphincter.
b. trimming in most modern poultry houses the chances of cannibalism developing are so high that beak trimming is almost a necessity, especially if the birds are to be reared in full light. Light-restricted accommodation greatly reduces the prevalence of this vice. A temporary trim is done at a few days of age but a permanent trim is necessary later. Special instruments, utilizing a hot, cutting blade cautery, are used and the operation must be done by an expert or badly deformed beaks result and the birds are unable to feed properly. Alternatives to trimming include the fitting of spectacles or pick guards but these are expensive, time-consuming to put on and not feasible for birds in cages.
beaker a round laboratory vessel of various materials, usually with parallel sides and often with a pouring spout.

beam a unidirectional emission of electromagnetic radiation. See also X-RAY.
external b. therapy radiotherapy in which the source is at a distance from the patient, e.g. orthovoltage, cesium-137, cobalt-60 or linear accelerator.
b. limitation restriction of the divergent beam as it appears from the tube window by a lead plate or cone or a light beam diaphragm located at the window.
primary b. the radiation beam as it passes through the window of the x-ray tube and before it is modified by extra-tube devices.

bean see EGG tooth.

beans see PHASEOLUS and VICIA.

bear see URSUS, BRUNUS EDWARDII and KOALA. Species of less legitimate lineage include Pooh, Paddington and Brideshead bears.

bear cat see ARCTICTIS *binturong*. Called also binturong.

bear foot HELLEBORUS *viridis*.

bear grass see NOLINA.

beard 1. in goats and dogs, beards are conventional collections of chin hairs; seen only in certain dog breeds such as Afghan hounds and Bearded collies. 2. in turkeys, beards are an agglomeration of modified feathers, or hair/feathers, consisting of individual filaments that arise from individual beard papillae. Called also barba.

beard tongue see PENSTEMON.

Bearded collie a medium- to large-sized, gray, fawn, blue, brown or black dog with harsh, strong medium to long hair, particularly around the face and under the chin, giving the name. The body is longer than it is high, in a ratio of 5 to 4. Called also the Highland collie, the Mountain collie or the Hairy Mou'ed collie.

bearded dragon see AMPHIBOLURUS BARBATUS.

bearded pig SUS *barbatus*.

bearing 1. the female genital tract. 2. a piece of harness.
lose the b. uterine PROLAPSE.
b. retainer device for retaining a replaced uterine or vaginal PROLAPSE.
b. trouble see vaginal PROLAPSE.

beat a throb or pulsation, as of the heart or of an artery.
apex b. the palpable shock caused by the apex of the heart beating against the chest wall with each systole and felt over the apex of the heart, normally in the fifth left intercostal space. May be replaced by a thrill.
capture b's occasional ventricular responses to a sinus impulse that reaches the atrioventricular node in a nonrefractory phase.
ectopic b. a heartbeat originating at some point other than the sinus node.
escaped b's heartbeats that follow an abnormally long pause.
forced b. an extrasystole produced by artificial stimulation of the heart.
fusion b. in electrocardiography, the complex resulting when an ectopic ventricular beat coincides with normal conduction to the ventricle.
premature b. an extrasystole.

Beauceron see BERGER DE BEAUCE.

beaver a large, 2 ft, aquatic rodent with webbed feet, a broad flat tail and thick fur. It lives in lodges constructed of timber and mud. It dams streams by accumulating logs. Called also *Castor canadensis*. There is also a European beaver, *C. fiber*.

Beaver scalpel detachable handle and blades in various shapes designed for use in ophthalmic surgery.

bechic pertaining to cough.

Bechtol screw a bone screw with a buttress thread used in compression plating of bones. See also SCREW.

Becker's suture a multilayer pattern for closure of the linear alba in horses.

Beck's triad rising venous pressure, falling arterial pressure, and small quiet heart; characteristic of cardiac compression.

beclomethasone dipropionate a glucocorticoid, commonly used as an inhalant.

becquerel the SI unit of radioactivity, defined as the quantity of a radionuclide that undergoes one decay per second (s^{-1}). One becquerel equals 3.7×10^{-11} Ci. Abbreviated Bq. Supersedes the CURIE.

bed 1. a supporting structure or tissue. 2. a couch or support for the body during sleep.
b. bugs see CIMEX LECTULARIUS.
capillary b. the capillaries of a tissue, area or organ considered collectively, and their volume capacity.
nail b. the area of modified epidermis beneath the claw, hoof or nail.

bedding materials used to provide comfort, conservation of body heat, protection of bony prominences and ease of cleaning. The materials vary widely, each having advantages. The need is for cost-effectiveness, softness with durability, freedom from dust or poisonous components, and springiness and avoidance of compaction. Things to avoid are palatability, e.g. salty sand, good oatstraw containing a lot of grain, shavings and sawdust from timber treated with wood preservatives or irritant resins, e.g. black walnut shavings. Some of the materials used are cereal straws, ferns or bracken harvested for the purpose, peat moss, sawdust and shavings, shredded paper, especially newsprint, sand, mats made from reconstituted rubber and indoor–outdoor carpet. The latter is a practicable solution for animals that have difficulty rising either because of infirmity or because of slipperiness of the flooring.
b. deprivation stress factor in farm animals housed in winter, also late pregnant companion animals.
b. down for a horse means removal of any manure from the stall, teasing out and topping up the bedding with fresh straw where necessary, and filling the water pail and the hay rack.
eating b. results from boredom, perversion of appetite or hunger. The latter is important in horses immediately after a general anesthetic for which they have been prestarved. The animals are only part-conscious but are hungry. They may eat a lot of indigestible roughage and develop colic due to impaction of the colon. Eating of salty sand may cause sand colic.

bedewing subepithelial edema of the cornea.

Bedlington terrier a small, soft-coated terrier, distinguished by its Roman nose and roached back which are accentuated by trimming and grooming for purposes of showing. Originally used for hunting small game, dog fighting and racing. The breed is subject to inherited retinal dysplasia and copper-associated hepatopathy.
B. t. copper-associated hepatopathy an inherited copper storage disease in which Bedlington terriers homozygous for the trait accumulate copper in their liver and suffer a slowly progressive hepatopathy. Clinical signs referable to liver disease develop in young to older adult dogs. The disease is incurable, but may be managed with D-penicillamine or other decoppering agents. Called also Bedlington terrier liver disease.

B. t. liver disease see Bedlington terrier copper-associated hepatopathy (above).
Bedsonia an obsolete name for CHLAMYDIA.
bedsore see DECUBITUS ulcer.
bee sting injury caused by the venom of a honey bee (*Apis mellifera*). Multiple stings cause local swelling, pain and excitement, and may cause dyspnea if the head is affected. A systemic effect, including diarrhea, hemoglobinuria, jaundice, tachycardia and prostration, may be observed in horses.
NOTE: a singular STING in a horse has quite a different meaning.
beech see FAGUS.
beef 1. the meat of cattle other than the young calf. It may be bullock, yearling, bull, cow beef or beef treated in various ways including corned, biltong, jerked or its origin may be specified, e.g. grass-fed, lot-fed. See also MEAT. 2. pertaining to cattle used for the production of beef.
baby b. slaughter cattle weighing 700–1000 lb at 9 to 15 months of age and grading good or better for quality.
block b. beef suitable for sale as blocks for conversion at the retail site into consumer cuts.
boning b. beef suited for manufacturing and processing.
b. breeds include ABERDEEN ANGUS, AFRIKANDER, AQUITAINE BLOND, BEEVBILDE, BELGIAN blue, BELTED GALLOWAY, BONSMARA, BORAN, BRAFORD, BRAHMAN, BRANGUS, BRAUNVIEH, CHARBRAY, CHAROLAIS, CHIANA, CHIANGUS, DEVON, DRAKENSBERGER, DROUGHTMASTER, FULANI, GALLOWAY, GELBVIEH, HARIANA, HEREFORD, JAPANESE BLACK, LIMOUSIN, MAINE-ANJOU, MEUSE-RHINE-YSSEL, MURRAY GREY, N'DAMA, PINZGAU, polled Hereford, ROMAGNA, SANTA GERTRUDIS, SALERS, SHORTHORN, SIMMENTAL, SOUTH DEVON, TEXAS LONGHORN, WEST HIGHLAND and many other less well known indigenous breeds.
b. feedlot see FEEDLOT.
b. grading grading of carcass beef according to quality for the information of the consumer and to provide the trade with a basis for pricing. The grade allotted depends on local requirements for consumers but usually takes into account marbling with fat, absence of excess fat, age and cutability.
hamburger b. see HAMBURGER BEEF.
b. herd comprises the bulls, the mature cows, the heifers yet to calve for the first time, the yearlings including bred heifers and calves not yet weaned. Where calves are not sold off for fattening elsewhere there will also be a bullock group.
b. herd computer simulation model see COMPUTER simulation model.
b. industry includes the beef production, breeding, fattening, marketing, slaughtering and processing and sale of the end product.
b. measles see TAENIA *saginata*.
b. production systems include extensive grazing, intensive grazing, feedlot, cow–calf operations or suckler herds, breeding herds.
b. production targets see performance TARGET.
b. tapeworm see TAENIA *saginata*.
Beef Shorthorn the beef variety of the SHORTHORN breed of cattle.
beefalo a cattle–buffalo hybrid of 37% buffalo, 37% Charolais and 25% Hereford which has achieved only passing fame.
beefling a fat young cattle beast weighing about 500 kg at 1.5 to 2 years of age.
beefy in dog conformation, used to describe overdevelopment of musculature in the hindquarters.
beeper a mobile or static device which emits an auditory warning signal, usually one stimulated by a telemetered signal.
beesbossie [Af.] see CHRYSOCOMA TENUIFOLIA.
beeskaroo [Af.] see CHRYSOCOMA TENUIFOLIA.
beesmelkbos [Af.] EUPHORBIA *mauritanica*.
beestings, biestings, beastings colostrum, usually of a cow.
beet see BETA *vulgaris*.
b. pulp the residue of the roots when the juice is extracted. Highly regarded as a feed supplement for extra energy in high producing cows. Called also beets.
b. tops the foliage of the beet plant, used as green feed but has a high oxalate content.
beetles members of the insect order Coleoptera. They are common intermediate hosts for tapeworms.
darkling b. this and other mealworms are common inhabitants of poultry houses and are suspected of aiding in the transmission of Marek's disease and other virus diseases and of attacking the skin of all types of birds. Their other importance is as a food source for captive reptiles and the like.
beetroot see BETA *vulgaris*.
beevbilde an African crossbred type of beef cattle. Includes Red Lincoln, Shorthorn and Aberdeen Angus blood.
beggar tick see BIDENS FRONDOSA.
behavior the activity or pattern of activity of the patient; can be modified by training and medication; used clinically as a measure of cerebral activity.
abnormal b. includes any activity judged to be outside the normal behavior pattern for animals of that particular class and age, including the vices, the fixed patterns of abnormality.
aggressive b. is common in animals as part of the establishment of territorial rights by males, as competition for sexual favors, because of fear of the unknown, and as maternal protection of young. In companion animals, aggression and dominance directed against humans can also be learned. See also AGGRESSION.
auditory b. the use of the voice to communicate is poorly developed in animals but is used for example in the various voices used by cattle including mooing, lowing, bellowing. Is used most extensively by animals in communicating between mother and young and in courtship.
automatistic b. see stereotypic behavior (below).
communicative b. the behavioral patterns that result in communication between animals. Includes auditory, visual and chemical patterns.
destructive b. involves digging or the destruction of items, such as furniture, doors, or toys, by chewing. Causes include separation anxiety, fear-induced aggression and play aggression.
elimination b. the ritual and method of passing urine and feces, particularly as seen in dogs and cats. This includes searching for the site, pre-elimination behavior of sniffing, scratching, etc., posture and post-elimination action such as scratching the ground or covering feces with dirt. Housetraining involves modification of this behavior.
hallucinatory b. behavior which suggests dementia. This may be inherent or acquired, e.g. shying at nonexistent objects in cows with nervous acetonemia, biting at imaginary flies by dogs.
ingestive b. includes overeating, inadequate intake of food, predation, wool sucking, pica, coprophagia, garbage eating and food-related aggression.
b. modification the use of learning techniques to alter behavior.
predatory b. chasing and killing is commonly dis-

played by cats in catching birds and rodents. Dogs, particularly in packs, may show predatory behavior in threatening and killing of livestock and, in some instances, humans.

sexual b. includes courtship and the mating act. Much of the behavior is visual including posture, feather fluffing, tail carriage; some of it is auditory, especially in cats, but chemical communication via PHEROMONES is the clincher.

social b. behavior relative to others in the group. Includes establishment of the peck order, bulling by steers in feedlots, crowd pressure in the feeding of large groups of pigs, cannibalism in overcrowded communities, even self-immolation in lemming communities. The social stress that may follow abnormal group behavior may result in lowered production, reduction in disease resistance, or the expression of actual disease, e.g. esophagogastric ulcer of pigs.

stereotypic b. constant and repetitive actions, such as vocalization, grooming, walking or weaving, which would otherwise be seen normally in the species. See also OBSESSIVE–COMPULSIVE BEHAVIOR.

thermoregulatory b. actions such as seeking cool places, lapping water, huddling are self-explanatory examples.

visual b. body language for animals. Posture, gait, other body movements all convey information about the animal.

behavioral pertaining to behavior.

b. disorders see VICE.

b. seizure see psychomotor SEIZURE.

b. therapy aims to modify patterns of behavior so that they are acceptable to the owner.

Bejuro marrullero URECHITES LUTEA.

bel a unit used to express the ratio of two powers, usually electric or acoustic powers; an increase of 1 bel in intensity approximately doubles loudness of most sounds (see also DECIBEL).

belching see ERUCTATION.

belemnoid 1. dart-shaped. 2. the styloid process.

Belgian having some relationship to Belgium.

B. barge dog see SCHIPPERKE.

B. black pied cattle black, Belgian dairy cattle.

B. blue dual-purpose cattle; blue, white or blue roan. Bred by crossing Dutch Friesian with British Shorthorn. Calves are large and dystocia common.

B. canary one of the oldest breeds of canaries, popular in the Victorian era. Characterized by a straight, upright back, but lowered head and neck so the shoulders are the highest point.

B. cattle dog see BOUVIER DES FLANDRES.

B. fancy long, slim canaries with flat chests, long necks and tail feathers, with an unusual posture of the head drooping down and a semicircular silhouette. Called also Slims, Scottish Fancy.

B. hare not a hare at all, but a breed of rabbit. It has a long, fine body and a deep red, tan or chestnut agouti coat.

B. horse heavy draft horse, mostly red-roan or chestnut but may be bay, brown, dun or gray; 16.1 to 17 hands high. A basic breed for many draft breeds. Called also Brabant. Full name is Belgian Heavy Draft. Affected by congenital cataracts and aniridia, which are inherited as a dominant trait.

B. Malinois, B. Tervuren two varieties of Belgian sheep herding dogs, recognized in the United States as separate breeds. See Belgian shepherd dog (below).

B. red cattle red, dual-purpose cattle from Belgium.

B. red pied cattle red and white, dual-purpose Belgian cattle.

B. sheep dog see Belgian shepherd dog (below).

B. shepherd dog there are several varieties in this breed. All are medium-sized with erect ears and are used as sheepdogs, guard dogs and for police work. The *Groenendael*, the most common variety, has a long, straight, smooth black coat. In the United States, it is recognized as a separate breed and called the Belgian sheepdog. The *Malinois* has a short, red, fawn or gray coat with black mask and frosting on the muzzle. It is called the Belgian Malinois in the United States. The *Tervueren* has a long, red, fawn or gray coat and is called the Belgian Tervueren in the United States. The *Laekenois* has a short, wiry reddish-fawn coat with black shading.

Bell–Magendie law the commonly accepted principle that the dorsal roots of spinal nerves contain only afferent or sensory fibers and that the ventral roots carry only efferent or motor ones. The law is generally valid but many of the fibers in the ventral roots are in fact afferent.

bell-mare a quiet old horse used to carry a bell at night so that horses can be located easily in scrub, in the dark or in a big paddock.

bell stage the period when the cap of enamel organ on the developing tooth is converted to a bell shape in cross section.

bell vine IPOMOEA *plebeia*.

bell-wether a tame wether which will lead a flock to a desired destination. Found usually at abattoirs and sale yards.

bella sombra PHYTOLACCA *dioica*.

belladonna *Atropa belladonna* (deadly nightshade), a plant that is the source of various alkaloids, e.g. atropine, hyoscyamine, etc.

b. leaf the dried leaves and fruiting tops of *Atropa belladonna*, used as an anticholinergic in the management of gastrointestinal disorders.

b. poisoning a severe toxic condition due to overdosage of belladonna or accidental ingestion of large amounts of the drug. Signs include dryness of the mouth, thirst, dilated pupils, tachycardia, fever and stupor.

bellies wool from the belly of the sheep.

pork b. a popular fictional commodity in futures markets on the stock exchange.

bellow one of the voices of cattle. Usually refers to the arrogant call of the bull used to announce territorial rights. Abnormalities of the voice include hoarseness as in rabies, or continuous repetition as in nervous acetonemia. See also LOW, MOO.

bellowing see BELLOW.

b. continuously in bovine rabies, continues until pharyngeal paralysis supervenes.

b. soundlessly cattle sffected by rabies in its late stages may make all movements as though bellowing but no sound happens, usually accompanied by inability to swallow and later by drooling of saliva.

bellows a term used to refer to the action produced by an intact thorax and diaphragm in inspiration and expiration.

b. disruption injury, usually by trauma, that disrupts the effectiveness of the thorax and diaphragm in moving air, e.g. puncture wounds of the thorax, flail chest and rupture of the diaphragm.

belly 1. the softer, ventral part of the abdomen. 2. the fleshy, contractile part of a muscle.

b. board a board attached to a cable or wire fence to ensure that cattle see the fence and do not injure themselves charging into it.

bellyache bush JATROPHA *gossypifolia*.

bellyband a part of the cart harness which is continuous with the backband and keeps the shafts from lifting the backband off.
Belted Galloway a breed of beef cattle, a variant of the Galloway breed. It is polled and black except for a genetically dominant wide band of white completely encircling its trunk behind the elbow.
belton a coat color pattern seen in the English setter dog consisting of ticking or roan in any one of several colors.
Beltsville No. 1 black-and-white pig with moderately lop ears.
Beltsville No. 2 red pig with white underline, and short, erect ears.
beluga the arctic dolphin. See DELPHINAPTERUS LEUCAS.
bemegride a respiratory analeptic and non-specific barbiturate antagonist.
benazepril an angiotensin converting enzyme inhibitor, similar to enalapril, used in the treatment of heart failure.
Bence Jones protein immunoglobulin light chain dimers found in the serum and urine of patients and animals with gammopathies, usually myelomas.
benchmark a point of reference about which comparisons can be made.
bendiocarb a carbamate pesticide.
Bendixen's key a hematological key used in the diagnosis of bovine viral leukosis. It is based on absolute lymphocyte counts in relation to age and classifies animals as normal, suspect or positive for the disease. It is not used widely as persistent lymphocytosis is not universally accepted as a preclinical sign of bovine viral leukosis nor is it restricted to that disease.
bendroflumethiazide, bendrofluazide a thiazide diuretic and antihypertensive; it enhances the excretion of sodium and chloride.
bends decompression sickness; a condition resulting from a too-rapid decrease in atmospheric pressure, as when a deep-sea diver is brought too hastily to the surface. The term bends is derived from the bodily contortions its victims undergo when atmospheric pressure is abruptly changed from a high pressure to a relatively lower one. A form of altitude sickness suffered by aviators who ascend too rapidly to high altitudes is similar to bends. Bends may also be a complication in a type of oxygen therapy called HYPERBARIC oxygenation, in which the patient is placed in a high-pressure chamber to increase the oxygen content of its blood. Likely to be an uncommon diagnosis in animals.
Benedenia a genus of the class of monogenetic Trematoda in the order Capsalidae; it is an important oral and cutaneous fluke parasite of aquarium, cultured and marine fish.
Benedict's solution, Benedict's reagent a chemical solution used to determine the presence of glucose and other reducing substances in the urine.
Benedinia see NEOBENEDINIA.
benefit–cost analysis a technique of economic evaluation, particularly for complex projects over a long period of time and involving substantial capital, that takes into account social costs and benefits as well as financial considerations.
benefit–cost ratio the ratio of the net present values of measurable benefits to costs. Used in benefit–cost analysis.
Bengal a breed of cats developed from crossing Asian leopard cats with domestic cats. It has a long, muscular body, small rounded ears, large oval eyes and a short coat with large tabby-like markings. The breed is affected by entropion.
Bengal goat small to dwarf milk and meat goat, usually black, also gray, brown or white; prolific, bearded, short coat and ears. Called also Black Bengal.
benign not malignant; not recurrent; favorable for recovery.
b. enzootic paresis see porcine viral ENCEPHALOMYELITIS.
b. fibrillators horses with a history of poor performance in races which suffer an attack of atrial fibrillation during or immediately after a race which soon recovers spontaneously so that the abnormality often goes undetected.
b. footrot occurs under very wet conditions. Caused by *Dichelobacter nodosus* of low virulence. There is dermatitis of the interdigital skin and minimal underrunning of horn at the heel. See also INTERDIGITAL dermatitis.
benoxaprofen a prostaglandin and leukotriene inhibitor used in the treatment of canine enterotoxemia.
benoxinate hydrochloride a surface anesthetic for the eye.
benthos bottom of the sea or other body of water; said of cyanobacteria which grow on submerged rocks in alpine lakes and cause sudden death in cattle at pasture during summer months.
bentiromide a synthetic peptide (*N*-benzoyl-L-tyrosyl-*p*-aminobenzoic acid) used in the BT-PABA TEST to assess chymotrypsin activity in the small intestine.
bentiromide test see BT-PABA TEST.
bentiromide/xylose test a test to assess digestion and absorption; indirectly measures exocrine pancreatic function (bentiromide; called also BT-PABA) and the absorptive surface (xylose) of the small intestine. See also PARA-AMINOBENZOIC ACID.
bentleg see BOWIE.
bentonite a naturally occurring pure clay capable of absorbing much moisture and swelling considerably. Used as a compacting and dispersing agent in the manufacture of fodder pellets and cat litter. Chemically and nutritionally inert.
b. flocculation test a superseded test for hydatidosis in humans.
sodium b. used as a binder in pellet manufacture. A refined form of clay.
benzalkonium chloride a quaternary ammonium compound used as a surface disinfectant and detergent and as a topical antiseptic and antimicrobial preservative. See also ZEPHIRAN.
benzathine an ammonium base which when combined with penicillin compounds prolongs their sojourn in tissues. The most common combinations are benzathine cloxacillin, used in the treatment of bovine mastitis, and benzathine penicillin.
benzcoumarins see clover UROLITH.
benzedrine see AMPHETAMINE.
benzene a liquid hydrocarbon, C_6H_6, from coal tar; used as a solvent.
b. hexachloride a chlorinated hydrocarbon. The gamma isomer was used extensively as an insecticide. Called also Gammexane, LINDANE.
b. hexachloride poisoning see CHLORINATED HYDROCARBONS.
b. ring the closed hexagon of carbon atoms in benzene, from which the different benzene compounds are derived by replacement of the hydrogen atoms.
benzestrol a synthetic estrogen, derived from diethylstilbestrol.

benzethonium chloride a synthetic quaternary ammonium compound used as a local anti-infective and as a detergent and disinfectant.

benzidine a compound used as a test for traces of blood (benzidine test).

benzimidazole a group of compounds with excellent anthelmintic properties. They all have the same central chemical structure—1,2-diaminobenzene. Some of the better known pharmaceutical compounds are THIABENDAZOLE, ALBENDAZOLE, CAMBENDAZOLE, FENBENDAZOLE, MEBENDAZOLE, OXFENDAZOLE, OXIBENDAZOLE and PARBENDAZOLE.

benzoate a salt of benzoic acid.

benzocaine a local anesthetic for topical use.

benzodiazepine any of a group of drugs having similar molecular structure. A drug in this group that has significant use in veterinary medicine is diazepam (Valium).

benzodioxans a class of synthetic α-receptor blocking agents used to lower blood pressure.

benzoic acid an acid from benzoin and other resins and from coal tar, used as an antifungal agent in pharmaceutical preparations and as a germicide. The sodium salt of benzoic acid, sodium benzoate, is used as an antifungal agent in pharmaceutical preparations, and may be used as a test for liver function. It was at one time used as a food preservative although now replaced in pet foods because of its toxicity in cats.

benzoin a balsamic resin from *Styrax benzoin* and other *Styrax* species, used chiefly as a topical protectant and antiseptic. Benzoin acts as an expectorant and thus is sometimes used in steam inhalations in treating respiratory disorders.

benzonatate a non-narcotic antitussive drug that depresses cough without affecting respiration.

benzothiadiazide see THIAZIDE.

benzoyl the acyl radical formed from benzoic acid, C_6H_5CO–.

b. peroxide dibenzoyl peroxide, a topical keratolytic with antibacterial and antipruritic properties, used in the treatment of skin diseases.

benzthiazide a thiazide diuretic. Called also benzothiadiazide. See also THIAZIDE.

benzydroflumethiazide see BENDROFLUMETHIAZIDE.

benzyl the hydrocarbon radical, C_7H_7.

b. alcohol a colorless liquid used as a bacteriostatic in solutions for injection, and also topically as a local anesthetic.

b. benzoate a clear, oily liquid used as a topical scabicide and with dimercaprol as an antidote in metal poisoning. Toxic in cats.

benzylpenicillin see PENICILLIN G.

bephenium an anthelmintic used as the embonate and hydroxynaphthoate.

BER basal energy requirement.

Berber sheep Moroccan carpetwool sheep, white, black or white with black head.

berberine a poisonous pyridine alkaloid found in the weeds *Argemone, Berberis, Mahonia* spp.

Berberis genus in the plant family Berberidaceae; contains berberine, a pyridine alkaloid; causes cardiomyopathy and congestive heart failure. Called also barberries.

Bergamasco a medium to large-sized Italian sheepdog with a long black or gray coat of harsh texture which forms into strands or loose mats.

Bergamo basic Lop-eared Alpine type of sheep; polled, used for meat and carpetwool. Origin of many other breeds of this type, found in the Alpine region of Central Europe.

Berge nerve block a technique for retrobulbar anesthesia of the eye in the horse.

Berger de Beauce a large French sheepdog, also used for military work. It is related to the Briard. It has a short coat of black with tan markings, or harlequin. The ears are usually cropped. Double dewclaws are required on the rear legs. Called also Beuceron, French shorthaired shepherd, Bas rouge.

Berger de Brie see BRIARD.

Bergmann's glia a specialized form of astrocytes in the Purkinje cell layer of the cerebellum.

Bergmeister's papilla a vestigial lesion of the eye due to incomplete atrophy of the posterior segment mesoderm. It is a cone of glial tissue with a vascular core which extends from the optic disk for a few millimeters into the vitreous humor in cattle.

bergslankop URGINEA *capitata*.

beriberi the name given to thiamin deficiency in humans. See THIAMIN nutritional deficiency.

Berkefeld's filter a filter composed of diatomaceous earth, impermeable to ordinary bacteria.

berkelium a chemical element, atomic number 97, atomic weight 247, symbol Bk. See Table 6.

Berkshire a sometime breed of pigs bred chiefly for pork. Characterized by a dished face and a black coat with white points. A variant with a longer body than the British breed is the Canadian Berkshire.

Berkson's bias a type of selection bias which may occur in case-control studies which are based entirely on hospital studies.

Bermuda buttercup OXALIS *pes-caprae*.

Bermuda grass CYNODON *dactylon*.

Bermuda oxalis OXALIS *pres-caprae*.

Berne virus see TOROVIRUS.

Bernese canary an uncommon breed; it is yellow or variegated, with smooth plumage.

Bernese mountain dog a large, sturdy, longhaired black dog with white feet, tail tip and chest markings, and brown or tan markings. The coat is thick and slightly wavy. It is a Swiss breed originally used as a cart dog. Called also Swiss mountain dog, although it is only one of four varieties. The breed is affected by malignant histiocytosis, hip dysplasia, elbow dysplasia and hypomyelinogenesis. Called also Bernese sennenhund.

Bernese sennenhund see BERNESE MOUNTAIN DOG.

Bernoulli principle a principle which relates to the flow of fluids through tubes: the total hydraulic energy of fluid moving along a tube is constant so that if the tube dilates and causes the velocity to decrease, the kinetic energy involved in moving the fluid is reduced resulting in an increase in the lateral pressure on the vessel wall. This accounts for the tendency for aneurysms to enlarge and for vessels to dilate below a constriction.

Berrichon du cher a French breed of milking sheep.

berrigan EREMOPHILA *longifolia*.

berry cottonbush see ENCHYLAENA TOMENTOSA.

Berry–Dedrick phenomenon the occurrence of typical myxoma in rabbits when injected with a mixture of myxomatosis virus that has been inactivated by heat and viable fibroma virus. The explanation is that the nucleic acid of the inactivated myxomavirus is incorporated into the protein coat of the fibromavirus. The hybrid particles which result retain the coding of the myxomavirus and cause myxomatosis.

berry poison GASTROLOBIUM *parvifolium*.

Bersama abyssinica a small African tree of the plant family Melicanthaceae; ingestion of the leaves causes salivation, profuse diarrhea, collapse and death; may contain cardiac glycosides.

Berteroa incana toxic plant in Brassicacae family; suspected of containing SMCO; causes hemolytic anemia and hemoglobinuria in ruminants and laminitis and abortion in horses. Called also hoary alyssum.

Bertiella a genus of nonpathogenic tapeworm of the family Anoplocephalidae. Includes *B. mucronata, B. studeri* (primates), *B. obesa* (koala).

bertielliasis infestation with *Bertiella* spp. tapeworms. Occurs in primates, possums, koalas and occasionally in humans and dogs.

Berula erecta toxic plant, a member of the Apiaceae family. Causes diarrhea, enteritis, milk taint. Called also water parsnip.

beryllium a chemical element, atomic number 4, atomic weight 9.012, symbol Be. See Table 6.

b. sulfate used as a vaccine adjuvant. Causes local granuloma formation which is believed to enhance antibody formation by stimulating T lymphocytes.

besembos [Af.] CROTALARIA *spartioides*.

Besnier–Boeck disease see SARCOID (1).

Besnoitia a genus of sporozoan parasites in the family Sarcocystidae. There are a number of species that are found only in wild animals. Horses and cattle are affected by disease in their role as intermediate hosts. In many of the species the definitive host is the cat. In the others the definitive host has not been identified.

B. bennetti causes BESNOITIOSIS of horses and donkeys.

B. besnoiti causes BESNOITIOSIS of cattle.

B. darlingi found in opossums, possibly lizards.

B. wallacei found in cats.

besnoitiosis the cutaneous form of besnoitiosis in horses and burros, caused by *Besnoitia bennetti*; characterized by a widespread, serious dermatitis. The disease in cattle, caused by *B. besnoiti*, is a systemic one manifested by swelling of the lymph nodes, subcutaneous swellings, diarrhea and abortion.

Besser–Lowry–Brock unit a unit used in the measurement of enzyme activity for acid or alkaline phosphatase.

best fit when making a diagnosis, the technique of finding amongst the diseases on the shortlist the one that is the best fit to the syndrome observed.

best linear unbiased prediction (BLUP) acronym for a statistical method of predicting the breeding values of animals. Fixed effects of environment and genetics on observed phenotypic values are estimated simultaneously and, therefore, genetic differences between herds are accounted for. BLUP animal models are now used in many countries for a number of species, including dairy and beef cattle, swine, sheep and fish.

besylate USAN contraction for benzenesulfonate.

Beta a genus of the Polygonaceae family.

B. vulgaris this species includes the large fodder roots. They provide a massive source of feed energy but they can cause poisoning if used unintelligently, e.g. (1) carbohydrate engorgement and lactic acidosis if too many are fed; (2) partly cooked mangels grown on high nitrate soils may cause primary nitrite poisoning; (3) the tops may contain toxic amounts of oxalate; (4) a sole diet of beet pulp is thought to cause a nutritional deficiency of vitamin A in cattle leading to blindness and encephalopathy. Called also fodder beet, sugar beet, mangels, mangolds, mangelwurzel, beetroot.

beta the second letter of the Greek alphabet, Β or β; used to denote the second position in a chemical classification system. Often used in names of chemical compounds to distinguish one of two or more isomers or to indicate the position of substituent atoms or groups in certain compounds. Also used to distinguish types of radioactive decay; brain rhythms or waves; adrenergic receptors; secretory cells of the various organs of the body that stain with basic dyes, such as the beta cells of the pancreas; and the type of hemolysis induced by bacteria that results in a zone of complete hemolysis when grown on blood agar, except for staphylococci.

b. adrenergic see ADRENERGIC.

b.-adrenergic receptors, β-adrenergic receptors specific sites on effector cells that respond to epinephrine. There are two types: β_1-receptors, found in the heart and small intestine, and β_2-receptors, found in the bronchi, blood vessels and uterus.

b. agonists see ADRENERGIC.

b. barrels a form of secondary structure of a polypeptide in which β strands of amino acids are wound into a super secondary structure; usually interconnected by α helical regions of the polypeptide on the outside of the molecule.

b.-blocker a drug that blocks the action of epinephrine at beta-adrenergic receptors on cells of effector organs. There are two types of these receptors: β_1-receptors in the myocardium and β_2-receptors in the bronchial and vascular smooth muscles. The principal effects of beta-adrenergic stimulation are increased heart rate and contractility, vasodilation of the arterioles that supply the skeletal muscles, and relaxation of bronchial muscles.

b. brain waves those having a frequency of more than 10 hertz (pulsations per second); seen during wakefulness. See also ELECTROENCEPHALOGRAPHY.

b.-carboline indoleamine alkaloid poisoning causes a nervous syndrome of hyper- or hypomotility, muscle tremor, flexed paresis of fore- or hindlimbs, hypermetria, walking backwards, convulsions. A plant poison found in *Peganum, Tribulus, Kallstroemia* spp.

b. carbon carbon-3 of a molecule or the carbon atom two on from the function group of a molecule, the carbon(s) of which are not included in the lettering.

b.-endorphin hormone secreted by central nervous system, hypothalamus, gastrointestinal tract. See also ENDORPHIN.

b. fibrillosis see AMYLOIDOSIS.

b.-folded domains compact, locally folded region of tertiary structure containing the β-sheets or β-turns.

b. hemolysin is a sphingomyelinase and is produced by staphylococci. It produces partial hemolysis of sheep and cattle erythrocytes. It appears to have little pathogenic effect. See also beta HEMOLYSIS.

b.-hydroxy-beta-methylglutaryl coenzyme A 1. intermediate in the formation of ketones. 2. key starting compound in the synthesis of cholesterol.

b.-hydroxybutyrate salt of the major circulating ketone body in animals, formed from the reduction of ACETOACETIC ACID.

b.-hydroxybutyrate dehydrogenase mitochondrial enzyme catalyzing the NADH-linked-reduction of acetoacetate to β-hydroxybutyrate.

b.-ketobutyric acid ACETOACETIC ACID.

b. particle an electron emitted from a nucleus.

b. radiation see RADIATION injury, RADIOTHERAPY.

b. sheet (β-sheet) a common structural feature of many proteins in which the single polypeptide chain is folded back and forth upon itself with each folded section running in an opposite direction to its nearest neighbors. The folded sections are held together by hydrogen bonds and the arrangement which occurs particularly in the core of proteins, confers great stability on the molecule.

b. subunit second-named chain (or subunit) occurring in the functional organization of macromolecules, usually proteins, containing two or more chains.

beta-carotene see CAROTENE.

beta-responsive sympathomimetic drugs drugs which cause bronchial dilation and cardiac stimulation.

Betadine a proprietary name for povidone-iodine.

Betaherpesvirinae one of three subfamilies within the family HERPESVIRIDAE. Called also CYTOMEGALOVIRUS.

betaine the carboxylic acid derived by oxidation of choline; it acts as a transmethylating metabolic intermediate.

betamethasone a long-acting synthetic glucocorticoid, used as an anti-inflammatory.

betatron an apparatus for accelerating electrons to millions of electron volts by magnetic induction.

betaxolol a topical sympatholytic agent used to reduce intraocular pressure in the treatment of glaucoma.

betazole a histamine analog used in gastric function tests to stimulate gastric secretion. Called also ametazole, gastramine.

bethanechol a choline ester with parasympathomimetic effects similar to acetylcholine; primarily a muscarinic agonist with little effect on nicotinic receptors. The chloride salt is used for urinary retention.

Betta splendens brightly colored tropical freshwater fish of the family Anabantidae; adult males have to be kept in separate tanks because of their aggressive behavior. Called also SIAMESE FIGHTING FISH.

Betz cells large pyramidal cells forming a layer in restricted parts of the cerebral cortex.

Beuceron see BERGER DE BEAUCE.

beukesbossie [Af.] see LIPPIA REHMANNII.

Beveren a large Belgian breed of fur rabbits, blue, black, brown or white with a dense, silky coat of short (1 to 1.5 in) fur, a pronounced Roman nose, big ears and a broad muzzle.

bevy a flock of birds.

bezoar a mass formed in the stomach by compaction of repeatedly ingested material that does not pass into the intestine. See also PHYTOBEZOAR, TRICHOBEZOAR.

Bezold–Jarisch reflex reflex cardiac slowing, hypotension and apnea caused by intravenous injection of veratrine, nicotine and some antihistamines.

BFU-E burst forming unit-ERYTHROID.

BGP see OSTEOCALCIN.

Bhalfilaria ladamii the only species in the genus *Bhalfilaria* which is in the family Filariidae. It is to be found in the heart of chickens in some parts of India.

BHC, γ-BHC see BENZENE hexachloride.

Bhotia pony Indian mountain riding and pack pony, white or bay; similar to Tibetan pony.

BHP blood hydrostatic pressure; the pressure exerted by the blood cells and plasma in the capillaries.

BHS beta-hemolytic streptococci.

BHV2 bovine herpesvirus-2.

Bi chemical symbol, *bismuth.*

bi- word element. [L.] *two.*

***bi* syndrome** *bi* in acupuncture terminology means obstruction; it may be wandering, painful, fixed, febrile.

biangled tube an x-ray tube with a rotating anode in which the surface of the anode disk has two target surfaces which are at different angles to the electron beam.

biarticular affecting two joints.

biarticulate having two joints.

bias any systematic error in the design, conduct or analysis of a study which results in estimates which depart from true values. An unbiased study is free from systematic error. Many types of bias have been named, but three general types can be identified, selection bias, information bias and CONFOUNDING. **Selection bias** is a systematic error in a study caused by the individuals selected into the study being different from the entire target population in an important way. See also BERKSON'S BIAS. **Information bias** is a systematic error in a study caused by errors in the data which is collected in the study, or in the analysis of the data.

bible meatworkers' name for omasum.

bibliographical pertaining to the literature of a subject.

b. tools the ways in which a bibliography can be approached or managed. These include current literature scans, article indexes, compilations of abstracts, lists of current contents, abstracting journals, lists of titles, subject reviews, bibliographies, lists of headings, lists of headwords and synonyms, computerized databases and thesauruses.

bicameral having two chambers or cavities.

bicapsular having two capsules.

bicarbonate any salt containing the HCO_3^- anion.

blood b. the bicarbonate of the blood plasma, an important parameter of ACID–BASE BALANCE measured in BLOOD GAS ANALYSIS. Called also plasma bicarbonate.

b. buffering major body buffering system in ACID–BASE BALANCE.

plasma b. see blood bicarbonate (above).

b. of soda sodium bicarbonate.

bicarotid trunk rupture a rare cause of sudden death in horses.

bicaudal, bicaudate having two tails.

Bicaulus a genus of nematode worms in the family Protostrongylidae. Now included in the genus *Varestrongylus.* Includes *B. sagitattus, B. schulzi* (sheep, goat, deer; lungs).

bicellular made up of two cells.

bicephalus a two-headed monster.

biceps a muscle having two heads. There is a biceps muscle in both fore- and hindlimbs. See Table 13. See also BICIPITAL.

b. brachii is a large fusiform muscle lying on the cranial surface of the humerus. Its function is to flex the elbow and integrate the actions of the shoulder and elbow. A medial displacement of the tendon of origin has been reported in dogs, causing a weight-bearing lameness.

b. femoris a large muscle of the caudolateral part of the thigh. Its function is to extend the hindlimb when propelling the body, during rearing or kicking. All of the joints are affected except those of the digit.

Rupture of the muscle causes acute hindlimb lameness in cattle. Resembles an intermittent upward fixation of the patella, with extension of the stifle and hock.

b. reflex is elicited in dogs by striking a finger placed on the biceps tendon on the craniomedial aspect of the elbow. An active reflex indicates intact spinal cord segments and nerve roots C6–8 and musculocutaneous nerve. It becomes exaggerated in disease of the upper motor neuron.

b. tendon ossification causes lameness in the horse. Is radiographically apparent.

bichloride a chloride containing two equivalents of chlorine.

Bichon frise a small lively dog with a fine, silky, pure white coat that forms soft corkscrew curls, giving a fluffy appearance. The tail is carried over the back and the topknot gives a rounded appearance to the head.

bicipital having two heads; pertaining to a BICEPS muscle.

b. bursa lies between the tendon of the biceps brachii muscle and the bicipital groove of the humerus. See also intertuberal BURSA.

b. bursitis inflammation of the bicipital bursa over the point of the shoulder where the tendon of the biceps bends over the humerus. Usually follows trauma and is characterized by a reduced stride, circumduction and dropped elbow. Forced extension of the limb and deep palpation of the joint causes pain.

b. tendon tendon of the biceps muscle.

bicolor a coat color of two colors, usually black with tan markings but may be other combinations such as ticking on a white background.

biconcave having two concave surfaces.

biconvex having two convex surfaces.

bicornate, bicornuate, bicornual having two horns or cornua, e.g. bicornuate uterus.

bicorporate having two bodies.

bicuspid 1. having two cusps. 2. bicuspid (mitral) valve. 3. in humans, a premolar tooth.

b.i.d. [L.] *bis in die* (twice a day). Called also bid.

Bidder's organ a vestigial ovary found in toads.

Bidens frondosa a North american plant in the Asteraceae family; may cause nitrite poisoning in ruminants because of a high content of nitrate. Called also beggar tick.

bidirectional operates in both directions, e.g. a computer printer which prints alternate lines in the opposite direction. Called also boustrophedonic, but only by pedants.

biduous lasting 2 days.

Biebrich scarlet see SCARLET RED.

Bier technique intravenous injection of a local anesthetic into a portion of the body isolated by a tourniquet, e.g. a distal limb, to anesthetize sensory motor nerves to the whole area. Called also intravenous regional analgesia.

bifid cleft into two parts or branches.

Bifidobacterium a genus of gram-positive obligately anerobic lactobacilli commonly occurring in the feces.

biforate having two perforations or foramina.

bifunctional enzyme an enzyme containing two distinct catalytic capacities in the same polypeptide chain, e.g. phosphofructokinase II and fructose-2,6-bisphosphatase, which controls the concentration of fructose-2,6-bisP, the major allosteric regulator of glycolysis (+ve) and gluconeogenesis (–ve).

bifurcate divided into two branches.

bifurcation 1. a division into two branches. 2. the point at which division into two branches occurs.

tracheal b. termination of the trachea, where it divides into two principal bronchi.

Big bend loco ASTRAGALUS *mollisimus* var. *earlei*.

Big bend lupine LUPINUS *leucopsis*.

big-dog little-dog syndrome injuries of the cervical region incurred by small dogs when attacked by large dogs that pick them up by the neck and shake them violently.

big-knee see CAPRINE arthritis–encephalitis.

big sage *Artemisia nova*.

big trefoil LOTUS *major*.

Bigelowia rusbeyi HAPLOPAPPUS *heterophyllus*.

bigeminy the condition of occurring in twos, especially the occurrence of two pulse beats in rapid succession.

ventricular b. an electrocardiographic tracing showing the pairing of sinus beat and a ventricular premature contraction.

bighead a general swelling of the head.

equine b. see OSTEODYSTROPHIA FIBROSA.

ovine b. a form of malignant edema due to *Clostridium novyi* in rams, usually the result of fighting. Called also swelled head.

yellow b. a syndrome of photosensitive dermatitis, causing edema of the ears and face, and a concurrent jaundice in sheep. Usually found in association with poisoning with millet or other *Panicum* spp. grasses, or *Tribulus terrestris*; called also geeldikkop, dikoor.

bighead carp HYPOPHTHALMICHTHYS *nobilis*.

Bighorn sheep a tall (up to 3 ft), heavy (up to 300 lb body weight) wild sheep that lives in inaccessible mountain country where it exercises its principal achievement of prodigious leaping and climbing. Called also *Ovis canadensis*. Several regional varieties, e.g. *O. c. californiana*, Californian bighorn sheep.

bigleg see sporadic LYMPHANGITIS.

biglycan a small chondroitin sulfate proteoglycan found in mineralized bone.

Big'n blue see AMERICAN BLUE GASCON HOUND.

biguanides a class of disinfectants, the most common one being CHLORHEXIDINE.

bike see SULKY.

Bikukulla see DICENTRA.

bilateral having two sides; pertaining to both sides.

bilayer a membrane layer two molecules thick.

phospholipid b. a layer containing two phospholipid molecules which is the basic structural unit of all biological membranes.

bile a clear yellow, orange or green fluid produced by the liver. It is concentrated and stored in the gallbladder, and is poured into the small intestine via the bile ducts when needed for digestion. Bile helps in alkalinizing the intestinal contents and plays a role in the digestion and absorption of fat; its chief constitutents are conjugated bile salts, cholesterol, phospholipid, bilirubin and electrolytes. See also BILE DUCT, BILIARY.

b. acids steroid acids derived from cholesterol; classified as primary, those synthesized in the liver, e.g. cholic and chenodeoxycholic acid, or secondary, those produced from primary bile acids by intestinal bacteria and returned to the liver by enterohepatic circulation, e.g. deoxycholic and lithocholic acid.

b. acid assay are used in the diagnosis of liver disease and portacaval shunts when there are increased levels in the blood.

b. lake bile duct obstruction may cause distension and rupture of biliary canaliculi. Small bile lakes result causing focal hepatic necrosis.

b. passages bile canaliculi drain into bile ductules and interlobular ducts. These unite to form a series of hepatic ducts which carry the bile to the porta where they unite to form the common hepatic duct. This duct receives a cystic duct from the gallbladder (absent in the horse) and thence becomes the BILE DUCT.

b. peritonitis leakage of bile from the common bile duct or gallbladder may occur as a result of trauma, including perforation during percutaneous needle biopsy of the liver, and (rarely) erosion from biliary calculi. A chemical peritonitis results and may be fatal unless surgical repair is accomplished.

b. pigment any one of the coloring matters of the bile; they are BILIRUBIN, biliverdin, bilifuscin, biliprasin, choleprasin, bilihumin and bilicyanin. See also UROBILINOGEN, STERCOBILIN.

b. pleuritis inflammation of the pleura resulting from perforating thoracic trauma with hepatodiaphragmatic fistula or iatrogenically from percutaneous liver biopsy techniques.

b. reflux usually refers to movement of bile from the duodenum into the stomach where it may alter the gastric mucosal barrier causing gastritis and ulceration.

b. salts see TAUROCHOLATE, CHENODEOXYCHOLIC ACID, GLYCOCHOLIC ACID.

white b. 1. bile containing much mucin. 2. bile trapped in obstructed system for a long period and from which pigments have been resorbed.

bile duct 1. generally, any of the biliary passages. 2. specifically the terminal segment of the biliary tree extending from the union of the common hepatic duct and cystic duct to the major duodenal papilla. See also BILE passages.

b. d. atresia if it is extensive it causes jaundice and steatorrhea soon after birth. It is observed rarely in kittens and puppies.

b. d. calculi see CHOLELITHIASIS.

b. d. canaliculi formed between adjacent hepatocytes these are the smallest components of the biliary system; they open into biliary ductules.

b. d. carcinoma see CHOLANGIOCELLULAR carcinoma.

b. d. cysts occur in all species and are probably derived from occluded or atretic embryonic bile ducts.

b. d. ductule bile duct.

b. d. dyskinesia a much-argued diagnosis in human medicine. The diagnosis assumes that there is a failure of biliary flow into the intestine for other than physical reasons. The hypothesis likens the problem to that of irritable colon. There is no proof of the existence of the malfunction in humans, much less in animals.

b. d. fibrosis a common severe lesion, accompanied by mineralization, as a result of infestation by *Fasciola hepatica*.

b. d. hyperplasia may be part of a general reaction of the liver but is most important as a purely cholangiolar proliferation, usually as a result of exposure to a poison such as BUTTER YELLOW.

b. d. inflammation see CHOLANGIOHEPATITIS.

b. d. obstruction see BILIARY obstruction.

b. d. proliferation see bile duct hyperplasia (above).

b. d. radiology see CHOLANGIOGRAPHY.

b. d. rupture/perforation most ruptures are traumatic and result in leakage of bile into the peritoneal cavity. See also biliary PERITONITIS.

b. d. tumors see CHOLANGIOCELLULAR.

bilharziasis see SCHISTOSOMIASIS.

Bilharziella a genus of the family Schistosomatidae.

B. polonica a trematode parasite found in the abdominal blood vessels of ducks.

bilharziosis see SCHISTOSOMIASIS.

bili- word element. [L.] *bile*.

biliary pertaining to the bile, to the bile ducts, or to the gallbladder. See also BILE DUCT.

b. excretion removal in the bile of substances including drugs, toxins, hormones or pigments, or their breakdown products. These are delivered to the duodenum and removed in the feces.

b. fever see BABESIOSIS.

b. fibrosis one of the three forms of hepatic fibrosis; largely confined to the portal triads; see also BILE DUCT fibrosis.

b. infarct areas of hepatic fibrosis that physically resemble vascular infarcts but are related to damaged bile ducts.

interlobular b. duct see BILE DUCT.

b. obstruction obstruction of biliary ducts may be intra- or extrahepatic, and intraluminal (calculi) or by external compression by tumor mass or cicatricial contraction, or more commonly in food animals by migrating ascarid larvae in the bile ducts or by cholangitis caused by *Fasciola hepatica* or *Dichrocoelium dendriticum*. Jaundice is the outstanding clinical sign of the condition. See also CHOLESTASIS.

b. salts see bile SALT.

b. stones see CHOLELITHIASIS.

b. tract the organs, ducts, etc., participating in secretion (the liver), storage (the gallbladder, if present), and delivery (hepatic and bile ducts) of bile into the duodenum.

biligenesis production of bile.

biligenic producing bile.

bililith gallstone.

bililithiasis see CHOLELITHIASIS.

bilious vomiting syndrome duodenogastric reflux of bile; early morning vomiting in dogs, believed to be due to a mild gastritis caused by reflux of bile during sleep.

biliousness a symptom complex in humans comprising nausea, abdominal discomfort, headache and constipation, formerly attributed to excessive bile secretion.

bilirachia the presence of bile pigments in the spinal fluid.

bilirubin an orange bile pigment produced by the breakdown of heme and reduction of biliverdin; it normally circulates in plasma and is taken up by liver cells and conjugated to form bilirubin diglucuronide, the water-soluble pigment excreted in the bile. Failure of the liver cells to excrete bile, or obstruction of the BILE DUCTS, can cause an increased amount of bilirubin in the body fluids and thus lead to obstructive or regurgitation jaundice.

Another type of jaundice results from excessive destruction of erythrocytes (hemolytic or retention jaundice). The more rapid the destruction of red blood cells and the degradation of hemoglobin, the greater the amount of bilirubin in the body fluids.

Most bilirubin is excreted in the feces. A small amount is excreted in the urine as urobilinogen.

conjugated b. bilirubin that has been conjugated, mainly to glucuronic acid, in the liver and gives a direct result to the VAN DEN BERGH TEST. High blood levels indicate obstructive or hepatocellular origin of the jaundice.

b. diglucuronide see conjugated bilirubin (above).

b. toxicity see KERNICTERUS.

unconjugated b. bilirubin that has not been conjugated in the liver. It gives an indirect reaction to the VAN DEN BERGH TEST. A high level of it in the blood is indicative of hemolysis or a lack of bilirubin clearance by the liver.

bilirubinemia the presence of bilirubin in the blood.

bilirubinuria the presence of bilirubin in the urine. In most species this is in the conjugated form. Not normally found in the horse, sheep, pig and cat. High levels are usually indicative of hepatic disease, intra- or extrahepatic biliary obstruction.

biliuria the presence of bile acids in the urine.

biliverdin a green bile pigment formed by catabolism of hemoglobin and converted to bilirubin in the liver.

bill see BEAK.

Billroth anastomosis see GASTRODUODENAL anastomosis.
billy adult male goat.
bilobate having two lobes.
bilobed having two lobes.
bilobular having two lobules.
bilocular having two compartments.
biloma an encapsulated collection of bile in the peritoneal cavity.
biltong strips of beef, or other meat, which are cured briefly in salt, marinaded in vinegar and then air-dried. The resulting dried meat is used as a snack or as a subsistence ration. Called also jerked beef.
bimanual with both hands.
bimastoid pertaining to both mastoid processes.
bimodal distribution a distribution with two peaks separated by a region of low frequency of observations.
binary made up of two elements, or of two equal parts; denoting a number system with a base of two.
b. code the basic code of computer machine languages in which all characters are defined in terms of 1 and 0.
b. fission the halving of the nucleus and then of the cytoplasm of the cell, as in protozoa.
b. scale a numerical scale with a radix of two in which 2 is 10, 3 is 11, 4 is 100, etc.
binaural pertaining to both ears.
binauricular pertaining to both auricles of the ears.
binder 1. a girdle or large bandage for support of the abdomen. 2. fibers in a wool fleece which bind the staples together; absence of them produces a locky fleece.
binding 1. holding separate units together. 2. in meat hygiene terms, the capacity to absorb and retain water.
b. element a specific sequence in DNA, usually less than 10 nucleotides, to which a particular protein binds; the tertiary structure of the sequence also influences the binding.
b. quality a measurement of the binding capacity of a sample, e.g. of meat.
b. test is used to measure amounts of antigen or antibody by measuring the amount to which it is bound in an immune complex either directly (primary), after separation by precipitation, agglutination or complement fixation (secondary) or the in vivo effects (tertiary).
binding out in contracts between partners or between principals and assistants in practices these are clauses which bind one or other of the parties to refrain from practicing in the practice area for a specified time if they should opt out of the partnership.
Bingley terrier an early name for the Airedale terrier; taken from the name of a town in Yorkshire, England.
binocular 1. pertaining to both eyes. 2. having two eyepieces, as in a microscope.
b. field the field of vision, simultaneously received by both eyes. Varies between animal species, depending on the placement of the eyes in the skull. Widest in the cat (90°), 60–70° in the horse and 15° in poultry.
binomial composed of two terms, e.g. names of organisms formed by combination of genus and species names.
b. distribution categorization of a group into two mutually exclusive subgroups, e.g. sick and not sick.
b. population a population which can be divided into a binomial distribution.
binotic see BINAURAL.
binovular pertaining to or derived from two distinct ova.
b. twins twins derived from two ova, that is, not identical or monozygotic TWINS. See also DIZYGOTIC.
binturong see ARCTICTIS *binturong*.
binuclear having two nuclei.
binucleation formation of two nuclei within a cell through division of the nucleus without division of the cytoplasm.
binucleolate having two nucleoli.
bio- word element. [Gr.] *life, living*.
bioaccumulation process producing an increase in the concentration of chemicals (usually toxins) in the tissues of organisms with each increase in the trophic level in the food chain. Examples include chlorinated hydrocarbons which reach their greatest concentrations in predatory birds and pelicans, and CIGUATERA in which the toxins are concentrated in large predatory fish such as gropers, barracudas and mackerel.
bioacoustics the science dealing with the communicating sounds made by animals.
bioactive having an effect on or eliciting a response from living tissue.
b. ration animal feed containing selected animal tissues, e.g. liver, spleen, embryonic calf.
bioaeration a modification of the activated sludge method of purifying sewage.
bioamine biogenic amine.
bioaminergic of or pertaining to neurons that secrete biogenic amines.
bioassay determination of the active power of a drug sample by comparing its effects on a live animal or an isolated organ preparation with those of a reference standard.
bioavailability the degree to which a drug or other substance becomes available to the target tissue after administration.
biobullet a technique and equipment for vaccinating and treating wild animals without catching them. Consists of hollow bullets made of hydroxypropylcellulose which melts in the warmth of living tissue. Bullet discharged from a 'gun' has low impact velocity and poor penetration. The payload of each bullet is about 250 mg.
biochanin A the 4-methyl ether of genistein, an estrogenic substance found in rye grasses and clovers.
biochemical oxygen demand the amount of oxygen required in a specified period to decompose organic matter at a temperature of 68°F (20°C). Used to assess sewage effluent. Called also BOD.
biochemistry the chemistry of living organisms and of their chemical constituents and vital processes.
biocidal destructive to living organisms.
b. sutures sutures impregnated with biocidal material.
biocide destructive to organisms including bacteria (bactericide), fungi (fungicide), amebae (amebicide), viruses (viricide).
bioclimatogram a graph representing the sum of two climatic variables, e.g. temperature, rainfall for a particular geographical locality for a specified period, with measurements taken at regular intervals, usually monthly. The common usage is to superimpose biological data, such as fungal spore counts on pasture, on the graph.
bioclimatology the science devoted to the study of the effects on living organisms of conditions of the natural environment (rainfall, daylight, temperature, air movement) prevailing in specific regions of the earth. See also BIOMETEOROLOGY.
biocompatibility the quality of not having toxic or injurious effects on biological systems.

biodegradable susceptible to degradation by biological processes, as by bacterial or other enzymatic action.
biodegradation the series of processes by which living systems render chemicals less noxious to the environment.
biodynamics the scientific study of the nature and determinants of the behavior of all organisms, including humans.
bioelectricity the electrical phenomena that appear in living tissues, as that generated by muscle and nerve.
bioenergetics section of biochemistry concerned with the mechanisms whereby the energy made released from the oxidation of substrates or the absorption of light can be used to drive thermodynamically unfavorable reactions such as the synthesis of ATP from ADP and Pi, or the accumulation of ions across membranes.
bioequivalence the relationship between two preparations of the same drug in the same dosage form that have a similar bioavailability.
biogenesis 1. origin of life, or of living organisms. 2. the theory that living organisms originate only from other living organisms.
biogenic having the property of originating in a biological process.
b. amine an amine neurotransmitter, such as epinephrine, norepinephrine, serotonin or dopamine.
endogenous b. amines occur naturally in the body, e.g. epinephrine, norepinephrine.
biogeography scientific study of the geographic distribution of living organisms.
bioglass a glass-ceramic biomaterial used for implants.
bioimplant denoting a prosthesis made of biosynthetic material.
biokinematics the study of the movements of the animal body. See also BIOKINETICS.
biokinetics 1. the study of the forces involved in movements of the body; the motions caused by the operation of an unbalanced system of forces. 2. the science of the movement of tissue and related phenomena that occur during the development of organisms.
biolistics the use of DNA-coated pellets, fired at high speed, to place DNA into plant and animal cells.
biologic see BIOLOGICAL.
b. response modifiers therapeutic agents used to increase or optimize immune responses. Includes immunomodulators, immunoaugmentators, immunoadjuvants, immunostimulators and immunopotentiators.
biological 1. pertaining to biology. 2. a medicinal preparation made from living organisms and their products; these include serums, vaccines, etc.
b. clock the physiological mechanisms which govern the rhythmic occurrence of certain biochemical, physiological and behavioral phenomena in living organisms. See also biological RHYTHM.
b. control control of a parasite by making use of its natural enemies, especially other pests. The target may also be a vector or a reservoir for infection.
b. data usually comprise a list of vital statistics about an animal or plant species, recording such things as preferred growth medium, temperature and humidity and details of the internal milieu including blood pH, normal blood electrolytes and the like.
b. environment includes the influence of all biological factors such as warmth, moisture and humidity, but also the plant ecosystem in which the animal lives and the associated populations of vertebrates and invertebrates that may compete for food and space, and may also act as reservoirs for infectious diseases.
b. filters are used for the treatment of sewage effluent. They comprise a column of stones or plastic pieces which become covered with bacteria which degrade the organic matter in the effluent.
b. significance is an estimate of the biological importance of a statistical or apparent causal association between two variables, e.g. feed supply and the occurrence of bovine acetonemia. The estimation takes into account the possible biological relationship between the two; an estimate of statistical significance would take only the mathematical relationship into account.
b. value relationship between the amount of nutrient absorbed and the amount utilized by the body. Expressed as a percentage. Called also BV.
biologist a specialist in biology.
biology scientific study of living organisms.
See also BIOLOGICAL.
radiation b. scientific study of the effects of ionizing radiation on living organisms.
bioluminescence chemoluminescence occurring in living cells.
biomarker a biological unit used as an indirect indicator of the impact of pollutants on biota, e.g. an enzyme such as mixed function oxygenase levels, immune status of animals in the receiving environment.
biomass the amount or entire assemblage of living organisms of a particular region, considered collectively.
biomaterial synthetic materials, including metals, ceramics and polymers. See also biological IMPLANT.
biome a large, distinct, easily differentiated community of organisms in a major ecological region.
biomechanics the application of mechanical laws to living structures.
biomedicine clinical medicine based on the principles of the natural sciences (e.g. biology, biochemistry).
biomembrane any membrane, e.g. the cell membrane, of an organism.
biometeorology that branch of epidemiology that deals with the effects of physical environmental factors such as rate of air exchange, barometric pressure and humidity on living organisms.
biometrics, biometry the application of statistical methods to biological data.
biomicroscope a microscope for examining living tissue in the body. See also slit LAMP.
biomicroscopy microscopic examination of living tissue in the body.
biomolecule a molecule produced by living cells, e.g. a protein, carbohydrate, lipid or nucleic acid.
bionecrosis see NECROBIOSIS.
bionics scientific study of functions, characteristics and phenomena observed in the living world, and application of knowledge gained to nonliving systems.
biophase the period during which an effective concentration of a drug is maintained in the vicinity of its site of action.
biophasic pertaining to the biophase of a drug.
b. availability the characteristic of a drug which determines its biophase.
b. concentration the concentration of a drug at the site at which it exerts its effect, that is in the immediate vicinity of its receptor site.
biophysics the science dealing with the application of physical methods and theories to biological problems.

biophysiology that portion of biology including organogenesis, morphology and physiology.

bioplasm see PLASMOGEN.

biopolymer any protein or nucleic acid produced by a living organism.

biopsy removal and examination, usually microscopic, of tissue from the living body. Biopsies are usually done to determine whether a tumor is malignant or benign; however, a biopsy may be a useful diagnostic aid in other disease processes such as infections.

aspiration b. biopsy in which tissue is obtained by application of suction through a needle attached to a syringe.

bite b. instrumental removal of a fragment of tissue.

bone marrow b. obtaining a sample of bone marrow, usually by needle aspiration, from a long bone, rib or sternum, for cytological examination.

brush b. removal of cells and tissue fragments using a brush with stiff bristles (introduced through an endoscope). Effective in obtaining tissue samples from inaccessible places such as the renal pelvis.

closed b. one carried out without access through an open incision such as a laparotomy. An example is a percutaneous, fine needle aspirate.

cone b. biopsy in which an inverted cone of tissue is excised, as from the uterine cervix.

cytological b. obtaining specimens of cells by various methods including irrigation of a hollow tube.

b. dart an alternative to immobilization of large and wild animals; a dart which cuts a skin bipsy, then falls out. Limited to use for superficial lesions.

endoscopic b. removal of tissue by appropriate instruments through an endoscope.

excisional b. biopsy of tissue removed from the body by surgical cutting.

exploratory b. a combination of exploratory surgery to determine size and location of a lesion and the taking of a biopsy.

fine needle b. see needle biopsy (below).

hepatic b. may be by transperitoneal incision, more commonly by percutaneous needle or trocar and cannula technique.

incisional b. biopsy of a selected portion of a lesion.

needle b. biopsy in which tissue is obtained by puncture of a tumor, the tissue within the lumen of the needle being detached by rotation, and the needle withdrawn.

punch b. see PUNCH biopsy.

Robson–Heggers b. a procedure for the collection of a piece of tissue from an infected wound in order to determine the extent and the nature of the infection.

sternal b. biopsy of bone marrow of the sternum removed by puncture or trephining (see also STERNAL puncture).

surface b. sample of cells scraped from the surface of a lesion or obtained by impression smears.

surgical b. one obtained during a surgical procedure.

synovial b. by a needle biopsy technique or through an arthrotomy incision using special forceps for a bite biopsy.

total b. obtained by removal of the entire lesion. May be for therapeutic as well as diagnostic purposes.

ultrasound-guided b. use of ultrasonography to guide the passage of a needle or biopsy instrument into an internal organ or lesion.

bioptome a cutting instrument for taking biopsy specimens.

bioreactor a container in which living organisms carry out a biological reaction.

bioreversible capable of being changed back to the original biologically active chemical form by processes within the organism; said of drugs.

biorhythm see biological RHYTHM.

BIOS acronym for Basic Input–Output System; that part of the computer operating system which communicates between the keyboard, the screen, the printer and other peripheral devices.

biosafety the safe handling of biological materials, particularly infectious agents which are classified on the basis of degree of risk to humans working with them and includes definition of biosafety levels for handling such agents. Level 1: standard microbiological practices; Level 2: Level 1 plus laboratory coats, decontamination of waste, restricted access, gloves, biohazard warning signs; Level 3: Level 2 practices plus special clothing and controlled access; Level 4: Level 3 practices plus change room access where all street clothing and accessories are removed and replaced with laboratory clothing or special half or full suits with independent air supply; all waste is decontaminated and personnel shower on exit.

bioscience the study of biology wherein all the applicable sciences (physics, chemistry, etc.) are applied.

biosecurity security from transmission of infectious diseases, parasites and pests.

biosphere 1. that part of the universe in which living organisms are known to exist, comprising the atmosphere, hydrosphere and lithosphere. 2. the sphere of action between an organism and its environment.

biostatics the science of the structure of organisms in relation to their function.

biostatistics VITAL statistics.

biosynthesis creation of a compound by physiological processes in a living organism.

Biot's respirations a type of respiration associated with spinal meningitis and other central nervous system disorders; respirations are faster and deeper than normal, interspersed with abrupt pauses in breathing. Called also Biot's respirations.

biota all the living organisms of a particular area; the combined flora and fauna of a region.

biotechnology the application for industrial purposes of scientific, biological principles. The most modern examples are the use of recombinant DNA technology and genetic engineering to manufacture a wide variety of biologically useful substances such as vaccines and hormones by expression of cloned genes in various host cell systems including bacteria, yeast and insect cells.

biotelemetry the recording and measuring of certain vital phenomena occurring in living organisms that are at a distance from the recording device.

biotic 1. pertaining to life or living organisms. 2. pertaining to the biota.

b. community the assemblage of living things, including animals, plants and bacteria, which inhabit a specific biotope.

b. potential the theoretical reproductive potential of a population when unimpeded by the environment.

biotin a member of the vitamin B complex, required by or occurring in all forms of life tested; prosthetic group of carboxylase enzymes. Called also vitamin H, coenzyme R.

b. nutritional deficiency natural animal diets are unlikely to be deficient in biotin. Experimental deficiency causes paralysis in calves. In pigs the syndrome includes alopecia, dermatitis and cracking of the hooves. The vitamin may be an important factor in the maintenance of pig hoof health. See also porcine FOOTROT. Deficiency in dogs and cats is associated with dry scurfy skin, alopecia, especially around the eyes, and a papulocrustaceous dermatitis. It can be caused by a diet with very high levels of uncooked egg whites. See also AVIDIN.

biotope an area of land surface that provides uniform conditions over its entire surface for animal and plant life.

biotoxicology scientific study of poisons produced by living organisms, their cause, detection and effects, and treatment of conditions produced by them.

biotoxin a poisonous substance produced by a living organism.

biotransformation the series of chemical alterations of a compound (e.g. a drug) occurring within the body, as by enzymatic activity. The metabolism of a drug may produce products that have different effects to those of the parent drug. This biotransformation may differ markedly between animal species and affect the dose rate to be used, or the usefulness of the drug.

neonatal b. is marked by a deficiency of some enzymes necessary for the biotransformation of drugs.

biotype a group of individuals having the same genotype. Breeds of animals are obvious biotypes. See also BIOVAR.

biovar a group of strains of a species of microorganisms having differentiable biochemical or physiological characteristics.

biovular see BINOVULAR.

biparental derived from two parents, male and female.

biparous producing two ova or offspring at one time.

bipenniform doubly feather-shaped; said of muscles whose fibers are arranged on each side of a tendon like barbs on a feather shaft.

biphenyl polybrominated and polychlorinated biphenyls are widely used industrial chemicals, as flame retardants, heat transfer agents and electrical insulators.

b. poisoning these chemicals are not known to produce illness in the average environment, but they accumulate in fat and have a very slow rate of excretion and biodegradability. Experimental poisoning causes diarrhea, poor weight gain, growth retardation and abortion.

bipolar 1. having two poles. 2. pertaining to both poles.

b. neurons one of the types of cells in the retina.

b. staining a characteristic of some bacteria, such as *Pasteurella* spp.

Bipolaris 1. a fungus which elaborates a toxin (sterigmatocystin) capable of producing hepatic carcinoma; includes *B. spicifera*. 2. a fungal cause of cutaneous chromomycosis in animals; the imperfect state of *Cochliobolus* spp. Called also *Drechslera*, *Curvularia* and *Helminthosporium*.

bipotentiality ability to develop or act in either of two different ways.

biproduct by-product.

BIPS barium impregnated polyethylene sphere.

bipyridyl herbicides see PARAQUAT, DIQUAT.

biramous having two branches.

Birbeck granule a 'tennis-racquet' organelle characteristic of human Langerhans cells; in animals occur only in Langerhans cells in cattle.

birch sawfly see ARGE PULLATA.

birchwood a wood whose shavings are favored in Europe for the smoking of meats.

bird any feathered vertebrate. See also FEATHER, AVIAN and under specific groupings such as COMPANION ANIMAL, GAME, RAPTOR, RATITE birds and WATERFOWL.

b. bug a number of bugs in the family Cimicidae (order Hemiptera) which infest birds. See HAEMATOSIPHON, OECIACUS VICARIUS, ORNITHODORUS.

b. cherry *Prunus pennsylvanica*, *P. padus*.

b. dog a dog trained to hunt birds.

domesticated b. includes groups of birds brought under close control by humans, for purposes of communication (e.g. pigeons), clothing and furnishing (e.g. duck, peacock), sport (e.g. hawks), garden ornaments (e.g. peacock), companionship (e.g. canary) and food (e.g. commercial poultry, turkey, duck, goose used for meat and eggs).

b.-fancier's lung a pulmonary disease in humans caused by an acquired inhalant hypersensitivity to birds usually kept as pets or commercially so that large numbers and high exposure is likely. The antigen is believed to be in the dander or droppings of pigeons, budgerigars, chickens and turkey. Called also bird-breeder's lung, pigeon-breeder's lung. See also FARMER'S LUNG.

b. flea see CERATOPHYLLUS.

b. louse members of the order MALLOPHAGA. Includes *Amyrsidea*, *Anaticola*, *Anatoecus*, *Bonomiella*, *Campanulotes*, *Chelopistes*, *Ciconiphilus*, *Clayia*, *Coloceras*, *Colpocephalum*, *Columbicola*, *Cuclogaster*, *Gonioctes*, *Goniodes*, *Hohorstiella*, *Holomenopon*, *Lagopoecus*, *Lipeurus*, *Menacanthus*, *Menopon*, *Numidicola*, *Ornithobius*, *Oxylipeurus*, *Physconelloides*, *Somaphantus*, *Trinoton*.

b. malaria see PLASMODIUM.

b. of prey see RAPTOR.

b. repellent materials used to repel birds and avoid losses to crops. Usually refers to chemicals which are mixed with grain. If mammals ingest the baits accidentally they may be poisoned. See also 4-AMINOPYRIDINE.

b. tick see HAEMAPHYSALIS *chordeilis*, ARGAS.

b. tongue lethal autosomal recessive trait described in dogs in which the tongue is narrow and folded on itself medially. Affected pups are unable to swallow and die within 3 days of birth.

bird-flower *Crotalaria laburnifolia*.

bird of paradise disease see CAESALPINIA.

bird-tongue dogs lethal, inherited defect of the glossopharynx in Basset hounds. The tongue is very narrow with fimbriated edges which fold medially on the dorsum. Sucking and swallowing are difficult.

Bird ventilator an automatic or patient-triggered machine used in veterinary anesthesia by interposing a bag-in-bottle.

birdsfoot trefoil see LOTUS.

Birdsville disease see INDIGOFERA *linnaei*.

Birdsville indigo see INDIGOFERA *linnaei*.

birefractive doubly refractive.

birefringence the quality of transmitting light unequally in different directions.

Birman a longhaired breed of cat with blue eyes and a light body with darker points (ears, face, legs and tail) in colors similar to the Siamese. The paws are white ('gloves'). Called also Sacred Cat of Burma.

Birnaviridae a family of nonenveloped, icosahedral viruses, containing a genome of two segments of double-stranded RNA. They cause infectious bursal disease in chickens and infectious pancreatic necrosis in trout.

birnavirus a member of the family BIRNAVIRIDAE.

birth a coming into being; the act or process of being born. See also PARTURITION.

b. canal the canal through which the fetus passes in birth; comprising the uterus, cervix, vagina and vulva.

b. cohort see COHORT.
b. control a term rarely used in dealing with animals. Instead see population CONTROL, CONTRACEPTION.
b. defects see CONGENITAL defects.
b. difficulties dystocia.
b. injury occurs to the fetus during birth. Includes rib fracture and meningeal hemorrhage.
b. interval the interval between succeeding parturitions. See also CALVING interval.
multiple b. the birth of two or more offspring produced in the same gestation period.
b. order the chronological order of births in a multiple birth. May have significance in causing stillbirths if the intervals between births are prolonged because of inertia.
premature b. expulsion of the fetus from the uterus before termination of the normal gestation period, but after independent existence has become a possibility. In humans prematurity is defined as a pregnancy of less than 37 weeks in a pregnancy normally lasting 40 weeks.
b. process comprises maturation of the fetus, relaxation of the bony pelvis and associated ligaments, softening and relaxation of the cervix, vagina, vulva and perineum, correct disposition of the fetus, contractions of the uterine myometrium and finally the only component under voluntary control, contraction of the abdominal muscles.
b. rate the number of births during one year for the total population (crude birth rate), for the female population (refined birth rate), or for the female population of reproductive age (true birth rate). Not a term much used with reference to animals. See CALVING, LAMBING rate.
b. size stature, including height at withers, crown to tail head length at birth.
b. weight the weight at birth. A significant determinant of survival in any species and of the occurrence of dystocia. See also PROLONGED GESTATION.

birth-injured fetus includes peroneal nerve paralysis, sciatic nerve injury, hip or other joint traumatic dislocation, vertebral or rib fracture, intracranial or other internal hemorrhage, liver rupture, subcutaneous edema.

birthwort ARISTOLOCHIA *clematitis*.

BIS-GMA a popular dental composite resin material.

bis in die [L.] *twice a day;* abbreviated b.i.d.

bisacodyl a diphenylmethane stimulant cathartic.

bisacromial pertaining to the two acromial processes.

bisalbuminemia a congenital abnormality marked by the presence of two distinct serum albumins that differ in mobility on electrophoresis.

biscuit of hay see HAYFLAKE.

bisection division into two parts by cutting.

bisexual 1. having gonads of both sexes. 2. hermaphrodite. 3. having both active and passive sexual interests or characteristics. 4. capable of the function of both sexes. 5. both heterosexual and homosexual. 6. a patient which is both heterosexual and homosexual. 7. of, relating to, or involving both sexes, as bisexual reproduction.

bisexuality 1. the condition of being bisexual or of being a bisexual. 2. hermaphroditism.

bisferious dicrotic; having two beats.

bishoping altering the table of the incisor teeth in a horse so that the horse appears younger. A hollow is gouged and the lining burned with a hot iron or stained with silver nitrate to give the appearance of an infundibulum.

bishop's weed see AMMI.

bishydroxycoumarin dicoumarol.

***N*-bis(2-hydroxypropyl)nitrosamine** a chemical capable of increasing the rate of occurrence of thyroidal neoplasms.

bisiliac pertaining to the two iliac bones or to any two corresponding points on them.

bismuth a chemical element, atomic number 83, atomic weight 208.980, symbol Bi. See Table 6. Several insoluble salts, including the subcarbonate and subnitrate, have been used in the management of inflammatory diseases of the stomach and intestines. Toxic doses cause kidney damage.
b. glycollylarsanilate see GLYCOBIARSOL.
b. subgallate used topically in wound powders and in the treatment of metritis.
b. subsalicylate, b. salicylate an insoluble salt, used orally in the treatment of diarrhea and as an antacid. There is liberation of salicylic acid which acts against prostaglandin synthetase.

bismuthosis chronic bismuth poisoning, with anuria, stomatitis, dermatitis and diarrhea.

Bison a genus of the family Bovidae. Have massive development of forequarters, covered with shaggy hair and topped by a large hump on the neck.
B. bison North American bison, a typical member of the bison group, the coarsest and most hairy of them.
B. bonasus the almost extinct European bison, a smaller, less hairy, more graceful version of *B. bison*.

bison-cattle hybrid see BEEFALO.

2,3-bisphosphoglycerate, diphosphoglycerate a product of glucose metabolism; binds strongly to deoxyhemoglobin. High concentrations are found in erythrocytes. Regulates oxygen-carrying capacity of hemoglobin.
b. mutase an enzyme in the Embden–Meyerhof pathway of glycolysis in eyrthrocytes. Inherited deficiency results in a hemolytic anemia. Called also diphosphoglycerate mutase.
b. pathway the sequence of reactions in erythrocytes which conduct the conversion of glucose to energy. The essential part of the cycle is 2,3-bisphosphoglycerate. Called also Rapoport–Luebering cycle.

bisphosphonates calcium-regulating drugs which inhibit bone resorption; used in the treatment of hypercalcemia and osteoporosis in humans. Previously called diphosphonates and biphosphonates.

bistoury a long, narrow, straight or curved surgical knife used in opening sinuses and fistulae, incising abscesses, etc.
Udall's teat b. designed for opening stenosed teat sphincters. The point is blunt and rounded, the cutting edge is inset from the true edge of the blade and is about 0.5 in long. The bistoury is inserted into the canal and withdrawn sharply so as to incise the scar tissue vertically. Three or four incisions are made in this way.

bisulfate an acid sulfate.

bit 1. the detachable piercing piece of a drill. 2. the metal part of the bridle that goes into the horse's mouth and over the tongue; used to restrain and direct the horse by exerting pressure on the attached reins. There are many patented designs, each with its devotees. The simplest is a plain bar but the common ones are jointed in the middle. The variations include side bars and curb chains which allow greater pressure to be put on the animal's jaw. 3. the smallest unit of information in a computer, either a 0 or a 1. A combination of bits is used to make a byte.
circular b. encircles the lower jaw and is connected by a standing martingale to the girth. It prevents the

horse throwing up its head and rearing. Used also in a head harness for leading an active stallion.

snaffle b. any bit jointed in the middle.

bitch female dog. See also DOG.

brood b. any female dog used for breeding.

puppy b. a female dog from 6 to 12 months of age; used to define a group for competition within the showring.

bite 1. seizure with the teeth. 2. a wound or puncture made by a living organism. 3. the position of upper and lower teeth in relation to each other when the mouth is closed. See also BITING.

animal b. trauma caused by teeth and usually heavily contaminated with microorganisms. In countries where rabies is present the additional consideration is to ensure that the biter is not rabid, or if there is uncertainty to decide on whether postbite treatment or vaccination would be desirable. See also CAT-bite abscess, CAT-SCRATCH DISEASE, FIGHTING.

dog b. see animal bite (above).

insect b. depending on the nature of the insect and the site, the tissue response may be minimal to extensive, particularly when a hypersensitivity reaction is involved. Pruritus is also variable.

open b. upper and lower incisors fail to meet when the mouth is closed.

overshot b. see BRACHYGNATHIA.

pincer b. upper and lower incisors make contact on their edges rather than overlapping when the mouth is closed.

reverse scissor b. the labial surface of the lower incisors makes contact with the lingual surface of the upper incisors when the mouth is closed.

scissor b. the lingual surface of the upper incisors contacts the labial surface of the lower incisors when the mouth is closed. Generally, a normal bite in carnivores.

b. wound it is often necessary to diagnose that a wound has in fact been caused by a bite. This may be aided by observation of typical puncture wounds, perhaps with extravasations of blood in the subcutaneous tissues, by parallel rake marks, by a matching pair of wounds made by the upper and lower jaws of the biter.

bitemporal pertaining to both temples or temporal bones.

bithionol a bacteriostatic agent especially effective against gram-positive cocci; formerly used in the formulation of surgical soaps. Also has anthelmintic and fungicidal properties.

b. sulfoxide an effective cestocide. Also used as a fasciolicide, usually in combination with other compounds because of its poor efficiency against immature flukes. It is now superseded as an anthelmintic.

Bithynia a genus of snails that act as intermediate hosts for the miracidia of the *Opisthorchis* spp. of bile duct flukes.

biting pertaining to the characteristic behavior of performing a bite.

b. louse see species of the insect suborder MALLOPHAGA.

b. midge insects of the family CERATOPOGONIDAE. Called also punkies, no-see-ums, sandflies.

b. pattern the pattern of distribution of bites, or of diseases transmitted by insect bites, which may suggest the identity of the biter.

Bitis arietans see puff ADDER.

bitrochanteric pertaining to both trochanters on one femur or to both greater trochanters.

bitter 1. an austere and unpalatable taste like that of quinine. 2. a medicinal and culinary agent used as a tonic, alterative or appetizer.

b. almond a variety of *Prunus amygdalus*, the almond tree. Grown for the production of almond oil. The kernel of its seed contains sufficient cyanogenetic glycoside to be a possible cause of cyanide poisoning. The smell of bitter almonds is often quoted as being a characteristic finding in cases of cyanide poisoning in animals.

b. bark see ALSTONIA *constricta*.

b. melon CITRULLUS *lanatus*.

b. rubberweed HYMENOXYS *odorata*.

b. sneezeweed HELENIUM *amarum*.

b. vetch ERVUM *ervilia*.

bitterappel SOLANUM *incanum*, *S. kwebense*.

bitterbos see BITTERBUSH.

bitterbush see CHRYSOCOMA TENUIFOLIA. Called also bitterbos.

bitterkaroo [Af.] see CHRYSOCOMA TENUIFOLIA.

bitters reflex sialogogues. Included in the group are gentian, quassia, nux vomica and quinine.

bittersweet SOLANUM *dulcamara*. Called also woody nightshade.

bitterweed see HYMENOXYS *odorata*, HELENIUM.

bitumen a series of natural and artificial dry petroleum products. When combined with pitch and used as a flooring it may contain sufficient phenol to cause poisoning in pigs fed on the floors.

biuret a urea derivative; its presence is detected after addition of sodium hydroxide and copper sulfate solutions by a pinkish-violet color (protein test) or a pink and finally a bluish color (urea test).

bivalent 1. having a valence of two. 2. denoting homologous chromosomes associated in pairs during the first meiotic prophase.

bivalve shellfish members of the Class Bivalvia. Molluscs enclosed between two shells which are hinged together. Includes oysters, clams, arkshells, mussels. Called also lamellibranch.

bivariate statistic a numerical value which indicates the relationship between two individual variables, e.g. correlation between fiber intake and butterfat content of milk.

biventral 1. having two bellies. 2. digastric muscle.

biventricular pertaining to or affecting both ventricles of the heart.

Bivitellobilharzia a genus of the family Schistosomatidae of blood flukes. Includes *B. loxodontae*, *B. nairi* (elephant; portal vein).

bizygomatic pertaining to the two most prominent points of the two zygomatic arches.

Bk chemical symbol, *berkelium*.

black 1. without color, at the opposite end of the spectrum to white; the color of soot. 2. a universally accepted coat color. In horses, solid black with no pattern in it, the muzzle is black, and there may be white markings on the lower limbs and the head.

black acacia see ROBINIA PSEUDOACACIA.

Black and tan coonhound a medium to large shorthaired, scent hunting dog developed in the United States. It has a black coat and tan markings on the face, legs, chest and toes; the ears are large and pendulous and the tail is long. The breed is affected by hip dysplasia, polyradiculoneuritis and hemophilia B.

Black and tan terrier see ENGLISH TOY TERRIER.

black bean see CASTANOSPERMUM AUSTRALE, ERYTHROPHLEUM *chlorostachys*.

black beef see DARK cutting beef. Called also DFB.

Black Bengal see BENGAL GOAT.

black-berry nightshade SOLANUM *nigrum*.

black bindweed FALLOPIA *convolvulus*.

black blowfly see PHORMIA.

black bryony see TAMUS COMMUNIS.

black Celebes ape see CYNOPITHECUS NIGER. Called also Celebes macaque.
black cherry PRUNUS *serotina*.
black cohosh see ACTAEA *spicata*.
black crumbweed CHENOPODIUM *melanocarpum*.
black death see PLAGUE.
black death disease high mortality disease in farmed shrimp caused by ascorbic acid deficiency. Juvenile shrimp develop large, black, necrotic foci in the gills, subcutis, walls of the stomach and hindgut.
black disease see INFECTIOUS necrotic hepatitis.
black elder SAMBUCUS *nigra*.
black-eyed Susan RUDBECKIA.
black fell terrier see PATTERDALE TERRIER.
black fever see LEISHMANIASIS.
black fly a term which covers a number of genera and species. In some areas in the summer months they cause a great deal of insect worry to animals. The annoyance may be sufficiently severe to result in animals being injured or even killed while stampeding. They also play a part in the transmission of *Onchocerca* spp. Called also buffalo gnat, sandfly, CNEPHIA, *Austrosimulium pestilens*, *A. bancrofti*. See also SIMULIUM *articum*, SIMULIUM *ornatum*.
black-footed ferret see FERRET.
black-footed penguin see PENGUIN.
black gill disease nonspecific term for dark gills in shrimp; causes include fouling of the water with sediments, *Fusarium solani* infection, cadmium poisoning and ciliate (apostome) infection.
black hellebore HELLEBORUS *niger*.
black henbane see HYOSCYAMUS NIGER.
black laurel LEUCOTHOE *davisiae*.
black-legged tick see IXODES.
black livers see LIPOFUSCINOSIS.
black locust see ROBINIA PSEUDOACACIA.
black mastitis see black MASTITIS.
black mustard SINAPIS *nigra*.
black nightshade SOLANUM *nigrum*.
black patch disease a fungus disease of legumes caused by *Rhizoctonia leguminicola*.
black patch necrosis darkening of skin between caudal and marginal fin rays in farmed Dover Sole infected with *Flexibacter columnaris*-like bacteria. Affected skin swells then sloughs, followed by deep ulceration and death.
black pigweed TRIANTHEMA *portulacastrum*.
black pith a butcher's term for melanosis of the meninges.
black pox see BLACK SPOT.
black puff-ball SCLERODERMA *citrinum*.
black quarter see BLACKLEG.
black rat see black RAT.
black roly-poly SCLEROLAENA *muricata*.
black sally wattle see ACACIA *salicina*.
black scour worm see TRICHOSTRONGYLUS.
black scours see WINTER DYSENTERY, SWINE dysentery.
black snake see PSEUDECHIS *porphyriacus*. Called also red-bellied black snake.
Papuan b. s. see PSEUDECHIS *papuanus*.
black soil blindness mycotoxicosis of cattle in northern Australia caused by grazing *Astrebla* spp. (Mitchell grass) pasture in which the seed heads and other parts of the plants are parasitized by coral-like fungal bodies produced by *Corallocytostroma* spp. Characterized by blindness, sudden death, rumenitis and nephrosis and its restriction to high rainfall periods on the black soil plains on which the grass dominates the pasture.
black soil itch see EUTROMBICULA *sarcina*.
black spot 1. lesions on the teats of cows and almost always confined to the tip and including the orifice of the teat sinus. They are deep ulcers containing granulation tissue and usually a black spot. Milk flow is impeded and the lesion is very painful. They are caused by excessive suction during milking although *Staphylococcus aureus* is usually recoverable from the lesions. Called also black pox. 2. a fungal infection of chilled beef caused by *Cladosporium herbarum* and characterized by black spots on the surface of the meat.
black spot disease see POSTHODIPLOSTOMUM *cuticula*.
black-striped wallaby MACROPUS *dorsalis*.
black-tailed deer see ODOCOILEUS *hemionus columbiana*.
black thorn + Molopo spp. moth cocoon fiber see ACACIA *mellifera*.
black vomit see HEMATEMESIS.
black walnut see JUGLANS NIGRA.
black water see AZOTURIA.
black wattle ACACIA *cunninghamii*, *A. salicina*.
black whip snake see DEMANSIA *olivaceae*.
black widow spider see LATRODECTUS *mactans*.
blackboy see XANTHORRHOEA.
blackbuck see INDIAN ANTELOPE.
Blackfaced mountain sheep carpetwool English and Scottish sheep; black or mottled face and legs.
blackhead[1] comedo; a plug of keratin and sebum within the dilated orifice of a hair follicle. The color of blackheads is caused not by dirt but by the discoloring effect of air on the sebum in the clogged pore. Infection may cause the comedo to develop into a pustule or BOIL.
blackhead[2] a disease of birds especially turkeys caused by the protozoan parasite HISTOMONAS *meleagridis* and characterized by necrotic lesions in the liver and inflammation and distension of the cecum. Earth worms are important vectors in the life cycle of the parasite.
Blackhead Persian South African, hairy (woolless), fat-rumped, polled mutton sheep; origin of several other similar breeds.
blackleaf 40 a commercially available concentrate of nicotine sulfate used as a parasiticide in horticulture and containing 40% of alkaloidal nicotine.
blackleg an acute, infectious myositis principally of cattle, caused by *Clostridium chauvoei*. The lesion arises without the need for any external injury. The animal is profoundly toxemic with a high fever and usually a very swollen painful thigh. The skin is gangrenous, and emphysema can be palpated in the subcutis. Death occurs in 12 to 36 hours.
pseudo-b. see MALIGNANT edema. Called also gas gangrene.
stable b. see MALIGNANT edema. Called also gas gangrene.
blacktail condition a disease of fish caused by a protozoan parasite, *Myxosoma* spp., which destroys cartilage in the vertebral column, causing abnormal activity of caudal pigment cells and black discoloration of the tail.
blacktongue a prominent feature of the severe stomatitis that occurs in dogs from NIACIN nutritional deficiency. Recognition that this condition was responsive to niacin led to identification of the cause of the human disease pellagra.
blackwater fever see BABESIOSIS.
blackwood see ACACIA *melanoxylon*.
BLAD bovine LEUKOCYTE adhesion deficiency.
bladder a membranous sac serving as a receptacle. See also GALLBLADDER, URINARY BLADDER.

b. meridian points acupuncture points on the bladder meridian.

bladder dock RUMEX *vesicarius*.

bladder worm see CYSTICERCUS *tenuicollis*. Called also long-necked bladder worm.

bladderpod SESBANIA *vesicaria*.

blade scalpel.

b. method a method of castrating very young pigs in which the skin and fascia in the inguinal area are incised with a scalpel blade to gain access to the spermatic cord.

Blakistonia one of the genera of TRAPDOOR SPIDERS.

Blalock Alfred Blalock, an American surgeon.

B. anastomosis a technique for repair of tetralogy of Fallot in which there is an end-to-side anastomosis of the subclavian and pulmonary arteries.

B. ligation a technique for placement of a ligature around the aorta to isolate the ductus arteriosus in the surgical repair of patent ductus arteriosus.

blanch to become pale.

blanket a large area of color, usually over the back, neck and sides, in the coat of dogs.

blanket dry-period treatment treatment of all quarters in all cows in the herd; compare with selective dry period treatment. See also DRY PERIOD treatment.

blanket therapy treatment of all animals in the group used usually as a protective measure against infection, or because a large proportion are suspected to be infected and it is more cost-effective to treat all of them than to test and treat selectively.

Blaschenausschlag [Ger.] *blister rash;* see infectious pustular VULVOVAGINITIS.

blast 1. an immature stage in cellular development before appearance of the definitive characteristics of the cell; used also as a word termination, as in ameloblast, etc. 2. the wave of air pressure produced by the detonation of high-explosive bombs or shells or by other explosions; it causes pulmonary damage and hemorrhage (lung blast, blast chest), laceration of other thoracic and abdominal viscera, ruptured eardrums, and effects in the central nervous system.

b. cells the precursor cells of bone marrow. See also MYELOBLAST, MONOBLAST, ERYTHROBLAST, MEGAKARYOBLAST.

blast freezing a method of freezing poultry in which the carcasses are subjected to temperatures of –40°F in a blast tunnel for 2 to 3 hours.

blast(o)- word element. [Gr.] *a bud, budding*.

blastema 1. the primitive substance from which cells are formed. 2. a group of cells that will give rise to a new individual, in asexual reproduction, or to an organ or part, in either normal development or in regeneration.

blastocele the fluid-filled central cavity of the blastula.

blastoconidia the unit of asexual reproduction produced by budding; seen in yeasts such as *Candida* and *Cryptococcus* spp. Called also blastospore.

blastocyst the mammalian conceptus in the post-morula stage, consisting of the trophoblast, an inner cell mass, and a central, fluid-filled cavity.

Blastocystis hominis a cause of diarrhea in the great apes.

blastocyte an undifferentiated embryonic cell.

blastocytoma see BLASTOMA.

blastoderm the layer of cells forming the wall of the blastula.

blastodisk the convex structure formed by the blastomeres at the animal pole of an ovum undergoing incomplete cleavage.

blastogenesis 1. development of an individual from a blastema, i.e. by asexual reproduction. 2. transmission of inherited characters by the germ plasm. 3. morphological transformation of small lymphocytes into larger cells resembling blast cells on exposure to phytohemagglutin, or to antigens to which the donor is immunized.

blastoid transformation called also mitosis.

blastoma a neoplasm composed of embryonic cells derived from the blastema of an organ or tissue.

blastomatosis the formation of blastomas; tumor formation.

blastomere one of the cells produced by cleavage of a fertilized ovum.

Blastomyces a genus of pathogenic fungi growing as mycelial forms at room temperature and as yeastlike forms at body temperature; applied to the yeasts pathogenic for humans and animals.

B. brasiliensis see PARACOCCIDIOIDES *brasiliensis*.

B. coccidioides former name for *Coccidioides immitis*.

B. dermatitidis the species causing North American BLASTOMYCOSIS. Called also *Ajellomyces* spp.

blastomycete any organism of the genus *Blastomyces*; also, any yeastlike organism.

blastomycin a sterile broth filtrate from cultures of *Blastomyces dermatitidis*, used intradermally as a diagnostic test for blastomycosis but results in dogs are unreliable as the test may be negative in advanced cases and there can be cross-reaction with *Histoplasma* spp.

blastomycosis 1. a disseminated or localized infection with *Blastomyces* spp. 2. infection with any yeastlike organism.

cheloidal b. an unsightly but innocuous disease of bottlenosed dolphins and humans. Characterized by the presence of red, hard, smooth cutaneous nodules. Caused by infection with a fungus, *Loboa loboi*.

cutaneous b. the skin form of North American blastomycosis.

disseminated b. North American blastomycosis in which lesions are present in most internal parenchymatous organs.

equine b. see EPIZOOTIC lymphangitis.

European b. see CRYPTOCOCCOSIS.

keloidal b. see cheloidal blastomycosis (above).

North American b. infection by *Blastomyces dermatitidis* which causes primary granulomatous or pyogranulomatous lesions in the lungs. Secondarily, lesions may occur in the skin, eyes, bone and elsewhere. A disease of dogs, cats and humans. Food animals in the same environment are not reported to be affected. Although the disease was originally recorded in North America and is endemic in some areas of the USA, it is now known to occur in Central and South America.

South American b. see PARACOCCIDIOIDOMYCOSIS.

blastopore the opening of the archenteron to the exterior of the embryo at the gastrula stage. Called also archistome, anus of Rusconi.

blastospore a spore formed by budding, as in yeast. Called also blastoconidia.

blastula the usually spherical body produced by cleavage of a fertilized ovum, consisting of a single layer of cells (blastoderm) surrounding a fluid-filled cavity (blastocoele); it follows the morula stage.

blastulation conversion of the morula to the blastula by development of a blastocele.

blaze a broad white stripe down the face, wider than the nasal bones and including the forehead and all or part of the muzzle. Used in the description of horses.

bleach see SODIUM hypochlorite.
bleaching powder calcium hypochlorite used as a bleaching and disinfectant agent. Called also chlorinated lime (chloride of lime) and used in error in whitewash. Causes skin and eye irritation and enteritis if ingested.
bleb a large flaccid vesicle, usually at least 0.5 inch in diameter.
pulmonary b. small pocket of air under the visceral pleura; may be congenital or acquired.
Blechnum a genus of toxic ferns in family Blechaceae; contains an unidentified toxin; causes diarrhea. Called also bungwall fern.
bleed see BLEEDING.
bleeder 1. the popular term for an animal who bleeds freely, especially one suffering from a condition in which the blood fails to clot properly such as in HEMOPHILIA. In horses the term means one which bleeds from the nostrils during a race. Such horses are not allowed to participate in races. See also EPISTAXIS. 2. any large blood vessel cut during surgery.
bleeding 1. the escape of blood, as from an injured vessel. See also HEMORRHAGE. 2. the purposeful withdrawal of blood from a vessel of the body; venesection; phlebotomy. See also BLOOD SAMPLING.
b. disorders see HEMORRHAGIC disease, COAGULOPATHY.
incomplete b. the carcass of an animal slaughtered for meat which is incompletely bled out has a darker meat and more blood in vessels and the heart cavities than a properly slaughtered animal. This gives it an appearance resembling a fevered carcass.
occult b. escape of blood in such small quantity that it can be detected only by chemical tests or by microscopic or spectroscopic examination.
b. time the time required for a small pinpoint wound to cease bleeding. If done properly, the test can be helpful in determining the functional capacity of platelets and of vasoconstriction.
bleeding heart DICENTRA *spectabilis*.
bleeding-out an abattoir practice to confer pale color and good preservation of meat; the jugular vein of the already dead animal is severed and the carcass hung to give maximum opportunity for the venous system to be evacuated.
blended rations all of the components of the ration, including roughage, concentrates and mineral and vitamin mix, are mixed together.
Blenheim spaniel see KING CHARLES SPANIEL.
Blenkinsop shoe a special horseshoe designed to prevent slipping and stumbling. The shoe is very thin and wide, and the toe is turned so that a half of its surface does not bear.
blennadenitis inflammation of mucous glands.
blenn(o)- word element. [Gr.] *mucus*.
blennogenic producing mucus.
blennoid resembling mucus.
blennorrhagia any excessive discharge of mucus; blenorrhea.
blennorrhea any free discharge of mucus.
inclusion b. inclusion conjunctivitis.
blennostasis suppression of an abnormal mucous discharge, or correction of an excessive one.
blennothorax an accumulation of mucus in the chest.
blennuria mucus in the urine.
bleomycin a polypeptide antibiotic mixture having ANTINEOPLASTIC properties, obtained from cultures of *Streptomyces verticellus*. Evidence indicates that bleomycin inhibits cell division, thymidine incorporation into DNA, and DNA synthesis. Has been used in dogs and cats in the treatment of squamous cell carcinoma, but side-effects, including pneumonia or pulmonary scarring, limit its use.
blepharadenitis inflammation of the meibomian glands.
blepharal pertaining to the eyelids.
blepharectomy partial or complete excision of an eyelid.
blepharism spasm of the eyelid; continuous blinking.
blepharitis inflammation of the eyelids. May be an extension of skin disease elsewhere on the face or body producing a blepharitis with similar characteristics, e.g. seborrheic, ulcerative, mycotic, etc.
angular b. inflammation involving the outer angle of the eyelids.
blephar(o)- word element. [Gr.] *eyelid, eyelash*.
blepharoadenitis see BLEPHARADENITIS.
blepharoatheroma an encysted tumor or sebaceous cyst of an eyelid.
blepharochalasis loss of elasticity of the skin of the upper eyelid.
blepharoclonus clonus involving the eyelids; abnormal reflex blinking.
blepharoconjunctivitis inflammation of the eyelids and conjunctiva.
blepharodermatomycosis fungal infection of the eyelids; mycotic blepharitis.
blepharoedema swelling of the eyelids.
blepharoncus a tumor on the eyelid.
blepharophimosis contraction of the palpebral fissures. May be acquired or occur congenitally, as in some dog breeds where it may be associated with microphthalmia. If the globe is normal size, entropion can result.
blepharoplasty plastic surgery of an eyelid. Most often done to correct entropion or ectropion in dogs.
Wharton–Jones b. a V to Y technique for the correction of broad-based cicatricial ectropion.
V to Y b. a technique for correction of mild ectropion.
Y to V b. a technique for correction of mild central entropion of the upper or lower eyelids.
blepharoplegia paralysis of an eyelid.
blepharoptosis drooping of an upper eyelid; ptosis.
blepharorrhaphy 1. suture of an eyelid. 2. tarsorrhaphy.
blepharospasm spasm of the orbicularis oculi muscle of the eyelid.
blepharostat an instrument for holding the eyelids apart.
blepharostenosis see BLEPHAROPHIMOSIS.
blepharosynechia growing together or adhesion of the eyelids.
blepharotomy surgical incision of an eyelid; tarsotomy.
Bleue du Nord CENTRAL AND UPPER BELGIAN breed of cattle.
blight see INFECTIOUS bovine keratoconjunctivitis.
blind not having the sense of sight. See also BLINDNESS.
double b. trial an experiment in which the identity of the animals in the treatment and control groups is unknown to the experimenter and in addition the assessment of the results is done without the animals' identities being known to the experimenter. Called also blind study.
b. experiment the identities of the animals that are in the treatment and the control groups are unknown to the experimenter until the end of the trial.
b. snakes see TYPHLOPID.
b. spot the area marking the site of entrance of the optic nerve on the retina; it is not sensitive to light.
b. staggers see DUMMY.

b. study see double blind trial (above).
b. teat see blind TEAT.

blind fouls footrot in cattle in which the infected tissue is fully contained without discharge to the exterior; causes severe pain. See also bovine FOOTROT.

blind grass see STYPANDRA GLAUCA. Called also candyup poison.

blind loop syndrome a profound toxemia caused by the proliferation of gram-negative bacteria in a bowel segment in which there is local stasis and recirculation of bowel contents. Called also stagnant loop syndrome.

blind quarter a quarter of an udder that produces no milk whilst the other quarters are lactating. See also blind TEAT.

blindfolding covering a horse's eyes with a blindfold as a means of restraint. Most horses when blindfolded can be persuaded to load onto trailers which they refuse to do without the blindfold. Of some but more limited use in other species. A comparable device used in pigs, a bucket placed over the head, causes the pig to walk backwards. Provided the rear of the pig is pointed in the correct direction this is a worthwhile last try in getting a large pig to go where you want it to go.

blinding a condition imposed on a study which is intended to keep knowledge of the treatment assignment of individual patients from a specified set of observers. Used to reduce information bias. **Single blind**: the owner of the patient is unaware of the treatment assignment but the veterinarian is aware. **Double blind**: both the owner of the patient and the veterinarian are unaware of the treatment assignments of the patients. **Triple blind**: the owners of the patients, the veterinarian and the person analyzing the results of the study are all unaware of the treatment assignments. Called also masking.

blindness lack or loss of ability to see. Diagnosed in an animal on the absence of a menace reflex, walking into obstructions and failure to indicate awareness of a soundless movement in its visual field, e.g. a falling cotton ball or feather.
Appaloosa night b. see APPALOOSA.
bright b. toxic retinopathy in sheep grazing bracken; characterized by blindness, dilated pupils, poor pupillary light reflex, retinal degeneration.
central b. due to a lesion of the optic cortex; the pupillary light reflex still functions. Called also cortical blindness.
cortical b. see central blindness (above).
day b. defective vision in bright light. See also HEMERALOPIA.
inherited congenital b. occurs in a number of breeds of cattle in which there are several defects in the eyes including irideremia, microphakia, ectopia lentis and cataract.
night b. failure or imperfection of vision in conditions of diminished illumination; a characteristic of progressive retinal atrophy.
peripheral b. blindness due to a lesion in the optical apparatus peripheral to the optical cortex, including lesions in the optic chiasma, optic nerve, retina, anterior and posterior chambers, lens and cornea. With the exception of obvious lesions in the eyeball this is characterized by dilatation of the pupil and absence of the pupillary light reflex.

blink the involuntary movement of one or both eyelids of both eyes simultaneously. The frequency varies between species. Cats blink the least, with the possible exception of owls. In birds it is the lower eyelid which is moved up to meet the upper lid. In mammals the upper eyelid is moved down to meet the lower lid. The blink is a part of several reflexes including the palpebral, conjunctival and menace reflexes.
b. reflex see BLINK response.
b. response absent in lesions of the ophthalmic branch of the trigeminal nerve. Called also blink reflex.

blinkers 1. rigid pieces of leather fitted to a head harness at a point where they will obstruct the horse's lateral vision. 2. a more sophisticated piece of harness worn by expensive horses consisting of a canvas head-covering with holes for the ears to protrude and two apertures for the eyes. These have saucer-shaped flaps which prevent the horse from seeing sideways. Called also winkers.

blinking a normal function having the effect of maintaining the tear film over the cornea, clearing debris and promoting clearance of tears into the lacrimal duct. Excessive blinking may be due to conjunctival irritation, to a state of enhanced irritability, or generalized muscle tetany.

blister 1. a vesicle, especially a bulla, a lesion of the skin. 2. a paste containing an irritant such as cantharides used to plaster onto a horse's leg to produce counterirritation and encourage healing of a strained tendon or ligament.
b. beetle see EPICAUTA VITTATA.
blood b. a vesicle having bloody contents, as may be caused by a pinch or bruise.
b. fly see CANTHARIS VESICATORIA.
internal b. see SCLEROSING AGENTS.

blisterweed see THAMNOSMA TEXANA.

bloat 1. tympany of the rumen, abomasum, stomach or cecum. See also RUMINAL tympany. 2. enteritis in young rabbits accompanied by distension of the abdomen.
gastric b. see gastric dilatation COLIC, GASTRIC dilatation–volvulus.
b. line appears at the point at which the cervical esophagus becomes the thoracic. At this line the engorged esophageal mucosa of the neck becomes the pallid mucosa of the thorax.
primary b. ruminal tympany caused by frothiness of the ruminal contents.
secondary b. ruminal tympany secondary to physical or functional obstruction of the esophagus.
b. whistle a device for temporarily relieving a cow with chronic bloat from dangerous overdistension. The bottom half of the device shaped as a flanged cannula is slipped into the rumen through a slit incision in the left flank. The small end of the cannula protrudes through the abdominal wall and is secured into place by slipping the top half of the device over it and screwing it tight.

block 1. an obstruction or stoppage. 2. regional anesthesia. 3. in computer terms means to highlight a block of text which will then be modified by the next command, e.g. delete, bold.
Arthur b. see segmental dorsolumbar EPIDURAL block.
bundle-branch b. a form of HEART BLOCK involving obstruction in one of the branches in the bundle of His.
field b. regional anesthesia obtained by blocking conduction in nerves with chemical or physical agents.
b. grazing see rotational GRAZING.
heart b. impairment of conduction in heart excitation; often applied specifically to atrioventricular heart block. See also HEART BLOCK.

b. mating mating of all the females in a group during a brief period, e.g. within the span of three estral cycles; a characteristic of seasonal animal farming.

metabolic b. the blocking of a biosynthetic pathway due to a genetic enzyme defect or to inhibition of an enzyme by a drug or other substance.

nerve b. regional anesthesia secured by injection of an anesthetic in close proximity to the appropriate nerve.

paracervical b. anesthesia of the inferior hypogastric plexus and ganglia produced by injection of the local anesthetic into the lateral fornices of the vagina.

parasacral b. regional anesthesia produced by injection of a local anesthetic around the sacral nerves as they emerge from the sacral foramina.

presacral b. anesthesia produced by injection of the local anesthetic into the sacral nerves on the anterior aspect of the sacrum.

ring b. regional anesthesia by the injection of local anesthetic in a complete circle around a limb of a horse, or the teat of a cow.

sacral b. anesthesia produced by injection of the local anesthetic into the extradural space of the spinal canal.

saddle b. the production of anesthesia in a region corresponding roughly with the areas of the buttocks, perineum and inner aspects of the thighs, by introducing the anesthetic agent low in the dural sac.

sinus b. sinus arrest.

vagal b., vagus nerve b. blocking of vagal impulses by injection of a solution of local anesthetic into the vagus nerve at its exit from the skull.

block calving a breeding management system in which all of the cows in a herd, or an area, are encouraged to calve at approximately the same time. Has the effect of concentrating all of the calving and puerperal problems at one time and having all of the cows begin and terminate their lactations together. Has the disadvantage that the herd's period of maximum productivity is also concentrated, making it subject to much greater risk of loss. Is the opposite of year-round calving. Called also seasonal calving.

blockade 1. in pharmacology, the blocking of the effect of a neurotransmitter or hormone by a drug. 2. in histochemistry, a chemical reaction that modifies certain chemical groups and blocks a specific staining method.

adrenergic b. see ADRENERGIC blockade.

cholinergic b. see CHOLINERGIC blockade.

narcotic b. inhibition of the euphoric effects of narcotic drugs by the use of other drugs, such as methadone, in the treatment of addiction.

sympathetic b. block of nerve impulse transmission between a preganglionic sympathetic fiber and the ganglion cell.

blockage of intestine, urethra, etc. See obstruction under anatomical location, e.g. intestinal, urethral.

blocker something that blocks or obstructs passage, activity, etc.

α-b., alpha-b. a drug that induces ADRENERGIC blockade at α-adrenergic receptors.

β-b., beta-b. a drug that induces adrenergic blockade at either β_1- or β_2-adrenergic receptors, or both (see also BETA-blocker).

calcium channel b. a drug that selectively inhibits the influx of calcium ions through a specific ion channel of cardiac muscle and smooth muscle cells (see also CALCIUM CHANNEL BLOCKER).

H_2-receptor b. a drug, such as cimetidine that inhibits the secretion of gastric acid stimulated by histamine, pentagastrin, food and insulin, and also basal secretion; used in the treatment of peptic ulcer.

blocking 1. interruption of an afferent nerve pathway (see BLOCK). 2. inhibition of an intracellular biosynthetic process; metabolic block.

b. agents see under ALPHA, ADRENERGIC, BLOCKADE, BLOCKER, GANGLIONIC, MUSCARINIC.

b. antibody see blocking ANTIBODY.

Blond D'Aquitaine see AQUITAINE BLOND.

blood the red fluid that circulates through the heart, arteries, capillaries and veins carrying nutrients and oxygen to the body tissues and metabolites away from them. It consists of a yellow, protein-rich fluid, the plasma, and the cellular elements including leukocytes, erythrocytes and platelets. It has a high viscosity and osmotic tension and clots on exposure to air and to damaged tissue. It has an essential role in the maintenance of fluid balance.

In an emergency, blood cells and antibodies carried in the blood are brought to a point of infection, or blood-clotting substances are carried to a break in a blood vessel. The blood carries hormones from the endocrine glands to the organs they influence. And it helps in the regulation of body temperature by carrying excess heat from the interior of the body to the surface layers of the skin, where the heat is dissipated to the surrounding air. See also BLOODY.

arterial b. oxygenated blood in the arterial side of the circulation between the cardiac ventricles and the capillaries.

b. buffers substances which enable the blood to absorb much acidity without significant change in pH. The principal ones are the bicarbonate and hemoglobin buffers.

central b. blood from the pulmonary venous system; sometimes applied to splanchnic blood, or blood obtained from chambers of the heart or from bone marrow.

central venous b. unoxygenated blood collected centrally from the right atrium or venae cavae.

citrated b. blood treated with sodium citrate to prevent its coagulation.

b. clotting cascade see COAGULATION cascade.

cord b. that contained in the umbilical vessels at the time of delivery of the fetus.

defibrinated b. whole blood from which fibrin has been separated during the clotting process.

extracorporeal b. flow see EXTRACORPOREAL circulation.

b. in feces see MELENA.

b. islet aggregates of splanchnic mesoderm on the surface of the yolk sac and allantois; the first blood cells in the embryo.

b. lactate this estimation has good predictive value in a number of diseases, e.g. intestinal obstruction in horses.

b. in milk appears as clots or as diffuse red tint. Common only in recently calved cows or after trauma. Of no disease significance but renders the milk unsuitable for sale.

occult b. that present in such small amounts as to be detectable only by chemical tests or by spectroscopic or microscopic examination. See also OCCULT blood test.

b. osmolality see serum OSMOLALITY.

peripheral b. that obtained from the circulation remote from the heart; the blood in the systemic circulation.

selective b. agar see blood AGAR.

shunted b. blood which is not oxygenated in the lung because it passes through unaerated tissue.

sludged b. blood in which the red cells have become aggregated into clumps and is most marked where the flow rate is slowest, i.e. in the capillaries.

b. solutes see individual elements, metabolic products, hormones and the like.

stiff b. agar see blood AGAR.

b. substitutes synthetic substances that may be used in place of blood or its components include dextran, hydroxyethyl starch, polyvinylpyrrolidone, gelatin and perfluorocarbon.

b. urea nitrogen (BUN) see UREA nitrogen.

b. urea test see UREA nitrogen.

b. in urine see HEMATURIA.

venous b. blood which has passed through the capillaries and discharged its oxygen load to tissues and relieved the tissue load of carbon dioxide by absorbing it, and is on its way to the lungs to reverse these processes; is dark red in color due to the high concentration of reduced hemoglobin.

b. volume expanders are used in the treatment of shock to restore tissue perfusion. Various fluids including whole blood, plasma, crystalloids and colloids may be used.

b. in vomitus see HEMATEMESIS.

whole b. that from which none of the elements has been removed, especially that drawn from a selected donor under aseptic conditions, containing citrate ion or heparin, and used as a blood replenisher.

blood bank a place of storage for blood.

blood barriers see BARRIER, BLOOD–BRAIN BARRIER.

blood blister intracutaneous hematoma.

blood–brain barrier (BBB) the barrier separating the blood from the brain parenchyma everywhere except in the hypothalamus. It is permeable to water, oxygen, carbon dioxide and nonionic solutes, such as glucose, alcohol and general anesthetics, and is only slightly permeable to electrolytes and other ionic substances. Some small molecules, e.g. amino acids, are taken up across the barrier by specific transport mechanisms.

blood cells See ERYTHROCYTE and LEUKOCYTE. Platelets are classed separately.

blood–cerebrospinal fluid barrier see blood–CSF BARRIER.

blood chemistry see individual elements, solutes and physical chemical characteristics.

blood clot see CLOT.

blood clotting see CLOTTING.

blood count the number of blood cells in a given sample of blood, usually expressed as the number of cells per liter of blood (RBCs × 10^{12}/l, WBCs and platelets 10^9/l). A differential white cell count determines the number of various types of leukocytes in a sampling of blood. The cell count is useful in the diagnosis of various blood dyscrasias, infections or other abnormal conditions of the body and is one of the most common tests done on the blood.

blood culture the collection of blood, using sterile equipment and technique, into a suitable culture medium, usually a broth, and its incubation prior to an appropriate bacteriological examination. Because the bacteremia in many cases is intermittent it is necessary to take a number of samples at intervals of several hours.

blood cysts an abattoir term describing freely bleeding cavernous hemangiomas in the skin of poultry carcasses.

blood dyscrasia see DYSCRASIA.

blood flow the movement of blood through the vessels. It is pulsatile in the large arteries, diminishing in amplitude as it approaches the capillaries. In the veins it is nonpulsatile. The flow in arteries is the result of ventricular ejection; in the veins it is a result of a number of factors including respiratory movement, muscle compression and the small residuum of arterial pressure.

laminar b. f. blood flowing through a large blood vessel moves forward in a series of concentric laminae that slide over each other like a telescoping radio aerial. The central lamina moves fastest; the outer layer may be stationary.

turbulent b. f. created when blood flows through a small caliber orifice. Is the cause of murmurs in the heart and large arteries.

blood fluke see SCHISTOSOMA and other less common genera of the family Schistosomatidae.

blood-forming organs see BONE MARROW, LYMPHOID tissue.

blood gas analysis laboratory study of arterial and venous blood for the purpose of measuring oxygen and carbon dioxide levels and pressure or tension, and hydrogen ion concentration (pH). Analyses of blood gases provide the following information:

$P_a\text{O}_2$—partial pressure (P) of oxygen (O_2) in the arterial blood (a); SaO_2—percentage of available hemoglobin that is saturated (Sa) with oxygen (O_2); $P_a\text{CO}_2$—partial pressure (P) of carbon dioxide (CO_2) in the arterial blood (a); pH—an expression of the extent to which the blood is alkaline or acidic; HCO_3^-—the level of plasma bicarbonate, TCO_2, base excess, base deficit.

These parameters are important tools for assessment of a patient's ACID–BASE BALANCE They reflect the ability of the lungs to exchange oxygen and carbon dioxide, the ability of the kidneys to control the retention or elimination of bicarbonate, and the effectiveness of the heart as a pump. Because the lungs and kidneys act as important regulators of the respiratory and metabolic acid–base balance, assessment of the status of a patient with any disorder of respiration and metabolism includes periodic blood gas measurements.

blood group the phenotype of erythrocytes defined by one or more cellular antigenic structural groupings under the control of allelic genes. The identification of specific blood groups is little used in veterinary medicine, except for the identification of parents, usually in horses and farm animals, and for purposes of selecting blood donors. For blood transfusions the usual practice is to carry out direct matching tests to avoid problems created by incompatibility. For blood group systems, see Table 7.

blood-horse see THOROUGHBRED.

blood lily see HAEMANTHUS MULTIFLORUS.

blood meal 1. an epidemiological term meaning the stomach contents of a blood-sucking insect which can be used to study the spread of specific infections. 2. a protein supplement containing 80 to 85% of protein. Is too unpalatable to constitute a large proportion of the diet.

blood nodule the cutaneous nodule produced by infestation with *Parafilaria* spp. in cattle and horses. In the warmer part of the year the nodules enlarge, burst and bleed and the eggs are released by the resident female, the microfilariae hatch and are picked up by a fly feeding on the blood.

blood packed cell volume see HEMATOCRIT.

blood parasites a term of little meaning. Includes those parasites which pass most of their lives in the vascular system, e.g. BABESIA, THEILERIA, TRYPANOSOMA, DIROFILARIA, and others.

blood $P\text{CO}_2$ see BLOOD GAS ANALYSIS.

blood pH see BLOOD GAS ANALYSIS.

blood plasma the liquid phase of the blood, obtained by sedimentation or centrifugation of blood treated with anticoagulant. Is the equivalent of serum plus fibrinogen and consists of water, proteins, electrolytes and other solutes.

blood poisoning the term used by lay persons to refer to the presence of infective agents (bacteria) or their toxins in the bloodstream, i.e. septic shock or septicemia. The condition is characterized by elevated body temperature, chills and weakness. Small abscesses may form on the surface of the body and red and blue streaks become apparent along the pathway of surface blood vessels leading to and from the site of the primary infection. A blood culture confirms the diagnosis and helps identify the most effective anti-infective drug for therapy.

Blood poisoning is a serious disease that must be treated promptly. Otherwise, the process of infection leads to circulatory collapse, profound shock and death.

blood pressure the pressure of the blood in the blood vessels. The term usually refers to the pressure of the blood within the arteries, or arterial blood pressure. This pressure is determined by several interrelated factors, including the pumping action of the heart, the resistance to the flow of blood in the arterioles, the elasticity of the walls of the main arteries, the blood volume and extracellular fluid volume, and the blood's viscosity, or thickness.

Relatively simple Doppler instruments can provide accurate blood pressure measurements in dogs and cats. The systolic pressure in dogs is 132±22 mmHg; in cats it is 108±23 mmHg. Thoroughbreds have been shown to be 112/77 mmHg. Indwelling catheters can be used in dogs to monitor CENTRAL venous pressure.

arterial b. p. the common measure of blood pressure. The measurement in animal patients must be by a method that does not require entrance to an artery, i.e. noninvasive. Standard methods use an inflatable cuff around a limb, around the tail in the horse, and measurement of the air pressure required to obliterate the pulse wave—the systolic blood pressure, and permit the re-entry of the pulse wave—the diastolic blood pressure.

b. p. homeostasis the maintenance of a steady state of blood pressure. The mechanisms involved include the baroreceptor mechanism, the chemoreceptor mechanism, the ischemic response of the central nervous system (the Cushing response), the renin–angiotensin vasoconstrictor and the renin–angiotensin–aldosterone system, the capillary fluid-shift mechanism, the regulation of body fluid level by the kidney and the stress–relaxation mechanism of the arterial wall.

b. p. impedance the resistance to pulsatile flow, as in arteries.

pulmonary wedge b. p. see wedge PRESSURE.

b. p. regulation the complex regulatory system which controls arterial blood pressure is dependent on sensory inputs related to cardiac output, peripheral resistance to blood flow at the arterioles, the viscosity of the blood, the volume of blood in the arterial system, the elasticity of the arterial walls. Changes in blood pressure are brought about by the control exerted on the same physiological mechanisms.

venous b. p. see CENTRAL venous pressure.

blood products by-products of the meat industry consisting largely of blood or its derivatives.

edible b. p. used as blood in a preparation of blood or black pudding. Or separated by centrifugation of citrated blood into plasma and cells. The cells are used in blood sausage and the dried plasma as a binding agent in sausages.

inedible b. p. usually contains extraneous water or fat, making it unsuitable for freeze drying for human consumption because of hemolysis. Used in the manufacture of meat and blood meals for animal feed.

blood progesterone the level of progesterone in the blood; used as a means of early pregnancy diagnosis in cows and ewes. See also PROGESTERONE, PREGNANCY tests.

blood sampling laboratory examination of samples of blood. These are usually collected from an appropriate vein, but arterial samples are required for some special techniques. Collection is by a closed method, either a hypodermic syringe or a vacuumized container. The site of collection varies with the species and the circumstances. The sample may be clotted, for serum estimations, or collected with an anticoagulant for examinations on plasma or whole blood.

blood serum the residual fluid of blood after clotting has occurred. It is plasma after the fibrinogen has been removed. It contains solutes of proteins, electrolytes, waste products, dissolved gases, hormones, enzymes, antibodies and water.

blood sinus an endothelial-lined, blood-filled cavity between the external sheath and the outer connective tissue capsule of the hair follicles associated with tactile hairs such as whiskers and vibrissae which are found on the muzzle, chin and above the eyes in many species. See also tactile HAIR.

blood splashes an abattoir term meaning large hemorrhages in muscles usually due to poor slaughtering technique.

blood spots spots of blood in hen eggs; an esthetic problem to the breakfast eater. They are of no disease significance and can be prevented by increasing the content of vitamin A in the diet. This is an effective preventive even in those families of birds which appear to have an inherited susceptibility to the defect.

blood-stained milk see BLOOD in milk.

blood-stock horses bred and kept for racing. Includes Thoroughbreds, Standardbreds, Trotters.

blood supply the volume of blood supplied to an organ or part during a particular time period. Usually a subjective estimate by a surgeon in determining whether the blood supply is adequate to maintain viability. A retrospective assessment is a common exercise in pathology.

blood transfusion see TRANSFUSION.

b. transfusion reaction see TRANSFUSION reaction.

blood type 1. blood group. 2. the phenotype of an individual with respect to a blood group system.

blood urea see blood UREA/nitrogen.

blood vessel any of the vessels conveying the blood; an artery, arteriole, vein, venule, sinusoid or capillary.

b. v. calcification in animals usually part of a generalized calcification syndrome; see CALCIFICATION.

b. v. congenital defect see arteriovenous ANEURYSM, PORTACAVAL shunt, PATENT ductus arteriosus, AORTIC coarctation.

coronary b. v. see CORONARY arteries.

b. v. disease includes ARTERITIS, PHLEBITIS, LYMPHANGITIS.

pulmonary b. v's see Table 9 (arteries), Table 15 (veins).

shunt b. v. include naturally-occurring arteriovenous

anastomoses and those caused by accidental injury or by congenital defect.

b. v. stenosis narrowing of the lumen caused by fibrous tissue contraction in the walls, or compression by other adjoining tissues, or congenital defect.

blood volume the total quantity of blood in the body. The regulation of blood volume in the circulatory system is affected by the intrinsic mechanism for fluid exchange at the capillary membranes and by hormonal influences and nervous reflexes that affect the excretion of fluids by the kidneys. A rapid decrease in the blood volume, as in hemorrhage, greatly reduces the cardiac output and creates a condition called SHOCK or circulatory shock. Conversely, an increase in blood volume, as when there is retention of water and salt in the body because of renal failure, results in an increase in cardiac output. The eventual outcome of this situation is increased arterial blood pressure.

Measurement of blood volume is accomplished by using substances that combine with red blood cells, for example, iron, chromium and phosphate, or substances that combine with plasma proteins. In either case the measurement of the blood volume is based on the 'dilution' principle. That is, the volume of any fluid compartment can be measured if a given amount of a substance is dispersed evenly in the fluid within the compartment, and then the extent of dilution of the substance is measured.

decreased b. v. caused by uncompensated blood loss, dehydration, water deprivation.

blood warts see congenital MELANOMA of pigs.

blood worms the large strongyles of horses. See STRONGYLUS *vulgaris*, STRONGYLUS *edentatus*, STRONGYLUS *equinus*.

Bloodhound a large, heavy bodied dog with loose skin folds around the face and head, and very long, pendulous ears. The coat is short and usually black and tan or red. The breed has a reputation as a scent hunter and is often used in the search for lost persons. Ectropion and entropion are common in the breed. Called also St. Hubert hound.

bloodstream the blood flowing through the CIRCULATORY system in the living body.

b. cooling part of cardipulmonary bypass procedures.

bloodworm a parasitic worm of cyprinid fish. Called also PHILOMETRA *abdominalis*.

bloody, blood in pertaining to or deriving from blood.

b. feces see DYSENTERY, MELENA.

b. guts see PROLIFERATIVE hemorrhagic enteropathy.

b. milk see HEMOLACTIA.

b. urine see HEMATURIA.

b. vomit see HEMATEMESIS.

bloom 1. the general appearance of the surface. In carcass meat it is the glistening, transparent effect and the gentle pink color that gives a good bloom to the carcass. It is the result of proper tissue hydration coupled with the correct proportions of fat, connective tissue and superficial layers of muscle. 2. appearance of the haircoat, usually taken to mean the gloss, luster and quality. 3. on stagnant water the collection of colored algae is called water bloom (see ALGAE, ALGAL poisoning).

bloomkoolbossie [Af.] see SALSOLA TUBERCULATIFORMIS.

blot analysis see BLOTTING.

blotting a technique used for the detection of DNA, RNA or protein. See NORTHERN BLOT, SOUTHERN BLOT, WESTERN BLOT. Called also blot analysis.

Blount staple a vitallium braced surgical staple for epiphyseal fixation. See also epiphyseal STAPLES.

blow dart a syringe-like implement with dart overtones delivered from a gun and propelled by compressed air, or carbon dioxide or an explosive charge, or from a mouth operated blowgun. The dart-like tail helps to maintain direction in what is a very low velocity flight. When the needle of the dart is driven into the skin of the target animal the piston is driven forward by the deceleration and discharges the contents of the syringe into the target's tissues. Used primarily to immobilize wild fauna.

blow-in a client who attends the surgery without an appointment when an appointment system is specified as the method of operation.

blowaway grass AGROSTIS *avenacea*.

blower can in the meat trade a term meaning a can of preserved food which has undergone sufficient bacterial contamination to distend the can.

blowfly a member of the family Calliphoridae of insects.

b. strike invasion of skin or exposed mucosae by blowfly larvae. See also cutaneous MYIASIS.

blowgun BLOW DART.

blowhole the anterior nares of whales and dolphins.

blowing 1. infestation of dead or living material with blowfly maggots. 2. subcutaneous inflation of a carcass of meat with compressed air in an attempt to facilitate skinning with least damage. Forbidden in most countries.

blowing check blowing down a stomach tube which has been passed into the cervical esophagus of a horse and checking that the tube is in the correct place by observing the passage of a large bubble of air. In cattle the check is to auscultate the rumen in order to hear a loud bubbling sound as an indication that the tube is in the esophagus.

blown grass AGROSTIS *avenacea*.

blowout with reference to hens, prolapse of the oviduct through the vent.

blowpipe 1. a tube through which a current of air is forced upon a flame to concentrate and intensify the heat. 2. a long tube through which blow darts are launched in wildlife capture.

b. dart see BLOW DART.

blows 1. distension of the cecum in rabbits. 2. the successive strips of wool removed by the shearing blades, e.g. 'beaten by a blow'.

blue 1. a color between green and violet in the visible spectrum; the color of the clear sky. 2. a silver-gray coat color. A description often used in dogs and cats, and some breeds of cattle.

Blue Andalusian a breed of chickens in which the typical blue color of the feathers occurs only in the heterozygotes; an example of co-dominant gene action.

blue bitou see CASTALIS SPECTABILIS.

blue-black a color mid-way between blue and black.

b.-b. ink used to stain fungal elements in diagnostic specimens.

blue breast(s) severe mastitis of rabbit with obvious cyanosis of the skin of the mammae. Called also caked udder.

blue catfish ICTALURUS *fircatus*.

blue comb disease turkey CORONAVIRUS enteritis.

blue couch grass CYNODON *incompletus*.

blue Doberman syndrome see color mutant ALOPECIA.

blue dog disease see color mutant ALOPECIA.

blue ear disease see PORCINE reproductive and respiratory syndrome.

blue-eared pheasant *Crossoptilon auritum*. See PHEASANT.
blue-eared pig disease see PORCINE reproductive and respiratory syndrome.
blue eye the common name given to edema of the cornea. It is occasionally used more specifically in reference to the reaction that may occur in dogs convalescing from infectious canine hepatitis or that have recently been immunized with a modified live virus hepatitis vaccine.
porcine b. e. see PARAMYXOVIRUS encephalomyelitis.
blue eye disease see PARAMYXOVIRUS encephalomyelitis.
blue ferret syndrome a bluish discoloration of the abdominal skin which sometimes appears after clipping; the condition resolves as hair regrowth occurs.
blue flag IRIS *versicolor*.
blue flax lily see DIANELLA REVOLUTA.
blue fur disease moist dermatitis infected with *Pseudomonas aeruginosa*; causes blue-green pigmentation of the fur in rabbits and rodents.
Blue-gray cattle a cross between a beef Shorthorn and either an Aberdeen Angus or a Galloway.
blue-green algae see ALGAL poisoning.
blue heliotrope HELIOTROPIUM *amplexicaule*.
blue hyacinth SCILLA *natalensis*.
blue line an undulating line between the superficial layer of an articular cartilage and its deeper mineralized layer. Called also tidemark.
blue loco ASTRAGALUS *diphysus*.
blue louse LINOGNATHUS *ovillus*.
blue meat meat discolored by superficial contamination by *Pseudomonas cyanogenus*.
blue nevus see blue NEVUS.
blue panic grass see PANICUM ANTIDOTALE.
blue periwinkle VINCA *major*.
blue pig root SISYRINCHIUM.
blue pimpernel ANAGALLIS *arvensis* var. *caerulea*.
blue-point see POINTS.
Blue Rex see REX.
blue-roan see ROAN.
blue rod see MORGANIA FLORIBUNDA.
blue rush JUNCUS *inflexus*.
blue sac disease a disease of young trout and other salmonid species; thought to be caused by unsuitable hatchery water.
blue shell syndrome a disorder of farmed panaeid shrimp, which develop a pale blue coloration on particular diets but respond to supplementation with carotene or vitamin A.
blue slime disease a disease manifested by a bluish film of tenacious mucus over the entire body of farmed brown trout and other salmonids; caused by a dietary deficiency of biotin and accompanied by hyperplastic goblet cells in the epidermis.
blue spot disease a herpesvirus infection of northern pike causing blue-white, flat, granular, epidermal lesions up to 10 mm diameter on dorsal skin and fins.
blue squill SCILLA *natalensis*.
blue tick see BOOPHILUS DECOLORATUS.
blue tulp MORAEA.
Blue V dye a blue dye used to color reject wheat which is unsuitable for human food consumption. If fed to chickens it causes green gizzard syndrome—the color changes at the low pH.
blue vitriol copper sulfate.
blue wildebeeste see CONNOCHAETES TAURINUS.
blue wing disease gangrenous dermatitis of turkeys caused by *Clostridium septicum*, *C. perfringens* type A and *Staphylococcus aureus*, in combination or singly. Infection occurs subsequent to injury, trauma during mating, vaccination, blood sampling or artificial insemination. Signs include a short course of about 24 hours, severe toxemia and heavy mortality in birds with moist areas of skin gangrene.
bluebag gangrenous mastitis of ewes caused by PASTEURELLA *multocida*.
bluebell (South Africa) SCILLA *nonscripta*.
bluebonnet or lupin; see LUPINUS.
bluebottle 1. the stinging Portuguese man-of-war (PHYSALIA PHYSALIS). 2. bluebottle or blowfly. See CALLIPHORIDAE.
bluebush pea CROTALARIA *eremaea*.
bluecomb a coronaviral disease of turkeys. See TRANSMISSIBLE gastroenteritis (2).
bluegrass see POA.
bluenose a name used in the UK for a photosensitive dermatitis of the horse's face marked by a cyanotic appearance in the early stages of skin which later sloughs. The disease occurs in the spring and may be accompanied by such a severe edema that it resembles purpura hemorrhagica.
bluesedge see ANDROPOGON.
bluestem see ANDROPOGON.
bluestone copper sulfate.
Bluetick coonhound a large hound-type dog with large ears and a short, dense tricolor coat with heavy black ticking in white areas.
bluetongue an infectious disease of sheep and rarely cattle caused by an orbivirus of which there are at least 20 identified serotypes. The infection is transmitted by insects and causes an acute, seriously debilitating disease. It is characterized by an erosive stomatitis and rhinitis, and lameness due to a coronitis and laminitis. Congenital infections with wild or vaccine virus may result in defects in the nervous system, the type and severity depending on the stage of gestation.
b. virus a member of the family *Reoviridae*, genus *Orbivirus* cultivatable on eggs or tissue culture, and found in many serotypes. Causes bluetongue in sheep and other ruminants.
blunt end the end of a DNA molecule in which both strands are of the same length.
b. e. ligation the joining of nucleotides at the end of two duplex DNA molecules.
BLUP best linear unbiased prediction.
blur lack of clarity in the radiograph caused by movement of the x-ray tube, subject or film during exposure.
BLV bovine leukemia virus.
BM abbreviation for bowel movement; used in medical records.
BMC see BOVINE malignant catarrh.
BMCC bulk MILK CELL COUNTS.
BMR basal metabolic rate.
BMU basic metabolic unit or BONE remodeling unit.
boa constrictor see CONSTRICTOR CONSTRICTOR.
boar a male pig more than 6 months old and destined for use as a sire.
b. shield a strong, oval layer of cartilage which develops over the shoulders of adult boars. Is a protective mechanism in boar fights. When cooked it becomes gelatinous.
b.–sow ratio the number of boars required to maintain a sow herd at full piglet-producing performance.
b. taint an odor specific to fresh boar meat, especially from adult boars, and said to resemble stale urine, is strongest immediately after slaughter, fades during storage but returns on frying or boiling. Some diners prefer the redolent rashers.
wild b. SUS *scrofa*.

board spleen a meat inspection term for an enlarged firm spleen caused by chronic infection.

boarding kennels a commercial establishment which provides accommodation, feeding and general care for dogs and cats on a short term, usually weekly, basis. Well-run institutions cater only for healthy animals with a good vaccination record.

bob veal calf calf 1–3 weeks old, sold for baby veal, often the male calves from dairy farms; average weight 150 lb (68 kg).

bobbejaantou see CYNANCHUM.

bobby calf a calf slaughtered while only a few days old.

bobcat see LYNX. Called also bay lynx.

bobtail a short tail, either natural or docked. Seen naturally in some species, e.g. bobcat, and some dog breeds, e.g. Schipperke and Old English sheepdog.

b. disease loss of the long hairs of the mane and tail in chronic selenium poisoning in horses. Other signs are emaciation, poor haircoat and defects of hoof growth.

BOD see BIOCHEMICAL OXYGEN DEMAND.

Bodansky unit a unit of measurement for alkaline phosphatase activity in the blood.

bodian classification a system of classification of neurons based on where the nerve cell is in relation to the axon proper and the dendritic and telodendritic zones of the typical axons.

body 1. the trunk, or animal frame, with its organs. 2. the largest and most important part of any organ. 3. any mass or collection of material.

acetone b's see KETONE bodies.

b. cavity see CAVITY.

ellipsoid b. formed in degenerating myelin sheaths. Each contains a fragment of myelin apparently undergoing enzymatic digestion around a fragment of degenerating axon.

fimbriate b. see CORPUS fimbriatum.

b. fluids see body FLUIDS.

gelatinous b. a 3–5 mm glycogen-rich body in the dorsal surface of the lumbosacral enlargement of the spinal cord in birds.

geniculate b's (lateral) two metathalamus eminences, one on each side just lateral to the medial geniculate bodies, marking the termination of the optic tract.

geniculate b's (medial) two metathalamus eminences, one on each side, just lateral to the superior colliculi, concerned with hearing.

Heinz b., Heinz–Ehrlich b. a dark staining refractile body of erythrocytes, consisting of denatured hemoglobin. See also Heinz body ANEMIA.

Howell's b's see HOWELL–JOLLY BODIES.

b. louse MENACANTHUS.

mamillary b. either of the pair of small spherical masses in the interpeduncular fossa of the midbrain, forming part of the hypothalamus.

b. mass see body WEIGHT.

multilamellar b. any of the osmiophilic, lipid-rich, layered bodies found in the type II alveolar cells of the lung.

Negri b's eosinophilic, oval or round inclusion bodies in the cytoplasm of neurones of animals dead of rabies.

olivary b. see OLIVE (2).

Pappenheimer b. dark, basophilic, iron-containing granules seen in erythrocytes (siderocytes). Occur in hemolytic anemia.

para-aortic b's enclaves of chromaffin cells near the sympathetic ganglia along the abdominal aorta, which secrete catecholamines during prenatal and early postnatal life, aiding the adrenal medulla. Tumors of these structures produce clinical signs similar to those of PHEOCHROMOCYTOMA.

paracloacal vascular b. a small patch of vascular tissue in the wall of the urodeum in birds.

phallic b. pair of bodies flanking the phallus of the male bird; participate in the insemination of the hen.

pituitary b. pituitary gland.

quadrigeminal b's see CORPORA quadrigemina.

striate b. see CORPUS striatum.

b. surface area (BSA) the total surface area of the body. Used to calculate drug dosages, particularly in the use of toxic drugs such as those used in cancer chemotherapy. This minimizes errors introduced by variations in distribution, metabolism and excretion of the drug. Several equations can be used to express the area, based on body weight, but conversion tables are usually used. See Table 21.

trapezoid b. transverse ridge crossing the ventral surface of the medulla oblongata.

vitreous b. the transparent gel filling the posterior segment of the eyeball between the lens and retina. Called also vitreous and vitreous humor.

b. weight see body WEIGHT.

wolffian b. see MESONEPHROS.

body-brush a wide, flat grooming brush with a strap across the back and short vegetable fibers.

body condition score an assessment of the animal's weight for age and weight for height ratios, and its relative proportions of muscle and fat. The assessment is made by eye, on the basis of amount of tissue cover between the points of the hip, over the transverse processes of the lumbar vertebrae, the cover over the ribs and the pin bones below the tail. Each animal is graded by comparison with animals pictured on the chart. The grading may be in a score of 5 or a score of 8.

body-fold dermatitis see fold DERMATITIS, INTERTRIGO.

body language the expression of feelings by means of postures or gestures. Flamboyant body language is characteristic of primates but most animal species use gestures to demonstrate their attitudes to other animals and to the environment generally.

body mange see PSOROPTIC MANGE in particular, but the term could refer to any mange.

body-section technique see TOMOGRAPHY.

Boer a dual-purpose South African goat, the common goat of that country, with lop ears, of many colors.

bog asphodel NARTHECIUM *ossifragum*.

bog-crook see PHOSPHORUS nutritional deficiency.

bog-lame see PHOSPHORUS nutritional deficiency.

bog laurel KALMIA *polifolia* var. *microphylla*.

bog spavin chronic synovitis of the tibiotarsal joint which causes an obvious distension of the capsule of the joint. Called also tarsal hydrarthrosis.

boggabri *Amaranthus mitchellii*, *Chenopodium carinatum*.

Bohemian terrier see CZESKY TERRIER.

Bohr effect displacement of the oxyhemoglobin dissociation curve by a change in carbon dioxide tension.

Bohr equation used to estimate the dead-space volume of the lungs.

boid snake members of the Boidae family, the boas, which kill prey by constriction.

Boidae a family of nonpoisonous constrictors, commonly called pythons, varying in length from 12 to 25 ft.

Boiga a genus of the Boiginae family of tree snakes.

B. dendrophila a glossy black 7 ft long tree snake;

aggressive and venomous. Called also mangrove snake.

B. irregularis a brown tree snake with very low toxicity of its venom.

boil a painful nodule formed in the skin by circumscribed inflammation of the corium and subcutaneous tissue, enclosing a central slough or 'core'. Called also furuncle.

saddle b's deep-seated subcutaneous abscesses under the saddle place. Associated usually with poor grooming technique.

shoe b. see elbow HYGROMA.

boiling bringing to the boil.

b. fowl a mature hen of about 2 years of age, suitable for eating but requires prolonged cooking.

b. test meat that has a taint or which is beginning to decompose can have its bad odor intensified, for the purpose of convincing the doubters, by boiling a sample of it. Meat that is less than 24 hours old does not perform well in this test.

Bokhara clover MELILOTUS *alba*.

boksuring RUMEX *acetosella*.

Boley gauge a caliper used for measuring the size of teeth.

Bollinger bodies inclusion bodies in epithelial cells infected with the fowlpox virus.

bologna bull said of a mature entire bull sold for meat. The market for such animals is good because of the high proportion of the carcass that is lean meat suitable for conversion into mince or bologna.

Bolognese a small (5–9 lb) bichon-type dog with a distinctive coat which is long and flocked without curls.

bolometer 1. an instrument for measuring the force of the heartbeat. 2. an instrument for measuring minute degrees of radiant heat.

bolting 1. of a horse, escaping from restraint at full gallop. 2. of a horse, eating its food greedily and rapidly.

bolus 1. a rounded mass of food or pharmaceutical preparation ready to be swallowed, or such a mass passing through the gastrointestinal tract. In previous times most medication for horses was given by bolus. Called also ball. 2. a concentrated mass of pharmaceutical preparation, e.g. an opaque contrast medium, given intravenously. 3. a mass of scattering material, such as wax or paraffin, placed between the radiation source and the skin to achieve a precalculated isodose pattern in the tissue irradiated.

alimentary b. the mass of food, made ready by mastication, that enters the esophagus at one swallow.

physic b. see PHYSIC (2).

purging b. an oldtime treatment for equine colic. Usually contained aloes or istin.

Bolz technique conservative technique for surgical retraction of an equine penis affected by paraphimosis.

boma confinement confinement of the flock or herd, including captive wild animals being held for transport to zoos, to the boma (enclosure, corral), traditionally constructed of thorn bushes; contemporary facilities are made of conventional yard posts and rails.

bomb calorimeter see CALORIMETER.

bomb fly see HYPODERMA.

Bombay an uncommon breed of cat which is the result of crossing Burmese and black American Shorthairs. It has short black hair and deep copper-colored eyes.

bombesin a tetradecapeptide found in the brain and gut.

bona fide client a client to whom service has been provided during the previous 2 years.

bonamiasis important protozoan disease affecting hemocytes of flat oysters worldwide.

Bonasa umbellus see RUFFED GROUSE.

bond the linkage between atoms or radicals of a chemical compound, or the symbol representing this linkage and indicating the number and attachment of the valencies of an atom in constitutional formulas, e.g. H–O–H, H–C≡C–H and can be represented by a pair of dots between atoms, e.g. H:O:H, H:C:::C:H.

coordinate covalent b. a covalent bond in which one of the bonded atoms furnishes both of the shared electrons.

covalent b. a chemical bond between two atoms or radicals formed by the sharing of a pair (single bond), two pairs (double bond) or three pairs of electrons (triple bond).

disulfide b. a strong covalent bond, –S–S–, important in linking polypeptide chains in proteins, the linkage arising as a result of the oxidation of the sulfhydryl (SH) groups of two molecules of cysteine.

high-energy phosphate b. an energy-rich phosphate linkage present in adenosine triphosphate (ATP), phosphocreatine and certain other biological molecules. On hydrolysis at pH 7 it yields about 8000 calories per mole, in contrast to the 3000 calories yielded by phosphate esters. The bond stores energy that is used to drive biochemical processes, such as the synthesis of macromolecules, contraction of muscles, and the production of the electrical potentials for nerve conduction.

high-energy sulfur b. an energy-rich sulfur linkage, the most important of which occurs in the acetyl-CoA molecule, the main source of energy in fatty acid biosynthesis.

human–animal b. the psychological interdependence between humans and companion animals.

hydrogen b. a weak, primarily electrostatic, bond between a hydrogen atom bound to a highly electronegative element (such as oxygen or nitrogen) in a given molecule, or part of a molecule, and a second highly electronegative atom in another molecule or in a different part of the same molecule.

ionic b. a chemical bond in which electrons are transferred from one atom to another so that one bears a positive and the other a negative charge, the attraction between these opposite charges forming the bond.

peptide b. the –CO–NH– linkage formed between the carboxyl group of one amino acid and the amino group of another; it is an amide linkage joining amino acids to form peptides.

phosphoanhydride b. a high energy bond present in ATP.

phosphodiester b. links between nucleotides in nucleic acids.

bonding 1. the development of a close emotional tie to a mate, offspring or parent, or between human and animal. See also human–animal BOND. 2. structural uniting between physical materials.

dental b. in restorative dentistry, the important process of adhering material to the tooth surface.

mother–young b. established by the pair staying in close proximity to each other, by intuitive vocal calls, by physical licking by the dam, and sucking by the neonate.

bone 1. the hard, rigid form of connective tissue constituting most of the skeleton of most vertebrates, composed chiefly of an organic component of collagenous matrix and cells and a mineral component of calcium phosphate and other salts. 2. any distinct piece of the skeleton of the body. For a named list of bones see Table 10. 3. describes conformation, substance, thickness and quality of bone structure in an animal, e.g. an animal with good bone. See also OSSEOUS.

b. ash analysis of the degree of mineralization of bone is done by an ash analysis in which the bone is heated at 600°C until there is no further weight loss.

b. atrophy see OSTEOPOROSIS.

brittle b's see OSTEOGENESIS imperfecta.

b. callus see CALLUS (2).

cancellated b., cancellous b. bone composed of thin intersecting lamellae, usually found internal to compact bone. Called also spongy bone.

cartilage b. bone developing within cartilage, ossification taking place within a cartilage model. Called also endochondral ossification.

b. cells see OSTEOCYTE, OSTEOCLAST, OSTEOBLAST.

cheek b. see ZYGOMATIC bone.

chevron b. see HEMAL arch.

chondroid b. has histological characteristics of both cartilage and bone; may develop in response to tensions from frequently changing directions.

b. clamp strongly built, handheld, tong-like instrument with outcurving blades making a circle when closed for grasping a piece of bone shaft. The handles are ratcheted to give a firm grasp, and the faces of the blades have deep, crossways grooves.

compact b. bone substance that is dense and noncancellous.

cortical b. the compact bone of the shaft of a bone that surrounds the marrow cavity.

b. cyst a discrete, grossly visible cavity, filled with fluid and often lined by a membrane. It may be located under cartilage (subchondral), be a single cavity (unicameral), filled with blood (aneurysmal) or contain epidermal cells (epidermoid).

decalcified b. a material for bone grafting. Prepared by treatment with hydrochloric acid, bone morphogenic protein is retained.

b. density the degree of mineralization, usually demonstrable in radiographs.

b. discoloration continuous intake of tetracycline colors bone of growing animals yellow; inherited or acquired porphyria discolors bone red-brown.

ectopic b. bone which develops in abnormal sites. Needs to be differentiated from ectopic ossification and ectopic mineralization.

endochondral b. bone formed by the ossification of cartilage. The means of lengthening of long bones. See also enchondral OSSIFICATION.

entoglossal b. the bone in a bird's tongue.

b. file, b. rasp see bone RASP.

flat b. one whose thickness is slight, sometimes consisting of only a thin layer of compact bone, or of two layers with intervening cancellated bone and marrow; usually curved rather than flat.

b. flour finely ground bone used as a mineral supplement in animal feed to supply additional calcium and phosphorus. Needs to be properly sterilized.

b. fragility the ease with which bone fractures depends to a large extent on the density of its compact bone, that is its degree of mineralization, which in turn depends on a number of factors including age, nutritional adequacy, state of pregnancy and lactation and exposure to weight bearing.

b. G1a protein see OSTEOCALCIN.

b. infection see OSTEITIS, OSTEOMYELITIS, OSTEOARTHRITIS.

intramembranous b. bone formed within membrane or under the periosteum.

jugal b. see ZYGOMATIC bone.

lamellar b. mature bone in which the collagen fibers are in an orderly layered arrangement producing lamellae.

laminar b. the formation of bone by the periosteum in layers, sometimes more than one layer at a time, to supplement the diaphyseal expansion of the bone. Is marked in farm animals and large dogs, and serves to accommodate the skeleton to the very rapid growth of the musculature.

lingual b. see HYOID bone.

long b. one whose length usually exceeds its breadth and thickness and which usually bears epiphyses at each extremity during growth.

malar b. see ZYGOMATIC bone.

marble b's see OSTEOPETROSIS.

mastoid b. the posterior part of the petrous temporal bone; the mastoid process.

b. matrix the intercellular component of bone. It includes COLLAGEN and amorphous ground substance consisting mostly of mucopolysaccharides (chondroitin sulfate).

b. meal a product made from meatless bones which are crushed and sterilized. The bones are derived from boning plants and retail outlets. The bonemeal is used as stock feed, fertilizer and in a number of industries. Care is needed in its preparation and in the selection of the bones because of the high risk of transmitting diseases including anthrax, salmonellosis, tuberculosis. A coarse grade of bone flour (see above).

membrane b. bone that develops within a connective tissue membrane.

metaplastic b. bone formed by connective tissue by redifferentiation of mesenchymal cells.

b. mineral principally calcium and phosphorus but includes also magnesium and, to a lesser extent, potassium and fluorine. Consisting mainly of hydrated calcium phosphate (apatite) and calcium carbonate.

b. modeling the sum of the activities of the endosteum and periosteum of bone to produce bone forms.

b. neoplasm includes fibroma, fibrosarcoma, chondroma, osteochondroma, chondrosarcoma, osteoma, osteosarcoma.

pelvic b. hip bone.

perilacunar b. low density bone around the lacunae of bone which contains much amorphous mineral. In this form the mineral is labile and therefore important in the maintenance of calcium homeostasis.

periosteal b. bone deposition by the periosteum in successive laminae; the bone formation in new bone and in a callus, beginning as fibrocellular tissue forming from the endosteum and periosteum, followed by calcification and bone formation.

b. pinning see PINNING.

pneumatic b. bone that contains air-filled spaces.

premaxillary b. see PREMAXILLA.

pterygoid b. a small skull bone that articulates with the sphenoid.

b. remodeling unit osteoclasts, osteoblasts and their progenitors, the basal metabolic unit of bone.

b. sand remnants of bone trabeculae destroyed in osteomyelitis and sequestered in pus.

b. sealant a composition of beeswax and isopropylpalmitate used to seal the cut end of bone and stop the oozing of blood.

shin b. see TIBIA and CANNON BONE.

short b. one of approximately equal length, width and thickness, usually without epiphyses.

solid b. compact bone.
spongy b. cancellous bone.
b. structural unit see BASIC multicell unit.
sutural b's variable and irregularly shaped bones in the sutures between the bones of the skull.
b. tumor includes cartilage-forming tumors (chondroma, osteochondroma, chondrosarcoma, multilobular tumor) and bone-forming tumors (osteoma, osteosarcoma).
tympanic b. the part of the temporal bone surrounding the middle ear.
b. wax see bone sealant (above).
wormian b's sutural bones.
woven b. primitive bone with coarse collagen bundles arranged in a disorderly fashion and replaced subsequently by lamellar bone.

bone marrow the soft, organic material in the cavities of bones, a network of blood vessels and special connective tissue fibers that hold together a composite of fat and blood-producing cells.

The chief function of bone marrow is to manufacture erythrocytes, leukocytes and platelets. These blood cells normally do not enter the bloodstream until they are fully developed, so that the bone marrow contains cells in all stages of development. If the body's demand for white cells is increased because of infection, the bone marrow responds immediately by increasing production. The same is true if more red blood cells are needed, as in hemorrhage or anemia.

There are two types of bone marrow, red and yellow. The former produces the blood cells; the latter, which is mainly formed of fatty tissue, normally has no blood cell-producing function.
b. m. aplasia any of the three cell lines may be singularly aplastic but a pancytopenic abnormality is most common. See also aplastic ANEMIA.
b. m. aspiration see bone marrow BIOPSY.
congenital b. m. hypoplasia see OSTEOPETROSIS.
b. m.-derived cells see B LYMPHOCYTE.
b. m. displacement see MYELOPHTHISIS.
b. m. dyscrasia abnormal cell production by the bone marrow. Occurs in some dog breeds, especially Poodles, in which there are maturation abnormalities of erythrocytes with macrocytosis and hypersegmented neutrophils.
b. m. spaces the cavities in cancellous bone that are usually filled with bone marrow.
b. m. suppression some drugs and infectious agents can cause reduced erythropoiesis, myelopoiesis and megakaryocytopoiesis. See also ANEMIA, PANCYTOPENIA.
toxic b. m. arrest see resurgence GRANULOPOIESIS.
b. m. transplantation the transfer of bone marrow from a normal, antigenically matched individual to another, usually for treatment of aplastic anemia, immunodeficiency or metabolic disorders.

bonelet an ossicle or small bone.

Boneliota fungillae an obsolete term; see AVIPOXVIRUS.

bong dok pu see LIGULARIA AMPLEXICAULLIS.

bongo the antelope *Boocercus eurycerus*.

boning the preparation of meat for human consumption by removing the bones from the carcass.
hot b. the boning process is carried out immediately, before the carcass has had time to cool and the meat to set.

bonnet monkey see MACAQUE.

Bonomiella columbae a species of pigeon louse.

Bonsmara a red breed of beef cattle bred in South Africa from Africander, Shorthorn and Hereford breeds.

bont tick see AMBLYOMMA HEBRAEUM.

bony pelvis the ring of bone formed by the sacrum and the first few coccygeal vertebrae as the roof, the pubis and ischia as the floor and the ilia and the acetabular part of the ischia as the walls.

bony spiral lamina bony projection of the modiolus which supports the membranous subdivisions of the cochlea in the internal ear.

boobialla see MYOPORUM.

book louse see PSOCID. The intermediate hosts of *Avitellina* spp. tapeworms.

book scorpion a member of the order Chelonethida of the Arachnida class. Called also false scorpion.

booklice see PSOCOPTERA.

boonaree ALECTRYON *oleifolius*.

boonery ALCETRYON *oleifolius*.

Boophane disticha African plant in the family Liliaceae (Amaryllidaceae); contains an alkaloid buphanine which has been used as an arrow poison. Its risk as a poison plant for grazing animals is unknown.

Boophilus a genus of ticks in the family Ixodidae.
B. annulatus a one-host tick which transmits *Babesia bigemina*. Called also North American tick.
B. calcaratus a tick that transmits *Anaplasma marginale*, *Babesia bigemina* and *B. berbera*.
B. decoloratus a one-host tick that transmits *Anaplasma marginale*, *Babesia bigemina*, *B. ovis*, *B. trautmanni* and *Borrelia theileri*.
B. microplus a one-host tick that transmits *Anaplasma marginale*, *Babesia bovis*, *B. bigemina* and *Coxiella burnettii*.

Booponus a genus of flies of the family Calliphoridae.
B. intonsus the maggots of this fly cause myiasis and skin damage on the lower parts of the legs of ruminants. Called also foot maggot.

Booroola gene see MERINO.

Booroola merino prolific strain of merino sheep with the outstanding characteristic of freedom from pigmented wool; developed in Australia from a mutant strain.

booster dose see booster DOSE.

booster theory one of the theories to explain the mechanism by which calcium and phosphorus are precipitated out of solution and deposited on the matrix of bone.

boot 1. an encasement for the foot; a protective casing or sheath. 2. to start up a computer and bring it to a state of readiness to receive commands. Called also initializing, 'boot the system'.
bell b. see brush boot (below).
brush b., brushing b. a rubber cover worn over the hoof by pacing and trotting horses to prevent damage to the inside of the opposite cannon bone. Called also bell boot.

bootstrap a method for estimating parameters by repeatedly drawing random samples, with replacement, from the collected observations.

bopple nut tree see MACADAMIA.

Boraginaceae a plant family which contains the well-known poisonous plants *Heliotropum*, *Echium*, *Amsinckia* and *Trichodesma* spp. Common source of pyrrolizidine alkaloids.

Boran a variety of *Bos indicus* milking cattle bred in central and northern Africa. Horned, white or gray, sometimes pied or red.

borate any salt of boric acid.

borax sodium borate. Poisoning occurs only in animals that eat relatively large amounts. Signs include diarrhea, prostration and convulsions.

borborygmus a rumbling noise caused by propulsion of gas through the intestines. See also BOWEL sounds.

Bordeaux mixture a fungicide used on grape vines consisting of copper sulfate, calcium hydroxide and water. It has also been used in the treatment of ringworm in cattle. It can cause copper poisoning.

border a boundary line, edge or surface.

basal b. of the lung the caudal border, where the lung border moves backwards and forwards on the diaphragm.

brush b. a specialization of the free surface of a cell, consisting of minute cylindrical processes (microvilli) that greatly increase the surface area.

Border collie a medium sized (30–45 lb), working sheepdog with a moderately long, usually black and white coat. There is a smooth-coated variety. Used extensively in the United Kingdom and Australia. The breed is subject to central progressive retinal atrophy and ceroid lipofuscinosis.

border disease an infectious disease of sheep, named for the Anglo-Scottish border area, caused by intrauterine infection with a togavirus closely related to the bovine virus diarrhea virus. The congenital signs that identify the presence of the disease are an abnormally hairy birth coat, gross tremor of skeletal muscle, poor growth, a variety of skeletal deformities and defective myelination in the central nervous system. Called also hairy shaker disease.

Border fancy a popular breed of canaries, originating from the Anglo-Scottish border area. They are semi-erect and close feathered.

Border Leicester a British breed of meat sheep with long, coarse wool, no horns, a prominent Roman nose and a head which is completely free of wool. Much favored as a part of a crossbreeding program to produce fatlamb mothers.

Border terrier a small (10–12 lb) terrier with a short, harsh red or tan coat; the small v-shaped ears are dropped and the tail is moderately short. Bred for hunting foxes. Congenital ventricular septal defects are found in the breed.

Bordet–Gengou phenomenon see COMPLEMENT fixation tests.

Bordetella a genus of gram-negative bacteria which cause respiratory disease in a number of species.

B. avium the cause of turkey coryza. Previously called *Alcaligenes fecalis*.

B. bronchiseptica a small, gram-negative, motile bacillus. A normal inhabitant of the respiratory tract in humans, dogs and pigs, but also causes pneumonia, stillbirths, abortions canine infectious tracheobronchitis (see KENNEL COUGH) and ATROPHIC rhinitis in pigs.

B. parapertussis implicated in pneumonia in sheep, in association with *Pasteurella haemolytica*.

B. pertussis the cause of whooping cough in humans. Used as an adjuvant for immunostimulation.

bordetellosis an inclusive name for diseases caused by *Bordetella bronchiseptica*. It includes chronic bronchitis and some case of suppurative bronchopneumonia associated with distemper in dogs, canine infectious tracheobronchitis, atrophic rhinitis, septicemia and suppurative bronchopneumonia in pigs.

bore water water accumulated in aquifers below the earth's surface but available for farm use by sinking a bore pipe into the aquifer. May discharge to the surface (artesian bore) or need to be pumped to the surface (subartesian bore).

boredom state of mind caused by a lack of space in animal accommodation because there is insufficient room for young animals to play. If severe, animals may develop vices. See also TAIL biting, EAR sucking, CRIB-biting and PICA.

b. barking an unsatisfactory habit of some dogs, usually those left alone while their owners are at work. Unnoticed by the owner, but very annoying to neighbors.

boree see ACACIA *cana*.

Borgia's bouquet PIMELEA *trichostachya*.

boric acid, boracic acid has weak bacteriostatic, fungistatic and astringent activity, used topically and commonly as a buffer in eye-drops. Also used as an insecticide.

boring 1. a gait in a horse in which the horse leans heavily on the bit. 2. in racing, movement of a horse to put lateral pressure on another horse racing beside it.

borism poisoning by a boron compound.

Borna disease a geographically restricted virus disease of horses and occasionally sheep, characterized by a uniformly fatal encephalomyelitis. Clinically it is characterized by pharyngeal paralysis, muscle tremor, lethargy and flaccid paralysis. The causative virus is a non-segmented, negative-stranded RNA virus with a nuclear site of replication and transcription of its genome. It is noncytolytic and highly neurotropic and is the prototype and only member thus far identified of the family *Bornaviridae*, in the order *Mononegavirales*. Serologic evidence indicates that the host range of Borna disease virus or an antigenically related virus is wide and the virus has been linked to psychiatric illnesses in humans. Called also Near Eastern equine encephalomyelitis.

borogluconate a substance whose calcium salt is used in the treatment of milk fever in cows, hypocalcemia in ewes and eclampsia in the bitch. It has the virtue of being nonirritant and can be administered subcutaneously as well as intravenously.

boron a chemical element, atomic number 5, atomic weight 10.811, symbol B. See Table 6.

Borrel bodies individual fowlpox virus particles visible under the light microscope.

Borrelia a genus of spiral, gram-negative bacteria. The spirals have a long amplitude and are irregular.

B. anserina causes fowl SPIROCHETOSIS.

B. burgdorferi causes LYME DISEASE in humans and animals.

B. recurrentis causes relapsing fever in humans, and a subclinical disease in Virginia opossum, one of the major reservoirs of the disease.

B. suilla not an accredited species. Originally identified as a cause of ULCERATIVE granuloma of swine.

B. theileri cause of THEILERIASIS in cattle, sheep and horses.

borreliosis infection with *Borrelia* spp.; see also LYME DISEASE.

Borzoi a tall (28–31 inches), thin hound with a long, silky flat coat of any color but usually predominantly white. A coursing sight hound, it is also known as the Russian wolfhound.

Bos a genus of cattle of the family Bovidae which includes buffalo, bison and many other wild ruminants.

***B. banteng* (*B. javanicus, B. sondaicus*)** a member of the wild cattle group of the family Bovidae. Brown or black with white stockings and rump patch.

B. gaurus a long-horned, dark-colored with light belly and stockings, wild cattle. Tall, 6 ft at shoulder, and unsuited to domestication.

B. indicus the zebu species. Called also Brahman (USA), Afrikaner (Africa). They are much prized for their hardiness in hot climates and because of their resistance to tick infestation. They have been crossbred extensively to produce new breeds including Santa Gertrudis, Brangus, Droughtmaster, Braford.

B. mutus see YAK.

B. taurindicus crossbred zebu and British breed cattle, usually as more or less fixed breeds with an official studbook.

B. taurus the common domestic cattle of Europe. Docile and productive they represent man's most effective symbiosis with animals. They provide draft, meat, milk products, leather and many by-products.

BOSCC bovine ocular squamous cell carcinoma.

Boselaphus tragocamelus see NILGAI.

bosganna see SALSOLA *tuberculatiformis*.

bosluisbessie [Af.] see FADOGIA HOMBLEI.

boss 1. a rounded eminence as at the base of a horn. 2. the dominant cow in a herd.

bosselated marked or covered with bosses.

bossy 1. in dog conformation, used to describe overdevelopment of the shoulder muscles. 2. vernacular pet name for a cow.

Boston terrier a small, shorthaired lively dog with a short nose, prominent eyes, erect ears and a short tapered or screw tail. It has a very short, smooth coat in brindle or black, with white markings. The breed originated in the United States late in the 19th century. Predisposed to hyperadrenocorticism, mast cell tumors, heart base tumors, persistent right aortic arch, hemivertebrae, cataracts and sebaceous gland tumors.

bot fly the flies that produce the maggots known as BOTS and the diseases referred to as GASTEROPHILOSIS and NASAL bot fly infestation.

b. f. infestation see GASTEROPHILOSIS.

bothria two longitudinal grooves on the scolex of e.g. *Diphyllobothrium* spp.

Bothriocephalus a genus of tapeworms in the order Pseudophyllidae. Occur, but appear to have little pathogenicity, in many wild fish. Includes *B. acheilognathi* (carp, goldfish).

botryoid shaped like a bunch of grapes.

b. rhabdomyosarcoma see URINARY BLADDER tumors.

botryomycosis a chronic, suppurative granulomatous disease usually caused by *Staphylococcus aureus* but other organisms may be involved. The lesions begin at a cutaneous wound and usually invade deeper tissues including muscle and bone. See also SPLENDORE–HOEPPLI MATERIAL.

Botrytis a common fungal cause of spoilage in stored meat.

bots maggots of flies which infest animals, especially horses and sheep. The term bot is also loosely used to include the invasive maggots such as those of *Cuterebra* and *Wohlfahrtia* spp.

horse b. see GASTEROPHILUS.

sheep nasal b. see OESTRUS *ovis*.

bottle jaw the accumulation of edema fluid in the intermandibular space. Occurs more readily in animals grazing at pasture than in those feeding from mangers because of the effect of gravity in producing dependent edema.

bottle-nosed dolphin see DOLPHIN.

bottle rearing the rearing of newborn animals by feeding natural milk or a prepared formula from a bottle equipped with a rubber nipple.

bottle tree see BRACHYCHITON *rupestris*.

botuliform sausage-shaped.

botulin see BOTULINUM TOXIN.

botulinal pertaining to *Clostridium botulinum* or to its toxin.

botulinum toxin a neurotoxin produced by *Clostridium botulinum*; causes botulism. Eight antigenically distinct types are recognized: A, B, C, C2, D, E, F and G.

botulism a highly fatal toxemia caused by the ingestion of the toxin of *Clostridium botulinum*. The toxin is preformed as a result of proliferation of the bacteria in decomposing animal matter. The clinical picture includes the development of flaccid paralysis over a period of 1 to 3 days, the animal becoming recumbent and being unable to eat or drink, but being fully conscious. Death is caused by respiratory paralysis. Called also western duck disease, limberneck.

wound b. a form resulting from infection of a wound with *Clostridium botulinum*. Called also toxicoinfectious botulism.

bougie a slender, flexible, hollow or solid, cylindrical instrument for introduction into the urethra or other tubular organ, usually for calibrating or dilating constricted areas.

filiform b. a bougie of very slender caliber.

soluble b. a bougie composed of a substance that becomes fluid in situ.

bougienage passage of a bougie.

bouhite see MAEDI. Called also *la bouhite*.

Bouin's fixative a tissue preservative composed of saturated picric acid, formaldehyde and glacial acetic acid. Particularly suitable for trichrome connective tissue stains.

bouncing bet see SAPONARIA.

bound said of electrolytes and hormones circulating in the blood, i.e. bound to protein molecules and not immediately available functionally. See also UNBOUND.

bounding a gait in which the animal progresses in a series of bounds instead of a normal walking or running gait.

bouquet a structure resembling a cluster of flowers.

Bourdon pressure gauge see Bourdon FLOWMETER.

Bourgelatia a genus of the family Chabertiidae of nematodes. Includes *B. diducta* (pig intestine).

Boussingaultia baselloides see ANREDERA CORDIFOLIA. Called also *Boussingaultia gracilis* var. *pseudobaselloides*.

boustrophedonic see BIDIRECTIONAL.

bouton [Fr.] *button*.

b. terminal the swollen end of an axon that contributes to a synapse.

boutonneuse fever a tick-borne rickettsial disease of humans, endemic in the Mediterranean area caused by *Rickettsia conorii*. Dogs are sometimes infected and may be a reservoir for the disease.

Bouvier des Flandres a medium to large dog of compact build, with a coarse, fawn or gray coat, and a docked or naturally short tail. The coat forms a characteristic beard and mustache. The breed is affected by an inherited laryngeal paralysis. Called also Belgian cattle dog.

Bovicola a genus of lice of the superfamily Ischnocera. Also called DAMALINIA. Includes *B. painei* (goat).

Bovidae a family of ruminants including cattle, buffalo and bison.

Bovimyces pleuropneumoniae see MYCOPLASMA *mycoides* subsp. *mycoides* (small colony type).

bovine pertaining to, characteristic of, or derived from the ox or cattle, members of the family Bovidae. See also CATTLE.

b. atypical interstitial pneumonia see ATYPICAL INTERSTITIAL PNEUMONIA.

b. bonkers see AMMONIATED FORAGE POISONING.

b. cutaneous angiomatosis see ANGIOMATOSIS.

b. enzootic hematuria see ENZOOTIC HEMATURIA.

b. ephemeral fever see EPHEMERAL FEVER.

epidemic b. abortion see epizootic bovine ABORTION.

b. epizootic fever see EPHEMERAL FEVER.

b. exfoliative dermatitis widespread dermatitis including vesicles on the muzzle in very young calves; recovers sponaneously.

b. familial convulsions and ataxia see FAMILIAL convulsions and ataxia of cattle.

b. farmer's lung see ATYPICAL INTERSTITIAL PNEUMONIA.

b. herpesviruses bovine herpesviruses 1, 2, 4 and 5. See HERPESVIRIDAE.

b. hysteria see AMMONIATED FORAGE POISONING.

b. immunodeficiency virus a lentivirus which causes leukopenia followed by persistent leukocytosis when inoculated into calves. The prevalence and significance of natural infection are unknown.

b. leukocyte adhesion deficiency see bovine LEUKOCYTE adhesion deficiency.

b. leukosis see bovine viral leukosis (below).

b. lymphomatosis see bovine viral leukosis (below).

b. lymphosarcoma see bovine viral leukosis (below).

b. malignant catarrh an acute highly infectious, fatal herpesvirus disease of cattle characterized by an erosive stomatitis and gastroenteritis, erosions on the mucosa of the upper respiratory tract, keratoconjunctivitis, encephalitis, and laymphadenopathy. There are at least two viruses involved. A wildebeest-associated form of the disease is caused by alcephaline herpesvirus 1, and a sheep-associated disease caused by a poorly characterized virus, presumably ovine herpesvirus 1, transmitted to cattle by lambing ewes which themselves show no clinical signs of disease.

b. mucosal disease see bovine virus diarrhea (below).

b. papular stomatitis see bovine PAPULAR stomatitis.

b. petechial fever an apparently infectious disease of ruminants in Kenya, caused by a rickettsia of the genus *Ehrlichia*, and manifested by fever and submucosal and serosal hemorrhages. There may be epistaxis and other evidence of a bleeding tendency. The disease has a strong similarity to TICKBORNE FEVER. The method of transmission is unknown. Called also Ondiri disease.

b. polyomavirus a virus not known to be pathogenic; up to 60% of cattle sera have antibody to the virus.

b. pneumonic pasteurellosis see pneumonic PASTEURELLOSIS.

b. protozoal abortion see NEOSPOROSIS.

b. pulmonary emphysema see ATYPICAL INTERSTITIAL PNEUMONIA.

b. respiratory disease a group of undifferentiated diseases of young cattle characterized by dyspnea, coughing, nasal discharge, evidence of pneumonia on auscultation of the lungs, and nonspecific signs as a result of the toxemia of infection and tissue destruction. Because of the complexity of the differential diagnosis of these diseases, it has become common practice to devise treatments and control programs which will deal satisfactorily with them as a group. Called also shipping fever.

b. respiratory syncytial virus a member of the family *Paramyxoviridae*, genus *Pneumovirus* which causes one of the more virulent forms of enzootic calf pneumonia. Many calves in the group are affected, there is severe dyspnea, and extensive involvement of the lungs. The mortality rate is high.

sporadic b. encephalomyelitis see sporadic bovine ENCEPHALOMYELITIS.

b. viral leukosis a highly fatal, systemic, malignant neoplasm of the reticuloendothelial system of cattle. It is characterized by tumors composed of aggregations of neoplastic lymphocytes in almost any organ with a great variety of clinical syndromes resulting. The causative retrovirus is transmitted in a number of ways, including insect vectors, but only to cattle over about 1.5 years of age. There is a significant component of genetic susceptibility in the etiology of the disease and many animals may receive the virus but not become infected. In those that do, the infection persists for life. One group of these cattle are seropositive and may not progress further. A second group are seropositive and develop a persistent lymphocytosis, a benign disease without further progress. The third group is the one in which the cattle develop malignant tumors, lymphosarcomas, and demonstrate any one or a combination of syndromes. These include abomasal obstruction and ulcer, congestive heart failure, posterior paralysis, pharyngeal obstruction, protrusion of the eyeball, and a cutaneous form with multiple nodes and plaques in the skin. There is also a sporadic occurrence in young cattle, a juvenile form in calves less than 6 months old, and a thymic form in yearlings. The disease is always fatal, often within a few weeks. Called also bovine lymphosarcoma, enzootic bovine leukosis.

b. virus diarrhea an infectious disease of cattle caused by a pestivirus. Clinical disease is sporadic and is seen only in young animals. The syndrome includes diarrhea, erosive stomatitis and rhinitis, often with similar lesions at all mucocutaneous and skin–horn junctions. Congenital defects occur in the offspring of females which become infected during pregnancy but do not themselves show clinical signs. The best known defect is cerebellar agenesis. Called also mucosal disease.

bovine leukemia virus see BOVINE viral leukosis.

bovine spongiform encephalopathy a prion disease of cattle, also known as mad cow disease. Called also BSE. It emerged as a new disease of cattle in the United Kingdom beginning in the mid 1980s following changes in the processing of offal that initially included sheep offal presumed to contain the sheep scrapie prion. Contaminated meat meal was then fed to cattle as a protein supplement. Other species fed BSE-infected bovine tissues, including Felidae and other ruminants in zoological collections and domestic cats, also developed spongiform encephalopathy. Suspected to be the cause of a variant form of Creutzfeldt–Jakob disease (vCJD) in humans. The pathogenesis and clinical course of BSE in cattle is similar to scrapie in sheep. The occurrence of BSE in cattle outside the United Kingdom has been traced to either movement of cattle or contaminated feed. The incidence of clinical cases peaked between 1992 and 1994 in the United Kingdom and vigorous efforts are being made, at a very high cost, to eradicate the disease. See also SCRAPIE.

bovovaccine a vaccine consisting of live, virulent human tubercle bacilli used to protect cattle against bovine tuberculosis. It was effective but was discontinued because it caused the excretion of live organisms in the milk!

bowel the INTESTINE.

b. edema see EDEMA disease.

b. entrapment see INTESTINAL strangulation.

hemorrhagic b. syndrome see PROLIFERATIVE hemorrhagic enteropathy.

b. sounds relatively high-pitched abdominal sounds caused by the propulsion of the intestinal contents through the lower alimentary tract. Auscultation of bowel sounds is best accomplished by using a diaphragm-type stethoscope rather than a bell-shaped one. Normal bowel sounds are characterized by bubbling and gurgling noises that vary in frequency, intensity and pitch. In the presence of distension from flatus, the sounds are hyperresonant and can be heard over the entire abdomen.

b. training see HOUSETRAINING.

Bowenia a genus of Australian cycads in the plant family Stangeriaceae; contain cycad glucoside causing a staggers syndrome in cattle. Includes *B. serrulata* (Byfield fern), *B. spectabilis* (zamia fern).

Bowen's disease in humans, multiple cutaneous squamous cell carcinomas in situ; reported in dogs and cats. There are hyperkeratotic, hyperpigmented plaques.

bowie a disease of young lambs characterized by lateral curvature of the long bones of the front limbs. The lambs become so lame that they lose condition and are markedly deformed by the age of 8 weeks. The cause is unknown.

bowleg an outward curvature of one or both legs near the knee; genu varum.

Bowman–Heidenhain theory the early theory of renal function which incorporated both glomerular and tubular secretory functions, as well as glomerular filtration and tubular reabsorption.

Bowman's capsule a two-layered cellular envelope enclosing the tuft of capillaries constituting the glomerulus of the kidney; called also glomerular capsule, malpighian capsule.

Bowman's disk one of the flat, disklike plates making up a striated muscle fiber.

Bowman's glands small mucous glands in olfactory mucosa; called also olfactory glands.

Bowman's membrane see CORNEAL laminae.

Bowman's space the cavity within the glomerular capsule in which glomerular filtrate collects.

box 1. an ornamental shrub. See BUXUS SEMPERVIRENS. 2. accommodation for a single horse averaging 10 ft × 12 ft in dimensions. Called also loose box. 3. to mix groups of sheep (box them up). 4. a repeating sequence of nucleotides that forms a transcription or a regulatory signal.

CAT b. a sequence associated with polymerase II activity.

Hogness b. see Pribnow box (below).

Pribnow b. the sequence of 5 to 10 bases in the promotor region of *Escherichia coli* genes. It is a variant of a basic sequence TATAATG. See also TATA box (below).

TATA b. a eukaryotic DNA sequence usually TATAAATA, similar to the Pribnow box of *Escherichia coli*, occurring in the promotor region 25 to 30 bases upstream from the transcriptional start site and required for mRNA chain initiation.

box and whisker plot, boxplot a graphical method of displaying the distribution of a variable.

box jellyfish members of the order Cubomedusae in the class Schyphozoa. They carry potent venom sufficient to kill an adult human. There are no records of animal mortality. Called also sea wasp.

box restraint see squeeze CAGE.

boxed beef the alternative to carcass meat. Major cuts, often deboned, are packed in sealed plastic bags and packed in strong cardboard boxes.

boxed horse colic a disorder of horses which come off pasture into boxes or stalls and on a diet in which roughage is lacking, encouraging them to eat bedding, causing impaction colic.

Boxer a medium-sized, short-nosed dog with a short brown coat and white and black markings around the face, chest and legs. It has a tail docked to a short length and, where practiced, the ears are cropped. The breed is predisposed to aortic and carotid body tumors, congenital heart defects, CARDIOMYOPATHY, gingival hyperplasia, skin tumors (particularly mastocytomas, melanomas and histiocytomas), brain tumors, corneal ulceration, histiocytic ulcerative colitis and an inherited AXONOPATHY.

B. ulcer see refractory ULCER.

boxwood see BUXUS SEMPERVIRENS.

Boyden chamber an instrument for assessing the in vitro chemotactic activity of neutrophils.

Boykin spaniel an American breed, originating in South Carolina as a turkey and waterfowl hunting dog. Medium-sized (30–38 lb), it has a wavy or curly, liver-colored coat.

Boyle's law at a constant temperature and mass the volume of a perfect gas varies inversely with pressure; that is, as increasing pressure is applied, the volume decreases. Conversely, as pressure is reduced, volume is increased.

Boynton tissue vaccine an obsolete term for an inactivated tissue vaccine used in pigs to prevent hog cholera.

boys and girls MERCURIALIS *annua*.

BP 1. blood pressure. 2. boiling point. 3. British Pharmacopoeia.

BP-6 a mixture of polybrominated biphenyls used as a flame retardant.

bp base pair.

b.p. boiling point.

Bq becquerel.

Br chemical symbol, *bromine*.

Brabancon see BRUSSELS GRIFFON.

Brabant disease trichlorethylene-extracted SOYBEAN meal poisoning.

Brabant mastitis test an early version of the California mastitis test based on the development of a gel in the sample as an indicator of the number of tissue cells present.

brace 1. an orthopedic appliance or apparatus (orthosis), usually made of metal or leather, applied to the body, particularly the trunk and lower extremities. Has limitations in animals as compared to humans. Used mainly for support for the lower limbs of horses. 2. the stance from which a polo shot is played. 3. a pair of animals.

brachial pertaining to the forelimb.

b. avulsion see brachial plexus AVULSION.

b. block regional anesthesia applied to the brachial plexus for the purpose of anesthetizing the forelimb.

b. paralysis injury to the brachial plexus causes paralysis and atrophy in the front limbs. See also brachial plexus AVULSION.

b. plexus a nerve plexus originating from the ventral branches of the last four cervical and the first thoracic spinal nerves. It gives off the principal nerves to the shoulder and forelimbs.

b. plexus neuritis occurs rarely in dogs. Characterized by an acute onset of pain and weakness in the forelimbs. There is hyporeflexia, neurogenic atrophy and loss of sensation.

brachialgia pain in the arm.

brachialis tendon the tendon of insertion of the brachialis muscle. A surgical procedure transposes this or the biceps tendon to the olecranon as a treatment for paralysis from brachial avulsion, but only if the musculocutaneous nerve function is still present.

Brachiaria a genus of the grass family Poaceae; contain steroidal saponins; manifested clinically by photosensitization. Includes *B. brizantha* (signal grass,

St. Lucia grass), *B. decumbens* (signal grass), *B. humidicola* (Koronivia grass), *B. radicans* (tanner grass), *B. ruziziensis*. Unidentified species (called also Brazilian tanner grass) may cause nitrite poisoning.

B. mutica the grass is not normally poisonous but may contain enough oxalate to cause osteodystrophy fibrosa in horses at pasture. Called also para grass.

brachi(o)- word element. [L., Gr.] *arm*.

brachiocephalic pertaining to the proximal forelimb and head.

brachiocrural pertaining to the arm and leg.

brachiocubital pertaining to the arm and elbow.

Brachionus plicatilis euryhaline zooplanktonic species, 125–300 μm in size, used as live food for larval marine fish. Called also rotifer.

brachium pl. *brachia* [L.] 1. the arm; specifically from the shoulder to elbow. Called also thoracic limb. 2. any armlike process or structure.

b. colliculi caudalis fibers from the caudal colliculus which enter the medial geniculate body and form part of the auditory pathway.

b. colliculi caudalis et rostralis the bridging fibers between the colliculi and the geniculate bodies.

b. conjunctivum the rostral cerebellar peduncle. A fibrous band extending from each hemisphere of the cerebellum upward over the pons, the two joining to form the sides and part of the roof of the fourth ventricle.

b. pontis the brachium of the pons, the middle cerebellar peduncle.

brachy- word element. [Gr.] *short*.

Brachyachne genus of Australian grasses, members of the family Poaceae. Cause cyanide poisoning. Includes *B. convergens* (Gulf star or spider grass), *B. tenella* (slender native couch grass).

brachybasia a slow, shuffling, short-stepped gait.

brachycardia see BRADYCARDIA.

brachycephalic having a short wide head.

b. breeds those dog breeds with very short faces, e.g. Boxer, Bulldog, King Charles spaniel, Pekingese, Pug. Associated with this type of skull, these breeds suffer from anomalies of the upper respiratory tract such as stenotic nares, elongated soft palate, and everted laryngeal saccules, and associated disorders, e.g. facial fold dermatitis. They are also predisposed to neoplasms of chemoreceptor tissue.

b. obstructive syndrome any of several upper airway disorders, prevalent in brachycephalic dogs, may lead to elongation and thickening of the soft palate, chronic pharyngitis and tonsillitis, inflammation and decreased diameter of the larynx and trachea. Conditions which predispose are everted laryngeal saccules, laryngeal collapse, stenotic nares.

brachycephaly the state of being brachycephalic.

Brachycera an order of large flies; includes *Brachycera ovis* (sheep), *B. bovis* (cattle). Includes TABANUS spp. flies.

brachyceros European cattle type derived from *Bos taurus brachyceros*; small, red, brown or black with short horns and deep forehead. Called also Celtic Red.

brachycheilia shortness of the lip.

Brachychiton Australian tree genus, members of the family Sterculiaceae. Valuable fodder trees in drought time but can poison sheep and cattle, the seeds being most poisonous. Toxin unidentified. Includes *B. populneum* (kurrajong tree).

B. rupestris may cause nitrate–nitrite poisoning. Called also bottle tree.

Brachycladium spiciferum an obsolete name for BIPOLARIS *spicifera*.

brachydactyly abnormal shortness of the digits.

Brachyglottis New Zealand shrub member of the plant family Asteraceae (Compositae).

B. repanda causes ataxia and recumbency. Called also rangiora.

brachygnathia abnormal shortness of the mandible resulting in a maxilla that is longer. Called also overshot, parrot mouth.

brachygnathism see BRACHYGNATHIA.

Brachylaemidae a family of trematodes that infest birds and mammals.

brachymetacarpia abnormal shortness of the metacarpal bones.

brachymetatarsia abnormal shortness of the metatarsal bones.

brachyodont see brachyodont TEETH.

brachyphalangia abnormal shortness of one of the phalanges.

brachytherapy a form of radiotherapy in which the source of radiation is applied in or on the patient in one prolonged dose, using surface applicators, needles, seeds or suspensions for use in serous cavities.

brachyury shortness of the tail, as in some Manx cats.

bracken see PTERIDIUM.

brackets in orthodontics, metal devices bonded onto teeth for attachment of elastic bands to reposition teeth.

Braco Italiano a powerful, muscular, medium to large-sized (55–88 lb) gun dog with fine, short coat in orange or chestnut with white or orange or chestnut with white, or orange or chestnut roan.

bradsot see BRAXY.

brady- word element. [Gr.] *slow*.

bradyacusia dullness of hearing.

bradyarrhythmia bradycardia associated with arrhythmia. Includes sinus BRADYCARDIA, SINOATRIAL block, ATRIAL standstill and atrioventricular HEART BLOCK.

Bradybaena terrestrial snail, the intermediate host for the pancreatic flukes *Eurytrema* spp.

bradycardia slowness of the heartbeat, in dogs and cats to less than 60 beats per minute.

sinus b. a slow sinus rhythm, characterized by normal electrocardiographic complexes in a normal rhythm or a sinus arrhythmia. A normal finding, most commonly seen in large breeds of dogs or athletic animals.

b.-tachycardia syndrome see SICK sinus syndrome.

bradykinesia abnormal slowness of movement; sluggishness of physical and mental responses.

bradykinin a nonapeptide kinin formed from a plasma protein, high-molecular-weight (HMW) kininogen, by the action of kallikrein; it is a very powerful vasodilator that increases capillary permeability and, in addition, constricts smooth muscle and stimulates pain receptors.

bradyphagia abnormal slowness of eating.

bradypnea respirations that are regular in rhythm but slower than normal in rate. This is normal during sleep; otherwise it is associated with disturbance in the brain's respiratory control center, as when the center is affected by opiate narcotics, a tumor, a metabolic disorder or a respiratory decompensation mechanism.

Bradypus tridactylus see SLOTH.

bradyspermatism abnormally slow ejaculation of semen.

bradysphygmia abnormal slowness of the pulse.

bradystalsis abnormal slowness of peristalsis.

bradytachycardia alternating attacks of bradycardia and tachycardia.

bradytocia slow parturition.

bradyuria slow discharge of urine.

bradyzoite small comma-shaped form of *Toxoplasma gondii* found in tissues enclosed in a pseudocyst; assumed to be slow-growing form of the parasite.

Braford a white-faced breed of red beef cattle produced by crossbreeding between Hereford and Brahman breeds.

Brahma heavy Asiatic breed of poultry with black or white body plumage, silver-gray head and neck, beak and legs yellow, heavy leg feather.

Brahman silver-gray, humped cattle created as a breed in the southern USA from cattle imported from India at the beginning of the 20th century. As a breed they may have had minor infusions of blood from the British breeds.

brailing a technique for temporarily preventing flight in game birds by the use of leather straps.

brain encephalon; that part of the central nervous system contained within the cranium, comprising the forebrain, midbrain and hindbrain, and developed from the embryonic neural tube. It is connected at its base with the spinal cord. The brain is a mass of soft, pinkish gray nerve tissue. For specific brain diseases see under headings relating to etiology and lesion.

b. abscess common signs caused by an abscess in the brain are circling, rotation of the head, abnormal reflexes in one eye. The CSF may show evidence of infection.

b. aneurysm see berry ANEURYSM.

b. anoxia acute or chronic insufficiency of the blood supply to the brain causes anoxia which causes clinical signs that vary with the severity of the deprivation. Acute anoxia causes muscle tremor, recumbency, convulsions and death or recovery if the anoxia is relieved soon enough. Chronic anoxia causes lethargy, weakness, blindness and sometimes convulsions. In either case there may be permanent damage.

b. case the cranium.

b. cestodal cyst see COENUROSIS.

b. coup lesion a derivation from CONTRECOUP.

b. death irreversible coma.

b. decompression relieving the pressure within the cranial vault. This may be done surgically by opening the cranium, or medically by administering hypertonic solutions of slowly metabolized materials, such as mannitol, intravenously.

b. edema an important part of a number of acute diseases, e.g. lead poisoning, encephalitis, salt poisoning in swine, polioencephalomalacia of ruminants and hypoxia due to any cause. Clinically manifested by blindness, opisthotonos, nystagmus, recumbency and tonic convulsions. Inherited in polled and horned Herefords; calves are recumbent at birth and are never able to stand but consciousness is normal. See also NEURAXIAL EDEMA.

b. ependymal lining see EPENDYMA.

b. hematoma may occur with trauma, in extradural, subdural or intraparenchymal locations. They can cause progressive increase in intracranial pressure and eventually death.

b. hemorrhage intracranial hemorrhage affecting the brain usually follows traumatic injury but spontaneous hemorrhage may result from an intrinsic vascular lesion. Loss of consciousness is a common sign followed by residual signs depending on the locality and size of the hemorrhage. Ataxia and convulsions are common sequelae.

b. herniation displacement of brain from the cranial vault through the foramina (tentorial notch or foramen magnum) or ventral to dural septae. The usual causes are brain edema or hemorrhage with resulting increase in intracranial pressure.

b. hypoxia see brain anoxia (above).

b. infarction see feline ischemic ENCEPHALOPATHY.

b. inflammation see ENCEPHALITIS, ENCEPHALOMYELITIS, MENINGOENCEPHALITIS.

b. ischemia see brain anoxia (above).

b. laceration occurs in cranial trauma that fractures the skull, causes severe acceleration or deceleration, or penetrates the skull and brain tissue.

b. necrosis see ENCEPHALOMALACIA.

b. pigmentation occurs in PHALARIS spp. poisoning; a characteristic greenish brown color grossly of the gray matter in brainstem nuclei and spinal cord, caused by a suspected lysosomal storage of granules of pigment material; usually associated with some degree of Wallerian degeneration within spinal cord tracts.

b. sand see ACERVULI.

b. scanning a radiographic, magnetic or nuclear medical procedure for the detection of brain tumors, abscesses, hematomas and other intracranial lesions. Not widely used in veterinary medicine because of the expensive equipment required.

b. spongy degeneration see BOVINE SPONGIFORM ENCEPHALOPATHY.

b. staggers see DUMMY.

b. trauma injury to the brain, including that caused by migrating worm larvae, will have diffuse effects including the development of edema, and local effects due to pressure by displaced bone or to hemorrhage. Initial shock, manifested as unconsciousness, is likely to be followed by residual localizing signs, e.g. facial paralysis, head rotation.

b. tumors cause signs suggestive of local space-occupying lesion in the cranial cavity, including the increased intracranial pressure syndrome, blindness with disturbance of ocular reflexes, head rotation, circling and jacksonian epileptic episodes.

b. ventricles see third, fourth, fifth VENTRICLE.

brain–allergy axis the observation that stress and conditioned reflexes can affect immune responsiveness and histamine release; postulated as a factor in allergic disease.

brain–blood–cerebrospinal fluid barrier see blood–CSF BARRIER.

brainstem the stemlike portion of the brain connecting the cerebral hemispheres with the spinal cord, and comprising the pons, medulla oblongata and midbrain; considered by some to include the diencephalon. See also RETICULAR activating system, ascending RETICULAR formation, THALAMUS.

b. auditory evoked response see brainstem auditory EVOKED RESPONSE.

b. hemorrhage results from cranial trauma and characteristically causes unconsciousness with varying types and degrees of motor paralysis and irregularities of respiration, depending on the site.

b. reticular formation see RETICULAR activating system.

Brambell Committee a technical committee set up by HM Government in the UK to *Inquire into the Welfare of Animals Kept Under Intensive Livestock Husbandry Systems*. The common usage name of the committee derived from its chairman Professor F.W.R. Brambell. Its report was published in 1965 and was the formal beginning of the age of animal welfare.

bran the outer layers of cereal grain seeds plus the inner, protein-rich aleurone layer. A bulky, slightly laxative food, highly prized as a supplementary feed for horses and cattle, and a basic feed for poultry. It has a high concentration of phosphorus but is low in calcium.

b. disease see OSTEODYSTROPHIA FIBROSA, HYPERPARATHYROIDISM.

b. mash an important item in the traditional mystique of nursing sick horses. Two double handfuls of bran and a tablespoon of salt are quickly mixed with sufficient boiling water to make a crumbly mash. This is covered with a sack for 15 minutes and then fed. The aroma is delicious.

bran-like epithelial scales, resembling flakes of bran, dusted over the surface of the skin.

branch 1. ramus; a division or offshoot from a main stem, especially of blood vessels, nerves or lymphatics. 2. the bearing surface of the horseshoe that supports the wall of the hoof. There is a lateral and a medial branch.

bundle b. a branch of the bundle of His.

communicating gray b. postganglionic nerve fibers coursing between the sympathetic ganglia and the spinal nerves; destined for skin glands, blood vessels and the like; join spinal and cranial nerves.

communicating white b. preganglionic fibers of the sympathetic system originate in the lateral columns of the spinal cord and pass to the spinal nerves and then, via the communicating white fibers, to the ganglia of the sympathetic trunk.

branch practice the term has two meanings. 1. a separate enterprise connected to the parent practice only by having a common ownership. 2. a subsidiary practice utilizing the resources and staff of the parent practice. Usually attended only at specified, limited hours, with the opportunity for a client to go to the parent practice in an emergency. This is really a branch premises.

branch premises see BRANCH PRACTICE.

branched-chain ketoaciduria see MAPLE SYRUP URINE DISEASE.

branched onion weed TRACHYANDRA *divaricata.*

branchiae gills of fish and their homologs in other vertebrate embryos.

branchial, branchiogenic, branchiogenous pertaining to, or resembling, gills of a fish or derivatives of homologous parts in higher forms.

b. arches paired arched columns that bear the gills in lower aquatic vertebrates and which, in embryos of higher vertebrates, become modified into structures of the face, mandible, ear and neck.

b. clefts the clefts between the branchial arches of the embryo, formed by rupture of the membrane separating corresponding entodermal pouch and ectodermal groove.

b. cyst a cyst formed deep within the neck from an incompletely closed branchial cleft, usually located between the second and third branchial arches. The branchial arches develop during early embryonic life and are separated by four clefts. As the fetus develops, these arches grow to form structures within the head and neck. Two of the arches grow together and enclose the cervical sinus, a cavity in the neck. A branchial cyst may develop within the cervical sinus. Called also branchiogenic or branchiogenous cyst. Seen rarely in dogs as a slowly developing swelling in the pharyngeal area, filled with saliva.

b. groove an external furrow lined with ectoderm, occurring in the embryo between two branchial arches.

branchiomerism the segmental arrangement of the branchial arches.

Branchiomyces a fungus which causes necrosis of gill tissue in warm water fish.

brand a mark put on the skin of animals as a means of identification. In livestock several methods are used. Fire-branding with a hot iron is the traditional method for horses and cattle but is being supplanted by the much superior FREEZE BRANDING. For sheep the branding of the surface of the fleece with tar or paint has been used for a long time but may have very damaging effects on the fleece and has been replaced by special branding formulations. See also TATTOOING.

b. cancer a mass of granulation tissue at the site of a fire-brand. Is usually chronic inflammatory tissue.

b. register a list of brands and owners maintained by a statutory authority to facilitate legal identification of animals.

Brangus a polled, black breed of beef cattle produced by crossbreeding of Brahman and Angus cattle. The breed retains many of the characteristics of its parents, including persistent frenulum and a resulting difficulty in mating.

Branhamella a genus of aerobic, nonmotile, nonspore-forming cocci. Several species are found in the upper respiratory tract and conjunctiva of humans and many animal species.

Branham's sign, Branham test, Branham reflex bradycardia produced by digital closure of an artery proximal to an arteriovenous fistula.

Brassica a genus of plants of the Brassicaceae (Cruciferae) family containing a large number of cultivated plants eaten by humans and food animals. Poisoning with them is rare but under particular growing conditions and if the diet consists almost entirely of the one plant some massive outbreaks of poisoning can occur.

Poisoning syndromes attributed to *Brassica* spp. include hemolytic anemia (kale anemia) caused by SMCO, goiter from glucosinolates, nitrate/nitrite, photosensitization, blindness (polioencephalomalacia), respiratory distress and rumen stasis.

Includes *B. campestris* (*B. rapa*), *B. hirta* (*Sinapis alba*), *B. juncea* (Indian or leaf mustard), *B. kaber* (*Sinapis arvensis*), *B. napus* var. *napus* (*B. napus*), *B. sinapistrum* (*Sinapis arvensis*).

B. alba annual weed; the seed is used, together with that of *B. nigra*, to make commercial mustard. The seed, stubble or plant in pod can cause gastroenteritis with signs of abdominal pain, salivation and diarrhea. The toxin is a mixture of isothiocyanates called mustard oil. The enzyme myrosinase is needed to activate the oil and produce irritant effect. Oil cake containing the oil may be nontoxic because myrosinase is inactivated but can become toxic if animal has access to alternative source of the enzyme simultaneously.

B. napobrassica swede turnip.

B. napus rape or canola.

B. nigra seeds are used in mixtures with *B. alba* in the manufacture of commercial mustard powder. Can cause poisoning as for *B. alba* (see above).

B. oleracea the commercial vegetables and cultivated fodder plants. Includes *B. o.* var. *acephala* (kale, cole, chou moellier), *B. o.* var. *botrytis* (cauliflower), *B. o.* var. *capitata* (cabbage), *B. o.* var. *gemmifera* (Brussel sprouts), *B. o.* var. *italica* (broccoli, calabrese).

B. rapa turnip.

Brassica rapa* subsp. *campestris turnip rape.

Braunvieh group of gray-brown, dual-purpose cattle breeds including Brown Swiss, Austrian brown, German brown etc. etc. Called also Brown mountain.

braxy an infectious disease of sheep caused by *Clostridium septicum* and characterized by a profound toxemia resulting from invasion of the abomasal wall by the clostridia. The lesion in the wall of the abomasum is thought to derive from damage by frosted grass, the disease being restricted in its occurrence to times of heavy frost.

Brazilian glory pea SESBANIA *punicea*.

Brazilian groundnut poisoning see AFLATOXICOSIS.

Brazilian lucerne see STYLO.

Brazilian nightshade SOLANUM *seaforthianum*.

Brazilian tanner grass see BRACHIARIA.

BRD bovine respiratory disease.

breach of contract failure to complete an agreed task. If a breach of contract can be proved the aggrieved person is entitled to compensation for loss incurred. Alternative penalties may be that the contract be completed or that other tasks be completed.

bread and butter pericarditis a pericarditis lesion in which the visceral and parietal epicardia are adherent and when drawn apart leave a felted, shaggy appearance on both surfaces. Called also cor villosum, shaggy heart.

break a discontinuity, e.g. the change in coat color from puppies to adults.

wool b. horizontal bands of weakness in wool or haircoats may result in a 'break' in the wool and loss of the fleece, or a significant downgrading of its value. The weakness is usually the result of a period of disturbed metabolism, e.g. a severe attack of disease, or of poor nutrition.

breakdown 1. sudden appearance of disease in an individual or herd/flock in which immunity had previously appeared adequate. The term is used especially in relation to breakdowns after vaccination, e.g. hog cholera, infectious avian laryngotracheitis, erysipelas. Also in individual animals which harbor inactive lesions which suddenly break down or metastasize and cause widespread lesions, e.g. in tuberculosis, contagious bovine pleuropneumonia. 2. acute onset of lameness in a racing horse.

breaking-in the training of a horse to be bridled, saddled, ridden and, in some horses, to be harnessed to vehicles and draw loads. Called also schooling.

breast in horses and birds used only in the singular and refers to the anterior parts of the pectoral region. Used synonymously with brisket in ruminants. See also MAMMARY gland, UDDER.

b. blisters a disease of commercial, housed poultry and turkeys comprising abscesses in the area of the carina of the sternum. They may contain pus or clear to blood-stained fluid. Usually relatable to environmental trauma.

blue b. mastitis in domestic rabbits caused by *Streptococcus*, *Staphylococcus* or *Pasteurella* spp. The mammary glands are hot, hard and swollen and there is a severe systemic illness. The glands develop a blue color due to local cyanosis.

b. boil deep abscesses in the anterior parts of the pectoral muscles in the horse. See also pectoral ABSCESS. Called also equine sternal granuloma.

b. muscles well-developed muscles for wing movement of birds composed mostly of the pectoral and supracoracoid muscles.

breastplate 1. for use with a saddle, a strap attached to the girth at its lowest point, which then passes between the forelimbs, passes upwards and divides to pass on either side of the neck and to meet at the withers after attaching to the front edge of the saddle. Designed to prevent the girth of saddle slipping backwards especially in a herring-gutted horse. 2. in harness, a broad strap, usually padded, which runs horizontally across the chest just below the neck. Behind the shoulders it is attached to the backstrap, which prevents it from falling down, and to the breeching which goes around the thighs of the horse. The breastplate keeps the harness from sliding back along the horse.

breath the air taken in and expelled by the expansion and contraction of the thorax.

bad b. see breath odor (below).

b. odor characteristic for a species, reflecting their diet. Abnormal or unpleasant odors may be caused by diseased or necrotic tissue in the respiratory or upper gastrointestinal tracts, including mouth and nasal cavity. Diseased teeth are a common cause in dogs and cats. In addition, certain metabolic diseases may produce distinctive breath odor, e.g. ketoacidosis, uremia.

b. sounds can be heard with a stethoscope on the chest and trachea. The normal sounds are the normally very faint vesicular murmur and the louder, tubular sounding bronchial tones. They are made by the air passing through the tubes of the bronchi. Adventitious (abnormal) sounds are the RALE, RHONCHUS, grunt, FRICTION rub, laryngeal stertor, WHEEZE and peristaltic sounds. Bronchovesicular sounds are intermediate between the two in character and site of origin. The vesicular sounds and the BRONCHIAL tones may be increased to the point of being an abnormality. Abnormal sounds are caused by narrowing of the tubes, collection of exudate in them or inflammation of the pleural surfaces.

b. volume may be assessed by observation of degree of chest movement and volume of expired air as felt by the hand. A respirometer is more accurate but is not available nor satisfactory for clinical use with animals unless the subject is trained to use one.

breathing the alternate inspiration and expiration of air into and out of the lungs (see also RESPIRATION).

costal b. see costal RESPIRATION.

intermittent positive-pressure b. (IPPB) the active inflation of the lungs during inspiration under positive pressure from a cycling valve.

periodic b. see PERIODIC breathing, BIOT'S RESPIRATIONS, CHEYNE–STOKES RESPIRATION.

breathlessness see DYSPNEA, HYPERPNEA, TACHYPNEA.

Breda virus see TOROVIRUS.

breech, britch the buttocks of an animal; the backs of the thighs.

b. presentation presentation of the buttocks of the fetus during parturition. See also PRESENTATION.

breeching part of a set of cart harness. A broad strap running horizontally across the backs of the thighs and attached in front to the shafts. Essential in the backing of the vehicle.

breed a group of related animals which are genotypically and phenotypically sufficiently similar to produce physically similar offspring when they are mated with each other. In most countries each breed is managed by a breed society which maintains a register of the animals that are members of the breed, and which animals shall be admitted to the register. The breed society also sets the standards for physical appearance that must be attained. See specific breed name for further descriptions and under species for list of breeds.

b. class averages the average production performance for all animals in the breed, arranged in groups according to age and sex.

commercial b. the breed is at the level where commercial herds are breeding them for the sale market as egg-layers or wool producers rather than as foundation stock to produce the sale article.

b. comparisons comparisons of productivity between populations each of which consists entirely of members of one breed.

b. complementation the practice of combining breeds in a breeding program so as to maximize the genetic merit of offspring for total productivity; implies use of breeds which tend to cancel out the undesirable elements in their genetic makeup.

b. multiplier second echelon in the breeding industry; the stud breeder producing usually sires and, to a lesser extent, dams of superior merit for commercial flocks or herds.

b. nucleus a stud producing its own male and female herd replacements, without the introduction of outside blood; supplies the multiplier.

b. preservation when superior breeds appear the superseded breeds are often in danger of extinction; preservation of genes which may be desirable at a later time dictates that the superseded breed be maintained in its pure state.

b. structure see traditional BREED pyramid.

traditional b. pyramid the supply structure of three echelons, each larger than the one before, within each breed; shape like a pyramid with the breed nucleus at the top, supplying to the second echelon, the multiplier, in turn supplying sires to commercial herds.

b. true to produce offspring that are very similar to the parent(s); refers to homozygotes.

breeder 1. a person with an animal enterprise involving the multiplication of the herd, flock or group. 2. a female animal used basically for the production of saleable young.

b. bull a bull sold specifically as a sire with an implied guarantee of fertility. Such bulls are usually replaced free of charge with a comparable animal by the vendor if the bull is not a fertile calf getter.

b. flock a flock of hens producing fertile eggs for hatching purposes.

breeding 1. pedigree. 2. the physical act of mating. 3. capable of being used for reproduction. 4. controlled propagation of animals or plants.

artificial b. see ARTIFICIAL INSEMINATION.

b. bitch a sexually entire bitch to be used for breeding.

b. bulls bulls used for paddock mating.

close b. see INBREEDING.

controlled b. 1. the animals are mated in such a way that the offspring can be guaranteed to be the progeny of the animals concerned, the number of matings can be counted and the use of the animals for breeding is tightly controlled. See also hand MATING. 2. controlled mating in that the occurrence of the estrus cycle, the probability of ovulation and fertilization and the termination are controlled by manipulation of the dam's internal hormonal environment.

b. display behavior likely to attract an animal of the opposite sex to mate. Used almost exclusively in relation to birds.

b. examination postpartum examination of cow to ascertain readiness for next mating; includes rectal examination of uterus and ovaries, vaginoscopic examination, possibly sample of cervical mucus for laboratory examination; in bulls the examination is for BREEDING soundness.

b. herds herds used for breeding in contrast to fattening herds.

b. history lifetime history of all events in a female's reproductive history, including postpartum and premating examinations.

b. injuries incurred during mating and as a result of it. Examples are penile hematoma and vaginal rupture.

line b. breeding of animals with the same blood lines but not closely related.

optimal b. time the time during the estral period when a mating is most likely to be fertile.

b. organizations bodies which advise on and assist in breeding programs, e.g. artificial insemination and embryo transfer centers, cow evaluation and mating advisory services, breed society classification programs, dairy herd improvement programs and the like.

b. problems see ABORTION, MUMMIFICATION, STILLBIRTH, no visible ESTRUS, FAILURE to conceive.

b. programs arrangement of matings on a farm to produce the desired effect in terms of cows in milk at a particular season, lambs being born when the weather is most clement, lowering the micron count of the wool by mating ewes with a low micron ram and so on.

pyramid b. system see PYRAMID breed structure.

b. record see BREEDING history.

b. season those parts of the year in which animals mate. This may be artificially arranged by humans. In animals that are not controlled there are periods of the year when they are more sexually active.

b. soundness the ability of the animal to mate and to initiate reproduction. In agricultural animals where the objective is to limit the number of sires, breeding soundness also embraces the ability to mate effectively on a large number of occasions over a brief period of time.

b. soundness examination conducted on behalf of intending vendors and purchasers, or before a limited breeding season in which high reproductive efficiency is desired. Should include perusal of results of previous reproductive performance, physical examination of the animal, especially of the genitalia, collection and examination of samples where these are an integral part of an examination for specific diseases of reproduction, e.g. blood test for brucellosis, preputial or vaginal swab examination for campylobacteriosis, and in the male a collection and examination of semen and a serving capacity test. The latter has not received universal acceptance, at least not in the form in which it is presently performed.

b. stock livestock used for breeding.

b. wheel a system of recording reproductive events on a disk which rotates once each year. The relationship between the expected calvings, the number of infertile matings and the required milk flow and feed need is readily understood from the overall pattern on the disk.

breeding value the sum of gene effects of a breeding animal as measured by the performance of its progeny.

aggregate b. v. see true breeding value (below).

estimated b. v. an estimate of the ability of an individual to produce superior offspring; based on one or more measurements of performance, using phenotypic values, taken on the animal itself or, more commonly, on a number of its relatives.

true b. v. genetic merit of an individual which can be conceptually defined as twice the average deviation of its offspring from the population mean when mated randomly to an infinite population.

true overall b. v. the true, overall breeding value arrived at by the addition of the true breeding values for each selection objective with each true breeding value multiplied by the relevant net economic value.

Breed's direct smear method a method of counting the total bacterial population of a sample, most commonly milk.

breelya GASTROLOBIUM *laytonii*.

breeze fly see TABANUS.

bremsstrahlung braking radiation produced by the electrons being decelerated in the target of the x-ray tube. These rays of mixed wavelengths form the heterogeneous part of the x-ray beam.

Breton horse heavy French draft or meat horse.

bretylium tosylate an adrenergic neuronal-blocking agent used as a ventricular antiarrhythmic and a chemical defibrillator in cardiopulmonary resuscitation.

brevicollis shortness of the neck.

brewer's grains the residue of the cereal grains after most of the starch has been fermented away. It is a highly palatable and nutritious feed much sought after for dairy cows because of its high protein content. It may be fed dried or wet, but wet grains must be fed fresh. If allowed to ferment it may develop sufficient lactic acid to cause lactic acidosis. Clinical signs are dehydration, rumen stasis, smelly diarrhea.

brewer's yeast a by-product of brewing. The yeast bodies of *Saccharomyces cerevisiae* are harvested and dried. It is an excellent source of vitamin B_1 (thiamin) and protein. Often fed as a supplement to dogs and cats.

Breynia oblongifolia member of plant family Euphorbiaceae; can cause cyanide poisoning. Called also coffee bush.

BRF the ratio of bulls to cows. Targets vary widely depending on circumstances and efficiency required.

Briard a large (75 lb), muscular dog with medium-length, slightly wavy, black, fawn or gray coat which covers the face and forms a beard and mustache. There are supposed to be double dewclaws on the hindfeet. The breed is predisposed to a progressive retinal atrophy. Called also Berger de Brie.

brick feed compacted into a solid mass weighing up to 2 lb. Bricks provide an alternative to pellets and have the advantage that they have to be eaten slowly.

brickworks a possible source of fluorine emitted in smoke and a health hazard for animals grazing local pastures.

Bridelia trees in a genus of the family Euphorbiaceae. Can cause cyanide poisoning. Includes *B. ovata*, *B. exalta*, *B. leichhardtii* (scrub ironbark).

bridge 1. pons. 2. a protoplasmic structure uniting adjacent elements of a cell, similar in plants and animals. 3. dental prosthesis for the replacement of missing teeth.

disulfide b. disulfide bond.

β-γ bridging one of the dysproteinemias in which there is no clear separation electrophoretically between the β_2 and γ_1 globulins. The cause is an increase in IgA or IgM, or both, and this is almost pathognomonic for chronic active hepatitis.

bridle injury chafing caused by a too tight or badly made bridle.

bright term used to describe wool which is free from discoloration.

bright-blindness see bright BLINDNESS.

brightness said of a fleece of wool, a desirable characteristic found in superior fleeces. Consists of a white color and good light reflection.

brilliant green an antiseptic dye used topically.

brim the anterior edge of the pubic bones; the attachment of the linea alba and the ventral abdominal muscles. Called also pecten pubis.

brindle a pattern of coat pigmentation in which darker hairs form bands on a lighter background. A common coat color in Great Danes and Boston terriers.

brine a salt solution used in the curing of meat. Standard ingredients are sodium chloride (15 to 30%) and sodium nitrate (0.15 to 1.50%) but many other ingredients may be added for special effects.

b. shrimp see ARTEMIA.

b. staining caused by leaky pipes carrying coolant in meat storage cold rooms. The coolant is usually calcium chloride and the stain is a pale green.

brisement [Fr.] *a crushing*, especially the breaking up of an ankylosis.

brisket the mass of connective tissue and fat covering the anterior part of the chest in ruminants. Lies at the most ventral part of the neck, between the front legs and covering the anterior end of the sternum.

b. disease see ALTITUDE SICKNESS.

b. edema an important indication of generalized edema due to congestive heart failure or hypoproteinemia. Also caused by local venous obstruction, e.g. due to thymic lymphosarcoma or injury due to sharp edges or too high fronts on feed troughs.

bristle 1. the thick strong animal fibers collected at commercial abattoirs for use in brushes. 2. the sharp serrated awns of grass and some cereal seeds that confer a capacity to penetrate normal skin and mucosa and to cause ulcerative stomatitis, grass seed abscess and the like.

bristle grass SETARIA *lutescens*.

bristling see HACKLES.

britch vernacular for BREECH.

British Alpine British milking goat, black with white facial stripes and light points. May be horned or polled.

British antilewisite BAL; see DIMERCAPROL.

British black see LARGE BLACK.

British bulldog see BULLDOG (2).

British dog tick see IXODES *canisuga*.

British Friesian cattle similar to and originating from Dutch Friesians.

British longwool see ENGLISH LONGWOOL.

British mandrake BRYONIA *dioica*.

British Pharmacopoeia a publication of the General Medical Council (UK) describing and establishing standards for medicines, preparations, materials and articles used in the practice of medicine, surgery and midwifery.

British saddleback pig black meat pig with white belt behind the shoulders; produced by crossing Essex and Wessex saddleback.

British shorthair a type of shorthaired cat with a large, round head and stocky body; includes many different varieties based on color of haircoat. It is contrasted with the 'foreign' shorthair type, with a slim body and almond-shaped, slanted eyes, that includes the Russian blue, Abyssinian and Somali breeds. The breed is affected by neonatal erythrolysis and hemophilia B.

British thermal unit BTU, a unit of heat being the amount necessary to raise the temperature of 1 pound of water from 39 to 40°F, generally considered the equivalent of 252 calories.

British Veterinary Association a voluntary professional organization which has the objective of maintaining the highest possible status of the British veterinary profession.

British Veterinary Codex pharmaceutical guide book for veterinarians published by the Council of the Pharmaceutical Society of Great Britain; contains information relating to substances and preparations of veterinary importance contained in the British Pharmacopoeia.

British white a dairy and beef breed of cattle, polled, white with black points, produced in the UK by crossing Wild white and Swedish mountain breeds.

Brittany bassett see BASSET FAUVE DE BRETAGNE.

Brittany spaniel a medium-sized (35–40 lb) dog with a flat, usually orange and white coat, pendulous ears and a naturally short tail. Although a spaniel, it points game like a setter. The breed suffers from an inherited complement deficiency and a spinal muscular atrophy. Called also Epagneul Breton.

brivudine a halogenated thymidine, similar to acyclovir but with lower toxicity and increased activity against herpesviruses. Called also bromovinyl deosyuridine.

broad said of wool in a fleece which is coarser than normal for the class of sheep.

broad beans see VICIA faba.

broad fish tapeworm see DIPHYLLOBOTHRIUM LATUM.

broad headed snake see HOPLOCEPHALUS BUNGAROIDES.

broad ligament see broad LIGAMENT.

broadleaf lupine LUPINUS *latifolius*.

broadleaf milkweed ASCLEPIAS *latifolia*.

broadleaf vetch see VICIA *villosa*.

Broca band a fiber bundle of the primordial rhinencephalon, close to the anterior perforated substance.

broccoli BRASSICA *oleracea* var. *italica*.

Brock procedure a surgical technique for correction of pulmonic stenosis in which there is excision of the fibromuscular obstruction in the right ventricle using a rongeur inserted through the wall of the right ventricle.

brodifacoum a second generation derivative of dicoumarol, used as an anticoagulant rodenticide. It is more potent, with longer lasting effects, than warfarin. Poisoning in dogs requires treatment with vitamin K_1 for at least 3 weeks.

Brodmann's areas specific occipital and preoccipital areas of the human cerebral cortex, distinguished by differences in the arrangement of their six cellular layers, and identified by number. They are considered to be the seat of specific functions of the brain.

broiler a young (about 8 weeks old) male or female chicken weighing 3 to 3.5 lb.

broken back a focal alopecia located in the center of the back of guinea pigs; associated with stress or pregnancy.

broken colored coat color in a horse, usually piebald or skewbald but includes any other mixture of large patches of contrasting colors.

broken down carpus see dropped CARPUS.

broken head see HYDROTOEA *irritans*.

broken hock in racing Greyhounds, fracture of the scaphoid.

broken mouth the dentition in a sheep when some of the incisors have been lost or badly worn and irregular so that they are unlikely to be able to graze effectively. Caused usually by old age and hard grazing conditions.

broken penis see PENILE hematoma.

broken-up face in dog conformation, a very short nose, deep stop with wrinkle, and an undershot jaw; seen in Pekingese and Bulldogs.

broken wind see pulmonary EMPHYSEMA, CHRONIC obstructive pulmonary disease.

broken wool see wool BREAK.

bromacil a methyluracil herbicide with moderate toxicity for sheep. Signs include bloat, incoordination, depression and anorexia.

bromadiolone a second generation derivative of dicoumarol, with greater potency and longer activity, used as an anticoagulant rodenticide; a cause of poisoning in dog.

bromegrass BROMUS *inermis*.

bromelains a group of proteolytic and milk-clotting enzymes derived from the pineapple plant, *Ananas sativus*. They are used as anti-inflammatory agents.

bromethalin a non-anticoagulant rodenticide that acts by uncoupling of oxidative phosphorylation, resulting in cerebral and spinal cord edema. It is very toxic to nontarget species such as dogs and cats.

bromhexine hydrochloride an expectorant and mucolytic.

bromhidrosis the secretion of foul-smelling perspiration.

bromide any binary compound of bromine. Bromides produce depression of the central nervous system, and were once widely used for their sedative effect. Potassium bromide is used in the treatment of intractable epilepsy. See also BROMINISM.

bromidrosis bromhidrosis.

bromine a chemical element, atomic number 35, atomic weight 79.909, symbol Br. See Table 6.

brominism poisoning by excessive use of bromine or its compounds. This condition occurs when the bromine concentration in the body fluids is high enough to have a toxic and depressant action on the central nervous system.

bromism see BROMINISM.

bromocresol green used as an indicator in the dye test for determination of serum albumin.

bromocriptine a dopamine agonist; as a derivative of ergot alkaloids it is a luteolytic and arbortifacient which suppresses prolactin secretion and lowers plasma ACTH levels. Used as an abortifacient and in the treatment of pituitary-dependant hyperadrenocorticism.

bromocyclen, bromociclen a halogenated hydrocarbon used as an acaricide. Causes vomiting and convulsions if taken orally.

bromoethane see METHYL bromide.

bromophenophos, bromofenofos an organophosphorus compound used to treat FASCIOLA *hepatica* infections in cattle.

bromophos-ethyl an organophosphate insecticide used principally as an acaricide.

bromosulfothalein see SULFOBROMOPHTHALEIN.

bromovinyl deosyuridine see BRIVUDINE.

brompheniramine a histamine H_1-receptor antagonist used in the treatment of hypersensitivity reactions and allergic skin diseases.

bromsalans biphenolic compounds used as fasciolicides; includes DIBROMSALAN and tribromsalan. They are very effective against juvenile flukes.

Bromsulphalein trademark for SULFOBROMOPHTHALEIN.

Bromus a genus of valuable fodder grasses in the family Poaceae. Includes *B. inermis* (smooth bromegrass), *B. catharticus* (*B. unioloides*, prairie grass).

bronch- prefix meaning bronchus.

bronchadenitis inflammation of the bronchial glands.

bronchi plural of *bronchus*.

bronchial pertaining to or affecting one or more bronchi.

b. calculus a hard concretion formed in a bronchus by accretion about an inorganic nucleus or from calcified portions of lung tissue or adjacent lymph nodes.

b. edema mucosal edema occurs in response to irritation and inflammation of tracheobronchial epithelium. Contributes to increased airway resistance.

feline b. asthma a syndrome in cats characterized by acute episodes of coughing and dyspnea with wheezing. Usually recurrent and believed to be due to allergic reaction. Similar to allergic asthma in humans.

b. hypoplasia swollen spongy tissue or cystic, lobulated tissue replaces lobes of normal lung tissue because of the impediment to air flow caused by dilated or collapsed hypoplastic bronchi; probably the basic defect in adenomatoid hamartoma or congenital adenomatoid malformation.

b. pattern bronchi become more prominent in x-rays because they become more dense than surrounding air-filled lung tissue. Caused by peribronchial infiltration, fluid within the bronchus and calcification of the bronchial cartilage. Seen in chronic bronchitis and bronchiectasis.

b. spasm bronchospasm.

b. tones are the sounds made by the respired air as it passes through the larger air passages of normal lungs. They are best heard over the bifurcation of the trachea. They are harsher and louder than the vesicular murmur, the normal sounds produced in the parenchyma of the lung.

b. tree the bronchi and their branching subdivisions.

b. tumors see PULMONARY neoplasm.

bronchiarctia bronchostenosis.

bronchidesmus ligaments that attach the pessulus of the avian syrinx to the esophagus and pericardium.

bronchiectasis chronic dilatation of the bronchi and bronchioles with secondary infection, usually involving the dependant parts of the lung. The condition may occur as a congenital malformation of the alveoli with resultant dilatation of the terminal bronchi. Most often it is an acquired disease secondary to partial obstruction of the bronchi with necrotizing infection. Primary diseases leading to bronchiectasis include chronic bronchitis, neoplasia or aspirated foreign body.

bronchiloquy high-pitched pectoriloquy due to lung consolidation.

bronchiocele dilatation or swelling of a bronchiole.

bronchiogenic bronchogenic.

bronchiolar pertaining to or emanating from the bronchioles.

b. microlithiasis see MICROLITHIASIS.

b. tumors see PULMONARY neoplasm.

bronchiole one of the successively smaller channels (1 mm or less) into which the bronchi divide.

respiratory b. the final branch of a bronchiole, communicating directly with the alveolar ducts; a subdivision of a terminal bronchiole, it has alveolar outcroppings and itself divides into several alveolar ducts.

bronchiolectasis dilatation of the bronchioles. See also BRONCHIECTASIS.

bronchiolitis inflammation of the bronchioles; bronchopneumonia. See also CHRONIC obstructive pulmonary disease.

catarrhal b. acute, mild irritation of the mucosa with excess mucus production, necrosis of epithelial cells, and transient exudation of leukocytes into the lumen.

chronic b.-emphysema complex, horses see CHRONIC obstructive pulmonary disease.

b. fibrosa obliterans see obliterative bronchiolitis (below).

obliterative b. response to necrosis of the lining epithelium at the bronchiolar–alveolar junction and subsequent fibroblastic organization of the fibrin exudation, obliterating the bronchiolar lumen.

purulent b. more severe than catarrhal; a viscid exudate characterized by a predominance of neutrophils, with mucus and sloughed epithelial cells.

ulcerative b. inflammation characterized by the loss of large areas of epithelium with exposure of the underlying tissue and the development of ulcers.

vesicular b. bronchopneumonia.

bronchioloalveolar portals points which mark the transition from cuboidal bronchiolar epithelium to squamous alveolar lining cells in the respiratory bronchioles.

bronchiolus pl. *bronchioli* [L.] bronchiole.

bronchiospasm bronchospasm.

bronchiostenosis bronchostenosis.

bronchitis inflammation of one or more bronchi. Signs of acute bronchitis include fever and an irritating cough.

Bronchitis may be either an acute or chronic disorder and frequently involves the trachea as well as the bronchi (tracheobronchitis). The acute stage of the disease often is an extension of an upper respiratory infection which is usually viral in origin. Causes other than infectious agents are physical and chemical irritants that are inhaled in air polluted by dust, industrial fumes and powdered feeds. The important clinical signs indicative of bronchitis are cough and the ease of stimulating a cough by compression of the trachea, and bronchial tones on auscultation of the base of the lungs. At necropsy the case may be classified as catarrhal, eosinophilic, fibronecrotic, purulent or ulcerative.

avian infectious b. caused by coronavirus. There are many serotypes. Causes gasping and rales, heavy mortality and rapid spread in young birds up to 4 weeks of age. Called also gasping disease.

infectious equine b. see EQUINE influenza.

parasitic b. see LUNGWORM.

bronchoalveolar pertaining to alveoli and bronchi.

bronchocandidiasis candidiasis of the respiratory tree.

bronchocavernous both bronchial and cavitary.

bronchocele localized dilatation of a bronchus.

bronchoconstriction bronchostenosis.

bronchoconstrictor 1. narrowing the lumina of the air passages of the lungs. 2. an agent that causes such constriction.

bronchodilatation a dilated state of a bronchus, or the site at which a bronchus is dilated.

bronchodilator 1. expanding the lumina of the air passages of the lungs. 2. an agent that causes dilatation of the bronchi. Epinephrine is one of the most powerful bronchodilators and can be administered by injection or by aerosol. Some drugs used to enlarge the lumen of the bronchi and thereby facilitate breathing and removal of secretions are albuterol, ipratropium and aminophylline.

b.-antitussive combination see ANTITUSSIVE–bronchodilator combination.

bronchoesophageal pertaining to or communicating with a bronchus and the esophagus.

bronchoesophagology the branch of medicine concerned with the air passages (bronchi) and esophagus.

bronchoesophagoscopy instrumental examination of the bronchi and esophagus.

bronchofiberoscopy examination of the bronchi through a bronchofiberscope.

bronchofiberscope a flexible bronchoscope utilizing fiberoptics.

bronchogenic, bronchogenous originating in the bronchi.

b. abscess occasional cases in most species, many caused by *Actinomyces pyogenes*; clinical cases show chronic cough, wasting, rarely cause erosion of blood vessel and fatal intrapulmonary hemorrhage and nasal bleeding.

b. tumors see PULMONARY neoplasm.

bronchogram the film obtained by bronchography.

air b. air-filled bronchi seen as radiolucent, branching bands within pulmonary densities. Indicates involvement of lung parenchyma.

bronchography radiography of the lungs after instillation of an opaque medium in the bronchi.

broncholith a bronchial calculus.

broncholithiasis a condition in which calculi are present within the lumen of the tracheobronchial tree.

bronchology the study and treatment of diseases of the tracheobronchial tree.

bronchomalacia a deficiency in the cartilaginous wall of the trachea or a bronchus that may lead to atelectasis or obstructive emphysema.

bronchomoniliasis see BRONCHOCANDIDIASIS.

bronchomotor affecting the caliber of the bronchi.

b. tone tone of the bronchial muscles as in BRONCHOSPASM.

bronchomucotropic augmenting secretion by the respiratory mucosa.

bronchopancreatic communicating with a bronchus and the pancreas, as a bronchopancreatic fistula.

bronchopathy any disease of the bronchi.

bronchoplasty plastic surgery of a bronchus; surgical closure of a bronchial fistula.

bronchoplegia paralysis of the muscles of the walls of the bronchial tubes.

bronchopleural pertaining to a bronchus and the pleura, or communicating with a bronchus and the pleural cavity, e.g. by a bronchopleural fistula.

bronchopneumonia inflammation of the bronchi and lungs, usually beginning in the terminal bronchioles. Predominantly the result of aerogenous infection. Marked by a patchy and variegated appearance of gross lesions and involvement of the ventral parts of anterior lobes of the lungs. Called also lobular pneumonia. See also PNEUMONIA.

bronchopneumopathy disease of the bronchi and lung tissue.

bronchopulmonary pertaining to the bronchi and lungs.

congenital b. foregut malformation accessory lungs which communicate with the intestine.

b. segment one of the smaller divisions of the lobe of a lung, separated from others by a connective tissue septum and supplied by its own branch of the bronchus leading to the particular lobe.

bronchorrhagia hemorrhage from the bronchi.

bronchorrhaphy suture of a bronchus.

bronchorrhea excessive discharge of mucus from the bronchi.

bronchoscope an endoscope especially designed for passage through the trachea to permit inspection of the interior of the tracheobronchial tree and carrying out of endobronchial diagnostic and therapeutic maneuvers, such as taking specimens for culture and biopsy and removing foreign bodies.

fiberoptic b. bronchofiberscope.

bronchoscopy inspection of the interior of the tracheobronchial tree through a bronchoscope. Bronchoscopy is used as a diagnostic aid and therapeutically.

As an aid to diagnosis the bronchoscope allows for visualization of the bronchial mucosa and removal of tissue for biopsy. Bronchial washings and collection of secretions are done at the time of bronchoscopy to obtain samples for culture and cytological examination. Therapeutically, the bronchoscope permits removal of foreign bodies that have been aspirated into the bronchial tree.

fiberoptic b. bronchofiberoscopy.

bronchospasm bronchial spasm; spasmodic contraction of the muscular coat of the smaller divisions of the bronchi, such as occurs in asthma.

bronchospirography the recording of bronchospirometry results.

bronchospirometry determination of vital capacity, oxygen intake and carbon dioxide excretion of a single lung, or simultaneous measurements of the function of each lung separately.

differential b. measurement of the function of each lung separately.

bronchostaxis bleeding from the bronchial wall.

bronchostenosis stricture or cicatricial diminution of the caliber of a bronchial tube.

spasmodic b. a spasmodic contraction of the walls of the bronchi.

bronchostomy surgical creation of an opening through the chest wall into the bronchus.

Bronchostrongylus see TROGLOSTRONGYLUS.

bronchotomy incision of a bronchus.

bronchotracheal pertaining to the bronchi and trachea.

bronchovesicular pertaining to the bronchi and alveoli.

b. breath sounds see BREATH sounds.

bronchus pl. *bronchi* [L.] any of the larger passages conveying air to (right or left principal bronchus) and within the lungs (lobar and segmental bronchi). See also RESPIRATION, BRONCHIAL.

b. clamp like a bowel clamp but with solid straight blades. Has ratcheted handles.

tracheal b. a lobar bronchus originating directly from the trachea in pigs and cattle, and which aerates the cranial lobe of the right lung.

bronchus-associated lymphoid tissue see bronchus-associated LYMPHOID tissue.

bronopol a preservative used in milk samples intended for butter fat estimation; the reject milk fed to calves causes erosive abomasitis and death due to peritonitis.

Bronzewing standard domestic turkey; black with bronzing on neck and back, and bronze barring on tail, which has a wide, white end-stripe. The female has white end-stripes on breast, back and wing bows, and secondary bows. Shanks are blackish-pink. Called also Australian bronze, American bronze.

bronzing syndrome a dermatosis seen in Dalmation dogs and believed to be associated with the peculiarities of uric acid metabolism in that breed. There is discoloration of the coat and secondary bacterial infection in the skin.

brood offspring or pertaining to offspring.

b. mare a mare dedicated to the production of foals.

brood capsule 1. a capsule containing a number of protoscolices which float freely within an *Echinococcus granulosus* cyst. 2. clusters of chondrocytes which are undergoing proliferation in cartilage.

brooder stage two of the usual bird rearing sequence. After hatching the baby birds are put into a brooder house, usually with a heat source attached, for rearing. Also used as a management strategy for baby pigs which are weaned early, at 3 weeks.

b. pneumonia respiratory tract infection of young birds with the fungus *Aspergillus fumigatus*. Called also aspergillosis.

broodfish mature fish used for the production of eggs or sperm. Called also spawners.

broodiness see AVIAN broodiness.

brooding patches, brood patches patches of the skin on the undersurface of the body of hen birds which become highly vascular during brooding; this facilitates the transfer of heat from the hen to the eggs.

broody see AVIAN broodiness.

brook trout SALVELINUS *fontinalis*.

Brooklynella an ectoparasitic ciliated protozoon that causes severe lesions on the gills of marine fish kept in aquaria.

brooklynellosis disease of marine fish caused by infestation with *Brooklynella* spp., a unicellular ciliate. Characterized by hyperplasia of the gill epithelium and clinically by respiratory embarrassment.

broom common names for bushy plants with long stiff stems. Includes *Cytisus scoparius* (common broom), *Spartium junceum* (Spanish broom), *Senecio spartioides* (broom groundsel), *Sorghum bicolor* (broom millet), *Gutierrezia microcephala* (broom snakeweed).

broom bush PIMELEA *trichostachya*.

broom rape see OROBANCHE MINOR.

broomcorn millet see PANICUM *miliaceum*.

broomweed GUTIERREZIA *microcephala*.

broth liquid MEDIA for culturing microorganisms.

cooked meat b. a medium useful for culturing anaerobic bacteria.

enrichment b. one modified to permit growth by selected bacteria. An example is selenite broth, which is selective for salmonellae.

brother-brother GASTROLOBIUM *tetragonophyllum*.

Broughton pea SWAINSONA *procumbens*.

brow the forehead, or either lateral half of it.

brown 1. a composite color, therefore variable from creamy to dark brown which is almost black, made from black, red and yellow. 2. a coat color; in horses a brown coat with a tan muzzle; a few hairs of another color may be scattered through the coat creating a brown roan (white admixture), brown chestnut (admixture of chestnut), etc. A brown-ticked gray is a gray horse with wheat grain sized patches of brown hairs scattered through the coat; in cattle a rich creamy brown as in Brown Swiss and many other indigenous breeds.

brown adipose tissue see brown ADIPOSE tissue.

Brown–Adson forceps standard tissue forceps with the opposing blade surfaces covered with long, needle-like teeth.

Brown Atlas cattle brown, brachyceros type, multipurpose cattle from North Africa.

brown atrophy see XANTHOSIS.

brown blood disease brown discoloration of normally red gill tissues due to the formation of methemoglobin in nitrite poisoning in cultured fish. See also NITRITE poisoning.

brown chicken louse see GONIODES *dissimilis*.

brown dog tick see RHIPICEPHALUS *sanguineus*.

brown ear tick see RHIPICEPHALUS *appendiculatus*.

brown fat see brown ADIPOSE tissue.

brown fat disease a brown-yellow discoloration of fat in pigs caused by the feeding of fish meal.

Brown forceps long-handled tissue forceps with the opposing blade surfaces in the form of two longitudinal rows of fine teeth. Similar to Brown–Adson forceps. Designed for handling thoracic tissues.

brown hypertrophy of the cere a condition in birds especially budgerigars, less commonly other psittacines, characterized by hyperplasia, cornification and keratinization of the cere. It may occlude the nares and cause beak breathing.

brown lick stain seen on the upper lip of dogs, caused by continuous licking, often of preputial or vulvar discharge.

Brown mountain cattle see BRAUNVIEH.

brown nose a form of photosensitive dermatitis in cattle, with the most obvious lesion on the muzzle.

brown pigmentation of all tissues. See XANTHOSIS.

Brown–Séquard's syndrome paralysis and loss of discriminatory and joint sensation on one side of the body and of pain and temperature sensation on the other, due to a lesion involving one side of the spinal cord. Seen in primates but not so evident in domestic animals because of bilateral spinal sensory afferent pathways.

brown snake see DEMANSIA *textilis*.

king b. s. see PSEUDECHIS *australis*.

brown stomach worm OSTERTAGIA *ostertagi* and TELADORSAGIA *circumcincta*.

Brown Swiss cattle a café-au-lait colored, heavy boned, heavyweight and heavy milking breed of dairy cattle. A derived breed is the American brown Swiss.

brown-tail moth see PORTHESIA CHRYSORRHOEA.

brown tree snake see BOIGA *irregularis*.

brown trout *Salmo trutta*.

Brown urethroplasty technique see Brown URETHROPLASTY technique.

brown winter tick see DERMACENTOR *nigrolineatus*.

browse 1. bushes and shrubs that goats and many wild herbivores eat in preference to grass and clover; they are said to browse instead of graze. 2. the bushy plants that goats eat; the counterpart of pasture. 3. term for scanning through information in a computer program.

browser animal species which eat browse rather than grass and herbs.

BRSV bovine respiratory syncytial virus.

Bruce County Project a Canadian developmental project which shipped feeder calves from the west to small farm feedlots in eastern Canada for fattening and sale in the eastern market. There was only one throughput of calves per year. A successful feeding and disease prevention program was developed.

Bruce effect the manipulation of pregnancy by pheromones. For example the termination of pregnancy in a recently bred mouse by placing it in a cage with a strange male.

Brucella a genus of gram-negative rods in seven species and several biotypes. The cause of many serious diseases in animals, including BRUCELLOSIS.

B. abortus a short rod or coccobacillus which causes BRUCELLOSIS in cattle and horses, and is a serious zoonosis. Two strains of reduced virulence and used for vaccination in cattle are Strain 19 and Strain 45/20.

B. canis a similar organism to the other brucellae except that it is inhibited in growth by a 10% concentration of CO_2, a cultural enhancement for the other species. Causes BRUCELLOSIS in dogs.

B. melitensis a rod so short that it is easily mistaken for a coccus with the same characteristics as the other brucellae. Causes BRUCELLOSIS in goats and Malta fever in humans, a serious zoonosis.

B. neotomae found only in the desert wood rat in the USA.

B. ovis has staining and cultural characteristics similar to the other brucellae. Causes BRUCELLOSIS in rams.

B. suis a typical brucella in morphology and cultural and staining characteristics. Causes BRUCELLOSIS in pigs and is a significant zoonosis.

Brucellergen trademark for a solution of nucleoproteins derived from *Brucella;* used in a skin test for brucella infection.

brucellosis infection by *Brucella* spp. It causes different syndromes in each animal species. (1) Bovine brucellosis, caused by *B. abortus*, is characterized by abortion in late pregnancy and subsequent infertility. (2) Ovine brucellosis, caused by *B. ovis*, is characterized by epididymitis in rams and resulting infertility. (3) Brucellosis in pigs, caused by *B. suis*, is a chronic disease manifested by infertility and abortion in sows, orchitis in boars and heavy piglet mortality. (4) Caprine brucellosis, caused by *B. melitensis*, is manifested principally by abortion although other signs including loss of weight, mastitis, lameness and orchitis are also reported. (5) There is no specific brucella organism in horses but *B. abortus* occurs not infrequently as a bursitis in FISTULOUS withers and POLL evil. (6) In dogs, *B. canis* causes late abortions in bitches, and infertility and scrotal dermatitis in males.

b. testing the eradication of bovine and porcine brucellosis has been a target for human public health and veterinary authorities for 50 years and has reached a stage of virtual eradication in most developed countries. During that time the veterinary profession has been involved in testing many millions of individual animals so that a test and slaughter eradication program could be implemented. The standard test has been the tube agglutination test with some assistance from screening tests such as the ABR or milk ring test and the card agglutination test.

Bruch's membrane the complex basal lamina separating the choroid from the retinal pigment epithelium.

brucine a strychnine-like alkaloid contained in nux vomica and STRYCHNOS spp.

Brücke's muscle a group of fibers in the eye which tense the choroid or pull the ciliary body forward when they contract.

Brugia a genus of the family Onchocercidae of worms. Includes *B. celonensis*, *B. malayi*, *B. pahangi*, *B. patei*, *B. timori* and others.

In tropical countries *Brugia* spp. are parasitic in the lymphatics of primates, carnivores and insectivores; parasitized animals may act as reservoirs for human infection. Transmission is via mosquitoes.

Brugmansia genus of the plant family Solanaceae. Contains shrubby species also known as *Datura candida* (angel's trumpet) and others in garden cultivation (*D. sanguinea*, *D. suaveolens*). Contain tropane alkaloids, neurotoxic hallucinogens.

Bruhner's method a method of suturing the vulva to retain a prolapsed organ. Consists of a buried suture running the full circle of the vulva and exiting to be tied at the ventral commissure. Needs a special long sharp needle such as a GERLACH NEEDLE.

bruise superficial discoloration due to hemorrhage into the tissues from ruptured blood vessels beneath the skin surface, without the skin itself being broken; called also CONTUSION.

bruised sole injury to the laminae of the horse's foot, caused by stepping on a sharp object. The lesion is usually at the edge of the sole and is discolored and painful. Lameness varies in keeping with the extent and duration of the lesion.

bruising discoloration and actual hemorrhage at the site of injury, and a serious disadvantage in the meat trade. In the first 12 hours after injury the bruise is bright red, at 24 hours it is dark red, at 24 to 36 hours it loses its firm consistency and becomes watery and at 3 or more days it is an orange-red color and has a soapy feel.

bruit [Fr.] a sound or murmur heard in auscultation, especially an abnormal one.

aneurysmal b. a blowing sound heard over an aneurysm.

cardiac b. see heart MURMUR.

placental b. a soft, blowing auscultatory sound supposed to be produced by the blood current in the placenta. Called also placental souffle.

brumby Australian feral horse, usually of poor quality physically and in temperament. Any color, up to 15 hands high. Descendants of escaped domestic horses.

Brumptia bicanda intestinal trematode in the rhinoceros.

Brun bone curette the standard equipment for curetting bone. Shaped like a miniature ice cream scoop it has very sharp and durable edges and a hand-filling, bulbous handle.

Brunner's glands glands in the submucosa of the duodenum, opening into the small intestine; called also duodenal glands.

Brunn's nest groups of proliferating epithelial cells in the submucosa of the urinary tract. They are a reaction to injury and may lead to the development of cystic ureteritis, pyelitis or cystitis.

Brunsfelsia South American plant genus in the family Solanaceae; contain an unidentified toxin; cause a syndrome of tremor and convulsions in dogs eating the plant's fruits. Includes *B. australis* (*B. bonodora*), *B. calycina* var. *floribunda*.

Brunus edwardii the urban, companion animal bear, much admired for its low food requirements and excellent house training, a high emotional output and complete freedom from disease. Called also *Ursus theodorus* (USA) and Pooh, Paddington or Brideshead bear (UK).

brush a bushy tail in dogs.

brush border a specialization of the free surface of a cell, consisting of minute cylindrical processes (microvilli) that greatly increase the surface area.

b. b. enzymes include maltase, lactase, α-dextrinase and peptidases. Deficiencies of these enzymes may be primary or, more often, secondary to other intestinal disease.

brushing striking of the medial aspect of the fetlock and coronet of the horse by the hoof of the opposite limb of a pair. See also CUTTING.

b. boot see brush BOOT.

Brussels griffon a small (8–10 lb) dog with a large head, very short nose, prominent chin and erect, folded-over ears. The haircoat is short, usually wiry, and red, black or black and tan. A smooth coated variety is called the Petite Brabancon.

Brussels sprouts BRASSICA *oleracea* var. *gemmifera*.

Bruton's agammaglobulinemia see Bruton's AGAMMAGLOBULINEMIA.

bruxism gnashing, grinding or clenching the teeth, common only in cattle. Repeated and continuous grinding of the teeth over a long period of time can wear down and loosen teeth and cause bone loss. It is a sign of subacute abdominal pain and encephalopathy, including hepatic encephalopathy.

bryonetin a glycoside in BRYONIA *dioica* which may be the cause of the plant's drastic purgative action.

Bryonia a genus of the plant family Cucurbitaceae. Contains a toxic oil bryonin. Causes diarrhea in cattle and purgation or constipation, sweating, diuresis and convulsions in horses. Includes *B. dioica* (*B. cretica* var. *dioica*, white bryony).

bryonidin, bryonin, bryonol one of the glycosides in *Bryonia dioica* and possibly the cause of the plant's purgative effect.

Bryophyllum genus of African and Madagascan plants in the family Crassulaceae. Contain bufadienolide, cardiac glycosides; causes dyspnea, diarrhea, cardiomyopathy. Includes *B. daigremontium*, *B. daigremontium* × *B. tubiflorum*, *B. fedtschenkoi*, *B. proliferum*. Called also *Kalanchoe*.

B. pinnatum *B. calycinum*, *Cotyledon pinnata*, live-leaf-of-resurrection plant.

B. tubiflorum *B. delagoense* (and its hybrid with *B. daigremontianum*). Called also mother-of-millions.

BSA body surface area.

BSE 1. bovine spongiform encephalopathy. 2. breeding soundness examination.

BSP Bromsulphalein, a dye used in the study of liver function. See also SULFOBROMOPHTHALEIN clearance test.

BT-PABA test a test which assesses chymotrypsin activity in the small intestine. Oral administration of the synthetic peptide BENTIROMIDE is followed by measurement of free *p*-aminobenzoic acid in the urine or blood.

BTU British thermal unit.

BTV bluetongue virus.

Bubalus bubalis the domestic buffalo of Europe; black cattle-like ruminants with very short hair, backswept horns and a liking for marshes in which they wallow. Called also water buffalo, carabao, arna, Indian buffalo.

bubble form region of a double-strand DNA that separates earlier than others, to form 'bubbles' when the heat is increased, because of lower G and C content.

bubble vaporizer see bubble VAPORIZER.

bubo an enlarged and inflamed lymph node, particularly in the axilla or groin, resulting from absorption of infective material and occurring in various diseases, e.g. tuberculosis.

indolent b. a hard, nearly painless bubo that shows no tendency to break.

bubonalgia pain in the groin.

bubonic characterized by or pertaining to buboes.

b. plague a highly contagious and severe disease caused by the bacillus *Yersinia pestis* carried in infected rats and transmitted to humans by fleas. See also PLAGUE.

bubonocele inguinal or femoral hernia forming a swelling in the groin.

bucardia extreme enlargement of the heart as in cor bovinum.

bucc- prefix meaning cheek.

bucca [L.] *the cheek* pl. *buccae*.

buccal pertaining to or directed toward the cheek.

b. cavity see MOUTH.

b. horsepox see HORSEPOX.

b. mucosa bleeding time see BLEEDING time.

bucco- word element. [L.] *cheek*.

buccopharyngeal pertaining to or emanating from the mouth and pharynx. Called also oropharyngeal.

b. antiseptics these agents are widely used in human medicine but find little acceptance in the veterinary pharmaceutical field because of their difficulty of application.

imperforate b. membrane a congenital defect of imperforation of the buccopharyngeal membrane. It prevents the animal from breathing through the nostrils and is incompatible with life. Called also choanal atresia.

b. membrane a membrane present in fetal life which separates the nasal cavities from the pharynx.

buccostomy surgical creation of fistulae from the buccal cavity as a prophylactic against crib-biting. Unlikely to be acceptable to today's public because of mutilatory overtones.

buccotomy a surgical incision through the cheek to gain access to an intraoral procedure. Usually performed in herbivores.

Bucephalus trematode parasite causing parasitic castration of clams and scallops.

buchu dried leaves of several *Barosma* spp. plants; contains disophenol, diosmin. A weak diuretic and urinary antiseptic.

buck 1. adult male goat. Unlikely to be kept for any purpose other than an active breeding life, and then only at a distance. 2. breeding male of most small, wild ruminant species, including roe, fallow, muntjac and Chinese water deer. In larger deer species is called bull. 3. the violent actions performed by a horse attempting to dislodge a rider. In rodeo contests steers and bulls may also be engaged in riding-bucking contests with human riders.

buck knees a condition in which the carpus appears to be overextended when viewed from the side.

buckbush GYROSTEMON *australasicus*, SALSOLA *kali*.

bucked shins a front limb lameness in 2- or 3-year-old Thoroughbred and racing Quarter horses. The metacarpal bone is painful on manual compression and the lameness is thought to be due to microfractures in the bone as a result of compression of the bone during exercise at high speed. There is a local periostitis.

bucket-fed see PAIL-FED.

bucket handle a term used to describe a form of injury, e.g. meniscal tears, or surgical technique that creates and utilizes a band of tissue, e.g. repair of eyelid defects and covering of corneal lesions.

buckeye see AESCULUS.

buckjump riding contests at rodeos in which riders attempt to sit out bucks by horses or cattle.

buckle fern see DRYOPTERIS.

buckley centaury CENTAURIUM *calycosum*.

buckling the process or an instance of becoming crumpled or warped.

scleral b. a technique for repair of detachment of the retina, in which indentations or infoldings of the sclera are made over the tears in the retina so as to promote adherence of the retina to the choroid.

buckskin body coat color in horses, varies from yellow to almost brown; the points, including mane, tail, lower limbs are brown to black.

buckthorn see KARWINSKIA HUMBOLDTIANA, RHAMNUS.

buckwheat see FAGOPYRUM SAGITTATUM.

Bucky band a compression band strapped across the animal's abdomen and tightened to reduce the thickness of tissue and to check respiratory movement during a radiographic procedure.

Bucky grid a grid used in radiography to prevent the scattered rays reaching the film, thus aiding clarity and definition of the picture. Called also Potter–Bucky grid.

Bucky tray a sliding metal tray under the radiographic table which holds the grid and the cassette. Called also Potter–Bucky tray.

bucnemia an obsolete term describing diffuse, tense, inflammatory swelling of the leg.

bud a structure resembling the bud of a plant, especially a protuberance in the embryo from which an organ or part develops.

end b. the remnant of the embryonic primitive knot,

from which arises the tail and caudal part of the trunk.
horn b. bilateral cranial protuberances, destined to develop to a fighting horn or antler stage.
limb b. one of the four lateral swellings appearing in vertebrate embryos, which develop into the two pairs of limbs.
tail b. 1. the primordium of the caudal appendage. 2. end bud.
taste b's end organs of the gustatory nerve containing the receptor surfaces for the sense of TASTE.
ureteric b. an outgrowth of the mesonephric duct giving rise to all but the nephrons of the permanent kidney.
b. of urethra bulb of urethra.

Budd–Chiari-like syndrome obstruction of hepatic venous outflow, caused by mechanical obstruction between the hepatic sinusoids and the heart. In dogs, causes include obstructive lesions in the caudal right atrium, caudal vena cava and the hepatic veins.

budding gemmation; asexual reproduction in which a portion of the cell body is thrust out and then becomes separated, forming a new individual.
b. virions viruses that acquire their envelope by budding through modified regions of host cell membranes.

budgee grass CYNODON *nlemfuensis*.

budgerigar, budgie see MELOPSITTACUS UNDULATUS.
b. fledgling disease a polyomavirus infection of young psittacines that causes failure of feather growth, hepatic and renal necrosis, and sometimes death.

budget a detailed financial statement of predicted costs and income for a business, e.g. a farm.
cash flow b. a budget setting out the expected cash receipts and cash payments associated with a business, enterprise or activity, e.g. a farm.
control b. periodic comparison between expected financial performance of a business or enterprise, e.g. a farm, as indicated by the prior budget and actual performance.
development b. a budget used when planning major changes in a business such as a farm, especially when full capacity is not expected to be attained for a long period.
finance b. one devoted to the borrowings which need to be made to maintain financial viability of a business such as a farm, and which shows expected cash flows, especially the financial outlay required to pay interest and capital returns.
parametric b. one which takes into account varying prices and yields.
partial b. one in which only the variable costs and income are entered. Fixed items such as rent and irrigation charges are not entered.

Budyonny horse chestnut or bay Russian light horse.

bufadienolide group of toxic cardiac glycosides found mainly in members of Crassulaceae family, e.g. *Cotyledon*, *Tylecodon*, *Bryophyllum* spp. Found also in skin and skin glands of toads, e.g. *Bufo marinus*. Those in *Cotyledon* and *Tylecodon* are cumulative and and produce krimpsiekte (COTYLEDONOSIS).

buffalo 1. water buffalo—see BUBALUS BUBALIS. Called also carabao, Indian buffalo, arna, European domestic buffalo. 2. Dwarf or Asiatic buffalo—see ANOA. 3. South African buffalo—SYNCERUS CAFFER. 4. American buffalo; is really a bison—see BISON *bison*.

buffalo bunchgrass PASPALUM *conjugatum*.

buffalo burr SOLANUM *rostratum*.

buffalo fly see HAEMATOBIA *exigua*.

buffalo gnat see BLACK FLY.

buffalo leprosy see ulcerative LYMPHANGITIS.

buffalo louse see HAEMATOPINUS *tuberculatus*.

buffalopox a disease caused by a virus which is antigenically identical to COWPOX virus; it is clinically the same as cowpox.

buffel grass see CENCHRUS CILIARIS.

buffer[1] 1. a substance that, by its presence in solution, increases the amount of acid or alkali necessary to produce a unit change in pH. 2. a storage device or area of limited capacity in a computer used for temporary storage of information going in or out of the computer.
isohydric b. systems all of the buffer systems in the extracellular fluid act in unison so that when e.g. extra acid is added all of the buffer systems will buffer some of the additional hydrogen ions. This is the isohydric principle and the buffer systems involved are the isohydric buffers.
b. pairs the pairs of compounds which, in themselves, serve as a buffer system. There are a number of such pairs in the blood and the sum of the blood's buffering capacity is the sum of these individual pairs.
radiology b. a chemical constituent of developer and fixer to keep the pH constant.
b. salt see buffer SALT.
b. systems a system consists of a weak acid and a conjugate base, e.g. a mixture of carbonic acid and bicarbonate ions. When one is present the addition of more acid or base will raise or lower the pH much less than if no buffer were present. The principal buffer systems are the bicarbonate, plasma protein, phosphate and hemoglobin buffers. See also HENDERSON–HASSELBALCH EQUATION.
b. titration curve mathematical calculations used to predict buffering capacity and bicarbonate concentration under various values of carbon dioxide tension.

buffer[2] a double-ended horse shoeing implement designed to be hit with a shoeing hammer. At one end is a broad-bladed chisel face for opening clinches. At the other end is a pointed punch for driving through the shoe nailholes.

buffering the action produced by a buffer.
b. agents amongst other uses these substances play a part in dairy cattle nutrition by helping to prevent damaging ruminal acidity on high grain rations. Sodium bicarbonate and magnesium oxide are the preparations most commonly used.

buffing striking the posteromedial aspect of a front hoof with the opposite hoof of the pair. A perfect situation for applying a buffing boot.
b. boot see brush BOOT.

buffy coat reddish gray layer consisting of white blood cells and platelets, observed above packed red cells in centrifuged blood.

Bufo a genus of toads of the family Bufonidae; these amphibians carry toxins in parotid glands in their skin. Dogs or cats which mouth them are poisoned. There are a number of toxins including the cardiotoxic bufogenins, bufotoxin, bufotenins, catecholamines and serotonin. The toxicity of each species depends on the mix and concentration of toxins. Species include *B. alvarius*, *B. canorus*, *B. exsul*, *B. ictericus*, *B. koynayensis*, *B. marinus*, *B. regularis*, *B. vulgaris*.
B. marinus the giant tropical toad. Introduced into many areas such as Australia and Hawaii to control insect pests. Absorption of the toxins through the oral mucosa of dogs, and less often cats, results in varying degrees of salivation, pulmonary edema, car-

diac arrhythmias, cyanosis and seizures which may culminate in death of the animal.

B. regularis African toad.

B. vulgaris causes excess salivation and distress if caught by a dog. Called also common toad.

bufodienolide a toad toxin. Called also bufogenin.

bufogenin a toad toxin. Called also bufadeniolide.

bufotalin a toxin causing vomiting and cardiac arrest. Present in the skin and saliva of BUFO *vulgaris*.

bufotenine a toad toxin. A specific basic pressor principle used as a hallucinogen in experimental medicine.

bufotoxin any toxin isolated from the skin of a toad.

bug 1. a member of the family Cimicidae in the order Hemiptera and includes the blood-sucking bugs. See HAEMATOSIPHON and OECIACUS VICARIUS. 2. an error in computer hardware or software. It is the object of validation periods for these devices that they be used extensively so that the bugs can be detected and eliminated.

Bugloooides arvensis see LITHOSPERMUM ARVENSE.

Buhner method a method for retaining a prolapsed vagina. A circumferential suture is placed deeply down each side of the vulva commencing at an incision dorsal to the vulva and exiting below it. This is repeated on the other side and the suture is then drawn tight and tied. Requires a special needle with the eye in the point, and a special braided tubular suture.

buiatrics the study of cattle and their diseases.

building covenant see COVENANT.

bulb 1. a rounded mass or enlargement. 2. medulla oblongata.

aortic b. the enlargement of the aorta at its point of origin from the heart.

auditory b. the membranous labyrinth and cochlea.

eye b. the eyeball.

gustatory b's taste buds.

hair b. the bulbous expansion at the proximal end of a hair, in which the hair shaft is generated.

heel b. the swollen part of the hoof wall and adjacent soft tissue at the back of the hoof characterized by a periople which is wider than at any other part of the hoof.

Krause's b's see BULBOID CORPUSCLE.

olfactory b. see OLFACTORY bulb.

penile b. see PENILE bulb.

taste b's taste buds.

urethral b. the enlarged proximal part of the corpus spongiosum.

vestibular b., vestibulovaginal b. a body consisting of paired masses of erectile tissue, situated one on either side of the vaginal orifice.

bulbar pertaining to a bulb; pertaining to or involving the medulla oblongata, as bulbar paralysis.

infectious b. necrosis one of the several forms taken by foot abscess in sheep. See also FOOT abscess.

infectious b. paralysis see AUJESZKY'S DISEASE.

b. paralysis originates from the medulla oblongata. The pyramidal and extrapyramidal tracts pass from the midbrain through the medulla and are susceptible to damage by agents that operate in the area. Paralysis of this type has the characteristics of an upper motor lesion with muscle tone and local tendon reflexes retained.

bulbiform bulb-shaped.

Bulbine plant genus in the Liliaceae family; some contain an unidentified toxin; causes vomiting, diarrhea, abdominal pain. Includes *B. bulbosa* (native leek), *B. semibarbata*.

Bulbinella ornithogaloides ORNITHOGALUM *ornithogaloides*.

bulbitis inflammation of the bulb of the urethra.

bulbocapnine isoquinoline alkaloid found in *Corydalis flavula*, *Dicentra spectabilis*. Causes a transient syndrome of frenzy, convulsions, tremor, opisthotonos, salivation, vomiting.

bulbocavernous glands relating to the bulb of the penis.

b. glands see BULBOURETHRAL glands.

b. muscle see Table 13.

bulbogastrone a gastrointestinal hormone.

bulboid corpuscle small encapsulated nerve endings occurring in the mucous membrane and skin. Called also Krause's bulbs.

bulbospongiosus reflex see BULBOURETHRAL reflex.

bulbourethral pertaining to the bulb of the urethra.

b. glands two glands on either side of the male pelvic urethra. Absent from the dog, and large in the boar. Called also bulbocavernous glands and Cowper's glands.

b. reflex mild pressure on the glans penis in a male dog causes contraction of the external anal sphincter. It tests function of the pudendal nerve and the S1 to S3 spinal cord segments. Called also bulbospongiosus reflex.

bulbous having the form or nature of a bulb; bearing or arising from a bulb.

b. buttercup RANUNCULUS *bulbosa*.

bulboventricle middle region of the embryonic tubular heart between the aorta and the atrium.

bulbus pl. *bulbi* [L.] bulb.

b. aortae the swollen, first part of the aorta, between the atria; swollen because of the sinuses above each of the three cusps of the aortic valves.

b. cordis the outflow tract of the embryonic heart between the primitive ventricle and the aorta.

b. glandis the bulb of the dog's penis; the proximal portion which enlarges greatly during erection and is the part responsible for preventing withdrawal during ejaculation.

b. oculi the EYEBALL.

b. pili see hair BULB.

b. rectricum a well-organized fibroadipose mass in a muscular envelope into which the retrices (tail feathers of birds) are embedded. It occupies a trough-shaped socket bounded by the caudal vertebrae and the intrinsic tail muscles.

Bulgarian brown cattle brown, dual-purpose, Bulgarian cattle.

bulging eye disease see UITPEULOOG.

bulimia abnormal increase in the sensation of hunger. Because of its subjectivity the diagnosis could only be assumed in an animal.

Bulinus water snail, intermediate host for paramphistomes and other trematodes.

bulk forming agents see bulk LAXATIVE.

bulk laxative see LAXATIVE.

bulk milk cell counts see MILK CELL COUNTS.

bull 1. a male bovine animal of breeding age, usually over one year of age. Until recent times the use classification for such an animal would be breeding. The present acceptance of bull beef by consumers adds this use to what was previously a limited range of life styles. See also BREEDER bull. See Table 20. 2. adult male of most wild ruminants except for small deer in which the male is called buck. Includes wapiti, moose, elk, reindeer. 3. adult male cetaceans and pinnipeds. See Table 20.

b. battery rarely used term for the total serving capacity of the bulls in a herd. Is the number of bulls multiplied by the length of the breeding season.

b. beef from entire males instead of the fatter steer or bullock.

b. calf male young entire bovine animal up to stage of yearling.

b.–cow ratio usually refers to paddock mating of beef cattle and reflects the desire of the farmer to achieve high fertility and over what period the breeding program can be allowed to continue. The proportion of bulls needed will also depend on their age, testicular size and serving capacity.

b. leader a pole about 6 ft (2 m) long with a spring clip on the end to snare the bull's nose ring. Enables the handler to keep the bull moving forward without any risk that the bull can come too close.

proven b. one whose progeny have achieved the production target set as desirable by the registering breed authority.

b. rotation changing the bull out of a group of cows and replacing him with a different bull at short intervals. The objective is to ensure a high mating rate or to mark the calves by using a bull of a different breed.

b. test station an establishment run by government or cooperative farmer organization which houses young bulls and measures rate of body weight gain under standard conditions of feeding and housing. A good rate of gain under these conditions does not guarantee a similar performance at pasture.

Bull and terrier dog an early name for the Staffordshire terrier.

bull-bred herd a herd in which the cows are mated to bulls; compare with artificially bred. Called also naturally bred.

bull-dogging the rodeo sport of jumping from the back of a running horse and catching a running calf or steer around the neck and wrestling it to the ground by grasping the horns and twisting the head.

bull's-eye lesion see TARGET lesion.

bull nettle SOLANUM *carolinense.*

Bull terrier a medium-sized (50–60 lb), very solidly built dog with narrow, deeply sunken triangular eyes, thick neck; the face has a distinctive flat profile without a stop. The dog was originally bred for pit fighting. There are two varieties, all-white or colored, which is any other, including spotted, than white. In some countries, a miniature variety is also recognized as a separate breed. The breed is subject to congenital renal disease, lethal acrodermatitis, and the white variety may be affected by congenital deafnesss.

bull thistle see SILYBUM *marianum.*

bulla pl. *bullae* [L.] a blister; a circumscribed, fluid-containing, elevated lesion of the skin, usually more than 5 mm in diameter.

emphysematous b. spherical air-filled cavities in the interlobular spaces and under the pleura, often in large numbers, as part of a general state of pulmonary emphysema.

lacrimal b. a large extension of the thin bony wall of the maxillary sinus in the ox, which bulges into the ventral part of the orbit. There is a small lacrimal bulla also in the pig.

osseous b. see tympanic bulla (below).

tympanic b. a thin-walled bony capsule which houses an extension of the cavity of the middle ear, the tympanic cavity.

Bullamon lucerne PSORALEA *patens.*

Bulldog a medium-sized (40–55 lb), thickset dog with very characteristic build and appearance. The head, with a very short face, neck and forequarters, are massive in proportion to the rest of the body and the legs are relatively short. The tail is naturally short. The breed is predisposed to cleft lip and palate, hemivertebra, hydrocephalus, congenital heart defects, spina bifida and upper respiratory structural abnormalities. Called also British bulldog. See also FRENCH BULLDOG.

American b. a larger dog with longer legs and longer nose than the (British) bulldog. It is said to resemble more closely the earlier version of that breed, as it was when brought to the Americas in colonial times.

bulldog see NOSE lead.

bulldog calves calves that are characterized by short limbs and neck and a swollen cranium with a short, depressed face, with a protruding tongue and cleft palate. There is severe chondrodystrophy and hydrocephalus. The condition is inherited in several breeds of cattle but is very common in Dexters. Called also chondrodystrophic dwarfism with hydrocephalus.

bulldog clamp springloaded crossover clamps used in surgery to clamp off small arteries. They open when squeezed and the serrated-face clamp blades shut when the squeeze is relaxed. See also GLOVER BULLDOG CLAMP.

bulldog twitch an appliance designed for application to a horse's nose for purposes of restraint. Consists of two bars, usually metal, hinged at one end. The jaw is clamped shut with a piece of muzzle in it. The other end is then fixed, usually with a ratchet device.

buller steer in groups of feedlot steers, a steer which submits to mounting by the others. Believed to be sometimes due to estrogen implants.

bullet 1. projectile for a humane killer that uses a conventional or free bullet. 2. a metallic, bullet-shaped mass given orally so as to lodge in the reticulum and discharge its critical component over a long period. Bullets containing cobalt selenium or magnesium are in use. Called also reticular retention bullets. 3. in computer terms, a symbol, commonly a filled circle, used to mark the beginning of each item in a list.

magnesium reticular b. heavy pellets delivering about 1 g magnesium daily administered orally to cattle as a prevention against hypomagnesemia; the 'bullets' lodge in the reticulum and are retained there until they dissolve completely.

bullfrog see RANA *catesbeiana.*

bulling acting like a bull. Said of cows when they mount other cows that are in standing estrus. The buller may be a cow with adrenal virilism which always acts in this manner or it may be a cow about to come into estrus. Said also of steers in a feedlot.

bullmask a mask made of leather or aluminum, which is tied across the bull's face. It has downward looking, horizontal slits, like fixed venetian blinds, which prevent the bull looking forward to attack but permits looking down to graze.

Bullmastiff a large (100–130 lb), powerfully built dog with a large, square head, short muzzle, thick neck, deep chest and tapered tail. The coat is very short and brindle, fawn or red. The breed was developed from the Mastiff and the Bulldog. It is affected by a familial ataxia and entropion.

bullnose see NECROTIC rhinitis.

bullock a mature castrated male cattle destined for meat production or draft.

bullosis the production of, or a condition characterized by, bullous lesions.

bullous pertaining to or characterized by bullae.

b. emphysema pulmonary emphysema characterized by the presence of subpleural and interlobular bullae.

b. epidermolysis see EPIDERMOLYSIS bullosa.

b. pemphigoid see bullous PEMPHIGOID.

bullrout a poisonous scorpion or wasp fish. See NOTESTHES ROBUSTA.
BULLSEARCH a computer program comprising a genetic evaluation database which, in return for inputs of herd qualities and objectives, advises intending user breeders about a pool of bulls known to provide the selected genetic criteria.
bully board plywood or plexiglass shields, similar to those used by riot police, used in the handling and management of animals which are difficult to catch and restrain, e.g. pigs, ostriches, deer.
Bulnesia sarmientii South American plant in the family Zygophyllaceae; toxin thought to be a saponin, causes enteritis, convulsions, pruritus. Called also Palo santo tree.
bulrush ORNITHOGALUM *conicum* subsp. *conicum*.
bulrush millet PENNISETUM *glaucum*.
bumblefoot inflammation of the ball of the foot of birds and guinea pigs caused usually by infection with *Staphylococcus* spp.
bumetanide a loop diuretic, with actions similar to furosemide.
bumps a term used to describe a variety of papulonodular dermatoses in horses, including 'heat bumps', 'feed bumps', 'protein bumps', 'wheat bumps' and others. No specific disease or etiology has been assigned to the term and veterinary dermatologists wish it would disappear from use.
BUN blood urea nitrogen. See UREA nitrogen.
BUN : creatinine ratio see CREATININE : blood urea nitrogen ratio.
bunamidine a cestocide used extensively for the treatment of tapeworms in dogs and cats. Used usually as the hydrochloride in dogs and cats and as the hydroxynaphthoate in sheep and goats.
bunch group of deer hinds.
bunchflower MELANTHRIUM *virginicum*.
Bundaberg disease see EPIZOOTIC ulcerative syndrome.
bundle a collection of fibers or strands, as of muscle fibers, or a fasciculus or band of nerve fibers.
accessory b. of Kent bundle of His.
atrioventricular b. bundle of His.
Bachmann b. a large muscle bundle between the right and left atria, thought to serve as a specialized conduction pathway.
b. branch see bundle BRANCH.
fundamental b. that part of the white matter of the spinal cord bordering the gray matter and containing fibers that travel for a distance of only a few segments of the cord, Called also ground bundle.
b. of His a band of atypical cardiac muscle connecting the atria with the ventricles of the heart; called also atrioventricular bundle.
His b. degeneration associated with sudden unexpected death or periods of viciousness; most common in Doberman and German shepherd dogs.
His b. stenosis inherited in Pug dogs; associated with syncope and sudden death.
Keith's b. a bundle of fibers in the wall of the atrium of the heart between the venae cavae.
medial forebrain b. a group of nerve fibers connecting the midbrain tegmentum and elements of the limbic system.
sinoatrial b. Keith's bundle.
Thorel's b. a bundle of muscle fibers in the human heart connecting the sinoatrial and atrioventricular nodes.
uncinate b. the sharply bent bundle that connects the frontal lobe of the brain with the temporal and occipital lobes.
b. of Vicq d'Azyr a band of fibers from the mamillary body to the anterior nucleus of the thalamus.
Bungner's bands proliferating Schwann cells in nervous tissue may appear as bands of spindle-shaped cells resembling fibroblasts.
bungwall fern BLECHNUM.
buninalike body inclusion body in degenerating nerve cells in horses with some of the pathological characteristics of Bunina bodies in humans.
bunk, bunker large storage bin.
b. forage forage, usually ensilage stored in a large storage bunk and made available to cattle or other livestock along a face of the storage.
Bunnell suture pattern one designed for tendon repair. Most of the path of the suture is intratendinous and it crosses the defect through the cut surfaces on either side and the ends are tied within the defect.
bunny hopping an abnormal gait in which dogs use their hindlegs simultaneously and symmetrically, rather than advancing one at a time and the legs tend to be greatly extended behind the body before being moved forward. A clinical feature of spinal dysraphism.
bunodont having cheek teeth with low, rounded cusps on the occlusal surface of the crown, as in mammals with mixed diet, such as swine and humans.
bunostomiasis infestation with the hookworms *Bunostomum phlebotomum* in cattle and *B. trigonocephalum* in sheep causing anemia and anasarca due to blood loss, together with poor growth. Called also hookworm disease.
Bunostomum a genus of hookworms of the family of Ancylostomatidae. Includes *B. phlebotomum* (*Bos indicus* and *Bos taurus* cattle), *B. trigonocephalum* (sheep, goat, deer).
bunting a behavior of cats in which they rub or push their face against objects, probably depositing glandular secretions; a form of olfactory communication.
b. order the equivalent to peck order of birds in the species that assert themselves by bunting with the head. It is the form of behavior by which Felidae establish themselves in the hierarchy of their social group.
Bunyaviridae a family of viruses comprising five genera: *Bunyavirus*, which includes Akabane and California encephalitis, *Phlebovirus*, which includes Rift Valley fever virus, *Nairovirus*, which includes Nairobi sheep disease and CRIMEAN–CONGO HEMORRHAGIC FEVER viruses, *Uukuvirus*, which does not contain pathogenic viruses, and *Hantavirus*, which infects rodents and causes hemorrhagic fever with renal syndrome in humans.
bunyavirus a virus in the family BUNYAVIRIDAE.
bunyip a mythical animal denizen of Australian swamps. Its ogreish reputation makes it a threatening figure to children.
buphanine a toxic alkaloid in the plant *Boophane disticha*, which has been used as an arrow poison.
buphthalmia 1. autosomal recessive trait in rabbits, causes unilateral or bilateral enlargement of the eyeball with secondary changes in the cornea. 2. see BUPHTHALMOS, HYDROPHTHALMOS.
buphthalmos abnormal enlargement of the eyes; see GLAUCOMA.
bupivacaine hydrochloride a local anesthetic used for peripheral nerve block, infiltration, and sympathetic, caudal or epidural block.
buprenorphine an analgesic and opiate antagonist. Its analgesic effects are much greater and last much longer than those of morphine.

buquinolate a quinolone cocciostat used in poultry.

bur a surgical instrument used to ream out the lining of a cavity, for example the lateral ventricle of horses in the operation for roaring, or to debride bone or teeth. A long stem with a round or oval head carrying rasp-like teeth. See also BURR.

finishing b. for shaping and smoothing composite or amalgam when used for filling teeth.

Burdizzo emasculatome an instrument designed for bloodless emasculation in all species but most adaptable to ruminants because of the extended scrotal neck in these species. The spermatic cord is crushed percutaneously by a double actioned forcing together of blunt blades which also have rounded edges so that the skin is not damaged. The instrument works because of the different strengths of the cord and the skin.

burdock see ARCTIUM LAPPA.

burette, buret a glass tube with a capacity of the order of 25 to 100 ml and graduation intervals of 0.05 to 0.1 ml, with stopcock attachment, used to deliver an accurately measured quantity of liquid.

burial see CARCASS disposal.

Burke's lupine LUPINUS *burkei.*

Burkholderia a genus of gram-negative, aerobic, rod-shaped bacteria.

B. mallei the causative agent of GLANDERS, a disease of horses that is communicable to humans. Previously called *Pseudomonas mallei.*

B. pseudomallei the causative agent of MELIOIDOSIS, a disease of rodents occasionally transmitted to all domestic animal species and humans. Formerly called *Pseudomonas pseudomallei.*

Burkitt's lymphoma, Burkitt's tumor a form of undifferentiated malignant lymphoma in humans and primates, especially marmosets and some gibbons. Usually found in central Africa, but also reported from other areas, and manifested most often as a large osteolytic lesion in the jaw or as an abdominal mass; called also African lymphoma.

The Epstein–Barr virus (EB virus), a gammaherpesvirus, has been isolated from Burkitt's lymphoma cells in culture, and has been implicated as a causative agent. The same virus causes the relatively benign, though debilitating, disease infectious mononucleosis (glandular fever) of humans.

Burley tobacco see NICOTIANA *tabacum.*

Burmese a medium-sized, shorthaired breed of cats. Originally it was always a solid brown color with golden yellow eyes. There are now numerous variations in color, including champagne, blue and platinum. The breed is affected by primary endocardial fibroelastosis, meningoencephalocele and lethal mid-facial malformations.

Burmilla a breed of cats developed from crossing Chinchillas and Lilac Burmese. It has the body of the Burmese with a short, close-lying coat in many colors.

burn injury to tissues caused by contact with dry heat (fire), moist heat (steam or liquid), chemicals, electricity, lightning or radiation. The damage done by a burn includes shock due to the tissue damage, severe dehydration due to the loss of the protective effect of the skin, infection of the burn site, damage to lungs and eyes by exposure to high temperatures and smoke and debris, damage to external somatic addenda including vulva, teats, prepuce, scrotum. The critical decision in a burn case is whether to allow the animal a faint chance of recovery and therefore to continue with treatment. See also BUSHFIRE INJURY.

friction b. the skin is damaged by the heat created by friction as by a rope burn, or when a dog is dragged by its lead behind a car.

full thickness b. involves all of the epidermis and the dermis and may include underlying structures, as well. In alternative classification, it is equivalent to third- and fourth-degree burns.

partial thickness b. involves part or all of the epidermis. Generally, equivalent to first- and second-degree burns.

solar b. sunburn is noticeable mainly in white pigs, white cats and in dogs with little or no pigmentation on the nose (areas not protected by haircoat) or following close clipping. Of little importance in pigs, other than esthetic importance, but in dogs and cats causes actinic dermatitis, which occasionally precedes the development of squamous cell carcinoma. See also solar DERMATITIS, PHOTOSENSITIVE dermatitis.

sole b. damage caused to the sensitive laminae of the feet by the prolonged application of an overheated horseshoe during a shoeing session. The horse is very lame and part of the hoof may subsequently slough.

burning bush see KOCHIA SCOPARIA.

Burow's solution a preparation of aluminum subacetate, glacial acetic acid and water; used topically on the skin as an astringent, and as a topical antiseptic and antipruritic in various skin disorders. Called also aluminum acetate solution.

burr 1. a plant seed capsule carrying many hooked structures which catch in animal coats thus promoting dissemination of the plant. The word is also used as a collective name for plants that carry burrs, e.g. Noogoora burr, Buffalo burr, burr medic, burr trefoil. 2. a surgical instrument. See BUR. 3. the irregular cartilage formation seen inside a dog's ear.

b. buttercup RANUNCULUS *testiculatus.*

b. tongue physical injury to tongue by foreign bodies especially plant awns and burrs.

burr clover MEDICAGO *minima.*

burr medic MEDICAGO *polymorpha.*

burr trefoil MEDICAGO *polymorpha.*

burrawang palm see MACROZAMIA.

burrhole the hole made surgically in bone to allow access to tissues below. Connecting a series of holes facilitates removal of a bone flap.

burro the Spanish word for DONKEY; commonly used in North and South America.

burrow weed HAPLOPAPPUS *heterophyllus.*

burrowing spiders spiders of the family Theraphosidae.

burry said of wool when it contains plant burrs, the adherent seed pods, usually of *Medicago polymorpha.*

bursa pl. *bursae, bursas* [L.] a small fluid-filled sac or saclike cavity situated in places in tissues where friction would otherwise occur.

Bursae function to facilitate the gliding of skin, muscles or tendons over bony or ligamentous surfaces. They are numerous and are found throughout the body; the most important are located at the shoulder, elbow, knee and hip. Inflammation of a bursa is known as BURSITIS. See also BURSAL.

atlantal b. lies between the ligamentum nuchae and the dorsal arch of the atlas. Called also cranial nuchal subligamental bursa.

axial b. under the ligamentum nuchae and over the axis. Called also the caudal nuchal subligamental bursa.

bicipital b. intertuberal bursa. See BICIPITAL bursa.

calcanean b. large bursa on the summit of the calcaneus where the superficial digital flexor muscle tendon is partly inserted as it passes distally to the foot; in the horse there may be an additional small subcutaneous bursa over the tendon at this site; its inflammation causes 'capped hock'.

cloacal b. bursa of Fabricius.

copulatory b. embraces the female nematode during copulation; the structure is useful for the identification of some species of nematodes.

cranial nuchal subligamental b. see nuchal bursa (below).

b.-dependent lymphocytes see B LYMPHOCYTE.

b. equivalent tissue an unidentified component of the lymphoid system, analogous to the bursa of Fabricius in birds, which is considered to be the primary site of the origin of B lymphocytes.

b. of Fabricius an epithelial outgrowth of the cloaca in birds, which develops in a manner similar to that of the thymus, atrophying after 5 or 6 months and persisting as a fibrous remnant in sexually mature birds. It contains lymphoid follicles, and before involution is a site of formation of B lymphocytes associated with humoral or antibody IMMUNITY.

May be very large in young chickens and compress the cloaca dorsally. It opens into the proctodeum, the most caudal of the three chambers of the cloaca.

infracardiac b. a small, serous membrane lined pouch ventral to the aorta and to the right of the esophagus and within the caudal mediastinum.

infraspinatus b. a bursa beneath the superficial tendon of the infraspinatus muscle as it crosses the greater tubercle of the humerus.

intertuberal b. lies between the tendon of the biceps brachialis muscle and the brachial groove of the humerus. Called also bicipital bursa.

intertubercular b. a bursa over the intertubercular groove of the humerus and beneath the tendon of the biceps brachii muscle, in horses and cattle.

b. mucosa, synovial b. a closed synovial sac interposed between surfaces that glide upon each other; it may be subcutaneous, submuscular, subfascial or subtendinous in location.

navicular b. lies between the navicular bone and the deep digital flexor muscle. Called also bursa podotrochlearis manus/pes.

nuchal b. a bursa above the dorsal arch of the atlas and beneath the funicular part of the ligamentum nuchae.

omental b. the potential cavity contained within the greater omentum. It communicates with the rest of the peritoneal cavity through the epiploic foramen (of Winslow).

ovarian b. see OVARIAN bursa.

b. podotrochlearis manus see navicular bursa (above).

subcutaneous b. bursae which develop in subcutaneous sites over any bony prominence, e.g. coxal tuber, olecranon.

supraspinous b. between the funicular and lamellar parts of the ligamentum nuchae and over the spine of the second thoracic vertebra of horses.

synovial b. see bursa mucosa (above).

testicular b. the space between the body of the epididymis and the testis created by the partly free body of the epididymis relative to its close attachment to the testis.

triceps b. beneath the tendon of the triceps brachii muscle as it passes over the summit of the olecranon. Called also tricipital bursa.

tricipital b. see triceps bursa (above).

trochanteric b. over the greater trochanter between the tendon of the accessory gluteal muscle and the trochanteric cartilage.

bursal emanating from or pertaining to bursa.

infectious b. disease a disease of 3- to 6-week-old chickens caused by a BIRNAVIRUS which primarily and selectively destroys B lymphocytes in the bursa of Fabricius resulting in a secondary immunodeficiency. Clinical signs are variable and include diarrhea, feather ruffling and droopiness. Death is often a consequence of septicemia associated with normally nonpathogenic strains of bacteria such as *Escherichia coli* or *Salmonella* spp. The morbidity in an initial outbreak will be 100% and the mortality up to 30%. Called also Gumboro disease, infectious avian nephrosis.

bursatti, bursattee, bursati see SWAMP CANCER.

bursectomy excision of a bursa.

neonatal b. an experimental procedure that removes the bursa of Fabricius, either surgically, hormonally or through infection with the virus of infectious bursal disease. The resulting immunodeficient chick is useful in immunological studies because of the loss of B lymphocytes.

bursitis inflammation of a bursa. Acute bursitis comes on suddenly; severe pain and limitation of motion of the affected joint are the principal signs. See also HYGROMA, intra-abdominal ABSCESS.

Chronic bursitis may follow the acute attacks. There is continued pain and limitation of motion around the joint.

atlantal b. see POLL evil.

carpal b. see carpal HYGROMA.

trochanteric b. inflammation, in the horse, of the bursa between the tendon of the middle gluteal muscle and the major trochanter of the femur or its cartilage. Causes lameness and atrophy of muscles in long-standing cases. Called also whirlbone lameness.

bursolith a calculus in a bursa.

bursopathy any disease of a bursa.

bursotomy incision of a bursa.

burst-forming unit-erythroid see burst forming unit-ERYTHROID.

Burttia prunoides a poisonous African shrub in the family Connaraceae; contains an unidentified toxin; causes sudden death in ruminants. Signs include bloat, salivation, running in circles, abdominal pain, convulsions and death.

bush-baby see GALAGO.

bush fly see MUSCA.

bush-foot see porcine FOOTROT.

bush pig *Portamochoerus porcus*, an animal similar to wild boar with a long snout, pointed ears, big bristles and a mane.

bush sickness see COBALT nutritional deficiency.

bushbuck an antelope, TRAGELAPHUS *scriptus*.

bushfire injury injuries sustained by animals in bushfires have special characteristics compared with fires in buildings. Depending on the nature of the material which burns, there may be injuries chiefly of the feet, limbs and underline, for example in a grass fire or in a hardwood forest fire where litter on the forest floor is the prime source of flame. Alternatively, there may be burning of the entire body in a softwood forest fire. For similar reasons there may be very few survivors or many survivors with either superficial or severe injuries. Called also forest fire injury.

bushman's poison see ACOKANTHERA.

business a commercial enterprise trading in goods or services which incurs expenditure, earns income and trades, hopefully, at a profit.

b. directory lists the names of all businesses operating in a particular area as an aid to consumers. It is now customary to list professional practices in the same directory.

b. names must be registered with a statutory bureau which controls the use of all business names and with the professional registering authority. Both of these organizations are tightly selective of the names that can be used. In the veterinary profession they are literally practice names.

b. nuisance anything done which interferes with the reasonable use of a person's business premises, e.g. traffic blocking access, noise or smell offensive to customers or workers, health risks because of poor sanitation or hygiene.

buspirone an anxiolytic agent.

buss disease see sporadic bovine ENCEPHALOMYELITIS.

Busse–Buschke disease see CRYPTOCOCCOSIS.

busulfan an alkylating antineoplastic agent used in the treatment of chronic granulocytic leukemia.

butacaine a local anesthetic; the sulfate salt is used as a topical anesthetic in the eye and on mucous membranes, in solution or ointment.

butalbital an intermediate-acting barbiturate used as a sedative and hypnotic.

butamben a local anesthetic used topically for the treatment of painful skin conditions.

b. picrate the picrate adds antiseptic activity; used as a topical ointment for the treatment of burns.

butamisole an anthelmintic used as the hydrochloride. Administered by injection in dogs for the treatment of *Trichuris vulpis* and *Ancylostoma caninum*.

butane an aliphatic hydrocarbon, C_4H_{10}, from petroleum.

1,3-butanediol an alkydiol with affinity for liver alcohol dehydrogenase, used in the treatment of ethylene glycol toxicity.

butanol-extractable iodine a method of estimating thyroid function by estimating the amount of protein-bound iodine in the plasma.

butcher's jelly lumps of hemorrhagic edema around sites damaged by larvae of *Hypoderma* spp.

butcher's joints the joints (integrated masses of similar kinds of meat from adjoining muscle masses and still in one piece) as prepared by the meat trade. Carcass meat is sold with the bone in or boned out and in primal cuts of fore- and hindquarters. The retail butcher reduces these to subprimal cuts from which standardized joints or cuts are prepared ready for sale to the consumer.

butenyl isothiocyanate a substance found in some samples of rapeseed and thought to be involved in causing the sudden deaths associated with feeding this material.

Buteo buteo a large predator bird that stalks terrestrial prey rather than other birds, and may eat carrion or vegetable matter. Called also buzzard.

Butler gag a gag similar to the HAUPTNER MOUTH GAG except that it can be fitted only so that the handle of the screw is below the bottom jaw. In the Hauptner, the body of the appliance fits over the maxilla and the handle points upwards.

butobarbital, butobarbitone a short- to intermediate-acting barbiturate; the sodium salt is used as a sedative and hypnotic.

butoconazole an imidazole antifungal used topically, effective particularly against *Candida*.

butopyronoxyl an insect repellent effective against ticks.

butorphanol tartrate a synthetic opioid with both agonist and antiagonist activities. It is used as an analgesic and antitussive.

butt 1. recognized pack for presentation of wool for sale; similar to but smaller than the standard bale; usually an incompletely filled bale. 2. see BUTTING.

butter bean PHASEOLUS *lunatus*.

butter yellow *p*-dimethylaminoazobenzene. Used as a laboratory agent. It is a carcinogen and is the type poison for causing hyperplasia of bile ducts involving the smaller interlobular bile ducts and the intralobular cholangioles.

buttercup see RANUNCULUS.

buttercup comb the kind of comb on a domestic chicken that is split longitudinally.

butterfat globules in the milk of all species. It can be separated to make butter. The nutritional value and the price of milk are judged on, among other things, the butterfat content of the milk. A dramatic drop in the content in milk of butterfat may be caused by a too low fiber content of the diet.

butterfly dog see PAPILLON.

butterfly flag DIPLARRENA *moraea*.

buttermilk residual fluid after removal of fat from milk in butter manufacture; a protein-rich supplement fed to pigs.

butting a form of fighting which is characteristic of ruminants in which the antagonists rush at each other at speed with heads lowered and attempt to meet squarely at the poll or forehead. The victor holds his ground. Sometimes an act of aggression against humans.

buttock either of the two fleshy prominences formed by the gluteal muscles on either side of the tail. Called also nates.

button 1. a knoblike elevation or structure. 2. in computer use means a graphic representation of a button used to indicate that selection of the item so marked will select the option, or the command to activate the option or to execute the command. 3. an appliance used in surgical anastomosis of the intestine (Murphy's button).

b. tumor see HISTIOCYTOMA.

b. ulcer craterous mucosal defects, the edges of which are raised above the surrounding mucosa. The original necrotic center of the lesion is shed leaving a deep ulcer. They are characteristic lesions in the cecum and colon of pigs with subacute salmonellosis. The lesions are usually few in number, small and deep.

button grass see DACTYLOCTENIUM RADULANS.

button weed see IXIOLAENA BREVICOMPTA.

buttress foot see PYRAMIDAL disease.

butyl a hydrocarbon radical, C_4H_9.

b. aminobenzoate see BUTAMBEN.

b. chloride has been used as an anthelmintic but causes poisoning similar to that caused by CARBON TETRACHLORIDE.

***n*-butyl chloride** a superseded anthelmintic with activity against ascarids, hookworms and whipworms in dogs.

butynorate a drug recommended for the treatment of avian coccidiosis.

Butynvibrio fibrisolvens one of the common bacteria in the rumen.

butyraceous of a buttery consistency.

butyrate a salt of butyric acid.

butyric acid a saturated 4-carbon fatty acid found in butter.

butyroid resembling butter.

butyrophenone a chemical class of major tranquilizers which includes droperidol and azaperone.

butyrous resembling butter.

butyryl CoA the first reduced intermediate in synthesis of fatty acids.

butyrylcholinesterase the cholinesterase of plasma (a pseudocholinesterase), which is different from the cholinesterase of the myoneural junctions (acetylcholinesterase).
buxine one of the toxic alkaloids in *Buxus sempervirens*.
buxinidine one of the toxic alkaloids in *Buxus sempervirens*.
Buxus sempervirens an ornamental and hedge shrub in the family Buxaceae; causes severe pain, dysentery, convulsions and death from asphyxia in horses. Pigs and cattle develop hemorrhagic enteritis. Called also box.
buzzard see BUTEO BUTEO.
BVA see BRITISH VETERINARY ASSOCIATION.
BVD see BOVINE virus diarrhea.
BVD/MD bovine virus diarrhea/mucosal disease. See BOVINE virus diarrhea.
BVDV bovine virus diarrhea virus.
BVL bovine viral leukosis.
BVP bovine viral papillomatosis.
BW abbreviation for body weight; used in medical records.
BWD bacillary white diarrhea. See PULLORUM DISEASE.
by-products materials generated incidentally to the production of a principal product in an industry or industrial enterprise. In the meat industry by-products include blood, bone, fat, bristle, hair, wool, hide, skin, hoof, horn and offal products prepared in various ways for use as human or animal food, for pharmaceutical and cosmetics and so on.
Byelorussian having some association with Byelorussia.
B. harness horse multiuse horse, including milk and meat, light draft, coach-horse.
B. red cattle red, dairy cattle from Byelorussia.
Byfield fern BOWENIA *serrulata*.
bypass an auxiliary flow; a shunt; a surgically created pathway circumventing the normal anatomical pathway, as an intestinal bypass.
cardiopulmonary b. diversion of the flow of blood from the entrance to the right atrium directly to the aorta, usually via a pump oxygenator, avoiding both the heart and the lungs; a form of extracorporeal circulation used mainly in experimental animals in the investigation of cardiac prosthetic devices. Called also CPB.
Byssochlamys nivea a fungus capable of producing PATULIN.
byte usually 8 bits; one letter usually requires one byte to store in a computer. Used to express the storage capacity of computer devices; the standard unit is a megabyte; gigabyte disks are commonplace.

C

C chemical symbol, *carbon*; cathode (cathodal); Celsius or centigrade (scale); cervical; clearance; clonus; closure; contraction; cylinder; cytosine; in the electrocardiogram, C stands for chest (precordial) LEAD[2]; symbol for *complement*.
C3 the third component of complement; a β protein. Split into two fragments, C3a and C3b, by C3 convertase which is triggered via the classical or alternative pathway of complement activation. An inherited deficiency occurs in Brittany spaniels and very low serum levels occur in some Finnish-Landrace lambs. See also COMPLEMENT.
C_L lung compliance.
C_T thoracic compliance.
C_{LT} total lung–thorax compliance.
c symbol, *centi-*.
C aberration an abnormal chromosome resulting from the loss, duplication or rearrangement of genetic material.
C banding production of one of the reproducible banding patterns on particular chromosomes by staining the karyotype with Giemsa.
C-bands bands produced in chromosomes after special fixing and staining techniques have been applied. The bands are produced by staining of DNA which has not been removed because it is protected by a nonhistone protein–DNA interaction at the centromere.
C cell a cell type of the thyroid gland, situated between or within the walls of follicles, with numerous small membrane-limited secretory granules in the cytoplasm. The source of calcitonin. Called also parafollicular cell.
C c. tumors (ultimobranchial) adenomas and carcinomas occur most frequently in aged bulls, associated with vertebral osteophytes, osteosclerosis, ankylosis and spondylosis. Believed to be associated with the long-term intake of a diet high in calcium.
C_H domains C_{H1}, C_{H2}, C_{H3} regions of the heavy chain of immunoglobulins with amino acid sequences that are constant in different antibodies of the same class.
C_L domain the region of light chain immunoglobulins that is constant in different antibodies of the same class.
C effects genetic speak for the common environment, e.g. the milk supply to a litter of pigs.
C fibers nerve fibers with the slowest conduction speeds; are very slow-conducting, unmyelinated nerve fibers, principally postganglionic sympathetic fibers.
C_1-inactivator one of the six major protease inhibitors of blood; it inhibits clotting factors XIa, XIIa and plasma kallikrein, but not Xa and plasmin.
C_6 oxidative pathway see GLUCURONATE PATHWAY.
C-peptide the central connecting polypeptide which is part of the proinsulin molecule. It is released when the two chains of insulin are cleaved off of the single chain looped polypeptide of proinsulin.
C protein a skeletal muscle contractile protein involved in the assembly of myosin.
C-reactive protein a serum protein produced in response to inflammation, infection or tissue damage; abbreviated CRP. It is immunosuppressive, promotes phagocytosis, inhibits platelets and activates complement.
C region see CONSTANT DOMAINS.
C-terminal the end of the peptide chain carrying the free alpha-carboxyl group of the last amino acid, conventionally written to the right.
C-type particle a crescent-shaped formation on the cell membrane of cells associated with the budding of so named C type retroviruses.
C-type virus a type of retrovirus, the oncoviruses.
C value amount of DNA in the haploid genome of a species.
CA cardiac arrest.
Ca chemical symbol, *calcium*; cathode (cathodal); cancer.
Ca-EDTA calcium ethylenediamine tetra-acetic acid. See EDETATE.

Ca^{2}+ calcium ions.
Ca^{2}+-ATPase calcium pump involved in the transport of calcium ions against a concentration gradient across a membrane barrier. The transport requires energy from the hydrolysis of ATP.
CAB Commonwealth Agricultural Bureaux.
Caballonema a genus of the subfamily Cyathostominae, small strongyles, cyathostomes of equids. Distribution is limited to the USSR and China.
cabbage a plant whose leaves may cause hemolytic anemia if eaten in large quantities. See BRASSICA *oleracea*. The seeds contain an antithyroid agent progoitrin which, on conversion to an active form (oxazolidone), causes growth inhibition in chickens.
cabbage poison VELLEIA *discophora*.
cabergoline a dopamine antagonist that suppresses progesterone. Used to cause abortion in the bitch.
cable snare see HOG holder.
Cacajao see UAKARI.
cacao see THEOBROMA CACAO.
Cacatua roseicapilla see GALAH.
cacesthesia disordered sensibility.
cache in computer usage is a section of random access memory in which recently accessed information can be stored in anticipation of early future use.
Cache Valley virus one of the California serotype bunyaviruses associated with equine viral encephalomyelitis.
cachectin tumor necrosis factor.
cachet [Fr.] a dish-shaped wafer or capsule enclosing a dose of medicine.
cachexia a profound and marked state of constitutional disorder; general ill health and malnutrition. See also EMACIATION.
cardiac c. severe wasting that occurs in association with chronic cardiac insufficiency. The result of anorexia, malabsorption and poor tissue perfusion with cellular anoxia.
pituitary c. that due to diminution or absence of pituitary function. Manifested by progressive loss of body weight associated with muscle atrophy due to lack of protein anabolism in the absence of growth hormone.
cac(o)- word element. [Gr.] *bad, ill.*
cacodylic acid pharmaceutical aliphatic organic arsenical; see also organic ARSENICAL.
cacomelia congenital deformity of a limb.
cacomistle a wild animal like a raccoon. Called also *Jemtinki sumichrasti.*
cacosmia foul odor; stench.
cactinomycin an antibiotic of the actinomycin complex produced by several species of *Streptomyces*. It is a combination of actinomycin D (dactinomycin), actinomycin C_2 and C_3; used as an antineoplastic agent.
cacumen pl. *cacumina* [L.] 1. the top or apex of an organ. 2. the top of a plant. 3. the anterior and upper part of the monticulus cerebelli; called also culmen.
Cadaba rotundifolia African plant in the Capparidaceae family; toxin unidentified; causes diarrhea, salivation, dyspnea, liver and kidney damage.
cadaver a dead body; generally applied to a body preserved for anatomical study.
c. disposal a serious problem in veterinary practice in the absence of a local government incinerator. Incineration and burial are the only satisfactory methods.
cadaverine a relatively nontoxic ptomaine, $C_5H_{14}N_2$, formed by decarboxylation of lysine.
cadence the rhythm of a horse's gait. The walk is a four beat cadence, the trot is two beat, the canter has three beats and the gallop has four.
cadherins calcium-dependent cell-adhesion molecules.
cadmium chemical element, atomic number 48, symbol Cd; its salts are poisonous. See Table 6. Poisoning in animals may be caused by aerial pollution of pastures or by accidental ingestion of fungicides or anthelmintics which contain the element. Nephropathy, anemia, bone demineralization and poor hair, skin and hoof growth result.
c. anthranilate no longer widely used as an anthelmintic for pigs because of its toxicity.
c. chloride causes bleaching of teeth, anemia, cardiac hypertrophy and bone marrow hyperplasia.
c. oxide a toxic compound used at one time as an anthelmintic for pigs.
caduceus the wand of Hermes or Mercury consisting of a winged staff with two serpents entwined; used as a symbol of the medical profession and as the emblem of most military Medical Corps. Another symbol of medicine is the staff of Æsculapius, which is the official insignia of the American Medical Association. The American Veterinary Medical Association uses a modification of the caduceus as an emblem. The staff is unwinged, there is a single serpent instead of two, and a large V is imprinted over the whole.
An adaptation of the caduceus, with only one snake winding itself around the staff is the emblem of the Veterinary Corps of the US Army.
CAE CAPRINE arthritis–encephalitis.
caecal see CECAL.
caecum see CECUM.
caeruloplasmin see CERULOPLASMIN.
Caesalpinia toxic plant in family Caesalpiniaceae; contains tannins; causes vomiting, diarrhea. Called also bird of paradise tree.
caesarean cesarean.
caesium cesium.
CAEV caprine arthritis–encephalitis virus.
cafe bravo [Span.] PALICOUREA *marcgravii.*
cafezinho PALICOUREA *marcgravii.*
caffeine a central nervous system stimulant from coffee, tea, guarana and maté; it also acts as a mild diuretic. The production of more effective drugs has led to caffeine being discarded as an analeptic. It has even been bypassed by the persons who dope horses, especially because it is readily detectable in urine for up to 10 days after its administration.
caffeinism an agitated state induced by excessive ingestion of caffeine.
cafta see CATHA *edulis.*
cage an animal or bird enclosure with the walls made of rods or mesh to provide maximum restraint with greatest ventilation, reduction in weight, visibility and access to the inhabitant.
c. birds companion birds that are customarily kept in cages to restrain and protect them.
c. biter syndrome damage caused to the teeth of caged exotic animals, particularly large cats, from aggressive biting on the cage wire or bars.
c. layer fatigue birds housed in cages may reach a stage where they are unable to stand up straight. They also develop very fragile bones. This problem is a common target for animal welfare complaints. It is a cause of wastage because of the rate of culling and because of splintering of bones and a resulting downgrading of carcasses at slaughter. Called also cage layer osteoporosis.
c. layer osteoporosis removal of medullary and

cortical bone from laying hens being fed a diet deficient in calcium. See also cage layer fatigue (above).
c. paralysis see THIAMIN nutritional deficiency.
c. rearing pigs that are weaned very early, e.g. at 3 weeks, are reared artificially in cages.
squeeze c. cage with one wall capable of being moved inwards, usually by mechanical means, so that the inhabitant can be restrained sufficiently to prevent its movement and to allow access to suitable sites for the administration of injections. An essential piece of equipment for veterinarians working at zoos, circuses and game farms.

cage-side tests various clinicopathologic testing procedures which may be carried out at the location of the animal's cage; includes rapid semiquantitative tests of hemostatic disorders such as buccal mucosa bleeding time and activated coagulation time. The equivalent of bed-side tests for human patients.

caged birds see CAGE birds.

caiman crocodilian reptile of the family Alligatoridae, very similar to alligators; resident in Central and South America. Genus name is *Caiman*, e.g. *C. sclerops* the spectacled caiman.

caimanpox causes typical pox lesions on the skin of young caimans.

Cairina moschata see MUSCOVY.

Cairn terrier a small (13–14 lb) active terrier with medium-length shaggy, weather-resistant, double coat, short tail, erect ears and dark eyes giving a foxy appearance. Cream, wheaten, red, gray, nearly black and brindle colors are found. The breed is subject to inherited globoid cell leukodystrophy, craniomandibular osteopathy, hemophilia and factor IX deficiency.

Cakala technique see PARAVERTEBRAL block.

cake the residuum after extraction of oil from oil seeds, used extensively as a protein supplement to diets of all housed animal species.
c. poisoning varies with the seed, linseed cake may cause cyanide poisoning, cottonseed cake may cause gossypol poisoning.

Cal kilocalorie.

cal calorie.

-cal suffix meaning pertaining to.

calabrese *Brassica oleracea* var. *italica* (Italian broccoli).

Caladium cultivated, ornamental plant genus in the family Araceae; contains calcium oxalate raphide crystals, causing erosive stomatitis, salivation.

calamary member of the Despinidae family of octopuses (class Cephalopoda).

calamine a preparation of zinc carbonate with with a small amount of ferric oxide; the lotion is used topically as protectant and astringent.

calamus in the shape of a reed or pen.
c. scriptorius reed-shaped portion of the floor of the fourth ventricle of the brain situated between the restiform bodies.

Calandrinia genus of the plant family Portulacaceae.
C. balonensis*, *C. polyandra used commonly as feed for cattle and sheep grazed extensively in arid and semi-arid areas of Australia, these plants have a high oxalate content and are suspected of causing deaths in wethers due to obstructive urolithiasis. Called also parakeelia, parakeelya.

calbindin a calcium-binding protein involved in facilitating the absorption of calcium from the intestine and its reabsorption from the glomerular filtrate in the renal tubules and the deposition of calcium in mineralized tissues; two identified forms of the protein are calbindin-D9k and calbindin-D28k.

calcaneal arising from or pertaining to the calcaneus.
c. epiphysis avulsion occurs in young animals in association with avulsion of the gastrocnemius tendon.
common c. tendon see ACHILLES TENDON.

calcaneal tendon see ACHILLES TENDON.

calcaneoapophysitis inflammation of the posterior part of the calcaneus, marked by pain and swelling.

calcaneoastragaloid pertaining to the calcaneus and talus (astragalus).

calcaneodynia pain in the heel.

calcaneoquartal joint the articulation of the calcaneus with the fourth tarsal bone.

calcaneum see CALCANEUS.

calcaneus, calcaneum the irregular quadrangular bone at the back of the tarsus. One of the two tarsal bones in the proximal row of bones of the hock joint and, because of its calcaneal tuber and the muscles attached to it, acts as a lever to extend the hock joint. Called also heel bone, os calcis, and fibular tarsal bone. See also Table 10.

calcar a spur or spur-shaped structure.
c. avis the lower of two medial elevations in the lateral cerebral ventricle, produced by the lateral extension of the calcarine sulcus; called also hippocampus minor.
c. metacarpale, c. metatarsale see ERGOT[2].

calcareous pertaining to or containing lime; chalky.

calcarine 1. spur-shaped. 2. pertaining to the calcar avis.
c. sulcus a sulcus of the medial surface of the occipital lobe, separating the cuneus from the lingual gyrus.

calcariuria the presence of lime (calcium) salts in the urine.

calcemia excessive calcium in the blood; hypercalcemia.

calcibilia the presence of calcium in the bile.

calcic of or pertaining to lime or calcium.

calcifediol nonproprietary name for 25-hydroxycholecalciferol, used as a calcium regulator in the treatment and management of metabolic bone disease or hypocalcemia associated with chronic renal failure.

calciferol VITAMIN D_2; ergocalciferol.
c.-25-hydroxylase a hepatic microsomal enzyme which controls the conversion of cholecalciferol to 25-hydroxycholecalciferol.

calcific forming lime.

calcification the deposit of calcium salts in a tissue. The normal absorption of calcium is facilitated by parathyroid hormone and by vitamin D. In poisoning with CALCINOGENIC glycosides and when there are increased amounts of parathyroid hormone in the blood (as in HYPERPARATHYROIDISM), there is deposition of calcium in the soft tissue. (In hyperparathyroidism secondary to renal disease there is deposition in the alveoli of the lungs, the renal tubules, beneath the parietal pleura, the gastric mucosa, and the arterial walls.) Normally calcium is deposited in the bone matrix to insure stability and strength of the bone. In OSTEOMALACIA there is an excess of unmineralized osteoid because the aged well-mineralized bone is replaced by a matrix that is inadequately mineralized.
dystrophic c. the deposition of calcium in abnormal tissue without abnormalities of blood calcium.
metastatic c. deposition of calcium in tissues as a result of abnormalities of calcium and phosphorus levels in the blood and tissue fluids.
nutritional c. calcification in soft tissues as a result of an increased intake of calcium.

soft tissue c. see metastatic calcification (above), dystrophic calcification (above).

calcify to mineralize by the deposition of calcium salts.

calcifying mineralized.

c. aponeurotic fibroma locally aggressive nodular masses that involve membranous bones, particularly those of the canine skull (zygomatic arch), and rarely metastasize. See also MULTILOBULAR chondroma and osteoma.

c. epithelial odontogenic tumor rare lesion in dogs and cats; epithelial, gingival masses susceptible to surgical excision.

c. epithelioma see PILOMATRIXOMA.

c. epithelioma of Malherbe see PILOMATRIXOMA.

calcined magnesite the mineral magnesite which has been reduced to a powder by heating, i.e. calcined. It is used as a dietary supplement for cattle and sheep to prevent hypomagnesemia. Used for top-dressing pasture with a similar objective. Contains about 90% magnesium oxide.

calcinogenic conducive to calcinosis.

c. glycoside toxic glycosides with their aglycone an analog of vitamin D_3. Found in plants including *Solanum malacoxylon, Cestrum diurnum, Solanum linneanum, Trisetum flavescens, Nierembergia veitchii.*

calcinosis a condition characterized by abnormal deposition of calcium salts in the tissues.

c. circumscripta localized deposition of calcium in small nodules in subcutaneous tissues, tongue or attached to tendons or joint capsules. Called also tumoral calcinosis.

c. cutis cutaneous mineralization, a characteristic lesion in dogs with hyperadrenocorticism. Lesions are commonest on the dorsal midline, ventral abdomen and inguinal region. The skin is usually thin and atrophic.

enzootic c. calcinosis occurring in larger numbers of animals in a local population than chance warrants. Usually a plant poisoning. May be caused by the following calcinogenic plants: SOLANUM *malacoxylon, S. linneanum,* CESTRUM *diurnum,* NIEREMBERGIA VEITCHII and TRISETUM FLAVESCENS. Manifested clinically by chronic wasting, reluctance to walk and constant shifting of weight from limb to limb. Called also *enteque seco.*

multicentric periarticular c. described in Hungarian vizsla dogs in association with a renal tubular defect in phosphorus transport, causing progressive lameness.

pulmonary c. see MICROLITHIASIS.

tumoral c. circumscribed, hard swellings with a granular radiopacity, usually immovable and located in horses on the lateral aspect of the proximal tibia.

c. universalis widespread deposition of calcium in nodules or plaques in the dermis, panniculus and muscles.

calcipenia deficiency of calcium in the system.

calcipexis, calcipexy fixation of calcium in the tissues.

calciphilia a tendency to calcification.

calciphylaxis the formation of calcified tissue in response to administration of a challenging agent after induction of a hypersensitive state.

calciprivia deprivation or loss of calcium.

calcitonin a polypeptide hormone secreted by the parafollicular or C cells of the thyroid gland, which is involved in plasma calcium homeostasis. It acts to decrease the rate of bone resorption. Called also thyrocalcitonin.

c. gene-related peptides potent vasodilators widely distributed in periadventitial nerves of blood vessels, sinoatrial and atrioventricular nodes, sensory neurons and the central nervous system generally.

c.-secreting cells parafollicular cells of the thyroid gland.

calcitriol a nonproprietary name for 1,25-DIHYDROXYCHOLECALCIFEROL; used as a calcium regulator in the management of hypocalcemia.

calcium a chemical element, atomic number 20, atomic weight 40.08, symbol Ca. See Table 6. Calcium is the most abundant mineral in the body. In combination with phosphorus it forms calcium phosphate, the dense, hard material of the bones and teeth. It is an important cation in intra- and extracellular fluid and is essential to the normal clotting of blood, the maintenance of a normal heartbeat, and the initiation of neuromuscular and metabolic activities.

Within the body fluids calcium exists in three forms. Protein-bound calcium accounts for about 47% of the calcium in plasma; most of it in this form is bound to albumin. Another 47% of plasma calcium is ionized. About 6% is complexed with phosphate, citrate and other anions.

Ionized calcium is physiologically active. One of its most important physiological functions is control of the permeability of cell membranes. Parathyroid hormone, which causes transfer of exchangeable calcium from bone into the bloodstream, and calcitriol maintain calcium homeostasis by preventing either calcium deficit or excess.

c. arsenate used extensively as a spray in orchards, constituting a poison hazard for livestock.

avian c. poisoning excess calcium in the avian diet, especially in diets low in phosphorus causes nephrosis, visceral gout and urolithiasis.

c. balance the balance between calcium intake and losses in feces and urine.

c. borogluconate see BOROGLUCONATE.

c. carbonate an insoluble salt occurring naturally in bone, shells and chalk. A common form of supplementary calcium in dogs and cats on meat-based diets, used because of its high concentration of calcium (40%) and absence of phosphorus.

c. challenge test an intravenous infusion of calcium will cause increased levels of gastrin in dogs with a gastrinoma. Often used in combination with a SECRETIN test.

c. channels see CHANNEL.

c. chloride a salt used in solution to restore electrolyte balance, to treat hypocalcemia and as an antidote to magnesium poisoning. Is highly irritant and has been discarded generally in favor of less irritating substances, e.g. calcium borogluconate.

c. cyanamide agricultural fertilizer capable of being toxic.

c. cytosolic see CYTOSOL.

diffusible c. see calcium (above).

c. edetate (Ca-EDTA) calcium ethylenediamine tetra-acetic acid; the disodium and dipotassium salts are commonly used as anticoagulants in the preservation of blood samples for hematology. A chelating agent, used parenterally in the treatment of lead poisoning. See also EDETATE.

excess c. in all species may cause HYPERCALCITONISM with decreased osteoclastic activity and skeletal remodeling. In dogs, disorders of enchondral ossification with curved radius and osteochondrosis have been demonstrated; secondary iron deficiency anemia occurs in piglets.

c. fluoride naturally occurring mineral. Called also fluorspar, fluorite.

c. gel contains high levels of calcium; given to cows as a drench or in the feed as a prophylaxis against milk fever.
c. gluconate a calcium replenisher and antidote to fluoride or oxalate poisoning.
c. gout see CALCINOSIS circumscripta.
c. homeostasis maintenance of normal calcium metabolism by the combined effects of adequate alimentary intake, renal excretion, parathyroid hormone involvement, 1,25 dihydroxycholecalciferol (or calcitriol) and calcitonin, plasma protein binding and deposition in tissues.
c. hydroxide an astringent compound used topically in solution or lotions; in dentistry used to encourage deposition of secondary dentine. Called also slaked lime. In solution, called lime water.
idiopathic c. phosphate deposition thought to be inherited as an autosomal dominant trait in Great Danes commencing in puppies about 5 weeks old, characterised by incoordination with deformity and displacement of the 7th cervical vertebra and mineral deposits in the intervertebral joints, in serous and synovial membranes and mineralization in most other tissues.
c. lactate used for supplementing the diet with calcium; contains 18% calcium. As calcium sodium lacate, containing 8% calcium, it is more soluble and can be used in drinking water.
c. levulinate a calcium compound used parenterally in the treatment of hypocalcemia; contains 14.8% calcium.
c. mandelate administered orally and used as a urinary antiseptic.
c. nitrate used as an additive during cheese making to control fermentation. Whey from this cheese may cause nitrate poisoning in pigs.
nondiffusible c. protein-bound fractions of plasma calcium.
c. nutritional deficiency nutritional deficiency of calcium is rarely primary except in carnivores on an all-meat diet. Secondary deficiency is usually the result of diets having too high a content of phosphorus. The outcome of either deficiency may be nutritional HYPERPARATHYROIDISM, RICKETS, OSTEOMALACIA, OSTEODYSTROPHY in horse and pigs, and degenerative ARTHROPATHY of cattle, depending on the species, age of the animal and availability of vitamin D. Hypocalcemia may not occur because of the activity of parathyroid hormone, but classical tetany and recumbency can occur if the deficiency is prolonged or if they are precipitated by some other factor.
c. oxalate a compound occurring in the urine in crystals and in certain calculi. See also oxalate UROLITH.
c. oxide alkaline and capable of causing gastroenteritis. There is a high concentration in BASIC slag and this may contribute to that poisoning.
c. pantothenate a calcium salt of the dextrorotatory isomer of pantothenic acid; used as a growth-promoting vitamin.
c. phosphate one of three salts containing calcium and the phosphate radical: dibasic and tribasic calcium phosphate are used as sources of calcium; monobasic calcium phosphate is used in fertilizer and as a calcium and phosphorus supplement. An important constituent of UROLITHS.
c. : phosphorus ratio the ratio of calcium to phosphorus in the diet, 1 : 1 to 1 : 2 is usually considered to be adequate for proper calcium nutritional status in most animal species. Diets outside this range are likely to cause osteodystrophies. Animals grazing phosphorus-deficient pasture, and those being intensively fed on grain rations which have an abnormally high phosphorus content, are the principal subjects. Horses on heavy grain diets and dogs and cats on meat diets without calcium supplementation are also targets for the disease.
c. polycarbophil a hydrophilic agent used as a bulk laxative in the treatment of constipation and diarrhea.
c. polysulfide see LIME-SULFUR.
c. propionate see PROPIONIC ACID.
protein bound c. biologically inert fraction of plasma calcium; most is bound to albumin and globulins with a small fraction complexed to organic and inorganic acids.
c. silicophosphate crystals of this mineral are thought to contribute physically to the gastroenteritis caused by BASIC slag poisoning.
c. sulfate the main component of plaster of Paris; also used as a dietary source of calcium and inorganic sulfate sulfur.
c. sulfide, c. polysulfide lime-sulfur.
c. supplements include calcium carbonate, gluconate, lactate and phosphate; bone flour, bone meal, ground limestone, chalk.
c. tungstate screens cards coated with calcium tungstate crystals are used to sandwich film in a light-tight cassette. They fluoresce when exposed to x-rays and, together with the beam, affect the film emulsion. They reduce the exposure factor required.
urinary c. calciuria.

calcium-binding protein see CALBINDIN.

calcium channel blocker a drug, such as nifedipine or verapamil, that selectively blocks the influx of calcium ions through a specific ion channel (the slow channel or calcium channel) of cardiac muscle and smooth muscle cells; used in the treatment of cardiac arrhythmias. Calcium channel blockers act to control arrhythmias by slowing the rate of sinoatrial (SA) node discharge and the conduction velocity through the atrioventricular (AV) node. Called also calcium blocker, calcium antagonist.

calciuria calcium in the urine.

calcofluor white stain used to produce fluorescence of fungal elements for ultraviolet microscopy.

calcospherite one of the minute globular bodies formed during calcification by chemical union of calcium particles and albuminous matter of cells.

calculator electronic instrument for doing mathematical calculations.
programmable c. one with an electronic circuitry that enables the operator to initiate the performance of a series of related mathematical calculations by a single command.

calculifragous breaking up calculi.

calculogenesis the formation of calculi.

calculolytic lysis of calculi, usually in the urinary tract.
c. diet see calculolytic DIET.

calculosis a condition characterized by the presence of calculi. Called also lithiasis.

calculus pl. *calculi* [L.] an abnormal concretion, usually composed of mineral salts, occurring within the animal body, chiefly in the hollow organs or their passages. Called also stones, as in kidney stones (UROLITHIASIS) and GALLSTONES. See also HIPPOMANES.
biliary c. a gallstone.
bronchial c. see BRONCHIAL calculus.
dental c. mineralized deposits of calcium phosphate

and carbonate, with organic matter, deposited on tooth surfaces. Found commonly in dogs and cats, sometimes in horses, rarely in sheep. May initiate caries and peridontal disease.

lung c. a concretion formed in the bronchi. See also BRONCHIAL calculus.

pancreatic c. very small (4 to 5 mm) calculi in pancreatic ducts, rare and of no pathogenic importance.

prostatic c. concretions of calcium phosphates and carbonates in the prostatic ducts are rare and of no clinical significance.

renal c. see UROLITHIASIS.

salivary c. white, hard, laminated concretions in the salivary duct; a sialolith. Occurs most commonly in horses.

urethral c. a calculus lodged in the urethra causes obstruction of the urethra with a potential for causing rupture of the bladder or perforation of the urethra and leaking of urine into subcutaneous or retroperitoneal sites. See also UROLITH, UROLITHIASIS.

urinary c. a calculus in any part of the urinary tract. See UROLITHIASIS.

vesical c. a urolith in the urinary bladder.

CALD chronic active liver disease.

calefacient causing a sensation of warmth; an agent that so acts.

calendar charts wall charts or wheels which are valuable management tools because they depict the reproductive and lactation status of each cow or sow in the herd at any given time.

Calendula plant genus in the family Asteraceae; cause cyanide poisoning; include *C. cuneata*, *C. viscosa* (both = *Dimorphotheca cuneata*).

calf 1. bovine young less than one year old. 2. young of other species including elephant, larger deer, e.g. red, Japanese sika, wapiti, elk, moose, reindeer, and also pinnipeds and cetaceans. 3. in dogs refers to the region of the hindlimb between the stifle and the hock.

bull c. male entire bovine under one year of age.

c. crop the group of calves born to a herd of cows during one breeding season.

c. crop percentage the percentage of calves born to the cows bred or exposed to breeding bulls.

c. diarrhea see CALF SCOURS.

fetal c. includes unborn and stillborn calves. Can be identified by the presence of atelectasis of the entire lungs, patency of the umbilical vessels which also contain unclotted blood, sodden quality of the skin, high water and nil fat content of the tissues, absence of milk from the gut. Called also slink. See also SLINK CALVES.

c. puller see FETAL extractor.

c. starter artificial feeding of calves includes liquid milk replacer and dry calf starter, the latter being provided from about one week of age. At 3 to 6 weeks the calf is able to exist solely on starter and the milk replacer or milk can be discontinued. Calf starters vary a great deal in composition, quality and price. They need to have a high digestibility coefficient, a high energy content and at least 18% crude protein.

calf-bed uterus of a cow.

calf diphtheria see calf DIPHTHERIA, FUSOBACTERIUM *necrophorum*.

calf-kneed a defect of conformation in horses; the cannon is set back behind the line of the radius.

calf lymphosarcoma see BOVINE viral leukosis.

calf pneumonia a group of diseases of calves caused primarily by viruses, often complicated by secondary bacterial invasion. The viruses include parainfluenza-3 (PI-3), respiratory syncytial virus (RSV), an adenovirus, a reovirus, bovine herpesvirus 1 and bovine rhinovirus. *Chlamydia* and *Mycoplasma* spp. are also causative agents. The clinical syndrome is the same with any of the viruses: fever, increased respiratory rate, hacking cough, overloud breath sounds on auscultation of the lungs. The calves show remarkably little toxemia. If secondary bacterial pneumonia follows the additional signs are toxemia, gurgling or squeaky breath sounds, and a fatal outcome. See also ENZOOTIC pneumonia.

calf scours diarrhea of calves, of most importance in the newborn because of their susceptibility to dehydration and toxemia. See COLIBACILLOSIS, COCCIDIOSIS, CRYPTOSPORIDIOSIS, CORONAVIRIDAE, ROTAVIRUS, SALMONELLOSIS, dietary DIARRHEA.

calfeteria farmyard equipment containing a tank, or tanks, for milk which supplies multiple teats on the exterior to provide sucking points for multiple calves.

calfkill KALMIA *angustifolia*.

caliber the diameter of the lumen of a canal or tube.

calibration determination of the accuracy of an instrument, usually by measurement of its variation from a standard, to ascertain necessary correction factors.

calibrator an instrument for dilating a tubular structure or for determining the caliber of such a structure.

calibre see CALIBER.

calicectasis dilatation of a calix of the kidney.

calicectomy excision of a calix of the kidney.

calices plural of *calix*.

Caliciviridae a family of viruses that are about 35 nm in diameter, with a capsid, composed of a single major capsid protein of about 60 kilodaltons that carries 32 shallow, cup-like circular indentations and a single-stranded, plus sense RNA genome of about 8 kilobases. There are at least five groups (possibly genera); includes feline calicivirus, vesicular exanthema of swine virus, San Miguel sealion virus, rabbit hemorrhagic disease, and the human viruses, Norwalk and related viruses and hepatitis E virus.

Calicivirus a genus of viruses in the family CALICIVIRIDAE.

calicivirus a virus in the genus *Calicivirus*.

canine c. has been isolated from the feces of dogs with diarrhea; the significance is unknown.

feline c. infection a common cause of upper respiratory disease and ulcerative glossitis in cats. Affected cats show varying degrees of ocular and nasal discharge, coughing and sneezing. Pneumonia sometimes occurs, mainly in young or debilitated cats. Ulceration of the tongue and palate is a regular feature of the disease, but lips, nares and skin are also sometimes involved. Lameness, diarrhea and seizures have also rarely been associated with calicivirus infection. Many recovered cats remain carriers of the virus, shedding infectious organisms from the pharynx. Most of these are asymptomatic, but some may have chronic oral lesions. Feline calicivirus has also been associated with FELINE urological syndrome, but its role in that disorder remains unclear. See also FELINE viral respiratory disease complex.

porcine c. the cause of VESICULAR exanthema of swine.

rabbit c. the cause of RABBIT HEMORRHAGIC DISEASE.

calico bush KALMIA *latifolia*.

calico cat see TORTOISESHELL.

Calicophoron stomach flukes of ruminants. Species include *C. calicophorum*, *C. cauliorchis*, *C. ijimai* and *C. raja*. See also PARAMPHISTOMOSIS.

caliculus a small cup or cup-shaped structure.
c. gustatorius see TASTE.
California black-legged tick see IXODES *pacificus*.
California buckeye tree AESCULUS *californica*.
California chicory see RAFINESQUIA CALIFORNICA.
California disease see COCCIDIOIDOMYCOSIS.
California encephalitis an encephalitis of humans caused by the La Crosse virus isolated from mosquitoes in California. Occurs experimentally in small laboratory rodents when the virus is injected intracerebrally. Suspected of natural passage through wild and domestic mammals.
California encephalomyelitis virus group mosquito-transmitted viruses of the family *Bunyaviridae*; can cause acute encephalitis in horses. Type viruses are Snowshoe hare and Jamestown Canyon; associated viruses are Main Drain and Cache Valley.
California eyeworm see THELAZIA *californiensis*.
California mastitis test an indirect test for bovine mastitis based on the presence of a high leukocyte count in mastitic milk. The test can be used in the milking shed or in the laboratory and as a test for individual quarters, or cows, or as a herd test. There is a good correlation between the results obtained and the actual leukocyte count and with the productivity of the quarter. It has faded in importance with the introduction of milk cell counts carried out electronically on automated equipment. See also BRABANT MASTITIS TEST.
California oat grass see DANTHONIA.
California poppy see ESCHSCHOLTZIA CALIFORNICA.
California rose bay RHODODENDRON *macrophyllum*.
California spangled a recently developed breed of cats, derived from Siamese, Manx and domestic cats. Its main feature is a short, spotted coat.
Californian burr *Xanthium strumarium* complex.
Californian rabbit popular as a fancy rabbit and for commercial purposes; it is white with black or chocolate points.
californium a chemical element, atomic number 98, atomic weight 249, symbol Cf. See Table 6.
calipers instrument with two bent or curved legs used to measure thickness or diameter of a solid, or the internal dimensions of a hollow object.
electronic c. used in ultrasonography to measure the distance between two points or the circumference of an object.
calix pl. *calices* [L.] a cuplike organ or cavity, e.g. one of the recesses of the kidney pelvis which enclose the tips of the pyramids; ovarian calix in birds comparable to the ovulation fossa in mammals.
calkins turned down portion of the heel of a horseshoe, designed to reduce slipping on worn stones or icy surfaces. Called also calks, frost studs.
calks see CALKINS.
Call–Exner body secretory globule resembling an ovum found in abortive follicles in ovarian neoplasms with tumor cells radially arranged around eosinophilic material.
calla lily see ZANTEDESCHIA AETHIOPICA.
Callicarpa longifolia Australian plant in the family Verbenaceae; an unidentified toxin causes hepatitis and photosensitization.
Callicebus see TITI MONKEY.
calling a lay term referring to the vocalization of a female cat in estrus and the associated, characteristic behavior that includes rolling, treading with the front feet and elevation of the hindquarters. Often misinterpreted by an inexperienced owner as signs of pain or illness.
Callionymidae family of fish containing only the poisonous stinkfish.
Calliphora a genus of flies which includes *C. augur*, *C. australis*, *C. erythrocephala*, *C. fallax*, *C. hilli*, *C. novica*, *C. stygia* and *C. vomitoria*. They may initiate blowfly strike in sheep but they mainly assume importance in sheep that are already infested.
calliphorid pertaining to blowflies.
calliphorid flies see BLOWFLY.
Calliphoridae the family containing most of the important blowflies, including *Calliphora*, *Chrysomyia*, *Lucilia*, *Callitroga* and *Phormia* spp.
Calliphorinae the blowfly subfamily.
calliphorine myiasis see cutaneous MYIASIS.
Callithrix monkeys of the marmoset and tamarin group.
Callitroga a genus of screw-worms which includes *C. americana*, *C. hominivorax* and *C. macellaria* (called also *Cochliomyia hominivorax* and *C. macellaria*). See under cutaneous MYIASIS.
Callorhinus ursinus northern fur seal.
callosity a callus.
callosum corpus callosum.
callous of the nature of a callus; hard.
callus 1. localized hyperplasia of the horny layer of the epidermis due to pressure or friction. In dogs, these often form over pressure points such as the elbow, hock and (in some breeds) sternum, particularly if the animal is sleeping on a hard surface. 2. an unorganized network of woven bone formed about the ends of a broken bone; it is absorbed as repair is completed (provisional callus), and ultimately replaced by true bone (definitive callus).
bridging c. bridging the callus gap.
external c. around the outside of a fracture.
hard c. fully mineralized.
hypertrophic c. a form of delayed healing in which fibrocartilage forms between fracture fragments, resulting in a false callus. Called also elephant's foot callus.
internal c. between the ends of fractured bones.
periosteal c. new bone formed by the proliferation of periosteal osteogenic cells.
provisional c. a subsequently remodeled callus.
c. pyoderma secondary bacterial infection, particularly of pressure point calluses in dogs; can be extensive with deep pyogenic inflammation.
soft c. the originating fibobrocellular tissue before calcification.
sternal c. may develop over a prominent sternum in some breeds of dogs, particularly Dachshunds, in response to pressure.
temporary c. see provisional callus (above).
calmative 1. sedative; allaying excitement. 2. an agent having such effects.
Calmette–Guérin bacillus see BCG.
calmodulin a calcium-binding protein concerned in the response of muscle fibers and other cells to calcium.
calomel see MERCUROUS chloride.
calor [L.] *heat;* one of the cardinal signs of inflammation.
caloric pertaining to heat or to calories.
c. density measure of the energy contained in food, usually quantified as calories or joules, per unit mass of food.
c. exhaustion see HYPOGLYCEMIA.
c. homeostasis process of regulation of energy intake from food to sustain energy balance.
c. intake measure of amount of food energy as calories eaten by an animal.
c. requirements see ENERGY requirements.
c. test irrigation of the external ear canal with hot or

very cold water will stimulate the flow of endolymph and will cause nystagmus if the vestibular system and brainstem are intact.

calorie any of several units of heat defined as the amount of heat required to raise the temperature of 1 gram of water by 1 degree Celsius (1°C) at a specified temperature. The calorie used in chemistry and biochemistry is equal to 4.184 joules. Symbol cal.

In referring to the energy content of foods it is customary to use the 'large calorie', which is equal to 1 kilocalorie (kcal), 1000 cal. Every bodily process—the building up of cells, motion of the muscles, the maintenance of body temperature—requires energy, and the body derives this energy from the food it consumes. Digestive processes reduce food to usable fuel, which the body burns in the complex chemical reactions that sustain life.

calorific generating heat measurable in calories.

calorigenic effect see SPECIFIC dynamic action.

calorimeter an instrument for measuring the amount of heat produced in any system or organism. The material is burned in the calorimeter and the heat energy produced is measured.

calorimetry measurement of the heat eliminated or stored in any system.

direct c. measurement of heat actually produced by the organism which is confined in a sealed chamber or calorimeter.

indirect c. estimation of the heat produced by means of the respiratory differences of oxygen and carbon dioxide in the inspired and expired air.

Calotis scapigera Australian plant in the family Asteraceae; contains cyanogenetic glycosides and is capable of causing cyanide poisoning; called also tufted burr daisy.

calotrope *Calotropis procera*.

Calotropis procera Australian plant in the family Asclepiadaceae; probably poisonous through cardiac glycosides. Called also caltrops, king's crown, rubber tree.

calsequestrin a calcium ion binding protein effecting a sequestration of calcium ions within the smooth endoplasmic reticulum.

Caltha palustris a toxic plant in the family Ranunculaceae; contains a vesicant substance protoanemonin. Ingestion of the plant causes stomatitis, salivation, diarrhea and abdominal pain. Called also marsh marigold, cowslip, kingcup.

caltrops see TRIBULUS *terrestris*.

calvaria, calvarium the domelike superior portion of the cranium, comprising the superior portions of the frontal, parietal and occipital bones.

calve act of parturition by a cow or other mammal producing a calf as offspring.

Calvé–Perthes disease see LEGG–CALVÉ–PERTHES DISEASE.

Calvin cycle see dark REACTION.

calving act of parturition in a bovine female, and presumably in any animal that bears a calf as its newborn. See also BLOCK CALVING, EASE OF CALVING.

c.–to-conception interval interval between calving and the next conception date.

difficult c. see DYSTOCIA.

c. facilities yards, crush, chute, hot and cold water, shelter, all the resources necessary for capturing and restraining a cow while helping her to deliver a calf.

c.-to-first-estrus interval interval between calving and the first observed estrus. Data used as a measure of reproductive performance, especially dairy herds where block mating needs to be completed in as brief an interval as possible.

c.-to-first-service interval alternative to calving-to-first-estrus interval but does not take into account any deferral of mating for managerial reasons.

c. grounds cows that are run on very extensive grazing may need to be under close surveillance by calving time. A small area of land can be enclosed or the herd herded into it—the calving ground.

c. index any method of expressing reproductive efficiency on the basis of the number of calves produced. May refer to the average calving interval or to the percentage of calves produced by the mated group of cows.

c. induction see PARTURITION induction.

c. injury damage to the uterus, vagina and vulva or surrounding tissues, especially obturator and sciatic nerves, caused by the parturition process.

c. interval the average time interval between successive calvings.

c. pad a small area specifically prepared with sand or limestone base and bedding of material such as rice hulls or sawdust, where all cows are located for calving. Allows intense supervision of periparturient and calving cows.

c. paralysis see MATERNAL obstetric paralysis.

c. pattern of a herd is a chronological list of calving dates. In seasonally calving herds a compact list indicates high fertility, a stretched out list indicates an indifferent fertility level.

c. percentage see CALF crop percentage.

c. record a record of the reproductive efficiency of each dam in the form of dates, events and procedures related to reproductive function.

c. season season of the year at which the herd, or other population of cows, calves, e.g. spring calving.

seasonal c. when the cows in a herd calve at about the same time. Thus spring calving, autumn calving. Usually used as a management tool to take maximum advantage of seasonal feed supplies or climate.

year-round c. herd management system in which cows are mated so that some cows in the herd will calve at all times of the year thus maintaining a regular milk supply for a fresh milk supply.

calx 1. lime or chalk. 2. heel.

Calycanthus australiensis see IDIOSPERMUM AUSTRALIENSE.

calyculus caliculus.

calyx calix.

major c. a fusion of minor calyxes.

minor c. the cup-shaped dilation of the intrarenal ureter; the space into which a single papilla of a multiple-lobed kidney protrudes.

CAM cell-adhesion molecule.

CAMAL see CORNELL alternate-month accelerated lambing system.

Camallanus nematode genus which infests freshwater turtles and aquarium fish.

camarillo a part albino type of horse found only in California; has white hair, pink skin and black eyes.

cambendazole an efficient broad-spectrum anthelmintic. See also ALBENDAZOLE.

Cambridge ventilator a powerful machine used in anesthetizing large animals. A hydraulically compressed bellows drives a 'bag-in-bottle' arrangement.

camel humped members of the Camelidae family of exotic ruminants.

Arabian c. called also *Camelus dromedarius*, or single-humped camel.

bactrian c. two-humped camel. Called also *Camelus bactrianus*, dromedary.

c. bush TRICHODESMA *zeylanica*.

dromedary c. one-humped camel. Called also *Camelus dromedarius*.

c. poison GYROSTEMON spp., ERYTHROPHLEUM *chlorostachys*, TRICHODESMA *zeylanica*.

single-humped c. see Arabian camel (above).

c. thorn ACACIA *erioloba*.

c. thorn + molopo moth *Acacia erioloba* + Gonometa spp.

camelid members of the family Camelidae; includes camels and the South American camelids—alpaca, guanaco, llama, vicuna.

Camelidae one of the six families of ruminants in the order ARTIODACTYLA.

Camellia includes *Camellia japonica*, *C. susanqua*; one of the two plants known to reflect the fluorine content of the soil on which it grows (the other is the tea plant (*C. sinensis*)). It may contain as much as 2000 ppm of fluorine.

Camelostrongylus a genus of the family Trichostrongylidae of intestinal helminths. Includes *Camelostrongylus mentulatus* (sheep, camel, wild ruminants).

camelpox a disease of particularly young camels caused by camelpox virus in the genus *Orthopoxvirus*. The lesions are typical of pox lesions and occur on the hairless parts of the body. The disease is transmissible to humans.

Camelus genus of two-toed ungulates in the family Camelidae. Includes *C. bactrianus* (bactrian camel), *C. dromedarius* (dromedary, one-humped or Arabian camel).

cameo in some countries a recognized color variety of longhaired cats with copper-colored eyes and a coat color that is basically a silver, cream or white undercoat with red tips that vary in intensity on different parts of the body.

camera pl. *camerae;* a cavity or chamber.

c. anterior bulbi anterior chamber of the eye.

c. posterior bulbi posterior chamber of the eye; small annular space between the posterior surface of the iris and the anterior surface of the lens, and bounded peripherally by the ciliary processes.

c. vitrea bulbi vitreous chamber of the eye, between the crystalline lens and the retina, that contains the vitreous body.

Cammerer rotation fork an instrument used to rotate a fetus which is badly presented. Each arm of the fork carries a canvas cuff for fixation of the limbs to the crutch. The external end of the device is a long crossbar to facilitate the rotation.

camomile see CHAMOMILE.

cAMP cyclic ADENOSINE monophosphate.

cAMP–CAP complex catabolite *a*ctivator *p*rotein binds to cAMP as a first step in the switch from glucose metabolism to lactose metabolism in *Escherichia coli*.

cAMP-dependent protein kinase a tetrameric protein composed of two regulatory subunits that bind cAMP, and two catalytic subunits that catalyze the transfer of a phosphoryl group from ATP to a target enzyme.

CAMP phenomenon a cultural phenomenon produced by most streptococci in Lancefield Group B. Called after the originators Christie, Atkins and Muench-Petersen. These streptococci hemolyze red cells in sheep blood agar plates but only in the presence of beta toxin of staphylococci. The phenomenon is used to presumptively diagnose the presence of *Streptococcus agalactiae* in mastitic cow's milk. Similar synergism in hemolytic activity is observed between *Rhodococcus equi* and *Corynebacterium pseudotuberculosis*, beta toxin of staphylococci or *Listeria monocytogenes*, and can be used for presumptive diagnosis of these species.

Campanulotes a genus of bird lice. Includes *Campanulotes bidentatus compar* (small pigeon louse).

camphechlor see TOXAPHENE.

camphor a ketone derived from the cinnamon tree, *Cinnamomum camphora*, or produced synthetically; used externally as an antiphlogistic and antiseptic; applied in liniments as a counterirritant; administered as a steam inhalant as an expectorant.

Campolino horse bay, sorrel or chestnut light Brazilian horse, bred from native horse with imported breeds.

Camponotus ant genus second intermediate host to the flukes *Dicrocoelium* spp.

camptodactyly permanent flexion of one or more digits.

camptomelia bending of the limbs, producing permanent bowing or curving of the affected part.

Camptotheca acuminata Asian plant in the family Nyssaceae; contains an alkaloid campothecin; causes diarrhea, dysentery.

Campylobacter a genus of bacteria, family Spirillaceae, made up of gram-negative, non-spore-forming, motile, comma-shaped rods, which are microaerophilic to anaerobic. Members of the genus were previously classified as *Vibrio* spp. and many of the diseases caused by these species are still referred to as vibriosis.

C. coli a commensal of the gastrointestinal tract of poulty, pigs and humans; can cause enteritis in pigs and humans.

C. fetus* subsp. *fetus causes ovine genital campylobacteriosis and abortion in sheep and cattle.

C. fetus* subsp. *venerealis causes bovine VIBRIOSIS, also known as epizootic bovine infertility.

C. hyointestinalis*, *C. mucosalis associated with the porcine intestinal ADENOMATOSIS complex, PROLIFERATIVE hemorrhagic enteropathy, NECROTIC enteritis.

C. jejuni causes abortion in sheep and enteritis in dogs, cats and other animals. An important food-borne cause of enteritis in humans, and the cause of avian vibrionic HEPATITIS.

C. sputorum* subsp. *bubulus*, *C. sputorum* biovar *fecalis found in cattle and sheep, but not known to cause disease.

C. upsaliensis may be associated with diarrhea in dogs and humans.

campylobacteriosis disease caused by infection with *Campylobacter* spp. Includes bovine VIBRIOSIS, VIBRIONIC abortion of sheep, enteritis of dogs.

avian c. Caused by *Campylobacter coli*, *C. jejuni*, *C. laridis*. Characterized by depression, diarrhea.

bovine genital c. see bovine VIBRIOSIS.

campylognathia curved jaw, a rare congenital defect in calves.

Canaan dog a medium-sized (35–55 lb), spitz-type dog with a sandy to red brown, white or black coat, with white markings. The tail is curled over the body.

Canada garlic ALLIUM *canadense*.

Canada thistle see CIRSIUM ARVENSE.

Canadian a black or brown breed of dairy cattle, bred in Canada from cattle imported from France in the late 17th century. Called also Quebec Jersey.

Canadian bluegrass see POA.

Canadian casting a method for casting a horse. One front limb is tied up with a kneestrap. The hindlimbs are pulled from under the horse by a system of sidelines and hobblestraps.

Canadian hairless cat a type of cat derived from a mutant cat with a generalized absence of hair that is transmitted as a recessive trait. Now being promoted as a distinct breed. Called Sphinx cat in the United States. See also ALOPECIA universalis.

Canadian horsepox a chronic pustular dermatitis caused by *Corynebacterium pseudotuberculosis*. The infection is spread on the harness with most lesions occurring on the harness sites. They are 0.5 to 1 inch in diameter and painful to touch. Called also acne contagiosa equi and contagious equine pustular dermatitis.

Canadian Kennel Club the principal body for registration of purebred dogs in Canada.

canal a relatively narrow tubular passage or channel.

accessory c. see lateral canal (below).

alar c. in the body of the basisphenoid bone, transmits the maxillary artery.

alimentary c. the digestive tube from mouth to anus. See also ALIMENTARY canal.

anal c. the terminal portion of the alimentary canal, from the rectum to the anus.

atrioventricular c. the common canal connecting the primitive atrium and ventricle; it sometimes persists as a congenital anomaly.

birth c. the canal through which the fetus passes in birth.

carotid c. one in the pars petrosa of the temporal bone, transmitting the internal carotid artery to the cranial cavity.

carpal c. on the palmar surface of the equine carpus where the carpal groove is converted into a canal by the flexor retinaculum which stretches from the accessory carpal bone to the medial side of the carpus. It houses the flexor tendons.

central brain c. lumen of the neural tube of the embryo within the brain.

cervical c. the part of the uterine cavity lying within the cervix.

condyloid c. in the occipital bone; transmits a vein.

c. of Corti a space between the outer and inner rods of Corti.

external ear c. the canal from the external auditory meatus to the eardrum.

facial c. osseous tube in the temporal bone that transmits the facial nerve.

femoral c. in the groin on the medial aspect of the thigh; contains the femoral artery and vein.

c's of Gartner in the ventral wall of the vagina; they are remnants of the mesonephric ducts and very variable in their occurrence. Called also ductus epoophori longitudinales.

haversian c. see HAVERSIAN canal.

c's of Hering openings between the bile canaliculi and the cholangioles, the terminal ducts of the biliary duct system. Called also CHOLANGIOLE.

hyaloid c. central canal of the vitreous humor running from the lens to the optic disk.

hypoglossal c. an opening in the occipital bone, transmitting the hypoglossal nerve and a branch of the posterior meningeal artery; called also anterior condyloid foramen.

infraorbital c. a canal running obliquely from the front of the orbit to the side of the muzzle, transmitting the infraorbital vessels and nerve. In the horse it passes through the maxillary sinus.

inguinal c. the oblique passage in the caudal abdominal wall on either side, through which passes the round ligament of the uterus in some females such as the bitch and the spermatic cord in the males.

intestinal c. small and large intestines.

lacrimal c. the nasolacrimal canal.

lateral c. a small canal in the root of a tooth which emerges on the side, rather than the apex. Called also accessory canal.

mandibular c. a passageway within the mandible for conduction of the inferior alveolar vessels and nerve; the inferior alveolar nerve enters the mandibular canal through the mandibular foramen and exits at the mental foramen supplying nerves to the lower cheek teeth in passing.

medullary c. 1. vertebral canal. 2. the cavity, containing marrow, in the diaphysis of a long bone; called also marrow or medullary cavity.

metatarsal c. formed by the metatarsal fascia on the plantar aspect of the chief metatarsal bone of the horse; transmits the tendons of the digital flexor muscles.

modiolar c. in the cochlea of the internal ear; it transmits blood vessels and nerves to the cochlea.

nasolacrimal c. in the maxilla it transmits the nasolacrimal duct.

nutrient c's large vascular canals through the cortex of bones. See also HAVERSIAN canal.

omasal c. the direct passage through the omasum from the reticulum to the abomasum.

optic c. a passage for the optic nerve through the cranium into the orbit.

palatine c. formed by the maxilla and the palatine bone; transmits the palatine artery and nerve.

pterygoid c. in the basisphenoid bone; contains the pterygoid nerve.

root c. see ROOT canal.

sacral c. the part of the vertebral canal through the sacrum.

Schlemm's c. the venous sinus of the sclera, a circular canal at the junction of the sclera and cornea that receives the aqueous humour. Called also scleral venous sinus.

semicircular c's the canals (anterior, lateral and posterior) of the bony labyrinth of the ear. See also SEMICIRCULAR canals.

spinal c., vertebral c. the canal formed by the series of vertebral foramina together, enclosing the spinal cord and meninges.

supraorbital c. in the frontal bone; transmits the frontal vein, passing through the zygomatic process to the orbital cavity.

tarsal c. formed by the plantar annular ligament of the tarsus which roofs over the tarsal groove; transmits the deep digital flexor tendon and plantar vessels.

triosseus c. the foramen at the junction of the coracoid, clavicle and scapula which transmits the tendon of a flight muscle, the supracoracoideus, in the avian skeleton.

vertebral c. spinal canal.

Volkmann's c's canals communicating with the haversian canals, for passage of blood vessels through bone from the periosteum.

canaliculus pl. *canaliculi* [L.] an extremely narrow tubular passage or channel.

bile c. fine tubular channels forming a three-dimensional network within the parenchyma of the liver. They join to form the bile ductules and eventually the hepatic duct.

bone c. branching tubular passages radiating like wheel spokes from each bone lacuna to connect with the canaliculi of adjacent lacunae, and with the haversian canal.

dentinal c. in the tooth dentine; converge towards the pulp of the tooth.

intracellular c. intracellular connection between apical plasmalemma and cytoplasm proper of the parietal cells in the gastric mucosa.

lacrimal c. the short passage in an eyelid, beginning

at the lacrimal point and draining tears from the lacrimal lake to the lacrimal sac; called also lacrimal duct. See also LACRIMAL apparatus.

mastoid c. a small channel in the temporal bone transmitting the tympanic branch of the vagus nerve.

secretory c. small canals in serous glandular epithelial cells connecting the cells with the luminal surface.

canalis pl. *canales* [L.] a canal or channel.

canalization 1. the formation of canals, natural or morbid. 2. the surgical establishment of canals for drainage.

canaloplasty plastic reconstruction of a passage, as of the external acoustic meatus.

canary see SERINUS *canaria*.

c. cholera see avian PSEUDOTUBERCULOSIS.

c. stain bright yellow stain in a wool fleece caused by bacterial growth. Not removable by usual industrial process.

canary cholera see avian PSEUDOTUBERCULOSIS.

canary grass PHALARIS *minor*, *P. canariensis*.

canarypox a disease caused by a poxvirus in the genus *Avipoxvirus*; it spreads slowly amongst canaries, finches and some other passerines. Characteristic pox lesions occur on eyelids, skin of the head, beak commissures and sometimes on the oral and pharyngeal mucosae. There is blepharitis and pruritus of the eyelids. Morbidity and mortality are very high.

Canavalia ensiformis a member of the plant family Fabaceae; seeds of this plant are used as stock feed but are toxic if fed in amounts in excess of 4% of the animal's body weight. Signs include diarrhea, stiffness and inability to eat or drink. Called also jack bean.

canavalin toxic amino acid in *Canavalia* spp.

canavanase see ARGINASE.

canavanine toxic amino acid in *Canavalia* spp.

cancellated having a lattice-like structure.

cancellous of a reticular, spongy or lattice-like structure; said mainly of bone tissue.

cancellus pl. *cancelli* [L.] the lattice-like structure in bone; any structure arranged like a lattice.

cancer any malignant, cellular tumor.

The term *cancer* encompasses a group of neoplastic diseases in which there is a transformation of normal body cells into malignant ones. This probably involves some change in the genetic material of the cells, deoxyribonucleic acid (DNA), perhaps as a result of faulty repair of damage to the cell caused by carcinogenic agents or ionizing radiation. The altered cells pass on inappropriate genetic information to their progeny cells and begin to proliferate in an abnormal and destructive way. Normally, the cells of which body tissues are made are regularly replaced by new growth, which stops when the cells are replaced; new cells form to repair tissue damage and stop forming when healing is complete. Why they stop forming is unknown, but clearly the body in its normal processes regulates cell growth. In cancer, cell growth is unregulated.

As the cancer cells continue to proliferate, the mass of abnormal tissue that they form enlarges, ulcerates, and begins to shed cells that spread the disease locally or to distant sites. This migration is called *metastasis*. Some cells invade neighboring tissues, destroying and displacing normal cells and taking their place. Others can enter the blood and lymphatic vessels and are carried along in the fluid to other parts of the body. Another way in which malignancy can be spread is by entering a body cavity by diffusion and coming in contact with a healthy organ.

See also TUMOR, NEOPLASM, NEOPLASIA. For individual cancers see under specific types. Cancers of specific organs or tissues are not listed.

cancer eye see ocular SQUAMOUS cell carcinoma.

canceremia the presence of cancer cells in the blood.

cancericidal destructive to cancer cells.

cancerigenic giving rise to a malignant tumor.

cancriform resembling cancer.

cancroid 1. cancer-like. 2. a skin cancer of a low grade of malignancy.

candela the SI unit of luminous intensity. Abbreviated cd.

candelabra tree EUPHORBIA *ingens*.

candicidin a fungicidal, fungistatic antibiotic derived from *Streptomyces griseus* with activity against *Candida albicans* and other fungal infections.

Candida a genus of yeast, commonly part of the normal flora of the mouth, skin, intestinal tract and vagina, but can cause a variety of diseases. Most infections are associated with predisposing factors, particularly immune suppression. Only *C. albicans* is commonly associated with disease. See also CANDIDIASIS.

C. albicans causes thrush in the mouth, crop, proventriculus and the gizzard of birds, and stomatitis, pneumonia and miscellaneous infections in other species. See CANDIDIASIS. Previously called *Monilia albicans*.

C. guilliermondii, C. krusei, C. pseudotropicalis, C. rugosa, C. tropicalis have been associated with mastitis in cattle.

C. parapsilosis associated with necrotizing placentitis and abortion in cattle.

candidamycosis see CANDIDIASIS.

candidate stem cell a stem cell in the hemopoietic system whose function is only assumed.

candidemia the presence in the blood of fungi of the genus *Candida*.

candidiasis, candidosis infection by fungi of the genus *Candida*, generally *C. albicans*. Three specific syndromes are recorded as being caused by *C. albicans*: (1) mycotic stomatitis of baby pigs which can spread to the lower alimentary tract and cause fatal enteritis; (2) chronic pneumonia in cattle in feedlots; (3) thrush-like lesions in the mouth of many species and esophagus, crop, proventriculus and gizzard of birds. Many other secondary infections occur, e.g. keratoconjunctivitis, stomatitis, bovine mastitis, esophagitis and ulcerative dermatitis in dogs. *Candida* is a common pathogen in immunosuppressed dogs or cats.

candidin a skin test antigen derived from *Candida albicans*, used in testing for the development of delayed-type hypersensitivity to the microorganism. Little used in veterinary medicine.

candidosis see CANDIDIASIS.

candiduria the presence of *Candida* organisms in the urine.

candle nut tree ALEURITES *moluccana*.

candling said of eggs; holding a hen's egg up to a lighted candle in a darkened room to detect a developing embryo.

candyup poison STYPANDRA GLAUCA.

cane toad see BUFO.

canecutter's disease see LEPTOSPIROSIS.

canicola fever canine LEPTOSPIROSIS due to *Leptospira canicola*.

Canidae a family which includes 14 genera; the two commonest are the dogs (*Canis* spp.) and the foxes (*Vulpes* spp.). Includes exotic Canidae, e.g. dingo.

canine 1. pertaining to or characteristic of dogs. 2. pertaining to a canine tooth (cuspid). See also TEETH, DOG.

c. acidophil-cell hepatitis an acute or chronic hepatitis reported in dogs in Great Britain, distinct from that caused by infectious canine hepatitis virus, characterized by the histopathologic presence of acidophil cells. Chronic active hepatitis and sometimes hepatocellular carcinoma may occur. The cause is unknown, but a viral etiology is suspected.

c. adenovirus type 1 (CAV-1) causes infectious canine HEPATITIS; type 2 (CAV-2) is one cause of canine respiratory disease complex (KENNEL COUGH).

c. babesiosis hemolytic disease of dogs caused by *Babesia canis* or *B. gibsoni*, transmitted by a tick, and characterized by anemia and hemoglobinuria. Called also tick fever, malignant jaundice.

c. erythrocyte antigen (CEA) nomenclature revised to dog erythrocyte ANTIGEN (DEA).

c. gastrointestinal hemorrhage syndrome see canine hemorrhagic GASTROENTERITIS.

c. herpesvirus infection a cause of a generalized, acute, rapidly fatal disease in neonatal puppies. In puppies older than 3 weeks and adults, mild to inapparent upper respiratory disease or vesicular genital lesions occur. The difference in age susceptibility is attributed to the temperature-dependent growth characteristics of the virus in that the optimum temperature for viral replication is about 91°F (33°C) so that puppies that are hypothermic develop severe, often fatal disease. Recovered puppies or dogs may have persistence of the virus in the genital or respiratory tracts.

c. hip dysplasia see HIP dysplasia.

c. hypertrophic osteodystrophy see hypertrophic OSTEODYSTROPHY.

c. hypoxic rhabdomyolysis see EXERTIONAL rhabdomyolysis.

infectious c. hepatitis see infectious canine HEPATITIS.

c. juvenile cellulitis see juvenile PYODERMA.

c. juvenile osteodystrophy see nutritional secondary HYPERPARATHYROIDISM.

c. laryngotracheitis see KENNEL COUGH.

c. nasal mites see PNEUMONYSSUS *caninum*.

c. papillomatosis see canine viral PAPILLOMATOSIS.

c. respiratory disease see canine DISTEMPER, KENNEL COUGH.

c. rickettsiosis see canine EHRLICHIOSIS.

c. secretory alloantigen see canine secretory ALLOANTIGEN system.

c. tracheobronchitis see KENNEL COUGH.

c. tropical pancytopenia see canine EHRLICHIOSIS.

c. venereal tumor see canine transmissible VENEREAL tumor.

c. viral hepatitis see infectious canine HEPATITIS.

c. viral papillomatosis see canine viral PAPILLOMATOSIS.

canine chorea see MYOCLONUS.

canine tooth see canine TEETH.

Canis a genus in the animal family Canidae. Includes the domestic dog (*C. familiaris*), wolf (*C. lupus*), red wolf (*Canis rufus*), Oriental jackal (*C. aureus*), coyote (*C. latrans*), dingo (*C. antarcticus* syn. *C. dingo*).

canities grayness of the hair.

canker ulceration, especially (1) of the lip or oral mucosa; (2) in horses of the horn of the sole of the foot; (3) often used erroneously to describe otitis externa.

avian c. disease of birds caused by *Trichomonas gallinae* and characterized by accumulations of caseous material in the throat.

ear c. see EAR canker.

equine c. chronic hypertrophy and necrosis of the horn-producing tissues of the horse's foot, usually a hindfoot. The horn is shed or easily removed from a swollen and necrotic corium. There is lameness and a penetrating foul odor.

lapine c. inflammation of the ears of rabbits caused by the mites *Psoroptes communis* or *Chorioptes cuniculi.* The ear canal is filled with an accumulation of serum and sebaceous material.

cannabidiol a physiologically inactive principle from *Cannabis*; its tetrahydro derivatives are active. Has been used as an anticonvulsant.

cannabinoid any of the active principles of *Cannabis*, including tetrahydrocannabinol, cannabinol and cannabidiol.

cannabis the dried flowering tops of CANNABIS SATIVA plants which have euphoric principles (tetrahydrocannabinols) and alkaloids (cannabinoids); grown commercially for the production of cannabis; classified as a hallucinogen and prepared as bhang, ganja, hashish and marihuana. It has excellent activity as a hypnotic and analgesic, especially in horses, but narcotic control regulations severely restrict use. Called also Indian hemp.

c. poisoning dogs show incoordination, alternating somnolence and hyperactivity, salivation and muscular weakness.

Cannabis sativa plant member of family Cannabidaceae; called also Indian hemp, hemp, 'grass'.

canned food food sterilized by heat in a closed, durable container such as tin and aluminum cans, flexible aluminum foil and thermoplastic containers including squeeze tubes. Technically, the processes used are highly efficient and used universally. Problems occur rarely but their identification is an important part of food hygiene. The problems arise either with the sterilization of the container or its contents, or because the container leaks after closure, permitting infection to occur. If the contained material contains toxins when it is first added to the can they will still be there when the can is opened.

cannibalism the eating of flesh of living members of the same or similar species. It is common only in pigs and chickens and is due partly to boredom because of the confined space in which the animals are kept. See also INFANTOPHAGIA.

cannon atrial waves, cannon A waves waves seen occasionally in the jugular vein of an animal with severe cardiac arrhythmia. When the atria and ventricles contract simultaneously a very large pressure wave runs up the vein.

cannon bone the 3rd metacarpal (metatarsal) of the horse, or the 3rd and 4th metacarpals (metatarsals) of ruminants.

cannon keratosis bilateral areas of alopecia, scaling and crusting on the anterior surface of the hind cannons. A persistent lesion in mares and stallions. Called also stud crud.

cannula a tube for insertion into a duct or cavity; during insertion its lumen may be occupied by a trocar.

nasal c. a means of delivering oxygen to dogs or cats over a long period.

cannulate to introduce a cannula, which may be left in place.

cannulation introduction of a cannula into a tubelike organ or body cavity.

umbilical vein c. a technique used especially for neonatal collapsed primates which need long-term fluid therapy.

canola see BRASSICA *napus*.

Canpak system continuous, conveyorized system of

line-slaughtering for use in a modern abattoir developed by Canada Packers in Toronto.

canter a gallop at an easy pace. The rhythm is three-time, first one hind, then the opposite hind with the diagonal fore, then the opposite fore, the leading limb.

collected c. the same action as a canter or gallop but at a very slow pace usually with the head carried high, with almost exaggerated movements but little forward progress, ideal for the showring.

canthal ligament bands of fibrous tissue at the corners of the eye which bind the eyelids to the skull; deficient function at the lateral canthal ligament in St. Bernard, English bulldog or Cocker spaniel causes combined ectropion at the central lid and entropion at the lateral canthus; repaired by use of a prosthetic ligament.

cantharides substance obtained from dried beetles (*Cantharis vesicatoria*) and used topically as a counterirritant. African cattle have been poisoned by drinking water contaminated by flies. They show excitement, diarrhea and nephritis. Called also blistering beetle, Spanish fly.

cantharidin the most active principle of CANTHARIDES with similar activity. Preparations containing cantharidin are used topically as a vesicant to remove warts and were popular at one time as rubefacients for horses.

Cantharis vesicatoria the source of commercial cantharides. Called also Spanish fly, *Lytta vesicatoria.*

canthaxanthin a carotenoid used as a coloring agent; also administered orally in humans to produce artificial suntan, and to canaries carrying the RED FACTOR to produce a stronger red color.

canthectomy excision of a canthus.

canthi see CANTHUS.

canthitis inflammation of a canthus.

Canthium vaccinifolium a toxic plant of the family Rubiaceae; causes cyanide poisoning.

cantholysis surgical section of a canthus or a canthal ligament.

canthoplasty plastic surgery of a canthus.

canthorrhaphy the suturing of the palpebral fissure at either canthus.

canthotomy incision of a canthus.

canthus pl. *canthi;* the angular junction of the eyelids at either corner of the eyes, the angles of the palpebral fissure, the medial and lateral canthi.

medial c. the medial angle formed by the eyelids.

recessed medial c. syndrome in many brachycephalic breeds, a deeply recessed medial canthus leads to medial entropion.

cantle the back-most part of the saddle seat; the place to grasp when mounting.

Cantonese pig black and white, meat and lard pig.

canudo IPOMOEA *fistulosa.*

canvassing making personal representation to individual persons to solicit their custom. Usually used in a political sense but also used in the sense of TOUTING for professional patronage, considered to be an unethical practice in most countries.

CAP 1. chloroacetophenone; a gas used for riot control in humans. Causes weeping, the so-called tear-gas. Animals exposed to this lacrimator will also be affected. 2. catabolite gene activator protein.

cap 1. the top, to top. 2. an oval or thumb-nail shaped area of light-colored feathers covering the crown of lizard canaries.

dental c. 1. residual deciduous teeth sitting on top of erupting permanent teeth. 2. a crown prosthesis.

dental c. stage the earliest stage in the development of the tooth, in the form of a tooth bud growing out of the primitive dental lamina.

spermatozoal c. invests the head of the spermatozoa. Called also acrosomal cap, head cap.

CAP binding protein *c*atabolite *a*ctivator *p*rotein, a regulatory protein in the switch from glucose to lactose metabolism in *Escherichia coli* that binds to the same sequence recognition site, located immediately in front of the *lac* operator sequence, as RNA polymerase.

cap-Chur one of the original capture darts which inject medicament explosively and are retained in tissue by a barbed needle; have the difficulty of failure to recover the dart.

cap structures of RNA a distinctive formation at the 5′ terminus of mRNA, consisting of an inverted methylated base attached via 5′-phosphate-5′-phosphate bonds rather than the usual internucleotide 3′,5′-phosphodiester linkages between adjacent riboses.

capacitance 1. the property of being able to store an electric charge. 2. the ratio of charge to potential in a conductor.

capacitation the physiological changes the spermatozoa must undergo in the female tract or in vitro before being capable of penetrating the ovum.

capacitor a device for holding and storing charges of electricity.

capacity the power to hold, retain, or contain, or the ability to absorb; usually expressed numerically as the measure of such ability.

carrying c. see CARRYING CAPACITY.

closing c. (CC) the volume of gas in the lungs at the time of airway closure. See also CLOSING VOLUME.

forced vital c. the maximal volume of gas that can be exhaled from full inspiration exhaling as forcefully and rapidly as possible. See also PULMONARY function tests.

functional residual c. the amount of gas remaining at the end of normal quiet respiration.

heat c. thermal capacity.

inspiratory c. the volume of gas that can be taken into the lungs in a full inspiration, starting from the resting inspiratory position; equal to the tidal volume plus the inspiratory reserve volume.

maximal breathing c. maximal voluntary ventilation.

thermal c. the amount of heat absorbed by a body in being raised 1°C.

total lung c. the amount of gas contained in the lung at the end of a maximal inspiration.

virus neutralizing c. the ability of a serum to inhibit the infectivity of a virus.

vital c. the volume of gas that can be expelled from the lungs from a position of full inspiration, with no limit to duration of expiration; equal to inspiratory capacity plus expiratory reserve volume.

Caparsolate a proprietary name for THIACETARSAMIDE SODIUM.

Cape Barren goose large gray and white Australian goose; *Cereopsis novaehollandiae.*

Cape honey flower MELIANTHUS *comosus.*

Cape hyacinth see LIDNERIA CLAVATA.

Cape khaki weed see DITTRICHIA GRAVEOLENS.

Cape lilac MELIA *azederach.*

Cape poison onion see ORNITHOGLOSSUM VIRIDE.

Cape slangkop see ORNITHOGLOSSUM VIRIDE.

Cape spinach see EMEX AUSTRALIS.

Cape tulip see HOMERIA.

caper spurge EUPHORBIA *lathyrus.*

capeweed see ARCTOTHECA CALENDULA.

capillarectasia dilatation of capillaries.

Capillaria a genus of parasitic nematodes of the subfamily Capillariinae and most commonly parasitic in birds. They cause capillariasis.

Those found in birds include *C. anatis*, *C. annulata* (*C. contorta*), *C. caudinflata*, *C. obsignata*.

Those found in mammals include *C. aerophila*, *C. bilobata*, *C. bovis*, *C. brevipes*, *C. didelphis*, *C. entomelas*, *C. erinacea*, *C. feliscati* (in cats), *C. hepatica*, *C. megrelica*, *C. mucronata*, *C. philippinensis*, *C. plica*, *C. putorii*.

There are others which occur in small rodents and in fish.

capillariasis infection with nematodes of the genus *Capillaria*. In birds the disease is manifested by chronic gastroenteritis and the affected birds are emaciated. The disease in mammals may be enteritis with diarrhea (*C. bovis*, *C. entomelas*), cystitis (*C. felis cati*, *C. plica*), hepatitis (*C. hepatica*) or bronchopneumonia (*C. aerophila*, *C. didelphis*).

capillarid a member of the family Capillariidae.

capillariomotor pertaining to the functional activity of the capillaries.

capillaritis inflammation of the capillaries.

capillarity the action by which the surface of a liquid where it is in contact with a solid, as in a capillary tube, is elevated or depressed.

capillary 1. pertaining to or resembling a hair. 2. one of the minute vessels connecting arterioles and venules, the walls of which act as a membrane for interchange of various substances between the blood and tissue fluid. (See CIRCULATORY system.) The walls consist of thin endothelial cells through which dissolved substances and fluids can pass. At the arterial end, the blood pressure within the capillary is generally higher than the pressure in the surrounding tissues, and the blood fluid and some dissolved solid substances pass outward through the capillary wall. At the venous end of the capillary, the pressure within the tissues is generally higher, and waste material and fluids from the tissues pass into the capillary, to be carried away for disposal. See STARLING'S HYPOTHESIS.

continuous c. a capillary with no pores or other interruptions in the endothelial walls, e.g. in muscle, lung, nervous system.

fenestrated c's capillaries with pores are scattered throughout the endothelial walls, e.g. in endocrine glands, intestines, kidneys.

c. fragility see capillary FRAGILITY.

lymph c. the smallest lymphatic vessel. Consist of an endothelial tube embedded in connective tissue.

perforated c. see fenestrated CAPILLARY (above).

c. permeability ability of large molecules to pass out of the capillary lumen into surrounding tissue spaces; inflammation, allergy, poisoning, burns cause increased permeability resulting in plasma leakage and edema in surrounding tissues.

c. refill time (CRT) the time required for mucosa (oral in horse or dog, vaginal in cow, sheep) which has been blanched by finger pressure to return to a normal pink color. Failure to return promptly is an indication of peripheral circulatory failure, due for example to dehydration or hypovolemic shock.

sinus c's part of the vasculature of avian skin. Occur together with standard capillaries but they are larger in diameter and may have some smooth muscle cells associated with the endothelial cells.

sinusoidal c's large and irregularly shaped; occur in endocrine glands, aortic and carotid bodies.

capillus pl. *capilli* [L.] a hair; used in the plural to designate an aggregation of hairs.

capital 1. items which are not consumed in a business such as a farm. Includes land, money, nondisposable equipment and fixed improvements. 2. pertaining to the head.

c. femoral epiphysis epiphysis of the head of the femur; its detachment represents a specific syndrome in pigs.

fixed c. nonconsumables that cannot be removed, e.g. buildings, water supply system, fencing and land. Called also fixed improvements.

c. gains the increase in cash value of fixed capital items due to an increase in their new market price.

c. investment money invested in fixed capital items, generally accepted as having a useful life of greater than one year, and which contributes to the profitability of an enterprise such as a farm.

working c. capital required for the everyday operation of a farm or any other business enterprise.

capitation the annual fee paid to a professional person of any sort as payment for providing services on a continuous basis. The fee paid is based on the number of animal participants in the scheme—the capitation fee.

capitular pertaining to a capitulum or the head of a bone.

capitulum pl. *capitula* [L.] a small eminence on a bone, as on the distal end of the humerus, by which it articulates with another bone.

c. humeri the small articular part of the lateral distal end of the humerus that articulates with the radius.

vertebral c. one of the articular prominences at the vertebral end of a rib.

capn- prefix meaning carbon dioxide.

Capnocytophaga a genus of small anaerobic, gram-negative, rod-shaped bacteria that are commensals of the mouth and nasopharynx of dogs and cats and have been implicated in septicemia, meningitis, endocarditis and have been isolated from dog and cat bite wounds in humans; they closely resemble *Bacteroides ochraceus*. Formerly called DF-2 and DF-2-like.

capnogram 1. a radiograph of the abdominal cavity taken with negative contrast in the perioneal cavity. See also PNEUMOPERITONEUM. 2. continuous measurement of carbon dioxide concentrations in the exhaled air especially of anesthetized animals.

capnography the technique of taking capnograms.

capon castrated male fowl, larger than broiler, weighing up to 7 lb; produced either by administration of estrogenic substances or by surgical excision of the testicles.

caponization technique of creating a capon.

caponizing castration by surgical removal of testicles through a surgical incision behind the last rib of a male bird; chemical castration is also practiced, usually by the implantation of a pellet containing stilbestrol or hexestrol.

capotement [Fr.] a splashing sound heard in dilatation of the stomach.

Capparis tomentosa African plant in the family Capparidaceae; contains an unidentified hepatoxin; causes hepatic insufficiency, jaundice, photosensitization and encephalopathy. Called also hekkabit, gulum.

capped elbow see elbow HYGROMA.

capped hock see hock HYGROMA.

cappie see DOUBLE scalp.

capping the provision of a protective or obstructive covering.

c. phenomenon the movement of anitibody-induced clustering of plasma membrane molecules (patching) to a single pole of the cell.

pulp c. the covering of an exposed dental pulp with some material to provide protection against external influences and to encourage healing.

Capra genus of wild goats and ibexes, e.g. *C. falconeri* (markhor) and *C. ibex* (Alpine ibex).

Capreolus capreolus see ROE DEER.

capreomycin sulfate a polypeptide antibiotic produced by *Streptomyces capreolus*, which is active against human strains of *Mycobacterium tuberculosis* and sometimes considered for the treatment of mycobacterial infections in animals.

capric acid, *n*-capric acid a 10-carbon fatty acid that occurs in butter. Called also decanoic acid.

caprine pertaining to or emanating from goats.

c. arthritis–encephalitis a multisystem disease of goats involving synovial lined connective tissue, caused by a a member of the family *Retroviridae*, subfamily *Lentivirinae*. It causes chronic arthritis in adults and leukoencephalomyelitis, characterized by ataxia, proprioceptive loss and paralysis, in young kids. There is also a clinically inapparent interstitial pneumonia. Called also big knee, caprine leukoencephalomyelitis.

c. encephalomyelitis see CAPRINE arthritis–encephalitis.

c. enzootic nasal granuloma infectious disease of goats and sheep caused by a retrovirus; characterized clinically by sero-mucoid nasal discharge, cough, dyspnea, stertor, emaciation, death; enzootic in the flock.

c. herpesvirus the cause of caprine LEUKOENCEPHALOMYELITIS.

c. idiopathic dermatitis alopecic, exudative dermatitis of pygmy goats of all ages affecting head, perineum, ventral abdomen.

caprinized vaccine see caprinized VACCINE.

Capripoxvirus a genus of viruses in the family *Poxviridae*.

caproate any salt or ester of caproic acid (hexanoic acid).

caprolactum see VETAFIL.

Capromyces see MYCOPLASMA.

caprylic acid a fatty acid used in the local treatment of fungal infections.

capsalid fluke see NEOBENEDINIA.

capsid the shell of protein that protects the nucleic acid of a virus; it is composed of individual morphological units called capsomers. For icosahedral viruses, there are two kinds of capsomers called pentamers, which occupy the 12 corner positions of the icosahedral shell, and hexamers, which occupy the face and edges. The number of hexamers varies between different viruses. The capsomers of helical viruses are composed of a single polypeptide and are also called protomers. All viruses of animals, except for poxviruses which have a complex structure, are minimally composed of a nucleocapsid which is the capsid surrounding the nucleic acid. In addition some viruses have an envelope surrounding the nucleocapsid.

capsitis inflammation of the capsule of the crystalline lens.

capsomer, capsomere a morphological unit of the capsid of a virus.

capsula pl. *capsulae* [L.] capsule.

capsular plexus terminal branches of the renal interlobular arteries which continue to the surface and terminate beneath the capsule of the kidney in the form of a plexus.

capsulation enclosure in a capsule.

capsule 1. an enclosing structure, as a soluble container enclosing a dose of medicine. 2. a cartilaginous, fatty, fibrous or membranous structure enveloping another structure, organ or part.

adipose renal c. the investment of fat surrounding the fibrous capsule of the kidney, continuous at the hilus with the fat in the renal sinus.

articular c. the saclike envelope that encloses the cavity of a synovial joint by attaching to the circumference of the articular end of each involved bone.

bacterial c. a gelatinous layer of polysaccharide surrounding a bacterial cell, usually polysaccharide but sometimes polypeptide in nature; it inhibits phagocytosis and is associated with the virulence of pathogenic bacteria.

Bowman's c. glomerular capsule.

brain c's two layers of white matter in the substance of the brain. See also external capsule (below) and internal capsule (below).

external c. the layer of white fibers between the putamen and claustrum.

fibrous renal c. the connective tissue investment of the kidney, which continues through the hilus to line the renal sinus.

Glisson's c. a sheath of connective tissue accompanying the hepatic ducts and vessels within the liver.

glomerular c. the globular dilatation forming the beginning of a uriniferous tubule within the kidney, and surrounding the glomerulus. Called also Bowman's capsule and malpighian capsule.

heart c. pericardium.

internal c. the fanlike mass of white fibers separating the lentiform nucleus laterally from the head of the caudate nucleus, the dorsal thalamus, and the tail of the caudate nucleus medially.

joint c. articular capsule.

lens c. the elastic sac enclosing the lens of the eye.

malpighian c. see glomerular capsule (above).

Tenon's c. the connective tissue enveloping the posterior eyeball. Called also vagina bulbi.

capsulectomy excision of a capsule, especially a joint capsule or lens capsule.

capsulitis inflammation of a capsule, as that of the lens.

capsulolenticular pertaining to the lens of the eye and its capsule.

capsuloma a capsular or subcapsular tumor of the kidney.

capsuloplasty plastic repair of a joint capsule.

capsulorrhaphy suture of a joint capsule.

capsulotomy incision of a capsule, as that of the lens or of a joint.

captan group of organic sulfur compounds used as fungicides, including topical treatment of dermatophytosis. Poisoning of birds causes loss of egg production, anorexia and slow growth.

captive said of naturally wild or feral animals kept in captivity for educational and scientific investigation with no attempt being made to domesticate them.

captive bolt pistol a handheld weapon used for euthanasia of large animals. The muzzle is placed against the subject's forehead. When the trigger is pulled, or the firing pin struck a sharp blow, a 3 cm rod, 1 cm diameter exits sharply from the muzzle and pierces the skull and damages the brain. The rod does not leave the weapon and there is no possible risk of injuring a bystander.

captive breeding mating programs designed for use with animals kept in captivity. See also hand MATING.

captopril an angiotensin-converting enzyme (ACE) inhibitor used as a vasodilator in the treatment of congestive heart failure, mitral regurgitation and hypertension. Now aften replaced by newer ACE inhibitors such as enalapril, lisinopril.

capture the snaring and restraint of an escaped domesticated animal or a feral animal. It requires safety for the captor and the subject. Includes physical means of trap cages, the thrown lariat, a handheld net for small companion animals. Thrownets for birds are still favored by lay persons. Veterinarians are more inclined to use immobilizing agents delivered by darts from bows and arrows or from dart guns. See also RESTRAINT.

c.-mark-release-recapture technique for establishing the nature of animal movements and the size of populations.

c. shock syndrome in recently captured animals with death 1–6 hours after capture. Signs include shallow, rapid respiration, tachycardia, physical collapse, hyperthermia, small pulse, elevated CPK levels, general vascular congestion at necropsy.

c. stress syndrome STRESS syndrome in wild animals in captivity.

capture myopathy see EXERTIONAL rhabdomyolysis.

capture–recapture method a method of estimating the prevalence of a condition in a population. Initially used in populations of wild animals, which were captured, marked, released and recaptured, but the same statistical process is now used in other types of population.

capuchin monkey one of the New World monkeys used commonly as a laboratory primate. Gregarious, arboreal and diurnal, they are popular pets and weigh up to 10 lb. Called also *Cebus* spp., ringtail or organ-grinder monkey.

caput pl. *capita;* the head; a general term applied to the expanded or chief extremity of an organ or part.

c. mallei head of the malleus in the middle ear.

c. mandibulae the head of the mandible that articulates with the squamous part of the temporal bone.

c. stapedis the head of the stapes in the middle ear.

capybara the largest rodent, the size of a small pig, 100 lb and 3 ft tall. It is largely aquatic and easily domesticated. Called also carpincho, *Hydrochoerus hydrochaeris*.

CAR congenital articular rigidity.

car exhaust fumes see CARBON MONOXIDE poisoning, LEAD[1] poisoning.

car sickness see MOTION SICKNESS.

carabao see BUBALUS BUBALIS.

caracal long-legged desert cat, related to the lynx; fawn color with black tips; *Caracal caracal.*

caracara a group of predatory birds in the family Falconidae that are characterized by long legs and reddish skin on the cheeks and throat. Called also carrion hawks. The common caracara, *Polyborus plancus*, is found in North and South America.

caracul see KARAKUL.

caramiphen ethanedisulfonate an anticholinergic and antitussive, also used in respiratory disease and the treatment of organophosphorus poisoning.

carapace the dorsal shell of turtles and tortoises. Abnormalities are caused by trauma, dietary deficiencies (particularly nutritional hyperparathyroidism), infections, environmental factors and tumors.

Carassius auratus see GOLDFISH.

Carassius carassius farmed finfish in family Cyprinidae; called also crucian carp. See Table 23.

carazolol a β-blocker administered at the beginning of parturition in sows to hasten delivery, shorten parturition and reduce prevalence of mastitis–metritis–agalactia.

carbachol a potent choline ester with muscarinic and nicotinic effects including defecation, slowing of the heart, urination and respiratory restriction due to bronchiolar constriction.

carbadox a substituted quinoxaline antibiotic used as feed additive in the prevention of swine dysentery and growth promotant, subject to regulations on drug withdrawal periods.

carbamates effective insecticides which exert their effect by temporarily inhibiting cholinesterase activity. They are also capable of poisoning. Clinical signs are pupillary constriction, muscle tremor, salivation, ataxia and dyspnea.

carbamazepine an anticonvulsant and analgesic used in the treatment of pain and for control of partial or generalized tonic–clonic seizures, often in combination with other drugs.

carbamide urea in anhydrous, lyophilized, sterile powder form; injected intravenously in dextrose or invert sugar solution to induce an osmotic diuresis in the treatment of cerebral edema and glaucoma. Now largely superseded by more effective agents.

c. peroxide urea hydrogen peroxide; a ceruminolytic agent used in cleaning ear canals.

carbaminohemoglobin a combination of carbon dioxide and hemoglobin, CO_2HHb, being one of the forms in which carbon dioxide exists in the blood.

carbamoyl the radical NH_2–CO–.

c. phosphate synthetases enzymes catalyzing the synthesis of carbamoyl phosphate. Carbamoyl-phosphate synthetase I is the starting enzyme of the urea cycle. Carbamoyl-phosphate synthetase II is the starting enzyme of pyrimidine synthesis.

carbamoyltransferase see ornithine carbamoyl TRANSFERASE.

carbamylcholine chloride see CARBACHOL.

carbamylmethylcholine see BETHANECHOL.

carbanilides drugs, e.g. imidocarb, with therapeutic efficiency against *Babesia* spp.

carbapenems β-lactam resistant antibiotics, including IMIPENEM and meropenem, which are effective against a wide range of bacteria.

carbarsone an arsenical compound once used as a feed additive for the prevention of histomoniasis in chickens and turkeys.

carbaryl carbamate insecticide used widely in companion animals to control ectoparasites.

carbaspirin calcium, carbasalate calcium an analgesic and antipyretic, metabolized to aspirin with similar effects.

carbenicillin an extended-spectrum penicillin, prepared as both the disodium and the potassium salt, particularly effective against gram-negative bacteria, including some strains of *Pseudomonas aeruginosa* and *Proteus* spp. Carbenicillin indanyl is suitable for oral administration.

carbimazole an antithyroid drug, metabolized to METHIMAZOLE; used in the treatment of feline hyperthyroidism.

carbofuran a carbamate acaricide and nematocide.

carbohydrase any of a group of enzymes that catalyze the hydrolysis of higher carbohydrates to lower forms.

carbohydrate a compound of carbon, hydrogen and oxygen, the latter two usually in the proportions of water $(CH_2O)_n$. They are classified into mono-, di-, tri-, poly- and heterosaccharides. Carbohydrates in food are an important and immediate source of energy for the body; 1 gram of carbohydrate yields 3.75 calories (16 kilojoules). They are present, at least in small quantities, in most foods, but the chief sources are the sugars and starches of plants. Herbivores are able to utilize the insoluble polysaccharides (crude fiber) because of bacterial conversion to volatile fatty acids by fermentation in the rumen and cecum.

Carbohydrates may be stored in the body as glycogen for future use. If they are eaten in excessive amounts they are converted to and stored as fat. Rapid ingestion of very large amounts in ruminants and horses causes CARBOHYDRATE ENGORGEMENT.

complex c. polysaccharides containing either α- and β-type glycosidic bonds. Usually occurring in mixtures in food.

dietary c. the carbohydrate components of food.

c. loading depletion/repletion means of maximally loading glycogen into type II muscle for increased power of muscle contraction.

c. loss glucose loss in urine due to diabetes mellitus or chronic renal disease.

c. metabolism series of related enzymic reactions involved in the synthesis and catabolism of carbohydrates.

c. tolerance test see GLUCOSE tolerance test.

carbohydrate engorgement engorgement by ruminants and horses on carbohydrate-rich food which results in fermentation in the rumen, or stomach in the case of horses, with the production of large amounts of lactic acid. Absorption of the acid results in the development of a lactic acidemia. Retention in the alimentary tract causes osmotic withdrawal of fluid from the body tissues and severe dehydration. The resulting clinical syndrome includes abdominal enlargement, hypovolemic shock, ruminal stasis, severe toxemia, weakness, recumbency and a very high mortality rate. The pH of the ruminal contents is usually less than 5. Absorption causes severe systemic acidosis. Horses also suffer dehydration and lactic acidosis after engorgement on grain. Laminitis is an additional sequel. Called also grain engorgement, rumen overload, maize crop engorgement, grape engorgement.

carbohydraturia excess of carbohydrates in the urine.

carbolic acid the common or trivial name for PHENOL a caustic poison obtained by distillation of coal tar or produced synthetically; used as an antiseptic and disinfectant, e.g. in some of the early cattle and sheep dips.

carbolic dip see CARBOLIC ACID.

carbolineum a disinfectant used as a spray for poultry houses. Excessive use causes damage and irritation to the wattles and comb, and acute hepatic inefficiency.

carbolism PHENOL (carbolic acid) poisoning.

carbomycin a macrolide antibiotic used as a feed additive and growth promotant.

carbon a chemical element, atomic number 6, atomic weight 12.011, symbol C. See Table 6.

asymmetric c. atom one bonded to four different atoms. See also ISOMER.

c. fiber made by the pyrolization of polymer fibers at very high temperatures and used in various forms as soft tissue implants, particularly in tendon and ligament repair.

c. fixation see dark REACTION.

carbon dioxide an odorless, colorless gas, CO_2, resulting from oxidation of carbons, formed in the tissues and eliminated by the lungs; used with oxygen to stimulate respiration and in solid form (carbon dioxide snow—see below) as an escharotic, as a gas to euthanize laboratory rabbits and rodents.

c. d. anesthesia exposure of pigs for 45 seconds in a mixture of 60 to 70% CO_2 in air is an adequate preslaughter anesthetic for pigs.

c. d. combining power the ability of blood plasma to combine with carbon dioxide; indicative of the alkali reserve and a measure of the acid–base balance of the blood.

c. d. content the amount of carbonic acid and bicarbonate in the blood; reported in millimoles per liter.

c. d. dissociation curve a graph demonstrating the relationship between the blood content of CO_2 and the $P\text{CO}_2$.

c. d. narcosis respiratory acidosis.

c. d. snow solid carbon dioxide, formed by rapid evaporation of liquid carbon dioxide; it gives a temperature of about −110°F (−79°C), and is used as an escharotic in various skin diseases. Called also dry ice.

c. d. tension the partial pressure of carbon dioxide in the blood; noted as $P\text{CO}_2$ in BLOOD GAS ANALYSIS. See also RESPIRATION.

c. d. transport carbon dioxide passes from tissues to blood by diffusion, in the blood by solution and via reactions within plasma and erythrocytes, from blood to pulmonary alveoli by diffusion.

carbon dioxide–bicarbonate buffer system major body buffering system for acid–base balance.

carbon dioxide–oxygen therapy administration of a mixture of carbon dioxide and oxygen (commonly 5% CO_2 and 95% O_2, or 10% CO_2 and 90% O_2); used for improvement of cerebral blood flow or stimulation of deep breathing. Carbon dioxide acts by stimulating the respiratory center; it also increases heart rate and blood pressure.

carbon disulfide an inflammable, volatile liquid used for treatment of bot fly larvae in the stomach of horses. Administered by stomach tube. Mixed with air it is dangerously explosive. Excess doses cause excitement, weakness and collapse.

carbon fiber implants implants used to strengthen tendons damaged due to sprain or transection. The implantation is done surgically.

carbon monoxide a colorless, odorless, tasteless gas, CO, formed by burning carbon or organic fuels with a scanty supply of oxygen; inhalation causes central nervous system damage and asphyxiation. Carbon monoxide is present in the exhaust of petrol engines, in the smoke of wood and coal fires, in manufactured gas such as that used in the household, and wherever carbon burns without a sufficient supply of oxygen. Used as a euthanizing agent for dogs and laboratory animals.

c. m. poisoning poisoning by carbon monoxide; one of the most common types of gas poisoning. When carbon monoxide is inhaled, it comes in contact with the blood and combines with hemoglobin. Since carbon monoxide combines more readily with hemoglobin than does oxygen, it takes the place of oxygen in the erythrocytes, and the tissues are thus deprived of their normal oxygen supply. Death from asphyxia results if a large enough quantity of carbon monoxide is inhaled. Because death is very sudden, carbon monoxide has been used as a euthanatizing agent for dogs in large numbers. It is not widely used because of the danger to human attendants and the difficulty in maintaining a CO generator in good condition for long periods.

carbon tetrachloride a clear, colorless, mobile liquid; the inhalation of its vapors can depress central nervous system activity and cause degeneration of the liver and kidneys. It has now been replaced as a fasciolicide so that poisoning by it is not as common as it used to be. It is a potent hepatoxin especially in sheep, in which it can cause serious losses at dose rates which on most occasions are innocuous, and in cattle when it is administered by mouth instead of by injection.

carbonate a salt of carbonic acid.

c. calculi see carbonate UROLITH.

carbonic acid aqueous solution of carbon dioxide, H_2CO_3.

c. a. anhydrase see CARBONIC ANHYDRASE.

carbonic anhydrase an enzyme which catalyzes the reversible conversion of carbon dioxide to bicarbonate ions and thus facilitates the transport and elimination of carbon dioxide from tissues. The enzyme is also important in making adequate calcium available for the deposition of shells on birds' eggs.

c. a. inhibitor diuretics diuretics such as acetazolamide exert their effect on tubular resorption in the kidney by inhibiting carbonic anhydrase. These compounds are used preferentially for the treatment of chronic glaucoma because the formation of aqueous humor is highly dependent on carbonic anhydrase.

carbonuria the presence in the urine of carbon dioxide or other carbon compounds.

carbonyl the bivalent organic radical, C=O or C:O, characteristic of aldehydes, ketones, carboxylic acid and esters.

carbophenothion an organophosphorus insecticide used on plants and animals; it is effective but has the usual potential toxicity of this group. In some countries, its use is not permitted on food producing animals.

carboplatin a cisplatin analog, but with fewer side-effects. Under investigation in the treatment of cancer in dogs. Myelosuppression limits the dose that can be used.

γ-carboxy glutamic acid-containing protein one of the proteins found in bone.

carboxy-lyase any of a group of lyases that catalyze the removal of a carboxyl group; it includes the carboxylases and decarboxylases.

carboxyatractyloside hepatic toxin in the cotyledons of XANTHIUM *pungens* and in *Cestrum, Wedelia* spp.

carboxyhemoglobin hemoglobin combined with carbon monoxide, which occupies the sites on the hemoglobin molecule that normally bind with oxygen and which is not readily displaced from the molecule; exposure to carbon monoxide thus results in cellular anoxia. See also HEMOGLOBIN.

carboxyhemoglobinemia excessive concentrations of carbon monoxide in the blood.

carboxyl the monovalent radical, –COOH, found in those organic acids termed carboxylic acids.

carboxylase an enzyme that catalyzes the removal of carbon dioxide from the carboxyl group of alpha amino keto acids.

carboxylation the addition of a carboxyl group, as to pyruvate to form oxaloacetate.

carboxylesterase an enzyme that catalyzes the hydrolysis of the esters of carboxylic acids.

carboxylic acid an organic compound containing the carboxy group (–COOH), which is weakly ionized in solution forming a carboxylate ion ($-COO^-$).

carboxyltransferase an enzyme that catalyzes carboxylation.

carboxymethylcellulose sodium a hygroscopic powder that forms an emollient gel; used as a bulk laxative. See also METHYLCELLULOSE.

carboxymyoglobin a compound formed from myoglobin on exposure to carbon monoxide.

carboxypenicillin a group of antipseudomonal penicillins which include carbenicillin and ticarcillin.

carboxypeptidase an exopeptidase enzyme secreted by the pancreas that acts only on the peptide linkage of a terminal amino acid containing a free carboxyl group; includes carboxypeptidases A and B.

Carbozoo anthrax vaccine to which saponin has been added as an adjuvant.

carbuncle a focus of infection in the skin consisting of multiple abscesses and sinuses.

carcase see CARCASS.

carcass, carcase 1. the body of an animal killed for meat. The head, the legs below the knees and hocks, the tail, the skin and most of the viscera are removed. The kidneys are left in and in most instances the body is split down the middle through the sternum and the vertebral bodies. Pig carcasses are dehaired (see below). Bird carcasses are not split; the feathers are removed after scalding but the skin is not removed and no viscera are left in place. In New York dressed poultry the viscera are left in. 2. the body of any dead animal.

c. condemnation meat inspection is carried out on the live animal and on viscera but the principal activity is during the carcass stage. If specific abnormalities are found which indicate that the carcass, or part of it, is unfit for human consumption it is condemned. It may be used for other purposes, e.g. after special processing inclusion in animal feeds.

c. contamination bacterial contamination of the carcass is a serious cause of deterioration of meat during storage. It is contributed to by having the animal come onto the abattoir floor with the hair and hide badly contaminated, by careless handling of the hide and the viscera, especially the alimentary tract, contamination of the water in scalding tanks for birds and pigs, and by lack of personal hygiene on the part of abattoir workers.

c. dehairing pig carcasses are not skinned. They are scalded and the bristles and superficial layers of skin scraped off. The scalding vat can be a source of serious contamination.

c. differentiation identification of the species, sex and age of a carcass is an important function of meat hygiene because of the need to guarantee the authenticity of the description of meat at the retail point. Much of this can be done on gross examination but final determination may require laboratory tests, especially in cases where fraudulent substitution is suspected.

c. disposal is necessary in an abattoir for condemned carcasses. Complete incineration is necessary in cases of highly infectious disease. Heat treatment sufficient to sterilize the tissues is carried out on less dangerous materials, leading to the preparation of animal feeds or agricultural fertilizer.

At practice premises the problem is a serious one if local government provisions do not include incineration of animal material. On site incineration may be prohibited by local legislation and the need to avoid unpleasant smells. Burial is satisfactory but tedious.

c. dressing removal of the hide, appendages and viscera.

c. drip see WEEPING.

c. electrical stimulation a method of tenderizing meat by the application of electrical stimulation so as to cause muscle contraction, lowering of pH and faster autolysis.

fevered c. congestion of the vessels so that the surfaces of tissues have a redder appearance, and individual vessels are more readily seen.

c. merit scale used in assessing carcass traits.
c. setting rigor mortis. The muscles are hard, the joints fixed, muscle tissue loses its translucence. Proper setting is an indication of satisfactory preparation for storage of the meat without deterioration.
c. traits criteria used in assessing quality of a carcass. Important in determining price, suitability of breeding program, value of sire. Includes length, weight, proportion of fat and lean, distribution of fat, relative size of valuable cuts.
c. yield proportion of the animal's liveweight salvaged at carcass point. Called also dressed weight, killing out percentage.

carcin- prefix meaning cancer.

carcinoembryonic antigen an oncofetal glycoprotein antigen found in colonic adenocarcinoma and other cancers and in certain nonmalignant conditions. See also oncofetal ANTIGEN. Called also CEA.

carcinogen a substance that causes cancer.

carcinogenesis production of cancer.

carcinogenic having a capacity for carcinogenesis.

carcinogenicity the ability or tendency to produce cancer.

carcinoid a tumor of the gastrointestinal tract formed from the endocrine (argentaffin) cells of the mucosal lining of a variety of organs including the stomach and intestine. In dogs they occur in the duodenum, colon and rectum, producing the carcinoid syndrome. Called also argentaffinoma, argentaffin tumor.
goblet-cell c. a rare tumor recorded in a dog; more common in human appendix; has characterisitics of carcinoid and adenocarcinoma. Called also adenocarcinoid.
hepatic c. a rare tumor originating from neuroectodermal tissue in the liver.

carcinolysis destruction of cancer cells.

carcinoma a malignant new growth made up of epithelial cells tending to infiltrate surrounding tissues and to give rise to metastases. A form of CANCER, carcinoma makes up the majority of the cases of malignancy of the mammary gland, uterus, intestinal tract, skin and tongue.
acinic cell c. locally invasive salivary gland tumors of dogs, and rarely other species, composed of glandular epithelium in an acinar pattern;
adenocystic c., adenoid cystic c. carcinoma marked by cylinders or bands of hyaline or mucinous stroma separated or surrounded by nests or cords of small epithelial cells, occurring in the mammary and salivary glands, and mucous glands of the respiratory tract. Called also cylindroma.
alveolar c. alveolar adenocarcinoma.
apocrine c. see APOCRINE tumors.
basal cell c. an epithelial tumor of the skin that seldom metastasizes but has potential for local invasion and destruction. Common in dogs and cats.
basosquamous c. carcinoma that histologically exhibits both basal and squamous elements.
bronchogenic c. carcinoma of the lung, so called because it arises from the epithelium of the bronchial tree.
cholangiocellular c. primary carcinoma of the liver originating in bile duct cells.
chorionic c. choriocarcinoma.
colloid c. mucinous carcinoma.
cylindrical cell c. carcinoma in which the cells are cylindrical or nearly so.
embryonal c. a highly malignant primitive form of carcinoma, probably of germinal cell or teratomatous derivation, usually arising in a gonad.
epidermoid c. that in which the cells tend to differentiate in the same way as those of the epidermis; i.e. they tend to form prickle cells and undergo cornification.
giant cell c. carcinoma containing many giant cells.
hepatocellular c. primary carcinoma of the liver cells.
Hürthle cell c. see HÜRTHLE CELL tumor.
c. in situ a neoplastic entity wherein the tumor cells have not invaded the basement membrane but are still confined to the epithelium of origin; popularly applied to such cells in the uterine cervix.
large-cell c. a bronchogenic tumor of undifferentiated (anaplastic) cells of large size.
medullary c. that composed mainly of epithelial elements with little or no stroma.
mucinous c. adenocarcinoma producing significant amounts of mucin.
oat-cell c. small-cell carcinoma.
papillary c. carcinoma in which there are papillary excrescences; called also papillocarcinoma.
scirrhous c. carcinoma with a hard structure owing to the formation of dense connective tissue in the stroma.
c. simplex an undifferentiated carcinoma.
c. of skin squamous cell carcinomas occur on the third eyelid, cornea or the eyelid of cattle and horses, on the penis and prepuce of horses, from the mucosa of the frontal sinus to invade the horn core of cattle (called also horn cancer), on the ears of sheep, on the vulva of ewes when the tail is docked too short. In goats the ears, udder, base of the horn and perineum are also susceptible sites. The tumors grow rapidly, show considerable invasiveness and often metastasize to local lymph nodes. In dogs and cats, squamous cell carcinomas are common, particularly on the face and pinnae of white cats. See also squamous cell carcinoma (below).
small-cell c. a radiosensitive tumor composed of clusters of small, oval, undifferentiated cells that have hyperchromatic nuclei and scant cytoplasm and are typically bronchogenic. Called also oat-cell carcinoma.
spindle cell c. squamous cell carcinoma marked by fusiform development or rapidly proliferating cells.
stomach c. squamous cell carcinomas occur in the stomach of the horse and the bovine rumen. The associated clinical syndrome in the horse is one of indigestion and weight loss. Metastasis occurs commonly. In cows there may be vagus indigestion or chronic tympany of the rumen.
transitional cell c. occurs mainly in the urinary bladder of older dogs. Several structural types may be observed: papillary, polypoid, fungoid or sessile. Metastasis to regional lymph nodes and lungs is possible.
udder c. occurs rarely in mares and doe goats.

carcinomatosis the condition of widespread dissemination of cancer throughout the body. Sometimes used to refer to widespread neoplastic involvement of an organ, e.g. abdominal carcinomatosis.

carcinomatous pertaining to or of the nature of cancer; malignant.

carcinophilia special affinity for cancerous tissue.

carcinosarcoma a malignant tumor composed of carcinomatous and sarcomatous tissues.
embryonal c. a rapidly developing, malignant mixed tumor of the kidneys, made up of embryonal elements.

carcinosis carcinomatosis.
miliary c. that marked by development of numerous nodules.

Carcopithecus see VERVET MONKEY.

card a computer's printed circuit board for a function such as a driver for a CD-ROM, fax machine. The board is plugged into an expansion slot and can be added to an existing computer or removed for replacement.

card files small cards used to store information in filing systems. They have the value of keeping information brief and in small packages. They can also be scanned visually with a minimum of fuss. By means of punch marks along the edges or at fixed locations in the center the cards can be sorted into categories with respect to one or a series of variables. Card systems were the forerunners of the computer and, given the availability of the latter, it seems unlikely that they still persist.

card test a test in which the reagent or antigen, usually dyed, is impregnated into absorbent paper. The subject specimen of urine, blood, plasma or serum is placed on the impregnated card and a color or similarly easily seen change is recorded.

brucellosis c. t. the reagent is dyed antigen consisting of a whole-cell suspension of *Brucella abortus* strain 1119-3. The antibody whose presence is under test is in plasma collected from the subject animals and extracted rapidly from the blood by the use of a special clumping agent. Only a positive or negative result is recorded.

cardenolide one of the two groups of naturally occurring CARDIAC glycosides; found in plants including *Digitalis, Nerium, Thevetia, Cryptostegia, Euonymus, Gomphocarpus, Asclepias, Corchorus, Convallaria, Gerbera, Adonis, Acokanthera* spp. Those from *Digitalis* spp. are used medicinally.

carder a grooming device consisting of a small, flat board with multiple, fine wire teeth on one side, and a short handle. It is used to comb out hair mats from the coats of dogs. Called also slicker brush.

cardia 1. the cardiac opening. 2. the cardiac part of the stomach; that part of the stomach surrounding the esophagogastric junction, distinguished by the presence of cardiac glands.

cardiac 1. pertaining to the heart. See also HEART. 2. pertaining to the gastric cardia.

c. afterload the impedance to ventricular emptying presented by aortic pressure.

c. area see PRECORDIUM.

c. biopsy an uncommon clinical procedure. May be performed via thoracotomy or with a biopsy catheter introduced intravenously.

c. catheterization the insertion of a catheter into a vein or artery and guiding it into the interior of the heart for purposes of measuring cardiac output, determining the oxygen content of blood in the heart chambers, and evaluating the structural components of the heart.

c. compensation in cardiac disease the compensation for the inefficiency of the heart's pump action by enlisting the various reserves of the heart such as hypertrophy, enlargement, increase in rate, so as to maintain circulatory equilibrium and prevent the appearance of signs of congestive heart failure.

c. compression an emergency measure to empty the ventricles of the heart in an effort to circulate the blood, and also to stimulate the heart so that it will resume its pumping action. Involves the application of pressure through the thoracic wall. More commonly used in animals than other forms of cardiac massage.

c. conducting cells specialized cardiac fibers modified to conduct impulses from the A-V node via the septum to the ventricles. Called also Purkinje fibers.

c. conducting system the cardiac tissue responsible for electrical conduction, made up of the sinoatrial node, the atrioventricular node, and the atrioventricular bundle and cardiac conducting fibers.

c. depressor nerve a branch of the vagus nerve composed of afferent nerve fibers which arise around the base of the heart; called also aortic nerve.

c. dilatation the heart volume is increased but the effective mass of cardiac muscle is not. A dilated heart has lost some of its reserve.

c. dullness the area of the chest wall over which a dull sound, indicating the position of the heart, can be elicited by percussion.

c. failure see HEART FAILURE.

c. fibrillation see ventricular FIBRILLATION.

c. fibrosis see cardiac CIRRHOSIS.

c. flow load the work required of the heart can be increased by a need for an increased flow rate of blood, e.g. when there is an anastomosis, congenital arteriovenous defect, portosystemic shunt.

c. function curves statistical curves used in modeling the cardiovascular functions, relating e.g. venous return to cardiac output.

c. glands in the cardiac region of the gastric wall; branched, tubular, coiled, mucus-secreting.

c. glycosides the glycosides of *Digitalis purpurea* (digitoxin, gitalin and gitoxin) and digoxin (from *D. lanata*). Strophanthin and ouabain are glycosides found in *Strophanthus* spp. Other cardiac glycosides are present in the skin of toads (*Bufo maritimus, B. vulgaris*), but are of toxicological rather than therapeutic interest.

c. horse sickness see AFRICAN HORSE SICKNESS.

c. hypertrophy enlargement of the heart coincident with an increase in muscle mass; an indication of response to an increase in load which may or may not be associated with disease. It is an expression of cardiac compensation but some of the cardiac reserve has been lost.

c. impulse see cardiac IMPULSE. Called also apex beat.

c. index cardiac output divided by the animal's body surface area in m^2. The normal range for dogs is 1.8–3.5 l/m^2.

left-sided c. enlargement may involve either the left ventricle or atrium, or both, and can be demonstrated on radiographs and electrocardiography. Seen most commonly in mitral valvular disease in dogs.

c. massage manual massage of the heart or stimulation with an electrical current through an open thoracic wall. The term is sometimes used interchangeably with cardiac compression.

c. mucosa the most cranial of the gastric mucosae; secretes only mucus, except in pigs, in which the area covered by this mucosa is much larger than in the other species and bicarbonate is also secreted.

c. murmur see heart MURMUR.

c. output the volume of blood pumped per unit of time. May be calculated by oxygen consumption measurement or determined by dilution of indocyanine green or cold saline, using catheters with thermistors placed intravenously (thermodilution method). It can be estimated clinically by measuring heart rate, pulse quality or pressure, and assessment of tissue perfusion, e.g. capillary refill time.

c. pacing employing cardiac pacemakers to control heart rate.

c. preload ventricular end-diastolic volume.

c. pressure load the stress of working against an elevated blood pressure in the arterial circuit; one of

the two major groups of causes of heart disease; the other is flow load.
c. racing syndrome a disease of companion birds manifested by a sudden increase in heart rate, up to 1000/min, in the period immediately after being restrained. Death occurs within a few seconds.
c. reserve the reserve mechanisms in the heart to compensate for defects which could make the heart's pumping action ineffective. The reserve mechanisms include hypertrophy, enlargement, increase in heart rate and an increase in stroke volume, a result of the increase in muscle mass and the enlargement of the ventricles.
right-sided c. enlargement may involve either the right ventricle or atrium. Occurs in heartworm disease in dogs.
c. rupture penetration of the myocardium by a reticular foreign body in cows, or rupture of a patch of chronic fibrotic myocarditis in horses, causes cardiac tamponade and sudden death.
c. size may increase as a result of hypertrophy, dilatation or a combination of the two. A common belief with some scientific support is that performance of horses in sprint races is closely related to heart size.
c. stroke volume the amount of blood ejected with each systole.
c. thrill see THRILL.
c. valve fenestration the valve surface is incomplete, creating a lattice effect; mostly congenital defects in foals.
c. valve hematocysts congenital, blood-filled cysts on the atrioventricular valves considered to be of no pathogenic significance.
c. valve laceration tearing of the valve tissue or attachment to myocardium may occur spontaneously or as a sequel to endocarditis; adds a significant additional flow load to the heart.
c. valve rupture see cardiac valve laceration (above).
c. valves heart valves formed by evaginations of the cardiac and vascular endothelium supported by connective tissue; includes atrioventricular and semilunar valves on both sides of the heart.
c. valvular disease see VALVULAR disease.
c. vascular shunts includes patent foramen ovale, ventricular septal defect, tetralogy of Fallot, patent ductus arteriosus.
c. work includes **effective** work—that needed for the onward propulsion of blood through the correct channels against arterial pressure, **total** work—includes all of the work performed by the heart including some involved in moving blood in the wrong direction.

cardialgia cardiodynia.
Cardigan Welsh corgi see WELSH CORGI.
cardinal flower LOBELIA *berlandieri.*
cardinal signs the most important clinical signs—temperature, pulse rate, respiration rate.
carding industrial process which flattens wool, draws fibers into a continuous sliver.
c. wool see carding WOOL.
cardi(o)- word element. [Gr.] *heart.*
cardioaccelerator quickening the heart action; an agent that so acts.
cardioactive having an effect on the heart.
cardioangiography the technology of radiological examination of the heart and blood vessels. It requires sophisticated equipment and technique because of the speed with which the injected radiopaque material passes through the heart. Called also angiocardiography.
cardioangiology the study of the diseases of the heart and blood vessels.
cardiocele hernial protrusion of the heart through a fissure of the diaphragm or through a wound.
cardiocentesis surgical puncture into the pericardial space and aspiration of fluid for therapeutic or diagnostic purposes. Therapeutically, the procedure is used as an emergency measure to relieve life-threatening cardiac tamponade. Other clinical situations in which cardiocentesis may be employed include pericardial effusion, traumatic perforation or rupture of the myocardium, and effusion secondary to a tumor or thoracic injury.
cardiochalasia relaxation or incompetence of the sphincter action of the cardiac opening of the stomach.
cardiocirculatory pertaining to blood flow through the heart and vascular system.
cardiodiaphragmatic pertaining to the heart and the diaphragm.
cardiodilator an instrument for dilating the cardia.
cardiodiosis dilatation of the cardiac opening of the stomach.
cardiodynamics study of the forces involved in the heart's action.
cardiodynia pain in the heart.
cardioesophageal pertaining to the cardia of the stomach and the esophagus, as the cardioesophageal junction or sphincter.
Cardiofilaria pavlovsky a tissue-invading filaroid worm found in many birds but appearing to cause little if any disease.
cardiogenesis development of the heart in the embryo.
cardiogenic originating in the heart.
c. plate the mesodermal primordium of the heart.
cardiogram a tracing of a cardiac event produced by cardiography. See also ELECTROCARDIOGRAM.
cardiograph an instrument for recording some element of the heartbeat.
cardiography the graphic recording of a physical or functional aspect of the heart, e.g. echocardiography, electrocardiography, kinetocardiography, phonocardiography, vibrocardiography.
apex c. graphic recording of low-frequency pulsations at the chest wall over the apex of the heart.
ultrasonic c. echocardiography.
vector c. see VECTORCARDIOGRAPHY.
cardiohepatic pertaining to the heart and liver.
cardioinhibitor an agent that restrains the heart's action.
cardiokinetic 1. exciting or stimulating the heart. 2. an agent that excites or stimulates the heart.
cardiokymography the recording of the motion of the heart by means of the electrokymograph.
cardiologist a physician who specializes in the diagnosis and treatment of heart disease.
cardiology study of the heart and its functions.
cardiolysis the operation of freeing the heart from its adhesions to the sternal periosteum.
cardiomalacia morbid softening of the muscular substance of the heart.
cardiomegaly enlargement of the heart.
cardiomelanosis melanosis of the heart.
cardiomotility the movement of the heart; motility of the heart.
cardiomyoliposis fatty degeneration of the heart muscle.
cardiomyopathy a general diagnostic term designating primary myocardial disease of unknown cause.
Boxer c. a dilated cardiomyopathy, believed to be

inherited, is seen in adult Boxers that show syncope, episodic weakness, arrhythmias, and left or biventricular heart failure.

congestive c. a syndrome characterized by cardiac enlargement, especially of the left ventricle, poor myocardial contractility, and congestive heart failure. Occurs most commonly in young to middle-aged dogs of the large and giant breeds with rapidly developing signs of biventricular failure, atrial fibrillation and occasionally systolic murmurs. Cats usually show acute signs of cardiac failure with pleural effusion but not ascites, and sometimes thromboembolism. Called also dilated cardiomyopathy.

Doberman c. a distinctive cardiomyopathy is seen in Doberman pinscher dogs, often presenting as an acute pulmonary edema, cardiogenic shock and sometimes sudden death.

hypertrophic c. occurs most commonly in cats, sometimes secondary to HYPERTHYROIDISM, occasionally in dogs and rarely in cattle in association with generalized GLYCOGENOSIS. There is myocardial hypertrophy, primarily in the left ventricle and ventricular septum, resulting in increased resistance to filling and sometimes an outflow obstruction. In cats there is often an associated aortic thromboembolism.

infiltrative c. myocardial disease secondary to deposition in the heart tissue of abnormal substances such as amyloid or neoplastic infiltration.

inherited c. occurs in calves and probably in the other species. In calves it causes death due to acute heart failure up to the age of 3 months. Recorded in polled Hereford and Japanese black cattle. There may be a brief period of dyspnea and blood-stained frothy nasal discharge before death. Myocardial degeneration is obvious at necropsy.

occult c. in the subclinical stage, but detectable with echocardiography and ambulatory electrocardiographic recording methods.

restrictive c. impaired left ventricular compliance reduces ventricular filling. Uncommon in animals but seen most often in cats, caused by endomyocardial fibrosis or abnormal left ventricular moderator bands. Called also obliterative cardiomyopathy.

cardiomyopexy surgical removal of the epicardium and application of a pedicled flap of adjacent muscle to the denuded myocardium and pericardium, as a means of supplying collateral circulation to the heart.

cardionatrin see ATRIAL natriuretic factor.

cardionector the conduction system of the heart, comprising the sinoatrial node, bundle of His and atrioventricular node.

cardionephric pertaining to the heart and kidney.

cardioneural pertaining to the heart and nervous system.

cardio-omentopexy suture of a portion of the omentum to the heart.

cardiopathy any disorder or disease of the heart.

cardiopericardiopexy surgical establishment of adhesive pericarditis, to provide ancillary blood supply to the myocardium.

cardiopericarditis inflammation of the heart and pericardium.

cardiophrenic pertaining to the heart and diaphragm.

c. angle viewed on radiographs as the angle formed by shadows of the diaphragm and the heart. Alterations may be used to assess changes in the size and position of the heart.

c. ligament see phrenicocardial LIGAMENT.

cardioplasty plastic surgery of the esophagus and stomach. Sometimes performed in the management of megaesophagus in dogs.

cardioplegia arrest of myocardial contraction, as by use of chemical compounds or cold in cardiac surgery.

cardiopneumatic pertaining to the heart and respiration.

cardiopneumograph an apparatus for registering cardiopneumatic movements.

cardioptosis downward displacement of the heart.

cardiopulmonary pertaining to the heart and lungs.

c. arrest (CPA) cessation of effective external respiration and beating of the heart. The common causes in animals are inadequate ventilation, caused by general anesthetic, thoracic trauma, airway obstruction, and impediments to movement of the lung, thoracic wall or diaphragm, acidemia, hypotension, electrolyte imbalance, or extreme changes in body temperature (hypothermia, hyperthermia).

c. resuscitation (CPR) the re-establishment of heart and lung action. The basic steps are: *A*irway, *B*reathing, *C*irculation. A patent airway must be established and maintained; any obstruction is relieved and an endotracheal or tracheostomy tube inserted. Adequate ventilation with oxygen is provided by intermittent positive pressure and, if required, cardiac (chest) compression or massage is commenced.

cardiopuncture cardiocentesis.

cardiopyloric pertaining to the cardiac opening of the stomach and the pylorus.

cardiorenal pertaining to the heart and kidneys.

cardiorrhaphy suture of the heart muscle.

cardiorrhexis rupture of the heart.

cardiosclerosis fibrous induration of the heart.

cardioselective having greater activity on heart tissue than on other tissue.

cardiospasm see ACHALASIA.

cardiosphygmograph a combination of the cardiograph and sphygmograph for recording the movements of the heart and an arterial pulse.

cardiosplenopexy suture of the parenchyma of the spleen to the denuded surface of the heart for revascularization of the myocardium.

cardiotachometer an instrument for continuously portraying or recording the heart rate.

cardiotachometry continuous recording of the heart rate for long periods.

cardiotherapy the treatment of diseases of the heart.

cardiotomy 1. surgical incision of the heart. 2. surgical incision into the cardia.

cardiotonic having a tonic effect on the heart; an agent that so acts.

cardiotoxic having a poisonous or deleterious effect upon the heart.

c. glycosides see CARDIAC glycosides.

cardiovalvular pertaining to the valves of the heart.

cardiovalvulotome an instrument for incising a heart valve.

cardiovascular pertaining to the heart and blood vessels.

c. accident includes AORTIC rupture, MARFAN'S SYNDROME, acute HEART FAILURE, CARDIAC valve rupture, cardiac TAMPONADE.

c. collapse see circulatory COLLAPSE.

c. reserve see CARDIAC reserve.

c. system see CIRCULATORY system.

cardioversion the delivery of a direct current shock synchronized with the QRS COMPLEX to the myocardium as an elective treatment to end tachydysrhythmias; called also countershock and precordial shock. Used in humans, it has been also been effectively used in dogs with atrial fibrillation and ventricular tachycardias.

cardioverter an energy-storage capacitor-discharge type of condenser that is discharged with an inductance; it delivers a direct-current shock which restores normal rhythm of the heart.

Cardiovirus one of the genera of viruses in the family *Picornaviridae*. Includes encephalomyocarditis (EMC) virus which causes disease in rodents, pigs, humans and some exotic species.

carditis inflammation of the heart; MYOCARDITIS.

cardivalvulitis inflammation of the heart valves.

Carduelis cannabina see LINNET.

Carduus a genus of thistles in the plant family Asteraceae (Compositae); has a high nitrate content, causing nitrite poisoning in ruminants. Includes *C. pycnocephalus*, *C. tenuifloris* (slender or winged thistle).

careless weed AMARANTHUS *reflexus*.

Carelian bear dog a Finnish dog breed used for hunting elk; named after a territory (Karelia) on the Russian–Finnish border. It is a large dog with a short, harsh black coat and white markings on the face, throat, chest, feet and tail tip. The tail is carried over the back and the ears are erect.

caret 1. the symbol ^ above a number indicating the expected value or expected frequency. 2. used to indicate exponentiation in many computer languages, e.g. 100=10^2 or ten squared.

Carex vulpina European plant in family Cyperaceae of sedges; contains cyanogenetic glucosides.

carfentanil an opioid analgesic; a very potent derivative of fentanyl used mainly in the capture of wild animals.

caribou *Rangifer tarandus caribou* (called also *Rangifer arcticus*). See REINDEER.

Carica papaya pawpaw tree, source of the proteolytic enzyme papain.

caries decay, as of bone or teeth.

dental c. demineralization and loss of substance of the hard tissues of the teeth, leading to continued destruction of enamel and dentine, and cavitation of the tooth. It is a very rare disease in animals. Occurs occasionally in sheep. May occur as pits or fissures. Called also a cavity.

carina pl. *carinae* [L.] a ridgelike structure.

c. apex the most cranial point of the keel of the sternum of birds.

sternal c. the keel of the sternum, as in birds and horses.

c. tracheae a ridge between the openings of the right and left principal bronchi.

carinate said of birds, having a carina or keeled sternum.

Carissa see ACOKANTHERA.

Carmalt forceps conventional ratcheted, box-jointed hemostat forceps with grooves on the blade surfaces that run in the same direction as the length of the blades.

carminative 1. relieving flatulence. 2. an agent that relieves flatulence.

carmustine a nitrosourea, used as an ANTINEOPLASTIC agent. Called also BCNU.

Carmyerius a genus of rumen (digenetic trematode) fluke found in Asia; member of the family Paramphistomatidae. Includes *Carmyerius gregarius*, *C. spatiosus* (small rumen flukes of Asia).

carnassial tooth a large, shearing cheek tooth; the upper fourth premolar and lower first molar in dogs and the upper third premolar and lower first molar in cats. Called also sectorial tooth.

c. abscess abscess at the root of a carnassial tooth. See MALAR abscess.

carnification development of fleshy fibrous tissue in the lung.

carnitine coenzyme of fatty acid oxidation and acetyl transfer; often designated vitamin B_T, due to its vitamin role in *Tenebrio* sp. Present in high concentrations (5% dry weight) in meat extracts.

c. acetyltransferase enzyme associated with buffering of acetyl groups from acetyl CoA.

c. deficiency associated with myocardial disease in dogs, particularly Boxers.

carnivore any animal, particularly mammals of the order Carnivora, that eats primarily flesh. Includes cats, dogs, bears, etc.

carnosinase an enzyme that hydrolyzes carnosine (amino-acyl-L-histidine) and other dipeptides containing L-histidine into their constituent amino acids.

carnosine a dipeptide composed of beta-alanine and histidine, found in skeletal muscle of vertebrates.

caroline jessamine see GELSEMIUM SEMPERVIRENS.

carotenase an enzyme that converts provitamin A carotenoids into vitamin A; not present in cats.

carotene a yellow or red pigment from carrots, sweet potatoes, milk and body fat, egg yolk, etc.; it is a chromolipoid hydrocarbon existing in several forms. α-, β- and γ-carotene are provitamins which can be converted into vitamin A in the body by all animals except cats. β-carotene is the most important because of a quantitatively greater activity.

β-carotene see CAROTENE.

carotenemia the presence of high levels of carotene in the blood.

carotenodermia yellowness of the skin due to carotenemia.

carotenoid 1. any member of a group of red, orange or yellow pigmented polyisoprenoid lipids found in carrots, sweet potatoes, green leaves and some animal tissues; examples are the carotenes, lycopene and xanthophyll. 2. marked by yellow color. 3. lipochrome.

c. pigments contribute to the yellow staining of fatty tissues especially in horses, Channel Island breeds of cattle and old cats.

carotenosis deposition of carotene in tissues, especially the skin.

caroticotympanic pertaining to the carotid canal and the tympanum of the middle ear.

carotid relating to the carotid artery, the principal artery of the neck. See Table 9.

c. body a small neurovascular structure lying in the bifurcation of the common carotid arteries, containing chemoreceptors that monitor oxygen content in blood and help to regulate respiration. Called also glomus caroticum.

c. body tumors usually unilateral nonfunctional adenoma, chemodectoma, nonchromaffin paraganglioma, or locally invasive carcinoma which may cause deviation of the trachea.

c. canal transmits the internal carotid artery to the cranial cavity through the pars petrosa of the temporal bone.

c. sheath contains the common carotid artery, internal jugular vein and vagosympathetic trunk.

c. sinus a dilatation of the proximal portion of the internal carotid or distal portion of the common carotid artery, containing in its wall pressoreceptors which are stimulated by changes in blood pressure.

c. sinus reflex slowing of the heart rate when pressure is applied over the carotid sinus.

c. sinus syndrome syncope sometimes associated

with convulsive seizures due to overactivity of the carotid sinus reflex.

carotidynia tenderness along the course of the carotid artery.

carp a freshwater fish used extensively for human food in some countries, a pest in others. There are many varieties, including decorative ones. See also SILVER, COMMON, BIGHEAD, MUD, CARASSIUS CARASSIUS, CTENOPHARYNGODON EDELLA. Called also *Cyprinus carpio*, *C. cyprinus*.

c.-dropsy complex the cause is unknown; the clinical syndrome includes ascites and exophthalmos.

c. erythrodermatitis see ERYTHRODERMATITIS.

c. pox an infectious disease of carp probably caused by a virus.

carpal pertaining to the carpus.

c. bones are located between the radius and ulna and metacarpals. Typically, there are six to eight bones, depending on the animal species, arranged in two rows and numbered from medial to lateral. See Table 10.

c. canal syndrome see carpal tunnel syndrome (below).

c. flexion posture at parturition the fetus is presented with the carpal joints flexed, thus increasing the diameter of initial parts entering the pelvic canal, resulting in dystocia in some patients.

c. fracture see CHIP FRACTURES, slab FRACTURE.

c. instability/flexion syndrome seen in young puppies, particularly Doberman pinschers and Shar peis; the carpi remain slightly flexed when standing and the paws are deviated inwards.

c. organ a group of vibrissae located on the posterior aspect of the forelimbs of cats, sensitive to touch. See also TACTILE hair organ.

c. pad see FOOTPAD.

c. sheath common synovial sheath in the forelimb of the horse, shared by the superficial and deep flexor tendons as they pass through the carpal canal.

c. tunnel the osseofibrous passage for the flexor tendons and median nerve, formed by the flexor retinaculum and the carpal bones.

c. tunnel syndrome a complex of signs resulting from compression of the median nerve in the carpal tunnel. In horses there is lameness with pain on extreme carpal flexion. There are no lesions on the anterior carpal bones.

carpal joint a series of joints that includes the antebrachiocarpal, formed by the distal ends of the radius/ulna and the proximal carpal row, the intercarpal joint between the two rows of carpal bones, the carpometacarpal joint(s) between the distal row of carpal bones and the metacarpal bone(s). The joint capsule is continuous throughout all of the joints and has three major sacs, the radiocarpal, the intercarpal and the carpometacarpal sacs. Called also the knee. See also CARPUS.

c. j. luxation a major injury in horses while racing, usually involving fractures of carpal bones and rupture of ligaments. The animal is unable to bear weight on the leg and there is excessive mobility and crepitus. In dogs and cats, violent hyperextension of the carpus damages soft tissue support for the joint so that the animal walks with the carpus on or near the ground.

c. j. osteochondrosis osteochondrosis dissecans and subchondral cysts occur in the carpal joints of horses, causing lameness, pain on passive extension and sometimes distension of the joint capsule.

c. j. subluxation may occur in the dog as a result of trauma but is also recorded as a familial disease associated with the simultaneous occurrence of hemophilia A.

Carpathian brown cattle dark brown to gray dual purpose cattle from Ukraine.

carpectomy excision of a carpal bone.

carpet snake a large python, a member of the subfamily Pythoninae of the family Boidae. They are not venomous and are often kept as pets. They are also useful in rodent control.

carpet weed KALLSTROEMIA *hirsutissima*.

Carpetmaster a New Zealand carpetwool sheep derived by mutation from the Perendale. It has a white face, dark hooves, and wool of 35 to 45 microns.

carpetwool see carpet WOOL.

carpetwool sheep breeds used extensively for the production of wool for carpet manufacture include Carpetmaster, Elliottdale, fat-tailed breeds generally, Scottish blackface, Swaledale, Tukidale.

carpincho see CAPYBARA.

carpitis common acute or chronic inflammation of the joint capsule of the carpus and the associated structures in horses. There is pain and swelling and there may be exostoses in chronic cases. Called also popped knee in horses.

Carpoglyphus a genus of the insect family of Acaridae. Includes *Carpoglyphus lactis* (the cause of dried fruit mite dermatitis).

carpometacarpal pertaining to the carpus and metacarpus.

c. joint the articulation between the distal row of carpal bones and the metacarpals in which there is very limited movement.

carpopedal affecting the carpus and foot.

carpophalangeal pertaining to the carpus and phalanges.

carpus the segment of the limb between the radius and ulna and metacarpus, made up of six to eight bones, depending on the animal species, arranged in two rows and numbered from medial to lateral. Called also the knee in horses and cattle and the wrist in dogs and cats. See also Table 10.

dropped c., broken-down c. hyperextension injury in the dog or cat that results in weight-bearing on the carpus and metacarpals.

Carré's disease see canine DISTEMPER.

carriage dog see DALMATIAN.

carrier 1. an animal which harbors a disease organism in its body without manifest signs, thus acting as a carrier or distributor of infection. A carrier may be one with a latent infection and which appears healthy. Other types of carriers are the incubatory carrier, when the animal is not yet showing clinical signs, or a convalescent carrier when it has passed the clinical stage. 2. a heterozygote, i.e. an animal which carries a recessive gene, autosomal or sex-linked, together with its normal allele. 3. an edible material used in the formulation of processed feeds. The carrier is used to absorb or attach other ingredients by impregnation or coating so that they are evenly mixed throughout the feed.

c. detection in genetic terms the detection of a heterozygote which carries the gene which is under investigation.

c. effect use of a hapten conjugated to a carrier protein in a primary immune response will result in a secondary immune response to the same combination, but not to the hapten alone or in association with a different carrier protein.

c. register in genetic terms is a list of all the animals which have produced an affected offspring.

c. state the state of being a carrier of an infectious disease or of a genetic defect.

c. test herd a herd consisting entirely of known carriers of a gene which is under investigation; a definition which could be extended to include a herd comprising only individuals known to carry a specific infectious agent.

carrier-free a term denoting a radioisotope of an element in pure form, i.e. essentially undiluted with a stable isotope carrier.

carrier-mediated transport movement which occurs across membranes, such as the blood–brain barrier and the gastrointestinal mucosa. Inherent in the mechanism is a rapidly reversible reaction between the substance being transported and components of the membrane. The membrane component is the 'carrier'. The mechanism is also characterized by (1) being saturable; (2) like substances being able to compete for the services of the carrier so that competitive inhibition occurs.

There are two forms of carrier-mediated transport, active transport and facilitated diffusion. The rapid transfer of drug metabolites into urine is by active transport. Entry of glucose into most cells is by facilitated diffusion but its passage across the gastrointestinal mucosa is by active transport. Active transport requires a direct expenditure of energy, whereas facilitated diffusion is not energy dependent. Active transport can move substances against a concentration gradient, facilitated diffusion cannot.

carrier protein membrane proteins that have a high affinity for particular solutes, e.g. glucose, and which facilitate the passage of these solutes through membrane barriers. See also CARRIER-MEDIATED TRANSPORT.

carrion eating a species trait, or a sign of nutritional deficiency usually phosphorus.

carrion hawk see CARACARA.

Carrion's disease see BARTONELLA.

carrot bush MYOPORUM *deserti*.

carrying capacity the number of animal units that a farm or area will carry on a year round basis, including that needed for conservation of winter feed. Usually stated as dry cows or dry sheep equivalents per hectare.

cart wheeled vehicle without motor power.

paraplegic c. a two-wheeled cart into which a paraplegic dog can be strapped so that its hindquarters are supported and its front limbs rest normally on the ground and provide a motor system. Used for short periods to give the animal exercise.

cartilage a specialized, gristly connective tissue present in both mature animals and embryos, providing a model in which most of the bones develop, and constituting an important part of the organism's growth mechanism; the three most important types are hyaline cartilage, elastic cartilage and fibrocartilage. Also, a general term for a mass of such tissue in a particular site in the body.

alar c's the cartilages of the wings of the nose.

annular ear c. a ring of cartilage interposed between the rolled-up auricular cartilage and the skull.

arthrodial c., articular c. that clothing the articular surfaces of synovial joints.

arytenoid c's two pyramid-shaped cartilages of the larynx.

auricular c. cartilage of the pinna and much of the external ear canal.

c. canals tunnels containing blood vessels incorporated in developing cartilage.

connecting c. that connecting the surfaces of an immovable joint.

costal c. a bar of hyaline cartilage that attaches a rib to the sternum in the case of true ribs, or to the immediately cranial rib in the case of the anterior false ribs.

cricoid c. a ringlike cartilage forming the caudal part of the larynx.

diarthrodial c. articular cartilage.

distal phalangeal c. the ungual cartilages of the third phalanx in the horse lie mostly against the hoof wall but can be palpated if ossified. See also SIDEBONE.

elastic c. cartilage that is more opaque, flexible and elastic than hyaline cartilage, and is further distinguished by its yellow color. The ground substance is penetrated in all directions by frequently branching fibers that give all of the reactions for elastin.

c. emboli see fibrocartilaginous embolic MYELOPATHY.

ensiform c. xiphoid process.

fibrous c. fibrocartilage.

floating c. a detached portion of semilunar cartilage in the stifle joint.

hoof c. see distal phalangeal cartilage (above).

hyaline c. flexible, somewhat elastic, semitransparent cartilage with an opalescent bluish tint, composed of a basophilic fibril-containing substance with cavities in which the chondrocytes occur.

interarytenoid c. an occasional cartilage located between the two arytenoid cartilages.

nasal c. rostral end to the internasal septum, separating the nasal cavities and anchoring the other cartilages around the nostrils.

parapatellar c. cartilaginous plates medial and lateral to the patella in some species, e.g. dogs.

permanent c. cartilage that does not normally become ossified.

retained enchondral c. cores occur in ulnar metaphysis and lateral femoral condyles of young, giant breed dogs. Visible radiographically as radiolucent inverted cones, extending into the metaphysis, they are often associated with growth deformities such as forelimb valgus and genu valgum.

reticular c. elastic cartilage.

scapular c. dorsal extension of the scapula in ungulates; tends to calcify with age.

c. scissors used for ear cropping in dogs.

semilunar c. one of the two intra-articular cartilages of the stifle joint.

temporary c. cartilage that is normally destined to be replaced by bone.

thyroid c. the unpaired cartilage of the larynx to which the vocal folds attach.

tibial c. the bed of cartilage located on the caudal surface of the intertarsal joint of birds; the tendons of the digital flexors pass through it.

ungual c. see distal phalangeal cartilage (above).

vomeronasal c. either of the two narrow strips of cartilage, one on each side, of the nasal septum supporting the vomeronasal organ.

xiphoid c. posterior continuation of the sternum; supports the anterior abdominal wall, especially the linea alba.

yellow c. elastic cartilage.

cartilage-forming tumor tumors containing principally cartilage; some contain bone. Only a small proportion of skeletal neoplasms, except in sheep, are cartilaginous.

cartilaginiform resembling cartilage.

cartilaginous consisting of, or of the nature of, cartilage.

c. joint the bones of the joint are joined together by fibrocartilage or hyaline cartilage. See SYNCHONDROSIS, SYMPHYSIS.

c. metaplasia occurs in normal tendons; is classified as abnormal only when the metaplasia is bony.
multiple c. exostosis see multiple cartilaginous EXOSTOSIS.
c. osteoid degenerate cartilage which has lost its basophilic quality and stains like osteoid.
c. tumor see CARTILAGE-FORMING TUMOR.

cartogram a map showing the distribution of a population by area.

cartography map making.
epidemiological c. making maps which show epidemiological data about distribution of disease or its causes by land area.

cartridge plug-in units for use in a computer and using memory chips and circuitry to provide such things as print fonts to the computer.

cartwheel flower plant see HERACLEUM MANTEGAZZIANUM.

carumonam sodium a monobactam antibiotic, very resistant to β-lactamase, with activity against gram-negative bacteria, including most *Pseudomonas aeruginosa*.

caruncle a small fleshy eminence, often abnormal.
hymenal c's small elevations of mucous membrane around the vaginal opening, being relics of the ruptured hymen, especially of women.
lacrimal c. the eminence at the medial angle of the eye.
maternal c. see uterine caruncle (below).
sublingual c. an eminence on either side of the frenulum of the tongue (frenulum linguae), on which the major duct of the sublingual gland and the duct of the submandibular gland open.
uterine c. fleshy masses on the wall of the uterus of pregnant ruminants. The placenta is attached only at these points. There are about 100 of them and they are very much smaller in the nonpregnant female.

caruncula pl. *carunculae* [L.] caruncle.

carunculitis inflammation of the uterine caruncles in ruminants.

Cary-Blair medium a transport medium for anaerobic bacteria.

caryo- for words beginning thus, see those beginning *karyo-*.

Caryophanon see SIMONSIELLA.

Caryophyllaeus a genus of the family of cestodes Caryophyllaeidae. Includes *Caryophyllaeus fimbriceps*, *C. laticeps* (carp).

Caryospora apicomplexan protozoan parasites affecting mostly reptiles and raptors.
C. bigenetica an occasional cause of pyogranulomatous dermatitis in puppies.

caryosporiosis infection by a species of coccidia in the genus *Caryospora*.

casanthranol a purified mixture of the anthranol glycosides derived from cascara sagrada; used as a laxative.

cascade 1. a series of steps or stages (as of a physiological process) which, once initiated, continues to the final step by virtue of each step being triggered by the preceding one, sometimes with cumulative effect. For example, the coagulation cascade. 2. in computer terminology is a display system which presents a series of document windows in an overlapping format, e.g. an additional list of menu items opening from a single menu item.

cascado [Indonesian] a bovine dermatitis caused by *Stephanofilaria dedoesi*.

cascara, cascara sagrada dried bark of *Rhamnus purshiana*, used as an irritant cathartic.

case in epidemiology, an animal which has the specified disease or condition which is under investigation.
c. abstract a structured summary of a case report suitable for computer entry; permits machine sorting and retrieval and leads an investigator to the original paper records on which detailed descriptions must be based.
c.-control sampling selection of cases as a sample to use in a case-control study (below).
c.-control study a retrospective, analytical, epidemiological study. A group of pre-existing cases of the disease are matched with a selected group of control animals that do not have the disease so that the presence or otherwise of an hypothesized disease determinant can be ascertained in both groups.
c. fatality rate the proportion of cases with a specified condition which die within a specified time.
c. finding the strategy of surveying a population to find the sick animals that are the foci of infection; an essential early step in the eradication of any disease.
c. history the collected data concerning an individual, contact and related animals, environment and management procedures, including any past medical history and any other information that may be useful in analyzing and diagnosing the case or for instructional or research purposes.
index c. the first case recorded in an outbreak.
c. management care of a sick animal including specific and supportive medication, surgical intervention, housing, bedding, nutrition, restraint, collection of specimens for submission to laboratory or stall-side tests.
c. population the group of animals in the total population which are sick or infected, as distinct from the control population, which are not sick or infected.
c. recording entry in records of the clinical findings of individual sick animals. May be structured or unstructured, paper or machine, with or without the accounting record for the case.

caseation 1. the precipitation of casein. 2. a form of necrosis in which tissue is changed into a dry, amorphous mass resembling cheese.

casein a phosphoprotein, the principal protein of milk, the basis of curd and of cheese. Called also caseinogen.
c. clot the insoluble form of caseinogen produced by the action of rennin in the presence of calcium.
c. digestion an identifying characteristic of *Corynebacterium renale* when grown on milk agar.

caseinogen outside North America, the term for casein.

caseopurulent the lesion is partly cheesy, partly purulent, or consistently of a consistency midway between the two.

caseous resembling cheese or curd; cheesy.

caseous lymphadenitis a chronic disease of sheep and goats caused by *Corynebacterium pseudotuberculosis* and characterized by caseopurulent abscesses in lymph nodes but with little effect on general health.

cash flow the movement of cash in and out of a business enterprise such as a farm or a veterinary practice. Becomes a realizable estimation in today's world of computers and spreadsheet programs.

cash transaction any transaction between parties in which there is a direct transfer of money by currency, check or credit card.

cashmere, cashmere wool fine, downy hair fiber from the Kashmiri goat.

cashmere goat see CENTRAL ASIATIC PASHMINA.

casings for sausage see SAUSAGE CASING.

Caslick E.A. Caslick, a veterinarian who pioneered in

the field of equine reproduction in the early 20th century.

C. operation a means of reducing the mucocutaneous cleft of the vulva to prevent the aspiration of air and thus reduce the amount of infection and inflammation in the urogenital tract. The simplest version of the operation is the suturing together of the lips of the vulva, after removal of a narrow strip of mucosa, over most of their length.

Casoni's test a test for hydatid infection used in humans. The production of a wheal and flare reaction at the site of intradermal injection indicates infection.

cassaine cardiotoxic alkaloid in the bark of *Erythrophloeum guineense* tree. Causes anorexia, defective vision, increased heart sounds and dyspnea.

cassava see MANIHOT ESCULENTA.

cassette 1. a light-proof housing for x-ray film, containing front and back intensifying screens, between which the film is placed and held during exposure. Although it is usual to have two screens, there may be only one where there is a special need for a high detail picture. 2. a magazine for film or magnetic tape.

c. grid composed of alternating strips of lead and radiotranslucent material such as aluminum. Placed on top of the cassette it permits the passage only of the x-rays that are passing directly to the film. Scattered rays are absorbed by the lead and this reduces the effect of scatter on the film and provides a more clearcut image.

c. holder a radiolucent holder, into which the cassette fits, is on a long handle permitting the person holding the cassette to stay well clear of the x-ray beam.

c. tunnel a device which enables the operator to pass a number of cassettes past the x-ray beam and the grid without the need to open and reload cassettes.

Cassia legume genus of the Caesalpiniaceae family of plants; contain anthraquinone glycosides which causes diarrhea and myopathy. Includes *C. acutiflora* (senna), *C. arachoides*, *C. barclayana*, *C. didymobotrya*, *C. floribunda*, *C. obtusiflora* (sicklepod), *C. roemeriana*. Many species in the genus have been reclassified as *Senna* spp.

C. occidentalis causes degeneration of striated muscle with a consequent myoglobinuria and atrophy of skeletal muscles and cardiomyopathy of sufficient extent to cause death. Called also coffee senna, wild coffee.

Cassine buchanani African plant in the family Celestraceae; an unknown toxin causes nephrosis. Called also *Elaeodendron buchananii*.

Cassou artificial insemination gun an instrument used for artificial insemination and embryo transfer. Consists of a very narrow diameter stainless steel plunger with a knob handle. The plunger is fitted into a plastic straw from which the semen or embryo is expelled.

cassowary a large Australian ratite bird with a brightly colored head and neck and a bony helmet on top of its head. Called also *Casuaris* spp.

cast 1. a positive copy of an object, e.g. a mold of a hollow organ (a renal tubule, bronchiole, etc.), formed of effused plastic matter and extruded from the body, as a urinary cast; named according to constituents, as epithelial, fatty, waxy, etc. 2. a restraint procedure used in horses and cattle, and occasionally in large beasts such as elephants, to pull them to the ground so that surgical procedures can be performed. Used less nowadays than previously because of the advent of new anesthetic techniques. There are many techniques and special harnesses for special purposes. 3. an animal lies down but is unable to right itself into a position of sternal recumbency so that it can rise, e.g. a horse in a loose box when it is lying too close to a wall, a sheep in heavy fleece in wet weather. When helped to the sternal posture the animal is able to rise. 4. to form an object in a mold, as a replica of teeth made in an impression. 5. a stiff dressing or casing, usually made of plaster of Paris, used to immobilize body parts. More modern, lightweight casts are made of polyurethane resins. 6. strabismus. 7. culled, e.g. cast for age. 8. shedding of velvet by deer stags and bucks.

full leg c. see long-leg cast (below).

half c. see walking cast (below).

long-leg c. a rigid material, usually plaster of Paris, is applied from the toes to as high as possible over the humerus or femur. Used for immobilization of fractures of the radius, ulna or tibia.

renal c's see urinary casts (below).

stone c. a reproduction of the jaw and dentition made from powdered gypsum stone and water in an impression mold.

urinary c's precipitates of mucoprotein or plasma protein in the shape of the renal tubular laminae in which they form, often with cellular elements. Observed in the examination of urinary sediment, they indicate renal tubular or epithelial damage. Hyaline casts are composed of mucoproteins or plasma proteins without formed cellular elements. Waxy, granular, epithelial, erythrocyte and leukocyte casts may occur, each representing a type of cellular reaction or stage of degeneration within the cast. Fatty casts are formed from degenerating tubular epithelial cells and, particularly in cats, lipid in these cells. Casts may dissolve in alkaline urine. Called also cylindroids.

walking c. one that does not extend above the elbow or stifle, thereby permitting movement of those joints so that the animal can walk on the leg. Suitable for fractures of the metacarpus or metatarsus.

Castalis spectabilis African member of the plant family Asteraceae; causes cyanide poisoning. Called also *Dimorphotheca spectabilis*, blue bitou, Transvaal bitou.

castanospermine pyrrolizidine alkaloid in the ripe seeds of *Castanosperma australe*. Powerful inhibitor of mononuclear cell beta-glucosidase which is however not the cause of the seeds' toxicity.

Castanospermum australe Australian tree in the legume family Fabaceae; contains CASTANOSPERMINE and an unidentified toxin which causes diarrhea and enteritis. Called also Moreton Bay chestnut, black bean.

casters the small rubber wheels on surgical trolleys, patient stretchers, mobile equipment.

conductive c. the casters are impregnated with carbon to facilitate the dispersal of static electricity from equipment. This is enhanced if the floor also has a conductive covering.

Castilleja a North American genus of the plant family Scrophulariaceae; selenium converter plants which selectively absorb selenium from the soil. Called also paintbrushes.

casting the technique of using a rope or a special harness designed for the purpose to make an animal fall to the ground or onto a specially prepared area. Used for large animals especially horses and cattle.

c. bed the area designated for a cast animal to fall. It is usually cushioned with straw or, in the case of a permanent facility, rubber or other synthetic padding.

Burley c. method one that uses a rope centered over the shoulders, crossed between the front legs, crossed over the back and then passed between the hindlegs, avoiding the scrotum or udder and with traction backwards. Used in cattle.

half hitches c. method suitable only for cattle; a non-slip knot is applied around the neck and half-hitches are placed behind the front legs and around the flanks. Traction is applied backwards.

c. harness an arrangement of leather or webbing straps, ropes and rings is applied to the hindlegs below the pasterns with ropes running forward through a shoulder harness. Traction on the ropes pulls the legs forward and the horse falls to one side. The ropes are used to tie the legs in a convenient position. Not suitable for use with cattle.

c. pen used at abattoirs to restrain animals that are to be slaughtered according to the Jewish law. It is a restraint cage or cradle which enables the operator to tip the animal onto its back so that it can be slaughtered while it is still conscious.

castor bean see RICINUS COMMUNIS.

castor bean tick see IXODES *ricinus*.

Castor canadensis (syn. *C. fiber*) see BEAVER.

castor oil a fixed oil obtained from the seed of the castor bean plant (RICINUS COMMUNIS); it has an irritant effect on the intestines and acts as a powerful purgative. Castor oil is also used externally as an emollient in seborrheic dermatitis and other skin diseases.

c. o. plant see RICINUS COMMUNIS.

false c. o. plant see DATURA.

Castor Rex see REX (2).

castrate 1. to deprive of the gonads, rendering the animal incapable of reproduction. 2. a castrated animal.

The strictly correct usage of the word is to apply it to animals of both sexes. Common usage is to restrict its use to the male.

castration excision of the gonads, or their destruction, as by radiation or parasites.

Burdizzo c. see BURDIZZO EMASCULATOME.

closed c. see covered castration (below).

covered c. the covering of the scrotal sac is incised and the testicle released still enclosed in its tunica vaginalis. The cord is ligatured and the testicle and its enveloping tunic removed in toto. Preferred for adult stallions or when the inguinal canal is considered to be sufficiently enlarged to permit eventration. Called also closed castration.

elastrator c. see ELASTRATOR.

female c. removal of the ovaries, or bilateral OOPHORECTOMY; spaying.

male c. removal of the testes, or bilateral ORCHIECTOMY.

mutilatory c. castration of companion animal males is thought by some to be an unnecessary mutilation. The view applies particularly to dogs. In the conflict between the animal liberators and those concerned with restraining the growth of the cat and dog populations, the zero population growth advocates hold most of the cards.

open c. incision through the tunica vaginalis. Compare with covered castration (above).

prepubertal c. in sheep, castration of males before puberty may result in a greater risk of subsequent obstructive urolithiasis because of failure of the urethra to fully develop its potential for dilatation.

c.-responsive dermatosis some dogs with hyposomatotropism or growth hormone-responsive dermatosis will regrow hair after castration. The etiology is unclear.

standing c. one done under sedation with local anesthetic with the animal standing. Most commonly done in horses.

Castroviejo ophthalmic instruments a series of ophthalmic surgical instruments including corneal scissors, forceps and trephines, razor blade holder, eyelid speculum and needle holder.

casualty an accident; an accidental wound; death or disablement from an accident; also the animal so injured.

c. slaughter abattoir slaughtering of injured or sick animals. Rarely done these days because of the difficulty of getting cattle with fractured or dislocated limbs onto the abattoir floor. The modern, highly automated meat packing plant is not geared to such interruptions.

Casuaris see CASSOWARY.

CAT computerized axial tomography. See computed TOMOGRAPHY.

cat any member of the family Felidae, including the domestic cat, *Felis catus*, and many exotic (here taken to mean nondomestic or zoological, rather than extraterritorial) species. See also FELINE.

c.-bite abscess a common sequela to a frequent injury. Particularly during the mating season, but also at other times, cats are likely to inflict or be subjected to bites or scratches during fighting or even vigorous play with each other. These contaminated puncture wounds, which are prone to abscessation, can be located anywhere on the body, but most often occur at the tail base, lower limbs and around the head and neck. *Pasteurella* spp., *Bacteroides* spp., fusiform bacilli and β-hemolytic streptococci are commonly involved.

c. breeds are generally of two groups, the longhair and shorthair types. Within these, there are numerous specific breeds whose differences may be great, in conformation, color and certain distinctive features, or slight, on the basis of coat and/or eye coloring.

The longhaired breeds, also called Persians, are of short, stocky (cobby) build with broad, short heads, small ears, large round eyes, and short, thick legs. One variety, the PEKE-FACED, has an extremely short nose. There are some specific breed types, but in general, they are divided on the basis of coat color, sometimes qualified by pattern of pigmentation or eye color, and the list is very long. The major groups are: solid colors (black, blue-eyed white, orange-eyed white, odd-eyed white, blue, chocolate, lilac, red, cream), broken colors (tabbies, TORTOISESHELL, cream, bicolors and harlequin), shaded colors (SMOKE, CHINCHILLA, silver and CAMEO), HIMALAYAN (1)/COLORPOINT (various colors). Additional longhaired breeds are the ANGORA, BIRMAN, BALINESE, CYMRIC, JAVANESE, MAINE COON, ORIENTAL LONGHAIR, RAGDOLL and TURKISH VAN.

The shorthaired breeds include: ABYSSINIAN, AMERICAN CURL, BENGAL, BOMBAY, BRITISH SHORTHAIR, BURMESE, CALIFORNIA SPANGLED, EXOTIC SHORTHAIR, HAVANA BROWN, KORAT, MANX (may be longhair or shorthair), ORIENTAL (many different color groups), REX, RUSSIAN BLUE, SIAMESE (further divided on the basis of color in their points), SINGAPURA, SOMALI and TONKINESE.

In addition, there is the CANADIAN HAIRLESS or Sphinx cat which is hairless.

c. fancy a term used in reference to breeders, registration bodies, clubs and societies, and any other groups sharing a common interest in cats (cat fanciers).

c. fever see FELINE panleukopenia.

c. flu see FELINE viral respiratory disease complex, feline CALICIVIRUS infection, feline viral RHINOTRACHEITIS.

c. foot in dog conformation describes a round, compact, foot with tightly bunched, arched toes.

c. fur mite see LYNXACARUS *radovsky*.

c. leprosy a granulomatous skin infection associated with *Mycobacterium lepraemurium*, the rat leprosy bacillus, hence the name. Infection is commonly believed to be the result of a rat bite. Single or multiple, painless, sometimes ulcerated nodular lesions are usually located around the head or on limbs. The organisms can be seen with acid-fast stains on direct smears or in biopsy material. Where possible, surgical excision is usually curative.

c. plague see FELINE panleukopenia.

pouting c. see fat-CHIN.

c. pox see COWPOX.

scabby c. disease feline miliary DERMATITIS.

c. scratch fever see CAT-SCRATCH DISEASE.

swimming c. see TURKISH VAN.

cat-bite fever an infectious disease of humans transmitted by the bite of a cat, caused by *Pasteurella multocida* and marked by the formation of an abscess at the site of inoculation. NOTE: Not to be confused with CAT-SCRATCH DISEASE.

cat flea CTENOCEPHALIDES *felis*.

cat-scratch disease a benign, subacute, regional lymphadenitis of humans believed to be caused by *Bartonella henselae* and usually associated with a scratch or bite of a cat or a scratch from a surface contaminated by a cat. Called also benign lymphoreticulosis. Not to be confused with CAT-BITE FEVER.

cat(a)- word element. [Gr.] *down, lower, under, against, along with, very.*

catabasis the stage of decline of a disease.

catabiosis the natural senescence of cells.

catabolic see CATABOLISM.

catabolin one of the monokine group of substances which stimulates bone resorption but only in the presence of osteoblasts. Called also IL-1, interleukin-1.

catabolism any destructive process by which complex substances are converted by living cells into simpler compounds, with release of energy. See also METABOLISM.

catabolite a compound produced in catabolism.

catacrotism a pulse anomaly in which a small additional wave or notch appears in the descending limb of the pulse tracing.

catadicrotism a pulse anomaly in which two small additional waves or notches appear in the descending limb of the pulse tracing.

catadromy migration of fish, as subadults or adults, from fresh to sea water.

catagen a transitional stage in the cycle of hair growth between active growth (anagen) and resting (telogen).

catagenesis involution or retrogression.

Catagonus wagneri Chacoan peccary.

Catahoula, Catahoula hog dog, Catahoula leopard dog an American dog breed, named after a parish in Louisiana where it was used to herd hogs, but is now used for cattle. It is a large dog with a short, merle and black and tan coat.

Catalan ass a Spanish black, dark gray or brown donkey with paler underline.

catalase a heme-containing enzyme that specifically catalyzes the decomposition of hydrogen peroxide and is found in almost all cells except certain anaerobic bacteria. The reaction can be used as a test in the identification of bacteria.

catalepsy a condition of diminished responsiveness usually characterized by a trancelike state and constantly maintained immobility, often with flexibilitas cerea (a waxy rigidity of muscles). In humans, the patient with catalepsy may remain in one position for minutes, days, or even longer.

cataleptiform resembling catalepsy.

catalysis increase in the velocity of a chemical reaction or process produced by the presence of a substance that is not consumed in the net chemical reaction or process; negative catalysis denotes the slowing down or inhibition of a reaction or process by the presence of such a substance.

covalent c. one type of enzyme reaction with substrates to form very unstable, covalently joined enzyme–substrate complexes which undergo further reaction the products.

catalyst any substance that brings about catalysis.

catalytic constant first-order rate constant (k_{cat}) reflecting the turnover number of the enzyme, or the number of molecules of substrate converted to product per unit time, when the enzyme is working at maximum efficiency. Called also turnover number.

catalyze to cause or produce catalysis.

catamnesis the follow-up history of a patient after it is discharged from treatment or a hospital.

catamnestic pertaining to catamnesis.

cataphora lethargy with intervals of imperfect waking.

cataphoresis introduction of ions of soluble salts through the intact skin by means of electrical current. Called also iontophoresis.

cataphoria a downward turning of the visual axes of both eyes after visual functional stimuli have been removed.

cataphylaxis movement of leukocytes and antibodies to the site of an infection.

cataplasia atrophy with tissues reverting to earlier, or more embryonic conditions.

cataplasm see POULTICE.

cataplexy a condition, often associated with NARCOLEPSY; marked by abrupt attacks of a loss of voluntary muscular function (flaccid paralysis), except those controlling respiration and eye movement. Observed in dogs, cats and horses, especially Shetland ponies. In dogs these have been precipitated by extreme excitement, vigorous physical or sexual activity. Usually of short duration. Most cases are idiopathic, but can be associated with lesions of the brainstem.

food-elicited c. test cataleptic dogs demonstrate repeated attacks of catalepsy when presented with several individual pieces of food.

cataract opacity of the lens of the eye or its capsule or both. Cataract may result from injuries to the eye, exposure to great heat or radiation, or inherited factors. Rare in cattle and swine, common in dogs. Treatment consists of surgical removal of the lens (lens extraction or cataract extraction). May affect the entire lens or be localized, e.g. posterior polar cataract.

acquired c. any non-congenital cataract; usually the result of trauma, systemic disease or another eye disorder.

after-c. 1. any membrane of the pupillary area after extraction or absorption of the lens. 2. secondary cataract (below).

capsular c. one consisting of an opacity of the capsule of the lens.
complicated c. a cataract occurring secondarily to other intraocular disease.
congenital c. present at birth; often not progressive. See also WHITE EYE CALF SYNDROME.
cortical c. an opacity in the cortex of the lens. The common form of cataract in dogs; inherited in many breeds, often in association with progressive RETINAL atrophy.
developmental c. one that occurs at any age before the animal becomes an adult.
diabetic c. one associated with diabetes mellitus.
electric c. one caused by electrical current as in electrocution.
embryonal c. one caused by prenatal influences.
focal ring c. a perinuclear opacity with normal lens fibers surrounding it. Usually the result of an in utero or neonatal insult to the lens.
galactosemic c. see GALACTOSEMIA.
hyaloid c. a focal opacity at the point where the hyaloid artery meets the posterior lens capsule. See also MITTENDORF'S DOT.
hypermature c. one in which the lens has begun to liquefy.
immature c. incomplete opacity.
incipient c. a very early stage of development with no impairment of vision.
inherited c. occurs in a number of breeds of cattle, often in combination with other abnormalities of the eye. Affected calves are usually normal in other respects and can be reared if the inconvenience of their blindness can be overcome. Also occurs in dogs, often with late onset and in association with other inherited ocular defects such as progressive retinal atrophy.
intumescent c. a mature cataract that has become swollen.
juvenile c. one developing in very young animals, for example dogs less than 6 months of age.
lenticular c. opacity of the lens not affecting the capsule.
mature c. one in which the lens is completely opaque.
morgagnian c. liquefaction, except the nucleus which drops to the bottom of the lens, and shrinkage of the capsule.
nuclear c. one involving the nucleus of the lens; the common form of congenital cataracts.
nuclear Y c. a form of congenital cataract in which small opacities outline the Y suture of the nucleus.
nutritional c. see GALACTOSEMIA.
radiation c. one caused by radiation, as in radiotherapy.
reduplication c. a capsular opacity covered by another layer of epithelium.
secondary c. 1. one that forms after most of the lens has been removed. 2. complicated cataract.
senile c. occurs in the aged of all species, preceded by nuclear SCLEROSIS.
subcapsular c. may be anterior or posterior. Inherited in several breeds of dogs.
toxic c. one caused by exposure to a toxic substance.
traumatic c. one caused by trauma.

cataracta [L.] *cataract.*

cataractogenic tending to induce the formation of cataracts.

catarrh inflammation of a mucous membrane (particularly of the head and throat), with free discharge.
bovine malignant c. see BOVINE malignant catarrh.
nasal c. see NASAL catarrh of rabbits.

catarrhal having the characteristic of catarrh.
bovine c. fever see BOVINE malignant catarrh.
ovine c. fever see BLUETONGUE.

catastrophe theory the mathematical basis for the study of large changes in a total system which may result from small changes in a critical variable in the system.

catatricrotism a pulse anomaly in which three small additional waves or notches appear in the descending limb of the pulse tracing.

Catatropis a genus of intestinal flukes (digenetic trematodes) of the family Notocotylidae. Includes *Catatropis verrucosa* (avian ceca).

catching pens small enclosures in the shearing shed from which the sheep are dragged onto the shearing floor to be shorn.

catchment area the region from which the data in a particular study are drawn.

catclaw ACACIA *gregii.*

catechol a compound, *o*-dehydroxybenzene, used as a reagent and comprising the aromatic portion in the synthesis of catecholamines.

catecholamine any of a group of sympathomimetic amines (including dopamine, epinephrine and norepinephrine), the aromatic portion of whose molecule is catechol.

The catecholamines play an important role in the body's physiological response to stress. Their release at sympathetic nerve endings increases the rate and force of muscular contraction of the heart, thereby increasing cardiac output; constricts peripheral blood vessels, resulting in elevated blood pressure; elevates blood glucose levels by hepatic and skeletal muscle glycogenolysis; and promotes an increase in blood lipids by increasing the catabolism of fats.
c.-depleting agents cause depletion of neuronal stores of norepinephrine, thereby reducing adrenergic responses, e.g. reserpine.

catecholaminergic activated by or secreting catecholamines.
c. receptor there are a variety of receptors that react differently with each of the catecholamine agonists and antagonists. It is therefore possible to blockade these receptors selectively.

catechu a powerful astringent formerly used internally for the treatment of diarrhea. Contains 25 to 35% catechutannic acid. Prepared from the heartwood of the leguminous tree *Acacia catechu.*

categorical data data relating to category such as qualitative data, e.g. dog, cat, female. It may be nominal when a name is used, e.g. location, breed, or ordinal when a range of categories is used, e.g. calf, yearling, cow.

caterpillar the larval stage of insects of the Lepidoptera family.
army c. see PSEUDOLETIA SEPARATA.
c. cell see ANITSCHKOW CELL.
hairy c. see HAIRY caterpillars.

catfish primitive, eel-like, freshwater fish; naked or covered with spines or plates but not scales. Members of the suborder *Siluroidea,* catfish are divided into many families, genera and species, e.g. blue, bullhead, channel, electric.

catgut an absorbable sterile strand derived from the intestinal submucosa of sheep and fixed in formalin, used as a surgical ligature and suture.
chromic c. treated with basic chromate salts; the suture does not absorb as much water as ordinary catgut and has a longer life and is stronger than the untreated product.

Catha edulis plant of the family Celastraceae. A

small, rare African tree. Contains an unidentified toxin which causes depression, muscle spasms and dysentery. The leaves are chewed by humans for their narcotic effect. Called also khat, gat, caffa.

Cathaemasiidae a family of alimentary tract flukes (digenetic trematodes) of birds.

Catharanthus a genus of the plant family of Apocynaceae; contains an unidentified toxin which causes incoordination and convulsions; includes *C. pusilla* (milagaipoondu), *C. roseus*.

C. roseus souce of vincine alkaloids used in cancer chemotherapy; called also Madagascan periwinkle.

catharsis a cleansing or purgation.

Cathartes aura see VULTURE.

cathartic 1. causing bowel evacuation, usually of liquid feces; an agent that so acts. 2. producing catharsis.

bulk c. one stimulating bowel evacuation by increasing fecal volume.

irritant c. contact irritants that directly or indirectly cause diarrhea. May cause superpurgation in susceptible animals, especially horses. Drastic purgatives such as croton oil are no longer used. Castor oil, danthron, senna and cascara are still used, but much less than more bland agents such as mineral oil.

lubricant c. one that acts by softening the feces and reducing friction between them and the intestinal wall.

osmotic c. agents which retain water into the intestinal lumen, thereby producing liquid feces; includes saline cathartics (below).

saline c. one that increases fluidity of intestinal contents by retention of water by osmotic forces, and indirectly increases motor activity.

stimulant c. one that directly increases motor activity of the intestinal tract.

cathepsin a proteinase found in most cells, which takes part in cell autolysis and self-digestion of tissues.

c. D an acid hydrolase isolated from cartilage which plays a part in the endogenous degradation of proteoglycans in degenerative diseases of joints.

catheter a tubular, flexible instrument, passed through body channels for withdrawal of fluids from (or introduction of fluids into) a body cavity.

angiographic c. one through which a contrast medium is injected for visualization of the vascular system of an organ. Such catheters may have preformed ends to facilitate selective locating (as in a renal or coronary vessel) from a remote entry site. They may be named according to the site of entry and destination, such as *femoral–renal* and *brachial–coronary*.

arterial c. one inserted into an artery and utilized as part of a catheter–transducer–monitor system to continuously observe the BLOOD PRESSURE of critically ill patients. An arterial catheter also may be inserted for x-ray studies of the arterial system and for delivery of chemotherapeutic agents directly into the arterial supply of malignant tumors.

cardiac c. a long, fine catheter especially designed for passage, usually through a peripheral blood vessel, into the chambers of the heart under fluoroscopic control. See also CARDIAC catheterization.

cardiac biopsy c. introduced intravenously under the direction of fluoroscopy, can be positioned in the right or left ventricle and an endocardial biopsy obtained.

central venous c. a long, fine catheter inserted into a vein for the purpose of administering through a large blood vessel parenteral fluids (as in parenteral NUTRITION), antibiotics and other therapeutic agents. This type of catheter is also used in the measurement of CENTRAL venous pressure. See also CENTRAL venous catheterization.

column disk c. an indwelling device for continuous peritoneal dialysis. It is implanted within the peritoneal cavity, resting against the body wall. The attached Silastic tubing is used for infusing and draining the dialysate at intervals.

double-lumen c. one having two channels; one for injection and one for removal of fluid.

c. drainage a catheter left in place to keep the bladder drained. Preferably should have a one-way valve to avoid aspiration of air and infection.

elbowed c. a catheter bent at an angle near the beak.

indwelling c. one especially designed so that it is held in place in the urethra for the purpose of draining urine from the bladder.

intravenous c. a large-bore sharp needle housed with an indwelling stilette, inside a thin-walled plastic tube. An incision is made over the filled vein, the needle-cannula inserted, the stilette withdrawn, then the needle, leaving the plastic cannula in situ.

self-retaining c. one constructed to remain in the bladder, effecting constant drainage.

tracheal c. one with small holes at the terminal 1 inch, especially designed for removal of secretions during tracheal SUCTIONING.

ureteral c. a long, extremely small gauge catheter designed for insertion directly into a ureter.

urethral c. any of various types of catheters designed for insertion via the urethra into the urinary bladder. See also CATHETERIZATION.

catheterization passage of a catheter into a body channel or cavity. See also CARDIAC catheterization and CENTRAL venous catheterization. The most common usage of the term is in reference to the introduction of a catheter via the urethra into the urinary bladder.

balloon c. see balloon VALVULOPLASTY.

catheterize to introduce a catheter into a body cavity, usually into the urinary bladder for the withdrawal of urine.

cathode 1. the negative electrode, from which electrons are emitted and to which positive ions are attracted. 2. the electrode through which current leaves a nerve or other substance.

c. beam, c. ray the beam of electrons, accompanied by high electrical potential which flows from the cathode to the anode in the x-ray tube and interacts with the tungsten target to produce x-rays.

c. filament the source of electrons in the cathode tube that interacts with the anode target to produce x-rays.

cathodic pertaining to or emanating from a cathode.

cathomycin see NOVOBIOCIN.

cation a positively charged ion.

c.–anion balance the balance in serum or plasma between the anions and cations must equilibrate near to the level of 155 mEq/l. Estimation of any imbalance, usually by chloride and bicarbonate measurement, is basic to any determination of acid–base abnormality.

c. channels channels through selectively permeable membranes via which only cations can migrate.

c.-exchange resin ion-exchange resin.

cation-exchange chromatography see ion-exchange CHROMATOGRAPHY.

cationic having qualities dependent on having free cations available.

c. detergents are wetting agents that disrupt or damage cell membranes, denature proteins and inactivate enzymes. Examples are the quaternary ammonium compounds.

catnip a plant in the mint family (*Nepeta cataria*) that contains the volatile terpenoid, nepetalactone. It has distinctive aromatic qualities that are particularly attractive to cats, inducing behavior that is variously described as sexual, playful, and sometimes as hallucinatory. Often included in stuffed toys marketed for the domestic cat.

Catostomus commersoni the common sucker fish, a secondary host for *Metorchis conjunctus*, a fluke of cats and dogs.

catpox a poxvirus infection of cats in the UK, believed to be the cowpox virus, characterized by multiple nodules and ulcerated lesions of the skin, mainly on the head, face, ears, neck and forelimbs. Occasionally there is conjunctivitis and oral ulceration and rarely generalized infection with fatal respiratory involvement.

catsear HYPOCHOERIS RADICATA.

catshead, catshead burr TRIBULUS *terrestris*.

cattalo produced in Canada by mating British beef bulls to bison cows. See also BEEFALO.

cattery a housing facility for cats; usually for boarding or breeding.

cattle members of the Bovidae family. There are wild cattle (*Bibos* spp.) including Banteng, Gaur and Gayal. They resemble domestic cattle but have a hump on their back. Domestic cattle are all members of the *Bos* genus. There are two species: *Bos taurus* or European or British breeds of cattle, and *Bos indicus* the Zebu or oriental domestic cattle. The common breeds of each are set out below. Interbreeding between the species is common, the offspring being called taurindicus or zeboid cattle.

beef c. breeds of cattle bred especially for the economic production of meat. See BEEF breeds.

c. breeding herds commercial cattle herds which produce beef calves for sale to fatteners.

commercial c. cattle used to produce milk or meat for the general market.

dairy c. cattle used solely for the production of dairy products. Called also milk or milch cows. See DAIRY breeds.

c. dog dogs used to herd and work cattle. See AUSTRALIAN cattle dog, WORKING DOGS.

dual-purpose c. most breeds of cattle in continental Europe are of this type. They produce heavy yields of milk and are also good carcass cattle. See DUAL-PURPOSE.

c. grubs see HYPODERMA. Called also warble fly.

c. louse see HAEMATOPINUS and LINOGNATHUS.

pedigree c. cattle that are registered in a recognized stud book.

purebred c. cattle produced by matings between members of the same breed, not necessarily pedigreed cattle.

stud c. pedigree cattle maintained as a separate herd, whose offspring are ofen sold as breeders, forming a major source of income for the enterprise.

c. tick any one of a large variety of tick species, the title being used locally to designate the preponderant species.

young c. farmers' term for weaned calves, yearlings and 2-year old-cattle.

cattle grid see STOCK guard.

cattle plague see RINDERPEST.

cattle tick fever see BABESIOSIS. Called also Texas fever, redwater fever.

Caucasian brown cattle brown with dark markings, dual-purpose cattle from Russia.

cauda pl. *caudae* [L.] a tail or tail-like appendage.

c. equina the collection of spinal roots that stream caudally from the end of the spinal cord and occupy the vertebral canal.

c. equina compression see LUMBOSACRAL stenosis.

c. equina syndrome see CAUDA EQUINA NEURITIS.

c. helicis caudal process of the helix of the ear of the dog.

cauda equina neuritis a nonsuppurative inflammation of the nerve trunks of the cauda equina in horses. It is characterized by paralysis of the tail, slackness of the anus and rectum which may lead to fecal incontinence, paralysis of the bladder sometimes with urinary incontinence, paresthesia or anesthesia of the tail and perineum, and incoordination of the hindlimbs. There may also be involvement of isolated cranial nerves. It is believed to be an immune-mediated disorder. Called also polyneuritis equi.

caudad directed toward the tail or distal end; opposite of cephalad.

caudal 1. pertaining to a cauda. 2. situated more towards the cauda, or tail, than some specified reference point; toward the inferior (in humans) or hinder (in animals) end of the body. See also POSTERIOR.

c. anesthesia a type of regional anesthesia in which the anesthetizing solution is injected into the caudal area of the spinal canal through the caudal end of the sacrum and tail. It affects the caudal nerve roots, and renders the cervix, vagina and perineum insensitive to pain.

c. cervical instability see WOBBLER SYNDROME. Called also caudal cervical malformation–malarticulation.

c. cervical malformation/malarticulation caudal cervical instability (see WOBBLER SYNDROME).

c. fold test the single intradermal (SID) fold tuberculin test for tuberculosis.

c. impression of liver the renal impression.

c. sheath part of the maturation process of spermatid to spermatozoa; a caudal sheath of microtubules develops at the caudal edge of the head cap. Called also manchette.

c. tailfold when the cow's tail is lifted there are two, rarely a single central, folds of skin from the edges of the ventral surface of the tail to beside the anus. The site of injection and a control for the single intradermal test. See also caudal fold test (above).

c. tract usually refers to the tubular part of the female genital tract.

c. vena cava see VENA cava.

c. vena caval thrombosis thrombosis of the caudal vena cava arises from an hepatic abscess. The commonest result is the subsequent shedding of emboli and the development of a chronic pulmonary disease often terminated by massive pulmonary hemorrhage and bleeding to death through the mouth and nostrils. Others suffer a chronic course with anemia, dyspnea and persistent cough and are euthanatized because of cachexia and prolonged distress.

caudate having a tail.

caudatum the caudate nucleus.

caudectomy sophisticated version of tail docking as practiced in dogs.

caul, caul fat meat hygiene term for the omentum and its contained fat depots.

cauliflower BRASSICA *oleracea* var. *botrytis*.

c. saltwort SALSOLA *tuberculatiformis*.

causal relating to or emanating from cause.

c. association a noxious agent is said to have a causal association with a particular disease when it can be shown that it plays some role in producing the occurrence of the disease. Generally both biological information and statistical information are combined to infer causal associations.

c. inference preliminary diagnosis.

c. modeling construction of models which set out the various relationships between causal agents and the initiation of a disease.

causality the relationship between cause and effects.

principle of c. the postulate that every phenomenon has a cause or causes, i.e. that events do not occur at random but in accordance with physical laws so that, in principle, causes can be found for each effect.

causation the relation of cause to effect.

c. analysis comparison of the rate of occurrence of the disease in animals which were exposed to the suspected agent to the occurrence rate in animals which were not so exposed.

cause in diseases, an agent, event, condition or characteristic which plays an essential role in producing an occurrence of the disease. Because there is nowadays much less certainty about what actually establishes a disease state it is becoming more common to use terms such as disease determinants, causal association, causal relationship. KOCH's postulates are no longer the sole criterion used in establishing causality.

constitutional c. an inherent characteristic of the patient. Usually a systemic defect, e.g. protoporphyria.

direct c. there must be no known variable intervening between the suspect factor and the disease.

endogenous c. the cause comes from within the patient. See also constitutional cause (above).

exogenous c. the cause comes from outside the patient, e.g. a virus infection.

indirect c. all causes other than the direct cause (see above).

host c. see endogenous cause (above).

necessary c. a factor which must be present to produce disease; the disease does not occur unless the factor was or is present.

precipitating c. the trigger mechanism that initiates the commencement of the disease state.

predisposing c. a mechanism that makes a patient more susceptible to the precipitating cause.

primary c. the principal factor in causing the disease.

secondary c. a factor that assists the primary cause. A cause of secondary importance.

specific c. the single cause in a single cause–single disease relationship.

sufficient c. a minimal set of conditions and events which inevitably produce disease.

caustic 1. burning or corrosive; destructive to tissue. 2. having a burning taste. 3. a corrosive or escharotic agent.

c. bush SARCOSTEMMA *australe*, *S. viminale*.

bottle tree c. EREMOPHILA spp.

c. creeper EUPHORBIA *drummondii*, SARCOSTEMMA *viminale*.

lunar c. toughened silver nitrate.

c. pencil see SILVER nitrate (toughened).

c. plant SARCOSTEMMA *australe*.

c. potash potassium hydroxide.

c. soda sodium hydroxide.

c. treated grain grain treated with caustic to improve its digestibility; can cause abomasal ulcer and interstitial nephritis in cattle.

c. treated roughage roughage treated with caustic to improve its digestibility; can cause interstitial nephritis when fed to cows over long periods.

c. vine SARCOSTEMMA *australe*, *S. viminale*. Called also caustic bush.

c. weed EUPHORBIA *drummondii*.

cauterant 1. any caustic material or application. 2. caustic.

cauterization destruction of tissue with a cautery.

cautery 1. the application of a caustic agent, a hot instrument, an electric current, or other agent to destroy tissue. 2. an agent so used.

cold c. cauterization by carbon dioxide, called also cryocautery.

cava [L.] 1. plural of *cavum*. 2. a vena cava.

cavagram a radiograph of a vena cava.

caval syndrome syndrome caused by the presence of large number of heartworms (*Dirofilaria immitis*) in the posterior vena cava which may lead to the sudden onset of signs of hemolytic anemia and liver failure, often without preceding cardiopulmonary signs. Disseminated intravascular coagulopathy is a common complication and the mortality rate is high. Called also vena caval syndrome.

cavaletti a small, portable jump for schooling horses. Constructed of light poles, 4 to 6 ft long, resting on a cross of timber at each end so that the pole is 12 to 18 inches above the ground.

Cavalier King Charles spaniel a small (10–18 lb) dog with prominent eyes, short nose and floppy ears. The haircoat is long and silky. Several colors or combinations are recognized: black and tan, ruby (rich chestnut red), Blenheim (white with chestnut red patches), and tricolor (called Prince Charles in the United States) (white with black patches and tan markings). Similar to, but larger than, the KING CHARLES SPANIEL, and with a longer nose (at least 1.5 inches long). The breed suffers from cardiac valvular disease.

cave sickness histoplasmosis.

caveola pl. *caveolae* [L.] one of the minute pits or incuppings of the cell membrane formed during pinocytosis.

caveolae membrane-lined cavities.

thymic c. large, membrane-lined cavities in the outer cortex of the thymus in which marrow-derived lymphocytes develop sophisticated lymphogenous traits.

caveolated cell flask-shaped cells characterized by an apical tubulovesical system or tuft which are scattered through the epithelial cells of the small intestine. Their function is unknown. Called also tuft cells.

caverna pl. *cavernae* [L.] a cavity.

cavernitis inflammation of the corpora cavernosa or corpus spongiosum of the penis.

cavernoma cavernous hemangioma. See also HEMANGIOMA.

cavernosal venal shunt vascular shunt between the corpus cavernosum penis and the exterior circulation of the penis. Too many of them results in inability to erect the penis.

cavernositis cavernitis.

cavernosogram a radiographic picture of the vascular system in a penis. Radiopaque material is injected into the corpus cavernosum penis and a series of radiographs taken.

cavernostomy operative drainage of a pulmonary abscess of the lung.

cavernous pertaining to a hollow, or containing hollow spaces.

c. hemangioma see TELANGIECTASIA.

c. sinus see cavernous SINUS.

cavesson a leather head harness including a cheek strap that goes over the poll and supports a noseband that usually goes right around the head, and a brow band. Used as a point of attachment for a martingale or a leading shank. See also NOSEBAND.

Cavia a genus of the rodent family of Caviidae, the guinea pigs.
C. porcellus see GUINEA PIG.
Caviacoptes caviae see TRIXACARUS *caviae*.
cavitary characterized by the presence of a cavity or cavities.
cavitas pl. *cavitates* [L.] cavity.
cavitate formation of cavities.
cavitation the formation of cavities; also, a cavity.
cavitis inflammation of a vena cava.
cavity 1. a hollow or space, or a potentional space, within the body (e.g. abdominal cavity) or one of its organs (e.g. cranial cavity). 2. in teeth, the lesion produced by dental CARIES.
absorption c's cavities in developing compact bone due to osteoclastic erosion, usually occurring in the areas laid down first.
amniotic c. the closed sac between the embryo and the amnion, containing the amniotic fluid.
cranial c. the space enclosed by the bones of the cranium.
dental c. 1. the central space, often branched or multiple in compound teeth, of each tooth; carries the nerve and blood supplies to the teeth. 2. the defect caused by decay on a tooth surface. Called also CARIES.
glenoid c. a depression in the ventral angle of the scapula for articulation with the humerus.
infraglottic c. the space in the larynx caudal to the vocal folds; reflects the shape of the cricoid cartilage.
medullary (marrow) c. the cavity, containing marrow, in the diaphysis of a long bone; called also medullary canal.
nasal c. the proximal part of the respiratory tract, within the nose, bisected by the nasal septum and extending from the nares to the pharynx. Much of the cavity is occupied by the turbinate bones or conchae which also divide it into dorsal, medial and ventral meatuses. The common meatus is the narrow, vertical passage close to the nasal septum. The rostral end of the cavity just inside the nostril is the nasal vestibule, and the caudal part opening into the pharynx is the nasopharyngeal meatus.
oral c. the cavity of the mouth, made up of a vestibule and oral cavity proper.
pelvic c. the space within the walls of the pelvis.
pericardial c. the potential space between the epicardium and the parietal layer of the serous pericardium.
peritoneal c. the potential space between the parietal and the visceral peritoneum.
pleural c. the potential space between the parietal and the visceral pleura.
pulp c. the pulp-filled central chamber in a tooth; called also dental cavity.
serous c. a celomic cavity, like that enclosed by the pericardium, peritoneum or pleura, not communicating with the outside of the body and lined with a serous membrane, i.e. one which secretes a serous fluid.
tension c. cavities of the lung in which the air pressure is greater than that of the atmosphere.
thoracic c. the body cavity situated between the neck and the diaphragm.
tympanic c. the cavity of the middle ear.
uterine c. the space within the uterus communicating on either side with the uterine tubes and caudally with the vagina.
cavography radiography of the vena cava.
cavum pl. *cava* [L.] cavity.
c. conchae that part of the ear canal supported by the deeper, conchal part of the auricular cartilage.
cavus [L.] *hollow*.
cavvy, cavy the group of saddle horses on a cattle ranch used to work cattle. Called also remuda.
cavy a GUINEA PIG, *Cavia porcellus*.
spotted c. see cavy (above).
cayenne tick see AMBLYOMMA *cajennense*.
cayuse the strong, hardy pony used by American Indians.
CBC complete blood (cell) count. See also BLOOD COUNT.
CBG corticosteroid-binding globulin.
CBH cutaneous basophil hypersensitivity.
CBP competitive protein binding.
CBPP see CONTAGIOUS bovine pleuropneumonia.
CC medical record abbreviation for chief complaint.
cc cubic centimeter.
CCK, CCK–PZ see CHOLECYSTOKININN.
CCl_4 see CARBON TETRACHLORIDE.
c.cm. cubic centimeter.
CCNU see LOMUSTINE.
CCPP contagious caprine pleuropneumonia.
CCS canine Cushing's syndrome.
CCU critical care unit.
CCV canine coronavirus.
CD[1] 1. canine distemper. 2. curative dose; that which is sufficient to restore normal health.
CD[2] cluster of differentiation or cell differentiation glycoproteins.
CD antigen a group of cell surface molecules which act as markers on T lymphocytes.
CD3 found on T helper (Th) and T cytotoxic (Tc) lymphocytes; associated with signal transduction.
CD4 found on T helper lymphocytes; an adhesion molecule that binds to class II MHC molecules.
CD8 found on T cytotoxic and variably on NK lymphocytes; an adhesion molecule that binds to class I MHC molecules.
CD_{50} median curative dose.
C.D. Companion Dog; the first level degree or title earned in obedience trials.
Cd 1. chemical symbol, *cadmium*. 2. caudal or coccygeal.
cd see CANDELA.
CD-ROM *C*ompact *D*isk-*R*ead *O*nly *M*emory. Massive data storage, a disk can hold as much as 650 megabytes of information, equal to half a billion text characters, but can only be read, not edited.
CD virus canine DISTEMPER virus.
CDAA allidochlor.
CDEC sulfallate.
Cdk cyclin-dependent protein kinase.
cDNA 1. complementary DNA. 2. copy DNA.
CDP cytidine diphosphate.
CDR complementary-determining regions of an antibody.
CDS method calibrated dichotomous sensitivity test; a form of the disk diffusion antimicrobial sensitivity test.
CDV canine distemper virus.
C.D.X. Companion Dog Excellent; the second level degree or title, after C.D., earned in obedience trials.
CE continuing education, client education.
Ce chemical symbol, *cerium*.
ce- for words beginning thus, see also those beginning *coe-*.
CEA carcinoembryonic antigen; collie eye anomaly; previously, canine erythrocyte antigen, which is now replaced by dog erythrocyte antigen (DEA).
Cebalges members of Psoroptidae family of mange mites. Includes *Cebalges gaudi* (primates).
Cebidae a family of non-human primates that includes New World monkeys.

cebocephalia congenital deformity of the head resembling a monkey; the nose is defective and the eyes close together. Called also cebocephaly.

cebocephaly see CEBOCEPHALIA.

Cebus see CAPUCHIN MONKEY.

ceca plural of CECUM.

cecal arising from or pertaining to the CECUM.

c. blackhead see HISTOMONAS *meleagridis*.

chicken c. worms *Heterakis*, *Subulura* spp., *Strongyloides avium*, *Trichostrongylus tenuis*, *Aulonocephalus lindquisti*.

c. coccidiosis see COCCIDIOSIS.

c. coliform granuloma a nodular condition of the intestines, liver and cecum.

c. dilatation a disease of cows which occurs soon after calving characterized by moderate abdominal pain, reduction in fecal volume, and a distended viscus in the upper right flank detectable externally or by rectal examination. Called also cecal dilatation and torsion but the circulation of the organ is rarely compromised. In horses it is usually part of tympany of the large intestine. See flatulent COLIC.

c. dilatation and torsion see cecal dilatation (above).

c. impaction in the horse can prove to be a serious problem because of the difficulty of moving a large volume of dry ingesta from such a large atonic viscus. The clinical picture is one of continuous low-grade colic with scant feces. A feature of mucoid enteropathy in rabbits.

c. inflammation see CECITIS.

c. intussusception see intestinal obstruction COLIC, INTUSSUSCEPTION.

c. inversion see cecocolic INTUSSUSCEPTION.

c. rupture is a specific entity in horses because it occurs during the act of foaling. Death occurs very quickly due to toxic shock.

c. torsion in cows is part of the syndrome of cecal dilatation. In horses constitutes a very serious threat to life. See also intestinal obstruction COLIC, RED GUT SYNDROME.

c. tympany see cecal dilatation (above), flatulent COLIC. Also occurs as an independent entity in young foals and causes acute colic with abdominal distension. The cause is unknown. It also occurs in newborn foals in conjunction with retained MECONIUM.

cecectomy excision of the cecum.

cecilian limbless, wormlike amphibian in the order Apoda.

cecitis inflammation of the cecum; occurs commonly as a part of a general inflammation of the bowel. The most common cause in dogs is infestation with whipworms (*Trichuris vulpis*). Called also typhlitis.

ceco- word element. [L.] *cecum*.

cecocele a hernia containing part of the cecum.

cecocolic pertaining to the cecum and the colon.

c. intussusception see cecocolic INTUSSUSCEPTION.

c. ostium opening between cecum and colon. Called also cecocolic ostium.

cecocolopexy an operation for fixation or suspension of the cecum and ascending colon.

cecocolostomy surgical anastomosis of the cecum and the colon.

cecoileostomy ileocecostomy; surgical anastomosis of the ileum to the cecum.

cecopexy fixation or suspension of the cecum to correct excessive mobility.

cecoplication plication of the cecal wall to correct ptosis or dilatation. An inverting stitch, e.g. Lembert, will also plicate the cecum. This could be used over a weakened wall which is still viable, e.g. needle decompression site.

cecorrhaphy suture or repair of the cecum.

cecostomy surgical creation of an artificial opening or fistula into the cecum.

cecotomy incision of the cecum.

cecotroph soft fecal pellets, ingested by rabbits directly from the anus during the night and early morning.

cecotrophy ingestion of cecotrophs; occurs in rabbits. See COPROPHAGY.

cecum 1. the first or proximal part of the large intestine, forming a dilated pouch distal to the ileum and proximal to the colon. There is a great deal of variation in the relative size between species. The dog's cecum is a small, coiled organ. In the horse it is a very large fermentation chamber stretching from the upper right flank to the xiphoid process of the sternum. Birds are different again. They have a double cecum which appears to compensate digestively for the absence of a significant colon. 2. any blind pouch. See also CECAL.

c. cupulare one of the blind ends of the cochlear duct of the inner ear; attached to the cupula of the cochlea.

c. vestibulare the other blind end of the cochlear duct of the inner ear; begins in the cochlear recess of the vestibule of the osseous labyrinth.

cecum–colon appertaining to the cecum and colon together.

c.–c. rupture rupture of the dorsal sac of the cecum or the colon in mares at foaling.

c.–c. tympany idiopathic in foals.

cefaclor a second generation CEPHALOSPORIN antibiotic, administered orally. Not widely used in veterinary medicine.

cefadroxil a first generation CEPHALOSPORIN antibiotic.

cefamandole a second generation CEPHALOSPORIN antibiotic.

cefapirin see CEPHAPIRIN.

cefazolin a first generation CEPHALOSPORIN antibiotic, given by injection; it has a long half-life.

cefixime a third generation CEPHALOSPORIN antibiotic.

cefmenoxime a third generation CEPHALOSPORIN antibiotic.

cefmetazole a second generation CEPHALOSPORIN antibiotic.

cefoperazone a third generation CEPHALOSPORIN antibiotic.

cefotaxime a third generation CEPHALOSPORIN antibiotic.

cefotetan a second generation CEPHALOSPORIN antibiotic.

cefoxitin sodium a second generation CEPHALOSPORIN antibiotic, especially effective against gram–negative organisms, with strong resistance to degradation by β-lactamase.

cefsulodin a second generation CEPHALOSPORIN antibiotic with a narrow range of activity.

ceftazidime a third generation CEPHALOSPORIN antibiotic, active mainly against gram-negative bacteria and particularly *Pseudomonas*.

ceftiofur a third generation CEPHALOSPORIN antibiotic.

ceftizoxime a third generation CEPHALOSPORIN antibiotic.

ceftriaxone a third generation CEPHALOSPORIN antibiotic.

cefuroxime a second generation CEPHALOSPORIN antibiotic.

cegadera see HETEROPHYLLAEA PUSTULATA.

celandine poppy see CHELIDONIUM MAJUS.
-cele word element. [Gr.] *tumor, hernia;* in American English, may also mean 'cavity'.
Celebes macaque see CYNOPITHECUS NIGER.
celery see APIUM GRAVEOLENS.
c. buttercup RANUNCULUS *sceleratus*.
c. leaved crowsfoot RANUNCULUS *sceleratus*.
celiac pertaining to the abdomen.
c. disease a malabsorption syndrome in humans characterized by marked atrophy and loss of function of the villi of the jejunum (and rarely, the cecum). Called also celiac sprue, gluten-induced enteropathy, nontropical sprue, and adult, childhood or infantile celiac disease. Occasionally suspected as the cause of villous atrophy in dogs.
celiac artery see Table 9.
celiacomesenteric ganglion the autonomic ganglion enmeshed in the celiacomesenteric plexus; located at origins of celiac and cranial mesenteric arteries.
celiectomy 1. excision of the celiac branches of the vagus nerve. 2. excision of an abdominal organ.
celio- abdominal. [Gr.] *abdomen, through the abdominal wall, cavity, hollow.*
celiocentesis puncture into the abdominal cavity.
celiocolpotomy incision into the abdomen through the vagina.
celioenterotomy incision through the abdominal wall into the intestine.
celiogastrotomy incision through the abdominal wall into the stomach.
celiography radiography of the abdomen.
celioma any tumor of the abdomen.
celiomyomectomy myomectomy by abdominal incision.
celiomyositis inflammation of the abdominal muscles.
celioparacentesis paracentesis of the abdominal cavity; more often the term abdominocentesis is used.
celiopathy any abdominal disease.
celiorrhaphy suture of the abdominal wall.
celioschisis, celoschisis congenital fissure of the abdominal wall.
celiotomy incision into the abdominal cavity.
vaginal c. incision into the abdominal cavity through the vagina.
cell 1. the basic structural unit of living organisms. 2. a small more or less enclosed space, e.g. at the intersection of a row and a column in a computer spreadsheet.

All living cells arise from other cells, either by division of one cell to make two, as in MITOSIS and MEIOSIS, or by fusion of two cells to make one, as in the union of the sperm and ovum to make the zygote in sexual reproduction.

All cells are bounded by a structure called the *cell membrane* or *plasma membrane*, which is a *lipid bilayer* composed of two layers of phospholipids. Each layer is one molecule thick with the charged, hydrophilic end of the lipid molecules on the surface of the membrane and the uncharged hydrophobic fatty acid tails in the interior of the membrane.

Cells are divided into two classes, eukaryotic cells and prokaryotic cells:

Eukaryotic cells have a true nucleus, which contains the genetic material, composed of the *chromosomes*, each of which is a long linear DEOXYRIBONUCLEIC ACID (DNA) molecule associated with protein. The nucleus is bounded by a nuclear membrane, which is composed of two lipid bilayer membranes.

Prokaryotic cells, the bacteria, have no nucleus, and their genetic material, consisting of a single circular naked DNA molecule, is not separated from the rest of the cell by a nuclear membrane.

Eukaryotic cells are larger and more complex than prokaryotic cells. They also have membrane-bounded structures, such as mitochondria, chloroplasts, Golgi apparatus, endoplasmic reticulum and lysosomes, that prokaryotic cells lack.

The contents of a cell are referred to collectively as the *protoplasm*. In eukaryotic cells the contents of the nucleus are referred to as *nucleoplasm* and the rest of the protoplasm as the *cytoplasm*.

The lipid bilayer of eukaryotic cells is impermeable to many substances, such as ions, sugars and amino acids; however, membrane proteins selectively move specific substances through the cell membrane by active or passive transport. Water, gases such as oxygen and carbon dioxide, and nonpolar compounds pass through the cell membrane by *diffusion*. Materials can also be engulfed and taken into the cell enclosed in a portion of the cell membrane. This is called *phagocytosis* when solids are ingested and *pinocytosis* when liquids are ingested. The reverse process is called *exocytosis*. All of these processes permit the cell to maintain an internal environment different from its exterior. See also body FLUIDS.

The cells of the body differentiate during development into many specialized types with specific tasks to perform. Cells are organized into tissues and tissues into organs. Embedded in the cell membrane are a wide range of molecules that vary with the cell type and are typically composed of proteins or glycoproteins that have a cytoplasmic transmembrane and external domains. These molecules serve as cell receptors and are involved in signal transduction for a wide range of ligands, including hormones, cytokines and incidentally serve as receptors for viruses and drugs.

See also BETZ CELLS, GAUCHER'S CELLS, GOLGI'S CELLS, HELA CELLS, HÜRTHLE CELL, KUPFFER'S CELLS, MERKEL CELL, MESANGIAL cell, NEUROENDOCRINE cell,
accessory c's macrophages involved in the processing and presentation of antigens making them immunogenic.
acinar c., acinous c. any of the cells lining an acinus, especially applied to the zymogen-secreting cells of the pancreatic acini.
adherent c. one that adheres to the glass or plastic container in cell cultures, to form the monolayer. See also CELL CULTURE.
alpha c's 1. cells in the islets of Langerhans that secrete glucagon. 2. acidophilic cells of the anterior pituitary.
APUD c's see APUD CELLS.
argentaffin c's enterochromaffin cells containing cytoplasmic granules capable of reducing silver compounds, located throughout the gastrointestinal tract, chiefly in the basilar portions of the gastric glands and the crypts of Lieberkühn. They secrete serotonin.
band c. an immature neutrophil in which the nucleus is not lobulated but is in the form of a continuous band, horseshoe shaped, twisted or coiled. Called also band-form granulocyte and stab cell.
basal c. an early keratinocyte, present in the basal layer of the epidermis.
basket c's cells in the cerebellar cortex whose axons carry basket-like groups of fibrils which enclose the cell body of each Purkinje cell.
beta c's 1. basophilic cells in the pancreas that secrete insulin and make up most of the bulk of the

islets of Langerhans; they contain granules that are soluble in alcohol. 2. basophilic cells of the anterior pituitary.
blood c. one of the formed elements of the blood. See also BLOOD.
c. body the nucleus of the cell and the adjacent cytoplasm in cells which have processes, e.g. neurons which consist of a cell body, an axon and dendrites.
bone c. a nucleated cell in the lacunae of bone. Called also osteocyte.
cartilage c. chondrocyte.
chromaffin c's cells whose cytoplasm shows fine brown granules when stained with potassium bichromate, occurring in the adrenal medulla and in scattered groups in various organs and throughout the body.
cleavage c. any of the cells derived from the fertilized ovum by mitosis; a blastomere.
c. count see ERYTHROCYTE, LEUKOCYTE, MILK CELL COUNTS.
c. culture see CELL CULTURE.
c. cycle see cell CYCLE.
daughter c. a cell formed by division of a mother cell.
c. dehydration fluid loss from cells due to elevation of the osmotic pressure of blood and tissue fluid; a potent stimulus to thirst.
dendritic c. macrophage-like cells with long, filamentous processes located in the cortex of lymph nodes and the skin. Important in antigen trapping, processing and presentation. See also LANGERHANS' CELL.
c. differentiation the process whereby cells become specialized usually with concurrent loss of reproductive capacity.
embryonic stem c. a stem cell of fetal origin. See stem cell (below).
epithelioid c. enlarged macrophages with enlarged lysosomes and much endoplasmic reticulum. May fuse to form multinucleated giant cell (below).
epsilon c. one of the groups of acidophilic cells in the adenohypophysis. Contains granules that stain with azocarmine dye.
foam c. a cell with a vacuolated appearance due to the presence of complex lipoids; seen in xanthoma.
c. fusion see SYNCYTIAL giant cell.
ganglion c. a large nerve cell, especially one of those of the spinal ganglia.
germ c. see GERM cell.
giant c. a very large, multinucleate cell; applied to megakaryocytes of bone marrow, to giant cells formed by coalescence and fusion of macrophages occurring in infectious granulomas and about foreign bodies, and to certain cancer cells.
glial c's neuroglial cells.
goblet c. a unicellular mucous gland found in the epithelium of various mucous membranes, especially that of the respiratory passages and intestines.
granular c. one containing granules, such as a keratinocyte in the stratum granulosum of the epidermis, when it contains a dense collection of darkly staining granules.
gustatory c. see TASTE bud.
heart failure c's, heart lesion c's iron-containing, rust-colored macrophages found in the pulmonary alveoli in congestive heart failure.
helmet c. schistocyte.
helper c. a subset of T lymphocytes which cooperate with B and other T lymphocytes for the synthesis of antibodies to many antigens; they play an integral role in immunoregulation.
hybrid c. a mononucleate cell produced from a binucleate heterokaryon after the latter undergoes mitosis. Such cells are initially unstable, tending to lose randomly some of the double complement of chromosomes. Used for mapping genes to particular chromosomes. See also HETEROKARYON, HYBRIDOMA.
immunologically competent c. see IMMUNOCYTE.
interstitial c's the cells of the connective tissue of the ovary or of the testis (Leydig's cells) which furnish the internal secretion of those structures, i.e. testosterone.
islet c's cells composing the islets of Langerhans in the pancreas. See alpha cells, beta cells (above).
juxtaglomerular c's specialized cells, containing secretory granules, located in the tunica media of the afferent glomerular arterioles. They cause aldosterone production by secreting the enzyme renin and play a role in the regulation of blood pressure and fluid balance.
K c's, killer c's T lymphocytes or null lymphocytes that have cytotoxic activity against target cells coated with specific IgG antibody.
lacis c. accumulation of cells between the arterioles at the glomerular hilus. Called also granular cell.
lacunar c. precursor of the malignant interdigitating reticular cell in Hodgkin-like lymphoma in humans.
LE c. a mature neutrophilic polymorphonuclear leukocyte characteristic of lupus erythematosus. See also LUPUS ERYTHEMATOSUS (LE) cell.
Leydig's c's interstitial cells of the testis, which secrete testosterone.
c. line see CELL CULTURE.
lutein c's the plump, pale-staining, polyhedral cells of the corpus luteum.
lymph c. lymphocyte.
lymphoid c's lymphocytes and plasma cells.
mast c. a connective tissue cell that has basophilic, metachromatic cytoplasmic granules that contain histamine, heparin, hyaluronic acid, slow-reacting substance of anaphylaxis (SRS-A), and, in some species, serotonin. Have Fc receptors specific for IgE in the cell membrane.
c.-mediated immune reaction see cellular IMMUNITY.
c. migration movement of cells from their place of origin to other tissues; one of the fundamental processes of development.
microglial c. see MICROGLIA. See also neuroglia cells (below).
milk c. count see MILK CELL COUNTS.
mother c. a cell that divides to form new, or daughter, cells.
Mott c. a plasma cell with large, clear cytoplasmic pockets.
natural killer c's, NK c's cells capable of mediating cytotoxic reactions without themselves being specifically sensitized against the target.
nerve c. any cell of the nervous system; a NEURON.
c. nests see ISOGENOUS GROUPS.
neuroglia c's, neuroglial c's see NEUROGLIA.
null c's lymphocyte-like cells that lack specific antigen receptors and other surface markers characteristic of B and T lymphocytes; they include K and NK cells; their numbers are elevated in active systemic lupus erythematosus and other disease states.
olfactory c's a set of specialized cells of the mucous membrane of the nose; the receptors for smell.
parafollicular c's see C CELL.
Pick's c's round, oval or polyhedral cells with foamy, lipid-containing cytoplasm found in the bone marrow and spleen in Niemann–Pick disease.

plasma c. a spherical or ellipsoidal cell with a single, eccentrically placed nucleus containing dense masses of chromatin in a wheel-spoke arrangement, an area of perinuclear clearing which contains the Golgi apparatus, and generally abundant cytoplasm. Plasma cells are produced by cell division of B lymphocytes following antigen stimulation and are involved in the synthesis and release of antibody. Called also plasmacyte and plasmocyte.
prickle c. a dividing keratinocyte of the prickle-cell layer of the epidermis, with delicate radiating process connecting with other similar cells.
prokaryotic c. see PROKARYOTE.
Purkinje's c's large branching cells of the middle layer of the cerebellar cortex.
red c., red blood c. erythrocyte.
Reed–Sternberg c's giant histiocytic cells, typically multinucleate, which are the common histological characteristic of Hodgkin's disease in humans.
reticular c's the cells forming the reticular fibers of connective tissue; those forming the framework of lymph nodes, bone marrow and spleen. They are weakly phagocytic, stromal in origin and are distinct from the monocyte–macrophage system.
reticuloendothelial c. a cell of the RETICULOENDOTHELIAL SYSTEM.
Schwann c. any of the large nucleated cells whose cell membrane spirally enwraps the axons of myelinated peripheral neurons supplying the myelin sheath between two nodes of Ranvier.
Sertoli c's elongated cells in the tubules of the testes to which the spermatids become attached; they provide support, protection and, apparently, nutrition until the spermatids are transformed into mature spermatozoa.
sickle c. a crescentic or sickle-shaped erythrocyte seen in some humans and deer. The abnormal shape caused by the presence of varying proportions of hemoglobin S.
signet-ring c. a cell in which the nucleus has been pressed to one side by an accumulation of intracytoplasmic mucin.
somatic c's the cells of the body other than the germ cells.
c. sorting see FLUORESCENCE-activated cell sorter.
c. specialization conversion of a simple cell type into a specialized cell type capable of a special function, e.g. a secretory cell; a major part of the growth of an embryo and the differentiation of basic mesenchymal tissue into specialized organs.
spindle c. spindle shaped cells of the dermis or subcutis; principal component of spindle cell tumors.
spur c. spiculed mature erythrocyte.
squamous c's flat, scalelike epithelial cells.
stab c. see band cell (above).
stellate c. any star-shaped cell, as a Kupffer cell or astrocyte, having many filaments extending in all directions.
stem c. 1. any precursor cell. 2. a primitive hematopoietic cell that is capable of self-replicating or differentiating into precursor cells of erythrocytes or any of the leukocytes.
stipple c. an erythrocyte containing granules that take a basic or bluish stain with Wright's stain.
suppressor c's a not well defined subset of T lymphocytes that are reported to inhibit antibody and cell-mediated immune responses. They may play a role in immunoregulation, and are believed to be abnormal in various autoimmune and other immunological disease states. See also T LYMPHOCYTES.
target c. 1. an abnormally thin erythrocyte showing, when stained, a dark center and a peripheral ring of hemoglobin, separated by a pale, unstained zone containing less hemoglobin; seen in various anemias and other disorders. Called also codocyte. 2. any cell selectively affected by a particular agent, such as a hormone or drug. 3. cell containing nonself antigens in its cell membranes that is a target for nonimmune and immune cytolysis, e.g. virus-infected or tumor cell.
taste c's cells in the taste buds associated with the nerves of taste.
totipotential c. an embryonic cell that is capable of developing into any type of body cell.
Türk's c. a lymphocyte with increased basophilia.
visual c's the neuroepithelial elements of the retina.
white c., white blood c. leukocyte.

011A cell suggested common progenitor cell for type 2 astrocyte and the oligodendrocyte.

cell-adhesion molecule membrane proteins expressed by endothelial cells which regulate the movement of molecules and leukocytes from the blood to tissues.

cell culture the artificial culture of living tissue outside a living body. Animal cells were originally grown in culture as *explant cultures*, i.e. small pieces of tissue. If pieces of tissue are treated with enzymes such as trypsin, single cell suspensions can be obtained which will settle onto glass or plastic surfaces and grow to form a *monolayer cell culture*. *Primary cell cultures* can be passaged to form *secondary cell cultures*. Cells in culture can be passaged a finite number of times before reaching a crisis which can be compared with AGING. The number of passages, before reaching crisis, has been termed the Hayflick limit and is related to the longevity of the species from which the tissue was originally derived. Within the Hayflick limit the cells are referred to as a *cell strain*. Cells that survive the crisis and continue to grow are referred to as a *cell line*. Cell lines can also be derived directly from cancer cells. There are many properties that distinguish cell lines from cell strains, including altered chromosome number, changes at the cell membrane, and reduced requirement for certain growth factors.

cell division the process by which cells reproduce; fission of a cell.

cell-mediated effected by cellular rather than chemical elements.
c.-m. hypersensitivity see delayed HYPERSENSITIVITY.
c.-m. immunity see cellular IMMUNITY.
c.-m. lympholysis assay a test of cell-mediated immunity in which activated cytoxic T lymphocytes cause lysis of ^{51}Cr-labeled target cells.

cellobiase an enzyme associated with bacteria and protozoa (particularly in ruminants) catalyzing the hydrolysis of $\beta 1 \rightarrow 4$ glycosidic bonds of the disaccharide, cellobiose. See also GLUCOSIDASE.

cellobiose a simple polysaccharide composed of two molecules of glucose and formed by the digestion of cellulose by cellulase.

cellular pertaining to, or made up of, cells.
c. genetics see CYTOGENETICS.

cellularity the state of a tissue or other mass as regards the number of its constituent cells.

cellules claveleuses mononuclear cells that accumulate in the dermis in lesions of sheeppox. They are virus-infected cells and their cytoplasm contains one or more eosinophilic inclusion bodies.

cellulicidal destroying cells.

cellulitis a diffuse inflammatory process within solid tissues, characterized by edema, redness, pain and interference with function. It may be caused by infection with streptococci, staphylococci or other organisms.

Cellulitis usually occurs in the loose tissues beneath the skin, but may also occur in tissues beneath mucous membranes or around muscle bundles or surrounding organs.

anerobic c. see MALIGNANT edema.

canine juvenile c. see juvenile PYODERMA.

epidemic equine c. see EQUINE viral arteritis, EQUINE influenza.

periapical c. see APICAL abscess.

periesophageal c. caused by perforation of the esophagus and establishment of a mixed infection into the tissues surrounding the esophagus.

cellulofibrous partly cellular and partly fibrous.

celluloneuritis inflammation of neurons.

cellulose a polysaccharide containing $\beta 1 \rightarrow 4$ linked glucose carbohydrate forming the skeleton of most plant structures and plant cells. In herbivores, digested by bacteria in the rumen or cecum, primarily to volatile fatty acids which can be used as a source of energy.

absorbable c. an absorbable oxidation product of cellulose, applied locally to stop bleeding. Called also oxidized cellulose.

c. acetate the most popular support field used in the electrophoresis of proteins.

oxidized c. see absorbable cellulose (above).

cellulose digestion test the time required for a thread of cotton to be digested, or for particulate material in a strained sample of ruminal fluid to achieve flotation, are used as laboratory tests of ruminal function.

cellulytic breakdown of cellulose, e.g. by hydrolysis. Occurs at a sufficient level to provide a source of energy only in ruminants and species with a large intestine adapted to fermentation.

c. bacteria bacteria in the rumen which digest cellulose to volatile fatty acids especially acetic, butyric and propionic.

celo- cavity. [Gr.] *cavity*.

CELO virus chicken embryo lethal orphan virus. See QUAIL bronchitis.

celoblastula the common type of blastula, consisting of a hollow sphere composed of blastomeres.

celom body cavity, especially the original cavity in the mammalian embryo between the somatopleure and splanchnopleure, which is both intra- and extraembryonic; the principal cavities of the trunk, the pericardial, pleural and peritoneal sacs, arise from the intraembryonic portion.

c. partitioning separation of the pleural and pericardial sacs in the embryo is established by the pleuropericardial septum formed by the fusion and extension of the pleuropericardial folds.

celoscope an endoscope for use in celoscopy.

celoscopy examination of a body cavity, especially the abdominal cavity, through a celoscope.

celosoma, celosomia congenital fissure or absence of the sternum, with hernial protrusion of the viscera.

celosomy a developmental anomaly characterized by protrusion of the viscera from and their presence outside the body cavity.

celothelioma mesothelioma.

Celsius scale a temperature scale with the ice point at 0 and the normal boiling point of water at 100 degrees (100°C). For equivalents of Celsius and Fahrenheit temperatures, see Tables 5 and 18.

Celsius thermometer a centigrade thermometer employing the Celsius scale. The abbreviation 100°C should be read as 'one hundred degrees Celsius'.

Celtic pony group of pony breeds including CONNEMARA, ICELAND, SHETLAND.

Celtic red see BRACHYCEROS.

CEM contagious equine metritis.

CEM selective medium chocolate agar made with Eugon agar and 5% horse blood; used to cultivate *Taylorella equigenitalis*.

cement 1. a substance that produces a solid union between two surfaces. 2. cementum.

bone c. usually an acrylic compound used in fracture repair and positioning of bone pins.

dental c. materials used to affix dental restorations and to fill cavities.

glass ionomer c. a material used for restorative dentistry. In veterinary dentistry, these are used for treatment of neck lesions on feline teeth and filling access holes after endodontic procedures.

c. lines basophilic lines in histological sections of bone that represent highly mineralized connective tissue that binds the elements of the bone together.

cementasome see KERATINOSOME.

cementicle a small, discrete globular mass of cementum in the region of a tooth root.

cementoblast a large cuboidal cell, found between fibers on the surface of cementum, which is active in the formation of cementum.

cementoblastoma an odontogenic fibroma whose cells are developing into cementoblasts and in which there is only a small proportion of calcified tissue.

cementoclasia disintegration of the cementum of a tooth.

cementoclast phagocytes of dental cement. See also OSTEOCLAST.

cementocyte a cell found in lacunae of cellular cementum, frequently having long processes radiating from the cell body toward the periodontal surface of the cementum.

cemento-enamel junction a line on the surface of a tooth where the enamel on the crown meets the cementum on the root. Called also cervical line, neck.

cementogenesis development of cementum on the root dentine of a tooth.

cementoma a mass of cementum lying free at the apex of a tooth, probably a reaction to injury.

cementosis proliferation of cementum.

cementosome see KERATINOSOME.

cementum the bonelike connective tissue covering the root of a tooth and assisting in tooth support.

Cenchrus ciliaris a grass of the family Poaceae; called also buffel grass. Ingestion of this grass plant by horses can cause osteodystrophia fibrosa because most of the calcium in the grass is in the form of oxalate crystals and unavailable for absorption. In very lush pasture can cause acute oxalate poisoning in sheep, but only if they are very hungry.

cenosis a morbid discharge.

cenosite coinosite.

censor a member of a committee on ethics or for critical examination of a medical or other society.

censoring in epidemiology, a loss of information from a study, whether by subjects dropping out of the study or because of infrequent measurement.

census measurement of a parameter of population by total counts of individuals—a full muster.

centaur a mythological race of savage men who lived in Greece. They were depicted as men from the head to the loins and horses from there back. A common emblem for veterinary organizations.

Centaurea a genus of thistles of the Asteraceae family of plants; contain sesquiterpene lactones which cause nigropallidal encephalomalacia in horses. Includes *C. melitensis* (Maltese cockspur), *C. repens* (*C. picris*, Russian or creeping knapweed, hard heads), *C. solstitialis* (yellow star or St. Barnaby's thistle).

Centaurium a genus of plants in family Gentianaceae. Contain an unidentified toxin which causes diarrhea, hepatic damage and nephrosis. Includes *C. beyrichii* (mountain pink, rock centaury), *C. calycosum* (mountain pink).

Centella uniflora New Zealand plant member of the family Apiaceae; contains an unidentified toxin which causes convulsions and recumbency, and liver and kidney damage. Called also centella.

center a point from which a process starts, especially a plexus or ganglion giving off nerves that control a function.

accelerating c. one in the brainstem involved in acceleration of heart action.

appetite c. located in the hypothalamus; controls appetite.

auditory c. the center for hearing, in the more anterior of the transverse temporal gyri.

cardioinhibitory c. one in the medulla oblongata that exerts an inhibitory influence on the heart.

deglutition c. a nerve center in the medulla oblongata that controls swallowing.

diaphragmatic c. see DIAPHRAGMATIC tendon.

emetic c. located in the reticular formation of the brainstem, this center controls vomiting.

eructation c. controls eructation in ruminants; located in the medulla oblongata.

expiratory c. one of the four respiratory centers (see below).

germinal c. the area in the center of a lymph node containing aggregations of actively proliferating lymphocytes.

gustatory c. the cerebral center supposed to control taste.

inspiratory respiratory c. one of the four respiratory centers.

lymph node germinal c. centers in lymph nodes where lymphocytes are produced.

medullary respiratory c. the center in the medulla oblongata that coordinates respiratory movements.

motor c. any center that originates, controls, inhibits or maintains motor impulses.

nerve c. a collection of nerve cells in the central nervous system that are associated together in the performance of some particular function.

c. of ossification see OSSIFICATION center.

perineal c. see PERINEAL body.

reflex c. any nerve center at which afferent sensory information is converted into efferent motor impulses.

respiratory c's a series of the centers (the apneustic, pneumotaxic and medullary respiratory centers) in the medulla and pons that coordinate respiratory movements.

c.-surround retinal organization the arrangement of cells in the receptive field of the retina; the sensitivity of a certain spot in the retina is affected by what is occurring in adjacent areas.

swallowing c. deglutition center.

thermoregulatory c's hypothalamic centers regulating the conservation and dissipation of heat.

vasomotor c. a combination of two centers in the reticular formation of the brainstem; includes a pressor and a depressor center.

vomiting c. see emetic center (above).

Center for Veterinary Medicine a body within the Food and Drug Administration of the Unites States Food and Drug Administration, concerned with ensuring safety of animal feeds and drugs.

center-tie a method for tethering cows in fixed stalls in barns. A chain is fixed overhead and to the center of the front edge of the feedtrough. The cow is attached to this by a curved yoke that slides up and down the chain.

centerencephalic pertaining to the center of the encephalon.

c. system the neurons in the central core of the brainstem from the thalamus down to the medulla oblongata, connecting the two hemispheres of the brain.

centering aid a device used when radiographing a part to ensure that the center of the beam of the x-ray will pass through the part at the correct angle and that the part will be in the center of the beam. Modern machines must all have a light beam diaphragm which acts as the centering aid as well as the beam collimator.

Centers for Disease Control an agency of the US Department of Health and Human Services, located in Atlanta, Georgia, which serves as a center for the control, prevention and investigation of diseases; abbreviated CDC.

-centesis word element. [Gr.] *puncture and aspiration of.*

centi- word element. [L.] *hundred;* usually used in naming units of measurement to indicate one-hundredth (10^{-2}) of the unit designated by the root with which it is combined, e.g. centigram. Symbol c.

centigrade having 100 gradations (steps or degrees), as the Celsius scale; abbreviated C. For equivalents of Celsius and Fahrenheit temperatures, see Tables 5 and 18.

centigram one-hundredth of a gram; abbreviated cg.

centiliter one-hundredth of a liter; abbreviated cl.

centimeter one-hundredth of a meter, or approximately 0.3937 inch; abbreviated cm.

cubic c. a unit of capacity, being that of a cube 1 cm on a side; abbreviated cm^3, cu.cm. or cc.

centimorgan a measure of the degree of recombination between two genes. One centimorgan is approximately 1000 kilobases. Named after T.H. Morgan. See also GENETIC map.

centipedes many-legged members of the class Chilopoda of the phylum Arthropoda. They are relatively harmless, but some of the 1500 species can inflict a painful bite to humans and it seems reasonable to assume that bites to animals could happen.

centrad toward a center.

central pertaining to a center; located at the midpoint.

c. artery of the optic nerve, the source of the retinal artery. See also Table 9.

c. channel the fast-flowing channel through the capillary bed, the rate controlled by the metarterioles which exert a sphincter-like action on the system.

c. convulsions convulsions arising from stimulation of the central nervous system, as distinct from those caused by lesions elsewhere.

c. cord syndrome injury to the central portion of the cervical spinal cord resulting in disproportionately more weakness or paralysis in the forelimbs than in the hindlimbs; pathological change is caused by hemorrhage or edema.

c. diabetes insipidus see DIABETES INSIPIDUS.

c. European tick-borne encephalitis see ENCEPHALITIS.

c. layer central of the three layers of gray matter in the cerebellum; the principal cell type is piriform.

c. nervous system see central NERVOUS system.
c. peripheral neuropathy see Boxer progressive AXONOPATHY.
c. processing unit electronic circuitry that makes up the operating mechanism of a computer. Attached to it are the monitor, the keyboard and the printer. Called also CPU.
c. progressive retinal atrophy see central progressive RETINAL atrophy.
c. projection law the laws of physics applied to the primary x-ray beam of photons, e.g. the closer the object being x-rayed is to the film the sharper will be its definition.
c. respiratory oscillator pool of nerve cells in the pons and medulla oblongata which are responsible for the rhythmic to-and-fro movements of respiration.
c. retinal degeneration see RETINAL.
c. sulcus fissure of Rolando.
c. tarsal bone the bone of the hock which lies between the proximal and distal rows of tarsal bones of tarsal bones.
c. tendon of diaphragm see DIAPHRAGMATIC tendon.
c. vein the centrally placed drainage vessel of each hepatic lobule, receiving blood from the hepatic sinusoids.
c. venous catheterization insertion of an indwelling catheter into a central vein for the purpose of administering fluid and medications and for the measurement of central venous pressure (see below).
c. venous pressure (CVP) the pressure of blood in the right atrium, measured by an in situ catheter in the right atrium, is a much better guide of the degree of vasogenic peripheral failure than is arterial blood pressure. The technique is used mainly in dogs and cats.

Central and Upper Belgian a white, blue pied or blue breed of dairy cattle produced in Belgium by crossing Shorthorn and Friesian with local red cattle.

Central Asiatic Pashmina a white or black-and-white goat, maintained for its haircoat, which produces cashmere fiber. Called also cashmere or Kashmiri goat.

Central Europe tickborne fever see Russian spring–summer ENCEPHALITIS.

central ray the center of the area of radiation created as the x-ray beam diverges. The further from the center of the ray one is, the more distortion there is and, if the beam is not correctly centered over the part to be viewed, there will be more distortion still. The central point is the point of minimum distortion.

centric pertaining to a center.
chromosome c. fusion replacement of two chromosomes by one produced by fusion of the centromeres of two acrocentric chromosomes. Called also Robertsonian translocation.

centriciput the central part of the upper surface of the head, located between the occiput and sinciput.

centrifugal moving away from a center.

centrifugate material subjected to centrifugation.

centrifugation the process of separating lighter portions of a solution, mixture or suspension from the heavier portions by centrifugal force.
density gradient c. a procedure for separating particles such as viruses or ribosomes or molecules such as DNA in which the sample is placed on a preformed gradient such as sucrose or cesium chloride. Upon centrifugation either by rate zonal or equilibrium procedures, the macromolecules are 'banded' in the gradient and can be collected as a pure fraction.

centrifuge 1. to rotate, in a suitable container, at extremely high speed, to cause the deposition of solids in solution. 2. a laboratory device for subjecting substances in solution to relative centrifugal force up to 25,000 times gravity.

centrilobular pertaining to the central portion of a lobule.
c. necrosis necrosis restricted to the hepatocytes immediately surrounding the central venule. Called also periacinar necrosis.

centriole either of the two cylindrical organelles located in the centrosome and containing nine triplets of microtubules arrayed around their edges; centrioles migrate to opposite poles of the cell during cell division and serve to organize the spindles. They are capable of independent replication and of migrating to form basal bodies.

centripetal moving toward a center.

centro- word element. [L., Gr.] *center, central location.*

centrokinesia movement originating from central stimulation.

centromere the clear constricted portion of the chromosome at which the chromatids are joined and by which the chromosome is attached to the spindle during cell division.

Centropogon australis a venomous fish of the family Scorpaenidae. Called also sixteen spined fortescue.

Centrorhynchus thorny-headed worms of reptiles. See also MACRACANTHORHYNCHUS.

centrosclerosis osteosclerosis of the marrow cavity of a bone.

centrosome a specialized area of condensed cytoplasm containing the centrioles and playing an important part in mitosis.

centrosphere centrosome.

centrostaltic pertaining to a center of motion.

centrum pl. *centra* [L.] 1. a center. 2. the body of a vertebra.
c. commune the solar plexus.

Centruroides see SCORPION.

century plant see AGAVE *americana*.

cenuriasis see COENUROSIS.

Cephaelis a South American plant genus of the family Rubiaceae whose root contains emetine, a powerful emetic, which at one time was used pharmaceutically. Poisoning may occur and is manifested by persistent, violent vomiting. Includes *Cephaelis ipecacuanha* (*C. acuminata*); called also ipecac, ipecacuanha.

cephalad toward the head.

cephaledema edema of the head.

cephalexin a first generation CEPHALOSPORIN antibiotic which is effective following oral administration. It is widely used in bacterial infections of the skin in dogs and cats.

cephalhematocele a hematocele under the pericranium, communicating with the sinuses of the dura mater.

cephalhematoma a localized effusion of blood beneath the periosteum of the skull of the newborn, due to disruption of the vessels during parturition.

cephalic pertaining to the head, or to the head end of the body.
c. index the width of the skull divided by the length. Sometimes expressed as 100 times the breadth divided by the length.
c. vein the vein on the cranial aspect of the forearm of most domestic mammals; much favored for intravenous injection in dogs; see Table 15.

cephalin a group of phospholipids found particularly in the brain and other nerve tissue.

cephalitis encephalitis.
cephal(o)- word element. [Gr.] *head.*
cephalocele protrusion of a part of the cranial contents. See also ENCEPHALOCELE.
cephalocentesis surgical puncture of the head.
cephalodactyly malformation of the head and digits.
cephalogyric pertaining to turning motions of the head.
cephalohematoma cephalhematoma.
cephalomelus a monster with an accessory limb growing from the head.
cephalomotor moving the head; pertaining to motions of the head.
Cephalomyia see RHINOESTRUS.
cephalonia a condition in which the head is abnormally enlarged, with sclerotic hyperplasia of the brain.
cephalonium a first generation CEPHALOSPORIN, used in intramammary and topical preparations.
cephalopagus see CRANIOPAGUS.
cephalopathy any disease of the head.
cephalopelvic pertaining to the head of the fetus and the pelvis of the dam.
c. disproportion the head of the fetus is disproportionately large and will not pass through the pelvis of the dam. Caused usually by hydrocephalus.
Cephalophus see DUIKER.
Cephalopina titillator see CEPHALOPSIS *titillator.*
cephalopods members of the class Cephalopoda, including cuttle fish, squid and octopus.
Cephalopsis a member of the genus of flies in the family Oestridae.
C. titillator nasal bot fly of camels. The larvae inhabit the nasal sinuses.
cephaloridine a first generation CEPHALOSPORIN antibiotic.
cephalosporinase an enzyme that hydrolyzes the –CO–NH– bond in the lactam ring of cephalosporin, converting it to an inactive product.
cephalosporins a group of broad-spectrum, semisynthetic antibiotics, derived from *Cephalosporium,* a genus of soil-inhabiting fungi, which share the nucleus 7-aminocephalosporanic acid. Cephalosporins named before 1975 are spelled with 'ph', while those named later are spelled with 'f'.

First generation preparations (cefaclor, cephazolin, cefadroxil, cephalexin, cephaloglycin, cephaloridine, cephalothin, cephapirin, cephradine) are active mainly against gram-positive bacteria. *Second generation* preparations (cephamandole and cefoxitin) have a broader spectrum of activity and *third generation* preparations (cefoperazone, cefotaxime and moxalactam) are active mainly against gram-negative organisms, including *Pseudomonas aeruginosa.*

In a more recently introduced system of classification, cephalosporins are grouped according to their route of administration and antimicrobial activity. The orally active cephalosporins, with fair activity against gram-positive bacteria and modest activity against gram-negative, but not *Pseudomonas,* form one group. Included are cephalexin, cephadrine, cefadroxil, cefachlor and cephaloglycin.

Those active by parenteral administration are placed into four groups: Group I, which includes cefapirin, cefacetrile, cephaloridine, cephalothin and cephazolin, has high activity against gram-positive bacteria and moderate activity against gram-negative, but not *Pseudomonas*; Group II, which includes cefamandole, cefmenoxime, cefotaxime, cefotiam, ceftiofur, cefuroxime and cefotriaxone, has high activity against Enterobacteriaceae; Group III, which includes cefulodin, ceftazidime and cefoperazone, has high activity against *Pseudomonas* and other gram-negative bacteria; Group IV, which includes cefoxitin, loxalactam, cefmetazole and cefotetan, is resistant to β-lactamase.
Cephalosporium acremonium the bacteria which produces the natural cephalosporin antibiotics.
cephalothin a first generation CEPHALOSPORIN antibiotic. Sensitive organisms include many penicillin-resistant staphylococci.
cephalothoracic pertaining to the head and thorax.
cephalothoracopagus a twin monster united at the head, neck and thorax.
cephalotomy 1. the cutting up of the fetal head to facilitate delivery. 2. dissection of the fetal head.
Cephalotrichum a genus of fungi reported to infect subcutaneous tissue in dogs and cats.
cephalotrypesis trephination of the skull.
cephamycins semisynthetic, β-lactam antibiotics produced by *Streptomyces* spp.; includes CEFOXITIN SODIUM, CEFMETAZOLE and CEFOTETAN.
cephapirin a first generation CEPHALOSPORIN antibiotic, resistant to β-lactamase. Most commonly used as an intramammary infusion in cows.
cephazolin see CEFAZOLIN.
Cephenemyia a genus of bot flies in the family Oestridae. Includes *Cephenemyia apicata, C. auribarbis, C. jellisoni, C. phobifer, C. pratti, C. stimulator, C. trompe, C. ulrichi* (nasal cavities of wild mammals).
cephradine a first generation CEPHALOSPORIN antibiotic with a spectrum of activity similar to cephalexin.
cera [L.] *wax.*
ceramic implant see biological IMPLANT.
ceramidase an enzyme occurring in most mammalian tissue that catalyzes the reversible acylation–deacylation of ceramides.
ceramide any of a group of naturally occurring sphingolipids in which the NH_2 group of sphingosine is acylated with a fatty acyl CoA derivative to form *N*-acylsphingosine.
c. glucoside the major sphingolipid accumulated in GAUCHER'S DISEASE.
c. lactosidosis a sphingolipidosis in which ceramide lactoside accumulates in neural and visceral tissues owing to a deficiency of a β-galactosidase.
cerate a medicinal preparation for external use, compounded of fat or wax, or both, intermediate in consistency between an ointment and a plaster.
cerato- for words beginning thus, see also those beginning *kerato-.*
Ceratocephalus testiculatus see RANUNCULUS.
Ceratocystis perfect state of the fungus *Sporothrix schenckii* often found growing on parsnip roots; induces production of a furocoumarin which causes primary photosensitization.
ceratohyoid short rods of the hyoid bone. Connects the body of the hyoid bone to the epihyoid (dog, cat, ruminants, pig) or stylohyoid (horse).
Ceratomyxa a genus in the class Myxosporea; may or may not be true protozoa.
C. shasta important parasite of young salmonids limited in occurrence to the Columbia river basin. Causes severe losses in young fish in culture ponds. Signs include swelling at vent, distended abdomen and subcutaneous boils.
Ceratophyllus a genus of fleas in the order Siphonaptera. Includes *Ceratophyllus columbae, C. (Nosopsyllus) fasciatus, C. gallinae, C. garei, C. niger* (Western chicken flea—rodents and wild birds).
Ceratopogonidae a family of biting midges; the most important genus is CULICOIDES.

Ceratostomella fimbriata a fungus that grows on green celery stalks; induces production of a furocoumarin which causes primary photosensitization.

Ceratotherium simum white rhinoceros.

Cerbera manghas plant in the family Apocynaceae; contains a cardenolide cardiac glycoside which can cause sudden death.

cercaria pl. *cercariae* [Gr.] the final, free-swimming larval stage of a trematode parasite.

cercarial pertaining to or emanating from cercariae.

c. dermatitis see TRICHOBILHARZIA.

cerclage [Fr.] encircling of a part with a wire ring or loop, as for fixation of fragments in a fractured bone.

Cercocarpus a North American genus of the Rosaceae plant family; includes *C. breviflorus*, *C. montanus*; contains cyanogenetic glycosides and may cause cyanide poisoning. Called also mountain mahogany.

Cercocebus albigena see MANGABEYS.

Cercopethididae a family of nonhuman primates that includes Old World monkeys.

Cercopithecus a genus of Old World monkeys in the family Cercopithecidae; includes macaques, baboons, and vervet and talapoin (*Cercopithecus talapoin*) monkeys.

cercus a bristle-like structure.

cere the firm, fleshy bond lying across the base of the beak of birds. Most obvious in the pigeon as a white, saddle-like object. The cere is blue in male budgerigars and light brown to pink in females, so offering a convenient means of sexing these birds. The color may fade in males with testicular tumors.

c. hypertrophy occurs in psittacine birds, particularly budgerigars; overgrowth may occlude the nares. Called also brown hypertrophy of the cere.

cereal cultivated grain crops of barley, wheat, rye and oats, members of the plant family Poaceae (Graminae). See also BARLEY, WHEAT, RYE, OAT.

c. crop oats, wheat, barley, rye crops used as grazing when immature or failed and short. Usually used when other feed is short and livestock are hungry. Hypomagnesemia, nitrate/nitrite poisoning and photosensitization may occur on immature green crops and lactic acid indigestion due to ingestion of grain on stunted mature crops.

c. mite see TYROGLYPHUS.

cerebellar pertaining to the cerebellum.

c. abiotrophy occurs in cattle, pigs and dogs. Affected young are normal at birth but at an early age ataxia and signs of cerebellar dysfunction appear, often progressing to complete immobilization. Cerebral function is usually normal. An inherited basis is suspected. In Kerry blue terriers, it is inherited as an autosomal recessive trait. Called also cerebellar neuronal abiotrophy.

c. agenesis absence of the cerebellum due to its non-appearance in the embryo.

c. aplasia see cerebellar atrophy (below).

c. ataxia the incoordination of gait characterized by exaggerated movements. There is no paresis. There is exaggerated strength and distance of movement—hypermetria. Caused usually by damage to the cerebellum or to the spinocerebellar tracts. May be congenital due to cerebellar atrophy or acquired due to inflammation or malacia of the cerebellum.

c. atrophy degeneration and loss of cells—Purkinje and granular cells of the cerebellum. Present at birth or soon after, is congenital in sheep, cattle, Arab horses, dogs and cats. Some of the diseases are inherited, some are known to be due to virus infection in utero, e.g. bovine virus diarrhea, feline panleukopenia. Some are in fact abiotrophies, premature aging of tissues. In the latter the animals are normal at birth but develop classical signs later. Segmental atrophy occurs in pigs but is asymptomatic.

c. coning see cerebellar lipping (below), BRAIN herniation.

c. cortex the superficial gray matter of the cerebellum.

c. dysfunction see cerebellar ataxia (above).

c. dysmelinogenesis recorded in Chow Chow dogs; characterized by congenital head tremor.

feline c. ataxia see FELINE panleukopenia.

c. hypomyelinogenesis abnormally reduced myelination in the cerebellum; characterized clinically by severe neonatal tremor.

c. hypoplasia deficiency of cells of the cerebellum, the degree and distribution of which is variable. See cerebellar atrophy (above).

inherited c. defects includes cerebellar abiotrophy, atrophy, agenesis, hypoplasia, neuraxonal dystrophy.

c. lipping caused by diffuse cerebral edema. The vermis of the cerebellum protrudes through the foramen magnum and lies like a tongue over the medulla.

c. neuronal abiotrophy see cerebellar abiotrophy (above).

c. neuraxonal dystrophy reported in collie sheepdogs. The lesion is limited to axons and there are no lesions in the cerebellar folial neurons.

c. syndrome see cerebellar ataxia (above).

cerebellitis inflammation of the cerebellum.

cerebello-olivary conducting or passing from the cerebellum to the olivary nucleus.

cerebellomedullary cistern see CISTERNA cerebellomedullaris.

cerebellopontine conducting or passing from the cerebellum to the pons varolii.

c. abscess usually complications of otitis media generated by pharyngeal infection. See also BRAIN abscess.

cerebelloreticular tract part of the reticular formation, matched by a reverse pathway of reticulocerebellar tract, and therefore of the modulating mechanism of the integration centers in the brain.

cerebellum the part of the metencephalon situated on the back of the brainstem, to which it is attached by three cerebellar peduncles on each side; it consists of a median lobe (vermis) and two lateral lobes (the hemispheres). Structures in the cerebellum include CINGULUM, cerebellar CORTEX, CULMEN, PYRAMID of cerebellum, UVULA and VERMIS. See also BRAIN.

vestibular c. see ARCHICEREBELLUM.

cerebral pertaining to the cerebrum. See also BRAIN.

c. circulation arterial blood supply reaches the anterior, middle and posterior cerebral arteries via the circle of Willis, in some species originating directly from the internal carotid and basilar arteries, in others via an interposed *rete mirabile.* See also BLOOD–BRAIN BARRIER, blood–CSF BARRIER, CEREBROSPINAL fluid.

c. contusion contusion of the brain following a HEAD injury. See also cerebral CONTUSION.

c. cortex the convoluted layer of gray matter covering the cerebral hemispheres, which governs thought, memory, sensation and voluntary movement. See also BRAIN, PYRAMIDAL tracts, EXTRAPYRAMIDAL system.

c. cortical dysplasia encompasses a range of disorders including neuronal heterotopia, microgyria, ulegyria, lissencephaly, pachygyria.

c. diencephalic syndrome the clinical signs associated with lesions of the cerebral cortex and diencephalon. They include behavioral or mental change, abnormal movements such as circling and head pressing, deficits in contralateral postural responses and sometimes visual impairment.

c. dura mater the membranous cover around the brain. Endosteal and meningeal layers are separated only by the cranial venous sinuses. Continuous with the spinal cord dura and the sheaths of the spinal nerves. Has three internal folds which separate sections of the brain. See FALX cerebri, TENTORIUM cerebelli, SELLA turcica.

c. edema, cytotoxic caused by neurotoxins, this edema is intracellular.

c. edema, generalized when all cerebral tissues are affected as in disturbances which create marked differences from normal of sodium and potassium ion concentration in tissues.

c. edema, interstitial edema of the central white matter as in hydrocephalus affecting the brain and hydromyelia affecting the spinal cord.

c. edema, vasogenic when the edema is intercellular and due usually to damage to the vascular endothelium.

c. flush the congestion of the cerebral vessels causing a pink coloration; of infections by *Babesia bovis* and *B. bigemina* it is the former in which the cerebral flush occurs.

c. gyri convolutions on the surface of the cerebrum.

c. hemisphere symmetrical right and left halves of the cerebrum divided by the longitudinal fissure.

c. peduncle see cerebral PEDUNCLE.

c. pia mater thin connective tissue membrane that lies closely against the cerebral surface and carries blood vessels into the tissues of the brain.

c. piriform lobe on the floor of the brain medial to the lateral olfactory tract.

c. pole frontal (rostral) and occipital (caudal) poles of the cerebrum.

c. substantia nigra occupies the interior of the cerebral peduncles.

c. theileriosis infection with *Theileria parva* or aberrant forms of *T. taurotragi* originating from the eland. Called also TURNING SICKNESS.

c. vascular accident (CVA) a disorder of the blood vessels serving the cerebrum, resulting from an impaired blood supply to parts of the brain. Called stroke in humans.

c. ventriculography see VENTRICULOGRAPHY.

cerebration functional activity of the brain.

cerebritis inflammation of the cerebrum.

cerebroangiography see cerebral ARTERIOGRAPHY.

cerebrocerebellar pertaining to the cerebrum and the cerebellum.

cerebrocortical pertaining to the cerebral cortex.

c. malacia see POLIOENCEPHALOMALACIA.

c. necrosis see POLIOENCEPHALOMALACIA.

cerebroid resembling brain substance.

cerebroma any abnormal mass of brain substance.

cerebromalacia abnormal softening of the substance of the cerebrum. See also LEUKOENCEPHALOMALACIA, POLIOENCEPHALOMALACIA.

cerebromeningitis meningoencephalitis.

cerebronic acid a fatty acid derived from sphingomyelin, which is the principal hydroxy saturated acid from the brain.

cerebropathy any brain disorder.

cerebrophysiology the physiology of the brain.

cerebropontile pertaining to the cerebrum and pons.

cerebrosclerosis morbid hardening of the substance of the cerebrum.

cerebroside a general designation for sphingolipids in which sphingosine is combined with galactose or glucose; found chiefly in nervous tissue.

cerebrosis any disease of the cerebrum.

cerebrospinal pertaining to the brain and spinal cord.

c. abscess see BRAIN abscess.

c. angiopathy is thought to be a sequel to subclinical edema disease due to an *Escherichia coli* toxemia of pigs. The disease is sporadic within a group and is characterized by incoordination, apathy, aimless walking and circling. Emaciation occurs rapidly and most affected animals are euthanatized on humanitarian grounds.

c. dysmyelinogenesis a characteristic lesion in the brain of newborn piglets affected by congenital tremor caused by swine fever infection of the dam during early pregnancy. See also CONGENITAL TREMOR SYNDROME of piglets.

c. embolism uncommon in animals. May result from marrow escaping into the circulation from a fracture site, or cartilage from a nucleus pulposus disruption. Usually in a ventral spinal artery causing a sudden onset of paralysis.

c. fluid (CSF) the fluid within the subarachnoid space, the central canal of the spinal cord, and the four ventricles of the brain. The fluid is formed continuously by the choroid plexus in the ventricles, and is reabsorbed into the blood by the arachnoid villi at approximately the same rate at which it is produced.

Examination of the CSF for the presence of abnormal or excessive numbers of cells, protein content, pressure is an important source of information about the nervous system.

c. fluid–blood barrier CSF passes into the CSF system (brain ventricles, the central canal of the spinal cord and the subarachnoid space) at the choroid plexus and passes out of the subarachnoid space into the sagittal sinus. The confining membranes of the system control selectively the passage of certain materials between it and the brain tissue (CSF–brain barrier) and between it and the blood (CSF–blood barrier).

c. fluid–brain barrier see cerebrospinal fluid–blood barrier (above).

c. nematodiasis invasion of the central nervous system by the microfilaria of *Setaria labiatopapillosa* (*S. digitata*) in most species causes an acute focal encephalomyelomalacia. The clinical picture is one of incoordination, then paralysis of the limbs, especially the hinds. *S. equina* may cause endophthalmitis in horses by similar invasion.

c. thrombosis see cerebrospinal embolism (above).

c. vasculitis see VASCULITIS.

cerebrotomy anatomy or dissection of the brain.

cerebrovascular pertaining to the blood vessels of the cerebrum or brain.

c. accident cerebral vascular accident. See also BRAIN hemorrhage, BRAIN hematoma.

cerebrum the main portion of the brain, occupying the front part of the cranial cavity; its two cerebral hemispheres are united by the corpus callosum. The term is sometimes applied to the postembryonic forebrain and midbrain together or to the entire brain. See also BRAIN.

Cereopsis novaehollandiae see CAPE BARREN GOOSE.

cerium a chemical element, atomic number 58, atomic weight 140.12, symbol Ce. See also Table 6.

ceroid an insoluble polymer of oxidized lipid and protein; an acid-fast, sudanophilic, pigment found in the liver, the nervous system and muscle. See also ceroid LIPOFUSCINOSIS.

ceroid lipofuscinosis see ceroid LIPOFUSCINOSIS.
certain safety factor margin of safety of a drug measured from the ratio of the median lethal dose and the median effective dose. Called also therapeutic index, LD_{50}/ED_{50}.
certainty confidence in a certain event or outcome occurring; a subjective judgment by a decision maker. The sure thing, the guaranteed happening, the certain winner.
c. equivalent the estimated value of a doubtful happening if it happened; used to help decision making in risky ventures.
c. required refers to the making of a diagnosis. The criterion on which a decision can be made about how far to go in the investigation of a case is the degree of certainty required.
certificate written certification of an examination, treatment, necropsy carried out by a veterinarian. Because the certificates are often the instruments on which compensation is made and lawsuits decided they are very important to the reputation of the veterinarian who prepares them and to the profession and its status in the community. The two areas of common error are the incomplete certificate that omits critical matters, especially the accurate identification of the patient, and the omission of the required entries which are left for the owner to complete, providing an opportunity and temptation to defraud.
ceruletide a compound isolated from the skin of an Australian frog, with activity similar to gastrin and pancreozymin. It causes contraction of the gallbladder and relaxation of the sphincter of Oddi. Used in humans to treat paralytic ileus and in radiography during cholecystography.
ceruloplasmin an alpha$_2$-globulin of the plasma, being the form in which most of the plasma copper is transported. Used as a measure of the copper status of animals.
cerumen a waxy secretion of the glands of the external acoustic meatus; ear wax.
c. glands modified sweat glands in the epithelial lining of the external auditory meatus.
ceruminolysis dissolution or disintegration of cerumen in the external acoustic meatus. The therapeutic effect of some medications used in the treatment of otitis externa.
ceruminosis excessive or disordered secretion of cerumen.
cervical pertaining to the neck or to the cervix.
c. ankylosis ankylosis of the intervertebral joints. See also HYPERVITAMINOSIS A.
c. aplasia segmental aplasia of the genital tract may be manifested by the absence or deformity of the cervix. Infertility is absolute. Diagnosis in large animals can be performed by rectal palpation; small animals may require surgical exploration.
c. cirrhosis caused by severe laceration at parturition; a rare cause of dystocia.
c. curve one of the vertebral curves of the body.
c. dislocation satisfactory method of euthanasia for laboratory mice, immature rats and poultry. Must be performed by an experienced person in order to achieve rapid and humane death.
c. fixation suturing of the cervix through the vaginal floor to the prepubic tendon. Used in the treatment of vaginal prolapse in cows.
c. incompetence damage to the cervix during parturition in the mare may cause its deformity and render it incapable of effectively closing off the uterus from the vagina. Infection of the uterus and infertility result.
incomplete c. dilation incomplete dilation of the cervix during parturition in adult cows, less commonly in heifers, may necessitate obstetrical, even cesarean, assistance; thought to be hormonal. See also RINGWOMB in ewes.
c. inflammation see CERVICITIS.
c. instability, c. malformation, c. malarticulation see canine WOBBLER SYNDROME.
c. line lesions lesions of the tooth neck characterized by progressive, subgingival, osteoclastic resorption. These occur commonly in cats.
c. lymphadenitis infection with abscessation of cervical lymph nodes in guinea pigs; usually caused by *Streptococcus zooepidemicus*.
c. massage suitable for use only in cows. The fetus is pulled up into the cervix and light traction maintained while a well-lubricated hand is pushed gently between the cervix and the fetus. This is done repeatedly and continued if there is no evidence of trauma. The cervix may dilate sufficiently to allow normal delivery of the calf.
c. mucus from the cervix. Its presence in liberal amounts is used as an indication of estrus.
c. paralysis inability to lift the head, usually accompanied by paralysis of all four limbs.
c. plexus see cervical PLEXUS.
c. rib a supernumerary rib arising from a cervical vertebra.
c. spinal cord lesion includes fracture–dislocation, cervical vertebral abscess, compression due to exostosis, spinal myelitis and myelacia, congenital lesions including spinal canal stenosis.
c. spine cervical vertebrae.
c. spondylolisthesis, spondylopathy see canine WOBBLER SYNDROME.
c. spondylosis see cervical ankylosis (above).
c. static stenosis one of the two syndromes listed under cervical vertebral stenotic myelopathy; characterized by compression of the cord at C5 to C7 in large male horses 1–4 years of age; the position of the neck is immaterial; the resulting syndrome is characterized by an insidious onset of ataxia. See also ENZOOTIC equine incoordination.
c. stenotic myelopathy focal myelopathy caused by compression of the spinal cord by excessive flexion of the neck in patients, especially dogs, in which there is a pre-existing narrowing of one of the two vertebral foramina in one or more vertebrae, especially cervical vertebrae. See also degenerative MYELOENCEPHALOPATHY.
c. swab swab of the os cervix for bacterial and virological examination for pathogens likely to affect fertility adversely. Used in fertility examination of cases of prolonged infertility in ruminants. See also UTERINE swab.
c. syndrome clinical signs caused by a lesion of the spinal cord between C1 and C5. They include tetraparesis to tetraplegia or hemiparesis to hemiplegia, hyperreflexia, hypertonia, depressed postural responses and sometimes cervical pain.
c. trauma most common are lacerations during parturition; resulting adhesions and fibrosis may cause subsequent dystocia.
c. vertebrae the skeleton of the neck, in most mammals comprising seven vertebrae, in birds up to 25.
c. vertebra fracture in horses occurs as a result of head-on collisions at speed; causes recumbency and inability to move limbs voluntarily, but there is full consciousness and patient can eat and drink if assisted.
c. vertebral stenotic myelopathy one of the causes

of incoordination in young horses. See also ENZOOTIC equine incoordination.
cervical abscess of pigs streptococcal abscess of the lymph nodes of the throat; a specific disease of pigs which exerts its importance at slaughter because of the rejection of affected parts. The cause is infection with beta-hemolytic streptococci of Lancefield Group E.
cervicectomy excision of the cervix uteri.
cervicitis inflammation of the cervix uteri.
cervic(o)- word element. [L.] *neck, cervix.*
cervicobrachialgia pain in the neck radiating to the forelimb, due to compression of nerve roots of the cervical spinal cord.
cervicocolpitis inflammation of the cervix uteri and vagina.
cervicofacial pertaining to the neck and face.
cervicofemoral angle the angle at which the neck of the femur joins the shaft. Called also the angle of inclination. Important in assessment for hip dysplasia in dogs.
cervicopexy suture of the uterine cervix to the prepubic tendon to retain a previously prolapsed cervix.
cervicoplasty plastic surgery on the neck.
cervicospinal arthropathy see CERVICAL vertebral stenotic myelopathy.
cervicothoracic ganglia the staging post for most sympathetic nerve impulses going to the heart; called also stellate ganglia.
cervicothoracic syndrome the clinical signs associated with lesions of the spinal cord from C6 to T2. Includes tetraparesis to tetraplegia or hemiparesis to hemiplegia, muscle atrophy in the forelimbs, depressed postural responses, and hypalgesia to analgesia caudal to the level of the lesion. Horner's syndrome is sometimes present.
cervicotomy incision of the circular muscle layers of the cervix to permit the passage of a normal sized fetus through a stenosed cervix. Performed only in the cow and not conducive to subsequent fertility.
cervicovaginal pertaining to the cervix and the vagina.
cervicovesical relating to the cervix uteri and urinary bladder.
cervid a member of the family Cervidae, deer, elk, reindeer, moose, wapiti, muntjacs and sikas.
Cervidae the family of the order Artiodactyla or ruminants, which contains the true deer including elk and moose.
cervix pl. *cervices;* neck; the front portion of the neck (collum), or a constricted part of an organ (e.g. cervix uteri, see below).
double c. incomplete fusion of the müllerian ducts leads to duplication of all or parts of the female genital tract. In cows one of these is a duplication of the cervix but with only one uterus. More common is a double external os but a single internal os. Both represent an inconvenience at artificial insemination and are detectable on rectal or vaginal examination.
c. uteri the narrow caudal end of the uterus that opens into the vagina.
c. vesicae the caudal constricted part of the urinary bladder, proximal to the opening of the urethra.
Cervus a genus of true deer in the family Cervidae. Includes *C. canadensis* (wapiti), *C. elaphus* (red deer) and *C. elaphus nannodes* (tule elk).
cesarean section delivery of a fetus by incision through the abdominal wall and uterus. The procedure takes its name from the Latin word *caedere*, to cut, and has no relation to the birth of Caesar as is sometimes believed.
cesarotomy see CESAREAN SECTION.
cesium a chemical element, atomic number 55, atomic weight 132.905, symbol Cs. See Table 6.
c.-137 a product of atomic fission by explosion or breakdown of a reactor. It is feared as a pollutant because of its very long half-life.
cesspit a pit to retain the sediment, usually fecal, of a drain.
cestocidal destructive to cestodes.
cestocide an agent that destroys cestodes.
cestodal cysts the larval (metacestode) stage of cestodes in mammal hosts, e.g. *Echinococcus* spp. cysts in humans, *Cysticercus tenuicollis* cysts in sheep.
cestode 1. any individual of the class Eucestoda. 2. cestoid.
cestodiasis infestation with tapeworms.
cestodology the scientific study of cestodes.
cestoid resembling a tapeworm.
Cestrum a genus of shrubs in the family Solanaceae. (1) *C. aurantiacum* (orange-flowered cestrum), *C. corymbosum* var. *hirsutum*, *C. elegans* (*C. newelii*, *C. purpureum*), *C. fasciculatum* (red cestrum), *C. hartwegii*, *C. laevigatum* (inkberry bush), *C. nocturnum* (night-flowering cestrum), *C. parqui* (green cestrum) cause liver necrosis. The toxin is a carboxyatractyloside.
(2) *C. diurnum* (jasmine, wild jasmine) causes generalized calcinosis through a calcinogenic glycoside. See also ENZOOTIC calcinosis.
Cetacaine a combination local anesthetic containing tetracaine, benzocaine and butamben used topically on mucous membranes.
cetacean includes the marine mammals of the order Odontoceti, the whales and their congeners, the dolphins, grampuses and porpoises.
cetalkonium chloride a cationic quaternary ammonium surfactant, used as a topical anti-infective and disinfectant.
Cetonia aurata see MACRODACTYLUS SUBSPINOSUS.
cetrimonium bromide a quaternary ammonium antiseptic and detergent, applied topically to the skin to cleanse wounds, as a preoperative disinfectant; also used to cleanse utensils and to store surgical instruments.
cetylpyridinium chloride a cationic disinfectant used as a local anti-infective applied topically to intact skin or mucous membrane.
cevadine one of the alkaloids of *Veratrum californicum* but not one known to be implicated in the production of congenital defects that occur in sheep fed on this plant.
cevitamic acid see ASCORBIC ACID.
Ceylonocotyle a genus of flukes (digenetic trematodes) in the family Paramphistomatidae. Includes *Ceylonocotyle scoliocoelium*, *C. streptocoelium* (rumen, reticulum). See under PARAMPHISTOMOSIS.
CF see FOLINIC ACID.
Cf chemical symbol, *californium.*
CFT complement fixation test.
CFU see COLONY-forming units.
cg centigram.
cGMP 3′5′ cyclic guanosine monophosphate; essential in regulation of sodium channels of the retina. Decrease in cGMP concentration leads to hyperpolarization of the retinal membrane.
CGS, c.g.s. centimeter–gram–second (system), a system of measurements based on the centimeter as the unit of length, the gram as the unit of mass, and the second as the unit of time.
Ch. a prefix denoting Champion; used on dog titles to designate one that has accrued the specified number of points in competitions.

CH_{50} the dose of complement that lyses 50% of a red cell suspension.

Chabertia a genus of nematodes in the superfamily Strongyloidea. *Chabertia ovina* (colon of ruminants). See CHABERTIASIS.

chabertiasis infestation with *Chabertia ovina*. Characterized by weight loss and the passage of soft feces containing much mucus. Called also chabertiosis.

chabertiosis see CHABERTIASIS.

chaerophyllin toxic principle in *Chaerophyllum*.

Chaerophyllum a genus in the plant family Apiaceae. Contains a toxin chaerophyllin capable of causing diarrhea and incoordination. Includes *C. sylvestre*, *C. temulentum* (rough or wild chervil, ass's parsley).

chaeta see SETA.

chafe to irritate the skin by friction, usually from harness, or the rubbing together of body surfaces, such as the thighs, when they are damp with perspiration, or the rubbing together of opposing skin folds.

chaff 1. chaffed hay; called also chop. 2. the winnowings from a threshing, consisting of awns, husks, glumes and other relatively indigestible materials.

Chagas' disease, Chagas–Cruz disease see TRYPANOSOMA *cruzi*, American TRYPANOSOMIASIS.

chagoma skin tumor in trypanosomiasis due to *Trypanosoma cruzi*.

Chailletia cymosa DICHAPETALUM *cymosum*.

chain a collection of objects linked together in linear fashion, or end to end, as the assemblage of atoms or radicals in a chemical compound, or an assemblage of individual bacterial cells.

c. binomial model model of an outbreak of an infectious disease in which the outbreak is depicted as a series of steps with a binomial statement of the probability of an outcome at each step.

branched c. an open chain of atoms, usually carbon, with one or more side chains attached to it.

heavy c. any of the large polypeptide chains of five classes that, paired with the light chains, make up the antibody molecule. Heavy chains bear the antigenic determinants that differentiate the immunoglobulin classes. See also HEAVY-CHAIN DISEASE.

J c. a polypeptide occurring in polymeric IgM and IgA molecules.

light c. either of the two small polypeptide chains (molecular weight 22,000) that, when linked to heavy chains by disulfide bonds, make up the antibody molecule; they are of two types, kappa and lambda, which are unrelated to immunoglobulin class differences.

light c. disease the overproduction of immunoglobulin light chain molecules by certain B cell tumors (plasmacytomas). See monoclonal GAMMOPATHY.

obstetric c. used in obstetrics in cattle and horses to snare extremities and for traction. Made of rustproof metal with links designed not to kink or to jam. They have a loop link at each end to facilitate single-handed formation of a loop. The links are shaped so that the ring-grip handles used for traction will grip at any point and stay put with the strongest pull.

c. shank a leather lead with a short section of chain at the proximal end. It can be placed over the horse's nose, through the mouth or across the upper gum for greater control.

side c. a chain of atoms attached to a larger chain or to a ring.

stallion c. strong chain, 1–2 ft (0.5 m) long, at the end of a solid lead. For leading a stallion with little chance of his biting through the lead.

c. termination method See SANGER–COULSON METHOD.

chalasia relaxation of a bodily opening, such as the cardiac sphincter. See also MEGAESOPHAGUS.

chalazae strands of albumen which come from each pole of a bird's egg and suspend the yolk in the approximate center of the egg. The chalazae are often twisted because of rotation of the yolk.

chalazion a small eyelid mass resulting from chronic inflammation of a meibomian gland. Called also meibomian cyst.

chalcosis copper deposits in tissue.

challenge feeding a system of feeding dairy cows which provides more feed than is justified by the level of the individual cow's milk production. In the early part of the lactation the cow is challenged to produce more milk and in many instances does so. If the cow does not respond the level of feeding is reduced. Called also lead feeding because the cow is led to produce more heavily.

chalone a group of tissue-specific, water-soluble substances that are produced within a tissue and that inhibit mitosis of the cells of that tissue and whose action is reversible.

chalybeate containing or charged with iron.

Chamaeleo the genus of chameleons. Includes *C. dilepis*, *C jacksonii*.

chamber an enclosed space.

anterior c. the part of the aqueous humor-containing space of the eyeball between the cornea and iris.

hyperbaric c. an enclosed space in which gas (oxygen) can be raised to greater than atmospheric pressure. See also HYPERBARIC oxygenation.

ionization c. see IONIZATION chamber.

posterior c. that part of the aqueous humor-containing space of the eyeball between the iris and the lens.

vitreous c. the vitreous humor-containing space in the eyeball, bounded anteriorly by the lens and ciliary body and posteriorly by the posterior wall of the eyeball.

chambering a technique of modifying the padding in harness over a gall or other sore spot. The stuffing is worked away with an awl or needle and stitched to the felt to stop it from working back into the cavity.

chameleon lizard member of the genus *Chameleo*.

chamois 1. sheepskin specially impregnated with fish oil to make it pliable; used for cleaning. 2. an agile goat-antelope; *Rupicapra rupicapra*.

c. contagious ecthyma virus see contagious ECTHYMA.

chamomile, camomile derived from flowerheads of two species of Compositae; used for its anti-inflammatory and antiseborrheic activity, usually topically but also administered orally as a tea for indigestion and in the treatment of calf scours.

champignon streptococcosis of the stump of the spermatic cord. Usually refers to castration of the horse.

chancre the 2 to 4 in, hard, hot, painful lesion which develops at the site of tsetse-fly bites when the fly is a transmitter of trypanosomiasis. In human medicine, refers to the primary lesion of syphilis.

chandelier plant see BRYOPHYLLUM *tubiflorum*.

Chandlurella quiscali a nematode parasite found in the emu.

channel in biophysical terms these are the 'pores' in semipermeable membranes through which specific physicochemical units, e.g. cations, calcium ions, can pass; the rate of passage of some channels may be much slower than others, hence there is an expansive nomenclature, e.g. slow calcium channel, fast calcium channel.

channel aeration a modification of the ACTIVATED

sludge method of disposing of sewage. The sewage is aerated in a long channel rather than in a lagoon.

channel catfish see ICTALURUS *punctatus*.

c. c. virus disease acute herpesvirus disease of young catfish fry. There is ascites, exophthalmos and hemorrhage in the fins. Widespread in North America.

Channos channos Asian wild fish used as human food. See also Table 23.

chaperone a family of proteins that aid in the folding of target proteins.

chaperonin a class of CHAPERONE proteins.

char arctic and subarctic species of the fish genus SALVELINUS.

characin a carnivorous fish belonging to the order Cyprinoidea. Includes piranha.

character a quality or attribute indicative of the nature of an object or an organism. 1. in genetics, the expression of a gene or group of genes as seen in a phenotype. 2. in computers, a single letter, number, space punctuation, or special character or symbol. 3. in wool the evenness of the crimp.

acquired c. a noninheritable modification produced in an animal as a result of its own activities or of environmental influences.

c. data alphanumeric data.

dominant c. a mendelian character that is expressed when it is transmitted by a single gene.

mendelian c's in genetics, the separate and distinct traits exhibited by an animal or plant and dependent on the genetic constitution of the organism.

primary sex c's those characters of the male and female directly concerned in reproduction.

recessive c. a mendelian character that is expressed only when transmitted by both genes (one from each parent) determining the trait.

secondary sex c's those characters specific to the male and female but not directly concerned in reproduction.

sex-conditioned c., sex-influenced c. an autosomal trait whose full expression is conditioned by the sex of the individual, e.g. human baldness.

sex-linked c. one transmitted consistently to individuals of one sex only, being carried in the sex chromosome.

characteristic 1. character. 2. typical of an individual or other entity. See also CHARACTER.

c. curve the photographic characteristics of an emulsion on an x-ray film based on plotting the density of the image obtained against the logarithm of the exposure under specified conditions of development.

c. radiation nearly homogeneous radiation produced in the target of the x-ray tube when orbital electrons are knocked out and replaced by electrons from outer shells.

c. x-rays see characteristic radiation (above).

charadriiform a member of the order Charadriiformes of shore birds including waders and gulls.

charbon [Fr.] see ANTHRAX.

Charbray a taurindicus breed of beef cattle, white to light red in color, produced by crossing Brahman and Charolais.

Charchesium polysinum a protozoa which parasitizes the skin of tadpoles. Lesions may cover the gills and cause asphyxia.

charcoal carbon prepared by charring wood or other organic material.

activated c. the residue of destructive distillation of various organic materials, treated to increase its adsorptive power; used as a general purpose antidote.

Charcot–Bottcher crystals characteristic intracellular cytoplasmic crystals which occur in normal canine Sertoli cells, but do not occur in Sertoli cell tumors.

Charcot triad biliary colic, jaundice and fever, three signs associated with acute cholecystitis.

charlatan a pretender to knowledge or skills not possessed; in veterinary medicine, a quack.

Charles' law at a constant pressure the volume of a given mass of perfect gas varies directly with the absolute temperature.

charlier shoe a special horseshoe which fits into a groove taken out of the bearing surface of the hoof wall. There is no toe clip and the shoe is narrow and light in weight. It is not a work shoe but intended to protect the hoof while the horse is resting for a period. Called also periplantar shoe.

charlock SINAPIS *arvensis*.

Charolais a white or cream breed of cattle with pink mucosae, produced in central France and used for dairy, beef or draft purposes.

Charollaise sheep meat and wool polled sheep, originated from Leicester longwool plus local breed.

charque South American dried salted beef.

chart a record of data in graphic or tabular form.

pedigree c. a graph showing various descendants of a common ancestor, used to indicate those affected by genetically determined disease.

charting the keeping of a clinical record of the important facts about a patient and the progress of its illness. The patient's chart most often contains a medical history, a nursing history, results of physical examinations, laboratory reports, results of special diagnostic tests, and the observations of the nursing staff. See also problem-oriented MEDICAL record.

Chartreux an old French breed of cats; it has a blue-gray, medium-length, double coat.

chase pursuit of a lure on a racetrack or of a dragged hare in a field by a Greyhound.

chaser a secondary or follow-up breeding male put in with a herd of cows or ewes when the fertility of the first stud is suspect.

Chastek paralysis, Chastek's paralysis see THIAMIN nutritional deficiency.

chauffage [Fr.] treatment with a low-heated cautery that is passed to and fro close to the tissue.

check ligament one of the two ligamentous accessory heads to the digital flexors of the horse. See also SUSPENSORY ligament.

c. l. desmotomy a treatment for contracted flexor tendons in horses.

check rein see check REIN.

checkerboard the pattern of a chess or draft board; used in many circumstances to display the results of mixing a specific number of variables. The variables are listed in columns designated along the horizontal border and the same or different variables in lines along the vertical border; the results of each mixing are recorded in the box where the columns and lines carrying the ingredients of the mix intersect.

checkpoint points in the cell cycle of eukaryotic cells which prevent progress until each stage is satisfactorily completed.

Chediak–Higashi syndrome an inherited disease in humans, cattle, Aleutian mink, white tigers and killer whales. There is dilution of color in the hair and ciliary processes of the eye, with large granules, believed to be lysosomes, in all cell types and particularly noticeable in circulating neutrophils and eosinophils. Leukocytes are defective in chemotaxis and intracellular killing. Affected individuals suffer from an increased susceptibility to infection and bleeding tendencies caused by a platelet storage defect.

cheek the fleshy portion of either side of the face, forming the sides of the mouth and continuing rostrally to the lips. Attached to alveolar borders of maxillae and mandibles. Called also bucca.

cleft c. facial cleft caused by developmental failure of union between the maxillary and primitive frontonasal processes.

c. pouches evaginations of the oral cavity extending alongside the head and neck, as far as the scapulae, in hamsters. Used to transport food. In experimental studies tissues in these pouches demonstrate immunologial tolerance to grafted tissues.

c. swelling caused usually by osteomyelitis of the jaw bones, local neoplasia, packing of food in a chronically malfunctioning cheek or a large foreign body stuck in the cheek space.

c. teeth molars and premolars.

cheese a food produced industrially by the precipitation of milk protein and capable of acting as a vector of animal disease caused by resistant bacteria but especially by viruses, especially foot-and-mouth disease.

c. fly infests cheese but of esthetic importance only. Called also cheese skipper, *Piophila casei*.

c. mite TYROGLYPHUS *siro*.

cheese-washer's lung a hypersensitivity pneumonitis of humans caused by inhalation of *Penicillin caseii* spores present in cheese casings.

cheeseweed see MALVA PARVIFLORA.

cheesewood ALSTONIA *scholaris*.

cheesy gland chronic disease characterized by hard swelling of one or more peripheral lymph nodes containing semiliquid to caseous pus; may rupture spontaneously or be lacerated during shearing and discharge pus to the exterior; colloquial for caseous lymphadenitis in sheep and goats.

cheetah see ACINONYX JUBATUS.

Cheilanthes a fern member of the family Sinopteridaceae; known toxic components include ptaquiloside and thiaminase. Called also cloak ferns, rock ferns.

C. distans, C. tenuifolia a rock fern that causes incoordination and somnolence in sheep.

C. sieberi has caused hemorrhagic disease, polioencephalomalacia and enzootic hematuria. Called also rock or mulga fern.

C. sieberi* subsp. *sieberi *C. sieberi*.

C. sinuata causes polioencephalomalacia ('jimmies') in grazing ruminants. Called also jimmy fern.

cheilectropion eversion of the lip.

cheilitis inflammation of the lips.

cheil(o)- word element. [Gr.] *lip*.

cheilognathopalatoschisis cleft of the lip, upper jaw, and hard and soft palates.

cheilognathoschisis cleft of the upper lip and jaw.

cheiloplasty surgical repair of a lip defect.

cheilorrhaphy suture of the lip; surgical repair of a harelip.

cheiloschisis see CLEFT lip.

cheilosis fissuring and dry scaling of the lips and angles of the mouth, a characteristic of riboflavin deficiency.

Cheilospirura a genus of nematodes of the family Acuariidae.

C. hamulosa found in the gizzard of fowls and turkeys. Heavy infestations cause emaciation, weakness and anemia. Called also *Acuaria*.

cheilotomy incision of the lip.

chelate to combine with a metal in complexes in which the metal is part of a ring; by extension, a chemical compound in which a metallic ion is sequestered and firmly bound into a ring within the chelating molecule. Chelates are used in treatment of metal poisoning.

chelating agent a substance which combines with a metallic ion to produce an inert chelate, e.g. ethylenediamine tetra-acetic acid, penicillamine.

chelerythrine a toxic alkaloid found in the plant CHELIDONIUM MAJUS.

chelicerae pair of movable oral appendages adapted for cutting carried by acarids, including ticks.

chelidonine a toxic alkaloid found in the plant CHELIDONIUM MAJUS.

Chelidonium majus temperate zone plant of the family Papaveraceae; contains the isoquinoline alkaloid chelidonine; causes vomiting, colic and diarrhea, possibly somnolence. Called also greater celandine, celandine poppy.

chelonethida false scorpion. A member of the order Pseudoscorpionidae of the class Arachnida.

Chelonia marine turtles; in the family Chelonidae.

C. mydas green turtle.

chelonian member of the order Chelonia of the class Reptilia. Includes tortoise, terrapin, turtle, sea turtle.

Chelopistes a genus of the superfamily Ischnocera of lice. Includes *C. meleagridis* (turkeys).

chemabrasion superficial destruction of the epidermis and the upper layer of the dermis by application of a cauterant to the skin.

chemexfoliation chemabrasion.

chemical 1. pertaining to chemistry. 2. a substance composed of chemical elements, or obtained by chemical processes. See also TOXIN.

c. adjuvant a chemical added to another to improve its activity. For example, mineral gels added to vaccines. May also be a chemical added to feed to improve digestion, e.g. monensin in ruminants. These are more commonly referred to as ADDITIVES. See also ADJUVANT.

agricultural c. chemical used in agriculture. Includes pesticides, anthelmintics, fertilizers, algaecides, herbicides, soil fumigants and the like.

c. environment that part of the animals' environment that is composed of chemicals. For farm livestock this includes fertilizers, defoliants, worm drenches, insect sprays, adjuvants to feed. For companion animals see household chemical (below).

household c. the roster of chemicals that one can expect to find in the average household. Includes insect sprays and repellents, snail bait, rodenticide, garden sprays, human medicines and the like.

c. pneumonitis results from aspiration of gastric acids.

c. senses see OLFACTION (2), TASTE.

c. shearing causing the fleece of sheep to be shed by the administration of a chemical substance to the sheep. Cyclophosphamide and MIMOSINE have been used experimentally but there is no commercially available system.

c. spoilage occurs in preserved foods, especially canned ones. Is usually the result of interaction between the contents and an imperfect container. There may be gas produced, e.g. hydrogen swells, or discoloration of the tin.

c. warfare agents used include: (1) systemic poisons, e.g. hydrocyanic acid; (2) lung irritants, e.g. chlorine, phosgene; (3) lacrimators (weeping stimulators), e.g. CN, CAP, CS; (4) sternutators (sneeze stimulators); (5) vesicants, e.g. mustards, nitrogen mustards, arsenic mustards and nettle gases; (6) nerve gases, e.g. organophosphorus compounds.

cheminosis any disease due to chemical agents.
chemiosmosis a process in which a proton gradient across a mitochondrial membrane and ATP synthesis pump metabolites across a membrane.
chemist 1. an expert in chemistry. 2. sometimes used as an abbreviation for pharmaceutical chemist or pharmacist.
chemistry the science that treats of the elements and atomic relations of matter, and of the various compounds of the elements.
colloid c. chemistry dealing with the nature and composition of colloids.
inorganic c. the branch of chemistry dealing with inorganic compounds.
organic c. the branch of chemistry dealing with organic compounds, those characterized by carbon–carbon bonds, i.e. all compounds containing carbon except oxides of carbon, carbides and carbonates.
chem(o)- word element. [Gr.] *chemical, chemistry*.
chemoattractant a chemical (chemotactic) agent that induces an organism or a cell, a leukocyte, to migrate toward it.
chemoautotroph a chemoautotrophic organism.
chemocautery cauterization by application of a caustic substance.
chemodectoma nonchromaffin paraganglionoma: any tumor of the chemoreceptor system, e.g. a carotid body tumor, AORTIC body tumor. Brachycephalic breeds of dogs are predisposed, possibly due to genetic factors and chronic hypoxia.
chemohormonal pertaining to drugs having hormonal activity.
chemoimmunization used in the control of protozoal diseases; consists of simultaneous administration of virulent protozoa and an appropriate babesicide.
chemokines a large family of *chemo*tactic cyto*kines* which stimulate leukocyte movement.
chemokinesis the ability to stimulate movement of leukocytes.
chemolithotroph an organism that derives its energy from oxidation of inorganic compounds and its carbon from carbon dioxide.
chemolithotrophic deriving energy from the oxidation of reduced inorganic compounds such as ferrous iron, ammonia, hydrogen sulfide or hydrogen; said of bacteria.
chemoluminescence the emission of light by chemical reactions, most commonly oxidation. (1) Used as a measure of metabolic activity of phagocytic cells, e.g. neutrophils, monocytes and macrophages. (2) A developing technique for marking the state of preservation of food. As the food deteriorates it begins to emit fluorescent light.
chemolysis chemical decomposition.
chemonucleolysis dissolution of a portion of the nucleus pulposus of an intervertebral disk by injection of a chemolytic agent for treatment of a herniated intervertebral disk.
chemo-organotroph an organism that derives its energy and carbon from organic compounds.
chemo-organotrophic deriving energy from the oxidation of organic compounds; said of bacteria.
chemopallidectomy destruction of tissue of the globus pallidus by a chemical agent.
chemoprophylaxis prevention of disease by chemical means.
chemoreception the physiological reception of chemical stimuli.
chemoreceptor any of the special cells or organs adapted for excitation by chemical substances and located outside the central nervous system. There are chemoreceptors in the large arteries of the thorax and the neck; called carotid and aortic bodies. These receptors are responsive to changes in the oxygen, carbon dioxide and hydrogen ion concentration in the blood. When oxygen concentration falls below normal in the arterial blood, the chemoreceptors send impulses to stimulate the respiratory center so that there will be an increase in alveolar ventilation, and consequently, an increase in the intake of oxygen by the lungs.

Other chemoreceptors are the taste buds, which are sensitive to chemicals in the mouth, and the olfactory cells of the nose, which detect certain chemicals in the air.
c. trigger zone (CTZ) located in the floor of the fourth ventricle; sensitive to motion, uremia, apomorphine. Activation stimulates neurons of the emetic center.
c. tumors see CHEMODECTOMA.
chemoreflex a physiological reflex initiated by a chemical substance.
chemosensitive sensitive to changes in chemical composition.
chemosensory relating to the perception of chemical substances, as in odor detection.
chemosis marked edema of the conjunctiva of the eye.
chemostat a vessel that provides constant growth conditions for bacteria.
chemosterilants chemicals used to render an animal sterile. To date, used principally in creating sterile male insects in the control of single mating insects such as screw-worm.
chemosurgery the destruction of tissue by chemical agents for therapeutic purposes; originally applied to chemical fixation of malignant, gangrenous or infected tissue, with use of frozen sections to facilitate systematic microscopic control of its excision.
chemosynthesis the building up of chemical compounds under the influence of chemical stimulation, specifically the formation of carbohydrates from carbon dioxide and water as a result of energy derived from chemical reactions.
chemotactic factor soluble molecules which attract and guide the movement of cells such as phagocytes in the inflammatory response.
chemotaxin a substance, e.g. a complement component, that induces chemotaxis.
chemotaxis taxis or directional movement in response to the influence of chemical stimulation.
leukocyte c. the response of leukocytes to products formed in immunological reactions, wherein leukocytes are attracted to and accumulate at the site of the reaction; a part of the inflammatory response. See also INFLAMMATION.
chemotherapy the treatment of illness by chemical means; that is, by medication.
cancer c. the use of antineoplastic agents in the treatment of malignant growths; usually employed because treatment by other means, such as surgical removal, is not possible. A variety of malignancies in dogs and cats have been successfully managed with some of the chemotherapeutic agents used in the treatment of cancer in humans.
combination c. several drugs are used in parallel or in sequence. A common procedure in human cancer therapy.
multimodal c. chemotherapy combined with other forms of treatment, e.g. surgical excision.
chemotic 1. pertaining to or affected with chemosis.

2. an agent that increases lymph production in the ocular conjunctiva.

chemotrophic deriving energy from the oxidation of organic (chemo-organotrophic) or inorganic (chemolithotrophic) compounds; said of bacteria.

chemotropism tropism in response to the influence of chemical stimulation.

chenodeoxycholic acid a primary bile acid, $C_{24}H_{40}O_4$, administered as an anticholelithogenic agent. Called also chenodiol.

chenodiol see CHENODEOXYCHOLIC ACID.

Chenopodium a plant genus of the Chenopodiaceae family; many plants in the genus contain oxalates and can cause oxalate poisoning. Includes *C. album* (fat hen, lambsquarters, white goosefoot), *C. atriplicinum* (*Scleroblitum atriplclinum*, lambstongue). Other plants can cause cyanide poisoning, e.g. *C. carinatum* (green crumbweed, Boggabri), *C. glaucum* (oak-leaved goosefoot), *C. melanocarpum* (black crumbweed), *C. rhadinostachyum* (*Dysphania radinostachya*, *C. chenostachyum*, mouse-tailed crumbweed).

C. ambrosioides contains wormseed oil; used as an anthelmintic. Capable of causing gastroenteritis. Called also *C. antheminticum* var. *ambrosioides*, wormseed.

Cherax American crayfish. See Table 23.

cherry PRUNUS *cerasus*, PRUNUS *laurocerasus*, SOLANUM *pseudocapsicum*.

cherry eye an eversion of the nictitating membrane (third eyelid) caused by hypertrophy and prolapse of the gland of the third eyelid, over the free margin of the membrane. Called also follicular ophthalmitis.

cherry laurel PRUNUS *laurocerasus*.

cherry-pie LANTANA *camara*.

chervil see CHAEROPHYLLUM.

Chesapeake Bay retriever a medium-sized, muscular dog with short, thick, water-repellent coat with woolly undercoat. The color is distinctive, from dark brown to faded tan or 'deadgrass'. Hereditary cataracts occur in the breed.

chest see THORAX, THORACIC, FLAIL chest.

c. compression a means of external cardiac massage; most likely to be effective in small dogs and cats, but very difficult in large animals.

c. wound common in horses and cattle, damage to the underlying chest wall with communication to the pleural cavity and pneumothorax is the main danger.

Chester White pig a fat, white breed of meat pigs developed in the USA. Known originally as Chester County White, and subsequently as Ohio Improved Chester.

chestnut 1. flattened, oval masses of horn on the medial surface of the forearm and the hock of the horse. Those on the forelimb are just proximal to the carpus, those on the hindlimb are at the distal end of the tarsus. In donkeys the hindlimb chestnut is very small, in mules it is absent. They are regarded as being vestiges of the carpal and tarsal pads. 2. fruit of the chestnut tree *Castanea sativa*. 3. a popular coat color in horses. A deep reddish brown varying from a red dominance or light chestnut, to a heavier brown tone, liver or deep chestnut. Mixed with white hairs is a chestnut roan.

c. oak QUERCUS *prinus*.

c. rule mating two chestnut horses will not produce offspring with black, gray, brown or bay coat colors.

c. slough occurs in cattle when limb badly swollen or injured in grass fire.

Cheviot long-woolled, meat sheep from the UK, characterized by a prominent roman nose, woolless face, polled head and medium-quality wool.

chevrotain mouse deer which comprise the Tragulidae, one of the six families of ruminants in the order Artiodactyla. They are very small (6 to 10 inches high), hornless and have protruding canine teeth which serve as tusks. Includes *Tragulus*, *Hyemoschus* spp.

chewing see MASTICATION.

c. disease see NIGROPALLIDAL ENCEPHALOMALACIA.

chewing the cud see RUMINATION.

Chewing's fescue FESTUCA *rubra commutata*.

Cheyletiella a genus of mites in the family Cheyletidae. Cause a mild, scaling dermatitis in dogs and cats, a more severe, pruritic dermatitis, mainly on the back of rabbits, and intensely pruritic vesicles in humans. Host specificity is not certain; in general *C. blakei* infests cats, *C. parasitovorax* infests rabbits and hares, and *C. yasguri* infests dogs.

cheyletiellosis infestation by *Cheyletiella* spp. Called also cheyletiella dermatitis, 'walking' dandruff.

Cheyletoides uncinata SYRINGOPHILUS *uncinatus*.

Cheyletus eruditus housedust mite capable of causing dermatitis in indoor companion animals.

Cheyne–Stokes respiration breathing characterized by rhythmic waxing and waning of the depth of respiration; the patient breathes deeply for a short time and then breathes very slightly or stops breathing altogether. The pattern occurs over and over again every 45 seconds to 3 minutes. Periodic breathing of this type is caused by disease affecting the respiratory centers.

CHF congestive heart failure.

ch'i see QI.

chi-square distribution in statistical terms this is said of a variable with K degrees of freedom if it is distributed like the sum of the squares of K independent random variables each of which has a normal distribution with mean zero and variance of 1.

chi-squared test one of the statistical techniques for determining (1) if there are significant differences between two or more series of frequencies or proportions and (2) whether one series of proportions is significantly different from a control series. Pearson's chi-square is used for unmatched data and McNemar's chi-square for matched data.

Chiana a very tall, white with black points and mucosae, breed of dairy cattle, used also for draft. Called also Chianina.

Chiangus a black, polled beef breed of cattle produced by crossing Chianina and Angus cattle.

Chianina cattle Italian spelling for the CHIANA breed of white with black points, meat cattle.

chiasm a decussation or Y-shaped crossing.

optic c. a structure in the forebrain formed by the decussation of fibers of the optic nerve from each half of each retina.

chiasma pl. *chiasmata* [L., Gr.] chiasm; in genetics, the points at which members of a chromosome pair are in contact during the prophase of meiosis and because of which recombination, or crossing over, occurs on separation.

c. formation the process by which a chiasma is formed; it is the cytological basis of genetic recombination, or crossing over.

c. syndrome optic atrophy with bilateral hemianopia.

chibata ARRABIDEA *bilabiata*.

Chicago disease blastomycosis.

chick abbreviation for CHICKEN (1).

chicken 1. a young domestic fowl up to the age at which the bird can survive without supplementary heat and feed. In some poultry industries that is about 4 weeks. However, the endpoint varies with the type of husbandry practiced. In the North American poultry industry a chicken is any domestic fowl up to about 20 weeks of age. 2. any young bird.

c. anemia virus see CIRCOVIRIDAE.

c. body louse MENACANTHUS *stramineus*.

c. bronchitis see avian infectious BRONCHITIS.

day old c's newly hatched chicks are delivered in large flat cardboard boxes from the multiplier to the broiler grower—the universal means of shipping live chickens.

c. edema disease a disease of broiler chickens fed on a diet containing fat contaminated by one of several toxic factors which cause hepatic necrosis. It is manifested clinically by drooping, dyspnea, death. At necropsy there are large accumulations of fluid in body cavities and a swollen liver and kidneys. The disease is caused by a toxic fat containing dioxin added to the ration of the birds. Called also toxic fat disease.

c. embryo chondrodystrophy caused by nutritional deficiency of manganese. Characterized by short, thick legs, short wings, parrot beak, retarded down and body growth.

c. embryo lethal organ (CELO) virus see QUAIL bronchitis.

c.-fat clot clots that develop after death; largely devoid of red blood cells. More common in animals that have had anemia or in which blood sedimentation was increased. Seen more often in horses than in other species.

c. fluff louse GONIOCOTES *gallinae*.

c. head louse see CYCLOTOGASTER HETEROGRAPHA.

c. hemorrhagic syndrome see INCLUSION BODY hepatitis.

infectious c. anemia bone marrow hypoplasia with thymic and bursal atrophy in young chicks caused by a circovirus. The disease is characterized by weakness, pallor and a high mortality rate. Secondary bacterial, viral and fungal infections are commonplace including hemorrhagic syndrome, anemia dermatitis and blue wing disease.

c. louse see MENOPON *pallidum*, MENACANTHUS *stramineus*.

c. mite see DERMANYSSUS GALLINAE.

c. pox see AVIPOXVIRUS.

c. sexing usually carried out on day-old chickens by examining inside the vent for small eminences. Up to 1000 chickens can be sexed per hour with 98% accuracy.

sticky c. sticky, edematous chickens caused by hatching at too low or too high humidities.

chickling vetch LATHYRUS *sativus*.

chickpea a drought-resistant legume with a 20% protein content in the seeds. Used for livestock and human consumption. Called also *Cicer arietinum*, gram, garbanzo.

chickweed common name for a number of plants, e.g. *Stellaria media*.

tropical c. DRYMARIA *diandra*.

chiclero ulcer leishmaniasis, particularly *L. braziliensis*.

chicory see CICHORIUM INTYBUS.

chief cells the zymogenic or peptic cells of the gastric mucosa which secrete pepsinogen.

chief complaint the most apparent clinical sign in a patient's illness. Called also cardinal sign, key sign.

chigger the six-legged red larva of mites of the family Trombiculidae. See TROMBICULA, TROMBICULOSIS. Some species are vectors of the rickettsiae of scrub typhus of humans. Called also chigger mite, harvest mite and red bug.

chigoe the sand flea, *Tunga penetrans*, of tropical and subtropical American and Africa. Called also chigger or chigoe flea. Not to be confused with chigger mites. See also CHIGGER.

Chihuahua a very small (1–6 lb) dog originating in Mexico. It has a prominent, domed skull, erect ears and medium-length tail carried over the back. There are long-coated and smooth-coated varieties in many colors. The breed is predisposed to hydrocephalus and the presence of an open fontanelle (molera) is allowed for in the breed standard.

chill see RIGOR, HYPOTHERMIA.

Chillagoe horse disease esophageal ulceration caused by *Crotalaria aridicola* or *C. medicaginea* (in Australia).

chilled meat meat preserved by chilling to and maintaining at no more than 45°F (7°C), 37°F (3°C) for offal, immediately after slaughter. Quick chilling has many advantages and maintenance of a low humidity is favored because of the prevention of mold growth.

Chilodenella a genus of ciliates in the phylum Ciliophora which occur in fish and amphipods.

C. cyprini, C. hexasticha found in fish; the former causes a serious loss of skin at the gills.

chilodenellosis disease of freshwater fish caused by the unicellular ciliate *Chilodenella* spp. Characterized by hyperplasia of the epithelium of the gill and difficult respiration, and infection of the skin.

Chilomastix a genus of parasitic protozoa found in the intestines of vertebrates. Members of the order Trichomonadida.

C. bettencourti, C. caprae, C. cuniculi, C. equi, C. gallinarum, C. intestinalis, C. wenrichi nonpathogenic protozoa found in the ceca of, respectively, rodents, goats, rabbits, horses, chickens, turkeys and guinea pigs.

Chilomitus nonpathogenic protozoa of the order Trichomonadida.

C. caviae, C. connexus found in the cecum of the guinea pig.

Chilopoda a class of the phylum Arthropoda embracing the centipedes. See also MYRIAPODA.

chimera, chimaera 1. a mythological, fire-spouting monster with a lion's head, goat's body and serpent's tail. 2. an animal whose body contains different cell populations derived from different zygotes of the same or different species, occurring spontaneously or produced artificially; i.e. an individual composed of a mixture of genetically different cells.

c. protein see fusion PROTEIN.

chimeric protein see fusion PROTEIN.

chimerism the state of being a chimera; the presence in an animal of cells of different origin, e.g. XX/XY chimerism.

blood c. twins that have a common circulation develop immune tolerance. Each of them is then a chimera. When the twins are of opposite sex, the female twin may be a FREEMARTIN. Sterilization of the female is brought about by the transfer of H-Y antigen to the female gonad.

chimpanzee *Pan troglodytes* or *Pan satyrus*; a large anthropoid ape with the most highly developed brain of all animals other than humans. Dark colored, 5 to 6 ft high, with large out-turned ears, they are arboreal and live in families.

chin the anterior prominence of the lower jaw; the mentum.

fat-c., c. edema lower lip swelling or nodules; part of the feline EOSINOPHILIC granuloma complex.

stripped c. see labial AVULSION.

chin-ball a ball worn in a harness fitted to a ram at mating time; it rotates through a reservoir of brightly colored paste which is smeared onto the rump of ewes which stand for the ram in its early seeking activity of resting its chin on the ewe just prior to mounting.

China clay see KAOLIN.

china eye see china EYE.

chinaberry MELIA *azederach*.

chincherinchee, chinkerinchee see ORNITHOGALUM.

Chinchilla member of the Chinchillidae family of the order Rodentia.

C. brevicaudata called also short-tailed chinchilla.

chinchilla 1. small, South American rodent, valued for its silver-gray fur. Called also *Chinchilla laniger*. 2. a breed of cat; see CHINCHILLA CAT. 3. a breed of rabbit; see CHINCHILLA RABBIT.

Chinchilla cat a coat color variety of longhaired cats that consists of white hairs with black tips.

Chinchilla laniger see CHINCHILLA.

Chinchilla rabbit a rabbit whose silky coat closely resembles that of the real *Chinchilla laniger*; popular for fur and meat, as well as exhibition.

Chinchilla Rex see REX (2) rabbit.

chine the animal's backline.

Chinese black and white cattle black and white, Chinese, dual-purpose cattle, originated from Dutch Holstein.

Chinese blister fly see MYLABRIS PHALERATA.

Chinese blistering beetle see MYLABRIS PHALERATA.

Chinese crested a very small (6 to 12 lb), fine-boned dog with a hairless body. Small numbers of long hairs are present on the lower legs, tail and the head where they are called the 'crest'. The hairlessness is a dominant trait and specimens of the breed are heterozygotes, the homozygous dominant state being lethal prenatally. The longhaired offspring (homozygous recessive) of crosses are called 'powderpuffs'.

Chinese hawthorn see PHOTINIA.

Chinese liver fluke CLONORCHIS *sinensis*.

Chinese river dolphin *Lipotes vexillifer*. See Chinese river DOLPHIN.

Chinese Shar pei see SHAR PEI.

Chinese tallow tree see SAPIUM SEBIFERUM.

Chinese tallow wood see SAPIUM SEBIFERUM.

Chinese yellow Chinese draft cattle of zebu origin. Usually yellow, also brown, red or black in color.

Chinook salmon ONCORHYNCHUS *tshawytscha*.

chintz cat see TORTOISESHELL.

chip complicated electronic circuits etched on silicon chips; the building blocks of modern electronics. See also COMPUTER.

chip fractures small pieces of bone which are chipped off a bone, causing minor but sometimes significant lameness, pain and swelling. In horses, usually involve one of the carpal bones.

chipmunk a terrestrial rodent similar to a squirrel but lacking the bushy tail, silky coat and tufted ears. Has longitudinal stripes along its back. Called also *Eutamius* spp. and *Tamias striatus*.

Chippendale legs a term used in dogs to describe front legs that turn out at the elbows and feet, but with the carpi close together, resembling Chippendale-style furniture legs.

Chiracanthrium nutrix a European spider which may cause poisoning.

Chirodiscoides cutaneous mite of the suborder Sarcoptiformes. Includes *Chirodiscoides caviae* (guinea pigs).

Chirodropsidae a family in the order Cubomedusae of jellyfish. Contains the stinging sea wasps and box jellyfish.

Chirodropus one of the four genera of the family Chirodropsidae, containing the poisonous box jellyfish.

Chironex one of the four genera in the family Chirodropsidae, the box jellyfish.

C. fleckeri a poisonous, stinging jellyfish which may weigh 4 to 7 lb and measure 6 to 7 inches across and 8 inches deep. These animals possess a remarkable stinging device and a most potent, agonizingly painful and rapidly lethal poison.

Chiropotes see SAKI.

chiropractic, chiropracty a system of treating disease by manipulation of the vertebral column. Chiropractic is based on the theory that most diseases are caused by pressure on the nerves because of faulty alignment of the bones, especially the vertebrae, and that the nerves are thus prevented from transmitting to various organs of the body the neural impulses for proper functioning. Medical science has never found a scientific basis for this theory. Veterinary science has a small number of persons, sometimes without any formal training or qualifications, who practice this art.

Acting on the theory that the pinching of nerves is the critical factor in the pathogenesis of disease, the chiropractor manipulates various parts of the spine in treating the complaint. If the patient is suffering from a displaced vertebra, the manipulation may bring relief. If they have some other disorder or disease, however, manipulation will have little if any effect.

In the eyes of the law persons who practice chiropractic may not be practicing medicine or veterinary science because the subject is not one of the subjects taught in the formal schools, so that the practitioners may be immune from prosecution for illegal practice. This view avoids the truth that the diagnosis of the diseases of animals is always by definition veterinary medicine or veterinary science.

chiropractor a practitioner in chiropractic.

chiropracty see CHIROPRACTIC.

Chiropsalmus one of the four genera comprising the poisonous Chirodropsidae family of box jellyfish.

Chiropsoides one of the four genera comprising the family of Chirodropsidae, or poisonous box jellyfish.

Chiroptera the order which comprises all of the 178 genera in 16 families of bats. Characterized by their ability to fly with the aid of an alar membrane which is attached to all four limbs and tail. They are fast fliers with a special sensory system to enable them to fly at their preferred time, dusk.

There are three groups, insectivorous e.g. *Macrotus* spp., fruit-eating e.g. *Pteropus* (called also flying foxes), and blood-drinking or vampire bats e.g. *Desmodus*, better known by their association with Nosferatu than as carriers of the rabies virus. (Much of the mythology of vampirism can be explained within the parameters of rabies epidemiology). Both fruit-eating and vampire bats are known to be involved in the spread of rabies and similar BAT rabies viruses.

chirurgenic arising as a result of a surgical procedure.

chirurgery see SURGERY.

chisel an instrument designed to be driven by a hammer to pare away at a surface. It has a cutting edge across the distal end with a bevel on one of its sides.

army c. a heavyweight steel chisel used for paring of the surface of bones.

obstetric c's have been largely discarded because of the danger associated with their use in fetotomy. A semisharp spatula may be used for the same purposes.

symphysiotomy c. used to divide the pubis at the pubic symphysis in immature heifers carrying large calves. The chisel point is angled inward toward the center of the blade so that the cutting surface will stay on the bone when it disappears from view.

chital see AXIS DEER.

chitin a horny polysaccharide of *N*-acetylglucosamine, the principal constituent of shells of arthropods and shards of beetles, and found in certain fungi.

chitinoclastic destructive of chitin.

chitinous made of CHITIN.

chitterlings cross-sectional rings of the large intestine of the pig; usually deepfried quickly to a crackling, crisp delicacy.

chives ALLIUM *schoenoprasm*.

chlamydemia the presence of chlamydiae in the blood.

Chlamydia a genus of bacteria comprising three species: *C. trachomatis* and *C. pneumoniae*, which do not infect animals but cause a number of serious diseases in humans, and *C. psittaci*, which causes many important diseases of animals described generally as CHLAMYDIOSIS. The organisms are obligate intracellular parasites that are totally dependent on the host cell for energy in the form of adenosine triphosphate (ATP), which they cannot synthesize. Outside of a host they exist as 300 nm diameter elementary bodies, which have a rigid cell wall and are unable to grow or divide. The elementary bodies attach to host cells and are taken in by phagocytosis. Inside the phagosome they become reticulate or initial bodies, which have flexible cell walls and grow and divide. After about 40 hours nascent elementary bodies are formed, the host cell is lysed, and the elementary bodies are released.

The organisms pass through filters that exclude other bacteria, are cultivable only in cell cultures and the yolk sac of chick embryos. The elementary bodies (LCL bodies) are gram-negative, nonmotile bacteria.

chlamydia pl. *chlamydiae;* any member of the genus *Chlamydia.*

Chlamydiaceae a family of bacteria containing a single genus, *Chlamydia.*

chlamydial pertaining to *Chlamydia* spp.

c. abortion abortion in cats, cows, ewes, goat does caused by *Chlamydia psittaci.*

c. ovine abortion late abortion in ewes caused by *Chlamydia psittaci* (*C. ovis*).

chlamydiosis any disease or infection caused by *Chlamydia psittaci*; takes many forms including: PSITTACOSIS and ORNITHOSIS in birds, placentopathy manifested by abortion in enzootic ovine ABORTION, and epizootic bovine ABORTION, sporadic bovine ENCEPHALOMYELITIS, pneumonitis in all species except pig, conjunctivitis in sheep, cats and laboratory rodents, POLYARTHRITIS in sheep, cattle, horse, enteritis in cattle and lagomorphs, and septicemia in EPIZOOTIC chlamydiosis in lagomorphs.

Chlamydonema see PHYSALOPTERA *praeputialis.*

chlamydospore a thick-walled intercalary or terminal asexual fungal spore formed by the rounding-up of a cell; it is not shed. Formed by differentiation of hyphae; seen in *Candida* and *Histoplasma* spp.

chloasma see MELASMA.

chloral 1. an oily liquid with a pungent, irritating odor, prepared by the mutual action of alcohol and chlorine; used in the manufacture of chloral hydrate and DDT. 2. vernacular contraction of the term chloral hydrate.

c. betaine formed by the reaction of chloral hydrate with betaine; used as a sedative.

c. hydrate rarely if ever used in small animals. Widely used as a hypnotic, analgesic and anesthetic agent in large animals, especially in horses. Has many disadvantages and has been superseded by many much more satisfactory preparations. Its continued use is a matter of economics. Chloral hydrate may be administered orally but is erratic and slow-acting in its effects by this route. Intravenously the effects are immediate; injection outside the vein causes a very severe cellulitis usually terminating in an extensive slough of tissue.

Chloral hydrate is a poor analgesic and severely depressant of respiratory and vasomotor centers in the medulla.

c. hydrate and guaiacol glyceryl ether used as an anesthetic combination in horses; combines muscular relaxation with hypnotic effect.

c. hydrate and magnesium sulfate an anesthetic preparation used in horses. Combines the hypnotic effect of chloral and the neuromuscular blocking effect of magnesium.

c. hydrate, magnesium sulfate and pentobarbital sodium see EQUITHESIN.

α-chloralose a compound with anesthetic properties but not used in clinical work because of the poor level of anesthesia induced, the prolonged recovery period and the inconvenience of having to prepare the solution, by mixing equal quantities of glucose and chloral hydrate, and heating, just before use. There are two isomers. Only the α-chloralose has anesthetic properties.

chloramben a hormonal herbicide, relatively nontoxic if used correctly. Massive doses cause anorexia, weight loss, limb weakness and recumbency.

chlorambucil a nitrogen mustard derivative used as an antineoplastic agent.

chloramine, chloramine T a chlorine disinfectant, used for wound treatment, in drinking water.

chloramine B sodium benzenesulfocholoramine.

chloramphenicol a broad-spectrum antibiotic with specific therapeutic activity against gram-positive and gram-negative bacteria, rickettsiae, chlamydiae and anaplasmae. Side-effects in animals are uncommon, but its use in food-producing animals is discouraged or prohibited because of the danger of residues to humans. The palmitate preparation is a suspension administered orally and chloramphenicol sodium succinate is water soluble for parenteral use.

chlorate as sodium or potassium chlorate, one of the original chemical herbicides but now largely superseded. Animals may be poisoned if they eat pasture or plant contaminated by the spray or the dry powder. It may also be administered accidentally because of its similarity to sodium chloride. Causes gastroenteritis with diarrhea, nitrite poisoning with anoxia and intravascular hemolysis resulting in anemic anoxia.

chlorazanil hydrochloride an aminouracil diuretic.

chlorazepate dipotassium an anxiolytic drug used in dogs.

chlorbenside an acaricide used to spray trees and crops; has low toxicity but heavy, continued use may cause hepatic insufficiency.

chlorbenzoic acid a hormonal herbicide, safe for animals if used according to instructions. Heavy dosing may cause anorexia, weight loss and muscle weakness.

chlorbutol see CHLOROBUTANOL.

chlorcyclizine an antihistamine and fungistatic agent, used as the hydrochloride salt.

chlordane see CHLORINATED HYDROCARBONS.

chlordiazepoxide an early benzodiazapene derivative; used as a tranquilizer with activity similar to diazepam.

Chlorella a green alga, thought to be the origin of the achloric alga *Prototheca* spp., a sometime animal pathogen. See PROTOTHECA.

chloremia 1. chlorosis. 2. hyperchloremia.

chlorfenethol an acaricide used on agricultural crops and trees. It has a low toxicity but can cause depression, diarrhea, dyspnea, salivation and lacrimation.

chlorfenvinphos an organophosphorus insecticide used in the control of ectoparasites in large and small animals.

chlorhexidine a bisbiguanide antiseptic with antibacterial, antifungal and some antiviral activity; used in skin cleansers for surgical scrub, preoperative skin preparation, cleansing skin wounds and teat dips. Used as the acetate, gluconate or hydrochloride salts. Proprietary names are Hibitane, Nolvasan.

c. digluconate used as a sclerosing agent for chemical vasectomy in dogs.

c. teat dip 0.5 to 1.0% chlorhexidine in polyvinylpyrrolidone or as 0.3% solution in water.

chlorhydria an excess of hydrochloric acid in the stomach.

chloride 1. a salt of hydrochloric acid; any binary compound of chlorine. 2. the principal anion in extracellular fluid and gastric juice.

Because of its domination of the anions in extracellular and intravascular fluid, it has profound importance for acid–base balance and for the regulation of osmotic pressure in these fluid compartments.

c. pump an active secretory process at a barrier membrane that facilitates the transfer of chloride ions across the membrane.

c. shift diffusion of chloride ions from the plasma into the erythrocytes to compensate for the loss of bicarbonate ions from the cells as a result of carbon dioxide metabolism. Called also Hamburger shift.

chloridorrhea diarrhea with an excess of chlorides in the stool.

chloriduria an excess of chlorides in the urine.

chlorinated charged with chlorine.

c. acids some, e.g. trichlorbenzoic acid, sodium chloroacetate, sodium trichloroacetate, are used as weedkillers and are relatively harmless as far as animals are concerned.

c. hydrocarbons see CHLORINATED HYDROCARBONS.

c. lime bleaching powder.

c. naphthalene see CHLORINATED NAPHTHALENES.

c. phenols see BIPHENYL.

chlorinated hydrocarbons insecticidal substances which are no longer recommended for use on food animals because of their persistence in animal tissues and entry into the human food chain. Many of them still find industrial and nonanimal use and poisoning of animals can occur. Poisoning is manifested by nervous excitement, tremor, convulsions and death. Includes aldrin, benzene hexachloride, chlordane, DDD, DDT, heptachlor, isodrin, lindane, methoxychlor.

chlorinated naphthalenes additives to lubricants, fire-retardants and insulants. They are poisonous and on low level intake over long periods cause hypovitaminosis A manifested by cutaneous hyperkeratosis, emaciation and death. See also HYPERKERATOSIS.

chlorine a gaseous chemical element, atomic number 17, atomic weight 35.453, symbol Cl. See Table 6. It is a disinfectant, decolorizer and irritant poison. It is used for disinfecting, fumigating and bleaching, either in an aqueous solution or in the form of chlorinated lime. See also HYPOCHLORITE, CHLORAMINE.

c. dioxide used in the aging of flour to make it more suitable for baking. Process does not produce toxic amino acid derivatives as other agents do. See also AGENE PROCESS.

c. disinfectants compounds which have a high content of free chlorine and exert a disinfectant effect by releasing the chlorine.

c. gas liberated from chlorine disinfectants and in factory effluents. Causes irritation to respiratory mucosa up to the point of pulmonary edema.

Chloriopsoroptes a genus of mange mites in the family Psoroptidae. Includes *Chloriopsoroptes kenyensis* (African buffalo).

Chloris a genus of grasses in the family Poaceae; some cause cyanide poisoning. Includes *C. distichophylla*, *C. gayana*, *C. truncata*, *C. ventricosa*. Called also windmill grass.

C. truncata causes photosensitization, possibly through steroidal saponins. Called also windmill grass.

chlorite a salt of chlorous acid; disinfectant and bleaching agent.

chlorleukemia see CHLOROLEUKEMIA.

chlormadinone acetate a progestagen with antigonadotropic, antiestrogenic and antiandrogenic activity. Used to synchronize estrus in cows and ewes, and for prevention of estrus in small animals.

chlormequat chloride a low toxicity herbicide.

chlormerodrin a mercurial diuretic.

c. Hg-197 chlormerodrin tagged with radioactive mercury (^{197}Hg); used as diagnostic aid in renal function determination.

c. Hg-203 chlormerodrin tagged with radioactive mercury (^{203}Hg); used as a diagnostic aid in renal function determination.

chlormezanone a nonbarbiturate sedative, used as a muscle relaxant and tranquilizer.

chloro-acetotoluidine (2-chloro-4-acetotoluidine) poisoning used commercially to poison bird pests.

chloro-p-toluidine (3-chloro-p-toluidine) poisoning used commercially to poison bird pests.

chloroanisoles substances liberated from wood preservatives by bacteria when shavings of the wood are used in deep litter. They taint meat of animals housed on the litter.

chloroazodin a chlorine-releasing antiseptic and disinfectant, similar to chloramine T.

chlorobenzilate an insecticide used on agricultural crops and plants. Has low toxicity if handled properly.

chlorobutanol, chlorbutol an antimicrobial preservative in pharmaceutical preparations.

chlorodyne an antiquated remedy for diarrhea in humans and dogs. Similar to tinct. chlor. et morphinae co.

1-(2-chloroethyl)-3-cyclohexyl-1-nitrosourea (CCNU) see LOMUSTINE.

chloroform $CHCl_3$; a liquid with an ethereal odor and sweet taste, used as a solvent; once used widely as an inhalation anesthetic and analgesic, and as an antitussive, carminative and counterirritant. An effective but dangerous anesthetic used commonly at one time especially in horses. Requires a proper mask. Prolonged anesthesia often results in severe liver damage.

chlorolabe the pigment in retinal cones that is more sensitive to the green portion of the spectrum than are the other pigments (cyanolabe and erythrolabe).

chloroleukemia myelogenous leukemia or granulocytic leukemia in which no specific tumor masses are observed at autopsy, but the body organs and fluids show a definite green color due to myeloperoxidase (especially in the pig).

chloroma, chlorolymphosarcoma a malignant, green-colored tumor arising from myeloid tissue, associated with myelogenous leukemia, and occurring anywhere in the body. See also GRANULOCYTIC sarcoma, eosinophilic LEUKEMIA.

Chloromycetin trademark for preparations of CHLORAMPHENICOL, a broad-spectrum antibiotic.

chloromyeloma chloroma with multiple growths in bone marrow.

chloropexia the fixation of chlorine in body tissues.

chlorophacinone an anticoagulant rodenticide.

chlorophenols compounds used as fungicides, including timber preservation, as herbicides and in termite control. They are quite poisonous. See TRICHLOROPHENOL, PENTACHLOROPHENOL.

chlorophyll any of a group of green pigments, containing a magnesium–porphyrin complex, that are involved in oxygen-producing photosynthesis in plants. Preparations of water-soluble chlorophyll derivatives are applied topically for deodorization of skin lesions and to stimulate healing. It is also administered orally to deodorize ulcerative lesions and the urine and feces.

A chlorophyll metabolite, PHYLLOERYTHRIN, is the common photodynamic agent in pastured animals with liver damage. The phylloerythrin accumulates because its excretory pathway is the biliary system.

chloropicrin a disinfectant for use on cereal grains. Can cause intense lacrimation if inhaled. Taken orally it causes vomiting, colic and diarrhea. Called also trichloronitromethane.

chloroprivic deprived of chlorides; due to loss of chlorides.

chloroprocaine a local anesthetic, used as the hydrochloride salt.

chloroquine an antiprotozoal agent, used in the treatment of avian malaria, anaplasmosis and theileriosis in cattle and amebiasis in non-human primates.

c. poisoning the drug has an affinity for melanin and ocular tissues with melanin; causes a drug-induced retinopathy.

chlorothiazide a thiazide diuretic. Called also Diuril.

chloroxylenol a chlorinated phenolic antiseptic, used in presurgical preparation of skin, cleaning wounds and in the treatment of bacterial, fungal and yeast infections of the skin and claws.

Chlorozophora plicata African plant in family Euphorbiaceae; contains an unidentified toxin; causes dyspnea, diarrhea and pulmonary edema. Called also terba.

chlorphenesin carbamate a centrally acting skeletal muscle relaxant, similar in action to mephenesin, used in the treatment of skeletal muscle spasms and trauma to tendons and ligaments.

chlorpheniramine a histamine H_1-receptor antagonist, used as the maleate salt in the treatment of hypersensitivity reactions and as an antipruritic.

chlorphenoxy herbicide includes 2,4-D and 2,4,5-T.

chlorpromazine a phenothiazine used as an antipsychotic agent and antiemetic. It has been largely superseded in veterinary work by acetylpromazine. Its principal use was as premedication for anesthesia.

chlorpropamide a first generation sulfonylurea derivative, used as an oral hypoglycemic drug in the treatment of diabetes mellitus.

chlorpropham a thiocarbamate herbicide of low toxicity for animals if used according to instructions. Can cause muscle weakness, anorexia, weight and hair loss.

chlorprothixene a thioxanthene derivative, related to the phenothiazine tranquilizers. Used as a tranquilizer, especially in pigs.

chlorpyrifos an organophosphorus insecticide used widely for the control of ectoparasites on animals and in the treatment of their environment.

chlortetracycline a broad-spectrum antibiotic obtained from *Streptomyces aureofaciens*, used in the form of the hydrochloride salt as an antibacterial (effective against both gram-positive and gram-negative bacteria) and as a feed additive to promote growth in calves, pigs and poultry. See also TETRACYCLINE.

chloruresis excretion of chlorides in the urine.

chloruria an excess of chlorides in the urine.

chlorzoxazone a skeletal muscle relaxant.

chloxyle see HEXACHLOROPARAXYLENE.

choana pl. *choanae* [L.] 1. any funnel-shaped cavity or infundibulum. 2. *choanae*, the paired openings between the nasal cavity and the nasopharynx.

choanal pertaining to or arising from the choanae.

c. atresia see imperforate BUCCOPHARYNGEAL membrane.

c. slit the sagittal slit in the hard palate of the normal bird.

c. stenosis choanal atresia.

Choanotaenia a genus of non-pathogenic tapeworms in the family Dilepididae. Includes *C. infundibulum* (fowl and turkey intestine).

chocolate a medium-brown (milk chocolate) coat color of cats seen on the extremities of chocolate-pointed Siamese and Colorpoints and, uncommonly, as a variety of Burmese.

chocolate engorgement overeating of chocolate; causes death in dogs due to THEOBROMINE poisoning. Called also CACAO poisoning.

chocolate-point see POINTS.

Choeropsis liberiensis see HIPPOPOTAMUS.

Choix fever Rocky Mountain spotted fever.

choke to interrupt respiration by obstruction or compression, or the condition resulting from such interruption. See also ESOPHAGEAL obstruction.

c. chain a string of metal links which, when looped through an end link, forms a noose. It is commonly used as a collar for dogs, particularly in training or for control of large, strong or unruly dogs as tension on the attached lead tightens the noose around the dog's neck giving great control.

c. chain injury soft tissue injury and fracture on luxation of the hyoid apparatus can occur with excessive force. Choke chains may also become imbedded in the tissues of growing dogs.

chokecherry PRUNUS *virginiana*.

choking pertaining to choke. Used to describe a syndrome in horses with dorsal SOFT PALATE displacement. A clinical sign of laryngeal disease.

cholagogue an agent that stimulates gallbladder contraction to promote bile flow.

cholangiectasis dilatation of a bile duct.

cholangiocarcinoma see cholangiocellular CARCINOMA.

cholangiocellular pertaining to the bile ducts.

c. adenoma solid or cystic; may be neoplastic or congenital or acquired cystic lesions.

c. carcinoma multiple, firm, white tumors occurring usually in dogs and cats. Capsular lesions have a typical umbilication of their serosal surface. Metastatic spread is constant. Called also bile duct carcinoma.

c. cystadenoma a variety of bile duct adenoma in

which the tumor is composed of multilocular cystic structures lined with epithelium resembling that of bile ducts.

cholangioenterostomy surgical anastomosis of a bile duct to the intestine.

cholangiogastrostomy surgical anastomosis of a bile duct to the stomach.

cholangiogram the film obtained by cholangiography.

cholangiography x-ray examination of the bile ducts, using a radiopaque dye given intravenously or orally, as contrast medium. Little used in veterinary medicine.

cholangiohepatitis inflammation of the biliary system and, by extension, of the periportal hepatic parenchyma. In large animals, it is nearly always the result of parasitic infestation, sometimes complicated by the presence of bacteria; sporidesmin, the toxin of *Pithomyces chartarum*, causes a specific cholangiohepatitis. Crystal-associated cholangiohepatopathy has a similar pathogenesis. Primary bacterial cholangiohepatitis is uncommon in animals. In cats, a cholangiohepatitis of unknown etiology occurs, often in association with a low-grade interstitial pancreatitis.

cholangiohepatoma primary carcinoma of the liver of mixed liver cell and bile duct cell origin.

cholangiohepatopathy disease of the liver parenchyma associated with and probably derived from disease of the biliary system. The best known is CRYSTAL-ASSOCIATED CHOLANGIOHEPATOPATHY.

cholangiolar pertaining to or emanating from the tissues of the biliary system.

cholangiole one of the fine terminal elements of the bile duct system.

cholangiolitis inflammation of the cholangioles.

cholangioma cholangiocellular carcinoma.

cholangiostomy fistulization of a bile duct.

cholangiotomy incision into a bile duct.

cholangitis inflammation of a bile duct.

chronic c.–cholangiohepatitis a fairly well-defined entity of mature cats, sometimes associated with pancreatitis; the inflammatory portal infiltrate is largely lymphocytic; regresses after prednisolone therapy. See also CHOLANGIOHEPATITIS.

hyperplastic c. see FASCIOLIASIS.

cholanopoiesis the synthesis of bile acids or of their conjugates and salts by the liver.

cholanopoietic 1. promoting cholanopoiesis. 2. an agent that promotes cholanopoiesis.

cholate a salt or ester of cholic acid.

chole- word element. [Gr.] *bile.*

cholecalciferol vitamin D_3, an oil-soluble antirachitic vitamin. See also VITAMIN D.

cholecystagogue an agent that promotes evacuation of the gallbladder.

cholecystalgia biliary colic.

cholecystectasia distension of the gallbladder.

cholecystectomy excision of the gallbladder.

cholecystenterostomy see CHOLECYSTOENTEROSTOMY.

cholecystic pertaining to the gallbladder.

cholecystitis inflammation of the GALLBLADDER.

cholecystoduodenostomy surgical anastomosis of the gallbladder and the duodenum.

cholecystoenterostomy surgical anastomosis of the gallbladder and intestinal tract, usually indicated if the common bile duct has been disrupted by injury or neoplasia and, as is the case in dogs and cats, repair or CHOLEDOCHOENTEROSTOMY is technically impractical. See also CHOLECYSTODUODENOSTOMY, CHOLECYSTOJEJUNOSTOMY.

cholecystogram a radiograph of the gallbladder.

cholecystography radiography of the gallbladder and bile ducts, using a radiopaque dye as contrast medium.

cholecystojejunostomy surgical anastomosis of the gallbladder and jejunum.

cholecystokinin a gastrointestinal hormone liberated from the intestinal mucosa in response to arrival of the products of digestion from the stomach. It stimulates secretion of pancreatic enzymes and gallbladder contraction. Abbreviated CCK, CCK–PZ. Called also cholecystokinin–pancreozymin, pancreozymin.

cholecystokinin–pancreozymin see CHOLECYSTOKININ.

cholecystolithiasis cholelithiasis.

cholecystotomy incision of the gallbladder.

choledochal pertaining to the bile duct.

choledochitis inflammation of the common bile duct.

choledocho- word element. [Gr.] *common bile duct.*

choledochoduodenostomy surgical anastomosis of the bile duct and the duodenum. Not commonly performed in animals.

choledochoenterostomy surgical anastomosis of the common bile duct to the intestine.

choledochogastrostomy surgical anastomosis of the common bile duct to the stomach.

choledochography radiology of the common bile duct.

choledocholithiasis calculi in the common bile duct.

choledochoplasty plastic repair of the common bile duct.

choledochotomy incision into the common bile duct.

choledochus the ductus choledochus, or bile duct.

choleic pertaining to the bile.

cholejejunoduodenostomy surgical anastomosis of the gallbladder, jejunum and duodenum.

cholelith see GALLSTONE.

cholelithiasis the presence or formation of gallstones. Rare in animals, they are usually found in the gallbladder probably secondary to mild cholecystitis. Usually asymptomatic, but occasionally they may cause obstruction of bile ducts or lead to erosion and perforation of the gallbladder with peritonitis. Calcareous stones may form in the bile ducts of cattle with DISTOMIASIS.

obstructive c. blockage of the common bile duct by a gallstone; characterized clinically by severe jaundice, abdominal pain.

cholelithotomy incision of the biliary tract for removal of gallstones.

cholelithotripsy, cholelithotrity crushing of a gallstone.

cholemesis vomiting of bile.

cholemia bile or bile pigment in the blood.

cholemic pertaining to or emanating from the bile.

c. nephrosis renal tubular nephrosis caused by a high concentration of bilirubin in the urine and subsequently in the tubular epithelium.

choleperitoneum the presence of bile in the peritoneum.

cholepoiesis the formation of bile in the liver.

choleresis the secretion of bile by the liver.

choleretic 1. stimulating bile production by the liver. 2. an agent that stimulates bile production by the liver.

cholestasis stoppage or suppression of bile flow, due to factors within (intrahepatic cholestasis) or outside the liver (extrahepatic cholestasis) resulting in regurgitation of biliary substances into the blood and jaundice.

cholesteatoma a cystlike mass with a lining of stratified squamous epithelium, filled with desquamating debris frequently including cholesterol, which occurs in the meninges, central nervous system and bones of the skull, but most commonly in the choroid plexus of the ventricles, and especially in horses and other Equidae. Causes signs of increased intracranial pressure, initial excitement followed by somnolence and apathy. Hydrocephalus may be the end-stage.

cholesteatosis fatty degeneration due to cholesterol esters.

cholesteremia hypercholesterolemia.

cholesterol a steroid alcohol found in animal fats and oils, bile, blood, brain tissue, milk, egg yolk, myelin sheaths of nerve fibers, liver, kidneys and adrenal glands. It is a necessary component of all cell surface and intracellular membranes and a constituent of myelin in nervous tissue; it is a precursor of bile acids and steroid hormones, and it occurs in the most common type of gallstone, in atheroma of the arteries, in various cysts, and in carcinomatous tissue. Most of the body's cholesterol is synthesized, but some is obtained in the diet.

The preoccupation in human medicine with the relationship between cholesterol and the development of atheromatous plaques in the coronary arteries is not reflected in veterinary medicine. The importance of cholesterol to the veterinarian is limited to the measurement of blood cholesterol levels as an indicator of liver disease or thyroid activity.

c. pneumonia see endogenous-lipid PNEUMONIA.

cholesterolemia hypercholesterolemia.

cholesterolosis bulbi cholesterol crystals in the vitreous.

cholesteroluria the presence of cholesterol in the urine.

cholesterosis a condition in which cholesterol is deposited in tissues in abnormal amounts.

cholestiatosis see CHOLESTEATOMA.

cholestyramine a bile-acid binding resin used to treat hyperlipidemia and as an absorbent to prevent intestinal absorption of toxins.

choletherapy treatment by administration of bile salts.

choleuria choluria.

cholic acid a major bile acid formed in the liver from cholesterol that plays, with other bile acids, an important role in digestion.

choline a quaternary amine which occurs in the phospholipid phosphatidylcholine and the neurotransmitter acetylcholine, and is an important methyl donor in intermediary metabolism. It was formerly considered to be a B-vitamin and was used to treat fatty degeneration of the liver.

c. acetylase, c. acetyltransferase an enzyme that brings about the synthesis of acetylcholine.

c. esters choline has some of the activity of a cholineric drug but the effect is multiplied many times over by combining it with an acid, e.g. acetic acid, to form an ester, e.g. acetylcholine. Other choline esters with important pharmacological activity are CARBACHOL, BETHANECHOL, METHACHOLINE.

c. nutritional deficiency requirements for choline are largely dependent on the amount of methionine in the diet. In dogs and cats, under normal circumstances, deficiency is unlikely, but choline is a dietary essential for pigs and young calves. Incoordination, weakness, dyspnea and hock swelling occur in experimental deficiency, but there is little evidence of naturally occurring disease. Poultry fed diets deficient in choline develop PEROSIS.

c. salicylate the choline salt of salicylic acid, which has analgesic, antipyretic and anti-inflammatory properties.

c. theophyllinate a theophylline derivative used as a bronchodilator. Called also oxtriphylline.

cholinergic 1. parasympathomimetic; activated or transmitted by acetylcholine; said of nerve fibers that liberate acetylcholine at a synapse when a nerve impulse passes, i.e. the parasympathetic fibers. 2. an agent that resembles acetylcholine or simulates its action.

c. blockade selective inhibition of cholinergic nerve impulses at autonomic ganglionic synapses, postganglionic parasympathetic effectors, or neuromuscular junctions.

c. neurotransmission that form of neurotransmission which depends on the production of acetylcholine at synapses.

c. receptors receptor sites on effector organs or at nerve synapses that are stimulated by acetylcholine released by the nerve terminal. There are two types: muscarinic receptors, present primarily on autonomic effector cells, and nicotinic receptors, present primarily on autonomic ganglion cells and on the motor end plates of skeletal muscle.

cholinesterase an enzyme that splits acetylcholine into acetic acid and choline. Called also acetylcholinesterase.

This enzyme is present throughout the body, but is particularly important at the neuromuscular junction, where the nerve fibers terminate. Acetylcholine is released when a nerve impulse reaches a neuromuscular junction. It diffuses across the synaptic cleft and binds to cholinergic receptors on the muscle fibers, causing them to contract. Cholinesterase splits acetylcholine into its components, thus stopping stimulation of the muscle fibers. The end products of the metabolism of acetylcholine are taken up by nerve fibers and resynthesized into acetylcholine.

c. inhibitor the drugs neostigmine, physostigmine and pyridostigmine inhibit cholinesterase. These drugs are used to treat MYASTHENIA gravis, a disease in which the cholinergic receptors are attacked by autoantibodies. The drugs extend the effect of acetylcholine on the muscle fiber.

c. reactivator choline-reactivating oximes are effective antidotes in organophosphorus insecticide poisoning, a state of acetylcholine excess because of cholinesterase inhibition. 2-PAM (2-pyridine aldoxime methchloride) is the most popular oxime for this purpose.

cholinoceptive pertaining to the sites on effector organs that are acted upon by cholinergic transmitters.

cholinoceptor cholinergic receptor.

cholinolytic 1. blocking the action of acetylcholine, or of cholinergic agents. 2. an agent that blocks the action of acetylcholine in cholinergic areas, i.e. areas supplied by parasympathetic nerves and voluntary muscles.

cholinomimetic having an action similar to that of acetylcholine; called also PARASYMPATHOMIMETIC.

c. alkaloids naturally occurring plant alkaloids which have cholinomimetic actions are ARECOLINE, PILOCARPINE, MUSCARINE.

chol(o)- word element. [Gr.] *bile*.

Choloepus didactylus see SLOTH.

cholohemothorax the presence of bile and blood in the thorax.

chololithiasis cholelithiasis.
cholothorax cholohemothorax.
choluria the presence of bile in the urine; discoloration of the urine with bile pigments.
Chondodendron one of the sources of curare.
chondral pertaining to cartilage.
chondralgia pain in a cartilage.
chondrectomy excision of a cartilage.
chondrification conversion into cartilage.
chondrio- word element. [Gr.] *cartilage, granule.*
chondritis inflammation of a cartilage.
chondro prefix meaning cartilage.
chondr(o)- word element. [Gr.] *cartilage.*
chondroadenoma adenochondroma.
chondroangioma a benign mesenchymoma containing chondromatous and angiomatous elements.
chondroblast an immature cartilage-producing cell.
chondroblastoma a benign tumor arising from young chondroblasts in the epiphysis of a bone.
chondrocalcin a calcium-binding protein found in the parts of the skeleton where bone proliferation or remodeling are taking place.
chondrocalcinosis deposition of calcium salts in the cartilage of joints.
chondroclast a giant cell believed to be concerned in absorption of cartilage.
chondrocostal pertaining to the ribs and costal cartilages.
chondrocranium the cartilaginous cranial structure of the embryo in early pregnancy when it is a unified cartilaginous mass without clear boundaries indicating the limits of future bones.
chondrocyte a mature cartilage cell embedded in a lacuna within the cartilage matrix.
Chondrodendron plant genus in the family Menispermaceae from which CURARE is extracted.
chondrodynia pain in a cartilage.
chondrodysplasia abnormal growth of cartilage; may be used to include achondroplasia. Causes disproportionate dwarfism and occurs as an inherited trait in cattle (Dexter, Telemark lethal and 'snorter'), sheep (Ançon and Cheviot) and dogs (Alaskan malamute, miniature poodles and Norwegian elkhound). See also ACHONDROPLASIA, ENCHONDROMATOSIS.
deforming hereditary c. inherited chondrodysplastic defects characterized by skeletal deformity, e.g. chondrodysplastic dwarfism.
chondrodysplastic dwarf see CHONDRODYSPLASIA.
chondrodystrophia, chondrodystrophy a disorder of cartilage formation.
c. fetalis see EPIPHYSEAL dysplasia.
chondrodystrophoid having chondrodystrophy as a characteristic.
c. breeds in dogs, e.g. Dachshund, Bulldog, Bassett hound, the features of chondrodystrophy are established as the breed type. Angular deformities of the limbs and degeneration of the mucinous nucleus pulposus of the intervertebral disk at an early age are unfortunate accompaniments of this trait.
chondrodystrophy any disorder of cartilage formation. See also CHONDRODYSPLASIA.
chicken embryo c. see CHICKEN embryo chondrodystrophy.
chondroendothelioma an endothelioma containing cartilage tissue.
chondroepiphyseal pertaining to epiphyseal cartilage.
chondroepiphysitis inflammation of the epiphyseal cartilages.
chondrofibroma a fibroma with cartilaginous elements.
chondrogenesis formation of cartilage.
chondrogenic giving rise to or forming cartilage.
chondroid resembling cartilage.
chondroitin sulfate a glycosaminoglycan (mucopolysaccharide) which is widespread in connective tissue, particularly cartilage, and in the cornea.
chondrolipoma a tumor containing cartilaginous and fatty tissue.
chondroma a tumor or tumor-like growth of cartilage cells. It may remain in the interior arising from the cartilage of the medullary cavity (true chondroma, or enchondroma), or may develop on the surface of a cartilage and project under the periosteum of a bone (ecchondroma, or ecchondrosis).
c. rodens see MULTILOBULAR chondroma and osteoma.
chondromalacia abnormal softening of cartilage.
chondromatosis formation of multiple chondromas.
synovial c. a rare condition in which cartilage is formed in the synovial membrane of joints, tendon sheaths or bursae, sometimes becoming detached and producing a number of loose bodies.
chondromatous pertaining to or of the nature of cartilage.
c. hamartoma a congenital anomaly of the lung. See also HAMARTOMA.
chondromere a cartilaginous vertebra of the fetal vertebral column.
chondrometaplasia a condition characterized by metaplastic activity of the chondroblasts.
chondromyoma a benign tumor with myomatous and cartilaginous elements.
chondromyxoma myxoma with cartilaginous elements.
chondromyxosarcoma a sarcoma containing cartilaginous and mucous tissue.
chondronectin a glycoprotein found in cartilage.
chondro-osseous composed of cartilage and bone.
chondropathy any disease of cartilage.
chondroplasia the formation of cartilage by specialized cells (chondrocytes).
chondroplast chondroblast.
chondroplasty plastic repair of cartilage.
chondroporosis the formation of sinuses or spaces in cartilage.
chondrosarcoma a malignant tumor derived from cartilage cells or their precursors.
chondrosis the formation of cartilage.
chondrosteoma a cartilage capped by knobby projection of the sternal surface of endochondral bone. They may recur singly or multicentrically (multiple cartilaginous EXOSTOSES). Inherited as an autosomal dominant trait in horses, dogs and humans.
chondrosternal pertaining to the costal cartilages and sternum.
c. depression see PECTUS excavatum.
chondrotomy the dissection or the surgical division of cartilage.
chondroxiphoid pertaining to the xiphoid cartilage.
Choniangium a genus of roundworms of the family Strongylidae. Includes *Choniangium epistomum*, *C. magnostomum* (Indian elephant cecum).
chook chicken.
chop chopped hay; used extensively when pastured animals need supplementary roughage and are required to eat the meal provided in a short time. Housed animals receive the same supply in the form of hay in a rack or net. Called also chaff.
green c. green feed that has been put through a chopper or forage harvester.
chord cord.

chorda pl. *chordae* [L.] a cord or sinew.
c. magna Achilles tendon.
c. tendineae tendinous cords connecting the two atrioventricular valves to the appropriate papillary muscles in the heart ventricles.
c. tendineae rupture causes acute, massive, cardiac insufficiency leading to congestive heart failure and an early death; called also detachment.
c. tympani a nerve originating from the facial nerve, distributed to the submandibular, sublingual and lingual glands and the anterior two-thirds of the tongue; it is a parasympathetic and special sensory nerve.
c. umbilicalis umbilical cord.
c. vocalis vocal cord.
chordal tissue the tissue of the notochord.
Chordata a phylum of the animal kingdom comprising all animals having a notochord during some developmental stage.
chordate 1. an animal of the Chordata. 2. having a notochord.
chordectomy excision of a vocal cord.
chordee downward deflection of the penis, due to a congenital anomaly (hypospadias) or to urethral infection.
chorditis inflammation of vocal or spermatic cords.
chordoma a malignant tumor arising from embryonic remains of the notochord.
chordotomy CORDOTOMY (2).
chorea in humans the ceaseless occurrence of rapid, jerky involuntary movements, but the term is usually applied to the MYOCLONUS seen in dogs associated with infection by distemper virus.
choreiform resembling chorea.
chorioadenoma adenoma of the chorion.
chorioallantoic vesicle the vesicle formed in early pregnancy around the embryo by the chorion; contains the allantoic sac, the yolk sac, the allantoic fluid and the embryo. Palpation of the sac is the basis of early manual pregnancy diagnosis in cows and mares.
chorioallantois an extraembryonic structure formed by union of the chorion and allantois, which by means of vessels in the associated mesoderm serves in gas exchange; in many mammals, it forms the placenta.
chorioamnionitis inflammation of the fetal membranes.
chorioamniotic folds a pair of folds consisting of extraembryonic somatopleure which grow out from the vitelline membrane and meet over the top of the embryo, fusing to complete the chorion and the amnion.
chorioangioma an angioma of the chorion.
choriocapillaris the capillary layer of the choroid, the lamina choriocapillaris.
choriocarcinoma a malignant neoplasm of trophoblastic cells formed by abnormal proliferation of the placental epithelium, without production of chorionic villi.
choriocele protrusion of the chorion through an aperture.
chorioepithelioma choriocarcinoma.
choriogenesis the development of the chorion.
chorioid choroid.
chorioma any trophoblastic proliferation, benign or malignant.
choriomeningitis cerebral meningitis with inflammation of the choroid plexus.
lymphocytic c. see LYMPHOCYTIC choriomeningitis.
chorion the outermost of the fetal membranes, composed of trophoblast lined with mesoderm; it develops villi, becomes vascularized by allantoic vessels, and forms the fetal part of the placenta.
c. frondosum the part of the chorion covered by villi.
c. laeve the nonvillous, membranous part of the chorion.
chorionic pertaining to the chorion.
c. girdle a circular band of cells of placental origin that invade the endometrium and form the endometrial cups in the mare.
c. girdle cells see chorionic girdle (above).
c. gonadotropin a hormone with properties similar to those of luteinizing hormone; it is secreted in large amounts by the placenta during gestation. It stimulates the formation of interstitial cells in the testes of the fetus and causes the secretion of testosterone. It is found in substantial amounts in the urine of pregnant mares (pregnant mares serum gonadotropin—PMSG) and pregnant women (human chorionic gonadotropin—HCG). It is used as an aid in the treatments to induce ovulation and the synchronization of estrus.
c. somatomammotropin see PLACENTAL lactogen.
c. vesicle the early embryonic vesicle before the allantois has developed and encircled the embryo to form the chorioallantoic vesicle and supplant it.
choriopmalaria see AVIAN malaria.
Chorioptes a genus of mange mites of the family Psoroptidae.
C. bovis found on the pasterns of horses and cattle, on the scrotum of sheep and on the perineal region of cattle. Causes CHORIOPTIC MANGE.
C. texanus occurs on goats and reindeer.
chorioptic mange the common form of mange in cattle and horses caused by *Chorioptes bovis*. Cattle show small scabs on the perineum, tailhead and back of the udder without irritation. Horses show severe dermatitis behind the pastern with severe itching at first and then soreness. Sheep show a scaly dermatitis on the legs and on the scrotum of the ram, and may suffer from infertility. Called also leg mange, tail mange, symbiotic mange.
chorioretinal pertaining to the choroid and retina.
c. dysplasia abnormal development of the choroid and retinal occurs in COLLIE eye anomaly.
chorioretinitis inflammation of the choroid and retina. Occurs in canine DISTEMPER and HAEMOPHILUS *somnus* septicemia.
congenital c. reported in foals born to mares that had respiratory disease during pregnancy.
septic c. seen in calves with OMPHALOPHLEBITIS.
chorioretinopathy a noninflammatory process involving both the choroid and retina.
post-traumatic c. occurs in young horses after trauma or severe blood loss. There is proliferation of pigment and retinal atrophy with blindness.
chorista defective development due to, or marked by, displacement of the primordium, the earliest sign of development of an organ.
choristoma a mass of histologically normal tissue in an abnormal location.
choroid the middle, vascular coat of the eye, between the sclera and the retina.
It contains an abundant supply of blood vessels and a large amount of brown pigment which serves to reduce reflection or diffusion of light when it falls on the retina. Adequate nutrition of the eye is dependent upon blood vessels in the choroid. See also TAPETUM, LAMINA cribrosa, LAMINA basilaris, VASCULAR lamina.
c. ependyma the ependymal cells which embrace choroid vessels to make up the choroid plexus.
c. inflammation see CHOROIDITIS.
c. plexus see choroid PLEXUS.

choroidal pertaining to or emanating from the choroid.
c. hypoplasia a not uncommon lesion in the dog, as part of COLLIE eye anomaly, and also in association with inherited coat color dilution characteristics, e.g. blue merles, harlequins.
choroidea choroid.
choroiditis inflammation of the choroid.
choroidocapillary layer one of the five laminae in the choroid coat of the eye.
choroidocyclitis inflammation of the choroid and ciliary processes.
choroidoiritis inflammation of the choroid and iris.
choroidoretinitis inflammation of the choroid and retina.
chou moellier BRASSICA *oleracea* var. *acephala*.
Chow Chow a medium-sized dog with a distinctive short-coupled body, erect ears and very thick, medium length coat; a smooth, short-coated variety is recognized in the United Kingdom. The breed is distinguished by a blue-black coloring on the tongue and much of the mouth. It is subject to myotonia congenita, believed to be inherited as an autosomal recessive trait, dysmyelinogenesis and a tyrosinase deficiency, and is predisposed to malignant melanomas and entropion.
CHR canine hypoxic rhabdomyolysis.
christmas bells see BRYOPHYLLUM *tubiflorum*.
Christmas berry see PHOTINIA.
Christmas disease (hemophilia B) a hereditary hemorrhagic diathesis clinically similar to, but less common than, hemophilia A (classic hemophilia), caused by deficiency of clotting factor IX (Christmas factor, plasma THROMBOPLASTIN component). It is an X chromosome-linked trait and occurs in human males, some breeds of dogs and British shorthaired cats. It is a mild to moderate disease in Cairn terrier, American Cocker spaniel and French bulldog, and a severe disease in Coonhounds, St. Bernards and Alaskan malamutes. Carrier females can be easily identified by quantitative coagulation assays.
Christmas factor clotting factor IX; deficiency is the cause of CHRISTMAS DISEASE (hemophilia B). See also plasma THROMBOPLASTIN component.
Christmas lily see LILIUM LONGIFLORUM.
Christmas rose HELLEBORUS *niger*.
chromaffin taking up and staining strongly with chromium salts.
c. reaction application of Zenker's solution to the flat cut surface of freshly excised chromaffin tumor forms a dark pigment within 20 minutes.
c. tissue a tissue composed largely of chromaffin cells, well supplied with nerves and vessels; it occurs in the adrenal medulla and also forms the paraganglia of the body, e.g. the carotid bodies, along with the sympathetic nerves, and in other organs.
chromaffinoma 1. any tumor containing chromaffin cells. 2. pheochromocytoma.
chromaphilic substance granular cytoplasmic reticulum and ribosomes found in nerve cell bodies; called also chromaphilic bodies or Nissl substance.
chromate any salt of chromic acid.
c. poisoning occurs accidentally as a result of exposure to chromate residues. Signs are abdominal pain, diarrhea and severe dehydration.
chromatic 1. pertaining to color; stainable with dyes. 2. pertaining to chromatin.
chromatid either of two parallel filaments joined at the centromere which make up a chromosome, and which divide in cell division, each going to a different pole of the dividing cell and each becoming a chromosome of one of the two daughter cells.
sister c. a chromatid formed by a replicating chromosome during interphase; because they are derived from the one homolog and joined at the center they are exact copies of each other.
chromatin the substance of the chromosomes, composed of nucleic acids and basic proteins (histones), the material in the nucleus that stains with basic dyes.
sex c. Barr body; the persistent mass of the material of the inactivated X chromosome in cells of normal females. See also DRUMSTICK.
chromatin-negative lacking sex chromatin; characteristic of the nuclei of cells in a normal male.
chromatin-positive containing sex chromatin; characteristic of the nuclei of cells in a normal female.
chromat(o)- word element. [Gr.] *color, chromatin.*
chromatogenous producing color or coloring matter.
chromatogram the record produced by chromatography.
chromatograph 1. to analyze by chromatography. 2. the apparatus used in chromatography.
chromatography a technique for analysis of chemical substances. The term *chromatography* literally means color writing, and denotes a method by which the substance to be analyzed is poured into a vertical glass tube containing an adsorbent, the various components of the substance moving through the adsorbent at different rates, according to their degree of attraction to it, and producing bands of color at different levels of the adsorption column. The term has been extended to include other methods utilizing the same principle, although no colors are produced in the column.

The mobile phase of chromatography refers to the fluid that carries the mixture of substances in the sample through the adsorptive material. The stationary phase (or adsorbent) refers to the solid material that takes up the particles of the substance passing through it. Kaolin, alumina, silica and activated charcoal have been used as adsorbing substances or stationary phases.

Classification of chromatographic techniques tends to be confusing because it may be based on the type of stationary phase, the nature of the adsorptive force, the nature of the mobile phase, or the method by which the mobile phase is introduced.

The technique is a valuable tool for the research biochemist and is readily adaptable to investigations conducted in the clinical laboratory. For example, chromatography is used to detect and identify in body fluids certain sugars and amino acids associated with inborn errors of metabolism.
adsorption c. that in which the stationary phase is an adsorbent.
affinity c. a method of chromatography that utilizes the biologically important binding interactions that occur on protein surfaces. For example, an enzyme substrate is covalently coupled to an inert matrix such as a polysaccharide bead. The enzyme can be bound to the bead and thereby separated when present in very low concentration in a very complex mixture of other macromolecules.
column c. the technique in which the various solutes of a solution are allowed to travel down a column, the individual components being adsorbed by the stationary phase. The most strongly adsorbed component will remain near the top of the column; the other components will pass to positions farther and farther down the column according to their affinity for the adsorbent. If the individual components are

naturally colored, they will form a series of colored bands or zones.

Column chromatography has been employed to separate vitamins, steroids, hormones and alkaloids and to determine the amount of these substances in samples of body fluids.

exclusion c. that in which the stationary phase is a gel having a closely controlled pore size. Molecules are separated based on molecular size and shape, smaller molecules being temporarily retained in the pores.

gas c. a type of chromatography in which the mobile phase is an inert gas. Volatile components of the sample are separated in the column and measured by a detector. The method has been applied in the clinical laboratory to separate and quantify steroids, barbiturates and lipids.

gas–liquid c. gas chromatography in which the substances to be separated are moved by an inert gas along a tube filled with a finely divided inert solid coated with a nonvolatile substance; each component migrates at a rate determined by its solubility in the stationary phase and its vapor pressure.

gel-filtration c., gel-permeation chromatography exclusion chromatography.

high performance liquid c. (HPLC) a miniaturized method in which the solution to be analyzed is passed, under high pressure, through a long, thin column packed with tiny beads such that analyses are completed in minutes rather than hours and with improved resolution.

ion-exchange c. that utilizing resins to which are coupled either cations or anions that will exchange with other cations or anions in the material passed through their meshwork.

molecular sieve c. exclusion chromatography.

paper c. a form of chromatography in which a sheet of special paper is substituted for the adsorption column. After separation of the components as a consequence of their differential migratory velocities, they are stained to make the chromatogram visible. In the clinical laboratory paper chromatography is employed to detect and identify sugars and amino acids.

partition c. a form of separation of solutes utilizing the partition of the solutes between two liquid phases, namely the original solvent and the film of solvent on the adsorption column.

thin-layer c. that in which the stationary phase is a thin layer of an adsorbent such as silica gel coated on a flat plate. It is otherwise similar to paper chromatography.

chromatolysis 1. the solution and disintegration of the chromatin of cell nuclei. 2. disintegration of the Nissl bodies of a neuron as a result of injury, fatigue or exhaustion.

chromatophil a cell or structure that stains easily.

chromatophore any pigmentary cell or color-producing plastid.

chromatophoroma see malignant MELANOMA.

chromatosome the basic nucleoprotein structural unit which consists of 166 base pairs of DNA and associated histone proteins.

chromaturia abnormal coloration of the urine.

chrome–arsenic–copper a very popular wood preservative. Treated pine is also a very popular material for the construction of horse yards. It is virtually nonpoisonous but horses with pica could nibble enough of the soft timber to be poisoned.

chromhidrosis secretion of colored sweat.

chromic acid 1. a dibasic acid, H_2CrO_4; its salts are called chromates. 2. chromium trioxide.

chromidium pl. *chromidia;* a granule of extranuclear chromatin in the cytoplasm of a cell.

chromidrosis see CHROMHIDROSIS.

chromium a chemical element, atomic number 24, atomic weight 51.996, symbol Cr. See Table 6.

c.-51 a radioisotope of chromium having a half-life of 27.8 days; used to label red blood cells to determine red cell volume and red cell survival time. Symbol ^{51}Cr. See also CR^{51} EDTA.

c. nutritional deficiency possibly causally related to the onset of diabetes mellitus in primates.

c. trioxide possibly carcinogenic in humans. See also CHROMATE.

chrom(o)- word element. [Gr.] *color.*

chromo body large, sclerotic bodies seen in subcutaneous microabscesses in chromoblastomycosis.

Chromobacterium violaceum a gram-negative bacteria found in tropical and subtropical areas. It is associated with pneumonia and other infections in several species.

chromoblast an embryonic cell that develops into a pigment cell.

chromoblastomycosis infections of skin and subcutaneous tissues caused by dematiaceous fungi.

chromoclastogenic giving rise to or inducing chromosomal disruption or damage.

chromocystoscopy cystoscopy of the ureteral orifices after oral administration of a dye which is excreted in the urine.

chromocyte any colored cell or pigmented corpuscle.

chromodacryorrhea bloody tears; seen with obstruction or disease of the nasolacrimal duct or sialodacryoadenitis, when excessive porphyrins are secreted with tears; a cause of skin irritation on the face of cats and gerbils.

chromogen any substance giving origin to a coloring matter.

chromogenesis the formation of color or pigment.

chromogenic producing color or pigment.

chromogranin A see PARATHYROID secretory protein.

chromolysis see CHROMATOLYSIS.

chromomere 1. any of the beadlike granules occurring in series along a chromonema. 2. granulomere.

chromomycosis a subcutaneous mycotic infection caused by a deeply pigmented fungus, e.g. CURVULARIA and PHIALOPHORA.

chromonema pl. *chromonemata* [Gr.] the coiled central thread of a chromatid along which lie the chromomeres.

chromophil any easily stainable structure.

chromophobe any cell, structure or tissue that does not stain readily; applied especially to the chromophobe cells of the anterior lobe of the pituitary gland.

c. adenoma a nonfunctional pituitary tumor of the pars distalis is hormonally inactive but commonly causes clinical signs by compression of the pituitary gland and other nearby structures. Clinical signs include incoordination, weakness and exercise intolerance, muscle atrophy, sexual inactivity, blindness and dilatation and fixation of the pupils.

c. carcinoma rare nonfunctional pituitary tumors are usually large and invasive causing destruction of the pars distalis leading to panhypopituitarism and diabetes insipidus. There is extensive invasion of the brain and cranial bones, and metastases to spleen and liver and to regional lymph nodes may occur.

chromophobia the quality of staining poorly with dyes.

chromophore any chemical group whose presence gives a decided color to a compound and which unites with certain other groups (auxochromes) to form dyes; called also color radical.

chromophoric 1. bearing color. 2. pertaining to a chromophore.

chromoprotein a protein combined with a pigment, e.g. hemoglobin.

chromoscopy the diagnosis of renal function by the color of urine following the administration of dyes.

gastric c. diagnosis of gastric function by the color of the gastric contents: a test for achylia gastrica.

chromosomal emanating from or pertaining to chromosome.

c. aberration see chromosomal abnormality (below).

c. abnormality abnormal karyotype; abnormalities can be detected before birth by means of amniocentesis, or after birth, but many are probably never observed because they cause death and disposal of the fetus. The abnormalities are either of number, or of composition of the individual chromosomes. Monosomy and trisomy are examples of numerical abnormalities. Translocations are examples of abnormalities of structure where parts of one chromosome have been transferred to another. The cause of these abnormalities is not known. Their importance is that many of them are linked with structural or functional defects of the animal body. The best known ones in veterinary medicine are those that are related to infertility, e.g. translocation 1/29, translocation 27/29.

c. analysis fetal cells obtained by AMNIOCENTESIS or lymphocytes from a blood sample can be cultured in the laboratory until they divide. Cell division is arrested in mid-metaphase by the drug Colcemid, a derivative of colchicine. The chromosomes can be stained by one of several techniques that produce a distinct pattern of light and dark bands along the chromosomes, and each chromosome can be recognized by its size and banding pattern. The chromosomal characteristics of an animal are referred to as its *karyotype*. This also refers to a photomicrograph of a cell nucleus that is cut apart and rearranged so that the individual chromosomes are in order and labeled. The autosomes are numbered roughly in order of decreasing length. The sex chromosomes are labeled X and Y. Karyotyping is useful in determining the presence of chromosome defects.

c. banding see BANDING (2).

c. chimerism see CHIMERA.

c. crossover see CROSSOVER.

c. deletion in genetics, loss from a chromosome of genetic material.

c. inversion see INVERSION (2).

c. linkage see LINKAGE (2).

c. mapping see GENETIC map.

c. non-disjunction failure of the chromatids or chromosomes to separate (disjoin) during meiosis.

c. replication see REPLICATION.

c. walking a technique for identification and isolation of contiguous sequences of genomic DNA.

c. X inactivation only one of a pair of female (X) chromosomes in the one cell is active, the other is inactivated.

chromosome in animal cells, a structure in the nucleus, containing a linear thread of DEOXYRIBONUCLEIC ACID (DNA), which transmits genetic information and is associated with RIBONUCLEIC ACID and histones.

During cell division the material composing the chromosome is compactly coiled, making it visible with appropriate staining and permitting its movement in the cell with minimal entanglement. Each organism of a species is normally characterized by the same number of chromosomes in its somatic cells. The diploid numbers (number of total chromosomes per cell) are cattle—60, sheep—54, horse—64, donkey—62, pig—38, dog—78, cat—38, human—46. The chromosomes are arranged in pairs and one of the pairs is the sex chromosomes (XX or XY), which determines the sex of the organism. See also HEREDITY.

compound c. a genetic engineering procedure which produces two chromosomes in one of which the left arms of the two original chromosomes are joined together and the two original right arms are also joined together; used in genetic control of insect populations.

homologous c's the chromosomes of a matching pair in the diploid complement that contain alleles of specific genes.

lampbrush c. so named because of the bristling appearance given them by many open loops of chromatin along the extended chromosome.

ring c. a chromosome in which both ends have been lost (deletion) and the two broken ends have reunited to form a ring-shaped figure.

sex c's the chromosomes responsible for determination of the sex of the individual that develops from a zygote, in mammals constituting an unequal pair, the X and the Y chromosome.

somatic c. autosome.

submetacentric c. see SUBMETACENTRIC.

W c. sex chromosome in animals such as poultry in which the female is the heterogametic state, the male has the ZZ genotype and the female the ZW genotype.

X c. the female sex chromosome, being carried by half the male gametes and all female gametes; female diploid cells have two X chromosomes, the male has the XY genotype.

Y c. the male sex chromosome, being carried by half the male gametes and none of the female gametes; male diploid cells have an X and a Y chromosome; females carry the XX genotype.

Z c. sex chromosome in animals, such as poultry, in which the female is the heterogametic sex; the male has the ZZ genotype and the female the ZW genotype.

chronaxie, chronaxy the minimum time at which an electric current must flow at a voltage twice the rheobase to cause a muscle to contract.

chronic persisting for a long time; the period is undefined and varies with circumstances; usually more than one week. US National Center for Health Statistics defines it as a condition of 3 months duration or longer. Also has the sense of the disease showing little change or very slow progression over a long period.

c. obstructive pulmonary disease (COPD) is primarily a disease of the horse. It is a well-identified and common syndrome of chronic respiratory disease. Clinical signs include chronic cough, loud abnormal breath sounds and a double expiratory effort. The disease is a combination of chronic bronchitis and bronchiolitis complicated by pulmonary emphysema. Called also heaves, broken wind.

c. respiratory disease a disease of chickens caused by infection with *Mycoplasma gallisepticum*. It is characterized by coughing, nasal discharge, respiratory rales, a long course and the complication of airsacculitis. There is a loss of egg production and wastage by culling of carcasses at the abattoir but mortality is low.

chron(o)- word element. [Gr.] *time.*
chronobiology the scientific study of the effect of time on living systems and of biological rhythms.
chronograph an instrument for recording small intervals of time.
chronological tactics techniques of planning experiments or analyzing retrospective data in order to make the most use of the passage of time, e.g. analysis of the relationship between a prior disease and a subsequent outcome.
chronotropic affecting the time or rate.
chronotropism interference with regularity of a periodical movement, such as the heart's action.
chronotropy affecting a time or rate, as in heart rate.
Chrosperma muscaetoxicum see AMIANTHIUM MUSCAETOXICUM.
Chrozophora spicata toxic African plant, member of the Euphorbiaceae family. Causes incoordination, diarrhea, and fatal pulmonary edema. The toxin has not been identified. Called also terba.
Chrysanthemum plant genus in the family Asteraceae; contains sesquiterpene lactones; causes contact dermatitis. Garden plants called also feverfew, marguerite.
C. cinerariaefolium the plant from which pyrethrum is extracted. Called also *Pyrethrum cinerarifolia.*
chrysanthemum-faced dog an early name for the Shih tzu.
Chrysemys picta painted turtle.
chrysiasis deposition of gold in living tissue.
chrys(o)- word element. [Gr.] *gold.*
Chrysocoma tenuifolia Southern African plant in the Asteraceae family; contains an unidentified toxin causing diarrhea, dermatitis, intestinal obstruction, myelomalacia in three syndromes, kaalsiekte (in lambs), lakseersiekte (adults), valsiekte. Called also bitterbush, beesbossie, beeskaroo, bitterkaroo, bitterbos. See also LAKSEERSIEKTE, KAALSIEKTE, VALSIEKTE.
chrysoderma permanent pigmentation of the skin due to gold deposit.
Chrysolina quadrigemina a beetle used in the biological control of St. Johns wort—*Hypericum perforatum.*
Chrysolophus the genus of pheasants; includes *C. amherstiae* (Lady Amherst's pheasant), *C. pictus* (golden pheasant).
Chrysomya a genus of flies of the family Calliphoridae. See also SCREW-WORM.
C. albiceps, C. bezziana, C. chloropyga, C. mallochi, C. rufifacies cause cutaneous MYIASIS. See also LUCILIA, CALLITROGA and PHORMIA.
Chrysomyia see CHRYSOMYA.
Chrysops a genus of blood-sucking tropical flies of the family Tabanidae. *C. discalis* (deer fly), a vector of tularemia in the western USA, and *C. silacea*, an intermediate host of *Loa loa*, a filarial parasite. Called also chrysops flies.
C. discalis, C. dimidiata, C. silacea these flies cause painful bites and worry livestock when they are about. They also mechanically transmit anthrax, anaplasmosis, the virus of infectious equine anemia, tularemia and the larvae of the filariid parasite *Loa loa.* A number of trypanosome species are also transmitted mechanically by this important means.
Chrysosporium saprophytic soil fungal organisms, which when inhaled have been the cause of granulomatous inflammation of the lungs (adiaspiromycosis). Formerly *Emmonsia.* The main species are *C. parvum* var. *parvum* (*E. parva*) and *C. parvum* var. *crescens* (*E. crescens*).
chrysotherapy the use of gold salts in the treatment of disease, e.g. autoimmune skin diseases and rheumatoid arthritis in dogs. They have antimicrobial, anti-inflammatory, anti-immunological and antienzymatic activity.
chthonophagia the habit of eating clay or earth; geophagia.
chuck a hand grip to be attached to intramedullary pins to enable the surgeon to rotate or drive them into bone.
chukka, chukker a term used in polo; a polo match is divided into six chukkas of 7 minutes each.
chun see TSUN.
churchyard yew *Taxus baccata* var. *fastigiata.*
chute 1. a device used to restrain large animals especially cattle and horses. It is a small stall into which the animal is encouraged to walk. The head is fixed, in cattle by a head bail, the back is closed and the animal can then be examined or treated. The quality of the chute depends on its freedom from injury to the animal and the operator and the accessibility of the animal for the procedures to be conducted. Speed of throughput is also an important consideration when large numbers are to be handled in repetitive treatments and quick-release gates are an essential part of the unit. Called also stocks, crush. 2. a similar crate or stall at a rodeo in which a wild animal can be saddled and mounted before being released to buck with the rider. See also RESTRAINING CHUTE.
CHV canine herpesvirus; caprine herpesvirus.
chylangioma a tumor of intestinal lymph vessels filled with chyle.
chyle the milky fluid taken up by the lacteals from the intestine during digestion, consisting of lymph and triglyceride fat (chylomicrons) in a stable emulsion, and conveyed by the thoracic duct to empty into the venous system.
chylemia the presence of chyle in the blood.
chylifaction, chylification the formation of chyle. Called also chylopoiesis.
chyliform resembling chyle.
chylo- prefix meaning chyle.
chyloabdomen chyloperitoneum.
chylocele distension of the tunica vaginalis testis with effused chyle.
chylofibrosis pleural fibrosis resulting from chylothorax.
chyloid resembling chyle.
c. effusion effusions, usually pleural, with a milky appearance, containing cholesterols or protein–lecithin compounds but not chylomicron globules, may be mistaken as chylous by their gross appearance. Seen in cats with cardiomyopathy or cardiac disease. Called also pseudochylous effusion.
chylomediastinum the presence of effused chyle in the mediastinum.
chylomicron a stable droplet containing principally triglyceride fat, but also cholesterol, phospholipids and protein; found in intestinal lymphatics (lacteals) and blood during and after meals.
c. test in chilled serum, chylomicrons rise to form a creamy top layer and the serum clears; very low-density lipoproteins remain dispersed and the serum is turbid. Called also the refrigeration test.
chylomicronemia an excess of chylomicrons in the blood.
chylopericardium the presence of effused chyle in the pericardium.
chyloperitoneum the presence of effused chyle in the peritoneal cavity.

chylopleura chylothorax.
chylopneumothorax the presence of effused chyle and air in the pleural cavity.
chylopoiesis production of chyle.
chylothorax the presence of effused chyle in the pleural cavity. Occurs most commonly in dogs and cats, caused by traumatic injury to the thoracic duct, neoplasms in the cranial mediastinum, or a congenital abnormality of the duct.
chylous pertaining to, mingled with, or of the nature of chyle.
c. ascites distension of the abdomen with chyle.
c. effusion accumulation of chyle, usually in a cavity, e.g. pleural cavity.
c. hydrothorax see CHYLOTHORAX.
chyluria the presence of chyle in the urine, giving it a milky appearance, due to obstruction of lymph flow, which causes rupture of lymph vessels into the renal pelves, ureters, bladder or urethra.
chyme the semifluid, homogeneous, creamy or gruel-like material produced by action of the gastric juice on ingested food and discharged through the pylorus into the duodenum.
chymification conversion of food into chyme; gastric digestion.
chymodenin a polypeptide secreted by the duodenum that specifically stimulates pancreatic secretion of chymotrypsinogen.
chymopapain a proteolytic enzyme (a sulfhydryl proteinase) from the tropical tree *Carica papaya*, used in chemonucleolysis.
chymosin the milk-curdling enzyme found in the abomasal juice of preweaned calves (before pepsin formation); a preparation from the stomach of the calf is used to coagulate milk protein in the preparation of junket and thus to facilitate its digestion. Rennin catalyzes the conversion of caseinogen from a soluble to an insoluble form (casein or curd). Called also rennin. See also RENNET.
chymotrypsin an endopeptidase with action similar to that of trypsin, produced in the intestine by activation of chymotrypsinogen from the exocrine pancreas; a product crystallized from an extract of the pancreas of the ox has been used clinically as an anti-inflammatory agent and for enzymatic zonulolysis and débridement.
c. test a test of pancreatic exocrine efficiency depending on the presence of chymotrypsin to split a peptide–para-aminobenzoic acid compound.
chymotrypsinogen the inactive precursor of chymotrypsin, the form in which it is secreted by the pancreas.
Ci curie. See BECQUEREL.
CI 634 see TILETAMINE.
CIA colony inhibiting activity.
cib. [L.] *cibus* (food); used in prescription writing, e.g. post cib. = after meals.
CIC circulating immune complexes.
cicatrectomy excision of a cicatrix.
cicatricial pertaining to a cicatrix.
c. tissue the dense fibrous tissue forming a cicatrix, derived directly from granulation tissue. Called also scar tissue.
cicatrix pl. *cicatrices* [L.] the fibrous tissue left after the healing of a wound; a scar.
cicatrization the formation of a cicatrix or scar; scarring. Surgical cicatrization, performed by injection of a strongly irritating substance such as iodine, is used in horses to tighten the patellar ligaments in the treatment for patellar luxation.
Cicer arietinum see CHICKPEA.
Cicherelli rongeur a rongeur with tapered jaws and a sharp tip; used in neurosurgery.
Cichorium intybus member of the Asteraceae plant family; the roots contain an unidentified toxin which causes salivation, diarrhea in cattle. Called also chicory.
ciclopirax olamine a wide-spectrum antifungal drug used topically to treat *Candida* and fungal infections of the skin.
Ciconiphilus pectiniventris a louse of duck and geese.
Cicuta a genus of the plant family Apiaceae; these plants contain a toxic alcohol, cicutoxin, which causes sudden death in grazing livestock, often within minutes of being eaten. Roots and tubers are most toxic. Clinical signs include diarrhea, frothing at the mouth and convulsions. Includes *C. bolanderi* (water hemlock), *C. bulbifera*, *C. californica*, *C. curtisii*, *C. douglasii*, *C. maculata*, *C. mackenziana*, *C. occidentalis*, *C. vagans* (cowbane), *C. virosa*.
cicutoxin toxic alcohol separable from plant material of CICUTA.
CID combined immune deficiency; cytomegalic inclusion body disease.
-cide word element. [L.] *destruction or killing* (homicide); *an agent that kills or destroys* (germicide).
CIE counter immunoelectrophoresis.
CIF clone-inhibiting factor.
ciguatera poisoning by consumption of the flesh or viscera of sporadically toxic tropical predatory fish of a wide range of species. The causative heat-stable toxins (ciguatoxin, maitotoxin and others) originate in the dinoflagellate (*Gambierdiscus toxicus*) and possibly others or from associated bacterial microflora. The toxins are subject to bioaccumulation in fish which eat the dinoflagellates, and subsequently in the predators. Growth of the dinoflagellates is promoted by the destruction of their coral reef habitat. Poisoning characterized by vomiting, diarrhea and paresis in cats, dogs, humans. See also LYNGBYA.
cilastatin an inhibitor of dehydropeptidase I, an enzyme found in renal tubules. Used in association with the antibiotic, imipenem, to prevent its inactivation.
cilia [L.] plural of *cilium*. 1. the eyelashes. 2. minute hairlike processes that extend from a cell surface, composed of nine pairs of microtubules around a core of two microtubules. They beat rhythmically to move the cell or to move fluid or mucus over the surface. Of particular importance in the respiratory epithelium, contributing greatly to the MUCOCILIARY escalator.
c.-associated respiratory (CAR) bacillus gram-negative bacterium associated with severe respiratory disease in rats and possibly mice; usually associated with *Mycoplasma pulmonis* infection.
conjunctival c. see ectopic cilia (below).
ectopic c. arise from the conjunctival surface of the eyelids and cause corneal irritation.
eyelid c. the eyelashes; smaller and shorter on the lower lids and may be absent altogether in dogs and pigs. There are also longer tactile hairs on the external surface of the eyelids.
immotile c. syndrome see IMMOTILE CILIA SYNDROME.
ciliariscope an instrument for examining the ciliary region of the eye.
ciliarotomy surgical division of the ciliary zone.
ciliary pertaining to or resembling cilia; used particulary in reference to certain eye structures, such as the ciliary body or muscles.

c. adenomas arise from the non-pigmented inner layer of the ciliary epithelium; cause hyphema or glaucoma.
c. body the thickened part of the vascular tunic of the eye, connecting choroid and iris, made up of the ciliary muscle and the ciliary processes. The processes radiate from the ciliary muscle and give attachments to ligaments supporting the lens of the eye.
c. body inflammation see CYCLITIS.
c. epithelium rostral continuation of the pars ciliaris retinae; non-pigmented, non-neural cells.
c. flush
c. glands sweat glands which have become arrested in their development, situated at the edge of the eyelids. Called also Moll's glands.
c. inflammation cyclitis.
c. injection peripheral hyperemia of the anterior ciliary vessels which produces a deep red or rose color of the corneal stroma, and must be distinguished from hyperemia of the conjunctival vessels. May spread to the perilimbic corneal tissue. Called also ciliary flush.
c. muscle the smooth (mammals) or striated (birds) muscle that forms the main part of the ciliary body and and functions in accommodation of the eye.
primary c. dyskinesia abnormality of ciliary function leading to diseases of respiratory and reproductive tracts including sinusitis and bronchiectasis. May be associated with cardiac displacement. See also KARTAGENER'S SYNDROME.
c. process folded structures on the posterior aspect of the ciliary body.
c. reflex movements of the pupil in accommodation.
c. zonules continuations of the ciliary processes of the ciliary body connecting it to the lens. They are in close contact with the hyaloid membrane of the vitreous body.

Ciliata a class of protozoa (subphylum Ciliophora) whose members possess cilia during the life cycle; a few species are parasitic.

ciliate 1. having cilia. 2. any member of the class Ciliata; in veterinary medicine the important group is the ciliate protozoa.

ciliated provided with cilia.

ciliectomy 1. excision of a portion of the ciliary body. 2. excision of the portion of the eyelid containing the roots of the eyelashes.

cili(o)- word element. [L.] *cilia, ciliary (body)*.

Ciliophora a subphylum of Protozoa, including two major groups, the ciliates and suctorians, and distinguished from the other subphyla by the presence of cilia at some stage during the organism's life cycle.

ciliospinal pertaining to the ciliary body and the spinal cord.
c. reflex dilatation of the pupil when the skin of the neck is stimulated painfully.

cilium pl. *cilia* [L.] see CILIA.

cillosis spasmodic quivering of the eyelid.

cilofungin an antifungal agent, effective aginst yeasts, especially *Candida albicans*.

cimbia a white band running across the ventral surface of the crus cerebri.

cimetidine a histamine H_2-receptor antagonist that inhibits the action of histamine at cell surface receptors of the gastric parietal cells and reduces basal gastric acid secretion and secretion stimulated by food, histamine, gastrin and insulin. It is used for short-term treatment of peptic ulcer and for treatment of pathological hypersecretory conditions.

Cimex a genus of the insect family Cimicidae.
***C. hemipterus* (*C. rotundatus*)** parasitic bugs of poultry.
C. lectularius blood-sucking insects parasitizing humans for the most part but can affect pigeons and poultry. Called also bed bugs.

cinch a saddle girth on an American stock saddle. Tightens with a knot on a ring instead of with straps and buckles.

cinchocaine see DIBUCAINE.

cinchona bark dried bark of the stem or root of various South American trees of the genus *Cinchona*. It is the source of quinine, cinchonine and cinchonidine. Used as a bitter and antipyretic.

cine- word element. [Gr.] *movement;* see also words beginning *kine-*.

cineangiocardiography the photographic recording of image intensification fluoroscopy of the heart and great vessels by motion picture techniques.

cineangiography the photographic recording of fluoroscopic images of the blood vessels by motion picture techniques.

cinefluorography see CINERADIOGRAPHY.

cinemicrography the making of motion pictures of a small object through the lens system of a microscope.

cineole see EUCALYPTOL.

cineradiography the making of a motion picture record of successive images appearing in image intensification fluoroscopy.

cinerea the gray matter of the nervous system.

cinerolone one of the ketoalcohols in *Chrysanthemum cinerariaefolium* that combines with carboxylic acids to produce pyrethrins.

cinesi- for words beginning thus, see those beginning *kinesi-*.

cineto- for words beginning thus, see those beginning *kineto-*.

cingulate gyrus the gyrus marking the presence of the cingulum, the medial olfactory tract.

cingulum pl. *cingula* [L.] 1. an encircling part or structure; a girdle. 2. a bundle of association fibers partly encircling the corpus callosum not far from the median plane, interrelating the cingulate and hippocampal gyri. 3. the ridge at the base of the crown of some teeth. 4. an annular band at the vestibulovaginal junction in the female genital tract; may be the site of a vestigial hymen.
c. membri pelvini see PELVIC girdle.
c. membri thoracici see shoulder GIRDLE.

Cinnamomum camphora see CAMPHOR.

cinnamon a herbal preparation obtained from the bark of *Cinnamomum* spp. It is used as an astringent in the treatment of diarrhea and flatulence. Cinnamon oil, sometimes used as a name for Cassia Oil, has similar activity, but contains cinnamaldehyde, which has been associated with hypersensitivity reactions.

cinoxacin a quinolone antibiotic with activity similar to nalidixic acid. Used in urinary tract infections and bacterial prostatitis in dogs.

ciodrin an organophosphorus insecticide for use on animals as a powder or spray.

Cionella lubrica a terrestrial snail, the first intermediate host of DICROCOELIUM *dendriticum*.

ciprofloxacin a fluoroquinolone antibiotic with particularly good activity against gram-negative bacteria, including Enterobacteriaceae and *Pseudomonas aeruginosa*. It is used mainly in urinary tract infections.

circadian denoting a period of about 24 hours.
c. clock the daily rhythm of physiological activity as expressed by the Chinese circadian clock. This explains the flow of energy or *Qi* through the body, via the meridians, each meridian having two hours of

maximum and two of minimum function in every day.

c. rhythm the regular recurrence of certain phenomena in cycles of approximately 24 hours, e.g. biological activities that occur at about the same time each day (or night) regardless of constant darkness or other conditions of illumination.

circannual occurring rhythmically every year.

circhoral pertaining to biological rhythms.

circinate resembling a ring or circle.

circle a round figure, structure or part.

c. block see ring BLOCK.

ciliary arterial c. formed from the anterior ciliary arteries; lies within the ciliary muscle.

iridial arterial c. formed from the posterior long ciliary arteries and supplying blood to the iris.

iridial vascular c. a ring of vessels formed by the anterior ciliary arteries; provide fine branches to the iris and ciliary body.

c. of safety see FLIGHT DISTANCE.

c. system see breathing CIRCUIT.

c. test walking a horse in a small circle, first one direction then the other, is used in a neurological examination to detect ataxia and abnormalities in proprioception.

c. of Willis anastomotic loop of vessels near the base of the brain. See cerebral ARTERIAL circle.

circling persistent walking in circles; it may be caused by deviation of the head because of a bend in the neck, or be due to rotation of the head, e.g. caused by listeriosis or brain abscess. A sign of unilateral vestibular disease or cerebral lesion (toward the side of the lesion; adverse syndrome).

c. disease see LISTERIOSIS.

Circoviridae a name proposed for a new family of viruses that may include porcine circovirus, chicken anemia virus, pigeon circovirus, and psittacine BEAK and feather disease virus. The three viruses are not uniform in their properties. They are the smallest animal viruses, 17 to 24 nm in diameter, and contain a single-stranded circular DNA genome composed of about 2500 nucleotides. Circoviruses replicate in the nucleus of cells and are assumed to be dependent on the host cell for many functions required for viral replication and probably, like parvoviruses, replicate in cells that are in the S-phase of the cell cycle.

circovirus a virus in the family *Circoviridae*.

circuit a round course, or course followed by, for example, electrical current, anesthetic gas, a traveling judge.

Bain coaxial c. a variant of the T-piece circuit of delivery of anesthetic gas in which the fresh gas passes up a central tube and the expired gas passes out through the outer sleeve.

breathing c. of an anesthetic machine is the pathway by which the volatile anesthetic agent and oxygen are conveyed to the patient and carbon dioxide is removed. The two methods for removal of carbon dioxide are that of venting all expired gases to the exterior, and the method of absorbing the CO_2 chemically and rebreathing the expired gas. The two basic circuits are the open circuit in which the patient has access to environmental air as well as the anesthetic–oxygen mixture and exhales into the environment, and the closed system in which all gases are rebreathed. The latter may be a to-and-fro system or a circle system, the latter based on the use of unidirectional valves to ensure that the gases always pass in the correct direction. See also Bain coaxial circuit (above), circle breathing circuit (below), coaxial circuit (below), Lack circuit (below), Magill circuit (below), SCHIMMELBUSCH MASK, T-piece circuit (below).

circle breathing c. in an anesthetic machine; the flow of gases is directed by an inclusion in the system of two unidirectional valves, one in an expiratory and one in an inspiratory tube. The rebreathing bag and the canister of sodalime for CO_2 absorption are located between the two tubes.

coaxial c. a system for the delivery of gaseous anesthetic which has separate conduits for fresh gas and expired air and is essentially the same as the T-piece system except that one conduit is inside the other. An attractive system because the exhaust gases can be ducted to the exterior.

Lack c. a coaxial breathing circuit used in anesthesia. Fresh gas flows up the outer sleeve, expired air and gas pass down the inner tube.

Magill c. a breathing circuit used in anesthesia. It includes a reservoir bag, wide-bore corrugated tubing and a spring-loaded expiratory valve. It is a semi-closed system in which rebreathing is prevented by having the gas flow rate from the cylinders slightly in excess of the patient's minute respiratory volume.

Mapleson c. an anesthetic breathing circuit in which the fresh gas flow is used to remove exhaled carbon dioxide. The Mapleson A circuit is called also the Magill circuit (above), Mapleson D circuit is called also the Bain circuit (above), and the JACKSON-REES T-PIECE is the Mapleson F circuit.

non-rebreathing c. anesthetic breathing circuits in which exhaled gases are discharged to the environment and do not pass back to the patient. See Magill circuit (above).

parallel c. a variation on the Bain and Lack circuits (above) in which there are two tubes running side by side instead of one inside the other.

rebreathing c. anesthetic breathing circuits in which the exhaled gas is recirculated to the patient with CO_2 removed.

T-piece c. a breathing circuit used in anesthesia. Shaped like a T. The exhaled gases are passed into a reservoir tube from which they are pushed by fresh gas from the anesthetic machine as it passes from the stem to the other arm of the T during expiration. There are no valves.

x-ray c. a complete path along which an electrical current flows. In its simplest form it includes a source of electrons (power source), a load or resistance, and a conductor.

circulation movement in a regular or circuitous course, returning to the point of origin, as the circulation of the blood through the heart and blood vessels. See also CIRCULATORY system.

antegrade c. circulation in the normal direction of flow.

artificial c. is maintained in cardiopulmonary arrest by cardiac compression.

collateral c. circulation carried on through secondary channels after obstruction of the principal channel supplying the part.

coronary c. that within the coronary vessels, which supply the muscle of the heart.

cutaneous c. cutaneous vessels are innervated by sympathetic adrenergic vasoconstrictor fibers; vasodilation is an important mechanism for losing heat after the body has been warmed.

enterohepatic c. the cycle in which bile salts and other substances excreted by the liver in the bile are absorbed by the intestinal mucosa and returned to the liver via the portal circulation.

extracorporeal c. circulation of blood outside the

body, as through a HEMODIALYZER or an EXTRACORPOREAL circulatory support unit.

fetal c. circulation of blood through the body of the fetus and to and from the placenta through the umbilical cord. See also FETAL circulation.

hepatic c. includes the hepatic arterial blood supply and the supply from the portal vein; drainage is via the hepatic veins to the caudal vena cava.

lymph c. see LYMPH.

maternal c. the circulation of the dam during pregnancy, including especially that of the uterus.

micro-c. see MICROCIRCULATION.

neonatal c. circulation in the newborn immediately after birth; the umbilical vessels contract forcing blood into the fetal veins; the foramen ovale closes, the ductus arteriosus narrows and eventually closes at day 1 to 2 after birth.

ocular c. consists of the uveal and retinal blood vessels supported by the aqueous humor and vitreous body.

placental c. consists of the umbilical arteries, the vessels of the placenta proper and the umbilical veins; approximates the fetal corporeal circulation in volume.

portal c. a general term denoting the circulation of blood through larger vessels from the capillaries of one organ to those of another; applied especially to the passage of blood from the gastrointestinal tract, pancreas and spleen through the portal vein to the liver.

pulmonary c. the flow of blood from the right ventricle through the pulmonary artery to the lungs, where carbon dioxide is exchanged for oxygen, and back through the pulmonary vein to the left atrium. See also PULMONARY circulation.

splenic c. flow of blood through the splenic artery and arterioles to either the capillaries, e.g. white pulp, or the highly permeable sinuses of the red pulp. Splenic venous blood drains into the portal vein and passes through the liver before re-entering the general circulation.

systemic c. the flow of blood from the left ventricle through the aorta, carrying oxygen and nutrient material to all the tissues of the body, and returning through the superior and inferior venae cavae to the right atrium.

c. time the time required for blood to flow between two given points. It is determined by injecting a substance into a vein and then measuring the time required for it to reach a specific site.

circulatory pertaining to circulation.

c. arrest see cardiac ARREST.

c. collapse SHOCK; circulatory insufficiency without congestive heart failure.

c. failure includes cardiac or central circulatory failure and peripheral circulatory failure. Although the mechanisms, causes and clinical syndromes are different the pathogenesis is the same: the circulatory system fails to maintain the supply of oxygen and other nutrients to the tissues and to remove the carbon dioxide and other metabolites from them. The failure may be hypovolemic, distributive.

c. response changes in the cardiac and vascular functions in response to such factors as emotional stress, physical exercise, temperature change.

c. shock see SHOCK.

c. support see EXTRACORPOREAL circulation.

c. system the major system concerned with the movement of blood and lymph; it consists of the heart and blood vessels. The circulatory system transports to the tissues and organs of the body the oxygen, nutritive substances, immune substances, hormones and chemicals necessary for normal function and activities; it also carries away waste products and carbon dioxide. It helps to regulate body temperature and helps maintain normal water and electrolyte balance.

The rate of blood flow through the vessels depends upon several factors: force of the heartbeat, rate of the heartbeat, venous return and control of the arterioles and capillaries by chemical, neural and thermal stimuli.

circulus see CIRCLE.

c. arteriosus cerebri the ring of arteries which serves as the major source of blood supply to the brain; a circle around the stalk of the pituitary gland ventral to thalamus; previously called circle of Willis.

circum- word element. [L.] *around.*

circumanal gland sebaceous glands in the skin around the anus of dogs. See PERIANAL gland.

circumcise to perform circumcision. See also PREPUTIAL prolapse.

circumcision surgical removal of part of the prepuce. Performed only to repair a prolapse of the prepuce, encountered in all species but especially in *Bos indicus* cattle. Called also posthioplasty.

circumclusion compression of an artery by a wire and pin.

circumduction circular movement of a limb or of the eye.

circumflex curved like a bow.

circumscribed bounded or limited; confined to a limited space.

circumvallate surrounded by a ridge or trench, as the vallate (circumvallate) papillae.

Circus see HARRIER (2).

cirrhosis a liver disease characterized pathologically by the loss of the normal microscopic lobular architecture and regenerative replacement of necrotic parenchymal tissue with fibrous bands of connective tissue which eventually constrict and partition the organ into irregular nodules. The term is sometimes used to refer to chronic interstitial inflammation of any organ.

cardiac c. fibrosis or scarring of the liver resulting from the anoxia and centrilobular necrosis associated with the passive congestion of congestive heart failure.

cirripede see BARNACLE.

cirrus coarse hairs, longer than those in the normal coat and less coarse than tactile hairs.

c. capitis hairs of the forelock.

c. caudae hairs of the tail.

c. metacarpeus frontlimb feather.

c. metatarseus hindlimb feather.

Cirsium arvense plant member of the family Asteraceae; may cause nitrate–nitrite poisoning. Called also Canada thistle.

cis [L.] in organic chemistry, having certain atoms or radicals on the same side; in genetics, having the two mutant genes of a pseudoallele on the same chromosome. Compare *trans.* See also *cis-trans* TEST.

***c.* acting** in molecular biology, a sequence or regulatory protein that is part of the same DNA molecule as the gene of interest. See also TRANS acting.

***c.*-acting mutation** in the lactose operon a mutation in the attenuator region that disrupts base pairing in the double-stranded portion of the termination hair pin and permits the RNA polymerase to 'read through' the termination signal.

***c.*-dominant mutation** occurs in regulatory sequences that are recognized by DNA binding proteins that affect only adjacent genes on the same DNA molecule.

cis-active a DNA sequence that controls a gene on the same chromosome.

cis face the proximal (or forming or *cis*) face of the Golgi apparatus.

cisapride a substituted benzamide, similar to metoclopramide, which stimulates gastrointestinal motility. Used as an antiemetic by promoting gastric emptying.

cisplatin, *cis*-platinum a platinum-containing complex used as an antineoplastic agent whose main mode of action resembles that of alkylating agents—production of cross-links between the two strands of DNA in the double helix so that DNA cannot be replicated and the cells cannot divide.

Cissus quadrangularis African plant in family Vitaceae; contains unidentified toxin causing gastroenteritis.

cistern a closed space serving as a reservoir for lymph or other body fluids, especially one of the enlarged subarachnoid spaces containing cerebrospinal fluid.

cisterna pl. *cisternae;* cistern.

c. cerebellomedullaris, c. magna the enlarged subarachnoid space between the caudal surface of the cerebellum and the dorsal surface of the medulla oblongata.

c. chyli the dilated portion of the thoracic duct at its origin in the lumbar region. Called also receptaculum chyli.

c. magna see cisterna cerebellomedullaris (above).

cisternal pertaining to a cistern, especially the cisterna cerebellomedullaris.

c. puncture puncture of the cisterna cerebellomedullaris (magna) with a hollow needle inserted through the aperture between the occipital crest and the anterior edge of the atlas. A sample of CSF may be collected, contrast medium injected or pressure measured. See also SPINAL puncture.

c. space a channel between opposing layers of a highly convoluted single membrane in the endoplasmic reticulum of all cells.

c. tap see cisternal puncture (above).

cisternography radiography of the basal cistern of the brain after subarachnoid injection of a contrast medium.

cistron a DNA segment corresponding to one polypeptide chain plus the start-and-stop codon. The smallest unit of genetic material that must be intact to function as a transmitter of genetic information; as traditionaly construed, approximately synonymous with gene.

citrate any salt of citric acid. Citrate is the first intermediate of the citric acid cycle and tricarboxylic acid (TCA) cycle. It also plays an important role in fatty acid synthesis which takes place in the cytoplasm. It acts as a carrier of acetyl-CoA, the construction material for fatty acids. The movement is assisted by two enzymes, citrate-condensing enzyme, which catalyzes the condensation of the acetyl unit with oxaloacetate in the mitochondria, and citrate-cleavage enzyme (citrate lyase), which catalyzes the release of the acetyl radical in the cytoplasm of the cell.

c. cleavage enzyme important enzyme in fatty acid synthesis from glucose; catalyzes the split of citrate to acetyl CoA and oxaloacetate.

c. synthase first enzyme of the TCA cycle catalyzing the formation of citrate from acetyl CoA and oxaloacetate.

citreoviridin the metabolite of *Penicillium citreoviride* thought to be the cause of yellow rice poisoning, manifested in humans and experimental animals by respiratory and circulatory failure, paralysis, convulsions and death. Identical to beriberi, originally considered to be a thiamin nutritional deficiency.

citric acid a tricarboxylic acid occurring in citrus fruits and acting as an antiscorbutic and diuretic. It functions as an anticoagulant in the blood preservatives, acid citrate dextrose and citrate phosphate dextrose. See also CITRATE.

c. a. cycle see TRICARBOXYLIC ACID CYCLE.

citrinin mycotoxin produced by the fungi *Penicillium viridicatum*, *P. palitans* and *Aspergillus ochraceus*; causes tremor, recumbency, convulsions, nephrosis.

Citrobacter a genus of gram-negative, lactose fermenting rods, members of the Enterobacteriaceae. Found in water, feces and urine, and not considered to be animal pathogens.

C. freundii have been identified as the cause of SEPTICEMIC cutaneous ulcerative disease of turtles. The disease is characterized by cutaneous hemorrhage and ulceration, loss of claws and digits, flaccidity and paralysis.

citronella oil a volatile oil obtained from the grass *Cymbopogon nardus* or *C. winterianus*. Used as an insect repellent.

citrovorum factor see FOLINIC ACID.

citrulline an alpha amino acid involved in the urea cycle.

c. phosphorylase see ornithine carbamoyl TRANSFERASE.

citrullinemia a disease caused by a defect of urea metabolism resulting in a marked low level of citrulline. Caused by an inherited deficiency of arginosuccinate synthetase; reported in dogs and cattle. In cattle, it is characterized clinically by a sudden onset of depression, recumbency, opisthotonos and seizures in previously normal calves of up to 3 days of age.

citrullinuria the presence in the urine of large amounts of citrulline, with increased levels also in both plasma and cerebrospinal fluid.

Citrullus genus of plants in family Cucurbitaceae; contains cucurbitacin, colocynthin, tetracyclic terpenes causing diarrhea; includes *C. colocynthis* (*C. vulgaris*), *C. lanatus*.

citrus fruit taint a common taint when meat and citrus fruit are stored close to one another, especially if the fruit rots.

cittosis see PICA.

Cittotaenia a tapeworm genus of the family Anoplocephalidae.

C. denticulata heavy infestations cause digestive disturbances, emaciation and some deaths in rabbits and hares.

Civatte body see APOPTOTIC BODY.

civet a large cat-like animal but with short legs and a long muzzle and without retractile claws. The family Viverridae includes civets and genets; the civets are characterized by the secretion of a valuable scent from their anal glands, and are kept in captivity so that the scent can be harvested. They are nocturnal, carnivorous and largely arboreal. Common genera are *Civettictis*, *Viverra* and *Genetta*, but there are many other genera of civets. Also the spotted skunk, a completely unrelated animal, is known as a civet in the USA.

civil law the form of law which is conducted inquisitorially with the judge asking all of the questions and deciding the outcome. The basis of European law. The opposite to English law, which is adversarial in its approach.

CK CREATINE kinase.
Cl chemical symbol, *chlorine.*
Cl–/HCO_3– exchanger transport of anions, particularly in erythrocytes by facilitated diffusion carried out by band-3 protein, catalyzing the exchange of bicarbonate anion from inside the cell for a chloride anion outside the cell.
Cladophora a genus of algae found in large numbers in the gills of fish dead of asphyxia.
cladosporiosis any infection with the fungus *Cladosporium* spp.
Cladosporium a genus of dematiaceous fungi.
C. carrionii an agent of chromoblastomycosis. Nominated also as one of the causes of hyphomycosis in animals.
***C. herbarum*,** causes black spot on meat in cold storage, growing at a temperature of 18°F (–8°C); spores are a common allergen.
C. trichoides a cause of phaeohyphomycosis.
Cladotaenia a genus of cestodes found in wild birds; larval stages in the livers of rodents.
clam there are a large number of clams; one which is cultivated commercially is VENERUPIS *japonica*.
clam digger's itch SCHISTOSOME dermatitis.
clamp a device for compressing a part or structure.
beam c. a scissors-like instrument originally used to pick up large blocks of ice. Consists of two inward pointing, sharp pointed hooks, pivoting around a pin at their middle, like scissors, and connected to each other at their blunt ends by a short chain. As beam hooks the points of the two blades are hooked into an overhead beam and a weight such as an animal's limb hung from the connecting chain. The animal's weight ensures that the clamp bites deeply.
silage c. a mass of ensilage held together at the sides between solid walls but open at the ends.
surgical c. a surgical instrument designed to compress a part, e.g. umbilicus.
vascular occluding c. used to completely or partially occlude the flow of blood in vessels.
vulvar c. various designs are available but all have as their objective the physical prevention of a prolapse of the vagina or uterus.
Claoxylon australe plant member of the family Euphorbiaceae; may cause nitrate–nitrite poisoning.
clapotement [Fr.] a splashing sound, as in succussion.
Clara cell nonciliated, secretory bronchiolar epithelial cells; function as stem cells for repair in the bronchioles and can divide into ciliated or nonciliated bronchiolar cells.
Clarence River snake see TROPIDECHIS CARINATUS.
clarificant a substance that clears a liquid of turbidity.
clarithromycin a macrolide antibiotic derived from erythromycin, with similar properties.
clasmatocyte monocytic leukocytes other than lymphocytes, monocytes and macrophages in synovial fluid.
clasp-knife release sudden release from rigidity in a limb when passive flexion is attempted.
class 1. a group of similar objects or values selected as a part of a classification. 2. a taxonomic category subordinate to a phylum and superior to an order. 3. a group of variables all of which show a value falling between certain limits.
c. action an exemplary court case fought on behalf of a number of litigants who can expect to be treated in the same way as the contesting litigant.
c. limits the highest and lowest values eligible to be included in a class when data are being classified or grouped.
c. mark the value selected to represent all of the values in a class. It may be the median or average value.
c. midpoint the average of the upper and lower limits of a class.
c. switching when a B lymphocyte changes over from producing one type of immunoglobulins to another.
classic hemophilia see HEMOPHILIA A.
classical, classic the first recognized form of the item; serving as a standard model or guide. See also classical CONDITIONING, EAST COAST FEVER, HOG cholera.
c. conditioning see CONDITIONING.
c. pathway one of the two pathways of complement activation, initiated by antigen–antibody complexes and involving C1, C2 and C4. It leads to activation of C3 and the terminal pathway. See also alternate COMPLEMENT pathway.
classification division of diagnoses, diseases, pathological findings, microbiological findings into categories or classes. See also NOMENCLATURE.
virus c. see Table 8.1.
classing categorizing according to quality, usually relative to a prestated set of rules, e.g. wool classing, sheep classing, cow classing. In some breed stud books animals may have to pass specific tests to be admitted to a special register of superior animals.
bulk wool c. small amounts of wool from small flocks are mixed together in a wool store to make a useful sized lot, then classed lines.
sheep c. classifying sheep and drafting into classes on the basis of wool yield, wool quality and conformation. Carried out as a basis for making up mating groups or groups of sheep for sale when even lines are required by purchasers.
wool c. grading of the wool into even lines based on type, fiber diameter, yield after cleaning, and eventual commercial value.
clastic 1. undergoing or causing division. 2. separable into parts.
clastogenic giving rise to or inducing disruption or breakages, as of chromosomes.
clathrate 1. having the shape or appearance of a lattice; pertaining to clathrate compounds. 2. *clathrate compounds*, inclusion complexes in which molecules of one type are trapped within cavities of the crystalline lattice of another substance.
clathrin a highly conserved, fibrous protein, mol. wt 180,000, which forms a characteristic polyhedral coat on the surface of coated pits and coated vesicles.
Clathrocystis see MICROCYSTIS.
claudication limping or lameness.
intermittent c. a complex of signs characterized by absence of pain or discomfort in a limb when at rest, the commencement of pain, tension and weakness after walking is begun, intensification of the condition until walking is impossible, and the disappearance of signs after the limb has been at rest. It is seen in occlusive arterial disease of the limbs, e.g. iliac thrombosis.
venous c. intermittent claudication caused by venous stasis.
claustrum pl. *claustra* [L.] the thin layer of gray matter lateral to the external capsule of the brain, separating it from the white matter of the insula.
Clavamox, Clavulox proprietary names for products containing amoxicillin and clavulanic acid which are used widely in veterinary therapeutics.
Clavaria a genus of mushrooms in the Basidiomycetes class of fungi. Thought to be the cause of fatal poisoning in cattle manifested clinically by mucosal

erosions, ocular lesions and abortion. Loss of hair and hooves and nervous signs are also attributed to them.

clavate club-shaped, as in the microconidia of *Microsporum nanum*.

Clavibacter toxicus bacterial species (formerly *Corynebacterium rathei*) that grows in galls caused by grass nematodes (*Anguina* spp.) on the seedheads of some temperate zone pasture grasses, e.g. *Agrostis avenacea*, *Lolium rigidum*, *Polypogon monspeliensis*, and produces a highly potent toxin (corynetoxin = tunicamycin) which causes sudden death in cattle.

Claviceps the ergot fungi, members of the Ascomycetes class. Parasites of seedheads of various plants.

C. cinerea this ergot causes the same poisoning syndrome as paspalum ergot. See PASPALUM ERGOT.

C. fusiformis this ergot grows on bulrush millet (*Pennisetum typhoides*) and causes agalactia in sows fed on it. Called also millet ergot.

C. paspali see PASPALUM ERGOT and PASPALUM STAGGERS.

C. purpurea the cause of rye ERGOT.

claviceptaceous emanating from or pertaining to *Claviceps* spp. fungi.

Clavicipitaceae a family of fungi to which *Claviceps* spp. belong. Members have long tubular asci and threadlike ascospores.

clavicipitaceous belonging to the Clavicipitaceae family of fungi.

clavicle the collar bone; reduced or absent from many domestic animals but present in animals that can grasp with their forelimbs such as the cat and primates. See also CLAVICULAR INTERSECTION.

clavicular intersection a vestigial clavicle. A small tendinous band embedded in the brachiocephalic muscle near the point of the shoulder in animals such as the horse and dog.

clavulanic acid, clavulanate a beta-lactam product of *Streptomyces* spp. It binds irreversibly and inhibits β-lactamase produced by many organisms. Used commonly in combination with AMOXICILLIN.

clavus a corn or callus.

claw 1. integumentary appendages at the extremities of the digits of carnivores and some other animals. Because of their sharp ends they are effective in their role of holding and tearing prey. They are sheathed by the action of elastic ligaments unless the flexor muscles are tensed, but can be actively retracted in Felidae, except the cheetah. 2. an alternative name for a digit in cloven-footed animals such as cattle, sheep, goats and pigs. 3. metal manifold in a milking machine cluster which connects the teat cups and the milk line; carries the air admission hole which allows the controlled entry of air from the environment to the vacuum unit of the milking machine.

c. amputation a surgical procedure that removes one digit of cattle, usually as a salvage procedure in septic pedal arthritis.

dew c. see DEWCLAW.

c. fold the skin fold covering the base of the nail in dogs and cats.

c. fracture fractures of the third phalanx in cattle occur uncommonly, usually due to trauma, nutritional disease and penetrating wounds.

ingrown c. likely to develop in Felidae denied the opportunity to rake with their claws, and in Canidae, especially dewclaws.

overgrown c. common in old inactive birds. Causes difficulty in moving.

clay pigeon target used at gun clubs. It causes poisoning in pigs at pasture which eat the targets. The coal tar pitch used as a binder causes severe hepatic necrosis. See also COAL TAR PITCH.

clay pipestem fibrosis fibrosis caused by *Schistosoma* spp. in the portal triads.

Clayia theresae guinea fowl lice.

Claytonia perfoliata see MONTIA PERFOLIATA.

clean pasture pasture that has been rested from grazing by the same, or parasitologically similar, species for a long, but variable period, the time depending on the parasite concerned and the climate. The pasture rarely if ever becomes completely clean, but it should be relatively so in terms of being a source of infection.

cleaning 1. a major part of sanitation procedures in veterinary preventive medicine because of the heavy contamination of animal accommodation by feces and urine, and in abattoirs because of the rapid accumulation of fat. High pressure cleaning with hot water and detergents is the only practicable procedure but brings its own attendant problems of disposal of effluent. 2. colloquial term for placenta of mare or cow.

cleanings see PLACENTA.

clear canary one with no dark colored feathering seen on the surface as the bird stands normally on its perch. Regarded as a desirable trait in classifying canary features.

clear cells cells with vacuolated cytoplasm and only the basal nucleus and cytoplasmic outline visible which are found in renal carcinoma.

clear-eyed blindness see bright BLINDNESS.

clear layer STRATUM lucidum.

clearance the act of clearing; it is a primary pharmacokinetic parameter which describes irreversible removal of a drug from the body by all processes and is made up of renal clearance and metabolic clearance.

blood-urea c. the volume of the blood cleared of urea per minute by renal elimination.

Bromsulphalein c. see SULFOBROMOPHTHALEIN clearance test.

creatinine c. see CREATININE.

inulin c. see INULIN clearance.

c. time the time required for a drug to be eliminated after administration. Eliminated means to the point where it can no longer be detected. Of most importance in avoiding drug residues in food animals and charges of doping in sports animals.

urea c. blood-urea clearance.

clearing clarification.

c. agent added to skin scrapings to digest keratin and permit better visualization of ectoparasites or fungal hyphae and spores. Potassium hydroxide is used most commonly.

c. time in radiographic processing is the time required for the fixative to dissolve away the 'milkiness' of developed halides on the film.

cleat, cleave claw of any cloven-footed animal.

cleavage 1. division into distinct parts, e.g. the double helix. 2. the early successive splitting of a fertilized ovum into smaller cells (blastomeres) by mitosis. See also HOLOBLASTIC, MEROBLASTIC.

c. site the places on a strand of DNA where the restriction enzyme cleaves the DNA.

cleave[1] in molecular biology, to break bonds in DNA or protein.

cleave[2] see CLEAT.

cleft a fissure or longitudinal opening, especially one occurring during embryonic development.

branchial c's the slit-like openings in the gills of fish between the branchial arches; also, the homologous branchial grooves between the branchial arches of mammalian embryos.

c. chin occasionally seen in cattle particularly Herefords. There is a notch at the mandibular symphysis and the central incisors may be directed centrally.

frog c. the sagittal cleft in the frog of the horse's foot.

glottic c. entrance to the larynx; called also rima glottidis.

infundibular c. common opening of the auditory tubes in birds.

interdigital c. separates the hooves.

c. lip a defect in fusion between the central prolabium and one or both lateral mesodermal masses. Most common in dogs of the brachycephalic breeds; may be inherited or caused by environmental factors. Often combined with defects in the palate. Called also primary cleft palate, harelip, cheiloschisis.

Congenital fissure, or split, may involve the hard or soft palate. A common cause of nasal regurgitation in neonates, especially foals. Known to be inherited in some breeds of cattle and dogs, particularly brachycephalic breeds. Called also secondary cleft palate, palatoschisis.

c. palate see cleft lip (above).

Rathke c. see RATHKE'S POUCH.

c. tongue the anterior portion is divided by a longitudinal cleft.

Cleiodiscus a genus of the family Dactylogyridae of monogenetic flukes which infest the gills of fish.

clemastine fumarate a histamine H_1-receptor antagonist used in the treatment of allergic disorders.

Clematis a genus of the plant family Ranunculaceae; contains toxin protoanemonin causing anorexia, thirst, violent diarrhea, convulsions when ingested, lacrimation, rhinorrhea when inhaled, vesication when rubbed on; includes *C. aristata*, *C. glycinoides*, *C. microphylla*, *C. vitalba* (travellers' joy).

Clemmys freshwater turtles or tortoises in the family Emydidae; includes *C. marmorata* (Pacific pond turtle), *C. leprosa* (Spanish terrapin).

clenbuterol a long-acting, β_2-adrenergic agonist. Causes bronchodilatation, decreases bronchial secretion and impedes uterine contraction. Used in the treatment of equine COPD.

clenches the turned down portions of the nails used to keep horseshoes in place. Where the nails come out of the hoof wall they are twisted off and turned down as clenches to prevent the nails from working out. Called also clinches.

Cleome serrulata toxic plant in the family Capparidaceae; may cause nitrate–nitrite poisoning; called also Rocky Mountain bee plant.

Clethra arborea toxic plant in family Clethraceae; contains andromedotoxin; causes diarrhea and sudden death. Called also lily-of-the valley tree.

Clethrionomys see VOLE.

Cleveland Bay English coach horse used for driving. Bay the only color, 16 to 16.2 hands high.

click 1. a brief, sharp sound, especially any of the short, dry clicking heart sounds during systole, indicative of various heart conditions. 2. pressing and releasing the computer mouse button.

click–murmur syndrome mitral valve prolapse.

clicking the sound made by a horse when the shoe of the hindfoot hits the shoe of the front foot while it is trotting. Called also forging.

Clidemia hirta plant in family Melatostomataceae; contains toxic tannins; causes hepatitis, nephrosis and weight loss. Called also harendong.

clidinium bromide a quaternary ammomium compound with anticholinergic activity. Used in the treatment of irritable bowel syndrome in dogs.

client a person whose animal(s) the veterinarian in question has had in his/her care during a finite period. The court usually operates on the basis that one or two years is sufficient to establish a continuing relationship.

c. files the clinical and financial and other records that a veterinarian maintains as a permanent history of his/her association with each of his/her clients and their animals.

c. rights a client is entitled to receive service from his/her regular veterinarian unless he/she has been advised that the client/doctor relationship has been terminated, that is assuming that the client is a bona fide one. A client is also entitled to be served or be advised that service is not available at the usual address but a comparable service is available at another practice and that arrangements have been made with that practice. As to quality of service, the client can expect to receive service of the quality that would be provided by any other veterinarian—the 'reasonable man' policy.

c. target what the owner is trying to achieve by consulting the veterinarian.

climate the total environmental effect of ambient temperature, barometric pressure, radiation, oxygen concentration, water precipitation, humidity, wind speed, wind direction and sunlight hours or cloud cover. Called also weather.

c. classes includes tropical, semitropical, desert, arid, semiarid, temperate, subarctic, arctic, polar.

c. impact includes overall statements of total effect of climate such as WIND-chill index, TEMPERATURE–HUMIDITY INDEX, effective TEMPERATURE.

climatic pertaining to or emanating from climate.

c. stress deleterious physical effects of climate on animals.

c. type see CLIMATE classes.

climatogram the elements of the climate, e.g. temperature, rainfall, are plotted against each other graphically. Establishes the type of climate such as winter rainfall. See also BIOCLIMATOGRAM.

climatological sheath an enclosed climatic area, e.g. a calf barn which is protected against the variations in the external climate. May be man-made or naturally occurring.

climatotherapy treatment of disease by means of a favorable climate, e.g. moving horses with anhidrosis from tropical climates, cattle with altitude disease to lower altitudes.

climax the period of greatest intensity, as in the course of a disease.

climazolam a potent benzodiazapine used as an anxiolytic, sedative and immobilizing agent.

climbing lily GLORIOSA *superba*.

climbing nightshade SOLANUM *dulcamara*.

clinches see CLENCHES.

clindamycin a semisynthetic bacteriostatic antibiotic derivative of lincomycin with improved activity against anaerobic bacteria. It also has some antiprotozoal activity.

clindamycin-associated colitis produced experimentally in horses and characterized by the presence of *Clostridium cadaveris*.

clinic 1. historically—a clinical lecture; examination of patients before a class of students; instruction at the bedside. 2. classically—an establishment where patients are admitted for special study and treatment by a group of physicians practicing medicine together. 3. realistically—is used in most veterinary contexts to describe an establishment conducted by a veterinarian at which patients are examined and treated as outpatients, in contrast to a hospital where patients are admitted for treatment.

clinical 1. pertaining to a clinic or to the bedside and therefore carried out on the living animal. 2. pertaining to or founded on actual observation and treatment of patients, as distinguished from theoretical or experimental. 3. productive of clinical signs; thus clinical disease as distinct from subclinical.

c. data storage storage of clinical data about patients; may be paper or computerized.

c. decision analysis the application of clinical, epidemiological and other data to influence outome probability and alternative decisions in such areas as surgery and pharmaceutical treatment.

c. epidemiologist an epidemiologist who sees patients and herds in a clinical capacity but with an epidemiological viewpoint. An investigator of clinical problems affecting populations.

c. epidemiology the application by a veterinarian who provides direct patient care of epidemiological methods to the study of diagnosis and therapeutics in order to promote efficiency in clinical care.

c. examination an examination of a patient including taking the history, physical examination by palpation, auscultation and percussion, clinicopathological examination and examination of the environment.

c. judgment exerted while the patient is still alive; the critical decisions made on the basis of scientific observations but with the added skill provided by long experience of similar cases. To this must be added an innate ability to make balanced judgments based not only on the state of the animal and its predictable future but also on some consideration for the patient's overall well-being and the client's financial status and degree of psychological, or in some cases actual, dependence on the patient.

c. nomenclature a catalog of the names given to diseases and problems of animals; usually alphabetical, may be numerical. Should contain keywords (including key diagnoses and key signs) and synonyms with each list related to the other. Because of the need to sort banks of clinical data into categories it is essential that recording be accurate and that the catalog be limited—a policy of limited vocabulary.

c. pathologist a veterinarian skilled in clinical pathology.

c. pathology the examination of diseased tissues, fluids or other materials from a living patient, using all of the techniques available including chemistry, hematology, enzymology, cytology, microbiology, parasitology, protozoology, immunology and histopathology.

c. pharmacology the study of the actions and metabolism of drugs in living animals.

c. policies professional rules of thumb which are used to decide on the management of a case when there are no research results on which to base decisions. They are policies originated by the senior members of the profession, especially those in academic posts.

c. propedeutics preliminary training in the clinical sciences; the introduction to veterinary medicine, surgery and animal reproduction.

c. qualifiers adjectives used to qualify diagnoses using terms from within a group of standard variables, e.g. chronic or acute, ovine or bovine, benign or malignant, clinical or latent.

c. record the record, made at the time, of clinical examinations, treatments and advice given, complete with dates, names of individuals concerned and drugs or tests used. The record is desirable for the purpose of evaluating the patient's progress, and essential from the legal point of view if arguments should arise about competence or justness of charges made.

c. signs the abnormalities of structure or function observed in the patient by the veterinarian or the client. These are customarily graded according to severity, e.g. severe, moderate, mild, and according to speed of onset and progress, e.g. peracute, acute, subacute, chronic, intermittent.

c. trials a planned experiment, conducted in the field, designed to test the efficacy of a treatment in herds of animals by comparing the outcome under the test treatment with that observed in a comparable group of animal herds receiving a control treatment.

c. vocabulary a catalog of terms approved for use in the description of clinical signs and problems, and for the definition of diagnoses and diseases.

clinically in terms used to express the results of a clinical examination.

c. dead as far as can be ascertained by a clinical examination the patient is dead. There is no pulse, no respiratory movement and no corneal reflex.

c. normal the patient is normal in all clinical parameters.

clinician a veterinarian skilled in working at first hand with sick animals in clinical surroundings, which may be in a closed environment such as a hospital, or in a field environment. May be medically, surgically or reproductively inclined.

clinicopathological pertaining to clinical pathology, i.e. to both signs of disease and its pathology.

Clinistix a commercially available product for rapid qualitative and quantitative detection of glucose in urine. It consists of a plastic strip with an impregnated paper tip which turns purple if glucose is present.

clinocephaly congenital flatness or concavity of the vertex of the head.

clinodactyly permanent deviation or deflection of one or more digits.

Clinostomum complanatum*, *C. marginatum flukes in the Clinostomidae family. Parasitize fauces of piscivorous birds. The first hosts are snails, the second are fish which infest the birds when they are eaten.

clioquinol see IODOCHLORHYDROXYQUIN.

clioxanide an anthelmintic used specifically as a flukicide. Because of its large dose size and greater variability in efficacy depending on whether the dose goes into the rumen or not, it has been largely superseded.

CLIP corticotropin-like intermediary peptide.

clip 1. a metallic device for approximating the edges of a wound or for the prevention of bleeding from small individual blood vessels. 2. the small, upturned flange on the front of the front shoe, on the sides of the hind shoe of a set of horseshoes, which helps to prevent lateral movement of the attached shoe. 3. to remove the wool of a sheep by cutting with shears, usually hand shears. 4. the total wool produced by a flock or a farm at one shearing.

c. suture see MICHEL clip.

Versa c. a hemostatic clip or staple applied with a special forceps.

clipping cutting of the hair or wool coat with clippers which may be equipped with blades of different sizes, depending on the purpose and degree of hair removal required. Fine-toothed blades are used in surgical preparation of the skin; coarse blades give various cosmetic results.

c. machine usually refers to electric clippers.

clition the midpoint of the anterior border of the clivus.

Clitocybe genus of toxic Basidiomycete mushrooms; contain an unidentified toxin; causes diarrhea, vomiting. Includes *C. discolor*, *C. rivulosa*.

clitoral pertaining to or emanating from the clitoris.

c. hypertrophy may occur in Cushing's syndrome as a result of increased androgens produced by a hyperplastic or neoplastic adrenal cortex.

c. sinus three to five of these cavities invade the glans of the clitoris in the mare; are the site of infection in contagious metritis in this species and require the excision of the clitoris for importation into some countries.

c. sinusectomy ablation of the clitoral sinus, e.g. of mares as a treatment for contagious equine metritis.

clitorectomy see CLITORIDECTOMY.

clitoridectomy excision of the clitoris.

clitoriditis see CLITORITIS.

clitoridotomy incision of the clitoris.

clitorimegaly enlargement of the clitoris.

clitoris the small, elongated, erectile body in the female; it occupies the clitoral fossa in the ventral commissure of the vulva where it is attached to the ischial arch by two crura. It is homologous with the penis in the male.

enlarged c. as seen in masculinized patients.

clitorism 1. hypertrophy of the clitoris. 2. persistent erection of the clitoris.

clitoritis inflammation of the clitoris.

clitoromegaly clitorimegaly.

clitoroplasty plastic surgery of the clitoris.

clivia African plant in the family Liliaceae; the bulbs of the plant contain toxic lycorine.

clivus pl. *clivi* [L.] a bony surface in the posterior cranial fossa sloping forward from the foramen magnum to the dorsum sellae.

cloaca pl. *cloacae* [L.] 1. a common passage for fecal, urinary and reproductive discharge in most lower vertebrates. 2. the terminal end of the hindgut before division into rectum, bladder and genital primordia in mammalian embryos. 3. an opening in the involucrum of a necrosed bone.

avian c. in birds the cloaca is divided into three poorly defined compartments: a coprodeum or a continuation of the rectum, a urodeum into which the urogenital ducts open (in the female the left genital duct is the oviduct) and the proctodeum which carries the cloacal bursa and the proctodeal glands.

common c. the urorectal septum fails to develop; defecation and urination share a common cavity. Seen in Manx cat.

cloacal emanating from or pertaining to cloaca.

c. kiss the contact which occurs during insemination in birds when the vent of the female is everted exposing the cloacal mucosa against which the phallus of the male is pressed.

c. membrane caudal boundary of the cloaca; membranous in the embryo, ruptured during organogenesis.

cloacitis inflammation of the cloaca.

cloacogenic originating from the cloaca or from persisting cloacal remnants; said of a group of rare transitional-cell nonkeratinizing epidermoid anal cancers.

cloak fern see CHEILANTHES.

clofazimine a human antileprosy drug used in the treatment of feline leprosy.

clofibrate an antihyperlipidemic drug.

cloisonne kidney a nonclinical condition of the kidney in goats in which the cortices are brown or black due to ferritin and hemosiderin deposits in the basement membranes of tubular epithelium.

clomiphene citrate a fertility drug that stimulates secretion of pituitary gonadotropin by blocking estrogen receptors in the pituitary and hypothalamus; used to stimulate ovulation.

clomipramine hydrochloride a tricyclic antidepressant.

clonal referring to a clone.

c. expansion occurs, for example, when B cells, under the influence of T cell interleukins, differentiate into two separate populations and, after several transformations produce sensitized B lymphocytes and plasma cells.

clonal selection theory a onetime theory now accepted as an established part of immunological dogma. Each lymphocyte during its development is committed to respond to one antigenic determinant. Accordingly each lymphocyte has a single type of antigen-specific receptor on its surface. Following contact with antigen, a single lymphocyte expands to form a clone of cells.

clonality the ability to form clones.

clonazepam a benzodiazepine derivative used as an oral anticonvulsant.

clone 1. the genetically identical or closely similar progeny produced by the natural or artificial asexual reproduction of a single organism, cell or gene, e.g. plant cuttings, a cell culture descended from a single cell, or genes reproduced by recombinant DNA technology. 2. to establish or produce such a line of progeny.

c. bank see GENE bank.

c. site the site where insertion of the transfer DNA segment may occur on a cloning vector.

clonic pertaining to or characterized by clonus, e.g. clonic convulsions.

c.-tonic a seizure in which there are clonic and tonic phases with jerking and flexing of muscular alternating with relaxation.

clonicity the condition of being clonic.

clonicotonic both clonic and tonic.

clonidine a centrally acting, α-adrenergic, antihypertensive agent; known to stimulate growth hormone release in dogs.

c. stimulation test used in the diagnosis of pituitary dwarfism. Administration of clonidine causes a marked increase in blood levels of growth hormone in normal dogs.

c. suppression test used in the diagnosis of pheochromocytoma in humans. Normally, clonidine suppresses the release of catecholamines, but it does not have this effect on tumor function.

cloning see RECOMBINANT DNA technology.

directional c. the insertion of a segment of foreign DNA which has a defined polarity, e.g. different restriction enzyme sites at each end, into a plasmid vector.

clonism a succession of clonic spasms.

clonogenic giving rise to a clone of cells.

clonograph an instrument for recording spasmodic movements of parts and tendon reflexes.

clonorchiasis see OPISTHORCHIASIS.

Clonorchis a genus of liver flukes in the family Opisthorchiidae.

***C. sinensis* (syn. *Opisthorchis sinensis*)** found in bile ducts, sometimes pancreatic ducts and duodenum in dogs, cats, pigs, some small wild mammals and humans. Causes diarrhea, abdominal pain, jaundice and ascites in humans. Called also oriental or Chinese liver fluke.

clonospasm clonic spasm.

clonotype the phenotype of a clone of cells.

clonus alternate involuntary muscular contraction and relaxation in rapid succession. A sign of upper motor neuron disease.

clopidol a pyridinol coccidiostat used in poultry.

cloprostenol a prostaglandin analog used in cattle for the treatment of misalliance, termination of pregnancy, treatment of pyometron and fetal mummification, cows with retained corpora lutea which are failing to come into estrus, and for estrus synchronization in embryo transplantation programs.

Cloquet's canal a tubular structure containing remnants of the primary vitreous, located between the posterior aspect of the lens and the retina in the vicinity of the optic disk.

clorazepate a benzodiazepine compound used in the treatment of seizures in dogs.

Clorox commercial name for a sodium hypochlorite preparation marketed as household bleach, but also used for disinfection.

clorsulon a benzenesulfonamide anthelmintic and flukacide used in cattle and sheep.

closantel an anthelmintic effective against *Fasciola hepatica*, *Haemonchus contortus* and nasal bots. Has a long residual effect on *H. contortus*.

close command to exit from a dialog box, a window or an application.

close-coupled a characteristic of conformation, used usually to refer to a horse, meaning that the body is short and compact with no weakness in the loin; the costal arch to stifle distance is short and the flank region well muscled.

close junction one of the complex structural alterations between adjacent cells. In contradistinction from tight junction the two cells are separated by 20 nm of intercellular space; composed of hexagonal subunits, the connexons.

close-up dry cow see dry COW.

closed-circle anesthesia see circle breathing CIRCUIT.

closed nucleus breeding schemes genetic programs in which no genetic material is introduced to the breeding population.

closeout, closure the finalization of a feeding program in a feedlot. The cattle are sold and a balance sheet is struck which includes the costs of feeding and housing or confining them.

closing volume the volume of gas in the lungs in excess of the residual volume (RV) at the time when small airways in the dependent portions of the lungs close during maximal exhalation; abbreviated CV. CV normally increases with age and is also increased in obstructive airways disease. It can be used to detect the disease in high-risk patients before clinical signs appear. The closing capacity (CC) is equal to CV plus RV.

clostridia members of the genus *Clostridium*.

enterotoxic c. produce enterotoxins. See also ENTEROTOXEMIA.

histotoxic c. are invasive and cause extensive destruction of muscle and connective tissue and are characterized by the formation of gas. Include *C. chauvoei*, *C. colinum*, *C. hemolyticum*, *C. novyi*, *C. perfringens* type A and C, *C. septicum* and *C. sordellii*.

neurotoxic c. produce neurotoxins. Include *C. botulinum*, *C. tetani*.

clostridial pertaining to or emanating from infection by *Clostridium* spp.

c. dermatomyositis see MALIGNANT edema.

c. enteritis see ENTEROTOXEMIA.

c. food poisoning diarrhea in humans caused by ingestion of preformed toxin produced by *C. perfringens* type A.

c. gangrenous dermatitis see BLUE WING DISEASE.

c. gas gangrene see histotoxic CLOSTRIDIA.

c. hemoglobinuria see BACILLARY hemoglobinuria.

c. intestinal hemorrhage syndrome of dogs see canine hemorrhagic GASTROENTERITIS.

c. myositis see BLACKLEG.

c. necrotic enteritis caused in birds by *Clostridium perfingens* types A and C. Characterized by short course with severe depression, diarrhea and high mortality and necropsy findings of pseudomembranous enteritis.

c. swelled head see ovine BIGHEAD.

c. ulcerative enteritis a disease of quail caused by *Clostridium colinum*. Characterized in young quail by acute hemorrhagic enteritis and very high case fatality and morbidity rates. Necrosis and ulceration of the intestinal wall occur in birds which survive for several days.

clostridiosis any disease caused by *Clostridium* spp.

intestinal c. see INTESTINAL clostridiosis.

Clostridium a genus of anaerobic spore-forming bacteria of the family Bacillaceae. Most are gram-positive rods.

C. bifermentans, C. sordelli see MALIGNANT edema.

C. botulinum see BOTULISM.

C. butyricum involved in the spoilage of meat.

C. cadaveris may be associated with colitis X in horses.

C. chauvoei formerly called *C. feseri*. See BLACKLEG.

C. colinum cause of ulcerative ENTERITIS and liver necrosis in quail, turkeys, grouse, partridge and chickens. Not an accredited species.

C. difficile see antibiotic-associated COLITIS.

C. feseri now called *C. chauvoei* (above).

C. haemolyticum formerly called *C. novyi* type D. See BACILLARY hemoglobinuria.

C. histolyticum a species found in feces, soil and sometimes wound infections. An important cause of meat spoilage.

C. nigrificans a thermophilic spoiler of canned meat producing hydrogen sulfide gas and causing purple staining of the inside of the can. Now called *Desulfotomaculum nigrificans*.

C. novyi see INFECTIOUS necrotic hepatitis. See also *C. haemolyticum* (above). Previously called *C. oedematiens*. type A causes MALIGNANT edema in cattle and sheep, and big head in rams, type B causes INFECTIOUS necrotic hepatitis (black disease), and type C has been associated with osteomyelitis in buffalo.

C. overgrowth see BACTERIAL overgrowth.

C. parabotulinum a proteolytic subgroup of *C. botulinum*; not a valid species.

C. perfringens cause of ENTEROTOXEMIA. Type A causes MALIGNANT edema, type B causes dysentery in lambs and enterotoxemia, type C causes struck in sheep and necrotic enteritis in piglets, type D causes enterotoxemia and type E causes necrotic enteritis.

C. putrefaciens causes deep bone taint in hams. See also *C. putrificum* (below).

C. putrificum a cause of bone taint in cured hams. There is no detectable abnormality on the surface of the ham.

C. septicum formerly called *C. septique*. See MALIGNANT edema, BRAXY.

C. sordelli cause of a small proportion of cases of gas gangrene in ruminants.

C. spiroforme associated with enteritis and enterocolitis in rabbits, guinea pigs and foals.

C. sporogenes an apathogenic clostridium often found in lesions of gas gangrene.

C. tetani a common inhabitant of soil and human and horse intestines, and the cause of TETANUS in humans and domestic animals.

C. villosum found in fight abscesses and pleurisy in cats.

C. welchii see *C. perfringens* (above).

clostridium pl. *clostridia* [Gr.] any individual of the genus *Clostridium.*

closure usually refers to suturing of a surgical incision.

clot 1. a semisolidified mass, as of blood or lymph. 2. to form such a mass.

dilute whole blood c. retraction test an indirect measure of fibrinolytic activity. Whole blood is diluted with saline, chilled, then warmed. The time for clot retraction, and later clot lysis, is measured.

c. formation a complex interaction, part of the phenomenon of blood clotting. The process is irreversible but the clot may be dissolved naturally.

c. lysis the time required for a clot to lyse at 98.6°F (37°C) is a reflection of the plasmin content of the blood. Clot retraction and fibrinogen content of the blood sample are also influential.

c. retraction the drawing away of a blood clot from a vessel wall, a function of thrombasthenin, released by blood platelets.

c. retraction test a test for platelet numbers and function. Clotted whole blood should retract away from the sides of a glass tube in 1 to 2 hours.

cloth chewing a vice, usually of cats and Siamese in particular. Believed to be an abnormal extension of sucking behavior. See also WOOL sucking.

cloth of gold *Baileya multiradiata.*

clothing artificial covering for protection or decoration or as a livery.

animal c. includes rugs for cattle and horses and for Sharlea sheep in sheds. For dogs there is a great variety of decorative clothing limited only by the imagination of the owner. Pleasure horses are also likely to have a wardrobe of rugs including a lightweight cooling-off rug and a waterproof mackintosh, a hood to cover the head and neck, a cap to cover the head only, hoof boots of various sorts, protective leg bandages, a tail sock and eye goggles.

protective c. for the veterinarian; this includes coveralls, rubber knee boots, rubber or plastic sleeves and gloves, obstetric gowns, surgical gowns, caps, masks and overshoes.

clotrimazole a synthetic imidazole derivative with antifungal activity, similar to ketoconazole; applied topically in the treatment of diseases caused by dermatophytes and yeasts.

clotting the formation of a jellylike substance over the ends or within the walls of a blood vessel, with resultant stoppage of the blood flow. Clotting is one of the natural defense mechanisms of the body when injury occurs. A clot will usually form within 5 minutes after a blood vessel wall has been damaged. The clotting mechanism is triggered by the platelets, which disintegrate as they pass over rough places in the injured surface. As they disintegrate they release serotonin and thromboplastin. Serotonin causes constriction of the blood vessels and reduction of local blood pressure. Thromboplastin unites with calcium ions and other substances which promote the formation of fibrin. When examined under a microscope, a clot consists of a mesh of fine threads of fibrin in which are embedded erythrocytes and leukocytes, small amounts of fluid (serum), and platelets.

c. defects see COAGULOPATHY.

c. factors a series of plasma proteins which are related through a complex cascade of enzyme-catalyzed reactions involving the sequential cleavage of large protein molecules to produce peptides, each of which converts an inactive zymogen precursor (factor II) into an active enzyme (Iia) leading to the formation of a fibrin clot. They are designated by Roman numerals, and an additional 'a' to indicate the activated state. They are: factor I (FIBRINOGEN), factor II (PROTHROMBIN), factor III (tissue THROMBOPLASTIN), factor IV (CALCIUM), factor V (proaccelerin), factor VI (no longer considered active in hemostasis), factor VII (PROCONVERTIN), factor VIII (ANTIHEMOPHILIC factor), factor IX (plasma THROMBOPLASTIN component; Christmas factor), factor X (STUART FACTOR), factor XI (plasma THROMBOPLASTIN antecedent), factor XII (HAGEMAN FACTOR), factor XIII (fibrin stabilizing FACTOR).

c. time the time required for blood to clot in a glass tube; a measure of the intrinsic system of coagulation. In the Lee–White method, blood in test tubes is maintained at a constant temperature and examined regularly until clotting occurs; the test can be also be performed in capillary tubes. Called also coagulation time. Less sensitive and now less often used than the activated COAGULATION time.

tissue c. factor clotting factor III; tissue THROMBOPLASTIN.

cloudburst a problem in doe goats. Pseudopregnancy is terminated by the sudden evacuation of a large volume of fluid from the uterus. Abdominal distension subsides and the doe begins an indifferent lactation.

clouded leopard see clouded LEOPARD.

cloudy swelling see cloudy SWELLING.

clove hitch see MILLER'S SUTURE TIE.

clover members of plant family Fabaceae; essential legume component of improved and irrigated pastures, and highly adapted to haymaking. Some annuals, e.g. sweet clover, are used as forage crops. They provide a large bulk of fiber and energy and a high content of protein and calcium. They play a part in preventing hypomagnesemia in cattle on pasture. Common varieties, including species and cultivars, are: *Trifolium hybridum* (alsike), *T. repens* (ladino), *T. pratense* (red), *T. fragiferum* (strawberry), *T. subterraneum* (subterranean), *Melilotus alba* (sweet), *T. repens* (white).

c. disease see ESTROGENISM.

c. poisoning clovers can cause poisoning in a number of ways. They are important in their contribution to the occurrence of ruminal tympany, of urolithiasis, and chronic copper poisoning. Individual poisonous plant species are sweet clover which contains dicoumarol, alsike clover which is reputed to be hepatoxic, and white clover, ladino, red and particularly subterranean clovers which contain estrogenic substances.

c. stone see clover UROLITHS.

c. tree GOODIA *lotifolia.*

Cloward technique a subtotal laminectomy for the treatment of vertebral body malformations and spinal cord trauma causing compression of the cervical spinal cord in the horse.

cloxacillin a semisynthetic penicillin, resistant to β-lactamase and active against gram-positive bacteria.

club colony so-called sulfur granules in lesions of actinomycosis and botryomycosis which consist of central colonies of *Actinomyces bovis* or *Staphylococcus* *aureus* surrounded by club-shaped structures of reactive protein.

clubbed down a condition in chickens suffering from a nutritional deficiency of riboflavin: the erupting feathers do not rupture the feather sheaths properly, causing the feathers to have a coiled structure.

clubbing and necrosis syndrome disease of unknown etiology affecting the gills of Atlantic salmon.

clubfoot see DACTYLOMEGALY.

Clumber spaniel a heavy, powerfully built dog with long body, short legs and very large head. The coat is flat, silky and white with small lemon-colored markings mainly around the head.

clumping the aggregation of particles, such as bacteria or other cells, into irregular masses.

Clun Forest sheep English shortwool, meat sheep with brown face and legs.

cluneal pertaining to the buttocks.

clunis pl. *clunes* [L.] buttock.

cluster 1. in epidemiological terms a naturally occurring group of similar units, e.g. animals which resemble each other, with respect to one or more variables, more than animals in different groups do, or a group of cases of a single disease in time or space. 2. assembly of claw and teat cups, as part of a milking machine.

c. analysis 1. statistical methods used to group variables or observations into strongly interrelated subgroups. 2. a statistical analysis of the relationships between clusters in time and/or space.

c. fly see POLLENIA *rudis*.

c. sampling see cluster SAMPLING.

clustered dock RUMEX *conglomeratus*.

clustering the gathering together of disease events. The clustering may be in space, geographical clustering, or in time, temporal clustering. See also CLUSTER.

clutch 1. the number of eggs laid by a hen on consecutive days in an uninterrupted series. Clutch lengths vary from 2 to 6 days but may be as many as 360. 2. a setting of eggs. 3. a group of chickens hatched by a hen from a setting of eggs.

Clydesdale Scottish medium to heavy draft horse, bay, brown or black in color, usually with white on the face and limbs, about 16.2 hands high. Very well behaved and showy because of eager action, white points and long leg feather.

clysis the administration other than orally of any of several solutions to replace lost body fluid, supply nutriment, or raise blood pressure; also, the solution so administered.

clyster an enema.

Cm chemical symbol, *curium*.

cM centimorgan.

cm centimeter.

cm^2 square centimeter.

cm^3 cubic centimeter.

cmH_2O centimeters of water.

CMI cell-mediated immunity.

CML cell-mediated lympholysis.

CMM cervical malformation and malarticulation.

c.mm. cubic millimeter.

CMP cytidine monophosphate.

CMT California mastitis test.

CMV cytomegalovirus.

cnemial pertaining to the shin.

Cnemidocoptes a genus of the family Sarcoptidae of mites. Called also *Knemidocoptes*.

C. jamaicensis causes scaly leg in a Jamaican wild bird.

C. laevis gallinae causes depluming itch of fowl, pheasants and geese.

C. laevis laevis causes depluming scabies in pigeons.

C. mutans causes scaly leg in fowls and turkeys.

C. pilae causes scaly leg and a crumbly, honeycomb-like mass at the cere of the budgerigar or parakeet, called scaly face.

cnemidocoptic mange a series of diseases of birds including scaly leg of poultry (*Cnemidocoptes mutans*), depluming itch of poultry (*C. gallinae*) and scaly face and tassel foot of cage birds (*C. pilae*).

Cnephia small black flies which cause intense livestock worry. Called also black fly. Includes *Cnephia pecuarum*.

Cnidaria a phylum of lowly animals including hydroids and hydromedusae (class Hydrozoa), true jellyfish and free-swimming medusae (class Scyphozoa) and sea anemones, sea pens and corals (class Anthozoa). Previously called Coelenterata and that name is still widely used.

cnidia see NEMATOCYSTS.

CNS central nervous system.

Co chemical symbol, *cobalt*.

co-dominance where both alleles of a pair are fully expressed in the heterozygote; called also incomplete dominance.

co-dominant gene action see CO-DOMINANCE.

CO_2 see CARBON DIOXIDE.

CO_2 content see CARBON DIOXIDE content.

CO_2 pistol a weapon for firing darts containing immobilizing agents at animals. Powered by compressed CO_2 and effective only at very short ranges—ranges at which cordite powered projectiles would cause trauma.

CoA coenzyme A.

COAD chronic obstructive airways disease. See CHRONIC obstructive pulmonary disease.

coadaptation the mutual, correlated, adaptive changes in two interdependent organs.

coagglutination the aggregation of particulate antigens combined with agglutinins of more than one specificity.

coagglutinin partial agglutinin.

coagulability the state of being capable of forming or of being formed into clots.

coagulant promoting, accelerating, or making possible coagulation of blood; also, an agent that so acts.

coagulase an antigenic substance of bacterial origin, produced chiefly by staphylococci, which may be causally related to thrombus formation.

c. test enzymatic conversion of fibrinogen in rabbit plasma to fibrin is used as a means of identifying pathogenic species of staphylococci. The test may be carried out rapidly on a slide or in several hours or overnight in a tube. Most coagulase-positive staphyloccoci are pathogenic; coagulase-negative ones commonly are not.

coagulate 1. to cause to clot. 2. to become clotted.

coagulation 1. formation of a clot. 2. in surgery, the disruption of tissue by physical means to form an amorphous residuum, as in electrocoagulation and photocoagulation.

activated c. time (ACT) a test of the intrinsic or common pathway of coagulation, using diatomaceous earth as an activating agent to hasten coagulation of whole blood, the time being measured. More sensitive than Lee–White or capillary tube tests. See also CLOTTING time.

c. cascade the sequence of enzymatic reactions leading to the formation of a blood clot. Each is initiated by the preceding and, in turn, produces the enzyme that catalyzes the next with an amplification of the process as it progresses.

cerebrospinal c. normal CSF does not coagulate. Inflammation of the meninges or contamination of the fluid by blood, possibly during collection, can cause coagulation in a sample.

c. defects see COAGULOPATHY.

disseminated intravascular c. (DIC) widespread formation of thromboses in the microcirculation, mainly within the capillaries. It is a secondary complication of a wide variety of disorders all of which activate in some way the intrinsic coagulation sequence. Paradoxically, the intravascular clotting ultimately produces hemorrhage because of rapid consumption of fibrinogen, platelets, prothrombin, and clotting factors V, VIII and X. Because of this pathology, DIC is sometimes called defibrination syndrome or consumption coagulopathy. Called also diffuse intravascular coagulation.

c. factors see CLOTTING factors. PLATELET factors also play a role in coagulation. They are designated by Arabic numerals from 1 to 4.

c. inhibitors these systems prevent widescale intravascular coagulation as a result of minor injury. The important systems are C_1-INACTIVATOR, antithrombin III, ALPHA$_1$-ANTITRYPSIN, (ALPHA)$_2$-MACROGLOBULIN, factor XIa inhibitor, LIPOPROTEIN factor Xa inhibitor.

c. necrosis see COAGULATIVE NECROSIS.

c. pathways the coagulation cascade can follow alternative routes depending on the initiating factor. The *extrinsic* pathway is initiated by tissue thromboplastin (factor III) and involves calcium ions and factor VII. In the *intrinsic* pathway, factors XII, XI, IX and VIII are activated by exposure to subendothelial collagen or foreign surfaces. Both pathways lead to the activation of factor X and proceed along the *common* pathway, involving factors V, II, I and XIII, to the formation of a fibrin clot.

c. proteins see CLOTTING factors.

synovial c. normal synovial fluid does not clot, but gels on standing (thixotropism). It contains no fibrinogen, nor any of the coagulation factors. Clotting is an indication of damage to the synovial membrane.

c. tests are used to determine the integrity of the coagulation pathways, and platelet function. In general, the common tests for the intrinsic or common pathways are the activated partial thromboplastin time (APTT) and activated coagulation time (ACT). One-stage prothrombin time (OSPT) is usually used to evaluate the extrinsic or common pathways, and platelet count, clot retraction, bleeding time and activated coagulation time reflect platelet numbers and function.

c. time see CLOTTING time.

coagulative necrosis necrotic tissue which is firm, retains its architectural pattern and is dense in comparison to surrounding tissue. See also liquefactive NECROSIS, Zenker's NECROSIS.

coagulopathy any disorder of blood coagulation. See also HEMOPHILIA.

consumption c. a bleeding tendency due to a reduction in clotting factors caused by their utilization. See also disseminated intravascular COAGULATION.

disseminated intravascular c. (DIC) see disseminated intravascular COAGULATION.

hepatic c. impaired synthesis of most clotting factors, including factors I, II, V, VII, IX and X, as well as other substances involved in the fibrinolytic system, in severe liver disease can cause significant abnormalities in coagulation.

coagulum pl. *coagula* [L.] a clot.

coal dust causes black discoloration in lungs and bronchial lymph nodes in animals living in urban areas where coal is used for energy. Called anthracosis.

coal gas a cause of poisoning where coal gas is still used because of its carbon monoxide content. Other heating gases are less poisonous and produce carbon monoxide only if they are burned in an inadequate oxygen supply. See also CARBON MONOXIDE.

coal oil bush see TETRADYMIA GLABRATA.

coal tar a by-product obtained in destructive distillation of bituminous coal or wood; useful for its keratolytic, keratoplastic and antiseborrheic effects in ointments and shampoos for the treatment of skin disease.

coal tar creosote see CREOSOTE.

coal tar pitch a cause of severe hepatic necrosis in pigs that nibble at pitch-coated pens and floors. The syndrome includes anemia, jaundice and emaciation.

coalescence a fusion or blending of parts.

coapt to approximate, as the edges of a wound.

coaptation having been coapted.

external c. for fractures by the use of external appliances, e.g. various splints, and casts.

coarctate 1. to press close together; contract. 2. pressed close together; restrained.

coarctation stricture or narrowing.

c. of aorta a localized malformation characterized by deformity of the tunica media of the aorta, causing narrowing, usually severe, of the lumen of the vessel. See also AORTIC coarctation.

reversed c. pulseless disease.

coast disease a combination of copper and cobalt nutritional deficiencies. See COPPER, COBALT.

coast myall ACACIA *glaucescens*.

coastal fever see EAST COAST FEVER.

coat 1. haircoat—the overall coating of hair on all our species of domestic animals. 2. a membrane or other tissue covering or lining an organ; in anatomic nomenclature called also tunica.

c. licking excessive self-grooming in farm animals, commonly a manifestation of nutritional deficiency, e.g. salt deficiency.

coat color the overall or main color of the animal. If the points are distinctively colored that is also noted, e.g. black with white points.

cat c. c. besides the conventional black, white, gray, orange, there are BLUE, LILAC, SEAL (2), CHOCOLATE, TORTOISESHELL (tortie), BICOLOR, CHINCHILLA CAT, SMOKE, CAMEO, pewter.

dog c. c. besides the conventional black, brown, white, gray, there are BADGER (1), BELTON, BLANKET, BLUE, BRINDLE, DEADGRASS, DAPPLE, GRIZZLE, HARLEQUIN, MERLE, ROAN, LIVER (2), PIED, SABLE (1), SADDLE (2), TICKING, TRICOLOR, WHEATEN.

horse c. c. see BAY, CHESTNUT, CREMELLO, BROWN, BLACK, GRAY, PALOMINO, CREAM (3), DUN, PIEBALD, SKEWBALD, ROAN.

coated pits regions of the cell membrane which are coated with bristle-like structures on their cytoplasmic surface and are involved in endocytosis. The coated pit is pinched off to form a coated vesicle, which is involved in intracellular vesicle transport between the cell's organelles.

coati Central and South American, long-snouted members of the Procyonidae, a family which also contains raccoons and kinkajous. Includes *Nasua rufa* (ring-tailed coati) and *N. narica* (coatimundi).

coatimundi a raccoon-like (procyonid) animal with a long, upright tail and long snout. It can climb easily and eats birds, lizards and insects. Called also coati, *Nasua nasua*.

coaxial circuit see coaxial CIRCUIT.

cob 1. a short-legged, thickset, strong type of horse, usually 13.2 to 14.2 hands high but not more than 15.2. Useful as a light cart horse or for riding as a means of transportation and for heavyweight riders wanting a steady rather than a flashy ride. Produced by mating polo pony stallions to carriage or light draft horses. 2. the central stem of a cob of CORN (3); common as a cause of esophageal and intestinal obstruction in dogs. 3. male swan.

cobalamin, cobalamine a cobalt-containing complex common to all members of the vitamin B_{12} group.

cobalt a chemical element, atomic number 27, atomic weight 58.933, symbol Co. A component of vitamin B_{12}. See Table 6.

c.-57 a radioisotope of cobalt having a half-life of 270 days; used as a label for cyanocobalamin. Symbol ^{57}Co.

c.-60 a radioisotope of cobalt having a half-life of 5.27 years and a principal gamma ray energy of 1.33 MeV; used as a radiation therapy source. Symbol ^{60}Co.

c. nutritional deficiency causes anorexia and poor weight gain. Identification of the disease is based on chemical analysis of pasture and soil and biochemical analysis of animal tissues and fluids. Called also enzootic marasmus, Grand Traverse disease and other regional names.

c. poisoning accidental overdosing with cobalt causes listlessness, weight loss and incoordination.

cobblerfish a venomous fish. See GYMNOPISTES MARMORATUS. Called also South Australian cobbler.

Cobboldia a genus of parasitic flies whose maggots inhabit the alimentary tract or tissues of mammalian hosts; members of the family Gasterophilidae. Includes *Cobboldia elephantis* (Indian elephant), *C. loxodontis* (African elephant, rhinoceros).

cobby in conformation, a short and sturdy build; said of horses, dogs and cats.

COBOL a computer language generally used in commercial applications; acronym for Common Business Oriented Language.

cobra a venomous snake of the family Elapidae. Called also *Naja* spp.

c. venom a component, cobra venom factor, causes depletion of complement and is used experimentally to reproduce genetic complement deficiencies. Pharmaceutical preparations have been used intralesionally in ACRAL lick dermatitis to cause a local hypalgesia.

cobweb spiders members of the dipneumonomorph spiders in the family Theridiidae. Includes the redback or black widow spider.

coca see COCAINE.

cocaine an alkaloid obtained from the leaves of various species of *Erythroxylon* (coca plants) or produced synthetically; used as an indirect-acting sympathomimetic and as a short-acting topical anesthetic for surgery of mucous membranes. Called also coca. Almost entirely replaced by synthetic analgesics because of the problems that arise through human addiction to cocaine. It is a controlled substance of the highest priority in most countries.

cocarcinogen an agent that increases the effect of a carcinogen by direct concurrent local effect on the tissue.

cocarcinogenesis the development, according to one theory, of cancer only in preconditioned cells as a result of conditions favorable to its growth.

cocci [L.] plural of *coccus*.

Coccidia a group of sporozoa in the family Eimeriidae commonly parasitic in epithelial cells of the intestinal tract, but also found in the liver and other organs; it includes three genera, EIMERIA, ISOSPORA and CYSTOISOSPORA.

coccidia plural of coccidium.

coccidial of, pertaining to, or caused by Coccidia.

coccidian 1. pertaining to Coccidia. 2. any member of the Coccidia; coccidium.

coccidioidal pertaining to or emanating from COCCIDIOIDES.

c. granuloma the lesions of the generalized disease, COCCIDIOIDOMYCOSIS, are granulomas, occurring mostly in the lung, but also bone and skin.

Coccidioides a genus of pathogenic fungi.

C. immitis the etiological agent of COCCIDIOIDOMYCOSIS. A common infection in desert rats whose feces act as the vehicle for spread of the infection.

coccidioidin a sterile preparation containing by-products of growth products of *Coccidioides immitis*, injected intradermally as a test for coccidioidomycosis.

coccidioidoma residual pulmonary granuloma or granulomas seen radiographically as solid round foci in coccidioidomycosis.

coccidioidomycosis a fungal disease of humans and animals caused by infection with *Coccidioides immitis*. This fungus grows in hot, dry areas, especially in the southwestern USA, Mexico, and parts of Central and South America. It is characterized by granulomatous lesions, especially in the respiratory system and bones, which resemble tuberculosis in cattle and caseous lymphadenitis in sheep. In dogs, the predominant lesions are in bone, lungs and skin. In endemic areas, many people and animals experience asymptomatic or mild, undiagnosed respiratory infection. Dissemination is more common in some races of humans and in dogs, Boxers and Doberman pinschers. Called also San Joaquin Valley fever, valley fever, desert fever.

coccidioidosis coccidioidomycosis.

coccidiomycosis coccidioidomycosis.

coccidiosis infection by coccidia causes enteritis in all species. The clinical picture varies between species. In calves it is a serious diarrhea and dysentery and death may occur because of the blood and protein loss and the dehydration. In sheep the effects are poor production and poor weight gain, although diarrhea and dysentery may occur. The clinical disease is rare in pigs and horses but outbreaks, similar clinically to those in cattle, may occur in young animals. In dogs and cats, infection is most common in young puppies and kittens where it can be the cause of severe diarrhea and even death. Adults usually experience only mild and self-limiting infections. All poultry species suffer severe outbreaks of the disease characterized by diarrhea and dysentery. Subclinical infections causing reduced productivity are a feature of the disease in birds. Affected fish are cachectic and trail long mucoid fecal casts.

The disease in all species except fish is caused by EIMERIA, ISOSPORA or CYSTOISOSPORA. In fish the species involved is *Eimeria* (*Epieimeria*), *Goussia*, *Cryptosporidium* spp.

nervous c. a small number of calves in an outbreak of classical coccidiosis may develop severe nervous signs including hyperesthesia, nystagmus, tremor, orthotonus and convulsions and die within a few hours. There is no detectable lesion in the brain.

coccidiostatic drugs drugs which control coccidiosis. The greatest importance of coccidiosis is in the chicken industry and many agents have been developed in an attempt to reduce losses. The important drugs or groups of drugs for this purpose are CLOPIDOL, QUINOLONES, MONENSIN, LASALOCID, SALINOMYCIN, ROBENIDINE, AMPROLIUM, DINITOLMIDE, NICARBAZIN, SULFONAMIDES and HALOFUGINONE.

coccidiostats see COCCIDIOSTATIC DRUGS.

Coccidium see EIMERIA, ISOSPORA, SARCOCYSTIS, TOXOPLASMA, HAMMONDIA, BESNOITIA, CRYPTOSPORIDIUM.

coccobacilliform bodies bacterial units with the physical characteristics of coccobacilli often associated with cultures of mycoplasma.

coccobacillus an oval bacterial cell intermediate between the coccus and bacillus forms.

coccoid resembling a coccus.

coccus pl. *cocci* [L.] a spherical bacterium, usually slightly less than 1 μm in diameter, belonging to the Micrococcaceae family. It is one of the three basic forms of bacteria, the other two being bacillus (rod-shaped) and spirillum (spiral-shaped). Almost all of the pathogenic cocci are either staphylococci, which occur in clusters, or streptococci, which occur in short or long chains. Both staphylococci and streptococci are gram-positive and do not form spores.

coccyge- prefix meaning coccyx or tail.

coccygeal pertaining to or located in the region of the tail.

c. muscle see Table 13.2.

c. vertebrae called also caudal vertebrae; see Table 10.

coccygectomy excision of the tail.

coccygeus pertaining to the tail.

c. muscle forms part of the pelvic diaphragm; important in the cause and surgical repair of perineal hernia in dogs.

coccygodynia pain in the tail.

coccygotomy incision of the tail.

coccyx collection of fused coccygeal vertebrae found in humans and apes.

Cochin heavy Asiatic breed of poultry; black, white or buff; yellow beak and legs, heavy leg feathers. Weighs up to 13 lb. Called also Cochin-China.

Cochin-China see COCHIN.

cochle- prefix meaning cochlea.

cochlea a spiral tube forming part of the inner ear, shaped like a snail shell, which is the essential organ of hearing.

The cochlea is filled with fluid and is connected with the middle ear by two membrane-covered openings, the oval window (fenestra vestibuli) and the round window (fenestra cochleae). Inside the cochlea is the organ of Corti, a structure of highly specialized cells that translate sound vibrations into nerve impulses. The cells of this organ have tiny hairlike strands (cilia) that protrude into the fluid of the cochlea.

Sound vibrations are relayed from the tympanic membrane (eardrum) by the ear ossicles in the middle ear to the oval window of the cochlea, where they set up corresponding vibrations in the fluid of the cochlea. These vibrations move the cilia of the organ of Corti, which then sends nerve impulses to the brain. Called also osseus cochlea. See also HEARING.

tibial c. articular surface of the distal extremity of the tibia.

cochlear pertaining to or emanating from the cochlea.

c. duct the coiled portion of the membranous labyrinth located inside the cochlea; contains endolymph.

c. nerve see Table 14.

Cochlearia armoracia see ARMORACIA RUSTICANS.

cochleariform spoon-shaped.

cochleitis inflammation of the cochlea.

cochleosaccular pertaining to the cochlear duct and saccule.

c. degeneration degeneration of the membranous cochlea including the organ of Corti, the saccular macula, and the walls of the cochlear and saccular membranous labyrinth, and degeneration of the neurons in the spiral ganglion. The defect is inherited as deafness associated with incomplete pigmentation of the haircoat and the ocular uvea and occurs in cats, dogs and probably cattle. See also WAARDENBURG'S SYNDROME.

cochleotopic relating to the organization of the auditory pathways and auditory area of the brain.

cochleovestibular pertaining to the cochlea and vestibule of the ear.

Cochliomyia a genus of the fly family of insects Calliphoridae. See CALLITROGA. Includes *C. hominivorax*, *C. macellaria*.

Cochlosoma a protozoan parasite of the family Cochlosomatidae.

C. anatis found in the large intestine of domestic and wild ducks and turkeys. May cause a catarrhal enteritis and diarrhea.

cock male bird.

c. fighting contests, usually with wagering riding on them, between adult male birds of fighting stock; frowned on in most developed countries because the fights are to the death.

cock-throttled heavy-jowled giving the head a heavy appearance.

Cockapoo a non-recognized dog breed, popular in the USA, produced by crossing a Cocker spaniel and a Poodle.

cockatiel small, canary-sized Australian parrot, crested and brown with a yellow head. Popular as cage pets because of their speed in learning to converse with humans and engaging personalities. Called also quarrian, *Nymphicus hollandicus*.

cockatoo a group of birds in the family Psittacidae, characterized by a topknot of erectile feathers. Includes the *Kakatoe* and *Microglossus* genera. There are many species with different colors.

c. beak and feather disease see PSITTACINE beak and feather disease.

Cocker spaniel a small to medium-sized dog with long hair, particularly under the body and from behind the legs, a short, docked tail, and low set, long ears. There are two varieties, usually regarded as distinct breeds: The *English Cocker spaniel* is larger and taller (15 to 16 inches), and a longer muzzle, somewhat like that of a setter. The *American Cocker spaniel* is smaller (14 to 15 inches tall), has a short muzzle, large, prominent eyes and profuse coat. The breeds are, among other things, affected by an inherited renal cortical dysplasia, seborrhea, glaucoma, progressive retinal atrophy, cataracts, neuronal ceroid lipofuscinosis, hemophilia A, factor X deficiency, patent ductus arteriosus and intervertebral disk disease.

cockerel young male domestic fowl, older than 4 weeks, up to sexual maturity at about 5 months.

cockle 1. a dermatitis of sheep consisting of inflammatory nodules, especially on the neck and shoulders. The cause is thought to be parasitic. 2. see AGROSTEMMA.

cockleburr see XANTHIUM.
cockles SAPONARIA *officinalis*.
cockroaches insects which may carry *Salmonella* spp. in their gut and play a part in the spread of the disease.
cock's comb AMARANTHUS *hybridus*.
cock's weed AMARANTHUS *deflexus*.
cocksfoot see DACTYLIS GLOMERATA.
cockspur thistle CENTAUREA *melitensis*.
cocoa a cooking ingredient derived from CACAO.
coconut fruit of the coconut palm.
c. meal residue after the extraction of coconut oil and used as a protein supplement in livestock diets.
c. oil a natural source of fatty acids of short and medium length.
cod scrotum and contents.
c. fat a mass of fat around the inguinal part of the cord; reaches its greatest development in castrated ruminants.
c. lock wool from the scrotum; usually heavily stained with yolk.
cod liver oil an oil pressed from the fresh liver of the cod and purified. It is one of the best-known natural sources of vitamin D, and a rich source of vitamin A. Because cod liver oil is more easily absorbed than other oils, it was formerly widely used as a nutrient and tonic, but it is rarely used today since more efficient sources are available.

The oil has a fishy odor, especially in pork, when the animals are fed on cheap grades of the oil before slaughter. The fat is most tainted and is discolored brown.

The oil gives its name to a form of aspiration or lipid pneumonia caused by overzealous and inefficient oral dosing of cats with the oil.

c. l. o. poisoning premixed animal feeds in which cod liver oil has been incorporated are damaged if they are exposed to air. The oil rancidifies and the oxidation destroys the vitamin E in the feed. Cod liver oil also contains a muscle damage agent. Excessive supplementation in young puppies and kittens can also lead to hypervitaminosis A and D.
code 1. a set of rules governing one's conduct. Called also ethical code. 2. a system by which information can be communicated. 3. a set of alphabetical or numerical markers which are an index to a much larger bank of information. 4. in the computer medium refers to hidden markers which govern how documents will appear on the screen and in print; called also tag.
c. of ethics see code of ETHICS.
genetic c. the arrangement of nucleotides in the polynucleotide chain of a chromosome that governs the transmission of genetic information to proteins, i.e. determines the sequence of amino acids in the polypeptide chain making up each protein synthesized by the cell. See also GENETIC code.
object c. a computer term; the code of a program in machine language, i.e. a series of 0's and 1's.
operation c. a computer term; the part of a computer program which determines which function to perform, e.g. add, subtract.
c. of practice/conduct a document produced by an authoritative body to provide a guide to people in their conduct relative to, for example, animal welfare, or their practice, for example, in the housing and feeding of pigs. It is the sort of document that is used when testing in a practical situation rules which are planned to be included in subsequent legislation.
source c. a computer term; a computer program is written in a computer language, e.g. BASIC, using a code of source symbols which are understood by the programmer. The object code is generated from the source code by a COMPILER OR INTERPRETER.
codeine an alkaloid obtained from opium or prepared from morphine by methylation; used as the phosphate or sulfate salt for analgesia and as an antitussive.
Codex Alimentarius a document entitled 'Recommended International Codes of Hygienic Practice for Fresh Meat, for Ante-Mortem and Post-Mortem Inspection of Slaughter Animals and for Processed Meat Products' published by FAO/WHO in 1976.
coding strand one of the two strands of DNA that is transcribed. Called also sense strand.
Codiostomum a genus of the nematode family of Strongylidae.
C. struthionis strongylid nematode found in the large intestine of the ostrich. Heavy infestations are likely to be dangerous.
Codman's spur see CODMAN'S TRIANGLE.
Codman's triangle a localized, triangular ridge of new bone formed where periosteum is elevated. Associated with neoplasms, particularly osteosarcoma and osteomyelitis lesions. Called also Codman's spur.
codocyte target cell.
codon a triplet in a chain of nucleic acids in mRNA that specifies the order in which amino acids are added. The codon triplet pairs with a sequence of three complementary nucleotides, called the anticodon, present in the anticodon arm of tRNA. Called also triplet. See also DEOXYRIBONUCLEIC ACID.
start c. see INITIATION codon.
stop c's three codons, UAG, UAA and UGA, also referred to as amber, ochre and opal codons, in mRNA which terminate translation.
termination c. see stop codons (above).
coefficient 1. an expression of the change or effect produced by the variation in certain factors, or of the ratio between two different quantities. 2. in chemistry, a number or figure put before a chemical formula to indicate how many times the formula is to be multiplied.
absorption c. 1. the fraction of a beam of radiation that is absorbed in passing through a unit length of absorbing material. 2. a number indicating the volume of a gas absorbed by a unit volume of a liquid at 32°F (0°C) and at a pressure of 760 mmHg.
alienation c. a measure of the *lack* of association between two variables. Called also the coefficient of nondetermination.
Bunsen c. see absorption coefficient (2) (above).
contingency c. a measure of association between qualitative assessments of two variables.
correlation c. a measure of association which indicates the degree to which two or more sets of observations fit a linear relationship. Denoted by 'r', it can vary from −1.0 to 1.0.
determination c. the coefficient of determination is the square of the correlation coefficient (r^2). It describes the proportion of the variation of one of the correlated variables, explainable by the variation of the other variable. The value of the coefficient must lie between 0 and 1.
digestibility c. percentage of the food ingested that is absorbed.
disarray c. the measure of the degree of discord between two variables.
friction c. the effect that the material in a surface has on the frictional force created by the application of a

force to the surface: S = f × N, where S = friction, f = friction coefficient, N = reaction to the vertical application of a given force. In a normal joint the f value is very small (0.008).

c. of nondetermination see alienation COEFFICIENT.

-coele word element; for words beginning thus see words beginning *-cele*. [Gr.] *cavity, space*.

Coelenterata a phylum of invertebrates including the hydras, jellyfish, sea anemones and corals. The most modern nomenclature is CNIDARIA.

coelenterate 1. pertaining or belonging to Coelenterata. 2. an individual member of the phylum Coelenterata.

coelenteron the digestive cavity of coelenterates. Has a single opening into which all food is taken and through which all waste products are ejected.

coeli(o)- word element. See CELIO-.

coelo- for words beginning thus, see words beginning *celo-*.

Coelogenys see PACA.

Coelosphaerium genus of toxic cyanobacteria in water bloom; causes sudden death, hepatitis.

coelozoic inhabiting the intestinal canal of the body; said of parasites.

coenurosis infection with the intermediate stage of *Taenia multiceps* which invades the brain and spinal cord of sheep and causes a variety of syndromes characteristic of slowly developing space-occupying lesions of the nervous system. Ataxia, head-pressing, somnolence and occasional convulsions are common signs of brain involvement. Paralysis and recumbency are the usual signs in spinal cord involvement. Called also gid, sturdy.

Coenurus a metacestode, a larval stage (metacestode) of a tapeworm belonging to the genus *Taenia* (*Multiceps*).

C. cerebralis metacestode of *Taenia multiceps* found in the brain and spinal cord of sheep, but in other organs of goats. See also COENUROSIS.

C. serialis metacestode of the tapeworm *Taenia serialis* of dogs and foxes found in the subcutaneous tissues and muscles of the intermediate host, a lagomorph.

coenzyme an organic molecule, usually containing phosphorus and some vitamins, often separable from the enzyme protein but essential as a cosubstrate in catalysis; a coenzyme and an apoenzyme must unite in order to function (as a holoenzyme).

c. A essential for carbohydrate and fat metabolism; among its constituents are pantothenic acid and a terminal SH group, which forms thioester linkages with various acids, e.g. acetic acid (acetyl-CoA) and fatty acids (acyl-CoA); abbreviated CoA.

c. A acetoacetyl see ACETOACETYL COA.

c. A acetyl see ACETYL COA.

c. Q any of a group of related quinones with isoprenoid units in the side chains (the ubiquinones), occurring in the lipid fraction of mitochondria and serving, along with the cytochromes, as an intermediate in electron transport; they are similar in structure to vitamin K_1.

c. R see BIOTIN.

coerulein a decapeptide; a potent stimulator of pancreatic and other exocrine secretions.

cofactor an element or principle, e.g. a coenzyme, with which another must unite in order to function.

ristocetin c. see RISTOCETIN cofactor.

COFAL test the complement fixation test for avian LEUKOSIS.

coffee bean see SESBANIA.

coffee bush see BREYNIA OBLONGIFOLIA.

coffee grounds a term used to describe vomited blood. See HEMATEMESIS.

coffee senna see CASSIA *occidentalis*.

coffee tree GYMNOCLADUS *dioica*.

coffee weed *Sesbania* spp.; called also coffee bean, rattlebrush.

coffin pertaining to the coffin bone.

c. bone distal phalanx in the horse.

c. joint distal interphalangeal joint, between the second and third phalanx, in the horse.

cog-wheel respiration jerky auscultation sounds, with a clicking sound on inspiration; due to swelling of the bronchial mucosa.

cogener see CONGENER.

cogenic genetic differences between individuals at a locus.

Coggins test the agar-gel, double diffusion immunodiffusion test for detection of antibodies to EQUINE infectious anemia virus.

cognate cooperation cooperation between T and B lymphocytes when both recognize epitopes on the same antigen.

cohesion the force causing various particles to unite.

cohesive end single-strand extension on each end of a duplex DNA molecule that is usually produced by restriction endonuclease digestion and which facilitates ligation of two similarly cut DNA molecules. Called also sticky ends.

Cohnheim's theory 1. the emigration of leukocytes is the essential feature of inflammation. 2. tumors develop from embryonic rests which do not participate in the formation of normal surrounding tissue.

Coho salmon ONCORHYNCHUS *kisutch*.

cohort in epidemiology a group of individuals who share a characteristic acquired at the same time. The term usually refers to a birth cohort, which contains animals born in a specified time period.

c. studies a prospective or follow-up, analytical, epidemiological study. The investigation identifies a group of animals which have the hypothesized cause and which are free of the disease of interest, and a comparison group of animals which are free of the hypothesized cause. Both groups, the cohorts, are followed over time to determine the incidence rates of the disease in question in each of the two groups.

coil a winding structure or spiral; called also helix.

coin test an auscultatory test for pulmonary consolidation in which a coin is used as a pleximeter. A sound is produced by striking the coin with a hard object such as a screwdiver used as a plexor. The coin is placed over the area to be examined. If the lung below is consolidated the sound produced by striking the coin is transmitted with greater clarity than if it were filled with air. Obviously designed for the farmyard veterinarian. The companion animal specialist will use a proper plexor hammer and diascope.

coital exanthema see infectious pustular VULVOVAGINITIS. Called also coital vesicular exanthema.

bovine c. vesicular exanthema see infectious pustular VULVOVAGINITIS.

equine c. e. venereal disease of the skin of the genitalia and perineum in stallions and mares caused by equine herpesvirus 3. Characterized by discomfort and discharge locally and the presence of vesicopustular lesions on the penis, prepuce, vulva and vaginal mucosa, and sometimes on the mare's teats and the lips of the foal at foot.

coital vesicular exanthema see infectious pustular VULVOVAGINITIS. Called also coital exanthema.

coition coitus.

coitus sexual union by vagina between male and female. See also MATING.

Coix lachryma-jobi a robust, tropical grass with shiny grains like tears. Grown as a fodder crop. Called also adlay, Job's tears.

Coke's hartebeest *Alcelaphus caama.*

col a slight depression in the underlying interdental papilla where two teeth contact each other.

colation the process of straining or filtration, or the product of such a process.

Colbred a crossbred meat sheep produced by crossing the European East Friesland breed with three British breeds, Border Leicester, Dorset Horn and Clun Forest. The characteristics of the breed are a high twinning rate and a high milk yield.

colcemid a compound related in structure and function to COLCHICINE.

colchiceine one of the two poisonous alkaloids in COLCHICUM AUTUMNALE. See also COLCHICINE.

colchicine a water-soluble antimitotic drug that blocks the addition of tubulin subunits to the ends of existing microtubules, preventing spindle formation. It is a poisonous alkaloid from COLCHICUM AUTUMNALE which causes violent purgation, abdominal pain and is often fatal. In research it is used to induce polyploidy by delaying mitosis. In humans it is used in the treatment of gout. See also COLCHICEINE.

Colchicum autumnale toxic plant in the family Liliaceae; a cultivated plant that does survive also in the wild. Causes severe, often fatal, enteritis, characterized by diarrhea and abdominal pain. It contains two poisonous alkaloids, colchicine and colchiceine. Called also meadow saffron, saffron, autumn crocus.

COLD chronic obstructive lung disease. See CHRONIC obstructive pulmonary disease (COPD).

cold 1. an acute disease of the upper respiratory tract characterized by cough, sneezing, running at the eyes and nose and mild fever, similar to the common cold of humans, occurring in captive primates. 2. a relatively low temperature; the lack of heat. A total absence of heat is absolute zero, at which all molecular motion ceases. See also HYPOTHERMIA.

c. acclimation short-term adjustments to carbohydrate and fat metabolism in response to exposure to low environmental temperatures.

c. acclimatization heat production is not increased, but heat loss is reduced by changes in haircoat and vascular supply to the skin.

c. applications the primary effect of cold on the surface of the body is constriction of the blood vessels. Cold also causes contraction of the involuntary muscles of the skin. These actions result in a reduced blood supply to the skin and produce a marked pallor. If cold is prolonged there may be damage to the tissues because of the decreased blood supply.

The secondary effects of cold are the opposite of its primary action. There is increased cell activity, dilatation of the blood vessels, and increased sensitivity of the nerve endings.

c. barn see cold housing (below).

c. cow syndrome see SHOCK.

c.-enrichment a procedure that promotes growth of some bacteria during laboratory isolation. Suspensions of specimens are held at refrigerator temperatures for extended periods before being cultured. Recommended for recovery of *Listeria monocytogenes* from neural listeriosis and *Yersinia* spp.

c. exposure see HYPOTHERMIA.

c. hemagglutinin disease see cold AGGLUTININ disease.

c. housing thin-walled, uninsulated barns with no central heating.

c. injury includes HYPOTHERMIA and FROSTBITE.

c.-nosed refers to a hound which is able to follow a cold (very old) scent.

c. receptors receptors in the skin which are sensitive to low temperatures.

c. rooms walk-in refrigerator; temperature used varies with material stored, e.g. meat needs 32°F to 45°F (0°C to 7°C), offal needs less than 28°F (−2°C).

c.-shoeing fitting a horseshoe without heating it in a forge and shaping it exactly to the foot. See also SHOEING.

c. shortening shrinkage of meat when temperature is excessively low in early stages of chilling.

c. steel surgery that using unheated cutting instruments; the normal surgical procedure in contrast to electrosurgery or cryosurgery.

c. storage for meat to be stored for more than 72 hours the chilling temperature should be between 30°F and 23°F (−1 and 5°C) and the humidity less than 90%.

c. store taint cut lean surfaces of chilled meat are covered with a brown slime and have a sour smell caused by growth of the bacteria *Achromobacter* spp.

c. stress occurs at temperatures less than 50°F (10°C), varying with chill factor, wetness, protection from wind.

c. therapy see CRYOSURGERY, therapeutic HYPOTHERMIA.

c. water hemolytic anemia see cold ANEMIA.

cold-blooded poikilothermic.

cold-insoluble globulin see FIBRONECTIN.

coldblood horses with no Arab blood in their ancestry; generally the draft breeds, Clydesdale, Shire, Percheron, Rhenish, Black Forest, Schleswig, South German.

coldwater disease a disease of fish kept in temperate water; caused by the bacteria *Cytophaga psychrophila* when the tank water temperature is maintained at too low a level. Called also peduncle disease. See also RAINBOW TROUT fry syndrome.

cole BRASSICA *napa* subsp. *campestris.*

Cole endotracheal tube see Cole-pattern ENDOTRACHEAL tube.

Cole infant tube a very small diameter uncuffed endotracheal tube suitable for use in a small animal.

colectomy excision of the colon or of a portion of it.

Coleoptera an order in the class Insecta—the beetles.

Coleosporium solidagensis toxic fungal rust occurs on *Solidago* spp. (goldenrod).

Colesiota conjunctivae a rickettsia, cause of ovine contagious OPHTHALMIA. They appear as purplish-red, small ovoid or short rod-shaped organisms in the cytoplasm of conjunctival cells harvested by scraping and stained with Giemsa.

colibacillary enterotoxemia see COLIBACILLOSIS.

colibacillemia the presence of *Escherichia coli* in the blood.

colibacillosis infection with *Escherichia coli*; takes many forms, some of them septicemic, some toxemic due to absorption of the enterotoxin and some locally toxigenic. See also COLIFORM mastitis, MASTITIS–METRITIS–AGALACTIA of sows, neonatal colibacillosis (below), COLIFORM gastroenteritis of weaned pigs, EDEMA disease, CEREBROSPINAL angiopathy, COLIGRANULOMA.

enteric c. the form of colibacillosis characterized by varying degrees of diarrhea. It occurs in all species, especially in the very young less than one week old. In pigs it occurs also immediately after weaning.

Specific serotypes, distinct from those that cause septicemia, cause this enteric form of the disease. The cardinal sign is diarrhea, varying from pasty to profuse and watery, foul smelling and pale in color. Most affected calves continue to feed and recover spontaneously in a few days. The others become anorexic, dehydrated and weak and die in 3 to 5 days. In newborn pigs the disease is much more serious and the majority of piglets die. In weaned pigs the situation is the same with many pigs dying quickly before other signs become evident. The critical clinical sign is a profuse diarrhea with death due to dehydration and electrolyte losses. The enteric form of the disease is uncommon in foals and lambs where the septicemic form prevails.

enterotoxemic c. toxin produced by a specific serotype is absorbed from the gut and exerts its toxicity on remote tissues. See also EDEMA disease. Called also enterotoxic colibacillosis.

neonatal c. a highly fatal form of colibacillosis which can occur in the young of all species during the first 48 hours of life. A high prevalence is usually associated with a low intake of colostrum and colostral antibodies and the presence of pathogenic serotypes. The disease may take the form of a septicemia or a profound endotoxemia or be limited to the gut lumen and cause severe diarrhea.

post-weaning c. post-weaning COLIFORM gastroenteritis.

septicemic c. invasion of the systemic circulation, with the probability of infection of all tissues, with *Escherichia coli.* The source of infection may be mastitis, metritis, cystitis, omphalophlebitis or enteritis. Characterized clinically by toxic shock, cardiovascular collapse, hypothermia, coma, a short course and a high mortality rate. Survivors may develop disease due to localization in joints, meninges, etc. Commonest in foals, calves and piglets.

colibacilluria the presence of *Escherichia coli* in the urine.

colibacillus see ESCHERICHIA coli.

Colibri forceps corneal forceps with very narrow blades and fine points which may be straight or angled. The blades may meet or overlap.

colic 1. pertaining to the colon. 2. a syndrome caused by severe paroxysmal pain due to disease of an abdominal organ. Usually due to alimentary tract disease, and rarely to infection or calculus in the urinary tract involving the renal pelvis, ureter, bladder or urethra.

bovine c. is characterized mainly by recurrent bouts of downwards arching of the back, restless walking, looking at the flank, lying down, rolling, and getting up again. Colic is evident for a few hours only and is followed by spontaneous recovery in most cases. These cases are probably caused by intestinal spasm.

The next most common cause is intestinal obstruction by PHYTOBEZOAR, VOLVULUS, STRANGULATION (2), or INTUSSUSCEPTION. In these the colic disappears but no feces are passed for some days. Rectal examination reveals scant, pasty gray or blood-stained feces, and possibly the presence of distended loops of intestine. Enterotomy or enterectomy is essential for survival. Rare cases also occur due to renal infarction or to ureteric obstruction.

colon impaction c. impaction of the colon on a diet high in tough fiber is common in horses and pigs. There is mild abdominal pain and hard fecal masses are passed. See also MECONIUM ileus, impaction colic (below).

equine c. most cases are due to intestinal disease. Characteristic signs are bouts of pain marked by pawing, looking at the flank, lying down and getting up restlessly, rolling; the gut sounds are either absent or excessive. Mild cases recover spontaneously or after medical treatment for gut spasm or impaction with dry feed. Life-threatened cases have shock, circulatory collapse and usually positive findings on abdominal paracentesis. Surgery is often obligatory. Acute colic is also an important part of the syndrome in acute enteritis and colitis in which diarrhea is a paramount sign. Peritonitis is usually manifested as subacute colic.

flatulent c. of horses is due to gas accumulation in the large intestine when grazing on lush pasture. There is severe pain, obvious distension of the abdomen, and the rectum is obstructed by distended loops of bowel. Sporadic cases occur as a result of partial obstruction of the intestine by fibrous adhesions. Trocarization through the flank or rectum is often necessary. Called also tympanitic colic. Previously called intestinal meteorismus.

gastric dilatation c. of horses due to gastric dilatation is a severe acute disease due to gorging on hay or grain, especially immediately after racing, or due to lipoma causing strangulation at the pylorus. Regurgitation through the nostrils or the discharge of large quantities of fluid gastric contents through a nasal tube is a frequent sign. Death is common as a result of gastric rupture.

impaction c. in horses is due to dry or indigestible feed, or bad teeth, or in foals by the retention of meconium. Subacute pain bouts occur at long intervals and over several days; death in untreated cases is due to exhaustion. Effective treatment is large oral doses of mineral oil (paraffin) administered by nasal tube. See also colon impaction colic (above).

intestinal obstruction c. in horses is caused by intestinal obstruction consisting mostly of acute life-threatening cases due to intussusception, strangulation or volvulus, usually affecting the small intestine, although sometimes it is the cecum or colon. Typical signs are shock, absence of gut sounds, very severe pain, short course, positive findings of blood-stained fluid on paracentesis, distended loops of gut on rectal examination and death due to shock and dehydration unless the blockage is relieved by surgery.

Less severe cases are caused by impaction of the ileocecal valve by undigested fine fiber or grain, by sand accumulation, obstruction by phytobezoars, enteroliths or linear foreign bodies, usually in the small colon. See also under ENTEROLITH, PHYTOBEZOAR, linear FOREIGN BODY, VOLVULUS, INTUSSUSCEPTION, STRANGULATION.

lead c. colic due to lead poisoning.

recurrent c. equine colic that recurs at intervals of weeks or months. Due usually to repeated dietary indiscretions or to a persisting defect, e.g. bad teeth, verminous aneurysm.

renal c. intermittent and acute pain usually resulting from the presence of one or more calculi in the kidney or ureter.

sand c. is caused by the ingestion of soil or sand and can be an acute syndrome due to ileocecal valve impaction or chronic mild pain with diarrhea for a period of months.

spasmodic c. this form of colic in horses is often due to excitement. Bouts of sharp pain are accompanied by loud, frequent gut sounds, and spontaneous recovery is usual within an hour. Occasional cases develop volvulus during bouts of rolling.

thromboembolic c. is caused by infarction of a section of gut wall or by stimulation by migrating strongyle larvae and may appear as intermittent spasmodic colic or subacute colic for a number of days followed by development of peritonitis. See also STRONGYLOSIS.

tympanitic c. see flatulent COLIC.

colicky pertaining to or affected by colic.

colicoplegia combined colic and paralysis in humans produced by lead poisoning.

coliform pertaining to fermentative gram-negative enteric bacilli, sometimes restricted to those fermenting lactose, i.e. *Escherichia*, *Klebsiella*, *Enterobacter* and *Citrobacter*. A wider range is also used and includes *Pseudomonas aeruginosa*, *Pasteurella* spp., and *Aerobacter aerogenes*.

avian c. septicemia a disease of chickens, ducklings and young turkeys causing heavy mortality. Characterized at autopsy by fibrinous exudates on the surface of all viscera and *E. coli* in all organs.

c. gastroenteritis a disease of recently weaned pigs characterized by sudden death or severe diarrhea and caused by pathogenic serotypes of *E. coli*. The pigs often die of dehydration and toxemia. Those that survive have lost a lot of condition. Called also post-weaning diarrhea.

c. mastitis peracute bovine mastitis caused by *E. coli* and characterized by minor enlargement and inflammation of the udder, thin serous milk containing small flakes. There is profound shock, the mortality rate is high and the quarter is lost. See also MASTITIS–METRITIS–AGALACTIA of sows.

c. pyometra the more severe form of pyometra in bitches and queens, characterized by severe toxemia and a fetid, viscous, red-brown uterine exudate.

c. septicemia see septicemic COLIBACILLOSIS.

c. septicemia, ducks manifested by moist granular to curd-like exudate in the pericardial sac, pleural and peritoneal cavities and air sacs.

coligranuloma a disease of birds caused by *Escherichia coli* and characterized by granulomas in the intestinal wall, liver and lungs. Called also Hjärre's disease.

Colinus virginianus see QUAIL.

coliplication coloplication.

colipuncture colocentesis.

colisepsis infection with *Escherichia coli*.

colisepticemia septicemia due to *Escherichia coli*.

colistimethate an antibiotic prepared from COLISTIN.

colistin a polymyxin antibiotic, active against gram-negative organisms and used in the treatment of urinary tract infections. Called also polymyxin E.

colitides plural of *colitis;* inflammatory disorders of the colon considered collectively.

colitis pl. *colitides;* inflammation of the colon. There are many types of colitis, each having different etiologies. The differential diagnosis involves the clinical history, fecal examinations, proctoscopy, radiological studies such as barium enemas, and sometimes biopsy.

antibiotic-associated c. colitis associated with antimicrobial therapy occurs in humans and animals. It can range from mild nonspecific colitis and diarrhea to severe fulminant pseudomembranous colitis (see below) with profuse watery diarrhea. The inflammation may be caused by a toxin produced by *Clostridium difficile*, a microorganism that is not normally present in the resident bowel flora. Presumably, the disruption of the normal flora allows the growth of *C. difficile*.

ciliate c. colitis in primates caused by *Troglodytella* spp. and characterized by diarrhea.

c. cystica profunda dilated, grossly visible colonic glands protrude through the muscularis mucosae into the submucosa; no specific cause attributed; an incidental necropsy finding, especially in pigs.

eosinophilic ulcerative c. occurs in humans and dogs, either as a primary disease or as part of an eosinophilic gastroenteritis. Characterized histologically by eosinophilic infiltration of the lamina propria and submucosa. May be caused by hypersensitivity reactions, parasites or foreign body reactions.

granulomatous c. see histiocytic ulcerative colitis (below).

histiocytic ulcerative c. a chronic, debilitating inflammation of the colon occurring predominantly in young Boxer dogs. Affected dogs have a chronic hemorrhagic diarrhea with tenesmus, and occasionally vomiting, inappetence and weight loss. Colonic mucosa is thickened, friable and ulcerated. Macrophages containing PAS-positive granules are found in the mucosa and submucosa. The cause of this disease is unknown. It is similar, but not identical to, ulcerative colitis, granulomatous colitis and Whipple's disease of humans.

idiopathic c. a disease similar to histiocytic ulcerative colitis (above), occurring predominantly in dogs other than Boxers and lacking the PAS-positive granules in histiocytes.

mucous c. see irritable COLON syndrome.

plasmacytic–lymphocytic c. mucosal infiltration by plasmacytes and lymphocytes associated with sign of colitis in dogs. Dietary hypersensitivity is considered an important cause.

pseudomembranous c. a severe acute inflammation of the bowel mucosa, with the formation of pseudomembranous plaques. It is most commonly associated with antimicrobial therapy (see antibiotic-associated colitis (above)). Called also pseudomembranous enterocolitis.

psychologically induced c. see irritable COLON syndrome.

uremic c. an outstanding lesion in cattle dying of uremia.

c.-X a peracute colitis of horses, sometimes occurring as outbreaks, characterized by a short course of about 24 hours, profuse diarrhea, sometimes with colic and dysentery and profound dehydration. The cause is unknown and the outcome invariably fatal.

colitoxicosis toxemia caused by absorption of *Escherichia coli* toxin from the intestine; it affects newborn animals within the first week of life and pigs after weaning. Older animals are affected from other sites such as mammary gland or uterus. The common syndrome, especially in calves, is collapse with circulatory failure, hypothermia and death within about 6 hours. In weanling pigs the outstanding feature is edema of the eyelids and other sites. A high morbidity and mortality are usual in a group of pigs which also show incoordination, weakness and paralysis. The course of the disease is about 24 hours. See also MASTITIS–METRITIS–AGALACTIA, COLIFORM mastitis.

colitoxin a toxin from *Escherichia coli*.

coliuria the presence of *Escherichia coli* in the urine.

collagen a fibrous structural protein that constitutes the protein of the white fibers (collagenous fibers) of skin, tendon, bone cartilage and all other connective tissues. It also occurs dispersed in a gel to provide stiffening, as in the vitreous humor of the eye. It is made of monomers of tropocollagen.

Different types of collagen (types I, II, III, IV and V and others) occur in different locations and have differing chemical compositions and physical characteristics.

c. diseases a group of diseases having in common certain clinical and histological features that are manifestations of involvement of CONNECTIVE TISSUE, i.e. those tissues that provide the supportive framework (musculoskeletal structures) and protective covering (skin and mucous membranes and vessel linings) for the body.

The basic components of connective tissue are cells and extracellular protein fibers embedded in a matrix or ground substance of large carbohydrate molecules and carbohydrate–protein complexes called mucopolysaccharides.

For the sake of clarity and organization, collagen diseases may be divided into two major groups: (1) those that are genetically determined and are a result of structural and biochemical defects, and (2) those that are acquired and in which immmunological and inflammatory reactions are taking place within the tissues. Among the first group are those diseases caused by a lack of a specific enzyme necessary for proper storage and excretion of one or more mucopolysaccharides, such as Ehlers–Danlos syndrome. These disorders are distinguished by structural defects affecting the formation of collagen.

Acquired connective tissue diseases are believed to develop as a result of at least two causative factors: a genetic factor and an abnormal immunological response. Examples of collagen diseases that are most probably the result of an aberration of the immunological reactions that mitigate injury and inflammation of connective tissues are systemic lupus erythematosus, rheumatoid arthritis, polymyositis and dermatomyositis.

c. dysplasia see HEREDITARY collagen dysplasia.

c. fascicles interspersed with patches of cartilage in fibrous cartilage (fibrocartilage).

c. fibers the principal component of connective tissue, providing strength and resisting stretching; a structural protein in fiber form.

c. fibrils collagen fibers are composed of fibrils visible only by electron microscope.

c. footpad disorder footpads in young German shepherd dogs become soft, tender, depigmented and ulcerated. Some dogs later develop renal amyloidosis. The cause is unknown.

microcrystalline c. a surface hemostatic agent.

c. nevus see NEVUS.

c. sponge surgical sponge made of collagen; used to fill surgical space and to control hemorrhage. Is not absorbable but has enormous fluid absorption capacity and has excellent wet strength and is very pliable and easy to use.

c. suture an absorbable suture of natural material; made from bovine flexor tendon. May be plain or chromic.

collagenase an enzyme that catalyzes the degradation of collagen.

c. ulceration a rapidly spreading ulceration of the cornea triggered by the liberation of collagenase from necrotic cells.

collagenation the appearance of collagen in developing cartilage.

collagenic 1. producing collagen. 2. pertaining to collagen.

collagenitis inflammatory involvement of collagen fibers in the fibrous component of connective tissue.

collagenoblast a cell arising from a fibroblast and which, as it matures, is associated with collagen production; it may also form cartilage and bone by metaplasia.

collagenocyte a mature collagen-producing cell.

collagenogenic pertaining to or characterized by collagen production; forming collagen or collagen fibers. See also COLLAGENIC.

collagenolysis dissolution or digestion of collagen.

collagenosis see COLLAGEN diseases.

collagenous made of collagen.

c. nevus see NEVUS.

c. tissue composed of collagen, reticular and elastic fibers; may be loose or dense; the latter may be regular or irregular.

collapse 1. a state of extreme prostration and depression, with failure of circulation. 2. abnormal falling in of the walls of a part or organ.

circulatory c. SHOCK; circulatory insufficiency without congestive heart failure.

lung c. see ATELECTASIS.

collar a decoration or harness worn around the neck. The primary means of restraint for domestic dogs. Used in cats as ornaments or to carry identification. See also ELIZABETHAN COLLAR.

choke c. see CHOKE chain.

flea c. see FLEA collar.

c. galls friction sores caused by rubbing of a saddlery collar on a horse's shoulder.

horse c. part of draft, cart or buggy harness. Made of leather, stuffed and lined with felt, they are fitted to the neck of the horse. They carry the metal hames to which plow chains or leather traces are attached.

tube c. a rigid cylinder, usually fashioned from x-ray film, applied around the neck to prevent the animal or bird from turning around to traumatize parts of the body with their mouth or beak.

collared brown snake see DEMANSIA *nuchalis nuchalis*.

collared peccary TAYASSU *tajacu*.

collarette a small collar; see EPIDERMAL collarette, IRIS collarette.

collateral 1. secondary or accessory; not direct or immediate. 2. a side branch, as of a blood vessel or nerve. 3. security for a loan.

c. circulation see collateral VESSEL.

c. fissure a longitudinal fissure of the cerebral hemisphere between the fusiform and parahippocampal gyri. Called also collateral sulcus.

c. ligaments see LIGAMENT.

c. recruitment the utilization of many small arterial–capillary units in pulmonary tissue during exercise and increased cardiac output, for increased exchange of gases.

c. relationship where two individuals have a common ancestor.

c. sulcus see COLLATERAL fissure.

collected a term describing the balance of a horse and rider, or a horse alone, while moving; smooth coordination of all parts working in unison.

collecting duct system includes collecting tubules, both straight and arched, and papillary ducts.

c. tubule see collecting TUBULE.

collective noun a word used to indicate a group of things, e.g. animals as in gaggle of geese, pod of whales. See Table 20.

colliculectomy excision of the seminal colliculus.

colliculitis inflammation about the seminal colliculus.

colliculus pl. *colliculi;* a small elevation.

caudal c. see midbrain colliculus (below).

midbrain c. there are four colliculi in the tectum of the midbrain, two caudal (inferior) and two rostral (superior) containing the visual and auditory reflex centers. Called also corpora quadrigemina.

seminal c., c. seminalis a prominent portion of the male urethral crest, on either side of which, depending on the species, are the openings of the vasa deferens or ejaculatory ducts; called also verumontanum.

superior c. see midbrain colliculus (above).

Collie a large dog with a distinctive elongated, flat head and nose. There are two varieties, the rough-coated (longhaired) and the smooth-coated (shorthaired), which are regarded as separate breeds in the United Kingdom. In the more common rough Collie, a thick, long coat forms a ruff or mane around the neck and front of the chest. The breed originated in Scotland as shepherd's dog and the rough-coated variety is also called a Scotch collie. The breed suffers from inherited abnormalities in eye development, collectively called collie eye anomaly, inherited epilepsy, hemophilia A, patent ductus arteriosus, cerebellar degeneration and cyclic neutropenia. It is also predisposed to nasal solar dermatitis (so-called collie nose).

c. ectasia syndrome see collie eye anomaly (below).

c. eye anomaly an autosomal recessive inherited trait which results in incomplete closure of the embryonic fissure; seen almost exclusively in Collies, Border collies and Shetland sheepdogs. Associated defects include scleral ectasia, coloboma of the optic disk, retinal folds and detachment, and microphthalmia. Called also collie ectasia syndrome.

collie granuloma see NODULAR fasciitis.

miniature c. see SHETLAND SHEEPDOG.

c. nose a depigmenting, crusting dermatitis of the planum nasale, adjacent skin on the dorsum of the nose, and sometimes lip and eyelid margins. Occurs most commonly in sunny climates and in individual dogs with the greatest exposure to sunlight. Once believed to be a breed-specific disorder related to the long nose of collies, it is now known that several diseases produce similar clinical features and in many breeds. These include discoid and systemic LUPUS ERYTHEMATOSUS, PEMPHIGUS erythematosus and PEMPHIGUS foliaceus, as well as solar DERMATITIS.

collimation in microscopy, the process of making light rays parallel; the adjustment of two or more optical axes with respect to each other. In radiology, the restriction of the beam size to the area under investigation. This reduces the scattered radiation reaching the x-ray film and the exposure of attendants.

collimator a device, sometimes a diaphragm, or series of diaphragms, which control the direction and the dimensions of the x-ray beam.

collinearity very high correlation between variables.

colliquative characterized by excessive liquid discharge, or by liquefaction of tissue.

collisional interactions collisions which occur when an electronic target is bombarded with high energy electrons as in x-rays. The collisions result in heat loss.

collodiaphyseal pertaining to the neck and shaft of a long bone, especially the femur.

collodion a highly flammable syrupy liquid compounded of pyroxylin dissolved in ether and alcohol, which dries to a clear tenacious film; used as a topical protectant applied to the skin to close small wounds, abrasions and cuts, to hold surgical dressings in place, and to keep medications in contact with the skin.

flexible c. a mixture of collodion, camphor and castor oil; used topically as a protectant.

salicylic acid c. flexible collodion containing salicylic acid, used topically as a keratolytic.

colloid 1. gluelike. 2. the translucent, yellowish, gelatinous substance resulting from colloid degeneration. 3. a chemical system composed of a continuous medium (continuous phase) throughout which are distributed small particles, 1 to 1000 nm in size (disperse phase), which do not settle out under the influence of gravity. For example, if the disperse phase is a solid and the dispersing phase a liquid, the system is called a *sol*, such as glue. Milk is an example of an emulsion, in which both phases are liquid, one an oil and one water. Colloidal particles are not capable of passing through a semipermeable membrane, as in DIALYSIS. Solutes that can pass through a semipermeable membrane are sometimes called crystalloids.

stannous sulfur c. a sulfur colloid containing stannous ions formed by reacting sodium thiosulfate with hydrochloric acid, then adding stannous ions; a diagnostic aid in bone, liver and spleen imaging.

colloidal of the nature of a colloid.

c. bath a bath containing gelatin, bran, starch or similar substances, to relieve skin irritation and pruritus.

c. body a homogeneous, eosinophilic structure found in the lower epidermis and dermis in systemic or discoid lupus erythematosus and any other skin disease in which there is damage to the basal cells. They are formed from degenerated epidermal basal cells and contain immunoglobulin, complement, fibrin and glycoprotein. Called also Civatte body, hyaline body.

c. degeneration the assumption by the tissues of a gumlike or gelatinous character.

c. goiter see GOITER.

c. osmotic pressure largely the osmotic pressure exerted by plasma proteins; see also oncotic PRESSURE.

c. solution used in the management of shock to increase osmotic pressure and volume of plasma. Dextrans and plasma are examples.

colloidin a jelly-like principle produced in colloid degeneration.

colloquial disease name the name given to a disease in a particular district. The same disease may therefore have many names.

collum pl. *colla* [L.] the neck, or a necklike part such as the part just below the head of the humerus, penis, malleus, stapes or mandible. The collum of the omasum is its narrow fusion with the reticulum.

c. distortum torticollis.

c. valgum coxa valga.

collunarium a nosewash; a nasal douche.

collutorium a mouthwash. Called also collutory.

collutory see COLLUTORIUM.

collyria eyewash.

Collyriclum a trematode genus of the family Troglotrematidae. Includes *Collyriclum faba* (subcutaneous cysts in fowls, turkeys, wild birds).

collyrium an eyewash; a lotion for the eyes.

colobis see COLOBUS monkey.

colo- word element. [Gr.] *colon.*

coloboma an apparent absence or defect of some ocular tissue, usually due to failure of a part of the fetal fissure to close; it may affect the choroid, ciliary body, eyelid (palpebral coloboma, coloboma palpebrale), iris (coloboma iridis), lens (coloboma lentis), optic nerve or retina (coloboma retinae). Colobomas of the choroid are common in cattle, and have been observed in miniature swine. Colobomas of the optic disk are an inherited defect in several breeds of cattle.

atypical c. on occurring at a location other than the fetal fissure.
iris c. a full thickness defect in the iris. When it occurs at the base of the iris, it is called IRIDODIASTASIS.
optic nerve c. part of the scleral ectasia syndrome in dogs; also seen in Basenji dogs and Charolais cattle.
typical c. one occurring in or near to the fetal cleft.

colobomatous pertaining to or emanating from coloboma.

Colobus a leaf-eating monkey, 1.5 to 2.5 ft long, 15 to 18 lb, striking black and white coat color, white at birth.

Colocasia a genus of toxic plants in family Araceae. May cause cyanide poisoning, also oral irritation on ingestion because of presence of oxalate-rich raphide crystals. Includes *C. esculenta* (*C. antiquorum*). Called also taro, elephant ears.

colocecostomy cecocolostomy.

colocentesis surgical puncture of the colon.

Coloceras a genus of feather-eating lice of the family Philopteridae which infest pigeons and doves. Includes *Colocera damicorne* (pigeons).

coloclysis irrigation of the colon.

coloclyster an enema introduced into the colon through the rectum.

colocolostomy surgical formation of an anastomosis between two portions of the colon.

colocutaneous pertaining to the colon and skin, or communicating with the colon and the cutaneous surface of the body.

colocynth CITRULLUS *colocynthis*.

colocynthin plant toxin in *Citrullus* spp., causes diarrhea, enteritis.

Colocynthis vulgaris CITRULLUS *colocynthis*.

coloenteritis enterocolitis.

colofixation the fixation of the colon in cases of ptosis.

coloileal ileocolic.

colon the part of the large intestine extending from the cecum to the rectum. It has the same basic design in all species. There is an ascending colon which begins at the cecum, passes forward to the cranial part of the abdominal cavity then crosses to the left side as the transverse colon. It then turns caudally again to become the descending colon. In the caudal abdomen the colon curves to the midline and joins the rectum. See also COLONIC.

In herbivores and omnivores there is a variation on this general plan in that the ascending colon is greatly lengthened. In the ruminants and the pig this takes the form of a spiral colon of centrifugal and centripetal loops which occupies the right side of the abdomen. In the horse the ascending colon forms an uncoiled loop reflexed upon itself, beginning at the cecum as the right ventral colon, passing to the left ventral, to the left dorsal at the pelvic flexure, then to the right dorsal, then back into the standard pattern at the transverse colon. In the horse there is the additional oddity of a significant reduction in diameter at the small colon, the terminal part which joins the rectum.

ascending c. the first segment of the colon which is either a short, cranially directed segment, as in the dog, or greatly expanded to form the spiral colon in ruminants, or the great colon of horses (right ventral, sternal flexure, left ventral, pelvic flexure, left dorsal, diaphragmatic flexure, right dorsal colons).
coiled c. see spiral colon (below).
descending c. the third and last of the three main divisions of the colon which runs caudally and terminates in the rectum. It is not extensive in the horse, in which it has an unusually long mesentery and is known as the small colon.
floating c. small or descending colon in horses.
irritable c. syndrome stress and psychological factors can cause the frequent passage of soft to watery feces, often with mucus, in dogs. Called also mucous colitis, spastic colon, psychologically induced colitis, and irritable bowel. See also spasmodic COLIC.
large c. the ascending colon of the horse.
left c. displacement colic forward displacement of the left dorsal colon is an uncommon cause of moderate colic in the horse. Characteristic findings include a palpable medial displacement of the spleen and the absence of the pelvic flexure of the colon from its usual site in front of the pelvis. Surgical removal of the displaced colon from its entrapment across the top of the gastrosplenic ligament is the only effective treatment.
short c. see descending colon (above).
small c. see descending colon (above).
spiral c. ascending colon of ruminants.

colonic pertaining to or arising from the colon.
c. aganglionosis see colonic AGANGLIONOSIS.
c. atony see MEGACOLON.
c. atresia affected neonates appear normal at birth but develop abdominal distension quickly. No feces are passed and death occurs at about one week unless surgical repair is effected. The defect occurs sporadically in most species. In horses and cattle it can be inherited, but the cause is not determined in most cases.
c. bands see TENIA *coli*.
c. constriction due to contraction of peritoneal adhesions in horses; causes chronic or intermittent colic.
c. contraction permanent inability of colon to dilate due to congenital aganglionosis.
c. crypt straight tubular glands in the colonic mucosa.
c. entrapment see left colonic displacement (below).
c. foreign body foreign bodies, e.g. halter shanks, are found in the colon in horses, having passed the gastric sphincter and the ileocecal valve; quickly encrusted with salts.
c. impaction intractable constipation occurs in dogs and cats, primarily with obstruction by foreign material and secondarily when there is an obstruction to the normal passage of feces, including retention because of pain at defecation. See also colon impaction COLIC of horses.
c. infarction see thromboembolic COLIC.
c. ischemia deprivation of blood supply to all or part of the colon. See also INTESTINAL torsion, INTESTINAL strangulation, intestinal obstruction COLIC.
c. obstruction see colonic impaction (above), INTESTINAL obstruction.
right dorsal c. displacement displacement of the right dorsal colon in the horse to the area between the right body wall and the cecum, in an anterior direction so that the pelvic flexure comes to lie against the diaphragm.
c. rupture occurs, apparently spontaneously, in mares at foaling, death occurring soon afterwards.
c. torsion in horses, see under equine COLIC. In cattle, torsion of the coiled colon is an acute obstruction with coils of gas-distended colon visible in the right flank and palpable per rectum.

colonitis inflammation of the colon; colitis.

colonopathy any disease or disorder of the colon.

colonorrhagia hemorrhage from the colon.
colonorrhea mucous colitis.
colonoscope an elongated flexible fiberoptic endoscope which permits visual examination of the lining of the entire colon.
colonoscopy endoscopic examination of the colon, either transabdominally during laparotomy, or transanally by means of a colonoscope.
colony a discrete group of organisms, as a single cluster of bacteria in a culture that was produced from a single starting bacterium.
c.-forming units colonies of pluripotent stem cells located and quantified in the spleen. Colonies grown in vitro interact with erythropoietin to give rise to morphologically identifiable erythroid cells.
c.-stimulating factors cytokines produced by lymphocytes and mononuclear phagocytes which stimulate the growth and differentiation of hematopoietic cells. Includes granulocyte–macrophage colony-stimulating factor, monocyte–macrophage colony-stimulating factor and granulocyte colony-stimulating factor.
colony-inhibiting activity limits the proliferating activity of the colony-forming (granulocyte-monocyte series) units in erythropoiesis.
colopexy surgical fixation or suspension of the colon, usually to the dorsolateral abdominal wall to prevent recurring rectal prolapse.
coloplication the operation of taking a reef or fold in the colon. An inverting stitch, e.g. Lembert, will also plicate the colon. This could be used over a weakened wall which is still viable, e.g. needle decompression site.
coloproctectomy surgical removal of the colon and rectum.
coloproctitis inflammation of the colon and rectum; colorectitis.
coloproctostomy anastomosis of the colon to the rectum.
coloptosis caudal displacement of the colon.
colopuncture colocentesis.
color 1. a property of a surface or substance due to absorption of certain light rays and reflection of others within the range of wavelengths (roughly 370 to 760 nm) adequate to excite the retinal receptors. 2. radiant energy within the range of adequate chromatic stimuli of the retina, i.e. between the infrared and ultraviolet. 3. a sensory impression of one of the rainbow hues.
broken c. in decribing coat color, a solid color broken up by another color, usually white.
coat c. see COAT COLOR.
c. dilution reduction of the concentration of the color pigment in tissue; most important in hair and other fiber coats, in the skin and in the ocular iris.
c. dilution alopecia see color mutant ALOPECIA.
c. flow Doppler see DOPPLER ULTRASOUND.
c. pigments the pigments influencing skin color are melanin, melanoid, oxygenated hemoglobin, reduced hemoglobin, carotene.
c. radical see CHROMOPHORE.
c. vision the domestic animal species have limited color vision, the best perception being in bright light. Birds probably have the best, cattle and sheep the least, if any.
color dilution alopecia see color mutant ALOPECIA.
color-marking bulls bulls fitted with chin-ball marking harness for the detection of cows in estrus.
Colorado rubber tree HYMENOXYS *richardsonii*, Colorado rubberweed.
Colorado rubberweed HYMENOXYS *richardsonii*.
Colorado tick fever a disease of humans caused by *Coltivirus*, transmitted from small mammals by the tick, *Dermacentor andersoni*.
colorectal pertaining to or of the nature of the colon and the rectum.
c. polyp benign or malignant; most commonly occurs at the anorectal junction in middle-aged dogs, causing diarrhea, dyschezia and rectal bleeding.
colorectitis inflammation of the colon and rectum; coloproctitis.
colorectostomy see COLOPROCTOSTOMY.
colorectum the distal portion of the colon and the rectum, regarded as a unit.
colored wool an inherited defect in sheep; tan or white; may be general or local, the latter producing badger face and spotted sheep.
colorimeter an instrument for measuring color differences; especially one for measuring the color of the blood in order to determine the proportion of hemoglobin.
colorimetry the science of measuring color by defining it and estimating its intensity.
Colorpoint in cats, a light-colored body with darker pigmentation on the ears, face, legs and tail (points), as seen in Siamese cats from which this was genetically derived. It has been developed in shorthair and longhair varieties. The colors and patterns developed by selective breeding appear to be endless.
C. longhair see HIMALAYAN.
C. shorthair essentially a Siamese cat with colored points other than the classic seal, chocolate, blue and lilac. In North America these are regarded as a separate breed, the Colorpoint shorthair, but in Britain they are regarded as separate varieties of Siamese.
colorrhaphy suture of the colon.
colorsided said of cattle of any breed that have head, back and underline, tail and legs of one, or a mixture of other colors and sides that are differently marked and colored, e.g. Banteng, Telemark.
coloscope see COLONOSCOPE.
coloscopy see COLONOSCOPY.
colostomy an artificial opening (stoma) created in the large intestine and brought to the surface of the abdomen for the purpose of evacuating the bowels; also the opening (stoma) so created. Has been used successfully in the treatment of rectal tears in horses.
colostral supplement products such as an ultrafiltrate of whey containing significant quantities of immunoglobulins are available for oral use as colostral supplements.
colostrogenesis secretion of colostrum.
colostrometer a hydrometer calibrated to read the immunoglobulin concentration in a sample of colostrum.
colostrum the thick, yellow secretion present in the mammary gland in increasing amounts for several days or weeks, depending on the species, before and for about a week after parturition. It is very rich in maternal antibodies and is essential in providing passive immunity to the neonate. An adequate amount of colostrum must be ingested during the first few hours after birth while the intestinal epithelium is still permeable to the large molecules of the immunoglobulins.

Immunoglobulin levels in colostrum vary between species and are much higher than those found later in the milk. The predominant immunoglobulin in colostrum is IgG. Called also beestings.
c.-induced anemia occurs in lambs fed cow colostrum; thought to be an immune-mediated hemolytic anemia.

synthetic c. although referred to as colostrum, formulas can only attempt to duplicate milk of a particular species since they are lacking in immunoglobulins. See MILK replacer.
c. vacuoles eosinophilic colostrum present in vacuoles in cytoplasm of intestinal epithelial cells in newborn animals.

colotomy incision of the colon.

colovaginal pertaining to or communicating with the colon and vagina.

colovesical pertaining to or communicating with the colon and urinary bladder.

colpalgia pain in the vagina.

colpatresia atresia, or occlusion of the vagina.

colpectasia distension or dilation of the vagina.

colpectomy excision of the vagina.

colpeurysis operative dilatation of the vagina.

colpitis inflammation of the vaginal mucosa; vaginitis.

colp(o)- word element. [Gr.] *vagina*.

colpocele see vaginal HERNIA.

Colpocephalum a genus of lice of the family Menoponidae. Includes *Colpocephalum tausi* (turkey), *Colpocephalum turbinatum* (pigeons).

colpocleisis surgical closure of the vaginal canal.

colpocystitis inflammation of the vagina and bladder.

colpocystocele hernia of the bladder into the vagina.

colpocytogram a differential listing of the cells observed in smears from the vaginal mucosa.

colpocytology the quantitative and differential study of cells exfoliated from the epithelium of the vagina.

colpoperineoplasty plastic repair of the vagina and perineum.

colpoperineorrhaphy suture of the ruptured vagina and perineum.

colpopexy suture of a relaxed vagina to the abdominal wall.

colpoplasty plastic surgery involving the vagina.

colpoptosis prolapse of the vagina.

colporrhaphy 1. suture of the vagina. 2. the operation of denuding and suturing the vaginal wall to narrow the vagina.

colporrhexis laceration of the vagina.

colposcope a speculum for examining the vagina and cervix by means of a magnifying lens.

colpospasm vaginal spasm.

colpostenosis contraction or narrowing of the vagina.

colpostenotomy a cutting operation for stricture of the vagina.

colposuspension a surgical procedure used in the treatment of urinary incontinence caused by urethral sphincter mechanism incompetence in female dogs. The procedure aims to move an intrapelvic bladder neck to an intra-abdominal position. Called also vaginal advancement.

colpotomy incision of the vagina with entry into the cul-de-sac.

colpoxerosis abnormal dryness of the vulva and vagina.

colt a young entire male horse up to 4 years of age; may be qualified, e.g. yearling colt; used also as an adjective, e.g. colt foal.

Coltivirus a genus in the family *Reoviridae* with only one member virus that causes Colorado tick fever in humans.

Colubridae a family of snakes in the class Reptilia. There are two subfamilies, the Colubrinae, which are aglyphous and therefore nonvenomous, and the Boiginae, which are rear-fanged but poisonous.

Colubrinae see COLUBRIDAE.

Columba palumbus see WOOD-PIGEON.

Columbia sheep medium wool, mutton type of polled American sheep.

Columbia SK virus a picornavirus in the genus *Cardiovirus* which causes encephalomyocarditis in zoo animals.

Columbicola a genus of lice in the superfamily Ischnocera. Includes *Columbicola columbae* (pigeons).

columbiformes see PIGEON.

columbine see AQUILEGIA VULGARIS.

Columbus fancy an American breed of canaries, derived from several English varieties. A medium to large-sized bird with either a smooth or crested head.

Columbus grass SORGHUM *almum*.

columella pl. *columellae* [L.] a little column.
c. auris a connecting rod between the avian eardrum and the perilymph of the inner ear via the rod's footplate.

column an anatomical part in the form of a pillar-like structure; anything resembling a pillar.
anal c's longitudinal folds of mucous membrane at the cranial half of the anal canal; called also rectal columns.
c. of Bertin extensions of renal cortex between the renal pyramids.
c. chromatography see CHROMATOGRAPHY.
dorsal c. the dorsal portion of the gray substance of the spinal cord, in transverse section seen as a horn.
gray c. the longitudinally oriented parts of the spinal cord in which the nerve cell bodies are found, comprising the gray matter of the spinal cord.
lateral c. the lateral portion of the gray substance of the spinal cord, in transverse section seen as a horn; present only in the thoracic and anterior lumbar regions.
rectal c's anal columns.
spinal c. the rigid structure in the midline of the back, composed of the vertebrae. Called also vertebral column. See also SPINE.
ventral c. the ventral portion of the gray substance of the spinal cord, in transverse section seen as a horn.

columna pl. *columnae* [L.] column.

columnaris disease a common disease of aquarium fish caused by infection with the bacteria *Flexibacter columnaris* (*Cytophaga columnaris*). It is characterized by circumscribed gray-white lesions on the skin about the head, gills and fins and on the body. Called also saddlepatch disease.

colza *Brassica rapa* subsp. *campestris*.

coma a state of unconsciousness from which the patient cannot be aroused, even by powerful stimuli.
alpha c. coma in which there are electroencephalographic findings of dominant alpha-wave activity.
diabetic c. the coma of severe diabetic ACIDOSIS. See also DIABETES MELLITUS.
hepatic c. results from reversible biochemical abnormalities of the cerebrum, caused by elevated blood levels of toxic substances such as ammonia, amino acids, short-chain fatty acids and beta hydroxylated biogenic amines that accumulate in severe liver disease. See also hepatic ENCEPHALOPATHY.
irreversible c. coma in which for a period of 24 hours there is complete nonreceptivity and nonresponsivity even to the most intensely painful stimuli, no spontaneous movement or breathing, absence of elicitable reflexes, and a flat electroencephalogram. Called also brain death.
myxedema c. the mental stupor caused by severe hypothyroidism; seen most often in Doberman pinchers, it is associated with hypoventilation, hypothermia, hypotension and bradycardia. Death may occur.

Comandra pallida North American plant in the family Santalaceae; a facultative selenium converter plant; a selenocompound causes poisoning in livestock. Called also bastard toadflax.

comatose pertaining to or affected with coma.

comb 1. a vascular, red cutaneous structure attached in a sagittal plane to the dorsum of the skull of domestic fowl. It consists of a base attached to the skull, a central mass called the body, a backward projecting blade and upward projecting points. 2. part of mechanical sheep shears. 3. see CTENIDIUM.

buttercup c. has no blade and is divided sagittally. It is cup-shaped with points arranged around the cup.

cushion c. a low, small, oval, smooth body with no points.

nasal c. the red, vascular structure across the base of the beak in the turkey. Called also snood, frontal process.

pea c. has three blades with a row of points arising from each.

rose c. a low elongated comb from which many small points arise. There is a backward projecting spike in lieu of a blade.

Silkie c. similar to the V-comb but without points.

single c. has all of the components without variation; the standard comb.

strawberry c. a small, oval, flattened comb with a wrinkled surface.

V-c. two large, conical points diverge from a sizeable body. Usually accompanies a crest of feathers.

combinatorial library in immunology, the ligation of cDNAs of light and heavy chains of immunoglobulins, each in a separate bacteriophage vector.

combined immune deficiency syndrome (disease) an inherited defect of immunity, including lack of immunoglobulin synthesis, absence of cell-mediated immunity, thymic hypoplasia and a marked reduction in the number of thymic, splenic and blood lymphocytes, which occurs in foals of Arab breeding. It is inherited as an autosomal recessive trait. Clinically the foal is normal at birth but as the passive antibody acquired from the mare declines the foal succumbs to a succession of respiratory infections characterized by nasal discharge, cough, dyspnea and noisy breath sounds. The disease is inexorably progressive and fatal. Called also CID and PSCID for primary severe CID.

combined movements involuntary movements of the head and limbs in which the components of the movement always occur in the same sequence and with the same force.

combing wool see combing WOOL.

Combretum platypetalum African plant in the family Combretaceae; the seeds cause vomiting, incoordination and paralysis in the pig. The foliage is not poisonous. Called also red wings.

combustion rapid oxidation with emission of heat.

Comeback Australian breed of wool sheep, bred by crossing Merino with Corriedale, Polwarth or Zenith sheep; wool is 21 to 25 microns. It is a registered breed, but the term is more commonly used in the sense of a type of sheep produced by crossbreeding a crossbred Merino back to Merino.

comedo pl. *comedones;* a blackhead; a plug of keratin and sebum within the dilated orifice of a hair follicle frequently containing bacteria. Found in feline and canine ACNE, HYPERADRENOCORTICISM, Schnauzer comedo syndrome (see below).

Schnauzer c. syndrome a condition in which numerous comedones form in the skin over the back of certain predisposed Schnauzer dogs, usually of the miniature variety. The cause is unknown but believed to be an inherited disorder of keratinization.

comedomastitis mammary duct ectasia.

comes pl. *comites* [L.] an artery or vein accompanying another vessel or nerve.

comet-tail in ultrasonography, a type of reverberation artifact, caused by a number of small, highly reflective interfaces, such as gas bubbles.

comfrey see SYMPHYTUM.

command an instruction which starts or stops a computer program.

c. points in acupuncture are specific points on each meridian which correspond to each of the five phases and each of the five elements.

Commelina cyanea ubiquitous urban weed; suspected to cause allergic dermatitis in dogs. Called also wandering jew.

commensal 1. living on or within another organism, and deriving benefit without harming or benefiting the host individual. 2. a parasitic organism that causes no harm to the host.

commensalism symbiosis in which one population (or individual) is benefited and the other is neither benefited nor harmed.

commingle to mingle together, e.g. cattle mingling with deer.

comminuted broken or crushed into small pieces, as a comminuted fracture.

comminution the act of breaking, or condition of being broken, into small fragments.

commissure, commissura a site of union of corresponding parts, as the angle of the lips or eyelids; used also with specific reference to the sites of junction between adjacent cusps of the heart valves.

brain c. the bands of fibers connecting the parts of the two cerebral hemispheres. They include the CORPUS callosum, the largest commissure, a rostral commissure which is part of the paleopallium and the fornical commissure which is related to the archipallium, the caudal collicular commissure which connects the caudal colliculi (corpora quadrigemina). Called also cerebral commissure.

cerebral c. see brain commissure (above).

fornical c. interconnection between the right and left hippocampi. Called also fornical commissure.

habenular c. interconnection between the right and left habenular nuclei.

middle c. a band of gray matter joining the optic thalami; it develops as a secondary adhesion and may be absent.

posterior c. a large fiber bundle crossing from one side of the cerebrum to the other dorsal to where the aqueduct opens into the third ventricle.

spinal cord c. the gray and white commissures which connect the two sides of the spinal cord.

commissurorrhaphy suture of the components of a commissure, to lessen the size of the orifice.

commissurotomy surgical incision or digital disruption of the components of a commissure to increase the size of the orifice.

mitral c. the breaking apart of the adherent leaves (commissure) of the mitral valve.

common a shared structure, function, disease. See also under specific name of the item, e.g. atrioventricular CANAL.

c. chemical sense mediated by the trigeminal nerve from chemical sense organs in the conjunctival sac and in the nasal and buccal cavities.

c. fee the fee for professional services agreed to formally or informally by a local group of the veterinary profession, usually determined by an interpractice survey of fees actually charged.

c. law the law of common usage, the practice or code which is usually followed. Based on decisions of the courts in individual cases. It is not written down as statutory law is.

c. pathway see COAGULATION pathways.

c. salt see SODIUM chloride.

c. source a point from which a number of animals are infected or affected. The point from which a common source or point epidemic begins.

c. stonecrop see SEDUM ACRE.

c. sucker a fish. See CATOSTOMUS COMMERSONI.

common carp see CYPRINUS CARPIO.

Commonwealth Agriculture Bureaux an information gathering and disseminating service for all matters agricultural and veterinary; abbreviated CAB. Communicates by traditional print and paper and electronically through its database for on-line consultation and general dial-up information service available through DIALOG, CAN/OLE, ESA/IRS, DIMDI and other services. CD-ROMs containing literature abstracts in a wide range of disciplines are also available for purchase. Periodical publications of major interest to veterinarians are Veterinary Bulletin, Index Veterinarius, Nutritional Abstracts and Reviews, Breeding Abstracts, Dairy Science Abstracts.

commonwealth weed SENECIO *bipinnattisectus*.

communicability transmissibility; ability to spread from infected to susceptible hosts.

c. period the time during which the patient is infectious to others.

communication communication between animals depends on sight and hearing and, especially in dogs, on the sense of smell. The matters about which animals communicate include (1) for recognition between dam and newborn; (2) for mating; (3) for initiating aggression or welcome; (4) for signaling danger or safety. See also VOCALIZATION.

auditory c. communication by all kinds of vocalization.

chemical c. communication by smell, especially by pheromones.

visual c. besides size and color other modes of visual communication which are of great importance in animal life include stance, demeanor, behavior, and the synthesis of all of these in 'body language'.

community a group of individuals living in an area, having a common interest, or belonging to the same organization.

c. adoption curve graphic display of the rate at which persons in a community adopt new techniques and strategies.

compact cattle dwarf cattle.

compaction packing together as in twin births when both fetuses engage the pelvis at the same time, in prolonged constipation in dogs, and in compaction of endochondral bone as a part of normal bone modeling.

companion animal dogs, cats, pleasure horses, birds, mice, guinea pigs and more exotic species kept by humans for company, amusement, psychological support, extrovert display and all of the other functions that humans need to share with animals of other species; companions who will not take emotional or psychological advantage of the person and will, for the most part, stay faithful.

companionship the faculty possessed by most truly domesticated animals. They are social creatures and have a great need for the companionship of other animals. Animals in groups are quieter and more productive as a rule.

comparative a study based on the use of comparison.

c. economic analysis comparison of the performance of an enterprise such as a farm with the performance of a peer group of enterprises.

c. medicine the study of human disease by comparison with the diseases of animals, depending largely on work with naturally occurring diseases of animals that are models for human diseases. May be confined to specialty areas, such as dermatology or ophthalmology. The reverse attitude also applies but not in the same positive sense that humans can be used as experimental animals.

comparison the basis of analytical epidemiology, the statistical comparison between groups.

c. groups the groups between which a statistical comparison is to be made.

c. population the population in which a comparison between groups is to be conducted. All of the groups to be used comprise the population.

compartment a part of the body as a whole and divided from the rest by a physical partition.

fluid c. that liquid part of the body excluded by cell membranes. Includes intravascular and intercellular compartments.

c. syndrome muscles which are contained in an aponeurotic sheath may be subjected to serious ischemia as a result of increase in the size of the muscle as a result of vigorous muscular activity.

compartmental muscle compression syndrome see COMPARTMENT syndrome.

compatibility having the quality of being COMPATIBLE.

compatible capable of existing together without adverse reaction. 1. in therapeutics drugs that can be administered together without reacting together so as to destroy each other's effectiveness. 2. in computer work the capacity of a machine to accept and process data prepared by another computer's software without the need for a code modification or conversion of the data. Much of the difficulty in transferring files between computers has been overcome in recent times by the software producers.

compensation the counterbalancing of any defect of structure or function. 1. in cardiology, the maintenance of an adequate blood flow without distressing signs. 2. in preventive medicine the payment of farmers for losses incurred by the destruction of their livestock when controlling an infectious disease.

depth-gain c. see TIME gain compensation.

compensatory pertaining to or emanating from compensation.

c. hypertrophy impaired function of one organ in a paired organ system or of part of an organ in a single organ system is followed by enlargement of the surviving organ or tissue so that functional capacity is maintained.

competent able.

c. bacterial cells able to take up DNA usually foreign and usually as a plasmid.

immune c. an individual with a fully functional immune system.

competitive the relationship in which two or more entities contend for association with another.

c. inhibitors compounds, usually structural analogs of the substrate, that bind reversibly to an enzyme and deny the substrates access to the active site.

c. protein binding binding proteins occur naturally and have affinity for other substances, for example sex hormone steroid-binding globulin. The property is made use of in the assay of such substances in body fluids and tissues. Called also CPB.

c. protein binding assay see competitive protein binding (above).

c. radioimmunoassay a technique utilizing isotope labeled antigen that competes with unlabeled antigen for union with specific antibody. A very sensitive assay, commonly used in detecting trace amounts of drugs.

compiler a computer program which converts the programmer's code to an executable program. See also INTERPRETER.

complement a complex series of enzymatic proteins occurring in normal serum that are triggered in a cascade manner by, and combine with, the antibody–antigen complexes, producing lysis when the antigen is an intact cell. Complement comprises 25 to 30 discrete proteins, labeled numerically as C1 to C9, and by letters, i.e. B, D, P, etc., and with C1 being divided into subcomponents C1q, C1r and C1s. Components C3 and C5 are involved in the generation of anaphylatoxin and in the promotion of leukocyte chemotaxis, the result of these two activities being the inflammatory response. C1 and C4 are involved in the neutralization of viruses. The components also combine in various sequences to participate in other biological activities, including antibody-mediated immune lysis, phagocytosis, opsonization and anaphylaxis. The complement system is known to be activated by the IMMUNOGLOBULINS IgM and IgG.

alternate c. pathway, alternative c. pathway the sequence in which complement components C3 and C5 to C9 are activated without participation by C1, C2 and C4 or the presence of an antibody–antigen complex.

c. cascade the sequence of reactions, each being the catalyst for the next, that leads to the terminal complement pathway and cell lysis. There are two pathways for activation of C3, the 'classical' (below) and the 'alternate' (above).

classical c. pathway the one in which all of the complement components C1 to C9 participate and is triggered by antibody–antigen complexes.

c. deficiency various complement components may be deficient without serious effects on the host. C3 deficiency is most severe and occurs in humans, Brittany spaniels and Finnish-Landrace lambs. Increased susceptibility to infections results.

c. fixation tests utilize antibody–antigen reaction and result in hemolysis to determine the presence of various organisms in the blood. Involves two stages. In the first, also referred to as the test system, antigen is mixed usually with serial dilutions of a test serum in the presence of complement. If the serum contains antibody, i.e. is positive, an antibody–antigen complex is formed which also binds (fixes) complement. In the second stage, also called the indicator system, sheep red blood cells coated with specific, usually rabbit anti-sheep red blood cell antibody are added. The red blood cells are said to be sensitized. If antibody was not present in stage 1, then the free complement lyses the sensitized sheep red blood cells. The basis of many serological tests including those for glanders, tuberculosis and contagious bovine pleuropneumonia. Called also Bordet–Gengou phenomenon. See also IMMUNITY.

c. regulatory proteins a set of at least seven proteins that are present in plasma (C1 INH, C4b-binding protein, factor H and factor I) or present in cell membranes (decay-accelerating factor [DAF], membrane cofactor protein [MCP] and homologous restriction factor [HHF]) that modulate the complement proteins and protect 'innocent' bystander cells and tissues from complement damage.

terminal c. pathway the final stages of complement activation in which C5, C6, C7, C8 and C9 are activated; common to both the alternate and classical pathways.

complementarity the relationship between bases in the DNA double helix whereby every base on one strand is matched to a complementary hydrogen bonding base on the other strand.

complementation infection of the same cell by two viruses in which one provides a gene product which the other requires.

α-complementation a method for selecting bacteria that have been transformed with a plasmid vector in the pUC series which carries the *N*-terminal coding sequence for β-galactosidase of the *lac* operon.

complete including all of the subdivisions of the whole.

c. blood count (CBC) see BLOOD COUNT.

complex 1. the sum or combination of various things, like or unlike, as a complex of clinical signs. 2. that portion of an electrocardiographic tracing that represents the systole of an atrium or ventricle.

antibody–antigen c. a complex formed by the combining of antibody and antigen. Called also immune complex.

Golgi c. a complex cellular organelle involved in the synthesis of glycoproteins, lipoproteins, membrane-bound proteins and lysosomal enzymes. See also GOLGI APPARATUS.

immune c. antibody–antigen complex.

major histocompatibility c. (MHC) see major HISTOCOMPATIBILITY complex.

multienzyme c. the bringing together of all of the enzymes involved in a series of reactions such that the product of enzyme A is passed directly to enzyme B and so on to the final product.

olivary nuclear c. gray matter located in the medulla oblongata dorsal to the pyramidal tracts; an important part of the motor feedback regulatory mechanism.

primary c. the combination of a parenchymal pulmonary lesion and a corresponding lymph node focus, occurring in primary tuberculosis. Similar lesions may also be associated with other mycobacterial infections and with fungal infections.

compliance the quality of yielding to pressure or force without disruption, or an expression of the measure of ability to do so, as an expression of the distensibility of an air- or fluid-filled organ, e.g. the lung or urinary bladder, in terms of unit of volume per unit of pressure.

The compliance of the lungs (C_L) and thorax (C_T) determine the elastic resistance to ventilation. The total compliance of the lungs and thorax (C_{LT}) is given by the formula $1/C_{LT} = 1/C_L + 1/C_T$. C_L is measured by determining the intrapleural pressure at different end-inspiratory volumes. A balloon-tipped catheter is used to determine the intrapleural pressure, which is transmitted through the soft wall of the esophagus. C_L is usually divided by the functional residual capacity to give the specific compliance. Lung compliance is decreased in congestive heart failure and interstitial lung disease and increased in emphysema. C_{LT} can be measured by determining the change in lung volume for various amounts of pressure difference between the mouth and chest surface using a body plethysmograph.

blood vessel c. the ability of each blood vessel to expand, or contract, to best accommodate a particular volume, and a particular hydrostatic pressure of blood depends on the proportional composition, and the distribution, of its content of collagen, elastin, smooth muscle.

C. Policy Guide a 1984 addition to the (US) Federal Food, Drug amd Cosmetic Act which allows for the extralabel use of drug products, approved for use in other species, to be used in animals.

complication 1. a disease(s) concurrent with another disease. 2. the occurrence of two or more diseases in the same patient.

component therapy in transfusion medicine, use of just that component of blood which is required, e.g. whole blood, packed red blood cells, or plasma.

composite a variety of resins used in restorative dentistry.

composite milk samples a specimen is taken from each of the four quarters, or the two halves in ewes, does and mares, into the same sample bottle. Contrast with quarter samples.

compound 1. made up of diverse elements or ingredients. 2. a substance made up of two or more materials. 3. in chemistry, a substance made up of two or more elements in union. The elements are united chemically, which means that each of the original elements loses its individual characteristics once it has combined with the other element(s).

c. 469 see ISOFLURANE.

c. 1080 see SODIUM fluoroacetate.

c. 1081 see FLUOROACETAMIDE.

c. granular corpuscle see GITTER CELLS.

c. interest rate the interest rate charged when COMPOUNDING or DISCOUNTING borrowed or loaned money.

compounding the annual addition of earned interest to a capital sum of borrowed or loaned money at the existing market interest rate, including the interest earned by the accumulated interest; calculated future value of an existing capital sum.

compress a square of gauze or similar dressing, for application of pressure or medication to a restricted area, or for local applications of heat or cold.

compression 1. the act of pressing upon or together; the state of being pressed together. A specific example is compression plating in fracture repair. 2. in embryology, the shortening or omission of certain developmental stages. 3. see DATA compression.

c. band pulled tightly across an animal on an x-ray table to reduce thickness, restrict respiratory movement and restrain the patient. Both ends of the band are fixed to the table and there is a mechanism for tightening it. May be used to apply pressure to an organ such as the urinary bladder to impede filling with excreted dye, but in other applications has the disadvantage of distorting organs and their disposition.

c./distraction methods a stress-radiographic method of positioning dogs for the assessment of hip laxity for the diagnosis of hip dysplasia. One radiograph is taken with the femoral heads compressed into the acetabula. The other position is with maximal lateral displacement of the femoral heads using a special device for leverage.

c. plating an internal fixation method of treating fractures by the application of plates across the fracture lines and fixing them in place with specially designed screws. The objective is to provide extreme stability of the fracture. Properly designed plates of the correct size for the patient and the use of screws with maximum holding power make the system independent of any additional form of support.

c. plating device a device that is connected to an already fixed end of a compression plate and then connected to the other bone fragment so as to obtain as complete compression as possible. Not commonly used when modern dynamic compression plates are utilized.

spinal cord c. compression of the cord by a space-occupying lesion in the vertebral canal causes an upper MOTOR neuron syndrome below and a lower MOTOR neuron syndrome at the site of the lesion.

comprest cattle dwarf cattle.

compromised 1. lacking adequate resistance to infection, or lacking the ability to mount an adequate immune response, owing to a course of treatment, e.g. immunosuppressive drugs or infections, irradiation, or to an underlying disorder, e.g. leukemia. 2. lacking a sufficient blood supply to remain viable.

Compton effect one of the three kinds of interaction when ion-pair formation occurs as x-rays pass through an absorbing medium. The interacting photons pass on in a new direction (Compton scatter) having given up part of its energy in ionizing an atom in the absorbing medium (Compton absorption). Important in the upper range of x-ray energies used in veterinary radiography.

Compton metabolic profile test a test based on the concept that the nutritional status of an animal can be estimated by the chemical measurement of some of the components of the blood. It is used to determine the need for variation in the diet of the animal or herd and is thought to be more accurate and to be effective much earlier than the clinical assessments that are more customary as preventive measures. The testing procedure includes the collection of blood samples on a number of occasions during the year and from cows in various stages of nutritional and lactational stress. Only a small group of cows is examined and proper statistical precautions are taken to ensure that conclusions drawn will be valid. A large number of biochemical estimations are carried out on the blood samples, and in some instances on urine samples, so that the animals' nutritional and metabolic status with respect to most of the significant metabolites can be assessed.

compulsive the state of being subject to compulsion.

c. drinking see primary POLYDYPSIA.

c. rolling an involuntary movement in which the recumbent patient persists in rolling, always in the same direction, until it meets an obstruction.

c. walking affected animals walk oblivious to their surroundings. They appear to be blind, walk into objects, headpress against them and stay in this position for long periods, are oblivious to danger and may die of misadventure. They may attempt to climb a wall and fall over backwards. Common causes are hepatic encephalopathy and increased intracranial pressure.

computed tomography a radiological imaging technique that produces images of 'slices' through a patient's body. See also computed TOMOGRAPHY.

computer an electronic machine capable of giving effect to a logical series of stored commands in relation to the capture, storage, analysis and retrieval of data which may be numerical, alphabetical or a combination of the two. It consists of a central processing unit which performs calculations and comparisons between sets of data stored in the memory, and in external storage such as magnetic tape or disk drives and either fixed (hard) or floppy disks. It also communicates with a keyboard or mouse through which all new communication must go. Optional but highly desirable attachments are the visual display unit which displays all of the input and output, a printer so that a permanent record can be made, or a plotter, or laboratory recording equipment.

Using a MODEM it is now possible to connect a computer with other computers over the INTERNET and the WORLD WIBE WEB in what is a truly global information highway.

Almost all modern computers use a digital system of communication; some, especially in laboratories receiving data from transponders, use an analog system in which variables in mathematical problems are represented by physical quantities, e.g. voltages.

Mainframe computers are very large with immense storage and located centrally. They may be accessed from remote sites by telephonic means via modems or acoustic couplers from dumb terminals, or other computers. Minicomputers or stand-alone computers have a much smaller capacity. Those with smaller capacity still, and suitable for use as personal computers, or as office or practice computers, are called microcomputers. Their small size is dependent on the development of microchips carrying the electronic circuits within a very small space.

c. assisted diagnosis a list of possible diagnoses, possibly arranged in order of their probability, can be derived from a suitable computer program and database by feeding in the key clinical signs, clinical pathology findings and epidemiological data.

c. hard disks built-in disks complete with their own disk drives. Are not physically accessible. Usually have a capacity of a gigabyte compared to 1.4 megabyte on the largest floppy disks.

c. language the operation of the computer is carried out by means of a machine language consisting of binary instructions of 0's and 1's. The next level of language is assembly language in which each instruction is given as a mnemonic. Even this is tedious for programming, so that the average user writes programs in a high level language, in which a simple 'English-like' instruction translates into several, even many, machine instructions. Such translation is carried out by a program called a compiler or an interpreter. The common languages in use are BASIC, COBOL, FORTRAN and PASCAL (2). Still higher level languages, fourth general languages (4GLs), have been developed to further reduce the amount of programming required to do a given task.

c. operating system for a computer to do useful work it requires a set of instructions called a program. The master program that controls all of the computer's basic tasks is called the operating system. Other more specific programs make use of the operating system to perform their own functions.

personal c. a small microcomputer for personal and home use; available as desk-top, portable and laptop models.

c. program see computer PROGRAM.

c. simulation model a simulation model adapted for use on a computer. See also SIMULATION.

c. software computer programs and their attendant manuals, floppy disks.

c. storage information for subsequent access can be stored by the computer on floppy disks, hard disks, magnetic tape and now compact disks.

computerized adapted for analysis, storage and retrieval on a computer.

c. axial tomography see COMPUTED TOMOGRAPHY.

c. clinical data storage clinical data is keyed in in the examination room, the clinical pathology laboratory and the radiology section. It is then capable of analysis in terms of diagnosis, identity of the veterinarian, drugs used, inventory reset and accounts raised. Accounts can be made up and posted and a monthly statement of income and expenditure prepared.

c. transaxial tomography see computed TOMOGRAPHY.

Con A concancavalin A.

conacaste tree ENTEROLOBIUM *cyclocarpum*.

conarium see PINEAL body.

concanavalin either of two phytohemagglutinins isolated along with canavalin from the meal of the jack bean (*Canavalia ensiformis* and other species of *Canavalia*), which agglutinate the blood of mammals as a result of reaction with polyglucosans.

c. A binds to sugar residues on cell surfaces and stimulates T lymphocytes to proliferate; has also been shown to inhibit the growth of ascites tumors. Called also Con A.

concancavalin toxic amino acid (lectin) found in *Canavalia* spp.

concatemers intermediate structures formed during the replication of some DNA molecules in which up to 200 unit-length molecules are joined together to form giant molecules, which are subsequently cleaved to form unit-length molecules.

concave rounded and somewhat depressed or hollowed out.

c. face of the Golgi complex in the developing embryo is associated with maturing secretory vesicles.

c. shoe a horseshoe with its inner edge thicker than the outer so that the surface touching the ground is slightly smaller than the surface in contact with the hoof.

concaveation the induction of maternal behavior in virgin females or males when exposed to neonates.

concavity a depression or hollowed surface.

concealed heat a lay term used to describe a silent estrus or one lacking overt signs recognized by an owner.

conceive to become pregnant.

concentrate 1. to bring to a common center; to gather at one point. 2. to increase the strength by diminishing the bulk of, as of a liquid; to condense. 3. a drug or other preparation that has been strengthened by evaporation of its nonactive parts. 4. a carefully compounded mixture of micro- and macronutrients, largely vitamins and minerals, suitable for adding to a herbivore's meal and roughage diet which is probably lacking the supplements contained in the concentrate.

concentration 1. increase in strength by evaporation. 2. the ratio of the mass or volume of a solute to the mass or volume of the solution or solvent.

hydrogen ion c. an expression of the degree of acidity or alkalinity (pH) of a solution. See also ACID–BASE BALANCE.

mass c. the mass of a constituent substance divided by the volume of the mixture, as milligrams per liter (mg/l).

minimum effective c. the threshold level of a drug in plasma below which the efficiency of the drug as a treatment drops off sharply.

molar c. the amount of a constituent in moles (millimoles or micromoles) divided by the volume of the mixture, as millimoles per liter (mmol/l).

c. test a test of renal function based on the patient's ability to concentrate urine. See WATER deprivation test.

conception the onset of pregnancy, marked by implantation of the blastocyst; the formation of a viable zygote. See also REPRODUCTION.
c. efficiency see conception rate (below).
c. failure when conception begins but fails soon afterwards. One of the most common causes of reproductive wastage in dairy cows.
c. prevention prevention of the establishment of pregnancy by the use of teaser males in commercial herds or flocks, or progestagen implants in the control of female wild animals.
c. rate percentage of matings that result in conception.
C. Vessel in acupuncture one of the two major extra meridians, besides the 12 regular meridians.
conceptus the whole product of conception at any stage of development, from fertilization of the ovum to birth, including extraembryonic membranes as well as the embryo or fetus.
c. dropsy see fetal ASCITES, HYDRAMNIOS, HYDRALLANTOIS.
concha pl. *conchae* [L.] a shell-shaped structure.
c. of auricle the base of the auricle of the external ear, bounded anteriorly by the tragus and posteriorly by the antihelix.
ethmoidal c. a series of scroll-like bones which arise from the ethmoid bone, project into the nasal chambers and support the olfactory mucous membrane.
nasal c. one of two or three delicate, mucosa-covered turbinate bones occupying a large part of each half of the nasal cavity. See also Table 10.
conchitis inflammation of a concha.
conchotomy incision of a nasal concha.
Concinnum a genus of flukes of the family Dicrocoeliidae. Includes *Concinnum brumpti* (African apes—liver, pancreas), *C. procyonis* syn. *Eurytrema proctonis* (cats, foxes—pancreatic, biliary ducts), *C. ten* (wild carnivores).
conclination inward rotation of the upper pole of the vertical meridian of each eye.
concomitant variable see concomitant VARIABLE.
concordance in genetics, the occurrence of a given trait in both members of a twin pair.
concrescence a growing together of parts originally separate.
concrete mixture of cement and reinforcing gravel or stones used in the surfacing of yards, passageways, milking parlors and the like; critical to the good condition of feet and hooves of farm livestock. Excessive wear due to a too-abrasive surface causes FOOTROT of pigs and epidemic lameness in dairy herds.
concretio [L.] *concretion.*
c. cordis adhesive pericarditis in which the pericardial cavity is obliterated.
concretion 1. a calculus or inorganic mass in a natural cavity or in tissue. 2. abnormal union of adjacent parts. 3. a process of becoming harder or more solid.
concurrent simultaneous as in disease, infection, infestation.
concussion a violent jar or shock, or the condition that results from such an injury.
brain c. loss of consciousness, transient or prolonged, due to a blow to the head; breathing often is unusually rapid or slow. Outward evidence of the injury may include bleeding, sometimes from the nose, and contusions (bruises). There may be residual signs such as local paralysis on recovery.
spinal cord c. may lead to temporary paresis or spinal shock, with possible local paralysis continuing after partial recovery.
c. stunner a sharp blow to the head sufficient to cause stunning may be used as a prelude to euthanasia or, in laboratory animals, as a means of euthanasia on its own.
condemned meat meat classified at inspection as unfit for human consumption.
c. m. room the room in an abattoir allocated to the temporary storage, prior to disposal, of condemned meat and offal.
condensation 1. the act of rendering, or the process of becoming, more compact. 2. the process of passing from a gaseous to a liquid or solid phase. In animal housing this is a matter of great importance because of the need for a dry environment as a prevention against the spread of infection, especially those spread by inhalation.
condenser 1. a vessel or apparatus for condensing gases or vapors. 2. a device for illuminating microscopic objects. 3. a device for boosting the voltage in an electrical circuit.
c. discharge unit used to generate high voltages needed for diagnostic x-rays using standard 110/220 volt input. An advantage for mobile units. It discharges over a short period, which helps prevent movement blur.
condition 1. to train; to subject to conditioning. 2. state of the body in terms of amount of tissue carried. Spoken of as obese, fat, thin, emaciated. See also BODY CONDITION SCORE. 3. of wool; a qualitative assessment of the degree of waste included in the fleece, including yolk, plant fiber, dust.
body c. see condition (2) (above).
body c. scale see BODY CONDITION SCORE.
light c. see THINNESS.
c. scoring the allocation of a score to indicate an animal's body condition. See also BODY CONDITION SCORE.
conditional probability the probability that event A occurs, given that event B has occurred. Written $P(A|B)$.
conditioned educated by a conditioning process. See CONDITIONING.
c. reinforcer the pairing of a neutral stimulus with a primary, or natural, reinforcer.
c. response a response that does not occur naturally in the animal but that may be developed by regular association of some physiological function with an unrelated outside event, such as ringing of a bell or flashing of a light. Soon the physiological function starts whenever the outside event occurs. Called also conditioned reflex. See also CONDITIONING.
conditioner involved in improving physical condition.
livestock c. a person involved in special feeding programs for heavy producing dairy cows or animals being prepared for shows, exhibitions, fairs and sale. Usually done at the conditioner's premises because of the secret nature of the materials and procedures. Represents a potential health threat from infectious disease.
soil c. agents such as gypsum added to clay soil to improve its physical state.
conditioning 1. learning; behavior modification in animals. 2. preparation of young cattle for shipment and entry into a feedlot. The procedure varies but usually includes vaccination against potential pathogens, prophylactic treatment for worms and lice, administration of vitamins and when necessary feeding of antibiotics and introduction to the kind of diet likely to be fed. 3. tenderizing of meat by careful storage at an appropriate temperature for a sufficiently long period.
classical c. a form of learning in which a response is

elicited by a neutral stimulus which previously had been repeatedly presented in conjunction with the stimulus that originally elicited the response. Called also respondent conditioning, Pavlovian conditioning.

The concept had its beginnings in experimental techniques for the study of reflexes. The traditional procedure is based on the work of Ivan P. Pavlov, a Russian physiologist. In this technique the experimental subject is a dog that is harnessed in a sound-shielded room. The neutral stimulus is the sound of a metronome or bell which occurs each time the dog is presented with food, and the response is the production of saliva by the dog. Eventually the sound of the bell or metronome produces salivation, even though the stimulus that originally elicited the response (the food) is no longer presented.

instrumental c. takes place only after the subject performs a specific act that has been previously designated. The most common form of this conditioning uses an instrument such as a bar that must be pressed by the subject to achieve the delivery of food or other reward.

operant c. learning in which a particular response is elicited by a stimulus because that response produces desirable consequences (reward).

Pavlovian c. see classical conditioning (above).

respondent c. see classical conditioning (above).

conditions of employment that part of an employment that sets out the duties, responsibilities, hours of work, salary, leave and other privileges to be enjoyed by persons employed, for example a veterinary nurse, in private practice. Most professional organizations provide a pro forma of such an agreement.

condominium a centrally owned, usually cooperative, facility of feed mill, feed trucks, feed purchasing and health services but separate individual ownership of livestock, and usually the feedlot yards.

condor a voiceless, New World vulture; a diurnal bird of prey noted for its large size. Includes *Vultur gryphus* (Andean condor) and *Gymnogyps californianus* (Californian condor).

conduct behavior as a professional. Behaviour relative to a code of ethics agreed to by members of a professional organization.

c. conducive to unfairly attracting business see TOUTING.

unprofessional c. see MISCONDUCT.

conductance ability to conduct or transmit, as electricity or other energy or material; in studies of respiration, an expression of the amount of air reaching the alveoli per unit of time per unit of pressure, the reciprocal of resistance.

conduction, conductive conveyance of energy, as of heat, sound or electricity.

accessory tract atrioventricular c. permits a sinus impulse from the atria to ventricles to precede that carried by the normal atrioventricular conduction system. Arrhythmia results, the particular electrocardiographic characteristics depending on the pathway(s) involved. See also WOLFF–PARKINSON–WHITE SYNDROME.

aerial c., air c. conduction of sound waves to the organ of hearing through the air.

c. anesthesia local anesthesia produced by the injection of an anesthetic agent close to a nerve in order to prevent transmission of nerve impulses along it.

bone c. conduction of sound waves to the inner ear through the bones of the skull.

c. disorder abnormalities in the conduction pathways of the heart.

James accessory c. see JAMES FIBERS.

c. system the system comprises the sinoatrial and atrioventricular nodes, atrioventricular bundle and Purkinje fibers.

c. time an indicator of a peripheral nerve's ability to carry an impulse; measured during electromyography. A nerve that has undergone Wallerian degeneration is unable to carry an impulse. Severe loss of myelin results in a prolonged conduction time.

conductive having the quality of readily conducting electric current.

c. flooring flooring or floor covering made specially conductive to electrical current, usually by the inclusion of copper wiring that is earthed externally.

conductivity capacity for conduction.

conduit a channel for the passage of fluids or air.

ileal c. the surgical anastomosis of the ureters or a bowel segment to one end of a detached segment of ileum, the other end being used to form a stoma on the abdominal wall.

vascular c. artificial blood vessel; used in repair of pulmonic stenosis by providing a bypass of the obstruction and in correction of arteriovenous fistulae.

condylarthrosis a modification of the spheroidal form of synovial joint, in which the articular surfaces are ellipsoidal rather than spheroid.

condyle a rounded projection on a bone, usually for articulation with another bone; a knuckle.

c. fracture one involving a condyle, most commonly distal humerus or femur in small animals and distal cannon bone in horses.

occipital c. flanking the foramen magnum.

condylectomy excision of a condyle.

condylion the most lateral point on the surface of the head of the mandible.

condyloid resembling a condyle.

condyloma an elevated wartlike lesion of the skin.

c. acuminatum a small, pointed papilloma of viral origin.

canine c. see canine transmissible VENEREAL tumor.

condylotomy transection of a condyle.

condylus pl. *condyli* [L.] see CONDYLE.

Condy's crystals see PERMANGANATE.

cone 1. a solid figure or body having a circular base and tapering to a point, especially one of the conelike structures of the retina, which, with the retinal rods, form the light-sensitive elements of the retina. The cones make possible the perception of color. 2. in radiology, a conical or open-ended cylindrical structure used as an aid in producing high detail x-rays. 3. surgical cone.

c. cells (1) the commonest, if not the sole, photoreceptors in the central area of the retina, where the function of acute vision is located. See also cone (1) above.

c. down in radiology, to restrict the x-ray beam. See also COLLIMATION.

c. dysplasia (1) progressive dysplasia of retinal cones in Alaskan malamute dogs; causes impaired day vision from an early age. The rods are normal.

ether c. a cone-shaped device used over the face in administration of ether for anesthesia.

c. flower see RUDBECKIA.

c. of light the triangular reflection of light seen on the tympanic membrane.

pressure c. the area of compression exerted by a mass in the brain, as in transtentorial herniation.

retinal c's see cone (1) above.

c. shellfish see CONUS.

cone-nose bug see REDUVIID BUG.
conexus a connecting structure.
confidence degree of assurance.
c. interval a range of values about a sample statistic that has a specified probability of including the true value of the statistic.
c. level 1 minus the type 1 ERROR; the probability that the trial under consideration will show no significant difference when there is in fact no significant difference between the treatments.
c. limits the highest and lowest values in a confidence interval.
confidentiality secrecy relating to information. All clinical data have a degree of confidentiality, the level varying with the information and the circumstances.
configuration 1. in anatomical terms the general form of a body. 2. in chemistry, the arrangement in space of the atoms of a molecule. 3. in computer terminology the group of interconnected machines that make up a practical working unit. Comprises computer, disk drive(s), printer, visual display unit.
configure see INITIALIZE.
confinement restriction of animals' movements so that they are not allowed to range freely and graze pasture but are confined either outdoors or indoors, with food brought to them. The degree of confinement varies from tie-stalls for cows and farrowing crates for sows, to lounging barns and feedlots for cattle.
total c. animals housed at all times; a common practice in some tropical countries where protection from the heat and humidity may be essential for high-producing livestock; labor and engineering services are costly production items.
conflicts of interest the ethical situation that arises when, for example, a veterinarian who practices and also conducts a pharmacy finds that his/her enthusiasm for merchandising is competing with his/her professional interest in being as accurate as possible diagnostically.
confluence a running together; a meeting of streams.
c. of sinuses the dilated point of confluence of the superior sagittal, straight, occipital and two transverse sinuses of the dura mater.
conformation symmetry, size and shape of the various body regions relative to each other or the general appearance of the animal in terms of satisfying the observer's appreciation of what is a desirable appearance. Most breed societies issue lists of desirable and undesirable points of conformation. Most of them are desirable. Some are not and react adversely on the animals' well-being. Desirable conformation may also be indicated by diagrams or photographs.
Also may refer to the spatial arrangement of atoms in a molecule.
mitochondrial c. mitochondria may be in an abnormal state of condensed conformation, detected by comparison with mitochondria of orthodox status; orthodox conformation is linked to inactive oxidase phosphorylation, condensed to active phosphorylation.
confounding when the effects of two, or more, processes on results cannot be separated, the results are said to be confounded, a cause of bias in disease studies.
c. factor one which is distributed non-randomly with respect to the independent (exposure) or dependent (outcome) variable which is the subject of an enquiry.
congener something closely related to another thing, as a member of the same genus, a muscle having the same function as another, or a chemical compound closely related to another in composition and exerting similar or antagonistic effects, or something derived from the same source or stock.
congenic a genetic term usually used to refer to specially inbred strains of mice that differ only in restricted regions of the genome; used particularly in mapping major histocompatibility complex antigens.
congenital present at and existing from the time of birth.
c. articular rigidity see ARTHROGRYPOSIS.
c. defects abnormalities of structure or function which are present at birth. They may or may not be inherited. There are a number of diseases, for example the LYSOSOMAL storage diseases, which may be inherited or environmental in causation, in which the insult is supplied while the fetus is in utero, but the defect does not become apparent until some time after birth. By definition these are not congenital defects although the animal is born with the metabolic lesion in place. See also individual defects listed by organ or system.
c. erythropoietic porphyria see PORPHYRIA.
infectious c. tremor see CONGENITAL TREMOR SYNDROME of piglets.
c. loco a congenital, inherited disease of domestic chickens characterized by opisthotonos, orthotonos, inability to stand, violent somersaulting. Affected birds die of starvation and dehydration.
congenital reduced phalanges incomplete limbs in newborn animals; they may have an inherited defect or may have been exposed to a noxious environmental influence such as irradiation in early pregnancy.
inherited c. r. p. a variety of defects is recorded. In some animals the intermediate bones are missing, in others it is the extremities. In others there are defects in other organs such as cryptorchidism. Called also amputates. See also HEMIMELIA, TIBIAL.
congenital tremor syndrome a benign, congenital disease of piglets manifested by severe muscle tremor, especially when standing, and absent when asleep. There is no muscle weakness, the only deaths are due to crushing due to impairment of evasive actions. There are several causes including two inherited forms, two caused by intrauterine viral infections, one of them hog cholera. The histological proof is a dysmyelinogenesis. Called also myoclonia congenita, trembles.
congestion abnormal accumulation of blood in a part.
pulmonary c. see PULMONARY congestion.
udder c. see UDDER edema.
congestive pertaining to or associated with congestion. See also congestive HEART FAILURE.
conglobation the act of forming, or the state of being formed, into a rounded mass.
conglutinant promoting union, as of the lips of a wound.
conglutination 1. the adherence of tissues to each other. 2. agglutination of erythrocytes that is dependent upon both complement and antibodies.
conglutinin a serum protein found in Bovidae which can bind to fixed C3b and cause C3b-coated particles to clump.
Congo dog see BASENJI.
Congo floor maggot see AUCHMEROMYIA *luteola*.
Congo red a synthetic dye, a derivative of benzidine and naphthionic acid. It is used for differential staining of elastic fibers for microscopic examination. Amyloid is stained a light orange-red with Congo red

and exhibits apple green birefringence under polarized light. Amyloid in cats stains poorly. Congo red undergoes a change in hue with acidity and thus can be used as an indicator of pH, turning red in the presence of alkalis (bases) and blue when exposed to acids.

C. r. test a laboratory test used in the diagnosis of AMYLOIDOSIS, based on measuring the amount of injected dye that is removed by amyloid in the tissues of the human patient. Not now commonly used.

Congo virus disease a transient fever of cattle and goats caused by a not well characterized arbovirus transmitted by *Hyalomma* spp. ticks. The virus is similar to Crimean hemorrhagic fever virus of humans.

conhydrine one of the piperidine alkaloids in *Conium maculatum*. A highly fatal toxin causing paralysis of the skeletal musculature.

conical flukes see PARAMPHISTOMES.

coniceine one of the toxic piperidine alkaloids in CONIUM MACULATUM.

Conidae a family of univalve shellfish whose members can be very poisonous to humans. See also CONUS.

conidiobolomycosis infection by fungi of the genus *Conidiobolus*.

Conidiobolus a genus of soil-borne fungi.

***C. coronatus* (syn. *Entomophthora coronata*)** causes granuloma, which may ulcerate, on the nasal mucosa and skin. See also SWAMP CANCER, PHYCOMYCOSIS.

C. incongruus has caused an epidemic form of nasal granuloma in sheep characterized by disfiguring swellings of the nose, invasion of the local lymph nodes and involvement of the lungs causing death.

conidiophore a specialized hypha upon which conidia are formed.

conidium pl. *conidia;* an asexual spore of fungi borne on hyphae. There are many types of conidia, BLASTOCONIDIA, ARTHROCONIDIUM, ANNELLOCONIDIUM, PHIALOCONIDIUM, POROCONIDIA and ALEURIOCONIDIA.

coniine one of the toxic piperidine alkaloids in CONIUM MACULATUM.

coniofibrosis pneumoconiosis with exuberant growth of connective tissue in the lungs.

coniosis a diseased state due to inhalation of dust.

coniotoxicosis pneumoconiosis in which the irritant affects the tissues directly.

Conium maculatum a toxic plant in the Apiaceae family; this weed may affect animals which eat it while grazing or in hay. Principal signs are tremor, ataxia, respiratory failure and death. Diarrhea, vomition, frequent urination, congenital arthrogryposis and spinal curvature occur in piglets from sows fed on the plant. Called also poison hemlock.

conjoined joined together.

c. monsters two deformed fetuses fused together.

c. twins see conjoined TWINS.

conjugata conjugate diameter (diameter of space encircled by items joined together, e.g. pelvic diameter—the diameter of the pelvic inlet from the sacral promontory to the pelvic brim).

conjugate 1. paired, or equally coupled; working in union. 2. to link marker protein such as fluorescein or enzyme to an antibody molecule to detect antigen, as by IMMUNOFLUORESCENCE or immunoperoxidase staining. 3. a conjugate diameter of the pelvic inlet; used alone usually to denote the true conjugate diameter. See also pelvic DIAMETER.

c. acids conjugate pair of strong bases.

conjugation a joining. In unicellular organisms, a form of sexual reproduction in which two individuals join in temporary union to transfer genetic material. In biochemistry, the joining of a toxic substance with some natural substance of the body to form a detoxified product for elimination from the body.

conjunct rotation the complicated movement whereby alternate flexion, adduction, extension and abduction brings about rotation.

conjunctiva pl. *conjunctivae* [L.] the delicate membrane lining the eyelids and covering parts of the eyeball. Is in several parts, bulbar, fornical, marginal, nictital, palpebral and tarsal, named for anatomical reasons.

conjunctival pertaining to or emanating from conjunctiva.

congenital c. membrane partial or complete obstruction of the lacrimal puncta occurs when a conjunctival membrane or flap is present over the opening.

c. flap surgical movement and fixation of conjunctiva, either bulbar or palpebral, to cover defects in conjunctiva or, more commonly, to cover lacerations or nonhealing, progressive or deep ulcerations of the cornea especially those with desmetoceles. The flaps serve to protect the corneal lesion from eyelid trauma and encourage migration and proliferation of fibroblasts and blood vessels into the area. There are many techniques; some utilize the nictitating membrane.

c. grafts defects of conjunctiva may be grafted with conjunctiva obtained from elsewhere in the same eye or the opposite eye. Buccal mucosa has also been used for this purpose.

c. granuloma see NODULAR fasciitis.

c. sac the tear-filled space, lined by conjunctiva, between the eyelids and the eyeball.

c. squamous metaplasia CANCER EYE. See ocular SQUAMOUS cell carcinoma.

conjunctivitis inflammation of the conjunctiva. Extension of the inflammation to the cornea is common, hence KERATOCONJUNCTIVITIS. Individual cases may be due to trauma or to grass seed or other foreign body intrusion. The most serious conjunctivitides are the infectious ones, including those in which conjunctivitis is only an incidental lesion to more serious problems, e.g. rinderpest, bovine malignant catarrh, canine distemper, infectious bovine rhinotracheitis. The common specific conjunctivitides are *Moraxella bovis* infection in cattle, *Rickettsia conjunctivae* in sheep, goats and pigs, but there is no such infection in horses. In cats, feline herpesvirus and *Chlamydia* cause a conjunctivitis. Parasitic conjunctivitis may be caused by *Habronema* spp. in horses and *Thelazia* spp. in all species. Classical signs of the disease are ocular discharge, serous at first, purulent later, and blepharospasm. Both eyes may be affected. Under-running of the conjunctiva and permanent opacity, even rupture of the eyeball, may follow.

equine seasonal c. irritation caused by flies (*Musca domestica*) or release of *Habronema* larvae; called also summer conjunctivitis.

fetal c. present in many cases of intrauterine infection and the causative organism can be cultured from the site.

follicular c. proliferation of lymphoid tissue on the bulbar surface of the third eyelid, often extending to the adjacent bulbar and palpebral conjunctiva in response to any chronic inflammation or stimulation such as dust, entropion, ectropion, distichiasis or bacterial infection.

c. neonatorum neonatal kittens infected by feline herpesvirus may have severe ocular involvement, even before their eyelids become unsealed. Ulcerative keratitis and panophthalmitis are common sequelae.

primary c. caused by infectious agents, parasites or toxic agents affecting the conjunctiva in the first instance.

secondary c. associated with foreign bodies or diseases of the cornea, lacrimal system, eyelids, orbit, or body as a whole.

conjunctivobuccostomy, conjunctivoralostomy a surgical technique for treatment of epiphora due to obstructed lacrimal canaliculi. It involves the creation of a new drainage track from the conjunctival surface opening to the oral cavity between the upper lip and dental arcade.

conjunctivoma a tumor of the eyelid composed of conjunctival tissue.

conjunctivoplasty plastic repair of the conjunctiva.

conjunctivoralostomy conjunctivobuccostomy.

conjunctivorhinostomy a surgical technique for the treatment of obstruction of the lacrimal duct in which a new drainage track is created from the conjunctiva to the maxillary sinus or nasal cavity.

connect time the time period for which a user is connected to a computer. Used as the basis for charging for computer use, particularly for networking and dial-up computer services.

connecting tubules one of the collecting ductal systems in the kidney permitting nephrons to connect directly with cortical collecting ducts.

connection points see LUO POINTS.

connective tissue a fibrous type of body tissue with varied functions. The connective tissue system supports and connects internal organs, forms bones and the walls of blood vessels, attaches muscles to bones, and replaces tissues of other types following injury.

Connective tissue consists mainly of long fibers embedded in noncellular matter, the ground substance. The density of these fibers and the presence or absence of certain chemicals make some connective tissues soft and rubbery and others hard and rigid. Compared with most other kinds of tissue, connective tissue has few cells. The fibers contain a protein called collagen.

Connective tissue can develop in any part of the body, and the body uses this ability to help repair or replace damaged areas. Scar tissue is the most common form of this substitute. See also COLLAGEN diseases.

elastic c. t. found especially in supportive tissues, e.g. some ligaments, and tendons, e.g. nuchal ligament or tunica flava.

reticular c. t. a type of connective tissue found principally in myeloid and lymphatic organs; they account for reticular meshwork.

Connell suture pattern a technique for suture of the gut wall which resembles the CUSHING SUTURE PATTERN except that the suture goes through all layers of the gut wall. The suture goes through the wall from the serosa to the mucosa, then back from the mucosa to the serosa on the same side. The stitch then crosses the incision to the serosa on the other side and then repeats.

Connemara pony Irish riding pony, usually dun, or gray, black, bay or brown, 13 to 14 hands high.

connexons components of the gap junction spaces between nerve cells; metabolic substances pass between nerve cells via these links.

Connochaetes taurinus the African ungainly antelope with the body of an antelope and the head of a buffalo of the family Bovidae; called also blue wildebeest, brindle gnu, *Gorgon taurinus*.

Conn's syndrome see HYPERALDOSTERONISM.

Conocephalus grasshoppers, an intermediate host for the flukes in the genus *Eurytrema*.

conotruncal abnormalities congenital anomalies in the conotruncal septum in the developing embryo; TETRALOGY of Fallot (a combination of three such defects) is the only one recorded in animals.

consanguinity blood relationship; kinship.

conscious capable of responding to sensory stimuli; awake; aware.

consciousness the state of being conscious; responsiveness of the brain to impressions made by the senses. Altered states range from the normal, complete alertness to depression, confusion, delirium and finally loss of consciousness.

consensual excited by reflex stimulation.

c. light reflex application of a bright light to one eye causes reflex constriction of the pupil of the other, as well as the pupil of the first eye.

consent in law, voluntary agreement with an action proposed by another, e.g. agreement to treat, to euthanatize. Consent is an act of reason so that the person consenting must be sane and of sufficient age to be capable of giving consent. Written consent is an agreement in writing.

informed c. agreement to a proposition when the consenting person is in possession of all of the facts relevant to the decision. In the eyes of the law the consent of a client to a surgical operation, to a financial expenditure, to euthanasia carries no authority unless the client is fully informed about what is to be done and what the alternatives are. If this is not done the client is entitled to sue for damages if the outcome is unsatisfactory.

conserved DNA sequences clusters of nucleotides that occur more often than would be predicted by random chance; include a number of transcription start regions called PROMOTERS and many others.

consideration the essential element in all contracts; the return for the outlay. Wages, leave entitlements are considerations in a contract of appointment, even though many of them are unwritten. The provision of housing as part of an employment package is a consideration. The fee for surgery is the consideration in return for the surgery.

consignment sale auction sales of consignments of breeding cattle which are excess to the owner's requirements.

Consolida ajacis larkspur, *C. ambigua*. See DELPHINIUM.

consolidated statutes statutes produced by the periodic merging of related statutes in order to economize on the law's letters.

consolidation solidification; the process of becoming solidified or the condition of being solid; said especially of the lung as it fills with fibrinous exudate in pneumonia.

constant a datum, fact or principle that is not subject to change.

Michaelis c. (K_m) a dissociation constant for the substrate concentration in an enzymatic reaction.

c. (C) region see CONSTANT DOMAINS.

constant domains the C-terminal regions of heavy and light chains of immunoglobulins; they contain the amino acid sequences that are similar in different antibodies of the same class. See also C_H DOMAINS; C_L DOMAIN.

constipation a condition in which the alimentary transit time is prolonged in view of the amount and type of food being ingested in the preceding day or two. This means usually that the feces are hard, dry and of small bulk and are passed less frequently than expected. They may also be difficult to pass and this may cause some straining; on rectal examination the rectum will be full of hard, dry feces. In some cases a small amount of very thin, soupy feces will be passed even though there is a sizable mass in the rectum; this is soft contents being passed around an impacted fecal mass, and OBSTIPATION is said to be present.

dietary c. caused by ingestion of large amounts of foreign material such as bones, hair or fiber that mixes with feces to form hard, dry masses which are difficult or impossible to pass.

drug-induced c. may result from treatment with antimotility drugs.

endocrine c. may accompany some disorders of endocrine glands causing reduced gastrointestinal motility, e.g. hypothyroidism and hypercalcemia of hyperparathyroidism.

environmental c. conditions of management, particularly in dogs and cats, that inhibit freedom for defecation or present unsuitable conditions, such as soiled litter trays or restriction of a house-trained animal to a cage, may cause retention of feces with eventual drying and increased size of the fecal mass.

neurogenic c. disorders of innervation to the colon or hindquarters may cause an atonic colon or prevent an animal from assuming normal posture for defecation, thereby inhibiting the desire to defecate. This is seen particularly in painful intervertebral disk lesions or musculoskeletal injuries or lesions.

obstructive c. any impediment to the passage of feces, either within the colon, rectum or anus, or from compression by surrounding tissues can cause drying and enlargement of the fecal mass.

spastic c. see irritable COLON syndrome.

constitution 1. the makeup or functional habit of the body. 2. the order in which the atoms of a molecule are joined together.

constitutional 1. affecting the whole constitution of the body; not local. 2. pertaining to the constitution.

constitutive produced at a steady rate, independent of internal or external stimuli. Said of enzymes, RNA or protein by an organism.

constriction a narrowing or compression of a part; a stricture.

constrictive restricting movement or dilatation of an organ.

Constrictor constrictor a large, nonvenomous snake of the subfamily Pythoninae. Called also python, boa constrictor.

constrictor muscle plain muscle surrounding cylindrical organs at orifices.

c. pupillae muscle muscle constricting the pupil.

c. vestibuli muscle muscles constricting the vagina.

c. vulvae muscle muscle constricting the vulva.

constructive occupation activities provided for caged or confined animals to prevent them developing vices.

consult to give or seek advice. The client may consult the advice of the practitioner who may then consult a specialist or consultant.

consultant a physician or surgeon whose opinion on diagnosis or treatment is sought by the physician originally attending a patient.

c. practice to be in practice as a consultant and give specialist advice to other veterinarians. In many instances the consultant is also in practice as a general practitioner, something that is not allowed in human medicine.

consultation 1. the seeing of a patient by a general practitioner. 2. a deliberation of two or more physicians about diagnosis or treatment in a particular case.

consulting rooms the place of work of a private practitioner. They may be attached to a clinic or a hospital.

consumer affairs bureau a bureau conducted by government services to inquire into complaints about prices charged and quality of goods. Usually intended to deal with matters of trade but tend to invade professional territories, including veterinary practice.

consumerism a policy dedicated to promoting the interests of consumers as a whole.

consumption the act of consuming, or the process of being consumed, as in consumption coagulopathy where a failure to clot has been caused by a consumption of platelets. See also disseminated intravascular COAGULATION.

contact 1. a mutual touching of two bodies or animals. 2. an animal known to have been sufficiently near an infected animal to have been exposed to the transfer of infectious material.

c. activation the initiation of the intrinsic pathway of coagulation that occurs when whole blood contacts glass or similar surfaces; involves the conversion of factor XII into its active form, factor XIIa. This subsequently converts factor XI to XIa and so the COAGULATION cascade begins.

c. allergy see contact dermatitis (below).

bone c. repair repair of a fracture by contact apposition of the two fracture surfaces.

c. dermatitis is caused by direct contact between the skin and a substance which is irritating or to which the animal is allergic or sensitive. The reaction usually occurs only on that area of the body that has come into contact with the substance. See also ALLERGIC contact dermatitis.

direct c., immediate c. the contact, by sharing the same accommodation or pasture or group, of a healthy animal with an animal having a communicable disease, the disease being transmitted as a result. See also contact TRANSMISSION.

c. healing a form of primary bone healing at a fracture site where there is cortical bone in contact.

c. hypersensitivity see ALLERGIC contact dermatitis.

indirect c. that achieved through some intervening medium, as propagation of a communicable disease through the air or by means of fomites or another animal, e.g. an infection may be passed to animal A from animal B via animal C; animal C is an indirect contact.

c. irritant dermatitis skin disease produced by contact with an irritating substance; in contrast with allergic contact dermatitis, an immune reaction is not involved.

mediate c. indirect contact.

contactant an allergen capable of inducing delayed contact-type hypersensitivity of the epidermis after one or more episodes of contact.

contagion 1. the spread of disease from one animal to another. 2. a contagious disease.

contagious capable of being transmitted from animal to animal.

c. abortion see BRUCELLOSIS.

c. agalactia acute mastitis, arthritis and ophthalmitis with painful joint swelling in goats and sheep caused by *Mycoplasma agalactiae*. Abortion is common, the udder is permanently damaged and many animals die.

c. aphtha see FOOT-AND-MOUTH DISEASE.

c. avian epithelioma see FOWLPOX.

c. bovine pleuropneumonia a highly infectious septicemia with a principal localization in the lungs, caused by *Mycoplasma mycoides* var. *mycoides*. It occurs only in cattle. The cardinal signs are cough, fever, dyspnea, pleuritic friction sounds and gurgling breath sounds on auscultation of the lungs. The case fatality rate is high. An important epidemiological characteristic is the common occurrence of carrier animals with sequestra of infected material in the lungs.

c. bovine pyelonephritis infection of the urinary tract of cattle by *Corynebacterium cystitidis* with lesions in the kidney, ureters and bladder. Diagnostic signs are the passage of urine containing blood or discrete red cells and pus, dysuria and palpable abnormalities per rectum of affected organs. Culture of urine confirms the diagnosis.

c. caprine/ovine pleuropneumonia highly infectious and fatal pleuropneumonia of goats and sheep. *Mycoplasma mycoides* var. *mycoides* is generally considered to be the cause. The clinical picture includes a short course with cough, dyspnea, and abnormal lung and pleural sounds on auscultation.

c. ecthyma see contagious ECTHYMA.

c. epididymitis and vaginitis see EPIVAG.

equine c. acne see CANADIAN HORSEPOX.

c. equine metritis a highly contagious venereal disease resident in mares and transmitted by the stallion, which shows no clinical signs. It is caused by *Haemophilus equigenitalis*. Clinically there is a profuse purulent discharge from the vulva about a week after service, endometritis and cervicitis.

c. equine pustular dermatitis see CANADIAN HORSEPOX.

c. mastitis see MASTITIS.

c. ophthalmia see contagious OPHTHALMIA.

c. ovine foot rot see ovine FOOTROT.

c. ovine/caprine ophthalmia see contagious OPHTHALMIA.

c. ovine pustular dermatitis see contagious ECTHYMA.

c. porcine pyoderma an infectious disease of young sucking pigs characterized by pustules on the face and neck from which streptococci and staphylococci are isolatable. The disease develops from infection of bite wounds inflicted by piglets whose needle teeth have not been removed.

c. pustular stomatitis see HORSEPOX.

c. pyoderma see EXUDATIVE epidermitis.

c. venereal infection of sheep see ULCERATIVE dermatosis.

c. venereal tumor see canine transmissible VENEREAL tumor.

contaminant something that causes contamination.

contaminated waste milk milk kept from the milk vat because the cow or a quarter has been treated with an antibiotic and the withholding period has not expired.

contamination 1. the soiling or making inferior by contact or mixture, as by introduction of infectious organisms into a wound, into water, milk, food or onto the external surface of the body or on bandages and other dressings. 2. the deposition of radioactive material in any place where it is not desired.

continence the ability to exercise voluntary control over natural impulses, such as the urge to defecate or urinate.

Continental toy spaniels the European name for dogs recognized elsewhere as two varieties of the PAPILLON.

contingency a critical event such as birth or death or affliction with a particular disease.

c. coefficient see contingency COEFFICIENT.

c. table tabular classification of epidemiological data in horizontal lines and vertical rows, e.g. cause of death vertically and age horizontally, so that each patient appears only once.

continual throughput housing drafts of finished fattening or growing animals are moved out for sale or to other accommodation as they reach their target weight or age so that animals are leaving all the time and their replacements arrive at the same irregular intervals. Compare with all-in-all-out housing.

continuing care a professional convention that a veterinarian who is treating an animal is obliged to continue treating that case unless an arrangement is made with its custodian to transfer the care to another practitioner or to a specialist.

continuing education educational courses relating to veterinary science, provided by an institution or recognized organization which supplements, brings up to date and refreshes the information that the graduate veterinarian already has. In some countries and professions a specified amount of such education is required to be completed each year by each veterinarian who wishes to continue his/her registration.

continuous continuing indefinitely without the need for renewal.

c. clinical service veterinarians are required by convention to provide a service to their clients at all times, either directly or by referral to a comparable practice.

c. health assessment provided by a herd health program in which monthly visits to the farm by a veterinarian are a feature.

c. positive airway pressure (CPAP) see CONTINUOUS POSITIVE AIRWAY PRESSURE.

c. stationery paper folded fanwise with perforations at standard page sizes, with pinholes at the margins to facilitate use by tractor-driven printers.

c. variable see continuous VARIABLE.

c. wave Doppler see DOPPLER ULTRASOUND.

continuous positive airway pressure a method of medical gas administration in which gas is delivered to the patient at positive pressure in order to hold open alveoli that would normally close at the end of expiration and thereby increase oxygenation, preventing atelectasis, and reduce the work of breathing; abbreviated CPAP. It is used with patients who are breathing spontaneously. When the same principle is used in mechanical ventilation, it is called positive end-expiratory pressure.

continuous power system the dressing system in an abattoir in which the line is moving continuously. Suitable only for large abattoirs with a high kill rate.

contour feather see contour FEATHER.

contra- word element. [L.] *against, opposed.*

contra-aperture a second opening made in an abscess to facilitate the discharge of its contents. Called also counteropening.

Contracaecum a genus of roundworms in the family Anisakidae. Includes *Contracaecum microcephalum*, *C. spiculigerum* (wild birds), *C. osculatum* (in seals, other fish eaters).

contraception prevention of conception or impregnation. Little practiced in the animal world (except in dogs and cats), population control being effected by other means. Is used in some less-developed communities where cattle are used as draft animals.

immunological c. involves immune-mediated control of hormone or degeneration of reproductive tissues. Some methods investigated in dogs include immunization with bovine or ovine luteinizing hormone (LH) or gonadotropin so that cross-reacting antibodies neutralize the animal's own hormone. Antibodies to porcine zona pellucida antigens inhibit fertilization and implantation.

contraceptive 1. diminishing the likelihood of or preventing conception. 2. an agent that diminishes the likelihood of or prevents conception. See also CONTRACEPTION.

contracted having undergone contraction, especially in length.

c. foal syndrome a congenital disease of unknown origin in foals characterized by contractural deformities of axial and appendicular joints. Asymmetry of the skull, eventration of viscera, torticollis and scoliosis may also be present.

c. foot see contracted heels (see below).

c. heels the heels of affected horses are drawn in, the bars are almost parallel and the frog is much reduced in size. Lameness is a common accompaniment. Called also contracted hoof, contracted foot.

c. hooves see contracted heels (above).

c. tendon see TENDON contracture.

contractile having the power or tendency to contract in response to a suitable stimulus.

c. proteins myosin, the main constituent of thick filaments of muscle, and actin, main constituent of thin muscle filaments.

contractility a capacity for becoming short in response to suitable stimulus.

cardiac c. the inotropic state of the myocardium; a major determinant of cardiac output and an important factor in cardiac compensation.

contraction a drawing together; a shortening or shrinkage.

isovolumetric c. ventricular muscle contraction during early systole after closure of the atrioventricular valves and before the semilunar valves open; the muscle continues to contract, forcing up the ventricular pressure without any change in the ventricular volume.

muscle c. see MUSCLE.

myocardial c. individual myocardial cells transmit motor impulses across cell boundaries and act as a syncytium.

c. phase the stage in wound healing when there is centripetal movement of surrounding tissues and the area of the wound decreases. This is believed to be a cell-mediated phenomenon, involving myofibroblasts.

postural c. the state of muscular tension and contraction that just suffices to maintain the posture of the body.

striated muscle c. see MUSCLE.

tetanic c., tonic c. sustained muscular contraction with alternating relaxation.

contractor the role adopted by a veterinarian who employs others, especially technicians, to carry out specific tasks, e.g. mulesing of sheep, without being financially liable for the quality of their work.

contracts agreements between parties in which considerations or rewards are offered by all contracting parties. Contracts may be written, verbal or implied and all are binding, the degree lessening as the probability of misunderstanding increases. Salaries, continuity of employment, out-of-hours attendance, weekend work are some of the considerations offered in veterinary employment contracts.

binding-out c. one of the parties binds himself or herself not to participate in some activity, e.g. practice within a certain area, in return for some consideration such as being employed as an assistant.

implied c. leaving a patient in a veterinarian's care is an implied contract by the owner to pay the costs of the attention provided. This may be estimated beforehand and the veterinarian may be obliged to adhere to the estimate, especially if the difference is large. It depends on the firmness of the offer.

contractual veterinary fees see FEES.

contracture abnormal shortening of muscle tissue, rendering the muscle highly resistant to stretching. A contracture can lead to permanent disability. It can be caused by fibrosis of the tissues supporting the muscle or the joint, or by disorders of the muscle fibers themselves.

flexor c. joint fixed in flexion.

inherited multiple tendon c. see INHERITED MULTIPLE TENDON CONTRACTURE.

contrafissure a fracture in a part opposite the site of the blow.

contraindication any condition that renders a particular line of treatment improper or undesirable.

contralateral pertaining to, situated on, or affecting the opposite side.

contrast radiographically the degree of perceptible difference between two color tones. Black and white images on the one film is said to be high contrast; an all gray film has low or nil contrast.

c. agents Contrast agents are used for injection into the vascular system for either a local visualization of a system or organ or for outlining an excretory system. Radiolucent (negative) contrast media are gases such as air, oxygen or carbon dioxide. The radiopaque (positive) contrast media include the insoluble salt barium sulfate and a variety of organic iodine compounds.

Barium is used for gastrointestinal studies. Water-soluble, iodinated contrast media excreted by the kidneys are used for many procedures, including all types of angiography and for intravenous and retrograde urography. Those excreted by the liver are used for oral or intravenous cholangiography or cholecystography. New, nonirritant iodine compounds have been developed for myelography. Oily iodinated media are used for lymphangiography and bronchography.

double c. the use of two contrast agents or two routes of administration in the one patient. For example, radiopaque dye and then air in the urinary bladder.

c. materials see contrast agents (above).

c. medium a substance used in radiography to permit visualization of internal body structures. Called also contrast agent, contrast material.

negative c. a contrast material that is not radiopaque such as air or carbon dioxide.

c. pattern the pattern made by the contrast agent. Includes confined extension patterns in diverticula and similar confined spaces, and unconfined extensions, e.g. in bladder rupture.

positive c. the use of a contrast material that is radiopaque such as barium sulfate and iodinated products.

triple c. the use of three contrast media or routes in the one patient at the one time.

water-soluble c. agents agents used for injection into the vascular system for either a local visualization of a system or organ or for outlining an excretory system. In the past these have consisted mostly of iodine preparations which are irritant and cause tissue damage so that they must be injected intravenously. However, there are now available some recently developed water-soluble iodine preparations that are nonirritant and which can be used in myelography. See also CONTRAST.

contrecoup [Fr.] denoting an injury, as to the brain, occurring at a site opposite to the point of impact.

contributory negligence a common countersuit to a charge of negligence. For example, it could be alleged that a fatal outcome to a surgical operation on an animal, the basis for a suit alleging negligence, has been contributed to by the owners because they did not seek further assistance until it was too late.

control 1. the governing or limitation of certain objects or events. 2. a standard against which experimental observations may be evaluated, as a procedure identical to the experimental procedure except for the one factor being studied; a requirement of any planned experimental study. Also, any individual of the group exhibiting the standard characteristics.

disease c. restraining or reducing the prevalence of individual disease. Includes the range of strategies from limitation of occurrence to eradication. Implies legislative control of notifiable disease.

c. elements nucleotide sequences on DNA that usually precede (upstream) the sequences coding for the structural gene at which regulator proteins act.

c. factor in a comparison between diseases caused by a number of contributing factors it may be necessary to supply controls for one or more of these factors.

c. group the group of animals with which the experimental group is to be matched; the group which has not had its variables manipulated experimentally. The selection of the animals to be included in the two groups may be based on matching them with respect to age, to their history of nutrition or inheritance, or vaccination or prophylactic treatment. Called also controls.

ovulation c. prevention of ovulation by administration of progesterone or stimulation of ovulation by injection of follicle-stimulating hormone are examples.

paired c. comparison between the experimental and control groups is most accurate if the control animal for each experimental animal is selected to be as similar as possible, i.e. a paired control.

c. pole a pole with a noose at the end used to catch and restrain small animals.

c. population a large control group.

population c. a variety of techniques are used with CONTRACEPTION being least used. Permanent surgical interference is common in food, racing and companion animal groups, and termination of pregnancy and estrus synchronization, both by hormonal means, are also extensively practiced. Increasing the culling rate is the standard procedure for dealing with a feed shortage.

x-ray c. unit the controlling mechanisms in an x-ray machine. Include the voltmeter and voltage compensator control, the kilovoltage, milliameter and milliamperage selectors and the timer and exposure control button.

controlled subjected to control.

c. breeding manipulation of mating and conception so as take advantage of seasonal demands for products, most favorable time for fertility or survival of offspring or for the purpose of controlling the size of the population. Includes managemental deferral of breeding, permanent surgical interference with male or female tracts and temporary hormonal suppression of reproductive activity.

c. environment buildings in which all food and drinking water are supplied and ambient temperature, humidity, air movement and light provision are controlled.

c. experiment one in which the experimental group which is to be subjected to a treatment or change in management is matched with a group which is very similar in every way except with respect to the variable that is to be manipulated.

c. release glass bolus see soluble GLASS.

c. vocabulary a database in which the names of diagnoses or medicines, etc. are limited to avoid a continual expansion of the titles, making comparisons between groups difficult.

Controlled Substances Act the law that regulates the prescribing and dispensing of dangerous substances, especially psychoactive drugs, including narcotics, hallucinogens, depressants and stimulants.

contuse to bruise; to injure without breaking the skin.

contusion injury to tissues without breakage of skin; a bruise. In a contusion, blood from the broken vessels accumulates in surrounding tissues, producing pain, swelling and tenderness. In light-colored animals a discoloration may appear as a result of blood seepage under the surface of the skin.

Serious complications may develop in some cases of contusion. Normally blood is drawn off from the bruised area in a few days, but there is a possibility that blood clotted in the area will form a cyst or calcify and require surgical treatment. The contusion may also be complicated by infection.

cerebral c. contusion of the brain following a HEAD injury. It may occur with extradural or subdural collections of blood, in which case the patient may be left with neurological defects or EPILEPSY.

Conus a genus of shellfish in the family Conidae.

C. catus stings of these shellfish are lethal for humans.

conus pl. *coni* [L.] 1. a cone or cone-shaped structure. 2. posterior staphyloma of the myopic eye.

c. arteriosus the funnel-shaped portion of the right ventricle of the heart at the entrance to the pulmonary trunk.

c. medullaris the cone-shaped caudal end of the spinal cord; found at the level of the upper lumbar vertebrae in the human spine, but more caudally in domestic animals.

convalescence the stage of recovery from an illness, operation or injury.

convalescent 1. pertaining to or characterized by convalescence. 2. a patient who is recovering from a disease, operation or injury.

convallamarin one of the toxic cardiac glycosides in the plant CONVALLARIA MAJALIS.

Convallaria majalis a toxic plant of the family Liliaceae; contains cardiac glycosides; causes cardiomyopathy, sudden death, diarrhea. Called also lily-of-the-valley.

convallarin one of the cardiac glycosides in CONVALLARIA MAJALIS.

convalloside one of the cardiac glycosides in the plant CONVALLARIA MAJALIS.

convection the act of conveying or transmission; specifically, transmission of heat in a liquid or gas by circulation of heated particles.

convenience pet foods commercial pet foods.

convention nonlegal rules of conduct with respect to other persons generally. In a professional sense means rules of conduct in relation to clients.

convergence 1. a moving together, or inclination toward a common point; the coordinated movement of the two eyes toward fixation of the same near point. 2. the point of meeting of convergent lines.

conversational mode a dialog mode at a computer terminal at which the operator answers questions posed by the computer program. Used in decision tree diagnostic programs.

conversion 1. the act of changing into something of different form or properties. 2. manipulative correction of malposition of a fetal part during labor.

c. formulae formulae for conversion of one numerical mode of expression into a different mode, e.g. avoirdupois to metric weight.

c. ratio a measure of activity of the thyroid gland; it expresses the proportion of the total radioactivity of the plasma, subsequent to the injection of radioactive iodine, which is bound to protein (PROTEIN-BOUND iodine test).

convertase an enzyme that converts a substance to its active state.

converter plants plants which convert an element such as selenium from a source from which it is usually unavailable to a soluble form that other plants can use.

convex having a rounded, somewhat elevated surface.

c. face see CIS FACE.

c. sole see DROPPED sole.

convolution a tortuous irregularity or elevation caused by the infolding of a structure upon itself.

Convolvulus purpureus IPOMOEA *purpurea*.

convulsant a drug which causes convulsions.

convulsion a series of involuntary contractions of the voluntary muscles. Convulsive seizures are symptomatic of some neurological disorder; they are not in themselves a disease entity. In animals, they are most often caused by infectious agents and toxins. Convulsions are also produced by any of a number of metabolic disorders, such as hypoglycemia, hypocalcemia and hormonal imbalances; brain cell injury from head trauma, tumors and degenerative neural disease; anoxia and hemorrhage which deprive brain cells of vital substances; and acute cerebral edema which interferes with normal brain cell function. Epilepsy is also a cause of convulsions in dogs and cattle. Called also fit, ictus. See also SEIZURE.

inherited c. and ataxia of cattle see FAMILIAL convulsions and ataxia of cattle.

convulsive pertaining to, characterized by, or of the nature of a convulsion.

c. ergotism see ERGOT[1].

c. foal syndrome see NEONATAL maladjustment syndrome.

c. seizure see CONVULSION.

cooba, cooby see ACACIA *salicina*.

cook tree THEVETIA *peruviana*.

Cooktown ironwood ERYTHROPHLEUM *chlorostachys*.

Cooktown loquat see RHODOMYRTUS MACROCARPA.

Coolah grass see PANICUM *coloratum*.

coolant a substance used to cool a system to below a specified level by conducting heat generated by the system away from it.

Cooley forceps a type of surgical thumb forceps with longitudinal ribs.

cooling systems for housed animals include spraying of roofs with water, evaporative pads with fans, foggers and misters; for pastured animals shelter from the sun by trees or artificial shade devices and cooling ponds are used.

Coombs tests laboratory tests that reveal certain antibody–antigen reactions; used in differentiating between various types of hemolytic anemias, for determining minor blood types, and for testing for alloimmune hemolytic disease of the newborn. Called also antiglobulin test.

direct C. t. the test used to detect the presence of cell-bound antibodies that may damage erythrocytes but will not cause visible agglutination. The red cells are washed free of serum and unbound antibody, and antiglobulin (species-specific antiserum directed against antibodies) is added. Agglutination indicates the presence of antibody. Clinically its most important use is in the diagnosis of ALLOIMMUNE hemolytic anemia of the newborn (Rh disease in humans) and autoimmune hemolytic ANEMIA.

indirect C. t. detects antierythrocyte antibodies in the serum. Test serum is incubated with red blood cells. The cells are then washed and mixed with antiglobulin serum. Agglutination indicates the presence of antibody in test serum. Supernatant from colostrum may be used instead of serum.

coon see RACCOON.

c. foot conformation defect in a horse in which the pastern is too long and sloping.

Coonabarabran ataxia see TRIBULUS *terrestris*.

coonhound a term loosely applied to a number of varieties of hunting dogs in the southern United States, few of which are recognized as specific breeds. See BLACK AND TAN COONHOUND, BLUETICK COONHOUND, ENGLISH COONHOUND, REDBONE COONHOUND, TREEING WALKER COONHOUND.

c. paralysis see POLYRADICULONEURITIS.

coonties ZAMIA *integrifolia*.

cooperative breeding schemes see GROUP breeding schemes.

cooperativity interaction between some proteins in which the binding of one may increase or decrease binding of the other.

Cooperia a genus of intestinal worms in the family Trichostrongylidae. Principal infestations in sheep and goats, *C. punctata*, *C. oncophora*, *C. curticei*; in cattle, *C. oncophora*, *C. pectinata*, *C. punctata*; miscellaneous infections with other species in ruminants generally are *C. bisonis*, *C. spatulata*, *C. surnabada* (syn. *C. mcmasteri*). The worms inhabit the small intestine. See also COOPERIASIS.

Cooperia pedunculata North American plant in the Liliaceae family; contains furanocoumarin causing primary photosensitization. Both dead and green leaves are toxic. Called also giant prairie lily, thunder lily, *Zephranthes*.

cooperiasis infestation of sheep and cattle with *Cooperia* spp.; causes diarrhea and wasting. The mortality rate without treatment can be serious but the most important losses are caused by poor weight gains in the survivors. See also COOPERIA PEDUNCULATA.

Coopworth New Zealand bred low-care sheep with medium wool, used principally as a meat sheep; originated by crossbreeding of Romney Marsh and Border Leicester breeds.

coordinates of a point on a graph or grid map, the points on the horizontal and vertical axes which identify the location of the point on the graph/map.

coordination the harmonious functioning of interrelated organs and parts. Applied especially to the process of the motor apparatus of the brain which provides for the coworking of particular groups of muscles for the performance of definite adaptive useful responses.

c. defect lack of refinement in the coordination of complex movements such as walking or trotting.

COP colloid osmotic pressure.

COPD chronic obstructive pulmonary disease (COPD).

copepod a member of the subclass Copepoda of

marine invertebrate parasites. There are more than 4500 species. Includes *Cyclops* spp. intermediate host for *Spirometra erinacei*, *Diphyllobothrium latum*.

Coplin jars wide-mouthed glass jars, usually with vertically grooved interior walls, used for the storage or staining of slides containing blood smears or tissue sections.

copper a chemical element, atomic number 29, atomic weight 63.54, symbol Cu. See Table 6. It is necessary for bone formation and for the formation of blood because it occurs in several oxidative enzymes including one involved in the transformation of inorganic iron into hemoglobin.

c. acetoarsenite an oldfashioned green pigment used in plaster, wallpaper, etc. A possible cause of chronic arsenic poisoning in very old houses. Called also Paris green.

c.-associated hepatopathy see BEDLINGTON TERRIER copper-associated hepatopathy.

c. calcium edetate used as a prophylactic in lambs and calves against swayback and hypocuprosis. Overdosing causes liver damage and severe subcutaneous edema and ascites.

c.-chrome–arsenate poisoning the preservative in 'treated pine'. Nibbling the wood causes poisoning in confined animals.

copper–molybdenum–sulfate relationship molybdenum combines with sulfur in the rumen to form Cu–Mo–S complexes (copper–thiomolybdates) which reduce the availability of copper in the ingesta.

c. naphthenate a complex of copper and naphthenic acid, used as a fungicide and insecticide. A treatment for footrot in cattle and sheep, and for thrush in horses.

c. nutritional deficiency in ruminants this causes anemia and demyelination in the central nervous system. The deficiency may be primary or secondary due to intervention of high dietary intakes of sulfate and molybdenum. In pigs incoordination and anemia have been recorded. Horses appear unaffected. Called also enzootic ataxia, swayback, coast disease, pine, peat scours, teart, falling disease, hypocuprosis, licking sickness, liksucht. Copper deficiency is rare in dogs and cats and is most likely to occur from excessive supplementation with calcium, which reduces absorption of many minerals, including copper.

c. poisoning may be acute because of accidental administration of inorganic preparations of copper, usually as a worm drench. Chronic poisoning is usually due to grazing on pasture growing on soils naturally rich in copper. The prevalence may be increased by the presence of converter plants, especially subterranean clover, which have a high uptake of copper, or of plants which cause liver damage and the sudden discharge of large amounts of copper which have accumulated in the liver. Such plants are *Heliotropum, Senecio* and *Echium* spp. Copper compounds reported to have caused poisoning in animals include the subacetate, oxychloride, chloride, oxide, naphthenate, carbonate, arsenite, sulfate.

Acute poisoning is characterized by gastroenteritis; chronic poisoning is a syndrome of acute hemolytic anemia caused by a sudden elevation of blood copper levels. The obvious signs are jaundice, hemoglobinuria and pallor of mucosae. Poisoning by organic copper preparations administered therapeutically causes nephrosis and death due to uremia. Called also toxemic jaundice. See also BEDLINGTON TERRIER copper-associated hepatopathy.

c. storage disease see BEDLINGTON TERRIER copper-associated hepatopathy.

c. sulfate used as a parasiticide in aquariums and in the treatment of foot rot in cattle.

copper burr SCLEROLAENA *calcarata*.

copper–chrome–arsenate wood preservative a wood preservative. See also CHROME–ARSENIC–COPPER.

copper nose photosensitive dermatitis affecting the muzzle of cattle.

copperbottle see LUCILIA *cuprina*.

copperhead snakes light copper-brown to black venomous snakes. Called also *Denisonia superba*, *Austrelaps superba* or *Agkistrodon contortrix*.

copperweed see OXYTENIA ACEROSA.

copra meal see COCONUT meal.

copra mite see TYROPHAGUS *longior*.

copracrasia fecal incontinence.

copremesis the vomiting of fecal matter.

coproantibody an antibody (chiefly IgA) present in the intestinal tract, associated with immunity to enteric infection.

coproculture culture of the feces for the purpose of hatching parasite eggs and obtaining larvae for morphological identification.

coprodeum, coprodaeum the cranial or deepest compartment of the CLOACA of birds.

COPROgen see COPROPORPHYRINOGEN.

coprolith a hard fecal concretion in the intestine.

coprology the study of the feces.

coprophagia see COPROPHAGY.

coprophagy the ingestion of dung or feces; a vice in dogs; normal in rabbits. Called also cecotrophy.

coprophilia a preoccupation with feces.

coprophilic emanating from or pertaining to coprophilia.

coproporphyria porphyria marked by excessive excretion of coproporphyrin, chiefly in the feces.

coproporphyrin a porphyrin formed in the blood-forming organs and intestine and found in the urine and feces. There are two chemically distinct substances, coproporphyrins I and III.

coproporphyrinogen the fully reduced, colorless compound giving rise to coproporphyrin by oxidation.

coproporphyrinuria the presence of excess coproporphyrin in the urine.

coprostasis fecal impaction.

coprozoic living in fecal matter.

copse laurel DAPHNE *laureola*.

copula any connecting part or structure.

copulation sexual union or coitus; usually applied to animals other than humans.

c. behavior see MATING behavior.

c. tie GENITAL lock.

copulatory pertaining to or emanating from copulation.

c. apparatus those parts of the genital organs involved in copulation; the penis, vulva and vagina. Term used in relation to birds where genitalia are concealed.

c. inability the male is able to maintain an erection but unable to penetrate the female.

c. tie during the second stage of coitus the male dog dismounts and faces the opposite way to the bitch but they remain locked together by their genitals for some minutes. Called also GENITAL lock.

copy number the number of plasmid or other DNA molecules in a cell.

CoQ coenzyme Q (ubiquinone).

coquera local name for the disease caused by poisoning by the pods of PROSOPIS JULIFLORIA.

cor [L.] *cordis*. See also HEART.

c. adiposum a heart that has undergone fatty degeneration or that has an accumulation of fat around it.
c. biloculare congenital defect with only two chambers in the heart.
c. bovinum a greatly enlarged heart due to a hypertrophied left ventricle, an inappropriate term when said of cattle.
c. pulmonale right ventricular heart failure due to pulmonary hypertension secondary to disease of blood vessels of the lung; usually chronic and due to COPD or heartworm disease. Clinical signs are those of right-sided congestive heart failure.
c. rugosum see cor villosum (below).
c. triatriatum dexter a rare congenital anomaly in which the right atrium is divided into two chambers by a persistence of the right sinus venosus valve resulting in obstruction of venous return.
c. triloculare a congenital defect of a heart with three chambers, which may be one atrium or one ventricle.
c. villosum means hairy heart; when the epicardium is covered with shaggy fibrinous tags as a result of chronic pericarditis.

coracidium first larval stage of a pseudophyllidean cestode; this motile stage consists of a ciliated embryophore containing the oncosphere.

coracoid 1. like a crow's beak. 2. the stout bone of the avian shoulder that is braced against the sternum. 3. the coracoid process, a projection from the rim of the glenoid of the scapula.

Coragyps atratus see VULTURE.

coral berry see RIVINA HUMILIS.

coral bush JATROPHA *multifida*.

coral fungus see RAMARIA.

coral pea see ABRUS *precatorius*.

coral plant JATROPHA *multifida*.

Corallocytostroma fungus infesting Mitchell grass (*Astrebla* spp.) in northwest Australia causing BLACK SOIL BLINDNESS.

Corchorus olitorius tropical jute plant in family Tiliaceae; its seeds contaminate cereal grain; contain a cardiac glycoside; cause sudden death. Called also jute.

cord any long, cylindrical, flexible structure.
angiogenic c. the embryonic beginnings in the lateral mesenchyme of the dorsal aortae and aortic arches; at first solid they later become patent.
scirrhous c. enlargement of the stump of the spermatic cord, common only in pigs and horses, and usually obvious within a few weeks of castration. The swelling may cause lameness, is painful and may be accompanied by systemic signs of fever and toxemia. The lesion is a mass of fibrous tissue interspersed with small abscess cavities and sinus tracts.
spermatic c. the structure extending from the abdominal inguinal ring to the testis, comprising the pampiniform plexus, nerves, ductus deferens, cremaster muscle, vaginal tunics, testicular artery and other vessels.
spinal c. see SPINAL CORD.
umbilical c. the structure connecting the fetus and placenta, and containing the channels through which fetal blood passes to and from the placenta.
vocal c's see VOCAL cords.

cord factor a surface lipid, 6,6′,dimycoloyl-α,α′-D-trehalose, of *Mycobacterium* spp. Its pathogenic significance is now regarded as uncertain.

cordal pertaining to a cord; used specifically in referring to the vocal cords.

cordate heart-shaped.

cordectomy excision of a cord, as of a vocal cord.

cording-up see TYING-UP SYNDROME.

corditis inflammation of the spermatic cord.

cordopexy surgical fixation of a vocal cord.

Cordophilus see ELAEOPHORA.

cordotomy 1. section of a vocal cord. 2. surgical division of the anterolateral tracts of the spinal cord. Not usually carried out in veterinary surgery.

Cordylobia a genus of blowflies of the family Calliphoridae.
C. anthropophaga the maggot parasitizes humans, rodents, monkeys and dogs causing cutaneous lumps. Called also tumbu or skin-maggot fly.
C. rodhaini the maggot causes skin lesions in antelope, rodents and humans. Called also Lund's fly.

core-elective educational programs core subjects are taken by all students in the class, being considered to be essential to all studies in the curriculum; other subjects are thought to be not essential to all students and therefore offered for special interest selection (election).

core sample sample of wool collected by passing a sharp hollow instrument through the bale; the sample is examined for color, contaminants and fiber diameter and the bale is sold on the basis of the sample and the weight of the bale.

corectasis morbid dilatation of the pupil of the eye.

corectome a cutting instrument for iridectomy.

corectomy iridectomy.

corectopia abnormal location of the pupil of the eye.

coredialysis surgical separation of the external margin of the iris from the ciliary body.

corediastasis dilatation of the pupil.

coregonid a member of the fish family Coregonidae.

corelysis operative destruction of the pupil; especially detachment of adhesions of the pupillary margin of the iris from the lens.

coremorphosis surgical formation of an artificial pupil.

corenclisis see IRIDENCLEISIS.

core(o)- word element. [Gr.] *pupil of the eye.*

coreometer see PUPILLOMETER.

coreoplasty any plastic operation on the pupil.

corepressor a substance (e.g. the product of a metabolic pathway) that activates a repressor by combining with it.

coretomy see IRIDOTOMY.

Corgi see WELSH CORGI.

Cori cycle pathway by which muscle lactate contributes to blood glucose. Lactate formed in muscle by glycolysis is transported to the liver and resynthesized to glucose there. Called also lactic acid cycle.

Cori's disease see GLYCOGENOSIS type III.

Coriaria New Zealand plant genus of the plant family, Coriaraceae; all parts of the plant are poisonous and cause excitation, vomiting, convulsions, exhaustion and death. Tutin, the toxin in the plant, is passed to the meat of poisoned animals and to honey in the neighborhood of the plants. Includes *C. angustissima*, *C. arborea*, *C. kingiana*, *C. lurida*, *C. plumosa*, *C. pottsiana*, *C. pteroides*, *C. sarmentosa*. Called also tutu.

coriitis inflammation of the corium of the hoof; see LAMINITIS.

coriosis degeneration of the corium of the hoof; see LAMINITIS.

corium the dermis; true skin; the fibrous inner layer of the skin just beneath the epidermis, derived from the embryonic mesoderm, well supplied with nerves and blood vessels and containing hair roots and sebaceous and sweat glands. See also DERMIS.
coronary c. specialized corium at the coronary band of ungulates providing nourishment via papillae

which extend into the hoof. Separated from the skin by the perioplic corium.

cuneal c. corium of the frog of the equine hoof.

foot c. see cuneal corium (above).

laminar c. corium of the sensitive laminae of the hoof. Bears laminae which interdigitate with lamellae of the hoof wall. Supplies nutrition to the horn and to the white zone of interlamellar horn.

papillary c. see coronary corium (above).

perioplic c. continuous with the corium of the skin, forming a narrow band between the skin and the coronary corium.

solear c. the corium of the sole of the foot, supporting the horn of the sole.

corkscrew a deformity in which the affected part is spiraled like a corkscrew.

c. claw a probably heritable defect of the lateral claw, usually of the front feet, of cattle causing serious lameness. The third phalanx is small and the claw is long, thin and curls over the medial claw. It takes very little weight. Called also curved claw, curled toe.

c. penis a corkscrew twist of the anterior, free part of the penis occurs normally in the vagina when a bull makes an ejaculatory thrust. Premature corkscrew penis is an abnormality which prevents intromission. It is caused by insufficiency of the dorsal apical ligament of the penis, very rarely by trauma. Most common in polled beef breed bulls.

c. tail a short curled tail, sometimes with an abnormal setting at the butt, occurs in calves and dogs of the breeds with naturally short tails. In dogs it often leads to skin irritation with secondary pyoderma in the surrounding, deep fold of skin.

corkwood see DUBOISIA.

corky passion flower PASSIFLORA *suberosa*.

Cormo sheep bred in Tasmania, Australia by crossing fine-wool merinos with Corriedale or Polwarth sheep. Easy-care, plain-body, open-face sheep, with wool 21 to 23 microns.

cormorant a sombre, mostly black, coastal bird that dives for its prey. There are many species. Called also shag, *Phalacrocorax* and *Halietor* spp.

corn 1. a circumscribed hyperkeratosis of the footpad of dogs, sensitive to pressure. 2. a hematoma between the sensitive laminae and horn of the sole, usually between the frog and bar, in the hoof of the horse. It is painful on pressure and a cause of lameness. 3. in USA and elsewhere *Zea mays*, a member of the plant family Poaceae, grown as a cereal crop bearing seeds and used as a grain feed, green chop and ensilage. Used also for human consumption as meal or flour. The grain is deficient in most essential amino acids, especially lysine and tryptophan (high-lysine varieties are available), and in calcium and cannot be used as a complete ration in pigs. It may be fed whole, cracked, flaked, roasted, as dried or as high moisture corn (contains 25% moisture). Overeating of the grain by ruminants causes carbohydrate engorgement, and of moldy standing corn causes moldy corn poisoning. Called also maize. 4. in UK TRITICUM AESTIVUM is also called corn. 5. the name corn is also used with other cereals such as rye corn, barley corn.

c. cob see COB (2). Ground into a meal it is used as a roughage of very low nutritive value in ruminant diets. Of some value as a diluent in high grain diets.

c. cockle AGROSTEMMA *githago*.

c. oil rich source of unsaturated fatty acids, particularly linoleic acid.

wild c. see VERATRUM *californicum*.

corn gromwell see LITHOSPERMUM ARVENSE.

corn-lily see VERATRUM *californicum*.

corn poppy see PAPAVER *rhoeas*.

cornbind see FALLOPIA CONVOLVULUS.

corne- prefix meaning cornea.

cornea the clear, transparent anterior segment of the fibrous tunic of the EYE. The cornea is subject to injury by foreign bodies in the eye, and bacterial and viral infections. See also CORNEAL, KERATITIS, KERATOPATHY.

c. nigrum see CORNEAL sequestrum.

c. plana a congenital flattening of the cornea.

corneal pertaining to the CORNEA. See also KERATITIS, KERATOPATHY.

c. anomaly includes MICROCORNEA, coloboma, MEGALOCORNEA, DERMOID, congenital opacity.

c. black body see corneal sequestrum (below).

c. coloboma an uncommon congenital defect in the continuity of the cornea; may have concurrent herniation of the uveal tract. See also COLOBOMA.

c. dystrophy a developmental condition, inherited in some breeds of dogs and cats. May cause corneal edema and ulceration. See also KERATOPATHY.

c. ectasia see KERECTASIA.

c. edema occurs when fluid accumulates in the corneal stroma, disrupting the normal lamellar structure and causing a loss of transparency. Commonly called BLUE EYE.

c. erosion syndrome see refractory ULCER.

feline focal c. necrosis see corneal sequestrum (below).

c. hyaline membrane an abnormal, semitransparent membrane on the posterior surface of the cornea, attached to the endothelium. Can be associated with persistent pupillary membrane. Caused by inflammation or a developmental defect.

c. inflammation see KERATITIS.

inherited c. opacity congenital opacity of the cornea occurs in cattle. The animals are not completely blind and the rest of the eye is normal. Both eyes are affected. The lesion is an edema of the corneal lamellae.

c. laminae the limiting membranes that separate the bulk of the cornea from the covering epithelia; the anterior is Bowman's, the posterior is DESCEMET'S MEMBRANE.

c. lipidosis cholesterol crystals and lipid vacuoles may be found in the corneal stroma as a result of persistent hypercholesterolemia or chronic stromal inflammation.

melting c. see collagenase ULCER.

c. mummification see corneal sequestrum (below).

c. opacity see LEUKOMA, MACULA, NEBULA.

c. pigmentation results from chronic irritation. The melanin is in the superficial stroma and the basal layer of the corneal epithelium. See also superficial pigmentary KERATITIS.

c. reflex a reflex action of the eye resulting in automatic closing of the eyelids when the cornea is stimulated. The corneal reflex can be elicited in a normal animal by gently touching the cornea with a wisp of cotton. Absence of the corneal reflex indicates deep coma or injury of one of the nerves carrying the reflex arc.

c. ring abscess an infected corneal ulcer in which there is a surrounding zone of liquefaction encircled by a zone of neutrophils.

c. scar corneal opacity.

c. sequestrum a central, focal, dark necrotic plaque on the cornea of cats, especially Persians, associated with chronic ulcerative or inflammatory disease of

the cornea. Called also focal superficial necrosis, corneal mummification, keratitis nigrum.
c. shield protection used in the treatment of corneal ulcers or wounds; commercial products consisting of collagen which is dissolved in the tear film are claimed to enhance healing.
c. stromal depositions minerals, lipids or pigment deposited in the stroma following injury.
superficial c. erosion see refractory ULCER.
c. tattooing done mainly in horses to obscure unsightly scarring of the cornea.
c. transparency the quality of being able to see objects through the cornea; partly the result of the strict horizontal lamellal distribution of its collagen fibers, parallel to the corneal surface.
c. transplantation see KERATOPLASTY.
c. ulcer a defect in the corneal epithelium and some amount of stroma; may be caused by trauma, chronic irritation as from distichiasis, entropion or keratitis sicca, or infectious agents. Deep ulcers can lead to rupture of the cornea, the escape of aqueous humor and often prolapse of the iris with a secondary uveitis and endophthalmitis. See also ULCER.
c. vascularization results from inflammation of the cornea, the vessels growing in from the limbus. It is a necessary repair process but it reduces visual acuity.

corneitis keratitis.

Cornell named after New York State Veterinary College at Cornell University, NY, USA.
C. alternative-month accelerated lambing system enables each ewe to lamb three times in every 2 years. Called also CAMAL scheme; superseded by the STAR system (see below).
C. semen tests in vivo and in vitro tests to detect IBR virus contaminated semen samples.
C. STAR accelerated lambing system an advanced development of the Alternate Monthly Accelerated Lambing system; the ewes in this scheme are ecouraged to lamb five times in 3 years.
C. teat curette has a long thin neck and a flat blade with a blunt-ended turned around tip with a straight cutting edge. Designed for curetting back towards the operator.
C. technique see PARAVERTEBRAL block.

corneoconjunctival pertaining to the cornea and conjuctiva, as in a corneal flap which transposes tissue from the conjunctiva.

corneoiridial pertaining to the cornea and the iris.

corneoiritis inflammation of the cornea and iris; keratoiritis.

corneosclera the cornea and sclera regarded as one organ. See also CORNEOSCLERAL.

corneoscleral pertaining to or emanating from the CORNEOSCLERA.
c. junction the point at which the sclera's opaque, wavy fibers join the more neatly arranged and transparent corneal fibers. Called also limbus.
c. transposition the movement of part of the sclera to repair adjacent cornea; a keratoplasty technique.
c. trephination formation of a drainage hole through the corneoscleral junction into the anterior chamber to allow the outflow of aqueous humor into the subconjunctival vasculature and lymphatics. Used in the treatment of glaucoma.

corneoscleroconjunctival pertaining to the conjunctiva, cornea and sclera.

corneous hornlike or horny; consisting of keratin.

corniculate process hornlike process such as the process of the arytenoid cartilage.

cornification 1. conversion into keratin, or horn. 2. conversion of epithelium to the stratified squamous type.

cornified converted into horny tissue (keratin); keratinized.

Cornish a compact-bodied meat breed of poultry used extensively in crossbreeding for production of commercial meat strains. Dark, white, white-laced or red color, yellow skin and legs, brown eggs. Poor layers.

Cornish rex see REX.

cornstalk disease mycotoxic LEUKOENCEPHALOMALACIA.

cornstalk poisoning a poorly defined syndrome in cattle feeding on standing corn damaged by drought or early frost. The syndrome is one of nervous signs highlighted by dullness, weakness, recumbency, constriction of pupil and clonic convulsions before death.

cornu pl. *cornua* [L.] horn; a hornlike excrescence or projection; a structure that appears horn-shaped, especially in section. See also CORNUAL.
c. ammonis see HIPPOCAMPUS.
dorsal c. the dorsal protuberance of gray matter in the spinal cord. Called also dorsal horn.
lateral c. the lateral projection from the lateral intermediate substance of the spinal cord. It is prominent only in the thoracolumbar parts of the cord.
nasal c. the slender, ventral part of the comma-shaped alar cartilages that make up the support for the rim of the nostril.
thyroid cartilage c. there are rostral and caudal cornua borne on this cartilage.
uterine c. the horns of the uterus.
ventral c. the ventral horn of gray matter in the spinal cord. Contains the motor horn cells for the neurons of the peripheral nerves.

cornual, cornuate pertaining to a horn: (1) to the horns of the spinal cord, (2) to the horns of a cow, bull, buck or ram.
c. nerve block regional anesthesia applied to the base of the bovine frontal horn core for the purpose of performing a painless cornuectomy.

cornuectomy dehorning.

Corona a type of canary, which can be any breed; distinguished by a cap of feathers like an inverted saucer or a Beatles haircut. Called also Crested.

corona pl. *coronae* [L.] a crown; a crownlike eminence or encircling structure.
glans c. the prominent, denticulated margin of the glans penis in the stallion.
c. radiata 1. the radiating crown of projection fibers passing from the internal capsule to every part of the cerebral cortex. 2. an investing layer of radially elongated follicle cells surrounding the zona pellucida of the ovum.

coronary encircling in the manner of a crown. 1. a term applied to vessels, ligaments, nerves, the band at the skin–hoof junction. 2. blood vessels partially encircling the heart.
c. arteries two large arteries that branch from the ascending aorta and supply all of the heart muscle with blood. See also Table 9.
c. artery anomaly one or both arteries originate from the pulmonary artery instead of the aorta; anoxia of the myocardium leads to congestive heart failure.
c. artery laceration in foals during a difficult parturition and in cattle due to penetration by a reticular foreign body; sudden death due to cardiac tamponade.
c. artery rupture can result from perforation by a foreign body from the reticulum as part of the syn-

drome of traumatic reticular pericarditis. Cardiac tamponade results, causing acute or congestive heart failure.

c. band the junction of the skin and the horn of the hoof.

c. chemoreflex intravenous injection of chemicals such as veratridine causes cardiac slowing, hypotension and apnea due to reflex response by the myocardium. Called also Bezold–Jarisch reflex.

c. cushion the spongy, resilient hypodermis beneath the coronary corium of the hoof.

c. emboli lodgment of an embolus in a coronary artery is a rare occurrence in animals. Myocardial ischemia and asthenia result, the effect on the animal varying with the amount of muscle compromised.

c. occlusion the occlusion, or closing off, of a coronary artery. The occlusion may result from formation of a clot (thrombosis). Narrowing of the lumen of the blood vessels by the plaques of ATHEROSCLEROSIS, as occurs in humans, does not occur in animals. If there is adequate collateral circulation to the heart muscle at the time of the occlusion, there may be little or no damage to the myocardial cells. When occlusion is complete, however, with no blood being supplied to an area of the myocardium, MYOCARDIAL infarction results.

c. perfusion pressure the difference between aortic diastolic and right atrial diastolic pressure; a determinant of the blood flow to cardiac muscle.

c. thrombosis formation of a clot in a coronary artery. See also MYOCARDIAL infarction.

coronaviral pertaining to or emanating from any of the coronaviruses, e.g. coronaviral enteritis of dogs, coronaviral enteritis of turkeys.

Coronaviridae a family in the order *Nidovirales* of enveloped, single-stranded, plus sense RNA viruses about 100 nm in diameter. The envelope has prominent droplet-shaped spikes which resemble a solar corona. The one genus includes viruses that cause avian infectious bronchitis, hepatitis in mice, transmissible gastroenteritis in swine, canine coronavirus gastroenteritis, bovine coronavirus enteritis in neonatal calves, hemagglutinating encephalitis of pigs, feline infectious peritonitis, turkey bluecomb disease and respiratory infections in humans.

coronavirus a virus in the family CORONAVIRIDAE.

canine c. a cause of acute enteritis in dogs.

feline enteric c. a cause of mild enteritis in kittens. It is closely related to feline infectious peritonitis virus.

coronet see CORONARY band.

Coronilla varia plant in the legume family Fabaceae; may contain a nitrocompound which causes dyspnea, incoordination, hydrothorax and ascites. Called also crown vetch.

coronitis dermatitis of the skin at the coronet of the hooves; a cause of lameness. Because of the implications of vesicular disease any animal with coronitis must receive an oral examination. The lesions may be vesicles, erosions or granuloma.

coronoid process 1. a part of the mandible that projects into the temporal fossa and provides attachment for the temporal muscle. 2. the medial and lateral prominences located on either side of the trochlear notch of the ulna, forming part of the articular surface with the radius and humerus.

fragmented c. p. a developmental lesion of young, large breed dogs. Causes a weight-bearing lameness. May occur in association with osteochondritis dissecans of the medial humeral condyle. Called also ununited coronoid process, elbow dysplasia.

ununited c. p. see fragmented coronoid process (above).

coronoidectomy surgical removal of the coronoid process of the mandible.

coroscopy retinoscopy, or skiametry.

corotomy see IRIDOTOMY.

corpora plural form of CORPUS.

c. albicantia see CORPUS albicans.

c. arenacea sandy or gritty bodies, found in the pineal body; appear to be of glial or stromal origin; have the structure of hydroxyapatite crystals. Called also brain sand, acervuli, psammomas.

c. cavernosa penis see CORPUS cavernosum penis.

c. lutea see CORPUS luteum.

c. nigra see IRIDIAL granule.

c. quadrigemina four rounded eminences on the posterior surface of the mesencephalon. See also COLLICULUS.

corporate 1. emanating from or pertaining to a group activity. 2. emanating from or pertaining to a company constituted legally under a Companies Act or similar legislation.

c. advertising advertising on behalf of a group such as a profession or an association. It promotes the group and escapes the stigma of personal aggrandisement.

corporation a business entity such as a company incorporated under legislation, usually a Companies Act, which can make the shareholders legally responsible only for the profits and debts of the company. That is the shareholders are not personally responsible. It has been held for generations that members of professions could not practice as corporations because they would lose their personal responsibility to their clients. It is becoming more common for this rule to be discarded.

corpus pl. *corpora* [L.] body.

accessory c. lutea the corpora lutea which develop during early pregnancy in the mare and which follow the subsidence of the first corpus luteum.

c. albicans, corpord albicantia white fibrous tissue that replaces the regressing corpus luteum in the ovary in the latter half of pregnancy.

c. amygdaloideum a small mass of subcortical gray matter within the tip of the temporal lobe, anterior to the temporal horn of the lateral ventricle of the brain; it is part of the limbic system.

c. amylacea small hyaline masses of degenerate cells found in the prostate, thyroid, neuroglia and milk where they may be sufficient in a cow to block the teat sinus. They are formed by stasis of milk flow in a duct and inspissation of the fluids. Subsequently they may become detached and find their way to the teat.

c. atreticum scar in the ovary produced by atresia of a follicle when late in its development.

c. callosum an arched mass of white matter in the depths of the longitudinal fissure of the brain, and made up of transverse fibers connecting the cerebral hemispheres.

c. callosum agenesis all or part of the corpus may be absent and there may be additional associated defects.

c. cavernosum clitoridis one of the pair of erectile bodies of the clitoris.

c. cavernosum penis either of the two columns of erectile tissue forming the body of the penis or clitoris. See also corpus cavernosum PENIS.

c. cavernosum penis rupture common in bulls occurring during mating; commonly at the distal bend of the sigmoid flexure; result in hematoma and subsequent adhesions with inability to protrude the penis properly or angulation of the penis.

c. cavernosum urethrae see corpus spongiosum PENIS.

c. fimbriatum a band of white matter bordering the lateral edge of the temporal cornu of the lateral ventricle of the brain.

c. geniculatum see geniculate BODY lateral, and geniculate BODY medial.

c. hemorrhagicum 1. an ovarian follicle, especially one freshly ruptured, containing blood. 2. a corpus luteum containing a blood clot.

c. luteum a progesterone-secreting yellow glandular mass in the ovary formed from the wall of an ovarian follicle that has matured and discharged its ovum. See also OVULATION. In most animals that do not conceive the corpus luteum regresses quickly and a new follicle develops. The corpus luteum may be retained when there is uterine pathology which mimics pregnancy; no new follicle develops and the cow fails to come into heat. Called also retained corpus luteum. A similar clinical picture is observed with cystic corpora lutea.

c. spongiosum penis see corpus spongiosum PENIS.

c. striatum a subcortical mass of gray and white substance in front of and lateral to the thalamus in each cerebral hemisphere.

corpuscle any small mass or body.

blood c's formed elements in the BLOOD, i.e. erythrocytes and leukocytes.

bulbous c. temperature-sensitive nerve endorgan.

colostrum c's large rounded bodies in colostrum, containing droplets of fat and sometimes a nucleus.

compound granular c. see GITTER CELLS.

genital c. pressure receptor nerve-endings in the penis and clitoris.

Golgi–Mazzoni c. probably a pressure receptor; occur in hairless skin and associated mucosae, glans penis, foot pad of carnivores, hoof connective tissue.

c. of Grandry in the dermis of a duck's bill. See also corpuscle of Herbst (below).

c. of Herbst located in the dermis of the duck's bill these corpuscles are extremely sensitive to vibration.

lamellar c. pressure-sensitive nerve-endings. Called also Ruffini corpuscle.

malpighian c. see renal corpuscle (below).

Meissner c. touch-sensitive nerve receptors.

meniscoid c. touch-sensitive nerve endorgan.

pacinian c's see PACINIAN CORPUSCLE.

Purkinje's c's large, branched nerve cells composing the middle layer of the cortex of the cerebellum.

red blood c. erythrocyte.

renal c. a tuft of capillaries enveloped by the dilated end of a renal tubule. Constitutes the beginning of the structural unit of the kidney (nephron). Called also malpighian corpuscle.

Ruffini c. see lamellar corpuscle (above).

tactile c's medium-sized encapsulated nerve endings in the skin; called also tactile papillae.

white blood c. leukocyte.

corpuscular radiation radiation consisting of moving particles of matter, usually submolecular particles such as α-particles, protons and electrons.

corral a small fenced-in enclosure with high, wooden fences, suitable for holding cattle or horses.

c. system a management system in which range cattle are put into corrals and fed hay for a period when the environment is most inhospitable or at other times of stress, e.g. calving.

corrective pertaining to or emanating from the correction of a fault.

c. mating an approach to selection of dams and sires in which an undesirable trait in one parent is 'corrected' in the offspring by mating to a parent with an opposing or improved value for the characteristic.

correlated response change in an unselected character resulting from genetic selection of another character.

correlation 1. in neurology, the union of afferent impulses within a nerve center to bring about an appropriate response. 2. the degree to which statistical variables vary together.

c. coefficient see correlation COEFFICIENT.

correspondence the condition of being in agreement or conformity.

corridor disease a disease of cattle caused by *Theileria lawrenci*; clinically resembles EAST COAST FEVER.

Corriedale medium wool, meat sheep originated in New Zealand and Australia by crossbreeding Lincoln or Leicester with merino; wool 25 to 30 microns.

Corrigan's pulse a jerky pulse with full expansion and full collapse.

corrosive having a caustic and locally destructive effect; an agent having such effects.

c. sublimate mercuric chloride; oldfashioned use as caustic, disinfectant, antiseptic. Called also mercury bichloride.

Cortaderia selloana a perennial reed-like plant with a large, silvery inflorescence, up to 10 ft high; used mainly as an ornamental but also as supplement to pasture; grows best in warm climates. Very palatable. Called also pampas grass.

cortex pl. *cortices* [L.] an outer layer, as the bark of the trunk or root of a tree, or the outer layer of an organ or other structure, as distinguished from its inner substance.

adrenal c. the outer, firm layer comprising the larger part of the ADRENAL gland; it secretes a number of hormones. See CORTICOSTEROID, ALDOSTERONE, MINERALOCORTICOID, GLUCOCORTICOID.

cerebellar c. the superficial gray matter of the cerebellum.

cerebral c., c. cerebri the convoluted layer of gray matter covering each cerebral hemisphere. See also CEREBRAL cortex.

renal c. the smooth-textured outer layer of the kidney, composed mainly of renal corpuscles and convoluted tubules, extending in columns between the pyramids.

Corti's canal a space between the outer and inner rods of Corti.

Corti's ganglion the ganglion of the cochlear nerve, located within the modiolus, sending fibers peripherally to the organ of Corti and centrally to the cochlear nuclei of the brainstem. Called also spiral ganglion.

Corti's organ see ORGAN of Corti.

Corti's rods rodlike bodies in the inner ear, having their heads joined and their bases on the basilar membrane widely separated so as to form a spiral tunnel.

cortical pertaining to or emanating from a cortex, usually bone, cerebral or adrenal.

c. epilepsy see partial SEIZURE.

c. hyperplasia caused by chronic stimulation of the adrenal cortex by ACTH.

c. necrosis see POLIOENCEPHALOMALACIA.

c. sinus vascular sinuses in the cortex of a lymph node.

corticate having a cortex or bark.

corticectomy excision of an area of cerebral cortex,

as of a scar or microgyrus in the treatment of focal epilepsy. Not a procedure used in veterinary surgery.

corticifugal proceeding, conducting, or moving away from the cortex.

corticipetal proceeding, conducting, or moving toward the cortex.

corticoadrenal, adrenocortical pertaining to the adrenal cortex.

corticobulbar pertaining to or connecting the cerebral cortex and the medulla oblongata or brainstem.

corticoid corticosteroid; a hormone of the adrenal cortex, or other natural or synthetic compound with similar activity.

corticolytic drugs see ADRENOLYTIC.

corticopontine pertaining to or connecting the cerebral cortex and the pons.

corticoreticular tract part of the reticular formation and therefore a participant in the modulation of the integration systems in the brain.

corticospinal pertaining to or connecting the cerebral cortex and spinal cord.

c. tracts nerve fibers in these spinal cord motor tracts have their cell bodies in the cerebral cortex. Some have crossed to the opposite side of the cord from their side of origin, some are direct.

corticosteroid any of the hormones produced by the ADRENAL cortex; also, their synthetic equivalents. Called also adrenocortical hormone and adrenocorticosteroid. All the hormones are steroids having similar chemical structures, but quite different physiological effects. Generally they are divided into GLUCOCORTICOIDS (cortisol, or hydrocortisone, and corticosterone), MINERALOCORTICOIDS (aldosterone and desoxycorticosterone, and also corticosterone) and androgens.

c.-binding globulin α-globulin that binds unconjugated corticosteroid and transports it in the plasma; called also transcortin.

corticosteroid-induced joint disease degenerative joint disease caused by repeated injections of corticosteroid into joint cavities to control lameness.

corticosteroid-induced parturition see PARTURITION induction.

corticosteroid-induced photosensitization photosensitive dermatitis of the teats in cows injected with corticosteroids to terminate pregnancy.

corticosterone a steroid hormone of the adrenal cortex; it is usually classified as a GLUCOCORTICOID, but it also has slight MINERALOCORTICOID activity.

corticotomy removal of a piece of bone cortex, leaving the intramedullary blood supply intact.

corticotrop one of the types of secretory cells in the adrenohypophysis; secrete ACTH and beta-lipoprotein.

corticotrope a cell of the anterior pituitary gland that secretes ACTH.

corticotroph adenoma functional tumors of the pars intermedia or the pars distalis of the pituitary gland which cause a syndrome of cortisol excess in dogs. See CUSHING'S DISEASE.

corticotrophic see CORTICOTROPIC.

corticotrophin see CORTICOTROPIN.

corticotropic having a stimulating effect on the adrenal cortex; pertaining to corticotropin; adrenocorticotropic.

corticotropin 1. adrenocorticotropic hormone. See also ACTH. 2. a pharmaceutical preparation derived from the anterior pituitary of mammals and used to stimulate adrenal cortical activity in various conditions, such as allergy, hypersensitivity and rheumatoid arthritis. It has also been used experimentally in a large number of disorders.

c.-like intermediary peptide a polypeptide hormone of the intermediate pituitary; stimulates insulin release from the pancreas.

c.-releasing factor secreted by the hypothalamus and conveyed by local circulation to the corticotrophs in the pituitary which are then stimulated to produce ACTH. Called also corticotropin-releasing hormone (CRF).

cortilymph the fluid filling the intercellular spaces of the organ of Corti.

Cortinarius a genus of the Basidiomycetes fungi; contains a cyclic peptide, cortinarin, which causes kidney damage, uremia. Includes *C. orellanoides* (*C. speciocissimus*), *C. orellanus*, *C. splendens*.

cortisol a hormone from the adrenal cortex; the principal GLUCOCORTICOID. Called also 17-hydroxycorticosterone and, pharmaceutically, hydrocortisone. A synthetic preparation is used for its anti-inflammatory actions.

c.-binding globulin much plasma cortisol is bound to a α-globulin—transcortin, some to albumin. Much is free and in the form of a glycuronide or sulfate.

c.:corticosterone ratio the ratio between the two hormones is different between species and even between individual animals. There is also a circadian rhythm in the ratio which must therefore be interpreted with caution.

c.:creatinine (C/C) ratio measured in the urine as a screening test for hyperadrenocorticism.

c. hemisuccinate see HYDROCORTISONE.

c. response test see ACTH response test; DEXAMETHASONE suppression test.

cortisone a GLUCOCORTICOID with significant MINERALOCORTICOID activity, isolated from the adrenal cortex; used as an anti-inflammatory agent and for adrenal replacement therapy.

Corvus a genus of large, perching birds of the family Corvidae which includes jays, magpies, crows. They are omnivorous and may act as physical carriers of contagious disease because they will on occasion eat carrion.

Corydalis a genus of American plants in the family Fumariaceae; contains isoquinoline alkaloids which cause convulsions, vomiting and diarrhea. Includes *C. aurea*, *C. caseana*, *C. flavula*. Called also fitweed, fumatory.

corymbiform clustered; said of lesions grouped around a single, usually larger, lesion.

Corynebacteriaceae a family of bacteria, made up of usually nonmotile rods, sometimes showing marked variation in form and sometimes beaded or banded with metachromatic granules. Contains the genus *Corynebacterium*.

corynebacterial pertaining to or emanating from bacteria of the genus *Corynebacterium*.

c. lymphadenitis see CASEOUS LYMPHADENITIS.

c. mastitis a severe, acute mastitis in cows causing much suppuration, mammary abscessation and loss of the affected quarter. See also summer MASTITIS.

c. pneumonia an infectious disease of young foals caused by *Corynebacterium* (*Rhodococcus*) *equi* and characterized by suppurative lesions in many organs but with clinical manifestations of pneumonia. There is dyspnea, cough, grossly abnormal breath sounds and diarrhea in some cases and death in most.

c. pyelonephritis see CONTAGIOUS bovine pyelonephritis.

Corynebacterium a genus of bacteria of the family CORYNEBACTERIACEAE. They are gram-positive and show a variety of morphologies. They are short, slightly curved rods, sometimes club-shaped. Likely to be grouped into angled and palisade arrays of cells. The type species is *Corynebacterium diphtheriae*, the cause of diphtheria in humans.

C. bovis a common inhabitant of the bovine udder but not considered to be a pathogen. May have importance in protecting the udder from more damaging pathogens.

C. cystitidis causes CONTAGIOUS bovine pyelonephritis.

C. equi now called RHODOCOCCUS EQUI.

C. kutscheri causes systemic abscessation in rodents similar to caseous lymphadenitis in sheep. Previously called *C. murium*.

C. minutissimum found in wound infections in lambs.

C. parvum now called *Propionibacterium acnes*.

C. pseudotuberculosis cause of CASEOUS LYMPHADENITIS of sheep and goats, ulcerative LYMPHANGITIS, and CANADIAN HORSEPOX and PECTORAL abscesses of horses. Previously called *C. ovis*.

C. pyogenes now called *Actinomyces pyogenes*.

C. rathayi see CLAVIBACTER TOXICUS.

C. renale previously classified as types I, II and III, but now allocated separate names of *C. renale*, *C. pilosum* and *C. cystitidis*, respectively. Causes CONTAGIOUS bovine pyelonephritis, and BALANOPOSTHITIS of bulls, and plays a large part in causing ENZOOTIC balanoposthitis in sheep.

C. suis now called *Eubacterium suis*.

C. ulcerans an uncommon cause of subacute bovine mastitis.

coryneform denoting or resembling organisms of the family Corynebacteriaceae. See also DIPHTHEROID.

corynetoxins tunicaminyluracil toxins produced by CLAVIBACTER TOXICUS; see also TUNICAMYCIN.

Corynocarpus laevigatus New Zealand plant in family Corynocarpaceae; contains karakin, a nitrocompound, which causes incoordination and paralysis. Called also karaka tree.

Corynosoma a genus of acanthocephalan parasites of the family Polymorphidae. Called also thornyheaded worm.

C. semerme* and *C. strumosum nonpathogenic parasites in the intestines of dogs and foxes. Cause enteritis in mink.

Corythaeola cristata great blue turaco.

Corythaixoides go-away birds.

coryza profuse discharge from the mucous membrane of the nose.

infectious c. see FOWL coryza.

pigeon c. see PIGEON herpesvirus.

turkey c. an upper respiratory tract disease, probably caused by *Bordetella avium*, occurring in turkey poults under conditions of stress, particularly poor ventilation. There is sneezing, a mucoid rhinotracheitis and collapse of the trachea. Secondary airsacculitis and pericarditis are common. Mortality is often as high as 25%. Called also rhinotracheitis.

coryzavirus see RHINOVIRUS.

Coscoroba see SWAN.

cosmesis cosmetic therapy or procedures, such as tattooing. Also sometimes applied to such procedures when used for therapeutic purposes.

cosmetic 1. beautifying; tending to preserve, restore, or confer comeliness. 2. a beautifying substance or preparation.

c. operations see cosmetic surgery (below).

c. shell an artificial device, molded in the shape of a phthisic globe, and permanently placed over that globe to produce an improved appearance.

c. surgery surgery carried out purely to enhance the appearance of the animal. When it is for the purpose of enhancing or disguising its appearance in the show ring, this is considered unethical. The animal is not in a position to judge or to express an opinion and the question of beauty is adjudicated by the owner. Because animal fashions have sometimes tended to the bizarre there has been a marked turn in public opinion against cosmetic operations which are seen by some as unwarranted mutilations.

cosmic rays ionizing irradiation from outer space bombarding the earth and its atmosphere. They contribute to the background radiation that is always present at the earth's surface.

cosmid a class of plasmid-based vectors carrying the bacteriophage λ cos sequences required for packaging of DNA into phage particles. Used for cloning large DNA fragments (up to 45 kilobases). Recombinant molecules constructed using cosmids are incorporated into bacteriophage using in vitro packaging extracts and introduced with high efficiency into *Escherichia coli*.

Cosmocephalus obvelatus nematode found in the esophagus of newly captured rockhopper penguins.

cost–benefit analysis see BENEFIT–COST ANALYSIS.

cost-effective profitable; representing a return to investment of more than the cost.

cost-effectiveness pertaining to cost-effective.

c.-e. analysis a comparison of the relative cost-efficiencies of two or more ways of performing a task or achieving an objective.

cost function a mathematical formula created for the purpose of estimating a cost, e.g. the cost of making an observation when it varies from stratum to stratum of a collection of data.

costa pl. *costae* [L.] a rib.

costalgia pain in the ribs.

costectomy excision of a rib.

Costia a genus of flagellated protozoa in the family Tetramitidae. Called also *Ichthyoboda*.

C. necatrix* and *C. pyriformis parasites on the skin of freshwater fish.

costive 1. pertaining to, characterized by, or producing constipation. 2. an agent that depresses intestinal motility.

costiveness see CONSTIPATION.

cost(o)- word element. [L.] *rib*.

costocervical pertaining to the ribs and neck.

costochondral pertaining to a rib and its cartilage.

enlarged c. joints visible in thin animals, palpable in fat ones; symptomatic of rickets; called also rachitic rosary.

costophrenic pertaining to the ribs and diaphragm.

c. angle in radiographs, the angle between the ribs and the diaphragm. Details may be blurred by the presence of fluid in the pleural cavity.

costosternal pertaining to the ribs and sternum.

costotomy incision or division of a rib or costal cartilage.

costotransverse lying between the ribs and the transverse processes of the vertebrae.

costovertebral pertaining to a rib and a vertebra.

costoxiphoid connecting the ribs and xiphoid cartilage or process.

cosyntropin a synthetic corticotropin used in the screening of adrenal functional capacity on the basis of plasma cortisol response after intramuscular or intravenous injection. Called also tetracosactrin.

Coton de Tulear a small white dog with a long, fine white coat that has the texture of cotton.

cotransport the simultaneous movement of two substances across a membrane. See also ANTIPORT, SYMPORT.

co-trimoxazole an antibiotic preparation made up of a mixture of TRIMETHOPRIM and sulfamethoxazole.

cottage cheese a soft, uncured cheese made from soured skim milk; most of the lactose is removed with the whey. Used in low-residue diets for dogs and cats.

cotted said of wool which has become matted or felted while on the sheep, due usually to continuous wetting.

Cottoidei a suborder of the order Perciformes of fishes important because of the large number of poisonous species that it contains.

cotton see SUTURE (3, 4), GOSSYPIUM.

c. bush (commercial cotton) plant *Gossypium* spp. in the family Malvaceae; seeds contain gossypol, a toxic phenol which causes cardiomyopathy, hepatopathy and edema in all organs.

c. seed meal meal or cake residue after extrusion of oil; used as livestock feed but toxic because of presence of gossypol.

c. test a test of vision in animals; a piece of cotton is dropped within the field of vision. A dog or cat with normal vision will follow the cotton as it descends.

cotton fireweed SENECIO *quadridentatus*.

cotton-leaf physic nut JATROPHA *gossypifolia*.

cotton-topped marmoset *Saquinus oedipus*; see MARMOSET.

cotton underfur a condition of the coat of mink caused by feeding on particular fish, e.g. Pacific hake, whiting, which encourages the development of anemia.

cotton wool disease see COLUMNARIS DISEASE.

cotton-wool spot white or gray soft-edged opacities in the retina composed of cytoid bodies.

cottonseed seed of the cotton plant. Made into cake after oil extraction and used as feed for livestock.

c. cake or meal contains GOSSYPOL and causes hepatitis and degeneration of cardiac muscle. The clinical syndrome includes dullness, weakness, dyspnea and edema. Usually fed as decorticated cake because of the high fiber content of the raw product.

c. hulls winnowed from the cotton seeds and used as roughage for ruminants. Have negligible feed value but are an effective diluent for grain because of the ease with which they can be handled by mechanical equipment.

cottontail a wild rabbit, *Sylvilagus* spp.

Cotugnia a genus of tapeworms in the family Davaineidae. Includes *C. cuneata*, *C. digonopora*, *C. fastigata*. Found in the intestines of birds.

Cotula radiata see MATRICARIA NIGELLIFOLIA.

Coturnix coturnix see QUAIL.

Cotyledon African genus of the plant family Crassulaceae; contains bufadienolide, cardiac glycosides; causes krimpsiekte (cotyledonosis). Includes *C. orbiculata* (*C. decusata*, *C. leucophylla*), *C. umbilicus* (*Umbilicus rupestris*, navelwort, pennywort). Many species have been reclassified as *Tylecodon* spp.

cotyledon 1. any subdivision of the uterine surface of the human placenta. 2. discrete elevations of chorioallantoic tissue of the ruminant fetal membranes that adhere intimately with the maternal caruncles to form placentomes. See also CARUNCLE.

cotyledonary pertaining to or emanating from cotyledons.

c. placentation see PLACENTATION.

cotyledonosis poisoning of livestock in southern Africa by plants in the genera *Tylecodon* and *Cotyledon* spp containing cumulative BUFADIENOLIDE cardiac glycosides. Clinical signs include exercise intolerance, paresis, paralysis, torticollis, paralysis of the lower jaw and tongue, dysphagia, drooling of saliva, abdominal pain, convulsions and death within a few hours. No significant necropsy lesions. Secondary poisoning occurs in dogs and humans who eat meat from diseased animals. Called also KRIMPSIEKTE.

Cotylophoron cotylophoron see PARAMPHISTOMIASIS.

Cotylurus a genus of digenetic trematodes in the family Strigeidae; includes *C. cornutus*, *C. flabelliformis*, *C. platycephalus*, *C. variegatus*; parasitic in the intestines of wild birds.

couch grass CYNODON *dactylon*.

couch grass + *Balansia* spp. grazing fungus-infested grass causes staggers syndrome.

couching surgical displacement of the lens of the eye in cataract.

cougar a large, solid fawn-colored cat that resembles a short-legged maneless lion. Called also puma, mountain lion, *Panthera concolor* (syn. *Felis concolor*).

cough 1. a sudden noisy expulsion of air from the lungs. 2. to produce such an expulsion of air.

dry c. cough without expectoration.

goose honk c. a chronic, harsh, dry cough characteristic of collapsed trachea.

nocturnal c. in dogs associated with heart disease, psychogenic coughing or collapsed trachea.

productive c. cough attended with expectoration of material from the bronchi.

psychogenic c. dogs sometimes associate coughing with the attention received and develop it as a habit.

c. reflex 1. the sequence of events initiated by the sensitivity of the lining of the passageways of the lung and mediated by the medulla as a consequence of impulses transmitted by the vagus nerve, resulting in coughing, i.e. the clearing of the passageways of foreign matter. 2. the response elicited by applying pressure on a trachea. Increased with inflammation of the respiratory epithelium; decreased by cough suppressants and pain.

coughing pertaining to COUGH.

coughing up feed indicates a problem with the swallowing mechanism, either functional e.g. pharyngeal paralysis, or physical e.g. foreign body lodged in pharynx.

coulomb 1. the unit of electrical charge, defined as the quantity of electrical charge transferred by 1 ampere in 1 second. Symbol C. 2. the SI unit of exposure to radiation. 1 coulomb per kilogram = 3876 roentgen; abbreviated C/kg.

Coulter counter an instrument that counts particles in a fluid medium by electronic means. Can be calibrated to count cells in milk or a blood sample.

coumachlor a coumarin derivative used as a rodenticide; can cause poisoning in domestic animals which are likely to be exposed to it. Causes internal and external hemorrhages and the animal dies of anemia. Lameness and profuse hemorrhagic diarrhea also occur.

coumafuryl see FUMARIN.

coumaphos an organophosphorus insecticide and anthelmintic, effective against *Haemonchus*, *Trichostrongylus*, *Ostertagia*, *Cooperia* and *Trichuris* spp. in cattle and sheep.

coumarin 1. a principle extracted from the tonka bean, from which several anticoagulants are derived, that inhibits hepatic synthesis of vitamin K-dependent coagulation factors. 2. any of these derivatives. 3. see also DICOUMAROL.

coumarinic acid a substance whose lactone is coumarin, the anticoagulant.
coumarol see DICOUMAROL.
coumatetralyl a derivative of warfarin and used as a rodenticide. As a poison in domestic animals it causes the same disease as warfarin but is more dangerous because of its use in concentrated form. See also WARFARIN.
coumestans estrogenic substances found in *Medicago* spp., e.g. lucerne/alfalfa and barrel medic.
coumestrol an estrogenic substance occurring naturally in *Trifolium repens*, *T. fragiferum* and *Medicago sativa*. See ESTROGEN.
Councilman body see CYTOSEGRESOME FORMATIONS.
count a numerical computation or indication.
differential c. a count, on a stained blood smear, of the proportion of different types of leukocytes (or other cells), previously expressed in percentages but now usually reported in absolute numbers (10^9/l) for a better indication of abnormalities that may exist.
milk cell c. see MILK CELL COUNTS.
platelet c. the count of the total number of platelets per liter (10^9/l) of blood by counting the platelets in a counting chamber, a hematology analyzer, or by estimating the number on a stained blood smear.
sperm c. see SEMEN concentration.
total bacterial c. determination of the total number of bacteria in the sample examined microscopically, then a calculation of the number per ml. These do not distinguish between viable and non-viable organisms. See also BREED'S DIRECT SMEAR METHOD.
viable bacterial cell c. enumerating the number of viable bacteria present in a sample based on counting the number of colonies from a given dilution.
wool c. an arbitrary number given to wool to indicate its fiber diameter, e.g. 60's, based on an eyeball assessment of the number of hanks of yarn that could be spun from one pound of wool. Now superseded by measurement of the diameter, e.g. 20 microns.
worm c. a total worm count requires a freshly slaughtered cadaver, collection of intestinal or other fluid in an aliquot sample; in the case of lungs it is necessary to digest the tissue; counting actual worms and by multiplication measuring the total worm burden.
counter an instrument or apparatus by which numerical value is computed; in radiology, a device for enumerating ionizing events.
Coulter c. see COULTER COUNTER.
Geiger c., Geiger–Müller c. a radiation counter using a gas-filled tube that indicates the presence of ionizing particles.
scintillation c. a device for detecting beta and gamma rays, permitting determination of the concentration of radioisotopes in the body or other substance. It is more important for gamma rays, which are poorly measured by a Geiger counter.
counterconditioning a technique of changing an undesirable response of an animal to a stimulus by engaging the animal in another response that is incompatible with the first.
countercurrent flowing in an opposite direction.
c. exchanger a countercurrent system in which transport between the inflow and the outflow is passive.
c. multiplier a mechanism that enables a membrane to absorb much more solute than water so that the residual fluid has a lower osmotic pressure. The classical example of this phenomenon is the loop of Henle in the kidney. Called also countercurrent multiplier mechanism or system.
counterelectrophoresis see COUNTER IMMUNOELECTROPHORESIS.
counterextension traction in a proximal direction coincident with traction in opposition to it.
counter immunoelectrophoresis a laboratory technique in which an electric current is used to accelerate the migration of antibody and antigen through a buffered gel diffusion medium; abbreviated CIE. Antigens in a gel medium in which the pH is controlled are strongly negatively charged and will migrate rapidly across the electric field toward the anode. The antibody in such a medium is less negatively charged and will migrate in an opposite or 'counter' direction toward the cathode. If the antigen and antibody are specific for each other, they combine and form a distinct precipitin line. Was used for the rapid diagnosis of some bacterial, mycoplasma and viral infections.
counterincision a second incision made to promote drainage or to relieve tension on the edges of a wound.
counterirritant 1. producing counterirritation. 2. an agent that produces counterirritation. Blistering by application of a paste or liquid containing rubefacient agents such as cantharides or mercuric iodide, and firing, by burning the skin and superficial tissues with a hot iron, were used as counterirritants on the lower limbs of lame horses. Less traumatic measures are more commonly used nowadays.
counterirritation superficial irritation intended to relieve some other irritation.
counteropening a second incision made across from an earlier one to promote drainage. Called also contra-aperture.
counterpressure externally applied pressure used to control internal hemorrhage and in the treatment of shock. See also ANTISHOCK PNEUMATIC GARMENT.
counterpulsation technique for assisting the circulation by the use of an external pumping device synchronized with cardiac systole.
counterpuncture a second opening made opposite another.
countershock see CARDIOVERSION.
counterstain a stain applied to render the effects of another stain more discernible.
countertraction traction opposed to traction; used in reduction of fractures.
counting-out pen the pen in which each shearer's sheep are collected after shearing and then counted as a basis for payment of the shearer.
coupage percussion of the thorax to aid in the removal of secretions.
coupling 1. in an animal's conformation, the distance between the top of the scapulae to the hip joints. 2. in ultrasonography, the transmission of sounds from the transducer into the tissues being examined. A medium such as a gel or mineral oil is used to exclude air from between the two surfaces.
course 1. the series of events in a disease incident in a patient. It may be peracute, acute, subacute, chronic or intermittent. 2. to course a rabbit, hare or fox is to run it in view, the opposite of conventional hunting by scent. Is prevented by legislation in most countries.
acute c. 1 or 2 days.
chronic c. more than 1 week.
intermittent c. periods of normality of a few minutes or hours.
peracute c. a few hours.
recurrent c. periods of normality of weeks to months.
subacute c. up to a week.

course-work said of a postgraduate degree based on lectures and practical work in courses rather than research.

court the persons assembled under the authority of the law to administer justice. This includes the presiding magistrate or judge, the jury if any, the counsel and advisors and witnesses for both parties.

c. hierarchy the ascending levels of the courts providing a series of higher tribunals to which appeals from lower courts can be taken. The more serious and complicated the case, the higher up in the court hierarchy it goes for primary hearing.

courtesy title title used by the community to identify a member of a professional group, e.g. Doctor; not titles legally bestowed by organizations and institutions with legal authority to do so.

courtship paying attention to a member of the opposite sex with a view to mating; occurs in farm animals but is not highly developed other than estral display by the female and seeking by the male, activities that are rather more pragmatic than implied in the definition. In the much smaller mating groups that prevail in wild animals, fish and birds in the wild, courtship is often a very ritualistic and prolonged activity including changes in behavior and coloring aided by physical contact, and sometimes the preparation and use of a courtship pad, as in peafowls (peacocks) and Argus pheasants.

c. feeding see neurotic REGURGITATION.

covalence a chemical bond between two atoms in which electrons are shared between the two nuclei.

covariance the expected value of the product of the deviations of corresponding values of two random variables from their respective means.

c. method used for the calculation of relationship and inbreeding in large populations.

covariate predictors during the allocation of experimental units in a randomized design.

Covault spay hook a long, thin, probelike instrument with a curved end and a buttoned tip, used to hook around the uterus of a companion animal and to bring it into the incision where an ovariohysterectomy can be performed.

covenant a constraint placed by local government authority upon the use of land or buildings. Applies to such matters as size of lots, use to which land can be put, amount of land that can be covered by a building.

cover see MATING.

coveralls overalls with full cover for the arms, trunk and legs; popular protective clothing for veterinarians working on farms.

coverglass a thin glass that covers a mounted microscopical object or a culture. Called also coverslip.

covering 1. the illegal practice of using an unqualified employee to work in the guise of a qualified one. This is with particular reference to practicing medicine and surgery and administering anesthetics and making diagnoses. The employing veterinarian is guilty of covering, the employed person is guilty of practicing illegally. 2. mating. 3. the legal practice of providing relief services for a veterinarian who is absent from his or her practice.

coverslip see COVERGLASS.

coverts see REMEX.

cow bovine female after having had one calf. See also CATTLE. The term is also used to describe mature females of some other species, e.g. elk, moose, reindeer, wapiti, elephants.

brood c. used for breeding.

c. bush see LEUCAENA LEUCOCEPHALA.

c.–calf pair a breeding beef cow with calf at foot.

c. cockle see SAPONARIA.

c. cress SIUM *angustifolium.*

dry c. 1. a cow in the 2 to 3 month period between the end of lactation and the subsequent calving. Cows in which calving is imminent are close-up dry cows, or are freshening. 2. a mature cow which is not lactating whatever the reason.

dry c. therapy see DRY period treatment.

empty c. cow not in calf when she should be. Called also barren cow.

foundation c. one from which many of the animals in a herd or breed have originated.

fresh c. a cow recently calved.

c. index an estimate of the genetic ability of the cow to transmit to her offspring her capacity to produce milk and butterfat. The index is calculated on the basis of the cow's record of production, especially her deviation from herdmates, the herd's productivity status and the productivity proof of her sire.

c.-kick a forward kick with a hindlimb, dangerous to the mounting rider of a horse, or to the clinician examining a cow.

open c. cow not in calf, usually said of cows still to be bred.

c. parsnip see HERACLEUM MANTEGAZZIANUM.

c.-pony American stock horse, used for working cattle on the range.

c. pool a cooperative arrangement for milking cows in which a central unit cares for and milks cows or herds which belong to different owners.

c. wheat *Melampyrum arvense.*

cow-associated mastitis see contagious MASTITIS.

cow-day for one cow for one day. Used as a measure of pasture, the amount required to fully feed a cow for peak lactation for one day (approximately 30 lb dry matter of grass).

cowbane CICUTA *virosa.*

Cowdria ruminantium the cause of HEARTWATER. A rickettsia called also *Rickettsia ruminantium.*

cowdriosis see HEARTWATER.

cow-hocked a conformation defect in a horse. The points of the hock are close together, the fetlocks wider apart than normal.

cowmen men, although the term usually includes women, who work physically with cattle. Includes herdsmen, grooms, milkers.

cowpea see VIGNA UNGUICULATA.

cowperitis inflammation of the bulbourethral (Cowper's) glands.

Cowper's glands see BULBOURETHRAL glands.

cowpox a benign, contagious disease of cows characterized by the appearance of pox lesions on the teat and udder skin. The causative virus is in the genus *Orthopoxvirus.* Typical lesions are a patch of erythema, then a papule, followed by a vesicle, then a pustule and finally a scab. The disease is transmissible to humans and is now rare.

c. virus a poxvirus which is antigenically distinct from vaccinia virus and pseudocowpox virus. The characteristics of the virus are otherwise identical with the vaccinia virus. See also VACCINIA.

cowside the bovine equivalent of bedside, e.g. said of manner.

c. mastitis tests test carried out in the milking parlor, not back in the laboratory, e.g. California Mastitis Test.

cowslip see CALTHA PALUSTRIS.

cox- prefix meaning hip.

coxa pl. *coxae* [L.] the hip, loosely, the hip joint.

c. plana flattening of the head of the femur resulting from osteochondrosis of its epiphysis.

c. valga deformity of the hip joint with increase in the angle of inclination between the neck and shaft of the femur, producing a straighter bone.
c. vara deformity of the hip joint with decrease in the angle of inclination between the neck and shaft of the femur.
coxal tuber see TUBER coxae.
coxalgia 1. hip joint disease. 2. pain in the hip.
coxcomb AMARANTHUS *deflexus*, *A. hybridus*.
Coxiella a genus of microorganisms of the order Rickettsiales.
***C.* abortion** possibly an occasional cause of abortion in sheep.
C. burnetii the causative agent of Q FEVER of humans. Also infects the trophoblast cells of sheep and cattle without causing disease.
coxiellosis infection by members of the genus *Coxiella*.
coxitis inflammation of the hip joint.
coxodynia pain in the hip.
coxofemoral pertaining to the hip and thigh.
c. arthropathy see degenerative JOINT disease.
c. joint see HIP joint.
coxsackievirus one of a heterogeneous group of enteroviruses of humans; recovered from dogs with mild diarrhea. Called also Coxsackie virus. Coxsackievirus B7 is related antigenically to swine vesicular disease virus.
coyote a North American predatory wild dog. Called also *Canis latrans*.
coyote tobacco NICOTIANA *attenuata*.
coyotillo see KARWINSKIA HUMBOLDTIANA.
coypu a large chestnut brown, 14 inch long and 15 lb in weight, aquatic rodent which is farmed extensively for its fur. It is herbivorous, diurnal and very fertile. As a wild animal in countries where it has escaped, it has become a pest. Called also nutria, *Myocastor coypus*, swamp beaver.
CPA cardiopulmonary arrest.
CPAP continuous positive airway pressure.
CP:ATP ratio creatine phosphate:adenotriphosphate ratio.
CPB see cardiopulmonary BYPASS.
CPBA competitive protein-binding assay.
CPD citrate-phosphate-dextrose.
CPD solution an anticoagulant solution used for the collection of blood for purposes of storage and transfusion. See also ACD solution.
CPE cytopathic effect.
CPG central pattern generators.
CPI characters per inch, a criterion of printing by a computer printer—usually 10, sometimes 12 or 16.5.
CPiV canine parainfluenza virus.
CPK creatine phosphokinase.
c.p.m. counts per minute.
CPR see CARDIOPULMONARY resuscitation.
CPRA see central progressive RETINAL atrophy.
CPRP cardiopulmonary cerebroresuscitation.
CPS characters per second, as a criterion of the speed of computer printers.
c.p.s. cycles per second.
CPT 3-chloro-*p*-toluidine, an avicide.
CPU CENTRAL processing unit; see also COMPUTER.
CPV canine parvovirus.
CR see CONDITIONED response.
Cr chemical symbol, *chromium*.
Cr^{51} EDTA a compound used to assess permeability of intestinal mucosa; 24-hour excretion is measured following oral administration.
crab-eating macaque *Macaca fascicularis*. See also MACAQUE.
crab grass DIGITARIA spp., ELEUSINE *indica*.
crabs eye see ABRUS *precatorius*.
Crabtree effect the inhibition of oxygen consumption on the addition of glucose to tissues or microorganisms having a high rate of aerobic glycolysis; the converse of the Pasteur effect.
crack a discontinuity in a hard, brittle surface such as horn, hoof.
toe c. see SANDCRACK.
cracked said of grain; indicates grain that has been exposed to a combined breaking and crushing action.
cracked heels dermatitis in the hollow between the heels occurring most commonly in the hindlimbs. Causes quite severe lameness as the horse is first moved but improves quickly. Site is smelly, wet and tender. Caused by constant wetness and dirty stables. May be infected with *Fusobacterium necrophorum*. See also GREASY HEEL.
cracked pot sound the sharp, nonresonant note, like the noise made by striking a cracked pot, made by percussion of subcutaneous emphysema or an air-filled cavity in the lungs.
cracker of little worth; term used to describe old sheep in poor condition and with no teeth.
crackles a small, sharp sound heard on auscultation. Caused by dry, bristly hair and insufficient pressure on the stethoscope head. Also characteristic of emphysema, especially when it is subcutaneous. An early observation in pleurisy but disappears as exudate separates pleural surfaces. See also RALE.
cracklings proteinaceous residues after fat is melted and run off during offal processing. Called also greaves.
cradle a barred restraining device.
calf c. is interposed in a chute in a vertical position. The calf is driven in. It may be anything up to 6 months of age. One side of the cradle is movable and the calf is clamped in tightly. The cradle is then swiveled on its bottom hinge and the calf is upended so that it can be castrated, branded, dehorned.
neck c. a series of bars tied together like a nonrigid fence. Tied round the neck of a horse like a loose splint, it prevents the horse from biting or licking itself.
lamb c. the lamb is laid on its back in the device, its legs are clamped in position exposing scrotum and tail for castration and tail docking, and the perineal area to expose skin folds for mulesing.
Crambe abyssinica plant in the family Brassicaceae; contains a glucosinolate which causes weight loss in poultry when seed meal made from this plant is fed.
cramp a painful spasmodic muscular contraction.
Greyhound c. muscle spasms, particularly in the hindlegs, usually in unfit dogs, with excessive excitement, or high environmental temperatures.
heat c. a form of equine colic after vigorous exercise with heavy sweating. Caused by electrolyte loss. Signs include muscle tremor and rigidity.
raptor c. hypocalcemic, tetanic convulsions in raptor birds caused by a dietary deficiency of calcium.
Scottie c., Scotch c. an inherited defect in Scottish terriers that occurs as hyperkinetic episodes from an early age, but may only be precipitated by exercise or excitement. Some dogs show the disorder only infrequently during their otherwise normal lives. Affected dogs become stiff with hyperextension of the limbs which may prevent walking or cause brief cessation of respiratory movements. Caused by a deficiency of serotonin.
crampiness see inherited PERIODIC spasticity.
cramping see CRAMP.

crampy spasticity see inherited PERIODIC spasticity.
crane large, gray, brown and white, long-legged, long-necked birds, with a loud raucous call. Includes *Ballearica* spp. (e.g. *B. pavonina*, the eastern crowned crane), GRUS, *Bugeranus* spp. and *Anthropoides* spp. (e.g. *A. virgo*, the desmoiselle crane).
craniad in a cranial direction; toward the head end of the body.
cranial pertaining to the cranium or to the head end of the body. See also ANTERIOR, CRANIUM.
c. intestinal portal the entrance into the embryonic foregut from the expanded midgut.
c. nerve reflexes see specific nerves.
c. nerves nerves which are attached to the brain and pass through the openings of the skull. There are 12 pairs of cranial nerves, symmetrically arranged so that they are distributed mainly to the structures of the head and neck. See also specific nerves and Table 14.
c. tibial reflex percussing just below the lateral tibial condyle (cranial tibial muscle) normally causes a slight flexion of the tibiotarsal joint. A test of the integrity of spinal cord segments L6 to S2, sciatic and peroneal nerves. Exaggerated in spinal cord lesions above L6.
c. tumor see BRAIN tumors.
c. vena cava see Table 15.
cranial vena caval thrombosis syndrome in which pulmonary abscesses cause cough, hyperpnea and poor exercise tolerance. Jugular vein engorgement and local edema may also occur. See also CAVAL SYNDROME.
Craniata a subphylum of the phylum Chordata. Includes vertebrates with a distinct brain and brain box.
craniectomy excision of a segment of the skull.
crani(o)- word element. [L.] *skull.*
craniocaudal the direction of entry of the x-ray beam. The beam enters at the cranial end of the part being examined and exits at the caudal end.
c. view in a system of nomenclature of radiographic positioning used in animals, means the path that the beam takes from the x-ray tube to the film, passing from the head end of the animal towards its tail.
craniocele protrusion of part of the brain through the skull.
craniocerebral pertaining to the skull and cerebrum.
cranioclasis see CRANIOTOMY (2).
cranioclast an instrument for performing craniotomy (2).
craniodidymus a monster with two heads.
craniofacial of or pertaining to the cranium and face.
c. dysplasia inherited in cattle; characterized by convex nasal profile, shortened mandible, macroglossia.
c. index an indication of the shape of the skull. The formula is cranium length/facial length.
c. malformations any congenital deformity of the cranium or face including cyclopia, cebocephaly, cheiloschisis.
craniomalacia abnormal softness of the bones of the skull.
craniomandibular pertaining to or emanating from the cranium and face.
c. osteopathy a proliferative bone disease occurring predominantly in immature West Highland white and Scottish terriers, and infrequently in several other breeds. Symmetrical bony enlargements occur on the mandible, occipital and temporal bones, less often other bones of the skull, and rarely long bones. Affected dogs may have varying degrees of difficulty in opening the mouth, salivation and recurring fever. Called also craniomandibular hyperostosis, lion jaw.
craniometer an instrument for measuring the skull in craniometry.
craniometry a branch of morphometry, being the measurement of the dimensions and angles of a bony skull.
craniopagus a double monster joined at the head; called also cephalopagus.
craniopharyngeal pertaining to the cranium and pharynx.
c. duct the primordial outgrowth from the roof of the pharynx from which the posterior lobe of the pituitary gland is formed; a vestigial structure in most species; see also RATHKE'S POUCH.
c. duct cyst cysts from remnants of the distal craniopharyngeal duct are found close to the pituitary gland. Pressure on the gland and inflammation and subsequent fibrosis of it can cause a syndrome of adenohypophyseal hypofunction. There may be blindness, obesity and diabetes insipidus. Brachyocephalic breeds of dogs are predisposed.
craniopharyngioma a benign tumor arising from the cell rests derived from the infundibulum of the hypophysis or Rathke's pouch. Usually seen in young animals, they grow slowly. Their effects may be seen as a hypopituitarism, cranial nerve deficits or central nervous system dysfunction.
cranioplasty any plastic operation on the skull.
craniopuncture exploratory puncture of the brain.
craniorachischisis congenital fissure of the skull and vertebral column.
c. totalis failure of fusion of the entire neural tube.
craniosacral pertaining to the skull and sacrum.
c. outflow the parasympathetic outflow.
cranioschisis congenital fissure of the cranium due to sagittal failure of fusion of the cranial bones; see also inherited CRANIUM bifidum.
craniosclerosis abnormal calcification and thickening of the cranial bones.
cranioscopy diagnostic examination of the head.
craniospinal pertaining to the skull and spine.
craniostenosis deformity of the skull due to premature closure of the cranial sutures.
craniostosis congenital ossification of the cranial sutures.
craniosynostosis premature closure of the cranial sutures.
craniotabes reduction in mineralization of the skull, with abnormal softness of the bone, usually affecting the occipital and parietal bones along the lambdoidal sutures.
craniotome a cutting instrument used in craniotomy.
craniotomy 1. any operation on the cranium. 2. puncture of the skull and removal of its contents to decrease the size of the head of a dead fetus and facilitate delivery.
craniotympanic pertaining to the skull and tympanum.
cranium pl. *crania* [L.] the skeleton of the head, variously construed as including all of the bones of the head, all except the mandible, or the eight bones forming the vault lodging the brain. See also HEAD, SKULL, CRANIAL.
inherited c. bifidum a defect in the closure of the bones of the cranial vault causes exposure of the brain. Meningocele or encephalocele may be present. Affected animals do not survive. Called also cranioschisis.
crash cart a portable trolley containing all equipment and drugs required for cardiopulmonary resuscitation and emergency care.

Craspedia chrysantha Australian plant in the Asteraceae family; unidentified toxin causes blindness, abdominal pain, diarrhea. Called also golden billy buttons.

Crassostrea genus of farmed oysters in subclass Lamellibranchia; includes *C. angulata* (Portuguese oyster), *C. gigas* (Pacific cupped oyster), *C. virginicus* (American cupped oyster), *Saccostrea commercialis* (Sydney rock oyster). See Table 23.

crater an excavated area surrounded by an elevated margin, as caused by ulceration.

crateriform bowl-shaped, like a crater.

craterization excision of bone tissue to create a crater-like depression.

Craterostomum a genus of nematode worms of the family Strongylidae. Includes *Craterostomum acuticaudatum*, *C. tenuicauda* (in equine large intestine).

craw see CROP (2).

crayfish Includes many genera and species, many of them farmed, e.g. *Procambarus*, *Oronectes*, *Astacus*, *Pastifastacus* spp. Called also freshwater crayfish.

freshwater c. see crayfish (above).

c. plague epizootic disease of European crayfish (*Astacus astacus*) caused by *Aphanomyces astaci*. Affects also *Cherax* spp (American crayfish), *Pacifastacus leniusculus*.

crayon a soft color-marking material used in identification especially in sheep.

c.-marking marking of ewes by rams wearing crayons on their chests and held there by a harness. By changing the color of the crayon it is possible to date the reproductive events of the flock. See also TUPPING crayon.

crazy chick disease a disease of young (2 to 4 weeks old) chickens caused by vitamin E nutritional deficiency. Signs include incoordination, orthotonos, opisthotonos, clonic convulsions, death.

crazy cow syndrome a North American disease, caused by SOLANUM *dimidiatum*.

CRD 1. chronic respiratory disease. See CHRONIC respiratory disease of chickens, MURINE respiratory mycoplasmosis. 2. chronic renal disease.

cream 1. an oil and water emulsion used topically in the treatment of skin disease. 2. the natural rising of butterfat on stored cow's milk; also obtained by mechanical centrifugation. 3. an uncommon coat color in a horse, although some very light palominos would qualify. The horse is cream all over, including the MUZZLE (1), MANE and tail; the skin is unpigmented and the haircoat is cream. There is often a deficiency of pigment in the iris.

cold c. useful as an emollient to soften and hydrate the skin.

c. rinse hair conditioners that make the coat lie flat and comb easily.

creatinase an enzyme that catalyzes the decomposition of creatine into urea and ammonia.

creatine a nonprotein nitrogen substance synthesized in the body from three amino acids: arginine, glycine (aminoacetic acid) and methionine. Creatine readily combines with phosphate to form phosphocreatine, or creatine phosphate, which is present in muscle, where it serves as the storage form of high-energy phosphate necessary for intense muscle contraction.

c. kinase (CK) an organ-specific enzyme catalyzing the transfer of a phosphate group from phosphocreatine to ATP. It has three isoenzymes: CK_1, found primarily in the brain; CK_2, found in the myocardium; and CK_3, found in both skeletal muscle and the myocardium. In humans, the presence of CK_2 in the blood is useful in diagnosing a recent myocardial infarction, but in animals CK_3 is most commonly increased related to muscle damage. Called also creatine phosphokinase, Lohmann's enzyme.

c. phosphate see creatine (above).

c. phosphokinase called also CPK; see creatine kinase (above).

creatinemia excessive creatine in the blood.

creatinine a nitrogenous compound formed as the irreversible end product of creatine metabolism. It is formed in the muscle in relatively small amounts, passes into the blood and is excreted in the urine.

A laboratory test for the creatinine level in the blood may be used as a measurement of kidney function. Since creatinine is normally produced in fairly constant amounts as a result of the breakdown of phosphocreatine and is excreted in the urine, an elevation in the creatinine level in the blood indicates a disturbance in kidney function.

c.:blood urea nitrogen ratio determination of blood creatinine and blood urea nitrogen (BUN) and the relationship between them is an additional assessment of renal function. It may be useful in the differential diagnosis of azotemia and in monitoring renal disease when protein-restricted diets are being given.

c. clearance test a measure of renal function based on the rate at which ingested creatinine is filtered through the renal glomeruli.

c.:cortisol ratio see CORTISOL:creatinine ratio.

c.–protein ratio see PROTEIN–creatinine ratio.

urine c./serum c. ratio used to distinguish between prerenal and renal azotemia.

creatinuria an increased concentration of creatine in the urine. An excessive endogenous breakdown of muscle can cause this.

creatorrhea undigested muscle fibers in the feces; occurs with deficiency of trypsin in chronic exocrine pancreatic disease.

creep a barrier containing small apertures. Only the young animals of the group can penetrate the barrier. See also CREEPING.

c. barrier a barred barrier permitting maximum auditory, olfactory, visual and palpatory contact without domination. A useful technique in a primate colony.

c. feeding feed is placed on one side of the barrier and only the young can get access to it.

c. grazing a creep is placed across the entrance to the pasture and only animals small enough to penetrate the creep get access to the pasture.

c. ration a weaning diet, suitable for weaning the young, which are the only animals able to penetrate the creep.

creeper cows see DOWNER COW SYNDROME.

creeper pigs pigs which crawl along on their bellies; unable to stand, e.g. Pietrain creeper pigs.

creeping 1. gradual progression of a lesion or tissue growth. 2. prostrate growth pattern of a plant, e.g. c. buttercup (*Ranunculus repens*), c. caustic (*Euphorbia drummondii*), c. charlie (*Glechoma hederacea*), c. Crofton weed (*Eupatorium riparium*), c. indigo (*Indigofera spicata*), c. knapweed (*Acroptilon repens*), c. lantana (*Lantana montevidensis*), c. mallow (*Modiola carolinianum*), c. millotia (*Millotia greevesii*), c. oxalis (*Oxalis corniculata*), c. saltbush (*Atriplex semibaccata*).

c. eruption see cutaneous LARVA migrans.

c. substitution gradual penetration across a fracture site by osteogenic tissue followed by bone formation.

creeping Charlie see GLECHOMA HEDERACEA.

creeps see OSTEOMALACIA.

cremaster muscle a slip of muscle detached from

the internal oblique muscle and passing through the inguinal canal; attached to the vaginal tunics of the spermatic cord the muscles are effective in drawing up the testicles when injury threatens. See Table 13.

cremasteric pertaining to the cremaster muscle.

cremation disposal of a cadaver by total burning.

cremello creamy white coat color in horses; result of dilution of a yellow color. Like chestnuts cremellos are homozygous; heterozygotes are palominos.

Cremophor EL see EUGENOL.

crenate, crenated scalloped or notched.

crenation the formation of abnormal notching around the edge of an erythrocyte; the notched appearance of an erythrocyte due to its shrinkage after suspension in a hypertonic solution.

crenocyte a crenated erythrocyte.

Crenosoma a genus of lungworms of the family Crenosomatidae. Includes *Crenosoma mephiditis*, *C. petrowi*, *C. striatum* (wild animals), *C. vulpis* (in dogs, wild carnivores).

crenulation crenation.

creosol one of the active constituents of creosote.

creosote a mixture of phenols from wood tar; used externally as an antiseptic and internally in chronic bronchitis as an expectorant. A mixture of the carbonates of various constituents of creosote (creosote carbonate) is used the same as the base.

c.-treated timber treating timber with creosote is a common method of preservation. Use of the timber for housing while it is still wet may cause poisoning especially in young pigs. There may be local burning of the skin, oral, esophageal and gastric erosion, or degeneration of parenchymatous organs.

crepenynic acid fatty acid myotoxin found in *Ixiolaena brevicompta*.

Crepidostomum digenetic trematode parasite of salmonid and other fish. The genus is a member of the family Allocreadiidae.

crepitant having a dry, crackling sound.

crepitation a dry, crackling sound or sensation, such as that produced by the grating of the ends of a fractured bone.

respiratory c. a dry, crackling sound.

crepitus 1. the grating of fractured bone fragments against each other. 2. the crackling of joints. 3. the noise produced by pressure on tissues containing an abnormal amount of air or gas, as in cellular emphysema. 4. the discharge of flatus from the bowels. 5. crepitation. 6. a crepitant rale.

crepuscular active at twilight or just before dawn; said of animals or birds.

crescent 1. shaped like a new moon. 2. a crescent-shaped structure.

glomerular c. proliferation of parietal epithelial cells lining Bowman's capsule in the kidney; may protrude into Bowman's space and eventually lead to destruction of the glomerulus.

cresols 1. a group of phenols from coal or wood tar; includes *p*-cresol, *o*-cresol (2-methylphenol), *m*-phenol (3-methylphenol), *p*-phenol (4-methylphenol). 2. a preparation consisting of a mixture of isomeric cresol from coal tar or petroleum is used as a disinfectant.

c. poisoning the form of poisoning depends on the route of entry and the dose. There may be local corrosion, or cardiac depression, or liver damage with signs of jaundice, weakness, coma and death.

cress see LEPIDIUM SATIVUM.

crest 1. a projecting structure or ridge, especially one surmounting a bone or its border. 2. a term describing the upper margin of the neck; root of the mane in a horse. 3. in canaries, a crown of long feathers on the head, all radiating out from a central point; inherited as a dominant trait.

ampullary c. linear thickenings of the walls of the ampullae of the semicircular canals.

dental c. the maxillary ridge passing along the alveolar processes of the fetal maxillary bones.

epicondylar c. ridges which extend from the epicondyles of the humerus to the shaft.

ethmoid c. located on the inside surface of the nasal bones of the pig and dog.

external occipital c. an extension of the external occipital protuberance to which the ligamentum nuchae is attached.

facial c. the prominent crest on the external aspect of the maxilla of horses stretching from beneath the orbit to the middle of the molar teeth. The masseter muscle is attached to its ventral surface.

c. hair see MANE.

iliac c. the thickened cranial border of the ilium of dogs and cats.

neck c. the fatty, fibrous tissue above the nuchal ligament which gives the stallion's neck its characteristic elevated contour.

neural c. cords of nervous tissue which detaches from the developing spinal cord in the embryo; contribute tissue to the somatic and autonomic ganglia, and many other structures.

nuchal c. the thick, transverse crest on the occipital bone.

palatine c. a low transverse ridge on the palatine bones.

petrosal c. divides the cranial cavity into cerebellar and cerebral compartments.

renal c. the median ridge in the pelvis of many kidneys onto which papillary ducts open.

reticular c's the mucosal folds in the ruminant reticulum that form the cells of the honeycomb compartments of the walls.

sacral c's the median crest is the fused dorsal spines of the sacral vertebrae; the lateral sacral crest is the fused articular processes.

sagittal c. the ridge in the middle of the skull which extends forwards from the occipital protuberance; more pronounced in some species, breeds and individuals.

trochanteric c. a ridge which runs between the greater and lesser trochanters and forms the caudal wall of the trochanteric fossa.

urethral c. a longitudinal ridge in the roof of the pelvic urethra formed from two folds of urinary bladder mucosa which fuse after separate origins at the ureteric orifices.

vestibular c. divides the vestibule of the inner ear into the spherical and elliptical recesses.

Crested canary a breed developed from the Norwich canary, characterized by a narrow head and a very large crest.

crested dog's tail see CYNOSURUS CRISTATUS.

cresyl tolyl.

***m*-cresyl acetate** a topical antiseptic and antifungal effective against superficial yeast infections.

cresylic acid see CRESOLS.

cretin a patient exhibiting cretinism.

cretinism arrested physical and mental development with dystrophy of bones and soft tissues, resulting in disproportionate dwarfism. Due to congenital or early-onset hypothyroidism. Seen in foals and possibly is an unrecognized cause of neonatal deaths in other species.

cretinoid resembling a cretin, or suggestive of cretinism.
cretinous affected with cretinism.
Creutzfeldt–Jakob disease a human spongiform encephalopathy, a variant of which first recognized as affecting younger individuals is probably caused by the bovine spongiform encephalopathy prion.
crevice a fissure.
gingival c. the space between the cervical enamel of a tooth and the overlying unattached gingiva.
crevicular fluid produced by epithelium of the gingival crevice, it contains immunoglobulins and has antimicrobial properties.
CRH corticotropin releasing hormone.
CRI constant-rate infusion.
cria young offspring of camelids.
crib a rack or manger in a stable.
c.-biting a neurosis or acquired habit in stabled horses characterized by stereotypic behavior. The horse grasps a solid object with its incisor teeth, arches the neck, pulls upwards and backwards and swallows air. The consequences are eroded teeth, occasionally gastric distension and severe weight loss. Called also wind-sucking, cribbing.
c.-biting operation partial myectomy of the sternohyoideus muscle prevents ventral flexion of the head; not commonly performed. An alternative procedure involves neurectomy of the spinal accessory nerve.
cribber a horse with the vice of CRIB-biting.
cribbing see CRIB-biting.
cribriform perforated like a sieve.
c. plate see cribriform PLATE.
cricetine members of the subfamily Cricetinae, the New World rats and mice.
Cricetus small brown rodent with black underbelly. Nocturnal, burrower, hoarder, brief gestation period (15–16 days) and possesses a pair of capacious cheek pouches. Popular as a research animal and as a pet. Includes *Cricetus cricetus* (common hamster), *C. griseus* (Chinese hamster) and *Mesocricetus auratus* (golden or Syrian hamster).
cricoarytenoid pertaining to the cricoid and arytenoid cartilages.
c. muscle see Table 13.1E.
cricoesophageal pertaining to the cricoid cartilage and the esophagus.
cricoid 1. ring-shaped. 2. the cricoid cartilage.
c. cartilage a ringlike cartilage at the caudal part of the larynx.
cricoidectomy excision of the cricoid cartilage.
cricolaryngotomy a surgical procedure for reconstruction of the larynx in subglottic stenosis.
cricopharyngeal pertaining to the cricoid cartilage and pharynx.
c. dysphagia see cricopharyngeal ACHALASIA.
c. myotomy a surgical procedure for the treatment of cricopharyngeal achalasia; involves severance of the median raphe between cricopharyngeus muscles on the dorsal aspect of the larynx.
cricopharyngeus muscle see Table 13.1C.
cricothyreotomy incision through the cricoid and thyroid cartilages.
cricothyroid pertaining to the cricoid and thyroid cartilages.
c. ligament attaches the cricoid to the thyroid cartilage.
cricothyrotomy incision through the skin and cricothyroid membrane to secure a patent airway for emergency relief of upper airway obstruction.
cricotomy incision of the cricoid cartilage.
cricotracheal membrane the mucosal lining of the cricotracheal ligament.
cricotracheotomy incision of the trachea through the cricoid cartilage.
Crile hemostatic forceps standard type of hemostats with box joint, ratchet catch, long blades with cross ridging on the blade face.
Crimean-Congo hemorrhagic fever a zoonotic disease of humans, in central Asia through to eastern Europe, who are in contact with livestock. Caused by a bunyavirus, it is transmitted by ticks. The principal signs are fever, widespread hemorrhages and necrotizing hepatitis.
crimidine a rapidly acting convulsant used as a rodenticide. Attacks all species similarly except for poultry which simply become somnolent. Pyridoxine is a complete antidote. Called also castrix.
criminal law the law as defined in the Crimes Act, or similar relevant act, which defines what are criminal offences and therefore come within the scope of the Act. The attitude taken is that the part of the offended party in the confrontation to be enacted is the state acting as the champion of all the people.
crimp a regular wave formation of small dimensions, e.g. the crimp of wool fibers epitomized in the Merino breed and its derivatives.
c. marks marks made by wrinkling the x-ray film while holding it between the fingers.
crimped said of grain that has been passed through corrugated rollers after previous exposure to moist heat so that the grain is fractured but there is a minimum of dust.
crin- prefix meaning secrete.
Criniferoides go-away birds.
C. leucogaster white-bellied go-away birds.
crinkle bush see LOMATIA SILAIFOLIA.
crinogenic causing secretion in a gland.
crinophagy a process in which excessive amounts of hormone are fused with lysozymes to degrade the hormone.
Crinum a genus of cultivated ornamental plants of the family Liliaceae (Amaryllidaceae), some of which are known to cause collapse and death in sheep and goats. Called also spider lily.
Criollo native Spanish-American light horse or riding pony. Includes a number of ethnic varieties, e.g. Argentine Criollo. Any color, 13.3 to 15 hands high. Originated from a mixture of Arab, Barb and Andalusian.
cripples see OSTEOMALACIA.
crisis pl. *crises* [L.] 1. the turning point of a disease for better or worse; especially a sudden change, usually for the better, in the course of an acute disease. 2. a sudden paroxysmal intensification of signs in the course of a disease.
addisonian c. signs of severe depression, muscle weakness, vomiting and diarrhea accompanying an acute attack of adrenocortical insufficiency (Addison's disease). Called also adrenal crisis.
adrenal c. see addisonian crisis (above).
crispatine a hepatoxic alkaloid present in the plant CROTALARIA *crispata*.
crista see CREST (1).
c. ampullare see ampullary CREST.
cristobalite the form of silicate which is found in the granulomatous lesions in silicate pneumoconiosis in horses.
Critesion see HORDEUM.
Crithidia a genus, the trypanosomes, in the family Trypanosomatidae found in arthropods and other invertebrates.

C. luciliae commercial preparations of this organism are used as substrate in assays for serum antibodies against native DNA.

crithidial stage see EPIMASTIGOTE.

critical 1. a point at which one property or state changes to another property or state. 2. pertaining to a crisis in a disease.

c. care care of a patient in a life-threatening situation of an illness. Includes artificial life support system.

c. care unit see INTENSIVE care unit.

embryological c. period the period during the life of the embryo, specific for each body system, during which organ genesis takes place.

c. distance see FLIGHT DISTANCE.

c. point drying the technique used in preparing tissues for electron microscopy; to eliminate distortion due to surface tension.

c. temperature the body temperature above which the animal is said to be fevered. See body TEMPERATURE.

critical care patient care pertaining to a crisis in a disease.

c. c. medicine emergency care for victims of trauma or disease.

c. c. unit a unit in a hospital in which special patient care staff and units, including ECG, blood gas analysis apparatus, resuscitation and life support equipment are available and used.

Crivellia see PRZEVALSKIANA.

crock cull ewe; called also crone.

crocodile large aquatic reptile, member of the family Crocodylidae. Includes the Nile (*Crocodylus niloticus*), the Marsh or Mugger (*C. palustris*), the Estuarine or Saltwater (*C. porosus*), the American (*C. acutus*), New Guinea (*C. novaeguineae*) and the West African (*Osteolaemus tetraspis*) crocodile. Crocodile and alligator farms are now an established means of producing hides for commerce.

Crocodilia see CROCODILE.

crocodylia reptile member of the order Crocodilia. Includes the alligators, caimans, crocodiles and gavials.

Crocuta crocuta see HYENA.

Crofton weed AGERATINA *adenophora*.

Crohn's disease a regional, granulomatous enteritis of humans; equine granulomatous ENTERITIS, histiocytic ulcerative COLITIS of Boxer dogs, JOHNE'S DISEASE of cattle, and regional or terminal ILEITIS of pigs are similar diseases and all have been proposed as possible animal models.

cromoglycate see CROMOLYN.

cromolyn a mast cell stabilizer which, if administered prior to exposure to allergens, prevents degranulation and release of histamine in a hypersensitivity reaction. Administered as an aerosol for prophylaxis of bronchial asthma and allergic rhinitis. Investigated for use in the treatment of CHRONIC obstructive pulmonary disease in horses. Called also cromoglycate.

crone see CROCK.

crooked calf disease LUPINUS *angustifolius*. See also ARTHROGRYPOSIS.

crooked neck a disease of turkeys thought to be due to airsacculitis caused by *Mycoplasma meleagridis*. A similar syndrome in Brown Leghorn chickens is due to an inherited defect.

crooked toe disease a disease of young chickens and turkeys of unknown etiology. Only a few birds are affected. The phalanges are twisted so that the toes are bent laterally or medially and the birds have difficulty in walking. Must be differentiated from CURLED TOE PARALYSIS.

Crookes' tube the original x-ray tube; worked on the principle of ionization of gas within the tube,

crop 1. a saccular diverticulum of the esophagus just anterior to the entrance to the thorax. Present in all domestic birds. 2. domesticated plants sown and harvested for use by humans. 3. a cosmetic surgical procedure carried out on the ears of dogs of certain breeds. See EAR CROPPING.

c.-bound impaction of the crop in a bird.

c.-eared small eared.

c. flush 1. treatment of a sick bird by a flushing out, with normal saline via an esophageal tube, of food and debris from the crop. 2. see also crop wash (below).

impacted c. distension of the crop with undigested food.

c. milk crumbly material, composed of lipid-laden, desquamated epithelial cells mixed with food, elaborated by both male and female pigeons in the crop and regurgitated to feed the nestlings.

pendulous c. a condition of domesticated birds in which the crop becomes very distended and full of feed. Sporadic cases only, but there is an inherited predisposition to gross distension in turkeys. Called also impacted crop or crop bound.

c. residues the remains of a crop after the commercially sought part of it has been harvested, e.g. wheat stubble, pea haulms, oaten straw.

c. wash used in the differential diagnosis of trichomoniasis and candidiasis and to assess crop flora in birds with regurgitation and other signs referable to upper alimentary tract disease.

crosier unfolding (uncurling) new leaf on bracken and most ferns; inspiration for the tip of ecclesiastical staffs.

cross 1. a cross-shaped figure or structure. 2. any organism produced by mating genetically distinct individuals. See also CROSSBREEDING, CRUCIATE.

c.-cut grid see CROSS-HATCH GRID.

c. pregnancy the fetus is in the horn on the side opposite to the corpus luteum.

c. table see HORIZONTAL beam.

c. tie a common method of restraining a horse for simple procedures such as grooming. The horse is tied to a pillar on either side, the shorter and tighter the better and preferably from the cheek dees of a hackamore. The head should be kept high to avoid the horse lashing out with both feet at once.

cross country races races which feature jumps, water hazards and which test the horses' speed and stamina.

cross-eye STRABISMUS in which there is manifest deviation of the visual axis of one eye toward that of the other eye, resulting in diplopia. Called also esotropia and convergent strabismus.

cross-firing see FORGING.

cross-fostering the transfer of young from one dam to another, usually to equalize numbers in litters of approximately the same age. Commonly practiced in rearing piglets.

cross-hatch grid a grid used in radiography in which there are two sets of parallel strips at right angles to each other. Called also crossed grid.

cross-immunity a form of immunity in which immunity to one bacteria or virus is effective in protecting the animal against an antigenically similar but different organism, e.g. protection of cattle against bacillary hemoglobinuria (*Clostridium haemolyticum*) by vaccination against black disease (*C. novyi*) and measles virus vaccine used to immunize dogs against canine distemper. See also heterotypic VACCINE.

cross matching a procedure vital in blood transfusions and organ transplantation. The recipient's erythrocytes or leukocytes mixed with the donor's serum and vice versa. Absence of agglutination, hemolysis and cytotoxicity indicates that the donor and recipient are blood group compatible or histocompatible.

cross-over groups groups of animals which are being compared with respect to certain variables and in which the difference in variables can be transposed from one group to the other so that a cross-over experiment is conducted.

cross ratio see ODDS ratio. Called also approximate relative risk.

cross-reaction a reaction which occurs when surface antigenic determinants on different molecules of quite different sources are identical, so that antibody directed against one antigen also reacts with another.

cross-reactivity the degree to which an antibody participates in cross-reactions.

cross-regulation in the regulation of enzyme activity, the product of one pathway serves as an inhibitor or activator of an enzyme in another pathway.

cross-sectional study a study in which a statistically significant sample of a population is used to estimate the relationship between an outcome of interest and population variables as they exist at one particular time. Since both the outcome and the variables are measured at the one time these studies are not strong at showing cause–effect relationships.

cross species colostrum preserved colostrum fed to a young animal from other than a dam of the same species.

crossbite malocclusion.

anterior c. mandibular incisors are anterior to the maxillary incisors.

posterior c. mandibular premolars or molars are buccal to their opposing teeth.

crossbow a weapon used to fire darts filled with immobilizing agent at otherwise uncontrollable animals. Less dangerous than cordite guns and does not scare other animals because there is no noise.

crossbred progeny of a mating between two animals which are purebreds of different breeds, e.g. crossbred sheep are usually offspring of matings between merinos and British breeds.

crossbreeding hybridization; the mating of organisms of different strains or species, e.g. when animals of different breeds are mated. Practiced extensively in farm animals to capitalize on advantages conferred by HYBRID vigor.

crossed extensor reflex a reflex movement which occurs in response to a test of a flexor reflex, extension is elicited in the opposite limb. Seen in upper motor neuron disease.

crossed grid see CROSS-HATCH GRID.

crossed legs while standing or walking is a sign of paresis.

crossing see CROSSBREEDING.

crossing over the exchanging of material between homologous chromosomes, during the first meiotic division, resulting in new combinations of genes.

Crossoptilon auritum blue-eared PHEASANT.

crossover an exchange of material between two homologous chromosomes.

Crotalaria a plant genus of the legume family Fabaceae. There are many species and most of them are poisonous. They all contain pyrrolizidine alkaloids which cause damage in liver, lungs and in pigs in the kidney. Called also rattlepods. The diseases caused have many names including WALKABOUT, Kimberley horse disease, stywcsiekte and jaagsiekte.

Includes as causes of liver damage, lung damage and dummy syndrome in horses and cattle: *C. anagyroides*, *C. barkae* (*C. geminiflora*), *C. burkeana*, *C. crispata*, *C. dissitiflora* (gray rattlepod), *C. dura* (wild lucerne), *C. globifera* (wild lucerne), *C. goreensis* (Gambia pea), *C. juncea* (sunn hemp), *C. lachnocarpoides*, *C. mauensis*, *C. mesopontica*, *C. mitchelli*, *C. mucronata*, *C. novae-hollandiae*, *C. pallida*, *C. polysperma* (*C. saltiana*, *C. striata*), *C. retusa* (wedge-leafed rattlepod), *C. rhodesiae*, *C. rotundifolia*, *C. sagittalis*, *C. spectabilis* (*C. retzii*, *C. sericea*), *C. steudneri* (*C. hispida*), *C. zimmermannii*.

Includes as causes of esophageal ulceration in horses: *C. aridicola* (Chillagoe horse poison), *C. medicaginea* (*C. trifoliastrum*).

Includes as a cause of pulmonary edema: *C. eremaea*, *C. spartioides*, *C. pallida*.

Crotalidae a family of snakes with movable fangs (Solenoglypha). Includes pit vipers (*Bothrops* spp.) and rattlesnakes (*Crotalus* spp.).

Crotalus see RATTLESNAKE.

crotamiton an acaricide used in the topical treatment of scabies in dogs and cnemidocoptic mange in budgerigars.

Croton a genus of the plant family Euphorbiaceae. Contains croton oil, a violent and lethal purgative. Cake made from the seeds after extraction of the oil may also cause severe gastroenteritis. Includes *C. capitatus*, *C. texensis*, *C. tiglium*.

croton oil a very potent purgative oil extracted from the plant CROTON.

crotonyl isothiocyanate a highly poisonous substance found in the seeds of swedes and turnips. Causes severe gastroenteritis.

crotoxyphos an insecticide used for fly control and externally on livestock; a cholinesterase inhibitor. See ORGANOPHOSPHORUS COMPOUND.

croup 1. the muscular area around and above the base of the tail in the horse. 2. acute obstruction of the larynx caused usually by allergy or respiratory infection. Used with reference to children and chickens.

crow a bird in the genus CORVUS.

c. pick predatory gouging of eyes and other soft tissues from sick or weak lambs by crows. Wounds often infected with gas gangrene organisms.

crow garlic ALLIUM *vineale*.

crow poison see AMIANTHIUM MUSCAETOXICUM.

crowding panic state developed by chickens, adult birds, sheep in response to perceived attack; group piles up in a corner and many die of suffocation; in horses takes the form of squeezing an attendant against another horse or a stable wall, a common vice in horses which are permanently stabled.

c. stress constant low level stress due to insufficient accommodation space per animal.

crown 1. the topmost part of an organ or structure, e.g. the top of the head. 2. artificial crown on a tooth.

anatomical c. the enamel-covered part of a tooth.

ciliary c. the portion of the ciliary body of the eye that is located closest to the lens and bears the ciliary processes.

clinical c. the exposed part of a tooth within the mouth.

c. height reduction a dental procedure sometimes done on canine teeth in dogs for the treatment of malocclusion or to prevent injury from biting.

reserve c. in a hypsodont tooth, that part of the crown located in the alveolus.

crown beard see VERBESINA ENCELIOIDES.

crown-of-thorns see EUPHORBIA.
crown vetch see CORONILLA VARIA.
crownbeard see VERBESINA ENCELIOIDES.
crowsfoot grass, crowfoot grass ELEUSINE *indica*.
crozier see CROSIER.
CRP C-reactive protein; cyclic AMP-receptor protein.
CRT capillary refill time.
CRTZ chemoreceptor trigger zone.
crucian carp see CARASSIUS CARASSIUS.
cruciate shaped like a cross.
caudal (posterior) c. ligament complements the cranial cruciate ligament in providing a major part of the stability of the stifle joint. It originates from the lateral aspect of the medial femoral condyle, passes caudally and distally to insert on the medial side of the popliteal notch (tibia). Rupture is rare, except in association with cranial cruciate rupture, and results from severe injuries to the joint.
cranial (anterior) c. ligament part of the stifle joint, originates in a fossa on the caudal aspect of the medial side of the lateral femoral condyle. It runs cranially, medially and distally between the condyles of the femur to insert on the cranial intercondyloid area of the tibia. The ligament acts to limit cranial movement of the tibia relative to the femur, and when the joint is flexed to limit internal axial movement. Rupture of this ligament is common in dogs, causing lameness, often with joint effusion, and chronic arthritis. Surgical reconstruction or stabilization of the joint is recommended.
c. suture pattern an interrupted cross mattress suture to close wounds that are under a lot of tension. The needle is inserted through the tissue, across the wound, then back through the tissue on the other side, across the wound on the outside and advancing the needle to the next suture site where a second stitch is made in the same manner as the first. The two ends are then tied across the wound so as to create the cross shape.
crucible a vessel for melting refractory substances.
cruciform cross-shaped.
crude fat see crude FAT.
crude fiber see FIBER[2].
crude oil fossil oil as it is retrieved from its natural location.
c. o. poisoning crude oil is usually too unpalatable for livestock but cattle will drink it if they are salt hungry. The effects of ingesting large amounts are severe depression, incoordination and vomiting, leading to development of aspiration pneumonia and death.
crude protein see crude PROTEIN.
crude rate a measure of overall frequency which has not been adjusted for significant factors which might have influenced the rate.
cruel vine see ARAUJIA HORTORUM.
cruelty the infliction of pain or distress unnecessarily.
c. to animals an offence under the Protection of Animals Act or similar legislation. The definition of *unnecessary* varies between countries and from time to time in the one country. Under the impetus of a great body of community compassion the threhold has been greatly lowered in recent times. Determination of the prevailing standard of cruelty can only be decided by the courts.

It is now taken to include, besides physical assault and surgery without anesthesia, deprival of food, water and shelter. The worst kinds of cruelty are susceptible to the heaviest penalty, under the classification of aggravated cruelty.
crufomate an organophosphorus compound used as an anthelmintic and in the control of warble fly in cattle. Called also Montrel, Ruelene.
cruor a blood clot.
crupper the part of the harness of a horse which encircles the tail and prevents the harness from slipping forward.
crural pertaining to or emanating from a crus.
c. hernia see FEMORAL hernia.
crus pl. *crura* [L.] 1. shaped like the human leg. 2. a leglike part. Called also branch, e.g. the branches or crura of the atrioventricular bundle.
c. cerebri the ventral part of the cerebral peduncles comprising fiber tracts descending from the cerebral cortex to form the longitudinal fascicles of the pons.
clitoridal c. the continuation of the corpora cavernosa of the clitoris, diverging posteriorly to be attached to the sciatic arch.
diaphragmatic c. two fibromuscular bands that arise from the lumbar vertebrae and insert into the central tendon of the diaphragm.
fornical c. two flattened bands of white matter that unite to form the body of the fornix of the cerebrum.
penile c. the continuation of each corpus cavernosum of the penis, diverging caudally to be attached to the sciatic arch.
crush 1. a restraining device for large animals. See also CHUTE. 2. application of pressure so as to destroy the natural condition, shape or integrity of the parts. 3. see CRUSHING.
crush syndrome the edema, oliguria and other clinical signs of renal failure that follow crushing of a part, especially a large muscle mass, causing the release of myoglobin. See also lower nephron NEPHROSIS.
crushing deaths of newborn animals, especially those in litters, caused by the mother lying on them accidentally. Contributed to by weakness of the neonate or awkward accommodation. A problem in piglets and puppies. Called also overlying.
crust a formed outer layer, especially an outer layer of solid matter formed by drying of a bodily exudate or secretion. It may be serocellular or hemorrhagic.
palisading c. there are alternating layers of cellular debris and exudate; typical of fungal infections of the skin and dermatophilosis.
waxy c. typical of exudative epidermitis.
crusta pl. *crustae* [L.] a crust.
Crustacea a class of arthropods including the lobsters, crabs, shrimps, wood lice, water fleas and barnacles.
crustaceans members of the class CRUSTACEA. Includes amongst the aquatic crustaceans, shrimp, prawn, yabby, crab, lobster. May of them are now farmed commercially in enclosed waters.
parasitic c. small crustaceans or copepods are common parasites on the gills of aquarium and pond fish where they appear as white spots. The gills become obstructed and the fish die of anoxia.
crutch 1. the area of the skin from the anus ventrally to the scrotum in the male and to a comparable position in the female. 2. an instrument consisting of a long handle with a U shape at one end.
Kühn's c. see KÜHN'S CRUTCH.
repulsion c. used in obstetrics to repel a calf or foal fetus to enable malpositioned limbs to be repositioned.
Williams c. a repulsion crutch in which the U-shaped end has a screw-in sharp spike at the bottom of the U to prevent the crutch slipping off the calf while repelling it.

crutching shearing of the wool from the perineal region of the sheep as a protection against blowfly strike. Wool contaminated by dags of manure and by urine is a major attractant for blowflies. See also DAGGING.
crutchings the wool obtained by crutching.
cryalgesia pain on application of cold.
cry(o)- word element. [Gr.] *cold.*
cryoadhesion in contact freezing, the bond between a cryoprobe and the tissue being treated; facilitated by moisture on the tissue.
cryoanalgesia the relief of pain by the application of cold by cryoprobe to peripheral nerves.
cryobank a facility for freezing and preserving semen at low temperatures (usually –196.5 °C) for future use.
cryobiology the science dealing with the effect of low temperatures on biological systems.
cryocautery see cold CAUTERY.
cryoepilation use of a cryoprobe to destroy hair follicles in the treatment of distichiasis.
cryoextraction use of a cryoprobe to form an attachment to the lens in an intracapsular lens removal.
cryoextractor a cryoprobe used in cryoextraction.
cryofibrinogen an abnormal fibrinogen that precipitates at low temperatures and redissolves at 98.6°F (37°C).
cryofibrinogenemia the presence of cryofibrinogen in the blood.
cryogen substance used to lower temperature in tissue to be frozen, e.g. liquid nitrogen, Freon, carbon dioxide and nitrous oxide.
cryogenic producing low temperatures.
cryoglobulin an abnormal globulin that precipitates at low temperatures and redissolves at 98.6°F (37°C).
cryoglobulinemia the presence of cryoglobulin in the blood, which is precipitated in the microvasculature upon exposure to cold.
cryohypophysectomy destruction of the pituitary gland by the application of cold.
cryolite a naturally occurring mineral, sodium aluminum fluoride, May be a source of fluorine poisoning if the mineral is used industrially.
cryometer a thermometer for measuring very low temperature.
cryophilic, psychrophilic preferring or growing best at low temperatures.
cryophylactic resistant to very low temperatures; said of bacteria.
cryoprecipitate any precipitate that results from cooling.
cryopreservation maintenance of the viability of excised tissue or organs by storing at very low temperatures.
cryoprobe an instrument for applying extreme cold to tissue.
cryoprotectant substance added to living biological material, e.g. embryo, ova, spermatozoa, that is to be preserved in a viable state by freezing. The common substances are DMSO and glycerol.
cryoprotective capable of protecting against injury due to freezing, as glycerol protects frozen red blood cells.
cryoprotein a blood protein that precipitates on cooling.
cryoscopy examination of fluids based on the principle that the freezing point of a solution varies according to the amount and nature of the solute.
cryospray the use of a liquid nitrogen spray in cryosurgery.
cryostat 1. a device by which temperature can be maintained at a very low level. 2. in pathology and histology, a chamber containing a microtome for sectioning frozen tissue.
cryosurgery the destruction of tissue by application of extreme cold. Used in the treatment of certain malignant lesions of the skin and mucous membranes, anorectal lesions and in the removal of cataracts.
cryothalamectomy destruction of a portion of the thalamus by application of extreme cold.
cryotherapy the therapeutic use of cold. See also CRYOSURGERY, HYPOTHERMIA.
cryotolerant able to withstand very low temperatures.
cryotome rotary microtome in a frozen section environment.
cryotonsillectomy cryosurgical excision of the tonsils.
crypt a blind pit or tube on a free surface.
anal c's furrows, with pouchlike recesses at the caudal end, separating the rectal columns; called also anal sinuses.
c's of Lieberkühn the lumen of intestinal glands on the surface of the intestinal mucous membrane.
tongue c. deep, irregular invaginations from the surface of the lingual tonsil.
tonsillar c's epithelium-lined clefts in the palatine tonsils.
cryptectomy excision or obliteration of a crypt.
cryptitis inflammation of the mucous membrane of the anal crypts.
crypt(o)- word element. [Gr.] *concealed, pertaining to a crypt.*
Cryptobia a genus of biflagellate protozoa that parasitize fish, amphibians and other aquatic creatures.
C. borreli, C. brachialis, C. cyprini parasitic hemoflagellates of fish, transmitted by leeches.
Cryptocarya pleurosperma Australian tree in the family Lauraceae; the bark contains a very irritating alkaloid, cryptopleurine, and the leaves contain pleurospermine which is also vesicant and irritant. Called also poison walnut.
Cryptocaryon a ciliate protozoan.
C. irritans cause of 'white spot' skin and gill disease in saltwater fish.
cryptocephalus a monster with an inconspicuous head.
cryptococcosis infection by *Cryptococcus neoformans*, having a predilection for the brain and meninges but also invading the skin, nasal cavity, lungs, eyes and rarely other organs such as the udder. In animals it occurs most often in cats, but is recorded in most other species. Granulomas in the upper respiratory tract and meningoencephalitis are the clinical features. Called also European blastomycosis, torulosis.
Cryptococcus a genus of yeastlike fungi.
C. farciminosum see HISTOPLASMA *farciminosum*.
C. neoformans a species of worldwide distribution, causing CRYPTOCOCCOSIS in all species including humans; there are two biovars, *C.* var *neoformans*, and *C.* var *gattae*. Called also *Torula histolytica, Torulopsis neoformans*.
Cryptocotyle a genus of flukes (digenetic trematodes) in the family Heterophyidae.
C. concavium, C. jejuna, C. lingua intestinal flukes that can cause enteritis in fish-eating birds, dogs and other mammals. Fish are the intermediate hosts.
cryptodeterminant hidden determinant.
cryptodidymus a twin monster, one fetus being enclosed within the body of the other.
cryptogenic of obscure or doubtful origin.

cryptoglioma a stage of retinal glioma in which the eyeball shrinks, masking the presence of the growth.

cryptolith a concretion in a crypt.

cryptomerorachischisis see SPINA bifida occulta.

cryptophthalmia, cryptophthalmus congenital absence of the palpebral fissure, the skin extending from the forehead to the cheek, and the eye malformed or rudimentary.

cryptopodia swelling of the lower leg and foot, covering all but the sole of the foot.

cryptorchid an animal with undescended testes. Called also rig, ridgling.

cryptorchidectomy excision of an undescended testis. See also ORCHIECTOMY.

cryptorchidism the state of being a cryptorchid. An improperly developed testis may never leave the abdomen, and it may not produce the hormones that induce secondary sex characters. A testis lodged in the canal may well produce these secondary sex characters, but cannot produce spermatozoa. Failure of both testicles to descend is uncommon. Usually only one testis is involved and the other produces sufficient spermatozoa to render the animal fertile. Called also rig.

inherited c. there is some evidence that cryptorchidism can be inherited in most species.

cryptorchism see CRYPTORCHIDISM.

cryptosporidiosis infection with *Cryptosporidium* spp. In all species causes diarrhea in the newborn. The protozoan may depend on the prior presence of another pathogen, e.g. rotavirus, to exert its pathogenicity. The critical lesion in the disease is villous atrophy causing a malabsorption defect. Also infects trachea, cloaca, bursa of Fabricius, and conjunctival sacs of birds, the stomach of mice and snakes, the bile duct of monkeys, and immunodeficient foals. See also CRYPTOSPORIDIUM.

Cryptosporidium a coccidial protozoan parasite in most species. A member of the family Eimeriidae. Includes *C. bayleyi* in birds, *C. serpentis* in reptiles, *C. crotalis* in reptiles, *C. meleagridis* in birds, *C. muris* and *C. parvum* in mammals, and *C. nasorum* in fish.

Cryptostegia grandiflora plant of the family Asclepiadaceae family, originally from Madagascar; contains cardiac glycosides; causes sudden death after exercise in cattle. Called also rubber vine.

Cryptostemma calendula see ARCTOTHECA CALENDULA.

cryptotoxic a substance with toxic properties which are only exhibited in particular circumstances.

crystal a naturally produced angular solid of definite form.

c.-associated hepatopathy see CRYSTAL-ASSOCIATED CHOLANGIOHEPATOPATHY.

c.-induced arthritis see GOUT, PSEUDOGOUT.

piezoelectric c. the source of sound waves in ULTRASONOGRAPHY.

radiographic c's crystals on radiographs caused by faulty use of fixative, commonly excess acidity or insufficient washing of the film.

synovial c. see GOUT, PSEUDOGOUT.

tissue c. recognizable crystals in tissues occur in crystal-associated cholangiohepatopathy, zinc and oxalate poisoning.

urines c's see CRYSTALLURIA.

c. violet a brilliant organic deep purple dye.

c. violet vaccine an obsolete hog cholera vaccine.

crystal-associated cholangiohepatopathy hepatopathy characterized by crystals in large quantities in the biliary system; always a plant poisoning but the toxin may be from one occurring naturally in the plant, e.g. *Agave lecheguilla*, or one produced by a metabolite in the plant when it interacts with a toxic fungus, e.g. *Tribulus terrestris* and sporidesmin. The toxin is thought to be a steroidal sapogenin.

crystallin a globulin in the crystalline lens of the eye.

crystalline 1. resembling a crystal in nature or clearness. 2. pertaining to crystals.

c. lens the transparent organ behind the pupil of the eye. See also LENS.

crystallography the science dealing with the study of crystals.

x-ray c. the determination of the three-dimensional structure of molecules by means of diffraction patterns produced by x-rays.

crystalloid 1. resembling a crystal. 2. a noncolloid substance. Crystalloids form true solutions and therefore are capable of passing through a semipermeable membrane, as in DIALYSIS. The physical opposite of a crystalloid is a COLLOID (3), which does not dissolve and does not form true solutions.

c. particle a matrix particle in a single membrane contained in a peroxisome, when viewed through an electron microscope. Called also nucleoid.

c. solution contains electrolytes and nonelectrolytes which will diffuse into all body fluid compartments. Examples are Ringer's solution and 5% dextrose in water.

crystalluria the excretion of crystals in the urine, causing irritation of the kidney. See also STRUVITE, FELINE urological syndrome.

Cs chemical symbol, *cesium.*

CSA canine secretory alloantigen.

csA cyclosporin A.

CSF cerebrospinal fluid.

CSF-1 monocyte-macrophage colony-stimulating factor.

CSFs colony-stimulating factors.

CSK see chronic superficial KERATITIS.

CSM cerebrospinal meningitis.

CT computed tomography.

CT number the density assigned to a voxel in a CT (computed TOMOGRAPHY) scan on an arbitrary scale on which air has a density −1000; water, 0; and compact bone +1000. CT numbers are sometimes said to be expressed in 'Hounsfield units'.

CT 1341 see SAFFAN.

CTA medium a semisolid medium with crystine and trypticase. Used together with carbohydrate disks to demonstrate acid production in the identification of fastidious bacteria.

CTAT computerized transaxial tomography.

ctenidium a spine which occurs in rows on the heads of fleas; called also combs; useful for morphological identification.

Ctenizidae a family of venomous spiders. It contains *Atrax* spp., the funnel-web spider.

Ctenocephalides a genus of fleas of the order Siphonaptera. Includes *Ctenocephalides canis* (dogs and related species), *C. felis*, *C. f. felis*, *C. f. strongylus*, *C. f. damarensis* and *C. f. orientalis*; infest cats, dogs and related small animals.

Ctenomys talarum an arid-zone rodent which develops type 2 diabetes when fed laboratory chow ad lib.

Ctenopharyngodon edella farmed finfish in the family Cyprinidae. Called also grass carp. See Table 23.

CTL cytotoxic T lymphocyte.

CTP cytosine triphosphate.

CTP synthetase see CYTIDINE 5 -triphosphate.

Cu chemical symbol, *copper* (L. *cuprum*).

cu. cubic.

cu.cm cubic centimeter.
cu.mm cubic millimeter.
cub the newborn of a number of animal species as diverse as lion, fox and bear.
Cuban molasses–urea–bagasse a feedlot cattle feeding system based on using excess sugar cane residues. Bagasse is the fibrous residue of sugar cane after the sugar juice is expressed.
cubes feed for animals compressed into cubes. May be entirely concentrate but many nowadays are a complete ration including hammer-milled fiber. Are more expensive but reduce wastage and can be eaten more quickly than a milled grain mixture. See also pelleted FEED.
cubicles individual cow bed spaces separated by half height and half length partitions. Usually located in loose housing cow accommodation in which the cow is free to wander at will.
cubitus the forelimb distal to the humerus; includes the elbow, forearm, paw.
c. valgus a deformity of the elbow in which it deviates away from the midline of the body when extended.
c. varus a deformity of the elbow in which it deviates towards the midline of the body when extended.
cuboid resembling a cube; applied particularly to bones.
Cubomedusae an order of aquatic animals including sea wasps and box jellyfish, e.g. *Chironex fleckeri*.
Cuboni test a pregnancy test for use in mares and based on detection of estrogens in the urine. Suitable for use only in mares bred for at least 5 months.
cuckoopint ARUM *maculatum*.
cucumber *Cucumis sativus*.
Cucumis a genus in the plant family Cucurbitaceae. The cucumbers. Contain toxic tetracyclic triterpenes which cause enteritis and diarrhea, possibly blindness in horses. Includes *C. africanus*, *C. melo* var. *agrostis* (*C. picrocarpus*, *C. trigonus*, Ulcardo melon), *C. myriocarpus* (prickly paddymelon), *C. sativus*.
Cucurbita maxima squash, pumpkin.
cucurbitacins toxic tetracyclic triterpenes found in plants of the family Cucurbitaceae, e.g. squash, pumpkin, cucumber, melons. Called also 'bitter principle of the cucurbits'.
cucurbitine marginally effective anticestodal compound in pumpkin seed.
cud the bolus regurgitated by ruminants. It contains fiber, other food particles, rumen liquor and flora.
c. chewing after regurgitation, chewing on the remains of the regurgitus.
c. dropping a usually temporary condition in the cow in which each regurgitated bolus is rejected to the exterior. There is no other abnormality.
losing the c. the cow that has 'lost her cud' is not ruminating. This is a nonspecific sign of illness.
c. transfer a therapeutic practice of collecting fresh ruminal contents, from the mouth of a ruminating cow or by stomach tube from a rumen or from a freshly killed normal animal, and administering an infusion of it to a cow with ruminal stasis. The objective is to repopulate the recipient rumen with viable, normal ruminal flora.
cuddie trot the strange gait of a sheep with scrapie. It is an unsteady trot with the ears moving loosely up and down.
cudding chewing the cud. See also RUMINATION.
cuffing formation of a cufflike surrounding border, as of leukocytes about a blood vessel, observed in certain infections.
c. pneumonia chronic enzootic pneumonia of calves in which there is lymphofollicular cuffing of small airways.
cul-de-sac [Fr.] *a blind pouch.*
Douglas' c. a sac or recess formed by a fold of the peritoneum dipping down between the rectum and the uterus. Called also rectouterine excavation or pouch.
culard see MYOFIBER hyperplasia.
culdoscope an endoscope used in culdoscopy.
Culex a genus of mosquitoes found throughout the world; cause insect worry and many species transmit various disease-producing agents, e.g. microfilariae, apicomplexan parasites and viruses, such as those of Japanese encephalitis and equine encephalomyelitis.
C. pipiens transmits the virus of fowlpox.
C. pipiens quinquefasciatus a serious pest of poultry and carrier of a number of poultry diseases.
C. tarsalis transmits western equine encephalomyelitis.
C. tritaeniohynchus transmits Japanese encephalitis virus.
Culicidae see CULEX, ANOPHELES.
culicide an agent that destroys mosquitoes.
culicifuge an agent that repels mosquitoes.
culicine 1. any member of the genus *Culex* or related genera. 2. pertaining to, involving, or affecting mosquitoes of the genus *Culex* or related species.
culicoid see CULICOIDES.
Culicoides a large genus of biting midges belonging to the family Ceratopogonidae. They act as vectors of bluetongue, ephemeral fever, Akabane virus of cattle, epizootic hemorrhagic disease of deer, and African horse sickness and many are intermediate hosts of filarioid nematodes.

Many are causes of cutaneous hypersensitivity in horses (Queensland or sweet itch)—*C. brevitarsis*, *C. imicola*, *C. insignis*, *C. lupicaris*, *C. obsoletus*, *C. pulicaris*, *C. punctatus*, *C. spinosus*, *C. stellifer*, *C. varipennis*.
***C. brevitarsis* (*C. robertsi*)** one of the vectors of bluetongue virus and causes hypersensitivity to its bite. Called also Queensland itch. See also SWEET itch.
C. furens intermediate host of *Mansonella ozzardi*.
C. grahami intermediate host of *Dipetalonema perstans* and *D. streptocerca*.
C. nubeculosus intermediate host of *Onchocerca cervicalis*.
C. pungens intermediate host of *Onchocerca gibsoni*.
culicoides hypersensitivity see SWEET itch.
Culiseta a genus of mosquitoes, e.g. *C. melanura*, which act as vectors for equine encephalomyelitis.
C. melanura transmits American encephalomyelitis virus; does not feed on large mammals but does on water birds.
cull the act of CULLING. Called also cast.
culling removal of inferior animals from a group of breeding stock. The removal is premature, i.e. before completion of its life span, disposal of an animal from a herd or other group. In farm animals this means disposal because of their being superfluous to the needs of the group to maintain its size. Animals may be culled because of age, either because thay are too old or because they are very young and their retention would necessitate culling an older, more desirable animal. Animals may also be culled because of disease, failure to produce or reproduce, because of inherited defects or because of undesirable conformation or breed type. There are two general classes of culls, involuntary culls, e.g. deaths, and voluntary culls, e.g. age culls.

biological c. culling of animals on the biological grounds of incapacity to pass a productivity test.
c. program a set of rules for a manager to follow in carrying out culling within a herd.
c. rate the number of animals culled as a proportion of the number of animals from which the culling was done.
culls the animals extracted from a herd or flock by culling.
culmen pl. *culmina* [L.] 1. the anterior and upper part of the monticulus cerebelli; called also cacumen. 2. the median longitudinal ridge on a bird's beak.
culms the shoots and roots of sprouted grains in the brewing process. These are removed during brewing and are salvaged as a food supplement. Called also malt culms.
cultivar plant variety produced under cultivation.
cultivation the propagation of living organisms, applied especially to the growth of microorganisms or other cells in artificial media.
culture 1. the propagation of microorganisms or of living tissue cells in special media conducive to their growth. 2. to induce such propagation. 3. the product of such propagation.
anaerobic c. one carried out in the absence of air.
continuous flow c. the cultivation of bacteria in a continuous flow of fresh medium to maintain bacterial growth in logarithmic phase.
explant c. a small piece of tissue such as trachea or gut maintained in culture.
hanging-drop c. a culture in which the material to be cultivated is inoculated into a drop of fluid attached to a coverglass inverted over a hollow slide.
primary c. a cell or tissue culture started from material taken directly from an organism. Subsequent passages of cells are referred to as secondary cultures.
secondary c. a subculture derived from a primary culture.
slant c. one made on the surface of solidified medium in a tube which has been tilted when the agar was solidifying to provide a greater surface area for growth.
stab c. a culture into which the organisms are introduced by thrusting a needle deep into the medium.
streak c. one in which the medium is inoculated by drawing an infected wire loop across it.
suspension c. a culture in which cells multiply while suspended in a suitable liquid medium.
tissue c. the maintaining or growing of tissue, organ primordia, or the whole or part of an organ in vitro so as to preserve its architecture and function. Used loosely to refer to monolayer cell cultures. See explant culture (above).
type c. a culture of a species of microorganism usually maintained in a central reference collection of type or standard organisms.
cumulus pl. *cumuli* [L.] a small elevation.
c. oophorus a mass of follicular cells surrounding the ovum in the vesicular ovarian follicle. Called also discus oophorus, discus ovigerous, discus proligerous.
cunean pertaining to the cunean tendon.
c. bursa the bursa interposed between the cunean tendon and the tarsal bones on the medial aspect of the hock of the horse.
c. tendon the medial branch of the insertion of the tibialis cranialis muscle in the hindlimb of the horse.
c. tendon bursitis inflammation of the cunean bursa.
c. tendonectomy surgical excision of a section of the cunean tendon as a treatment for bone SPAVIN.
cuneate wedge-shaped.
c. tubercle a slight elevation in the medulla oblongata indicating the position of the cuneate nucleus of the lemniscal system.
cuneiform 1. wedge-shaped. 2. the first, second and third tarsal bones.
c. process processes of the arytenoid cartilage in dogs, or the epiglottic cartilages of horses.
cuneus pl. *cunei* [L.] a wedge-shaped lobule on the medial aspect of the occipital lobe of the cerebrum.
c. ungulae see FROG (2) of the horse's foot.
cuniculus pl. *cuniculi* [L.] a burrow in the skin made by the mange mite, *Sarcoptes scabiei.*
Cuniculus paca see PACA.
cunjevoi ALOCASIA *brisbanensis*.
cup a depression or hollow.
glaucomatous c. a depression of the optic disk due to persistently increased intraocular pressure, broader and deeper than a physiological cup, and occurring first at the temporal side of the disk.
optic c. an evagination of the optic vesicle, an outgrowth from the neural tube, which forms a cup, the forerunner of the eyeball.
physiological c. a slight depression sometimes observed in the optic disk.
tooth c. central depression on the occlusal surface of the horse's incisor teeth at the time of eruption; as the horse ages and the occlusal surface is eroded, the cup becomes smaller and eventually disappears; the reducing size is used in aging of horses by their teeth.
cupola cupula.
cupping the formation of a cup-shaped depression.
cupping vacuum therapy applying negative pressure to acupuncture points by the use of cups.
Cupressocyparis leylandii member of the plant family Cupressaceae; contains ISOCUPRESSIC ACID. May cause abortion in livestock. Called also Leyland cypress.
Cupressus genus of trees in the family Cupressaceae; the leaves contain isocupressic acid, and when fed to pregnant cattle cause abortion. The aborted fetus has a typical leukoencephalomalacia. Includes *C. macrocarpa*, *C. sempervirens*. Called also cypress (Monterey cypress).
cupric pertaining to or containing divalent COPPER.
c. complex see CUPRIMYXIN.
cuprimyxin a copper-containing antibacterial and antifungal agent for topical use.
cuproprotein copper bound to a protein, e.g. ceruloplasmin.
cuprous pertaining to or containing monovalent copper.
cupruresis the urinary excretion of copper.
cupula pl. *cupulae* [L.] a small, inverted cup or dome-shaped cap over a structure.
diaphragmatic c. the ventral dome of the diaphragm.
pleural c. the apex of each pleural sac lying at the cranial aperture of the thorax.
cupulolithiasis the presence of calculi in the cupula of the posterior semicircular duct.
cur a derogatory term for a mongrel dog.
curare any of a wide variety of highly toxic extracts from various botanical sources, including species of *Strychnos*, a genus of tropical trees; used originally as arrow poisons in South America. A form extracted from the shrub, *Chondrodendron tomentosum*, has been used as skeletal muscle relaxant. The active principle is *d*-tubocurarine.
curariform like curare in its action.

c. drugs these include *d*-tubocurarine, gallamine, decamethonium, succinylcholine (suxamethonium). Like curare they cause collapse due to neuromuscular paralysis but without loss of consciousness.

curarization administration of curare (usually tubocurarine) to induce muscle relaxation by its blocking activity at the neuromuscular junction.

curb 1. thickening of the plantar tarsal ligament in the hock of the horse. The ligament is obviously thickened a few inches below the point of the hock. Initially there is pain at the site, the horse is lame and at rest stands with the weight on the other leg. 2. that part of a curb bit in a bridle that provides the restraint additional to the bit itself. Includes the bars and chain. See also BIT (2).

c. reins the reins attached to the bars of a curb bit.

curby hocks hocks which are affected by CURB.

curcas bean JATROPHA *curcas*.

curcin a phytotoxin found in JATROPHA *curcas*.

curd the proteinaceous part of milk precipitated by rennin. Usually contains some fat when whole milk is used.

cure 1. the course of treatment of any disease, or of a special case. 2. the successful treatment of a disease or wound. 3. a system of treating diseases. 4. a medicine effective in treating a disease. 5. preserve meat by salting, smoking, pickling.

cured meat meat which has been treated with salt and nitrate or nitrite. The salt dehydrates the meat, the nitrate releases nitrous acid which converts myoglobin to nitrosomyoglobin which has an attractive pink color when cooked. The cooking process converts the nitrosomyoglobin to nitrosohemochrome. Salted meat is produced by simply adding salt.

Bacon, ham and other specialty cured meats are put through additional processes, especially smoking, to achieve special effects. See also BACON CURING, PICKLING.

curet see CURETTE.

curettage [Fr.] the cleansing of a diseased surface, as with a curette.

endometrial c. physical curettage of the uterus is not practiced in animals but chemical irritation achieves a similar effect and is used in cows. The commonest infusion is an iodine preparation such as Lugol's iodine.

subgingival c. aids in the treatment of periodontal disease; consists of removing inflammatory tissue under the free gingival margin and adjacent bony structures.

curette, curet 1. a spoon-shaped instrument for cleansing a diseased surface. 2. to use a curette.

bone c. there are a number of types, e.g. BRUN BONE CURETTE, NAIL-hole curette.

curettement curettage.

curie a non-SI unit of radioactivity, defined as the quantity of any radioactive nuclide in which the number of disintegrations per second is 3.7×10^{10}; abbreviated Ci. Now replaced by the BECQUEREL.

curie-hour a non-SI unit of dose equivalent to that obtained by exposure for one hour to radioactive material disintegrating at the rate of 3.7×10^{10} atoms per second.

curing said of meat. See CURED MEAT.

curium a chemical element, atomic number 96, atomic weight 247, symbol Cm. See Table 6.

curled (curly) dock RUMEX *crispus*.

curled St. Johns wort HYPERICUM *triquettrifolium*.

curled toe see CORKSCREW claw.

curled toe paralysis a disease of chickens caused by a nutritional deficiency of riboflavin. A complete deficiency of the vitamin causes early mortality before the deformity develops. The toes are curled inwards or under and the chicken has to stand and walk on its hocks. See also CROOKED TOE DISEASE.

curled tongue a deformity of the tongue in young turkey poults caused by a ration composed of finely ground feed fed as a dry powder. Feeding the same ration as a mash prevents the disease.

curly coat seen in some breeds of dogs, such as Curly coated retrievers, Irish water spaniels; reported as an inherited condition in some breeds of cattle, horses and pigs.

Curly coated retriever a medium-sized gun dog with distinctive black or liver coat in short, crisp curls over the entire body except the face.

curly toe paralysis see CURLED TOE PARALYSIS.

curracabah ACACIA *cunninghamii*.

currant-jelly clot the blood clot in the heart at post mortem that contains erythrocytes. Is indicative of clotting before sedimentation of the cells has occurred and of a sufficiency of red cells.

current that which flows; electric transmission in a circuit.

alternating c. a current that flows in opposite directions sinusoidally.

direct c. a current whose direction is always the same.

c. directory the directory in which a directory search will be conducted.

currycomb a flat toothed device used like a brush in grooming horses, principally for removing debris such as caked mud. Made usually of metal or hard rubber. Used in combination with a dandybrush or bodybrush.

Curschmann's spirals coiled, basophilic plugs of mucus formed in the lower airways and found in sputum and tracheal washings; indicate chronic obstruction.

cursed crowfoot RANUNCULUS *scleratus*.

cursor an indicator of the user's position on the computer monitor's screen.

cursorial adapted for running; said of certain birds and bones.

curvature a nonangular deviation from a normally straight course.

greater c. of reticulum in the cow lies against the diaphragm opposite the sixth and seventh ribs and faces left and ventrally.

greater c. of stomach the left or lateral border of the stomach, marking the junction of the parietal and visceral surfaces.

lesser c. of reticulum in the cow faces right and dorsally and lies against the omasum.

lesser c. of stomach the right or medial border of the stomach, marking the junction of the parietal and visceral surfaces.

spinal c. abnormal deviation of the vertebral column, as in KYPHOSIS, LORDOSIS and SCOLIOSIS.

curve a line that is not straight; the line representing varying values in a graph.

epidemic c. a graphical representation showing the number of new cases of the disease plotted against time. A decision on when the new infection rate creates an epidemic varies with the disease and the circumstances. The rate would need to be clearly in excess of its expected frequency.

fitted c. the theoretical frequency distribution whose closeness of fit to the subject data is under test.

freehand c. a line drawn in by hand on a scattergram to establish the relationship between two variables.

frequency c. a curve representing graphically the probabilities of different numbers of occurrences of an event.

logarithmic c. the curve which demonstrates the straightline relationship between two variables when both of them are scaled as logarithms.

log dose–response c. the standard way of presenting pharmacological data about a drug. The response is plotted against dose on a semilogarithmic graph. It has the advantage that a wide range of dose rates can be entered on the one graph.

plasma concentration–time c. the plasma concentration of a drug plotted against time.

semilogarithmic c. as for logarithmic curve except that only one of the variables is scaled as a logarithm. See also LOGARITHMIC relationship.

sigmoid c. an S-shaped curve. A common curve in biological distributions.

survivorship c. a graphic presentation of a life table. Obviously the proportion of survivors decreases with advancing age of the group.

vertebral c. the downward curve of the thoracolumbar region and that of the cervical region in some animals.

curved claw see CORKSCREW claw.

curvilinear a line appearing as a curve; nonlinear.

c. regression see curvilinear REGRESSION.

Curvularia a colored fungus associated with black-grain MYCETOMA.

curvus a deformity in which there is curvature. Seen in growth deformities of the radius and ulna in which premature closure of the distal ulnar physis and the radius continues to grow with a cranial bowing. See also VALGUS.

Cuscuta a genus of parasitic plants in the family Convolvulaceae; an unidentified toxin causes nervousness, staggering vomiting, diarrhea. Includes *C. campestris*, *C. epithymium*, *C. europea*, *C. trifolii*. Called also dodder.

Cushing's disease hyperadrenocorticism secondary to excessive pituitary excretion of adrenocorticotropic hormone; based on the original description by Dr. Harvey Cushing of humans with pituitary tumors, described as basophil adenomas of the pars distalis; now taken to include also the more common corticotroph adenomas (CUSHING-LIKE DISEASE). Called also pituitary-dependent HYPERADRENOCORTICISM.

Cushing-like disease a disease caused by functional corticotroph adenomas of the adenohypophysis which may give rise to clinical signs of cortisol excess; seen most commonly in dogs. See also CUSHING'S DISEASE.

Cushing phenomenon a sudden rise in intracranial pressure causes systemic hypertension.

Cushing suture pattern a fast, continuous, easy inverting suture pattern for making the external closure of an intestinal incision. Bites are taken parallel to the incision but the suture does not pass right through the wall into the lumen. The external part of each suture bite crosses the wound. It approximates the peritoneum.

Cushing's syndrome a group of signs produced by an excess of free circulating cortisol from the ADRENAL cortex. Causes are: (1) excessive secretion of adrenocorticotropic hormone (ACTH) from the pituitary gland, which may actually result from faulty release of corticotropin-releasing factor (CRF) from the hypothalamus or a functional tumor, usually corticotroph adenoma; (2) tumor of the adrenal cortex, causing hypersecretion of the glucocorticoids; (3) *iatrogenic* Cushing's syndrome resulting from excessive or prolonged administration of exogenous glucocorticoids; and in humans (4) ectopic production of ACTH by extrapituitary tumors. Most commonly seen in dogs (canine Cushing's syndrome; CCS), infrequently in aged horses and rarely in other species. See also HYPERADRENOCORTICISM.

Affected dogs show polyuria, polydipsia, polyphagia, muscle weakness and atrophy, pendulous abdomen, hair loss and an increased susceptibility to infection, particularly of the skin and urinary tract.

pseudo C. s. see GROWTH HORMONE-responsive dermatosis.

cushingoid resembling Cushing's syndrome, said of signs and clinical features. See also GROWTH HORMONE-responsive dermatosis.

cushion a term describing exceptional thickness of the upper lips or flews seen in some short-nosed breeds of dogs, e.g. Boxer, British bulldog.

cushion comb a small, low, oval comb with a smooth surface on a domestic fowl.

cusp a pointed or rounded projection, such as on the crown of a tooth, or a segment of a cardiac valve.

semilunar c. any of the semilunar segments of the aortic valve or the pulmonary valve.

cuspid 1. in the horse, pig, dog, and cat the fourth tooth on either side from the midline in each jaw; called also canine tooth. 2. having one cusp.

cuspis pl. *cuspides* [L.] a cusp.

custom done to the order of the customer on materials owned by the customer, e.g. custom FEEDLOT.

cuSum cumulative sum; sum of the data so far, updated as each item is collected.

cut 1. gelded; castrated. 2. of meat. The standard parts of a carcass of meat. Varies between countries. Includes sirloin, neck chops, silverside and so on. 3. incision made by any sharp edge. 4. yield of wool per head of sheep shorn.

c. proud a lay term and a lay operation used in horses. Intended to retain some stallion characteristics especially ramping and pseudo-aggression. The practice is to leave all of the spermatic cord and a little of the epididymis in the horse. There is no anatomical basis for the view that the practice has the desired effect, nor that the gelding that unintentionally has these characteristics loses them if the ends of his spermatic cords are further pruned.

speedy-c. see SPEEDY-CUTTING.

cut-and-fit ration balancing a trial and error method of designing a ration, adding and deleting different amounts and different source feeds until the target analysis is achieved.

cut back zone the proximal metaphysis of long bone where primary and secondary trabeculae are remodeled out of cortical bone, forming the cortex.

cutability said of meat; the proportion of boneless, trimmed, saleable retail cuts of meat obtained from a carcass.

cutaneous pertaining to the SKIN. See also under headings of individual diseases, e.g. cutaneous actinobacillosis.

idiopathic c. and renal glomerular disease a potentially fatal disease of unknown etiology which affects racing and training Greyounds. There is edema and erythema with well demarcated cutaneous ulceration on the distal extremities, especially in the hindlimbs, with thrombocytopenia and acute renal insufficiency. Called also Alabama rot, Greenetrack disease.

cutdown creation of a small incised opening, especially in the tissues over a vein (venous cutdown) to facilitate venipuncture and permit the passage of a needle or cannula for withdrawal of blood or administration of fluids.

Cuterebra large flies whose larvae are parasitic, mostly on wild rodents but cats and dogs are occasionally infected. The larvae burrow under the skin and cause cyst-like cavities. Called also cuterebra flies. Includes *C. americana*, *C. buccata*, *C. emasculator*, *C. lepivora*.

cuticle 1. a layer of more or less solid substance covering the free surface of an epithelial cell. 2. the narrow band of epidermis extending from the wall of the nail or claw, onto the surface; called also eponychium. 3. the layer of cells on the surface of a hair shaft or wool fiber. In wool it is the projection of the edge of cuticular plates that gives the fiber its unique felting property. 4. an extremely thin, transparent, proteinaceous covering over the eggshell of bird's eggs. It may contain pigment and is permeable to gases.

c. of koilin a tough membrane, usually greenish, and a carbohydrate–protein complex, produced by the solidification of the secretion of the tubular glands in the gizzard mucosa of birds; the cuticle protects the mucosa during its crushing operations.

Cutifilaria a genus of nematodes in the family Onchocercidae. Includes *Cutifilaria wenki* (deer, skin).

cutin 1. a waxy constituent of the cuticle of plants. 2. a preparation of ox serosa used as suture material and as a wound dressing.

cutireaction an inflammatory or irritative reaction of the skin, occurring in certain infectious diseases, or on application or injection of a preparation of the organism causing the disease.

cutis the outer protective covering of the body; the skin.

c. anserina transitory erection of the hair follicles due to contraction of the arrectores muscles, a reflection of sympathetic nerve discharge; goose flesh.

c. asthenia see cutaneous ASTHENIA.

c. hyperelastica see EHLERS–DANLOS SYNDROME.

cutleaf nightshade SOLANUM *triflorum*.

cutting 1. a gait defect in horses. See BRUSHING. 2. severing tissue, as with a blade, knife or scissors.

press c. a technique for making an incision with a scalpel blade in which there is increasing pressure in the same direction the blade is being moved.

slide c. pressure is applied at right angles to the movement of the blade. Safer and better controlled than press cutting when dissecting.

Cutting horse not a breed, but a class of horse used for working cattle on the range, in cattle camps and in yards. Several varieties exist, e.g. Canadian Cutting horse, American Cutting horse. See also AUSTRALIAN Stock horse.

cuttlefish a member of the Cephalopoda family of molluscs with a bony structure (gladius) internally. This boatlike structure is a common finding at the sea's edge and is much used as a dietary supplement and plaything for caged birds.

cuvette [Fr.] a glass container generally having well-defined characteristics (dimensions, optical properties), to contain solutions or suspensions for study.

cv. cultivar.

CVA cerebrovascular accident.

CVP central venous pressure.

cwt 112 pounds avoirdupois weight.

cyacetazide see CYANACETHYDRAZIDE.

cyadox a quinoxaline derivative, used as a growth promotant.

cyanacethydrazide an anthelmintic used in the treatment of lungworms. Poisoning is characterized by incoordination and convulsions. Pyridoxine is the antidote. Called also cyacetazide.

cyanamide in the form of calcium cyanamide, a fertilizer and may cause CYANIDE poisoning.

Cyanea giant blubber jellyfish in sea water and capable of stinging an animal. Member of the order Semaeostomae.

cyanhemoglobin a compound formed by the combination of hydrogen cyanide with hemoglobin. It gives the bright red color to the blood that is characteristic of peracute cyanide poisoning.

cyanide a binary compound of cyanogen. Some inorganic compounds, such as cyanide salts, potassium cyanide and sodium cyanide, are important in industry for extracting gold and silver from their ores and in electroplating. Other cyanide compounds are used in the manufacture of synthetic rubber and textiles. Cyanides are also used in pesticides.

There are many potential sources of cyanide in the environment of farm animals. Cyanide poisoning occurs most commonly when cattle gain access to a bulk supply of a cyanogenetic plant, e.g. sudan grass, immature sorghum. Typical clinical signs are dyspnea within a few minutes of getting access to the food, restlessness, recumbency and death within a matter of 15 minutes to 2 hours. The cyanide is not free in the plants but is combined with a glycoside radical and must be degraded by ruminal enzymes to release its HCN. Called also hydrocyanic acid. See CYANOGENETIC glycosides.

cyanmethemoglobin a compound formed by combination of hydrocyanic acid with methemoglobin. It is formed when methylene blue is administered as an antidote in cyanide poisoning. In laboratory methods, hemoglobin is converted to cyanmethemoglobin and measured spectrophotometrically.

cyanmetmyoglobin a compound formed from metmyoglobin by addition of the cyanide ion.

cyan(o)- word element. [Gr.] *blue*.

cyanoacrylate glue tissue adhesives used for treatment of minor wounds and abrasions, vascular and ophthalmic surgery, and hemostasis.

β-cyano-L-alanine a lathyrogenic agent in *Vicia* spp.

cyanobacteria photosynthezing bacteria of widely varying form and inhabiting many environments including marine and fresh water. They produce a green pigment which changes color to blue or blue-green when the bacteria are stressed or dying. Formerly classified as algae (division Cyanophyta) and known as blue-green algae. Some species are non-toxic, some produce hepatoxins, other produce neurotoxins, and still others produce dermatoxins. Toxic species include *Anabaena*, *Anabaenopsis*, *Aphanizomenon*, *Coelosphaerium*, *Cylindrospermopsis*, *Fischerella*, *Gloeotrichia*, *Gomphosphaeria*, *Haplosiphon*, *Hormothamnion*, *Lyngyba*, *Microcystis*, *Nodularia*, *Nostoc*, *Oscillatoria*, *Pseudoanabaena*, *Schizothrix*, *Seytonema*, *Synechococcus*, *Tolypothrix*, *Trichodesmium*. Called also cyanophytes. See also ALGAL poisoning.

cyanocobalamin see VITAMIN B_{12}.

cyanogen bromide reagent used to fragment peptide chains, since it cleaves only those peptide bonds in which methionine contributes the carbonyl group. Also used as coupling agent in affinity chromatography where it reacts with the Sepharose matrix forming a reactive product to which proteins, nucleic acids or other biopolymers can be coupled.

cyanogenesis cyanide production.

cyanogenetic, cyanogenic generating or giving rise to cyanide.

c. glycosides potentially poisonous cyanide radicals are found in plants in the form of cyanogenetic glycosides, in which form they are not poisonous. The glycosides may be broken down by plant enzymes or by rumen microorganisms and the material then releases its cyanide.

cyanolabe the pigment in retinal cones that is more sensitive to the blue range of the spectrum than are chlorolabe and erythrolabe.

cyanopenphas an organophosphate insecticide which causes delayed neurotoxicity in birds.

Cyanophyceae see CYANOBACTERIUM.

cyanophyte see CYANOBACTERIUM.

cyanopsin a visual pigment.

cyanosed see CYANOSIS.

cyanosis a bluish discoloration of the skin and mucous membranes due to excessive concentration of reduced hemoglobin in the blood. Used wrongly by clinicians describing skin lesions in pigs where there is severe congestion of cutaneous vessels and some leakage of blood into perivascular tissues.

central c. that due to arterial unsaturation, the aortic blood carrying reduced hemoglobin.

enterogenous c. a syndrome due to absorption of nitrites and sulfides from the intestine, principally marked by methemoglobinemia and/or sulfhemoglobinemia associated with cyanosis.

peripheral c. that due to an excessive amount of reduced hemoglobin in the venous blood as a result of extensive oxygen extraction at the capillary level.

Cyathocephalus a tapeworm genus of the family Cyathocephalidae.

C. truncatus a tapeworm of fish that can cause retardation of growth.

Cyathospirura a spiruroid nematode that causes granulomatous lesions in the stomachs of cats and foxes. Includes *C. seurati*.

Cyathostoma a genus of the roundworm family Syngamidae. Includes *Cyathostoma bronchialis*, *C. brantae*, *C. lari*, *C. variegatum* (birds, respiratory tract).

cyathostomiasis massive infestations of small strongyles, including CYATHOSTOMUM, CYLICOCYCLUS, CYLICODONTOPHORUS, CYLINDROPHARYNX, CYLICOSTEPHANUS, POTERIOSTOMUM, GYALOCEPHALUS and CABALLONEMA; they cause profuse diarrhea and death in some cases.

Cyathostominae a subfamily of the strongylid roundworms of horses which replaces the original genus of *Trichonema*. It includes the genera *Cyathostomum*, *Cylicocyclus*, *Cylicodontophorus*, *Cylicostephanus*, *Poteriostomum*, *Petrovinema*, *Gyalocephalus*, *Cylindropharynx* or *Caballonema*.

cyathostomosis disease state caused by *Cyathostomum* spp. infection.

Cyathostomum a genus of strongylid worms of the family Strongylidae.

C. catinatum, C. coronatum, C. labiatum, C. labratum, C. sagittatum, C. tetracanthum found in the large intestine of horses and other equids. Heavy infestations can cause severe diarrhea.

cybernetics the science of communication and control in the animal and in the machine.

cycad a member of the plant genus of CYCAS, dioecious, non-flowering woody plants (gymnosperms) which produce seeds in a woody cone consisting of exposed seed leaves (sporophylls), not enclosed in an ovary. The leaves are usually in a rosette at the top of the stem, which may be subterranean. Include *Bowenia*, *Cycas*, *Dioon*, *Encephalartos*, *Lepidozamia*, *Macrozamia*, *Zamia* spp.

c. glycoside group of glycosides including cycasin, macrozamin, found in cycad plants; oxidized in vivo to release toxin methylazoxymethanol (MAM).

Cycas one of the CYCAD genera from Australia, Asia, the Pacific and eastern Africa. Includes *C. armstrongii* (*C. lane-poolei*), *C. angulata*, *C. basaltica*, *C. media*, *C. circinalis*, *C. revoluta*. They contain the cycad glycoside cycasin. The leaves cause incoordination when eaten by cattle; see ZAMIA staggers. The seeds may also cause severe gastroenteritis and hepatic necrosis. Seeds of *C. circinalis* are also eaten by humans as guam and may cause a degenerative disease of the nervous system in them. Called also zamia.

cycasin a toxic glycoside found in *Cycas* spp. and other cycads.

cyclacillin, ciclacillin a semisynthetic penicillin of the ampicillin class.

Cyclamen europaeum a member of the plant family Primulaceae which contains cyclamin, a toxic glycoside.

cyclamin a toxic glycoside present in *Cyclamen europaeum*.

cyclarthrosis a pivot joint.

cyclase an enzyme that catalyzes the formation of a cyclic phosphodiester.

cycle a succession or recurring series of events.

cardiac c. a complete cardiac movement, or heartbeat, including systole, diastole, and the intervening pause.

The cycle includes eight separate phases: (1) isovolumetric contraction; (2) maximum ejection; (3) reduced ejection; (4) protodiastole (onset of ventricular relaxation); (5) isovolumetric relaxation; (6) rapid flow; (7) diastasis (onset of atrial contraction); (8) atrial systole.

cell c. the cycle of biochemical and morphological events occurring in a dividing cell population; it consists of the S phase, occurring toward the end of interphase, in which DNA is synthesized; the G_2 phase, for gap 2, the interval between S and M; the M phase, for mitosis, consisting of the four phases of mitosis; and the G_1 phase, which lasts from the end of M until the start of S phase of the next cycle. Fully differentiated cells are nondividing and are said to be in G_0.

citric acid c. see TRICARBOXYLIC ACID CYCLE.

estrus c. see ESTROUS cycle.

Krebs c. see TRICARBOXYLIC ACID CYCLE.

ovarian c. the sequence of physiological changes in the ovary involved in ovulation. See also OVULATION and REPRODUCTION.

reproductive c. the cycle of physiological changes in the reproductive organs, from the time of fertilization of the ovum through gestation and parturition. See also REPRODUCTION.

sex c., sexual c 1. the physiological changes recurring regularly in the reproductive organs of female mammals when pregnancy does not supervene. 2. the period of sexual reproduction in an organism that also reproduces asexually.

c. time the time in microseconds between successive accessions to a storage location in the main memory by the microprocessor of a computer; a measure of the speed of the processor.

tricarboxylic acid c. see TRICARBOXYLIC ACID CYCLE.

urea c. a cyclic series of reactions that produce urea, a major route for removal of the ammonia produced in the metabolism of amino acids in the liver and kidney. See also UREA.

cyclectomy 1. excision of a piece of the ciliary body. 2. excision of a portion of the ciliary border of the eyelid.

cyclic pertaining to or occurring in a cycle or cycles. The term is applied to chemical compounds that contain a ring of atoms in the nucleus.
c. adenosine monophosphate (AMP) see cyclic ADENOSINE monophosphate.
c. guanosine monophosphate (cGMP) see cyclic GUANOSINE monophosphate.
canine c. hematopoiesis an abnormality of hematopoietic stem cells that results in detectable, cyclic fluctuations in numbers of circulating neutrophils. Affected dogs have an increased susceptibility to infections. The condition is inherited as an autosomal recessive in collies where it is occurs with a distinctive silver-gray coat color; called also gray collie syndrome.
c. neutropenia see canine cyclic hematopoiesis (above).
c. non-breeder cows cows demonstrating estrus regularly but not being submitted for mating; deferral of mating.
c. nucleotide see cyclic NUCLEOTIDE.
cyclical occurring in cycles; statistically a periodic movement of a time series, e.g. recurrent epidemics.
cyclicity cycling of disease incidence, being seasonal (annual on a seasonal basis) or secular (long-term, greater than one year, e.g. outbreaks of ephemeral fever).
cyclicotomy see CYCLOTOMY.
cyclins a set of related proteins that regulate the passage of cells through the cell cycle by forming complexes with cyclin-dependent protein kinases.
c.-dependent protein kinase (Cdk) forms complexes with cyclins to become active in activating stages of the eukaryotic cell cycle.
cyclitic membrane a retrolental, fibrovascular membrane which stretches across the back of the lens and develops as a result of organization of inflammatory exudate in the posterior chamber of the eye.
cyclitis inflammation of the ciliary body.
cyclizine an antihistamine used in the form of the hydrochloride salt as an antinauseant to prevent motion sickness in dogs.
cycl(o)- word element. [Gr.] *round, recurring, ciliary body of the eye.*
cyclochlorotine a toxin produced by the fungus *Penicillium islandicum.* It is a hepatoxin and its metabolites are hepatocarcinogenic.
cyclochoroiditis inflammation of the ciliary body and choroid.
Cyclocoelidae a family of large flukes (digenetic trematodes) parasitic in body and nasal cavities, and air sacs of aquatic birds. Includes *Tracheophilus cymbius* (*Tracheophilus sisowi*) of ducks.
cyclocryotherapy freezing of the ciliary body; done in the treatment of glaucoma.
cyclodialysis creation of a communication between the anterior chamber of the eye and the suprachoroidal space, to allow alternative route of filtration for aqueous humor in glaucoma.
cyclodiathermy destruction of a portion of the ciliary body by diathermy to reduce aqueous formation in the treatment of glaucoma.
cyclohexamines, cyclohexylamines a group of dissociative anesthetics that includes phencyclidine and its analog, ketamine.
cycloheximide an antibiotic produced by *Streptomyces griseus* that inhibits protein synthesis. It is too toxic and nonselective for common clinical use, but is used in treatment of cancers and management of graft-versus-host reactions following transplantation. Also used agriculturally for the control of fungal diseases of plants and turf and as a bacterial inhibitor in selective media for culturing fungi.
cyclokeratitis inflammation of the cornea and ciliary body.
cycloleucine an amino acid important in the study of amino acid transport.
cyclomethycaine a topical anesthetic agent.
cyclonite a plastic explosive; also used as a rodenticide; toxic effects in humans and dogs manifested by convulsions.
cyclo-oxygenase important enzyme in the synthesis of prostaglandins. Called also prostaglandin synthetase.
cyclopamine a steroidal alkaloid in the plant *Veratrum californicum* responsible for the development of the cyclopian deformity caused by feeding the plant to pregnant ewes on the 14th day of pregnancy.
cyclopean, cyclopian pertaining to a cyclops.
c. deformity there are two identified causes in animals, poisoning of sheep by the plant VERATRUM *californicum,* and one of the two forms of inherited prolonged gestation in cattle.
cyclopegia partial fusion of the two eyeballs as a congenital defect.
cyclopentanoperhydrophenanthrene the steroid nucleus.
cyclopentolate in the hydrochloride form, an anticholinergic used as eyedrops to produce cycloplegia and mydriasis.
cyclophosphamide a neoplastic suppressant used in the treatment of lymphomas and leukemias.
Cyclophyllidea important order of cestodes in the class Cestoda, parasitic in birds and mammals.
cyclopia a developmental anomaly characterized by a single orbital fossa, with the globe absent or rudimentary, apparently normal, or duplicated, or the nose absent or present as a tubular appendix located above the orbit and absence of the maxillae. Important animal occurrences of cyclopia are in one of the forms of inherited PROLONGED GESTATION, and in poisoning by VERATRUM *californicum.*
cyclopiazonic acid a mycotoxin produced by *Aspergillus* and *Penicillium* spp. fungi growing on feedstuffs. Causes feed refusal in pigs but often combined with aflatoxin poisoning and more serious effects.
cycloplegia paralysis of the ciliary muscle; paralysis of accommodation.
cycloplegic 1. pertaining to, characterized by, or causing cycloplegia. 2. an agent that produces cycloplegia.
cycloposine one of the alkaloids in the plant *Veratrum californicum* responsible for the development of cyclopean deformities in sheep.
cyclopropane a powerful central nervous system depressant used as an inhalation ANESTHETIC. The drug can be given in small doses and is particularly useful in anesthetizing poor-risk patients. This gas is highly explosive and requires special handling and precautions against sparks or flames, which would result in an explosion. No longer used for safety reasons.
Cyclops a genus of minute crustaceans with terrestrial life cycles, some species of which act as hosts of *Diphyllobothrium* and *Dracunculus* spp. Called also water flea.
cyclops a monster exhibiting cyclopia.
cyclosis movement of the cytoplasm within a cell, without external deformation of the cell wall.
cyclosporin A see CYCLOSPORINE.
cyclosporine a neutral cyclic peptide, the major

metabolic product of the fungus *Tolypocladium inflatum*; a specific suppressor of the T lymphocyte response, important in tissue transplantation.

cyclothiazide a diuretic and antihypertensive agent.

Cyclotogaster heterographa a species belonging to the order Ischocera (insects). Called also head louse. Affects fowl and partridge.

cyclotomy incision of the ciliary muscle; cyclicotomy.

cyclotropia STRABISMUS in which there is permanent deviation of the eye around the anteroposterior axis in the presence of visual fusional stimuli, resulting in diplopia.

cyclozoonosis a zoonotic disease that requires at least two species of vertebrates as definitive and intermediate hosts. Examples are hydatid disease (*Echinococcus granulosus*) and trichinosis (*Trichinella spiralis*).

Cydonia oblonga the quince tree, a member of the Rosaceae family; can cause cyanide poisoning.

cyesis see PREGNANCY.

cyfluthrin a fluorinated pyrethroid, used in ear tags on cattle to control flies and ticks.

cygnet a young swan.

Cygnus see SWAN.

cygon see DIMETHOATE.

cyhalothrin a synthetic pyrethroid used to control lice and ked on sheep.

cyhexatin an acaricide used in horticulture and reputed to cause congenital defects in experimental animals.

Cylicocyclus one of the eight genera of the strongylid nematodes in the subfamily Cyathostominae. Includes *Cylicocyclus elongatus*, *C. insignis*, *C. leptostomus*, *C. nassatus*, *C. ultrajectinus* (found in large intestine of horses, other Equidae).

Cylicodontophorus one of the genera of nematodes within the strongylid subfamily Cyathostominae. Includes *Cylicodontophorus bicoronatus*, *C. euproctus*, *C. mettami* (found in horse large intestine).

Cylicospirura felineus a spiruroid worm associated with the formation of nodules in the stomach of domestic and wild felids.

Cylicostephanus one of the genera of strongylid nematodes in the subfamily Cyathostominae, previously included in the genus *Trichonema*. Found in the large intestine of horses and other equids are *C. calicatus*, *C. goldi*, *C. hybridus*, *C. longibursatus*, *C. minutus*.

cylicostomes see CYATHOSTOMINAE.

cylindroid 1. shaped like a cylinder. 2. a urinary CAST of various origins, which tapers to a slender tail that is often twisted or curled upon itself.

cylindroma adenocystic carcinoma.

Cylindropharynx a genus of strongylid nematodes in the subfamily Cyathostominae.

cylindrospermin hepatoxic alkaloid in *Cylindrospermopsis*.

Cylindrospermopsis raciborskii member of the cyanobacteria; contains the alkaloid hepatoxin cylindrospermin.

cylindruria the presence of cylindroids in the urine.

Cymbiforma see OGMOCOTYLE.

Cymopterus a genus of toxic plants in the family Apiaceae; contain furanocoumarins which cause primary photosensitization. Includes *C. longipes*, *C. watsonii*. Called also spring parsley.

Cymric a relatively new breed of cat which is really a longhaired MANX cat.

cynanchoside neurotoxin in *Cynanchum* spp. and possibly *Sarcostemma* spp.

Cynanchum South African genus of plants in the family Asclepiadaceae; contains an alkaloid cynanchoside which causes incoordination, tremor, paralysis. Includes *C. africanum*, *C. ellipticum*, *C. obtusifolium*. Called also monkey rope, klimp, bobbejantou.

cynapine toxic piperidine alkaloid in *Aethusa cynapium*.

Cynodon genus of grasses in the Poaceae family; they may contain cyanogenetic glycosides, and acute cyanide poisoning (geilsiekte) and goiter have been attributed to them. All of the grasses are very widespread and enjoy good reputations as pasture grass. Includes *C. aethiopicus* (Nkuru grass), *C. dactylon* (couch grass, Bermuda grass), *C. incompletus* (blue couch), *C. nlemfuensis* (*C. plectostachyus*, Naivasha stargrass).

C. dactylon* + *Balansia epichloe couch grass infested by the fungus causes incoordination.

Cynoglossum officinale a member of the plant family Boraginaceae; contains the hepatoxic pyrrolizidine alkaloids heliosupine and echinatine; called also houndstongue.

cynology study of dogs.

Cynomys ludovicianus see PRAIRIE dog.

Cynopithecus niger a black, 20 to 30 inches, 9 to 18 lb, monkey with pink ischial tuberosities. Called also *Celebes macaque*.

Cynosurus cristatus a host for *Claviceps purpurea*—rye ergot—and a potential source of ergot poisoning. Called also crested dog's tail.

cyotrophy nutrition of the fetus.

cypermethrin a synthetic pyrethroid used as an insecticide and acaricide.

cypress CUPRESSUS *macrocarpa*. Called also Monterey cypress.

cyprinid a member of the fish family Cyprinidae, including carp, tench, minnow, goldfish, barbel, chub, bream and many others.

Cyprinus carpio farmed finfish in family Cyprinidae. Called also common carp. See Table 23.

cyproheptadine a histamine and serotonin antagonist used as an antipruritic and antihistaminic. It has also been used in the treatment of pituitary-dependent hyperadrenocorticism.

Cyrnea a genus of spiruroid worms in the family Habronematidae.

C. colini, C. piliata found in the proventriculus and gizzard of birds.

cyromazine a triazine insect growth regulator, used as a feed additive for chickens to control fecal-feeding flies, and in Australia to control fly strike of sheep.

cyrtometer a device for measuring the curved surfaces of the body.

Cys cysteine.

cyst 1. a closed epithelium-lined sac or capsule containing a liquid or semi-solid substance. Most cysts are harmless but they occasionally may change into malignant growths, become infected, or obstruct a gland. There are four main types of cysts: retention cysts, exudation cysts, embryonic cysts and parasitic cysts. See also specific locations and organs. 2. a stage in the life cycle of certain parasites, during which they are enveloped in a protective wall. See also CYSTIC.

aneurysmal c. see BONE cyst.

blood c's these are found in the carcasses of poultry at meat inspection. They are small round cystic lesions containing blood. They are hemangiomas.

branchial c., branchiogenic c., branchiogenous c. one formed from an incompletely closed branchial cleft. See also BRANCHIAL cyst.

cervical c's retention cysts of glands in the uterine cervix in the cow, are palpable as fluctuating masses on rectal examination. Called also nabothian cyst or follicle.
chocolate c. one filled with hemosiderin following local hemorrhage.
cutaneous c. see EPIDERMAL cyst, DERMOID cyst, FOLLICULAR cyst, SEBACEOUS cyst.
daughter c. one that develops within a parent cyst, e.g. hydatid cyst.
dentigerous c. see DENTAL cyst.
echinococcus c. hydatid cyst.
embryonic c. one developing from bits of embryonic tissue that have been overgrown by other tissues, or from developing organs that normally disappear before birth. An example is a BRANCHIAL cyst.
epidermal inclusion c. see epithelial INCLUSION.
exudation c. a cyst formed by the slow seepage of an exudate into a closed cavity.
fatty c. formed when fat accumulates in large amounts and the cells break down forming a central mass of lipid surrounded by a multinuclear rim.
follicular c. one due to occlusion of the duct of a follicle or small gland, especially one formed by enlargement of a graafian follicle as a result of accumulated transudate.
Gartner's duct c. see cystic GARTNER'S DUCTS.
horn c. intracutaneous cystic accumulations of keratin. Seen in trichoepitheliomas and basal cell tumors. Called also keratin cyst.
hybrid c. one combining elements of epidermoid and trichilemmal cysts.
hydatid c. the larval stage (metacestode) of the tapeworms *Echinococcus granulosus* and *E. multilocularis*. See also HYDATID disease.
inclusion c. see EPIDERMAL cyst.
interdigital c's see PODODERMATITIS; interdigital PYODERMA.
keratin c. one arising in the pilosebaceous apparatus, lined by stratified squamous epithelium and containing largely macerated keratin and often sufficient sebum to render the contents greasy and often rancid.
lateral cervical c. see BRANCHIAL cyst.
luteal c's develop from ovarian follicles which fail to rupture but have a lining of luteal cells. Anestrus is the presenting clinical sign.
marine fish c's worldwide occurrence in fish of round nodules in fibrous capsules; the cause is unknown.
meibomian c. see CHALAZION.
mesenteric c. congenital, thin-walled cyst between the leaves of the mesentery; may enlarge and cause colic or even intestinal obstruction.
c. mites see LAMINOSIOPTES *cysticola*.
c. of Morgagni see MORGAGNI'S HYDATID.
nabothian c. see cervical cyst (above).
orbital c. see MUCOCELE.
ovarian c. see cystic OVARIAN disease.
parasitic c. one forming around larval parasites (tapeworms, amebae, trichinae) that enter the body.
pseudohorn c. invagination of hyperplastic epidermis; not a true cyst.
retention c. a tumor-like accumulation of a secretion formed when the outlet of a secreting gland is obstructed. These cysts may develop in any of the secretory glands—the mammae, pancreas, kidney, salivary or sebaceous glands, and mucous membranes. See also renal RETENTION cysts.
sarcosporidian c's cylindrical cysts (schizonts) containing bradyzoites, found in the muscles of those infected with *Sarcocystis* spp.
subconjunctival c., conjunctival c. misplaced secretory tissue which causes a slowly enlarging, fluctuant subconjunctival mass.
uveal c. an acquired or congenital structure which may arise from the iris or the ciliary body. Visible as a mass attached to the iris or may be floating freely in the anterior chamber. Those arising from the ciliary body may not be visible. Seen most commonly in horses. See also IRIS cyst.
vitelline c. a congenital cyst lined with ciliated epithelium occurring along the gastrointestinal canal; the remains of the omphalomesenteric duct.

cystacanth an intermediate stage of *Macracanthorhyncus* spp. in arthropods.

cystadenocarcinoma adenocarcinoma with extensive cyst formation.

cystadenoma cystoma blended with adenoma.
mucinous c. a multilocular, usually benign, tumor produced by ovarian epithelial cells and having mucin-filled cavities.
papillary c. any tumor producing patterns that are both papillary and cystic; called also papilloadenocystoma.
serous c. a cystic tumor of the ovary containing thin, clear yellow serum and some solid tissue.

cystalgia pain in the bladder.

cystathionase cystathionine β-synthase, the enzyme catalyzing the synthesis of cystathionine from homocysteine.

cystathionine key intermediate in the trans-sulfuration pathway from methionine to cysteine.

cystectasia dilatation of the bladder.

cystectomy 1. excision of a cyst. 2. excision or resection of the urinary bladder.

cysteine a sulfur-containing amino acid produced by enzymatic or acid hydrolysis of proteins, readily oxidized to cystine; sometimes found in urine.

cystencephalus a monster with a membranous sac in place of a brain.

cystic 1. pertaining to or containing cysts; see CYST. 2. pertaining to the urinary bladder or to the gallbladder.
c. calculus calculus in the urinary bladder.
c. corpus luteum the normal corpus luteum is solid. Some have a central cavity filled with fluid but this does not affect their function. See also LUTEAL cyst.
c. duct the excretory duct of the gallbladder. See also BILE DUCT.
c. endometritis see PYOMETRA.
c. eye the failure of the optic vesicle to come into close apposition to the cranial ectoderm during embryological development results in persistence of the vesicle and the formation of a cystic eye.
c. follicle see cystic FOLLICLE.
c. hyperplasia see cystic ENDOMETRIAL hyperplasia.
c. hyperplasia–pyometra complex the term applied to a series of endometrial changes leading to PYOMETRA in dogs; first cystic endometrial hyperplasia, then plasma cell infiltration of the endometrium during diestrus, followed by acute inflammatory reaction which then becomes chronic.
c. ovarian disease includes cystic FOLLICLE, LUTEAL cyst, cystic corpus luteum (above).
c. pancreatic duct a sometime congenital defect; occasionally associated with polycystic kidneys and cystic bile ducts.
c. placental mole results from the death of the fetus with the persistence of the fetal membranes.
c. prostatic hyperplasia caused by blockage of glandular ducts. Enlargement of the gland may cause constipation, possibly dysuria. The enlarged gland should be palpable per rectum.

c. rete tubules occur in the ovaries of cows, bitches, queens; may be sufficiently large to be mistaken for cystic follicles.

c. retinal degeneration see MICROCYSTOID RETINAL DEGENERATION.

c. right oviduct the right oviduct in birds regresses to a vestigial level in the adult; sometimes the regression is incomplete and a cyst develops.

cysticercoid a stage in the life cycle of pseudophyllidean cestodes. One of the forms of metacestodes in which there is a single, retracted scolex withdrawn into a small vesicle which has a very small cavity, e.g. *Dipylidium caninum*. Found in invertebrates such as oribatid mites, fleas, etc.

cysticercosis infection with cystercerci in the intermediate hosts of a number of species-specific cestodes. The disease is largely symptomless except for cysticercosis caused by *Cysticercus cellulosae*, but has some food hygiene importance. Called also sheep measles, beef measles. See CYSTICERCUS.

Cysticercus larval (metacestode) stage, consisting of an invaginated scolex surrounded by a fluid-filled cyst cavity, of cyclophyllidean cestodes in the family Taeniidae. The common ones are listed below.

C. bovis larval stage of TAENIA *saginata*, a tapeworm of humans. The cysticerci are found in the muscles and other tissues of cattle. Humans are infected by eating uncooked beef. Called also beef measles.

C. cellulosae larval stage of TAENIA *solium*, a tapeworm of humans. The cysticerci are found in the skeletal and cardiac muscles of the pig and in the muscles and central nervous system of humans. Humans are infested by eating uncooked pork. Called also pork measles.

C. fasciolaris the larval stage of TAENIA *taeniaeformis*, a tapeworm of cats and wild Felidae and related species. The cysticerci are in the liver of rodents.

C. ovis the larval stage of TAENIA *ovis*, a tapeworm of dogs and wild carnivores. The cysticerci are found in the skeletal and cardiac muscles of sheep and goats. Dogs are infected by ingesting raw infected meat.

C. pisiformis the larval stage of TAENIA *pisiformis*, a tapeworm of dogs and wild carnivores. The cysticerci are in the peritoneal cavity of rabbits and hares.

C. tarandi the larval stage of TAENIA *krabbei*, a cestode parasite of dogs and wild carnivores. The cysticerci are found in the muscles of wild ruminants.

C. tenuicollis the larval stage of the tapeworm TAENIA *hydatigena*, a tapeworm of dogs and wild carnivores. The cysticerci are found in the liver and on the peritoneum in sheep but also in other ruminants including wild ones and pigs. Infection in the dog occurs when infected offal is fed raw. Called also long-necked bladderworm.

cysticercus pl. *cysticerci* [Gr.] a larval form of tapeworm. See also CYSTICERCOSIS.

cystiform resembling a cyst.

cystigerous containing cysts.

cystine a naturally occurring amino acid, an important sulfur-containing component of the protein molecule. It is sometimes found in the urine and in the kidneys in the form of minute hexagonal crystals, frequently forming cystine calculus in the bladder.

c. calculi see cystine UROLITHS.

cystinemia the presence of cystine in the blood.

cystinuria a hereditary condition characterized by persistent excessive urinary excretion of cystine, lysine, ornithine and arginine, due to impairment of renal tubular reabsorption of these amino acids. The predominant clinical manifestation is the formation of urinary cystine calculi. See also UROLITHIASIS.

cystistaxis oozing of blood from the mucous membrane into the bladder.

cystitis inflammation of the urinary bladder. The condition may result from an ascending infection coming from the exterior of the body by way of the urethra, or it may be caused by an infection descending from the kidney. Often cystitis is not an isolated infection but is rather a result of some other physical condition. For example, urinary retention, calculi in the bladder, tumors, or neurological diseases impairing the normal function of the bladder may lead to cystitis.

Clinical signs include freqency, pain on urination, blood-stained urine, a thickened bladder wall. Significant clinical pathology findings include hematuria, a high cell count indicative of inflammation, and a positive bacterial culture.

c. cystica cystitis marked by the presence of submucosal cysts.

emphysematous c. an occasional complication of diabetes mellitus in dogs and cats, caused by gas-forming bacteria.

epizootic equine c. an Australian disease of horses similar to *Sorghum* spp. poisoning.

gangrenous c. results from severe inflammation and ischemia; the bladder wall is green to black.

c. glandularis mucin-secreting glands present in the mucosa in a case of cystitis.

hemorrhagic c. hemorrhage is the main clinical feature.

interstitial c. a lower urinary tract disease of women in which there is painful urination and hemorrhagic lesions in the bladder wall, but no cause can be diagnosed. A similar syndrome is believed to occur in cats.

polypoid c. the mucosa is folded with polypoid projections.

cystitis–ataxia syndrome principally a disease of horses grazing *Sorghum* spp.; characterized by incoordination, frequent urination, urine scalding of hind quarters; suspected cause is a chronic low-level intake of cyanogenetic glycosides. A similar syndrome seen in cattle and sheep grazing *Sorghum* spp.

cystitis–pyelonephritis combined cystitis and pyelonephritis; pyelonephritis often succeeding an initial cystitis.

cystitomy surgical division of the capsule of the crystalline lens.

cyst(o)- word element. [Gr.] *cyst, bladder.*

cystoadenocarcinoma adenocarcinoma associated with cysts.

cystocarcinoma carcinoma associated with cysts.

Cystocaulus a nematode genus of the family Protostrongylidae of worms. Includes *Cystocaulus nigrescens* (*C. ocreatus*) Found in the lungs of sheep and goats.

cystocele herniation of the urinary bladder into the vagina.

cystocentesis puncture of the bladder for the purpose of obtaining an uncontaminated urine sample. Usually performed through the abdominal wall in the suprapubic position. Called also vesicopuncture.

cystodynia pain in the bladder; cystalgia.

cystoelytroplasty surgical repair of a vesicovaginal fistula.

cystoepithelioma a tumor with cystic and epitheliomatous elements.

cystofibroma a fibroma containing cysts.

cystogastrostomy surgical anastomosis of a pancreatic cyst to the stomach for drainage.

cystogram the film obtained by cystography.

micturating c. see voiding cystogram (below).
retrograde c. a radiograph made while the bladder is being filled with contrast agent from the urethra.
voiding c. a radiograph of the urinary tract made while the animal is urinating. Called also micturating cystogram.
cystography radiography of the urinary bladder using a contrast medium, so that the outline of the organ can be seen clearly. This type of examination frequently is part of a complete x-ray study of the kidneys, urethra and ureters as well as the bladder. See also PYELOGRAPHY. It is useful in diagnosing tumors or other defects in the bladder wall, vesicoureteral reflux, or calculi or other pathological conditions of the bladder.
cystoid 1. resembling a cyst. 2. a cystlike, circumscribed collection of softened material, having no enclosing capsule.
Cystoisospora a new genus including many coccidia previously classified as *Isospora* spp. with indirect life cycles.
C. burrowsi, C. canis, C. heydorni, C. ohioensis, C. wallacei coccidia of dogs; may cause enteritis.
C. felis, C. rivolta coccidia of cats; may cause hemorrhagic enteritis.
cystojejunostomy surgical anastomosis of a pancreatic cyst to the jejunum.
cystolith a vesical calculus.
cystolithectomy surgical removal of a vesical calculus.
cystolithiasis formation of vesical calculi.
cystolithic pertaining to a vesical calculus.
cystolithotomy see CYSTOLITHECTOMY.
cystoma a tumor containing cysts of neoplastic origin; a cystic tumor.
cystometer an instrument for studying the neuromuscular mechanism of the bladder by means of measurements of pressure and capacity.
cystometrogram the record obtained by cystometrography.
cystometrography the graphic recording of intravesical volumes and pressures.
cystometry the study of bladder efficiency by means of the cystometer to measure pressures in the urinary bladder.
cystomorphous resembling a cyst or bladder.
cystopexy fixation of the bladder to the abdominal wall.
cystoplasty plastic repair of the bladder.
cystoplegia paralysis of the bladder.
cystoproctostomy surgical creation of a communication between the urinary bladder and the rectum.
cystoptosis prolapse of part of the inner coat of the bladder into the urethra.
cystopyelitis inflammation of the bladder and renal pelvis.
cystopyelonephritis combined cystitis and pyelonephritis.
cystorrhaphy suture of the bladder.
cystorrhea mucous discharge from the bladder.
cystorrhexia urinary bladder rupture.
cystoscope an endoscope especially designed for passing through the urethra into the bladder to permit visual inspection of the interior of that organ. It has an outer sheath with a lighting system, a telescope with forward or oblique viewing, and an obturator which can be removed to allow passage of various devices.
cystoscopy examination of the bladder by means of a cystoscope, which is introduced into the urinary meatus and passed through the urethra and into the bladder.

A catheter can be passed through the cystoscope into the bladder or, if necessary, beyond, into the ureters and kidneys. In this way samples of urine can be obtained for diagnostic purposes. Also, radiopaque fluids can be injected into the bladder or ureters for x-rays of the urinary tract. See also PYELOGRAPHY.
cystostomy surgical formation of an opening into the bladder.
cystotomy incision of the bladder. See also VESICOTOMY.
cystoureteritis inflammation involving the urinary bladder and ureters.
cystoureterogram a radiograph of the bladder and ureter.
cystourethrography radiography of the urinary bladder and urethra.
voiding c. x-ray studies taken while the animal is voiding urine.
cystourethroplasty surgical revision of the urinary bladder and urethra, usually applied to creation of a urethral sling in the treatment of urinary incontinence in dogs.
cystourethroscope an instrument for examining the posterior urethra and bladder.
Cyt cytosine.
cytapheresis a procedure in which cells of one or more kinds (leukocytes, platelets, etc.) are separated from whole blood and retained, the plasma and other formed elements being retransfused into the donor; it includes leukapheresis and thrombocytapheresis.
cytarabine an antimetabolite that inhibits DNA synthesis, and hence has antineoplastic and antiviral properties. Called also cytosine arabinoside, arabinosyl cytosine, ara-C.
Cytauxzoon a genus of protozoan parasites of the family Theileriidae.
C. felis causes a fatal disease of cats.
C. sylvicaprae, C. strepsicerosi, C. taurotragi these protozoa multiply by fission in erythrocytes. They have been observed in wild animals and in cats.
cytauxzoonosis a disease of cats caused by *Cytauxzoon* spp. transmitted probably by ixodid ticks and characterized by fever, anemia and jaundice.
-cyte word element. [Gr.] *a cell.*
cythioate an organophosphorus anthelmintic administered orally to dogs and cats for control of fleas.
cytidine a nucleoside, cytosine riboside; a constituent of RNA and cytidine nucleotides.
c. 5′-triphosphate CTP; pyrimidine-nucleotide base involved in the structure of the nucleic acids, DNA and RNA, in the activation of sugars, and in phospholipid synthesis.
cytisine the toxic quinolizidine alkaloid in laburnum (*Laburnum anagyroides*), *Retama retam* and broom (*Cytisus scoparius*) trees.
Cytisus genus of the Fabaceae legume family; contain the toxic alkaloid cytisine which causes excitement, incoordination, convulsions and death due to asphyxia. Includes *C. scoparius*, *C. multiflorus*, *C. proliferus*. Called also brooms.
cyt(o)- word element. [Gr.] *a cell.*
cytoanalyzer an electronic optical apparatus for the detection of malignant cells in smears.
cytochalasin any of a group of fungal metabolites that affect the motility of polymorphonuclear leukocytes.
cytochemistry the identification and localization of the different chemical compounds and their activities within the cell.
cytochrome any of a class of hemoproteins, widely

distributed in animal and plant tissue, whose main function is electron transport; distinguished according to their prosthetic group as *a*, *b*, *c* and *d*.

c. b_5 reductase a flavoprotein involved in the desaturation of fatty acids in the liver.

c. oxidase an *a* type cytochrome which contains copper and receives electrons from another cytochrome, of the *c* type, and transfers them to oxygen atoms allowing the oxygen to combine with hydrogen atoms to form water. A nutritional deficiency of copper leads to a general reduction in metabolic rate because of the absence of cytochrome oxidase *a*.

c. system the sum of cytochromes which play a part in the body's metabolic processes. Includes the cytochrome oxidases and cytochrome reductases.

cytocidal causing cell destruction.

cytocide an agent that destroys cells.

cytoclasis the destruction of cells.

cytodiagnosis diagnosis based on examination of cells.

cytodifferentiation the development of specialized structures and functions in embryonic cells.

cytodistal denoting that part of an axon remote from the cell body.

Cytodites a genus of mites; parasites in the air sacs of birds, the air sac mite; usually do not have any pathogenic effect. Includes *Cytodites nudus*.

Cytoecetes a genus of rickettsiae.

C. bovis, C. phagocytophila the cause of tickborne fever of sheep, transmitted by *Ixodes ricinus*. Called also *Rickettsia phagocytophila* or *Ehrlichia phagocytophila*.

C. ondiri the cause of bovine petechial fever or Ondiri disease transmitted by an unidentified insect vector.

C. phagocytophila see *C. bovis* (above).

cytofilaments elements of the cytoplasmic skeleton; other elements are microtubules, filaments and cytoplasmic inclusions.

cytogenesis the origin and development of the cell.

cytogenetic pertaining to or originating from the origin and development of the cell.

c. defects abnormalities in the composition of the chromosomes in an individual animal. These can be detected in the fetus by the study of amniotic fluid obtained by abdominocentesis but has limitations in animals that bear litters. Prenatal sex determination is also possible by this means.

c. infertility infertility related to chromosomal abnormality.

cytogenetics that branch of genetics devoted to the cellular constituents concerned in heredity, i.e. the chromosomes; the combined sciences of genetics and cytology.

clinical c. the branch of cytogenetics concerned with relations between chromosomal abnormalities and pathological conditions.

cytogenic 1. pertaining to cytogenesis. 2. forming or producing cells.

cytoglycopenia deficient glucose content of the body or blood cells.

cytohistogenesis development of the structure of cells.

cytohistology the combination of cytological and histological methods.

cytoid resembles a cell.

cytokine soluble biological messenger proteins controlling macrophages and lymphocytes taking part in cell-mediated immune reaction. See also MONOKINE and LYMPHOKINE.

cytokinesis the division of the cytoplasm between daughter cells in MITOSIS or MEIOSIS.

Cytoleichus see CYTODITES.

cytolemma of the oocyte, the limiting membrane of the yolk of a bird's egg; the plasma membrane.

cytolisin toxic agent in snake venom; causes cell destruction, including platelets, leading to intravascular coagulation.

cytological, cytologic pertaining to cytology.

c. examination examination of material for purposes of cytology. Carried out on cerebrospinal fluid, joint fluid, aspirates of body cavities and cystic lesions. Includes total and differential counts.

cytologist a specialist in cytology.

cytology the study of cells, their origin, structure, function and pathology.

aspiration biopsy c. (ABC) the microscopic study of cells obtained from superficial or internal lesions by suction through a fine needle.

brush c. examination of cells obtained from a mucosal surface using a cytological brush.

exfoliative c. microscopic examination of cells desquamated from a body surface or lesion as a means of detecting malignancy and microbiological changes, to measure hormonal levels, etc. Such cells may be obtained by such procedures as aspiration, washing, smear and scraping, and the technique may be applied to vaginal secretions, urine, abdominal fluid, prostatic secretion, etc.

cytolysin a substance or antibody which causes cytolysis.

cytolysis the dissolution of cells.

immune c. cell lysis produced by antibody with the participation of complement.

cytolysosomes cytolysosomes are formed when products of cytoplasmic degeneration are engulfed by primary lysosomes; they are finally digested and the residual body which remains is extruded from the cell.

cytolytic pertaining to or emanating from cytolysis.

c. reactivity type II hypersensitivity.

cytomegalic a state of cytomegaly.

c. inclusion body disease a disease of young pigs. See INCLUSION BODY rhinitis.

cytomegalovirus herpesvirus provisionally placed in the subfamily *Betaherpesvirinae*, they infect humans, monkeys, pigs and rodents in which they appear to establish life-long infections. The viruses are highly host specific, slow growing, remain highly cell-associated and produce large intranuclear inclusion bodies in enlarged cells. Diseases produced by cytomegaloviruses are subtle.

equine c. see EQUINE herpesvirus 2.

mouse c. causes subclinical infection of submaxillary salivary glands and other tissues in wild mice.

porcine c. causes INCLUSION body rhinitis and a generalized infection in young pigs.

cytomegaly unique and marked enlargement of cells; a characteristic of cytomegaloviruses; occurs also in cells infected with one strain of an ovine adenovirus.

cytometaplasia change in function or form of cells.

cytometer a device for counting cells.

cytometry the counting of blood cells.

cytomorphology the morphology of body cells.

cytomorphosis the changes through which cells pass in development.

cyton cell body of a neuron; called also soma.

cytopathic pertaining to or characterized by pathological changes in cells.

cytopathogenesis production of pathological changes in cells.

cytopathogenic pertaining to or emanating from cytopathogenesis.
c. effect having a destructive effect on cells. See also CYTOLYTIC.
cytopathological, cytopathologic relating to cytopathology; denoting the changes in cells in disease.
cytopathologist an expert in the study of cells in disease; a cellular pathologist.
cytopathology the study of cells in disease; cellular pathology.
cytopenia deficiency in the cells of the blood.
Cytophaga a genus of gram-negative, gliding, rod-shaped bacteria.
C. columnaria the cause of columnaris disease in salmonid fish, associated with increased water temperature. Characterized by white necrotic plaques overlaying skin ulcers. Previously called *Flexibacter columnaris*.
C. johnsonae see FALSE COLUMNARIS DISEASE.
C. psychrophila causes peduncle or cold water disease of Brook trout. Predisposed to by subnormal water temperature.
cytophagy the ingestion of cells by phagocytes.
cytophilic having an affinity for cells.
c. antibody see cytotropic ANTIBODY.
cytophylaxis 1. the protection of cells against cytolysis. 2. increase in cellular activity.
cytopipette a pipette for taking cytological smears.
cytoplasm the protoplasm of a cell surrounding the nucleus (nucleoplasm).
cytoplasmic pertaining to or included in cytoplasm.
c. inclusions include secretory inclusions (enzymes, acids, proteins, mucosubstances), nutritive inclusions (glycogen, lipids), pigment granules (melanin, lipofuscin, hemosiderin). See also INCLUSION BODY.
c. inheritance the cytoplasmic organelles, chloroplasts and mitochondria contain DNA which contains a number of genes. These extrachromosomal genes are transmitted to daughter cells via cytoplasm. Called also maternal inheritance.
c. nuclear inclusion see INCLUSION BODY.
c. skeleton includes microtubules, centrioles, cilia, flagellae.
cytoplasmolysis lysis or digestion of the cytoplasm of cells as part of the death of tissues.
cytosegresome formations spherical, refractile, eosinophilic structures which develop in hepatic cells that have been injured by sublethal noxa such as hypoxia, nutritional deficiencies and hepatoxins. Called also Councilman bodies, hepatocellular acidophilic bodies.
cytosine a pyrimidine base found in the NUCLEIC ACIDS, DEOXYRIBONUCLEIC ACID (DNA) and RIBONUCLEIC ACID (RNA).
c. arabinoside see CYTARABINE.
cytoskeleton a conspicuous internal reinforcement in the cytoplasm of a cell, consisting of tonofibrils, filaments of the terminal web, and other microfilaments.
cytosol the liquid medium of the cytoplasm, e.g. cytoplasm minus organelles and nonmembranous insoluble components.
cytosome the body of a cell apart from its nucleus.
cytostasis inhibition of cell proliferation.
cytostatic 1. suppressing the growth and multiplication of cells. 2. an agent that so acts.
cytotaxis the movement and arrangement of cells with respect to a specific source of stimulation.
cytotaxonomy study of the relationships between and the classification of organisms.
cytotechnologist a medical laboratory technologist specializing in cytology.
cytothesis restitution of cells to their normal condition.
cytotoxic having a deleterious effect upon cells.
c. antibody see cytotoxic ANTIBODY.
c. drugs generally refers to those used in chemotherapy of neoplasms, e.g. cyclophosphamide, vincristine, etc.
c. T lymphocyte see T LYMPHOCYTE.
cytotoxicity destruction of cells; used to describe lysis of cells by immune mechanisms. See also ANTIBODY-dependent cell-mediated cytotoxicity (ADCC).
cytotoxin a toxin having a specific toxic action on cells of special organs.
cytotrophoblast the cellular (inner) layer of the trophoblast.
cytotropism 1. cell movement in response to external stimulation. 2. the tendency of viruses, bacteria, drugs, etc., to be attracted to and exert their effect upon certain cells of the body.
cytula the impregnated ovum.
cyturia the presence of cells of any sort in the urine.
Czech pied cattle red and white, pied, dual purpose cattle from former Czechoslovakia.
Czerny–Lembert suture a combination of the Czerny and Lembert suture patterns. The Czerny suture, which may be interrupted or continuous, is buried by a seromuscular Lembert layer.
Czerny suture 1. an intestinal suture in which the thread is passed through the mucosa only. 2. union of a ruptured tendon by splitting one of the ends and suturing the other into the split.
Czesky terrier a long, low set terrier with pendulous ears, long tail and wavy, silky coat of gray-blue or light brown with yellow and gray markings; clipped to a short length, except on the upper part of the head, lower legs, over the ribs and the belly. A Czechoslovakian breed, developed from Scottish and Sealyham terriers. Called also Bohemian terrier.

D

D chemical symbol, *deuterium*.
2,4-D see 2,4-DICHLOROPHENOXYACETIC ACID.
d symbol, *deci-*; 2′-deoxyribo.
d- prefix, *dextro-*.
d-amino acid oxidase an active enzyme, widespread in animal tissues, but of little known significance in animals; capable of oxidative deamination of amino acids, but d-amino acids are almost completely absent from animal tissues.
D gene segment see diversity GENE.
D-loop a structure produced during the initial stages of the replication of a circular DNA molecule as a result of strand displacement, by the leading strand, of the unreplicated lagging strand.
4D meat meat from animals which are dead, diseased, dying or have been destroyed. Usually salvaged for rendering.
dacarbazine an alkylating and antimetabolite, cell-cycle nonspecific antineoplastic agent. Abbreviated DTIC.
Dacelo novaeguineae see KOOKABURRA.

Dachshund a small (approximately 20–25 lb) breed of dog characterized by its long body, deep chest and very short legs. A German breed, the name means 'badger dog' and it was bred for hunting small game. There are three coat types: smooth (or shorthaired), longhaired and wire-haired, found in black, shades of brown, brindled and dappled. A miniature variety (less than 10 lb) is also bred in all three coat types. The breed is predisposed to intervertebral disk protrusion, acanthosis nigricans, cystinuria and diabetes mellitus.
Dacron polyethylene terephthalate, a polyester synthetic material used widely for vascular prostheses.
dacryagogue 1. an agent that induces a flow of tears. 2. a lacrimal duct.
dacry(o)- word element. [Gr.] *tears* or the lacrimal apparatus of the eye.
dacryoadenalgia pain in a lacrimal gland.
dacryoadenectomy excision of a lacrimal gland.
dacryoadenitis inflammation of a lacrimal gland.
dacryoblennorrhea mucous flow from the lacrimal apparatus.
dacryocele see DACRYOCYSTOCELE.
dacryocyst see LACRIMAL sac.
dacryocystalgia pain in the lacrimal sac. Called also dacryoadenalgia.
dacryocystectomy excision of the wall of the lacrimal sac.
dacryocystitis, dacrocystitis inflammation of the lacrimal sac.
dacryocystoblennorrhea chronic catarrhal inflammation of the lacrimal sac, with constriction of the lacrimal gland.
dacryocystocele hernial protrusion of the lacrimal sac; dacryocele.
dacryocystoptosis prolapse of the lacrimal sac.
dacryocystorhinography radiography of the nasolacrimal duct.
dacryocystorhinostenosis narrowing of the duct leading from the lacrimal sac to the nasal cavity.
dacryocystorhinostomy surgical creation of an opening between the lacrimal sac and nasal cavity.
dacryocystorhinotomy passage of a probe through the lacrimal sac into the nasal cavity.
dacryocystostenosis narrowing of the lacrimal sac.
dacryocystostomy surgical creation of a new opening into the lacrimal sac with drainage.
dacryocystotomy incision of the lacrimal sac and duct.
dacryocyte a red blood cell with a single, tear-shaped spicule; observed in fragmentation anemia and myelofibrosis.
dacryohemorrhea the discharge of tears mixed with blood.
dacryolith a lacrimal calculus.
dacryolithiasis the presence of dacryoliths.
dacryoma a tumor-like swelling due to obstruction of the lacrimal duct.
dacryon the point where the lacrimal, frontal and maxillary bones meet.
dacryops distension of the lacrimal duct with fluid.
dacryopyorrhea the discharge of tears mixed with pus.
dacryorrhea excessive flow of tears.
dacryoscintigraphy scintigraphy of the lacrimal ducts.
dacryosolenitis inflammation of a lacrimal duct.
dacryostenosis stricture or narrowing of a lacrimal duct.
dacryosyrinx 1. lacrimal duct. 2. a lacrimal fistula. 3. a syringe for irrigating the lacrimal ducts.
dactinomycin an antibiotic of the actinomycin complex (actinomycin D), produced by several species of *Streptomyces*; used as an antineoplastic agent.
dactyl a digit.
Dactylaria gallopava a thermophilic dematiaceous hyphomycete known to cause encephalitis in chicken and poults. Called also dactylariosis.
dactylariosis a fungal encephalitis of birds caused by *Dactylaria gallopava*.
Dactylis glomerata a valuable temperate region pasture grass which contains a lamb growth inhibitor. Called also cocksfoot, orchard grass.
dactylitis inflammation of a digit.
dactyl(o)- word element. [Gr.] *a digit*.
Dactyloctenium radulans Australian grass of the family Poaceae. Can sometimes contain toxic levels of nitrate, but is still a valuable pasture plant. Called also button or finger grass, *Eleusine aegyptica*, *E. radulans*.
dactylogryposis permanent flexion of the digits.
Dactylogyrus a genus of monogenetic flukes of the family Dactylogyridae that infest fish.
D. extensus, D. vastator cause an important parasitic disease of the gills of marine and freshwater fish.
dactylolysis 1. surgical correction of syndactyly. 2. loss or amputation of a digit.
dactylomegaly abnormally large digits.
dactylus pl. *dactyli* [L.] a digit.
daddy-long-legs see HARVESTMEN.
DAF DECAY-accelerating factor.
daffodil see NARCISSUS.
d. tree THEVETIA *peruviana*.
daft lamb see CEREBELLAR atrophy.
dagging removal of lumps of wool matted together with feces (dags) from the perineal region of the sheep.
dags locks or staples of wool in the crutch that are heavily fouled with caked feces.
daidzein an estrogenic plant isoflavone.
daily pull and dead records a daily account kept in a feedlot of the deaths and the animals pulled out of each pen because of illness or injury.
dairy 1. a retail outlet for milk products. 2. the feeding and milking sheds on a dairy farm. 3. pertaining to or emanating from an animal or other thing concerned in the production of milk, e.g. dairy goat, dairy cleanser.
d. barn standard indoor housing in temperate and subarctic northern hemisphere countries; a common plan is to have animal housed on the ground floor and grain and hay on the top floor from which it is delivered to the animals below; the cows are tied in stanchions and milked on the spot or roam free and are milked in a parlor.
d. breeds see AUSTRALIAN Shorthorn, AYRSHIRE, BROWN SWISS CATTLE, DAIRY SHORTHORN, JERSEY, GUERNSEY, HOLSTEIN-FRIESIAN, RED POLL, AUSTRALIAN Milking Zebu, BRITISH WHITE, DEXTER, JAMAICA HOPE, MILKING SHORTHORN.
d. calf calf of a mating between a bull and a cow, both of dairy breeds.
d. cow cow of a breed specifically defined as being for milk production, as distinct from a beef or dual purpose breed.
d. farmer a farmer whose major enterprise is dairy farming.
d. herd includes milking cows, dry cows, heifers (maiden and in-calf), calves and, where needed, bulls. Called also milking herd, dry herd, followers.
d. herd improvement a centralized system, usually sponsored by a government or a farmer-owned

erative, for recording milk yield and assessing the productive status of individual cows. Recommendations are then made relative to culling or mating program for the individual cows. The central database provides information on which analyses of performance can be made relative to a multiplicity of variables, such as herd size, breed, times per day milking.

d. industry includes the farms, the milk collecting and handling services, the processors, manufacturers and retailers and the private and government organizations involved in a coordinating or controlling function with respect to the harvesting and disposal of dairy products.

d. sanitizers disinfectants suitable for use in an environment and in a situation in which contamination of the human food chain is likely to occur.

Dairy shorthorn the dairy variety of the SHORTHORN breed of cattle. Called also Milking shorthorn.

dairyCHAMP a computer program designed to aid dairy herd health and production management. Originates from the University of Minnesota.

dairyCOMP an on-farm computer program devised to participate in dairy herd health management.

dairying 1. the occupation of being a dairy farmer. 2. the practice of running a dairy farm.

seasonal d. breeding the herd as a block so as to have the herd calve when feed supplies are good.

year-round d. a management system in which cows are bred to calve so that there is a constant influx of freshly calved cows.

dairyMAN a dairy computer program designed to aid dairy herd health and production management. Originates from Massey University, New Zealand.

DAISY acronym for Dairy Information System—a well-known herd health program and dairy information management system. Designed at Reading University, UK.

daisy wheel the printing head of an early model of letter quality printer.

Dakin's solution an aqueous solution containing sodium hypochlorite and sodium bicarbonate; used in enormous quantities when veterinary surgery was a barnyard and kitchen table practice, and infected wounds were the norm. It was in general use as a local antibacterial and to irrigate wounds.

DALA delta-amino levulinic acid.

dalapon a chlorinated acid used as a herbicide; experimentally high doses cause abortions and weak lambs; nontoxic at normal concentrations.

Dales pony English heavy miniature horse, 14 to 14.2 hands high, usually black or dark brown, sometimes gray.

Dall sheep *Ovis dalli*; a medium-sized wild sheep.

Dallas grass PASPALUM *dilatatum*.

Dalmatian, Dalmatian coach hound a medium-sized, shorthaired dog distinguished by its white color with black or brown spots distributed uniformly over the entire body. The breed has a unique protein metabolism that results in high levels of uric acid excretion into the urine. As a result the breed is predisposed to urate uroliths and some dermatoses believed to be associated with this metabolic characteristic. It also is affected by inherited deafness and a cavitating leukodystrophy. Called also English coach dog, Carriage dog, Plum pudding dog, Fire house dog and Spotted Dick.

Dalmatian insect powder see PYRETHRUM.

Dalmeny disease see SARCOCYSTOSIS.

dalton an arbitrary unit of mass, being one-twelfth the mass of the nuclide of carbon-12, equivalent to 1.657×10^{-24} g. Called also atomic mass unit.

Dalton's law the pressure exerted by a mixture of nonreacting gases is equal to the sum of the partial pressures of the separate components.

dam female parent.

d. line characteristics contributed to the offspring of a cross mating by the dam.

d.–offspring bond the close relationship of seeking, suckling and protecting imprinted at birth by sight, taste and smell. Called also maternal bond.

dam-family average the average performance of the full-sib family of which the subject is a member.

Dama a genus of true deer in the family Cervidae. Called also *Odocoileus*.

D. dama see FALLOW DEER.

D. hemionus see MULE DEER.

damages money paid to the victor in a court case in which loss of property or income is alleged, covered by the law of torts. Simple damages are assessed on the value of the actual loss. Punitive or exemplary damages are in excess of simple damages and are awarded as a punishment against the loser in the suit if it is judged that the tort was an aggravated one, and that the defendant has been, for example, wilfully and recklessly neglectful.

Damalinia a genus of mammal lice of the superfamily Ischnocera. Called also *Bovicola*. Includes *Damalinia bovis* (cattle), *D. caprae* (goats), *D. crassiceps* (goats), *D. equi* syn. *D. pilosus* (horses), *D. limbata* (Angora goats), *D. ovis* (sheep).

Damaliscus lunatus medium-sized, short-horned, East African antelope; called also topi.

DAMN IT acronym for a clinical investigation plan, based on probable pathophysiologic causes of the disease present. It consists of **D**egenerative, developmental; **A**llergic, autoimmune; **M**etabolic, mechanical; **N**utritional, neoplastic; **I**nflammatory, immune-mediated, iatrogenic, ischemic, idiopathic; **T**oxic, traumatic.

damping 1. steady diminution of the amplitude of successive vibrations of a specific form of energy, as of electricity. 2. sprinkling a feed with water to reduce dust and inhalation of dust as a prevention of chronic obstructive respiratory disease in horses and dust tracheitis in feedlot steers.

danazol an attenuated androgen that suppresses the ovarian–pituitary axis by inhibiting the release of gonadotropins from the pituitary gland. In animals, it has been used in the treatment of immune-mediated disorders, including anemia and thrombocytopenia.

dancing pigs see CONGENITAL TREMOR SYNDROME.

dandelion see TARAXACUM OFFICINALE.

dander small scales from the hair or feathers of animals, which may be a cause of allergy in sensitive persons.

Dandie Dinmont terrier a small dog with pendulous ears and a medium length, crisp coat in colors described as mustard (fawn to reddish brown) or pepper (dark bluish black to light silvery gray). The legs are short, with the front being shorter than the rear so the shoulder height is about 10 inches. The large head is accentuated by a fluffy topknot.

dandruff excessive scaling from the skin or, in humans, scalp.

walking d. cheyletiellosis.

dandy-brush a grooming brush of stiff whisk fiber.

Dandy–Walker syndrome congenital hydrocephalus due to obstruction of the foramina of Magendie and Luschka. A deformity in humans also recorded in dogs and sheep. Called also Dandy–Walker malformation.

danewort SAMBUCUS *ebulus*.

dangerous wild animals animals that may be specified by local legislation as requiring a license if they are to be kept by a private person and outside circuses or zoos, which are legislated for separately.
Danish black pied cattle Danish black and white dairy cattle, originated from Dutch Friesian.
Danish hobbles see ABILDGAARD METHOD.
Danish red cattle Danish red dairy cattle.
Danish Swine Slaughter Data System a centralized, computer-based system by which pig health can be monitored via an abattoir meat inspection service. There is a standard list of diagnostic codes which ensures compatibility of results over a number of operators.
danofloxacin antimicrobial agent of the fluoroquinolone group with a wide range of activity against bacteria and mycoplasmas.
dan's cabbage SENECIO *latifolius*, *S. isatideus*.
Danthonia widespread, perennial bunchgrass and a palatable pasture grass. Called also California oatgrass.
danthron a by-product of the dye industry used as a purgative, especially in horses. Called also dihydroxyanthraquinone. Veterinary practice with horses has veered away from these relatively violent purges and depends on mineral oil or liquid paraffin to treat constipation.
dantrolene skeletal muscle relaxant producing its effect primarily on the neuromuscular junction and the muscle tissue, and only secondarily on the central nervous system.
Daphne a genus of plants in the family Thymelaceae; contain dihydroxycoumarin glycosides, e.g. daphnetin; these are very toxic and cause severe irritation to the gut, leading to severe enteritis, vomiting and diarrhea. Includes *D. cneorum*, *D. genka*, *D. laureola*, *D. mezereum*. Called also spurge laurel, mezereon, garland flower, wood or copse laurel, wild pepper, spurge olive.
daphnetin toxic dihydroxycoumarin glycoside found in *Daphne* spp.
Daphnia pulex a water flea, one of the intermediate hosts of *Echinuria uncinata*, a roundworm of ducks.
daphnin a nontoxic glycoside in DAPHNE. Called also mezerein.
dapple a spotted, mottled or irregularly pigmented coat color pattern, usually with darker colors on a lighter background, Seen in some Dachshunds. A similar pigmentation pattern in longhaired dog breeds such as collies is usually called MERLE. Also occurs commonly in horses of any color, but is most striking in grays. May be noticeable only when the coat is short.
dapsone an antibacterial used in humans for the treatment of leprosy and malaria. Used in cats to treat mycobacterial infections, particularly feline leprosy, caused by *Mycobacterium lepraemurium*.
dark approaching black; reflecting little light.
d. cutting beef the meat is much darker than normal on its cut surface; caused by preslaughter stress. Called also dark, firm dry muscle, DFD.
d. firm, dry muscle see dark cutting beef (above).
d. film x-ray film that has been overexposed, or grossly overdeveloped.
film d. spots caused by developer splashing on the x-ray film causing prolonged local development.
d. room a room dedicated to the processing of film; must be light-proof, temperature stable and fitted with water and power.
dark neuron shrunken basophilic neurons are considered to be artefacts.
Darling's disease histoplasmosis.
Darling pea specifically *Swainsona greyana* but used to refer to any *Swainsona* spp.
darnel see LOLIUM *temulentum*.
Darrow's solution a mixture of potassium chloride, sodium chloride and sodium lactate; used in fluid therapy to repair a potassium deficit. Called also lactated potassium saline injection.
dart see BLOW DART.
d. gun see BLOW DART.
Dartmoor pony English heavy pony, 12.2 hands high, bay, black or brown.
dartoid resembling the dartos.
dartos the contractile tissue under the skin of the scrotum; called also tunica dartos.
darwinism the theory of evolution according to which higher organisms have been developed from lower ones through the influence of natural selection.
dassies see HYRAX.
Dasyprocta aguti see AGOUTI.
Dasypsyllus gallinulae a species of flea in the order Siphonaptera. It is found on wild birds.
Dasypus novemcinctus nine-banded armadillo, a member of the family Dasypodidae characterized by a covering of bony plates or a leathery carapace. It is a plantigrade, insectivorous, burrowing animal with the remarkable characteristic of always bearing four monozygous offspring. There are a number of other genera of similar armadillos. Armadillos are valued as experimental hosts in studies of leprosy.
dasyurids carnivorous marsupials in the family Dasyuridae. Includes Tasmanian devil (*Sarcophilus harrisii*), the Tasmanian tiger (*Thylacinus cynocephalus*), the smaller Australian Eastern native cat (*Dasyurus quoll*) and marsupial rats (*Phascogale* spp.).
data plural of *datum*. A collection of information or facts See also INFORMATION.
d. accessibility see data ACCESSIBILITY.
d. adjustment for useful results data often need to be modified before analysis; for example for age, for sex or for difficulty or for number of attempts.
d. analysis submission of data to statistical analysis; includes sorting into categories and determining relationships between variables.
d. bank an obsolete term meaning database.
d. capture a mechanism for collecting specified segments or categories of data from a stream of automatically recorded data some of which may be irrelevant for the specific purpose.
categorical d. are qualitative and suited to classification into categories. Further divisible into nominal (names), ordinal (levels of quality, development), dichotomized (mutually exclusive).
d. compression technique for reducing the size of a data file for storage; the original file is obtained by reversing the compression procedure.
continuous d. data which have an infinite number of possible values.
diagnostic d. lists of diagnoses and data of clinical signs, clinical pathology results and pathology lesions used in the making of diagnoses.
dimensional d. numerical or quantitative data. May be explicit and therefore continuous, or grouped into approximate groups, e.g. nearest whole number, i.e. discrete data.
discrete d. data that have finite (usually whole integer) value and therefore fall naturally into groups of similar values; opposite to continuous data.
d. file a collection of like data kept together for ease of retrieval. May be kept in a manilla folder or on a computer disk.

d. handling the capture, collection, storage, archiving, analysis and retrieval of data. Categorized into systems such as manual, card, computerized.
incidence d. data related to the occurrence of specific disease incidents.
non-normal d. data whose frequency distribution is markedly different to that of normal data (see below).
normal d. data which manifests graphically as a bell-shaped curve distributed symmetrically about the peak value.
ordinal d. a type of data containing limited categories with a ranking from the lowest to the highest, e.g. very= mild, moderate, severe.
paired d. see PAIRED data.
passive d. data acquired from records collected for some other purpose.
pre-existing d. data in existence before the commencement of a study. Of limited value unless they are exactly the data required, have been collected adequately, and a group of pre-existing controls with their corresponding data can be identified.
prevalence d. disease occurrences are recorded against the size of the population at risk at the time.
d. processing see data PROCESSING.
raw d. data as they are collected and before any calculation, ordering, etc. has been done.
screening d. data obtained by periodic diagnostic testing of randomly selected samples of a population.
secondary d. the use of data for purposes other than that for which it was intended.
sentinel d. data collected from SENTINEL animals or other recording units.
d. set see MODEM.
d. source the collecting agency.

database an accumulation of data stored in such a way that any part of the contents can be found and retrieved accurately and quickly, modified and then returned to its storage place. The size of the storage can be massive, provided the computer program can deal with it adequately.
d. management system a management system as a computer program designed to effectively and accurately store, access and update a database.

Datisca glomerata North American plant in the family Datiscaceae; contains an unidentified toxin which causes diarrhea, enteritis. Called also durango root.

Datura a genus of toxic plants in the family Solanaceae; contain tropane alkaloids including hyoscine (scopolamine), hyoscyamine, atropine which cause excitement, restlessness, pupillary dilation, dryness of the oral mucosa. Poisoning in animals is rare and usually results from eating crushed seeds. Includes *D. candida* (*Brugmansia*, angel's trumpet), *D. ferox* (false castor oil plant, thorn apple), *D. inoxia*, *D. leichhardtii*, *D. metel*, *D. meteloides*, *D. sanguinea* (*Brugmansia sanguinea*), *D. suaveolens* (*Brugmansia suaveolens*), *D. wrightii*.
D. stramonium is also reported to cause arthrogryposis in piglets when fed to their dams. Fortunately the plant is very unpalatable. Called also devil's food, devil's trumpet, false castor oil plant, Jamestown lily, Jamestown weed, jimson weed, mad apple, thorn apple.

Daubentonia the plant genus *Sesbania* spp.

Daubentonia madagascariensis AYE-AYE (a primate).

Daubentoniidae a family of primates containing only one member, the Aye-aye (*Daubentonia madagascariensis*), a furry, cat-sized, nocturnal, tree-climbing creature.

Daucus carota plant in the family Apiaceae; mildly poisonous but a common plant causing few problems. Called also Queen Anne's lace, wild carrot.

daughter 1. female offspring. 2. arising from cell division, as a daughter cell. 3. product of the decay or radioactive disintegration of a radionuclide. Usually formed as a result of successive transformations in a series. See also DECAY (3).
d. cyst see daughter CYST.

daunomycin see DAUNORUBICIN.

daunorubicin an anthracycline antibiotic produced by a strain of *Streptomyces coeruleorubidus* that is closely related to DOXORUBICIN and has antimitotic, cytotoxic and immunosuppressive effects.

Davainea a genus of tapeworms of the family Davaineidae.
D. proglottina causes severe enteritis in fowls and other gallinaceous birds.

Davis forceps thumb-operated tissue forceps with a special atraumatic grasping surface to its blades—a hollow surrounded by shallow ridges. Designed for handling lung.

Davison–Danielli membrane model first generally accepted model of membrane structure proposing a lipid bilayer as the basis of the structure.

day blindness see HEMERALOPIA.

day-blooming jessamine CESTRUM *diurnum*.

day length the number of daylight hours per day, increasing towards midsummer and the reverse towards midwinter. The effective trigger in the commencement and cessation of the breeding seasons in those species that demonstrate seasonal breeding.

day lily see HEMEROCALLIS.

day-old chicks the standard output from the hatchery for broiler growers and egg producers in the poultry industry.

days open the period between calving and conception in cows. Called also calving-to-conception interval.

2,4-DB 4-(2,4-dichlorophenoxy) butanoic acid; a phenoxyacid herbicide, not poisonous in its own right but may cause damaged plants to have higher than normal concentrations of nitrate.

DCT dry cow treatment.

DD dichlorodiphenyldichloroethane, an insecticide; see CHLORINATED HYDROCARBONS.

DDAVP see DESMOPRESSIN.

DDP diamminedichloroplatinum, a heavy metal complex; used as an antineoplastic agent. See also CISPLATIN.

DDT dichlorodiphenyltrichloroethane, a powerful insect poison; see CHLORINATED HYDROCARBONS.

DDVP see DICHLORVOS.

DDx abbreviation for differential diagnosis; used in medical records.

de- word element. [L.] *down from;* sometimes negative or privative, and often intensive.

de Bruin spatula a small hand-sized obstetric spatula used to skin a fetus in utero in a cow.

de Vita pin a bone pin used to stabilize hip luxations by being placed ventral to the ischial tuberosity, dorsal to the femoral neck, and into the ilium. It forms an extension of the dorsal and lateral acetabular rim.

DEA dog erythrocyte antigen.

dead destitute of life. The state of DEATH.
d. wool wool plucked from dead sheep in the field. See also FELL-MONGERING.

dead animal disposal in most intensive farming areas, dead stock facilities (knackery yards in some countries) and rendering works are markets for cadavers. In extensive farming areas burning or burial are desirable but natural decay is a common outcome.

dead mans fingers OENANTHE *crocata*.
dead nettle see LAMIUM AMPLEXICAULE.
deadgrass a coat color of pale yellow to tan, associated with the Chesapeake Bay retriever breed of dogs.
deadly nightshade *Atropa belladonna*. Commonly confused with *Solanum* spp.
deaf lacking the sense of hearing or not having the full power of hearing; exhibiting DEAFNESS.
deafness lack or loss, complete or partial, of the sense of HEARING.
conductive d. sound vibrations are interrupted in the outer or middle ear and do not reach the inner ear and its nerve endings.
congenital d. infrequent in dogs and cats, not recorded in other species. In most cases is due to cochlear duct degeneration. See also inherited deafness (below).
cortical d. that due to disease of the cortical centers of the cerebrum.
inherited d. occurs in some blue-eyed white cats and in some dog breeds; particularly common in the Dalmatian. In some cases it is associated with coat coloration, e.g. white Bull terriers, merle collies and Old English sheepdogs.
nerve d. due to degeneration of the acoustic sensory organ. Most common in dogs at an early age and associated with incomplete pigmentation of the haircoat and the uvea, in animals with a white or merle coat color. Occurs also in mink, cats and mice.
sensorineural d. due to damage of the inner ear nerve endings, the cochlear portion of the eighth cranial nerve, the vestibulocochlear nerve, or the cortical hearing center. See also nerve deafness (above).
toxic d. overdosing with aminoglycoside antibiotics causes deafness.
transmission d. conductive hearing loss.
deamidase an enzyme that splits amides to form a carboxylic acid and ammonia.
deamidization liberation of the ammonia from an amide.
deaminase an enzyme causing deamination, or removal of an amino group from organic compounds, named according to its substrate as adenosine deaminase, cytidine deaminase, guanine deaminase, etc.
deamination removal of the amino group, $-NH_2$, from a compound.
deAngelis technique a method for extra-articular reconstruction of the cranial cruciate ligament which involves placement of an imbrication suture from the lateral femero-fabella ligament to the distal patellar tendon.
death the cessation of all physical and chemical processes that invariably occurs in all living organisms. Even in humans there is at present no standardized diagnosis of clinical death. The existing procedure, and the one recommended for use in animals, is to declare the animal dead when brain death has occurred. Brain death has occurred when the animal is in a deep irreversible coma. The criteria on which a diagnosis of brain death can be made are: (1) absolute unresponsiveness to externally applied stimuli; (2) cessation of movement and breathing, including no spontaneous breathing for 3 minutes after an artificial respirator has been turned off; and (3) complete absence of cephalic reflexes. The pupils of the eyes must be dilated and unresponsive to direct light.
d. adder see death ADDER.
d. agony involuntary movements of all parts of the body in the few moments before death.
d. camas see ZIGADENUS.
d. cap a mushroom, AMANITA *phalloides*.
clinical d. the absence of heartbeat (no pulse can be felt) and cessation of breathing.
d. rate the number of deaths per stated number of animals in a specified region in a specified, usually annual, time period.
DeBakey an illustrious American cardiovascular surgeon.
D. bulldog clamps surgical instruments designed for temporary occlusion of large blood vessels.
D. tissue forceps delicate surgical thumb forceps with longitudinal ribs, designed for delicate, nontraumatic vascular surgery.
debarking surgical removal of all or part of the vocal cords; practiced in the dog to reduce a barking nuisance. Called also devocalization.
debeaking removal of part of the beak, usually the front third of the upper beak, of domestic fowls as a prevention against cannibalism in birds in intensive housing. See also CANNIBALISM.
debilitation being in a state of DEBILITY.
debility lack or loss of strength; weakness.
debleating resection of the vocal cords in a pet goat or sheep which has become a noise nuisance in an urban environment.
deboned carcass meat from which the bone has been removed.
debrancher enzyme an enzyme involved in the glycogenolytic process of releasing glucose from glycogen. A deficiency of the enzyme results in accumulation of glycogen in tissues. Both are characteristics of type III glycogen storage diseases.
débride [Fr.] to remove by débridement.
débridement [Fr.] the removal of all foreign material and all contaminated and devitalized tissues from or adjacent to a traumatic or infected lesion until surrounding healthy tissue is exposed.
block d. a method in which the wound is packed with gauze or toweling, sutured together and then the entire mass is removed surgically. Usually reserved for badly damaged tissues.
enzymatic d. use of enzymes such as trypsin and CHYMOTRYPSIN, usually applied topically, to achieve débridement.
debris devitalized tissue or foreign matter.
debt something owed.
bad d. see BAD DEBT.
oxygen d. the extra oxygen that must be used in the oxidative energy processes after a period of strenuous exercise to reconvert lactic acid to glucose and decomposed ATP and creatine phosphate to their original states.
d. serving capacity annual cash flow from an enterprise which is available to service loans, that is before deducting the payment of interest on loans and repayment of loan capital.
debug removal of an error in the computer software or hardware. See also BUG (2).
debulking removal of excess bulk of tissue from a lesion either to assist in healing or as an adjunct to chemotherapy.
DEC diethylcarbamazine.
deca-, deka- word element. [Gr.] *ten* used in naming units of measurement to indicate a quantity 10 times the unit designated by the root with which it is combined.
decalcification 1. the process of removing calcareous matter. 2. the loss of calcium salts from bone or teeth.
decalcify to deprive of calcium or its salts.

decamethonium a muscle relaxant used in surgical anesthesia in the form of its bromide or iodide salt.

decamethonium bromide a depolarizing neuromuscular blocking agent.

decannulation the removal of a cannula.

decanoate a salt of DECANOIC ACID.

decanoic acid one of the saturated fatty acids found in the endosperm of the coconut (*Cocos nucifera*), in coconut oil and in other seed oils. Used in diets for patients with fat malabsorption syndromes. Called also *n*-capric acid.

decantation the pouring of a clear supernatant liquid from a sediment.

decapeptide a polypeptide consisting of a chain of ten amino acids.

decapitation removal of the head, as of an animal, fetus or bone.

Decapoda an order in the class of Cephalopoda. All of its genera are composed of species with ten legs, e.g. the ten-legged squid, cuttlefish and calamaries.

decapsulation removal of a capsule, especially the renal capsule.

decarboxylase any of the lyase class of enzymes that catalyze the removal of a carbon dioxide molecule from a compound.

d. test tests for the identification of bacteria, based on the production of ammonia from lysine, ornithine or arginine. In a positive result, the alkaline product is indicated by bromocresol purple.

decarboxylation removal of the carboxyl group from a compound.

decay 1. the gradual decomposition of dead organic matter. 2. the process or stage of decline, as in old age. 3. in radioactivity terminology the disintegration of the nucleus of an inactive nuclide by the spontaneous emission of alpha or beta particles. Called also radioactive disintegration. Substances produced by the disintegrations are called DAUGHTER (3) compounds.

d.-accelerating factor a membrane-associated protein found on many cells, including peripheral blood cells, that inhibits the activity of complement.

decerebellate an animal from which the cerebellum has been removed, experimentally or, an unlikely event, accidentally.

decerebrate to eliminate cerebral function by transecting the brainstem or by ligating the common carotid arteries and basilar artery at the center of the pons; an animal so prepared, or a brain-damaged animal with similar neurological signs.

d. rigidity rigid extension of the limbs as a result of decerebration; also occurs as a result of lesions in the upper brainstem.

decerebration the act of decerebrating.

decholesterolization reduction of cholesterol levels in the blood.

deci- word element. [L.] *one-tenth;* used to indicate one-tenth (10^{-1}) of the unit designated by the root with which it is combined.

decibel a unit used to express the ratio of two powers, usually electric or acoustic powers, equal to one-tenth of a bel; one decibel equals approximately the smallest difference in acoustic power the human ear can detect. Abbreviated dB or db. See also BEL.

decidua a name applied to the human and primate endometrium during pregnancy, all of which except for the deepest layer is shed after birth of the young. Called also the decidual, or deciduous, membrane.

basal d., decidua basalis that portion on which the implanted ovum rests.

capsular d., decidua capsularis that portion directly overlying the implanted ovum and facing the uterine cavity.

parietal d. the decidua exclusive of the area occupied by the implanted ovum. Called also true decidua, decidua verra.

true d. see parietal decidua.

d. verra see parietal decidua.

deciduate, deciduous, decidual characterized by shedding, e.g. teeth, placenta.

d. placenta, deciduate membrane endothelial and hemochorial PLACENTAS.

deciduation the shedding of the decidua.

deciduitis a bacterial disease leading to changes in the decidua.

deciduoma an intrauterine mass containing decidual cells.

deciduosis the presence of decidual tissue or of tissue resembling the endometrium of human or primate pregnancy in an ectopic site.

deciduous falling off; subject to being shed, as deciduous TEETH.

decile one of the groups when a series of ranked data is divided into ten equal parts, or dividing points between such groups. See also QUARTILE.

decision a choice between a number of possible answers to a question.

d. analysis a systematic approach to decision making under conditions of imperfect knowledge; a practical application of probability theory. Used to calculate the optimal strategy from among a series of alternative strategies. May be expressed graphically in the form of a decision tree (below).

d. making making a decision can be done in three principal ways and many variations and mixtures of the methods: (1) rote, the decision is made on the basis of a set of rules and no selectivity is required; (2) intuitive, decisions are made on the basis of cerebrally stored information and reasoning systems which permit a fast response. The increasing complexity of veterinary clinical questions increases the probability of error; (3) decision analysis, a means of solving complicated problems by including all of the factors that could possibly affect the outcome of the analysis in a series of sequential questions. This gives each of the factors an opportunity of affecting the outcome. The chance of error by omission can be eliminated but the process is prolonged.

d. support systems computer programs used to assist decision making in particular fields of work, e.g. the management of patients in intensive care.

d. theory the theoretical basis for decision analysis.

d. tree a diagrammatic representation of the possible outcomes and events used in decision analysis. The questions to be asked in an analysis of a question are arranged as a series of nodes each with a yes and no branch, creating an arborization effect. The sequential steps proceed with each step depending on the decision made in the preceding step.

decking multiple decks in animal accommodation or transportation facilities. Common for young animals, chiefly piglets, commercial poultry, laboratory animals, cats and dogs.

declawing surgical removal of the claws of Felidae and Canidae. Not a universally accepted procedure except where there are specific health implications for the patient. Can happen accidentally in penned wildlife, e.g. anteaters. Called also onychectomy.

declive a slope or a slanting surface. The part of the vermis of the cerebellum just caudal to the primary fissure.

declivis [L.] *declive.*

decoction a medicine prepared by steeping the raw material in boiling water. The only common decoction is tea.

decoloration 1. removal of color; bleaching. 2. lack or loss of color.

decolorizer an agent that removes color, bleaches.

decombing surgical removal of the comb in the chicken or young bird to facilitate protrusion of the head through the bars of a battery cage. Pendulous wattles may be treated in the same way.

decompensation failure of compensation.

cardiac d. inability of the heart to maintain adequate circulation; it is marked by dyspnea, venous engorgement, cyanosis and edema.

decomposition 1. biologically speaking, the separation of compound bodies into their constituent principles; the natural process of biodegradation of animal and plant materials. Its occurrence in human and animal foods is a constant threat and preventing it is the prime objective of the food hygienist. 2. statistically speaking, the removal of accountable influences on a set of data so that only variation due to random error remains.

decompression 1. the return to normal environmental pressure after exposure to greatly increased pressure. 2. the artificial lowering of barometric pressure, e.g. to simulate high altitude.

cerebral d. removal of a flap of the skull and incision of the dura mater for the purpose of relieving intracranial pressure. Decompression can also be accomplished by the intravenous injection of hypertonic solutions, e.g. mannitol, usually accompanied by parenteral corticosteroids.

gastric d. by stomach tube or transperitoneal tap. An essential part of treatment for acute gastric dilatation in dogs and horses.

decongestant 1. tending to reduce congestion or swelling. 2. an agent that reduces congestion or swelling, usually of the nasal membranes. Decongestants may be inhaled, administered as spray or nose drops, or used orally in liquid or tablet form. The medication acts by reducing swelling of the nasal membranes and thus opening up the nasal passages. Among the leading medications used as decongestants are epinephrine, ephedrine and phenylephrine. Antihistamines, alone or in combination with decongestants, may also be effective.

decongestive reducing congestion.

decontamination the freeing of a patient or an object of some contaminating substance such as war gas, radioactive material, etc.

decoppering agents drugs which promote excretion of copper; includes D-penicillamine, trientine (2,2,2-tetramine) and 2,3,2-tetramine.

decoquinate a quinolone anticoccidial which is nontoxic but subject to a high rate of development of resistant coccidia.

decorin a small chondroitin sulfate proteoglycan found in bone, thought to be involved in the organization and mineralization of bone.

decortication, decortification 1. removal of the outer covering from a plant, seed or root. 2. removal of portions of the cortical substance of a structure or organ.

decrement the recovery after a fever; the excessive stored heat is dissipated by vasodilatation and sweating, and heat production is reduced by relaxation of muscles. Called also defervescence.

decremental conduction a phenomenon which occurs in the cardiac AV node when, during complete AV block, continued stimulation causes a slowing and diminished amplitude of phase 0 in the AV nodal cells until a nonpropagated local response occurs.

decrudescence diminution or abatement of the intensity of clinical signs.

Decrusia a genus of strongylid worms from the family Strongylidae. Includes *Decrusia additicta* (found in the large intestine of Indian elephants).

decubital ulcers see DECUBITUS ulcer.

decubitus pl. *decubitus*. 1. the act of lying down; the position assumed in lying down. 2. a decubitus ulcer.

dorsal d. lying on the back.

lateral d. lying on one side, designated right lateral decubitus when the subject lies on the right side and left lateral decubitus when it lies on the left side.

d. ulcer an ulcer due to local interference with the circulation; called also pressure sore. The ulcer usually occurs over a bony prominence such as that of the sacrum, hip, heel, shoulder or elbow. Excessive or prolonged pressure produced by the weight of the body or limb is the primary cause.

ventral d. lying on the stomach.

decussate 1. to cross especially in the form of Y. 2. crossed especially like the letter Y.

decussatio nervorum trochlearium the decussation of the trochlear nerve.

decussation a crossing over; the intercrossing of fellow parts or structures especially in the form of a Y.

d. of pyramids the anterior part of the lower medulla oblongata in which some of the fibers of each pyramid intersect as they cross the midline and descend as the lateral corticospinal tracts.

dedicated line a telephone line provided specifically for the use of a particular computer.

dedifferentiation regression from a more specialized or complex form to a simpler state.

dedrobenzperidol see DROPERIDOL.

dee a metal part shaped like a capital D and used in harness to make a T junction.

deep freeze see FREEZER.

deep litter a husbandry system used in most species but especially in poultry. Any form of bedding is used but short material such as shavings or sawdust is most easily handled. After an initial shallow layer is fouled, more litter is added to cover the droppings. Additions are continued daily until the end of the housing period when the entire bed is removed. Properly cared for the system is clean and warm and easy on labor.

deep pectoral myopathy a disease of turkey and broiler breeders in which the breast muscles become necrotic and turn a green color. Apparently caused by faulty blood supply and resulting muscle ischemia. Called also degenerative myopathy of turkeys, Oregon disease, green muscle disease.

deer the Cervidae family. Includes 17 genera and 53 species. The principal members are deer, elk, reindeer, wapitii, muntjack and sika. The common species are: black-tailed deer (ODOCOILEUS *hemionus columbiana*), Columbian white-tailed deer (*Odocoileus virginianus, Dama virginianus*); CHEVROTAIN (*Tragulus* spp.); MULE DEER (*Odocoileus hemionus*); MUNTJAC (*Muntiacus* spp.); PÈRE DAVID'S DEER (*Elaphurus davidianus*); FALLOW DEER (*Dama dama*); ROE DEER (*Capreolus capreolus*); AXIS DEER (*Axis axis*); REINDEER or CARIBOU (*Rangifer tarandus*); RED DEER (*Cervus elaphus*); SAMBAR DEER (*Rusa unicolor*); WAPITI (*Cervus canadensis*) called also American elk; HOG DEER (*Axis porcinus*); AMERICAN MOOSE (*Alces americana*).

deer fly see CHRYSOPS.

deer fly fever see TULAREMIA.

Deerhound see SCOTTISH DEERHOUND.
deermouse see PEROMYSCUS LEUCOPUS.
DEET diethyltoluamide.
defaecate see DEFECATE.
defatted 1. fat is removed from the tissue by fat solvents. 2. deprived of fat as a food.
default the action taken by the computer program if the user fails to enter a more specific request to a question posed by the program.
defaunate elimination of microscopic fauna, especially protozoa, in the rumen and cecum, with depressing effects on digestion.
defeathering plucking of feathers from bird carcasses after immersion momentarily in boiling water. Final treatment of poultry is singeing. Ducks are waxed.
defecate the act of DEFECATION.
defecation elimination of wastes and undigested food, as feces, from the rectum.
defect an imperfection, failure or absence.
filling d. an interruption in the contour of the inner surface of viscus revealed by contrast radiography, indicating excess tissue or substance on or in the wall of the organ, foreign body or other space-occupying lesions.
septal d. a defect in the cardiac septum resulting in an abnormal communication between opposite chambers of the heart. See also AORTIC septal defect, ATRIAL septal defect and VENTRICULAR septal defect.
defective interfering virus viral particles containing subgenomic amounts of nucleic acid usually produced following infection of cells at high multiplicity and which interfere with the replication of complete virions.
defective virus one unable to replicate on its own and needing to be complemented by a 'helper' virus for replication.
defeminization loss of female sexual characteristics.
defense 1. against infection, including hematological and immunological systems. 2. behavior directed to protection of the individual from injury.
d. mechanisms means by which the host repels invading organisms; externally, these include the barrier provided by the skin and epithelial lining of the gastrointestinal, genitourinary and respiratory tracts, together with their secretions and normal microflora, and internally, phagocytic cells, humoral and cellular immunity.
d. reaction the physiological reaction to emotional stress, particularly fear, includes tachycardia, increased cardiac output, vasodilation in skeletal muscle, elevation of blood pressure. Behavioral responses include alerting and aggressive behavior.
deferens [L.] *deferent.*
deferent conducting or progressing away, as from a center or specific site of reference.
d. duct see DUCTUS deferens.
deferentectomy excision of a ductus deferens.
deferential pertaining to the ductus deferens.
deferentitis inflammation of the ductus deferens.
deferoxamine, desferrioxamine an iron chelating compound used as the mesylate to treat iron poisoning.
deferral days an important item in dairy cow fertility data; management needs may dictate that cows are not to be bred at their first or subsequent estrus; such delays should not be counted into the average calving-to-mating interval.
deferred grazing see deferred GRAZING.
defervescence the period of abatement of fever. Called also decrement.
defibrillation 1. termination of atrial or ventricular fibrillation, usually by electric shock. 2. separation of tissue fibers by blunt dissection.

Defibrillation by precordial shock is accomplished by delivering a nonsynchronized direct current to the myocardium. It is an emergency procedure, used to terminate a life-threatening ventricular arrhythmia. The electric shock is delivered by means of metal paddles applied directly to the heart muscle, as in cardiac surgery, or by placing the paddles on the chest (closed defibrillation).

The high-voltage electrical current delivered during precordial shock causes complete depolarization of the heart muscle, disrupting all of the electrical circuits that are activating the heart muscle and causing ventricular fibrillation. This allows the heart's natural pacemaker to regain control and regulation of the heart rate and rhythm.

chemical d. where electrical equipment is not available for defibrillation, some combinations of drugs have been used. These include potassium chloride followed by calcium chloride or potassium chloride and acetylcholine.
defibrillator an apparatus used to produce defibrillation by application of brief electroshock to the heart, directly or through electrodes placed on the chest wall.
defibrination the destruction or removal of fibrin, as from the blood.
d. syndrome see disseminated intravascular COAGULATION.
deficiency a lack or shortage; a condition characterized by the presence of less than the normal or necessary supply or competence.
antidiuretic hormone d. see DIABETES INSIPIDUS.
clotting factor d. see CLOTTING.
Hageman factor d. see CLOTTING.
nutritional d. see under specific nutritional factors.
Stuart factor d. see CLOTTING.
deficient a state of being in deficit.
deficit a lack or deficiency.
oxygen d. a lack of OXYGEN, as in hypoxia or anoxia.
defining criterion the hallmark of each disease; a characteristic lesion or result of a clinicopathological test or clinical sign without which the diagnosis cannot be made. Called also key sign.
definition establishment of a clear boundary, a clear line of demarcation.
clinical d. an accurate description of the disease in terms of clinical signs and clinicopathological findings.
epidemiological d. an accurate description of the disease in terms of its epidemiological parameters of when, where, why and how it has occurred.
genetic d. an accurate description of a disease in terms of the familial relationships between affected animals.
radiographic d. a sharp line of demarcation between radiographic densities. A gradual merging of densities creates blurring of the image.
definitive host the host in which the infectious agent in question undergoes the adult and sexual stage of its reproduction. Called also final host.
deflation receptor receptors in the upper airways that are part of the HERING–BREUER REFLEXES.
defleecing see CHEMICAL shearing.
deflighting removing the ability of birds to fly; can be effected by monthly clipping of the flight feathers on one or both wings, temporarily by bandaging one wing in a flexed position, or permanently by PINIONING or PATAGIECTOMY.
defluorination reduction of the fluorine content of a feed to below the level accepted as being nontoxic.

defluvium [L.] a falling out, as of the hair.
defluxion 1. a sudden disappearance. 2. a copious discharge, as of catarrh. 3. a falling out, as of hair. See also ANAGEN defluxion, TELOGEN defluxion.
defoliant a chemical used to remove the leaves from plants to facilitate mechanical harvesting. The early defoliants, especially arsenical compounds, presented serious hazards if the plants were later fed to livestock or if the spray drifted to nearby pasture paddocks. Modern defoliants are nontoxic if used according to manufacturer's recommendations. See MCPA, TRIBUTYL TRIPHOSPHOROTRITHIOITE, THIDIAZURON.
deformability the ability of cells, such as erythrocytes, to change shape as they pass through narrow spaces, such as the microvasculature.
deformation 1. deformity, especially an alteration in shape or structure. 2. the process of adapting in shape or form.
deforming cervical spondylosis see HYPERVITAMINOSIS A.
deformity distortion of any part or general disfigurement of the body; malformation.
deformylase a prokaryotic enzyme that removes the formyl group from amino acids, e.g. the methionine coded by the initiation codon AUG.
degenerate 1. to change from a higher to a lower form. 2. characterized by degeneration.
degeneration deterioration; change from a higher to a lower form, especially change of tissue to a lower or less functionally active form. When there is chemical change of the tissue itself it is true degeneration; when the change consists in the deposit of abnormal matter in the tissues, it is infiltration. See also WALLERIAN DEGENERATION, Zenker's NECROSIS.
albuminoid d. cloudy swelling, an early stage of degenerative change characterized by swollen, parboiled-appearing tissues which revert to normal when the cause is removed.
ballooning d. swelling of the cytoplasm in epidermal cells without vacuolization, enlarged or condensed nuclei and acantholysis. A characteristic of viral infections of the skin. Called also koilocytosis.
caseous d. CASEATION (2).
colloid d. degeneration with conversion of the tissues into a gelatinous or gumlike material.
cystic d. degeneration with formation of cysts.
fatty d. deposit of fat globules in a tissue.
feathery d. said of hepatocytes; a hydropic change in hepatocytes which have suffered long-term exposure to cholestasis.
fibrinoid d. deposition or replacement with eosinophilic fibrillar or granular substance resembling fibrin.
fibroid d. degeneration into fibrous tissue.
hyaline d. a regressive change in cells in which the cytoplasm takes on a homogeneous, glassy appearance; also used loosely to describe the histological appearance of tissues. Called also hyalinosis.
hydropic d. see HYDROPIC degeneration.
macular d. degenerative changes in the macula retinae.
mucoid d. degeneration with increased mucin which can be epithelial or mesenchymal in origin.
mucous d. degeneration with accumulation of mucus in epithelial tissues. Called also myxomatous degeneration.
myxomatous d. see mucous degeneration (above).
reticular d. extreme intracellular edema of epidermal cells, resulting in rupture and multilocular intraepidermal vesicles with septae formed by the remaining cell walls. Seen in acute inflammatory dermatoses.
spongy d. on microscopic examination has the physical appearance of a sponge. Usually applied to tissue of the central nervous system, caused by the loss of myelin.
degenerative pertaining to or emanating from degeneration. See also ARTHROPATHY, AXONOPATHY, ENCEPHALOMALACIA, degenerative JOINT disease, MYELOENCEPHALOPATHY, MYOPATHY, OSTEOARTHRITIS.
avian d. joint disease common in coxofemoral joints of mature male turkeys and meat chickens.
d. disease a disease in which the sole pathogenesis is degeneration; that is without the intervention of other pathogeneses, e.g. inflammation, traumatic injury, neoplasia.
d. joint disease see degenerative JOINT disease.
d. left shift an increase in immature neutrophilic granulocytes, in excess of mature cells of the series, with a normal or increased white blood cell count. A poor prognostic sign, indicating an inability of the bone marrow to respond adequately to infection.
d. myopathy due to ischemia in well-conditioned cattle which are recumbent for 24 hours or more; affected muscles are pale, the serum creatine phosphokinase and glutamic-oxaloacetic transaminase levels are markedly elevated for brief periods; commonly the condition is irreversible.
d. myopathy of turkeys see DEEP PECTORAL MYOPATHY.
d. osteoarthritis probably inherited in cattle; degeneration with erosion of joint surfaces, especially the stifle joint, and especially in Holstein-Friesian and Jersey cattle. Lameness develops gradually in adults, accompanied by local muscle atrophy, joint enlargement.
d. pannus see chronic superficial KERATITIS.
degloving the avulsion of skin from underlying structures, usually a result of trauma. Besides the possibility of injury to other structures, there may be a problem with viability of the skin involved.
deglutition the act of swallowing. There are differences in the mechanism between birds and mammals. Most birds cannot swallow without raising their heads.
degradation conversion of a chemical compound to one less complex, as by splitting off one or more groups of atoms.
degranulation the loss of granules; usually refers to the secretory granules in certain cells, e.g. pituitary chromophobes, acidophils and basophils. In basophils and mast cells, it is associated with the release of active substances from the cells and is characteristic of type I immediate HYPERSENSITIVITY.
degreasing agent one used to remove excessive sebaceous secretions and scale from the skin; shampoos containing selenium sulfide or benzoyl peroxide are examples.
degree 1. a grade or rank awarded scholars by a college or university. 2. a unit of measure of temperature. 3. a unit of measure of arcs and angles, one degree being 1/360 of a circle.
degrees of freedom used to define statistical distributions of several tests, usually based on the number of data items less the number of parameters estimated.
degu a South American rodent of the family Octodontidae.
degustation the act or function of tasting.
dehairing removal of hairs and bristles of pigs by a scraper after scalding in a tank or a steam cabinet.
dehiscence a splitting open, as in a surgical wound.
dehorner instrument for removing the horns.

Barnes d. two sharp-edged scoops hinged together. Opening them forcefully brings the cutting edges together. Suitable for calves up to 3 to 4 months of age.

hot cautery d. an electrically heated instrument that resembles a round soldering iron with a flat, indented head. The iron is heated to red heat and placed over the horn to burn a ring of skin at the base of the horn. The horn is not removed but is allowed to slough. Satisfactory for use in calves up to 2 months of age.

Keystone d. a guillotine type instrument with detachable blades. Has handles 3 feet long and is capable of chopping off the largest cow horns and most bull horns.

tube d. a metal tube with a very sharp edge at one end and a wooden round palm-fitting handle at the other. The tube is placed over the horn and rotated to isolate the horn skin. The tube edge is then used as a gouge to remove the horn. A hole in the side of the tube permits the debris to be removed. For use in calves up to 2 to 3 months of age.

dehorning the removal of horns either by caustic paste or electrocautery when very young or by surgical amputation with a DEHORNER or saw at any age. Special care is needed with goats because of their extreme reaction of shock.

d. nerve block see CORNUAL nerve block.

dehull to remove the outer covering of a seed used as feed. Improves the nutrient value of the grain. The hulls may be used separately as a roughage supplement.

dehumidifier an apparatus for reducing the content of moisture in the atmosphere.

dehydratase any enzyme of the lyase class that catalyzes the removal of H_2O, leaving double bonds (or adding groups to double bonds).

dehydrate 1. to undergo the process of dehydration. 2. reduce the moisture content of a feed by drying.

dehydrating agent agent used in the clearing and mounting of tissue slides for microscopic examination, e.g. ethanol, butanol, isopropanol.

dehydration the state when the body loses more water than it takes in. There is a negative fluid balance, so that the circulating blood volume decreases and tissue fluids are reduced and tissues are dehydrated. The clinical syndrome of dehydration includes loosening and wrinkling of the skin, and a bad skin-tenting reaction, in which a pinched-up fold of skin takes longer than normal to disappear; there is usually evidence of the cause of the dehydration, e.g. vomiting, polyuria. Clinical pathological tests are essential to determine the severity of the dehydration.

cellular d. caused by increased osmoconcentration of the extracellular fluid.

dehydrocholesterol 7-dehydrocholesterol; a sterol found in the skin which, when properly irradiated by ultraviolet rays, forms vitamin D.

activated 7-d. cholecalciferol.

dehydrocholic acid a semisynthetic bile acid used to increase output of bile by the liver and the filling of the gallbladder. Preparations of this acid are used to aid the digestion of fats and increase absorption of fat-soluble vitamins.

11-dehydrocorticosterone one of the least active of the glucocorticosteroids produced by the adrenal cortex.

dehydroepiandrosterone an androgen occurring in normal human urine and synthesized from cholesterol.

dehydrogenase an enzyme that mobilizes the hydrogen of a substrate so that it can pass to a hydrogen acceptor, such as NAD+ or FAD+.

alcohol d. dimeric enzyme protein of the liver catalyzing the NAD+- linked dehydrogenation of ethanol to acetaldehyde.

glucose-6-phosphate d. see GLUCOSE-6-phosphate dehydrogenase.

glutamate d. (GD), glutamic d. an enzyme that catalyzes the reversible reaction of glutamic acid into 2-oxoglutaric acid and ammonia. High concentrations occur in the liver of sheep, cattle, horses and dogs. Serum levels are useful in detecting hepatocellular damage in ruminants.

L-iditol d. (ID) a liver specific enzyme; serum determinations have been used in the horse to detect hepatocellular damage. Called also sorbitol dehydrogenase, SDH.

isocitrate d. (ICD) an enzyme found in high concentrations in many tissues. Two major forms of the enzyme, an NAD+-dependent ICD associated with the mitochondrial TCA cycle and a NADP+-dependent ICD associated with fat synthesis in adipose tissue and lactating mammary gland of ruminants or with steroidogenesis in endocrine tissues. Serum levels have been used to detect hepatocellular damage, but it is not highly specific.

lactate d. (LDH), lactic acid d. an enzyme that catalyzes the interconversion of lactate and pyruvate. It is widespread in tissues and is particularly abundant in kidney, skeletal muscle, liver and myocardium. It appears in elevated concentrations when these tissues are injured. See also MOUSE lactic dehydrogenase elevating virus.

lactate d. agent see PESTIVIRUS.

polyol d. see L-iditol dehydrogenase (above).

sorbitol d. (SDH) see L-iditol dehydrogenase (above).

dehydrogenate to remove hydrogen from.

dehydrongaione the hepatoxin found in *Myoporum* spp.

dehydropiandrosterone weak androgen secreted by the testes and ovary.

dehydroretinal the aldehyde of dehydroretinol, derived from the visual pigment porphyropsin, found in freshwater fishes and certain vertebrates and amphibians; its metabolic role is analogous to that of rhodopsin in other animals.

dehydroretinol vitamin A_2, the form, $C_{20}H_{28}O$, of vitamin A found in the retina and liver of freshwater fishes and certain invertebrates and amphibians; it differs from retinol (vitamin A_1) in having one more conjugated double bond and has approximately one-third the biological activity of retinol. Called also retinol$_2$.

Deinocerites a mosquito, vector of the virus of equine encephalomyelitis.

deiodinase an enzyme that deiodinates two of the iodinated amino acids (iodothyrosines) within the thyroid gland. Selenium-dependent deiodinase I converts thyroxine (T4) to triiodothyronine (T3), the more active thyroid hormone.

deionization the production of a mineral-free state by the removal of ions.

Deiter's nucleus lateral vestibular nucleus in the brainstem.

dejecta excrement.

delacrimation excessive flow of tears.

delactation 1. weaning. 2. cessation of lactation.

Delafondia see STRONGYLUS.

delay phenomenon a method of improving survival of skin grafts by raising large flaps in several stages before they are transferred.

delayed prolonged beyond the time normally required.

d. hypersensitivity see delayed HYPERSENSITIVITY.

d. neurotoxic effects a characteristic effect of the neurotoxins in industrial triaryl phosphates.

d. ovulation individual cows appear to have a prolonged follicular phase in their estral cycle, usually about 48 hours.

d. primary closure the surgical closing of a wound several days after the injury because the wound was initially too contaminated to close. Union of the wound closed in this manner is called healing by third intention.

delead, de-lead to induce the removal of lead from tissues and its excretion in the urine by the administration of chelating agents.

deleterious injurious; harmful.

deletion in genetics, loss of genetic material from a chromosome.

Deletrocephalus nematode genus of the superfamily Strongyloidea. Placed in the family Deletrocephalidae; found in the large intestine of the rhea.

Delhi boil see LEISHMANIASIS.

deliquescence the condition of becoming moist or liquified as a result of absorption of water from the air.

deliver 1. to aid in parturition. 2. to remove, as a fetus, placenta or lens of the eye.

delivery expulsion or extraction of the young and fetal membranes at birth.

abdominal d. delivery of a neonate through an incision made into the uterus through the abdominal wall (CESAREAN SECTION).

d. per vaginam normal birth, the fetus being delivered through the vagina; in contrast to a cesarean delivery.

dell a small depression or dimple.

dellen saucer-shaped excavations at the periphery of the cornea, usually on the temporal side.

delmadinone acetate a progesterone with antiestrogen and antiandrogen activity; used to suppress estrus and prevent pregnancy in dogs and cats.

delomorphous having definitely formed and well-defined limits, as a cell or tissue.

Delosperma genus of African plants in family Aizoaceae; contains soluble oxalates which cause nephrosis, edema.

Delphinapterus leucas a small 10 to 13 ft, 1000 to 1500 lb whale with a rounded head and no dorsal fin. A member of the family Monodontidae. Called also arctic dolphin, beluga whale, sea canary, white whale.

delphinine the best known toxic alkaloid in *Delphinium* plants.

Delphinium a genus of the plant family Ranunculaceae which includes the domesticated plants, delphinium and larkspur. One of the commonest causes of plant poisoning in North America.

They contain a number of toxic diterpenoid alkaloids, especially delphinine. Cause uneasiness, stiff gait, straddled posture and sudden collapse. Animals may die from respiratory paralysis or inhalation of regurgitated ruminal contents.

Include *D. andersonii*, *D. barbeyi*, *D. brownii*, *D. geyeri*, *D. glaucum*, *D. glauscens*, *D. nelsonii* (*D. bicolor*, *D. menziesii*), *D. nuttallianum*, *D. occidentale* (*D. cucullatum*, *D. scopulorum*), *D. parryi*, *D. ramosum* (*D. elongatum*), *D. recurvatum* (*D. hesperium*), *D. robustum*, *D. tricorne*, *D. trolliform*, *D. vestitum*, *D. virescens* (*D. camporum*).

Delphinus delphis see DOLPHIN.

delrad an algicide used in water supplies but is nontoxic at the concentrations used. Poisoning can occur with high doses.

delta 1. the fourth letter of the Greek alphabet, Δ or δ; used in chemical names to denote the fourth of a series of isomeric compounds or the carbon atom fourth from the carboxyl group, or to denote the fourth of any series. 2. a triangular area.

d. T lymphocyte see T LYMPHOCYTE.

delta-aminolevulinic acid see δ-AMINOLEVULINIC ACID.

delta-aminolevulinic acid dehydratase an enzyme of which the concentration in erythrocytes is a widely used indicator of the level of lead poisoning in animals.

delta-lysin one of the toxins produced by *Staphylococcus aureus*. Causes dermonecrosis and destroys leukocytes. Called also delta-toxin.

delta-toxin DELTA-LYSIN of *Staphylococcus aureus*.

delta virus hepatitis D virus.

deltoid 1. triangular. 2. the deltoid muscle.

d. muscle a lateral muscle of the shoulder, between the scapula and the humerus that helps flex the shoulder and abducts the arm. See also Table 13.

demand the predicted amount of a product or service which will be sold at a stated price.

d. elasticity the responsiveness with which the demand for a product or service, for example for veterinary services, varies with its price. If there is great flexibility there is elasticity. When the demand is the same irrespective of the price there is inelasticity.

Demansia a genus of venomous snakes.

D. nuchalis affinis as for *D. textilis* (below). Called also dugite, spotted brown snake.

D. nuchalis nuchalis similar to *D. textilis*. Called also gwardar, western brown snake, *Pseudonaja nuchalis*.

***D. olivaceae* (syn. *D. psammophis olivacea*)** a thin, poisonous snake up to 7 ft long. Called also black whip snake.

D. textilis the Australian brown snake with a powerful toxin and a willingness to attack. Envenomation is characterized by clinical signs of drowsiness, drooping of lips and eyelids, inability to swallow, labored abdominal respiration, muscle tremor, recumbency and pupillary dilatation in some cases. Called also common brown snake.

dematiaceous darkly pigmented; said of some fungi.

deme a population of animals with very similar physical characteristics, which interbreed and occupy a limited geographic region. Called also a genetic population.

demeanor behavior towards others; body language.

demecarium a cholinergic agonist, used topically in the management of glaucoma and as lacrimomimetics; it is more potent and has longer activity than pilocarpine.

demeclocycline a broad-spectrum tetracyclic antibiotic produced by a mutant strain of *Streptomyces aureofaciens*.

demecolcine a cytotoxic alkaloid derived from *Colchicum autumnale*. It is used in CHROMOSOME analysis to arrest cell division in mid-metaphase so that the chromosomes can be stained by one of several techniques that produce a distinct pattern of light and dark bands along the chromosomes, and each chromosome can be recognized by its size and banding pattern.

dementia loss of intellectual capacity accompanied usually by irrational behavior.

demephion an organophosphorus compound used as an insecticide and acaricide.

Demerol a proprietary name for meperidine.
demeton an organophosphorus insecticide used as a treatment for sucking lice. Consists of a mixture of two compounds and toxicity varies a good deal depending on their relative concentrations.
demilune crescent shaped.
serous d. serous fluid-producing cells in glands; small canals connect the serous cells with the luminal surface.
demineralization excessive elimination of mineral or organic salts from the tissues of the body.
demodectic mange mange which in all species is caused by species-specific *Demodex* spp. Characterized by folliculitis with hair loss and often pustule formation anywhere on the body although the head, face, neck and shoulders are most often affected. The cause of wastage due to the disease in large animals, mainly cattle, goats and pigs, is the reduced value of the hide or pelt.
The disease is most common in dogs where it is associated with an abnormality of cell-mediated immunity. Most often, there are one or a few areas of hair loss in young dogs (localized) which will heal spontaneously, although treatment is often given. Occasionally the disease is generalized, severe and resistant to all treatment. Examination of a skin scraping confirms the diagnosis. Called also follicular mange, red mange, demodicosis.
Demodex a genus of mites parasitic within the hair follicles of the host; a member of the family Demodicidae. Some of the more common species are: *Demodex aries* (found in sheep); *D. bovis* (infests cattle); *D. caballi* (infests horses); *D. canis* (infests dogs); *D. caprae* syn. *D. capri* (infests goats); *D. cati* (infests cats), *D. criceti* (infests hamsters); *D. equi* (infests horses); *D. folliculorum* (infests humans); *D. ghanensis* (infests cattle); *D. muscardini* (infests dormice); *D. ovis* (infests sheep); *D. phylloides* (infests pigs).
demodicosis demodectic mange.
demogram a report of demographic results, usually in grid form.
demographics the graphic representation of demographic results.
demography the statistical science dealing with populations, including matters of health, disease, births and mortality. Strictly speaking the word refers to human populations but common usage includes lower animal populations.
demucosation removal of the mucous membrane from a part.
demulcent 1. soothing; bland. 2. a soothing mucilaginous or oily medicine or application.
alimentary d. substances of high molecular mass and good solubility that lubricate, coat and protect the mucosa of the upper alimentary tract. Usually they mask unpleasant tastes, stabilize emulsions, and act as suspension agents. Methyl cellulose, gum tragacanth, agar, mineral oil and propylene glycol are used for this purpose.
demyelinate to destroy or remove the myelin sheath of a nerve or nerves.
demyelination destruction, removal, or loss of the myelin sheath of a nerve or nerves.
demyelinization see DEMYELINATION.
denarcotize to deprive of narcotics or of narcotic properties.
denasality hyponasality.
denaturant a denaturing agent.
denaturation 1. a change in the usual nature of a substance, as by the addition of methanol or acetone to alcohol to render it unfit for drinking. 2. in proteins and nucleic acids produced by heat or certain chemicals, usually results in loss of function. In proteins, various noncovalent bonds are disrupted resulting in unfolding of the polypeptide chain; in nucleic acids hydrogen bonds between nucleotides are disrupted converting double-stranded molecules or parts of them into single-stranded forms.
protein d. any nonproteolytic change in the chemistry, composition or structure of a native protein which causes it to lose some or all of its unique or specific characteristics.
denature to deprive a substance of its natural qualities, e.g. by heating a protein to destroy its specific biological activity.
dendraxon a nerve cell whose axon splits up into terminal filaments immediately after leaving the cell.
dendric pertaining to a dendrite.
dendriform tree-shaped.
dendrite any of the threadlike extensions of the cytoplasm of a neuron; dendrites, which typically branch into treelike processes, compose most of the receptive surface of a neuron.
dendritic 1. branched like a tree. 2. pertaining to or possessing dendrites.
d. cell see dendritic CELL.
d. reticular cell cells in lymph nodes participating in the provision of immune responses.
d. zone region of the neuron subjected to excitatory and inhibitory stimulation.
Dendritobilharzia a genus of digenetic trematodes in the family Schistosomatidae.
D. pulverulenta found in the dorsal aorta of swans.
dendr(o)- word element. [Gr.] *tree, treelike.*
Dendroaspis see MAMBA.
dendrochiotoxicosis see DENDROCHIUM TOXICUM.
Dendrochium toxicum toxic fungus which parasitizes stored grain; contains an unidentified toxin which causes a blood dyscrasia and degenerative visceral lesions.
Dendrocnide genus of Australian rainforest trees in family Urticaraciae. Stinging hairs on the foliage cause severe irritation and vesication of skin on contact; contains a toxic peptide moroidin. Includes *D. excelsa*, *D. moroides*, *D. photinophylla*. Called also *Laportea* spp., stinger, gympie.
dendrodendritic see dendrodendritic SYNAPSE.
Dendrohyrax see HYRAX.
dendroid branched like a tree.
Dendromus see common MOUSE. Called also banana mouse.
dendron dendrite.
Dendronessa galericulata mandarin duck. See AIX GALERICULATA.
denervation interruption of the nerve connection to an organ or part.
d. atrophy reduction in muscle fiber diameter as a result of discontinuation of nerve supply; always accompanied by paralysis; also called neurogenic atrophy.
Denisonia superba see COPPERHEAD SNAKES.
Denman Island disease severe disease of Pacific oysters in British Columbia, especially in the vicinity of Denman Island. See also MIKROCYTOSIS.
denominator the bottom line of a fraction; the base population on which population rates such as birth and death rates are calculated.
dens pl. *dentes* [L.] a tooth or toothlike structure. The axis has a dens or odontoid process which protrudes from the cranial part of the body of the axis and articulates with the ventral arch of the atlas.

d. en dente a malformed tooth consisting of an invagination of the enamel, dentine and pulp within the tooth bud, appearing as a tooth within a tooth.

d. hypoplasia see ATLANTOAXIAL subluxation.

d. lupinus first premolar tooth in the horse. Always vestigial, often missing. Called also wolf tooth.

dense bars optically dense structures which occur in series aligned along the presynaptic membrane in neuromuscular junctions and contribute to active zones in muscle–nerve relationships.

dense bodies round, amorphous bodies scattered through the cytoplasm of smooth muscle fibers; they appear to be points of attachment for myofilaments.

densimeter, densitometer 1. an instrument for determining density or specific gravity of a liquid. 2. an instrument used for measuring photographic transmission and/or reflection density.

densitometry determination of variations in density by comparison with that of another material or with a certain standard.

density 1. the ratio of the mass of a substance to its volume. 2. the quality of being compact. 3. the quantity of matter in a given space. 4. the quantity of electricity in a given area, volume or time. 5. the degree of film blackening in an area of a photograph or radiograph.

disk d. a measure of the amount of information that can be stored on a computer disk.

population d. number of animals per unit of area; important in relation to the rate of spread of disease.

d. sampling see SAMPLING.

Densovirus a genus of viruses in the family PARVOVIRIDAE that infect insects.

dental pertaining to the TEETH.

d. abscess see ALVEOLAR abscess, MALAR abscess.

d. aging telling the age of an animal by its teeth. Significant especially in horses, cattle and sheep. See also AGE determination.

d. arcade the complete array of teeth in the form of an arch. There is an upper and a lower arcade, except in ruminants where the incisor sector of the upper arcade is absent.

d. attrition occlusal wear of a tooth, as a result of tooth to tooth contact as in mastication; physiological rather than pathological.

d. bud the dental laminae, focal thickenings of the oral mucosae of the developing embryo, invaginate to form dental buds, the early stage of the enamel organ of the embryonic teeth.

d. caps a condensation of the oral epithelium of the embryo's dental lamina establishes the cap stage of the developing tooth.

d. chisel see dental hoe (below).

d. claw an instrument used often for scaling teeth in dogs and cats. It has a thick, sickle-shaped end.

d. cyst may be odontogenic, containing cell rests of dental tissue, or dentigerous, in which all or part of a tooth is in the cyst. Causes a local swelling of the jaw which may be visible externally. Called also dentigerous cyst.

d. discoloration occurs as a result of medication with tetracyclines when the teeth are still in the development stage, in cases of porphyrinuria, and in small discrete lesions in association with fluorosis, again when the poisoning occurred in the pre-eruption stage. Congenital absence of dentine and enamel, as occurs in calves, causes the teeth to look pink because of their vascularity.

d. fistula caused by the spread of alveolar periostitis or abscess. The fistula discharges from the tooth root to the side of the face below the eye, the maxillary sinus or the nasal cavity. Called also MALAR abscess, gum boil.

d. fluorosis see FLUOROSIS.

d. formula an alphanumeric system for listing the number, type (I = incisor, C = canine, P = premolar, M = molar), and position (upper or lower) of teeth: ox and sheep $2(I^0_4\ C^0_0\ P^3_3\ M^3_3) = 32$; horse $2(I^3_3\ C^1_1\ P^4_3\ M^3_3) = 42$; pig $2(I^3_3\ C^1_1\ P^4_4\ M^3_3) = 44$; dog $2(I^3_3\ C^1_1\ P^4_4\ M^2_3) = 42$; cat $2(I^3_3\ C^1_1\ P^3_2\ M^1_1) = 30$.

d. fracture/fissure usually the result of traumatic injury. Causes great discomfort, unwillingness to close the jaw or chew; often the mouth sags open and saliva is allowed to drool.

d. hoe an instrument commonly used in veterinary dentistry. It has a broad end with a beveled edge. Called also dental chisel.

d. impaction failure of teeth to erupt out of the alveolar bone or through the gum.

d. irregular wear see WAVE MOUTH.

d. lamina in the embryonic oral mucosa dental lamina form as local thickenings of the epithelium; they invaginate to form dental buds, later the enamel organ. See also DENTAL bud.

d. luxation includes loosening of teeth through to complete avulsion.

d. malocclusion see MALOCCLUSION.

d. mirror a small round mirror set at an angle on one end of a handle, used in dental examinations to reflect images from intraoral surfaces.

d. numbering systems see PALMER'S DENTAL NOTATION, FÉDÉRATION DENTAIRE INTERNATIONALE SYSTEM, TRIADAN SYSTEM.

d. occlusion see OCCLUSION (2).

d. pad the thick layer of connective tissue that replaces the upper incisor teeth in the ruminant; a rostral projection of the hard palate.

d. papillary mesenchyme the tissue which converts the dental cap stage of the growing tooth to the bell stage by covering it with enamel.

d. pellicle a thin, acellular membrane of salivary proteins adsorbed to the enamel or cementum.

d. plaque a dense mass of bacteria in an intercellular matrix, adhering to the surface of the tooth. It is important in that it initiates caries and periodontitis. A precursor of calculus. See also bacterial PLAQUE.

d. pulp the sensitive content of the cavity of the tooth carrying its nerve and blood supply.

d. records contain the history of dental treatment given, generally recorded on diagrams or charts of the mouth, showing position of individual teeth, gingiva and occlusion.

d. resorption may occur if the tooth pulp is traumatized, by osteoclastic action inside the tooth or outside, in the alveolar bone.

d. sac the remains of the dental follicle at the apex of immature teeth.

d. star the mark on the occlusal surface of a tooth, especially horse incisors, which is caused by the appearance of secondary dentine, contributed by the pulp cavity, as the tooth wears.

d. tartar see dental calculus (above).

dentalgia toothache.

dentate notched, toothed; tooth-shaped.

dentia a condition relating to development or eruption of the teeth.

d. precox premature eruption of the teeth.

d. tarda delayed eruption of the teeth, beyond the usual time for their appearance.

dentibuccal pertaining to the cheek and teeth.

denticle 1. a small toothlike process. 2. a distinct calcified mass within the pulp chamber or in the dentine of a tooth.

dentification formation of tooth substance.

dentigerous bearing teeth.

d. cyst see DENTAL cyst.

dentilabial pertaining to the teeth and lips.

dentilingual pertaining to the teeth and tongue.

dentin see DENTINE.

secondary d. the dentin added during the post-erupted life of the tooth.

dentinal pertaining to dentin.

d. fibers fibers contained in predentin but displaced by dentin as it is deposited, the fibers leaving apical processes of odontocytes behind, contained in dentinal tubules through which nerves also pass; called also odontoblastic processes.

d. tubules see dentinal fibers (above).

dentine one of the hard tissues of the teeth which constitutes most of its bulk. Lies between the pulp cavity and the enamel, and where it is not covered by enamel is covered by cementum, the third hard substance of the tooth.

sclerotic d. a dense clear dentine formed when the dentinal tubules are filled with mineralized material.

secondary d. dentine laid down in later development of a tooth, helping to avoid the exposure of the tooth pulp. It is often pigmented and is responsible for the appearance of the dental star.

dentinoblastoma see DENTINOMA.

dentinoenamel junction the junction where dense, acellular enamel, being deposited by ameloblasts, meets the retreating ameloblastic front.

dentinogenesis the formation of dentine.

d. imperfecta disorder of tooth development characterized by discoloration and early wear of all teeth.

dentinoma a tumor of odontogenic origin and consisting mainly of dentine.

dentinosteoid a tumor composed of or containing dentine and bone.

dentinum see DENTINE.

dentistry that branch of the healing arts concerned with the teeth and associated structures of the oral cavity, including prevention, diagnosis and treatment of diseases of the teeth.

conservative d. involved with the preservation of natural teeth.

restorative d. the repair of defects or injury to teeth.

dentition the teeth in the dental arch; ordinarily used to designate the natural teeth in position in the alveoli.

deciduous d. the complement of teeth that erupt first and are later succeeded by the permanent teeth.

mixed d. the complement of teeth in the jaws after eruption of some of the permanent teeth, but before all the deciduous teeth are shed.

permanent d. the complement of teeth that normally erupt after the deciduous teeth and that are never shed except in old age.

dent(o)- word element. [L.] *tooth, toothlike.*

dentoalveolar pertaining to a tooth and its alveolus.

d. abscess see ALVEOLAR abscess.

dentoalveolitis periodontitis.

dentofacial of or pertaining to the teeth and alveolar process and the face.

dentulous having natural teeth.

denture a complement of teeth, either natural or artificial; ordinarily used to designate an artificial replacement for the natural teeth and adjacent tissues. Isolated reports of use in dogs.

denucleation deprivation of the nucleus.

denudation the stripping or laying bare of any part.

deodorant 1. destroying or masking odors. 2. an agent that masks offensive odors.

deodorize to neutralize or absorb odor.

deodorizer a deodorizing agent.

deorsumversion the turning downward of a part, especially of the eyes.

deossification loss or removal of the mineral elements of bone.

deoxidation the removal of oxygen from a chemical compound.

deoxy- a chemical prefix designating a compound containing one less atom of oxygen than the reference substance. For words beinning thus, see also those beginning *desoxy-*.

deoxycholate any salt of deoxycholic acid.

deoxycholic acid one of the bile acids, capable of forming soluble, diffusible complexes with fatty acids, and thereby allowing for their absorption in the small intestine.

11-deoxycorticosterone, desoxycorticosterone, deoxycortone one of the mineralocorticoids, adrenocortical steroids which lack a substituent at C-11; has a greater effect on electrolyte metabolism than glucocorticoids. Available pharmaceutically as the acetate (DOCA), which is short-acting, and the pivalate, a slow release form for use in the treatment of hypoadrenocorticism.

deoxygenation the act of depriving of oxygen.

2-deoxy-D-glucose an antimetabolite of glucose with antiviral activity; it acts by inhibiting the glycosylation of glycoproteins and glycolipids; it has been investigated for treatment of herpesvirus infections.

deoxyhemoglobin hemoglobin not combined with oxygen, formed when oxyhemoglobin releases its oxygen to the tissues.

deoxynivalenol trichothecene toxin produced by the fungus *Fusarium graminearum* and other fungi. Called also DON, food refusal factor, emetic factor, vomitoxin.

deoxyribonuclease an enzyme that catalyzes the hydrolysis (depolymerization) of deoxyribonucleic acid (DNA). Abbreviated DNase.

deoxyribonucleic acid a NUCLEIC ACID occurring in cells as the basic structure of the GENES. DNA is present in all body cells of every species, including unicellular organisms and DNA viruses. The structure of DNA was first described in 1953 by J.D. Watson and F.H.C. Crick.

DNA molecules are long linear polymers of small molecules called *nucleotides*, each of which consists of one molecule of the five-carbon sugar *deoxyribose* bonded to a *phosphate* group and to one of four heterocyclic nitrogenous compounds referred to as *bases.* A single strand of DNA is made by linking the nucleotides together in a chain with bonds between the sugar and phosphate groups of adjacent nucleotides. It thus consists of a backbone of alternating sugar and phosphate groups with a base attached to each sugar as a side chain. The four bases are two purines, *adenine* (A) and *guanine* (G), and two pyrimidines, *cytosine* (C) and *thymine* (T). Single-stranded DNA can be synthesized with any specified sequence of bases, but in living cells the base sequence has a meaning; it specifies the amino acid sequence of all of the polypeptides and proteins made by the cell. And since all of the enzymes that catalyze biochemical reactions are proteins, the DNA contains the specifications for all of the biochemistry and structure of the cell.

The chemical basis of the genetic code lies in the ability of the bases to form hydrogen bonds with each other. Unlike the covalent bonds holding together the atoms of a single strand of DNA, hydrogen bonds are weak and easily broken and reformed. Hydrogen bonding is governed by the base pairing rule: A always bonds with T, and C always bonds with G. A and T (or C and G) are called *complementary bases*. The genetic information is read and preserved by the matching up of complementary bases.

In cells, the DNA is double-stranded. The configuration of the DNA molecule resembles a ladder in which the sides are the sugar–phosphate backbones, which are antiparallel (they run in opposite directions), and the rungs are hydrogen-bonded complementary bases; thus, the entire sequence along the two strands is complementary. This whole structure is twisted so that the two strands form a double helix. Once before each cell division, a group of proteins splits the two strands apart, and as complementary nucleotides bond to the bases of each strand they are jointed to form a new strand. This process is called *replication*. It results in the exact duplication of the DNA molecule, because each strand serves as a *template* (pattern) for the synthesis of its complementary strand. When the cell divides, one copy goes to each daughter cell. Thus, the genetic information is passed on from generation to generation without change except for rare mutations, which result from copying errors or incorrectly repaired breaks in the DNA molecule that change the base sequence.

The reading of the genetic code involves two processes: *transcription* and *translation*. In transcription, a length of DNA is used as a template to make a complementary strand of *messenger RNA* (mRNA). RNA (ribonucleic acid) is a nuceic acid like DNA. The only differences are that the sugar, ribose, has an extra oxygen atom, and the pyrimidine base, *uracil* (U), which also pairs with adenine, replaces thymine. In translation, the mRNA molecule is read by a structure called a ribosome, which produces the polypeptide specified by the mRNA message.

The genetic code is a triplet code. Every triplet of bases along the strand specifies a single amino acid. There are 64 possible triplets (codons) that can be formed from the four bases. Each one specifies that one of 20 different amino acids be inserted in a growing polypeptide chain or marks either the start or the end of a chain.

Two other types of RNA are involved in translation. *Ribosomal RNA* (rRNA) forms a large part of the ribosome. *Transfer RNA* (tRNA) is the means by which codons are matched with amino acids. tRNAs are small molecules with several self-complementary sections so that they fold up into a compact structure owing to bonding between complementary bases. One end of the molecule is a three-base anticodon, which bonds to its complementary codon on mRNA molecules. The other end is recognized by a specific enzyme which attaches the correct amino acid to it. During translation, the ribosome proceeds along the mRNA molecule and, as each codon is matched by a specific tRNA, the amino acid it carries is transferred to the growing polypeptide chain, and the process is repeated until the 'stop' codon is reached. Like the mRNA molecules, rRNA and tRNA molecules are formed on DNA templates; the genetic material contains not only the information for polypeptide sequences but also for rRNA and tRNA sequences.

The chromosomes of mammalian cells contain 3×10^9 base pairs which is enough to code for the 100,000 or so enzymes and structural proteins. Less than 10% of the DNA codes for proteins and RNA, the rest is noncoding, also referred to as 'junk' DNA, and is of uncertain purpose. DNA is the molecule that directs all of the activities of living cells, including its own reproduction and perpetuation in generation after generation.

deoxyribonucleoprotein a nucleoprotein in which the sugar is D-2-deoxyribose.

deoxyribonucleoside a nucleoside having a purine or pyrimidine base bonded to deoxyribose.

deoxyribonucleotide a nucleotide having a purine or pyrimidine base bonded to deoxyribose, which in turn is bonded to a phosphate group.

deoxyribose an aldopentose found in deoxyribonucleic acid, deoxyribonucleotides and deoxyribonucleosides.

depasture to feed livestock by grazing them on pasture.

Dependovirus a genus of viruses in the family PARVOVIRIDAE that includes the ADENO-ASSOCIATED VIRUSES.

dephosphophosphorylase the less active form of the regulatory hydrolytic enzyme involved in the phosphorolytic breakdown of glycogen to glucose.

dephosphorylation hydrolytic removal of a phosphate group from an organic molecule.

depigmentation removal of pigment; usually refers to melanin. See also HYPOPIGMENTATION.

nasal d. occurs in dogs with a normal, darkly pigmented nasal planum at birth which later fades to brown or a pale gray-white. Called also Dudley nose, the cause is unknown, but it may be a form of vitiligo. A seasonal loss of pigmentation, usually during winter months, occurs in some breeds, including Siberian huskies, Golden retrievers, Labrador retrievers and Bernese mountain dogs. Called also snow nose.

depilate to remove hair.

depilation removal of hair by the roots. See also EPILATION.

chemical d. the use of chemicals applied externally or internally to remove hair. See also CHEMICAL shearing.

depilatory 1. having the power to remove hair. 2. an agent that removes or destroys the hair.

depletion syndrome chronic water and electrolyte deficits.

depluming removing the feathers of birds.

d. itch CNEMIDOCOPTES *laevis gallinae*. Called also depluming mite, depluming scabies.

d. mite CNEMIDOCOPTES *laevis gallinae*.

d. scabies see depluming itch (above).

depolarization the process or act of neutralizing polarity as in the decrease of membrane potential.

myocardial d. the conducted cardiac impulse transiently reverses membrane polarity. In this depolarized phase the myocardium is incapable of further contraction.

depolarize the act of depolarization.

depolarizing agent a drug that causes depolarization. Usually applied to those used to produce neuromuscular block and muscle paralysis.

depolymerization the conversion of a compound into one of smaller molecular weight and different physical properties without changing the percentage relations of the elements composing it.

depopulation removal of all animals from the particular environment.

herd d. disposal of all animals in the herd.

deposit 1. sediment or dregs. 2. extraneous inorganic matter collected in the tissues or in an organ of the body.

depot a body area in which a substance, e.g. a drug, can be accumulated, deposited or stored and from which it can be distributed.

fat d. a site in the body in which large quantities of fat are stored, as in adipose tissue.

depraved appetite see PICA.

depreciation the decline in value over time of capital items.

l-deprenyl a monoamine oxidase inhibitor used in the treatment of pituitary-dependent hyperadrenocorticism in dogs. Called also selegiline hydrochloride.

depressant 1. diminishing any function or activity. 2. an agent that retards any function, especially a drug that acts on the central nervous system to depress activity at all levels by stabilizing neuronal membranes. CNS depressants, e.g. barbiturates and inhalational anesthetics, are used as sedatives, hypnotics and anesthetics.

depressed carried below the normal level; associated with depression.

depression 1. a hollow or depressed area. 2. a lowering or decrease of functional activity. 3. decreased interest in surroundings, decreased response to external stimuli. The least degree in a range of depressive mental states. See also SOMNOLENCE, LASSITUDE, NARCOLEPSY, CATALEPSY, SYNCOPE, COMA.

d. fracture important in the skull where they may penetrate brain tissue, introduce infection, or cause pressure on the brain because of hemorrhage or hematoma formation.

depressive mental states include SOMNOLENCE, LASSITUDE, CATALEPSY, NARCOLEPSY, SYNCOPE, COMA.

depressomotor 1. retarding or abating motor activity. 2. an agent that so acts.

depressor anything that depresses, as a muscle, agent or instrument, or an afferent nerve, whose stimulation causes a fall in blood pressure.

tongue d. an instrument for pressing down the tongue, usually for purposes of visualizing the soft palate and posterior pharynx.

deprivation loss or absence of parts, organs, powers or things that are needed.

d. test see WATER deprivation test.

deradelphus a twin monster fused at or near the navel, and having one head.

derangement 1. mental disorder. 2. disarrangement of a part or organ.

deregistration removal of right to practice by local registering body, usually as a disciplinary measure because of professional misconduct, possibly because of inability to perform because of psychiatric problem.

derencephalus a monster with a rudimentary skull and bifid cervical vertebrae, the brain resting in the bifurcation.

derepression 1. elevation of the level of an enzyme above the normal, either by lowering the corepressor concentration or by a mutation that decreases the formation of aporepressor or the response to the complete repressor. 2. the inhibition of the repressor substance produced by the regulator genes with the result that the operator gene is free to initiate the process of polypeptide formation.

Derf needle holder a fine instrument used in ophthalmic surgery.

derm- prefix meaning dermis or skin.

derma the corium, or true skin.

dermabrasion PLANING of the skin done by mechanical means, e.g. sandpaper, wire brushes, etc.

Dermacentor a genus of ticks parasitic on various animals, and vectors of disease-producing microorganisms; member of the family Ixodidae.

D. albipictus a one-host tick that transmits anaplasmosis and possibly Rocky Mountain spotted fever. Parasitizes moose mostly but also other wild ruminants and pastured livestock. Called also moose tick, winter tick.

D. andersoni a species of tick common in the western USA, parasitic on numerous wild mammals, most domestic animals, and humans. It is a vector of Rocky Mountain spotted fever, tularemia, Colorado tick fever, and Q fever in the USA, and is one of the causes of tick paralysis in USA.

D. halli, D. marginatus, D. nuttalli, D. silvarum miscellaneous ticks of little importance to animals.

D. nigrolineatus a one-host tick occurring mostly on white-tailed deer, but also on pastured livestock. Called also brown winter tick.

D. nitens a one-host tick that parasitizes horses mostly and is the vector of equine piroplasmosis; predisposes animals to screw-worm attack. Called also tropical horse tick, *Anocentor nitens*.

D. occidentalis a three-host tick found on many animals. Immature forms are on rodents. Transmits anaplasmosis, Colorado tick fever, Q fever, tularemia, causes tick paralysis. Called also Pacific Coast tick.

D. parumapterus a vector of Rocky Mountain spotted fever.

D. reticulatus a three-host tick that transmits equine piroplasmosis.

D. variabilis a three-host tick that transmits *Anaplasma marginale* in cattle, tularemia in humans, is the chief vector of Rocky Mountain spotted fever in the central and eastern USA and causes tick paralysis in the dog. The dog is the principal host of the adult forms, but also parasitic on cattle, horses, rabbits and humans. Called also American dog tick.

D. venustus see *Dermacentor andersoni* (above).

dermal pertaining to the true SKIN, or corium.

d. asthenia called also dermal fragility syndrome; see cutaneous ASTHENIA.

d. fragility syndrome see dermal asthenia.

d. melanocytosis the malignant neoplastic form of melanoma in horses with multiple lesions in the skin and in internal organs; common, and usually fatal, in gray horses and mules.

d. network sensory nerves of the dermis.

d. papillae fingerlike processes invading the epidermis from the dermis.

Dermanyssidae family of parasitic mites. Includes *Dermanyssus*, *Ornithonyssus* and *Pneumonyssus* spp.

Dermanyssus gallinae a member of the genus of the Dermanyssidae family of mites.

A major parasite of domestic fowls but also occurs on other birds including aviary and wild colonies. Causes death due to anemia. A vector for spirochetosis of fowls and possibly the equine encephalitides. A common chance parasite of humans from heavy infestations in urban bird colonies. Called also red mite.

dermatan sulfate a component of the acellular ground substance of skin.

dermatic dermal.

dermatitides plural of *dermatitis*; inflammatory conditions of the skin considered collectively.

dermatitis inflammation of the skin. Dermatitis can result from various animal, vegetable and chemical substances, from heat or cold, from mechanical irritation, from certain forms of malnutrition, or from infectious disease.

actinobacillary d. rare disease in cattle; large ulcers discharging yellow pus or nodules, on lymphatics with local lymph node enlargement.

acute moist d. a superficial bacterial infection of the skin, usually caused by self-trauma, i.e. scratching, rubbing, biting. In dogs, ectoparasites, otitis, anal sacculitis and pruritic skin diseases are common precipitating causes. Affected skin is moist, weeping, and has a covering of matted haircoat and dried exudate. *Staphylococcus* spp. are usually present. Called also pyotraumatic dermatitis, 'hot spots'.
allergic contact d. see ALLERGIC contact dermatitis.
allergic inhalant d. see canine ATOPY.
atopic d. see canine ATOPY.
cercarial d. see TRICHOBILHARZIA.
cheyletiella d. see CHEYLETIELLA.
contagious pustular d. of sheep see contagious ECTHYMA.
coronet d. part of several infectious mucosal diseases of cattle; also in equine pemphigus.
d. crustosa exudative epidermitis.
elaeophorial d. see ELAEOPHORIASIS.
equine contagious pustular d. see CANADIAN HORSEPOX.
equine exfoliative eosinophilic d. characterized by infiltration of eosinophils and granulomatous inflammation with ulcerative stomatitis and wasting; suspected of being a hypersensitivity to *Strongylus equinus* larvae.
equine staphylococcal d. see EQUINE staphylococcal dermatitis.
exudative d. of pigs see EXUDATIVE epidermitis.
feline miliary d. a papular, crusting skin disease located predominantly on the back, with varying degrees of pruritus. Ectoparasites, food and drug allergy, and infection by fungi or bacteria are among the many possible causes. Called also scabby cat disease.
feline psychogenic d. see idopathic HYPERESTHESIA syndrome.
feline solar d. see solar dermatitis (below).
fibrosing d. dermatitis sufficiently severe to affect deep layers of the dermis results in scarring of the skin due to excessive fibrous tissue formation.
filarial d. see STEPHANOFILAROSIS.
fold d. moisture, friction and secondary infection in body folds such as facial fold in brachycephalic dog breeds, tail fold in dog breeds with extremely short, often screw, tails, lip fold in spaniel breeds, perivulvar fold in obese bitches, and all over the body in the Shar pei.
grain itch mite d. a transient, superficial dermatitis, mostly about the head in horses; may be all over the body in pigs. Caused by PEDICULOIDES VENTRICOSUS or TYROGLYPHUS.
granular d. swamp cancer.
d. herpetiformis chronic dermatitis in humans marked by successive crops of grouped, symmetrical, erythematous, papular, vesicular, eczematous or bullous lesions, accompanied by itching and burning; a granular deposition of IgA immunoglobulin around the lesion almost always occurs. Occurs rarely in dogs.
idiopathic caprine d. alopecic, exudative dermatitis of pygmy goats.
infectious d. of piglets see CONTAGIOUS porcine pyoderma.
inhalant d. see canine ATOPY.
interdigital d. see INTERDIGITAL dermatitis.
interface d. a histopathological pattern of inflammatory skin disease with the dermoepidermal junction obscured by hydropic degeneration and/or lichenoid cellular infiltrate.
intertriginous d. see fold DERMATITIS.
intraepidermal pustular d. see equine ALLERGIC dermatitis.
lipfold d. see fold dermatitis (above).
***Malassezia* d.** a pruritic, seborrheic skin disease of dogs, particularly some breeds including West Highland white terriers, Shetland sheepdogs, Poodles, and Cocker spaniels, and rarely cats, caused by colonization of the skin by the yeast, *Malassezia pachydermatis*. There is usually an underlying cause such as atopy or bacterial pyoderma.
mammary pustular d. see MAMMARY pustular dermatitis.
d. medicamentosa an eruption or solitary skin lesion caused by a drug taken internally.
miliary d. see feline miliary dermatitis (above).
moist d. of rabbits the rabbit's pendulous dewlap keeps getting wet and develops a moist dermatitis as a result. Called also slobbers, wet dewlap.
mycotic d. see MYCOTIC dermatitis.
nasal solar d. see solar dermatitis (below), COLLIE nose.
ovine interdigital d. see ovine FOOTROT.
ovine staphylococcal d. ulcerative dermatitis of the face of adult sheep and young lambs caused by a dermatopathic strain of *Staphylococcus aureus*. Called also ovine staphylococcal pyoderma.
pastern d. see GREASY HEEL.
pelodera d. caused by larvae of the free-living nematode *Pelodera strongyloides* and characterized by alopecia, itching, thick, scurfy skin and 0.5 inch diameter pustules which contain the larvae.
photocontact d. allergic contact dermatitis caused by the action of sunlight on skin sensitized by contact with a substance capable of causing this reaction.
photosensitive d. see PHOTOSENSITIVE dermatitis.
plastic dish d. a contact dermatitis caused by plastic feeding dishes to which a dog is allergic.
porcine juvenile pustular psoriasiform d. a disease of pigs, most commonly white breeds such as Landrace, up to 3 months old characterized by circular lesions 1 inch diameter which often coalesce to produce large irregular lesions. The central area of the lesion is an area of comparatively normal skin, covered by thin brown scales and surrounded by a very narrow, 1 to 2 mm raised zone of erythema. There is no irritation or no bristle loss and spontaneous recovery is usual. The etiology is unknown. Called also pityriasis rosea, pseudoringworm.
potato d. see POTATO dermatitis.
primary-irritant d. contact dermatitis (see above) induced by a substance acting as an irritant rather than as a sensitizer or allergen.
proliferative d. see strawberry FOOTROT.
pyotraumatic d. see acute moist dermatitis (above).
d.–pyrexia–hemorrhage syndrome a pruritic, papulocrustous dermatitis in dairy cows which is accompanied by fever and hemorrage from the nose and anus. It is believed to be caused by a toxin.
rhabditic d. see pelodera dermatitis (above).
seasonal allergic d. see ATOPY, equine ALLERGIC dermatitis.
seborrheic d., d. seborrheica a chronic, usually pruritic, dermatitis with erythema, dry, moist or greasy scaling, and yellow crusted patches on various areas, with exfoliation of an excessive amount of dry scales (dandruff) or encrustations of sebum on the skin. See also EXUDATIVE epidermitis (pigs), GREASY HEEL (horses), FLEXURAL seborrhea (cows).
solar d. a chronic, inflammatory reaction on white or lightly pigmented and exposed skin caused by sunlight. Most commonly seen on the ear tips, nose and

eyelids of white cats and the nose of collie dogs or related breeds. Squamous cell carcinomas sometimes develop in affected skin. Called also nasal solar dermatitis, actinic dermatitis. See also COLLIE nose.

spongiotic d. perivascular inflammation with spongiosis.

summer d. see equine ALLERGIC dermatitis.

superficial pustular d. immature dogs may develop pustules on the inguinal or axillary skin, often in association with poor nutrition, systemic infection, or parasitism. In kittens, these may occur on the neck, caused by 'mouthing' by the queen.

trefoil d. see TREFOIL dermatitis.

tyroglyphid d. see TYROGLYPHUS.

unilateral papular d. a disease of horses characterized by the appearance of many nodules or papules on one side of the neck and body. The lesions are eosinophilic folliculitis and perifolliculitis. The etiology and the unilateral distribution of the lesions are unexplained.

ventral midline d. small ulcers with hemorrhagic crusts and hair loss, located on the abdomen, particularly around the umbilicus, of horses; caused by biting flies and gnats.

vesicular d. see avian VESICULAR dermatitis.

viral contagious d. see contagious ECTHYMA.

viral papular d. see EQUINE papular dermatitis.

x-ray d. radiodermatitis.

dermat(o)- word element. [Gr.] *skin.*

Dermatobia a genus of bot flies in the family Cuterebridae. Includes *Dermatobia hominis*, the larvae of which are parasitic in the skin of humans, mammals and birds causing subcutaneous swellings with central holes. A major parasite of cattle in South America.

dermatocele a disorder in which the skin and subcutaneous tissue hypertrophy so that the skin hangs in loose folds.

dermatofibroma a fibrous tumor-like nodule of the skin.

dermatofibrosarcoma a fibrosarcoma of the skin.

dermatofibrosis a syndrome inherited as a dominant trait in German shepherd dogs in which multiple, firm cutaneous and subcutaneous nodules of mature fibrous tissue, up to 2 inches in diameter, develop in middle age. Affected animals show a high incidence of renal adenocarcinoma and females have multiple uterine and vaginal leiomyomas. Called also nodular dermatofibrosis.

dermatoglyphics the surface features of skin, including wrinkles, folds, ridges and furrows.

dermatographia dermatographism.

dermatographism urticaria due to physical allergy in which a pale, raised welt or wheal with a red flare on each side is elicited by stroking or scratching the skin with a dull instrument.

dermatoheteroplasty the grafting of skin derived from an animal of another species.

dermatohistopathology the histopathological study of the skin.

dermatological, dermatologic pertaining to dermatology; of or affecting the skin.

dermatologist a veterinarian who specializes in dermatology.

dermatology the specialty concerned with the diagnosis and treatment of skin diseases.

dermatomal pertaining to a dermatome.

d. mapping designation of regions of the body, the extent of each corresponding to the distribution of the dorsal root axons.

dermatome 1. an instrument for cutting thin skin slices for grafting. 2. the area of skin supplied with afferent nerve fibers by a single dorsal spinal root. 3. the lateral part of an embryonic somite.

Brown d. an electric or pneumatic instrument used for cutting split-thickness skin grafts.

dermatomegaly see DERMATOCELE.

dermatomere a segment of the embryonic integument.

dermatomycosis a fungal infection of the skin or of its appendages by a fungus other than the dermatophytes, *Microsporum*, *Trichophyton* or *Epidermophyton*.

dermatomyoma a dermal leiomyoma.

dermatomyositis an acute, subacute or chronic disease of humans, marked by nonsuppurative inflammation of the skin, subcutaneous tissue and muscles, with necrosis of muscle fibers.

canine familial d. an inherited disease found mainly in Collies and Shetland sheepdogs. Starting at a young age, there is hair loss, alopecia, scaling, crusting and sometimes ulceration on the face, ear tips, pressure areas over the carpus and tarsus, and the tail. Myositis may be severe, causing a stiff gait, difficulty in chewing and atrophy, or be unrecognized except by biopsy.

dermatopathic, dermopathic of the nature of or pertaining to dermatopathy.

dermatopathology pathology that is especially concerned with lesions of the skin.

dermatopathy any disease of the skin; dermopathy.

Dermatophagoides a genus of mites of the family Epidermoptidae. Includes *Dermatophagoides farinae*, *D. pteronyssinus* (housedust mites).

dermatophilosis a group of diseases caused by *Dermatophilus* spp. Includes MYCOTIC dermatitis, strawberry FOOTROT.

Dermatophilus a genus of bacteria in the family Dermatophilaceae.

D. chelonae causes skin lesions in turtles.

D. congolensis gram-positive, tapering filaments with right-angled branching, producing coccoid cells and flagellated, motile zoospores. Causes MYCOTIC dermatitis, strawberry FOOTROT, streptothricosis. Has many synonyms including *D. dermatonomus*, *D. pedis*, *Polysepta*, *Nocardia*, *Streptothrix* spp.

dermatophyte fungi parasitic upon the skin, including *Microsporum*, *Trichophyton*, and *Epidermophyton* spp. Occasional pathogens are *Keratinomyces allejoi* in horses and *Scopulariopsis brevicaulis* in cattle.

d. test medium (DTM) a special culture medium for fungi containing phenol red as an indicator. Pathogenic fungi produce alkali during growth causing the medium to turn red.

dermatophytid a secondary skin eruption which is an expression of hypersensitivity to a dermatophyte, occurring on an area remote from the site of infection. Called also an 'id' reaction.

dermatophytosis fungal infection of the skin caused by one of the pathogenic genera, *Microsporum*, *Trichophyton* or *Epidermophyton*; see also RINGWORM.

dermatoplasty a plastic operation on the skin; operative replacement of lost skin.

dermatorrhagiae parasitaire [Fr.] parafilariasis.

dermatosclerosis see SCLERODERMA.

dermatosis pl *dermatoses*; any skin disorder, especially one not characterized by inflammation.

d. erythematosa a disease of unknown etiology which occurs in pigs, mainly the white varieties; there is nonpruritic, acute erythema over large areas of the body and spontaneous recovery occurs in a matter of days.

exfoliative d. one involving severe desquamation;

includes drug reaction, contact hypersensitivity, autoimmune diseases, cutaneous lymphomas and parapsoriasis.
generic dog food d. see GENERIC pet food.
growth hormone-responsive d. see GROWTH HORMONE-responsive dermatosis.
hereditary lupoid d. a scaling and crusting skin disease seen from a young age in German shorthaired pointers.
infantile pustular d. pustules, depression and anorexia in neonatal puppies; the etiology is unknown.
invisible d. skin diseases which are evident clinically, but the histopathology is consistent with normal skin.
linear IgA d. a rare, immune-mediated skin disease of Dachshunds in which immunoglobulin A is deposited at the basement membrane zone. There are pustules, with alopecia, hyperpigmentation, scaling and crusting.
linear preputial d. a narrow line of hyperpigmentation along the midline between the prepuce and scrotum is considered a marker for testicular neoplasia in dogs.
psychogenic d. one caused by self-trauma for which no cause is known; in dogs and cats, boredom, overcrowding or confinement are often associated. See idopathic HYPERESTHESIA syndrome, ACRAL lick dermatitis, FLANK sucking, TAIL sucking.
seborrheic d. see seborrheic DERMATITIS.
subcorneal pustular d. a very rare skin disorder of dogs in which short-lived, sterile, superficial pustules form, particularly on the head and trunk. Pruritus is variable. The cause is unknown.
ulcerative d. see ULCERATIVE dermatosis.
d. vegetans an inherited skin disease of Landrace pigs. Young piglets may be affected at birth or develop at an early age an erythematous, papular dermatitis, mainly on the ventral abdomen and medial thighs. There is also erythema and edema of the coronary bands and subsequent deformities of the foot. Pneumonia develops before death.
zinc-responsive d. a breed-related form occurs in Siberian huskies and several other Artic breeds, and a dermatosis can occur in puppies of any breed if their diet is deficient in zinc or absorption is impaired by excessive supplementation of calcium. There is scaling and crusting, especially over pressure points and footpads. See also PARAKERATOSIS for a similar disease in pigs and a familial one in cattle.

dermatosparaxia fragility of skin and subcutaneous tissue rendering the skin very stretchable. Most common in inherited defects in cattle and dogs. See also EHLERS–DANLOS SYNDROME.

dermatosparaxis an inherited defect in collagen synthesis caused by a deficiency of procollagen peptidase. Results in fragility, hyperelasticity and laxity of the skin. Occurs in cattle, some breeds of sheep, and Himalayan cats. Called also Ehlers–Danlos syndrome, hyperelastosis cutis, cutaneous ASTHENIA.

dermatotherapy treatment of skin diseases.

dermatotropic having a specific affinity for the skin.
d. bovine herpesvirus see LUMPY skin disease.

Dermatoxys a genus of nematodes in the family Oxyuridae. Includes *Dermatoxys veligera* (occurs in the large intestine of rabbits and hares).

dermatozoon any animal parasite on the skin; an ectoparasite.

Dermestes a genus of beetles in the order Coleoptera.
D. lardarius destroys stored grain, meat, hides and accumulated droppings of pigeons. The larvae may attack pigeon fledglings. Called also larder beetle.

dermis the corium; the principal layer of skin between the epidermis and the subcutaneous tissue; made up mostly of a network of collagen fibers but also containing nerves, blood vessels, cells and other fibers. It is divided into papillary and reticular parts, and when tanned forms leather.
hoof d. a greatly modified dermis, continuous at the coronet with the common dermis of the skin; the modified dermis supports the horn of the hoof.

dermoabrasion removal of the superficial layers of hypertrophic epidermis with a wire brush.

dermoblast the part of the mesoderm which develops into the true skin.

Dermocystidium a protozoan parasite which causes cysts in the skin of fish and amphibians.
D. ranae parasitizes the grass frog (*Rana temporaria*).

dermoepidermal pertaining to the dermis and the epidermis.
d. junction is straight compared to the undulating border in humans; consists of lamina lucida externa, lamina densa, lamina lucida interna and anchoring filaments.

Dermoglyphus a genus of the Dermoglyphidae family of mites. Includes *Dermoglyphus elongatus*, *D. minor* (found in the feather shafts of birds but cause no lesion).

dermogram a diagram illustrating sequential stages in the development of a skin disease, or various changes which may occur, as a cross-section of the skin.

dermographia see DERMATOGRAPHISM.

dermographism see DERMATOGRAPHISM.

dermoid 1. skinlike. 2. a dermoid cyst.
d. cyst a tumor of developmental origin consisting of a fibrous wall lined with stratified epithelium and containing hair follicles, sweat glands, sebaceous glands, nerve elements and teeth; a teratoma. Occurs in subcutaneous sites, in the ovary and various locations in the eye, including cornea, conjunctiva and eyelids.
ocular d. dermoid on the eyelid, cornea or conjunctiva.
ovarian d. when these cysts occur in the ovary they may present no signs but their long pedicles may cause twisting, resulting in acute abdominal pain.
d. sinus an inherited abnormality in Rhodesian Ridgeback dogs in which a neural tube, which is an invagination of the skin, connects the skin with the dura mater in the vertebral canal or to an intervening structure. Characterized by the presence of a tuft of hair protruding from each sinus and sometimes complicated by infection with drainage.

dermoidectomy excision of a dermoid cyst.

dermolipoma a congenital, yellow-colored growth of fatty tissue occurring under the bulbar conjunctiva.

dermomycosis see DERMATOMYCOSIS.

dermonecrosis necrosis of the skin.

dermopathy any skin disease; dermatopathy.

dermophyte see DERMATOPHYTE.

dermosynovitis inflammation of the skin overlying an inflamed bursa or tendon sheath.

dermotropic see DERMATOTROPIC.

dermovascular pertaining to the skin and blood vessels of the skin.

derodidymus a monster with two heads; dicephalus.

derriengue [Span.] posterior incoordination of cattle in South America (1) poisoned by *Zamia* spp., (2) affected by paralytic rabies.

derris powdered root of plants of the genus *Derris* of the family Leguminosae. Used as an insecticide and source of rotenone and rotenoid compounds. See also ROTENONE.

Derry's disease type 2, GM_1 gangliosidosis.
Derzsy's disease see GOOSE hepatitis.
DES diethylstilbestrol.
desaturase an enzyme capable of catalyzing desaturation of fatty acids.
desaturation insertion of double bonds; process of insertion of double bonds in the carboxyl end of fatty acids.
descemetocele herniation of Descemet's membrane, usually through a corneal wound or deep ulceration.
Descemet's membrane the posterior lining membrane of the cornea, a thin hyaline membrane between the substantia propria and the endothelial layer. In buphthalmos, stretching of the globe may be accompanied by tears in Descemet's membrane, called Descemet's streaks.
descensus pl. *descensus* [L.] downward displacement or prolapse.
d. testis normal migration of the testis from its fetal position in the abdominal cavity to its location within the scrotum.
d. uteri prolapse of the uterus.
descenting surgical excision of the sebaceous glands on the top of the head of the male goat or the anal sacs of the skunk in order to eliminate the unpleasant odors each gives off.
Deschamps aneurysm needle a long thin instrument with a palm-held handle and a thin needle-like extension which at its tip bends laterally at right angles and then describes a semicircle in the same plane. The tip has a needle eye and a pointed but not sharp end. It is designed to place ligatures around vessels in poorly accessible sites.
descriptive epidemiology see descriptive EPIDEMIOLOGY.
descriptive statistics see STATISTICS.
Descurainia pinnata a plant member of the Brassicaceae family, a mustard; an unidentified toxin causes impaired vision, inability to swallow, paresis of tongue and muscles of mastication. Called also tansy mustard.
desensitization the prevention or reduction of immediate hypersensitivity reactions mediated by IgE by the administration of graded doses of allergen; hyposensitization. See also IMMUNOTHERAPY.
extinction d. see EXTINCTION.
desensitize 1. to deprive of sensation. 2. to subject to desensitization.
desert baileya *Baileya multiradiata*.
desert bighorn sheep *Ovis canadensis cremnobates*. See BIGHORN SHEEP.
desert death adder see desert death ADDER.
desert fever the primary form of COCCIDIOIDOMYCOSIS. Called also desert rheumatism.
desert poison bush GASTROLOBIUM *grandiflorum*.
desert rheumatism see DESERT FEVER.
desert rice flower PIMELEA *simplex*, *P. trichostachya*.
desert tobacco NICOTIANA *trigonophylla*.
desert tortoise see GOPHERUS AGASSIZII.
desex removal of the organs of generation, the ovaries or testes.
desferrioxamine see DEFEROXAMINE.
desflurane a gaseous anesthetic agent similar to isoflurane.
desiccant 1. promoting dryness. 2. an agent that promotes dryness.
desiccate to render thoroughly dry.
desiccation the act of drying.
d. keratitis see KERATOCONJUNCTIVITIS sicca.
designated persons staff in a radiology unit who are in frequent contact with x-rays and who are allotted a higher Dose Equivalent Limit of radiation than other persons; abbreviated DPs. It is expected that the DPs will have been instructed in all matters related to radiation safety.
deslanoside a rapid-acting cardiotonic glycoside obtained from lanatoside C.
Desmarres forceps forceps for grasping chalazions. Thumb-operated spring forceps with large oval tips to the blades, one a solid plate the other a circle. The blades can be clamped shut with a thumbscrew.
Desmarres retractors handheld eyelid retractors consisting of a handle and a bent spoon tip which curves back on itself.
desm(o)- word element. [Gr.] *ligament*.
desmin protein found in muscle cells that forms intermediate filaments.
desmitis inflammation of a ligament.
desmocollins one of the glycoproteins found in the core of desmosomes; responsible for adhesive recognition between cells.
desmocranium the mass of mesoderm at the cranial end of the notochord in the early embryo, forming the earliest stage of the skull.
Desmodus rotundus murinus vampire bat of Central and South America. Important as long-term vectors of rabies virus. See also DERRIENGUE.
desmogleins one of the glycoproteins found in the core of deamosomes; responsible for adhesive recognition between cells.
desmography a description of ligaments.
desmoid 1. fibrous or fibroid. 2. a fibromatous tumor arising in a muscle sheath; it resembles a fibrosarcoma. Called also desmoid, desmoma.
desmology the science of ligaments.
desmolysis acantholysis.
desmoma see DESMOID (2).
desmopathy any disease of the ligaments.
desmoplasia the formation and development of fibrous tissue, usually indicating that caused by neoplastic processes.
desmopressin a synthetic analog of 8-arginine vasopressin; the acetate (DDAVP) is used for antidiuretic replacement therapy in the management of central diabetes insipidus and for the temporary polyuria and polydipsia associated with trauma to or surgery in the pituitary region.
desmorrhexis rupture of a ligament.
prepubic d. rupture of the prepubic ligament.
desmosine special amino acid, derived from four lysine residues, and found only in elastin. Allows elastin to stretch reversibly in all directions.
desmosome the 'spot-welds' which provide one of the structural units that bind epithelial cells together. Half units are called hemidesmosomes.
d. core a dense core of glycoproteins filling the space between cells which are adhered by desmosomes.
half d's structures which provide points of adhesion to anchor cytoskeletal elements to basal cell membranes. Called also hemidesmosomes.
desmotomy the cutting or division of ligaments. See also PATELLAR ligament desmotomy, CHECK LIGAMENT desmotomy.
desnooding surgical removal of the snood in the turkey to prevent cannibalism and the creation of a portal of entry for erysipelas infection.
desonide a synthetic corticosteroid used as a topical anti-inflammatory agent in the treatment of steroid-responsive dermatoses.
desorb to remove a substance from the state of absorption or adsorption.

desorption the process or state of being desorbed.
desoximetasone, desoxymethasone an anti-inflammatory, antipruritic and vasoconstrictive corticosteroid used topically to relieve inflammation in corticosteroid-responsive dermatoses.
desoxy- for words beginning thus, see also those beginning *deoxy-*.
desoxymethasone see DESOXIMETASONE.
desquamation the shedding of epithelial elements, chiefly of the skin, in scales or sheets.
destruction of living animals; see EUTHANASIA.
desulfhydrase an enzyme that splits cysteine into hydrogen sulfide, ammonia and pyruvic acid.
detachment the condition of being separated or disconnected.
retinal d. separation of the inner layers of the retina from the pigment epithelium, which remains attached to the choroid. Retinal detachment occurs most often as a result of degenerative changes in the peripheral retina and vitreous body, which produce holes or tears in the retina that can range from minute breaks no larger than 0.1 mm to extensive holes that extend over the entire fundus. Causes include trauma to the eyeball, severe contusions, inflammatory lesions and sometimes ocular surgery.
rhegmatogenous d. retinal detachment with holes.
nonrhegmatogenous d. retinal detachment with no holes present.
detail in radiological terms means ease of defining structures visually. Depends on degree of contrast, sharpness of edges and absence of fogging or other obscuring defect.
detergent 1. purifying, cleansing. 2. an agent that purifies or cleanses.
anionic d. a substance which when dissolved contributes a hydrophobic ion which carries a negative charge to the solution. Soap is an example.
cationic d. the dissociated substance produces a positively charged hydrophobic ion. The quarternary ammonium compounds are the best known examples. They are innocuous if properly diluted but the concentrates are very poisonous.
nonionic surface-acting d. e.g. the polyoxyethylenes are regarded as nonpoisonous.
detergescence the state of relative dehydration that contributes greatly to the transparency of the cornea; maintained by several active mechanisms, especially the sodium-pump of endothelium and epithelium.
determinant a factor that establishes or changes the nature of an entity or event. The factor may be environmental, be a part of the host or its defenses, be single or multiple and be immediate or remote.
allotypic d. an antigenic determinant which varies among members of the same species.
antigenic d. a structural component of an antigen against which immune responses are made and to which antibody or T cell receptor binds; an antigen such as a protein has many antigenic determinants. Called also epitope.
disease d's factors which affect the occurrence or rate of ocurrence of a disease.
hidden d. an antigenic determinant located in an unexposed region of a molecule so that it is prevented from interacting with receptors on lymphocytes, or with antibody molecules, and is unable to induce an immune response; it may appear following stereochemical alterations of molecular structure.
isotypic d. one that occurs in all individuals of the same species.
determination the establishment of the exact nature of an entity or event. See also AGE determination, SEX determination.
d. coefficient see determination COEFFICIENT.
embryonic d. the loss of pluripotentiality in any embryonic part and its start on the way to an unalterable fate.
determinism the theory that all phenomena are the result of antecedent conditions and that nothing occurs by chance.
deterministic model one in which each variable changes according to a mathematical formula, rather than with a random component. See also COMPUTER simulation model.
detomidine a potent α_2-adrenoceptor agonist, used as a sedative and analgesic, particularly in horses and cattle.
detorsion rod an obstetrical instrument used to assist in the correction of uterine torsion in the cow. It is a meter long rod with a bar handle for applying torque. At the other end is a double prong with an eyelet at the end of each prong. Each of the two presenting limbs is fixed to one of the prongs by rope or chain and the fetus can then be rotated along its long axis by rotating the handle.
detoxicate detoxify.
detoxification, detoxication 1. reduction of the toxic properties of a substance. 2. treatment designed to assist in recovery from the toxic effects of a drug.
metabolic d. reduction of the toxic properties of a substance by chemical changes induced in the body, producing a compound which is less poisonous or more readily eliminated.
detoxify to subject to detoxification.
detrition the wearing away, as of teeth, by friction.
detritus particulate matter produced by or remaining after the wearing away or disintegration of a substance or tissue.
d. cysts occur in arthritis where there is hemorrhage and necrotic bone.
detruncation decapitation, especially of the fetus.
detrusor a general term for a muscle that expresses a substance. The detrusor muscle of the bladder squeezes urine towards the outlet.
detumescence the subsidence of congestion and swelling.
detusking removal of part or all of the tusks of a boar to prevent injury to other pigs and people.
deuterium the mass 2 isotope of hydrogen, symbol ^2H or D; it is available as a gas or heavy water and is used as a tracer or indicator in studying metabolism.
deuterohemophilia a group of hemorrhagic disorders resembling classical hemophilia, due to coagulation factor deficiencies or to the action of certain anticoagulants.
Deuteromycetes a class (Fungi Imperfecti) which contains many of the fungi pathogenic for humans and animals.
Deuteromycota the phylum of fungi known as Fungi Imperfecti, containing *Cryptococcus*, *Candida* and some *Microsporum* and *Trichophyton* spp.
deuteropathy a disease that is secondary to another disease.
deuteroporphyrin III the protoporphyrin of heme, the only known naturally occurring isomer of etioporphyrin III.
devascularization interruption of circulation of blood to a part due to obstruction or destruction of blood vessels supplying it.
developer develops the latent image on the exposed x-ray film. A standard developer is a mixture of Metol and hydroquinone.

developing agent see DEVELOPER.

development the process of growth and differentiation.

developmental pertaining to development.

d. anomaly absence, deformity or excess of body parts as the result of faulty development of the embryo. Called also developmental defect.

d. defect see developmental anomaly (above).

deviant varying from a determinable standard.

deviation variation from the regular standard or course. 1. In ophthalmology, a tendency for the visual axes of the eye to fall out of alignment owing to muscular imbalance. 2. in statistics the difference between the predicted value of a variable and the actual value.

standard d. a measure of statistical dispersion. See STANDARD deviation.

devil's pertaining to the devil; said of something evil.

d. apple SOLANUM *capsicoides*.

d. bit see SCABIOSA SUCCISA.

d. droppings see ASAFETIDA.

d. fig SOLANUM *torvum*.

d. fish giant squid of the family Architeuthidae, presenting no danger to humans or animals, despite generations of fictive folk lore.

d. food DATURA *stramonium*.

d. grip a conformation defect in sheep in which the thorax is pinched in behind the shoulders. Reputed to make affected sheep more susceptible to fleece rot and blowfly strike.

d. ivy see DATURA.

d. thorn see TRIBULUS *terrestris*.

d. trumpet DATURA *stramonium*.

devocalization surgical interference with the voice-producing mechanism to prevent annoying noise made by the animal. In the dog and sealion the operation is a resection of the vocal cords. Equine devocalization was an important procedure for mounted units in wartime; it was a ventriculectomy with added cord resection for a greater level of muting. In the peacock devocalization is carried out by scarification of the mucosa of the syrinx.

Devon a cherry red breed of dairy cattle, bred in the UK. See also SOUTH DEVON.

Devon rex see REX.

Dewar flask an insulated container for the storage of cryogenic liquids such as liquid nitrogen.

dewattling surgical removal of the wattles from a chicken. See also DECOMBING.

dewclaw 1. the rudimentary first digit of dogs and cats, found on the inner side of the front legs, above the weight-bearing digits. These are commonly removed from puppies at an early age because of the susceptibility to injury throughout life. Occasionally found on the hindlegs of some dogs and in some breeds this is required, e.g. the Great Pyrenees dog and Briard in which double rear dewclaws must be present. 2. the accessory claws of the ruminant foot.

d. slough sequel to laminitis, severe edema of the lower extremity, severe coronitis.

dewlap loose skin under the throat and neck which may be pendulous in some species or breeds, e.g. Bloodhounds, Indian cattle, rabbits.

deworming preparations see ANTHELMINTIC.

dexamethasone a synthetic glucocorticoid used primarily as an anti-inflammatory agent in various conditions, including autoimmune diseases, hypersensitivity reactions and shock; it is also used in a screening test for the diagnosis of CUSHING'S SYNDROME, and for the termination of pregnancy in cattle.

d. suppression test the determination of blood cortisol levels before and after administration of dexamethasone assists in diagnosing Cushing's syndrome and identifying the cause, depending on the protocol and dose used. Dexamethasone suppresses pituitary secretion of ACTH in normal animals and therefore the blood level of cortisol is decreased; low doses do not suppress cortisol levels in dogs with pituitary-dependent Cushing's syndrome, high doses do. Cortisol production by functional adrenal tumors is not affected by dexamethasone.

dexbrompheniramine the dextrorotatory isomer of BROMPHENIRAMINE, used as an antihistaminic in the form of the maleate salt.

dexchlorpheniramine the dextrorotatory form of chlorpheniramine used as an antihistaminic in the form of the maleate salt.

Dexon trademark for a synthetic suture material, polyglycolic acid, a polymer that is completely absorbable and nonirritating.

dexpanthenol the D-isomer of panthenol, a coenzyme A precursor with cholinergic activity. Used to increase peristalsis in atony and paralysis of the lower intestine and as an antiflatulent; also used topically to stimulate skin healing in various skin diseases.

Dexter a red or black, short-legged breed of cattle used for dairy or beef purposes, produced in Ireland. Called also Dexter-Kerry. They are achondroplastic and the breed has a number of inherited defects, including bulldog calves.

dexter [L.] *right, on the right side.*

Dexter-Kerry see DEXTER.

dextran a water-soluble polysaccharide of glucose (dextrose) produced by the action of *Leuconostoc mesenteroides* on sucrose; used as a plasma volume extender. Several preparations of dextran are used as anticoagulants.

d. 40 used as an adjuvant in blood transfusion, an anticoagulant.

d. sulfate used as an anticoagulant and recently investigated for its antiviral activity.

dextranomer small beads of highly hydrophilic dextran polymers used in débridement of secreting wounds, such as venous stasis ulcers; the sterilized beads are poured over secreting wounds to absorb wound exudates and prevent crust formation.

dextriferron a complex of ferric hydroxide and partially hydrolyzed dextrin used in the treatment of iron-deficiency anemia.

dextrin any of a range of glucose polymers of varying sizes formed during the hydrolysis of starch.

limit d. a by-product of glycogenolysis.

dextrin-1,6-glucosidase dextrin 6-glucanohydrolase: an enzyme that catalyzes the hydrolysis of α-1,6-glucan links in dextrins containing short 1,6-linked side chains.

dextrinose see ISOMALTOSE.

dextrinosis a condition characterized by accumulation in the tissues of an abnormal polysaccharide.

dextrinuria presence of dextrin in the urine.

dextr(o)- word element. [L.] *right.*

dextroaorta dextropositioned aorta; a congenital anomaly in which the aorta develops from the embryonic right fourth aortic arch instead of the left. The left subclavian artery then crosses over the esophagus, forming a vascular ring and a cause of regurgitation in the neonate.

dextrocardia location of the heart in the right side of the thorax, the apex pointing to the right.

mirror-image d. location of the heart in the right side of the chest, the atria being transposed and the right ventricle lying anteriorly and to the left of the left ventricle.

dextromethorphan a synthetic morphine derivative used as an antitussive in the form of the hydrobromide salt.

dextroposition displacement to the right.

dextropropoxyphene see PROPOXYPHENE.

dextrorotatory turning the plane of polarization, or rays of light, to the right.

dextrose an old chemical name for D-glucose, an important energy source for all tissues and the sole energy source for the brain in some species such as the sheep. The term dextrose continues to be used to refer to glucose solutions administered intravenously for fluid or nutrient replacement. See also GLUCOSE.

dextrosuria the presence of dextrose in the urine; called also glucosuria.

dextrothyroxine sodium the dextrorotatory isomer of thyroxine used as an antihyperlipoproteinemic in the treatment of hyperlipemia.

dextroversion 1. version to the right, especially movement of the eyes to the right. 2. location of the heart in the right chest, the left ventricle remaining in the normal position on the left, but lying anterior to the right ventricle.

DF degrees of freedom.

DF-2 see CAPNOCYTOPHAGA.

DFA test direct immunofluorescent antibody test.

DFB acronym for dark, firm, dry meat. Called also DARK cutting beef.

DFP di-isopropylfluorophosphate. See ISOFLUROPHATE.

DHAP dihydroxyacetone phosphate, an intermediate of glycolysis formed as an end product of the aldol cleavage of fructose-1,6-bisphosphate.

24,25-DHCC 24,25-dihydroxycholecalciferol; a metabolite in calcium metabolism, formed in the kidney from 25-hydroxycholecalciferol by the activation of a 24-hydroxylase. See also DIHYDROXYCHOLECALCIFEROL.

***dhfr* gene** see *dhfr* GENE.

DHI see DAIRY herd improvement.

DHIA Dairy Herd Improvement Association. Most developed countries have a DHIA dedicated to improving the productivity of their dairy cattle. Membership is optional but fees are low because of heavy government subsidy. See also DAIRY herd improvement.

Dhobie itch see equine ALLERGIC dermatitis.

dhrek see MELIA *azederach.*

dhurrin a cyanogenetic glycoside in sorghum.

di- word element. [Gr., L.] *two.*

2,6-di-iodo-4-nitrophenol see DISOPHENOL.

dia- word element. [Gr.] *through, between, apart, across, completely.*

diabetes a general term referring to a variety of disorders characterized by polyuria and polydipsia. See DIABETES MELLITUS and DIABETES INSIPIDUS.

diabetes insipidus a metabolic disorder due to injury of the neurohypophyseal system, which results in a deficient quantity of antidiuretic hormone (ADH or vasopressin) being released or produced, resulting in failure of tubular reabsorption of water in the kidney. As a consequence, there is the passage of a large amount of urine having a low specific gravity, and great thirst. It may be acquired through infection, neoplasm or trauma to the posterior lobe of the pituitary gland or it may be inherited or idiopathic. Called also central diabetes insipidus.

dipsogenic d. i. see psychogenic diabetes insipidus (below).

nephrogenic d. i. a rare form of diabetes insipidus, resulting from failure of the renal tubules to reabsorb water; there is excessive production of antidiuretic hormone but the tubules fail to respond to it.

psychogenic d. i. a primary polydipsia resulting from a disorder of thirst control, or as a behavioral problem. The polyuria is secondary to the excessive water intake. Called also dipsogenic diabetes insipidus.

diabetes mellitus a broadly applied term used to denote a complex group of syndromes that have in common a disturbance in the oxidation and utilization of glucose, which is secondary to a malfunction of the beta cells of the pancreas, whose function is the production and release of INSULIN. Because insulin is involved in the metabolism of carbohydrates, proteins and fats, diabetes is not limited to a disturbance of glucose homeostasis alone.

Diabetes mellitus has been recorded in all species but is most commonly seen in middle-aged to older, obese, female dogs. A familial predisposition has been suggested. It is possible to identify two types of diabetes, corresponding to the disease in humans, depending on the response to an intravenous glucose tolerance test. Type I is insulin-dependent and comparable to the juvenile onset form of the disease in children in which there is an absolute deficiency of insulin—there is a very low initial blood insulin level and a low response to the injected glucose. This form is seen in a number of dog breeds, particularly the Keeshond, Doberman pinscher, German shepherd dog, Poodle, Golden retriever and Labrador retriever.

Type II is non-insulin-dependent, similar to the adult onset diabetes in humans due to pancreatic damage—there is a high or normal initial blood insulin level and no increase in insulin levels as a result of the glucose load. It is the form seen most often in cats.

brittle d. m. diabetes mellitus that is difficult to control, characterized by unexplained oscillation between hypoglycemia and diabetic ketoacidosis.

gestational d. m. diabetes mellitus in which onset or recognition of impaired glucose tolerance occurs during pregnancy.

hyperosmolar d. m. a syndrome of marked hyperglycemia and hyperosmolarity with central nervous signs, resembling diabetic coma.

insulin-dependent d. m. (IDDM) due to deficient secretion of insulin by the beta cells of the pancreas. See diabetes mellitus type I (above).

juvenile d. m. develops in the young; see diabetes mellitus type I (above).

non-insulin-dependent d. m. (NIDDM) the secretion of insulin is unimpaired but the response of tissue receptors is diminished. See diabetes mellitus type II (above).

secondary d. m. hyperglycemia may occur in association with pancreatitis, hyperadrenocorticism, acromegaly, and treatment with glucocorticoids or progesterone.

steroid d. m. altered carbohydrate tolerance is induced by glucocorticoids and progestogens. Hyperglycemia and diabetes mellitus can be associated with the administration of such drugs or hyperadrenocorticism.

diabetic pertaining to or characterized by diabetes.

diabetogenic producing diabetes.

diabetogenous caused by diabetes.

diabrotic 1. ulcerative; caustic. 2. a corrosive or escharotic substance.

diacetoxyscirpenol non-macrocyclic trichothecene

mycotoxin from the fungi *Fusarium* spp. Causes emesis, voracious appetite, frequent passage of normal feces, and posterior paresis in pigs.

diacetylmorphine see HEROIN.

diacrisis 1. diagnosis. 2. a disease characterized by a morbid state of the secretions. 3. a critical discharge or excretion.

diacritic diagnostic; distinguishing.

sn-1,2-diacylglycerol second messenger produced from the action of an agonist via G-proteins activating phospholipase C leading to the hydrolysis of phosphatidylinositol 4,5-bisphosphate to sn-1,2-diacylglycerol and inositol 1,4,5-trisphosphate. sn-1,2-Diacylglycerol subsequently activates protein kinase C by greatly increasing the affinity of the enzyme for calcium ions.

diadochokinesia the function of arresting one motor impulse and substituting one that is diametrically opposite.

diadromy migration of fish in either direction, from fresh to sea water or the reverse.

diagnose to identify or recognize a disease.

diagnosis a name given to a disease so that each veterinarian means the same syndrome as every other veterinarian. It is then possible to prescribe for and make a prognosis about any one case on the basis of the outcomes in a series of animals with the same diagnosis. A diagnosis may be the name of a disease with a specific etiology, or one which is only a description of the morphological identity of the disease, a pathoanatomical diagnosis, or be a syndrome which is a description of the total symptomatology, or a single clinical sign.

clinical d. diagnosis based on clinical signs and laboratory findings during life.

computer assisted d. a computer program identifies the diseases that fit the identified abnormalities best.

differential d. the determination of which one of several diseases may be producing the signs observed.

etiological d. identifies the specific cause of the disease.

pathoanatomical d. diagnosis to the point of identifying the system and organ involved and the nature of the lesion, but short of identifying the cause.

physical d. diagnosis based on information obtained by inspection, palpation, percussion and auscultation.

radiological d. a good radiological report does more than report findings. It interprets these findings if possible up to the point of making a pathoanatomical diagnosis (see above).

veterinary d. diagnosis performed by a veterinarian and based on information gleaned from a variety of sources, including (1) findings from a physical examination, (2) interview with the owner or custodian of the animal, (3) veterinary history of the patient and its cohorts and (4) paraclinical findings as reported by pertinent laboratory tests and radiological studies.

diagnostic pertaining to or emanating from the making of a diagnosis.

d. codes alphanumeric codes used to identify diagnoses for the purposes of computer storage. The codes can be entirely alphabetical, and therefore much more user-friendly, but the number of diagnoses that the system can hold is limited. Completely numeric code systems offer limitless volumetric capacity, a disadvantage in a working hospital.

d. data data with finite values as opposed to continuous data, e.g. the number of puppies born per litter.

d. disciplines the disciplines applied to the making of diagnoses. Includes clinical medicine, surgery and reproduction and also epidemiology, pathology, microbiology, parasitology and toxicology.

d. hypotheses preliminary list of potential diagnoses.

d. kits commercially available tests used in the diagnosis of disease. Most are intended for biochemical estimation or the qualitative detection of antigen or antibody. Many are based on an ELISA.

d. plan in problem-oriented diagnosis, the systematic outline of procedures and tests to be undertaken in making a diagnosis.

d. points in acupuncture terminology include ASSOCIATION points (back *Shu* points and ALARM POINTS, front *Mu* points).

d. test tests likely to provide information which aids in the making of a diagnosis.

d. trail a standard procedure for making a clinical and laboratory examination so that nothing is omitted and so that the procedure can be checked or repeated.

diagnostician an expert in diagnosis.

diagnostics 1. the science and practice of diagnosis of disease. 2. a set of routines on a computer disk used to detect errors in the software when there is a system malfunction.

diagonal gait see diagonal GAIT.

diakinesis in cell division the stage of first meiotic prophase, in which the nucleolus and nuclear envelope disappear and the spindle fibers form.

dial-up a method of accessing a distant computer system by using a standard telephone line. Requires the use of a modem.

d. information service information is stored in a central database in a computer and can be accessed by telephone, although the user commonly has restricted access to some parts of the base. For higher fees it is possible to access more and more valuable information. Called also on-line information service.

di-allate a thiocarbamate herbicide; chronic poisoning causes anorexia, weight loss and alopecia. See also TRI-ALLATE.

di-allylacetamide a weedkiller. Acute poisoning is unlikely because of the large dose required. Chronic toxicity is possible.

DIALOG a comprehensive veterinary on-line service with information covering all diseases in all animal species since 1972. Put up by CAB. Available internationally via Lockheed's DIALOG system in California, USA.

dialog box window within a program which displays, in attention-catching boxes, messages, especially warnings, which direct the user to select and implement commands by pressing the appropriate command button.

Dialopsis africana African tree in the family Sapindaceae; contains a toxic saponin; plant causes diarrhea and dysentery in browsing ruminants.

dialysance the minute rate of net exchange of solute molecules passing through a membrane in dialysis.

dialysate the material passing through the membrane in dialysis. In peritoneal dialysis, the fluid infused and later removed from the peritoneal cavity.

dialysis the diffusion of solute molecules through a semipermeable membrane, passing from the side of higher concentration to that of the lower; a method sometimes used in cases of defective renal function to remove from the blood elements that are normally excreted in the urine (hemodialysis). The principles of dialysis are utilized in renal dialysis with a hemodialyzer (HEMODIALYSIS) and in PERITONEAL dialysis.

extracorporeal d. dialysis by a hemodialyzer. See HEMODIALYSIS.

peritoneal d. dialysis through the peritoneum, the dialyzing solution being introduced into and removed from the peritoneal cavity, as either a continuous or an intermittent procedure. See also PERITONEAL dialysis.

dialyzer an apparatus for performing dialysis; a hemodialyzer.

diameter the length of a straight line passing through the center of a circle and connecting opposite points on its circumference; hence the distance between the two specified opposite points on the periphery of a structure such as the cranium or pelvis.

cranial d's, craniometric d's imaginary lines connecting points on opposite surfaces of the cranium.

pelvic d. any of the diameters of the pelvis; any measurement that expresses the diameter of the birth canal in the female.

diamfenetide, diamphenethide a fasciolicide used in sheep; effective against immature flukes but with diminishing activity as the fluke ages. An effective compound for use in prophylactic programs against *Fasciola hepatica*.

diamide 1. compound containing two amido groups. 2. hydrazine.

diamidine 1. a compound that contains two amino acids. 2. a group of antiprotozoal drugs; includes phenamidine, pentamidine, diminazene and imidocarb.

diaminobutyric acid a neurotoxin in LATHYRUS *hirsutus*.

diaminodiphenoxyalkane a schistosomicidal drug; causes degeneration of pigmented retinal epithelium.

diaminophenylsulfone see DAPSONE.

3,4-diaminopyridine a parasympathomimetic agent, similar to 4-aminopyridine.

diaminopyrimidines synthetic antimicrobial agents that act as competitive antagonists in the conversion of folic acid to folinic acid. Examples are trimethoprim and pyrimethamine. Usually combined with a sulfonamide, providing a sequential blockade in nucleic acid synthesis.

diamniotic having or developing within separate amniotic cavities, as diamniotic twins.

diamond skin disease see swine ERYSIPELAS.

diamond snake a python, member of the subfamily Pythoninae, nonvenomous but a potent rodent controller.

Diamond's medium a culture medium especially suitable for culturing cervicovaginal mucus for the isolation of *Trichomonas foetus*.

diamorphine see HEROIN.

diamphenethide see DIAMFENETIDE.

Dianella revoluta plant in the family Liliaceae; contains stypandrol, a naphthoquinone, which causes encephalomalacia, neuronopathy and blindness, paresis, paralysis. No cases of poisoning with this plant appear to have been recorded. Called also blue flax lily.

dianthrone group of primary photosensitizing plant toxins, includes hypericin. Called also helianthrone.

diapause a state of inactivity and arrested development accompanied by greatly reduced metabolism, as in many eggs, insect pupae and plant seeds. It is a mechanism for surviving adverse weather conditions.

diapedesis the outward passage of blood cells through intact vessel walls.

diaphanoscope an instrument for transilluminating a body cavity.

diaphemetric pertaining to measurement of tactile sensibility.

diaphoresis perspiration, especially profuse perspiration.

diaphoretic 1. pertaining to, characterized by, or promoting diaphoresis. 2. an agent that promotes diaphoresis.

diaphragm 1. the musculomembranous partition separating the thoracic and abdominal cavities. On its sides, it is attached to the caudal ribs; ventrally to the sternum; at the back, to the spine. The esophagus, the aorta and vena cava, and nerves pass through the diaphragm. When relaxed, the diaphragm is convex but it flattens and moves caudally as it contracts during inhalation, thereby enlarging the chest cavity and allowing for expansion of the lungs. See also RESPIRATION. 2. any separating membrane or structure. 3. a disk with one or more openings or with an adjustable opening, mounted in relation to a lens, by which part of the light may be excluded from the area.

See also DIAPHRAGMATIC.

Potter–Bucky d. see Potter–Bucky GRID.

lightbeam d. an adjustable diaphragm which is used to cone down a light beam that indicates the dimensions of an x-ray beam and marks the position of the central ray.

pelvic d. the portion of the caudal wall of the pelvis formed by the coccygeus muscles, the levator ani muscles and fascia.

slit d. see FILTRATION membrane.

urogenital d. the musculomembranous layer superficial to the pelvic diaphragm, extending between the ischiopubic rami and surrounding the urogenital ducts.

diaphragma sellae a sheet of dura separating the pituitary gland in its fossa from the brain above.

diaphragmatic pertaining to the diaphragm.

d. abscess in the cow produces a syndrome of humped back, pain on percussion over the xiphoid area, fever and leukocytosis.

d. hernia in cattle, cases resulting from traumatic reticulitis show chronic ruminal tympany, distension, emaciation, anterior displacement of the heart with systolic murmur. Congenital cases in calves and those in cows due to trauma show dyspnea, displacement of the heart, and gut sounds audible in the chest. Horse cases are usually traumatic in origin and result in an acute onset of severe colic with no good distinguishing signs. In dogs and cats, uncommonly congenital but a common sequela to trauma with signs of dyspnea and pleural effusion. See also PERITONEOPERICARDIAL hernia.

d. rupture see diaphragmatic hernia (above).

d. septal defects include pleuroperitoneal and pericardioperitoneal defects.

synchronous d. flutter violent, unilateral hiccoughs occur with each heartbeat, sometimes with muscle tetany reminiscent of LACTATION TETANY; some cases of that disease also have flutter. Acid–base imbalance is present in most cases. Recovery is spontaneous and following treatment with calcium solutions.

d. tendon the heart-shaped tendinous center of the diaphragm.

diaphragmatocele see DIAPHRAGMATIC hernia.

diaphragmitis inflammation of the diaphragm.

diaphyseal pertaining to or affecting the shaft of a long bone (diaphysis).

d. aclasis see multiple cartilaginous EXOSTOSIS, inherited multiple EXOSTOSIS.

d. dysplasia see juvenile HYPEROSTOSIS.

diaphysectomy excision of part of a diaphysis.

diaphysial diaphyseal.

diaphysis pl. *diaphyses*. 1. the portion of a long bone between the ends or extremities, which are usually articular, and wider than the shaft; it consists of a tube of compact bone, enclosing the medullary cavity. Called also shaft. 2. the portion of a bone formed from a primary center of ossification.

diaplasis the setting of a fracture or reduction of a dislocation.

diapophysis a transverse process of a vertebra.

Diaporthe toxica see PHOMOPSIS LEPTOSTROMIFORMIS.

diapositive mask a mask used in subtraction radiography. It is prepared from a scout film of the site and masks out the high density shadows so that the one created by a contrast radiograph will be highlighted.

Diaptomus gracilis a diaptomid copepod, a first intermediate host of the cestode DIPHYLLOBOTHRIUM *latum*.

diapyesis suppuration.

diarrhea rapid movement of fecal matter through the intestine resulting in poor absorption of water, nutritive elements and electrolytes, and producing abnormally frequent evacuation of watery droppings.

The major causes are local irritation of the intestinal mucosa by infectious or chemical agents (gastroenteritis). In all types of diarrhea there is rapid evacuation of water and electrolytes resulting in a loss of these essential substances. Potassium supply especially is depleted by diarrhea, thus producing ACIDOSIS as well as FLUID VOLUME DEFICIT.

acute idiopathic d. acute diarrhea syndromes in horses which are not diagnosable, such as SALMONELLOSIS, STRONGYLOSIS, CYATHOSTOMIASIS, Potomac horse fever, COLITIS-X, antibiotic-induced diarrhea (above), INTESTINAL clostridiosis.

acute undifferentiated d. of the horse severe, acute diarrhea likely to be fatal may be related to stress or antibiotic therapy. See also COLITIS-X, INTESTINAL clostridiosis, SALMONELLOSIS.

bovine virus d. see BOVINE virus diarrhea.

campylobacter d. watery diarrhea without other obvious signs and without other obvious cause in yearling sheep, calves and foals. *Campylobacter fetus* subspp. *jejuni* and *intestinalis* have been suggested as causes. See also WINTER DYSENTERY.

chronic undifferentiated d. of the horse chronic, very watery diarrhea for very long periods but the horse has normal appetite and loses weight only gradually. Esthetically very displeasing to pleasure horse owners. Irreversible but not usually fatal.

ciliate d. colitis caused by TROGLODYTELLA in primates.

dietary d. a result of dietary indiscretion; occurs in all species. It is caused by the chemical or physical nature of the ingested material. The commonest occurrence of the syndrome is in newborn animals, especially those who ingest too much milk. There is often a history of access to an oversupply of milk or of a recent change of source to an over-rich milk replacer or indigestible components in replacer. It is also caused by too-rapid drinking. Affected animals are bright and alert and have a normal appetite but the feces are voluminous, soft to fluid and evil-smelling. Secondary bacterial enteritis may ensue but most cases recover spontaneously when the diet is adjusted. Scavenging dogs and cats ('garbage eaters') commonly ingest food that is spoiled or to which they are unaccustomed, resulting in various degrees of vomiting or diarrhea. Called also dietetic scours.

effusion d. caused by an increase in the transepithelial hydrostatic pressure gradient, such as occurs in congestive heart failure and hepatic portal hypertension.

epizootic porcine d. at least two types of epidemic diarrhea occur in pigs which are not transmissible gastroenteritis or due to other known cause.

large bowel d. in dogs and cats, signs referable to the site of enteric disease responsible for the diarrhea being the large intestine include tenesmus, mucus, hematochezia, and increased frequency of defecation.

malabsorptive d. villous atrophy, such as occurs with some viral infections, causes malabsorption diarrhea because of the reduction in area of absorptive intestinal epithelium.

nursery d. see NURSERY diarrhea.

osmotic d. an overload of unabsorbed osmotically active particles will attract and retain water, increasing fecal volume and causing diarrhea. Associated with maldigestion, malabsorption, overeating, excessive carbohydrates or fats. The basis for the laxative effect of magnesium sulfate, sodium sulfate or sodium phosphate.

psychogenic d. see irritable COLON syndrome.

secretory d. derangement of normal secretory and absorptive functions of intestinal epithelium such as occurs with bacterial enterotoxins may result in excessive secretion and a resulting diarrhea. *Escherichia coli* is the prime example of an infection with this effect.

small bowel d. in dogs and cats, signs referable to the site of enteric disease responsible for the diarrhea being the small intestine include lack of tenesmus or mucus, increased fecal volume, melena and weight loss.

undifferentiated d. of the newborn the situation in which a newborn animal (less than 7 days old) has life-threatening acute diarrhea. There is insufficient time and it would cost too much to differentiate between all of the possible causes. Added to this is the common occurrence in which there are two or more agents present, often acting in concert. Because of the need to treat these cases urgently and effectively if their lives are to be saved it has become the practice to group them together for the purposes of treatment and prognosis.

diarrheogenic giving rise to diarrhea.

diarrhoea see DIARRHEA.

diarthric pertaining to or affecting two different joints; biarticular; diarticular.

diarthrodial of the nature of a diarthrosis.

d. joint see DIARTHROSIS.

diarthrosis pl. *diarthroses* [Gr.] a specialized form of articulation in which there is more or less free movement, the union of the bony elements being surrounded by an articular capsule enclosing a cavity lined by synovial membrane; called also synovial joint.

d. rotatoria a joint characterized by mobility in a rotary direction.

diarticular pertaining to two joints; diarthric.

diaschisis loss of function and electrical activity in an area of the brain due to a lesion in a remote area that is neuronally connected with it.

diascopy a special technique for examination of erythematous skin lesions. If a clear glass slide, pressed over the lesion, causes the color to fade, there is vascular engorgement; if it does not fade, it is hemorrhage in the skin.

diastase a combination of enzymes produced during germination of seeds, and contained in malt; it converts starch into maltose and then into dextrose.

diastasis 1. dislocation or separation of two normally attached bones between which there is no true joint. Also, an abnormally large separation between associated bones, as between the ribs. 2. diastasis cordis, the rest period of the cardiac cycle, occurring just before systole.

diastema a space or cleft, e.g. the space in the dental arch between the incisors and canines and cheek teeth. Called also interdental space.

diastematocrania congenital longitudinal fissure of the cranium.

diastematomyelia abnormal congenital length-wise division of the spinal cord by a bony spicule or fibrous band protruding from a vertebra or two, into two halves, each of the halves being surrounded by a dural sac.

diastematopyelia congenital median fissure of the pelvis.

diastole the phase of the cardiac cycle in which the heart relaxes between contractions; specifically, the period when the two ventricles are dilated by the blood flowing into them. See also BLOOD PRESSURE and HEART.

diastrophic bent or curved; said of structures, such as bones, deformed in such manner.

diataxia ataxia affecting both sides of the body.

diathermal, diathermic pertaining to diathermy; permeable by heat waves.

diathermy the use of high-frequency electrical currents as a form of physical therapy and in surgical procedures.

Diathermy is used in physical therapy to deliver moderate heat directly to pathological lesions in the deeper tissues of the body. Surgically, the extreme heat that can be produced by diathermy may be used to destroy neoplasms, warts and infected tissues, and to cauterize blood vessels to prevent excessive bleeding. The technique is particularly valuable in neurosurgery and surgery of the eye. See also ELECTROSURGERY.

surgical d. electrosurgery.

diathesis an unusual constitutional susceptibility or predisposition to a particular disease, e.g. bleeding diathesis, EXUDATIVE diathesis.

diatomic 1. containing two atoms. 2. dibasic.

diatoms a series of unicellular algae, microscopic in size, with cell walls containing silica. Members of the family Diatomaceae. Their remains accumulate as geological deposits and are mined. See diatomaceous EARTH.

diatrizoate the most commonly used water-soluble, iodinated, radiopaque x-ray contrast medium.

diaveridine a folic acid antagonist used as a synergist with sulfonamides against *Eimeria* spp.

diazemuls see DIAZEPAM.

diazepam a benzodiazepine tranquilizer used as an antianxiety agent, a skeletal muscle relaxant, anticonvulsant, and as an appetite stimulant.

diazinon an organophosphorus insecticide, used in ear tags for cattle and in flea collars and rinses for dogs. Called also dimpylate. See also ORGANOPHOSPHORUS COMPOUND.

diazo- the group $-N_2-$.

diazotize to introduce the diazo group into a compound.

diazoxide an oral agent that inhibits insulin release, enhances glycogenolysis and inhibits the uptake of glucose; used to treat hypoglycemia due to hyperinsulinism.

dibasic containing two replaceable hydrogen atoms, or furnishing two hydrogen ions.

dibenzazepine derivative a group of α-blocking agents, e.g. azapetine.

Dibothriocephalus see DIPHYLLOBOTHRIUM.

dibromoethane a fungistat used to protect stored grain from weevils which causes fatal edema, fibrosis and alveolar epithelialization of the lungs when eaten by livestock.

dibromsalan one of two bromsalans (the other is tribromsalan) which, mixed in a variety of proportions, are used as treatments for liver flukes. See also BROMSALANS.

dibucaine a long-acting local anesthetic used topically and intraspinally in the form of the base and as the hydrochloride salt; the latter is also used intramuscularly for infiltration anesthesia. Called also cinchocaine. Has a special characteristic of needing only a small dose (about one-fortieth the dose of procaine).

dibutyltin dilaurate a coccidiostat used in commercial poultry.

d. d. poisoning feeding to calves in error causes diarrhea and polyuria.

DIC disseminated intravascular COAGULATION.

dicamba a benzoic acid herbicide of very low toxicity. Very large doses cause anorexia, weight loss and stiffness of the hindlimbs.

dicarboxylic acid any organic molecule containing two carboxyl groups.

dicelous, dicoelus 1. hollowed on each of two sides. 2. having two cavities.

Dicentra a genus of the Fumariaceae family of plants; contain an isoquinoline alkaloid which causes a syndrome of diarrhea, incoordination and other nervous signs. Includes *D. cucullaria* (dutchman's breeches), *D. canadensis* (squirrel corn), *D. eximia* (wild bleeding heart), *D. formosa* (western bleeding heart), *D. spectabilis* (dutchman's breeches, wild bleeding heart). Called also *Bikukulla* spp.

dicephalous having two heads.

dicephalus a monster with two heads.

Dicerorhinus see RHINOCEROS.

Diceros see RHINOCEROS.

D. bicornis black rhinoceros.

Dichapetalum African genus of the plant family Dichapetalaceae; contain high levels of fluoroacetate; cause very sudden death, preceded in some cases by momentary tremor. Includes *D. braunii*, *D. cymosum* (*D. venenatum*, poison leaf, gibflaar), *D. deflexum*, *D. guineense*, *D. heudelotii*, *D. macrocarpum*, *D. michelsonii*, *D. mossambicense*, *D. ruhlandiii*, *D. stuhlmanii*, *D. tomentosum*, *D. toxicarium* (ratsbane).

Dichelobacter nodosus causative bacteria of infectious footrot of sheep and goats. Called also *Bacteroides nodosus*.

dichlone a fungicide, algacide and herbicide used to treat seeds and water.

dichloralphenazone a complex of chloral and phenazone, a sedative and hypnotic.

dichlormate a carbamate organic herbicide; has low toxicity but in very large doses causes diarrhea, abdominal pain and bloat in cattle.

dichloro-diphenyl-trichloroethane DDT.

dichloroethylsulfide a chemical warfare agent. Called also mustard gas.

dichloroformoxime a gas which causes painful skin irritation. Used as a crowd harrassing agent. Called also nettle gas.

dichlorophen a phenol derivative used as a teniacide; superseded except in combination with piperazine and other compounds.

2,4-dichlorophenoxyacetic acid a herbicide not known to be toxic at normal use rates in agriculture.

Spraying may increase nitrate content of sprayed plants to toxic levels. Called also 2,4-D.

S-dichlorovinyl-L-cysteine a compound thought to be the toxic agent in trichlorethylene-extracted SOYBEAN meal poisoning.

dichlorovos an organophosphorus compound. See DICHLORVOS.

dichlorphenamide a carbonic anhydrase inhibitor used to reduce intraocular pressure in glaucoma.

dichlorvos a broad-spectrum organophosphorus insecticide and anthelmintic. Can be combined with polyvinyl chloride resin and when administered orally or in collars or ear tags to give a slow release effect.

dichoptic said of eyes which are widely separated, e.g. in some insects.

dichorial, dichorionic having two distinct chorions; said of dizygotic twins.

Dichrocephalia chrysanthemifolia small perennial African shrub, in the family Asteraceae; contains an unidentified toxin; plant toxic only when there are green shoots. An unidentified toxin causes diarrhea and abortion.

dichroic characterized by dichroism.

dichroism the quality or condition of showing one color in reflected and another in transmitted light.

dichromate a salt containing the bivalent Cr_2O_7 radical.

dichromatic pertaining to or characterized by dichromatism.

dichromatism 1. the quality of existing in or exhibiting two different colors. 2. dichromatopsia.

Dickinson–Nunamaker procedure a surgical technique for intra-articular reconstruction of the cranial cruciate ligament which involves a modification of the Paatsama procedure in which the fascia graft based on the craniolateral tibia is placed directly into the joint and emerges through a tunnel in the lateral femoral condyle before being sutured to itself.

diclofenac a nonsteroidal anti-inflammatory agent, used topically in ophthalmic diseases.

dicloxacillin a semisynthetic penicillinase-resistant penicillin used primarily in the treatment of infections due to penicillinase-resistant staphylococci.

dicoria double pupil.

dicoumarol, dicumarol a potent anticoagulant that acts by inhibiting the synthesis of vitamin K-dependent clotting factors (prothrombin and factors VII, IX and X) in the liver; used in the prevention and treatment of thromboembolic disorders. Produced naturally by conversion of nontoxic coumarin in moldy sweet clover hay or sweet vernal hay. Eating the hay causes blood loss due to spontaneous hemorrhage. Formerly called bishydroxycoumarin. See also MELILOTUS, ANTHOXANTHUM ODORATUM.

dicrocoeliasis hepatic fascioliasis due to infection with DICROCOELIUM *dendriticum*.

Dicrocoelium a genus of flukes (digenetic trematodes) in the family Dicrocoeliidae.

***D. dendriticum* (syn. *D. lanceolatum*)** a liver fluke that infects most domestic and many wild animals and has been reported in humans. Heavy infestation causes cirrhosis and biliary obstruction and a clinical syndrome of edema, anemia and emaciation.

D. hospes occurs in the bile ducts of cattle in Africa.

dicrotic having the characteristic of dicrotism, e.g. the dicrotic notch of the pulse.

dicrotism the occurrence of two sphygmographic waves or elevations to one beat of the pulse.

dictyate a stage in the development of oocytes which are arrested at the same stage of meiotic prophase; the stage varies between species.

Dictyocaulus a genus of lungworms in the family Dictyocaulidae. Includes *D. arnfieldi* (see below) and *D. cameli* (camels), *D. eckerti* (deer), *D. filaria* (see below), *D. viviparus* (see below).

D. arnfieldi primarily a lungworm of donkeys but has little clinical effect in them. The infestation in horses is also clinically innocuous and the worms do not usually mature in this species.

D. filaria lungworms that cause a chronic disease in small ruminants. Clinical signs are limited to persistent cough, moderate dyspnea and loss of condition. Young sheep and goats may be severely affected, occasionally fatally.

D. viviparus the common lungworm of cattle causes several serious diseases including verminous pneumonia, acute interstitial pneumonia and secondary bacterial pneumonia. The infestation is widespread and affects mainly young cattle. Massive larval intakes can cause a high mortality due to a peracute syndrome of interstitial pneumonia. More moderate infestations cause a syndrome of paroxysmal coughing, moderate dyspnea and loss of condition. A few calves may die as a result of a secondary bacterial pneumonia. Warm moist autumnal conditions are most conducive to serious outbreaks.

dictyoma see DIKTYOMA.

dictyosome see GOLGI STACK.

dicyclomine an anticholinergic; the hydrochloride is used as a gastrointestinal antispasmodic.

didactylism the presence of only two digits on the paws of a usually five-toed animal.

didelphia the condition of having a double uterus.

Didelphis see OPOSSUM.

dideoxynucleotide a synthetic molecule used in enzymatic DNA sequencing.

didymalgia pain in a testis.

didymitis inflammation of a testis.

Didymotheca cupressiformis see GYROSTEMON *tepperi*.

didymous occurring in pairs.

didymus a testis; also used as a word termination designating a fetus with duplication of parts or one consisting of conjoined symmetrical twins.

diecious sexually distinct; denoting species in which male and female genitals do not occur in the same individual. In botany, having staminate and pistillate flowers on separate plants.

Dieffenbach forceps small, thumb-operated spring forceps that cross over so that releasing the blades causes the tips to close.

Dieffenbachia a genus of the plant family Araceae; contains insoluble raphide oxalate crystals, and possibly other toxins, which cause severe irritation of the oral mucosa, especially swelling of the tongue. Includes *D. maculata*, *D. picta*, *D. seguinae*. Called also dumbcane.

diehard nickname for the Scottish terrier.

dieldrin see CHLORINATED HYDROCARBONS.

dielectric said of an insulating substance through which an electric force acts by induction but not conduction.

diembryony the production of two embryos from a single egg.

diencephalic pertaining to or arising from the diencephalon.

d. infundibulum funnel-shaped diverticulum of the third ventricle which contributes to the formation of the caudal surface of the adenohypophysis, the distal part forming the neurohypophysis.

d. syndrome an uncommon paraneoplastic syndrome seen in dogs in which a tumor in the diencephalon is associated with abnormalities of the hypothalamus, hypophysis, including high levels of growth hormone, and autonomic nervous system.

diencephalon 1. the caudal part of the forebrain, consisting of the hypothalamus, thalamus, metathalamus and epithalamus; the subthalamus is often considered to be a distinct division. 2. the more caudal of the two brain vesicles formed by specialization of the prosencephalon in the developing embryo. See also BRAINSTEM.

dienestrol a synthetic derivative of diethylstilbestrol.

Dientamoeba a genus of amebas commonly found in the colon and appendix of primates and of humans.

D. fragilis occurs in the cecum of humans and monkeys. A species that has been associated with diarrhea but its pathogenicity is unclear.

dieresis 1. the division or separation of parts normally united. 2. the surgical separation of parts.

diesel oil a common fuel on farms. Grazing ruminants are most likely to be poisoned by diesel fuel, especially cattle who find petroleum products palatable. Obvious clinical signs are anorexia, mild bloat, vomiting and aspiration pneumonia. The feces are oily and have a characteristic smell.

diesoline see DIESEL OIL.

diestral shift in vaginal cytology of the bitch, the rapid change from predominantly superficial epithelial cells to parabasilar cells which occurs at the end of estrus and the beginning of diestrus.

diestrus the resting period between estral periods of animals. The female rejects the male, blood levels of estrogens are minimal and progesterone levels are high. This provides a physiological state in the uterus which is most conducive for implantation and growth of the developing fetus. Diestrus is terminated by luteolytic factors, such as prostaglandin $F_{2[alpha]}$ secreted by the endometrium, if pregnancy does not occur.

diet the customary amount and kind of food and drink taken by an animal from day to day; more narrowly, a diet planned to meet specific requirements of the animal, including or excluding certain foods. See also WINTER DIET.

acid d. diets of low alkalinity which are fed to cows to prevent milk fever. The diet in the 4 weeks preceding parturition, which is ordinarily highly alkaline, is supplemented with calcium chloride, and aluminum and magnesium sulfates, to reduce this alkalinity.

bland d. one that is free from any irritating or stimulating foods.

calcium homeostatic d. a diet aimed at maintaining normal blood levels of calcium in recently calved cows.

calculolytic d. formulated to aid in the dissolution of struvite uroliths. Usually provides a low intake of protein, restricts phosphorus and magnesium, and acidifies the urine. Additional salt may also be included. These have been used successfully in dogs and cats.

computerized d. a computer can be programmed to prepare a least cost diet from a database of ingredients which includes percentages of the known macro- and micronutrients.

deficient d. see NUTRITIONAL deficiency disease.

drought feeding d. see DROUGHT FEEDING.

elemental d. contains nutrients as small molecular weight compounds, i.e. proteins as amino acids or peptides, carbohydrates as oligosaccharides or monosaccharides, and fats as medium-chain triglycerides. Used in the treatment of gastrointestinal disease. Called also monomeric diet.

elimination d. one for diagnosing food allergy, based on the sequential omission of foods which might cause the clinical signs in the patient.

geriatric d. may vary in composition; generally, they are formulated to provide lower energy intake and increased digestibility.

gluten-free d. one without wheat, rye, barley, buckwheat, or oats or related products.

high-calorie d., high-energy d. one that furnishes more calories than needed for maintenance; used to increase body condition, in recovery from illness and for maintenance under stressful conditions.

high-fiber d. one relatively high in dietary fiber; in dogs and cats, used in the management of large and small bowel diarrhea, diabetes mellitus, constipation and obesity.

high-protein d. one containing large amounts of protein; used in the management of dogs and cats recovering from illness.

home-prepared d. one prepared in the home kitchen, in contrast with commercially prepared pet foods.

hypoallergenic d. one formulated to avoid suspected allergens; usually used in the management of allergic skin or bowel disease.

liquid d. a diet limited to liquids or to foods that can be changed to a liquid state.

low-calorie d. one containing fewer calories than needed to maintain weight; normally used in management of obesity in dogs and cats.

low-fat d. one containing limited amounts of fat; used in the management of pancreatic disease, bowel disease, and obesity in dogs and cats.

low-fiber d. see low-residue diet (below).

low purine d. in dogs and cats, generally a low-meat diet.

low-residue d. one with a minimum of cellulose and fiber and restriction of connective tissue found in certain cuts of meat. It is prescribed for irritations of the intestinal tract, after surgery of the large intestine, in partial intestinal obstruction, or when limited bowel movements are desirable. Called also low-fiber diet.

low vitamin A d. one containing low levels of vitamin A; in dog and cat diets, this would mean little or no organ meats. The only probable indication for such a diet is in the treatment of hypervitaminosis A.

lower urinary tract disease d. one that promotes acidification of the urine and containing restricted magnesium and phosphorus, and sometimes increased salt.

monomeric d. see elemental diet (above).

phosphate-restricted d. one containing restricted amounts of phosphorus; used in the management of chronic renal disease.

polymeric d. meal replacement diets; fed to animals with almost normal gastrointestinal function. Proteins, fats and carbohydrates are present in high molecular weight forms.

sodium-restricted d. used in management of congestive heart failure and systemic hypertension in dogs and cats.

dietary 1. pertaining to diet. 2. a course or system of diet.

d. hepatic necrosis see HEPATOSIS dietetica.

d. indigestion see INDIGESTION.

d. mineral tolerance levels of minerals in the diet which animals will tolerate without impairing their productivity.

d. requirement the amount of each dietary constituent required in the diet for the animal to produce efficiently. In some individuals the requirements are abnormally high compared to the rest of the population.

dietetic pertaining to diet or proper food.

d. microangiopathy occurs in pigs on diets deficient in selenium and vitamin E.

d. scours see dietary DIARRHEA.

dietetics the science of diet and nutrition.

diethyl ether see ETHER (1).

diethylcarbamazine an antifilarial agent used in dogs as the citrate salt for the prevention of heartworm. Used also for the treatment of ascarids in dogs and immature lungworms in cattle and sheep.

diethyldithiocarbamate a carbamate insecticide; causes spinal cord tract degeneration in chickens.

diethylene glycol antifreezing agent. Causes poisoning similar to ETHYLENE glycol.

diethylenetriamine penta-acetic acid a chelating agent (abbreviated DTPA); used in nuclear medicine in preparing radiopharmaceuticals, e.g. ^{99m}Tc-DTPA. Called also pentetic acid.

diethylstilbestrol a synthetic nonsteroidal estrogen; abbreviated DES. In cattle used to treat infertility and as a stimulant to weight gain by increasing muscular development. Its use is limited as a weight gain stimulant because of the possible entry of the compound into the human food chain. Excessive, long-term administration causes anal prolapse, abortion, fracture of the pelvis and nymphomaniac behavior. Sometimes used in dogs to treat misalliance and urinary incontinence, but limited by its myelotoxic effects.

diethylthiambutene hydrochloride an analgesic with an effect like that of morphine. Highly toxic to cats. Can cause convulsions if injected intravenously. Called also Themalon.

diethyltoluamide an insect repellent used on dogs and cats. Toxicity has been reported with vomiting, tremors and seizures. Called also DEET.

dietitian one who is concerned with the promotion of good health through proper diet and with the therapeutic use of diet in the treatment of disease.

dietotherapy the scientific regulation of diet in treating disease, especially important in patients with inborn errors of metabolism and various other metabolic diseases.

difenacoum a potent, synthetic anticoagulant rodenticide with prolonged antagonism of vitamin K.

difenoxin a meperidine derivative used to control diarrhea.

Diff-Quik stain a commercial name for a Romanowsky stain which can be applied rapidly to smears of aspirated cells or exudate.

difference in mathematical terms the result after subtracting one value from another; the difference may be negative or positive.

differential exhibiting or depending on a difference.

d. absorption see differential ABSORPTION.

d. cell count see differential COUNT.

d. diagnosis the differences between diseases in terms of clinical signs and epidemiological parameters; used as a basis for selecting as a diagnosis the one with the best fit to those seen in the subject.

d. leukocyte count see differential COUNT.

d. milk cell counts count of cells in a milk sample including individual counts of somatic cells and individual leukocyte types.

d. thromboplastin time used in differentiating the cause of hemophilia. Reagents containing either factor VIII or factor IX are added in the partial thromboplastin time test to demonstrate which factor corrects the prolonged clotting time.

differentiation 1. the distinguishing of one thing from another. 2. the act or process of acquiring completely individual characteristics, such as occurs in the progressive diversification of cells and tissues in the embryo, e.g. sex differentiation. 3. increase in morphological or chemical heterogeneity.

diffraction the bending or breaking up of a ray of light into its component parts.

x-ray d. a method used to determine the three-dimensional structure of the single object, e.g. protein molecule, that composes the crystal. Based on recording and analyzing the diffraction pattern of an x-ray beam passing through a crystalline structure, either organic or inorganic.

diffusate material that has diffused through a membrane.

diffuse 1. not definitely limited or localized. 2. to pass through or to spread widely through a tissue or substance.

d. intravascular coagulation see disseminated intravascular COAGULATION.

d. placentation see PLACENTATION.

diffuse interstitial pulmonary fibrosis see interstitial PNEUMONIA.

diffusing capacity the rate at which a gas diffuses across the alveolar–capillary membrane per unit difference in the partial pressure of the gas across the membrane, expressed in ml/min/mmHg. Because of their high affinity for hemoglobin both oxygen and carbon monoxide are limited in their rate of diffusion by their diffusing capacity.

diffusion 1. the state or process of being widely spread. 2. the spontaneous mixing of the molecules or ions of two or more substances resulting from random thermal motion; its rate is proportional to the concentrations of the substances and it increases with the temperature.

In the body fluids the molecules of water, gases, and the ions of substances in solution are in constant motion. As each molecule moves about, it bounces off other molecules and loses some of its energy to each molecule it hits, but at the same time it gains energy from the molecules that collide with it.

The rate of diffusion is influenced by the size of the molecules; larger molecules move less rapidly, because they require more energy to move about. Molecules of a solution of higher concentration move more rapidly toward those of a solution of lesser concentration; in other words, the rate of movement from higher to lower concentration is greater than the movement in the opposite direction.

d. coefficient the number of milliliters of a gas that will diffuse at a distance of 0.001 mm over a square centimeter surface per minute, at 1 atmosphere of pressure. The diffusion coefficient for any given gas is proportional to the solubility and molecular weight of the gas. The diffusion coefficient for oxygen is 1.0, for carbon dioxide it is 20.3, and for nitrogen it is 0.53. The diffusion capacity of a gas varies directly with the diffusion coefficient.

facilitated d. mechanisms in intestinal absorption which assist the passage of those products of digestion, which cannot occur by simple diffusion, across the intestinal cell membranes. They include a carrier mechanism involving proteins, and active transport which provides energy from the breakdown of high-energy phosphate bonds.

Fick's first law of d. see FICK'S FIRST LAW OF DIFFUSION.

d. hypoxia a transient hypoxic episode after the cessation of nitrous oxide anesthesia if air is inhaled instead of pure oxygen; caused by the rapid diffusion of nitrous oxide out into the alveoli diluting the oxygen that is there.

diflorasone diacetate a corticosteroid used topically in treatment of inflammatory skin diseases.

diflubenzuron an ectoparasiticide similar to LUFENURON.

diflunisal a salicylic acid derivative that, like aspirin, has analgesic and anti-inflammatory properties.

difluoromethylornithine EFLORNITHINE hydrochloride.

difluorotetrachloroethane see TETRACHLORODIFLUORETHANE.

digastric 1. having two bellies. 2. digastric muscle. See Table 13.

Digenea a subclass of trematodes that includes most of the flukes of veterinary importance.

digenean pertaining to or of the nature of members of the fluke subclass Digenea.

digenetic 1. having two stages of multiplication, one sexual in the mature forms, the other asexual in the larval stages. 2. belonging to the subclass of flukes Digenea.

d. trematodes see DIGENEA.

DiGeorge's syndrome an immunodeficiency syndrome in humans and mice, associated with thymic hypoplasia or aplasia and absence of T lymphocytes, resulting from a congenital absence of the third and fourth branchial pouches.

digesta alimentary tract contents undergoing digestion.

digestant 1. assisting or stimulating digestion. 2. an agent capable of aiding digestion.

digestibility the proportion of a feed or diet which can be digested by the normal animal of the subject species.

d. coefficient see digestibility COEFFICIENT.

digestible having the quality of being able to be digested.

d. energy the proportion of the potential energy in a feed which is in fact digested.

d. protein see digestible PROTEIN.

total d. nutrients see TOTAL DIGESTIBLE NUTRIENTS.

digestion 1. the act or process of converting food into chemical substances that can be absorbed into the blood and utilized by the body tissues. 2. the subjection of a substance to prolonged heat and moisture, so as to disintegrate and soften it.

Digestion is accomplished by physically breaking down, churning, diluting and dissolving the food substances, and also by splitting them chemically into simpler compounds. Carbohydrates are eventually broken down to monosaccharides (simple sugars); proteins are broken down into amino acids; and fats are absorbed as fatty acids, monoglycerides and glycerol (glycerin).

The digestive process takes place in the alimentary canal or DIGESTIVE system. The salivary glands, liver, gallbladder and pancreas are located outside the alimentary canal, but they are considered accessory organs of digestion because their secretions provide essential enzymes and other substances.

avian d. differs markedly from mammals in the mouth; there are no teeth, dental functions being performed by the beak and the muscular gizzard; the esophagus, in other than owls and insectivorous species, has one or two crops, dilations where ingesta are held temporarily.

enzymatic d. most digestive processes in monogastric animals are enzymatic brought about by enzymes secreted into the lumen of the gastrointestinal tract and enzymes located at the brush borders of the intestinal epithelium.

d. error any disruption of the normal digestive process; caused by abnormal ingesta, either chemically or physically, or by an error in the physiological and biochemical processes which constitute digestion.

gastric d. digestion by the action of gastric juice.

impaired d. see MALDIGESTION.

intestinal d. digestion by the action of intestinal juices, bile and pancreatic juice.

luminal phase d. the stage of the digestion of fats that goes on in the lumen of the intestine; as distinct from the mucosal phase that occurs in the epithelial cells.

pancreatic d. digestion by the action of pancreatic juice.

peptic d. gastric digestion by pepsin.

primary d. digestion occurring in the gastrointestinal tract.

ruminant d. characterized by the fermentative functions that are carried on in the forestomachs. Cellulose is readily digested with the output of short-chain fatty acids being the chief energy source for the animal. Nonprotein nitrogen is utilized by the ruminal bacteria for the manufacture of protein which is later available for the satisfaction of the animal's protein needs.

salivary d. the change of starch into maltose by the saliva; most marked in humans.

d. tests see STARCH digestion test, LACTOSE digestion test, GELATIN digestion test.

digestive pertaining to digestion.

d. enzymes include **salivary** (amylase), **gastric** (pepsin), **pancreatic** (trypsin, chymotrypsin, amylase, lipase), **small intestinal mucosa** (carbohydrases including isomaltase, lactase, maltase, sucrase, trehalase).

d. inoculant administered mostly to neonates primarily to provide an inoculum of beneficial bacteria and protozoa essential to proper digestion and usually picked up from the environment. In many commercial products the irresistible temptation to include other materials, including dietary essential vitamins and minerals, clouds the effect of the inoculant, and may, as in iron poisoning in foals, cause disaster.

d. system the organs that have as their particular function the ingestion, digestion and absorption of food or nutritive elements. They include the mouth, teeth, tongue, pharynx, esophagus, stomach and intestines. The accessory organs of digestion, which contribute secretions important to digestion, include the salivary glands, pancreas, liver and gallbladder. Birds have an unusual system in that there are no teeth and no soft palate in most. There is a pregastric buffer, the crop; the stomach is separated into two organs, one secretory and one muscular, and the large intestine is replaced by a dual cecum. The rectum empties into a cloaca which is shared with the urogenital tract. The ruminant system is complicated by the presence of the forestomachs, the reticulum, rumen and omasum, and there are no upper incisor teeth. The peculiarities of horses are the greatly distended large intestine and the absence of a gallbladder.

d. tract the digestive system less the ancillary organs of salivary glands, liver and pancreas; the luminal organs through which food passes. See also ALIMENTARY canal.

digit 1. a toe in cats, dogs and chickens, a foot in the horse, a claw or cleat in cattle, sheep, goats and pigs. Called also a cleat in sheep. 2. any of the ten numerals in the series 0 to 9.

digital emanating from or pertaining to the digit.

d. cushion a wedge-shaped mass of white and elastic fibers mixed with some fat and islands of cartilage overlying the frog of the horse's hoof and acting as a shock absorbing mechanism.

d. dermatitis herd lameness characterized by round, painful, raised lesion on the back of the pastern, most commonly on hindlimb of cattle, especially heifers. Invasive spirochete in lesion; responds well to antibiotic treatment.

d. nerve block local anesthesia of a digit, effected by a ring block in which a transverse plane is infiltrated, a local intravenous injection, or by a local block of individual nerves. The latter is more prone to failure if the anatomy of the part is not well established.

d. pad see FOOTPAD.

regional intravenous d. nerve block local anesthesia procured by ligaturing the digit and injecting the local anesthetic. The anesthetic is left confined to the digit for the duration of the ligaturing. A preferred technique for cattle digital surgery.

d. sheath a common synovial sheath shared, in ruminants and horses, by the superficial and deep digital flexor tendons.

digitalin a mixture of digitalis glycosides extracted from the seeds of *Digitalis purpurea*.

Digitalis a genus of herbs in the family Scrophulariaceae; contains digitalis-related (cardenolide) cardiac glycosides, e.g. digoxin, lanatoside. Includes *D. lanata* (woolly foxglove), *D. purpurea* (purple foxglove). Sources of commercial digitalis.

digitalis dried leaf of *Digitalis purpurea*; used as a cardiotonic agent. All drugs prepared from this digitalis leaf are members of the same group and principles of administration are the same. The drugs vary according to speed of action and potency. Digitalis can be very effective in the treatment of various cardiac conditions, but its therapeutic range is very narrow; a therapeutic dose is only about one-third less than the dose that will induce toxicity. Toxicity is manifested by vomiting, diarrhea, cardiac irregularity and heart failure.

d. glycosides DIGITOXIN, DIGOXIN.

digitalization the administration of digitalis in a dosage schedule designed to produce and then maintain optimal therapeutic concentrations of its cardiotonic glycosides.

Digitaria grass genus containing a large number of valuable species in the family Poaceae. Contains cyanogenetic glycosides, can cause cyanide, and possibly oxalate, poisoning. Includes *D. eriantha* (*D. decumbens*), *D. didactyla*, *D. saginata*, *D. sanguinalis*. Called also crabgrass, pangola grass, summer grass.

D. exilis seed is used for human and animal food, and the plant for pasture or hay. Called also hungry rice, acha.

digitation 1. a finger-like process. 2. surgical creation of a functioning digit by making a cleft between two adjacent metacarpal bones, after amputation of some or all of the digits.

digitiform finger-like.

digitigrade a form of locomotion in which the animal walks only on its digits, e.g. dogs, contrasted with plantigrade, in which the animal walks on its metatarsi, metacarpi, e.g. bears, humans.

digitonin a saponin in *Digitalis purpurea*. It has no effect on heart muscle.

digitoxigenin a metabolic product of the cardioactive alkaloids, digitoxin and gitoxin.

digitoxin a cardiotonic glycoside obtained from *Digitalis purpurea* and other species of the same genus; used in the treatment of congestive heart failure.

digitoxose a desoxy sugar, a metabolic product of digitoxin and gitoxin.

diglossia bifid tongue.

diglyceride a glyceride containing two fatty acid molecules in ester linkage.

dignathus a fetus with two lower jaws.

digoxin a cardiotonic glycoside obtained from the leaves of *Digitalis lanata*; used in the treatment of congestive heart failure.

DiGuglielmo's syndrome erythroleukemia.

digyny fertilization of one ovum by more than one spermatozoon.

dihematoporphyrin ether a photosensitizing agent used in photodynamic treatment of neoplasms.

dihydrocodeine an opioid analgesic and antitussive.

dihydrocodeinone see HYDROCODONE.

dihydroergotamine hydrogenated ergotamine, an alpha-adrenergic blocking agent and vasoconstrictor.

dihydrofolate reductase enzyme catalyzing the conversion of folate to 5,6,7,8-tetrahydrofolate, which is the key carrier of one-carbon units in purine and pyridime synthesis, the pathway for the breakdown of histidine and the synthesis of *S*-adenosylmethionine from *S*-adenosylhomocysteine. This enzyme is the target for methotrexate, which inhibits enzyme action, a key means of inducing remissions in acute leukemias.

dihydrolipoic acid an essential coenzyme of pyruvic oxidase.

dihydrostreptomycin an aminoglycoside antibiotic produced by the hydrogenation of STREPTOMYCIN; ototoxic with damage to sensory end organs.

dihydrotachysterol a synthetic steroid derived from tachysterol; an antihypocalcemic agent used in the treatment of hypoparathyroidism.

dihydrotestosterone reduced, more active form of testosterone in males; associated with follicular atresia in the female.

dihydroxyanthraquinone see DANTHRON.

dihydroxycholecalciferol a group of active metabolites of cholecalciferol (vitamin D_3) numbered according to the carbon atom(s) on which a hydroxyl group is substituted. 1,25-Dihydroxycholecalciferol (calcitriol) is the most active derivative; the 25-hydroxylation occurs in the liver under the influence of substrate concentration whereas the second 1-hydroxylation occurs in the kidney mitochondria under regulation by parathyroid hormone in response to decreases in plasma calcium concentration. 1α,25-Dihydroxycholecalciferol acts like a steroid hormone stimulating calcium absorption from the small intestine and calcium mobilization from bone.

dihydroxycoumarin glycoside a group of plant toxins including daphnin and daphnetin in *Daphne* spp. and other plants.

3,4-dihydroxyphenylalanine dopa.

1,25-dihydroxyvitamin D_3 see DIHYDROXYCHOLECALCIFEROL.

1,25-dihydroxyvitamin D_3 glycoside the calcinogenic agent in SOLANUM *malacoxylon* and related plants.

diiodohydroxyquinoline see IODOQUINOL.

di-iodotyrosine, diiodotyrosine a step in the pathway to the formation of thyroglobulin in the thyroid gland. I_2 conjugates with tyrosine to form compounds which are then coupled to form thyronines, the principal thyroid hormones.

di-isopropyl phosphorofluoridate, diisopropyl phosphorofluoridate an ophthalmic cholinergic used as a miotic; called also isoflurophate.
dikkop cardiac form of AFRICAN HORSE SICKNESS.
dikoor see yellow BIGHEAD.
diktyoma a tumor of the ciliary epithelium resembling embryonic retinal tissue in structure.
Dikukulla canadensis DICENTRA *canadensis*.
dilaceration a tearing apart, as of a cataract. In dentistry, an abnormal angulation or curve in the root or crown of a formed tooth.
dilan a chlorinated hydrocarbon used as an insecticide.
dilatation, dilation 1. the condition, as of an orifice or tubular structure, of being dilated or stretched beyond normal dimensions. 2. the act of dilating or stretching. See under anatomical location, e.g. esophageal, cardiac, intestinal, gastric, pupillary.
  d.–torsion syndrome see GASTRIC dilatation–volvulus.
dilated a state of dilatation.
  d. cardiomyopathy see congestive CARDIOMYOPATHY.
  d. pupil syndrome see feline DYSAUTONOMIA (Key–Gaskell syndrome).
dilation see DILATATION.
dilator a structure (muscle) that dilates, or an instrument used to dilate.
  d. pupillae muscle dilator muscle of the pupil.
diltiazem a calcium-channel blocking agent used to produce peripheral and coronary vasodilation in the management of heart disease.
diluent 1. diluting. 2. an agent that dilutes or renders less potent or irritant.
  semen d. see semen EXTENDER.
dilution 1. reduction of concentration of an active substance by admixture of a neutral agent. 2. a substance that has undergone dilution.
  limit d. a method of obtaining a pure culture of bacteria or virus by subculturing from the highest dilution in which the organism is demonstrably present.
  serial d. 1. the progressive dilution of a substance or infectious agent in a series of tubes or wells in a tray in predetermined ratios, e.g. 2-fold or 10-fold dilution steps. 2. a method of obtaining a pure bacterial culture by rapid transfer of a small amount of material from one nutrient medium to a succeeding one of the same volume.
dimenhydrinate an antihistamine used as an antinauseant and antiemetic.
dimensional data see dimensional DATA.
dimer chemical compound formed by the union of two identical molecules.
dimercaprol a chelating agent used in the treatment of heavy metal poisoning. The drug forms a relatively stable compound with arsenic, mercury, gold and certain other metals, thus protecting the vital enzyme systems of the cells against the effects of the metals. It is sometimes diluted with water and used to wash the stomach, some of the solution being permitted to remain in the stomach. At the dose levels required for effect in ruminants at the level of poison dose experienced in agriculture, dimercaprol is itself poisonous. The drug has a very disagreeable skunklike odor and should be handled carefully to avoid spilling. Called also British antilewisite, BAL, dimercaptopropanol.
dimercaptopropanol see DIMERCAPROL.
dimethicone a silicone oil used as a skin protective and as an antifoaming agent in the treatment of frothy bloat in ruminants.
  activated d. see SIMETHICONE.
dimethindene an antihistaminic, used as the maleate salt.
dimethisoquin a local anesthetic; used topically to relieve pain and pruritus.
dimethoate an organophosphorus contact insecticide used principally as a premise spray; capable of causing poisoning. Chronic intake causes salivation and diarrhea in calves.
dimethyl ether of *d*-tubocurarine a little-used muscle relaxant used as an adjunct to general anesthesia.
dimethyl phthalate an insect repellent, sometimes used topically on dogs to discourage licking of skin lesions. Abbreviated DMP.
dimethyl sulfoxide see DMSO.
***p*-dimethylaminoazobenzene** see BUTTER YELLOW.
dimethyldisulfide a hemolytic agent produced in the rumen by bacterial action on *S*-methylcysteine sulfoxide; present in *Brassica* spp. plants.
dimethylnitrosamine a potent hepatoxin in HERRING MEAL. Chronic poisoning causes changes reminiscent of neoplasia and the substance is now regarded as a carcinogen.
dimethylnortestosterone see MIBOLERONE.
dimethylpolysiloxane dimethicone.
dimethyltryptamine 1. a group of alkaloids found in the grass *Phalaris aquatica* and known to be closely associated with the acute form of poisoning with this plant. 2. a hallucinogenic substance derived from the plant *Prestonia amazonica*; abbreviated DMT.
dimetilan a chlorinated hydrocarbon used as insecticide.
dimetria a condition characterized by a double uterus.
dimetridazole a nitrothiazole compound used therapeutically and prophylactically in histomoniasis in turkeys. Poisoning is manifested by infertility and hepatic and renal insufficiency.
dimidium bromide a compound used in the treatment of trypanosomiasis.
diminazene a diamidine antiprotozoal agent used as the aceturate.
diminishing returns the characteristic of any production system in which increases in variable inputs result in increasing reduction of total output. An indicator of when to stop making additional inputs to the system, when the input exceeds the additional output.
dimmed the less dense than normal appearance of an option in a menu, usually in the shape of an icon or button, which is not available at the particular time.
Dimorphandra South American genus of plants in the legume family Cesalpiniaceae; contain an unidentified toxin which causes nephrosis in cattle. Includes *D. gardneriana*, *D. mollis* (faveira).
dimorphic see dimorphic FUNGUS.
dimorphism the quality of existing in two distinct forms.
  sexual d. 1. physical or behavioral differences associated with sex; males and females of the same species are different in appearance. 2. having some properties of both sexes, as in the early embryo and in some hermaphrodites.
Dimorphotheca see OSTEOSPERMUM.
dimple see MYOTONIC dimple.
dimpylate see DIAZINON.
Dina parva a leech found in the nasal cavity of aquatic birds.
Dingmann clamp a heavy-duty bone and cartilage clamp; scissor action with ratcheted handles and curved, heavily serrated blade faces which enclose an oval space when closed.

dingo Australian wild dog (*Canis antarticas*, *C. dingo*), 20 inches high, 30 inches long, and weight 50 lb, whole colored yellow, sable, red. Large pricked ears. Predatory on sheep flocks and calves, possibly small humans.
dingy used as a description of fleece wool; the wool is lacking in brightness.
dinitolmide a nitrobenzamide anticoccidial agent used in poultry.
dinitro compounds a group of herbicides including 2,4-DINITROPHENOL, DINITRO-ORTHOCRESOL and DINOSEB. They are relatively nontoxic at recommended dose rates. Signs of poisoning include dyspnea, sweating, thirst, weakness, prostration and death.
dinitro herbicide effective herbicides, nontoxic unless administered in concentrate form or if the material as supplied contains a toxic contaminant.
dinitro-*o*-toluamide a toxic coccidiostat; can cause ataxia, torticollis and reduced growth.
dinitro-orthophenol relatively nontoxic wood preservative.
dinitroaniline a group of herbicides of low toxicity for animals. Accidental poisoning causes diarrhea, nervousness and failure to gain weight.
3,5-dinitrobenzamide a coccidiostat used in poultry. Called also nitromide.
dinitrochlorobenzene a hapten whose application to the skin results in a contact hypersensitivity; abbreviated DNCB. Sometimes used to test for type IV or delayed type hypersensitivity reactions.
dinitrocresol see DINITRO-ORTHOCRESOL.
dinitro-orthocresol a valuable herbicide but it can cause deaths in animals exposed to high doses by inhalation, percutaneous absorption or ingestion; abbreviated DNOC. Signs of poisoning include restlessness, sweating, dyspnea and collapse. Ruminants are also subject to intravascular hemolysis, methemoglobinemia and hypoproteinemia. Chronic poisoning causes cataracts.
2,4-dinitrophenol, dinitrophenol 1. DNP; an inhibitor of oxidative phosphorylation. Acts by uncoupling electron flow from phosphorylation. Used as a haptenic immunogen in immunology. 2. a herbicide toxic to animals. Effects are similar to those of DINITRO-ORTHOCRESOL. See also DINITRO COMPOUNDS.
4-dinitrophenol relatively nontoxic herbicide and insecticide.
dinitrotoluidine chemical compounds used as insecticides and herbicides; toxic to fish if they pollute streams.
dinkum oil eucalyptus oil.
Dinobdella a member of the genus *Limnatis* of leeches of the class Hirudinea.
D. ferox found in the pharynx of ruminants and the upper respiratory tract of dogs, monkeys and humans.
dinobdelliasis infestation of all animal species with nasal leeches (*Dinobdella ferox*).
dinoflagellates minute aquatic protozoa; they produce red pigment and toxins which are taken up by shellfish without apparent ill effect, but the toxin is not metabolized and the shellfish may poison animals if eaten.
dinoprost prostaglandin $F_{2[alpha]}$; stimulates contraction of the myometrium and luteolysis. Used as the tromethamine and administered intra-amniotically to induce abortion.
dinoseb a phthalmic acid derivative herbicide which may cause poisoning in range chickens when used at standard dose rates. Includes dinoseb 136.
dinsed an anticoccidial agent used in mixtures for the control of coccidiosis in chickens.
Dioctophyme a genus of nematode worms in the family Dioctophymidae. Includes *Dioctophyme renale*, a very large nematode found in the kidneys and other organs of dogs and wild carnivores and occasionally ruminants. May be severely destructive and cause fatal uremia.
dioctophymosis infection with the kidney worm DIOCTOPHYME *renale*.
dioctyl calcium sulfosuccinate docusate calcium; a surfactant used as a wetting agent and nonlaxative fecal softener.
dioctyl sodium sulfosuccinate docusate sodium; abbreviated DSS. Used pharmacologically as a fecal softener, wetting agent and cathartic. Overdosing in horses for the treatment of impaction colic can cause deaths preceded by paralytic ileus, severe dehydration and diarrhea.
diode a piece of equipment with two terminals which carries electrical current in one direction only.
Diodontidae a family of venomous fishes. Called also toadfish.
dioestrus see DIESTRUS.
diol an organic compound containing two hydroxy groups, a dihydric alcohol. Called also glycol.
Diomedea see ALBATROSS.
Dioon edule Central American cycad in the family Zamiaceae; contains a cycad glycoside causing diarrhea, posterior ataxia and hepatic necrosis in cattle.
diopter a unit adopted for calibration of lenses, being the reciprocal of the focal length when expressed in meters; symbol D.
dioptric pertaining to refraction or to transmitted and refracted light; refracting.
dioptrics the science of refracted light.
Diorchis nyrocae a common cestode of ducks in the family Hymenolepididae.
Dioscorea a plant genus with edible roots in the family Dioscoreaceae. Some species are poisonous due to their content of dioscorine, an alkaloid with an action like picrotoxin. Called also yams. See also TAMUS COMMUNIS.
dioscorine an alkaloid in the plants of *Dioscorea* spp. Has an action similar to picrotoxin.
dioxacarb a carbamate pesticide.
dioxathion an organophosphorus insecticide used as a spray or dip mainly against ticks. The toxic level is about four times the no-effect concentration.
dioxin a highly toxic and teratogenic chlorinated hydrocarbon that is a trace contaminant in the herbicide 2,4,5-T. Acute poisoning causes vomiting, abortion, anestrus. Chronic poisoning causes liver damage, especially in dogs. Congenital defects caused include cranio-facial deformity and anasarca. It is excreted in the milk.
dioxygenases enzymes which incorporate both atoms of O_2 into one substrate. Less common than mono-oxygenases. Important example is the 15-15′-dioxygenase enzyme in the small intestine which cleaves plant carotenoids containing provitamin A activity, such as β-carotene, into retinal. This enzyme is absent from felines, such as the cat, and is the reason cats are dependent on animal sources of vitamin A.
dip 1. plunge (vat) or spray dip installations in which insecticide solutions are applied to animals, especially cattle and sheep. 2. the dipping solutions, commonly sodium arsenite, rotenone, synthetic pyrethroids and organophosphorus preparations. 3. to submit animals to DIPPING. 4. see TEAT DIP.

d. stain wool fiber stained by improper dipping procedure.

dipalmityl lecithin a surfactant present in the lungs of most species and necessary for normal respiratory function produced by alveolar type II cells.

dipalmitylphosphatidylcholine principal constituent of the phospholipid surfactant in the lungs, the absence of which plays a large part in the development of the acidophilic hyaline membranes which characterize the pulmonary lesions in neonatal respiratory distress syndrome in foals and piglets. See NEONATAL maladjustment syndrome.

Dipcadi African plant genus in the family Liliaceae; contain an unidentified toxin which causes head pressing, aimless wandering, diarrhea, enteritis. Includes *D. glaucum* (*D. gracilipes*, *D. longibracteatum*, wild or poison onion, malkop-ui).

dipeptidase a proteolytic enzyme occurring in the pancreatic secretion of chickens, and the intestinal brush border of mammals.

dipeptidyl aminopeptidase IV a digestive enzyme of the small intestine enterocytes (brush border).

diperodon a surface anesthetic and analgesic; used as the hydrochloride salt.

dipes having two hindlimbs.

Dipetalonema a genus of filarioid parasites of the superfamily Filarioidea.

D. dracunculoides found in peritoneal membranes of dogs and humans.

D. evansi found in spermatic and pulmonary artery of camels.

D. gracile, D. marmosetae, D. obtusa, D. tamarinae found in the peritoneal cavity of primates.

D. grassii occurs in the subcutaneous tissue of dogs.

D. loxodontis found in the African elephant. Called also *Loxodontofilaria loxodontis*.

D. odendhali found in the subcutaneous and intermuscular tissues of California sealion.

D. perstans, D. streptocerca these species are primarily parasitic in humans, other primates serving as reservoir hosts.

D. reconditum found in body cavities, connective tissue and kidney of dogs.

D. spirocauda found in the right heart and pulmonary artery of seals.

diphacinone an inandione derivative rodenticide, similar in effect to warfarin, but with prolonged activity. See also PINDONE.

diphallia the state of DIPHALLUS.

diphallus a developmental anomaly characterized by duplication of the penis.

diphasic occurring in two phases.

d. milk fever a disease of humans transmitted via the milk of goats and caused by the tickborne encephalitis virus. Called also Russian spring–summer encephalitis. *Ixodes ricinus* is the vector and goats and other ruminants are inapparent reservoirs.

diphemanil an anticholinergic drug used as the methyl sulfate to inhibit gastric motility and secretion, relieve pylorospasm, control sweating and relieve pruritus.

diphenadione an indandione type anticoagulant used as a rodenticide and as a counter to vampire bat predation. Effects are similar to those of warfarin but cardiopulmonary and neurological damage also occur. See also PINDONE.

diphenamid an amide type of herbicide with very low toxicity if used at recommended concentrations. Poisoning causes anorexia, weight loss and posterior paresis.

diphenhydramine an antihistamine used as the hydrochloride in treatment of allergic disorders and also for its sedative, antiemetic, antitussive, local anesthetic, and anticholinergic effects. Well known as Benadryl.

diphenidol used as the hydrochloride for control of nausea and vomiting; it has an antivertigo effect on the vestibular apparatus, inhibiting the chemoreceptor trigger zone to control nausea and vomiting, thus preventing motion sickness.

diphenoxylate a derivative of meperidine with little analgesic effect, but used as the hydrochloride for the management of diarrhea.

diphenylamine 1. a larvicide used in mixtures applied topically to screw-worm lesions. 2. a common contaminant in phenothiazine and may cause clotting defects after dosing with phenothiazine. 3. used in a field test for nitrate/nitrite poisoning.

diphenylhydantoin see PHENYTOIN.

diphenylthiocarbazone 1. a chelating agent used in the treatment of thallium poisoning, but has its own toxicity, causing blindness in dogs. 2. a very sensitive test agent for small amounts of metals, e.g. lead. Called also dithizon.

diphenytoin see PHENYTOIN.

2,3-diphosphoglycerate see 2,3-BISPHOSPHOGLYCERATE.

diphosphonate see BISPHOSPHONATES.

diphosphopyridine nucleotide one of the two growth factors released from erythrocytes during the preparation of chocolate agar. Called also V-factor. Now called nicotinamide-adenine dinucleotide (NAD).

diphosphoric acid see PYROPHOSPHORIC ACID.

diphthamide an amino acid residue formed by post-translational modification of histidine. There is ADP-ribosylation of elongation factor 2 (EF2) protein; the mode of action of diphtheria toxin whereby translation of mRNA is blocked.

diphtheria a human disease caused by *Corynebacterium diphtheriae*. There is no counterpart in animals but the name diphtheria is used in diseases that have some clinical similarity to it.

avian d. see FOWLPOX.

calf d. a severe, often fatal necrosis of the pharynx and larynx in calves up to 3 months of age caused by *Fusobacterium necrophorum*. The disease is commonly associated with poor hygienic management, especially in the feeding of milk or milk substitutes, but some losses occur in well-managed calf units, and severe outbreaks can also occur in yearling cattle in feedlots. Characteristic clinical signs include high fever, moist painful cough, severe dyspnea, nasal discharge, pain on external palpation of the larynx and a foul smell on the breath. See also ORAL necrobacillosis.

diphtheritic pertaining to features of the human disease, diphtheria.

d. inflammation an adherent membrane, consisting of necrosis of the superficial layers of the mucosa combined with inflammatory exudate, is formed on the mucosa.

d. membrane the peculiar membrane characteristic of diphtheria in humans and in other species. The term is used to describe membranes with a similar appearance in other disease conditions. See also diphtheritic INFLAMMATION.

diphtheroid 1. resembling the diphtheria bacillus *Corynebacterium diphtheriae*. See also CORYNEFORM. 2. pseudodiphtheria.

diphydont see DIPHYODONT.

diphyllobothriasis infection with *Diphyllobothrium* spp.

Diphyllobothrium a genus of long TAPEWORMS in the family Diphyllobothriidae.

D. dalliae, D. dendriticum, D. pacificum, D. strictum, D. minus, D. ursi are all tapeworms of fish-eating mammals including humans.

D. erinacei SPIROMETRA *erinacei.*

D. latum the broad or fish tapeworm, a species found in the small intestines of humans, dogs, cats and other fish-eating mammals.

diphyodont having two dentitions, a deciduous and a permanent.

diphyodonty the condition of having a single replacement set of teeth after a first erupted set.

dipivefrin an epinephrine prodrug used as the hydrochloride in ophthalmic drops to treat open-angle glaucoma.

Diplarrena Southern Australian genus of plants in the family Iridaceae; probably contains cardiac glycosides; causes hemorrhagic diarrhea. Includes *D. moraea*. Called also butterfly flag, native lily.

diplegia paralysis of like parts on either side of the body.

diplobacillus a short, rod-shaped organism occurring in pairs; diplobacterium.

diplobacterium see DIPLOBACILLUS.

diploblastic having two germ layers.

diplocardia a condition in which the heart appears to be partly divided by a central fissure.

Diplococcus former name for a genus of bacteria (tribe Streptococcaceae). The species have been assigned other names. See STREPTOCOCCUS *pneumoniae.*

diplococcus pl. *diplococci*. Any of the spherical bacteria occurring usually in pairs as a result of incomplete separation after cell division in a single plane.

diplocoria double pupil.

Diplocyclos palmatus African vine in the family Cucurbitaceae; may contain cucurbitacins; causes severe diarrhea.

Diplodia maydis a toxic fungus which grows on corn grain; causes incoordination and paresis in cattle in southern Africa which are pastured on crops carrying infected cobs. Called also *D. zeae, Stenocarpella maydis.*

diplodiosis poisoning caused by DIPLODIA MAYDIS.

diploë the spongy layer between the inner and outer compact layers of the flat bones of the skull.

diplogenesis the production of a double monster.

Diplogonoporus a genus of tapeworms in the family Diphyllobothriidae. Includes *D. grandis*, found as tapeworm of humans, probably an accidental final host. The real host is probably a seal.

diploid 1. having a pair of each chromosome characteristic of a species, i.e. genomes in which chromosomes occur in pairs. 2. a diploid individual or cell.

human d. cell vaccine see human diploid cell VACCINE.

d. karyotype a karyotype consisting of chromsomes in pairs.

diploidy the state of being diploid.

Diplolophium africanum a toxic plant in the family Apiaceae; contains an unidentified toxin and, if ingested in large quantities when it is green, causes dyspnea, salivation, abdominal pain, staggering and death.

diplomyelia lengthwise fissure and seeming doubleness of the spinal cord.

diplonema the double chromosomes in the diplotene stage.

diploneural having a double nerve supply.

diplopia seeing two images; double vision.

Diplopoda see MYRIAPODA.

Diplopylidium a genus of tapeworms found in dogs and cats. Belongs to the family Dipylidiidae.

diplosomatia a condition in which complete twins are joined at some of their body parts.

diplosomia see DIPLOSOMATIA.

Diplostomum a genus of digenetic trematodes of the family Diplostomatidae.

D. spathaceum found in the intestines of gulls. A cause of cataracts in fish and heavy infestations may cause severe mortalities.

diplotene the stage of the first meiotic prophase, following the pachytene, in which the two chromosomes in each bivalent begin to repel one another and a split occurs between the chromosomes.

Diplozoon a genus of monogean trematode parasites in the family Diplozooidae.

D. barbi, D. paradoxus found on the gills of freshwater fish. They cause damage to the gills and predispose to bacterial infection.

Dipluridae a family of spiders. Includes the funnel-web spider.

dipnoi, dipnoë lungfish. Fish that breathe through gills when in water but through lungs when out of it. Their peculiarity is that their nasal cavities, which are blind-ended, olfactory organs in most fish, connect with the roof of the mouth.

Dipodomys deserti see kangaroo RAT.

dipole 1. a molecule having charges of equal and opposite sign. 2. a pair of electric charges or magnetic poles separated by a short distance.

dipped back conformation in an animal in which the normal dip between withers and croup is exaggerated. Called also swayback.

dipping application of insecticide in large volume, dilute solution over the entire body for the purpose of controlling external parasites. It may be done in a plunge bath where the animal is totally immersed and must swim to the other end, or by spray dip where the animal passes through a battery of sprays that apply spray under pressure from every direction. Local application of insecticide for local effect is also carried out by jetting, and general effects are also obtained by insecticides applied as pour-ons. See also DIP, TEAT dipping.

d. cage the beasts are put into the cage one at a time and lowered into a small vat of insecticide.

d. vat a deep, long trough which is filled with insecticide and the animals are forced to swim through it. Called also plunge dip.

diprenorphine an analgesic antagonist used principally to reverse the effects of etorphine in captured wild animals. The reversal is complete and very quick. Called also Revivon.

diprivan see PROPOFOL.

diprophylline a theophylline derivative used as a bronchodilator. Called also dyphylline.

diprosopus a monster with varying degrees of duplication of the face.

dipsotherapy the therapeutic limitation of the amounts of fluids ingested.

dipsticks absorbent paper strips impregnated with reagents for testing urine or other fluid for their content of electrolytes, other solutes and blood. The container is usually provided with a color matching scale so that a rough quantitative estimation can be made.

Diptera an order of insects with two wings, including flies, gnats and mosquitoes.

dipterous 1. having two wings. 2. pertaining to insects of the order Diptera.

dipygus a fetus with a double pelvis.
dipylidiasis infection with *Dipylidium caninum*.
Dipylidium a genus of TAPEWORMS of the family Dipylidiidae. Besides those listed below, includes *D. gracile*, *D. compactum*, *D. diffusum*, *D. buencaminoi* (syn. *D. caninum*), *D. sexcoronatum* (cats).
D. caninum the dog tapeworm, parasitic in dogs and cats and occasionally found in humans. Esthetically unattractive but causes little damage other than anal irritation.
dipyridamole a coronary vasodilator with antiplatelet activity.
dipyridyl compounds highly toxic herbicides. See DIQUAT, PARAQUAT.
dipyrone an analgesic and antipyretic agent, used also as an antispasmodic in equine colic. Overdosing may cause defective blood clotting, leukopenia and agranulocytosis, hemolytic anemia and convulsive episodes.
diquat a hormone weedkiller which may poison animals, particularly those grazing pasture contaminated by the agent. Lesions in fatal cases include pulmonary emphysema, enteritis, abomasitis and hepatic and myocardial degeneration. Clinical signs include diarrhea and a high mortality rate.
direct without intervening steps.
d. antiglobulin test see direct COOMBS TEST.
d. capture ELISA mastitis test measures polymorphonuclear antigens in milk sample as an indication of elevated milk cell counts and therefore presence of mastitis.
d. contact see direct CONTACT.
d. costs see VARIABLE costs.
d. effect the effect of one variable on another without passing through a third variable.
d. immunofluorescence testing see FLUORESCENCE microscopy.
d. oxidative pathway see pentose phosphate PATHWAY.
d. relationship see direct RELATIONSHIP.
direction orientation within the body.
caudal d. towards the tail end of the body.
cranial d. towards the head end of the body.
distal d. distant from the long axis of the body.
dorsal d. 1. the surface directed towards the back or spine. 2. the extensor surface of the distal limbs.
lateral d. the surface directed away from the median plane.
medial d. towards the median plane (a vertical plane passing through the body from nose tip to tail tip).
palmar d. the flexor aspect of the foot, below the carpus, the surface directed towards the ground.
plantar d below the tarsus, the surface directed towards the ground.
proximal d. closer to the long axis of the body.
rostral d. towards the head or mouth.
ventral d. the surface directed towards the belly or ground.
director a long, slender, grooved instrument for guiding a knife or other surgical instrument.
directory the internal list of files on a computer disk or other media.
Dirofilaria a genus of nematode parasites of the superfamily Filarioidea.
D. acutiuscula causes swelling in the subcutaneous fascia of the dorsolumbar area of the peccary.
D. conjunctivae a zoonotic infection on the eyelids of humans, due to infestation of wildlife.
D. corynodes occurs in monkeys.
D. immitis occurs in dog, cat, fox and wolf and has been recorded in humans and many other species. Transmitted by the intermediate hosts, *Culex*, *Aedes*, *Anopheles* and other mosquito genera. Found in the blood vessels, especially the heart and the pulmonary artery. Causes HEARTWORM disease.
D. reconditum found in subcutaneous tissues of dogs.
D. repens occurs in the subcutaneous tissues of the dog and cat, and occasionally humans.
D. roemeri see PELECITUS ROEMERI.
D. striata found in the bobcat.
D. tenuis found in subcutaneous tissues of raccoons and humans.
D. ursi occurs in black bears.
dirofilariasis infection with nematodes of the genus *Dirofilaria*. Includes subcutaneous swellings. See also HEARTWORM disease.
dirty mare syndrome the vaginal discharge seen in nonspecific metritis in the mare, which may be caused by a number of bacteria and opportunist fungi.
dirty puppy syndrome see congenital SEBORRHEA.
dirty tail disease ascending urinary tract disease caused by *Chlamydia* spp. in koalas.
dis- word element. [L.] *reversal, separation*. [Gr.] *duplication*.
disability 1. inability to function normally, physically or mentally; incapacity. 2. anything that causes disability.
disaccharidase any of a group of enzymes which are components of the brush border of the intestinal epithelium and which hydrolyze disaccharides to monosaccharides. They include lactase, maltase, sucrase and galactosidase. Enteric infections may cause a temporary deficiency of lactase leading to the development of an osmotic-type diarrhea.
disaccharide any of a class of sugars each molecule of which yields two molecules of monosaccharide on hydrolysis.
disarming removal of the crown of the canine teeth in primates. Includes denervation of the pulp cavity.
disarray coefficient see disarray COEFFICIENT.
disarticulation amputation or separation at a joint.
disaster medicine the practice of veterinary medicine under circumstances resulting from natural disasters. Appropriate planning usually includes provisions for emergency treatment of animal injuries, control of and temporary housing of displaced animals, reuniting lost animals with their owners, and contributions to management of public health.
disbudding removal of the immature horns in young ruminants. This is a much simpler and less traumatic operation than removal of the adult horns and is usually done without an anesthetic. The usual technique is a dehorning tube or set of scoops. A hot iron has some exponents. See DEHORNING.
disc see DISK.
disc- for words beginning thus, see words beginning *disk-*.
discharge 1. a setting free, or liberation. 2. material or force set free. 3. an excretion or substance evacuated.
ocular d. a sign of conjunctivitis; green or yellow discharge is indicative of cellular content and inflammatory response.
discission incision, or cutting into, as of a soft cataract.
d.-aspiration a surgical technique for removal of soft cataracts in which abnormal lens material is broken into small pieces and removed by aspiration. Similar to phacofragmentation.

Discocotyle a genus of monogenetic trematode parasites of the family Discocotylidae.

D. sagittata a significant parasite of fish causing serious mortalities due to damage to the gills.

discocyte a discoid-shaped red blood cell, seen normally in dogs.

discoid 1. disk-shaped. 2. a disk-like medicated tablet.

d. lupus erythematosus see LUPUS ERYTHEMATOSUS.

d. meniscus an abnormality of the meniscus, usually lateral, in the stifle joint, reported in dogs. Instead of being semilunar in shape it is discoid; the frequency, clinical significance and cause are unclear.

discontinuous variable see discrete VARIABLE.

discoplacenta a disc-shaped placenta.

discordance the occurrence of a given trait in only one member of a twin pair.

discounted cash flow future cash flow discounted now by the interest which would be earned by investing the money in the interim.

discounting estimating the present value of a future sum; it is estimation of compound interest in reverse.

d. factor value used to estimate present value of a future cash flow; the future sum is multiplied by the discounting factor to calculate its present value.

discreditable conduct conduct by a professional person which is likely to bring sufficient discredit to the profession generally that the public's confidence in it is reduced. Penalties imposed by the registering authority may be as severe as deregistration.

discrete made up of separated parts; characterized by lesions that do not become blended.

discretizing measurements modification of measurement data (e.g. body weight to the nearest kg) to make classification into discrete groups possible.

discus pl. *disci* [L.] 1. see DISK[1]. 2. vernacular term for the fish *Symphysodon discus*; see Table 23.

d. oophorus see CUMULUS oophorus.

d. ovigerus see CUMULUS oophorus.

d. proligerus see CUMULUS oophorus.

disease traditionally defined as a finite abnormality of structure or function with an identifiable pathological or clinicopathological basis, and with a recognizable syndrome or constellation of clinical signs.

This definition has long since been widened to embrace subclinical diseases in which there is no tangible clinical syndrome but which are identifiable by chemical, hematological, biophysical, microbiological or immunological means. The definition is used even more widely to include failure to produce at expected levels in the presence of normal levels of nutritional supply and environmental quality. It is to be expected that the detection of residues of disqualifying chemicals in foods of animal origin will also come to be included within the scope of disease.

For specific diseases see under the specific name, e.g. Aujeszky's disease, Bang's disease, foot-and-mouth disease.

air-borne d. the causative agent is transmitted via the air without the need for intervention by other medium. See also WIND-BORNE DISEASE.

d. carrier see CARRIER, VECTOR.

clinical d. see CLINICAL (3).

d. cluster a group of animals with the same disease occurs at an unusual level of prevalence for the population as a whole. The cluster may be in space, with high concentrations in particular localities, or in time, with high concentrations in particular seasons or in particular years.

communicable d. infectious disease in which the causative agents may pass or be carried from one animal to another directly or indirectly on inanimate objects or via vectors.

complicating d. one that occurs in the course of some other disease as a complication.

constitutional d. one involving a system of organs or one with widespread signs.

contagious d. see communicable disease (above).

d. control reducing the prevalence of a disease in a population, including eradication, by chemical, pharmaceutical, quarantine, management including culling, or other means or combinations of means.

d. control programs organized routines specifying agents, administration, time and personnel allocations, community support, funding, participation of corporate or government agencies, animal and animal product disposal.

deficiency d. a condition due to dietary or metabolic deficiency, including all diseases caused by an insufficient supply of essential nutrients.

degenerative joint d. see degenerative JOINT disease, OSTEOARTHRITIS.

demyelinating d. any condition characterized by destruction of myelin.

d. determinant any variable associated with a disease which, if removed or altered, results in a change in the incidence of the disease.

egg-borne d. an infectious disease of birds in which the agent is spread via the egg.

endemic d. see ENDEMIC.

environmental d. control control by changing the environment, e.g. draining a swamp, ventilating a barn.

epidemic d. see EPIDEMIC.

etiological d. classification diseases arranged in the order of their etiological agents, e.g. bacterial, mycoplasma.

exotic d. a disease that does not occur in the subject country. Said of infectious diseases that may be introduced, e.g. rabies is exotic to the UK, contagious bovine pleuropneumonia is exotic to the USA.

focal d. a localized disease.

fulminant d. an explosive outbreak in a group or a rapidly developing, peracute development of a disease in an individual. Called also fulminating.

functional d. any disease involving body functions but not associated with detectable organic lesion or change.

generalized d. one involving all or many body systems; often said of infectious diseases in which there is spread via the bloodstream. See also systemic disease (below).

glycogen d. any of a group of genetically determined disorders of glycogen metabolism, marked by abnormal storage of glycogen in the body tissues. See also GLYCOGEN STORAGE DISEASE.

heavy chain d. see HEAVY-CHAIN DISEASE.

hemolytic d. of newborn see ALLOIMMUNE hemolytic anemia of the newborn.

hemorrhagic d. of newborn see neonatal HEMORRHAGIC disease.

d. history that part of a patient's history which relates only to the disease from which the patient is suffering.

holoendemic d. most animals in the population are affected.

hyperendemic d. the rate of infection is steady but high.

hypoendemic d the rate of infection is steady and only a few animals are infected.

immune complex d. see IMMUNE complex disease.

infectious d. one caused by small living organisms

including viruses, bacteria, fungi, protozoa and metazoan parasites. It may be contagious in origin, result from nosocomial infections or be due to endogenous microflora of the nose and throat, skin or bowel. See also communicable disease (above).

manifestational d. classification diseases arranged in the order of their clinical signs, epidemiological characteristics, necropsy lesions, e.g. sudden death diseases.

mesoendemic d. the disease occurs at an even rate and a moderate proportion of animals are infected.

metabolic d. see METABOLIC diseases.

molecular d. any disease in which the pathogenesis can be traced to a single, precise chemical alteration, usually of a protein, which is either abnormal in structure or present in reduced amounts. The corresponding defect in the DNA coding for the protein may also be known.

multicausal d. 1. a number of causative agents are needed to combine to cause the disease. 2. the same disease can be caused by a number of different agents.

multifactorial d. see multicausal disease (above).

new d. disease not previously recorded. May be variants on an existing disease, e.g. infectious bovine rhinotracheitis, or escapes from other species, e.g. the Marburg virus disease of humans.

notifiable d. a disease of which any occurrence is required by law to be notified to government authorities.

organic d. see ORGANIC disease.

pandemic d. a very widespread epidemic involving several countries or an entire continent.

quarantinable d. a disease which the law requires to be restricted in its spread by putting the affected animals, farms or properties on which it occurs in quarantine.

reportable d. see notifiable disease (above).

d. reservoir any animal or fomite in which an infectious disease agent is preserved in a viable state or multiplies and upon which it may depend for survival.

secondary d. 1. a disease subsequent to or a consequence of another disease or condition. 2. a condition due to introduction of incompatible, immunologically competent cells into a host rendered incapable of rejecting them by heavy exposure to ionizing radiation.

self-limited d. see SELF-LIMITED.

sex-limited d. disease limited in its occurrence to one or other sex. See also SEX-LINKED.

sexually transmitted d. (STD) a disease that can be acquired by sexual intercourse. See also venereal disease (below).

slaughter d. control see SLAUGHTER (2).

sporadic d. occurring singly and haphazardly; widely scattered; not epidemic or endemic. See also sporadic bovine ENCEPHALOMYELITIS, SPORADIC LEUKOSIS, SPORADIC LYMPHANGITIS.

storage d. see STORAGE DISEASE.

d. syndrome see SYNDROME.

systemic d. sufficiently widespread in the body to cause clinical signs referable to any organ or system, and in which localization of infection may occur in any organ.

d. wastage loss of income generated by production of milk, eggs, fiber, or loss of capital value because of diminution in the patient's value.

wasting d. any disease marked especially by progressive emaciation and weakness.

zoonotic d. disease capable of spread from animals to humans. See also ZOONOSIS.

disease-free animals a term for animals born and reared in an uninfected environment from uninfected parents and guaranteed to be free of infection. More guarded titles are usual, e.g. SPECIFIC PATHOGEN FREE, hysterectomy produced, artificially reared.

disengagement emergence of the fetus, or part thereof, from the vaginal canal.

disequilibrium unstable equilibrium.

dish development development of radiographic film in the simplest equipment, developing trays.

dished face less than normal growth of the facial bones so that the lateral silhouette of the face is depressed. Called also stag face.

dishing a fault in a horse's gait in which one or both forefeet is thrown outwards when moving forward.

dishorning see DEHORNING.

disinfect to free from pathogenic organisms, or to render them inert.

disinfectant 1. freeing from infection. 2. an agent that destroys infection-producing organisms. Heat and certain other physical agents such as live steam can be disinfectants, but in common usage the term is reserved for chemical substances such as mercury bichloride or phenol. Disinfectants are usually applied to inanimate objects since they are too strong to be used on living tissues. Chemical disinfectants are not always effective against spore-forming bacteria.

disinfection the act of disinfecting.

terminal d. disinfection of a loose box or cage and its contents at the termination of a disease.

disinfestants see INSECTICIDE.

disinfestation destruction of insects, rodents or other animal forms present on the animal or its harness or in its surroundings, and which may transmit disease.

disintegrant an agent used in pharmaceutical preparation of tablets, which causes them to disintegrate and release their medicinal substances on contact with moisture.

disjunction the act or state of being disjoined. In genetics, the moving apart of bivalent chromosomes at the first anaphase of meiosis.

disk[1] a circular or rounded flat plate. See also INTERVERTEBRAL disk.

articular d. a pad of fibrocartilage or dense fibrous tissue present in some synovial joints. As specialized intra-articular structures they differ from articular plates in that they have nerve and blood supplies.

choked d. papilledema.

embryonic d. a flattish area in a cleaved ovum in which the first traces of the embryo are seen. Called also germinal disk.

d. explosion the lesion produced by a sudden extrusion of non-degenerate nucleus pulposus from intervertebral disks into the cervical vertebral canal as a result of trauma.

germinal d. the embryo in a hen egg.

intra-articular d. articular disk.

olfactory d. these develop on the ventrolateral aspects of the head early in fetal development. They deepen, are surrounded by the developing nasal processes, then break through into the oral cavity and become the nasal cavities.

slipped d. the popular name for prolapse of the nucleus of an INTERVERTEBRAL disk.

disk[2] the information storage medium used in most computers. There are a variety of disks, some based on magnetized media, others using optical technology. Hard disks are made of aluminum, some are portable but most are fixed. Floppy disks or diskettes can be removed from the computer and are the principal medium for the transfer of small volumes of data between computers. Magnetic tapes are used for large volumes.

Data is stored usually in blocks of 256 bytes, the blocks being sectors of circular tracks recorded magnetically onto the disk. In some cases the sectors are determined by the hardware (hard-sectored), in others by the software (soft-sectored). In either case the blocks must be written onto the disk before it can be used, a process known as formatting.

The major advantage of disks over magnetic tape is the short time needed to retrieve any particular piece of data from them.

compact d. digitally encoded disk, usually 12 cm diameter. Used for the recording and reproduction of sound and more recently for the storage and reproduction of very large amounts of data, and of text, often extensively illustrated by graphics and photographs, and linked to a sound producing unit.

d. corruption disturbance of the electronic signals on a computer disk so that its stored information is lost, is inaccessible, partly or wholly, or is inaccessible without further modification.

d. drive the hardware that includes the read–write head and the motor that rotates the disk.

d. operating system the program that operates the housekeeping and communications necessary between the processor of the computer and its peripheral devices.

disk-diffusion test see ANTIMICROBIAL sensitivity test.

diskectomy excision of an intervertebral disk.

diskette the standard portable, 3.125 inch diameter disk originally of black vinyl; now enclosed in a rigid cover. May store information on one or both sides and in single, double or quad density. Their capacity varies is usually 1.4 megabytes.

diskiform in the shape of a disk.

diskitis inflammation of a disk, especially of an intervertebral disk.

diskogenic caused by derangement of an intervertebral disk.

diskography radiography of the vertebral column after injection of radiopaque material into an intervertebral disk.

diskolysis lysis of an intervertebral disk. See also INTERVERTEBRAL disk disease.

diskospondylitis a destructive, inflammatory and proliferative process involving intervertebral disks, their associated end-plates and vertebral bodies; best described in pigs and dogs.

dislocation 1. displacement of a bone from a joint. Signs include loss of motion, temporary paralysis of the involved joint, pain and swelling, and sometimes shock. Some dislocations, especially of the hip, are congenital, usually resulting from a faulty construction of the joint. 2. displacement of the lens in the eye. See LENS luxation.

complete d. one in which the surfaces are entirely separated.

compound d. one in which the joint communicates with the outside air through a wound.

pathological d. one due to disease of the joint or to paralysis of the muscles.

simple d. one in which there is no communication with the air through a wound.

dismemberment amputation of a limb or a portion of it.

dismutase any of a group of enzymes that have the ability to catalyze the reaction of two molecules of the same compound to yield two molecules in different oxidation states.

disodium EDTA see EDETATE.

disomus a double-bodied monster.

disophenol an injectable anthelmintic for hookworms in cats and dogs and *Haemonchus contortus* in sheep; abbreviated DNP. larger than normal doses cause somnolence, prostration and sometimes death. Transient cataract is also recorded as a toxic sequel See also NITROPHENOL.

disoprofol see PROPOFOL.

disopyramide an antiarrhythmic agent used for suppression and prevention of recurrence of both unifocal premature ventricular contractions and those of multifocal origin, paired premature ventricular contractions, and episodes of ventricular tachycardia that are not persistent.

disorder a derangement or abnormality of function. Used as a euphemism when it is not certain that the abnormality is in fact a disease, or when public relations suggest that the word disease is likely to be inflammatory or upsetting.

disorganization the process of destruction of any organic tissue; any profound change in the tissues of an organ or structure which causes the loss of most or all of its proper characters.

disorientation the patient appears to suffer a loss of proper bearings, or a state of mental confusion as to time, place or identity.

cetacean d. see PINNIPED stranding.

dispensary 1. a place for dispensation of free or low-cost medical treatment. 2. any place where drugs or medicines are actually dispensed.

dispensatory a book that describes medicines and their preparation and uses.

D. of the United States of America a collection of monographs on unofficial drugs and drugs recognized by the Pharmacopeia of the United States, the Pharmacopoeia of Great Britain, and the National Formulary, also on general tests, processes, reagents, and solutions of the USP and NF, as well as drugs used in veterinary medicine.

dispensing provision of drugs or medicines as set out properly on a lawful prescription. A prescription can only be filled, the drugs supplied, by a registered pharmacist, veterinarian, dentist or member of the medical profession. The law requires that a prescription be written only for patients that are in the veterinarian's care.

dispermy the fertilization of one egg by two sperm.

dispersal sale sale of an entire herd or flock; implies that the breeder is not retaining breeding animals and that the purchaser will now have the advantage of controlling that genotype.

disperse to scatter the component parts, as of a tumor or the fine particles in a colloid system; also, the particles so dispersed.

dispersion 1. the act of scattering or separating; the condition of being scattered. 2. the incorporation of one substance into another. 3. a colloid solution.

Dispharynx see SYNHIMANTUS.

displaced see DISPLACEMENT.

displacement removal to an abnormal location or position.

d. of abomasum see left, right ABOMASAL displacement.

fracture d. the movement of fractured bone fragments away from their relatively normal alignment.

inherited d. of molar teeth see inherited displacement of MOLAR teeth.

left dorsal colon d. see left COLON displacement colic.

liver d. see LIVER displacement.

display font the appearance of the font on the computer screen, which may be different to the printed font.

disposition setting in place.

d. curve the graphic representation of changes in the blood concentration of a drug after administration.

drug d. getting a drug into its appropriate position in the body and in an appropriate concentration.

disproportion a lack of the proper relationship between two elements or factors.

fetopelvic d. abnormally large size of the fetus in relation to the maternal pelvis, leading to difficulties in delivery.

dissect to cut apart, or separate; especially, the exposure of structures of a cadaver for anatomical study.

dissecting aneurysm see dissecting ANEURYSM.

dissection 1. the act of dissecting. 2. a part or whole of an organism prepared by dissecting. 3. passage of blood between layers of the wall of a blood vessel.

blunt d. separation of tissues along natural lines of cleavage, by means of a blunt instrument or finger.

sharp d. separation of tissues by means of the sharp edge of a knife or scalpel, or with scissors.

water beam d. the use of a high-pressure jet of saline to remove parenchymal cells, retaining more resistant structures such as ducts, capsule and vessels.

disseminated scattered; distributed over a considerable area.

d. intravascular coagulation (DIC) see disseminated intravascular COAGULATION.

d. visceral coccidiosis of cranes causes granulomatous nodules in many organs in sandhill cranes; caused by *Eimeria* spp. penetrating the blood or lymphatic system from the intestine and dissemination results.

Disse's space small lymph-carrying spaces between the liver sinusoids and hepatocytes.

dissociation the act of separating or the state of being separated.

atrial d. independent beating of the left and right atria, each with normal rhythm or with various combinations of normal rhythm, atrial flutter or atrial fibrillation.

atrioventricular d. independent pacemakers in the atria and ventricles.

d. constant the tendency of a solute to dissociate in solution.

hepatocyte d. hepatocytes becomes detached from their neighboring cells, either generally or locally; a feature of death of the patient.

dissolution 1. the process in which one substance is dissolved in another. 2. separation of a compound into its components by chemical action. 3. liquefaction. 4. death.

dissolve 1. to cause a substance to pass into solution. 2. to pass into solution.

distad in a distal direction.

distaff the female line in the pedigree of an animal.

distal remote; farther from any point of reference. See also DIRECTION.

d. convoluted tubule the part of the renal tubular system interposed between the nephron loop and the arched collecting tubule. See also convoluted TUBULES.

d. interphalangeal joints see Table 11.

d. phalanx third phalanx.

d. sesamoid navicular bone in the horse.

d. tarsal bones the tarsal bones adjacent to the metatarsals.

distance the measure of space intervening between two objects or two points of reference.

critical d. see FLIGHT DISTANCE.

focal–film d. the distance between the anode of the x-ray tube and the film; an important exposure value.

fright d. see FLIGHT DISTANCE.

guard d. see FLIGHT DISTANCE.

interocclusal d. the distance between the occluding surfaces of the maxillary and mandibular teeth with the mandible in physiological rest position.

interocular d. the distance between the eyes, usually used in reference to the interpupillary distance (the distance between the two pupils when the visual axes are parallel).

distemper a name for several infectious diseases of animals.

avian d. see NEWCASTLE DISEASE.

canine d. an acute virus disease of dogs caused by a morbillivirus, and characterized by high morbidity and high mortality, ocular and nasal discharge, vomiting, diarrhea, coughing, dyspnea and seizures. In addition, some dogs develop 'hard pads' (hyperkeratosis of the footpads), persistent muscle twitches (CHOREA), optic neuritis and later retinal atrophy, enamel hypoplasia (distemper teeth—see below), or a chronic encephalitis. Interstitial pneumonia and demyelinating encephalomyelitis are common pathological features. Also occurs in other Canidae as well as Procyonidae, Ursidae, Mustelidae and Hyaenidae. The disease can be prevented by vaccination at a young age. Called also Carré's disease.

equine d. see STRANGLES.

feline d. see FELINE panleukopenia.

phocine d. a disease first observed in European harbor seals in 1988 caused by a morbillivirus; clinical signs are similar to those of distemper.

d. teeth the pitted, discolored teeth that may result when young dogs are infected with distemper virus prior to the eruption of their permanent teeth. Other insults to enamel formation at this age may also be responsible for this defect.

distension the state of being distended, or stretched out or enlarged; the act of distending. For individual local distensions see the location, e.g. abomasal distension.

distichia the presence of a double row of eyelashes, one or both of which are turned against the eyeball.

distichiasis the condition caused by having distichia and characterized by severe, chronic conjunctival injury leading to conjunctivitis, blepharospasm and keratitis.

distillate a product of distillation.

distillation vaporization; the process of vaporizing and condensing a substance to purify the substance or to separate a volatile substance from less volatile substances.

fractional d. separation of volatilizable substances into a number of fractions, based on their different boiling points.

distiller's pertaining to the by-products of the distillation of spirits.

d. grains one of the residues of fermentation for the production of spirits. Contains most of the protein of the original grain and is an excellent supplement to diets of heavy milking cows.

d. solubles the dehydrated thin stillage from whisky manufacture. Contains a high concentration of B vitamins.

distobuccal pertaining to or formed by the distal and buccal surfaces of a tooth, or by the distal and buccal walls of a tooth cavity.

distocclusion malrelation of the dental arches, with

the lower jaw in a distal or caudal position in relation to the upper.

distomatosis see FASCIOLIASIS.

distomiasis infection due to trematodes or flukes. See also FASCIOLIASIS.

Distomum hepaticum see FASCIOLA *hepatica*.

distortion the state of being twisted out of normal shape or position.

distraction 1. diversion of attention. 2. separation of joint surfaces without rupture of their binding ligaments and without displacement. 3. surgical separation of the two parts of a bone after it is transected.

d. index a measure of hip laxity in which the degree of subluxation demonstrated radiographically when some stress is applied to the femurs is assessed as an indicator of hip dysplasia in dogs.

d. osteogenesis the development of new bone growth in an area subjected to gradual tension stress by the deliberate separation of fragments by traction.

distress physical or mental anguish or suffering.

distribution the arrangement of numerical data. The arrangement may be in accordance with magnitude, a frequency distribution, or in relation to geographical location, a spatial distribution.

age d. see AGE distribution.

bimodal d. the distribution has two regions of high frequency of observations separated by a zone of low frequency.

binomial d. a probability distribution associated with two mutually exclusive outcomes.

cluster d. a nonrandom distribution with observations aggregating about geographic or temporal variables. May be deceptive and merely reflect the distribution of an uneven population.

frequency d. a table or graph of the frequency of occurrence of each value of a variable.

Gaussian d. see normal distribution (below).

hypergeometric d. may apply to sampling without replacement of a finite population.

lognormal d. a distribution which is normal when the log values of the variable are considered.

normal d. a graph of the distribution appears as a bell-shaped curve which is symmetrical on the two sides of the vertical axis through the peak of the curve. Called also gaussian distribution.

parent d. the distribution (population) that was originally sampled.

Poisson d. see POISSON DISTRIBUTION.

regular d. distributed at regular intervals of time or space; all values within its given interval are equally likely.

sex d. an increase in frequency in one sex, which includes neutered males and neutered females. Called also sex-linked or sex-associated.

skewed d. a distribution in which the curve illustrating it is not symmetrical but has a long tail on one or other side og the graph.

spatial d. variations in distribution related to position in space, e.g. close to the door of a barn.

***t*-d.** see *t*-TEST.

temporal d. variation in distribution related to time, e.g. occurrence of disease incidents after visits by veterinarians, inseminators, feed salesmen.

distributive circulatory failure see vasogenic SHOCK.

disturbance a departure or divergence from that which is considered normal.

disulfoton an organophosphorus pesticide.

DIT di-iodotyrosine.

ditch millet PASPALUM *scrobiculatum*.

diterpene highly irritant plant diterpenoid esters, e.g. daphnane, tigliane, ingemane.

diterpenoid alkaloid a group of complex plant chemicals with similar structure to that of a terpene. Includes well-known toxins, e.g. aconitine, barbitine, lycoctinine, delphine, heteratisine.

dithiazanine a broad-spectrum anthelmintic and microfilaricide used for the treatment of heartworm in dogs; also used for treatment of *Strongyloides* and *Spirocerca* spp. Called also dizan.

dithiocarbamates fungal seed dressing unlikely to be poisonous for animals.

dithiosemicarbazone one of a series of these compounds, Gloxazone, is used as a treatment for *Anaplasma marginale*. It has the virtue of incomplete sterilization, encouraging the development of premunition.

dithizon see DIPHENYLTHIOCARBAZONE.

Dittrichia graveolens plant in the family Asteraceae; contains a toxic oil and causes dermatitis, diarrhea, enteritis. Called also *Inula graveolens*, stinkwort, cape khaki weed.

di-ureido isobutane a nitrogen-rich industrial by-product, used as a feed supplement but can be poisonous to ruminants if fed in more than small amounts and in a diet deficient in carbohydrate; abbreviated DUIB. The toxic effect is that of ammonia poisoning as experienced with urea feeding. See also UREA.

diurese the act of effecting diuresis.

diuresis increased excretion of the urine.

cold d. occurs in hypothermia as a result of peripheral vasoconstriction, hyperglycemia and decreased renal tubular absorption.

osmotic d. due to increased concentration of solutes which are not reabsorbed in the proximal tubules and which, by osmotic pressure, cause water to be retained. See also osmotic DIURETIC.

postobstruction d. due to the diuretic effect of urea and electrolytes retained during the period of obstruction.

water d. ingestion and excretion of an excess of water, without a corresponding amount of sodium; involves expansion of plasma volume, increased left atrial pressure and inhibition of ADH. See also OBLIGATORY water diuresis.

diuretic 1. increasing urine excretion or the amount of urine. 2. an agent that promotes urine secretion.

aldosterone antagonist d. affects tubular function by blocking the sodium retention activity of aldosterone. See also SPIRONOLACTONE.

aminouracil d's heterocyclic compounds similar to xanthines and with similar effects. See xanthine diuretics (below).

benzothiazide d's exert their effect on the proximal part of the renal tubule preventing resorption of sodium. Called also thiazide diuretics. The best known members of the group are chlorothiazide and its derivatives.

carbonic anhydrase inhibitor d's inhibit carbonic anhydrase activity and inhibit ion exchange mechanisms especially that of sodium and potassium ions. See also ACETAZOLAMIDE.

loop of Henle d's affect the resorption of sodium in the ascending loop of Henle. Called also loop diuretic. See also FUROSEMIDE, ETHACRYNATE SODIUM.

mercurial d. now largely displaced; the mode of action is to interfere with tubular enzyme systems so that tubular resorption is blocked. Overuse causes permanent renal damage.

osmotic d's produce a very rapid loss of sodium and water by inhibiting their reabsorption in the kidney tubules and the loop of Henle. Mannitol is clinically the most useful of these diuretics, but it has some serious side-effects, such as pulmonary edema and congestive heart failure.

potassium-retaining d's appear to act directly on renal tubular function. See also TRIAMTERENE.

xanthine d's have effect of stimulating cardiac activity but also have a direct effect on the renal tubules. See also THEOPHYLLINE.

Diuril see CHLOROTHIAZIDE.

diurnal pertaining to or occurring during the daytime, or period of light.

diuron a phenylurea herbicide of low toxicity but capable of poisoning animals if given in very large amounts. Causes anorexia, weight loss and muscular weakness.

divalent 1. bivalent. 2. carrying an electronic charge of two units.

divalproex a salt of VALPROIC ACID.

divergence a moving apart, or inclination away from a common point.

diverticular pertaining to or resembling a diverticulum.

diverticulectomy excision of a diverticulum.

diverticulitis inflammation of a diverticulum, especially inflammation involving diverticula of the intestine. Weakness of the muscles of the bowel leads to the formation of diverticula, small blind pouches lined by intestinal mucosa in the lining and wall, usually following blood vessels. Inflammation may occur as a result of collections of bacteria or other irritating agents trapped in the pouches and perforation may occur. In horses and pigs these are associated with muscular hypertrophy of the small intestine.

d. and ileitis see porcine intestinal ADENOMATOSIS.

diverticulogram a radiograph of a diverticulum.

diverticulosis the presence of diverticula in the absence of inflammation. See DIVERTICULITIS.

diverticulum pl. *diverticula* [L.] a circumscribed pouch or sac occurring normally or created by herniation of the lining mucous membrane through a defect in the muscular coat of a tubular organ.

auditory tube d. see GUTTURAL POUCH.

dorsal urethra d. a small pouch dorsal to the urethra in the male ruminant.

esophageal d. a congenital or acquired localized dilatation or outpouching of the esophageal wall in which food and liquids may accumulate. *Pulsion* (or pressure) diverticula result from increased intraluminal pressure and protrusion of mucosa through the muscular wall. *Traction* diverticula are created by periesophageal inflammation, fibrosis and adhesions to surrounding structures. Vascular ring anomalies are a common cause of anterior thoracic esophageal diverticula in dogs.

Clinical signs include dysphagia and regurgitation, and esophageal obstruction by impacted food may occur.

intestinal d. a pouch or sac formed by hernial protrusion of the mucous membrane through a defect in the muscular coat of the intestine.

nasal d. the part of the horse's nostril dorsal to the alar fold leads into this blind pouch, which is lined with skin. Called also false nostril.

pressure d. see esophageal diverticulum (above).

pulsion d. see esophageal diverticulum (above).

rectal d. weakness and rupture of the muscular layer of the rectal wall allows formation of a pocket. Most commonly seen in dogs in association with perineal hernia. There is straining and an obvious bulge beside the anus.

stomach d. a small pouch at the left end of the pig's stomach, close to the esophageal entry into the stomach.

suburethral d. lies below the opening of the urethra of the cow.

traction d. see esophageal diverticulum (above).

d. tubae auditivae see GUTTURAL POUCH.

diving the act of submerging underwater; diving by fish and amphibians creates an obvious need for mechanisms that allow them to be submerged under water for long periods. Most mammalian and avian orders also have aquatic species that have a similar need. Diving reflexes operate as soon as nostrils are submerged and include oxygen conservation, respiratory arrest, intense peripheral vasoconstriction, bradycardia and compression of the chest with almost complete evacuation of the lungs.

division the act of separating into parts.

cell d. fission of a cell, the process by which cells reproduce.

divulsion the act of separating or pulling apart.

divulsor an instrument for dilating the urethra.

dizygotic, dizygous pertaining to or derived from two separate zygotes (fertilized ova); said of TWINS.

DJD degenerative JOINT disease, OSTEOARTHRITIS.

dk symbol, *deka-*.

DL chemical prefix (small capitals) denoting that the substance is an equimolecular mixture of two catamorphs, one of which corresponds in configuration to D-glyceraldehyde, the other to L-glyceraldehyde.

D_LCO diffusing capacity of the lung for carbon monoxide.

D_LO_2 diffusing capacity of the lung for oxygen.

dl decaliter (the unit of volume).

DLA dog leukocyte antigen.

DLE discoid LUPUS ERYTHEMATOSUS.

DM 1. dry matter. 2. one of the arsenical smokes used in crowd control. A sternutator and causes lacrimation, sneezing and vomiting. Called also adamsite.

DMI dry matter intake.

DMNA dimethylnitrosamine.

DMSA dimercaptosuccinic acid.

DMSO dimethyl sulfoxide, an industrial solvent that has the ability to penetrate plant and animal tissues and to preserve living cells during freezing. It has bacteriostatic, anti-inflammatory, analgesic, radioprotective, fibrinolytic and vasodilative properties, and inhibits cholinesterase and granulation tissue. DMSO also has been used as an agent to increase the penetrability of other substances. Only approved for veterinary use, it has found varied applications as a topical treatment for musculoskeletal conditions in horses and skin diseases, mainly in dogs.

DMT dimethyltryptamine.

DNA DEOXYRIBONUCLEIC ACID.

DNA binding proteins are of two general types, histone proteins which are part of the unit structure of chromosomes called NUCLEOSOMES and nonhistone proteins which are present in small amounts and include regulatory proteins.

chromosomal DNA see CHROMOSOME.

circular DNA a DNA molecule that is a closed-ring structure, found in mitochondria, prokaryote chromosomes, plasmids, and certain viruses.

closed DNA complexes the first of two kinetically distinct steps required for RNA polymerase to initiate transcription in which the RNA polymerase holoenzyme binds electrostatically to the promoter DNA.

DNA construct a DNA molecule which has been inserted into a cloning vector.

copy DNA a DNA copy of mRNA which contains only regulatory and coding sequences, i.e. introns have been removed. mRNA is copied into double-stranded DNA using reverse transcriptase; the cDNA can then be cloned and amplified and introduced into an expression vector (plasmid or phage) and its protein product produced in either bacterial, yeast, insect or mammalian cells. Called also cDNA.

DNA deletion see DELETION.

DNA double helix see double HELIX.

duplex DNA double-stranded DNA.

end labeling DNA methods for labeling DNA with radioisotopes or other detectable marker molecules at the ends using the terminal transferase 3′-labeling or polynucleotide kinase for 5′-labeling.

episomal DNA that present in a cell as extra chromosomal; exemplified by plasmids of prokaryotic cells. See PLASMID.

eukaryotic DNA see DEOXYRIBONUCLEIC ACID.

exogenous DNA the DNA that has been introduced into a host by cloning.

DNA fingerprint see RESTRICTION FRAGMENT LENGTH POLYMORPHISM.

DNA glycosylases enzymes involved in the excision-repair mechanisms for DNA.

heteroduplex DNA duplex DNA with each strand from a different origin.

DNA library a collection of cloned DNA molecules from a genome.

DNA ligase an enzyme that seals nicks in the DNA helix, joins Okazaki fragments together during DNA replication and is essential in recombinant DNA technology for DNA cloning.

mobile DNA a sequence present in the variable locations on the chromosome. Called also jumping genes. See also RETROTRANSPOSON and transposable GENETIC elements.

open DNA complex a local opening of about 10 base pairs formed at the transcription initiation site following the electrostatic binding of RNA polymerase holoenzyme to the promoter region.

DNA polymerase of *Escherichia coli*; has three distinct enzymatic activities: (a) a 5′ to 3′ polymerase activity which, under the direction of a template DNA, catalyzes the addition of mononucleotide units, produced from deoxynucleoside 5′-triphosphates, to the 3′-hydroxyl terminus of a primer chain; (b) a 5′ to 3′ exonuclease active only on duplex DNA; (c) a 3′ to 5′ exonuclease primarily active on single-stranded DNA which can selectively remove mismatched terminal nucleotides, thus carrying out a proofreading function. Additionally it catalyzes both the pyrophosphorolysis of DNA, a reaction which is the reverse of polymerization, and pyrophosphate exchange which represents a repetitive sequence of nucleotide addition and pyrophosphorolysis.

DNA probe see PROBE (2).

DNA repair a series of enzymatic mechanisms whereby errors or damage to one of the two DNA strands are removed by excision and replaced by correct nucleotides using the undamaged strand as template. The mechanisms include removal of lesions of depurination and DNA glycosylases which recognize altered bases.

repeat DNA, repetitive DNA includes (a) satellite DNA and so-called (b) interspersed repeated DNA sequences. The latter are interspread throughout the chromosomes in hundreds of thousands of individual copies, each about 300 nucleotides long; they are, unlike satellite DNA, transcribed.

satellite DNA serially repeated DNA sequences of one or a few nucleotides with a repeat length of up to 250 nucleotides that are not transcribed and commonly located in the heterochromatin associated with the centrometric regions of chromosomes.

selfish DNA a mobile DNA element that appears to have no function except to replicate itself. Part of junk DNA.

DNA sequencing determining the order of nucleotides in DNA from which amino acid in a polypeptide chain can be predicted.

single-copy DNA the fraction of DNA that contains most of the protein-coding genes and reassociates most slowly.

single-stranded DNA produced when double-stranded DNA is denatured or found naturally in some viruses.

spacer DNA single-copy DNA sequences which do not encode proteins or functional RNA molecules.

supercoiled DNA the double helix is itself twisted.

superhelical DNA a twisted structure formed by circular DNA molecules. See also supercoiled DNA (above).

DNA transcription see DEOXYRIBONUCLEIC ACID.

DNA translation see DEOXYRIBONUCLEIC ACID.

unique DNA DNA sequences that occur only once in the haploid genome.

DNA viruses viruses with a double or singlestrand of DNA. Viruses contain a single molecule of DNA as their genetic material. All are double-stranded DNA genomes except parvoviruses and circoviruses which are single-stranded and hepadnaviruses which are partially double-stranded: *Poxviridae*—includes poxvirus; African swine fever virus, which is unclassified; *Herpesviridae*—includes many species of herpesvirus; *Adenoviridae*—includes adenovirus; *Papovaviridae*—includes papillomavirus; *Parvoviridae*—includes parvovirus; *Circoviridae*—includes circovirus; *Hepadnaviridae*—includes human hepatitis B, duck hepatitis, woodchuck hepatitis viruses.

Z-DNA an alternative structural form of DNA which differs from the more commonly occurring B- and related A-form in that the helix is left handed compared with the right hand helixes of B- and A-forms. Z is for zig-zag. The functional significance of Z-DNA is unknown.

DNase *d*eoxyribo*n*ucle*ase*. Group A streptococci elaborate DNases and commercially available DNase agar may be used to identify pathogenic species.

DNCB dinitrochlorobenzene.

DNOC dinitro-orthocresol.

DNP 2,4-dinitrophenol.

DOA dead on admission (arrival).

DOB abbreviation for date of birth; used in medical records.

Doberman pinscher, Dobermann a medium-sized (66–88 lb), lean, muscular dog with very short hair that is usually black with brown markings around the face and on the legs, but occasionally has a brown or blue body color. The tail is docked to a short length and where practiced, the normally pendant ears are cropped. The breed is often used for police or guard work. It is subject to spondylolisthesis (wobbler syndrome), color mutant alopecia, generalized demodecosis, chronic active hepatitis, cardiomyopathy, von Willebrand's disease, and degeneration of the bundle of His.

dancing D. disease a very slowly progressive, painless neuromuscular disease in which affected dogs periodically flex one hindleg when standing. Hindleg weakness and atrophy of the gastrocnemius muscle eventually develops. In some cases both hindlegs are affected with flexion and extension of alternating hindlegs, hence the name.

miniature D. p. see MINIATURE PINSCHER.

dobutamine a synthetic catecholamine used as the

hydrochloride and administered parenterally for inotropic support in short-term treatment of cardiac decompensation due to depressed contractility resulting either from organic heart disease or from cardiac surgical procedures.

DOC doxycorticosterone.

DOCA deoxycortosterone acetate.

dock[1] 1. the amputation of a tail. Commonly performed in dogs, usually in accordance with breed standards that strictly define length, particularly in the spaniel and terrier breeds. Also occasionally done in some draft and harness horses. In both species, the practice is now being viewed as unnecessary and discouraged by many authorities. A universal procedure in lambs, carried out by farmers. 2. the solid part of a horse's tail.

dock[2] group of plants the family Polygonaceae. Called also dock sorrel, *Rumex* spp.

docking tail amputation. See DOCK[1].

docking protein SRP receptor.

doctor 1. a practitioner of the healing arts, as one graduated from a college of medicine, osteopathy, dentistry or veterinary medicine and licensed to practice. 2. a holder of a diploma of the highest degree from a university, qualified as a specialist in a particular field of learning.

docusates anionic surfactants used as the calcium, sodium or potassium salts as fecal softeners.

dodder see CUSCUTA.

doddler calf a congenital defect of the nervous system in Hereford calves produced by the inheritance of an autosomal recessive trait. It is characterized by continuous clonic convulsions, nystagmus and pupillary dilatation, all of which are present at birth. The disease is inevitably lethal.

dodine dodecylguanidine acetate, an agricultural fungicide; causes irritation of skin and mucosae; ingestion causes vomiting and diarrhea.

doe an adult female goat or deer; amongst deer it is especially common usage in the roe, fallow, muntjac and Chinese water deer species. In the larger species the term cow is used.

Doehle body accumulations of residual endoplasmic reticulum found in mature neutrophils of patients with severe toxemia.

doenca da sono [Span.] *trypanosomiasis*.

dog 1. a member of the Canidae family of the order Carnivora. Includes the domestic dog, *Canis familiaris*, many wild dogs, foxes, fennecs, jackals and wolves. 2. the term is also used by dog people to mean the entire male dog. There is no other name for him as there is in the other species. See also CANINE.

assistance d. those trained to be of assistance to handicapped or diasabled people. The most familiar ones are guide dogs and hearing dogs, but others may be trained to assist people confined to wheelchairs or with other types of limited mobility.

d.-catcher a loop of rope at the end of a pole, with the end of the rope at the holding end of the pole. The loop goes over the dog's head and is pulled tight.

domestic d. classified as HOUND, GUN dogs, TERRIERS, NONSPORTING DOG, WORKING DOGS, DRAFT animals, TOY BREEDS.

Breeds of dogs are listed below:

AFFENPINSCHER, AFGHAN HOUND, AIREDALE TERRIER, AKITA INU, ALASKAN MALAMUTE, AMERICAN COCKER SPANIEL, AMERICAN PIT BULL TERRIER, AMERICAN STAFFORDSHIRE TERRIER, AMERICAN WATER SPANIEL, ANATOLIAN SHEPHERD DOG, APPENZELLER, AUSTRALIAN cattle dog, AUSTRALIAN kelpie, AUSTRALIAN silky terrier, AUSTRALIAN terrier.

BASENJI, BASSET FAUVE DE BRETAGNE, BASSET HOUND, BEAGLE, BEARDED COLLIE, BEDLINGTON TERRIER, BELGIAN SHEPHERD DOG (sheepdog) (Groenendael, Malinois and Tervueren), BERGAMASCO, BERGER DE BEAUCE, BERNESE MOUNTAIN DOG, BICHON FRISE, BLACK AND TAN COONHOUND, BLOODHOUND, BLUETICK COONHOUND, BOLOGNESE, BORDER COLLIE, BORDER TERRIER, BORZOI, BOSTON TERRIER, BOUVIER DES FLANDRES, BOXER, BOYKIN SPANIEL, BRACO ITALIANO, BRIARD, BRITTANY SPANIEL, BRUSSELLS GRIFFON, BULL MASTIFF, BULL TERRIER, BULLDOG, BULLMASTIFF.

CAIRN TERRIER, CANAAN DOG, CARELIAN BEAR DOG, CATAHOULA, CAVALIER KING CHARLES SPANIEL, CHESAPEAKE BAY RETRIEVER, CHIHUAHUA, CHINESE CRESTED, CHOW CHOW, CLUMBER SPANIEL, COCKER SPANIEL, COLLIE, COONHOUND, COTON DE TULEAR, CURLY COATED RETRIEVER, CZESKY TERRIER.

DACHSHUND, DALMATIAN, DANDIE DINMONT TERRIER, DEERHOUND, DOBERMANN PINSCHER, DOGUE DE BORDEAUX, DUNKER.

ELKHOUND, ENGLISH SETTER, ENGLISH SPRINGER SPANIEL, ENGLISH TOY TERRIER, ESKIMO DOG, ESTRELA MOUNTAIN DOG.

FIELD SPANIEL, FINNISH LAPPHUND, FINNISH SPITZ, FLAT COATED RETRIEVER, FOX TERRIER, FOXHOUND, FRENCH BULLDOG.

GERMAN PINSCHER, GERMAN SHEPHERD DOG, GERMAN SHORTHAIRED POINTER, GERMAN SPITZ, GERMAN WIREHAIRED POINTER, GLEN OF IMAAL TERRIER, GOLDEN RETRIEVER, GORDON SETTER, GRAND BASSET GRIFFON BENDEEN, GRAND BLEU DE GASCOIGNE, GREAT DANE, GREAT PYRENEES, GREATER SWISS MOUNTAIN DOG, GREYHOUND, GRIFFON BRUXELLOIS.

HAMILTONSTOVARE, HARRIER, HOVAWART, IBIZAN HOUND, IRISH SETTER, IRISH TERRIER, IRISH WATER SPANIEL, IRISH WOLFHOUND, ITALIAN GREYHOUND, JACK RUSSELL TERRIER, JAPANESE CHIN, JAPANESE SPITZ.

KEESHOND, KERRY BLUE TERRIER, KING CHARLES SPANIEL, KOMONDOR, KOOIKERHONDJE, KUVASZ, LABRADOR RETRIEVER, LAKELAND TERRIER, LANCASHIRE HEELER, LARGE MUNSTERLANDER, LEONBERGER, LHASA APSO, LOWCHEN, LUNDEHUND, MALTESE, MANCHESTER TERRIER, MAREMMA SHEEPDOG, MASTIFF, MEXICAN HAIRLESS, MINIATURE PINSCHER.

NEOPOLITAN MASTIFF, NEWFOUNDLAND, NIPPON INU, NORFOLK TERRIER, NORWEGIAN BUHUND, NORWEGIAN ELKHOUND, NORWICH TERRIER, NOVA SCOTIA DUCK TOLLING RETRIEVER, OLD ENGLISH SHEEPDOG, OTTER HOUND, PAPILLON, PARSON JACK RUSSELL TERRIER, PEKINGESE, PETIT BASSET GRIFFON VENEEN, PHARAOH HOUND, PLOTT HOUND, POINTER, POLISH LOWLAND SHEEPDOG, POMERANIAN, POODLE, PORTUGESE WATER DOG, PUG, PULI.

REDBONE COONHOUND, RHODESIAN RIDGEBACK, ROTTWEILER, ST. BERNARD, SALUKI, SAMOYED, SCHIPPERKE, SCHNAUZER, SCOTTISH DEERHOUND, SCOTTISH TERRIER, SEALYHAM TERRIER, SEGUGIO ITALIANO, SHAR PEI, SHETLAND SHEEPDOG, SHIBA INU, SHIH TZU, SIBERIAN HUSKY, SKYE TERRIER, SLOUGHI, SOFT COATED WHEATEN TERRIER, SPINONI ITALIANI, STAFFORDSHIRE BULL TERRIER, STUMPY-TAIL CATTLE DOG, SUSSEX SPANIEL, SWEDISH LAPLAND DOG, SWEDISH VALLHUND.

TIBETAN MASTIFF, TIBETAN SPANIEL, TIBETAN TERRIER, TREEING WALKER COONHOUND, VIZSLA, WALKER HOUND, WEIMARANER, WELSH CORGI, WELSH SPRINGER SPANIEL, WELSH TERRIER, WEST HIGHLAND WHITE TERRIER, WHIPPET, WIREHAIRED POINTING GRIFFON, YORKSHIRE TERRIER.

d. erythrocyte antigen (DEA) see blood group ANTIGEN.

d. flea CTENOCEPHALIDES *canis*.

guide d. one trained as an aid to the mobility of a visually impaired person. Guide dogs do not 'take' their owners to specific destinations, but respond to commands given for directions. They are of particular value in avoidance of obstacles, both on the ground and overhead. Many breeds have been used for this purpose, but German shepherd dogs and Labrador retrievers are the most common. Called also seeing-eye dogs.

hearing d. one trained to respond to certain sounds such as a telephone bell or door knocker and to alert a person with impaired hearing.

d. kennel a small box-like unit for housing a single dog, or an establishment that boards dogs, or breeds them or maintains a colony, e.g. a pack of hounds, or a stable of Greyhounds.

d. leukocyte antigen (DLA) complex the major histocompatibility complex in dogs.

d. murrain chronic selenium poisoning in pastured ruminants. An Irish expression.

d. pox a papular balanoposthitis and vaginitis described in young dogs; a viral etiology is suspected, but has never been confirmed.

seeing-eye d. see guide dog (above).

d. tick varies with the country: American d. tick, see DERMACENTOR *variabilis*; Australian d. tick, see IXODES *holocyclus*; British d. tick, see IXODES *canisuga*; brown d. tick, see RHIPICEPHALUS *sanguineus*; yellow d. tick, see HAEMAPHYSALIS *leachi leachi*.

wild d. includes dingo, Siberian wild dog, the South American bush dog, the maned wolf, Cordillera fox, crab-eating fox, Azara's fox. See also FOX, JACKAL, WOLF.

dog-ear a defect in skin created when an elliptical surgical incision is too short or one side is longer than the other.

dog's mercury see MERCURIALIS.

dog-sitting posture sitting on the haunches like a dog. When cattle or horses sit for long periods on their haunches with the foreparts of their body off the ground and their forelimbs extended like a dog, and if there is difficulty in rising, there may be a musculoskeletal problem in the area of the pelvis and caudal vertebral column. This dog-sitting posture adopted for short periods by horses and associated with other signs indicative of abdominal pain is usually associated with impaction of the large bowel and pressure on the diaphragm.

dogbane see APOCYNUM *cannabinum*.

Dogue de Bordeaux a French breed of dogs, resembling the Bull mastiff. The head is massive with a short nose; the coat is short and dark auburn or fawn in color. Called also French mastiff.

dol a unit of pain intensity.

dola see LIGULARIA AMPLEXICAULIS.

DOLD diffuse obstructive lung disease. See CHRONIC obstructive pulmonary disease.

Dole pony a small Norwegian horse, 14.2 to 15.2 hands high, most of which are black or brown. Called also Dole-Gudsbrandsdal.

D. p. trotter a pony related to Dole pony but lighter in weight and used for harness racing.

dolich(o)- word element. [Gr.] *long*.

dolichocephalic having a narrow, long head. Characteristic of some dog breeds, e.g. Collie, Borzoi, Greyhound.

dolichofacial having a long face.

dolichol special lipid molecule that links oligosaccharide to asparagine residues in proteins via a pyrophosphate bridge; an example of protein glycosylation.

dolichopellic having a long pelvis from front to back.

dolicomorphic having a long, thin, asthenic body type.

dollar spots subcutaneous plaques characteristic of the second stage of dourine caused by *Trypanosoma equiperdum*. See DOURINE.

doll's eye the fixation of the eye in midorbit, unresponsive to vestibular stimulation. Seen in brainstem injury.

d. e. reflex symmetrical deviation of the eyes when the head is moved in different positions, always returning to center. Abnormalities are caused by lesions of the inner ear or brainstem, especially the pons and midbrain. Called also oculocephalogyric reflex, oculovestibulocephalic reflex. Called also doll's head reflex.

doll's eyes see ACTAEA *spicata*.

doll's head reflex see DOLL'S EYE.

dolomite a limestone with a high concentration of magnesium. Used as a mineral supplement for animals. Called also dolomitic limestone.

dolophine see METHADONE.

dolor [L.] *pain;* one of the cardinal signs of inflammation.

dolorific producing pain.

dolorimeter an instrument for measuring pain in dols.

dolphin a member of the suborder Odonotoceti of the order Cetacea, the whales. Includes the Amazon and Ganges freshwater dolphins, the common dolphin (*Delphinus delphis*) and the bottle-nosed dolphins (*Tursiops truncatus*), and the Arctic dolphin, more commonly called the beluga whale. Others include Chinese river dolphin (*Lipotes vexillifer*).

domain 1. region of a protein with a characteristic tertiary structure and function; homologous domains may occur on different proteins. 2. regions of the heavy chain of immunoglobulins. See $C_{1/2}$ DOMAIN, $C_{5/8}$ DOMAIN.

transmembrane d. for any membrane-bound protein or glycoprotein, those amino acid sequences that traverse and are present in the cell membrane. In receptor biology, transmembrane domains are distinguished from the extracellular ligand binding domains, cytoplasmic domains, and from immunological domains.

domed forehead bulging of the forehead; in the newborn it is usually indicative of congenital hydrocephalus or of achondroplastic disease as in dwarfism. See also MENINGOCELE.

domestic pertaining to an environment managed by humans.

d. animals animals accustomed to living in a domestic environment.

d. cat often used to describe mongrel or crossbred cats, either shorthaired or longhaired.

d. markets local markets; usually refers to markets in the same country.

domiciliary pertaining to a household.

d. calls professional veterinary calls made to patients at their owners' residences. Called also house calls.

d. practice the practitioner does not possess a fixed professional premises but makes all of his/her calls at the owners' houses.

dominance 1. the supremacy, or superior manifestation, in a specific situation of one of two or more competitive or mutually antagonistic factors or animals. 2. in genetics, alleles which fully express their phenotype when present in the heterozygous state.

d. aggression behavior by an animal that asserts its dominance over another or a human, such as competing for food, resisting control measures, or assuming dominant postures.

d. deviation a deviation from gene additive action due to dominance.

incomplete d. when a heterozygote displays the effects of two alleles at the same location; the alleles are said to be incompletely dominant or co-dominant.

location dependent d. behavior in which an animal is dominant when in its home territory, but it becomes subordinate outside that territory.

d. relationship probability of relatives having the same genotype.

dominant 1. exerting a ruling or controlling influence; in genetics, capable of expression when carried by only one of a pair of homologous chromosomes. 2. a dominant allele or trait. If a defect, appearance in all heterozygotes and homozygotes tends toward the trait being self-limiting because of culling or death. See also GENE, DOMINANCE.

d. X-linked inheritance see X-LINKED.

domination the relationship between animals and humans in which little consideration is given to the rights of the animals. The prevailing sentiment is one of proprietary domination.

domperidone a dopamine antagonist used as an antiemetic.

DON see DEOXYNIVALENOL.

Don horse golden chestnut Russian light horse.

Donati vertical mattress suture a variation on the vertical mattress suture pattern in which the suture material penetrates the skin on only one side. On the other side it is intracutaneous.

donkey a member of the family Equidae, descended from the wild ass of which there are still many varieties. Characteristically gray to sable in color, short of stature, long, floppy-eared and with a bray as a call instead of a whinny. Many have a dorsal and shoulder stripes. The male participates in the development of the mule and the female in the production of the hinny. Males are jacks, females are jennies. Called also ass, burro.

d. foot an upright, narrow foot with a small sole area and usually a poorly developed frog. Works well on a donkey but in a horse expected to do fast, hard work it causes chronic mild lameness. All four feet are affected.

donkey-heeled shoe a horseshoe with the lateral heel carried out and away from the hoof. Used on a pigeon-toed horse to help keep the feet away from each other and prevent brushing.

Donnan's equilibrium the state of equilibrium that exists at a semipermeable membrane when it separates two solutions containing electrolytes, the ions of some of which are able to permeate the membrane and the others not. The distribution of the ions in the two solutions becomes complicated so that an electrical potential develops between the two sides of the membrane and the two solutions have different osmotic pressures. Called also Gibbs–Donnan phenomenon.

donor 1. an organism that supplies living tissue to be used in another body, as an animal which furnishes blood for transfusion, or an organ for transplantation. 2. a substance or compound that contributes part of itself to another substance (acceptor).

dont- prefix meaning teeth.

doolan see ACACIA *salicina*.

door the movable barrier, usually hinged, that closes a passageway normally used for entering and leaving an enclosure.

dog/cat d. usually consists of a hinged flap covering an opening just large enough for the animal to pass through, within an existing window or door. Intended for use of the animal at will, but excluding larger intruders.

dopa L-3,4-dihydroxyphenylalanine. Key intermediate in two pathways; the production of melanins from tyrosine catalyzed by the copper-containing enzyme, tyrosinase, to produce dopa, or the biosynthesis of catecholamines catalyzed by the action of tyrosine. It is used in manganese poisoning. Called also L-dopa and levodopa.

dopamine a compound, hydroxytyramine, produced by the decarboxylation of dopa; an intermediate product in the synthesis of norepinephrine. It is a neurotransmitter in the central nervous system; administered intravenously to correct hemodynamic imbalance in shock syndrome.

d. agonist used to terminate pregnancy. See BROMOCRIPTINE, CABERGOLINE.

d. [beta]-hydroxylase enzyme catalyzing the synthesis of norepinephrine from dopamine. A copper-containing mono-oxygenase requiring vitamin C (ascorbic acid).

dopaminergic activated or transmitted by dopamine; pertaining to tissues or organs affected by dopamine.

DOPC deoxycorticosterone pivilate.

doping the illicit administration of drugs or other agents to racing animals with the intention of altering their physical performance, either adversely or positively. Called also sting.

doppellender, doppellendigkeit [Ger.] see MYOFIBER hyperplasia.

doppellendigkeit see MYOFIBER hyperplasia.

Doppler an Austrian physicist and mathematician.

duplex D. imaging see DOPPLER ULTRASOUND.

D. effect the relationship of the apparent frequency of waves, as of sound, light and radio waves, to the relative motion of the source of the waves and the observer, the frequency increasing as the two approach each other and decreasing as they move apart.

The Doppler effect can be experienced when a train whistle or automobile horn produces a continuous sound as it approaches and passes a listener. The pitch of the sound suddenly falls as the source passes the listener.

D. shift the change in frequency that occurs when high frequency sound waves are reflected from a moving surface; the basis for DOPPLER ULTRASOUND.

Doppler-shift sphygmomanometer an instrument that replaces auscultation of the artery for the appearance and disappearance of Korotkoff sounds by an ultrasound flowmeter.

Doppler ultrasound that in which measurement and a visual record are made of the shift in frequency of a continuous ultrasonic wave proportional to the blood-flow velocity in underlying vessels; used in diagnosis of extracranial occlusive vascular disease. It is also used in detection of the fetal heartbeat or of the velocity of movement of a structure, such as the beating heart.

color flow D. u. a form of pulse wave Doppler in which the energy of the returning echoes is displayed as an assigned color; by convention echoes representing flow towards the transducer are seen as shades of red, and those representing flow away from the transducer are seen as shades of blue. The color display is usually superimposed on the B-mode image, thus allowing simultaneous visualization of anatomy and flow dynamics.

continuous wave D. u. a technique in which the transducer emits and receives the ultrasound beam continuously, enabling the measurement of high velocity blood flow, such as occurs through heart valve stenoses.

duplex D. u. a form of image display in which both spectral and color flow images are seen simultaneously. This facilitates accurate anatomical location of the blood flow under investigation.

D. u. flowmeter a device for measuring blood flow that transmits sound at a frequency of several megahertz downstream along the flowing blood. Some of the sound waves are reflected by the moving red blood cells back toward the transducer. The difference in pitch between the transmitted and reflected sounds is produced as an audible tone and is proportional to the velocity of blood flow. The flowmeter can be incorporated into a stethoscope so that qualitative and quantitative measurements of the flow of blood through arteries and veins can be obtained. The Doppler flowmeter is capable of recording very rapid pulsatile changes in flow as well as steady flow.

pulse wave D. u. a technique in which the transducer emits ultrasound in pulses. Blood flow velocities so measured are limited to around the physiologic range (up to approximately 1.5 meters/second) but the depth from which the returning echoes originate can be accurately determined.

spectral D. u. a form of ultrasound image display in which the spectrum of flow velocities is represented graphically on the Y-axis and time on the X-axis; both pulse wave and continuous wave Doppler are displayed in this way.

dorcas gazelle a small North African gazelle; called also *Gazella dorcas*.

Dormer South African dual-purpose sheep with fleece of 22 to 24 micron fiber diameter. Produced by crossing Merino and Dorset Horn breeds.

dormitory effect the apparent influence on promoting estrus in queens when they are housed with others who are cycling.

dormouse see GLIS.

dornase a shortened term for *de*oxy*r*ibo*n*ucle*ase*; also a word termination, as in strepto*dornase.*

Doronicum hungaricum European plant in the family Asteraceae; contains an unidentified toxin which causes paralysis and convulsions. Called also wild sunflower.

Dorper South African meat sheep bred by crossing BLACKHEAD PERSIAN with DORSET HORN sheep; white with black head, black feet, and a hairy, carpetwool fleece.

dorsad toward the back.

dorsal directed toward or situated on the back surface, the surface facing away from the ground; opposite the ventral.

d. column system the sensory tracts in the dorsal funiculus of the spinal cord, consisting of the fasciculus gracilis and fasciculus cuneatus.

d. metacarpal disease a range of compressive stress lesions of the cortex of the third metacarpal bone of young racing horses; includes bucked shins, incomplete cortical fracture.

d. recumbency see dorsal RECUMBENCY.

d. respiratory group that part of the respiratory center which is located in the dorsal medulla oblongata.

d. stripe the dark brown mark that runs along the middle of the back from the poll to the butt of the tail in donkeys, mules, yellow dun horses and primitive horses and ponies.

dorsalgia pain in the back.

dorsalis [L.] *dorsal.*

Dorset Down English short wool, meat sheep, polled, with brown face and legs.

Dorset horn short wool, meat sheep, with large, curled horns; widely used as fat lamb sire. Wool is medium-fine at 27 microns.

dorsiflexion backward flexion or bending, as of the neck.

dors(o)- word element. [L.] *the back, the dorsal aspect.*

dorsocephalad toward the back of the head.

dorsolateral pertaining to the back and side.

d. tract a group of nerve fibers in the lateral funiculus of the spinal cord that cap the dorsal column.

dorsopalmar the passage of an x-ray beam from the dorsal aspect of the forelimb to the palmar aspect. Its use is limited to the carpus and below.

dorsoplantar passage of an x-ray beam from the dorsal aspect of the hindlimb to the plantar aspect. Its use is limited to the hock and below.

dorsoventral 1. pertaining to the back and belly surfaces of a body. 2. passing from the back to the belly surface.

d. view in radiology, passage of the x-ray beam from the dorsum of the animal to the ventral side of the body.

dorsum pl. *dorsa* [L.] 1. the back; the superior surface of a body or body part, as of the paw or foot. 2. the aspect of an anatomical structure or part corresponding in position to the back; posterior in the human.

DOS DISK operating system.

dosage 1. in pharmaceutical terms is the determination and regulation of the size, frequency and number of doses. 2. genetically speaking refers to the amount of gene product in each cell.

d. compensation compensation by random X-inactivation, of the dosage of gene material in the cells of males and females carrying X-linked genes.

dose the quantity to be administered at one time, as a specified amount of medication or a given quantity of radiation.

absorbed d. that amount of energy from ionizing radiations absorbed per unit mass of matter, expressed in Grays.

air d. the intensity of an x- or gamma-ray beam in air, expressed in coulombs per kilogram.

booster d. an amount of immunogen (vaccine, toxoid or other antigen preparation), sometimes smaller than the original amount, injected at an appropriate interval after primary immunization to enhance and sustain the immune response to that immunogen.

curative d. (CD) a dose that is sufficient to restore normal health.

divided d. a fraction of the total quantity of a drug prescribed to be given at intervals, usually during a 24-hour period.

d. equivalent limits the limits of ionizing radiation set for radiation workers and the general public by the International Commission on Radiological Protection. For radiology workers this limit for the whole body is 50 mSv.

fatal d. lethal dose.

infectious d. 50 (ID_{50}) that amount of pathogenic microorganisms that will produce infection in 50% of the test subjects.

infective d. (ID) that amount of pathogenic microorganisms that will cause infection in susceptible subjects.

lethal d. (LD) the amount of toxin or drug that will kill an animal.

d. level the amount administered per unit of body weight.

loading d. the initial large dose of a drug given to bring tissue and fluid levels to an effective concentration quickly. Called also priming dose.
maintenance d. the smaller doses given to maintain effective levels in body fluids and tissues after the loading dose has achieved the concentration desired.
maximum permissible d. see dose equivalent limits (above).
median curative d. (CD_{50}) a dose that abolishes signs in 50% of test animals.
median effective d. (MED) the dose that produces the desired effect in 50% of the test animals.
median lethal d. (MD_{50}) the quantity of an agent that will kill 50% of the test subjects; in radiology, the amount of radiation that will kill, within a specified period, 50% of individuals in a large group or population.
minimum lethal d. (MLD) the lowest dose which kills all of the test subjects.
d. rate the amount administered per unit of time.
d. response 1. the incremental change in the subject per unit of additional dose. The response as a function of the dose. 2. the frequency of occurrence of a disease as the intake of the suspected risk factor increases. The relationship is expressed by the proximity of the illustrative curve to the expected relationship.
skin d. 1. the air dose of radiation at the skin surface, comprising the primary radiation plus backscatter. 2. the absorbed dose in the skin.
tolerance d. the largest quantity of an agent that may be administered without harm.

dose-related see DOSE response.
dosimeter an instrument used to detect and measure exposure to radiation.
dosimetry scientific determination of amount, rate and distribution of radiation emitted from a source of ionizing radiation.
dosing injuries injuries inflicted on patients with dosing equipment. Includes buccal and pharyngeal injuries with balling guns, dosing syringes, drenching guns, esophageal and nasal tubes, gags and specula.
dot matrix see dot matrix PRINTER.
double two of them.
d. burst stimulation a technique of nerve stimulation in which two short tetanic stimuli are applied and the response pattern used to monitor neuromuscular blockade during anesthesia.
d. cervix see double CERVIX.
d. click pressing and releasing the mouse button twice in quick succession.
d. diffusion precipitin test see IMMUNODIFFUSION.
d. fleece 2 years' growth of wool.
d. gee see EMEX AUSTRALIS.
d. muscling see MYOFIBER hyperplasia.
d. pregnancy see SUPERFETATION.
d. reciprocal plot a graphical technique for analyzing drug antagonisms by plotting the effect against the dose. Called also Lineweaver–Burk plot.
d. scalp palpable thinning of the cranial bones in young sheep on inadequate diet.
d.-stranded (ds) nucleic acid occurring as a two-strand helix.

double-blind study a study of the effects of a specific agent in which neither the administrator nor the recipient, at the time of administration, knows whether the active or an inert substance is given.
double-seeded emu bush see GYROSTEMON *tepperi*.
douche [Fr.] a stream of water or air directed against a part of the body or into a cavity.
air d. a current of air blown into a cavity, particularly into the tympanum to open the eustachian tube.
vaginal d. irrigation of the vagina to cleanse the area, to apply medicated solutions to the vaginal mucosa and the cervix.

dough stage a stage in the maturation of a cereal crop when the seeds are soft and immature but fully formed. This is the optimum time to convert the crop into hay or ensilage.
Douglas spurred lupin LUPINUS *laxiflorus*.
dourine a sexually transmitted trypanosomiasis of horses caused by *Trypanosoma equiperdum*, characterized by inflammation of the external genitalia, edema of the ventral abdominal wall, muscle weakness and incoordination. Severe loss of condition may be followed by emaciation to the point where euthanasia is necessary. Urticaria-like plaques called dollar spots occur on the skin in some forms of the disease.
douroucouli see OWL MONKEY.
dove a bird which together with the pigeon forms the large bird family Columbidae. There appears not to be a clearcut distinction between the two groups and some types have alternative names, one of them a pigeon, the other one a dove. They vary in color, but mostly within the range of gray, through cream and light brown to a deep beige, sometimes with markings. The legs are clean of feathers.
dowel a slim cylinder of bone consisting of two plates of cortical bone separated by an internal sandwich of cancellous bone. Used for fusing bones or reconstructing large bones.
down feather small feathers whose barbs do not unite to form a closed vane, thus giving it a fluffy appearance.
down regulation means of controlling hormone action where the number of hormone receptors at the cell surface is decreased by internalization of the receptor complex.
down time the periods when a computer is not available for use, usually because of hardware or software malfunction.
downer cow syndrome a commonly fatal condition of dairy cows closely associated with the unsuccessful treatment of cases of hypocalcemic parturient paresis. At postmortem examination there is a variety of contributing lesions including especially ischemic necrosis of the muscles of the thigh, damage to major nerves to the hindlimb, traumatic separation of muscles and tendons, hip dislocation and hepatic and myocardial degeneration.
downhill vagina the cranial vagina is lower than the vestibule so that drainage is inadequate.
Downs sheep a group of breeds of British shortwool or mutton breeds of sheep with colored faces. All are polled and have some Southdown blood. Includes Dorset Down, Southdown, Oxford Down, Suffolk, Hampshire, Shropshire.
downstream a term used in molecular biology to describe nucleotides of a nucleic acid molecule which lie in the 3′ direction from a particular reference point, such as the site of initiation of transcription. See also UPSTREAM.
doxapram hydrochloride a respiratory stimulant which acts upon peripheral chemoreceptors. It is commonly used to reverse sedation induced by xylazine, although the antagonism is not specific.
doxepin a tricyclic antidepressant and potent histamine H_1-receptor blocker, similar to amitriptyline, used in the treatment of psychogenic dermatitis in dogs and cats.
doxorubicin an antineoplastic antibiotic, which binds to DNA and inhibits synthesis of nucleic acids and cell division. It is used intravenously to produce

regression in various neoplastic conditions. The side-effects include bone marrow depression, alopecia and cardiac toxicity. Called also adriamycin. See also anthracycline ANTIBIOTIC.

doxycycline a second-generation, lipid-soluble tetracycline derivative with greater activity against anaerobes and intracellular bacteria, and a longer half-life. Used as the monohydrate.

doxylamine an antihistamine used in the treatment of allergic reactions and laminitis in cattle and horses.

Doyen forceps lightly compressive, long-bladed, curved forceps with rachet handle designed for intestinal compression. The blade faces are lightly grooved along their length. Called also Gillman forceps.

Doyle's disease see NEWCASTLE DISEASE.

DPG diphosphoglycerate.

dpi dots per inch, a measure of the density, and therefore the clarity, of print of each character.

DPN diphosphopyridine nucleotide.

Dr. Doctor.

dr. dram.

Dr. Larson's teat tube a plastic, self-retaining tube with a blunt end and side holes which acts as a permanent drain for the quarter. It has a screw-on cap so that the drainage can be arrested. Good for retaining patency after teat surgery.

Drabkin's solution a solution used in a technique for hemoglobin estimation.

drachm dram.

dracunculiasis, dracunculosis infection and infestation by nematodes of the genus *Dracunculus*.

Dracunculus a genus of spiruroid nematode parasites in the family Dracunculidae. Includes *D. alii*, *D. dahomensis*, *D. globocephalus*, *D. ophidensis* (all in reptiles), *D. fuelliborni* (in opossum); *D. lutrae* (in otter),

D. insignis a spiruroid worm infesting dogs and wild carnivores. Causes cutaneous lesions and ulcers, sometimes internal lesions, e.g. in heart and vertebral column. Called also dragon, fiery dragon, guinea worm.

D. medinensis a thread-like worm widely distributed in North America, Africa, the Near East, East Indies and India; frequently found in the subcutaneous and intermuscular tissues of humans and also in dogs, sometimes horses and cattle. Causes cutaneous nodules and subsequently ulcers.

draft[1] a potion or dose.

draft[2] 1. the hauling of vehicles, implements and other loads. 2. separation of a group of animals into different classifications, e.g. those for sale and those to be kept for breeding. Commonly a procedure performed in a drafting race or chute, and through a drafting gate.

d. animals includes dogs, horses and other Equidae, oxen, reindeer, yak, elephant, water buffalo.

draft horses see DRAFT animals.

drag technique used to move an object or some text. The object is selected by clicking the mouse button and holding it down over the subject. Still holding the button down the mouse is moved to the new location for the subject and the button released, thus completing the maneuver.

Dräger tonometer instrument for the measurement of intraocular pressure.

Dräger vaporizer a copper kettle halothane vaporizer; is temperature compensating and calibrated to deliver concentrations of halothane from 0 to 5%. See also NORTH AMERICAN Dräger.

dragon see DRACUNCULUS *insignis*.

Drahthaar an early name for the German wirehaired pointer.

drain 1. to withdraw liquid gradually. 2. any device by which a channel or open area may be established for exit of fluids or purulent material from a cavity wound, or infected area. See also WOUND healing.

cigarette d. a drain made by drawing a small strip of gauze or surgical sponge into a tube of gutta-percha or rubber.

Penrose d. a thin tube of latex rubber; secretions drain around, not through this tube.

sump d. a drainage system in which a small air tube is located inside the lumen or wall of a larger tube that drains fluid from a cavity.

underwater d. the external opening of the drainage tube is immersed in a sealed container of water; used for drains from the pleural cavity to collect drainage yet maintain a mild negative pressure.

drainage systematic withdrawal of fluids and discharges from a wound, sore or cavity.

d. angle IRIDOCORNEAL angle.

capillary d. that effected by strands of hair, catgut, spun glass, or other material of small caliber which acts by capillary attraction.

closed d. drainage of an empyema cavity carried out with protection against the entrance of outside air into the pleural cavity.

open d. drainage of an empyema cavity through an opening in the chest wall into which one or more rubber drainage tubes are inserted, the opening not being sealed against the entrance of outside air.

peritoneal d. drainage of the peritoneum; limited by the rapid formation of adhesions and can only be accomplished with lavage or through an open cavity.

suction d. a source of continuous or intermittent negative pressure is used to maintain drainage in various sites, particularly negative pressure in the pleural cavity. A syringe and valve, one-way valve, vacuum tube or underwater drain can be used for this purpose.

d. systems see DRAIN.

tidal d. drainage of the urinary bladder by an apparatus that alternately fills the bladder to a predetermined pressure and empties it by a combination of siphonage and gravity flow.

d. tubes see DRAIN.

drake 1. male duck. 2. LOLIUM *temulentum*.

Drakensberger a black breed of cattle used for meat and dairying, produced in South Africa by crossing Friesian with Africander. Called also Black Africander.

dram, drachm a unit of weight in the avoirdupois (27.344 grains, $\frac{1}{16}$ ounce) or apothecaries' (60 grains, $\frac{1}{8}$ ounce) system; symbol ʒ.

fluid d. a unit of liquid measure of the apothecaries' system, containing 60 minims, and equivalent to 3.697 ml. See also Table 4.3. Abbreviated fl. dr.

drape the cloth used to cover the animal for surgery leaving exposed only that part of the body that has been aseptically prepared and is actually required for the surgical procedure. Applying the drapes is called draping.

draping covering the animal with sterile drapes for surgery leaving exposed only that part of the body that has been aseptically prepared and is actually required for the surgical procedure.

Draschia a genus of the worm family of Habronematidae. Includes *D. megastoma* (syn. *Habronema megastoma*) found in intramural nodules in the stomach wall of horses.

drastics a term used to describe highly irritant laxatives.

drawer sign see ANTERIOR (cranial) drawer sign.

drawing knife see hoof KNIFE.

Drechslera genus of fungi; includes *D. biseptata*, *D. campanulata*, *D. rostrata*, *D. spicifera*. Called also *Bipolaris* spp.

D. rostrata a fungus isolated from nasal cavities of cattle affected by ENZOOTIC nasal granuloma. Now called *Exserohilum rostratum*.

D. spiciferum an obsolete name for *Bipolaris spicifera*. The imperfect state of *Cochliobolus spicifera*. Associated with phaeohyphomycosis in animals.

drench 1. to give medicines in liquid form by mouth and forcing the animal to drink. See also DRENCHING. 2. medicines given as a drench.

drenching farmer's term for the administration of medicines as solutions or suspensions in water by mouth with a drench bottle, gun or funnel.

d. bit to be included in a bridle as a bit. Has a hollow tube instead of a solid bit, with perforations, and an inlet to which a funnel is fitted. The drench material is poured into the funnel and exits into the mouth.

d. gun injury laceration of the oral mucosa or fauces with the nozzle of the gun, due usually to over-vigorous attempts to use the gun as a device to open the jaws.

drepanocyte a sickle cell.

drepanocytosis occurrence of drepanocytes (sickle cells) in the blood.

dressage the dressing of a riding horse as distinct from the training of a racing horse. The term has come to include formal training and competition in a standard arena and with standard furniture for jumps and a standard layout for the course to be followed. The formal training comprises a complex series of exercises in deportment for the horse and rider. They require great precision in execution so that the quintessence of the training is the lightness of the commands and controls and the degree to which the horse and rider are collected in their movements.

dressed seed corn cereal grain intended for seed and treated with antifungal agents; it is often fed to livestock when it is not needed for seed and may cause poisoning. See SEED dressing.

dressed weight weight of a carcass of an animal being prepared for use as meat; the head, lower limbs, skin (with the exception of poultry which have, however, been defeathered) and viscera (except kidney) have been removed.

dressing 1. any of various materials used for covering and protecting a wound. A pressure dressing is used for maintaining constant pressure, as in the control of bleeding. A protective dressing is applied to shield a part from injury or from septic infection. 2. of a carcass of meat see CARCASS dressing.

biological d. skin grafts.

dry d. support and pressure bandages not applied to moist wounds.

occlusive d. plastic film placed over medication that has been applied to the skin enhances absorption by trapping moisture, raising skin temperature and concentrating the medication.

d. percentage see CARCASS yield.

wet d. soaking of a bulky dressing to aid in cleansing, drainage and débridement of a wound. May be applied intermittently or continuously.

dressing-out percentage see CARCASS yield.

DRG see DORSAL respiratory group.

dribblers steers in feedlots with incomplete urethral obstruction by urinary calculi so that they pass small amounts of urine frequently. In some of these cases the calculus has an irregular shape and permits the passage of some urine.

dried fruit mite itch see CARPOGLYPHUS.

drift chance variation; in genetics, the random changes in gene frequencies in a population.

antigenic d. see ANTIGENIC drift.

d. lambing a strategy in which ewes which have lambed are periodically removed from a flock of lambing ewes by moving the unlambed ewes on to the next paddock or field.

drifting sideways the patient moves gradually to one side when attempting to walk in a straight line.

drill 1. one of the Old World monkeys; resembles the mandrill but has a black face. Called also *Mandrillus leucophaeus*. 2. in dentistry, a mechanical device used for removing tooth structure. See also BUR.

drinking water supply of water available to animals for drinking supplied via nipples, in troughs, dams, ponds and larger natural water sources; an insufficient supply leads to dehydration; it can be the source of infection, e.g. leptospirosis, salmonellosis, or of poisoning, e.g. fluorine, sodium chloride.

Drinkwater mouth gag a mouth gag for use in cattle and horses. Made of cast aluminum, it consists of two wedges, one for each side of the mouth, which are pushed up between the upper and lower molars. The reflex clamping of the jaws ensures that they are retained. Gives excellent access to the pharynx and the incisors are in full view.

drip the slow, drop-by-drop infusion of a liquid.

postnasal d. drainage of excessive mucous or mucopurulent discharge from the postnasal region into the pharynx.

d. rate pumps a mechanical device used to deliver a constant rate of intravenous fluids. It applies pressure to the fluid line through a set of rollers.

dripping 1. continuous discharge of an exudate or secretion. 2. rendered beef fat.

drive 1. motivation; determination to pursue a course of action or achieve a specific target. 2. the mechanical device in a computer which drives the program and the data base past the reading head of the computer, e.g. hard disk drive, floppy disk drive, magnetic tape drive.

drive census collection of data about a population by herding them all together, making a complete muster for an area.

driver a program used to control a peripheral device such as a a printer.

driving disease see ovine PULMONARY adenomatosis.

Dromaius novae-hollandiae see EMU.

dromedary see CAMELUS *dromedarius*.

dromotropic pertaining to dromotropy.

dromotropy affecting conductivity of a nerve fiber; it may be positive or negative.

Droncit a proprietary name for PRAZIQUANTEL.

dronkgras see MELICA DECUMBENS.

drooling the discharge of saliva from the mouth. A normal feature in some breeds of dogs such as St. Bernard, Newfoundland and English bulldog, presumably because of their loose, pendulous lips. In other dogs and in cats it can be a sign of abnormalities of swallowing, painful oral lesions, diseased teeth, or disorders of salivary glands with hypersialosis.

drooping quarters see GOOSE-RUMPED.

drop 1. a minute sphere of liquid as it hangs or falls. 2. a descent or falling below the usual position.

droperidol a tranquilizer of the butyrophenone series, used as a narcoleptic preanesthetic and, in combination with fentanyl citrate, as a neuroleptanalgesic.

droplet very small drop of fluid.

d. nuclei the finite particles of matter which are transmitted from animal to animal.

dropout a patient which becomes inaccessible or ineligible to follow-up procedures.

dropped said of an anatomical part that has fallen below its usual position.

d. elbow results from injury to the axillary and/or thoracodorsal nerves and paralysis of the flexors of the shoulder. Occurs in injuries to the brachial plexus or its roots, such as avulsion. See also RADIAL paralysis.

d. jaw see MANDIBULAR neurapraxia.

d. monkey muscle separation of the triceps muscle from the scapula in a Greyhound.

d. muscle rupture of the gracilis muscle.

d. sole a lesion only in the horse. The horn of the sole becomes detached from its sensitive laminae and drops to the point where the concavity of the normal sole is flat. Can occur acutely due to edema of the part or because of acute laminitis, or chronically, usually due to recurrent minor episodes of laminitis.

d. toe rupture of the extensor tendons and dorsal elastic ligament of a toe in a dog; especially common in racing Greyhounds.

d. udder see MAMMARY suspensory ligament rupture.

d. wrist ventriflexion and weakness of the hand in primates with severe demineralization because of dietary deficiency of vitamin D alone or in combination with calcium.

dropper 1. a pipette or tube for dispensing liquids in drops. 2. a wooden or metal spreader holding the wires in a farm fence apart.

droppings a term commonly applied to feces, particularly from birds.

dropsical affected with or pertaining to dropsy.

dropsy an abnormal accumulation of serous fluid in a body cavity or in the cellular tissues; called also hydrops, edema. See also EDEMA.

fetal d. includes ascites, hydrothorax or local due to lymph node agenesis; causes dystocia.

fetal sacs d. see HYDRALLANTOIS, HYDRAMNIOS.

placenta d. usually accompanies a placentitis.

tropical fish d. caused by *Aeromonas liquefaciens*. Begins as cutaneous erythema, followed by abdominal distension.

dropwort see OENANTHE.

Drosanthemum genus of southern African plants in the family Aizoaceae; contain soluble oxalates which may cause nephrosis.

Drosera genus of insectivorous plants in family Droseraceae; some species may cause cyanide poisoning. Called also sundews.

drought feeding feeding of cattle and sheep on minimal diets to maintain life during periods of poor rainfall and pasture growth. Requires judgment to avoid animals reaching an irreversible stage of thinness.

drought-resistant pasture types or animal breeds which survive better than others during periods of low rainfall.

Droughtmaster a red, polled or horned breed of beef cattle produced in Australia by crossing Brahman and Shorthorn breeds.

droving 1. moving cattle or sheep from one place to another by driving them slowly on foot along roadways or stock routes. 2. in less temperate climates the same exercise conducted by truck is called droving.

drowning death from suffocation resulting from aspiration of water or other substance or fluid. Drowning occurs because the liquid prevents breathing.

dry-d. asphyxiation, but with little or no inhalation of water as a result of persistent laryngospasm.

near-d. see NEAR-DROWNING.

secondary d. pulmonary edema may occur some time after a near-drowning due to loss of surfactant.

drug 1. any medicinal substance. 2. a narcotic. 3. to administer a drug.

d. administration includes aerosol, oral, transtracheal infusion, subcutaneous, intramuscular, intravenous, intrauterine, intraperitoneal, intra-articular, intramammary, intrathecal, subconjunctival, percutaneous, percutaneous intraruminal, gas inhalation. Mass medication is per feed or drinking water or, in the case of captive fish, in the tank water. For feral animals individual dosing by projectile dart is usual, for group therapy administration by bait is possible.

d. allergy immune-mediated hypersensitivity to a drug molecule. Includes anaphylaxis, cutaneous reaction.

animal d. a drug specifically tested for, and recommended for use in, animals. A legal point of importance if an animal dies as a result of an unusual or allergic reaction to medication with a drug not licensed for use in animals.

d. augmented swine dysentery pigs receiving prophylactic medication are more severely affected than untreated pigs.

bactericidal/bacteriostatic d. see ANTIBIOTIC.

d. binding binding of a drug to a large molecule in the tissues or fluids, e.g. binding to protein in the blood, may affect the metabolism of the drug, especially its rate of excretion.

chemotherapeutic d. see CHEMOTHERAPY.

d. combinations a pharmaceutical strategy of combining several drugs into one formulation to provide for a specific requirement, e.g. an antibiotic combined with an anti-inflammatory agent in a mastitis ointment. Has the disadvantage that the dose of one drug is determined by the dose of the other.

controlled d. availability and use of the drug is controlled by law. The control is at various levels of severity depending on the degree of danger associated with the uncontrolled use of each drug.

d. delayed swine dysentery swine dysentery appears several days after treatment is discontinued.

d. delayed-augmented swine dysentery after successful treatment during an attack of swine dysentery a more severe form of the disease occurs after treatment ceases.

d. diminished swine dysentery the disease is reduced in severity as a result of treatment but is not eliminated.

d. eruption an eruption or solitary skin lesion caused by a drug. See also DERMATITIS medicamentosa.

d. hypersensitivity see drug allergy (above).

mutagenic d's those that affect the DNA of the target organism have the hazard of creating new races of microorganisms with increased pathogenicity.

d. residue the amount of the drug that can be detected in tissues at specified times after administration of the drug ceases. See also drug tolerance (below).

d. resistance said mainly of antibacterial drugs and of microorganisms that are unaffected by the drug whilst most organisms of its species are susceptible. The resistance may be inherent or secondary to frequent exposure at sublethal levels. Resistance of an animal to a specific drug, e.g. to insulin, can also occur in this way.

d. resistant swine dysentery medication of the feed is not an effective procedure and diarrhea and deaths occur.

d. safety margin the magnitude of the difference between the dose required to produce a maximum therapeutic effect and that which produces a toxic effect. Registering authorities require this information.

d. selectivity capacity to produce a single effect.

teratogenic d. produces a toxic effect on the fetus at a particular phase of development producing a malformation.

drug-induced caused by the administration of a drug. See also IATROGENIC.

drug–nutrient interaction alterations in nutritional status can affect drug metabolism; some drugs can affect nutritional status.

druggist pharmacist.

drumhead cabbage BRASSICA *oleracea* var. *capitata*.

drumstick a spherical shape with a single, long extension or conversely, a long stick with a knob on the end.

d. lobe a lobe attached by a thin strand of nuclear membrane to the nucleus of a varying percentage of neutrophils in females. Contains the Barr body. Called also sex bud.

d. spore the characteristic spherical, terminal spore of *Clostridium tetani.*

druse crystals a crust of small crystals lining the sides of a cavity.

drusen 1. hyaline excrescences in Bruch's membrane, the inner layer of the choroid of the eye, usually due to aging. 2. rosettes of granules occurring in the lesions of actinomycosis. Called also sulfur granules.

dry a state of dehydration or relative deficiency of water.

d. bench 1. that part of a radiographic dark room where film and cassettes are handled, i.e. there is no chance of film being contaminated by chemicals. 2. a slang expression for simulated research work, for reported experiments that were not actually done.

d. coat syndrome see ANHIDROSIS.

d. eye see KERATOCONJUNCTIVITIS sicca.

d. feeding the entire ration is made up of dried stored grain or hay.

d. food the meal or biscuit type dog and cat foods that contain approximately 10% water. Economical, easily transported and stored; in many countries, this is the most commonly used form of mass produced pet food.

d. ice solidified carbon dioxide; in an icebox, it produces temperatures of about −76°F (−60°C).

d. lot the livestock, usually cattle, are kept in a small area with a firm floor but no roof or walls. All food and water are brought to them. Refers usually to dairy herds. See also FEEDLOT.

d. mash a method of feeding poultry. Essentially a mixture of grain and supplements.

d. rales see RALE.

dry herd see DAIRY herd.

dry matter plant or animal tissue residue after it has been heated to a constant weight and all of the moisture in the sample has been driven off by gentle heat.

d. m. basis a method of expressing the concentration of a nutrient or poison in a feed, by expressing its concentration in terms of the dry matter content.

d. m. intake the feed intake, usually per day, expressed in terms of its dry matter content.

dry period the period during the lactation cycle when the cow is not lactating, i.e. the period between the end of one lactation and the beginning of the next.

d. p. colostrum see dry period secretion (below).

d. p. secretion after lactation ceases in normal cows the milk in the udder changes to a thin watery fluid, then disappears altogether in some, then a thick, honey-like secretion appears, then to a very thick opalescent colostrum and finally the normal custard-like colostrum.

d. p. treatment treatment of the udder of dairy cows during the dry (nonlactating) period. This is an important part of most bovine mastitis control programs in the removal of subclinical infections which have established during the lactation, and reduction of new infections occurring during the dry period. This is effected by treating each quarter of the udder with a long-acting, broad-spectrum antibiotic preparation immediately after the last milking of a lactation. The strategy is highly effective against the common contagious bacterial causes of mastitis, including *Staphylococcus aureus*, *Streptococcus agalactiae*.

The possibility exists that the sterilizing effect that the technique has on the udder may increase its sensitivity to other infections. In order to avoid this it is recommended that only those cows that show evidence of mastitis be treated in this way. This also greatly reduces the cost of the operation in those herds in which the incidence of the disease is low.

dry sheep equivalent a unit of animal feed based on how much more or less feed each animal requires compared with that required by one dry (not lactating) sheep; abbreviated DSE. The same system can be used to estimate the nutritive value of a paddock of pasture or a shed full of hay. Based on the figure of a daily requirement for 7.2 megajoules of metabolizable energy for a 2-year-old dry sheep weighing 45 kg; e.g. a dairy cow milking 20 kg milk/day has a dry sheep equivalent of 23; a beef calf of 200 kg body weight has a DSE of 4.

dryfarming farming without the aid of irrigation.

drying off the management technique of ceasing to milk cows that are still lactating. Dairy herd management is greatly facilitated if cows can be dried off abruptly when the milk yield has fallen below a profitable level or the ensuing parturition is close. Cows with subclinical mastitis are likely to suffer an attack of clinical mastitis if milking is ceased abruptly, especially if the milk yield is still high. The risks of new infections during the dry period are also greater with abrupt drying off and this may be significant if the prevalence of quarter infection in the herd is high. Precautions against these problems include a short period of once-daily milking and severe restriction of food and water intake, and use of dry period treatment. Another problem arising at drying off, or at cessation of milking to improve the appearance of the cow, is that of anaphylaxis or milk ALLERGY. This takes the form of urticaria and dyspnea about 24 hours after milking is stopped.

d. o. anaphylaxis see milk ALLERGY.

d. o. chronic quarters infusion of an escharotic agent, e.g. silver nitrate, copper sulfate solution into the individual chronically affected quarter, leaving it for a short period, then evacuating the quarter and if necessary perfusing it with normal saline.

drylot see DRY lot.

Drymaria a plant genus of the family Caryophyllaceae; contain an unknown toxin which causes tremor, diarrhea and liver and kidney lesions. Includes *D. arenarioides* (alfombrilla), *D. cordata*, *D. diandra* (tropical chickweed), *D. pachyphylla* (drymary).

drymary DRYMARIA *pachyphylla*.

Dryopteris a genus of the fern family Aspleniaceae; rhizomes contain a toxin thought to be a thiaminase and which causes somnolence, stumbling gait and blindness due to encephalopathy in sheep and cattle. Includes *D. borreri*, *D. filix-mas*. Called also male fern.

Drysdale New Zealand carpetwool sheep derived from ROMNEY MARSH by mutation; wool fiber diameter 35 to 45 microns, white face and dark hooves; rams are horned, ewes polled.

ds double-stranded; used in reference to nucleic acid.
DSE dry sheep equivalent.
DSMA disodium monomethanearsonate; an organic arsenical herbicide. Can cause poisoning similar to inorganic arsenic. See also ARSENIC poisoning.
DTH delayed type hypersensitivity.
DTIC dacarbazine.
DTM dermatophyte test medium.
DTPA diethylenetriamine penta-acetic acid.
Du Du see GOVERNING VESSEL.
dual-purpose applies to any animal but usually refers to cattle (meat and milk), sheep (wool and meat) and fowl (eggs and meat). Dual-purpose cattle breeds include DAIRY SHORTHORN, DEXTER, MEUSE-RHINE-YSSEL, RED POLL, SIMMENTAL, SOUTH DEVON and WELSH BLACK.
dubbeltjie [Af.] see TRIBULUS *terrestris*.
dubbing removal of most of the comb of day-old chickens. See also DECOMBING.
Dubin–Johnson syndrome hereditary chronic nonhemolytic jaundice thought to be due to defective excretion of conjugated bilirubin and certain other organic anions by the liver; a brown coarsely granular pigment in hepatic cells is pathognomonic. A very similar disease occurs in Corriedale and Southdown sheep. See also inherited PHOTOSENSITIZATION.
Duboisia Australian genus of the plant family Solanaceae; contain the piperidine alkaloids nicotine and nor-nicotine, and high concentrations of pyridine alkaloids, e.g. hyoscine, hyoscyamine, with atropine-like actions. Signs include somnolence, tremor, thirst, dilatation of pupil, incoordination. Include *D. hopwoodii* (pituri, pitchery), *D. leichhardtii*, *D. myoporoides* (corkwood).
Duchenne dystrophy a human disease; called also pseudohypertrophic muscular dystrophy.
duck a member of the family Anatidae which includes many genera of ducks, geese and swans. See ANAS PLATYRHYNCHOS, AYLESBURY, ROUEN, INDIAN RUNNER, KHAKI CAMPBELL, PEKIN, MUSCOVY.
d. bush, d. plant *Gomphocarpus physocarpus*. See also ASCLEPIAS.
d. hepatitis a highly infectious and fatal disease of young ducklings caused by an enterovirus, and characterized by hepatitis of sufficient severity to kill the birds within a few hours of signs of illness first being observed.
d. louse *Anaticola crassicornis* (slender duck louse), *Trinoton querquedulae* (large duck louse).
new d. disease see PASTEURELLA *anatipestifer*.
d. plague see duck PLAGUE.
d. septicemia see PASTEURELLA *anatipestifer*.
d. sickness type C botulism.
d. virus enteritis see duck PLAGUE.
duck-billed platypus see PLATYPUS.
duckbill see PLATYPUS.
duckling baby duck.
duckmole see PLATYPUS.
duct a passage with well-defined walls, especially a tubular structure for the passage of excretions or secretions. See also DUCTUS.
accessory pancreatic d. the duct of the dorsal pancreatic primordium that opens on the minor duodenal papilla. Called also Santorini's duct or duct of Santorini.
allantoic d. see URACHUS.
alveolar d. one of the final branches of the bronchial tree consisting of a tube whose walls are composed of alveoli.
bile d., biliary d. the passages for the conveyance of bile in and from the liver. See also BILE DUCT.
cochlear d. a spiral membranous tube in the bony canal of the cochlea divided into the scala tympani, scala vestibuli and spiral lamina.
common bile d. a duct formed by the union of the cystic and hepatic ducts. See also BILE DUCT.
cystic d. the passage connecting the gallbladder neck and the bile duct.
efferent d. any duct that gives outlet to a glandular secretion.
ejaculatory d. the duct formed by union of the ductus deferens and the duct of the seminal vesicles, opening into the prostatic urethra on the colliculus seminalis. Found in the horse and ruminants.
endolymphatic d. a canal connecting the membranous labyrinth of the ear with the endolymphatic sac.
epididymal d. developed from the first part of the mesonephric duct.
excretory d. one through which the secretion is conveyed from a gland.
d. of Gartner see GARTNER'S DUCTS.
hepatic d. the excretory duct of the liver, or one of its branches in the lobes of the liver. See also BILE DUCT.
incisive d. one of a pair of ducts perforating the palate and which communicate between the mouth and the nasal cavity; they are thought to conduct chemicals for olfactory appraisal by the vomeronasal organ.
intralobar d. ducts within lobes which provide drainage for secretions of lobes of glands.
intralobular d. ducts found within lobules which provide drainage for secretions of lobules of glands.
lacrimal d. one of the excretory ducts of the lacrimal gland. See also LACRIMAL apparatus.
lacrimonasal d. nasolacrimal duct.
lactiferous d. ducts conveying the milk secreted by the lobes of the mammary gland to the lactiferous sinuses or to the teats.
lobar d. drains the secretions from the lobes of gland, connecting with the main excretory duct.
lobular d. drains the secretions of lobules of glands.
lymphatic d. larger lymph drainage vessels, e.g. thoracic duct.
lymphatic d. (left) thoracic duct.
lymphatic d. (right) a vessel draining lymph from the cranial right side of the body, receiving lymph from the right subclavian, jugular and mediastinal trunks when those vessels do not open independently into the right brachiocephalic vein.
mammary d. lactiferous ducts.
mandibular d. drainage duct of the mandibular salivary gland.
mesonephric d. see MESONEPHRIC duct.
metanephric d. the embryonic ureter.
müllerian d. see MÜLLERIAN DUCT.
nasal d. the duct leading from the lacrimal sac, opening on the floor of the nasal vestibule. Called also nasolacrimal duct. See also LACRIMAL apparatus.
nasolacrimal d. see nasal duct (above).
nasopalatine d. see incisive duct (above).
pancreatic d. the main excretory duct of the pancreas, which usually opens with the bile duct on the major duodenal papilla; may be a single duct, or two ducts which join, or two independent ducts opening into opposite sides of the intestine. See also BILE DUCT. Called also Wirsung's duct.
papillary d's (kidney) the straight excretory or collecting portions of the renal tubules, which descend through the renal medulla to a renal papilla or renal crest.
papillary d. (teat) see TEAT CANAL.

paramesonephric d. MÜLLERIAN DUCT.
parotid d. the duct by which the parotid gland empties into the mouth vestibule opposite the upper molars. See also PAROTID glands.
perilymphatic d. see AQUEDUCT of cochlea.
pronephric d. the early embryonic duct from the primitive kidney which leads into the mesonephric duct in the embryo's later stages.
prostatic d's minute ducts from the prostate, opening into or near the prostatic sinuses on the dorsal wall of the urethra.
salivary d's the ducts of the salivary glands.
semicircular d's the long ducts of the membranous labyrinth of the ear.
sublingual d. the excretory ducts of the sublingual salivary glands.
submandibular d. the duct that drains the submandibular gland and opens at the sublingual caruncle. Called also submaxillary duct.
submaxillary d. submandibular duct (above).
tear d. nasolacrimal duct.
thoracic d. a duct beginning in the cisterna chyli and emptying into the venous system at the junction of the left subclavian and left jugular veins. It acts as a channel for the collection of lymph from the portions of the body caudal to the diaphragm and from the left side of the body cranial to the diaphragm.
thyroglossal d. the transient, non-patent duct, from the thyroid gland to the floor of the pharynx which is the legacy of the development of the thyroid from the floor of the pharynx.
vitelline d. see MECKEL'S diverticulum.

ductile susceptible of being drawn out without breaking.

ductless having no excretory duct.
d. glands the endocrine glands.

ductule a minute duct.
d. efferent seminiferous tubules open into a rete testis which drains through these efferent ductules which pierce the testicular capsule and join the head of the epididymis.

ductuli biliferi smaller bile ducts accompanying the branches of the portal vein.

ductuli efferentes connect the rete testis with the ductus epididymis.

ductulus pl. *ductuli* [L.] ductule.

ductus pl. *ductus* [L.] duct.
d. arteriosus a fetal blood vessel that joins the aorta and pulmonary artery. Abnormal persistence of an open lumen after birth results in a PATENT ductus arteriosus. Called also persistent or patent ductus arteriosus.
d. choledochus see BILE DUCT.
d. deferens the excretory duct of the testis, which in horses and ruminants joins the excretory duct of the seminal vesicle to form the ejaculatory duct; called also vas deferens.
d. epididymis the duct which, in combination with connective tissue and muscle, forms the head, body and tail of the epididymis and continues as the ductus deferens.
d. epoophori longitudinales see GARTNER'S DUCTS.
d. reuniens the joining channel between the cochlea and sacculus of the membranous labyrinth of the inner ear.
d. venosus a major blood channel that develops through the embryonic liver from the left umbilical vein to the caudal vena cava and closes within a few days after birth. If it remains patent, a congenital PORTACAVAL anastamosis is created.

Dugaldia hoopesii HELENIUM *hoopesii*.

dugaldin a toxic glycoside in HELENIUM.

Dugbe virus a tickborne virus infection of cattle in West Africa. A bunyavirus related to the virus of Nairobi sheep disease.

dugite the spotted brown snake. See DEMANSIA *nuchalis affinis*.

dugong a sirenian animal belonging to the family Dugongidae. Massive (10 to 13 ft long, weighing 600 lb) fusiform silhouette, forelimbs well developed but no hindlimbs or dorsal fin. Called also *Dugong dugon*.

Duhring's disease dermatitis herpetiformis.

DUIB di-ureido isobutane.

duiker, duyker small (up to 50 lb) antelope. Includes gray duiker (*Sylvicapre grimmia*) and *Cephalophus* spp.

duinebos CROTALARIA *spartioides*.

duinsiekte [Af.] 'dune disease', a manifestation of pyrrolizidine alkaloidosis caused by *Crotalaria spartioides* poisoning.

dulaa a saclike pouch of the soft palate, capable of being inflated, everted through the mouth and gargled through by the male camel when in rut.

Dulbecco's medium a phosphate buffered saline diluent used for the storage of fertilized sheep and goat ova.

dullness 1. a quality of sound elicited by percussion, being short and high-pitched with little resonance. 2. a state of consciousness in which the animal's movements are sluggish and its response to external stimuli is one of indifference.
cardiac d. the area of the precordium over which a dull percussion sound is elicited.

dumb mute. Commonly said of animals generally but their capacity for vocal communication makes it necessary on occasion to mute the mute. See DEVOCALIZATION.
d. terminal see TERMINAL.

dumbcane DIEFFENBACHIA *seguinae*.

dumdum fever see LEISHMANIASIS.

dummy state of depressed consciousness in which the still mobile animal walks continuously and compulsively, head down, stumbling gait, walking into fixed objects, head presses when it meets a fixed object, when trapped in a narrow place is incapable of backing out, walks into human habitation which it would ordinarily shun. May walk in circles. Does not respond to ordinary stimuli, does not eat or drink. Caused by encephalitis, hepatic encephalopathy, subacute lead poisoning. Called also blind staggers, dummy syndrome. See also NEONATAL maladjustment syndrome.
d. calf syndrome thought to be a behavior problem inherited in some breeds; the newborn calf is bright and alert but lacks teat seeking and teat sucking reflexes.
d. disease said of lambs born with hydranencephaly due to intrauterine infection with bluetongue virus, usually the vaccine strain.

dumping 1. shortening the toe of the hoof by rasping down the outside wall; creates a weakness of the wall and is a defect in a shod horse. 2. heavy mechanical compression of a standard bale of wool to about half of its normal size and clamping by metal bands; used to facilitate export shipment.

dumping syndrome a complex of vasomotor signs associated with eating and the rapid emptying of hyperosmolar gastric contents into the proximal small intestine; believed to be due to the shift of fluid into the gut lumen, intestinal distension and contraction of plasma volume.

DUMPS inherited deficiency of the enzyme UMP synthase which participates in the reaction which converts orotate to uridine 5′-monophosphate.

dun a coat color, generally a yellow varying from gray-yellow to light yellow, always with a brown stripe from the wither to the tail butt.

Duncan applicator a device used for the control of ticks in game animals; as the animal licks bait feed in the center of the device it receives a dose of pour-on insecticide.

duncecap larkspur DELPHINIUM *occidentale*.

dune bush CROTALARIA *spartioides*.

dung feces. Called also manure, droppings.

Dunker a medium-sized scenthound, popular in Norway. It is a powerfully built dog with a short coat, pendulous ears and long tail. The short coat may be tan with black saddle and white markings, or the black may be splotched (merled). Called also Norwegian hound.

dunkop the pulmonary form of AFRICAN HORSE SICKNESS.

dunsiekte [Af.] dummy syndrome due to hepatic insufficiency and caused by pyrrolizidine alkalosis. Called also 'thin disease'. See SENECIO.

duodenal of or pertaining to the duodenum.

d. glands glands in the submucosa of the duodenum, opening into the small intestine; called also Brunner's glands.

d. reflux retrograde movement of duodenal contents, either into the stomach where it has been incriminated as a cause of vomiting and gastric hyposecretion, or into the pancreatic duct and parenchyma as a factor in the etiology of acute pancreatitis.

d. stenosis occurs in young foals up to 4 months old. Characterized by salivation, mild colic, regurgitation and unthriftiness.

d. ulcer peptic ulcer of the duodenum. See also ULCER.

duodenectomy excision of the duodenum, total or partial.

duodenitis inflammation of the duodenum. A cause of colic in horses; a high case fatality rate.

duodenocholedochotomy incision of the duodenum and common bile duct.

duodenoenterostomy anastomosis of the duodenum to some other part of the small intestine.

duodenography radiography of the duodenum.

duodenohepatic pertaining to the duodenum and liver.

duodenoileostomy anastomosis of the duodenum to the ileum.

duodenojejunostomy anastomosis of the duodenum to the jejunum.

duodenorrhaphy suture of the duodenum.

duodenoscopy examination of the duodenum by an endoscope.

duodenostomy surgical formation of a permanent opening into the duodenum. May be for the purpose of introducing a tube for post-pyloric feeding.

duodenotomy incision of the duodenum.

duodenum the first or proximal portion of the small intestine, extending from the pylorus to the jejunum. It plays an important role in digestion of food because the bile and pancreatic ducts empty into it. See also DIGESTIVE system.

duplex DNA double-stranded DNA.

duplication a doubling; in genetics, the presence of an extra segment of chromosome.

dupp a syllable used to represent, or mimic the second sound heard at the apex of the heart in auscultation. See also HEART SOUNDS.

dura mater [L.] the outermost, toughest and most fibrous of the three membranes (meninges) covering the brain and spinal cord.

dural pertaining to the dura mater.

d. ossification see dural OSSIFICATION.

d. sinuses, d. venous sinuses venous spaces between the layers of dura which collect cerebrospinal fluid and return it to the vascular system.

durango root see DATISCA GLOMERATA.

Durham tube an inverted glass tube in bacterial carbohydrate fermentation tests. Used to detect gas production.

Durham's tube a jointed tracheotomy tube.

Durikainema macropti nematode parasite in the venous system of some kangaroo species.

duroarachnitis inflammation of the dura mater and arachnoid.

Duroc Jersey red pigs with prick ears lopped over halfway up. Produced by the merging of two breeds, Duroc and Jersey, in USA. Called also Duroc.

durotomy incision of the dura mater.

Dursban 44 see CHLORPYRIFOS.

durum a class of WHEAT producing hard flour.

dust heavy dust such as in dust storms or volcanic fallout may contaminate animal feed sufficiently to cause sand colic in horses. Ruminants seem not to be much affected.

d. balls equine intestinal foreign bodies composed of plant fibers with a superficial coating of dense minerals. Because of their light weight they are often evacuated with the feces.

d. inhalation important risk factor in etiology of coccidioidomycosis (corral dust), chronic obstructive pulmonary disease in horses (feed dust in stables).

d. mite see HOUSEDUST MITE.

d. rhinotracheitis dusty feed fed in a confined space such as a stable can cause chronic coughing due to rhinotracheitis in cattle.

dusting powders a popular form of applying antibacterial materials onto animal wounds, external parasiticides onto skin generally, and ophthalmic preparations for large animals that present difficulties in restraint.

dusty miller SENECIO *cineraria*.

Dutch black pied cattle black and white dual-purpose cattle from Holland.

Dutch rabbit a very hardy, trouble-free, breed of rabbits with white saddle, feet and face markings and almost any other color elsewhere, including tortoiseshell, chocolate and yellow. It is a small, less than 5 lb rabbit with a dense coat of fine fur.

dutchman's breeches DICENTRA *cucullaria*, *D. spectabilis*, THAMNOSMA TEXANA.

dutchman's pipe ARISTOLOCHIA *elegans*.

Duttonella a subgenus of the genus *Trypanosoma*. Includes *Trypanosoma vivax* and *T. uniforme*.

Duvenhage virus a rabies-like virus isolated from fruit-eating bats in which it causes a disease similar to rabies.

Duverny's glands see BARTHOLIN'S GLANDS.

DV dorsoventral.

DVM Doctor of Veterinary Medicine.

dwarf an abnormally undersized animal or plant. See also DWARFISM.

d. bay DAPHNE *mezereum*.

d. cattle see DWARFISM.

d. Darling pea SWAINSONA *luteola*.

dolichocephalic d. dwarf with a long, narrow head.

d. elder SAMBUCUS *ebulus*.

d. goat a dwarf variety of any of the standard goat breeds; the best known is a dwarf of West African breed.

d. laurel KALMIA *angustifolia*.
proportional d. see PROPORTIONAL dwarf.
d. tapeworm see HYMENOLEPIS *nana*.

dwarfing genes alleles at different loci in chicken chromosomes that generate chickens with a much lower body weight at maturity.

dwarfism the state of being a dwarf; underdevelopment of the body. Dwarfism may be the result of a developmental anomaly, of nutritional or hormone deficiencies, or of other diseases. See also ACHONDROPLASIA, CRETINISM.
achondroplastic d. an inherited defect in cattle caused by defective cartilage growth which is effectively lethal because the calves do not grow well and die before 6 months of age. Typical signs are short legs, large, wide, short head, protruding lower jaw, depression of the maxilla with obstruction of respiration and stertorous breathing. The tongue protrudes and the eyes bulge, the abdomen is distended and there is chronic bloat. Urine levels of glycosaminoglycans are much higher than normal in some of the calves. Called also snorter dwarfs. The condition has also been seen in dogs and cats.
chondrodystrophic d. with hydrocephalus see BULLDOG CALVES.
constitutional d. a proportional dwarfism due to a generalized genetic defect.
disproportionate d. the skeleton is dystrophic, the soft tissues are normal. The animal is pot-bellied, dyspneic and the tongue protrudes. Characteristic of achondroplastic and chondrodystrophic dwarfs.
German shepherd dog d. an inherited juvenile panhypopituitarism caused by a defect in differentiation of the oropharyngeal ectoderm of Rathke's pouch. Affected puppies appear normal at birth but soon show a reduced rate of growth, retention of deciduous teeth and puppy hair, alopecia, delayed closure of epiphyseal growth plates, infantile genitalia and shortened life span.
pituitary d. see German shepherd dog dwarfism (above).
primordial d. general proportional dwarfism of all organs of the kind that has produced Kerry cattle and Miniature pinschers.
proportional d. primordial dwarfism (above).
thyroid d. hypothyroidism in an immature animal causes retarded growth and development of bones with disproportionate dwarfism. See CRETINISM.

dwarfism–joint hypermobility inherited disproportionate dwarfism in some cattle breeds with abnormal joint mobility caused by a collagen defect in joint cartilage.

dwelling an abnormality of gait in a horse in which there is a momentary hesitation before the foot is placed on the ground.

Dx abbreviation for diagnosis; used in medical records.

Dy chemical symbol, *dysprosium*.

dyclonine hydrochloride a bactericidal and fungicidal topical anesthetic agent.

dye any of various colored substances containing auxochromes and thus capable of coloring substances to which they are applied; used for staining and coloring, as test reagents, and as therapeutic agents.
acridine d. acriflavine and proflavine are antiseptic dyes.
azo d. dyes like scarlet red and phenazopyridine are used as antiseptics to be applied topically or as urinary antiseptics.
diagnostic d. several diagnostic test procedures involve the administration of a dye and determination of the rate of excretion, either by measuring levels remaining in the body or amounts excreted in the urine, feces, etc. Examples are the bromsulfthalein (BSP) test for liver function, and the phenolsulfonphthalein (PSP) renal function test.
d. dilution method the standard method of measuring circulating plasma volume; based on the degree of dilution of a physiologically inert dye injected intravenously.
vital d. see vital STAIN.

dyeberry PHYTOLACCA *octandra*.

dyhydrose tropicale see SWEATING sickness.

dying-back disease axonal degeneration which selectively involves distal parts of long fibers first, then slowly spreads to more proximal parts. See LARYNGEAL paralysis.

dying back neuropathy distal axonal degeneration.

dynamic pertaining to or manifesting force.
d. compression plates used in orthopedic surgery. See COMPRESSION plating.

dynamics 1. the scientific study of forces in action; a phase of mechanics. 2. the motivating or driving forces, physical or moral, in any field.

dynamite a commercially available explosive containing ammonium nitrate, which has caused nitrate poisoning in cattle.

dynamization a strategy for promoting bone healing in fractures by allowing some movement or compressive loading.

dynamograph a self-registering dynamometer.

dynamometer an instrument for measuring the force of muscular contraction.

dyne the metric unit of force, being that amount which would, during each second, produce an acceleration of 1 cm per second in a particle of 1 gram mass.

dynein a protein from the microtubules of cilia and flagella which functions as an ATP-splitting enzyme and is essential to the motility of cilia and flagella.

dyphylline see DIPROPHYLLINE.

dys- prefix. [Gr.] *bad, difficult, disordered.*

dysadrenalism, dysadrenia any disorder of adrenal function, whether of decreased or heightened function.

dysarthrosis 1. deformity or malformation of a joint. 2. dysarthria.

dysautonomia dysfunction of the autonomic nervous system. See also GRASS sickness.
feline d. a dysfunction of the autonomic nervous system in cats characterized by constipation, megaesophagus with regurgitation, dilated pupils, protrusion of the nictitating membranes, dry nasal and buccal mucosae, reduced laryngeal secretions and bradycardia. Seen almost exclusively in the United Kingdom; the cause is unknown. Called also Key–Gaskell syndrome, dilated pupil syndrome, feline autonomic polyganglionopathy.

dysbacteriosis 1. possibly a bacterial disease; classified as a bacterial disease but its authentication is dubious. 2. disease caused by an imbalance of the normal flora of the organ or part of the organ.

dysbarism any clinical syndrome caused by difference between the surrounding atmospheric pressure and the total gas pressure in the various tissues, fluids and cavities of the body, including such conditions as barosinusitis, barotitis media, or expansion of gases in the hollow viscera.

dysbasia difficulty in walking, especially that due to a nervous lesion.

dysbetalipoproteinemia the accumulation of abnormal β-lipoproteins in the blood.

dyscephaly malformation of the cranium and bones of the face.

dyschezia difficult or painful evacuation of feces from the rectum.
dyscholia a disordered condition of the bile.
dyschondroplasia see ENCHONDROMATOSIS.
tibial d. a mass of hypertrophic cartilage develops in the proximal end of the tibiotarsal bone in young broilers and turkeys. May cause lameness and limb deformity.
dyschromia any disorder of pigmentation of the skin or hair.
dyscoria abnormality in shape or form of the pupil or in the reaction of the two pupils.
dyscorticism disordered functioning of the adrenal cortex.
dyscrasia a morbid condition, usually referring to an imbalance of component elements.
blood d. any abnormal or pathological condition of the blood.
dysecdysis abnormal shedding of the skin of reptiles, usually due to undernutrition or too cold or too dry environment.
dysembryoma see TERATOMA.
dysentery any of a number of disorders marked by inflammation of the intestine, especially of the colon, with abdominal pain, tenesmus, and frequent stools often containing blood and mucus. The causative agent may be chemical irritants, bacteria, protozoa, viruses or parasitic worms.
See also LAMB dysentery, SWINE dysentery, WINTER DYSENTERY, COCCIDIOSIS, SALMONELLOSIS, canine PARVOVIRUS, COLITIS-X, TRICHURIASIS, ENTAMOEBA *histolytica* infection.
amebic d. see AMEBIC dysentery.
bacillary d. see SHIGELLOSIS.
dyserythropoiesis defective red cell formation.
d. dyskeratosis–progressive alopecia probably inherited congenital anemia of Polled Hereford cattle.
dysesthesia 1. impairment of any sense. 2. abnormal perception of a sensory stimulus. Assumed to occur in animals.
dysfibrinogenemia the presence of abnormal fibrinogens in the body. An inherited dysfibrinogenemia occurs in humans and has been reported in a collie dog.
dysfunction disturbance, impairment or abnormality of functioning of an organ.
dysgalactia disordered milk secretion.
dysgammaglobulinemia a selective deficiency of one or more, but not all, class of immunoglobulin. A HEREDITARY dysgammaglobulinemia has been recorded in chickens.
dysgenesis defective development; malformation.
dysgenic genetically harmful.
dysgerminoma a solid, often radiosensitive, malignant ovarian neoplasm derived from undifferentiated germinal cells; the counterpart of seminoma of the testis.
dysglycemia any disorder of blood sugar metabolism.
dysgnathia any oral abnormality extending beyond the teeth to involve the maxilla or mandible, or both.
dysgonic seeding badly; said of bacterial cultures that grow poorly.
dyshematopoiesis defective blood formation.
dyshesion 1. disordered cell adherence. 2. loss of intercellular cohesion; a characteristic of malignancy.
dyshidrosis any disorder of the eccrine sweat glands.
dyskaryosis abnormality of the nucleus of a cell.
dyskeratoma a dyskeratotic tumor.
warty d. benign proliferation of the epithelium seen in dogs; the lesions are wart-like papules with a hyperkeratotic, umbilicated center.
dyskeratosis abnormal, premature or imperfect keratinization of the keratinocytes as in primary seborrhea.
dyskeratotic pertaining to or of the nature of dyskeratosis.
d. alopecia deficiency of hair fibers in skin affected by dyskeratosis.
dyskinesia impairment of the power of voluntary movement.
ciliary d. see primary CILIARY dyskinesia.
dyslipoproteinemia an abnormal distribution of lipoproteins in the blood.
dyslochia disordered lochial discharge.
dysmaturity the condition of being small or immature for gestational age; said of fetuses that are the product of a pregnancy involving placental dysfunction.
dysmelia malformation of a limb or limbs due to disturbance in embryonic development.
dysmetria inability to properly direct or limit motions. A characteristic of cerebellar lesions.
dysmorphism 1. appearing under different morphological forms. 2. an abnormality in morphological development.
dysmorphogenesis giving rise to dysmorphism.
dysmyelination see HYPOMYELINATION.
dysmyelinogenesis any abnormality of myelin formation. Includes hypomyelinogenesis, as occurs in congenital tremor of piglets, and puppies and calves.
dysmyelopoiesis see MYELODYSPLASIA.
dysmyelopoietic syndromes see MYELODYSPLASIA.
dysmyotonia muscular dystonia; abnormal tonicity.
dysodontiasis defective, delayed, or difficult eruption of the teeth.
dysontogenesis defective embryonic development.
dysorexia impaired or deranged appetite.
dysostosis defective ossification; a defect in the normal ossification of fetal cartilages.
dyspancreatism disorder of function of the pancreas.
dyspepsia specifically, impairment of digestion, but commonly applied to subjective feelings of indigestion in humans.
dysphagia difficulty in swallowing.
cricopharyngeal d. see cricopharyngeal ACHALASIA.
esophageal d. difficulty in swallowing due to esophageal malfunction.
gastroesophageal d. impaired passage of the bolus through the caudal esophageal sphincter.
neuropathic d. may be caused by lesions of the glossopharyngeal or vagus nerves or associated nuclei of the caudal medulla oblongata.
oropharyngeal d. abnormalities in mastication and pharyngeal contraction may be caused by hypoglossal nerve dysfunction, polyneuropathy, polymyositis, meningitis, brainstem lesions and generalized neuromuscular disease.
Dysphania rhadinostachya Australian plant in the family Chenopodiaceae; may cause cyanide poisoning; called also *Chenopodium chenostachyum*, *C. rhadinostachyum*, red or mouse-tailed crumbweed.
dyspigmentation any abnormality of pigmentation of the skin or hair.
dysplasia an abnormality of development; in pathology an alteration in size, shape and organization of adult cells.
black hair follicular d. a familial disorder of hair follicles in dogs, occurring only in areas with black pigmentation. Affected dogs have a normal haircoat except in black areas where hair growth is thin and the skin scaly.
canine hip d. see HIP dysplasia.

occipital d. congenital enlargement of the foramen magnum, sometimes associated with hydrocephalus or cerebellar herniation or spina bifida. Observed most often in toy breeds of dogs.

dysplastic emanating from or pertaining to abnormality of development.

dyspnea labored or difficult breathing; a sign of a variety of disorders and is primarily an indication of inadequate ventilation, or of insufficient amounts of oxygen in the circulating blood.

dyspnoea dyspnea.

dyspoiesis a disorder of formation; as of blood cells.

dyspragia painful performance of any function.

dyspraxia partial loss of ability to perform coordinated movements.

dysprosium a chemical element, atomic number 66, atomic weight 162.50, symbol Dy. See Table 6.

dysproteinemia disorder of the protein content of the blood. This may be associated with clotting defects due to concurrent thrombocytopenia or to coating of the platelet with the abnormal protein.

dysraphism incomplete closure of a raphe, e.g. of the neural tube. The defect may be complete or partial.

spinal d. an inherited defect in Weimaraner dogs and reported in many other breeds. From an early age, affected puppies show varying degrees of 'bunny hopping', symmetrical and simultaneous use of the back legs, often overextending them before stepping forward. More severe defects have associated musculoskeletal abnormalities and may be a cause of perinatal death.

dysrhythmia disturbance of rhythm.

dysspermia impairment of the spermatozoa, or of the semen.

dysstasia difficulty in standing.

dyssynergia muscular incoordination.

detrusor-sphincter d. see detrusor-urethral dyssynergia (below).

detrusor-urethral d. a disorder of micturition caused by a lack of coordination between contraction of the detrusor muscle and relaxation of the urethra.

dystectia defective closure of the neural tube.

dysthrombopoiesis defective platelet formation, such as occurs in systemic lupus erythematosus, with histological changes evident in the platelets.

dysthyroid, dysthyroidal denoting defective functioning of the thyroid gland.

dystocia difficult parturition to the point of needing human intervention.

maternal d. that due to some condition inherent in the dam.

placental d. difficult delivery of the placenta.

d. rate number of assisted births per hundred births.

d. risk the incidence of dystocia is enhanced by many factors including inherited large fetal size, especially in some breeds, high feeding level of the dam during pregnancy, inherited small diameter pelvic canal, youth of the dam, male calves compared to females, the occurrence of multiple births and congenital abnormalities which increase fetal size.

dystokia see DYSTOCIA.

dystonia abnormality of muscular tonus.

dystopia malposition; displacement.

dystrophia [Gr.] *dystrophy*.

d. adiposogenitalis see ADIPOSOGENITAL DYSTROPHY.

d. epithelialis corneae dystrophy of the corneal epithelium, with erosions.

d. ungulae see SEEDY TOE.

dystrophic pertaining to or emanating from dystrophia.

d. calcification mineralization of soft tissues can occur in HYPERADRENOCORTICISM, VITAMIN D toxicity, and HYPERVITAMINOSIS A. See also CALCIFICATION.

dystrophin a membrane-associated protein, deficient in some types of muscular dystrophy.

dystrophy any disorder due to defective or faulty nutrition. See also CORNEAL dystrophy, MUSCULAR dystrophy.

bone d. see OSTEODYSTROPHIA FIBROSA, OSTEOMALACIA, RICKETS, OSTEOPOROSIS.

Duchenne d. see Duchenne MUSCULAR dystrophy.

muscular d. includes ENZOOTIC muscular dystrophy of cattle, sheep, pigs and foals, all of dietary origin, and some probably familial diseases in cattle, sheep and dogs. See also MUSCULAR dystrophy.

dysuria painful or difficult urination.

Dz abbreviation for disease; used in medical records.

dzo any cross between cattle and yak. Called also zho, zo.

E

E symbol, *exa-*; electromotive force; eye.

e- for words beginning thus, see also those beginning *oe-*.

E-mail a system of sending mail from one computer to another possibly using internal computer networks and dialing connections to the Internet or to a dedicated system in which the message is transmitted via a modem and a standard voice telephone line to a server operated by a commercial communications provider. The server connects with other host servers and thence host computers. Connections between servers are arranged through public access networks such as the Internet or closed networks which are accessible only by fee-paying members.

EAE experimental allergic encephalomyelitis.

EAEC enteroadherent *Escherichia coli*.

eagle raptor bird of the families Falconidae and Accipitridae. Includes the harpy eagle (*Harpia harpyja*), golden eagle (*Aquila chrysaetos*), tawny eagle (*Aquila rapax*) and bald eagle (*Haliaeetus leucocephalus*).

EAN experimental allergic NEURITIS.

ear the organ of hearing and of equilibrium. The ear is made up of the outer (external) ear, the middle ear and the inner (internal) ear. The anatomical parts of all three can be found under their specific names. See also AURICULAR, AUDITORY, EXTERNAL EAR.

The outer ear consists of the auricle, or pinna, and the external acoustic meatus. The auricle collects sound waves and directs them to the external acoustic meatus which conducts them to the tympanum.

The tympanic membrane (eardrum) separates the outer ear from the middle ear. In the middle ear are the three ossicles, the malleus (hammer), incus (anvil), and stapes (stirrup), so called because of their resemblance to these objects. These three small bones form a chain across the middle ear from the tympanum to the oval window of the inner ear. The middle ear is connected to the nasopharynx by the auditory tube, through which the air pressure on the inner side of the eardrum is equalized with the air pressure on its outside surface. Two muscles attached to the ossicles contract when loud noises strike the tympanic membrane, limiting its vibration and thus protecting it and the inner ear from damage.

In the inner ear (or labyrinth) is the cochlea, containing the nerves that transmit the electrical impulses stimulated by sound to the brain. The inner ear also contains the SEMICIRCULAR canals, which are essential for the sense of balance. When a sound strikes the ear it causes the tympanic membrane to vibrate. The ossicles function as levers, gearing down the motion of the tympanic membrane, and passing the vibrations on to the cochlea. From there the vestibulocochlear (eighth cranial) nerve transmits the vibrations, translated into nerve impulses, to the auditory center in the brain. See also HEARING.

e. alopecia see pinnal ALOPECIA.

broken e. deformed or misshapen ears, as a result of injury or congenital defect. Most often of concern in dog breeds that are supposed to have erect or specifically defined ear conformation, e.g. Collie, German shepherd dog, Chihuahua.

button e. in dogs, an ear flap lying close to the head, and pointing toward the eye. Seen in fox terriers.

e. cancer a squamous cell carcinoma of the ear of sheep. The lesion commences around the free edge and then invades the entire ear.

e. canker a lay term applied generally to OTITIS externa but sometimes specifically to that caused by ear mites.

e. carriage drooped, erect, alert, all indicative of mental state or state of muscle tone. Also a specified feature of breed standards for dogs.

e. cartilage see auricular CARTILAGE.

e. chewing a vice of confined pigs due largely to boredom and overcrowding.

e. cyst a misplaced tooth germ or ear tooth in horses; occur unilaterally at the base of the ear, attached to the temporal bone. Called also heterotopic polyodontia.

drop e. an ear that is normally not erect; the end folds over or droops forward. Seen in many dog breeds.

drooping e. inability of the ear to remain in an upright position in those species in which that is the norm. It may be a congenital abnormality, due to injury that has damaged the cartilage, or a sign of neurological deficit.

e. hematoma see AURICULAR hematoma.

e. mange see PSOROPTIC MANGE, OTODECTES *cynotis*, RAILLIETIA.

e. margin dermatosis crusts, scabs and sometimes ulcerations, may occur at the edges of the external ear flap in dogs. Usually a form of seborrhea.

e. mark patterned pieces of cartilage punched out as a means of identification. Very popular at one time with intricate codes to identify age and family groups of pigs. Marks nicked out of the edges but also the centers of the ears.

e. mites see PSOROPTES *cuniculi*, RAILLIETIA *auris*, RAILLIETIA *caprae*.

e. notch see ear mark (above).

e. pinna see PINNA.

e. plaque hypertrophic dermatitis appearing as small (0.5 inch diameter) plaques on the inner surface of the ear pinna in horses. They are scaly, slightly papillomatous, painless and alopecic. The cause is unknown.

e. punch alligator forceps with cup-shaped opposing blades up to 1.5 inch diameter. A biopsy instrument for use in the depths of the ear canal.

e. resection see lateral ear RESECTION, vertical ear canal RESECTION.

e. rigid ear pricked and patient unable to move them; indicative of general skeletal muscle tetany.

e. sloughing result of phlebitis and venous thrombosis occurring in many septicemias. It is most common in pigs where it begins as purple discoloration of the ears and surrounding skin. Also part of the response in peripheral gangrene syndrome caused by ingestion of the fungus CLAVICEPS *purpurea*.

spinose e. tick see OTOBIUS *megnini*.

e. sucking a vice occurring in penned pigs and calves caused by boredom. Has no serious effect unless it leads to cannibalism in pigs.

e. tag a technique of animal identification favored in sheep and cattle. Has the disadvantage that tags are often lost. This can be avoided by putting duplicates in each ear. The need to catch the animal to read the tag is overcome by using large placard type tags. For cattle being worked through a chute, tail tags are more convenient. Insecticides can be incorporated into the tag to provide protection against horn fly and head fly.

e. tick see OTOBIUS *megnini*.

e. tipping clipping off the tip of the external ear so that the animal can be identified from a distance. Limited categories available.

e. tip necrosis a common problem in individual pig herds; sporadic cases usually related to frostbite, thrombosis after septicemic disease; herd problems may be due to ergot poisoning, an ear-sucking habit.

e. tooth see POLYODONTIA.

e. trimming see ear cropping (above).

e. twitch a rope twitch is twisted onto an ear instead of the muzzle.

ear cropping a cosmetic surgical procedure carried out on dogs of certain breeds, including Boxer, Great Dane, Schnauzer, Doberman pinscher and Bouvier des Flandres, that removes approximately one-third of the ear flap and braces the remainder so it stands erect. Practiced widely in the USA, but considered inhumane and an unethical procedure in most of the British Commonwealth countries.

e. c. clamps clamps consisting of two aluminum bars with thumbscrews at both ends to screw the bars together, with the part of the ear to be cropped protruding from the edge. They act as a template for cropping the ears of dogs in the correct shape.

eardrum see TYMPANIC membrane.

earle loco ASTRAGALUS *mollissimus*.

early at or near the beginning.

e. bloom the stage at which to cut alfalfa for hay; when 10% of the crop is in bloom.

e. breeding 1. in seasonal breeding management systems it is customary to commence mating on a specific day in the expectation that the offspring will be born at a time to take most advantage of a seasonal peak of pasture. Early mating, before the recommended day, may be because of an expected poor level of fertility or similar overriding factor. 2. mating before the recommended age for that particular class or breed of stock; usually to maximize the productive life of the individual animal.

e. fetal recovery the use of embryo transfer in test matings to increase the speed of the program and reduce the time required in gestation to determine the constitution of the fetus.

e. genes genes expressed during early development of the fetus.

e. pregnancy hormone (factor) identified in mice and several other species including sheep, cattle, pigs, humans; appears in the blood within a few hours of conception and persists for several weeks; identifiable by laboratory test.

early warning system a specific procedure for the early detection of any departure from normal frequencies of clinical cases or serological reactors of specific diseases by monitoring a sample of the population at risk.

earmark taking a piece out of the edge or center of the ear with a punch as an identification mark. The shape of the mark may be registerable under local legislation.

earsore dermatitis around the ear of water buffalo caused by *Stephanofilaria zaheeri*.

earth 1. soil; softer part of the land, as distinct from rock. 2. metallic oxides in the form of unchangeable powder.

diatomaceous e. a fine white powder composed of the siliceous skeletons of diatoms; used in treating diarrhea and as a feed additive. Called also infusorial earth, purified siliceous earth.

infusorial e. see diatomaceous earth (above).

siliceous e. see diatomaceous earth (above).

earth-eating most commonly associated with nutritional deficiency of sodium chloride. See also PICA.

earthing the safety device of connecting an electrical system in a building to the earth, especially in a milking shed. Failure of the connection causes electrification of parts of the building. This may cause poor milk letdown, restlessness, convulsions or sudden death depending on the strength of the current and the completeness of the animals' contact with the floor. See also ELECTROCUTION, FREE electricity.

earthworm the common oligochete worm of the genera *Lumbricus*, *Allobophora*, *Eisenia* etc.; they act as intermediate hosts for a number of internal parasites of livestock, and are reputed to bring anthrax spores to the surface and precipitate an outbreak of the disease.

earwax see CERUMEN.

e. remover various proprietary mixtures are used to aid in the removal of cerumen in the treatment of OTITIS externa.

earworm infestation of the ears of cattle by RHABDITIS *bovis*, often complicated by blowfly infestation.

ease of calving thought to be an inherited trait due to pelvic canal dimensions in the dam, and fetal size in the sire. See also DYSTOCIA.

ease of fracture bones fracture easily due to local weakness of structure and calcification due to osteomyelitis or generalized osteoporosis.

East African sleeping sickness a disease of humans caused by *Trypanosoma rhodesiense*. The parasite is infectious for many animal species which act as reservoirs for humans. The disease is fatal in humans if it is not treated. Keratitis and encephalitis occur in goats and sheep, facial paralysis and emaciation in horses.

East African swine fever see AFRICAN SWINE FEVER.

East Coast fever a disease of cattle caused by THEILERIA *parva* and transmitted by the tick RHIPICEPHALUS *appendiculatus*. Other ticks are known to be capable of transmitting the infection. Resident and zebu cattle are resistant to infection. Clinical signs in susceptible animals are high fever, lymphadenopathy, nasal discharge, lacrimation, diarrhea and dysentery. The mortality rate is high.

East Friesian, East Friesland marsh-type dairy sheep, polled, with a woolless rat-tail.

East–West front in dog conformation, front feet turned outwards.

easter flower see ANEMONE.

easter lily see LILIUM LONGIFLORUM.

easter rose HELLEBORUS *niger*.

Eastern encephalitis see equine viral ENCEPHALOMYELITIS.

Eastern equine encephalomyelitis see ENCEPHALOMYELITIS.

Eastern gray kangaroo MACROPUS *giganteus*.

eastern hemlock CICUTA *maculata*.

eastern whorled milkweed ASCLEPIAS *verticillata*.

Easton's syrup an antique proprietary medicine from the era of empirical remedies and nonspecific stimulants. Contains strychnine (renowned as a stimulant), iron phosphate (listed as a brain food) and quinine (appetite and general stimulant). Available also as tablets.

easy-care sheep sheep of any breed but selected for ease of lambing. Is a response to the need to reduce labor inputs into sheep husbandry.

easy keeper an animal of any species that grows or fattens on a smaller intake than average.

eating combined prehension, mastication and swallowing.

e. disorders see ANOREXIA, REGURGITATION, QUIDDING, DYSPHAGIA, POLYPHAGIA, PICA.

Ebert technique a technique for forming a conjunctival flap by suturing the nictitating membrane across the eye. Used in treatment of corneal ulcer in the horse.

EBHS European brown hare syndrome.

Ebola virus see FILOVIRIDAE.

Ebstein's anomaly a malformation of the tricuspid valve, usually associated with an atrial septal defect, characterized by a downward displacement of the base of the valves.

eburnation conversion of bone into a hard, ivory-like mass.

EBV estimated BREEDING VALUE.

E&C euthanasia and cremation.

ec- prefix meaning outward.

ecaudate tailless.

Ecballium elaterium toxic plant in the family Cucurbitaceae; contains cucurbitacins, which cause diarrhea and enteritis. Called also squirting cucumber.

ecbolic oxytocic.

ecchondroma, ecchondrosis a hyperplastic growth of cartilaginous tissue on the surface of a cartilage or projecting under the periosteum of a bone.

ecchymoma swelling due to blood extravasation.

ecchymosis pl. *ecchymoses* [Gr.] a hemorrhagic spot, larger than a petechia, in the skin or mucous membrane, forming a nonelevated, rounded or irregular, blue or purplish patch.

ecchymotic hemorrhage see ECCHYMOSIS.

eccrine exocrine, with special reference to glands that secrete their product without loss of cytoplasm. See SWEAT glands.

e. tumors adenomas and adenocarcinomas occur rarely.

eccritic 1. promoting excretion. 2. an agent that promotes excretion.

eccyesis ectopic pregnancy.

ecdysis shedding of the external layers of the skin—only the epidermis participates. Is controlled by the endocrine glands. May be complete or incomplete due usually to poor nutrition. Called also exuviate. See also DYSECDYSIS.

ECF extracellular fluid.

ECF-A eosinophil chemotactic factor of anaphylaxis.

ECG electrocardiogram. Called also EKG.

eCG equine chorionic gonadotropin. Called also pregnant mare serum gonadotropin.

echidna an Australian terrestrial anteater; a burrower with a long snout and tongue. A monotreme. Called also spiny anteater, *Tachyglossus* and *Zaglossus* spp. Includes long-nosed echidna (*Zaglossus bruijni*), short-nosed echidna (*Tachyglossus aculeatus*).

Echidnophaga a genus of fleas that remain attached to the host for long periods. Includes *E. myrmecobii* (in rabbits), *E. perilis* (in rats).

E. gallinacea causes insect worry and blood loss in poultry. Does not transmit disease in animals but may transmit endemic murine typhus to humans. Called also stickfast flea.

echimidine one of the toxic pyrrolizidine alkaloids in *Echium plantagineum*.

echinatine a toxic alkaloid in *Cynoglossum officinale*.

Echinochasmus a genus of flukes of the family Echinostomatidae. Includes *E. perfoliatus* (in intestines of carnivores).

Echinochloa genus of grasses in the family Poaceae. Mostly good forage plants but linked anecdotally with outbreaks of primary photosensitization, in grazing ruminants. Toxin unidentified but some plants contain high concentrations of nitrate. Includes *E. crus-galli* (barnyard grass, Japanese millet), *E. pyramidalis* (antelope grass), *E. utilis*.

echinococcosis an infection of humans and animals, usually of the liver or lungs, caused by the larval stage (hydatid cysts) of TAPEWORMS of the genus *Echinococcus*, marked by the development of expanding cysts. See also HYDATID disease.

Echinococcus a genus of small TAPEWORMS of the family Taeniidae.

E. granulosus a species parasitic in dogs and wolves and occasionally in cats; its larvae may develop in ungulates and macropods, forming hydatid cysts in the liver, lungs, kidneys and other organs.

E. multilocularis a species whose adult stage usually parasitizes the fox, dog and cat. It resembles *E. granulosus*, but the larvae form alveolar or multilocular rather than unilocular cysts and occur principally in rodents but can infect humans.

E. oligarthus occurs in wild cats with larval stages in rodents.

E. vogeli occurs in domestic and wild dogs with intermediate stages in rodents and humans.

echinocyte a crenated erythrocyte with 10 to 30 spicules; resembles a sea urchin.

Echinolaelaps echidninus the spiny rat mite, transmitter of *Hepatozoon* spp., the protozoan blood parasite. A mite of the Gamasidae family. Called also lelapid mite.

Echinoparyphium a genus of the fluke family Echinostomatidae.

E. paraulum see ECHINOSTOMA *revolutum*.

E. recurvatum occurs in the small intestine of doves, pigeons and domesticated birds, and can cause emaciation and anemia.

Echinophthirius lice of pinnipeds (seals, walrus and sealions).

E. horridus cause pruritus and self-injury.

Echinopogon genus of grasses in the Poaceae family; contains an unidentified toxin which causes incoordination, convulsions and distressed breathing. Includes *E. ovatus*, *E. caespitosa*, *E. mauritanica*. Called also rough-bearded grass.

Echinorhynchus salmonis acanthocephalan parasite of freshwater and marine fish. Found in the intestine of salmonids.

Echinostoma a genus of flukes in the family Echinostomatidae. Includes, besides those listed below, *Echinostoma aphylactum*, *E. caproni*, *E. hortense*, *E. jassyenese*, *E. lindoensis*, *E. suinum*.

E. iliocanum found in the intestine of dogs, rodents and humans and may cause enteritis.

***E. revolutum* (syn. *E. paraulum*)** found in the rectum and ceca of birds and in humans. Severe infestations may cause enteritis.

Echinostomatidae a family of flukes (digenetic trmatodes) found in birds.

echinulate having small spikes or prickles.

Echinuria a genus of spiruroid worms of the family Acuaridae. Includes *E. uncinata* (infests the upper alimentary tract of birds, causing caseous nodules in the wall of the esophagus).

Echium a genus of the Boraginaceae family of plants; contains a series of hepatotoxic pyrrolizidine alkaloids and continued ingestion of the plants causes chronic liver damage. The plant also contributes to the development of toxemic jaundice, the end-stage of chronic copper poisoning in sheep. Includes *E. plantagineum* (*E. lycopsis*), *E. sericeum*, *E. vulgare*. Called also Paterson's curse, Salvation Jane, Viper's buglos, Lady Campbell weed.

echiumidine one of the hepatoxic pyrrolizidine alkaloids in *Echium plantagineum*.

echo a reflected sound; the basis for ECHOCARDIOGRAPHY and ULTRASONOGRAPHY.

echo-ranging in ultrasonography, determination of the position or depth of a body structure on the basis of the time interval between the moment an ultrasonic pulse is transmitted and the moment its echo is received.

echocardiogram the record produced by echocardiography.

echocardiography recording of the position and motion of the heart walls or internal structures of the heart and neighboring tissue by the echo obtained from beams of ultrasonic waves directed through the chest wall.

Echocardiography is based on the same principle as the oceanographic technique of depth-sounding; that is, it utilizes ultrasound to delineate anatomical structures by recording on a graph the echoes from the heart structures. It is particularly useful in demonstrating, without danger to the patient, valvular and other structural deformities of the heart which formerly required CARDIAC catheterization or some other elaborate procedure for accurate diagnosis. See also ULTRASONOGRAPHY.

contrast e. microbubbles in liquid are used as a vascular contrast medium. When injected intravenously in a selected or non-selected location, these can be tracked to demonstrate abnormalities of blood flow.

transesophageal e. the ultrasound probe is mounted on a flexible endoscope and is positioned in the esophagus over the base of the heart, thus enabling unique viewing projections of structures in this area.

echocontrast agents see contrast ECHOCARDIOGRAPHY.

echoencephalogram the record produced by echoencephalography.

echoencephalography a diagnostic technique in which pulses of ultrasonic waves are beamed through the head from both sides, and echoes from the midline structures of the brain are recorded graphically; shifts from any midline may indicate a centrally placed mass.

echogenic in ultrasonography, giving rise to reflections (echoes) of ultrasound waves; hyperechoic.

echogenicity the characteristic ability of a tissue or substance to reflect sound waves and produce echoes. Bone and gas are most echogenic and fluids such as urine and bile the least. Organ parenchyma and soft tissues are intermediate, but each differs slightly from the other and relative characteristics are known.

echogram the record made by echography.

echography ultrasonography; the use of ultrasound as a diagnostic aid. Ultrasound waves are directed at the tissues, and a record is made, as on an oscilloscope, of the waves reflected back through the tissues, which indicate interfaces of different acoustic densities and thus differentiate between solid and cystic structures.

echolucent permitting the passage of ultrasonic waves without giving rise to echoes, the representative areas appearing black on the sonogram.

echophonocardiography the combined use of echocardiography and phonocardiography.

echopoor hypoechoic.

echothiophate iodide a cholinesterase inhibitor used to reduce intraocular pressure in glaucoma.

echovirus some viruses, which were originally considered nonpathogenic, in the family *Picornaviridae*, genus *Enterovirus*. The name is derived from the first letters of the description '*e*nteric *c*ytopathogenic *h*uman *o*rphan', but similar viruses ECBO and ECPO (for bovine and porcine, respectively, and other species) are also recognized. At the time of the isolation of the viruses the diseases they caused were not known, hence the term 'orphan', but it is now known that some of these viruses produce many different types of human disease, especially aseptic meningitis, and diarrhea and various respiratory diseases. The members of the group are now included in the enteroviruses.

Eck's fistula an artificial communication made between the portal vein and the vena cava.

eclabium eversion of a lip.

eclampsia a syndrome including convulsions and coma occurring in animals soon after birth of the young.

bitch e. see puerperal TETANY.

guinea pig e. see PREGNANCY toxemia (3) and KETOSIS.

mare e. see LACTATION TETANY (2).

puerperal e. see puerperal TETANY.

sow e. a poorly defined condition of older sows after farrowing which responds to treatment with calcium and magnesium.

eclamptogenic causing eclampsia.

eclectus parrot *Eclectus roratus.*

Eclectus roratus small, wax-billed parrot in the famoly Lorius; the males are green, the females winered; called also eclectus parrot.

eclipse period the time interval between viral penetration and the production of progeny virions.

ecological emanating from or pertaining to ecology.

e. biome see BIOME.

e. climax the state of balance in an ecosystem when its inhabitants have established their permanent relationships with each other.

e. fallacy bias following misinterpretation that ecological factors affect all individuals equally.

e. imbalance the naturally occurring changes in the environment, e.g. bushfires, floods, volcanic fallout, which leave it unbalanced with respect to the type and quality of the feed they provide.

e. interface the border between two ecosystems.

e. mosaic a pattern of interspersed ecosystems.

e. niche 1. the position occupied by an organism in relation to other organisms and to the environment. 2. a particular part of an ecological environment in which a particular plant or animal species prospers. It is the set of terms, in relation to food and water supply and relationship with predators and disease and with competitors, by which the organism achieves its full biological potential.

ecologist a person skilled in ecology.

ecology the science of organisms as affected by environmental factors; the study of the environment and the life history of organisms.

econazole an imidazole antifungal agent related to miconazole; used topically as the nitrate in the treatment of fungal infections of the skin.

economic dealing with costs and profits.

e. analysis estimation of income and expenditure in a series of segments so that the profitable and losing sections can be identified.

e. indices indexes of profitability of a project.

economies of scale reduced cost of production per unit as the number of units produced increases.

EcoR1 EcoR1 restriction endonuclease.

ecosystem the fundamental unit in ecology, comprising the living organisms and the nonliving elements interacting in a certain defined area. In more sophisticated terms, a biotic community living in its biotope.

ecotaxis the movement or 'homing' of a circulating cell, e.g. a lymphocyte, to a specific anatomical compartment.

ecotype a breed or race within a species adapted to a specific environment.

écraseur [Fr.] a crushing instrument with a loop of chain or wire which is placed over a part or organ, and can then can be tightened, creating or encircling a pedicle, and by further tightening remove the part by dividing it from its base.

ECSU extracorporeal circulatory support unit.

ECT electroconvulsive therapy.

ectasia expansion, dilatation or distension.

ectasis see ECTASIA.

-ectasis suffix meaning expansion.

ectental pertaining to the ectoderm and entoderm, and to their line of junction.

ecthyma a shallowly eruptive form of impetigo.

contagious e. a specific dermatitis of sheep caused by a poxvirus in the genus *Parapoxvirus*. The virus is strongly antigenic and an attack of the disease or vaccination provides long-lasting immunity. If the flock has previously been exposed the disease is restricted in occurrence to lambs and young sheep. The characteristic lesions occur mostly on the lips and the skin around the mouth, but have appeared wherever skin contact has been made with a source of infective virus, e.g. ear tagging, tail docking. Lesions are first papules, then crusts, and finally discrete thick tenacious scabs over vigorous granulation tissue. Very young lambs develop an extensive form of the disease involving even the alimentary tract. Occasional older sheep also have extensive lesions on other skin areas such as the coronets, and at the other mucocutaneous junctions. The disease is transmissible to humans. Called also orf, scabby mouth, contagious pustular dermatitis.

ect(o)- word element. [Gr.] *external, outside.*

ectoantigen 1. an antigen that seems to be loosely attached to the outside of bacteria. 2. an antigen formed in the ectoplasm (cell membrane) of a bacterium.

ectoblast the ectoderm.

ectocardia congenital displacement of the heart; exocardia.
ectocervix portio vaginalis.
ectoderm the outermost of the three primitive germ layers of the embryo; from it are derived the epidermis and epidermal derivatives, such as the claws, hair and glands of the skin, the nervous system, external sense organs (eye, ear, etc.) and mucous membrane of the mouth and anus.
ectodermosis a disorder based on congenital maldevelopment of organs derived from the ectoderm.
ectoentad from without inward.
ectoenzyme an extracellular enzyme.
ectogenous originating outside the organism.
ectoglobular formed outside the blood cells.
ectomere one of the blastomeres taking part in formation of the ectoderm.
-ectomy word element. [Gr.] *excision, surgical removal.*
ectoparasite a parasite living on the surface of the host's body.
ectoparasitism the state in which the ectoparasite is living on the surface of the host's body.
ectophyte a plant parasite living on the surface of the host's body.
ectopia [L.] *ectopy.*
e. cordis congenital displacement of the heart outside the thoracic cavity.
e. lentis congenital displacement of the lens away from its usual site attached to the ciliary body. Occurs as one of a series of defects in an inherited syndrome of cattle. The other defects are irideremia, microphakia and cataract. The calves are normal in other respects.
ectopic 1. pertaining to or characterized by ectopy. 2. located away from normal position. 3. arising or produced at an abnormal site or in a tissue where it is not normally found. See also specific sites or structures.
e. ACTH syndrome production of ACTH by nonpituitary tumors occurs in humans and is a cause of adrenal hyperplasia and hyperadrenocorticism. It has not been reported in animals.
e. endocrinopathy production of hormones by nonendocrinal, usually neoplastic, tissues. The most common example in animals is pseudohyperparathyroidism in dogs caused by a variety of tumors, particularly apocrine adenocarcinomas of the anal sacs and lymphosarcoma.
e. heart see ECTOPIA cordis.
e. kidney usually an unascended kidney.
e. lens see ECTOPIA lentis.
e. mineralization deposition of calcium salts of phosphate, silicate, etc. in unusual situations, e.g. calcifying myopathy in horses. See also MINERALIZATION.
e. ossification see ectopic mineralization (above).
e. teeth see DENTAL cyst.
ectoplacental cone a syncytial body formed in the murine trophoblast; an essential component of the nidation process in this species.
ectoplasm an old-fashioned term which referred to a peripheral band of gel-like cytoplasm, free of organelles, found in free and motile cells.
ectopy displacement or malposition, especially if congenital.
ectosteal pertaining to or situated on the outside of a bone.
ectostosis ossification beneath the perichondrium of a cartilage or the periosteum of a bone.
ectothrix a fungus that grows inside the shaft of a hair, but produces a conspicuous external sheath of spores.
ectoturbinates papyraceous bones in the nasal cavity which are interleaved with endoturbinates.
ectozoon ectoparasite.
ectro- word element. [Gr.] *miscarriage, congenital absence.*
ectrodactylia inherited, congenital skeletal defect in pups and kittens; there is incomplete fusion of the three rays that develop from the forelimb bud in the embryo; the paw is split up the middle as far as the metacarpals or to the carpus in some. Called also split-hand deformity.
ectrodactyly see ECTRODACTYLIA.
ectrogeny congenital absence or defect of a part.
ectromelia 1. gross hypoplasia or aplasia of one or more long bones of one or more limbs. 2. a generalized poxvirus disease of mice resembling smallpox in humans. Used in studies as a model of generalized virus infections.
ectromelus an animal with rudimentary limbs.
ectropion eversion or turning outward, as of the margin of an eyelid.
cicatricial e. caused by contraction of scar tissue following injury or surgery to the eyelid.
congenital e. most commonly seen in some breeds of dogs, such as St. Bernard, Bloodhound and spaniels where it may be considered normal. Called also heritable ectropion.
heritable e. see congenital ectropion (above).
intermittent acquired e., physiological e. may occur in some dogs intermittently for unknown reasons.
physiological e. see intermittent acquired ectropion (above).
ectrosyndactyly a condition in which some digits are absent and those that remain are webbed.
eczema 1. a general term for any superficial inflammatory process involving primarily the epidermis, marked early by redness, itching, minute papules and vesicles, weeping, oozing and crusting, and later by scaling, lichenification and often pigmentation. 2. atopic dermatitis.
facial e. see FACIAL eczema.
miliary e. see feline miliary DERMATITIS.
moist e. see acute moist DERMATITIS.
nasal e. see solar DERMATITIS. Called also Collie nose.
watery e. EXUDATIVE epidermitis.
eczematoid resembling eczema.
eczematous characterized by or of the nature of eczema.
E&D euthanasia and disposal.
ED_{50} median effective dose.
EDB ethylene dibromide; a grain fumigant toxic to chickens.
EDDI ethylene diamine dihydroiodide.
edema an abnormal accumulation of fluid in the cavities and intercellular spaces of the body.

Edema can be caused by a variety of factors, including hypoproteinemia, in which a lowered concentration of plasma proteins decreases the osmotic pressure, thereby permitting passage of abnormal amounts of fluid out of the blood vessels and into the tissue spaces. Some other causes are poor lymphatic drainage, increased capillary permeability (as in inflammation), and congestive HEART FAILURE. See also ANASARCA, ASCITES, HYDROTHORAX, HYDROPERICARDIUM and anatomically located edemas, e.g. brain, corneal, pulmonary edema.

angioneurotic e. see ANGIOEDEMA.
cardiac e. is part of the syndrome of congestive heart failure. It comprises 'bottle jaw', jugular vein

engorgement, edema of the brisket and underline, and ascites, hydrothorax and hydropericardium. See also congestive HEART FAILURE.

dependent e. edema affecting most severely the lowermost parts of the body.

e. disease 1. in **pigs** a highly fatal disease of young pigs in the weaner and grower age groups characterized by incoordination, a hoarseness of voice, weakness, flaccid paralysis and blindness. Edema of the eyelids, face and ears is diagnostic but is seldom visible on clinical examination. The course is short, often less than 24 hours, and many pigs are just found dead. The disease is attributed to an enterotoxemia caused by the opportunistic proliferation of specific serotypes of *Escherichia coli* in an intestinal environment brought about by a change to a diet more dense in carbohydrates. Called also gut edema, bowel edema. 2. in **goats** a disease caused by *Mycoplasma* F38; a fatal cellulitis.

gravitational e. see dependent edema (above).

gut e. see EDEMA disease.

hepatic e. edema is a common accompaniment of hepatic disease because of the decline in production of plasma proteins and a fall in the blood's hydrostatic pressure. Ascites may occur independently because of portal hypertension when there is severe liver disease and obstruction to blood flow in the portal vein.

laryngeal e. see LARYNGEAL edema.

leg e. a disease of market age turkeys of unknown cause and characterized by edema of the legs and focal muscle necrosis.

low-pressure e. noncardiogenic pulmonary edema. See acute RESPIRATORY distress syndrome.

e. neonatorum edema of the newborn. See LYMPHATIC vessel obstruction.

pitting e. edema in which pressure by the clinician's finger leaves a persistent depression in the tissues.

subcutaneous e. may be generalized and constitute ANASARCA. Local areas of edema occur in such other conditions as ANGIOEDEMA and URTICARIA, edematous plaques in dourine and infectious equine anemia, and in purpura hemorrhagica.

vasogenic e. that characterized by increased permeability of capillary endothelial cells; the most common form of brain edema.

edemagen an irritant that elicits edema by causing capillary damage but not the cellular response of true inflammation.

edematogenic producing or causing edema.

Edentata an order of mammals that includes anteaters, armadillos, sloths.

edentate 1. an animal without teeth, e.g. giant anteater. 2. used in the proper sense a member of the animal order Edentata, including anteaters and sloths.

edentia absence of the teeth.

edentulous without teeth.

edetate any salt of ethylenediamine tetra-acetic acid (EDTA), including *edetate disodium calcium*, used in the diagnosis and treatment of lead poisoning, and *edetate disodium*, used in the treatment of poisoning with lead and other heavy metals, and, because of its affinity for calcium, in the treatment of hypercalcemia.

edetic acid ethylenediamine tetra-acetic acid (EDTA).

EDIM epizootic diarrhea of infant mice. See MURINE epizootic diarrhea.

Edles Warmblut horse German light horse.

EDP electronic data processing.

EDRF endothelium-derived relaxing factor.

edrophonium a cholinergic used in the form of the chloride salt as a curare antagonist; used in the edrophonium challenge test to diagnose myasthenia gravis. See also TENSILON.

EDS see EGG drop syndrome.

EDTA ethylenediamine tetra-acetic acid. See EDETATE.

Edwards medium selective for streptococci, which show ESCULIN hydrolysis.

Edwardsiella a genus of bacteria of the family Enterobacteriaceae. Inhabits the intestines of snakes; found also in water.

E. ictaluri causes enteric septicemia in catfish.

***E. tarda* (syn. *E. anguillimortifera*)** causes edwardsiellosis, septicemia in catfish and eels, characterized by the appearance of evil-smelling, gas-filled cavities in muscle. Also a reported cause of diarrhea in dogs, pigs and calves.

edwardsiellosis disease caused by infestation with *Edwardsiella tarda*.

EEE eastern equine encephalomyelitis.

EEG electroencephalogram.

eel elongated, serpent-like fish with no scales. Most are marine species but there are some freshwater types. They are members of the order Apodes and constitute a number of suborders.

e. rhabdovirus several isolates from eels have not been shown to be associated with disease in eels, but some are pathogenic for trout and salmon.

e. stomatopapilloma thought to be a viral infection.

e. stripe see DORSAL stripe.

EENT eye–ear–nose–throat.

EF elongation factor.

ef- prefix meaning away from or outward.

EF-4 eugonic fermenter-4.

EFA essential fatty acid.

EFF Elokomin fluke fever.

effacement the obliteration of form or features; applied to the cervix uteri during labor when it is so changed that only the ostium uteri remains.

effect a result produced by an action. The relationship between the two can be expressed in linear form. The total association between them may be the sum of a number of effects. The effect may be direct when it is exerted without being transmitted through intervening factors, or indirect when it is. It may also be a spurious effect when the observed changes are due to causes and correlations common to both.

additive e. the combined effect produced by the action of two or more agents, being equal to the sum of their separate effects.

Coolidge e. the stimulation of sexual behavior in a male animal upon exposure to a new female.

cumulative e. cumulation action.

experimenter e's demand characteristics; the characteristics supplied by the experimental subject in response to what it perceives are the demands of the experimenter.

e. modifier a factor which modifies the effect of a causal factor under study. Called also interaction.

position e. in genetics, the changed effect produced by alteration of the relative positions of various genes on the chromosomes.

pressure e. the sum of the changes that are due to obstruction of tissue drainage by pressure.

side e. a consequence other than that for which an agent is used, especially an adverse effect on another organ system.

effective exerting a measurable effect.

e. circulating volume that part of the blood volume that is effectively perfusing the tissues at a particular time.

e. focus see effective FOCAL SPOT.
e. refractory period time interval during which the effector cell remains unresponsive after a previous reaction to a stimulus: see also REFRACTORY period.
e. temperature an expression of the temperature combined with humidity and wind speed.
effectiveness the ability to produce a specific result or to exert a specific measurable influence.
relative biological e. an expression of the effectiveness of other types of radiation in comparison with that of gamma or x-rays.
effector 1. a muscle or gland that contracts or secretes, respectively, in direct response to nerve impulses. 2. a molecule that binds to an enzyme with an effect on its catalytic activity, i.e. either an activator or inhibitor.
allosteric e. one that binds to an enzyme at a site other than the active site.
e. cell cell in the immune system that mediates an immune function.
effemination feminization.
efferent conducting or progressing away from a center or specific site of reference, as an efferent nerve.
e. arterioles see efferent ARTERIOLE.
e. ductules conducting tubules from the rete testis to the head of the epididymis, forming part of the transport mechanism for spermatozoa in the testis.
[gamma] e's small nerves supplying intrafusal muscle fibers.
e. nerve any nerve that carries impulses from the central nervous system toward the periphery, as a motor nerve. See also NEURON.
efficacy intrinsic activity; is equal to the magnitude of the maximal response.
efficiency 1. in clinical practice equals the effect achieved in relation to the expenditure and effort expended. 2. in physiological terms, efficiency of any organ or tissue is equal to the ratio of useful energy produced to total energy expended.
effleurage [Fr.] stroking movement in massage.
efflorescence 1. the quality of being efflorescent. 2. a rash or eruption.
efflorescent becoming powdery by losing the water of crystallization.
effluent waste from an abattoir carried away in liquid form. Disposal is a major problem because of the need to avoid pollution of waterways. See AEROBIC effluent treatment, ANAEROBIC effluent treatment.
effluvium pl. *effluvia* [L.] 1. an outflowing or shedding, as of the hair. 2. an exhalation or emanation, especially one of noxious nature.
anagen e. see ANAGEN defluxion.
effusion 1. escape of a fluid into a part; exudation or transudation. See also specific anatomic sites. 2. an exudate or transudate.
eflornithine an antiprotozoal agent, used as the hydrochloride in trypanosomiasis and PNEUMOCYSTIS *carinii* pneumonia.
EGD esophagogastroduodenoscopy.
egesta undigested material discharged from the body.
egestion the casting out of undigested material.
egg 1. an ovum; a female gamete. 2. an oocyte. 3. a female reproductive cell at any stage before fertilization and its derivatives after fertilization and even after some development. 4. hen egg, consisting of a blastodisk, remnant of the nucleus in a mass of white yolk sitting on top of the yellow yolk, the yolk suspended by two twisted strands of mucin-like protein, the chalazae, from the two poles of the egg, two yolk membranes that separate the yolk from the albumen, the albumen or white of the egg, which is in four separate layers of liquid and jelly material, two thin shell membranes and an eggshell. See also AVIAN oogenesis. 5. helminth egg.
e. bound a disease of cage birds, birds in zoological collections and in fish. In birds the hen may show pain and be straining and the egg may be palpable. The syndrome is comparable with dystocia in a viviparous animal. In fish the only sign is the wrinkled, shriveled eggs.
e. count counting of helminth eggs as an estimate of the parasite status in the animal or group. Flotation techniques and special counting chambers are used. The results are expressed as eggs per gram of feces or e.p.g.
e. dipping dipping of hatchery eggs in antibiotic solutions, especially erythromycin or tylosin, to prevent the transmission of infections from adults to chickens.
e. drop syndrome first observed in 1976 the disease is caused by an adenovirus and characterized by the hens laying a reduced number of thin-shelled or shell-less eggs. Subsequently the egg yield is reduced.
e. eating a vice which begins without apparent reason. A high rate of egg breaking in the unit encourages birds to begin. Many techniques are used in prevention but frequent egg removal is essential.
e. heating heating eggs in a hot-air incubator for 12–14 hours to reduce the transmission of infection on the egg exterior.
e. peritonitis see egg PERITONITIS.
e. retention see egg bound (above).
e. shell secreted around the egg mass and membranes during its last 15 hours in the uterus; composed of calcium carbonate and a glycoprotein matrix; surrounded by the cuticle.
thin-shelled e. occurs in egg drop syndrome (see above), DDT poisoning. The shell of the egg is very thin, often missing altogether.
e. tooth the additional tip to the beak in birds that is used by the hatching chick to peck out the circular hatch of shell to allow it to emerge. The egg tooth drops off in a few days. Called also bean.
e. transmission transmission of disease from hen to chicken and between chickens via infection in the egg, e.g. *Mycoplasma gallisepticum*, *M. meleagridis*.
e. white injury the effects of biotin deficiency induced by feeding of raw egg whites (albumen). The factor responsible is avidin which binds biotin, preventing absorption.
e. yield in domestic fowl the normal annual average over a large, national population is about 130 eggs per bird; good units average 200.
Eggers bone plate slotted contact plate for orthopedic use in stainless steel or vitallium. Fitted with matching screws.
eggplant SOLANUM *melongena*.
egobronchophony, egophony increased vocal resonance with a high-pitched bleating quality of the transmitted voice or other sound, detected by auscultation of the lungs, especially over lung tissue compressed by pleural effusion.
egophony egobronchophony.
egret wading birds of the order Ciconiiformes and particularly of the genus *Egretta* with long legs and bills; highly prized for ornamental plumage. The cattle egret is a separate species, *Ardeola bis*.
Egyptian buffalo an Indian buffalo breed, gray-black in color, used for milk and draft. Has short curved horns.
Egyptian mau a medium-sized, muscular breed of cats with green eyes and a medium length, patterned coat which is a mixture of spots and stripes.

EHD epizootic hemorrhagic disease.

EHDV epizootic hemorrhagic disease virus.

EHEC enterohemorrhagic *Escherichia coli.*

Ehlers–Danlos syndrome a congenital hereditary syndrome of joint hyperextensibility, hyperelasticity and fragility of the skin, poor wound healing leaving parchment-like scars, capillary fragility and subcutaneous nodules after trauma. Called also cutis hyperelastica, cutaneous asthenia, hereditary collagen dysplasia.

In humans a series of these disorders, listed as Ehlers–Danlos syndrome Type I to Type VII, represent different errors in collagen synthesis and maintenance with subsequent variations in clinical and pathological manifestations.

Ehmer sling a style of bandage used in dogs and cats that holds the hindleg in flexion with the hip in abduction and internal rotation. Commonly used after reduction of hip luxation.

Ehretia membranifolia member of the Boraginaceae plant family; may cause nitrate–nitrite poisoning.

Ehrlichia a genus of the order *Rickettsiales*. Intracellular parasites of white blood cells. See RICKETTSIA.

E. bovis causes benign bovine rickettsiosis.

E. canis causes canine EHRLICHIOSIS.

E. equi causes equine EHRLICHIOSIS. Called also Potomac fever.

E. ondiri causes ONDIRI DISEASE. Called also bovine petechial fever. See also JEMBRANA DISEASE.

E. ovina causes benign ovine rickettsiosis.

E. phagocytophilia CYTOECETES *phagocytophila.*

E. platys causes infectious cyclic thrombocytopenia in dogs.

E. risticii the cause of equine intestinal EHRLICHIOSIS.

ehrlichial colitis see equine intestinal EHRLICHIOSIS.

ehrlichiosis the disease caused by infection with the rickettsial agent *Ehrlichia* spp.

canine e. caused by *Ehrlichia canis* which is transmitted by the brown dog tick, *Rhipicephalus sanguineus.* The disease is characterized by pancytopenia and bleeding tendencies, particularly epistaxis. Called also tropical canine pancytopenia, canine hemorrhagic fever, tracker dog disease, canine rickettsiosis, canine tick typhus, Nairobi bleeding disease, Lahore canine fever. Clinical signs may be potentiated by simultaneous infection with *E. platys.*

equine e. is an infectious disease caused by *Ehrlichia equi.* The clinical syndrome comprises high fever, hemolytic anemia, incoordination, edema of the extremities and a marked leukopenia. The disease bears a strong resemblance to equine infectious anemia.

equine intestinal e. a highly fatal enterocolitis of horses caused by *Ehrlichia risticii.* Characterized by high fever, leukopenia and acute diarrhea. Called also Potomac horse fever, equine monocytic ehrlichiosis.

ehrlichosis see EHRLICHIOSIS.

Ehrlich's test used to examine urine for the presence of urobilinogen; based on the use of Ehrlich's diazo reagent, a sodium *p*-diazobenzenesulfonate solution.

EHV equine herpesvirus.

EHV1, EHV2, EHV3, EHV4, EHV5 see EQUINE herpesvirus.

EIA equine infectious anemia.

eicosanoids a family of compounds derived from arachidonic acid (eicosatetraenoic acid). Includes prostaglandins, prostacyclin and thromboxanes, the principal mediators of inflammation.

eicosapentaenoic acid a 20-carbon polyunsaturated fatty acid with five double bonds; a precursor of 1, 2 and 3 series prostaglandins.

eicosatetraenoic acid arachidonic acid.

EIEC enteroinvasive *Escherichia coli.*

eigenvalues statistical term meaning latent root.

eight conditions an acupuncture term for one of the ways of making a diagnosis. Each of the conditions is expressed as a pair of opposites, *Yin* and *Yang*, internal and external, hot and cold, deficiency and excess.

Eimeria a genus of protozoan parasites in the family Eimeriidae. There are many species (see below), mostly in birds and herbivores. They are the principal cause of COCCIDIOSIS, which also has other causes. See CYSTOISOSPORA, ISOSPORA, TYZZERIA, WENYONELLA.

Commonly listed *Eimeria* spp. and their hosts are listed below:

E. abramovi—wild duck, geese; *E. acervulina*—domestic poultry, quail; *E. adenoeides*—turkey; *E. ahsata*—sheep, goats; *E. alabamensis*—cattle; *E. alijevi*—goats; *E. alpacae*—llama, alpaca; *E. anatis*—mallard, domestic duck; *E. ankarensis*—water buffalo; *E. anseris*—domestic geese, wild geese; *E. apsheronica*-goats; *E. arkhari*—sheep, goats; *E. arloingi*—sheep, goat; *E. auburnensis*—cattle; *E. augusta*—grouse; *E. aurata*—fish; *E. azerbaidschanica*—water buffalo.

E. bactriani—one- and two-humped camel; *E. bakuensis*—sheep; *E. bareillyi*—water buffalo; *E. battakhi*—domestic duck; *E. bombayansis*—zebu cattle; *E. bonasae*—grouse; *E. boschadis*—wild duck, geese; *E. bovis*—cattle, zebu, water buffalo; *E. brantae*—wild duck, geese; *E. brasiliensis*—cattle, zebu, water buffalo; *E. brinkmanni*—rock ptarmigan; *E. brunetti*—domestic poultry; *E. bucephalae*—wild duck, geese; *E. bukidnonensis*—cattle, zebu, buffalo.

E. cameli—one- and two-humped camels; *E. canadensis*—domestic cattle, zebu, bison, water buffalo; *E. canis*—dogs and cats; *E. caprina*—goats; *E. caprovina*—goats; *E. carinii*—rats; *E. carpelli*—fish; *E.caviae*—guinea pig; *E. cerdonis*—pig; *E. christenseni*—domestic goat; *E. christianseni*—mute swan; *E. clarkei*—lesser snow goose; *E. coecicola*—rabbit; *E. colchici*—pheasant; *E. columbae*—pigeon; *E. columbarum*—rock dove; *E. coturnicus*—quail; *E. crandallis*—domestic sheep, small wild ruminants; *E. cylindrica*—domestic cattle, zebu, water buffalo; *E. cyprini*—fish.

E. danailovi—mallard; *E. danielle*—domestic sheep; *E. debliecki*—pig; *E. dispersa*—turkey; *E. dolichotis*—Patagonian cavey; *E. dromedarii*—one- and two-humped camels.

E. ellipsoidalis—domestic cattle, zebu, European bison, water buffalo; *E. elongata*—domestic rabbit; *E. exigua*—rabbits, Greenland hare.

E. falciformis—mouse; *E. fanthami*—rock ptarmigan; *E. farri*—white fronted goose; *E. faurei*—sheep, small wild ruminants; *E. ferrisi*-mouse; *E. fulva*—wild geese.

E. gallopavonis—turkey; *E. gilruthi*—sheep, goat; *E. gokaki*—buffalo; *E. gonzalei*—sheep; *E. gorakhpuri*—guinea fowl; *E. granulosa*—domestic and wild sheep; *E. grenieri*—guinea fowl; *E. guevarai*—pig.

E. hagani—poultry; *E. hasei*—rats; *E. hawkinsi*—sheep, goat; *E. hermani*—wild geese; *E. hindlei*—mouse; *E. hirci*—goats.

E. illinoisensis—cattle; *E. innocua*—turkey; *E. intestinalis*—rabbit; *E. intricata*—sheep, wild small ruminants; *E. irresidua*—rabbit, jackrabbit.

E. jolchijevi—goats; *E. keilini*—mouse; *E. kocharli*—goats; *E. kofoidi*—partridge; *E. koganae*—wild duck, geese; *E. kosti*-cattle; *E. kotlani*—domestic geese; *E. krijgsmanni*—mouse.

E. labbeana—pigeons; *E. lagopodi*—ptarmigan; *E. lamae*—alpaca; *E. langeroni*—pheasant; *E. leuckarti*—horse; *E. lyruri*—partridge.

E. macusaniensis—llama, alpaca; *E. magna*—rabbit, hare; *E. magnalabia*—wild geese; *E. mandali*—peafowl; *E. marsica*—sheep; *E. matsubayashii*—domestic rabbit; *E. maxima*—poultry; *E. mayurai*—peafowl; *E. media*—domestic and wild rabbit; *E. megalostromata*—pheasant; *E. meleagridis*—turkey; *E. meleagrimitis*—domestic turkey; *E. mitis*—poultry; *E. mivati*—domestic fowl; *E. miyairii*—rat; *E. mundaragi*—cattle, zebu; *E. musculi*—mouse.

E. nadsoni—grouse; *E. nagpurensis*—rabbit; *E. necatrix*—domestic fowl; *E. neodebliecki*—pig, wild pig; *E. neoleporis*—rabbit; *E. nieschultzi*—rat; *E. ninakohlyakimovae*—sheep, goat and small wild ruminants; *E. nocens*—domestic and wild geese; *E. nochti*—rat; *E. norvegicus*—rat; *E. numida*—guinea fowl.

E. ovina—domestic sheep, small wild ruminants; *E. ovoidalis*—buffalo.

E. pacifica—pheasant; *E. pallida*—domestic sheep and goat; *E. parva*—domestic sheep and goat, small wild ruminants; *E. parvula*—goose; *E. pavonina*—peafowl; *E. pavonis*—peafowl; *E. pelleryi*—bactrian camel; *E. pellita*—cattle; *E. perforans*—rabbit, hare; *E. perminuta*—pig; *E. peruviana*—llama; *E. phasiani*—pheasant; *E. piriformis*—domestic rabbit; *E. polita*—pig; *E. porci*—pig; *E. praecox*—poultry; *E. procera*—partridge; *E. punctata*—sheep; *E. punoensis*—alpaca.

E. rajasthani—dromedary; *E. ratti*—rat.

E. saitamae—duck; *E. scabra*—domestic and wild pig; *E. schachdagica*—duck; *E. schueffneri*—mouse; *E. scrofae*—pig; *E. separata*—rat; *E. solipedum*—horse; *E. somateriae*—wild duck; *E. spinosa*—pig; *E. stiedae*—rabbit, hare; *E. stigmosa*—domestic goose; *E. striata*—wild goose; *E. subepithelialis*—carp; *E. subrotunda*—turkey; *E. subspherica*—cattle, zebu, water buffalo; *E. suis*—domestic pig.

E. tenella—domestic poultry; *E. tetricis*—grouse; *E. thianethi*—buffalo; *E. tropicalis*—pigeon; *E. truncata*—domestic and wild goose; *E. truttae*—salmon.

E. uniungulati—horse, mule; *E. weybridgensis*—sheep; *E. wyomingensis*—cattle, zebu, water buffalo; *E. zuernii*—cattle, zebu, water buffalo.

einsteinium a chemical element, atomic number 99, atomic weight 254, symbol Es. See Table 6.

Einthoven Dutch physiologist, discoverer of the electrocardiogram.

E.'s law the potential differences between the bipolar leads measured simultaneously will, at any given moment, have the values II = I + III.

E. triangle an equilateral triangle used as a model of the standard limb leads used in electrocardiography.

EIPH exercise induced pulmonary hemorrhage. See EPISTAXIS.

Eisenmenger German physician (1864–1932).

E. complex interventricular septal defect.

E. syndrome the clinical syndrome caused by the Eisenmenger complex, a ventricular septal defect with pulmonary hypertension and cyanosis due to right-to-left (reversed) shunt of blood. Sometimes defined as pulmonary hypertension (pulmonary vascular disease) and cyanosis with the shunt being at the atrial, ventricular, or great vessel area. Characterized by exercise intolerance, cyanosis, anasarca, palpable thrill and auscultatable cardiac murmur.

ejaculate 1. to expel an ejaculate. 2. the products of an ejaculation. See also EJACULATION.

ejaculatio ejaculation.

ejaculation forcible, sudden expulsion; especially expulsion of semen from the male urethra, a reflex action that occurs as a result of sexual stimulation. Includes lubricating fluid from bulbourethral glands, prostatic and seminal vesicular fluids and semen. Called also seminal ejaculation.

electrical e. see ELECTROEJACULATION.

incomplete e. the process of ejaculation of semen is not completed and semen does not reach the external urethral orifice, due usually to a defect in the sympathetic innervation of the region.

retrograde e. after intercourse, in which no semen is ejaculated from the external urethral orifice, semen is found in the urinary bladder.

ejecta refuse cast off from the body.

ejection forcible expulsion through a narrow orifice.

e. fraction of the cardiac stroke volume equals the ratio of the stroke volume to the end-diastolic volume.

milk e. see LETDOWN.

ventricular e. time that part of the cardiac ventricular contraction time when blood is actually discharged through the semilunar valves.

ejection fraction in echocardiography, the fractional volume of blood leaving the left ventricle in systole.

EKG, ECG electrocardiogram.

ekoa see LEUCAENA LEUCOCEPHALA.

EKY electrokymogram.

El Guedda see HEMORRHAGIC septicemia.

elaborate to produce complex substances out of simpler materials.

elaboration the process of producing complex substances out of simpler materials.

Elaeodendron buchananii African tree in family Celastraceae, whose leaves, if ingested, cause death after a clinical illness with signs of dyspnea, incoordination and diarrhea in those animals that live for several days. A causative toxin has not been identified. Called also *Cassine buchananii*, *Elaeodendron kiniense*.

Elaeophora a genus of filariid nematodes in the family Onchocercidae.

E. bohmi found in the arteries and veins of the extremities of horses. Called also *Onchocerca bohmi*.

E. poeli found in the aorta of cattle and other ruminants.

E. sagittus found in bovine hearts. Called also *Cordophilus sagittus*.

E. schneideri found in arteries of deer, elk and sheep; causes ELAEOPHORIASIS.

elaeophoriasis dermatitis caused by vascular lesions of infestation with microfilariae of *Elaeophora schneideri*. The parasite can also cause rhinitis, keratoconjunctivitis and stomatitis in sheep infected by bites of horse flies. This and other species may also cause sporadic cases of disease due to vascular obstruction.

elaeophorosis see ELAEOPHORIASIS.

Elam gag a gag used in horses and cattle to obtain access to the interior of the mouth. Shaped like a stringless tennis racquet with two horizontal bars, one of which can be moved by manipulating a screw drive. The gag is inserted in the mouth in a horizontal position and immediately brought to the vertical position with the bars located caudad to the incisor teeth. The bars are now screwed apart giving unimpeded access to the interior of the mouth.

eland large (1000 to 2000 lb) true antelopes, capable of domestication and favored for game ranches. Called also *Taurotragus oryx*.

elandsboontjie see ELEPHANTORRHIZA ELEPHANTINA.
elaphostrongyliasis infestation with *Paraelaphostrongylus tenuis*. See NEUROFILARIASIS.
Elaphostrongylus a genus of metastrongylid nematodes of the family Protostrongylidae.
E. cervi found in connective tissue and central nervous system of deer. Causes CEREBROSPINAL nematodiasis.
E. panticola found in the brain of deer.
E. rangiferi occurs in the central nervous system and muscles of reindeer. See also CEREBROSPINAL nematodiasis.
E. tenuis see PARELAPHOSTRONGYLUS *tenuis*.
Elaphurus davidianus see PÈRE DAVID'S DEER.
Elaphus maximus Asian or Indian elephant.
elapid see ELAPINE.
Elapidae a family of venomous front-fanged snakes; includes cobras, kraits, mambas, coral snakes and hamadryads. Their poison is largely neurotoxic.
elapine a snake belonging to the ELAPIDAE family.
elasmobranch members of the class Elasmobranchii; includes sharks and rays.
elastance the quality of recoiling on removal of pressure without disruption, or an expression of the measure of the ability to do so in terms of unit of volume change per unit of pressure change; it is the reciprocal of compliance.
elastase an enzyme capable of catalyzing the digestion of elastic tissue.
elastic capable of resuming normal shape after distortion.
e. bands used in orthodontics as a means of moving teeth.
e. modulus the constant or scale factor which defines quantitatively the relationship between the deformation of the vascular wall (or other elastic medium) and the deforming force.
e. ring castration see ELASTRATOR.
e. tissue connective tissue made up of yellow elastic fibers, frequently massed into sheets.
elasticity the quality of being elastic.
demand e. see DEMAND elasticity.
blood vessel e. a composite value of the combined elasticities of the smooth muscle, collagen and elastin of which the walls are composed.
elastin a yellow scleroprotein, the essential constituent of elastic connective tissue; it is brittle when dry, but flexible and elastic when moist.
elastofibroma a tumor consisting of both elastin and fibrous elements.
elastolysis the digestion of elastic substance or tissue.
elastoma a tumor or focal excess of elastic tissue fibers or abnormal collagen fibers of the skin.
elastometer an instrument for measuring the elasticity of tissues.
elastorrhexis a rupture of fibers composing elastic tissue.
elastosis 1. degeneration of elastic tissue. 2. degenerative changes in the dermal connective tissue with increased amounts of elastotic material. 3. any disturbance of the dermal connective tissue.
solar e. see SOLAR elastosis.
elastotic 1. pertaining to or characterized by elastosis. 2. resembling elastic tissue; having the staining properties of elastin.
elastration see ELASTRATOR.
elastrator an implement used for castration and tail docking by applying elastrator rings to animals. Closing the handles of this double-action, scissor-like instrument opens the jaws and dilates the rubber ring. This is slipped over the scrotum or tail and the handles released. The ring is now in place and the tool is withdrawn.
e. ring a specially constructed, thick and very strong rubber ring for use in an elastrator. Has sufficient strength to close off all the blood vessels to a part and cause it to slough.
elbow 1. the bend of the lower forelimb. 2. the joint connecting the humerus, radius and ulna. It is one of the body's more versatile joints, with a combined hinge and rotating action allowing the limb to bend and paw to make a half turn. The flexibility of the elbow and shoulder joints together permits a nearly infinite variety of paw movements. In ungulates the elbow is a simple hinge.
e. abduction in the standing posture the elbows are constantly abducted from the chest; usually a posture indicative of pleural pain.
e. dysplasia includes the developmental defects, ununited anconeal process and fragmented (ununited) coronoid process, which occur in young, actively growing, large breed dogs, causing lameness and later arthritis of the elbow.
e. flexion a frequent malposition of a forelimb causing dystocia in cows. The foot is presented but is a long way back from the one on the opposite limb. The flexed limb increases the diameter of the fetus significantly.
e. luxation uncommon in most species because of the innate stability of the elbow joint; can be congenital or caused by trauma, sometimes associated with fractures.
elder see SAMBUCUS.
elderberry see SAMBUCUS.
elderly animals see GERIATRIC.
ELE equine leukoencephalomalacia.
elective non-urgent; at an elected time, e.g. of surgery.
electric generating or powered by electricity. See also ELECTRICAL.
e. clippers see CLIPPING.
electrical producing, produced by or powered by electricity.
e. anesthesia see electrical IMMOBILIZATION.
e. analgesia see electrical IMMOBILIZATION.
e. axis in electrocardiographic work is the direction of the electrical forces in the heart at a given moment in the cardiac cycle. See also MEAN electrical axis.
e. conductivity in milk increases with an increase in the severity of inflammation of the mammary tissue. Used as a mastitis detection device.
e. fences temporary fences, usually one or two strands of wire, electrified by low voltage batteries, used to confine cattle, pigs or horses to specified sections of a pasture. Similar wires are added to wooden and other fences to prevent animals rubbing against them.
e. ignition sources electric power outlets, switches and electrical equipment in the surgery can be the cause of explosion if flammable anesthetic agents or oxygen are being used.
e. injuries shock caused by the passage of electric current passing through the body can cause irritation, unconsciousness, burns or immediate death depending on the voltage, the amperage of the current, the efficiency of the patient as an earth contact and the duration of the shock. Signs and the fatal outcome are due to paralysis of medullary centers in the medulla oblongata. Burns when they occur are usually at the points of contact between the animal and the earth. High voltage current will cause sudden death (electrocution). Low voltage house current will

knock a cow down and may cause death, trickle current loss will cause cows to bellow and to kick. Lower voltage current still has been associated with a high prevalence rate of mastitis. See also LIGHTNING strike.

Household pets, particularly puppies and kittens, most often are injured from chewing on electrical cords. If not electrocuted, they incur burns of the mouth or lips that vary from small, punctate lesions to large areas. These are caused by coagulation and necrosis and do not become apparent until 2 to 3 weeks after the incident, making the diagnosis very difficult. Pulmonary edema is also a major feature of electrical injury in dogs and cats and it can be the cause of death.

e. point finding identification of acupuncture points by the use of an electrical point finder; this measures the resistance of the skin to the flow of electricity; it is much lower over acupuncture points.

e. stimulators battery-powered instruments which generate a current sufficient to stimulate acupuncture points.

e. stunning the passage of a low voltage electrical current through the brain to cause unconsciousness. The current is passed through a pair of tongs clamped to the head like a pair of earphones. Used mostly for pigs and poultry but also for lambs and calves. The tongs should be applied for at least 10 seconds and the amperage not less than 250 milliamps and the voltage not less than 75 volts. See also STUNNING.

e. wiring see electrical injuries (above), EARTHING, FREE electricity.

electro- word element. [Gr.] *electricity*.

electroacupuncture passing electrical energy through acupuncture needles to acupoints; the energy supply is from a special device.

electroaffinity see ELECTRONEGATIVITY.

electroanalgesia the reduction of pain by electrical stimulation of a peripheral nerve or the dorsal column of the spinal cord.

electroanesthesia see electrical IMMOBILIZATION, ELECTRONARCOSIS.

electrocardiogram the record produced by ELECTROCARDIOGRAPHY; a tracing representing the heart's electrical action derived by amplification of the minutely small electrical impulses normally generated by the heart. Called also ECG and EKG.

electrocardiograph the apparatus used in electrocardiography.

electrocardiographic emanating from or pertaining to electrocardiography.

e. monitoring maintenance of a more or less continuous surveillance of a patient's cardiac status by means of electrocardiography.

electrocardiography the graphic recording from the body surface of the potential of electric currents generated by the heart, as a means of studying the action of the heart muscle.

With the modern electrocardiograph, the current that accompanies the action of the heart is amplified 3000 times or more, and it moves a small, sensitively balanced lever in contact with moving paper. The pattern of heart waves that is traced on the paper indicates the heart's rhythm and other actions.

The normal electrocardiogram is composed of a P wave, Q, R and S waves known as the QRS COMPLEX, or QRS wave, and a T wave. The P wave occurs at the beginning of each contraction of the atria. The QRS wave occurs at the beginning of each contraction of the ventricles. The T wave seen in a normal electrocardiogram occurs as the ventricles recover electrically and prepare for the next contraction. There is a refractory period after each P wave and QRS complex during which the muscle is inexcitable; this period is usually about 0.30 second.

The electric impulses in the heart muscle are picked up and conducted to the electrocardiograph by electrodes or leads connected to the body by small metal plates or other methods. The metal plates are moistened with a conductive paste and attached to the limbs and chest (cardiac area) of the animal.

electrocautery cauterization of tissue by means of an electrode that consists of a red hot piece of metal, such as a wire, held in a holder, and is heated by either direct or alternating current. The term *electrocautery* is used to refer to both the procedure and the instrument used in the procedure.

electrochemical emanating from or pertaining to electrochemistry.

e. equivalent the atomic weight divided by the ionic valence of an electrolyte. Provides a quantitative indication of the combining properties of an electrolyte solution. The relationship between weight per volume and milliequivalents can be expressed as:

$$\frac{\text{mg/100 ml}}{\text{atomic weight}} \times \text{valence} \times 10 = \text{mEq/l}$$

e. gradient the differences in electrochemial potential between two points.

intestinal e. gradient electrical potential differences and ion concentration differences across the external membrane of the intestinal mucosa arising from the active transport of most electrolytes and some nonelectrolytes across the membrane.

electrochemistry the study of chemical changes produced by electric action.

electrocoagulation a method of electrosurgery used to coagulate tissue, which employs moderately damped or modulated undamped alternating current, and requires both an active concentrating electrode and an inactive dispersing electrode. See also ELECTROSURGERY.

electrocochleography measurement of electrical potentials of the eighth cranial nerve in response to acoustic stimuli applied by an electrode to the external acoustic canal, promontory or tympanic membrane.

electrocontractility contractility in response to electric stimulation.

electrocorticography electroencephalography with the electrodes applied directly to the cerebral cortex.

electrocution causing death by the passage of an electric current through the body of the patient. May be intentional, as a means of euthanasia, or accidental by lightning strike or electrical current. See ELECTRICAL injuries.

electrode either of two terminals of an electrically conducting system or cell.

active e. therapeutic electrode.

calomel e. one capable of both collecting and giving up chloride ions in neutral or acidic aqueous media, consisting of mercury in contact with mercurous chloride; used as a reference electrode in pH measurements.

depolarizing e. an electrode that has a resistance greater than that of the portion of the body enclosed in the circuit.

hydrogen e. an electrode made by depositing platinum black on platinum and then allowing it to absorb hydrogen gas to saturation; used in determination of hydrogen ion concentration.

indifferent e. one larger than a therapeutic electrode, dispersing electrical stimulation over a larger area.

point e. an electrode having on one end a metallic point; used in applying current.

therapeutic e. one smaller than an indifferent electrode, producing electrical stimulation in a concentrated area; called also active electrode.

electrodermal pertaining to the electrical properties of the skin, especially to changes in its resistance.

electrodesiccation a method of electrosurgery that desiccates tissue by dehydration. A highly or moderately damped alternating electrical current is radiated through a monoterminal active electrode that is applied directly to or inserted into the tissue being treated. See also ELECTROSURGERY.

electrodiagnosis the use of electrical recording devices such as ELECTROMYOGRAPHY, ELECTROENCEPHALOGRAPHY, CYSTOMETROGRAPHY, ELECTROCARDIOGRAPHY, in making a clinical diagnosis.

electrodialyzer a blood dialyzer utilizing an applied electric field and semipermeable membranes for separating the colloids from the solution.

electroejaculation a method used for the collection of semen for artificial insemination or for examination. Electrical stimulation has to be provided by electrodes applied to the lumbar sympathetic nerves to promote semen emission and to the pelvic splanchnic and internal pudendal nerves to promote ejaculation and erection of the penis. The electrodes are contained in a probe placed in the rectum.

electroejaculator a device consisting of a rectal probe and a power control system which gives stepwise control over the current applied, and a stimulator control which permits variation within the steps. Probes vary in their construction and a good design will direct stimulation at the relevant nerves, reducing the stimulation of the back and the hindlimbs.

electroencephalogram the record produced by ELECTROENCEPHALOGRAPHY; a tracing of the electric impulses of the brain. Called also EEG.

electroencephalograph the instrument used in electroencephalography.

electroencephalography the recording of changes in electric potentials in various areas of the brain by means of electrodes placed on the head or on or in the brain itself, and connected to an amplifier, which augments the impulses more than a million times. The impulses are of sufficient magnitude to move an electromagnetic pen that records the brain waves.

electroendosmosis osmosis under the influence of an electronic field as in electrophoresis.

electroepilation use of electrosurgical methods, such as electrocautery or diathermy, for destroying hair follicles; used in the treatment of distichiasis.

electrofulguration a method of electrosurgery used to produce superficial desiccation of tissue, which employs a highly or moderately damped alternating electrical current that is radiated through a monoterminal active electrode that is held close to the patient so that sparks spray over the lesion being treated. See also ELECTROSURGERY.

electrogastrograph an instrument for recording the electrical activity of the stomach by means of swallowed gastric electrodes.

electrogastrography the recording of the electrical activity of the stomach as measured between its lumen and the body surface.

electrogoniometer an instrument for measuring angles, e.g. the angle of a joint. Used in gait research. See also GONIOMETER.

electrogoniometry the science of measuring angles and the changes in them. Much used in the study of gait.

electrogram any record produced by changes in electric potential.

His bundle e. an intracardiac electrocardiogram of potentials in the bundle of His, done through a cardiac catheter.

electrohemostasis arrest of hemorrhage by electrocautery.

electrohysterography the recording of changes in electric potential associated with contractions of the uterine muscle.

electro-immobilization see electrical IMMOBILIZATION.

electroimmunoassay see IMMUNOELECTROPHORESIS.

electroimmunodiffusion see IMMUNOELECTROPHORESIS.

electroincision cutting of tissue by an electrosurgical device.

electrokymogram the record produced by electrokymography.

electrokymograph the instrument used in electrokymography.

electrokymography the photography on x-ray film of the motion of the heart or of other moving structures which can be visualized radiographically.

electrolysis destruction by passage of a galvanic current, as in disintegration of a chemical compound in solution or destruction of hairs such as cilia from eyelids in distichiasis or trichiasis.

electrolyte a chemical substance which, when dissolved in water or melted, dissociates into electrically charged particles (*ions*), and thus is capable of conducting an electric current. The principal positively charged ions in the body fluids (*cations*) are sodium ($Na+$), potassium ($K+$), calcium (Ca^2+), and magnesium (Mg^2+). The most important negatively charged ions (*anions*) are chloride (Cl^-), bicarbonate (HCO^3-), and phosphate ($PO_4{}^3-$). These electrolytes are involved in metabolic activities and are essential to the normal function of all cells. Concentration gradients of sodium and potassium across the cell membrane produce the membrane potential and provide the means by which electrochemical impulses are transmitted in nerve and muscle fibers.

The concentration of the various electrolytes in body fluids is maintained within a narrow range. However, the optimal concentrations differ in the extracellular fluid and intracellular fluid. An electrolyte imbalance exists when the serum concentration of an electrolyte is either too high or too low.

Stability of the electrolyte balance depends on adequate intake of water and the electrolytes, and on homeostatic mechanisms within the body that regulate the absorption, distribution and excretion of water and its dissolved particles.

The effects of an electrolyte imbalance are not isolated to a particular organ or system. In general, however, imbalances in CALCIUM concentrations affect the bones, kidney and gastrointestinal tract. Calcium also influences the permeability of cell membranes and thereby regulates neuromuscular activity. SODIUM affects the osmolality of blood and therefore influences blood volume and pressure and the retention or loss of interstitial fluid. POTASSIUM affects muscular activities, notably those of the heart, intestines and respiratory tract, and also affects neural stimulation of the skeletal muscles.

e. clearance ratio see FRACTIONAL excretion tests.

e. disturbances include hyper- and hypo-potassemia, natremia, phosphatemia, calcemia, chloremia.

e. fluid balance balance between fluid and electrolytes.

e. homeostasis maintenance of the osmotic pressure of the blood and tissue fluids by the maintenance of a proper balance between the normal electrolytes in the fluid, and at the same time maintaining adequate concentrations of calcium and magnesium and the proper acid–base balance.

e. solution therapy see FLUID therapy.

electrolytic pertaining to electrolysis or to an electrolyte.

electromagnet a piece of metal rendered temporarily magnetic by passage of electricity through a coil surrounding it.

electromagnetic pertaining to or emanating from electromagnetism.

e. flowmeter measures the electromagnetic force generated when the blood flowing through a vessel of known diameter passes through a magnetic field at right angles to the magnetic lines of force.

e. radiation transport of energy through space. Examples are x-rays, radio waves.

e. receptors receptors which perceive electromagnetic stimuli.

electromagnetism magnetism developed by an electric current.

electromechanical coupling the coupling which transforms an electrical impulse into a mechanical action, e.g. in smooth muscle.

electromechanical dissociation when the electrical impulse passes through the system but no movement occurs, e.g. in ECG recordings.

electromotive force the force that, by reason of differences in potential, causes a flow of electricity from one place to another, giving rise to an electric current.

electromyogram the record obtained by electromyography. Abbreviated EMG.

electromyograph the instrument used in electromyography. Abbreviated EMG.

electromyography the recording and study of the intrinsic electrical properties of skeletal muscle; abbreviated EMG.

When it is at rest, normal muscle is electrically silent, but when the muscle is active, an electrical current is generated. In electromyography the electrical impulses are picked up by needle electrodes inserted into the muscle and amplified on an oscilloscope screen in the form of wavelike tracings.

electron any of the negatively charged particles arranged in orbits around the nucleus of an atom and determining all of the atom's physical and chemical properties except mass and radioactivity. Electrons flowing in a conductor constitute an electric current; when ejected from a radioactive substance, they constitute the beta particles.

e. acceptor see OXIDANT.

e. beam the stream of electrons that flows from the anode to the cathode in the x-ray tube and then interacts with the tungsten target to produce x-rays.

e. carrier a molecule associated with membrane-bound proteins that accepts and transfers electrons.

e. donor see REDUCTANT.

e. micrographs photographic images of electron microscopic fields.

e. microscope see electron MICROSCOPE.

e. microscopy technology of using an electron microscope.

electron-dense in electron microscopy, having a density that prevents electrons from penetrating.

electronarcosis narcosis produced by passage of an electric current through electrodes placed on the head.

electronegative bearing a negative electric charge or an excess of electrons.

electronegativity the relative power of an atom to attract electrons.

electroneurography the measurement of the conduction velocity and latency of peripheral nerves.

electroneuromyography electromyography in which the nerve of the muscle under study is stimulated by application of an electric current.

electronic pertaining to or carrying electrons.

e. identification systems electronic devices, such as transponders, carried by animals and which trigger off sensitometers, thus recording the animal's feed consumption, milk yield and identity.

e. mail the sending of messages by electronic means, e.g. telex, facsimile transmitters, acoustic couplers, modems and dial-up information systems.

e. scanning one of the two forms of electronic microscopy. See also transmission electronic MICROSCOPE; useful for ascertaining spatial relationships.

e. spreadsheet see SPREADSHEET.

e. stylus see LIGHT pen.

e. timer essential for accurate timing in radiology when short exposure times are being used.

electronystagmography electroencephalographic recordings of eye movements that provide objective documentation of induced and spontaneous nystagmus.

electro-oculography measurement of retinal function by recording changes in steady, resting electric potentials of the eye with electrodes placed near the canthi. Useful in studies of eye movements and retinal function.

electropexy electric shock. See also ELECTRICAL stunning.

electropherogram electrophoretogram.

electrophile a chemical compound that serves as an electron acceptor in a chemical reaction.

electrophoresis the movement of charged particles suspended in a liquid through various media, e.g. paper, cellulose acetate, gel, liquid, under the influence of an applied electric field.

The various charged particles of a particular substance migrate in a definite and characteristic direction—toward either the anode or the cathode—and at a characteristic speed. This principle has been widely used in the separation of proteins and nucleic acids and is therefore valuable in the study of diseases in which the serum and plasma proteins are altered. See also IMMUNOELECTROPHORESIS.

SDS–polyacrylamide gel e. (SDS–PAGE) a procedure that revolutionized the analysis of complex mixtures of proteins. The proteins are solubilized by the powerful, negatively charged detergent sodium dodoecyl sulfate (SDS) which causes proteins to unfold into extended, single polypeptide chains. A reducing agent such as mercaptoethanol is usually added to break disulfide bonds. The constituent polypeptides are then electrophoresed through an inert matrix of highly cross-linked gel of polyacrylamide. The pore size of the gel can be varied by altering the concentration of polyacrylamide.

two-dimensional gel e. a SDS–polyacrylamide gel electrophoresis run, first in one direction, then again at right angles. In the first dimension an isoelectric-focusing gel is run and in the second dimension the proteins are separated in SDS–PAGE. A greater number of individually different proteins can be resolved in a highly repeatable fingerprint-like pattern.

electrophoretogram the recording produced by bands of material as they have been separated on the support medium by the electrophoresis process.
electrophysiologic testing see ELECTROMYOGRAPHY, ELECTROCARDIOGRAPHY.
electrophysiology study of the electrical phenomena involved in physiological processes.
electroplectic emanating from or pertaining to electroplexy.
e. fit the extensor tonus or tetanic fit experienced by most animals that are stunned for slaughter by electric shock.
electroporation the use of high-voltage electrical impulse to create pores through a cell membrane and allow uptake of DNA into a cell.
electropositive bearing a positive electric charge.
electroreceptors nerve endings which perceive differences in voltage fields; a feature of fish and monotremes.
electroresection electrosection.
electroretinogram the record obtained by electroretinography; abbreviated ERG.
electroretinograph an instrument for measuring the electrical response of the retina to light stimulation.
electroretinography the recording of electrical changes in the retina in response to stimulation by light.
electroscission cutting of tissue by means of electrosurgery.
electroscope an instrument for measuring radiation intensity which really measures the electrical charge.
electrosection a method of electrosurgery used to incise or excise tissue, which employs a slightly damped, modulated undamped, or undamped alternating electrical current, and requires both an active concentrating electrode and an inactive dispersing electrode. Called also electroresection. See also ELECTROSURGERY.
electrostatic pertaining to static electricity.
e. unit a measure of electrical energy; abbreviated e.s.u. 1 e.s.u. = 2.08×10^9 electrons. Relative to radiological output 1 roentgen (R) = amount of x- or gamma radiation which produces 1 e.s.u./ml in dry air. See also COULOMB (2).
electrostimulation electric stimulation of tissues.
electrostimulator a device used as a form of physiotherapy. It delivers electrical impulses via needles inserted in tissues or clamps applied to the skin. An alternative to acupuncture.
electrostriatogram an electroencephalogram showing differences in electric potential recorded at various levels of the corpus striatum.
electrosurgery the use of high-frequency alternating current to remove, incise or destroy tissue. This is accomplished by converting the electrical energy into heat through tissue resistance to the passage of the electrical current. Called also surgical diathermy.

Two types of current are utilized in electrosurgery, damped and undamped; a damped current destroys and coagulates tissue and stops bleeding, and undamped current destroys minimal tissue and incises tissue. Basically, there are four types of electrosurgical techniques: electrodesiccation, electrofulguration, electrocoagulation and electrosection.
electrotaxis taxis in response to electric stimuli.
electrotherapeutics see ELECTROTHERAPY.
electrotherapy treatment of disease by means of electricity. See also DIATHERMY.
electrothermal therapy the use of heat to destroy cells, particularly in tumors.
electrotonic 1. pertaining to electrotonus. 2. denoting the direct spread of current in tissues by electrical conduction, without the generation of new current by action potentials.
e. junctions see GAP JUNCTIONS.
electrotonus the altered electrical state of a nerve or muscle cell when a constant electric current is passed through it.
electroureterography electromyography in which the action potentials produced by peristalsis of the ureter are recorded.
electrovalence the number of charges an atom acquires in a chemical reaction by gain or loss of electrons.
electroversion the act of electrically terminating a cardiac dysrhythmia.
electrovert to apply electricity to the heart or precordium to depolarize the heart and terminate a cardiac dysrhythmia. See also DEFIBRILLATION, CARDIOVERSION.
electuary a medicinal preparation consisting of a powdered drug made into a paste with honey or syrup.
eledoisin a decapeptide from the posterior salivary gland of a species of snail (*Eledone*), which is a precursor of a large group of biologically active peptides; it has vasodilator, hypotensive and extravascular smooth muscle stimulant properties.
eleidin a substance, allied to keratin, found in the cells of the stratum lucidum of the skin.
element 1. any of the primary parts or constituents of a thing. 2. in chemistry, a simple substance that cannot be decomposed by ordinary chemical means; the basic 'stuff' of which all matter is composed.

Chemical elements are made up of atoms. Each atom consists of a nucleus with a cloud of negatively charged particles (ELECTRONS) revolving around it. The two major components of the nucleus are protons and neutrons. The number of protons in the atoms of a particular element is always the same, and therefore the physical and chemical properties of the element are always the same. It is possible, however, for a chemical element to exist in several different forms, the difference depending on the number of neutrons in the nucleus of its atoms. Different forms of the same element are called isotopes.

There are at least 105 different chemical elements known. Table 6 lists the elements, and the symbol, atomic weight and atomic number of each. The atomic number of an element is determined by the number of protons in the nucleus of an atom of the element. The mass number of an isotope is determined by the total number of neutrons and protons in the nucleus.
formed e's (of the blood) erythrocytes, leukocytes and platelets.
e. points see HORARY POINTS.
trace e. a chemical element present or needed in extremely small amount by plants and animals, such as manganese, copper, cobalt, zinc, iron. See also TRACE ELEMENT.
elemental emanating from or pertaining to elements.
e. diet see elemental DIET.
elementary not resolvable into simpler parts.
e. body 1. the constituent parts of inclusion bodies. Considered to be virus particles. See also INCLUSION BODY. 2. basic extracellular infectious unit of *Chlamydia* spp.
ele(o)- word element. [Gr.] *oil*.
eleoma a tumor or swelling caused by injection of oil into the tissues.
elephant a member of the order Proboscidae.

Includes the African elephant, *Loxodonta africana*, and the Indian elephant, *Elephas maximus*.

e. foot callus see hypertrophic CALLUS.

Northern e. seal see MIROUNGA ANGUSTIROSTRIS.

e. skin disease see BESNOITIOSIS.

e. throat bot fly see PHARYNGOBOLUS.

elephant ears ALOCASIA spp., COLOCASIA *esculenta*.

elephant grass see PENNISETUM *purpureum*.

Elephantorrhiza elephantina African plant in the legume family Mimosaceae; contains toxic tannins which cause diarrhea. Called also elandsboontjie.

Elephas maximus Asian or Indian elephant.

Eleusine grasses in the family Poaceae; some species, e.g. *E. indica*, are capable of causing nitrite or cyanide poisoning; includes *E. aegyptica*, *E. indica* (crowfoot or crab grass), *E. radulans*. See DACTYLOCTENIUM RADULANS.

elevator 1. dental elevator used to loosen tooth in socket. 2. rib elevator, usually combined with a periosteum stripper, e.g. Sayre double-ended PERIOSTEAL elevator, Matson rib stripper and elevator.

elimination 1. discharge from the body of indigestible materials and of waste products of body metabolism. See also elimination BEHAVIOR, DEFECATION, URINATION. 2. of a disease; equivalent to eradication.

ELISA *e*nzyme-*l*inked *i*mmuno*s*orbent *a*ssay. A type of primary binding test used to detect and measure either antigen or antibody. Either antigen or antibody is bound to a solid substrate (polystyrene surface), and a second antibody to which enzyme is conjugated is added, followed by a substrate for the enzyme.

elixir a clear, sweetened, usually hydroalcoholic liquid containing flavoring substances and sometimes active medicinal ingredients, for oral use.

Elizabethan collar a rigid material fashioned so as to project outward from around the neck of a dog or cat and prevent the mouth or teeth from damaging skin, casts or dressings on the legs or body. X-ray film or heavy plastic sheeting are usually used for this purpose. Also used in birds.

reversed E. c. in birds, reversing the collar permits better movement and is better tolerated.

E. c. test improvement of alopecia or traumatic skin lesions after placement of an Elizabethan collar for a short period of time will identify the cause as self trauma or excessive grooming.

elk a large deer; there are two species, the European elk (*Alces alces*) and the American moose (*A. americana*). The largest deer, 6 ft high at the withers and 2000 lb in weight, with a prominent Roman nose, an overhanging upper lip and a beard hanging from the lower jaw, brown body hair and white on the legs. The bulls have palmate antlers, the cows have no antlers.

e. lip a blemish in a horse, a heavy, overhanging top lip.

Elkhound see NORWEGIAN elkhound.

Ellangowan poison bush MYOPORUM *deserti*.

-elle suffix meaning a small.

Elliottdale Australian carpetwool sheep, derived from the ROMNEY MARSH by mutation; wool of 35 to 45 microns, white face and dark hooves; mostly polled.

ellipsoid body see ellipsoid BODY.

elliptical excision surgical undermining of the edges of a wound that is too wide to be sutured. Frees up the edges so that they can be approximated.

elliptocyte an oval-shaped erythrocyte.

elliptone an insecticidal substance, other than rotenone, found in derris root.

Ellis pin a device used in fracture repair which has threads at the tip, designed to engage only the opposite cortex of the bone in which it is inserted.

elodont a tooth that increases in length throughout its life.

Elokomin fluke fever a disease of Canidae, ferrets, bears and raccoons caused by a rickettsia-like agent, possibly a strain of *Neorickettsia helminthoeca*, transmitted by a fluke, *Nanophyetus salmincola*. Fish are the intermediate host and dogs are infected by eating the fish. Clinical signs are similar to, but milder, than those of SALMON poisoning.

elongation 1. in protein synthesis, cyclic process of growth of a polypeptide chain from mRNA attached to ribosomes. Requires mRNA, ribosomes, activated aminoacyl-tRNA, elongation factor EF-Tu activated with GTP. 2. in fatty acids, a process of adding carbon from acetyl CoA to a lengthening acyl chain. Mechanism for achieving diversity of fatty acids in biological systems.

e. factor one in a group of proteins involved in the elongation of polypeptide chains during protein synthesis.

Elschnig–O'Brien forceps very fine, toothed forceps used in ophthalmic surgery.

Elso heel an inherited spastic paresis of calves that develops after birth. Signs are stiffness of one or both hindlimbs on rising but with the stiffness passing after a few minutes. Affected animals have to be destroyed at about 12 months of age because of irreversible changes in the muscles of the affected limbs. No lesion has yet been identified as being involved in the pathogenesis of the disease. Called also inherited spastic paresis.

eluate the substance separated out by, or the product of, elution or elutriation.

eluent the solution used in elution.

elution in chemistry, separation of material by washing; the process of pulverizing substances and mixing them with water in order to separate the heavier constituents, which settle out in solution, from the lighter.

elutriation purification of a substance by dissolving it in a solvent and pouring off the solution, thus separating it from the undissolved foreign material.

EM electron microscope.

emaciation excessive leanness; a wasted condition of the body; generally taken to mean that the body weight is less than 50% of the normal expected for a comparable normal animal.

emanation that which is given off, such as a gaseous disintegration product given off from radioactive substances, or an effluvium.

emasculation removal of the penis or testes.

emasculatome instrument for bloodless castration of cattle or sheep. Works on the principle of crushing spermatic cord without breaking the skin of the neck of the scrotum. Several types available. See BURDIZZO EMASCULATOME.

emasculator instrument for simultaneous crushing and cutting of exposed spermatic cord in open castration. Cutting the cord is simple, crushing the vessels so that hemorrhage is avoided in a mature stallion is much more difficult. Crushing is effected by having one or a series of opposing ridged surfaces on the horse side of the cutting edge. Complexity of crushing apparatus varies from a single crushing face, e.g. the Frank emasculator, to a multiple with ratchet handle so that the apparatus can be left in place for a short time, e.g. the REIMER EMASCULATOR.

embalming treatment of a dead body to retard decomposition.

embarrass to impede the function of; to obstruct.

Embden–Meyerhof pathway the series of enzymatic reactions in the anaerobic conversion of glucose to lactic acid, resulting in energy in the form of adenosine triphosphate (ATP).

embedding fixation of tissue in a firm medium, in order to keep it intact during cutting of thin sections for pathological examination.

embole the reducing of a dislocated joint.

embolectomy surgical removal of an embolus.

emboli plural of *embolus*.

embolic pertaining to embolism or an embolus.

e. endarteritis see ENDARTERITIS.

e. glomerulitis glomerular inflammation as a result of lodgment of an infected embolus, e.g. in cases of endocarditis.

fibrocartilaginous e. myelopathy necrotizing myelopathy as a result of vascular obstruction by a fibrocartilaginous embolus.

e. pneumonia see embolic PNEUMONIA.

embolism the sudden blocking of an artery by a clot of foreign material (embolus) that has been brought to its site of lodgment by the blood current. The obstructing material is most often a blood clot, but may be a fat globule, air bubble, piece of tissue, e.g. degenerated intervertebral disk, or clump of bacteria. It may therefore be the site of origin of a shower of microabscesses or a neoplastic metastasis. See also saddle THROMBUS, ILIAC artery thrombosis.

air e. air injected accidentally into veins which may cause temporary paralysis or dyspnea, or may be fatal if the embolism occurs in the heart or brain. It has been used as a method of performing EUTHANASIA but is too uncertain and inhumane to be recommended.

cerebral e. embolism of a cerebral artery; one of the causes of CEREBRAL vascular accident.

renal e. embolism in the kidney causes no observable clinical effect unless it involves a very large area, when toxemia may result and be followed by uremia.

embolization 1. the process or condition of becoming an embolus. 2. therapeutic introduction of a substance into a vessel in order to occlude it.

embolus pl. *emboli* [Gr.] a clot or other plug, usually part or all of a thrombus, brought by the blood from another vessel and forced into a smaller one, thus obstructing circulation. See also EMBOLISM.

fibrocartilaginous e. see fibrocartilaginous embolic MYELOPATHY.

saddle e. one situated at the bifurcation of a large artery, usually the terminal aorta, blocking both branches. See also saddle THROMBUS.

embrocation see LINIMENT.

embryectomy excision of an extrauterine embryo or fetus.

embryo a new organism in the earliest stage of development, i.e. from the time that the fertilized embryo begins to develop a long axis up to the time that the major structures have begun to develop, when it becomes a fetus.

e. collection collection of an embryo from the genital tract for the purposes of embryo transfer; surgical and nonsurgical techniques available.

e. cryopreservation preservation of embryos by freezing.

hexacanth e. the larva present in the cestode egg when it escapes from the uterus of the adult tapeworm. Called also oncosphere.

e. micromanipulation handling of an embryo under a microscope, for examination, dissection.

e. transfer collection of fertilized ova from one female before they become implanted and transfer to another female to complete the gestation. The donor is usually superovulated and then inseminated. Collection may be surgical via a laparotomy or nonsurgical by flushing through the cervix. Collected embryos must be stored carefully. They are evaluated in terms of fertilization, possibly cleaved artificially to create clones, and washed to eliminate the possibility of transferring infection with the embryo. Long-term storage by freezing is a practicable procedure.The recipient needs to be in appropriate stage of uterine receptivity, effected by synchronizing the estrus cycle with that of the donor.

e. transplant see embryo transfer (above).

embryocardia a clinical sign in which the heart sounds resemble those of the fetus, there being very little difference in the quality of the first and second sounds.

embryoctony destruction of the living embryo or fetus.

embryogenesis the process of embryo formation. See EMBRYO.

embryological patterning during embryonic growth the establishment of groups of cells in the proper relationship to each other and to surrounding tissues.

embryologist an expert in embryology.

embryology the science of the development of the individual animal during the embryonic stage and, by extension, in several or even all preceding and subsequent stages of the life cycle.

embryoma a general term applied to neoplasms thought to be derived from embryonic cells or tissues, including dermoid cysts, teratomas, embryonal carcinomas.

embryonal emanating from or pertaining to embryo.

e. nephroma see NEPHROBLASTOMA.

embryonated said of an egg which contains an embryo.

embryonic emanating from or pertaining to embryo. See also EMBRYO.

e. death see early EMBRYONIC mortality (below).

e. disk larger cells of the mammalian blastocyst which develop into the embryo.

early e. mortality death of the embryo, i.e. before it becomes a fetus; a principal cause of temporary infertility in farm livestock. Amongst causes are errors in timing of insemination, chromosomal defects, asynchronous development of the endometrium.

e. period see EMBRYO.

e. regulation ability of embryonic tissues to recognize changes in their size and location and to make the necessary adjustments to form the disk-shaped assembly of appropriate structures.

e. stem cell stem CELL of fetal origin.

e. vesicle see CHORIONIC vesicle.

embryonization reversion of a tissue or cell to the embryonic form.

embryonoid resembling an embryo.

embryopathy a morbid condition of the embryo or a disorder resulting from abnormal embryonic development, with consequent congenital anomalies.

embryophore the thick layer of the tapeworm egg, which surrounds the oncosphere.

embryoplastic pertaining to or concerned in formation of an embryo.

embryotome see FETOTOME.

embryotomy dismemberment of the fetus in difficult labor in which a normal delivery is impossible.

embryotoxicity toxic to embryos.

embryotoxin a substance poisonous to embryos.

embryotroph the total nutriment (histotroph and hemotroph) made available to the embryo.

embryotrophy the nutrition of the early embryo.
embryulcus a blunt hook for removal of the fetus from the uterus.
Emden an upright, white goose with orange beak and legs, blue eyes.
emedullate to remove bone marrow.
emerald green cheap green pigment containing arsenic and capable of causing poisoning.
emergency a sudden and unexpected occurrence which requires urgent attention. Most veterinary practice is based on the need to take care of animal emergencies in medicine, surgery and reproduction. See also VETERINARY emergency service.
e. care delivery of urgent treatment to an animal, either as a temporary measure until full investigation and treatment is practical, or as a life-saving measure. See also CRITICAL CARE.
e. slaughter a desirable procedure if animals are to be dealt with humanely and farmers protected against avoidable financial loss. Sheep and cattle burned in bush fires are a case in point. Emergency slaughter of animals with unspecified illness is a common source of food poisoning unless the animals are submitted to rigorous meat inspection.
emergent 1. coming out from a cavity or other part. 2. coming on suddenly.
emesis the act of vomiting. Also used as a word termination, as in *hematemesis*.
emetic 1. causing vomiting. 2. an agent that causes vomiting. A strong solution of salt (1 tablespoon to 1 cup of water), mustard water (1 tablespoon to 1 cup of water), and powdered ipecac or ipecac syrup are examples of emetics. In dogs, commonly in need of such treatment, apomorphine may be used.
e. factor an agent, probably deoxynivalenol, produced by *Fusarium graminearum* and found in mold-affected grain. Causes vomiting and food rejection in pigs fed the grain. Called also vomitoxin.
emetine an alkaloid derived from ipecac or produced synthetically. Its hydrochloride salt is used as an antiamebic.
emetocathartic 1. both emetic and cathartic. 2. an emetocathartic agent.
Emex australis Australian plant in the family Polygonaceae; contains sufficient oxalate to cause poisoning but field occurrences are rare. Called also spiny emex, double gee, Cape spinach, prickly jack.
EMF electromotive force.
EMG electromyogram, electromyograph, electromyography.
-emia [Gr.] *condition of the blood.*
emigration the escape of leukocytes through the walls of small blood vessels; diapedesis.
Emilia sonchifolia African plant in the family Asteraceae; can cause nitrate–nitrite poisoning.
eminence a projection or boss.
iliopubic e. on the leading edge of the pubis; an attachment point for abdominal muscles.
eminentia pl. *eminentiae* [L.] see EMINENCE.
emiocytosis a form of glandular secretion in which granules storing the secretory product are released through the plasma membrane into the extracellular space. Seen in insulin secretion by beta cells of the pancreas.
emissarium a vein that connects an intracranial venous sinus with a vein outside the cranium.
emissary affording an outlet, referring especially to the venous outlets from the dural sinuses through the skull.
emission a discharge.
EMMA Engstrom Multigas Monitor for anesthesia.
emmetropia proper coordination of the refractive system and the focal length of the eyeball so that the focused image falls exactly on the retina.
Emmonsia a genus of fungi. See CHRYSOSPORIUM.
EMO vaporizer Epstein–Macintosh–Oxford vaporizer, designed to deliver ether anesthesia.
emodin a purgative glycoside found in the plant RHAMNUS.
emollient 1. soothing and softening, as an emollient bath given for various skin disorders. 2. an agent that softens or soothes the skin, or soothes an irritated internal surface.
emotion aroused state involving intense feeling, autonomic activation and related behavior. Animals have emotions insofar as they are motivated to behave by what they perceive and much of the reaction is learned rather than intuitive. The reactions are based on rewarding and adversive properties of stimuli from the external environment. The center for the control of emotional behavior is the limbic system of the brain.
emphysema a pathological accumulation of air in tissues. The air may derive from a skin laceration and be drawn in by the movements of muscles. A discontinuity of the tracheal mucosa is a common cause, either by way of laceration or ulceration. Extension from a pulmonary lesion is also common. The syndrome resulting depends on the location of the air. See also pulmonary emphysema and subcutaneous emphysema (below).
acute bovine pulmonary e. see ATYPICAL INTERSTITIAL PNEUMONIA.
alveolar e. see pulmonary EMPHYSEMA.
bullous e. emphysema in which bullae form in areas of lung tissue so that these areas do not contribute to respiration.
conjunctival e. may occur after head trauma which permits escape of air from the paranasal sinuses.
fetal e. see emphysematous/putrescent FETUS.
generalized e. widespread distribution of air, including subcutaneous tissues, seen with pneumomediastinum.
hypoplastic e. pulmonary emphysema due to a developmental abnormality, resulting in a reduced number of alveoli, which are abnormally large.
interlobular e. accumulation of air in the septa between lobules of the lungs.
interstitial e. presence of air in the peribronchial and interstitial tissues of the lungs.
intestinal e. a condition marked by accumulation of gas under the tunica serosa of the intestine.
lobar e. emphysema involving less than all the lobes of the affected lung.
mediastinal e. see PNEUMOMEDIASTINUM.
orbital e. may occur after trauma to the head which permits escape of air from the paranasal sinuses; appears as swelling with crepitus under the conjunctiva or periocular skin.
panacinar e., panlobular e. generalized obstructive emphysema affecting all lung segments, with atrophy and dilatation of the alveoli and destruction of the vascular bed.
pulmonary e. distension of the lung caused by overdistension of alveoli and rupture of alveolar walls (alveolar emphysema) and in some cases escape of air into the interstitial spaces (interstitial emphysema). It is a common pathological finding in many diseases of the lung in all species, but also occurs independently, especially in horses, as a principal lesion in CHRONIC obstructive pulmonary disease. It is also a prominent lesion in bovine ATYPICAL INTERSTITIAL PNEUMONIA.

It is always secondary to a primary lesion which effectively traps an excessive amount of air in the alveoli. It is characterized clinically by cough, dyspnea, forced expiratory effort and poor work tolerance. A double expiratory effort is a characteristic sign—hence broken wind.

subconjunctival e. occurs with fractures involving the paranasal sinuses.

subcutaneous e. air or gas in the subcutaneous tissues. The characteristic lesion is a soft, mobile swelling which crackles like stiff paper when palpated. There is no pain, nor heat and no ill effects unless the pharyngeal area is sufficiently involved to cause asphyxia.

surgical e. subcutaneous emphysema following operation.

unilateral e. emphysema affecting only one lung, frequently due to congenital defects in circulation.

vesicular e. see panacinar emphysema (above).

emphysematous of the nature of or affected with emphysema.

e. gangrene see BLACKLEG.

empiricism skill or knowledge based entirely on experience; compare with rationalism.

emprosthotonos tetanic downward flexure of the head and tail and upward flexure of the back.

empty said of a female of breeding age; nonpregnant.

α-adrenergic receptors see ADRENERGIC receptors.

empty-sella syndrome a syndrome in which the pituitary fossa appears to be empty but the pituitary gland is present in a flattened form.

emptying time the time taken for stomach contents to be passed into the duodenum; influenced by gastric motility and activity of the pyloric sphincter.

empyema accumulation of pus in a body cavity, particularly the presence of a purulent exudate within the pleural cavity (pyothorax). It occurs as an occasional complication of pleuritis or some other respiratory disease. Signs include dyspnea, coughing, chest pain, malaise and fever. Thoracentesis may be done to confirm the diagnosis and determine the specific causative organism. Said also of nasal sinus, joint cavity, epidural space. See also GUTTURAL POUCH empyema, PYOTHORAX.

empyesis a pustular eruption.

emu a large flightless bird, hence a ratite, native to Australia; up to 6 ft high and weighing up to 100 lb; *Dromaius novae-hollandiae*.

emulgent 1. effecting a straining or purifying process. 2. a renal artery or vein. 3. a medicine that stimulates bile or urine flow.

emulsifier a substance used to make an emulsion.

emulsion a mixture of two immiscible liquids, one being dispersed throughout the other in small droplets; a colloid system in which both the dispersed phase and the dispersion medium are liquids. Margarine, cold cream and various medicated ointments are emulsions. In some emulsions the suspended particles tend to join together and settle out; hence the container must be shaken each time the emulsion is used.

x-ray e. radiation-sensitive coating of an x-ray film consisting of a suspension of finely divided grains of silver halide in gelatin.

emulsoid a colloid system in which the dispersion medium is liquid, usually water, and the disperse phase consists of highly complex organic substances, such as starch or glue, which absorb much water, swell, and become distributed throughout the dispersion medium.

emunctory 1. excretory or cleansing. 2. an excretory organ or duct.

Emydidae see TURTLE.

en- prefix meaning inward.

en bloc resection see en bloc RESECTION.

enalapril an angiotensin converting enzyme (ACE) inhibitor, used as the maleate in the management of heart failure by reducing systemic blood pressure and producing diuresis.

enamel the white, compact and very hard substance covering and protecting the dentine of the crown of a tooth.

e. bulge the area of greatest diameter of a tooth, just external to the gum line, which acts to deflect food from the free gingival margin and the gingival crevice.

e. epithelium epithelium which creates a bell-shaped enamel organ, surrounding the dental papilla; the internal epithelium consists of columnar ameloblasts which secrete enamel.

e. hypoplasia incomplete or partial development; a common defect in dogs.

inherited e. defect an inherited absence of enamel from all teeth combined with excessive flexibility of joints in Holstein–Friesian cattle. The teeth are pink and obviously deficient in substance. A defect in collagen formation is probable.

e. layer the outermost layer of cells of the enamel organ.

mottled e. dental fluorosis; defective enamel, with a chalky white appearance or brownish stain, caused by excessive amounts of fluorine in drinking water and food preparations during the period of enamel calcification.

e. organ an epithelial cap over a dental papilla that develops into the enamel-producing organ. The shape of the enamel organ determines the shape of the tooth.

e. points sharp projections of enamel at the junction of the buccal and occlusal surfaces of a tooth. Seen most commonly in horses.

e. rods progressively mineralized glycoproteinaceous tubules, the basic structural units of enamel; enamel is acellular and consists of interrod material and rods,

e. spot remnant of the enamel cup in the center of an incisor tooth table in a horse.

e. works factories manufacturing enamels or using them extensively; sources of fluorine for pollution of pasture and water.

enameloblastoma see AMELOBLASTOMA.

enanthema an eruption upon a mucous surface.

enantiomorph one of a pair of isomeric substances, the molecular structures of which are mirror opposites of each other.

enarthrodial having the nature of an ENARTHROSIS.

enarthrosis a joint in which the rounded head of one bone is received into a socket in another, permitting motion in any direction; called also ball-and-socket joint.

encainide an antiarrhythmic drug that blocks Na+ conduction; used as the hydrochloride in the treatment of ventricular arrhythmias.

encapsulation enclosure within a capsule.

Encephalartos hildebrandtii one of many African cycadsplant of this genus in family Zamiaceae. Meal made from the seeds contains cycad glycoside and causes liver, kidney and heart damage.

encephalic 1. pertaining to the brain. 2. within the skull.

encephalitides plural of *encephalitis*.

encephalitis inflammation of the brain. Changes in vessel walls, as well as of nervous tissue, are almost a constant feature of encephalitis.

There are many types of encephalitis, depending on the causative agent and the structures involved. A large percentage of the cases are caused by viruses, some of them, e.g. equine encephalomyelitis, being transmitted from animals to humans. Clinically encephalitis is characterized by initial signs of nervous irritation including muscle tremor, excitement and convulsions, followed by a stage of loss of function characterized by weakness, paralysis, coma and death. The more acute and serious symptoms may include fever, delirium, convulsions, coma, and, in a significant number of patients, death.

Many encephalitides are accompanied by involvement of the spinal cord and are more correctly classified as encephalomyelitides. See also ENCEPHALOMYELITIS.

The etiologically or geographically specific diseases are listed under their specific titles. Human pathogens which sometimes infect animals include Central European, Far Eastern Russian tick-borne encephalitides, Omsk hemorrhagic fever, Kyasanur forest disease. Viruses isolated from asymptomatic cases of encephalomyelitis include Kunjun virus.

acute disseminated e. postinfection encephalitis.

arthropod-borne e. a group of viral encephalitides of humans in which animals play some epidemiological part. See TOGAVIRIDAE, FLAVIVIRIDAE.

canine distemper e. a demyelinating encephalitis, most severe in the cerebellum and optic tracts, is a feature of infection by canine distemper virus.

demyelinating e. seen in certain viral infections, e.g. canine distemper, caprine arthritis–encephalitis and visna of sheep.

equine herpesvirus e. that caused by some strains of equine herpesvirus 1. The lesions differ from other herpesvirus encephalidities in other species in that there are thrombi in small blood vessels, probably caused by viral antigen–antibody complexes and consequent anoxic changes, including loss of neurons.

granulomatous e. see granulomatous MENINGOENCEPHALOMYELITIS.

histiocytic e. see granulomatous MENINGOENCEPHALOMYELITIS.

Israeli turkey e. see Israeli turkey ENCEPHALOMYELITIS.

Japanese B e. believed to be primarily a disease of birds that are the source of infection for animals, including humans, pigs and horses. Transmission is by mosquito. Affected horses show a wide variety of signs including incoordination, excitability and blindness. Most cases recover. Ruminants show little clinical effect. Pigs are a major source of virus and extensive losses occur by way of encephalitis in young pigs and abortion and stillbirth in adult sows.

Murray Valley e. there is tentative evidence of clinically inapparent infection of horses in Australia with this flavivirus virus during an epidemic of the disease in humans.

old dog e. a chronic, progressive, sclerosing panencephalitis in mature dogs; characterized by motor and mental deterioration, blindness, pacing and circling. Believed to be caused by distemper virus, but there are distinct differences from distemper encephalitis.

Ontario e. see hemagglutinating ENCEPHALOMYELITIS virus disease of pigs.

postinfection e. an acute disease of the central nervous system seen in patients convalescing from infectious, usually viral, diseases.

postvaccinal e. acute encephalitis sometimes occurring after vaccination, mediated by immune mechanisms.

Powassan e. a tick-borne flavivirus disease of humans with serological but no clinical evidence of infection in nearby goats.

Pug e. see Pug MENINGOENCEPHALITIS.

Ross River e. there is tentative evidence of clinically inapparent infection of horses in Australia with the causative mosquito-borne alphavirus virus of this human disease.

Russian spring–summer e. a similar and probably identical disease to the flavivirus that causes louping ill of sheep, occurring in central Europe. It is a disease of humans occurring in epidemics related to the prevalence of vector ticks in forests where the disease is most common. Lesions are present in organs other than the brain. The severity varies from mild to fatal.

St. Louis e. an arthropod-borne flavivirus infection, first observed in 1932 in Illinois. It is a serious pathogen of humans, but does not cause disease in animals.

toxoplasma e. see TOXOPLASMOSIS.

encephalitis virus disease important emerging disease or diseases of larval marine fish; occur worldwide and often cause mass mortality. Typical pathology is vacuolation of cells of the brain and retina. Caused by nodaviruses (previously called picorna-like viruses).

Encephalitozoon a genus of protozoa in the class Microsporea.

E. cuniculi occurs in rodents, dogs, primates and humans. Has a similar physical appearance and pathogenetic effect to toxoplasmosis. Causes ENCEPHALITOZOONOSIS.

encephalitozoonosis a disease caused by *Encephalitozoon cuniculi* in rabbits; characterized clinically by paralysis and lesions in the brain.

encephal(o)- word element. [Gr.] *brain.*

encephalocele hernial protrusion of brain substance through a congenital or traumatic opening of the skull.

encephalocystocele hernial protrusion of the brain distended by fluid.

encephalogram the film obtained by encephalography.

encephalography radiography demonstrating the intracranial fluid-containing spaces after the withdrawal of cerebrospinal fluid and introduction of air or water-soluble contrast media. Called also pneumoencephalography, ventriculography, cerebral ventriculography.

encephaloid 1. resembling the brain or brain substance. 2. medullary carcinoma.

encephalolith a brain calculus.

encephalology the sum of knowledge regarding the brain, its functions and its diseases.

encephaloma 1. any swelling or tumor of the brain. 2. medullary carcinoma.

encephalomalacia literally, softening of the brain but the term is used to include degenerative diseases of the brain generally. Leukoencephalomalacia refers to the white matter, polioencephalomalacia to the gray matter. The syndrome associated with encephalomalacia is primarily one of loss of function including somnolence, blindness, ataxia, head pressing, circling and terminal coma.

degenerative e. includes NIGROPALLIDAL ENCEPHALOMALACIA, LEUKOENCEPHALOMALACIA.

focal symmetrical e. a subacute form of enterotoxemia due to *Clostridium welchii* type D in sheep which are partly immune to the toxin. Clinical signs are the dummy syndrome of aimless wandering, head pressing, blindness and incoordination. Most affected sheep die after an illness of about 7 days.

nigropallidal e. see NIGROPALLIDAL ENCEPHALOMALACIA.

encephalomeningitis see MENINGOENCEPHALITIS; inflammation of the brain and meninges.

encephalomeningocele meningocephalocele; protrusion of the brain and meninges through a defect in the skull.

encephalomeningopathy meningoencephalopathy; disease involving the brain and meninges.

encephalomere one of the segments making up the embryonic brain.

encephalometer an instrument used in locating certain of the brain regions.

encephalomyelitides plural of *encephalomyelitis*.

encephalomyelitis inflammation of both the brain (encephalitis) and spinal cord (myelitis). The pathogenesis and clinical picture are similar to those of encephalitis. The pathological lesions, however, include a significant involvement of the spinal cord. Many of the causes are viral as they are in encephalitis.

arthropod-borne e. a number of viral agents responsible for causing encephalomyelitis are transmitted by arthropods. See ARBOVIRUS.

avian e. caused by an enterovirus this disease affects young birds up to few weeks old. There is an obvious tremor of the neck, followed by weakness and incoordination and finally paralysis and death.

equine protozoal e. called also equine protozoal myeloencephalitis; originally ascribed to *Toxoplasma* spp. infection; now regarded as infection by *Sarcocystis neurona*.

equine viral e. there are three known serotypes of the family *Togaviridae*, genus *Alphavirus* that cause encephalomyelitis of horses and which occur only in the Americas and are transmitted by mosquitoes. The horse is a terminal host for the eastern and western serotypes; the reservoir of the infection is probably birds and other native fauna. For the Venezuelan virus the horse is also a donor host along with birds and other fauna. The disease has great zoonotic significance because of its high prevalence in epidemic years, and significant mortality rate in humans. Clinical signs in horses include initial excitement, muscle tremor, walking in circles, followed by a paralytic phase including somnolence, staggering, dropping of the head and finally recumbency. Most infections are subclinical.

experimental allergic e. inoculation of animals with brain tissue in Freund's complete adjuvant produces an autoimmune encephalomyelitis. Called also EAE.

granulomatous e. a disease marked by granulomatous inflammation and necrosis of the walls of the cerebral and spinal ventricles.

hemagglutinating e. virus disease of pigs a disease of sucking pigs caused by a hemagglutinating coronavirus characterized by the occurrence of two different clinical forms of the disease. They are probably the extremes of a clinical spectrum of one disease because both may be seen in the one outbreak in one piggery. The encephalitic form is characterized by incoordination, convulsions and death in 2–3 days. In the other form the principal signs are vomiting, inability to drink and severe dehydration and emaciation—hence vomiting and wasting disease. Called also Ontario encephalitis.

Israeli turkey e. nonsuppurative encephalomyelitis of turkeys caused by a flavivirus and carried by insects, probably mosquitoes. Manifested by a progressive paralysis.

mouse e. virus see THEILER'S DISEASE.

Near Eastern equine e. the cause is a virus, antigenically identical with the Borna disease virus, which normally infects birds, but in its transport by a vector tick it infects horses. The disease is clinically indistinguishable from BORNA DISEASE.

ovine e. see LOUPING ILL.

porcine viral e. a series of antigenically different enteroviruses capable of causing porcine encephalomyelitis; the virulence of the viruses and the severity of the diseases that they cause varies. Clinically the disease is characterized by a syndrome comprising hyperesthesia, paresis and convulsions but the severity is very much less in older pigs than in baby pigs. Adult pigs are commonly infected but show no clinical signs. Also known as Teschen disease, Talfan disease, poliomyelitis suum.

postinfectious e. inflammation of the brain and spinal cord following vaccination or infection. Was commonly seen after the administration of earlier rabies vaccines containing brain tissue.

postvaccinal e. see postinfectious encephalomyelitis (above).

sporadic bovine e. caused by *Chlamydia psittaci* and characterized by inflammation of vessel walls, serous membranes and synoviae, with incidental involvement of nervous tissue in some cases. Clinically there is high fever and weakness, circling and knuckling in some. At necropsy there is fibrinous peritonitis, pleurisy and pericarditis—hence serositis—as well as encephalomyelitis. Called also transmissible serositis, Buss disease, SBE.

encephalomyeloneuropathy a disease involving the brain, spinal cord and nerves.

encephalomyelopathy a disease involving the brain and spinal cord.

encephalomyeloradiculitis inflammation of the brain, spinal cord and spinal nerve roots.

encephalomyeloradiculopathy a disease involving the brain, spinal cord and spinal nerve roots.

encephalomyocarditis inflammation of the brain and cardiac muscle; abbreviated EMC.

e. virus disease of pigs a sporadic disease of pigs caused by a picornavirus which is primarily a pathogen of rodents but which infects other species including humans. Affected pigs are most commonly found dead of heart failure without having displayed clinical signs. Longer surviving pigs show tremor, incoordination and dyspnea. There is a characteristic myocarditis evident at necropsy.

encephalon the brain; with the spinal cord (medulla spinalis) constituting the central nervous system.

encephalopathy any degenerative disease of the brain.

biliary e., bilirubin e. kernicterus.

feline ischemic e. an acute, ischemic cerebral necrosis causing various degrees of cerebral dysfunction including depression, ataxia, circling, behavioral changes, blindness and seizures.

hepatic e. severe hepatic insufficiency may induce a syndrome of excitability, tremor, compulsive walking, head pressing, and apparent blindness, followed by coma and convulsions, a dummy syndrome. The probable pathogenesis of this hepatic encephalopathy is the accumulation of ammonia, because of the failure of the liver to metabolize it, and the development of a spongy degeneration of the brain as a direct result of the hyperammonemia. A similar pathogenesis is hypothesized for the genesis of a cerebrotoxi-

cant in companion animals with congenital defects in hepatic vasculature. See also PORTACAVAL shunt, HEPATITIS.
hypernatremic e. a severe hemorrhagic encephalopathy induced by the hyperosmolarity accompanying hypernatremia and dehydration.
lead e. brain disease caused by lead poisoning.
e.–microphthalmia syndrome an inherited disorder in HEREFORD cattle with ocular and neurological defects and muscular dystrophy. Affected calves are blind and unable to stand.
portosystemic e. hepatic encephalopathy.
transmissible mink e. transmissible disease of mink which resembles scrapie in sheep. There is a very long incubation period, hyperirritability, biting, paralysis, coma and death. The scrapie agent is believed to be the cause.
encephalopuncture surgical puncture of the brain.
encephalopyosis suppuration or abscess of the brain.
encephalorrhagia hemorrhage within or from the brain.
encephalosclerosis hardening of the brain.
encephalosis any organic brain disease.
encephalotomy 1. craniotomy (2). 2. dissection or anatomy of the brain.
encephalotrophy atrophy of the brain.
enchondral situated, formed or occurring within cartilage.
e. ossification see enchondral OSSIFICATION.
retained e. cartilage cores see retained enchondral CARTILAGE cores.
enchondroma a benign growth of cartilage arising in the metaphysis of a bone.
enchondromatosis a condition in humans characterized by hamartomatous proliferation of cartilage cells within the metaphysis of several bones, causing thinning of the overlying cortex and distortion of the growth in length. Called also dyschondroplasia, Ollier's disease.
enchondrosarcoma central chondrosarcoma.
Enchylaena tomentosa Australian plant in the family Chenopodiaceae. Contains high concentrations of soluble oxalate and may cause poisoning. Called also Barrier salt bush, ruby salt bush, berry cotton bush.
enclave tissue detached from its normal connection and enclosed within another organ.
enclitic having the planes of the fetal head inclined to those of the maternal pelvis.
encode to code. See GENETIC code.
encopresis incontinence of feces not due to organic defect or illness.
encysted enclosed in a sac, bladder or cyst.
end-artery an artery that does not anastomose with other arteries.
end-bulb one of the small encapsulated bodies at the end of sensory nerve fibers in skin, mucous membranes, muscles and other areas. They are called also Krause's bulbs or corpuscles.
end-feet button- or knob-like terminal enlargements of naked nerve fibers which end in a synapse with dendrites of another cell.
END method the *E*xaltation of *N*ewcastle *D*isease virus method; a Japanese technique for indirectly detecting the presence of hog cholera virus.
end organ one of the larger, encapsulated endings of sensory nerves.
end pieces the distal portion of the spermatozoon consisting of irregularly arranged microtubules.
end-plate a flattened discoid expansion at the neuromuscular junction, where a myelinated motor nerve fiber joins a skeletal muscle fiber.
e.-p. potential created by acetylcholine causing depolarization of the muscle cell membrane.
end-stage a pathologist's term for any organ in the final stages of functional life. Said of kidney, liver, muscle, joint.
end-tidal at the end of a respiratory cycle. Said of the carbon dioxide concentration.
end-to-end a pattern of anastomosis in which severed ends are matched and united, in contrast with other patterns such as end-to-side or side-to-side. Usually applied to anastomosis of the intestine.
endadelphos a monster in which a parasitic twin is enclosed within the body of the other twin (the autosite).
Endamoeba a genus of amebae parasitic in the intestines of invertebrates. They differ from *Entamoeba* spp. because they lack a central endosome.
endangered species species of animals (and plants) whose existence on earth is threatened, principally by the activities of humans.
endangiitis inflammation of the endangium.
endangium tunica intima (inner coat) of a blood vessel.
endaortitis inflammation of the membrane lining the aorta.
endarterectomy excision of thickened atheromatous areas of the innermost coat of an artery.
carotid e. endarterectomy within an extracranial carotid artery, usually within the common carotid. See also carotid ENDARTERECTOMY.
endarterial within an artery.
endarteritis inflammation of the innermost coat (tunica intima) of an artery.
e. obliterans a form in which the lumen of the smaller vessels becomes narrowed or obliterated as a result of proliferation of the tissue of the intimal layer.
endaural within the ear.
endbrain see TELENCEPHALON.
endectocides systemically administered parasiticides; includes ivermectin and milbemycin.
endemic present in a predictable, continuous pattern in an animal community at all times; said of a disease which is clustered in space but not in time. See also ENZOOTIC.
e. erosive stomatitis resembles bovine papular stomatitis. Recorded in Africa as spreading to and from cattle and humans.
endemiology the science dealing with all the factors relating to the occurrence of endemic disease.
endemoepidemic endemic, but occasionally becoming epidemic.
endergonic characterized or accompanied by the absorption of energy; requiring the input of free energy.
ending a termination, especially the peripheral termination of a nerve or nerve fiber.
end(o)- word element. [Gr.] *within, inward.*
endoaneurysmorrhaphy opening of an aneurysmal sac and suture of the orifices.
endoangiitis endangiitis.
endoarteritis see ENDARTERITIS.
endoblast entoderm.
endobronchial pertaining to or emanating from the lining of the bronchi.
e. intubation incorrect positioning of an endotracheal tube; a cause of inadequate delivery of gaseous anesthesia, hyperventilation, hypoxia and cyanosis.
endobronchitis inflammation of the epithelial lining of the bronchi.

endocardial 1. situated or occurring within the heart. 2. pertaining to the endocardium.

e. cushions elevations on the atrioventricular canal of the embryonic heart which later help partition the heart. Defective development contributes to several cardiac anomalies, including ventricular septal defect and ATRIOVENTRICULARIS COMMUNIS.

e. fibroelastosis the accumulation of collagen and elastic fibers in the endocardium, together with left ventricular hypertrophy dilatation, is an inherited, primary cardiac anomaly in Burmese cats.

e. fibrosis occurs with cardiac dilatation or hypertrophy. In cats, leads to restrictive CARDIOMYOPATHY.

e. splitting a complication of chronic valvular insufficiency and congestive cardiomyopathy in dogs. May be partial or full thickness; can occur on the interatrial septum, producing an acquired septal defect, or elsewhere causing hemopericardium.

e. tube formed from the cardiogenic plate in the developing embryo, this forms the primordium of the truncus arteriosus, the atrium and the ventricles; it is later invested by the myocardium.

endocardiosis common cause of cardiac disease in the dog. Characterized by chronic fibrosis and nodular thickening of the free edges of the atrioventicular valves. In the worst cases the valve cusps are distorted converting a minor leak into a massive incompetence. Leads to congestive heart failure. There is no specific cause.

endocarditis exudative and proliferative inflammatory alterations of the endocardium, characterized by the presence of vegetations on the surface of the endocardium or in the endocardium itself, and most commonly involving a heart valve, but also affecting the inner lining of the cardiac chambers or the endocardium elsewhere.

Lesions on the valves may interfere with the ejection of blood from the heart by causing insufficiency or stenosis of the valves. Murmurs associated with the heart sounds are the major manifestation and if interference with the blood flow is sufficiently severe congestive heart failure develops. The further hazard with endocarditis, especially if it is bacterial in origin, is that of septic emboli in the lungs or in the other organs.

bacterial e. infectious endocarditis, acute or subacute, caused by various bacteria, including streptococci, staphylococci, enterococci and gram-negative bacilli. Of particular interest in animals is the predilection of *Erysipelothrix rhusiopathiae* to cause endocarditis, epecially in pigs.

ductal e. due to thrombosis in a persistent ductus arteriosus with resulting mural inflammation.

infectious e., infective e. that due to infection with microorganisms, especially bacteria and fungi.

mural e. that affecting the lining of the walls of the heart chambers only.

nonbacterial thrombotic e. that in which the vegetations, single or multiple, consist of fibrin and other blood elements.

parietal e. mural endocarditis.

tuberculous e. that resulting from extension of a tuberculous infection from the pericardium and myocardium.

valvular e. that affecting the membrane over the heart valves only.

vegetative e. endocarditis, infectious or noninfectious, the characteristic lesions of which are vegetations or verrucae on the endocardium. Called also verrucous endocarditis.

verrucous e.

endocardium the endothelial lining membrane of the cavities of the heart and the connective tissue bed on which it lies.

endocervicitis inflammation of the endocervix.

endocervix 1. the mucous membrane lining the canal of the cervix uteri. 2. the region of the opening of the cervix uteri into the uterine cavity.

endochondral see ENCHONDRAL.

e. ossification see enchondral OSSIFICATION.

endochondroma tumor arising from cartilage within the medullary cavity.

endochromatosis condition in which there are multiple endochromas; a similar developmental abnormality occurs in humans.

endocolitis inflammation of the mucous membrane of the colon.

Endoconidium temulentum an incomplete fungus that grows on the grass LOLIUM *temulentum* or darnel grass and may be responsible for the grass's toxic effects.

endocranial within the cranium.

endocranitis inflammation of endocranium.

endocranium the endosteal layer of the dura mater of the brain.

endocrine 1. secreting internally. 2. pertaining to internal secretions; hormonal.

e. cell are either gathered together in specific endocrine glands or scattered diffusely through other tissue, e.g. in the walls of the gastrointestinal tract and the pancreas in which the cells are clustered together into islands.

e. dermatosis skin changes accompanying many diseases of the endocrine glands such as hypothyroidism, hyperadrenocorticism and hypopituitarism.

e. glands included are the pituitary, thyroid, parathyroid and adrenal glands, gonads, pancreas and paraganglia.

e. system organs or groups of cells that secrete regulatory substances that are released directly into the circulation (HORMONE). The endocrine or hormonal system and the nervous system are the two major control systems of the body, and their functions are interrelated. Hormonal activity is mostly concerned with regulating metabolic activities by controlling the rates at which chemical reactions take place within cells, the transport of substances across the cell membrane, and activities related to growth and reproduction. The word hormone is applied to substances released by the endocrine glands that have physiological effects on target organs (which can be other endocrine glands) and tissues distant from the gland. There are, however, local hormones (autacoids) secreted at the site of the tissue being affected, for example, acetylcholine and serotonin.

e. tumor adenoma or carcinoma; usually only one cell type, that of the normal tissue, but may be more than one type of cell capable of secreting more than one hormone.

endocrinism endocrinopathy.

endocrinologist an individual skilled in endocrinology, and in the diagnosis and treatment of disorders of the glands of internal secretion, i.e. the endocrine glands.

endocrinology study of the endocrine system.

endocrinopathy any disease due to disorder of the endocrine system.

endocrinotherapy treatment of disease by the administration of endocrine preparations; hormonotherapy.

endocrinous of or pertaining to an internal secretion (hormone) or to a gland producing such a secretion, i.e. to an endocrine gland.

endocystitis inflammation of the bladder mucosa.
endocytosis the uptake by a cell of material from the environment by invagination of the plasma membrane; it includes both phagocytosis and pinocytosis.
endoderm see ENTODERM.
endodermal pertaining to or emanating from endoderm.
e. sinus tumor see YOLK sac tumor.
endodontia see ENDODONTICS.
endodontic pertaining to or emanating from the pulp cavity of the tooth.
e. file an instrument used in the débridement of root canals.
endodontics the branch of dentistry concerned with the etiology, prevention, diagnosis and treatment of conditions that affect the tooth pulp, root and periapical tissues.
endodontium dental pulp.
endodyogeny asexual multiplication in protozoa in which two daughter cells are formed within the parent cell. Occurs for example in *Toxoplasma* and *Sarcocystis* spp.
endoenteritis inflammation of the intestinal mucosa.
endogamy fertilization by union of separate cells having the same chromatin ancestry.
endogenous produced within or caused by factors within the organism.
e. analgesic system includes the secretion by the brain of ENDORPHINS in response to the central perception of pain.
e. calcium calcium contributed to the feces by the intestinal secretions.
e. feline oncornavirus see RD114 VIRUS.
e. magnesium magnesium contributed to the feces by the intestinal secretions.
e. pain caused by factors within the body, e.g. stretching of mesentery.
e. sarcoma virus see FELINE sarcoma virus.
endointoxication poisoning by an endogenous toxin.
endolaryngeal situated on or occurring within the larynx.
Endolimax a genus of amebas found in the colon of humans, other mammals, birds, amphibians and cockroaches; none of them appear to be pathogenic.
E. caviae found in guinea pigs.
E. nana found in humans and monkeys.
E. ratti found in rats.
endolymph the fluid within the membranous labyrinth of the ear.
endolymphatic pertaining to or emanating from the endolymph.
e. duct connects the saccule of the membranous labyrinth of the internal ear to the endolymphatic sac.
endometrial pertaining to or emanating from the endometrium.
e. biopsy punch biopsy specimens obtained in the mare and cow by passing the instrument through the cervix and controlling the site of the biopsy by a hand in the rectum.
e. cups ulcer-like structures in the endometrium of the pregnant mare. They are produced by the fetus but become detached from it. Their function is to produce equine gonadotropin, formerly PMSG.
e. curettage débridement of the endometrium by metal curette is not practiced in animals but a chemical equivalent, by the infusion of irritant substances, is used instead.
e. cyst in cows and ewes near caruncles; develop during uterine involution due to adhesions from the caruncle; no clinical importance.
cystic e. hyperplasia pathological hyperplasia of endometrium, as distinct from the physiological state, due in most instances to excessive and prolonged estrogenic stimulation; characterized by thickening of the endometrium, development of mucus-filled glands and the accumulation of mucus in the lumen of the uterus. Associated with cystic ovarian disease in cows. In ewes it is usually due to prolonged low level intake of phyto-estrogens, e.g. on subterranean clover pasture. It may be a precursor of or associated with pyometra, especially in the dog where the hormonal cause is progesterone. See also PYOMETRA.
e. folds in the mare these run the length of the uterus as observed by fiberscope.
e. glands provide uterine fluid (histotrophe) on which the developing fetus depends for subsistence during its first few days of existence.
e. hyperplasia with pyometra see cystic ENDOMETRIAL hyperplasia.
e. polyp found in the bitch and may cause prolapse of the affected horn with the polyp visible in the vagina.
e. regeneration postpartum return to normal of the endometrium, e.g. in cows by the sloughing of superficial layers of caruncles.
endometriosis a condition in which tissue more or less perfectly resembling the uterine mucous membrane occurs aberrantly in various locations in the pelvic cavity. See also uterine ADENOMYOSIS.
endometritis inflammation of the endometrium. See also METRITIS.
hyperplastic e. see PYOMETRA.
puerperal e. endometritis following parturition.
purulent e. characterized by a small accumulation of pus in the uterus and a discharge, which may be intermittent, of thick pus from the vulva.
syncytial e. a benign tumor-like lesion with infiltration of the uterine wall by large syncytial trophoblastic cells.
tuberculous e. inflammation of the endometrium, usually also involving the uterine tubes, due to infection by *Mycobacterium bovis*, with the presence of tubercles.
endometrium the mucous membrane lining the uterus.
endomitosis mitosis taking place without dissolution of the nuclear membrane, and not followed by cytoplasmic division, resulting in doubling of the number of chromosomes within the nucleus.
endomyocardial fibrosis see restrictive CARDIOMYOPATHY.
endomyocarditis inflammation of the endocardium and myocardium.
endomysium the sheath of delicate reticular fibrils that surrounds each muscle fiber.
endoneuritis inflammation of the endoneurium.
endoneurium the interstitial connective tissue in a peripheral nerve, separating individual nerve fibers.
endonuclease a nuclease that cleaves internal bonds of polynucleotides.
restriction e. see RESTRICTION ENDONUCLEASE.
endoparasite a parasite that lives within the body of the host.
endopelvic within the pelvis.
endopeptidase a peptidase capable of acting on any peptide linkage in a peptide chain.
endopericarditis inflammation of the endocardium and pericardium.
endoperimyocarditis inflammation of the endocardium, pericardium and myocardium.

endoperitonitis inflammation of the serous lining of the peritoneal cavity.
endophlebitis inflammation of the intima of a vein.
endophthalmitis inflammation of the ocular cavities and their adjacent structures.
lens-induced e. see phacoanaphylactic endophthalmitis (see below).
nonsuppurative e. may be caused by trauma to the eye, or secondary to severe corneal inflammation.
phacoanaphylactic e. hypersensitivity to lens material. Called also lens-induced endophthalmitis.
starch e. inflammation caused by starch from surgical gloves.
suppurative e. caused by foreign bodies or infectious agents, which may be associated with systemic infection.
endophyte a parasitic plant living within its host's body.
endophytic 1. pertaining to an endophyte. 2. growing inward; proliferating on the interior of an organ or structure.
e. fungus fungal species living as symbionts within the tissues of pasture grasses including *Acremonium* spp. in *Festuca* and *Lolium* spp.
endoplasm central cytoplasm, full of organelles.
endoplasmic pertaining to or arising from endoplasm.
e. ribosomes small, cytoplasmic granules consisting of approximately 60% RNA and 40% protein.
endopolyogeny asexual reproduction in protozoa in which new progeny are produced by budding within the parent cell.
endoreduplication replication of chromosomes without subsequent cell division.
endorphin one of a group of opiate-like peptides produced naturally by the body at neural synapses at various points in the central nervous system pathways where they modulate the transmission of pain perceptions. The term *endorphin* was coined by combining the words *endogenous* and *morphine.* Like morphine, endorphins raise the pain threshold and produce sedation and euphoria; the effects are blocked by naloxone, a narcotic antagonist.
endosalpingitis inflammation of the endosalpinx.
endosalpingoma adenomyoma of the uterine tube.
endosalpinx the mucous membrane lining the oviduct (uterine tube).
endoscope an instrument used for direct visual inspection of hollow organs or body cavities. Specially designed endoscopes are used for such examinations as BRONCHOSCOPY, CYSTOSCOPY, GASTROSCOPY and PROCTOSCOPY.

Although the design of an endoscope may vary according to its specific use, all endoscopes have similar working elements. The viewing part (scope) may be a hollow metal or fiber tube fitted with a lens system that permits viewing in a variety of directions. The endoscope also has a light source, power cord and power source. Accessories that might be used with an endoscope for diagnostic or therapeutic purposes include suction tip, tubes and suction pump; forceps for removal of biopsy tissue or a foreign body; and electrode tip for cauterization.
endoscopy visual examination of interior structures of the body with an endoscope.
endosepsis septicemia originating from causes inside the body.
endoskeleton the cartilaginous and bony skeleton of the body, exclusive of that part of the skeleton of dermal origin.
endosmosis inward osmosis; inward passage of liquid through a membrane of a cell or cavity, by which one fluid passes through a septum into a cavity that contains fluid of a different density.
endosome intracellular vesicles formed from the cell membrane which are involved in intracellular transport.
endosteal 1. pertaining to the endosteum. 2. occurring or located within a bone.
e. lining cells cover the internal surfaces of the compact bone, trabecular bone and osteonal canals.
endosteitis inflammation of the endosteum.
endosteoma a tumor in the medullary cavity of a bone.
endosteum the tissue lining the medullary cavity of a bone.
cortical e. endosteal lining to cortical bone; delimits the marrow cavity.
osteonal e. endosteal lining of the osteonal canals.
trabecular e. the endosteum which coats the interior surfaces of the trabeculae.
endostoma see ENDOSTEOMA.
endostoses bony outgrowths on the medullary surface of long bones. Called also enostosis.
endosulfan an organochlorine insecticide. See CHLORINATED HYDROCARBONS.
endotendineum the delicate connective tissue separating the secondary bundles (fascicles) of a tendon.
endotendon, endotenon fine connective tissue between the strands in a tendon.
endothelia [Gr.] plural of *endothelium.*
endothelial pertaining to or made up of endothelium.
e tissue special connective tissue lining blood and lymph spaces.
e. tumors many caused by fowl leukosis virus; mesothelioma may also result.
endothelin see ENDOTHELIUM-DERIVED constricting factor.
endotheliochorial see PLACENTA.
endotheliocyte a large mononuclear phagocytic wandering cell of the circulating blood and tissues. Called also endothelial leukocyte.
endothelioid resembling endothelium.
endothelioma a tumor arising from the endothelial lining of blood vessels.
endotheliosis proliferation of endothelial elements.
endothelium pl. *endothelia* [Gr.] the layer of epithelial cells that lines the cavities of the heart and of the blood and lymph vessels, sometimes applied to other internal epithelial surfaces.
corneal e. lines the inner surface of the cornea, between the corneal stroma and aqueous humor; called also the posterior epithelium.
endothelium-derived derived from endothelium.
e.-d. vasoactive substances substances produced by or released from endothelial cells which regulate vascular smooth muscle or other regulatory mechanism; include prostacyclin and other prostanoids, angiotensin, and relaxing or constricting factors.
e.-d. constricting factor vasoconstrictive peptides isolated from vascular endothelial cells which are actively vasoconstrictive; **endothelin** (ET) is the most active of them.
e.-d. relaxing factor several are known; nitrous oxide is one of the chief mediators, probably derived from L-arginine.
endothermal, endothermic 1. characterized by the absorption of heat. 2. pertaining to endothermy.
endothermy see DIATHERMY.
endothrix a dermatophyte whose growth and spore production are confined chiefly within the shaft of a hair.

endotoxemia the presence of endotoxins in the blood.

endotoxic pertaining to or possessing endotoxin.

e. shock see TOXEMIC shock.

endotoxin a heat-stable toxin present in the intact bacterial cell but not in cell-free filtrates of cultures of intact bacteria. It is the lipopolysaccharide (LPS) of gram-negative outer membranes. Also called O antigen. It is pyrogenic and increases capillary permeability through stimulation of tumor necrosis factor alpha release.

endotracheal within the trachea.

Cole-pattern e. tube one with a tapered shape with no cuff; designed to be fitted with a wider shoulder at the larynx and narrow end in the trachea. Used in horses.

e. intubation an AIRWAY catheter inserted in the trachea during endotracheal INTUBATION to assure patency of the upper airway by allowing for removal of secretions and maintenance of an adequate air passage. In animals, endotracheal intubation is usually accomplished through the mouth using an orotracheal tube.

nasal e. tube an endotracheal tube designed to be passed through the nasal cavity into the trachea. It usually has a thin wall.

reinforced e. tube a spiral wire or nylon strip is incorporated into the wall to reduce the risk of collapse or kinking.

e. tube a variety of endotracheal tubes is available. The tubes are almost always 'cuffed' to allow for their use with a mechanical ventilator. The cuff is a rubber balloon-like device that fits over the lower end of the tube. It is attached to a narrow tube that extends outside the body and allows for inflation of the cuff. Once the cuff is inflated there is no flow of air through the trachea other than that going through the endotracheal tube.

endovasculitis see ENDANGIITIS.

endrin a highly toxic insecticide of the chlorinated hydrocarbon group. See CHLORINATED HYDROCARBONS.

endurance rides equine performance tests requiring contestants to complete a course of 80 to 150 km in 1 to 2 days. They create special problems in equine sports medicine. These include the exhausted horse syndrome, evidence of impending pulmonary edema, heat exhaustion, exertional rhabdomyolysis and a variety of disturbances of acid–base balance. The problem for the veterinarian is to decide whether horses should be allowed to continue in the contest. See also EXHAUSTION syndrome.

Endymion nonscriptus see SCILLA.

enema 1. introduction of fluid into the rectum. 2. a solution introduced into the rectum to promote evacuation of feces or as a means of administering nutrient or medicinal substances, or opaque material in radiological examination of the lower intestinal tract. See also BARIUM study.

through-and-through e. an extensive enema in which a large volume of fluid is slowly introduced into the rectum, massaged through the intestines, and finally emerges from the duodenum to cause vomiting of intestinal contents. Sometimes advocated for complete clearing of the intestinal tract in cases of ingested poisons.

enemata plural of *enema*.

energy power that may be translated into motion, overcoming resistance, or effecting physical change; the ability to do work. Energy assumes several forms; it may be thermal (in the form of heat), electrical, mechanical, chemical, radiant or kinetic. In doing work, the energy is changed from one form to another or to several forms. In these changes some of the energy is 'lost' in the sense that it cannot be recaptured and used again. Usually there is loss in the form of heat, which escapes or is dissipated unused. All energy changes give off a certain amount of the energy as heat.

All activities of the body require energy, and all needs are met by the consumption of food containing energy in chemical form. The animal diet comprises three main sources of energy: carbohydrates, proteins and fats. Of these three, carbohydrates most readily provide the kind of energy needed to activate muscles. Proteins work to build and restore body tissues. The body transforms chemical energy derived from food by the process of METABOLISM, an activity that takes place in the individual cell. Molecules of the food substances providing energy pass through the cell membrane. Inside the cell, chemical reactions occur that produce the new forms of energy and yield by-products such as water and waste materials. See also ADENOSINE.

dietary e. the total energy intake in the diet is the gross energy. Digestible energy is gross energy less fecal energy. Metabolizable energy is digestible energy less that lost in fermentation in the gut, energy lost in urine. Net energy is metabolizable energy less energy used in SPECIFIC dynamic action response. Expressed as joules, calories or occasionally therms (1 calorie=4.18 joule).

e. density see CALORIC density.

e. feeds feeds with a high carbohydrate content and therefore low fiber (<18%) and protein (<20%) contents.

free e. the energy equal to the maximum amount of work that can be obtained from a process occurring under conditions of fixed temperature and pressure.

nuclear e. energy that can be liberated by changes in the nucleus of an atom (as by fission of a heavy nucleus or by fusion of light nuclei into heavier ones with accompanying loss of mass).

nutritional e. deficiency causes loss of body weight, milk, egg and wool production. Continued for long periods or severe restriction causes particular metabolic upsets in pregnant and lactating ewes and cows—see PREGNANCY toxemia, ACETONEMIA (2); in neonates, HYPOGLYCEMIA. In others causes EMACIATION, INANITION, STARVATION.

e. production production of ATP through oxidative phosphorylation or anaerobic glycolysis.

e. requirements generally vary between species and particularly between individuals. They are determined by many factors, especially age, level of activity, physiological status and body size, specifically body surface area. The *basal energy requirement* (BER) is the level required by a healthy animal at complete rest in a neutral environmental temperature. It can be calculated by using several formulae, based on body weight or body surface area, which is then used in the further calculation of the *maintenance energy requirement* (MER) which takes into account the individual animal's level of activity or disease status.

e. reserves any reduced carbon stored in compounds such as fatty acids in triacylglycerols of adipose tissue, glucose in glycogen, and amino acids in protein releases energy, ultimately in the form of ATP on oxidation of the carbon.

e. transfer conversion of energy from one form usually chemical in the form of ATP to another usually chemical, but can be electrical, mechanical or heat energy.

enervation 1. lack of nervous energy. 2. removal of a nerve or a section of a nerve.
enflagellation the formation of flagella; flagellation.
enflurane a fluorinated ether, similar in action to halothane, used for general inhalation anesthesia.
ENG enzootic nasal granuloma.
engastrius a double monster in which one fetus is contained within the abdomen of the other.
engine oil a cause of poisoning. See SUMP OIL.
English bobtail see OLD ENGLISH SHEEPDOG.
English bulldog see BULLDOG.
English coach dog see DALMATIAN.
English cocker spaniel see COCKER SPANIEL.
English coonhound despite the name, a breed developed and recognized in the United States. A medium-sized, hound type dog with a short, usually redticked coat, and a long slender tail.
English forceps heavy duty, thumb-operated standard tissue forceps with large, strong teeth at the blade tips.
English foxhound see FOXHOUND.
English Game a long-legged, long-necked meat fowl with a wide, shallow body, long, muscular legs and muscular wings. Multicolored, mostly red, brown and white; originated from fighting birds.
English ivy see HEDERA HELIX.
English Leicester see LEICESTER.
English longwool a class of sheep; includes Romney Marsh, Leicester, Lincoln (Lincoln longwool) and Border Leicester. Called also British longwool.
English oak QUERCUS *petraea*, *Q. robur*.
English pointer see POINTER.
English rabbit a hardy breed of domestic rabbits resembling the Dutch but up to 9 lb in weight. It is basically a white rabbit with other colors, including chocolate, blue, black, gray and tortoiseshell, on the body, ears, muzzle and around the eyes.
English setter a medium-weight, tall, lean, deep-chested dog with a long, silky coat that is most profuse under the neck, trunk, tail and behind the legs. The coat is basically white with black, liver, lemon or orange spots and flecks. The breed is predisposed to neuronal ceroid lipofuscinosis (juvenile amaurotic familial idiocy), entropion and progressive retinal atrophy.
English springer spaniel a medium-sized, compact dog with floppy ears, short, docked tail and a long, flat, silky coat in brown and white or black and white, that is most profuse under the neck and body, and behind the legs. The breed is affected by an inherited storage disease (fucosidosis), cutaneous asthenia, factor XI deficiency, retinal dysplasia and cataracts.
English toy spaniel see KING CHARLES SPANIEL.
English toy terrier a very small (7–9 lb), lean, short-coated black and tan dog with erect, 'candle-flame' shaped ears and a tapered tail. Called also Black and tan terrier.
English yew TAXUS *baccata*.
engorgement distension.
carbohydrate e. see CARBOHYDRATE ENGORGEMENT.
equine wheat e. see CARBOHYDRATE ENGORGEMENT.
vascular e. local congestion; distension with fluids; hyperemia.
Engstrom Multigas Monitor a monitoring system for all halogenated hydrocarbon anesthetics which makes possible accurate continuous estimation of the concentration of anesthetic. The system uses a quartz crystal detector sensitive to anesthetic vapors.
enhancement immunologically speaking, ways of increasing the level of an immune response. Immunoenhancement.
tumor e. successful establishment and prolongation of survival time of a transplanted tumor allograft, as a result of binding of specific antibody which acts to mask tumor specific antigens on the surface of the tumor cells.
enhancer see enhancer SEQUENCE.
Enhydra see OTTER.
enilconazole a broad-spectrum imidazole antifungal agent particularly useful in the treatment of canine nasal aspergillosis.
enkatarrhaphy the operation of burying a structure by suturing together the sides of tissues adjacent to it.
enkephalin either of two naturally occurring pentapeptides (methionine enkephalin and leucine enkephalin) isolated from the brain, which have potent opiate-like effects and probably serve as neurotransmitters. They are classified as ENDORPHINS.
enol one of two tautomeric forms of a substance, the other being the keto form; the enol is formed from the keto by migration of hydrogen from the adjacent carbon atom to the carbonyl group.
enolase an enzyme in glycolytic systems that changes phosphoglyceric acid into phosphopyruvic acid.
enophthalmos a backward displacement of the eyeball into the orbit.
enostosis a bony growth within a bone cavity or on the internal surface of the bone cortex. See also PANOSTEITIS.
enoxacin a fluoroquinolone antibiotic, similar to ciprofloxacin.
enoxolone see GLYCYRRHETINIC ACID.
enrobing the process of spraying additional ingredients, usually fat and palatability enhancers, on the outside of extruded, dry-type pet foods.
enrofloxacin a fluoroquinolone antibiotic, similar to ciprofloxacin, useful against a wide spectrum of aerobic bacteria, but particularly gram-negative bacteria and mycoplasma. Marketed for veterinary use only as Baytril.
ENS enteric nervous system.
ensiform sword-shaped; xiphoid.
e. cartilage the xiphoid cartilage.
ensilage stored green feed preserved by encouraging primary fermentation to a sufficient level of acetic acid. Good ensilage keeps well for several years and has high nutritive value and palatability. Some silage adjuvants are available to encourage proper fermentation. Called also silage. See also PYREXIA–pruritus–hemorrhage syndrome.
ensiled pertaining to or emanating from ensilage.
ensomphalus a double monster with blended bodies, two separate navels and two umbilical cords.
enstrophe inversion; especially of the margin of the eyelids.
ENT ear, nose and throat.
entactin an adhesive glycoprotein contributing to the cell-to-basal membrane and lamina-to-matrix interfaces.
entad toward a center; inwardly.
ental inner; central.
Entameba a genus of amebas parasitic in the intestines of vertebrates. Member of the family Endamoebidae.
E. bovis found in cattle; nonpathogenic.
E. bubalis an ameba with a single nucleus in the cysts in its trophozoite.
***E. canibuccalis* (syn. *E. gingivalis*)** in the mouth of cats, dogs, humans and primates; nonpathogenic.
E. caviae found in guinea pigs; nonpathogenic.
E. coli a nonpathogenic form found in the intestinal tract of humans. Its importance is that it may be confused with the pathogenic *E. histolytica*.

E. cuniculi found in large bowel of rabbits.
E. equi found in horses.
E. equibuccalis nonpathogenic; found in the mouths of horses.
E. gedoelsti found in horse large intestine; nonpathogenic.
E. hartmanni found in large intestine of humans and the colons of dogs; nonpathogenic.
E. histolytica a species causing AMEBIC dysentery and abscess of the liver in humans. Found also in monkey, dog, cat, rat, pig.
E. invadens cause of entamebiasis in reptiles. See AMEBIASIS.
E. moshkovskii found in sewage. Resembles *E. histolytica.*
E. muris found in large intestine of rats and mice; nonpathogenic.
E. ovis found in sheep.
E. ranarum found in tadpoles.
E. suigingivalis found in the mouths of pigs.
E. suis found in swine.
E. wenyoni an entameba with eight-nucleated cysts in the trophozoite.

entamebiasis infection by *Entamoeba* spp. Occurs in most animal species but clinical illness is evident only in humans in the form of amebic dysentery caused by *E. histolytica.*

Entandrophragma cylindricum African tree in the family Meliaceae whose wood shavings, when used as bedding, have caused balanoposthitis in rams. Sawdust from this tree, used as litter for chickens, has caused hyperkeratosis, weight loss, nervous signs and collapse. Called also redwood.

entasia a constrictive spasm; tonic spasm.

ENTEC enterotoxigenic *Escherichia coli.*

enteque seco [Span.] see ENZOOTIC calcinosis.

enteral within, by way of, or pertaining to the intestine.
e. feeding delivery of nutrients directly into the stomach, duodenum or jejunum. Called also enteral nutrition.
e. nutrition see enteral feeding (above).
e. tube the feeding tube positioned in the alimentary tract for administration of nutrients. See also ENTEROSTOMY tube.

enteralgia pain in the intestine. Called also COLIC.

enterectomy excision of a portion of the intestine.

enterelcosis ulceration of the intestine.

enteric pertaining to the small intestine.
e. bacteria straight gram-negative rods, members of the family ENTEROBACTERIACEAE.
e.-coated designating a special coating applied to tablets or capsules which prevents release and absorption of their contents until they reach the intestine.
e. fever see SALMONELLOSIS.
e. protein loss see protein-losing ENTEROPATHY.

enteritis inflammation of the intestinal mucosa resulting in clinical signs of diarrhea, sometimes dysentery, abdominal pain and dehydration and electrolyte loss and imbalance. In more severe cases there is much mucus in the feces and in the worst ones there are shreds or even sheets of exfoliated mucosa. Gastritis is commonly an accompanying lesion. Vomiting may be a concurrent sign in monogastric animals. The causes are many and include bacteria, viruses, chemicals, damaged feedstuffs and nematode parasites and protozoa. Descriptions of those diseases will be found under the headings of their causative agents, e.g. rotavirus, coronavirus, enterovirus, *Salmonella.* There is a further list of diseases in which diarrhea is the cardinal sign but in which there are no lesions of enteritis. These are the enteropathies. See also ENTEROPATHY.
canine viral e. common causes in dogs are canine parvoviruses, coronavirus and rotavirus. Other viruses isolated from dogs with enteritis but of unknown clinical significance are astrovirus, calicivirus and parainfluenza virus.
equine chronic eosinophilic e. part of a multisystemic epitheliotropic syndrome including pancreatitis and dermatitis.
feline e. see FELINE panleukopenia.
granulomatous e. horses with this disease continue to lose condition over a long period and most have diarrhea and edema. There is a hypoproteinemia and protein loss in the feces. In dogs, the changes are similar, but may be segmental and can be the cause of partial obstruction.
hemocytic e. enteritis of shrimps associated with blooms of some blue-green algae.
lymphocytic–plasmacytic e. infiltration of the lamina propria with lymphocytes and plasma cells can be a nonspecific response to chronic inflammation, but is classified by some as a primary, immune-mediated disease of the intestine causing malabsorption, chronic watery diarrhea and sometimes a protein-losing enteropathy.
mink e. see MINK enteritis.
necrotic e. see NECROTIC enteritis.
parvoviral e. canine PARVOVIRUS.
phlegmonous e. a condition with clinical signs resembling those of peritonitis, which may be secondary to other intestinal diseases, e.g. chronic obstruction, strangulated hernia, carcinoma.
proximal e. duodenitis.
regional e. see terminal ILEITIS.
turkey coronaviral e. acute, highly infectious disease of turkeys of all ages characterized by inappetence, wet droppings, weight loss and heavy mortality is caused by a coronavirus. Called also bluecomb disease.
turkey hemorrhagic e. caused by an adenovirus this disease affects turkey poults over 4 weeks old and is characterized by bloody droppings and sudden death. An epidemic disease now very widespread.
ulcerative e. an acute disease of chickens, poults and game birds caused by *Clostridium colinum.* It is characterized by rapid spread of an acute symptomless disease. Quail show watery white droppings. Lesions include hemorrhagic enteritis in acute cases with ulceration the major finding in subacute cases. The morbidity in quail may be 100%, in chickens it is nearer 10%. Called also quail disease.

enter(o)- word element. [Gr.] *intestine.*

enteroanastomosis see ENTEROENTEROSTOMY.

Enterobacter a genus of straight gram-negative rods, lactose-fermenting bacteria of the tribe Klebsielleae of the family Enterobacteriaceae. Found chiefly in the environment in water and soil but are common invaders of tissues in contaminated wounds of animals and in opportunistic infections such as cystitis and pyelonephritis in cattle. *E. aerogenes* (syn. *Klebsiella mobilis*) is occasionally a cause of bovine mastitis, uterine infections in mares and the mastitis–metritis–agalactia syndrome in sows.
E. cloacae occasionally isolated from dogs and cats with septicemia.

Enterobacteriaceae a family of gram-negative, rod-shaped bacteria (order Eubacteriales) occurring as plant or animal parasites or as saprophytes. Includes the lactose-fermenting genera of *Escherichia,*

Enterobacter, *Serratia* and *Klebsiella*, and the apathogenic genera, *Citrobacter* and *Erwinia*. Also includes the nonlactose fermenters with pathogenic significance, *Salmonella*, *Proteus* and *Yersinia*.

enterobiasis infection with nematodes of the genus *Enterobius*, especially *E. vermicularis*. A disease of humans that also occurs in primates, causing perianal irritation and aggressive behavior.

Enterobius a genus of nematodes of the family Oxyuridae. Includes *E. vermicularis*, the human pinworm; causes ENTEROBIASIS.

enterocele 1. intestinal hernia. 2. the body cavity formed by outpouchings from the archenteron.

enterocentesis surgical puncture of the intestine.

enteroception reception of sensory stimuli in the walls of hollow internal organs.

enterochromaffin pertaining to intestine and chromaffin.

e. cells epithelial cells of the intestinal mucosa which stain with chromium salts; they usually contain serotonin.

e. tumor see CARCINOID.

enteroclysis the injection of liquids into the intestine.

enterococci bacteria in the genus *Enterococcus*.

Enterococcus a group of streptococci, mostly of Lancefield Group D. *E. durans* (previously *Streptococcus durans*), *E. faecalis* (previously *S. faecalis*) and *E. faecium* (previously *S. faecium*) are a cause of avian STREPTOCOCCOSIS. Mostly they are found in the feces of animals and may be involved in opportunist infections. *E. avium* (previously *S. avium*) is of unknown pathogenicity.

E. seriolicida an important pathogen for Japanese yellowtail and rainbow trout. Called also *Lactococcus parviae* and *Streptococcus* spp. biovar 1.

enterocolectomy resection of part of the intestine, including the ileum, cecum and colon.

enterocolitis inflammation of the small intestine and colon. Classifications include eosinophilic, granulomatous, hemorrhagic, plasmacytic, pseudomembranous, ulcerative.

antibiotic-associated e. that in which treatment with antibiotics alters the bowel flora and results in diarrhea or pseudomembranous enterocolitis.

hemorrhagic e. enterocolitis characterized by hemorrhagic breakdown of the intestinal mucosa, with inflammatory cell infiltration.

pseudomembranous e. an acute inflammation of the bowel mucosa, with the formation of pseudomembranous plaques, usually associated with antimicrobial therapy.

ulcerative e. ulcers of the enteric mucosa resulting from bacterial or fungal infection of pre-existing erosions; can also result from tannin poisoning as in horses which consume foliage of oak trees.

enterocolostomy surgical anastomosis of the small intestine to the colon.

enterocrinin a hormone found in the canine small intestine and may stimulate intestinal juice secretion.

enterocutaneous pertaining to or communicating with the intestine and the skin, or surface of the body.

enterocyst a cyst proceeding from subperitoneal tissue.

enterocystocele hernia of the bladder and intestine.

enterocystoma see vitelline CYST.

enterocyte the predominant cells in the small intestinal mucosa. They are tall columnar cells and responsible for the final digestion and absorption of nutrients, electrolytes and water.

enterodynia pain in the intestine.

enteroendocrine pertaining to intestinal hormones.

e. cells cells of the intestinal mucosa that produce hormones such as secretin and cholecystokinin.

enteroenterostomy surgical anastomosis between two segments of the intestine.

enteroepiplocele hernia of the intestine and omentum.

enterogastritis inflammation of the small intestine and stomach.

enterogastrone an uncharacterized hormone of the duodenum which has been suggested to mediate the humoral inhibition of gastric secretion and motility produced by ingestion of fat. Called also anthelone E.

enterogenous 1. arising from the primitive foregut. 2. originating within the small intestine.

enteroglucagon the hyperglycemic, glycogenolytic substance isolable from the intestinal mucosa.

enterogram an instrumental tracing of the movements of the intestine.

enterohepatic pertaining to the liver and the intestine.

enterohepatitis inflammation of the intestine and liver.

infectious e. a disease of poultry. See HISTOMONIASIS.

enterohepatocele an umbilical hernia containing intestine and liver.

enterohydrocele hernia with hydrocele.

enteroinsular axis the relationship between insulin secretion and the entrance of a glucose load into the intestine. The response to a glucose meal taken orally is much greater than if the glucose is given intravenously.

enterokinase the intestinal hormone that activates trypsinogen into becoming active trypsin.

enterokinesia peristalsis.

enterokinetic pertaining to or stimulating peristalsis.

enterolike viruses see INFECTIOUS stunting syndrome.

enterolith a calculus in the intestine; they achieve their greatest importance in horses where they can cause obstruction of the large intestine. In most cases the resulting attacks of colic are recurrent. The enteroliths are smooth, lamellated objects consisting of ammonium magnesium phosphate and occur in mature animals.

Enterolobium central American genus of plants in the family Mimosaceae. Includes *E. cyclocarpum* (conocaste tree), *E. contortisiliquum* (timbauba), *E. gummiferum* (tamboril da campo); no specific toxin identified, but cases of illness show hepatogenous photosensitization.

enterolysis surgical separation of intestinal adhesions.

enteromegaly enlargement of the intestines.

enteromerocele femoral hernia.

Enteromonas a genus of the family Monocercomonadidae of protozoa. None appears to have pathogenic effects.

E. caviae found in the cecum of the guinea pig.

E. hominis found in the cecum of humans, primates and rodents.

E. suis found in the cecum of pigs.

enteromycosis fungal disease of the intestine.

enteron the gut or alimentary canal; usually used in medicine with specific reference to the small intestine.

enteroparesis relaxation of the intestine resulting in dilatation.

enteropathogen a microorganism with pathogenicity for the intestine. Includes enterobacteria, enterococci, corynebacteria, *Mycobacterium paratuberculosis*, *Serpulina hyodysenteriae*, *Lawsonia intracellularis*, campylobacter, clostridia, coronavirus, rotavirus, torovirus, calicivirus, astrovirus, canine parvovirus, bovine virus diarrhea virus, rinderpest virus, bovine malignant catarrh virus, coccidia, cryptosporidia.

enteropathogenesis the production of disease or disorder of the intestine.

enteropathogenic having pathogenicity for the intestine.

e. *Escherichia coli* strains of *E. coli* which cause enteritis by close association with enteric cells. Includes attaching and effacing *E. coli*.

enteropathy any disease of the intestine. Includes enteritis plus those diseases in which there is no physical lesion of enteritis but in which there is severe diarrhea.

cystic mucinous e. see lymphocytic–plasmacytic ENTERITIS.

gluten e. celiac disease. See wheat-sensitive enteropathy (below).

mucoid e. a secretory diarrhea of rabbits, of unknown cause; characterized by occurrence of mucoid diarrhea, abdominal distension, cecal impaction, constipation, depression and hypothermia in rabbits of weaning age and older.

mycotic e. one caused by a fungal agent; see HISTOPLASMOSIS, PHYCOMYCOSIS, CANDIDIASIS.

porcine proliferative e. see PROLIFERATIVE hemorrhagic enteropathy.

protein-losing e. (PLE) a nonspecific term referring to conditions associated with excessive loss of plasma proteins into the intestinal lumen. Associated with a variety of systemic and bowel disorders, including congestive heart failure, gastric ulceration, gastric tumors, intestinal mucosal ulceration and lymphatic disorders.

rabbit e. complex term used to designate a number of poorly defined diarrheal conditions of rabbits; includes mucoid enteropathy and nonspecific enteropathy.

wheat-sensitive e. an hereditary sensitivity to gluten, seen in Irish setters. There is diarrhea and poor growth in young dogs.

enteropeptidase an enzyme of the intestinal juice which activates the proteolytic enzyme of the pancreatic juice by converting trypsinogen into trypsin.

enteropexy surgical fixation of the intestine to the abdominal wall.

enteroplasty plastic repair of the intestine.

enteroplegia see PARALYTIC ileus.

enteroplication surgical procedure for treatment of intussusception and prevention of obstructive adhesions following abdominal surgery; adjacent loops of intestine are sutured to each other.

enteroptosis abnormal downward displacement of the intestine.

enterorrhagia intestinal hemorrhage.

enterorrhaphy suture of the intestine.

enterorrhexis rupture of the intestine.

enteroscope an instrument for inspecting the inside of the intestine.

enterosepsis sepsis developed from the intestinal contents.

enterospasm intestinal colic.

enterostasis intestinal stasis.

enterostenosis narrowing or stricture of the intestine.

enterostomal relating to or having undergone an enterostomy.

enterostomy the artificial formation of a permanent opening into the intestine through the abdominal wall. See also COLOSTOMY, ILEOSTOMY, DUODENOSTOMY, JEJUNOSTOMY.

e. tube one introduced through a surgical opening in the small intestine (duodenostomy or jejunostomy). May be for purposes of introducing food past the pylorus, or for collection of intestinal contents.

enterosystemic the relationship between the intestine and the systemic circulation.

e. fluid cycle the net movement of fluid into and out of the gut lumen every 24 hours. The volume of the exchange is large and a temporary suspension of it can cause fatal dehydration in a horse in 24 hours. The volume depends very much on the diet, being much larger on a high-fiber diet such as in herbivores.

enterotomy incision of the intestine.

enterotoxemia a condition characterized by the presence in the blood of toxins produced in the intestines.

***Clostridium welchii* e.** all of the types of *C. welchii* cause profound enteroxemia with sudden death as the principal manifestation. The postmortem lesions in type D (pulpy kidney disease) enterotoxemia are minimal especially if the course is short. In types A, B, C and E there is a severe enteritis with diarrhea and dysentery. The diseases are most common in young rapidly growing ruminants but foals and piglets are sometimes affected.

coliform e. see *Escherichia coli* enterotoxemia (below).

***Escherichia coli* e.** calves with an enteric infection with the relevant serotype of *E. coli* show sudden collapse, subnormal temperature, coma, slow irregular heart rate, collapse of veins and pale mucosae. The course is short and affected calves die within 2–6 hours. Postmortem lesions are limited to flaccidity of the intestines and the presence of thin, yellow contents.

enterotoxemic jaundice an acute disease of lambs reported in the Western United States in which there is hemoglobinuria, anemia and jaundice. It is caused by *Clostridium perfringens* type A, alpha toxin. Called also yellow lamb disease.

enterotoxic of the nature of or pertaining to enterotoxin.

e. bacteria bacteria capable of producing enterotoxins.

e. colibacillosis a severe toxemia caused by enterotoxic strains of *Escherichia coli*; characterized by collapse, low body temperature, coma, and slow irregular heart rate.

enterotoxicosis intoxication by enterotoxins.

enterotoxigenic producing, produced by, or pertaining to production of enterotoxin.

e. colibacillosis see *Escherichia coli* ENTEROTOXEMIA. Called also enterotoxic colibacillosis.

e. *Escherichia coli* cause diarrhea due to attachment by specific fimbriae and production of enterotoxin see K88 ANTIGEN, K88 ESCHERICHIA COLI SCOURS, K99 ANTIGEN.

enterotoxin 1. a toxin specific for the cells of the intestinal mucosa. 2. a toxin arising in the intestine.

enterotoxism autointoxication of enteric origin.

enterotropic affecting the intestines.

enterovaginal pertaining to or communicating with the intestine and the vagina, as an enterovaginal fistula.

enterovenous communicating between the intestinal lumen and the lumen of a vein.

enterovesical pertaining to or communicating with the intestine and urinary bladder.

Enterovirus a genus of the family *Picornaviridae*. The genus includes the important animal pathogens of porcine poliomyelitis (Teschen disease), possibly SMEDI disease (see porcine PARVOVIRUS), avian encephalomyelitis (epidemic tremor), duckling hepatitis, turkey hepatitis. Equine and bovine enteroviruses of doubtful pathogenicity have also been isolated. Human enteroviruses, e.g. Coxsackie virus, ECHO virus, are also isolated occasionally from animals without appearing to cause disease.

enterovirus a virus in the genus *Enterovirus*.

e. encephalitis several porcine enteroviruses cause highly transmissible encephalitides. See also porcine viral ENCEPHALOMYELITIS (Teschen disease, Talfan disease, poliomyelitis suum).

enterozoon an animal parasite in the intestines.

enterprise a definable system which produces a commodity or groups of related commodities. On a farm there may be only one or several, e.g. grass seed production, lamb production, fat sheep sales, wool production, wheat production.

enthalpy the bond energy in a biochemical reaction.

enthesiophyte calcification of a muscle attachment or ligament at the point of its insertion into the bone.

enthesis 1. the use of artificial material in the repair of a defect or deformity of the body. 2. the site of attachment of a muscle or ligament to bone.

enthetobiosis a term suggested to denote the dependency of an organism on a mechanical device implanted within the body, for example, dependency of a patient on an electronic cardiac pacemaker to regulate the heartbeat. The relationship between the organism and the device is critical. Called also epenthetobiosis.

entire a term used in reference to an uncastrated animal, male or female.

entire-leaved thorn apple DATURA *metel*.

ento- word element. [Gr.] *within, inner*.

entoblast the entoderm.

entocele an internal hernia.

entochoroidea the inner layer of the choroid of the eye.

entoderm the innermost of the three primitive germ layers of the embryo; from it are derived the epithelium of the pharynx, respiratory tract (except the nose), digestive tract, bladder and urethra.

entoectad from within outward.

Entoloma lividum a mushroom which causes severe gastroenteritis in humans.

entomere a blastomere normally destined to become entoderm.

entomology that branch of biology concerned with the study of insects.

Entomophthora a genus of phycomycetous fungi. See SWAMP CANCER and CONIDIOBOLUS *coronatus*.

entomophthoromycosis infection caused by *Entomophthora* spp. See SWAMP CANCER.

entomopoxvirus a group of poxviruses recovered from insects.

Entonyssus an entonyssid mite of snakes.

Entophionyssus an entonyssid mite of snakes.

entopic occurring in the proper place.

entoptic originating within the eye.

entoptoscopy inspection of the interior of the eye.

entoretina the nervous or inner layer of the retina.

entotic situated in or originating within the ear.

entozoon an internal animal parasite.

entrainement the phenomenon in which a species of bacteria growing close to another may acquire some of the characteristics of the second species. See also RECOMBINATION.

entraining loading horses, cattle or any other livestock onto a train.

entrapment the state of being trapped.

bowel e. the intestine is caught up in adhesions or peritoneal ligaments. Obstruction, with or without compromise of the blood supply to the incarcerated loop, follows.

epiglottic e. see EPIGLOTTIC.

legal e. the legal device by which a suspect is tempted to infringe the law or rules while under observation.

Entrefino Spanish meat and medium wool sheep, white, polled; includes many Spanish breeds. It is a class of sheep rather than a single breed.

entropion inversion, or the turning inward, as of the margin of an eyelid. Causes irritation, blepharospasm, keratitis. May be congenital or acquired.

anatomic e. see conformational entropion (below).

cicatricial e. caused by scarring of the eyelid or conjunctiva following injury or inflammation.

conformational e. a conformational feature of some dog breeds, including Shar peis, Chow Chows, and St. Bernards, which either have excessive and thick skin on the face, or deeply set eyes. Called also anatomic entropion.

geriatric e. occurs in older dogs because of temporal muscle atrophy, loss of retrobulbar tissue or general debilitation.

inherited congenital e. occurs in sheep, cattle, miniature pigs and some breeds of dogs.

lateral e. affects the lateral part of the eyelids. Involvement of both upper and lower eyelids may be caused by inadequate function of the retractor anguli oculi muscle.

medial e. seen most often in brachycephalic dogs.

neonatal e. seen in Shar pei puppies, because of their thick skin and enophthalmos. Temporary surgical correction is required at an early age. Newborn lambs, calves and goats may also be affected.

spastic e. due to spasticity of the orbicularis oculi muscle caused by painful conditions of the eye, such as ulcerative keratitis, distichiasis or foreign bodies.

uveal e., e. uveae infolding of the pupillary border and adherence to the anterior surface of the iris.

entropy 1. in thermodynamics, a measure of the part of the internal energy of a system that is unavailable to do work. In any spontaneous process, such as the flow of heat from a hot region to a cold region, entropy always increases. 2. in information theory, the negative of information, a measure of the disorder or randomness in a physical system. The theory of statistical mechanics proves that this concept is equivalent to entropy as defined in thermodynamics.

entry box the area in a dialog box in which the user can type a response to a question posed by the program.

enucleate to remove whole and clean, as the eye from its socket.

enucleation removal of an organ or other mass intact from its supporting tissues, as of the eyeball from the orbit.

lateral subconjunctival e. involves a lateral canthotomy and a subconjunctival approach to the globe, extraocular muscles and optic nerve.

transpalpebral e. removal of eyelids, conjunctiva and extraocular muscles along with eyeball.

enuresis see INCONTINENCE.

***env* gene** a gene which encodes a protein precursor for the envelope proteins, found in the retroviral genome.

envelope an encompassing structure or membrane. In

virology, a bilayer lipoprotein membrane with glycoprotein spikes surrounding the nucleocapsid and usually furnished, at least partially, by the host cell. In bacteriology, the cell wall and the plasma membrane considered together.

nuclear e. the condensed double layer of lipids and proteins enclosing the cell nucleus and separating it from the cytoplasm; its two concentric membranes, inner and outer, are separated by a perinuclear space.

envenomation the poisonous effects caused by the bites, stings or effluvia of insects and other arthropods, or the bites of snakes.

environment the sum total of all the conditions and elements that make up the surroundings and influence the development of an animal. The environment of animals is often assumed to comprise only physical, chemical and biological factors but society is gradually coming to appreciate that there is also an emotional and psychological side to the life of all animals.

environmental pertaining to or emanating from the environment.

e. injuries include burns, electrical injuries, frostbite, heat stroke.

e. mastitis mastitis caused by *Escherichia coli*, *Klebsiella* spp., *Aerobacter aerogenes*.

permanent e. factors factors which affect all measures of performance equally and through the patient's lifetime, e.g. fulltime at pasture, tropical climate.

e. pollution the presence of offensive, but not necessarily infectious, matter in the environment. For example, pollution may be by specific organic or inorganic chemicals, by physical agents such as dust, volcanic fallout, smoke, automobile fumes, radioactive material and animal feces and urine. Each of these items and noise pollution is dealt with under specific headings.

e. stress see STRESS (2).

temporary e. factors risk factors which may vary widely, e.g. nutrition, pregnancy status, disease.

e. variance that portion of the phenotypic variance caused by differences in the environment to which the individuals have been exposed.

environmentalist a person with an interest and knowledge about the interaction of humans and animals with the environment.

enzootic peculiar to or present constantly in a location. See also ENDEMIC.

e. arthrogryposis/hydranencephaly infection of the pregnant cow, ewe or goat doe with the Akabane virus causes congenital defects of the nervous system of the fetus.

e. ataxia a disease of unweaned lambs caused by a nutritional deficiency of copper and characterized by an absence of myelin in tissues of the central nervous system, and a clinical picture of incoordination and terminally recumbency and death from starvation. Called also Gingin rickets, renguera, swayback, lamkruis.

e. balanoposthitis an endemic inflammation of the prepuce and penis of castrated male sheep. It is caused by *Corynebacterium renale* but the clinical disease appears only when there is lush pasture and a consequent high alkalinization of the urine, and also a high intake of estrogens from the pasture. There is a concurrent vulvitis in ewes and bulls may be affected. There is swelling, scabby ulceration and inflammation of the exterior and the interior of the prepuce and the glans penis. Affected wethers dribble urine, show pain at the site and may become flyblown. Called also pizzle rot, sheath rot.

e. bovine adenomatosis see ATYPICAL INTERSTITIAL PNEUMONIA.

e. bovine arthrogryposis see AKABANE VIRUS disease.

e. bovine leukopsis see BOVINE viral leukosis.

e. calcinosis a poisoning by the plant *Solanum malacoxylon* causes a significant increase in calcium absorption and deposition in tissues. The characteristic clinical signs are stiffness of the limbs and the back, and unwillingness to stand up if lying down, or to lie down if standing up. Identical diseases are caused by a grass *Trisetum flavescens*, and by herbs *Nierembergia veitchii*, *Solanum linneaneum*, *S. torvum* and *Cestrum diurnum*. Called also enteque seco, Manchester wasting disease, Naalehu, espichamento.

e. equine ataxia see enzootic equine incoordination (below).

e. equine incoordination a series of diseases with very strong clinical similarity. The syndrome is one of chronic incoordination in young horses associated with a variety of pathological processes in the cervical spinal cord. These include a degenerative myeloencephalopathy of unknown origin, compression of the cord by overflexion of the neck, or by stenosis of the vertebral canal, and an inflammatory lesion in the cord caused by *Sarcocystis* spp. Affected horses are quite unsafe to ride even though some of them do not get to be too badly affected. Surgical intervention in appropriate cases is now a practical reality. Called also wobbler.

e. ethmoidal tumor this disease has been a problem in cattle in Brazil and Sweden. Epistaxis and nasal obstruction are the important findings. The paranasal sinuses may also be invaded.

e. hematuria a disease characterized by hemangiomatous lesions in the bladder of cattle, causing the intermittent passage of heavily blood-stained urine. The blood loss may be sufficiently severe to cause a fatal hemorrhagic anemia. Caused by chronic intake of ptaquiloside from *Pteridium* spp., *Cheilanthes sieberi*, *Onychium contiguum*; most cases are obviously related to the long-term ingestion of bracken. See also PTERIDIUM AQUILINUM.

e. icterus a syndrome which includes the hepatopathies of grazing animals. Includes FACIAL eczema, TOXEMIC jaundice and toxipathic HEPATITIS.

e. intestinal adenocarcinoma a disease of sheep in New Zealand, Iceland, Norway and of cows in New Zealand.

e. marasmus see COBALT nutritional deficiency.

e. muscular dystrophy a disease which is due to a nutritional deficiency of vitamin E or selenium and occurs in calves, lambs and foals. There is a sudden onset, commonly after exercise. The calf may drop dead or show dyspnea, a frothy nasal discharge and a rapid and irregular heartbeat, all signs of acute heart failure. Less acute cases show recumbency with inability to rise, and increased respiratory rate. Less severe cases still are able to stand and walk but are weak and dyspneic. Although the pathogenesis is an acute myopathy there is no myoglobinuria except in unusual circumstances in yearling male cattle.

e. nasal granuloma a form of chronic nasal obstruction which occurs most commonly in dairy cows of the Channel Islands breeds. The disease is a chronic dyspnea with stertorous breathing due to partial obstruction of both nasal cavities by eosinophilic granulomas about 4 mm in diameter on the mucosa just inside the nostril. The disease is thought to have an allergic origin. Called also allergic rhinitis, atopic rhinitis. See also CAPRINE enzootic nasal granuloma.

e. nodular thelitis of alpine cows in Switzerland; characterized by nodular lesions in the teat wall.
e. ovine abortion caused by *Chlamydia* spp. The abortion occurs during the last month of pregnancy and the ewe is not sick beforehand, with the placenta often retained afterwards. Metritis may also occur. See also CHLAMYDIAL abortion.
e. pneumonia a group of pneumonic diseases which affect young animals. They are principally of viral origin, although mycoplasmas also play a part, and are only mildly pathogenic unless secondary bacterial invasion intervenes. In calves parainfluenza-3 virus, respiratory syncytial virus, adenovirus, bovine herpesvirus 1, rhinovirus, reovirus and mycoplasmas and *Chlamydia* sp. are causes. In lambs the list of causes is the same. In pigs there is only one agent, *Mycoplasma hyopneumoniae* (syn. *M. suipneumoniae*). The importance of these diseases is not the wastage that they cause in their own right, although there is sometimes a significant loss of productivity and occasional cases of severe illness and even death, but the losses that occur when lethal bacterial pneumonia supervenes.
e. posthitis see enzootic balanoposthitis (above).
e. staphylococcosis a septicemia of lambs caused by *Staphylococcus aureus*; the spread of the disease is facilitated in some way by tick bites. The lambs are affected soon after birth and die quickly of septicemia or develop arthritis and meningitis later. Called also tick pyemia.

enzootische herztod see PORCINE stress syndrome.

enzygotic developed from one zygote.

enzymatic of, relating to, caused by, or of the nature of an enzyme.

enzyme any protein that acts as a catalyst, increasing the rate at which a chemical reaction occurs. The animal body probably contains about 10,000 different enzymes. At body temperature, very few biochemical reactions proceed at a significant rate without the presence of an enzyme. Like all catalysts, an enzyme does not control the direction of the reaction; it increases the rates of the forward and reverse reactions proportionally.
activating e. one that activates a given amino acid by attaching it to the corresponding transfer ribonucleic acid.
e. assays several enzymes are important in clinical pathology. Enzymes characteristic of a tissue are released into the blood when the tissue is damaged, and enzyme levels in the blood can aid in the diagnosis or monitoring of specific diseases. Lipase and amylase levels are useful in pancreatic diseases; alkaline phosphatase (ALP), aspartate aminotransferase (AST) and alanine aminotransferase (ALT) in liver diseases; and lactate dehydrogenase (LD), AST and creatine kinase (CK) in muscle disease. ALP is also released in bone diseases. Many enzymes have different forms (*isoenzymes*) in different organs. The isoenzymes can be separated by electrophoresis in order to determine the origin of the enzyme. Isoenzymes of LD, CK and ALP have the most clinical utility.
brancher e., branching e. amylo-(1,4→1,6)-transglycosylase; important in the synthesis of the branched glycogen molecule. Absence of the enzyme causes an increase in the length of the glucose chains and a decrease in the number of branch points in the glycogen molecules.
congenital e. deficiency in humans hundreds of genetic diseases that result from deficiency of a single enzyme are now known. Many of these diseases fall into two large classes. The *aminoacidopathies*, e.g. phenylketonuria (PKU), result from deficiency of an enzyme in the major pathway for the metabolism of a specific amino acid. The amino acid accumulates in the blood, and it or its metabolites are excreted in the urine. The *lysomal storage diseases*, e.g. GANGLIOSIDOSIS, MANNOSIDOSIS, result from deficiency of a lysomal enzyme and the accumulation of the substance degraded by that enzyme in lysosomes of cells throughout the body. The stored material is usually a complex substance, such as glycogen, a sphingolipid or a mucopolysaccharide. Many similar diseases are now identified in animals and are to be found under the specific name of each disease.
constitutive e. one produced by a microorganism regardless of the presence or absence of the specific substrate acted upon.
core e. the smallest aggregate of an enzyme's subunits that has enzymatic activity.
debrancher e., debranching e. dextrin-1,6-glucosidase: an enzyme that acts to move glucose residues of the glycogen molecule, and is important in glycogenolysis.
induced e., inducible e. one whose production requires or is stimulated by a specific small molecule, the inducer, which is the substrate of the enzyme or a compound structurally related to it.
e. induction the effect some compounds such as phenobarbitone and phenytoin have in increasing the activity of microsomal hepatic enzymes. This may cause alterations in the metabolism of concurrently administered drugs.
microsomal e's those associated with the endoplasmic reticulum of cells, particularly of the liver.
proteolytic e. one that catalyzes the hydrolysis of proteins and various split products of proteins, the final product being small peptides and amino acids.
repressible e. one whose rate of production is decreased as the concentration of certain metabolites is increased.
respiratory e's enzymes of the mitochondria, e.g. cytochrome oxidase, which serve as catalysts for cellular oxidations.
restriction e's see RESTRICTION ENDONUCLEASE.

enzyme-linked immunoabsorbent assay see ELISA.

enzymic enzymatic.

enzymology the study of enzymes and enzymatic action.

enzymopathy an inborn error of metabolism consisting of defective or absent enzymes, as in the glycogenoses or the mucopolysaccharidoses.

EOD abbreviation for every other day; used in medical records.

EOG electro-oculogram; electro-olfactogram.

Eohippus the oldest known ancestor of the horse. A short, 25–50 cm high, rodent-like animal with four toes on each forefoot and three on each hind. Each toe had a hoof. The *Eohippus* survived by its speed. See also MESOHIPPUS.

Eomenacanthus see MENACANTHUS.

EOSCC equine ocular SQUAMOUS cell carcinoma.

eosin any of a class of rose-colored stains or dyes, all being bromine derivatives of fluorescein; eosin Y, the sodium salt of tetrabromofluorescein, is much used in histological and laboratory procedures. See also hematoxylin and eosin STAIN.

eosin- prefix meaning red.

eosinopenia abnormal deficiency of eosinophils in the blood. Commonly associated with stress or the administration of corticosteroids.

eosinophil an element readily stained by eosin; specifically, a granular leukocyte with a nucleus that usually has two lobes connected by a thread of chromatin, and cytoplasm containing coarse, round or rod-shaped, eosinophilic granules (lysosomes) of uniform size.

eosinophilia 1. the formation and accumulation of an abnormally large number of eosinophils in the blood. 2. the condition of being readily stained with eosin.

eosinophilic staining readily with eosin; pertaining to eosinophils or to eosinophilia.

cartilaginous e. streaks streaks of eosinophilic matrix in cartilage. Some are normal zones of development, others represent areas of matrix degeneration and osteochondrosis.

e. chemotactic factor a primary mediator of type I anaphylactic hypersensitivity, it is an acidic peptide (molecular weight 500) released by mast cells, which attracts eosinophils to areas where it is present.

equine e. chronic dermatitis acanthosis and hyperkeratosis accompanied by eosinophilic granulomas in pancreas and other epithelial organs.

feline e. granuloma complex a collective name given to the lesions of eosinophilic ulcer, eosinophilic plaque (below), and linear granuloma because of similarities in histopathology, clinical course and occasionally simultaneous occurrence in the cat.

e. granuloma nodules or plaques that occur on skin or oral mucosa of dogs. Usually not pruritic, but oral lesions can cause some difficulties in eating. The cause is unknown. See also feline eosinophilic granuloma complex (above), EQUINE nodular collagenolytic granuloma.

e. intestinal granuloma see ANGIOSTRONGYLUS *costaricensis*.

e. lung disease see PIE SYNDROME.

e. meningitis see GNATHOSTOMA *spinigerum*.

e. meningoencephalitis see SODIUM chloride poisoning, ANGIOSTRONGYLUS *cantonensis*.

e. myocarditis in cattle may be observed in normal animals at slaughter. Histologically there is a predominant eosinophil invasion of the heart muscle. May be accompanied by similar lesions in skeletal muscles.

e. plaque well-defined, raised, ulcerated and extremely pruritic lesions that occur on the skin of cats, usually on the abdomen or hindlegs. There are large numbers of eosinophils present in the dermis and sometimes peripheral blood. See also eosinophilic granuloma (above), feline eosinophilic granuloma complex (above).

e. pneumonia see PIE SYNDROME.

e. ulcer a well-defined ulceration, usually on the upper lip of cats overlying the canine tooth, which is shallow initially but can become extremely erosive and sometimes neoplastic. Mildly irritating to the cat. Called also indolent ulcer, rodent ulcer. See also feline eosinophilic granuloma complex (above).

eosinopoiesis formation of eosinophils.

Epagneul Breton see BRITTANY SPANIEL.

epallobiosis dependency on an external life-support system, as on an EXTRACORPOREAL circulatory support unit or hemodialyzer. See HEMODIALYSIS.

epaxial situated above or upon an axis.

EPEC enteropathogenic *Escherichia coli*.

epencephalon 1. cerebellum. 2. metencephalon.

ependyma the cells lining the cerebral ventricles and the central canal of the spinal cord; principal source of cerebrospinal fluid, mostly from where the ependyma covers the choroid plexuses.

ependymal emanating from or pertaining to ependyma.

e. cells squamous-to-columnar cell lining of the spinal central canal and the four ventricles of the brain; supports the choroid plexuses.

ependymitis inflammation of the ependyma.

ependymoma fleshy masses protruding into the third ventricles, the central canal in the medullary region or the central spinal canal; arise from the ependyma.

epenthetobiosis see ENTHETOBIOSIS.

Eperythrozoon a genus of microorganisms of the family Anaplasmataceae in the order Rickettsiales. They are small prokaryotic forms occurring on the surface of erythrocytes and may also be found free in the plasma.

E. coccoides found in mice, may cause anemia.

E. felis see HAEMOBARTONELLA felis.

E. ovis found in sheep; often an inapparent infection but may cause anemia and jaundice in an acute episode or chronic poor condition.

E. parvum found in pig; usually nonpathogenic.

E. suis found in pig; causes icteroanemia and may cause heavy mortality in piglets.

E. teganodes found in cattle; nonpathogenic; remarkable because it is found only in the plasma and not attached to erythrocytes.

E. wenyoni found in cattle. May cause fever and anemia but usually nonpathogenic.

eperythrozoonosis infection with *Eperythrozoon* spp. The infection is mostly innocuous but in times of stress, e.g. in the presence of another disease, it may cause an acute anemia with fever. There is no hemoglobinuria. The infection is spread by insects and the disease may be seasonal as a result. In many cases the disease is a subacute one with illthrift as the main presenting sign.

EPF early pregnancy factor.

EPH early pregnancy hormone.

ephapse a point of lateral contact (other than a synapse) between nerve fibers across which impulses are conducted directly through the nerve membranes.

ephebogenesis the bodily changes occurring at sexual maturity.

Ephedra viridis North American member of the plant family Ephedraceae; contains an unidentified toxin which causes diarrhea and vomiting in ruminants.

ephedrine an adrenergic alkaloid obtained from several species of the shrub *Ephedra* or produced synthetically; used as the hydrochloride as a bronchodilator, antiallergic, central nervous system stimulant, mydriatic, pressor agent, and for stimulation of the α-adrenergic receptors in the treatment of certain types of urinary incontinence.

ephemeral fever an infectious disease of cattle caused by an arthropod-borne rhabdovirus, and is characterized by inflammation of mesodermal tissues. Clinically there is fever, muscle stiffness and shivering, lameness, enlargement of lymph nodes and recumbency. The disease is a nonfatal one and has an average course of 3 days—hence 3-day fever. The virus is transmitted by insect vectors, e.g. the sandfly, *Ceratopogonidae* spp. Called also 3-day sickness.

EPI exocrine pancreatic insufficiency.

epi- word element. [Gr.] *upon*.

epibiotic fouling fouling of external surfaces of mainly shellfish but sometimes finfish, with living organisms, principally protozoa of the genera *Zoothanium*, *Epistilis*, *Vorticella*.

epiblast layer of cells roofing over the blastocoel in the avian embryo.

epiblepharon a developmental anomaly in which a

horizontal fold of skin stretches across the border of the eyelid, pressing the lashes against the eyeball.

epibulbar situated upon the eyeball.

epicanthus a vertical fold of skin on either side of the nose.

epicardia the lower portion of the esophagus, extending from the esophageal hiatus to the cardia, the upper orifice of the stomach.

epicardial pertaining to the visceral pericardium (epicardium) or to the epicardia.

e. receptors receptors in the left ventricle adapted to respond to stretch and chemical stimulants.

epicardium the inner layer of the serous pericardium, which is in contact with the heart.

Epicauta vittata an insect which may infest hay and cause colic and frequent urination in horses. Contains the vesicant substance cantharidin. Called also blister beetle.

epiceras, epikeras a thin layer of skin covering the junction between the base of a horn and the surrounding skin, similar to the periople of the hoof.

Epichloë typhina fungus found on tall fescue grass and possibly implicated in causing poisoning. See also FESTUCA.

epichorion the portion of the uterine mucosa enclosing the implanted conceptus.

epicillin an aminopenicillin antibiotic.

epicondyle an eminence upon a bone, above its condyle, as in the distal extremity of the humerus and femur.

epicondylitis inflammation of an epicondyle or of tissues adjoining the humeral epicondyle.

epicranium the structures collectively that cover the skull.

epicritic determining accurately; said of cutaneous nerve fibers sensitive to fine variations of touch or temperature.

epicyte cell membrane.

epidemic a level of disease occurrence in an animal population which is significantly greater than usual; only occasionally present in the population, widely diffused and rapidly spreading. The disease is clustered in space and time. The word has common usage in veterinary science in preference to the more accurate, epizootic.

common source e. see point epidemic (below).

e. curve see epidemic CURVE.

e. diarrhea of infant mice see MURINE epizootic diarrhea.

e. hyperthermia poisoning by *Acremonium coenophialu*; called also fescue summer toxicosis.

multiple event e. when the epidemic begins at about the same time in a number of places, e.g. when a poisoned batch of feed is supplied to a number of farms.

point e. when the epidemic begins at one central point, with a large number of animals coming in contact with the source over a short time; a very rapid form of spread with a number of cases presenting with the same stage of the disease at the one time, indicating the single source of the pathogen.

propagated e., propagative e., propagating e. outbreaks in which the disease propagates in one or more initial cases and then spreads to others, a relatively slow method of spread.

e. tremor see avian ENCEPHALOMYELITIS.

e. typhus see RICKETTSIA *prowazeki*.

epidemicity the quality of being widely diffused and rapidly spreading throughout a population.

epidemiogenesis the escalation of a communicable disease to epidemic proportions.

epidemiological emanating from or pertaining to epidemiology.

e. associations the associative relationships between the frequency of occurrence of a disease and its determinants, its predisposing and precipitating causes.

e. intelligence all of the epidemiological information about a disease occurrence. Includes information gathering over a short period at the time of an outbreak and the more prolonged follow-up of surveillance afterwards.

e. model see COMPUTER simulation model.

e. techniques include CASE-control study, CLINICAL trials, COHORT studies.

epidemiologist an expert in epidemiology.

epidemiology 1. the study of the relationships of various factors determining the frequency and distribution of diseases in a community. 2. the field of veterinary medicine dealing with the determination of specific causes of localized outbreaks of infection, toxic poisoning, or other disease of recognized etiology. 3. the study of disease in communities. 4. Called also epizootiology.

analytical e. statistical analysis of epidemiological data in an attempt to establish relationships between causative factors and incidence of disease.

descriptive e. information about the occurrence of a disease, some of it mathematical, but with no attempt to establish relationships between cause and effect.

experimental e. prospective population experiments designed to test epidemiological hypotheses, and usually attempt to relate the postulated cause to the observed effect. Trials of new anthelmintics are an example.

gum-boots e. see shoe-leather epidemiology (below).

landscape e. epidemiology of a disease in relation to the entire ecosystem under study.

observational e. based on clinical and field observations, not on experiments.

shoe-leather e. epidemiology conducted as a field study. Called also gum-boots epidemiology.

theoretical e. the use of mathematical models to explain and examine aspects of epidemiology, e.g. computer simulation models of outbreaks.

epidermal pertaining to or emanating from epidermis.

e. appendage see HAIR, CLAW, HOOF, HORN, CHESTNUT (1), ERGOT[2], DEWCLAW, COMB, WATTLE, SPUR (3), PAD, FOOTPAD, BEAK, frontal PROCESS, FEATHER (1), CERE, SCALE, FIN, ANTLER, BRISTLE (1), WOOL, MOHAIR, CASHMERE, ANGORA.

e. clefts slit-like discontinuities in the epidermis that do not contain fluid.

e. collarette a feature of a skin lesion, consisting of an encircling rim of epidermal scale with the free edge toward the central area. May represent the margins of an earlier bulla, vesicle or pustule. Characteristic of bullous pemphigoid.

e. crust a consolidated mass of cellular debris, dried exudate, serum, hair, epidermophytic hyphae. Usually is dry and crumbly but in parakeratosis may have a greasy feel about it.

e. cyst, epidermoid cyst an intradermal or subcutaneous cyst containing keratinizing squamous epithelium. It arises from occluded hair follicles. Called also infundibular cyst, wen.

e. dysplasia abnormal development of individual cells of the epidermis. In West Highland white terriers, a familial skin disease characterized by seborrhea, pruritus, alopecia and lichenification from an early age. Infection by *Malassezia* spp. is a common feature. See also INHERITED EPIDERMAL DYSPLASIA of calves.

e. growth factor a potent growth factor for both epithelial and fibroblast cells.
e. lacunae see epidermal clefts (above).
e. laminae structures formed of epidermal pegs; part of the interdigitating structure between the dermis and the epidermis. Called also epidermal ridges.
e. limbi the layer of soft, light-colored horn that covers the outer side of the coronary border and merges with the horn of the hoof.
e.-melanin unit a melanocyte and adjacent keratinocytes.
e. necrolysis see toxic epidermal NECROLYSIS.
e. nibbles focal areas of epidermal edema, eosinophils and necrosis; suggestive of ectoparasite injury to the skin.
e. papilla a knob-like projection of the epidermis into the dermis; a touch receptor. Called also tylotrich pad and haarscheiben.
e. pegs see RETE pegs.
e. renewal time see KERATINOCYTE transit time.
e. ridge see RETE ridge.

epidermis the outermost and nonvascular layer of the skin, derived from the embryonic ectoderm, the thickness varying between species and in different locations on the body. There are generally five layers, from within outward: (1) *basal layer* (stratum basale), composed of columnar cells arranged perpendicularly; (2) *prickle-cell* or *spinous layer* (stratum spinosum), composed of flattened polyhedral cells with short processes or spines; (3) *granular layer* (stratum granulosum), composed of flattened granular cells; (4) *clear layer* (stratum lucidum), composed of several layers of clear, transparent cells in which the nuclei are indistinct or absent; and (5) *horny layer* (stratum corneum), composed of flattened, cornified, non-nucleated cells. The clear layer is only present in certain areas such as the footpads of dogs and cats and the planum nasale.
limbic e. transitional epithelium between limb skin and hoof horn; covers the limbic corium.
perioplic e. see limbic epidermis (above).
tubular e. covering of the corium of the hoof coronet; produces the tubular horn of the hoof wall.

epidermitis inflammation of the epidermis.
peracute e. see EXUDATIVE epidermitis.

epidermodysplasia see EPIDERMAL dysplasia.

epidermoid 1. resembling the epidermis. 2. any tumor occurring at a noncutaneous site and formed by inclusion of epidermal cells.
e. carcinoma see SQUAMOUS cell carcinoma.
e. cysts occur in dogs and humans and represent sections of epidermal tissue isolated during the closure of the neural tube.

epidermoidoma a cerebral or meningeal tumor formed by inclusion of ectodermal elements at the time of closure of the neural groove.

epidermolysis a loosened state of the epidermis with formation of blebs and bullae either spontaneously or at the site of trauma.
e. bullosa a hereditary disease of humans, Collie dogs, Shetland sheepdogs, Suffolk, South Dorset Down and Scottish blackface sheep, and Simmental and Brangus calves. Characterized by epidermal bullae, particularly on areas of pressure or trauma and in sheep in the mouth and on woolless skin. There may be shedding of hooves and horns. Called also red foot disease.
congenital bovine e. ulcers on lips, gums, tongue, muzzle and limb extremities at birth; skin lesions may be local alopecia without ulceration; resembles epidermolysus bullosa simplex in humans; an autosomal dominant recorded in Simmentals.

epidermomycosis see DERMATOPHYTOSIS.

epidermophytid dermatophytid.

epidermophytin a filtrate of *Epidermophyton* spp. cultures that induces a hypersensitivity reaction of the tuberculin type when used in humans.

Epidermophyton a genus of dermatophytic fungi. *E. floccosum* is a common cause of fungal skin and nail infections in humans; rare in animals.

epidermophytosis a fungal skin infection, especially one due to *Epidermophyton floccosum*. The common form is athlete's foot in humans, but the infection has been identified in the dog, mule and goat. Called also dermatophytosis.

epidermopoiesis formation of the epidermis.

Epidermoptes a genus of parasitic mites of the family Epidermoptidae. Includes *E. bifurcatus (E. bifurcata)*, *E. bilobatus*; found on the skin of birds; capable of causing allergy in humans. May coexist with fungal infections, e.g. *Lophophyton* spp.

epidermotropic predilection for epidermis.
e. lymphoma see EPITHELIOTROPIC lymphoma.

epididymal emanating from or pertaining to the epididymis.
e. inflammation see EPIDIDYMITIS.
e. segmental aplasia a defect in mesonephric development in which part of the epididymis is missing. A cause of infertility in male dogs manifested by azoospermia. Usually unilateral in bulls and rams; probably inherited.
e. sperm granulomas see sperm GRANULOMA.
e. stagnation a condition in stallions in which peak fertility is maintained only by frequent ejaculation.

epididymectomy excision of the epididymis.

epididymis pl. *epididymides* [Gr.] an elongated, cordlike structure along the attached border of the testis, whose coiled duct provides for the storage, transport and maturation of spermatozoa.

epididymitis inflammation of the epididymis. Nonspecific epididymitis may result from an infection in the urinary tract, especially in the prostate. Rarely it may be traced to an infection elsewhere in the body. Specific epididymitides are those caused by *Actinobacillus seminis* and by *Brucella ovis*, both in rams, by *B. canis* in dogs, and the virus of epivag, bovine viral epididymitis and vaginitis in bulls.

epididymitis–orchitis see EPIDIDYMO-ORCHITIS.

epididymitis-vaginitis inflammation of the epididymis and the tunica vaginalis.

epididymo–orchitis inflammation of the epididymis and testis.

epididymotomy incision of the epididymis.

epididymovasostomy surgical anastomosis of the epididymis to the ductus deferens.

epidural pertaining to or emanating from the dura mater.
e. abscess see BRAIN abscess, SPINAL abscess.
e. anesthesia produced by injecting local anesthetic agent into the epidural space of the spinal canal at the first or second intercoccygeal space. Injection of a small amount of anesthetic agent produces anesthesia of the perineum without paralysis of the hindlimbs, a low epidural. Injection of a large volume at the same site produces a high epidural. The same effect is achieved by injecting the anesthetic at the lumbosacral or first interlumbar space. Called also extradural anesthesia, or analgesia, extradural block, epidural block.
e. block see epidural anesthesia (above).
segmental dorsolumbar e. block injection of local anesthetic into the epidural space between the first two lumbar vertebrae produces anesthesia of both

flanks. Used for standing abdominal surgery in horses or cattle.

epidurography radiography of the spine after a radiopaque medium has been injected into the epidural space.

epigastralgia pain in the epigastrium.

epigastrium the cranial and middle region of the abdomen, located within the sternal angle.

epigenesis the development of an organism from an undifferentiated cell, consisting in the successive formation and development of organs and parts that do not preexist in the fertilized egg.

epigenetic theory proposes that the form and tissues of an organism arise in a sequential and organized manner from the undifferentiated contents of the fertilized egg.

epiglottal swelling the enlargements which appear on the floor of the pharynx of the embryo and subsequently take part in the formation of the lateral ventricles.

epiglottic pertaining to or emanating from the epiglottis.

e. cartilage attached to the thyroid cartilage of the larynx by the thyroepiglottic ligament; it is the structural basis of the epiglottis.

e. cysts see PHARYNGEAL cyst.

e. entrapment the epiglottis is trapped by the aryteno-epiglottic fold and fails to function normally. Affected horses show exercise intolerance, noisy breathing, coughing and a characteristic appearance of the laryngeal opening viewed through a fiberscope.

e. hypoplasia a smaller than normal epiglottis is often associated with dorsal displacement of the soft palate in horses, resulting in respiratory embarrassment during exercise.

epiglottis the lidlike cartilaginous structure guarding the entrance to the larynx.

The muscular action of swallowing closes the opening to the trachea by placing the larynx against the epiglottis. This prevents food and drink from entering the larynx and trachea, directing it instead into the esophagus.

epihyoid middle of the chain of hyoid bones; it articulates with the stylohyoid and the ceratohyoid.

epikeras see EPICERAS.

epilate to remove hair.

epilation the removal of hair by the roots.

cryosurgical e. see CRYOEPILATION.

electric e. see ELECTROEPILATION.

epilemma endoneurium.

epilepsy paroxysmal transient disturbances of nervous system function resulting from abnormal electrical activity of the brain. It is not a specific disease, but rather a group of signs that are manifestations of any of a number of conditions that overstimulate the brain. Such signs include episodic impairment or loss of consciousness, abnormal motor phenomena or convulsions, psychic or sensory disturbances or perturbation of the autonomic nervous system. The term is often used interchangeably with SEIZURES or convulsions.

There are several methods for classifying the various types of epilepsy. On the basis of origin, epilepsy is idiopathic (cryptogenic, essential, genetic) or symptomatic (acquired, organic). Symptomatic epilepsy has a physical cause, for example, brain tumor, injury to the brain at birth, a wound or blow to the head, or an endocrine disorder.

autonomic e. see visceral epilepsy (below).

cortical e. seizures originating from a discrete focus in the cerebrum. Called also partial seizures.

idiopathic e. no cause can be diagnosed during life and no lesions are demonstrable at autopsy. The diagnosis is made by ruling out all extracranial and other intracranial causes. In dogs, this disorder occurs most frequently in certain breeds, particularly German shepherd dogs, miniature poodles, Keeshonds, Tervuren shepherds and Beagles, in which it is regarded as an inherited trait. Generalized seizures begin occurring at a young age, typically from 1 to 3 years; the affected dog is otherwise normal. Called also true epilepsy.

In affected cattle seizures occur from 2 to 3 months of age. A form of idiopathic epilepsy has been recorded in horses.

Jacksonian e. see JACKSONIAN EPILEPSY.

myoclonic e. see GLYCOPROTEINOSIS.

visceral e. a visceral response to a focus of irritation in the cerebral cortex, usually vomiting and diarrhea. Called also autonomic epilepsy.

epileptic 1. pertaining to or affected with epilepsy. 2. a patient affected with epilepsy.

e. seizure a clonic–tonic convulsion during an epileptic attack.

epileptiform 1. resembling epilepsy or its manifestations. 2. occurring in severe or sudden paroxysms.

epileptogenic causing an epileptic seizure, e.g. an epileptogenic scar in the cerebral cortex, or more significantly in the cerebrum and its proximate meningeal tissue.

epileptoid see EPILEPTIFORM.

epimastigote a developmental stage in trypanosomes. The undulating membrane is shortened and the axoneme and the kinetoplast are anterior to the nucleus; in the previous stage they are near the tail and behind the nucleus. This stage occurs usually in the arthropod host. Called also crithidial stage.

epimer one of two or more isomers which differ only in the configuration about one carbon atom.

epimerase an isomerase that catalyzes the inversion of asymmetric groups in substrates (epimers) having more than one center of asymmetry.

epimere the dorsal portion of a somite, from which is formed muscles innervated by the dorsal ramus of a spinal nerve.

epimerite an organelle of certain protozoa by which they attach themselves to epithelial cells.

epimerization the changing of one epimeric form of a compound into another, as by enzymatic action.

epimorphosis the regeneration of a piece of an organism by proliferation at the cut surface.

epimyocardial receptors pressure receptors in the left ventricle concerned with regulation of the blood volume.

epimysial sheath see EPIMYSIUM.

epimysium the fibrous sheath around an entire skeletal muscle.

epinephrectomy see ADRENALECTOMY.

epinephrine a hormone produced by the medulla of the ADRENAL glands; called also adrenaline. Its function is to aid in the regulation of the sympathetic branch of the AUTONOMIC nervous system. At times when an animal is highly stimulated, as by fear, anger or some challenging situation, extra amounts of epinephrine are released into the bloodstream, preparing the body for energetic action. Epinephrine is a powerful vasopressor which increases blood pressure and increases the heart rate and cardiac output. It also increases glycogenolysis and the release of glucose from the liver.

epineural situated upon a neural arch.

e. capping the surgical procedure of folding the

epineurium over the proximal end of a transected nerve and suturing it in place helps to prevent the development of painful neuroma.

epineurium the sheath of a peripheral nerve.

epiphora an abnormal overflow of tears down the face, due usually to stricture of the nasolacrimal duct. Called also illacrimation.

epiphyseal emanating from or pertaining to the epiphysis.

e. aseptic necrosis caused by (1) idiopathic primary necrosis of the epiphysis in growing small-breed dogs (Legg–Calvé–Perthes disease); (2) fracture of the femoral neck; or (3) epiphyseal slippage, particularly of the femoral head in young dogs, cats, pigs, calves and foals. The disease has a characteristic radiographic appearance.

e. cartilage between the epiphysis and the diaphysis of long bones; growth at the cartilage is responsible for continuing growth of the bone; when growth ceases the cartilage disappear. Called also growth plate, physis.

e. detachment see EPIPHYSIOLYSIS.

e. dysplasia an inherited defect of dogs characterized by very short limbs and early degenerative arthropathy. Called also chondrodystrophia fetalis and pseudoachondroplastic dysplasia of Miniature poodles. A similar histological lesion occurs in multiple epiphyseal dysplasia in Beagles.

e. fracture one involving the epiphysis. See also SALTER CLASSIFICATION.

e. plate the thin plate of cartilage between the epiphysis and the shaft of a long bone; it is the site of growth in length and is obliterated by epiphyseal closure. Called also growth plate, physis.

e. scar on radiographs, the radiodense band seen at the junction of the epiphysis and metaphysis, which represents the closed physis.

epiphysiolysis separation of the epiphysis from the diaphysis of a bone. It is a traumatic lesion originating from a defect in the growth plate, often osteochondrosis.

femoral head e. disease of 5–12 month old pigs, characterized by hindlimb lameness followed in a few days by inability to stand on the hindlimbs.

epiphysis pl. *epiphyses* [Gr.] 1. the end of a long bone, usually wider than the shaft, and either entirely cartilaginous or separated from the shaft by a cartilaginous disk. 2. part of a bone formed from a secondary center of ossification, commonly found at the ends of long bones, on the margins of flat bones, and at tubercles and processes; during the period of growth epiphyses are separated from the main portion of the bone by cartilage.

e. cerebri pineal body.

epiphysitis a lesion observed radiologically at the epiphyses of long bones and the ends of ribs of animals affected by osteodystrophy. Clinically there is swelling of the bone and there may be subsequent epiphysiolysis or separation of the femoral head. See also OSTEODYSTROPHY, PHYSEAL dysplasia.

epipial situated upon the pia mater.

epiplocele see OMENTAL hernia.

epiploenterocele a hernia containing intestine and omentum.

epiplomerocele a femoral hernia containing omentum.

epiplomphalocele an umbilical hernia containing omentum.

epiploon pl. *epiploa* [Gr.] the greater omentum.

Epipremnum pinnatum* cv. *aureum plant in family Araceae; contains oxalate raphide crystals; causes stomatitis, salivation. Called also devil's ivy, money plant.

epirubicin an anthracycline antibiotic similar to DOXORUBICIN, used as an antineoplastic agent.

episclera the loose, highly vascular connective tissue on the surface of the sclera; blends with Tenon's capsule.

episcleral 1. overlying the sclera. 2. pertaining to the episclera.

e. space narrow space between the deep muscular fascia and the eyeball.

episcleritis inflammation of the episclera and adjacent tissues.

nodular granulomatous e. see NODULAR fasciitis.

episioperineoplasty plastic repair of the vulva and perineum.

episioperineorrhaphy suture of the vulva and perineum.

episioplasty plastic repair of the vulva.

episiorrhaphy 1. suture of the labia majora. 2. suture of a lacerated perineum.

episiostenosis narrowing of the vulvar orifice.

episiotomy surgical incision into the perineum and vagina for obstetrical purposes.

episode a noteworthy happening occurring in the course of a continuous series of events.

episodic muscular weakness see HYPERKALEMIC PERIODIC PARALYSIS.

episome any accessory extrachromosomal replicating genetic element that can exist either autonomously or integrated with the chromosome. See also PLASMID.

epispadia see EPISPADIAS.

epispadias a congenital malformation with absence of the upper wall of the urethra, occurring in both sexes, but more commonly in the male, the urethral opening being located anywhere on the dorsum of the penis.

epispastic substance producing blisters on the skin. Called also vesicant.

episplenitis inflammation of the capsule of the spleen.

epistasis non-allelic masking of one gene by another, e.g. the masking of the black gene by the orange gene in tortoiseshell cats.

epistatic deviation deviation from normal additive gene action due to epistasis.

epistaxis bleeding from the nose. This is usually from damaged vessels in the nasal mucosa but can also be due to an increased fragility of capillaries or bleeding tendencies, particularly thrombocytopenia. Injury may be due to erosion or ulceration of the mucosa by a systemic disease, e.g. glanders in the horse, or by a local disease of the mucosa, e.g. allergic rhinitis, trauma to the face or to the head generally, in which case the bleeding is likely to be due to a serious lesion, or to foreign bodies up the nose, a common cause.

Bleeding from the nose originating from sites other than the nasal mucosa is a common and serious occurrence in all species but particularly in the horse because of its implication for safety while racing. The passage of large amounts of blood suddenly is usually associated with pulmonary hemorrhage and is often fatal in horses and cattle. In horses this usually occurs during hard exercise. When the bleeding in the horse occurs at rest the origin is commonly from the guttural pouch and due to mycotic erosion of the blood vessels there. See also GUTTURAL POUCH mycosis, PULMONARY hemorrhage.

episternal 1. situated on or over the sternum. 2. pertaining to the episternum.

episternum the manubrium, or cranial segment of the sternum.

epistropheus see AXIS (2).

Epistylis a genus of ciliated protozoan parasites in the phylum Ciliophora. Found commonly on the skin of freshwater fish; usually nonpathogenic.

epitendineum the fibrous sheath covering a tendon.

epitenon outer or parietal layers of tendons.

epithalamus the part of the diencephalon just superior and posterior to the thalamus, comprising the pineal body and adjacent structures; considered by some to include the stria medullaris.

epithelial pertaining to or composed of epithelium.

e. root sheath a fold of gingival epithelium which grows down into the dental alveolus and surrounds the tooth root.

e. tissue a general name for tissues not derived from the mesoderm.

epithelialization healing by the growth of epithelium over a denuded surface.

adnexal e. partial-thickness loss of epidermis can be re-epithelialized by epithelial cells from the remaining portions of adnexal structures.

epithelialize to cover with epithelium.

epitheliitis inflammation of the epithelium.

epitheliochorial see PLACENTA.

epitheliocystis disease of aquarium and marine fish caused by a chlamydia and characterized by small vesicles in the epidermal cells of the gills and skin.

epitheliogenesis development of the epithelium.

e. imperfecta congenital absence of the skin and commonly also the mucosae; an inherited defect in most animal species. It is incompatible with life. Called also aplasia cutis.

e. imperfecta linguae bovis see SMOOTH tongue.

epithelioid resembling epithelium.

e. cells histiocytes with elongated or oval vesicular nuclei and finely granular eosinophilic cytoplasm; seen in epithelioid sarcoma.

epitheliolysis destruction of epithelial tissue.

epithelioma any tumor derived from epithelium.

e. adenoides cysticum see TRICHOEPITHELIOMA.

basal cell e. see BASAL cell tumors.

benign calcifying e. see PILOMATRIXOMA.

intracutaneous cornifying e. a benign skin tumor of dogs that consists of a keratin-filled cyst, usually opening to the surface of the skin through a pore. Occasionally, and particularly in some breeds, tumors may be multiple or recurring.

e. of Malherbe see PILOMATRIXOMA.

sebaceous e. a benign tumor of sebaceous glands that is histologically similar to basal cell tumor.

epitheliosis proliferation of conjunctival epithelium, forming trachoma-like granules.

bovine e. see BOVINE malignant catarrh.

epitheliotropic having a special affinity for epithelial cells.

e. lymphoma closely resembles the same disease in humans. Occurs in older dogs in the form of exfoliative dermatitis, dermal plaques, nodules and ulcers.

epithelium pl. *epithelia* [Gr.] the cellular covering of internal and external surfaces of the body, including the lining of vessels and other small cavities. It consists of cells joined by small amounts of cementing substances. Epithelium is classified into types on the basis of the number of layers deep and the shape of the superficial cells. Standard classifications include ciliated (cilia attached), columnar (taller than wide), cuboidal (same height as width), pseudostratified (single layer but because of varying cell height appears to be more than one), simple (one cell layer), squamous (flattened, plate-like cells), stratified (more than one layer), transitional (variable number of layers apparent). Other types are listed below.

anterior e. the thin layer of stratified squamous cells that form the outermost layer of the cornea.

corneal e. see anterior epithelium (above).

germinal e. thickened peritoneal epithelium covering the gonad from earliest development; formerly thought to give rise to germ cells.

glandular e. that composed of secreting cells.

lens e. cuboidal epithelium covering the lens.

pigmentary e., pigmented e. that made of cells containing granules of pigment.

posterior e. the single layer of epithelial cells on the back of the cornea, between stroma and aqueous humour; the corneal endothelium.

retinal pigment e. see RETINA.

sense e., sensory e. see NEUROEPITHELIUM (1).

epithelization epithelialization.

epitonic abnormally tense or tonic.

epitope see antigenic DETERMINANT.

continuous e. contiguous amino acid sequences in a linear array.

discontinuous e. one in which amino acids are in close proximity in the folded protein, but distant when unfolded.

epitrichium see PERIDERM.

epitrochlea the medial condyle of the humerus.

epitympanic emanating from or pertaining to the eardrum.

e. recess see ATTIC.

epitympanum the upper part of the tympanum.

epivag an incompletely defined venereal disease of cattle, probably caused by a herpesvirus. Cows develop a profuse purulent vaginal discharge with spread of the infection to the uterus and rendering many cows sterile because of damage to the fallopian tube and bursa. Initially in bulls there is swelling followed by fibrosis of the epididymis; associated lesions include abscess formation, ampullitis, seminal vesiculitis and degeneration of the testicles. Recorded only in Africa.

epivaginitis see EPIVAG.

epizoic pertaining to or caused by an epizoon.

epizoon pl. *epizoa* [Gr.] an external animal parasite.

epizootic a disease which attacks many subjects in a region at the same time but is only occasionally present in the population; when it occurs it is widely diffused and rapidly spreading. The rarely used equivalent of epidemic in veterinary medicine.

e. cellulitis see EQUINE viral rhinopneumonitis.

e. cellulitis-pinkeye see EQUINE viral arteritis.

e. chlamydiosis a disease of rabbits, hares, deer mice, squirrels and muskrats caused by *Chlamydia* spp. and characterized by septicemia, fever, diarrhea.

e. diarrhea of infant mice see MURINE epizootic diarrhea.

e. hematopoietic necrosis reported only in Australian redfin perch and rainbow trout; characterized by massive mortalities in juvenile perch but dribbling mortalities in trout; caused by an iridovirus. May have originated in amphibians.

e. hemorrhagic disease of deer is caused by an orbivirus antigenically similar to the virus of Ibaraki disease, a bluetongue-like disease of cattle. The disease is clinically similar to bluetongue in sheep and causes very heavy mortalities in deer herds.

e. hemorrhagic septicemia see HEMORRHAGIC septicemia.

e. lymphangitis a chronic, contagious disease of horses caused by *Histoplasma farciminosum* (or

Blastomyces, Cryptococcus, Saccharomyces, Zymonema). It is characterized by suppurative lymphangitis, lymphadenitis and cutaneous ulcers. Lesions may also occur on the muzzle and nasal mucosa, in the eye causing keratitis, and also in the lungs causing pneumonia. The disease is an important one on its own account but it also has importance because of its similarity to glanders. Called also pseudoglanders.

e. pneumoenteritis see CHRONIC respiratory disease. Called also CRD.

e. ulcerative syndrome important cause of loss in ornamental fish and foodfish; extensive ulceration causes loss of fins, tail, jaw, and penetrates the abdominal wall. The cause has not been identified.

epizootiology with reference to animal diseases is the rarely used, etymologically proper, equivalent of EPIDEMIOLOGY.

EPN ethyl *p*-nitrophenyl benzenethiophosphanate; a nonsystemic organophosphorus insecticide and acaricide.

EPO see ERYTHROPOIETIN.

Epomidiostomum a genus of nematode worms in the family Amidostomidae. The worms cause hemorrhage and necrosis in the proventriculus and the stomach and gizzard. Includes, in geese, ducks and swans, *E. crispinum, E. skrjabini, E. uncinatum, E. vogelsangi.*

epontol see EUGENOL.

eponychium 1. the narrow band of epidermis extending from the claw wall onto the claw surface; commonly called cuticle. 2. the horny fetal epidermis at the site of the future claw.

eponym a name or phrase formed from or including a person's name, e.g. Theiler's disease, Cowper's gland, Aschheim–Zondek test.

epoophoron a vestigial structure associated with the ovary; originates from the cranial mesonephric tubules and cysts of it may resemble ovarian cysts.

epoprostenol see PROSTACYCLIN.

epornithic an epidemic in a population of birds.

epornithology the scientific study of those diseases of birds which occur in a community sporadically but with high morbidity: the study of avian epidemics.

epostane an antiprogesterone agent used to terminate pregnancy in dogs and to induce farrowing in sows.

epoxide any compound containing a three-membered ring of two carbon atoms and one oxygen atom, e.g. oxirane.

epoxy 1. containing one atom of oxygen bound to two different carbon atoms. 2. a resin composed of epoxy polymers and characterized by adhesiveness, flexibility and resistance to chemical actions.

epoxyscillirosidin toxic cardiac glycoside in HOMERIA *glauca*.

epsilon the fifth letter of the Greek alphabet ε.

e.-aminocaproic acid see ε-AMINOCAPROIC ACID.

e. cell see epsilon CELL.

epsiprantel a tapeworm anthelmintic.

Epsom salts magnesium sulfate, a cathartic.

EPSP excitatory postsynaptic potential.

Epstein–Barr virus see BURKITT'S LYMPHOMA.

EPTC *S*-ethyldipropylthiocarbamate; a thiocarbamate herbicide.

epulides see EPULIS.

epulis pl. *epulides* [Gr.] a benign tumor of mixed cell origin arising from periodontal squamous cell residues.

acanthomatous e. a locally invasive, sometimes recurrent, tumor of the gums of dogs and sometimes cats. Called also oral adamantinoma.

giant-cell e. see periodontal fibromatous epulis (below).

ossifying e. has a greater abundance of hard tissue, osteoid, bone and cementum than fibromatous epulides.

periodontal fibromatous e. firm, nodular benign structures on the lingual or labial gum margins, resembling normal gingiva in color and texture. Common in dogs, particularly the brachycephalic breeds. Considered by some to be hyperplastic rather than neoplastic. Called also giant-cell epulis.

epulosis a scarring over; cicatrization.

Eq equivalent; see chemical EQUIVALENT.

equatorial the circle which divides the spherical object into two equal halves.

e. region the middle piece; said of spindle muscle fibers.

equestrian a rider of horses.

equid see EQUIDAE.

Equidae a family of mammals, members of which have a single functional digit although the second and third digits persist as splint bones. Includes horses, wild horses, asses (donkeys) and zebras. Quaggas were a member of the family but are now extinct.

equilenin one of two estrogens produced by the pregnant mare which are unique to Equidae. Both have unsaturated B rings.

equilibration the achievement of a balance between opposing elements or forces.

equilibrium a state of balance between opposing forces or influences. In the body, equilibrium may be chemical or physical. A state of *chemical equilibrium* is reached when the body tissues contain the proper proportions of various salts and water. See also ACID–BASE BALANCE and FLUID BALANCE. *Physical equilibrium*, such as the state of balance required for walking or standing, is achieved by a very complex interplay of opposing sets of muscles. The labyrinth of the inner ear contains the semicircular canals, or organs of balance, and relays to the brain information about the body's position and also the direction of body motions. *Genetic equilibrium* is achieved when the allelic frequencies do not change from generation to generation.

e. dialysis a technique for determining the affinity of an antibody for an antigen.

e. disturbances see POSTURE, posture BALANCE.

dynamic e. the condition of balance between varying, shifting and opposing forces that is characteristic of living processes.

equilin one of two estrogens produced by the pregnant mare that are unique to Equidae. They have unsaturated B rings.

equimarginal returns a technique of financial management in which units of capital are allocated to variable inputs of the various enterprises in a business, such as a farm, in sequence from the most to the least profitable until capital is exhausted.

equine pertaining to, characteristic of, or derived from the horse.

e. abortion infectious causes include equine herpesvirus 1, equine viral arteritis, *Salmonella abortusequi*. See also equine VIRAL abortion.

acute e. respiratory syndrome see equine morbillivirus (below) and ACUTE EQUINE RESPIRATORY SYNDROME.

e. adenovirus see equine ADENOVIRUS (types 1 and 2).

e. allergic rhinitis seasonal occurrence, acute onset, sneezing, nasal discharge, nose rubbing, no mucosal lesion; common cause of head shaking.

e. alphaherpesvirus see HERPESVIRIDAE.

e. arteritis see equine viral arteritis (below).
e. babesiosis see BABESIOSIS.
e. biliary fever see BABESIOSIS.
e. chorionic gonadatropin see PREGNANT mare serum gonadatropin.
e. coital exanthema see equine COITAL EXANTHEMA.
e. colic see equine COLIC.
contagious e. metritis called also CEM; see CONTAGIOUS equine metritis.
e. ehrlichial colitis see equine intestinal EHRLICHIOSIS.
e. ehrlichiosis see equine EHRLICHIOSIS.
e. encephalitis see BORNA DISEASE, equine viral ENCEPHALOMYELITIS, equine herpesvirus 1 (below).
e. encephalosis a disease in horses in South Africa, caused by an orbivirus, distinct from African horse sickness. It is characterized by abortion and encephalitis.
e. eosinophilic granuloma see equine nodular collagenolytic granuloma (below).
e. epidemic cough see equine influenza (below).
e. farcy see GLANDERS.
e. herpesvirus 1 (EHV1) the major cause of equine viral abortion (see also equine VIRAL abortion) and an encephalomyelitis. The latter is characterized by nervous signs varying from mild ataxia to enforced recumbency. Also causes respiratory disease (rhinopneumonitis), but the distinctly different equine herpesvirus 4, is more commonly identified as the cause of rhinopneumonitis and rarely abortion. A paralytic syndrome also occurs but usually in horses that are reinfected or, in a few instances, have been vaccinated. The disease may be a transitory incoordination or a permanent recumbency necessitating euthanasia. The virus may also cause viremia in newborn foals, the foals showing severe mental depression—sleepy foals.
e. herpesvirus 2 (EHV2) a very common infection of horses, often asymptomatic but also associated with a variety of signs including pharyngitis, malaise and coughing. Formerly called equine cytomegalovirus or slowly growing equine herpesvirus, but now known to be a gammaherpesvirus 2 genus.
e. herpesvirus 3 (EHV3) see equine COITAL EXANTHEMA.
e. herpesvirus 4 (EHV4) a major cause of equine viral rhinopneumonitis (below).
e. herpesvirus 5 (EHV5) a member of the gammaherpesvirus 2 genus distinctly different from EHV2.
e. histoplasmosis see EPIZOOTIC lymphangitis.
e. incoordination see ENZOOTIC equine incoordination.
e. infectious anemia (EIA) is caused by a nononcogenic retrovirus in the subfamily *Lentivirinae*. After an initial acute attack of fever, weakness to the point of incoordination, jaundice, petechiation of the mucosae and conjunctivae and ventral edema, there are alternating periods of normality and illness that may continue for many years. During ensuing attacks there is a gradual development of anemia, emaciation and cardiac insufficiency. The disease is contagious to all Equidae and is spread by biting flies and mosquitoes. Spread by veterinary equipment has occurred frequently in the past.
infectious e. bronchitis see equine influenza (below).
e. influenza an infectious disease of the upper respiratory tract of horses of all ages, and caused by members of the family *Orthomyxoviridae*, genus A. The identified viruses are influenza A/Equi Prague/56 (H7N7) and A/Equi-2/Miami/63 (H3N8). The clinical signs typical of the infection are a minor fever and a persistent, long-term cough which prevents the horse being exercised. Droplet infection is highly effective and the disease has the capacity to reach epidemic proportions quickly and disrupt racing and other equine activities. The course is about 3 weeks and there are usually no serious sequelae if the horse is cared for properly. Formerly called with some uncertainty also equine infectious bronchitis, Hoppengarten cough, laryngotracheobronchitis, shipping fever. Effective inactivated vaccines are available although the duration of protective immunity to infection is short. The viruses do not show the same degree of antigenic change (drift and shift) evident in human influenza A viruses.
e. laryngeal hemiplegia see LARYNGEAL hemiplegia.
e. linear keratosis vertical linear areas of alopecia, scaling and crust formation on the sides of the neck, shoulder and chest.
e. lipemia see equine HYPERLIPEMIA.
e. monocytic ehrlichiosis see equine intestinal EHRLICHIOSIS.
e. morbillivirus a virus which in morphology and nucleotide sequence is similar to morbilliviruses and parainfluenza virus but will probably be assigned to a new genus in the family *Paramyxovirinae*. The virus causes fatal illness in horses and humans following 'natural' infection, and of guinea pigs and cats following experimental inoculation. See ACUTE EQUINE RESPIRATORY SYNDROME.
e. nodular collagenolytic granuloma firm subcutaneous nodules 0.5 to 5 mm diameter on the side of the neck, withers and back. They are eosinophilic granulomas and the cause is not known.
e. papular dermatitis a transient skin disease of horses which may be caused by a virus. Begins with 0.25 to 1 inch diameter papules which subsequently crust over and then become alopecic. A number of horses are likely to be affected at the one time and an insect vector is suspected.
e. parainfluenza 3 see PARAINFLUENZAVIRUS 3.
e. plague see AFRICAN HORSE SICKNESS.
e. recurrent ophthalmia see periodic OPHTHALMIA.
e. reovirus see REOVIRUS.
e. rhinopneumonitis see equine viral rhinopneumonitis (below).
e. rhinovirus 1 and 2 (ERhV1, ERhV2) members of the family *Picornaviridae*, they cause an upper respiratory tract infection in horses with laryngitis and a copious sometimes purulent nasal discharge. ERhV1 is most closely related to aphthoviruses and ERhV2 shows some similarity to cardioviruses. Infection with ERhV1 is accompanied by viremia and systemic signs including fever.
e. sarcoid a common transplantable cutaneous neoplasm in horses. The cause is unknown but similar lesions can be caused by the intracutaneous injection of bovine papilloma virus. Lesions are hairless fibroid tumor masses that frequently ulcerate, look like large warts, often recur after excision, and occur most commonly on the lower legs but can occur on any part of the body. See also SARCOID.
e. sensory ataxia see ENZOOTIC equine incoordination.
e. serum hepatitis see POSTVACCINAL hepatitis.
e. spinal ataxia see equine protozoal ENCEPHALOMYELITIS.
e. sports medicine all aspects of equine medicine which touch on quality of performance by show, event or racing horses; particular attention paid to diseases of the respiratory, cardiovascular and musculoskeletal systems.

e. staphylococcal dermatitis a contagious but low prevalence equine dermatitis from which *Staphylococcus aureus* can be isolated regularly. Small, painful nodules appear under the harness; subsequently become pustular and rupture. Called also saddle scab, tail pyoderma.

e. sternal granuloma see BREAST boil.

e. tropical lichen see equine ALLERGIC dermatitis.

e. viral abortion see equine herpesvirus 1 (above).

e. viral arteritis (EVA) a member of the family *Arteriviridae*, genus *Arterivirus*, causes this acute, severe infection of the upper respiratory tract of horses of all ages. Clinically the disease is more severe than the URTIs, the signs including abortion, conjunctivitis with edema of the conjunctiva, spasm of the eyelids and a profuse discharge. Coughing is severe and there is edema of the legs and ventral abdominal wall.

e. viral encephalomyelitis see equine viral ENCEPHALOMYELITIS.

e. viral rhinopneumonitis (EVR) predominantly caused by equine herpesvirus 4. Occasionally this virus has caused abortion, but EHV1 is the predominant cause of abortion. The rhinopneumonitis is manifested by a cough, serous nasal discharge, mild conjunctivitis and fever. Abortion, when it occurs, does so in the last few months of pregnancy and the mare is not systemically ill at that time.

e. zygomycosis see SWAMP CANCER.

equinovalgus a deformity of the lower limb in which the flexor tendons are contracted and the fetlock is straight or knuckled over in front.

equinovarus talipes equinovarus; a foot deformity in which the heel is turned inward and the foot is plantar flexed.

equipotential having similar and equal power or capability.

equipotentiality the quality or state of having similar and equal power; the capacity for developing in the same way and to the same extent.

Equisetum genus of the fern ally family Equisetaceae; These plants have a high content of thiaminase, and horses which eat a lot of them, usually in their hay, develop thiamin deficiency. This is characterized by incoordination, falling, bradycardia and severe cardiac irregularity. Response to treatment with thiamin is rapid and complete.

Includes *E. arvense*, *E. hyemale*, *E. laevigatum*, *E. limosum*, *E. palustre*, *E. ramosissimum*. Called also horsetails, foxtails, marestails.

equitation the art of horsemanship.

Equithesin a mixture of chloral hydrate, magnesium sulfate and pentobarbital used as an anesthetic, especially for horses. Thirty years ago this was the preferred equine anesthetic. It was very safe, the dose rate was easy to adjust and the anesthesia was good and could be maintained for several hours. It had the disadvantage of having to be freshly mixed just before use.

equity 1. a justifiable share; one likely to be recognized as a fair share in an equity court. 2. total assets less total liabilities.

e. capital the value of the capital involved in the enterprise. Includes assets less liabilities, expressed as a fixed sum.

percentage e. absolute equity expressed as a proportion of the total worth of the enterprise.

equivalence zone a variable ratio of antigen and antibody which results in precipitation in which there is no unbound antibody or antigen.

equivalency the combining power of an electrolyte. See also EQUIVALENT.

equivalent 1. of equal force, power, value, etc. 2. something that has equivalent properties. 3. chemical equivalent.

chemical e. that weight in grams of a substance that will produce or react with 1 mole of hydrogen ion or 1 mole of electrons. Symbol Eq. The concentrations of electrolytes are often specified in milliequivalents per liter (mEq/l).

epilepsy e. any disturbance, mental or physical, that may take the place of an epileptic seizure.

temperature e. see Table 5.

equol isoflavan.

equulosis the disease caused by infection with *Actinobacillus equuli.* See also SHIGELLOSIS.

Equus see EQUUS.

E. burchelli common ZEBRA.

E. caballus the modern horse.

E. grevyi Grevyi's ZEBRA.

E. przewalskii see MONGOLIAN WILD HORSE.

E. zebra see ZEBRA.

equus the final stage of the evolution of the horse. The evolution appears to have been direct beginning with *Eohippus*, through *Miohippus* and *Merychippus* to *Pliohippus* and finally to *Equus.*

Er chemical symbol, *erbium.*

ER bodies erythrocyte refractile bodies; see Heinz BODY.

eradication extermination of an infectious agent so that no further cases of the related disease can occur.

virtual e. reduction of the frequency of occurrence of a disease to an arbitrary level which is considered to be not a threat to the animal population at risk.

erasion removal by scraping or curettage.

Erb–Goldflam disease myasthenia gravis.

erbium a chemical element, atomic number 68, atomic weight 167.26, symbol Er. See Table 6.

Erb's dystrophy a human condition; called also pseudohypertrophic muscular dystrophy.

Erechtites see SENECIO.

erect position the patient is held upright standing on its hindlegs.

erectile capable of erection.

e. tissue spongy tissue that expands and becomes firm when filled with blood, e.g. corpus cavernosum of the penis.

erection the condition of becoming rigid and elevated, as erectile tissue when filled with blood; applied especially to the swelling and rigidity that occur in the penis as a result of sexual or other types of stimulation. Impulses received by the nervous system stimulate a flow of blood from the arteries leading to the penis, where the erectile tissue fills with blood, and the penis becomes firm and erect. Erection makes possible the transmission of semen into the body of the female. See REPRODUCTION.

persistent e. see PRIAPISM.

erector [L.] a structure that erects, as a muscle that holds up or raises a part.

Eremocarpus setigerus North American plant in the family Euphorbiaceae; contains large proportion of indigestible roughage which causes abomasal impaction, regurgitation, vomiting. Called also turkey mullein.

Eremophila an Australian plant genus of the Myoporaceae family; *E. maculata* contains cyanogenetic glycosides and can cause hydrocyanic acid poisoning. Toxic species include *E. latrobei*, *E. longifolia*, *E. maculata* (native fuchsia).

erethism excessive irritability or sensitivity to stimulation.

erethisophrenia exaggerated mental excitability.

ERG electroretinogram.
erg a unit of work or energy, equivalent to 1.0×10^{-7} joules, to 2.4×10^{-8} calories, or to 0.624×10^{12} electron volts.
erg- prefix meaning work.
ergasia any mentally integrated function, activity, reaction or attitude of an individual.
Ergasilus a miniature crustacean of the subclass Copepoda.
E. sieboldi found as parasites on the gills of many freshwater fish causing impairment of the respiration, growth and sexual maturation. Heavy infestations can kill the host fish.
ergocalciferol vitamin D_2; an oil-soluble antirachitic vitamin. See also VITAMIN D.
ergograph an instrument for measuring work done in muscular action.
ergometrine see ERGONOVINE.
ergonomics the science of relating the physiological and anatomical characteristics of the working or racing animal to the physical aspects of its working environment.
ergonovine one of the alkaloids from ERGOT[I] or produced synthetically, used as an oxytocic.
ergosterol a sterol occurring in animal and plant tissues which on ultraviolet irradiation becomes a potent antirachitic substance, vitamin D_2 (ergocalciferol).
ergot[1] the dried sclerotia of the fungi *Claviceps* spp. parasitic on grass seed heads.
e. alkaloids clavine alkaloids, lysergic acid and its amides and ergot peptide alkaloids (ergotamine, ergosine, ergocristine etc.).
bulrush millet e. *Claviceps fusiformis* parasitizes bulrush millet (*Pennisetum glaucum*) and causes agalactia and piglet loss in sows. Called also munga ergot.
paspalum e. *Claviceps paspali* is an ergot fungus that parasitizes *Paspalum* spp. Animals eating the infected plants are poisoned; the clinical syndrome consisting of gross incoordination is indistinguishable from cerebellar ataxia. Recovery is quick and complete if the animals are removed from the contaminated pasture.
rye e. *Claviceps purpurea*, the ergot of rye, infests cereal rye and other grasses including *Lolium* spp. It contains a number of alkaloids one of which, ergonovine (ergometrine), is extracted and used pharmaceutically as an oxytocin. Livestock and humans fed on contaminated grain or seed from affected crops develop chronic ergotism, the classical syndrome of gangrene of the extremities in cold weather or hyperthermia in hot conditions. Central nervous system stimulation, characterized by drowsiness, incoordination and convulsions, occurs if large amounts of the ergot are taken. Abortion is a constant sign of the poisoning in humans but does not occur in any of the domestic animals.
ergot[2] the small mass of horn in a small bunch of hair on the palmar or plantar aspects of the fetlock of the horse. Regarded as the vestige of the metacarpal or metatarsal pads.
e. ligament shimmering band of connective tissue connecting the fetlock ergot to the distal parts of the pastern in the horse. It is easily confused with the digital nerves during neurectomy.
ergotamine an alkaloid derived from rye ergot; the tartrate is used as an oxytocic.
ergotherapy treatment of disease by physical effort.
ergothioneine a sulfur-containing base, present in significant quantities in the semen of the boar and the stallion, which is thought to protect spermatozoa against oxidizing agents. In other species this role is played by ascorbic acid.
ergotism see rye ERGOT[I].
ergotoxin a mixture of alkaloids extracted from *Claviceps purpurea.* Has vasoconstrictor and ecbolic actions.
ergovaline ergot alkaloid found in ACREMONIUM *coenophialum.*
ERhV equine rhinovirus.
Erinaceus see HEDGEHOG.
Eriobotrya japonica tree in the family Rosaceae, has edible fruits the seeds of which contain sufficient cyanide to cause poisoning if eaten in quantity. Called also loquat.
Eriocephalus ericoides, E. glaber African plant in the Asteraceae family; causes pyloric obstruction because of high content of indigestible fiber.
Eristalis a genus of flies in the family Syrphidae whose maggots breed in drains. Called filth flies, rat-tailed maggots.
ermine 1. the European stoat, *Mustela erminea.* 2. the pelt of *Mustela erminea.*
e. marks small brown or black spots on a white section of coat surrounding one or more coronets; resembles ermine.
Ermine Rex a rabbit; see REX (2).
Erodium two Australian species of the genus, belonging to the family Geraniaceae, *E. cicutarium* and *E. moschatum* are alleged to cause photosensitization without there being a hepatic lesion; no specific toxin has been identified. Called also storksbill.
Erophaca baetica ASTRAGALUS *lusitanicus.*
erosion an eating or gnawing away; a shallow or superficial ulceration; in dentistry, the wasting away or loss of substance of a tooth by a chemical process that does not involve known bacterial action.
erosive stomatitis a disease of the mouth characterized by the presence of discrete, superficial ulcers or erosions of the mucosal surface, as in bovine mucosal disease, rinderpest and mucosal disease of cattle. Secondary ulcerative stomatitis is common.
endemic e. s. of cattle recorded in Africa. Similar to and may be identical with bovine PAPULAR stomatitis.
ERPF effective renal plasma flow.
errhine promoting a nasal discharge; an agent that so acts.
Errington's disease a disease of snowshoe hare, rabbit and muskrat characterized by hemorrhagic enteritis and focal hepatic necrosis. The cause is not defined but *Clostridium welchii*, *Francisella tularensis* and *Leptospira* spp. have all been implicated.
error 1. the wrong answer in an experiment or result to a questionnaire. 2. malfunction in a computer or program.
experimental e. of two types, errors of objectivity when the experimenter knows the groups and the expected result, and errors of detection or measurement due to inadequate technique or the uneven application of measuring techniques.
e. message displayed on the computer screen when a malfunction or an error is detected. The messages are renowned for their cryptic style.
random e. error which occurs due to chance, such as sampling error.
sampling e. one due to the fact that the result obtained from a sample is only an estimate of that obtained from using the entire population.
systematic e. when the error is applied to all results, i.e. those due to bias.
e. types I and II in making a statistical test, you can

reject the null hypothesis when it is true (type I) or accept the null hypothesis when it is false (type II).

eructate performance of the act of eructation.

eructation the oral ejection of gas or air from the stomach; belching. A normal activity for ruminants who void gases, principally methane, produced by fermentation in the rumen. Interference with eructation in those species causes ruminal tympany or BLOAT (1).

eruption 1. the act of breaking out, appearing or becoming visible, as eruption of the teeth. 2. visible efflorescent lesions of the skin due to disease, with redness, prominence, or both; a rash.

creeping e. see cutaneous LARVA migrans.

drug e. see DRUG eruption.

tooth e. used in veterinary medicine as a guide to an animal's age.

grouped tooth e. permanent posterior teeth erupting side by side with no replacement horizontally.

sequential tooth e. permanent posterior teeth replaced by craniad movement of caudal teeth; seen in macropods and elephants.

tooth e. times see Table 19.

ERV expiratory reserve volume.

erva cafe [Span.] PALICOUREA *marcgravii.*

erva de rato [Span.] PALICOUREA *marcgravii.*

Ervum a genus of the plant family Leguminosae; contains an unidentified toxin which causes depression, vomiting, incoordination, coma in pigs. Includes *E. ervilia* (bastard lentil, bitter vetch), *E. lens* (*Lens culinaris, L. esculenta* lentil).

Erwinia a genus of plant pathogens and saprophytes. See also ENTEROBACTERIACEAE.

Erysimum cheiranthoides toxic plant in the family Brassicaceae; contains mustard oil glucosinolates which cause stomatitis, vomiting, diarrhea. Called also wormseed mustard.

erysipelas 1. infection with *Erysipelothrix rhusiopathiae*; occurs rarely in cattle and sheep, principally as an arthritis and laminitis, occasionally as a systemic infection. It is a common and serious infection in pigs and turkeys. In pigs it may be a septicemia with characteristic diamond-shaped skin lesions, or a chronic disease manifested principally as arthritis, sometimes as endocarditis. Turkeys are the only bird species affected at a significant level. In them the disease is manifested as a septicemia with no diagnostic signs. 2. An erythematous–edematous lesion, commonly on the hand, resulting from contact with infected meat, hides or bones; the usual lesion in humans and is called erysipeloid.

erysipelatous pertaining to or of the nature of erysipelas.

erysipeloid see ERYSIPELOTHRIX.

Erysipelothrix a genus of bacteria containing a single species; short gram-positive rods which show remarkable longevity in alkaline soils. Once the infection appears on a farm it is likely to recur.

E. rhusiopathiae the causative organism of swine ERYSIPELAS, which also infects sheep, turkeys and rats. Formerly called *E. insidiosa.*

erythema redness of the skin caused by congestion of the capillaries in the lower layers of the skin. It occurs with any skin injury, infection or inflammation.

e. ab igne that due to exposure to radiant heat.

e. chronicum migrans the early skin rash at the site of the tick bite which infects humans with *Borellia burgdorferi* (Lyme disease); rarely seen in dogs.

e. multiforme a disease of unknown etiology, but is sometimes drug-related; presumed to be immune-mediated. It occurs in all species and is characterized by an acute onset of erythematous macules, papules, vesicles or bullae. There may also be fever, depression and anorexia.

e. multiforme major a rapidly fulminating, ulcerative form of erythema multiforme with involvement of oral mucosa and systemic signs.

necrolytic migratory e. in humans, a skin disease associated with glucagon-secreting tumors of the pancreas. The same association has not been observed in dogs, but disease of the liver and pancreas is often present. There are vesicles and crusted, ulcerated lesions, mainly on the face, mucocutaneous areas, distal limbs and feet.

e. nodosum a rare disorder in dogs characterized by fever, depression, arthralgia and septal panniculitis.

toxic e., e. toxicum a generalized erythematous or erythematomacular eruption due to administration of a drug or to bacterial toxins or other toxic substances.

erythematous characterized by erythema.

Erythizon dorsatum see PORCUPINE.

erythremia see POLYCYTHEMIA.

erythremic myelosis a myeloproliferative disorder of cats, rarely other species, manifested by marked anemia but with marked anisocytosis without an accompanying polychromasia. Large numbers of rubricytes can be found in the bone marrow and sometimes in the circulation. The condition has been compared to Di Guglielmo syndrome in humans. Feline leukemia virus has been implicated in the etiology.

blast form of e. m. previously called reticuloendotheliosis, the predominant cell type is more primitive.

erythritol the sugar present in high concentration in the genital tract of the male and the pregnant female and enhances the growth of *Brucella abortus,* which preferentially utilizes erythritol.

erythr(o)- word element. [Gr.] *red, erythrocyte.*

erythroblast originally, any nucleated erythrocyte, but now more generally used to designate the nucleated precursor from which an erythrocyte develops.

basophilic e. see NORMOBLAST.

orthochromatic e. see NORMOBLAST, METARUBRICYTE.

polychromatophilic e. see NORMOBLAST.

erythroblastemia the presence in the peripheral blood of abnormally large numbers of nucleated red cells; erythroblastosis.

erythroblastic of, or relating to erythroblasts.

e. islets a bone marrow unit consisting of a central macrophage and surrounding erythroblasts and in which differentiation of erythroblasts takes place.

erythroblastoma a tumor-like mass composed of nucleated red cells.

erythroblastopenia abnormal deficiency of erythroblasts.

erythroblastosis the presence of erythroblasts in the circulating blood.

avian e. caused by the viruses of the leukosis/sarcoma group. Manifested by weakness, pallor, comb cyanosis, diarrhea and spontaneous hemorrhage.

e. fetalis, e. neonatorum see neonatal HEMORRHAGIC disease, ALLOIMMUNE hemolytic anemia of the newborn.

Erythrocebus patas see PATAS MONKEY.

erythrochromia hemorrhagic, red pigmentation of the cerebrospinal fluid.

erythroclasia splitting up of erythrocytes.

erythroclasis fragmentation of the red blood cells.

erythrocuprin see CERULOPLASMIN.

erythrocytapheresis the withdrawal of blood, separation and retention of red blood cells, and retransfusion of the remainder into the donor.

erythrocyte a red BLOOD cell, or corpuscle; one of the formed elements in the peripheral blood. For immature forms see NORMOBLAST, METARUBRICYTE. In most mammals mature erythrocytes are biconcave disks that have no nuclei. The degree of concavity varies between species, as does the size. Birds have nucleated, oval erythrocytes. The cell consists mainly of hemoglobin and a supporting framework, called the stroma. Erythrocyte formation (erythropoiesis) takes place in the red bone marrow in the adult, and in the liver, spleen and bone marrow of the fetus. Erythrocyte formation requires an ample supply of certain dietary elements such as iron, cobalt and copper, amino acids and certain vitamins.

e. antigen see blood group ANTIGEN and BLOOD GROUP.

e. casts see urinary CAST.

e. count see BLOOD COUNT.

e. ghosts in new methylene blue, erythrocytes fail to take up stain and appear only as a pale outline.

hypochromatic e. see HYPOCHROMIA (2).

e. indices calculated values for the mean corpuscular volume (MCV), mean corpuscular hemoglobin (MCH), and mean corpuscular hemoglobin concentration (MCHC), taken from the hematocrit, hemoglobin concentration and red blood cell count. Used in determining the likely etiology of anemias and other abnormalities of the erythron. Called also mean cell constants.

matchstick e. describes the appearance of sickled deer erythrocytes containing hemoglobin II.

normochromic e. see NORMOCHROMIA.

e. refractile bodies (ERF) a term usually used to describe Heinz bodies in the erythrocytes of cats. Sometimes restricted in definition to the smaller (Heinz) bodies that are normally found in up to 10% of feline erythrocytes, as distinct from larger bodies associated with hemolytic anemia.

e. sedimentation rate (ESR) an expression of the extent of settling of erythrocytes in a column of fresh citrated or otherwise treated blood, per unit of time. Of greatest diagnostic value in dogs as horses normally have a greatly accelerated rate and ruminants show none except in very extreme circumstances. In the dog, ESR is elevated with inflammatory processes. See also SEDIMENTATION rate.

e. tonicity the degree of distension of the erythrocyte. This is dependent on the osmotic pressure of the cell's contents compared with that of the plasma. If it is greater, water will pass into the cell and it may rupture. If it is less, water passes out of the cell which shrinks and becomes crenated.

e. volume mean corpuscular volume (MCV); see erythrocyte indices (above).

erythrocythemia an increase in the number of erythrocytes in the blood, as in erythrocytosis.

erythrocytic 1. pertaining to, characterized by, or of the nature of erythrocytes. 2. pertaining to the erythrocytic series.

erythrocyto-opsonin see HEMOPSONIN.

erythrocytolysin a substance that produces erythrocytolysis.

erythrocytolysis dissolution of erythrocytes and escape of hemoglobin.

erythrocytorrhexis a morphological change in erythrocytes, consisting in the escape from the cells of round, shiny granules and splitting off of particles; called also plasmorrhexis.

erythrocytosis increase in the total red cell mass secondary to any of a number of nonhematogenic systemic disorders in response to a known stimulus (secondary polycythemia), in contrast to primary polycythemia (polycythemia vera).

e. stimulating factor a lipid isolated from the plasma of anemic animals; distinct from erythropoietin, causes production of microcytes without increasing hemoglobin. Its role in disease is unknown.

stress e. an apparent polycythemia resulting from diminished plasma volume.

erythroderma abnormal redness of the skin over widespread areas of the body.

exfoliative e. reported in a single cow and her calves; believed to be an immune-mediated disorder associated with colostrum.

lymphomatous e. widespread redness of the skin associated with lymphoma.

maculopapular e. a reddish eruption composed of maculae and papules.

erythrodermatitis a disease of pond fish caused by *Aeromonas salmonicida* and characterized by ulcers of the skin and a high mortality rate. Called also carp erythrodermatitis.

erythrodontia reddish-brown pigmentation of the teeth.

erythrogenesis the production of erythrocytes.

erythrogenic 1. producing erythrocytes. 2. producing or causing erythema.

erythrogenin see ERYTHROPOIETIN.

erythrogonium see PROMEGALOBLAST.

erythroid 1. of a red color; reddish. 2. pertaining to the developmental series of cells ending in erythrocytes.

e. aplasia see pure red cell APLASIA.

burst forming unit-e. produced in in vitro cultures of erythroid stem cells. It has low sensitivity to erythropoietin and gives rise to colony forming unit-erythroid which, with erythropoietin, gives rise to erythroid cells.

e. hypoplasia see hypoplastic ANEMIA.

e. leukosis see avian ERYTHROBLASTOSIS.

erythrokeratodermia a reddening and hyperkeratosis of the skin.

erythrokinetics the quantitative, dynamic study of in vivo production and destruction of erythrocytes.

erythroleukemia a malignant blood dyscrasia of dogs and cats; one of the myeloproliferative disorders, with atypical erythroblasts and myeloblasts in the peripheral blood.

erythroleukosis see avian ERYTHROBLASTOSIS.

erythrolysis erythrocytolysis; dissolution of erythrocytes and escape of hemoglobin.

erythromycin a broad-spectrum antibiotic produced by a strain of *Streptomyces erythreus.* It is effective against a wide variety of organisms, including gram-negative and gram-positive bacteria. The stearate can be given orally; the lactobionate is a soluble salt which can be administered intravenously.

erythron the circulating erythrocytes in the blood, their precursors, and all the body elements concerned in their production.

erythroneocytosis the presence of immature erythrocytes in the blood.

erythropenia deficiency in the number of erythrocytes.

erythrophage a phagocyte that ingests erythrocytes.

erythrophagia, erythrophagocytosis phagocytosis of erythrocytes.

erythropheresis see ERYTHROCYTAPHERESIS.

erythrophil 1. a cell or other element that stains easily with red. 2. erythrophilous.

erythrophilous easily staining red.
erythrophleine alkaloid esters of diterpenoid acids, the toxic agent in the tree *Erythrophleum chlorostachys*.
Erythrophleum a plant genus of the Caesalpiniaceae family from Africa, Asia and Australia; contain diterpenoid alkaloids, e.g. erythrophleine, cause a clinical syndrome of tremor, ataxia, increased intensity of the heart sounds, dyspnea and sudden death. Includes *E. africanum*, *E. chlorostachys* (Cooktown ironwood tree, camel poison), *E. guineense* (sassy bark).
erythrophthisis a condition characterized by severe impairment of the restorative power of the erythrocyte-forming tissues.
erythropoiesis the formation of erythrocytes. Called also hematopoiesis.
balanced e. balanced progressive development of the nucleus and the cytosol of the erythrocytes.
ineffective e. hemopoietic production which does not result in the functional release of new erythrocytes.
erythropoietic emanating from or pertaining to erythropoiesis.
e. porphyria porphyria of genetic origin; a manifestation of involvement of erythropoietic tissue.
e. protoporphyria protoporphyria of genetic origin in which the defect in porphyrin metabolism is in the erythropoietic tissue. In the bovine disease the deficiency is of heme synthetase (ferrochelatase).
erythropoietin a glycoprotein hormone secreted mainly by the kidney. A profactor, erythropoietinogen, is first produced in the liver, transferred to the kidney and converted to active erythropoietin in the kidney. The erythropoietin acts on stem cells of the bone marrow to stimulate red blood cell production (erythropoiesis). Called also erythropoietin stimulating factor, erythrogenin.
recombinant e. used to treat dogs and cats with nonregenerative anemia of renal disease; animals develop antibodies to the human product.
e. stimulating factor see erythropoietin (above).
erythropoietinogen precursor of ERYTHROPOIETIN.
erythrosine depresses thyroid function by inhibiting 5′-deiodinase.
erythrosis 1. reddish or purplish discoloration of the skin and mucous membranes, as in polycythemia vera. 2. hyperplasia of the hematopoietic tissue.
erythrostasis the stoppage of erythrocytes in the capillaries, as in disseminated intravascular coagulation.
Erythroxylum coca a South American plant in family Erythroxylaceae from which cocaine is extracted. *E. bolivianum* is also used.
erythruria excretion of red urine.
Es chemical symbol, *einsteinium*.
escape 1. the act of becoming free. 2. a keyboard control key on a computer which enables the operator to stop any routine in a computer program.
vagal e. the exhaustion of or adaptation to neural chemical mediators in the regulation of systemic arterial pressure.
ventricular e. extrasystole in which a ventricular pacemaker becomes effective before the sinoatrial pacemaker; it usually occurs with slow sinus rates and often, but not necessarily, with increased vagal tone.
eschar a deep cutaneous slough such as that produced by a thermal burn, a corrosive action, a decubitus ulcer, a saddle gall or setfast.
escharotic 1. capable of producing an eschar; corrosive. 2. a corrosive or caustic agent.
escharotomy surgical incision of the eschar and superficial fascia of a circumferentially burned limb in order to permit the cut edges to separate and restore blood flow to unburned tissue distal to the eschar. Edema may form beneath the inelastic eschar of a full-thickness burn and compress arteries, thus impairing blood flow and necessitating an escharotomy. The incision is protected from infection with the same antimicrobial agent being used on the burn wound.
Escherichia a genus of widely distributed gram-negative bacteria in the family Enterobacteriaceae.
E. coli a species constituting the greater part of the normal intestinal flora of animals. The organism most used in recombinant DNA work. Pathogenic strains a cause of urinary tract infections, epidemic diarrheal diseases, especially in newborn animals and late respiratory disease in broiler chickens. Also a common opportunistic pathogen. See COLIBACILLOSIS, COLIFORM mastitis, COLIFORM gastroenteritis, avian COLIFORM septicemia, MASTITIS–METRITIS–AGALACTIA. See also ENTEROPATHOGENIC, ENTEROTOXIGENIC.
***E. coli* J5 vaccine** vaccine prepared from *E. coli* mutant; provides protection against coliform mastitis in cows.
Eschscholtzia californica a North American plant in the Papaveraceae family. It could be poisonous because of its high content of isoquinoline alkaloids. Called also California poppy.
escorcin a brown powder prepared from a substance extracted from the horse chestnut; used in detecting corneal and conjunctival lesions.
esculin, aesculin a hydroxycoumarin glycoside found in the bark of *Aesculus* spp. Together with ferric citrate, it is used in a broth for the identification of some bacteria which cause hydrolysis and a color change. Also causes animal poisoning; see AESCULUS.
escutcheon the shield-like pattern of distribution of the haircoat in the area below the vulva, down to the top of the udder, in the cow. The escutcheon itself is composed of hairs which lie vertically downwards; its edges consist of a well-demarcated ridge created when this vertically inclined hair meets the horizontally inclined hair of the lateral aspect of the thigh. Wishful-thinking herdsmen used to read predictions of milking capacity into the shape of the escutcheon of a dairy cow.
eserine see PHYSOSTIGMINE.
-esis word element. [Gr.] *state, condition*.
Eskimo dog 1. a term sometimes applied to any of the Arctic breeds of dogs, such as Samoyed, Alaskan malamute and Siberian Husky. 2. a recognized dog breed in the United Kingdom. It is a large (60–100 lb), powerful dog with a heavy, thick double coat in any color. The head is broad, ears short and erect, and tail large and bushy. Called also Husky, Esquimaux, Canadian Eskimo dog. In the United States called the American eskimo dog, which also comes in miniature and toy varieties; always white or cream.
Esmarch having to do with Johann Esmarch, a 19th century German surgeon.
E's bandage an India rubber bandage applied upward around (from the distal part to the proximal) a part in order to expel blood from it; the part is often elevated as the elastic pressure is applied.
E. plaster shears, scissors see PLASTER shears.
esmolol a short-acting β-receptor blocking agent, used as the hydrochloride to treat cardiac arrhythmias.
eso- word element. [Gr.] *within*.
esoethmoiditis inflammation of the ethmoid sinuses.

esogastritis inflammation of the gastric mucosa.

esophageal of or pertaining to the esophagus.

e. achalasia see MEGAESOPHAGUS.

e. anomalies very rare; include atresia, duplication, segmental aplasia, esophagorespiratory fistulae, diverticula, epithelial inclusion cysts.

e. atresia congenital lack of continuity of the esophagus, commonly accompanied by tracheoesophageal fistula, and characterized by accumulations of mucus in the nasopharynx, gagging, vomiting when fed, cyanosis and dyspnea. Treatment is by surgical repair by esophageal anastomosis and division of the fistula.

e. distension may result from acute or chronic obstruction of the esophagus, or from defective innervation. See also MEGAESOPHAGUS.

e. duplication may be tubular and communicate with the effective esophagus, or cystic appearing as a cystic mass close to the functioning esophagus.

e. ectasia see MEGAESOPHAGUS.

e. enlargement clinically visible enlargement as seen in esophageal diverticulum, stenosis, paralysis, cardial obstruction.

e. fibrosis a cause of acquired megaesophagus; usually caused by trauma or spontaneous ulceration.

e. groove see RETICULAR groove.

e. groove lesion includes granuloma, papilloma, foreign body lodgment; cause of obstructive bloat.

e. hyperkeratosis hyperkeratotic thickening of the esophageal mucosa due usually to hypovitaminosis A or chlorinated naphthalene poisoning.

e. inflammation see ESOPHAGITIS.

e. motility disorders see MEGAESOPHAGUS.

e. neoplasm very rare except for papilloma and fibropapilloma; causes chronic esophageal obstruction.

e. obstruction acute obstruction is manifested by inability to swallow, regurgitation of saliva, food and water through the nose and much discomfort expressed by retching movements and pawing at the throat. Ruminants develop ruminal tympany. Chronic obstruction shows the same syndrome but with a gradual development and a tendency to develop aspiration pneumonia.

e. osteosarcoma occurs in dogs in association with the parasite *Spirocerca lupi*.

e. papilloma a cause of obstructive bloat.

e. paralysis causes esophageal obstruction.

e. perforation causes local cellulitis and compression-obstruction of esophagus.

e. pulsion diverticulum a diverticulum that pushes outwards causing pressure on surrounding organs and tissues.

e. segmental aplasia causes esophageal obstruction in neonates.

e. stenosis, e. stricture causes esophageal obstruction; may be partial, permitting passage of liquids.

e. tube see NASOGASTRIC tube.

e. ulcer usually associated with pressure necrosis due to prolonged obstruction and injury by a solid foreign body or, rarely equine dysautonomia or *Gasterophilus* spp. infestation.

e. varices distended veins at the gastric cardia causing dysphagia.

esophagectasia dilatation of the esophagus.

esophagectomy excision of a portion of the esophagus.

esophagism spasm of the esophagus.

esophagismus see ESOPHAGISM.

esophagitis inflammation of the esophagus. Primary esophagitis, caused by physical irritants, causes spasm and obstruction, with pain on swallowing or palpation, profuse salivation, regurgitation of slimy, blood-stained saliva and feed, and may lead to stricture formation. Esophagitis also occurs commonly in ruminants as a secondary lesion in diseases characterized by erosive and vesicular lesions of the alimentary tract. Gastric reflux, invasion of the esophageal wall by *Hypoderma* spp., thallotoxicosis and paraquat poisoning are other causes.

peptic e. inflammation of the esophagus due to a reflux of acid and pepsin from the stomach; occurs particularly in dogs and cats while under general anesthesia. Called also reflux esophagitis.

reflux e. see peptic esophagitis (above).

esophagobronchial pertaining to or communicating with the esophagus and a bronchus, e.g. esophagobronchial fistula.

esophagocele abnormal distension of the esophagus; protrusion of the esophageal mucosa through a rupture in the muscular coat.

esophagocoloplasty excision of a portion of the esophagus and its replacement by a segment of the colon.

esophagodynia pain in the esophagus.

esophagoenterostomy surgical formation of an anastomosis between the esophagus and the small intestine.

esophagoesophagostomy anastomosis between two formerly remote parts of the esophagus.

esophagogastrectomy excision of the esophagus and stomach.

esophagogastric pertaining to the esophagus and the stomach.

e. ulcer rapidly growing penned pigs on heavy concentrate diets develop esophagogastric ulcers which may bleed and cause sudden death from hemorrhagic anemia.

esophagogastroanastomosis esophagogastrostomy.

esophagogastroduodenoscopy endoscopic examination of the esophagus, stomach and duodenum.

esophagogastroplasty plastic repair of the esophagus and stomach. See also CARDIOPLASTY.

esophagogastroscopy endoscopic inspection of the esophagus and stomach.

esophagogastrostomy anastomosis of the esophagus to the stomach.

esophagogram a contrast radiograph of the esophagus.

esophagography radiography of the esophagus.

esophagojejunostomy anastomosis of the esophagus to the jejunum.

esophagomalacia softening of the walls of the esophagus.

esophagometer an instrument for measuring the esophagus.

esophagomyotomy incision through the muscular coat of the esophagus. See also Heller's MYOTOMY.

esophagoplasty plastic repair of the esophagus.

esophagoplication infolding of the wall of an esophageal pouch.

esophagoptosis prolapse of the esophagus.

esophagopulmonary pertaining to the esophagus and lungs, e.g. esophagopulmonary fistula.

esophagorespiratory pertaining to or communicating with the esophagus and respiratory tract (trachea or a bronchus).

e. fistula between the esophagus and trachea.

esophagorespiratory fistula congenital or acquired, the latter usually after traumatic injury; characterized by gastric inflation and aspiration pneumonia.

esophagoscope an endoscope for examination of the esophagus.

esophagoscopy direct visual examination of the esophagus with an esophagoscope. Esophagoscopy usually is done as a diagnostic procedure for the purpose of locating and inspecting a disorder of the esophagus. After the esophagoscope has been inserted it is possible to obtain samples of tissue for microscopic study. In some instances the esophagoscope can be used to remove a foreign object that has become lodged in the esophagus.

esophagostenosis stricture of the esophagus.

esophagostomiasis infestation with *Oesophagostomum* spp.

esophagostomosis infestation with *Oesophagostomum* spp. worms; causes necrotic nodules in the wall of the intestine. The resulting clinical syndrome includes poor condition and the passage of soft droppings containing more than normal amounts of mucus.

esophagostomy the creation of an artificial opening into the esophagus.

cervical e. one performed in cervical section of esophagus, often for purposes of placing an indwelling feeding tube when oral alimentation is impossible because of injury or surgery.

esophagotomy incision of the esophagus.

esophagotracheal pertaining to or communicating with the esophagus and trachea, e.g. esophagotracheal fistula.

esophagram see ESOPHAGOGRAM.

esophagus the musculomembranous passage extending from the pharynx to the stomach, consisting of an outer fibrous coat, a muscular layer (all striated in dogs and ruminants, plus some smooth muscle in cats, pigs and horses), a submucous layer, and an inner mucous membrane. Each end is equipped with a functional sphincter although these are not distinct anatomically.

esophoria heterophoria in which there is deviation of the visual axis of one eye toward that of the other eye in the absence of visual fusional stimuli.

esosphenoiditis osteomyelitis of the sphenoid bone.

esotropia STRABISMUS in which there is deviation of the visual axis of one eye toward that of the other eye, resulting in diplopia. Called also cross-eye and convergent strabismus. Commonly seen in Siamese cats.

Esox a large predatory freshwater fish in the suborder *Esocoidea*. The two common species are *Esox lucius* (northern pike) and *Esox americanus* (pikerel), both popular sporting fish. Called also pike.

espichamento [Span.] see ENZOOTIC calcinosis.

esponja swamp cancer.

espundia leishmaniasis, particularly *L. braziliensis*.

ESR erythrocyte sedimentation rate.

essence 1. the distinctive or individual principle of anything. 2. a mixture of alcohol with a volatile oil.

essential 1. constituting the necessary or inherent part of a thing; giving a substance its peculiar and necessary qualities. 2. indispensable; required in the diet, as essential fatty acids. 3. idiopathic; self-existing; having no obvious external exciting cause.

e. fatty acids (EFAs) the unsaturated fatty acids, linoleic and α-linolenic, cannot be synthesized by animals but are essential nutrients that must be supplied in the diet.

e. fatty acid deficiency in dogs and cats, there is scaling, alopecia and seborrhea. Poor wound healing, immunosuppression and infertility have also been reported.

Essig wiring technique a method of stabilizing alveolar fractures using wire looped around a group of teeth with secondary wires looped around individual teeth.

ester chemical combination of an alcohol and an acid. In domestic animals the most common linkage is glycerol with fatty acid to form glycerides.

esterase any enzyme that catalyzes the hydrolysis of esters into its alcohol and acid.

lipid e. an enzyme found in pancreatic secretions which requires bile acids to be active.

esteratic site that part of a cholinesterase macromolecule that recognizes and binds acetylcholine. This combination results in the hydrolysis of the acetylcholine.

esterification conversion of an acid into an ester by combination with an alcohol and removal of a molecule of water.

esterify to combine with an alcohol with elimination of a molecule of water, forming an ester.

esterolysis the hydrolysis of an ester into its alcohol and acid.

esterophilic site that part of a cholinergic receptor macromolecule which attracts the ester part of acetylcholine. Hydrolysis of the acetylcholine does not occur at this location.

esthematology esthesiology.

esthes- prefix meaning sensation.

esthesiogenic producing sensation.

esthesiology the scientific study or description of the sense organs and sensations.

esthesiometer an instrument for measuring tactile sensibility; tactometer.

esthesioneuroblastoma see OLFACTORY neuroblastoma.

esthesioneurocytoma see OLFACTORY neuroblastoma.

esthesioneuroepithelioma see OLFACTORY neuroblastoma.

esthesioneurosis any disorder of the sensory nerves.

esthesiophysiology the physiology of sensation and sense organs.

esthesodic conducting or pertaining to conduction of sensory impulses.

estil see EUGENOL.

estimate a measurement which is believed likely to incorporate a degree of error.

estimated breeding value see estimated BREEDING VALUE.

estimated transmitting ability an estimate of an animal's ability to transmit its phenotypic value or performance—its breeding value. Called also ETA.

estival, aestival pertaining to, or occurring in, summer.

estivation the dormant state in which certain animals pass the summer. The opposite of hibernation.

estivoautumnal, aestivoautumnal occurring in summer and autumn.

estradiol the female steroid hormone produced by the mature ovarian follicle and the adrenal cortex and responsible for sexual receptivity at the time of estrus. Is the dominant estrogenic hormone in the nonpregnant animal. In the pregnant animal the dominant hormone is estrone; called also estradiol-17β; commercial products include estradiol benzoate and the cyprionate.

e. cyclopentyl propionate a pharmaceutical preparation used in dogs; recorded as a cause of hyperestrogenism.

estral see ESTROUS.

estranes parent structure of hormones involved in female reproductive processes, including estradiol-17β, estrone.

Estrela mountain dog a large, powerful, mastiff type dog with a powerful head, small ears, short, thick neck and long tail. The coat may be short or long, and fawn, brindle or wolf gray in color. Named after the Estrela mountain range in Portugal. Called also Portuguese sheepdog.

estrin estrogen.

estrinization production of the cellular changes in the vaginal epithelium characteristic of estrus.

estriol a relatively weak ESTROGEN, being a metabolic product of estradiol and estrone found in high concentration in the urine of women.

estrogen a generic term for estrus-producing compounds; the naturally occurring female sex hormones include ESTRADIOL, ESTRIOL and ESTRONE.

In animals the estrogens are formed in the ovary, adrenal cortex, testis and fetoplacental unit, and are responsible for female secondary sex characteristic development, and act on the female genitalia to produce an environment suitable for fertilization, implantation and nutrition of the early embryo. A very important function is the creation of a state of sexual receptivity in the female.

conjugated e's a mixture of sulfate esters of estrogenic substances, principally estrone and equilin; the uses are those of estrogens.

esterified e's a mixture of esters of estrogenic substances, principally estrone; the uses are those of estrogens.

fungal e. *Fusarium graminearum* (*F. roseum*) produces zearalenone which has estrogenic activity.

placental e. see estrogen (above).

plant e. subterranean and red clover may contain significant amounts of an isoflavone, genistein, with estrogenic activity. See also ESTROGENISM.

e. poisoning see ESTROGENISM.

e.-responsive dermatosis a bilaterally symmetrical alopecia, sometimes with seborrhea, seen in spayed bitches; responsive to treatment with estrogens such as diethylstilbestrol.

estrogen-induced stimulated by high blood levels of estrogen.

e.-i. transdifferentation a persistent high estrogen intake causes male behavior in ewes and secondary sex characters, e.g. mammary gland and teat hypertrophy, in wethers, and changes in the promotion of development of endometrial-type glands in the cervix.

e.-i. uroliths diets high in estrogens thought to contribute to the development of uroliths by increasing the rate of epithelial desquamation in the urinary tract, thus facilitating the formation of a nidus around which concretion of salts can then develop.

estrogenic estrus-producing; having the properties of, or properties similar to, an estrogen.

e. substances are used in treatment of animals for diseases of the reproductive tract. In some countries they are still used as growth promotants in food animals. They also occur naturally in cultivated plants, e.g. subterranean clover, in fungi growing on plants and plant products, e.g. *Fusarium graminearum, F. roseum*. Poisoning with estrogens can occur in any of these circumstances. The clinical signs are, in general terms, feminization of males, and in females nymphomaniac activity and infertility due to endometrial changes, prolapse of the cervix and uterus and maternal dystocia due to uterine inertia. See also TRIFOLIUM, FUSARIOTOXICOSIS, GROWTH promotants.

estrogenism the disease state caused by the continued ingestion of low but toxic levels of estrogens. This may be iatrogenic in origin in companion animals but the most important occurrence is in farm animals pastured on plants containing phytoestrogens. The signs are those related to endometrial hyperplasia and vaginal tumefaction, including long-term infertility and rectal prolapse, especially in pigs, uterine prolapse, especially in ewes, and feminization of male castrates.

Dogs are particularly susceptible to the myelotoxic effects of estrogens and high dose or prolonged administration causes severe bone marrow depression with thrombocytopenia, then leukopenia and anemia.

estrone an oxidation product of estradiol, and androstenedione in the animal body; less active than estradiol and produced in greater quantities in the pregnant female.

e. sulfate test 1. a pregnancy diagnosis carried out on cow's milk; has very high accuracy but impractical because of lateness of applicability, e.g. maximum at day 105 of pregnancy. 2. a test using serum which detects the presence of a retained testicle in horses with no testicles in the scrotum but which are demonstrating sexual behavior.

estrophilin a cell protein that acts as a receptor for estrogen, found in estrogenic target tissue and in estrogen-dependent tumors and metastases.

estropipate a preparation of piperazine estrone sulfate used therapeutically for its estrogenic activity.

estrous pertaining to or emanating from ESTRUS.

e. cycle one of the two types of reproductive cycles, the other is the menstrual cycle of humans and primates. Regularly occurring periods during which the female is sexually active and receptive, ESTRUS, separated by periods in which there is no sexual receptivity. This period is divided, on the basis of ovarian activity into metestrus (early corpus luteum development), diestrus (mature corpus luteum) and proestrus (period of follicle development). The details of estral activity are summarized in Table 17.

estruation see ESTRUS.

estrum see ESTRUS.

estrus the time during the reproductive cycle in animals when the female displays interest in mating and in most species will stand to be mounted by both sexes and mated by males. In most cases the animal is about to or has just ovulated, and is therefore pregnable, but some, including pregnant ones, may not be in true estrus.

At the time of estrus there are behavioral signs and changes in the external genitalia. In cows these include the passage of very clear mucus, swelling of the lips of the vulva and hoof brush marks on the side of the rump. Mares show frequent urination with squatting, elevation of the tail, swelling and winking of the vulva and rhythmic extrusion of the clitoris. Ewes are not demonstrative other than positioning themselves close to the rams or teasers. Goat does bleat a lot, rub themselves against fixed objects and hold their tail high, urinate frequently and evert the clitoris. Bitches wander away, stand with their tails held to one side and are attractive and receptive to males. Queens may be very demonstrative, especially Siamese. They rub against anything, crawl with their belly close to the floor, roll and vocalize with a deep, throaty growl.

e. detection in natural mating the male is, in most situations, the best possible detector. In artificial breeding or in hand mating the need to pick cows which are on heat is of paramount importance. Techniques available include the use of infertile teasers combined with heat mount detectors, tail paint, chin ball or siresine harnesses. In dairy herds it is usual to dispense with the teasers and depend on other cows to pick out and mount the cows that are in heat.

In sheep crayon or paint marking harnesses are used. In mares individual teasing with a pony or similar manageable male is used. In the other species detection is by simple visualization.

e. expectancy chart a wall chart for use at the dairy which points out those cows which are due to come into estrus during the next day or two and need to be observed closely.

false e. behavioral and external genital signs of estrus without ovulation occurring.

e. induction see estrus synchronization (below).

no visible e. abbreviated NVO (to accommodate the British spelling of oestrus) or NVE. Diagnosis indicating reproductive inefficiency; applied to cows which are not observed as being in estrus for a variable period, usually 50 days, after calving. Includes cows with anestrus due to various causes and failure of staff to observe or record estrus. A percentage of more than 10% of cows in a herd which have no visible estrus is an indication of a herd problem.

silent e. ovulation occurs, as detected by palpation or estrogen levels in the blood in the absence of behavioral signs.

e. suppression prevention of estral activity in companion animals without spaying them is practiced frequently. A variety of progestins are available and, at times, intravaginal and intrauterine devices have been used for this purpose. See also CONTRACEPTION.

e. synchronization aimed at having all of the animals in estrus, and later calving or lambing, at the same time. Prostaglandin injection is a common technique used to induce estrus in cows.

unexpressed e. see silent estrus (above).

e.s.u. electrostatic unit.

ETA estimated transmitting ability.

etching see ACID ETCH TECHNIQUE.

ETEC enterotoxigenic *Escherichia coli*.

ethacrynate sodium the sodium salt of ethacrynic acid used intravenously as a diuretic; effective in promoting sodium and chloride excretion.

ethambutol a tuberculostatic agent.

ethanol the major ingredient of alcoholic beverages; called also ethyl ALCOHOL and grain alcohol.

20% e. administered intravenously it can be used in the treatment of ethylene glycol poisoning in dogs. Pets may be poisoned by consumption of ethanol, usually in the form of alcoholic beverages. Signs include an initial period of excitement and incoordination, followed by stupor, coma, respiratory failure and seizures.

e. gel test used to detect the presence of fibrinogen-split products in a blood sample; based on the separation of the split products from fibrinogen by the use of ethanol.

ethanolamine a colorless, moderately viscous liquid with an ammoniacal odor contained in cephalins and phospholipids, and derived metabolically by decarboxylation of serine.

e. phosphotransferase an enzyme of the endoplasmic reticulum, particularly in the liver, that catalyzes the biosynthesis of phosphatidylethanolamine.

ethaverine an analog of papaverine used as an antispasmodic and smooth muscle relaxant.

ethene see ETHYLENE.

ether 1. diethyl ether: a colorless, transparent, very volatile, highly inflammable liquid with a characteristic odor; given by inhalation to produce general ANESTHESIA. 2. any organic compound containing an oxygen atom bonded to two carbon atoms.

spiritus e. nit. used as a stimulant for depressed animals, both as an inhalant and in oral drenches.

vinyl e. a clear colorless liquid used as an inhalation anesthetic.

ethereal 1. pertaining to, prepared with, containing or resembling ether. 2. evanescent; delicate.

e. sulfates an important detoxication process in the liver is the formation of these sulfates that are more readily excreted than the parent compounds.

etherization induction of anesthesia by means of ether.

ethics rules or principles which govern right conduct. Each practitioner, upon entering a profession, is invested with the responsibility to adhere to the standards of ethical practice and conduct set by the profession.

code of e. the written rules of ethics.

veterinary e. the values and guidelines governing decisions in veterinary practice.

ethidium see HOMIDIUM.

ethinamate a short-acting, nonbarbiturate sedative.

ethinylestradiol see ESTRADIOL.

ethiofencarb a carbamate pesticide.

ethmo- prefix meaning ethmoid or sieve.

ethmocarditis inflammation of the connective tissue of the heart.

ethmoid 1. sievelike; cribriform. 2. the ethmoid bone.

e. bone the sievelike bone that forms a roof for the nasal fossae and part of the floor of the rostral cranial fossa. See also Table 10.

e. sinus see CONCHA.

ethmoidal pertaining to the ethmoid bone.

enzootic e. tumor see ENZOOTIC ethmoidal tumor.

e. foramen carries the ethmoidal nerve as it re-enters the cranial cavity.

e. hematoma see PROGRESSIVE nasal hematoma.

ethmoidectomy excision of the ethmoid cells or of a portion of the ethmoid bone.

ethmoiditis inflammation of the ethmoid bone or ethmoid sinuses.

ethmoidotomy incision into the ethmoid sinus.

ethmoturbinal relating to or consisting of the ethmoturbinates.

ethmoturbinate the scroll-like, papyraceous parts of the ethmoid bone occupying the caudal part of the nasal fossae.

e. tumors reportedly endemic in sheep, and less so in cattle. They are adenopapillomas or locally invasive adenocarcinomas of nasal epithelium.

ethnoveterinary medicine the folk beliefs, knowledge, skills, methods and practices relating to the health care of animals. Includes medicinal and spiritual aspects, but more commonly taken to mean the use of medicinal plants.

ethologist a person skilled in ethology.

ethology the scientific study of animal behavior, particularly in the natural state.

ethopabate a supplementary drug that improves the coccidiostatic effect of amprolium.

ethosuximide a succinide derivative used as an anticonvulsant. See SUCCINIMIDES.

ethoxyquin an antioxidant added to animal feeds to prevent loss of fat, vitamins A and E, and to prevent avian encephalomalacia.

ethoxzolamide a carbonic anhydrase inhibitor diuretic, used mainly to reduce intraocular pressure in glaucoma.

ethyl the monovalent radical, C_2H_5.

e. alcohol see ethyl ALCOHOL; called also ethanol and grain alcohol.

e. aminobenzoate see BENZOCAINE.

e. carbamate see URETHANE.

e. chloride a local anesthetic applied topically to intact skin. It has a very low boiling point and the skin is temporarily frozen and insensitive to pain.

e. lactate an antibacterial agent used in shampoos.

ethylene a colorless, highly flammable gas with a slightly sweet taste and odor, used as an inhalation anesthetic to induce general ANESTHESIA.

e. dibromide (EDB) grain fumigant. Treated seed seriously reduces egg production when fed to hens in very small amounts.

e. dichloride industrial fumigant; causes respiratory and ophthalmic irritation, narcosis, disturbance of equilibrium.

e. glycol antifreeze; palatable enough for animals to drink in quantity. Causes ataxia, depression, coma, polydipsia, vomiting and convulsions due to formation of oxalate crystals in brain blood vessels and renal tubules.

e. oxide a fumigant used for foodstuffs, surgical equipment and as an agricultural fungicide. It is a gaseous, flammable alkylating agent with a broad spectrum of activity, being sporicidal and viricidal. It is used (mixed with CO_2 or fluorocarbons because it is explosive above 3%) for disinfecting and sterilizing equipment and instruments that are used in the hospital, surgery, dentistry, and the pharmaceutical and other industries, and that are thermolabile or will be adversely affected by immersion in water or other media. Its optimal germicidal effect occurs after a 3-hour exposure at 86°F (30°C). Its vapor is irritating to eyes and respiratory mucosa and can cause serious pulmonary edema. Called also oxirane.

ethylenediamine in complex with theophylline, it forms aminophylline.

e. dihydrochloride a urinary acidifier.

e. dihydroiodide used in livestock as an expectorant, anti-inflammatory agent and iodine supplement. Can cause poisoning if taken in excess. Signs include nasal and ocular discharge, dyspnea and cough.

e. tetra-acetic acid see EDETATE.

ethylenimine an industrial chemical known to be a carcinogen.

ethylisobutrazine hydrochloride a neuroleptic tranquilizer; a phenothiazine derivative.

ethylmercuri-toluene sulfonanilide a fungicidal agent used in agriculture. Capable of causing organic mercury poisoning.

ethylmercury an organic radical used extensively in agriculture as a basis for fungicides.

e. chloride this antifungal seed dressing is capable of causing organic MERCURY poisoning.

e. iodide used in agriculture as a fungicidal seed dressing. Can cause mercury poisoning.

e. phosphate used as a fungistatic seed dressing; seed consumed by animals or humans causes organic mercury poisoning.

ethylnoradrenaline see ETHYLNOREPINEPHRINE.

ethylnorepinephrine, ethylnoradrenaline a synthetic adrenergic brochodilator. See also NOREPINEPHRINE.

ethynyl the group –C≡CH, when it occurs in organic compounds.

etidocaine a local anesthetic of the amide type used for percutaneous infiltration anesthesia, peripheral nerve block, and caudal and epidural block.

etidronate a bone calcium regulator.

etiolation blanching or paleness of a plant grown in the dark; due to lack of chlorophyll.

etiological pertaining to ETIOLOGY.

e. diagnosis the name of a disease which includes the identification of the causative agent, e.g. *Streptococcus agalactiae* mastitis.

e. factors risk factors contributing to the cause of a disease.

etiology literally the science dealing with causes of disease; common usage is the causes of diseases.

etioporphyrin a synthetic porphyrin used as a basis for the classification of porphyrins.

etiquette the rules of decorous behavior. In a professional sense this includes behavior towards clients and colleagues which is in the best interests of the patients.

etomidate an intravenous, nonbarbiturate, fast-inducing anesthetic with no analgesic effect. Also causes suppression of adrenal steroidogenesis and may be used in the treatment of hyperadrenocorticism.

etoposide a derivative of podophyllotoxin with antineoplastic activity; used in the treatment of leukemias.

etorphine a very potent, semisynthetic analgesic usually used in heavy dosage to avoid side-effects and then reversed with diprenorphine. Used mostly as an immobilizer for free-ranging wild animals, usually in combination with hyoscine and acepromazine.

etretinate a synthetic retinoid, used orally in the treatment of skin diseases, particularly keratinization disorders. Like other synthetic retinoids, it is teratogenic and has a very long half-life.

Eu chemical symbol, *europium*.

eu- word element. [Gr.] *normal, good, well, easy*.

Eubacterium a genus of gram-negative, rod-shaped bacteria found in the intestinal tract as parasites, and as saprophytes in soil and water. Belong to the family Lactobacillaceae. Found sporadically in purulent lesions but are probably secondary invaders.

E. suis causes PYELONEPHRITIS and cystitis in swine. Previously called *Corynebacterium suis*.

Eubothrium a genus of tapeworms of the family Amphicotylidae. Found in wild and captive salmonids.

eucalyptol a colorless liquid obtained from eucalyptus oil and other sources; used as an expectorant, flavoring agent and local anesthetic. Called also cineole.

Eucalyptus genus of Australian trees in the family Myrtaceae, widely planted throughout the world. Two species *E. cladocalyx* (sugar gum) and *E. viminalis* (manna gum) may contain toxic amounts of cyanogenic glycosides. Called also gum trees.

E. melanophloia host tree larvae of Australian sawfly (*Lophyrotoma interrupta*) which may poison sheep and cattle. Called also silver-leaf ironbark.

eucalyptus oil a volatile oil from fresh leaf of species of *Eucalyptus*, the chief constituent of which is eucalyptol.

eucaryosis see EUKARYOSIS.

Eucaryotae a kingdom of organisms that includes higher plants and animals, fungi, protozoa and most algae (except blue-green algae), all of which are made up of eukaryotic cells. See also EUKARYOTE.

eucaryotic see EUKARYOTIC.

Eucestoda one of the two classes of cestodes. Includes the true tapeworms identified by having a holdfast organ or scolex, usually a segmented body, and a life cycle which includes an intermediate host.

euchlorhydria the presence of the normal amount of hydrochloric acid in the gastric juice.

eucholia normal condition of the bile.
euchromatin that state of chromatin in which it stains lightly, is genetically active, and is considered to be partially or fully uncoiled.
Eucoleus aerophilus CAPILLARIA *aerophila*.
Eucotylidae a family of flukes (digenetic trematodes) found in the kidney of birds. Includes genera of *Tanaisia* spp. and *Eucotyle* spp. Neither appears to have significant pathogenicity.
eucrasia 1. a state of health; proper balance of different factors constituting a healthy state. 2. a state in which the body reacts normally to ingested or injected drugs, proteins, etc.
eudiemorrhysis the normal flow of blood through the capillaries.
eudipsia ordinary, normal thirst.
Eudyptula minor prebreeding penguins.
euesthesia a normal state of the senses.
euflavine, euflavin see ACRIFLAVINE.
eugenol the chief constituent of clove oil; also obtained from other sources. Used as a dental topical analgesic and antiseptic. Derivatives have been used as intravenous anesthetics but the extremely short action and side-effects limit use.
euglobulin one of a class of globulins characterized by being insoluble in water but soluble in saline solutions.
e. lysis test used to differentiate between types of pathological fibrinolysis.
euglycemia a normal level of glucose in the blood.
eugonic growing luxuriantly; said of bacterial cultures.
Eugonic Fermenter-4 a group of unclassified gram-negative, rod-shaped bacteria isolated from cases of multifocal interstitial pneumonia in miscellaneous carnivora.
Euhopllopsyllus glacialis lynx a flea that parasitizes wild felines.
eukaryon 1. a highly organized nucleus bounded by a nuclear membrane, a characteristic of cells of higher organisms. 2. eukaryote.
eukaryosis the state of having a true nucleus.
Eukaryotae see EUCARYOTAE.
eukaryote an organism of the Eucaryotae, whose cells have a true nucleus bounded by a nuclear membrane and containing the CHROMOSOMES and which divide by MITOSIS. Eukaryotic cells also contain membrane-bound organelles, such as mitochondria, chloroplasts, lysosomes and the Golgi apparatus. Plants and animals, protozoa, fungi and algae (except blue-green algae) are eukaryotes. Other organisms (the bacteria) are prokaryotes.
eukaryotic pertaining to EUKARYOSIS.
e. cells see CELL.
e. transcription see DEOXYRIBONUCLEIC ACID.
eukinesia normal or proper motor function or activity.
Eulaelaps a genus of lelaptid mites in the family Gamasidae.
E. stabularis a parasite of small mammals found in poultry houses, feed stores and such places where they cause irritation to workers. A vector for *Francisella tularensis*.
eulaminate having the normal number of laminae, as certain areas of the cerebral cortex.
eumelanin black to brown pigment produced by melanin. See also PHEOMELANIN.
eumelanosome pigment granules containing eumelanin, produced within cells by melanosomes.
Eumetopius see SEALION.
eumetria a normal condition of nerve impulse, so that a voluntary movement just reaches the intended goal; the proper range of movement.
eumycetoma see MYCETOMA.
eunuchoid an animal which resembles a human eunuch. Said of an entire male which appears to lack characteristics indicating male virility including aggressive posturing and vocalizing, large, heavy-featured head, dished face with heavy brows, shaggy forelock, heavy shoulders with a finer boned hindquarter. High serving capacity is also a good recommendation.

Males with the chromosome anomaly XXY, the classical aneuploidy, are usually eunuchoid and scrotal formation may be defective.
e. syndrome a state of decreased aggression, disinterest, and loss of stamina in working dogs after ovariectomy.
eunuchoidism deficiency of the testes or of their secretion, with impaired sexual power and eunuchoid signs.
hypergonadotropic e. that associated with secretion of high levels of gonadotropins, as in Klinefelter's syndrome.
hypogonadotropic e. that due to lack of gonadotropin secretion.
Euonymus europaeus plant in the family Celastraceae; contains a toxic cardiac glycoside, evonoside, with a digitalis-like action. Called also spindle tree, skewer wood.
eupancreatism normal functioning of the pancreas.
Euparyphium see ECHINOSTOMA.
Eupatorium a plant genus of the Asteraceae family; contains mostly unidentified toxins. Includes *E. wrightii*.
E. adenophorum in Australia and Hawaii, pulmonary fibrosis is the principal lesion, and dyspnea and cough the cardinal signs in poisoning of horses by these plants. Called also Numinbah horse sickness, Tallebudgera horse disease.
E. rugosum, E. ageratoides, E. urticaefolium poisoning causes tremor, dyspnea, paralysis and recumbency and can be fatal. The toxic alcohol that it contains is passed through the milk of cows and can poison persons who drink it. Called also white snakeroot.
eupepsia good digestion; the presence of a normal amount of pepsin in the gastric juice.
Euphorbia a genus of the plant family Euphorbiaceae; contains diterpenes which cause enteritis and diarrhea. Some species are suspected of containing cyanogenic glycosides. Toxic species include *E. boophthona* (Gascoyne spurge), *E. characias*, *E. drummondii* (mat spurge, caustic creeper), *E. helioscopia* (sun spurge), *E. hydnorae*, *E. mauritanica*, *E. melanostica* (yellow milk bush), *E. phymatoclada*, *E. ingens* (candelabra tree), *E. lathyrus* (caper spurge), *E. marginata* (snow-on-the-mountain), *E. milii* (crown-of-thorns), *E. peplus* (petty spurge), *E. prostrata*, *E. pulcherrima* (poinsettia), *E. tirucalli*.
euplastic readily becoming organized; adapted to tissue formation.
euploid 1. having a balanced set or sets of chromosomes, in any number. 2. a euploid individual or cell.
euploidy the state of being euploid.
eupnea normal, quiet breathing.
eupraxia intactness of reproduction of coordinated movements.
eurhythmia regularity of the pulse.
European emanating from or pertaining to Europe.
E. bat lyssavirus see LYSSAVIRUS.
E. beech tree FAGUS *sylvaticus*.

E. blastomycosis see CRYPTOCOCCOSIS.
E. brown hare syndrome a highly fatal necrotizing hepatitis caused by a calicivirus, occurs naturally and only in *Lepus europeus* (European hare) and *Lepus timidus* (Northern hare). Proposed as a possible progenitor virus for rabbit calicivirus. See also RABBIT HEMORRHAGIC DISEASE.
E. buffalo the true buffalo of the Old World (*Bubalus bubalis*), not the BISON. Includes many breeds and varieties. Used for milk, meat and draft. Dark gray to black in color, often with white on the head, tail and feet. Called also Indian buffalo.
E. cattle breeds include AQUITAINE BLOND, BELGIAN blue, BROWN SWISS, CENTRAL AND UPPER BELGIAN, CHAROLAIS, CHIANA, FRIESIAN, HOLSTEIN–FRIESIAN, LIMOUSIN, MAINE-ANJOU, MARCHE, PIEDMONT, PINZGAU, ROMAGNA, SIMMENTAL, STEPPE.
E. chick flea CERATOPHYLLUS *gallinae*.
E. feedlot see European FEEDLOT.
E. harvest mite see TROMBICULA *autumnalis*.
E. mistletoe see VISCUM ALBUM.
E. oak QUERCUS *robur*.
E. rabbit flea see SPILOPSYLLUS CUNICULI.
E. swine fever see HOG cholera.
E. yew TAXUS *baccata*.

europium a chemical element, atomic number 63, atomic weight 151.96, symbol Eu. See Table 6.

eury- word element. [Gr.] *wide, broad*.

euryblepharon a symmetrical enlargement of the palpebral fissure.
congenital e. seen in brachycephalic dogs; in association with shallow orbits, the eyes are prominent and subject to exposure keratitis.
transient juvenile e. occurs in young German shepherd dogs and usually resolves in several months. It gives the appearance of exophthalmos. No other abnormalities are present.

eurycephalic having a wide head.

euryhaline species of fish capable of osmoregulation in waters over a range of salinities.

Euryhelmis a genus of intestinal flukes (digenetic trematodes) in the family Heterophyidae.
E. monorchis found in mink.
E. squamula found in wild carnivora. Causes fatal hemorrhagic enteritis in mink.

Eurytrema a genus of flukes (digenetic trematodes) in the family Dicrocoeliidae.
E. brumpti CONCINNUM *brumpti*.
E. coelomaticum, E. pancreaticum found in pancreatic ducts of sheep and cattle.
E. fastosum found in the pancreatic and biliary ducts of carnivores.
E. ovis found in the perirectal fat of sheep.
E. procyonis CONCINNUM *procyonis*.

Euschongastia a genus of mites in the family Trombiculidae.
E. latchmani causes trombiculidiasis in cats.

eustachian tube see PHARYNGOTYMPANIC TUBE.

eustachitis inflammation of the pharyngotympanic tube; not likely to be made as a clinical diagnosis in animals but is a common accompaniment of the more severe syndrome of otitis media.

Eustachys distichophylla CHLORIS *distichophylla*.

eustress a stress which is beneficial to the animal.

Eustrongylides a genus of nematodes in the family Dioctophymatidae. Found in birds and wild and cultured fish.
E. papillosus found in the esophagus and proventriculus of ducks and geese. Can cause extensive nodule formation.
E. tubifex found in the intestine of anatine birds.

Eutamius, Tamius see CHIPMUNK.

euthanasia 1. an easy or painless death. 2. the deliberate ending of life of an animal suffering from an incurable disease; called also mercy killing, to put down, to put to sleep.

For the individual animal intravenous injection of a massive dose of barbiturate is best. Any narcotizing drug creates difficulties if the carcass is to be disposed of for pet meat. In those cases shooting with a bullet or captive bolt pistol is recommended because of the speed of the despatch. For large numbers of animals at a pound or shelter, injection procedures are still superior to the bulk methods which all have the fallibility of poorly managed and supervised machinery. Carbon monoxide is very fast but dangerous to the operators of the cabinet. Electrocution cannot be performed en masse and gassing with carbon monoxide or lowering of the atmospheric pressure are not really quick enough. Small laboratory animals are still despatched by a sharp blow to the head and birds by guillotine or separation of the cervical vertebrae.
electrical e. uses mains electrical current passed through the subject's body via clips applied to the skin of the ear and the tail. Not much employed because of danger to human operators, likelihood of equipment failure and need for close contact with device.

euthanasiate see EUTHANATIZE.

euthanatize to perform EUTHANASIA. Called also euthanize.

euthanize see EUTHANATIZE.

euthermic characterized by the proper temperatures; promoting warmth.

euthyroid having a normally functioning thyroid gland.
e. sick syndrome a euthyroid state in which extrathyroidal factors cause a reduction of serum T_3 or T_4 and elevation of reverse T_3 levels. Seen in patients with systemic illness, trauma, fever, starvation, treatment with glucocorticoids, etc. May be a protective metabolic effect.

euthyroidism state of normal thyroid function.

eutocia normal parturition.

Eutrombicula a subgenus of mites in the mite genus *Trombicula* of the family Trombiculidae. See also CHIGGER.
E. alfreddugesi the common chigger of the USA; called also *Trombicula alfreddugesi*. Causes dermatitis in most species.
E. sarcina causes leg itch and black soil itch of sheep, manifested by dermatitis on the lower limbs up to about the fetlock.

eutrophia a state of normal (good) nutrition.

eutrophication the accidental or deliberate promotion of excessive growth (multiplication) of one kind of organism to the disadvantage of other organisms in the same ecosystem.

eV electron volt.

EVA equine viral arteritis.

evacuant 1. promoting evacuation. 2. an agent that promotes evacuation.

evacuation 1. an emptying or removal, especially the removal of any material from the body by discharge through a natural or artificial passage. 2. material discharged from the body, especially the discharge from the bowels.

evagination an outpouching of a layer or part.

evaluation a critical appraisal or assessment; a judgment of the value, worth, character or effectiveness of that which is being assessed.

Evans blue an odorless green, bluish green, or brown powder dye, used as a diagnostic aid in estimation of blood volume. The dye is injected into the bloodstream and after a sufficient period of time samples of the blood are taken to determine the degree of dilution of the dye. Called also azovan blue.

Evans' syndrome immune-mediated hemolytic anemia concurrent with immune-mediated thrombocytopenia.

evaporated reduced in volume by evaporation; concentrated to a denser form.

evaporative pertaining to evaporation.

e. loss loss of body water by evaporation of water from the body to the air; a heat control mechanism and a factor in water balance studies.

evapotranspiration loss of water from the soil by direct loss plus loss through evaporation of moisture by plants growing on the soil.

Eve tonsil snare a wire loop protruding from a long, hollow tube and a three-finger operated system for closing the snare, the loop. The mechanism may have a ratchet to ensure that the closure of the loop is maintained until the tonsil is removed.

evening primrose oil one of the few plant oils containing γ-linolenic acid. Obtained from seeds of *Oenothera biennis*, it is used for its anti-inflammatory effects in the treatment of skin diseases.

evening trumpetflower see GELSEMIUM SEMPERVIRENS.

event 1. an equine contest other than a race, e.g. a 3-day event. 2. in statistics the outcome of a random experiment.

e. diary pocket diary designed for farmer use to record all events necessary to complete farm records kept for health and production surveillance purposes.

e. horse a horse suitable for use in 3-day events and similar contests.

eventration 1. protrusion of the bowels through the abdomen. 2. removal of the abdominal viscera.

diaphragmatic e. elevation of the dome of the diaphragm into the thoracic cavity, usually due to phrenic nerve paralysis.

evergreen chloris CHLORIS *distichophylla*.

everlasting pea LATHYRUS *sylvestris*, *L. latifolius*.

everman's lupine LUPINUS *evermannii*.

evernazione a method of killing an animal for slaughter. A short two-edged knife is plunged into the neck at the atlanto-occipital joint, severing the medulla oblongata. Called also neck stab.

eversion a turning inside out; a turning outward, e.g. of the uterus, the third eyelid. See under each anatomical location.

evert to turn inside out; to turn outward.

evidence any thing properly presented to a court which will assist it to make a decision in a case. Testimony is evidence given orally.

evisceration extrusion of the viscera, or internal organs; disembowelment.

ocular e. removal of the contents of the eyeball, leaving the sclera.

orbital e. see ENUCLEATION.

evoked potential see EVOKED RESPONSE.

evoked response a technique for the detection of low amplitude electrical activity in response to stimuli for the purpose of evaluating sensory mechanisms. Called also evoked potential.

brainstem auditory e. r. (BAER) variations in electromyographic or electroencephalographic recordings in response to sound stimuli. Used to evaluate brainstem lesions and hearing in dogs.

visual e. r's electrical potentials to flash or pattern displays that are recorded over the occipital lobe region.

evolution the process of development in which an organ or organism becomes more and more complex by the differentiation of its parts; a continuous and progressive change according to certain laws and by means of resident forces.

convergent e. the development, in animals that are only distantly related, of similar structures or functions in adaptation to similar environment.

divergent e. the development of different characteristics in animals that were closely related in response to being placed in different environments.

evonoside a cardiac glycoside found in the plant *Euronymus europaeus*.

evulsion extraction by force.

ewe a female sheep of breeding age. May be qualified as maiden ewes, not yet bred, or ewe lambs, up to one year.

dry e. 1. a ewe without milk whatever the reason. 2. female sheep of breeding age without a lamb at foot.

ewe-necked a defect in conformation in a horse. The topline of the neck is concave when viewed from the side.

ex- word element. [L.] *away from, without, outside;* sometimes used to denote *completely*.

ex vivo outside the living body; denoting removal of an organ (e.g. the kidney) for reparative surgery, after which it is returned to the original site.

exacerbation increase in severity of a disease or any of its clinical signs.

examination inspection or investigation, especially as a means of diagnosing disease, qualified according to the methods used, as physical, cystoscopic, etc.

breeding soundness e. of a male usually, although it could be a practical request in a female, requiring ideally a physical clinical examination, a special physical examination of the reproductive system, a field and a laboratory examination of semen and for evidence of freedom from venereal disease, and a test of serving efficiency.

necropsy e. see NECROPSY. Called also postmortem, autopsy.

postnatal e. usually of cows to ensure that the uterus is clean and the ovaries cycling so that the next pregnancy can commence without delay.

presale e. may be at any level. In horses usually a clinical physical examination, a special examination of the limbs and the gaits of the animal. Companion animals are usually examined for general health and special attention for any defect that could be heritable.

exanthem any cutaneous eruptive disease or fever.

exanthema pl. *exanthemata* [Gr.] see EXANTHEM. See also VESICULAR exanthema of swine, COITAL EXANTHEMA.

exanthematous characterized by or of the nature of an eruption or rash.

exarticulation amputation at a joint; partial removal of a joint.

excavatio see EXCAVATION.

excavation 1. the act of hollowing out. 2. a hollowed-out space, or pouchlike cavity.

atrophic e. cupping of the optic disk, due to atrophy of the optic nerve fibers.

optic disk e. a normally occurring depression in the center of the optic disk.

rectovesical e. the space between the rectum and bladder in the peritoneal cavity of the male.

vesicouterine e. the space between the bladder and uterus in the peritoneal cavity of the female.

excavator a scoop or gouge for surgical use.
excerebration removal of the brain.
exchange diffusion a carrier transport mechanism across a membrane. The transport is faster than can be explained by simple diffusion but does not result in net transport.
exchange transfusion see exchange TRANSFUSION.
excipient any more or less inert substance added to a drug to give suitable consistency or form to the drug; a vehicle.
excise to remove by cutting.
excision removal, as of an organ, by cutting which may be by steel scalpel, CRYOSURGERY or ELECTROSURGERY.
e. DNA repair comprises four distinct sequential steps—incision, in which the damaged base is recognized, excision, resynthesis and ligation.
e. en bloc see en bloc RESECTION.
radical e. extensive removal, usually of a tumor mass, which includes surrounding tissues which might be involved and sometimes regional lymph nodes as well.
shave e. biopsy of superficial lesions of the gingival mucosa can be performed with a scalpel blade, slicing off a thin layer from the surface, without the need for sutures to close the defect.
excitability readiness to respond to a stimulus; irritability.
excitant an agent producing excitation of the vital functions, or of those of the brain.
excitation an act of irritation or stimulation; a condition of being excited or of responding to a stimulus; the addition of energy, as the excitation of a molecule by absorption of photons.
e.-conduction-contraction in the stimulation of muscle contraction this is the coupling which occurs at the sarcolemma–sarcoplasmic reticulum junction. Mediated by the release of calcium ions in the aqueous sarcoplasm.
e.-contraction coupling conversion of an excitation stimulus into contraction of the effector muscle fiber; ionic calcium is the link between the two.
indirect e. electrostimulation of a muscle by placing the electrode on its nerve.
e.-secretion in the stimulation of muscular contraction this is the stimulation of secretion of acetylcholine from the vesicles in the cholinergic nerve terminals into the synaptic cleft at the nerve–muscle junction.
e. signs see IRRITATION nervous signs.
excitement a mental state of greater excitation than normal, but less than frenzy. To be distinguished from, but similar to, the increased motor activity state of restlessness.
excitomotor tending to produce motion or motor function; an agent that so acts.
excitosecretory producing increased secretion.
excitotoxicity exaggerated and continuous stimulation by a neurotransmitter, especially in those neuronal systems which use glutamate as the transmitter.
excitovascular causing vascular changes.
exclave a detached part of an organ.
exclusion a shutting out or elimination; surgical isolation of a part, as of a segment of intestine, without removal from the body.
e. principle it is possible to prove from a parentage test that a particular animal is not the true parent but it is impossible to prove that a particular animal is a parent.
Excoecaria Asian and Australian trees in the family Euphorbiaceae; their milky sap is very irritating and causes intense pain in the eye or on other tender parts. Cause poisoning of livestock. No specific toxin has been identified. Includes *E. agallochia* (river poison tree, milky mangrove), *E. dallychyana* (gutta-percha).
excoriation superficial traumatic abrasions and scratches which remove some of the skin substance. Commonly caused in animals by rubbing or scratching pruritic skin.
excrement fecal matter; matter cast out as waste from the body.
excrementitious pertaining to or of the nature of excrement.
excrescence an abnormal outgrowth; a projection of morbid origin.
excreta excretion products; waste material excreted or eliminated from the body, including FECES, URINE and SWEAT. Mucus and carbon dioxide also can be considered excreta. The organs of excretion are the intestinal tract, kidneys, lungs and skin.
excrete to throw off or eliminate, as waste matter, by a normal discharge.
excretion 1. the act, process or function of excreting. 2. material that is excreted.

Ordinarily, what is meant by excretion is the evacuation of feces. Technically, excretion can refer to the expulsion of any matter, whether from a single cell or from the entire body, or to the matter excreted.
virus e. see SHEDDING.
excretory pertaining to excretion.
e. behavior see elimination BEHAVIOR.
e. urography see descending UROGRAPHY.
exculpatory clause a clause in an agreement that excuses the signatory from any blame, e.g. in an admission to hospital certificate. Legal opinion is that these have very little use as a defense against a suit for damages based on negligence.
excursion a range of movement regularly repeated in performance of a function, e.g. excursion of the jaws in mastication.
excystation escape from a cyst or envelope, as in that stage in the life cycle of parasites occurring after the cystic form has been swallowed by the host.
execution the actual performance of the steps as set out in a program.
exemplary damages the result of a judgment in court proceedings in which the person against whom the judgment is made is required to pay more than the assessed loss and is required to pay an additional sum as a punishment or as an example. Such a decision is rare and made only in circumstances where the person has been wilfully or recklessly neglectful.
exencephaly a congenital defect in which the brain is completely exposed or protrudes through a defect in the cranial vault.
exenteration surgical removal of all of the internal organs, for example of the eye or pelvic cavity.
ocular e. removal of the globe, adnexa and associated structures. See also transpalpebral ENUCLEATION.
exercise performance of physical exertion to obtain food or to achieve normal functions such as reproduction, for pleasure and for improvement of health or correction of physical deformity.
active e. motion imparted to a part by voluntary contraction and relaxation of its controlling muscles.
e. conditioning repeated exercise to condition an animal for a better performance at another time depends on an improvement in cardiovascular responses, splenic contraction and muscle, ligament and tendon responses.

corrective e. therapeutic exercise.
e. fatigue poor exercise tolerance.
e. intolerance manifested by a disinclination to move quickly in the absence of any apparent physical lameness or incoordination and respiratory distress on exercise.
passive e. motion imparted to a segment of the body by a therapist, machine or other outside force.
e. physiology includes the integrated physiological responses to exercise plus physical conditioning by training.
e. testing a technique for evaluating circulatory response to physical stress; called also stress testing. The procedure involves continuous electrocardiographic monitoring during physical exercise, the objective being to increase the intensity of physical exertion until a target heart rate is reached or signs of cardiac ischemia appear.
therapeutic e. the scientific use of bodily movement to restore normal function in diseased or injured tissues or to maintain a state of well-being. Called also corrective exercise.
e. tolerance one of the ways to measure cardiac and circulatory system efficiency is to measure the response of the cardiac and respiratory systems to graded exercise. In most animals such tests must be subjective because no data are available on normal responses. In horses tests are available for assessment of cardiopulmonary disease and as a measure of fitness.

exercising exercise as part of a training program. See EXERCISE conditioning.

exeresis surgical removal, or excision.

exergonic accompanied by the release of free energy.

exertional emanating from or pertaining to exertion.
e. rhabdomyolysis occurs as an acute recumbency or immobility state when muscle masses disrupt during exercise. Occurs as equine paralytic myoglobinuria in horses after unaccustomed exercise while on a heavy carbohydrate diet, in sheep and cattle after violent physical exercise, in racing greyhounds and as capture or transport myopathy in deer and other wildlife. Called also azoturia, Monday morning disease, tying up syndrome, capture myopathy.

exflagellation the protrusion or formation of flagelliform microgametes from a microgametocyte in some sporozoa.

exfoliation a falling off in scales or layers.

exhalation 1. the giving off of watery or other vapor, or of an effluvium. 2. a vapor or other substance exhaled or given off. 3. the act of breathing out.

exhaust fumes fumes given off by vehicles; contain some carbon monoxide, the amount varying with the efficiency of combustion in the particular engine. In most engines the use of exhaust fumes for euthanasia is not recommended because it operates partly on the carbon dioxide content, and if the content is high the animal dies slowly of asphyxia. Car exhaust fumes also contain significant amounts of lead, if the petrol/gasoline is still leaded, and foliage receiving a lot of exhaust deposit can cause lead poisoning in animals eating it. See also LEAD[1] poisoning.

exhausted horse syndrome see EXHAUSTION syndrome.

exhaustion privation of energy with consequent inability to respond to stimuli; lassitude.
heat e. an effect of excessive exposure to heat. See also HEAT exhaustion.
physical e. occurs most commonly in horses engaged in endurance or marathon events. Also in males engaged in territorial combats; bulls and boars are the usual combatants. There are some lacerations but exhaustion is the main problem. Manifested by lethargy, dehydration, hyperthermia, hyperpnea, tachycardia, muscle tremor and some muscle spasm, restlessness, anal relaxation, unwillingness to stand, fidgeting while down, pale cyanotic mucosa and poor capillary refill time.
e. syndrome in a fit horse normal levels of function in the cardiopulmonary system should be regained within 30 to 60 minutes of stopping work. This is unlikely with horses that are exhausted and which have the following clinical signs—lethargy, dehydration, hyperthermia, hyperpnea, tachycardia, muscle tremor, restlessness, relaxation of the anal sphincter, reluctance to stand, pale mucosa, poor capillary refill and a respiratory to cardiac rate ratio of greater than 2 : 1. Called also exhausted horse syndrome.

Exmoor pony English riding pony. Bay, brown or mousy dun, with no white markings; 12.2 to 12.3 hands high.

exo- word element. [Gr.] *outside of, outward.*

exocardia congenital displacement of the heart; ectocardia.

exocardial situated, occurring, or developed outside the heart.

exocolitis inflammation of the outer coat of the colon.

exocrine 1. secreting externally via a duct. 2. denoting such a gland or its secretion.

exocytosis 1. the discharge from a cell of particles that are too large to diffuse through the plasma membrane; the opposite of endocytosis. 2. the aggregation of migrating leukocytes in the epidermis as part of the inflammatory response.

exodeviation a turning outward; in ophthalmology, exotropia.

exodontia removal of teeth.

exodontics that branch of dentistry dealing with extraction of teeth.

exoenzyme an enzyme that acts outside the cell that secretes it.

exoerythrocytic occurring or situated outside the red blood cells (erythrocytes), a term applied to a stage in the development of protozoan parasites that takes place in cells other than erythrocytes.

exogamy protozoan fertilization by union of elements that are not derived from the same cell.

exogenous originating outside or caused by factors outside the organism.
e. fecal contents e.g. calcium taken in with the diet but not absorbed; is distinct from endogenous calcium which is contributed by the body.
e. photodynamic agent agent contributed by the environment; may be a primary agent or a hepatoxin.

exomphalos 1. hernia of the abdominal viscera into the umbilical cord. 2. congenital umbilical hernia.

exon regions of a primary RNA transcript in eukaryotic cells that are coding and are joined together when introns are spliced-out, to make the functional mRNA.

exonuclease a nuclease that cleaves single mononucleotides from the end of a polynucleotide chain.
e. III one from *E. coli* that removes nucleotides from the 3′ ends of double-stranded DNA.

exopeptidase a proteolytic enzyme whose action is limited to terminal peptide linkages.

Exophiala a genus of dematiaceous fungi that cause mycetomas and pheohyphomycosis including cutaneous and systemic lesions, in fish and captive frogs and toads. Includes *E. pisciphilus, E. salmonis.*

exophthalmometry measurement of the extent of protrusion of the eyeball in exophthalmos.

exophthalmos abnormal protrusion of the eye.
congenital e. seen in brachycephalic breeds with shallow orbits; see also EURYBLEPHARON.
inherited e. exophthalmos with strabismus is inherited in cattle.
ophthalmoplegic e. inability to move the eye because of exophthalmos.
pulsating e. due to an arteriovenous fistula of the orbit.
exophytic growing outward; in oncology, proliferating externally or on the surface epithelium of an organ or other structure in which the growth originated.
exoplasm the plasma membrane.
e. face the side of a membrane facing away from cytosol.
exorbitism protrusion of the eyeball.
exormia a papular skin eruption.
exoserosis an oozing of serum or exudate.
exoskeleton an external hard framework, as a crustacean's shell, that supports and protects the soft tissues of lower animals, derived from the ectoderm. In vertebrates the term is sometimes applied to structures produced by the epidermis, as hair, claws, hoofs, teeth, etc.
exosmosis osmosis or diffusion from within outward.
exostosis pl. *exostoses* [Gr.] a benign new growth projecting from a bone surface and characteristically capped by cartilage.
e. cartilaginea a variety of osteoma consisting of a layer of cartilage developing beneath the periosteum of a bone.
inherited multiple e. a benign hereditary disorder in horses. The lesions are visible externally but appear to cause little inconvenience. Similar to multiple cartilaginous exostoses (see below) in dogs and cats.
multiple cartilaginous e's multiple bony exostoses in bones formed by enchondral ossification are seen in young dogs, usually on vertebrae, ribs and long bones. Adult cats are infrequently affected, and mainly on cranial bones. The bony enlargements are painless, but may cause musculoskeletal or neurological dysfunction. Neoplastic transformation has been reported. An hereditary basis is suspected in dogs. Called also diaphyseal aclasis, metaphyseal aclasis, osteochondromatosis, and in horses, inherited multiple exostosis (see above). See also OSTEOPHYTE.
periarticular e. occurs in any joint injury, commencing as cartilaginous osteophytes within a few days of the injury occurring.
exothermal, exothermic marked or accompanied by the evolution of heat; liberating heat or energy.
exotic not native, not indigenous.
Exotic shorthair a cat breed derived from crossing American shorthair cats with Persians. It closely resembles the Persian ancestors, with small ears, large round eyes, and a short nose. It has a medium-length coat in many different colors.
exotoxigenic caused by an exotoxin.
e. organism those capable of producing exotoxins, e.g. *Clostridium* spp.
exotoxin a potent toxin formed and secreted by the bacterial cell, and found free in the surrounding medium.
Exotoxins are generally heat labile, and are protein in nature. Many can be detoxified with retention of antigenicity by treatment with formaldehyde (toxoid). Many are important virulence factors in pathogenic bacteria.
exotropia STRABISMUS in which there is permanent deviation of the visual axis of one eye away from that of the other, resulting in diplopia. Called also divergent strabismus and walleye.
expanded memory one method of using memory exceeding 1.0 megabyte.
expanded pet food a form of dry pet food production in which the ingredients are cooked, then forced through a die under pressure, resulting in expansion.
expander something that enlarges or prolongs; extender.
plasma volume e. a substance that can be transfused to maintain fluid volume of the blood in event of great necessity, supplemental to the use of whole blood and plasma. Called also artificial plasma extender and plasma volume extender.
expectation of life an epidemiological expression of the probability of dying between one age and the next. Based on the human cohort life table which describes the actual mortality experience of a group of animals which were all born at the same time.
expected in statistics refers to the expectation as predicted by the relevant formula or model.
e. frequency see expected FREQUENCY.
e. monetary value a method of estimating the value of uncertain outcomes, in which both the value of the outcome and the probability of the outcome are combined.
e. value see expected VALUE.
expectorant 1. promoting expectoration. 2. an agent that promotes expectoration.
liquefying e. an expectorant that promotes the ejection of mucus from the respiratory tract by decreasing its viscosity.
expectoration 1. the coughing up and swallowing of material from the lungs, bronchi and trachea. In humans the coughed up material is discarded by spitting. 2. sputum.
expeller process use of a screw press to extract oil from seeds. Alternatives are extraction by hydraulic press and chemical extraction.
experiment a study involving a comparison group in which the investigator intentionally alters one or more risk factors in order to discover or demonstrate some fact or general truth.
control e. one made under standard conditions, to test the correctness of other observations.
controlled e. one in which an exact replica of the animals experimented on are kept without any treatment in order to show what changes occurred in normal animals, reinforcing the view that the observed changes in the experimental animals were in fact the result of the treatment administered.
factorial e. one set up in such a way that all levels of each intervention or treatment occur with each level of response.
field e. one carried out in normal circumstances and environment, e.g. on the farm or in the cattery rather than in an experimental institution where many of the factors affecting the occurrence or severity of a disease may not operate.
laboratory e. carried out in a laboratory where conditions can be almost completely controlled.
latin square e. a method of laying out a field experiment in such a way as to avoid bias by physical location.
prospective e. those carried out to see what happens if certain influences are applied to an animal or a group of animals. Retrospective experiments are those which set out to explain events that have already been observed.
experimental emanating from or pertaining to experiment.
e. animals animals kept expressly for the purposes of conducting experiments on them. Called also LABORATORY animals.

e. design the method of allocating experimental units to treatment groups in an experiment; many complicated and sophisticated designs are available, e.g. balanced, unbalanced, crossover, factorial, randomized, non-random, split-plot.
e. epidemiology the study of changes effected in populations by changes made in the factors affecting their performance, behavior or health.
e. model experiment carried out using a model of a real system which contains some of the risk factors which apply in the real state; the model is a simplification of real life.
e. study a study in which all of the risk factors are under the direct control of the investigator.

expert computer system software applications which use inference and symbolic representation to perform analysis and reasoning functions rather than the strictly numerical approach of conventional programs.

expirate exhaled air or gas.
single e. the gas exhaled at a single expiration.

expiration 1. the act of breathing out, or expelling air from the lungs. 2. termination, or death.

expiratory relating to or employed in the expiration of air from the lungs.
e. center the nerve center in the descending reticular formation which terminates inspiration and triggers the commencement of expiratory movements.
e. groan a groan with each expiration; usually an expression of severe pain or extreme fatigue.
e. reserve volume the volume of air which the patient can still exhale after the tidal volume has been exhaled.

expire 1. to breathe out. 2. to die.

explant 1. to take from the body and place in an artificial medium for growth. 2. tissue taken from the body and grown in an artificial medium.

exploration investigation or examination for diagnostic purposes.

explosive substance used for causing explosions. They may be accessible to animals and cause poisoning.
plastic e. poisoning see CYCLONITE. Called also PE4.

exponential growth strictly speaking that of a population where rate of growth is proportional to its population size, but is often used to mean an ever increasing growth.

export to transport, secrete or excrete protein out of the cell.

exposure 1. the act of laying open, as surgical exposure. 2. the condition of being subjected to something, as to infectious agents or extremes of weather or radiation, which may have a harmful effect. 3. in radiology, a measure of the amount of ionizing radiation at the surface of the irradiated object, e.g. the body.
e. button of an x-ray machine. Usually on a 4 to 5 ft cable so that the operator can stand at a distance away from the primary beam. Combined with a timing device that is preset and controls the exposure time. The button is usually a two-stage mechanism, the first causing preheating of the cathode filament and/or rotating the anode, the second closing the electrical circuit and the creation of the x-ray beam.
e. chart a chart set up after a preliminary trial that sets out the best arrangement of exposure factors for a particular set of radiological equipment in order to obtain the best results.
climatic e. exposure to the weather without provision of shelter. See HYPOTHERMIA, HYPERTHERMIA.
e. error under- or overexposure in radiography causing inferior contrast and detail.
e. factors the milliampere-seconds and kilovoltage for radiography of a particular animal. The factors are influenced by the speed of the film to be used, the anode to film distance, the grid to be used and the size of the subject. The exposure factors should be kept constant as far as possible.
e. latitude degree of over- or underexposure tolerable in a correctly developed film to still produce an acceptable radiographic image.
provocative e. in testing for possible hypersensitivity, the exposure to a suspected offensive agent to see if there is a recurrence of clinical signs.
e. time in radiography variable but fastest is best with animals because of the difficulty of holding the animal quite still or of delaying its breathing for any length of time. The milliamperage used should be as high as possible to keep the exposure time short.

expression 1. the aspect or appearance of the face as determined by the physical or emotional state. 2. the act of squeezing out or evacuating by pressure. 3. the manifestation of a heritable trait in an individual carrying the gene or genes which determine it.
e. library a number of different DNA molecules cloned into a single expression vector.
e. vector a cloning vector that carries a gene into the host cell and promotes its expression.

expressivity the extent to which a heritable trait is manifested by an individual carrying the principal gene or genes that determine it. Called also genetic expressivity.

expulsive driving or forcing out; tending to expel.

exsanguination extensive blood loss due to internal or external hemorrhage.

exsection see EXCISION.

Exserohilum rostratum a dematiaceous fungus which causes PHAEOHYPHOMYCOSIS.

exsheathing fluid fluid secreted by strongylid larvae preparatory to shedding the current larval stage sheath.

exsheathment shedding of the retained sheath of the second larval stage of strongyle nematodes before the parasitic stage of its existence can begin.

exsiccation the act of drying out; in chemistry, the deprival of a crystalline substance of its water of crystallization.

exstrophy the turning inside out of an organ.
bladder e. congenital absence of a portion of the abdominal wall and bladder wall, the bladder appearing to be turned inside out, with the internal surface of the posterior wall showing through the opening in the anterior wall.
cloaca e. a developmental anomaly in which two segments of bladder (hemibladders) are separated by an area of intestine with a mucosal surface, which appears as a large red tumor in the midline of the lower abdomen.

ext. external; extract.

extended memory one of the methods for using memory in excess of 1 MB.

extender something that enlarges or prolongs; expander.
artificial plasma e. see plasma volume EXPANDER.
semen e. a diluent for semen. The commonest one for bull semen is skim or homogenized milk containing 7% glycerol.

extensibility index a measure of the ability of skin to stretch, calculated by lifting a fold of skin over the lumbar spine to its maximum distance. This distance is divided by the body length, times 100. Used to evaluate cutaneous asthenia in dogs and cats.

extension 1. the movement by which the two ends of any jointed part are drawn away from each other. 2. a movement bringing the members of a limb into or toward a straight condition.

nail e. extension exerted on the distal fragment of a fractured bone by means of a nail or pin (Steinmann pin) driven into the fragment.

extensive grazing a system of grazing management based on a low carrying capacity on unimproved native pasture without irrigation and usually in area of medium to low rainfall.

extensor [L.] any muscle that extends a joint. See Table 13 for list of all muscles.

crossed e. reflex see CROSSED EXTENSOR REFLEX.

e. postural thrust a postural reflex reaction tested in small animals by lifting the patient off the ground, then lowering it to see whether the hindlegs are extended to make contact and support weight and several short steps are taken to maintain posture. Called also extensor reaction.

e. process disease see PYRAMIDAL disease.

e. reaction see EXTENSOR postural thrust.

e. rigidity see under upper MOTOR NEURON.

exteriorize to transpose an internal organ to the exterior of the body.

extermination mass killing of animals or other pests. Implies complete destruction of the species or other group.

extern a veterinary student or graduate in veterinary science who assists in patient care in the hospital but does not reside there.

external situated or occurring on the outside, toward or near the outside; lateral.

e. elastic membrane a condensation of elastic fibers separating the media of blood vessels from the adventitia.

e. environment environment outside the animal; includes ambient temperature, wind chill factor, bedding adequacy, stall space, feed and water supply.

e. germinal layer the superficial layer of proliferating neuroepithelial cells on the surface of the embryonic cerebellum.

e. inguinal ring abdominal RING (external).

e. parasites see under individual listings for insects, insect larvae and helminths.

e. root sheath epithelial layer acting as a sheath to the root of hairs; continuous with the germinal matrix at the base of the developing follicle.

external ear the outer ear; includes the AURICLE (1) or pinna and the external auditory meatus that carries the sound waves picked up by the auricle to the eardrum or tympanic membrane.

e. e. canal the tubular part of the auricle.

e. e. canal inflammation see OTITIS externa.

e. e. hematoma see AURICULAR hematoma.

e. e. marginal dermatosis see EAR margin dermatosis.

externalities side-effects, either harmful or beneficial, borne by those not directly involved in the production of a commodity.

externalize see EXTERIORIZE.

externship holding the position of an EXTERN.

externus external; denoting a structure farther from the center of an organ or cavity.

exteroceptor a sensory nerve ending stimulated by the immediate external environment, such as those in the skin and mucous membranes.

exterofective responding to external stimuli; a term applied to the cerebrospinal nervous system.

extima outermost; the outermost coat of a blood vessel; the adventitia.

extinction the disappearance of a conditioned response as a result of nonreinforcement.

extirpation complete removal or eradication of an organ or tissue.

extorsion rotation of the pupil, observed only in animals with horizontal pupils such as cattle and sheep. Caused by paralysis of the dorsal oblique muscle, as seen in polioencephalomalacia of ruminants.

extra- word element. [L.] *outside, beyond the scope of, in addition.*

extra-articular situated or occurring outside a joint.

extra-label use of a drug in a way or for a purpose not specified on the label, or more practically the documents provided by the manufacturer. In the case of an adverse reaction the responsibility for any loss incurred rests with the veterinarian, not the manufacturer. Extra-label use is common in veterinary practice because of the large number of animal species being treated and because many of the diseases encountered in companion animals require drugs which have been registered for use only in humans.

extra-orbital muscles the muscles of the eyeball which lie outside the orbit.

extra points most acupuncture points are found along the meridians; a few, called *extra* points, are not on meridians but have special effects on nearby organs.

extracapsular situated or occurring outside a capsule.

e. cataract extraction removal of the lens, together with the anterior lens capsule, but sparing the posterior capsule.

open sky e. extraction one in which the intact lens is removed through a large anterior capsulectomy and corneal incision.

extracellular situated or occurring outside a cell or cells.

e. constituents all of the constituents of the body outside the cells; include water, electrolytes, protein, glucose, enzymes, hormones.

e. fluid all of the body fluid lying outside the cells. Includes intravascular fluid or plasma and the interstitial fluid. That part of the extracellular fluid that is in special cavities which have special characteristics, e.g. synovial fluid, urine, aqueous humor of eye, are called TRANSCELLULAR FLUIDS.

e. matrix the network of proteins and carbohydrates that surround a cell or fill the intercellular spaces.

e. space see INTERCELLULAR.

extracorporeal situated or occurring outside the body.

e. circulation the circulation of blood outside the body, as through a HEMODIALYZER for removal of substances usually excreted in the urine, or through an extracorporeal circulatory support unit for carbon dioxide–oxygen exchange (see below).

e. circulatory support unit a heart–lung machine. In animals used mainly in the investigation of cardiac prosthetic devices.

extracorticospinal outside the corticospinal tract.

extracranial external to the cranial vault.

e. convulsions when the cause of the convulsions is external to the brain, e.g. hypocalcemic tetanic convulsions.

e. meningioma anaplastic, locally aggressive tumors in the paranasal region and the orbit.

extract a concentrated preparation of a vegetable or animal drug.

allergen e. an extract usually containing protein of any substance (plant, food, insect, etc) to which an animal may be allergic.

cell-free e. the solution obtained by rupturing cells and removing all particulate matter.
crude e. usually of cells when they are suspended in buffer and broken up and nothing is removed.

extraction 1. the process or act of pulling or drawing out. 2. the preparation of an extract.
breech e. extraction of a fetus from the uterus in cases of breech presentation.
flap e. removal of a cataract by making a flap in the cornea.
e. forceps concave beaks to grasp teeth.
vacuum e. removal of the contents of a body cavity by application of a vacuum.

extractive any substance present in an organized tissue, or in a mixture in a small quantity, and requiring extraction by a special method.

extractor an instrument for removing a calculus or foreign body.

extradural situated or occurring outside the dura mater. See also EPIDURAL.

extraembryonic external to the embryo proper, as the extraembryonic celom or the extraembryonic membranes.
e. membranes the fetal membranes, chorion, amnion, allantois, yolk sac; term used mostly in the early embryonic period.

extrafusal situated outside a striated muscle spindle.

extragenic occurring outside a gene, or in a gene other than the one in question.

extralemniscal system a secondary (besides the lemniscal system) spinothalamic sensory system which conveys information from peripheral sensors to the thalamus, on cruder levels of touch and pressure, pain and temperature.

extramastoiditis inflammation of tissues adjoining the mastoid process.

extramedullary situated or occurring outside any of the medullas including the medulla oblongata and the medullary cavities of the bones.
e. hematopoiesis see extramedullary HEMATOPOIESIS.

extramural situated or occurring outside the wall of an organ or structure.

extraocular situated or occurring outside the eye.

extraosseous occurring outside a bone or bones.

extraplacental outside of or independent of the placenta.

extrapleural situated or occurring outside the pleural cavity.

extrapolation inference of a value on the basis of that which is known or has been observed; usually applied to estimation beyond the range of observed data as opposed to interpolation between data points.

extrapulmonary not connected with the lungs.

extrapyramidal outside the pyramidal tracts.
e. disease, e. syndrome any of a group of clinical disorders marked by abnormal involuntary movements, alterations in muscle tone, and postural disturbances.
e. motor system see extrapyramidal system (below).
e. system a functional, rather than anatomical, unit comprising the nuclei and fibers (excluding those of the pyramidal tract) involved in motor activities; they control and coordinate especially the postural, static, supporting and locomotor mechanisms. It includes the corpus striatum, subthalamic nucleus, substantia nigra and red nucleus, along with their interconnections with the reticular formation, cerebellum and cerebrum; some authorities include the cerebellum and vestibular nuclei. Called also extrapyramidal motor system.

extrascleral situated or occurring outside the sclera of the orbit.
e. prosthesis see ocular PROSTHESIS.

extrasystole a premature cardiac contraction that is independent of the normal rhythm and arises in response to an impulse outside the sinoatrial node.
atrial e. premature beat arising from stimuli discharged in atrial wall ectopic to atrial pacemaker and may or may not initiate cardiac irregularity.
atrioventricular e. one in which the stimulus is thought to arise in the atrioventricular node.
interpolated e. a contraction taking place between two normal heartbeats.
nodal e. atrioventricular extrasystole.
retrograde e. a premature ventricular contraction followed by a premature atrial contraction, due to transmission of the stimulus backward, usually over the bundle of His.
triggered e. cardiac ectopic beats triggered by afterdepolarizations.
ventricular e. one in which either a pacemaker or a re-entry site is in the ventricular structure.

extratubal situated or occurring outside a tube.

extrauterine situated or occurring outside the uterus.
e. pregnancy ectopic pregnancy.

extravasation 1. a discharge or escape, as of blood, from a vessel into the tissues; blood or other substance so discharged. 2. the process of being extravasated.

extravascular situated or occurring outside a vessel or the vessels.

extraversion see EXTROVERSION.

extremitas pl. *extremitates* [L.] extremity.

extremity 1. the distal or terminal portion of elongated or pointed structures. 2. the limb, tail, ear.

extrinsic of external origin.
e. allergic alveolitis see hypersensitivity PNEUMONITIS.
e. factor see extrinsic FACTOR.
e. incubation period the period between infection of the arthropod insect vector and the vector's ability to infect the next vertebrate host.
e. pathway see COAGULATION pathways.
e. protein see MEMBRANE proteins.

extroversion a turning inside out; exstrophy.

extrude to force out, or to occupy a position distal to that normally occupied. In feed preparation to force through a die under pressure.

extrusion a pushing out; e.g. an orthodontic procedure which makes a tooth emerge further from its alveolus.

extubation removal of a tube used in intubation.

exuberant copious or excessive in production; showing excessive proliferation.

exudate a fluid with a high content of protein and cellular debris which has escaped from blood vessels and has been deposited in tissues or on tissue surfaces, usually as a result of inflammation. It may be septic or nonseptic. See also EXUDATIVE.

exudation 1. the escape of fluid, cells or cellular debris from blood vessels and deposition in or on the tissue. 2. exudate.

exudative of or pertaining to a process of exudation.
e. diathesis a disease of young pigs and chickens caused by a nutritional deficiency of vitamin E. Characterized by severe edema of the subcutaneous tissues.
e. epidermitis a disease of young pigs caused by *Staphylococcus hyicus* (*S. hyos*) and characterized by an acute generalized seborrheic dermatitis. Called also greasy pig disease.
e. muscle see PORCINE stress syndrome.

exumbilication 1. marked protrusion of the navel. 2. umbilical hernia.
exuviae the shed skin, e.g. of a snake or other reptile.
exuviate to cast off or shed skin.
eyas a nestling raptor bird to be trained as a hawking bird.
eye the organ of vision. In the embryo the eye develops as a direct extension of the brain, and thus is a very delicate organ. To protect the eye the bones of the skull are shaped so that an orbital cavity protects the dorsal aspect of each eyeball. In addition, the conjunctival sac covers the front of the eyeball and lines the upper and lower eyelids. Tears from the lacrimal duct constantly wash the eye to remove foreign objects, and the lids and eyelashes aid in protecting the front of the eye.

The eyeball has three coats. The cornea is the clear transparent layer on the front of the eyeball. It is a continuation of the sclera (the white of the eye), the tough outer coat that helps protect the delicate mechanism of the eye. The choroid is the middle layer and contains blood vessels. The third layer, the retina, contains rods and cones, which are specialized cells that are sensitive to light. Behind the cornea and in front of the lens is the iris, the circular pigmented band around the pupil. The iris works much like the diaphragm in a camera, widening or narrowing the pupil to adjust to different light conditions.

The optic nerve, which transmits the nerve impulses from the retina to the visual center of the brain, contains nerve fibers from the many nerve cells in the retina. The small spot where it leaves the retina does not have any light-sensitive cells, and is called the blind spot.

e. adnexa include orbital fascia, ocular muscles, eyelids, tunica conjunctiva, lacrimal apparatus and, in the pig, the orbital ligament.
almond-shaped e. observed with dehydration in birds, where the eyeball is sunken, particularly in raptors which normally have a prominent, round globe.
blue e. a common term for corneal edema. See also BLUE EYE.
cherry e. see CHERRY EYE.
china e. one with a blue iris.
cross e. esotropia.
diamond-shaped e. seen in dogs with sunken eyes and loose skin in the eyelids which drop inwards, such as St. Bernards and Newfoundland. Often contributes to entropion.
e. drop vestibular nerve lesion will cause the eye on the affected side to deviate downward more than the opposite eye when the head is lifted.
dry e. see KERATOCONJUNCTIVITIS sicca.
fatty e. permanent protrusion of the lower conjunctival sac; thought to be inherited in some breeds of guinea pigs.
mirror e. term for congenital cataracts in guinea pigs.
pink e. pinkeye.
e. preservation reflex see MENACE REFLEX.
red e. an eye showing dilation of conjunctival, episcleral or ciliary blood vessels.
e. reflexes includes eye preservation (menace), pupillary light, consensual light reflexes.
e. specialist see OPHTHALMOLOGIST.
e. teeth see canine TEETH.
wall e., walleye the irregular distribution of melanin in a blue iris. Seen commonly in dogs with merle coat color and Siberian huskies. Called also HETEROCHROMIA iridis. In humans, the term refers to EXOTROPIA, or divergent strabismus. See also WALLEYE.
e. wash various medicated solutions used to flush the eye; called also collyria.
watch e. one with an iris containing blue and yellow or brown pigment.
e. worm see THELAZIA, ONCHOCERCA.
eye fluke *Diplostomum* spp. larvae in the eyes of freshwater fish.
eyeball the ball or globe of the eye.
e. equator an imaginary line drawn around the eyeball midway between the poles.
e. fundus the depths of the eyeball viewed from the pupil.
e. meridians imaginary lines drawn round the eyeball joining the two poles.
e. oscillation see NYSTAGMUS.
e. size abnormal includes macrophthalmia, microphthalmia.
eyeground the fundus of the eye as seen with an ophthalmoscope.
eyehooks obstetrical instruments which provide an attachment to the head for purposes of traction. The hook may be a single with a long (3 ft) handle manipulated from outside the cow or mare, for which these instruments are designed. There are also small (2 to 3 inch) hooks used in pairs hung facing each other on a loop of cord. Each hook is placed in the medial canthus of one of the eye and traction applied; the traction serves to pull the hooks together and deeper into the eye sockets.
eyelash cilium; one of the hairs growing on the edge of an eyelid.
eyelid either of two movable cutaneous folds (upper and lower) protecting the anterior surface of the eyeball. Most mammals and birds have a third eyelid that moves across the eye from the medial canthus.
e. abnormality includes entropion, ectropion, ptosis.
e. coloboma a congenital, full thickness defect of varying degrees in an eyelid margin.
e. drooping see PTOSIS.
e. eversion see ECTROPION.
e. inflammation see BLEPHARITIS.
e. inversion see ENTROPION.
premature opening e. opening of eyelids in puppies and kittens before the normal age of 7 to 10 days may result in exposure keratitis because of inadequate production of tears.
e. snapping winking.
e. speculum an instrument used to keep the eyelids apart.
third e. see MEMBRANA nictitans.
eyepiece the lens or system of lenses of a microscope (or telescope) nearest the user's eye, serving to further magnify the image produced by the objective.

F

F chemical symbol, *fluorine*; Fahrenheit; field of vision; formula; French (catheter size); statistical symbol for variance ratio.
F-2 toxin ZEARALENONE.
F distribution the distribution of the ratio of two independent quantities each of which is distributed like a variance in a normally distributed sample. Called also variance ratio distribution.

F–J hybrid see JERSIAN.
F_1 first filial generation, a term used in genetics. See also FIRST CROSS.
F_2 second filial generation, the progeny produced by the mating of F_1 generations.
F and R force and rhythm (of pulse).
F_{cells} factor the ratio of total body hematocrit to venous hematocrit; increased when the spleen is engorged with erythrocytes and decreased when the spleen has contracted, discharging erythrocytes into the circulation.
F4 see K88 ANTIGEN.
F wave see WAVE F.
F5 see K99 ANTIGEN.
f symbol, *femto-*.
FA fluorescent antibody. See IMMUNOFLUORESCENCE.
Fab fragment a portion of an immunoglobulin molecule usually obtained by papain digestion, containing one light chain and part of a heavy chain with a single antigen-combining site.
$F(ab)_{'2}$ fragment a portion of an IgG molecule, produced by pepsin digestion, that contains two Fab fragments, that is two light chains and portions of two heavy chains, joined by disulfide bonds in the hinge region. Contains two antigen-combining sites.
faba beans see VICIA *faba*.
fabella pl. *fabellae* [L.] a sesamoid bone in the origin of the gastrocnemius muscle. Present in carnivores; most species have two that articulate with the femoral condyles. See Table 10.
fabrication breaking down of a carcass of meat into consumer cuts or boned meat.
Fabricius an Italian anatomist and surgeon. See BURSA of Fabricius.
face 1. the anterior aspect of the head from the forehead to the chin, inclusive. 2. any presenting aspect or surface.
f. fly see MUSCA *autumnalis*.
f. louse LINOGNATHUS *ovillus*.
f. mask used in the semi-open method of anesthesia which ensures that all of the inspired air and gas passes through a mask and is exited to the atmosphere. Several patent masks are available for use in animals, e.g. Cox and Schimmelbush masks.
facet a small, plane surface on a hard body such as a bone.
facetectomy excision of the articular facet of a vertebra.
facial of or pertaining to the face.
f. abscess see MALAR abscess.
f. cleft very uncommon congenital defect of failure of closure at various facial sites, e.g. cleft from corner of mouth to ear on the same side.
f. dermatitis see CONTAGIOUS porcine pyoderma.
f. eczema hepatogenous photosensitization in sheep and cattle, by the ingestion of sporidesmin from the the fungus *Pithomyces chartarum*. It grows best on litter in pasture composed of plants with heavy leaf growth, e.g. perennial rye and white clover. Many animals die early because of the hepatic insufficiency combined with the widespread tissue damage.
f. fold dermatitis see fold DERMATITIS.
f. hyperostosis see HYPERPARATHYROIDISM.
f. nerve the seventh cranial nerve; its motor fibers supply the muscles of facial expression. These are a complex group of cutaneous muscles that move the eyebrows, eyelids, ears, corners of the mouth, and other parts of the face. The sensory fibers of the facial nerve provide a sense of taste in the forward two-thirds of the tongue, and also supply the submaxillary, sublingual and lacrimal glands for secretion. See also Table 14.
f. nerve root granuloma chronic, inflammatory disease in calves characterized by space-occupying, granulomatous lesions on the facial and vestibulocochlear nerves and clinical signs of facial paralysis and balance abnormalities.
f. paralysis characterized by unilateral signs related to facial movements and asymmetry of the face. There is droopiness of the ear and an inability to move it, drooping of the eyelid, sagging and drooping of the lower lip and deviation of the nose to the normal side.
f. sinus see MALAR abscess.
f. sinusitis infection and inflammation occurs secondarily to rhinitis or to damage to a horn or dehorning. Neoplasia of a horn core may extend into the sinus.
facies facial expression.
facilitation hastening or assistance of a natural process; the increased excitability of a neuron after stimulation by a subthreshold presynaptic impulse. The resistance is diminished so that second application of the stimulus evokes the reaction more easily.
facilitative in pharmacology, denoting a reaction arising as an indirect result of drug action, such as development of an infection after the normal microflora has been altered by an antibiotic.
faci(o)- word element. [L.] *face*.
faciobrachial pertaining to the face and upper front limbs.
faciocervical pertaining to the face and neck.
faciolingual pertaining to the face and tongue.
facioplasty restorative or plastic surgery of the face.
facioplegia see FACIAL paralysis.
FACS FLUORESCENCE-activated cell sorter.
facsimile in data communications, transmission of written or pictorial matter over a conventional telephone line by one page at a time.
facteur thymique sérique a peptide secreted by thymic epithelial cells; abbreviated FTS.
factitial artificially produced; produced unintentionally.
factitious artificial; not natural.
factor an agent or element that contributes to the production of a result. In epidemiology and statistics called also a VARIABLE because the factor may have a number of values. In an experiment a factor is a type of treatment and in the experiment the factor will be represented in different groups by different values. Such a factor may originate spontaneously or be introduced by an investigator.
f. analysis a statistical method for analyzing the correlations between several variables.
antihemorrhagic f. vitamin K.
antinuclear f. (ANF) antinuclear antibody.
antirachitic f. vitamin D.
f. B a complement component (C3 proactivator) that participates in the alternate complement pathway.
C3 nephritic f. a gamma globulin that is not an immunoglobulin, which is found in the plasma of certain individuals with membranoproliferative glomerulonephritis associated with hypocomplementemia; it initiates the alternate complement pathway.
citrovorum f. folinic acid.
clotting f's, coagulation f's factors essential to normal blood clotting, whose absence, diminution or excess may lead to abnormality of the clotting mechanism. See also CLOTTING factors.
f. D a factor that, when activated, serves as a serine esterase in the alternate complement pathway.
extrinsic f. a hematopoietic vitamin that combines with intrinsic factor for absorption from the intestine

and is needed for erythrocyte maturation; called also cyanocobalamin and vitamin B_{12}.

F f., fertility f. the plasmid that determines the mating type of conjugating bacteria, being present in the donor (male) bacterium and absent in the recipient (female).

f's I to XIII see CLOTTING factors and names of individual factors.

f. VIII activity a test for HEMOPHILIA A; activity is measured in biologic assays using factor VIII-deficient plasma as the substrate.

f. VIII-related antigen von Willebrand antigen.

f. IX deficiency see plasma THROMBOPLASTIN component (PTC).

f. IX complex a sterile, freeze-dried powder containing coagulation factors II, VII, IX and X.

factor X deficiency see STUART FACTOR.

factor XI deficiency see plasma THROMBOPLASTIN antecedent (PTA).

f. XII deficiency see HAGEMAN FACTOR.

fibrin stabilizing f. factor XIII, one of the blood clotting factors that converts soluble fibrin monomer to insoluble, stable fibrin polymer.

intrinsic f. a glycoprotein secreted by the parietal cells of the gastric glands, necessary for the absorption of VITAMIN B_{12} (cyanocobalamin, extrinsic factor). Its absence in humans results in pernicious anemia. Porcine stomach is a very rich source.

LE f. an immunoglobulin (a 7S antibody) that reacts with leukocyte nuclei, found in the serum in systemic lupus erythematosus.

f. loading a relationship between observable manifestations (or variables) and the underlying factors affecting the variables.

lymph node permeability f. (LNPF) a substance from normal lymph nodes which produces vascular permeability.

lymphocyte transforming f. (LTF) a lymphokine causing transformation and clonal expansion of lymphocytes.

osteoclast activating f. substance produced by lymphocytes which facilitates bone resorption.

platelet f's factors important in hemostasis that are contained in or attached to the platelets. See also PLATELET factors.

platelet-activating f. (PAF) an immunologically produced substance which leads to clumping and degranulation of blood platelets.

R f., resistance f. a bacterial plasmid (R plasmid) which carries genes for antimicrobial resistance; it can be transmitted to other bacterial cells by conjugation, as well as to daughter cells.

release f. a protein that binds directly to any stop CODON that reaches the A site on the ribosome.

releasing f's factors elaborated in one structure (as in the hypothalamus) that effect the release of hormones from another structure (as from the anterior pituitary gland), including corticotropin releasing factor, melanocyte-stimulating hormone releasing factor and prolactin releasing factor. Applied to substances of unknown chemical structure, while substances of established chemical identity are called *releasing hormones*.

transfer f. (TF) a factor released from sensitized lymphocytes that has the capacity to transfer delayed hypersensitivity to a normal (nonsensitized) animal. See also TRANSFER FACTOR.

factorial experiment see factorial EXPERIMENT.

f. design a design for an experiment in which all levels of each controlled variable is included with all levels of the others.

factory farming a farming system in which industrial procedures are utilized, e.g. animals in crates moving past a fixed feeding point at prearranged intervals, battery accommodation, debeaking, single animal accommodation with no physical contact between animals.

facultative not obligatory; pertaining to or characterized by the ability to adjust to particular circumstances or to assume a particular role. See also ACCUMULATOR PLANTS.

faculty 1. a normal power or function, especially of the human mind. 2. the teaching staff and the facilities of an institute of learning, especially a university department.

f. in the field members of the veterinary profession who are formally associated with the university faculty so that they participate in the instruction of undergraduates who see practice with them. This supplements the somewhat narrower education provided by the university teaching hospital.

FAD 1. oxidized form of FLAVIN adenine dinucleotide. 2. flea allergy dermatitis.

fadge a horse gait. See FOXTROT.

$FADH_2$ reduced form of flavin adenine dinucleotide.

fading fading skin coloring. See Arabian fading syndrome (below). Declining in body condition, general health, activity and productivity.

Arabian f. syndrome general health is unimpaired. Affected horses, usually Arabians, gradually lose their skin coloring on round, depigmented macules and multiple patches, most obviously around the muzzle and the perineum. It is a noninflammatory leukoderma. The cause is unknown. See also VITILIGO. Called also pinky syndrome, lavender foal.

f. chick syndrome in ostriches, used to describe any chick that is failing to gain weight and grow.

f. horse syndrome see Arabian fading syndrome (above).

f. kitten/puppy syndrome apparently normal young are born, but within the first week or two of life individuals within the litter gradually weaken and die. Not a specific disorder, but generally applied to infectious causes.

f. pig syndrome see NEONATAL hypoglycemia.

Fadogia homblei a South African plant, member of the family Rubiaceae, and contains an uncharacterized myocardial toxin which causes myocarditis and sudden death (gousiekte). Called also *F. fragrans*, *F. monticola*, *F. oleoides*, wild date, bosluisbessie, wildedadel.

faex [L.] see FECES.

fagopyrin a red, fluorescent pigment of the helianthrone family, present in *Fagopyrum sagittatum* (buckwheat), and causing primary photosensitization.

fagopyrism see FAGOPYRUM SAGITTATUM.

Fagopyrum sagittatum a plant of the Polygonaceae family; contains fagopyrin which causes photosensitization. Called also *F. esculentum*, *F. syggitum*, *Polygonum sagittatum*, buckwheat.

Fagus a genus of trees in the family Fagaceae; the residue (or mast) of the fruits or beech nuts are made into a cake after their oil is expressed. The cake and the nuts may cause poisoning, manifested by severe abdominal pain, convulsions and death. Includes *F. grandifolium* (American beech), *F. sylvaticus* (European beech).

Fahrenheit scale a temperature scale with the ice point at 32 degrees (32°F) and the normal boiling point of water at 212 degrees (212°F). For equivalents of Fahrenheit and Celsius temperatures, see Table 5.

Fahrenheit thermometer a thermometer employing the Fahrenheit scale. The abbreviation 100°F should be read as 'one hundred degrees Fahrenheit'.

FAHRMX a computer program developed at the University of Michigan, USA that analyzes epidemiological data so that analyses are retrievable as well as raw data.

FAIDS feline acquired immune deficiency syndrome. See FELINE leukemia virus.

failure inability to perform or to function properly.

f. to conceive said of cows which return to estrus after mating.

kidney f. see RENAL failure.

respiratory f. called also ventilatory failure; see RESPIRATORY failure.

f. to thrive used generally to describe young animals which are not gaining weight or growing; can be due to disease or management problems. In llamas, used to describe a specific syndrome in which the young are normal in early age, but later stop growing. Rickets is one possible cause, but there may be others.

faint temporary loss of consciousness due to generalized cerebral ischemia; syncope. The term is not generally applied to animals.

fainting see SYNCOPE.

fairy clubs RAMARIA mushrooms.

fairy flax LINUM *catharticum*.

fairy grass AGROSTIS *avenacea*.

faking improper alteration of the appearance of a horse for purpose of fraud. Refers usually to teeth. See also BISHOPING.

Falabella Argentinian miniature horse, less than 7 hands high, with a spotted coat color in most animals; a curiosity.

falcial pertaining to a falx.

falciform sickle-shaped.

f. ligament a sickle-shaped sagittal fold of peritoneum that helps to attach the liver to the diaphragm and separates the right and left lobes of the liver.

Falco a genus of the family Falconidae (birds of prey). Includes *F. biarmicus*—lanner falcon, *F. columbaris*—kestrel, pigeon hawk or merlin, *F. mexicanus*—prairie falcon, *F. peregrinus*—peregrine falcon, *F. rusticolus*—gyrfalcon, *F. sparverius*—American kestrel, *F. tinnunculus*—Old World kestrel.

falcon a bird of prey. See FALCO.

falconiform a strong, fierce and large, diurnal bird of prey, of the order Falconiformes. Prey is warm-blooded vertebrates, fish, reptiles and amphibians; some eat carrion. With the nocturnal predators, the falconiforms comprise the raptors. The group includes Old World and New World vultures, hawks, harriers, eagles, sea-eagles, buzzards, osprey, falcons and secretary bird.

falconry the sport of hunting with trained falcons.

falcular see FALCIFORM.

Falculifer a genus of the family of mites Dermoglyphidae.

F. clornutus, F. rostratus feather mite of pigeons.

fall in dog conformation, hair that hangs over the face.

fall fever see LEPTOSPIROSIS.

falling while walking is a common clinical sign in severe ataxia and incoordination due to any cause.

f. disease severe nutritional deficiency of copper in cattle which causes sudden death due to myocardial degeneration.

f. easily involuntary falling down.

f. to one side involuntary falling down, always to one side.

Fallopia convolvulus plant in the family Polygonaceae; contains an unidentified toxin which causes hepatogenous photosensitization; called also *Polygonum convolvulus*, cornbind, black bindweed.

fallopian tube called also uterine tube. See OVIDUCT.

Fallot's tetralogy see TETRALOGY of Fallot.

fallout the settling to the earth's surface of radioactive fission products from the atmosphere after a nuclear explosion.

fallow a pale cream, light fawn, or pale yellow coat color in dogs.

fallow deer a small, 150 lb, fawn deer with white spots and a white spot bordered with black on each buttock. Called also *Dama dama*.

false said of diseases or plants that have a superficial resemblance to another plant or disease.

f. acacia see ROBINIA PSEUDOACACIA.

f. blackleg cellulitis and myositis caused by *Clostridium septicum* and *C. novyi*. More commonly called malignant edema. Characterized by high fever, severe toxemia and local swelling around a wound with subsequent local gangrene and a high mortality rate.

f. blusher see AMANITA *pantherina*—a mushroom.

f. buckbush see GYROSTEMON *australasicus*.

f. bursa see HYGROMA.

f. castor oil plant DATURA *stramonium*, *D. ferox*.

f. columnaris disease similar to COLUMNARIS DISEASE but caused by infection with the bacteria *Cytophaga johnsonae*. Characterized by skin erosion especially at the fins and jaws.

f. distemper a disease of horses with some similarity to strangles. See pectoral ABSCESS.

f. garlic ALLIUM *vineale*.

f. gid see OESTRUS *ovis*.

f. hellebore VERATRUM *californicum*, *V. viride*.

f. indigo see BAPTISIA LEUCANTHA.

f. joint a fracture in a long bone that does not heal; the ends callus over and there is mobility at the point.

f. layer a hen with all the appearances and the behavior of a laying hen but which does not lay any eggs. There is a defect in ovum entrapment and the eggs are discharged into the peritoneal cavity although egg peritonitis is not apparent.

f. lupine THERMOPSIS *montana*, *T. rhombifolia*.

f. negative when the result of a test in a patient is negative when the disease or condition which is the subject of the search is present.

f. positive see FALSE-POSITIVE.

f. quarter a condition of the horse's hoof in which a serious injury to the coronet causes an overgrowth of horn which overlaps the normal wall.

f. scorpions members of the order Pseudoscorpiones. Nonvenomous arachnids called also book scorpions.

false-positive 1. denoting a test result that wrongly assigns a patient to a diagnostic or other category. 2. a patient so categorized. 3. an instance of a false-positive result.

falsification a deliberate misstatement or misrepresentation.

falx pl. *falces* [L.] a sickle-shaped structure.

f. cerebelli the fold of dura mater separating the cerebellar hemispheres.

f. cerebri a sickle-shaped fold of dura mater in the longitudinal fissure, which separates the two cerebral hemispheres.

familial occurring in or affecting members of a closely related group of animals more than would be expected by chance.

f. aggregations groups of diseased animals concentrated in related groups of animals. Called also familial clusters.

Basenji f. anemia see familial nonspherocytic ANEMIA of Basenji dogs.

f. cluster see familial aggregations (above).

f. convulsions and ataxia of cattle an inherited, congenital disease of Aberdeen Angus calves characterized by intermittent tetanic convulsions which are replaced as the calf gets older by incoordination and then paralysis in older animals. The characteristic lesion is a selective cerebellar cortical degeneration.

f. disease diseases which occur at a higher than expected frequency in closely related groups of animals, where the relationship is a shared environment or an inheritance.

f. glomerulonephritis of Dobermans characterized by development of signs in dogs less than a year old but cases may survive for some years; the histopathological lesion is a membranoproliferative glomerulonephritis.

f. renal disease includes familial glomerulonephritis, nephropathy, juvenile nephropathy, all of dogs, familial glomerulonephritis of Finnish-Landrace sheep, progressive renal fibrosis of mutant Southdown sheep.

family 1. a group of animals related by blood or their inheritance. 2. a taxonomic category below an order and above a genus.

f. farm traditional basis of agriculture being gradually overcome in developed countries by amalgamation into larger farms dedicated to business efficiency.

f. selection selection of individuals to be used in a breeding program based on the merits of sibs or half sibs.

famophos see FAMPHUR.

famotidine a histamine H_2-receptor antagonist, similar to CIMETIDINE.

famphur an organophosphorus insecticide used in cattle, sheep and goats. Called also famophos.

Fanconi's syndrome 1. a rare hereditary disorder in humans, characterized by hypoplasia of the bone marrow, and patchy brown discoloration of the skin due to the deposition of melanin, and associated with multiple congenital anomalies of the musculoskeletal and genitourinary systems. 2. a general term for a group of diseases marked by dysfunction of the proximal renal tubules with multiple defects in reabsorption. Occurs as an inherited disorder in Basenji dogs. There is increased urinary excretion of glucose (in the absence of diabetes mellitus), phosphorus, sodium, uric acid and amino acids, and metabolic acidosis.

F.-like syndrome a reversible renal tubular dysfunction reportedly induced by outdated tetracycline antibiotics.

fancy in the name of canary breeds, refers to a special, cultivated show type of bird, rather than the ordinary type. In dog and cat circles, it refers to the entire following of breeders, owners and admirers.

fang 1. a sharp or pointed tooth. 2. a root of a tooth.

f. hole see DENTAL star.

Fannia a genus of flies in the family Muscidae that pupate in feces.

F. australis may cause tertiary blowfly strike.

F. benjamini cause insect worry.

F. canicularis, F. scalaris may cause urogenital myiasis.

fantail a horse's tail cut and pulled so that it protrudes only a few inches beyond the end of the butt.

fanweed see THLASPI ARVENSE.

FAO Food and Agriculture Organization of the United Nations.

Far Eastern tick-borne encephalitis a human disease but transmissible to animals; caused by a *Flavivirus* closely related antigenically to the louping ill virus.

far eastern tick-borne fevers febrile illnesses of humans and animals caused by a group of tick-borne flaviviruses; includes Russian spring–summer ENCEPHALITIS.

Farabeuf retractor a hand- and finger-held surgical instrument with flat blades, one each end, designed for holding back tissues in deep cavities.

FARAD Food Animal Residue Avoidance Database. A cooperative effort of the Universities of California, Florida and North Carolina State University, with primary files maintained and archived at Oregon State University.

farad the unit of electric capacity; capacity to hold 1 coulomb with a potential of 1 volt. Symbol F.

faradic currents see FARADISM.

faradism a method of passive exercise which can be applied locally to stimulate nerves and muscles. The faradic current applied can be varied as to pulse, wave form, voltage and location.

farcin-de-boeuf see bovine FARCY.

farcy the more chronic and constitutional form of GLANDERS. Called also glanders.

bovine f. a purulent lymphadenitis and lymphangitis of cattle caused by *Nocardia farcinica* with *Mycobacterium farcinogenes* also playing a role. The lesions are mostly on the lower limbs but in occasional cases spread to the lungs. The animal's general health is not usually impaired but it may react positively to the tuberculin test.

f. buds cutaneous nodules seen in equine glanders.

f. cords see farcy pipes (below).

Japanese f. epizootic lymphangitis.

Neapolitan f. see EPIZOOTIC lymphangitis.

f. pipes the enlarged subcutaneous lymphatic vessels seen in equine glanders. Called also farcy cords.

farm agricultural enterprise based on land use.

f. animal animals used for the production of human and animal food and feed, fiber, skin and hide and, to the extent that they are used in farm work, bullocks and horses used in the hauling of freight and for transport.

f. chemical includes fertilizers, insectides, herbicides, medicines, bird repellents, poison baits: a common source of poisoning for farm animals.

dry f. a farm dependent on rainfall as its water resource—no irrigation is available.

irrigation f. a farm with a significant part of its area under irrigation.

pasture f. a farm whose principal resource is pasture for grazing animals.

f. profile a description of the resources and practices on a farm drawn up so that an assessor can estimate the financial viability and potential of the unit.

f. visits see VETERINARY farm visits.

farm-unit surveillance system a surveillance system set up on a farm in which the farmer records specifically requested types of data relating to health and productivity.

farmer–feeder a farmer with his or her own feedlot or other fattening facility in which he/she fattens cattle or sheep reared on the home farm. Numbers are small, usually less than 1000 head of cattle at a time.

farmer's lung a subacute, immediate immune complex, hypersensitivity pneumonitis of humans caused by inhalation of dust from moldy hay, particularly the organism *Micropolyspora faeni*. The disease has some similarity to ATYPICAL INTERSTITIAL PNEUMONIA in cattle. See also BIRD-fancier's lung.

farmyard pox a general term used to describe the several pox-type lesions humans may acquire while working with animals; includes vaccinia, cowpox, goatpox, pseudocowpox, bovine papular stomatitis, horsepox, contagious viral pustular dermatitis (contagious ecthyma, orf).

Farquharson operation a technique for submucous resection of the prolapsed vagina which excises devitalized tissues and takes a tuck in the length of the vagina. A transverse, crescent-shaped piece of mucosa is stripped away and the edges of the incision sown together.

Farr test a radioimmunoassay for DNA antibodies in the context of autoimmune disease.

farrier a person skilled in the techniques of making, fitting and remodeling horseshoes, including hot and cold fitting, orthopedic shoeing.

farriery the techniques used by a farrier. Part of the occupation of blacksmith.

farrow see FARROWING.

farrow-to-finish a pig raising system in which piglets are born, reared, weaned, grown, fattened in the one unit. Contrast with piglets moving to other operators at each major stage of their development.

farrow-to-wean a pig raising system in which piglets are born and reared up to weaning in the one unit, then moved to the care of specialist growers and fatteners.

farrowing the act of parturition in the sow; giving birth to a litter of piglets at term, average the 115th day after conception.

batch f. a group of sows due to farrow at about the same time are moved into the farrowing facility at the same time and kept there until all are farrowed; they are then moved out; the facility is then thoroughly sanitized ready for the next batch.

f. crate cage-like, open pipework unit large enough to hold a sow but too narrow to permit it to turn around. Maximizes use of space and mechanical services, minimizes labor and feed wastage, reduces crushing losses.

f. fever see MASTITIS–METRITIS–AGALACTIA.

f. house a specialist accommodation unit devoted to the care of sows at farrowing.

f. hysteria affected gilts restless at farrowing savage piglets without cannibalizing them. Mortality rate very high. Likely to recur at next farrowing and gilt or sow should be culled.

induced f. hormonal initiation of parturition before full term, usually with a prostaglandin.

f. interval interval between litters; 6 months is the objective.

isolated f. program sows are farrowed in isolation as a means of preventing the spread of enzootic diseases, especially atrophic rhinitis and enzootic pneumonia.

f. rate the number of sows that farrow divided by the number mated.

Fartlek training a form of physical training used in humans and applicable to Greyhounds and horses. Involves exercising over long distances continuously but with variation in the speed of movement.

fascia pl. *fasciae* [L.] a sheet or band of fibrous tissue such as lies deep to the skin or invests muscles and various body organs.

f. adherens one of the methods of attachment of actin filaments to the sarcolemma in cardiac muscle; a continuous zone of attachment.

aponeurotic f. a dense, firm, fibrous membrane investing the trunk and limbs and giving off sheaths to the various muscles. Called also deep fascia.

f. cribrosa the superficial fascia of the thigh covering the saphenous opening.

croup and thigh f. extensive sheets between muscle masses giving appearance of distinct molding of muscles, especially when horses in hard training; gives extensive attachments to muscle fascicles and serves as an energy store.

crural f. the investing fascia of the leg.

deep f. aponeurotic fascia.

endothoracic f. that beneath the serous lining of the thoracic cavity.

extrapleural f. a prolongation of the endothoracic fascia sometimes found at the root of the neck, important as possibly modifying the auscultatory sounds at the apex of the lung.

iliac f. covers the iliopsoas muscle below the wing of the ilium.

f. lata the external investing fascia of the thigh. An implant of this fascia is used in operation to correct penile deviation in the bull and for reconstruction of a ruptured anterior (cranial) cruciate ligament in dogs.

leg f. a colloquial, non-anatomic term for the extensive fascia, especially in horses, which converts the upper limb into a series of osteofascial compartments. Consists of a superficial layer continuous with the thigh fascia, a middle layer formed by extensive aponeuroses, e.g. tensor facia lata, biceps, semitendinosus, gracilis, sartorius muscles, and a deep layer between muscles and attaching them to the tibia.

orbital f. three layers connecting muscles to bone, the eyeball and eyelids.

spermatic f. dense fascia surrounding the spermatic cord and testes; internal to the tunica dartos; in layers corresponding to the layers of abdominal muscle; an internal layer adherent to the tunica vaginalis and an external layer adherent to the skin.

superficial f. 1. a fascial sheet lying directly beneath the skin. 2. subcutaneous tissue.

thyrolaryngeal f. the fascia covering the thyroid gland and attached to the cricoid cartilage.

transverse f. that between the transversalis muscle and the peritoneum.

fascial sling see COLPOSUSPENSION.

fascicle a small bundle or cluster, especially of nerve or muscle fibers.

fascicular clustered together; pertaining to or arranged in bundles or clusters; pertaining to a fascicle.

f. block see HEMIBLOCK.

fasciculated clustered together or occurring in bundles, or fasciculi.

fasciculation 1. the formation of fasicles. 2. a small local involuntary muscular contraction visible under the skin, representing spontaneous discharge of a number of fibers innervated by a single motor nerve filament.

fasciculus pl. *fasciculi* [L.] fascicle.

f. arcuatus a tract of nerve fibers joining the frontal area with the temporal, occipital and parietal regions of the cerebrum.

f. atrioventricularis see BUNDLE of His.

central nervous system f. a tract of nerve fibers of a common origin but usually identifiable only by experimental means.

f. cuneatus of medulla oblongata the continuation into the medulla oblongata of the fasciculus cuneatus of the spinal cord.

f. cuneatus of spinal cord the lateral portion of the dorsal funiculus of the spinal cord, composed of ascending fibers that end in the nucleus cuneatus.

f. gracilis of medulla oblongata the continuation into the medulla oblongata of the fasciculus gracilis of the spinal cord.

f. gracilis of spinal cord the median portion of the dorsal funiculus of the spinal cord, composed of ascending fibers that end in the nucleus gracilis.

f. lenticularis a nerve bundle that connects the pallidum with the cerebrum and the brainstem.

f. longitudinalis the dorsal and medial part of this bundle of nerve fibers connects the vestibular apparatus with the oculomotor and trochlear motor nuclei as well as the medullary and spinal neurons responsible for the movements of the head and neck.

f. occipitofrontalis ventralis a nerve tract which connects the frontal cortex with the occipital lobe.

uncinate f. a tract of nerve fibers that connects the frontal and temporal lobes of the cerebral cortex.

fasciectomy excision of fascia.

fasciitis inflammation of a fascia.

necrotizing f. a gas-forming, fulminating, necrotic infection of the superficial and deep fascia, resulting in thrombosis of the subcutaneous vessels and gangrene of the underlying tissues. It is usually caused by multiple pathogens.

nodular f., proliferative f. see NODULAR fasciitis.

fasciodesis suture of a fascia to skeletal attachment.

Fasciola a genus of flukes in the family Fasciolidae.

F. gigantica found in the liver of domestic livestock and is the common liver fluke of Africa. Similar anatomically to *F. hepatica* but much larger. Causes FASCIOLIASIS.

F. hepatica found in the liver parenchyma and bile ducts of sheep, cattle and most other domesticated species and humans. In humans and horses, the unusual hosts, the flukes may be in lungs or other unusual sites and they are often in the lungs of cattle. Causes FASCIOLIASIS.

F. jacksoni found in elephants. Causes a disease similar to ovine FASCIOLIASIS.

fasciola pl. *fasciolae* [L.] 1. a small band or striplike structure. 2. a small bandage.

fascioliasis the disease caused by infestation with FASCIOLA. Called also distomatosis, distomiasis.

hepatic f. acute or chronic hepatic insufficiency results. Acute fascioliasis in sheep is characterized by sudden death due to blood loss from the liver. Chronic fascioliasis in sheep and cattle causes anemia, weight loss, submandibular edema and mucosal pallor. The livers are badly damaged due to fibrosis and cholangitis and are a cause of loss at abattoirs. See also INFECTIOUS necrotic hepatitis, BACILLARY hemoglobinuria.

f.–ostertagiasis complex a disease of cattle in which the diarrhea of ostertagiasis is accompanied by the anemia of fascioliasis.

fasciolicidal lethal for *Fasciola* spp.

f. drugs includes drugs effective against mature flukes, including halogenated hydrocarbons, e.g. carbon tetrachloride, the substituted salicylanilides, e.g. bromsalans, closantel, rafoxanide, oxyclozanide, the substituted phenols, e.g. nitroxynil, and the benzimidazoles, e.g. albendazole, and drugs affecting immature flukes, e.g. diamphenethide and trichlorbendazole.

fasciolicide fasciolicidal.

Fascioloides a genus of flukes of the family Fasciolidae.

F. magna found in the liver and rarely the lung of cattle, sheep, deer, pig and horse and in many wild ruminants in North America and Europe. Sheep are the only species which appear to suffer ill effects because of damage to the liver by the unrestricted migration of the flukes in this species. In the other host species the flukes are enclosed in cysts.

fasciolopsiasis infection with *Fasciolopsis* spp. Principally a disease of humans manifested by intestinal inflammation and ulceration.

Fasciolopsis a genus of trematodes of the family Fasciolidae.

F. buski the largest of the intestinal flukes; found in the small intestines of humans and pigs throughout Asia. Causes FASCIOLOPSIASIS.

fascioplasty plastic repair of a fascia.

fasciorrhaphy repair of a lacerated fascia.

fasciotomy incision of a fascia.

fast 1. immovable or unchangeable; resistant to the action of a specific drug, stain or destaining agent. 2. quick.

f. death factor in algal poisoning caused by cyanobacteria of water bloom; microcystin, a cyclic decapeptide.

f. feathering at one day of age, chicks with the gene K+ at the Z-linked feathering locus have longer primary feathers than those with the K^s gene. The difference can be used to determine sex at an early age. See also Z-LINKED SEXING.

f. muscles muscles which respond to stimulation quickly and have a fast rate of contraction. They tend to be 'white' muscles but the association is not absolute.

f. twitch muscle fibers fast twitch glycolytic cells adapted for rapid contraction for short periods, obtaining energy almost exclusively by anaerobic metabolism.

fastigium [L.] 1. the highest point in the roof of the fourth ventricle of the brain. 2. the acme, or highest point. For example in fever: the high point of constant temperature between the increment and the decrement.

fasting abstaining from eating; animals do not voluntarily abstain from food and cannot be said to fast. The closest similarities are in highly strung animals such as merino weaners when under stress, and the food aversion created by some fungal toxins.

preoperative f. that imposed for some hours before surgery to minimize the risk of aspiration of food from the stomach.

fat 1. the adipose or fatty tissue of the body. 2. neutral fat; a triglyceride (or triacylglycerol), which is an ester of fatty acids and glycerol (a trihydric alcohol). Each fat molecule contains one glycerol residue connected by ester linkages to three fatty acid residues, which may be the same or different. The fatty acids may have no double bonds in the carbon chain (saturated fatty acids), one double bond (monounsaturated), or two or more double bonds (polyunsaturated).

f. absorption test assesses the absorptive capacity of the small intestine, quantitatively by measuring serum lipid levels or qualitatively by PLASMA turbidity, at timed intervals after the oral administration of fats.

animal f. a most important abattoir by-product providing edible fat for the human food chain. Products include oleo oil and oleo stearin used in margarine manufacture and dripping for commercial baking. Nonedible fats go to leather dressings, glycerol manufacture and lubricants. Beef and pork fat are the valuable ones, mutton fat having too strong a flavor for edible fat.

boiling (burning) f. see ACROLEIN poisoning.
f. cattle a class of beef cattle of any age but usually greater than one year, well-covered and judged ready for slaughter to provide prime cuts of beef.
f. cow syndrome a syndrome of anorexia and ketonuria that occurs in overfat cows at calving. Precipitated by events that interfere with the cow's feed intake for even short periods. A poor response to treatment and many cows die.
crude f. that part of a feed that is extractable by ether. Includes fat, oil, wax, resin and some pigments.
dietary f. a rich source of energy for carnivores and omnivores and to a limited extent ruminants. Are usually too expensive for widespread use other than as excipients. They aid in the formation of pellets and in reducing dustiness. Their problem is a tendency to rancidification unless an antioxidant is added.
f. embolism lesion created by a fat embolus.
f. embolus globules of fat, sufficient to act as emboli occur usually after trauma or surgery, but can also occur in hyperlipemia, myositis and atherosclerosis.
leaf f. the best edible fat from a pig carcass, from under the peritoneum.
f. marbling deposition of fat between muscle fibers. A highly desirable characteristic in beef. Is a guarantee of a carcass from a young animal.
f. necrosis necrosis in which fat is broken down into fatty acids and glycerol, usually occurring in subcutaneous tissue as a result of trauma. See also LIPOMATOSIS.
orbital f. fat located deep to the eyeball; substantial amounts provide good shock-absorbent surroundings.
perivaginal f. prolapse during a difficult parturition in a fat cow or heifer perivaginal fat is pushed caudally and bursts through the vaginal wall into the vagina.
f. phanaerosis conversion in the tissues of invisible fatty substances into fat which can be stained and thus become visible.
f. prolapse see perivaginal fat prolapse (above).
f. sheep a class of meat sheep of any age but usually greater than one year, well-covered and judged ready for slaughter to provide prime cuts of mutton.

fat-granule cell see GITTER CELLS.

fat hen CHENOPODIUM *album*.

fat lazy cat syndrome see FELINE urological syndrome.

fat-rumped sheep a class of sheep, mostly Russian, similar to fat-tailed sheep but the large depot of fat is on the rump instead of the tail and although most of them are carpetwool sheep some are of merino type with fine wool. Some breeds are Chuntuk, Kazakh, Jaidara.

fat-soluble said of substances that occur naturally in fats and are soluble in fat solvents but not in water.

fat-tailed sheep a class of carpetwool sheep with large deposits of fat in the tail and on the posterior thighs; heavyweight (rams weigh up to 400 lb), with high productivity of meat and tallow and a capacity to walk long distances on nomadic treks. Their fat tails may be either broad or S-shaped and weigh as much as 80 lb. Many breeds of this type exist in Europe, Asia and Africa. Popular breeds are Gissar (syn. Hissar), Edil'baev, Tadzhik, Saradzhin.

fatal causing death; deadly; mortal; lethal.

fatality rate see CASE fatality rate.

fatigability easy susceptibility to fatigue.

fatigue a state of increased discomfort and decreased efficiency resulting from prolonged exertion; a generalized feeling of tiredness or exhaustion; loss of power or capacity to respond to stimulation. Fatigue is a normal reaction to intense physical exertion, emotional strain or lack of rest. Fatigue that is not relieved by rest may have a more serious origin. It may be a sign of generally poor physical condition or of specific disease.

fattening operations farm animal enterprises in which animals in store or light body condition are fed intensively so as to produce carcasses carrying a good proportion of fat.

fatty pertaining to or characterized by fat. See also ADIPOSE.
f. acids organic compounds of carbon, hydrogen and oxygen that are esterified with glycerol to form fat. All fats are esters of fatty acids and glycerol, the fatty acids accounting for 90% of the molecule of most natural fats. A fatty acid consists of a long chain of carbon atoms with a carboxylic acid group at one end. *Saturated* fatty acids have no double bonds in the carbon chain. The medium and long chain fatty acids are solid at room temperature and are the components of the common animal fats, such as butter and lard. *Unsaturated* fatty acids contain one or more double bonds. The unsaturated fatty acids are liquid at room temperature and are found in oils such as olive oil and linseed oil. *Polyunsaturated* fatty acids have two or more double bonds.
Volatile fatty acids (VFAs) including acetic, butyric and propionic acids are produced in large quantities in the rumen by the fermentative digestion of cellulose. Much of the energy consumption of ruminants comes from these VFAs in the situation in which other animals use glucose. See also 3-omega fatty acid (below).
f. acid nutritional deficiency a secondary deficiency occurs in pigs on high-calcium diets. This may have a connection with parakeratosis of pigs caused by zinc deficiency and calcium excess in the diet. Requirements for dietary fat in dogs and cats are usually expressed as the essential LINOLEIC ACID and ARACHIDONIC ACID.
f. acid synthase in bacteria, a multiprotein complex; in mammals, a single multifunctional protein important in the synthesis of palmitate as a major source of fatty acids.
f. acyl CoA generic term for long hydrocarbon chains, generally between C12 and C20, linked via thioester to coenzyme A.
f. acyl CoA:cholesterol acyltransferase enzyme (ACAT) catalyzing the transfer of fatty acyl group to cholesterol, irreversible physiologically. Its action regulates the number of LDL receptors by converting excess cholesterol (which inhibits LDL receptors) to cholesterol esters.
branched chain f. acids fatty acids usually containing a methyl branch; lowers the melting point compared with the equivalent straight chain fatty acid.
f. casts see urinary CAST.
f. degeneration deposit of fat globules in a tissue.
essential f. acids (EFA) ESSENTIAL fatty acids.
f. liver accumulation of fat in a liver beyond the level which is normally encountered may be a result of a normal physiological response to increased peripheral lipolysis, obesity or the action of hepatotoxins.
f. liver disease see FAT cow syndrome.
f. liver syndrome 1. a disease of laying birds housed in battery cages. The cause is unknown. Affected birds are significantly heavier, there is a fall in egg production and they die acutely of liver rupture. The liver is greasy, mushy in consistency and yellow in

color. 2. a severe fatty accumulation in the liver and hypertriglyceridemia that may develop in obese cats that are anorexic. There is jaundice, weight loss, neurological signs and a high mortality. Called also idiopathic feline hepatic lipidosis.

omega-3 (n-3) f. acids include α-linolenic acid, eicosapentanoic acid, docosahexanoic acid. High concentrations found in cold water marine (fish) oils.

omega-6 (n-6) f. acids found in terrestrial plants, including safflower oil, corn oil and evening primrose oil, which is a rich source of linoleic and arachidonic acids.

f. tissue connective tissue made of fat cells in a meshwork of areolar tissue.

fatty liver-hemorrhagic syndrome a disorder that occurs as sporadic outbreaks in laying hens, especially those in cages. Hens are found dead with pale heads; large clots of blood in the abdomen have originated from the fatty liver; cause unknown.

fatty liver/kidney syndrome a biotin-responsive condition in broiler chickens characterized by slow growth, hypoglycemia and fatty infiltration of liver and kidney.

fauces the passage from the mouth to the pharynx.

faucitis inflammation of the fauces.

faveira plant poisoning caused by DIMORPHANDRA *mollis*.

faveolate honeycombed; alveolate.

faveolus see FOVEOLA.

favoring an animal is said to be favoring a leg when it avoids putting all of its weight on the limb. A part of being lame in a limb.

favus a disease of fowls caused by *Microsporum gallinae*. Small white patches appear on the comb, then coalesce and thicken. If lesions spread to feathered parts typical favus shield-like scabs are formed. In long-standing cases scabs on the skin of the neck may be packed close together and, with their depressed centers, give a honeycomb appearance, hence the name honeycomb ringworm.

fawn young of the small deer species. See also Table 20.

fawn Irish setter syndrome see color mutant ALOPECIA.

FAX facsimile transmission.

fazadinium bromide a nondepolarizing neuromuscular blocking agent which has some undesirable side-effects in dogs and cats and is not recommended.

Fc fragment a portion of an immunoglobulin molecule, produced by papain digestion, with parts of two heavy chains. It has no antigen-combining sites, but contributes to a number of effector functions such as the binding of antibody to Fc receptors on a variety of cells, the transfer of antibody from the circulation into colostrum, the transfer across the gut of the newborn, and the binding of complement.

5FC 5-flucytosine.

FCA Freund's complete adjuvant.

FCV feline calicivirus.

FD fatal (lethal) dose; focal distance.

FDA US Food and Drug Administration.

FD&C Red No. 3 see ERYTHROSINE.

FDP fibrin (fibrinogen) degradation product.

Fe chemical symbol, *iron* (L. *ferrum*).

fear a normal emotional response to consciously recognized external sources of danger such as those often associated with loud noises, threatening gestures, strange people and thunderstorms; it is manifested in animals by flight, by attack or by cringing.

feather 1. skin appendages of all birds. Comprise a central shaft with a flat vane on either side. The shaft consists of the calamus, embedded in the feather follicle, and the rachis which is outside the follicle. The calamus has an opening at each end, the superior and inferior umbilicus. The inferior umbilicus contains the dermal papilla which produces the pulp which continues up the interior of the calamus to end at and pass out through the superior umbilicus. Each feather has two parts, the mainfeather and a small afterfeather which is attached at the superior umbilicus. Barbs and barbules form the bulk of the vane.

Contour feathers are large feathers that give the bird its shape. *Down* feathers are very small feathers. Semiplume feathers are intermediate in size between contour and down. Filoplume feathers are hairlike and remain after other feathers are plucked. They have only one small tuft of barbs. Specialized additional feathers include auricular feathers, around the ear lobes, oil gland feathers, at the oil gland on the tail, bristle feathers on the eyelids and powder feathers in aquatic birds. Remiges are the large flight feathers of the wing and rectrices the very long contour feathers coming from the side of the tail. These are the longest feathers of all in the domestic fowl.

The feather coat consists of feather tracts (see below) or pterylae that are well defined and carry contour feathers and semiplumes. They are separated by unfeathered tracts called apteria. The distribution of special feathers of particular colors in particular pterylae is what gives the breeds their distinctive appearance. The feather coat is divided up into regions that include hackle, cape, cushion, saddle, wing bars, wing fronts and wing bows.

2. long hairs on the fetlocks of draft breeds of horses and in dogs, on the ventral body, caudal aspect of the legs, and ventral tail of spaniels and setters.

3. hair-streams that produce feather-like marks, in the haircoat of an animal.

f. clipping clipping the flight feathers with tin shears will prevent flight for several months.

f. coat the total feather covering of a bird. Called also ptilosis.

contour f. the externally visible feathers which determine the bird's silhouette and the contours of the wings, body and tail.

f. cushion the plumage from the pelvic tract of the hen, forming the back cover.

f. cysts contain unerupted feathers and keratinous debris that may form large cutaneous lumps.

f. disease an idiopathic disease of all varieties of cockatoos, lovebirds and budgerigars as young birds and characterized by a chronic, progressive, symmetrical loss of feathers, elongation of toenails and upper beak, which later becomes necrotic and sloughs off. Called also psittacine beak and feather syndrome.

filoplume f. hairlike feathers, commonest on neck, head.

flight f. the strong feathers on the wings and tail of birds used in flight. Called also remiges (plural), remex (singular).

f. follicle a small tubular invagination of the skin with a fleshy dermal papilla at the bottom from which the feather grows. The papilla is inserted in the opening at the end of the quill.

f. mites mites that live on and in feathers, often in enormous numbers but have little pathogenicity. Include the genera of *Analges* and *Megninia* of the family Analgesidae and the genus *Dermoglyphus* of the family Dermoglyphidae. Other miscellaneous genera are *Syringophilus*, *Falculifer*, *Freyana*, *Pterolichus*, *Pteronyssus*.

f. muscles similar to erector pili muscles of mammals; attached to the sides of the follicle; capable of elevating or lowering entire groups of feathers.

f. picking a vice thought to be due to insecurity and manifested by the bird pecking off its own feathers. If blood is drawn cannibalism may develop.

primary f. flight feathers on the wings of birds.

psittacine beak and f. disease see PSITTACINE beak and feather disease.

f. pulling see feather picking (above).

f. pulp remnants of vascular tissue contained in the core of each feather.

saddle f. the plumage covering the back of male birds.

f. syndrome see PSITTACINE beak and feather disease.

f. tract area of the skin of a bird in which feathers grow. They are well defined and separated by unfeathered areas called apteria.

feathering a digital stroking of the vagina, done in whelping bitches to stimulate contractions and straining.

febantel an imidazothiazole anthelmintic used in sheep, cattle and horses. Has a wide spectrum of efficiency against nematodes and is safe for use in all stages of pregnancy but should not be used within 7 days of bromsalans.

febricide lowering bodily temperature; an agent that so acts.

febrifacient producing fever.

febrifuge an agent that reduces body temperature in fever; antipyretic.

febrile pertaining to fever; feverish.

fecal pertaining to or of the nature of feces.

f. bilirubin bilirubin in feces should be reduced to urobilinogen and its presence is suggestive of abnormality. See also BILIRUBIN.

f. consistency classified as watery, soft, normal, dry and firm, scybalous.

f. eating see COPROPHAGY.

f. egg count see EGG count.

f. examination for worms adult worms in anthelmintic trials are collected in sieves after sampling of fecal output. Fecal larvae are counted by special techniques, e.g. BAERMANN TECHNIQUE.

f. fat normally a small amount in feces. Large amounts in feces of carnivores indicates malabsorption or maldigestion, suggestive of deficiency of bile or pancreatic or intestinal lipase. May cause clinical STEATORRHEA.

f. hemagglutination see HEMAGGLUTINATION test.

f. marking see MARKING (2).

f. output see fecal volume (below).

f. pellets an indication of normal health in sheep and goats, most rodents and wild ruminants. Horse balls are an equine approximation of pellets.

f. porphyria abnormally high quantities in feces are indicative of the presence of porphyria or protoporphyria.

f. smudge pattern the pattern of feces wiped on the buttocks of calves by their tails is used as an indication of the type of abnormality of the feces and of the gut.

f. softeners agents that act against excessive drying of feces in the colon, aiding defecation. Psyllium hydrophilic mucilloid, methylcellulose and dioctyl sodium succinate are examples.

total f. fat a determination of the amount of fat found in a 24-hour sample. Used to identify maldigestion or malabsorption of fat.

f. trypsin may be measured qualitatively or quantitatively to diagnose exocrine pancreatic insufficiency.

f. volume varies a great deal depending on food and water intake. Otherwise is an indicator of digestive efficiency. Also expressed as fecal volume.

f. water varies with water intake and composition of feed, especially in herbivores. Otherwise an indicator of absorptive capacity of intestine, or enteropathy or use of purgatives.

fecalith a mass of very hard feces requiring surgical removal. Strictly speaking is a mineralized concretion around a fecal mass.

fecaloid resembling feces.

fecaloma a tumor-like accumulation of feces in the rectum; stercoroma.

fecaluria the presence of fecal matter in the urine.

feces [L.] plural of *faex;* body waste discharged from the intestine; called also stool, excreta or excrement. The feces are formed in the colon and pass down into the rectum by the process of peristalsis. When the rectum is sufficiently distended, nerve endings in its wall signal a need for evacuation, which is made possible by a voluntary relaxation of the sphincter muscles around the outer part of the anus.

acholic f. see ACHOLIA.

black f. is usually MELENA due to the presence of digested blood pigments. Caused also by black pigments such as iron preparations and charcoal used in the treatment of diarrhea and poisonings.

bloody f. see MELENA.

watery f. diarrheic feces with a high water content.

Fechner's law a natural law relating the frequency of discharge from a nerve receptor to the strength of the stimulus. This law states that the response, or sensation, is linearly related to the logarithm of the stimulus.

feculent 1. having dregs or sediment. 2. excrementitious.

fecundity the ability to produce offspring frequently and in large numbers. In demography, the physiological ability to reproduce, as opposed to fertility.

f. gene as found in the Booroola strain of merino sheep; causes increased ovulation rate.

FECV feline enteric coronavirus.

Federal Food, Drug and Cosmetic Act a regulation in the United States which requires all drugs used in animals to be approved by the Food and Drug Administration.

Federal Insecticide, Fungicide and Rodenticide Act regulations administered by the (US) Environmental Protection Agency which regulate dispensing and use of pesticides.

Fédération Cynologique Internationale an authority representing numerous countries, mainly in Europe, which sets standards and recognizes dog breeds.

Fédération Dentaire Internationale System numbers are used to record the quadrant, the position of teeth and whether they are primary or secondary teeth.

Fédération Équestre Internationale an organization that produces a set of rules for the conduct of equestrian contests.

feed materials of nutritional value fed to animals. Each species has a normal diet composed of feeds or feedstuffs which are appropriate to its kind of alimentary tract and which are economically sensible as well as being nutritious and palatable. Agricultural animals at pasture have a diet which is very variable and subject to naturally occurring nutritional deficiencies. See also RATION.

f. additives pharmaceutical or nutritional substances that are not natural feedstuffs are added to made-up and stored feeds for various purposes, chiefly to control infectious disease or to promote growth. Improper use may cause poisoning in the subject animals or undesirable residues in food for human consumption produced by the animals. The use of additives in this way is strictly controlled by legislation in most countries. Some of them require a prescription by a veterinarian to comply with local poisons laws. See also mass MEDICATION, GROWTH promotants.

f. beets varieties of *Beta vulgaris* developed specifically to provide feed for cattle.

f. blocks nutritional materials pressed into a block form which animals lick or nibble. Used usually as a vehicle for protein and mineral–vitamin mixes with a variable amount of carbohydrate in the form of cereal grain or molasses.

f. budget comparison of feed required with feed available and likely to be grown during the time of the budget projection.

f. bunk see FEEDBUNK.

compound f. a mixture of macro- and micronutrients in appropriate concentrations to be added to grain or concentrate mixtures to provide an adequate diet for high producing animals.

f. concentrates one method of supplying supplements and additives is to prepare a mix of these substances which is added to the basic ration. These mixes are called concentrates and, because they usually have a high content of cereal grains, mixes that contain only grain are also called concentrates.

f. conversion units of production (e.g. lb or kg weight gain) per unit of feed fed (lb or kg weight of feed fed) during a specified time period.

f. conversion rate the number of pounds or kilograms of the ration needed to produce 1 pound or kilogram of animal under standard conditions.

f. deprivation complete or partial withholding of feed.

forage f. hay, ensilage, green chop. Any feed with a high cellulose content relative to other nutrients.

f. grade said of a consignment of grain. Suitable for animal feed but not for human consumption.

f. grain cereal and other grains used as animal feed. Includes wheat, barley, oats, rye, maize, sorghum.

pelleted f. concentrated foods made into pellets. Have the advantages of ease of handling, lack of dust and waste, and a standard composition of the pellets. They have the disadvantage of additional cost and the potential danger of destruction of vitamins by heat or compression during processing. A common feeding technique in poultry and rabbits. See also ruminal PARAKERATOSIS.

f. poisoning a group of acute illnesses due to ingestion of contaminated food. It may result from allergy, toxemia from foods such as those inherently poisonous or those contaminated by poisons, foods containing poisons formed by bacteria or bloodborne infections. Food poisoning usually causes inflammation of the gastrointestinal tract (gastroenteritis).

f. refusal the patient is hungry but refuses to eat the particular feed.

f. residues materials left over from some treatment of pasture or crop, or of animal material from animals that have been treated with for example a chlorinated hydrocarbon. The residues may be toxic to the animals or their risk may be that of subsequent passage to the human food chain.

f. standards a set of tables which include the amounts of each dietary constituent required by each age and class of animal for maintenance and for different levels of production. When complemented by tables of composition of feeds it is then possible to accurately formulate rations for individual or groups of animals, a process essential for operation of a least-cost ration feeding program.

f. supplements nutritive materials which are feedstuffs in their own right and which are added to a basic diet such as pasture to supplement its deficiencies. Includes trace elements and macrofeeds such as protein supplements.

f. antibiotic supplement antibiotics fed to supply undefined growth promotion factors to farm animals. Called also feed probiotic supplements.

f. probiotic supplement see feed antibiotic supplement (above).

f. utilization proportion of a feed which can be utilized by the patient for bodily functions; abnormality may be a characteristic of the feed or of the patient's digestive or metabolic processes.

feedback the return of some of the output of a system as input so as to exert some control in the process.

Feedback controls are a type of self-regulating mechanism by which certain activities are sustained within prescribed ranges. For example, the serum concentration of oxygen is affected in part by the rate and depth of respirations and is, therefore, an output of the respiratory system. If the concentration of oxygen drops below normal, this information is transmitted as *input* to the respiratory control center. The control center is thereby stimulated to increase the rate of respirations in order to return the oxygen concentration in the blood to within normal range.

This series of events is an example of *negative feedback*, which always causes the controller to respond in a manner that opposes a deviation from the normal level (setpoint). It is, therefore, a corrective action that returns a factor within the system to a normal range. *Positive feedback* tends to increase a deviation from the setpoint. In other words, positive feedback reinforces and accelerates either an excess or deficit of a factor within the system. See also HOMEOSTASIS.

feedbunk a bulk store of feed from which the herd or group can eat, thus avoiding rehandling. Requires a suitable means of controlling the amount to be eaten per day and avoiding wastage.

feeder abbreviation for self-feeders. Used in feeding groups of animals at intervals of several days. Feed has to be dry and comminuted so that it will run down the spouts from the hopper into the troughs.

magnetic f. a self-feeding device in which a feed hopper is triggered to deliver a particular quantity of feed depending on the signal received from a transponder worn by an individual cow. The feeders are normally closed and will open only for cows carrying the transponder, and deliver either a set amount of feed to all cows or an amount specified in the particular cow's signal.

feeder livestock cattle, lambs or pigs being prepared for entry to or being fattened in a feedlot. Where livestock are fattened on pasture the term refers to castrated males, spayed heifers and cull animals offered for sale to farmers who will put them on good pasture for 3 to 9 months until they fatten. Called also store.

feedforward the anticipatory effect that one intermediate in a metabolic or endocrine control system exerts on another intermediate further along in the pathway; such effect may be positive or negative.

feeding the taking or giving of food.

artificial f. feeding of a neonate with food other than its dam's milk.

f. behavior difficulty in prehension, quidding, regurgitation through the nostrils, coughing and aspiration are all abnormalities of feeding behavior of clinical importance.

challenge f. animals are fed more feed than their present production or growth justifies in an attempt to elicit higher production still.

enteral f. see ENTERAL feeding.

force f. administration of food by force to animals who cannot or will not receive it, e.g. anorexic animals or weak neonates.

intravenous f. administration of nutrient fluids through a vein. See also INTRAVENOUS infusion.

lead f. see challenge feeding (above).

f. module a concentrated source of one type of nutrient, e.g. carbohydrate, fat or protein.

orphan f. diets for newborn animals which have lost their dams; milk replacers.

f. pattern 1. the procedure adopted by an animal while eating a meal. May consist of eating concentrates before roughage. Includes nibbling, gorging and sham feeding. See also feeding behavior (above). 2. the program of feeding adopted by the animal's custodian. Includes single, large meals, frequent, small snacks.

pellet f. the ration is converted into pellets, logs or bricks. Has the advantage of reducing wastage and facilitating feeding especially with automatic feeders. There is the additional cost of manufacturing.

restricted f. used in times of shortage, e.g. during a drought or as a management tool to modify the carcass, especially its fat content, or the milk yield at drying off. Restraint in feeding for animals that receive only stored feeds is simple. There are difficulties in animals that are at pasture or in feedlots on self-feeders. For pastured animals strip GRAZING is the accepted strategy. In feedlots it is customary to add a feed-aversion agent such as salt or flowers of sulfur to grain ration.

silo f. feed stored in a silo is augered out to surrounding troughs. May be grain or ensilage.

f. trial assessment of the performance of a particular feed, determined by any of several parameters, e.g. body weight (loss or gain), digestibility, growth rate, palatability, of the feed being fed over a set period of time.

tube f. feeding of liquids and semisolid foods through an esophageal or gastric tube.

feedlot a management system in which naturally grazing animals are confined to a small area which produces no feed and are fed on stored feeds. See also DRY lot.

backgrounding f. a feedlot for the purpose of introducing young cattle to feedlot feeding.

backup f. one that is not always in use but which is established to utilize sporadic overruns of grain which are not economic to sell as food grain.

beef f. for the fattening of cattle. Many systems are used depending on feedlot costs, feed costs, availability of cattle, age at which cattle are available, value of output.

f. bloat ruminal tympany as an endemic problem in cattle on high-grain diets in feedlots. Cause not properly understood and control inadequate other than increasing the ration's content of fiber.

f. consultant specialist, paid advisors in areas such as nutrition, health, milling, feed mixing, environment protection.

custom f. the feedlot operator does not own the cattle but charges a daily per head rate for accommodating and feeding cattle that belong to someone else.

European f. completely housed, usually over a cesspit, often completely controlled climatically and feeding a ration franchised by a central feed compounder. Based on veal calf and bull beef production.

farm f. a temporary feedlot maintained on a grain farm and used only when the prices of cattle and grain make feedlotting the most profitable option.

permanent f. outdoor, large-scale feedlot utilizing steers from 6 to 18 months of age in short or long keep systems. Feed is cereal grain 75% and roughage 25% although programs vary enormously. Based on utilization of large volumes of cheap grain or other similar feeds such as brewer's or distiller's grains, beet pulp, orange pulp. A popular management unit in North America.

f. pneumonia see pneumonic PASTEURELLOSIS.

feedlotted the processing of animals through a feedlot.

feedstuff see FEED.

fees veterinarians' charges rendered to clients for services. They include charges for such things as hospitalization, mileage, drugs supplied and materials and services used. These are quite separate from, and should be recorded so, the professional fees charged for examination, diagnosis, advice on prognosis and prevention and treatment including surgery and obstetrics.

Justifiable professional fees are based on the amount of time spent on the case, with a varying fee per hour depending on the difficulty and complexity of the problem, and on the specialist superiority of the veterinarian. Most veterinarians charge on a fee for service basis, including procedure-based fees for individual surgical procedures, but large animal practices sometimes arrange fees with individual clients on a contractual basis with agreement on an hourly fee or a fee per head per year.

feet see FOOT.

FEF forced expiratory flow rate.

feg aftermath.

Fehling's solution a solution used in clinical pathology as a test for glucose in solutions such as urine. (1) 34.66 g cupric sulfate in water to make 500 ml; (2) 173 g crystallized potassium and sodium tartrate and 50 g sodium hydroxide in water to make 500 ml; mix equal volumes of (1) and (2) at time of use.

FEI Fédération Équestre Internationale.

fel abbreviation for feline.

f. d l allergen airborne feline saliva allergen.

Felicola subrostratus a biting louse of the superfamily Ischnocera. Found on cats.

Felidae the family of cats; includes the domestic CAT (*Felis catus*) and feral cats of approximately the same dimensions. There are a large number of breeds of the former (see under CAT) and a larger number of genera of the latter. See also LION, TIGER, LEOPARD, LYNX, mountain LION, JAGUAR, OCELOT, cheetah (ACINONYX JUBATUS).

felids cats.

feline of, or pertaining to, members of the family Felidae. See also CAT.

f. agranulocytosis see feline panleukopenia (below).

f. actinic dermatitis see solar DERMATITIS.

f. ataxia called also feline cerebellar ataxia; see feline panleukopenia (below).

f. atypical mycobacterial granulomas see opportunist MYCOBACTERIAL granuloma.

f. autonomic polyganglionopathy see feline DYSAUTONOMIA.

f. cerebellar ataxia see feline panleukopenia (below).

f. corneal necrosis see CORNEAL sequestrum.
f. cowpox see COWPOX.
f. distemper see feline panleukopenia (below).
f. endocrine alopecia see feline acquired symmetric ALOPECIA.
f. enteric coronavirus (FECV) see feline enteric CORONAVIRUS.
f. enteritis see feline panleukopenia (below).
f. granulomatous disease see feline infectious peritonitis (below).
f. herpesvirus the cause of feline viral RHINOTRACHEITIS.
f. immunodeficiency virus a common lentivirus infection of cats considered to share many features in common with human immunodeficiency virus and human AIDS. Initial infection is accompanied by fever and lymphadenopathy which is followed by a long (several years) incubation period and then the gradual onset of a wide range of clinical signs that include fever, lymphadenopathy, anemia, lethargy, weight loss and nonspecific behavioral changes. Secondary bacterial, fungal and protozoal infections are common in more advanced stages. Cat bite wounds and saliva contribute to horizontal spread; there is a higher incidence of FIV antibody in male than female cats.
f. inappropriate elimination see elimination BEHAVIOR.
f. infectious anemia (FIA) a hemolytic anemia caused by the red blood cell parasite, *Haemobartonella* (*Eperythrozoon*) *felis*. Infected cats experience a progressive, usually cyclic, decrease in numbers of red blood cells, weight loss, splenomegaly and occasionally icterus. The causative agent can be demonstrated in blood smears. Called also hemobartonellosis.
f. infectious peritonitis (FIP) a progressive disease of the domestic cat and other Felidae caused by a coronavirus. The disease is characterized by an insidious onset, fever, weight loss, and any of a wide variety of clinical signs reflecting the highly variable distribution of vasculitis, granulomatous lesions and effusions. Immune complexes are believed to be important in the pathogenesis of this disease. In the *wet* form, there are peritoneal or pleural effusions, or both. In the *dry* form, typical pyogranulomas occur in almost any location. Anemia, hypergammaglobulinemia and elevated antibody titer to coronavirus assist in making a diagnosis. Called also feline granulomatous disease, feline infectious vasculitis.
f. infectious vasculitis see feline infectious peritonitis (above).
f. influenza see feline viral respiratory disease complex (below).
f. keratitis nigra see CORNEAL sequestrum.
f. lentivirus infection see feline immunodeficiency virus (above).
f. leprosy a granulomatous skin disease of cats believed to be associated with *Mycobacterium lepraemurium* infection. Single or multiple, sometimes ulcerated, lesions occur most often on the face, head or legs. Believed to be caused by contact with rodents.
f. leukemia virus (FeLV) an oncornavirus, antigenically related to other leukemia viruses; exists in three subtypes, A, B and C. Subclinical infection occurs in many cats, but some become persistently viremic carriers, shedding the virus in saliva and urine. The virus causes neoplastic (lymphosarcoma and other lymphoid tumors and myeloproliferative disease) and many non-neoplastic (bone marrow suppression, including nonregenerative anemia, thymic atrophy and immunosuppression) diseases and is associated with reproductive failure, glomerulonephritis and autoimmune hemolytic anemia. The immunosuppression predisposes to a very wide spectrum of disease, particularly the infectious agents of feline infectious anemia, feline infectious peritonitis, viral respiratory disease, stomatitis, abscess, etc.
f. mammary fibroadenomatosis see feline MAMMARY hypertrophy.
f. mammary fibroadenomatous hyperplasia see feline MAMMARY hypertrophy.
f. mammary fibroepithelial hyperplasia see feline MAMMARY hypertrophy.
f. mammary hypertrophy see feline MAMMARY hypertrophy.
f. oncornavirus cell membrane antigen (FOCMA) see feline oncornavirus cell membrane ANTIGEN.
f. panleukopenia (FPL) an acute disease, particularly of young cats, caused by feline parvovirus. Clinical signs are depression, vomiting, diarrhea and marked dehydration. There is a panleukopenia of varying severity that aids in diagnosis. Intrauterine or perinatal infection may cause fetal death, abortion, neonatal deaths, and a degeneration of the external layer of the cerebellum that results in a cerebellar ataxia in surviving kittens. Most infections are subclinical, but in clinical cases mortality is high. The disease can be prevented by vaccination at an early age. All felids, mustelids and procyonids are also susceptible to feline panleukopenia virus infection.
f. parvovirus see feline panleukopenia (above).
f. picornavirus see feline CALICIVIRUS infection.
f. pneumonitis infection by *Chlamydia psittaci* causes a chronic, often recurrent, conjunctivitis and infrequently lower respiratory disease. See also feline viral respiratory disease complex (below).
f. restraint bag a bag made of heavy canvas, about 12 in × 6 in with zippers at strategic points so that a cat can be popped in, with its head free, and one limb at a time exteriorized.
f. retroviral test tests for feline leukemia virus and feline immunodeficiency virus; combined tests are available.
f. rhinotracheitis see feline viral RHINOTRACHEITIS.
f. sarcoma virus (FeSV) a recombinant virus in the family *Retroviridae* formed from feline leukemia virus and cat cellular DNA *onc* gene sequences. It is the cause of multicentric fibrosarcomas in cats.
f. syncytia-forming virus (FeSFV) see foaming VIRUS, RETROVIRIDAE.
f. T-lymphotropic virus an earlier name for feline immunodeficiency virus (above).
f. ulcerative stomatitis an inflammatory disease of the oral mucosa, particularly the fauces, hard palate, gingiva and gums. The cause is unknown, but feline calicivirus is sometimes isolated, and immunosuppression may predispose.
f. upper respiratory disease (FURD) see feline viral respiratory disease complex (below).
f. urological syndrome (FUS) a collection of clinical signs which typically includes hematuria, dysuria, and partial or complete obstruction of the urinary tract by uroliths, microcalculi or excessive amounts of struvite crystals. The cause is unknown but appears to be multifactorial, with mineral and water content of the diet, urinary pH and water turnover having some effect on the development of the disease. Called also the fat, lazy cat syndrome.
f. viral respiratory disease complex mild to severe upper respiratory infection characterized by a high morbidity, low mortality, fever, ocular and nasal discharges, sneezing, coughing and ulcerations of the

tongue. Feline herpesvirus and feline calicivirus are the most common etiological agents, occurring with about equal frequency; rarely *Chlamydia psittaci* or mycoplasmas are involved. It is often not possible to identify the causative agent on the basis of clinical signs, but in general calicivirus is associated with a milder illness, marked by ulcerations of the tongue, lips, nasal philtrum, and sometimes skin, while feline herpesvirus causes a more severe disease with sneezing, coughing and ocular lesions that include chemosis, keratitis and corneal ulceration. Lower respiratory disease occasionally occurs, most often in kittens. Vaccines are available to prevent these infections. See also feline CALICIVIRUS infection, feline viral RHINOTRACHEITIS. Called also cat flu, feline influenza.

f. viral rhinotracheitis (FVR) see feline viral RHINOTRACHEITIS.

felinine an amino acid in the urine of cats. Its role in the metabolism in cats and its significance in the urine are unknown.

Felis a genus of cats in the family Felidae. Includes the leopard cat (*F. bengalensis*), domestic cat (*F. catus*), mountain lion (*Panthera concolor*, syn. *F. concolor*), ocelot (*Panthera pardalis*, syn. *F. pardalis*) and many other wild cats.

Fell pony an English riding pony similar to the Dales pony but smaller. Black, brown, bay and occasionally gray; 13 to 14 hands high.

fellmonger strictly a person who harvests wool from hides or dead sheep; common usage is person who deals in hides or skins of animals, especially sheepskins.

fellmongering removal of wool from hides by bacterial action or treatment with chemicals. Called also sweating.

felt woollen fabric used as lining for harness.

felting the property of wool by which fibers interlock and form a compact mass.

feltwork a complex of closely interwoven fibers, as of nerve fibers.

FeLV feline leukemia virus.

female 1. an individual of the sex that produces ova or bears young. 2. feminine.

f. genital system anomalies includes hermaphroditism, freemartinism, ovarian hypogenesis and aplasia, imperforate hymen, segmental aplasia of the paramesonephric duct, including uterus unicornis, uterus didelphys double cervix, cervical diverticula.

f. pseudohermaphrodite see PSEUDOHERMAPHRODITISM.

feminine pertaining to the female sex, or having qualities normally characteristic of the female.

feminism the appearance or existence of female secondary sex characters in the male.

feminization 1. the normal induction or development of female sex characters. 2. the induction or development of female secondary sex characters in the male, e.g. in testicular SERTOLI CELL tumor.

testicular f. a condition in which the subject is phenotypically female, but lacks nuclear sex chromatin and is of XY chromosomal sex.

feminizing syndrome recognized rarely and usually in dogs. Some cases caused by Sertoli-cell tumor of a testicle. Manifested by attractiveness to other males, symmetrical alopecia, atrophy of the penis and unaffected testis, mammary enlargement, swelling of the prepuce and prostate, and lack of libido. Other cases are idiopathic.

femoral pertaining to the femur or to the thigh.

f. artery the chief artery of the thigh. See Table 9.

f. canal the passage that conducts the femoral vessels from the abdomen to the thigh.

f. epiphyseolysis occurs in pigs 5 to 12 months old. There is moderate lameness in one or both hindlimbs. The onset is sudden and often precipitated by physical effort; it worsens within a few days so that the pig cannot use the limb. There is crepitus at the hip joint. There is an underlying osteochondrosis.

f. head rounded proximal articulating extremity of the femur; participates in the hip joint.

f. head necrosis see LEGG–CALVÉ–PERTHES DISEASE.

f. hernia protrusion of a loop of intestine into the femoral canal, a tubular passageway that carries nerves and blood vessels to the thigh.

f. ligament ligament of the femoral head which runs from the depths of the acetabulum (hip socket) to the pit (fossa) in the head of the femur. See Table 12.

f. nerve the largest branch of the lumbar plexus. See Table 14.

f. slipped head see FEMORAL epiphyseolysis.

f. vein the chief vein of the thigh. See Table 15.

femorocele see FEMORAL hernia.

femoropatellar pertaining to or emanating from the femur and the patella.

femorotibial pertaining to or arising from the femur and the tibia.

f. osteoarthrosis a degenerative joint disease of cattle affecting especially the stifle joint. See also inherited OSTEOARTHRITIS.

femto- a combining form used in naming units of measurement to indicate one-thousand-million-millionth (10^{-15}) of the unit designated by the root with which it is combined.

femur pl. *femora* [L.] 1. the thigh bone, extending from the pelvis to the stifle. The greater and lesser trochanters are the two processes (prominences) at the proximal end of the femur. 2. the thigh.

fenbendazole a broad-spectrum, benzimidazole anthelmintic for use against nematodes in sheep, cattle and horses; can be acutely poisonous in cattle if administered with or within a few days of bromsalans (Fascol) having been administered as a treatment for liver fluke.

fence an outdoor partition made of timber, wire or other material effective in keeping animals apart.

introductory f. one that will keep animals apart but which is pervious enough, e.g. made of wire netting, that there is plenty of opportunity for visual, olfactory and licking contact of new introductions before actually co-mingling them.

fenchlorphos an organophosphorus insecticide suitable for use as a systemic treatment for warble fly larvae. Is an anticholinesterase and capable of being poisonous.

fenestra pl. *fenestrae* [L.] a window-like opening.

f. cochleae a round opening in the inner wall of the middle ear covered by the secondary tympanic membrane; called also round window.

sternal f. large openings in the caudal edge of the sternum of birds.

f. vestibuli an oval opening in the inner wall of the middle ear, which is closed by the stapes; called also oval window.

fenestrate to pierce with one or more openings.

fenestration 1. the act of perforating or the condition of being perforated. 2. the surgical creation of a new opening in the labyrinth of the ear for the restoration of hearing in otosclerosis.

aortopulmonary f. aortic septal defect.

f. heart valves naturally occurring fenestrations are

common in horses and cause development of cardiac murmurs, especially audible in foals. They appear to be congenital and to exert no significant deleterious effect.

fenitrothion an organophosphorus contact insecticide used in agriculture. Has a low toxicity for animals.

Fenn effect the proportionality between work done by a muscle contraction and the shortening heat (heat produced by the muscle contraction).

fennec small, large-eared, nocturnal desert fox from North Africa and Arabia. Sandy buff-color; hairy soles of feet to facilitate walking on sand. Called also *Fennicus zerda*.

Fennicus zerda see FENNEC.

fenoprofen a nonsteroidal anti-inflammatory drug.

fenoprop a phenoxyacid herbicide of very low direct toxicity but capable of causing indirect nitrite poisoning by altering the metabolism of treated plants.

fenoxycarb a carbamate insecticide, with ovicidal and larvicidal activity against fleas.

fenprostalene a prostaglandin $F_{2[alpha]}$ used to cause abortion and synchronize estrus in cattle.

fentanyl a piperidine derivative; the citrate salt is used as a narcotic analgesic, and in combination with droperidol or butyrophenone as a neuroleptanalgesic.

fenthion an organophosphorus insecticide used topically. Used on cattle as a pour-on, dust or spray to control grubs, and in dogs as a spot dermal application that is effective against fleas for 2 to 3 weeks.

fenugreek see TRIGONELLA FOENUM-GRAECUM.

fenuron a phenylurea type herbicide with very low toxicity for animals.

fenvalerate a synthetic pyrethroid insecticide used in ear tags for the control of head fly and ear ticks on cattle and topically on many species for control of fleas, flies, tick and lice.

fer-de-lance virus a myxovirus-like agent isolated from snakes with respiratory disease.

feral untamed; often used in the sense of having escaped from domesticity and run wild.

Ferguson's reflex abdominal muscle contraction stage of parturition initiated by stretching of pelvic soft tissues.

Fergusson angiotribe heavy duty scissor-type forceps with ratchet handles and blade faces that are cross-hatched and have a matching longitudinal male–female groove running their length. Designed for hemostasis and prevention of subsequent bleeding.

ferkelgrippe [Ger.] see SWINE influenza.

ferment 1. to undergo fermentation. 2. any substance that causes fermentation.

fermentation the anerobic enzymatic conversion of organic compounds, especially carbohydrates, to simpler compounds, especially to lactic acid or ethyl alcohol, producing energy in the form of ATP. An essential part of the digestion that goes on in the rumen and in the colon and cecum of horses. Used commercially in the preparation of alcoholic beverages and the generation of by-products used as animal feed. Also the basic process in the manufacture of antibiotics.

batch f. one of the methods used in the industrial production of microorganisms, where the sterile growth medium is inoculated with the microorganisms and no additional growth medium is added.

fermium a chemical element, atomic number 100, atomic weight 253, symbol Fm. See Table 6.

fern a terrestrial vascular plant of the order Filicales; reproduction is through spores. A few ferns are poisonous. See PTERIDIUM AQUILINUM, EQUISETUM, CHEILANTHES, DRYOPTERIS. Called also pteridophyte.

fern-leaved lomatia see LOMATIA SILAIFOLIA.

ferning the appearance of a fernlike pattern in a dried specimen of cervical mucus, an indication of the presence of estrogen.

-ferous word element. [L.] *bearing, producing*.

ferredoxin a nonheme iron-containing protein having a very low redox potential; the ferredoxins participate in electron transport in photosynthesis, nitrogen fixation and various other biological processes.

ferret a member of the family Mustelidae. The common ferret (*Mustela putorius furo*) is an albino variant of the European polecat *M. putorius putorius*. It has yellow-brown fur and pinkish-red eyes. The polecat-ferret has brown fur. A North American native, the black-footed ferret (*M. nigripes*) has a black face mask and brown-black markings on the tail and feet. The female ferret is called a *jill*, the male a *hob*, and the offspring, kittens. Ferrets are highly susceptible to infection by the canine distemper virus.

ferric containing iron in its plus-three oxidation state, Fe(III) (sometimes designated $Fe^{3}+$).

f. chloride $FeCl_3$, used as a reagent and topically as an astringent and antiseptic.

f. cyanoferrate, f. hexacyanoferrate see PRUSSIAN BLUE.

f. oxide see SACCHARATED IRON.

Ferris–Smith forceps thumb forceps; the tips of the blade faces are cross-hatched with grooves and have several prominent teeth for secure grasping of tissues.

ferritin the iron–apoferritin complex, one of the forms in which iron is stored in the body.

ferrochelatase an enzyme involved in the incorporation of elemental iron into the hemoglobin synthesis cycle. Called also heme synthetase.

ferrocyanide an organic compound used in industry that is reputed to be virtually harmless in spite of its cyanide content.

ferrokinetics the turnover or rate of change of iron in the body.

ferroprotein a protein combined with an iron-containing radical; ferroproteins are respiratory carriers.

ferrotherapy therapeutic use of iron and iron compounds.

ferrous containing iron in its plus-two oxidation state, Fe(II) (sometimes designated $Fe^{2}+$).

f. fumarate the anhydrous salt of a combination of ferrous iron and fumaric acid; used as a hematinic.

f. gluconate a hematinic that is less irritating to the gastrointestinal tract than other hematinics, and generally used as a substitute when ferrous sulfate cannot be tolerated.

f. selinite is insoluble and soils rich in iron oxide tend to be nontoxic because of the formation of this compound.

f. sulfate the most widely used hematinic for the treatment of iron-deficiency anemia. It is believed to be less irritating than equivalent amounts of ferric salts and is more effective.

ferroxidase a substance that oxidizes iron thus facilitating the transfer of iron to transferrin.

ferruginous bodies fine fibers coated with amorphous protein and ferritin, found in lungs, and usually taken as evidence of exposure to asbestos inhalation. May be associated with the occurrence of mesotheliomas.

ferrum [L.] *iron* (symbol Fe).

fertility the capacity to conceive or to induce conception. In commercial animals includes the ability to reproduce prolifically which can be defined in terms of expectations for each species; there is a continuous spectrum from very high to very low or absent fertility. See also INFERTILITY.

f. index takes into account pregnancy rate to first service, services per conception, calving to conception interval, culling rate.

fertilization in animal reproduction, the process by which the spermatozoon unites with the ovum. By this event, also called conception, the male and female gametes unite to form a single-celled zygote. When one spermatozoon penetrates the ovum a reaction occurs which prevents any further spermatozoa entering. The nuclei of the spermatozoon and the ovum fuse in a process called syngamy and fertilization is complete.

Spermatozoa lodged in the female reproductive tract maintain their fertility for 5 days in mares, up to 90 hours in bitches and for 24 to 48 hours in cow, ewe, sow. In the female, the ovulated ovum remains viable in the tract for 12 to 18 hours.

in vitro f. union of male and female germ cells outside the body, in an artificial environment.

fertilizer material added to soil to improve its fertility by adding to its chemical composition. Usually infers a chemical agent such as superphosphate but blood and bone and kelp humus are included also. Some of them, e.g. calcium cyanamide, ammonium sulfate, urea, can cause poisoning.

Ferula a plant genus in the family Apiaceae; contain coumarin and cause hemorrhagic diathesis; includes *F. asafoetida*, *F. communis* (giant fennel *F. communis* var. *brevifolia*).

fervescence increase of fever or body temperature.

fescue see FESTUCA.

f. foot caused under conditions of low ambient temperature by interference with the peripheral vasculature by ergot alkaloids produced by *Acremonium coenophialum* infesting tall fescue grass; characterized by dry gangrene of the extremities, especially the feet, causing severe lameness, often commencing as long as several weeks after ingestion of infected grass. Infestation with *Claviceps purpurea*, or possibly other related fungi may also cause the disease. Accompanied by severe lameness.

f. summer toxicosis hyperthermia and loss of milk production in dairy cattle caused, under conditions of high ambient temperature, by heavy infestation with the endophytic fungus *Acremonium coenophialum* of tall fescue grass. Called also summer slump.

FeSFV feline syncytia-forming virus. See also RETROVIRIDAE.

fesselo see FISTULOUS withers.

fester to suppurate superficially.

festinant accelerating.

festoon a dermal papilla denuded of epithelial cells protruding into a vesicle or bulla. Seen in bullous pemphigoid and drug eruptions.

Festuca pasture grasses, members of the family Poaceae; toxic when infested with endophytic fungi or grass nematodes. Includes *F. arundinacea* (*F. elatior* var. *arundinacea*, tall fescue) with *Acremonium coenophialum* (causes fescue summer toxicosis and fescue foot); *F. rubra* var. *commutata* (Chewing's fescue) + Anguina agrostis nematodes + Clavibacter toxicus causes tunicaminyluracil poisoning.

FeSV feline sarcoma virus.

fetal of or pertaining to a fetus or to the period of its development.

f. age age of the fetus; this may be determined by its crown to rump length, and various other surface features such as hair follicles and eyelids.

f. alcohol syndrome in humans and laboratory animals; in laboratory animals manifested by small head and nose, narrow forehead, short palpebral fissures, long thin upper lip.

f. circulation the circulation of blood through the body of the fetus and to and from the placenta through the umbilical cord. Oxygenated blood from the placenta is carried to the fetus by the umbilical vein. The blood from the fetus is returned to the placenta by two umbilical arteries. Oxygenation of the fetal blood and disposal of its waste products is carried on through the placenta. When the lungs begin to function at birth some of the fetal vessels, such as the ductus arteriosus, and the fetal passages, such as the foramen ovale, begin to fall into disuse. This is a gradual process of fibrosis that takes place in the period after birth.

f. crowding too much fetal tissue in the uterus. May cause fetal retardation in some; also papyraceous fetus. Thought to cause some of the minor congenital deformities, e.g. carpal flexion in calves, facial distortion in foals.

f. death results in resorption, mummification or discharge to the exterior.

f. death ratio see fetal death RATIO.

f. dimensions crown to rump (tail head) length; varies with species; useful as a guide to pregnancy duration.

f. disease disease of the fetus in utero.

f. dropsy in cattle may be due to inherited defect of lymph nodes and lymphatic drainage.

f. dystocia dystocia caused by some characteristic of the fetus, e.g. size, monstrosity, dropsy.

f. early death see early EMBRYONIC mortality.

f. extractor a device consisting of a breech bar that fits across the back of the cow's thighs below the vulva, with a 6 ft long rod with a ratchet running its length. A small tractor is levered along the ratchet and exerts traction on the calf via obstetric chains fitted to its feet. Has the advantages of a block and tackle but with the mobility of being fixed to the cow.

f. fluids the amniotic and allantoic fluids.

f. giantism due to PROLONGED GESTATION, although all prolonged gestations are not giants. Inherited in Holstein cows.

f. hepatitis focal or diffuse lesions in the fetal liver caused by bacteria or viruses, e.g. Tyzzer's disease, equine herpesvirus 1.

f. maceration sterile necrosis and dissolution of the fetus. May be ejected in this form or go on to mummification.

f. malposition presentation of the fetal parts in inappropriate positions for the easiest passage through the cervix, e.g. retention of the head, breech presentation.

f. maternal rotation alteration of the longitudinal relationship of the fetus to the dam effected per vaginam by manipulation with the hand or an obstetric crutch, or externally by casting the dam and rolling her from side to side while the fetus is held in position via a hand in the vagina.

f. membranes the membranes which protect the embryo and provide for its nutrition, respiration and excretion; the yolk sac (umbilical vesicle), allantois, amnion, chorion, decidua and PLACENTA. See also extraembryonic MEMBRANES, PLACENTA.

f. membrane expulsion occurs usually at the birth or less commonly within 12 hours; expulsion is by means of separation of the uterine attachment and contraction and involution of the uterine wall.

f. membrane retention see retained PLACENTA.

f. membrane slip the sensation of a thread or edge of tissue slipping through the fingers when the amni-

otic vesicle in an early pregnant bovine uterus is grasped between the thumb and forefinger; the best indicator in a manual check for pregnancy until the time when cotyledons can be palpated.
f. mobility fetal movements during pregnancy.
f. mole see MOLE.
f. monstrosities see MONSTER, MONSTROSITY.
f. position position of the fetus within the dam, described in terms of the dorsum of the fetus and the sector of the circumference of the dam's pelvis, e.g. dorsosacral, dorsoventral.
f. posture relationship of the movable extremities or appendages of the fetus to each other and the rest of the fetus, e.g. flexed neck.
f. presentation see PRESENTATION.
f. rotation a method of correcting uterine torsion in cows; the fetus is reached manually via the vagina. and the fetus rotated around its long axis using a firm grasp on the upper part of a limb as a handle; the uterus, clinging to the fetus, rotates with it, undoing the torsion. Requires a fresh parturition, a slim but strong forearm and a nice appreciation of the physical law of torque.
f. resorption early death of the embryo during the fetal period with lysis and complete resorption of all of the products of the conception. The dam resumes normal estral cyclicity after a period of anestrus while there is maternal recognition of the pregnancy See also early EMBRYONIC mortality.
f. sex diagnosis the karyotype of the fetus is determined from fetal cells collected from the amniotic fluid by amniocentesis.
fetal age estimation see AGING.
fetalization 1. continuation into extrauterine life of characteristics of fetal existence. 2. changes to the alveolar epithelium causing changes to the lung giving it the appearance of fetal lung.
fetation 1. development of the fetus. 2. pregnancy.
feterita a variety of grain sorghum used as feed.
feticide destruction of the fetus.
fetid having a rank, disagreeable smell.
fetlock a term used for the metacarpo- and metatarsophalangeal joint of large animals and sometimes dogs.
f. flexion test passive flexion of the fetlock to determine if there is limitation of movement or pain with passive movement.
f. knuckling fetlock flexes when the patient puts weight on the limb.
fetography radiography of the fetus in utero.
fetology the study of the fetus in utero.
fetomaternal disproportion a condition in which the fetus is too large, relative to the diameter of the dam's pelvic canal.
fetometry measurement of the dimensions of the fetus.
fetopelvic pertaining to both the fetus and the pelvis, especially at the time of parturition.
f. disproportion the pelvis is unusually small or the fetus unusually large. Causes dystocia, in the absence of any obstruction from the cervix or vagina.
fetoplacental pertaining to the fetus and placenta.
f. unit the fetus and the placenta as a single physiological unit; the conceptus.
α-fetoprotein alpha-fetoprotein.
fetor stench or offensive odor.
f. oris halitosis.
fetoscope 1. a specially designed stethoscope for listening to the fetal heartbeat. 2. an endoscope for viewing the fetus in utero.
fetoscopy viewing of the fetus in utero by means of the fetoscope.
fetotome an instrument designed for use in cows and mares for the purpose of dissecting a dead fetus in utero when normal delivery is impossible and cesarean section inadvisable. There are a number of special instruments all based on fetotomy wire saws passed through metal tubes about 3 ft long. These are threaded external to the cow by passing the wire saw out of the end of one tube, into the uterus and around the part to be amputated, out of the uterus and into the other tube. The two ends of the saw are brought out of the far ends of the tubes and special handles are attached. The tubes are inserted into the uterus and pushed hard up against the skin. Rapid see-sawing with the saw completes the task.
fetotomy dissection of a dead fetus in utero. Applicable particularly to cows because of the size of the uterus and the opportunity to introduce instruments to the full depth of the fetus.
percutaneous f. the fetus is dissected through the skin using first a knife to open the skin followed by a fetotome. It is faster than a subcutaneous approach but offers more risk to the uterine wall.
subcutaneous f. the fetus is entered between the first ribs and the thoracic cage destroyed within the skin. The fetus is extracted when its mass has been reduced by this internal demolition and removal.
fetus [L.] the developing young in the uterus, specifically the unborn offspring in the postembryonic (see also EMBRYO) period, after major anatomical structures have been outlined.
anomalous f. a fetus with one or more congenital defects.
calcified f. lithopedion; a fetus that has become calcified.
emphysematous/putrescent f. due usually to death of the fetus at parturition; the fetus has been dead for several days, decomposition has occurred and gas has been produced and can be palpated as subcutaneous crepitus; presents a major obstetrical difficulty because of the increased size of the fetus and its extreme dryness due to lack of fetal fluids. The conceptus has a putrid and persistent odor.
f. in fetu a small, imperfect fetus, incapable of independent life, contained within the body of another fetus.
mummified f. see MUMMIFICATION.
oversized f. commonly the result of very good feeding in the last trimester of pregnancy and often the cause of dystocia in beef heifers. See also fetal GIANTISM.
f. papyraceus a fetus flattened by being pressed against the uterine wall by a living twin.
parasitic f. an incomplete minor fetus attached to a larger, more completely developed fetus, or autosite.
FEV forced expiratory volume.
fever 1. an abnormally high body temperature; pyrexia. See also HYPERTHERMIA. 2. any disease characterized by marked increase of body temperature. See body TEMPERATURE.

For diseases characterized by fever, see the eponymic or descriptive name: e.g. AFRICAN SWINE, BOVINE petechial, CANICOLA, CAT-SCRATCH disease, DESERT, EPHEMERAL, equine intestinal EHRLICHIOSIS, HOG CHOLERA, MALIGNANT CATARRHAL, MALTA, MEDITERRANEAN COAST, Q, RIFT VALLEY, ROCKY MOUNTAIN SPOTTED, Russian spring–summer ENCEPHALITIS, TICKBORNE, TULAREMIA, UNDULANT. MILK FEVER is not accompanied by pyrexia.
aseptic f. fever associated with aseptic wounds, presumably due to the disintegration of leukocytes or to the absorption of avascular or traumatized tissue.

central f. sustained fever resulting from damage to the thermoregulatory centers of the hypothalamus.
chemical f. fever caused by the intake of a sterile substance, e.g. the injection of a foreign protein, the administration of dinitrophenols.
continued f., continuous f. persistently elevated body temperature, showing no or little variation and never falling to normal during any 24-hour period.
intermittent f. an attack of fever, with recurring paroxysms of elevated temperature separated by intervals during which the temperature is normal.
remittent f. elevated body temperature showing fluctuation each day, but never falling to normal.
septic f. see SEPTIC fever.
f. of unknown origin (FUO) a recognized clinical syndrome of persistently (>2 weeks) elevated body temperature (>104°F) and without other signs. Causes include infections, neoplasia, immune-mediated diseases, and drug reactions.

fever tree ALBIZIA *tanganyicensis* or *A. versicolor*.

feverfew TANACETUM (*Chrysanthemum*) *parthenium*.

FFD film-focal distance.

FIA feline infectious anemia.

fiber[1] an elongated threadlike anatomical structure.
A f's myelinated fibers of the somatic nervous system having a diameter of 1 to 22 μm and a conduction velocity of 5 to 120 meters per second.
accelerating f's, accelerator f's adrenergic fibers that transmit the impulses which accelerate the heartbeat.
adrenergic f's nerve fibers that liberate epinephrine-like substances at the time of passage of nerve impulses across a synapse.
alpha f's motor and proprioceptive fibers of the A type having conduction velocities of 70 to 120 meters per second and ranging from 13 to 22 μm in diameter.
arcuate f's any of the bow-shaped fibers in the brain, such as those connecting adjacent gyri in the cerebral cortex, or the external or internal arcuate fibers of the medulla oblongata.
association f's nerve fibers that interconnect portions of the cerebral cortex within a hemisphere. Short association fibers interconnect neighboring gyri; long fibers interconnect more widely separated gyri and are arranged into bundles or fasciculi.
B f's myelinated preganglionic autonomic axons having a fiber diameter less than 3 μm and a conduction velocity of 3 to 15 meters per second.
binding f's the fibers holding staples of wool in a fleece together so that the fleece can be handled as a unit.
beta f's touch and temperature fibers of the A type having conduction velocities of 30 to 70 meters per second and ranging from 8 to 13 μm in diameter.
C f's unmyelinated postganglionic fibers of the autonomic nervous system; also, the unmyelinated fibers at the dorsal roots and at free nerve endings having a diameter of 0.3 to 1.3 μm and a conduction velocity of 0.6 to 2.3 meters per second.
cholinergic f's nerve fibers that liberate acetylcholine at the synapse.
circular f's fibers running in a circle, e.g. in the ciliary muscle of the eye around the corneoscleral junction.
collagen f's, collagenic f's, collagenous f's the soft, flexible, white fibers that are the most characteristic constituent of all types of connective tissue, consisting of the protein collagen, and composed of bundles of fibrils that are in turn made up of smaller units (microfibrils) that show a characteristic cross-banding with a major periodicity of 65 nm.
depressor f's nerve fibers which, when stimulated reflexly, cause a diminished vasomotor tone and thereby a decrease in arterial pressure.
elastic f's yellowish fibers of elastic quality traversing the intercellular substance of connective tissue.
gamma f's fibers that conduct touch and pressure impulses and innervate the intrafusal fibers of the muscle spindle; they conduct at velocities of 15 to 40 meters per second and range from 3 to 7 μm in diameter.
gray f's unmyelinated nerve fibers found largely in the sympathetic nerves.
intrafusal f's modified muscle fibers which, surrounded by fluid and enclosed in a connective tissue envelope, compose the muscle spindle.
James f's auxiliary conduction fibers from the atrium to the ventricle that bypass the A-V bundle. See also MAHAIM FIBERS.
light f's muscle fibers poor in sarcoplasm and more transparent than dark fibers.
Mahaim f's see MAHAIM FIBERS.
medullated f's myelinated fibers.
meridianal f's fibers of the ciliary muscle of the eye, running in an anterior-posterior direction.
motor f's nerve fibers transmitting motor impulses to a muscle.
muscle f. see MUSCLE.
myelinated f's grayish-white nerve fibers encased in a myelin sheath.
nerve f. a slender process of a neuron, especially the prolonged axon which conducts nerve impulses away from the cell; classified on the basis of the presence or absence of a myelin sheath as myelinated or unmyelinated.
nonmedullated f's unmyelinated fibers.
osteogenetic f's, osteogenic f's precollagenous fibers formed by osteoblasts and becoming the fibrous component of bone matrix.
postganglionic f's nerve fibers passing to involuntary muscle and gland cells, the cell bodies of which lie in the autonomic ganglia.
preganglionic f's nerve fibers passing to the autonomic ganglia, the cell bodies of which lie in the brain or spinal cord.
pressor f's nerve fibers which, when stimulated reflexly, cause or increase vasomotor tone.
projection f's bundles of axons that connect the cerebral cortex with the subcortical centers, brainstem and spinal cord.
Purkinje's f's modified cardiac muscle fibers in the subendothelial tissue concerned with conducting impulses in the heart.
radicular f's fibers in the roots of the spinal nerves.
reticular f's immature connective tissue fibers, staining with silver, forming the reticular framework of lymphoid and myeloid tissue, and occurring in interstitial tissue of glandular organs, the papillary layer of the skin, and elsewhere.
Sharpey's f's 1. collagenous fibers that pass from the periosteum and are embedded in the outer circumferential and interstitial lamellae of bone. 2. terminal portions of principal fibers that insert into the cementum of a tooth.
spindle f's the microtubules radiating from the centrioles during mitosis and forming a spindle-shaped configuration.
unmyelinated f's nerve fibers that lack a myelin sheath.
zonular f. extensions of the ciliary processes attaching to the lens suspending it around its periphery.

fiber[2] dietary fiber; that portion of ingested foodstuffs that cannot be broken down by intestinal enzymes and juices of monogastric animals and, therefore, passes through the small intestine and colon undigested. It is composed of cellulose, which is the 'skeleton' of plants, hemicellulose, gums, lignin, pectin and other carbohydrates indigestible by members of animal species other than Equidae and ruminants.

Dietary fiber is not to be confused with 'crude fiber', which is the term used in tables listing the composition of foods. Crude fiber is mainly lignin and cellulose and is the residue remaining after a food has been subjected to a standardized treatment with dilute acid and alkali. Crude fiber measurements usually underestimate actual total dietary fiber by at least 50%.

Plant fiber is essential in the diet of herbivores. Too much causes impaction of horse intestines and cattle rumens. Too little causes faulty ruminal function including ruminal tympany and ruminal lactic acidosis; a deficiency also causes an unacceptably low level of fat in cow's milk. See also impaction COLIC, ILEOCECAL valve impaction, RUMINAL tympany, low-fat MILK, PHYTOBEZOAR.

acid-detergent f. a modification of the procedure used to estimate crude fiber in animal feeds; it omits the alkali step, reducing loss of carbohydrates and giving a more accurate estimation. Estimates the proportion of dry matter which is insoluble in acid detergent, i.e. the cellulose and lignin in the sample. The normal range in farm animal feeds is 250–450 g/kg DM. The target for high quality grass silage is 350g ADF/kg DM.

f. balls see PHYTOBEZOAR, PHYTOTRICHOBEZOARS.

crude f. a laboratory estimate of the cellulose, hemicellulose and lignin content of a feed. It gives no indication of the digestibility of the feed. The sample is boiled gently in weak acid, then in weak alkali and the residue washed.

insoluble f. has little water-holding capacity and is not degraded in the intestine; includes celluloses, some hemicelluloses and lignin. Wheat bran and other cereal grains, and vegetables are sources.

neutral-detergent f. a modification of the procedure used in determination of crude fiber. See crude fiber (above); it retains hemicellulose and gives a more accurate estimation.

soluble f. forms viscous solutions in water because of its great water-holding capacity and it is easily degraded by intestinal bacteria; includes pectin, vegetable gums and some hemicelluloses.

fiber-illuminated transmitting light by means of bundles of glass or plastic fibers, utilizing a lens system to transmit the image; said of endoscopes of such design.

fibercolonoscope a fiberscope for viewing the colon.

fibergastroscope a fiberscope for viewing the stomach.

fiberglass cast a cast made of a water activated polyurethane resin incorporated into a bandage; used for fractured limbs. Has the virtues of very light weight, great strength and very quick setting.

fiberoptic pertaining to fiberoptics; coated with flexible glass or plastic fibers having special optical properties and orientation.

fiberoptics the transmission of an image along flexible bundles of glass or plastic fibers each of which carries an element of the image.

fiberoptiscope see FIBERSCOPE.

fiberscope a flexible endoscope whose lumen is coated with fiberoptic glass or plastic fibers having special optical properties. Called also fiberoptiscope.

fibra pl. *fibrae* [L.] fiber.

fibre see FIBER.

fibril a minute fiber or filament.

fibrillar center of a nucleolus; contains DNA not undergoing transcription.

fibrillation 1. a small, local, involuntary, muscular contraction, due to spontaneous activation of single muscle cells or muscle fibers. 2. the quality of being made up of fibrils. 3. the initial degenerative changes in osteoarthritis, marked by softening of the articular cartilage and development of vertical clefts between groups of cartilage cells.

atrial f. a cardiac arrhythmia marked by rapid randomized contractions of the atrial myocardium, causing a totally irregular, often rapid, ventricular rate. There is no synchronous atrial contraction and the ventricles beat irregularly. The heartbeat is irregular, the pulse is irregular in rhythm and amplitude. Common in the horse; an affected animal can still race but the performance is poor. Occurs in dogs in association with cardiac disease, particularly idiopathic congestive cardiomyopathy, and electrolyte disturbances.

ventricular f. a cardiac arrhythmia marked by fibrillatory contractions of the ventricular muscle due to rapid repetitive excitation of myocardial fibers without coordinated ventricular contraction. Ventricular fibrillation is a frequent cause of cardiac ARREST. An apparatus called a defibrillator sometimes is used to alleviate fibrillation. The defibrillator delivers an electric shock to the heart muscle, depolarizing the muscle and ending the irregular contractions. The heart is then able to resume normal, regular contractions.

fibrillogenesis the formation and development of fibrils.

fibrin an insoluble protein that is essential to CLOTTING of blood, formed from fibrinogen by action of thrombin.

f.–fibrinogen degradation products (FDPs) the breakdown products of fibrin and fibrinogen, resulting from activation of the fibrinolytic system, they inhibit fibrin formation and platelet adherence. Elevated levels are found in the blood and urine in association with disseminated intravascular coagulation and detection is a test for that condition.

f.–fibrinogen split products see fibrin–fibrinogen degradation products (above).

f. foam a clot promoting surgical material for application to oozing surfaces. Strips of fine white sponge to be soaked in thrombin solution before application.

f. glue a mixture of bovine thrombin and concentrated fibrinogen. It may be used topically or by injection in management of hemostasis.

f. plate method a method of measuring fibrinolytic activity by incubating a fibrin clot with test serum in a Petri dish.

soluble f. monomers a stage in the clot formation process of producing insoluble fibrin monomers.

f. stabilizing factor see fibrin stabilizing FACTOR.

fibrinocellular made up of fibrin and cells.

fibrinogen a high-molecular-weight protein in the blood plasma that by the action of thrombin is converted into fibrin; called also clotting factor I. In the CLOTTING mechanism, fibrin threads form a meshwork for the basis of a blood clot. Most of the fibrinogen in the circulating blood is formed in the liver. Elevations in the blood are nonspecific indicators of inflammatory disease.

f. deficiency may be due to AFIBRINOGENEMIA, HYPOFIBRINOGENEMIA or DYSFIBRINOGENEMIA.
f. degradation products (FDPs) see FIBRIN–fibrinogen degradation products.
f. split products see FIBRIN–fibrinogen degradation products.
fibrinogenemia see HYPERFIBRINOGENEMIA.
fibrinogenolysis the proteolytic destruction of fibrinogen in the circulating blood.
fibrinogenopenia decreased fibrinogen in the blood.
fibrinohemorrhagic a combination of fibrinous and hemorrhagic; said of discharge or exudate.
fibrinoid 1. resembling fibrin. 2. a homogeneous, eosinophilic, relatively acellular refractile substance with some of the staining properties of fibrin.
fibrinoligase clotting factor XIIIa, associated with fibrin-stabilizing factor (factor XIII) in the conversion of soluble fibrin monomer to insoluble, stable fibrin polymer.
fibrinolysin 1. plasmin. 2. a preparation of proteolytic enzyme formed from profibrinolysin (plasminogen) by action of physical agents or by specific bacterial kinases; used to promote dissolution of thrombi.
fibrinolysis the dissolution of fibrin by enzymatic action.
pathological f. see primary fibrinolysis (below).
primary f. occurs with an excess of activators or decreased plasma inhibitors that cause hyperplasminemia, as in severe liver disease, heat stroke and malignancy.
secondary f. is a response to the widespread formation of microthrombi as in disseminated intravascular coagulation.
fibrinolytic pertaining to or emanating from fibrinolysis.
f. agent substances that stimulate or inhibit fibrinolysis.
f. inhibitors include ε-aminocaproic acid and antiplasmin-α_1.
f. mechanism an ordered sequence of interactions between an enzyme and a cofactor on a specific substrate; the components of the process include plasminogen, tissue plasminogen activator, urokinase and kallikrein.
f. stimulators includes hormones (e.g. corticosteroids), enzymes (e.g. streptokinase) and others such as epinephrine.
f. system tests ways of examining the system include clot lysis time, euglobulin lysis time, fibrin plate test.
fibrinopenia deficiency of fibrinogen in the blood.
fibrinopeptide either of two peptides (A and B) split off from fibrinogen during blood CLOTTING by the action of thrombin.
fibrinoscopy see INOSCOPY.
fibrinous pertaining to or of the nature of fibrin.
fibrinuria discharge of fibrin in the urine.
fibr(o)- word element. [L.] *fiber, fibrous.*
fibroadenoma adenoma containing fibrous elements. See also feline MAMMARY hypertrophy.
fibroadipose both fibrous and fatty.
fibroameloblastoma see ameloblastic FIBROMA.
fibroangioma an angioma containing much fibrous tissue.
fibroareolar both fibrous and areolar.
Fibrobacter succinogenes one of the bacteria involved in ruminal fermentation.
fibroblast an immature fiber-producing cell of connective tissue capable of differentiating into a chondroblast, collagenoblast or osteoblast. Called also fibrocyte.
fibroblastoma any tumor arising from fibroblasts; now classified as fibromas and or fibrosarcomas.
perineural f. schwannoma.
fibrocalcific pertaining to or characterized by partially calcified fibrous tissue.
fibrocarcinoma scirrhous carcinoma.
fibrocartilage cartilage made up of thick, compact collagenous bundles, separated by narrow clefts containing the typical cartilage cells (chondrocytes).
f. embolic myelopathy see fibrocartilaginous embolic MYELOPATHY.
middle phalangeal complementary f. forms a bearing surface for the deep flexor tendon on the proximo-palmar surface of the bone in horses.
parapatellar f. medial extension of the patella.
fibrochondritis inflammation of fibrocartilage.
fibrochondroma chondroma containing areas of fibrosis.
fibrocollagenous both fibrous and collagenous.
fibrocyst cystic fibroma.
fibrocystic characterized by an overgrowth of fibrous tissue and the development of cystic spaces, especially in a gland.
fibrocystoma cystic fibroma.
fibrocyte a cell that produces fibrous tissue; called also FIBROBLAST.
fibrodysplasia fibrous dysplasia.
f. ossificans see MYOSITIS ossificans.
fibroelastic both fibrous and elastic.
fibroelastosis overgrowth of fibroelastic elements.
endocardial f. see ENDOCARDIAL fibroelastosis.
fibroenchondroma enchondroma containing fibrous elements.
fibroepithelioma a tumor composed of both fibrous and epithelial elements.
fibroglia border fibrils in close relation to the surface of fibroblasts.
fibroglioma a glioma containing excessive fibrous tissue.
fibrohistiocytic having fibrous and histiocytic elements.
fibroid 1. having a fibrous structure; resembling a fibroma. 2. fibroma.
f. tumor fibroma.
fibroleiomyoma mixed fibrous and smooth muscle tumors of the lower reproductive tract of intact females.
fibrolipoma a lipoma containing excessive fibrous tissue.
fibroma a tumor composed mainly of fibrous or fully developed connective tissue. Their common association with particular sites, e.g. nasal, genital, laryngeal, falx cerebri, results in some well-identified clinical syndromes. See also INTERDIGITAL fibroma, MYXOMATOSIS.
ameloblastic f. an odontogenic fibroma, marked by simultaneous proliferation of both epithelial and mesenchymal tissue, without formation of enamel or dentine. A rare tumor recorded in calves and young cats. It behaves like an ameloblastoma. Called also fibroameloblastoma.
cementifying f. cementoblastoma; a tumor usually occurring in the mandible consisting of fibroblastic tissue containing masses of cementum-like tissue.
chondromyxoid f. of bone a benign slowly growing tumor of chondroblastic origin, usually affecting the long bones.
cystic f. one that has undergone cystic degeneration.
f. myxomatodes myxofibroma; a fibroma containing myxomatous tissue.
nonossifying f. a rare benign tumor of bone derived from fibrous tissue in the bone cortex.

nonosteogenic f. a degenerative and proliferative lesion of the medullary and cortical tissues of bone.
odontogenic f. a benign tumor of the jaw arising from the embryonic portion of the tooth germ, the dental papilla, or dental follicle, or later from the periodontal membrane.
ossifying f., ossifying f. of bone a benign, relatively slow-growing, central bone tumor, usually of the jaws, especially the mandible, which is composed of fibrous connective tissue within which bone is formed.
Shope rabbit f. a transmissible disease of rabbits caused by a poxvirus found only in the tumors. The virus is closely related to that of myxomatosis. Clinically there are one or more subcutaneous tumors which grow rapidly and then regress in the domestic rabbit but grow very slowly in the cottontail rabbit. Fibroma virus has been used as a vaccine against myxomatosis. See also BERRY–DEDRICK PHENOMENON.
soft f. see fibrovascular PAPILLOMA.
squirrel f. see SQUIRREL fibroma.

fibromatoid resembling fibroma; fibroma-like.

fibromatosis 1. the presence of multiple fibromas. 2. the formation of a fibrous, tumor-like nodule arising from the deep fascia, with a tendency to local recurrence.
f. gingivae, gingival f. see EPULIS.

fibromatous pertaining to or of the nature of fibroma.
f. epulis see EPULIS.

fibromuscular both fibrous and muscular.

fibromyitis inflammation of muscle with fibrous degeneration.

fibromyoma a myoma containing fibrous elements, a leiomyoma.

fibromyomectomy excision of a fibromyoma (leiomyoma).

fibromyositis inflammation of fibromuscular tissue.

fibromyxoma a fibroma containing myxomatous tissue; myxofibroma.

fibromyxosarcoma a sarcoma containing fibrous and mucous elements.

fibronecrotic a lesion covered with a thick, yellow membrane composed of exudate and firmly attached to the tissue beneath.

fibronectin an adhesive glycoprotein; one form circulates in plasma, acting as an opsonin, another is a cell-surface protein which mediates cellular adhesive interactions.

fibroneuroma see NEUROFIBROMA.

fibropapilloma the common wart composed of epithelial and connective tissue. In most animal species caused by a species-specific papovavirus. In cattle, five 'strains' are proposed, three causing lesions on teats, one on skin generally and one on anogenital skin. The lesions are fleshy masses with intact covering unless abraded; they may be sessile or pedunculated. See also PAPILLOMA, FIBROMA.
genital f. see genital PAPILLOMATOSIS.
transmissible f. caused by fibropapillomatosis type 2 on the penis of the bull; transmitted by coitus.

fibroplasia the formation of fibrous tissue, as in the healing of a wound.

fibropruritic nodule multiple, small cutaneous nodules located mainly over back; seen in dogs with chronic flea bite hypersensitivity.

fibrosarcoma a sarcoma arising from collagen-producing fibroblasts. They occur in many organs and cause well-identified syndromes, e.g. oral, nasal, gastric.
odontogenic f. a malignant tumor of the jaws, originating from one of the mesenchymal components of the tooth or tooth germ.

fibroserous composed of both fibrous and serous elements.

fibrosis formation of fibrous tissue; fibroid degeneration.
postfibrinous f. that occurring in tissues in which fibrin has been previously deposited.
proliferative f. that in which the fibrous elements continue to proliferate after the original causative factor has ceased to operate.

fibrothorax adhesion of the two pleural layers, the lung being covered by thick nonexpansible fibrous tissue.

fibrous composed of or containing fibers.
f. bone see woven BONE.
cardiac f. skeleton includes a ring around each of the atrioventricular valves and each of the great arteries leaving the heart; between the rings are the right and left fibrous trigones.
f. dysplasia localized overgrowth of fibrous tissue in bone.
f. feeds feeds high in fiber, cellulose and lignin.
f. growth plates growth plates composed of fibrocartilage such as that for the tibial tubercle.
f. histiocytoma see MALIGNANT fibrous histiocytoma.
f. hyperplasia indistinguishable clinically from fibromatous epulis.
f. joint 1. a joint whose bony elements are united with fibrous tissue. See SUTURE (1), SYNDESMOSIS. 2. stiffness in a joint due to fibrous tissue reaction in the joint capsule and other supporting structures.
f. osteodystrophy see OSTEODYSTROPHIA FIBROSA.
f. rings bands of fibrous tissue surrounding the semilunar valves of the aorta and pulmonary artery and the atrioventricular valves.
f. tissue the common connective tissue of the body, composed of yellow or white parallel elastic and collagen fibers.

fibrovascular both fibrous and vascular.
f. papilloma see MALIGNANT fibrous histiocytoma.

fibroxanthoma a xanthoma with a significant accumulation of fibrous elements.

fibula the lateral and smaller of the two bones of the hind shank. In the horse, ox and sheep, the shaft is vestigial or not present and the ends are fused with the tibia. In the pig, the bone is complete but the ends are free until several years of age when they fuse with the tibia. See also Table 10.

fibular pertaining to the fibula.
f. nerve see PERONEAL nerve and Table 14.
f. nerve block see PERONEAL nerve block.
f. tarsal bone see Table 10. Called also calcaneus.

ficin a highly active, crystallizable proteinase from the sap of fig trees, which catalyzes the hydrolysis of many proteins at acid (4.1) pH, the clotting of milk, and digestion of some living worms, e.g. whipworms. Ficin is used as a protein digestant and to enhance the agglutination of red blood cells by IgG. It also shows esterase activity.

Fick principle the amount of a substance taken up by the circulation per unit of time equals the arterial level of the substance minus the venous level multiplied by the blood flow. Used to measure cardiac output.

Fick's first law of diffusion an equation describing the rate of movement of solutes by diffusion from a higher to a lower concentration.

Ficus tsiela Indian tree in the family Moraceae; contains an unidentified toxin which causes hepatitis and hepatic encephalopathy.

fiddle front in dogs, front legs with the elbov

feet turned out, but carpi close together. Called also Chippendale legs, French front.

fiddle-head large, plain, coarse head on a horse.

fiddleneck see AMSINCKIA.

fido, phideaux term of endearment addressed to a dog.

fiducial pertaining to trust or reliance; in statistics has much the same meaning as confidence.

field 1. an area or open space, such as an operative field or visual field. 2. a range of specialization in knowledge, study or occupation. 3. in embryology, the developing region within a range of modifying factors. 4. in computer work an element of a data RECORD; a specified space in a storage facility.

auditory f. the space or range within which stimuli will be perceived as sound.

f. beans see PHASEOLUS.

f. experiments experiments conducted on large groups of animals in conditions thought to be average for the particular type of commercial operation.

f. fungi fungi that attack plants that grow in the field. See also STORAGE FUNGI.

high-power f. the area of a slide visible under the high magnification system of a microscope.

individuation f. a region in which an organizer influences adjacent tissue to become a part of a total embryo.

low-power f. the area of a slide visible under the low magnification system of a microscope.

morphogenetic f. an embryonic region out of which definite structures normally develop.

f. nettle see STACHYS ARVENSIS.

f. pea PISUM *sativum*.

f. penny-cress see THLASPI ARVENSE.

f. poppy see PAPAVER *rhoeas*.

sequential f. trial a trial to which additional segments are added as results are obtained in original segments, e.g. concentrating efforts on aspects of the work which appear to be promising.

f. trial see field experiments (above).

visual f. the area within which stimuli will produce the sensation of sight with the eye in a straight-ahead position.

Field spaniel a medium-sized (35–50 lb), muscular gun dog with the general spaniel characteristics of pendulous ears, docked tail, and flat or wavy coat with feathering on the legs, ears and under the body, in solid colors, usually liver or black. The nose is characteristically very long, which supposedly gives it great scenting ability.

fierce thornapple DATURA *ferox*.

fiery dragon guinea worm. See DRACUNCULUS *insignis*.

Fife fancy a miniature version of the Border fancy canary (maximum 4.5 inches long).

fig *Ficus* spp. See FICUS TSIELA.

Figge's model a mathematical formula, used to estimate non-respiratory acid–base disorders, using serum electrolyte levels and $P\text{CO}_2$.

figging, fidding see GINGERING.

fight-or-flight reaction coordinated result of increased secretion of adrenal medullary hormones and of stimulation and resulting increased activity of the sympathetic nervous system. Creates the optimum situation for the survival of the individual by fighting the adversary or fleeing from it. The reaction comprises constriction of the blood vessels of alimentary tract and skin but dilatation of those to skeletal muscles; increased cardiac rate and output, and coronary dilatation occur; also elevation of the blood sugar levels and metabolic rate, dilatation of the pupils, evacuation of blood from the spleen, bronchodilatation, piloerection and decrease in coagulation time.

fighting often a problem of animal welfare and of financial loss in animals kept in close confinement. Due partly to boredom but also to overcrowding, incorrect sex ratios and lack of amenities. May result in deaths, septic wounds and subsequent amyloidosis.

Fighting bull a special breed of black or dark brown, rarely gray, red or pied, horned cattle, bred in some parts of Spain and Portugal. Called also toro de lidia and ganado bravo.

FIGLU formiminoglutamic acid.

figworts *Scrophularia* spp. See SCROPHULARIA AQUATICA.

fila [L.] plural of *filum*.

filaceous composed of filaments.

filaggrin an intermediate filament-associated protein which is involved in cross-linking of keratin; the main constituent of keratohyalin in the granular layer of the epidermis.

filament a delicate fiber or thread.

beard f. structures of the beard of the male turkey are neither hairs nor feathers but have some of the characteristics of both.

f. control in an x-ray machine this controls the filament current in the x-ray tube. The size of the current and its duration are controlled in this way.

f. current in an x-ray machine the strength of the current to the filament is varied by the use of a filament or stepdown transformer.

f. focal spot size the focal spot of the x-ray beam should be as small as possible to give maximum sharpness and clarity. Its size is determined by the size of the filament opposite that generates the beam, the anode angle and other factors.

intermediate f. non-contractile elements in the supportive structure of cytoplasm.

filamentous composed of long, threadlike structures.

f. body see COLLOIDAL body.

Filaria genus of filarid nematodes in superfamily Filarioididea. Includes *F. haemorrhagica* (syn. *Parafilaria multipapillosa*), *F. taxidea*.

F. taxidea a nematode worm reputed to cause filarial dermatitis in the badger.

filaria pl. *filariae* [L.] a nematode worm of the superfamily Filarioididea.

filarial pertaining to or emanating from filariae.

f. dermatitis see cutaneous STEPHANOFILAROSIS.

f. dermatosis see ELAEOPHORIASIS.

f. uveitis see ONCHOCERCIASIS.

filariasis infection with filarial nematodes. See also FILARIAL.

hemorrhagic f. see PARAFILARIA *multipapillosa*.

ocular f. the occurrence of filariae, particularly of *Dirofilaria immitis* in dogs, in the anterior chamber or vitreous body.

filaricide an agent that destroys filariae.

filarid any filaria.

filariform resembling filariae; threadlike.

Filarinema species of trichostrongylid nematodes in free-living kangaroos.

Filaroides a genus of worms in the family Filaroididae and the superfamily Metastrongyloidea. They are parasites of the respiratory tract of mammals.

F. bronchialis occurs in mink and polecats.

F. cebus, F. gordius found in the lungs of capuchin and squirrel monkeys.

F. hirthi found in the lungs of dogs.

F. martis found in the lungs and blood vessels of mink and other Mustelidae.

F. milksi found in the lungs of dogs.
F. osleri see OSLERUS *osleri*.
F. pilbarensis found in Australian marsupials.
F. rostratus may cause tracheobronchitis in cats.

file a group of data in a computer storage system that can be dealt with as a single unit. It can be retrieved and stored, deleted, or modified en bloc.
dental f. used in endodontics to smooth the pulp chamber.
f. extension optional three letter suffix attached, after a period, at the end of a computer file name and used as a means of categorizing the file as e.g. a data file, or a program.
input f. the file to be processed by a program.
f. name the name given to each file by the user to enable the program being used to access, open and then save the file.
output f. the results of a program.
text f. a file saved in ASCII file format and containing text, spaces and returns but no formatting codes.

file snake aquatic snake with a stout body and very rough skin like a file. Belongs to the subfamily Acrochordinae. Called also *Mehelya*.

filial generation any generation following the parental generation.

Filicollis a genus of small cylindrical worms (acanthocephalans) in the family Polymorphidae and the order Palaeacanthocephala.
F. anatis found in the intestine of wild and domestic aquatic birds. Causes emaciation and some deaths due to peritonitis as a result of perforation of the bowel wall. Called also thorny-headed worm.

filiform 1. threadlike. 2. an extremely slender bougie.

filing teeth filing or rasping the sharp points off the molar teeth of a horse.

fill see GUTFILL.

filled legs minor edema of the lower limbs of a horse due to lack of exercise. A peculiarity of some horses.

fillet 1. a loop, as of cord or tape, for making traction. 2. in the nervous system, a long band of nerve fibers. 3. the psoas major and iliacus muscles.
f. technique a surgical procedure for subtotal prostatectomy in which the prostatic urethra is preserved and postsurgical complications from urinary incontinence are minimized.

filly young female horse up to first breeding or 4 years, then a maiden mare. Called filly foal up to weaning, then weanling filly to 1 year, then yearling filly to 2 years.

film 1. a thin layer or coating. 2. a thin sheet of material (e.g. gelatin, cellulose acetate) specially treated for use in photography or radiography; used also to designate the sheet after exposure to the energy to which it is sensitive.
f. badge a radiographic film worn as a badge and used for detection and approximate measurement of radiographic exposure of personnel.
f. changing device enables the radiographer to change films quickly when a series of shots is being used, e.g. angiography.
copy f. film with a special reversal emulsion so that a contact print can be made with white light. Called also duplicating film.
dental f. nonscreen film used in dental radiography.
duplicating f. see copy film (above).
flat f. a film lacking in radiographic contrast.
gelatin f. a sterile, nonantigenic, absorbable, water-insoluble coating used as an aid in surgical closure and repair of defects in the dura mater and pleura and as a local hemostatic.
f. label details of the animal examined and when and where the examination took place. Usually made on the x-ray by photographic means or by using radiopaque tape.
f. marker any device, usually lead letters, placed on the film to indicate which part of the animal was examined and the projection used.
nonscreen f. film for getting very fine detail, used without a cassette and requiring long exposure time. This film is now banned in some parts of the world.
plain f. an x-ray film taken without contrast medium or other special effects. Often an exploratory or scout film.
spot f. a radiograph of a small anatomic area obtained (1) by rapid exposure during fluoroscopy to provide a permanent record of a transiently observed abnormality, or (2) by limitation of radiation passing through the area to improve definition and detail of the image produced.
standard f. fine-grain, medium-speed with wide tolerance for exposure times.
x-ray f. film sensitized to x-rays, either before or after exposure.

Filobasidiella neoformans a fungus in the class Basidiomycetes; the perfect state of *Cryptococcus neoformans*.

filoplume hairlike feathers with only one small tuft of barbs; they remain after other feathers are plucked.

Filoviridae a family of viruses; very long, up to 970 nm × 80 nm, filamentous rods; sometimes more compact convoluted forms are recognized, which are enveloped and have a helical nucleocapsid and a single-strand RNA genome. The two viruses in the family, Marburg and Ebola, are endemic in certain African countries and produce highly fatal hemorrhagic fevers in humans, including laboratory workers handling infected monkeys, which are believed to be the reservoirs.

filovirus members of the family *Filoviridae*.

filter a device for eliminating certain elements, as (1) particles of certain size from a solution, (2) bacteria and fungi from suspensions of virus, or (3) rays of certain wavelength from a stream of radiant energy.
bacteria-proof f. see BERKEFELD'S FILTER, PASTEUR–CHAMBERLAND FILTER, MILLIPORE FILTER.
Wood's f. a nickel-oxide filter that holds back all but a few violet rays and passes ultraviolet rays of about 365 nm. See also WOOD'S LIGHT.
x-ray f. see GRID (1).

filterable, filtrable capable of passing through the pores of a filter.

filth fly see ERISTALIS.

filtrate a liquid that has passed through a filter.
glomerular f. the filtrate that passes from the lumen of the glomerular capillary to the space of Bowman's capsule.

filtration passage through a filter or through a material that prevents passage of certain molecules, e.g. capillary wall, blood–brain barrier, radiographic grid.
f. angle developmental or acquired distortion of this part of the eye is the common cause of glaucoma. It is the space bounded by the sclera externally, the ciliary muscle posteriorly, the root of the iris medially and the anterior chamber of the eye anteriorly. Within the space is the filtering mechanism, a mass of anastomosing mesodermal spindle cells with many perforations between them.
f. barrier the physiological function which limits the passage of small molecules through the renal corpuscle.
glomerular f. the process by which glomerular filtrate is formed, involving the balance of pressures across the walls of the glomerular capillaries.

inherent f. attenuation of the primary x-ray beam as a result of its passage out of the x-ray tube through the insulating medium and tube window.

f. membrane the membrane which stretches across the filtration slits in the renal corpuscle.

f. pressure the net driving force which pushes fluid into tissue spaces and out of vascular sites; the net result between capillary osmotic pressure and intravascular hydrostatic pressure.

f. slits openings in the glomerular corpuscle which are part of the filtration process in the renal glomerulus.

filum pl. *fila* [L.] a threadlike structure or part.

f. durae matris spinalis encloses the filum terminale (see below).

f. olfactoria fibers that pass from the olfactory lobe of the brain to the ethmoid plate through which they pass.

f. reticulare fibers of the dorsal nerve root which spread out in a fanlike pattern to enter the spinal cord along a dorsolateral groove.

f. terminale a slender, threadlike prolongation of the spinal cord from the conus medullaris to the sacrum and tail.

fimbria pl. *fimbriae* [L.] 1. a fringe, border or edge; a fringelike structure. 2. one of the minute filamentous appendages of certain bacteria; associated with antigenic properties of the cell surface. See also PILUS, ADHESIN.

f. hippocampi the band of white matter along the median edge of the ventricular surface of the hippocampus.

ovarian f. occur together with the fimbriae of the uterine horn. Located in the ovulation fossa.

uterine tube f. the numerous divergent fringelike processes on the distal part of the infundibulum of the uterine tube.

fimbrial pertaining to or emanating from fimbriae.

f. cysts cysts in the region of the ovulation fossa; appear to cause no impediment to fertility except in very old mares where they may obstruct ovulation. If the cysts are in ovarian tissue they are known as ovarian cysts; if they are in the connective tissue at the base of the fimbriae they are called fimbrial cysts.

Fimbriaria a genus of tapeworms that belong to the family Fimbriariidae.

F. fasciolaris an unusual tapeworm found in the small intestine of chickens and anserine birds.

fimbriate fringed.

fimbriated fringed; bordered by slender processes.

fin winglike structure attached to the body of fish and cetaceans; used for steering and propulsion during progress through the water.

f. rot a disease of aquarium fish characterized by thickening followed by necrosis of the fin and tail tissues, commencing at the edges, caused by *Haemophilus piscum* and *Aeromonas* spp. May be bracketed with fin rot/tail rot/snout erosion. Often associated with suboptimal cultural conditions. Mixed populations of opportunistic bacteria are usually present.

final common path see GSE.

final host see DEFINITIVE HOST.

finasteride an inhibitor of 5-α reductase, which is responsible for conversion of testosterone to dihydrotestosterone in the prostate; used in the treatment of canine benign prostatic hyperplasia.

finch a bird in the family Fringillidae; includes about 125 species, many of them companion birds such as the common canary, linnets, goldfinches, the zebra and Bengalese finches.

fine-leaved water dropwort OENANTHE *aquatica*.

fine-wool a class of wool sheep, only Merinos qualify, characterized by fiber diameter of 19 microns, spinning quality of 70's, yield of 6 lb.

fines particles that will pass through a sieve of mesh size smaller than that specified.

finfish fish with fins, that is teleosts, elasmobranches, holocephalids, agnathids and cephalochordates; also a fish marketer's term used to include that section of marketable fish which is neither shellfish nor molluscs.

finger cherry see RHODOMYRTUS MACROCARPA.

finger grass see DACTYLOCTENIUM RADULANS.

finger hakea see HAKEA.

finger plakkie COTYLEDON *orbiculata*.

fingerling young fish.

fingerprint see RESTRICTION FRAGMENT LENGTH POLYMORPHISM.

finish said of animals offered for sale prior to slaughter; is the degree of fatness short of obesity.

finite population see finite POPULATION.

Finney's pyloroplasty enlargement of the pyloric canal by establishment of an inverted U-shaped anastomosis between the stomach and duodenum after longitudinal incision.

Finnish-Landrace sheep dual-purpose, short-tailed sheep; polled, white, occasionally black, brown or gray.

F.-L. glomerulopathy an inherited disease found in lambs less than 4 months old. Many are found dead. Enlarged kidneys are palpable and there is a high BUN level and proteinuria. Most cases are in purebred Finnish-Landrace lambs but cases have occurred in crossbred lambs. The pathogenetic basis of the disease is a mesangiocapillary glomerulitis caused by the deposition of immune complexes in the walls of the renal capillaries.

Finnish Lapphund a medium-sized spitz-type dog with a profuse, long coat of any color. The tail is curved over the back. Very similar to, but smaller than, the Swedish Lapphund.

Finnish spitz a small (25–35 lb), lively dog with alert expression, narrow muzzle, small, pointed, erect ears, and a red to gold colored coat that is medium length on the body but long and dense on the shoulders, thighs and tail.

Finochietto rib spreader two broad, curved-outward blades which are mounted on a ratcheted bar. Spreading of the ribs can be achieved by inserting the blades through the thoracotomy incision and spreading them manually.

fins see FRILLED.

FIP feline infectious peritonitis.

FIPV feline infectious peritonitis virus.

fire naked flame.

f. ant *Solenopsis invicta*; bites can cause severe conjunctivitis and corneal ulcers.

f. brand see BRAND.

f. engine practice see fire engine PRACTICE.

f. fish members of the fish family Scorpaenidae, or scorpion fish which cause intense skin irritation.

f. injury see BURN, BUSHFIRE INJURY.

f. retardant chemicals used to proof timber or fabric against fire. Many of these agents are poisonous. The best known are polybrominated and polychlorinated BIPHENYLS.

fire cherry PRUNUS *pennsylvanica*.

firehouse dog see DALMATIAN.

fireweed SENECIO spp., e.g. *S. lautus*, *S. linearifolius*, *S. madagascariensis*.

firing an oldfashioned technique for applying long-term counterirritation to a part, usually a lower limb, in an attempt to encourage healing of a damaged ligament or tendon. A red hot iron is applied to an area of anesthetized skin and a pattern of holes of lines drawn over the area. The firing could be deep, point firing, or superficial, line firing. Enforced rest results because of the soreness of the part, but the benefits of this method of treatment are questioned.

f. irons specially designed irons, including those for pin and line firing, to be used on a horse's limbs.

firmware computer software integral to the control of a peripheral device and stored in Read Only Memory (ROM).

first aid emergency care and treatment of an injured patient before complete medical and surgical treatment can be secured.

first-calf said of heifers aged about 2 years usually, with their first calf just born.

first cross the F_1 generation; the first generation of crosses between animals of two pure breeds.

first-lactation female livestock during their first lactation; a term reserved usually for cattle.

first law of thermodynamics law dealing with the transformation of energy. States that energy can neither be created nor destroyed, only converted from one form to another.

first-opinion cases patients making their first visit to a veterinarian for a current disease problem. Difficult cases may be passed to a consultant for a second opinion. See also CONSULTATION.

first-pass effect the metabolism of orally administered drugs by gastrointestinal and hepatic enzymes, resulting in a significant reduction of the amount of unmetabolized drug reaching the systemic circulation.

first phalanx see proximal phalanx in Table 10.

first-set reaction, phenomenon rejection of a first allograft is slow, taking about 10 days, in contrast to a second-set reaction. See also REJECTION.

first-stage said of larva; the first of several larval stages.

Fischoederius a genus of digenetic trematodes in the family Paramphistomatidae.

F. cobboldi, F. elongatus found in the rumen of cattle and other bovids.

fish members of the classes Cephalochordata (lancelets), Agnatha (hagfish and lampreys), Elasmobranchii (sharks and rays), Holocephali (ghost sharks), Osteichthyes (bony fish), Gastropoda (gastropods), Pelecypoda (bivalves), Cephalopoda (cephalopods), Crustacea (crustaceans).

f. handler's disease erysipeloid.

f. liver oils used in animal diets because of their high content of vitamin A and D. Should be stabilized to avoid loss of vitamins in storage and need an antioxidant to avoid rancidification and loss of vitamin E. May also cause tainting of animal foods. See also COD LIVER OIL, omega-3 FATTY acids.

f. meal a protein feed supplement rich in calcium, phosphorus and having a good iodine content. Made from inedible fish residues from the canning and fresh fish industries. May taint animal products. Toxic amines produced by bacterial spoilage cause gizzard erosion and fatal hemorrhage in birds.

f. mouth used to describe gaping wounds of the skin.

f. mouthing a surgical technique for anastomosing two pieces of bowel when one is moderately larger in diameter than the other. The smaller diameter is made wider by slitting it longitudinally down the sides so that it opens like a fish's mouth.

f. poisoning see DIODONTIDAE, TETRAODONTIDAE.

f. scale disease, f. skin disease see inherited congenital ICHTHYOSIS.

f. solubles dehydrated fishwater from oil extraction and fishmeal industries.

f. tuberculosis disease of aquarium fish caused by *Mycobacterium* spp. Causes weight loss, exophthalmos, cutaneous ulcers and pallor. At necropsy there are internal granulomas. The acid-fast organisms can be found in the ulcers. Also found in a variety of cultured species including shrimps.

f. viruses includes rhabdoviruses and birnavirus.

fish kill mass death of many fish, usually in a restricted area.

Fisher's exact test a statistical test for association in a two-by-two table based on the exact hypergeometric distribution of the frequencies within the table.

fissalo see FISTULOUS withers.

fission 1. the act of splitting. 2. asexual reproduction in which the cell divides into two (binary fission) or more (multiple fission) daughter parts, each of which becomes an individual organism. 3. nuclear fission; the splitting of the atomic nucleus, with release of energy.

fissiparous propagated by fission.

fissula pl. *fissulae* [L.] a small cleft.

fissura pl. *fissurae* [L.] fissure.

fissure 1. a narrow slit or cleft, especially one of the deeper or more constant furrows separating the gyri of the brain. 2. in dermatology a deep crack in the skin, often through a scab, which penetrates into the subcutis.

abdominal f. a congenital cleft in the abdominal wall.

anal f., f. in ano a painful linear ulcer at the margin of the anus.

f. of Bichat transverse fissure (2).

branchial f. branchial cleft.

central f. fissure of Rolando.

collateral f. a longitudinal fissure on the ventral surface of the cerebral hemisphere between the fusiform gyrus and the hippocampal gyrus.

dorsal median f. 1. a shallow vertical groove in the closed part of the medulla oblongata, continuous with the dorsal median sulcus of the spinal cord. 2. a shallow vertical groove dividing the spinal cord throughout its whole length in the midline dorsally. Called also dorsal median sulcus.

ear f. a split in the margin of the pinna which can gradually become larger from continued trauma.

hippocampal f. one extending from the splenium of the corpus callosum almost to the tip of the temporal lobe; called also hippocampal sulcus.

interhemispheric f. the fissure between the two cerebral hemisphere in birds.

interincisive f. fissure between the two incisive bones at the rostral end of the pig's face.

laryngeal f. the dorsal laryngeal furrow.

ligamentum teres f. on the diaphragmatic surface of the liver; houses the ligamentum teres.

longitudinal f. the deep fissure between the cerebral hemispheres.

macropalpebral f. an enlarged palpebral fissure.

optic f. a ventral fissure in the developing optic cup through which blood vessels pass to the enclosed mesenchyme.

orbital f. see orbital FORAMEN.

palatine f. a pair of fissures perforating the rostral extremity of the palate.

palpebral f. the opening between the eyelids.

perianal f. see PERIANAL fistula.

petrotympanic f. the CHORDA tympani, on its way to

merge with the lingual branch of the mandibular nerve, passes across the tympanic cavity and emerges at the petrotympanic fissure.

portal f. porta hepatis.

presylvian f. the ventral branch of the fissure of Sylvius.

Rolando's f., f. of Rolando a groove running obliquely across the superolateral surface of the cerebral hemisphere, separating the frontal from the parietal lobe. Called also central fissure and central sulcus.

round ligament f. one on the visceral surface of the liver, lodging the round ligament in the adult.

sylvian f., f. of Sylvius one extending laterally between the temporal and frontal lobes, and turning dorsally between the temporal and parietal lobes of the brain.

transverse f. 1. porta hepatis. 2. the transverse cerebral fissure between the diencephalon and the cerebral hemispheres; called also fissure of Bichat.

tympano-occipital f. on the ventral surface of the skull, near the confluence of the osseous bulla and the occipital bone, this pair of fissures serve as conduits for the glossopharyngeal, vagal and accessory nerves in species without a jugular foramen.

ventral median f. a longitudinal furrow along the midline of the ventral surface of the spinal cord and medulla oblongata.

zygal f. a cerebral fissure consisting of two branches connected by a stem.

fistula pl. *fistulae, fistulas;* any abnormal, tubelike passage within body tissue, usually between two internal organs, or leading from an internal organ to the body surface. Some fistulae are created surgically, for diagnostic or therapeutic purposes; others occur as a result of injury or as congenital abnormalities. See also ARTERIOVENOUS fistula.

blind f. one open at one end only, opening on the skin (external blind fistula) or on an internal surface (internal blind fistula).

branchial f. a persisting branchial cleft.

complete f. one extending from the skin to an internal body cavity.

craniosinus f. one between the cerebral space and one of the sinuses, permitting escape of cerebrospinal fluid into the nose.

crop f. the crop communicates with the skin on the neck of the bird.

enterocutaneous f. one in which there is communication between the intestinal tract and the skin. Some fistulae are created surgically, with gastrostomy, esophagostomy or colostomy. Others may result from surgical trauma, breakdown of an intestinal anastomosis, or erosions around a surgical drain or tube.

esophageal f. communication between the esophagus and some portion of the respiratory tract, e.g. trachea, bronchi or pulmonary tissue. May be congenital or acquired as a result of trauma or inflammatory lesions, particularly esophageal foreign bodies.

fecal f. a colonic fistula opening on the external surface of the body and discharging feces.

foreign body f. remnant of a foreign body impalation or a grass seed are the common causes. Fistula drains continuously.

gastric f. an abnormal passage communicating with the stomach; often applied to an artificially created opening, through the abdominal wall, into the stomach.

horseshoe f. a semicircular fistulous tract about the anus, with both openings on the skin.

incomplete f. blind fistula.

lateral cervical f. see BRANCHIAL cyst.

oroantral f. between the oral cavity and a sinus. In dogs, usually involves the maxillary sinus and is caused by periodontal disease of the fourth premolars and first molars.

oronasal f. between the nasal and oral cavities. Occurs most commonly in dogs with advanced periodontal disease of the maxillary canine tooth, but can result from disease of canines and premolars. It may also occur after tooth extraction, particularly in dogs, leading to the passage of food into the nasal cavity and a secondary chronic rhinitis and nasal discharge.

ruminal f. created surgically in left upper flank. May occur accidentally due to persistence of trocar puncture for treatment of bloat.

salivary f. usually discharges saliva on to the side of the face but may discharge into the mouth. Usually due to laceration of the duct by trauma.

umbilical f. an abnormal passage communicating with the gut or the urachus at the umbilicus.

urachal f. persistence of the urachal canal with communication between the urinary bladder and umbilicus. See also persistent URACHUS.

fistulation see FISTULIZATION.

fistulectomy excision of a fistula.

fistulization 1. the process of becoming fistulous. 2. surgical creation of a fistula.

fistulogram radiograph after infusion of the sinus tract with radiopaque material.

fistulography contrast study of a fistula.

fistulotomy incision of a fistula.

fistulous pertaining to or of the nature of a fistula.

f. withers one or more sinuses discharge at the withers from an infected supraspinous bursa between the ligamentum nuchae and the tips of the dorsal spinous processes of the anterior thoracic vertebrae. *Brucella bovis* is a common cause of the bursitis. *Actinomyces bovis* is a common accompaniment to the brucellosis.

fit 1. an episode characterized by inappropriate and involuntary motor activity. In humans there are similar psychic disturbances as well. The most common manifestation is a convulsion; similar involuntary movements of restricted parts of the body would also fit this description. Called also convulsion, seizure. 2. the quality of similarity between two sets of data.

goodness of f. the degree of similarity between two sets of data, e.g. the frequencies of two attributes; a test for the significance of the similarity.

FITC fluorescein isothiocyanate; used as a fluorescent label for proteins, especially antibodies.

fitch 1. the European polecat, *Mustela putorius putorius*; farmed for its fur. 2. pelt of the polecat.

fitness good health; equine and canine sports medicine devote much enthusiasm to the measurement of fitness, the ability to perform work, or physical activity, well. Besides actual tests of performance there are biochemical, hematological and electrocardiographic tests which can be of assistance. Radiographic examination of skeletal features has special application to racing animals. Includes fitness for performing, racing or for draft work.

f. prediction the art of predicting whether a horse will win a particular race; a combination of knowing the horse's racing form, fitness, owner and trainer intentions, jockey competence, suitability of the track.

fitted curve see fitted CURVE.

fitting preparation of animals for special occasions of stress, e.g. parturition, exhibition at fairs and shows. Includes additional feed, exercise, grooming, handling.

fitweed see CORYDALIS.

Fitzgerald factor a high-molecular-weight kininogen; a blood clotting factor.
Fitzwygram shoe a horseshoe with a triangular cross-section so that only a rim acts as a ground surface.
FIV feline immunodeficiency virus.
five element theory a major influence in Chinese traditional medicine; the theory is that everything in the universe is the product of change and movement of the five elements, wood, fire, earth, metal, water, as concepts not as objects.
five-gaited said of a horse capable of performing five gaits, i.e. walk, trot, canter, FOXTROT and RACK.
five point program see NIRD MASTITIS control program.
fixateur a device for holding fragments in a fixed position, e.g. for a fractured bone or luxated joint.
fixation 1. the act or operation of holding, suturing or fastening in a fixed position, e.g. in orthopedic surgery. 2. the condition of being held in a fixed position. 3. in microscopy, the treatment of material so that its structure can be examined in detail with minimal alteration from the normal state, and also to provide information concerning the chemical properties (as of cell constituents) by interpretation of fixation reactions. 4. in chemistry, the process whereby a substance is removed from the gaseous or solution phase and localized. 5. in film processing, the chemical removal of all undeveloped salts of the film emulsion, as on x-ray films. 6. in genetic terms means the attainment, by selection, of homozygosity in a population with respect to one or more favorable genes.
circular external skeletal f. see ILIZAROV EXTERNAL RING SKELETAL FIXATION.
complement f., f. of complement see COMPLEMENT fixation tests.
external skeletal f. a method of immobilizing fracture fragments using percutaneous pins that penetrate the bone and are stabilized, one to the other, by one or more external connecting rods.
fixative an agent such as formalin used in preserving a histological or pathological specimen so as to maintain the normal structure of its constituent elements.
fixed costs the costs which are not affected by the size and the output of the enterprises in a business, such as a farm. Called also overhead costs. Includes interest on mortgage, rates, taxes.
fixed-dose combination drugs commercially available drug preparations containing several remedies. Veterinary therapeutic supply lists contain many examples of combinations of antibiotics. These preparations contain their drugs in fixed combinations and therefore have some advantages and some disadvantages. The advantages are that a broad spectrum of antibiotic activity can be achieved, an important feature in veterinary work because so many infections are mixed ones, and the possibility of resistant bacterial populations emerging is reduced.

One disadvantage is that the drugs in the combination may be antagonistic. The antibiotics most likely to demonstrate this activity are the tetracyclines, the macrolides and chloramphenicol. The principal disadvantage is that the dose rate of each of the component drugs is dictated by the content of the other drugs present, a serious matter if the causative bacteria and its sensitivity are known.
fixed-length records see fixed-length RECORD.
fixed model see MODEL 1.
fixer in the processing of a radiological film the developed image is put into fixer (sodium or ammonium thiosulfate) to dissolve the unexposed silver halide and to harden the film.
f. fog careless or inefficient handling of the fixer bath will seriously compromise the clarity of the film being taken by creating a fog effect.
fixing removal of the undeveloped silver halide from the emulsion on a radiographic film after the exposed crystals have been developed.
Fjord pony Norwegian pony, dun with dark mane, back stripe and tail; 13 to 14.2 hands high. Descendant of the Mongolian wild horse.
flaccid weak, lax, soft; applied especially to muscles.
flaccidity quality of lack of tone of muscular or vascular organ or tissue.
flag[1] see UDDER edema.
flag[2] signal placed on an individual record in a data file that will alert the operator that there is something special about this record, e.g. that the cow has had milk fever previously.
flag iris IRIS *missouriensis*.
flagella see FLAGELLUM.
flagellar of or pertaining to a flagellum.
Flagellaria indica plant in family Flagellariaceae; can cause cyanide poisoning.
flagellate 1. any microorganism having flagella. 2. any protozoon of the subphylum Mastigophora. 3. having flagella.
flagelliform shaped like a flagellum or lash.
flagellosis infection with flagellate protozoa.
flagellum pl. *flagella* [L.] a long, mobile, whiplike appendage arising from a basal body at the surface of a cell, serving as a locomotor organelle; the only known example in biology of a rotatory motion. In eukaryotic cells, flagella contain nine pairs of microtubules arrayed around a central pair; in bacteria, they contain tightly wound strands of flagellin.
flail exhibiting abnormal or pathological mobility, as flail chest or flail joint.
f. chest a loss of stability of the chest wall due to multiple rib fractures or detachment of the sternum from the ribs as a result of a severe crushing chest injury. The loose chest segment moves in a direction which is the reverse of normal; that is, the segment moves inward during inspiration and outward during expiration (PARADOXICAL respiration). Other manifestations of flail chest include shortness of breath, cyanosis, and extreme pain in the area of trauma.
f. joint an unusually movable joint.
f. segment the portion of skin, chest-wall or other structure lacking stability.
flake an epidermal scale.
flaked grain see flaked GRAIN.
flame 1. the luminous, irregular appearance usually accompanying combustion, or an appearance resembling it. 2. to render sterile by exposure to a flame.
f. cell the excretory cell in cestodes and trematodes; their number and arrangement is a basis for identification.
f. figure in skin lesions such as insect bite reactions, eosinophilic granulomas; characterized by areas of altered collagen surrounded by eosinophils and eosinophilic cytoplasmic granules.
f. follicle inactive hair follicles with excessive trichilemmal keratinization.
f. retardants see FIRE retardant.
flame lily GLORIOSA *superba*.
flamingo see PHOENICOPTERUS RUBER.
flank the side of the body between the ribs and ilium.
f. fat thickness of the flank fold; a measure favored by cattle buyers as an indicator of the probable level of fat in the animal.

f. laparotomy a common procedure for exploration of the abdomen in cattle. Also a preliminary to resection of intestine, rumenotomy. Has the virtue that surgery can be performed with the animal standing.

f. sucking 1. a vice in dairy calves being reared on bucket or nipple feeders when sucking time does not satisfy sucking reflex. 2. a vice in dogs, particularly common in Doberman pinschers, once believed to be due to whipworm infestation but now considered a psychogenic disorder, possibly a manifestation of psychomotor epilepsy.

f. watching the patient spreads all four limbs and turns the head and neck into one flank; posture adopted, especially by horses, in cases of subacute abdominal pain; the tendency is for the patient to look repeatedly at the one side.

flanking method of restraint in calves. The animal is thrown by the operator reaching across the animal's back, grasping the loose flank and lifting it off its feet.

flanking regions noncoding sequences on either side of the coding region of a gene that contain various regulatory sequences (motifs).

flap 1. a mass of tissue for GRAFTING (1), usually including skin, only partially removed from one part of the body so that it retains its own blood supply during transfer to another site. See also specific sites, such as CONJUNCTIVAL. 2. an uncontrolled movement.

advancement f. release of a portion of tissue and reattachment at an advanced position.

antral f. in circumcostal gastropexy or belt loop gastropexy a seromuscular flap from the pyloric antrum is passed under a rib or strip of abdominal wall muscle and sutured back to its position on the stomach.

bone f. a surgical procedure in which a flap is created in a flat bone by leaving one side of a rectangle cut in the bone intact. Used for gaining access to a cavity, e.g. a sinus, with minimum disfigurement.

buccal f. a section of mucosa released from mucosa of the gum and lip used to close oronasal fistulas.

cartilage f. a detached piece of cartilage as a result of osteochondrosis dissecans, seen particularly in the shoulder of dogs.

free f. an island flap detached from the body and reattached at the distant recipient site by microvascular anastomosis.

f.-imprint interlocking processes in adult cortical lens fibers.

ischial-pubic f. to increase exposure for surgery in the colorectal region, osteotomies of the pubic and ischial bones may be required. The bone flap created is reflected and replaced at the conclusion of the surgical procedure.

island f. a flap consisting of skin and subcutaneous tissue, with a pedicle made up of only the nutrient vessels.

mucoperiosteal f. a section of oral mucosa, gingiva and underlying periosteum in periodontal surgery and tooth extractions.

mucosal f. used in repair of defects in the oral cavity such as oronasal fistula and those created by excision of tumor and bone.

myocutaneous f. a compound flap of skin and muscle with adequate vascularity to permit sufficient tissue to be transferred to the recipient site.

pedicle f. see pedicle GRAFT.

overlapping f. a technique for repair of cleft soft palate with two flaps, one on the oral side and one on the nasal side, and with the assistance of relaxing incisions these are overlapped to ensure an adequate seal.

rope f. one made by elevating a long strip of tissue from its bed except at its two ends, the cut edges then being sutured together to form a tube. Called also tubed graft.

rotation f. see pedicle GRAFT.

skin f. a standard technique in skin grafting; based on the part isolation of a graft by creation of a flap which retains its original circulation while becoming established at the new site on the new blood supply. Many types of flap are used, e.g. axial pattern, bipedicle, composite, delayed tube, direct, interpolating, reverse saphenous conduit. See also skin GRAFT.

sliding f. technique for closing skin wounds where there is a large deficiency of skin. Includes sliding-H flap and Z-flap or Z-plasty. Skin around the defect is separated from its subcutis and the defect repaired by strategic additional incisions and the use of tension sutures.

tracheal f. a method of placing a tracheostomy tube which will minimize the subsequent formation of excessive granulation tissue. The opening is made by cutting a flap across two tracheal rings and reflecting it to permit entry of the tube. After extubation, the flap is replaced.

tube f., tunnel f. rope flap.

flap-necked chameleon *Chamaeleo dilepis*.

flare a diffuse area of redness on the skin around the point of application of an irritant, due to vasomotor reaction.

flashing erratic swimming; said of fish in aquaria.

flask a laboratory vessel, usually of glass and with a constricted neck.

flat billy buttons see IXIOLAENA BREVICOMPTA.

flat cat syndrome a term descriptive of the extreme depression and reluctance to rise, seen in cats from different causes, but usually those involving dehydration or shock such as feline panleukopenia or snake bite.

Flat-coated retriever a medium-sized, black or liver colored dog with a flat, long coat, but feathered legs and tail. The ears are pendulous and the tail is long.

flat feet lack of flexor tone in the paw of a dog so that the phalanges are flatter to the ground; said particularly of Greyhounds.

flat oysters *Ostrea* spp.

flat pea LATHYRUS *sylvestris*.

flat-pod pea LATHYRUS *cicera*.

flat puppy syndrome dorsoventral compression of the thorax with legs spread to the sides, sometimes with rotation of the humeral, radial and femoral articulations; observed in puppies of 2 to 4 weeks of age. The cause is unknown, but rapid weight gain, as occurs in offspring of bitches with abundant milk and few puppies, may account for some cases. An hereditary predisposition has been suggested in some breeds. Many affected puppies recover with normal conformation and use of the legs with only minor therapy. Called also swimmer pups.

flat race a race without obstacles for the horses to jump.

flat sour see BACILLUS *circulans*.

flat-topped thorn ACACIA *sieberana*.

flat warts see AURICULAR plaque.

flatfish fish with severely flattened bodies, having both eyes on one side and swim on one side; includes halibut, flounder, sole; generally considered to mean members of the order Pleuronectiformes.

flatness a peculiar sound lacking resonance, heard on percussing an abnormally solid part.

flatulence excessive formation of gases in the stomach or intestine, released through the anus.

flatulent characterized by flatulence; distended with gas.
flatus 1. gas or air in the gastrointestinal tract. 2. gas or air expelled through the anus.
flatweed see HYPOCHOERIS RADICATA.
flatworm any worm of the phylum Platyhelminthes—the flukes or trematodes, and the cestodes or tapeworms of domestic animals.
Flaujeac factor a high-molecular-weight kininogen, a blood clotting factor.
flavin any of a group of water-soluble yellow pigments widely distributed in animals and plants, including riboflavin and yellow enzymes.
f. adenine dinucleotide (FAD) a coenzyme that is a condensation product of riboflavin phosphate and adenylic acid; it forms the prosthetic group of certain enzymes, including D-amino acid oxidase and xanthine oxidase, and is important in electron transport in mitochondria.
f.-linked dehydrogenases class of dehydrogenases with prosthetic groups containing either flavin mononucleotide or flavin adenine dinucleotide tightly bound to the enzyme structure. Example is succinate dehydrogenase of the TCA cycle.
f. mononucleotide (FMN) a derivative of riboflavin consisting of a three-ring system (isoalloxazine) attached to an alcohol (ribitol); it acts as a coenzyme for a number of oxidative enzymes, including L-amino acid oxidase and cytochrome C reductase.
flavine compounds antiseptic compounds derived from aniline dye manufacture, including acriflavine, euflavine, proflavine.
Flaviviridae viruses that were formerly a genus of the family *Togaviridae*, now an independent family comprising two genera, *Flavivirus* and *Pestivirus*, and a third proposed genus containing human hepatitis C virus. They are single-stranded, plus sense RNA viruses. The type species of the genus *Flavivirus*, which are arthropod borne viruses, is the yellow fever virus of humans (flavi = yellow); other viruses cause encephalitis in humans and some cause encephalitis in animals. Amongst the viruses in the genus which affect animals are: St. Louis encephalitis—a disease of humans but the virus has been isolated from animals; JAPANESE B ENCEPHALITIS VIRUS; California encephalitis of humans, but viremia detectable in feral animals; LOUPING ILL; Central European tick-borne fever and Murray Valley encephalitis, both diseases of humans and the viruses that occur in small ruminants; WESSELSBRON DISEASE, Israeli turkey MENINGOENCEPHALITIS; Powassan disease; and the Tahyna virus. The genus PESTIVIRUS includes hog cholera, bovine virus diarrhea–mucosal disease and ovine border disease viruses. Not arthropod borne.
flavivirus a virus in the family *Flaviviridae*.
flav(o)- word element. [L.] *yellow*.
Flavobacterium a genus of glucose-non-fermenting gram-negative bacteria characteristically producing yellow, orange, red or yellow-brown pigmentation, found in soil and water; some species are said to be pathogenic.
F. branchiophilia cause of chronic proliferative inflammation in the gills of salmonid fish. Called also bacterial gill disease.
flavoenzyme any enzyme containing a flavin nucleotide (FMN or FAD) as a prosthetic group.
flavokinase see RIBOFLAVIN kinase.
flavoprotein Fp; a conjugated protein containing a flavin nucleotide.
flavoxate a smooth muscle relaxant; the hydrochloride is used as a urinary tract spasmolytic.
flax *Linum usitatissimum* (cultivated flax, linseed) and *L. catharticum* (purging flax).
dwarf bay f. DAPHNE *mezereum*.
flax-leaf rice-flower PIMELEA *linifolia*.
flaxweed PIMELEA *simplex*, *P. trichostachya*.
flay to strip off the skin.
fl.dr. fluid dram.
flea a small, wingless, blood-sucking insect. Many fleas are ectoparasites and may act as disease carriers. They are members of the order Siphonaptera. The common recorded species and their principal hosts are listed below:
Ctenocephalides felis—cat, dog, rarely humans, primates, rodents; *C. canis*—dog, fox; *Archaeopsylla erinacei*—hedgehogs; *Spilopsyllus cuniculi*—rabbit, hare; *Leptopsylla segnis*—house mouse, rat, wild rodents; *Ceratophyllus* (*Nosopsyllus*) *fasciatus*—rat, house mouse; *Xenopsylla cheopis*—rodents (the plague flea); *Pulex irritans*—humans; *Tunga penetrans*—humans; *Ceratophyllus gallinae*—chickens (European chicken flea); *C. columbae*—pigeons; *C. garei*—water fowl; *C. niger* (Western chicken flea) *Dasypsyllus gallinulae*—wild birds; *Echidnophaga gallinacea*—chickens (stick-fast or sticktight flea); *E. perilis* and *E. myrmecobii*—rabbits; *Vermipsylla ioffi*, *V. perplexa*, *V. alacurt*, *V. dorcadia*—ruminants and horses.
f. allergy dermatitis the inflammatory lesions and self-trauma caused by a hypersensitivity to flea bites. In dogs, this is usually centered on the back over the lumbosacral spine, around the tail base, and inside the hindlegs. Secondary infection is common.
f. antigen see flea ANTIGEN.
f. collar a collar (or tag) impregnated with insecticide, hung around the animal's neck. There is a slow release of the active ingredient, either as a vapor or powder, to kill ectoparasites on the body.
f. collar dermatitis a contact dermatitis in dogs and cats caused by the insecticide-impregnated polyvinyl chloride collars marketed for flea control. Although the initial and most severe skin reaction occurs where direct contact is made, surrounding skin may also become involved. Correct use of the collars minimizes this risk.
f. dip any of the external parasiticides applied to dogs as a rinse; dipping is not a practical form of application in most companion animals.
flea-bite dermatitis see FLEA allergy dermatitis.
flea-bitten a coat color marking seen in horses; a gray coat is flecked with hairs of another color.
fleam a medieval lancet used for drawing blood in the blood-letting therapeutic procedure. A straight metal bar with a downward protruding, small, sharp, fixed blade. The blade was poised over a distended vein and given a sharp thump with a hardwood mallet held in the other hand.
fleawort INULA *conyza*, SENECIO *integrifolius*, PLANTAGO *psyllium*.
flecainide an antiarrhythmic drug that blocks Na+ conduction; used in the treatment of ventricular arrhythmias.
fledgling period period of immaturity before the bird is fully feathered; varies widely from pigeons at 10 to 35 days to the Californian condor at 180 to 210 days.
fleece the wool covering of the sheep shorn off as one piece, except for the scraps at the legs, face and crutch.
double f. two-year growth of wool in the one fleece.
f. fly strike see cutaneous MYIASIS.
f. rot a dermatitis of sheep caused by prolonged wetting of the skin leading to exudation, the formation of crusts and the matting together of the wool fibers.

Discoloration of the matted wool by the growth of chromogenic bacteria is a common accompaniment. The damaged fleece loses much of its commercial value.

tender f. a staple of the wool will break easily across the fibers with only moderate tension having been applied.

f. weight the weight of wool produced by a sheep in a year.

f. worm see cutaneous MYIASIS.

flehmen the ritual of urine sniffing; a behavioral component of libido in the male animal. The animal appears to be carrying out a test for odor in the urine. He sniffs the urine or the perineum, then extends the head, dilates the nostrils, and lifts and curls the upper lip. See also GAPE.

Flemish giant largest of the rabbit breeds; it can weigh as much as 15 lb. Gray is the most common of many colors; the body is broad, long and heavy-boned.

fleroxacin a fluoroquinolone antibiotic, similar to ciprofloxacin.

flesh the soft muscular tissue of the animal body.

f. flies large blowflies of the subfamily Sarcophaginae and the genera *Sarcophaga* and *Wohlfahrtia*.

f. marks patches on a horse's skin where there is no normal skin pigment.

milky f. myoliquefaction observed at necropsy in teleosts; caused by infection with myxosporeans of the genera *Kudoa*, *Unicapsula*, *Chloromyxum*, *Henneguya*. Also thought to be sometimes associated with infections by microsporidia.

proud f. exuberant amounts of soft, edematous, unhealthy-looking granulation tissue developing during healing of large surface wounds.

f. side the rough side of leather or skin; the side that was undermost in the live state.

fleshy prawn PENAEUS *chinensis*.

Fletcher factor a prekallikrein involved in blood coagulation; acts by enhancing the activity of Hageman factor (factor XII).

F. f. deficiency a rare coagulation disorder in dogs and cats.

Fletcher twitch a compact nose twitch for horses. Consists of a cord loop attached to a hollow metal cap that can be screwed to the end of any wooden handle.

flews a term used to describe the fleshy, pendulous upper lip of some dogs such as the Bloodhound.

flex to bend or put in a state of flexion.

Flexibacter members of the *Cytophaga/Flexibacter* group of long, flexuous, gram-negative bacteria; common cause of superficial infections. Includes *F. columnaris* (*Cytophaga columnaris*, see COLUMNARIS DISEASE), *F. maritimus* (see MARINE FLEXIBACTER DISEASE). See also CYTOPHAGA.

flexibilitas [L.] *flexibility*.

flexibility the state of being unusually pliant.

flexion the act of bending or the condition of being bent.

f. reflex see FLEXOR reflex.

Flexispira rappini highly motile, flagellar, rod-shaped bacterium closely related to *Helicobacter* spp. In pregnant ewes causes fetal mummification, abortion (but not outbreaks), weak lambs, and lambs with hepatitis. Not a completely classified organism.

flexor any muscle that flexes a joint. See Table 13.

f. reflex a spinal reflex in which a painful (pressure) stimulus applied to a toe, coronary band or heel bulb, results in a flexion, or withdrawal, of the leg. A test of the integrity of the reflex arc and sensory pathways. Called also withdrawal reflex.

f. retinaculum any bracelet-like band of fibrous tissue on the flexor surface of a joint, e.g. transverse palmar carpal ligament.

f. spasm see MYOCLONUS.

f. tendon tendons of the superficial and deep digital flexor muscles, situated behind the metacarpal or metatarsal bones.

flexuose winding or wavy.

flexura pl. *flexurae* [L.] see FLEXURE.

f. centralis central flexure of the spiral colon of ruminants.

f. portalis the first curve in the duodenum.

flexural pertaining to the flexure of a joint.

f. deformity fixation of joints in flexion. In the newborn called contracted calves or foals.

f. seborrhea dermatitis with heavy outpouring of sebaceous exudate. If allowed to stay wet becomes rancid and develops offensive odor. Common sites for lesion are between halves of udder, between udder and medial aspect of thigh and in axilla. Common only in freshly calved cows.

flexure a bend or fold; a curvation.

brain f. as head folding occurs in the developing embryo midbrain; cervical and pontine flexures also occur in the brain.

caudal f. the bend in the lumbosacral region of the embryo.

cephalic f. the curve in the midbrain of the embryo.

cervical f. a bend in the neural tube of the embryo at the junction of the brain and spinal cord.

cranial f. the anterior of the two ventral flexures of the developing embryo.

diaphragmatic f. the flexure between the left and right dorsal colons in the horse.

pelvic f. where the left ventral colon in the horse is flexed upward to become the left dorsal colon; there is a sharp reduction in the diameter of the colon at this flexure and the contents become much firmer, less fluid.

sigmoid f. the flattened loop of colon, immediately succeeding the cecum in ruminants.

sternal f. where the right ventral colon in the horse turns to become the left ventral colon.

flight control see DEFLIGHTING.

flight distance the distance that agricultural and wild animals like to keep between themselves and a threat of danger. The distance varies with the degree of wildness of the animals and the circumstances. Called also the circle of safety, critical, fright or guard distance. Important in planning animal handling facilities, yards, zoos and the like. Neglect of the need to provide adequate space in which an animal can escape will lead to them damaging themselves by running into fences.

flight range the distance that an insect or bird is capable of flying. An important factor in the spread of disease by vectors or mechanical spreaders.

flightless see RATITE.

Flinders poppy PIMELEA *decora*.

flipper fin-like structures of pinnipeds.

flipper can in food inspection a can of food in which the lid flips into a blown position when the can is knocked but the bulge can be suppressed with light pressure. A can in the early stages of spoilage.

float 1. an instrument used in the filing or rasping of a horse's premolar and molar teeth. Handles are 24 to 28 in (60 to 70 cm) with a broad head into which an interchangeable rasp can be screwed. Some rasps work when pulled toward the operator, others work only when pushed away. Short-handled floats with the heads set at an angle are used for the front upper molars. 2. in British countries, the term for a road vehicle used for the transport of large animals, usually horses or cattle. A low-level float may be an independent unit towed behind another vehicle. A high-level float is standard-truck height and an integral part of the vehicle.

floater a small opacity in the vitreous.

floating vernacular for filing or rasping a horse's molar teeth.

floating kidney excessive mobility of the kidney; called also hypermobile kidney. Nephroptosis refers to a dropping of the kidney from its normal position.

floccose see FLOCCULENT.

flocculation a colloid phenomenon in which the disperse phase separates in discrete, usually visible, particles rather than in a continuous mass, as in coagulation.

flocculent woolly, containing downy or flaky shreds; said of bacterial growth composed of short, curved chains, variously oriented.

flocculonodular lobe posterior lobe of the cerebellum, comprising the nodulus and the paired lateral flocculi; involved in the maintenance of balance.

flocculus pl. *flocculi* [L.] 1. a small tuft or mass, as of wool or other fibrous material. 2. a small mass on the lower side of each cerebellar hemisphere, continuous with the nodule of the vermis.

flock 1. a group of one species of animal or bird which eats or travels or is kept together, e.g. flock of sheep, of wild geese. 2. wool or cotton particles or debris used as stuffing or packing.

f. ewe not a stud ewe; a ewe kept for breeding or wool production.

f. ram a ram mated to flock ewes.

flocking 1. counterpart of herding but for a flock. 2. precipitation, usually by the addition of a chemical, of protein in a solution for the purpose of clarifying it.

Flomasta ventilator used in anesthetizing smaller animals. It is operated by the gas-flow from the anesthetic apparatus to which it is attached.

flood natural disaster important in the spread of animal disease and insects and disruption of quarantine areas.

f. fever see LEPTOSPIROSIS.

f. plain staggers Australian (north-western New South Wales) syndrome caused by tunicaminyluracils produced in seedhead galls on *Agrostis avenacea*, the galls produced by *Anguina funesta* (grass nematodes) and infected by *Clavibacter toxicus*. Clinically the disease is characterized by convulsions precipitated by driving and often death during the convulsion. Hypermetric ataxia is characteristic in less severe cases. Cattle are most affected, sheep and horses less frequently.

flooding a technique of training or behavior modification in which an extreme version of a feared stimulus is applied and continued until the fear response is diminished.

floor ground surface within a building.

f. feeding used in large-scale pig-raising enterprises where many pigs must be fed during a short period. Requires that pigs be trained to defecate only in their dunging area. Probably increases the chances of disease spread, even in minimal disease herds.

f. licking sometimes the preliminary behavior in partial seizures.

f. quality physical qualities which make a floor good for animals include non-slipperiness, warmth, freedom from abrasiveness with resulting injuries to hooves and the skin of the lower limbs, ease of cleaning and disinfection.

f. space the amount of floor space that each animal needs. An important characteristic in the design of animal accommodation because of the need to economize on building costs and mechanical services maintenance.

f. sweepings in feed mills and feed mixing and processing plants this is the floor residue. Collected periodically. Most likely to be contaminated with rodent droppings, weed seeds, rodent control agents and such like.

floppy disk see DISKETTE.

flora the collective plant organisms of a given locality.

intestinal f. the microorganisms normally residing within the lumen of the intestine. Ecology is influenced by age, physiological state and environment of the host.

rumen f. includes bacteria and protozoa in about equal volumes but the bacteria in much greater numbers, and fungi. The important protozoa are ciliated anaerobes.

Florestina tripteris North American plant in the family Asteraceae; can cause cyanide poisoning.

florfenicol an antimicrobial agent, closely related to chloramphenicol, but free of the ability to induce aplastic anemia in humans.

Florida arrowroots ZAMIA *integrifolia*.

Florida fungus see acid-fast KERATOPATHY.

Florida horse leech see SWAMP CANCER.

Florida spots see acid-fast KERATOPATHY.

flotation tank a once-popular, but now little used, technique of suspending a horse in a harness in a tank filled with water for long periods while a limb bone fracture healed; still used for brief periods of several days for lesser injuries.

flounder members of the families Bothidae and Pleuronectidae; flatfish with eyes on the same side of the head.

f. ulcer disease progressive and sometimes fatal ulceration in greenback flounder and probably other species of flatfish. Caused by *Aeromonas salmonicida*. See also atypical AEROMONAS *salmonicida*.

flour mite a mite capable of causing dermatitis. See TYROGLYPHUS (*Acarus*), TYROPHAGUS, GLYCYPHAGUS, SUIDASIA NESBITTI, CARPOGLYPHUS.

Flourensia cernua an American plant in the family Asteraceae; may contain sesquiterpenes which cause abdominal pain, respiratory distress, enteritis and liver damage. Called also tarbush.

flow chart a graphic representation, using boxes and lines, of the sequence of a program of work from commencement to completion. The original documentation for a computer program.

flow cytometry a technique used to identify and separate different types of cells based on detecting and measuring the fluorescence emitted with a laser light beam. See also FLUORESCENCE microscopy.

flow receptors bursts of impulses fired by flow receptors in urethra when urine commences to flow, initiating reflexes which contract the bladder and further relax its sphincter.

flower spray endings afferent secondary nerve endings attached to muscle fibers; function uncertain but probably to transmit information about muscle length to the CNS.

flowers of sulfur commercial grade sulfur, commonly used by animal owners as a parasiticide dressing; also administered orally for the same purpose; overdosing causes gastroenteritis.

flowload the load placed on the heart by the need for an increase in the volume of blood discharged per minute, e.g. A-V valve insufficiency. Called also pressure load.

flowmeter an apparatus for measuring the rate of flow of liquids or gases.

Bourdon f. based on the straightening of a flexible metal tube as gas pressure increases. Has limitations, especially at very low flow rates.

floxacillin see FLUCLOXACILLIN.

floxuridine a derivative of 5-fluorouracil used as an antiviral and antineoplastic agent; abbreviated FUDR.

Floydia praealata Australian rainforest tree in the family Proteaceae. Kernels of the nuts on this tree may contain toxic amounts of cyanogenic glycosides.

fl.oz. fluid ounce.

fluanisone a butyrophenone tranquilizer used in combination with fentanyl for neuroleptanalgesia in animals.

flucloxacillin a penicillinase-resistant antibiotic; an isoxazolyl derivative of penicillin.

fluconazole a triazole antifungal agent, used particularly in the treatment of cryptococcosis.

fluctuation 1. a variation, as about a fixed variation or mass. 2. a wavelike motion in a fluid-filled cavity.

5-flucytosine a fluorinated pyrimidine used as a systemic antifungal agent in the treatment of severe candidal and cryptococcal infections.

fludrocortisone a synthetic adrenal corticoid with effects similar to those of hydrocortisone and desoxycorticosterone. Used as an acetate.

fludroxycortide see FLURANDRENOLONE.

flue see UNDERFLUE.

flufenamic acid an anti-inflammatory, analgesic, serotonin antagonist; little used in animals because of toxic effects.

fluff louse see GONIOCOTES *gallinae*.

flugestone acetate, flurogestone acetate a steroid used in the synchronization of estrus in ewes; used in progesterone impregnated vaginal pessaries or tampons.

fluid 1. a liquid or gas; any liquid of the body. 2. composed of molecules which freely change their relative positions without separation of the mass.

allantoic f. the fluid contained within the allantois.

amniotic f. the fluid within the amnion that bathes the developing fetus and protects it from mechanical injury.

ascitic f. see ASCITES.

f. balance a state in which the volume of body water and its solutes (electrolytes and nonelectrolytes) are within normal limits and there is normal distribution of fluids within the intracellular and extracellular compartments. The total volume of body fluids should be about 60% of the body weight, and it should be distributed so that one-third is extracellular fluid and two-thirds intracellular fluid. Although this distribution remains constant in a healthy animal, there is continuous movement of fluid into and out of the various compartments. See also DEHYDRATION, WATER intoxication.

body f's the fluids within the body, composed of water, electrolytes and nonelectrolytes. The volume and distribution of body fluids vary with age, sex and amount of adipose tissue. Throughout life there is a slow decline in the volume of body fluids; obesity decreases the relative amount of water in the body.

Although the body fluids are continuously in motion, moving in and out of the cells, tissue spaces and vascular system, physiologists consider them to be 'compartmentalized'. Fluid within the cell membranes is called *intracellular* fluid and comprises about two-thirds of the total body fluids. The remaining one-third is outside the cell and is called *extracellular* fluid. The extracellular fluid can be further divided into tissue fluid (*interstitial* fluid), which is found in the spaces between the blood vessels and surrounding cells, and intravascular fluid, which is the fluid component of blood.

The maintenance of a proper balance between the intracellular and extracellular fluid volumes is essential to health. In patients with HEART FAILURE and renal failure the balance becomes upset, producing either localized or generalized EDEMA. Excessive fluid loss produces fluid volume deficit causing cellular dehydration and impaired cellular function.

Bouin's f. a histological fixative.

cerebrospinal f. the fluid contained within the ventricles of the brain, the subarachnoid space, and the central canal of the spinal cord. See also CEREBROSPINAL fluid.

f. dram see fluid DRAM.

f. extract a liquid preparation of a vegetable drug, containing alcohol as a solvent or preservative, or both, of such strength that each milliliter contains the therapeutic constituents of 1 gram of the standard drug it represents.

fetal f. allantoic plus amniotic fluids.

interstitial f. the extracellular fluid bathing the cells in most tissues, excluding the fluid within the lymph and blood vessels.

isotonic f. having the same tonicity or osmotic pressure as blood.

lacrimal f. aqueous fluid secreted by the lacrimal glands; called also tears.

f. line in radiographs, the interface between fluid and gas, as in the gastrointestinal tract, will show as a straight line.

f. loss by vomiting, diarrhea, polyuria, water deprivation. See DEHYDRATION.

f. mosaic model the modern concept of the structure of a biological membrane developed by S.J. Singer and G.L. Nicolson. In it the membrane consists of protein molecules partly embedded in a discontinuous bilayer of phospholipids that form the matrix of a mosaic of functional cell units.

f. ounce see fluid OUNCE.

pericardial, pleural, peritoneal f. normally present in amounts sufficient only to lubricate the movement of viscera within the respective cavities. Composition similar to blood serum.

f. replacement see fluid therapy (below).

f. restriction the limitation of oral fluid intake to a prescribed amount for each 24-hour period.

f. retention see EDEMA.

spinal f. the fluid within the spinal canal.

f. splashing sounds audible when gas and fluid are free in a cavity, e.g. abomasum in cases of abomasal displacement; can be elicited by shaking a small animal or part of a large animal (i.e. succussion) or by simultaneous percussion and auscultation.

synovial f. synovia.

f. therapy aims to replace fluids lost by disease process or by restriction of intake, or to maintain a high rate of fluid excretion to ensure removal of toxins, or to administer therapeutic or anesthetic agents slowly over a long period. The amounts and route of administration vary with the need of the patient. Normal solutions include 5% dextrose and Ringer's solution; alkalinizing fluids include lactated Ringer's and 1.3% sodium bicarbonate; acidifying solutions include isotonic saline and 1.9% ammonium chloride.

f. thrill see THRILL.

f. volume deficit an imbalance in fluid volume in which there is loss of fluid from the body not compensated for by an adequate intake of water. The major causes are: (1) insufficient fluid intake, and (2) excessive fluid loss from vomiting, diarrhea, suctioning of gastric contents, or drainage through operative wounds, burns or fistulae. Decreased volume in the intravascular compartment is called *hypovolemia*. Because water moves freely between the compartments, extracellular fluid deficit causes intracellular fluid deficit (cellular dehydration), which leaves the cells without adequate water to carry on normal function.

f. volume excess an overabundance of water in the interstitial fluid spaces or body cavities (edema) or an excess of fluid within the blood vessels (hypervolemia) and water intoxication.

Factors that contribute to the accumulation of edematous fluid are: (1) dilatation of the arteries, as occurs in the inflammatory process; (2) reduced effective osmotic pressure, as in hypoproteinemia, lymphatic obstruction and increased capillary permeability; (3) increased venous pressure, as in congestive heart failure, thrombophlebitis and cirrhosis of the liver; and (4) retention of sodium due to increased reabsorption of sodium by the renal tubules.

f. wave see THRILL.

fluid–electrolyte disturbance see DEHYDRATION, WATER intoxication.

fluidrachm fluid dram.

fluke[1] a helminth organism of the class Trematoda in the phylum Platyhelminthes, characterized by a body that is usually flat and often leaflike. Trematodes can infect the blood, liver, intestines and lungs. All of the species that infect domestic animals are in the subclass Digenea, that is they are digenetic flukes. Members of the subclass Monogenea occur on the gills or scales of fish.

blood f. see SCHISTOSOMA.

common liver f. see FASCIOLA *hepatica*.

conical f. PARAMPHISTOMUM, *Cotylophoron*, CALICOPHORON.

giant liver f. see FASCIOLA *gigantica*.

lancet f. see DICROCOELIUM *dendriticum*.

large liver f. see FASCIOLOIDES *magna*.

lesser liver f. see DICROCOELIUM *dendriticum*.

liver f. FASCIOLA *hepatica*, *F. gigantica*, FASCIOLOIDES *magna*, DICROCOELIUM *dendriticum*.

lung f. see PARAGONIMUS; includes also *Dasymetra*, *Stomatrema* etc., which infest the mouths of reptiles and can be found in the lungs.

pancreatic f. see EURYTREMA.

stomach f. PARAMPHISTOMUM, *Cotylophoron*, CALICOPHORON.

fluke[2] each half of the tail of a whale or dolphin.

fluke disease see hepatic FASCIOLIASIS, PARAMPHISTOMIASIS.

flukicide an agent that destroys flukes.

flumazenil a benzodiazepine antagonist.

flumen pl. *flumina* [L.] a stream. See also FLUMINA PILORUM.

flumenazil a benzodiazepine antagonist, used to reverse sedation produced by that group of tranquilizers.

flumequine a quinolone antibiotic effective against Enterobacteriaceae.

flumethasone a long-acting glucocorticoid; the pivalate is used topically in the treatment of skin diseases.

flumethrin a synthetic pyrethroid insecticide.

flumina pilorum hair streams; the direction of the hair flow.

flunixin meglumine a prostaglandin inhibitor; a nonsteroidal anti-inflammatory agent with potent analgesic and antipyretic activity; particularly effective in visceral pain and is used in the treatment of equine colic.

fluocinolone acetonide a corticosteroid anti-inflammatory used topically in the treatment of skin diseases and inflammation of anal sacs. Called also Synalar.

fluocinonide an ester of fluocinolone acetonide used topically in the treatment of certain dermatoses.

fluopromazine see TRIFLUPROMAZINE.

fluorapatite a fluorine-bearing mineral in rock phosphate. Contributes to local fluorine poisoning and also to distant sites if the rock phosphate is mined for livestock feeding as a dietary phosphorus supplement.

fluorescein a fluorescing dye, an acid fluorochrome; the sodium salt is used in solution to reveal corneal lesions and as a test of circulation in the retina and extremities. The isothiocyanate derivative (FITC) is used for labeling of immunoglobulins in various IMMUNOFLUORESCENCE techniques.

f. strips sterilized applicators impregnated with fluorescein for use in ophthalmic tests.

fluorescence the property of emitting light while exposed to light, the wavelength of the emitted light being longer than that of the absorbed light.

f.-activated cell sorter (FACS) an instrument for analysis (FACscan) and separating mixed populations of cells after labeling individual cell-specific surface antigens with fluorescent antibody. The individual cells in droplets are passed through a laser beam; the droplet is deflected into one of two or more collection vessels depending upon which fluorescent antibody is bound to its surface. Two or more different fluorescent antibodies are used.

f. microscopy the use of techniques for conjugating antibodies with fluorescent dyes in order to identify specific microorganisms or tissue constituents using a fluorescence microscope. Fluorescent antibody (FA) techniques can be used in place of time-consuming culture methods for identifying bacteria and viruses. There are two major types of FA techniques, direct and indirect, both of which are based on the antigen–antibody reaction in which the antibody attaches itself to its specific antigen.

In the *direct* fluorescent antibody (DFA) method, the antibody is bound to the antigen, for example, a bacterial cell in a smear, and cannot be easily removed by elution (washing). The antibody remains attached to the cell after all other serum proteins have been washed away. Since the antibody has been rendered fluorescent by conjugation with fluorescein or another dye, the outline of the bacterial cell that it coats can readily be seen with a special microscope.

In the *indirect* method (IFA), the specific antibody is allowed to react with the antigen. The slide is then washed and treated with a labeled antibody to the specific antibody. For example, if the specific antibody was raised in a rabbit, it is then treated with fluorescein-labeled anti-rabbit globulin, which results in a combination of this labeled antibody with the rabbit immunoglobulin already attached to the antigen.

Fluorescent antibody studies have been used in the detection of numerous bacterial, viral, fungal and protozoan infections and in the identification and localization of many tissue antigens.

fluorescent having the quality of fluorescence.
f. antibody see FLUORESCENCE microscopy.
f. antibody test see FLUORESCENCE microscopy.
f. bone marker tetracycline is used experimentally to mark bone for procedures such as measuring rate of growth of bone.
f. crystals phosphors used in radiographic intensifying screens. A fine grade of crystals improves the definition of the image obtained but significantly slows the speed of the film. Calcium tungstate was commonly used as the phosphor but is gradually being replaced by rare earths.
f. dye used in fluorescent staining and FLUORESCENCE microscopy.
f. screen used as a fluoroscopic screen.
f. staining use of a fluorescent dye linked to an antibody forms the basis for FLUORESCENCE microscopy.

fluoridation treatment with fluorides; the addition of fluorides to drinking water as a measure to reduce the incidence of dental caries in humans.

fluoride any binary compound of fluorine. See also FLUORINE.

fluorimeter see FLUOROMETER.

fluorimetry see FLUOROMETRY.

fluorinated material to which a fluoride has been added, e.g. water for human consumption treated as a prophylaxis against tooth decay.

fluorine a chemical element, atomic number 9, atomic weight 18.998, symbol F. See Table 6.
f. poisoning see FLUOROSIS.

fluorite a fluorine-bearing rock mineral. Called also fluorspar, calcium fluoride.

fluoroacetamide a rodenticide, also used in control of rabbits. Odorless, tasteless and soluble in water and has excellent credentials as a rodenticide but is dangerous for other species including farm livestock and even humans. Signs of poisoning in dogs include extreme excitation, hyperirritability, crazy running and tonic–clonic convulsions. In horses and ruminants there are no signs of nervous excitation, death occurring as a result of cardiac failure manifested by tachycardia and cardiac arrhythmia. Called also Compound 1081.

fluoroacetate a rodenticide used on an extensive scale in agriculture, in the form of the sodium salt. It also occurs as a natural component in the plants *Gastrolobium grandiflorum* and *Oxylobium* spp. and in *Acacia georginea*. The clinical syndrome is the same as for FLUOROACETAMIDE poisoning.

fluoroacetic acid a potent cardiac poison found in DICHAPETALUM spp., GASTROLOBIUM spp., ACACIA *georginae*, PALICOUREA spp.

fluoroapatite see APATITE.

fluorochrome a fluorescent compound, as a dye, used to mark protein with a fluorescent label. See also FLUORESCEIN.

fluorocitrate a metabolic product of fluoroacetic acid which inhibits aconitase and causes the tissue build-up of citrate, the pathogenesis of fluoroacetate poisoning.

fluorocitric acid see FLUOROCITRATE.

fluorocytes nucleated cells of the erythrocyte series present in the bone marrow. They fluoresce under the fluorescence microscope because of the presence of porphyrin in the nuclei.

5-fluorocytosine see 5-FLUCYTOSINE.

fluorodeoxyuridine see FLOXURIDINE.

fluorography see PHOTOFLUOROGRAPHY.

fluorometer the instrument used in fluorometry, consisting of an energy source (e.g. a mercury arc lamp or xenon lamp) to induce fluorescence, monochromators for selection of the wavelength, and a detector.

fluorometholone a topical anti-inflammatory glucocorticoid.

fluorometry an analytical technique for identifying minute amounts of a substance by detection and measurement of the characteristic wavelength of the light it emits during fluorescence.

fluoro-oleic acid the toxin in the seeds of the plant DICHAPETALUM *toxicarium* (ratsbane).

fluorophotometry the measurement of light given off by fluorescent substances.
vitreous f. the measurement of light given off by intravenously injected fluorescein that has leaked through the retinal vessels into the vitreous; done to detect the breakdown of the blood–retinal barrier.

fluoroquinolone a group of antibiotics which exert their antimicrobial effects by inhibiting bacterial DNA gyrase. They are effective primarily against gram-negative organisms. Includes CIPROFLOXACIN, NORFLOXACIN, ENROFLOXACIN.

fluororadiography see PHOTOFLUOROGRAPHY.

fluoroscope an instrument for visual observation of the form and motion of the deep structures of the body by means of x-ray. The patient is put into position so that the part to be viewed is placed between an x-ray tube and a fluorescent screen. The x-rays from the tube pass through the body and project the bones and organs as shadowy images on the screen. Examination by this method is called fluoroscopy, but the image is viewed on a separate television monitor and not on the fluorescent screen. See also IMAGE intensification.

The advantage of the fluoroscope is that the action of joints, organs and entire systems of the body can be observed directly. The use of radiopaque media aids in this process. See also BARIUM study.

fluoroscopy examination by means of the fluoroscope, a fluoroscopic screen set up to produce a visual image.

fluorosis a condition due to ingestion of excessive amounts of fluorine or its compounds. Fluorine poisoning usually takes a chronic form in animals which are exposed to small amounts in their drinking water or food over long periods. Clinical signs include excessive wear and mottling of developing teeth, lameness due to osteoporosis and unthriftiness. Acute fluorosis caused by factory effluent is characterized by gastroenteritis, tetany and death.

5-fluorouracil an antimetabolite used as an antineoplastic agent. See also FLOXURIDINE.

fluorspar see FLUORITE.

Fluothane a proprietary name for HALOTHANE.

fluoxetine a serotonin inhibitor, used as an antidepressant. Called also Prozac.

fluoxymesterone an anabolic androgenic steroid.

fluphenazine a piperazine-phenothiazine tranquilizer, used as the enanthate ester and hydrochloride salt.

fluprostenol a prostaglandin analog used in mares to synchronize estrus.

flurandrenolone, flurandrenolide a glucocorticoid used topically in the treatment of certain skin diseases. Called also fludroxycortide.

flurazepam a benzodiazepine hypnotic and sedative, usually used as the hydrochloride salt,

flurbiprofen a nonsteroidal anti-inflammatory agent used in musculoskeletal disorders and as the sodium salt topically in ocular inflammation.

Flury strain a high egg passage of rabies virus used in some vaccines for animals.

flushing a sudden increase in flow.

f. agents water under pressure, sterile saline and Ringer's solution are used to irrigate and cleanse wounds. Various antiseptic compounds, in dilute solutions, have the added advantage of antibacterial effects and some, with detergent action, are more efficient in removing necrotic tissues and debris, but they may be irritating and delay healing.

nutritional f. an abrupt and sizable increase in nutritional status practiced as a management tactic, usually prior to the mating period in order to improve semen characteristics in the male and ovulation and conception rates in the female. Most attention is given to the protein concentration of the ration.

flutamide a nonsteroidal drug with antiandrogen effects; used in the treatment of prostatic hyperplasia in dogs.

flutter a rapid vibration or pulsation.

atrial f. cardiac arrhythmia in which the atrial contractions are rapid (200–320 per minute), but regular.

diaphragmatic f. peculiar wavelike fibrillations of the diaphragm of unknown cause. See also synchronous DIAPHRAGMATIC flutter.

impure f. atrial flutter in which the atrial rhythm is irregular.

mediastinal f. abnormal mobility of the mediastinum during respiration.

pure f. atrial flutter in which the atrial rhythm is regular.

f. valve in an intravenous infusion apparatus, a floating bead in the fluid chamber that allows air to enter the system but prevents fluid from escaping. Its movement is often viewed as an indicator of the speed of fluid infusion, but it is inaccurate.

ventricular f. a possible transition stage between ventricular tachycardia and ventricular fibrillation, the electrocardiogram showing rapid, uniform, and virtually regular oscillations, 250 or more per minute.

flutter–fibrillation impure flutters that vary from moment to moment in their resemblance to flutter or fibrillation, respectively.

flux 1. an excessive flow or discharge. 2. matter discharged.

bloody f. dysentery.

fly members of the order Diptera. See BLACK FLY, BLOWFLY, BOT FLY, CHRYSOPS, CNEPHIA, CORDYLOBIA, CUTEREBRA, ERISTALIS, FLESH flies, HAEMATOBIA, HIPPOBOSCA, HYDROTOEA, HYPODERMA, MUSCA, PHORMIA, PIGEON fly, SANDFLY, SCREW-WORM, SIMULIUM, STOMOXYS CALCITRANS, TABANUS, TORSALO GRUB, TSETSE, WARBLES.

f. agaric a mushroom. See AMANITA.

f. biting, f. catching behavior by dogs that looks like an attempt to catch a nonexistent flying object, hence the name. When repeated or continual, believed to be a form of partial seizure or hallucinations.

f. control limitation of fly population by disposal of rotting animal tissue, use of insecticides in sprays, back applicators, impregnated ear tags or pet collars, liberation of sterilized males, fly traps.

f. dermatitis biting flies will inflict skin damage on the face and particularly ear tips of outdoor dogs, causing bleeding, dried crusts and moderate irritation that sometimes leads to the development of auricular hematomas. Also reported to be a common problem in zoo bears.

ear tip f. bite see fly dermatitis (above).

forest f. see HYDROTOEA *irritans*.

head f. see HYDROTOEA *irritans*.

horn f. see HAEMATOBIA.

louse f. see HIPPOBOSCA.

f. poison see AMIANTHIUM MUSCAETOXICUM.

sand f. see PHLEBOTOMUS.

stable f. see STOMOXYS CALCITRANS.

f. strike cutaneous MYIASIS.

f. worry all fly infestations cause worry to their host animals. Heavy infestations with black flies in horses and buffalo flies in cattle may cause deaths from worry, blood loss, interference with grazing and intercurrent disease. See also fly dermatitis (above).

fly poison see AMIANTHIUM MUSCAETOXICUM.

flyblown infested with fly maggots, usually BLOWFLY larvae.

flying fox includes gray-headed flying fox; see CHIROPTERA.

flying fox lyssavirus disease a disease identified in 1996 in Australian fruit-eating flying foxes (*Pteropus* spp.) in which it is presumed endemic and in which it may cause encephalitis; the virus, of the genus *Lyssavirus* and the family RHABDOVIRIDAE, has also caused fatal rabies-like illness in persons working closely with infected bats.

Fm chemical symbol, *fermium*.

FMD foot-and-mouth disease.

FMDV foot-and-mouth disease virus.

FMN oxidized form of flavin mononucleotide.

$FMNH_2$ reduced form of flavin mononucleotide.

foal a junior horse from birth to one year. May be filly foal, colt foal.

f. ataxia see ENZOOTIC equine incoordination.

contracted f. congenital flexion contracture of the distal limb joints, plus torticollis, scoliosis, skull distortion; cause unknown.

f. hemolytic disease see ALLOIMMUNE hemolytic anemia of the newborn.

f. heat the first estrus after foaling. Usually commences at the 7th to 15th day.

f. heat diarrhea a transient attack of diarrhea in the foal at the time of the mare's foaling heat, ascribed to excitement and subtle changes in composition of the milk.

f. MAC test a field test on blood to detect low blood levels of immunoglobulins (IgG) in foals.

f. mortality deaths in foals as a group; include congenital defects, immaturity, foaling injury, septicemia, joint ill, enteritis, shigellosis, barkers and wanderers, isoimmune hemolytic anemia.

f. restraint generally achieved by holding against a wall and using one arm under the neck and the other hand lifting the tail.

f. septicemia common causes, usually from intrauterine infection contracted through the cervix of the dam, are *Actinobacillus equuli*, *Klebsiella pneumoniae*, *Staphylococcus aureus*, *Pseudomonas aeruginosa*, *Escherichia coli* and β-hemolytic streptococci.

foaling parturition in the mare.

f. induction bringing on the birth of the foal, usually via the injection of oxytocin.

f. injuries includes first-degree injury to the perineum, involving the mucosa of the roof of the vestibule and the dorsal commissure of the vulva. Second-degree injuries involve disruption of the musculature of the vulva and vaginal vestibule but there is no rectal lesion. Third-degree lacerations are those where the rectal wall is ruptured creating either a rectovaginal fistula, or a complete rupture of the rectovaginal septum out to and including the perineal skin.

foam frothy liquid, e.g. from the nostrils of an animal with terminal pulmonary edema, in the rumen of the cow with frothy bloat.

f. cell vacuolated histiocytes.

f. cell pneumonia see endogenous lipid PNEUMONIA.

f. test fresh urine is shaken vigorously. A yellow-green foam is indicative of bilirubinuria.

focal 1. limited to a small area or volume. 2. pertaining to or emanating from focus.

f. distance see focal–film DISTANCE.

f. length the distance between the lens and an object from which all rays of light are brought to a focus.

f. liver disease widely disseminated micro-abscesses or abscesses, migration paths of helminth larvae.

f. macular melanosis dark colored spots on the skin, not elevated above the skin surface but apt to be confused with melanosis.

f. myelitis–encephalitis widely disseminated inflammatory lesions, usually the result of blood-borne infection, in brain and spinal cord.

f. symmetrical encephalomalacia see focal symmetrical ENCEPHALOMALACIA.

f. symmetrical spinal poliomalacia see focal symmetrical spinal POLIOMALACIA.

f. zone in ultrasound, the area of the transducer where the sound beam is most sharply focussed and where the area under examination will give the best image.

focal spot the area on the target of the x-ray tube which the electron stream strikes and from which x-rays are emitted. Called also focus. The larger the area of the focal spot, the poorer is the detail in the x-ray image.

actual f. s. the actual area of the focal spot on the radiographic target as viewed at right angles to the plane of the target.

broad f. s. a relative term which refers to the effective dimension of the x-ray focal spot usually greater than 1 mm^2. See also fine focal spot (below).

effective f. s. the face of the anode that carries the target in an x-ray tube is slanted from the vertical to increase the volume of the target but to reduce the size of the origin of the x-ray beam.

f. s.–film distance see focal–film DISTANCE.

fine f. s. a focal spot of less than 1 mm^2 which is used in radiography studies where high detail is required.

f. s.–skin distance distance from the film spot to the skin of a patient receiving radiation therapy.

FOCMA feline oncornavirus-associated cell membrane ANTIGEN.

focus pl. *foci* [L.] 1. the point of convergence of light rays, x-rays or sound waves. 2. the chief center of a morbid process. See also focal spot.

focusing the act of converging at a point.

isoelectric f. electrophoresis in which the protein mixture is subjected to an electric field in a gel medium in which a pH gradient has been established; each protein then migrates until it reaches the site at which the pH is equal to its isoelectric point.

fodder feed for herbivorous animals, usually used to describe dried leafy material such as hay. See also FORAGE.

f. beet a root crop grown solely as a source of feed for cattle, possibly sheep. Lactic acidosis, OXALATE and NITRITE poisoning are all possible with fodder beet feeding. See also BETA *vulgaris*, CARBOHYDRATE ENGORGEMENT.

f. crop crops being grown for hay, e.g. oats, barley, wheat. Can also be used for grazing and may cause hypomagnesemia or nitrite poisoning. The group of diseases is known as CEREAL crop poisoning.

f. poisoning an all-embracing term used with reference to sickness occurring in animals being fed hay which is often moldy or damaged in some way. See also MYCOTOXICOSIS.

f. radish see RAPHANUS *sativus*.

f. sorghum SORGHUM *bicolor*.

Foerster sponge forceps used to hold swabs or sponges for mopping up the site. Scissor-type operation with ratcheted handles. The blades are loops with serrated opposing faces. May be straight or, for better visibility of the site, curved.

fog 1. a colloid system in which the dispersion medium is a gas and the dispersed particles are liquid. 2. regrowth after harvesting of a cereal crop. Called also aftermath, feg. 3. obscuring opacity on an x-ray film.

basic f. blackening of an unexposed x-ray film after development.

f. fever see ATYPICAL INTERSTITIAL PNEUMONIA.

x-ray f. local or general exposure to extraneous radiation, light or chemical action which is additional to the true photographic image. Leads to spoiling of the x-ray image.

foggage aftermath; stubble regrowth or grass grown for winter feed.

folacin see FOLIC ACID.

folate the generic term for FOLIC ACID and related compounds.

fold[1] 1. in anatomical terms a plica; a thin, recurved margin or doubling. 2. the big skin folds down the front of a merino ram's neck.

alar f. see ALAR fold.

amniotic f. the folded edge of the amnion where it rises over and finally encloses the embryo.

anal f. in the developing embryo the cloacal folds divide into the dorsal anal folds, forming the rectum and anus, and the urogenital folds.

cecocolic f. connects the right ventral colon with the cecum in the horse.

circular f's the permanent transverse folds of the luminal surface of the small intestine.

coprourodeal f. annular fold separating the coprodeum from the urodeum in the cloaca of birds.

f. dermatitis see fold DERMATITIS.

duodenocolic f. in the horse connects the small colon with the terminal part of the duodenum.

facial f. the deep wrinkles of skin over the nose of brachycephalic dogs and cats. A distinctive feature of the breeds concerned, but often a site of fold DERMATITIS. The hairs also become a source of irritation to the cornea.

flank f. skin fold from the lower, lateral abdominal wall to the hindlimb at the region of the stifle.

gastric f's see GASTRIC folds.

gastropancreatic f. in the horse connects the stomach and duodenum to the liver, vena cava and pancreas.

genital f. a transverse peritoneal fold in the pelvis that supports the vas deferens in the male and is the broad ligament of the uterus in the female.

glossoepiglottic f. extends from the root of the tongue to the base of the epiglottis.

gluteal f. the crease separating the buttocks from the thigh, usually absent from domestic mammals.

head f. a fold of blastoderm at the cephalic end of the developing embryo.

ileocecal f. a short mesenteric fold connecting the ileum and the cecum, and which is used to define the ileum in domestic animals.

lacrimal f. a fold of mucous membrane at the rostral opening of the nasolacrimal duct.

mucosal f., mucous f. a fold of mucous membrane.

nail f. the fold of palmar skin around the base and sides of the nail or claw.

neural f. one of the paired folds lying on either side of the neural plate that form the neural tube in the developing embryo.

preputial f. the telescopic fold of preputial skin which invests the glans of the stallion's unengorged penis. In the mare, a mucosal fold covering most of the clitoris.

pterygomandibular f. the fold of mucosa which runs from the lower to upper jaw on the same side of the mouth and caudal to the last molar tooth.

rumenoreticular f. on the internal ventral wall of the rumenoreticulum and separating the rumen from the reticulum.

tail f. 1. a fold of the blastoderm at the caudal end of the developing embryo. 2. the skin, usually on an obese dog, around the very short tail such as seen on British bulldogs. May be the site of fold DERMATITIS. 3. site for injection of tuberculin in SID test for tuberculosis in cattle. See also CAUDAL tailfold.

urogenital f. the transverse peritoneal fold which, in the male, carries the seminal vesicles, the deferent duct and the uterus masculinus.

uroproctodeal f. in the bird separates the urodeum from the proctodeum.

ventricular f., vestibular f. a false vocal cord.

vesical f. paired lateral folds of peritoneum containing the bladder's round ligaments.

vestigial f. a pericardial fold enclosing the remnant of the embryonic left anterior cardinal vein.

vocal f's see VOCAL cords.

fold^2 a pasture management system in which animals are run at pasture during the day and locked up at night in a portable pen or shed in the pasture. Also used to mean temporary subdivision of a paddock.

fold-back DNA a single strand of DNA, folded back upon itself, resulting in a hydrogen-bonded region. Also referred to as hairpin structures.

Foley catheter a soft rubber retention catheter with an inflatable bulb on the end.

folia cerebelli the divisions of the cerebellar cortex.

foliar pertaining to or having the quality of leaves.

folic acid one of the vitamins of the B complex. Folic acid is involved in the synthesis of amino acids and DNA; its deficiency causes megaloblastic anemia. Folic acid is supplied in adequate amounts by natural pasture plants and most diets for dogs and cats. Possibly required in greater amounts in racing horses confined to stables. Called also vitamin B_c, pteroylmonoglutamic acid.

f. a. antagonist a compound such as trimethoprim or methotrexate which acts as an antimetabolite of folic acid, interfering with DNA replication and cell division by inhibiting the enzyme dihydrofolate reductase.

folinic acid 5-formyltetrahydrofolic acid, a metabolically active derivative of folic acid used to treat folic acid deficiency and as an antidote to folic acid antagonists. Called also citrovorum factor, CF, leucovorin, 5-formyltetrahydropteroylglutamic acid.

folium pl. *folia* [L.] a leaflike structure, especially one of the leaflike subdivisions of the cerebellar cortex.

folivore eats foliage; includes arboreal folivores—animals whose diet consists largely of tree foliage.

follicle a sac or pouchlike depression or cavity.

atretic f. an involuted ovarian follicle.

conjunctival f. focal accumulations of hypertrophied lymphoid tissue in conjunctiva, indicative of an inflammatory reaction.

cystic f. ovarian follicle that has not ruptured, is grossly enlarged, may be multiple and on both ovaries. Caused by insufficient luteinizing hormone. Affected cows may be nymphomaniac in behavior, but most are anestrous and anovulatory.

dental f. the structure within the substance of the jaws enclosing a tooth before its eruption; the dental sac and its contents.

gastric f. lymphoid masses in the gastric mucosa.

graafian f. a maturing ovarian follicle among whose cells fluid has begun to accumulate, leading to the formation of a single cavity and leaving the ovum located in the cumulus oophorus; called also vesicular ovarian follicle.

hair f. see HAIR follicle.

lymph f., lymphatic f 1. a small collection of actively proliferating lymphocytes in the cortex of a lymph node. 2. a small collection of lymphoid tissue in the mucous membrane of the gastrointestinal tract; such collections may occur singly (solitary lymphatic follicle) or closely packed together (aggregated lymphatic follicles).

ovarian f. the ovum and its encasing cells, at any stage of its development.

primary ovarian f. an immature ovarian follicle consisting of an immature ovum and the few specialized epithelial cells surrounding it.

primordial f. an ovarian follicle consisting of an ovum enclosed by a single layer of cells.

sebaceous f. a hair follicle with a relatively large sebaceous gland, producing a relatively insignificant hair.

solitary f. 1. areas of concentrated lymphatic tissue in the mucosa of the colon. 2. small lymph follicles scattered throughout the mucosa and submucosa of the small intestine. Called also solitary glands.

thyroid f. discrete cystlike units filled with a colloid substance, constituting the lobules of the thyroid gland.

vesicular ovarian f. graafian follicle.

wool f. site of origin of wool fiber.

follicle-stimulating hormone one of the gonadotropic hormones of the anterior lobe of the PITUITARY gland that stimulates the growth of graafian follicles in the ovary, and stimulates spermatogenesis in the testis. Abbreviated FSH.

f.-s. h. and luteinizing-hormone releasing h. (FSH/LH-RH) gonadotropin releasing hormone.

follicle-stimulating hormone releasing hormone a hormone produced in the hypothalamus and transported by the pituitary portal circulation to the anterior lobe of the pituitary gland where it stimulates the secretion of FSH or LH. Called also luteinizing-hormone releasing hormone, gonadotropin releasing hormone (GnRH). Abbreviated FSH-RH. See also FOLLICULAR.

follicular pertaining to or emanating from a follicle.

f. antrum spaces formed by the confluence of small lakes of follicular liquid in the ovary.

canine hereditary black hair f. dysplasia see black hair follicular DYSPLASIA.

cyclic f. dysplasia see seasonal flank ALOPECIA.

f. cyst 1. see cystic FOLLICLE. 2. retention cysts in the hair follicles are common, resembling pustules.

f. dysplasia syndrome in Siberian huskies; a late-appearing, symmetrical alopecia, affecting mostly the guard hairs.

f. hyalinosis see INTRAFOLLICULAR hyalinosis.

f. mange see DEMODECTIC MANGE.

f. pharyngitis chronic disease in young racing horses; of importance as a disruption of training; characterized by frequent cough, dyspnea with exercise, poor exercise tolerance.

f. phase see PROLIFERATIVE phase.

f. plug formed by excessive keratin in an inactive hair follicle.

folliculi ovarici vesiculosi a follicle containing oocytes, the early stage of ovarian follicles.

folliculitis inflammation of a follicle(s); used ordinarily in reference to hair follicles, but sometimes in relation to follicles of other kinds.

eosinophilic f. a feature of hypersensitivity reactions in the skin.

nasal f. see nasal PYODERMA.

pyotraumatic f. see acute moist DERMATITIS.

sterile eosinophilic f. usually nonpruritic, papular, crusted lesions with alopecia on the head, neck and trunk. The cause is unknown. In dogs, lesions occur mainly on the ears. In horses and cats, it is believed to be a hypersensitivity reaction to insect bites or other allergens.

folliculogenesis growth and development of the primordial follicle in the ovary. The maximal number of oocytes that the female will ever have are present in the ovary at birth.

folliculoma granulosa–theca cell tumor.

folliculosis see follicular CONJUNCTIVITIS.

folliculostatin a hormone produced by the ovarian granulosa cells; has a negative feedback influence on FSH production.

folliculus pl. *folliculi* [L.] follicle.

follistatin a gonadal peptide hormone isolated from the ovarian follicular fluid. Suppresses FSH secretion.

follow-up subsequent.

f. plan plan of action subsequent to the initial procedure, e.g. course of therapy, surgical procedure preventive program.

f. studies ascertaining what happened to a particular patient or group after a significant lapse of time.

followers see DAIRY herd.

fomentation treatment by warm, moist applications; also, the substance thus applied. Hosing down with cold water is referred to as cold fomentation.

fomes pl. *fomites* [L.] an inanimate object or material on which disease-producing agents may be conveyed, e.g. feces, bedding, harness.

fomites see FOMES.

Fonsecaea a genus of fungi that causes CHROMOMYCOSIS in humans and rarely animals.

font, fount the size and style of a type face.

fixed pitch f. every letter is allocated the same horizontal space. Called also monospaced font. See also proportionally spaced font (below).

monospaced f. see fixed pitch font (above).

proportionally spaced f. narrow letters such as 'i' are allocated less space than medium letters such as 'b' which have less space than wide letters such as 'W'. Called also variable pitch font.

variable pitch f. see proportionally spaced font (above).

Fontan procedure a method for repair of pulmonic stenosis in which a valved conduit is placed between the right atrium and the pulmonic artery.

fontanelle, fontanel a soft spot; skin and membrane-covered spaces remaining at the junction of the sutures, especially between the frontal and parietal bones in the incompletely covered skull of the fetus or neonate. This fontanelle usually closes after birth but in hydrocephalus and in some miniature breeds of dogs, particularly Chihuahuas, it may remain open. Called also fonticulus, molera.

fonticulus see FONTANELLE.

food materials taken into the body by mouth which provide nourishment in the form of energy or in the building of tissues. Common usage is to use the term in relation to humans and dogs and cats and to use feed for the other animals but the rule is not absolute. See also DIET, RATION, FEED.

f. additive nonfood materials added to a diet to enhance or limit a body function, e.g. growth, to control infection or to physically alter the food to facilitate handling or processing or preserving. See food ADDITIVE.

f. allergy an immune-mediated reaction to a food or food additive; clinical signs are most commonly demonstrated in the alimentary tract or skin but may affect any system and in any hypersensitivity mode. Commonly diagnosed in dogs, occasionally in horses, but rarely in the other species. Called food hypersensitivity. See also DERMATITIS, PRURITUS, ANGIOEDEMA, URTICARIA, GASTROENTERITIS.

f. anaphylaxis an acute allergic response to a food or food additive, with systemic signs typical of anaphylaxis in the species concerned. See also systemic ANAPHYLAXIS.

f. animals animals used in the production of food for humans. Includes, in common usage, the species and breeds that also supply fiber and hides for human use. Use of this term has spawned a rash of new knowledge disciplines such as food animal medicine, food animal ophthalmology, and new service areas such as food animal practice.

f. bumps see URTICARIA.

f. chain the path taken by a raw food product from the farm or other producing unit to the table of the consumer. Includes sale, transport, storage, processing, packaging and retail sale and all of the points of risk at which the food may become contaminated or spoiled or corrupted in some way.

f. contaminants include bacteria, parasites and toxic residues.

f. conversion ratio efficiency in converting the food into energy or tissue; a characteristic of the food relating largely to digestibility.

f. exchanges foods of approximately equivalent levels of energy, proteins, fats and carbohydrates, which may be exchanged or substituted in a diet without significant alteration to its nutritional balance.

generic f. see GENERIC pet food.

f. hypersensitivity see food allergy (above).

f. idiosyncrasy an adverse reaction to ingested food by an individual, not mediated by immune mechanisms; may be due to an enzyme defect.

f. intake amount of food taken in a unit of time, usually daily.

f. intolerance an abnormal physiologic response to food which is not immune-mediated.

f. legislation the content, purity and public health connotations of animal foods are usually controlled by local legislation.

manufactured f. those commercially formulated and prepared; includes stock feeds, particularly supplements and pellets, canned and dry dog and cat foods.

f. marker inert material included in food to measure speed of passage of food through alimentary tract.

pet f. usually refers to commercially prepared food such as canned, semimoist, dry, kibbled, biscuits, loaves, and butcher's scraps in various forms provided for dogs and cats.

plant-based f. usual in livestock, but in carnivores it refers to mixed-source diets with a high plant-origin carbohydrate content; a common formula in commercially prepared pet foods.

f. poisoning a group of acute illnesses due to ingestion of a specific toxin in the food. Usually causes gastroenteritis and vomiting and diarrhea.

f. refusal syndrome observed mostly in pigs; refusal to eat a particular feed or meal but willing to eat other feeds. See also FOOD REFUSAL FACTOR, DEOXYNIVALENOL, VOMITOXIN.

f. rewards the many types of food items owners and

trainers use to reward their dogs or cats for behavior that pleases them; may be a part of training and behavior modification programs, but is often done simply as a result of the owner's affection for the pet.

f. specific dynamic action see SPECIFIC dynamic action.

f. toxicity may be the result of toxins or microorganisms contaminating the food or excessive levels of a nutrient, such as vitamin A.

Food and Agriculture Organization an instrumentality of the United Nations coordinating activities in the fields of food animal health and production and in agriculture generally. For the most part its activities have been directed to carrying the agricultural technology of developed countries to developing ones. Abbreviated FAO.

Food and Drug Administration a US regulatory agency responsible for regulating the safety of foods and drugs. Abbreviated FDA.

food-producing animals see FOOD animals.

food refusal factor one or more factors in mycotoxins, especially from *Fusarium* spp., which cause affected pigs to refuse to eat without other signs of illness. See DEOXYNIVALENOL, VOMITOXIN.

foodborne infection or other damaging agent transmitted via the animal's (or human's) food chain.

fool's a look-alike; commonly mistaken for.

f. mushroom AMANITA *verna.*

f. parsley AETHUSA *cynapium.*

f. watercress SIUM *angustifolium.*

foot the distal part of the primate leg, upon which the individual stands and walks. Used loosely also in lieu of hoof, paw.

f. abscess in all species has characteristics of local inflammation. Special disease in sheep—abscess under horn either at toe or heel. Caused by *Fusobacterium necrophorum.* Severe lameness with pus discharging at coronet. Slow outbreaks occur in wet years. Footrot in pigs is really a foot abscess. See also porcine FOOTROT. Called also toe abscess, heel abscess.

at f. used to describe a female of breeding age accompanied by its unweaned offspring, e.g. ewe with a lamb at foot.

f. bath used in the control of footrot in sheep and cattle. Made of concrete or metal, preferably not metal because of the corrosive nature of copper sulfate solution. Deep enough to accommodate a 4 inch depth of solution, wide enough so that animals can stand on all four hooves in comfort, with a side fence to ensure that they do actually stand in the bath, and long enough to accommodate five to 10 animals, which need to stand in the solution for about 10 minutes. Solutions used include copper sulfate or formalin. In dairy cattle the foot bath may be at the entrance to the milking parlor so that cows walk through it twice each day.

f. laminae includes primary (insensitive) laminae of cornified material and secondary (sensitive) laminae comprising nerve endings, germinal epithelium and dermal structures in the horse's hoof.

f. licking although it can result from various causes of irritation, through contact, this is a common clinical sign of ATOPY in dogs.

f. louse LINOGNATHUS *pedalis.*

Madura f. see MADUROMYCOSIS.

f. maggot the larvae of the fly BOOPONUS *intonsus.*

f. mange see CHORIOPTES.

f. processes large cytoplasmic processes extending from the internal lining epithelium of the glomerular capsule of the kidney and terminate on the basement membrane.

f. scald dermatitis of the skin of the sheep's interdigital cleft. There is minor lifting of horn at the horn–skin junction but there is no underrunning and no odor. Avirulent strains of *Dichelobacter nodosus* are the cause; the introduction of virulent *D. nodosus* will result in severe footrot. Called also benign footrot.

slew f. in dog conformation, a turned out foot.

f. stomping gerbils stomp their rear feet to signal territorialism; sheep do it with their front hooves as a threatening gesture, especially to flocking dogs.

foot-and-mouth disease an extremely contagious, acute disease of all cloven-footed animal species. It is caused by members of the genus *Aphthovirus* in the family *Picornaviridae* which has seven serotypes and at least 80 subserotypes. Clinically there is a syndrome of fever and vesicular lesions in the mouth and around the coronets. The first sign is often lameness. Spread is very rapid and the virus is very resistant so that the infection is readily transmitted on inanimate objects. The disease is not fatal except occasionally in calves, where it also produces a myocarditis, but herd productivity is reduced disastrously. Called also FMD, aftosa.

f. d. virus (FMDV) a picornavirus, seven serotypes, at least 80 subtypes, affecting all ruminants, pigs, hedgehogs and elephants. The virus is extremely acid-labile but survives well in offal, particularly glandular tissue and bone marrow which were commonly fed as garbage to pigs resulting in outbreaks of disease.

foot–nape fetus posture a cause of dystocia in mares; the foal's front feet are displaced dorsally so that they come to lie over the top of the neck.

foot-pound the amount of energy necessary to raise 1 pound of mass a distance of 1 foot.

foothill abortion see epizootic bovine ABORTION.

footpad the thick, spongy structure located on each digit, and under the metacarpal– and metatarsal–phalangeal joints, and the carpus of dogs and cats. The skin is thickened, tough, and may be hyperpigmented and the hypodermis contains large amounts of adipose tissue. Important in birds, in which they are commonly damaged.

f. abscess caused by wound infection in fowls; painful and swollen.

collagen f. disorder see COLLAGEN footpad disorder.

f. hyperkeratosis see digital HYPERKERATOSIS, nasal HYPERKERATOSIS, HARDPAD.

footplate the flat portion of the stapes, which is set into the oval window on the medial wall of the middle ear.

footprinting a technique for identification of protein-binding regions on DNA, based on the principle that segments with bound protein are resistant to endonuclease activity and these can be demonstrated as missing bands in gel electrophoresis.

footrot a disease of the foot characterized by dermatitis of the interdigital skin and with some underrunning of the horn, especially at the heel. Infection under the horn is common. Most forms of the disease are infectious and caused by bacteria. Called also pododermatitis.

bovine f. the probable cause is *Fusobacterium necrophorum.* There is severe dermatitis in the cleft of the foot initially and severe lameness. Further spread to deep structures of the foot, requiring amputation of a claw, may occur. Called also foul-in-the-foot, fouls.

ovine f. is caused by *Dichelobacter nodosus.* A highly contagious inflammation of the skin–horn junction followed by underrunning of the horn and inflammation of the sensitive laminae of the foot. Lameness is severe and may affect all four feet.

porcine f. a noncontagious infection of the sensitive tissues of the foot caused by abrasive wearing of the horn, usually on the lateral aspect of the lateral digit, and the introduction of a mixed infection. There is abscess formation with scanty pus discharging at the coronet. Can cause severe lameness and a permanently deformed claw in some. Common in pigs housed on abrasive floors. A nutritional deficiency of biotin is thought by some to play a predisposing role or at least that provision of the vitamin has a preventive effect. See also FOOT abscess.

stable f. *Bacteroides* spp. are the probable cause of minor outbreaks of this horn junction dermatitis which occurs in housed cattle. There is a bad odor, underrunning of the horn and a sebaceous exudate. Secondary infection of the deep structures may occur.

strawberry f. is a proliferative dermatitis of the skin of the back of the pastern of sheep caused by *Dermatophilus congolensis* (*D. pedis*). It does not resemble any of the other footrots. Called also proliferative dermatitis.

forage strictly speaking, dried winter feed, usually hay. Used also to include ensilage and even pasture so that the term becomes synonymous with ROUGHAGE. See also BUNK forage.

f. mites see TROMBICULA.

f. poisoning the forage contains a toxic agent. See FOOD poisoning.

foramen pl. *foramina* [L.] a natural opening or passage, especially one into or through a bone.

alar f. a foramen which perforates the wing of the atlas in some species and transmits the vertebral artery; appears as a notch in dogs.

apical f. the opening at or near the apex of the root of a tooth and into the dental cavity.

auditory f. (external) the external acoustic meatus.

auditory f. (internal) the passage for the auditory (vestibulocochlear) and facial nerves in the pars petrosa of the temporal bone. Called also internal acoustic meatus.

caudal palatine f. the caudal opening into the greater palatine canal.

caval f. one of the three openings in the diaphragm; situated in the central tendinous part of the diaphragm; called also vena caval foramen, foramen venae cavae.

cecal f., f. cecum a blind opening between the frontal crest and the crista galli.

f. cecum linguae an occasional finding in humans; marks the boundary of the caudal and rostral contributions to the tongue, the site of the origin of the thyroid gland; called also cecum foramen.

condyloid f. (anterior) hypoglossal canal.

condyloid f. (posterior) condylar canal.

epiploic f. an opening connecting the omental bursa with the rest of the abdominal cavity; situated on the visceral surface of the liver dorsal to the portal fissure. Called also foramen of Winslow.

e. f. hernia strangulation rare cause of acute intestinal obstruction in horses.

incisive f. one of the openings of the incisive canals into the incisive fossa of the hard palate.

infraorbital f. the facial opening of the infraorbital canal, a prominent feature of the lateral aspect of the face; provides a point of emergence for the infraorbital nerve.

interventricular f. a passage from the third to the lateral ventricle of the brain.

intervertebral f. a passage for a spinal nerve and vessels formed by notches on the pedicles of adjacent vertebrae.

jugular f. an opening formed by the jugular notches of the temporal and occipital bones.

f. lacerum the irregular gap between the basioccipital, petrous temporal and sphenoid wing bones, making up a large, membrane-covered foramen in horses, but reduced to a slit in other domestic mammals.

f. magnum a large opening in the occipital bone, between the cranial cavity and spinal canal.

f. magnum herniation see transtentorial HERNIATION.

mandibular f. in the medial surface of the mandible; inferior alveolar vessels and nerve enter here.

maxillary f. one of the foraminae ventral to the orbit; leads to the infraorbital canal.

mental f. foramina on the lateral aspect of the mandible from which the inferior alveolar nerve and blood vessels emerge to supply the chin.

mastoid f. an opening in the temporal bone behind the mastoid process.

f. of Monro interventricular foramen.

nutrient f. the entrance for the nutrient artery of a bone.

obturator f. the large opening between the pubic bone and the ischium.

optic f. the opening into the optic canal.

orbital f. transmits ophthalmic branch of trigeminal, oculomotor, abducent and trochlear nerves. Called also orbital fissure.

orbitorotundum f. the copy, in pigs and ruminants, of the orbital foramen in other species.

f. ovale 1. the septal opening in the fetal heart that provides a communication between the atria. The opening closes at birth; failure to close results in ATRIAL septal defect. 2. an aperture in the great wing of the sphenoid for vessels and nerves.

palatine f. (anterior) greater and lesser foramina in the hard palate for conduction of palatine vessels.

pneumatic f. apertures in avian bones which connect with air sacs making pneumatization of bone marrow cavities possible.

f. primum opening in the septum primum between the two atria of the embryonic heart; called also ostium primum.

retroarticular f. the external opening of the temporal canal just caudal to the zygomatic arch; this foramen provides an exit for a large vein, the transverse sinus which drains the cranial cavity.

f. rotundum, round f. a round opening in the great wing of the sphenoid for the exit of the maxillary branch of the trigeminal nerve from the cranial cavity; in ruminants it is combined with the orbital fissure.

round f. see foramen rotundum (above).

sacral f. (dorsal) passage on the dorsal surface of the sacrum for the dorsal branches of the sacral nerves.

sacral f. (ventral) passage on the pelvic surface of the sacrum for the ventral branches of the sacral nerves.

Scarpa's f. an opening behind the upper medial incisor, for the nasopalatine nerve.

sciatic f. either of two foramina, the greater and the lesser sciatic foramina, formed by the sacrotuberal and sacrospinous ligaments in the sciatic notches of the hip bone.

f. secundum the second of the two orifices to perforate the septum primum between the cardiac atria; forms through cell death. Called also ostium secundum.

sphenopalatine f. a space between the orbital and

sphenoidal processes of the palatine bone, opening into the nasal cavity and transmitting the sphenopalatine artery and the nasal nerves.
spinous f. a hole in the great wing of the sphenoid for the middle meningeal artery.
stylomastoid f. the opening of the facial canal, adjacent to the ear from which the facial nerve emerges.
supracondylar f. a fissure in the mediodistal part of the humerus in cats through which the median nerve and vessels pass.
supraorbital f. passage in the frontal bone for the supraorbital vessels and nerve; often present as a notch bridged only by fibrous tissue.
thebesian f. minute openings in the walls of the heart through which the smallest cardiac veins (thebesian veins) empty into the cardiac chambers.
transverse f. the passage in either transverse process of a cervical vertebra that, in the first six vertebrae, transmits the vertebral vessels.
f. triosseum the hole between the ends of the avian clavicle, coracoid and scapula that transmits the tendon of the supracoracoid muscle and serves as a fulcrum to lever the wing upwards.
vena cava f. an opening in the diaphragm for the caudal vena cava.
vertebral f. 1. the large opening in a vertebra formed by its body and its neural arch. 2. transverse foramen.
f. of Vesalius an occasional opening medial to the foramen ovale of the sphenoid, for passage of a vein from the cavernous sinus.
f. of Winslow epiploic foramen.

forb native, nongrass, broadleaf, herbaceous range plants eaten by livestock. Responsible for a great deal of animal production in arid and semiarid regions. Includes saltbush, sage, shinoak.

Forbes' disease glycogenosis type III.

force energy or power; that which originates or arrests motion or other activity.
electromotive f. the force that, by reason of differences in potential, causes a flow of electricity from one place to another, giving rise to an electric current.
moment of f. the effect of a force exerted on a lever and about a fixed point.
reserve f. energy above that required for normal functioning. In the heart it is the power that will take care of the additional circulatory burden imposed by bodily exertion.
shearing f. a force exerted perpendicularly to a horizontal surface.
Van der Waals f's the relatively weak, short-range forces of attraction existing between atoms and molecules, which results in the attraction of nonpolar organic compounds to each other (hydrophobic bonding).

forced done by force.
f. feeding see force FEEDING, intravenous ALIMENTATION.

forceps pl. *forcipes* [L.] a two-bladed instrument with a handle for compressing or grasping tissues in surgical operations, and for handling sterile dressings, etc.
alligator f. strong toothed forceps having a double clamp. Long-handled with short jaws at the end of a long shank. Designed for grasping in an enclosed space, e.g. removing grass seeds from ear canals.
bayonet f. a forceps whose blades are offset from the axis of the handle.
bone-cutting f. have cutting blades and may be double-action.
bone-holding f. designed to grip bones or fragments.
capsule f. a forceps for removing the lens capsule in cataract.
clamp f. a forceps-like clamp with an automatic lock, for compressing arteries, etc.
dressing f. finger- and thumb-operated spring forceps used for general grasping of tissues, dressings; there is a great variety of tips available to the blades. Called also thumb forceps.
grasping f. includes tissue, sponge, towel, vulsellum forceps.
hemostatic f. used to clamp the ends of vessels and establish hemostasis or to cross clamp a vascular pedicle. See also CRILE HEMOSTATIC FORCEPS, HALSTED mosquito forceps, KELLY–MURPHY FORCEPS, ROCHESTER–CARMALT FORCEPS.
obstetric f. forceps for extracting the fetal head from the maternal passages.
rongeur f. a forceps designed for use in cutting bone.
sponge f. see FOERSTER SPONGE FORCEPS.
thumb f. for holding tissue with the left hand while using another instrument in the right hand (or vice versa for the sinistral surgeon). Called also tissue forceps.
tissue f. includes ADSON TISSUE FORCEPS, alligator forceps (see above), ALLIS TISSUE FORCEPS, BABCOCK FORCEPS, KNOWLES FORCEPS, RIGHTANGLE FORCEPS, VULSELLA.
towel f. spring clips with middle crossover and spring at end. Inward curving, sharp pointed tips. Used to fix drapes to tissue with minimal trauma. Also usable as light tissue forceps or rib approximators in small animals.
transfer f. a sterile grasping instrument, used to move surgical instruments, blades, needles and suture material to the instrument table at surgery.

Ford suture pattern an interlocking suture pattern; modification of the simple continuous stitch. The emerging, across-the-wound lap goes back through the preceding beside-the-wound lap before continuing to the next entry point for another across-the-wound lap.

fore front, e.g. forelimb.
f. cannon the third metacarpal bone of the horse.

forearm the part of the foreleg supported by the radius and ulna, between the elbow and the carpus.

forebrain see PROSENCEPHALON.

foregut the endodermal canal of the embryo cephalic to the junction of the yolk stalk, giving rise to the pharynx, lung, esophagus, stomach, liver and most of the small intestine.

forehand the head, neck, shoulders, withers and forelimbs of the horse.

forehead the region between the eyes and the ears; supported by the frontal and parietal bones.
domed f. forehead bulges; may be soft and fluid-filled; a problem only in neonates.

foreign body plant or mineral matter which finds its way into organs and tissues. The syndromes caused are described elsewhere under the specific organ or cavity, e.g. oral, gastric, corneal.
constricting f. b. elastic bands, cords and collars that have become too small which may become embedded in skin and subcutaneous tissues to the point of disappearing. Some objects are placed maliciously on the scrotum, tail, neck, ears or muzzle of dogs and cats.
esophageal f. b. causes complete, where obstruction is by a solid object, blockage of ingesta or regurgitus, or partial, e.g. wire lodged across lumen, when fluid and gas may pass unimpaired.
f. b. giant cell see giant CELL.

f.-b. glossitis inflammation of the tongue due to penetration or laceration by a foreign body.
linear f. b. twine, fishing line, and mane hair has the effect of telescoping/pleating a length of intestine and causing obstruction without compromising the blood supply to the part but with the probability of cutting into the mucosa and possibly through the bowel wall. The characteristic radiographic appearance of intestinal pleating assists in diagnosis.
penetrating f. b's long thin foreign bodies, e.g. those penetrating the reticular wall in traumatic reticuloperitonitis, or the sole of the horse's foot.
rectal f. b. objects passing through the intestinal tract may cause proctitis and difficulties in passing through the anus with straining and blood in the feces. Malicious insertion may cause penetration of the rectal wall and death from peritonitis.

foreign dyes dyes introduced into the body, usually for the purpose of making a physiological measurement, e.g. bromsulfthalein (BSP), Evans blue, indocyanine green, rose bengal, phenoltetrachlorphthalein, occasionally as treatment, e.g. methylene blue for nitrite poisoning.

foreignness a characteristic required for antigens, to be recognized as not a normal self constituent.

forelegs see FORELIMB.
inherited thick f. juvenile HYPEROSTOSIS (inherited thick forelegs) of pigs.

forelimb the front limb.
f. paralysis see BRACHIAL paralysis.
f. restraint hold restraint of a horse by holding a forelimb tightly flexed at the knee, either manually using an assistant, or by a tightly buckled strap; suitable only for simple procedures.

forelock in maned animals the most anterior part of the mane, hanging down between the ears and onto the forehead. In sheep refers to the wool in a similar situation.

foremilk the first few streams of milk at any milking time. After the first squirt of milk is discarded the rest of the foremilk is suitable as a source of material for laboratory examination for the presence of mastitis organisms.

forensic pertaining to, or applied in legal proceedings in courts of law.

forepaw the distal part of the front limb, including the carpus, metacarpals and phalanges, as in dogs and cats.

forequarter the quarter of an animal carcass that includes a forelimb; in the live animal refers to the part of the animal forward of the elbow, excluding the neck and head.

forest pertaining to or emanating from the forest.
f. fire injury see BUSHFIRE INJURY.
f. primrose HYPERICUM *revolutum*.
f. tsetses GLOSSINA *brevipalpis*, *G. fusca*.

forestomachs the first three compartments of the ruminant stomach, namely the reticulum, rumen and omasum; the gut compartment in which the major part of digestion in ruminants takes place, largely by fermentation. Called also proventriculus.

forge the fire equipped with forced-draft bellows used by a farrier for rapid heating of horseshoes for hot-shoeing.

forging an abnormality of gait in the horse in which the toe of a hind hoof hits the opposite front hoof while the horse is moving at the trot. Called also clicking or cross-firing.

form 1. species, kind or variety. 2. a structured document or computer screen for the collection of information. 3. particular shape of a lesion or syndrome of a disease, e.g. forms of BOVINE malignant catarrh.
f. tractor the wheels with pins on a printer using continuous stationery which engage the holes in computer paper or forms and advance them past the printing head. Their other function is to ensure that the paper is kept absolutely straight.

formaldehyde a gaseous compound with strongly disinfectant properties. It is used in solution (formol) for disinfection of excreta and utensils and also in the preparation of toxoids from toxins, and as a gas for the fumigation of hatching eggs. As formalin also used in the treatment of grain and forage and causes enteritis if the feed is improperly mixed.
f. hypersensitivity causes an allergic contact dermatitis.
f.-malachite green a treatment for external parasites in aquarium fish.

formalin a 37% solution of formaldehyde used as a fixative and, diluted to 10%, as a treatment and prevention for ovine footrot. Also used for the treatment of fungal diseases of fish but may be toxic if contaminated with paraformaldehyde.
f. ether sedimentation of feces a method of flotation of *Giardia* cysts.
f. treated grain fed to cows to produce dairy foods with a high concentration of polyunsaturated fats. May cause rumenitis and diarrhea if improperly prepared.

formamidase an enzyme which catalyzes the hydrolysis of formylkynurenine to kynurenine and formate in tryptophan metabolism.

formamidines a group of acaricidal compounds, used as plant sprays and topically on animals. See also AMITRAZ.

format 1. the initial preparation of a disk for use in a computer. 2. the layout or the laying out of a word-processing document.

formatio pl. *formationes* [L.] formation.

formation 1. the process of giving shape or form; the creation of an entity, or of a structure of definite shape. 2. a structure of definite shape.

formatting see DISK[2].

formic acid a colorless, pungent liquid with vesicant properties, from nettles and ants and other insects; derivable from oxalic acid and from glycerin and from the oxidation of formaldehyde.

Formica fusca an ant, second intermediate host for *Dicrocoelium dendriticum*.

formiciasis a morbid condition caused by ant bites.

formiminoglutamic acid a product of histidine metabolism. High levels in ruminant urine suggest possibility of nutritional deficiency of cobalt. Called also FIGLU.

formol formaldehyde solution.
f. cresol antiseptic solution used in endodontics.

formononetin an isoflavone found in clovers which is converted in the rumen into a potent estrogen, equol. Formononetin itself has no estrogenic potency.

Formston–McCunn method an out-dated surgical technique for lateral ear resection in which two Carmalt hemostat forceps are applied over the lateral wall of the external ear canal with curved tips facing and the U-shaped section of cartilage between them is removed.

formula pl. *formulae, formulas* [L.] an expression, using numbers or symbols, of the composition of, or of directions for preparing, a compound, such as a medicine, or of a procedure to follow to obtain a desired result, or of a single concept.
chemical f. a combination of symbols used to express the chemical components of a substance.
dental f. see DENTAL formula.

empirical f. a chemical formula that expresses the proportions of the elements present in a substance.
gait f. sets out the times that the feet are individually in contact with the ground while the animal is moving.
molecular f. a chemical formula expressing the number of atoms of each element present in a substance, without indicating how they are linked.
spatial f., stereochemical f. a chemical formula giving the numbers of atoms of each element present in a molecule of a substance, which atom is linked to which, the types of linkages involved, and the relative positions of the atoms in space.
structural f. a chemical formula showing the spatial arrangement of the atoms and the linkage of every atom.
vertebral f. sets out the number of vertebrae in each of the sections of the spinal column.

formula-fed 1. veal calves fed a liquid milk diet indoors, >3 weeks old, weigh 150 to 400 lb (68 to 182 kg). 2. any neonate fed on reconstituted milk products or replacer by bucket or bottle.

formulary a collection of formulae.
National F. a book of standards for certain pharmaceuticals and preparations not included in the USP; revised every 5 years, and recognized in the USA as a book of official standards by the Pure Food and Drug Act of 1906. Abbreviated NF.

formulation a fixed recipe for the preparation of a medicine or a commercial feed.

formyl the radical, HCO or H·C:O–, of formic acid.

***N*-formyl loline alkaloids** suspected of vasoconstrictive toxicity in seeds of *Festuca arundinacea.*

fornical pertaining to a fornix.

fornix pl. *fornices* [L.] an archlike structure or the vaultlike space created by such a structure.
cerebral f. either of a pair of arched fiber tracts that unite under the corpus callosum, so that together they comprise two columns, a body, and two crura.
conjunctival f. line of reflexion of the conjunctiva from the eyelid to the eyeball.
hippocampal f. a thick bundle of nerve fibers leaving the hippocampus to enter the hypothalamus, terminating in the mamillary body.
telencephalic f. see cerebral fornix (above).
vaginal f. the annular recess around the outside of the cervix.

Forssell technique either of two equine surgical procedures. One is for the correction of rectovaginal fistula, the other for the correction of the crib-biting/windsucking vice.

Forssman antigen see Forssman ANTIGEN.

Fort Bragg fever leptospirosis.

Fort William disease a name given to infection by the MINK enteritis virus.

fortescue a venomous fish. See CENTROPOGON AUSTRALIS.

Forthane a proprietary name for ISOFLURANE.

FORTRAN a computer language used for scientific applications.

forward a term used in animal husbandry to mean close to, usually close to parturition, e.g. forward ewes are those close to lambing.

forward-motility protein present in the epididymis; confers motility on the spermatozoon.

foscarnet a pyrophosphate analog used as an antiviral agent against herpesviruses.

fosfomycin a phosphonic acid compound with antibacterial activity.

fosmidomycin a phosphonic acid compound, similar to fosfomycin, produced by *Streptomyces lavendulae,* with antibacterial activity.

fossa pl. *fossae* [L.] a trench or channel; a hollow or depressed area.
acetabular f. the nonarticular part of the acetabulum.
amygdaloid f. the depression in which the palatine tonsil is lodged in some species.
cerebral f. any of the depressions on the floor of the cranial cavity.
lateral cerebral f. see VALLECULA sylvii.
f. clitoridis the cavity in which the glans clitoridis resides.
condylar f., condyloid f. either of depressions lateral to the occipital condyles.
coronoid f. a depression in the humerus for the coronoid process of the ulna. Called also radial fossa.
cranial f. any one of the three hollows (rostral, middle and caudal) in the base of the cranium for the lobes of the brain.
ethmoid f. the hollow in the cribriform plate of the ethmoid bones, for the olfactory bulb.
f. glandis depression at the end of the stallion glans penis, housing the urethral process; it harbors smegma and potential pathogens.
glenoid f. mandibular fossa.
hyaloid f. a depression in the front of the vitreous body, lodging the lens.
hypophyseal f., hypophysial f. a depression in the sphenoid lodging the pituitary gland; called also pituitary fossa.
infratemporal f. an irregularly shaped cavity medial or deep to the zygomatic arch.
intercrural f. the fossa between the cerebral peduncles.
interpeduncular f. a triangular depression between the *crura cerebri.*
ischiorectal f. a potential space between the pelvic diaphragm, the ischium and the skin.
lacrimal sac f. excavated from the lacrimal bone and housing the lacrimal sac.
lingual f. the transverse groove on the dorsum of the bovine tongue between the torus and the tip.
mandibular f. a depression in the pars squamosa of the temporal bone at the base of the zygomatic process, in which the condyle of the mandible rests; called also glenoid fossa.
nasal f. the right or left half of the nasal cavity.
f. nudatae see synovial fossa (below).
olecranon f. between the epicondylar crests at the distal end of the humerus; receives the anconeal process of the ulna.
f. ovalis cordis a fossa in the right atrium of the heart; the remains of the fetal foramen ovale.
ovarian f. a shallow depression on the surface of the mare's ovary. Called also ovulation fossa.
paralumbar f. the hollow of the flank, bounded dorsally by the transverse processes of the lumbar vertebrae, cranially by the last rib and caudally by the muscles of the thigh.
pituitary f. hypophyseal fossa.
radial f. see coronoid FOSSA.
rhomboidal f. floor of the fourth ventricle.
supracondylar f. the depression between the condyles of the femur.
supraspinous f. a depression cranial to the spine of the scapula.
synovial f. depressed, cartilage-free islands in large articular cartilages; no function has been determined for them. Called also fossa nudatae.
temporal f. an area on the side of the cranium bounded by the temporal line and the zygomatic arch, lodging the temporal muscle.

trochanteric f. the deep fossa at the proximal end of the femur between the greater and lesser trochanters.
fossette 1. a small depression. 2. a small, deep corneal ulcer.
fossula pl. *fossulae* [L.] a small fossa.
foster standing in for, surrogate.
f. mother an adoptive dam that accepts the offspring of another for purposes of feeding. Usually planned because of the death or lack of milk in the natural dam.
f. practice associated with a university veterinary school as a teaching practice.
fostering practice of putting newborn to suck on a lactating female, not the neonate's natural mother.
Fouchet's test a test for bile pigments, suitable for use on serum or urine.
foul a recognized classification of markings in canaries; it refers to a pattern of white feathers among the flight feathers and otherwise dark plumage.
foul-in-the-foot see FOOTROT. Called also foul-of-the-foot.
foulage [Fr.] kneading and pressing of the muscles in massage.
foulfoot see FOOTROT.
fouls see FOOTROT.
found dead a classification that means that the animal was found dead but may not have been attended for some time. It signifies that no signs of illness were observed—a very different category from SUDDEN DEATH.
foundation cow see foundation COW.
founder see LAMINITIS.
founder effect extreme genetic drift that occurs when a new population is based on only a few individuals ('founders'). Called also founder principle.
founder principle see FOUNDER EFFECT.
four-chamber method a method of postmortem dissection of the heart in which it is bisected from apex to base, exposing all chambers. Good for visualizing the ventricular septum and ventricular free wall in dogs and cats with cardiomyopathy.
four-in-hand a special coach harness for driving four horses accurately and with minimum coach sway. The front horses are harnessed to the centerpole, the back horses are hitched to the forepart of the carriage proper. The driver has four sets of reins arranged so that a change of direction is signaled to both lead horses at once and not by one horse pulling the other.
four-letter genetic code alphabet the genetic code is 'written' in a linear sequence in four letters corresponding to two purines, A and G (adenine and guanine), and two pyrimidines, C and T (cytosine and thymine); in mRNA, U (uracil) replaces T. The words of the alphabet comprise 3 letters, thus there are 4^3=64 permutations or words which are called codons. 61 of the 64 codons code for 1 of 20 amino acids. Since more than one codon codes for a particular amino acid the code is said to be redundant. Four of the 64 codons punctuate the message; one, AUG, is the start signal and three, UAG, UAA and UGA, are stop signals.
four-stitch interrupted suture an old term for interrupted horizontal MATTRESS SUTURE PATTERN.
four tooth young sheep with four permanent central incisors erupted; approximately two years old.
four-way cross the mating of the crossbred progeny of two separate lots of two-way cross parents to produce a marketable line of progeny.
four wing saltbush ARTEMISIA *canescens*.
fovea pl. *foveae* [L.] a small pit or depression, usually in a bone, e.g. in the center of the articular surface of the head of the femur; often used alone to indicate the central fovea of the retina.
central f. of retina, f. centralis retinae a small pit in the center of the macula lutea of the human and avian eye, composed of slim, elongated cones; it is the area of clearest vision.
foveate pitted.
foveation formation of pits on a surface, as on the skin; a pitted condition.
foveola pl. *foveolae* [L.] a minute pit or depression.
fowl domestic fowl. A member of the genus *Gallus* of the family Phasianidae, the pheasant family. Characterized by a fleshy comb, earlobes below the eyes and wattles from below the beak, long, drooping hackle feathers on the neck of the cock, pendent, lancet-shaped covert feathers on the wings, upward curving sickle feathers in the tail of the male, jointed spurs on the legs of the cock bird and well-marked sexual dimorphism.

There are many breeds of domestic fowl but they have diminished in importance with the expansion of the broiler and egg industries, most enterprises carrying their own genetic strains identified by code numbers. Some of the more common breeds are identified under the headings: BRAHMA, COCHIN, CORNISH, ENGLISH GAME, LANGSHAN, MINORCA, ORPINGTON (Buff and Black), PLYMOUTH ROCK, RHODE ISLAND RED, SILKIE, SUSSEX, WHITE LEGHORN, WYANDOTTE and many breeds of BANTAM.

For most entries relating to fowls see under AVIAN.
f. cholera a contagious widespread disease of fowls caused by *Pasteurella multocida* and manifested by septicemia with sudden onset, rapid spread, short course and high mortality. There may be diarrhea and dyspnea.
f. coryza a serious, widespread, respiratory disease of fowls caused by *Haemophilus paragallinarum* and characterized by acute inflammation of the upper respiratory tract and air sacs. It is characterized by an acute onset of mucoid or serous nasal discharge, facial edema and conjunctivitis, swollen wattles, diarrhea, reduced feed intake and a heavy culling rate.
f. manna grass GLYCERIA *striata*.
f. paralysis see MAREK'S DISEASE.
f. paratyphoid an important cause of wastage in commercial birds, especially turkeys occurring as outbreaks of severe enteritis in young birds caused by *Salmonella* spp. including over 100 species.
f. pest see NEWCASTLE DISEASE.
f. plague see AVIAN influenza.
f. pox see FOWLPOX.
f. tick see ARGAS *persicus*.
f. typhoid a disease of fowl and turkeys caused by *Salmonella gallinarum*. It affects only adult hens and is rare in modern, hygienically managed commercial flocks. There is weakness, diarrhea and anemia. The course is short and case mortality is high.
Fowler's solution an old-time tonic of potassium arsenite solution, composed of arsenic trioxide, potassium bicarbonate, hydroxide or carbonate, and water.
fowlpox a slow-spreading disease of fowl and turkeys caused by the avian poxvirus and characterized by pox lesions on the skin of the head, and on the neck in turkeys. Involvement of eyelids causes lacrimation and accumulation of caseous material in the conjunctival sac. Lesions may also be present in the mouth, esophagus and upper respiratory tract. Transmitted by mosquitoes or by contact.
fox a member of the same family as dogs, wolves and

jackals, the family Canidae, but has characteristic long body and short legs, pointed snout, big, erect ears, oval pupils and long bushy tail. The type species is the Old World red fox (*Vulpes vulpes*). See also KIT, FENNEC.

arctic f. a farmed blue or white fox. Called also *Alopex lagopus*.

f. encephalitis see infectious canine HEPATITIS.

gray f. gray to black, omnivorous wild fox. Called also *Urocyon cinereoargenteus*.

kit f. small, yellow-brown fox similar to the red fox. Called also *Vulpes velox*, *V. inacrotis*.

Old World red f. see red fox (below).

f. rabies the fox is an important reservoir host for rabies, particularly in eastern and western Europe where it is endemic.

red f. the common, sandy to red brown fox with black legs and backs of ears, white underparts, sharp muzzle, large erect ears. Mostly nocturnal, lives in burrows. Called also *Vulpes vulpes*, Old World red fox.

silver f. a farmed fox with a lustrous black coat with white tips along the back; a variant of the red fox (see above).

South American f. a group of specialized wild dogs, not true foxes, of South America. Includes crab-eating fox and maned wolf.

Fox rabbit a popular exhibition breed, weighing 5 to 7 lb; it has a ticked coat in blue, black, chocolate or lilac.

Fox terrier a small active dog with narrow head, ears that fold over, and a tail docked to three-quarters its original length. The short hair may be smooth or wiry, the two varieties usually being regarded as separate breeds (smooth fox terrier and wire fox terrier). In addition, in the United States, the United Kennel Club recognizes the Toy Fox Terrier (called also AmerToy). The breed(s) is predisposed to atopic dermatitis, glaucoma, lens luxation and an hereditary ataxia.

foxglove DIGITALIS *purpurea*.

Foxhound a medium- to large-sized muscular dog with pendulous ears, long tapered tail and short coat, in the usual hound colors of black, brown and white. The ears are traditionally shortened surgically by several inches ('rounding'). English and American varieties are recognized as separate breeds in the United States. The American variety is leggier and lighter in weight.

foxtail grass see SETARIA^2 *lutescens*, HORDEUM.

foxtails 1. a name given to plant awns of the HORDEUM in the western USA. 2. *Equisetum* spp.

foxtrot one of the two artificial gaits of the FIVE-GAITED horse. A four-beat gait midway in speed between a walk and a trot. There is a great deal of similarity with several other gaits such as amble, fadge, slow pace, stepping pace, running walk, jog, hound jog. A breed of pleasure horse which is highly proficient at the foxtrot is the Fox Trotting Horse.

Fp flavoprotein.

FPL feline panleukopenia.

FPV feline panleukopenia virus.

Fr chemical symbol, *francium*.

fraction size expressed as a relative part of a unit.

attributable f. the proportion of disease in the exposed group which is caused by the factor.

fractional size expressed as a relative part of a unit.

f. catabolic rate the percentage of an available pool of body component, e.g. protein, iron, which is replaced, transferred or lost per unit of time. Takes account of the size of the pool of available metabolite in determining the absolute amount of it which is lost or transferred. Same principle applies in fractional transfer rate.

f. excretion tests, f. clearance tests measures of urine electrolyte clearance ratios to assess renal function. They express the proportion of a substance excreted in the urine, compared with the amount filtered by the glomerulus.

fractionated radiotherapy a radiation dose divided and given over a number of treatments.

fractionation 1. in radiotherapy, division of the total dose of radiation into small doses given at intervals. 2. in chemistry, separation of a substance into components, as by distillation or crystallization. 3. in histology, isolation of components of living cells by differential centrifugation.

fracture 1. the breaking of a part, especially a bone. 2. a break in the continuity of bone. Fractures may be caused by trauma, by twisting due to muscle spasm, or indirect loss of leverage or by disease that results in decalcification of the bone.

avulsion f. separation of a small fragment of bone cortex at the site of attachment of a ligament or tendon.

blow-out f. fracture of the orbital floor caused by a sudden increase of intraorbital pressure due to traumatic force; the orbital contents herniate into the maxillary sinus so that the inferior rectus or inferior oblique muscle may become incarcerated in the fracture site, producing diplopia on looking up.

capillary f. one that appears on a radiograph as a fine, hairlike line, the segments of bone not being separated; sometimes seen in fractures of the skull.

closed f. one that does not produce an open wound.

comminuted f. one in which the bone is splintered or crushed.

complete f. one involving the entire cross-section of the bone.

compound f. see open fracture (below).

compression f. one produced by compression.

contaminated f. see open fracture (below).

depressed f. fracture of the skull in which a fragment is depressed. See also DEPRESSION fracture.

direct f. one at the site of injury.

dislocation f. fracture of a bone near an articulation with concomitant dislocation of that joint.

double f. fracture of a bone in two places.

fissure f. a crack extending from a surface into, but not through, a long bone.

greenstick f. one in which one side of a bone is broken, the other being bent.

impacted f. fracture in which one fragment is firmly driven into the other.

incomplete f. one that does not involve the complete cross-section of the bone.

indirect f. one at a point distant from the site of injury.

interperiosteal f. greenstick or incomplete fracture.

intrauterine f. fracture of a fetal bone incurred in utero.

lead pipe f. one in which the bone cortex is slightly compressed and bulged on one side with a slight crack on the other side of the bone.

malunion f. a large space between the displaced ends of the bone has been filled by new bone.

nonunion f. there is still a wide translucent space between the ends of the broken bone.

oblique f. a common type, usually seen in the shaft of a long bone, such as the femur, tibia or humerus.

open f. one in which a wound through the adjacent or overlying soft tissues communicates with the site of the break; called also compound fracture. A classification system has been used which is based on the mechanism of injury and the extent of tissue damage. In *type I*, a bone fragment was briefly forced through the skin leaving a communicating wound; *type II* fractures are caused by impact and there is damage to overlying tissues and exposure of the bone; in *type III*, there is extensive damage and loss of overlying tissues, including shearing and degloving wounds, with loss of vascular supply.

pathological f. one due to weakening of the bone structure by pathological processes, such as neoplasia, osteomalacia or osteomyelitis.

pertrochanteric f. fracture of the femur passing through the greater trochanter.

Salter f. see SALTER CLASSIFICATION.

saucer f. creates a saucer-shaped fragment; caused usually by direct trauma at midshaft in a long bone. Likely to create a sequestrum.

simple f. closed fracture.

slab f. one in which a flat piece of underlying bone or tooth is separated or lost. Common in carpal bones of horses and in teeth.

spiral f. one in which the bone has been twisted apart.

spontaneous f. pathological fracture.

sprain f. the separation of a tendon from its insertion, taking with it a piece of bone. See also avulsion fracture (above).

stellate f. one with a central point of injury, from which radiate numerous fissures.

stress f. fracture produced by the stress created by the pull of muscles without the intervention of trauma or extreme weight-bearing.

trabecular f. there is no discontinuity of the bone as a whole but microscopic examination shows fractured trabeculae.

transverse f. one at right angles to the axis of the bone.

trophic f. one due to a nutritional (trophic) disturbance.

fracture–dislocation a fracture of a bone near a joint, also involving dislocation.

fragiligraph an instrument that records the results of a mechanical OSMOTIC fragility test for erythrocytes.

fragilitas [L.] *fragility*.

f. crinium a brittleness of the hair.

f. ossium congenita osteogenesis imperfecta.

fragility susceptibility, or lack of resistance, to influences capable of causing disruption of continuity or integrity.

f. of blood see erythrocyte fragility (below).

capillary f. abnormal susceptibility of capillary walls to rupture.

erythrocyte f. susceptibility of erythrocytes to hemolysis when subjected to mechanical trauma (mechanical fragility) or when exposed to increasingly hypotonic saline solutions (osmotic fragility). A test of erythrocyte osmotic fragility is used in diagnosing hemolytic anemia. Called also fragility of blood.

fragmentation division into small pieces.

frame 1. a rigid supporting structure. 2. a structure for immobilizing a part.

f. shift mutation see frame shift MUTATION.

framework region (FR) less variable sequences in the variable regions of immunoglobulin molecules which are located between the hypervariable or complementary determining regions (CDRs).

framycetin an aminoglycoside antibiotic derived from *Streptomyces decaris*, which is a major component of neomycin. Used, usually in combination with other antibacterial agents, in topical preparations. Called also neomycin B.

Francisella a genus of very small gram-negative bacteria.

F. tularensis biotype A is the etiological agent of tularemia; biotype B is less virulent. Formerly called *Pasteurella tularensis*.

francisia BRUNSFELSIA *australis*.

francium a chemical element, atomic number 87, atomic weight 223, symbol Fr. See Table 6.

francolin large game birds resembling partridges: called also *Francolinus*.

Francolinus see FRANCOLIN.

Frangula alnus RHAMNUS *frangula*.

Frank emasculator a single crush emasculator with a thumbscrew at the joint.

Frank–Starling mechanism an intrinsic adaptive response which serves to adjust each ventricular output to its inflow by increasing the force of contraction of the myocardium proportionally to any increase in the length of the muscle fibers.

Franklin–Silverman biopsy needle used for obtaining biopsy specimens of the liver, kidney, prostate. Consists of a stylet that fits inside a needle split along its length and which spreads open when not confined within the third part of the appliance, the cannula. The split needle and stylet are longer than the cannula, and are protruded beyond it in the suspect tissue and withdrawn into it to harvest the specimen.

Franseria discolor North American plant in the family Asteraceae; may cause nitrate–nitrite poisoning. Called also white ragweed.

Fratercula a genus of puffins, fish eating birds from the northern subarctic region.

F. arctica Atlantic puffin.

F. corniculata horned puffin.

Fraunhofer zone in ultrasonography, the area of the sound beam beyond the focal zone where the beam diverges and resolution decreases.

Fraxinus excelsior European tree in the plant family of Oleaceae; contains an indigestible fiber which causes ruminal impaction, abdominal pain, incoordination and collapse in cows. Called also ash tree.

Frazier–Ferguson suction tube an instrument for removing fluid or blood from a surgical site. It has a compression hole near the handle which can be covered to modify the degree of suction.

Frazier retractor an instrument designed for use in spinal laminectomies. Consists of two opposed sets of curled hands which slide along a bar to which they can be fixed by thumbscrews.

FRC see FUNCTIONAL residual capacity.

Fredet–Ramstedt operation see RAMSTEDT OPERATION.

free not tied; unconfined.

f. bullet humane killer see HUMANE killer.

f. electricity the presence of uncontrolled electrical current in solid materials at low amperages and voltages, usually due to faulty wiring and poor earthing (grounding) of the electrical power system. It causes restlessness, and failure of letdown of milk. In some cases when the circumstances are suitable there may be stunning of animals and rarely fatal electrocution.

f. fatty acids most fatty acids in the body are combined with alcohols in the form of triglycerides. Free fatty acids are produced during digestion and metabolism but most of them in the circulation are combined with protein during this phase.

f. fluid fluid in the body, other than in the alimentary or urinary tracts, which is not part of tissue fluid but free in a body cavity or as a discrete mass in an organ.

f. gas bloat see RUMINAL tympany.

f. hormone hypothesis the unbound fraction of hormone is the indicator of what is available to tissues, available for metabolism and excretion. See also free THYROXINE.

f. return a return of service for a mare to the same stallion in the next season if she does not produce a live foal.

f. stall housing cow accommodation in which there are enough stalls for each cow to have one but the cows are not tied in; they are free to lie down in a cubicle or to feed or to seek other cows coming on heat.

f. T_4 index see free THYROXINE.

f. water clearance the capacity to excrete urine of lower osmolality than plasma, thus avoiding depletion of salt reserves.

free-choice the animals are free to eat as much as they like of two or more feeds which are available.

free-living running uncontrolled on range.

free-ranging running uncontrolled on range.

freemartin a sterile female born co-twin with a male. Occurs most commonly in cattle, very rarely in sheep, and apparently not at all in the other species. Male hormones produced by the male calf share the common circulation and inhibit the normal development of genitalia of the female. The female is also an erythrocytic chimera and can be diagnosed as a freemartin by this means. It can also be diagnosed by cytogenetic techniques. It produces white cells with XY as well as cells with XX chromosomes. Structural changes of nonpatent vagina, small vulva, cordlike uterus and hypoplastic ovaries are diagnostic but inconsistent. Some freemartins are quite normal clinically but all are sterile.

freemartinism the state of being a freemartin.

Freer periosteal elevator a double-ended instrument used in orthopedic surgery.

freeway space space between opposing premolars when the mouth is closed.

freeze branding branding animals by depigmentation of the haircoat with supercooled instruments. The carefully gauged degree of cold application causes selective destruction of the pigment-producing cells, the melanocytes.

freeze-drying 1. a method of tissue preparation in which the tissue specimen is frozen and then dehydrated at low temperature in a high vacuum. See also LYOPHILIZATION. 2. a process of removing water from frozen foods or vaccines. The material must be powdered, sliced or diced and be stored in moisture-proof containers.

freeze-etching a method used to study unfixed cells by electron microscopy, in which the object to be studied is placed in 20% glycerol, frozen at −148°F (−100°C), and then mounted on a chilled holder.

freeze-fracturing a method used to examine cell structure in electron microscopy in which the specimen is frozen in liquid N_2 (−196 °C) in the presence of a cryprotectant (antifreeze) to prevent distortion; the frozen block is then cracked such that the fracture line passes through the hydrophobic middle of the lipid bilayers, thereby exposing the interior of the cell membranes. The resulting structure is then shadowed with platinum, the organic matter is dissolved away, and the replica is floated off and viewed in the electron microscope. A closely related technique is freeze-etch electron microscopy.

freeze frame a facility on an ultrasound machine which permits an image to be held on a screen.

freeze-substitution a modification of freeze-drying in which the ice within the frozen tissue is replaced by alcohol or other solvents at a very low temperature.

freeze–thaw cycle in cryosurgery, the process of rapid freeze and slow thaw that results in cell death. Often repeated a set number of times according to the size and nature of lesion being treated.

freezer the compartment in which meat and offal are stored at freezing temperatures of 10 to 16°F (−12 to −9°C) although there is a trend to lower temperatures of 0 to −22°F (−18 to −30°C).

f. burn discoloration of offal due to dehydration at very low temperatures. The tissue is withered, yellow and unpalatable and is condemned.

sharp f. a freezing chamber kept at the lower temperature range of 0 to −22°F (−18 to −30°C).

freezing reducing the temperature of materials to the freezing point of water so that they are frozen solid. Used in the preservation of food, the preparation of material for histopathological examination and in cryosurgery.

f. point the temperature at which a liquid begins to freeze; for water, the freezing point is 32°F (0°C).

quick f. greatly improves the quality of meat because of reduced ice crystal formation.

skin f. see CRYOSURGERY.

Freibank system a German system of handling meat products of inferior quality from a health point of view. Similar provisions apply in many countries. Meat from carcasses of late pregnant or recently calved cows, from carcasses affected by local lymph node involvement with tuberculosis or caseous lymphadenitis or tissue parasites not communicable to humans is released under special licenses that require its treatment by heat before sale.

fremitus a vibration perceptible on palpation or auscultation, e.g. palpable in the middle uterine artery in late pregnant cows, palpable in a grossly enlarged thyroid gland affected by goiter.

French Alpine goat polled, mostly chamois-colored, dairy goat.

French bean see PHASEOLUS.

French brown cattle French brown dual purpose cattle originated from Brown Swiss.

French bulldog a small, compact dog with large, domed head, very short nose, prominent 'bat' ears (broad based and erect), and a small, short tail that is straight or kinked. The hair is short and fawn, brindle or pied (brindle with white). The breed is predisposed to hemivertebrae and factor IX deficiency.

French front see FIDDLE FRONT.

French gauge a standard set of diameters for round objects such as needles, catheters, rubber tubing. Range from gauge 3 (1 mm) to gauge 34 (11.3 mm). Each gauge unit is approximately equivalent to 0.33 mm diameter.

French honeysuckle see GALEGA OFFICINALIS.

French lilac see GALEGA OFFICINALIS.

French millet see PANICUM *miliaceum*.

French molt a disease of companion birds, especially budgerigars, characterized by breaking of flight and tail feathers of immature birds about to leave the nest. See also PSITTACINE beak and feather disease.

French poodle see POODLE.

French scale see FRENCH GAUGE.

French shorthaired shepherd see BERGER DE BEAUCE.

French straws 0.25 ml diameter plastic straw to contain extended bull semen and to be used in a special inseminating device. Characteristic is the small diameter compared with the USA straw.

frenectomy excision of a frenum (frenulum).

mandibular f. releases the frenulum attaching the lower lip to the mandibular gingiva near the first premolar tooth; performed to reduce food accumulation in the vicinity.

Frenkelia a genus of protozoa in the family Sarcocystidae. Cysts are found in the brain and spinal cord of birds of prey, the intermediate hosts are the prey.

F. clethrionomyobuteonis the hosts are *Buteo* (buzzard) and *Microtus* (vole).

frenoplasty the correction of an abnormally attached frenum by surgically repositioning it.

frenotomy the cutting of a frenum (frenulum).

frenulum pl. *frenula* [L.] a small fold of integument or mucous membrane that limits the movements of an organ or part.

clitoridal f. a fold from the clitoridal fossa to the clitoris.

f. linguae frenulum of tongue.

lingual f. the vertical fold of mucous membrane under the tongue, attaching it to the floor of the mouth; called also frenulum linguae.

f. of lip a median fold of mucous membrane connecting the inside of each lip to the corresponding gum.

penile preputial f. thin ventral sheet of preputal skin and connective tissue forming a fold under the penis and connecting its ventral raphe with the preputial mucosa. Normally breaks down at the approach of puberty. Persistence of a part of the frenulum causes deviation and incomplete protrusion of the penis and inability to mate, is an inherited defect in cattle. Most cases can be satisfactorily corrected surgically.

superior medullary velum f. a band lying in the superior medullary velum at its attachment to the inferior colliculi in the brain.

frenum pl. *frena* [L.] a restraining structure or part; see FRENULUM.

frenzy the most severe of the excitation mental states. The animal's movements are violent and uncontrolled and are dangerous to attendants and other animals, and to the affected animal, which often injures itself. There may be aggressive physical attacks.

Freon trademark for a series of fluoridated hydrocarbons used primarily in refrigeration.

F. 112 a flukicide in sheep. See TETRACHLORODIFLUORETHANE.

frequency 1. the number of occurrences of a periodic process in a unit of time. 2. in statistics, the number of occurrences of a determinable entity per unit of time or of population.

cumulative f. the graph of its cumulative frequencies.

f. distribution see frequency DISTRIBUTION.

expected f. the expected number of occurrences.

observed f. the actual frequency; as opposed to the expected frequency.

relative f. the number of observations of a particular, nominated value expressed usually as a proportion of the total frequency.

total f. the total number of observations in the set of data.

ultrasound f. see ULTRASOUND.

frescon see 4-TRITYLMORPHOLINE.

fresh cows cows recently calved and still in their first flush of lactation, that is within 2 weeks, possibly 4 weeks since calving.

freshness the degree to which meat, or other biological material, approximates the state it was in at the time of slaughter or harvest. In meat freshness is determined by the developing acidity due to proteolytic degeneration of the muscle fibers and the oxidation of the fat.

f. meters several commercial instruments are available. They depend on the measurement of the pH of the surface of the meat.

Fresnel zone in ultrasonography, the area of the sound beam between the transducer and the focal zone in which complex diffraction patterns occur.

Freund's complete adjuvant a water-in-oil emulsion with killed mycobacteria organisms. See also MURAMYL DIPEPTIDE.

Freund's incomplete adjuvant Freund's adjuvant without the mycobacteria component.

Freyana a genus of mites in the family Dermoglyphidae.

F. chanayi found on the feathers of turkeys.

FRF follicle-stimulating hormone releasing factor.

friable easily pulverized or crumbled.

friar's balsam a complex mixture of natural medicaments including benzoin, storax, balsam of Peru, balsam of Tolu, aloe, myrrh, angelica and alcohol. Called also balsam traumatic.

fribby fleece wool containing an excessive number of sweat points.

fribs small pieces of wool, e.g. second cuts, on the outside of the main fleece.

Frick speculum a simple metal tube 20 inches × 1.5 inches diameter with ferruled strengthened ends; used to reach the pharynx of the cow and to pass a stomach tube without fear of damage by the cow's teeth.

friction the act of rubbing.

f. coefficient see friction COEFFICIENT.

f. injury caused most commonly by automobile trauma in dogs and cats in which the animal has been dragged along the road or pavement, causing avulsion of tissue, from skin through to ligaments, tendons, muscles and bone. See also friction BURN.

f. rub sound heard on auscultation caused by rubbing together of two inflamed surfaces, e.g. pleuritic friction rub. See also PLEURAL friction rub.

frictional pertaining to or emanating from friction.

f. acanthosis see ACANTHOSIS nigricans.

Friedman test a modification of the ASCHHEIM–ZONDEK TEST for pregnancy in the mare based on the use of a rabbit instead of mice. Little used because of the cost of the rabbit.

friendly neighbor BRYOPHYLLUM *tubiflorum*.

Friesian a breed of dairy cattle. See HOLSTEIN–FRIESIAN.

F. horse Dutch light horse used for driving and riding. Black with no markings, 15 hands high. A muscular horse with feather on the lower limbs.

Friesland cattle a South African adaptation of Friesian cattle.

fright disease see canine HYSTERIA.

frigorific producing coldness.

frijolito *Sophora* spp. See SOPHORA SECUNDIFLORA.

frilled a mutation producing a specific form of feathering in different areas of the body of canaries. There may be curled feathers on the shoulders and wings (mantle), on the breast (jabot), or on the flanks (fins). Frilled breeds include the North Dutch frill, South Dutch frill, Parisian frill, Milan frill, Swiss frill, Gibber Italicus, and Gibboso Espagnole.

frilling separation of the photographic emulsion from the film base commencing at the edges of the film. Usually caused by prolonged immersion in a liquid at too high a temperature.

Frills see FRILLED.

fringed tapeworm see THYSANOSOMA ACTINIOIDES.

Fringillidae see FINCH.

Fritillaria meleagris toxic plant in the family Liliaceae; reputed to contain a poisonous alkaloid. Called also fritillary, snake's head.

fritillary see FRITILLARIA MELEAGRIS.

frog 1. amphibious, poikilothermic animal. See also RANA. 2. v-shaped pad of soft horn between the bars on the sole of the horse's hoof.

f. legs BRYOPHYLLUM *tubiflorum*.

f.-leg position one of the positions used when x-raying dogs for hip dysplasia. The dog is in dorsal recumbency and the hindlegs are held in a fully flexed, abducted position.

leopard f. member of the animal order Anura of the class Amphibia. Called also *Rana pipiens*.

f. mouth see PHILYDRUM LANGUINOSUM.

f. pad leather pad nailed onto horse hoof above the shoe to protect the frog.

f. posture the hindlimbs trail behind in a recumbent animal that scrambles forwards with the front limbs. Characteristic of bilateral hip luxation and compression of the lumbar spinal cord.

frog-stay an internal spine of hoof horn projecting from the frog upward into the digital cushion.

Fröhlich's syndrome see ADIPOSOGENITAL DYSTROPHY.

front *Mu* points see ALARM points.

frontad toward a front, or frontal aspect.

frontal 1. pertaining to the face and forehead. 2. denoting a plane passing through the body from side to side. In quadrupeds it is synonymous with a transverse plane while in bipeds it is synonymous with a coronal plane.

f. abscess in cattle usually results from infection of a dehorning wound, in sheep from infection by *Oestrus ovis*.

f. bone the paired bones constituting the upper part of the face. See also Table 10.

f. lobe the rostral (anterior) portion of the cerebral hemisphere.

f. nerve block see SUPRAORBITAL nerve block.

f. plane see dorsal PLANE.

f. process see COMB.

f. sinus see frontal SINUS.

f. sinusitis inflammation of the frontal sinus; commonly a sequel to infection of a dehorning wound. occurs as a chronic disease of unknown origin in bighorn sheep running at range in the wild.

frontalis [L.] *frontal*.

f. muscle cutaneous muscle stretching over the forehead into the upper eyelid.

frost 1. a deposit of frozen dew. 2. a deposit resembling frozen dew or vapor.

f. (1) studs large-headed horseshoe nails that protrude below the horseshoe, or special studs fitted to the shoe itself, that give better grip on the ice. Called also calks, calkins, cogs.

urea f. (2) the appearance on the skin of salt crystals left by evaporation of the sweat in urhidrosis.

frostbite injury to tissues due to exposure to extreme cold. Not a common occurrence in free-living animals in the wild but is observed in poorly housed captive animals and birds. May cause whole-body freezing or gangrene of extremities including deer antlers. Deer forms are probably the most susceptible animals. Gangrene of the extremities, especially in pigs, and of the comb in chickens does occur in the domestic species but only if they are in poor condition and are caught outside in a storm.

frosting the slight graying of the haircoat around the face, particularly muzzle, in dogs with aging and as a regular feature of some breeds such as the Belgian shepherd dog.

frosty face sheep's face covered by harsh, chalky white hairs.

frothing at mouth profuse salivation, frothed with air, during jaw champing as part of involuntary movements. Contrast with an outpouring of fine froth from the nostrils and mouth in the terminal stages of pulmonary edema.

frothy bloat see RUMINAL tympany.

frounce casous accumulations in the throat of hawks. See also avian TRICHOMONIASIS.

frozen said of material kept at less than 0°C. Biological materials are frozen solid because of their high water content.

f. embryo see EMBRYO transfer.

f. meat meat preserved at low temperatures in a FREEZER.

f. section a specimen of tissue that has been quick-frozen, cut by microtome, and stained immediately for rapid diagnosis of possible malignant lesions. A specimen processed in this manner is not satisfactory for detailed study of the cells, but it is valuable because it is quick and gives the surgeon immediate information regarding the malignancy of a piece of tissue.

f. semen see SEMEN.

fructofuranose the combining and more reactive form of fructose, containing a furanose ring structure.

β-fructofuranosidase an enzyme occurring in yeasts and other organisms that catalyzes the hydrolysis of sugars with a terminal unsubstituted β-D-fructofuranosyl residue.

fructokinase an enzyme that catalyzes the transfer of a high-energy phosphate group to D-fructose, to form fructose-1-phosphate.

fructolysis the conversion of fructose to lactate.

fructosamine a glycated serum protein complex which reflects average blood glucose concentration over the previous 1–3 weeks; used in the management of insulin therapy for diabetes mellitus.

fructose a hexose sugar found in honey and many sweet fruits; called also levulose and fruit sugar. It is used in solution as a fluid and nutrient replenisher.

f. 1,6-bisphosphatase key regulatory enzyme of gluconeogenesis.

f. 1,6-bisphosphate aldolase cleavage enzyme taking hexose-phosphates to triose-phosphates.

f. 1,6-diphosphatase a pacemaker or rate-limiting enzyme in the liver; participates in the control of the rate of hepatic metabolism.

f. 2,6-bisphosphatase part of multifunctional enzyme that regulates the concentration of the key positive allosteric effector of glycolysis, fructose 2,6-bisphosphate.

f. 1-phosphate aldolase cleaves fructose 1-phosphate to dihydroxyacetone phosphate; sometimes called aldolase B.

f. 6-phosphate key intermediate of glycolysis.

f. tolerance test a little used test of liver function.

fructosemia the presence of fructose in the blood, as in fructose intolerance.

fructoside a compound which bears the same relation to fructose as a glucoside does to glucose.

fructosuria the presence of fructose in the urine.

fructosyl a radical of fructose.

frugivorous fruit-eating.

fruit bat see CHIROPTERA.

frusemide see FUROSEMIDE.

FRV feline rhinotracheitis virus.

fry newly hatched fish. Called also larvae.
advanced f. young fish in the post-yolk stage. Called also alevin.
FSE focal symmetrical ENCEPHALOMALACIA.
FSH see FOLLICLE-STIMULATING HORMONE.
FSH/LH-RH FOLLICLE-STIMULATING HORMONE RELEASING HORMONE and LUTEINIZING HORMONE releasing hormone.
FSH-RH FOLLICLE-STIMULATING HORMONE RELEASING HORMONE.
FSP fibrin/fibrinogen split products.
FTC failure to conceive.
FTLV feline T-lymphotropic virus.
FTS facteur thymique sérique.
***fu* organs** having *yang*, a positive, active quality.
fuchsin any of several red to purple dyes.
acid f. a mixture of sulfonated fuchsins; used in various complex stains.
basic f. a histological stain, a mixture of pararosaniline, rosaniline and magenta II. Also, a mixture of rosaniline and pararosaniline hydrochlorides used as a local anti-infective.
fucose a monosaccharide occurring as L-fucose in a number of mucopolysaccharides and mucoproteins.
fucosidase an enzyme occurring in two forms that catalyzes the hydrolysis of fucoside to an alcohol and fucose. See also (ALPHA)-FUCOSIDOSIS.
fucoside an acetal derivative of fucose.
α-fucosidosis an hereditary disease of humans and English springer spaniel dogs, due to deficient activity of the enzyme α-L-fucosidase and resulting in accumulation of fucose in all tissues; marked by progressive cerebral degeneration, various neurological defects, and emaciation within the first 2 years of life.
FUDR see FLOXURIDINE.
fuel oils see OIL.
-fugal word element. [L.] *driving away, fleeing from, repelling.*
fuh see ONYCHIUM CONTIGUUM.
Fulani a cattle-owning tribe in West Africa. Many varieties of zebu cattle are included in the general category of Fulani. See SUDANESE FULANI CATTLE.
fulgurate 1. to come and go like a flash of lightning. 2. to destroy by contact with electric sparks generated by a high-frequency current.
fulguration destruction of living tissue by electric sparks generated by a high-frequency current.
full bloom the stage of a crop when two-thirds of the plants are in flower; the crop is mature.
full-feed the level of feeding at which the animals are eating as much feed as they can safely eat.
full mouth the stage of development of an animal that has all of its incisors erupted and in wear, e.g. 6 years on the average in horses, 5 years in cattle, 4 years in sheep.
full-sib full brother or full sister; individuals with both parents in common.
full text reports unabridged versions; raw data plus analyses.
full-thickness graft see full-thickness GRAFT.
full wave rectification rectification of the power supply to an x-ray tube that makes it possible for the reverse cycle, as well as the forward cycle, of the mains current coming to the tube to be utilized.
fullered said of a horseshoe with one or more grooves in the length of the shoe's ground surface. The nail holes are made in these grooves.
fullering the groove in the ground surface of the horseshoe. The nail holes are punched in it.
fuller's earth an absorbent, commonly used in dusting powders.
fulminate to occur suddenly with great intensity.
fulminating see fulminant DISEASE.
fulvine one of the toxic alkaloids in *Crotalaria* spp.
fumagillin an antibiotic produced by *Aspergillus fumigatus.* Used in bees to control the parasite, *Nosema.*
fumarase an enzyme that catalyzes the interconversion of fumarate and malate.
fumarate a salt of fumaric acid.
Fumaria officinalis toxic plant in the family Fumariaceae; reputed to cause poisoning in farm livestock. Called also fumitory.
fumaric acid an unsaturated dibasic acid; it is the *trans*-isomer of maleic acid and an intermediate in the tricarboxylic acid cycle.
fumarin a coumarin analog used as a rodenticide. Called also coumafuryl. See also WARFARIN.
fumatory, fumitory CORYDALIS, FUMARIA OFFICINALIS.
fumes odorous gases and other volatile materials; inhalation of irritating fumes causes coughing and, if sufficiently severe, irreversible pulmonary edema.
fumigation exposure to disinfecting fumes, e.g. formaldehyde.
fumitoxin toxic substance found in *Aspergillus fumigatus.*
fumitremorgen toxic substance isolated from *Aspergillus fumigatus.* Causes ataxia, lethargy, hypersensitivity and frenzy in horses.
fumonisin neurotoxic, pneumotoxic and hepatotoxic mycotoxins in *Fusarium moniliforme.*
function 1. the special, normal or proper action of any part or organ. 2. a variable quantity whose value at any time can be determined by the value at that time of some other variable because there is a fixed mathematical relationship between them. The first variable is said to be a function of the second.
f. abnormality the basis of all disease; structural abnormalities are important only insofar as they impede normal function.
f. keys special keys on a computer keyboard whose functions often have nothing to do with the names written on them. The computer program in operation often controls the functions performed by these keys.
f. tests tests which assess the efficiency of functions of the organ, e.g. liver function, renal function tests, glucose tolerance, xylose absorption tests.
functional pertaining to or fulfilling a function; affecting the function but not the structure. A common qualification when no lesion is found to explain or justify a diagnosis.
f. alveolar emphysema reversible, uncomplicated bronchiolitis.
f. blindness blindness in the absence of a lesion, e.g. in nervous acetonemia, pregnancy toxemia.
f. colic colic in the absence of a structural fault, e.g. spasmodic colic, paralytic ileus.
f. disease a disease involving body functions but having no known organic basis.
f. ileus see PARALYTIC ileus.
f. residual capacity (FRC) the amount of air remaining in the lungs at the end of a normal expiration. Called also FRC, functional residual capacity.
f. tumors those producing an active substance, usually found in glandular tissue, e.g. pituitary, pancreas, thyroid, parathyroid. Because such activity is autonomous and not subject to the normal feedback mechanisms, a syndrome resembling hyperactivity of the gland results, e.g. primary hyperparathyoidism, hyperthyroidism.
fundament 1. a base or foundation, as the breech or rump. 2. the anus and parts adjacent to it.

fundamental number the total number of major chromosome arms; is constant across most species.
fundectomy excision of the fundus of an organ, as of the stomach.
fundiform shaped like a loop or sling.
fundoplication mobilization of the lower end of the esophagus and plication of the fundus of the stomach up around it, in the treatment of gastroesophageal reflux disease. Two modifications of this procedure are the Belsey and Nissen fundoplication techniques.
fundus pl. *fundi* [L.] the bottom or base of an organ, or the part of a hollow organ farthest from its mouth.
f. of bladder the depths or cranial part of the urinary bladder.
f. camera used to photograph the fundus of the eye.
f. of eye the back portion of the interior of the eyeball, visible through the pupil by use of the ophthalmoscope.
f. of gallbladder the dilated portion of the gallbladder.
nasal f. the caudal extremity of the nasal cavity, occupied by the ethmoid bone.
nontapetal f. the nonreflective portion.
ocular f. see fundus of eye (above).
f. reticuli sulci floor of the reticular groove.
f. of stomach the part of the stomach to the left and above the level of the opening between the stomach and esophagus.
tigroid f. one lacking pigment so that underlying choroid vessels are visible as irregular stripes.
f. tympani the floor of the tympanic cavity.
unpigmented nontapetal f. lack of pigment permits larger blood vessels of the choroid to appear on fundoscopic examination. Seen in Siamese cats, dogs with merle coat color and Appaloosa horses.
f. uteri the part of the uterus between the cervix and the horns of the uterus.
funduscope see OPHTHALMOSCOPE.
funduscopy examination of the eye with a funduscope.
fundusectomy excision of the fundus of the stomach.
fungal pertaining to or caused by a fungus.
f. disease the three principal manifestations are the skin infections, the dermatophytoses, systemic infections such as coccidioidomycoses, and the mycotoxicoses, the fungal poisonings.
f. hypersensitivity may occur in animals; possibly the cause of fungal KERION.
f. hyphae see HYPHA.
f. infection see MYCOSIS.
f. mastitis see Table 16.
f. slide culture a method of culturing fungi that allows good visualization of conidia for identification purposes.
f. toxins there are a large number of known poisonous fungi, some of which grow on living plants, many of them visible on the outside of the plant, many of them growing inside the plant and therefore not visible. Many more grow on stored feed such as grain and hay. The best known fungal toxins include aflatoxin, citrinin, ergotamine, fumonisins, ergovaline, ochratoxin, phomopsin, slaframine, sporidesmin, trichothecenes (e.g. satratoxin, deoxynivalenol), zearalenone.
fungate to produce fungus-like growths; to grow rapidly, like a fungus.
fungemia the presence of fungi in the bloodstream.
fungi [L.] plural of *fungus*.
Fungi Imperfecti one of the six phyla of fungi. Called also Deuteromycota. Fungi in this phylum have septate hyphae but their method of reproduction has not been identified.
fungicide an agent that destroys fungi.
fungiform shaped like a fungus, or mushroom.
fungistasis inhibition of the growth of fungi.
fungistat a substance that checks the growth of fungi.
fungitoxic exerting a toxic effect upon fungi.
fungoid resembling a fungus.
chignon f. a nodular growth on the hair.
fungosity a fungoid growth or excrescence.
fungous of the nature of, caused by, or resembling a fungus.
funguria fungi in the urine.
fungus pl. *fungi* [L.] a general term for a group of eukaryotic organisms (mushrooms, yeasts, molds, etc.) marked by the absence of chlorophyll, the presence of a rigid cell wall in some stage of the life cycle, and reproduction by means of spores. Fungi are present in the soil, air and water, but only a few species can cause disease. Among the fungal diseases (mycoses) are HISTOPLASMOSIS, COCCIDIOIDOMYCOSIS and RINGWORM. Although the fungal diseases develop slowly, are difficult to diagnose, and are resistant to treatment, they are rarely fatal.

Another important section of the disease spectrum caused by fungi is the mycotoxicoses, e.g. FACIAL eczema, RYEGRASS staggers, mushroom poisoning—AMANITA, RAMARIA, CLAVARIA, CORTINARIUS, CLITOCYBE, INOCYBE, PSILOCYBE, SCLERODERMIA.
dimorphic f. those with two growth forms, molds or yeasts, depending on whether they are grown on artificial media or occur in the environment or in tissues or alternatively, depending on the incubation temperature. Included are *Sporothrix schenckii*, *Blastomyces dermatitidis*, *Histoplasma capsulatum*, *Coccidioides immitis* and *Paracoccidioides brasiliensis*. These organisms typically cause deep or systemic mycoses in animals and humans.
funicle funiculus.
funiculi plural of funiculus.
funiculitis 1. inflammation of the spermatic cord. 2. inflammation of that portion of a spinal nerve root which lies within the intervertebral canal.
funiculoepididymitis inflammation of the spermatic cord and the epididymis.
funiculus pl. *funiculi* [L.] a cord; a cordlike structure or part, especially one of the large bundles of nerve tracts making up the white matter of the spinal cord.
dorsal f. the white substance of the spinal cord lying on either side between the dorsal median septum and the dorsal root.
lateral f., f. lateralis the lateral mass of fibers on either side of the spinal cord, between the dorsolateral and ventrolateral sulci.
f. spermaticus see SPERMATIC cord.
f. spinalis see SPINAL CORD.
ventral f the white substance of the spinal cord lying on either side between the ventral median fissure and the ventrolateral sulcus.
funiform resembling a rope or cord.
funnel-web spider see ATRAX *robustus*.
Funtumia latifolia an African wood. When the fungus *Fusarium solani* grows on the shavings of this wood chickens housed on the shavings and sawdust have undergone sex changes.
FUO fever of unknown origin.
fur short, very fine and soft hair. Valuable as pelts for use in cold climate and high fashion garments.
f. animal animals bred or trapped in the wild for their pelts. Includes mink, sable, otter, lapin, ermine, marten.

f. ball accumulations of fur, swallowed during the natural grooming procedures of cats, can be a cause of vomiting, enteritis and uncommonly intestinal obstruction. Most troublesome in longhaired cats and those with skin disease that prompts more grooming.
f.-bearing animal see fur animal (above).
f. clipping chewing of fur by captive mink rendering the pelt useless. A vice apparently caused by cage boredom.
f. mite see LYNXACARUS *radovsky*.
f. seal alopecia caused in captive seals by overgrooming, a displacement activity. Alopecia occurs on the head and the posterior body, the easiest places for the seal to scratch.

furaltadone a nitrofuran antibiotic, used locally in the treatment of mastitis and in ear drops.

furano-sesquiterpenes, furanosesquiterpenes toxic essential oils, e.g. ngaione, myodesmone.

furanocoumarin naturally occurring photodynamic substances in plants and probably fungi. See also FUROCOUMARIN.

furanosesquiterpenoid pertaining to furanosesquiterpenes.

furazolidone a nitrofuran antibiotic, used as a local antibacterial and antiprotozoal. Used in poultry and swine as a feed additive to treat bacterial and protozoal intestinal infections. Calves fed low levels of furazolidone over long periods develop a leukopenia, petechial hemorrhages everywhere and are susceptible to infection. It is usually a sequel to prophylactic feeding of antibiotics. See also GRANULOCYTOPENIC calf disease.

furcal forked.

furcation the area where roots join the crown in a tooth with multiple roots.
f. exposure a classification of the degree of exposure accessible with a periodontal probe. Used in periodontal charting.

furcula the united clavicles in birds; a spring-like connection between the two shoulder joints; called also wishbone.

furfuraceous fine and loose; said of scales resembling dandruff or bran.

furious rabies see RABIES.

furlong 220 yards, 0.125 of a mile.

furnishings the extra type or quantity of hair on the head, tail, ears or legs, specified for a particular breed. For example, the feathers in setters, the beard in Bearded collies, the eyebrows in Schnauzers.

furocoumarin photosensitizing substances which occur normally in some plants such as *Ammi majus* and *Cymopterus watsonii*, and in others only if they are infected with bacteria or fungi. The furocoumarins are endogenous photodynamic agents which have the capacity to cause photosensitive keratoconjunctivitis. See also PHYTOALLEXIN.

furosemide, frusemide a diuretic that acts by blocking reabsorption of sodium and chloride in the ascending loop of Henle.

furrow a groove or trench.
atrioventricular f. the transverse groove marking off the atria of the heart from the ventricles.
gluteal f. the furrow that separates the buttocks.

Furstenberg's rosette see ROSETTE of Furstenberg.

furuncle a focal suppurative inflammation of the skin and subcutaneous tissues, enclosing a central slough or 'core'; called also boil.

furunculoid resembling a furuncle or boil.

furunculosis 1. the persistent sequential occurrence of furuncles over a period of weeks or months. 2. the simultaneous occurrence of a number of furuncles.
anal f. see PERIANAL fistula.
muzzle f. see nasal PYODERMA.
salmonid f. caused by *Aeromonas salmonicida*; characterized by bacteremia, septicemia and sometimes accompanied by deep necrotic lesions on the sides and backs of fish.

furze see ULEX EUROPAEUS.

FUS feline urological syndrome.

fusaric acid mycotoxin produced by *Fusarium moniliforme*; causes depression and vomiting in pigs.

fusariomycosis infection by fungi in the genus *Fusarium*.

fusariotoxicosis poisoning caused by ingesting feed contaminated by the fungi FUSARIUM spp. or their toxins. Includes loss of appetite and milk production, diarrhea, staggers.

Fusarium a genus of fungi; some species are plant pathogens and some are opportunistic infectious agents of humans and animals. Many also produce trichothecene toxins which cause poisoning of animals if the infected material, usually stored feed, is eaten.
F. acuminatum, F. culmorum, F. equiseti on maize crop causes inappetence, food rejection, diarrhea and incoordination in cattle.
F. graminearum* (*Gibberella zeae*), *F. roseum associated with moldy maize or barley grain and produces an estrogenic mycotoxin, zearalenone, which may cause signs of estrogenism, especially vulvovaginitis, in pigs.
F. moniliforme cause leukoencephalomalacia in horses, pulmonary edema in pigs.
F. roseum see *F. graminearum* (above).
F. scirpi causes diarrhea, staggers and food rejection in cattle.
F. solani, F. javanicum 1. growing on sweet potatoes this fungus produces bovine atypical interstitial pneumonia. 2. as an environmental fungus causing melanized granulomas (black gill disease) in shrimps, especially *Penaeus japonicus*.
F. sporotrichiella causes a fatal hemorrhagic disease of sheep.
F. sporotrichioides, F. tricinctum 1. causes poor weight gain, necrotic mouth lesions and deaths in turkeys and chickens. 2. causes a hemorrhagic syndrome in cattle and pigs, similar to stachybotrytoxicosis.

fusarochromanone a lethal mycotoxin found in *Fusarium roseum*; causes dyschondroplasia in broiler chickens.

fuschia bush see EREMOPHILA.

fuscin a brown pigment of the retinal epithelium.

fusidic acid a lipophilic steroid antibioitic, the product of *Fusidium coccineum*; mainly active against gram-positive bacteria.

fusiform spindle-shaped.

Fusiformis see FUSOBACTERIUM.

fusimotor denoting motor nerve fibers (of gamma motoneurons) that innervate intrafusal fibers of the muscle spindle.

fusion 1. the act or process of melting. 2. the merging or coherence of adjacent parts or bodies. 3. the operative formation of an ankylosis or arthrosis.
diaphyseal–epiphyseal f. operative establishment of bony union between the epiphysis and diaphysis of a bone.
nerve f. nerve anastomosis done to induce regeneration for resupplying empty tracts of a nerve with new growth of fibers.
nuclear f. the fusion of two atomic nuclei to form a single heavier nucleus, resulting in the release of enormous amounts of energy.

spinal f. surgical creation of ankylosis between contiguous vertebrae; spondylosyndesis.

fusional marked by fusion.

f. defects congenital defects marked by incomplete fusion of body parts, e.g. spina bifida.

Fusobacterium a genus of anaerobic non-spore-forming, gram-negative bacteria found as normal flora in the mouth and large bowel, and often in necrotic tissue, probably as secondary invaders.

F. necrophorum found in abscesses of the liver, lungs and other tissues and in chronic ulcer of the colon. A common major participant in bovine footrot, calf diphtheria, ruminal necrobacillosis, hepatic abscesses and thrush in horses. Synergistic with *Dichelobacter nodosus* in ovine footrot.

F. nodosus see DICHELOBACTER NODOSUS.

F. russii reported as a cause of soft tissue infections in cats.

fusocellular having spindle-shaped cells.

fusospirochetal of or caused by fusiform bacilli and spirochetes.

fusospirochetosis see VINCENT'S ANGINA.

futures quantities of a specified product at a specified level of quality guaranteed for delivery at a specified future date, and as specified in a contract tradable in a futures market. By purchasing at today's prices it is possible to make big profits in the future if the estimate is correct. There is the equivalent danger that prices will fall. The attractiveness in futures trading is that only a small proportion of the original purchase price needs to paid immediately.

FVC forced vital capacity.

FVIII-C factor VIII-coagulant.

FVR feline viral rhinotracheitis.

G

G symbol for *giga;* gingival; glucose; gonidial; guanine.

g 1. gravity; the unit of force exerted upon a body during acceleration and deceleration. 2. gram (or grams).

G banding the technique of demonstrating G BANDS.

G bands in cytogenetics the pattern of bands produced by staining the chromosomes with Giemsa after fixing the proteins to prevent them binding with dye.

G-CSF granulocyte-colony stimulating factor.

G protein a regulatory protein which becomes activated when bound to GTP and is involved in signal transduction.

G_1 phase, G_1 period see cell CYCLE.

G_2 phase, G_2 period see cell CYCLE.

G6PD glucose-6-phosphate dehydrogenase.

Ga chemical symbol, *gallium*.

GABA gamma-aminobutyric acid.

gad fly see HYPODERMA.

Russian g. f. see RHINOESTRUS *purpureus*.

Gadd technique a modification of the episioplasty procedure for second degree perineal lacerations. A triangular piece of mucous membrane is removed from the dorsal vestibule. The vestibular mucosa is then apposed, then the perineal body is reconstructed with a series of interrupted absorbable sutures, before the skin is closed.

gadding restlessness and excitement in horses, to a lesser extent cattle, because of the presence of biting flies, more specifically warble flies in cattle and bot flies in horses.

gadolinium a chemical element, atomic number 64, atomic weight 157.25, symbol Gd. See Table 6.

Gaertner's canal see GARTNER'S DUCTS.

gag 1. a surgical device for holding the mouth open. See also MOUTH speculum. 2. to retch, or strive to vomit.

mouth g. (1) see DRINKWATER MOUTH GAG, HAUSSMAN–DUNN GAG, SPRING GAG, VARNELL GAG, PROBANG.

g. (2) reflex elevation of the soft palate and retching elicited by touching the back of the tongue or the wall of the pharynx; called also pharyngeal reflex.

***gag* gene** a gene which encodes precursors of internal virion proteins found in the retroviral genome.

Gage excavator a long, thin, handheld instrument consisting of a handle, a thin neck and a slightly curved, rounded blade that slips between the vertebrae and scoops out degenerated disk material. Used in the fenestration of intervertebral disks in dogs.

Gage knife an instrument similar to the GAGE EXCAVATOR except that the blade is straight and has a cutting edge.

gagging the swallowing–vomiting activity of the gag reflex.

GAGs glycosaminoglycans.

Gaigeria a genus of hookworms in the family Ancylostomatidae.

G. pachyscelis occurs in the duodenum of the goat and sheep. A voracious blood-sucker and an infestation of as few as 24 can be fatal.

gain increase in body weight. See also GROWTH rate, gain RATIO.

g. controls see TIME gain compensation.

gait the manner or style of locomotion. Often used in assessing horses and dogs. See also ATAXIA, DYSMETRIA, INCOORDINATION, SPASTIC, STRINGHALT, WALK, TROT, CANTER, GALLOP (2), CADENCE, FIVE-GAITED.

g. analysis evaluation of the manner or style of walking, usually done by observing the animal as it walks or trots in a straight line. The normal forward step consists of two phases: the *stance phase*, during which one or more legs and feet are bearing most or all of the body weight, and the *swing phase*, during which the other feet are not touching the walking surface and the body weight is borne by the others. In a complete two-step cycle all feet are in contact with the ground at the same time for about 25% of the time. This part of the cycle is called the *double-support phase*.

An analysis of each component of the three phases of ambulation is an essential part of the diagnosis of various neurological disorders and the assessment of patient progress during rehabilitation and recovery from the effects of a neurological disease, a musculoskeletal injury or disease process, or amputation of a lower extremity.

antalgic g. a limp adopted so as to avoid pain on weight-bearing structures, characterized by a very short stance phase.

ataxic g. an unsteady, uncoordinated walk, employing a wide base.

diagonal g. one in which a forelimb is moved in unison with its opposite hindlimb, e.g. trot.

double-step g. a gait in which there is a noticeable difference in the length or timing of alternate steps.

high stepping g. may be normal in some fancy gaited horses. In others it may be a sign of blindness or poor proprioception, usually because of a defect in the sensory nervous system. It may also be a manifestation of hypermetria.

horse g. there are three natural gaits, WALK, TROT, CANTER and two artificial gaits, the FOXTROT, RACK. There are a number of other less well-defined gaits similar to foxtrot.

spastic g. a walk in which the legs move in a stiff manner, the toes seeming to drag and catch.

staggery g. see STAGGERS.

waddling g. exaggerated alternation of lateral trunk movements with an exaggerated elevation of the hip, suggesting the gait of a duck.

gaited see FIVE-GAITED.

Gal galactose.

GAL virus Gallus adeno-like virus; the *Aviadenovirus* genus.

galactagogue 1. promoting the flow of milk. 2. an agent that promotes the flow of milk.

galactans an ingredient of the toxins of *Mycoplasma* spp.

galactemia the presence of milk in the blood.

galactic 1. pertaining to milk. 2. galactagogue.

galactischia suppression of milk secretion.

galact(o)- word element. [Gr.] *milk*.

galactoblast a colostrum corpuscle in the acini of the mammary gland.

galactobolic of or relating to the action of neurohypophyseal peptides which contract the mammary myoepithelium and cause ejection of milk.

galactocele 1. a milk-containing, cystic enlargement of the mammary gland. 2. hydrocele filled with milky fluid.

galactocerebrosidase an enzyme that catalyzes the hydrolytic cleavage of galactose from galactocerebroside. Deficiency results in accumulation of galactocerebroside in tissues (globoid cell LEUKODYSTROPHY). Called also galactosylceramidase, galactosylceramide β-galactosidase.

galactocerebroside a glycosphingolipid with a galactose unit. Called also galactolipid. See globoid cell LEUKODYSTROPHY.

galactocerebrosidosis see globoid cell LEUKODYSTROPHY.

galactography radiography of the mammary ducts after injection of a radiopaque substance into the duct system.

galactokinase an enzyme that catalyzes the first step in the metabolism of galactose, the transfer of a phosphate group from ATP to galactose, producing galactose-1-phosphate.

g. deficiency see GALACTOSEMIA.

galactolipid, galactolipin see GALACTOCEREBROSIDE.

galactoma galactocele (1).

galactophore 1. galactophorous. 2. a milk duct.

galactophoritis inflammation of the milk ducts.

galactophorous conveying milk.

galactophygous arresting the flow of milk.

galactoplania secretion of milk in some abnormal part.

galactopoiesis the production of milk by the mammary glands.

galactopoietic 1. pertaining to, marked by, or promoting milk production. 2. an agent that promotes milk flow.

galactorrhea excessive or spontaneous milk flow; persistent secretion of milk irrespective of nursing; lactorrhea. May occur in dogs with severe hypothyroidism, due to hyperprolactinemia, pseudocyesis, or trauma to the mammary gland.

galactosamine an amino derivative of galactose.

galactose a monosaccharide derived from lactose. D-galactose is found in lactose, cerebrosides of the brain, raffinose of the sugar beet, and in many gums and seaweeds; L-galactose is found in flaxseed mucilage.

g. 1-phosphate uridylyl transferase involved in the metabolism of galactose to glycogen. Congenital galactosemia of humans and macropods is associated with a deficiency of this enzyme.

g. tolerance test a laboratory test done to determine the liver's ability to convert the sugar galactose into glycogen. Not much used in animals.

galactosemia a biochemical disorder in which there is a deficiency of enzymes necessary for proper metabolism of galactose. The condition is inherited in humans in two forms, due to deficiency of either galactokinase or galactose-1-phosphate uridyltransferase. Adult macropods are normally deficient in these enzymes.

Normally the sugar derived from lactose in milk is changed by enzymatic action into glucose. When the conversion of galactose to glucose does not take place, the galactose accumulates in the tissues and blood, typically causing cataract formation; commonly seen in young macropods reared on cow's milk.

galactosidase an enzyme that catalyzes the conversion of galactoside to galactose; it occurs in two forms: α-galactosidase (melibiase) and β-galactosidase (lactase). In deficiency states gangliosides (galactose-containing cerebrosides) accumulate in tissues. See also GM_1 GANGLIOSIDOSIS.

β-galactosidase a lysosome hydrolase.

galactoside a glycoside containing galactose.

galactosis the formation of milk by the lacteal glands.

galactostasis 1. cessation of milk secretion. 2. abnormal collection of milk in the mammary glands.

galactosuria the presence of galactose in the urine.

galactosylceramidase see GALACTOCEREBROSIDASE.

galactosylceramide see GALACTOCEREBROSIDASE.

galactosylhydroxylase-transferase an enzyme which contributes to glycolization.

galactotherapy treatment of sucking neonates by medication given to the dam.

galacturia chyluria; the discharge of urine with a milky appearance.

Galago gregarious, nocturnal, arboreal, monkeylike prosimians, up to a foot long; silver-gray, brown or black. Includes bush-baby, great galago and other species.

galah Australian bird, gray above, pink below. Noisy and a pest in grain crops because of large numbers. Called also *Cacatua roseicapilla*, roseate cockatoo.

Galanthus nivalis European plant in the family Liliaceae; bulbs cause salivation, vomiting and diarrhea. Called also snowdrop.

Galba the host snail for the intermediate stages of *Fasciola hepatica* in North America.

galea pl. *galeae* [L.] a helmet-shaped structure.

g. aponeurotica aponeurosis connecting the frontal and occipital bellies of the primate occipitofrontal muscle.

g. capitis the cap over the head of the spermatozoon. Called also acrosomal vesicle.

g. glandis the diminutive caplike glans of the ruminant penis.

Galega officinalis European plant in the legume family Fabaceae; contains galegine, which causes sudden death from hydrothorax and pulmonary edema. Called also goats' rue, French lilac or honeysuckle.

galena a mineral containing lead.

Galenia genus of African plants in family Aizoaceae; includes *G. africana*—contains an unidentified cardiotoxin which causes waterpens, a cardiomyopathy, liver fibrosis and ascites, and *G. pubescens*—may cause nitrate–nitrite poisoning.

galenicals, galenics medicines prepared according to the formulae of Galen. The term is now used to denote standard preparations containing one or several organic ingredients, as contrasted with pure chemical substances.

Galeopsis a European genus of the plant family Lamiaceae. Seeds of these plants contain an unidentified toxin which causes anorexia, anasarca and jaundice. Called also hedge nettle, hemp nettle.

galeta grass *Hilaria jamesii*, commonly infested with *Claviceps cinerea*, which causes poisoning.

Galiceno small, solid-colored (any color) pleasure horse of Mexican origin.

Galician Blond cattle Spanish cream to red-brown meat cattle.

Galician sheep prolific Spanish meat and medium-wool sheep, mostly polled.

gall 1. the bile. 2. a sore caused by chafing; said commonly of horses. 3. an excrescence on a plant, e.g. on the seedheads of *Lolium rigidum*, caused by plant nematodes and causing poisoning. 4. an extract of galls. Used in medicine as a bitter.

girth g. see GIRTH gall.

saddle g. see SADDLE sore.

g. sickness see ANAPLASMOSIS.

gallamine a competitive neuromuscular blocking agent used as a muscle relaxant. Used as the triethiodide. It competes with acetylcholine for the cholinergic receptors at the postsynaptic membrane.

gallate antioxidant used in food preservation, especially in foods containing oils and fats. Includes propyl, octyl and dodecylgallate.

gallbladder the pear-shaped reservoir for bile attached to the visceral surface or between the lobes of the liver in all domestic animal species except the horse. It serves as a storage place for bile. The gallbladder may be subject to such disorders as inflammation and the formation of GALLSTONE.

g. cystic mucosal hyperplasia hyperplasia of the mucus-secreting glands in the gallbladder and larger bile ducts.

g. edema a gross lesion in many cases of infectious canine hepatitis.

g. inflammation cholecystitis.

g. meridian points acupuncture points on the gallbladder MERIDIAN.

g. paralysis a specific abnormality in lantadene poisoning. The gallbladder is grossly distended and full of viscid, pale bile.

g. radiography see CHOLECYSTOGRAPHY.

galliform see GALLINACEOUS.

gallinaceous, galliform belonging to the genus *Gallus*, hence domestic and wild fowl.

gallium a chemical element, atomic number 31, atomic weight 69.72, symbol Ga. See Table 6.

g.-67 a radioisotope of gallium having a half-life of 78.1 hours; used in the imaging of soft tissue tumors.

g. nitrate used in the treatment of hypercalcemia.

g. scan a nuclear medicine procedure using the radioisotope gallium-67 in the form of gallium citrate. Gallium has a high affinity for certain tumors and also for non-neoplastic lesions, such as abscesses. Gallium scans are particularly useful in the staging of lymphomas, and in localizing occult abscesses.

gallon a unit of liquid measure; 4 quarts. The Imperial gallon equals 4.546 liters and the American gallon equals 3.785 liters.

gallop 1. a disordered rhythm of the heart. See also gallop RHYTHM. 2. the horse's fastest gait. All four hooves are off the ground at the one time and the rhythm is one of four beats. The sequence of contact by the hooves is near hind, off hind, near fore, then off fore (when the off fore is the leading limb).

diastolic g. see gallop RHYTHM.

gallotannic acid see TANNIC ACID.

Galloway a polled, black-brown breed of dairy cattle originating in Scotland.

G. pony a now extinct Scottish pony. Nowadays the term is used to identify a show class of pony which is greater than 14 hands high but not more than 14.2 hands high.

gallstone a stonelike mass that forms in the gallbladder. See CHOLELITHIASIS.

Gallus a genus of birds of the pheasant family Phasianidae. Includes the domestic fowl. See also FOWL.

G. domesticus see *Gallus gallus* (below).

G. gallus the Red Junglefowl, the progenitor of the domestic fowl. Also the domestic fowl, itself sometimes called *G. domestica.*

GALT gut-associated LYMPHOID tissue.

Galt trephine a 0.75 inch cylinder with a saw-toothed cutting edge at one end and grinding ridges down the outside with a crossbar handle at the other end for excision of a plate of bone. The center of the cutting circle has a sharp-pointed pin which prevents the trephine from moving laterally while cutting and fixes the trephined bone disk so that it does not fall into a cavity.

Galtonia clavata see LIDNERIA CLAVATA.

galtonian inheritance based on a multilocal system of character definition so that progeny present a continuous series of a characteristic rather than specific classes, e.g. a range of body weights rather than giants and dwarfs.

Galumna mites which act as intermediate hosts for *Moniezia* spp. tapeworms.

galvanic current a steady direct electric current.

galvanocontractility contractility in response to stimulation by galvanic current.

galvanometer an instrument for measuring current by electromagnetic action.

galvanopalpation testing of nerves of the skin by means of galvanic current.

Galvayne's groove a vertical goove in the labial surface of the upper corner incisor tooth in the horse. It appears at the gum margin at 10 years of age, is halfway to the end of the tooth at 15 years, has reached the end at 20 years, has disappeared from the top of the tooth at 25 years and has disappeared completely at 30 years. The ages quoted are subject to variation.

Galvayne's twitch a twitch for restraint; made by passing a loop of soft rope around the poll and into the mouth under the top lip and in front of the upper incisor teeth.

Galway sheep polled, Irish meat and longwool sheep.

Gambardella technique a modification of the lateral imbrication approach to extra-articular reconstruction of the cranial cruciate ligament in dogs. Nonabsorbable sutures are placed between the distal patellar tendon and the proximal femorofabellar fascia and the lateral collateral ligament.

Gambee suture pattern a rapidly inserted, interrupted suture used to close a bowel anastomosis with one layer of stitches. The suture goes from serous to mucosal surface, back into the mucosa on the same side of the incision, out into the middle of the cut surface to be approximated, across the incision into the wound edge opposite, down into gut lumen, back through the mucosa and through the wall to the serous surface and a tie with the tail of the suture across the incision.

Gambel's oak QUERCUS *gambelii*.

gambia pea CROTALARIA *goreensis*.

Gambian sleeping sickness see TRYPANOSOMA *gambiense*.

Gambierdiscus toxicus marine dinoflagellate; the main source of toxins responsible for CIGUATERA.

gambrel the bracket-shaped piece of iron rod on which a sheep carcass is traditionally hung to cool and set.

Gambusia small, 1 inch long, pale fish which eat mosquito larvae and are used in their control.

Game broad-breasted, brightly colored breed of table poultry used widely in breeding hybrid table poultry.

game birds or animals hunted and killed in the chase, i.e. for sport. Used also in respect of animals hunted for provisions and skins. Said of animals and birds, hence game birds, etc.

g. animals includes deer and other similar large ruminants, wild pig and the group of largely African animals classed as 'big game'. Game fish are marlin, tuna and other big marine fish rather than the smaller freshwater fish of rod and reel devotees.

g. birds birds originally hunted but nowadays also farmed. Includes pheasants, quail, partridge, francolin, jungle fowl, guinea fowl.

g. farm farm dedicated to keeping game animals, usually exotic ones, in the wild in conditions as nearly natural as possible. In most instances they are a hobby or for relaxation and entertainment. They are really private zoos or zoological gardens.

g. fish fish hunted for sport.

g. meat meat from slaughtered game animals.

g. ranch see game farm (above).

Game cock closest domestic fowl variety to the ancestral Red Junglefowl. Used in cockfighting. A tall, upright, gaudily colored bird with a fearsome hooked beak and spurs. The head and neck and tail coverts are bright yellow, the back and the wings are brown, the breast is black. The beak is brown and the feet are slate-colored.

game theory a branch of mathematical logic which deals with all of the possible reactions to a particular strategy used mainly in systems analysis.

gamefowl see GAME COCK.

gamete a haploid germ cell; one of two cells, male (spermatozoon) and female (ovum), whose union is necessary in sexual reproduction to initiate the development of a new individual.

gametocyte an oocyte or spermatocyte; a cell that produces gametes.

gametogenesis the development of the male and female sex cells (gametes).

gametogony 1. the development of merozoites into male and female gametes, which later fuse to form a zygote. 2. reproduction by means of gametes.

gamma 1. the third letter of the Greek alphabet, Γ or γ. 2. used in names of chemical compounds to distinguish one of three or more isomers or to indicate the position of substituting atoms or groups. 3. used in sensitometry to denote the straight line of a characteristic curve. The greater the film contrast the higher the gamma.

g. benzene hexachloride see CHLORINATED HYDROCARBONS.

g. delta T lymphocyte see T LYMPHOCYTE.

g. globulin a class of plasma proteins composed almost entirely of IMMUNOGLOBULINS, the proteins that function as antibodies. Gamma globulins, immunoglobulins, antibodies and antiserum are often used synonomously and interchangeably. See also ANTIBODY.

Commercial preparations of gamma globulin are derived from blood serum of several species and are used for prevention, modification and treatment of various infectious diseases. This type of gamma globulin, which is an immune serum, contains a wide range of antibodies, depending on its method of production, and it provides passive immunity for several weeks. In cattle, its most common use is in the newborn orphan which receives no colostrum. In dogs and cats, it has been used in the prophylaxis, and occasionally treatment, of viral infections.

The production of gamma globulin may be increased in the body by the invasion of harmful microorganisms. An abnormal amount of gamma globulin in the blood, a condition known as hypergammaglobulinemia, may be indicative of a chronic infection or certain malignant blood diseases. There is also a rare inherited condition, AGAMMAGLOBINEMIA, in which the body is unable to produce gamma globulin. Animals suffering from this condition are extremely susceptible to infection.

g. glutamyl transferase (GGT) see gamma glutamyl TRANSFERASE.

gamma-aminobutyric acid an amino acid that is one of the principal inhibitory neurotransmitters in the central nervous system. Abbreviated GABA. Avermectins act by stimulating the presynaptic release of GABA and enhancing its binding to the postsynaptic receptors.

Gamma–Gandy body, Gandy–Gamma nodule an organizing focus of hemosiderin, deposited in a congested spleen. Called also siderotic nodule.

gamma rigidity see DECEREBRATE rigidity.

gamma subunit third-named chain (or subunit) occurring in the functional organization of macromolecules, usually proteins, containing three or more chains.

gammaglobulinopathy see GAMMOPATHY.

Gammaherpesvirinae one of three subfamilies within the family HERPESVIRIDAE, some members of which are associated with tumor formation; divided into gamma 1 viruses, which include Epstein–Barr virus, and gamma 2 viruses, which include herpesvirus saimiri, equine herpsvirus 2 and bovine herpesvirus 4.

Gammarus water crustaceans; intermediate hosts for *Tetrameres* spp. worms.

gammexane see LINDANE.

gammopathy abnormal proliferation of the B lymphocytes resulting in abnormal levels of immunoglobulin production; the gammopathies include multiple myeloma, macroglobulinemia and Hodgkin's disease. Called also gammaglobulinopathy.

monoclonal g. an increased production of one type of immunoglobulin by a single clone of cells. The abnormal protein produced is called *paraprotein* or *M component* and may be composed of whole immunoglobulin molecules or subunits, light-chains (Bence Jones proteins) or heavy-chains. Occurs in myelomas, lymphoproliferative neoplasms, and occasionally chronic inflammatory or immune-mediated diseases. Greatly elevated serum levels of protein may result in a hyperviscosity syndrome.

polyclonal g. a hypergammaglobulinemia resulting

from an increased production of several different immunoglobulins and usually attributable to persistent, high level exposure to antigens; occur in a wide variety of infectious, inflammatory, and immune-mediated diseases. Examples in animals are feline infectious peritonitis, canine ehrlichiosis, Aleutian mink disease and equine infectious anemia.

gamogenesis sexual reproduction.

gamont gametocyte.

ganado bravo [Span.] see FIGHTING BULL.

ganciclovir a synthetic nucleoside analog of guanine with antiviral activity against herpesviruses, especially cytomegalovirus.

ganglial pertaining to a ganglion.

gangliated provided with ganglia; ganglionated.

gangliectomy excision of a ganglion; ganglionectomy.

gangliform having the form of a ganglion.

gangliitis see GANGLIONITIS.

gangli(o)- word element. [Gr.] *ganglion.*

ganglioblast an embryonic cell of the cerebrospinal ganglia.

gangliocyte a ganglion cell.

gangliocytoma see GANGLIONEUROMA.

ganglioform gangliform.

ganglioglioma a glioma rich in mature neurons or ganglion cells.

ganglioglioneuroma see GANGLIONEUROMA.

ganglioma see GANGLIONEUROMA.

ganglion pl. *ganglia, ganglions* [Gr.] a knot or knotlike mass; a general term to designate a group of nerve cell bodies, located outside the central nervous system. Occasionally applied to certain nuclear groups within the brain or spinal cord, e.g. basal ganglia.

aorticorenal g. small sympathetic ganglia supplying nerve fibers to the kidneys.

Arnold's g. see otic ganglion (below).

autonomic g. aggregations of cell bodies of neurons of the autonomic nervous system; the parasympathetic and the sympathetic ganglia combined.

basal g. subcortical masses of gray matter embedded in each cerebral hemisphere, comprising the corpus striatum (caudate and lentiform nuclei), amygdaloid body and claustrum. Other structures have also been considered to be part of the basal ganglia. Called also basal nuclei.

cardiac g. ganglia of the superficial cardiac plexus found close to the aortic arch.

celiac g. two large sympathetic ganglia, found on either side of the celiac artery, supplying nerve fibers to the viscera supplied by that artery; sensory and parasympathetic fibers also pass through the ganglia.

cephalic g. parasympathetic ganglia in the head, consisting of the ciliary, otic, pterygopalatine and submandibular ganglia.

cerebrospinal g. those associated with the cranial and spinal nerves.

cervical g. 1. any of the three ganglia (cranial, middle and caudal) of the sympathetic trunk found near the base of the skull and inside the thoracic inlet. 2. one near the cervix uteri.

cervicothoracic g. a ganglion on the sympathetic trunk formed by a union of the caudal cervical and one or more thoracic ganglia. Called also stellate ganglion.

ciliary g. a parasympathetic ganglion in the posterior part of the orbit supplied by the oculomotor nerve.

Corti's g. spiral ganglion.

dorsal root g. spinal ganglion.

false g. an enlargement on a nerve that does not have a true ganglionic structure.

gasserian g. trigeminal ganglion.

geniculate g. the sensory ganglion of the facial nerve, on the geniculum of the facial nerve.

g. impar the single ganglion commonly found where the sympathetic trunks of the two sides unite.

jugular g. 1. the proximal ganglion of the vagus nerve. 2. the proximal (superior) ganglion of the glossopharyngeal nerve.

lumbar g. the ganglia on the lumbar part of the sympathetic trunk.

otic g. a parasympathetic ganglion next to the medial surface of the mandibular nerve, just ventral to the foramen ovale. Its postganglionic fibers supply the parotid gland. Called also Arnold's ganglion.

parasympathetic g. aggregations of cell bodies of cholinergic neurons of the parasympathetic nervous system; these ganglia are located near to or within the wall of the organs being innervated.

petrous g. the distal ganglion of the glossopharyngeal nerve.

pterygopalatine g. a parasympathetic ganglion in a fossa in the sphenoid bone, formed by postganglionic cell bodies that synapse with preganglionic fibers from the facial nerve via the nerve of the pterygopalatine canal. Called also sphenopalatine ganglion.

sacral g. those of the sacral part of the sympathetic trunk.

semilunar g. trigeminal ganglion.

sensory g. any of the ganglia of the peripheral nervous system that transmit sensory impulses; also, the collective masses of nerve cell bodies in the brain subserving sensory functions.

simple g. a cystic tumor in a tendon sheath.

sphenopalatine g. pterygopalatine ganglion.

spinal g. ganglia on the dorsal root of each spinal nerve.

spiral g. the ganglion on the cochlear nerve, located within the modiolus, sending fibers peripherally to the organ of Corti and centrally to the cochlear nuclei of the brainstem. Called also Corti's ganglion.

stellate g. cervicothoracic ganglion.

sympathetic g. aggregations of cell bodies of adrenergic neurons of the sympathetic nervous system; these ganglia are arranged in chainlike fashion on either side of the spinal cord.

thoracic g. the ganglia on the thoracic portion of the sympathetic trunk.

trigeminal g. a ganglion on the sensory root of the fifth cranial nerve. Called also gasserian ganglion and semilunar ganglion.

tympanic g. an enlargement on the tympanic branch of the glossopharyngeal nerve.

vestibular g. the sensory ganglion of the vestibular part of the eighth cranial nerve, located in the dorsal part of the lateral end of the internal acoustic meatus.

Walther's g. ganglion impar.

Wrisberg's g. cardiac ganglia.

ganglion blocking blocking of transmission through the autonomic ganglia.

autonomic g. b. agents substances such as nicotine which block transmission across sympathetic ganglia by blocking the nicotinic receptors in the ganglion, reducing transmission to about 20% of normal.

synthetic g. b. agents include methonium compounds (e.g. hexamethonium, trimethidinium) and other unrelated compounds, e.g. mecamylamine. Have the advantage of avoiding side-effects of nicotine.

ganglionated provided with ganglia; gangliated.

ganglionectomy excision of a ganglion; gangliectomy.

ganglioneuritis see GANGLIONITIS.
ganglioneuroma a rare benign neoplasm composed of nerve fibers and ganglion and Schwann cells. Generally, these occur in dogs, intracranially in the brain or cranial nerve ganglia, or rarely in the adrenal medulla or autonomic ganglia. See also NEUROBLASTOMA.
ganglionic pertaining to a ganglion.
g. blockade inhibition by drugs of nerve impulse transmission at autonomic ganglionic synapses.
g. blocking agent see GANGLION BLOCKING.
ganglionitis inflammation of a ganglion; gangliitis.
myoenteric g. causes chronic intestinal pseudoobstruction in horses.
ganglionostomy surgical creation of an opening into a cystic tumor on a tendon sheath or aponeurosis.
ganglioplegic 1. blocking transmission of impulses through the sympathetic and parasympathetic ganglia. 2. an agent that so acts.
ganglioradiculitis inflammation of spinal ganglia and nerve roots. Clinical signs in affected dogs include sensory deficits, ataxia, hypermetria, megaesophagus, dysphonia and Horner's syndrome. Siberian huskies are predisposed.
ganglioside a class of galactose-containing cerebrosides found in central nervous system tissues; they are glycolipids of the basic composition ceramide-glucose-galactose-*N*-acetyl neuraminic acid. The form GM_1 accumulates in tissues in generalized GANGLIOSIDOSIS as observed in Friesian cattle, dogs and cats. The form GM_2 accumulates in a similar disease of Yorkshire pigs, dogs and cats.
gangliosidosis a group of inherited lipid storage disorders marked by accumulation of gangliosides in tissues due to an enzyme defect. Characterized by progressive neuromuscular dysfunction and impaired growth from an early age.
GM_1 g. a defect of β-galactosidase which causes accumulation of galactoside GM_1. Identified in Friesian cattle, dogs and cats.
GM_2 g. a defect of hexosaminidase A in dogs and pigs, and hexosaminidase A and B in cats. Analogous to the similar diseases in humans, which are called also Sandhoff's disease, Tay–Sachs disease and Bernheimer–Seitelberger disease.
gangrene the death of body tissue, generally in considerable mass, usually associated with loss of vascular (nutritive) supply, and followed by bacterial invasion and putrefaction. Although it usually affects the extremities, gangrene sometimes may involve the internal organs. Signs depend on the site and include fever, pain, darkening of the skin, and an unpleasant odor. If the condition involves an internal organ, it is generally attended by pain and collapse.
dry g. occurs gradually and results from slow reduction of the blood flow in the arteries. There is no subsequent bacterial decomposition; the tissues become dry and shriveled. It occurs only in the extremities, and usually because of gradual diminution of the blood supply. Signs include gradual shrinking of the tissue, which becomes cold and lacking in pulse, and turns first brown and then black. Usually a line of demarcation is formed where the gangrene stops, owing to the fact that the tissue above this line continues to receive an adequate supply of blood.
gas g. results from dirty lacerated wounds infected by anaerobic bacteria, especially species of *Clostridium.* It is an acute, severe, painful condition in which muscles and subcutaneous tissues become filled with gas and a serosanguineous exudate.
internal g. in strangulated HERNIA, a loop of intestine is caught in the bulge and its blood supply is cut off; gangrene may occur in that section of tissue. Thrombosis of the mesenteric artery may result in gangrene of a section of intestine. Gangrene can be a rare complication of lung abscess in pneumonia.
moist g. caused by sudden stoppage of blood, resulting from burning by heat or acid, severe freezing, physical accident that destroys the tissue, a tourniquet that has been left on too long, or a clot or another embolism. At first, tissue affected by moist gangrene has the color of a bad bruise, smells atrociously, is swollen, and often blistered. The gangrene is likely to spread with great speed. Toxins are formed in the affected tissues and absorbed.
segmental g. gangrene of a section of an organ, e.g. of part of an elephant's ear, as a result of sectional compromising of blood supply.
gangrenous pertaining to, marked by, or of the nature of gangrene.
g. cellulitis gangrenous necrosis of the skin of the thorax and thighs of chickens of 1 to 4 months of age caused by *Clostridium septicum* and other clostridia. Most affected birds die and the mortality rate in a flock may be as high as 60%. Called also necrotic dermatitis, gangrenous dermatitis.
g. coryza see BOVINE malignant catarrh.
g. dermatitis see GANGRENOUS cellulitis.
g. ergotism see rye ERGOT[1].
Ganjam virus a member of the family *Bunyaviridae*, genus *Nairovirus* causing a tickborne virus infection of sheep and goats in India.
ganskweek see LASIOSPERMUM BIPINNATUM.
gantho metho SENECIO *raphanifolius.*
gantho metho ajang SENECIO *biligulatus.*
gap junctions regions of high and special ionic permeability between closely apposed cells. They are places at which cells exchange molecules of large size and provide an avenue by which developing cells can influence each other. Called also nexus.
neuronal g. j. very tight contacts between some neurons permitting the almost instant transmission of impulses from one neuron to the other; structural elements extend across the gap conferring a continuity of cytoplasm between the cells.
gape a behavioral response shown by cats in recognition of urine odor. After sniffing, the cat flicks the tongue against the hard palate, opens its mouth, licks the nose, and has a fixed gaze. This may be similar to the FLEHMEN reaction.
gapes see SYNGAMUS *trachea.*
gapeworm see SYNGAMUS *trachea.*
garbage-eating scavenging by dogs and cats involving ingestion of spoiled food, excessive quantities of unusual foods, and bones, resulting in gastroenteritis.
garbancillo ASTRAGALUS *wootoni.*
garbanzo see CHICKPEA.
garden grown in gardens; cultivated.
g. bean see PHASEOLUS.
g. lupin LUPINUS *polyphyllus.*
g. nightshade SOLANUM *nigrum.*
g. pea PISUM *sativum.*
gare long, hairy, non-serrated fibers in the fleece of some crossbred sheep; usually in breech wool; the fibers cannot be dyed or spun.
gargaloo PARSONSIA *eucalyptophylla.*
garget 1. mastitis. 2. PHYTOLACCA *americana.*
gargoylism MUCOPOLYSACCHARIDOSIS I; Hurler's syndrome.
garland flower see DAPHNE.
garlic ALLIUM *sativum.*
garron a type of large, sturdy pony bred in Scotland;

originated in cross between Percheron and Highland pony. Also used generally to describe the native ponies of Scotland and Ireland.

Gartner's ducts remnants of the embryonic mesonephric ducts, sometimes found on the floor of the vagina, which often open into the vestibule.

cystic G. d. cystlike structures in the floor of the vagina.

gas any elastic aeriform fluid in which the molecules are widely separated from each other and so have free paths.

alveolar g. the gas in the alveoli of the lungs, where gaseous exchange with the capillary blood takes place. See also OXYGEN, CARBON DIOXIDE.

blood g. see BLOOD GAS ANALYSIS.

g. bubble disease a disease of fish in tanks in which the water is supersaturated with oxygen or nitrogen. Gas embolism develops in the gills. Air bubbles can be seen in the gills, eyes and under the skin and the fish show bizarre nervous behavior.

g. cap a cap of gas above fluid or solid contents in a hollow viscus, e.g. in a static rumen. Seen radiologically in distended intestinal loops in paralytical ileus.

g. edema disease see BLUE WING DISEASE.

g. exchange gases move by simple diffusion in response to pressure differences; net diffusion occurs from areas of high pressure to areas of lower pressure irrespective of whether the gas is present as a gas or in solution or gases moving from gas to solution or vice versa. The rate of exchange of gases in body tissues, e.g. between alveolar space and erythrocyte, is influenced by many other factors, especially the diffusion distance and the solubility of the gas.

g. inhalation irritant gases, e.g. manure gas, cause pulmonary edema.

laughing g. nitrous oxide.

manure g. poisoning see MANURE pit gas poisoning.

tear g. a gas that produces severe lacrimation by irritating the conjunctivae. See LACRIMATOR.

g. transport relates to the efficiency of transport of gas, e.g. oxygen, by the patient as a whole. The efficiency of gas transport varies widely between normal individuals and between species, e.g. athletic breeds of horses and dogs have much faster gas transport systems than human athletes; the efficiency of gas transport in the individual depends largely on the rapidity of increase in minute ventilation, plus a similar rate of increase in cardiac output.

g. tube see CROOKES' TUBE.

Gascoyne spurge EUPHORBIA *boophthona*.

gaskin the muscular portion of the hindleg between the stifle and hock, corresponding to the human calf. The term is used in horses and sometimes dogs.

gasoline poisoning see OIL products.

gasping disease see avian infectious BRONCHITIS.

gasserian ganglion see trigeminal GANGLION.

gaster [Gr.] see STOMACH.

gasterophiliasis gasterophilosis.

gasterophilosis the disease caused by infestation with *Gasterophilus* spp. Sporadic cases of abscess formation, even rupture of the stomach wall with local peritonitis, occur but the infestation, though dramatic, is virtually nonpathogenic.

Gasterophilus a genus of flies, the horse bot flies, the larvae of which develop in the gastrointestinal tract of horses and may sometimes infect humans. A member of the family Gasterophilidae.

G. equi see *G. intestinalis* (below).

G. haemorrhoidalis eggs are laid around the mouth and on the cheeks; the larvae are found in the mucosa of the tongue and establish finally in the stomach.

G. inermis eggs are laid around the mouth and on the cheeks; the larvae are found in the cheek mucosa and settle finally in the rectum.

***G. intestinalis* (syn. *G. equi*)** the eggs are laid near the front fetlocks and up the legs as far as the shoulder; the larvae are found in the mucosa of the tongue and subsequently at the gastric cardia.

***G. nasalis* (syn. *G. veterinus*)** the larvae are laid in the intermandibular space; larvae are found at the pylorus and in the duodenum.

G. nigricornis an uncommon horse bot fly.

G. pecorum the eggs are laid on plants, the larvae are found in the mucosa of the cheeks and eventually gastric pylorus.

G. veterinus see *G. nasalis* (above).

gasteropod see GASTROPOD.

gastradenitis inflammation of the gastric glands.

gastralgia pain in the stomach; gastric colic.

gastrectasis distension of the stomach.

gastrectomy excision of the stomach (total gastrectomy) or a portion of it (partial or subtotal gastrectomy).

gastric pertaining to, affecting, or originating in the stomach.

g. acid see gastric juice (below).

g. atony a large distended stomach lacking in tone as seen in a horse that is a windsucker and continuously swallows air. Predisposes to chronic indigestion.

g. cicatricial contraction in horses causes constriction of the stomach and subsequent dilatation of the dorsal sac.

g. dilatation see gastric dilatation COLIC.

g. dilatation–displacement see gastric dilatation–volvulus (below).

g. dilatation–volvulus (GDV) a syndrome of gastric dilatation leading to volvulus, seen most often in deep-chested, large breed dogs. The etiology is unclear, but aerophagia or overeating are important factors. Gastric hemorrhage and ulceration, hypotensive, hypovolemic shock, and severe electrolyte disturbances contribute to the high mortality. Surgical intervention is often required, cardiac dysrhythmias complicate recovery, and recurrences are common. Called also gastric dilatation–displacement, bloat.

g. distension in pigs commonly results in vomiting.

g. edema an accompaniment of edema in most organs in cases where edema is widespread; as a sole lesion is significant in the abomasum in cases of arsenic poisoning, ostertagiasis and in edema disease in pigs.

g. emptying time the time taken for the stomach to begin to empty of contents; demonstrated in contrast radiography. Delayed in gastric retention due to dysfunction of the pylorus, abnormalities of gastric motility, foreign bodies and systemic diseases.

g. fluid see gastric juice (below).

g. folds folds in the gastric mucosa and part of the submucosa oriented in the direction of the long axis of the stomach, as they are in the abomasum; they may be few and simple or numerous and tortuous, as in the dog.

g. foreign body occurs most commonly in dogs, causing vomiting. Occasionally it may pass into the small intestine, causing partial or complete obstruction with more severe signs of dehydration, shock, and sometimes perforation with peritonitis. A variety of objects may be swallowed, e.g. needles, balls, children's toys, bones, fish hooks and socks, to name a few.

g. habronemiasis see HABRONEMIASIS.
g. hemorrhage caused by gastric ulcer or foreign body. May cause sudden death due to exsanguination, as in pigs with esophagogastric ulcer, or anemia with melena.
g. hormones see GASTROINTESTINAL hormones.
g. impaction in horses fed a diet of coarse indigestible roughage; a cause of subacute colic.
g. inhibitory polypeptide (GIP) a tentative gut hormone secreted by the mucosa of the small intestine and playing a part in controlling gastric (inhibition) and intestinal (stimulation) secretion and insulin release (stimulation).
g. intubation see INTUBATION.
g. juice the secretion of glands in the walls of the stomach for use in digestion. Its essential ingredients are pepsin, an enzyme that breaks down proteins in food, and hydrochloric acid, which destroys bacteria and is of assistance in the digestive process.
g. motility varies between the three regions of the stomach, being most active in the antrum, has a basic slow wave motility and a capacity to increase in response to the fullness of the stomach and to decrease with a rise in acidity of the duodenal contents.
g. mucosa secretes pepsin (as pepsinogen), hydrochloric acid.
g. neoplasia includes adenocarcinoma, carcinoma, benign adenomatous polyps, leiomyomas, plasmacytoma, squamous cell carcinoma.
g. outlet obstruction see PYLORIC obstruction, PYLORIC outflow failure.
g. peptidases includes pepsin A, trypsin, chymotrypsin, elastase, carboxypeptidase A, carboxypeptidase B.
g. perforation in horses occurs secondarily to lesions of the stomach wall, especially squamous cell carcinoma; causes a local peritonitis, often with extension to the spleen.
g. pits multiple small depressions in the gastric area of the stomach; a gastric gland opens into the bottom of each pit.
g. rotation rotations of the stomach in the embryonic abdomen between its first appearance and its final disposition. In simple-stomached animals such as dogs two rotations are recognized, from the axial tube ventrally and to the left.
g. rupture causes sudden cessation of abdominal pain caused by distension; acute endotoxic shock and peracute, diffuse peritonitis kill the animal within a few hours.
g. squamous-cell carcinoma the commonest gastric neoplasm in horses. Seen usually in the advanced stages of anorexia and weight loss. Characterized by a fungating mass in the pars esophagea often with secondary implants locally, sometimes widespread in other organs.
g. torsion in sows, predisposed by large, sloppy meal and great excitement at feeding time leading to very fast eating. There is a short course with death due to shock and infarction of the stomach wall. See also gastric dilatation–volvulus (above).
g. ulcer an ulcer of the inner wall of the stomach. It occurs in all species at a low level but causes little disease. Esophagogastric ulcer in pigs may reach epidemic proportions in some piggeries and cause serious mortalities due to blood loss. Called also gastric mucosal ulceration.
g. venous infarction gross lesions of bright red to dark red mucosa; occur in many septicemias, viremias and toxemias in horses and pigs.
g. waves peristaltic waves, the pacemakers for antral peristalsis.

gastricism gastric disorder.

gastricsin a proteolytic enzyme isolated from gastric juice; its precursor is pepsinogen but differs from pepsin in molecular weight and in the N terminal amino acid.

gastrin a polypeptide hormone secreted by certain cells of the pylorus, which strongly stimulates secretion of gastric acid and pepsinogen, and weakly stimulates secretion of pancreatic enzymes and gallbladder contraction.
g. assay plasma levels are elevated in gastrointestinal disease and other systemic diseases.

gastrinoma a gastrin-secreting, non-beta islet cell tumor of the pancreas, associated with ZOLLINGER–ELLISON SYNDROME.

gastritis inflammation of the lining of the stomach. Gastritis is one of the most common stomach disorders, and occurs in acute, chronic and toxic forms. Its clinical manifestation is vomiting. In veterinary medicine, the pathogenesis, clinical findings and postmortem lesions are poorly defined and are, in many cases, based on functional rather than on structural changes.
acute g. severe gastritis caused by food poisoning, overeating or bacterial or viral infection, and often accompanied by enteritis. The outstanding sign of acute gastritis is abdominal pain.
atrophic g. an immune-mediated disorder described in dogs with systemic lupus erythematosus; associated with antiparietal antibodies.
chronic g. an inflammation of the stomach that may occur repeatedly or continue over a period of time.
chronic atrophic g. rare in dogs; associated with mucosal thinning, loss of parietal cells, mucosal metaplasia and atrophy of gastric glands.
emphysematous g. inflammation of the gastric wall by *Clostridium perfringens*.
eosinophilic g. diffuse infiltration or discrete nodules of eosinophils in the stomach wall occur rarely in dogs. May be immune-mediated, due to allergy or parasites.
giant hypertrophic g. excessive proliferation of the gastric mucosa, producing diffuse thickening of the wall; inflammatory changes may be associated. Weight loss, vomiting, diarrhea, hematemesis and hypoalbuminemia occur. Occurs in humans, dogs (particularly Basenjis), mice and nonhuman primates. Called also Ménétrier's disease.
granulomatous g. see gastric HABRONEMIASIS.
histiocytic g. rare cases occur in dogs in association with amyloidosis.
hypertrophic glandular g. see giant hypertrophic gastritis (above).
infarctive g. seen rarely in dogs, usually associated with fungal infection.
toxic g. gastritis resulting from ingestion of a corrosive substance such as a strong acid or poison. There is cramping stomach pain, accompanied by diarrhea and vomiting. The vomitus may be bloody. The victim may collapse.

gastr(o)- word element. [Gr.] *stomach.*

gastroanastomosis see GASTROGASTROSTOMY.

gastrocamera a small camera which can be passed down the esophagus to photograph the inside of the stomach.

gastrocardiac pertaining to the stomach and the heart.

gastrocele hernial protrusion of the stomach or of a gastric pouch.

gastrocentesis percutaneous, transabdominal needle puncture of the stomach to temporarily relieve gastric dilatation prior to more permanent correction of the displacement.

gastrocnemius muscle see Table 13.

g. m. rupture, g. m. avulsion the muscle may have torn away from its insertion, in which case the tendon will be slack, or it may be a complete or partial separation of the belly of the muscle, when the muscle will be swollen and hard. There is a special case in the cow at calving. The cow may be unable to rise. If it does get up the hock is much closer to the ground than normal and the cow may be able to take weight on the leg only if the point of the hock reaches the ground.

slipped g. m. tendon see TENDON luxation.

g. m. tendon the tendon of the gastrocnemius muscle. More accurately the ACHILLES TENDON.

g. m. tendon rupture see gastrocnemius muscle rupture (above). A high incidence may occur in flocks of meat birds but rarely in turkeys.

gastrocnemius reflex a spinal reflex, elicited by tapping the gastrocnemius tendon. A normal response is extension of the hock. Depressed by lesions in the spinal cord from L6 to S2 and of the sciatic and peroneal nerves; increased in spinal cord lesions above L6.

gastrocolic pertaining to or communicating with the stomach and colon.

g. ligament tension usually the result of displacement of the left dorsal colon so that it lies across the ligament; causes reflex dilation of the stomach.

g. reflex distension of the stomach leads to rectal contractions and defecation.

gastrocolitis inflammation of the stomach and colon.

gastrocolostomy surgical anastomosis of the stomach to the colon.

gastrocolotomy incision into the stomach and colon.

gastrocutaneous pertaining to the stomach and skin, or communicating with the stomach and the cutaneous surface of the body, as a gastrocutaneous fistula.

gastrodiaphany examination of the stomach by transillumination of its walls with a small electric lamp passed down the esophagus.

gastrodidymus symmetrical conjoined twins joined in the abdominal region.

Gastrodiscoides a genus of intestinal flukes (digenetic trematodes) in the family Paramphistomatidae.

***G. hominis* (syn. *Gastrodiscus hominis*)** a natural parasite of the colon of the pig but found also in the human cecum.

Gastrodiscus a genus of intestinal flukes (digenetic trematodes) in the family Paramphistomatidae.

G. aegyptiacus found in the intestines of horse, pig and wart hog.

G. hominis see GASTRODISCOIDES *hominis*.

G. secundus found in the colon of horse and elephant.

gastroduodenal pertaining to the stomach and duodenum.

g. anastomosis may be required when lesions in the region of the lesser curvature of the stomach, pyloric antrum and pylorus are surgically removed. Two techniques used are the Billroth type I procedure, when the pancreatic and bile ducts are not involved, and Billroth type II, in which the pancreatic ducts are ligated, the gallbladder is anastomosed to the duodenum, and the stomach is anastomosed to the duodenum or jejunum.

g. junction at the pyloric sphincter.

gastroduodenitis inflammation of the stomach and duodenum.

gastroduodenoscopy endoscopic examination of the stomach and duodenum.

gastroduodenostomy anastomosis of the stomach to a formerly remote part of the duodenum. See GASTRODUODENAL anastomosis (Billroth type I).

gastrodynia pain in the stomach.

gastroenteralgia pain in the stomach and intestines.

gastroenteric pertaining to the stomach and intestines.

gastroenteritis inflammation of the lining of the stomach and intestine. The clinical manifestations are vomiting and diarrhea. See also GASTRITIS.

canine hemorrhagic g. an acute syndrome of vomiting and bloody diarrhea with dehydration and marked hemoconcentration. If not treated vigorously, it may lead to circulatory failure and death in a short time. The cause is unknown.

eosinophilic g. a chronic segmental disease of the alimentary tract characterized by a variety of signs depending on the location of the lesion but including vomiting, or diarrhea or melena or hematochezia. Occurs in dogs, particularly German shepherd dogs, rarely in cats, and in horses. Diarrhea, weight loss and a protein-losing enteropathy result. A hypersensitivity to ingested allergens is the suggested cause. The diagnostic lesion is the aggregation of eosinophils in the intestinal wall. See also eosinophilic GASTRITIS.

transmissible viral g. of pigs see TRANSMISSIBLE gastroenteritis.

gastroenteroanastomosis surgical anastomosis of the stomach to the small intestine.

gastroenterocolitis inflammation of the stomach, small intestine and colon.

gastroenterologist a physician specializing in gastroenterology.

gastroenterology the study of the stomach and intestine and their diseases.

gastroenteropancreatic the unity of the gut and the pancreas.

g. cells produce peptide hormones which help coordinate the physiological processes of digestion and carbohydrate metabolism. The cells are located in the intestinal mucosa and in the islets of Langerhans in the pancreas. The hormones produced include insulin, serotonin, glucagon, somatostatin.

gastroenteropathy any disease of the stomach and intestine.

protein-losing g. see protein-losing ENTEROPATHY.

gastroenteroptosis downward displacement or prolapse of the stomach and intestine.

gastroenterostomy surgical anastomosis of the stomach to the intestine.

gastroenterotomy incision into the stomach and intestine.

gastroepiploic artery see Table 9.

g. a. rupture may be caused by foreign body perforation in traumatic reticulitis in cattle. Causes death due to acute hemorrhagic anemia.

gastroesophageal pertaining to the stomach and esophagus. See also ULCER.

g. reflux see peptic ESOPHAGITIS.

gastroesophagitis inflammation of the stomach and esophagus.

gastroesophagostomy surgical anastomosis between the stomach and esophagus.

gastroferrin an iron-binding protein found in gastric juice.

gastrofiberscope a fiberscope for viewing the stomach.

gastrogastrostomy surgical creation of an anastomosis of two previously remote portions of the stomach, such as anastomosis between the pyloric and cardiac ends of the stomach.
gastrogavage artificial feeding through a tube passed into the stomach.
gastrogenic originating in the stomach.
gastrogram gastric x-ray. See also PNEUMOGASTROGRAM.
gastrograph an instrument for registering motions of the stomach.
gastrography contrast radiography of the stomach.
double contrast g. radiography of the stomach taken after administration of barium, then air. Useful in evaluating details of the gastric mucosa.
gastrohepatic pertaining to the stomach and liver.
gastrohepatitis inflammation of the stomach and liver.
gastroileac pertaining to the stomach and ileum.
gastroileitis inflammation of the stomach and ileum.
gastroileostomy surgical anastomosis of the stomach to the ileum.
gastrointestinal pertaining to the stomach and intestine.
g. foreign body see INTESTINAL obstruction.
g. hormones hormones secreted by the gastrointestinal epithelium that affect the function of the tract itself and of its allied organs, e.g. gastrin, glucagon, enteroglucagon, somatostatin, secretin, cholecystokinin-pancreozymin, motilin, gastric inhibitory polypeptide, vasoactive intestinal polypeptide.
g. series a radiological examination of the upper gastrointestinal tract using barium as the contrast medium for a series of x-ray films. Called also a barium meal. See BARIUM study.
g. tract the stomach and intestines in continuity. See also DIGESTIVE system.
gastrojejunal pertaining to the stomach and jejunum.
g. constipation constipation occurring reflexly as a result of disease somewhere in the alimentary tract.
gastrojejunocolic pertaining to the stomach, jejunum and colon.
gastrojejunostomy anastomosis of the stomach to a formerly remote part of the duodenum. See GASTRODUODENAL anastomosis (Billroth type II).
gastrolienal pertaining to the stomach and spleen; gastrosplenic.
gastrolith a calculus in the stomach.
gastrolithiasis the presence or formation of gastroliths.
Gastrolobium a genus of Australian plants in the Fabaceae family, with numerous toxic species. All but one occur in south-western Australia. The toxic principle is monofluoroacetic acid and all species cause sudden death due to cardiomyopathy and heart failure.

G. appressum, *G. bennettsianum*, *G. bilobum*, *G. callistachys*, *G. calycinum*, *G. crassifolium*, *G. densifolium*, *G. floribundum*, *G. forrestii*, *G. glaucum*, *G. grandiflorum*, *G. graniticum*, *G. hamulosum*, *G. heterophyllum*, *G. laytonii*, *G. microcarpum*, *G. ovalifolium*, *G. oxyloboides*, *G. parviflorum*, *G. parvifolium*, *G. polystachyum*, *G. propinquum*, *G. pycnostachyum*, *G. racemosum*, *G. rotundifolium*, *G. spectabile*, *G. spinosum*, *G. stenophyllum*, *G. tetragonophyllum*, *G. tomentosum*, *G. trilobum*, *G. velutinum* and *G. villosum* are shrubs of various heights and habits. All have a common name including the word poison, e.g. heart-leaf poison bush. Several were previously classified as *Oxylobium* spp.
gastrology study of the stomach and its diseases.
gastrolysis surgical division of perigastric adhesions to mobilize the stomach.
gastromalacia softening of the wall of the stomach.
gastromegaly enlargement of the stomach.
gastromycosis fungal infection of the stomach.
gastromyxorrhea excessive secretion of mucus by the stomach.
gastroparalysis paralysis of the stomach; gastroplegia.
gastropathy any disease of the stomach.
chronic hypertrophic pyloric g. a syndrome of pyloric obstruction in dogs. See also giant hypertrophic GASTRITIS.
gastropexy surgical fixation of the stomach, most commonly to the abdominal wall as a means of preventing recurrence of gastric volvulus.
belt-loop g. a modification of the circumcostal technique in which the seromuscular gastric flap is passed around a loop of transverse abdominal muscle instead of a rib.
circumcostal g. fixation by a flap of gastric serosa and muscularis anchored around a rib.
permanent incisional g. edges of an incision into the seromuscular layers of the pyloric antrum are sutured to an incision into the peritoneum and internal fascia of the rectus abdominal or transverse abdominal muscles.
tube g. a method using a Foley catheter placed in the pyloric antrum and through the abdominal wall in the right paracostal area during the postsurgical period.
Gastrophilus see GASTEROPHILUS.
gastrophrenic pertaining to the stomach and diaphragm.
g. ligament binds the left crus of the diaphragm to the fundus of the stomach.
gastroplasty plastic repair of the stomach.
gastroplegia gastroparalysis.
gastroplication treatment of gastric dilatation by stitching a fold in the stomach wall.
gastropod univalve shellfish, e.g. snail, whelk, cone.
gastroptosis downward displacement of the stomach.
gastropulmonary pertaining to the stomach and lungs.
gastropylorectomy excision of the pyloric part of the stomach.
gastropyloric pertaining to the stomach and pylorus.
gastrorrhagia hemorrhage from the stomach.
gastrorrhaphy suture of the stomach.
gastrorrhea excessive secretion by the glands of the stomach.
gastroschisis a congenital fissure of the abdominal wall.
gastroscope an endoscope especially designed for passage into the stomach to permit examination of its interior. The gastroscope is a hollow, cylindrical tube fitted with special lenses and lights. The newer types of gastroscope are made of glass fiber (fiberscope) which is more flexible. Each glass fiber reflects light and creates a mirror effect, making it possible to 'go around corners', and facilitating visualization of the curvature of the stomach.
gastroscopy inspection of the interior of the stomach with a gastroscope.
gastrospasm spasm of the stomach.
gastrosplenic pertaining to the stomach and spleen; gastrolienal.
gastrostaxis the oozing of blood from the stomach mucosa.
gastrostenosis contraction or shrinkage of the stomach.

gastrostogavage feeding through a gastric fistula.
gastrostolavage irrigation of the stomach through a gastric fistula.
gastrostomy the creation of an opening into the stomach.
 blind g. placement of a gastric feeding tube without laparatomy or endoscope, simply by manipulating the end of the tube through the stomach and body wall.
 percutaneous g. used for placement of a gastric feeding tube. An endoscope is used to position an incision through the body wall and stomach wall, to grasp and withdraw a suture inserted through the opening and to guide the placement of the tube which is pulled back into the stomach and through the opening by traction on the suture which has been attached to the distal end of the tube.
 tube g. as part of the surgical correction of gastric dilatation–volvulus, an inflatable catheter can be used to maintain traction on the stomach, provide fixation, and allow decompression.
gastrothoracopagus symmetrical conjoined twins joined at the abdomen and thorax.
Gastrothylax a genus of stomach flukes (digenetic trematodes) in the family Paramphistomatidae.
 G. crumenifer an elongated circular fluke found in the rumen and reticulum in sheep, cattle, zebu and buffalo.
gastrotomy incision into the stomach.
gastrotropic having affinity for or exerting a special effect on the stomach.
gastrotympanites tympanitic distension of the stomach.
gastrula an embryo in the stage following the blastula stage; the simplest type consists of two layers of cells, the ectoderm and entoderm, which have invaginated to form the archenteron and an opening, the blastopore.
gastrulation the process by which a blastula becomes a gastrula or, in forms without a true blastula, the process by which three germ cell layers are acquired.
gat see CATHA EDULIS.
gate control a theory of physiological control of pain based on the proposal that pain impulses are mediated in the substantia gelatinosa of the spinal cord and the dorsal horns act as 'gates' that control the entry of pain signals into the central pain pathways.
gathered nail a nail gathered up and penetrating the sole of the horse's hoof. See HOOF abscess, TETANUS. Called also nail prick.
gating alteration of the transport function through a mucosa; can be effected by means of a chemical agent (chemical gating) or because of a change in electrical potential (electrical gating).
Gaucher's cells large, foamy macrophages characteristic of Gaucher's disease which accumulate in many tissues; they result from accumulated glucocerebroside due to deficiency in β-GLUCOCEREBROSIDASE.
Gaucher's disease a hereditary disorder of glucocerebroside metabolism, marked by the presence of Gaucher's cells in many tissues. Occurs in dogs (Australian silky terriers), sheep, pigs and mice. See also GLUCOCEREBROSIDE, GAUCHER'S CELLS.
gaunt thin plus obvious diminution in abdominal size, indicative of reduced feed intake leading to reduced gut fill.
Gaur see BOS *gaurus*.
gauze a light, open-meshed fabric of muslin or similar material.
 absorbent g. white cotton cloth of various thread counts and weights, supplied in various lengths and widths and in different forms (rolls or folds).
 g. mask see SURGICAL mask.
 petrolatum g. a sterile material produced by saturation of sterile absorbent gauze with sterile white petrolatum.
 zinc gelatin impregnated g. absorbent gauze impregnated with zinc gelatin.
gavage [Fr.] 1. forced feeding or irrigation through a tube passed into the stomach. See also tube FEEDING, gastric LAVAGE. 2. superalimentation.
gavial, gharial a member of the crocodile family, e.g. Indian gavial (*Gavialis gangeticus*).
gazehound a sight-hunting hound such as the Greyhound.
Gazella see GAZELLE.
gazelle very fast-moving, sandy-colored, small, wild ruminant with white rump and lyre-shaped, long horns. There are many species including impala and springbok. Called also *Gazella* spp.
 g. hound see SALUKI.
GD glutamate dehydrogenase.
Gd chemical symbol, *gadolinium.*
GDP guanosine diphosphate.
GDV gastric dilatation/volvulus.
Ge chemical symbol, *germanium.*
gearing ratio of debt to equity.
Gedoelstia a genus of flies of the family Oestridae.
 G. cristata larvae are deposited in the eye and pass via a vein to the cardiovascular system. Larvae migrate up the trachea to the nasal cavity. Aberrant infection occurs in domestic ruminants; the usual hosts are wild ruminants.
 G. hassleri larvae of this fly are deposited in the conjunctival sac and migrate to the nasal cavity via blood vessels, meninges and subdural space in hartebeeste and wildebeeste, but without causing clinical illness. Aberrant infection occurs in domestic ruminants causing severe ocular and neural disease. Called also ophthalmomyiasis, uitpeuloog, gedoelstial myiasis.
gedoelstial myiasis infestation with the larvae of the fly *Gedoelstia* spp.
geeldikkop [Af.] see yellow BIGHEAD.
geese domestic geese which were derived from the wild goose *Anser anser.* There are many other species in this genus and in the other genus of geese, the *Branta* spp. of which *Branta canadensis* is typical.
Geiger counter, Geiger–Müller counter an amplifying device that indicates the presence of ionizing particles emitted by a substance; used as a means of determining the presence of radioactivity.
Geigeria a genus of plants in the family Asteraceae. Contain sesquiterpene lactones which cause vermeersiekte—degeneration of skeletal muscles manifested as stiffness and paralysis, plus brain and spinal cord damage. There is also esophageal dilation and vomition. Includes *G. aspera* var. *aspera*, *G. burkei* subsp. *burkei* var. *zeyheri*, *G. filifolia*, *G. ornativa* (*G. africana*), *G. passerinoides*, *G. pectidae*.
geilsiekte [Af.] plant-associated cyanide poisoning; literal translation = lush pasture sickness.
gel a colloid that is firm in consistency, although containing much liquid; a colloid in a gelatinous form.
 coupling g. see COUPLING.
 g. diffusion technique see IMMUNODIFFUSION.
gelatin a substance obtained by partial hydrolysis of collagen derived from skin, white connective tissue, and bones of animals; used as a suspending agent for various drugs or in manufacture of capsules and suppositories; suggested for intravenous use as a plasma substitute, and has been used as an adjuvant protein

food. In absorbable film and sponge, it is used in surgical procedures.

g. digestion test a tube test for the presence of fecal proteases; used in the diagnosis of exocrine pancreatic insufficiency.

g. liquefaction test a biochemical test used for the identification of several bacterial species. Detects the ability of the organism to produce substances which hydrolyze gelatin.

g. sponge a spongy form of denatured gelatin, soaked with thrombin and used as a hemostatic.

zinc g. a preparation of zinc oxide, gelatin, glycerin and purified water, applied topically as a protective.

gelatinize to convert into a jelly, or to become converted into gelatin. Feed grains are said to be gelatinized when they are treated by a combination of moisture, heat and pressure so as to rupture their starch granules.

gelatinoid resembling gelatin.

gelatinous like jelly or softened gelatin.

gelation conversion of a sol into a gel.

Gelbvieh cream to red and yellow dual-purpose breed of cattle. Called also German Yellow, Austrian Yellow.

geld see ALTER.

gelding castrated male horse.

gelosis a hard, swollen lump in a tissue, especially in muscle.

Gelpi retractor a self-retaining, small spreader suitable for small sites such as for perineal surgery in dogs or laryngotomy in horses. Two blades, hinged in the middle, separate as the handles are closed and are held open by a rachet. The blades turn down at right angles at their tips, and are bowed towards each other so that they push the edges of the incision apart and retain themselves in it.

gelsemine a toxic indole alkaloid in the plant *Gelsemium sempervirens*; has similar pharmacological actions to nicotine.

Gelsemium sempervirens temperate zone garden plant in the family Loganiaceae; poisoning by the plant is manifested by incoordination, pupillary dilatation and convulsions. The toxin is the indole alkaloid gelsemine. Called also yellow jessamine, Carolina jessamine, evening trumpetflower.

Gély's suture pattern a continuous series of cross stitches for wounds of the intestine, made with a thread having a needle at each end.

gemastocyte see gemistocytic ASTROCYTE.

gemellology the scientific study of twins and twinning.

geminate paired; occurring in twos.

gemination the abnormal tooth formation as a result of an unsuccessful attempt at forming two separate teeth. There is usually a longitudinal groove.

gemistocyte plump astrocyte produced as a reaction to severe injury.

gemmation development of a new organism from a protuberance on the cell body of the parent, a form of asexual reproduction; called also budding.

gemmule 1. a reproductive bud; the immediate product of gemmation. 2. any of the little spinelike processes on the dendrites of a nerve cell.

gemsbok a medium-sized antelope. Called also *Oryx gazella*.

-gen word element. [Gr.] *an agent that produces.*

genal pertaining to the cheek; buccal.

gender sex; the category to which an individual is assigned on the basis of sex.

gene the unit of heredity most simply defined as a specific segment of DNA, usually in the order of 1000 nucleotides, that specifies a single polypeptide. Many phenotypic characteristics are determined by a single gene, while others are multigenic. Genes are specifically located in linear order along the single DNA molecule that makes up each chromosome. All eukaryotic cells contain a diploid (2n) set of chromosomes so that two copies of each gene, one derived from each parent, are present in each cell; the two copies often specify a different phenotype, i.e. the polypeptide will have a somewhat different amino acid composition. These alternative forms of gene, both within and between individuals, are called alleles. Genes determine the physical (structural genes), the biochemical (enzymes), physiological and behavioral characteristics of an animal.

The formation of gametes (sperm, ova) involves a process of meiosis, which allows crossing over between four pairs of chromosomes, two derived from each parent, which means that new forms of a particular chromosome are created. Gamete formation also results in cells (gametes) with a haploid (n) set of chromosomes that in fertilization creates a new individual, which is a recombinant of 2n chromosomes, half derived by way of the ovum from the mother and half via the spermatozoa from the father.

Changes in the nucleotide sequence of a gene, either by substitution of a different nucleotide or by deletion or insertion of other nucleotides, constitute mutations which add to the diversity of animal species by creating different alleles and can be used as a basis for genetic selection of different phenotypes. Some mutations, be they a single base change in a single gene or a major deletion, are lethal.

g. action the way in which genes exert their effects on tissues or processes, e.g by being dominant or recessive, or partially so, being absent, being sex-linked, being involved in chromosomal aberrations.

allelic g's different forms of a particular gene usually situated at the same position (locus) in a pair of chromosomes.

g. amplification see gene duplication (below).

g. bank the collection of DNA sequences in a given genome. Called also gene library.

barring g. responsible for the barred pattern on the feathers of Barred Plymouth Rock birds.

g. box see BOX (4).

g. clone see CLONE.

g. cluster a group of related genes derived from a common ancestral gene, located closely together on the same chromosome. Called also multigene family.

complementary g's two independent pairs of nonallelic genes, neither of which is functional without the other.

g. conversion a non-reciprocal exchange of DNA elements during meiosis which results in a functional rearrangement of chromosomal DNA.

***dhfr* g.** dihydrofolate reductase gene; an enzyme required to maintain cellular concentrations of H_2 folate for nucleotide biosynthesis, and which has been used as a 'selective marker'; cells lacking the enzyme only survive in media containing thymidine, glycine and purines; mutant cells (dhfr) transfected with DNA that is dhfr′ can be selectively grown in medium lacking these elements.

diversity (D) g. genes located in diversity (D) segment; contribute to the hypervariable region of immunoglobulins.

dominant g. one that produces an effect (the phenotype) in the organism regardless of the state of the corresponding allele. Examples of traits determined

by dominant genes are short hair in cats and black coat color in dogs.
g. duplication as a result of non-homologous recombination, a chromosome carries two or more copies of a gene.
g. expression see EXPRESSION (3).
g. frequency the proportion of the substances or animals in the group which carry a particular gene.
holandric g's genes located on the Y chromosome and appearing only in male offspring.
immune response (Ir) g's genes of the major histocompatibility complex (MHC) that govern the immune response to individual immunogens.
jumping g. see mobile DNA.
g. knockout replacement of a normal gene with a mutant allele, as in gene knockout mice.
lethal g. one whose presence brings about the death of the organism or permits survival only under certain conditions.
g. library see gene bank (above).
g. locus see LOCUS.
mutant g. one that has undergone a detectable mutation.
non-protein encoding g. the final products of some genes are RNA molecules rather than proteins.
overlapping g's when more than one mRNA is transcribed from the same DNA sequence; the mRNAs may be in the same reading frame but of different size or they may be in different reading frames.
g. pool total of all genes possessed by all members of the population which are capable of reproducing during their lifetime.
g. probe see PROBE (2).
recessive g. one that produces an effect in the organism only when it is transmitted by both parents, i.e. only when the individual is homozygous.
regulator g., repressor g. one that synthesizes repressor, a substance which, through interaction with the operator gene, switches off the activity of the structural genes associated with it in the operon.
reporter g. one that produces products which can be measured and therefore used as an indicator of whether a DNA construct has successfully been transferred.
sex-linked g. one that is carried on a sex chromosome, especially an X chromosome.
g. splicing see SPLICING.
structural g. nucleotide sequences coding for proteins.
g. therapy the insertion of functional genes into cells of the host in order to alter its phenotype, usually used to treat an inherited defect.
g. transcription see TRANSCRIPTION.
g. transfer see RECOMBINATION.

genera [L.] plural of *genus*.

general in a clinical context means whole of body.
g. clinical assessment an overall statement on the patient's state of health.
g. clinical examination a complete clinical examination including all body systems.
g. populations include all classes and levels of animals (or plants) without any attempt to categorize them.

general adaptation syndrome the syndrome described in humans as a consequence of continued stress. There is no identified counterpart in animals.

generalization forming general propositions from particular cases or clinical signs.

generalized glycogenosis see bovine generalized GLYCOGENOSIS.

generalized Shwartzman-like reaction a reaction characterized by disseminated intravascular coagulation; caused by oliguric renal failure in cases of septicemia or endotoxemia in parturient cows; see also SHWARTZMAN PHENOMENON.

generalized tremor syndrome see SHAKER DOGS.

generation 1. the process of reproduction. 2. a class composed of all individuals removed by the same number of successive ancestors from a common predecessor, or occupying positions on the same level in a genealogical (pedigree) chart. Said also of antibiotics or other chemicals derived from parent compounds.
alternate g. reproduction by alternate asexual and sexual means in an animal or plant species.
asexual g. production of a new organism not originating from union of gametes. Called also direct generation.
direct g. see asexual generation (above).
filial g. (first) the first generation offspring of two parents; symbol F_1.
filial g. (second) all of the offspring produced by two individuals of the first filial generation; symbol F_2.
g. interval the mean age of the parents when the animals that are to replace them are born.
parental g. the generation with which a particular genetic study is begun; symbol P_1.
sexual g. production of a new organism from the zygote formed by the union of gametes.
spontaneous g. the discredited concept of continuous generation of living organisms from nonliving matter.
g. time 1. in epidemiological terms the time required between infection occurring and the patient reaching full infectivity. 2. in histological terms the time required to complete one full cell cycle; average of 20 hours for mammalian cells.

generative pertaining to reproduction.

generator something that produces or causes to exist; a machine that converts mechanical to electrical energy.
pulse g. the power source for a cardiac pacemaker system, usually powered by a lithium battery, supplying impulses to the implanted electrodes, either at a fixed rate or in a programmed pattern.

generic 1. pertaining to a genus. 2. nonproprietary; denoting a drug name not protected by a trademark, usually descriptive of the drug's chemical structure.
g. pet food commercially prepared pet foods without a brand name; usually of low cost and possibly of poor quality. High levels of calcium in generic dog foods have reportedly been the cause of copper, zinc and iodine deficiency in a syndrome called generic dog food disease.

genesiology the sum of what is known concerning generation.

genesis creation; origination; used as a word termination joined to an element indicating the thing created, e.g. carcinogenesis.

genet 1. a small, 16 to 20 inch long without the tail, arboreal and terrestrial, nocturnal, carnivorous animal. It has a long tail and a spotted and striped coat. It is the *Genetta* spp. of the family Viverridae. 2. see JENNY.

genetic 1. pertaining to reproduction or to birth or origin. 2. inherited.
g. abnormality inherited defect, which may or may not be congenital.
g. analysis analysis of breeding and pedigree records to establish degrees of relationship between single animals and groups of animals. Segregation analysis with full-sibling families is an obvious technique.

g. code the manner in which the arrangement of nucleotides in the polynucleotide chain of a chromosome governs the transmission of genetic information to proteins, i.e. determines the sequence of amino acids in the polypeptide chain making up each protein synthesized by the cell. Genetic information is coded in DNA by means of four bases (two purines: adenine and guanine; and two pyrimidines: thymine and cystosine). Each adjacent sequence of three bases (a codon) determines which of the 20 amino acids will be inserted into the nascent polypeptide.

g. complementation see COMPLEMENTATION.

g. control of inherited disease consists of preventing carrier animals from contributing their genes to succeeding generations of the population of which they are members.

g. correlation a change in an unselected character resulting from selection of another character during a breeding program.

g. defects defects of function or structure passed on from parents to offspring. Inherited defects.

g. determination see broad-sense HERITABILITY.

g. disease resistance inherited resistance to diseases caused by non-hereditary risk factors.

g. dominance see DOMINANCE (2).

g. drift see ANTIGENIC drift.

g. engineering the manipulation of genes by recombinant DNA technologies to produce chromosomal combinations that are unlikely to occur by natural means, for example the introduction of genes for insulin into a yeast cell which then produces insulin which can be purified and used as a therapeutic substance. See also RECOMBINANT DNA technology.

g. etiology disease caused by inheritance of specific disease without the intervention of other risk factors; established by strongly positive relationship in terms of genes held in common between the affected patient and other affected individuals.

g. evaluation assessment, for predictive purposes, of productive improvement or conformational characteristics, of the gain to be derived by the use of the animal in question in a breeding program.

g. expressivity see EXPRESSIVITY.

g. heterogeneity demonstrated by the way in which more than one disease with identical clinical signs can be inherited.

g. immunization use of a cloned genetically engineered gene with an encoded antigen to immunize the host against that antigen. See also DNA VACCINE.

g. map the linear arrangement of genes along a chromosome. Called also linkage map.

g. merit inherited productivity or performance qualities.

mobile g. elements see transposable genetic elements (below).

g. penetrance see PENETRANCE.

g. production potential inherited productivity but still influenced by environmental risk factors.

g. resistance genetically determined resistance to specified infectious agents.

g. selection selection of animals as breeding stock on the basis of known inherited characteristics.

transposable g. elements pieces of DNA varying in length from a few hundred to tens of thousands of base pairs found in both prokaryotic and eukaryotic cells that move from place to place in the chromosomes of a single cell; some are viruses. Called also mobile genetic elements or transposons.

g. variance that portion of the phenotypic variance of a trait in a population which can be attributed to genetic difference amongst individuals.

geneticist a specialist in genetics.

genetics the branch of biology dealing with the phenomena of heredity and the laws governing it. Expressed in other definitions, e.g. POPULATION genetics.

biochemical g. the science concerned with the chemical and physical nature of genes and the mechanism by which they control the development and maintenance of the organism.

The field of biochemical or molecular genetics is relatively new and is increasingly used to define the cause of many inherited diseases. These diseases usually result from defective protein synthesis, such as HEMOPHILIA A and IMMUNODEFICIENCY, and more than 200 so-called 'inborn errors' of metabolism identified thus far in animals, such as MANNOSIDOSIS and GALACTOSEMIA, in which lack or alteration of a specific enzyme prohibits proper metabolism of carbohydrates, proteins or fats and thus produces clinical signs.

clinical g. the study of the possible genetic factors influencing the occurrence of a pathological condition. In addition to the diseases mentioned under biochemical genetics, other aspects of clinical genetics include the study of chromosomal aberrations, such as those that cause testicular hypoplasia, and immunogenetics, or the genetic aspects of the IMMUNE response and the transmission of genetic factors from generation to generation.

molecular g. the study of the molecular structure of genes, involving DNA and RNA. See also DEOXYRIBONUCLEIC ACID.

genetotrophic disease caused by the inheritance of a higher requirement than normal for a specific metabolite.

Genetta see GENET (1).

genial pertaining to the chin.

genic pertaining to or caused by the genes.

-genic word element. [Gr.] *giving rise to, causing.*

genicular pertaining to the knee.

geniculate bent, like a knee.

g. body see geniculate BODY (lateral).

g. ganglion see geniculate GANGLION.

geniculum pl. *genicula* [L.] a little knee; a sharp kneelike bend in a small structure or organ.

genioplasty plastic surgery of the chin.

Genista see CYTISUS.

genistein an isoflavone with estrogenic properties and found in subterranean and other clovers.

genital pl. *genitalia* 1. pertaining to reproduction, or the REPRODUCTIVE organs. 2. *genitals*, the REPRODUCTIVE organs, especially the external genital organs.

g. bursatti see SWAMP CANCER.

g. campylobacteriosis see bovine VIBRIOSIS.

g. ducts male—efferent ductules, ductus epididymis, ductus deferens; female—uterine tubes (fallopian tubes, oviducts), uterus, vagina.

g. lock the joining together of the dog and the bitch during coitus in which the enlarged penile bulb of the dog is held tightly in the bitch's vagina. The dog normally dismounts and stands back-to-back with the bitch, with the penis still locked in the vagina. Called also the 'tie'.

g. mycoplasmosis see GRANULAR vaginitis.

g. organs see PENIS, VULVA, etc.

g. ridge bilateral thickenings in the roof of the embryo's celom which are the primordia of the gonads.

g. squamous cell carcinoma squamous cell carcinoma of the penis and prepuce and of the vulva.

g. system the reproductive system including ovaries,

ovarian bursa, uterine tubes, uterus, cervix, vagina, vulva, vestibular glands of the female and testicles, epididymis, vas deferens, penis, prostate, seminal vesicles, bulbourethral glands, prepuce and scrotum of the male.
g. tract from the ovaries to the vulva, from the testicles to the external urethral meatus.
g. tubercle the eminence in the embryo which develops into the clitoris or penis.
g.–urinary system the combined urinary and reproductive systems.
g. vibriosis see bovine VIBRIOSIS.
g. warts see genital PAPILLOMATOSIS.
genitalia see GENITAL system.
external g. vulva of the female, testes, penis of the male.
genito- word element. [L.] relating to the organs of reproduction.
genitocrural pertaining to the genitalia and the leg or shank.
genitofemoral pertaining to the genitalia and the thigh.
genitoplasty plastic surgery on the reproductive (genital) organs.
genitourinary pertaining to the genitalia and urinary apparatus; urogenital.
g. system the organs of reproduction, together with the organs concerned with production and excretion of urine; called also urogenital, genitourinary system.
genocopy an animal whose phenotype mimics that of another genotype but whose character is determined by a distinct assortment of genes.
genodermatosis a genetic disorder of the skin, usually generalized.
genome all of the genes carried by a gamete, i.e. the complete set of hereditary factors contained in the chromosomal DNA. For some viruses, the genome is RNA.
diploid g. having two genetically identical RNA molecules of RNA, characteristic of retroviruses.
integrated g. the integration of the viral DNA into the cellular DNA of the host, as occurs in some kinds of persistent infections and the induction of tumors.
segmented g. the genome is composed of separate segments. A characteristic of some viruses.
genomic pertaining to a genome.
g. clone see CLONE.
g. DNA the DNA sequences making up the genome of an individual.
g. library see GENE bank.
genotype 1. the entire genetic constitution of an individual; also, the alleles present at one or more specific loci. 2. the type species of a genus.
g. frequency the proportion of the population which have the same genetic constitution.
genotypic emanating from or pertaining to genotype.
g. selection selection of breeding stock on the basis of known inherited characteristics.
g. value value of the effect of all the individual's genes which affect the trait in question.
g. variance the measure of the differences in genotype between individuals, i.e. the differences between individuals in factors which are determined the moment they are conceived.
-genous word element. [Gr.] *arising or resulting from, produced by.*
gentamicin, gentamycin an antibiotic complex elaborated by fungi of the genus *Mircromonospora*, effective against many gram-negative bacteria, especially *Pseudomonas* species, as well as certain gram-positive bacteria, especially *Staphylococcus aureus*. As with other aminoglycoside antibiotics gentamicin is ototoxic and nephrotoxic. Used as the sulfate.
gentian the dried rhizome and roots of *Gentiana lutea*; has been used as a bitter tonic.
g. violet an antibacterial, antifungal and anthelmintic dye, derived from triphenylmethane; applied topically in the treatment of infections of the skin and mucous membranes associated with gram-positive bacteria and molds, and at one time administered orally for the treatment of pinworm and liver fluke infections in humans. Called also crystal violet, methylrosaniline chloride.
gentianophilic staining readily with gentian violet.
gentianophobic not staining with gentian violet.
gentle to accustom a young horse to be caught, handled, haltered and led but not broken in to saddle or harness.
genu pl. *genua* [L.] the knee.
g. extrorsum bowleg.
g. of facial nerve the bend in the facial nerve at the lateral end of the internal acoustic meatus.
g. introrsum knock-knee.
g. recurvatum hyperextensibility of the knee joint.
g. valgum knock-knee.
g. varum bowleg.
genus pl. *genera* [L.] a taxonomic category (taxon) subordinate to a tribe (or subtribe) and superior to a species (or subgenus).
geo- word element. [Gr.] *the earth, the soil.*
***Geochelone* spp.** a genus of tortoises. Includes *G. carbonaria* (South American red-footed tortoise), *G. chilensis* (Argentine tortoise).
geode a dilated lymph space.
geographic pertaining to geography.
g. epidemiology the effect of climate, terrain, population of humans and animals, industrial enterprises on animal disease. Includes the zoogeography of the subject species itself, plus that of carrier species, and vectors and intermediate hosts, especially mobile ones such as insects. The distribution and concentration of poisonous plants and the use of specific management techniques which put the animals at greater risk are also important.
g. ulcer see geographic ULCER.
geomedicine the branch of medicine dealing with the influence of climatic and environmental conditions on health. See also GEOGRAPHIC epidemiology.
geometric mean see geometric MEAN.
Geomys see GOPHER.
geophagia, geophagism the habit of eating clay or earth (soil); chthonophagia.
geophilic soil-loving; said of certain fungi found in soil.
Georgina gidgee see ACACIA *georginae.*
Georgina gidyea see ACACIA *georginae.*
geotaxis see GEOTROPISM.
Geotrichia see MICROCYSTIS.
geotrichosis a candidiasis-like infection due to *Geotrichum candidum*, which may attack the bronchi, lungs, mouth or intestinal tract.
Geotrichum a genus of yeastlike fungi. See HYALOHYPHOMYCOSIS.
G. candidum a species found in feces and in dairy products. Causes a systemic infection, especially in animals in captivity, and has been associated with necrosis of the scales in snakes. May be associated with bovine mastitis. See also GEOTRICHOSIS.
geotropism a tendency of growth or movement toward or away from the earth; the influence of gravity on growth.
GEP gastroenteropancreatic.

ger-, gero-, geronto- word element. [Gr.] *old age, the aged.*

geratic pertaining to old age.

geratology, gereology the science dealing with old age. See also GERIATRICS.

gerbil *Gerbillus* spp. or *Tatera* spp.

Mongolian g. *Meriones unguiculatus*; a small rodent, native to desert regions in Mongolia and China, related to the gerbil. Typically has an agouti coat but other colors have been developed. Have fully furred tails, ears and footpads. Called also jird.

Gerbillus see GERBIL.

gerenuk a tall antelope with a long, thin neck which it uses to maximum effect while browsing. Called also *Litocranius walleri* and giraffe-necked gazelle.

Gerhardt's test a test for ketone bodies in the urine, using ferric chloride.

geriatric pertaining to or emanating from geriatrics.

canine g. syndrome see canine idiopathic VESTIBULAR syndrome.

geriatrician a specialist in geriatrics.

geriatrics the branch of medicine dealing with the problems of aging and diseases of the older animal; usually dealing with companion animals.

Gerlach needle a needle designed for inserting buried, perivaginal sutures in cows. Consists of a loop large enough to fill the palm, a shank about 4 inches long and a slightly scooped, flattened point with an eyehole large enough to take tape. Reminiscent of a bagneedle.

germ 1. old-fashioned and lay term for a pathogenic microorganism. 2. living substance capable of developing into an organ, part or organism as a whole; a primordium. Commonly used to refer to the embryos of wheat grains which are removed during milling and sold separately as wheat germ.

g. cell direct descendants of the primordial cells which originate from the yolk sac endoderm and migrate to the gonadal ridges of the embryo, where they give rise to either ova or spermatozoa. Called also gonocytes, sex cells.

g. cell tumor a rare tumor in dogs, similar to more common lesions in humans. Similar to pituitary adenomas in distribution and cellular characteristics.

g. line the genetic material as it is transferred via the gametes, before being modified by somatic recombination or mutation.

g. line cells gametes.

g. line transmission a mode of transmission, particularly of retroviruses, whereby the genome of the virus is integrated into the chromosomal DNA and transmitted via gametes to offspring.

g. plasma evaluation program a planned imvestigative, large scale breeding program aimed at accumulating comparative information on the relative performance of various breeds and crossbreeds of agricultural animals.

g. theory 1. all organisms are developed from a cell. 2. infectious diseases are of microbial origin.

g. tube a tube-like structure that develops during the growth of some fungi and becomes a hypha; a feature of the yeast, *Candida albicans.*

wheat g. see WHEAT germ.

germ free animal see AXENIC.

German black pied cattle German adaptation of Friesian dairy cattle.

German blackheaded mutton sheep polled, meat, shortwool German sheep originated from British downs breeds sheep.

German brown cattle German adaptation of Brown Swiss cattle.

German mastiff see GREAT DANE.

German pinscher a medium-sized (25–35 lb), compact dog with a short, smooth coat in black or shades of gray, red or brown. The ears may be erect or dropped, but usually cropped, and the tail is docked to a short length. Called also Standard Pinscher.

German roller a breed of canaries descended from the Hartz Mountain Roller canary. See ROLLER.

German shepherd dog a large muscular dog with medium length, double coat of tan and black, erect ears and bushy tail. The breed has been used widely as a working dog in police and military activities and as a guide dog for the blind. It is predisposed to epilepsy, giant axonal neuropathy, pituitary dwarfism, hip dysplasia, pyoderma, anal furunculosis, pancreatic insufficiency, pannus, persistent right aortic arch, subaortic stenosis, eosinophilic myositis and von Willebrand's disease. Called also Alsatian.

German shorthaired pointer a medium- to large-sized gun dog with pendulous ears, docked tail and very short haircoat that is liver- or black-colored in solid, spotted or ticked patterns. It is used as a retriever and pointer. The breed is affected by an inherited GM_2 gangliosidosis.

German spitz a spitz-type dog with a broad head, small, triangular erect ears, a curled tail and an abundant coat that stands out. Several sizes are recognized.

German whiteheaded mutton sheep polled, meat sheep originated from British Cotswold and Marsh sheep plus Texel.

German wirehaired pointer a medium- to large-sized gun dog with a harsh, medium length coat in solid liver or liver or black with white spots or ticking. The ears are pendant and the tail is docked to half its length. Called also Griffon (wire-haired pointer).

German yellow see GELBVIEH.

germanium a chemical element, atomic number 32, atomic weight 72.59, symbol Ge. See Table 6.

germicidal destructive to pathogenic microorganisms.

germicide an agent that destroys pathogenic microorganisms.

germinal pertaining to or of the nature of a germ cell or the primitive stage of development.

g. crescent the region of development of primary germ cells in the avian embryo.

g. inclusion cyst see OVARIAN serous inclusion cyst.

germination the sprouting of a seed or spore or of a plant embryo.

germinative pertaining to germination or to a germ cell.

germinoma a neoplasm of germ tissue (testis or ovum), e.g. a seminoma.

geroderma, gerodermia dystrophy of the skin and genitals, giving the appearance of old age.

geromarasmus the emaciation sometimes characteristic of old age.

gerontal pertaining to old age.

Gerstmann–Strausser disease a human disease, like Kuru and Creutzfeldt–Jakob disease, similar in brain pathology to scrapie.

gestagen any hormone with progestational activity.

gestation the period of development of the young in viviparous animals, from the time of fertilization of the ovum to birth. See also PREGNANCY.

g. period the duration of pregnancy in the domestic animal species are: cow—273 to 292 days (*Bos taurus*), 271 to 310 days (*Bos indicus*); mare—333 to 346 days; ass—365 to 375 days; ewe—143 to 147 days (meat sheep), 147 to 155 days (merino); goat doe—146 to 155 days; sow—111 to 116 days; bitch—58 to 68 days; queen—61 to 70 days.

In laboratory and quasi-pet animals: guinea pig 59–72 days, gerbil 24–26 days, hamster 15.5–16 days, mouse 19–21 days, rat 21–23 days, rabbit 29–35 days.
perpetual g. chart a table based on the average gestation period of the particular species, e.g. 63 days for bitches, that plots the anticipated date of parturition against the breeding (conception) date. Designed to be independent of the year so it is valid indefinitely.
prolonged g. see PROLONGED GESTATION.
gestational pertaining to or emanating from gestation.
g. age the age of the fetus in terms of time lapse, e.g. three month fetus, or in terms of proportion of total gestational duration, e.g. first trimester fetus.
g. failure termination by fetal death and resorption, abortion, miscarriage.
gestosis any toxemic manifestation in pregnancy.
get the total offspring of an individual male; refers usually to a stallion.
Getah virus a member of the family *Togaviridae*, genus *Alphavirus*, transmitted by mosquitoes. It causes a highly infectious disease of horses manifested clinically by fever, mucosal exanthema and edema of the limbs.
GeV gigaelectron volt.
GFR glomerular filtration rate.
GGT γ-glutamyl transferase.
GH growth hormone.
GH-RH growth hormone releasing hormone.
gharial see GAVIAL.
gherkin CUCUMIS *sativus*.
ghost cell see SHADOW CELL.
ghost weed EUPHORBIA *marginata*.
GI gastrointestinal; globin (zinc) insulin.
giant of very large stature or dimensions.
g. breeds in dogs this includes the very largest breeds, generally in excess of 100 lb body weight, e.g. Great Dane, Irish wolfhound, Mastiff, St. Bernard, Deerhound, Great Pyrenees and Borzoi. See also DOG.
g. buttercup RANUNCULUS *acris*.
g. fennel FERULA *communis*.
g. forest hog see HYLOCHOERUS MEINERTZHAGENI.
g. hogweed see HERACLEUM MANTEGAZZIANUM.
g. kidney worm DIOCTOPHYME *renale*.
g. liver fluke see FASCIOLA *gigantica*, FASCIOLOIDES *magna*.
g. panic see BRACHIARIA *mutica*.
g. pigweed TRIANTHEMA *portulacastrum*.
g. prairie lily COOPERIA PEDUNCULATA.
g. schizonts up to 300 μm diameter in sheep and goats, as part of the life cycle of *Eimeria* spp.
G. Schnauzer see SCHNAUZER.
g. sea perch see LATES CALCARIFER.
g. sensitive plant MIMOSA *invisa*.
g. star grass CYNODON *nlemfuensis*.
g. taro ALOCASIA *brisbanensis*.
g. tiger prawn PENAEUS *monodon*. See Table 23.
giant cell 1. very large cells in normal tissue, e.g. megakaryocytes in bone marrow. 2. multinucleate macrophages found around foreign bodies and in granulomas. Three variants of multinucleated giant cells are recognized—Langhans, Touton and foreign body. Differentiation is based on the distribution of their nuclei.
g. c. epulis peripheral giant cell granulomas appearing as bright red, smooth gingival masses in cats and dogs; includes hyperplastic epithelium and many giant cells in densely cellular stroma.
extraskeletal g. c. tumor see MALIGNANT fibrous histiocytoma.
epidermal multinucleated g. c. found in viral infections and chronic, pruritic dermatoses characterized by epidermal hyperplasia or dyskeratosis.
giant-cell tumor 1. a rare bone tumor of dogs and cats with benign and malignant variants arising from primitive stromal elements of the bone marrow, composed of a spindle cell stroma containing multinucleated giant cells resembling osteoclasts. 2. carcinoma of the thyroid, a highly malignant undifferentiated neoplasm derived from poorly differentiated thyroid follicular cells. 3. giant cell epulis. See peripheral giant cell reparative GRANULOMA.
giantism 1. gigantism. 2. excessive size, as of cells or nuclei.
fetal g. occurs in one of the inherited forms of PROLONGED GESTATION in cattle.
Giardia a genus of flagellate protozoa parasitic in the intestines of most animals. They are capable of causing protracted, intermittent diarrhea suggestive of malabsorption, sometimes dysentery, but many infections may be innocuous. Includes *G. bovis* (cattle), *G. canis* (dogs), *G. caprae* (goats), *G. cati* or *G. felis* (cats), *G. caviae* (guinea pigs), *G. chinchillae* (chinchillas), *G. duodenalis* (rabbits), *G. equi* (horses), *G. felis* (cats), *G. intestinalis* (*G. lamblia*; found in humans, pigs, budgerigars, monkeys), *G. muris* (mice, rats).
giardiasis infection with GIARDIA protozoa. Infection in dogs and cats is common with subclinical to severe disease resulting. There may be profuse watery diarrhea with borborygmus. Chronic small bowel diarrhea can also result, with weight loss and signs of malabsorption. Transmission to humans can occur.
gibata ARRABIDEA *bilabiata*.
Gibber Italicus a closely inbred Italian canary breed. It has a distinctive stance, erect with stiff legs and the head thrust forward, forming a figure seven. The plumage is scanty with frills on the shoulders, breast and flanks. The breast bone is exposed and the thighs largely unfeathered.
gibberellins tremorgen toxins produced by *Fusarium* spp.
gibbon slender, tailless, noisy, arboreal ape, about 3 ft high and weighing about 15 lb. The least anthropoid of the anthropoid apes, in the family Pongidae. Called also *Hylobates* spp.
Gibbose Espagnole a canary breed similar to the Gibber Italicus, with an even more exaggerated posture. The neck is very long and the head is held very low.
gibbosity the condition of being humped; kyphosis.
gibbous humped; protuberant.
Gibbs–Donnan equilibrium see DONNAN'S EQUILIBRIUM.
Gibbs–Donnan phenomenon see DONNAN'S EQUILIBRIUM.
gibbus a hump.
Giberella see FUSARIUM.
gibflaar fluoroacetate poisoning caused by the ingestion of *Dichapetalum* spp.
Gibraltar fever see BRUCELLOSIS.
gid see COENUROSIS.
Giemsa stain a solution containing azure II-eosin, azure II, glycerin and methanol; used for staining protozoan parasites, *Leptospira*, *Borrelia*, viral inclusion bodies and *Rickettsia*.
Gierke's disease, von Gierke's disease see GLYCOGENOSIS type I.
gifappel SOLANUM *incanum*.

gifblaar DICHAPETALUM *cymosum*.
gifbossie THESIUM *namaquense*.
gig see SULKY.
giga- word element. [Gr.] *huge;* used in naming units of measurement to designate an amount 10^9 times the size of the unit to which it is joined, e.g. gigameter (10^9 meters); symbol G.
g.-bytes 10^9 bytes.
gigantism abnormal overgrowth of the body or a part; excessive size and stature. The condition results from overproduction of growth hormone before the epiphyseal plates have closed. The opposite condition, DWARFISM, is caused by underproduction of the same hormone. Overproduction of growth hormone in adults causes ACROMEGALY.
Gigantobilharzia a genus of blood flukes in the family Schistosomatidae which inhabit the blood vessels of their hosts. Found in birds.
Gigantocotyle a genus of flukes (digenetic trematodes) in the family Paramphistomatidae.
G. explanatum found in the duodenum, bile ducts and gallbladder of cattle and buffalo.
Gigli wire saw a very strong wire saw used in orthopedics. Also suited to performing fetotomies on fetal calves and foals. Used to remove horns and digits in digital amputations in ruminants.
GIH growth hormone release inhibiting hormone; see SOMATOSTATIN.
Gila monster *Heloderma suspectum,* a poisonous, legged reptile, colored brown with orange spots and a skin covered with large beadlike tubercles. Venom injected by bites causes local pain and swelling that is soon followed by vomiting, shock and depression of the central nervous system.
Gilbert's syndrome benign hereditary hyperbilirubinemia of humans marked by mild intermittent jaundice and often by fatigue, weakness and abdominal pain. A comparable disease has been identified in mutant Southdown sheep. See inherited PHOTOSENSITIZATION.
Gilchrist's disease see North American BLASTOMYCOSIS.
gill external breathing apparatus of fish. Very susceptible to a wide range of diseases.
g. disease an infectious disease of aquarium and salmonid species of fish caused by *Flavobacterium bronchiophila*. Also in *Crassostrea angulata* caused by an iridovirus and in larval shrimp caused usually by a *Leucothrix* spp. bacterium. Chronic, proliferative inflammation causes the gill filaments to be swollen and may be clubbed or fused. Called also bacterial gill disease.
g. parasites the following external parasites are commonly found on the gills, and elsewhere on the skin, in aquarium fish: *Gyrodactylus elegans*—a monogenetic fluke; *Diplozoon barbi*, *D. paradoxum*—monogenetic flukes; *Ergasilus sieboldi*—crustaceans. Freshly caught seahorses may carry the crustacean *Argulus* spp. Pond fish may carry the anchor worm *Lernaea* spp. These are all visible with the naked eye and can be removed manually.
gill-flirter see RECTOVAGINAL fistula.
Gillies needle holder a needle holder with scissors incorporated into the blades.
gilt a female breeding pig that has not yet had a litter of piglets.
g. anestrus failure of gilts to show the first estrus at a sufficiently early age. Being confined and with no boar in the environment plus failure of the attendant to recognize estrus behavior are significant contributors to the total loss.

Gimenez stain a carbol fuschin stain, counterstained with malachite green, to demonstrate rickettsiae and chlamydia.
gimmer a ewe that has not yet borne a lamb.
ginger produced from the rhizomes of *Zingiber officinale*; used as a carminative, stimulant and antiemetic.
gingering the practice of putting something irritating in the vagina of a mare at sale time to ginger her up; causes an elevation of the tail and a smarter appearance generally. In males the same effect may be attempted by putting the irritant in the rectum but the rapid evacuation from that site would reduce the severity of the irritation. Substances used are a clove of ginger or onion, pepper, etc. Done with some discretion it should not do a great deal of harm but would be considered to be an act of cruelty in any civilized community.
Gingin rickets see ENZOOTIC ataxia.
gingiva pl. *gingivae* [L.] the gum.
alveolar g. the portion overlying the alveolar process and firmly attached to it.
areolar g. the portion attached to the alveolar process by loose areolar connective tissue.
free g. the portion that surrounds the tooth and is not directly attached to the tooth surface.
gingival pertaining to or emanating from the gum.
g. hypertrophy, g. hyperplasia general or local gum overgrowth which may be severe enough to cover the crowns of the teeth and prevent the mouth from being closed. Common only in dogs. May be localized to one or several teeth, resulting in discrete, tumorlike masses (epulis), or diffuse, affecting the gums at all teeth locations. The latter form is familial in Boxer dogs and inherited as a recessive trait in Swedish silver foxes.
g. index a graded assessment of gingival health used in periodontal charting.
g. pocket see PERIODONTAL pocket.
g. recession the free gingival margin may recede towards the tooth root in association with resorption of alveolar and supporting bone in periodontal disease in dogs and cats. The cemento-enamel junction and root surface become exposed contributing to progression of dental disease.
g. vascular hamartoma rare congenital vascular anomaly on the gums of calves; lobulated masses covered with mucosa but may be traumatized; consist of vascular channels.
gingivalgia pain in the gingiva.
gingivectomy surgical excision of all loose infected and diseased gingival tissue to eradicate periodontal infection and reduce the depth of the gingival sulcus.
gingivitis a general term for inflammation of the gums, of which bleeding is one of the primary signs. Other signs include swelling, redness, pain and difficulty in chewing. There are numerous causes for this condition, and it can lead to a more serious disorder, PERIODONTITIS. One of the most common causes of gingivitis is the accumulation of food particles in the crevices between the gums and the teeth.
feline plasma cell g.–pharyngitis, feline plasma cell-lymphocytic g.–pharyngitis a chronic inflammatory disease of the mouth in cats, characterized by proliferative and ulcerative lesions of the gums and palatine fossa. There is often anorexia and a fetid odor to the breath. The cause is unknown.
necrotizing ulcerative g. a gingival infection marked by redness and swelling, necrosis, pain, hemorrhage, a necrotic odor and often a pseudomembrane. Extension to the oral mucosa is called necrotizing ulcerative gingivostomatitis.

gingivo- word element. [L.] *gingival*.
gingivoglossitis inflammation of the gingiva and tongue.
gingivolabial pertaining to the gums and lips.
gingivoplasty surgical remodeling of the gingiva.
gingivosis a chronic, diffuse inflammation of the gums, with desquamation of the papillary epithelium and mucous membrane.
gingivostomatitis inflammation of the gingiva and oral mucosa.
necrotizing ulcerative g. that due to extension to the oral mucosa of necrotizing ulcerative gingivitis.
ginglymus a joint that allows movement in one plane, as does a door hinge; called also hinge joint.
ginseng a mixture of saponins from the dried root of *Panax* sp; reputed to have a wide range of pharmacologic properties. Used variously as a stimulant, a sedative and to increase stamina and resistance to disease.
GIP gastric inhibitory polypeptide.
gir cattle Indian, mottled red and white multi-purpose cattle.
Giraffa camelopardalis see GIRAFFE.
giraffe the long-necked ruminant member of the family Giraffidae which it shares with the okapi. Its horns are bony outgrowths covered with skin. Called also *Giraffa camelopardalis*.
giraffe-necked gazelle see GERENUK.
giraffid member of the Giraffidae family; includes giraffes and okapi.
girdle an encircling or confining structure.
pelvic g. see PELVIC girdle.
shoulder g. the incomplete bony ring made up of the scapulae, clavicles and coracoids (when present) sometimes incorporating the manubrium of the sternum. Called also pectoral or thoracic girdle.
Girella nigricans opal-eye fish, carrier of the SMSV-7 strain of the San Miguel sealion virus, capable of producing lesions identical to those of vesicular exanthema disease when injected into pigs.
girth 1. the greatest circumference of the chest in horses and dogs, just behind the withers, shoulder and elbow. 2. the leather strap that completes the enclosure of the horse's girth by the saddle and keeps the saddle in place. There are a multitude of patterns all designed to prevent slipping and avoid causing girth galls.
g. (2) gall a skin abrasion on the chest just behind the elbow of a horse caused by pressure or movement of the girth while being ridden. Caused by sharp edges of the girth, girth adjusted too tightly or too loosely or a poor conformation of the horse.
g. (2) itch dermatitis behind the elbow in the horse. Due usually to ringworm, the infection being transmitted by the girth strap.
gitalin amorphous gitalin; a mixture of digitalis glycosides used as a cardiotonic in congestive heart failure and cardiac arrhythmias.
githagenin a toxic saponin found in the plant *Agrostemma githago*.
gitoxigenin a steroid aglycone, the hydrolysis product of gitoxin in the body.
gitoxin one of the cardiac glycosides of *Digitalis purpurea*.
gitter cells microglial phagocytic cells of the central nervous system which are laden with degenerating myelin. The cells are spherical with a bubbly margin and with a reduced nucleus. Called also compound granular corpuscles, scavenger cells, Hortega cells, fat-granule cell.
giving set fluid administration apparatus, usually including the plastic bag containing the mixture to be infused and a long, flexible clear plastic tube to be connected to the needle or catheter. There is also usually a chamber built into the line where a pool of fluid collects and maintains a steady flow, free of air bubbles.
gizzard the muscular stomach of the bird, separated from the more cranial proventriculus or glandular stomach by a constriction. Called also ventriculus.
green g. gizzard stained by a dye used in feed wheat that makes it unsaleable as human food.
g. impaction can cause heavy mortality in young turkey poults; the gizzard is impacted with fibrous material, thought due to eating litter.
g. myopathy occurs as part of a vitamin E–selenium nutritional deficiency.
g. strongyles see AMIDOSTOMUM *anseris*.
g. worms *Habronema incertum* causes sudden death or chronic watery diarrhea in companion birds.
glabrous smooth and bare.
gladdon IRIS *foetidissima*.
gladiolus a decorative floral plant of which the corms may be poisonous and cause diarrhea. Called also *Gladiolus* spp.
glairy slimy, resembling white of an egg.
gland an aggregation of cells specialized to secrete or excrete materials not related to their ordinary metabolic needs. Glands are divided into two main groups, endocrine and exocrine.

Specific glands will be found under their individual names.
accessory genital g's glands other than the gonads, intimately associated with the reproductive organs, especially of the male, in which they include vesicular glands (seminal vesicles), ampullary glands, prostate, bulbourethral glands, coagulating glands. Called also ACCESSORY sex glands.
accessory sex g. see accessory genital glands (above).
acinous g. one made up of one or more oval or spherical sacs (acini).
alveolar g. one whose secretory units consist of saclike dilatations with a distinct lumen.
alveolar–tubular g. gland composed of a mixture of alveolar and tubular structures.
ampullary g. fusiform enlargement of the deferent duct, as it passes across the bladder wall, due to proliferation of glandular tissue in the regionally folded mucosa.
anal g's small glands in the anal columnar mucosal cells plus larger and more numerous circumanal glands in the surrounding skin.
apocrine g. one whose discharged secretion contains part of the secreting cells.
avian stomach g's mucosal and submucosal glands in the stomach of birds; the submucosal glands are thought to secrete both acidic and enzymic substances.
bronchial g's glands which contain a mixture of serous and mucus-secreting cells found in the bronchial mucosa.
buccal g's buccal salivary glands lying in the submucosal tissues of the cheek and sometimes the orbit and whose ducts secrete directly into the buccal cavity.
cardiac g. one of the three (the other two are the pyloric and proper gastric or fundic) types of gland in the stomach wall and capable of secretion into the gastric juices; this gland secretes only mucus.
carpal g's cutaneous, 'marking' glands found on the medial aspect of the carpus in the pig; although pre-

sent in both sexes are thought to be used to mark mated females.
circumoral g's large glands in the lips of cats; used to mark territory either directly by the familiar fawning head rub, or indirectly by rubbing the secretion of the gland onto the fur during grooming.
ceruminous g's cerumin-secreting glands in the skin of the external auditory canal.
compound g. one made up of a number of smaller units whose excretory ducts combine to form ducts of progressively higher order.
deep (lacrimal) g., g. of the third eyelid an additional lacrimal gland found in the skin of the cartilaginous support of the third eyelid.
ductless g's endocrine glands.
eccrine g. a gland that secretes its product without loss of cytoplasm, such as the sweat glands on dog footpads or human skin.
endocrine g's or ductless glands, discharge their secretions (hormones) directly into the blood; they include the adrenal, pituitary, thyroid and parathyroid glands, the islets of Langerhans in the pancreas, the gonads and the pineal body.
exocrine g's discharge through ducts opening on an external or internal surface of the body; include the salivary, sebaceous and sweat glands, the liver, the gastric glands, the pancreas, the intestinal, mammary and lacrimal glands, and the prostate.
fundic g's, fundus g's numerous, tubular glands in the mucosa of the stomach that contain the cells which produce acid and pepsin. According to the species, they are usually found in the body and occasionally in the fundus.
gustatory g. branched, tubuloalveolar serous glands which open into large lingual papillae.
hematopoietic g. glandlike body, e.g. the spleen, that takes a part in blood formation.
hemolymph g. small node resembling lymph node but red or brown in color and containing blood sinuses instead of or alongside lymph spaces. Common in ruminants and some rodents and typically located along the large arteries.
Harderian g. see HARDERIAN GLAND.
haversian g. fold on synovial surface regarded as secretor of synovia.
holocrine g. one whose discharged secretion contains the entire secreting cells as in sebaceous glands.
horn g. a scent gland found caudomedial to the horn base in goats of both sexes; increase in size and activity in breeding season. Produce the pungent secretion so characteristic of goats, described best as the distilled essence of reek.
infraorbital g's special sebaceous glands which line the infraorbital sinus (pouch) in sheep.
inguinal g's the collection of special tubular and sebaceous glands which line the inguinal pouch (sinus) in sheep.
interdigital g's special sebaceous and tubular glands in the interdigital sinus (pouch) in sheep.
intestinal g's microscopic tubular glands which lie in the mucosa of the gut and secrete intestinal juice into the lumen of the small intestine.
labial g's minor salivary glands; mucous in small ruminants, serous in others.
lateral nasal g's a local glandular thickening of the mucosa lining the maxillary sinus of dogs and some other species; this tissue is largely responsible for the continually wet nose of the dog.
lingual g. minor salivary glands, mixed serous and mucous in cattle and horses, mucous in sheep, cats, dogs.
lymph g's lymph nodes; they are not glands in the true sense.
male sex g. see TESTIS, accessory genital glands (above).
mammary g. the milk-secreting organ of female mammals, existing also in a rudimentary state in the male. See also UDDER, BREAST.
mandibular salivary g's major salivary glands; large and with long salivary ducts to deliver secretion into the mouth.
marrow-lymph g. hemolymph gland having a marrow-like tissue.
meibomian g. sebaceous follicle between the cartilage and conjunctiva of the eyelids. Called also tarsal gland.
mental g. a focal specialization of glands in the skin of the pig, caudal to the mandibular symphysis. It is a round raised nevus-like structure composed of sebaceous and apocrine glands with coarse bristles.
merocrine g. one whose discharged secretion contains no part of the secreting cells.
mixed g's 1. seromucous glands. 2. glands that have both exocrine and endocrine portions.
molar salivary g. unique gland in felids; predominantly mucoid cells with a few serous.
Moll's g's, g's of Moll see MOLL'S GLANDS.
multicellular g's glands which occur as sheets of epithelial cells with secretory function, e.g. gastric and intestinal mucosae.
multilobular proventricular g's in the glandular stomach of the bird these glands appear to secrete both pepsin and hydrochloric acid.
nasal g's small glands scattered throughout the nasal mucosa.
nasolabial g. see NASOLABIAL gland.
olfactory g's seromucous glands located beneath the olfactory epithelium; their secretion keeps the local mucosa moist.
palatine salivary g. a minor salivary gland containing serous or mucoid or mixed secretory cells.
palpebral g. see meibomian gland (above).
parotid salivary g. a major salivary gland usually containing serous secretory cells; in carnivores there may also be a few mucus-secreting cells.
preen g. see uropygial gland (below).
preputial g's sebaceous and apocrine sweat glands within the prepuce; sometimes aggregated into discrete sacs (musk deer) or diverticula (pigs); their secretions combine with desquamated epithelial cells to produce smegma.
proctodaeal g's mucous glands containing lymphoid tissue located in the proctodeum of male and female birds.
proper gastric g. the main digestive glands of the stomach; found in different parts of the stomach in different species but usually in the body of the stomach; secrete pepsin and hydrochloric acid; open into microscopic pits and clefts.
scent g. secrete pheromones which play such a large part in olfactory communication between animals. Located in a variety of places, e.g. in the elephant they are behind the eyes, in the musk deer they are in the belly wall.
seminal g. see seminal VESICLE.
sentinel g. an enlarged lymph node, considered to be pathognomonic of some pathological condition elsewhere.
sex g's, sexual g's gonads. See OVARY, TESTIS.
shell g. the caudal portion of the uterus in the female bird in which the egg is held while the shell is secreted.

simple g. one with a nonbranching duct.
sine ductibus g. ductless gland.
solitary g's solitary follicles.
sperm host g. in the vagina of birds; store and nourish visiting spermatozoa which are released when oviposition occurs.
splenolymph g's hemolymph glands having more of the splenic type of tissue.
sublingual salivary g. a major salivary gland; predominantly mucous cells in ruminants, swine, rodents; mixed serous and mucoid cells in small carnivores and horses.
submental g's a group of sebaceous glands in the intermandibular space in cats.
submucosal intestinal g's simple, branched, tubuloacinar glands; mucous in ruminants and dogs, mixed serous and mucous in cats and serous in horses and dogs; in carnivores and small ruminants confined to the proximal or middle parts of the duodenum, extend to jejunum in large ruminants, horses, pigs.
submucosal stomach g. large, numerous, branched, compound, tubular gland in birds; thought to secrete both acid and enzymatic products.
sudoriferous g's, sudoriparous g's sweat glands.
supracaudal g. scent producing cells found only in dogs and cats; in dogs confined to a small area at the base of the tail, in cats extend along the dorsal surface of most of the tail; called also tail gland.
suprarenal g. see ADRENAL GLAND.
tail g. see supracaudal gland (above).
target g. one specifically affected by a hormone.
tarsal g. see meibomian gland (above).
third eyelid g. a secondary lacrimal gland; a second, deeper gland occurs in pigs and cattle.
tubular g. any gland made up of or containing a tubule or tubules.
ultimobranchial g. tissue from the fourth pharyngeal pouch which in mammals is absorbed into the thyroid gland. In fish, amphibians, reptiles and birds the tissue forms separate glands containing calcitonin.
unicellular g. a single cell that functions as a gland, e.g. a goblet cell.
urethral g's accessory sex glands in males; secrete serous and mucoid liquids into the urethra to nourish and activate spermatozoa.
uropygial g. the oil or preen gland of birds is attached to the tail and consists of a bilobed simple tubular, holocrine gland.
vesicular g. see seminal VESICLE.
vestibular g's major and minor mucus-producing glands in the vestibule of the vulva.
Wolfring g's small tubuloalveolar glands in subconjunctival tissue above the upper border of the tarsal plate; open onto conjunctiva.
g's of Zeis, Zeis g's prominent sebaceous sweat glands on the eyelid margins, associated with hair follicles of cilia. See also external HORDEOLUM.
Zuckerkandl g. two large bodies included with the paraganglia along the abdominal aorta.
zygomatic salivary g. a unique salivary gland in small carnivores; contains mainly mucous cells with a few serous cells; a modified dorsal buccal gland.

glanders a contagious disease of all solipeds caused by *Burkholderia (Pseudomonas) mallei* and transmissible to humans. It occurs in a chronic or acute form, both of which are inexorably fatal. It is characterized by the development of ulcers or nodules on the skin and in the respiratory tract. In the acute form the critical lesion is bronchopneumonia. See also FARCY.

glandilemma the capsule or outer envelope of a gland.

glandula pl. *glandulae* [L.] gland.

glandular 1. pertaining to or of the nature of a gland. 2. pertaining to the glans penis.
g. organs organs consisting principally of glands.

glandule a small gland.

glans pl. *glandes* [L.] a small, rounded mass or glandlike body.
g. clitoridis the erectile tissue on the free end of the clitoris.
g. penis the cap-shaped expansion of the corpus spongiosum at the end of the penis.

glanular pertaining to the glans penis or to the glans clitoris.

Glanzmann–Naegeli syndrome see THROMBASTHENIA.

Glanzmann's disease thrombasthenia.

Glasgow Coma Scale see TRAUMA score.

glass 1. a hard, brittle, often transparent material, usually consisting of the fused amorphous silicates of potassium or sodium, and of calcium, with silica in excess. 2. a container, usually cylindrical, made from glass.
g. embolism small particles of glass from a vial may be injected suspended in a fluid.
ground g. may be used in an attempt to poison animals maliciously but has little effect. May cause transient enteritis.
g. housing glass cover of the x-ray tube; contains the anode and cathode and the vacuum that makes generation and control of the x-ray beam possible.
soluble g. glass in which the magnesium and calcium content have been modified from that in normal glass so that it is much more soluble in water or ruminal contents. Used in the form of a reticular retention bolus as a vehicle for therapeutic agents such as antibiotics or anthelmintics which are delivered to the animal over a period of weeks or months.

glass-eye see WALLEYE (3).

Glässer's disease a contagious disease of young pigs caused by *Haemophilus* spp. and occurring in outbreaks with an acute syndrome characterized by polyarthritis, pericarditis, pleurisy and peritonitis.

Glassman intestinal forceps non-crushing forceps used in holding sections of viable bowel during anastomosis procedures.

glassy membrane basement membrane in hair follicles, separating connective tissue and follicular epithelium.

Glauber's salt sodium sulfate, used as a saline purgative.

Glaucium corniculatum plant in the family Papaveraceae; may cause nitrate–nitrite poisoning.

glaucoma a group of diseases of the eye characterized by increased intraocular pressure, resulting in pathological changes in the optic disk and typical visual field defects, and eventually blindness if not treated successfully. Uncommon in domestic animals, except in dogs where several breeds are predisposed.

The normal eye is filled with aqueous humor in an amount carefully regulated to maintain the shape of the eyeball. In glaucoma, the balance of this fluid is disturbed; fluid is formed more rapidly than it leaves the eye, and pressure builds up. The increased pressure damages the retina. If not relieved by proper treatment, the pressure will eventually damage the optic nerve, causing blindness.
absolute g. end-stage glaucoma with buphthalmos and severe degenerative changes.
aphakic g. forward displacement of the posterior

lens capsule and vitreous body with incarceration in the pupil; usually occurs after cataract surgery.

closed-angle g. one in which the iridocorneal angle is obstructed, either due to collapse or interference with drainage by the iris or connective tissue. The cause may be congenital (GONIODYSGENESIS) or acquired, due to an abnormality of the lens, anterior chamber or iris.

congenital g. that due to defective development of the structures in and around the anterior chamber of the eye, and resulting in impairment of drainage. See also GONIODYSGENESIS.

narrow-angle g. a form of primary glaucoma caused by abnormal development of the iridocorneal angle. See also GONIODYSGENESIS.

open-angle g. a form of glaucoma in which there is no detectable abnormality of the iridocorneal angle, but drainage is obstructed by elements in the aqueous humor, luxation of the lens, or elevated episcleral venous pressure. In some cases, particularly in predisposed breeds of dogs such as beagles, no contributing factors are detectable.

phacolytic g. leakage of lens material from a hypermature cataract causes anterior uveitis that impedes aqueous outflow.

primary g. increased intraocular pressure occurring in an eye with no other eye disease being present.

secondary g. increased intraocular pressure due to disease or injury to the eye.

Glc glucose.

GLDH glutamate dehydrogenase.

Glechoma hederacea toxic plant in the family Lamiaceae; contains an unknown toxin which causes pulmonary edema and emphysema. Called also *Nepeta hederacea*, creeping charlie, ground ivy.

gleet a chronic discharge, especially one that is mucoid or purulent, e.g. vent gleet of fowls, nasal gleet.

Glen of Imaal terrier a small active dog with short legs, broad head, folded ears, and a harsh, medium-length blue or wheaten coat.

glenoid resembling a pit or socket.

g. cavity a depression in the ventral angle of the scapula for articulation with the humerus.

g. cavity dysplasia may be a contributing cause of scapulohumeral luxations, particularly in small and toy breeds of dogs.

g. fossa a depression in the temporal bone in which the condyle of the lower jaw rests; called also mandibular fossa.

g. lip a ring of fibrocartilage joined to the rim of the glenoid cavity.

Gleotrichia see GLOEOTRICHIA.

glia neuroglia; the supporting cells of the central nervous system, made up of astrocytes, oligodendrocytes and microglia.

gliacyte a cell of the glia or neuroglia.

glial of or pertaining to glia or neuroglia.

g. limitans a dense network of glial processes at the pia mater.

g. nodule foci of microglia about degenerating neurons.

g. shrubbery an accumulation of glial nodules around degenerating Purkinje cells in the molecular layer of the cerebellum.

glibenclamide see GLYBURIDE.

glicentin a hormone, function unknown, in the intestinal wall of chickens.

glider gliding marsupials equipped with lateral membranes connecting the fore and hindlimbs; includes *Petaurus breviceps* (sugar glider), *Petauroides volans* (greater glider) and *Acrobates pygmaeus* (feather-tailed glider).

glioblast spongioblast.

glioblastoma an undifferentiated malignant astrocytoma.

g. multiforme a rapidly growing tumor, usually of the cerebral hemispheres, often supratentorial.

Gliocladium a common fungal contaminant.

glioma a tumor composed of neuroglia in any of its states of development; sometimes extended to include all intrinsic neoplasms of the brain and spinal cord, such as astrocytoma, ependymoma, mixed glioma, etc.

g. retinae see RETINOBLASTOMA.

gliomatosis excessive development of the neuroglia, especially of the spinal cord, in certain cases of syringomyelia.

gliosis an excess of astroglia in damaged areas of the central nervous system.

glipizide a second generation sulfonylurea derivative, used as an oral hypoglycemia agent in the treatment of diabetes mellitus, most commonly in cats.

Gliricola a genus of biting lice of the suborder Amblycera.

G. pistoi found on New World primates.

G. porcelli found on guinea pigs and rodents.

Glis one of the genera into which the dormouse is classified. The others are *Eliomys*, *Muscardinus*, *Graphiurus*, *Platacanthomys*, *Typhlomys*. The dormouse is a small yellow-gray with light underside, arboreal animal intermediate between squirrels and rats. It is nocturnal and vegetarian.

Glishrocaryon genus of Australian plants in the Haloragidaceae family; contains cyanogenetic glucosides. Includes *G. aureum*, *G. roei*. Called also *Loudinia* spp., yellow pop flower.

glissonian pertaining to the capsule of the liver—Glisson's capsule, e.g. glissonian cirrhosis.

glissonitis inflammation of Glisson's capsule.

Glisson's capsule a sheath of connective tissue enclosing the hepatic artery, hepatic duct and portal vein.

glitch 1. slang for an unexplained error or problem in any information medium, but used usually in reference to a computer program. 2. a sudden electronic surge that causes problems in electronic devices.

Gln glutamine.

global search a computer technique of searching, in a single pass, a number of files to find a specified character string.

globe see GLOBUS.

optic g. see EYEBALL.

globeflower see TROLLIUS EUROPAEUS.

globi plural of *globus*.

Globicephala a genus of whale, the pilot whales. There are several species. They are black, 20 to 30 ft long with protuberant foreheads and a small beaklike muzzle.

globidiosis a name formerly given to a disease thought to be caused by GLOBIDIUM. Abomasal and cutaneous forms were described. These are now classified as EIMERIA and BESNOITIA respectively.

Globidium a poorly defined genus of protozoa; nowadays classified as EIMERIA.

G. gilruthi in goats, sheep.

G. leuckarti infestation with this parasite may cause diarrhea, but is rarely pathogenic in young horses. Called also *Eimeria leuckarti*.

globin the protein constituent of hemoglobin; also, any member of a group of proteins similar to the typical globin.

Globocephaloides a genus of nematodes in the trichostrongyloid family Herpetostrongyloidae.

G. trifidospicularis a blood-sucking parasite in the small intestine of the gray kangaroo, *Macropus giganteus*.

Globocephalus a genus of blood-sucking nematodes in the subfamily Ancylostominae; occur in the intestine of pigs and probably cause anemia if the infestation is heavy. Includes *G. longemucronatus*, *G. samoensis*, *G. urosubulatus*, *G. versteri*.

globoid cell leukodystrophy see globoid cell LEUKODYSTROPHY.

globular resembling a globe.

g. heart a spherical cardiac silhouette, usually greatly enlarged and lacking the detailed outline of the right and left atria and apex. Characteristic of pericardial effusion and cardiomyopathy.

g. nematode see TETRAMERES *americana*.

globule a small spherical mass; a little globe or pellet, as of medicine. See also MORGAGNIAN GLOBULE.

g. leukocyte mononuclear cell with large eosinophilic cytoplasmic granules found in the intestinal epithelium.

globulin a general term for proteins that are insoluble in water or highly concentrated salt solutions but soluble in moderately concentrated salt solutions. All plasma proteins except albumin and prealbumin are globulins. The plasma globulins can be separated into five fractions by serum protein electrophoresis (SPE). In order of decreasing electrophoretic mobility these fractions are the $alpha_1$, $alpha_2$, $beta_1$ and $beta_2$ globulins, and the gamma globulins.

The globulins include carrier proteins, which transport specific substances; acute phase reactants, which are involved in the inflammatory process; clotting factors; complement components; and immunoglobulins. Examples are transferrin, a $beta_1$ globulin that transports iron, and $alpha_1$-antitrypsin, an acute phase reactant that inhibits serum proteases. The GAMMA globulin fraction is almost entirely composed of IMMUNOGLOBULINS.

accelerator g. a substance present in plasma, but not in serum, that functions in the formation of intrinsic and extrinsic thromboplastin; called also CLOTTING factor V.

antihemophilic g. (AHG) CLOTTING factor VIII.

antilymphocyte g. (ALG) a substance used as an immunosuppressive agent in organ transplantation, usually in combination with immunosuppressive drugs; it is the gamma globulin fraction of ANTILYMPHOCYTE SERUM.

immune g. a sterile solution containing antibodies normally present in blood, derived from donor animals, sometimes after hyperimmunization with certain microorganisms; used for passive immunization against some infectious diseases and in the treatment of gamma globulin deficiency.

serum g. the fraction of proteins precipitated from blood serum by half saturation with ammonium sulfate; the principal groups include the α-, β- and γ-globulins.

globulinuria the presence of globulins in the urine.

globus pl. *globi* [L.] a sphere or ball; a spherical mass.

g. pallidus the smaller and more medial part of the lentiform nucleus of the brain.

Glock forceps large, ratchet-handled, scissor-action uterine forceps with large round blades for grasping and holding up an exteriorized bovine uterus.

Gloeotrichia a genus of Cyanobacteria including toxic species which contain microcystins.

glomangioma a painful, benign tumor developing as a result of hypertrophy of a GLOMUS.

glomectomy excision of a glomus.

glomera plural of *glomus*.

glomerular pertaining to or of the nature of a glomerulus, especially a renal glomerulus.

g. basement membrane the structure located between endothelial cells of renal capillaries and the visceral epithelial cells of the glomerulus. It functions as a barrier to filtration of large molecules.

g. capsule Bowman's capsule.

g. crescent see glomerular CRESCENT.

g. diseases see GLOMERULONEPHRITIS, GLOMERULONEPHROPATHY, GLOMERULOPATHY.

g. filtrate the acellular low-protein ultrafiltrate of plasma that passes the glomerulus.

g. filtration see GLOMERULUS.

g. filtration rate varies widely depending on diet. It is the ability of the renal tubules to vary their absorbing capacity that ensures there is no great electrolyte loss during the periods of high rates of glomerular filtration.

g. lipidosis characterized by the presence of large foam cells in glomerular tufts in dogs. They appear to have no disease significance.

g. permeability in normal subjects the capillary endothelium of the glomerulus, by virtue of its fenestration, is permeable to all blood constituents except blood cells and colloids so that the glomerular filtrate has a close similarity to plasma and interstitial fluid but has a lower protein concentration than both of them.

glomeruli plural of *glomerulus*.

glomerulitis inflammation of the glomeruli of the kidney.

glomerulocystic disease a disease of newborn animals characterized by minute cysts present in Bowman's capsules. In puppies they may be the cause of uremia; in foals their pathogenesis is unknown and their significance appears to be nil.

glomerulonephritis a variety of NEPHRITIS characterized by inflammation of the capillary loops in the glomeruli of the kidney with secondary tubulointerstitial and vascular changes. It occurs in acute, subacute and chronic forms and may be secondary to infection or immune mechanisms.

immune-mediated g. caused by deposition of immune complexes on the glomerular basement membrane or autoantibodies against the glomerular basement membrane.

lobular g. a form in which all glomeruli are affected, with accentuation of the lobulation of the glomerular tufts; it is marked by constant proteinuria and microscopic hematuria.

membranoproliferative g., mesangiocapillary g. a chronic, slowly progressive glomerulonephritis in which the glomeruli are enlarged as a result of proliferation of mesangial cells and irregular thickening of the capillary walls, which narrows the capillary lumina; the onset is sudden, with hematuria, proteinuria or nephrotic syndrome and a persistent reduction in serum complement levels and deposition of activated complement components in the glomerular capillaries. Occurs in Finnish-Landrace sheep and is the most common glomerulopathy seen in dogs.

membranous g. diffuse and irregular thickening of the basement membrane where there is diffuse granular deposition of immunoglobulin and complement. The most common type of glomerular disease in cats.

mesangioproliferative g. see membranoproliferative glomerulonephritis (above).

proliferative g. glomerular changes are principally those of cellular proliferation.

glomerulonephropathy any noninflammatory disease of the renal glomeruli.

glomerulopathy any disease, especially any noninflammatory disease, of the renal glomeruli.

Finnish-Landrace g. see membranoproliferative GLOMERULONEPHRITIS.

Samoyed hereditary g. inherited as an X-linked dominant trait it affects males more severely and earlier than females; wasting and proteinuria are characteristic; males are dead by 15 months of age.

glomerulopressin hepatic-derived renal vasodilator.

glomerulosa the outer layer of the adrenal cortex, the zona glomerulosa.

glomerulosclerosis progressive hyalinization such that glomeruli become shrunken, eosinophilic and hypocellular masses.

intercapillary g. see KIMMELSTIEL–WILSON SYNDROME.

glomerulotubular pertaining to the glomeruli and the tubules.

g. imbalance when the rate of tubular resorption does not balance the glomerular filtration rate, so that there is polyuria or oliguria and possibly electrolyte loss.

glomerulus pl. *glomeruli* [L.] a small tuft or cluster.

cerebellar g. termination sites for dendrites and axons of cerebellar and medullary and spinal nerve fibers.

olfactory g. termination points of olfactory nerves in the olfactory lobes.

renal g. a small convoluted mass of capillaries, a network of vascular tufts, encased in the malpighian or Bowman's capsule.

The glomerulus is an integral part of the NEPHRON, the basic unit of the KIDNEY. Each nephron is capable of forming urine by itself, and each kidney has many nephrons. The specific function of each glomerulus is to bring blood (and the waste products it carries) to the nephron. As the blood flows through the glomerulus, about one-fifth of the plasma passes through the glomerular membrane, collects in the malpighian capsule, and then flows through the renal tubules. Much of this fluid passes back into the blood via the small capillaries around the tubules (peritubular capillaries). The continuous filtration of fluid from the glomeruli and its reabsorption into the peritubular capillaries is made possible by a high pressure in the glomerular capillary bed and a low pressure in the peritubular bed.

Any disease of the glomeruli, such as acute or chronic glomerulonephritis, must be considered serious because it interferes with the basic functions of the kidneys; that is, filtration of liquids and excretion of certain end products of metabolism and excess sodium, potassium and chloride ions that may accumulate in the blood.

glomoid resembling a glomus.

glomus pl. *glomera* [L.] a small histologically recognizable body composed primarily of fine arterioles connecting directly with veins, and having a rich nerve supply.

g. caroticum carotid body.

g. cell a specialized cell of the carotid body.

g. choroideum an enlargement of the choroid plexus of the lateral ventricle.

g. tumor neoplasm of one of the chemoreceptors. Tumors of the glomus jugulare have been reported in a dog.

Gloriosa garden plant of the family Liliaceae; contains a colchicine-like toxin which causes excitement, diarrhea and alopecia. Includes *G. carsoni*, *G. simplex*, *G. superba*. Called also glory lily, flame lily.

glory lily GLORIOSA *superba*.

glossal pertaining to the tongue.

glossalgia pain in the tongue.

glossectomy excision of all or a portion of the tongue.

Glossina a genus of biting flies in the family Glossinidae. It includes the tsetse flies, which serve as vectors of trypanosomes causing various forms of TRYPANOSOMIASIS in humans and animals. Listed species of tsetse flies are *G. brevipalpis*, *G. fusca* (forest tsetse), *G. longipalpis*, *G. morsitans* (savannah tsetse), *G. pallidipes*, *G. palpalis* (riverine tsetse), *G. tachinoides*.

glossitis inflammation of the tongue.

gloss(o)- word element. [Gr.] *tongue*.

glossocele swelling and protrusion of the tongue.

glossodynia pain in the tongue.

glossology 1. the sum of knowledge regarding the tongue. 2. a treatise on nomenclature.

glossopathy any disease of the tongue.

glossopharyngeal pertaining to the tongue and pharynx.

g. nerve the ninth cranial nerve; it supplies the carotid sinus, mucous membrane, muscles of the pharynx, soft palate and caudal part of the tongue, and the taste buds in the caudal part of the tongue. By serving the carotid sinus, the glossopharyngeal nerve provides for reflex control of the heart. It is also responsible for the swallowing reflex, for stimulating secretions of the parotid glands, and for the sense of taste in the caudal part of the tongue. Lesions of the nerve cause dysphagia or inability to swallow, regurgitation through the nostrils and sometimes abnormality of the voice and interference with respiration. See also Table 14.

glossoplasty plastic surgery of the tongue.

glossoplegia paralysis of the tongue.

glossorrhaphy suture of the tongue.

glossospasm spasm of the tongue.

glossotomy incision of the tongue.

glossotrichia hairy tongue; elongation of papillae because of improper keratinization or desquamation of epithelial cells.

Gloster fancy a recently developed, very popular canary. The breed occurs in a crested variety, known as Corona, and a plain, smooth head variety, called Consort.

glottic pertaining to (1) the glottis, or (2) the tongue.

g. stenosis see LARYNGEAL stenosis.

Glottidium vesicarium SESBANIA *vesicaria*.

glottis pl. *glottides* [Gr.] the vocal apparatus of the larynx, consisting of the true vocal cords (vocal folds) and the opening between them.

g. stenosis may follow trauma, including tissue damage associated with use of an endotracheal tube, and leads to the formation of granulation tissue, scarring and laryngeal stenosis.

Gloucester Old Spot pig rare, black and white, spotted meat pig from UK; almost extinct.

glove a covering garment for the hand with a separate sheath for each finger.

lead g. for protection of the animal holder during radiography. Fabric gloves lined with thin lead/rubber sheet with a minimum lead equivalent of 0.25 mm.

g. powders are used to assist in the wearing of surgical gloves but materials used may cause foreign body reactions in tissues. For this reason talcum powder has largely been replaced by less irritating corn starch and rice starch.

surgical g. latex rubber, sterilized or capable of sterilization, thin enough not to interfere with touch sensation or digital dexterity, disposable or reusable.

Glover bulldog clamp for temporary occlusion of vascular structures, this type of clamp has a tension-adjusting screw so pressure can be controlled.

gloving the procedure of donning sterile rubber gloves, in such a way as to preserve asepsis of the operator, before each surgical procedure.

gloxazone see DITHIOSEMICARBAZONE.

Glu glutamate.

glucagon a polypeptide hormone secreted by the alpha cells of the islets of Langerhans in response to hypoglycemia or to stimulation by growth hormone. It increases blood glucose concentration by stimulating glycogenolysis in the liver and is administered to relieve hypoglycemic coma from any cause, especially hyperinsulinism.

g. diabetes glucagon elevates blood glucose levels and may contribute to the severity of diabetes if there is already an insulin deficit but it is not necessary to, nor sufficient for, the development of diabetes.

g. stimulation test a provocative test of growth hormone (GH) function in which the fasting serum level of GH is measured before and after administration of glucagon.

g. tolerance test evaluates the insulin response to elevation of blood glucose induced by administration of glucagon. Used in diagnosing hyperinsulinism.

glucagonoma a glucagon-secreting tumor of the alpha cells of the islets of Langerhans.

gluc(o)- word element. [Gr.] *sweetness, glucose;* see also words beginning *glyco-*.

glucoamylase see AMYLASE.

β-glucocerebrosidase an enzyme that catalyzes the hydrolytic cleavage of glucose from glucocerebroside. A deficiency results in accumulation of glucocerebroside in tissues (GAUCHER'S DISEASE). Called also glucosylceramidase, cerebroside β-glucosidase.

glucocerebroside a cerebroside containing a glucose sugar; it accumulates in the tissues in GAUCHER'S DISEASE (glucocerebrosidosis).

glucocerebrosidosis see GAUCHER'S DISEASE.

glucocorticoid any corticoid substance that increases gluconeogenesis, raising the concentration of liver glycogen and blood sugar, i.e. cortisol (hydrocortisone), cortisone and corticosterone. These substances are widely used as anti-inflammatory agents; they are effective at terminating pregnancy if it is in the late stages and they are used as a management tool in cattle for that purpose.

glucocorticosteroid see GLUCOCORTICOID.

glucofuranose a form of glucose in which carbon atoms 1 and 4 are bridged by an oxygen atom.

glucogenesis the formation of glucose by the breakdown of glycogen.

glucogenic giving rise to or producing sugar.

glucokinase an enzyme that in the presence of ATP catalyzes glucose to glucose-6-phosphate.

glucokinetic mobilizing sugar so as to maintain the sugar level of the body.

gluconate the salts of gluconic acid; used as alkalinizing agents in fluid therapy. They have the virtue of being metabolized to bicarbonate slowly and having a prolonged effect.

gluconeogenesis the synthesis of glucose from noncarbohydrate sources, such as amino acids, propionate and glycerol. It occurs primarily in the liver and kidneys whenever the supply of carbohydrates is insufficient to meet the body's metabolic demands or in the rumen by the action of bacteria in well-fed ruminants. Gluconeogenesis is stimulated by cortisol and other GLUCOCORTICOIDS and by glucagon. Formerly called glyconeogenesis.

gluconeogenic pertaining to gluconeogenesis.

glucophore the group of atoms in a molecule that gives the compound a sweet taste.

glucoprivation a lack of utilizable glucose.

glucopyranose the principal form of glucose in which carbon atoms 1 and 5 are bridged by an oxygen atom.

glucosamine an amino derivative of glucose occurring in many glycoproteins and mucopolysaccharides.

***N*-acetyl-β-glucosaminidase** one of the substances stored in mast cells; contributes to the hydrolysis of connective tissue GAGs.

glucose, D-glucose a simple sugar, a monosaccharide in certain foodstuffs, especially fruit, and in normal blood; the major source of energy for many living organisms. See also DEXTROSE.

Glucose, whose molecular formula is $C_6H_{12}O_6$, is the end product of carbohydrate digestion; other monosaccharides (fructose and galactose) are largely converted into glucose. Glucose is the only monosaccharide present in significant amounts in the body fluids. The oxidation of glucose produces energy for the body cells; the rate of metabolism is controlled by a number of hormones the most important of which are insulin and glucagon. Glucose that is not needed for energy is stored in the form of glycogen as a source of potential energy, readily available when needed. Most of the glycogen is stored in the liver and muscle cells. When these and other body cells are saturated with glycogen, the excess glucose is converted into fat and stored as adipose tissue. See also HYPOGLYCEMIA, HYPERGLYCEMIA.

[1-^{14}C]-g. radioactive glucose used experimentally.

liquid g. a thick syrupy, sweet liquid, consisting chiefly of dextrose, with dextrins, maltose and water, obtained by incomplete hydrolysis of starch; used as a flavoring agent, as a food, and in the treatment of dehydration.

g.-1-phosphate an intermediate in carbohydrate metabolism.

g.-6-phosphatase a liver (and kidney) enzyme that irreversibly cleaves glucose-6-phosphate to free glucose and phosphate; important in glucose homeostasis.

g.-6-phosphate an intermediate in carbohydrate metabolism.

g.-6-phosphate dehydrogenase (G6PD) a regulatory enzyme in the metabolism of glucose-6-phosphate. A deficiency of the enzyme in the erythrocyte results in a hemolytic anemia; an inherited abnormality in humans, rats and mice and acquired in animals in phenothiazine toxicity and ingestion of kale.

g. phosphate isomerase converts glucose-6-phosphate to fructose-6-phosphate and the reverse reaction.

g. suppression test suppression of blood levels of growth hormone by the intravenous administration of glucose is used to diagnose acromegaly.

g. tolerance factor (GTF) a naturally occurring substance containing chromium which potentiates the effects of insulin.

g. tolerance test a test of the body's ability to utilize carbohydrates. It is often used to detect abnormalities of carbohydrate metabolism such as occur in diabetes mellitus, hypoglycemia, and liver and adrenocortical dysfunction. If administered orally, it may also be used to assess the absorptive capacity of the small intestine.

glucosidase an enzyme of the hydrolase class that cleaves the glucosidic bond between two glucose molecules, occurring as α-, β- and α-1,3-glucosidase; α-glucosidase (maltase) occurs in intestinal juice, and β-glucosidase (cellobiase) in the kidney, liver and intestinal mucosa.

1,6-glucosidase an intestinal mucosal digestive enzyme concerned in the digestion of 1,6-glucosides.

α-glucosidase deficiency see GLYCOPROTEINOSIS.

glucosidic pertaining to glucoside.

glucosinolates substances in *Brassica* spp. crops which are degraded in the rumen to thiocyanates which may cause congenital goiter by interfering with the absorption of iodine.

glucosteroid see GLUCOCORTICOID.

glucosuria 1. the presence of glucose in the urine. 2. dextrosuria. Called also glycosuria.

renal g. glucosuria due to an inherited inability of renal tubules to reabsorb glucose completely.

glucosylceramidase see (BETA)-GLUCOCEREBROSIDASE.

glucosylceramidosis glucocerebrosidosis. See GAUCHER'S DISEASE.

glucuronate pathway one of the alternatives to the Embden–Meyerhof pathway of glycolysis, of oxidation of glucose-6-phosphate. See also the pentose phosphate PATHWAY.

glucuronic acid a uronic acid formed by oxidation of C-6 of glucose to a carboxy group; it occurs in proteoglycans (mucopolysaccharides), and is conjugated in the liver with many natural and foreign compounds or their metabolites, forming glucuronides, which are excreted in the urine.

g. a. pathway see GLUCURONATE PATHWAY.

β-glucuronidase an enzyme which attacks glycosidic linkages in natural and synthetic glucuronides; occurs in the spleen, liver and endocrine glands.

g. deficiency is the basis for MUCOPOLYSACCHARIDOSIS type VII in humans, dogs and inbred mice.

glucuronide any glycosidic conjugate of glucuronic acid; glucuronides, which are generally inactive, constitute the major proportion of the metabolites of many phenols, alcohols and carboxylic acids.

Glugea a genus of protozoa in the class Microsporea. Found in the tissues of fish. They cause large cysts, called glugea-cysts or xenomas, which result in deformity or intestinal obstruction. Includes *G. anomala*, *G. hertwigi*, *G. stephani*.

glutamate Glu; the anionic form of glutamic acid; in biochemistry, the term is often used interchangeably with glutamic acid.

g. dehydrogenase (GD) see glutamate DEHYDROGENASE.

glutamic acid a dibasic nonessential amino acid occurring in proteins. It is also an inhibitory neurotransmitter in the central nervous system. Its hydrochloride salt is used as a gastric acidifier. The monosodium salt (sodium glutamate; SMG) is used in treating encephalopathies associated with hepatic disease, and to enhance the flavor of foods and tobacco.

glutamic-oxaloacetic transaminase abbreviated GOT; see ASPARTATE AMINOTRANSFERASE.

glutamic-pyruvic transaminase abbreviated GPT; see ALANINE AMINOTRANSFERASE.

glutaminase an enzyme that hydrolyzes the splitting of glutamine into glutamate and ammonia.

glutamine Gln; an amide of glutamic acid, an amino acid occurring in proteins; it is an important carrier of ammonia to the kidney where it is released by glutaminase.

g. synthetase enzyme catalyzing the synthesis of the amino acid, glutamine from glutamate ammonia and ATP. Major means of detoxifying ammonia from amino acid catabolism in peripheral tissues and then transporting the ammonia as the amido-N in glutamine to the liver of kidney.

β-(γ-L-glutamyl) aminopropionitrile the form in which the toxin of lathyrism—β-aminopropionitrile—is found in plants.

L-glutamyl-β-cyanoalanine a lathyrogen.

γ-glutamyl cycle a mechanism involved in the transport of certain amino acids into cells in such tissues as the intestine, brain and kidney.

γ-glutamyl transpeptidase see gamma glutamyl TRANSFERASE.

glutaral see GLUTARALDEHYDE.

glutaraldehyde a disinfectant used in aqueous solution for sterilization of non-heat-resistant equipment; also used topically as an anhidrotic and as a tissue fixative for light and electron microscopy.

g. coagulation test a test used for the detection of hypogammaglobulinemia in calves.

glutathione reduced glutathione (GSH), a tripeptide containing glutamic acid, cysteine and glycine, which serves as a reducing agent in many biochemical reactions, being converted to oxidized glutathione (GSSG) in which the cysteine residues of two glutathione molecules are connected by a disulfide bridge. Reduced glutathione is important in protecting erythrocytes from oxidation and hemolysis; deficiency causes sensitivity to oxidant drugs.

g. peroxidase a selenium-containing enzyme whose blood level is a good indicator of the selenium status of the animal; occurs in a plasma form, an enzyme with specificity for phospholipids, and an intracellular form. Called also GPx.

g. reductase a flavin enzyme involved in the defense of the erythrocyte against hemolysis. A partial deficiency occurs relatively frequently but is due to a deficiency of riboflavin; called also GR.

glutathionuria the excretion of excessive amounts of glutathione in the urine.

gluteal pertaining to the buttocks.

g. muscles three muscles which extend, abduct, and rotate the thigh; the superficial, middle and deep gluteals. See also Table 13.

g. nerves nerves that innervate the gluteal muscles. See also Table 14.

gluten the protein of wheat and other grains that gives dough its tough, elastic character.

g. sensitivity called also gluten enteropathy. See wheat-sensitive ENTEROPATHY.

glutinous adhesive; sticky.

glutitis inflammation of the gluteal muscles.

L-glutamate dehydrogenase an enzyme involved in oxidative deamination of amino acids. Is spread widely in animal tissues.

Gly glycine.

glyburide a second generation sulfonylurea used as an oral hypoglycemic agent in the treatment of diabetes mellitus.

glycan polysaccharide.

glycemia the presence of glucose in the blood.

glycemic pertaining to the level of glucose in the blood.

g. control indicators in addition to periodic measurement of blood glucose levels, management of diabetes mellitus can be assessed by measurement of glycosylated hemoglobin or fructosamine.

g. index the area under the curve in a blood glucose response test.
glyceraldehyde a compound, glyceric aldehyde, formed by the oxidation of glycerol.
g. phosphate dehydrogenase an enzyme of the glycolytic pathway.
Glyceria genus of grasses of the Poaceae family; cause cyanide poisoning. Includes *G. maxima* (*G. aquatica*, reed sweet grass), *G. striata* (fowl manna grass).
glyceride an organic acid ester of glycerin, designated, according to the number of ester linkages, as a mono, di- or triglyceride.
glycerin a clear, colorless, syrupy liquid, used as a humectant and as a solvent for drugs; it is a trihydric sugar alcohol, being the alcoholic component of triglycerides. Called also glycerol.
glycerine see GLYCERIN.
glycerokinase hepatic enzyme catalyzing the phosphorylation of glycerol to glycerol-3-phosphate which can then enter the glycolysis pathway, or more usually gluconeogenesis.
glycerol a trihydric sugar alcohol, $CH_2OH{\cdot}CHOH{\cdot}CH_2OH$, which is a component of triglycerides. Pharmaceutical preparations are called glycerin.
g. guaiacolate see GLYCERYL guaiacolate.
g. 3-phosphate dehydrogenase two enzymes, an NAD+-dependent form in the cytosol and an FAD-dependent form present in the inner mitochondrial membrane. These two enzymes complete the transfer of reducing power generated as NADH+H+ during glycolysis through to $FADH_2$ which can enter complex II of the oxidative phosphorylation sequence. This process is called the glycerophosphate shuttle.
g. phosphate shuttle main means for the transfer of reducing power generated in the cytosol as NADH+H+ to the mitochondrion as $FADH_2$ so that ATP can be generated in oxidative phosphorylation. There is the loss of one potential ATP as a consequence of this shuttle. Commonly found in the brain.
glycerolipid one of the two dominant 'families' of lipids, derived from a glycerol base.
glycerolize to treat with or preserve in glycerol, as in the exposure of red blood cells to glycerol solution so that glycerol diffuses into the cells before they are frozen for preservation.
glycerophosphatase see ALKALINE phosphatase.
glyceryl the mono-, di- or trivalent radical formed by the removal of hydrogen from one, two or three of the hydroxy groups of glycerol.
g. guaiacolate a centrally acting muscle relaxant very popular as an additive in anesthesia, especially in horses.
g. trinitrate see NITROGLYCERIN.
g. trioleate see OLEIN.
glycine a nonessential amino acid, $H_2N{\cdot}CH_2{\cdot}COOH$, occurring as a constituent of proteins and functioning as an inhibitory neurotransmitter in the central nervous system; used as a gastric antacid and dietary supplement, and in the treatment of various myopathies. Called also aminoacetic acid. Abbreviation gly.
[^{15}N]-g. radioactive glycine used experimentally.
g. tolerance test has been used as a liver function test in cows but not a generally used one.
Glycine max see SOYBEAN.
glyco- word element. [Gr.] *sweetness, glucose;* see also words beginning *gluco-*.
glycoaldehyde an intermediate stage in the metabolism of ethylene glycol to oxalate, the toxic end product of poisoning by the glycol.
glycobiarsol an organic arsenic derivative with anthelmintic and antiprotozoal activity. Used in the treatment of whipworm (*Trichuris vulpis*) infections in dogs. Called also bismuth glycollylarsanilate.
glycocalyx the glycoprotein–polysaccharide covering that surrounds many cells.
glycocholate a salt of GLYCOCHOLIC ACID.
glycocholic acid a conjugated form of one of the bile acids that yields glycine and cholic acid on hydrolysis.
glycoconjugates secondary bile acids linked to glycine in the liver and secreted into bile.
glycogen a polysaccharide, the chief carbohydrate storage material in animals. It is formed and stored in the liver and muscles (phosphorylytically cleaved to glucose-1-phosphate). Called also animal starch.
g. granules electron-dense accumulation of glycogen molecules.
g. nephrosis deposition of glycogen in the renal tubles in diabetes mellitus but without apparent effect on renal function.
g. phosphorylase glycogen phosphorylase the major enzyme in glycogenolysis, leading to the release of glucose 1-phosphate from glycogen. This enzyme is activated by phosphorylation from ATP by glycogen phosphorylase kinase, activated by cAMP-dependent protein kinase or by Ca^2+ via calmodulin, or inhibited by hydrolysis of the phosphate by glycogen phosphorylase phosphatase.
g. synthase an enzyme in the glycogenesis process.
glycogen storage disease any of a group of genetically determined disorders of glycogen metabolism, marked by abnormal storage of glycogen in the body tissues. Includes Pompe's disease, Cori's disease, phosphofructokinase deficiency. See also GLYCOGENOSIS.
glycogenase an enzyme that splits glycogen into dextrin and maltose.
glycogenesis the conversion of glucose to glycogen for storage in the liver and muscle.
glycogenic pertaining to, characterized by, or promoting glycogenesis; pertaining to glycogen.
glycogenolysis the splitting up of glycogen in the liver or muscle, yielding glucose-1-phosphate.
muscle g. metabolic process under the regulatory control of adrenergic hormones or calcium ions for providing a rapid supply of ATP for muscle contraction and movement, particular for type II fibers. See also GLYCOGEN phosphorylase.
glycogenosis pl. *glycogenoses;* any genetically determined disorder of glycogen metabolism, marked by abnormal storage of glycogen in the tissues of the body. See also GLYCOGEN STORAGE DISEASE.
bovine generalized g. an inherited glycogen storage disease of Shorthorn and Brahman cattle resembling glycogenosis type II (Pompe's disease) of humans, caused by a deficiency of α-1,4-glucosidase. Widespread accumulation of glycogen occurs in the nervous system and muscles, leading to poor growth, incoordination, muscle weakness and eventually recumbency. There is also cardiomyopathy and often left-sided heart failure.
g. type I in humans, a deficiency of the hepatic enzyme glucose-6-phosphatase resulting in liver and kidney involvement, with hepatomegaly, hypoglycemia, hyperuricemia and gout. A similar condition has been observed in young dogs with hypoglycemia that does not respond to glucagon. Called also Gierke's disease or von Gierke's disease.

g. type II see bovine generalized glycogenosis (above). Also reported in sheep, cats, dogs and quail. Called also Pompe's disease.

g. type III an inherited deficiency of amylo-1,6-glucosidase causing neurological deterioration, hepatomegaly and retarded growth in German shepherd dogs from an early age. Called also Cori's disease, Forbes' disease, limit dextrinosis.

g. type VII see PHOSPHOFRUCTOSEKINASE deficiency.

glycohemoglobin see glycosylated HEMOGLOBIN.

glycol see ETHYLENE, POLYETHYLENE, PROPYLENE GLYCOL.

glycolic acid the primary toxic metabolic product of ethylene glycol.

glycolipid a lipid containing carbohydrate groups, often galactose but also glucose, inositol or others; the glycolipids include the cerebrosides.

glycolysis the enzymatic conversion of glucose to lactate or pyruvate, resulting in chemical bond energy stored in the form of ATP, as occurs in all tissues.

glyconeogenesis see GLUCONEOGENESIS.

glyconucleoprotein nucleoprotein bearing carbohydrate groups.

glycopenia a deficiency of sugar in the tissues.

glycopeptide any of a class of peptides that contain carbohydrates, including those that contain amino sugars.

glycopexis fixation or storing of sugar or glycogen.

glycophilia a condition in which a small amount of glucose produces hyperglycemia.

glycophorin a protein that projects through the thickness of the cell membrane of erythrocytes; it is attached to oligosaccharides at the outer cell membrane surface and to contractile proteins (spectrin and actin) at the cytoplasmic surface.

glycoprotein any of a class of conjugated proteins consisting of a compound of protein with a carbohydrate group.

g. deficiency an inherited disorder in dogs in which there is defective phagocytic function. Affected dogs have a marked, persistent neutrophilia and are susceptible to infections.

alpha-2HS glycoprotein serum protein important in bone resorption.

glycoproteinosis intracytoplasmic accumulations of a complex of glycoprotein and acid mucopolysaccharide in the central nervous system (PAS positive Lafora bodies), associated with seizures in familial progressive myoclonic epilepsy (Lafora's disease) in humans, and also reported in dogs.

glycoptyalism see GLYCOSIALIA.

glycopyrrolate, glycopyrronium an anticholinergic used to reduce gastric acid secretion and hypermotility.

glycorrhachia the presence of sugar in the cerebrospinal fluid.

glycorrhea any sugary discharge from the body.

glycosamine an amino sugar.

glycosaminoglycan any of the carbohydrates containing amino sugars occurring in proteoglycans, e.g. hyaluronic acid or chondroitin sulfate. These substances are secreted in very much greater quantities in the urine of achondroplastic dwarf calves than in other urines. This suggests that the disease is an inherited defect of metabolism similar to the mucopolysaccharidoses of humans. See also GLYCOGENOSIS.

g. polysulfate an antiarthritic compound which affects synovial membrane activity, increasing viscosity of synovial fluid.

glycosaminolipid any of a class of lipids that contain amino sugars.

glycosecretory concerned in secretion of glycogen.

glycosialia glucose in the saliva; glycoptyalism.

glycosialorrhea excessive flow of saliva containing sugar.

glycosidase any of a large group of hydrolytic enzymes acting on glycosyl compounds.

glycoside any compound containing a carbohydrate moiety (sugar), particularly any such natural product in plants, convertible, by hydrolytic cleavage, into a sugar and a nonsugar component (aglycone), and named specifically after the sugar contained, as glucoside (glucose), pentoside (pentose), fructoside (fructose), etc.

cardiac g. any one of a group of glycosides occurring in certain plants (e.g. *Digitalis*) having a characteristic action on the contractile force of the heart muscle. See also CARDENOLIDE, BUFADIENOLIDE.

glycosidic bond the covalent bond between two monosaccharides to form a disaccharide.

***N*-g. b., linkage** a type of carbohydrate–protein covalent linkage between an asparagine side chain amide and a sugar; type I linkage.

***O*-g. b., linkage** a type of carbohydrate–protein covalent linkage between a serine or threonine hydroxyl side chain amide and a sugar; type II linkage.

glycosphingolipid a sphingolipid containing the sugar glucose or galactose.

glycostatic tending to maintain a constant sugar level.

glycosuria see GLUCOSURIA.

glycosyl a radical derived from a carbohydrate.

g. transferases enzymes catalyzing the transfer of a monosaccharide unit from a nucleotide-linked sugar to the non-reducing end of an oligosaccharide chain, or to an appropriate functional group on a protein.

glycosylation the formation of linkages with glycosyl groups.

***N*-linked g.** attachment of oligosaccharides, synthesized on a dolichol-lipid platform to proteins through the amino acid asparagine spaced close to threonine or serine in the polypeptide sequence.

***O*-linked g.** attachment of groups of oligosaccharides directly to proteins through the hydroxyl group of threonine.

glycotropic having an affinity for sugar; causing hyperglycemia.

glycuresis the normal increase in the glucose content of the urine that follows an ordinary carbohydrate meal.

glycylglycine the simplest peptide; used in the synthesis of more complicated peptides.

Glycyphagus a genus of mites in the family Acaridae.

G. destructor a cause of hay itch.

G. domesticus very common as a parasite in stored food products and as a cause of dermatitis (grocer's itch) in humans.

glycyrrhetinic acid an extract of liquorice root. Reputed to have anti-inflammatory properties. Called also enoxolone.

glyoxylate a carbohydrate precursor.

g. pathway a pathway for the direct incorporation of acetate into a glucose precursor; operates in plants but not identified as an animal process.

glyphosate herbicide and desiccant for grains. Heavy doses to birds cause soft shells on their eggs.

Glyptauchen panduratus a poisonous fish with 17 dorsal spines. Called also goblin fish.

gm gram.

GM-CSF granulocyte–macrophage colony-stimulating factor.

GM$_1$ gangliosides see GANGLIOSIDE.
GM$_1$ gangliosidosis see GANGLIOSIDOSIS.
GM$_2$ gangliosidosis see GANGLIOSIDOSIS.
GMA glycol methacrylate.
GME granulomatous meningoencephalitis.
Gmelin test, Gmelin–Rosenbach test a test for the presence of bilirubin conjugates in feces and urine, based on the conversion of bilirubin to multicolored compounds by the addition of nitric acid.
GMP guanosine monophosphate.
Gnaphalium purpureum North American plant of the Asteraceae family; may cause nitrate–nitrite poisoning. Called also purple cudweed.
gnat see SIMULIUM, CNEPHIA.
gnathic pertaining to the jaw or cheeks.
gnathitis inflammation of the jaw.
gnath(o)- word element. [Gr.] *jaw*.
gnathocephalus a headless monster with jaws.
gnathodynamometer an instrument for measuring the force exerted in closing the jaws.
gnathology the science dealing with the masticatory apparatus as a whole.
gnathoplasty plastic repair of the jaw or cheek.
gnathoschisis congenital cleft of the upper jaw, as in cleft palate.
Gnathostoma a genus of spiruroid nematodes of the family Gnathostomatidae.
G. doloresi found in domestic and wild pigs.
G. hispidum adults found in the stomach of pigs and cause gastritis. Larvae migrate through the liver causing hepatitis.
G. nipponicum causes granuloma in the esophagus of weasels.
G. spinigerum found in the stomach of cats, dogs, mink, polecat and wild carnivora and erratically as a parasite under the skin of humans. Causes damage to liver and other organs while migrating, and establishes large cyst-like structures containing worms in the stomach wall.
gnathostomiasis infection with the nematodes *Gnathostoma* spp. contracted by eating the intermediate host, e.g. undercooked fish infected with the larvae of *G. spinigerum*. Includes gastritis and cysts in the stomach wall caused by the adults and hepatitis caused by the larvae.
Gnidia genus of small, African, woody plants in the family Thymelaeaceae which contain daphnetin and cause cardiomyopathy, nephrosis and enteritis. Contains *G. kraussiana*, *G. anthylloides*, *burchellii*, *G. latifolia*, *G. polycephala*. Called also *Lasiosiphon* spp., *Arthrosolen* spp., harpuisbos, januariebos.
gnosia the faculty of perceiving and recognizing.
gnotobiote a specially reared animal whose microflora and microfauna are known in complete detail. *Gnoto* is a Greek word for known, and *biota* is lifeforms, in this case microorganisms. See also GNOTOBIOTIC animal.
gnotobiotic pertaining to a gnotobiote or to gnotobiotics.
g. animal one that has been born germ free and then infected with known microorganisms. See also AXENIC and SPECIFIC PATHOGEN FREE.
gnotobiotics the science of rearing gnotobiotes. Also used in the more general sense of rearing specific pathogen free animals for use in a disease-free environment on commercial farms.
Gn-RH see GONADOTROPIN-RELEASING HORMONE.
GnRIF gonadotropin release inhibiting factor.
gnu a large, ungainly antelope with a head like a buffalo. Called also wildebeeste or *Gorgon taurinus*, *Connochaetes* spp.
go-away bird see MUSOPHAGID.
goad see PROD.
goanna a large carrion-eating MONITOR (3) lizard.
goat a small, horned ruminant used for milk, and angora and kashmir fibers. A variety of the species *Capra hircus* which also includes the wild goat. Common breeds of dairy goats are ANGLO-NUBIAN, BRITISH ALPINE, SAANEN, TOGGENBURG. Common indigenous goats, e.g. BOER, are usually dual or even multipurpose.
g. deodorizing performed on the bucks by removing an area of skin from medially and posteriorly to the horns. The scent is contained in sebaceous cells in areas of wrinkled, folded and hairless skin. There is another lesser smell in the urine of the buck.
g. doe mastitis see Table 16.
g. louse DAMALINIA *caprae*, biting louse; LINOGNATHUS *stenopsis*, sucking louse.
g. plague peste des petits ruminants.
g. pox see GOATPOX.
Rocky Mountain g. is really a goat-antelope, with a shaggy white coat and black horns.
g. sheep hybrids matings between the species are often fertile to the extent that an embryo is conceived but it invariably dies by about 60 days of pregnancy.
wild g. there are many genera of wild goats including ibex, steinbok and the true wild goat, *Capra hircus*, the progenitor of the domestic goat.
goat-antelopes small, wild ruminants, intermediate between goats and antelopes. Called also GORAL, takin, serow.
goatling young female goat between one and two years of age.
goatpox a disease caused by a poxvirus in the genus *Capripoxvirus* which includes the antigenically related sheeppox virus. Characterized by typical pox lesions on the hairless skin, especially the perineum. Kids may develop a severe systemic form with a high mortality rate.
goat's rue see GALEGA OFFICINALIS.
goatweed HYPERICUM *perforatum*.
gobbler male turkey. Called also tom.
goblet cell solitary mucus-secreting cell, especially of the intestinal and respiratory epithelium.
goblin fish see GLYPTAUCHEN PANDURATUS.
goeldi's monkey a small (about 8 oz, 8 inches long) monkey with thick soft brown to black hair. Arboreal and diurnal, they are sought after as research animals.
Goetze's suture pattern a special 6-bite suture pattern used in the one-stage repair of third-degree perineal laceration in the mare.
goggles see periocular LEUKOTRICHIA.
going sour development of bad temperament manifested by biting other horses while racing, savaging of attendants; worst problems are in mares with ovarian tumors.
goiter, goitre enlargement of the thyroid gland, causing a swelling in the front part of the neck.
adenomatous g. multilobular goiters cause thyroid enlargement in cats.
colloid g. is characterized by the presence of a large soft thyroid gland with its glandular space distended with colloid. Most cases occur in neonatal lambs, calves and kids which show a high rate of stillbirths and weakness and a high mortality rate. Enlarged thyroid glands and alopecia are good indicants of the existence of a nutritional deficiency of iodine, the usual cause of goiter in animals.
dyshormonogenetic g. an impairment in thyroglobulin synthesis is thought to be the cause of

inherited, congenital goiter recorded in sheep, cattle and goats. The thyroid gland is enlarged, there is a high neonatal mortality, a silky wool in sheep and a rough, sparse haircoat in goats. Called also inherited goiter.

goitrogen-induced g. there are a number of goitrogens in the environment of grazing animals. Their effect is almost entirely on the newborn. Common agents are low level intakes of cyanogenetic glycosides, e.g. in white clover, the glucosinolates in *Brassica* spp. plants, and mimosine in *Leucaena leucocephala.*

hyperplastic g. diffuse hyperplasia is the standard response to dietary iodine deficiency and to poisoning by plant goitrogens. It may also be caused by persistent exposure of the fetus to a high iodine intake of the dam. See also iodide goiter (below). Neonates are the usual subjects and the disease is manifested by clinical goiter, often sufficient to cause dystocia, and weak neonates with a high rate of stillbirths and deaths soon after birth.

inherited g. see dyshormonogenetic goiter (above).

iodide g. that occurring in reaction to iodides at high concentrations, due to inhibition of iodide organification.

nodular g. an endocrinologically inactive nodular enlargement of the thyroids in old dogs and horses. In old cats similar goiters sometimes develop functional adenomas.

goitrin the goitrogen produced by ruminal degradation of the glucosinolates in *Brassica* spp. plants. It prevents the organification of iodine by the thyroid.

goitrogen a goiter-producing agent. See also goitrogen-induced GOITER.

goitrogenesis the process of inducing goiter formation.

goitrogenic glucosinolates thiones and thiocyanates produced by metabolism of glucosinolates; potent goitrogens; see GOITRIN.

goitrogenicity the tendency to produce goiter.

gold a chemical element, atomic number 79, atomic weight 196.967, symbol Au. See Table 6. Gold and many of its compounds are used in human medicine and occasionally in veterinary medicine. See also CHRYSOTHERAPY.

g.-198 a radioisotope of gold having a half-life of 2.7 days and emitting gamma and beta radiation. Symbol ^{198}Au.

g. colloid scintiscan see SCINTISCAN.

g. dust a disease of aquarium fish caused by the flagellate protozoon *Oodinium limnecicum.* Affected fish develop a varnished look caused by a very heavy infestation of the protozoa on the skin and die within a few days.

g. standard the ultimate standard to which all endeavors aspire.

golden banner THERMOPSIS *rhombifolia.*

golden billy buttons see CRASPEDIA CHRYSANTHA.

golden chain see LABURNUM ANAGYROIDES. Called also golden rain.

golden glow see RUDBECKIA.

golden lion marmoset a gold to orange, longhaired monkey; up to 20 inches long and up to 1 lb weight. Called also *Leontideus rosalia.*

golden lion tamarin see LEONTOPITHECUS ROSALIA.

golden oat grass see TRISETUM FLAVESCENS. Called also yellow oat grass.

golden period in trauma surgery the period after the wound is inflicted during which primary intention healing is probable after suturing because the body's defenses can take care of the infection that has been introduced; considered to be less than 6 hours.

golden rain see LABURNUM ANAGYROIDES.

Golden retriever a medium- to large-sized gun dog with a flat or wavy, medium length coat in shades of gold or cream. The breed is predisposed to cataracts, progressive retinal atrophy, hypothyroidism, a congenital myopathy and von Willebrand's disease.

golden slipper the effect created by the convex yellow sole of the hoof of a stillborn or slink calf.

golden tip GOODIA *lotifolia.*

golden top see PSILOCYBE.

golden weed see OONOPSIS.

goldenrod see SOLIDAGO, HAPLOPAPPUS.

rust on g. see COLEOSPORIUM SOLIDAGENSIS.

goldfish the companion fish among the aquarium fishes. Gold dorsally shading to yellow on the belly. There are many fancy variants including the veiltail, the shubunkin and the lionhead. Called also *Carassius auratus.* See also Table 23.

g. ulcer disease ulcers scattered over the body caused by atypical *Aeromonas salmonicida*; encouraged by high water temperature and overcrowding. Called also GUD.

Goldie–Coldman hypothesis a theory relating drug resistance to spontaneous cell mutations; it is used to justify the use of multiple agents in chemotherapy of tumors.

Goldman equation quantifies the voltage potential of resting membranes.

golf ball a source of lead from the compound in the center that can poison dogs that chew them.

Golgi apparatus a complex intracellular organelle consisting mainly of a number of flattened sacs (cisternae) and associated vesicles, which is involved in the synthesis of glycoproteins, lipoproteins, membrane-bound proteins and lysosomal enzymes. The sacs form primary lysosomes and secretory vacuoles. Called also Golgi complex.

Golgi neurons 1. *Type I:* pyramidal cells with long axons, which leave the gray matter of the central nervous system, traverse the white matter, and terminate in the periphery. 2. *Type II:* stellate neurons with short axons in the cerebral and cerebellar cortices and in the retina.

Golgi stack the Golgi apparatus as seen in thin section electron micrographs of a cell; the set of flattened, disk-shaped cisternae resembling a stack of plates. Called also dictyosome.

Golgi tendon organ any of the mechanoreceptors arranged in series with muscle in the tendons of mammalian muscles, being the receptors for stimuli responsible for the lengthening reaction.

Golgi's cells Golgi neurons.

GoLIGHTLY see POLYETHYLENE glycol electrolyte solution.

Gomco pump standard suction kit including electric motor, pump and collecting jar.

gomdagga LANTANA *camara.*

Gomen disease cerebellar ataxia and degeneration in horses in New Caledonia apparently caused by an environmental toxin.

gomitoli a network of capillaries in the upper infundibular stem (of the hypothalamus), which surrounds terminal arterioles of the superior hypophyseal arteries and leads into the portal veins to the adenohypophysis.

gompertzian growth a pattern of cell growth in tumors in which there is increased doubling time and decreased growth fraction as a function of time.

Gomphocarpus synonym for some *Asclepias* spp. Includes *G. fruticosus, G. physocarpus.*

gomphosis a type of fibrous joint in which a conical process is inserted into a socket-like portion.
Gomphosphaeria genus of toxic cyanobacteria.
Gomphrena celosioides toxic plant of the Amaranthaceae family; contains an unidentified toxin which causes incoordination, frequent falling and dragging of the toes in horses. Recovery follows withdrawal of the plant from the diet. Called also soft khaki weed, gomphrena weed.
gomphrena weed see GOMPHRENA CELOSIOIDES.
gonad a sex gland; a gamete-producing gland; the OVARY in the female and the TESTIS in the male.
The ovary produces the ovum and the testis produces the spermatozoon. In addition, the gonads secrete hormones that influence the development of the reproductive organs and the physical traits that differentiate males from females, such as a crest and body form and size (the secondary sex characters). The hormones produced by the ovary include ESTROGEN and PROGESTERONE. The principal hormone produced by the testis is TESTOSTERONE.
hermaphroditic g's these gonads vary widely between combinations of male amd female tissues in an ovotestis, of which there may be one or two, to a testicle on one side and an ovary on the other.
indifferent g. the primordial stage of the embryonal gonad, before differentiation into a male or female organ.
gonadal pertaining to or arising from a gonad. See also TESTICULAR, OVARIAN.
g. cords cords formed by epithelial cells which migrate from the mesonephric tubules in the embryo to the gonadal ridge and establish the indifferent stage of gonadogenesis.
g. ridge the structures in the embryo to which the primordial germ cells migrate, and from which the gonads develop.
g. steroids see STEROID.
g. stromal tumor tumors of granulosa cells and thecal cells of the ovary.
gonadectomy removal of a gonad.
gonadoblastoma a rare, primary tumor of testicle or ovary containing, besides interstitial cells, germ cells, epithelial cells and granulosa cells.
gonadopathy any disease of the gonads.
gonadorelin gonadotropin-releasing hormone.
gonadotherapy treatment with gonadal hormones.
gonadotrope, gonadotrop, gonadotroph a basophilic cell of the anterior pituitary specialized to secrete follicle-stimulating hormone or luteinizing hormone.
gonadotroph gonadotrope.
gonadotrophic see GONADOTROPIC.
gonadotrophin see GONADOTROPIN.
gonadotropic stimulating the gonads; applied to hormones of the anterior PITUITARY gland which influence the gonads, including luteinizing and follicle-stimulating hormones, and human chorionic gonadotropin.
g. hormone one that has a stimulating influence on the gonads. Includes luteinizing and follicle-stimulating hormones from the pituitary gland and chorionic gonadotropin from pregnant mare's serum.
gonadotropin any hormone having a stimulating effect on the gonads. Two such hormones are secreted by the anterior pituitary: follicle-stimulating hormone and luteinizing hormone, both of which are active, but with differing effects, in the two sexes.
chorionic g. a gonad-stimulating hormone produced by cytotrophoblastic cells of the placenta; used in treatment of underdevelopment of the gonads and to induce ovulation. See also PREGNANCY tests.
g. release inhibiting factor pituitary hormone which inhibits the release of luteinizing hormone or follicle stimulating-hormone.
gonadotropin-releasing hormone a hormone produced in the hypothalamus and passed to the adenohypophysis via the hypophyseal portal vascular system, stimulating the release of the gonadotropins, especially luteinizing hormone. Abbreviated Gn-RH.
gonaduct the duct of a gonad; an oviduct or seminal duct.
gonalgia pain in the femorotibial joint.
gonangiectomy vasectomy.
gonarthritis inflammation of the femorotibial joint.
gonarthrotomy incision into the femorotibial joint.
Gonderi a genus of protozoa related to *Theileria*. See also GONDERIA MUTANS.
Gonderia mutans an alternative name for *Theileria mutans*.
gonecystis a seminal vesicle.
gonecystitis inflammation of a seminal vesicle.
gonecystolith a concretion in a seminal vesicle.
gonecystopyosis suppuration of a seminal vesicle.
Gonglyonema a genus of spiruroid nematodes in the superfamily Spiruroidea.
G. crami, G. ingluvicola found in the crop of domestic fowls.
G. minimum found in the esophagus of primates; may cause anemia, vomiting, gastritis and enteritis.
G. monnigi found in the rumen of sheep and goats.
G. neoplasticum found in the tongue, esophagus and stomach of laboratory rats and mice but causes little epithelial reaction.
***G. pulchrum* (syn. *G. scutatum*)** occurs in the esophageal mucosa of ruminants and occasionally in humans.
G. sumani found in the crop of domestic fowl.
G. verrucosum found in the rumen of ruminants.
gonidium pl. *gonidia* [Gr.] 1. the algal component of the thallus of a lichen. 2. a motile reproductive unit of certain nitrogen-fixing bacteria.
Goniocotes a genus of lice infesting the feathers of domestic fowl and guinea fowl. They belong to the superfamily Ischnocera.
***G. gallinae* (syn. *G. hologaster, Goniodes hologaster*)** found in the feathers of domestic fowl. Called also fluff lice.
G. hologaster see *G. gallinae* (above).
G. maculatus found in the feathers of guinea fowl.
Goniodes a genus of biting lice of the superfamily Ischnocera.
G. dissimilis on domestic fowl. Called also brown chicken louse.
***G. gigas* (syn. *Goniocotes gigas*)** called also large chicken louse.
***G. hologaster* (syn. *Goniocotes gallinae*)** see GONIOCOTES *gallinae*.
G. meleagridis see CHELOPISTES.
goniodysgenesis abnormal development of the iridocorneal filtration angle. A familial defect with glaucoma in Basset hounds.
gonioimplant an artificial device positioned in the anterior chamber to assist in drainage of aqueous humor.
goniolens a contact lens placed on the eye to allow direct or indirect ophthalmoscopic examination of the iridocorneal angle. See also GONIOSCOPY.
goniometer an instrument for measuring angles; the instrument used in GONIOMETRY.
goniometry the measurement of range of motion in a joint. The technique may be used as a diagnostic or

therapeutic measure to determine the functional status of a patient with a musculoskeletal or neurological disability. There is a variety of tools and techniques by which joint motion can be measured, but for most clinical purposes the simple universal goniometer is an adequate instrument. The system for recording measurements of range of motion may be somewhat complex or it may be based upon the simple technique of relating the degree of joint motion to a full circle (360 degrees).

gonion pl. *gonia* [Gr.] the most inferior, posterior and lateral point on the angle of the mandible.

goniopuncture insertion of a knife blade through the clear cornea, just within the limbus, across the anterior chamber of the eye and through the opposite corneoscleral wall, in treatment of glaucoma.

gonioscope an optical instrument for examining the angle of the anterior chamber of the eye and for demonstrating ocular motility and rotation.

gonioscopy examination of the angle of the anterior chamber of the eye with a gonioscope.

goniotomy an operation for glaucoma; it consists in opening Schlemm's canal under direct vision.

gonitis inflammation of the stifle (femorotibial) joint.

gono- word element. [Gr.] *seed, semen.*

gonochorist fish species in which the embryonic gonad subsequently divides into ovaries or testes; may be a differentiated gonochorist, in which the differentiation is direct, or an undifferentiated gonochorists, in which there is an intermediate stage of an ovary-like gonad, a situation quite different from hermaphrodites.

gonocyte the primitive reproductive cell of the embryo. See also GERM cell.

Gonometa an African moth which infests *Acacia erioloba* and *A. mellifera* producing very many cocoons of silk fiber which cause ruminal impaction in cattle browsing on the tree. Called also Molopo moth.

gonophore an accessory reproductive organ, such as the oviduct.

Gonyaulax poisonous dinoflagellate which render shellfish eating them poisonous to animals eating the shellfish.

gonycampsis abnormal curvature of the femorotibial joint.

gonyocele synovitis of the femorotibial joint.

gonyoncus tumor of the femorotibial joint.

gonys profile of the midline curvature of the lower beak of birds.

good samaritan law a law that provides protection against claims of malpractice for medical practitioners who render emergency care at the scene of an accident except when gross negligence or willful misconduct can be proved. Most states in the USA have passed such laws; all the laws cover doctors, and about half the laws cover nurses. It would be beneficial if similar laws were enacted to protect veterinarians and their patients.

Goodia a plant genus of the legume family Fabaceae; may cause cyanide poisoning. Includes *G. lotifolia* (clover-leaf poison, clover tree), *G. medicagena* (small golden tip).

Goodpasture's syndrome an autoimmune disease of humans in which glomerulonephritis and pulmonary hemorrhage are produced by complement-mediated tissue damage caused by antibodies directed against the glomerular and alveolar basement membranes. A proliferative glomerulonephritis associated with antiglomerular basement membrane antibodies, analogous to the renal component of Goodpasture's syndrome, occurs rarely in domestic animals; it has been reported in horses and is suspected to occur in dogs.

goose pl. *geese;* a web-footed, long-necked bird of the family Anatidae. Domestic geese were derived from the wild goose, *Anser anser*. There are many other species in this genus and in the other *Branta* genus of geese, of which *Branta canadensis* is typical.

Popular domestic breeds include EMDEN, TOULOUSE.

g. body louse see TRINOTON ANSERINUM.

g. enteritis a parvovirus infection.

g. hepatitis occurs only in goslings less than 4 weeks old and caused by goose parvovirus. Affected birds have conjunctivitis, nasal discharge and polydipsia, huddle together and die. Postmortem findings include hepatitis and myocarditis. Called also gosling hepatitis, gosling plague.

g. honk see goose honk COUGH.

g. influenza see PASTEURELLA *anatipestifer*. Called also infectious serositis, new duck disease.

g. parvovirus infection see goose hepatitis (above).

g. plague see goose hepatitis (above).

g. septicemia a fatal septicemia caused by *Borrelia* (*Treponema*) *anserina* and transmitted by the tick *Argas persicus*.

slender g. louse ANATICOLA *anseris*.

g. venereal disease an apparently infectious disease of ganders with an uncertain etiology, causing necrosis and scarring of the phallus, making reproduction impossible.

goose-rumped a defect in the conformation of the horse. The line from the top of the rump to the base of the tail is too steep and is insufficiently muscled. Called also drooping quarters.

goose-stepping an abnormality of gait manifested by balancing on one leg of a pair and swinging the opposite member through without flexing it. May be difficult to differentiate clinically from hypermetria because of the tendency in both abnormalities to overreach the target.

goosefoot several plants of the family Chenopodiaceae.

goosegrass ELEUSINE *indica*.

goosiekte PACHYSTIGMA poisoning.

gopher a small burrowing rodent. Called pocket gopher because of its habit of storing food in a cheek pouch. Species are *Thomomys talpoides* (gray gopher) and *Geomys* spp. (pocket gopher).

Gopherus agassizii desert tortoise.

goral an intermediate type between goat and antelope. Look, smell and climb like goats but have wide muzzles like antelopes and are not bearded. Called also *Naemorhedus* spp.

Gordon extender an adjustable metal frame designed to be used as a means of applying traction to a limb, or keeping it extended.

Gordon setter a medium- to large-sized, muscular gun dog with medium length hair that is longer under the neck and body, tail and behind the legs ('feathering'). The color is black with mahogany or chestnut brown markings. The breed is predisposed to progressive retinal atrophy.

Gorgon taurinus see GNU.

gorilla the biggest and strongest of the anthropoid apes; *Gorilla gorilla* of the family Pongidae. Up to 6 ft tall and 500 lb, mostly terrestrial, fruit-eating primate, with a ferocious appearance but gentle nature if unprovoked and a legendary involvement with human adventure. Include *G. g. beringei*, the mountain gorilla.

Gorki sheep polled Russian meat and shortwool

sheep; originated from local breeds plus Hampshire Down.

gorse see ULEX EUROPAEUS. Called also furze.

goshawk slate-blue, expert hunting hawk, 2 ft long with a 4 ft wingspan. A quick flyer that catches most of its prey on the wing. Called also *Accipiter gentilis.*

gosling a young goose.

g. hepatitis see GOOSE hepatitis.

g. plague see GOOSE hepatitis.

Gosset retractor a self-retaining retractor suitable for exposure of abdominal viscera. Two retractor blades are mounted on a bar and can be moved apart to open the incision. The blades are the standard P shape with a curved loop to provide retention.

Gossypium Includes *G. hirsutum* (*Gossypium arboreum, G. barbadense, G. herbaceum*), the commercial cotton plant of the family Malvaceae.

Cotton seeds are a residue of the cotton industry and, after extraction of the oil, the residual cottonseed cake is much valued as a protein supplement for livestock. The seeds contain gossypol, a toxic polyphenolic pigment, and unless the processing is appropriate the cake and meal can be very poisonous, causing severe myocardial necrosis and liver damage. Ruminants may be affected but the severest disease occurs in pigs. Clinically there is congestive heart failure and severe dyspnea. The cake is also very low in vitamin A and nutritional deficiency may result.

gossypol toxic phenolic pigment in the glands of seeds of GOSSYPIUM spp.

gossypurpurin a minor pigment found with gossypol and gossyverdurin in cottonseed feed products.

gossyverdurin a phenolic pigment found in cottonseed products together with gossypol and gossypurpurin. It is the most toxic of the three.

GOT glutamic–oxaloacetic transaminase.

Gotland pony Swedish pony; black, brown or bay.

goubos PACHYSTIGMA *pygmaeum.*

gouge a hollow chisel for cutting and removing bone. See also ALEXANDER GOUGE.

gousiekte Afrikaans name (quick sickness) for the disease of sheep and cattle caused by poisoning by PACHYSTIGMA, PAVETTA and FADOGIA HOMBLEI. A syndrome of sudden death caused by cardiomyopathy. The causative toxin has been isolated but not characterized.

gousiekteboom [Af.] PAVETTA *schumanniana*; called also gousiekte tree.

gousiektebossie PACHYSTIGMA *pygmaeum.*

gout a disorder of uric acid metabolism in which there is hyperuricemia and deposition of urates in and around the joints. Occurs in humans and anthropoid apes. Most animals possess the enzyme uricase that converts uric acid to allantoin. Dalmatian dogs excrete large amounts of uric acid in their urine, but the breed is not affected by gout. A disease called gout occurs in commercial chickens due to feeding of excessive amounts of protein.

articular g. caused by gross excesses of protein in the diet. A chronic disease manifested by swelling of the joints which contain a thick white fluid consisting largely of uric acid crystals.

visceral g. birds become weak and listless and die. The viscera are covered with a frosting of urea crystals. There is a primary renal disease and a fatal uremia. The high-protein diet exacerbates that original disease.

Governing Vessel in acupuncture one of the two major extra meridian vessels. Called also *Du.* The other is the Conception Vessel.

governmental veterinary services veterinary services provided by the public sector. In former communist and many Third World countries all veterinary as well as other professional services are provided by governments. In western countries it is usual to divide the services between government and the public sector. The dividing line is set at different levels in different countries and fluctuates depending on the socialist inclinations of the government of the day. At present there is a general move towards governments withdrawing from some of the field or towards setting up a government-owned 'consumer pays' service. In general governments accept responsibility for diseases and management systems that have implications for farmers over a wide area, or where losses are going to be more than an individual farmer can possibly bear, or when the country's or state's capacity to export animal products is threatened.

Gower's solution a diluting fluid for red cell counts; an isotonic solution containing sodium sulfate and glacial acetic acid.

gown protective garment, usually of fabric or paper; used in surgery as a barrier between the patient and the operating personnel.

GPT glutamic–pyruvic transaminase.

GPx see GLUTATHIONE peroxidase.

GR glutathione reductase.

gr. grain; approximately 65 mg.

Graaff–Reinet disease see MAEDI.

graafian follicle a small sac, embedded in the OVARY, that encloses an ovum. At sexual maturity each ovary has a large number of immature follicles, each of which contains an undeveloped egg cell. These structures are called primordial, or primitive, follicles. At varying intervals in the different animal species, one of these follicles develops to maturity, or ripens; as it does so the animal shows the signs of sexual receptivity known as ESTRUS.

As the follicle ripens, it increases in size. The ovum within becomes larger, the follicular wall becomes thicker, and fluid collects in the follicle and surrounds the egg. At this point, it is also known as a vesicular ovarian follicle. The follicle also secretes estradiol, the hormone that prepares the endometrium to receive a fertilized egg. As the follicle matures, it moves to the surface of the ovary and forms a projection. When fully mature, the graafian follicle breaks open and releases the ovum, which passes into the UTERINE tubes. This release of the ovum is called OVULATION.

The released ovum travels down the tube to the uterus. Meanwhile, the empty graafian follicle in the ovary becomes transformed into the corpus luteum, or yellow body, by becoming filled with cells containing a yellow substance. The corpus luteum secretes progesterone, a hormone that causes further change in the endometrium, allowing it to provide a good milieu in which a fertilized ovum can grow through the stages of gestation to become a fetus.

atretic g. f. a follicle which enlarges and then regresses without proceeding to ovulation; occurs normally in animals as waves of follicles developing and regressing during estrous cycles and sometimes during pregnancy; occurs also in seasonally anestrous females. Follicular atresia can be a disease when it occurs at a time when the female should be coming into estrus but is on an inadequate diet, or suffering from a debilitating primary disease. The effect is a failure of the animal to come into estrus and to be fertile.

cystic g. f. see cystic FOLLICLE.

gracile slender; delicate.
gracilis muscle a muscle which occupies the medial surface of the thigh; arises from the pelvic symphysis and inserts on the tibial crest. See Table 13.
g. muscle rupture a common injury in racing Greyhounds, causing lameness, inability to extend the stifle, and an obvious swelling in the medial thigh. Called also dropped muscle.
grackle a 10 inch long bird like a starling with iridescent black plumage, and a keel-like crease in its tail. Called also common grackle, American blackbird, *Quiscalus quiscala*.
Gracula religiosa see MYNAH BIRD.
grade progeny of a mating between a purebred and a crossbred animal.
g. up when an animal of inferior breeding and quality is bred to one of much superior standing.
gradient rate of increase or decrease of a variable value.
grading setting a numerical value, e.g. body condition scoring.
clinical sign g. giving a value to a clinical sign so that its relative importance in the diagnosis of a particular disease is given its appropriate weighting, a matter of some significance in computer-assisted diagnosis. The numerical value for a particular clinical sign may well vary widely for different diseases.
graduate 1. person who has received a degree from a university or college. 2. a measuring vessel marked by a series of lines.
g. programs educational programs for persons who already have their basic degree that entitles them to practice. Includes programs provided for persons attempting postgraduate research degrees, vocational diplomas and coursework masterates, and for refresher and update courses for professional veterinarians under the general heading of professional continuing education.
graduated marked by a succession of lines, steps or degrees.
Graefe ophthalmic instruments a series of instruments especially for ophthalmic surgery. Includes cataract knives, iris forceps, eyelid speculum and strabismus hook.
Graff–Reinert disease see MAEDI.
graft 1. any tissue or organ for implantation or transplantation. 2. to implant or transplant such tissue. See also FLAP (1), GRAFTING, ALLOGRAFT, XENOGRAFT.
autodermic g., autoepidermic g. a skin graft taken from the patient's own body.
autologous g., autoplastic g. a graft taken from another area of the patient's own body; an autograft.
avascular g. a graft of tissue in which not even transient vascularization is achieved.
g. bed site to which a graft is to be joined.
bone g. the transfer of living bone, usually for fracture repair or reconstructive surgery. Various types of bone grafts are identified, depending on their source and treatment, if any, e.g. cortical, autograft, allograft, cancellous, xenograft, isograft.
cable g. a nerve graft made up of several sections of nerve in the manner of a cable.
cutis g. dermal graft.
dermal g., dermic g. skin from which epidermis and subcutaneous fat have been removed, used instead of fascia in various plastic procedures.
g. enhancement prior exposure of the recipient to the donor's tissues may prolong survival of a graft.
epidermal g. a piece of epidermis implanted on a raw surface.
fascia g. a graft of tissue taken from the external investing fascia of the leg (fascia lata).
fascicular g. a nerve graft in which bundles of nerve fibers are approximated and sutured separately.
free g. a graft of tissue completely freed from its bed, in contrast to a flap.
full-thickness g. a skin graft consisting of the full thickness of the skin, with little or none of the subcutaneous tissue.
heterodermic g. see HETERODERMIC.
heterologous g., heteroplastic g. a graft of tissue transplanted between animals of different species; a heterograft or xenograft.
homologous g. a graft of tissue obtained from the body of another animal of the same species but with a genotype differing from that of the recipient; a homograft or allograft.
isologous g., isoplastic g. a graft of tissue transplanted between genetically identical individuals; an isograft.
lamellar g. replacement of the superficial layers of an opaque cornea by a thin layer of clear cornea from a donor eye.
mesh g. skin grafts in which multiple small incisions have been made to permit lateral stretching of the graft and to increase flexibility to facilitate placement in tricky sites.
omental g's free or attached segments of omentum used to cover suture lines following gastrointestinal or colonic surgery.
patch g. used in the surgical repair of defects in the pulmonary outflow tract. Allows for growth of the patient and enlarges the outflow tract.
pedicle g. a portion of skin and subcutaneous tissue with a vascular attachment moved from one part of the body to another. Grafted to the new site, they not only can survive because of their own vascular supply, they can improve circulation in the site. Called also pedicle flap.
penetrating g. a full-thickness corneal transplant.
periosteal g. a piece of periosteum to cover a denuded bone.
pinch g. a piece of skin graft about 6 mm in diameter, obtained by elevating the skin with a needle and slicing it off with a knife.
punch g. grafts are obtained by using a skin biopsy punch on the animal or on a piece of separated skin.
g. rejection see REJECTION.
seed g. small pieces of skin are imbedded in granulation tissue on the same patient.
sieve g. a skin graft from which tiny circular islands of skin are removed so that a larger denuded area can be covered, the sievelike portion being placed over one area, and the individual islands over surrounding or other denuded areas.
skin g. a piece of skin implanted to replace a lost part of the integument. Many types of graft are used and are included in this list.
split-skin g. a skin graft consisting of only a portion of the skin thickness.
sponge g. a bit of sponge inserted into a wound to promote the formation of granulations.
thick-split g. a skin graft cut in pieces, often including about two-thirds of the full thickness of the skin.
tubed g. see rope FLAP.
tunnel g. see rope FLAP.
vascular g. see vascular CONDUIT.
graft-versus-host disease a condition that occurs when immunologically competent cells or their precursors are transplanted into an immunologically incompetent recipient (host) that is not histocompatible with the donor. Because the host is immunodeficient, the graft is not rejected. Immunocompetent T

lymphocytes present in the donor tissue are activated and recognize the recipient's tissue as 'foreign' and react to them, producing clinical manifestations including edema, erythema, ulceration, loss of hair, and heart and joint lesions similar to those occurring in connective tissue disorders. Called also GVH disease or reaction, runting syndrome.

grafting 1. the implanting or transplanting of skin or other tissue from another part of the body or from another animal to serve as replacement for damaged or missing tissue. The purpose may be to encourage healing, to improve function, to act as a safeguard against infection, to improve appearance, or to replace a diseased body organ. See also TRANSPLANTATION. 2. of orphan calves. See FOSTERING.

Grahamella small intraerythrocytic rickettsiae parasitizing small mammals and turtles. They are transmitted by blood-sucking ectoparasites, especially fleas. Related to *Bartonella* spp.

Graham's law the rate of diffusion of a gas through porous membranes varies inversely with the square root of its density.

grain 1. a seed, especially of a cereal plant; for best results in feeding the seed may be ROLLED, CRACKED, flaked (below). 2. the twentieth part of a scruple: 0.065 g; abbreviated gr. See also Table 4.2. 3. the texture and patterned appearance of the outside of leather. 4. the size and nature of the crystals of the fluorescent salt used in intensifying screens and also the size and nature of silver halide crystals used in photographic emulsion.

g. engorgement see CARBOHYDRATE ENGORGEMENT.

flaked g. grain that has been cooked and then rolled flat. The digestibility is greatly enhanced but the process is costly.

g. fumigants substances used to fumigate silos full of grain to kill insect pests. Use of these agents other than as recommended by the makers may lead to poisoning. See also METHYL bromide.

high-moisture g. see MOIST grain storage.

g. itch mites see PEDICULOIDES VENTRICOSUS.

micronized g. heated in a dry heat then rolled.

g. overload see CARBOHYDRATE ENGORGEMENT.

popped g. grain passed across a heated plate and popped like popcorn.

g. rash grain itch mite DERMATITIS.

roasted g. roasted in dry heat but not popped.

g. screenings debris from a grain batch that is removed by passing it over a screen. Has some feeding value but this varies with the mix of contents.

g. sorghum *Sorghum bicolor (S. vulgare)*.

spent g. grain used in brewing or liquor production that has been exhausted of its carbohydrate; includes brewer's grains, distiller's grains.

sprouted g. see HYDROPONICS.

graininess a fault in x-ray films in which there is clumping together of the silver particles in the emulsion, causing the image to lose its homogeneous appearance and to give an impression of lumpiness.

grains grainlike masses of inspissated necrotic material and debris found in swamp cancer lesions. See also SWAMP CANCER, BREWER'S GRAINS, DISTILLER'S grains.

gram 1. the basic unit of mass (weight) of the metric system, being the equivalent of 15.432 grains; symbol g, sometimes abbreviated gm. See also Table 4.2 and SI UNITS. 2. see GRAM'S STAIN. 3. see CHICKPEA.

g. atomic weight the same numerically as the atomic weight of an element but expressed in grams.

g. molecular weight the same numerically as the molecular weight of the substance but expressed in grams.

gram- word element. [Gr.] *written, recorded.*

-gram word element. [Gr.] *written, recorded.*

gram-molecule see MOLE (2).

gram-negative said of bacteria that are decolorized by alcohol in Gram's method of staining (see GRAM'S STAIN), and are thus stained only with the counter stain (usually red). Gram-negative bacteria have a much thinner layer of peptidoglycan in the cell wall than Gram-positive bacteria.

gram-positive said of bacteria that resist decolorization by alcohol in Gram's method of staining (see GRAM'S STAIN) and thus retain the crystal violet–iodine complex and appear purple; a characteristic of bacteria whose cell wall is composed of a thick layer of peptidoglycan and teichoic acid.

Gram's stain a staining procedure in which bacteria are stained with crystal violet, treated with strong iodine solution, decolorized with ethanol or ethanol–acetone and counterstained with a contrasting dye, usually safranin. The iodine alters the structure of the cell wall in gram-positive bacteria so that the crystal violet is locked within the cell. Organisms that retain the crystal violet stain are deep purple in color and are classed as gram-positive and those losing the crystal violet stain are classified as gram-negative and are red in color.

gramicidin an antibacterial substance produced by the growth of *Bacillus brevis*, one of the two principal components of tyrothricin; called also gramicidin D. Gramicidin S is a closely related substance produced by a thermophilic strain of *B. brevis*.

gramine a toxic alkaloid in *Phalaris arundinacea*.

graminivorous feeding on grass and grass seeds and other grain.

Grammocephalus a genus of hookworms in the subfamily Bunostominae.

G. clathratus found in the bile ducts of the African elephant.

G. hybridatus found in the bile ducts of the Indian elephant.

G. intermedius found in the bile ducts of the rhinoceros.

G. varedatus found in the bile ducts of the Indian elephant.

grampus killer whale, *Orcinus orca*. The name is also used for Risso's dolphin, *Grampus griseus*.

Grand Basset Griffon Vendeen a hunting dog of medium height and with a rough, long coat of white with lemon, orange, tri-color or grizzle markings. See also PETIT BASSET GRIFFON VENEEN.

Grand Bleu de Gascoigne a medium- to large-sized hunting dog with a long head, wrinkled face, pendulous lips and a dewlap. The smooth coat is a distinctive color of black mottling on a white base, which gives the blue appearance. There are two black marks on the head, each covering an ear and eye, and one on the skull; tan markings are found on the cheeks, lips, inside the ears, on the legs and under the tail.

grand mal [Fr.] a major seizure attended by loss of consciousness and convulsive movements, as distinguished from petit mal, a minor seizure. See also EPILEPSY, SEIZURE.

Grand Traverse disease a disease of the Great Lakes region of the USA and Canada. See COBALT nutritional deficiency.

granddam mother of an animal's sire or dam.

grandparent generation first generation of a three generation breeding program.

grandsire sire of an animal's dam or sire.

granivorous feeding on grain.

granny bonnets AQUILEGIA VULGARIS, ISOTROPIS *cuneifolia*.

granny knot an insecure knot with the loose ends of the suture coming out from the loop one over and one under when they should be both under or both over.

Grant's capsule a electronic device for measuring arterial blood pressure.

granula iridica see IRIDIAL granule.

granular made up of or marked by the presence of granules or grains.

g. casts homogeneous urinary casts with a granular structure; composed of fractions of serum proteins.

g. cell myoblastoma rare tumor at the base of the tongue of the dog.

g. cell tumor a benign, circumscribed, tumor-like lesion of soft tissue, particularly of the lung of the horse, tongue of dogs, skin and muscle, composed of large cells with prominent granular cytoplasm; considered by some to arise from myoblasts (myoblastoma) and by others from neurogenic elements (granular cell schwannoma).

g. layer see STRATUM granulosum.

g. reticulum rough-surfaced endoplasmic reticulum.

g. vaginitis spherical, 1 mm diameter nodules on the vulvar mucosa of the cow and the penile skin of the bull. Appears to be a nonspecific hyperplasia of lymphoid tissue, but linked anecdotally with *Mycoplasma* spp. Called also granular vulvovaginitis.

g. venereal disease see granular vaginitis (above).

g. vulvitis part of a venereal disease caused by *Ureaplasma diversum* in cattle; other signs include embryonic death, abortion, dead or weak calves.

g. vulvovaginitis see granular vaginitis (above).

granulatio pl. *granulationes* [L.] a granule, or granular mass.

granulation 1. the division of a hard substance into small particles. 2. the formation in wounds of small, rounded masses of tissue during healing; also the mass so formed.

arachnoid g's enlarged arachnoid villi projecting into the venous sinuses and creating slight depressions on the inner surface of the cranium.

exuberant g's excessive proliferation of granulation tissue in the healing of a wound.

g. tissue the new tissue formed in repair of wounds of soft tissue, consisting of connective tissue cells and ingrowing young vessels. It ultimately forms the cicatrix; excessive granulation is a common cause of chronic failure of wounds on the lower limbs of horses to heal.

granule 1. a small particle or grain. 2. a small pill made of sucrose.

acidophil g's granules staining with acid dyes.

aleuronoid g's colorless myeloid colloidal bodies found in the base of pigment cells.

alpha g's 1. oval granules found in blood platelets; they are lysosomes containing acid phosphatase. 2. large granules in the alpha cells of the islets of Langerhans; they secrete glucagon. 3. acidophilic granules in the alpha cells of the adenohypophysis.

amphophil g's granules that stain with both acid and basic dyes.

azur g's, azurophil g's granules that stain easily with azure dyes; they are coarse, reddish granules and are seen in many lymphocytes.

basophil g's granules staining with basic dyes.

beta g's 1. granules in the beta cells of the islets of Langerhans that secrete insulin. 2. basophilic granules in the beta cells of the adenohypophysis.

g. cell the largest group of cells produced by the external germinal layer on the external surface of the embryonal cerebellum; they form the thick granular layer of the cerebellum; called also granule neurons.

chromatic g's, chromophilic g's see NISSL bodies.

cone g's the nuclei of the visual cells in the outer nuclear layer of the retina which are connected with the cones.

eosinophil g's those staining with eosin. See also alpha granules (above).

epsilon g. see neutrophil granules (below).

Grawitz's g's minute granules seen in the erythrocytes in the basophilia of lead poisoning.

iodophil g's granules staining brown with iodine, seen in polymorphonuclear leukocytes in various acute infectious diseases.

keratohyalin g. keratin precursor; in the stratum granulosum of the epithelium.

metachromatic g's granules present in mast cells and many bacterial cells, having an avidity for basic dyes and causing irregular staining of the cell.

mitochondrial g's organelles in osteoblasts through which temporary calcium ion sequestration can be effected.

g. neurons see granule cell (above).

neutrophil g's neutrophilic granules from the protoplasm of polymorphonuclear leukocytes; called also epsilon granules.

Nissl's g's see NISSL bodies.

oxyphil g's acidophil granules.

pigment g's small masses of coloring matter in pigment cells.

primary g's the peroxidase-positive granules of neutrophils, most prominent in the progranulocyte and early myelocyte stages.

rod g's the nuclei of the visual cells in the outer nuclear layer of the retina which are connected with the rods.

secondary g's the peroxidase-negative ('specific') granules seen in mature neutrophils.

seminal g's the small granular bodies in the semen.

sulfur g's see SULFUR granule.

toxic g's dark-staining granules in neutrophils that contain peroxidase and acid hydrolases. They occur in inflammatory reactions.

granuloadipose showing fatty degeneration containing granules of fat.

granuloblast myeloblast; an immature granulocyte.

granuloblastosis a superseded name for MYELOBLASTOSIS.

granulocyte any cell containing granules, especially a granular leukocyte.

band-form g. band cell.

g. colony-stimulating factor see COLONY-stimulating factors.

g.–macrophage colony-stimulating factor see COLONY-stimulating factors.

granulocytic pertaining to granulocytes.

g. leukemia see myelocytic LEUKEMIA.

g. sarcoma extramedullary growth of multiple, focal granulocytic neoplasm. They may be neutrophilic or eosinophilic. Lesions may be in any tissue but favor lung, gut and skin. They have a greenish color due to the exposure of myeloperoxidase to air. Called also chloroma.

granulocytopathy any disorder of the granulocytes.

bovine g. syndrome inherited in Holstein cattle as a recessive trait; chronic febrile disease with poor growth, emaciation, dermatitis, oral ulcers, lymph node enlargement, recurrent infestion, poor wound healing, anemia and marked leukocytosis.

canine g. syndrome an inherited disorder in Irish setters in which defective bactericidal function of neutrophils results in recurrent infections with neutrophilia.

granulocytopenia see AGRANULOCYTOSIS.
granulocytopenic pertaining to or emanating from granulocytopenia.
g. calf disease disease characterized by petechiae and necrotic lesions in the alimentary tract. The lesions in the mouth lead to hypersalivation, those in the nasal cavities to a nasal discharge. The depression of bone marrow is manifested by neutropenia and thrombocytopenia, leading to serious and often fatal secondary infections. The cause is unknown. See also FURAZOLIDONE, RADIOMIMETIC, RADIATION injury.
granulocytopoiesis the production of granulocytes.
granulocytosis an excess of granulocytes in the blood.
masked g. an increase in the total number of granulocytes but not the leukocyte count, resulting from an increase in the marginal pool.
paraneoplastic g. seen in association with neoplasia; the cause is unknown.
granulokinetics factors affecting cell production and migration.
granuloma a tumor-like mass or nodule of granulation tissue, with actively growing fibroblasts and capillary buds, consisting of a collection of modified macrophages resembling epithelial cells, surrounded by a rim of mononuclear cells, chiefly lymphocytes, and sometimes a center of giant multinucleate cells; it is due to a chronic inflammatory process associated with infectious disease or invasion by a foreign body.
acropruritic g. see ACRAL lick dermatitis.
apical g. modified granulation tissue containing elements of chronic inflammation located adjacent to the root apex of a tooth with infected necrotic pulp.
canine eosinophilic g. see EOSINOPHILIC granuloma.
cholesterol g. see CHOLESTEATOMA.
coccidioidal g. the secondary, progressive, chronic (granulomatous) stage of coccidioidomycosis.
dental g. one usually surrounded by a fibrous sac continuous with the periodontal ligament and attached to the root apex of a tooth.
enzootic nasal g. see ENZOOTIC nasal granuloma.
equine dermal g. see SWAMP CANCER.
feline lick g. see feline EOSINOPHILIC granuloma complex.
g. fissuratum a firm, whitish, fissured, fibrotic granuloma of the gum and buccal mucosa, occurring on an edentulous alveolar ridge and between the ridge and the cheek.
foreign body g. a localized histiocytic reaction to a foreign body in the tissue.
idiopathic sterile g's occur in dogs and cats; the lesions are painless and may become ulcerated and secondarily infected. An immune-mediated cause is suspected and the lesions often respond to treatment with corticosteroids or other immunomodulating drugs. Sometimes lesions regress spontaneously.
infectious g. infection by one of the systemic mycotic fungal agents which result in a granulomatous lesion in the skin.
intestinal eosinophilic g. see ANGIOSTRONGYLUS *costaricensis*.
linear g. well-delineated, elevated plaques with an eroded surface that occur in a linear pattern, usually on the caudal aspect of the hindleg(s) of cats. Pruritus is variable. Similar lesions may also occur in the oral cavity and on the lips. See also feline EOSINOPHILIC granuloma complex.
lipoid g. a granuloma containing lipoid cells; xanthoma.
lipophagic g. a granuloma attended by the loss of subcutaneous fat.
mycotic g. see SWAMP CANCER.
palisading g. one characterized by the arrangement of histiocytes surrounding a focus of fibrin, foreign material, degenerating collagen.
paracoccidioidal g. paracoccidioidomycosis.
peripheral giant cell reparative g. a pedunculated or sessile lesion of the gingivae or alveolar ridge, apparently arising from the periodontium or mucoperiosteum, and usually due to trauma. It is uncommon in humans and animals. Called also reparative granuloma of the jaw.
pressure point g. see PRESSURE points.
pyogenic g. a benign, solitary, nodule resembling granulation tissue, found anywhere on the body, commonly intraorally, usually at the site of trauma as a response of the tissues to a nonspecific infection.
reparative g. of the jaw see peripheral giant cell reparative granuloma (above).
sperm g. granuloma of the epididymis caused by leakage of spermatozoa from the efferent tubules or the epididymis into surrounding tissue. May be due to trauma, infection or to congenital defects in the duct system.
staphylococcal g. a large mass containing small abscesses, found in the wall of the uterus of the sow. See also BOTRYOMYCOSIS.
telangiectatic g. a form characterized by numerous dilated blood vessels.
tuberculous g. the lesion of tuberculosis and the prototype of granulomatous inflammation. It is composed of histiocytes and epithelioid cells surrounded by giant cells of the Langhans type, lymphocytes and fibroblasts. Bacteria are found in the cytoplasm of the epithelioid and giant cells.
ulcerative g. of swine see ULCERATIVE granuloma of swine.
venereal g. see canine transmissible VENEREAL tumor.
granulomatosis the formation of multiple granulomas.
lymphomatoid g. a lymphohistiocytic proliferative disorder in dogs, usually involving viscera but occasionally including skin lesions.
Wegener's g. a mononuclear granulomatous disease characterized by granulomatous inflammation and necrotizing vasculitis.
granulomatous composed of granulomas.
g. colitis see histiocytic ulcerative COLITIS.
g. encephalitis see granulomatous MENINGOENCEPHALOMYELITIS.
g. enteritis see granulomatous ENTERITIS.
equine generalized g. disease a generalized disease affecting skin and all internal organs and of unknown origin; characterized by exfoliative dermatitis, wasting, and granulomatous lesions internally; skin lesions are dermal granulomatous nodules plus superficial exfoliation.
g. meningoencephalomyelitis see granulomatous MENINGOENCEPHALOMYELITIS.
g. perineuritis see CAUDA EQUINA NEURITIS.
g. rhinitis see ENZOOTIC nasal granuloma.
g. skin disease see granular DERMATITIS.
g. synovitis/arthritis lesion characterized by granulomatous tissue on the synovial surface of the bones in the joint; may occur in systemic mycotic infections.
g. urethritis see granulomatous URETHRITIS.
granulomere the center portion of a platelet in a dry, stained blood smear, apparently filled with fine, purplish red granules.

granulopenia see AGRANULOCYTOSIS.
granuloplastic forming granules.
granulopoiesis the formation and development of granulocytes.
resurgence g. the cessation of granulopoiesis during systemic illness, followed by the release of immature granulocytes into the circulation. Seen in cats. Called also toxic bone marrow arrest.
granulopoietin an unidentified substance thought to regulate the rate of granulopoiesis.
granulosa cell tumor an ovarian stromal tumor originating in the solid mass of cells (granulosa cells) that surrounds the ovum in a developing graafian follicle. It may be associated with excessive production of estrogen, inducing endometrial hyperplasia and signs of hyperestrogenism. Most commonly observed in cows and mares, less commonly in the bitch, queen and ewe.
granulosa–theca cell tumor an ovarian tumor predominantly composed of either granulosa cells (follicular cells) or theca cells, and often associated with excessive production of estrogen, and in some cases androgens.
granulosis the formation of granules.
granum [L.] *grain;* very small particles.
grape lesions grapelike lesions on the pleura of cattle caused usually by tuberculosis.
grapes commercial table and wine grapes, or dried raisins, sultanas, currants.
g. engorgement see CARBOHYDRATE ENGORGEMENT.
graph 1. a diagram or curve representing varying relationships between sets of data. Includes bar, pie, line, scatter diagrams, population pyramids, frequency polygons. 2. Often used as a word ending denoting a recording instrument.
Graphidium a genus of nematodes in the family Trichostrongylidae.
G. strigosum found in the stomach and small intestines of rabbits and hares; may cause digestive upset and poor body condition.
-graphy word element. [Gr.] *writing or recording, a method of recording.*
grasping a similar equine neurosis to windsucking; the horse grasps a fixed object with its teeth, but does not swallow air.
grass plant members of the family Poaceae (Gramineae).
g. chinkerinchee ORNITHOGALUM *ornithogaloides.*
g. disease see GRASS sickness.
eating g. is commonly seen in dogs and cats, sometimes associated with gastrointestinal disease, but more often an innocuous habit. May be a cause or a means of easy vomiting when the stomach is empty.
elephant g. see PENNISETUM *purpureum.*
g. founder laminitis.
g. nematode see ANGUINA LOLII.
g. pea LATHYRUS *sativus.*
g. seed abscess a common lesion in cattle in summer when grazing dry, native grasses with serrated awns. Lesions occur on the sides of the face and in the parotid area. They are cold abscesses, slow-growing, firm, painless and without heat. They rarely rupture and cause little inconvenience. Their importance is the need to differentiate them from actinomycosis of the jaw.
g. seed awns see AWN.
g. seed nematode poisoning see ANGUINA LOLII.
g. sickness a dysautonomia of horses; a noninfectious disease of unknown etiology characterized by drooling of saliva from the nostrils, alimentary tract stasis, small hard feces and severe mental depression. The outcome is always fatal. There is a diagnostic degenerative lesion in the sympathetic ganglia.
g. staggers see LACTATION TETANY (2).
g. tetany see LACTATION TETANY (2).
g. vetchling LATHYRUS *nissolia.*
grass carp see CTENOPHARYNGODON IEDELLA.
grass-fed 1. veal calves >3 weeks old, weigh 150 to 400 lb (68 to 182 kg) and fed on solid feed. 2. animals which are full-time at pasture and have no other significant feed source.
grassland see GRAZING (2), PASTURE.
grasstree see XANTHORRHOEA.
grattage [Fr.] removal of granulations by scraping.
gratuitous inducers thiogalactosides such as isopropythiogalactoside (IPTG) fortuitously discovered in the study of the lactose operon, that act to induce β-galactosidase; they are not metabolized by the induced enzyme.
gravel calculus occurring in small particles.
Graves speculum standard duckbill vaginal speculum. Inserted closed, opened by an exterior screw device that separates two thin blades, semicircular in cross-section. The cervix can be viewed through the external ring of the instrument.
gravid pregnant; containing developing young.
gravida a pregnant female called gravida I (primigravida) during the first pregnancy, gravida II (secundigravida) during the second, and so on.
gravidic occurring in pregnancy.
gravidocardiac pertaining to heart disease during pregnancy.
gravimetric pertaining to measurement by weight; performed by weight, as the gravimetric method of drug assay.
gravity weight; tendency toward the center of the earth.
g. rail system a rail system for moving carcasses of meat about in an abattoir. Carcasses move from station to station by gravity; suited only to slow kill rates.
gray[1] the SI unit of absorbed radiation dose, defined as the transfer of 1 joule of energy per kilogram of absorbing material (1 J/kg); symbol Gy; 1 Gy equals 100 rad.
gray[2] 1. the color gray, intermediate between black and white. 2. common coat color in most species; to be classed as a gray a horse should have gray points and have an even color over the body. With black points they are steel grays, with a red tinge they are rusty grays, with small spots of dark hair through the coat they are flea-bitten grays; silver grays have white mane and tail.
Gray Alpine cattle gray Italian multipurpose cattle.
gray birch see BRIDELIA EXALTATA.
gray collie syndrome canine CYCLIC hematopoiesis.
gray crab disease infection of blue crabs by *Paramoeba perniciosa* causing gray translucency of ventral aspect of the body and limbs.
gray diarrhea disease of ranched mink clinically distinguished by a ravenous appetite and copious gray fetid diarrhea and death due to malnutrition; it has not been defined etiologically.
gray eye see MAREK'S DISEASE.
gray fever Q fever.
gray ghost see WEIMARANER.
gray matter gray areas of brain and spinal cord made up primarily of cell bodies and dendrites of nerve cells rather than myelinated axons. White matter or substance is the tissue composed primarily of myelinated, or medullated, fibers.

The bodies of the nerve cells are centered in the

gray matter. In the brain the gray matter may be external to white matter, e.g. cerebellum, or central to it, e.g. cerebrum. The cerebral cortex is composed of gray matter and there are some deep-seated nuclei too. In the spinal cord there is a central core of gray matter surrounded by white matter. On a cross-section of the spinal cord the gray matter follows the general pattern of the letter H.

gray meat fly see SARCOPHAGA *carnaria*.

gray patch disease fatal herpesvirus-associated disease of farmed green sea turtles characterized by papules and widespread gray plaques of epidermal necrosis.

gray pearl disease NEODIPLOSTOMUM *perlatum*.

gray powder an oldfashioned purgative containing elemental mercury.

gray rattlepod CROTALARIA *dissitiflora*.

gray rule gray horses must have at least one parent with a gray coat color.

gray scale a scale of intensities of the color gray. Of value in assessing radiographic and ultrasonographic results. See also B-mode ULTRASONOGRAPHY.

gray-scale imaging see gray-scale ULTRASONOGRAPHY.

gray Shirazi Iranian meat and carpetwool sheep, gray wool, similar to Karakul, polled or horned.

gray substance see GRAY MATTER.

gray swainson pea SWAINSONA *canescens*.

grayanotoxin the toxic tetracyclic polyol in plants of the Ericaceae family including rhododendron, azalea. Called also andromedotoxin or acetylandromedol.

grazing 1. actions of herbivorous animals eating growing pasture or cereal crop. 2. area of pasture or cereal crop to be used as standing feed. See also PASTURE.

g. behavior most grazing species prefer grazing in daylight hours and graze as a social or herd unit, all performing the same function at about the same time.

block g. see rotational GRAZING (below).

continuous g. the livestock are left in the field for long periods without rotation; a common practice in extensive farming systems where internal parasites are not a problem.

deferred g. a field is closed up and not used for grazing for the spring and summer but is then grazed as mature autumn feed. This may be a tactic to provide grazing at a time when pasture is usually in short supply, or it may be to allow a pasture to regenerate. Called also autumn saving.

g. fee see AGIST.

leader–follower g. the age group most susceptible to helminth infestation grazes the pasture first and are followed by the less susceptible older groups.

g. pattern the way in which each herbivorous species grazes a pasture, including closeness of cropping, preference for grass over clover over browse.

rented g. see AGIST.

rotational g. the herd or flock is moved frequently (days to weeks) from field to field in a management system aimed at reducing worm load and increasing production of dry matter. In many circumstances it does neither. Called also block grazing. See also ROTATION programs.

strip g. the field is grazed in strips which are changed every 1 to 3 days. This is done by careful placement of an electric fence so that the grazing strip is moved further and further away from the entrance to the field.

zero g. an animal husbandry strategy in which the plant material is harvested daily and fed to livestock in a dry lot. Avoids damage to pasture by cattle walking on it but requires much higher capital investment for harvesting machinery, construction and maintenance.

greasewood see SARCOBATUS VERMICULATUS.

greasy heel chronic, incapacitating dermatitis of the back of the pastern in horses. The cause is unknown but many cases occur in horses obliged to stand in unmucked out stables or in wet standing of any sort. There are horizontal fissures and a sebaceous exudate. The area is very painful to the touch.

greasy pig disease see EXUDATIVE epidermitis.

great ape one of the larger monkeys, usually the tailless ones; includes gorilla, orang-utan, chimpanzee.

great burdock see ARCTIUM LAPPA.

Great Dane a very large (28–32 inches tall) dog with broad head, small ears carried erect but folded over, a long neck and long tail. Called also German mastiff. The breed is predisposed to cystinuria, spondylolisthesis, osteochondrosis, hypertrophic osteodystrophy and gastric dilatation.

great-grandparent generation first generation of a four generation breeding program.

great laurel RHODODENDRON *maximum*.

Great Pyrenees a very large (90–140 lb), powerfully built dog with a medium to long, thick coat in white, sometimes with patches of badger, gray or pale yellow. The ears are small and the tail long. Characteristically, there are double dewclaws on the hindfeet. The breed is predisposed to osteochondrosis. Outside North America, called Pyrenean Mountain dog.

great water parsnip SIUM *latifolium*.

greater ammi AMMI *majus*.

greater celandine see CHELIDONIUM MAJUS.

greater kudu see KUDU.

greater spearwort RANUNCULUS *lingua*.

Greater Swiss mountain dog similar to the Bernese mountain dog, but larger, weighing approximately 130 lb.

greaves cracklings, an edible raw fat from the meat trade. The skimmings from the preparation of this fat are also called greaves. They represent a low grade of meat meal.

Greek Zackel sheep Greek milk, carpetwool or meat sheep, polled or horned, usually white with black or red spots on face and legs.

green 1. a composite color made by mixing blue and yellow; the color of young grass. 2. untrained.

green amaranth AMARANTHUS *viridis*.

green bottle fly see LUCILIA.

green cereal crop crop of young, green oats, wheat, barley, rye corn, used as grazing and to reduce an over-exuberant crop destined for grain production.

green cestrum CESTRUM *parqui*.

green crumbweed CHENOPODIUM *carinatum*.

green feed fresh green grass or other material cut and brought to the animal.

green frog *Rana clamitans*.

green gizzard see green GIZZARD.

green hellebore HELLEBORUS *viridis*.

green mother-of-millions see BRYOPHYLLUM *pinnatum*.

green muscle disease a disease of turkey breasts. See DEEP PECTORAL MYOPATHY.

green panic grass see PANICUM *maximum*.

green pea LATHYRUS *sativus*.

green struck see HEATED BEEF.

green veratrum see VERATRUM *viride*.

green vetch LATHYRUS *sativus*.

green water culture extensive culture of fish larvae in fertilized ponds carrying a phytoplankton bloom.

green wool see FLEECE rot.
greenback flounder see RHOMBOSOLEA TAPIRINA.
Greenetrack disease see idiopathic CUTANEOUS and renal glomerular disease.
greenstick fracture see greenstick FRACTURE.
gregarines low pathogenicity protozoans commonly infecting the gut of shrimps.
grenz rays very soft electromagnetic radiation of wavelengths about 2 Å.
grenz zone a zone of relatively normal collagen demarcating the boundary between normal epidermis and a dermal lesion such as a granuloma or a neoplasm.
Grevillea a large genus of Australian shrubs or small trees in the family Proteaceae; seeds and pods of a few species contain cyanogenetic glycosides but poisoning is not recorded; includes *G. banksii*, *G. helmsiae*, *G. robusta* (silky oak). Some species also have caustic resins on their seed pods, e.g. *G. pyramidalis*, *G. mimosoides*.
Grevyi's zebra called also *Equus grevyi*. See Grevyi's ZEBRA.
greyface a crossbred sheep of Border Leicester × Blackface breeding.
Greyhound a tall dog with very lean body, a distinctive deep chest and small abdomen, slender legs, small head and ears, long, arched neck and long, slender tail. The coat is very short and of any solid or spotted color. The breed has been used for racing for over 5000 years.
Arabian G. see SLOUGHI.
G. cramp see Greyhound CRAMP.
G. exertional rhabdomyolysis see EXERTIONAL rhabdomyolysis.
Persian G. see SALUKI.
G. polyarthritis an erosive arthritis, particularly affecting joints of the distal limbs, occurs in young Greyhounds. The cause is unknown.
Greyia brandegei a selenium converter plant in the family Polygonaceae.
GRH growth hormone releasing hormone.
grid 1. a grating; in radiology, a device consisting essentially of a series of narrow lead strips closely spaced on their edges and separated by spacers of low density material; used to reduce the amount of scattered radiation reaching the x-ray film. 2. a chart with horizontal and perpendicular lines for plotting curves.
g. cassette a radiographic cassette with a grid permanently installed in it.
g. cutoff excessive loss of radiation beam because of incorrect angulation between the tube and the lead strips.
g. diaphragm a grid interposed between the film and the x-ray beam. See also (1) above.
g. factor because of the filtering out of rays by the lead strips there is a loss of penetrating effect of the beam so that exposure time must be increased.
focused g. the lead strips in the grid are sloped slightly inwards at the top so that the apertures more closely approximate the angle taken by the rays in a diverging beam.
linear g. a cassette grid in which the radiopaque strips are parallel to each other.
g. map a map marked by a grid of numbered intersecting parallel lines making it possible to identify particular locations numerically.
movable g. one that moves during the exposure of the film to the x-ray beam: a Potter–Bucky grid.
nonfocused g. see parallel grid (below).
parallel g. the lead strips in the grid are parallel to each other and vertical to the plane of the film. This has the disadvantage that more diverging rays are absorbed by the grid at the edges of the film than at the center with a lowering of exposure there.
Potter–Bucky g. a focused grid moved mechanically across the x-ray beam. Suited only to large installations. Called also Bucky and Potter–Bucky diaphragm.
pseudo-focused g. something of the same effect as a focused grid is obtained by gradually lowering the height of the strips in the grid as they approach the edge of the grid.
g. ratio the ratio between the height of the strips to the distance separating them. The greater the ratio the more rays will be filtered out.
reciprocating g. one that moves during the exposure of the subject to the beam of radiation.
rotating g. one that moves while x-rays are being generated.
stationary g. one that is stationary while the film is being exposed so that there is a pattern of grid lines on the radiograph.
g. tube a special tube designed to take cineradiographic x-rays.
Griffon Bruxellois see BRUSSELS GRIFFON.
Griffon wire-haired see GERMAN WIREHAIRED POINTER.
grilse in the European terminology a salmon which has matured after only one winter in a salt water environment, whereas true salmon has passed two winters at sea. Many commercial farmed salmon are actually grilse.
Grindelia squarrosa North American selenium converter plant in the family Asteraceae. Other species in this genus may also have this characteristic. Called also gumweeds.
grinding of teeth see BRUXISM.
grip a grasping or clasping.
devil's g. see DEVIL'S grip.
fingertip g. a method of holding a scalpel between the thumb and other fingers with the palm over the handle.
palm g. a method of holding a scalpel under the palm with the thumb pressing on the top of the blade and the fingers curled under and around the handle.
pencil g. a method of holding a scalpel as a pencil between the thumb and first finger with the handle over the top of the space between them.
griseofulvin a fungistatic antibiotic produced by *Penicillium griseofulvum* used orally for treatment of fungal infections of the skin. Toxic effects include bone marrow suppression and teratogenicity.
grit a necessary part of the diet of birds especially layers. Plays a part in the trituration that goes on in the gizzard. Usually supplied as shellgrit or crushed limestone to add calcium to the diet.
g. pad a laceration of the pad permits entry of pieces of grit causing lameness in dogs, especially racing Greyhounds. The grit works its way through the pad and may even invade the flexor tendon.
grits very fine pieces of maize grain produced by crushing or kibbling. The bran and germ have been removed by sieving.
grizzle a bluish-gray or iron-gray coat color in dogs, consisting of a mixture of black and white hairs. In canaries, it describes light, grayish markings on the head, body, wings or tail.
groats grain which has been dehulled and the hulls winnowed off.
grocer's itch see GLYCYPHAGUS *domesticus*.
Groenendael see BELGIAN shepherd dog.

groin the junctional region between the abdomen and thigh; the inguinal region.

Gromark an easy-care breed of meat sheep, produced in Australia by crossing Border Leicester and Corriedale sheep.

grooming brushing and combing of the hair. A passive exercise in dogs and horses resulting in the development of a minor occupation of groom, institution of grooming parlor, and equipment. Cats and some dogs actively groom themselves. Cattle make some attempts at it, especially cows of their calves.

g. disorders grooming-type behavior that is damaging to the cat or objectionable to the owner; includes excessive grooming as a displacement activity associated with stress.

grootlamsiekte Afrikaans name for 'big lamb disease', the prolonged gestation in ewes caused by SALSOLA *tuberculata*.

groove a narrow, linear hollow or depression. Called also sulcus.

abomasal g. the third part of the gastric groove. Runs along the inside of the lesser curvature of the abomasum.

alar g. the slot-like part of the nostril of the dog beneath the wing of the nose; the homologous part in other animals.

atrioventricular g. see coronary groove (below).

branchial g. an external furrow lined with ectoderm, occurring in the embryo between two branchial arches.

carpal g. the bony part of the carpal tunnel on the palmar surfaces of the carpal bones.

coronary g. indicates, on the external surface of the heart, the demarcation of the atria from the ventricles. Called also atrioventricular groove.

esophageal g. a superseded name for RETICULAR groove.

gastric g. in the simple stomach runs along the lesser curvature of the internal surface from the cardia to the pylorus. In the ruminant it is divided into three parts, the reticular, omasal and abomasal grooves.

hoof g's coronet to sole grooves in ruminant hooves; demarcate horn of wall from horn of heel; the axial groove is a point of weakness and subject to injury.

humerus g. see intertubercular groove (below).

intermammary g. median groove which divides the mammary glands into left and right halves.

intertubercular g. separates the tubercles at the head of the humerus; called also humerus groove.

interventricular g. there are two of these, right and left, which are external indicators of the separation between the two ventricles. The two grooves do not quite meet at the apex.

jugular g. the furrow in the ventral part of the neck which accommodates the jugular vein just below the skin.

lacrimal g. on the nasal surface of the maxillary bone; houses the nasolacrimal duct.

laryngotracheal g. in fetal development this groove appears in the ventral wall of the pharynx and deepens and separates to form the trachea and lower respiratory tract.

left descending interventricular grooves see paraconal groove (below).

medullary g., neural g. that formed by the invagination of the neural plate of the embryo to form the neural tube.

omasal g. the middle segment of the gastric groove in the ruminant, between the reticulo-omasal and the omasoabomasal orifices.

optic g. on the internal surface of the presphenoid bone; occupied by the optic chiasma.

ossification g. see OSSIFICATION groove.

paraconal g. the fat and vessel-filled furrow on the left side of the heart, marking the division between the two ventricles; named from its position beside the conus arteriosus; called also left descending interventricular grooves.

paracuneal g. deep V-shaped furrows which separate the frog of the equine hoof from the bars and the sole.

rachitic g. a horizontal groove along the lower border of the thorax corresponding to the costal insertion of the diaphragm; seen in cases of advanced rickets.

g. of Ranvier see OSSIFICATION groove.

reticular g. see RETICULAR groove.

right descending interventricular groove see subsinuosal groove (below).

ruminoreticular g. the external demarcation of the division between the reticulum and the rumen.

subsinuosal g. fat and vessel-filled groove on the right side of the heart, marking the division between the two ventricles; named for its position beneath the sinus venosus; called also right descending interventricular groove.

grooved director a grooved metal probe used to direct another surgical instrument to a particular site which is out of view.

groover instrument for making grooves.

Hughes hoof g. like a bone curette except that instead of a spoon-shaped blade there is an open loop with one or both edges sharpened.

gross coarse or large; visible to the naked eye.

g. energy total energy of a feed as measured by direct calorimetry.

g. income total income before costs have been deducted.

g. margin total returns from an enterprise minus the variable costs incurred by the enterprise.

Grosspiculagia see OSTERTAGIA.

ground bundle see fundamental BUNDLE.

ground hemlock TAXUS *canadensis*.

ground-hog small, 1 to 2 ft long, 7 to 17 lb, yellow, brown, reddish rodent. They live in burrows, are diurnal, and have a well-known winter hibernation, and an even more notable spring awakening. Called also marmot, *Marmota monax*.

ground ivy see GLECHOMA *hederacea*.

ground-level climate the microclimate at the ground surface; critical to the welfare of insect intermediate stages, helminth larvae and fungal spores.

ground substance the amorphous, gel-like material in which connective tissue cells and fibers are embedded.

groundnut see PEANUT.

g. meal the cake remaining after expression of the oil from groundnuts is a valuable protein supplement but has a toxicity hazard if it contains aflatoxin due to infection of the cake or the original nuts with *Aspergillus flavus* fungus.

g. poisoning see AFLATOXICOSIS.

groundsel SENECIO *vulgaris*.

groundsel bush BACCHARIS *halimifolia*.

group 1. an assemblage of objects or animals having certain things in common. 2. a number of atoms forming a recognizable and usually transferable portion of a molecule.

azo g. the bivalent radical, –N=N–.

blood g's categories into which blood can be classified on the basis of agglutinogens. See also BLOOD GROUP.

g. breeding scheme method of selecting breeding stock in which a group of breeders cooperate to run an open nucleus breeding scheme; in return they receive a regular supply of breeding stock, mostly males, for use in their own herds or flocks. Called also cooperative breeding scheme.
g. medication see MASS medication.
g. practice see group PRACTICE.
prosthetic g. 1. an organic radical, nonprotein in nature, which together with a protein carrier forms an enzyme. 2. a cofactor tightly bound to an enzyme, i.e. it is an integral part of the enzyme and not readily dissociated from it. 3. a cofactor that may reversibly dissociate from the protein component of an enzyme; a coenzyme.
g. specific antigen see group specific ANTIGEN.
group-transfer denoting a chemical reaction (excluding oxidation and reduction) in which molecules exchange functional groups, a process catalyzed by enzymes called transferases.
grouse a group of related species of game birds in the family Tetraonidae. They are the red grouse (*Lagopus scoticus*), wood grouse (*Tetrao urogallus*), black grouse (*Lyrurus tetrix*), ruffed grouse (*Bonasas umbellus*), sage grouse (*Centrocercus urophasianus*) and the prairie chickens (*Tympanuchus* spp.).
g. disease see TRICHOSTRONGYLUS *tenuis*.
grow to increase in size and stature by natural development.
g. out to increase in size without fattening.
grower pig scours see NONSPECIFIC colitis.
growing-finishing pigs pigs in the 50 to 250 lb (25 to 100 kg) body weight class being grown and fattened for slaughter.
growing fork see REPLICATION fork.
growth 1. the progressive increase in size of a living thing, especially the process by which the body reaches its point of complete physical development. 2. an abnormal formation of tissue, such as a tumor.
g. arrest line a radiologically detectable line parallel to the growth plate in the metaphysis that indicates a temporary cessation of bone growth.
g. check an event or state, usually the result of inadquate nutrition, parasitism or other disease, which temporarily reduces or stops growth in a young animal. often followed by a period of compensatory GROWTH.
compensatory g. increased growth rate during a time period as a result of lower than normal growth rate during a previous period.
g. cone bulbous enlargement at the tip of every growing axonal fiber in the fetus, from which many long filapodia extend.
g. curve the curve obtained by plotting increase in size or numbers against the elapsed time.
g. disorders are sometimes traceable to excess or shortage of pituitary secretions, and may arise from hereditary defects or from glandular abnormalities. Abnormally large secretions of growth hormone can produce GIGANTISM. Failure of the pituitary gland to develop sufficiently or to secrete adequate amounts of growth hormone may result in DWARFISM. In adulthood, overproduction of growth hormone may lead to ACROMEGALY.
g. factor substances which act as local regulators of cell division and function; classified as autocrine (act on cells of the same class) or paracrine (act on cells of a different class).
hematopoietic g. factors see COLONY-stimulating factors.
one-step g. curve a plot typical of the rapid growth of a virus in cell culture when all cells are infected simultaneously.
g. plate the epiphyseal cartilage at which new bone formation occurs to lengthen long bones during their growth phase. Called also physis. See also EPIPHYSEAL plate.
g. promotants includes all agents used to increase the rate of body weight gain. Used principally in food animals but also in horses with a view to increasing muscle mass and physical performance, and in any species to hasten recuperation in animals debilitated by illness. Pharmaceutical preparations are principally anabolic steroids. Husbandry procedures include estrogen and zearalenone implants and dietary supplementation with antibiotics, monensin and, in the case of pigs, copper.
g. rate rate of increase in body weight per unit of time, e.g. lb/day in beef cattle.
recombinant g. factor recombinant growth hormone.
g. retardation stature smaller than normal; called also runt.
g. retardation lattice radiodense metaphyseal lines parallel to the epiphyseal plate developing in fetal bone.
transforming g. factor *[beta]* a family of extracellular signaling molecules important in the transformation of cells and in growth and development.
growth hormone a substance that stimulates growth, especially the polypeptide hormone secreted by the anterior lobe of the PITUITARY gland that directly influences protein, carbohydrate and lipid metabolism, and controls the rate of skeletal and visceral growth. The hormone acts on tissues via peripheral factors. Called also somatotropin, SOMATOMEDIN.
g. h. release inhibiting h. see SOMATOSTATIN.
g. h. releasing h. (GH-RH) a hormone elaborated by the hypothalamus, which stimulates the release of growth hormone from the pituitary gland. Called also somatocrinin.
g. h.-responsive dermatosis a rare, symmetrical alopecia and hyperpigmentation in dogs. The cause is unknown, but the condition is responsive to bovine or porcine growth hormone. Called also pseudo-Cushing's syndrome, hyposomatotropism, pituitary alopecia.
g. h. stimulation test see CLONIDINE stimulation test.
growthy said of an animal that is large for its age and appears to have potential for further rapid growth.
grub maggot-like or caterpillar-like insect larva; said of beetles and flies, most properly of beetles.
black g. metacercariae of digenetic flukes in the skin and/or musculature of finfish.
cattle g. see HYPODERMA.
head g. see OESTRUS *ovis*.
torsalo g. DERMATOBIA *hominis*.
white g. metacercariae of digenetic flukes in the skin and/or musculature of finfish.
yellow g. metacercariae of digenetic flukes in skin and/or musculature of finfish.
grubby gullets see grubby GULLET.
gruel a mixture made of ground feed mixed with water.
Gruenhagen's space a space created by the separation of the epithelium of the intestinal villi from the basement membrane as a result of ischemia. The epithelial cells have a normal appearance.
grumous lumpy or clotted.
grunt quick, sharp sound created by a forced expiration against a closed glottis; elicited by sharp pain. See also GRUNTING.

abdominal palpation g's, g. expiratory a grunt occurs with each expiration.
percussion g. grunt with each percussion over the sensitive area.
walking g. a grunt with each step while walking.

grunt test a clinical test in which a positive result is an audible grunt by the subject.
In cows the test is for traumatic reticuloperitonitis and can be conducted in several ways. The cow may be pinched over the withers by forcibly picking up a fold of skin. This causes a sharp depression of the back and pain resulting in a grunt. A second method is to lift sharply on a beam of wood held under the sternum behind the elbows. A third method is to punch the cow in the same spot and auscultate over the trachea.
In horses the test is for laryngeal hemiplegia. The subject is restrained against a wall so that it cannot jump away and a sharp, threatening gesture is made at the abdomen with a stick or crop.

grunting a forced expiration against a closed glottis. It is characteristic of painful and labored breathing and of expiratory effort due to any cause, e.g. emphysema.

Grus a genus of cranes. Includes *G. amogine* (Sarus crane), *G. canadensis* (sandhill crane).

gryposis abnormal curvature, as of the joints.

gs antigen group specific antigen.

GSA general somatic afferent system of nerves.

GSE general somatic efferent system.

GSH reduced GLUTATHIONE.

GSSG oxidized GLUTATHIONE.

GTF glucose tolerance factor.

GTP guanosine triphosphate.
GTP binding protein see G PROTEIN.

GTPase guanosine triphosphatase.

GU genitourinary.

Gua guanine.

guaiac test a tree resin from *Guajaaem officinale*; used in a test for occult blood in the feces.

guaiacol an extract of tar used as an expectorant.
g. glyceryl ether see GUAIFENESIN. Previously called glyceryl guaiacolate.

guaifenesin the glyceryl ester of guaiacol; used as an expectorant and as a muscle relaxant in anesthetic procedures.

guaiphenesin guaifenesin.

guajillo see ACACIA *berlandieri*.

guanaco a small cameloid. See LLAMA. Called also huanaco.

guanethidine an adrenergic-blocking agent.

guanidine the amidine of amino carbamic acid. The hydrochloride preparation is used to increase acetylcholine release in the treatment of myasthenia gravis and botulism.

guanidoacetic acid an intermediate product in the synthesis of creatine.

guanine G; a purine base, one of the fundamental components of nucleic acids (DNA and RNA).

guano compacted droppings of birds or bats used as fertilizer; a known carrier of disease, e.g. histoplasmosis.

guanosine a nucleoside, guanine riboside, one of the major constituents of nucleic acids.
cyclic g. monophosphate (cyclic GMP, cGMP) a cyclic 3′,5′-phosphate that acts as an intercellular second messenger mediating the activity of hormones and other substances; essential in vision where cGMP concentrations increase in the dark.
g. monophosphate a nucleotide important in metabolism and nucleic acid synthesis; called also GMP.
g. pentophosphate involved with guanosinetetraphosphate in the so called stringent response of bacteria in which, because the cell does not have a sufficient pool of amino acids to maintain protein synthesis, tRNA and rRNA synthesis is reduced by about 20-fold, which suspends many of the cells' activities until conditions improve.
g. tetraphosphate see guanosine pentophosphate (above).
g. triphosphate an energy-rich compound involved in several metabolic reactions; called also GTP.

guanylate cyclase enzyme catalyzing the synthesis of 3′5′ cyclic-GMP from GTP in photoreceptor cells of the retina in its dark state. cGMP binds to Na+-channels of the retinal cells, causing them to open.

guar gum an extract from seeds of the plant *Cyamopsis psoraloides*; used as a thickening agent, pharmaceutically as a tablet binder, and as a soluble fiber in the dietary management of diabetes mellitus.

guaranteed analysis see guaranteed ANALYSIS.

guard dog large, aggressive dog trained to attack intruders; usually German shepherd dogs, Dobermanns, Rottweilers, Bull terriers. See also DOG.

Guarnieri bodies large intracytoplasmic inclusion bodies originating from Paschen bodies, caused by infection with vaccinia or variola virus.

guayiga ZAMIA *pujilla*.

gubernaculum the embryonic structure that tows and guides the descending testis to its scrotal site.

GUD goldfish ulcer disease.

Gudden's atrophy degeneration of central nerve cells when the axon is damaged or infected by virus.

guenon a large group of related small monkeys of the genus CERCOPITHECUS. They vary greatly in their coloring and markings.

guereza a type of colobus monkey (*Colobus* spp.) of which there are a number of species, all beautifully colored and dramatically marked. Will not survive in captivity.

Guernsey a yellow-brown and white, horned breed of dairy cattle. One of the Channel Islands breeds, originating from the island of Guernsey in the English Channel.

Guest cannula a hollow needle within a stainless steel blunt-pointed cannula. They are introduced into a vein together and the needle withdrawn when blood flows. The cannula is left in situ.

guildford grass ROMULEA *rosea* var. *australis*.

Guillain–Barré syndrome a relatively rare disease of humans affecting the peripheral nervous system, especially the spinal nerves, but also the cranial nerves. Often observed after parenteral administration of drugs and vaccines. Pathological changes include demyelination, inflammation, edema and nerve root decompression. Called also acute idiopathic polyneuritis, postinfectious polyneuritis and Landry's paralysis. The cause is unknown but is believed to be related to an autoimmune mechanism. Idiopathic polyradiculoneuritis (coonhound paralysis) in dogs and cauda equina neuritis in horses are similar.

guillotine a surgical instrument with a sliding blade for excising a tonsil or a toenail.

guinea fowl *Numida meleagris*, the domesticated guinea fowl; there are a number of wild species, all in the bird family Numidinae. Pearly green plumage, long, shapely neck, featherless head and neck except where the head has either a crest of feathers or a bony casque, and a characteristic raucous call.
g. f. feather louse *Goniodes numidae* (guinea fowl feather louse), *Lipeurus numidae* (slender guinea fowl louse).

guinea grass see PANICUM *maximum*.
Guinea hog see miniature PIG.
guinea pig the domestic guinea pig, popular as a pet and as an experimental laboratory animal. Distinctive because of its requirement for a source of dietary vitamin C, long gestation period of 63 days and very mature young at birth. Comes in a great variety of broken and whole colors and color combinations, the most common being Himalayan (white with black points), tortoiseshell (patches of dark and light brown), tortoise and white, Dutch (white with brown or tan pattern), brindle, silver agouti (silver and gray underside), golden agouti (dark hair tipped with yellow), and albino (pure white with pink eyes). There are three varieties: English shorthaired—short, fine, glossy hair; Peruvian longhaired—long, silky hair obscures just where the vital structures of this guinea pig are; Abyssinian roughhaired—short, wiry coat composed of swirls or rosettes. Called also *Cavia porcellus*.
guinea worm see DRACUNCULUS *medinensis*.
gulah anatomical structure peculiar to the male dromedary; an inflated bladder, a diverticulum from the soft palate, which protrudes from the mouth of the sexually aroused male. Called also dulaa.
Gulf Coast coast of the Gulf of Mexico.
G. C. fungus see SWAMP CANCER.
G. C. tick see AMBLYOMMA *maculatum*.
gulf star grass BRACHYACHNE *convergens*.
gull member of the bird family Laridae. An effortless flier, webfooted, hookbeaked and an inhabitant of the shoreline.
gullet see ESOPHAGUS.
grubby g. gullets damaged by migrating *Hypoderma* spp.
g. worm see CAPILLARIA, ECHINURIA, GONGYLONEMA.
Gullstrand's slit lamp an apparatus for projecting a narrow flat beam of intense light into the eye. See also slit LAMP.
Gulo luscus see WOLVERINE.
gulping exaggerated, sometimes difficult, swallowing movements; seen in cats with laryngitis or esophagitis.
gulum see CAPPARIS TOMENTOSA.
gum 1. a mucilaginous excretion of various plants. 2. see GINGIVA.
g. arabic see ACACIA.
g. tragacanth see TRAGACANTH.
gum boil see DENTAL fistula.
gum-boots British for rubber over-boots. Called also wellingtons.
gum trees see EUCALYPTUS.
Gumboro disease infectious BURSAL disease of chickens.
gumma a soft, gummy tumor.
gummy an old sheep that has lost all of its incisor teeth.
gumweeds *Grindelia* spp. See GRINDELIA SQUARROSA.
gun 1. weapon for firing a projectile. 2. of the top rank, e.g. gun shearer.
balling g. see BALLING gun.
dart g. see BLOW DART.
g. dog one of the group of domestic dogs developed for use in hunting fowl. The dogs work with the hunter by detecting the scent of birds on the ground, then indicating their location (setters, pointers) or flushing them from the undergrowth, or by retrieving the fallen bird (retrievers). Called also sporting dogs.
drenching g. a handheld metal automatic syringe capable of delivering a preset dose of agent, most commonly an anthelmintic, and with a variable dose up to about 100 ml, via the mouth.
Günther's disease congenital erythropoietic porphyria.
L-gluonolactone oxidase hepatic, microsomal enzyme necessary for the formation of vitamin C in the body; lacked by humans, some primates and guinea pigs, which therefore need a dietary source of the vitamin.
guppy a small aquarium fish up to 1.5 inches long in many color combinations. Called also *Poecilia reticulata*.
Gurltia a genus of worms in the family Angiostrongylidae found in the veins of the leptomeninges of Felidae.
G. paralysans found in the thigh veins of cats; may cause paralysis.
gustation the act of tasting or the sense of taste.
gut 1. the bowel or intestine. 2. the primitive digestive tube, consisting of the fore-, mid- and hindgut. 3. catgut.
g.-associated lymphoid tissue (GALT) see gut-associated LYMPHOID tissue.
g. edema see EDEMA disease.
g. sweetbread see PANCREAS.
g.-tie see pelvic HERNIA.
gutfill the amount of an animal's total body weight that is composed of food, digesta and feces. This is very variable and can greatly influence an animal's body weight. This is most important in ruminants and to a lesser extent in horses.
Gutierrezia a North American plant genus of the family Asteraceae.
G. microcephala*, *G. sarothrae contains a toxic saponin which causes an acute illness with sudden death and lesions of gastroenteritis, hepatitis and nephritis. Chronic poisoning causes a syndrome of abortion, stillbirth and retained placenta. Converter plants for selenium. Called also *Xanthocephalum lucidum*, *X. sarothrae*, perennial broomweed, slinkweed, snakeweed, turpentine weed.
gutta pl. *guttae* [L.] a drop.
gutta-percha the coagulated latex of a number of tropical trees of the family Sapotaceae; used as a dental cement and in splints.
gutta-percha tree EXCOECARIA *dallachyana*.
guttat. [L.] *guttatim* (drop by drop).
guttate resembling a drop.
guttatim [L.] *drop by drop*.
guttering the cutting of a gutter-like excision in bone.
guttery part of an abattoir used to empty gut of contents. Called also gut and tripe room.
guttural pertaining to the throat.
guttural pouch a large air-filled sac that develops as a ventral diverticulum of the auditory tube in the horse. Located dorsal to the pharynx the paired sacs cause swelling in the parotid region when distended. Several large vessels and nerves run over its surface and are vulnerable to pathology of the pouch.
g. p. empyema causes local swelling visible in the throat region, dysphagia and a purulent nasal discharge.
g. p. mycosis may result in erosion of the internal carotid artery and sudden, spontaneous nose-bleeding which may cause exsanguination. Dysphagia, abnormal respiratory sounds and Horner's syndrome also occur.
g. p. tympany occurs mainly in foals during the first few days of life. Causes enormous swelling of the throat but little distress.
GVA general visceral afferent system of nerves.
GVE general visceral efferent system of nerves.
GVH graft-versus-host.

GVHD graft-versus-host-disease.
gwardar see the snake DEMANSIA *nuchalis nuchalis*.
Gy gray.
Gyalocephalus a genus of nematodes in the subfamily Cyathostominae.
G. capitatus a rare finding in the large intestine of horses. May contribute to the clinical signs of CYATHOSTOMIASIS.
Gymnocladus a North American genus of trees in the legume family Caesalpiniaceae; contains an unidentified toxin which causes intense gastrointestinal inflammation. Includes *G. dioica* (*G. canadensis*). Called also Kentucky coffee tree.
Gymnogyps californianus see CONDOR.
Gymnopistes marmoratus a venomous fish in the family Scorpaenidae. Called also South Australian cobbler.
Gymnorhina see MAGPIE.
gymnospore a spore without a protective envelope.
gympie DENDROCNIDE *moroides*.
gyn-, gyne-, gyno- word element. [Gr.] *woman*.
Gynandriris setifolia African plant member of the family Iridaceae; contains a bufadeniolide cardiac glycoside which causes cardiac irregularity, sudden death. Called also thread iris.
gynandrism 1. hermaphroditism. 2. female pseudohermaphroditism.
gynandroblastoma an ovarian tumor containing elements of both arrhenoblastoma and granulosa cell tumor; it produces both androgenic and estrogenic effects.
gynandroid a hermaphrodite or a female pseudohermaphrodite.
gynandromorph an organism exhibiting gynandromorphism.
gynandromorphism the presence of chromosomes of both sexes in different tissues of the body, which produces a mosaic of male and female sex characteristics.
gynecomastia abnormal enlargement of the mammary glands in the male, even to the point of secreting milk; usually the result of endocrine influences such as in the feminizing syndrome associated with functional Sertoli cell tumors of the testes.
gynogenesis development of an egg that is stimulated by a sperm in the absence of any participation of the sperm nucleus.
gynoplastics plastic or reconstructive surgery of female reproductive organs.
Gypius fulvus see VULTURE.
gypsum native calcium sulfate, which, when calcined, becomes plaster of Paris; used in making plaster casts for fractures.
gyrase one of the type II topoisomerases involved in the supercoiling of double-stranded circular DNA molecules.
gyrate convoluted; ring- or spiral-shaped.
g. atrophy atrophy of the choroid and retina; an inherited, progressive disease causing blindness in humans, caused by a deficiency of ornithine-δ-aminotransferase. Has been reported in a cat.
gyration revolution about a fixed center.
gyre gyrus.
gyrectomy excision or resection of a cerebral gyrus, or a portion of the cerebral cortex.
Gyrencephala a group of higher mammals, including humans, having a brain marked by convolutions.
gyrencephalic pertaining to the members of the family Gyrencephala; having a brain marked by convolutions.
gyrfalcon the most popular bird for hunting by falconry. A large white to gray bird, very discriminating hunter and kills only while in flight. Called also *Falco rusticolus*.
Gyrodactylus see DACTYLOGYRUS.
G. elegans a common monogenetic trematode parasite of fish and found attached to their skin.
G. salavis important trematode pathogen of wild Atlantic salmon in Scandinavia. Spread by hatchery-reared salmonids.
Gyromitra esculenta a mushroom poisonous to humans when fresh.
Gyropus ovalis a louse parasite of guinea pigs and other rodents. A member of the superfamily Amblycera.
gyrospasm rotatory spasm of the head.
Gyrostemon a genus of Australian plants in the family Gyrostemonaceae; contains an unidentified toxin which is reputed to cause pulmonary edema in horses and nervous signs in camels. Includes *G. australasicus*, *G. ramulosus*. Called also camel poison.
G. tepperi contains an unidentified toxin which causes incoordination and cystitis. Called also *Didymotheca cupressiformis*, double-seeded emu bush.
Gyrostigma a genus of stomach flukes.
G. conjugens found in the forestomachs of the black rhinoceros.
G. pavesii found in the forestomachs of the white rhinoceros.
Gyrotheca tinctoria see LACHNANTHES TINCTORIA.
gyrus pl. *gyri* [L.] one of the many convolutions of the surface of the brain caused by infolding of the cortex (gyri cerebri), separated by fissures or sulci. These are not defined here. The list usually includes: g. ambiens, gyri breves insulae, g. callosus, g. centrifugales, g. centripetales, gyri cerebri, g. fasciolaris, g. lunaris and the cingulate, coronal, dentate, ectomarginal, ectosylvian, genual, marginal, occipital, parahippocampal, postcruciate, postsplenial, precruciate, prorean, splenial, suprasplenial and sylvian gyri.
cerebral gyri, gyri cerebri the tortuous elevations (convolutions) on the surface of the cerebral hemisphere, caused by infolding of the cortex and separated by fissures or sulci.

H

H chemical symbol, *hydrogen;* [L.] *hora* (hour).
H+ symbol, *hydrogen ion*.
h symbol, *hecto-*.
H & E hematoxylin and eosin (stain).
H-2 complex the major HISTOCOMPATIBILITY complex in the mouse.
H antigen see H ANTIGEN.
H band a zone across the center of the sarcomeres of skeletal muscle cells.
H chain see heavy CHAIN.
H-plasty placement of skin flaps in which two single pedicle advancement flaps, opposite each other, form an H pattern when closed. This may be more effective than a single, longer flap in closing a large area.
H_2-receptor see histamine RECEPTOR.
H-wave reflex in nerve conduction studies by electromyography, a pattern of recording which evaluates both afferent and efferent pathways.

H-Y factor a cell-surface component on intermediate mesodermal cells carrying a Y chromosome; the H-Y factor is an obligatory component in the transformation in the embryo of the indifferent gonad into a testis.
H_2O_2 hydrogen peroxide.
H_4folate see TETRAHYDROFOLATE.
HA hemagglutinin.
Ha chemical symbol, *hahnium.*
Haalstra's method a laboratory procedure for isolating *Dermatophilus congolensis* from infectious material, based on chemotaxis stimulated by carbon dioxide.
haarscheiben tylotrich pad.
HABA 2-(4′-hydroxyazobenzene) benzoic acid.
habena the peduncle of the pineal body.
habenula pl. *habenulae* [L.] 1. any frenulum, especially one of a series of structures in the cochlea. 2. a triangular area in the dorsomedial aspect of the thalamus rostral to the pineal gland.
habit 1. an action that has become automatic or characteristic by repetition. 2. predisposition; bodily temperament.
habitat the environment inhabited by a specific organism or animal.
habituation 1. the gradual adaptation to a stimulus or to the environment. 2. the extinction of a conditioned reflex by repetition of the conditioned stimulus; called also negative adaptation.
habitus [L.] *habit, body conformation.*
Habronema a genus of nematodes in the order Spirurida.
H. incertum found in the proventriculus and gizzard of companion birds causing chronic digestive upset and diarrhea. Also causes sudden death. Called also *Spiroptera incerta.*
H. khalili found in the large intestine of elephant and rhinoceros.
H. majus* (syn. *H. microstoma*), *H. muscae parasites in the stomach of horses.
H. megastoma DRASCHIA *megastoma.*
H. microstoma see *H. majus* (above).
habronemiasis a disease of horses caused by the nematodes *Habronema muscae*, *H. majus* (*H. microstoma*) and *Draschia megastoma.*
conjunctival h. granulomatous lesions caused by invasion by *Habronema* spp. larvae occurring on the third eyelid, or the eyelid proper, or on the conjunctiva of the medial canthus.
cutaneous h. is manifested by granulomatous lesions caused by the invasion of skin wounds or excoriations by the larvae of *Habronema* spp. and *Draschia megastoma*. See also SWAMP CANCER. Called also summer sore, bursati, granular dermatitis and jack sores.
gastric h. large granulomatous masses in the gastric mucosa caused by invasion by *Draschia megastoma* larvae. They are usually clinically silent unless perforation of the gastric wall occurs. The larvae of *Habronema majus* and *H. muscae* cause mild gastritis but without the formation of tumors.
HACCP hazard analysis critical control points.
hachement [Fr.] a hacking or chopping stroke in massage.
hack 1. a recognized style of horse and not a breed. Not to be confused with Hackney, the breed of harness horses. Mostly Thoroughbreds, sometimes with some Arab or Quarter horse blood. Any color, usually 14.2 to 15.2 hands high, may be lightweight or heavyweight. 2. to go for a ride. 3. to manipulate a computer program, especially to gain unauthorized access to data.
hackamore a single-rein bitless bridle for a horse.
hacker a computer enthusiast, especially one who gains unauthorized access to data.
hackles the hairs over the neck and back that are elevated by arrector pili muscles in response to fright or anger. A mechanism to threaten opponents, perhaps by appearing larger.
h. feathers the feathers of the dorsal cervical tract of the domestic fowl that cover the dorsal and lateral parts of the neck. In the rooster they are often large and colorful and are erected as a sign of aggression.
Hackney 1. an English breed of light horses used for driving; bay, brown, black or chestnut, usually with white markings, 15 to 16 hands high. 2. an English breed of ponies, similar to the horse but 12.2 to 14.2 hands high.
H. pony small version of the Hackney.
Hadenvirus see bovine PARVOVIRUS.
haem see HEME.
haem- for words beginning thus see also those beginning hem-.
Haemadipsa a genus of leeches in the class Hirudinea. Small, 1 to 1.5 inches, but heavy infestations can cause anemia.
Haemanthus multiflorus African plant of family Liliaceae; may contain a cardiac glycoside which causes cardiac irregularity and sudden death. Called also blood lily.
Haemaphysalis a large genus of small ticks in the family Ixodidae.
H. bancrofti found on cattle and marsupials. Called also wallaby tick.
H. bispinosa found on cattle.
***H. chordeilis* (syn. *H. cinnabarina*, *H. punctata*)** found on birds.
H. cinnabarina punctata found on most mammals and on birds. Implicated in the transmission of *Babesia bigemina*, *B. motasi*, *Anaplasma centrale*, *A. marginale.*
H. humerosa transmits Q fever.
H. inermis a widespread tick.
H. leachi leachi occurs on domestic carnivora and rodents. Called also yellow dog tick. Transmits canine piroplasmosis, *Rickettsia conori* and *Coxiella burnetii.*
H. leachi mushami occurs on small carnivora.
H. leporispalustris found on rabbits, other small mammals and birds. Transmits *Coxiella burnetii*, *Francisella tularensis* Called also rabbit tick.
H. longicornis a three-host tick found on most mammals including humans. Transmits *Theileria* spp. and *Coxiella burnetii.*
H. otophila found on rodents. May transmit *Francisella tularensis.*
H. parmata found on carnivora and antelope.
H. punctata see *H. cinnabarina punctata* (above).
Haematobia a genus of small, gray, blood-sucking flies. Called also *Lyperosia* spp., *Haematobosca* spp.
H. atripalpis a vector for *Parafilaria bovicola.*
***H. exigua* (syn. *Siphona* spp.)** a parasite of buffalo and cattle. Transmits *Trypanosoma evansi*, *Habronema majus*. Called also buffalo fly.
H. irritans found on cattle, occasionally other mammals. Creates skin lesions around horns, and along neck and back, often invaded by screw-worms. Transmits *Stephanofilaria stilesi*. Called also horn fly.
H. minuta as for *H. exigua.*
H. stimulans a pest of cattle.
Haematobosca see HAEMATOBIA.
Haematomyzus exotic, rare lice of aberrant constitution. The only genus in the family Rhynchophthirina.

H. elephantis found on elephants.
H. hopkinsi found on wart hogs.

Haematopinus a genus of sucking lice in the order Phthiraptera.
H. asini found on horses.
H. bufali found on buffalo.
H. eurysternus found on cattle. Called also short-nosed cattle lice.
H. quadripertusus found on cattle.
H. suis the large pig louse.
H. trichechi found on walrus.
H. tuberculatus found on cattle, camel, yak and buffalo.

Haematopota large, blood-sucking flies predatory on vertebrates. A genus of the family Tabanidae. They are mechanical transmitters of anthrax, equine infectious anemia, anaplasmosis and *Trypanosoma evansi*. Cyclical transmitters of *Trypanosoma theileri*. Cause significant insect worry to horses. Includes *H. pluvialis*.

Haematosiphon a genus of blood-sucking, true bugs of the family Cimicidae which includes, for example, the bed bug of humans.
H. indora a serious parasite of domestic poultry in Central America.
H. nodorus the most important species of bird bugs; infests poultry, turkeys and some wild birds.

Haematoxenus a genus of nonpathogenic protozoan parasites in the family Theileriidae.
H. separatus found in sheep. Transmitted by *Rhipicephalus evertsi*.
H. veliferus found in the bloodstream of cattle. Transmitted by *Amblyomma variegatum*.

haemo- word element. [Gr.] *blood*. See words beginning *hem-* and *hemato-*.

Haemobartonella a genus of parasitic microorganisms in the family Anaplasmataceae that parasitize the cell surface of erythrocytes. Only the infection in cats appears to result in a naturally occurring disease.
H. bovis found in cattle.
H. canis found in dogs but is nonpathogenic unless the dog is splenectomized.
H. felis found in cats and in animals whose resistance is reduced; causes FELINE infectious anemia. Called also *Eperythrozoon felis*.
H. muris found in rats, transmitted by lice; usually asymptomatic, but capable of causing a fatal anemia in animals subjected to splenectomy or immunosuppressed.
H. tyzzeri found in guinea pigs.

Haemodipsus a genus of lice in the family Hoplopleuridae.
H. ventricosus found on field rabbits; uncommon in laboratory animals.

Haemogamasus a genus of mites in the family Gamasidae.
H. pontiger found in bedding and on rodents and insectivorous animals.

Haemogregarina a genus of protozoa parasitic on fish. Includes coccidia that cause hepatic necrosis, castration and occlusion of the air bladder.
H. sachae participates in the production of a leech-vector-transmitted lymphoma in cultured turbot.

Haemolaelaps a genus of mites of the family Gamasidae.
H. casalis a mite infesting birds and their litter.

Haemonchus a genus of blood-sucking nematodes of the family Trichostrongylidae.
H. bedfordi found in African buffalo and some gazelles.
H. contortus found in the abomasum of most ruminants and the cause of serious losses in sheep from HAEMONCHOSIS. There have been attempts to subdivide the species, e.g. *H. contortus cayugensis*, but the differences between the subspecies have not been substantiated.
H. dinniki found in gazelles.
H. krugeri found in impala.
H. lawrenci found in duiker.
H. longistipes found in camel, dromedary.
H. mitchelli found in gazelle, eland, oryx.
H. placei the parasite of cattle which can cause hemonchosis in that species.
H. similis found in cattle and deer.
H. vegliai found in oryx, antelope.

haemophagous see HEMOPHAGOUS.

Haemophilus a genus of hemophilic gram-negative coccobacilli or rod-shaped bacteria.
H. agni see *H. somnus* (below).
H. bovis see MORAXELLA *bovis*.
H. equigenitalis see TAYLORELLA EQUIGENITALIS.
H. gallinarum now classified as *H. paragallinarum*.
H. haemoglobinophilus found on canine genitalia; sometimes linked to puppy mortality but not often a cause of disease.
H. influenzaemurium the cause of respiratory disease and conjunctivitis in mice.
H. ovis has been reported as a cause of bronchopneumonia in sheep.
H. paracuniculus may be associated with MUCOID enteropathy in rabbits.
H. paragallinarum the cause of FOWL coryza.
***H. parahemolyticus* (syn. *H. pleuropneumoniae*)** see ACTINOBACILLUS *pleuropneumoniae*.
H. parainfluenzae reputed to cause a syndrome in pigs similar to Glasser's disease (*H. suis*, *H. parasuis*).
H. parasuis a common concurrent infection with SWINE influenza virus and causes GLÄSSER'S DISEASE of swine.
H. piscium a cause of ulceration of the gills and mouth of trout.
H. somnus causes HEMOPHILOSIS. Includes organisms previously classified as *H. agni* and *Histophilus ovis*.
H. suis now classified as *H. parasuis* (above).

Haemoproteus a genus of protozoan blood parasites of the family Plasmodiidae. Cause of avian 'malaria'.
H. antigonis found in cranes.
H. canachites found in grouse; transmitted by *Culicoides* spp.
H. columbae found in pigeons, doves and some wild birds. Transmitted by hippoboscid flies. May cause anemia in baby pigeons.
H. danilewski found in wild birds.
H. lophortyx found in quail. Transmitted by biting flies. May cause anemia.
H. meleagridis occurs in turkeys.
H. nettionis found in ducks, geese, swans.
H. sacharovi found in doves. *Culicoides* spp. possibly the vector.

Haemorhedus see GORAL.

Haflinger horse chestnut, light mane and tail, riding and draft pony from Austria, Germany, Italy.

Hafnia a genus of gram-negative, rod-shaped bacteria, members of the family, Enterobacteriaceae; found in soil and feces.

hafnium a chemical element, atomic number 72, atomic weight 178.49, symbol Hf. See Table 6.

Hagedorn's needle see Hagedorn's NEEDLE.

Hageman factor factor XII, one of the blood CLOTTING factors. Deficiency occurs in humans and cats and is asymptomatic.

Hageman trait an asymptomatic coagulation deficiency caused by the inherited deficiency of clotting factor XII (Hageman FACTOR). Occurs in humans and cats.

haggis pig stomach filled with oatmeal, minced offal, suet and seasoning and cooked like a large sausage.

hahnium a chemical element, atomic number 105, atomic weight 260, symbol Ha. See Table 6.

Haight baby rib spreader a self-retaining retractor, designed for surgery on human infants, but useful in small animals.

Hainan pig small to dwarf, Chinese pig, black with white head and back, smooth skin, long head, prick ears.

Hainsworth's energy groups animals divided into groups on the basis of their mean core body temperature range; used for scaling dose rates of drugs for animals on the basis of body weight.

hair 1. a threadlike keratinized epidermal structure developing from a follicle sunk in the dermis, produced only by mammals and characteristic of that group of animals. Also, the aggregate of such hairs. 2. various other threadlike structures.

auditory h's hairlike attachments of the epithelial cells of the inner ear.

h. beds coat hairs occur in groups of about three primary follicles and a variable number of secondary follicles.

burrowing h. one that grows horizontally in the skin.

h. cells sensory neuroepithelial cells which have hairlike processes; found in organ of Corti, ampullary crests and utricle and saccule of the inner ear.

club h. a hair whose root is surrounded by a bulbous enlargement composed of keratinized cells, preliminary to normal loss of the hair from the follicle.

h. coat see COAT (1).

cover h. see guard hair (below).

h. follicle one of the tubular invaginations of the epidermis enclosing the hair roots and from which the hairs grow.

h. follicle unit see APOPILOSEBACEOUS COMPLEX.

h. granuloma granuloma in the esophageal wall caused by swallowed hairs acting as foreign bodies.

h. growth cycle a period of growth, called anagen, is followed by a transitional stage, called catagen, and then a period of inactivity in the hair follicle, called telogen, lasting until the cycle starts again. The duration of each stage varies with the species, anatomical location, genetic influence, and a variety of environmental and physiological factors.

guard h. the coarse, stiff and often longer and more prominent hairs in a haircoat with an undercoat. For example, the darkly colored, outer hairs of a German shepherd dog. Called also primary hair, master hair, cover hair.

ingrown h. one that has curved and re-entered the skin.

lanugo h. the fine hair on the body of the fetus.

master h. see guard hair (above).

primary h. see guard hair (above).

ringed h. see THRIX annulata.

secondary h. finer and growing from a more superficial follicle than a guard hair; forms the undercoat.

sensory h's hairlike projections on the surface of sensory epithelial cells.

sinus h. the vibrissae or whiskers located on the muzzle and face of many species has an endothelium-lined blood sinus between the inner and outer layers of the dermal portion of the follicle with a rich nerve supply. This structure serves to increase sensory perception.

specialized h. includes auditory, guard, sensory, tactile, taste, tylotrich hairs (see this list).

h. streams the hairs in the coat of animals are inclined in one or other direction so that collectively they create streams that meet at vortices or cowlicks.

tactile h's hairs particularly sensitive to touch.

taste h's short hairlike processes projecting freely into the lumen of the pit of a taste bud from the peripheral ends of the taste cells.

tipped h. one with a different, usually darker, color at the tip; seen in Chinchilla cats.

tylotrich h. special hairs that act as rapid-adapting mechanoreceptors; large, primary follicles with a ring of neurovascular tissue around them. Always associated with a tylotrich pad, a local area of epidermal thickening with a layer of highly vascular and well-innervated connective tissue below.

hairball see TRICHOBEZOAR.

hairiness see HIRSUTISM.

hairlessness see ALOPECIA, HYPOTRICHOSIS, SEMIHAIRLESSNESS.

hairpin a secondary structure that occurs in single-strand RNA during protein synthesis in which the strand turns back on itself. The structure is the result of base pairing and hydrogen bond formation.

hairworms see CAPILLARIA.

hairy characterized by a covering of hairs.

h. angels' trumpet DATURA *metel*.

h. caltrop KALLSTROEMIA *hirsutissima*.

h. caterpillars elongated mucosal erosions occur in mouths of horses grazing pasture infested with hairy caterpillars. See also EROSIVE STOMATITIS.

h. cell leukemia a condition of humans, of which a counterpart is seen in cats. Previous name was reticuloendotheliosis.

h. gousiektebossie PACHYSTIGMA *pygmaeum*.

h. millet see PANICUM *effusum*.

h. panic grass see PANICUM *effusum*.

h. shakers see BORDER DISEASE.

h. thornapple DATURA *metel*.

h. vetch see VICIA *villosa*.

Hairy moustached collie see BEARDED COLLIE.

Hakea genus of plants in family Proteaceae; some species contain cyanogenic glycosides. Includes *H. dactyloides* (finger hakea), *H. salicifolia* (*H. saligna*, willow-leaved hakea).

Halal slaughter see MUSLIM SLAUGHTER.

Halarachne a genus of mites in the family Halarachnidae found in the nostrils of sealion and seal.

halcinonide a topical corticosteroid used in the treatment of skin diseases.

Haldane effect oxygen loss from hemoglobin makes the hemoglobin more basic and enhances the absorption of CO_2.

Halerpestis cymbalaria RANUNCULUS *cymbalaria*.

half-bred the progeny of the first cross between animals of two pure breeds, the F_1 generation. Often used locally without identifying the parentage, e.g. Cheviot ewe × Border Leicester ram.

half-hitch knot a style of surgical knot, consisting of one straight strand with the other thrown over, back over itself, under the original strand and back through the loop created by the earlier steps. It is the basis for square, granny and surgeon's knots, depending on how the hitches are thrown.

half-life the time in which the radioactivity usually associated with a particular isotope is reduced by half through radioactive decay.

half-pin splint see half-pin SPLINT.

half-sib see half SIBLING.

half-value layer the thickness of a given substance which, when introduced in the path of a given beam of rays, will reduce its intensity by a half.

half-wave rectification rectification of the power supply to an x-ray machine so that the forward phase of the cycle can be utilized and in the reverse phase no current flows across the tube.

halfmoon locoweed ASTRAGALUS *allochrous*, *A. argillophilus*.

Haliaeeatus leucocephala bald eagle.

Halicephalobus see MICRONEMA, e.g. *M. delatrix*.

halide a compound of a halogen with an element or radical.

Haliotis a marine shelled snail; grown commercially in culture-based coastal fisheries. Called also abalone. See Table 23.

Haliotrema a genus of flukes (monogenetic trematodes) parasitic on fish.

halisteresis deficiency of mineral salts (calcium) in a part, as in osteomalacia.

halitosis offensive odor of the breath.

halitus an expired breath.

hallucinogen an agent capable of producing hallucinations or false sensory perceptions. Unlikely to have any use in animals.

haloalkylamine derivatives a group of synthetic α-blocking agents including phenoxybenzamine, dibenamine.

Halobacterium obligate halophiles which spoil meat of high salt content.

haloduric organisms bacteria which are tolerant to high concentrations of salt and can survive on and cause spoilage of salted meats.

halofuginone a coccidiostat used in poultry; derived from ornamental hydrangeas.

halogen an element of group VII of the periodic table, the members of which form similar (saltlike) compounds in combination with sodium. The halogens are bromine, chlorine, fluorine, iodine and astatine.

halogenated pertaining to a substance to which a halogen is added.

h. salicylanilides. see RAFOXANIDE, CLIOXANIDE.

halogenation the process of adding a molecule of a halogen to each double bond of an unsaturated fatty acid. Forms a basis for the measurement of a food's content of unsaturated fatty acids.

halogeton *Halogeton glomeratus*.

Halogeton glomeratus toxic plant of the family Polygonaceae: contains oxalate in sufficient quantities to cause poisoning. Called also halogeton.

haloperidol a dopamine antagonist in the brain, used as a neuroleptoanalgesic agent.

halophil, halophile a halophilic microorganism.

halophilic pertaining to or characterized by an affinity for salt; requiring a high concentration of salt for optimal growth.

haloprogin a synthetic broad-spectrum topical antifungal.

Haloragis a genus of shrubs in the family Haloragidaceae.

H. heterophylla contains sufficient cyanogenetic glycoside to cause poisoning. Called also raspwort, raspweed.

H. odontocarpa an unidentified substance in the plant causes red coloration of the urine of cattle eating it.

halostachine an alkaloid found in *Lolium perenne* and thought at one time to be involved in causing rye grass staggers.

halothane a colorless, mobile, nonflammable, heavy liquid used by inhalation to produce general ANESTHESIA.

h. test pigs susceptible to malignant hyperthermia experience an attack of the disease if anesthetized with halothane.

haloxon an organophosphorus anthelmintic once used against nematodes of the abomasum and small intestine in ruminants. Not recommended for use in pigs or horses, in which it has caused laryngeal paralysis, and is very toxic for geese.

halquinol a topical hydroxyquinoline antibiotic and amebicide, but also used orally in calves to treat diarrhea.

Halsey needle holder a conventional needle holder but with smooth blade faces; designed for ophthalmic surgery.

Halsted pertaining to William Halsted, an American surgeon of the late 19th and early 20th centuries.

H. mosquito forceps popular, fine-pointed, ratcheted hemostats used to crush very small vessels.

H. suture pattern an interrupted suture pattern most useful in the suturing of friable tissues. The needle is passed in and out of the skin on one side of the incision, then across the incision and the suture is repeated on the other side. A pass is made at right angles to the suture and then a repeat of the stitch made back acoss the incision and the two ends tied.

halter the simplest form of restraint for the head of farm animals. Comprises a poll strap, a nose band and a halter shank that brings the ends of the nose band together under the mandible. Made of leather or cotton or manila rope.

h. broken said of a young animal that has been taught to allow itself to be caught, haltered and led but not broken in to saddle or cart.

h. classes show classes in which entrant horses are required only to be halter broken.

haltere knob-like relics of the second pair of wings in the insect genus Diptera.

ham, hams the musculature of the upper thigh; common usage implies the cured upper thigh of a full-grown pig.

h. beetle the 0.5 inch long larvae of the beetle which infest hams. Called also *Dermestes lardarius*.

h. curing see CURED MEAT.

h. fly the larvae or skippers, because of their habit of leaping long distances, of the fly *Piophila casei* which invade cured ham.

Hamadan ass a white, Iranian donkey.

hamamelis see WITCH HAZEL.

hamartia a defect of tissue combination in development.

hamartoblastoma a tumor developing from a hamartoma.

hamartoma a benign tumor-like nodule composed of an overgrowth of mature cells and tissues normally present in the affected part, but often with one element predominating.

h. adenomatoid see BRONCHIAL hypoplasia.

gingival h. pink, lobulated, often pedunculated masses on the gums of newborn calves; soon become inflamed and ulcerated resembling chronic granulation tissue.

lymphangiomatous h. a lymphangioma occurring as a congenital malformation.

vascular h. tumor mass, usually dermal, consisting of primitive to well formed blood vessels.

hamartomatous pertaining to a disturbance in growth of a tissue in which the cells of a circumscribed area outstrip those of the surrounding areas.

hamate 1. hooked. 2. the fourth carpal bone.

Hambletonian one of the very early and important sires in the Standardbred breed of racing horses.

hamburger beef lean beef with up to 12% fat prepared from cull cows, reject bulls and grass-fed other cattle. Called also manufacturing beef.

Hamburger shift see CHLORIDE shift.

hames linked metal, curved bars that fit around the horse collar and serve as the attachment for the trace chains and traces.

Hamilton hound see HAMILTONSTOVARE.

Hamiltonstovare a medium-sized, muscular hunting dog with black and tan short coat and white on the muzzle, neck and tail. It has a narrow head, folded ears and a long tail. Called also Hamilton hound.

hammer the malleus, the largest of the three bones of the middle ear.

h. stunning a blow in the center of the forehead with a 4 to 5 lb hammer on a handle 3 ft long; used as a means of stunning an ox before opening its jugular vein and letting it bleed out.

hammer-milled feed processed through a hammermill, a piece of farming machinery which combines a cutting and crushing action aimed at improving the digestibility and conversion efficiency of the feed.

hammerhead RNA structure a folding arrangement for autocleavage of RNA found in the RNA genomes of some viruses.

Hammondia a genus of protozoa in the family Eimeriidae.

H. hammondi nonpathogenic, found in the intestine of cats. The oocysts, shed in feces, are identical to those of *Toxoplasma gondii*.

H. heydorni nonpathogenic, found in dogs.

Hampshire a black pig with a white belt, originating in the USA.

Hampshire Down an English short-woolled meat sheep, polled, black-brown face and legs. The wool is of a characteristic Downs type of 26 to 28 microns.

Hampton line in contrast radiography of gastric ulceration, a radiolucent line across the ulcer crater at the level of the original gastric lumen, caused by undermining of the surrounding mucosal edge.

hamster see CRICETUS.

hamstring 1. the two tendons behind the knee or stifle and their associated muscles (biceps femoris, semitendinosus and semimembranosus). 2. the Achilles tendon. A hamstrung animal has this tendon ruptured.

hamulus any hook-shaped process.

cochlear h. the hooklike process at the end of the cochlea of the internal ear.

pterygoid h. the ventral extremity of the pterygoid bone around which the tendon of the tensor veli palatini is reflected.

Han sheep prolific Chinese meat and carpetwool sheep; fat-tailed variants.

hanahiri LEUCOTHOE *grayana*.

hand 1. unit of measurement of height in a horse; hands high, abbreviated hh. 1 hand = 4 inches = 10.16 cm. 2. the terminal part of an upper extremity of a primate.

h. gallop a restrained gallop at less than top speed.

h. milking see HANDMILKING.

hand-feeding 1. feeding stored feeds to livestock, especially pastured animals in drought, flood or other stringent times. 2. newborn animals without a dam to suck being fed by dropper, bottle or spoon. Called also hand-rearing. See also ARTIFICIAL rearing.

hand-foot-and-mouth disease a mild, highly infectious virus disease of children, with vesicular lesions in the mouth and on the hands and feet. Not related to any disease of animals. Included here for comparative purposes only.

hand-rearing rearing a neonate with milk in a bottle or bucket; standard practice with orphans, early-weaned calves.

hand tie suture tie made manually rather than with instruments.

handle the degree of softness of fleece wool.

handled said of a horse that has been caught, led, groomed. See also GENTLE.

handlers persons involved in the handling of, for example, circus animals. Includes grooms, milkers, herdsmen, strappers. Used mostly in referring to persons handling animals for show or auction.

handmilking milking with the fingers; two basic techniques are used; the preferred technique is to occlude the top of the teat with thumb and forefinger and then progressively close the fingers down the teat, then release the fingers to allow the teat to refill with milk; the second method, referred to as stripping, consists of running the thumb and forefinger, or two fingers, down the length of the teat; contrast with machine milking.

handpiece sheep SHEARS.

handslip a term describing a training method in which a racing Greyhound is urged to chase and then slipped out of its collar by hand. Used in training for moderately fast work short of full galloping and chasing a lure.

hanekam AMARANTHUS *deflexus*.

hang an unscheduled stop in a computer program due usually to a software error. It is usually necessary to reboot.

Hanger–Rose antigen a preparation of infective material, presumably including antigen derived from *Bartonella henseae*, obtained from patients with CAT-SCRATCH DISEASE. It is used as an intradermal test for the disease.

hangers used for hanging x-ray films to dry. There is a clip type, with a clip at each corner, and a channel type in which the film sits in channels in the sides of the frame.

hangnail excessive growth and cracking of the cuticle on the feet of elephants.

Hannemania chigger mites infesting amphibians especially frogs. Cause red spots and vesicles.

Hanover a German light horse used mostly for riding, with an excellent record in equitation and dressage. Bay, brown, chestnut or black, 16.2 to 17 hands high. Called also, apparently incorrectly, Hanoverian.

Hanover technique a technique for correction of abomasal displacement by right flank laparotomy, replacement of abomasum and omentopexy by fixation in the flank.

Hanoverian see HANOVER.

Hansen's bacillus *Mycobacterium leprae*, the causative agent of human leprosy. Does not infect animals, except the nine-banded armadillo under experimental circumstances. Included here for reassurance.

Hansen's classification a system of describing INTERVERTEBRAL disk protrusions. Type I is a complete rupture of the annulus with an extrusion of the nucleus pulposus into the vertebral canal. Seen in chondrodystrophoid breeds in which there is chondroid metaplasia of the intervertebral disk. Type II protrusions occur in nonchondrodystrophoid breeds, usually as a feature of advancing age, are the result of fibrinoid metaplasia, and consist of partial rupture of the annular bands and a domelike bulging of the dorsal annulus.

Hantavirus a genus of viruses in the family BUNYAVIRIDAE.

hao chen the characteristic fine-caliber acupuncture needle.

HAP hydroxyapatite.

Hapalochlaena maculosa small, highly poisonous bane of surf beaches; called also blue-ringed octopus; has blue rings on the tentacles which show up when it is handled; injects a paralyzing toxin as it bites and causes deaths in humans and could, one supposes, do the same to animals. Called also *Octopus maculatus*.

haploid having half the number of chromosomes characteristically found in the somatic (diploid) cells of an organism; typical of the gametes of a species whose union restores the diploid number.

h. karyotype see HAPLOTYPE.

haploidentity the condition of having the same antigenic phenotype at certain specified loci; said of donor–recipient combinations in transplantation studies.

haploidy the state of being haploid.

haplomycosis a fungal disease caused by EMMONSIA.

Haplopappus a North American genus in the plant family Asteraceae (Compositae); plants contain a toxic alcohol, tremetol, and ingestion of the plant over a period causes a stiff gait, severe tremor and final collapse and death. Includes *H. fruticosus, H. hartwegii, H. heterophyllus, H. tenuisectus*. Called also *Isocoma wrightii, Bigelowia rusbeyi*, jimmy weed, rayless goldenrod, burrow weed. See also EUPATORIUM *rugosum*.

Haplosporangium see EMMONSIA.

haplosporidiosis protozoan infection of hemocytes and organs of oysters and clams in the USA. Includes *H. nelsoni*.

Haplosporidium genus of parasitic protozoa in the order Balanosporida found in segmented worms and leeches (annelids).

H. nelsoni cause of multinucleate sphere unknown (MSX) disease in the American oyster.

haplotype the group of alleles of linked genes contributed by either parent; the haploid genetic constitution contributed by either parent.

hapten, haptene a small-molecular-weight either inorganic or organic molecule that alone is not antigenic but which when linked to a carrier protein, e.g. albumin, is antigenic; the antibody so produced will react with the hapten alone.

haptic tactile.

haptoglobin a group of serum alpha$_2$ globulin glycoproteins, produced by the liver, that bind free hemoglobin; important in acute phase reactions (response). The different types, genetically determined, are distinguished electrophoretically.

haptoglobulin HAPTOGLOBIN.

haptor posterior disk of a monogenetic trematode.

Harbin white pig a white, meat pig produced in China from local pigs crossed with Large White imports.

harbinger medic MEDICAGO *littoralis*.

harbor seal the common seal, 5 to 6 ft long, up to 300 lb body weight, and a good performer in captive aquatic shows. Called also *Phoca vitulina*.

hard copy printed version of a disk file, program output etc.

hard disk see DISK.

hard heads see CENTAUREA REPENS.

hard milker a cow hard to milk from all quarters because of the small caliber of the teat canals or stenosis of the sphincters.

hard palate that part of the roof of the mouth supported by the palatine processes of the incisive and maxillae and the horizontal plates of the palatine bones. See also PALATE.

hard rush JUNCUS *inflexus*.

hard-sectored see DISK.

hard tick see hard TICK.

hard udder see CAPRINE arthritis–encephalitis.

hard x-rays x-rays of shorter wavelength.

hardener a substance used to harden the gelatin of the emulsion on an x-ray film.

Harderian gland the part of the third eyelid that lies between the cartilage of the third eyelid and the cornea.

Harder's gland a portion of the third eyelid located deep within the orbit. Found in pigs.

hardkeeper an animal that is difficult to fatten.

hardmouthed said of a horse that is hard to restrain with the average bit.

hardpad hyperkeratosis of the footpads and the planum nasale; often associated with distemper infection in dogs.

hardship lines horizontal lines in the horn of hoofs; farmer belief is that they are caused by serious illness or feed deprivation.

hardware 1. metallic foreign bodies in the reticulum of ruminants, especially in dairy cattle, and the cause of traumatic reticulitis. 2. the physical mechanical parts of a computer. See COMPUTER hardware.

h. disease TRAUMATIC reticuloperitonitis.

Hardy–Weinberg law states that in an infinitely large, closed population, in which random mating occurs, both gene frequencies and genotype frequencies will remain constant.

hare see LEPUS.

calling h. see PIKA.

h. fibroma a poxvirus disease of hares, caused by a leporipoxvirus, characterized by the formation of fibromas.

harelip congenitally CLEFT lip.

inherited h. can be an inherited defect in many species; in cattle it can be combined with cryptorchidism; in sheep it may be bilateral.

harendong see CLIDEMIA HIRTA.

Hariana Indian gray-white shorthorn-type draft cattle.

Harleco apparatus an instrument for assessing acid–base status of a patient by measuring the total CO_2 content of the blood.

harlequin 1. a coat color pattern that consists of irregular patches, usually gray, blue or black, on a white background. Common in Great Danes. 2. a breed of fancy rabbit with harlequin coat pattern in several colors.

harmaline see HARMINE.

harmel PEGANUM *harmala*.

harmine one of the β-carboline alkaloids found in the plant family Zygophyllaceae, e.g. *Peganum* spp., *Tribulus* spp.; a central nervous system stimulant.

harmless snakes see SNAKE.

harmol one of the toxic β-carboline indoleamine alkaloids in the plants *Peganum, Tribulus, Kallstroemia* spp.

harmonic mean see harmonic MEAN.

harness a series of leather or webbing straps fitted together like the skeleton of a garment. Used to attach the draft animal to a waggon or a buggy, even to a saddle or a marking crayon or chin ball harness.

h. galls cutaneous plaques of fibrous tissue where harness rubs.

harpuisbos GNIDIA (*Lasiosiphon*) *burchellii*.

Harrier a medium-sized, muscular, shorthaired dog with straight legs, level back and square chest. It is a scent hound and is said to be a small replica of the English Foxhound.

harrier substantive name of hawk-like bird, called also *Circus* spp.

Harrington rod a threaded metal rod used to connect distraction hooks in the stabilization of cervical vertebral instability.

Harrison's groove a horizontal groove along the posterior border of the thorax corresponding to the costal insertion of the diaphragm; seen in rickets.

Harrison's test a test for the presence of bilirubin in feces; the addition of Fouchet's reagent to a 1:20 dilution of feces causes a blue color in a positive test.

hart male deer at 5 years. Called also stag.

hartebeest medium-sized antelope with long legs and lyre-shaped horns. Called also *Alcelaphus caama*, *A. buselaphus*.

Hartenstein's gland the popliteal lymph node, e.g. in the pig.

Hartertia a genus of nematodes of the family Spirocercidae.

H. gallinarum found in the intestine of fowls and wild bustards. Can cause emaciation, weakness and diarrhea. Transmits *Histomonas meleagridis*.

Hartmannella a protozoan parasite, free-living and thought not to be pathogenic, although they were at one time listed as being so.

Hartmann's solution a solution containing sodium chloride, sodium lactate, and phosphates of calcium and potassium; used intravenously as a systemic alkalizer and as a fluid and electrolyte replenisher.

harvest pertaining to or emanating from grain or cereal crops or the harvesting of them.

h. fever a disease of humans caused by *Leptospira* spp.

h. mites are pests of grain and hay where they are predators on arthropods. The larvae ordinarily parasitize rodents but can infest other animals including humans. The infections are self-limiting but can cause dermatitis of the face and the lower limbs. The lesions are itchy, small scabs, which cause rubbing and stamping of the feet. In pigs the lesions are distributed over most of the body. Called also chigger mites, grain mites, *Pyemotes ventricosus*, *Neotrombicula autumnalis*, *Eutrombicula alfreddugesi*, *E. splendens*, *E. batatas*, *Lepotrombidium* spp., *Schoengastia* spp.

harvestmen arachnids of the order Opiliones (or Phalangida) with very long legs and small round bodies. Predatory and carnivorous but not venomous. Called also daddy-long-legs.

Hashimoto's disease a progressive disease of the thyroid gland with degeneration of its epithelial elements and replacement by lymphoid and fibrous tissue; called also struma lymphomatosis, Hashimoto's thyroiditis. Similar to lymphocytic THYROIDITIS in dogs.

hashish dried flowering or fruiting tops of the plant *Cannabis sativa*. Animals that eat it show nervous signs of incoordination, and sleepiness, sometimes alternating with periods of excitement.

Hassall's corpuscles bodies of epithelial cells found in the medulla of the thymus.

hatchability the percentage of eggs set to hatch that in fact hatch. Governed by many factors especially nutritional adequacy.

hatchery a commercial establishment dedicated to the hatching of bird eggs to provide day old chicks and poults to the poultry industry.

hatching assisted close surveillance of valuable eggs, e.g. ostrich in an incubator, to ensure that environmental conditions are as close as possible to those specified for the particular clutch.

haulms dead, dry aerial parts of plants after their seed, e.g. beans, or tubers, e.g. potatoes, have been harvested.

haunch 1. in conformation terms, the region of the iliac crests. 2. in the meat trade, the leg and loin.

Hauptner mouth gag a speculum for opening the mouth of horses or cows. Consists of two dental plates into which the incisors fit (the dental pad in the upper jaw of the cow). The bottom plate is fixed, the top plate can be moved away from the bottom one, thus opening the mouth, by twisting a screw-threaded handle which passes through a metal arch that goes over the nose and is fixed to the bottom plate.

Haussman–Dunn gag a speculum for examining the mouth cavity of cattle and sheep. Two horizontal plates accommodate the upper and lower dental arcades (upper dental pad in cattle). They are carried on ratcheted scissor-type mechanisms supported up each side of the face by a poll strap. When levered open the plates stay open until the ratchet is released. Gives excellent access to the mouth but excludes incisor teeth.

haustra plural of *haustrum*.

haustration 1. the formation of a haustrum. 2. a haustrum.

haustrum pl. *haustra* [L.] one of the pouches of the large intestine, produced by the puckering action of the tenia coli and responsible for circular muscle fibers at 0.5 to 1 inch distances, and responsible for the sacculated appearance of the large intestines of horses and pigs.

hauteur machine-estimated mean fiber length in a top of wool; the basis for the pricing of tops.

Havana a dark chocolate-colored meat and fur rabbit weighing about 6 lb.

Havana brown a medium-sized, slender cat with rich, mahogany brown short hair, including their whiskers, green eyes and pink footpads.

Haverhill fever STREPTOBACILLUS *moniliformis*.

haversian named after the English physician and anatomist Clopton Havers, 1650–1702.

h. canal any of the anastomosing axial channels of the haversian system in compact bone, containing blood and lymph vessels, and nerves.

h. glands synovial villi.

h. system the basic unit of compact bone consisting of a haversian canal and its concentrically arranged cylindrical lamellae. Called also osteon.

haw, haw-eyedness a lay term used by dog owners, with various meanings. Can be used to refer to a sagging of the lower eyelid that exposes palpebral conjunctiva; an ectropion. In veterinary medicine it has been applied to a protrusion of the nictitating membrane (third eyelid) which may occur with dehydration, a loss of mass behind the globe such as atrophy of temporal muscles, or in cats particularly with sympathetic stimulation or irritation. May be associated with enlargement and prolapse of the gland of the third eyelid, called CHERRY EYE.

h's syndrome bilateral protrusion of the nictitating membranes.

hawk bird of prey in the subfamily Accipitridae. Includes genera of *Accipiter* (goshawk and European sparrowhawk). The unrelated American sparrowhawk (*Falco sparverius*) is a member of the falcon family.

hay dried green grass (meadow hay) or cereal crop (wheat, oats or barley hay) or legume crop (lucerne, alfalfa) used as feed for housed animals in the winter time and for supplementary feeding of pastured animals when there is need.

h. itch see GLYCYPHAGUS *destructor*.
h. net a wide-mesh string net to be filled, and hung in a loose box, to provide day-long nibbling for a confined horse.
Hayem's solution an isotonic fluid used for diluting blood samples in red blood cell counts. Contains mercuric chloride, sodium sulfate and sodium chloride.
hayflake a 1 to 2 inch thick flake of hay from a rectangular bale. Called also biscuit of hay.
Hayflick limit see CELL CULTURE.
Hayflick's medium a broth or agar medium for the cultivation of ureaplasmas.
haylage a feed that is halfway between hay and silage. The feed is cut when green, chopped small (0.5 to 1 inch) wilted and then stored in a special airtight tower silo.
Hay's sulfur test, Haye's sulfur test a test for the presence of bile salts.
haysickness chronic obstructive pulmonary disease of horses.
hazard a risk.
h. analysis critical control points a systematic procedure used to identify specific hazards (for example in food production) and establish control systems that focus on preventive measures rather than rely on end-product testing.
chemical h. a chemical capable of causing poisoning is on the premises and represents a potential threat.
radiation h. radioactive material is on the premises and represents a potential threat to animals in that environment.
Hb hemoglobin.
Hb-meter hemoglobinometer.
HBC a definition for medical records to denote 'hit by car'.
HbCo carbon monoxide hemoglobin.
HbO_2 oxyhemoglobin.
HC hog cholera.
HCB hexachlorobenzene.
25-HCC 25-hydroxycholecalciferol.
HCDD hexachloro-dibenzo-*p*-dioxin, a contaminant of 2,4,5-T, one of the plant hormone weedkillers; a teratogen.
HCG, hCG human chorionic gonadotropin.
γ-HCH hexachlorocyclohexane; see LINDANE.
HCl hydrochloric acid.
HCN hydrocyanic acid.
HCO_3^- bicarbonate ion; main body buffer for acid–base balance.
HDL high-density lipoprotein.
He chemical symbol, *helium*.
he- for words beginning thus, see also those beginning *hae-*.
head 1. the anterior or superior part of a structure or organism, in vertebrates containing the brain and the organs of special sense. See also SKULL, CAPUT. 2. one animal; used in reference to farm livestock, e.g. ten head of cattle. 3. the part of a disk or tape drive which reads and writes data to the medium.
articular h. an eminence on a bone by which it articulates with another bone.
h. bail see HEADSTOCK.
h. bob the patient is unable to keep the head still while at rest, it makes an involuntary, usually at regular intervals, short, quick downward movement then recovers.
h. bot see CEPHENEMYIA.
h. cap of spermatozoon, formed by the collapse of the acrosomial vesicle over the nucleus.
h. carriage includes at attention, drooping, rotated, deviated.
h. catarrh BOVINE malignant catarrh.
h. clamp see HEADSTOCK.
h. collar a leather halter-like piece of harness consisting of a poll strap, nose band and usually a rope shank.
h. cover hood or cap used by surgical personnel to reduce contamination of the surgical area by hair and associated flora.
h. crash a serious equipment malfunction in computer disk drive causing loss of data and damage to the disk.
h. deviation the poll–nose axis is turned laterally so that the animal walks in circles but there is no disturbance of balance. Occurs in lesions of the neck and of the cerebral cortex.
fetal h. lateral deviation the fetal head is deviated laterally to lie against the shoulder of the fetus, the front feet and the lateral aspect of the neck being presented to the pelvic inlet; a dystocia which can only be relieved by repulsion of the fetus and the return of the head to between the front feet.
fetal h. ventral deviation the head of the fetus is flexed ventrally so that the fore feet and the dorsum of the neck are presented to the pelvic inlet; a dystocia which can only be relieved by repulsion of the fetus and lifting of the head into the pelvic canal.
h. grit jaundice, photosensitization and hepatic injury in lambs caused by *Narthecium ossifragum* poisoning.
h. injury traumatic injury to the head resulting from a fall or violent blow. Such an injury may be open or closed and may involve a brain CONCUSSION, skull fracture, or contusions of the brain.
h. mange see NOTOEDRIC MANGE.
nerve h. the optic disk.
h. nod see head bob (above).
h. picking a form of cannibalism in which birds pick at and injure each other's wattles, combs, eyes; beak trimming reduces the problem but does not prevent the vice.
h. posture see head carriage (above).
h. pressing persistent pushing with the head against a fixed object. Part of the dummy syndrome as in hepatic encephalopathy or encephalitis.
h. process the elongating cephalic tissues which represent the first step in the development of the fetal body.
h. rotation twisting of the head around the axis from the poll to the nose. To be differentiated from deviation of the head. Caused usually by lesions of the vestibular apparatus on one side. The animal walks in circles and has problems maintaining its balance.
h. shaking common in dogs and cats with acute inflammation or foreign bodies in the external ear canal. May be a cause of auricular hematoma.
h. shy said of a horse that tries to avoid having its head handled or its headstall put on.
h. stall see head collar (above).
h. tilt includes rotation and deviation.
h. tremor a feature of cerebellar lesions.
h. twist injury injury to cervical vertebrae may occur in horses as a result of a fall with the head and neck under the body.
h.'s zones in acupuncture the zones of human skin which are responsive to abnormalities in each of the vital organs.
head and eye form BMC see BOVINE malignant catarrh.
head-down disease a poisoning of rabbits by *Asclepias eriocarpa* usually present in the hay being

fed. Affected rabbits have paralysis of the neck and incoordination.

head fly see HYDROTOEA *irritans*.

head louse see CYCLOTOGASTER HETEROGRAPHUS.

head–neck deviation lateral deviation of the head and neck.

headstock substantial wooden or metal fixed apparatus for restraining a cow by the neck in a crush, milking parlor or feed stalls. There is a bar or tongue which is swiveled at the bottom and can be opened at the top. When the animal puts its head into the open space the tongue is closed tight enough to prevent the beast getting its head out. The tongue has a quick release catch so that it can be opened quickly in an emergency. Called also head bail, neck yoke, head clamp.

healing the restoration of structure and function of injured or diseased tissues. The healing processes include blood clotting, tissue mending, scarring and bone healing. See also WOUND healing.

h. by first intention *per primam;* union of accurately coapted edges of a wound, with an irreducible minimum of granulation tissue.

h. by second intention *per secundam;* union by adhesion of granulating surfaces.

h. by third intention *per tertiam;* union of a wound that is closed surgically several days after the injury. See also DELAYED primary closure.

health a state of physical and psychological well-being and of productivity including reproduction.

h. indices easily observed parameters that can be used as a guide to the animal's or group's state of health. Most obvious are food intake and fecal output. In agricultural animals there are additional monitoring guides such as body weight, milk yield, racing performance, egg yield, freedom of wool from breaks, feed conversion efficiency and so on.

h. management a system of preventive medicine that takes into account the whole animal, and the total influences including social, with respect to relationships with others in the herd or flock, psychological and environmental factors that affect health, including nutrition, exercise, housing, freedom from crowding and boredom and from physical or psychological harassment or cruelty.

repeated periodic h. care periodic examination of an individual or herd, exemplified in modern herd health programs.

veterinary public h. the field of veterinary medicine that is concerned with safeguarding and improving the health of the human community as a whole by controlling diseases of animals that are communicable to humans or which affect the human food chain to the detriment of the health of the consumers.

health care system an organized plan of health services by which health care is made available to the animal population and financed by government or private enterprise or both. A health care system embraces the following: (1) health care services available to individual animals and to groups through private practices and government veterinary officer services in veterinary clinics, laboratories and hospitals and the clients' own homes and on farms, in stables and other group animal facilities; (2) the veterinary preventive medical services needed to maintain a healthy environment; for example, control of medicine and food supplies, regulation of drugs, and control of the movement of animals intended to protect a given population; and (3) teaching and research activities related to the prevention and treatment of disease.

health/production programs coordinated health and production management programs for animal farming enterprises which utilize all disease control techniques which are relevant and cost-effective and integrate these with breeding, feeding and housing strategies. See also HERD health program.

healthy 1. a state of being in good health. 2. pertaining to, characterized by, or promoting health.

hearing the sense by which sounds are perceived, by conversion of sound waves into nerves impulses, which are then interpreted by the brain. Also, the capacity to perceive sound. The organ of hearing is the EAR, which is divided into three sections, the outer, middle and inner ear. Each plays a special role in hearing. Connecting the middle ear with the nasopharynx is the pharyngotympanic canal, through which air enters to equalize the pressure on both sides of the TYMPANIC membrane (eardrum).

h. aid an instrument to amplify sounds for the hard of hearing. These have been fitted to dogs, but are not normally offered in veterinary practice.

h. tests are difficult to administer and interpret in any other than laboratory-trained animals or without specialized electronic equipment such as an impedance audiometer or electroencephalograph with which AUDITORY cortical evoked responses can be measured.

h. dog a dog trained to respond to sounds such as a telephone ring or door bell; used to assist hearing impaired humans.

hearing loss partial or complete loss of hearing; see also DEAFNESS.

heart the hollow muscular organ lying on the sternum that serves as a pump controlling the blood flow in two circuits, the pulmonary and the systemic. See also CIRCULATORY system.

artificial h. a mechanical device that replaces the heart by using pulsating air to pump blood to the body. Successfully placed in calves, sheep and dogs as experimental models for the subsequent use of such methods in humans.

h. attack see MYOCARDIAL infarction.

h. bones ossicles in the fibrous skeletal ring which surrounds the aortic orifice of the heart in cattle and occasionally in other species; called also ossa cordis.

h. conducting system consists of the sinoatrial node, the atrioventricular node, the atrioventricular bundle and its two crura.

cyanotic h. malformations insufficient oxygenated hemoglobin is received in the peripheral capillary beds resulting in blue discoloration of tissues, and an incapacity of the body to maintain a life-sustaining level of activity.

h. disease an all-embracing term including those diseases in which there is intrinsic disease of the heart such as uremia, valvular disease, African horse sickness, vitamin E–selenium nutritional deficiency, inherited cardiomyopathies of dogs and cattle, altitude disease, canine parvovirus infection, and in a number of plant and other poisonings. See also MULBERRY HEART DISEASE.

h. failure cells hemosiderin-laden macrophages present in the pulmonary alveoli in cases of congestive heart failure.

h. malformations includes ectopia cordis, patent foramen ovale, ventricular septal defects such as Fallot's tetralogy, Eisenmenger complex, patent ductus arteriosus, aortic coarctation, right aortic arch persistence, truncus arteriosus persistence, fibroelastosis, subvalvular aortic stenosis, anomalous origin of carotid arteries, transposition of great vessels, pulmonic stenosis, aortic stenosis.

h. massage see cardiac MASSAGE.
h. meridian points acupuncture points along the heart meridian.
h. rate the number of contractions of the cardiac ventricles per unit of time. For normal rates see PULSE rate.
h. score a concept which sets out that performance in racing horses is related to heart size, now a well-established relationship, and that heart size can be estimated in the living horse by the measurement of the QRS interval.
h. sounds see HEART SOUNDS, heart MURMUR.
h. strain is an unpopular concept in any medical science but overtrained horses which perform poorly do have a high incidence of abnormal T waves.
h. valve anomalies failure of complete development of atrioventricular or semilunar valves results in stenosis or incompetence of the valves and often congestive heart failure.
h. valve hematoma congenital, usually multiple lesions on the edges of atrioventricular valves, mostly in calves; disappear spontaneously in most cases.
h. valve thrombosis common lesion on the free edges of valves, often the source of widespread emboli; on healing leave scarred, insufficient valves.
h. valves flaps of endothelial connective tissue that guard the entrance into and exit from the ventricles and bring about unidirectional blood flow. Include the atrioventricular and semilunar valves, the proper closure of which is essential to maintain circulatory equilibrium, can be diseased and cause heart failure. See also heart MURMUR, ENDOCARDITIS, ENDOCARDIOSIS.

heart-base tumor aortic body tumors, but generally includes adenomas and carcinomas of ectopic thyroid tissue.

heart block impairment of conduction in heart excitation; often applied specifically to atrioventricular heart block.

When isolated impulses from the atria fail to reach the ventricles, heartbeats are missed and the block is called incomplete. When no impulses reach the ventricles from the atria the heart block is complete, with the result that the atria and the ventricles beat at separate rates. In this case the beats remain regular but the rate of the ventricular beats is greatly slowed down.

atrioventricular (A-V) h. b. a form in which the blocking is at the atrioventricular junction. It is *first degree* when A-V conduction time is prolonged; *second degree* (partial heart block) when some but not all atrial impulses reach the ventricle; *third degree* (complete heart block) when no atrial impulses at all reach the ventricle, and the atria and ventricles act independently of each other.
bundle-branch h. b. a form in which one ventricle is excited before the other because of absence of conduction in one of the branches of the bundle of His.
complete h. b. see atrioventricular heart block (above).
fascicular h. b. one originating on one of the two divisions of the left bundle branch. See also HEMIBLOCK.
interventricular h. b. bundle-branch heart block.
Mobitz h. b's variations of second-degree heart blocks. See also WENCKEBACH'S PHENOMENON.
sinoatrial h. b. partial or complete impairment of conduction from the sinoatrial node to the atria, resulting in delay or absence of an atrial beat.

heart failure inability of the heart to maintain a circulation sufficient to meet the body's needs; most often applied to myocardial failure affecting the right or left ventricle.
acute h. f. sudden cardiac arrest such as occurs in anesthetic death and cardiac myopathy of various kinds. It causes death by acute anoxia of tissues especially brain. The clinical syndrome varies between a brief convulsion and the development of PULMONARY edema.
backward h. f. a concept of heart failure emphasizing the contribution of passive engorgement of the systemic venous system as a cause.
congestive h. f. (CHF) that which occurs as a result of impaired pumping capability of the heart and is associated with abnormal retention of water and sodium. The condition ranges from mild congestion with few symptoms to life-threatening fluid overload and total heart failure.

CHF results in an inadequate supply of blood and oxygen to the body's cells. The decreased cardiac output causes an increase in the blood volume within the vascular system. Congestion within the blood vessels interferes with the movement of body fluids in and out of the various fluid compartments, and they accumulate in the tissue spaces, causing edema.

There are three general kinds of pathological conditions that can bring about CHF: (1) *ventricular failure*, in which the contractions of the ventricles become weak and ineffective, as in myocardial ischemia from coronary artery disease; (2) *mechanical failure* of the ventricles to fill with blood during the diastole phase of the cardiac cycle, which can occur when the mitral valve is narrowed or when there is an accumulation of fluid within the pericardial sac (cardiac tamponade) pressing against the ventricles, preventing them from accepting a full load of blood; and (3) an *overload* of blood in the ventricles during the systole phase of the cycle. High blood pressure, aortic stenosis and aortic valvular regurgitation are some of the conditions that can cause ventricular overload.
decompensated h. f. see congestive heart failure (above).
forward h. f. a concept of heart failure emphasizing the inadequacy of cardiac output as the primary cause and considering venous distension to be secondary.
high output h. f. that in which cardiac output remains high, associated with anemia, emphysema, etc.
left-sided h. f., left ventricular h. f. failure of the left ventricle to maintain a normal output of blood. Since the left ventricle does not empty completely, it cannot accept blood returning from the lungs via the pulmonary veins. The pulmonary veins become engorged and fluid seeps out through the veins and collects in the pleural cavity. Pulmonary edema and pleural effusion result. In many cases heart failure begins on the left side and eventually involves both sides of the heart.
low-output h. f. that in which cardiac output is diminished, associated with cardiovascular diseases.
right-sided h. f., right ventricular h. f. failure of proper functioning of the right ventricle, with subsequent engorgement of the systemic veins, producing pitting edema, enlargement of the liver, and ascites.

heart-leaf poison GASTROLOBIUM *bilobum* (in Western Australia), *G. grandiflorum* (in Queensland).

heart–lung unit see EXTRACORPOREAL circulatory support unit.

heart sounds the sounds heard on the surface of the chest in the heart region. They are amplified by and heard more distinctly through a stethoscope. These sounds are caused by the vibrations of the normal cardiac cycle. They may be produced by muscular action, valvular actions, motion of the heart, and blood as it passes through the heart.

The first heart sound (S_1) is heard as a firm but not sharp 'lubb' sound. It consists of four components: a low-frequency, indistinct vibration caused by ventricular contraction; a louder sound of higher frequency caused by closure of the mitral and tricuspid valves; a vibration caused by opening of the semilunar valves and early ejection of blood from the ventricles; and a low-pitched vibration produced by rapid ejection.

The second heart sound (S_2) is shorter and higher pitched than the first, is heard as a 'dupp' and is produced by closure of the aortic and pulmonary valves.

The third heart sound (S_3) is very faint and is caused by blood rushing into the ventricles.

The fourth heart sound (S_4) is rarely audible in a normal heart but can be demonstrated on graphic records. It is short and of low frequency and intensity, and is caused by atrial contraction. The vibrations arise from atrial muscle and from blood flow into, and distension of, the ventricles.

muffled h. s. the heart sounds are normal in outline but muffled, due usually to the presence of fluid between the heart and the stethoscope.

heartbeat the cycle of contraction of the heart muscle, during which the chambers of the heart contract. The beat begins with a rhythmic impulse in the sinoatrial node, which serves as a pacemaker for the heart. See also HEART.

heartwater a disease of cattle, sheep, goats and wild ungulates caused by *Cowdria ruminantium*, transmitted by the *Amblyomma* spp. ticks. In domestic animals it causes high fever and sudden death, or a less acute form manifested by incoordination, circling, blind charging, convulsions and death from encephalitis.

heartworm the common name for DIROFILARIA *immitis*.

h. dermatitis cutaneous dirofilariasis; a variety of skin lesions have been seen in dogs infested by *Dirofilaria immitis,* including hypersensitivity reactions, pyogranulomas and seborrheic dermatitis.

h. disease the syndrome of pulmonary artery disease with hypertension, heart failure (primarily cor pulmonale), and occasionally liver failure and interstitial, tubular and glomerular renal lesions caused by infestation by *Dirofilaria immitis*. Many species may be infected, but dogs are most commonly affected by chronic cough, weight loss and ultimately congestive heart failure. Infestation by the parasite, and the disease, can be prevented with appropriate prophylactic chemotherapy. Called also dirofilariasis. See also OCCULT heartworm infection, CAVAL SYNDROME.

heat[1] energy that raises the temperature of a body or substance; also, the rise of the temperature itself. Heat is associated with molecular motion, and is generated in various ways, including combustion, friction, chemical action and radiation. The total absence of heat is absolute zero, at which all molecular activity ceases.

h. balance balance between heat loss and heat production; its maintenance is critical to the patient's survival.

h. bumps see URTICARIA.

h. exhaustion a disorder resulting from overexposure to heat or to the sun. Long exposure to extreme heat or too much activity under a hot sun causes excessive sweating which removes large quantities of salt and fluid from the body. When the amount of salt and fluid in the body falls too far below normal, heat exhaustion may result. The same disease in birds is called heat prostration (below). See also heat stroke (below).

h. increment see SPECIFIC dynamic action.

latent h. the heat that a body may absorb without changing its temperature.

h. loss body heat can be lost by conduction, convection, evaporation and radiation; evaporation is the critical one during exercise and in hot environments.

h. prostration caused by exposure to high ambient temperature, especially if the humidity causes hyperthermia in birds. This is exacerbated by their poor heat loss mechanisms.

h. regulation is one of the functions of the hypothalamus and consists of a balancing of the body's heat loss and heat gain by regulation of respiration, skin temperature, sweating and muscle tone.

h. shock proteins proteins expressed by heat shock (*hsp*) genes as a result of exposure to increased temperature or other stress. See also heat shock response (below).

h. shock response decreased transcription and translation activity caused by the synthesis of heat shock proteins by an organism as a result of exposure to increased temperatures or other stress.

specific h. the number of calories required to raise the temperature of 1 g of a particular substance one degree centigrade.

h. stress exposure of the animal to high ambient temperatures.

h. stroke elevation of body temperature above physiologically active levels due to the production of excessive heat, exposure to excessive ambient temperatures or failure to lose heat. Characterized by restlessness, followed by dullness, weakness and recumbency. There is severe hyperthermia, the animal seeks cool places, is dyspneic and lapses into a coma terminally.

h. teratogenicity is observed only in experimental application of high temperatures in early pregnancy. Observed defects are of the central nervous system, and of the limbs including arthrogryposis and selective shortening.

h. therapy see HYPERTHERMIA.

h. tolerance in animals is their ability to function well under high environmental temperatures. This capacity varies widely between species and breeds. Much of the difference is due to variations in the capacity to increase heat loss under conditions of heat stress.

h. weaning the weaning of commercial chickens away from an artificial heat source at about 4 weeks of age.

heat[2] estrus in female animals.

h. detection identifying cows in heat has become one of the most critical techniques in modern dairy farming. As well as acute observation by farmers a number of devices are used as aids, e.g. tail paint, several kinds of color-change patches that are glued onto the cow's tailhead, and devices worn by infertile males that mark the cows.

heat-labile toxins one of two plasmid-encoded toxins produced by *Escherichia coli.*

heat-stable toxin one of two plasmid-encoded toxins produced by *Escherichia coli.*

heated beef deterioration in quality of sides of meat or game which are hung too close together so that they do not cool down quickly after slaughter. Called also sour side, green struck.

heath 1. a large area of open scrubland. 2. a member of the plant family Ericaceae; see HEATHER.

Heath sheep a European class of sheep, including many ethnic varieties; a black, horned carpetwool sheep.

heather a member of the plant family Ericaceae; called also heath. None of the native heathers of the UK, e.g. *Erica cinerea*, *E. (Calluna) vulgaris*, are poisonous but the exotic shrubs, *Andromeda* (see PIERIS) and KALMIA, are.

heather blindness contagious OPHTHALMIA of sheep.

heavenly bamboo see NANDINA DOMESTICA.

heaves see CHRONIC obstructive pulmonary disease.

h. line the visible groove between the aponeurotic and muscular parts of the external oblique muscle caused by the persistent double expiratory effort, with maximum abdominal muscle input, imposed by the poor respiratory gas exchange in this disease.

heavy having great weight.

h. chain see heavy CHAIN.

h. chain switch see CLASS switching.

h. grain feeding feeding of cereal grain feeds at levels in excess of conventional practice is frequently followed by carbohydrate engorgement, rumenitis and hepatic abscessation. Persistent feeding at levels less than those conducive to lactic acidosis is thought to contribute to the development of left displacement of the abomasum.

h. horse breeds includes CLYDESDALE, SHIRE, SUFFOLK HORSE, BELGIAN, PERCHERON.

h. metals lead, mercury, silver, zinc, copper, arsenic, iron.

h. veal calves fed on hard feed, weigh >400 lb (182 kg), aged >3 weeks Called also western veal calves.

heavy-chain disease a monoclonal gammopathy in which the heavy chain fragment alone is produced in large amounts and can be detected in both serum and urine.

hebetic pertaining to sexual maturity.

hecatomeric having processes that divide in two, one going to each side of the spinal cord; said of certain neurons.

hecto- word element. [Fr.] *hundred;* used in naming units of measurement to designate an amount 100 times (10^2) the size of the unit to which it is joined, e.g. hectoliter (100 liters); symbol h.

Hedera helix a member of the plant family Araliaceae. May contain a toxic saponin which causes milk fever-like recumbency in cattle. Called also ivy, common ivy.

hedge nettle see GALEOPSIS.

hedge pink SAPONARIA *officinalis*.

hedgehog nocturnal, insectivorous and immune to snakebite, this spiny animal plays a beneficial role in an environment by controlling some pests. Called also *Erinaceus erinaceus*, a member of the family Erinaceidae.

h. fleas see FLEA.

h. grass see ECHINOPOGON.

h. tick see IXODES *hexagonus*.

hedging insuring against making a loss whilst holding stocks of a commodity. Usually achieved by taking an opposite position on the futures market.

Hedycarya arborea New Zealand plant in the family Monomiaceae; contains an unidentified toxin which causes weight loss. Called also pigeonwood.

heel 1. (rare) in cats and dogs, the hock joint or tarsus. 2. in ungulates, the place at the rear of the hoof or claw where horn and skin meet and where the wall of the hoof turns horizontally to become the sole.

h. abscess one of the forms taken by foot abscess in sheep. There is pain and swelling at the affected heel, and separation and discharge of pus occurs at the skin–horn junction. The abscess is caused by infection with *Fusobacterium necrophorum* and *Corynebacterium pyogenes,* the infection resulting from an extension of the infection from an interdigital dermatitis.

h. bug see TROMBICULA *autumnalis.*

h. bulb necrosis see infectious BULBAR necrosis.

contracted h. the heels of the affected hoof are closer together than normal, the frog is narrow and shrunken and the bars form a narrower angle than in the normal hoof. The horse is usually lame on the leg.

h. easing trimming the foot so that the heels can spread more.

h. effect unequal distribution of the x-ray beam intensity emitted from the x-ray tube. Due to angulation of the target, the distribution of the beam intensity decreases rapidly towards the anode due to absorption of the x-ray beam by the target and anode material.

h. fly see HYPODERMA.

sheared h. vertical separation occurs between the heels of a horse's hoof causing lameness. A chronic condition due usually to overuse of one heel because of a conformational imbalance.

heft Irish name for ovine ILLTHRIFT.

heifer young female cattle up to the birth of first calf or in the lactation following the first calving. May be qualified as replacement, to enter the herd as a replacement for a culled cow, pregnant, maiden or spayed heifer. A springing heifer is in the last one or two weeks of pregnancy.

Heimlich valve a valve placed on an indwelling catheter to prevent reflux of air into cavity being evacuated, as in drainage of the pleural cavity.

Heineke–Mikulicz pyloroplasty enlargement of a pyloric stricture by incising the pylorus longitudinally and suturing the incision transversely.

Heinz body see Heinz BODY.

Heinz–Ehrlich body see Heinz BODY.

hekkabit see CAPPARIS TOMENTOSA.

Heko-Heko see PORCINE reproduction and respiratory syndrome.

HeLa cells cells of the first continuously cultured carcinoma strain, descended from a human cervical carcinoma; used in the study of life processes, including viruses, at the cell level.

helcoid like an ulcer.

helenalin a sesquiterpene, a toxin in the plant *Helenium microcephalum.*

Helenium North American genus of plants in the Asteraceae family; contain sesquiterpene lactones which cause a syndrome of abdominal pain, vomiting, diarrhea, lncoordination, dyspnea. Includes *H. amarum* (*H. tenuifolium*), *H. autumnale* (sneezeweed, bitter weed), *H. flexuosum* (*H. nudiflorum*), *H. hoopesii* (orange sneezeweed), *H. integrifolium*, *H. microcephalum* (small head sneezeweed). *H. amarum* imparts a bitter taste to the milk of cattle which eat it. Called also *Dugaldia* spp., sneezeweed.

helianthrone see DIANTHRONE.

Helianthus annuus toxic plant in the family Asteraceae; causes nitrate–nitrite poisoning. Called also summer flower.

helical shaped like a HELIX.

helicase an enzyme involved in DNA replication, responsible for unwinding the double helix.

Helichrysum genus in the plant family Asteraceae; in southern Africa *H. argyrosphaerum* contains an unidentified toxin which causes blindness and paresis resulting from degenerative lesions in the brain. In

Australia *H. blandowskianum* (*Argentipallium blandowskianum*, everlasting woolly daisy) is hepatoxic but the toxin is unknown.

helicine spiral.

h. arteries spiral arteries opening into the cavernous tissue of the penis; have an important role in enhancing erection and failitating detumescence.

Helicobacter microaerophilic, curved to spiral-shaped, gram-negative bacteria associated with gastritis and peptic ulcer disease in humans. The type species is *H. pylori*. It may also be involved in the etiology of gastric neoplasia.

H. acinonys, H. canis, H. felis, H. heilmannii, H. mustelae isolates from the stomach of cheetahs, dogs, cats, dogs and ferrets, respectively. It is likely that they may be responsible for gastric disease in these species.

helicoid coiled; spiral.

helicopodia helicopod gait; a dragging, shuffling gait in which the feet describe half circles.

helicopter disease see INFECTIOUS stunting syndrome.

helicotrema the passage that connects the scala tympani and the scala vestibuli at the apex of the cochlea in the internal ear.

Helictometra giardi see THYSANIEZIA *giardi*.

heli(o)- word element. [Gr.] *sun*.

heliosupine toxic alkaloid in CYNOGLOSSUM OFFICINALE.

heliotrine toxic pyrrolizidine alkaloid in HELIOTROPIUM *europaeum*.

heliotrope HELIOTROPIUM *europaeum*.

Heliotropium plant genus of the Boraginaceae family; contains pyrrolizidine alkaloids; causes hepatic injury and a syndrome of depression, jaundice and photosensitization. Also a significant contributor to the development of toxemic jaundice in sheep; may also cause sufficient intravascular hemolysis to result in hemoglobinuria and hemolytic anemia. Includes *H. amplexicaule*, *H. europaeum*, *H. ovalifolium*. Called also heliotrope.

helium a chemical element, atomic number 2, atomic weight 4.003, symbol He. See Table 6.

Helium is a chemically inert element that is odorless, tasteless and noncombustible. Because of its low density it is easily moved through the air passages and therefore requires little effort in breathing on the part of the patient who is in respiratory distress. Although helium itself has no chemical therapeutic value, when combined with oxygen it facilitates the delivery of this gas to the lungs (see HELIUM–OXYGEN THERAPY).

helium–oxygen therapy the administration of a mixture of helium and oxygen (commonly 80% He and 20% O_2 or 70% He and 30% O_2); used in humans in the management of airway obstruction associated with bronchospasm or bronchial asthma. The He–O_2 mixture is about one-third the density of air. This reduces turbulent flow and the patient effort required for ventilation.

helix 1. a coiled structure. 2. the free margin of the pinna of the ear.

α-h., alpha-h. the folding arrangement of parts of protein molecules in which a single polypeptide chain forms a right-handed helix.

h. destabilizing proteins proteins that bind in a cooperative manner to DNA single-strands during DNA replication and help open up the replication fork. Called also single-strand DNA binding proteins.

double h. the native state of DEOXYRIBONUCLEIC ACID (DNA), in which two antiparallel chains with complementary nucleotide sequences are wound around each other. The DNA molecule consists of two sugar-phosphate strands with the nucleotide base pairs stacked between them. The orientation of the two strands is antiparallel, i.e. 5′→3′ directions are opposite. Called also Watson–Crick helix.

helix-to-coil transition phenomenon observed in melting or denaturation of double-stranded helical DNA; as the temperature increases there is bubble formation produced by the initial separation of relatively high adenine and thymine pairs; the single strands within the bubbles, and later in the completely separated single strands, form coils.

hellebore HELLEBORUS spp., VERATRUM *californicum*, *V. album*, *V. viride*.

Helleborus European plant genus in the Ranunculaceae family; contains a protoanemonin glycoside hellebrin causing diarrhea, dysentery, abdominal pain, and cardiac glycosides which cause sudden death. Includes *H. argutifolius* (*H. corsicus*), *H. foetidus* (stinking hellebore, setterwort), *H. niger* (Christmas rose), *H. orientalis*, *H. viridis* (green hellebore).

hellebrigenin a cardiotoxic aglycone in the plants *Helleborus* spp.

hellebrin a cardiotoxic, protoanemonin glycoside in the plants *Helleborus* spp.

Heller and Paul anticoagulant a balanced mixture of potassium and ammonium oxalates used to prevent coagulation of blood samples collected for cell counts.

Heller's operation called also Heller's esophagomyotomy. See CARDIOPLASTY.

helminth a parasitic worm; a nematode, cestode or trematode.

helminthagogue anthelmintic; vermifuge; an agent that expels worms or intestinal animal parasites.

helminthemesis the vomiting of worms.

helminthiasis, helminthosis disease caused by an helmintic infection which may take any one of a number of forms. Worms living virtually free in the gut lumen, e.g. *Moniezia*, are relatively nonpathogenic, those that suck blood may cause anemia, those causing mucosal damage, e.g. *Ostertagia* spp., are followed by inappetence, malabsorption, a protein-losing enteropathy. A group that burrows into the gastrointestinal wall, e.g. *Oesophagostomum* spp., cause physical disturbances to gut function. Some species, e.g. *Strongylus vulgaris*, migrate through other tissues and cause clinical signs related to that migration.

helminthology the scientific study of parasitic worms.

helminthoma a tumor caused by a parasitic worm.

helminthosis see HELMINTHIASIS.

Helminthosporium genus of toxic fungi.

H. biseptatum a fungus growing on onion grass (*Romulea bulbocodium*) and thought to contribute to its toxicity. Also found in maduromycosis lesions. Called also *Drechslera* spp.

H. spiciferum BIPOLARIS *spicifera*.

helmintic pertaining to or emanating from helminths.

h. immunity antibodies produced by the host to antigens in the worm's exsheathing fluid, and enzymes produced by the worm; these are thought to damage the worms and encourage their expulsion.

heloma a corn.

helotomy excision or paring of a corn or callus.

helper assisting; symbiotic.

h. lymphocytes see helper LYMPHOCYTE.

h. substance soluble proteins that regulate the

responses of other cells to antigens. More properly called CYTOKINE; see also LYMPHOKINE.
h. T cells see helper LYMPHOCYTE.
h. virus one that helps a defective virus to complete its replication cycle in infected cells.
helvellic acid one of the toxins in the large fungus *Gyromitra esculenta*.
hem- word element. [Gr.] *blood*. See also words beginning *hemato-* and *hemo-*.
hemacytometer see HEMOCYTOMETER.
hemadsorption the adherence of red cells to other cells, particles or surfaces. Hemadsorption and hemadsorption inhibition are used for the assay of some viruses and their specific antibodies, e.g. paramyxovirus.
hemadynamometer an instrument for measuring blood pressure.
hemadynamometry measurement of blood pressure.
hemagglutinating encephalomyelitis virus disease see hemagglutinating ENCEPHALOMYELITIS virus disease of pigs.
hemagglutination agglutination of erythrocytes usually by either antibodies, viruses or certain plant lectins; abbreviated HA.
indirect h. test see hemagglutination inhibition test (below).
h. inhibition (HI) test an assay for the presence of specific antiviral antibodies in a test serum. The serum, usually a twofold dilution series, is mixed with a standard number, usually 4 to 8 HA units, of virus and incubated prior to the addition of a standard suspension of erythrocytes. The highest dilution of serum that inhibits hemagglutination is the HI titer of the serum.
passive h. test see passive AGGLUTINATION test.
h. (HA) test hemagglutinating viruses directly agglutinate erythrocytes by binding to specific receptor sites on the surface of the erythrocyte and this characteristic can be used in detection, identification and quantitation of the virus.
h. viruses viruses capable of agglutinating red blood cells of a variety of animals, e.g. adenoviruses, parvoviruses, togaviruses, some coronaviruses, picornaviruses, orthomyxoviruses and paramyxoviruses. Useful in classifying viruses and assaying amounts of virus and antibody. See also HEMADSORPTION.
hemagglutinin a substance that causes agglutination of erythrocytes. See HEMAGGLUTINATION.
cold h. one that acts only at temperatures near 39.2°F (4°C).
warm h. one that acts only at temperatures near 98.6°F (37°C).
hemal pertaining to blood or blood vessels.
h. arch small, v-shaped bones attached to the caudal ends of the ventral surface of several caudal (coccygeal) vertebrae where they protect several coccygeal vessels; they are small in dogs, absent in horses and cattle, large in kangaroos and whales.
h. node occur under the peritoneum along the vertebral column, in some viscera, near the spleen and kidneys and in the jugular furrow in ruminants; resemble lymph nodes but their sinuses are filled with blood. Have functions probably like those of the spleen. Called also hemolymph node.
hemalomyelia see progressive hemorrhagic MYELOMALACIA.
hemanalysis analysis of the blood.
hemangiectasis dilatation of blood vessels.
hemangioblast a mesodermal cell that gives rise to both vascular endothelium and hemocytoblasts.
hemangioendothelioma a hemangioma in which endothelial cells are the predominant component.
malignant h. see HEMANGIOSARCOMA.
hemangioepithelioma hemangiosarcoma.
hemangioma a benign tumor made up of newly formed blood vessels, clustered together. In animals they occur mostly on the skin and in the spleen. In birds, they may be caused by leukosis virus. See also bovine cutaneous ANGIOMATOSIS, HEMANGIOMATOSIS, TELANGIECTASIA.
disseminated cavernous h. multiple, small hemangiomatous tumors found in skin and internal organs; in calves and pigs rarely.
verrucous h. hemangioma in superficial dermis; induce epithelial hyperplasia.
hemangiomatosis the presence of multiple hemangiomas.
hemangiopericytoma a tumor composed of spindle cells with a rich vascular network, which apparently arises from pericytes. See also SCHWANNOMA.
hemangiosarcoma a malignant tumor of endothelial cells characterized by extensive metastasis, being cavitatious and bleeding profusely if cut. Occurs in spleen, liver, skin, right atrium and muscle. It can cause severe hemorrhagic anemia by bleeding internally. Common in German shepherd dogs. Called also angiosarcoma.
hemapheresis any procedure in which blood is withdrawn, a portion (plasma, leukocytes, platelets, etc.) is separated and retained, and the remainder is retransfused into the donor.
hemarthros, hemarthrosis blood in a joint cavity.
hematemesis the vomiting of blood. The appearance of the vomitus depends on the amount and character of the gastric contents at the time blood is vomited and on the length of time the blood has been in the stomach. Gastric acids change bright red blood to a brownish color and the vomitus is often described as 'coffee-ground' in color. Bright red blood in the vomitus indicates a fresh hemorrhage and little contact of the blood with gastric juices.
hematencephalon effusion of blood into the brain.
hemathermous warm-blooded; hematothermal.
hematic 1. pertaining to the blood. 2. hematinic.
h. fetal mummification a form of mummification in which degenerated blood, resembling melted chocolate has accumulated between the chorion and the uterus.
hematidrosis excretion of bloody sweat.
hematin a compound formed by the oxidation of heme from the ferrous Fe(II) to the ferric Fe(III) state; it does not combine with oxygen.
h. methods basic method of estimating hemoglobin content of blood by converting it to acid hematin and doing a colorimetric estimation. See also HEMOGLOBINOMETER.
hematin pigment crystalline brown deposits, mostly in vessels, formed by the action of formic acid on hemoglobin and accepted as a postmortem artifact; likely to be confused with hemosiderin.
hematinemia the presence of heme in the blood.
hematinic 1. improving the quality of the blood. 2. an agent that improves the quality of the blood, increasing the hemoglobin level and the number of erythrocytes; examples are iron preparations, liver extract and the B complex vitamins.
hematinuria the presence of heme in the urine.
hemat(o)- word element. [Gr.] *blood*. See also words beginning *hem-* and *hemo-*.
hematobilia bleeding into the biliary passages.
hematoblast see HEMOCYTOBLASTS.
hematocele an effusion of blood into a cavity, especially into the tunica vaginalis testis.

hematochezia blood in the feces.
hematochromatosis hemochromatosis.
hematochyluria the discharge of blood and chyle in the urine.
hematocrit the volume percentage of erythrocytes in whole blood; also, the apparatus or procedures used in its determination. The hematocrit (which means, literally, 'to separate blood') is determined by centrifuging a blood sample to separate the cellular elements from the plasma; the results of the test indicate the ratio of cell volume to plasma volume (packed cell volume, PCV) and are expressed as milliliters of packed cells per 100 ml of blood, or in volumes per 100 ml. The hematocrit, in conjunction with other hematological tests, provides information about the size, functioning capacity and number of erythrocytes. See also WINTROBE METHOD.
hematocyst effusion of blood into the bladder or in a cyst.
hematocyturia the presence of erythrocytes in the urine.
hematogenic 1. hematopoietic. 2. hematogenous.
h. peripheral circulatory failure peripheral circulatory failure due to loss of blood volume, either by loss of whole blood, or serum or water. See also CIRCULATORY failure.
hematogenous produced by or derived from the blood; disseminated through the bloodstream or by the circulation.
hematogone a lymphocyte-like cell appearing in the bone marrow as a nucleus without a cell cytoplasm. Considered to be a blood cell precursor.
hematoid like blood.
hematoidin a substance apparently chemically identical with bilirubin but formed in the tissues from hemoglobin, particularly under conditions of reduced oxygen tension.
hematolactia see HEMOLACTIA.
hematological, hematologic pertaining to or emanating from blood cells.
h. tests total and differential white cell counts, hematocrit estimation, erythrocyte count.
hematologist a specialist in hematology.
hematology the science dealing with the morphology of blood and blood-forming tissues, and with their physiology and pathology.
h. reference values normal numbers per unit volume of each cell included in a blood COUNT. See Tables 1.1 and 1.2.
hematolymphangioma a tumor composed of blood and lymph vessels.
hematolysis see HEMOLYSIS.
hematoma a localized collection of extravasated blood, usually clotted, in an organ, space or tissue. Contusions (bruises) are familiar forms of hematoma that are seldom serious. Hematomas can occur almost anywhere on the body; they are almost always present with a fracture and are especially serious when they occur inside the skull, where they may produce local pressure on the brain. In minor injuries the blood is absorbed unless infection develops.
For regional hematomas of individual importance see under anatomical name, e.g. ear, penile, vaginal, brain, ethmoid.
hematomediastinum effusion of blood into the mediastinum.
hematometry measurement of hemoglobin and estimation of the percentage of various cells of the blood.
hematomphalocele an umbilical hernia containing blood.
hematomyelia hemorrhage into the substance of the spinal cord. See also progressive hemorrhagic MYELOMALACIA.
hematomyelitis acute myelitis with bloody effusion into the spinal cord.
hematomyelopore formation of canals in the spinal cord due to hemorrhage.
hematonephrosis the presence of blood in the renal pelvis.
hematopathology the study of diseases of the blood; hemopathology.
hematopedesis see HEMODIAPEDESIS.
hematophagous subsisting on blood, e.g. hematophagous flies.
hematophilia see HEMOPHILIA.
hematopoiesis the formation and development of blood cells, usually taking place in the bone marrow.
cyclic h. of collies see canine CYCLIC hematopoiesis.
h. depression a significant finding in cases of endotoxemia.
extramedullary h. the formation of and development of blood cells outside the bone marrow, as in the spleen, liver and lymph nodes.
fetal h. in embryogenesis migration of stem cells from the yolk sac blood islands sets up hematopoiesis in thymus, lymph nodes, liver and spleen. When fetal bone develops a marrow cavity hematopoiesis is similarly established. At birth hematopoiesis is largely medullary.
regenerative h. increased hematopoietic activity in response to a need for more cells; indicated by the presence of a higher than normal proportion of immature forms in the peripheral blood.
hematopoietic 1. pertaining to or affecting the formation of blood cells. 2. an agent that promotes the formation of blood cells.
h. dysplasia dyshematopoiesis.
h. system organs and tissues involved in the production of blood cells; includes bone marrow, spleen, thymus, lymph nodes.
hematopoietic necrosis see INFECTIOUS hematopoietic necrosis of fish.
hematoporphyria a constitutional state marked by abnormal quantity of porphyrin (uroporphyrin and coproporphyrin) in the tissues and secreted in the urine, pigmentation of the mucosae (and later of the bones), sensitivity of the skin to light, vomiting, and intestinal disturbance; see PORPHYRIA.
hematoporphyrin an iron-free derivative of heme, a product of the decomposition of hemoglobin.
hematoporphyrinemia hematoporphyrin in the blood.
hematoporphyrinuria hematoporphyrin in the urine. See also bovine congenital erythropoietic PORPHYRIA.
hematorrhachis hemorrhage into the vertebral canal.
hematorrhea copious hemorrhage.
hematosalpinx an accumulation of blood in the uterine tube.
hematoscheocele an accumulation of blood within the scrotum.
hematospermatocele a spermatocele containing blood.
hematospermia blood in the semen.
hematosteon hemorrhage into the medullary cavity of a bone.
hematothorax see HEMOTHORAX.
hematotoxic 1. pertaining to blood poisoning. 2. poisonous to the blood and hematopoietic system.
hematotrachelos distension of the cervix uteri with blood.
hematotropic having a special affinity for or exerting a specific effect on the blood or blood cells.

hematotympanum hemorrhage into the middle ear.
hematoxylin an acid coloring matter obtained from the wood of a tree (*Haematoxylon campechianum*); used as a stain for histological specimens and as an indicator. See also hematoxylin and eosin STAIN.
hematozoa plural of HEMATOZOON.
hematozoon any animal microorganism living in the blood; refers usually to protozoa.
hematuria the discharge of blood in the urine. The urine may be slightly blood tinged, grossly bloody, or a smoky brown color.
enzootic h. see ENZOOTIC hematuria.
heme the nonprotein, insoluble, iron protoporphyrin constituent of hemoglobin, of various other respiratory pigments, and of many cells, both animal and vegetable. It is an iron compound of protoporphyrin and so constitutes the pigment portion or protein-free part of the hemoglobin molecule, and is responsible for its oxygen-carrying properties.
h. pigment nephropathy see HEMOGLOBINURIC nephrosis.
h. synthetase the rate-controlling enzyme for the synthesis of heme.
hememelis witch hazel.
hemeralopia day blindness; defective vision in a bright light due to a degeneration or absence of cones. An inherited defect in Alaskan malamutes and miniature poodles.
hemerocallin see STYPANDROL.
Hemerocallis plant genus in the family Liliaceae; contains a naphthaquinone (stypandrol) which causes neuropathy and encephalomalacia experimentally but no natural cases have been recorded. Called also day lily.
hemi- word element. [Gr.] *half*.
hemiacardius an unequal twin in which the heart is rudimentary, its circulation being assisted by the other twin.
hemiacetal formed by nucleophilic addition of an alcohol to the carbonyl group of an aldehyde. Most open-chain hemiacetals are not stable, but cyclic hemiacetals of the type present in aldehyde sugars such as glucose are more stable.
hemiamyosthenia lack of muscular power on one side of the body.
hemianacusia loss of hearing in one ear.
hemianalgesia analgesia on one side of the body.
hemianencephaly congenital absence of one side of the brain.
hemianesthesia anesthesia of one side of the body.
hemianopia blindness in half of the visual field. Occurs with unilateral lesions of the optic tracts.
hemianopsia hemianopia.
hemiataxia ataxia on one side of the body.
hemiathetosis athetosis of one side of the body.
hemiatrophy atrophy of one side of the body or one half of an organ of part.
hemiaxial at any oblique angle to the long axis of the body or a part.
hemiballism, hemiballismus violent motor restlessness of half of the body, most marked in the upper extremity.
hemibladder a half bladder; a developmental anomaly in which the bladder is formed as two physically separated parts, each with its own ureter.
hemiblock failure in conduction of cardiac impulse in either of the two main divisions (fascicles) of the left branch of the bundle of His; the interruption may occur in either the anterior or posterior division. Called also fascicular block.
hemic pertaining to blood.
h. murmur caused by a reduction in viscosity of the blood such as occurs in a blood loss anemia. The murmur is soft and waxes and wanes with respiration reaching its loudest at the peak of inspiration. See also heart MURMUR.
hemic–lymphatic system the combined blood and lymphatic systems; the secondary defense system of the body, after the skin and mucosae.
hemicardia the presence of only one side of a four-chambered heart.
hemicellulose structural polysaccharide of plants. Consists of β1,4-linked pentose sugars, mainly xylose.
hemicephalia congenital absence of the cerebrum.
hemicephalus a fetus exhibiting hemicephalia.
hemicerclage wire use of a cerclage wire to stabilize fragments in a fractured bone, especially useful for transverse irregular or short oblique fractures.
hemicholinium competes with choline for choline uptake into cholinergic neurons; results in the gradual development of paralysis.
hemichorea chorea affecting only one side of the body.
hemicolectomy excision of approximately half of the colon.
hemicrania a developmental anomaly with absence of half of the cranium.
hemicraniosis hyperostosis of one side of the cranium and face.
hemidesmosome see half DESMOSOME.
hemidiaphoresis sweating on one side of the body only.
hemidiaphragm see diaphragmatic CRUS.
hemidysesthesia a disorder of sensation affecting only one side of the body.
hemidystrophy unequal development of the two sides of the body.
hemiectromelia a developmental anomaly with imperfect limbs on one side of the body.
hemiepilepsy epilepsy affecting one side of the body.
hemifacial affecting one side of the face.
h. spasm hypertonicity of facial muscles may occur with increased irritability of the facial nerve as in otitis media or lesions of the brainstem.
hemigastrectomy excision of half of the stomach.
hemiglossectomy excision of part of the tongue.
hemiglossitis inflammation of half of the tongue.
hemignathia a developmental anomaly characterized by partial or complete lack of the lower jaw on one side.
hemihidrosis sweating on one side of the body only.
hemihypalgesia diminished sensitivity to pain on one side of the body.
hemihyperesthesia increased sensitivity of one side of the body.
hemihyperhidrosis excessive sweating on one side of the body.
hemihyperplasia overdevelopment of one side of the body or of half of an organ or part.
hemihypertonia increased muscle tone on one side of the body.
hemihypertrophy overgrowth of one side of the body or of a part.
hemihypesthesia diminished sensitivity on one side of the body.
hemihypoplasia underdevelopment of one side of the body or of half of an organ or part.
hemihypotonia diminished muscle tone on one side of the body.
hemilaminectomy removal of a vertebral lamina on one side only.

hemilaryngectomy excision of one lateral half of the larynx.
hemilateral affecting one side of the body only.
hemilesion a lesion on one side of the spinal cord.
hemimandibulectomy surgical removal of the mandible on one side.
hemimaxillectomy surgical removal of one entire side of the upper jaw, including the premaxilla, maxilla and hard palate. Usually carried out in removal of neoplasms.
hemimelia congenital absence of all or part of the distal half of a limb.
inherited tibial h. only the first and second phalanges of each limb are missing in this inherited defect in cattle.
radial h. see RADIAL hemimelia.
hemimelus an individual exhibiting hemimelia.
hemin porphyrin required by some bacterial species for growth. Called also X factor.
heminephrectomy excision of part (half) of a kidney.
hemiopia hemianopia.
hemipagus twin fetuses joined laterally at the thorax.
hemiparalysis paralysis of one side of the body.
hemiparanesthesia anesthesia of the posterior half of one side.
hemiparaplegia paralysis of the posterior half of one side.
hemiparesis paresis affecting one side of the body.
hemiparesthesia perverted sensation on one side.
hemiparetic 1. pertaining to hemiparesis. 2. a patient affected with hemiparesis.
hemipenes paired, vascular, eversible sacs which open into the posterior cloaca in snakes and lizards. The two hemipenes are brought together to act as a penis and are inserted into the cloaca of the female during copulation.
hemipeptone a form of peptone obtained from pepsin digestion.
hemiplegia paralysis of one side of the body; usually caused by a brain lesion, such as a tumor.
Hemiptera an order of arthropods (class Insecta); includes some 30,000 species, known as the true bugs; characterized by having mouthparts adapted to piercing or sucking, and usually having two pairs of wings.
hemirachischisis fissure of the vertebral column without prolapse of the spinal cord.
hemisacralization fusion of the last lumbar vertebra to the first segment of the sacrum on only one side.
hemisection division into two equal parts; bisection.
hemispasm spasm affecting only one side.
hemisphere half of a spherical or roughly spherical structure or organ.
cerebral h. one of the paired structures constituting the largest part of the brain, which together comprise the extensive cerebral cortex, centrum semiovale, basal ganglia and rhinencephalon, and contain the lateral ventricle. See also BRAIN.
hemispherium pl. *hemispheria* [L.] hemisphere.
hemistanding a postural reaction that tests the animal's ability to support weight on the thoracic and pelvic limbs on one side.
hemithorax one side of the chest; the cavity lateral to the mediastinum.
hemithyroidectomy excision of one lobe of the thyroid.
Hemitragus see TAHR.
hemivertebra a developmental anomaly in which one side of a vertebra is incompletely developed. Occurs commonly in British bulldogs, Boston terriers and the Pug without clinical effects, but occasionally leads to invertebral disk herniation, vertebral luxation or spinal cord compression.
hemivertebrata an inappropriate name for hemichordata.
hemiwalking a postural response in which walking is forced on the thoracic and pelvic limbs of one side.
hemizygosity the state of having only one of a pair of alleles transmitting a specific character.
hemizygote an animal exhibiting hemizygosity.
hemlock there are a number of weeds in different genera that go by this name.
poison h. see CONIUM MACULATUM.
water h. see CICUTA.
h. water dropwort OENANTHE *crocata*.
hemo- word element. [Gr.] *blood.* See also words beginning *hemato-* and *hem-*.
hemoacupuncture venipuncture (bleeding).
hemobartonellosis infection by *Hemobartonella* spp. in which parasitized erythrocytes are preferentially removed from the circulation by phagocytic cells and an anemia develops. Diagnosis depends on observation of the characteristic rod-shaped and ring-shaped organisms around the periphery of the red cells. See also FELINE infectious anemia.
hemobilia see HEMATOBILIA.
hemoblast see HEMOCYTOBLASTS.
hemoblastosis a general term for proliferative disorders of the blood-forming tissues.
hemocatheresis the destruction of erythrocytes.
hemocele the body cavity in insects comparable to the celom in mammals; between the gut and the body wall.
hemochorial a deciduate placenta characteristic of humans, many other primates and rodents. At parturition the maternal vascular endothelium of the uterus is shed, as well as uterine epithelium so that the chorionic cells are in direct contact with maternal blood.
hemochromatosis a condition observed in sheep and cattle which have been exposed to high intakes of iron in their rations; the liver is enlarged and brown, the hepatic lymph nodes are brown; large amounts of iron are stored in liver and lymph nodes. Seen also in ostriches.
hemoclasis destruction of erythrocytes.
hemoconcentration increase in the proportion of formed elements in the blood, as a result of a decrease in its fluid content, e.g. in clinical dehydration.
hemoconia pl. *hemoconiae* [L.] small, round or dumbbell-shaped bodies exhibiting brownian movement, observed in blood platelets in darkfield microscopy of a wet film of blood.
hemoconiosis presence in blood of excessive amounts of hemoconia.
hemocyst congenital hematoma on the margin of an atrioventricular valve.
hemocyte a blood cell.
hemocytoblastoma a tumor containing all the cells typical of bone marrow.
hemocytoblasts the central cells of the cell groups known as cell islands, which develop on the surface of the yolk sac and the allantois. The cell islands eventually form the endothelial lining of vessels, the hemocytoblasts form blood cells.
hemocytocatheresis destruction of erythrocytes.
hemocytogenesis formation of blood cells; hematopoiesis.
hemocytology the study of blood cells.
hemocytolysis see HEMOLYSIS.
hemocytometer an instrument used in counting blood cells, commonly applied to a combination of

counting chambers with coverglasses and pipettes for erythrocytes and leukocytes, all meeting established specifications.

hemocytometry the technique of counting blood cells.

hemocytotripsis disintegration of blood cells by pressure.

hemodiagnosis diagnosis by examination of the blood.

hemodializer, hemodialyser an apparatus by which HEMODIALYSIS may be performed, blood being separated by a semipermeable membrane from a solution of such composition as to secure diffusion of certain elements out of the blood. Popularly called artificial kidney.

hemodialysis removal of certain elements from the blood by virtue of difference in rates of their diffusion through a semipermeable membrane while the blood is being circulated outside the body. The procedure is used to remove toxic wastes from the blood of a patient with acute or chronic renal failure. See also KIDNEY.

hemodiapedesis extravasation of blood through the skin without there being any obvious discontinuity.

hemodilution increase in the fluid content of blood, resulting in diminution of the concentration of formed elements.

hemodynamics the study of the forces and physical mechanisms concerned with the circulation of the blood.

hemoendothelial denoting a type of placenta in which maternal blood comes in contact with the endothelium of chorionic vessels, e.g. rabbit, rat and mouse.

hemofiltration the removal of waste products from the blood by passing the blood through extracorporeal filters.

hemoflagellate any flagellate protozoan parasitic in the blood. See also TRYPANOSOMA.

hemofuscin a brownish-yellow pigment resulting from hemoglobin decomposition; it gives urine a deep ruddy color.

hemogenesis the formation of blood; hematogenesis.

hemogenic pertaining to production of blood.

hemoglobin an allosteric protein found in erythrocytes that transports molecular oxygen (O_2) in the blood. Symbol Hb.

Oxygenated hemoglobin (*oxyhemoglobin*) is bright red in color; hemoglobin unbound to oxygen (*deoxyhemoglobin*) is darker. This accounts for the bright red color of arterial blood, in which the hemoglobin is about 97% saturated with oxygen. Venous blood is darker because it is only about 20–70% saturated, depending on how much oxygen is being used by the tissues.

The affinity of hemoglobin for carbon monoxide is 210 times as strong as its affinity for oxygen. The complex formed (*carboxyhemoglobin*) cannot transport oxygen. Thus, carbon monoxide poisoning results in hypoxia and asphyxiation.

Another form of hemoglobin that cannot transport oxygen is *methemoglobin*, in which the iron atom is oxidized to the +3 oxidation state. During the life span of a red cell, hemoglobin is slowly oxidized to methemoglobin. At least four different enzyme systems can convert methemoglobin back to hemoglobin. When these are defective or overloaded, methemoglobinemia, in which high methemoglobin levels cause dyspnea and cyanosis, may result.

As red cells wear out or are damaged, they are ingested by macrophages of the reticuloendothelial system. The porphyrin ring of heme is converted to the bile pigment bilirubin, which is excreted by the liver. The iron is transported to the bone marrow to be incorporated in the hemoglobin of newly formed erythrocytes.

h. A_{1c} see glycosylated HEMOGLOBIN.

carcass h. tests include hemoglobin extraction test, hemoglobin–pseudoperoxidase test. Used on suspect meat to determine if it has been properly bled out; poor bleeding is an indication of fever or septicemia.

h. concentration varies with the hematocrit; determined by several methods. Assesses the oxygen-carrying capacity of blood.

cyanotic h. malformations insufficient oxygenated hemoglobin is received in the peripheral capillary beds resulting in blue discoloration of tissues, and an incapacity of the body to maintain a life-sustaining level of activity.

glycosylated h. hemoglobin A with a glucose moiety attached to the amino terminal valine of the beta chain. This type of hemoglobin is made at a slow constant rate during the life span of the erythrocyte. Increased levels correlate with glucose intolerance in diabetes. With adequate insulin treatment, levels return to the normal range and periodic assays can be helpful in evaluating effective control of diabetes mellitus. Called also hemoglobin A_{1c}.

glycosylated h. test measurement of the percentage of hemoglobin A molecules that formed a stable ketoamine linkage between the amino terminal valine residue of the beta chain and a glucose moiety; used to assess diabetic control.

h.–oxygen dissociation curve the incremental increase in oxygen saturation of the hemoglobin with each unit increase of the partial pressure of oxygen in the blood. Any factor that shifts the curve to the right will automatically reduce the concentration of O_2 held by the hemoglobin and increase the rate of its delivery to tissues.

urine h. see HEMOGLOBINURIA.

h. variants the globin part of hemoglobin is composed of a large number of amino acids and the hemoglobins are therefore susceptible to a great many variations. In humans a large number of variants have been identified but only a few in animals and none are deleterious. The identified ones are the three adult hemoglobin types, HbA, HbB and HbC. There is also an embryonic, HbE, and a fetal hemoglobin, HbF.

hemoglobinemia presence of excessive hemoglobin in the blood plasma.

hemoglobinolysis the splitting up of hemoglobin.

hemoglobinometer a laboratory instrument for colorimetric determination of the hemoglobin content of the blood; abbreviated Hb-meter.

Sahli h. is based on the separation of globin from hemoglobin by treatment with hydrochloric acid to produce acid hematin which is measured by colorimetry.

Spencer h. measures oxyhemoglobin by light absorption using a green filter.

hemoglobinometry the technique of using a hemoglobinometer to estimate the hemoglobin content of a sample of blood.

hemoglobinopathy any hematological disorder due to alteration in the genetically determined molecular structure of hemoglobin, with characteristic clinical and laboratory abnormalities and often overt anemia. There are many such diseases in humans but none have yet been identified in animals.

hemoglobinous containing hemoglobin.

hemoglobinuria the presence of free hemoglobin in the urine. In true hemoglobinuria the protein has originated from erythrocytes hemolyzed within the vascular system. In false hemoglobinuria it comes from erythrocytes in the urine that have hemolyzed there, leaving red cell envelopes in the urinary sediment. In both forms the urine is colored dark red to almost black.

bacillary h. is an acute, highly fatal toxemia of cattle and sheep caused by *Clostridium haemolyticum* (*C. novyi* type D). It is characterized by hemoglobinuria, jaundice and sudden death with large, usually single infarcts in the liver.

cold h. intravascular hemolysis occurs in the blood vessels in the intestinal wall immediately after the calf, rarely an adult, has drunk a large amount of very cold water after a period of deprivation. Transient hemoglobinuria may occur. See also cold ANEMIA.

false h. when lysis of erythrocytes occurs after the urine is passed.

postparturient h. see POSTPARTURIENT hemoglobinuria.

hemoglobinuric pertaining to or emanating from hemoglobin.

h. nephrosis is the result of intravascular hemolysis and the excretion of large quantities of hemoglobin in the urine. The epithelial cells and lumina of the tubules become packed with hemoglobin resulting in renal failure. See also NEPHROSIS.

hemogram a graphic or tabular representation of the differential blood count.

hemohistioblast the hypothetical stem cell from which all blood cells are derived.

hemoid resembling blood.

hemokinesis the flow of blood in the body.

hemolactia blood in the milk. Can occur transitorily in the cow at any time as a result of acute trauma such as a kick in the udder. Immediately after calving it is usually the result of rupture of many small congested blood vessels. Severity varies from large clots and frank blood to a pale pink tinge.

hemolith a concretion in the walls of a blood vessel.

hemolymph 1. blood and lymph. 2. the bloodlike fluid of invertebrates having open blood–vascular systems.

h. node see HEMAL node.

hemolymphangioma see HEMATOLYMPHANGIOMA.

hemolymphatic system the combined blood and lymph systems.

hemolysate the product resulting from hemolysis.

hemolysin a substance that liberates hemoglobin from erythrocytes by interrupting their structural integrity.

hemolysis rupture of erythrocytes with release of hemoglobin.

In a transfusion reaction or in alloimmune hemolytic anemia antibody mediated lysis of red blood cells involves triggering of the complement cascade. Red blood cells also clump together. The agglutinated cells become trapped in the smaller vessels or are phagocytosed and eventually disintegrate.

Some microbes form substances called hemolysins that have the specific action of destroying red blood cells; beta-hemolytic streptococci are an example.

Intravenous administration of a hypotonic solution or plain distilled water will cause the red cells to fill with fluid until their membranes rupture and the cells are destroyed.

Wherever either in vitro or in vivo IgG or IgM antibodies are bound to red blood cell antigens in the presence of complement, the complement cascade is triggered the final products of which include enzymes that result in holes being 'punched' in the wall of the red blood cell, allowing hemoglobin to escape and which is observed as lysis.

Snake venoms and certain plant substances may cause hemolysis. A great variety of chemical agents can lead to destruction of erythrocytes if there is exposure to a sufficiently high concentration of the substance. These chemical hemolytics include copper.

A disorder of the immune response in which antibodies are made to 'self' red blood cell antigens resulting in the lysis of the cells. See also autoimmune hemolytic ANEMIA.

alpha (α) h. a characteristic of some bacteria, especially streptococci, manifested by a zone of greenish coloration of cleared agar around a colony of the bacteria on a blood–agar plate. Note that α-hemolysis of staphylococci causes complete lysis. See also STREPTOCOCCUS.

beta (β) h. complete hemolysis of sheep and ox erythrocytes by bacteria in culture media. Note that β-hemolysin of staphylococci causes incomplete hemolysis.

blood transfusion h. see TRANSFUSION reaction.

differential h. a technique for identification of chimerism, e.g. freemartin calves. Antisera against a single blood group causes only partial hemolysis of the blood composed of two cell populations with different blood cell antigens.

double h. two types of hemolysis produced on blood agar by alpha and beta lysins found in *Staphylococcus aureus* and *S. intermedius*.

extravascular h. the hemolysis which occurs when fragments of erythrocytes and the majority of aged erythrocytes are phagocytosed directly by the cells of the mononuclear phagocytic system.

h. fever the rise in body temperature which accompanies each hemolytic incidence of significant size.

fragmentation h. see microangiopathic ANEMIA.

h. inhibition test a serological test used in the diagnosis of *Corynebacterium pseudotuberculosis* infection.

intravascular h. disruption of red blood cells occurs while they are within blood vessels.

microangiopathic h. fragmentation hemolysis often associated with microvascular injury, as in disseminated intravascular coagulation, and resulting from a primary disease.

target h. see double hemolysis (above).

hemolytic pertaining to, characterized by, or producing hemolysis.

h. anemia anemia caused by the increased destruction of erythrocytes which may occur in the vascular system—*intravascular* hemolysis, or due to phagocytosis by the monocyte–macrophage system—*extravascular* or intracellular hemolysis. It may result from incompatibility (see ALLOIMMUNE hemolytic anemia of the newborn), from mismatched blood transfusions, from poisons such as copper, organic agents in plants such as kale, from nutritional deficiencies such as phosphorus and from protozoan infections such as BABESIOSIS. Hemolytic anemia may also occur as a result of a disorder of the IMMUNE response in which B cell-produced antibodies fail to recognize erythrocytes that are 'self' and directly attack and destroy them. In addition to the usual signs of anemia, the patient may also exhibit jaundice.

h. component a degree of extravascular hemolysis in association with other types of anemia.

h. disease of the newborn see ALLOIMMUNE hemolytic anemia of the newborn.

h. enterotoxemia a little reported disease recorded mostly in Australia in sheep, cattle and foals; a highly fatal hemolytic anemia associated with a heavy population of *Clostridium perfringens* type A in the intestines.

h. plaque assay see PLAQUE assay.

h.–uremic syndrome a microangiopathic hemolytic anemia with thrombocytopenia and severe involvement of renal vasculature which leads to acute renal failure. In humans associated with verocytoxin-producing bacteria such as *Escherichia coli*, *Shigella* and some *Salmonella*; usually associated with the ingestion of poorly cooked meat. A similar clinical syndrome has been reported in cows, horses and dogs.

hemolyze to subject to or to undergo hemolysis.

hemomediastinum an effusion of blood into the mediastinum.

hemomelasma ilei small, up to 1 by 2 inches, slightly elevated, red-brown plaques, under the serosa of the terminal small intestine; caused by migrating larvae of *Strongylus* spp. in horses.

hemonchosis infestation with the abomasal worms *Haemonchus contortus* and *H. placei.* The disease in sheep, goats and cattle is characterized by acute anemia, anasarca and death due to anemic anoxia. See also HAEMONCHUS.

hemonephrosis effused blood in the renal pelvis; hematonephrosis.

hemoparasite an animal parasite, specifically a hemoflagellate or filarid worm, living in the blood of a vertebrate, e.g. *Babesia* spp., *Eperythrozoon* spp., *Trypanosoma* spp.

hemopathology the study of diseases of the blood.

hemopathy any disease of the blood.

hemoperfusion the passage of blood through an extracorporeal adsorptive system to remove compounds of larger molecular size than those removed by hemodialysis.

hemopericardium an effusion of blood in the pericardial cavity, caused by rupture of the atrium, perforation of the ventricle or rupture of a coronary artery. It is usually manifested by very sudden death.

hemoperitoneum an effusion of blood in the peritoneal cavity.

hemopexin a heme-binding serum protein.

hemopexis coagulation of blood.

hemophagocyte a cell that destroys blood corpuscles.

hemophagous feeding on blood.

h. zone marginal hematomas seen as circumferential bands in zonary placentas; thought to contribute to the needs of the fetus for iron.

hemophil 1. thriving on blood. 2. a microorganism that grows best in media containing hemoglobin.

hemophilia a condition characterized by impaired coagulability of the blood, and a strong tendency to bleed. See also deficiency of the following clotting factors, AFIBRINOGENEMIA and HYPOPROTHROMBINEMIA, and PROCONVERTIN, STUART FACTOR, plasma THROMBOPLASTIN antecedent, HAGEMAN FACTOR and fibrin stabilizing FACTOR.

h. A classical hemophilia, due to deficiency of clotting factor VIII-C; occurs in dogs, horses and cats and is transmitted by the female to the male as a sex-linked recessive abnormality.

h. B a form similar to classical hemophilia but due to a deficiency of clotting factor IX; called also CHRISTMAS DISEASE and factor IX deficiency. Occurs in dogs and cats.

h. C in dogs an autosomal dominant form due to deficiency of clotting factor XI (plasma thromboplastin antecedent). Called also factor XI deficiency. The disease also occurs in cattle but the clinical disease is minor and it is inherited as a recessive character.

double h. dogs with both hemophilia A and hemophilia B have been produced experimentally.

vascular h. deficiency of clotting factor VIII and factor VIII-related antigen occurs in many breeds of dogs, particularly Doberman Pinschers, and in rabbits and pigs. See also VON WILLEBRAND'S DISEASE.

hemophiliac an animal affected with hemophilia.

hemophilic 1. pertaining to hemophilia. 2. in bacteriology, growing well on culture media containing blood or having a nutritional requirement for constituents of fresh blood.

h. arthropathy bleeding into a joint due to hemophilia.

hemophilioid resembling classical hemophilia clinically, but not due solely to clotting factor VIII deficiency.

hemophilosis a septicemic disease of cattle caused by *Haemophilus somnus* characterized by an acute illness with a short course and a high mortality rate. In survivors there are residual lesions, especially hemorrhagic infarcts in the brain, and synovitis, pleurisy and pneumonia. Clinical signs vary widely but predominant signs are blindness due to ophthalmitis, weakness, ataxia and recumbency. Called also thromboembolic or thrombotic meningoencephalomyelitis.

Hemophilus see HAEMOPHILUS.

hemophoric conveying blood.

hemophthalmia extravasation of blood inside the eye.

hemopleura see HEMOTHORAX.

hemopneumopericardium effused blood and air in the pericardium.

hemopneumothorax an accumulation of blood and air in the pleural cavity.

hemopoiesis see HEMATOPOIESIS.

hemoprecipitin a precipitin specific for blood.

hemoprotein a conjugated protein whose nonprotein portion is heme.

hemopsonin an opsonin that renders erythrocytes more liable to phagocytosis. Called also erythrocytoopsonin.

hemoptysis coughing and spitting of blood as a result of bleeding from any part of the respiratory tract. In true hemoptysis the sputum is bright red and frothy with air bubbles; it must not be confused with the dark red or black color of hematemesis.

Hemoptysis is a most unusual sign in animals, most aspirated blood being swallowed. Anything more profuse than that may gush from the nostrils and the mouth but that can hardly be classified as spitting.

endemic h. schistosomiasis.

hemorrhage the escape of blood from a ruptured vessel. Hemorrhage can be external, internal, or into the skin or other tissues. Blood from an artery is bright red in color and comes in spurts; that from a vein is dark red and comes in a steady flow.

Hemorrhages in particular anatomical sites may be found under their specific anatomical headings.

alimentary tract h. includes hematochezia, melena.

cancer-associated h. see paraneoplastic hemorrhage (below).

capillary h. oozing of blood from minute vessels.

cerebral h. see BRAIN hemorrhage.

concealed h. internal hemorrhage.

ecchymotic h. see ECCHYMOSIS.

exercise-induced pulmonary h. see exercise-induced PULMONARY hemorrhage.

fibrinolytic h. that due to abnormalities in the fibrinolytic system and not dependent on hypofibrinogenemia.
internal h. that which occurs into cavities, e.g. hemoperitoneum, or into tissues, e.g. vulvar hematoma in mares. The only evidence of illness may be extreme pallor and weakness. There may be moderate dyspnea and other signs related to the distension of individual organs.
h. intra-abdominal see HEMOPERITONEUM.
intra-articular h. see HEMARTHROS.
intracranial h. bleeding within the cranium, which may be extradural, subdural, subarachnoid or cerebral.
intraocular h. see HYPHEMA.
mesenteric h. uncommon syndrome caused by leakage of blood into the potential space between the two serosal layers of the mesentery. An extensive hemorrhage causes severe abdominal pain, shock, some blood-staining of peritoneal fluid and leakage of blood into the intestinal lumen.
paraneoplastic h. a variety of hemostatic disorders develop in association with neoplasia in animals and may result in disseminated intravascular coagulation and hemorrhage. Called also cancer-associated hemorrhage.
peritoneal h. see HEMOPERITONEUM.
petechial h. subcutaneous hemorrhage occurring in minute spots.
postpartum h. that which follows soon after parturition.
primary h. that which soon follows an injury.
secondary h. that which follows an injury after a considerable lapse of time.
subcutaneous h. causes a soft, painless fluctuating swelling capable of being moved easily. Paracentesis reveals the presence of whole blood.

hemorrhagenic causing hemorrhage.

hemorrhagic pertaining to or characterized by hemorrhage.
h. bowel disease of swine see PROLIFERATIVE hemorrhagic enteropathy.
canine h. fever see canine EHRLICHIOSIS.
h. diathesis a tendency to bleed due to any one or a combination of clotting defects. Occurs, for example, in diseases of liver in which there may be defects in the prothombin complex, or in fibrinogen or thromboplastin availability. See HEMOPHILIA, PURPURA hemorrhagica, disseminated intravascular COAGULATION.
h. disease an undifferentiated disease manifested by unprovoked hemorrhage and caused by any one of a number of factors. See also HEMOPHILIA, EPIZOOTIC hemorrhagic disease of deer, WARFARIN, canine EHRLICHIOSIS, hemorrhagic syndrome (below).
h. disease of the newborn see neonatal hemorrhagic disease (below).
h. enteritis an acute, highly fatal disease of turkeys over 4 weeks of age characterized by bloody droppings, a short course and a high prevalence and caused by an adenovirus.
h. enterotoxemia profound toxemia accompanied by hemorrhagic enteritis. It is caused by *Clostridium welchii* types A, B, C and E.
h. foal enteritis see antibiotic-associated COLITIS.
neonatal h. disease hemorrhagic disease of the newborn; may be due to maternal isoimmunization, e.g. in pigs. See also UMBILICAL hemorrhage.
h. septicemia a septicemic pasteurellosis of cattle and other ruminants, rarely of pigs and horses. It is caused by *Pasteurella multocida* type 1 (or B) rarely D or E, and characterized by a sudden onset of high fever, dyspnea, salivation, hot painful subcutaneous swellings and submucosal petechiae and death in about 24 hours. Called also septicemic pasteurellosis, el guedda.

Occurs also in finfish, caused by opportunist bacteria including *Aeromonas*, *Pseudomonas* spp.
h. shock see SHOCK.
h. syndrome a widespread disease of domestic fowl causing significant losses due to death in birds about 5 to 9 weeks of age. The cause may be multifactorial but a viruses are suspected to play an important role. Characterized by clinical anemia, leukopenia, anemia and hemorrhages in all tissues.

hemorrhagin a cytolysin present in snake venoms. An endotheliotoxin which causes serious damage to blood vessels.

hemorrhea hematorrhea.

hemorrheology the scientific study of the deformation and flow properties of cellular and plasmatic components of blood in macroscopic, microscopic and submicroscopic dimensions and the rheological properties of vessel structure with which the blood comes in direct contact.

hemosiderin an insoluble form of intracellular storage iron, visible microscopically both with and without the use of special stains.

hemosiderinuria the presence of hemosiderin in the urine.

hemosiderosis a focal or general increase in tissue iron (hemosiderin) stores without associated tissue damage.
pulmonary h. the deposition of abnormal amounts of hemosiderin in the lungs, due to bleeding into the lung interstitium.

hemospermia, haemospermia blood in the semen.

hemosporidia see BABESIA, THEILERIA, PLASMODIUM, HAEMOPROTEUS, LEUCOCYTOZOON.

hemostasis arrest of the escape of blood by either natural (clot formation or vessel spasm) or artificial (compression or ligation) means, or the interruption of blood flow to a part, or the artificial stimulation of clotting, e.g. electrocautery, topical collagen.

hemostat 1. a small surgical clamp for constricting blood vessels. 2. an antihemorrhagic agent.

hemostatic 1. checking blood flow. 2. an agent that checks the flow of blood.
h. defects see COAGULOPATHY.
h. plug see CLOTTING.

hemostyptic see HEMOSTATIC.

hemotherapy the use of blood in treating disease.

hemothorax collection of blood in the pleural cavity which can cause collapse of the lung and dyspnea, absence of breath sounds and pallor of mucosae.

hemotoxic see HEMATOTOXIC.

hemotoxin an exotoxin characterized by hemolytic activity.

hemotroph the sum total of the nutritive material from the circulating blood of the maternal body, utilized by the early embryo. It is absorbed directly from the maternal blood by the allantochorion or vitellochorion.

hemp see CANNABIS SATIVA.

hemp nettle see GALEOPSIS.

hen 1. a mature, egg-laying bird, or bird of egg-laying age that is temporarily not laying eggs; in most cases a female bird more than 5 months old. 2. an adult, female bird.

hen-and-chickens see BRYOPHYLLUM *tubiflorum*.

hen harrier see HARRIER. Called also marsh hawk.

henbane see HYOSCYAMUS NIGER.

henbit see LAMIUM AMPLEXICAULE.

Henderson–Hasselbalch equation an equation by which the pH of a buffer solution, blood plasma being such a one, can be determined:

$$pH = pK' + \log \frac{[BA]}{[HA]}$$

where pK′ is the negative log of the dissociation constant of a weak acid in a buffer solution, [HA] is the concentration in the buffer solution of the weak acid and [BA] is the concentration of a salt of that acid.

Henle named after F.G.J. Henle, a German anatomist and histologist.

H's chromoreaction a color change to dark brown within 20 minutes of applying Zenker solution to the cut surface of a pheochromocytoma.

H's fissure spaces filled with connective tissue between the muscular fibers of the heart.

H.–Koch's postulates used in the evaluation of a microorganism as the cause of a disease. See KOCH'S postulates.

H's layer outermost layer of the inner root sheath of the hair follicle.

H's ligament lateral expansion of the lateral edge of the rectus abdominis muscle which attaches to the pubic bone.

H's loop U-shaped loop of the uriniferous tubule of the kidney.

H's membrane inner layer of choroid (basal lamina) in contact with the retina.

H's sheath the endoneurium, especially the delicate continuation around terminal branches of nerve fibers.

H's tubules straight ascending and descending portions of a renal tubule forming Henle's loop.

Henneguya a genus of protozoa causing disease in free-living fish. Genus of class Myxosporea, the myxosporids.

H. exilis causes cysts in the gills of channel catfish and death due to suffocation.

H. zschokkei causes boil disease in salmonid fishes.

Henning plaster spreader heavy duty pivoted instrument. Closing the handles forces open the large, square, flat blades that have been inserted in the cut already made in the plaster cast that is to be removed.

Henrici test a field test for the detection of cyanide compounds in food material.

Henry's law the solubility of a gas in a liquid solution is proportional to the partial pressure of the gas.

Hensen's node the primitive knot in the early embryo from which the notochord develops. It establishes the longitudinal axis and the polarity of the embryo. Called also primitive node, primitive knot.

HEP high egg passage, with reference to virus attentuation usually for vaccine production.

Hepadnaviridae a family of viruses that are icosahedral with a circular, partially double-strand DNA genome. The prototype virus causes serum hepatitis or hepatitis B and hepatocellular carcinoma in humans; related viruses cause hepatitis and hepatocellular carcinoma in ducks, woodchucks, ground squirrels and dogs.

hepadnavirus a virus in the family *Hepadnaviridae*.

hepar [L.] *liver*.

heparan sulfate a sulfated mucopolysaccharide structurally related to heparin, which occurs normally in the liver, aorta and lung; it is an accumulation product in several mucopolysaccharidoses.

heparin an acid mucopolysaccharide present in many tissues, especially the liver and lungs, and having potent ANTICOAGULANT properties. It also has lipotrophic properties, promoting transfer of fat from blood to the fat depots by activation of lipoprotein lipase. Also, a mixture of active principles capable of prolonging blood clotting time, obtained from domestic animals; used in the prophylaxis and treatment of disorders in which there is excessive or undesirable clotting and as a preservative for blood specimens.

heparinize to treat with heparin.

hepatalgia pain in the liver.

hepatatrophia atrophy of the liver.

hepatectomize to deprive of the liver by surgical removal.

hepatectomy surgical excision of liver tissue.

hepatic emanating from or pertaining to liver.

h. abscess common in cattle as a sequel to rumenitis; characterized by fever, leukocytosis and pain on percussion over the liver.

h. acinus see liver ACINUS.

h. angle the angle made by the caudolateral border of the caudate liver lobe on abdominal radiography.

h. arterioportal fistula shunt between the hepatic artery and the portal vein.

h. atrophy and nodular regeneration a disease of dogs, due to unknown cause but possibly a toxin, characterized by nodular regenerative hyperplasia and atrophy of severely fatty hepatocellular parenchyma and gradually developing, always fatal, liver insufficiency.

h. cell hepatocyte.

h. cirrhosis diffuse hepatic fibrosis associated with the formation of structurally abnormal, regenerative, parenchymal nodules. Initiated by hepatocyte necrosis.

h. coccidiosis spoken of but recorded only once in a calf.

h. congestion a common feature of congestive heart failure and other circulatory embarrassments of venous drainage of the liver; occurs also in anaphylaxis.

diffuse h. fibrosis results from continued, chronic hepatic injury or the summation of repeated bouts of zonal necrosis; the resulting fibrosis links portal areas and hepatic venules and bisects liver lobules.

h. distomatosis infection of the liver with flukes, e.g. *Fasciola hepatica*, *Fascioloides magna*, *Metorchus conjunctus*. See also FASCIOLIASIS.

h. diverticulum an outgrowth of the embryonic duodenum; it divides into a pars hepatica and a pars cystica, forerunners of the liver and the gallbladder respectively.

h. duct see hepatic DUCT.

h. fibrosis a reaction to chronic injury to the liver; includes biliary fibrosis, postnecrotic scarring, diffuse hepatic fibrosis and periacinar fibrosis.

h. injury see HEPATITIS.

h. jaundice jaundice caused by disease of hepatic parenchyma in contrast to hemolytic and obstructive jaundice.

h. lipidosis see FATTY liver.

h. microsomal enzymes see microsomal ENZYMES.

h. necrosis death of hepatic parenchyma which may be single cell (necrobiosis), or multicell in piecemeal, focal, periacinar, midzonal, periportal or paracentral locations. Massive necrosis refers to events in individual acini in which all hepatocytes are dead.

omphalogenic h. abscess abscess resulting from infection of the umbilicus and direct vascular extension to the liver.

h. periacinar fibrosis fibrosis limited to the zones around hepatic venules; a response to congestive heart failure or to intoxication.

h. photosensitization see secondary PHOTOSENSITIZATION.
h. sinusoids the intralobular vascular supply system; lined by endothelial cells and stellate macrophages.
hepatic(o)- word element. [Gr.] *hepatic duct.*
hepaticoduodenostomy anastomosis of the hepatic duct to the duodenum.
hepaticoenterostomy anastomosis of the hepatic duct to the intestine (duodenum or jejunum).
hepaticogastrostomy anastomosis of the hepatic duct to the stomach.
hepaticojejunostomy anastomosis of the hepatic duct to the jejunum.
Hepaticola hepatica CAPILLARIA *hepatica.*
hepaticolithotomy incision of the hepatic duct with removal of calculi.
hepaticolithotripsy the crushing of a calculus in the hepatic duct.
hepaticostomy fistulization of the hepatic duct.
hepaticotomy incision of the hepatic duct.
hepatin glycogen.
hepatitis inflammation of the liver which may be toxic or infectious in origin; characterized by signs due to diffuse injury to the liver. See also LIVER dysfunction. There are a number of etiologically specific hepatitides which are listed under their individual headings. They are avian VIBRIONIC hepatitis, infectious canine hepatitis (see below), INFECTIOUS necrotic hepatitis, DUCK hepatitis, TURKEY hepatitis, INCLUSION BODY hepatitis, MOUSE hepatitis, POSTVACCINAL hepatitis, TOXEMIC jaundice, and those caused by FASCIOLA and FASCIOLOIDES, CYSTICERCUS, and plant toxins including PYRROLIZIDINE alkaloids, SPORIDESMIN, AFLATOXIN. See also HEPATOSIS dietetica.
h. A, B, C, D and E viruses causes of hepatitis in humans and some nonhuman primates.
avian vibrionic h. a disease of domesticated poultry which has disappeared from those areas in the USA which were its sole habitat. Vibrio-like organisms were isolated from the outbreaks which occurred.
cholangiolitic h. see CHOLANGIOHEPATITIS.
chronic active h. a chronic inflammatory liver disease in humans, probably of several types with different causes, but with distinctive histopathological features of piecemeal necrosis, bridging fibrosis and active cirrhosis. A similar, but not identical disease of unknown etiology has been described in dogs.
copper-induced h. see BEDLINGTON TERRIER copper-associated hepatopathy.
duck h. see DUCK hepatitis.
gosling h. see GOOSE hepatitis.
infectious canine h. an acute, highly contagious disease, occurring mainly in young dogs, caused by canine adenovirus type 1. Many dogs experience subclinical infections. Those with clinical signs show fever, depression, vomiting and abdominal pain. The course is short and in severe cases death occurs within a few days. Peracute infections occur in very young puppies. Mild infections may cause only vague signs of malaise and anorexia and many cases are not diagnosed. Dogs recovering from infection sometimes develop corneal edema ('blue eye'). A chronic hepatitis is reported as an occasional sequela. The disease can be prevented by vaccination.
mouse h. a coronavirus disease which causes heavy losses in baby mice. It is characterized by tremor, jaundice and hemoglobinuria.
mycotic h. commonly caused in cattle by extension from mycotic rumenitis due to lactic acid indigestion and damage to ruminal epithelium.
necrotic h. see INFECTIOUS necrotic hepatitis.
toxipathic h. hepatitis caused by toxins, especially ingested plant toxins, e.g. some pyrrolizidine alkaloids, sporidesmin, aflatoxin.
trophopathic h. see TROPHOPATHIC hepatitis.
turkey h. see TURKEY hepatitis.
h. X a hepatoxic disease of dogs and pigs caused by aflatoxins. See also MYCOTOXICOSIS.
hepatitis cysticercosa damage to the liver caused by migrating cestode larvae, including oncospheres and post-oncopheral stages, cysticerca in much the same way as migrating fluke larvae cause damage.
hepatization transformation into a liverlike mass, especially the solidified state of the lung in lobar pneumonia. The early stage, in which the pulmonary exudate is blood-stained, is called red hepatization. The later stage, in which the red cells disintegrate and a fibrinosuppurative exudate persists, is called gray hepatization.
hepat(o)- word element. [Gr.] *liver.*
hepatobiliary pertaining to or emanating from the liver, bile ducts and gallbladder.
h. system the liver, bile ducts and, in most species, gallbladder.
hepatoblastoma a malignant intrahepatic tumor consisting chiefly of embryonic tissue.
hepatocarcinogen a substance capable of causing hepatic neoplasia.
hepatocarcinoma hepatocellular carcinoma; carcinoma derived from the parenchymal cells of the liver (hepatocytes).
hepatocele hernia of the liver.
hepatocellular pertaining to or affecting liver cells.
h. adenoma tumor is usually single, may be lobulated, sessile; no acinar development and no ductal system.
h. fusion there is fusion then disappearance of adjacent hepatic cell membranes giving the tissue a syncytial appearance.
h. jaundice jaundice arising because of damage to hepatic cells.
hepatocerebral disease acute hepatic necrosis accompanied by spongiform changes in white matter of the brain, e.g. in poisoning by *Helichrysum* spp.
hepatocholangiocarcinoma cholangiohepatoma.
hepatocholangitis inflammation of the liver and bile ducts.
hepatocirrhosis cirrhosis of the liver.
hepatocutaneous syndrome see necrolytic migratory ERYTHEMA.
hepatocystic pertaining to the liver and gallbladder.
Hepatocystis a genus of intra-erythrocytic protozoan parasites in the family Plasmodiidae.
H. kochi the common malarial parasite of many primates. Rarely causes disease but may cause white to gray nodular foci on the liver.
hepatocyte a liver cell.
h. acidophilic body see CYTOSEGRESOME FORMATIONS.
hepatodiaphragmatic pertaining to the liver and the diaphragm.
hepatodynia pain in the liver.
hepatoencephalopathy hepatic ENCEPHALOPATHY.
hepatogastric pertaining to the liver and stomach.
hepatogenic 1. giving rise to or forming liver tissue. 2. hepatogenous.
hepatogenous 1. originating in or caused by the liver. 2. hepatogenic.
h. chronic copper poisoning copper accumulates in liver cells damaged by ingested hepatoxic agents in plants, e.g. *Heliotropum europaeum.*
hepatogram 1. a tracing of the liver pulse in the sphygmogram. 2. a radiograph of the liver.

hepatography 1. a treatise on the liver. 2. radiography of the liver. 3. the recording of the liver pulse.
hepatoid resembling the liver in its structure.
h. cells polygonal cells with abundant eosinophilic cytoplasm and small, round nucleus, resembling a hepatocyte and found in perianal glands of dogs.
h. gland see PERIANAL gland.
hepatojugular pertaining to the liver and jugular vein.
h. reflux distension of the jugular vein induced by manual pressure over the liver; it suggests insufficiency of the right heart.
hepatolenticular degeneration Wilson's disease.
hepatolienography radiography of the liver and spleen.
hepatolith a calculus in the liver.
hepatolithectomy removal of a calculus from the liver.
hepatolithiasis the presence of calculi in the biliary ducts of the liver.
hepatology the scientific study of the liver and its diseases.
hepatolysin a cytolysin destructive to liver cells.
hepatolysis destruction of the liver cells.
hepatoma any tumor of the liver, especially hepatocellular carcinoma (malignant hepatoma).
hepatomalacia softening of the liver.
hepatomegaly enlargement of the liver.
hepatomelanosis melanosis of the liver.
hepatometry measurement of the dimensions of the liver; often performed radiographically; valuable provided accurate criteria are available as a base for comparison.
hepatomphalocele umbilical hernia with liver involvement in the hernial sac.
hepatomycotoxins fungal toxins with hepatotoxic characteristics.
hepatonephric pertaining to the liver and kidney.
hepatopancreatic involving the pancreas and the liver.
h. necrosis see NECROTIZING hepatopancreatitis.
h. parvovirus disease usually multifactorial in etiology, including parvovirus and bacteria, in juvenile *Penaeus* spp.
hepatopathy any disease of the liver.
hepatopexy surgical fixation of a displaced liver to the abdominal wall.
hepatopleural pertaining to the liver and pleura or pleural cavity.
hepatopneumonic pertaining to, affecting, or communicating with the liver and lungs.
hepatoportal pertaining to the portal system of the liver.
hepatopulmonary hepatopneumonic.
hepatorenal pertaining to the liver and kidneys.
h. syndromes diseases in which there is concurrent involvement of both liver and kidneys. This may be the result of a toxin such as carbon tetrachloride which simultaneously damages both organs, or as a result of hepatic injury causing, for example, a cholemic nephrosis.
hepatorrhaphy suture of the liver.
hepatorrhexis rupture of the liver.
hepatoscan scintigraphy of the liver.
hepatoscopy examination of the liver.
hepatosis any functional disorder of the liver.
h. dietetica a degenerative disease of the liver of pigs due to a nutritional deficiency of vitamin E or selenium. There is massive hepatic necrosis; sudden death is the only clinical abnormality.
fatty h. see FATTY liver.
serous h. veno-occlusive disease of the liver.
hepatosplenitis inflammation of the liver and spleen.
h. infectiosa strigum acute viral hepatitis of owls caused by *Herpesvirus stringis* and characterized by sudden death and autopsy lesions of miliary necrotic foci in the liver, spleen and bone marrow.
hepatosplenography radiography of the liver and spleen.
hepatosplenomegaly enlargement of the liver and spleen.
hepatotherapy administration of liver or liver extract for its pharmacological effect rather than its nutritional value as a protein.
hepatotomy incision of the liver.
hepatotoxemia septicemia originating in the liver.
hepatotoxic causing liver damage.
hepatotoxin a toxin that destroys liver cells.
fungal h. includes some of the most potent hepatotoxins, e.g. sporidesmin, aflatoxin, rubratoxin, and the toxin of *Phomopsis leptostromiformis*, a fungus growing on lupins.
hepatotrophic having a specific effect on the liver or exerting a specific effect on it.
Hepatovirus a genus of single-stranded, plus sense RNA viruses in the family PICORNAVIRIDAE. It includes human and simian hepatitis A viruses.
hepatoxicity the quality of a substance which makes it toxic to liver cells.
hepatoxin substance toxic to hepatic cells.
Hepatozoon a genus of protozoan parasites in the family Haemogregarinidae.
H. canis found in dogs and other canines and in cats, in circulating leukocytes and bone marrow cells. Transmitted by the tick *Rhipicephalus sanguineus*. Causes intermittent fever, anemia, loss of weight, splenomegaly and posterior paralysis, but many infected animals are clinically normal.
H. cuniculi occurs in rabbits.
H. griseisciuri occurs in gray squirrels.
H. muris occurs in rats and transmitted by rat mites.
H. musculi found in white mice.
hepatozoonosis infection with the protozoa HEPATOZOON.
hepta- word element. [Gr.] *seven*.
heptachlor a CHLORINATED HYDROCARBON insecticide.
heptose a sugar whose molecule contains seven carbon atoms.
Heracleum mantegazzianum European plant in the family Apiaceae; contains furocoumarins which cause primary photosensitization. Called also cow parsnip, giant hogweed.
herb a flowering plant with one or more stems that does not persist as a plant but dies back to ground level each year.
h. Christopher see ACTAEA *spicata*.
herbage standing growing nonwoody plants, mostly annuals and especially grasses.
h. larval counts harvesting of a representative sample of herbage, washing it and sieving off larvae for the purpose of assessing levels of contamination of pasture with infective larvae of strongylid nematodes.
herbal medicine use of naturally occurring substances, usually of plant origin, in the prevention and treatment of disease. Certain of these herbal substances or their preparations which contain contaminants are capable of inducing toxicosis if used incorrectly or to excess.
herbicide a substance that destroys weeds. A large number of chemical compounds are used as general and selective herbicides. Most of them have very low toxicity because their availability to animals on

recently sprayed pasture is an obvious toxic hazard. Most poisoning incidents arise when animals have accidental access to large volumes of the agent, e.g. if there has been a spillage. The well-known herbicide groupings are bipyridyls, chlorinated acids, dinitro compounds, phenoxyacid derivatives, thiocarbamates and triazines.

herbivore one of the Herbivora; animals that subsist in their natural state entirely by eating plants and plant products. In confined management systems foods of animal origin may be included in their diets, e.g. meat meal, fish meal.

herbology use of Chinese herbs in medicine.

herd a group of animals, usually cattle, or pigs, or related wild animal species, which live a collective life together. This may be a natural pattern of behavior or be imposed by a human operated management system.

h. abnormality an abnormality detectable only by examination of epidemiological data, e.g. milk yield per hectare, conception rate to first service.

h. composition includes bulls (where applicable), cows in milk, dry cows, heifers not yet calved, bred heifers, virgin heifers, yearlings, calves weaned and suckers or at foot. Called also herd structure.

h. diagnosis a diagnosis made to fit a herd problem which may be, for example, a low reproduction rate, or wool yield, or win rate at the races.

dairy h. herd used exclusively for milk production.

h. epidemic an epidemic confined to one herd.

h. fertility control scheme programs based on surveillance of all reproduction data and comparison of indexes with preset targets. Correction of inefficiencies may be implemented by the farmer but diagnosis of the cause and treatments and prophylaxes are largely the province of the veterinarian.

h. health program a health management system based on periodic visits to the herd by a veterinarian to check the status of a series of identifiable health parameters including production, reproductive efficiency, mastitis prevalence, calf survival, cow culling and mortality rate, fecal egg counts. Superior programs also include production management so that genetics, nutrition, housing, disease control and financial management are coordinated in a whole-farm approach.

h. immunity a level of resistance in a herd or flock which is sufficient to prevent the entry of a particular disease into, or its spread within, the herd. The resistance may be innate, a genetically based resistance, or acquired as a result of previous exposure to the particular agent or of vaccination. The general usage of the term relates to the prevention of spread of infection at an epidemic level. So that in a herd in which there are 70 to 80% of immune animals there may be sporadic cases but the prevalence is unlikely to be significant. The same comments apply to larger populations, e.g. a wild animal or companion animal population which is really not managed as a herd.

h. level test test performed on the entire herd or an adequate sample of it.

h. sampling examination, either physical or clinical pathological, of a herd to determine the herd status in a particular epidemiological parameter.

h. size a critical factor in planning for productivity efficiency. May be quoted as the number of animals of a particular age or stage of production, e.g. milking cows, assuming that other, usually young, stock are also carried on the farm.

h. structure see herd composition (above).

h. udder health status of the herd with respect to the prevalence of quarter infection, clinical mastitis, teat lesions.

herding 1. natural congregation of animals into groups; see also FLOCKING. 2. management of animals into large groups or herds by humans to facilitate animal husbandry procedures.

hereditary transmissible or transmitted from parent to offspring; genetically determined.

h. ataxia occurs in smooth-haired Fox terriers and Jack Russell terriers and is progressive over a long period, commencing at 2 to 4 months of age; characterized by symmetrical demyelination within the spinal cord.

h. collagen dysplasia a group of diseases which occur in most species and are characterized by looseness and stretchability of the skin, often accompanied by laxity of the joints and occasionally by absence of the tooth enamel. The inherited defect is one of deficient collagen synthesis. See also DERMATOSPARAXIS, EHLERS–DANLOS SYNDROME. Called also hyperelastosis cutis, rubber-puppy syndrome.

h. defect anatomical or functional defect conditioned in its appearance by inherited factors.

h. melanoma benign, heritable, cutaneous tumor of pigs.

h. thrombopathias an inherited bleeding tendency in which the platelets do not function properly. Recorded in cattle and dogs.

heredity the transmission of genetic traits from parents to offspring. The hereditary material is DNA in the ovum and sperm, so that the offspring's heredity is determined at the moment of conception.

Inside the nucleus of each germ cell are structures called *chromosomes.* A chromosome is composed of DEOXYRIBONUCLEIC ACID (DNA) which is associated with histone proteins. Genes are segments of the DNA molecule; there are an estimated 100,000 GENES in each cell. Most genes carry code for a specific protein which may be recognized as a specific hereditary trait. These traits are physical, biochemical and physiological. Thus genes affect not only the physical appearance of an animal but also its behavior, physiological makeup, its tendency to develop certain diseases, and the daily activities of all the cells of its body. See also INHERITANCE.

heredofamilial occurring in certain families under circumstances that implicate a hereditary basis.

Hereford a breed of beef cattle, red with white head, underline and legs. There are polled and horned varieties.

H. encephalopathy–microphthalmia syndrome originally called inherited hydrocephalus. Inherited as a single autosomal recessive. Characterized by a domed skull, skeletal muscle degeneration, small palpebral fisures and orbits, retinal dysplasia, vitreous liquefaction, uveal malformation, microphakia, bilateral microphthalmia.

H. pig red pig with white head, legs, belly and tail, originating in the USA.

Herellea a genus of nonmotile, paired, gram-negative enteric bacilli. Now classified as *Acinetobacter.*

Hering–Breuer reflexes inflation and deflation reflexes that help regulate the rhythmic ventilation of the lungs, thereby preventing overdistension and extreme deflation. These reflexes arise outside the respiratory center in the brain; that is, the receptor sites are located in the respiratory tract, mainly in the bronchi and bronchioles. They are activated by either a stretching or a nonstretching and compression of the lung; the impulses are transmitted from the receptor sites through the vagus nerve to the brainstem and thence to the respiratory center.

The *inflation* reflex acts to inhibit inspiration and thereby prevents further inflation. When the lung tissue is stretched by inflation, the stretch receptors respond by sending impulses to the respiratory center, which in turn slows down inspiration. As the expiratory phase begins, the receptors are no longer stretched, impulses are no longer sent, and inspiration can begin again. This is called the Hering–Breuer *deflation* reflex. It is also believed that in addition to the cessation of impulses from the stretch receptors, there may be an activation of compression receptors which transmit impulses that inhibit expiration, thus allowing inspiration to begin.

heritability 1. the proportion of total variation in the population that can be attributed to variation in genetic factors. 2. the degree to which inheritance plays a part in the etiology of a disease.

broad-sense h. the degree to which a trait is genetically determined, expressed as the ratio of the total genetic variance to the phenotypic variance (V_G/V_P).

narrow sense h. the degree to which a trait is passed from parent to offspring expressed as the ratio of the additive genetic variance to the total phenotypic variance (V_A/V_P).

Hermann's tortoise TESTUDO *hermanni*.

hermaphrodism hermaphroditism.

hermaphrodite an individual whose body contains tissue of both male and female gonads. The ovaries and testes may be present as separate organs, or ovarian and testicular tissue may be combined in the same organ (ovotestis). The ovarian and testicular tissues may be present at the same time (synchronous hermaphrodite) or sequentially (when the sex organs appear one after the other; protandrous when the testes come first, protogynous when the ovaries appear first) See also HERMAPHRODITISM.

hermaphroditism a state characterized by the presence of both ovarian and testicular tissue and of ambiguous morphological criteria of sex. Hermaphroditism is not to be confused with pseudohermaphroditism, in which an individual with only one kind of gonad possesses reproductive organs that reflect some characteristics of the opposite sex, owing to improper balance of male and female hormones or other endocrine disorder.

bilateral h. that in which gonadal tissue typical of both sexes occurs on each side of the body.

false h. pseudohermaphroditism.

lateral h. presence of gonadal tissue typical of one sex on one side of the body and tissue typical of the other sex on the opposite side.

sequential h. see HERMAPHRODITE.

synchronous h. see HERMAPHRODITE.

transverse h. that in which the external genital organs are typical of one sex and the gonads typical of the other sex.

true h. coexistence in the same animal of both ovarian and testicular tissue, with somatic characters typical of both sexes.

unilateral h. presence of gonadal tissue typical of both sexes on one side and of only an ovary or a testis on the other.

hermetic impervious to the air.

hernia the abnormal protrusion of part of an organ or tissue through the structures normally containing it.

In this condition, a weak spot or other abnormal opening in a body wall permits part of the organ to bulge through. A hernia may develop in various parts of the body; most commonly in the region of the abdomen.

A layman's term for hernia is rupture. A hernia is either acquired or congenital.

Anatomically specific hernias are listed under their individual sites.

caudal abdominal h's see INGUINAL, FEMORAL, scrotal hernias (below).

cerebral h. see BRAIN herniation.

cord h. a type of umbilical hernia in which the midgut has failed to return to the abdominal cavity during fetal development and remains within the umbilical cord.

crural h. femoral hernia.

external h. protrusion of abdominal contents through an opening in the abdominal wall.

false h. a structural defect with contents but without a peritoneal sac.

fat h. hernial protrusion of peritoneal fat through the abdominal wall or through the vulvar wall during a difficult calving.

incarcerated h. hernia so occluded that it cannot be returned by manipulation; it may or may not become strangulated.

incisional h. hernia after operation at the site of the surgical incision, owing to improper healing or to excessive strain on the healing tissue; such strain may be caused by excessive muscular effort, activity, or by obesity, which creates additional pressure on the weakened area.

inguinoscrotal h. see scrotal hernia (below).

irreducible h. incarcerated hernia.

mesenteric h. hernia of a loop of small intestine through a traumatic tear in the mesentery.

muscle h. the belly of the muscle protrudes through a tear in the fascia and epimysium.

paraesophageal h. hiatal hernia in which part or almost all of the stomach protrudes through the hiatus into the thorax to the left of the esophagus, with the gastroesophageal junction remaining in place.

pelvic h. hernia caused by a loop of intestine becoming incarcerated in a hiatus between the wall of the pelvis and the ductus deferens, caused by tearing of the fold of the ductus at castration. May occur many months after the castration operation. Can be resolved, if diagnosed early enough, by traction on the taut mesentary per rectum.

pericardial h. see PERITONEOPERICARDIAL hernia.

perineal h. see PERINEAL hernia.

prepubic h. the result of avulsion of the cranial pubic tendon.

reducible h. one that can be returned by manipulation.

scrotal h. inguinal hernia which has passed into the scrotum. When these become strangulated they cause severe abdominal pain and acute local swelling. In large animals the tightened spermatic cord can be felt disappearing into the inguinal canal. See also INTESTINAL obstruction.

sliding hiatal h. hiatal hernia in which the stomach and the cardioesophageal junction protrude into the caudal mediastinum; the protrusion, which may be fixed or intermittent, is partially covered by a peritoneal sac.

slip h., slipped h. sliding hernia.

strangulated h. one that is tightly constricted. As any hernia progresses and bulges out through the weak point in its containing wall, the opening in the wall tends to close behind it, forming a narrow neck. If this neck is pinched tight enough to cut off the venous return, the hernia will quickly swell and become strangulated. This is a very dangerous condition that can appear suddenly and requires immediate surgical attention. Unless the blood supply is restored promptly, gangrene can set in and may cause death.

traumatic h. protrusion of abdominal viscera into a subcutaneous site because of traumatic injury to the abdominal muscles.

uterine h. a gravid uterus can prolapse through an inguinal hernia in dogs and cats.

vaginal h. hernia into the vagina; called also colpocele.

ventral h. trauma with tearing of the body wall results in prolapse of abdominal contents into the subcutaneous tissue. Also reported in ewes from violent straining during parturition.

herniation abnormal protrusion of an organ or other body structure through a defect or natural opening in a covering membrane, muscle or bone. See also HERNIA and individual anatomical sites for hernia.

nucleus pulposus h. rupture or prolapse of the nucleus pulposus into the spinal canal, or against the spinal cord. See also INTERVERTEBRAL disk disease.

transtentorial h. downward displacement (caudal transtentorial herniation; uncal herniation) of the medial brain structures through the tentorial notch by a supratentorial mass, exerting pressure on the underlying structures, including the brainstem.

uncal h. transtentorial herniation.

hernioid resembling hernia.

herniology the study of hernia.

hernioplasty surgical repair of hernia, with reconstruction of tissue.

herniorrhaphy surgical repair of HERNIA, with suture of the defective tissue. When the weakened area is very large, hernioplasty is done and some type of strong synthetic material is sewn over the defect to reinforce the area.

heroin a highly addictive narcotic analgesic derived from morphine; called also diacetylmorphine, diamorphine. Its sale is prohibited in the USA and in many other countries of the world.

heron tall, elegant, fish-eating waterbird, with long legs and a long neck. They are mostly *Ardea* spp. of the family Ardeidae. Includes gray, purple, great blue and little blue herons.

herpes pigeon virus 1 a cause of respiratory disease.

herpes simiae herpes B virus, the cause of a herpes simplex-like disease in non-human primates and of a uniformly fatal encephalitis in humans.

herpes simplex virus a virus in the family HERPESVIRIDAE that causes oral and genital disease, occasionally encephalitis, in humans and monkeys and fatal disease in owl monkeys and tree shrews.

Herpestes ichneumon see MONGOOSE.

Herpesviridae a family of viruses, the members of which are about 150 nm in diameter, enveloped, with a nucleocapsid of about 100 nm in diameter, composed of 162 capsomers and contain a large, double-stranded DNA. The viruses replicate in the nucleus of the infected cell, where they induce the formation of a characteristic inclusion body; some also induce formation of a cytoplasmic inclusion body. The herpesviruses are classified into three subfamilies: (1) *Alphaherpesvirinae*, which are rapidly growing viruses that cause acute diseases, except Marek's disease which causes tumors in chickens; (2) *Betaherpesvirinae*, which are slow growing, highly cell-associated viruses, also called cytomegaloviruses, which produce subtle diseases with a prolonged clinical course; and (3) *Gammaherpesvirinae*, some of which produce low grade, prolonged clinical illness typified by infectious mononucleosus/glandular fever of humans, caused by Epstein–Barr virus, and probably a similar disease of horses caused by equine herpesvirus 2; the primate viruses are associated with tumors.

The important diseases of animals caused by herpesviruses are dealt with under their individual headings: AUJESZKY'S DISEASE, INFECTIOUS bovine rhinotracheitis, infectious pustular VULVOVAGINITIS, equine VIRAL abortion, EQUINE viral rhinopneumonitis, EQUINE coital exanthema, equine herpesvirus 2 infection, the Allerton form of LUMPY-skin disease, the generalized infection of cattle with bovine herpesvirus 2, BOVINE herpes mammillitis, the African 'wildebeest-associated' BOVINE malignant catarrh, CANINE herpesvirus respiratory, genital and neonatal infections, feline viral RHINOTRACHEITIS. In birds there are INFECTIOUS laryngotracheitis, PIGEON herpesvirus, duck PLAGUE and MAREK'S DISEASE.

herpesvirus a member of the family HERPESVIRIDAE.

h. hominus infects nonhuman primates.

h.-1 infection see Table 8.2.

h. paralysis disease of horses, commonly those reinfected with EHV1. Signs vary from slight ataxia to incoordination, recumbency and death.

h. saimiri has produced malignant lymphomas in some monkeys.

h. tamarinus a cause of inclusion body hepatitis in marmosets and owl monkeys.

herpetic pertaining to or of the nature of herpes; relating to or caused by herpesviruses.

herpetiform resembling herpes.

Herpetomonas a genus of protozoa in the family Trypanosomatidae. Found in invertebrates and of no veterinary importance.

Herpetosoma a subgenus of the genus *Trypanosoma*, containing nonpathogenic species of *T. lewisi*.

Herring bodies the accumulated neurosecretions and carrier molecules in the axons of magnocellular neurons of the neurohypophysis.

herring gull *Larus argentatus*. See also GULL.

herring-gutted gaunt or tucked-up appearance.

herring meal a protein feed supplement used in Scandinavia but some batches contain a potent hepatoxin, thought to be dimethylnitrosamine. A dummy syndrome develops after several weeks of eating the meal.

herring worm see ANISAKIS.

herringbone parlor see MILKING parlor.

Herrold's egg yolk medium a medium used for the cultivation of *Mycobacterium paratuberculosis*.

hersage [Fr.] surgical separation of the fibers of a peripheral nerve.

Hertia pallens South African plant in the Asteraciae family; contains an unidentified toxin which causes hepatitis, pulmonary edema, fibrosis and emphysema. Called also springbokbush.

Hertwig's epithelial root sheath an extension formed by the free edge of the enamel organ on the developing tooth which goes beyond the enamel–dentine junction and molds a dental papilla to form the root of the tooth.

hertz a unit of frequency, equal to one cycle per second; symbol, Hz.

herztod PORCINE stress syndrome.

hetacillin a semisynthetic penicillin, which is converted in the body to ampicillin, and has actions and uses similar to those of ampicillin. The potassium salt can be given orally.

hetastarch an artificial colloid produced by addition of hydroxyethyl ether groups into amylopectin; used as a plasma volume expander for treatment of shock.

heteradelphus a twin monster with one fetus more developed than the other.
Heterakis a genus of nematodes in the family Heterakidae.
H. beramporia found in nodules in the cecal wall of chickens.
H. brevispiculum a parasite of chickens and guinea fowl.
H. dispar found in goose and duck.
H. gallinae* (syn. *H. gallinarum*), *H. vesicularis*, *H. papillosa found in most species of domestic birds and some wild species. A vector for *Histomonas meleagridis*.
H. indica found in chickens.
H. isolonche found in pheasants, quail and other gallinaceous birds. Causes nodular typhlitis, diarrhea, emaciation and death.
H. linganensis found in chicken.
H. meleagris found in turkey.
H. pavonis found in peafowl and pheasant.
H. spumosa found in the cecum of rats.
heterergic having different effects; said of two drugs one of which produces a particular effect and the other does not.
heter(o)- word element. [Gr.] *other, dissimilar.*
heteroagglutination agglutination of particulate antigens of one kind by antibodies derived from a different antigen.
heteroagglutinin an agglutinin (antibody) that is capable of heteroagglutination.
heteroantibody an antibody combining with antigens originating from a species foreign to the antibody producer.
heteroantigen an antigen originating from a species foreign to the antibody producer.
heteroantiserum antiserum produced by injecting antigens into another member of a different species.
Heterobilharzia a genus of blood flukes (digenetic trematodes) in the family Schistosomatidae.
H. americanum occurs in raccoons, bobcats, dogs, other mammals.
heteroblastic originating in a different kind of tissue.
heterocaryon see HETEROKARYON.
heterocellular composed of cells of different kinds.
heterocephalus a monster with two unequal heads.
heterochromatin that state of chromatin in which it is dark-staining, genetically inactive, and tightly coiled.
heterochromia diversity of color in a part normally of one color.
h. iridis difference in color of the iris in the two eyes, or in different areas in the same iris. May occur with extraocular pigmentary defects. See also WALLEYE (3).
heterochromic pertaining to heterochromia.
heterochronia irregularity in time; occurrence at abnormal times.
heterochronic 1. pertaining to or characterized by heterochronia. 2. existing for different periods of time; showing a difference in ages.
heterochthonous originating in an area other than that in which it is found.
heterocyclic having or pertaining to a closed chain or ring formation that includes atoms of different elements.
heterocytotropic having an affinity for cells from different species.
Heterodendrum oleifolium ALECTRYON *oleifolius*.
heterodermic denoting a skin graft from an individual of another species.
heterodont having teeth of different shapes, as molars, incisors, etc.
heterodonty the state of having heterodont teeth.
Heterodoxus a genus of lice in the superfamily Amblycera.
H. longitarsus a louse of kangaroos.
H. macropus found on kangaroos and wallabies.
H. spiniger parasitizes dogs.
heteroduplex DNA see heteroduplex DNA.
heteroecious requiring different hosts in different stages of development; a characteristic of certain parasites.
heterogametic sex the sex which produces gametes containing dissimilar sex chromosomes, i.e. males in all mammalian species.
heterogamety production by an individual of one sex (as the human male) of unlike gametes with respect to the sex chromosomes.
heterogamy the conjugation of gametes differing in size and structure, to form the zygote from which the new organism develops.
heterogeneity the state of being heterogeneous.
heterogeneous not of uniform composition, quality or structure.
heterogenesis 1. alternation of generations; reproduction differing in character in successive generations. 2. asexual generation.
heterogenote a cell that has an additional genetic fragment, different from its intact genotype; usually resulting from transduction.
heterogenous of other origin; not originating in the body.
heterogony heterogenesis.
heterograft a graft of tissue transplanted between individuals of different species; a xenograft.
heterohemagglutination agglutination of erythrocytes by a hemagglutinin (antibody) derived from an individual of a different species.
heterohemagglutinin a hemagglutinin that agglutinates erythrocytes of animals of other species.
heterohemolysin a hemolysin that destroys erythrocytes of animals of other species than that of the animal in which it is formed.
heteroimmunity an immune state induced in an individual by immunization with cells of an animal of another species.
heterokaryon a single binucleate cell formed by fusing one cell with another. Fusion is usually accomplished by using inactivated parainfluenza virus or polyethylene glycol, both of which alter the cell membranes in such a way as to induce fusion.
heterokeratoplasty grafting of corneal tissue taken from an individual of another species.
heterokinesis the differential distribution of the sex chromosomes in the developing gametes of a heterogametic organism.
heterolateral relating to the opposite side; contralateral.
heterologous 1. made up of tissue not normal to the part. 2. derived from an individual of a different species.
heterolysin an antibody that lyses cells of species other than the one in which it is formed.
heterolysis destruction of cells of one species by lysin from another species.
heteromeric sending processes through one of the commissures to the white matter of the opposite side of the spinal cord.
heterometaplasia formation of tissue foreign to the part where it is formed.
heteromorphosis the development, in regeneration, of an organ or structure different from the one that was lost.

heteromorphous of abnormal shape or structure.

heteronomous subject to different laws; in biology, subject to different laws of growth or specialized along different lines.

hetero-osteoplasty osteoplasty with bone taken from an individual of another species.

heteropagus a conjoined twin monster consisting of unequally developed components.

heterophagosome an intracytoplasmic vacuole formed by phagocytosis or pinocytosis, which becomes fused with a lysosome, subjecting its contents to enzymatic digestion.

heterophagy the taking into a cell of exogenous material by phagocytosis or pinocytosis and the digestion of the ingested material after fusion of the newly formed vacuole with a lysosome.

heterophil 1. a finely granular polymorphonuclear leukocyte represented by neutrophils in humans, but characterized in other mammals by granules (lysosomes) that have variable sizes and staining characteristics. 2. heterophilic.

h. antigen see heterogenetic ANTIGEN.

heterophilic 1. having affinity for other antigens or antibodies besides the one for which it is specific, i.e. cross-reactive. 2. staining with a type of stain other than the usual one.

heterophonia any abnormality of the voice.

heterophoria latent strabismus.

heterophthalmia difference in the direction of the axes, or in the color, of the two eyes.

Heterophyes a genus of intestinal flukes (digenetic trematodes) of the family Heterophyidae. Other genera of this family infest birds, e.g. *Cryptocotyle* spp.

H. heterophyes found in the intestine of dogs, cats, foxes and humans. Regarded as having little pathogenicity.

heterophyiasis infection with *Heterophyes* spp. In dogs and cats, generally mild, but occasionally severe hemorrhagic diarrhea may occur.

Heterophyllaea pustulata South American plant in the family Rubiaceae; contains an unidentified toxin which causes photosensitization in cattle and sheep. Called also cegadera.

heteroplasia replacement of normal by abnormal tissues; malposition of normal cells.

heteroplasm heterologous tissue.

heteroplastic pertaining to or emanating from heteroplasia.

heteroplasty plastic repair with tissue derived from an individual of a different species.

heteroploid 1. characterized by heteroploidy. 2. an individual or cell with an abnormal number of chromosomes.

heteroploidy the state of having an abnormal number of chromosomes.

heteropyknosis 1. the quality of showing variations in density throughout. 2. a state of differential condensation observed in different chromosomes, or in different regions of the same chromosome; it may be attenuated (negative heteropyknosis) or accentuated (positive heteropyknosis).

heteroscedasticity an irregular scattering of values in a series of distributions; accompanied by a comparable scatter of variances.

heterosis the existence, in the first generation hybrid, of greater vigor than is shown by either parent.

heterotaxia abnormal position of viscera.

heterotonia a state characterized by variations in tension or tone.

heterotopia displacement or misplacement of parts.

heterotopic pertaining to heterotopia.

heterotransplant tissue taken from one individual and transplanted into one of a different species; a xenograft.

heterotrichosis growth of hairs of different colors on the body.

heterotroph a heterotrophic organism.

heterotrophic unable to synthesize metabolic products from inorganic materials; requiring complex organic substances (growth factors) for nutrition.

heteroxenous requiring more than one host to complete the life cycle.

h. apicomplexan protozoa includes *Besnoitia*, *Frenkelia*, *Hammondia*, *Sarcocystis*, *Toxoplasma*.

heterozygosity the state of having different alleles in regard to a given character.

heterozygote an individual exhibiting heterozygosity. Detection is critical in most programs to control genetic defects; methods used include karyotyping (rarely successful), test mating, blood typing, a full clinical pathology test spectrum, radiology.

heterozygous having different alleles at the one locus.

heuristic encouraging or promoting investigation; conducive to discovery.

Heuter–Volkmann principle within physiological limits, compressive forces stimulate accelerated growth of articular, epiphyseal, and/or physeal cartilage.

HEV hemagglutinating encephalomyelitis virus of pigs.

hex(a)- word element. [Gr.] *six*.

hexacanth embryo the infective stage (larvae, oncosphere) in a cestode egg after fertilization takes place.

hexachlorobenzene a fungistatic agent used in the preservation of stored grain. In very large doses it causes liver damage but its greater importance is as a contaminant of foods of animal origin. The substance is virtually undegradable and its presence in meat is a cause for its condemnation.

hexachlorocyclohexane a compound whose gamma isomer is gammexane or LINDANE.

hexachlorodibenzodioxin one of the suspected causes of CHICKEN edema disease of broiler chickens.

hexachloroethane an anthelmintic used in the treatment of fascioliasis. Poisoning manifested by narcosis, staggering and falling. Fatal cases in cattle have abomasitis and hepatic necrosis.

hexachlorohexahydrophenanthrene one of the possible causes of toxic fat disease of broiler chickens.

hexachloronaphthalene a high pressure lubricant capable of causing hyperkeratosis in cattle.

hexachloroparaxylene a chlorinated derivative of benzene used as a fasciolicide; effective only against adult flukes. Called also chloxyle.

hexachlorophene, hexachlorophane a compound used as a tenicide in poultry, a fasciolicide in cattle, and as a germicidal agent in soaps and dermatological preparations. Causes poisoning in sheep, cattle, cats and puppies at relatively small doses and the low safety margin has limited its use in other species. Signs of toxicity in cattle include nystagmus, tremor, opisthotonos; in sheep the signs are anorexia, diarrhea, recumbency and atrophy of seminiferous tubules. Dogs and cats may die suddenly after large doses, or show cerebellar signs with chronic exposure.

hexad 1. a group or combination of six similar or related entities. 2. an element with a valence of six.

hexadecimal a numbering system used in computer science; consists of 16 digits including numbers 0 through 9 and letters a through f.

hexafluorenium bromide a neuromuscular blocking agent used in anesthesiology to prolong and potentiate the skeletal muscle relaxing action of suxamethonium during surgery.

Hexamastix a genus of flagellated protozoa in the family Monocercomonadidae.

H. caviae, H. robustus found in the cecum of the guinea pig.

H. muris found in the cecum of rats and other rodents.

hexamethonium a ganglion-blocking quaternary ammonium compound.

hexamethylenetetramine methenamine.

hexamethylmelamine see ALTRETAMINE.

hexamine see METHENAMINE.

Hexamita a genus of flagellated protozoa in the family Hexamitidae.

H. columbae occurs in the small intestine of pigeons and may cause enteritis.

H. meleagridis a major parasite of turkeys in which it produces an enteritis, which may cause serious losses with a mortality rate of up to 80%. Can cause disease in other species of birds.

H. muris occurs in the intestines of rodents and causes enteritis.

H. pitheci occurs in the large intestine of rhesus and other monkeys.

H. salmonis found in the intestine of salmonids and may cause acute enteritis or may become systemic and cause death. *Hexamita*-like organisms can be associated with hole-in-the-head disease in aquarium fish, especially DISCUS and OSCAR.

H. truttae found in the intestines of fish; causes enteritis, peritonitis, cholecystitis in debilitated fish.

hexamitiasis an infectious catarrhal enteritis of turkey poults caused by the protozoan HEXAMITA *meleagridis*.

hexamitosis see HEXAMITA *salmonis*.

***N*-hexane** poisoning with the chemical can cause testicular atrophy.

2,5-hexanedione a neurotoxic hydrocarbon thought to be the principal toxin in *N*-hexane poisoning; causes Sertoli cell damage and testicular atrophy.

hexavalent having a valence of six.

hexestrol a derivative of diethylstilbestrol and used as an estrogen.

Hexham scent MELILOTUS *indica*.

hexobarbital sodium an ultra-short-acting barbiturate little used in veterinary anesthesia.

hexobarbitone hexobarbital.

hexocyclium methylsulfate an anticholinergic having antisecretory and antispasmodic activities; used in the management of peptic ulcer and other gastrointestinal disorders accompanied by hyperacidity, hypermotility and spasm.

hexokinase an enzyme that catalyzes the transfer of a high-energy phosphate group of ATP to a hexose sugar, usually D-glucose, producing D-glucose-6-phosphate.

hexosamine a nitrogenous sugar in which an amino group replaces a hydroxyl group.

hexosaminidase an enzyme that catalyzes the cleavage of hexose from ganglioside GM_2. Occurs in two forms, A and B. Deficiency occurs in GM_2 GANGLIOSIDOSIS of dogs, cats and pigs.

hexose a monosaccharide containing six carbon atoms in a molecule.

h. monophosphate shunt metabolic pathway starting from glucose-6-phosphate, and leading to the production of NADPH for reductive syntheses, ribose sugars for nucleic acid synthesis and for the diversification and rearrangement of sugars.

hexosephosphate an ester of hexose sugar with phosphoric acid and an important intermediate in carbohydrate metabolism.

hexylcaine a local anesthetic, used as the hydrochloride salt.

hexylresorcinol a superseded anthelmintic for intestinal roundworms and trematodes.

HF Hageman factor, or clotting factor XII.

Hf chemical symbol, *hafnium*.

HFOC hair-filled otic canals.

Hg chemical symbol, *mercury* (L. *hydrargyrum*).

Hgb hemoglobin.

HGE hemorrhagic gastroenteritis.

hh hands high. See also HAND (1).

HI hemagglutination inhibition.

5-HIAA 5-hydroxyindoleacetic acid.

hiatal pertaining to or emanating from esophageal HIATUS.

h. hernia, hiatus hernia protrusion of a structure, often a portion of the stomach, through the esophageal hiatus of the diaphragm.

hiatus pl. *hiatus* [L.] an aperture, gap, cleft or opening.

aortic h., h. aorticus the opening in the diaphragm through which the aorta and thoracic duct pass.

esophageal h. hernia see HIATAL hernia.

esophageal h., h. esophageus the opening in the diaphragm for the passage of the esophagus and the vagus nerves.

vena caval h. the opening in the diaphragm for the passage of the caudal vena cava; properly called foramen venae cavae.

hibernation the dormant state in which certain animals pass the winter, marked by narcosis and by sharp reduction in body temperature and metabolism.

artificial h. a state of reduced metabolism, muscle relaxation, and a twilight sleep resembling narcosis, produced by controlled inhibition of the sympathetic nervous system and causing attenuation of the homeostatic reactions of the organism. Induced hypothermia has had experimental use as an anesthetic medium for extensive surgical operations in humans.

hibernoma a rare benign subcutaneous tumor made up of large foamy polyhedral cells distended with multiple lipoid-filled vacuoles. A fetal fat cell lipoma.

Hibitane a proprietary name for chlorhexidine.

hiccup, hiccough spasmodic involuntary contraction of the diaphragm that results in uncontrolled breathing in of air; called also singultus. The peculiar noise of hiccups is produced by a beginning inspiration that is suddenly checked by closure of the glottis. Commonly seen in puppies. An unusual occurrence in horses affected by electrolyte imbalances, especially hypocalcemia. The clinical effect is hiccup with each cardiac cycle, often present on only one side of the diaphragm. See also synchronous DIAPHRAGMATIC flutter.

Hickey–Hare test hypertonic saline infusion test that induces plasma hyperosmolality. Used for distinguishing between different causes of polyuria and polydipsia.

Hickman navicular block a specially carved block of wood in which the horse is persuaded to rest its hoof while an x-ray is taken of the navicular bone.

hide raw or dressed skin of cattle, sheep or horse as removed at abattoir.

h. flayer handheld vibrating instrument for separating hide from carcass at the points where a knife would normally be used.

h. puller abattoir implement for pulling hides from carcasses at places where the hide pulls easily.

hidebound said of skin that is not easily lifted from the subcutaneous tissue. Occurs in emaciated animals because of the absence of fat and connective tissue rather than absence of fluid.
hidradenitis inflammation of the sweat glands.
hidradenocarcinoma carcinoma of the sweat gland.
hidradenoid resembling a sweat gland; having components resembling elements of a sweat gland.
hidradenoma a general term for tumors of the skin, the components of which resemble epithelial elements of sweat glands; they may be nodular (solid) or papillary.
hidr(o)- word element. [Gr.] *sweat*.
hidrocystoma a retention cyst of a sweat gland.
hidropoiesis the formation of sweat.
hidrorrhea profuse perspiration.
hidroschesis suppression of perspiration. Called also anhidrosis.
hidrosis sweating.
hidrotic pertaining to, characterized by, or causing sweating.
hieralgia pain in the sacrum.
hierarchy order of superiority; the arrangement of echelons of command.
court h. the way in which the courts in a country are arranged so that appeals can be carried from the lower to the higher courts.
hierolisthesis displacement of the sacrum.
high at a level higher than normal or optimal. Most such entries will be found under the noun that is qualified, e.g. blood pressure.
h. endothelial venule (HEV) specialized areas of vascular endothelium found in lymphoid organs, which express a variety of cell-adhesion molecules and are involved in lymphocyte extravasation.
h. kVp technique radiographic technique using upwards of 100 kVp for diagnostic examination.
h. radiation area areas of a building or yards where there is some risk of radiation injury to attendants. It should be labeled as a warning.
h. tension transformer an essential component of a radiography unit; produces current of sufficiently high voltage that x-rays can be produced, i.e. 40 kV and up.
h. voltage circuits the high voltage required by an x-ray tube is generated by a step-up transformer. By appropriate electrical circuitry the voltage can be increased from 110 to 220 volts up to 40 to 150 kV.
high-level language see COMPUTER language.
high-rise syndrome a variety of injuries, including traumatic cleft palate, hyperextension injuries, vertebral compression fractures and traumatic pancreatitis seen in dogs and cats falling from heights, particularly high-rise apartment buildings.
high-tailing a horse at a fast gallop with the tail held up straight.
Highland named after the Scottish highlands.
H. cattle red-brown, brindle, dun or black, long-haired beef cattle with long spreading horns; called also West Highland.
H. collie see BEARDED COLLIE.
H. garron see GARRON.
H. pony gray, dun, black or brown heavyweight pony with dorsal stripe, stands 12.3 to 14.2 hands high.
Highlands J virus an alphavirus that causes encephalitis in horses in North and South America.
hiking gait patellar luxation when the patella catches but does not lock. Seen in Standard-bred horses.
hilar echo an echogenic streak seen in the middle of the canine prostate gland, presumed to be periurethral fibrous tissue.
Hilaria grass genus in the family Poaceae; may be infested with CLAVICEPS *cinerea* which causes poisoning. Includes *H. jamesii* (galleta grass), *H mutica* (tobo grass). See also PASPALUM STAGGERS.
hilitis inflammation of a hilus.
hill sickness see COBALT nutritional deficiency.
hillock a small prominence or elevation.
hilum hilus.
hilus pl. *hili* [L.] a depression or pit on an organ, giving entrance and exit to vessels and nerves, e.g. the hilus of the kidney, lung, ovary, spleen.
HIM hematopoietic inductive environment.
Himalayan 1. a longhaired breed of cats with the short stature of the Persian and a temperature-dependent pigmentation pattern like the Siamese. Called also Colorpoint longhair. 2. a breed of white rabbits with pink eyes and black or blue points.
hind 1. emanating from or pertaining to HINDLIMB. 2. adult female deer, especially red and other large species.
blue h. a hind which has not borne young.
hindbrain the rhombencephalon, the portion of the brain developed from the most caudal of the three primary brain vesicles of the early embryo, comprising the metencephalon (cerebellum and pons) and myelencephalon (medulla).
hindgut the caudal portion of the embryonic gut which develops into the colon and the rectum.
hindlimb the pelvic limb; back leg.
hindquarter the rump and legs, i.e. the loin, pelvis, pelvic limb and associated musculature.
asymmetric h. see ASYMMETRIC HIND QUARTER SYNDROME.
hinge see hinge JOINT.
craniofacial h. flexible connection between the skull bones in many birds and reptiles which permit the upper jaw to be raised at the same time as the mandible is depressed; well developed between the nasal and frontal bones in psittacine birds.
hinge region a proline-rich portion of an immunoglobulin heavy chain between the Fc and Fab regions that confers mobility on the two Fab arms of the antibody molecule thereby allowing it to combine better with the two epitopes.
hinny progeny of a stallion and a jenny (female donkey), being more horselike in appearance than a mule.
horse h. a male hinny.
mare h. a female hinny, called also a molly.
hip 1. the region of the body around the articulation of the femur and the pelvis. 2. loosely, the hip joint.
h. bone os coxae, which comprises the ilium, ischium and pubis. See also Table 10.
h. dislocation manifested by inability to bear full weight on the limb, excessive mobility of the limb, crepitus at the joint, and in some cases shortening of the limb.
h. dysplasia (HD) is manifested (1) radiographically by a shallow acetabulum, a small, misshapen femoral head and sometimes osteophyes, and (2) clinically, by a lax joint, weak rump muscles with or without lameness. In dogs inheritance has a degree of influence on the occurrence of the disease. See also degenerative JOINT disease.
h. flexion posture posterior presentation of a fetus in the birth canal with the hocks flexed.
h. joint the ball-and-socket joint formed between the head of the femur and the acetabulum of the pelvis.
h. laxity subluxation of the coxofemoral articulation, a feature of hip dysplasia (above).
h. sling a metal clamplike device used to lift a

downner cow. Comprises two loops which fit over both iliac tuberosities (coxal tubers) and which are clamped together so that the cow is closely held. The sling is lifted with a block and tackle or by a frontend loader or hoist on a tractor.

total h. replacement replacement of the femoral head and acetabulum with prostheses that are cemented into the bone; called also total hip arthroplasty.

hiplock the point in a dystocia at which the front half of the calf's body has been delivered but further progress is prevented by the stifle joints of the fetus being stuck at the brim of the pelvis; the fetus is jammed at the hips.

Hippeastrum see AMARYLLIS.

hippo-harness stocks made from ropes for restraint of horses.

Hippobosca a genus of flies that cause fly worry for horses and cattle. Members of the family Hippoboscidae.

H. camelina attacks camels and horses.

H. capensis attacks dogs.

H. equina, H. maculata, H. rufipes attack cattle and horses usually; transmit *Trypanosoma theileri* to cattle and *Haemoproteus* spp. to birds. Called also horse louse fly.

hippoboscid fly see HIPPOBOSCA, LIPOPTENA, PSEUDOLYNCHIA, MELOPHAGUS.

Hippocampus see SEA horse.

hippocampus pl. *hippocampi* [L.] in evolutionary terms, an old part of the cerebral cortex that forms part of the floor of the lateral ventricle; identified by its white surface and convoluted appearance on section. It is examined for Negri bodies in suspected cases of rabies.

h. major hippocampus.

h. minor the lower of two medial elevations in the lateral cerebral ventricle.

hippoid horselike.

hippolasso a set of gear for a kicking horse. A breastplate is connected directly with a breeching, both being supported by straps over the back. When the horse kicks, the breeching pulls the breastplate back hard onto the chest.

hippomanes small (up to 1.5 inch thick and 8 inches diameter), circular, flat, smooth bodies found in the allantoic fluids especially in mares and cows. Called foal's bread or foal's tongue. On cut section they are semisolid, homogeneous, amber-colored.

hippophagy eating horsemeat.

hippopotamus the large piglike mammal in the family Hippopotamidae. There are two genera and two species *Hippopotamus amphibius*, the great African hippopotamus, and the pygmy hippopotamus (*Choeropsis liberiensis*).

Hippotragus equinus roan antelope.

hippulin a natural estrogen found in mare's urine.

hippurate hydrolysis a biochemical reaction used to identify bacteria. Particularly used for differentiation of streptococci causing bovine mastitis.

hippuria an excess of hippuric acid in urine.

hippuric acid a compound formed by conjugation of benzoic acid and glycine; it occurs in the urine of herbivorous animals, rarely in human urine.

h. acid test has been tested as a means of assessing hepatic efficiency but is not favored.

hippus abnormal exaggeration of the rhythmic contraction and dilatation of the pupil, independent of changes in illumination or in fixation of the eyes.

hiranolike body elongated eosinophilic cytoplasmic inclusion bodies in neurons; no apparent significance.

Hirschsprung's disease congenital absence of the parasympathetic nerve ganglia in the anorectum or proximal rectum, resulting in the absence of peristalsis in the affected portion of the colon and a consequent massive enlargement of the colon, constipation and obstruction. A disease of humans without a definite equivalent in domestic animals. See also MEGACOLON.

hirsute shaggy; hairy.

hirsutism, hirsuties abnormal hairiness. Seen in aged horses with functional pituitary neoplasms and hyperadrenocorticism.

hirudin the active principle of the buccal secretion of leeches; it prevents clotting of the blood.

hirudiniasis infestation by leeches.

Hirudo a genus of leeches in the class Hirudinea.

H. medicinalis up to 5 inches long and 1 inch diameter, this greenish leech may attach to animals. Used medicinally.

His histidine.

His–Purkinje system specialized conduction tissue in the AV node.

His's bundle see BUNDLE of His.

Hissar sheep prolific, brown, Russian fat-rumped, meat and carpetwool sheep.

histaminase an enzyme that inactivates histamine.

histamine an amine, $C_5H_9N_3$, produced by decarboxylation of histidine, found in all body tissues.

It induces capillary dilatation, which increases capillary permeability and lowers blood pressure; contraction of most smooth muscle tissue; increased gastric acid secretion; and acceleration of the heart rate. It is also a mediator of immediate hypersensitivity. There are two types of cellular receptors of histamine: H_1-receptors, which mediate contraction of smooth muscle and capillary dilatation; and H_2-receptors, which mediate acceleration of heart rate and promotion of gastric acid secretion. Both H_1- and H_2-receptors mediate the contraction of vascular smooth muscle. Histamine may also be a neurotransmitter in the central nervous system. It is used as a diagnostic aid in testing gastric secretion and in the diagnosis of pheochromocytoma.

There are two types of histamine antagonists that act at either the H_1- or the H_2-receptors. Drugs such as diphenhydramine and chlorpheniramine are referred to as ANTIHISTAMINES or H_1-blockers; they block the effects of histamine on vascular, bronchial and gastrointestinal smooth muscle and on capillary permeability. They are used for relief of allergic and gastrointestinal disorders. Drugs such as cimetidine (Tagamet) are referred to as H_2-blockers; they block the stimulation of gastric acid secretion and are used to treat gastrointestinal ulceration.

h.-containing foods some food sources, particularly some species of fish, have high levels of histamine; increased levels can also occur from improper storage which permits conversion of histidine to histamine, and an excessive carbohydrate content may promote bacterial growth, fermentation and production of histamine.

h.-releasing foods some foods can cause release of histamine from mast cells; these include egg white, shellfish and fish.

h. shock manipulation and particularly surgical trauma to large mast cell tumors may lead to decreased blood pressure and persistant bleeding caused by the release of histamine and vasoactive amines.

histaminemia histamine in the blood.

histaminergic pertaining to the effects of histamine at histamine receptors of target tissues.

histidase an enzyme of the liver that converts histidine to urocanic acid.

histidine His; a naturally occurring amino acid, essential for optimal growth of the young; its decarboxylation results in formation of histamine.

Histiocephalus spiruroid worms found in the gizzard of free-living birds; rarely pathogenic.

histiocyte a large phagocytic interstitial cell of the reticuloendothelial system; a macrophage.

histiocytic pertaining to histiocytes.

h. leukemia see malignant HISTIOCYTOSIS.

h. lymphocyte prolymphocyte.

h. lymphoma is not a tumor of the macrophage system but has large lymphoid cells with cytoplasmic vacuoles and does resemble a macrophage tumor.

h. ulcerative colitis see histiocytic ulcerative COLITIS.

histiocytoma a tumor containing histiocytes.

atypical h. Merkel cell tumor.

benign cutaneous h. multiple, dermal histiocytic nodules in young dogs; no clinical significance, eventually disappear.

transmissible h. canine transmissible venereal tumor.

histiocytosis a condition marked by the abnormal appearance of histiocytes in the blood.

cutaneous h. a benign proliferative disease in dogs, particularly Collies and Shetland sheepdogs. there are multiple plaques or nodules in the skin or subcutaneous tissue. The cause is unknown.

lipid h. Niemann–Pick disease.

malignant h. a systemic, progressive invasive proliferation of neoplastic histiocytes. Recognized as a familial disorder in Bernese mountain dogs with clinical signs of respiratory disease, involvement of the central nervous system, and anemia.

systemic h. a proliferative disorder of histiocytes with infiltrates in the skin and lymph nodes. Occurs in young Bernese mountain dogs.

histiogenic formed by the tissues.

histioid histoid.

hist(io)(o)- word element. [Gr.] *tissue*.

histoblast a tissue-forming cell.

histochemistry that branch of histology that deals with the identification of chemical components in cells and tissues.

histoclinical combining histological and clinical evaluation.

histocompatibility the quality of a cellular or tissue graft enabling it to be accepted and functional when transplanted to another animal.

h. antigen genetically determined antigens present on the cell membranes of nucleated cells of most tissues, which incite rejection when tissues are grafted to a different individual and thus determine the compatibility of tissues in transplantation. *Major* histocompatibility antigens exert the strongest effect on transplanted tissues, while the many *minor* histocompatibility antigens, such as blood group substances and the secretory alloantigen system, have a weaker, though often highly significant role in graft rejection.

h. genes genes that code for the histocompatibility antigens.

major h. complex (MHC) a cluster of loci on one autosomal chromosome containing the genes that code for the major histocompatibility antigens. The best studied MHC is the H_2 complex of the mouse followed by the HLA (*h*uman *l*eukocyte *a*ntigen) of humans. In other species it is further specified: the *d*og *l*eukocyte *a*ntigen (DLA), the *bo*vine *l*eukocyte *a*ntigen (BOLA), the *s*wine *l*eukocyte *a*ntigen (SLA), etc.

MHC class I is a polymorphic set of transmembrane heterodimeric proteins consisting of an α chain, encoded within the MHC gene complex, associated noncovalently with β_2-microglobulin expressed on nearly all nucleated cells and which form a trimeric complex with typically 9-mer peptides that are then transported and presented on the surface of the cells and serve as targets for cytotoxic T lymphocytes (CTL or Tc), CD8 cells. A major defense mechanism against viral infections.

MHC class II is a polymorphic set of transmembrane heterodimeric proteins that consist of noncovalently associated α and β proteins, both encoded within the MHC gene complex. They form a trimeric complex with antigenic peptides, which may be up to 35-mers, in antigen presenting cells which are then transported to the surface of the cell for presentation to T helper lymphocytes. The basis for all T lymphocyte responses.

histodialysis disintegration or breaking down of tissue.

histodifferentiation the acquisition of tissue characteristics by cell groups during development.

histogenesis differentiation of cells into the specialized tissues forming the various organs and parts of the body.

histogram a graph in which values found in a statistical study are represented by lines or symbols placed horizontally or vertically, to indicate frequency distribution.

histoid 1. developed from one kind of tissue. 2. resembling one of the tissues of the body.

histoincompatibility the quality of a cellular or tissue graft preventing its acceptance or functioning when transplanted to another animal; said of the relationship between the genotypes (histocompatibility genes) of donor and recipient in which a graft generally will be rejected because of allogeneic differences in the major histocompatibility antigens.

histokinesis movement in the tissues of the body.

histological technician a person trained in tissue processing technique (fixation, dehydration, embedding, sectioning, routine and special staining, and mounting of tissue specimens), and also in histology and histochemistry.

histologist one who specializes in histology.

histology that department of anatomy dealing with the minute structure, composition and function of tissues.

pathological h. the science of diseased tissues.

histolysis breaking down of tissues.

histoma any tissue tumor.

histomonad a member of the genus *Histomonas*.

Histomonas a genus of ameboid, single flagellate protozoa in the family Monocercomonadidae.

H. meleagridis found in many species of birds but important only in turkeys as cause of HISTOMONIASIS. Transmitted by the nematode *Heterakis gallinarum*. Chickens are resistant carriers.

H. wenrichi see PARAHISTOMONAS *wenrichi*.

histomoniasis a very widespread disease of gallinaceous birds, especially turkeys, caused by the protozoan parasite *Histomonas meleagridis*. It is characterized by ulceration of the cecal mucosa and necrotic foci in the liver.

histone a simple protein, soluble in water and insoluble in dilute ammonia, found combined as salts with acidic substances, such as in DNA where they have a structural and functional role.

h. acetylase, h. deacylase enzymes responsible for the reversible acylation of four lysine residues near the *N*-terminus of histone H_4.

histonuria histone in the urine.
histopathology pathological histology.
Histophilus ovis one of the causes of epididymitis in rams. Now classified as *Haemophilus somnus*.
histophysiology the correlation of function with the microscopic structures of cells and tissues.
Histoplasma a genus of fungi belonging to the phylum Ascomycota.
H. capsulatum a species of pathogenic fungi that cause HISTOPLASMOSIS. The fungi appear in tissues as small, single oval bodies.
H. farciminosum a similar fungus to *H. capsulatum*. Causes EPIZOOTIC lymphangitis of horses.
histoplasmin a preparation of growth products of *Histoplasma capsulatum*, injected intracutaneously as a test for histoplasmosis.
histoplasmoma a rounded granulomatous density of the lung in humans due to infection with *Histoplasma capsulatum*; seen radiographically as a coin-shaped lesion.
histoplasmosis a disease caused by inhalation of *Histoplasma capsulatum* carried on dust with a primary infection in the lung. Spread to other tissues results in the development of granulomatous enteritis, colitis, osteomyelitis and endophthalmitis. The syndrome includes heptomegaly, lymphadenopathy, anasarca and emaciation. It is particularly common in certain geographical regions, e.g. the Mississippi river system of the USA.
historical controls use of historical information as a comparison group in a study; that is a before and after comparison.
historrhexis the breaking up of tissue.
history in a clinical examination, the collection of facts about the clinical signs of the patient, its environment including feeding, vaccination status, exposure to infection, recorded and arranged in chronological order and in relation to each other.
histotechnologist a laboratory technologist that specializes in the preparation of tissue specimens.
histothrombin thrombin derived from connective tissue.
histotome a cutting instrument used in microtomy; microtome.
histotomy dissection of tissues; microtomy.
histotopy the relationship of the layers, tissues or coats of an organ to each other.
histotoxic poisonous to tissue.
h. hypoxia lower than normal oxygen content of tissue resulting from toxic effects on oxygen-binding enzyme systems.
histotrophe the sum total of nutritive material derived from maternal tissue other than the blood, utilized by the early embryo. A milky fluid containing the secretions and debris of the endometrial glands plus extravasated maternal blood. Called also uterine milk.
histotrophic 1. encouraging formation of tissue. 2. pertaining to histotrophe.
histotropic having affinity for tissue cells.
hitch to fasten by a knot, usually used to describe tying a horse to a post.
hitch up to harness a horse to a vehicle or implement.
Hitching gag a gag shaped like an F. The horizontal bars can be moved apart or together by a screwthread in the column of the F; they consist of hollowed-out plates, into which the incisor teeth fit.
hitching gait see HIKING GAIT.
Hitching hobble a hobble used for casting horses. It consists of leather straps with quick-release catches that fit around the pastern. The casting rope passes through a ring on each of the four hobbles and is fastened to the last one. Pulling the rope brings all four feet together and the horse falls.
Hitra disease hemorrhagic disease of Atlantic salmon caused by *Vibrio salmonicida*.
HIV-like viruses lentiviruses that cause disease resembling that caused by human immunodeficiency virus. Included are FELINE immunodeficiency virus, BOVINE immunodeficiency virus and EQUINE infectious anemia virus.
hive a well-defined, elevated, edematous skin lesion associated with an acute hypersensitivity reaction. Called also wheal. See also URTICARIA.
HJ bodies Howell–Jolly bodies.
Hjärre's disease see COLIGRANULOMA.
HLA (*h*uman *l*eukocyte *a*ntigen) the human major histocompatibility complex of antigens.
HMM heavy meromyosin.
HMWK high-molecular-weight KININOGEN.
hnRNA heterogeneous RNA (RIBONUCLEIC ACID).
Ho chemical symbol, *holmium*.
HOA see hypertrophic OSTEOPATHY.
Hoareosporidium a genus of coccidia in the family Eimiriidae.
H. pellerdyi found in the tissues of dogs; causes mild inflammation.
hoarseness a rough quality of the voice.
hoary alyssum see BERTEROA INCANA.
hob a male ferret.
hobble leather straps fastened around the pasterns of horses, mules and donkeys. Placed on all four legs and pulled together by a rope, it provides an effective means of casting the horse. Putting them on the two fore pasterns and fastening them by a short chain restricts the horse's movements so that it cannot run away but can still graze. Called also hopple.
breeding h's leather strap hobbles to tie the front feet together; used chiefly in mares to prevent escape from stallion.
crossed h. a rope is used to tie the forearm of the upper limb of a cast horse to the hindlimb above the hock. The hobbles on the pasterns can then be released and surgical work performed on the hoof.
hobby farm a small acreage of land used by a city dweller for weekend or summer relaxation.
h. f. malnutrition underfeeding of livestock because of owner's ignorance of animal's needs which a small hobby farm often cannot provide.
Hobday forceps obstetrical forceps for use in dogs and cats. Scissor-type forceps without ratchets, with slightly incurving loops instead of blades, to grasp a fetal head.
hock the ankle joint of quadripeds; the tarsus.
broken h. fracture of the central tarsal bone in racing Greyhounds.
capped h. see hock HYGROMA.
cow h. one that turns inward from an imaginary vertical line drawn from the tuber ischii to the hindfeet.
dropped h. walking with the hocks close to the ground. Seen in dogs and cats with muscle weakness, injury to the gastrocnemius tendon, and poor conformation.
h. flexion posture in a dystocia caused by a breech presentation with the flexed hocks being the first structures presented into the cervix, and the distal extremities of the hindlimbs retained.
h. flexion test see SPAVIN test.
point of h. the summit of the calcaneus.
sickle h. a more acute angulation of the hock joint than is normal for the species or breed. Instead of the

metatarsals being approximately vertical in a standing position, there is a greater slope.

straight h. a greater angle between the tibia and metatarsal bones at the hock joint; the opposite of sickle hock. A feature of some dog breeds, e.g. Chow Chows.

turkey h. enlargement hock enlargement with bowed legs appears in young turkey poults on diets low in vitamin E.

Hodgkin's disease a primary lymph node neoplastic disease of humans. Rarely in animals, mainly dogs, do lymphoid neoplasms satisfy the criteria, e.g. Reed–Sternberg cells, for diagnosis as Hodgkin's lymphoma.

hodoneuromere a segment of the embryonic trunk with its pair of nerves and their branches.

Hoeppli's reaction see SPLENDORE–HOEPPLI MATERIAL.

Hoffa procedure a technique for shortening of tendons in which a suture is placed across the tendon then stitched in and out lengthwise for a distance, then pulled up and tied. It results in a gathering and shortening of that portion of the tendon.

Hoflund syndrome see VAGUS indigestion.

hog[1] see also SWINE, PIG.

h. badger see hog BADGER.

h. cholera a highly infectious disease of pigs caused by a pestivirus and characterized in its classical form by high fever, lassitude, purple discoloration of abdominal skin, conjunctivitis and nervous signs including circling, incoordination, tremor and convulsions. Most affected pigs die at 5 to 7 days with a characteristic petechiation under the kidney capsule—turkey egg kidney. There is a second form, characterized by nervous signs and caused by a strain of virus of lower virulence. Other syndromes caused by low virulence strains are reproductive inefficiency and congenital defects including myotonia congenita. Called also swine fever.

h. holder a flexible wire cable is welded to one end of a strong steel tube, looped on itself and passed up the tube. At its emergence a crossbar handle is fixed. The loop is passed over the hog's upper snout and the cable is pulled tight. The person pulling on the holder pulls one way, the hog pulls the other and complete restraint is achieved, that is provided the hog does not decide to rush forwards.

pygmy h. SUS *salvanius.*

h.-tied all four feet are tied together so that the animal is unable to rise.

wart h. see WART HOG.

hog[2] to remove all of the hair in a mane of a horse.

hog deer short-legged (height up to 2 ft) Indian deer. Called also *Axis porcinus.*

hogg castrated male sheep usually 10 to 14 months old. Also used to describe an uncastrated male pig.

hogged mane a horse's mane from which all of the hair has been removed.

hogget hogg.

hogging clipping the mane.

Hogness box see Pribnow BOX.

hogweed see ZALEYA GALERICULATA.

hogwort CROTON *capitatus, C. texensis.*

Hohmann retractor a handheld surgical instrument designed for retracting tissues to expose bones during orthopedic surgery.

Hohorstiella lata a pigeon louse.

holandric inherited exclusively through the male descent; transmitted through genes located on the Y chromosome in mammals.

Holarctic a distribution including North America, Europe and northern Asia.

Holcus lanatus a grass in the plant family Poaceaeae. A common pasture grass of mediocre value which may contain cyanogenic glycosides. Selectively poor absorption of iodine and may predispose to goiter. Called also Yorkshire fog.

holding pen a pen, paddock or yard for holding a group of sheep or cattle temporarily, e.g. before slaughter, after shearing. A pen to which animals are added one by one until a group of sufficient size is accumulated.

holistic medicine an alternative approach to health care and prevention of disease which integrates the body as a whole, including mind and spirit, rather than separate systems. Includes homeopathy, naturopathy, hypnosis, iridology and psychic healing.

hollow 1. a depression. 2. contains a cavity.

h. back backbone has a downward curvature in the center.

h. horn a mythical disease of cattle in primitive communities; treated by removal of the horns.

h. wall SEEDY TOE.

holly see ILEX.

holmium a chemical element, atomic number 67, atomic weight 164.930, symbol Ho. See Table 6.

hol(o)- word element. [Gr.] *entire, whole.*

holoacardius an unequal twin fetus in which the heart is entirely absent.

holoblastic undergoing cleavage in which the entire ovum participates; completely dividing.

Holocalyx glaziovii South American tree in the legume family Fabaceae; contains an unidentified toxin in the regrowth from the stumps of this tree causing hepatic insufficiency and photosensitization. Called also alecrim.

holocrine wholly secretory; that type of glandular secretion in which the entire cell forms the secreted matter of the gland, as in the sebaceous glands; cf. apocrine and merocrine.

holodiastolic pertaining to the entire diastole.

holoendemic affecting practically all the animals of a particular region.

holoenzyme an enzyme which contains several different subunits and retains some activity even when one or more of the subunits is missing.

hologynic inherited exclusively through the female descent; transmitted through genes located on attached X chromosomes in mammals.

Holomenopon bird lice of the superfamily Amblycera.

H. leucoxanthum parasitizes ducks causing soiling and loss of waterproofing of feathers. Ducks may become chilled and die of pneumonia.

holometabolous characteristic of insects in the Diptera family consisting of egg, up to three larval stages, pupa and an adult stage which differs markedly from the earlier stages.

holomyarian arrangement of the somatic musculature in a group of trematodes, including *Trichuris* spp., which have their body cavity completely surrounded by longitudinal muscle cells.

holophytic one of the three forms of nutrition in Mastigophora protozoa. It comprises the synthesis of simple carbohydrates from carbon dioxide and water by chlorophyll contained in chloroplasts.

holoprosencephaly developmental failure of cleavage of the prosencephalon with a deficit in midline facial development and with cyclopia in the severe form.

holoprotein a complete protein with its prosthetic group.

holoptic said of eyes which are very close together as in some insects.

holorachischisis fissure of the entire vertebral column with prolapse of the spinal cord.
holosystolic pertaining to the entire systole.
h. murmur a heart murmur occurring throughout systole. Called also pansystolic.
holotopy relationship between an organ and the body as a whole.
holozoic one of the forms of nutrition of the Mastigophoran protozoa—comprising the capture and assimilation of organic materials in the environment.
Holstein German heavyweight riding and dressage horse. Initially a carriage horse. Bay, black or brown, 15.3 to 16.2 hands high. Called also Holsteiner, Warmblut, Warmblood.
Holstein–Friesian a breed of black-and-white dairy cattle bred in Canada and the USA from Friesian cattle from the Netherlands. A red-and-white variety is available. Called also Holstein, Friesian.
Holstein udder plague MASTITIS caused by *Corynebacterium pyogenes.*
holsteiner see HOLSTEIN.
Holter monitoring use of a portable electrocardiograph recording device (Holter harness); attached to the patient to obtain a 24 hour record of cardiac rhythm.
Holtz–Celsus procedure a surgical procedure for correction of congenital entropion involving clamping and excising an elliptical piece of skin from the lid margin.
Homalopsinae a subfamily of poisonous snakes which have poison fangs at the back of the mouth and are unlikely to be a serious threat to animals.
homaluria production and excretion of urine at a normal, even rate.
Homarus farmed lobsters in the family Nephropsidae; includes *Homarus vulgaris* (European lobster), *H. americanus* (American lobster). See Table 23.
homatropine an anticholinergic alkaloid obtained by the condensation of tropine and mandelic acid having anticholinergic effects similar to but weaker than those of atropine; used to produce parasympathetic blockade and as a mydriatic. The hydrobromide salt is used topically in ophthalmic drops and the methylbromide derivative is used orally for intestinal spasms.
homeo- word element. [Gr.] *similar, same, unchanging.*
homeokinesis achievement of equilibrium in body functions by dynamic processes.
homeomorphous of like form and structure.
homeopathy a system of therapeutics founded by Samuel Hahnemann (1755–1843) in which diseases are treated by drugs that are capable of producing in healthy animals signs like those of the disease to be treated, the drug being administered in minute doses.
homeoplasia formation of new tissue like that normal to the part.
homeostasis a tendency of biological systems to maintain stability while continually adjusting to conditions that are optimal for survival.

Homeostatic mechanisms are necessary for the body to regain its balance when disease or injury occurs and to maintain that balance if it is to remain healthy.

homeostatic pertaining to homeostasis.
homeotherapy treatment with a substance similar to the causative agent of the disease. See also HOMEOPATHY.
homeothermal homoiothermic.
homeothermism having the characteristic of being homeothermic or warm-blooded.
homergic having the same effect; said of two drugs each of which produces the same overt effect.
Homeria a South African plant genus of the family Iridaceae; contains bufadienolide cardiac glycosides which cause diarrhea, dysentery, tympany, stiff gait and sudden death. Includes *H. flaccida* (*H. aurantica, H. breynia, H. collina*), *H. glauca* (*H. natalensis*), *H. miniata, H. mossii, H. ochroleuca* (*H. lucasi*), *H. pallida, H. pura.* Called also native tulip, Cape tulip, Natal yellow tulp.
homidium 1. a trypanocide; used as the bromide or chloride salt. May cause transient hepatic insufficiency. Called also ethidium. 2. a dye much used for the staining of DNA fragments after electrophoretic separation in agarose gels. The molecule intercalates across the double helix and is detected by UV illumination.
homing the differential migration of lymphocyte subsets across venules and into lymphoid tissues. Called also trafficking.
homing pigeon see homing PIGEON.
hominy a by-product of the milling of maize; contains bran, germ and fragments of starchy material.
Homo the genus of primates containing the single living species *H. sapiens* (humans).
homo- 1. word element. [Gr.] *same, similar.* 2. chemical prefix indicating addition of one CH_2 group to the main compound.
homobiotics a factor affecting growth in biological systems which is normally present in those systems.
homocysteine key intermediate in the pathway of conversion of methionine to propionyl CoA.
homocystine a homolog of cystine which results from demethylation of methionine.
homocytotropic having an affinity for cells of animals of the same species.
homodimer a protein composed of two identical polypeptide chains.
homodont having all teeth of the same form, e.g. dolphin.
homodynamical structures structures found in a craniocaudal succession of similar segments of the body, e.g. the ribs, the vertebrae.
homogametic the sex which produces only one kind of sex chromosome, i.e. females in all mammals.
homogenate material obtained by homogenization.
homogeneity the state of being homogeneous.
homogeneous of uniform quality, composition or structure.
homogenesis reproduction by the same process in each generation.
homogenic homozygous.
homogenicity homogeneity.
homogenize to convert into material that is of uniform quality or consistency throughout; to render homogeneous.
homograft allograft.
homoiotherm an animal that exhibits homoiothermy; a so-called warm-blooded animal.
homoiothermy maintenance of a constant body temperature despite variation in environmental temperature.
homolateral ipsilateral; pertaining to or situated on the same side.
Homologaster a genus of paramphistomes found in ruminant large intestines in Asia.
homologous 1. corresponding in structure, position, origin, etc. 2. derived from an animal of the same species but of different genotype; allogeneic.

homologue 1. any homologous organ or part; that is, structures with a common evolutionary origin but not necessarily with a similar function. 2. in chemistry, one of a series of compounds distinguished by addition of a CH_2 group in successive members.

homology the state of being homologous. Refers also to homology of base sequences in different DNA molecules and the similarity between antigen and specific antibody.

serial h. craniocaudal succession of similar or homologous segments. See also METAMERE.

homolysin a lysin produced by injection into the body of an antigen derived from an animal of the same species.

homonomous subject to the same laws; in biology, subject to the same laws of growth or developed along the same line.

homonymous 1. having the same or corresponding sound or name. 2. standing in the same relation.

homophilic reacting only with specific antigen.

homoplastic 1. pertaining to homoplasty. 2. denoting organs or parts, as the wings of birds and insects, that resemble one another in structure and function but not in origin or development.

homoplasty 1. operative replacement of lost parts or tissues by similar parts from another individual of the same species. 2. similarity between organs or their parts not due to common ancestry.

homopolymeric tailing see TAILING (2).

homorganic produced by the same or by homologous organs.

homoscedasticity characterized by variances which do not differ greatly between distributions.

homosulfanilamide see MAFENIDE.

homotherm homoiotherm.

homotopic occurring at the same place upon the body.

homotype a part having reversed symmetry with its mate, as for example the paw.

homozygosis the formation of a zygote by the union of gametes that have one or more identical alleles.

homozygosity the state of having identical alleles in regard to a given character or characters.

homozygote an animal exhibiting homozygosity.

homozygous having the characteristic of homozygosity.

honda a quick release metal eyelet for the end of a lariat. When the restrained animal is no longer required it is not necessary to slacken off the loop and pull it over the head—a very great advantage when working with wild cattle or unbroken horses.

honey bear see KINKAJOU; called also *Potos flavus*.

honey bee called also *Apis mellifera*. See also BEE STING.

honey flower see LAMBERTIA *formosa*, MELIANTHUS.

honeycomb a mosaic of closely packed units with depressed centers giving a honeycomb appearance.

h. ringworm see FAVUS.

h. stomach reticulum.

honeysuckle see LAMBERTIA *formosa*.

honker syndrome disease of feedlot cattle caused by edema of the tracheal mucosa. Characterized by a loud sound like a goose honking at each inspiration.

hood an item of horse clothing. A cloth cover for the head; with eye and ear holes.

long h. covers the head and neck to the shoulders.

hooding controlling ratite birds with darkness by covering the head with a hood which covers the head and the cranial half of the neck without occluding the nostrils.

hoof the horny covering of the digit of ungulates. Consists of a wall, a sole and in the horse reflections of the wall which enclose a triangular frog. The hoof is attached to the underlying soft tissues by lamellae which interdigitate with similar lamellae in the soft tissues. The wall is composed of many minute horn tubes united by intertubular horn produced by a germinative layer at the coronary band where the skin and horn join. A thin, narrow band of soft, very light-colored horn called periople forms a flexible union between wall and skin. The wall is that part of the hoof extending from the coronet to the sole. It grows from the coronet and in horses takes about 1 year to reach the sole at the toe and some months fewer at the heel. The wall and the sole join at a visible band called the white line though this is often yellowish. These various parts of the hoof are described in more detail under their individual headings. See also CLEAT.

h. abscess results usually from a nailprick of the sole or from a cracked sole. The cavity of the abscess cannot be large because of the rigid nature of the tissues. Spread from the original site is via the potential space between the sensitive laminae and the hoof and eventually surfaces at the coronet with pus discharging from a sinus there. Causes severe lameness, and tetanus is a common accompaniment.

h. avulsion in cattle and horses the hoof it is usually the result of trauma and carries a very poor prognosis.

h. block see DIGITAL nerve block.

h. congenital absence with all four limbs affected, recorded in calves.

h. cutters pincer-like instruments with one blade sharp and chisel-pointed, the other square and acting as a block for the other to cut against. The good implements have a double-scissor action and detachable blades.

h. erosion occurs in association with interdigital dermatitis in cattle and contributes to lameness.

h. lameness lameness due to pain in the hoof; detected by tapping with a hammer or pinching with a hoof tester.

h. oil a mixture of 20 parts neat's-foot oil and 1 part Stockholm tar; used to prevent a horse's hooves from becoming dry and brittle.

h. overgrowth in old animals kept on very soft pasture or bedding; the hoof wall elongates and will eventually curl under so that the patient is walking on hoof wall instead of sole.

h. pick a pointed appliance in various shapes used to pick dirt and stones out of the grooves in the sole of a horse's hoof.

h. slough the wall and sole are detached from the sensitive laminae and the coronet and falls off. When the detachment is partial, the hoof is retained but is not viable and the patient gives the appearance of wearing slippers.

h. tester shaped like a pair of large pincers. One of the blades is placed on apparently normal hoof and the other on the part to be tested. If there is a flinch response when the handles are squeezed this is taken as an indication of pain at one of the pressure sites.

h. ulcer see PODODERMATITIS circumscripta.

worn h. excessive wear, e.g. that which occurs in pastured cows forced to walk twice daily along races floored with recently paved non-slip concrete; may expose sensitive tissue, causing herd level lameness in all four limbs.

hoof-and-mouth disease foot-and-mouth disease.

hoof cracks for single cracks in individual hooves see SANDCRACK, QUARTER crack. Multiple cracks in all hooves represent a response to a systemic state, usually nutritional deficiency, e.g. hypovitaminosis A in all species, hypobiotinosis A in pigs.

hook 1. metal instrument turned backwards on itself at one end. 2. the aggressive upward thrusting action of a cattle beast with its horns.

h. bone TUBER coxae.

obstetric h. see EYEHOOKS.

ovariectomy h. see spay hook (below).

spay h. a small 6 inch blunt-pointed hook for exteriorizing a uterine horn during a spay operation in a cat or dog. See also COVAULT SPAY HOOK and SNOOK HOOK.

Hook and Tucker Analyzer automatic analyzer of inhaled or exhaled anesthetic gases.

Hooke's law the law explaining linear behavior of elastic material.

hooklets the structure by which the distal barbules of bird feathers engage the indentations of the proximal barbules.

hookworm nematodes of the genera ANCYLOSTOMA, BUNOSTOMUM, GAIGERIA, NECATOR, UNCINARIA.

h. dermatitis penetration of the skin by third-stage larvae of the hookworm species causes an inflammatory reaction. Can occur in many species, but seen particularly in dogs on skin that comes in contact with the ground. See also cutaneous LARVA migrans.

h. disease see BUNOSTOMIASIS, ANCYLOSTOMIASIS, UNCINARIASIS.

hoose LUNGWORM disease.

Hoplocephalus bungaroides a venomous rock and tree-climbing snake with a noticeably broad head and striking yellow, crisscross markings on a black skin. Its venom carries a potent neurotoxin and the snake must be considered to be a toxic hazard.

Hoplodontophorus a nematode found in hyrax.

Hoplopleura a genus of sucking lice in the family Hoplopleuridae.

H. acanthopus, H. captiosa, H. pacifica. sucking lice of rodents.

Hoppengarten cough [Ger.] an upper respiratory tract infection of horses of indefinite etiology. See also EQUINE influenza.

hopping moving by quick springy leaps.

h. response a test of postural reactions. The animal is supported while three limbs are held off the ground and it is made to move forward, backward, and laterally on one leg at a time. Strength and coordination of the hopping movement is assessed.

hopples see HOBBLE.

horary points pertaining to an hour; in acupuncture refers to the way in which the five elements travel through the meridians in a circadian rhythm, increasing the sensitivity of the points on each meridian; called also element points.

hordenine toxic alkaloid in *Phalaris* spp.

hordeolum inflammation of one or more sebaceous glands of the eyelid.

external h. involves the glands of Zeis and Moll, forming an abscess on the eyelid margin. Called also sty.

internal h. involves the meibomian glands. See also CHALAZION.

Hordeum the barley genus of cereals and grasses in the family Poaceae.

H. geniculatum* (syn. *H. hystrix*), *H. jubatum*, *H. leporinum*, *H. murinum some of the grasses which are significant causes of grass seed injury and GRASS seed abscess; heavy seed content may cause feed refusal. Called also barley grass. The seeds are also called foxtails.

H. vulgare cereal barley, one of the cereal grains commonly involved in carbohydrate engorgement. The green crop if grazed may cause hypomagnesemia or nitrite poisoning.

horizontal parallel to the plane of the horizon.

h. beam positioning of a subject so that the x-ray beam needs to be directed horizontally. Used because of difficulty in positioning the animal for a dorsoventral shot, or because of interest in the position of fluid or gas.

h. mattress suture see MATTRESS SUTURE PATTERN.

Hormel pigs miniature breed used extensively in biomedical research; subject to congenital melanosis.

hormesis stimulation by a subinhibitory concentration of a toxic substance.

Hormodendrum see WANGIELLA.

hormonagogue an agent that increases the production of hormones.

hormonal emanating from or pertaining to hormones.

h. antibodies hormones can be used as antigens and antibodies produced against them so that reproductive functions can be retarded or enhanced.

h. dermatoses skin diseases caused by an abnormality of any of the many hormones that influence the skin and adnexa, particularly growth of hair. See also endocrine ALOPECIA.

h. hypersensitivity a papulocrustous dermatitis associated with hypersensitivity to endogenous gonadal hormones. Seen most commonly in bitches during stages of the estrus cycle.

h. pregnancy diagnosis performed commercially in cows by determining that progesterone levels in milk are maintained after mating instead of declining by the 20th day.

h. synergism when their combined effect is greater than the simple addition of each of their individual effects.

hormone a chemical transmitter substance produced by cells of the body and transported by the bloodstream and other means to the cells and organs which carry specific receptors for the hormone and on which it has a specific regulatory effect.

Hormones act as chemical messengers to body organs, stimulating certain life processes and retarding others. Growth, reproduction, control of metabolic processes, sexual attributes and behavior are dependent on hormones.

Hormones are produced by various organs and body tissues, but mainly by the ENDOCRINE glands, such as the pituitary, thyroid and gonads (testes and ovaries). Each gland apparently manufactures several kinds of hormones; the adrenal glands alone produce more than 25 varieties. The total number of hormones is still unknown, but each has its unique function and structure. After a hormone is discharged by its parent gland into the capillaries or the lymph, it may travel a circuitous path through the bloodstream to exert influence on cells, tissues and organs (target organs) far removed from its site of origin.

adrenomedullary h's substances secreted by the ADRENAL medulla, including epinephrine and norepinephrine.

androgenic h's the masculinizing hormones, androstenedione and testosterone.

h. assay modern techniques include the use of competitive protein binding assay and radioimmunoassay.

calciotropic h. any hormone which is specifically involved in the homeostatic regulation of serum calcium levels through their effects on bone and other organs, e.g. parathyroid hormone, calcitonin.

corpus luteum h. progesterone.
cortical h. corticosteroid.
ectopic h's those secreted by tumors of nonendocrine tissues but having the same physiological effects as their normally produced counterparts. It is not known exactly how the synthesis and secretion of endocrine hormones from nonendocrine tissues occurs. Most of these tumors are derived from tissues that have a common embryonic origin with endocrine tissues. When the cells undergo neoplastic transformation, they can revert to a more primitive stage of development and begin to synthesize hormones.
enteric h. hormone secreted by endocrine cells in the wall of the intestine or stomach or in the pancreas. Includes gastrin, cholecystokinin, secretin, gastric inhibitory polypeptide, enteroglucagon, motilin, neurotensin, 5-HT, substance P, pancreatic polypeptide, somatostatin.
estrogenic h's substances capable of producing certain biological effects, the most characteristic of which are the changes which occur in mammals at estrus; the naturally occurring estrogenic hormones are β-estradiol, estrone and estriol.
gonadal h's steroids in birds which affect development of the reproductive tubular system, head decorations, feathers, squawk, behavior.
h. herbicide substances sprayed on plants which exert a lethal hormonal effect on the entire plant. See also hormone weedkiller (below).
lactation h., lactogenic h. prolactin.
luteotropic h. (LTH) see LUTEOTROPIN.
neurohypophyseal h's those stored and released by the neurohypophysis, i.e. oxytocin and vasopressin.
peptide h's peptide molecules which exert their effects only on target cells that carry the hormone-specific receptors.
placental h. one secreted by the placenta, including chorionic gonadotropin, relaxin, and other substances having estrogenic, progestational or adrenocorticoid activity. See also PLACENTAL hormones.
progestational h's substances, including PROGESTERONE, that are concerned mainly with preparing the endometrium for nidation of the fertilized ovum if conception has occurred. See also PROGESTATIONAL agent.
h. receptors the presence of hormone-specific receptors on cells is the means of determining which cells respond to the circulating hormones. The number of receptors on each cell is one of the ways of regulating the degree of response.
reproductive h's see FOLLICLE-STIMULATING HORMONE, LUTEINIZING HORMONE, LUTEOTROPIC hormone, ESTROGEN, OXYTOCIN, PITUITRIN, PROGESTERONE, PROLACTIN, RELAXIN, STILBESTROL, TESTOSTERONE.
sex h's see SEX hormones.
somatotrophic h., somatotropic h. growth hormone.
somatotropin release inhibiting h. somatostatin.
somatotropin releasing h. (SRH) growth hormone releasing hormone.
thymic h. thymosin.
h. weedkiller includes 2,4-D, 2,4,5-T, MCP, silvex, dalapon. See also TCDD, HCDD and DIOXIN.

hormone–receptor complex hormone specifically bound to its receptor either on the plasma membrane or intracellularly.

hormone-sensitive triacylglycerol lipase enzyme catalyzing the hydrolytic release of fatty acid from carbon-1 or -3 of the glycerol moiety of triacylglycerols in white adipose tissue in response to epinephrine during stress or glucagon during fasting.

hormonogen prohormone.

hormonopoiesis the production of hormones.

hormonotherapy treatment by the use of hormones; endocrinotherapy.

horn 1. a pointed projection. 2. the processes carried on the foreheads of most ruminants and rhinoceroses including skin-covered bony knobs in giraffes, velvet-covered branched deciduous bony antlers of deer, branched deciduous keratinized processes in pronghorns and the familiar hollow horns of bovids. In these a horny sheath is composed of keratinized epithelial cells borne on a fibrous corium that is carried on a cornual process, an extension of the frontal bone. In mature cattle the cavity of the frontal sinus extends into the cornual process. Called also fighting horns.

Cattle and buffalo horns are classed as shorthorn (short, in-curving), lyre (see LYRATE), crescent or sickle (large, inward curving, downward inclined), long (long, handlebar configuration).
h. aging telling the age of a cattle beast by counting the rings at the base and adding one. Can give a guide but can also mislead. It is also capable of being faked and even obliterated by rasping or by dehorning.
h. amputation see DEHORNING.
h. button immature horn on the frontal bone of very young ruminants. Called also horn BUD.
h. core cancer, h. cancer is a squamous cell carcinoma of the mucosa of the frontal sinus which invades the horn core usually resulting in dehiscence of the horn. Has a very high prevalence in adult male cattle in India.
cicatricial h. a hard, dry outgrowth from a cicatrix, commonly scaly and rarely osseous.
cutaneous h. single or multiple firm projections ('horns') of keratin on the skin or footpads. They may originate from papillomas, keratoses or various skin tumors, particularly intracutaneous cornifying epithelioma, or in association with dermatophilosis or feline leukemia virus infection.
dorsal h. of spinal cord the horn-shaped structure seen in transverse section of the spinal cord, formed by the dorsal column of the cord.
h. fly see HAEMATOBIA *irritans*.
h. nerve block see CORNUAL nerve block.
overgrown h. malaligned shorthorn type horns which curve in too far and penetrate the skull, usually into a frontal sinus.
h. paste made of hoof raspings mixed with lard. Packed into the clefts beside the bars of the sole in the horse's foot before the taking of a radiograph; avoids the misleading opacities created by the clefts on radiographs. Now usually replaced by Playdo.
h. pearls microscopic structures found in some neoplasms of epithelial origin. Called also squamous or keratin pearls.
sebaceous h. a hard outgrowth of the contents of a sebaceous cyst.
h. shears devices used for removing horns. Most work as a guillotine and provide great leverage for cutting the horns at the base where a rim of skin can be included.
h. tubule basic structural element in many horny outgrowths; produced by a dermal papilla, it bears some resemblance to a hair and grows approximately vertical to the dermal surface; it is united by intertubular horn to neighboring tubules.
ventral h. cell diseases motor neuron diseases; rare

in animals, but hereditary spinal MUSCULAR atrophy of Brittany spaniels is an example.

ventral h. of spinal cord the horn-shaped structure seen in transverse section of the spinal cord, formed by the ventral column of the cord.

warty h. a hard, pointed outgrowth of a wart.

horneblende see ASBESTOS.

Horner's muscle a branch of the orbicularis oculi muscle which passes behind the lacrimal gland and contributes to the lacrimal pump.

Horner's syndrome enophthalmos, ptosis of the upper eyelid, slight elevation of the lower lid, constriction of the pupil, and narrowing of the palpebral fissure caused by paralysis of the cervical sympathetic nerve supply.

first order (central) H's s. caused by lesions within the parenchyma of the brain or spinal cord, before the synapse of sympathetic fibers within gray matter of thoracic segments T1 to T3.

second order (peripheral) H's s. involves the sympathetic trunk from its origin at T2 to T4 to the cranial cervical ganglion.

third order H's s. involves sympathetic fibers distal to the cranial cervical ganglion. Middle and inner ear disease can affect these fibers, which pass close to the tympanic bulla.

hornet members of the genus *Vespula* of wasps in the order Hymenoptera. Hornet venom contains histamine, serotonin, acetylcholine, hyaluronidase and phospholipase.

horror autotoxicus an old term that predicted the occurrence of diseases in which the rules guaranteeing self tolerance are broken.

horse[1] 1. the human race's martial, draft, racing, pleasure and companion animal of antiquity. Called also *Equus caballus*, a species sharing the genus with the ass, zebra and quagga. A member of the family Equidae in the order Perissodactyla, the odd-toed ungulates. 2. the word is also used to mean the entire male—the stallion.

Horses are classified in several ways: ancestry—warmblood, coldblood; use—draft, pony, carriage or carthorse, hack, polo pony, mustang, drafting or cutting horse, cowpony, jumper, hunter, standardbred, trotter, pacer, harness horse, eventer, dressage, rodeo, polocrosse, steeplechaser, remount, galloper; breeds—AMERICAN SADDLE HORSE, AMERICAN TROTTER, ANDALUSIAN, ANGLO-ARAB, APPALOOSA, ARAB, AUSTRALIAN pony, BARB, BELGIAN, CAMPOLINO, CLEVELAND BAY, CLYDESDALE, CONNEMARA PONY, CRIOLLO, DALES PONY, DARTMOOR PONY, DOLE PONY, EXMOOR PONY, FALABELLA, FELL PONY, FJORD PONY, Fox Trotting Horse, FRIESIAN, Galiceno, GALLOWAY pony, GOTLAND PONY, HACKNEY pony, HANOVER, HOLSTEIN, HIGHLAND pony, LIPITSA, LUSITANO, MORGAN HORSE, NEW FOREST pony, OVERO, Pasos (Paso fino, Peruvian Paso, American Paso Fino), Palomino, PERCHERON, QUARTER HORSE, SHETLAND PONY, SHIRE, STANDARDBRED, SUFFOLK HORSE, TENNESSEE WALKING HORSE, THOROUGHBRED, TIMOR PONY, TROTTER, WELSH PONY, Ysabella.

h. bots see GASTEROPHILUS.

h. coat colors see individual colors BAY, BLACK, BROWN, CHESTNUT (3), GRAY.

h. dentition see DENTAL formula.

h. louse fly see HIPPOBOSCA.

h. pox see HORSEPOX.

h.-sick said of a field that has had horses grazing on it for too long or at too heavy a stocking rate. The pasture is too rank and clumpy and the population of *Strongyle* spp. and other helminth larvae is likely to be high.

h. sickness AFRICAN HORSE SICKNESS.

h. sickness fever a clinically inapparent form of African horse sickness; usually a response in a vaccinated animal or one which is reinfected.

horse[2] adjective used to describe a coarse or free-growing weed. Includes *Oenanthe aquatica* (horse bane), *Parkinsonia aculeata* (horse bean), *Tetradymia* spp. (horse brush), *Aesculus hippocastanum* (horse chestnut), *Pennisetum glaucum* (horse millet), *Mentha longifolia* (horse mint), *Solanum carolinense* (horse nettle), *Amoracia rusticana* (horse nettle), *Equisetum arvense* (horse tails).

horse fly see TABANUS.

horsebreaker a person expert at BREAKING-IN horses.

horsebrush see TETRADYMIA GLABRATA.

horsechestnut see AESCULUS.

horsenettle SOLANUM *carolinense*.

horsepox a disease caused by a poxvirus in the genus Orthopoxvirus and characterized by typical pox lesions on the lower limbs or around the muzzle. See also POX. Called also Jenner's horsepox, contagious pustular stomatitis.

Canadian h. see CANADIAN HORSEPOX.

horseradish see AMORACIA RUSTICANS.

horseshoe see HORSESHOEING.

horseshoe crab amebocyte test a biological test using the amebocytes to test for the presence of endotoxin. Called also limulus test.

horseshoe kidney see horseshoe KIDNEY.

horseshoeing that part of the art of blacksmithing to do with making horseshoes, fitting them to hooves, trimming the hooves to fit the shoes. There are two main techniques, hot shoeing and cold shoeing, the former being done beside a forge. The shoes may be mild steel or aluminum in racing plates.

corrective h. shoes custom made to correct some defect in the horse's gait or conformation.

horsetails see EQUISETUM.

horsing the behavior of a mare which is displaying ESTRUS.

Hortega cell see GITTER CELLS.

hospital an institution for the care and treatment of sick and injured animals. In order to meet legal requirements in some countries it is necessary for the building to include ward accommodation for inpatients, a radiology facility and a clinical pathology laboratory.

teaching h. one that conducts formal educational programs or courses of instruction that lead to the granting of recognized certificates, diplomas or degrees or that are required for professional certification or licensure.

hospitalization 1. the placing of a patient in a hospital. 2. the period of confinement in a hospital.

host 1. an animal or plant that harbors and provides sustenance for another organism (the parasite). Includes paratenic, intermediate etc. 2. the recipient of an organ or other tissue derived from another organism (the donor). 3. said of computers; the computer that one dials up when operating from a remote terminal.

accidental h. one that accidentally harbors an organism that is not ordinarily parasitic in the particular species.

alternate h. intermediate host.

h. determinants characteristics in the host which determine its susceptibility to a disease, e.g. closeness to parturition and metabolic diseases.

h.–parasite reaction the inflammatory reaction that sometimes occurs around a parasite in tissues, e.g. a warble fly larva in the esophageal wall.

predilection h. the host preferred by a parasite.
primary h. definitive host.
reservoir h. an animal (or species) that is infected by a parasite, and which serves as a source of infection for humans or another species.
h. risk factors epidemiological factors contributing to the development of a disease and which are contributed by the host.
secondary h. intermediate host.
h. specificity the characteristic of a parasite that renders it capable of infecting only one or more specific hosts.
transfer h., transport h. one that is used until the appropriate definitive host is reached, but is not necessary to complete the life cycle of the parasite.
h. variable see host determinants (above).

host–agent balance the relationship between the host and the disease agent; determines whether the two live commensally or the host dies or masters the agent.

host–parasite relationship may be at any one of a series of classified levels in two groups, those of disease and symbiosis. In the disease category there are VELOGENIC, MESOGENIC and LENTIGENIC.

hot–cold hemolysis complete hemolysis of sheep and ox erythrocytes by bacteria in culture media after chilling of the culture. A feature of β-hemolysin in staphylococci.

hot needle used in acupuncture; the needle wrapped in cotton wool, dipped in alcohol and lit, the charred cotton removed and the needle applied to the acupuncture point.

hot packing application of hot packs made by frying oats in vinegar and enclosing them in cloth sacs; used as an adjunct to acupuncture.

hot spots acute moist DERMATITIS.

Hotis test an indirect test carried out on milk to detect the presence of mastitis. Bromcresol is added to a sample which is then incubated. A positive reaction is a change in color of the sample.

Hotz–Celsus operation a technique for repair of entropion involving resection of a portion of the eyelid and orbicularis muscle.

hound a hunting dog. There are two types: coursing hounds (Greyhound, Saluki, Afghan, Whippet) use their speed to hunt by eyesight, while tracking hounds (Bloodhound, Beagle, Foxhound) use scent.

hound's tongue see CYNOGLOSSUM OFFICINALE.

Hounsfield unit an arbitrary unit of x-ray attenuation used for CT scans. Each voxel is assigned a value on a scale in which air has a value of −1000; water, 0; and compact bone, +1000.

hour-glass spiders see LATRODECTUS.

hourly fees see FEES.

house fly see MUSCA *domestica*.

housebreaking HOUSETRAINING.

housedust mite a probable factor in the development of allergic skin diseases in dogs. See ALLODERMANYSSUS, DERMATOPHAGOIDES, CHEYLETUS ERUDITUS, TYROPHAGUS *farinae*.

household the occupants, contents and the interior of a house; the greater part of the environment of the average companion animal.
h. cluster a grouping of animals or occurrences of disease within a household as occurs with some infectious diseases such as feline leukemia virus-related disorders.
h. product poisoning poisoning by materials that are normal contents in the average person's house, e.g. cleaning fluids, proprietary medicines.
h. residency duration of a companion animal's stay in a household. Controlled by disease, age, age at acquisition, financial viability of the owner, habits and personality of the animal.

housekeeper contractions intestinal peristalsis that occurs when food is not present.

housekeeping computer terminology for tidying up storages, culling defunct files and records, backing-up.

housemouse mite ALLODERMANYSSUS *sanguineus*.

housesoiling inappropriate defecation or urination by dogs or cats. See also inappropriate MICTURITION.

housetraining training of a companion animal to defecate and urinate outside or in specifically designated places such as a litter tray.

housing animal accommodation of all kinds including zoo cages, hen batteries, sow crates, loose housing for cows, dry cow corrals, calf hutches and the like. Animal welfare considerations have made great changes in what is permissible in animal housing and codes of conduct are now available in most countries which specify areas, volumes of space, type of construction, furniture and feeding and watering facilities. See also ALL-IN-ALL-OUT HOUSING, CONTINUAL THROUGHPUT HOUSING.
h. stress stress imposed on naturally pastoral animals when they are housed; includes the risk factors of overcrowding, incorrect temperature, humidity, ventilation, noise, uncomfortable bedding, infrequent feeding, watering.

Houttuynia a genus of tapeworms in the family Davaineidae.
H. struthionis found in the intestine of the ostrich and rhea; causes unthriftiness and diarrhea in chicks.

Hovawart a medium-sized, muscular herding dog with a long black, gold or blond coat.

hoven RUMINAL tympany.

Howell–Jolly bodies small, round or oval bodies, probably nuclear remnants, seen in erythrocytes when stains are added to fresh blood and found in various anemias and after splenectomy or reduced splenic function.

howler monkey a bearded, black monkey with long prehensile tail, about the size of a large dog and noted for its loud voice created by an extraordinarily large and cavernous larynx. Called also *Alouatta* spp.

Hoya a genus of the plant family Asclepiadaceae; poisoning caused by an unidentified toxin; characterized clinically by staggering, falling, convulsions. Includes *H. australis*, *H. carna*. Called also wax flower.

Hp haptoglobin, a serum protein that binds free hemoglobin.

HPG human pituitary gonadotropin.

HPL human placental lactogen.

HPLC high performance liquid chromatography.

HPO 1. hyperbaric (high-pressure) oxygenation. 2. hypertrophic pulmonary osteodystrophy.

HPP hyperkalemic periodic paralysis.

HPR host parasite reaction.

HR heart rate.

hr hour.

HRF homologous restriction factor.

ht height.

5-HT serotonin (5-hydroxytryptamine).

HTLV-BLV retrovirus group human T-cell lymphotropic virus/bovine leukemia virus group of retroviruses that cause bovine leukemia.

HTML HYPERTEXT markup language.

huanaco see GUANACO.

huck towel small (16 × 32 inch) cotton surgical towel with typical honeycomb texture.

hucklebones the top of the hip bones; a term used in dog conformation.

Hughes nail-hole curette see NAIL-hole curette.
Hug's teat tumor extractor a long thin cylindrical instrument to be inserted into the teat of a cow for the removal, by a guillotine-like action, of a tumor on the interior wall. The instrument is inserted closed, is then opened and the tumor guillotined, and the guillotine closed again before removing the instrument.
Hulet's rod technique an aid to pregnancy diagnosis used in ewes and goats that are 70 to 100 days pregnant. The animal is fasted and laid on its back. The lubricated rod is passed 14 inches into the rectum and the end moved in an arc from the spine to the abdominal wall. The pregnant uterus can be felt by an external hand as the rod moves it up to the abdominal wall.
Hulse procedure a method of intra-articular surgical reconstruction of a cranial cruciate ligament in which a graft formed by part of the patellar tendon and part of the lateral retinaculum is placed under the intermeniscal ligament and over the top of the lateral femoral condyle.
human see HOMO-.
h. carriers humans who act as active carriers of diseases of animals and infect animals.
h. immunodeficiency virus includes HIV1 (more common) and HIV2 which are lentiviruses that cause acquired immunodeficiency disease (AIDS) in humans.
h. leukocyte antigen see major HISTOCOMPATIBILITY complex.
humane pertaining to the avoidance of infliction of pain, discomfort and harassment; used especially with regard to animals.
h. considerations subjects which need to be taken into account by persons who have animals in their care, e.g. freedom from disease, from hunger, water deprivation, exploitation while performing.
h. destruction see EUTHANASIA (2).
h. killer a firearm for fast euthanasia of animals of all types. The classical instrument, the Greenough humane killer, can be taken apart and stowed in a small space. The instruments are gunmetal tubes with a firing pin and a sloping head to ensure that the projectile enters at the correct angle. The projectile may be a captive bolt that protrudes about 1 inch when the weapon is fired with a blank shell. The alternative is a standard rifle shell which is fired in the normal way.
h. societies voluntary organizations that carry out a valuable public service by watching for abuses of the laws that protect animals against cruelty, and by promoting relevant educational programs.
h. twitch a twitch in which a slipknot is fastened over the lower jaw and the rope is passed back, through a ring in a surcingle, back along the other side of the neck and into the slipknot loop. Pulling on the rope pulls the head into the chest. Called also martingale twitch.
humbles liver, kidney and entrails of a deer obtained at a hunting kill. Made into a pie for the tenants; hence 'humble pie'.
humectant 1. moistening. 2. a moistening or diluent medicine.
humeral of or pertaining to the humerus.
h. condyle knuckle on the distal end of the humerus.
humeroradial pertaining to the humerus and radius.
humeroradioulnar pertaining to the humerus, radius and ulna.
h. joint elbow.
humeroscapular pertaining to the humerus and scapula.
humeroulnar pertaining to the humerus and ulna.
humerus the bone of the upper forelimb, extending from shoulder to elbow. It consists of a shaft and two enlarged extremities. The proximal end has a smooth round head that articulates with the scapula to form the shoulder joint. Just below the head are two rounded processes called the greater and lesser tubercles. The distal end of the humerus has a trochlea, which articulates with the ulna, and a capitulum, which articulates with the radius, at the elbow. See also Table 10.
humidifier an apparatus for controlling humidity by adding moisture to the air.
humidity the degree of moisture in the air.
h. therapy, humidification therapy the therapeutic use of water to prevent or correct a moisture deficit in the respiratory tract. Under normal conditions the respiratory tract is kept moist by humidifying mechanisms that allow for evaporation of water from the respiratory mucosa. If these mechanisms fail to work, are bypassed as in ENDOTRACHEAL intubation, or are inadequate to overcome the drying and irritating effects of therapeutic gases and mucosal crusting, some form of humidification must be provided.
hummel entire, naturally polled deer.
humor pl. *humores, humors* [L.] any fluid or semifluid in the body.
aqueous h. see AQUEOUS humor.
ocular h. either of the humors of the eye—aqueous or vitreous.
vitreous h. see VITREOUS humor.
humor- prefix meaning liquid.
humoral effects carried out via the fluids of the body.
h. acupuncture mechanisms thought to be β-endorphins released by the pituitary.
h. immunity immunity based on antibody. See humoral IMMUNITY.
hump of zebu cattle fleshy mass over the withers due mainly to enlargement of the rhomboideus muscles.
humpback see HUNCHBACK.
humpsore see STEPHANOFILAROSIS.
humpyback a syndrome affecting full-woolled sheep in summer in Australia; manifested by a hunched stance and poor exercise tolerance and death if driven hard; necropsy lesions include cardiomyopathy and degenerative lesions in the white matter of the spinal cord; etiology uncertain but ingestion of fruits of *Solanum esuriale* or foliage of *Malvastrum americanum* suspected.
hunchback a rounded deformity, or hump, of the back, or an animal with such a deformity. The condition is called also KYPHOSIS and is the result of an abnormal upward curvature of the spine.
Hungarian kuvasz see KUVASZ.
Hungarian pointer see VIZSLA.
Hungarian puli see PULI.
Hungarian vizsla see VIZSLA.
Hungarian wirehaired vizsla a dog breed similar to the VIZSLA, but the coat is harsh, short on the head and legs, and longer on the ears and body.
Hungate roll tube method standard procedure for culture of ruminal organisms.
hunger a craving, as for food. A localized subjective sensation, assumed to occur in animals, caused by emptiness and a resulting hypermotility of the stomach.
h. hollow paralumbar FOSSA in ruminants.
hungry rice see DIGITARIA *exilis*.
Huntaway a type of dog found in New Zealand, where they use barking sheepdog breeds or types to

round up sheep and return them to the hills; that is the dogs drive sheep away from the shepherd, instead of the customary activity of bringing them to the herder. There is not a recognized breed for the purpose; most are Airedale crossbreds.

hunter a horse used for hunting. A hunter can be any size or shape but is in most cases the product of mating a thoroughbred stallion to a draft mare. Their role is much wider than carrying a rider to a hunt; they are now the mainstay of the jumping and eventing scene.

h. clip the horse's long winter coat is clipped except for the limbs and saddle place.

Hunter burr XANTHIUM *italicum*.

Hurler's syndrome mucopolysaccharidosis I.

Hürthle cell large oxyphilic, eosinophilic cells found in the thyroid gland. They are metabolically altered follicular cells which accumulate large numbers of mitochondria. See also Hürthle cell tumor (below).

H. c. tumor a new growth of the thyroid gland composed wholly or predominantly of large cells (Hürthle cells) having abundant granular, eosinophilic cytoplasm. Such tumors are usually benign (Hürthle cell adenoma) but on occasion may be locally invasive or may rarely metastasize (Hürthle cell carcinoma, or malignant Hürthle cell tumor). Called also oxyphilic adenoma of thyroid gland.

HUS hemolytic uremic syndrome. See also HEMOGLOBINURIC nephrosis.

husbandry careful management of e.g. animals. Implies thrifty, humane, caring. See also ANIMAL HUSBANDRY.

husk see LUNGWORM disease.

Husky see SIBERIAN HUSKY.

hutch 1. standard cagelike accommodation for rabbits. 2. light, movable cabin for calves or pigs; to provide shelter and warmth for animals at pasture.

h. burn a disease of rabbits characterized by external inflammation of the external genitalia and the anus caused by constant wetness due to wet hutch floors.

Huxley's layer one of the three layers in the internal root sheath of the hair.

HVL HALF-VALUE LAYER.

Hx abbreviation for history; used in medical records.

H-Y antigen see H-Y ANTIGEN.

hyacinth see HYACINTHUS ORIENTALIS.

Hyacinthoides nonscripta SCILLA *nonscripta*.

Hyacinthus orientalis European plant of the family Liliaceae. The bulbs are poisonous to cattle. They may contain a cardiac glycoside and cause salivation, diarrhea, collapse and death. Called also hyacinth.

Hyaenanche globosa South African plant in the family Euphorbiaceae. Contains a toxic substance hyaenanchin. Called also hyena poison.

hyaenanchin a toxic substance present in the plant *Hyaenanche globosa*.

hyalin a translucent albuminoid substance obtainable from the products of amyloid degeneration.

hyaline glassy; pellucid.

h. body see APOPTOTIC BODY.

h. cartilage see hyaline CARTILAGE.

h. cast see urinary CAST.

h. degeneration see hyaline DEGENERATION.

h. globules composed of fibrin degradation products these contribute to the formation of microthrombi. Called also shock bodies.

h. membrane composed of fibrin and cell debris, this membrane lines the alveoli when there has been severe damage to the alveolar epithelium. See also hyaline MEMBRANE (3).

h. membrane disease a disorder of newborn animals, most commonly foals, characterized by the formation of a hyalin-like membrane lining the terminal respiratory passages. Neonates with this disease do not secrete adequate quantities of surfactant, which is secreted by type II alveolar epithelial cells, and decreases the surface tension of the fluids lining the alveoli and bronchioles. When the surface tension is kept low, air can pass through the fluids and into the alveoli. If the surface tension is not decreased by adequate supplies of surfactant, the alveoli cannot fill with air and there is partial or complete collapse of the lung (atelectasis). Thus the foal with hyaline membrane disease suffers from respiratory embarrassment with severe DYSPNEA. See also NEONATAL maladjustment syndrome.

hyalinization conversion into a substance resembling glass.

hyalinosis hyaline degeneration.

pulmonary h. multifocal accumulations of macrophages and giant cells which contain laminated PAS-positive hyaline material. Some deposits in the lungs of dogs are grossly visible subpleurally at the ventral borders of the lungs.

hyalinuria hyalin in the urine.

hyalitis inflammation of the vitreous body.

h. punctata a form marked by small opacities.

h. suppurativa purulent inflammation of the vitreous body.

hyal(o)- word element. [Gr.] *glassy*.

hyalocentesis aspiration of vitreous. See also vitreous PARACENTESIS.

hyalohyphomycosis includes the several types of opportunist infections caused by nonpigmented fungi. See PAECILOMYCOSIS, PSEUDALLESCHERIOSIS, GEOTRICHUM, ASPERGILLOSIS, PENICILLIOSIS.

hyaloid pellucid; like glass.

h. artery see persistent hyaloid artery (below).

persistent h. artery the embryonic artery that runs from the optic disk to the posterior lens capsule may persist; the site of attachment may form an opacity. See MITTENDORF'S DOT.

hyaloidocapsular ligament in humans this ligament performs a limited attachment of the lens to the vitreous body, permitting intracapsular removal of the lens.

hyalomere the pale, homogeneous portion of a blood platelet.

Hyalomma a genus of ticks in the family Ixodidae. The several stages of these ticks transmit *Babesia caballi*, *B. equi*, *Theileria parva*, *T. annulata*, *T. dispar*, *Coxiella burnetii*, *Rickettsia bovis* and *R. conori*. There are significant differences of opinion about the nomenclature of these ticks. A further subdivision creating new genera of *Hyalommina* and *Hyalommosta* is proposed. The currently listed species are: *Hyalomma anatolicum*, *H. detritum mauretanicum*, *H. detritum scupense* (*H. uralense*, *H. volgense*), *H. dromedarii*, *H. excavatum* (*H. anatolicum*), *H. impressum*, *H. plumbeum plumbeum* (*H. marginatum*), *H. truncatum* (*H. transiens*). See also SWEATING sickness.

Hyalommina suggested new genus, subdivision of *Hyalomma* spp.

Hyalommosta suggested new genus, subdivision of *Hyalomma* spp.

hyalonyxis the act of puncturing the vitreous body.

hyaloplasm see AXOPLASM.

hyaloserositis inflammation of serous membranes marked by conversion of the serous exudate into a pearly coating of the affected organ.

hyalosis degenerative changes in the vitreous humor.

asteroid h. the presence of spherical or star-shaped opacities in the vitreous humor.

hyaluronate salt of hyaluronic acid.

hyaluronic acid a sulfate-free mucopolysaccharide in the intercellular substance of various tissues, especially the skin; also isolated from the vitreous humor, synovial fluid, umbilical cord, etc. Used therapeutically in degenerative joint disease and in solution as a tear film replacement.

hyaluronidase an enzyme that catalyzes the hydrolysis of hyaluronic acid, the 'cement material' of connective tissues; it is found in leeches, snake and spider venom, in testes, and is produced by various pathogenic bacteria, enabling them to spread through tissue. A preparation from mammalian testes is used to promote absorption and diffusion of solutions injected subcutaneously. When hyaluronidase is mixed with fluids administered subcutaneously, absorption is more rapid and less uncomfortable. Hyaluronidase should not be given in areas where there is infection. Since it hastens absorption, it must be given with caution when administered with toxic drugs, as the toxic reaction can occur very rapidly.

Hybomitra a genus of the fly family Tabanidae. Called also horse fly. Capable of transmitting anthrax, anaplasmosis, tularemia and equine infectious anemia. They also cause significant insect worry and blood loss.

hybrid an offspring of parents of different strains, varieties or species.

h. mother-of-millions BRYOPHYLLUM *daigremontium* × *B. tubiflorum*.

h. vigor increased productivity and performance in the first generation of crossbred animals produced by the mating of dissimilar breeds. The gain is lost if the hybrids are interbred. Called also heterosis.

hybridization the production of hybrids.

in situ h. of nucleic acid a fragment of radioisotope or otherwise labeled DNA can be used as a probe to detect related nucleic acid sequences in cells or tissues. The method requires that both the probe and the cellular nucleic acid sequences be melted to single-stranded forms and then allowed to form either DNA:DNA or DNA:RNA double-stranded forms.

interspecies h. see interspecific HYBRIDOMA.

nucleic acid h. double-stranded DNA when heated in aqueous solution separates into two single strands in a process called denaturation or melting. The single strands readily reform a double helix when the solution is allowed to cool in a process called DNA renaturation. Hybridization will occur between any two single-stranded nucleic acid molecules (DNA:DNA, RNA:RNA, RNA:DNA) provided they have complementary nucleotide sequences. The degree of homology between any two nucleic acid molecules can be measured by the percentage of base pairing.

hybridoma a cell culture consisting of a clone of a hybrid cell formed by fusing cells of different kinds. Hybridomas formed from mouse B lymphocytes following inoculation of a particular antigen and myeloma cells are immortal and produce monoclonal antibodies to the inoculated antigen. Such antibodies have produced a revolution in the level at which antibody–antigen reactions can be analyzed leading to precise definition of important epitopes, to methods for purifying antigens, improved diagnostic methods and, it is anticipated, to new methods of therapy.

interspecific h. one formed by fusion of cells from two different species, such as mouse and rat or hamster.

hydatid 1. a hydatid cyst. 2. any cyst-like structure.

h. cyst the larval stage of the tapeworm *Echinococcus granulosus* or *E. multilocularis*, containing daughter cysts, each of which, if fertile, will have many protoscoleces; it is the cause of hydatid disease. Called also *Echinococcus* cyst and hydatid.

h. disease an infection in humans, sheep, cattle, pigs and horses, and occasionally in many other mammal species. The infection is usually of the liver or lungs, caused by larval forms (hydatid cysts) of TAPEWORMS of the genus *Echinococcus*, and characterized by the development of expanding cysts. In the infection caused by *E. granulosus*, single or multiple cysts that are unilocular in character are formed, and in that caused by *E. multilocularis*, the host's tissues are invaded and destroyed as the cyst(s) enlarge by peripheral budding. Called also echinococcosis.

false h. see CYSTICERCUS *tenuicollis*.

Morgagni's h. see MORGAGNI'S HYDATID.

sessile h. the hydatid of Morgagni connected with a testis.

stalked h. the hydatid of Morgagni connected with an oviduct.

hydatidiform resembling a hydatid.

hydatidocele a tumor of the scrotum containing hydatids.

hydatidoma a tumor containing hydatids.

hydatidosis hydatid disease.

hydatiduria excretion of hydatid cysts in the urine.

Hydatigera see TAENIA.

hydraeroperitoneum water and gas in the peritoneal cavity.

hydragogue 1. increasing the fluid content of the feces. 2. a purgative that causes evacuation of watery stools.

hydralazine an antihypertensive and vasodilator drug that relaxes arteriolar smooth muscle by direct action. It is used as the hydrochloride in peripheral vascular disease, thrombophlebitis and congestive heart failure.

hydrallantois a gross accumulation of fluid in the allantoic sac. Occurs in cows, rarely in mares. Causes dystocia, uterine inertia and death or abortion of the fetus.

hydramnios excess of amniotic fluid. Commonly associated with fetal deformity. A high incidence in cattle–bison hybrids. Occurs in cows and ewes.

hydranencephaly absence of the cerebral hemispheres, their normal site being occupied by cerebrospinal fluid.

arthrogryposis and h. occurs as a combined congenital defect in epidemic form in calves, lambs and kids. It may be caused by intrauterine viral infection with the Akabane and Aino viruses, by poisoning with fungi on lupins, and by inheritance of a conditioning factor. See also AKABANE VIRUS disease, AINO VIRUS disease.

Hydrangea a genus in the plant family Saxifragaceae; poisoning caused by an unidentified toxin characterized by transient diarrhea in animals eating the plants. Includes horticultural, wild hydrangeas. *H. arborescens*, *H. hortensis*, *H. macrophylla*, *H. quercifolia*.

hydrargyria chronic poisoning from mercury.

hydrargyrum [L.] *mercury* (symbol Hg).

hydrarthrosis an accumulation of watery fluid in the cavity of a joint.

hydrase, hydratase any enzyme that catalyzes the hydration–dehydration of C–O linkages.

hydrate 1. a compound of water with a radical. 2. a salt or other compound that contains water of crystallization.

hydration the absorption of or combination with water.

h. status the status of the fluid–electrolyte balance in a patient.

hydraulic fluid toxic because of its high content of industrial triaryl phosphate.

hydraulics the science dealing with the mechanics of liquids.

hydrazine a gaseous diamine, H_4N_2, or any of its substitution derivatives.

h. sulfate an inhibitor of gluconeogenesis; used as an appetite stimulant.

hydremia excess of water in the blood.

hydrencephalocele hernial protrusion of brain tissue containing fluid.

hydrencephalomeningocele hernial protrusion, through a cranial defect, of meninges containing cerebrospinal fluid and brain substance.

hydr(o)- word element. [Gr.] *hydrogen, water.*

hydrocalycosis a usually asymptomatic cystic dilatation of a major renal calix, lined by transitional epithelium, and due to obstruction of the infundibulum.

hydrocarbon an organic compound that contains carbon and hydrogen only.

alicyclic h. one that has cyclic structure and aliphatic properties.

aliphatic h. one that does not contain an aromatic ring.

aromatic h. one that has cyclic structure and a closed conjugated system of double bonds.

hydrocele a painless swelling of the scrotum caused by a collection of fluid in the tunica vaginalis testis, the outermost covering of the testes. Called also water seed.

hydrocelectomy excision of a hydrocele.

hydrocephalocele hydrencephalocele.

hydrocephaloid resembling hydrocephalus.

hydrocephalus a condition characterized by abnormal accumulation of cerebrospinal fluid within the cerebral ventricular system. As a consequence, the ventricles are enlarged and the brain is diminutive. Called also water on the brain.

Although hydrocephalus occurs occasionally in adults, it is usually associated with a congenital defect in offspring.

There are two types of hydrocephalus, the distinction being based on whether there is abnormal absorption of the cerebrospinal fluid or an obstruction to its flow. In *communicating hydrocephalus* there is some abnormality in the capacity to absorb fluid from the arachnoid space. There is no obstruction to the flow of fluid between the ventricles. In *noncommunicating hydrocephalus* there is an obstruction at some point in the ventricular system. The cause of noncommunicating hydrocephalus usually is a congenital abnormality, such as stenosis of the aqueduct of Sylvius, or congenital atresia of the foramina of the fourth ventricle. Infections, intraventricular hemorrhage, trauma and tumors can produce acquired communicating hydrocephalus.

There are three forms that occur in cattle: in one there is gross distension of the cranium with normal facial bones; in the second there is a similar enlargement of the cranium with an accompanying achondroplastic dishing of the face and foreshortening of the maxilla and a shortening of the limb bones—these are the classical 'bulldog' calves; in the third the cranium is normal in size but there is internal hydrocephalus and the calves are blind and imbecile. There are a number of inherited hydrocephalitides in cattle. The disease also occurs in pigs but the inheritance is complex in that it is exacerbated by a concurrent hypovitaminosis A.

In dogs and cats, hydrocephalus is common in some toy breeds such as the Chihuahua in which a domed cranium is a desirable feature of conformation. It also occurs less often in adults in association with brain tumors and from infections such as toxoplasmosis and feline infectious peritonitis.

compensatory h. cerebrospinal fluid occupies space vacated by brain parenchyma because of malformation or degeneration. Examples are seen in fetal infection by bluetongue virus or bovine virus diarrhea virus, severe polioencephalomalacia in cattle, and cerebral infarction in cats.

external h. the excess fluid is in the arachnoid space; rare in animals.

hypertensive h. accompanied by increased cerebrospinal fluid pressure.

internal h. the excess fluid is within the ventricular system; common in domestic animals and may be congenital or acquired.

normotensive h. accompanied by normal cerebrospinal fluid pressure.

hydrochloric acid HCl; a normal constituent of gastric juice in humans and other animals. The absence of free hydrochloric acid in the stomach, called achlorhydria, may be found with chronic gastritis. Called also gastric anacidity.

hydrochloride an addition salt of hydrochloric acid with an organic base.

hydrochlorothiazide a thiazide diuretic; sometimes used for an antidiuretic effect in the treatment of diabetes insipidus in dogs.

Hydrochoerus hydrochaeris see CAPYBARA.

hydrocholecystis distension of gallbladder with watery fluid.

hydrocholeresis secretion of bile relatively low in specific gravity, viscosity and total solid content.

hydrocholeretic 1. pertaining to or producing hydrocholeresis. 2. an agent that stimulates an increased output of bile of low specific gravity.

hydrocirsocele hydrocele with varicocele.

hydrocodone a synthetic narcotic analgesic similar to but more active than codeine; the bitartrate is used as an antitussive.

hydrocolloid a colloid in which water is the dispersion medium.

h. wound dressing impermeable to oxygen and carbon dioxide, the colloid interacts with tissue fluid to form a nonadhesive gel.

hydrocolpos collection of watery fluid in the vagina.

hydrocortisone the pharmaceutical term for cortisol, the principal GLUCOCORTICOID secreted by the adrenal gland; it is used in the treatment of inflammations, allergies, pruritus, collagen diseases, adrenocortical insufficiency, and certain neoplasms. The soluble salts, sodium succinate and sodium phosphate, are used intravenously in the treatment of shock.

hydrocyanic acid a volatile liquid that is extremely poisonous because it checks the oxidation process in protoplasm. See also CYANIDE.

hydrocyst a cyst with watery contents.

hydroeicosatetraenoic acid a product of the conversion of hydroperoxyeicosatetetraenoic acid; capable of causing bronchial spasm.

hydrofluoric acid a glass etching agent; is in the effluent gases from some industrial plants making bricks, pottery, working aluminum. Creates a toxic hazard associated with industry. See also FLUOROSIS.

hydrogel a gel that contains water.

hydrogen a chemical element, atomic number 1, atomic weight 1.00797, symbol H. See Table 6. It exists as the mass 1 isotope (protium, or light or ordinary hydrogen), mass 2 isotope (deuterium, heavy hydrogen), and mass 3 isotope (tritium).

h. bonding weak electrostatic attraction between one electronegative atom and the hydrogen atom covalently linked to a second electronegative atom.

h. cyanide hydrocyanic acid.

heavy h. hydrogen having double the mass of ordinary hydrogen; deuterium.

h. ion balance see ACID–BASE BALANCE.

h. ion concentration the degree of concentration of hydrogen ions (the acid element) in a solution. Its symbol is pH, and expresses the degree to which a solution is acidic or alkaline. The pH range extends from 0 to 14, pH 7 being neutral. A pH of less than 7 indicates acidity, above 7 indicates alkalinity. See also ACID–BASE BALANCE and PH.

h. peroxide H_2O_2, used in solution as an antibacterial agent. A 3% solution foams on touching skin or mucous membrane and appears to have a mechanical cleansing action.

h. peroxide-based teat dips see TEAT DIP.

h. sulfide an ill-smelling, colorless, poisonous gas, H_2S; much used as a chemical reagent. Hydrogen sulfide is often present in gases from oil wells and from manure vats under slatted floor barns. Poisoning of cattle causes diarrhea, dehydration, dyspnea and death in convulsions. The feces are black and the breath smells of hydrogen sulfide. Called also hydrosulfuric acid. See also MANURE pit gas poisoning.

h. swell defective canned meat can. Can is distended due to production of hydrogen as a result of corrosion of the can surface.

hydrogenase an enzyme that catalyzes the reduction of various substances by combining them with molecular hydrogen.

hydrogenate to cause to combine with hydrogen; to reduce with hydrogen.

hydrogenation the process or reaction of combining with hydrogen.

hydrokinetic relating to movement of water or other fluid, as in a whirlpool bath.

hydrokinetics the science dealing with fluids in motion.

hydrolase one of the six main classes of enzymes, comprising those that catalyze the hydrolysis of a compound.

hydro-lyase an enzyme that catalyzes the removal of a hydrogen atom and a hydroxyl group from the substrate molecule as water and the formation of a double bond.

hydrolysate any compound produced by hydrolysis.

protein h. a mixture of amino acids prepared by splitting a protein with acid, alkali or enzyme. Such preparations provide the nutritive equivalent of the original material in the form of its constituent amino acids and are used in special diets or for patients unable to take the ordinary food proteins.

hydrolysis the cleavage of a compound by the addition of water, the hydroxyl group being incorporated in one fragment and the hydrogen atom in the other.

hydrolyze to performance hydrolysis.

hydroma hygroma.

hydromedusa see MEDUSA.

hydromeningitis meningitis with serous effusion.

hydromeningocele protrusion of the meninges, containing fluid, through a defect in the skull or vertebral column.

hydrometer an instrument for determining the specific gravity of a fluid.

hydrometra collection of watery or mucoid fluid in the uterus.

hydrometrocolpos collection of watery fluid in the uterus and vagina.

hydrometry measurement of specific gravity with a hydrometer.

hydromicrocephaly smallness of the head with an abnormal amount of cerebrospinal fluid.

hydromorphone a hydrogenated ketone of morphine with effects similar to morphine but of shorter duration; the hydrochloride is used as an analgesic and cough suppressant.

hydromphalus a cystic accumulation of watery fluid at the umbilicus.

hydromyelia dilatation of the central canal of the spinal cord with an abnormal accumulation of fluid.

hydromyelomeningocele a defect of the spine marked by protrusion of the membranes and tissue of the spinal cord, forming a fluid-filled sac.

hydromyoma a leiomyoma with cystic degeneration.

hydronephrosis distension of the renal pelvis and calices with urine.

If it is allowed to progress, the functioning units of the kidney are destroyed. The collecting tubules dilate and the muscular walls of the renal pelvis and calices stretch, are replaced by fibrous tissue, and eventually form a large, fluid-filled, functionless sac. Caused usually by obstruction of a ureter.

Unilateral hydronephrosis is likely to go unobserved unless its size becomes apparent during a clinical examination. Bilateral involvement will present a picture of developing uremia.

capsular h. see feline PERIRENAL cysts.

hydronium the hydrated proton H_3O+; exists in aqueous solution, a combination of H+ and H_2O.

hydropericarditis pericarditis with watery effusion.

hydropericardium an excess of transudate in the pericardial cavity. The cardiac shadow is enlarged and distorted on radiography; its size encroaches on the area over which lung sounds can normally be heard.

hydroperitoneum a collection of fluid in the peritoneal cavity; ASCITES.

hydroperoxyeicosatetraenoic acid a conversion product of arachidonic acid.

Hydrophiidae see SEA snakes.

hydrophilia the property of absorbing water; having a strong affinity for water.

hydrophilic readily absorbing moisture; hygroscopic; having strongly polar groups that readily interact with water.

hydrophilous hydrophilic.

hydrophobia 1. fear of water. 2. rabies.

hydrophobic 1. pertaining to hydrophobia (RABIES). 2. repelling water; insoluble in water; not readily absorbing water.

h. interaction interaction of nonpolar (un-ionizable) hydrocarbon molecules forced together because of stronger water–water interaction.

h. signal peptides 15 to 30 amino acids located at or near the *N*-terminus of a protein that always includes a hydrophobic core of at least eight nonpolar amino acids, found in proteins that are synthesized on membrane bound ribosomes and destined for export from the cell.

hydrophthalmos distension of the eyeball in glaucoma of the young.

hydrophysometra collection of fluid and gas in the uterus.

hydropic affected with dropsy, or hydrops.
h. degeneration a general histopathological finding in which cells absorb much water, indicating ischemic or toxic injury or early autolysis.
hydropneumatosis collection of fluid and gas in the tissues.
hydropneumogony injection of air into a joint to detect the presence of effusion.
hydropneumopericardium fluid and gas in the pericardium.
hydropneumoperitoneum fluid and gas in the peritoneal cavity.
hydropneumothorax a collection of fluid and gas within the pleural cavity.
hydroponics a method of cultivating plant growth without soil. Based on use of a solution containing all essential plant nutrients. The plant material is harvested at about 2 weeks of age. The herbivore's equivalent of sprouts or shoots in the human diet. Called also sprouted grain.
hydropropulsion using water pressure as a force to move objects; used to dislodge calculi in the urethra.
hydrops [L.] abnormal accumulation of serous fluid in the tissues or in a body cavity; called also dropsy. See also HYDRAMNIOS (hydrops amnii), HYDRALLANTOIS (hydrops allantois).
fetal h., hydrops fetalis gross edema of the entire body of the newborn, in hemolytic disease of the newborn.
h. uteri see HYDRAMNIOS, HYDRALLANTOIS.
hydropyonephrosis urine and pus in the renal pelvis.
hydroquinone thought at one time to be the toxic component of *Xanthium* spp., a now discredited view.
hydrorrhea a copious watery discharge.
h. gravidarum watery discharge from the gravid uterus.
hydrosalpinx accumulation of watery fluid in a uterine tube.
hydrosarcocele hydrocele and sarcocele together.
hydroscheocele a scrotal hernia containing fluid.
hydrosol a colloid in which the dispersion medium is a liquid.
hydrostatic pertaining to a liquid in a state of equilibrium or the pressure exerted by a stationary fluid.
h. pressure a significant factor in intestinal absorption; the tissue fluid pressure against which osmosis has to achieve a positive gradient if small molecules are to pass the cell membranes and be absorbed.
hydrostatics the science of equilibrium of fluids.
hydrosyringomyelia distension of the central canal of the spinal cord, with the formation of cavities and degeneration.
hydrotaxis an orientation movement of motile organisms or cells in response to the influence of water or moisture.
hydrotherapy the external use of water in the treatment of disease and injury.

Because of its physical properties related to the conduction of heat, buoyancy and cleansing action, water is an ideal agent for applications of HEAT (1) and COLD (2) to obtain desired physiological effects, débridement of wounds that are extensive and not easily cleansed by other methods, and the implementation of programs of therapeutic EXERCISE. See also whirlpool BATH.

hydrothermal, hydrothermic relating to the temperature effects of water, as in hot baths.
hydrothionemia hydrogen sulfide in the blood.
hydrothionuria hydrogen sulfide in the urine.
hydrothorax the presence of noninflammatory serous fluid within the pleural cavity. The fluid in the pleural cavity causes compression of lung with resulting dyspnea and ventral absence of lung sounds.
Hydrotoea a genus of head flies in the family Muscidae. Their importance depends on their proclivity for sweat, blood and tears. They cause insect worry in all animal species and in lexicographers.
H. albipuncta, H. meteorica, H. occulta sweat flies of horses and humans.
H. dentipes a dung fly, not recorded as annoying animals.
H. irritans the sheep head fly; causes insect worry, some damage to the skin around the horns and may predispose sheep, and sometimes cattle, to blowfly strike. Implicated in the transmission of summer MASTITIS in cows.
hydrotropism a growth response of a nonmotile organism to the presence of water or moisture.
hydrotympanum a collection of serous fluid in the middle ear.
hydroureter distension of the ureter with fluid, due to obstruction.
hydrous containing water.
hydrovarium a collection of serous fluid in an ovary.
hydroxamic acid an inhibitor of urease and a chelating agent. See also ACETOHYDROXAMIC ACID.
hydroxide the OH^- anion or a compound containing the OH^- ion.
hydroxocobalamin, hydroxycobalamin an analog of cyanocobalamin (vitamin B_{12}) having exceptionally long-acting hematopoietic activity. Called also vitamin B-12b.
hydroxy- a chemical prefix indicating presence of the univalent radical –OH.
17-hydroxy-11-deoxycorticosterone adrenocortical steroid with most effect on electrolyte metabolism (mineralocorticoid).
4-hydroxy-3-nitrophenylarsonic acid see ROXARSONE
3-hydroxy-4(1H)-pyridone toxic degradation product of mimosine; found in the rumen. Called also 3-hydroxy-4-pyridone.
hydroxyanisole an antioxidant used in food preservation, usually as the butylated form.
hydroxyapatite the principal inorganic constituent of bone matrix and teeth, imparting rigidity to these structures, and consisting of hydrated calcium phosphate.
2-(4′-hydroxyazobenzene) benzoic acid an acid dye used at one time in the colorimetric assay of serum albumin, now superseded by other methods. Called also HABA.
hydroxybenzoate an antioxidant used in food preservation; the butylated product is the standard form of usage. Also used as a preservative in pharmaceutical preparations. Called also parabens.
3-hydroxybutyric acid, β-hydroxybutyric acid major ketone body in circulation; hydroxyacid rather than ketone; important source of energy for extrahepatic tissues (not the brain in sheep) during starvation or diabetes mellitus. Excreted in bovine ACETONEMIA, ovine and bovine PREGNANCY toxemia and diabetic ketoacidosis.
hydroxychloroquine a drug used as the sulfate salt in the treatment of lupus erythematosus, rheumatoid arthritis and giardiasis.
25-hydroxycholecalciferol a metabolically activated form of cholecalciferol synthesized in the liver.
11-hydroxycorticosteroids corticosteroids with a hydroxyl group in the 11 position, e.g. cortisol, corticosterone.
17-hydroxycorticosteroids (17-OHCS) adrenocor-

ticosteroid hormones with a hydroxyl group at C-17, with or without oxygen at C-11, e.g. cortisol, cortisone and 11-deoxycortisol.

urinary 17-h. determination of urinary 17-hydroxycorticosteroids is an indication of the plasma level of cortisol and the functional status of the adrenal cortex.

5-hydroxy-*N*,*N*-dimethyltryptamine a toxic indole alkaloid in *Phalaris aquatica* (*tuberosa*).

hydroxyethyl starch see HETASTARCH.

L-hydroxyethylamide one of the alkaloids of *Claviceps purpurea*.

hydroxyl the univalent radical –OH.

hydroxylase any enzyme that brings about the coupled oxidation of two donors, with incorporation of oxygen into one of them.

21-h. a partial deficiency of the enzyme, in Pomeranian dogs, is thought to cause a dermatosis; histopathological lesions are of cutaneous atrophy; clinical signs include bilateral alopecia of the trunk, caudal thighs, ventral neck.

hydroxylation addition of –OH groups to a molecule.

hydroxylysine a naturally occurring amino acid.

hydroxymethylglutaryl-CoA a regulatory enzyme involved in the maintenance of the level of cholesterol in cells; key intermediate in synthesis of cholesterol in cytosol; also produced in mitochondria during ketogenesis.

h.-reductase similarly involved in cholesterol metabolism and the regulation of its contents in tissues.

hydroxyphenobarbital a metabolic product of phenobarbital produced in the liver; has very little anticonvulsant activity.

hydroxyprogesterone progesterone derivative used in bitches to prevent estrus and to treat pseudopregnancy.

hydroxyproline Hyp; an amino acid derived from proline.

hydroxypropyl methylcellulose a compound applied topically to the conjunctiva to protect the cornea during certain ophthalmic procedures and to lubricate the cornea.

hydroxyquinolines 8-hydroxyquinoline and 8-hydroxyquinoline sulfate are used as topical antiseptics and disinfectants.

hydroxystilbamidine isethionate a systemic fungicide and antiprotozoal drug.

hydroxytetracycline see OXYTETRACYCLINE.

hydroxytoluene an antioxidant used in food preservation; used as the butylated form.

5-hydroxytryptamine serotonin.

hydroxyurea an ANTINEOPLASTIC agent that blocks the conversion of ribonucleotides to deoxyribonucleotides, thus stopping DNA synthesis.

γ-hydroxyvinylacrylic acid an acid whose lactone is PROTOANEMONIN.

hydroxyzine a piperazine derivative which acts to block histamine H_1-receptors. Used as a sedative and antipruritic.

Hydrozoa the class of aquatic jellyfishes to which the Portuguese-man-of-war belongs.

hydruria excretion of urine of low specific gravity.

hyena member of the family Hyaenidae. Carnivorous but only for carrion, these ugly, smelly animals with their raucous voices and hysterical-sounding laughter are offensive in most ways. They have four toes, low hindquarters relative to their strong forequarters, and rough coats consisting mostly of guardhairs. Called also *Crocuta crocuta* (spotted hyena) and *Hyaena hyaena*, *H. brunnea* (striped and brown hyenas respectively).

h. disease cattle disease of slow growth, underdevelopment of hindquarters, thick, stiff bristles along the back, aggressive behavior. A chondrodystrophy affecting hindlimb bones and lumbar vertebrae. The overall effect is to create a silhouette like that of a hyena. Cause unknown.

hyena poison see HYAENANCHE GLOBOSA.

hygiene 1. the science of health and its preservation. 2. a condition or practice, such as cleanliness, that is conducive to preservation of health.

hygienics a system of principles for promoting health.

hygienist a specialist in hygiene.

hygro- word element. [Gr.] *moisture*.

hygroma an accumulation of fluid in a sac, cyst or bursa.

carpal h. large fluid-filled subcutaneous sac on the anterior aspect of the carpus caused by trauma.

cystic h., h. cysticum an endothelium-lined, fluid-containing lesion of lymphatic origin.

elbow h. a fluid-filled, painless, subcutaneous swelling over the point of the elbow involving the formation of a false bursa. Occurs mainly in the large breeds of dogs and in horses where it is called shoe boil.

hock h. a swelling of the subcutaneous bursa over the tuber calcis. The initial soft fluctuating swelling is replaced by a firm fibrous capsule to form a hygroma.

perirenal h. see feline PERIRENAL cysts.

hygrometer an instrument for measuring atmospheric moisture.

hygromycin B an antibiotic produced by *Streptomyces hygroscopicus*; used for the control of ascariasis and esophagostomiasis in sows. The method of use is to feed it to sows over a period of several weeks, or continuously to growing pigs. Overdosing may cause deafness and cataracts. Used also for the control of *Ascaria*, *Capillaria* and *Heterakis* spp. in poultry.

hygroscopic readily absorbing moisture.

hygroscopicity the quality of being hygroscopic.

Hylobactidae a family of nonhuman primates which includes gibbons and siamangs.

Hylobates see GIBBON, SIAMANG.

Hylochoerus meinertzhageni the giant forest hog, a vector for African swine fever.

hymen the membranous fold partly or completely closing the vaginal orifice usually inconspicuous in domestic animals.

imperforate h., persistent hymen white heifer disease associated commonly with cattle with all-white coats but occurs also in cattle of other colors and sporadically in other species. The heifer comes on heat and may breed but with difficulty and with straining afterwards. On rectal examination there is a distended uterus. The membrane may be rupturable and the animal conceive but there may be other tubular defects and the animals are best discarded.

hymenectomy excision of the hymen.

hymenitis inflammation of the hymen.

hymenolepiasis infection due to species in the tapeworm genus of *Hymenolepis*.

Hymenolepis a genus of cyclophyllidean tapeworms of the family Hymenolepididae; mostly have little pathogenicity.

H. cantaniana found in small intestine of chickens and other birds.

H. carioca occurs in fowls.

H. diminuta occurs in wild rodents and in humans.

H. lanceolata found in ducks and geese.

H. microstoma found in duodenum, gallbladder and bile ducts of rodents.

H. nana occurs in primates, rodents and humans. Called also dwarf tapeworm.

Hymenoptera an order of the class Insecta. Includes the ants, wasps, hornets, bees, fireants and sawflies. Characterized by two pairs of shiny, membranous wings.
h. sting a cause of injury and sometimes serious toxic and hypersensitivity reactions, particularly in dogs, which may be local or systemic. See also BEE STING.
hymenotomy incision of the hymen.
hymenovin a toxic sesquiterpene lactone in *Hymenoxys odorata*. Called also hymenoxon.
hymenoxon hymenovin.
Hymenoxys a plant genus of the Asteraceae (Compositae) family; contain toxic sesquiterpene lactone; poisoning causes a syndrome called 'spewing sickness' consisting of gastroenteritis manifested by lethargy, salivation, vomiting, abdominal pain and diarrhea plus nervous signs of tremor, incoordination and convulsions in pastured animals which eat the plant. Includes *H. lemmoni*, *H. odorata*, *H. richardsonii* (*H. floribunda*). Called also *Actinea* spp., bitterweed, Colorado rubber weed, pingue.
hyoechoic producing a decreased amplitude of waves returned in ultrasonography; characteristic of fluid.
hyoepiglottidean pertaining to the hyoid bone and epiglottis.
hyoglossal pertaining to the hyoid bone and tongue or to the hyoglossal muscle (Table 13.1B) or nerve (Table 14).
hyoid 1. shaped like Greek letter upsilon (υ). 2. pertaining to the hyoid bone.
h. apparatus the suspensory mechanism for the tongue and larynx. Consists of the single basihyoid, and the paired thyrohyoid, ceratohyoid, epihyoid and stylohyoid bones and the tympanohyoid cartilages.
h. bone one or more of the bones of the hyoid apparatus, fused in some species (e.g. human) to form a horseshoe-shaped bone situated at the base of the tongue, just below the thyroid cartilage. See also Table 10.
hyoscine see SCOPOLAMINE.
hyoscyamine an anticholinergic alkaloid usually obtained from species of the plant *Hyoscyamus* and other solanaceous plants. It is the levorotatory component of atropine with actions and uses similar to those of atropine but with more potent effects.
Hyoscyamus niger a European plant in the family Solanaceae; contains sufficient hyoscyamine to cause poisoning; signs include restlessness, excitement, muscle tremor and dilatation of the pupils. Called also henbane.
hyostrongylosis disease of pigs caused by infestation with the worm *Hyostrongylus rubidus*. Characterized by loss of condition, anemia, diarrhea.
Hyostrongylus a genus of gastric nematodes in the family Trichostrongylidae.
H. rubidus causes hyostrongylosis in pigs. The worms are found in the stomach of the pig.
hyovertebrotomy a surgical approach to the guttural pouch of the horse for the purpose of ligating a leaking internal carotid artery. The approach is between the hyoid apparatus and the vertebral wing of the atlas.
Hyp hydroxyproline.
hyp- see HYPO-.
word element. [Gr.] *abnormally decreased, deficient, beneath, under*.
hypalgesia reduced sensitivity to pain.
hypamnios deficiency of amniotic fluid.
hypanakinesia hypokinesia.
HYPAR acronym for *hy*sterectomy *p*roduced *a*rtificially *r*eared pigs. See SPECIFIC PATHOGEN FREE.

hypaxial beneath an axis, as the axis of the vertebral column.
hyper- word element. [Gr.] *abnormally increased, excessive*.
hyperabsorption increased intestinal absorption of a substance.
hyperacid abnormally or excessively acid.
hyperacidity excessive acidity.
hyperactive exhibiting hyperactivity; hyperkinetic.
hyperactivity the state of being hyperactive. Seen in early stages of many poisonings causing nervous system excitation, early encephalitides, anoxia, water deprivation; also at weaning or temporary separation from young or herd. Also in canine and sow hysteria.
rumenoreticular h. a diagnostic sign in VAGUS indigestion.
hyperacute extremely acute; course of a few hours. Called also peracute.
hyperadenosis enlargement of glands.
hyperadiposis extreme fatness.
hyperadrenalcorticism hyperadrenocorticism.
hyperadrenalemia increased amount of adrenal secretion in the blood.
hyperadrenalism, hyperadrenia overactivity of the adrenal glands.
hyperadrenocorticalism hyperadrenocorticism.
hyperadrenocorticism disease caused by hyperactivity of the adrenal cortices. May be caused by a corticotropic adenoma of the pituitary or by overtreatment with corticosteroids. The clinical picture is that of CUSHING'S SYNDROME.
iatrogenic h. induced by the administration of corticosteroids in the treatment of inflammatory or immune-mediated diseases. Seen with increasing frequency in small animals, particularly dogs.
juvenile h. reported in dogs; likely to result in stunted growth in addition to other clinical signs of Cushing's syndrome.
pituitary-dependent h. (PDH) see CUSHING'S SYNDROME.
hyperadrenocorticoidism see HYPERADRENOCORTICISM.
hyperaggression furious aggressiveness, a normal state for some wild cats when captured. A clinical sign in ordinarily mild-mannered animals in furious rabies.
hyperalbuminemia excessive albumin content of the blood.
hyperaldosteronemia excess of aldosterone in the blood.
hyperaldosteronism an abnormality of electrolyte metabolism produced by excessive secretion of aldosterone; it may be primary (Conn's syndrome) or occur secondarily in response to extra-adrenal disease. There may be hypertension, hypokalemia, alkalosis, muscular weakness, polyuria and polydipsia. Called also aldosteronism.
hyperaldosteronuria excess of aldosterone in the urine.
hyperalgesia a state of abnormally increased sensitivity to pain or nociceptive stimuli, as occurs under the influence of low doses of barbiturate anesthetic drugs.
hyperalimentation a program of parenteral administration of all nutrients for patients with gastrointestinal dysfunction; called also total parenteral alimentation (TPA) and total parenteral nutrition (TPN).

Although the term *hyperalimentation* is commonly used to designate total or supplemental nutrition by intravenous feedings, it is not technically correct inasmuch as the procedure does not involve an abnormally increased or excessive amount of feeding. For more information, see parenteral NUTRITION, SUPERALIMENTATION.

enteral h. the use of a gastrointestinal tube.

hyperalkalinity excessive alkalinity.

hyperalphalipoproteinemia the presence of abnormally high levels of α-lipoproteins in the serum.

hyperammonemia, hyperammoniemia 1. the presence of ammonia in excess of the normal range of concentration of ammonia in the blood. 2. a metabolic disorder marked by elevated levels of ammonia or ammonium ion in the blood. One of the effects of severe hepatic dysfunction. May cause hepatic encephalopathy.

hyperammoniuria excess of ammonia in the urine.

hyperamylasemia abnormally high levels of amylase in the blood serum.

hyperanakinesia excessive motor activity.

hyperandrogenism a cause of perianal gland hyperplasia and tail gland hyperplasia in male dogs; seborrheic skin disease and alopecia may also occur.

hyperazotemia excess of nitrogenous matter in the blood.

hyperazoturia excess of nitrogenous matter in the urine.

hyperbaric characterized by greater than normal pressure or weight; applied to gases under greater than atmospheric pressure, or to a solution of greater specific gravity than another taken as a standard of reference.

h. oxygenation exposure to oxygen under conditions of greatly increased pressure; abbreviated HPO, for high-pressure oxygenation. This treatment is given to patients who, for various reasons, need more oxygen than they can take in by breathing while in the ordinary atmosphere, or even in an oxygen tent.

hyperbarism a condition due to exposure to ambient gas pressure or atmospheric pressures exceeding the pressure within the body.

hyperbetalipoproteinemia increased accumulation of β-lipoproteins in the blood.

hyperbilirubinemia excess of bilirubin in the blood; classified as conjugated or unconjugated according to the form of bilirubin present. See also JAUNDICE.

congenital h. see GILBERT'S SYNDROME.

hyperbrachycephalic having a very short, wide head.

hyperbradykininemia an excess of bradykinin in the blood.

hypercalcemia excess of calcium in the blood; calcemia due to overdosing with hypervitaminosis D, PSEUDOHYPERPARATHYROIDISM, osteolytic lesions, primary HYPERPARATHYROIDISM, some cases of renal failure, hemoconcentration, hypoadrenocorticism, disuse osteoporosis and some neoplasms.

malignancy-associated h. see PSEUDOHYPERPARATHYROIDISM.

hypercalcemic pertaining to hypercalcemia.

h. nephropathy continuous high blood levels of calcium reduce renal efficiency and may cause mineralization of tubules and then glomeruli.

hypercalcitonism a state in which a high blood calcitonin level is maintained because of abnormalities in the secretion of calcitonin. May be caused by a chronic overfeeding of calcium or functional medullary (C cell) thyroid neoplasms. Leads to a persistent hypocalcemia, arrested bone resorption and osteosclerosis. See also C CELL tumors.

nutritional secondary h. caused in ruminants by a prolonged high-calcium diet, of three to five times the recommended intake, and results in a blocking of normal bone resorption and the development of osteopetrosis and ankylosing spondylosis.

hypercalciuria excess of calcium in the urine.

absorptive h. caused by increased absorption of calcium from the intestine. Blood calcium levels are normal and parathyroid hormone levels are normal or low. May be caused by an excess of vitamin D or hypophosphatemia.

renal leak h. decreased renal resorption of calcium.

resorptive h. results from hypercalcemia with excessive calcium filtration and renal tubular resorption.

hypercapemia hypercapnia.

hypercapnia, hypercarbia excess of carbon dioxide in the blood, indicated by an elevated $P\text{CO}_2$ as determined by BLOOD GAS ANALYSIS, and resulting in respiratory ACIDOSIS.

hypercarbia hypercapnia.

hypercatabolism abnormally high rate of catabolism.

hypercatharsis excessive purgation.

hypercellularity abnormal increase in the number of cells present, as in bone marrow.

hypercementosis abnormal thickening of the cement of the teeth; may affect a few or most of the teeth; often associated with inflammation of the dental root.

hyperchloremia excess of chlorides in the blood; occurs as a result of fluid deficit for which the kidney attempts to compensate by reabsorbing large amounts of water and the chloride dissolved in it. The clinical signs of hyperchloremia are those of ACIDOSIS.

hyperchlorhydria excess of HYDROCHLORIC ACID in the gastric juice.

hyperchloridemia hyperchloremia.

hypercholesterolemia, hypercholesteremia an excess of cholesterol in the blood; a normal finding in lactating cows. Occurs in obstructive jaundice. See also HYPERLIPOPROTEINEMIA.

hypercholia excessive secretion of bile.

hyperchromatism 1. excessive pigmentation. 2. degeneration of cell nuclei, which become filled with particles of pigment, or chromatin. 3. increased staining capacity.

hyperchromatosis hyperchromatism.

hyperchromia 1. hyperchromatism. 2. abnormal increase in the hemoglobin content of erythrocytes.

hyperchylia excessive secretion of gastric juice.

hyperchylomicronemia the presence in the blood of an excessive number of particles of fat (chylomicrons).

hypercoagulability abnormally increased coagulability of the blood.

hypercoagulable characterized by increased coagulability.

hypercontracted sarcomeres basis of the eosinophilic bands seen in coagulative myocytolysis in damaged heart muscle.

hypercorticism hyperadrenocorticism.

hypercortisolism a state of excess production of cortisol; CUSHING'S SYNDROME.

hypercyanotic extremely cyanotic.

hypercythemia excess of erythrocytes in the blood.

hypercytosis an abnormally increased number of cells, especially of leukocytes.

hyperdactylism see POLYDACTYLISM.

hyperdactyly see POLYDACTYLISM.

hyperdicrotic markedly dicrotic.

hyperdistension excessive distension.

hyperdiuresis excessive secretion of urine.

hyperdontia the presence of supernumerary teeth.

hyperdynamia excessive muscular activity.
hyperdynamic endotoxemia the early phase of the disease characterized by increased heart rate and cardiac output; followed by a hypodynamic phase.
hyperechoic producing an increased amplitude of waves returned in ultrasonography; characteristic of bone and dense tumor tissue.
hyperelastosis cutis see HEREDITARY collagen dysplasia.
hyperemesis excessive vomiting.
hyperemia an excess of blood in a part.
active h., arterial h. that due to local or general relaxation of arterioles.
leptomeningeal h. congestion of the pia-arachnoid.
passive h. that due to obstruction to flow of blood from the area.
pulpal h. hyperemia of the tooth pulp.
reactive h. that due to increase in blood flow after its temporary interruption.
venous h. passive hyperemia.
hyperencephalus a monster with the cranial vault absent and the brain exposed.
hypereosinophilia an extreme degree of eosinophilia.
hypereosinophilic syndrome a group of disorders in humans characterized by greatly increased numbers of eosinophils in the blood, mimicking leukemia, and eosinophilic infiltration of many tissues. Eosinophilic enteritis, eosinophilic leukemia, and eosinophilic granuloma complex in cats are similar disorders.
hyperepinephrinemia excessive epinephrine in the blood.
hypererethism extreme irritability.
hyperergasia excessive functional activity.
hyperergia, hyperergy hypersensitivity to allergens.
hypererythrocythemia excess of erythrocytes in the blood; hypercythemia.
hyperesophoria deviation of the visual axes upward and inward.
hyperesthesia a state of abnormally increased sensitivity to stimuli.
h. syndrome used by some to describe a recurring illness with fever, anorexia, reluctance to move and pain on palpation of the abdomen and lumbar spine; of unknown etiology.
idiopathic h. syndrome dogs and especially cats may show an increased sensitivity to being touched or handled, with intense chewing or licking over the sensitive area, which is commonly the back or one or more limbs. No dermatitis is present initially, but it does develop with continuing self-trauma. The cause is usually unknown, but sensory neuropathies, psychogenic factors, arthritis, anal sac disease, tapeworm infestation and psychomotor epilepsy have been suggested. Called also ACRAL lick dermatitis, psychogenic ALOPECIA, feline hyperesthesia syndrome.
hyperesthetic a state of hyperesthesia.
hyperestrinism condition due to excessive secretion of estrin.
hyperestrogenism condition characterized by and caused by excessive secretion or intake of estrogen. See also FEMINIZING SYNDROME, ESTROGENISM.
hyperexcitability excessive mental and physical activity.
hyperexophoria deviation of the visual axes upward and outward.
hyperextensibility see cutaneous ASTHENIA.
hyperextension extension of a limb or part beyond the normal limit.
h. injury see dropped CARPUS.
spinal h. injury usually results in damage to the dorsal articular facets and rupture of the ventral annulus fibrosus with escape of the nucleus pulposus.
hyperferremia excess of iron in the blood.
hyperfibrinogenemia excessive fibrinogen in the blood; fibrinogenemia.
hyperfibrinolysis excessive FIBRINOLYSIS.
hyperfiltration theory increased glomerular capillary pressure and glomerular hypertrophy as adaptive mechanisms in response to increased dietary protein; suggested as a causative factor in progressive chronic renal failure.
hyperflexion flexion of a limb or part beyond the normal limit.
hyperfunction excessive functioning of a part or organ.
hypergalactia, hypergalactosis excessive secretion of milk.
hypergammaglobulinemia increased gamma globulins in the blood.
mink h. see ALEUTIAN MINK DISEASE.
monoclonal h. an increased level of homogeneous immunoglobulin molecules of a single specificity in the blood following proliferation of a clone of immunoglobulin-producing B lymphocytes. See also GAMMOPATHY.
hypergastrinemia an excess of gastrin in the blood. See also ZOLLINGER–ELLISON SYNDROME.
hypergenesis excessive development.
hypergenitalism hypergonadism.
hypergia diminished sensitivity to allergens. See HYPOSENSITIVITY (2), ANERGY.
hyperglandular marked by excessive glandular activity.
hyperglobulia excess of erythrocytes; erythrocytosis; polycythemia.
hyperglobulinemia excess of globulin in the blood.
monoclonal h. see monoclonal GAMMOPATHY.
polyclonal h. see polyclonal GAMMOPATHY.
hyperglucagonemia abnormally high levels of glucagon in the blood.
hyperglucocorticoidism hyperadrenocorticism.
hyperglycemia excess of glucose in the blood.
posthypoglycemic h. see SOMOGYI EFFECT.
hyperglycemic characterized by or causing hyperglycemia.
h. hyperosmolar nonketotic coma (HHNK) a metabolic derangement in which there is an abnormally high serum glucose level without ketoacidosis. It can occur as a complication of borderline and unrecognized DIABETES mellitus, in pancreatic disorders that interfere with the production of insulin, and in conditions marked by an excess of steroids, as in steroid therapy or acute stress conditions.

Hyperosmolality, resulting from the extremely high concentration of sugar in the blood, causes a shift of water from the intracellular fluid (the less concentrated solution) into the blood (the higher concentrated solution). This results in cellular dehydration. Another symptom of HHNK, polyuria, occurs because the high plasma osmolality prevents the normal osmotic return of water to the blood by the renal tubules, and it is excreted in the urine. This leads to a decreased blood volume, which severely hampers the kidney's excretion of glucose and a vicious cycle is begun.
hyperglycemic factor see GLUCAGON.
hyperglyceridemia excess of glycerides in the blood.
hyperglycinemia excessive glycine in the blood.
hyperglycinuria an excess of glycine in the urine.
hyperglycogenolysis excessive splitting up of glycogen (glycogenolysis).

hyperglycorrhachia excessive sugar in the cerebrospinal fluid.
hyperglycosuria extreme glycosuria.
hypergonadism abnormally increased functional activity of the gonads, with excessive growth and precocious sexual development.
hypergranulosis an increased thickness of the stratum granulosum. Seen in skin diseases with epidermal hyperplasia and orthokeratotic hyperkeratosis.
hyperhemoglobinemia an excess of hemoglobin in the blood.
hyperhidrosis excessive sweating.
bovine h. syndrome inherited in Shorthorn cattle and associated with conjunctivitis, pityriasis and digestive disturbances.
hyperhistaminemia an excess of histamine in the blood. See also ZOLLINGER–ELLISON SYNDROME.
paraneoplastic h. associated with mast cell tumors which may release histamine spontaneously or in response to manipulation of the tissue. Seen most commonly in dogs.
hyperhydration abnormally increased water content of the body.
hypericin the exogenous photodynamic agent in HYPERICUM *perforatum*—St. John's wort.
hypericism poisoning by HYPERICIN.
Hypericum a genus of the Clusiaceae (syn. Guttiferae) family of plants; contain the photosensitizing agent hypericin causing primary photosensitive dermatitis; includes *H. aethiopicum*, *H. lanceolatum*, *H. leucoptychodes*, *H. perforatum* (amber, goat weed, St. Johns wort, Klamath weed), *H. revolutum* (forest primrose), *H. triquetrifolium* (curled-leaved St. Johns wort).
hyperidrosis hyperhidrosis.
hyperimmune possessing very large quantities of specific antibodies in the serum.
h. serum serum especially prepared for temporary passive protection or treatment of animals. Commercial preparation is by repeated injections of the selected antigens.
hyperimmunization repeated injections of antigen leading to high levels of antibody.
hyperimmunoglobulinemia abnormally high levels of immunoglobulins in the serum. Called also hypergammaglobulinemia.
hyperinflation excessive inflation or expansion, as of the lungs; overinflation.
hyperinsulinism 1. excessive secretion of insulin by the pancreas, resulting in hypoglycemia. See also INSULINOMA. 2. insulin shock from overdosage of insulin.
hyperinvolution superinvolution.
hyperirritability pathological responsiveness to slight stimuli.
hyperisotonic denoting a solution containing more than 0.45% salt, in which erythrocytes become crenated as a result of exosmosis. Called also hypertonic.
hyperkalemia abnormally high potassium concentration in the blood, most often due to defective renal excretion, as in kidney disease, severe and extensive burns, intestinal obstruction, diabetes mellitus, acute renal failure and hypoadrenocorticism.

High blood potassium levels can produce electrocardiographic abnormalities evident first as elevated T waves and depressed P waves, and eventually by atrial asystole. Other clinical signs include muscular weakness and a slow irregular pulse. As the amount of serum potassium continues to rise there is potential for respiratory paralysis, asystole or ventricular fibrillation, and cardiac arrest.

hyperkalemic periodic paralysis inherited defect in Quarter horses, characterized by intermittent, self-limiting episodes of muscular fasciculation and weakness to the point of recumbency, accompanied by temporary hyperkalemia; called also episodic muscular weakness.
hyperkeratinization excessive development of keratin in the epidermis.
hyperkeratosis 1. hypertrophy of the horny layer (stratum corneum) of the skin, or any disease characterized by it; the hyperkeratoses may have distinctive formats, e.g. annular (ring formations), basket-weave, compact, laminated. 2. hypertrophy of the cornea.
bovine h. CHLORINATED NAPHTHALENE poisoning.
digital h. increased thickness of the keratinized epidermis of footpads in dogs and rarely cats. May be in response to trauma or associated with distemper (hardpad disease), or PEMPHIGUS foliaceus.
epidermolytic h. a form of ichthyosis in humans which is inherited as an autosomal dominant trait; there is severe degeneration of the granular layer of the epidermis.
juvenile h. a crusting dermatosis over bony prominences, face and chin of young dogs. See zinc-responsive DERMATOSIS.
nasal h. an abnormal thickening, sometimes with fissures, of the planum nasale of dogs. May occur in association with digital hyperkeratosis (see above) as a feature of distemper (hardpad disease). Also seen in PEMPHIGUS foliaceus and discoid LUPUS ERYTHEMATOSUS.
nasodigital h. see nasal hyperkeratosis, digital hyperkeratosis (above).
orthokeratotic h. hyperkeratosis with non-nucleated cells present.
parakeratotic h. hyperkeratosis with nucleated cells present; called also PARAKERATOSIS.
hyperketonemia abnormally increased concentration of ketone bodies in the blood.
hyperketonuria excessive ketone in the urine.
hyperketosis excessive formation of ketone.
hyperkinemia abnormally high cardiac output.
hyperkinesia abnormally increased motor function or activity. See also HYPERACTIVITY.
hyperkinesis hyperkinesia.
hyperkinetic pertaining to or marked by hyperkinesia.
h. episodes see Scottie CRAMP.
h. circulatory disorders cardiovascular disorders characterized by increased cardiac output; includes hyperthyroidism, chronic anemia and arteriovenous fistulas.
hyperlactatemia increased levels of lactic acid in the blood.
hyperlactation lactation in greater than normal amount or for a longer than normal period.
hyperleukocytosis excess of leukocytes in the blood.
hyperlipasemia excessive amounts of lipase in the blood.
hyperlipemia an excess of lipids in the blood.
equine h. a metabolic disease of pony mares in late pregnancy or early lactation. The serum has milky opalescence. Clinically there is lethargy progressing to coma, diarrhea and acidosis. Most cases terminate fatally.
hyperlipidemia a general term for elevated concentrations of any or all of the lipids in the plasma. See also HYPERLIPOPROTEINEMIA.
postprandial h. a normal increase following ingestion of food.
primary h. caused by decreased activity of lipoprotien lipase, it occurs in miniature Schnauzer dogs.

secondary h. may occur in association with diabetes mellitus, hypothyroidism, pancreatitis, hyperadrenocorticism, cholestatic liver disease and nephrotic syndrome.

hyperlipoproteinemia an excess of lipoproteins in the blood, which is due to a disorder of lipoprotein metabolism, and may be acquired or hereditary. The acquired form occurs secondarily to another disorder or as a result of environmental factors (e.g. diet) and occurs most commonly in dogs in association with primary hypothyroidism. The hereditary form in humans is classified into five major phenotypes based on clinical features, enzymatic abnormalities and serum lipoprotein electrophoretic patterns. In animals a familial form may occur in Beagles, miniature Schnauzers and cats. A heritable hyperlipoproteinemia occurs in a certain strain of White Leghorn chickens and a hypercholesterolemic strain of pigeons has been developed.

hyperliposis excess of fat in the blood serum or tissues.

hyperlithuria excess of uric (lithic) acid in the urine.

hyperlysinemia elevated levels of lysine in the blood.

hypermagnesemia an abnormally large magnesium content of the blood plasma.

hypermastia 1. excessive size of mammary glands. 2. the presence of one or more supernumerary mammary glands; polymastia.

hypermelanosis hyperpigmentation.

hypermetabolic state experiencing HYPERMETABOLISM.

hypermetabolism increased metabolism. Occurs during periods of stress and with many diseases. There is increased peripheral insulin resistance, increased protein catabolism and a negative nitrogen balance.

extrathyroidal h. abnormally elevated basal metabolism unassociated with thyroid disease.

hypermetria ataxia in which movements overreach the intended goal.

hypermetropia farsightedness; hyperopia. The opposite of myopia.

hypermineralized primer early, densely mineralized, woven bone.

hypermobility excessive mobility, as of a joint.

hypermotility excessive or abnormally increased motility.

gut h. decreased transit time for the entire alimentary tract.

intestinal h. is characterized by increase in gut sounds, spasms of pain, e.g. in spasmodic COLIC in horses and, in some cases, diarrhea.

hypermyotonia excessive muscular tonicity.

hypermyotrophy excessive development of muscular tissue.

hypernatremia an excess of SODIUM in the blood, indicative of water loss exceeding the sodium loss.

hypernatriuria excessive amounts of sodium in the urine.

hyperneocytosis leukocytosis with an excessive number of immature forms of leukocytes.

hypernephroma carcinoma of the kidney whose cells resemble those from the adrenal cortex.

hypernutrition overfeeding and its ill effects.

hyperonychia hypertrophy of the claws.

hyperopia hypermetropia.

hyperorchidism abnormally increased functional activity of the testes.

hyperorexia excessive appetite.

hyperorthocytosis leukocytosis with a normal proportion of the various forms of leukocytes.

hyperosmolality an increase in the osmolality of the body fluids.

hyperosmolar pertaining to or emanating from hyperosmolality.

h. nonketotic coma coma due to hyperosmolality, e.g. hyperglycemia in some diabetic patients. See also HYPERGLYCEMIC hyperosmolar nonketotic coma.

h. nonketotic diabetes diabetes characterized by high blood levels of glucose but without significantly increased blood levels of ketone bodies.

hyperosmolarity abnormally increased osmotic concentration of a solution.

hyperosmotic pertaining to hyperosmolarity.

h. state condition caused by the accumulation in the body of significant quantities of osmotically active solutes, e.g. hypernatremia, hyperglycemia. See also HYPEROSMOLALITY.

hyperostosis excessive growth of bony tissue.

craniomandibular h. see CRANIOMANDIBULAR osteopathy.

diffuse idiopathic skeletal h. occurs in dogs and pigs; cause unknown, possibly familial in pigs; extensive bone deposition around joints but articular surfaces not affected.

facial h. in hyperparathyroidism resorption of cancellous bone, particularly maxillae and mandibles, and the formation of poorly mineralized osteoid and excessive fibro-osseous tissue cause deformities of the face and head that are clinically obvious and may prevent closure of the mouth. Occurs in primary and secondary HYPERPARATHYROIDISM.

inherited congenital h. see juvenile hyperostosis (below).

juvenile h. a congenital defect of pigs. The legs of affected newborn pigs are swollen below the elbow. The piglets have difficulty standing and moving around. The bone is thick and the periosteum rough and there is extensive edema. Called also thick forelegs, inherited congenital hyperostosis.

hyperoxaluria an excess of oxalate in the urine; occurs in dogs in association with oxalate urolith formation.

primary h. inherited metabolic defect in cats. Characterized by heavy deposits of oxalates in renal tubules, leading to oxalate nephrosis and fatal uremia before the patient reaches a year of age.

hyperoxemia excessive acidity of the blood.

hyperoxia an abnormally increased supply or concentration of oxygen.

hyperparasite a parasite that preys on a parasite.

hyperparathormonemia increased level of parathyroid hormone in the blood.

hyperparathyroidism abnormally increased activity of the parathyroid gland. *Primary* hyperparathyroidism is associated with either neoplasia (chiefly adenomas) or hyperplasia.

An excess of parathyroid hormone leads to resorption of bone, increased resorption of calcium and increased excretion of phosphorus by the renal tubules, and increased absorption of calcium by the gastrointestinal mucosa. It may result in *kidney stones* and calcium deposits in the renal tubules; in generalized decalcification of bone (*osteoporosis*), resulting in pain and tenderness of bones and spontaneous fractures; and in *hypercalcemia*, leading to muscular weakness and gastrointestinal signs.

Secondary hyperparathyroidism develops as a compensatory mechanism when the serum calcium level is persistently below normal or serum phosphorus is elevated, as in chronic renal disease, insufficient calcium or excessive phosphorus in the diet, vitamin D deficiency, low-level soluble oxalate intoxication in horses, and intestinal malabsorption syndromes causing insufficient absorption of calcium and vitamin D.

See also PSEUDOHYPERPARATHYROIDISM.

nutritional secondary h. a disease of horses, pigs, goats, dogs, cats, and rarely cattle. It is most commonly caused by an excessive dietary intake of phosphorus in the absence of adequate calcium, which in horses is likely to be the result of a diet mainly of grain and in dogs and cats one predominantly of meat, but it may also result from other dietary causes of secondary hyperparathyroidism. In most species there is swelling of the maxillae and mandibles which is most marked in horses, loosening of teeth, shifting lameness, and particularly in dogs and cats, weight-bearing skeletal deformities (ANGEL WINGS) and folding or compression fractures. Called also miller's disease, bran disease, bighead, Siamese cat disease, paper-bone disease.

renal secondary h. caused by chronic renal dysfunction, mostly in dogs, sometimes in cats, in which there is a secondary hyperparathyroidism, caused by the retention of phosphates. There is demineralization of bones, particularly the maxillae and mandibles, with loosening of teeth and facial swelling. Clinical signs are often overshadowed by the effects of the renal failure. Called also rubber jaw, renal rickets, renal osteitis fibrosa.

hyperpathia abnormally exaggerated subjective response to painful stimuli.

h. test pressure over the transverse processes or dorsal spinous processes of the lumbar and thoracic vertebrae will cause tensing of the abdominal muscles at the level of a spinal cord lesion.

hyperpepsinia excessive secretion of pepsin in the stomach.

hyperperistalsis excessively active peristalsis.

hyperphagia ingestion of more than the normal amount of food.

hyperphalangism the presence of a supernumerary phalanx on a digit.

hyperphonesis intensification of the sound in auscultation or percussion.

hyperphoria permanent upward deviation of the visual axis of an eye in the absence of visual fusional stimuli. Called also heterophoria.

hyperphosphatasemia high levels of alkaline phosphatase in the blood.

hyperphosphatemia an excess of phosphates in the blood.

hyperphosphaturia an excess of phosphates in the urine.

hyperpigmentation abnormally increased pigmentation.

hyperpituitarism a condition due to pathologically increased PITUITARY gland activity, especially increased secretion of growth hormone, resulting in acromegaly or gigantism.

hyperplasia abnormal increase in volume of a tissue or organ caused by the formation and growth of new normal cells. Categorized as irregular, papillated, regular. See also MYOFIBER hyperplasia.

myofiber h. see MYOFIBER hyperplasia.

papillated epidermal h. increased thickness of the epidermis with projections above the surface of the skin.

pseudocarcinomatous epidermal h. extreme, irregular thickening of the epidermis with increased mitoses, squamous eddies, and horn pearls which may mimic squamous cell carcinoma.

psoriasiform h. has clubbed and fused rete ridges seen in epitheliotropic lymphoma, PSORIASIFORM-lichenoid dermatosis of English springer spaniel dogs, parapsoriasis and ACRAL lick dermatitis.

hyperplasmia 1. excess in the proportion of blood plasma to corpuscles. 2. increase in size of erythrocytes through absorption of plasma.

hyperplasminemia increased levels of plasmin in the blood.

hyperplastic characterized by a state of hyperplasia, e.g. hyperplastic enteritis, hyperplastic cholangitis, hyperplastic endometritis, hyperplastic gingivitis.

hyperploid 1. characterized by hyperploidy. 2. a hyperploid individual or cell.

hyperploidy the state of having more than the typical number of chromosomes in unbalanced sets.

hyperpnea abnormal increase in depth and rate of respiration but not to the point of being labored, the critical point for dyspnea.

hyperpnoea see HYPERPNEA.

hyperpolarization an increase in the amount of electrical charge on either side of a cell membrane so that there is an increase in the electric potential across the membrane.

hyperponesis excessive action-potential output from the motor and premotor areas of the cerebral cortex.

hyperposia abnormally increased ingestion of fluids for relatively brief periods.

hyperpotassemia excess of potassium in the blood. Occurs in renal failure, adrenocortical insufficiency and gastrointestinal disorders and contributes to reduced cardiac efficiency and muscle weakness. See also HYPERKALEMIA.

hyperpragic characterized by excessive activity.

hyperpraxia abnormal activity; restlessness.

hyperprogesteronism a state caused by excessive production or intake of progesterone, e.g. in retained or cystic corpora lutea. Some hyperprogestinic states are cystic glandular hyperplasia of the endometrium in bitches and pseudocyesis.

hyperproinsulinemia the presence of proinsulin in excess of normal concentrations in the blood.

hyperprolactinemia increased levels of prolactin in the blood; occurs in severe hypothyroidism, caused by excessive thyrotropin-releasing hormone. Galactorrhea and anestrus results.

hyperproteinemia an excess of protein in the blood.

hyperproteosis a condition due to excess of protein in the diet.

hyperptyalism abnormally increased secretion of saliva.

hyperpyrexia excessively high fever; hyperthermia.

See also FEVER (1).

malignant h. see PORCINE stress syndrome.

hyperreactive showing a greater than normal response to stimuli.

hyperreflexia exaggeration of reflexes.

detrusor h. involuntary contraction of the detrusor muscle; a cause of urge INCONTINENCE.

hyperreninemia elevated levels of renin in the blood.

hyperresonance exaggerated resonance on percussion.

hypersalemia abnormally increased content of salt in the blood.

hypersalivation abnormally increased secretion of saliva.

hypersecretion excessive secretion, e.g. of hormones.

hypersegmentation excessive subdivision into lobes or segments, e.g. hypersegmented neutrophils.

hypersensitivity 1. a state of altered reactivity in

which the body reacts with an exaggerated immune response to a foreign agent; ALLERGY is a synonym for hypersensitivity. ANAPHYLAXIS is a form of hypersensitivity.

There are four basic types of hypersensitivity reactions: *Type I* (called also immediate hypersensitivity) involves cell-fixed antibody, mainly IgE attached to mast cells or basophils. Antigen binding causes the cell to release vasoactive factors. The basis for anaphylaxis and atopy. *Type II* causes cell destruction (cytotoxicity) by the action of immunoglobulin with complement or cytotoxic cells. Seen in red blood cell transfusion reactions and in alloimmune hemolytic anemia. See also ANTIBODY-dependent cellular cytotoxicity. *Type III* (called also immune-complex or subacute hypersensitivity) causes tissue damage and inflammation by the deposition of antigen–antibody complexes that activate complement and attract polymorphonuclear cells. *Type IV* (called also delayed hypersensitivity) involves sensitized T lymphocytes that react with cell bound or associated antigen and release lymphokines, causing mononuclear cell accumulation, tissue damage and inflammation, typically manifesting at least 24 hours after exposure to the antigen.

2. a state of increased responsivity to physical stimuli.

h. angiitis variant of polyarteritis nodosa; a disease of small blood vessels in humans; called also leukocytoclastic vasculitis.

antibody-mediated h. types I, II and III hypersensitivity reactions. Called also immediate hypersensitivity.

bacterial h. immune responses to bacteria or bacterial products may contribute to the clinical features of some diseases, e.g. the anemia associated with salmonellosis, arthritis in erysipelas of pigs, intestinal lesions in Johne's disease, or be the principal cause as in staphylococcal hypersensitivity dermatitis in dogs.

contact h. a type IV reaction produced by contact of the skin with a low-molecular-weight chemical substance having the properties of a hapten in a sensitized individual; it includes ALLERGIC contact dermatitis.

cutaneous basophil h. a delayed inflammatory response characterized by large numbers of basophils.

cytotoxic h. type II hypersensitivity.

delayed h. type IV reaction. A slowly developing cell-mediated immune response in which T helper 1 lymphocytes respond to specific antigen by releasing cytokines, some of which activate macrophages, as occurs in tuberculin reaction, graft rejection, some autoimmune diseases, etc.

drug h. may be either an immediate (antibody mediated) or delayed type (T lymphocyte mediated) reaction. See also DRUG eruption.

flea bite h. see FLEA allergy dermatitis.

food h. hypersensitivity reaction to various dietary constituents has been the suspected cause of allergic dermatitis in most species, but conclusive evidence is often lacking. It may also result in diarrhea.

fungal h. may contribute to the clinical features of cutaneous fungal infections, particularly KERION formation. It is also the basis for skin testing for systemic mycoses, e.g. histoplasmin and coccidioidin.

helminth h. occurs, e.g. the self-cure phenomenon, and the allergic response of a sensitized animal to an invasion, e.g. of lungs, causes massive pulmonary edema.

immediate h. antibody-mediated hypersensitivity, i.e. types I, II and III, characterized by a response that appears within minutes to hours, resulting either from a release of histamine and other mediators of hypersensitivity from IgE-sensitized mast cells, causing increased vascular permeability, edema and smooth muscle contraction (type I), from antibody-mediated lysis of red blood cells (type II), or from immune complex mediated pathology (type III).

immune complex h. type III hypersensitivity (above).

mold h. see ACUTE bovine pulmonary emphysema–edema.

h. pneumonitis see hypersensitivity PNEUMONITIS.

staphylococcal h. see bacterial hypersensitivity (above).

h. threshold a theory that certain levels of allergens may be tolerated by some sensitized individuals without manifestations of disease, but a slight increase in the level precipitates clinical signs.

tuberculin type h. the classical T lymphocyte cell–mediated hypersensitivity associated with mycobacterium infection or immunization with antigens containing Freund's adjuvant.

hypersensitization the induction of hypersensitivity.

hypersexuality see MOUNTING behavior.

hypersialism hypersialosis.

hypersialosis excessive secretion of the salivary glands; in animals, drooling.

hypersomatotropism acromegaly.

hypersomnia pathologically excessive sleep or drowsiness.

hypersplenism a condition characterized by splenomegaly and exaggeration of the phagocytic function of the spleen, resulting in deficiency of peripheral blood elements, and often by hypercellularity of the bone marrow.

hypersthenia increased strength or tonicity.

hypersthenuria excessive osmolality of the urine.

hypertelorism abnormally increased distance between two organs or parts.

ocular h., orbital h. increase in the interocular distance.

hypertensinogen angiotensinogen.

hypertension persistently high blood pressure. Detected sporadically in animals partly due to the technical difficulties in diagnosis and the lack of recognizable signs. Greyhounds normally have a higher blood pressure than is found in crossbred dogs with features resembling essential hypertension in humans. Secondary hypertension due to advanced renal disease, hyperthyroidism and hyperadrenocorticism does occur in dogs and cats. Temporary episodes of hypertension occur in all animals suffering severe pain, and in horses with acute laminitis.

endocrine h. that occurring in association with diseases of the endocrine glands.

Goldblatt h. see Goldblatt KIDNEY.

inherited h. see rat hypertension (below).

neurogenic h. produced experimentally in laboratory animals by the imposition of surgical and psychological insults on the central nervous system.

ocular h. persistently elevated intraocular pressure in the absence of any other signs of glaucoma; it may or may not progress to chronic simple glaucoma.

portal h. abnormally increased pressure in the portal circulation caused by impedance of blood flow through a diseased liver or portal vein.

pulmonary h. results from high-pressure blood flow from the right ventricle or impedance to blood flow through the lungs or through the left heart. Chronic hypertension causes endothelial degeneration and fibroplasia of vessel walls. The end result may be cor pulmonale or pulmonary edema. See also ALTITUDE SICKNESS, COR pulmonale.

rat h. several strains of spontaneously hypertensive rats have been bred.

renal h. secondary hypertension.

systemic venous h. elevation of systemic venous pressure, usually detected by inspection of the jugular veins.

hypertensive characterized by or causing increased tension or pressure, as abnormally high blood pressure.

hypertensor a substance that raises the blood pressure.

hypertestosteronemia see HYPERANDROGENISM.

hypertext information which contains both formatting instructions and links to other documents.

h. markup language set of codes embedded in a hypertext document which give instructions to the browser about the formatting of the document. Called also HTML.

h. transfer protocol provides the set of rules used by one computer to obtain an HTML (hypertext markup language) document from another.

hyperthecosis hyperplasia and excessive luteinization of the cells of the inner stromal layer of the ovary.

hyperthelia the presence of supernumerary nipples or teats.

hyperthermalgesia abnormal sensitiveness to heat.

hyperthermia 1. greatly increased body temperature. May have effect as TERATOGEN. 2. heat therapy. Used in the treatment of tumors, often in conjunction with chemotherapy or radiation. Whole body, regional or localized hyperthermia is induced with electromagnetic radiation, radiofrequency current heating or ULTRASONIC heating.

epidemic h. poisoning by ACREMONIUM *corenophialum*.

idiopathic h. term applied in error to the effects of ergotism under conditions of high ambient temperature. See also rye ERGOT, ACREMONIUM *coenophialum*.

malignant h. a drug induced stress syndrome of pigs which have been treated with halothane or suxamethonium. Isolated cases have been reported in dogs and cats. The clinical syndrome includes muscle rigidity and hyperthermia. It is fatal and susceptibility to it is inherited. See also PORCINE stress syndrome.

hyperthermic ergotism a lesser syndrome in poisoning of cattle by *Claviceps purpurea* characterized by fever, salivation, dramatic fall in herd milk yield.

hyperthrombinemia an excess of thrombin in the blood.

hyperthymism excessive thymus activity.

hyperthyroidism excessive functional activity of the thyroid gland. Rare in animals except in aged dogs and cats where it is associated with functional thyroid neoplasms.

Affected animals show increased thirst, weight loss despite an increased appetite, restlessness and cardiac arrhythmias.

apathetic h. a small percentage of hyperthyroidic cats show, lethargy, depression and anorexia; may be due to associated dysfunction.

hyperthyroxinemia an excess of thyroxine in the blood.

hypertonia abnormally increased tonicity or strength.

h. oculi high intraocular pressure; glaucoma.

hypertonic 1. pertaining to or characterized by an increased tonicity or tension. 2. having an osmotic pressure greater than that of the solution with which it is compared.

h. dehydration occurs when the body loss or deprivation is of water only, i.e. there is no electrolyte loss.

h. saline test see HICKEY–HARE TEST.

hypertonicity the state or quality of being hypertonic.

hypertrichiasis, hypertrichosis excessive hairiness; hirsutism.

hypertriglyceridemia an excess of triglycerides in the blood; seen in fatty liver syndrome in cats.

hypertrophic characterized by a state of hypertrophy.

h. pulmonary osteoarthropathy see hypertrophic OSTEOPATHY.

h. scar a protruding scar resembling a fibroma or collagen nevus.

hypertrophy increase in volume of a tissue or organ produced entirely by enlargement of existing cells.

brown h. of cere CERE hypertrophy.

ventricular h. hypertrophy of the myocardium of a ventricle, causing abnormal deviation of the axis of the electrocardiogram.

hypertropia STRABISMUS in which there is permanent upward deviation of the visual axis of one eye.

hyperuricemia an excess of uric acid in the blood; found in Dalmatian dogs and selected strains of chickens.

hyperuricosuria an excess of uric acid in the urine.

hypervariable region regions present on light and heavy chains of immunoglobulins where most of the variation in amino acid sequences occurs. These are also sites of antigen binding.

hypervascular extremely vascular.

hyperventilation 1. increase of air in the lungs above the normal amount. 2. abnormally prolonged and deep breathing, usually associated with acute anxiety or emotional tension. A transient, respiratory ALKALOSIS commonly results from hyperventilation. More prolonged hyperventilation may be caused by disorders of the central nervous system, or by drugs.

h. syndrome nervous or hyperexcitable dogs may hyperventilate to the point of syncope.

hyperviscosity excessive viscosity, as of the blood.

h. syndrome increased viscosity of the blood occurs with IgM and IgA myelomas because of the high levels of macroglobulins; causes increased resistance to blood, hypoxia, organ failure, retinal lesions, abnormalities in platelet function, coagulation defects and cardiac failure.

hypervitaminosis a condition produced by ingestion or injection of excessive amounts of vitamins; symptom complexes are associated with excessive intake of vitamins A and D.

h. A occurs mainly in cats, and is caused by a long-term diet consisting almost entirely of liver. Affected cats show neck pain and stiffness caused by a deforming cervical spondylosis. Other joints may be similarly affected. There is also hyperesthesia, irritability, anorexia, weight loss, and sometimes neurological deficits. Premature loss of teeth has also been reported.

h. D caused by overdosing with vitamin D preparations as in milk fever prophylaxis and inappropriate treatment of disorders of dietary calcium and phosphorus, by errors in a diet mix, and oversupplementation of small puppies and kittens. Causes dystrophic soft tissue calcification, particularly nephrocalcinosis with subsequent renal failure. See also ENZOOTIC calcinosis.

hypervolemia abnormal increase in the volume of circulating fluid (plasma) in the body. See also FLUID volume excess.

hypesthesia abnormally diminished sensitiveness; hypoesthesia.

hypha pl. *hyphae* [L.] one of the filaments composing the mycelium of a fungus.
spiral h. hyphae which end in a coil; typical of *Trichophyton* spp.
hyphema, hyphemia hemorrhage into the anterior chamber of the eye.
hyphidrosis scanty sweating.
Hyphomyces destruens now called *Pythium insidiosum*.
Hyphomycetes the mycelial (hyphal) fungi, i.e. the molds.
hyphomycosis 1. infection with fungi of the genus *Hyphomyces*. 2. infection with hyphomycetes (imperfect fungi).
A skin disease of horses and mules caused by infection with *Hyphomyces destruens*. It is marked by the formation of subcutaneous abscesses which ulcerate leaving large, raw surfaces. See also SWAMP CANCER. Called also oomycosis.
hypnagogic producing sleep.
hypnagogue 1. hypnotic; inducing sleep. 2. an agent that produces sleep.
hypn(o)- word element. [Gr.] *sleep, hypnosis*.
hypnolepsy narcolepsy.
hypnosis an artificially induced state of passivity. In animals an immobility reflex can be induced with varying ease in the different species. It has some similarity to the hypnotic state in humans.
animal h. can be induced by dopamine-receptor blockers or by restraint or visual fixation; guinea pigs, rabbits and chickens are most susceptible.
hypnotic 1. pertaining to or inducing hypnosis or sleep. 2. an agent that induces sleep.
hypo 1. a colloquial abbreviation of hypodermic. 2. sodium thiosulfate, used as a photographic fixing agent.
hypo- word element. [Gr.] *abnormally decreased, deficient, beneath, under*.
hypoacidity decreased acidity.
hypoadrenal corticalism negative hormonal state in premature foals; conducive to early demise.
hypoadrenalism deficiency of adrenal activity, as in Addison's disease.
hypoadrenocorticism diminished hormone production from the cortex of the adrenal gland. In all species, injury to the gland may occur from hemorrhage, mineralization, amyloid deposition, or invasion by infectious agents but clinical signs of insufficiency rarely occur except in the dog.
immune-mediated h. see primary hypoadrenocorticism (see below).
primary h. occurs most often in dogs, usually the result of an idiopathic atrophy of the adrenal glands involving all layers of the cortex. Immune-mediated mechanisms are suspected. The clinical effects are related to insufficient production of mineralocorticoids causing hyponatremia, hypochloremia and hyperkalemia. Hypovolemia, prerenal azotemia and cardiac conduction abnormalities lead to weakness, vomiting, diarrhea and bradycardia. Deficiency of glucocorticoids may also cause hypoglycemia. Called also Addison's disease, immune-mediated hypoadrenocorticism.
secondary h. lesions of the pituitary and, more commonly in dogs, the long-term administration of corticosteroids which causes a reduced secretion of ACTH and leads to reduced synthesis and low blood levels of glucocorticoids. Mineralocorticoid levels remain normal.
hypoalbuminemia abnormally low levels of albumin in the blood.
hypoalbuminosis the condition of having an abnormally low level of albumin in the blood.
hypoaldosteronism deficiency of aldosterone in the body.
hypoalimentation insufficient nourishment.
hypoandrogenism a deficiency of androgens in the body leading to a lack of virility and sexual potency. See also FEMINIZING SYNDROME, TESTOSTERONE-responsive dermatosis.
hypoazoturia diminished nitrogenous material in the urine.
hypobaric characterized by less than normal pressure or weight; applied to gases under less than atmospheric pressure, or to solutions of lower specific gravity than another taken as a standard of reference.
hypobaropathy the disturbances experienced at high altitudes due to reduced air pressure and lack of oxygen; altitude sickness.
hypobasemia a low blood concentration of buffer bases.
hypobilirubinemia abnormally low level of bilirubin in the blood.
hypobiosis arrested stage of development, as of nematode larvae in the gut mucosa of the definitive host. See also DIAPAUSE.
hypobiotinosis experimental nutritional deficiency of biotin causes posterior paralysis in calves; natural deficiency causes lameness due to poor hoof horn in gilts and sows.
hypoblast the entoderm.
hypocalcemia total serum calcium levels are lower than normal; both ionized calcium (physiologically active form) and nonionized calcium are depressed.
acute puerperal h. called also bovine parturient hypocalcemia; see MILK fever.
bovine parturient h. see MILK fever.
nonparetic parturient h. milk fever without recumbency in recently calved cows; inappetence, drop in milk production, alimentary tract stasis, reduced rumination; responds to treatment with parenteral injections of calcium solution.
non-parturient h. hypocalcemia, with or without clinical signs of staggery gait, recumbency, ruminal response which responds to treatment with parenteral calcium, occurring as incidents detached from parturient ruminants. A standard experience as mare eclampsia. In ruminants occurs as part of acute oxalate poisoning, sudden change to lush feed in heavily milking cows.
nutritional h. occurs most commonly in dogs and cats fed all-meat diets. See also ALL-MEAT SYNDROME.
ovine h. occurs at a high morbidity rate in lactating ewes subjected to bad weather or any other cause of reduced feed intake. The syndrome is similar to that in MILK fever in cows, but occurs also in young sheep on meager rations, those grazing lush green cereal crops or pastures heavily contaminated by oxalate-bearing plants.
periparturient h. in ruminants hypocalcemia is most common in the immediate postparturient period due to the drain of lactation and inadequate parathyroid gland response and nutritional supply. In bitches and mares hypocalcemia occurs most commonly later in lactation. See also MILK fever, LACTATION TETANY (3), soluble OXALATE poisoning, puerperal TETANY.
renal h. chronic hypocalcemia due to chronic renal disease.
hypocalcemic emanating from hypocalcemia; state of elevation of blood calcium level.
h. factor see CALCITONIN.
h. paresis see MILK fever, ovine HYPOCALCEMIA.

h. tetany tetany of limbs, muscle tremor, tetanic convulsions occur in hypocalcemia in bitches and mares. See also ECLAMPSIA, LACTATION TETANY (2).
hypocalciuria an abnormally diminished amount of calcium in the urine.
hypocapemia hypocapnia.
hypocapnia diminished carbon dioxide in the blood.
hypocarbia hypocapnia.
hypocellularity abnormal decrease in the number of cells present, as in bone marrow.
hypochloremia an abnormally low level of chloride in the blood; clinical signs are those of ALKALOSIS. Occurs most commonly in enteritis, acute intestinal obstruction and continued vomiting and, in ruminants with abomasal dilatation, impaction and torsion. The hydrogen chloride and potassium ions normally absorbed by the small intestine are lost to the animal. A hypochloremic, hypokalemic alkalosis results.
hypochlorhydria deficiency of hydrochloric acid in the gastric juice.
hypochloridemia hypochloremia.
hypochlorite any salt of hydrochlorous acid. The sodium salt is used as a germicidal agent when mixed in dilute solution. See also SODIUM hypochlorite.
hypochlorization reduction of sodium chloride in the diet.
hypochlorous acid an unstable compound used as a disinfectant and bleaching agent.
hypochloruria diminished chloride content in the urine.
Hypochoeris radicata toxic plant in the family Asteraceae; contains an unidentified toxin; probably causes Australian stringhalt. Called also flatweed, catsear.
hypocholesterolemia, hypocholesteremia low level of cholesterol in the blood.
hypocholinosis see CHOLINE nutritional deficiency.
hypochondrium the cranial abdominal region on either side of the costal arch.
hypochondrodysplasia abnormal (deficient) cartilage growth. See also CHONDRODYSPLASIA.
hypochondroplasia chondrodysplasia.
hypochromasia 1. staining less intensely than normal. 2. decrease of hemoglobin in erythrocytes so that they are abnormally pale.
hypochromatism abnormally deficient pigmentation, especially deficiency of chromatin in a cell nucleus.
hypochromatosis the gradual fading and disappearance of the nucleus (the chromatin) of a cell.
hypochromia 1. hypochromatism. 2. decrease of hemoglobin in the erythrocytes so that they are abnormally pale.
hypochromic effect the decrease in the absorbance of UV (~260 nm) that accompanies the denaturation (melting) of DNA and used to monitor the process.
hypochylia deficiency of chyle.
hypocitruria abnormally low levels of citric acid in urine; observed in dogs in association with calcium oxalate uroliths.
hypocleidium the flattened plate in birds interposed between the clavicles at their ventral extremities, and connected to the sternum.
hypocomplementemia diminution of complement levels in the blood. An inherited defect in Finnish-Landrace sheep.
hypocorticism hypoadrenocorticism.
hypocortisolemia abnormally low level of cortisol in the blood.
hypocrinism a state due to deficient secretion of an endocrine gland.
hypocupremia abnormally diminished concentration of copper in the blood.
hypocuprosis disease state caused by abnormally low level of copper in the blood.
hypocyanocobalaminosis see VITAMIN B_{12}.
hypocythemia deficiency in the number of erythrocytes in the blood.
hypodactyly less than the usual number of digits on the limb extremity.
Hypoderaerum a genus of the family Echinostomatidae of flukes.
H. conoideum found in the terminal portion of the small intestine of pigeon, fowl and most aquatic birds. It causes localized enteritis in ducks.
Hypoderma a genus of flies, whose larvae invade tissues causing damage to tissue, and to the skin as they emerge through it. Members of the family Oestridae.
H. actaeon a central European fly.
H. aeratum found in sheep and goats,
***H. bovis, H. lineatum* (syn. *H. lineata*)** hairy flies about 0.5 inch long, which parasitize cattle, bison and rarely horses. The larvae cause warbles under the skin and an emission puncture to mar the hide of the animal.
H. capreola found in roe deer.
H. crossi found in goats and sheep.
H. diana found in red deer and roe deer.
H. moschiferi found in musk deer.
H. silenus attacks horses and goats.
hypodermiasis a creeping eruption of the skin in humans and cattle caused by the larvae of *Hypoderma* spp.
hypodermic 1. beneath the skin; injected into subcutaneous tissues. 2. a hypodermic, or subcutaneous, injection; a hypodermic syringe.
hypodermis subcutis.
hypodermoclysis the introduction into the subcutaneous tissues of fluids, especially physiological sodium chloride solution, in large quantity. The most common sites for insertion of the needles for hypodermoclysis are over the sides of the rib cages and the loose tissue in each upper flank. This method of introducing fluids into the body is contraindicated in cases of edema, and it may be complicated by abscess formation, puncture of a large blood vessel, and necrosis and sloughing of the tissues due to poor absorption. The enzyme hyaluronidase may be injected into the tubing at each injection site at the start of clysis, and sometimes an additional 1 ml is added to the solution to facilitate absorption. Called also subcutaneous infusion.
hypodipsia abnormally diminished thirst.
hypodontia partial anodontia.
hypodynamia abnormally diminished power.
hypodynamic shock the second phase of shock, after the hyperdynamic phase, manifested by systemic hypotension, reduced cardiac output, hypothermia, rapid irregular pulse, prolonged capillary refill time and pale mucosae.
hypoeccrisia abnormally diminished excretion.
hypoendocrinism insufficiency of endocrine gland activity.
hypoergasia abnormally decreased functional activity.
hypoergia 1. hypoergasia. 2. hyposensitivity to allergens.
hypoergic 1. less energetic than normal. 2. pertaining to or characterized by hypoergy.
hypoergy abnormally diminished reactivity; hyposensitivity.
hypoesophoria deviation of the visual axes downward and inward.

hypoesthesia a state of abnormally decreased sensitivity to stimuli; is only assumed in animals when there is an inadequate response to the application of a touch or pain stimulus which is a test of reflex arc integrity. An expression of pain by an animal in response to stimulation is accepted as evidence of central perception.

hypoestrinism a lower level than normal of estrogens in the body, e.g. in the spayed female. Normal estral activity is absent; in bitches there may be a socially distressing urinary incontinence.

hypoestrogenism hypoestrinism.

hypoexophoria deviation of the visual axes downward and laterally.

hypoferremia deficiency of iron in the blood.

hypofertility diminished reproductive capacity.

hypofibrinogenemia deficiency of fibrinogen in the blood. Has been reported as an inherited defect in St. Bernard dogs; is acquired in liver disease and as a sequel of disseminated intravascular COAGULATION.

hypoflexion reduced ability to flex a limb.

hypofolicosis see FOLIC ACID.

hypofunction diminished functioning.

hypogalactia deficiency of milk secretion.

hypogammaglobulinemia an immunological deficiency state marked by abnormally low levels of generally all classes of immunoglobulins, with increased susceptibility to infectious diseases. It may be primary (called also inherited), or secondary (called also acquired), or it may be physiological. The latter occurs in normal neonates. See also AGAMMAGLOBULINEMIA.

The young of most animal species are born hypogammaglobulinemic and remain so until they ingest maternal colostrum which has a high content of immunoglobulins. The ingestion must occur during the first 24–48 hours of life because the large molecules of the globulins are absorbed only during this period. Inadequate supply, or inadequate ingestion or absorption of the immunoglobulins results in prolonged hypogammaglobulinemia and puts the neonate at grave risk of life-threatening infections. This failure of passive antibody transfer is the most common immunodeficiency disease encountered in domestic animal species, especially foals and dairy calves.

transient h. occurs in some foals at 3 to 4 months of age because of a delayed onset of immunoglobulin synthesis.

hypogangliosis, hypoganglionosis deficiency in the number of myenteric ganglion cells, usually in the colon leading to the development of megacolon. See also AGANGLIONOSIS.

Clydesdale myenteric h. megacolon develops at about 4–9 months old. Possibly an inherited trait.

hypogastric pertaining to the hypogastrium.

h. nerve see Table 14.

hypogastrium the most caudal middle abdominal region.

hypogenesis defective development.

hypogenitalism lack of sexual development because of deficient activity of the gonads; hypogonadism.

hypoglobulinemia lower than normal levels of globulin in the blood.

hypoglossal situated beneath the tongue, as the hypoglossal nerve.

h. cord the large aggregation of myogenic cells which migrates from somites 3–5 to a location ventral to the pharynx, and forms the tongue.

h. nerve paralysis causes difficulty in prehension, deglutition and mastication. Unilateral lesions cause deviation of the protruded tongue toward the side of the lesion.

hypoglottis 1. the underside of the tongue. 2. ranula.

hypoglucagonemia abnormally reduced levels of glucagon in the blood.

hypoglycemia an abnormally low level of sugar (glucose) in the blood. The condition may result from an excessive rate of removal of glucose from the blood or from decreased secretion of glucose into the blood. Overproduction of insulin from the islets of Langerhans or an overdose of exogenous insulin can lead to increased utilization of glucose, so that glucose is removed from the blood at an accelerated rate. Tumors of the islands of Langerhans can increase the production of insulin and result in rapid removal of glucose from the blood. Because the liver is the source of most of the glucose entering the blood while an animal is fasting, damage to the liver cells can result in impaired ability to convert glycogen into glucose. If secretion of the adrenocortical hormones, especially the GLUCOCORTICOIDS, is deficient, the protein precursors of glucose are not available and the blood glucose level drops as the liver's glycogen supply is depleted.

In animals the clinical picture of hypoglycemia includes muscle weakness, lethargy and recumbency. Ketosis and acetonuria are usual. Profound hypoglycemia or a very rapid fall in blood sugar causes convulsions and final coma.

hunting dog h. a stress-related syndrome seen in dogs that are fasted before a hunt, later experiencing exhaustion and hypoglycemic seizures.

juvenile h. occurs in in young puppies, mainly of toy breeds, causing weakness, muscle tremors, ataxia and seizures. Often precipitated by excitement, anorexia, hypothermia or gastrointestinal disorders. The cause is unclear, but believed to be incomplete development of metabolic pathways for glucose production. Affected puppies usually become normal with maturity.

leucine-induced h. orally administered leucine causes a significant further hypoglycemia in patients with an existing hyperinsulinism due to islet cell tumor.

neonatal h. see NEONATAL hypoglycemia.

h. unresponsiveness the hypoglycemia induced by insulin fails to return to the normal level in the required time, usually because of hyperinsulinism, or hypopituitarism or hypoadrenalism.

hypoglycemic pertaining to, characterized by, or producing hypoglycemia.

h. crisis profound weakness and seizures may be caused by very low blood glucose levels. Untreated hyperinsulinism and overdosing with insulin in the treatment of diabetes mellitus are common causes.

h. encephalopathy degenerative lesions in brain tissue caused by prolonged hypoglycemia, as in pregnancy toxemia of ewes.

oral h. agents synthetic drugs that lower the blood sugar level. These drugs stimulate the synthesis and release of INSULIN from the beta cells of the islets of Langerhans in the pancreas, and are used to treat human patients with non-insulin-dependent DIABETES mellitus. They have limited use in dogs and cats with diabetes mellitus as they have nonfunctional beta cells that cannot produce insulin.

h. factor see INSULIN.

h. seizures see hypoglycemic crisis (above).

hypoglycogenolysis defective splitting up of glycogen in the body.

hypoglycorrhachia abnormally low sugar content in the cerebrospinal fluid.

hypogonadism decreased functional activity of the gonads, with reduced production of germ cells and/or hormones; may be associated with retardation of growth and sexual development.

hypogonadotropic relating to or caused by deficiency of gonadotropin.

hypogranulosis decreased thickness of the stratum granulosum.

hypohidrosis abnormally diminished secretion of sweat. See also ANHIDROSIS.

hypoinsulinism deficient secretion of insulin by the pancreas resulting in hyperglycemia.

hypokalemia abnormally low potassium concentration in the blood; it may result from potassium loss by renal secretion or via the gastrointestinal tract, as in vomiting and diarrhea. Other causes include uncontrolled diabetes mellitus and attendant polyuria, increased adrenocortical secretion, steroid therapy, diuretic therapy, and burns or other injuries that result in loss of potassium. A special circumstance in which hypokalemia occurs is dilatation and displacement of the abomasum in which large quantities of potassium accumulate. The clinical syndrome of hypokalemia includes muscle weakness, lethargy, recumbency and terminal coma. Called also hypopotassemia.

hypokalemic 1. pertaining to or characterized by hypokalemia. 2. an agent that lowers blood potassium levels.

feline h. polymyopathy seen in cats with severe potassium depletion, usually caused by renal dysfunction and excessive urinary potassium losses. There is generalized muscle weakness, characterized by ventroflexion of the neck; other signs include weight loss, chronic vomiting and constipation.

h. nephropathy chronic loss of potassium due to alimentary tract disease can cause vacuolar degeneration of renal tubular epithelium.

hypokeratosis a decreased thickness of the stratum corneum of the skin.

hypokinesia abnormally diminished motor activity.

hypolactasia deficiency of lactase activity in the intestines.

hypoleydigism abnormally diminished secretion of androgens by Leydig's cells.

hypolipidemic promoting the reduction of lipid concentrations in the serum.

hypolipoproteinemia the presence of lipoproteins below normal concentrations in the blood.

hypoluteoidism deficient progesterone production, a state incompatible with continued pregnancy.

hypomagnesemia abnormally low magnesium content of the blood, manifested clinically by neuromuscular excitability.

hypomagnesemic emanating from or pertaining to hypomagnesemia.

calf h. tetany a highly fatal disease of calves fed solely on a milk diet and therefore lacking in magnesium. Clinically there is muscle tremor, hypersensitivity to touch and convulsions. In between fits the calves may appear relatively normal. Death is common. Called also milk tetany.

h. tetany see LACTATION TETANY, calf hypomagnesemic tetany (above).

hypomania mania of a mild type.

hypomastia abnormal smallness of mammary glands.

hypomelanosis hypopigmentation.

hypomere 1. the ventrolateral portion of a myotome, forming muscles innervated by the ventral rami of the spinal nerves. 2. the lateral plate of mesoderm that develops into the walls of the body cavities.

hypometabolism decreased metabolism; low metabolic rate.

hypometria ataxia in which movements fall short of the intended goal.

hypomochlion center of rotation of a joint.

hypomotility deficient power of movement in any part.

gut h. prolonged transit time of ingesta through the gut.

hypomyelination abnormally reduced amount of myelin in nervous tissue.

hypomyelinogenesis inadequate synthesis of myelin; includes failure of formation of myelin, plus incomplete and delayed myelination of axons. It occurs in several species and may be caused by simple nutritional deficiency, by viral infection, or inherited defect. Occurs in several breeds of dogs including Samoyeds, Dalmatians, Chow Chows, Weimaraners, Bernese mountain dogs, English springer spaniels, in all of which it is inherited as an X-linked trait. See also HYPOMYELINOGENESIS CONGENITA (calves) and CONGENITAL TREMOR SYNDROME (piglets).

hypomyelinogenesis congenita a congenital disease of calves manifested by inability to rise, and severe muscle tremor with periods of spasticity. At postmortem examination there is a myelin deficiency especially in the cerebellum and brainstem. Bovine virus diarrhea virus infection during early pregnancy is a likely cause.

hypomyotonia deficient muscular tonicity.

hypomyxia decreased secretion of mucus.

hyponatremia deficiency of SODIUM in the blood; salt depletion. The common cause is loss of sodium from the intestinal tract due to diarrhea. Clinically there is muscle weakness, hypothermia and dehydration.

hyponeocytosis leukopenia with the presence of immature leukocytes in the blood.

hyponiacinosis see NIACIN nutritional deficiency.

hyponychium the thickened epidermis beneath the free distal end of the claw of a digit.

hypo-orchidism defective activity of the testes. See also TESTICULAR agenesis.

hypo-orthocytosis leukopenia with a normal proportion of the various forms of leukocytes.

hypo-osmolality a decrease in the osmolality of the body fluids.

hypo-osmotic pertaining to hypo-osmolality.

hypopancreatism diminished activity of the pancreas.

hypopantothenosis PANTOTHENIC ACID nutritional deficiency.

hypoparathyroidism the condition produced by greatly reduced function of the parathyroid glands or by the removal of these bodies. The lack of parathyroid hormone leads to a fall in serum calcium level, which may result in increased neuromuscular excitability and, ultimately, in tetany. There is also a rise in the plasma phosphate level, which results in a decrease in bone resorption and an increased density of bone.

iatrogenic h. usually due to accidental removal of the glands during thyroidectomy.

idiopathic h. recorded in dogs due usually to an immune-mediated diffuse lymphocytic parathyroiditis.

hypoperfusion decreased blood flood through an organ, as in circulatory shock; if prolonged, it may result in permanent cellular dysfunction and death.

hypophagia reduced food intake.

hypophalangism absence of a phalanx on a digit.

hypopharynx laryngopharynx.
hypophonesis diminution of the sound in auscultation or percussion.
hypophonia a weak voice due to incoordination of the vocal muscles.
hypophoria permanent downward deviation of the visual axis of an eye in the absence of visual fusional stimuli. Called also heterophoria.
hypophosphatemia a lower than normal level of inorganic phosphorus, present as phosphates, in the blood. May be due to nutritional deficiency, several different malignant neoplasms, and primary hyperparathyroidism or pseudohyperparathyroidism associated with hypercalcemia. See also RICKETS, OSTEOMALACIA, POSTPARTURIENT hemoglobinuria.
hypophosphaturia abnormally decreased levels of urinary phosphate.
hypophosphites substances, especially calcium and iron salts, which have been incorporated in patent medicine tonics for many years in the belief that they provide replacement materials for damaged nervous tissue.
hypophrenic caudal to the diaphragm.
Hypophthalmichthys genus of farmed finfish in the family Cyprinidae; includes *H. molitrix* (silver carp), *H. nobilis* (bighead carp). See Table 23.
hypophyseal, hypophysial pertaining to the hypophysis (PITUITARY).
h. base the pars tuberalis and the infundibular stalk of the pituitary gland.
h. portal system the vascular anatomy of the pituitary gland which provides the route for hypothalamic regulating hormones to enter and control the secretion of the adenohypophyseal hormones.
h. system the hypothalamus, the pituitary gland and the hypophyseoportal circulation.
hypophysectomy excision of the hypophysis, or pituitary gland. Surgical removal is a form of treatment for pituitary-dependent Cushing's syndrome in dogs.
hypophyseoportal system the portal system of the pituitary gland, in which hypothalamic venules connect with the sinusoidal capillaries of the anterior pituitary.
hypophysial see HYPOPHYSEAL.
hypophysioprivic due to deficiency of hormonal secretion of the hypophysis.
hypophysis pl. *hypophyses* [Gr.] see PITUITARY.
h. cerebri hypophysis.
h. sicca posterior pituitary.
hypopiesis abnormally low pressure, in particular, low blood pressure.
hypopigmentation abnormally decreased pigmentation.
acquired h. following skin injury in horses; hyperpigmentation the rule in other species. In dogs depigmentation, due to damage of basal keratinocytes, due usually to immune-mediated diseases, e.g. lupus erythematosus. Skin depigmentation, such as occurs in human vitiligo, is recorded in dogs and horses.
congenital h. see ALBINISM.
epidermal h. due to defective melanization as a result of defective melanocytes in the skin or to their damage or destruction after birth.
hair h. leukotrichia.
hereditary h. see ALBINISM; PIEBALDISM.
skin h. leukoderma.
hypopituitarism the condition resulting from diminution or cessation of hormonal secretion by the pituitary gland, especially the anterior pituitary. Signs vary with the degree of dysfunction; proportionate dwarfism in German shepherd dogs is one of the best-known syndromes.
hypoplasia, hypoplasty incomplete development or underdevelopment of an organ or tissue, e.g. cerebellar hypoplasia, bone marrow hypoplasia, gonadal hypoplasia, small intestinal mucosal hypoplasia.
hypoplastic characterized by hypoplasia, e.g. hypoplastic anemia.
h. left heart syndrome a congenital anomaly seen in cats in which there is mitral atresia and incomplete development of the left ventricle and aortic valve.
hypopnea abnormal decrease in depth and rate of respiration.
hypopolarization in neurochemical transmission of nerve impulses this is decreased polarity of the postsynaptic membrane, e.g. that caused by excitation from receptor stimulation.
hypoporosis deficient callus formation after bone fracture.
hypoposia abnormally diminished ingestion of fluids.
hypopotassemia hypokalemia.
hypopraxia abnormally diminished activity.
hypoproconvertinemia reduced levels of PROCONVERTIN (clotting factor VII) in the blood.
hypoprogesteronism the state of being deficient in progesterone; incompatible with sustained pregnancy.
hypoproteinemia deficiency of protein in the blood caused by inadequate intake or synthesis due to liver damage or to loss in protein losing enteropathy, renal disease or intestinal parasite infestation. Clinically represented by edema and emaciation. See also HYPOGAMMAGLOBULINEMIA.
hypoprothrombinemia deficiency of PROTHROMBIN in the blood.
hypoptyalism abnormally decreased secretion of saliva.
hypopyon pus in the anterior chamber of the eye.
hypopyridoxinosis PYRIDOXINE (vitamin B_6) deficiency.
hyporeactive showing less than normal response to stimuli.
hyporeflexia diminution or weakening of reflexes.
hyporeninemia low levels of renin in the blood.
hyporiboflavinosis see RIBOFLAVIN nutritional deficiency.
hyposalemia diminution of salt levels in the blood.
hyposalivation hypoptyalism.
hyposcleral beneath the sclera.
hyposecretion diminished secretion.
hyposensitivity 1. abnormally decreased sensitivity. 2. the state of being less sensitive to a specific allergen after repeated and gradually increasing doses of the particular allergen. This is believed to be due to an increase in circulating antibodies, particularly IgG to the allergen. The antibodies form complexes with the incoming allergen and prevent it from binding to IgE bound to mast cells.
hyposensitization the act or process of inducing hyposensitivity; desensitization. See also IMMUNOTHERAPY.
hyposmolarity abnormally decreased osmolar concentration of a solution.
hyposomatotropism deficient secretion of somatotropin (growth hormone) or secretion of inactive somatotropin, resulting in dwarfism.
hyposomia subnormal body development.
hypospadia hypospadias.
hypospadiac 1. pertaining to hypospadias. 2. an animal affected with hypospadias.
hypospadias a developmental anomaly in the male in

which the urethra opens on the underside of the penis or on the perineum.

hyposplenism diminished functioning of the spleen, resulting in an increase in peripheral blood elements.

hypostasis poor or stagnant circulation in a dependent part of the body or an organ.

hypostatic 1. pertaining to, due to, or associated with hypostasis. 2. abnormally static; said of certain inherited traits that are liable to be suppressed by other traits.

hyposthenia diminished strength or tonicity.

hyposthenuria excretion of urine of low specific gravity.

hypostome an appendage on the ventral aspect of the oral opening of some insects and arachnids.

hypostomia a developmental anomaly characterized by abnormal smallness of the mouth, the slit being vertical instead of horizontal.

hypostypsis moderate astringency.

hyposynergia defective coordination.

hypotelorism abnormally decreased distance between two organs or parts.

hypotension diminished tension; lowered blood pressure. In animals almost the only occurrence is in severe peripheral circulatory failure, especially traumatic, toxemic or anaphylactic shock.

postural h. a slight fall in systolic blood pressure is normal upon rising. Abnormal postural hypotension involves a decrease in both systolic and diastolic pressures with changes in heart rate.

hypotensive 1. characterized by or causing diminished tension or pressure, as abnormally low blood pressure. 2. an animal with abnormally low blood pressure.

h. shock see hypovolemic SHOCK.

hypotensor a substance that lowers the blood pressure.

hypothalamic pertaining to the hypothalamus.

h. hormones see HYPOTHALAMUS.

h.-pituitary-adrenocortical axis the complex system of interaction between the hypothalamus, pituitary gland and adrenal cortex that involves stimulation of synthesis and release by corticotropin-releasing factor and adrenocorticotropic hormone, and the negative feedback effect of cortisol.

h. secretory neurons are located in nuclei of the hypothalmus; they receive information from higher centers to regulate hormone secretion.

h. thermoregulatory mechanism receptive to stimulation by pyrogens to elevate the body temperature in fever.

hypothalamic–ovarian axis the operating relationship between the hypothalamus and the ovaries; optic and olfactory stimuli modulate the axis' activity.

hypothalamohypophyseal pertaining to the hypothalamus and pituitary complex.

h. portal system see HYPOPHYSEAL portal system.

h. syndrome disorder of pituitary and hypothalamus functions caused by an enlarging pituitary tumor compressing or infiltrating the overlying hypothalamus.

h. tract a tract of unmyelinated nerves connecting the hypothalamus and the hypophysis; their cell bodies are located in the supraoptic and paraventricular nuclei of the hypothalamus.

hypothalamus the portion of the diencephalon lying beneath the thalamus at the base of the cerebrum, and forming the floor and part of the lateral wall of the third ventricle. It includes the optic chiasm, mammillary bodies, tuber cinereum, infundibulum and hypophysis (pituitary gland), but for physiological purposes, the hypophysis is considered a distinct structure.

The hypothalamic nuclei activate, control and integrate many of the involuntary functions necessary for living. The various hypothalamic centers influence peripheral autonomic mechanisms, endocrine activity and many somatic functions, e.g. a general regulation of water balance, body temperature, sleep, thirst and hunger, and the development of secondary sex characteristics.

Because of its influence on the release and inhibition of pituitary hormones, the hypothalamus indirectly plays an important role in the regulation of protein, fat and carbohydrate metabolism, body fluid volume and electrolyte content, and internal secretion of endocrine hormones. The hormones synthesized and secreted by the special neurons of the hypothalamus are called *hypothalamic releasing* and *inhibiting hormones* or *factors*. They act directly on the tissues of the pituitary gland. Some of the major hypothalamic factors are: *thyroid-stimulating hormone releasing hormone* (TRH), which activates the release of the thyroid-stimulating hormone (TSH) from the anterior lobe of the pituitary gland; *corticotropin-releasing factor* (CRF); *growth hormone releasing factor* (GHRF); *gonadotropin releasing hormone* (GnRH); and *prolactin-inhibiting factor* (PIF). In addition, there are other stimulating and inhibiting factors that influence the release and retention of other anterior pituitary hormones.

The hypothalamic hormones or factors are secreted directly into the veins in the lower part of the hypothalamus and are transported directly to the tissues of the pituitary gland. This transportation network is called the *hypothalamic–hypophyseal portal system*. The secretion of the hypothalamic hormones is a part of a regulatory negative FEEDBACK system that continuously operates to maintain homeostasis.

hypothermia low body temperature.

Hypothermia may be symptomatic of a disease or disorder of the temperature-regulating mechanism of the body, may be due to exposure to cold, or may be induced for certain surgical procedures or as a therapeutic measure. Exposure to cold is well tolerated by animals except those that have poor peripheral circulation, e.g. cows with milk fever, animals under anesthesia and the newborn. Newborn piglets are particularly susceptible, but high mortalities may also occur in lambs during inclement weather and puppies deprived of warmth from the bitch. Even adult sheep may die of hypothermia if they are exposed to cold, wet, windy weather immediately after shearing.

induced h. deliberate reduction of the temperature of all or part of the body; sometimes used as an adjunct to anesthesia in surgical procedures involving a limb, and as a protective measure in cardiac and neurological surgery. The hypothermia may be continued only for the duration of the operation or it may be prolonged depending on the reason for its use.

neonatal h. a significant cause of loss especially in lambs born outdoors in changeable weather with a high chill factor combining low temperature, rain and wind and no shelter from the wind. Piglets are the neonates most susceptible to cold.

symptomatic h. pathological reduction of body temperature as a result of decreased heat production or increased heat loss. Hypothyroidism, severe blood loss with circulatory failure, and damage to the heat-producing cells of the hypothalamus can lead to decreased heat production.

therapeutic h. the application of cold to acute injuries induces vasoconstriction and limits edema and muscle spasm.

hypothesis a supposition that appears to explain a group of phenomena and is assumed as a basis of reasoning and experimentation.

h. testing a standard practice using statistical methods, usually analytical observational studies, to differentiate between two hypotheses. For example, the user assumes that vaccination against a particular disease reduces the prevalence of the disease, then tests that hypothesis.

h. testing sampling sampling of material or data for the purpose of testing a hypothesis.

hypothetico-deductive diagnosis method a method of building up diagnostic hypotheses suggested by the answers to questions to the client, then testing each hypothesis as it arises by further questions or by clinical examination or laboratory test until a single diagnosis or a short list of diagnostic possibilities remains.

hypothiaminosis see THIAMIN nutritional deficiency.

hypothrombinemia deficiency of thrombin in the blood, resulting in a tendency to bleed.

hypothymism diminished thymus activity.

hypothyroidism deficiency of THYROID gland activity, with underproduction of thyroxine, or the condition resulting from it. Common in adult dogs, particularly certain breeds, as a result of an idiopathic atrophy of the thyroid or a lymphocytic thyroiditis. Alopecia, weight gain, mental dullness, fatigue, cold intolerance, infertility and neurological deficits are seen. In food animals the syndrome is classical neonatal colloid goiter. See also GOITER.

autoimmune h. see lymphocytic THYROIDITIS.

congenital h. results from congenital thyroid dysgenesis, defective hormone synthesis or severe iodine deficiency. There is dwarfism, macroglossia and mental dullness.

iatrogenic h. may follow treatment for hyperparathyroidism in cats.

juvenile h. congenital hypothyroidism (above).

primary h. that resulting from disease of the thyroid glands.

secondary h. caused by a deficiency of thyroid-stimulating hormone, usually as a result of a lesion in the pituitary gland.

tertiary h. caused by a lack of synthesis or release of thyrotropin releasing hormone.

hypotonia abnormally decreased tonicity or strength.

ocular h. low intraocular pressure.

hypotonic 1. having an abnormally reduced tonicity or tension. 2. having an osmotic pressure lower than that of the solution with which it is compared.

h. dehydration occurs when there is secretory loss of sodium from the intestinal epithelium, e.g. salmonellosis, in osmolar excess of the concurrent fluid loss. See also DEHYDRATION.

hypotony hypotonia.

hypotoxicity abnormally reduced toxic quality.

hypotransferrinemia deficiency of transferrin in the blood.

hypotrichosis presence of less than the normal amount of hair. Called also alopecia.

canine hereditary h. see black hair follicular DYSPLASIA.

congenital h. absence of hair at birth. Occurs as an inherited trait in the hairless breeds of dogs and cats, Mexican hairless, Chinese crested and Sphinx, and sporadically in other breeds; has also been reported as an inherited condition in several breeds of cattle.

congenital h. universalis see ALOPECIA universalis.

inherited congenital h. partial or complete absence of haircoat at birth. Some may have had a partial haircoat and lost it subsequently. Tactile hairs and eyelashes are present. There may be other defects including absence of thyroid tissue. The affected animals may or may not be viable. Occurs in all species but most common in cattle and in some breeds of dogs. See also inherited symmetrical ALOPECIA.

lethal h. occurs in Holstein–Friesian cattle; affected calves die within hours.

tardive h. reported as a sex-linked trait in Holstein–Friesian cattle; affected females are normal until a few months of age when a progressive loss of hair occurs. They are otherwise normal.

viable h. an autosomal recessive trait in Guernsey, Jersey and Holstein–Friesian cattle. Affected calves are nearly hairless at birth, but later some hair grows on the thorax and abdomen.

hypotrophy abiotrophy.

hypotropia STRABISMUS in which there is permanent downward deviation of the visual axis of one eye.

hypotympanotomy surgical opening of the hypotympanum.

hypotympanum the lower part of the cavity of the middle ear, in the temporal bone.

hypouricemia deficiency of uric acid in the blood, along with xanthinuria, due to deficiency of xanthine oxidase, the enzyme required for conversion of hypoxanthine to xanthine and of xanthine to uric acid.

hypoventilation reduction in the amount of air entering the pulmonary alveoli.

hypovitaminosis a condition produced by lack of an essential vitamin. See under the name of each vitamin.

hypovolemia abnormally decreased volume of circulating fluid (plasma) in the body.

hypovolemic pertaining to hypovolemia. See also hypovolemic SHOCK, HYPOVOLEMIC CIRCULATORY FAILURE.

hypovolemic circulatory failure CIRCULATORY failure due to HYPOVOLEMIA.

hypovolia diminished water content or volume, as of extracellular fluid.

hypoxanthine an intermediate product of uric acid synthesis, formed from adenylic acid and itself a precursor of xanthine.

hypoxemia deficient oxygenation of the blood. The most reliable method for measuring the degree of hypoxemia is BLOOD GAS ANALYSIS to determine the partial pressure of oxygen in the arterial blood. Decreased oxygenation of the blood eventually leads to HYPOXIA.

hypoxia a broad term meaning diminished availability of oxygen to the body tissues.

Its causes are many and varied. There may be a deficiency of oxygen in the atmosphere, as in ALTITUDE SICKNESS, or a pulmonary disorder that interferes with adequate ventilation of the lungs. Anemia or circulatory deficiencies can lead to inadequate transport and delivery of oxygen to the tissues. Finally, edema or other abnormal conditions of the tissues themselves may impair the exchange of oxygen and carbon dioxide between the capillaries and the tissues. The effect of hypoxia is to reduce the functional activity of tissues. The initial response may be one of temporarily increased activity. Terminally the tissue may be irreparably damaged.

anemic h. due to inadequate supply of hemoglobin in the blood.

cerebral h. may be acute or chronic causing either a tremor–convulsion syndrome or one of longer term weakness, ataxia, apparent blindness and lethargy.
fetal h. occurs as a result of deprivation of the fetus of oxygen during parturition, because it is delayed or the umbilical cord pinched off. Clinically there is weakness, imbecility, disinclination to suck, possibly hypothermia. Foals experience a much more violent, convulsive or dummy syndrome. See also NEONATAL maladjustment syndrome. Called also intrapartum hypoxia.
intrapartum h. see fetal hypoxia (above).
ischemic h. insufficient oxygen in tissues because of an inadequate blood supply.
stagnant h. inadequate supply of oxygen to tissues because of slow rate of passage of the blood through the tissues.

hypoxic a state of hypoxia.
h. cell sensitizers compounds that selectively sensitize hypoxic tumor cells to the effects of radiation.
h. vasoconstriction reduced oxygen supply to tissues causes local vasoconstriction and diversion of the blood to other tissues.

hyps(o)- word element. [Gr.] *height*.

hypsodont having teeth all the same height.

Hyptiasmus a genus of flukes (digenetic trematodes) in the family Cyclocoelidae.
H. tumidus causes rhinitis and sinusitis in ducks and geese.

hyracoid resembling the rodent hyrax; members of the order Hyracoidea.

Hyraconema see SETARIA[1].

hyracotherium eohippus.

hyrax small herbivorous animal that lives in burrows. It has feet like those of a rhinoceros with five toes on the forefeet and three on the hind and with blunt nails. Called also dassie. Member of the genera *Procavia* or *Dendrohyrax* in the family Hyracoidea.

hysteratresia atresia of the uterus.

hysterectomy surgical removal of the UTERUS.
abdominal h. that performed through the abdominal wall.
cesarean h. cesarean section followed by removal of the uterus.
radical h. excision of the uterus, upper vagina, and parametrium.
subtotal h. that in which the cervix is left in place.
total h. that in which the uterus and cervix are completely excised.

hysterectomy produced artificially reared pigs called also HYPAR; see SPECIFIC PATHOGEN FREE.

hysteresis the failure of coincidence of two associated phenomena, such as that exhibited in the differing temperatures of gelation and of liquefaction of a reversible colloid.

hystereurynter an instrument for dilating the ostium uteri.

hystereurysis dilatation of the ostium uteri.

hysteria a state of excitement or tension in which there is a temporary loss of control over the emotions. The term is probably an inappropriate one for use in animals. It has common usage for conditions in which animals are assumed to have lost control of their emotions because of their atypical, excessively active behavior, e.g. a sow savaging her piglets at parturition. See also FARROWING hysteria.
canine h. a disease characterized by fits of frantic running, terminating in convulsions. Reported in dogs fed biscuits made of flour whitened by the agene process. The process is no longer used and the disease has disappeared.

hyster(o)- word element. [Gr.] *uterus, hysteria*.

hysterocatalepsy hysteria with cataleptic signs.

hysterocele hernia of the uterus.

hysterocleisis surgical closure of the ostium uteri.

hysteroepilepsy severe hysteria with epileptic convulsions.

hysterogenic causing hysterical phenomena or signs.

hysterography 1. the graphic recording of the strength of uterine contractions in labor. 2. radiography of the uterus after instillation of a contrast medium.

hysteroid resembling hysteria.

hysterolith a uterine calculus.

hysterolysis freeing of the uterus from adhesions.

hysterometer an instrument for measuring the uterus.

hysterometry measurement of the uterus.

hysteromyoma leiomyoma of the uterus.

hysteromyomectomy local excision of a leiomyoma of the uterus.

hysteromyotomy incision of the uterus for removal of a solid tumor.

hysteropathy any uterine disease; metropathy.

hysteropexy fixation of a displaced uterus by surgery.

hysteroptosis prolapse of the uterus.

hysterorrhaphy 1. suture of the uterus. 2. hysteropexy.

hysterorrhexis rupture of the uterus.

hysterosalpingography in animals, contrast radiography of the body and horns of the uterus; used in bitches to diagnose pyometritis.

hysterosalpingo-oophorectomy excision of the uterus, uterine tubes and ovaries; the common spay procedure in dogs and cats. See also OVARIOHYSTERECTOMY.

hysteroscope an endoscope used in direct visual examination of the canal of the uterine cervix and the cavity of the uterus.

hysterospasm spasm of the uterus.

hysterotomy incision of the uterus. See also CESAREAN SECTION.

hysterotrachelorrhaphy suture of the uterus and uterine cervix.

hysterotrachelotomy incision of the uterus and uterine cervix.

hysterotubography hysterosalpingography.

Hystrichis a genus of nematodes of the family Dioctophymatidae occurring in aquatic birds.
H. tricolor causes nodules and some destruction of tissue in the proventriculus of ducks.

hystricomorph resembling or of the rodent family Hystricidae, Old World porcupines.

Hystrix cristata see PORCUPINE.

Hz hertz; cycles per second.

I

I chemical symbol, *iodine* (L. *iodum*).

I_a antigen histocompatibility antigens found primarily on B lymphocytes but also on some macrophages, T lymphocytes and skin.

I band the lighter colored cross-striation of muscle fibers; composed of filaments of actin.

I-cell disease see MUCOLIPIDOSIS II.

-ia word element, *state; condition.*
-iasis word element. [Gr.] *condition, state.*
IATA International Air Transport Association, which sets the rules for air transport, including those concerning air transport of animals.
iatric pertaining to medicine or to a physician. Also loosely construed to include veterinary medicine and veterinary physicians, e.g. buiatrics.
iatr(o)- word element. [Gr.] *medicine, physician.*
iatrogenic resulting from the activity of a physician; said of any adverse condition in a patient resulting from treatment by a physician or surgeon, for instance, death after injection of an inappropriate solution or of an appropriate solution in an inappropriate manner, e.g. rapid injections of solutions of magnesium salts, unbuffered solutions of high alkalinity or acidity, or of a substance to which the animal is allergic. See also iatrogenic HYPERADRENOCORTICISM.
Ibaraki disease see IBARAKI VIRUS.
Ibaraki virus an orbivirus which causes a disease of cattle in Japan, similar to BLUETONGUE in sheep.
IBD 1. infectious bursal disease of chickens. 2. inflammatory bowel disease.
ibex wild goats of the genus *Capra* spp. includes Spanish ibex (*C. pyrenaica*), Siberian ibex (*C. ibex siberica*), Cretan wild goat (*C. aegagues cretica*).
Ibizan hound a medium-sized (22 to 27 in tall), very lean, muscular dog with a smooth or rough coat of white, chestnut or lion. The ears are large, thin and erect, the head long and flat, and the tail long and thin. The breed was an ancient Egyptian hunting dog.
IBK see INFECTIOUS bovine keratoconjunctivitis.
ibotenic acid the insecticidal agent in the mushroom AMANITA *muscaria.*
IBR see INFECTIOUS bovine rhinotracheitis.
IBR/IPV see INFECTIOUS bovine rhinotracheitis/infectious pustular VULVOVAGINITIS.
ibuprofen a nonsteroidal anti-inflammatory agent that possesses analgesic and antipyretic activities; used for symptomatic relief of rheumatoid arthritis and osteoarthritis in humans, but its use in dogs is limited by the occurrence of undesirable side-effects such as gastrointestinal hemorrhage.
IC inspiratory capacity.
i.c. medical record abbreviation for intracardiac.
-ic suffix meaning pertaining to.
-ical suffix meaning pertaining to.
ICAMs intercellular adhesion molecules.
ICD 1. International Classification of Diseases (of the World Health Organization). 2. intrauterine contraceptive device. 3. isocitrate dehydrogenase.
Iceland pony a pony derived from North British ponies; mostly chestnut, some brown, gray, black.
Iceland poppy see PAPAVER *nudicaule.*
Icelandic cattle usually polled, mostly red or red and white dairy cattle.
Icelandic pneumonia see MAEDI.
Icelandic sheep multipurpose, usually white with light brown head and legs; sometimes black, gray or pied; horned.
ICG indocyanine green.
ICH infectious canine hepatitis.
Ich see ICHTHYOPHTHIRIUS *multifiliis* and CRYPTOCARYON *irritans.*
ichor a watery discharge from wounds or sores.
ichorrhea copious discharge of ichor.
ichthammol an ammoniated coal tar product, used as an ointment in the treatment of acute, septic lesions such as cellulitis and abscesses.
ichthyismus ichthyotoxism.
Ichthyoboda a genus of small, flagellate protozoan parasites of the skin of freshwater and marine fish. Cause a steel-gray discoloration of the skin and often respiratory distress.
ichthyoid fishlike.
ichthyology the study of fishes.
ichthyophagous eating or subsisting on fish.
ichthyophoniasis see ICHTHYOPHONUS.
Ichthyophonus a genus of fungi causing ichthyophoniasis, cutaneous ulcers and cysts in most body organs, of aged aquarium and wild fish.
Ichthyophthirius a genus of protozoan parasites in the phylum Ciliophora.
I. multifiliis causes white spot disease or Ich in freshwater fish in aquariums and hatcheries. Characterized by white nodules on the skin; these may coalesce and cause sloughing of the skin and many affected fish die. Also affects the gills leading to respiratory distress.
ichthyosarcotoxin a toxin found in the flesh of poisonous fish.
ichthyosarcotoxism poisoning due to ingestion of poisonous fish, marked by various gastrointestinal and neurological disturbances.
ichthyosis any of several generalized skin disorders marked by dryness, roughness and scaliness, due to hypertrophy of the horny layer, resulting from excessive production or retention of keratin, or a molecular defect in the keratin.
inherited congenital i. alopecia and plates of horny epidermis over the entire skin surface. Seen in calves at birth and they are not viable. Also occurs in dogs. Called also fish scale disease.
Ichthyosporidium obligate, intracellular, protozoan parasites in the class Microsporea.
I. giganteum found in the connective tissue of the body wall of fish, causing large ventral swellings full of cysts.
ichthyotoxin any toxic substance derived from fish. See also ICHTHYOSARCOTOXIN.
ichthyotoxism any intoxication due to an ichthyotoxin.
icosahedral a regular polyhedron with 20 triangular faces, 12 corners and 30 sides, having cubic symmetry with 5:3:2-fold axes. A common structural form for the capsid of many viruses including herpesviruses, adenoviruses, parvoviruses, reoviruses, picornaviruses and retroviruses.
ICSH interstitial cell-stimulating hormone. See LUTEINIZING HORMONE.
ictal pertaining to, characterized by an acute epileptic seizure.
Ictalurus a genus of catfish, intermediate hosts for parasites of animals. See Table 23.
I. furcatus blue catfish.
I. melas black bullhead catfish, paratenic host for DIOCTOPHYME *renale.*
I. nebulosa the brown bullhead catfish, the paratenic host for DIOCTOPHYME *renale.*
I. punctatus finfish in family Ictaluridae. Called also channel catfish.
icteric pertaining to or affected with jaundice.
i. index is the density of color of the serum of an icteric patient compared to the standard solution. A rough measure of severity of hepatic insufficiency.
icteroanemia jaundice with mucosal pallor as in hemolytic anemia; see also EPERYTHROZOONOSIS.
icterogenic causing jaundice, e.g. icterogenic hepatopathy.
icterogenins pentacyclic triterpene acid hepatoxins

present in the plant LIPPIA *rehmanni*. Cause cholestasis and photosensitization.

icterohepatitis inflammation of the liver with marked jaundice.

icteroid resembling jaundice.

icterus see JAUNDICE.

ictus a seizure, stroke, blow, or sudden attack.

ICU see INTENSIVE care unit.

ID 1. infective dose. 2. L-iditol dehydrogenase.

ID_{50} median infective DOSE; the dose that will infect 50% of the experimental group.

Id idiotype.

id see DERMATOPHYTID.

-id [Gr.] a suffix meaning having the shape of, or resembling.

idarubicin an anthracycline antibiotic used as an antineoplastic agent; similar to doxorubicin.

idazoxan an α_2-adrenoceptor antagonist used to reverse xylazine.

-ide suffix indicating a binary compound.

identical by descent said of all genes which are copies of the same segment of DNA.

identical twins monozygotic TWINS.

identification a description of an animal sufficient to distinguish it from others. The means of identification include a written description, earmark, paint brand or paper or fabric applied by special adhesive, FREEZE BRANDING and fire branding (see BRAND), TATTOOING, neckbands, ankle bands, EAR tagging, TAIL tagging and TAIL painting, and ELECTRONIC identification systems including activated responders or transponders carried on the animal, often subcutaneously.

patient i. an adequate identification includes species and breed, sex, color and markings, brands and other distinguishing marks or attachments, whether horned or polled where appropriate, age, name or number used by the owner, and name and address of the owner or custodian.

identity the aggregate of characteristics by which an individual is recognized.

idio- word element. [Gr.] *self, peculiar to a substance or organism.*

idiocy a state of severe mental retardation, difficult to determine in an animal but typical examples are calves with hydranencephaly, yearling cattle with polioencephalomalacia.

juvenile amaurotic familial i. see AMAUROTIC familial idiocy.

Idiogenes a genus of tapeworms of bustards.

idiogram a drawing or photograph of the chromosomes of a particular cell.

idiopathic self-originated; occurring without known cause.

i. adrenocortical atrophy see primary HYPOADRENOCORTICISM.

i. disease without known cause.

i. hemorrhagic syndrome see canine EHRLICHIOSIS.

i. peripheral vestibular disease see canine idiopathic VESTIBULAR syndrome, feline ischemic ENCEPHALOPATHY.

i. polyneuritis see GUILLAIN–BARRÉ SYNDROME.

i. thrombocytopenia see immune-mediated THROMBOCYTOPENIA.

idiopathy an undiagnosed morbid state arising without known cause.

Idiospermum australiense Australian rainforest tree in the family Idiospermaceae; eating the fruit causes a syndrome of tetanic convulsions, hypersensitivity; called also idiot fruit.

idiosyncrasy 1. a habit or quality of body or behavior peculiar to any individual animal. 2. an abnormal susceptibility to an agent (e.g. a drug) that is peculiar to the individual animal.

idiot fruit see IDIOSPERMUM AUSTRALIENSE.

idiotope an antigenic determinant on the variable region of an antibody.

idiotrophic capable of selecting its own nourishment.

idiotype the antigenic characteristic of the variable region of an antibody. A set of idiotopes. Called also Id.

cross-reacting i. (IdX) one that is present on other immunoglobulins produced in response to the same antigen, permitting a cross reaction. See also CROSS-REACTION.

idioventricular pertaining to the cardiac ventricle alone.

L-iditol dehydrogenase see L-iditol DEHYDROGENASE.

IDL intermediate density lipoprotein.

idopsin a visual pigment in the cone membranous lamellae of the eye.

idoxuridine a pyrimidine analog that prevents replication of DNA viruses; used topically in infection by herpesviruses.

IDU see IDOXURIDINE.

iduronic acid part of the dermatan sulfate molecule.

iduronidase deficiency see MUCOPOLYSACCHARIDOSIS I.

alpha-L-iduronidase deficiency of the enzyme considered to be counterpart of mucopolysaccharidosis in cats and dogs; a neuronal storage disease.

IDV intermittent demand ventilation.

IF intermediate filaments.

IFA immunofluorescent antibody.

IFN interferon.

iforrestine heterocyclic nephrotoxin in *Isotropis* spp.

Ig immunoglobulin of any of the five classes: IgA, IgD, IgE, IgG and IgM.

IgA immunoglobulin A. See IMMUNOGLOBULIN.

IgD immunoglobulin D. See IMMUNOGLOBULIN.

IgE immunoglobulin E. See IMMUNOGLOBULIN.

IGF-I see SOMATOMEDIN C.

IgG immunoglobulin G. See IMMUNOGLOBULIN.

IgM immunoglobulin M. See IMMUNOGLOBULIN.

IgM deficiency occurs as an inherited defect and as part of the primary severe combined immunodeficiency in Quarter horses and Arab horses.

ignipuncture therapeutic puncture with hot needles.

Ignis sacer see rye ERGOT[1].

IGR insect growth regulator.

IHA isoimmune hemolytic anemia. See ALLOIMMUNE hemolytic anemia of the newborn.

IHA test indirect hemagglutination test.

IIT indirect IMMUNOFLUORESCENCE test.

IK immunoconglutinins.

IL interleukin.

IL-1 see INTERLEUKINS.

IL-I catabolin.

Ile isoleucine.

ileac 1. of the nature of ileus. 2. pertaining to the ileum.

ileal, ileac pertaining to the ileum.

i. atresia see inherited alimentary tract segmental ATRESIA.

i. conduit use of a segment of the ileum for the diversion of urinary flow from the ureters.

i. muscular hypertrophy a cause of chronic or intermittent colic of horses characterized by loud ileocecal gut sounds and a palpably enlarged terminal ileum on rectal examination. See also INTUSSUSCEPTION.

transmissible i. hypertrophy see WET TAIL.

ileitis inflammation of the ileum or distal portion of small intestine, manifested by chronic or intermittent diarrhea and weight loss.
granulomatous i. see granulomatous ENTERITIS.
proliferative i. a disease of pigs resembling Crohn's disease of humans. The terminal ileum is thick-walled, with ulceration and sometimes perforation so that acute peritonitis develops. There are no diagnostic signs. Called also diverticulitis and ileitis of pigs. See also ILEAL muscular hypertrophy.
regional i. see terminal ileitis (below).
terminal i. a disease of young animals including pigs, lambs and horses characterized by illthrift and sometimes diarrhea.
transmissible i. see WET TAIL.
ile(o)- word element. [L.] *ileum*.
ileocecal pertaining to the ileum and cecum.
i. valve the valve guarding the opening between the ileum and cecum; called also ileocolic valve.
i. valve frenulum see RETINACULUM morgagni.
i. valve impaction is common in horses as result of feeding on finely chopped indigestible roughage. Causes mild colic initially, followed by evidence of acute intestinal obstruction. Fatal without surgical correction. See also intestinal obstruction COLIC.
ileocecocolic, ileocaecocolic pertaining to the combined ileum, cecum and colon.
ileocecostomy surgical anastomosis of the ileum to the cecum.
ileocolic pertaining to the ileum and colon.
i. intussusception intussusception of the ileum through the ileocecal valve into the colon. May extend through the rectum, appearing as a rectal prolapse.
i. valve ileocecal valve.
ileocolitis inflammation of the ileum and colon.
ileocolostomy surgical anastomosis of the ileum to the colon.
ileocolotomy incision of the ileum and colon.
ileocystoplasty repair of the wall of the urinary bladder with an isolated segment of the wall of the ileum.
ileocystostomy use of an isolated segment of ileum to create a passage from the urinary bladder to an opening in the abdominal wall.
ileoileostomy surgical anastomosis between two parts of the ileum.
ileorectal pertaining to or communicating with the ileum and rectum.
ileorrhaphy suture of the ileum.
ileostomy an artificial opening (stoma) created in the small intestine (ileum) and brought to the surface of the abdomen for the purpose of evacuating feces.
urinary i. use of a segment of the ileum as a stoma for the diversion of urinary flow from the ureters. See also ileal CONDUIT.
ileotomy incision of the ileum.
ileum the distal portion of the small intestine, extending from the jejunum to the cecum. See also ILEAL.
duplex i. congenital duplication of the ileum.
i.–umbilicus fistula a persistent and patent Meckel's diverticulum.
ileus intestinal obstruction, especially functional obstruction or failure of peristalsis. It frequently accompanies peritonitis, and usually results from disturbances in neural stimulation of the bowel. In the horse it is a major problem in the recovery period after surgical treatment for colic. Called also paralytic, functional and adynamic ileus.
dynamic i. obstructive ileus.
mechanical i. obstructive ileus.
obstructive i. a physical lesion accounts for the intestinal distension.
sentinel loop i. a distended intestinal loop caused by localized paralytic ileus, usually resulting from local infection or pain.
Ilex a bush bearing berries containing saponins; cause vomiting, diarrhea. Called also holly.
iliac pertaining to the ilium.
i. artery thrombosis in horses an acute onset is characterized by severe pain, even recumbency, and marked reduction of the amplitude of the digital arterial pulse. The affected limb is cold and is not used. The chronic disease is characterized by increasing weakness of the affected limb as exercise progresses. In both forms there is a unilateral abnormality of the iliac artery palpable per rectum.

Dogs and, more commonly, cats are affected by thrombosis of the aorta (saddle thrombus) or an iliac artery, usually in association with cardiac disease. Depending on the rate of development, the affected limb becomes weak, cold and painful, the pulse is weak, and the animal becomes distressed. See also AORTIC embolism.
iliadelphus symmetrical conjoined twins united in the iliac region; iliopagus.
ilial iliac.
ili(o)- word element. [L.] *ilium*.
iliocaudal muscle the more cranial of the two of the levator ani muscles; it originates on the medial surface of the body of the ilium and inserts on the ventral aspect of the tail.
iliofemoral pertaining to the ilium and femur.
ilioinguinal pertaining to the iliac and inguinal regions.
iliolumbar pertaining to the iliac and lumbar regions.
iliopagus symmetrical conjoined twins united in the iliac region.
iliopectineal pertaining to the ilium and pubes.
iliotrochanteric pertaining to the ilium and femoral trochanters.
ilium pl. *ilia* [L.] the cranial portion of the hip bone. See also Table 10.
Ilizarov external ring skeletal fixation a device for stabilization of fractures using an external circular frame and a series of wires, nuts, bolts and rods.
illacrimation see EPIPHORA.
Illawarra cattle Australian red or red roan dairy cattle. Called also Australian milking shorthorn, Australian Illawarra shorthorn, AIS.
Illinois semen diluent used in the storage of boar semen; saturated with CO_2 it will store semen for 3 days. Called also Illinois Variable Temperature Semen Diluent.
Illinois sternal needle a needle with a screw-in stylet, large hub and guard used for aspiration of bone marrow.
illness a subjective state in a human marked by feelings of deviation from the normal healthy state; a term not thought to be applicable to animals.
illthrift failure to grow, increase in weight or maintain weight in the presence of apparently adequate food supplies and in the absence of recognizable disease. See also WEANER illthrift.
illumination the lighting up of a part, cavity, organ or object for inspection.
darkfield i., dark-ground i. the casting of peripheral light rays upon a microscopical object from the side, the center rays being blocked out; the object appears bright on a dark background.
illuminator the source of light for viewing an object.
ILT infectious laryngotracheitis.
IM intramuscularly.
im- a prefix, replacing *in-* before words beginning *b*, *m* and *p*.

image the picture reproduced on the x-ray film or by other radioimaging methods such as ultrasonography.
i. amplifier system includes amplifer and viewer or television camera and tape player.
i. display modes see ULTRASONOGRAPHY, A-mode, B-mode and M-mode.
i. formation exposure of the film to the x-ray beam ionizing radiation or to other radiant energy forms causes ionic changes in the silver bromide crystals in the film emulsion so that it acquires a silver atom. It is the deposition of reduced silver atoms in particles or zones that causes the black zones or foci on the film. The amount of silver deposited depends on the intensity of the initial radiation x-ray exposure.
i. intensification a technique used to increase the brightness of the image while maintaining its sharpness. Used particularly in fluoroscopy and viewing directly or indirectly through a television camera and monitor, cineradiography, videotape or split-film device.
latent i. the invisible picture on the film after it has been exposed to the x-ray beam. It requires exposure to a developer and fixer before the image is visible and permanent.
weak i. said of x-ray films which lack density due to underexposure, too brief period of development, insufficient developer or developer temperature too low.
imaging the production of diagnostic images, e.g., radiography, ultrasonography, or scintigraphy.
electrostatic i. a method of visualizing deep structures of the body, in which an electron beam is passed through the patient and the emerging beam strikes an electrostatically charged plate, dissipating the charge according to the strength of the beam. A film is then made from the plate.
nuclear i. see SCINTIGRAPHY.
organ i. outlining the size and location of organs by the injection of nuclides into the animal and observing their location by the use of a rectilinear scanner or a scintillation camera. See also SCINTIGRAPHY.
imago pl. *imagoes, imagines* [L.] the adult or definitive form of an insect.
imbalance lack of balance; especially lack of balance between muscles, as in insufficiency of ocular muscles.
autonomic i. defective coordination between the sympathetic and parasympathetic nervous systems, especially with respect to vasomotor activities.
sympathetic i. vagotonia.
vasomotor i. autonomic imbalance.
imbecile an animal in a continuous state of IMBECILITY.
imbecility a state of mind in which an animal does feeble, weak, absurd things and does not respond to usual environmental stimuli. Usually congenital. See also HYDRANENCEPHALY, ENCEPHALOPATHY.
imbibition absorption of a liquid.
imbricated overlapping like shingles or roof slates or tiles.
imbrication surgical pleating and folding of tissue to realign organs and provide extra support, e.g. chronically stretched joint capsule.
Flo i. a method for repair of cranial cruciate repair in the dog in which sutures are placed around the patellar tendon and the fabellae.
imidazathiazoles levamisole, tetramisole.
imidazoles a group of synthetic antifungal agents; includes CLOTRIMAZOLE, MICONAZOLE, ECONAZOLE and KETOCONAZOLE.
imidazothiazoles a group of broad-spectrum anthelmintics including BUTAMISOLE and LEVAMISOLE.
imide any compound containing the bivalent group –CONHCO–.
imidocarb an antiprotozoal agent, used as the hydrochloride or dipropionate, in the treatment of babesiosis and ehrlichiosis.
imino acid proline or hydroxyproline, the two amino acids in which the amino group is part of a closed ring.
imipenem one of the carbapenem group of antibiotics which are β-lactamase resistant. It has a very wide spectrum, but is inactivated by renal tubular enzymes and is given in association with cilastatin, which inhibits renal metabolism. Called also thienamycin.
imipramine a tricyclic antidepressant used in the treatment of behavior disorders and urinary incontinence in dogs.
immature unripe or not fully developed.
immediate direct, precipitating or primary; having no intermediate stage or mechanism, e.g. direct cause, immediate variant.
i.-type hypersensitivity reaction see immediate HYPERSENSITIVITY.
immersion 1. the plunging of a body into a liquid. 2. the use of the microscope with the object and object glass both covered with a liquid.
i. chilling method used for chilling poultry carcasses with iced water to ensure rapid cooling immediately after slaughter.
i. foot a condition similar to immersion foot in humans has been reported in cattle standing in cold water for days. There was erythema, edema and pain, followed by necrosis and sloughing of tissue.
i. syndrome vagal reflex, induced by contact with very cold water, causes cardiac arrest and death.
immiscible not susceptible to being mixed.
immobility standing still and disinclined to move, as in an animal suddenly blinded; responds to other stimuli unless immobility is part of a dummy syndrome when all stimuli are ignored.
immobilization the rendering of a part incapable of being moved.
i. band see COMPRESSION band.
electrical i. pulses of low voltage current are passed through the skin and through the body. It causes a tetanic immobilization but it is unknown whether or not it decreases pain perception.
immobilize to render incapable of being moved, as by a cast.
immobilizing drugs see MUSCLE RELAXANT.
Immobilon trade name for a muscle relaxant composed of a mixture of ETORPHINE and a phenothioazine tranquilizer such as ACEPROMAZINE or METHOTRIMEPRAZINE. Comes in two strengths, one for small animals and one for large animals.
immortality said of cell lines which are capable of undergoing an unlimited number of cell divisions.
immotile cilia syndrome congenital defect of ciliary movement recorded in dogs. See also primary CILIARY dyskinesia, KARTAGENER'S SYNDROME.
immune 1. being highly resistant to a disease because of the formation of humoral antibodies or the development of immunologically competent cells, or both, or as a result of some other mechanism, such as interferon activities in viral infections. 2. characterized by the development of antibodies or cellular IMMUNITY, or both, following exposure to antigen. 3. produced in response to antigen, such as immune serum globulin. The essential feature of antibody and

cell-mediated immunity is that they are highly antigen specific.
i. adherence the binding of antibody–antigen–complement complexes to complement receptors found on red blood cells.
i. complex see antibody–antigen COMPLEX.
i. complex disease disease induced by the deposition of or association with antigen–antibody–complement complexes in the microvasculature of tissues. Fixation of complement component C3 by the complexes initiates inflammation. See also SERUM sickness, HYPERSENSITIVITY.
i. complex reaction type III HYPERSENSITIVITY (1).
i. deficiency disease one in which animals have inadequate immune responses and so are more susceptible to infectious disease. The defect may be primary (inherited), or secondary (acquired) which usually develops after birth because of toxins or infectious agents. See also COMBINED IMMUNE DEFICIENCY SYNDROME, HYPOGAMMAGLOBULINEMIA, AGAMMAGLOBULINEMIA, inherited PARAKERATOSIS, CHEDIAK–HIGASHI SYNDROME and canine GRANULOCYTOPATHY syndrome.
i. hemolysis see immune-mediated hemolytic anemia (below).
i. interferon see INTERFERON.
i. modulator see IMMUNOMODULATION.
i. reaction immune response.
i. reaction fever aseptic fever occurring in anaphylaxis, angioedema.
i. response the specific response to substances interpreted by the body as not-self, the result being humoral and cellular IMMUNITY. The immune response depends on a functioning THYMUS and the conversion of stem cells to B and T lymphocytes. These B and T lymphocytes contribute to ANTIBODY production, cellular immunity and immunological memory. See also humoral IMMUNITY.
i. response (Ir) genes see immune response GENES.
i. surveillance the detection by lymphocytes, especially T lymphocytes, of new antigens, particularly on tumor cells.
i. system consists of the primary lymphoid organs (thymus and Bursa of Fabricius or its equivalent (bone marrow) in mammals) and secondary lymphoid organs (lymph nodes, spleen and other lymphoid tissue).
i. tolerance see immunological TOLERANCE.

immune-mediated caused by an unspecified immune reaction.
i.-m. contact hypersensitivity see ALLERGIC contact dermatitis.
i.-m. hemolytic anemia see autoimmune hemolytic ANEMIA; ALLOIMMUNE hemolytic anemia of the newborn.

immunifacient producing immunity; said of diseases, such as strangles and salmonellosis, that produce immunity against reinfection, which lasts for some time after an infection.

immunity 1. the condition of being immune; security against a particular disease; nonsusceptibility to the invasive or pathogenic effects of microorganisms or helminth parasites or to the toxic effect of antigenic substances. Called also functional or protective immunity. 2. responsiveness to antigen that leads to more rapid binding or elimination of antigen than in the nonimmune state; it includes both humoral and cell-mediated immunity (below). 3. the capacity to distinguish foreign material from *self*, and to neutralize, eliminate or metabolize that which is foreign (*non-self*) by the physiological mechanisms of the IMMUNE response.

The mechanisms of immunity are essentially concerned with the body's ability to recognize and dispose of substances which it interprets as foreign and sometimes harmful to its well-being. When such a substance enters the body, complex chemical and mechanical activities are set into motion to defend and protect the body's cells and tissues. The foreign substance, usually a protein, is called an ANTIGEN, that is, one which generates the production of an antagonist. The most readily recognized response to the antigen is the production of ANTIBODY. The antigen–antibody reaction is an essential component of the overall immune response. Of equal or greater importance to antibody, particularly for some antigens, is the development of so-called cell-mediated immune response, which involves clonal expansion of specifically reactive T lymphocytes including cytotoxic T lymphocytes (T_c lymphocytes) which play a major role in eliminating the foreign antigens that are cell associated.

Immunological responses in animals can be divided into two broad categories: humoral immunity, which refers to the production of antibody which becomes part of the body fluids (humors), especially serum, and cell-mediated or cellular immunity, which involves a variety of activities designed to destroy or at least contain cells that are recognized by the body as expressing foreign antigens on their cell surface, e.g. viral antigens. Both types of responses are mediated by lymphocytes that originate in the bone marrow as stem cells and later are converted into mature cells having specific properties and functions.
acquired i. antigen specific immunity attributable to the production of antibody and of specific immune T lymphocytes (responsible for cell-mediated immunity), following exposure to an antigen, or passive transfer of antibody or immune lymphoid cells (adoptive immunity).
active i. that which follows exposure to an antigen; acquired immunity attributable to the presence of antibody or of immune lymphoid cells formed in response to antigenic stimulus.
adoptive i. passive immunity of the cell-mediated type conferred by the administration of sensitized lymphocytes from an immune donor to a naive recipient.
artificial i. includes acquired (active) immunity produced by deliberate exposure to an antigen, such as a vaccine or the administration of antibody (passive).
cellular i. dependent upon T lymphocytes which are sensitized by first exposure to a specific antigen. Subsequent exposure stimulates the release of a group of substances known as lymphokines, such as interferon, and interleukins as well as direct killing by cytotoxic T lymphocytes.
functional i. see immunity (above).
humoral i. mediated by antibodies formed by antigen-specific B lymphocytes. Each B lymphocyte has monomeric IgM receptors which capture specific antigen, initiating production of the specific immunoglobulins. B lymphocytes activated by the presence of their specific antigen undergo transformation, lymphocyte blastogenesis, whereby they become metabolically active, divide, and some mature to plasma cells, which are major producers of antibodies. Some cells revert to small lymphocytes, 'memory' cells, and the expanded clone of these cells, on re-exposure to the antigen, undergo further lymphocyte blastogenesis, leading to further increased antibody production and numbers of memory cells.

There are two types of humoral immune response: primary and secondary. The primary response begins immediately after the inital contact with an antigen; the resulting antibody, predominantly IgM, appears 48 to 72 hours later. The secondary response occurs within 24 to 48 hours and produces large quantities of predominantly IgG. The secondary response persists much longer than the primary response and is the result of repeated contact with the antigens.

innate i., native i., natural i. natural immunity resulting from the genetic makeup of the host, before exposure to an antigen.

maternal i. that acquired by the neonate by transplacental transfer of immunoglobulins or from ingestion of colostrum or via the yolk sac in the case of birds. See also passive immunity (below).

natural i. see innate immunity (above).

passive i. the transfer of antibodies from a donor in which they were produced to a recipient for temporary immunity. Can be in the form of serum or colostrum or yolk. Significant transplacental transfer of antibodies is found in primates, but does not occur in domestic animals. Passive immunity in domestic mammals comes via the colostrum, with its high concentration of antibodies, and the more than normally pervious epithelium of the neonate's intestinal epithelium. In birds maternal antibody is transferred to the yolk, from where the developing chick embryo absorbs it from about day 11 of incubation. See also passive IMMUNIZATION.

protective i. see immunity (above).

immunization the process of rendering a subject immune, or of becoming immune. See also VACCINATION.

active i. stimulation with a specific antigen to promote an immune response. In the context of infectious diseases, the antigenic substances may include: (1) inactivated bacteria, as in BOTULISM immunization; (2) inactivated viruses, as in the canine PARVOVIRUS vaccination; (3) live attenuated viruses, e.g. RABIES virus, and (4) toxoids, chemically treated toxins produced by bacteria, as in immunization against TETANUS and PASTEURELLOSIS. Any of a vast number of foreign substances may induce an active immune response.

Since active immunization induces the body to produce its own antibodies and specifically reactive cells and to go on producing them, protection against disease will last several years, in some cases for life.

antihormone i. immunization against hormones, e.g. against androstenedione for the stimulation of ovulation in ewes, is now a commercial reality and promises to be a significant management tool in intensive animal production. See also immunological CONTRACEPTION.

deliberate i. the administration of an immunogen, usually by injection but sometimes orally or by inhalation, for the purpose of producing immunity.

natural i. stimulation of the immune system through exposure to antigens that have not been deliberately administered.

passive i. transient immunization produced by the introduction into the system of pre-formed antibody or specifically reactive lymphoid cells. The animal immunized is protected only as long as these antibodies or cells remain in the blood and are active—usually from 4 to 6 weeks. The immunity may be natural, as in the transfer of maternal antibody to offspring, or artificial, passive immunity following inoculation of antibodies or immune cells.

immunize to render immune.

immunoabsorbent a preparation of antigen attached to a solid support or antigen in an insoluble form, which absorbs homologous antibodies from a mixture of immunoglobulins. See IMMUNOSORBENT, ELISA.

immunoadjuvant see ADJUVANT.

immunoassay the quantitative determination of either antibody or antigen, e.g. hormones, drugs, vitamins, and specific proteins, by means of antigen–antibody interaction, as by agglutination, precipitation, ELISA, radioimmunoassay, etc.

immunoaugmenting to enhance immune response in a nonantigen specific manner by stimulating macrophage and reticuloendothelial function.

i. agents include BCG, mixed bacterial vaccine (MBV), and *Corynebacterium parvum*.

immunobiology that branch of biology dealing with immunological effects on such phenomena as infectious disease, growth and development, recognition phenomena, hypersensitivity, heredity, aging, cancer and transplantation.

immunoblast lymphoblast.

immunoblastic pertaining to or involving the stem cells (immunoblasts) of lymphoid tissue.

immunoblot see WESTERN BLOT.

immunochemistry the study of the chemical basis of immune phenomena and their interactions.

immunochemotherapy a combination of immunotherapy and chemotherapy.

immunocompetence the capacity to develop an immune response following exposure to antigen.

immunocomplex immune complex.

immunocompromised having reduced immune responsiveness as a result of inherited defects or infection, particularly by retroviruses and herpesviruses or by administration of immunosuppressive drugs, including antilymphocyte serum, by irradiation, by malnutrition, and by certain disease processes, e.g. cancer.

immunoconglutinin antibody formed against complement components that are part of an antibody–antigen complex, especially C3.

immunoconjugates monoclonal antibodies which are target-specific carriers for specific compounds such as plant or bacterial toxins, radionuclides, photoactive agents and chemotherapeutic drugs.

immunocyte any cell of the lymphoid series which can react with antigen to produce antibody or to participate in cell-mediated immunity; called also immunologically competent cell.

immunocytoadherence the aggregation of red cells to form rosettes around lymphocytes with surface immunoglobulins.

immunocytochemical staining use of antibody to detect and stain particular cell types, e.g. immunoperoxidase staining.

immunocytochemistry the application of immunochemical techniques to cytochemistry; includes direct and indirect fluorescent antibody techniques.

immunodeficiency a deficiency in the immune system, either that mediated by antibody or T lymphocytes, or both. See also AGAMMAGLOBULINEMIA, HYPOGAMMAGLOBULINEMIA, FELINE immunodeficiency virus, BOVINE immunodeficiency virus.

acquired i. see IMMUNE deficiency disease.

cancer-associated i. in general, associated with cachexia and debilitation, and also related to the type of neoplasia. Tumor-related effects on the immune system include impaired function of lymphocytes, altered cytokine production and activation of suppressor cell functions.

combined i. see COMBINED IMMUNE DEFICIENCY SYNDROME (DISEASE).

common variable i. a term encompassing a heterogeneous group of syndromes, which may be inherited or acquired, characterized by recurring persistent infections and deficiencies of some of the immunoglobulin classes.

congenital i. see IMMUNE deficiency disease.

i. disease see IMMUNE deficiency disease, COMBINED IMMUNE DEFICIENCY SYNDROME (DISEASE).

iatrogenic i. secondary IMMUNE deficiency disease.

severe combined i. see COMBINED IMMUNE DEFICIENCY SYNDROME (DISEASE).

X-linked i. an inherited form of severe combined immunodeficiency has been reported in dogs. Puppies fail to grow and die from overwhelming infections at an early age.

immunodepression an absence or deficient supply of the components of either humoral or cellular immunity, or both. See also AGAMMAGLOBULINEMIA, HYPOGAMMAGLOBULINEMIA, IMMUNODEFICIENCY.

immunodermatology the study of immunological phenomena as they affect skin disorders and their treatment or prophylaxis.

immunodiagnostic pertaining to diagnosis by immune reactions.

immunodiffusion the diffusion of antigen and antibody from separate wells, usually cut in agar, such that precipitation lines form in the agar between the wells.

radial i. (Mancini technique) antigen diffuses into the agar which contains specific antibody and a ring of precipitate is formed, the diameter of which is directly proportional to the concentration of the antigen and can thereby be used to quantitate the amount of antigen. A reverse radial immunodiffusion test, in which antigen is incorporated in the agar, can be used to quantitate the amount of antibody in a sample.

i. tests include double immunodiffusion (Ouchterloney technique) which is used in the COGGINS TEST for equine infectious anemia and single immunodiffusion (Oudin technique), as well as radial immunodiffusion.

immunodominance the property of an antigenic determinant that causes it to be responsible for the major immune response in a host.

immunoelectrophoresis separation, usually in an agar gel, of complex mixtures of antigens which then combine, following immunodiffusion, with antibody to form precipitation lines for each separated antigen.

counter i. antigen and antibody are placed in separate wells, close together and electric current is applied first in one direction then in the other. When they migrate and meet, a line of precipitin is formed.

rocket i. electrophoresis in which antigen migrates from a well through agar gel containing antiserum, forming cone-shaped (rocket) precipitin bands; the area under the cone is used to calculate the amount of antigen.

immunofiltration purification of antibodies by mixing with specific antigen, the antigen is then removed from the antibody by treatment with soluble carriers. Called also affinity purification of antibodies.

immunofluorescence a method of determining the location of antigen (or antibody) in a tissue section or smear using a specific antibody (or antigen) labeled with a fluorochrome. In the direct methods, the fluorochome is chemically linked to the specific antibody. In indirect methods, a labeled anti-immunoglobulin that binds to the specific antibody is used. See also FLUORESCENCE microscopy.

immunofluorescent having the characteristic of immunofluorescence.

i. antibody test see FLUORESCENCE microscopy.

i. microscopy see FLUORESCENCE microscopy.

immunogen substance that elicits an immune response.

immunogenetics the study of the genetic factors controlling the animal's immune response and the transmission of those factors from generation to generation.

immunogenic producing immunity; evoking an immune response.

immunogenicity the ability of a substance to provoke an immune response or the degree to which it provokes a response.

immunoglobulin a specialized class of serum proteins, which may occur naturally in serum, but are usually produced following exposure to an almost limitless (>10^7) number of antigens. Called also antibody. Immunoglobulins combine only with the antigen (or one closely related to it) that elicited their production. Immunoglobulins are major components of what is called the humoral IMMUNE response system. They are synthesized by B lymphocytes and their derivative plasma cells, and are found in the serum and in other body fluids and tissues, including the urine, spinal fluid, lymph nodes and spleen. See also IMMUNITY.

Immunoglobulin molecules consist of two kinds of polypeptide chains: heavy chains (H-chains) and light chains (L-chains). There are five antigenically different kinds of H-chains, designated γ, μ, α, δ and ε, and this difference is the basis for the classification of immunoglobulins. Classes vary in their chemical structure and in the number of antigen-binding sites.

The five classes of immunoglobulins (Ig) are: IgG, IgM, IgA, IgD and IgE. Only IgG, IgM and IgA are found in all species of domestic animals.

IgA is present in low concentrations in the serum, but it is the major immunoglobulin of secretions and has a major first-line defense role in infections that enter via mucosal surfaces. Two IgA molecules are linked by a polypeptide called the secretory piece and by a J chain. Secretory IgA is present in nonvascular fluids, such as saliva, bile, synovial fluid, and intestinal and respiratory tract secretions. Both secreted and circulating IgA types are known to have antiviral properties; their production is preferentially stimulated by local administration of antigens such as oral and aerosol immunizations.

IgD is found in trace quantities in the serum in humans and chickens. It is found on the surface of B lymphocytes. Its function is uncertain.

IgE, once called reaginic antibody, is present in very low levels in serum and is generally present in increased levels in individuals with allergy. It has not been found in the chicken. IgE binds to Fc receptors on the surface of cells particularly mast cells and basophils, via the Fc part of the molecule. Following exposure to antigen (allergen), and its binding to the Fab of two adjacent IgE molecules, perturbations of the cell membrane are produced, leading to the release of vasoactive amines, particularly histamine and serotonin, which are the mediators of anaphylaxis and atopic reactions, including urticaria, asthma, hayfever and gastroenteritis. Allergic reactions such as urticaria, atopy and anaphylactic shock are examples of IgE-mediated reactions. It is recognized in humans and dogs that there is an inherited (familial) predisposition for certain individuals to produce IgE.

IgG is the most abundant of the five classes of immunoglobulins, representing about 80% of serum immunoglobulin protein. It is the major antibody in the secondary humoral response of immunity, serves to activate the complement system, and is frequently involved in opsonization. IgG is the only immunoglobulin that crosses the placenta and is the major component of passive maternal antibody transfer via colostrum and yolk.

IgM is the first antibody produced in the primary immune response. It represents about 20% of serum antibodies. Like the IgG, IgM bound to antigen activates the complement system, and together these two classes of immunoglobulins serve as specific antitoxins against the toxins of diphtheria, tetanus, botulism and anthrax microorganisms, and snake venoms, and play a major role in defense against most infectious diseases.

colostral i. colostrum contains a high level of IgG for several days after parturition. Following ingestion, colostral IgG molecules are absorbed unchanged across the intestinal mucosa for the first 1 to 2 days in cattle, dog, pig and horse and for up to 4 days in the sheep and goat. IgA is also present in colostrum but is not translocated to the circulation of the suckling animal to any extent; it may provide some local gut immunity.

i. deficiency see IMMUNODEFICIENCY.

i. genes genes that code for the light and heavy chains of immunoglobulins.

secretory i. IgA.

i. superfamily immunoglobulins and a number of other proteins including T cell receptor, major histocompatibility molecules, T cell accessory proteins and some adhesion molecules that are structurally related to immunoglobulins.

immunogold a labeling technique for the detection and localization of particular antigens in a specimen. See also immunoelectron MICROSCOPY.

immunohistochemical denoting the application of antibody–antigen interactions to histochemical techniques, as in the use of immunofluorescence.

immunoincompetent lacking the ability or capacity to develop an immune response to antigenic challenge.

immunologic, immunological emanating from or pertaining to immunology.

i. competence see IMMUNOCOMPETENCE.

i. domains in cell receptor biology, the structure of receptors is conveniently considered in terms of three functional domains: transmembrane, ligand binding and innumological; the latter contain primary antigenic regions.

i. fertility control antihormone IMMUNIZATION.

i. incompetence immunoincompetence.

i. injury see IMMUNOPATHY.

i. reactions see IMMUNE response, IMMUNITY.

i. status a reference to IMMUNOCOMPETENCE of a host.

i. tolerance see immunological TOLERANCE.

immunologist a specialist in immunology.

immunology the scientific study of all aspects of immunity, including allergy, hypersensitivity, etc.

immunomodulating having the capacity for and used for IMMUNOMODULATION.

immunomodulation adjustment of the immune response to a desired level, as in immunopotentiation, immunosuppression, or induction of immunological tolerance.

immunomodulator agents that alter the immune response by suppression (IMMUNOSUPPRESSIVE) or enhancement (IMMUNOSTIMULANT).

immunopathogenesis the process of development of a disease in which an immune response or the products of an immune reaction are involved.

immunopathological emanating from or pertaining to immunopathogenesis.

immunopathology 1. that branch of biomedical science concerned with immune reactions associated with disease, whether the reactions be beneficial, without effect, or harmful. 2. the structural and functional manifestations of the immune response involved in a disease.

immunopathy any abnormal immune response. Includes: 1. deficient or absent response. See COMBINED IMMUNE DEFICIENCY SYNDROME (DISEASE). 2. excess production of gamma globulins (HYPERGAMMAGLOBULINEMIA), e.g. in the excessive proliferation of plasma cells in a multiple myeloma. 3. over-reaction to extrinsic antigens as in immediate and delayed type HYPERSENSITIVITY. 4. over-reaction to intrinsic antigens, abnormal response of the body to its own tissues, e.g. the AUTOIMMUNE diseases such as lupus erythematosus and thyroiditis.

immunoperoxidase staining a technique of histological staining that provides morphological details and immunological identification. Analogous to immunofluorescence techniques, but uses peroxidase conjugated to immunoglobulin instead of fluorescent dyes.

immunophysiology the physiology of immunological processes.

immunopotency the capacity of an individual antigenic determinant of an antigen molecule to initiate an immune response.

immunopotentiation accentuation of the response to an immunogen by administration of another substance, e.g. adjuvant, interleukin 2.

immunoprecipitation precipitation resulting from interaction of antibody and soluble antigen.

immunoproliferative characterized by the proliferation of the lymphoid cells producing immunoglobulins, as in the gammopathies.

i. disease see GAMMOPATHY, HYPERGAMMAGLOBULINEMIA.

immunoprophylaxis prevention of disease by the administration of vaccines or hyperimmune sera.

immunoradiometry the use of radiolabeled antibody (in the place of radiolabeled antigen) in radioimmunoassay techniques.

immunoreactant a substance exhibiting immunoreactivity.

immunoreactive exhibiting immunoreactivity.

immunoregulation the control of specific immune responses and interactions between B and T lymphocytes and macrophages.

immunoresponsiveness the capacity to react immunologically.

immunosorbent the binding of antigen or antibody to a solid support, usually a plastic surface at the bottom of a well in a microtiter plate or a latex particle. See also ELISA.

immunostimulant 1. stimulating an immune response. 2. an agent that stimulates an immune response.

immunostimulation stimulation of an immune response, e.g. by use of BCG vaccine, levamisole, thiabendazole.

immunosuppressant immunosuppressive.

immunosuppression diminished immune responsiveness; may occur following certain infections, notably viral infections such as retroviruses or herpesviruses (cytamegaloviruses), exposure to x-irradiation or toxic chemicals or be deliberately produced

in transplantation patients by drugs or antilymphocyte serum.
therapeutic i. treatment which suppresses immune function where it is contributing to the disease process. Includes immune-mediated diseases of the eye, hemopoietic system, skin, kidney and central nervous system.

immunosuppressive 1. pertaining to or inducing immunosuppression. 2. an agent that induces immunosuppression.

immunosurveillance the monitoring function of the immune system whereby it recognizes and reacts against aberrant cells arising within the body.

immunotherapy passive immunization of an animal by administration of preformed antibodies (serum or gamma globulin) actively produced in another individual; by extension, the term has come to include the use of immunopotentiators, replacement of immunocompetent lymphoid tissue (e.g. bone marrow or thymus), etc. Because the immune response is a process of surveillance, recognition and attack of foreign cells, immunotherapy has emerged as a promising mode of treatment for cancer.
Nonspecific immunotherapy relies on general immune stimulants to activate the whole immune system. In the past decade, immunotherapy against cancer has involved the use of the bacille Calmette–Guérin (BCG) vaccine (see BCG vaccine), which is evolved from strains of *Mycobacterium tuberculosis*, and is used to provide some immunity to tuberculosis. Recently, INTERFERON has been considered as a good prospect for converting inactive immune cells into active 'natural killers' that attack tumor cells directly.

immunotolerance see immunological TOLERANCE.

immunotoxin an antitoxin.

immunotransfusion transfusion of blood from a donor previously rendered immune to the disease affecting the recipient.

IMP inosine 5-monophosphate.

impacted being wedged in firmly. In obstetrics, denoting twins so situated during delivery that the pressure of one against the other prevents complete engagement of either. In gastroenterology denotes the formation of a mass of food or fecal material that cannot be moved caudally unless it is softened and reformed or broken up. Used also in relation to an impacted tooth or to describe a fracture.

impaction the condition of being impacted. Most commonly a condition in the alimentary tract of herbivores fed on roughage of poor digestibility. See also impactions of ANAL SACS of dogs, OVIDUCT of birds, SCENT glands of ruminants.
i. colic see impaction COLIC.
fecal i. a syndrome of moderate toxemia, an absence of fecal movements and straining in some cases. There is a collection of putty-like or hardened feces in the rectum or sigmoid. In horses fed on roughage of poor digestibility, the syndrome is one of colic due to impaction in the colon or cecum or both, or of the ileocecal valve. In cattle the syndrome is one of indigestion and ruminal stasis, less commonly abomasal impaction. In both syndromes there is a delayed passage of feces and palpably distended, firm viscera in appropriate locations. Each of these specific impactions is discussed under COLIC, ABOMASAL impaction, RUMINAL impaction, OMASAL impaction, CROP-bound and OVIDUCT impaction of birds.
i. large intestine see impaction COLIC.
teeth i. see impacted TEETH.

impala an extraordinarily agile antelope about 3 ft high, with long, lyre-shaped horns on the male. Called also *Aepyceros melampus*.

impalpable not detectable by touch.

impar not even; unequal; unpaired.

impatent not open; closed.

impedance obstruction or opposition to passage or flow, as of an electric current or other form of energy.
acoustic i. an expression of the opposition to passage of sound waves, being the product of the density of a substance and the velocity of sound in it.

imperfect state the asexual stage in the life cycle of fungi.

imperforate not open; abnormally closed. Common sites for atresia are anus, hymen, teat sphincter, lacrimal puncta.

impermeable not permitting passage, as for fluid.

impetigo usually a staphylococcal skin infection marked by vesicles or bullae that become pustular, rupture, and form yellow crusts. In animals a superficial infection of the face of newborn piglets, the abdominal skin of puppies, and one of the teats of cows, go under the name of impetigo. See also UDDER impetigo, CONTAGIOUS porcine pyoderma.
i. contagiosa see EXUDATIVE epidermitis.

implant 1. to insert or to graft (tissue or radioactive material) into intact tissues or a body cavity. 2. any material inserted or grafted into the body, e.g. carbon fiber, metal or plastic prostheses, hormone, electronic signal, growth promoter.
biological i. foreign materials placed in the body tissues for purposes of assisting in some function, either temporarily or permanently. May be made of soft tissues, synthetics, metals, or ceramics that are relatively inert and compatible with body tissues.

implantation 1. the insertion of an organ or tissue in a new site in the body. 2. the attachment and embedding of the fertilized ovum in the endometrium. 3. the insertion or grafting into the body of biological, living, inert or radioactive material.
embryo i. attachment of the trophoblast to the uterine lining. The form of attachment varies widely from superficial apposition to varying degrees of endometrial invasion.

implantology the science dealing with implants.

implied contract a contract assumed to have been drawn in spite of there being no written record nor any actual verbal agreement. An implied contract exists when a veterinarian examines and treats an animal. It is implied that the veterinarian will do his/her best and that the client will pay the fee charged.

implosion flooding.

impotence inability of the male to achieve or maintain an erection of sufficient rigidity to perform sexual intercourse successfully.

impotentia coeundi [L.] inability of the male animal to perform sexual intercourse.

impregnation 1. the act of fertilizing or rendering pregnant. 2. saturation.

impressio pl. *impressiones* [L.] impression (1).

impression 1. a slight indentation or depression, as one produced in the surface of one organ by pressure exerted by another. 2. a negative imprint of an object made in some plastic material that later solidifies. 3. an effect produced upon the mind, body or senses by some external stimulus or agent.
i. plate a plastic plate with a central well filled with agar that has a convex surface. The agar is pressed against the tissue to be examined bacteriologically.
dental i. a mold taken of the teeth or jaw and used in the fabrication of dental appliances to be used in restorative dentistry or orthodontics.

i. smear a sample of cells, microorganisms or fluids obtained by pressing against the surface of a specimen which may be tissue excised or in situ. Commonly used for cytology examination.

imprinting a kind of learning in the very young based mainly on maternal attachment and acquisition of basic behavior patterns.

improvement lag the time delay between improved performance in one tier of a breeding program until it appears in the next tier.

impulse 1. a sudden pushing force. 2. a sudden uncontrollable act. 3. a nerve impulse.

cardiac i. movement of the chest wall caused by the heartbeat. Called also APEX beat.

nerve i. the electrochemical process propagated along nerve fibers.

IMV intermittent mandatory ventilation.

In chemical symbol, *indium.*

in- 1. a prefix, *in, within* or *into.* 2. an intensive prefix. 3. a negative or privative prefix.

in extremis [L.] *at the point of death.*

in-hand being led; a show class of led horses.

in-pup pregnant; similarly with in-lamb, in-calf, in-foal.

in situ [L.] *in its normal place;* confined to the site of origin.

i. s. hybridization see in situ HYBRIDIZATION of nucleic acid.

in tela [L.] *in tissue;* relating especially to stained histological preparations.

in utero [L.] *within the uterus.*

in vitro [L.] literally *within a glass,* i.e. outside the living body; observable in a test tube; in an artificial environment.

in vivo [L.] *within the living body.*

inability to rise see RECUMBENCY.

inactin a quick-acting barbiturate, used as an induction agent.

inactivated rendered inactive; the activity is destroyed.

i. viruses treated so that they are no longer able to produce evidence of growth or damaging effect on tissue. Inactivation may be by physical means including heat, ultraviolet light, ultrasonic vibration, or by chemical treatment. Used in inactivated viral vaccines.

inactivation the destruction of activity, as of a virus, by the action of heat, chemical or other agent.

inanimate 1. without life. 2. lacking in animation.

inanition the exhausted state due to prolonged undernutrition; starvation.

inapparent not clearly seen.

i. infection infection without clinical signs.

inappetence partial lack of appetite or desire contrasted to ANOREXIA. Presence is inferred in animals which have depressed food intake.

inappropriate mating time at too young an age; too early in the lactation cycle; not an appropriate time to provide for a saleable young at yearling sales, major exhibitions at which entrants are grouped in age classes.

inarticulate not having joints; disjointed.

inassimilable not susceptible of being utilized as nutriment.

inborn congenital; inherited or acquired before birth.

i. error of metabolism congenital disorders of metabolism. Includes cystinuria, fucosidosis, citrullinemia, mannosidosis, tyrosinemia and glycogenosis.

inbred said of offspring produced by INBREEDING.

i. lines succeeding generations of animals all derived by breeding from the same group of closely related individuals.

inbreeding the mating of closely related organisms or of organisms having closely similar genetic constitutions.

i. coefficient the probability that the two genes present at a locus in that individual are identical by descent.

i. depression depression of performance caused by inbreeding.

incarceration unnatural retention or confinement of a part, e.g. of an intestinal loop.

incidence the rate at which a certain event occurs, as the number of new cases of a specific disease occurring during a certain period.

i. reporting schemes prospective gathering of epidemiological data on incidence of nominated diseases.

incident impinging upon, as incident radiation.

incineration the act of burning to ashes.

incipient beginning to exist; coming into existence.

incisal the cutting edge of an incisor or canine tooth.

incision 1. a cut or a wound made by a sharp instrument. 2. the act of cutting.

bold i. one described as firm and free in action so as to cut through the skin in a minimum of motions, rather than multiple short, light strokes.

grid i. a surgical approach through a flank incision in horses and cattle in which the several muscle layers are separated in the direction of their fibers, each of which is different, and the peritoneum is incised in a vertical direction. Called also a modified McBurney incision.

modified McBurney i. see grid incision (above).

paramedian i. one located near the midplane, most commonly parallel and close to the linea alba.

relaxing i. one made to allow movement of skin for closure of a wound or parallel incision.

stab i. made with the point of a scalpel.

incisive 1. having the power of cutting; sharp. 2. pertaining to the incisor teeth.

i. bone the bone bearing the incisors. Called also premaxilla. See Table 10.

incisor 1. adapted for cutting. 2. any one of the six (eight in ruminants but only in the lower jaw) front teeth of either jaw. See also TEETH.

incisure a cut, notch or incision.

inclusion 1. the act of enclosing or the condition of being enclosed. 2. anything that is enclosed; a cell inclusion.

epithelial i. probably endothelial displacements during embryonic development; epithelial cells in acinar or ductal structure enclosed in a layer of epithelial cells on a basement membrane.

cell i. a usually lifeless, often temporary, constituent in the cytoplasm of a cell.

chlamydial i. see ELEMENTARY body.

dental i. a tooth so surrounded with bony material that it is unable to erupt.

fetal i. a partially developed embryo enclosed within the body of its twin.

nutritive i's glycogen inclusions, visible only with electron microscope, include α-particles (rosettes) and β-particles (single particles).

inclusion body round, oval or irregular-shaped bodies in the cytoplasm and nucleus of cells, as in diseases due to viral infection, such as rabies, inclusion body rhinitis. May be acid-fast as in lead poisoning. See also BOLLINGER BODIES, BORREL BODIES, ELEMENTARY body (1), GUARNIERI BODIES, JOEST BODIES, Negri BODY, PASCHEN BODIES and type A, type B inclusion bodies (below).

falcon i. b. disease caused by a herpesvirus, the clinical signs include weakness, anorexia, diarrhea and a mortality rate of 100%. There is a profound leukopenia.

i. b. hepatitis a disease of young chickens caused by an adenovirus and characterized by jaundice and anemia. The mortality rate is about 25%. Called also chicken hemorrhagic syndrome.

i. b. rhinitis a disease of the upper respiratory tract of young pigs caused by a cytomegalovirus. Clinically there is paroxysmal sneezing, a serous, ocular and nasal discharge, and a benign course. It may be a precursor to atrophic rhinitis.

snake i. b. disease thought due to a virus; observed in many boid snakes; characterized by heavy mortality after signs of CNS disease; inclusion bodies in most tissues, especially brain.

type A i. b. found in chromatically disrupted nuclei with margination of the chromatin fragments and the inclusion body is amorphous or granular and acid-staining; characteristic of cells infected with, for example, herpesvirus and adenovirus.

type B i. b. the nucleus is still well organized, there is no margination of chromatin and the inclusion bodies are well defined; seen in cells infected with, for example, distemper virus.

incoagulability the state of being incapable of coagulation.

income financial return from a project or for help provided.

i. elasticity see DEMAND elasticity.

net i. gross income less costs.

i. over feed cost a rough indicator of the profitability of an animal enterprise based principally on fattening of young livestock, e.g. in a feedlot. The fixed costs are the depreciation on the installation and labor, the variable costs are the price of cattle and the feed.

incompatibility the quality of being incompatible.

drug i. may be *chemical*, i.e. the drugs react with each other and precipitate, produce gas or similar effect, or *pharmacological* in that the effects of the two on tissues are opposite, or *pharmaceutical*, e.g. immiscibility, insolubility.

incompatible not suitable for combination, simultaneous administration, or transplantation; mutually repellent.

incompetence 1. inability to function properly. 2. the legal term used in a suit charging that loss of an animal occurred because a veterinarian had a level of competence below that which could reasonably be expected. See also NEGLIGENCE.

incompetent 1. not able to function properly, e.g. incompetent cervix. 2. a veterinarian determined by the courts to be less competent than the community should reasonably expect.

incomplete base-pairing see MISMATCH (2).

incontinence 1. inability to control excretory functions. Food animals are not easy to classify with respect to their continence. Companion animals who suddenly lose their house training manners may be diagnosed as incontinent. See also URINARY incontinence. 2. immoderation or excess.

fecal i. the inability to retain feces until a coordinated and appropriate act of defecation. Characterized by a relaxed anal sphincter and fecal material dropping out at intervals. Can be caused by injury to the anal sphincter or its nerve supply, particularly spinal nerves S1 to S3. A feature of sacral agensis.

neurogenic i. see neurogenic URINARY BLADDER.

retention-overflow i. see atonic neurogenic URINARY BLADDER.

stress i. 1. involuntary urination when stressed; common in young puppies. 2. URETHRAL incompetence.

urge i. frequent urination of small amounts; detrusor HYPERREFLEXIA.

incoordination a lack of normal adjustment of muscular action so that the intended movement of the limb or other part is not made smoothly and harmoniously, and does not accurately achieve its objective. If the abnormality is hypermetric, the condition is referred to as ataxia. If it is inclined to weakness, e.g. knuckling at the turn, stumbling, failure to flex limbs properly, or to misdirection as in a proprioceptive deficit, it is called incoordination. The judgment is best made with the animal going at a good pace, preferably unrestrained, and on level going. A number of sophisticated techniques are available for the examination of the gaits of racing horses.

As affecting sphincters, especially of the alimentary tract, the term is used alternatively to achalasia.

enzootic equine i. see ENZOOTIC equine incoordination.

incorporation 1. the union of one substance with another, or with others, in a composite mass. 2. a legal procedure by which a veterinary practice is turned into a company. Unless the company is run entirely by veterinarians there is the risk that the professional ethic that the good of the patient is paramount may be overcome by a more profit-conscious set of rules. There are many advantages to incorporation in terms of financial security and adequacy of financial return to the veterinarian.

increment 1. an increase or addition; the amount by which a value or quantity is increased. 2. the early stage of fever, where the temperature is rising; clinically there is shivering, coldness of the skin, and absence of sweating.

incremental lines see VON EBNER'S LINES.

incrustation 1. the formation of a crust. 2. a crust, scab or scale.

incubate 1. to subject to or to undergo incubation. 2. material that has undergone incubation.

incubation 1. the provision of proper conditions for growth and development, as for bacterial or tissue cultures. 2. development of a disease by multiplication of an infectious agent within the host. 3. the development of the embryo in the eggs of oviparous animals. See also AVIAN incubation periods. 4. the maintenance of an artificial environment for a neonate, especially a premature one.

artificial i. use of a machine which warms, turns, humidifies bird eggs to incubate and eventually hatch them.

i. behavior see AVIAN broodiness; almost non-existent in egg-laying birds; persists in meat strains and turkeys.

i. period the interval between effective exposure to a pathogenic infectious agent, leading to the invasion of the body and the establishment of the infection, and the appearance of the first clinical signs of the disease in question. Incubation periods vary from a few days to several years, depending on the causative organism and type of disease. See also EXTRINSIC incubation period.

incubator an apparatus for maintaining optimal conditions (temperature, humidity, etc.) for growth and development, especially one used for cultures, and for hatching eggs.

incudal pertaining to the INCUS.

incudiform anvil-shaped.
incudomalleal pertaining to the incus and malleus.
incudostapedial pertaining to the incus and stapes.
incurable 1. not susceptible of being cured. 2. an animal with a disease that cannot be cured.
incus the middle of the three ossicles of the ear; called also anvil. See also Table 10.
indandione any of a group of synthetic anticoagulants derived from 1,3-indandione, including pindone and diphacinone, which impair the hepatic synthesis of the vitamin K-dependent coagulation factors (prothrombin, factors VII, IX and X). Used in human medicine as an anticoagulant and as a rodenticide in a manner similar to that of warfarin.
independence in statistical terms two variables are independent if the expected distribution of one variable is the same for each and every value of the other. Independence implies zero correlation, but the reverse is not necessarily true.
index pl. *indexes, indices* [L.] the numerical ratio of measurement of any part in comparison with a fixed standard.
i. case the first case of a disease in a group to be brought to the attention of the clinician.
Color I. a publication of the Society of Dyers and Colorists and the American Association of Textile Chemists and Colorists, containing an extensive list of dyes and dye intermediates. Each chemically distinct compound is identified by a specific number, the CI number, avoiding the confusion of trivial names used for dyes in the dye industry. The Royal Horticultural Society, London, produces a similar document to aid in the identification of flower colors.
erythrocyte i's see ERYTHROCYTE indices.
I. Medicus a monthly publication of the National Library of Medicine, in which the world's leading biomedical literature is indexed by author and subject.
opsonic i. a measure of opsonic activity determined by the ratio of the number of microorganisms phagocytized by normal leukocytes in the presence of serum from an animal infected by the microorganism, to the number phagocytized in serum from a normal animal.
phagocytic i. the average number of bacteria ingested per leukocyte of the patient's blood.
production i. a method of expressing production compared with a potential or target.
refractive i. the refractive power of a medium compared with that of air (assumed to be 1).
therapeutic i. originally, the ratio of the maximum tolerated dose to the minimum curative dose; now defined as the ratio of the median lethal dose (LD_{50}) to the median effective dose (ED_{50}). It is used in assessing the safety of a drug.
I. Veterinarius a periodic listing of all publications in the veterinary literature by the Commonwealth Agricultural Bureaux, United Kingdom. Also available on on-line data search.
vital i. the ratio of births to deaths within a given time in a population.
Indian antelope black antelope with spiral horns, white eyepatch and white underparts. Called also blackbuck, *Antilope cervicapra*.
Indian beech see PONGAMIA *glabra*.
Indian bulrush PENNISETUM *glaucum*.
Indian hemp see CANNABIS *sativa*.
Indian liquorice see ABRUS *precatorius*.
Indian millet PENNISETUM *glaucum*.
Indian mustard BRASSICA *juncea*.
Indian pea LATHYRUS *sativus*.
Indian poke see VERATRUM *viride*.
Indian runner an egg-laying duck which originated in Malaysia and China. There are five color varieties: fawn, white, fawn and white, black, and chocolate. The duck has an almost vertical stance and a characteristic running gait.
Indian tobacco LOBELIA *berlandieri*.
Indian turnip see ARISAEMA.
Indian walnut ALEURITES *moluccana*.
indican 1. a substance formed by decomposition of tryptophan in the intestines and excreted in the urine. 2. a yellow indoxyl glycoside from indigo plants.
indicant an indicator or signal. A clinical indicant is a clinical sign, an item of history, epidemiology or environmental peculiarity that suggests a particular diagnosis for inclusion in the list of possibles.
indicanuria an excess of indican in the urine. High levels are indicative of prolonged alimentary tract sojourn and increased absorption of this detoxification product of indole.
indication a sign or circumstance that points to or shows the cause, treatment, etc. of a disease. See also INDICANT.
indicator 1. a piece of information that suggests a suitable line of action, in diagnosis, treatment or control. 2. any substance that indicates the appearance or disappearance of a chemical by a color change or attainment of a certain pH.
i. plants plants (e.g. *Astragalus* and *Xylorrhiza* spp.) that prefer a higher than normal soil content of a particular element, e.g. selenium, copper. Their presence indicates a potentially poisonous pasture. Called also obligate ACCUMULATOR PLANTS.
indigestible fiber/roughage includes feeds such as straw, mature meadow hay, cereal stubble, browse comprising mostly woody shrubs; conducive to impaction (rumenoreticular in ruminants, large intestine in equidae).
indigestion lack or failure of digestive function; commonly used to denote vague abdominal discomfort after eating. In animals the use of the term is restricted to cattle. Manifested by ruminal stasis, anorexia, reduced fecal output. Usually due to dietary error. See also VAGUS indigestion.
indigitation intussusception (1).
Indigofera a genus of legumes in the Fabaceae family of plants; some species contain a hepatoxin, indospicine, a toxic amino acid; *I. australis* (native indigo), *I. linnaei*, *I. spicata* (*I. endecaphylla*, creeping indigo), *I. teysmannii*, *I. truxillensis*.
***I. linnaei* (*I. dominii*, *I. enneaphylla*)** a prostrate Australian herb which causes Birdsville horse disease, characterized by marked incoordination, frequent falling, emaciation and terminal convulsions. May be prevented by dietary supplementation with protein. There are no lesions specific to the disease. A nitrotoxin is suspected as the cause. Called also Birdsville indigo.
I. hochstetteri contains an unidentified toxin, causes incoordination, dyspnea, diarrhea.
indigotindisulfonate sodium a dye used as a diagnostic aid in renal disease.
indirect done through an intermediate animal or function.
i. advertising advertising about the veterinary profession which indirectly benefits individual veterinarians.
i. comparisons comparisons made between individuals or groups in different locations.
i. contact see indirect CONTACT.
i. fluorescent antibody see FLUORESCENCE microscopy.

i. repeat see INVERTED REPEAT.

i. selection improving one character while selecting on another.

i. social distance social distance is distance between contacts in an infectious disease; indirect social distance is distance between indirect contacts.

i. transmission of infection transmission of infection via another medium, e.g. housing or bedding, without the animals ever being close to each other.

indium a chemical element, atomic number 49, atomic weight 114.82, symbol In. See Table 6.

individual a unit member of a population; peculiar to an individual animal.

i. animal productivity production record of an individual animal.

i. cow lifetime record a cow's record of production or health or both kept as a continuing separate record.

i. distance the distance that a bird assumes as its private domain and inside which it will attack any intruder.

i. times e.g. cow-years at risk, dog-months of protection.

individuation 1. the process of developing individual characteristics. 2. differential regional activity in the embryo occurring in response to organizer influence.

indocyanine green a dye used intravenously as a diagnostic aid in the determination of blood volume, cardiac output and hepatic function.

Indofilaria a genus of filaroid nematodes in the family Filariidae.

I. patabiramani causes dermatitis in elephants.

indole a compound obtained from coal tar and indigo and produced by decomposition of tryptophan in the intestine, where it contributes to the peculiar odor of feces. It is excreted in the urine in the form of indican. 3-Methyl-indole and L-tryptophan are implicated in causing acute interstitial pneumonia in cattle.

i. alkaloids include β-carbolines, dimethyl tryptamines, hydroxy methyltryptamines, alstonines.

i. test a biochemical test for the identification of bacteria, based on the production of indole from tryptophan in the medium provided.

indolent causing little pain; slow growing.

i. ulcer see EOSINOPHILIC ulcer, refractory ULCER.

indolizidine alkaloid e.g. swainsonine (occurs in plants such as *Astragalus*, *Swainsonia* and *Oxytropis* spp.) and castanospermine (occurs in *Castanospermum* spp.). Inhibit α-mannosidase.

indomethacin an anti-inflammatory, analgesic and antipyretic agent, used in arthritic disorders and degenerative joint disease in humans, but is capable of causing serious gastrointestinal side-effects, particularly hemorrhage, in dogs and cats.

Indonesian fat-tailed sheep multipurpose, polled, short or long tails; indigenous to Indonesia.

indoor strictly in a human dwelling; more widely includes an animal dwelling.

i. environment the physical, social and psychological environment within a human dwelling that can influence the health of a companion animal. See also ENVIRONMENT.

i. lambing see SHED lambing.

indospicine a hepatoxic and teratogenic amino acid found in *Indigofera* spp. which competes with arginine in metabolic pathways.

indoxyl an oxidation product of indole formed in tryptophan decomposition, and excreted in the urine as indican.

indoxyluria an excess of indoxyl in the urine.

Indriidae a family of non-human primates that includes indrises.

induced induction.

i. ovulation ovulation in rabbits, cats, camels is induced by coitus; artifical induction by hormonal treatment.

inducer 1. in biosynthesis, a compound that induces synthesis of a specific enzyme or sequence of enzymes, by antagonizing the corresponding repressor, or by some other mechanism. 2. a substance that stimulates the production of interferon by a cell.

induction 1. the process or act of inducing, or causing to occur, especially the production of a specific morphogenetic effect in the embryo through evocators or organizers, or the production of anesthesia or unconsciousness or parturition by use of appropriate agents. 2. the generation of an electric current or magnetic properties in a body because of its proximity to an electrified or magnetized object.

i. period the time from exposure to a non-infectious agent to the first appearance of the disease. Analogous to the INCUBATION period but for non-infectious pathogenic agents.

inductive 1. eliciting a reaction within an organism. 2.

i. heating a form of radiofrequency HYPERTHERMIA that selectively heats muscle, blood and proteinaceous tissue, sparing fat and air-containing tissues.

i. interactions an established relationship between tissues manifested by the necessity for the action or presence of one tissue for the development of another tissue.

inductor a tissue elaborating a chemical substance that acts to determine the growth and differentiation of embryonic parts.

inductotherm an electrical instrument used in the treatment of sprained tendons in horses; produces high tissue temperatures by induction.

indurated hardened; abnormally hard.

induration the quality of being hard; the process of hardening; an abnormally hard spot or place.

black i. the hardening and pigmentation of the lung tissue, as in pneumonia.

brown i. 1. a deposit of altered blood pigment in the lung in pneumonia. 2. an increase of the pulmonary connective tissue and excessive pigmentation, due to chronic congestion from valvular heart disease, or to anthracosis.

cyanotic i. hardening of an organ from chronic venous congestion.

granular i. cirrhosis.

gray i. induration of lung tissue in or after pneumonia, without pigmentation.

red i. interstitial pneumonia in which the lung is red and congested.

indurative mastitis see CAPRINE arthritis–encephalitis; called also hard udder.

indusium griseum [L.] a thin layer of gray matter on the dorsal surface of the corpus callosum.

indwelling to occupy a space; in surgery, left in position; said particularly of catheters. See also indwelling CATHETER.

inelastic 1. tissue lacking in elasticity. 2. in financial terms, lack of response in a variable, e.g. inelastic demand, when the demand for, say, veterinary services is not reduced by a downturn in the local economy.

Inermicapsifer a genus of tapeworms in the family Anoplocephalidae.

I. cubensis, I. madagascariensis found in rodents and hyracoids and occasionally in humans.

inert inactive.

inertia inactivity, inability to move spontaneously.
colonic i. weak muscular activity of the colon, leading to distension of the organ and constipation.
i. time the time required to overcome the inertia of a muscle after reception of a stimulus from a nerve.
uterine i. sluggishness of uterine contractions in labor.

infamous conduct a phrase used in legislation governing the rules of professions. It is the most serious level of misconduct and defined as notoriously evil, vile and abominable.

infanticide see INFANTOPHAGIA.

infantilism reduced size, poor sexual development, poor mental development in adult companion animals.

infantophagia a form of pica manifested by the mother eating her newborn. In many cases in companion animals, particularly in rabbits, and possibly in pigs, the behavior is due to anxiety by the mother about a too close attendance by humans.

infarct a localized area of ischemic necrosis produced by occlusion of the arterial supply or the venous drainage of the part. Clinical signs depend on the size of the devitalized tissue and the organ affected.
anemic i. one due to sudden interruption of flow of arterial blood to the area.
hemorrhagic i. one that is red owing to oozing of erythrocytes into the injured area.

infarctectomy surgical removal of an infarct.

infarction 1. the formation of an infarct. 2. an infarct.
cardiac i. see myocardial infarction (below) and also MYOCARDIAL infarction.
cerebral i. an ischemic condition of the brain, causing a persistent focal neurological deficit in the area affected.
i. fever an aseptic fever caused by liberation of pyrogens from damaged tissue.
intestinal i. a common occurrence in horses due to occlusion of arteries by larvae of *Strongylus vulgaris*. Sections of intestine, sometimes very large ones, become devitalized leading to peritonitis and death.
May also result from torsion or strangulation. See also thromboembolic COLIC.
myocardial i. gross necrosis of the myocardium, due to interruption of the blood supply to the area. See also MYOCARDIAL infarction.
pulmonary i. localized necrosis of lung tissue, due to obstruction of the arterial blood supply.
renal i. is usually conical, anemic and multiple and may heal leaving a narrow scar. It is usually clinically inapparent unless the obstructing material is infected. This leads to the development of RENAL abscess or embolic NEPHRITIS, also usually without clinical signs unless the abscesses are large or numerous.
spinal cord i. caused sometimes by fibrocartilaginous emboli of prolapsed disk material, causing sudden loss of function of large sections of the spinal cord, leading to flaccid paralysis of the hindlimbs or of all four, depending on the site of the infarct.
splenic i. usually hemorrhagic; may be difficult to differentiate from subcapsular hematoma.
venous i. a thrombus in a vein may cause infarction, e.g. in the thigh muscles of downer cow, recumbent for long periods, or in the gastric mucosa of pigs, where it is a common finding in acute septicemia.

infection 1. invasion and multiplication of microorganisms in body tissues, especially that causing local cellular injury due to competitive metabolism, toxins, intracellular replication or antigen–antibody response. 2. an infectious disease.
acute i. short duration, of the order of several days.
airborne i. infection by inhalation of organisms suspended in air on water droplets or dust particles.
arrested i. restrained in its development by a capsule or adhesion but still containing infective material.
chronic i. long duration, of the order of weeks or months.
i. control the utilization of procedures and techniques in the surveillance, investigation and compilation of statistical data in order to reduce the spread of infection, particularly nosocomial infections.
cross i. infection transmitted between patients infected with different pathogenic microorganisms.
droplet i. infection due to inhalation of respiratory pathogens suspended on liquid particles exhaled by an animal that is already infected.
dustborne i. infection by inhalation of pathogens that have become affixed to particles of dust.
endogenous i. that due to reactivation of organisms present in a dormant focus, as occurs in tuberculosis, etc.
exogenous i. that caused by organisms not normally present in the body but which have gained entrance from the environment.
general i. see systemic infection (below).
latent i. the animal is infected but there are no clinical signs nor infectious agent detectable in discharges.
local i. has a common syndrome of varying degree, depending on the site and acuteness of the lesion and the type of microorganisms present, including fever, toxemia and leukocytosis with a left shift. The specific individual signs relate to the location of the lesion and the pressure it exerts on nearby organs. See also ABSCESS, CELLULITIS, PHLEGMON, OSTEOMYELITIS, OMPHALOPHLEBITIS, EMPYEMA, ADENITIS, METRITIS, MASTITIS, PERIPHLEBITIS.
masked i. an infection is known to occur but the infectious agent cannot be demonstrated, e.g. the sheep-associated bovine malignant catarrh virus.
mixed i. infection with more than one kind of organism at the same time.
nosocomial i. pertaining to or acquired in hospital.
opportunistic i. infection with organisms which are normally harmless but become pathogenic when the body's defense mechanisms are compromised.
patent i. one in which the infectious agent can be demonstrated in discharges of the patient.
persistent i. a characteristic of some viruses, particularly herpesviruses and lentiviruses, in which there may be long-lasting or life-long latent infections, with asymptomatic periods and recurring acute episodes of clinical disease (herpesviruses) or onset of severe clinical disease (lentiviruses).
pyogenic i. infection by pus-producing organisms.
secondary i. infection by a pathogen following an infection by a pathogen of another kind.
i. stones see struvite UROLITH.
subclinical i. infection associated with no detectable signs but caused by microorganisms capable of producing easily recognizable diseases, such as mastitis or brucellosis; often detected by the production of antibody, or by delayed hypersensitivity exhibited in a skin test reaction to such antigens as tuberculoprotein.
super i. a second infection occurs in an animal which is already experiencing an infection with another agent.
systemic i. the infection is widespread throughout the body and must be assumed to be in all organs.
terminal i. an acute infection occurring near the end of a disease and often causing death.

transmissible i. an infection capable of being transmitted from one animal to another. Called also contagious.

waterborne i. infection by microorganisms transmitted in water.

infectious caused by or capable of being communicated by infection.

i. avian nephritis caused by a picornavirus this disease of young chickens causes a transient unremarkable disease with lesions appearing in the kidney.

i. bovine cervicovaginitis thought to be due to a herpesvirus-4 infection, transmitted by coitus, causing sterility in a high percentage of cows and some bulls. Recorded only in South Africa. Called also epivag.

i. bovine keratoconjunctivitis the common infectious keratitis of cattle caused by *Haemophilus (Moraxella) bovis.* It occurs as outbreaks, characterized by ocular discharge, blepharospasm and pain. Underrunning of the conjunctiva leads to complications in a few cases. Called also pinkeye, blight, New Forest disease.

i. bovine meningoencephalomyelitis see HEMOPHILOSIS.

i. bovine rhinotracheitis (IBR) a highly infectious disease of cattle, particularly when crowded together as in feedlots, caused by bovine herpesvirus 1 and characterized by nasal discharge, rhinitis, tracheitis, conjunctivitis, fever and a short course unless complicated by other infections, particularly those leading to pneumonia. Less common forms of the disease include encephalitis in calves and a systemic infection in neonates, manifested by oral erosions and diarrhea. Infectious pustular vulvovaginitis is also caused by this virus. Called also rednose.

i. bulbar paralysis see AUJESZKY'S DISEASE.

i. caprine keratoconjunctivitis contagious ophthalmia caused by *Mycoplasma conjunctivae.*

i. coryza see FOWL coryza.

i. equine anemia see EQUINE infectious anemia.

i. equine bronchitis see EQUINE influenza.

i. equine cough see EQUINE influenza.

i. equine encephalomyelitis see equine viral ENCEPHALOMYELITIS.

i. hematopoietic necrosis of fish important rhabdoviral infection of *Onchorhyncus* spp. especially steelhead (anadromous rainbow trout).

i. hypodermal and hemopoietic necrosis parvovirus infection causing high mortalities in juvenile *Penaeus stylirostris* and runt deformity syndrome in *P. vanname.*

i. labial dermatitis see contagious ECTHYMA.

i. laryngotracheitis (ILT) a highly infectious disease of birds of all ages caused by avian herpesvirus 1 and characterized by a very rapid spread of respiratory distress, the signs including gasping, respiratory gurgling and rattling, and death often from asphyxiation because of massive pseudomembrane formation in the trachea. The mortality rate may be as high as 70%.

i. necrotic hepatitis an acute toxemia of cattle, sheep and pigs caused by *Clostridium novyi* which elaborates a toxin in necrotic infarcts in the liver. These infarcts are caused usually by larvae of *Fasciola hepatica.* Many affected animals are found dead. Clinical findings include severe depression, hypothermia and muffling of heart sounds. Called also black disease.

i. pancreatic necrosis of fish a disease of salmonids caused by a group of related birnaviruses. It is characterized by hemorrhages and anemia, and spiral swimming and abdominal distension in fry.

i. porcine dermatitis see CONTAGIOUS porcine pyoderma.

i. porcine polyarthritis see GLÄSSER'S DISEASE.

i. pustular vulvovaginitis see infectious pustular VULVOVAGINITIS.

i. salmon anemia severe disease of Atlantic salmon, reported only, to date, from Norway; characterized by liver necrosis caused by an unidentified virus.

i. serositis a septicemic disease of young ducks caused by *Pasteurella anatipestifer* and characterized by torticollis, head tremor, loss of balance and a high mortality rate.

i. sinusitis a contagious disease of turkeys caused by *Mycoplasma gallisepticum.* The same infection also causes CHRONIC respiratory disease of chickens. The disease in turkeys is characterized by swelling of the infraorbital sinuses, which are filled with thick exudate. The course is chronic and the death rate low but there is severe loss of condition and damage to the respiratory tract.

i. stunting syndrome caused by an enterolike virus this disease causes serious losses in the broiler industry; it is characterized by severe growth depression commencing at 1 week of age or earlier. Called also helicopter disease.

i. synovitis see infectious avian SYNOVITIS.

infective infectious, capable of producing infection; pertaining to or characterized by the presence of pathogens.

i. bulbar necrosis ovine FOOT abscess.

infectivity ability of an agent to infect.

inference a conclusion about a population derived from a sample of the population.

inferential statistics see inferential STATISTICS.

inferior situated below, or directed downward; the lower surface of a structure, or the lower of two (or more) similar structures. In bipeds, it is usually synonymous with caudal, in quadripeds with ventral.

infertility the inability to conceive and produce viable offspring. In agricultural animals there are requirements that the animals reproduce prolifically and at a particular time chosen to best suit the availability of feed. A decision as to when infertility can be said to be present varies with the species and with the mating pair, and also with the state of the environment. For example, a dairy cow mated three times without conceiving to proven fertile semen by artificial insemination or by natural breeding to a known fertile bull is judged to require treatment for infertility. Infertility is a diagnosis about a mating rather than an individual animal; the error may be with the male or the female and it may be permanent or temporary. As a herd problem it provides a major brake on production in all species. In many instances the problem is man-made and in many of those there is in fact nothing wrong with the animals but there is with the management program, especially the nutritional regimen, which affects a mating at a time when fertility is marginal.

infestation parasitic attack or subsistence on the skin and/or its appendages, as by insects, mites or ticks; sometimes used to denote parasitic invasion of the organs and tissues, as by helminths.

infiltrate 1. to penetrate the interstices of a tissue or substance. 2. material deposited by infiltration.

interstitial i. cellular infiltrate scattered evenly throughout the thickness of the dermis.

infiltration the diffusion or accumulation in a tissue or cells of substances not normal to it or in amounts in excess of the normal; also, the material so accumulated.

adipose i. fatty infiltration.
i. anesthesia the injection of a number of small amounts into the tissue around the operation site.
calcareous i. deposit of lime and magnesium salts in the tissues.
cellular i. the migration and accumulation of cells within the tissues.
fatty i. 1. a deposit of fat in tissues, especially between cells. 2. the presence of fat vacuoles in the cell cytoplasm.
urinous i. the extravasation of urine into a tissue.

infiltrative relating to or characterized by infiltration.
i. lipoma the tissue in the growth resembles normal fat but infiltrates and destroys muscle and connective tissue. Occurs in dogs.

infinite number a number so large as to be uncountable. Represented by ∞, frequently obtained by 'dividing' by zero.

infirm weak; feeble, as from disease or old age.

inflammation a localized protective response elicited by injury or destruction of tissues, which serves to destroy, dilute, or wall off both the injurious agent and the injured tissue.

The inflammatory response can be provoked by physical, chemical and biological agents, including mechanical trauma, exposure to excessive amounts of sunlight, x-rays and radioactive materials, corrosive chemicals, extremes of heat and cold, and infectious agents such as bacteria, viruses and other pathogenic microorganisms. Although these infectious agents can produce inflammation, infection and inflammation are not synonymous.

The classic signs of inflammation are *heat*, *redness*, *swelling*, *pain* and *loss of function*. These are manifestations of the physiological changes that occur during the inflammatory process. The three major components of this process are: (1) changes in the caliber of blood vessels and the rate of blood flow through them (hemodynamic changes); (2) increased capillary permeability; and (3) leukocytic exudation.

acute i. inflammation, usually of sudden onset, marked by the classic signs of heat, redness, swelling, pain and loss of function, and in which vascular and exudative processes predominate.
adhesive i. promotes adhesion of adjacent surfaces.
atrophic i. one that causes atrophy and deformity.
catarrhal i. a form affecting mainly a mucous surface, marked by a copious discharge of mucus and epithelial debris.
chronic i. prolonged and persistent inflammation marked chiefly by new connective tissue formation; it may be a continuation of an acute form or a prolonged low-grade form.
croupous i. a homogeneous layer of exudate lying close to but detached from the underlying inflamed tissue, which is comparatively unharmed; may form a fibrinous cast.
diphtheritic i. manifested by the development of a fibrinous exudate which is firmly attached to the underlying tissue, such that it cannot be removed except by tearing off a superficial layer.
exudative i. one in which the prominent feature is an exudate.
fibrinous i. one marked by an exudate of coagulated fibrin.
fibrous i. leads to the development of fibrous tissue.
granulomatous i. a form, usually chronic, attended by formation of granulomas.
hyperplastic i. leads to the development of new connective tissue.
hypertrophic i. leading to the enlargement of the affected tissues.
interstitial i. inflammation affecting chiefly the stroma of an organ.
obliterative i. inflammation within a vessel or viscus leading to occlusion of the lumen.
parenchymatous i. inflammation affecting chiefly the essential tissue elements of an organ.
productive i., proliferative i. one leading to the production of new connective tissue fibers.
pseudomembranous i. an acute inflammatory response to a powerful necrotizing toxin, e.g. *Fusobacterium necrophorum* toxin, characterized by formation on a mucosal surface of a *false* membrane composed of precipitated fibrin, necrotic epithelium and inflammatory leukocytes. See also diphtheritic inflammation (above).
purulent i. suppurative inflammation.
serous i. one producing a serous exudate.
specific i. one due to a particular microorganism.
toxic i. one due to a poison, e.g. a bacterial product.
traumatic i. one that follows a wound or injury.
ulcerative i. that in which necrosis on or near the surface leads to loss of tissue and creation of a local defect or ulcer.

inflammatory pertaining to or emanating from inflammation.
i. bowel disease an idiopathic disease of cats, principally, and dogs characterized by cyclic bouts of vomiting and or diarrhea which may continue over periods of years; see also lymphocytic–plasmacytic ENTERITIS.
i. edema a disease of the subcutis caused usually by *Clostridium* spp.
i. response see INFLAMMATION.

inflation see TEAT CUP LINER.
carcass i. pumping of air under the skin of a carcass of sheep or cattle to facilitate skinning. Universally discouraged, mostly forbidden for meat for human consumption.

inflection, inflexion the act of bending inward, or the state of being bent inward.

inflow–outflow method a technique for postmortem examination of the heart that preserves the atrioventricular valves.

influenza an acute viral infection of the respiratory tract, occurring usually in epidemics, and pandemics. Influenza viruses are single-stranded RNA viruses belonging to the family *Orthomyxoviridae*, which contains three genera termed A, B and C. All of the viruses of interest to veterinarians are influenza type A viruses and include those causing EQUINE influenza, SWINE influenza and AVIAN influenza (fowl plague).

Common usage is to diagnose influenza or 'flu' in many nonspecific respiratory infections in animals or those caused by other viruses, but this is etiologically incorrect. Typical examples are cat flu and goose influenza.

informatics information management; the technology of information storage, retrieval and transmission. Includes on-line access to and editing of data bases, facsimile transmission, optical reading and word processing. The application of electronics to information management has greatly expanded the opportunities for dealing with large amounts of data for research, clinical records, herd health programs and accounting for veterinarians.

information 1. data which has intrinsic value. 2. changes occurring in central neurons as a result of stimuli received from sensory neurons. The signals received are coded, selected, with some being discarded and some stored, analyzed and compared with similar data stored in memory, after packing and merging. Many of the processes used in the human brain have identical counterparts in computers and the handling of information in the two systems has a great deal of similarity.

i. base in computer terms this is the database (see DATA). In human terms it is human memory plus whatever resources of information there are, including paper and film, and tape and computer disks.

i. evaluation an essential step to avoid unnecessary storage and the utilization of erroneous information in drawing conclusions. The rating will depend on whether the information is experimentally derived, obtained by clinical experience, or procedures in between. It is necessary in many situations to utilize information with a low rating because of a lack of availability of better information. There must necessarily be a lower level of certainty in the conclusions based on such material.

infra- word element. [L.] *beneath.*

infra-axillary below the axilla.

infraclusion a condition in which the occluding surface of a tooth does not reach the normal occlusal plane and is out of contact with the opposing tooth.

infracostal behind a rib.

infraction incomplete bone fracture without displacement.

infradian pertaining to a period longer than 24 hours; applied to the cyclic behavior of certain phenomena in living organisms (infradian rhythm).

infrahyoid behind the hyoid bone.

inframaxillary beneath the maxilla.

infranuclear below a nucleus.

infraorbital lying under or on the floor of the orbit.

i. nerve block can be used for surgery about the upper lip and the nostrils. It requires locating the nerve where it emerges from the infraorbital foramen.

infrapatellar beneath the patella.

infrared denoting electromagnetic radiation of wavelength greater than that of the red end of the spectrum, having wavelengths of 0.75–1000 μm. Infrared rays are sometimes subdivided into long-wave or far infrared (about 3.0–1000 μm) and short-wave or near infrared (about 0.75–3.0 μm). They are capable of penetrating body tissues to a depth of 10 mm. Sources of infrared rays include heat lamps, hot water bottles, steam radiators and incandescent light bulbs.

Infrared rays are used therapeutically to promote muscle relaxation, to speed up the inflammatory process, and to increase circulation to a part of the body. See also HEAT.

infrascapular behind the scapula.

infrasonic below the frequency range of sound waves.

infraspinatus infraspinous.

i. muscle see Table 13.3.

infraspinous beneath or caudal to the spine of the scapula.

infrasternal caudal to the sternum.

infratentorial beneath the tentorium of the cerebellum.

infratrochlear beneath the trochlea.

infraversion 1. downward deviation of the eye. 2. infraclusion.

infundibular pertaining to any of the body's infundibula. See also INFUNDIBULUM.

i. cyst see EPIDERMAL cyst.

i. necrosis tooth necrosis, commencing in the tooth infundibulum, common in old horses.

i. process the central part of the posterior pituitary gland; called also pars nervosa.

i. recess the diverticulum off the third ventricle that occupies the infundibulum of the hypophysis.

i. stalk the stalk of the hypophysis; with the pars tuberalis comprises the hypophyseal base.

i. stenosis narrowing of the pulmonary artery just below the pulmonic valves; the stenosis is produced by a ring of connective tissue around the outflow tract of the right ventricle.

infundibuliform shaped like a funnel.

infundibuloma glioma of the infundibular stalk (of the pituitary).

infundibulum pl. *infundibula* [L.] 1. any funnel-shaped passage. 2. conus arteriosus of the heart.

cardiac i. CONUS arteriosus.

hypothalamic i. a hollow, funnel-shaped mass in front of the tuber cinereum, extending to the posterior lobe of the pituitary gland.

oviduct i. cranial end of the avian oviduct; captures the oocyte released from the ovary and, during a 15 minute sojourn, invests it with its chalaziferous layer and the thin layer of albumen around the yolk.

tooth i. an invagination of the enamel from the wearing service of a tooth, as found in ruminant cheek teeth and the incisive and upper grinder teeth of horses.

i. of uterine tube the distal, funnel-shaped portion of the uterine tube. In birds the left uterine tube is the functional one and has a large thin-walled infundibulum.

infusion 1. the steeping of a substance in water to obtain its soluble principles. 2. the product obtained by this process. 3. the slow therapeutic introduction of fluid other than blood into a vein. See also INTRAVENOUS infusion.

NOTE: An *infusion* flows in by gravity, an *injection* is forced in by a syringe, an *instillation* is dropped in, an *insufflation* is blown in, and an *infection* slips in unnoticed.

constant-rate i. the continuous intravenous administration of medication usually through an electronic delivery device, in order to maintain constant blood levels. Most suitable for use with rapid onset of action and short half-life.

intramammary i. material used to introduce medicaments, especially antibiotics, into the teat and udder sinuses for the treatment or prevention of mastitis. May be in liquid or thin paste form and usually prepackaged in tubes for the treatment of individual quarters. Contain antibiotics and adjuvants in a slow or fast-release base depending on objective, e.g. dry period or lactation period treatment. May contain dye to warn that milk may contain antibiotics. Specially prepared watery infusions of escharotic agents, e.g. silver nitrate, copper sulfate, may be used to dry off permanently a quarter that is chronically affected.

intrauterine i. administration of fluids for irrigative purposes.

subcutaneous i. administration of fluids directly into subcutaneous tissues for the purpose of providing hydration. See also HYPODERMOCLYSIS.

infusoria protozoa of the class Infusoria; microscopic, aquatic, with vibratile cilia. Found in ruminant forestomachs.

ingesta material taken into the body by mouth.

ingestant a substance that is or may be taken into the body by mouth or through the digestive system.

ingestion the taking of food, drugs, etc. into the body by mouth.

ingluvies the crop of a bird. Called also craw. Used also as a name for rumen.
ingluvitis inflammation of the ingluvies.
ingravescent gradually becoming more severe.
inguen pl. *inguina* [L.] the groin.
inguina the inguinal region.
inguinal pertaining to the groin.
i. abscess characterized by a history of prior castration and a syndrome of unilateral edema, pain and swelling in the inguinal region, possibly confirmable by rectal palpation.
i. canal the oblique passage in the ventral abdominal wall, through which passes the round ligament of the uterus in the female, and the spermatic cord in the male.
i. hernia hernia occurring in the groin, or inguen, where the abdominal folds of flesh meet the thighs. Protrusion of intestine, omentum and occasionally a gravid uterus, either directly through a weak point in the abdominal wall (direct inguinal hernia) or downward into the inguinal canal (indirect inguinal hernia; called also scrotal hernia in the male). A serious complication is incarceration with or without strangulation of the herniated viscus. Most commonly seen in bitches; occasionally a heritable trait in dogs and may be inherited in pigs and cattle.
i. ring there are two rings, one at the entrance and one at the exit of the inguinal canal. See also RING.
i. strangulation see INGUINAL hernia.
inhalant a substance that is or may be taken into the body by way of the nose and trachea, that is through the respiratory system, e.g. gaseous anesthetics.
canine i. dermatitis see ATOPY.
inhalation 1. the drawing of air or other substances into the lungs. 2. any drug or solution of drugs administered (as by means of nebulizers or aerosols) by the nasal or oral respiratory route.
i. injury bronchiolitis and pulmonary edema result from the inhalation of smoke.
i. pneumonia see ASPIRATION pneumonia.
inhaler an apparatus for administering vaporized or volatilized agents by inhalation, or for protecting the lungs from harmful substances in the air.
inherent existing as an inseparable part, congenital, innate, inherited, inborn, inbuilt, intrinsic.
inheritance 1. the acquisition of characters or qualities by transmission from parent to offspring. 2. that which is transmitted from parent to offspring. See also GENE, DEOXYRIBONUCLEIC ACID and HEREDITY.

Mendelian inheritance is the basis of all genetic practice, but it has limitations in explaining the small differences that occur in a range of offspring of similar and related matings. Galtonian genetics deals specifically with this problem and is better fitted as a tool in population genetics and in dealing with characters that are dependent on a number of chromosomal loci rather than on a single locus.

autosomal i. controlled by genes located on autosomes.
intermediate i. inheritance in which the phenotype of the heterozygote falls between that of either homozygote.
maternal i. the transmission of characters that are dependent on peculiarities of the egg cytoplasm produced, in turn, by nuclear genes.
X-linked i. see X-LINKED.
inherited received by inheritance.
i. achondroplastic dwarfism see achondroplastic DWARFISM.
i. combined immunodeficiency see COMBINED IMMUNE DEFICIENCY SYNDROME (DISEASE).
i. congenital defects inherited defects visible at birth.
i. defects conditions caused by genes which condition the structure or function of an organ or tissue.
i. diseases see INHERITED defects.
i. metabolic defects errors of metabolism conditioned by genes.
i. trait a distinguishing characteristic or quality received by inheritance.
inherited cerebellar atrophy see CEREBELLAR atrophy.
inherited congenital cerebellar hypoplasia see CEREBELLAR atrophy.
inherited epidermal dysplasia an hereditary disease of calves appearing at 1 to 2 months of age and characterized by alopecia, cracking and ulceration of skin in the axillae, flanks and at the limb joints. There is also emaciation, failure of horns to grow, elongation of the feet and hypersalivation. The calves are not viable. Called also baldy calves.
inherited multiple tendon contracture affected calves have congenital contractures in flexion or extension of limb joints, causing dystocia. Survival is not possible.
inherited osteoarthritis see inherited OSTEOARTHRITIS.
inherited thick forelegs see juvenile HYPEROSTOSIS.
inhibin a nonsteroid hormone originating in the seminiferous tubules and ovarian follicles and which regulates follicle-stimulating hormone secretion.
inhibited larval development see HYPOBIOSIS.
inhibiting factors inhibiting hormones secreted by hypothalamic neurosecretory cells.
inhibition arrest or restraint of a process.
competitive i. inhibition of enzyme activity by an inhibitor (a substrate analog) that competes with the substrate for binding sites on the enzymes.
contact i. inhibition of cell division and cell motility in normal animal cells when in close contact with each other.
end-product i. see feedback inhibition (below).
feedback i. a common way of regulating enzyme activity in which the reaction product (or in the case of a biosynthetic pathway, the product of the reaction sequence) inhibits the enzyme activity. Called also end-product inhibition.
neurological i. the intermittency of transmission of nervous impulses depends on variations in the balance between excitation and inhibition, the latter being either pre- or postsynaptic.
noncompetitive i. inhibition of enzyme activity by substances that combine with the enzyme at a site other than that utilized by the substrate.
inhibitor 1. any substance that interferes with a chemical reaction, growth or other biological activity. 2. a chemical substance that inhibits or checks the action of a tissue organizer or the growth of microorganisms. 3. an effector that reduces the catalytic activity of an enzyme.
coagulation i's CLOTTING factors.
fibrinolytic i's CLOTTING factors.
phosphodiesterase i. inhibits phosphodiesterase, which in turn inactivates cyclic adenosine monophosphate. The effect of the inhibitor is to increase the heart muscle content of cAMP.
reversible i's pharmaceutical inhibitors which have only a temporary effect, e.g. the cholinesterase inhibitors neostigmine, physostigmine.
inhibitory emanating from or pertaining to inhibition.
i. factor growth hormone a hypothalamic hormone released into the hypophyseal portal system.

inion the most prominent point on the external occipital protuberance.
iniopagus a twin monster joined at the occiput.
initial at the beginning.
i. plan problem-oriented MEDICAL record.
i. problem list problem-oriented MEDICAL record.
i. segment the first 50–100 μm of the axon; point of cell body emergence to point of myelin initiation.
initialize a computer term meaning to set up the basic conditions for the implementation of a program. Most hardware and software nowadays needs a once-only initialization or configuring, carried out by the formatting procedure.
initiation the beginning or introduction rites. In cell biology, the first stage of transcription.
i. codon the codon AUG which specifies the first amino acid, methionine, in protein synthesis. Called also initiator.
i. complex is formed at the initiation of protein synthesis and includes initiation factors, tRNA, mRNA and the ribosomal subunit.
i. factors (IF) a group of proteins that are required for initiation of protein synthesis to occur.
initiator see initiation.
initis inflammation of the substance of a muscle.
injected 1. introduced by injection. 2. congested.
injection 1. the forcing of a liquid into a part, as into the subcutaneous tissues, the vascular tree, or an organ. 2. a substance so forced or administered; in pharmacy, a solution of a medicament suitable for injection. 3. congestion. 4. immunizing substances, or inoculations, are generally given by injection. When a patient is unconscious, injection may be the only means of administering medication, and in some cases nourishment. Some medicines cannot be given by mouth because chemical action of the digestive juices or of hepatic enzymes would change or reduce their effectiveness, or because they would be removed from the body too quickly to have any effect. Certain potent medicines must be injected because they would irritate body tissues if administered any other way. A medication may be injected so that it will act more quickly.

In addition to the most common types of injections described below, injections are sometimes made under the conjunctiva, into arteries, bone marrow, the spine, the sternum, the pleural space of the chest region, the peritoneal cavity and joint spaces.
i. collar a collar carrying an injection device which can be triggered from a remote site.
epidural i. see EPIDURAL.
hypodermic i. subcutaneous injection.
intradermal i., intracutaneous i. injection of small amounts of material into the corium or substance of the skin. This method is used in diagnostic procedures and in administration of regional anesthetics, as well as in treatment procedures. In certain allergy tests, the allergen is injected intracutaneously. These injections are given in an area where the skin and hair are sparse, usually on the inner part of the thigh in dogs or the caudal fold in cows. A small-gauge needle is recommended and it is inserted at a 10- to 15-degree angle to the skin.
intramuscular i. injection into the substance of a muscle, usually the thigh or pectoral muscle, or the muscle of the neck or rump. Intramuscular injections are given when the substance is to be absorbed quickly. They should be given with extreme care, especially in the thigh, because the sciatic nerve may be injured or a large blood vessel may be entered if the injection is made without drawing back on the syringe first.
intraperitoneal i. liquid injection, usually of antibacterial agent, rarely anesthetic or euthanatizing agents, administered to obtain systemic blood levels of the agent; faster than subcutaneous or intramuscular injection and used when veins not accessible. The needle is introduced into the upper flank and the syringe plunger withdrawn to ensure that intestine has not been penetrated. The injected solution should run freely.
intratesticular i. a method of administering a general anesthetic agent to boars for castration.
intravenous i. an injection made into a vein. Intravenous injections are used when rapid absorption is called for, when fluid cannot be taken by mouth, or when the substance to be administered is too irritating to be injected into the skin or muscles. In certain diagnostic tests and x-ray examinations, a drug or dye may be administered intravenously. Blood transfusions also are given by this route. See also INTRAVENOUS infusion.
subarachnoid i. the risk of injection is greatest at the atlanto-occipital space where the vertebral venous plexus is most likely to be lacerated.
subcutaneous i. injection made into the subcutaneous tissues; called also hypodermic injection. Although usually fluid medications are injected, occasionally solid materials, such as steroid hormones, are administered subcutaneously in small, slowly absorbed pellets to prolong their effect. Subcutaneous injections may be given wherever there is subcutaneous tissue, usually in the loose skin on the side of the chest or in the flank. The amount injected should not exceed 2 ml for cats and small dogs, 5 ml for large dogs and 20 ml for horses. Cows are often given 200 ml because of their very loose skin. The needle is held at a 45-degree angle to the skin.
injection-site reactions apart from those caused by infection at the site there is a characteristic reaction in dogs and cats which is a germinal center created by the strong antigenic stimulus provided by the injection.
injury harm or hurt; a wound or maim; usually applied to damage inflicted on the body by an external force. See also BURN, ELECTRICAL injuries, FROSTBITE, HYPOTHERMIA, RADIATION injury.
casting i. in large animals while being cast with ropes or harness for treatment or examination; may be injury or even fracture of a limb bone, or injury to a nerve, especially facial or radial nerves.
racing i. includes stripping of the tendons of the rear limb by being galloped on, striking the flexor tendons of the forelimb with the toes of the hindlimb (forging or striking), or brushing, (hitting the inside of one lower forelimb by the other). Fractures, tendon ruptures, muscle and tendon sprains are all part of the racing hazard. Fracture or dislocation of cervical vertebrae are an especial hazard in hurdle races and steeplechases.
shoeing i. injury inflicted while shoeing; includes paring too much sole, exposing sensitive laminae, nailprick of sensitive laminae, and paring too much lateral wall, causing bleeding at the white line.
Injury Severity Score (ISS) a scoring system for assessing trauma; used in humans. Each injury is assigned a numerical value, based on severity and body region. The ISS is a sum of the scores squared, from the three regions with the highest scores.
inkanga SENECIO *isatideus*.
inkberry PHYTOLACCA *octandra*, *P. americana*, CESTRUM *laevigatum*.

inkweed DRYMARIA, PHYTOLACCA *octandra*.
inland pigweed PORTULACA *oleracea*.
inlet a means or route of entrance.
pelvic i. see PELVIC inlet.
INN International Nonproprietary Names.
innate inborn; hereditary; congenital.
inner ear see EAR.
innervation 1. the distribution or supply of nerves to a part. 2. the supply of nervous energy or of nerve stimulation sent to a part.
reciprocal i. the innervation of antagonistic muscles such that when one muscle is excited its antagonist is inhibited.
innidiation development of cells in a part to which they have been carried by metastasis.
innocent not malignant; benign.
i. bystander reaction when antibody attaches to antigen bound to erythrocytes, the erythrocytes are marked for complement mediated lysis and phagocytosis by reticuloendothelial cells, these 'innocent bystander' cells are protected from lysis by complement components.
innocuous harmless.
Innovar-Vet a proprietary name for a combination of DROPERIDOL and FENTANYL citrate.
innovators people who will try new things.
early i. important figures in the farming or client community because they are the leaders in the introduction of new techniques and management systems.
inochondritis inflammation of a fibrocartilage.
inoculability the state of being inoculable.
inoculable 1. susceptible of being inoculated; transmissible by inoculation. 2. not immune against a transmissible disease.
inoculation introduction of pathogenic microorganisms, infective material, serum, or other substances into tissues of living organisms or into culture media; introduction of a disease agent into a healthy animal to produce a mild form of the disease, followed by IMMUNITY.
inoculum material used in inoculation.
Inocybe a genus of macrofungus (i.e. mushroom/toadstool), in the order Cortinariaceae. Contains muscarine, causes vomiting and diarrhea. Includes *I. patouilliardii*, *I. phaecomis*.
inogenous produced from or forming tissue.
inoperable not susceptible to treatment by surgery.
inorganic 1. having no organs. 2. not of organic origin.
i. chemistry that branch of chemistry which deals with inorganic compounds, those not containing carbon and also carbides, oxides of carbon, and carbonates.
inoscopy the diagnosis of disease by artificial digestion and examination of the fibers or fibrinous matter of the sputum, blood, effusions, etc. Called also fibrinoscopy.
inosculation establishment of communication channels between blood vessels or tubular organs that lie next to one another.
inosemia 1. the presence of inositol in the blood. 2. an excess of fibrin in the blood.
inosine a purine nucleoside containing the base hypoxanthine and the sugar ribose, which occurs in transfer RNAs.
i. monophosphate (IMP) a nucleotide produced by the deamination of adenosine monophosphate (AMP) in the metabolism of purine nucleotides.
i. 5¸-monophosphate the first fully formed purine nucleotide in the pathway of purine synthesis. Called also IMP or inosinic acid.
inosinic acid see INOSINE 5¸-monophosphate.
inositol a cyclic sugar alcohol, $C_6H_{12}O_6$; usually referring to the most abundant isomer, *myo*-inositol, which is found in many plant and animal tissues.
i. 1,4,5-trisphosphate intracellular second messenger released from phosphatidyl 4,5-bisphosphate in response to agonist-dependent, GTP-G protein-activated phospholipase C. Called also IP_3. Causes release of Ca^2+ from intracellular stores, thereby activating calmodulin.
inosituria the presence of inositol in the urine.
inotrope a drug with positive INOTROPIC effects, e.g. dobutamine, digitalis, milrinone.
inotropic affecting the force of muscular contractions; commonly applied to drugs that increase contractility of cardiac muscle, e.g. digitalis glycosides.
inotropy the force of muscle contraction.
input information entered into a computer.
i.–output an all-embracing term to cover all of the peripheral equipment of a computer involved in input and output, and all of the data similarly involved; abbreviated IO, I/O.
input voltage regulation a voltage compensator on an x-ray machine that ensures consistent voltage input and therefore consistent beam output and radiographic images.
INRA cattle special strain of French double-muscled Charolais beef cattle.
insalubrious injurious to health.
inscriptio pl. *inscriptiones* [L.] inscription.
i. tendinea intersectio tendinea.
inscription 1. a mark or line. 2. that part of a prescription containing the names and amounts of the ingredients.
insect any individual of the class Insecta.
i. bites and stings injuries caused by the mouth parts and venom of insects and of certain related creatures, known as arachnids—spiders, scorpions, ticks—but popularly classified with insects. Bites and stings can be the cause of much discomfort. Usually there is no real danger, although a local infection can develop from scratching. Some insects, however, establish themselves on the skin as parasites, others inject poison, and still others transmit disease. See also BEE STING.
i. growth regulators (IGRs) substances found naturally in insects which regulate morphogenesis and reproduction; synthetic chemicals with similar activity are used topically and in the environment to control ectoparasites, particularly fleas, as a larvicide and ovicide. Called also juvenoids. See also METHOPRENE, FENOXYCARB.
i. larva the second stage in the standard insect life cycle, the maggot or caterpillar.
i. pupa stage 3 in the insect life cycle. Inert, dormant stage from which the adult emerges.
i. vector insects may carry infection mechanically on feet or mouthparts, by passage through the digestive tract but without the insect being infected, or by becoming an intermediate host with some part of the parasite's life cycle taking place in insect tissues.
i. worry swarms of biting insects cause sufficient worry to interfere with grazing and the animals lose weight.
Insecta a class of arthropods whose members are characterized by division of the body into three distinct regions: head, thorax, and abdomen, and have three pairs of legs.
insecticide an agent that kills insects. May be applied by POUR-ON technique, DIPPING, SPRAYDIP, JETTING, DUSTING POWDERS. Insecticides come in a wide vari-

ety of chemical compounds. See also PYRETHROIDS, ROTENONE, DERRIS, CHLORINATED HYDROCARBONS, ORGANOPHOSPHORUS COMPOUND, ARSENICAL, CARBAMATES, TRIAZINES. The toxicity of an insecticidal preparation may be greatly altered by the agents used as emulsifiers and solvents. Called also pesticide.

i. resistance insects exposed to one insecticide for long periods may develop a resistance to it and suffer no ill-effects when it is applied.

Insectivora the order of mammals containing insectivorous animals such as senrecs, moles, shrews and hedgehogs.

insectivorous eating insects to the extent that they are significant as a contributor to the patient's diet.

inseminate see INSEMINATION.

insemination the deposit of seminal fluid within the vagina, cervix or uterus.

artificial i. that done by artificial means, e.g. by pipette or straw through the cervix. See also ARTIFICIAL INSEMINATION.

surgical i. the semen is deposited in the uterus by injection through its wall, having first exposed the uterus by a laparotomy.

inseminator person employed to inseminate animals with live semen; restricted largely to work with cattle; in most countries inseminators are licensed as having been trained in the techniques and tested for proficiency.

i. efficiency efficiency as determined by the conceptions/insemination index derived from the insemination data and pregnancy diagnosis; inefficiency should be observed on more than one farm; poor results on one farm more likely to indicate an infertility problem.

insensible 1. devoid of sensibility or consciousness. 2. not perceptible to the senses.

i. sweating water lost by evaporation from the skin without the skin or hair becoming obviously wet.

insert a segment of DNA that has been spliced into a cloning vector.

insertion 1. the act of implanting, or condition of being implanted. 2. the site of attachment, as of a muscle to the bone that it moves.

i. sequence (IS) see transposable GENETIC elements.

velamentous i. attachment to a membrane, such as the umbilical cord to the fetal membranes.

insertional pertaining to 1. surgical or reproductive manipulation 2. molecular biological manipulation.

i. activity the electrical tracing produced in electromyography as a result of the insertion of the needle electrode.

i. inactivation in recombinant DNA technology, an early method for selecting ampicillin (amp+) and tetracycline (tet+) resistant *Escherichia coli* transformed with plasmids such as pBR 322; foreign DNA was cloned into the tet gene, thereby disrupting the gene and rendering the cell tet$^-$, which enabled selection when cells were plated onto amp and tet plates.

insidious coming on stealthily; a gradual and subtle development.

insoluble not susceptible to being dissolved.

insonate to expose to ultrasound waves.

insorption movement of a substance into the blood, especially from the gastrointestinal tract into the circulating blood.

inspection visual examination for detection of features or qualities perceptible to the eye.

antemortem i. see ANTEMORTEM inspection.

postmortem i. inspection of all organs and tissues for evidence of disease which would make the meat unsuitable for human nutrition.

inspersion sprinkling, as with powder.

inspirate the air inhaled at a single inspiration.

inspiration the drawing of air into the lungs.

inspiratory pertaining to or used in the inspiration of air into the lungs.

i. center one of the four respiratory centers in the reticular formation of the brainstem.

i.-inhibitory reflex see HERING–BREUER REFLEXES.

i. reserve volume the volume of air which the patient can still inhale after the completion of inhalation of the tidal volume.

inspissated being thickened, dried, or made less fluid by evaporation.

instar a stage between molts in the development of an insect in which it undergoes a metamorphosis and changes its shape to a degree away from the first instar and towards the final one. The number of instars in an insect's metamorphosis varies widely between species from 5 up to 20 or more.

instillation administration of a liquid drop by drop.

instinct a complex of unlearned responses characteristic of a species.

herd i. the instinct or urge to be one of a group and to conform to its patterns of behavior.

instrument a delicate tool.

i. milk an emulsion used as an instrument lubricant.

i. ties ties for knots in sutures made with instruments.

instrumentarium the equipment or instruments required for any particular operation or purpose; the physical adjuncts with which a veterinarian combats disease.

instrumentation work performed with instruments.

insudation 1. the accumulation, as in the kidney, of a substance derived from the blood. 2. the substance so accumulated.

insufficiency inability to perform properly an allotted function.

adrenal i. hypoadrenalism.

aortic i. inadequacy of the aortic valve, permitting blood to flow back into the left ventricle of the heart.

cardiac i. inability of the heart to perform its function properly; heart failure.

coronary i. decreased supply of blood to the myocardium resulting from constriction or obstruction of the coronary arteries, but not accompanied by necrosis of the myocardial cells. Called also ischemic myocardial necrosis.

hepatic i. inadequate liver function, short of hepatic failure.

ileocecal i. inability of the ileocecal valve to prevent backflow of contents from the cecum into the ileum.

pulmonary i. insufficiency of the pulmonary valve, permitting blood to flow into the right ventricle of the heart.

respiratory i. a condition in which respiratory function is inadequate to meet the body's needs when increased physical activity places extra demands on it. See also RESPIRATORY insufficiency.

thyroid i. hypothyroidism.

valvular i. failure of a cardiac valve to close perfectly, causing the blood to flow back through the orifice (valvular regurgitation); named, according to the valve affected, aortic, mitral, pulmonary or tricuspid insufficiency.

velopharyngeal i. failure of velopharyngeal closure due to cleft palate, muscular dysfunction, etc., resulting in defective swallowing with regurgitation through the nose.

venous i. inadequacy of the venous valves with impairment of venous drainage, resulting in edema.

insufflation 1. the blowing of a powder, vapor, or gas into a body cavity. 2. a drug administered by this method, especially a powder or aerosol carried into the respiratory passages.

tubal i. insufflation of carbon dioxide gas through the uterus into the uterine tubes as a test of their patency.

insufflator an instrument used in insufflation.

insula pl. *insulae* [L.] a triangular area of the cerebral cortex that forms the floor of the lateral cerebral fossa.

insular pertaining to the insula or to an island, as the islands of Langerhans.

insulating oil oil used to insulate the high tension transformer in an x-ray unit.

insulation 1. the surrounding of a space or body with material designed to prevent the entrance or escape of radiant energy. 2. the material so used.

insulin a double-chain peptide hormone formed from proinsulin in the beta cells of the pancreatic islets of Langerhans. Insulin promotes the storage of glucose and the uptake of amino acids, increases protein and lipid synthesis, and inhibits lipolysis and gluconeogenesis.

The secretion of endogenous insulin is a response of the beta cells to a stimulus. The primary stimulus is glucose; others are amino acids, particularly leucine, and the 'gut hormones', such as secretin, pancreozymin and gastrin. These chemicals play an important role in maintaining normal blood glucose levels by triggering the release of insulin after ingestion of a meal.

Commercially prepared insulin is available in various types, which differ in the speed with which they act and in the duration of their effectiveness. There are three main groups: rapid acting (regular or semilente), intermediate acting (isophane suspension or NPH, zinc suspension or lente), and long acting (protamine zinc suspension or PZI, or ultralente). Mixtures are also marketed.

i. deficiency diabetes mellitus.

i.-dextrose therapy a combination used in emergencies to lower blood potassium levels in acute hypoadrenocorticism.

i.:glucagon ratio ratio of insulin to glucagon; thought to determine the predominance of the action of one hormone over the other.

i.:glucose ratio a comparison of simultaneously obtained blood levels of immunoreactive insulin and plasma glucose. An increased ratio suggests an insulin-secreting tumor of the pancreas. A modification is the amended insulin:glucose ratio, based on the calculation:

$$\frac{\text{serum insulin } (\mu\text{U/ml}) \times 100}{\text{plasma glucose (mg/dl)} - 30}$$

immunoreactive i. radioimmunoassay methods are used in determining blood levels of insulin. Increased levels are found with hypoglycemia caused by functional islet cell tumors.

i. pump a device consisting of a syringe filled with a predetermined amount of short-acting insulin, a plastic cannula and a needle, and a pump that periodically delivers the desired amount of insulin. Sometimes used in humans, but of limited application in animals.

i. sensitivity test, i. response test used to differentiate diabetes mellitus from pituitary and adrenal diabetes. A test dose of exogenous insulin will produce a rapid and marked decrease in blood glucose if the pancreas is not secreting sufficient insulin. A much less dramatic response is produced if hyperglycemia is due to excessive secretion of either pituitary or adrenocortical hormones rather than insufficient insulin production.

i. syringe disposable syringe with a capacity of 1 ml or less and a fine gauge needle (27–29G) attached, and graduation markings corresponding to insulin units in standard preparations. Needles may also be treated to minimize pain on injection.

insulin-like growth factor one of the twenty or so substances, additional to the classic bone-regulating hormones, which exert an effect on bone cell metabolism. See also SOMATOMEDIN C.

insulinase an enzymatic activity in body tissues that destroys or inactivates insulin; this effect is probably due to several nonspecific proteases.

insulinemia the presence of insulin in the blood.

insulinogenesis the formation and release of insulin by the islets of Langerhans.

insulinogenic relating to insulinogenesis.

insulinoma a tumor of the beta cells of the islets of Langerhans; although usually benign, it is one of the chief causes of hypoglycemia.

insulitis cellular infiltration of the islets of Langerhans, possibly in response to invasion by an infectious agent.

insuloma insulinoma.

insulopenic diminishing, or pertaining to a decrease in, the level of circulating insulin.

insurance animals may be insured for loss of production, or for loss of life. Before insured animals are euthanatized or submitted to surgery or a course of medical treatment it is important that the insurer be consulted to ensure that the contract is not breached and that his or her equity in the asset is not put at unnecessary risk.

insusceptibility the state of being unaffected or uninfluenced; may result from genetic resistance or from immunity.

intact-nephron hypothesis the concept that each nephron is either a fully functional unit or does not function. Surviving nephrons can increase their functional capacity by undergoing hypertrophy. As further nephrons are destroyed in progressive renal disease the kidney's capacity to accommodate to emergencies diminishes and renal insufficiency begins to develop.

intake the substances, or the quantities thereof, taken in and utilized by the body. The record of intake and output is called FLUID balance record.

integer a whole number; not a fraction.

integral essential component, part of a whole.

i. membrane protein see MEMBRANE proteins.

i. proteins membrane proteins essential to the structure and function of membranes. See MEMBRANE proteins.

integrase an enzyme involved in the integration of some viruses, such as bacteriophage lambda, and some transposons into host cell chromosomal DNA.

integrated circuit a complete system of electronic units provided as a single unit.

integration 1. assimilation; anabolic action or activity. 2. the combining of different acts so that they cooperate toward a common end; coordination. 3. in bacterial genetics, assimilation of genetic material from one bacterium (donor) into the chromosome of another (recipient).

industrial i. integration of the various levels of an industry so that they are all working in unison, usually under the same ownership. Thus in the poultry industry it is commonplace for the same company to grow the feed, hatch the chickens, franchise feeders, slaughter the broiler output in their own plant and wholesale the dressed birds to retailers.

integrins a group of receptors that promote cell adhesion.

integument a covering or investment; the skin.

avian i. consists of a thin dry skin (dermis and epidermis) plus appendages (feathers, uropygial gland, comb, wattles, beak, leg scales, spurs, toepads).

common i. the skin and skin derivatives such as horn, hooves and feathers.

mammalian i. consists of epidermis, derived from ectoderm, and dermis and hypodermis, derived from mesoderm; specializations of the epidermis produce glands, hair, hooves, horn, callosities, pads.

integumentary 1. pertaining to or composed of skin. 2. serving as a covering.

i. system SKIN and its appendages.

integumentum [L.] *integument.*

intellect the mind, thinking faculty, or understanding. Not a highly developed function in animals.

intelligence 1. the ability to comprehend or understand. 2. information gathered about the state of affairs in a farming system, a disease occurrence study, a public health survey or a veterinary service.

intelligent terminal see TERMINAL (3).

intensification factor stated about an intensifying screen used in x-ray cassettes. The ratio of exposure required for a film to produce a given density when exposed to direct x-rays, and the exposure required to produce the same density when using intensifying screens.

intensifying screen calcium tungstate screens which fluoresce and transform the invisible x-ray image to a fluorescent blue or ultraviolet one. This reduces the exposure time a great deal. The image is intensified. Rare-earth intensifying screens are more modern and produce more intensification. They also produce different colored light, depending on the rare earth used.

rare-earth i. s. faster than the standard calcium tungstate screens but much more usable at high kV range. They require the use of special film and safelights.

intensimeter see INTENSIONOMETER.

intensionometer an ionometric instrument for measuring the intensity of x-rays. Two series of plates, separated by an air gap that serves as the dielectric, are connected to opposite terminals in a closed chamber. An electric circuit is completed when the air becomes ionized by the x-rays, and the difference in electric potential is registered by deflection of a galvanometer needle.

intensity the dose-rate (mA·s) of the beam of x-rays; the further the film is from the source of x-rays the less intense is the beam.

intensive of great force or intensity or concentration.

i. care unit (ICU) a hospital unit in which is concentrated special equipment and specially trained personnel for the care of seriously ill patients requiring immediate and continuous attention. Called also critical care unit (CCU).

i. lambing see SHED lambing.

i. livestock production production on small acreage with a high stocking rate, e.g. on irrigated pasture, in feedlots, fattening barns, chicken battery houses, Singaporean animal flats, Californian drylots.

i. husbandry systems see intensive livestock production (above).

intention a manner of HEALING, e.g. first intention when a surgical incision heals immediately, second intention when a gaping wound fills with granulation tissue and is then covered from the sides with epithelium. See also WOUND healing.

i. tremor tremor of the head or a limb which increases as the patient tries to perform a particular function, e.g. following a moving object by moving the head. See also intention TREMOR.

inter- word element. [L.] *between.*

inter-generational interval see GENERATION interval.

interaction 1. the quality, state or process of (two or more things) acting on each other. 2. in statistical terms, the response to one factor at any particular level, which differs according to the level of the other factor. 3. see EFFECT MODIFIER.

drug i. the action of one drug upon the effectiveness or toxicity of another (or others).

interactive characterized by INTERACTION.

i. program a computer program that requires responses from the user to continue operating, e.g. answering questions posed by the program.

interatrial between the atria of the heart.

i. foramen see FORAMEN ovale.

i. septal defects includes patent foramen ovale, persistent foramen primum, persistent foramen secundum.

i. septum primum one of the two membranous sheets which help to partition the two atria during development of the embryo.

i. septum secundum the second of the two membranous sheets which partially separate the two atrial chambers in the developing embryo.

interbrain 1. thalamencephalon. 2. diencephalon.

interbreed to breed between animal or plant species, breeds, families.

interbreeding crossbreeding, as between half-breds.

intercalary inserted between; interposed.

intercalated inserted between.

i. disk dark staining, transversely orientsd bands scattered through cardiac muscle fibers; points of end-to-end contact between contiguous myocardial fibers.

i. duct small tubules connecting alveoli of salivary glands to intralobular striated ducts and finally to excretory duct.

intercalation the insertion of certain organic compounds such as aridines and ethidium bromide that possess a planar aromatic ring structure of appropriate size and geometry so as to insert between base pairs in double-stranded DNA.

intercalving interval period between successive calves, a target of 1 year in many cattle enterprises. Calculated as an index for the herd but may not provide a full picture of reproductive efficiency if significant numbers of cows do not calve for a second time and are not included in the calculation.

intercapital ligament ligament connecting the pair of rib heads of the one thoracic segment by crossing the intervertebral space just dorsal to the intervertebral disk.

intercartilaginous between, or connecting, cartilages.

intercellular between the cells.

i. coupling regions of special and high ionic permeability at points of junction between closely apposed cells. These regions offer lower resistance to the passage of electric current and large molecules. This phenomenon is most apparent in the skin.

epidermal i. edema see SPONGIOSIS.

i. infection of ducks a disease principally of Muscovy ducks caused by an unidentified bacteria and accompanied by hyperemia and edema of the lungs.

i. substance extracellular material occurring in large amounts in connective tissue; includes the intercellular matrix composed of fibrous and amorphous (glycosaminoglycans, proteoglycans) components.

intercept in mathematical terms the points at which a curve cuts the two axes of a graph.

interchondral intercartilaginous.

intercondylar between two condyles.

i. eminences see intercondylar TUBERCLE.

i. fossa between the condyles on the distal end of the femur, on its posterior aspect.

intercostal between two ribs.

intercourse mutual exchange.

sexual i. coitus.

intercricothyrotomy incision of the larynx through the lower part of the fibroelastic membrane of the larynx (cricothyroid membrane); inferior laryngotomy.

intercritical denoting the period between attacks or bouts of a recurrent disease, e.g. equine infectious anemia.

intercurrent occurring during the course of.

i. disease a disease occurring during the course of another disease with which it has no connection.

interdental space see DIASTEMA.

interdigital between two digits.

i. cysts see interdigital PYODERMA, PODODERMATITIS.

i. dermatitis 1. the early lesion in the development of infectious footrot in sheep; called also sheep scald. 2. inflammatory, usually moist, skin disease between the toes in dogs and sometimes cats. May be due to any cause, but often associated with the pruritus of atopy and the dog's persistent licking, allergic contact dermatitis, or hookworm penetration.

i. fibroma a wart-like mass of fibrous tissue which develops in the anterior part of the interdigital cleft of cattle causing chronic lameness.

i. fibropapillomata are typical wart structures located at the posterior end of the interdigital cleft of cattle just above the heel bulbs, causing chronic lameness.

i. necrobacillosis bovine FOOTROT.

i. papillomatosis slowly spreading lameness in a large number of animals in a herd of cattle characterized by an erythematous, annular lesion in the midline on the back of the pastern, usually on one hindlimb of a cow, caused by an invasive spirochete.

interdigitation 1. an interlocking of parts by finger-like processes. 2. one of a set of finger-like processes.

interestrous between estral periods.

i. cycle the cycle of proestrus, estrus, metestrus, diestrus. See also Table 17.

i. interval the interval, in days, between estrus periods. See Table 17. An important figure in the differential diagnosis of infertility.

interface the point where two systems or structures meet.

chemical i. the boundary between two chemical systems or phases.

computer i. a cable which provides communication between two electronic devices such as a computer and a visual display screen.

i. dermatitis skin disease with histopathological changes, either hydropic degeneration or lichenoid cellular infiltrate or both, involving dermoepidermal junction.

ecological i. the boundary between ecosystems.

hydropic i. a type of interface dermatitis in which the main lesion at the dermoepidermal junction is hydropic degeneration.

lichenoid i. a type of interface dermatitis in which the main lesion at the dermoepidermal junction is like lichen.

interfascicular between adjacent fascicles.

interfemoral between the thighs.

interference in virology, the inhibition of viral replication by the presence of other viruses. Most instances of viral interference are mediated by INTERFERON (INF).

ultrasound i. lines in ultrasonography, white lines across the image, usually caused by poor contact between the skin and transducer.

interferon (INF) a natural glycoprotein cytokine released by cells invaded by viruses. Interferon is not itself an antiviral agent but rather acts as a stimulant to noninfected cells, causing them to synthesize another protein with antiviral characteristics, probably by initiating DNA-directed RNA synthesis and, thus, protein synthesis.

The natural production of interferon is not restricted to viral infections; it can be released in response to a wide variety of inducers, including certain nonviral and infectious agents such as rickettsiae, bacteria and synthetic double-strand RNA polymers.

Interferon acts as a regulator of cell growth and has a variety of effects on the immune system by either activating or suppressing selected components of the immune system. For example, interferon can activate macrophages and thereby increase phagocytosis, enhance some primary antibody responses and inhibit others, enhance the expression of major histocompatibility antigens, and affect the specific cytotoxicity of lymphocytes. In regard to cell growth, interferon has the ability to inhibit the proliferation of certain cells.

There are three major classes of interferon depending on the cell of origin: INF-α, which is produced by fibroblasts; INF-β, which is produced by nonlymphocyte leukocytes; and INF-γ, which is a lymphokine, produced by T lymphocytes and also called immune interferon.

interfibrillar between fibrils.

interfilar between or among the fibrils of a reticulum.

interfirm comparison a technique for assessing the financial profitability of a veterinary practice by comparing it on the basis of a number of criteria with other practices in similar situations. The practices are rated according to their performance in each area, e.g. percentage of potential income written off as bad debts, percentage of annual income on the sundry debtors ledger.

interictal occurring between attacks, fits or paroxysms.

interkinesis the period between the first and second divisions in meiosis.

interleukins (IL) a group of polypeptide cytokines that carry signals between cells in the immune system. The molecules are produced by the cells and bind to specific receptors on the surface of appropriate target cells.

Among the interleukins so far characterized are: IL1, which is released from macrophages, hence also called MONOKINE, and affects T lymphocytes; IL2, produced by T lymphocytes and affects T lymphocytes, also known as T lymphocyte growth factor; IL3, produced by B lymphocytes and affects B lymphocytes, also known as B lymphocyte growth factor; IL4, produced by helper T lymphocytes and acts on B lymphocytes; IL5, produced by T lymphocytes and acts on eosinophils; IL6, produced by mononuclear phagocytes and acts on hepatocytes and B lymphocytes; IL7, secreted by bone marrow and thymic stromal cells and induces stem cells to differentiate into progenitor T and B lymphocytes; IL8, secreted by macrophages and endothelial cells and chemotactically attracts neutrophils and induces their adherence to vascular endothelium and extravasation; IL9, secreted by T helper lymphocytes and acts as a mitogen for these cells; IL10, secreted by T helper 2 lymphocytes and acts on macrophages to suppress cytokine production and thus indirectly reduce cytokine production by T helper 1 lymphocytes; IL11, secreted by bone marrow stromal cells and promotes differentiation of progenitor B lymphocytes and megakaryocytes; induces hepatocytes to synthesize acute phase proteins and supports growth of plasmacytomas; IL12, produced by macrophages and B lymphocytes and acts synergistically with IL2 to induce cytotoxic T lymphocytes; also stimulates proliferation of natural killer (NK), lymphokine activated killer (LAK), and T helper 1 cells; IL13, produced by T helper lymphocytes and inhibits activation and release of inflammatory cytokines by macrophages; an important regulator of the inflammatory response. Interferons α, β, γ are also interleukins. There are others.

interlobar between lobes.

interlobular between lobules.

intermandibular between the rami of the mandible.

i. cellulitis see PHARYNGEAL phlegmon.

i. edema floppy, soft swelling, which pits on pressure, between the mandibles. Not to be confused with the normal floppiness of tissues in this region in most breeds of dairy cattle. See also BOTTLE JAW.

intermaxillary between the maxillae.

intermediate 1. between; intervening; resembling, in part, each of two extremes. 2. a substance formed in a chemical process that is essential to formation of the end-product of the process.

i. cell mass see NEPHROTOME.

i. filaments intracellular protein fibers which are part of the cytoskeleton in eukaryotic cells.

i. host especially in parasitology, a host in which the parasite undergoes a stage, usually the larval or nonsexual stage, in its development. The host may be an insect vector which also acts as the transmitting medium, or another insect or animal species which is a passive enhancer, the infection being spread by other means.

i. junction see ZONULA adherens.

i. mesoderm mesoderm located just lateral to the somites, uniting the paraxial and lateral plate mesoderm.

i. sheep footrot less underrunning of horn and less likelihood of resulting in chronic lesions than in virulent footrot.

intermedin melanocyte-stimulating hormone.

intermediolateral between the medial and lateral aspects of an organ or anatomical structure.

intermedius [L.] *intermediate;* denoting a structure lying between a lateral and a medial structure, etc.

intermeningeal between the meninges.

intermittent marked by alternating periods of activity and inactivity.

i. mandatory ventilation (IMV) see intermittent mandatory VENTILATION.

i. positive-pressure breathing (IPPB) a form of respiratory therapy utilizing a VENTILATOR for the treatment of patients with inadequate breathing. As the name implies, the treatment involves application of pressure only during the inspiratory phase, its purpose being to assist the patient to breathe more deeply. See also intermittent positive-pressure VENTILATION.

intermural between the walls of an organ or organs.

intermuscular between muscles.

intern a recent veterinary graduate serving and often residing in a hospital, with the objective of getting concentrated, supervised, postgraduate, in-service training in a particular field of veterinary science. Completion of a two-year program and assignments is usually rewarded with a certificate of performance or a diploma.

internal situated or occurring within or on the inside; in anatomy, many structures formerly called internal are now termed medial.

i. abdominal abscess see RETROPERITONEAL abscess.

i. carotid artery arteritis parasitic arteritis of the external carotid artery as it courses around the edge of the guttural pouch may lead to copious nasal bleeding in horses when the artery ruptures.

i. elastic membrane a condensation of elastic fibers separating the tunica intima from the tunica media.

i. environment within the animal; includes blood pressure, circulating blood volume, tissue fluid volume, blood sugar level, tidal air volume, glomerular filtration rate.

i. fixation immobilization of fractured bones by internal appliances as distinct from casts or external fixation. Includes intramedullary pins which run the length of the medullary cavity, transfixing pins that penetrate across the medullary cavity and are maintained in position by external bars or casts, and compression plating based on the use of special screws and plates.

i. hernia see HERNIA.

i. inguinal ring see abdominal RING (internal).

i. layer unshelled eggs are free in the peritoneal cavity, thought to have been delivered there by reverse peristalsis in the oviduct.

i. laying eggs are deposited in the peritoneal cavity and become walled off.

i. limiting membrane a persistent fibrillar condensation of the vitreous body of the eye; it covers the retina and ciliary body.

i. parasitic mites poultry cutaneous mites in a number of families are found in the trachea, air sacs and subcutaneous tissues. Includes *Cytodites, Epidermoptes*, *Laminosioptes*, *Pneumonyssus*, *Rivoltsia* and *Sternastoma* spp.

i. rate of return the interest rate needed to discount future income in order to equate it with the present investment in a program.

i. repeat repetitive base sequences within DNA which may be inverted (indirect) or non-inverted (direct).

i. root sheath connective tissue sheath around the hair follicle; this part of the sheath extends only to the opening of debaceous glands into the follicle. See also ROOT sheath cuticle.

turkey i. hemorrhage see dissecting ANEURYSM.

i. vomiting any reflux of intestinal contents which does not reach the mouth, e.g. abomasal reflux into the rumenoreticulum.

internatal between the buttocks.

International Committee on Veterinary Anatomical Nomenclature publisher of *Nomina Anatomica Veterinaria* (NAV), the internationally accepted list of veterinary anatomical terms.

International Nonproprietary Name (INN) the designations recommended by the World Health Organization for pharmaceuticals.

International System of Units see SI UNITS.
International two-digit system see FÉDÉRATION DENTAIRE INTERNATIONAL SYSTEM.
International Union of Directors of Zoological Gardens an organization that monitors studbooks and promotes communication between member zoos.
interneship internship.
internet network of computer networks spanning the globe. Provides ready access to services such as E-mail, bulletin boards, text and image libraries, message forums, news services and, almost synonymous with the Internet, the world wide web.
interneuron a neuron between the primary afferent neuron and the final motor neuron (motoneuron). Also any neuron whose processes lie entirely within a specific area, such as the olfactory lobe.
internist a specialist in internal medicine.
i. program a postgraduate training program suitable for an internist.
internode a space between two nodes.
internship the position held by an INTERN.
internuclear situated between nuclei or between nuclear layers of the retina.
internuncial transmitting impulses between two different parts.
internus [L.] *internal;* denoting a structure nearer to the center of an organ or part.
interoceptor a sensory nerve terminal located in and transmitting impulses from the viscera.
interofective affecting the interior of the organism—a term applied to the autonomic nervous system.
interolivary between the olivary bodies.
interorbital between the orbits.
interosseous between two bones.
i. tendon see SUSPENSORY ligament (1).
interpalpebral between the eyelids.
interparietal 1. intermural. 2. between the parietal bones.
interparoxysmal between paroxysms.
interpeduncular between two peduncles, e.g. cerebellar peduncles.
interphalangeal situated between two contiguous phalanges.
interphase the interval between two successive cell divisions, during which the chromosomes are not individually distinguishable. The long stage in the cell cycle between successive meioses.
interpolation 1. surgical transplantation of tissue. 2. use a range of values in order to determine the value of a function at a point within the range. See also EXTRAPOLATION.
interpretation the veterinarian's explanation of how the disease process is causing the observed signs and how the laboratory findings are caused by the causative agent.
clinical i. explaining all of the clinical signs observed in terms of the lesions thought to be present.
radiological i. explaining the observed changes seen in the radiograph.
interpreter a computer program that converts each command in source code to machine code, executes the command and then proceeds to the next command.
interproximal between two adjoining surfaces.
interpubic between the pubic bones.
interpupillary between the pupils.
interrod matrix formless material between the rods of enamel produced on the developing tooth.
interscapular between the scapulae.
intersectio pl. *intersectiones* [L.] intersection.
i. clavicularis see CLAVICULAR INTERSECTION.
i. tendinea, inscriptio tendinea a fibrous band traversing the belly of a muscle, dividing it into two parts.
intersection a site at which one structure crosses another.
i. tendinous irregular transverse septa divide the rectus abdominis muscle into a number of segments.
intersex 1. intersexuality. 2. an animal which exhibits intersexuality.
chromosomal i. includes all patients whose sexual abnormalities are due to sex chromosome abnormalities.
i. condition where there is ambiguity in the structure of the gonads, reproductive tract or external genitalia.
gonadal i. patients who have a normal male or female karyotype but whose gonads do not correspond to their chromosomal sex.
phenotypic i. patients with normal gonadal and chromosomal sex but their sex organs in whole or in part are abnormal; their other sexual characteristics may also be abnormal.
true i. a true HERMAPHRODITE.
intersexuality an intermingling, in varying degrees, of the characters of each sex, including physical form, reproductive tissue and sexual behavior, in one animal, as a result of some flaw in embryonic development. See also HERMAPHRODITISM and PSEUDOHERMAPHRODITISM.
interspace a space between similar structures.
interspecific hybridization the results of matings between members of different animal species.
interspersion pattern a form of moderately reiterated DNA consisting of alternating blocks of single copy sequence and moderately reiterated sequences.
intersphenoidal synchondrosis the cartilage joint, present during skull growth, between the presphenoid and basisphenoid bones;
interspinal between two spinous processes.
interstice an interval, space or gap in a tissue or structure.
interstitial pertaining to or situated between parts or in the interspaces of a tissue.
atypical i. pneumonia see ATYPICAL INTERSTITIAL PNEUMONIA.
i. cell adenoma see interstitial cell tumor (below).
i. cell-stimulating hormone luteinizing hormone.
i. cell the cells of the connective tissue of the ovary or the testis (Leydig's cells), which furnish the internal secretion of those structures.
i. cell tumor a common testicular tumor in old dogs. Most are benign and not associated with any major clinical disturbances but there may be concurrent perianal gland neoplasms, infertility and rarely feminization or viciousness. Called also Leydig cell tumor or interstitial cell adenoma.
i. edema edema of the interstitial interlobular tissue in the lung.
i. emphysema pulmonary emphysema with air accumulated in the interlobular connective tissue; characteristic of emphysema in cattle.
i. fluid the extracellular fluid bathing cells in most tissues, excluding the fluid within the lymph and blood vessels.
i. gland of the ovary, consisting of polyhedral epithelioid cells in the stroma of the ovary and have characteristics of cells which produce steroids.
i. nephritis see NEPHRITIS.
i. fluid pressure pressure exerted by the free interstitial fluid; if the pressure is negative this tends to suck

fluid out of the vascular system and into the tissue space; if the pressure is greater than the intravascular pressure fluid tends to move out of the tissue space.
i. pneumonia see PNEUMONIA.
i. space tissue space.
i. tissue connective tissue between the cellular elements of a structure.
interstitial–lymphatic flow system the system of drainage from the gel-like matrix of the tissue interstitium to the terminal lymphatics.
interstitium 1. interstice. 2. interstitial tissue.
intersucking a vice in calves and even in adult cattle of sucking one another's teats, and drinking the milk if it is available.
intertarsal between the rows of tarsal bones.
interthalamic adhesion the joining of the two thalami in the center of the third ventricle. Called also thalamic intermediate mass.
intertragic notch a small but palpable notch in the dorsal and more exposed edge of the auricular cartilage between the antitragus caudally and the tragus anteriorly.
intertransverse situated between or connecting the transverse processes of the vertebrae.
intertrigo an erythematous skin eruption occurring on apposed surfaces of the skin, as the creases of the neck, folds of the groin and axilla, and between pendulous mammary glands. It is caused by moisture, warmth, friction, sweat retention and infectious agents. Signs include moistness, redness, maceration, and sometimes erosions, fissures and exudations. It occurs in recently calved cows in good condition. See also fold DERMATITIS.
axillary i. lesions confined to the axilla.
intertrochanteric between the greater and lesser trochanters of the femur.
intertubular between tubules.
interureteral, interureteric between the ureters.
intervaginal between sheaths.
interval the space between two objects or parts; the lapse of time between two events. In statistical terms, the numerical distance between two values.
atrioventricular i., A-V i. see P–R interval (below).
cardioarterial i. the time between the apex beat and arterial pulsation.
P–R i. in electrocardiography, the time between the onset of the P wave (atrial activity) and the QRS complex (ventricular activity).
QRST i., Q–T i. the duration of ventricular electrical activity.
intervalvular between valves.
intervascular between blood vessels.
intervening sequence see INTRON.
intervention the act of intervening in a disease or epidemiological sequence.
i. strategy in the sequence of examination, diagnosis, treatment and control it is necessary, especially in herd problems, to design a strategy for intervening, either to test the hypothesis or to plan the treatment and control sequence which may require a change in the environment, the feeding regime or the breeding practices; for most efficient use of resources the intervention may need detailed planning.
i. study testing an hypothesized epidemiological cause–effect relationship by intervening in a population and modifying a supposed causal factor and measuring the effect of the change.
interventricular between the ventricles of the heart.
i. foramina communication openings between the third ventricle and the two lateral ventricles of the brain.
i. septal defect see VENTRICULAR septal defect.
intervertebral between two vertebrae.
i. disk the pad of fibrocartilage between the bodies of adjoining vertebrae made up of a pulpy center surrounded by a series of concentric fibrous rings. It is subject to degeneration, extrusion, protrusion and herniation resulting in the development of intervertebral disk disease (see below) known in humans as slipped DISK.
i. disk disease the syndrome of pain and neurological deficits, sometimes complete paralysis, resulting from displacement of part or all of the nucleus of an intervertebral disk. Seen most often in dogs, particularly those of chondrodystrophoid breeds such as Dachshund, Basset hound and Beagle. The most frequently involved disks are in the thoracolumbar region from T11 to L2, but those in the cervical and lumber spine are also commonly affected. See also HANSEN'S CLASSIFICATION.
i. disk space the space between vertebrae occupied by an intervertebral disk as seen on radiographs.
i. foramen see intervertebral FORAMEN.
intervillous between or among villi.
interwound turns in supercoiled DNA a structure produced by unfolding a toroidal turn along an axis which is distinct from the supercoil axis.
intestinal pertaining to the intestine.
i. accident sudden change in normal intestinal structure or disposition, e.g. intestinal VOLVULUS.
i. adenomatosis see porcine intestinal ADENOMATOSIS.
i. adhesions relics of inflammatory incidents binding loops of intestine together or to peritoneum; have the effect of obstruction or luminal constriction.
i. aganglionosis see colonic AGANGLIONOSIS.
i. amphistomiasis see PARAMPHISTOMIASIS.
i. arterial thromboembolism see VERMINOUS mesenteric arteritis.
i. atony occurs reflexly as a result of peritonitis, of severe inflammation or distension in other parts of the alimentary tract and abdominal viscera, or directly as a result of severe inflammation, as distinct from the early excitation or movement that occurs with mild or early inflammation. See also PARALYTIC ileus.
i. clostridiosis a rare disease of the horse manifested by an acute, highly fatal diarrhea associated with the presence in the gut of large numbers of *Clostridium welchii* type A.
i. compression by a tissue mass, e.g. tumor, organ enlargement, causing partial or complete obstruction.
i. constriction by adhesion, local blood clot causing partial or complete obstruction.
i. crypts simple, branched, tubular invaginations of mucosa at the base of the villi.
i. dilatation the causes of the dilatation are fluid, feces or flatus (gas). All cause pain of varying degree, and initially an increase in motility, followed by atony. In distension of long duration, e.g. with feces, the distended bowels are easily palpable and are usually the cause of some abdominal distension. In acute dilatation the distension and palpability of the loops of intestine are less obvious and later in their appearance than other signs.
i. displacement causing partial or complete obstruction, e.g. displacement of the colon in horses.
i. diverticulum may cause intestinal compression and obstruction, e.g. Meckel's diverticulum.
i. fibrinous casts gelatinous, sausage-shaped masses, like casts of the intestinal lumen, resulting

from severe inflammation and protein loss from the bowel wall.
i. fluids fluids in the lumen of the intestine; the balance between intake and absorption of these fluids determines the form of the feces; disruption can cause diarrhea or constipation.
i. foreign body has most importance as a cause of intestinal obstruction. It may also cause laceration and intestinal hemorrhage or penetration of the intestinal wall and the development of peritonitis.
i. granuloma resulting from chronic local inflammation; cause constriction of the intestinal lumen.
i. hemorrhage into the small intestine causes the appearance of red-black feces (melena); from the large intestine the appearance is typical of whole blood, which may be mixed homogeneously with feces or be scattered through them as clots.
i. hemorrhage syndrome PROLIFERATIVE hemorrhagic enteropathy.
i. hypermotility causes abdominal pain, increased gut sounds, diarrhea and decreased opportunity for the absorption of nutrients. It occurs as a result of irritation to the intestinal lining, as in enteritis, to stimulation of the parasympathetic nervous system by the use of parasympathomimetic drugs, or to changes in the composition of the gut contents such as occurs when there is a malabsorption problem.
i. hypersecretion occurs as a result of distension and as a major part of the response to enterotoxic *Escherichia coli* toxin. The effect is to increase the fluidity of the gut contents; diarrhea results.
i. hypomotility see ATONIA.
i. idiopathic muscular hypertrophy ILEAL muscular hypertrophy.
i. ileocecal valve impaction see intestinal obstruction COLIC.
i. impaction see impaction COLIC.
i. incarceration passage of a loop of intestine through a small orifice, e.g. inguinal canal, with resulting swelling, obstruction and occlusion of blood supply.
i. infarction may be nonstrangulating, presenting a clinical picture of subacute but still fatal colic, or strangulating, e.g. when torsion precedes the development of the infarct, a much more acute and potentially fatal situation; see thromboembolic COLIC, intestinal INFARCTION.
i. inflammation see ENTERITIS.
i. intramural hematoma causes a swelling in the bowel wall and partial obstruction of the lumen.
i. linear foreign body see linear FOREIGN BODY.
i. lipofuscinosis brown discoloration of the intestinal muscularis, especially the terminal small intestine.
i. obstruction any hindrance to the passage of the intestinal contents. Causes may be *acute*, such as those caused by foreign body, phytobezoar, intussusception, volvulus and strangulation. There is sudden onset of abdominal pain, cessation of feces evacuation, vomiting in dogs and cats, gastric distension in horses, rumen distension in ruminants, loops of intestine distended with fluid and gas palpable per rectum or visible radiographically, shock and dehydration. Obstruction may also be *chronic* and manifested by intermittent vomiting and abdominal pain, chronic intestinal distension, loud intestinal sounds, and palpable distended loops of intestine. See also intestinal obstruction COLIC.
i. parasitism infestation of the intestinal lumen and wall by nematodes, cestodes and immature trematodes.
i. polyp see POLYP; may cause intermittent bowel obstruction or erratic passage of feces.
porcine i. hemorrhagic syndrome see PROLIFERATIVE hemorrhagic enteropathy.
i. portals openings to the closed foregut and hindgut of the embryo.
i. pseudo-obstruction the patient presents a clinical picture of intestinal obstruction with no surgically correctable lesion, e.g. paralytic ileus.
i. reflux is part of the reaction to increased gut motility resulting in gastric dilatation and the vomiting of intestinal contents, even feces.
i. rupture can occur as a result of extreme distension. More commonly it follows compromise to a section of gut, e.g. strangulation, in which a necrotic section of gut wall collapses. The effects of perforation of the gut wall through a deep ulcer are similar but not so sudden. The result of a rupture is sudden death due to shock and endotoxemia. With a slower leak the result is an initial stage of acute peritonitis accompanied by fever and abdominal pain.
i. sclerosis mild to obvious bowel dilation with mononuclear inflammatory infiltrate in the smooth muscle fibers plus interstitial fibrosis and atrophy of smooth muscle cells.
i. secretory-absorptive imbalance includes excessive absorptive function, e.g. thrifty bowel syndrome, or over-secretion, the classical malabsorption syndrome, e.g. in enteric colibacillosis.
i. segmental ischemic necrosis of mares occurs spontaneously in the small colon of pregnant or postpartum mares; intestinal rupture and death follow quickly.
i. smooth muscle intrinsic disease see intestinal sclerosis (above).
i. spasm see HYPERMOTILITY.
i. stenosis constriction of the bowel lumen, as a result of incomplete aplasia, cicatricial contraction after injury or infection, leads to a syndrome of chronic or intermittent subacute abdominal pain.
i. strangulation occurs in an incarcerated hernia, umbilical, inguinal, mesenteric tear, uterine ligament, or a volvulus. There may be a double problem of acute intestinal obstruction plus an intestinal infarction characterized by profound shock and toxemia, paralytic ileus and a blood-stained paracentesis specimen. Less severe but still lethal strangulations occur as a result of tightening of a lipoma pedicle, displacement of dorsal colon in the horse over the gastrosplenic ligament.
i. torsion is a common cause of acute intestinal obstruction. There is an obstruction to the movements of contents and compromise to the circulation of the twisted segment.
i. tract the small and large intestines in continuity. The long, coiled tube of the intestine is the part of the digestive system where most of the digestion of food takes place. The small intestine has three parts: the duodenum, jejunum and ileum; the large intestine, the cecum, colon and rectum.
i. tympany is part of most cases of intestinal obstruction. Primary cases of intestinal tympany are rare and confined in their occurrence to the horse. See also flatulent COLIC.

intestine the part of the alimentary tract extending from the pyloric opening of the stomach to the anus. It is a musculomembranous tube lined with a secretory and/or absorptive mucosa, comprising the small intestine and large intestine; called also bowel and gut. See also INTESTINAL tract.
large i. CECUM (1), COLON, RECTUM.
small i. DUODENUM, JEJUNUM, ILEUM.

intestinum pl. *intestina* [L.] intestine.
i. crassum large intestine.
i. tenue small intestine.
intima the innermost coat of a blood vessel; called also tunica intima.
intimal pertaining to or emanating from vascular intima.
i. bodies irregular mineralized masses covered by endothelium and protruding into the lumen of small arteries and arterioles of horses, especially in the intestinal submucosa.
i. tracks aggregations of cellular debris, fibrin and inflammatory cells, especially eosinophils, in the form of tortuous tracks in the intima of arteries in horses; caused by migrating larvae of *Strongylus vulgaris*.
intimitis endarteritis; inflammation of the innermost coat of an artery.
intolerance inability to withstand or consume; inability to absorb or metabolize nutrients.
drug i. the state of reacting to the normal pharmacological doses of a drug with the signs of overdosage.
intoxication poisoning; the state of being poisoned.
intra- word element. [L.] *inside of, within.*
intra vitam [L.] *during life.*
intra-abdominal within the abdomen.
intra-aortic within the aorta.
i. balloon pump a mechanical aid to the circulatory function of the heart that acts to provide internal counterpulsation.
intra-arterial within an artery.
i. injection used as an intentional procedure in radiology; can occur accidentally during attempts at intravenous injection.
intra-articular within a joint.
intracanalicular within a canaliculus.
intracapsular within a capsule.
i. cataract extraction removal of the entire lens, together with the capsule. In animals, usually reserved for removal of luxated lenses.
intracardiac within the heart.
intracartilaginous within a cartilage.
intracellular within a cell or cells.
i. fluid fluid within cells.
intracervical within the canal of the cervix uteri.
intracisternal within a subarachnoid cistern.
intracornual within the horns of the uterus.
i. frenulum the division between the two horns visible internally through a fiberscope. Called also intercornual septum, velum uteri.
intracranial within the cranium.
i. abscess signs will vary depending on which parts of the brain are compressed and damaged. General signs include circling, rotation of the head and mental dullness. The CSF may contain inflammatory cells.
i. hemorrhage in the form of localizing hematomas with localizing signs occur very rarely in animals. May be multiple petechiae in asphyxial newborn lambs.
i. pressure (ICP) the pressure within the subarachnoidal fluid, which is present in the space between the skull and the brain. Intracranial pressure, like arterial blood pressure, can fluctuate markedly and quickly during straining to defecate. While signs of sustained increased intracranial pressure can be significant in the assessment of a patient with a neurological disorder, momentary increases in intracranial pressure are not in themselves necessarily detrimental.
i. tumors cause an increase in intracranial pressure and localizing signs, depending on the location of the tumor and the structures that are compressed.
intractable unmanageable, intolerable.
intracutaneous within the substance of the skin.
i. cornifying epithelioma see intracutaneous cornifying EPITHELIOMA.
i. injection see intradermal INJECTION.
i. test intradermal test. See SKIN test.
intracystic within a bladder or a cyst.
intradermal within the dermis.
i. test see SKIN test.
single i. test a test used in the field diagnosis of bovine tuberculosis. A small volume of tuberculin is injected intradermally, commonly in a tail fold, and observed at 72 to 96 hours for a significant increase in thickness of the skin. The tuberculin elicits a cell-mediated immune reaction at the site of injection in infected animals and the increased thickness of the skin is the consequence of infiltration into the site of T lymphocytes and activated macrophages.
intradermopalpebral test the intradermal injection of a test reagent into the skin of the eyelid. A positive reaction is a swollen eyelid with a conjunctival reaction and an ocular discharge. Used in horses for the mallein test for glanders and in tuberculin testing of nonhuman primates.
intraductal within a duct.
intradural within or beneath the dura mater.
intraepidermal within the epidermis.
intraepithelial within epithelial cells.
i. lumina, i. cysts intracellular vacuoles associated with epithelial hyperplasia in the epididymis; indicative of regeneration after previous damage.
intrafetal within the fetus.
i. fetotomy see subcutaneous FETOTOMY.
intrafollicular within (1) hair follicles or (2) follicles of the spleen.
i. hyalinosis the degenerating germinal centers in the spleen are replaced by a transudate of plasma proteins.
intrafusal pertaining to the striated fibers within a muscle spindle.
intragastric cooling a method for inducing hypothermia in preparation for cardiac surgery. Cold water is circulated through a balloon placed in the stomach.
intrahepatic within the liver.
i. primary cholestasis obstruction of bile flow by pathological changes in the liver parenchyma, especially fibrosis, causing obstruction to minute biliary canaliculi.
intralesional occurring in or introduced directly into a localized lesion.
intralobar within a lobe.
intralocular within the loculi of a structure.
intraluminal within the lumen of a tubular structure.
intramammary within or into the mammary gland.
i. devices plastic devices inserted in the teat cistern to cause an inflammatory reaction and restrict invasion of the quarter by bacteria; no great benefit recorded plus some disadvantages.
i. infusion intramammary INFUSION.
intramedullary within the spinal cord, medulla oblongata, or the marrow cavity of a bone.
i. administration see INTRAOSSEOUS catheterization.
i. pinning see INTERNAL fixation.
intramembranous within a membrane.
i. ossification see intramembranous OSSIFICATION.
intramolecular base pairing the secondary structure founding single-stranded RNA produced by hydrogen bonded base pairing interspersed with unpaired 'loop' and 'hairpin' structures.
intramural within the wall of an organ.

intramuscular within the substance of a muscle.
i. injection see intramuscular INJECTION.
intranasal neuroblastoma see OLFACTORY neuroblastoma.
intraocular within the eye.
i. hemorrhage see HYPHEMA.
i. pressure see intraocular PRESSURE, GLAUCOMA.
intraoperative occurring during a surgical operation.
intraoral within the mouth.
intraorbital within the orbit.
i. prosthesis see ocular PROSTHESIS.
intraosseous within a bone; sometimes used to refer to the bone marrow cavity in place of intramedullary.
i. catheterization percutaneous placement of an intravenous catheter into a marrow cavity provides an alternative route for the administration of fluids and medication when peripheral blood vessels are collapsed or inaccessible. In small animals, the femur is most often used.
intraparenchymal within the parenchyma of an organ.
i. mastitis treatment injection of an antibiotic preparation into a quarter via a long hypodermic needle inserted percutaneously into the glandular tissue.
intraparietal 1. intramural. 2. within the parietal region of the brain.
intrapartum occurring during parturition.
i. death stillbirth.
intraperiod lines the fused outer leaflets of contiguous plasma membranes produce the intraperiod lines in the neuronal myelin sheath.
intraperitoneal within the peritoneal cavity.
i. injection see intraperitoneal INJECTION.
intrapharyngeal within the pharynx.
i. ostium the aperture through which the rostral laryngeal cartilages protrude.
intrapleural within the pleura.
i. pressure the pressure in the pleural cavity; called also intrathoracic pressure.
intrapulmonary within the substance of the lung.
intrapulmonic pressure the pressure in the lung tissue and passages.
intrarenal urine reflux reflux of urine during urination which extends as far as the glomerulus.
intraretinal space the space separating the outer pigment epithelium and the inner neural retina of the optic cup. Called also opticoel, optic cup cavity.
intraruminal pellets bolus-sized medication dispensed orally via balling gun, destined for slow dissolution in the reticulorumen.
intrascleral within the sclera.
i. prosthesis see ocular PROSTHESIS.
intraspinal within the spinal column.
intrasternal within the sternum.
intrathecal within a sheath; through the theca of the spinal cord into the subarachnoid space.
intrathoracic within the thorax.
i. pressure see INTRAPLEURAL pressure.
intratracheal endotracheal.
i. therapy through an endotracheal tube or by percutaneous injection into the trachea for the delivery of antibiotics into the lungs.
intratubal within a tube.
intratympanic within the tympanic cavity.
intrauterine within the uterus.
i. contraceptive device a mechanical device inserted into the uterine cavity for the purpose of contraception. These devices, used in human gynecology, have been used in draft cattle in Asia for many years. Used occasionally also in dogs. Called also IUD.
i. growth retardation failure to grow properly in utero in stature, as measured by crown to rump measurement. Pituitary dwarfism in cattle and runting in piglets and puppies are typical examples.
i. medication medication applied to the uterus via a cervical catheter, or manually in the recently birthed mare, sow or cow.
i. therapy is a common practice in food animals. Infusion of fluid material or manual placement of solid materials are the usual methods employed. The method has the advantage of achieving maximum concentration of the medicament at the endometrium but only low concentrations are achieved in the deeper layers. See also INFUSION.
intravasation the entrance of foreign material into vessels.
intravascular within a vessel or vessels.
disseminated i. coagulation see disseminated intravascular COAGULATION.
i. fluid that part of the total body fluid that is within the vascular system.
i. space the space occupied by the blood.
intravenous within a vein.
i. feeding see intravenous infusion (below).
i. infusion administration of fluids through a vein; called also phleboclysis, venoclysis and intravenous feeding. This method of feeding is used most often when a patient is suffering from severe dehydration and does not drink fluids because it is unconscious, recovering from an operation, unable to swallow normally, or vomiting persistently. Prolonged feeding of patients with chronic intestinal dysfunction can be accomplished by total parenteral NUTRITION.
i. pyelography see PYELOGRAPHY.
intraventricular within a ventricle.
intravital occurring during life.
intrinsic situated entirely within, or pertaining exclusively to, a part.
i. factor see intrinsic FACTOR.
i. host determinants characteristics peculiar to the host that affect the spread and occurrence of a disease.
i. nerve some evidence exists for the presence of autonomous nerves, without connection to the CNS, in the adventitia of small arteries and arterioles.
i. pathway, i. system see COAGULATION pathways.
i. protein see MEMBRANE proteins.
introducer a heavy metal fist-sized instrument to which a wire saw can be attached to be introduced into the uterus of a cow or mare and dropped over the part to be sawed. The weight and shape of the introducer ensure that it is easily found and pulled out with the wire attached, so that the fetotome can then be threaded.
intromission the entrance of one part or object into another.
intron untranslated, intervening sequences that are interspersed between coding sequences of a particular gene of almost all eukaryocytic genes and which are excised from the primary RNA transcript to yield mRNA.
i.–exon junction introns are removed by the catalytic action of small nuclear riboproteins (snRNPs) which bind to special recognition sequences at the 5,(donor junction) and 3,(receptor junction) to form a complex called a SPLICEOSOME.
introsusception intussusception.
introversion the turning outside in, more or lees completely, of an organ.
intrusion an orthodontic procedure in which a tooth is made to move further into the alveolus.

intubate to perform intubation.
intubation the insertion of a tube, as into the larynx. The purpose of intubation varies with the location and type of tube inserted; generally the procedure is done to allow for drainage, to maintain an open airway, or for the administration of anesthetics or OXYGEN.
Intubation into the stomach or intestine is done to remove gastric or intestinal contents for the relief or prevention of distension, or to obtain a specimen for analysis, or to introduce drugs, medication, food or nutrients. A rubber or plastic nasogastric tube is introduced through the mouth or nose and into the stomach.
intumescence 1. a swelling, normal or abnormal. 2. the process of swelling.
brachial i. cervical enlargement of the spinal cord at C6 to T1.
cervical i. see brachial intumescence (above).
lumbar i. enlargement of the lumbar spinal cord at L4–S2.
intumescentiae thickenings, intumescences.
spinal cord i. spinal cord thickenings at regions providing nerve supply to fore- and hindlimbs and to the *conus medullaris*.
intussusception 1. prolapse of one part of the intestine into the lumen of an immediately adjacent part, causing INTESTINAL obstruction. 2. the reception into an organism of matter, such as food, and its transformation into new protoplasm.
Intestinal obstruction due to intussusception occurs sporadically in all species, and in series in cattle associated with intestinal polyposis and in sheep with esophagostomiasis. The intussusception may be of the small intestine into itself or into the colon through the ileocecal valve, and in cattle into the spiral colon.
cecocolic i. cecal inversion occurs uncommonly in dogs, with clinical signs of blood-stained feces and sometimes vomiting and weight loss. With a barium enema, radiographs may show a filling defect and 'accordion pleating' of the proximal colon.
gastroesophageal i. inversion of the stomach, and occasionally spleen and pancreas, into the esophagus. Occurs most commonly with megaesophagus.
intussusceptum the portion of intestine that has prolapsed in intussusception.
intussuscipiens the portion of the intestine containing the intussusceptum.
Inula plant genus in the family Asteraceae; contains an irritant, toxic oil, and carries physically injurious awns and spines.
I. conyza causes gastrointestinal disturbance and hepatic centrilobular necrosis. Called also fleawort, plowman's spikenard.
I. graveolens see DITTRICHIA GRAVEOLENS.
inulin a starch occurring in the rhizome of certain plants, which on hydrolysis yields fructose. It is used to measure glomerular function in tests of renal function.
i. clearance an expression of the renal efficiency in eliminating inulin from the blood, a measure of glomerular function.
inunction 1. the act of anointing or applying an ointment by friction. 2. an ointment made with lanolin as a menstruum.
invaginate to infold one portion of a structure within another portion.
invagination 1. the infolding of one part within another part of a structure, as of the blastula during gastrulation. 2. intussusception.
invasive 1. having the quality of invasiveness. 2. involving puncture or incision of the skin or insertion of an instrument or foreign material into the body; said of diagnostic techniques.
invasiveness 1. the ability of microorganisms to enter the body and spread in the tissues. 2. the ability to infiltrate and actively destroy surrounding tissue, a property of malignant tumors.
inventory a list of the names and numbers or volumes of the items in stock in a store, or files in a computer program directory.
i. management keeping the list up to date, ordering new stocks, maintaining an accurate price list.
inverse square law for a given exposure the amount of radiation falling on a given area of radiographic film varies inversely as the square of the distance of that area from the source of irradiation in the focal spot.
inversion 1. a turning inward, inside out, or other reversal of the normal relation of a part. 2. a chromosomal aberration due to the inverted reunion of the middle segment after breakage of a chromosome at two points, resulting in a change in sequence of genes or nucleotides.
paracentric i. the inverted segment does not include the chromosome's centromere; has exactly the same size and shape as a normal chromosome but will have different banding patterns.
pericentric i. an inversion in a chromosome in which the centromere is included in the inverted segment.
teat i. the tip is invaginated so that the orifice is closed by the act of sucking. Causes a problem to sucking pigs. Affected sows should be culled.
invert sugar see invert SUGAR.
invertebrate 1. having no vertebral column. 2. any animal that has no vertebral column.
inverted reverse in position, direction or order.
i. L block a pattern of local filtration anesthesia commonly used in laparotomy in the ox. A horizontal line of infiltration is made just ventral to the transverse processes of the lumbar vertebrae, a vertical one just caudal to the costal arch.
inverted repeat blocks of nucleotide sequence that are present in more than one copy, but in a reverse order, such as ABCDE and E,D,C,B,A,; they may be terminal or internal. Called also indirect repeat. See also PALINDROME.
invertose see invert SUGAR.
investment appraisal evaluation of the potential profitability of a proposed investment.
inveterate confirmed and chronic; long-established and difficult to cure.
involucrin a structural protein synthesized in the stratum spinosum of the epidermis.
involucrum pl. *involucra* [L.] a covering or sheath, as in encapsulation of a sequestrum.
involuntary performed independently of the will.
i. culling see CULLING.
i. movement includes convulsions and tremor and intermittent contractions of large muscle masses which result in movement of individual limbs or other parts of the body. See also STRINGHALT, CHOREA.
i. muscle plain muscle, not under voluntary control.
i. nervous system see autonomic NERVOUS system.
involution 1. a rolling or turning inward. 2. one of the movements involved in the gastrulation of many animals. 3. a retrograde change of the entire body or in a particular organ, as the retrograde changes in the female genital organs that result in normal size after delivery. 4. the progressive degeneration occurring

naturally with advancing age, resulting in shriveling of organs or tissues.

uterine i. reduction in size of the uterus in the period immediately after parturition.

inwintering housing animals for the winter.

IO, I/O see INPUT–output.

Io chemical symbol, *ionium*.

iocetamic acid a water-soluble, iodinated, radiopaque, x-ray contrast medium.

iodamide a water-soluble, radiopaque, iodinated radiographic contrast medium; used for intravenous excretory urography.

Iodamoeba a genus of amebae in the family Endamoebidae.

I. buetschlii parasitic and may cause intestinal ulceration in humans. Found also in pigs.

I. suis found in pigs.

iodide a binary compound of iodine or the I^- anion. Iodide inhibits the release of thyroxine from the thyroid gland. See also GOITER.

iodinated a compound into which iodine has been incorporated.

i. casein is used as a feed additive to increase milk production in dairy cows but can cause poisoning manifested by hyperpnea, cardiac arrhythmia, nervousness and diarrhea.

i. protein used as a feed additive to increase milk production in cows and growth rate in pigs.

iodination the incorporation or addition of iodine in a compound.

iodine a chemical element, atomic number 53, atomic weight 126.904, symbol I. See Table 6. Iodine is essential in nutrition, being especially prevalent in the colloid of the THYROID gland. It is used in the treatment of HYPOTHYROIDISM and as a topical antiseptic. Iodine is a frequent cause of poisoning. See also IODISM.

i.-125 a radioisotope of iodine having a half-life of 60 days and a principal gamma-ray photon energy of 28 keV; used as a label in radioimmunoassays and other in vitro tests, and also for thyroid imaging. Symbol ^{125}I.

^{123}i.-metaiodobenzylguanidine a radioisotope which concentrates in chromaffin cells; used in diagnostic scintigraphy, e.g. in cases of pheochromocytoma.

i.-131 a radioisotope of iodine having a half-life of 8.1 days and a principal gamma-ray photon energy of 364 keV; used in treatment of hyperthyroidism and carcinoma of the thyroid, in thyroid function testing, and in imaging of the thyroid gland and other organs. Symbol ^{131}I.

i. deficiency may occur in all species under certain conditions; in dogs and cats, a factor in all-meat diets. See also GOITER.

i. contrast agents iodine salts are opaque to x-rays; therefore they can be combined with other compounds and used as contrast media in diagnostic x-ray examinations.

i. nutritional deficiency is characterized by goiter, neonatal mortality and alopecia.

i. poisoning occurs usually due to accidental overdosing. It causes lacrimation, anorexia, coughing due to bronchopneumonia, and a heavy dandruff. Paradoxically, iodine excess may result in thyroid hyperplasia and goiter, especially in the young.

protein-bound i. a test of thyroid function. See also PROTEIN-BOUND iodine (PBI) test.

radioactive i. see iodine-125, iodine-131 (above).

i. residues in milk careless use of iodine-based teat dips results in unacceptable residues of iodine in milk.

i. solution contains 2% free iodine and 2.4% sodium iodide in an aqueous solution.

i. solution (strong) contains 5% free iodine and 10% potassium iodide in an aqueous solution.

tamed i. see IODOPHOR.

i. trapping the selective absorption of iodine from the circulation by the thyroid gland.

iodine-based teat dips see TEAT DIP.

iodinophilous easily stainable with iodine.

iodipamide a radiopaque medium used in the form of its meglumine and sodium salts in intravenous cholecystography.

iodism chronic poisoning by iodine or iodides, manifested by coryza, ptyalism, emaciation, weakness and skin eruptions.

iodized salt contains 200 mg potassium iodate per kg of salt.

iodo-casein IODINATED casein.

iodochlorhydroxyquin, iodochlorhydroxyquinoline a topical antifungal and antibacterial agent. Called also clioquinol. Most commonly known as Vioform.

iododerma any skin lesion resulting from iodism.

iodoform a topical anti-infective containing 97% iodine, used as a skin disinfectant and stimulant for wound healing.

iodohippurate an iodine-containing compound administered as a radiopaque medium in pyelography. When labeled with radioactive iodine, it may be used as a diagnostic aid in determination of renal function.

iodophilia a reaction shown by leukocytes in certain pathological conditions, as in toxemia and severe anemia, in which the polymorphonuclears show diffuse brownish coloration when treated with iodine or iodides.

iodophor name given to any product in which surface-acting agents, such as nonoxynol, act as carriers and solubilizing agents for iodine. Used as skin disinfectants, especially as teat dips in mastitis control. Called also tamed iodine.

iodophthalein see TETRAIODOPHENOLPHTHALEIN.

iodopsin a visual pigment.

iodoquinol an amebicide and antibiotic, used in the treatment of intestinal amebiasis and topically in shampoos for the treatment of seborrheic skin conditions in dogs.

iodotherapy treatment with iodine or iodides.

iodothyronine group name for the thyroid hormones triiodothyronine and tetraiodothyronine.

iodum [L.] *iodine*.

iohexol a non-ionic iodinated positive contrast agent used in contrast radiography.

ion an atom or group of atoms having a positive (cation) or negative (anion) electric charge by virtue of having gained or lost one or more electrons. Substances forming ions are ELECTROLYTES.

i. channel see CHANNEL.

dipolar i. zwitterion.

hydrogen i. the positively charged hydrogen atom (H+), present to excess in acid solutions.

i. pair the pair of ions created when an atom has had an electron removed by ionizing radiation.

i. pump see calcium PUMP, sodium PUMP.

i. trapping a strategy for treatment of poisonings based on the principle that cell membranes are less permeable to ionized compounds. With knowledge of the characteristics of the toxin, treatment can be given to alter the acid–base balance in favor of ionization.

ion-exchange resin a high-molecular-weight, insoluble polymer of simple organic compounds with the ability to exchange its attached ions for other ions in the surrounding medium. They are classified as cation- or anion-exchange resins, depending on which ions the resin exchanges. Cation-exchange resins are used to restrict sodium absorption in edematous states; anion-exchange resins are used as antacids in the treatment of ulcers. Ion-exchange resins may also be classified as carboxylic, sulfonic, etc., depending on the nature of the active groups. Used in biochemical extractions and purifications.

ionic pertaining to an ion or ions.

i. medication iontophoresis.

ionizable side-chain groups side-chains predominantly of amino acids capable of ionization in aqueous solution depending on pH. Lysine, arginine and histidine have basic ionizable side-chains and aspartate and glutamate have acidic ionizable side-chains.

ionization 1. the dissociation of a substance in solution into ions. 2. iontophoresis.

i. chamber an enclosure containing two or more electrodes between which an electric current may be passed when the enclosed gas is ionized by radiation; used for determining the intensity of x-rays and other rays.

ionize to convert into ions.

ionizing radiation high-energy radiation, such as x-rays and gamma-rays which react in a similar manner to produce ion pairs or IONIZATION. Gamma-rays are used in the control of growth of tumors and sterilization of food, in which they have some undesirable side-effects, e.g. they destroy the enzymes in meat that cause tenderizing; off-flavors are also a problem.

ionophore any molecule, as of a drug, that increases the permeability of cell membranes to a specific ion.

i. antibiotic monocarboxylic polyether antibiotics. They may be monovalent (e.g. monensin, salinomycin) or divalent (e.g. lasolocid). They facilitate transport of ions across biological membranes by forming lipid-soluble complexes with mono or divalent cations; latter day additions to the list include narasin, maduramycin,

i. poisoning see MONENSIN.

iontophoresis the introduction of ions of soluble salts into the body by an electric current as a form of therapy.

IOP intraocular pressure.

iopamidol a non-ionic iodinated positive contrast agent used in contrast radiography.

iophendylate a fat-soluble radiopaque contrast medium used in myelography.

iothalamate a radiopaque contrast medium used in angiography and urography.

IP intraperitoneal.

IP_3 see INOSITOL 1,4,5-trisphosphate.

ipecac the dried rhizome and roots of *Cephaelis ipecacuanha* or *Cephaelis acuminata;* used as an emetic or expectorant. Called also ipecacuanha; the common preparation is syrup of ipecac.

ipecacuanha see IPECAC.

Iphiona aucheri Asian plant in the family Asteraceae; contains a sesquiterpene lactone; causes hepatic necrosis.

ipodate a radiopaque contrast medium used in oral cholecystography.

4-ipomeanol a furanoterpene produced in sweet potatoes (*Ipomoea batatus*) by the fungus *Fusarium solani* (*F. javanicum*) which has the effect of damaging pulmonary epithelium and producing lesions characteristic of atypical interstitial pneumonia in cattle which consume moldy sweet potatoes. The toxin is produced from furanosesquiterpenoid PHYTOALLEXINS.

Ipomoea widespread genus of poisonous vines of the family Convolvulaceae; may contain various toxins including the indole alkaloid lysergic acid, furanoterpenes, indolizidine alkaloids (swainsonine). Includes *I. asarifolia* (salsa), *I. batatas* (commercial sweet potato) if infested with fungi *Fusarium solani*, *I.* sp. aff. *calobra* (weir vine), *I. carnea*, *I. fistulosa* (canudo), *I. muelleri* (native morning glory), *I. plebeia* (bell-vine), *I. purpurea* (purple-flowered morning glory).

IPPB intermittent positive-pressure breathing.

IPPV intermittent positive-pressure ventilation.

ipratropium a synthetic anticholinergic used as a bronchodilator; similar to atropine but with fewer side-effects.

ipronidazole a nitroimidazole derivative, similar to metronidazole, used in the treatment of histomoniasis in turkeys.

ipsi- word element. [L.] *same, self.*

ipsilateral on the same side.

IPSP inhibitory postsynaptic potential.

IPV see infectious pustular VULVOVAGINITIS.

Ir chemical symbol, *iridium.*

Ir gene immune response gene.

IRC inspiratory reserve capacity.

iridal pertaining to the iris.

iridauxesis thickening of the iris.

iridectomesodialysis excision and separation of adhesions around the inner edge of the iris.

iridectomy excision of part of the iris.

peripheral i. the peripheral or basal portion is removed.

sector i. a sector, from pupillary margin to base, is removed.

iridectropium eversion of the iris.

iridemia hemorrhage from the iris.

iridencleisis surgical incarceration of a slip of the iris within a corneal or limbal incision to act as a wick for aqueous drainage in glaucoma.

i.–cyclodialysis a surgical procedure used in the treatment of many types of glaucoma. Combines a posterior sclerectomy, CYCLODIALYSIS and trans-scleral iridencleisis.

irideremia congenital absence of the iris.

inherited i. occurs in cattle in association with other ocular defects.

irides plural of *iris.*

iridescence the condition of gleaming with bright and changing colors.

iridesis repositioning of the pupil by fixation of a sector of iris in a corneal or limbal incision.

iridial pertaining to the iris.

i. angle peripheral margin of the anterior chamber at the limbus.

i. angle meshwork see IRIDOCORNEAL meshwork.

i. granule proliferative, well-vacularized extensions of the iridial stroma and pigment epithelium appearing as black, cystic masses along the iridial margin in ruminants and horses. Called also corpora nigra, granula iridica.

i. stroma loose connective tissue, blood vessels, chromatophores, smooth muscle in the uveal tract of the eye.

iridic iridial.

iridin a cardiac glycoside found in the leaves of plants in the iris family (*Iris* spp.) and the roots of plants in the *Violaceae* family, the violets. Causes severe, often bloody, diarrhea.

iridium a chemical element, atomic number 77, atomic weight 192.2, symbol Ir. See Table 6.

irid(o)- word element. [Gr.] *iris of the eye.*

iridoavulsion complete tearing away of the iris from its periphery.

iridocapsular emanating from or pertaining to the iris and the lens capsule.
iridocapsulitis inflammation of the iris and lens capsule.
iridocele hernial protrusion of part of the iris through the cornea.
iridochoroiditis inflammation of the iris and choroid.
iridociliospasm spasm of the iris and ciliary body.
iridocoloboma congenital fissure or coloboma of the iris.
iridoconstrictor a muscle element or an agent that acts to constrict the pupil of the eye.
iridocorneal pertaining to the iris and the cornea.
i. angle where the base of the iris attaches to the peripheral cornea and sclera; the site of aqueous drainage from the anterior chamber.
i. meshwork solid trabeculae interspersed between fluid spaces, at the iridial angle of the eye. Called also iridial angle meshwork.
iridocyclectomy excision of part of the iris and of the ciliary body.
iridocyclitis inflammation of the iris and ciliary body. See also anterior UVEITIS.
heterochromic i. a unilateral low-grade form leading to depigmentation of the iris of the affected eye; called also heterochromic uveitis.
iridocyclochoroiditis inflammation of the iris, ciliary body and choroid.
iridocystectomy excision of part of the iris to form an artificial pupil.
iridodesis iridesis.
iridodialysis separation or loosening of the iris from its attachments.
iridodiastasis a defect in development of the base of the iris; a coloboma of the iris.
iridodilator a muscle element or an agent that acts to dilate the pupil of the eye.
iridodonesis tremulousness of the iris on movement of the eye, occurring in subluxation of the lens.
iridokeratitis inflammation of the iris and cornea.
iridokinesia, iridokinesis contraction and expansion of the iris.
iridoleptynsis thinning or atrophy of the iris.
iridology the study of the iris as associated with disease.
iridomalacia softening of the iris.
iridomesodialysis surgical loosening of adhesions around the inner edge of the iris.
iridomotor pertaining to movements of the iris.
iridoncus tumor or swelling of the iris.
iridoparalysis iridoplegia.
iridoperiphakitis inflammation of the lens capsule.
iridoplegia paralysis of the sphincter of the iris, with lack of contraction or dilatation of the pupil; called also iridoparalysis.
iridoptosis prolapse of the iris.
iridopupillary pertaining to the iris and pupil.
iridorhexis 1. rupture of iris. 2. the tearing away of the iris.
iridoschisis splitting of the mesodermal stroma of the iris into two layers, with fibrils of the anterior layer floating in the aqueous humor.
iridosclerotomy incision of the sclera and of the edge of the iris in glaucoma.
iridosteresis removal of all or part of the iris.
iridotasis stretching of the iris in treatment of glaucoma.
iridotomy incision of the iris.
Iridoviridae a family of large DNA viruses that are 180 nm in diameter, enveloped with an icosahedral nucleocapsid and contain a large, single, double-stranded DNA genome of 150 kilobases. They replicate in the cytoplasm of infected cells. Most infect larvae of insects, giving them an iridiscent appearance. African swine fever virus was once considered a member of the family.
iridovirus a virus in the family IRIDOVIRIDAE.
Iris a European plant genus of the Iridaceae family; contain cardiac glycosides. Cause sudden death, diarrhea. Includes *I. foetidissima* (wild iris), *I. germanica* (cultivated iris), *I. missouriensis*, *I. pseudacorus* (yellow flag), *I. versicolor*.
iris[1] pl. *irides* [Gr.] the disk-like, centrally perforated, pigmented membrane behind the cornea; the most anterior portion of the vascular tunic of the eye, it is made up of a flat band of circular muscular fibers surrounding the pupil, a thin layer of radial muscle fibers by which the pupil is dilated, and, posteriorly, two layers of pigmented epithelial cells. See also IRIDIAL, PUPIL.
angle of i. see filtration ANGLE.
i. annulus the inner, smooth, narrow section of iris is the *minor* iridial annulus; the wider, outer, plicated zone, the *major* iridial annulus.
Basenji mesodermal i. defect see persistent PUPILLARY membrane.
i. bombé the iris is bowed forward by increased pressure in the posterior chamber and may adhere to the cornea.
i. collarette short, threadlike projections from the minor arterial circle of the iris.
i. cyst may be congenital or developmental, following injury or inflammation. The cysts may detach and float free in the anterior or posterior chamber. They occur rarely in dogs and cats.
i. freckle an area of hyperpigmentation without hyperplasia of the melanocytes.
i. heterochromia see HETEROCHROMIA iridis.
i. hypopigmentation may be unilateral—called HETEROCHROMIA. The structures of the iris are normal, as is the rest of the eye, except for the tapetum, which may be hypoplastic.
i. hypoplasia a vestigial iris; usually the ciliary body is normal. The lens is cataractous and may be displaced.
i. inflammation see IRITIS.
i. nevus a benign melanotic tumor of the iris consisting of melanocytes.
i. prolapse protrusion of part of the iris through a perforation in the cornea or the sclera.
iris[2] see *Iris*.
Irish blue see KERRY BLUE TERRIER.
Irish red and white setter a red and white version of the Irish setter, recognized by the Kennel Club in the United Kingdom. The dog is slightly more athletic than the Irish setter and has a domed head.
Irish setter a medium to large, slim dog with a long head, pendulous ears and silky, chestnut to mahogany colored haircoat that is longest under the neck, body and tail, and behind the legs. Called also Red setter. The breed is predisposed to hypothyroidism, progressive retinal atrophy, rod-cone dysplasia, hemophilia A, ambylopia and epilepsy.
Irish terrier a small to medium sized, active dog with a long head, erect, folded ears, docked tail, and a hard, wiry coat in shades of red or wheaten. The breed is affected by cystinuria and congenital myotonia.
Irish water spaniel a medium to large, compact gun dog with long pendulous ears, somewhat domed head with prominent occiput, and a short, straight, tapered tail. The dark liver-colored coat is a breed

characteristic, consisting of dense, tight, crisp ringlets or 'curls' with a natural oiliness. It covers the legs and body, forming a well-defined topknot that comes down in a peak on the forehead. The tail has only short, straight hairs and is often referred to as a 'rattail'. The breed is used as a retriever and is reportedly very tolerant of cold water.

Irish wolfhound a very large (at least 100 lb in weight and 30 inches tall), muscular dog with a long head, small ears, long neck, long tail, and deep chest. One of the giant breeds. The coat is medium length, rough, and wiry, in beige, fawn, gray, brindle and other solid colors. The breed is affected by hygromas, portacaval shunts and hypothyroidism.

Irish yew TAXUS *baccata* var. *fastigiata*.

iritis inflammation of the iris. The condition may be acute, occurring suddenly with pronounced signs, or chronic, with less severe but longer-lasting signs.

serous i. iritis with a serous exudate.

iritoectomy surgical excision of deposits of aftercataract on the iris, together with iridectomy, to form an artificial pupil.

iritomy iridotomy.

iron a chemical element, atomic number 26, atomic weight 55.847, symbol Fe. See Table 6. Iron is chiefly important to the animal body because it is the main constituent of hemoglobin, cytochrome, and other components of respiratory enzyme systems. A constant although small intake of iron in food is needed to replace erythrocytes that are destroyed in the body processes.

i.-59 a radioisotope of iron having a half-life of 45 days; used in ferrokinetics tests to determine the rate at which iron is cleared from the plasma and incorporated in red cells. Symbol ^{59}Fe.

i. binding absorbed iron is rapidly and tightly bound to a specific transport protein, transferrin or siderophilin, from which it is discharged at iron receptor sites in the bone marrow.

i. dextran an injectable form of iron used in the prevention of iron deficiency. See iron poisoning (below).

i. galactan used as an injection vehicle for iron in young piglets.

i. nutritional deficiency is most common in piglets raised on sows kept indoors under artificial conditions. Clinical signs are pallor, dyspnea, edema of the head and a secondary diarrhea.

organic i. poisoning see iron poisoning (below).

i. overload storage of excessive iron in body tissues such as occurs in human idiopathic hemochromatosis is not recorded in animals, but overload may occur as a result of excessive therapy.

i. poisoning overdosing piglets with iron compounds by mouth causes diarrhea and death. Organic iron preparations, usually dextrans, injected in piglets can cause deaths acutely, within an hour or two of injection. At postmortem examination there is myonecrosis of skeletal muscle. Deaths have also occurred within a few minutes of intramuscular injection of organic iron preparations in horses. Sudden death due to massive liver damage also recorded in newborn foals dosed orally with ferrous fumarate with or without yeast in a paste. Asymmetry of the hindquarters in pigs is also recorded as a sequel of intramuscular injections of iron. See also ASYMMETRIC HIND QUARTER SYNDROME. Bore water often contains significant levels of iron and when used for fish culture in dams may cause mortalities.

i. pool a source of readily available iron for metabolic emergencies, probably located in the bone marrow.

i. storage disease hemochromatosis.

i.-sulfur proteins polypeptides that contain iron-sulfur centers capable of Fe_2S_2 or Fe_4S_4 stoichiometry and with standard reduction potential between NAD+ and ubiquinone. Critical components of many electron transport chains, e.g. in oxidative phosphorylation and photosynthesis.

total i.-binding capacity the serum iron plus the unbound iron-binding capacity of the serum.

i. turnover see iron TURNOVER.

unbound i.-binding capacity that portion of the plasma transferrin molecule that is not bound to Fe^{3}+.

i.-yeast paste highly hepatoxic in some newborn foals when fed as a dietary supplement.

iron grass see LOMANDRA LONGIFOLIA.

iron-poor diet reconstituted liquid milk replacer the common one; used to feed veal calves as a sole diet.

ironstone a natural ore which may contain significant amounts of fluorine and cause fluorosis in cattle grazing pastures in the vicinity of a factory which calcines the ore.

ironweed see AMSINCKIA, SIDERANTHUS.

irotomy iridotomy.

irradiate 1. to treat with x-rays or other form of radioactivity. 2. to expose to rays such as ultraviolet light. See also IRRADIATION.

irradiated yeast yeast that has been exposed to ultraviolet light to increase its vitamin D content.

irradiation exposure to radiant energy (heat, x-rays, etc.) for therapeutic or diagnostic purposes. See also RADIATION (3).

Irradiation of certain foods, including milk, kills harmful bacteria and prevents spoilage. X-ray photography is used in industrial research and in diagnosis of disorders within the body.

i. teratogen irradiation at the time of organogenesis which is capable of causing congenital defects such as ankylosis of limb joints and cleft palate.

irreducible not susceptible to reduction, as a fracture, hernia or chemical substance.

irregular pulse caused by cardiac arrhythmia or inadequate ventricular contractions failing to open aortic semilunar valves.

irrigant fluid used to irrigate cavities.

irrigation 1. washing of a body cavity or wound by a stream of water or other fluid. 2. artificial watering of agricultural crops and pasture by flood, furrow, drip or sprinkler system. This has a significant implication for animals both nutritionally and in terms of health because of the great change in the soil microclimate and the reaction of this on parasite larvae and fungi.

irritability 1. ability of an organism or a specific tissue to react to the environment. 2. the state of being abnormally responsive to slight stimuli, or unduly sensitive.

myotatic i. the ability of a muscle to contract in response to stretching.

irritable 1. capable of reacting to a stimulus. 2. abnormally sensitive to stimuli.

i. bowel syndrome see irritable COLON syndrome.

irritant 1. causing irritation. 2. an agent that causes irritation.

i. contact dermatitis see CONTACT dermatitis.

irritation 1. the act of stimulating. 2. a state of overexcitation and undue sensitivity.

i. nervous signs increased reactions of the effector organs including tetany, tremor, convulsions, hyperesthesia, parasthesia.

i. therapy local application of an irritant substance with the purpose of destroying tissue, e.g. podophyllum-tincture benzoini composita painted on warts or sarcoids to remove them. The treatment needs to be repeated on a number of occasions.

IRV inspiratory reserve volume.

IS element in DNA, an insertion sequence.

Isabella a light fawn coat color in dogs; seen in dilute red Doberman pinschers.

isabelline having a light brown, sandy color. A common coloration in desert animals.

ischemia deficiency of blood in a part, due to functional constriction or actual obstruction of a blood vessel.

cerebral i. BRAIN anoxia.

myocardial i. deficiency of blood supply to the heart muscle, due to obstruction or constriction of the coronary arteries.

renal i. severe or prolonged ischemia causes irreversible renal failure and death from uremia. Called also ischemic nephrosis.

ischemic emanating from or pertaining to ischemia.

i. encephalopathy see feline ischemic ENCEPHALOPATHY.

i. myelopathy see fibrocartilaginous embolic MYELOPATHY.

i. myonecrosis muscle necrosis due to interruption of the blood supply, as in prolonged recumbency of cows or in thrombus development. See DOWNER COW SYNDROME, ILIAC artery thrombosis.

i. necrosis necrosis of any tissue due to interruption of its blood supply.

i. nephrosis see renal ISCHEMIA.

ischiadic, ischial ischiatic.

ischial callosity leathery patches on the buttocks of Old World primates.

ischialgia pain in the ischium.

ischiatic pertaining to the ischium.

ischidrosis anhidrosis.

ischi(o)- word element. [Gr.] *ischium.*

ischiobulbar pertaining to the ischium and the bulb of the urethra.

ischiocapsular pertaining to the ischium and the capsular ligament of the hip joint.

ischiocavernosus muscle the principal muscle in the erection of the penis. See also Table 13.2.

ischiocele hernia through the sacrosciatic notch.

ischiococcygeal pertaining to the ischium and coccyx.

ischiodidymus conjoined twins united at the pelvis.

ischiodynia pain in the ischium.

ischiofemoral pertaining to the ischium and femur.

ischiohebotomy surgical division of the ischiopubic ramus and the cranial ramus of the pubis.

ischioneuralgia pain along the path of the sciatic nerve; sciatica.

ischiopagus conjoined twins fused at the ischial region.

ischiopubic pertaining to the ischium and pubis.

ischiorectal pertaining to the ischium and rectum.

ischiourethral pertaining to the ischium and the urethra.

i. muscle a slip of muscle arising on the ischium which, through venous compression, assists in the erection of the penis. See also Table 13.2.

ischium the caudal, dorsal portion of the hip bone. See Table 10. See also OS coxae.

ischuria retention or suppression of the urine.

ISCOM immune-stimulating complexes.

isepamicin an antibiotic derived from gentamicin and with similar activity.

isethionate USAN contraction for 2-hydroxyethanesulfonate.

Isfahan an unclassified vesiculovirus usually bracketed with vesicular stomatitis virus but much less virulent.

island a cluster of cells or an isolated piece of tissue.

blood i's aggregations of mesenchymal cells in the angioblast of the embryo, developing into vascular endothelium and blood cells.

i. of Calleja discrete group of very small nerve cells in the olfactory tubercle of the forebrain.

i's of Langerhans see ISLET of Langerhans.

i. outbreak outbreak limited to a specific population, usually a herd, caused often by a localized lack of immunity in a closed herd.

islet an island.

i. cell one of the cells making up the islet of Langerhans.

i. cell neoplasia occur mostly in old dogs and morphologically they occur as adenomas or adenocarcinomas. Functionally they appear only in the form of hyperinsulinism and hypoglycemia. Rarely there are gastrin-secreting tumors causing a ZOLLINGER–ELLISON SYNDROME.

i's of Langerhans irregular microscopic structures scattered throughout the pancreas and comprising its endocrine portion. They contain the *alpha cells*, which secrete the hyperglycemic factor glucagon; the *beta cells*, which secrete insulin, and whose degeneration is one of the causes of DIABETES MELLITUS; and the *delta cells*, which secrete somatostatin.

pancreatic i. see islets of Langerhans (above).

-ism suffix meaning a state, process or condition.

iso- word element. [Gr.] *equal, alike, same.*

isoagglutinin an agglutinin that acts on cells of individuals of the same species.

isoallele an allelic gene that is considered as being normal but can be distinguished from another allele by its differing phenotypic expression when in combination with a dominant mutant allele.

isoamylase 1. any of the several isoenzymes of α-amylase. 2. a hydrolase that catalyzes the hydrolysis of 1,6-α-glycosidic branch linkages in glycogen and amylopectin.

isoanaphylaxis anaphylaxis produced by serum from an individual of the same species. See also passive ANAPHYLAXIS.

isoantibody alloantibody.

isoantigen alloantigen.

isobar 1. one of two or more chemical species with the same atomic weight but different atomic numbers. 2. a line on a map or chart depicting the boundaries of an area of constant atmospheric pressure.

isocarb a carbamate pesticide.

isocellular made up of identical cells.

isochromatic of the same color throughout.

isochromatophil staining equally with the same stain.

isochromosome an abnormal chromosome having a median centromere and two identical arms, formed by transverse, rather than normal longitudinal, splitting of a replicating chromosome.

isochronic, isochronous performed in equal times; said of motions and vibrations occurring at the same time and being equal in duration.

isocil one of the methyluracil herbicides; access to recently sprayed pasture causes bloat, incoordination, anorexia in sheep.

isocitrate dehydrogenase see isocitrate DEHYDROGENASE.

isocitric acid an intermediate in the tricarboxylic acid cycle, formed from citric acid and is itself converted to 2-oxoglutaric acid.

Isocoma wrightii HAPLOPAPPUS *heterophyllus*.

isocoria equality of size of the pupils of the two eyes.
isocortex see NEOPALLIUM.
isocupressic acid toxin in *Pinus*, *Cupressocyparis*, *Cupressus* spp.; causes abortion in livestock; called also pine needle abortion.
Isocyamus delpini an ectoparasitic copepod that parasitizes the skin of whales. Called also whale lice.
isocytosis equality in size of cells, especially of erythrocytes.
isodactylism relatively even length of the digits.
isodemic said of maps constructed so that land areas are distorted to represent the area's population density.
isodiametric measuring the same in all diameters.
isodontic having all the teeth alike.
isodose in radiotherapy a radiation dose of equal intensity to more than one body area.
i. chart a diagram of depth dose measurement at various positions within an x-ray beam in which points of equal dose throughout the beam are joined to give isodose lines.
isodrin an insecticide containing CHLORINATED HYDROCARBONS; it may cause poisoning.
isoechoic returning waves of normal amplitude in ultrasonography.
isoelectric showing no variation in electric potential.
i. focusing an electrophoretic method for separating proteins in gels which depends on the fact that the net charge on the protein varies with the pH of the surrounding medium. At the isoelectric point the protein has no net charge and will not therefore migrate further in an electric field. The polyacrylamide gel is cast in a narrow tube that provides a pH gradient from top to bottom.
i. period the moment in muscular contraction when no deflection of the galvanometer is produced.
isoenzyme any of the several forms of an enzyme, all of which catalyze the same reaction, but which may differ in reaction rate, inhibition by various substances, electrophoretic mobility or immunological properties. Several enzymes, particularly alkaline phosphatase, lactate dehydrogenase and creatine kinase, have clinically important isoenzymes. Isoenzymes are separated by electrophoresis, and the pattern indicates which damaged organ has released the enzymes.
isoerythrolysis outdated term for alloimmune hemolytic anemia; the paradigm of Rh disease of humans.
neonatal i. ALLOIMMUNE hemolytic anemia of the newborn.
isoetharine a sympathomimetic amine having more effect on the β_2-adrenergic receptors of the bronchi and vascular smooth muscle than the β_1-adrenergic receptors of the heart; used as a bronchodilator in bronchial disease and for relief of bronchospasm in chronic obstructive pulmonary disease.
isoferritins the several forms in which ferritin occurs.
isoflavan estrogenic substance in plants. Called also equol.
isoflavone 3-phenyl-4H-1-benzopyran-4-one; many of the naturally occurring estrogenic substances in pasture plants are isoflavones.
isoflurane a chlorofluorocarbon used as an inhalational anesthetic; known also as Forthane or Forane.
isoflurophate an anticholinesterase inhibitor used as a miotic in glaucoma.
isoflurophosphate an organophosphorus insecticide which has the usual toxic effect of all of these compounds, that of being an anticholinesterase. It also causes demyelination of the peripheral nerves and the spinal cord.
isoforms isomeric forms of the same protein, with slightly different amino acid sequences, but with the same activity.
isogamety production by an individual of one sex of gametes identical with respect to the sex chromosome.
isogamy reproduction resulting from union of two gametes identical in size and structure, as in protozoa.
isogeneic having the same genetic constitution; syngeneic.
isogeneric of the same kind; belonging to the same species.
isogenesis similarity in the processes of development.
isogenous groups groups of cells developed from the same cell, e.g. clusters of chondrocytes. Called also cell nests.
isograft a graft between individuals of the same species that are genetically identical.
isohemagglutination agglutination of erythrocytes caused by an isohemagglutinin.
isohemagglutinin an isoantibody that agglutinates erythrocytes.
isohemolysin an isoantibody that causes hemolysis.
isohemolysis hemolysis produced by isohemolysin.
isohydric the principle underlying the series of reactions that occurs in erythrocytes and makes it possible for them to take up carbon dioxide and release oxygen without the production of excess hydrogen.
isohypercytosis increase in the number of leukocytes, with normal proportions of neutrophil cells.
isohypocytosis decrease in the number of leukocytes with the normal relation between the number of various forms.
isoimmune possessing antibodies to isoantigens.
i. hemolytic anemia see ALLOIMMUNE hemolytic anemia of the newborn.
i. hemorrhagic anemia see PURPURA hemorrhagica.
i. neonatal leukopenia recorded as a cause of immune deficiency in foals; antibodies to the sire's lymphocytes in the mare's serum.
i. thrombocytopenia see immune-mediated THROMBOCYTOPENIA.
isoimmunization alloimmunization.
i. of pregnancy see ALLOIMMUNIZATION of pregnancy.
isolate 1. to separate from others, or set apart. 2. a group of individuals prevented by geographic, genetic, ecological or social barriers from interbreeding with others of their kind. 3. a population of microorganisms that has been obtained in pure culture from a field case or location.
isolated soybean protein the pure protein that can be spun into a fiber and then, if it is colored and flavored, has a very close resemblance to meat.
isolation the act of isolating or state of being isolated, such as (1) the physiological separation of a part, as by tissue culture or by interposition of inert material; (2) the segregation of patients with a communicable disease; (3) the successive propagation of a growth of microorganisms until a pure culture is obtained; (4) the chemical extraction of an unknown substance in pure form from a tissue.
i. technique special precautionary measures and procedures used in the care of a patient with a communicable DISEASE.
isoleucine Ile; an amino acid produced by hydrolysis of fibrin and other proteins; essential amino acid for optimal growth of the young and for nitrogen equilibrium in adults.
isologous characterized by an identical genotype.

isolysin a lysin, usually antibody, acting on cells of animals of the same species as that from which it is derived.

isolysis lysis of cells by isolysins.

isomaltase an intestinal mucosal enzyme that hydrolyzes isomaltose.

isomaltose an isomeric form of maltose formed by the action of maltase on glucose. Found in beer, honey and other natural substances. Called also dextrinose.

isomer any compound exhibiting, or capable of exhibiting, isomerism.

isomerase a major class of enzymes comprising those that catalyze the process of isomerization, such as the interconversion of aldoses and ketoses.

1¸5 disulfide i. an enzyme that catalyzes disulfide bond formation by cross-linking certain cystine residues of polypeptides; occurs as a post-translational modification.

isomerism the possession by two or more distinct compounds of the same molecular formula, each molecule having the same number of atoms of each element, but in different arrangement.

isomerization the process whereby any isomer is converted into another isomer, usually requiring special conditions of temperature, pressure, or catalysts.

isometheptene a sympathomimetic drug, used parenterally as the hydrochloride or orally as the mucate, as a smooth muscle relaxant.

isometric maintaining, or pertaining to, the same length; of equal dimensions.

i. contraction muscle contraction without appreciable shortening or change in distance between its origin and insertion.

i. exercise active exercise performed against stable resistance, without change in the length of the muscle.

isomorbs lines on a map which join geographical points at which the morbidity rate for a particular disease is the same.

isomorphism identical in form; in genetics, referring to genotypes of polypoid organisms that produce similar gametes even though containing genes in different combinations on homologous chromosomes.

isomorts lines on a map which join geographical points at which the mortality rate for a particular disease is the same.

isoniazid an antibacterial compound used in treatment of tuberculosis and opportunistic mycobacterial infections.

isopathy the treatment of disease by means of products of the disease or with material from the affected organ.

isopleth lines on a map that join geographical points which have the same value for a particular continuous variable.

isopod member of the order Isopoda. Includes water slaters, woodlice. Suborders include Flabellifera (aquatic parasites in marine fish).

isopotential lines connecting points of equal electrical potential.

isoprecipitin an isoantibody that acts as a precipitin.

isoprenaline see ISOPROTERENOL.

isoprene hydrocarbon 2-methyl-1,3-butadiene; building block for many lipids including cholesterol, steroids and bile acids, the lipid-soluble vitamins, dolichol, coenzyme Q and many more terpenoid biomolecules.

isoprinosine an antiviral agent containing a mixture of inosine, dimethylaminoisopropanol and paracetamidobenzoic acid.

isopropamide an anticholinergic used in the form of the iodide to suppress gastric and pancreatic secretion.

isopropanol isopropyl alcohol.

isopropyl denotes the 1-methylethyl group, $-CH(CH_3)_2$.

i. alcohol rubbing alcohol, used as a solvent and rubefacient. Formed naturally in the rumen of the cow in nervous acetonemia.

i. isothiocyanate a cyanogenetic compound found in plants of *Brassica* spp. May cause acute deaths due to cyanide poisoning and also act as a goitrogen.

i. methanesulfonate an alkalizing agent that causes testicular degeneration.

isopropylarterenol see ISOPROTERENOL.

isoproterenol a synthetic cathecholamine and potent β-receptor agonist; it causes vasodilation and positive inotropic and chronotropic effects in the heart. Called also isoprenaline.

isopyknosis the quality of showing uniform density throughout, especially the uniformity of condensation observed in comparison of different chromosomes or in different areas of the same chromosome.

isoquant a curve showing the various combinations of two inputs which can be used to produce a specific level of output.

isoquinoline alkaloid includes berberine, bulbocaprine, chelidonine, corydaline.

isorrhea an equilibrium between the intake and output, by the body, of water and/or solutes.

isoschizomers restriction enzymes that have the same recognition sequence as another enzyme, which was the first enzyme discovered with that particular recognition sequence.

isosensitization allosensitization.

isosexual pertaining to or characteristic of the same sex.

isosmotic having the same osmotic pressure.

isosorbide an osmotic diuretic; the dinitrate of isosorbide is used as a coronary vasodilator.

Isospora a genus of apicomplexan parasites in the family Eimeriidae found mainly in dogs and cats. These protozoa develop intracellularly in the cells of the intestinal epithelium and some of them are associated with attacks of diarrhea. Includes *I. almaataensis* (pigs), *I. bahiensis* (dogs), *I. bigemina* (*Cystoisospora burrowsi*), *I. burrowsi* (*C. burrowsi*), *I. buteonis* (*raptor birds*), *I. canis* (*C. canis*), *I. felis* (*C. felis*), *I. heydoni* (*C. heydoni*), *I. neorivolta* (dog), *I. ohioensis* (*C. ohioensis*), *I. ratti* (rats), *I. rivolta* (*C. rivolta*), *I. suis* (pigs), *I. wallacei* (*Besnoitia wallacei*).

isospore 1. an isogamete of organisms that reproduce by spores. 2. an asexual spore produced by a homosporous organism.

isosthenuria maintenance of a constant osmolality of the urine, regardless of changes in osmotic pressure of the blood.

isotherm a line on a map or chart depicting the boundaries of an area in which the temperature is the same.

isothermal, isothermic having the same temperature.

isothiocyanate see ALLYL isothiocyanate.

isotone one of several nuclides having the same number of neutrons, but differing in number of protons in their nuclei.

isotonia 1. a condition of equal tone, tension or activity. 2. equality of osmotic pressure between two elements of a solution or between two different solutions.

isotonic 1. of equal tension. 2. denoting a solution in which body cells can be bathed without net flow of water across the semipermeable cell membrane; also, denoting a solution having the same tonicity as another solution with which it is compared.

i. contraction muscle contraction without appreciable change in the force of contraction; the distance between the muscle's origin and insertion becomes lessened.

i. dehydration occurs when the fluid lost is isotonic with serum, as in sweating, simple enteritis, nephrosis. There are therefore no errors of electrolyte balance likely to result.

i. saline aee NORMAL saline.

isotope a chemical element having the same atomic number as another (i.e. the same number of nuclear protons), but having a different atomic mass (i.e. a different number of nuclear neutrons).

radioactive i. one having an unstable nucleus and which emits characteristic radiation during its decay to a stable form. See also RADIOISOTOPE.

stable i. one that does not transmute into another element with emission of corpuscular or electromagnetic radiations.

isotretinoin a synthetic form of retinoic acid (13-*cis*-retinoic acid), used in dermatology for the treatment of disorders of keratinization. It is a potent teratogen.

isotropic 1. having the same value of a property, such as refractive index, in all directions, as in a cubic crystal or a piece of glass. 2. being singly refractive.

Isotropis a genus of Australian legumes in the family Fabaceae. They may contain a heterocyclic nephrotoxin, iforrestine. Many cases are characterized by sudden death with no lesions. Include *I. atropurpurea* (poison sage), *I. cuneifolia* (lamb poison, granny bonnets), *I. drummondii* (lamb poison), *I. foliosa*, *I. forrestii*, *I. juncea*, *I. wheeleri*.

isotropy the quality or condition of being isotropic.

isotype the antigenic variability between related proteins, e.g. between immunoglobulin classes of a single species.

isotypical of the same kind.

isoxsuprine a beta-adrenergic receptor agonist; the hydrochloride is used as a uterine relaxant and as a vasodilator.

isozyme isoenzyme.

Israel turkey encephalomyelitis see Israeli turkey ENCEPHALOMYELITIS.

Israeli Friesian Israeli version of black and white Dutch Friesian dairy cattle.

issue a discharge of pus, blood, or other matter; a suppurating lesion emitting such a discharge.

IST infectious sinusitis of turkeys.

-ist suffix meaning one who specializes in.

isthmectomy excision of an isthmus, especially of the isthmus of the thyroid.

Isthmiophora a genus of intestinal flukes in the family Echinostomatidae.

I. melis found in the intestine of cat, fox and many other small wild mammals, including mink. It is nonpathogenic except in mink, in which it causes a severe hemorrhagic enteritis.

isthmoparalysis, isthmoplegia paralysis of the isthmus faucium.

isthmus a narrow connection between two larger bodies or parts.

aortic i. that part of the aorta between the origin of the brachiocephalic trunk, or the left subclavian artery, and that of the ductus arteriosus which is partly constricted in the fetus; it marks the partial separation of fetal blood flow derived from right and left ventricles, and is most conspicuous in the newborn calf.

i. of auditory tube the narrowest part of the pharyngotympanic tube at the junction of its bony and cartilaginous parts. Called also isthmus of pharyngotympanic tube.

i. of fauces, i. faucium the constricted aperture between the cavity of the mouth and the pharynx.

oviduct i. the short slightly narrower section of the oviduct of the bird between the magnum and the uterus, where the shell membranes are laid down.

pharyngeal i. the aperture between the dorsal and ventral parts of the pharynx and separated by the free edge of the soft palate and the palatopharyngeal arch.

i. of pharyngotympanic tube see isthmus of auditory tube (above).

i. of rhombencephalon the narrow segment of the fetal brain, forming the plane of separation between the rhombencephalon and cerebrum.

i. of thyroid the band of tissue joining the lobes of the thyroid. It is fibrous in sheep and horses and glandular in dogs and cattle.

i. of uterine tube the narrower, thicker-walled portion of the uterine tube closest to the uterus.

isthmus-catagen cyst see TRICHILEMMAL cyst.

isuria excretion of urine at a uniform rate.

IT information technology.

i.t. medical record abbreviation for intratracheal.

Italian arum ARUM *italicum*.

Italian brown cattle Italian version of Brown Swiss dairy cattle.

Italian cockle burr XANTHIUM *strumarium*.

Italian greyhound a small (6–10 lb), very slender, shorthaired dog with deep chest and thin waist that make it appear to be a miniature Greyhound. It has a characteristic high-stepping gait.

Italian pointer see SPINONI ITALIANI.

Italian red pied cattle red, spotted dual-purpose cattle from Italy, originated from Simmental.

Italian ryegrass LOLIUM *multiflorum*.

Italian spinone see SPINONI ITALIANI.

itch a skin disease attended with itching.

girth i. see GIRTH itch.

grain i. pruritic dermatitis due to a mite, *Pyemotes ventricosus*, which preys on certain insect larvae which live on straw, grain and other plants.

ground i. the pruritic eruption caused by the entrance into the skin of the hookworm larvae. See also BUNOSTOMIASIS, ANCYLOSTOMIASIS, UNCINARIASIS.

mad i. see AUJESZKY'S DISEASE.

i. mite see PSORERGATES *ovis*.

Queensland i. see equine ALLERGIC dermatitis.

sweet i. see equine ALLERGIC dermatitis.

itchiness pruritus.

itching pruritus; an unpleasant cutaneous sensation, provoking the desire to scratch or rub the skin.

itchy leg see CHORIOPTES.

item in statistical terms a single observation.

iterate in computer terminology a term meaning to repeat automatically, but under control of a program, a series of processing steps until a predefined criterion is reached.

iteration automatic repetition of one cycle.

-itis pl. *-itides;* word element. [Gr.] *inflammation.*

ito cell see LIPOCYTE.

ITP 1. idiopathic thrombocytopenic purpura. 2. immune-mediated thrombocytopenia. 3. inosine triphosphate.

itraconazole a triazole antifungal agent, used parenterally in the treatment of cryptococcosis in cats.

IU 1. immunizing unit. 2. International Unit.

IUCD INTRAUTERINE contraceptive device.

IUD INTRAUTERINE contraceptive device.

IUDZG International Union of Directors of Zoological Gardens.

IV, i.v. intravenous, intravenously.

Iva angustifolia North American member of the

plant family Asteraceae; contains an unidentified toxin; causes abortion in cattle. Called also narrow-leaved sumpweed.

-ive suffix meaning pertaining to.

ivermectin an avermectin with broad activity against many helminths and arthropods. A broad-spectrum anthelmintic, acaricide and insecticide, used orally, subcutaneously and as a pour-on.

ivory exceptionally hard dentine which forms the tusks of elephants, walruses, hippopotami and some other animals.

IVP intravenous pyelography. See PYELOGRAPHY.

IVT intravenous transfusion.

ivy *Hedera helix*; called also English ivy.

ivy loop technique a method of stabilizing fractures of the mandible or maxilla by wiring around two adjacent teeth.

ivybush KALMIA *latifolia*.

I.W.S. International Wool Secretariat.

Ixiolaena brevicompta Australian plant in the family Asteraceae; toxin is crepenynic acid; causes dystrophy of skeletal and heart muscle and death. Affected sheep may fall dead when made to run. Others have low exercise tolerance and cardiac irregularity. Called also button weed, plains plover-daisy, flat billy-buttons.

Ixodes a genus of hard-bodied ticks in the family Ixodidae. Some species are vectors of disease.

I. angustus a dog tick.

I. canisuga a dog tick found also on foxes and occasionally other species in Europe.

I. cookei found on most species.

I. cornuatus found on dogs and other species in Australia; may cause paralysis.

I. dammini a three-host tick, important transmitter of *Borrelia burgdorferi* in the USA.

I. hexagonus the hedgehog tick, found also on dogs and other species in Europe.

I. holocyclus a tick of bandicoots in Australia; found also on other species. Transmits *Coxiella burnetii* and causes tick paralysis by a toxin secreted by its salivary glands. It also produces a cardiovascular component which causes intense vasoconstriction, high blood pressure and death.

I. kingi the rotund tick of dogs.

I. loricatus a very rare infestation in New World primates.

I. muris the mouse tick, found on dogs.

I. ornithorhynchi the platypus tick.

I. pacificus the California black-legged tick, found on most species.

I. persulcatus transmits *Babesia* spp.

I. pilosus bush, sour-veld or russet tick found on most species. Does not cause paralysis.

I. ricinus the castor-bean tick, found on many species of mammals and birds in Europe. Transmits *Babesia divergens*, *B. bovis*, *Anaplasma*, tick pyemia, *Coxiella burnetii*, several human encephalitides and also causes paralysis.

I. rubicundus infests most species but not cat, horse or bird. Causes paralysis.

I. rugosus found on dogs.

I. scapularis shoulder or black-legged tick; found on most species. May transmit anaplasmosis and tularemia.

I. sculptus found on dogs.

I. texanus found on dogs.

ixodiasis any disease or lesion due to tick bites; infestation with ticks.

ixodic pertaining to, or caused by, ticks.

ixodid a tick of the family Ixodidae.

Ixodidae a family of ticks comprising the hard-bodied ticks.

J

J symbol for *joule*.

J antigen the basis of the J BLOOD GROUP system in cattle.

J chain a small polypeptide that links (joins) monomeric components of IgM and IgA molecules; responsible for maintaining the polymeric form.

J genes genes coding for the J chain of IgM and IgA molecules.

J receptor see JUXTACAPILLARY receptor.

jaagsiekte [Af.] 1. see ovine PULMONARY adenomatosis. 2. pyrrolizidine alkaloidosis of horses caused by *Crotalaria dura*, *C. globifera*, *C. juncea*. Term means 'panting sickness' with reference to prominent lung lesions.

jaagsiektebossie CROTALARIA *dura*, *C. globifera*.

jabot see FRILLED.

jack 1. male donkey; called a stallion in Great Britain. 2. see TRACK LEG.

j. colt male donkey less than 3 years of age.

mule j. one bred to mares for the production of mules.

jack bean see CANAVALIA ENSIFORMIS.

jack-in-the-pulpit see ARISAEMA.

jack oak QUERCUS *marilandica*.

jack rabbit the common American Hare. Called also *Lepus californicus*.

Jack Russell terrier a small, very active dog, usually with a docked tail, and with a white coat with brown, lemon or black patches. In many countries, it is not officially recognized as a distinct breed and there is considerable variation between the many types of dogs called Jack Russell and PARSON JACK RUSSELL TERRIER, particularly in body size, length of legs, and texture and length of coat. The 'breed' is affected by an inherited form of myasthenia gravis and a progressive ataxia.

jack sores see cutaneous HABRONEMIASIS.

jackal member of the family Canidae, standing midway between the fox and the wolf in size and habits. It is slender, long-legged with a pointed muzzle, has a disagreeable yapping voice, is nocturnal and hunts in packs. It is a predator and a scavenger. Includes *Canis aureus*, the oriental jackal, and *C. mesomelas*, the black-backed jackal.

Jackson Rees T-piece a modification of a T-piece anesthesia CIRCUIT in which the breathing bag is attached to the end of the expiratory limb.

Jackson technique a method of ligating a patent ductus arteriosus that eliminates dissection around the medial side of the ductus.

Jacksonian epilepsy a form of EPILEPSY marked by clonic movements that start in one muscle group and spread systematically to adjacent groups.

Jackson's chameleon *Chamaeleo jacksonii*.

jackstones see silica UROLITHS.

jacobine a pyrrolizidine alkaloid found in the weed *Senecio jacobea*.

Jacob's sheep an ornamental fourhorned British sheep, which originally served a dual purpose. Spotted dark brown on face.

Jacobson's organ vomeronasal organ.
Jaculus jaculus see JERBOA.
Jaeger keratome an ophthalmic surgical knife with an angled, triangular, sharp-pointed blade.
Jafarabadi an Indian buffalo breed, used for dairying; usually black, with large drooping horns.
Jaffe reaction a method of creatinine assay based on the orange-red color produced by creatinine reacting with alkaline picrate.
Jaffe's test the alkaline picrate method for creatinine analysis.
jaguar the leopard of the New World. A very large yellow cat with black spots, four or five spots being arranged around a central one in a rosette formation, a good swimmer and an avid predator, even a man-eater. Called also *Panthera onca.*
jaguarundi a small, 3 ft long, American wild cat, slender, otter-like, gray or red. Called also *Panthera jaguarundi.*
Jakta slaughter see SIKH SLAUGHTER.
jalap the dried root of *Exogonium purga.* A violent cathartic long since purged from the pages of pharmacology textbooks.
Jamaica black a breed of polled, black beef cattle bred in Jamaica from Aberdeen Angus and Zebu cattle.
Jamaica Brahman cattle bred up from Ongole, Hissar and Mysore zebus.
Jamaica Hope a dairy breed produced in Jamaica from Jersey and Zebu breeds.
Jamaica red a red beef breed produced in Jamaica from Zebu, Red Poll and Devon cattle.
James fibers conduction fibers that originate in the atrial internodal tracts and pass to the ventriculum but bypass the AV node. Called also James accessory conduction.
Jamestown Canyon virus serotype of California group of viruses capable of causing equine encephalitis in horses.
Jamestown weed, Jamestown lily DATURA *stramonium.*
Jamshidi biopsy needle a tubular needle with a cone-shaped tip with cutting edge used for obtaining a bone-marrow core.
janet a female mule.
janiceps a double monster with one head and two opposite faces.
Jansen retractor a handheld retractor used in abdominal surgery.
januariebos GNIDIA *polycephala.*
January disease version of East Coast Fever, occurring in Central Africa, caused by *Theileria parva bovis* transmitted by *Rhipicephalus appendiculatus.*
Japanese Akita see AKITA.
Japanese amberjack SERIOLA *quinqueradiata.*
Japanese B encephalitis virus a member of the family *Flaviviridae* and transmitted by mosquitoes from asymptomatic avian reservoir hosts. A major cause of morbidity in humans and domestic animal species, particularly pigs, in which it causes abortion. See also Japanese B ENCEPHALITIS.
Japanese black breed of cattle developed by crossing one of the indigenous breeds of Japanese cattle with European cattle. Black, horned (some polled), small, fine-boned; used principally for meat, some draft, occasionally milk. Similar breeds are Japanese brown, Japanese polled.
Japanese bobtail a breed of cats with a very short tail which has a pompon or fluffy appearance. The coat is medium-length and comes in many colors.
Japanese brown cattle light grown to red-brown beef cattle bred from local cattle and Simmental and Devon.
Japanese chin, Japanese spaniel a very small (4–7 lb), lively dog with a large, rounded head, very short muzzle, large eyes, and profuse, long silky coat in black and white or red and white.
Japanese eel ANGUILLA *japonica.*
Japanese encephalitis see Japanese B ENCEPHALITIS.
Japanese killifish see MEDEHAS.
Japanese millet ECHINOCHLOA *utilis.*
Japanese pieris PIERIS *japonicum.*
Japanese poll cattle polled black meat cattle formed by crossing native cattle with Angus.
Japanese river fever see SCRUB typhus.
Japanese scallop see PECTEN YESSOENSIS.
Japanese Shiba inu a small, spitz-type dog with small eyes, erect ears and a dense, straight coat.
Japanese spaniel see JAPANESE CHIN.
Japanese spitz a small (13 lb), lively dog with a pointed muzzle, triangular-shaped, erect ears and a pure white coat, particularly thick on the neck, shoulders and tail.
Japanese yew TAXUS *cuspitata.*
jasmine CESTRUM *diurnum.*
Jatropha a genus of the plant family Euphorbiaceae; some plants contain unidentified purgatives and cause diarrhea. Includes *J. curcas* (physic or purging nut), *J. gossypifolia* (bellyache bush), *J. stimulosa* (spurge nettle); others cause cyanide poisoning, e.g. *J. multifida* (umbrella tree, coral bush).
jaundice yellowness of skin, sclerae, mucous membranes, and excretions due to hyperbilirubinemia and deposition of BILE pigments. Called also icterus. It is usually first noticeable in the sclera.

The pigment causing jaundice is called BILIRUBIN. It is derived from hemoglobin that is released when erythrocytes are hemolyzed and therefore is constantly being formed and introduced into the blood as worn-out or defective erythrocytes are destroyed by the body. Normally the liver cells absorb the bilirubin and secrete it along with other bile constituents. If the liver is diseased, or if the flow of bile is obstructed, or if destruction of erythrocytes is excessive, the bilirubin accumulates in the blood and eventually will produce jaundice. Determination of the level of bilirubin in the blood is of value in detecting elevated bilirubin levels at the earliest stages before jaundice appears, when liver disease or hemolytic anemia is suspected.

acholuric j. jaundice without bilirubinemia, associated with elevated unconjugated bilirubin that is not excreted by the kidney.
cholestatic j. that resulting from abnormality of bile flow in the liver.
hematogenous j. hemolytic jaundice.
hemolytic j. jaundice associated with HEMOLYTIC anemia in which most of the bilirubin is unconjugated. Called also retention jaundice, prehepatic jaundice.
hepatocellular j. jaundice caused by injury to or disease of the liver cells.
j. index see ICTERIC index.
nonhemolytic j. that due to an abnormality in bilirubin metabolism.
obstructive j. that due to blockage of the flow of bile, resulting in conjugated hyperbilirubinemia. Called also regurgitation jaundice.
physiological j. mild icterus neonatorum during the first few days after birth.
regurgitation j. obstructive jaundice (above).

toxic j. see hepatocellular jaundice (above).
Java barb see PUNTIUS JAVANICUS.
Java bean PHASEOLUS *lunatus*.
Javanese a breed of cat similar to the Siamese, except with a long fur lying close to the body, and a wider variety of colored points. The tail is long and thin with hair that spreads out like a plume.
jaw either of the two opposing bony structures (maxilla and mandible) of the mouth of vertebrates; they bear the teeth and are used for seizing prey, for biting, or for masticating food.
j. bone the mandible or maxilla, especially the mandible.
j. champing involuntary, rapid, repetitive clenching of the teeth; accompanied by frothing of saliva; frequently accompanies clonic convulsions.
j. chattering involuntary, rapid clicking together of the teeth without salivation and usually accompanied by generalized shivering; in animals, may be a sign of painful teeth.
dropped j. see MANDIBULAR neurapraxia.
j. locking a dislocation of the jaw, usually following wide opening, in which the mouth cannot be closed. See also TEMPOROMANDIBULAR dysplasia.
j. malapposition see MALOCCLUSION.
overshot j. see BRACHYGNATHIA.
pig j. see BRACHYGNATHIA.
j. retractor a dental gag used to keep the jaws of an animal as open as possible.
rubber j. see renal secondary HYPERPARATHYROIDISM.
undershot j. see UNDERSHOT.
jay see CORVUS.
jejunectomy excision of the jejunum.
jejunitis inflammation of the jejunum.
jejunocecostomy anastomosis of the jejunum to the cecum.
jejunocolostomy anastomosis of the jejunum to the colon.
jejunoileal pertaining to the jejunum and ileum; connecting the proximal jejunum with the distal ileum.
jejunoileitis inflammation of the jejunum and ileum.
jejunoileostomy surgical creation of an anastomosis between the proximal jejunum and the terminal ileum; anastomosis of the jejunum to the ileum.
jejunoileum the jejunum and the ileum considered as a single organ.
jejunojejunostomy surgical anastomosis between two portions of the jejunum.
jejunorrhaphy operative repair of the jejunum.
jejunostomy surgical creation of a permanent opening between the jejunum and the surface of the abdominal wall.
j. tube a surgically positioned tube in the jejunum, protruding through the skin; it is used for enteral feeding when it is necessary to bypass the upper gastrointestinal tract.
jejunotomy incision of the jejunum.
jejunum that part of the small intestine extending from the duodenum to the ileum.
jelly a soft, coherent, resilient substance; generally, a colloidal semisolid mass.
cardiac j. a gelatinous substance present between the endothelium and myocardium of the embryonic heart that transforms into the connective tissue of the endocardium.
Wharton's j. the soft, jelly-like intracellular substance of the umbilical cord.
jellyfish members of the class of aquatic animals the Scyphozoa, the true jellyfishes, in the phylum Cnidaria. All possess cnidia or stings and are capable of causing stings to animals.
Jembrana disease a highly fatal, infectious, generalized disease of cattle characterized by diarrhea, hemorrhages, rarely erosions in the mucosae, anemia and lymphadenopathy, and a high fever. The cause is probably an Ehrlichia carried by the tick *Boophilus microplus*. See also RINDERPEST.
Jemtinki sumichrasti see CACOMISTLE.
jennerian relating to Edward Jenner, who developed vaccination in England in 1796.
Jenner's horsepox see HORSEPOX.
jennet jenny.
jenny female donkey, called also jennet; called a mare in Great Britain.
j. filly one less than 3 years of age.
jequirity bean see ABRUS *precatorius*.
jerboa small, long-tailed rodent with long hindlimbs adapted to jumping. There are many species, including the Egyptian jerboa, *Jaculus jaculus*.
jerk a sudden reflex or involuntary movement.
ankle j. see GASTROCNEMIUS REFLEX.
biceps j. called also elbow jerk; see BICEPS reflex.
elbow j. see biceps jerk (above).
j. nystagmus see vestibular NYSTAGMUS.
patellar j. see PATELLAR reflex.
tendon j. see tendon REFLEX.
jerked beef see BILTONG. Called also jerky.
jerky see BILTONG.
Jersey a breed of fawn, mulberry or gray, dairy cattle often with black pigmentation of the skin.
Jersian a crossbreed produced by a Jersey bull on a Friesian cow. Called also F–J hybrid.
Jerusalem cherry SOLANUM *pseudocapsicum*.
Jerusalem thorn see PARKINSONIA ACULEATA.
jervine a poisonous substance contained in the root of VERATRUM *album*.
jessamine CESTRUM *diurnum*.
jesse, jess a leather strap placed around each shank of a hawk used for hunting, for the attachment of a leash.
jet lesion localized areas of subendocardial fibrosis, usually in the atria, thought to be due to abnormal jets of blood caused by valvular lesions.
jetting application of insecticide to sheep by use of a high-pressure spraying machine. The jets at the head of the handheld appliance are combed through the wool so that the jetted fluid penetrates to the skin. See also DIP, DIPPING.
jeukbol URGINEA *altissima*.
Jewish slaughter an abbatoir technique of killing in which the animal must be conscious; in some countries it is required to use a rotating casting pen to restrain the animals. The throat and its vessels must be severed with one thrust of a very sharp knife whose length is about twice as long as the width of the neck. Only cattle, calves, sheep, goats, deer, and poultry are allowed to be killed for Jewish consumption. Called also shechita.
jibbing a vice in which the horse refuses to move forwards and may run backwards when in harness. Called also balking.
jigger see TUNGA penetrans. Called also chigoe or jigger flea.
j. flea see TUNGA penetrans.
jill a female ferret.
jill flerted see RECTOVAGINAL fistula.
jimmies fits of trembling and convulsions suffered by sheep, cattle and goats which have eaten jimmy ferns, CHEILANTHES *sinnata*.
jimmy fern CHEILANTHES *sinnata*.
jimmy weed HAPLOPAPPUS *heterophyllus*.
Jimson weed DATURA *stramonium*.

jird *Meriones unguiculatus*; see Mongolian GERBIL.
jirvine one of the toxic alkaloids in the weeds of *Veratrum* spp.
Job's tears see COIX LACHRYMA-JOBI.
jockey itch see RINGWORM.
Joest bodies, Joest–Degen bodies intranuclear bodies, sometimes intracytoplasmic, found in neurons in the brains of animals with Borna disease.
johanneskruid HYPERICUM *aethiopicum*.
Johne's disease a specific, infectious disease of cattle, sheep and goats caused by *Mycobacterium paratuberculosis*. In cattle it is characterized by chronic diarrhea and thickening and corrugation of the intestinal wall. In all species there is progressive wasting.
johnin an extract of the culture of *Mycobacterium paratuberculosis* used in a cutaneous delayed hypersensitivity test for Johne's disease. A positive test is a thickening and edema at the site of injection 48 hours later.
johnny hairy-legs the house centipede (*Scutigera* spp.), which can inflict a painful bite. It is light brown, 2 inches long with 15 pairs of legs and runs like a spider with the body off the ground.
Johnson grass SORGHUM *halepense*.
joining mating, usually one male with a group of females.
j. (J) gene segment a variable coding sequence that codes for amino acids that link the variable and constant regions of immunoglobulins.
j. programs include special arrangements for the percentage of males used, periods males left in, a succession of males, use of teasers beforehand.
joint the site of the junction or union of two or more bones of the body. See also ARTHRITIS. The primary functions of joints are to provide motion and flexibility to the skeletal frame, or to allow growth.

Some joints are immovable, such as certain fixed joints where segments of bone are fused together in the skull. Other joints, such as those between the vertebrae, have extremely limited motion. However, most joints allow considerable motion.

Many joints have a complex internal structure. They are composed not merely of ends of bones but also of ligaments, which are tough whitish fibers binding the bones together; cartilage, which is connective tissue, covering and cushioning the bone ends; the articular capsule, a fibrous tissue that encloses the ends of the bones; and the synovial membrane, which lines the capsule and secretes a lubricating fluid (synovia).

Joints are classified by variations in structure that make different kinds of movement possible. The movable joints are usually subdivided into hinge, pivot, gliding, ball-and-socket, condyloid and saddle joints.

For a complete named list of joints in the body see Table 11.

arthrodial j. gliding joint.
ball-and-socket j. a synovial joint in which the rounded or spheroidal surface of one bone ('ball') moves within a cup-shaped depression ('socket') on another bone, allowing greater freedom of movement than any other type of joint. Called also spheroidal joint.
biaxial j. permits movement around two axes.
cartilaginous j. one in which the bones are united by cartilage, providing either slight flexible movement or allowing growth; it includes symphyses and synchondroses.
condyloid j. one in which an ovoid head of one bone moves in an elliptical cavity of another, permitting all movements except axial rotation. Called also condylar joint.
congenital j. disease see ARTICULAR rigidity, JOINT hypermobility, ARTHROGRYPOSIS, CONTRACTURE.
j. contracture see CONTRACTURE.
degenerative j. disease a disease of the joints of all species and all ages but reaching a particularly high prevalence in pen-fed young bulls in which it is characterized by the sudden onset of lameness in a hindlimb, with pain and crepitus in the hip joint and rapid wasting of the muscles of the croup and thigh. There is a family predisposition to this degenerative arthropathy; it is exacerbated by a diet high in phosphorus and low in calcium and dense in energy so that the bull has a high body weight and is growing fast. The onset is acute and often precipitated by fighting or mating. The disease may not develop until 3 or 4 years of age in bulls that are reared at pasture. Called also coxofemoral arthropathy. See also HIP dysplasia.
diarthrodial j. synovial joint.
j. disease see ARTHRITIS, ARTHROPATHY, JOINT-ILL, ANKYLOSIS, ARTICULAR rigidity.
ellipsoid j. circumference of the joint is an ellipse with the articular surfaces longer in one direction than the other.
j. enlargement includes arthritis, arthropathy, rickets.
facet j's the synovial joints of the vertebral column between the neural arches.
fibrocartilaginous j. a combination of fibrous and cartilaginous joints. Called also amphiarthrosis. Movement limited and variable.
fibrous j. one in which the bones are connected by fibrous tissue; it includes suture, syndesmosis and gomphosis.
j. fixation includes ankylosis, tendon contracture, arthrogryposis.
fixed j. see SYNARTHROSIS.
flail j. an unusually mobile joint.
fleshy j. see SARCOARTHROSIS.
j. fusion arthrodesis.
ginglymus j. see hinge joint (below).
gliding j. a synovial joint in which the opposed surfaces are flat or only slightly curved, so that the bones slide against each other in a simple and limited way. The synovial intervertebral joints are gliding joints, and many of the small bones of the carpus and tarsus meet in gliding joints. Called also arthrodial joint and plane joint.
hinge j. a synovial joint that allows movement in only one plane, through the presence of a pair of collateral ligaments that run on either side of the joint. Examples are the elbow and the interphalangeal joints of the digits. The jaw is primarily a hinge joint, but it can also move somewhat from side to side. The carpal and tarsal joints are hinge joints that also allow some rotary movement. Called also ginglymus.
hip j. the joint between the head of the femur and the acetabulum of the hip bone; loosely called hip.
hyaline cartilage j. see cartilaginous joint (above).
j. hyperextension joint can be extended beyond the normal position.
j. hypermobility usually a congenital defect with all joints affected. Degree varies from extreme, in which limbs can be tied in knots and animal unable to stand, to mild, in which the patient is able to walk but the gait is abnormal. There may be additional defects such as pink teeth lacking enamel and dermatosparaxis (hyperelastosis cutis). See also HEREDITARY collagen dysplasia.

knee j. 1. the joint between the femur and tibia, fibula and patella. 2. in large ungulates the compound joint between the radius, ulna, carpus and metacarpus.

j. mouse fragments of cartilage or bone that lie free in the joint space. See also joint MOUSE.

osseous j. inflexible joint composed of bone; called also synostosis.

pivot j. a joint in which one bone pivots within a bony or an osseoligamentous ring, allowing only rotary movement; an example is the joint between the first and second cervical vertebrae (the atlas and axis).

plane j. see gliding joint (above).

j. receptors sensory nerve endings capable of detecting the position or angle of the joint.

saddle j. the articulating surfaces are reciprocally saddle-shaped and permit movement of all kinds, though not rotation, e.g. interphalangeal joints in the dog.

spheroidal j. see ball-and-socket joint (above).

synarthrodial j. a fixed joint.

synovial j. a specialized form of articulation permitting more or less free movement, the union of the bony elements being surrounded by an articular capsule enclosing a cavity lined by synovial membrane. Called also diarthrosis and diarthrodial joint.

trochoid j. see pivot joint (above).

uniaxial j. permits movement in one direction only.

joint-ill a nonspecific, usually purulent and bacterial, arthritis of the newborn resulting from an omphalitis which is usually still in evidence. There is fever, toxemia and severe lameness. In many cases there are other, similar lesions in other organs.

joint-leaf rush JUNCUS *holoschoenus*.

jointed charlock see RAPHANUS RAPHANISTRUM.

JOINTEX Joint Exercise in Animal Health and Productivity; a 3-year survey of the effects of combined management and health advice to dairy farmers conducted in the UK in the late seventies.

Jonas splint a popular intramedullary fracture maintenance splint for dogs and cats which was excellent in principle but caused too many cases of latent osteomyelitis and is no longer in use.

Jones clamp a towel clamp with a crossover action, thumb operated and with sharp single teeth at the end of narrow blades.

Jones terrier an early name for the Norwich terrier.

jonquil see NARCISSUS.

josamycin a macrolide antibiotic similar in effect to erythromycin.

joule the SI unit of energy, being the work done by a force of 1 newton acting over a distance of 1 meter. Symbol J.

Joule–Thomson effect the principle of rapid gas expansion to achieve ultracold in cryoprobes used in cryosurgery.

jowl external throat or upper neck, especially if fat or loose skin is present. Anterior to the DEWLAP.

j. abscess see CERVICAL ABSCESS OF PIGS.

Joyeuxiella a genus of tapeworms of dogs and cats of the family Dipylidiidae.

juba mane, e.g. of the horse.

jugal, jugale pertaining to the cheek or zygomatic (cheek) bone.

j. arch avian homolog of the mammalian zygomatic arch.

j. point the point at the angle formed by the masseteric and maxillary edges of the zygomatic bone.

jugale JUGAL point.

Juglans nigra shavings of the wood of this North American tree in the family Juglandaceae contain a toxin juglone; used as bedding, have caused edema of the lower limbs and laminitis in horses. Called also black walnut.

juglone naphthoquinone resinoid from *Juglans nigra*.

jugular 1. pertaining to the neck. 2. one of the jugular veins.

j. furrow the groove on each side of the neck in which the jugular vein can be located. Lies dorsal to the trachea.

j. inlet the depression at the base of the neck where the jugular vein passes medial to the first rib. Examination of the inlet is valuable because it is possible to determine the activity and efficiency of the right atrium and the patency of the jugular vein by observing the movements of the vein's wall.

j. vein distension see jugular vein engorgement (below).

j. vein engorgement is a clinical indicator of obstruction to the return of blood to the right atrium, e.g. because of congestive heart failure or space-occupying lesion in the anterior thorax.

j. veins two pairs of large veins, internal and external, that return blood to the heart from the head and neck.

jugum pl. *juga* [L.] a depression or ridge connecting two structures.

j. alveolaris a ridge in the jawbone over the site of impending eruption of a tooth.

juice any fluid from animal or plant tissue.

gastric j. the liquid secretion of the gastric glands. See also GASTRIC juice.

intestinal j. the liquid secretion of glands in the intestinal lining.

pancreatic j. the enzyme-containing secretion of the pancreas, conducted through its ducts to the duodenum.

prostatic j. the liquid secretion of the prostate, which contributes to semen formation.

jumbey the name given in the West Indies to the disease caused in animals by the ingestion of LEUCAENA LEUCOCEPHALA.

Junco hyemalis slate-colored junco; sparrow-shaped bird inhabiting west coast of North America.

Junco pox a disease of *Junco hyemalis* (slate-colored junco of the west coast of USA and Canada) caused by an avian poxvirus similar to fowlpox virus.

junction the place of meeting or coming together.

cell j. specialized regions of the cell surface where adjacent eukaryotic cell membranes are joined. Functionally, there are three types: TIGHT JUNCTIONS (impermeable), GAP JUNCTIONS (communicating) and adhering junctions (DESMOSOMES).

corneoscleral j. see CORNEOSCLERAL junction.

costochondral j. the joint between the bony dorsal part of a rib and the ventral cartilaginous part.

ileocecocolic j. the T-junction between the ileum and the large intestine; in the cat the ileum and the colon merge end to end, the cecum enters from the side; in the horse the ileocecal and the cecocolic junctions are separated from each other.

mucocutaneous j. see MUCOCUTANEOUS margin.

neuromuscular j. see NEUROMUSCULAR junction.

sclerocorneal j. see CORNEOSCLERAL junction.

junctional pertaining to a junction or join.

j. complex an attachment point between epithelial cells composed of a number of complex structures, including DESMOSOMES and GAP JUNCTIONS.

j. diversity the diversity in the amino acid sequence of antibodies is, in part, due to the different amino acid sequences generated at the junctions of the variable and constant regions.

j. mechanobullous disease inherited defect of skin in Belgian foals, Angus and Simmental calves, Suffolk and South Dorset lambs. See EPIDERMOLYSIS bullosa.
junctional premature beats see PREMATURE heartbeats.
junctionopathy a disorder of the neuromuscular junction, e.g. botulism, tick paralysis, myasthenia gravis.
junctura pl. *juncturae* [L.] see JUNCTION, JOINT.
j. cranii articulations of the skull.
j. zygapophyseales synovial intervertebral joints.
Juncus a genus of plants in the rush family Juncaceae. Perennial herbaceous plants found in marshes, swamps and other poorly drained sites. Contain cyanogenetic glycosides and rarely cause poisoning. Includes *J. effusus*, *J. inflexus* (blue or hard rush), *J. glaucus* (*J. inflexus*), *J. holoschoenus*, *J. pauciflorus*, *J. prismatocarpus*.
juneberry see AMELANCHIER ALNIFOLIA.
junglefowl see GALLUS *gallus*.
juniper see JUNIPERUS.
juniperene an alkaloid found in *Juniperus* spp.
Juniperus a genus of coniferous trees in the plant family Cupressaceae; includes *J. communis*, *J. osteosperma*, *J. sabina*, *J. virginiana*; the leaves are reported to cause abortion in ewes.
jurisprudence the science of the law.
medical j. the science of the law as applied to the practice of medicine.
Jussiaea LUDWIGIA.
jute see CORCHORUS OLITORIUS.
juvenile 1. pertaining to young animals; young or immature. 2. a cell, tissue, disease or organism intermediate between the immature and mature forms.
j. aponeurotic fibroma see MULTILOBULAR chondroma and osteoma.
j. bovine leukosis see BOVINE viral leukosis.
j. cellulitis see juvenile PYODERMA.
j. osteoporosis see OSTEOGENESIS imperfecta.
j. pancreatic atrophy see PANCREATIC acinar atrophy.
j. sterile granulomatous dermatitis and lymphadenitis see juvenile PYODERMA.
juvenoids see INSECT growth regulators.
juxta- word element. [L.] *situated near, adjoining*.
juxta-articular near or in the region of a joint.
juxtacapillary close to a capillary.
j. receptor located in the lung, reportedly stimulated by lung congestion and edema. Called also J receptor.
juxtacortical next to the cortex of the bone. Called also parosteal.
j. osteosarcoma periosteal osteosarcoma.
juxtaglomerular near to or adjoining a glomerulus of the kidney.
j. apparatus, j. complex a group of structures adjoining a renal glomerulus and which includes afferent and efferent arterioles, macula densa, extraglomerula mesangium and the juxtaglomerular cells (modified afferent arteriolar smooth muscle cells).
juxtamedullary on the edge of or close to the renal medulla.
juxtaposition apposition; a placing side by side or close together; the condition of being side by side or close together.
juxtapyloric near the pylorus.
juxtaspinal near the vertebral column.
juxtavesical situated near or adjoining the urinary bladder.

K

K 1. chemical symbol, *potassium* (L. *kalium*); symbol for *kelvin*. 2. equilibrium constant. 3. 2^{10} or 1024—used to specify the size of a computer's memory (kilobytes), e.g. 128 K, and usually measured in increments of 8.
k symbol, *kilo-*.
K antigen see K ANTIGEN.
K cell killer cell.
K chain kappa chain.
K88 antigen a pilus antigen of *Escherichia coli*; provides adhesion of the bacteria to the epithelial lining of the intestine of piglets. Important in both neonatal and postweaning diarrhea. Called also F4.
K88 *Escherichia coli* scours the K88 antigen confers a potent pathogenicity on the serotypes of *E. coli* which carry it; the disease is an unusual form of neonatal scours in that some strains of *E. coli* lack the K88 antigen and that some families of pigs are not susceptible to the antigen.
K99 antigen pilus antigen of enterotoxigenic *Escherichia coli* of calves and piglets, responsible for adhesion of the bacterium to intestinal cells, which is essential for them to be pathogenic. Vaccines based on purified K99 antigen produced by recombinant DNA technology are used for the control of the disease. Called also F5.
kaalmelkbos EUPHORBIA *mauritanica*.
kaalsiekte [Af.] alopecia caused by *Chrysocoma tenuifolia* in lambs and kids; characterized by alopecia, pruritis, oculonasal discharge, alimentary tract obstruction by phytobezoar.
Kaeshi disease Ibaraki disease.
kaffir one of the types of grain SORGHUM.
kakiebos see TAGETES MINUTA.
kakosmia cacosmia.
kala-azar see LEISHMANIASIS.
Kalanchoe genus of African plants in family Crassulaceae. Classified as *Bryophyllum* spp. Includes *K. daigremontiana*, *K. integra*, *K. lanceolata*, *K. luerbitiana*, *K. paniculata*, *K. pentheri*, *K. pinnata*, *K. rotundifolia*, *K. K. spathulata*, *K. thyrsiflora*, *K. tubiflora*. Contain bufadienolide cardiac glycosides; may cause KRIMPSIEKTE.
kale see BRASSICA *oleracea*.
kalemia, kaliemia the presence of potassium in the blood. See also HYPERKALEMIA.
kaley pea see LATHYRUS *hirsutus*.
Kalicephalus a genus of hookworm of the family Diaphanocephalidae, found in snakes.
kaliopenia hypokalemia.
kalium [L.] *potassium* (symbol K).
kaliuresis excretion of potassium in the urine.
kaliuretic 1. pertaining to or promoting kaliuresis. 2. an agent that promotes kaliuresis.
kallidin kinin liberated by the action of kallikrein on a globulin of blood plasma. Kallidin I is the same as bradykinin; kallidin II is composed of bradykinin with a lysine added at the *N*-terminal.
kallikrein any of a group of proteolytic enzymes present in various glands, lymph, urine, blood plasma, etc., or produced directly from mast cells or basophils, or indirectly from activated platelets. The major action of kallikreins is the liberation of kinins from α-2-globulins (kininogens), and they hence have vasodilator and whealing actions.
k.–kinin system the enzyme system responsible for

capillary permeability and smooth muscle contraction.

kallikreinogen the inactive precursor of kallikrein which is normally present in blood.

Kallstroemia unidentified toxin in North American plants of this genus in the family Zygophyllaceae causes incoordination, weakness, convulsions. Includes *K. hirsutissima* (hairy caltrop), *K. parviflora* (warty caltrop).

Kalmia genus of North American trees in the family Ericaceae; contains the poisonous tetracyclic polyol, andromedotoxin; causes vomiting, incoordination, paralysis and hyperexcitability. Includes *K. angustifolia* (dwarf laurel), *K. latifolia* (mountain laurel), *K. polifolia* var. *microphylla* (hog laurel).

kamala an anticestodal agent derived from the plant *Mallotus philippinensis*; now replaced by better and safer compounds.

Kamer grip applied to the head of the foal or calf fetus for the purpose of rotating it. The palm is placed on the calf's forehead with the thumb and the little finger each in an eye socket. It is then possible to pull, repulse and rotate the head.

kanamycin an aminoglycoside antibiotic used as the sulfate; active against many gram-negative and acid-fast bacteria. Similar to amikacin.

kangaroo see MACROPUS.

k. apples SOLANUM *aviculare*, *S. laciniatum*, *S. simile*, *S. symonii*, *S. vescum*, *S. capsiciforme*.

k. posture see kangaroo POSTURE.

k. rat see kangaroo RAT.

kangaroo gait a syndrome observed in lactating sheep in New Zealand consisting of a polyneuropathy which selectively affects the radial nerves. It is manifested by an inability to advance the front feet in a coordinated way, resulting in a bounding gait similar to that of a kangaroo. Affected ewes recover at the end of lactation.

Kansas horse plague see equine viral ENCEPHALOMYELITIS.

Kansas thistle SOLANUM *rostratum*.

kao haole [Hawaiian] see LEUCAENA LEUCOCEPHALA.

kaolin native hydrated aluminum silicate; used externally as an adsorbent and protective and internally as a gastrointestinal adsorbent and demulcent in mild diarrhea. The basis of the antiphlogistine poultice. Called also China clay.

Kapp–Beck clamp a ratchet-handled, scissor-type forcep used as a coronary sinus clamp. Has delicate, curved, claw-like blades.

Kapp–Beck–Thomson clamp used as a bronchus clamp; ratchet-handled, scissor-type forceps with heavy blades, set at an angle to the handles and with grooved faces on the blades.

kappa the tenth letter of the Greek alphabet, Κ or κ.

k. (κ) chain one of the two light chains in IMMUNOGLOBULIN. The other is lambda (λ).

Karai virus a probable arbovirus isolated from Kenyan sheep which experience an unexplained mortality. Nearby *Rhipicephalus evertsi* ticks are suspected vectors.

karaka see CORYNOCARPUS LAEVIGATUS.

karakin toxic nitrocompound in *Corynocarpus laevigatus*.

Karakul an originally Russian breed of wool and milk sheep that produces the curly coated fleece so desired by hat and garment makers in Asia. There are many sub-breeds producing a variety of colored wools, varying from traditional black, through gray, brown, to rose, and occasionally spotted. The desirable wool is obtained only from the pelts of full-term, newborn lambs. Survival for a few days or prolongation of pregnancy seriously reduces the financial worth of the pelt. Called also caracul, Astrakhan.

karanja see PONGAMIA GLABRA.

karaya gum the dried gummy exudation from *Sterculia urens* or other species of *Sterculia*, which becomes gelatinous when moisture is added. It is available in rings that can be molded into any desired shape. Commonly used as an obstetrical lubricant. Called also sterculia gum.

Karelian bear dog see CARELIAN BEAR DOG.

karoo bietou *Dimorphotheca cuneata*. See also OSTEOSPERMUM.

Kartagener's syndrome a hereditary syndrome of humans consisting of dextrocardia, bronchiectasis and sinusitis. Cases of a similar disease are reported in dogs. The disease is primarily a defect in cilia motility. See also primary CILIARY dyskinesia.

Karwinskia humboldtiana North American plant in the family Rhamnaceae; contains an unidentified toxin; causes degeneration of skeletal muscles and axonal dystrophy in the cerebellum and spinal cord. The clinical picture includes hypersensitivity, tremor, ataxia, recumbency and absence of tendon reflexes. Called also coyotillo, buckthorn, tullidora.

karyo- word element. [Gr.] *nucleus*.

karyocyte a nucleated cell.

karyogenesis the formation of a cell nucleus.

karyogram a graphic representation of a KARYOTYPE.

karyokinesis division of the nucleus, usually an early stage in the process of cell division, or mitosis.

karyolymph the fluid portion of the nucleus of a cell, in which the other elements are dispersed.

karyolysis dissolution of the cell nucleus.

karyomorphism the shape of a cell nucleus.

karyon the nucleus of a cell.

karyophage a protozoon that phagocytizes the nucleus of the cell it infects.

karyoplasm nucleoplasm.

karyopyknosis shrinkage of a cell nucleus, with condensation of the chromatin.

karyorrhexis rupture of the cell nucleus in which the chromatin disintegrates into formless granules that are extruded from the cell.

karyosome any aggregation of chromatin within a cell.

karyotheca the nuclear membrane.

karyotype the chromosomal constitution of the cell nucleus; by extension, the photomicrograph of chromosomes arranged in numerical order.

karyotyping preparation of a KARYOTYPE.

Kasen disease see equine ALLERGIC dermatitis. Also sometimes attributed to *Onchocerca* spp. infestation.

Kashmiri a goat; see CENTRAL ASIATIC PASHMINA.

Kaswan technique a method or repair of third-eyelid prolapse. The third-eye lid is sutured to the rim of the orbit.

kat katal.

kata see PESTE DES PETITS RUMINANTS.

kat(a)- word element. [Gr.] *down, against*. See also words beginning *cat(a)-*.

katal the SI unit of measurement to express activities of all catalysts, including enzymes, being that amount of a catalyst that catalyzes a reaction rate of 1 mole of substrate per second. Symbol kat.

katathermometer a thermometer with a wet bulb and a dry bulb, for detecting cooling rates.

Katayama's disease schistosomiasis.

katipo see LATRODECTUS *mactans*.

kb kilobase; a thousand bases or nucleotides in a nucleic acid molecule. See also KBP.

kbp kilobase pair; for double-stranded nucleotides, a thousand nucleotide base pairs.
kcal kilocalorie.
KCS keratoconjunctivitis sicca.
44-kDa phosphoprotein see OSTEOPONTIN.
kebbing see ENZOOTIC ovine abortion.
ked see MELOPHAGUS *ovinus*.
keel 1. the ventrally directed large surface of the bird's sternum, the site of attachment of the major muscles of flight. Called also carina. 2. the prominent area over the sternum in Dachshunds.
keeled goosefoot see CHENOPODIUM *carinatum*.
keeling the marking of ewes by the ram when they are mated by the marking on the ewe of paint or chalk from the sternum of the ram.
keep 1. to feed, e.g. long-keep steer. 2. pasturage.
Keeshond a medium-sized, compact dog with very thick, medium length, ash gray haircoat that forms a characteristic ruff around the neck and is profuse on a tail that curls tightly over the back. The ears are small and erect and the face is fox-like. The breed is predisposed to atopy, epilepsy and heart defects.
keet a young guinea fowl.
Keith's bundle a bundle of fibers in the wall of the right atrium between the openings of the venae cavae; see also SINOATRIAL node. Called also sinoatrial bundle, Keith's node, Keith–Flack node.
Keith–Flack node see KEITH'S BUNDLE.
Keith's node see KEITH'S BUNDLE.
KELA test kinetics-based, enzyme-linked immunosorbent assay.
Keller spatula a 3 ft long obstetrical instrument used in the cow and mare to skin part of a fetus in utero prior to performing fetotomy. Has a long round handle and a grooved spatulate end which is used to perform blunt dissection of the skin, having first incised it with a palm knife. Pushing is generated outside the uterus by the operator who has one hand inside to direct the spatula.
Kellog's spurred lupin LUPINUS *caudatus*.
Kelly–Murphy forceps conventional small hemostats with ratcheted handles and straight or curved blades with fine grooves running crossways inside the tip.
kelp see SEAWEED.
kelsey milk vetch ASTRAGALUS *atropubescens*.
kemps coarse hair fibers, found in a wool fleece; a cause for severe downgrading of value. The fibers are hard, brittle, opaque and medullated. They are shed after a short growing period and lie loose in the wool fibers; they will not take dye and will not spin together.
Kennedy's syndrome ipsilateral optic nerve atrophy and contralateral papilledema, associated with pathology of the frontal lobe.
Kennel Club the principal body for maintaining stud books and registering purebred dogs in the Great Britain.
kennel cough a highly contagious, acute respiratory disease of dogs, commonly consisting of laryngitis, tracheitis and bronchitis. It may be caused by any one or a combination of several viruses, bacteria and mycoplasmas. Canine parainfluenza virus, canine adenoviruses types 1 and 2, canine herpesvirus and *Bordetella bronchiseptica* are the most common infectious agents. Affected dogs usually have a harsh, dry cough, and occasionally fever, serous nasal discharge and lymphadenopathy. Particularly in puppies, more severe illness sometimes occurs. Called also canine infectious tracheobronchitis, rhinotracheitis.
kennelitis social maladjustment toward humans, seen in young dogs raised in a kennel rather than with humans.
keno- word element. [Gr.] *empty*.
Kent accessory bundle, Kent's bundle the right- and left-sided myocardial conduction tissue bridge between the atria and the ventricles.
Kent Marsh see ROMNEY MARSH.
Kentucky coffee tree GYMNOCLADUS *dioica*.
Kenya Boran cattle an improved Kenyan version of Boran cattle.
Kenya SGPV Kenya sheep and goat poxvirus.
Kenya sheep/goat pox highly infectious disease of sheep and goats spread by contact; highly fatal in lambs; in adults a benign disease characterized by typical cutaneous pox lesions.
keraphyllocele keratoma.
kerasin a cerebroside from brain tissue, yielding galactose, sphingosine and lignoceric acid on hydrolysis.
keratalgia pain in the cornea.
keratan sulfate a glycosaminoglycan which exists as either of two sulfated mucopolysaccharides (I and II). Keratan sulfate is an important component of the proteoglycan of cartilage, and occurs in the cornea and the nucleus pulposus.
keratectasia protrusion of a thin, scarred cornea.
keratectomy excision of a portion of the cornea; kerectomy.
superficial k. involves removal of the corneal epithelium and anterior stroma, on either a specified portion the whole cornea.
keratic 1. pertaining to keratin. 2. pertaining to the cornea.
k. precipitates fibrous deposits on the posterior surface of the cornea, usually associated with uveitis. Called also KPs.
keratin a scleroprotein which is the principal constituent of epidermis, hair, nails, horny tissues, and the organic matrix of the enamel of the teeth. Its solution is sometimes used in coating pills when the latter are desired to pass through the stomach unchanged.
k. cyst see horn CYST.
k. pearl see HORN pearls.
k. tag see fibrovascular PAPILLOMA.
keratinase a proteolyic enzyme that hydrolyzes keratin.
keratinization the development of or conversion into keratin.
k. defects include hyperkeratosis, hypokeratosis, dyskeratosis. Diseases in which abnormal keratinization is an important feature include SEBORRHEA, VITAMIN A responsive dermatosis, nasodigital HYPERKERATOSIS, ACNE, PARAPSORIASIS.
keratinocyte the cell of the epidermis that synthesizes keratin, known in its successive stages in the various layers of the skin as basal cell, prickle cell and granular cell.
k. transit time the time required for a keratinocyte to move from its origin in the actively dividing cells of the stratum basale to the surface of the epidermis where it is shed. Called also epidermal renewal time. In the normal dog, this is approximately 22 days.
Keratinomyces see TRICHOPHYTON.
keratinosome small organelle in the intercellular space of the epidermis; it has a role in retaining water and in cell cohesion. Called also Odland's body; cementasome.
keratinous containing or of the nature of keratin.
keratitis inflammation of the cornea. Keratitis may be deep, when the infection causing it is carried in the blood or spreads to the cornea from other parts of the

eye, or superficial, caused by bacterial or viral infection, trauma, or by allergic reaction. The clinical signs include pain, blepharospasm, ocular discharge, and when chronic, pigmentation.

chronic superficial k. a progressive cellular infiltration with vascularization and eventually pigmentation of the cornea that usually commences at the temporal (lateral) quadrant and advances towards the center. The whole cornea may become involved. It occurs in dogs, particularly German shepherd dogs. The cause is unknown, but exposure to ultraviolet light may be a factor. Cellular infiltrates suggest immune mechanisms are involved in the pathogenesis. Called also CSK, degenerative pannus, Uberreiter's syndrome.

eosinophilic k. a superficial neovascularization and cellular infiltration of the cornea, beginning at the temporal limbus, in adult cats. Eosinophils and plasma cells are found in conjunctival or corneal scrapings and biopsies, and a peripheral eosinophilia is sometimes present. The cause is unknown, but it may be immune-mediated.

exposure k. keratitis resulting from ineffective or incomplete closure of the eyelids with drying of the corneal tear film. Occurs in paralysis of the eyelids, brachycephalic dogs with prominent globes, and cats during ketamine anesthesia. See also LAGOPHTHALMOS.

herpetic k. herpesvirus infections of the cornea occur in feline and bovine rhinotracheitis infections, and are suspected in dogs. In cats there may be ulcerative keratitis with dendritic ulcers; in cattle conjunctivitis is more common than keratitis.

infectious k. see THELAZIA, ONCHOCERCA, MORAXELLA *bovis*.

interstitial k. inflammation of the substantia propria, causing dense corneal clouding.

mycotic k. see KERATOMYCOSIS.

neurotrophic k., neuroparalytic k. a chronic keratopathy resulting from impairment of the sensory (trigeminal) innervation of the cornea.

k. nigrum see CORNEAL sequestrum.

k. sicca see KERATOCONJUNCTIVITIS sicca.

superficial diffuse k. see chronic superficial keratitis (above).

superficial pigmentary k. a pigmentation of epithelium and superficial stroma of the cornea, resulting from chronic keratitis from a variety of causes. Seen most commonly in brachycephalic dogs in which the contributing factors are exposure keratitis, distichiasis, irritation from the nasal folds and sometimes keratoconjunctivitis sicca.

superficial punctate k. a keratopathy with discrete opacities of the cornea, without ulceration. Can be caused by irritation.

ulcerative k. see CORNEAL ulcer.

kerat(o)- word element. [Gr.] *horny tissue, cornea.*

keratoacanthoma see intracutaneous cornifying EPITHELIOMA.

keratoblast flattened fibroblast contained in interfibrillar space in the cornea.

keratocele hernial protrusion of Descemet's membrane.

keratocentesis puncture of the cornea, keratonyxis.

keratoconjunctivitis inflammation of the cornea and conjunctiva.

chronic immune-mediated k. syndrome see chronic superficial KERATITIS.

infectious k. see also INFECTIOUS bovine keratoconjunctivitis. Caused by *Moraxella bovis*, *Histoplasma capsulatum*, *Chlamydia* spp., *Mycoplasma* spp.

proliferative k. see NODULAR fasciitis.

k. sicca a condition marked by hyperemia of the conjunctiva, thickening and drying of the corneal epithelium, secondary to quantitative and qualitative deficiencies in the tear film. Deep keratitis and corneal ulceration may occur. Often a tenacious, stringy mucoid discharge accumulates in the conjunctival sac. Called also dry eye.

keratoconus conical protrusion of the central part of the cornea.

keratocyte 1. a flattened connective tissue cell lying between the fibrous tissue lamellae which constitute the cornea. The keratocyte has branching processes that communicate with those of other keratocytes. 2. a red blood cell with notches that results in projections that look like horns. Keratocytes occur when fibrin is being deposited within blood vessels as in disseminated intravascular coagulation.

keratoderma hypertrophy of the horny layer of the skin.

keratodermia keratoderma.

keratogenesis the production of keratin; a function of keratinocytes in the epidermis.

keratogenous giving rise to a growth of horny material.

keratoglobus an anomaly in which the cornea is enlarged and globular in shape.

keratohelcosis ulceration of the cornea.

keratohemia deposition of blood in the cornea.

keratohyalin the substance in the granules in the stratum granulosum of the epidermis.

keratoid resembling horn or corneal tissue.

keratoiridoscope a compound microscope for examining the eye.

keratoiritis inflammation of the cornea and iris, corneoiritis.

keratoleptynsis removal of the anterior portion of the cornea and replacement with bulbar conjunctiva.

keratoleukoma a white opacity of the cornea.

keratolysis loosening or separation of the horny layer of the epidermis.

keratolytic 1. pertaining to or promoting keratolysis. 2. an agent that promotes keratolysis.

keratoma keratosis.

keratomalacia softening and necrosis of the cornea associated with vitamin A deficiency.

keratome a knife for incising the cornea.

keratometer an instrument for measuring the curves of the cornea.

keratometry measurement of corneal curves.

keratomycosis fungal disease of the cornea and usually conjunctiva. Occurs mainly in horses; introduced by foreign bodies.

keratonyxis puncture of the cornea; keratocentesis.

keratopathy noninflammatory disease of the cornea. See also CORNEAL.

acid-fast k. corneal opacities seen in dogs in tropical and subtropical areas of the United States; attributed to an unidentified mycotic or mycobacterial infection. Called also Florida spots, Florida fungus.

band k. subcorneal calcification associated with local ocular disease or systemic abnormalities of calcium or phosphorus metabolism.

bullous k. a nonspecific response of the cornea to inflammation in which vesicles and bullae occur.

lipid k. deposition of lipid in the stroma of the cornea. In the primary disease, there is no association with abnormalities of lipid metabolism or elevated blood lipid levels. In secondary disease, lipids are deposited in scars and previous corneal lesions, or in association with abnormalities of systemic lipid metabolism.

keratoplastic 1. pertaining to plastic surgery of the cornea. 2. promoting the production of keratin.

keratoplasty plastic surgery of the cornea; corneal grafting.

lamellar k. a partial thickness graft of the cornea; only epithelium and superficial stroma is removed and replaced by donor tissue as distinct from penetrating or full-thickness grafting.

optic k. transplantation of corneal material to replace scar tissue that interferes with vision.

penetrating k. a full thickness of the cornea is removed and replaced with donor tissue.

tectonic k. transplantation of corneal material to replace tissue that has been lost.

keratoprosthesis replacement of part of the cornea with a prosthesis; not commonly performed in animals.

keratorhexis, keratorrhexis rupture of the cornea.

keratoscleritis inflammation of cornea and sclera.

keratoscope an instrument for examining the cornea.

keratoscopy inspection of the cornea.

keratosis any horny growth on the skin, such as a wart or callosity; a firm, elevated, circumscribed area of excessive keratin production. Common in humans but uncommon in animals.

actinic k. varies from a sharply outlined verrucous or keratotic growth to poorly defined areas of erythema, which are premalignant lesions. Due to excessive exposure to the sun. Called also solar keratosis.

equine cannon k. see CANNON KERATOSIS.

linear k. see EQUINE linear keratosis.

k. pilaris hyperkeratosis limited to the hair follicles.

seborrheic k., k. seborrheica single or multiple elevated plaques and nodules often hyperpigmented with a hyperkeratotic greasy surface. They are benign, of unknown etiology, but have no connection with seborrhea. Occur in dogs and humans.

solar k. see actinic keratosis (above).

keratotomy incision of the cornea.

multiple punctate k. multiple, non-penetrating punctures of the corneal stroma to stimulate healing of refractory or recurrent corneal erosions.

Kerckring folds mucosal folds in the human small intestine which greatly increase the absorptive surface area of the organ.

kerectasia loss of substance and scarring of the cornea resulting in a thin layer of tissue that bulges from the surface.

kerectomy keratectomy.

kerion a boggy, exudative tumefaction covered with pustules, as may occur in dermatophyte infections.

Kern forceps heavyweight forceps with bowed jaws to encircle a bone and a crutch on the end of one of the handles to enable traction to be employed with the forceps.

kernel whole grains and the meats of nuts and stone fruit pips or pits.

kernicterus bilirubin toxicity; may occur with severe hyperbilirubinemia. Rarely observed in dogs and cats.

kerosene, kerosine see PARAFFIN (2).

kerosene grass ARISTIDA *contorta*.

Kerry blue terrier a medium-sized (33–40 lb) dog with a wavy haircoat that is black at birth but 'clears' to a gray blue by 18 months of age. The head is narrow and long, the ears erect and folded forward, and the docked tail is carried upright. Called also Irish blue terrier. The breed is predisposed to a cerebellar neuronal abiotrophy.

Kerry cattle see DEXTER.

kersey coarse, narrow cloth used for leg bandages in horses.

kestrel a falcon (*Falco tinnunculus*) with a special hovering flight and a high-pitched call. Reddish-brown with dark spots on the dorsal parts.

ketamine hydrochloride a nonbarbiturate anesthetic related to phencyclidine (PCP), which is administered intravenously or intramuscularly to produce dissociative anesthesia. It has serious limitations in usefulness in animals. It is used routinely in cats and nonhuman primates, in combination with other agents and for short-term procedures.

keto- word element, *ketone group*.

keto acids compounds containing both of the groups CO (carbonyl) and COOH (carboxyl).

ketoacidosis the accumulation of ketone bodies in the blood which results in metabolic acidosis. See also KETOSIS.

diabetic k. an overproduction and underutilization of ketone bodies in the diabetic results in ketosis. Ketonemia and ketonuria with accompanying loss of $Na+$ and $K+$, leads to a base deficit and acidosis.

ketoaciduria the presence of keto acids in the urine.

ketoconazole an imidazole antifungal agent, used orally and topically as the nitrate in the treatment of cutaneous and systemic fungal infections. It also inhibits steroidogenesis and has been used in the treatment of canine hyperadrenocorticism; infertility and teratogenicity may occur.

ketogenesis the production of ketone bodies.

ketogenic forming or capable of being converted into ketone bodies.

k. diet one containing large amounts of fat, with minimal amounts of protein and carbohydrate. The object of such a diet is to produce KETOSIS.

17-ketogenic steroid a marker used in the measurement of androgen excretion in the urine.

α-ketoglutarate a salt or anion of α-ketoglutaric acid.

α-k. dehydrogenase multienzyme complex catalyzing the oxidative decarboxylation of α-ketoglutarate to succinyl CoA in the TCA cycle.

α-ketoglutaric acid 2-oxoglutaric acid; intermediate of TCA cycle.

ketolysis the splitting up of ketone bodies.

ketone any compound containing the carbonyl group, CO, and having hydrocarbon groups attached to the carbonyl carbon, i.e. the carbonyl group is within a chain of carbon atoms.

k. bodies the substances acetone, acetoacetic acid and β-hydroxybutyric acid; except for acetone (which may arise spontaneously from acetoacetic acid), they are normal metabolic products usually derived from excess acetyl CoA from fatty acids within the liver, and are oxidized by the extrahepatic tissues; excessive production leads to urinary excretion of these bodies, as in diabetes mellitus. Called also acetone bodies. See also KETOSIS, ACETONEMIA, PREGNANCY toxemia.

k. pulegone see PENNYROYAL OIL.

ketonemia an excess of ketone bodies in the blood.

ketonuria an excess of ketone bodies in the urine.

ketoprofen a propionic acid, nonsteroidal anti-inflammatory agent; used also as an analgesic and antipyretic.

ketose any sugar that contains a ketone group.

ketosis 1. accumulation in the blood and tissues of large quantities of the KETONE bodies: β-hydroxybutyric acid, acetoacetic acid and acetone. Because the first two are acids, this results in metabolic acidosis. Thus, the condition is often referred to as ketoacidosis. 2. in ruminants is used synonymously with ACETONEMIA, PREGNANCY toxemia. See also FAT COW syndrome.

secondary k. acetonemia secondary to another condition which reduces the cow's feed intake.

ketosteroid a steroid having ketone groups on functional carbon atoms.

17-k's steroids found in normal urine and in excess in certain tumors, which have a ketone group on the 17th carbon atom, and include certain androgenic and adrenocortical hormones.

Ketostix a commercially available product for rapid detection of ketones in urine, serum or plasma. It consists of a plastic strip with an impregnated paper tip which turns buff pink to purple in a positive reaction.

Kety curves a mathematical description of the uptake of anesthetic gas under certain conditions.

keV kilo (1000) electron volts (3.82×10^{-17} calorie, or 1.6×10^{-9} erg).

Kew gardens spotted fever see RICKETTSIALPOX.

Key–Gaskell syndrome see feline DYSAUTONOMIA.

key indicants the important clinical signs, epidemiological characteristics and sequence of events in the history that can form the basis for a diagnosis.

key signs the important signs on which a diagnosis can be based. Equivalent to key words in literature searches.

Keyes punch a skin biopsy instrument similar to and used like a cork borer by pushing down on the palm-held handle and rotating the instrument so that its sharp, circular cutting edge cuts through the skin.

keystroke one stroke of a key on a computer keyboard.

keyword the significant word or words in a piece of information; often used to accurately store information and by which it can be retrieved.

kg kilogram.

17-KGS 17-ketosteroids.

Khaki Campbell English egg-laying duck. Khaki in color, head and neck green in the drake, with a dark green bill and deep orange legs. Bred by mating Rouen and a white Indian Runner.

khaki weed see DITTRICHIA GRAVEOLENS.

Khalilia a genus of strongyles in the family Strongylidae.

K. buta, K. pileata, K. sameera found in the large intestine of elephants.

khat see CATHA EDULIS.

Khawia a genus of tapeworms in the family Caryophyllaeidae.

K. sinensis causes hemorrhagic enteritis in carp.

kHz kilohertz.

kiawe bean see PROSOPIS JULIFLORA.

kibble baked dough that is crushed or cracked. Prepared usually by extruding and then heating-drying the dough. Used as dry food for dogs and cats.

kicking lashing out behind with the hindfeet. 1. a normal defense reaction in horses and cattle that are unused to human attendants. 2. a vice in some cattle and horses. 3. part of the normal behavior of trained mules and to a lesser extent donkeys.

k. at belly part of the syndrome of acute abdominal pain in horses, and to a lesser extent in ruminants; usually accompanied by crouching and other signs; not to be confused with TREADING.

kid young goat or roe deer up to about 4 months of age.

kidney either of the two organs in the lumbar region that filter the blood, excreting the end-products of body metabolism in the form of urine, and regulating the concentrations of hydrogen, sodium, potassium, phosphate and other ions in the extracellular fluid. Bean-shaped in the dog, cat, sheep and laboratory animals, lobed in the ox and some fetal animals such as the horse; irregularly lobed in birds. See also RENAL.

artificial k. an extracorporeal device used as a substitute for nonfunctioning kidneys to remove endogenous metabolites from the blood, or as an emergency measure to remove exogenous poisons such as barbiturates. Called also hemodialyzer.

balloon k. meat hygiene term for cystic kidney.

basal lamina k. part of the filtration barrier of the kidney; is much thicker than most basal laminae.

cake k. a solid, irregularly lobed organ of bizarre shape, formed by fusion of the two renal anlagen. Called also lump kidney.

cicatricial k. a shriveled, irregular and scarred kidney due to suppurative pyelonephritis.

contracted k. an atrophic kidney that may be scarred and granular.

duplicate k. occurs in most species, without apparent increase in total renal mass.

enlarged k. may be due to polycystic kidney disease, hydronephrosis, pyelonephritis or congenital absence of one kidney resulting in hypertrophy of the other.

fatty k. one affected with fatty degeneration.

floating k. one that is freely movable, especially a human kidney (normally more firmly fixed than those in quadripeds); called also hypermobile kidney. See also NEPHROPTOSIS.

fused k. a single anomalous organ developed as a result of fusion of the renal anlagen.

giant k. worm DIOCTOPHYME *renale*.

Goldblatt k. one with obstruction of its blood flow, resulting in renal hypertension. Produced experimentally in dogs.

horseshoe k. an anomalous organ resulting from fusion of the corresponding poles of the renal anlagen.

hypermobile k. one that is freely movable; called also floating kidney. See also NEPHROPTOSIS.

lump k. cake kidney.

k. meridian points acupuncture points on the kidney meridian.

pelvic k. a kidney which has failed to ascend from its primordial site to the roof of the abdomen.

polycystic k. disease the most common congenital renal defect but most cases are sporadic and do not cause clinical illness because there is still sufficient renal mass to avoid uremia. In some cases the enlarged kidney is detected incidentally during a clinical examination. Rarely both kidneys are badly involved and the animal is dead at birth or dies soon afterwards. In some cases, there are signs of progressive renal failure, perhaps not until later in life. The defect is inherited in Persian cats, Cairn terriers and pigs. In Cairn terriers, cysts may also occur in the liver. See also feline PERIRENAL cysts.

pulpy k. disease see *Clostridium welchii* ENTEROTOXEMIA.

k. scan radioimaging of a kidney by the use of a rectilinear scanner after the intravenous administration of a radiopaque material.

k. stones see UROLITHIASIS.

supernumerary k. additional kidneys which develop as a consequence of two ureteric buds arising from one mesonephric duct so that two kidneys develop on the one side.

k. transplant commonly and successfully performed in experimental dogs. Increasingly used as a therapeutic procedure in clinical veterinary medicine for renal failure in cats and dogs.

turkey egg k. a speckled pattern caused by hemorrhagic glomeruli in diseases such as porcine erysipelas.

wandering k. floating or hypermobile kidney. See also NEPHROPTOSIS.
waxy k. amyloid kidney.
white-spotted k. focal nonsuppurative interstitial nephritis, seen most commonly in calves.

kidney bean PHASEOLUS *vulgaris.*

Kienböck's unit a unit of x-ray exposure equal to 0.1 erythema dose; symbol X.

Kikuth's disease see CANARYPOX.

kikuyu grass see PENNISETUM *clandestinum.*

kill term used to describe heavy mortalities in wild fish or fauna, especially those in the wild, or at extensive range, and usually where the deaths are unexpected and generally not easily explained.

killed vaccine see dead VACCINE.

killer cell see K CELLS.

killer whale see killer WHALE.

killing-out percentage see CARCASS yield.

kilo- word element. [Gr.] *one thousand;* used in naming units of measurement to designate an amount 10^3 times the size of the unit to which it is joined; abbreviated k.

kilobase a unit of size for nucleic acids, being 1000 nucleotide bases for single-stranded nucleic acids or 1000 nucleotide base pairs in the case of double-stranded nucleic acids. Abbreviated kb or kbp.

kilobyte, k 1024 bytes of information or storage space.

kilocalorie a unit of heat equal to 1000 calories; symbol kcal or Cal.

kilogram a unit of mass (weight) of the metric system, 1000 grams; equivalent to 15,432 grains, or 2.205 pounds (avoirdupois) or 2.679 pounds (apothecaries' weight); abbreviated kg. See Table 4.1.
k. calorie large calorie. See also KILOCALORIE.

kilohertz one thousand (10^3) hertz; abbreviated kHz.

kilojoule 1000 joules.

kilometer one thousand (10^3) meters; 3280.83 feet; five-eighths of a mile; abbreviated km.

kilopascal one thousand (10^3) pascals; the metric unit of pressure; equal to 7 pounds per square inch; abbreviated kPa.

kilotex, ktex unit of measurement expressing thickness, e.g. of a staple of wool expressed as grams per meter; used an indication of the strength of the staple.

kilovolt one thousand (10^3) volts; abbreviated kV.
k. peak the maximal amount of voltage that an x-ray machine is using; abbreviated kVp.

kilovoltage in radiography, the x-ray tube peak voltage during an exposure, measured in kilovolts.

Kiluluma a genus of nematode parasite of the family Strongyldae, found in the intestine of rhinoceros.

Kimberley horse disease see WALKABOUT.
K. horse poison CROTALARIA *crispata.*

Kimberling–Rupp spaying device a guillotine-type device within a hollow tube for insertion into the abdominal cavity and trapping each ovary in turn. The cutting mechanism is operated from outside the abdomen.

kimberly couch grass BRACHYACHNE *convergens.*

Kimmelstiel–Wilson syndrome a degenerative complication of DIABETES MELLITUS in humans, with albuminuria, edema, hypertension, renal insufficiency and retinopathy. A small proportion of diabetic dogs have roughly similar lesions of diffuse or nodular hyaline deposits in glomeruli. The characteristic nodules are referred to as Kimmelstiel–Wilson nodules. Called also intercapillary glomerulosclerosis.

kinase 1. a subclass of the transferases, comprising the enzymes that catalyze the transfer of a high-energy group from a donor (usually ATP) to an acceptor, and named, according to the acceptor, as creatine kinase, fructokinase, etc. 2. an enzyme that activates a zymogen, and named, according to its source, as enterokinase, streptokinase, etc.
protein k's cellular enzymes which utilize ATP to phosphorylate proteins, usually at a selected OH group of serine, threonine or tyrosine residue in the protein, so as to increase or decrease the activity of the protein.
protein k. C membrane bound protein kinase designated C because it requires Ca^2+ and phosphatidyl serine for its activity. Activated by sn-1,2-diacylglycerol (DAG) produced from phosphatidyl inositol 4,5-bisphosphate. Phosphorylates target proteins such as the insulin receptor, β-adrenergic receptor, glucose transporter, HMG-CoA reductase, cytochrome P-450 and tyrosine hydroxylase.

kindle pregnancy in the rabbit, e.g. a doe in kindle.

kindling parturition in the doe rabbit.

kine- word element. [Gr.] *movement.* See also words beginning *cine-*.

kinematics that phase of mechanics which deals with the possible motions of a material body.

kinesalgia pain on muscular exertion.

kinesia motion sickness.

kinesialgia kinesalgia.

kinesiatrics see KINESITHERAPY.

kinesimeter 1. an instrument for quantitative measurement of motions. 2. an instrument for exploring the body surface to test cutaneous sensibility.

kinesin one of three mechanochemical proteins (the other two are myosin and dynesin) associated with the cytoskeleton that converts chemical energy into mechanical energy and is the driving force for the movement of vesicles and organelles along the microtubule.

kinesi(o)- word element. [Gr.] *movement.*

kinesiology scientific study of movement of body parts.

kinesis [Gr.] *movement,* e.g. the activity of an organism in response to a stimulus; the direction of the response is not controlled by the direction of the stimulus (in contrast to a taxis).

-kinesis word element. [Gr.] *movement, motion* (e.g. cytokinesis).

kinesitherapy treatment of disease by movements or exercise.

kinesthesia the sense by which position, weight and movement are perceived.

kinesthesis kinesthesia.

kinesthetic sensation sensory inputs which recognize the orientation of the different parts of the body in relation to other parts as well as the rates of movements of the body parts.

kinetic pertaining to or producing motion.
k. energy the energy of motion.

kinetics the scientific study of the turnover, or rate of change, of a specific factor in, or position of the body, commonly expressed as units of amount per unit time.
chemical k. the scientific study of the rates and mechanisms of chemical reactions.
locomotion k. study of the rates and mechanisms of the movement or progression of animals.

kinetocardiogram the record produced by kinetocardiography.

kinetocardiography the graphic recording of the slow vibrations of the cranial chest wall in the region of the heart, representing the absolute motion at a given point on the chest.

kinetochore a centromere.
kinetogenic causing or producing movement.
kinetoplast an accessory body found in many protozoa, primarily the Mastigophora; it contains DNA and replicates independently.
kinetosis any disorder due to unaccustomed motion. See also MOTION SICKNESS.
kinetotherapy kinesitherapy.
kinety a row of granules, each of them situated at the base of a cilium.
King–Armstrong unit a unit of measurement of phosphatase; one unit equals 1 mg phenol liberated in 30 min at 100°F (37.5°C) and pH 9. Now largely replaced by International Units.
king brown snake see PSEUDECHIS *australis*.
King Charles spaniel a small, compact dog with domed head, very short nose, pendulous ears and long, silky, wavy coat; four solid or broken-colored varieties are recognized: black and tan, ruby (rich chesnut red), Blenheim (white with chestnut red patches, one of which must be in a white blaze in the center of the skull and called the 'lozenge' or 'kissing spot'), and tricolor (called Prince Charles in the United States) (white with black patches and tan markings). Similar to, but smaller than, the CAVALIER KING CHARLES SPANIEL. In the USA, the breed is called the English toy spaniel.
king cup see CALTHA PALUSTRIS.
King Island melilot MELILOTUS *indica*.
kingdom one of the three major categories into which natural objects are usually classified: the animal (including all animals), plant (including all plants), and mineral (including all substances and objects without life). A fourth, the Protista, includes all single-celled organisms.
Kingman forceps alligator forceps in which the jaws are opened by a system of levers so that there is no increase in diameter of the long, thin stem. Only the blades open, and that by one lying flat and the other angling away from it, like an alligator jaw movement.
king's crown see CALOTROPIS PROCERA.
kinin any of a group of endogenous peptides that increase vascular permeability, elevate blood pressure, and induce smooth muscle contraction.
venom k. a peptide found in the venom of insects.
kininase an enzyme that rapidly inactivates kinin found in tissues and plasma. There are two types: kininase I, which is a carboxypeptidase; and kininase II, which is an angiotensin-converting enzyme.
kininogen an α_2-globulin of plasma that is a precursor of the kinins.
kininogenases see KALLIKREIN.
kinkajou a member of the Procyonidae family, the raccoons, with a long prehensile tail. It is arboreal, vegetarian and nocturnal, weighing up to 10 lb. It has short dense fur colored olive, yellow or red brown. Called also *Potos flavus*, night monkey, honey bear.
kinked tail a deformity in dogs and commonly Siamese cats. Caused by multiple coccygeal hemivertebrae. Occasional cases in calves, usually associated with other skeletal deformities.
kinky back a congenital deformity of chickens. See SPONDYLOLISTHESIS.
kinocilium pl. *kinocilia;* a motile, protoplasmic filament on the free surface of a cell.
kinship a group of animals of varying degrees of descent from a common ancestor.
kinyoun's carbolfuschsin stain acid-fast stain useful in microbiology for assistance in the diagnosis of diseases caused by mycobacteria and actinomycetes, and demonstration of coccidial oocysts.
kiowa bean see PROSOPIS JULIFLORIA.
Kirby–Bauer method a method for testing the antimicrobial susceptibility of bacteria based on the size of zones of inhibition of growth of a lawn culture around disks impregnated with the antimicrobial drug.
Kiricephalus a genus of pentastomid parasites of colubrid snakes.
Kirschner named after Martin Kirschner, a German surgeon, a name commonly associated with surgical equipment.
K. apparatus a system of stainless steel threaded fixation pins, interconnecting rods, clamps and nuts for external fixation of fractures.
K.–Ehmer splint an external splinting device based on transfixation pinning.
K. wire a steel wire for skeletal transfixture of fractured bones and for obtaining skeletal traction in fractures.
Kisenyi sheep disease a virus disease of the nervous system of sheep in Africa transmitted by the tick *Rhipicephalus appendiculatus*.
kiss marks in dogs, tan marks over the eyes and on the cheeks.
kissing bugs see TRIATOMA.
kissing spot see LOZENGE (3).
kit a newborn fox or mink.
kitasamycin a macrolide antibiotic, produced by *Streptomyces kitasatoensis*, with activity similar to erythromycin. Called also leucomycin.
kitchen deaths see POLYTETRAFLUOROETHYLENE.
kite a member of the family Accipitridae, subfamily Aegypiinae (Old World vultures), which steal prey from other raptors. They are slim, with long narrow wings and an elongated tail. There are a number of genera, e.g. *Milvus* and *Haliastur* spp.
kitten newborn or young cat or ferret.
k. mortality complex a general term applied to a syndrome involving death of young kittens, particularly in breeding establishments. It is etiologically nonspecific, but generally applies to infectious causes and has occasionally been specifically applied to feline infectious peritonitis virus.
kiwi rare ratite bird, peculiar to New Zealand. They are brown, tailless, virtually wingless and have plumage resembling hairs rather than feathers. They are nocturnal, about the size of a domestic fowl and have a distinctive cry from which its name derives. Called also *Apteryx* spp.
klaaslouwboss see ATHANASIA TRIFURCATA.
Klamath weed HYPERICUM *perforatum*.
klapperbos CROTALARIA *burkeana*.
Klebsiella a genus of gram-negative bacteria in the tribe Klebsiellae, family Enterobacteriaceae. Includes *K. mobilis* (syn. *Enterobacter aerogenes*).
K. pneumoniae carried in the vestibule of the vagina, urethra and clitoridal fossa of the mare as normal flora, but invasion of the cervix and uterus does occur, causing metritis and infertility. An occasional cause of bovine mastitis, hematogenous osteomyelitis originating in pulmonary lesions in cattle, bronchopneumonia in dogs, and pyothorax in horses.
kleingrass see PANICUM *coloratum*.
Klein's disease see FOWL typhoid.
Kleinshmidt preparation a method for observing nucleic acid molecules in the electron microscope. Molecules are first spread on the surface of a solution from which they are picked up on a grid and then shadowcast with a heavy metal.
Klenow fragment treatment of the enzyme DNA

polymerase 1 with subtilism produces two cleavage products, a small fragment which is unstable and a large fragment, called the Klenow fragment, which retains both the 5′-3′ polymerase and the 3′ exonuclease activities, but not the 5′ exonuclease activity, of the intact enzyme, together with the pyrophosphorolysis and pyrophosphate exchange activities. Used to synthesize DNA complementary to single-stranded DNA template by adding nucleotides to the free 3′-hydroxyl end of an annealed DNA primer.

klimp CYNANCHUM *africanum*, *C. ellipticum*, *C. obtusifolium*.

Klinefelter's syndrome a condition in humans characterized by the presence of small testes, with fibrosis and hyalinization of the seminiferous tubules, impairment of function and clumping of Leydig cells, and an increase in urinary gonadotropins, associated with an abnormality of the sex chromosomes. It is associated typically with an XXY chromosome complement. A similar condition is seen in male tortoiseshell and white cats, and has been recorded rarely in stallions, bulls, rams and dogs.

Klossiella a genus of coccidians in the family Eimeriidae.

K. boae found in the intestine of the boa constrictor. It may cause anorexia, restlessness, hemorrhagic enteritis and intussusception.

K. cobayae found in guinea pigs.

K. equi found in the kidneys of horses, donkeys, zebra and burro.

K. muris causes renal coccidiosis in mice.

km kilometer.

K_M constant substrate concentration that gives half maximal velocity of an enzymatic reaction. Measure of the affinity of enzyme and substrate with the higher the K_M, the lower the affinity. Called also Michaelis constant; Michaelis–Menten constant.

KMC kitten mortality complex.

knacker operator of a KNACKERY.

knackered slang for being so exhausted or decrepit that a horse is suitable only for the knacker's yard.

knackery an industrial establishment which converts animal remains into animal feed supplements and fertilizer. Accept living derelict, unwanted and recently dead animals for disposal. A favorite source of postmortem information on animals that have been under surveillance.

knapweed Russian knapweed (*Acroptilon repens*). See CENTAUREA.

knee in large animals, the carpus; in small animals, the stifle. See Table 11.

bench k. conformation defect in which the metacarpus is not centered symmetrically to the carpus.

blemished k. scarred or otherwise imperfect appearance.

broken k. used to mean that a horse has fallen and broken the skin over the carpus.

k. gall see knee thoroughpin (below).

k. jerk see PATELLAR reflex.

popped k. see CARPITIS.

k. spavin an old-fashioned name for chronic carpitis in horses.

k. strap a short strap used to strap up a horse's leg in a flexed position so that it is as immobile as a three-legged horse. A good form of restraint for a horse that is rearing.

k. thoroughpin distension of the carpal sheath in the horse. Visible as a fluid-filled distension at the back of the knee.

knee-cap an item of horse clothing; made of canvas or basil, it is wrapped around and strapped over the carpus for protection during traveling.

kneecap see PATELLA.

Knemidocoptes see CNEMIDOCOPTES.

knife a single-bladed cutting instrument other than a scalpel and usually designed for a special purpose.

castrating k. there are many straight bladed instruments available. A special hooked knife is popular for use with calves and lambs. It has a cutting edge which is bent down at right angles to form a shallow hook. The instrument is drawn towards the operator and provides much less risk to him/her. See also Newberry castrating knife (below).

drawing k. see hoof knife (below).

finger k. used in bovine obstetrics to cut the skin of a dead fetus. It consists of a flat palm-piece that lies flat against the palm of the hand and from which the hooked knife protrudes. The knife has a single finger ring on its spine, through which a finger is passed and over the front of the knife. The knife is passed into the uterus, and hooked into appropriate skin, which is cut by pulling backwards. Some knives have an eyelet to which a cord can be attached to facilitate this part of the task.

hoof k. a strong, slightly curved knife with its tip turned laterally on itself to form a tunnel. The flat part of the blade is used to trim the bottom of the hoof wall and the curved part to make grooves or cut holes. The standard knife is the Hauptner. The blade in some knives is sharpened on both edges. Called also hoof parer, drawing knife.

The Swiss hoof knife is a large, flattened loop turned down at right angles to the handle. It is for paring the sole and is drawn towards the operator with the lower front-edge sharpened. Special grooving knives are also available. See also Hughes hoof GROOVER.

Lichty's teat k. a narrow, 0.1 inch wide blade about 0.4 inch long, sharpened on one edge and with a rounded blunt point, which is inserted into the teat canal. A cut is made laterally through the overtight sphincter or scar tissue.

Newberry castrating k. a pincer-like instrument with a block at the end of one blade and a chisel-pointed knife on the other. When the sharp blade is closed on the exposed spermatic cord, it compresses the cord against the block.

palm k. a small version of the Stanley hobby knife, which can be carried into the uterus in the palm of the hand and the concealed blade opened. Cuts are made in the fetal skin in a normal cutting manner.

tenotomy k. has a blunt, rounded tip on the blade, which is curved slightly forward so that the knife can be inserted under the tendon without damage to local nerves and blood vessels and so that a cut can be made outwards without the tendon slipping off the knife. Called also a tenotome.

Wamberg spavin k. used for transecting the cunean tendon in a horse affected by spavin. Has a 1.5 inch blade on a curved neck so that the blade can be inserted under the tendon without being obstructed by the knuckles of the hand holding the handle.

knizocyte a red blood cell with two or more concavities (triconcave erythrocyte); associated with hemolytic anemia.

knock-knee the knees approximate and the fetlocks are wide apart. Called also genu valgum.

knocked-down hip fracture of the wing of the ilium. A common problem in cows due to injury during estrus. Also occurs in racing Greyhounds, significantly altering its conformation but not altering the gait.

knocked-up shoe a horseshoe designed to lift the medial aspect of the hoof and counter the tendency to brush one hoof against the medial aspect of the other leg. The bar of the inner wing of the shoe is higher and narrower than the lateral bar.

knocked-up toe see kicked-up TOE.

knopvelsiekte [Af.] see LUMPY skin disease.

knot 1. an intertwining of the ends or parts of one or more threads, sutures, or strips of cloth. See SQUARE KNOT, GRANNY KNOT, HALF-HITCH KNOT, PACKET KNOT and SURGEON'S KNOT. 2. in anatomy, a knob-like swelling or protuberance.

knotgrass POLYGONUM *persicaria*.

knothead MYELOCYTOMATOSIS of poultry.

Knott's test a technique for the detection of microfilariae, most often for the diagnosis of *Dirofilaria immitis* infection in dogs. The blood is hemolyzed and concentrated.

knotweed POLYGONUM *aviculare*.

Knowles forceps long-handled tissue forceps with ratcheted handles suitable for grasping the cervix of the mare and drawing it back into the vagina for suturing or other surgical treatment.

Knowles scissors bandage scissors with a knob on the end of the longer blade.

knuckle 1. the dorsal aspect of any human interphalangeal joint, or any similarly bent structure. 2. the swollen end of any long bone.

knuckled over see KNUCKLING.

knuckling a forward bending at the fetlock joint. May be a feature of the conformation or a sign of neurological deficit. Called also overshot fetlock.

k. over sometimes used synonymously with knuckling. Also refers to weightbearing on the dorsal surface of a flexed foot or paw; often a sign of deficit in normal proprioception that would reflexly cause a repositioning to the normal position.

ko cycle the cycle of control or destruction in acupuncture theory; a mechanism which ensures that no single element becomes too powerful.

koa haole [Hawaiian] see LEUCAENA LEUCOCEPHALA.

koala a small (10 to 15 lb) bear-like, marsupial creature of the family Phascolarctidae. The baby koala is very small when born and is subsequently carried in the mother's pouch and later on her back. Called also *Phascolarctos cinereus*.

kob a medium to large, semi-aquatic antelope related to the waterbuck. Called also *Kobus* spp.

Kobus see WATERBUCK.

Koch named after Robert Koch, a German bacteriologist.

K. blue spot, K. blue body see THEILERIASIS.

K. OT Koch's old tuberculin, used in the tuberculin test.

K. phenomenon the role of delayed type hypersensitivity in the pathogenesis of tuberculosis.

K's postulates a statement of the kind of experimental evidence required to establish the causative relation of a given microorganism to a given disease. The conditions are: (1) the microorganism must be present in every case of the disease; (2) it must be isolated and cultivated in pure culture; (3) inoculation of such culture must produce the disease in susceptible animals; (4) it must be observed in, and recovered from, the experimentally diseased animal.

Kocher forceps ratchet-handled, scissor-type, artery forceps with curved blades with cross-grooved faces. The tips of the blades have one pair of interlocking, sharp teeth.

Kochia scoparia North American small shrub of the family Chenopodiaceae; may cause polioencephalomalacia and hepatogenous photosensitization. Called also summer cypress, Mexican fireweed, burning bush.

Kodiak island disease congenital defects in calves caused by LUPINUS *sericeus*.

Koeppe's criterion a phenomenon which occurs in the determination of hematocrit by centrifugation. With complete packing of red blood cells the column becomes translucent.

KOH potassium hydroxide.

KOH-cleared specimens specimens of external parasites cleared of epithelial debris by potassium hydroxide solution.

kohlrabi BRASSICA *oleracea* var. *acephala*.

koilin cuticle see CUTICLE of koilin.

koilo- word element. [Gr.] *hollowed, concave*.

koilocytosis ballooning degeneration.

kolp- for words beginning thus, see those beginning *colp-*.

kolypeptic hindering or checking digestion.

Komondor a very large (80–150 lb), muscular dog with a distinctive white coat that forms long tassel-like cords, completely obscuring any details of conformation. The breed is a shepherding and guard dog of Asiatic origin.

Konratice virus a strain of porcine enterovirus isolated in Czechoslovakia from pigs with porcine viral ENCEPHALOMYELITIS (Teschen disease).

Kooikerhondje a small (20–24 lb), gun dog, approximately 14–16 inches in height, and a slightly longer body. The coat is medium long, wavy or straight, and white with orange-red patches and a white blaze. The tail is plumed.

kookaburra an arboreal, insectivorous and carnivorous bird of the kingfisher family (Alcedinidae) with an identifying, laugh-type call. Called also laughing jackass, *Dacelo novaeguineae*.

koolganna see SALSOLA *tuberculatiformis*.

Korat a breed of cats originating in Thailand. It has a short, silver-blue coat and large, green eyes. GM_1 gangliosidosis is reported to occur in the breed.

Korean lespedeza see LESPEDEZA STIPULACEA.

Korean Native cattle yellow-brown meat and draft cattle.

koronivia grass BRACHIARIA *humidicola*.

Korotkoff's sounds sounds heard during auscultatory determination of BLOOD PRESSURE in humans, thought to be produced by vibratory motion of the arterial wall as the artery suddenly distends when compressed by a pneumatic blood pressure cuff. Origin of the sound may be within the blood passing through the vessel or within the wall itself.

kosher slaughter see JEWISH SLAUGHTER.

Kotonkan virus a rabies-like virus of African origin.

Kovac's reagent a reagent used to detect the presence of indole. Used in the identification of bacteria.

kPa kilopascal.

KPs keratic precipitates.

Kr chemical symbol, *krypton*.

kraalbos [Af.] GALENIA *africana*.

Krabbe's disease see globoid cell LEUKODYSTROPHY.

kraurosis a dried, shriveled condition.

Krause named after W.J.F. Krause, a German anatomist.

K's bulb, K's corpuscle, K's endbulb see BULBOID CORPUSCLE.

K. glands mucous glands in the conjunctiva.

Krebs cycle see TRICARBOXYLIC ACID CYCLE.

kregda a severe pneumonia caused by *Mycoplasma ovipneumoniae* in sheep in Iceland and Switzerland.

Krey–Schottler hook a multiple jointed obstetric implement which approximates its two opposing hooks when these have been anchored in eye-sockets and the end ring is pulled. Excellent for applying traction to the head of a calf.

krimpsiekte [Af.] 'shrinking disease'; caused by poisoning by COTYLEDON and TYLECODON spp. plants. See COTYLEDONOSIS.

kryo-ichthyozoosis a disease of aquarium fish caused by a virus that survives only in cold water. The disease is manifested by awkward swimming action and death in 5 to 6 hours.

krypton a chemical element, atomic number 36, atomic weight 83.80, symbol Kr. See Table 6.

KSGPV Kenya sheeppox and goatpox virus, genomically identical with lumpy skin disease virus.

kudu a large, striking-looking antelope with very long, spiral horns, gray or tawny color with white stripes, called *Strepsiceros strepsiceros* and *S. imberbis*. Also greater kudu (*Tragelaphus strepsiceros*).

kudzu see PUERARIA LOBATA.

Kühn's crutch an obstetric instrument for use in large animals. It has a 3 feet long handle and a U-shaped endpiece with an eyelet for cord in the end of each arm. Suitable for trapping a limb and repelling or rotating all or part of a fetus.

Kuhnt–Helmbold operation a technique for repair of ectropion.

Kuhnt–Szymanowski operation a technique for repair of ectropion caused by a greatly elongated lower eyelid.

kulchitsky cell tumor see CARCINOID.

kumara IPOMOEA *batatas*.

kumri see CEREBROSPINAL nematodiasis.

Kundi a Pakistani breed of Murrah-type Indian buffalo. Black or brown in color, often with white on the head, tail and feet.

KuneKune pig indigenous, tasseled, fat pig of the Maori people; any color.

Kunjin virus a flavivirus isolated from cases of asymptomatic encephalomyelitis of calves. See also ENCEPHALITIS.

kunka caseous granules found in granulomatous lesions of habronemiasis.

kunkur, kunker see SWAMP CANCER.

Kuntscher nail an intramedullary splint with a hollow, slightly clover-leaf cross-section.

Kupffer's cells large, stellate or pyramidal, intensely phagocytic cells lining the walls of the hepatic sinusoids and forming part of the reticuloendothelial system.

kurdee see SAFFLOWER MEAL.

Kurdi a carpetwool, polled, fat-tailed, black sheep from the Middle East, with many ethnic varieties.

Kurloff bodies structures seen in the large mononuclear leukocytes of guinea pigs and related rodents. Their origin is uncertain.

kurrajong BRACHYCHITON *populneum*.

Kursteiner's cyst see PARATHYROID cyst.

kurtosis the quality of peakedness in a unimodal distribution. Abnormalities are leptokurtosis where values are clustered about the mean and the tails of the curve, and platykurtosis where the clustering produces a plateau-shaped curve.

kuru a chronic, progressive, uniformly fatal central nervous system prion disease of humans probably resembling the scrapie agent of sheep, and transmissible to nonhuman primates; seen only in the Fore and neighboring peoples of New Guinea. Believed to be transmitted by cannibalism.

Kussmaul's respiration a distressing dyspnea occurring in paroxysms, characteristic of diabetic acidosis and coma. Called also air hunger.

Kuvasz a large, sturdy Hungarian dog breed used for guarding livestock. It has a thick, pure white or ivory coat, dark eyes, small, pendulous ears and a moderately long tail.

kV kilovolt.

kVp KILOVOLT peak.

kwashiorkor protein-caloric malnutrition; a human condition.

Kyasanur Forest disease a highly fatal flavivirus disease of monkeys in the Kyasanur Forest of India, communicable to humans, in whom it produces hemorrhagic symptoms. See also ENCEPHALITIS.

kymatism MYOKYMIA; quivering of muscles.

kymogram the graphic record (tracing or film) produced by the kymograph.

kymograph an instrument for recording variations or undulations, arterial or other.

kymography the use of the kymograph.

kynocephalus a monster with a head like that of a dog.

kynurenine a metabolite of tryptophan found in microorganisms and in the urine of normal animals; it is a precursor of kynurenic acid and an intermediate in the conversion of tryptophan to niacin.

kyphos the hump in the spine in kyphosis.

kyphoscoliosis upward (kyphosis) and lateral (scoliosis) curvature of the spine.

kyphosis abnormally increased convexity in the curvature of the thoracic spine as viewed from the side.

kyrtorrhachic having a vertebral column in which the lumbar curvature is ventrally convex.

kyto- for words beginning thus, see those beginning *cyto-*.

L

L Latin; left; length; [L.] *libra* (pound, balance); licentiate; light sense; [L.] *limen* (boundary); liter; lumbar; coefficient of induction.

L_0 Ehrlich's symbol for a toxin–antitoxin mixture that is completely neutralized and will not kill an animal.

L+ Ehrlich's symbol for a toxin–antitoxin mixture that contains one fatal dose in excess and will kill the experimental animal.

L- chemical prefix (written as small capital) that specifies that the substance corresponds in chemical configuration to the standard substance L-glyceraldehyde. Carbohydrates are named by this method to distinguish them by their chemical composition. The opposite prefix is D-.

l liter.

l- chemical abbreviation, *levo-* (i.e. left or counterclockwise).

L antigen see L ANTIGEN.

L chain see light CHAIN.

L-form see L-form BACTERIA.

L genes class I MHC genes in mice.

L-plasty a technique for suturing a crescent-shaped skin defect by starting at one end, removing the excess that develops on the longer side by cutting a V, then closing as a right angle. A L-shaped incision results.

L-shaped rumen a chronically distended rumen which extends from the left abdomen to fill the right half as well.
La chemical symbol, *lanthanum*.
la bouhite [Fr.] see MAEDI.
LA test latex agglutination test.
la tremblante [Fr.] see SCRAPIE.
lab laboratory.
label something that identifies; an identifying mark, tag, etc.
radioactive l. radioactive tracer.
labeling to attach a label.
pulse-chase l. a method for following metabolic processes using radioisotopes. Typically a labeled precursor substance is present for a brief period (pulse) followed by a period in which it is present only in an unlabeled form (chase).
labellum mouthparts of insects; carry tubes for the passage of aspirated fluids.
labia [L.] plural of *labium*.
oral l. lips of the mouth; musculomembranous folds that surround the mouth.
pudendal l. lips of the vulva.
vulvar l. see VULVA.
labial pertaining to a lip, or labium.
l. ulcer see EOSINOPHILIC ulcer.
labile 1. gliding; moving from point to point over the surface; unstable; fluctuating. 2. chemically unstable.
lability the quality of being labile.
labio- word element. [L.] *lip*.
labiogingival lamina a thickening of the embryonal stomodeal ectoderm eventually forming the oral vestibule.
labioglossolaryngeal pertaining to the lips, tongue and larynx.
labioglossopharyngeal pertaining to the lips, tongue and pharynx.
labiogram imprint pattern taken from the muzzle of an animal; suggested as a means of identification. Called also nasolabiogram, nose print.
labiomental pertaining to the lips and chin.
labionasal pertaining to the lip and nose.
labiopalatine pertaining to the lips and palate.
labioplasty plastic repair of a lip; cheiloplasty.
labioscrotal swellings paired swellings flanking the developing genital tubercle and urogenital orifice prior to sex differentiation; destined to form the labia or scrotum.
Labiostrongylus the largest of the common nematodes in the stomach of macropods.
labium pl. *labia* [L.] a fleshy border or edge; a lip.
labor the function of the female organism by which the product of conception is expelled from the uterus through the vagina to the outside world.

Labor may be divided into three stages. The first stage (*dilatation*) begins with the onset of regular uterine contractions and ends when the cervical os is completely dilated and flush with the vagina, thus completing the birth canal. The second stage (*expulsion*) extends from the end of the first stage until the expulsion of the neonate is completed. The third stage (*placental*) extends from the expulsion of the neonate until the placenta and membrane are expelled and contraction of the uterus is completed. Called also parturition.

difficult l. see DYSTOCIA.
induced l. that which is brought on by extraneous means, e.g. by the use of drugs that cause uterine contractions; called also artificial labor.
laboratory a place equipped for making tests or doing experimental work.
l. animals the group of animals constantly used in laboratories for general research in all subjects. Includes rats, mice, rabbits and guinea pigs. In special-use laboratories additional animal species can be added, e.g. hamsters, nonhuman primates, amphibians, fowl, sheep and pigs.
clinical l. one for examination of materials derived from the animal body for the purpose of providing information on diagnosis, prevention or treatment of disease.
l. findings the results of laboratory examinations, usually with analyses and judgments.
maximum containment l. one designed and equipped to provide the highest level of security in the handling of infectious agents that are serious pathogens for humans and animals. See BIOSAFETY.
l. rat see Sprague–Dawley, Wistar and Long–Evans RAT.
labour see LABOR.
Labradoodle a hybrid name applied to dogs resulting from crossing Labrador retrievers and standard Poodles. Conformation and coat characteristics vary widely between those of the parents.
Labrador retriever a medium-sized, strongly built gun dog with broad head, drop ears, thick tapered tail, and short, very dense coat in black, yellow or chocolate. The medium length tail has a thick base and is covered in the thick coat, but not feathered; sometimes called an 'otter' tail. The breed is predisposed to inherited cataracts, progressive retinal atrophy, cystinuria, hemophilia A, osteochondrosis and hip dysplasia.
labriform milkweed ASCLEPIAS *labriformis*.
labrum pl. *labra* [L.] an edge, rim or lip, e.g. upper lip of insects.
acetabular l. the ring of fibrocartilage that is attached to and deepens the acetabulum; large and thick in the horse and cow. Called also acetabular glenoidal labrum.
acetabular glenoidal l. see acetabular labrum (above).
articular l. a fibrocartilaginous rim around the edge of some joint sockets such as the acetabulum and the glenoid.
laburnum *Laburnum anagyroides*.
Laburnum anagyroides plant member of the legume family Fabaceae; popular but very poisonous tree; the pods and seeds contain the quinolizidine alkaloid cytisine, which causes incoordination, excitement, sweating, convulsions and death. Vomiting also occurs in dogs. Called also laburnum, *Cytisus laburnum*, golden chain, golden rain.
labyrinth the system of interconnecting cavities or canals of the internal ear, consisting of the vestibule, cochlea and SEMICIRCULAR canals.

The cochlea is concerned with hearing, and the vestibule and semicircular canals with equilibrium (sense of balance).

bony l. the bony or osseous labyrinth is composed of a series of canals tunneled out of the temporal bone.
ethmoid l., ethmoidal l. either of the paired lateral masses of the ethmoid bone, consisting of numerous thin-walled cellular cavities, the ethmoidal cells.
membranous l. inside the osseous labyrinth is the membranous labyrinth, which conforms to the general shape of the osseous labyrinth but is smaller. A fluid called perilymph fills the space between the osseous and membranous labyrinths. Fluid inside the membranous labyrinth is called endolymph. These fluids play an important role in the transmission of sound waves and the maintenance of body balance.

osseous l. a complex excavation in the petrous part of the temporal bone which houses the membranous labyrinth.

labyrinthectomy excision of the labyrinth.

labyrinthine pertaining to or emanating from a labyrinth.

l. responses include righting and placing reflexes and nystagmus.

l. righting reflex the reflex which coordinates body movements so that a cat dropped from a height with its belly uppermost will rotate in flight so that its belly is closest to the ground.

labyrinthitis inflammation of the labyrinth; OTITIS interna.

labyrinthotomy incision of the labyrinth.

lac pl. *lacta* [L.] milk.

***lac* operon** the lactose operon, a nucleotide sequence in *Escherichia coli* that controls the synthesis of the enzyme β-galactosidase comprising binding sequence motifs for the cap protein, which activates transcription, the repressor protein, which inhibits transcription, and a region with which RNA polymerase interacts. The first, best studied and best understood model for gene regulation.

***lac* repressor** see *lac* REPRESSOR.

laceration 1. the act of tearing. 2. a wound produced by the tearing of body tissue, as distinguished from a cut or incision.

Lacerta a genus of the suborder Lacertilia and the family Lacertidae, the family of lizards. Agile, very fast moving four-legged reptiles with long pointed tails. Can inflict unpleasant bites but are not venomous. There are more than 150 species.

lacertilian see LIZARD.

lacertus pl. *lacerti* [L.] a name given to certain fibrous attachments of muscles.

l. fibrosus part of the antebrachial fascia extending from the biceps to the radial carpal extensor muscles and a significant part of the horse's stay apparatus.

Lachnanthes tinctoria a North American plant in the family Haemodoraceae. Reputed to cause dermatitis in white-skinned pigs and pink discoloration of their bones. Called also *L. caroliniana*, *Gyrotheca tinctoria*, redleg, redroot.

Lachnospira multiparus a bacterial digestive adjunct resident in rumens.

lachry- for words beginning thus see words beginning lacri-.

Lacombe a lop-eared bacon pig produced in Canada by crossing Landrace, Chester White and Berkshire pigs.

lacrim- prefix meaning tears.

lacrimal pertaining to tears.

l. apparatus a group of organs concerned with the production and drainage of tears; it is a nutritive and protective device that helps keep the eye moist and free of dust and other irritating particles. Includes lacrimal gland, accessory lacrimal glands, third eyelid glands and the nasolacrimal duct.

l. canaliculus the lacrimal duct within the eyelid.

l. caruncle the rounded, often pigmented swelling at the medial canthus of the eye.

l. cyst congenital displacement of lacrimal tissue results in subconjunctival cysts.

l. drainage system the structures concerned with tear collection; includes lacrimal lake, puncta, canaliculi, sac and nasolacrimal duct.

l. duct there are two of these minute ducts draining tears from the conjunctiva, via the lacrimal puncta, into the lacrimal sac. Called also lacrimal canaliculus.

l. duct irrigator a 20 gauge, blunt-pointed, straight or curved cannula with a needle attachment so that it can be attached directly to a syringe nozzle.

l. fossa fossa in the medial wall of the orbital rim which houses the lacrimal sac.

l. gland contained in a pad of fat in the dorsolateral part of the orbital cavity and drains into the conjunctival sac via many excretory ducts. The secretion is largely watery tears, but in the pig is mucus. May develop adenitis.

l. gland anomalies failure of patency of the duct, supernumerary opening of the duct and ductal ectasia recorded.

l. gland atrophy part of the syndrome of keratoconjunctivitis sicca.

imperforate l. puncta see imperforate PUNCTUM.

l. lake the recess between the lids at the nasal commissure of the eye where the tears collect.

l. pump contraction of the orbiculari oculi muscle creates pressure on the lacrimal sac which causes tears to drain from the lacrimal lake.

l. punctum there is one on each eyelid close to the medial canthus. Each drains tears from the conjunctival sac into the lacrimal duct in the same eyelid. The tears then pass to the lacrimal sac and into the nasolacrimal duct. See also PUNCTUM.

l. reflex tear production caused by irritation of the cornea and conjunctiva.

l. sac the distended proximal end of the nasolacrimal duct into which the lacrimal ducts empty.

l. sinus an excavation of the lacrimal bone which communicates with the maxillary sinus in some species.

l. system see lacrimal apparatus (above).

lacrimation secretion and discharge of tears.

lacrimator an agent, such as a gas, that induces the flow of tears.

lacrimatory causing a flow of tears.

lacrimonasal pertaining to the lacrimal sac and nose.

lacrimotomy incision of the lacrimal gland, duct or sac.

Lacroix operation a surgical procedure used to establish drainage of the external ear canal in dogs by the removal of a V-shaped segment of the lateral cartilaginous wall. See also ZEPP OPERATION.

lactacidemia an excess of lactic acid in the blood; lacticemia; lactic acidemia.

lactacidosis see LACTIC acidosis.

lactaciduria lactic acid in the urine.

lactagogue an agent that promotes the flow of milk; galactagogue.

lactam a cyclic amide formed from aminocarboxylic acids by elimination of water; lactams are isomeric with lactims, which are enol forms of lactams.

β-l. antibiotics includes the penicillins, cephalosporins, carbapenems and penems. See also β-lactam ring (below).

β-l. ring an integral part of the formula of β-lactam antibiotics. Disruption of the ring by β-lactamase produced by some bacteria, e.g. *Escherichia coli*, *Bacillus anthracis*, destroys the antimicrobial activity of the compound.

β-lactamase either of two enzymes: β-lactamase I is penicillinase; β-lactamase II is cephalosporinase.

lactase D-galactosidase; an enzyme in the intestinal mucosa that hydrolyzes lactose, producing glucose and galactose.

l. deficiency a deficiency of intestinal lactase, which causes abdominal distension and cramping and often diarrhea when milk is drunk.

lactate 1. any salt of lactic acid or the anion of lactic acid. 2. to secrete milk.

l. dehydrogenase called also LD, LDH; see lactate DEHYDROGENASE.
l. dehydrogenase test a high level in milk used as an indicator of the presence of mastitis in the quarter.
exercise blood l. exercise by a horse begins aerobically without any elevation of blood lactate levels; exercise at faster levels is eventually performed anaerobically and blood lactate levels rise steeply.
l. shuttle the production of lactate in resting muscle where adequate oxygenation is available; represents a mechanism for conserving glucose absorbed from the gut by allowing it to be converted to lactate by skeletal muscle and later used for work or transferred to the liver for glycogen synthesis.
l. T_m maximal tubular concentration of lactate.

lactated potassium saline see DARROW'S SOLUTION.

lactated Ringer's solution classical isotonic, balanced electrolyte solution with major electrolytes in the same concentration as in blood. Contains sodium, potassium, calcium, chloride, and bicarbonate as lactate.

lactating cows cows in milk; contrast with milking cows.

lactation 1. the secretion of milk by the mammary glands. 2. the period of weeks or months during which the dam lactates.
artificial l. see lactation induction (below).
current l. listing a list of all the cows in a herd which are currently being milked.
l. curves daily milk yield plotted along one abscissa of a graph, days along the other. Used to monitor peak MILK output and MILK persistency, especially to assess nutritional management.
early l. drop an unexpected downturn in the lactation curve of a dairy cow in early lactation.
l. failure see AGALACTIA.
l. hormone lactogenic hormone, or prolactin.
inappropriate l. see GALACTORRHEA.
l. induction in nonpregnant cows by the administration of hormones, usually a combination of estradiol and progesterone.
l. ketosis see ACETONEMIA.
l.–pregnancy cycle in dairy cows the cycle of the cow's year, commencing with calving and lactation onset, followed by conception, then drying off followed by calving again, all with impeccable timing, when aiming at a 365 day cycle.

lactation tetany 1. lactation tetany of ruminants is a highly fatal disease of recently calved, lactating cows and recently lambed ewes. The disease reaches serious levels of prevalence in animals grazing grass dominated pastures and cereal crops. It is characterized by hypomagnesemia and usually an accompanying hypocalcemia. Clinical highlights include tonic and clonic muscular spasms, and convulsions and death due to respiratory failure. 2. lactation tetany of mares is a similar disease clinically but occurs at the foaling heat or just after the foal is weaned. It is primarily a hypocalcemia, with hypomagnesemia an uncommon finding. The disease in cattle is called also hypomagnesemic tetany, grass tetany, grass staggers. 3. lactation tetany of dogs and cats, see puerperal TETANY.

lactational osteoporosis may facilitate fracture of the femur, vertebrae and phalanges in lactating sows fed diets deficient in calcium and normal to high phosphorus.

lacteal 1. pertaining to milk. 2. any of the intestinal lymphatics that transport chyle.

lactenin a bacteriostatic substance in milk.

lactescence resemblance to milk.

lactic pertaining to milk.
l. acid a compound formed in the body in metabolism of carbohydrate, by fermentation of carbohydrates in the rumen and by bacterial action on milk. The sodium salt of racemic or inactive lactic (sodium lactate) acid is used as an electrolyte and fluid replenisher.
l. acid cycle the metabolic system by which lactic acid produced by glycolysis in muscles is converted in the liver to glucose. Called also the Cori cycle.
l. acid indigestion see CARBOHYDRATE ENGORGEMENT.
l. acidemia lactacidemia.
l. acidosis the state in ruminants in which there is an excess of lactic acid and lactate in the body, due usually to unadapted grain feeding and carbohydrate engorgement.
ruminal l. acid the level is high in CARBOHYDRATE ENGORGEMENT.

D-lactic acidosis see lactic ACIDOSIS.

lacticemia lactacidemia.

lactiferous conveying milk.
l. ducts appearing first as epithelial diverticula which invade the mammary mesenchyme from the mammary buds, the precursors of the teats, these solid cords of cells later cavitate to produce lactiferous ducts.
l. sinus large cavity, continuous with the lactiferous ducts in mammary tissue, which serves as a reservoir for accumulated milk in the mammary gland until it is released at milking or suckling via the teat sinus and teat canal; is a combination of gland and teat sinuses.

lactifuge checking or stopping milk secretion; an agent that so acts.

lactigenous producing milk.

lactigerous see LACTIFEROUS.

lactim see LACTAM.

lactivorous feeding or subsisting upon milk.

lact(o)- word element. [L.] *milk*.

Lactobacillus a genus of gram-positive, rod-shaped bacteria, all of which are generally considered to be nonpathogenic, although they have been isolated from abscesses in cats. They produce lactic acid by fermentation and play a part in the development of lactic acidosis in ruminants fed on too much carbohydrate. See also YOGURT.

lactobacillus pl. *lactobacilli;* any individual organism of the genus *Lactobacillus.*

lactocele see GALACTOCELE.

Lactococcus parviae see ENTEROCOCCUS *seriolicida.*

lactoferrin an iron-binding protein found in neutrophils and bodily secretions (milk, tears, saliva, bile, etc.), having bactericidal activity, and acting as an inhibitor of colony formation by granulocytes and macrophages.

lactoflavin see RIBOFLAVIN.

lactogen any substance that enhances lactation.

lactogenesis the process of differentiation of cells of the mammary alveoli, as a consequence of which the alveolar cells develop the capacity to secrete milk.

lactogenic stimulating the production of milk.
l. hormone one of the gonadotropic hormones of the anterior pituitary; it stimulates and sustains lactation in postpartum animals, and shows luteotropic activity in certain mammals. Called also prolactin.

lactoglobulin a globulin occurring in milk.
immune l's antibodies (immunoglobulins) occurring in the colostrum of mammals.

lactolith see MILK stone.

lactone 1. an aromatic liquid from lactic acid. 2. a cyclic organic compound in which the chain is closed

by ester formation between a carboxyl and a hydroxyl group in the same molecule.
lactoperoxidase an enzyme found in milk that oxidizes thiocyanate to bacteriostatic products.
lactophenol cotton blue a preparation of phenol, lactic acid, glycerin, distilled water, and cotton blue dye, used to stain fungi in wet preparations.
lactorrhea excessive or spontaneous milk flow; persistent secretion of milk irrespective of nursing; galactorrhea.
lactose a sugar derived from milk, which on hydrolysis yields glucose and galactose.
l. digestion test oral test of foal's ability to digest milk sugar.
l. intolerance inability to digest lactose in the diet because of the lack of the enzyme lactase in the small intestine. Clinical consequences are intestinal discomfort and diarrhea.
l. tolerance test a monitor of intestinal epithelial damage, similar to the starch digestion test. The test measures the rise in blood glucose at timed intervals after oral administration of lactose; essentially a test of disaccharidase efficiency of the gut.
lactoside glycoside in which the sugar constituent is lactose.
lactosuria lactose in the urine.
lactotherapy treatment by milk diet.
lactotrope an acidophilic cell of the anterior pituitary that secretes prolactin.
lactotroph see LACTOTROPE.
lactotrophin, lactotropin see PROLACTIN.
Lactuca serriola plant in the family Asteraceae; toxin unidentified; young plants cause pulmonary emphysema manifested by dyspnea, weakness and death. Called also prickly lettuce.
lactulose a synthetic disaccharide used as a cathartic and to enhance the excretion of ammonia in the treatment of hepatic encephalopathy.
lacuna pl. *lacunae* [L.] 1. a small pit or hollow cavity. 2. a defect or gap, as in the field of vision (scotoma).
absorption l. a pit or groove in developing bone that is undergoing resorption; frequently found to contain osteoclasts.
bone l. a small cavity within the bone matrix, containing an osteocyte, and from which slender canaliculi radiate and penetrate the adjacent lamellae to anastomose with the canaliculi of neighboring lacunae, thus forming a system of cavities interconnected by minute canals.
cartilage l. any of the small cavities within the cartilage matrix, containing a chondrocyte.
Howship's l. the concave cavities which are formed by osteoclasts in the process of bone resorption.
osseous l. bone lacuna (see above).
osteocytic l. see bone lacuna (above).
urethral l. numerous small depressions or pits in the mucous membrane of the urethra.
vascular l. a breach in any membrane or other tissue which is navigated by blood vessels.
lacunule a minute lacuna.
lacus pl. *lacus* [L.] lake.
l. lacrimalis see LACRIMAL lake.
ladder diagram a method of interpreting cardiac arrhythmias by using the electrocardiogram with a diagram drawn from the important points of atrioventricular conduction.
ladino clover TRIFOLIUM *repens*.
Lady Campbell weed ECHIUM *plantagineum*.
Laekenois see BELGIAN shepherd dog.
Laelaptidae a family of mites, found as occasional infestations on chickens and pigeons.
laevo- see words commencing with *levo-*.
Lafora bodies large, cytoplasmic inclusion bodies in central neurons in normal dogs and in larger numbers in cases of neurological disease in young dogs. See also GLYCOPROTEINOSIS.
Lafora's disease see GLYCOPROTEINOSIS.
lag 1. the time elapsing between application of a stimulus and the resulting reaction. 2. the early period after inoculation of bacteria into a culture medium, in which the growth or cell division is slow.
l. screw a screw used in compression plating of bone fractures; it has U-shaped threads.
lagena 1. the curved, flask-shaped organ of hearing in vertebrates lower than mammals, corresponding to the cochlear duct. 2. the upper extremity of the cochlear duct.
lageniform flask-shaped.
Lagenorhyncus a genus that includes white-sided and white-nosed dolphins. See also DOLPHIN.
Lagochilascaris a genus of nematodes in the family Ascarididae.
L. minor found in wild felines and didelphoids (American opossums).
lagomorphs hares and rabbits, members of the order Lagomorpha.
lagophthalmos incomplete or defective closure of the eyelids.
geriatric l. may occur as a result of facial neuropathy or hypothyroidism.
l. keratitis see exposure KERATITIS.
Lagos virus a rhabdovirus found in bats that has serological similarities to, but significant differences from, the rabies virus.
Lagothrix see WOOLLY MONKEY.
Lahey forceps surgical forceps of several kinds.
L. hemostat forceps standard, straight or curved hemostats with ratcheted handles and cross-grooved blade faces.
L. traction forceps scissor-type forceps with ratcheted handles and in-turning, three-pronged blades that look like bent dinner forks.
lahiet el tis [Ar.] see PERRALDERIA CORONOPIFOLIA.
Lahore canine fever canine EHRLICHIOSIS.
Laikipia disease a progressive enzootic pneumonia of sheep which resembles maedi and jaagsiekte. Recorded only in Kenya. Called also laikipia disease.
lairage animal handling facilities at saleyards or abattoirs. Includes loading ramps, laneways, branding and injection chutes, weigh-scales, holding pens, drafting races, covered housing, waterpoints and feed bunkers.
LAK cells lymphokine-activated killer cells.
lake 1. to undergo separation of hemoglobin from erythrocytes. 2. a lacuna; a circumscribed collection of fluid in a hollow or depressed cavity.
lacrimal l. aee LACRIMAL lake.
lake trout SALVELINUS *namaycush*.
Lakeland terrier a small (17 lb) active dog with short, harsh coat in blue and tan or black and tan. The ears are small and folded over, the tail is docked to a medium length.
lakseersiekte [Af.] 'purging sickness' caused by ingestion of *Chrysocoma tenuifolia*; characterized by dysentery and rapid death.
lalobe see BALANITES AEGYPTICA.
Lama See LLAMA.
Lamarck's theory a discredited theory that acquired characteristics may be transmitted.
lamb young sheep still with its dam or up to 5 months of age. Qualified as ram or ewe lamb. In commercial usage may include much older animals, e.g in Europe.

l. dysentery a severe, highly fatal enteritis with diarrhea and dysentery in young lambs caused by *Clostridium welchii* type B.
l. industry includes stud flocks which produce rams of fat lamb breeds, e.g. Dorset Down, commercial farms breeding crossbred fat lamb mothers and fattening the lambs. The latter may be undertaken in feedlots or on special pasture fattening farms. Saleyards and sale rings, lamb abattoirs and wholesale outlets comprise the marketing side of the industry.
l. marking earmarking, castration and tail docking.
l. marking rate the percentage of lambs born which reach the stage of lamb marking. An index of lamb mortality rate.
l. poison see ISOTROPIS.
l's quarter CHENOPODIUM *album*.
l's tongue *Scleroblitum* (CHENOPODIUM) *atriplicinum*, PLANTAGO.

lamb mortality heavy death losses in a group of lambs.

lambda 1. the eleventh letter of the Greek alphabet, Λ or λ. 2. the point of union of the lambdoid and sagittal sutures of the cranium.
l. chain one of the two light chains of IMMUNOGLOBULINS; the other is κ.

lambdoid shaped like the Greek letter lambda, Λ or λ.

lambert crazyweed OXYTROPIS *lambertii*.

Lambertia Australian genus of shrubs in the family Proteaceae.
L. formosa has potential to be poisonous because of high content of cyanide. Called also honeysuckle, honeyflower, mountain devil.

lambing parturition in the ewe.
batch l. arranging for ewes to lamb in groups preselected on the basis of their breeding date. Maximizes use of labor in intensive lambing management aimed at minimizing losses of lambs at lambing.
drift l. as ewes in a big flock lamb they are moved off into other groups so that management can be intensified with the residue.
extensive l. the ewes are left to lamb unattended on extensive range. There is the least possible harassment, suitable for the timid merinos usually maintained in these conditions, but no opportunity to assist a ewe in trouble, an uncommon occurrence in this kind of sheep.
l. paralysis see MATERNAL obstetric paralysis.
l. rate numbers of lambs born per hundred ewes mated.
l. sickness see MILK fever.
l. stain a yellow-to-brown stain of the escutcheon and backs of the legs caused by placental fluids, an indication that the ewe has recently lambed. A valuable guide in the culling technique of wet-drying the ewes.

lambkill KALMIA *angustifolia*.

Lamblia see GIARDIA.

lambliasis giardiasis.

lambs' tail see ANREDERA CORDIFOLIA.

lame incapable of normal locomotion; deviation from the normal gait. The commonest cause of lameness in animals is pain in a limb or its supporting structures, but contractures of joints, and deformities and shortness of limbs are also causes.

lamella pl. *lamellae* [L.] 1. a thin scale or plate, as of bone. 2. a medicated disk or wafer to be inserted under the eyelid.
circumferential l. one of the bony plates that underlie the periosteum and endosteum.
concentric l. haversian lamella (see below).
endosteal l. one of the bony plates lying beneath the endosteum.
ground l. interstitial lamella (see below).
haversian l. one of the concentric bony plates surrounding a haversian canal.
intermediate l. one of the bony plates that fill in between the haversian systems; called also interstitial lamella.
interstitial l. see intermediate lamella (above).
intrasinusal l. incomplete partitions which divide the frontal sinus of the horse into a number of communicating diverticula.

lamellar pertaining to or emanating from lamella.
l. deflection the asymmetrical lateral force encounted when incising the cornea obliquely, which causes the incision to deviate towards a plane parallel to the lamellae.
l. phagosomes common degradation product in pigment epithelium.
l. suppuration pyogenic infection between the horn of the hoof and the sensitive laminae. See also HOOF abscess.

lamellibranch see BIVALVE.

lamellipodium pl. *lamellipodia* [L., Gr.] delicate sheetlike extension of cytoplasm that forms transient adhesions with the cell substrate and waves gently, enabling the cell to move along the substrate.

lameness the state of being lame.
complementary l. redistribution of weight from one painful leg can cause lameness in another, previously normal, leg.
fescue l. see FESTUCA.
regional l. lameness in a particular part of a limb, e.g. stifle lameness.
supporting leg l. discomfort is evident when the animal is standing or bearing weight on the leg.
swinging leg l. abnormality of movement, such as hitching or failure to flex a joint, is evident when the leg is in motion.
three-legged l. the animal does not put weight on one of its limbs.
weightbearing l. the lameness is not caused by movement of the limb but by putting weight on it.
whirlbone l. see trochanteric BURSITIS.

lamina pl. *laminae* [L.] a thin, flat plate or layer; a layer of a composite structure. Often used alone to mean a vertebral lamina.
l. basilaris the posterior wall of the cochlear duct, separating it from the scala tympani.
l. choroidocapillaris the inner layer of the choroid, composed of a single-layered network of small capillaries.
l. cribrosa 1. fascia cribrosa. 2. (of ethmoid bone) the sieve-like transverse plate of ethmoid bone forming the roof of the nasal cavity, and perforated by many foramina for passage of olfactory nerves. 3. (of sclera) the perforated part of the sclera through which pass the axons of the retinal ganglion cells to enter the optic nerve.
l. densa, l. dura a layer of dental alveolar bone containing more than usual amounts of highly calcified cementing substance, associated with periodontal fibers in the bone; causes lines of increased radiodensity in dental radiographs—hence the name.
epithelial l. the layer of ependymal cells covering the choroid plexus.
l. epithelialis mucosae the layer of epithelial cells on the surface of the mucosa.
l. femoralis that part of the aponeurosis of the external abdominal oblique muscle which continues the lateral lip of the superficial inguinal ring onto the

medial surface of the thigh in some species such as the horse.

l. fibroreticularis a thick layer of collagenous fibers projecting into the connective tissue space underlying the basement membrane.

l. fusca the loose connective tissue, deep, pigmentary layer of the sclera.

horny l. the laminae on the inside of the hoof which interdigitate with the sensitive laminae attached to the hoof corium.

l. limitans the layer of unmineralized matrix covering a bone surface that is not undergoing metabolic or structural change.

l. lucida the modified cell coat, appearing as a clear zone separating the basal lamina from the cell membrane.

l. mucosae includes laminae epithelialis mucosae (above), muscularis mucosae, propria mucosae (see below).

l. muscularis mucosae one or more smooth muscle layers, provides local mobility to the mucous membrane of organs; variable in occurrence.

omasal l. the leaves which line the internal aspect of the omasal wall; accounts for the colloquial name for the organ—bible; the religious connotation, if any, is unexplained.

l. propria, l. propria mucosae 1. the connective tissue layer of mucous membrane. 2. the middle fibrous layer of the tympanic membrane.

sensitive l. the laminae which interdigitate with the horny laminae of the hoof and which are made up of laminar corium plus a coat of not yet cornified epidermis.

spiral l., l. spiralis 1. a double plate of bone winding spirally around the modiolus, dividing the spiral canal of the cochlea into the scala tympani and scali vestibuli. 2. a bony projection on the outer wall of the cochlea in the lower part of the first turn.

terminal l. of hypothalamus the thin plate derived from the telencephalon, forming the anterior wall of the third ventricle of the cerebrum.

l. terminalis grisea thin plate forming the rostral wall of the third ventricle.

transverse l. separates the caudal part of the nasal cavity of the pig and dog into a ventral respiratory part and a dorsal olfactory part.

udder suspensory l. see UDDER suspensory apparatus.

vascular l. the vascular layer of the choroid of the eye; it lies between the suprachoroid and the choriocapillary layer.

vertebral l. either of the pair of broad plates of bone flaring out from the pedicles of the vertebral arches and fusing together at the midline to complete the dorsal part of the arch and provide a base for the spinous process.

laminagraphy see TOMOGRAPHY.

laminar made up of laminae or layers; pertaining to a lamina.

l. bone see laminar BONE.

l. cortical necrosis necrosis of the superficial layers of the cerebral cortex. See also POLIOENCEPHALOMALACIA.

l. dermis the sensitive laminae in the horse's hoof; interdigitate with the insensitive laminae on the inner aspect of the horn of the hoof.

l. flow the flow of liquid through a tube so that the fluid passes along in concentric layers which slide over each other.

laminated made up of laminae or thin layers.

lamination a laminar structure or arrangement.

laminectomy surgical excision of the dorsal arch of a vertebra. The procedure is most often performed to relieve the signs caused by a ruptured intervertebral disk or a space-occupying lesion that is compressing the spinal cord.

Funquist l. modifications of the procedure which include in type A, bilateral excision of both cranial and caudal articular processes and partial removal of the peduncles. In type B, these structures are preserved.

laminin a glycoprotein found in basement membrane.

laminitis a disease of horses, and rarely cattle, characterized by damage to the sensitive laminae of the hooves, and clinically by severe lameness, especially in the front hooves. There is heat and pain at the coronets and in bad cases protrusion of the third phalanx through the sole of the hoof. Most cases are caused by severe toxemia, as in engorgement on grain or metritis in the mare, and are called metabolic laminitis. Sporadic cases in heavily pregnant, overfat mares are referred to as puerperal laminitis. Some are caused by trauma, such as in pawing due to boredom or in horses transported over long distances without rest, and are called traumatic laminitis. Called also founder.

laminography a special technique of body-section radiography. See TOMOGRAPHY.

Laminosioptes a genus of mites in the family Laminosioptidae.

L. cysticola cause small, flat, oval nodules in the subcutaneous tissue of fowls. Called also cyst mites.

laminotomy transection of a vertebral lamina.

lamins fibrous proteins found in the polymeric network underlying the nuclear membrane.

Lamium amplexicaule toxic plant in family *Lamiaceae;* toxin unidentified; signs include hypersensitivity, tremor, incoordination, recumbency, sudden death. Called also henbit, dead nettle.

lamkruis [Af.] see SWAYBACK.

lamp an apparatus for furnishing heat or light.

slit l. one embodying a diaphragm containing a slit-like opening, by means of which a narrow, flat beam of intense light may be projected into the eye. It gives intense illumination so that microscopic study may be made of the conjunctiva, cornea, iris, lens and vitreous, the special feature being that it illuminates a section through the substance of these structures.

ultraviolet l. an electric light bulb that transmits ultraviolet rays; used as a therapeutic device. See also ULTRAVIOLET therapy.

lamp oil see PARAFFIN (2).

lampas inflammation of the mucosa of the hard palate, just posterior to the upper incisors. It may interfere with mastication and prehension. Called also palatitis.

lamtoro [Indonesian] the name given to the disease caused by the ingestion of *Leucaena leucocephala.*

lamziekte [Af.] *lame sickness;* botulism in cattle and sheep.

LANA test L-alanine-4-nitroanilide. A test for identification of gram-negative bacteria.

lanatoside C a glycoside obtained from *Digitalis lanata*, used as a cardiotonic like digitalis.

Lancashire an older British breed of canaries; it comes in crested (Coppies) and Plainhead varieties.

Lancashire heeler a small, low set cattle working dog which also hunts rabbits and rats like a terrier. The length of coat varies from season to season; the color is black with tan markings. Called also Ormskirk terrier or heeler.

lance 1. lancet. 2. to cut or incise with a lancet.

Lancefield classification the classification of streptococci into groups on the basis of cell wall antigen. Each group is indicated by a letter from A to V. Some species are antigenically heterogeneous.

lanceolate fluke see OPISTHORCHIS *tenuicollis*.

lancet a small, pointed, two-edged surgical knife.

l. fluke see DICROCOELIUM *dendriticum*.

Landrace a large white pig with ears pitched forwards and top edge level with topline of snout. There are many ethnic varieties. Originated in Denmark.

Landry's paralysis see GUILLAIN–BARRÉ SYNDROME.

landscape the position of a page of paper in which the longer margin is horizontal.

Landseer a black and white NEWFOUNDLAND dog, recognized as a separate breed in Europe.

Lane forceps designed for holding bones, these heavyweight forceps have long ratcheted handles and a curled-up handle end to facilitate traction. The blades enclose a diamond-shaped aperture when closed and have deep spikes.

Langat virus a tick-borne flavivirus isolated in Malaysia, closely related to other viruses that cause louping ill.

Langenbeck retractor a simple handheld instrument with a flat blade bent down at right angles to the handle. Useful for temporary retraction of soft tissue.

Langerhans' cell dendritic cell in the skin that functions in the processing of antigen. See also dendritic CELL.

Langerhans' islets see ISLETS of Langerhans.

Langhans' giant cell a multinucleated giant cell in which the nuclei form a circle or semicircle at the periphery of the cell.

langouste see PANULIRUS.

Langshan black dual-purpose poultry breed. There are two types: a smaller, egg-laying Chinese type; and a larger, Croad type used for meat production. All black in color, but with a bright green iridescence on the hackle, wing and tail feathers. Single comb, and feathers on legs.

language see COMPUTER language.

langur large, slim monkey without prehensile tail. Member of the genus *Presbytis* in the family Circopithecidae, the Old World monkeys.

Lankesterella a genus of protozooan parasites of lymphocytes and monocytes of birds.

lanolin wool fat or wool grease that is refined and incorporated into many commercial preparations. Lanolin is a by-product of the process that accompanies the removal of sheeps' wool from the pelt. In its crude form it is a greasy yellow wax of unpleasant odor which disappears when the lanolin is emulsified and made into salves, creams, ointments and cosmetics. Although lanolin is slightly antiseptic, it has no other medicinal benefits and is valuable principally because of the ease with which it penetrates the skin, and because it does not become rancid.

l. bush ZIERIA *smithii*.

lanosterol one of the substances formed during the synthesis of cholesterol.

lantadene lantadene A and B are triterpene cholestatic poisons in LANTANA *camara*.

Lantana genus of South American plants in the family Verbenaceae; some contain toxic triterpenes, lantadenes, potent hepatoxins; cause severe jaundice and photosensitization. Include *L. achyranthifolia*, *L. aculeata*, *L. camara*, *L. montevidensis* (*L. sellowiana*, creeping lantana), *L. ovatifolia*, *L. vetulina*; of these only *L. camara* is well recognized as being pathogenic. Sloughing skin of the muzzle leaves a raw pink surface giving rise to the name 'pink nose'.

lanthanum a chemical element, atomic number 57, atomic weight 138.91, symbol La. See Table 6.

lanugo see lanugo HAIR.

laparo- word element. [Gr.] *loin* or *flank, abdomen*.

laparocystidotomy incision of the urinary bladder through the abdominal wall.

laparohysterotomy see CESAREAN SECTION.

laparorrhaphy suture of the abdominal wall.

laparoscope an endoscope for examining the peritoneal cavity.

laparoscopic examination examination of the peritoneal cavity using a laparoscope.

laparoscopy examination of the peritoneal cavity by means of the laparoscope.

laparotomy incision through the flank or, more generally, through any part of the abdominal wall.

exploratory l. for the purpose of physically examining the contents of the peritoneal cavity.

l. grid see grid INCISION.

lapinization serial passage of a virus through rabbits to modify its characteristics. e.g. rinderpest virus.

lapinize to attenuate (as a virus for use as a vaccine) by serial passage through rabbits.

Laplace's law a law that, like the BERNOULLI PRINCIPLE, accounts for the higher wall tension in an arterial aneurysm.

Laportea moroides DENDROCNIDE *moroides*.

lappets lobe-like structures, e.g. the wattles of a fowl.

lard commercially retrieved pig fat.

larder beetle see DERMESTES *lardarius*.

large dimensionally big.

l. bietou *Dimorphotheca acuneata*. See also OSTEOSPERMUM.

l. chicken louse see GONIODES *gigas*.

l. intestine see CECUM (1), COLON, RECTUM.

l. leaved lupine LUPINUS *polyphyllus*.

l. liver fluke see FASCIOLOIDES *magna*, FASCIOLA *gigantica*.

l. roundworm in swine called *Ascaris suum*.

l. stomach worm see HAEMONCHUS.

l. strongyles in horses are *Strongylus vulgaris*, *S. edentatus*, *S. equinus*; in donkeys *S. asini*.

Large black a breed of black, lop-eared pig. Called also British black.

Large Munsterlander a medium to large sized, muscular gun dog with a medium length white coat with black patches, flecks or speckles. The tail may be long or docked and the ears are pendulous, lying close to the head. A smaller variety is recognized as a separate breed in Europe.

large-scale farms the modern trend to enlarge farms to reach optimal size as a business enterprise rather than as a unit size suited to single family management.

Large white pig a breed of white, prick-eared pig, with a long face and straight nose. Called also Large white Yorkshire.

Large white Ulster pig extinct meat and lard, lop-eared pig, from Northern Ireland.

Large White Yorkshire pig see LARGE WHITE PIG.

largemouth bass see MICROPTERUS SALMOIDES.

lariat lasso.

larkspur see DELPHINIUM.

Larus see SEAGULL.

larva an independent, immature stage in a life cycle in which the stage is unlike the parent and must undergo changes in form and size to reach the adult stage. There may be one or several, three is common, larval stages in the one life cycle. In fish larvae are also called fry.

l. currens a variant of larva migrans caused by

Strongyloides stercoralis, in which the linear progress of the lesions is much more rapid.
cutaneous l. migrans creeping eruption; a convoluted, thread-like skin eruption in humans and other species which appears to migrate; caused by the burrowing beneath the skin of roundworm larvae, particularly *Ancylostoma*, *Strongyloides* and *Gnathostoma* spp. *A. braziliense*, *A. caninum*, *B. phlebotomum* can cause the disease.
ocular l. migrans infection of the eye with the larvae of the roundworm *Toxocara canis* or *T. cati*, which may lodge in the choroid or retina or migrate to the vitreous; on the death of the larvae, a granulomatous inflammation occurs, the lesion varying from a translucent elevation of the retina to massive retinal detachment and pseudoglioma.
visceral l. migrans a condition due to prolonged migration of larvae of animal nematodes in human tissues other than skin, commonly caused by larvae of the roundworms *Toxocara canis* and *T. cati*.

larval 1. pertaining to larvae. 2. larvate.
l. migrans see cutaneous and visceral LARVA migrans.

larval mycosis opportunistic infections in larval crustaceans by marine water molds *Lagenidium* and *Sirolpidium* spp.

larvate masked; concealed: said of a disease or of a clinical sign of a disease.

larvicide an agent that kills insect larvae.

laryngalgia pain in the larynx.

laryngeal pertaining to the larynx.
l. adductory reflex, adduction test slapping of the saddle region of a horse just behind the withers causes a flickering, adductory movement of the contralateral arytenoid cartilage in normal horses. The movement of the cartilage can be viewed endoscopically. The reflex is abolished by damage to the adductory component of the recurrent laryngeal nerve, by lesions in the spinal cord in the anterior thoracic region and by excitement. Called also slap test.
l. airsacculitis inflammation of the large air sacs found attached to the larynx in great apes.
l. cartilage includes EPIGLOTTIS, THYROID, CRICOID, and the paired ARYTENOID cartilages.
l. chondritis necrosis and ulceration of laryngeal mucosa caudal to the vocal cords; seen in calves and especially in Texel and Southdown sheep.
l. chondroma can cause laryngeal obstruction in horses.
l. collapse a cause of upper airway obstruction, particularly in brachycephalic dogs.
l. congenital anomalies epiglottal hypoplasia (horse, pig) is a rare anomaly.
l. contact ulcers are ulcerative lesions which develop at the site of minor abrasions caused by frequent contact and rubbing of the epiglottis and arytenoid cartilages.
l. edema a part of acute inflammation of the laryngeal mucosa due to infection, allergy or inhalation of irritant materials. It causes obstruction to air flow, stertor, dyspnea and potentially asphyxia.
everted l. saccules the laryngeal saccules protrude into the lumen of the larynx, become edematous and cause upper airway obstruction with increased inspiratory effort.
l. fremitus a vibration palpable at the throat with partial obstruction of the larynx.
l. hemiplegia unilateral paralysis, called also roaring, is a common condition in horses, causing a reduction in exercise tolerance and a loud stertor at exercise. Bilateral paralysis causes a more severe but similar syndrome.
l. mound a conspicuous mound in the throat of birds; carries the entrance to the larynx.
l. necrobacillosis the principal lesion in calf diphtheria.
l. necrosis occurs in outbreaks in feedlot steers at the site of contact ulcers on the larynx. The common bacteria in the lesions is *Fusobacterium necrophorum*.
l. neoplasm includes chondroma, papilloma.
l. neuropathy dysfuction, most commonly unilateral hemiplegia, of the recurrent layngeal nerve; see ROARING.
l. obstruction may be acute or chronic, with signs varying to match. Stertor, inspiratory dyspnea and local signs, such as pain, swelling and the presence of foreign bodies, constitute the clinical syndrome.
l. papilloma occurs in feedlot steers at the site of contact ulcers on the larynx.
l. paralysis can result from lesions of the vagus or recurrent laryngeal nerves, and may be acquired or congenital. It is seen in association with hypothyroidism in dogs. An inherited laryngeal paralysis occurs in the Bouvier des Flandres breed of dogs, causing varying degrees of noisy respirations and upper airway obstruction from several months of age. In immature Dalmation dogs it is seen as part of a more widespread polyneuropathy with megaesophagus, neurologic deficits. See also laryngeal hemiplegia (above).
l. polyp recorded in horses in association with *Besnoitia* spp. infection.
l. pyriform recesses permit the grazing ruminant to breathe, and to sniff the air, while eating and ruminating.
l. saccule the lining of the laryngeal ventricle.
l. sounds the normal sounds of air going in and out past the larynx, as heard with a stethoscope. When there is stenosis the sounds are loud and harsh, also called stertor; with catarrhal inflammation they are gurgling.
l. spasm a reflex constriction of the larynx because of contact with foreign material being inhaled or during administration of a gaseous anesthetic, especially in cats. May cause asphyxiation.
l. sphincteric girdle the muscles that constrict the laryngeal opening, and the cricoarytenoid, transverse arytenoid and thyroarytenoid muscles.
l. stenosis may follow laryngeal surgery, injury (particularly prolonged intubation), or infection; granulation tissue and cartilage degeneration and collapse can cause a progressive reduction in the airway.
l. stertor loud breath sounds caused by a narrowing of the laryngeal lumen.
l. ulceration common subclinical lesion in feedlot cattle; lesions are at points of apposition of vocal processes and medial angles of arytenoid processes.
l. ventricle a bilateral outpocketing of the laryngeal mucosa in the dog, pig and horse. In the dog and the horse they are between the vocal and vestibular folds in the lateral walls of the laryngeal vestibule. In the pig they are in the lateral wall of the glottis.
l. ventriculectomy removal of the mucosa lining the relevant laryngeal ventricle as a treatment of laryngeal hemiplegia in horses.
l. vestibule the short space from the entrance to the larynx to the rima glottidis.

laryngectomy partial or total removal of the larynx by surgery.

laryngemphraxis obstruction or closure of the larynx.

laryngeoplasty plastic procedure on the larynx such as cricoarytenoid fixation with an elastic prosthesis for roaring in horses. See also LYCRA.

laryngismus spasm of the larynx.
l. stridulus sudden laryngeal spasm with crowing inspiration.
laryngitis inflammation of the mucous membrane of the larynx, characterized by cough, pain on palpation over the larynx, dysphagia, and possibly regurgitation through the nose; usually there are other signs of inflammation of the upper respiratory tract.
necrotic l. see calf DIPHTHERIA.
laryng(o)- word element. [Gr.] *larynx*.
laryngocele a congenital anomalous air sac communicating with a cavity of the larynx; it may produce a tumor-like lesion visible on the outside of the neck.
laryngocentesis surgical puncture of the larynx, with aspiration.
laryngoenteritis see FELINE panleukopenia.
laryngofissure median laryngotomy.
laryngogram a radiograph of the larynx.
laryngography radiography of the larynx.
laryngology that branch of the clinical sciences that has to do with the throat, pharynx, larynx, nasopharynx and tracheobronchial tree.
laryngopathy any disorder of the larynx.
laryngopharyngeal pertaining to the larynx and pharynx.
laryngopharyngitis inflammation of the larynx and pharynx.
laryngopharynx the caudal portion of the pharynx opening into the larynx and esophagus.
laryngophony the vocal sound heard in auscultating the larynx.
laryngoplegia paralysis of the larynx.
laryngorhinology the branch of the clinical sciences that deals with the larynx and nose.
laryngorrhaphy suture of the larynx.
laryngoscleroma scleroma of the larynx.
laryngoscope an endoscope equipped with a blade to depress the tongue, and light and mirrors for illumination and examination of the larynx.
Rowson l. one with a blade designed for use in large animals.
laryngoscopy direct visual examination of the larynx with a laryngoscope.
laryngospasm spasmodic closure of the larynx.
laryngostenosis narrowing or stricture of the larynx.
laryngostomy surgical creation of an artificial opening into the larynx.
laryngotomy incision of the larynx.
laryngotracheal pertaining to the larynx and trachea.
l. aspiration inhalation of oral, pharyngeal or gastric contents.
laryngotracheitis inflammation of the larynx and trachea.
infectious avian l. see INFECTIOUS laryngotracheitis (ILT).
laryngotracheobronchitis see EQUINE influenza.
laryngotracheotomy incision of the larynx and trachea.
laryngoxerosis dryness of the larynx.
larynx pl. *larynges* [Gr.] the muscular and cartilaginous structure, lined with mucous membrane, situated at the cranial end of the trachea and behind the root of the tongue and the hyoid bone. The larynx contains the vocal cords, and is responsible for vocalization; it is called also the voice box. It is part of the respiratory system, and air passes through the larynx as it travels from the pharynx to the trachea and back again on its way to and from the lungs.

The larynx is composed of nine cartilages (thyroid, cricoid and epiglottis, and the paired arytenoid, corniculate and cuneiform) held together by muscles and ligaments.
lasalocid a polyether ionophore related chemically to monensin, used as a growth promotant in cattle and coccidiostat in chickens. It is relatively nontoxic but gross overdosage of cattle causes acute heart failure. Horses are very susceptible and the use of the compound in them is prohibited. Animals may be found dead or show dyspnea, mucosal congestion, diarrhea and cardiac irregularity and tachycardia.
laser a device which generates an extremely intense, small and nearly nondivergent beam of monochromatic radiation in the visible region, with all the waves in phase; capable of mobilizing immense heat and power when focused at close range, it is used as a tool in surgery, in diagnosis, in physiological studies, in computer printers, and storage devices and in the long-distance transmission of information in a high capacity medium. Laser is an acronym for *l*ight *a*mplification by *s*timulated *e*mission of *r*adiation.

Used also as a modern version of acupuncture and considered to be the biggest breakthrough in that technology for 5000 years. It provides a quick, painless and noninvasive method of point stimulation.
argon l. used in ophthalmic surgery and in photodynamic surgery of the skin.
carbon dioxide l. used in microsurgery and ophthalmic procedures.
l. therapy in acupuncture the application of low intensity laser to acupuncture points.
lash the horsehair or thin leather tag attached to the end of a stockwhip and which is responsible for the pistol shot-like report produced by the gun whip crackers.
lasiocarpine one of the potent pyrrolizidine alkaloid hepatoxins in the plant *Heliotropum europaeum*.
Lasiosiphon see GNIDIA.
Lasiospermum bipinnatum South African plant in the family Asteraceae. It contains a furanosesquiterpene and causes photosensitization. Called also ganskweek.
Lasix a proprietary name for furosemide.
lasolocid see IONOPHORE.
Lassa fever virus a highly fatal, hemorrhagic disease of humans caused by an arenavirus transmitted from certain rodents.
lassitude weakness; exhaustion.
lasso stiff manila, cotton or rawhide rope suitable for making a noose at the end. Called also lariat. The loop is thrown around the animal's neck or one or more legs while working the cattle on the range or in stockyards. Usually used from horseback and exerting a strong pull by locking the rope around the horn on the pommel of the saddle, or by using a harness when working in yards. A quick-release HONDA used to make the loop is an advantage when loosing a wild animal.

The lasso is used while on foot by a horsebreaker wanting to reach the first hands-on step in the breaking-in process.
latamoxef see MOXALACTAM.
late bloom said of mature plants at the stage where the flowers have fallen off.
latebra part of a bird's egg. Includes a ball of white yolk in the center of the yellow yolk, connected by a neck to the latebral disk, an inverted cone of white yolk, lying under the blastodisk at the surface of the yellow yolk.
latency a state of being hidden.
latent dormant or concealed; not manifest; potential. See also latent IMAGE, INFECTION.

l. period a seemingly inactive period, as that between exposure of tissue to an injurious agent and the manifestations of response, or that between the instant of stimulation and the beginning of response. The latent period in virus replication defines the period from adsorption, penetration and uncoating of the virus until the first progeny virus are released from the cell.

laterad toward the lateral aspect.

lateral 1. denoting a position farther from the median plane or midline of the body or a structure; the side or outside. 2. pertaining to a side.

l. aids used by the rider to move a horse sideways; pressure by the neck rein and the thigh and calf on the same side at the same time.

l. body folds folds which commence at the head, then at the tail eventually meeting at the umbilicus; the folds gradually separate the embryo from the extraembryonic tissues.

l. collateral ligament lateral ligaments of many joints, e.g. the femorotibial articulation.

l. decubitus lateral recumbency.

l. geniculate nucleus a terminal and relay station for optical nerve fibers within the thalamus, beneath the lateral geniculate body.

l. mesoderm or lateral plate mesoderm; mesoderm which extends (a) around the embryonal gut and (b) inside the surface ectoderm to enclose the celom between these splanchnic and parietal layers respectively.

l. nasal process a process which borders the nasal pit, eventually the nostril, and which is derived from the embryo's frontonasal mesenchyme.

l. palatine processes processes which grow out from the maxillary processes and grow into the oronasal cavity, eventually fusing with each other and the medial palatine process and the nasal septum to form the embryo's hard palate.

lateralis [L.] *lateral.*

lateroduction movement of an eye to either side.

lateroflexion flexion to one side.

laterotorsion twisting of the vertical meridian of the eye to either side.

lateroversion abnormal turning to one side.

Lates calcarifer farmed finfish in the family Centropomatidae. Called also barramundi, giant sea perch. See Table 23.

lathyrism a morbid condition of humans marked by spastic paraplegia, pain, hyperesthesia and paresthesia, due to ingestion of the seeds of leguminous plants of the genus *Lathyrus*, which includes many kinds of peas.

In animals there are reports of two basic groups of disease, *neurolathyrism*, including transient laryngeal paralysis in horses associated with degenerative changes in the vagus and recurrent laryngeal nerves, and *osteolathyrism* manifested by a variety of skeletal changes. Hepatitis, splenitis and dissecting aortic aneurysm are also recorded.

lathyrogen plant toxin in *Lathyrus* spp. causing lathyrism; includes 3-aminopropionitrile.

lathyrogenic pertaining to or emanating from lathyrogen.

Lathyrus genus of plants in legume family Fabaceae; toxin is 3-aminopropionitrile; causes neurological disease, including excitability, convulsions and death without skeletal lesions; includes *L. angulatus*, *L. aphaca*, *L. cicera*, *L. clymenum*, *L. hookeri*, *L. latifolius*, *L. nissolia* (grass vetchling), *L. polymorphus* subsp. *incanus*, *L. pusillus* (singletary pea), *L. sativus*, *L. splendens* (Pride of California), *L. sylvestris*, *L. tingitatus* (Tangier pea).

L. hirsutus causes poisoning in cattle, the main sign being lameness due to pain in the feet. Called also Kaley pea, wild winter pea, Indian pea.

L. odoratus the ornamental sweetpea, of which the seeds cause skeletal abnormality when fed experimentally; may cause equine STRINGHALT.

Laticaudinae one of the two families of sea snakes. Includes *Laticauda colubrina*. Sea snakes are amongst the most venomous reptiles.

Latin terminology used originally as the international language of scholars, and persisted with in some areas, e.g. pharmacy. Its universal usage in botanical, bacteriological and parasitological nomenclature ensures its continuation.

latissimus [L.] *widest, a broad structure.*

l. dorsi the broad muscle of the back that serves to retract the forelimb.

latrodectism intoxication due to venom of spiders of the genus *Latrodectus.*

Latrodectus a genus of poisonous spiders belonging to the dipneumomorph family Theridiidae.

L. hasseltii the Australian redback spider, an ecological variant of *L. mactans* and with the same toxicity.

L. mactans a species found in the United States; commonly known as the black widow. In New Zealand called katipo. Satiny black with a broad sagittal red stripe in the female, which is venomous. Its bite may cause severe local pain and general paralysis.

lattice a pattern of regularly placed, narrow, intersecting strips, such as the geometric atomic arrangement in a crystal, as seen in x-ray analysis.

l. theory the interaction of multivalent antigen with multivalent antibody will, at optimum proportions of each (zone of equivalence), result in the formation of a lattice and a precipitate. In the zone of equivalence all antibody and antigen are bound in the lattice. With an excess of either antigen or antibody, the lattice is incomplete or disassembled so that the amount of precipitate is reduced; the basis for precipitin tests.

latus [L.] 1. broad, wide. 2. the side or flank.

Latvian brown cattle brown to dark red meat and draft cattle.

laudanum tincture of opium.

laughing gas nitrous oxide.

laughing jackass see KOOKABURRA.

Laurelia novae-zealandiae New Zealand plant of the family Monimiaceae; contains an unidentified toxin; causes tremor, sudden death. Called also pukatea.

lavage 1. irrigation or washing out of an organ or cavity, as of the stomach or intestine. 2. to wash out, or irrigate. See also WASH.

abdominal l. the infusion of saline into the peritoneal cavity, usually through a catheter inserted through the abdominal wall, for diagnostic purposes. The fluid returned may be examined for red blood cells, bacteria, enzymes, etc. Called also peritoneal lavage.

bronchoalveolar l. percutaneous entry of a catheter between tracheal rings, followed by infusion of a small volume of normal sterile saline which is then aspirated. The sample is submitted to microbiological and histopathological examination.

colonic l. irrigation of the colon, usually to remove ingested toxins.

gastric l. gastric lavage, or irrigation of the stomach, is usually done to remove ingested poisons. The solutions used for gastric lavage are physiological saline, 1% sodium bicarbonate, plain water or a specific antidote for the poison. A gastric tube is passed and then the irrigating fluid is funneled into the tube. It is allowed to flow into the stomach by gravity. The solution is removed by siphonage; when the funnel is lowered, the fluid flows out, bringing with it the contents of the stomach. Called also gavage.

ice water l. administration of ice water through a stomach tube is used in the treatment of acute upper gastrointestinal hemorrhage. There is a risk of inducing hypothermia.

ruminal l. used in the treatment of carbohydrate engorgement. Serial gavages are performed until the fluid comes back clear. A 2.5 in (6 cm) diameter Kingman tube is necessary if any bulk of material is to be retrieved and a hose from a tap is the only practical irrigating mechanism.

subpalpebral l. a method of medicating the eye, particularly useful in treating corneal ulcerations in horses. Tubing is inserted from the conjunctival sac through the upper eyelid and extended onto the head or neck. Medication can then be delivered continuously in a drip.

thoracic l. irrigation of a pleural sac via a paracentesis cannula.

lavender foal see Arabian FADING syndrome.

laventelbos LIPPIA *rhemannii.*

law 1. natural law; a uniform or constant fact or principle in nature. 2. legal law; the laws of persons, developed so that social contacts between individuals can be managed on a basis of mutual understanding and agreement.

adversarial l. (2) system arguments are settled by having each opponent, one of whom is often the state, argue his/her case before a court, which decides the outcome, often on the basis of precedent in previous similar cases.

l. (1) of the circle the radiographic principle on which localization of a radioopaque foreign body can be specified exactly. It depends on taking the x-rays at right angles to each other, a ventrodorsal and a lateral.

civil l. (2) see inquisitorial law (below).

common l. (2) the law of common usage, in which principles are derived from case law and the judgments made in actual cases.

English l. (2) the original common law system.

l. (1) of independent assortment the members of gene pairs segregate independently during meiosis. See also MENDEL'S LAWS.

inquisitorial l. (2) system the basis of Roman law. The court questions each of the adversaries in an argument and decides the outcome on the basis of the code layed down.

l. (1) of mass action the rate of a reversible reaction, in either direction, is proportional to the concentrations of the reacting substances.

private l. (2) law relating to the conduct of individuals, e.g. contract, divorce, matrimonial, property law.

public l. (2) the law relating to group conduct, especially the state and its criminal, industrial and constitutional law, but also corporation law.

Roman l. (2) law by application of an elaborate written code, the basis for most European law. It is an inquisitorial law system.

l. (1) of segregation in each generation the ratio of (1) pure dominants, (2) dominants giving descendants in the proportion of three dominants to one recessive, and (3) pure recessives is 1 : 2 : 1. This ratio follows from the fact that the two alleles of a gene cannot be a part of a single gamete, but must segregate to different gametes. See also MENDEL'S LAWS.

statute l. (2) that part of an English law system that is set down in statutes or law established by Act of Parliament of the day.

lawrencium a chemical element, atomic number 103, atomic weight 257, symbol Lw. See Table 6.

Lawsonia intracellulare bacterial cause of porcine proliferative enteropathy. An obligately intracellular gram-negative, curved rod; may also cause proliferative enteropathy in foals and white-tailed deer.

laxative a medicine that loosens the bowel contents and encourages evacuation. A laxative with a mild or gentle effect on the bowels is also known as an aperient; one with a strong effect is referred to as a CATHARTIC or a PURGATIVE.

bulk l. hydrophilic, indigestible substances that absorb water and swell to form an emollient gel. The distension of the intestine stimulates defecation.

contact l. see stimulant laxative.

emollient l. the fecal softeners; act without being changed and simply aid expulsion by softening and lubricating. Called also lubricant laxative.

lubricant l. see emollient laxative (above).

stimulant l. stimulate accumulation of water and electrolytes in the colon, increasing intestinal motility. Called also contact laxative.

laxator that which slackens or relaxes.

laxity looseness. Used to describe the hyperextensibility of skin, and sometimes joints, in cutaneous ASTHENIA and EHLERS–DANLOS SYNDROME.

layer 1. stratum; a sheetlike mass of tissue of nearly uniform thickness, several of which may be superimposed, one above the other, as in the epidermis. 2. a commercial fowl which is laying eggs, i.e. a female of more than about 5 months of age, up to the stage of being a 'spent hen' suitable only for slaughter.

basal l. 1. the deepest layer of the epidermis. See also STRATUM basale. 2. the deepest layer of the uterine mucosa.

blastodermic l. germ layer (see below).

clear l. stratum lucidum; the clear translucent layer of the epidermis, just beneath the horny layer.

columnar l. 1. layer of rods and cones. 2. mantle layer.

compact l. the layer of the endometrium nearest the surface, containing the necks of the uterine glands.

functional l. the compact and spongy layers of the endometrium considered together.

cerebellar ganglionic l. the thin middle gray layer of the cortex of the cerebellum, consisting of a single layer of Purkinje cells.

germ l. any of the three primary layers of cells formed in the early development of the embryo (ectoderm, entoderm and mesoderm), from which the organs and tissues develop.

germinative l. any proliferative layer such as the basal layer of the epidermis or the lower layer of the claw, from which the claw grows.

granular l. 1. the layer of epidermis between the clear and prickle-cell layers; called also stratum granulosum. 2. the deep layer of the cortex of the cerebellum. 3. the layer of follicle cells lining the theca of the vesicular ovarian follicle.

horny l. 1. stratum corneum; the outermost layer of the epidermis, consisting of dead and desquamating cells. 2. the outer, compact layer of the claw, etc.

keratohyaline l. granular layer (1).

mantle l. the middle layer of the wall of the primitive neural tube, containing primitive nerve cells and later forming the gray matter of the central nervous system.

nervous l. all of the retina except the pigment layer; the inner layer of the optic cup.

prickle-cell l. stratum spinosum; the layer of the epidermis between the granular and basal layers, marked by the presence of prickle cells.

l. of rods and cones a layer of the retina immediately beneath the pigment epithelium, between it and the external limiting membrane, containing the rods and cones.

spinous l. prickle-cell layer.

spongy l. the middle layer of the endometrium, containing the tortuous portions of the uterine glands.

subendocardial l. the layer of loose fibrous tissue uniting the endocardium and myocardium.

zonal l. of thalamus a layer of myelinated fibers covering the dorsal surface of the thalamus.

lazy leukocyte syndrome decreased responsiveness of leukocytes in chemotactic assays.

lb [L.] *libra* (pound); pound weight avoirdupois.

LCAT latex cryptococcal antigen test; antibody coated latex beads used to detect polysaccharide antigens of *Cryptococcus neoformans* in body fluids.

LCL bodies a collection of elementary bodies and other replicative forms observed particularly in hepatocytes prepared as impression smears; characteristic of psittacosis, caused by *Chlamydia psittaci.*

LCM lymphocytic choriomeningitis.

LCR ligase chain reaction. See also PCR.

LD 1. lethal dose. 2. lactate dehydrogenase.

LD_{50} median lethal dose; the dose that will kill 50% of the tested group.

LDA left displacement of the abomasum.

LDH lactic acid dehydrogenase; see lactate DEHYDROGENASE.

LDL low-density lipoprotein.

LDL receptors specialized receptor proteins for binding low-density lipoproteins; clustered on the plasma membrrane in a structure called a coated pit, an invagination containing the protein clathrin. On binding with LDL, the plasma membrane fuses near the receptor–LDL complex and the coated pit becomes an endocytotic vesicle which is transported into the cell, fuses with the lysosomes enabling contact between the LDL–receptor complex and hydrolytic enzymes of the lysosomes.

LE lupus erythematosus.

LE cell test see LUPUS ERYTHEMATOSUS phenomenon.

lead[1] a chemical element, atomic number 82, atomic weight 207.19, symbol Pb. See Table 6.

l. acetate sugar of lead, formed on lead paint surfaces after much weathering; it is palatable and attracts animals to lick the surface, causing lead poisoning.

l. acetate paper strips detect hydrogen sulfide gas formation and used as a test for *Brucella* spp.

l. arsenate used as an insecticidal and fungistatic spray in orchards; capable of causing arsenic poisoning.

l. carbonate white lead used in paints.

l. chromate used in paints as a hardener and coloring agent.

l. equivalent measurement of the protective efficiency of clothing and other materials against x-rays, in terms based on comparison with lead sheeting of specific thickness.

l. letters used as markers on x-ray films.

l. poisoning a form of poisoning caused by the presence of lead or lead salts in the body. Lead poisoning affects the brain, nervous system, blood and digestive system. It can be either chronic or acute. This is a common finding in cattle and in urban dogs because of the frequent presence of lead in the environment in lead paints, and the sweet taste of the paint when it is weathered.

Adult animals show a subacute syndrome of severe depression, aimless walking, blindness, complete ruminal stasis and a black diarrhea in small amounts. Calves show violent convulsions and death within a few hours.

Poisoning can result from swallowing paint flakes or chewing surfaces covered with lead-based paints, golf balls, newsprint, linoleum, fishing sinkers, or numerous other household objects containing lead. Clinical signs usually include abdominal pain, vomiting, diarrhea and seizures. Basophilic stippling of red blood cells, nucleated red blood cells, and a moderate anemia are characteristic.

l. protective clothing aprons and gloves containing lead and worn as protection against scattered x-irradiation.

red l. tri-plumbic tetroxide.

l. shot see LEAD poisoning.

l. sulfide form of lead found in the ore galena.

l. weights made of metallic lead, used in window sashes, can cause poisoning.

lead[2] 1. in electrocardiography, a specific array (pair) of electrodes used in recording changes in electric potential, created by the activity of an organ, such as the heart (electrocardiography) or brain (electroencephalography); applied also to the particular segment of the tracing produced by the potential registered through the specific electrodes; in electrocardiography, lead I records the potential differences between the two forelimbs, lead II between the right forelimb and left hindlimb, and lead III between the left forelimb and left hindlimb, and a fourth lead from various sites over the chest. 2. for attachment to a collar to facilitate walking a dog.

bipolar l. an array involving two electrodes placed at different body sites.

esophageal l. one attached to an electrode inserted in the esophagus.

l. feeding see challenge FEEDING.

invasive l's those placed within the body, e.g. esophageal and intracardiac leads. They may be more useful in identification of certain arrhythmias and in pacing the heart for diagnostic and therapeutic purposes.

orthogonal l's measures three axes, left to right, head to tail, and vertebral column to sternum.

precordial l's leads recording electric potential from various sites over the heart, designated V with a subscript numeral indicating the exact site.

l. time the time that must elapse between coming to a decision and actually putting the decision into operation.

unipolar l. an array of two electrodes, only one of which transmits potential variations.

lead tree see LEUCAENA *leucocephala*.

leaden entoloma a mushroom causing gastroenteritis in humans. Called also *Entoloma lividum*.

leader sequence the nontranslated section of mRNA before the coding region.

leading leg the last hoof to reach the ground in the three-beat cadence. The first is one of the hinds, then the other hind and its diagonal fore together, then the leading fore; the hoof that reaches out the furthest in front in the foot pattern.

leaf terminal outgrowths of plant foliage, usually flat green blades that conduct the plants' photosynthesis. Of the foliage it is much the most nutritious part and is often incorporated into special feeds, e.g. lucerne leaf meal.

l. intestinal impaction impaction of the cecum and colon in horses with access to indigestible tree leaves.

l. mustard BRASSICA *juncea.*

leafing separation, collapse and rounding of lung lobes caused by the presence of pleural effusion. Lung lobes appear as small, relatively radiolucent 'leaves' against a homogeneous background of pleural fluid.

lean tissue muscle tissue without fat.

leaning leaning against fixed objects, associated with frequent falling; an indication of loss of balance and of a lesion of the vestibular apparatus.

learning learning is remembering associations. A memory is essential to learning and animals have both a memory and the ability to learn in variable degrees. There are a number of ways in which learning can be achieved or facilitated: imprinting, especially of the neonate; conditioning, including simple association and instrumental and avoidance conditioning; operant conditioning; visceral learning; discriminative learning; generalization of stimuli; and habituation.

discriminative l. the basis of Pavlovian research; teaching animals to choose the correct behavioral response by a positively reinforcing reward when they do.

least cost ration the ration that fulfils all of the nutritional requirements of the particular group of animals but uses the mix of ingredients from the list of those available that costs the least.

least squares a method of regression analysis. The line on a graph that best summarizes the relationship between two variables is the one that ensures that there is the least value of the sum of the squares of the deviation between the fitted curve and each of the original data points.

leather 1. the ear flap; pinna. 2. a product made by tanning the dermal layer of ox hide, sheep pelt, pig skin, horse hide and other more exotic skins, including emu, ostrich, alligator and the like.

l. chewing common form of pica in horses kept indoors.

leather bottle lesion see LINITIS plastica.

lecheguilla see AGAVE *lecheguilla.*

lechiguana Brazilian disease of cattle characterized by multiple subcutaneous granuloma populated by *Pasteurella granulomatis.*

lecithin any of a group of phospholipids found in animal tissues, especially nerve tissue, the liver, semen and egg yolk, consisting of esters of glycerol with two molecules of long-chain aliphatic acids and one of phosphoric acid, the latter being esterified with the alcohol group of choline.

lecithinase an enzyme that splits lecithin. Called also phospholipase.

lecitho- word element. [Gr.] *the yolk of an egg, ovum.*

lecithoblast the primitive entoderm of a two-layered blastodisk.

lecithoprotein a combination of protein and lecithin; found in all cells of animal tissues.

lectin 1. hemagglutinating substances present in saline extracts of certain plant seeds, which agglutinate erythrocytes of certain blood groups or stimulate lymphocyte proliferation. 2. antinutritive factors in legume seeds; interfere with protein digestion in monogastric livestock.

LED light emitting diode.

Ledum genus of North American plants in family Ericaceae; toxin is andromedotoxin; causes sudden death, abdominal pain, vomiting, dullness, tremor, tenesmus, diarrhea, salivation; includes *L. columbianum* (Pacific labrador tea), *L. glandulosum* (Western labrador tea).

Lee biopsy needle a needle designed for cutting and aspiration of tissue for biopsy, particularly of aerated lung tissue.

lee waves waves on the sheltered side, away from the wind, of an obstruction; a meteorological wind phenomenon thought to play a part in abnormal downwind transmission of foot-and-mouth disease.

Lee–White clotting time see CLOTTING time.

leech 1. any of the annelids of the class Hirudinea, especially *Hirudo medicinalis*; some species are bloodsuckers, and used for drawing blood. 2. one of the granular bodies in swamp cancer. Called also grains.

equine l. see SWAMP CANCER.

left left-hand side. See specific sites, e.g. left atrium, displacement of abomasum, ventricle.

l. colon displacement causes colic in horses; caused by entrapment of the left colon behind the nephrosplenic ligament; requires surgical intervention; manifested clinically by absence of the pelvic flexure of the colon from the left ventral abdomen.

l. shift see SHIFT to the left.

l.-sided recurrent laryngeal neuropathy see LARYNGEAL hemiplegia.

leg strictly, the part of the limb supported by the tibia; generally, see LIMB (1), FORELIMB, HINDLIMB.

l. band plastic band worn around the pastern in cows. Makes identification easy in pit-type milking sheds, but a band is needed on each hindlimb and muddy lanes make the numbers difficult to read. Metal bands or rings are also placed on the legs of caged birds for identification purposes.

bow l. genu varum.

l. mange occurs in horses, cattle and sheep; caused by CHORIOPTES *bovis.*

milk l. severe lameness in senior dairy cows due to degenerative arthritis of the femorotibial joint. Presumed due to long-term negative calcium balance in heavy milking cows.

leg-itch mite of sheep; see EUTROMBICULA *sarcina.*

leg-twitch a tourniquet applied tightly above the knee or hock; usually causes complete immobilization of the leg. See also TWITCH (2).

leg weakness difficulty in rising, staggery gait.

l. w. of pigs a locomotor disability of pigs unassociated with infectious arthritis. It is a combination of noninfectious arthropathy and osteopathy, and is a significant cause of mandatory culling in pig herds. Included as causes of the syndrome are defects of conformation, osteochondrosis and arthrosis, epiphyseolysis, lumbar intervertebral disk degeneration, and spondylosis. The clinical syndrome varies from lameness to difficulty in rising, to recumbency. Characteristic signs are carrying of a hindleg, sitting on the haunches for long periods, and a shuffling gait.

l. w. of turkeys swelling of the hock and deformity of the tarsometatarsal bone in turkeys; it is of unknown etiology.

legal proper under the law.

l. consent a consent agreement signed by the owner or custodian, consent being to surgery, euthanasia, autopsy, or raising of fees. To be legal, the document needs to be dated, have an accurate description of the animal, an exact description of what is being agreed to, and must not deny the owner the right to proceed in litigation about the matter.

l. evidence anything properly submitted to a court that will enable it to make a proper judgment on a matter before it.

l. medicine see forensic VETERINARY MEDICINE.

Legg–Calvé–Perthes disease an idiopathic necrosis and lysis of the femoral head; occurs in young, small-breed dogs. Lameness of varying severity occurs and a degenerative arthropathy follows. Surgical removal of the femoral head is the usual treatment. Called also Legg's disease, Legg–Calvé disease, Perthes disease.

Legg's disease see LEGG–CALVE–PERTHE DISEASE.

leggy said of animals that appear to have legs longer than normal for the species, breed and age.

Leghorn see WHITE LEGHORN.

legislative action group a group of professional veterinarians prepared to lobby their individual legal representatives at short notice if a potential legislative action warrants intensive action.

legume 1. the pod or fruit of a leguminous plant, such as peas and beans. 2. a leguminous plant, i.e. a member of the family Leguminosae.

l. bloat frothy ruminal tympany in cattle grazing clover or lucerne.

Leicester an English longwool breed of polled, meat sheep, with wool 32 to 38 microns. It has been used to produce many subsidiary breeds, e.g. CORRIEDALE.

Leighton pin a metal pin used as an internal splint in the reduction of fractures of long bones. It is V-shaped in cross-section and has a shuttle device to assist in advancing the pin further into the bone.

leiodermia abnormal smoothness and glossiness of the skin.

leiomyoma a benign tumor derived from smooth muscle, most often of the uterus (leiomyoma uteri) but can occur in urinary bladder, upper intestinal tract and esophagus.

l. uteri leiomyoma of the UTERUS; called also colloquially, fibroids.

leiomyometaplasts gray to brown granules in the gut wall causing a poorly defined lesion known as brown gut.

leiomyosarcoma a sarcoma containing cells of smooth muscle.

Leiperia a genus of parasites in the class Pentastomida found in crocodiles.

Leipernema a genus of worms of the family Kathlaniidae.

L. galebi found in the intestine of Indian elephants.

L. leiperi found in the intestine of the African elephant and hippopotamus.

Leishman–Donovan bodies round or oval bodies found in reticuloendothelial cells, especially those of the spleen and liver, in visceral leishmaniasis; they are amastigote intracellular stages of *Leishmania donovani*. The term is also used to designate similar forms of *L. tropica* found in macrophages in lesions of cutaneous leishmaniasis.

Leishmania a genus of protozoan parasites transmitted by sandflies, which also act as intermediate hosts.

L. adleri found in lizards and other mammals.

L. aethiopica reservoir hosts are hyraxes.

L. brasiliensis brasiliensis reservoir hosts are forest rodents. Causes mucocutaneous leishmaniasis in humans.

L. brasiliensis guyanensis dogs are infected; in humans the disease is the cutaneous form in most cases.

L. brasiliensis panamensis reservoirs are sloths, kinkajous and many other forest animals.

L. chagasi causes visceral leishmaniasis in humans and dogs.

L. donovani causes visceral leishmaniasis in humans and in carnivores.

L. enriettii causes cutaneous leishmaniasis in guinea pigs.

L. infantum causes visceral leishmaniasis in dogs and other carnivores. In humans it is children who are most commonly affected.

L. major dogs and bush mammals are reservoir hosts. In humans this is the cause of oriental sore, the important cutaneous form of the disease.

L. mexicana amazonensis causes cutaneous leishmaniasis in humans. Rodents and bush animals are reservoir hosts.

L. mexicana mexicana reservoir hosts are rodents; causes cutaneous leishmaniasis in humans.

L. mexicana pifanoi causes chronic cutaneous leishmaniasis in humans.

L. peruviana causes cutaneous leishmaniasis in humans; probably infests dogs.

L. tropica causes cutaneous leishmaniasis in humans and dogs.

leishmaniasis infection by *Leishmania* spp.; occurs in humans, domestic Canidae and rodents, and is an important zoonosis throughout the world, except Australia. Three forms occur: (1) visceral (kala-azar, black fever, dumdum fever), caused by *L. donovani*; (2) cutaneous (Oriental sore, Bagdad boil, Aleppo button), caused by *L. tropica*; and (3) mucocutaneous, caused by *L. brasiliensis.* Visceral leishmaniasis in the dog is a chronic, debilitating disease with weight loss, enlargement of the liver and spleen, and polyarthritis. Chronic ulcerations of the skin occur in the cutaneous form.

leishmanoid like leishmaniasis.

lekkerruikpeul see ACACIA *nilotica* subsp. *kraussiana*.

lelapid mite see ECHINOLAELAPS ECHIDNINUS.

Lelystad virus the agent responsible for PORCINE reproductive and respiratory syndrome.

Lembert rongeur fine-pointed, single-action instrument for breaking off segments of bone. When lying flat the blades have a distinct curve to one side.

Lembert suture pattern the classical suture pattern for closing gut. The needle is directed to cross the incision, penetrating the serosa and muscularis but not the mucosa, then back out through the serosa, across the incision to repeat the maneuver on the other side. When the suture is tightened it is serosa that approximates. Can be continuous or interrupted.

lemming small, nocturnal rodent that conducts mass migrations every few years. Called also *Lemmus lemmus*.

l. fever see TULAREMIA.

lemmoblastic forming or developing into a neurolemma cell.

lemmocyte a cell that develops into a neurolemma cell.

Lemmus lemmuss see LEMMING.

lemniscal system one of the major sensory pathways ascending the spinal cord and into consciousness; conducts sensitive impulses relating to touch, pressure, vibration and joint proprioception via the dorsal funiculus and the medial lemniscus and thalamus before reaching the cortex.

lemniscus pl. *lemnisci* [L.] a ribbon or band; a band or bundle of nerve fibers in the central nervous system.

medial l. an ascending tract of sensory nerve fibers in the medulla oblongata.

Lempert rongeur a surgical forcep for cutting bone with tapered jaws and sharp points. Used in neurosurgery.

lemur monkey-like animals intermediate between monkeys and insectivorous animals. They have pointed snouts and fur-covered faces, long tails and soft fur. They are arboreal and nocturnal. There are many varieties in the genera *Lemur*, *Cheirogaleus* and *Microcebus*.

Lemuridae a family of nonhuman primates that includes the LEMUR.

length an expression of the longest dimension of an object, or of the measurement between its two ends.

crown–heel l. the distance from the crown of the head to the heel in embryos, fetuses and neonates.

crown–rump l. the distance from the crown of the head to the point of attachment of the tail.

lenperone an anxiolytic and antiemetic agent.

Lens includes *L. culinaris*, *L. esculenta*. See ERVUM.

lens 1. a piece of glass or other transparent material so shaped as to converge or scatter light rays. 2. crystalline lens; the transparent, biconvex body separating the posterior chamber and the vitreous body of the eye. The crystalline lens refracts (bends) light rays so that they are focused on the RETINA. In order for the eye to see objects close at hand, light rays from the objects must be bent more sharply to bring them to focus on the retina. See also LENTICULAR.

apochromatic l. one corrected for both chromatic and spherical aberration.

biconcave l. one concave on both faces.

biconvex l. one convex on both faces.

l. cells the only nucleated cells in the lens of the adult are those of the epithelium beneath the capsule on the rostral surface.

concave l. one with one or both (biconvex) faces curved like a section of the interior of a hollow sphere; it disperses light rays. Called also dispersing lens.

contact l's lenses that fit directly over the cornea of the eye; used in humans for correction of refractive errors but only rarely applied in animals and then for therapeutic purposes. They can be applied in cases of severe bullous keratopathy or, after saturation with antibiotic solution, the delivery of antibiotics in high concentration to the cornea.

converging l. one curved like the exterior of a hollow sphere; it brings light to a focus. Called also convex lens.

convex l. see converging lens (above).

convexoconcave l. one that has one convex and one concave face.

crystalline l. see lens (2) (above).

dispersing l. concave lens.

ectopic l. see ECTOPIA lentis.

l. fibers elongated, modified cells oriented meridianly in concentric layers; the most peripheral contain nuclei; they interlock with each other via the medium of ball and socket interdigitations and flaps and imprints.

l.-induced uveitis see phacolytic UVEITIS, phacoclastic UVEITIS.

l. induction see INDUCTIVE interactions.

intraocular l. plastic lenses placed within the lens capsule after cataract surgery.

intumescent l. see intumescent CATARACT.

l. luxation separation of the lens from its zonular attachments, allowing displacement and freedom to move in the posterior chamber, anterior chamber or occasionally the vitreous. Occurs most commonly in dogs and is a result of trauma or as a familial trait, particularly in wirehaired Fox terriers and Sealyham terriers, predisposing to glaucoma. Luxation can occur secondary to space-occupying intraocular tumors, enlargement of the globe in chronic glaucoma, or swelling of the lens as seen in intumescent cataract.

l. opacity cataract.

l. sclerosis see nuclear SCLEROSIS.

l. subluxation partial separation of zonular attachments, allowing some alteration in position but not movement into another chamber.

l. sutures structures formed by the contact between caudal and rostral lens fibers resulting in Y-shaped lens stars.

lens fluke see DIPLOSTOMUM *spathaceum*.

lent rose HELLEBORUS *niger*.

lentectomy excision of the lens of the eye.

lenten rose HELLEBORUS *orientalis*.

lenticonus a congenital conical bulging, anteriorly or posteriorly, of the lens of the eye.

lenticular 1. pertaining to or shaped like a lens. 2. pertaining to the lens of the eye. 3. pertaining to the lenticular nucleus. See also LENS.

lenticulostriate pertaining to the lenticular nucleus and corpus striatum.

lenticulothalamic relating to the lenticular nucleus and the thalamus.

lentiform lens-shaped.

lentigenic a host–parasite relationship in which the host shows little or no disease, the relationship persists for a very long time, and the host often survives or dies of intercurrent disease.

lentiginosis profusa characterized by black pigmented, slightly raised macules, called lentigines, mostly along the back, but generalized; occurs in young dogs, especially pugs.

lentiglobus exaggerated curvature of the lens of the eye, producing an anterior or posterior spherical bulging.

lentigo pl. *lentigines* [L.] a flat, brownish pigmented spot on the skin due to increased deposition of melanin and an increased number of melanocytes; a freckle.

orange cat l. lentigo simplex.

l. simplex pigmented macules develop in orange cats from about 1 year of age, mainly on the lips. They are of no significance. Called also orange cat lentigo.

lentil see ERVUM.

lentinan a plant extract that is a potent stimulator of the reticuloendothelial system; used as an immunomodulator.

Lentivirinae a subfamily of viruses in the family RETROVIRIDAE. It contains the viruses of MAEDI–visna, CAPRINE arthritis–encephalitis, EQUINE infectious anemia, and human immunodeficiency/AIDS.

lentivirus a member of the subfamily LENTIVIRINAE.

l. encephalitis see VISNA, CAPRINE arthritis–encephalitis.

feline T-lymphotropic l. see FELINE immunodeficiency virus.

lentogenic only marginally virulent. See also NEWCASTLE DISEASE.

Leon-Zamora ass a longhaired, black Spanish donkey, with paler underline and muzzle.

Leonberger a large (80–150 lb) muscular dog with a light yellow, golden or red-brown wavy coat which forms a mane at the throat and chest. It is webfooted.

Leontideus see GOLDEN LION MARMOSET.

Leontopithecus rosalia small monkey in the Callithricidae family; called also golden lion tamarin.

leopard a big, graceful, yellow cat with dark brown to black spots and a long, thin tail. It is spread widely through the world. Called also *Panthera pardus*.

l. cat FELIS *bengalensis*.

clouded l. the coat color is grayish but in other respects this cat resembles *Panthera pardus*. Called also *Neofelis nebulosa*.

snow l. dark spots on a white skin and a long, thick tail make this a very handsome cat. Called also *Uncia uncia*, ounce.

LEP low egg passage, with reference to virus attenuation usually for vaccine production.

Lepeophtherius salmonis the salmon louse.

lepidic pertaining to scales.

Lepidium sativum member of the plant family Brassicaceae. Called also cress, the salad vegetable; contains toxic amounts of mustard oil glucosinolates; causes unpalatability, diarrhea, milk taint.

lepidosis a scaly eruption.

Lepidozamia peroffskyana Australian cycad plant in the family Zamiaceae; contains cycad glycosides which may cause hepatic necrosis and ZAMIA staggers; called also *Macrozamia denisonii.*

Lepiota a genus of very large mushrooms called parasol mushrooms; cause abdominal pain and diarrhea in humans; includes *L. dolichaula*, *L. helveola*, *L. molybdites.*

Leporipoxvirus a genus of viruses in the family POXVIRIDAE.

Lepotrombidium see HARVEST mites.

lepra cells enlarged cells with foamy cytoplasm and containing many acid-fast bacilli; characteristic of murine leprosy.

leprosy a disease of humans caused by *Mycobacterium leprae* and manifested by granulomatous lesions of the peripheral nerves, skin and mucosae.

buffalo l. may be ulcerative lymphangitis caused by acid-fast bacilli.

feline l. see FELINE leprosy.

rat l. see RAT leprosy.

leptazol a convulsant analeptic. Called also pentylenetetrazol.

Lepte automnale see TROMBICULA *autumnalis.*

lepto- word element. [Gr.] *slender, delicate.*

leptocurare one of the two groups of neuroblocking agents, based on chemical structure. The other group is the pachycurares.

leptocyte a thin, flattened hypochromic erythrocyte with a normal diameter and decreased MCV. See also target CELL.

leptocytosis leptocytes in the blood.

leptokurtosis see KURTOSIS.

leptomeninges plural of *leptomeninx;* the two more delicate components of the meninges: the pia mater and arachnoid considered together; the pia-arachnoid.

leptomeningitis inflammation of the leptomeninges.

leptomeningopathy any disease of the leptomeninges.

leptomeninx see LEPTOMENINGES.

Leptomonas a genus of the protozoan family Trypanosomatidae, the members of which are found in invertebrates.

leptopellic having a narrow pelvis.

leptophonia weakness or feebleness of the voice.

Leptopsylla segnis a flea found on house mice, rats and field rodents.

Leptopus decaisnei Australian plant in family Euphorbiaceae; causes cyanide poisoning; called also *Andrachne decaisnei*, andrachne.

Leptospira a genus of thin, coiled, motile bacteria that cannot be visualized with conventional bacteriological staining methods. They are usually observed by dark-field microscopy or detected in tissue sections by special (silver) stains. There are 11 species, of which *L. interrogans*, *L. borgpetersenii*, *L. inadai*, *L. kirschneri*, *L. noguchii*, *L. weilii*, and *L. santarosei* are significant animal pathogens. Each species contains many serovars and different species may contain antigenically related serovars. Significant serovars include *L. interrogans* sv *canicola, grippotyphosa, hardjoprajitno, icterohaemorrhagiae, pomona* and *zanoni*, *L. borgpetersenii* sv *hardjobovis*, *L. kirschneri* sv *grippotyphosa.* Isolates can also be grouped on the basis of serogroups, which include Grippotyphosa, Pomona, Icterohaemorrhagiae, Canicola, Sejroe and Tarassovi. Serovars vary in their host specificity, their preferred host and their pathogenicity.

Two of the bacteria's characteristics, which are important in the epidemiology of the diseases that it causes, are its ability to survive in the environment in warm, moist and slightly alkaline conditions, and its survival in kidneys for long periods, with a resulting frequent and often long-term shedding in the urine.

Although the disease caused by each of the leptospirae has some differences in clinical and epidemiological manifestations in each of the species, there is still sufficient similarity for the diseases to be dealt with as LEPTOSPIROSIS.

leptospiremia the presence of leptospirae in the blood.

leptospires organisms in the genus LEPTOSPIRA.

leptospirosis an infectious disease of all species. The common causes are *Leptospira interrogans* serovars *pomona, hardjo, hyos, tarassovi, icterohaemorrhagiae, canicola* and many other less important varieties (see LEPTOSPIRA). In adult cattle the common syndromes are an abortion storm or a subacute febrile illness. In calves it is an acute hemolytic anemia with jaundice and hemoglobinuria and an interstitial nephritis. In sheep and goats there may be acute septicemia sometimes accompanied by abortion. In pigs it is usually a syndrome of abortion and stillbirths, although fatal septicemia may occur in piglets. In horses there is possibly an etiological relationship with periodic ophthalmia and with abortion. In dogs there may be peracute illness, which is frequently fatal, or acute illness with jaundice or acute nephritis. Vaccines are available for prevention of the infection.

leptospiruria leptospires are present in the urine.

leptotene the stage of meiosis in which the chromosomes are threadlike in shape.

Leptotrombidium genus of the family Trombiculidae. The mites act as vectors of the human scrub typhus agent.

Lepus a group of lagomorphs, members of the *Lepus* spp. of the family Leporidae. Differing from the rabbits who are in the same family, by the length of their ears, and because they do not burrow and they do not live in social groups as rabbits do. Includes *L. americanus* (snowshoe hare), *L. arcticus* (arctic hare), *L. californicus* (black-tailed jackrabbit), *L. europaeus* (European brown hare), *L. timidus* (mountain hare). Called also jack rabbit, hare.

Lernaea a genus of crustaceans in the class Crustacea which attach themselves to the skin of freshwater fish causing ulceration. Affected fish swim sluggishly and grow poorly, and the mortality may be heavy. *L. ciprinacea* is the common species. Called also anchor worms.

LES lower esophageal sphincter.

lesion any pathological or traumatic discontinuity of tissue or loss of function of a part. Lesion is a broad term, including wounds, sores, ulcers, tumors, cataracts and any other tissue damage. They range from the skin sores associated with eczema to the changes in lung tissue that occur in tuberculosis.

target l. see TARGET lesion.

Lespedeza stipulacea a legume in family Fabaceae, similar to alfalfa or lucerne in nutritional content but with the advantage that it will produce on relatively poor soil. There are annual and perennial varieties. Contains the toxin coumarin and moldy hay made from the crop causes a hemorrhagic disease. Called also Korean lespedeza.

lesser the smaller, less important, of two.

l. celandine RANUNCULUS *ficaria*.

l. hemlock AETHUSA *cynapium*.

l. liver fluke see DICROCOELIUM *dendriticum*.

l. loosestrife see LYTHRIUM HYSSOPIFOLIA.

l. mealworm see ALPHITOBIUS DIAPERINUS.

l. spearwort RANUNCULUS *flammaula*.

letdown 1. the sudden flush of milk flow that occurs when the calf begins to suck or when milking commences in a properly prepared cow. Depends for its occurrence on the release of oxytocin from the pituitary gland in response to massage of the teats and udder. Environmental stimuli such as free electricity and fear or excitement can block the response. Is also sometimes absent in freshly calved cows but the cycle can be triggered by an injection of oxytocin. 2. a horse in overfat condition is said to be letdown; the converse of tuckedup.

milk l. failure occurs sporadically in all species. May be due to painful conditions of the teat or sharp teeth of sucker. Anxiety, as in maiden heifers, can be a cause. Other cases occur without obvious reason and respond dramatically to a single injection of oxytocin.

lethal deadly; fatal.

l. trait an inherited characteristic that ensures the early death of the inheritor. See also inherited PARAKERATOSIS, and canine CYCLIC hematopoiesis.

l. trait A46 see inherited PARAKERATOSIS.

l. white the name given to the progeny of white horses in which the gene for the white character is dominant. Their progeny have a very high mortality rate. The same applies to the offspring of a mating of two OVERO horses; the defect in these is atresia of the intestine.

l. white foal disease see lethal white (above).

lethargy a condition of drowsiness or indifference.

Leu leucine.

leu-enkaphalin leucine ENKEPHALIN; abbreviated Leu-ENK.

Leucaena leucocephala tree in the legume family Mimosaceae; contains the toxic amino acid mimosine; causes hair loss, goiter, infertility and weight loss. Called also *L. glauca*, lead tree. The disease is called also ekoa, jumbey, koa haole, lamtoro.

leucenosis intoxication by plants of the genus *Leucaena*.

leucine Leu; a naturally occurring amino acid, essential for growth in the young and for nitrogen equilibrium in adults.

l. aminopeptidase a digestive enzyme of small intestine enterocytes (brush border).

DL-l. synthetic form of leucine.

l. enkephalin leu-enkephalin; see ENKEPHALIN.

L-l. natural form of leucine.

l. zipper a structured motif found in some DNA binding regulatory proteins formed from a region of α-helix containing at least four leucines, each separated by six amino acids from one another; the leucines align along one edge of the α-helix with one leucine at every second turn of the helix such that the leucine of one protein can interdigitate with the leucines of another protein in a zipper manner.

leuc(o)- for words beginning thus, see also those beginning *leuk(o)-*.

Leucochloridiomorpha a genus of intestinal flukes (digenetic trematodes).

L. constantiae found in the intestine of raccoons and the bursa of Fabricius in ducks.

leucocyte leukocyte.

Leucocytozoon a protozoan parasite of avian erythrocytes transmitted by the 'blackfly' *Simulium* spp. Infection causes the disease LEUCOCYTOZOONOSIS.

L. andrewsi see *L. caulleryi* (below).

L. bonasae found in grouse and ptarmigan.

***L. caulleryi* (*L. andrewsi*)** found in chickens; causes leucocytozoonosis.

L. grusi found in cranes.

L. mansoni found in grouse.

L. marchouxi found in doves and pigeons.

L. sabrazesi found in fowl.

L. sakharoffi found in crow and other wild birds.

L. schoutedeni chickens only in east Africa.

***L. simondi* (*L. anseris, L. anatis*)** found in ducks and geese.

L. smithi found in turkeys.

leucocytozoonosis an acute disease in young birds caused by infection with *Leucocytozoon* spp. and characterized by emaciation, weakness and debility. Death is usual within a few days and the mortality rate may be very high. In adult birds the course is longer and the signs may include dyspnea.

leucoencephalomalacia leukoencephalomalacia.

leucomycin see KITASAMYCIN.

Leuconostoc a genus of gram-positive, nonpathogenic, facultatively anaerobic bacteria spherical to lenticular in shape. They are of food hygiene importance because they cause slime on high sugar foods, cause taints and are salt-tolerant.

L. mesenteroides* subsp. *dextranicum*, subsp. *mesenteroides produce dextran which is the major component of the slime on foods.

Leucothoe a genus of plants in the family Ericaceae that contain the tetracyclic polyol andromedotoxin, which causes abdominal pain, vomiting and aspiration pneumonia, and sudden death due to respiratory failure. Include *L. davisiae*, *L. grayana*. Called also sierra or black laurel.

leucovorin see FOLINIC ACID.

leukapheresis the selective removal of leukocytes from withdrawn blood, which are then retransfused into the donor. See also PHERESIS.

Leukassay F test a commercial ELISA test for the detection of feline leukemia virus antigen in the blood of cats.

leukemia a progressive, malignant disease of the blood-forming organs, marked by distorted proliferation and development of leukocytes and their precursors in the blood and bone marrow. Signs include fever and enlargement of the lymph nodes, spleen and liver. The persistent lymphocytosis that occurs in some cattle is a response to infection with the bovine viral leukosis virus. Similarly, leukemia may occur in the lymphoproliferative and myeloproliferative diseases caused by feline leukemia virus in cats.

aleukemic l. leukemia in which the leukocyte count is normal or below normal.

avian l. see avian LEUKOSIS.

basophilic l., basophilocytic l. leukemia in which basophilic granulocytes predominate.

B-cell l. leukemia arising from B lymphocytes.

bovine l. see BOVINE viral leukosis.

l. cutis skin lesions associated with dissemination of systemic leukemia; they may be neoplastic or nonspecific.

embryonal l. stem cell leukemia.

eosinophilic l. occurs rarely in cats. There are large

numbers of eosinophils with infiltration of spleen, liver, lymph nodes and bone marrow.
feline l. complex the array of diseases associated with infection of cats by the feline leukemia virus; includes lymphoreticular neoplasms, myelodysplastic disorders and abnormalities of the immune system.
feline l. virus (FeLV) see FELINE leukemia virus.
granulocytic l. myelocytic leukemia.
leukopenic l. aleukemic leukemia.
lymphatic l., lymphoblastic l., lymphocytic l., lymphogenous l., lymphoid l. leukemia associated with hyperplasia and overactivity of the lymphoid tissue, in which the leukocytes are lymphocytes or lymphoblasts.
lymphosarcoma cell l. a form marked by large numbers of lymphosarcoma cells in the peripheral blood; depending on the degree of bone marrow involvement, it may be a variant of lymphosarcoma.
mast cell l. a form marked by overwhelming numbers of tissue mast cells in the peripheral blood.
megakaryoblastic l. a rare disease of young dogs, characterized by intestinal hemorrhage, anemia and a fatal outcome within a few weeks. There is a pancytopenia and marked thrombocytopenia.
megakaryocytic l. a form with numerous megakaryocytes in the spleen, bone marrow, and other tissues, but decreased numbers or abnormal thrombocytes in the peripheral blood, and anemia. Reported in dogs and cats. Called also megakaryocytic myelosis.
monocytic l. leukemia in which the predominating leukocytes are monocytes.
myeloblastic l. characterized by a predominance of immature myeloid series of cells in the blood; largely a disease of young male dogs and cats.
myelocytic l., myelogenous l., myeloid l. a form arising from myeloid tissue in which the granular polymorphonuclear leukocytes and their precursors predominate.
myelomonocytic l. concurrent neoplasia of the neutrophilic and monocytic cell lines with a monocytic leukemia, a high total leukocyte count, anemia and thrombocytopenia.
plasma cell l., plasmacyte l. a form in which the predominating cell in the peripheral blood is the plasma cell.
premyelocytic l. a form in which the predominant cells are premyeloblasts, rather than myeloblasts, often associated with abnormal bleeding secondary to thrombocytopenia, hypofibrinogenemia and decreased levels of clotting factor V.
promyelocytic l. characterized by a predominance of promyelocytes in peripheral blood and in the bone marrow. A disease of dogs and cats with bleeding tendencies, anemia and a susceptibility to septicemia with a fatal outcome within a few weeks.
stem cell l. leukemia in which the predominating cell is so immature and primitive that its classification is difficult.
subleukemic l. aleukemic leukemia.
undifferentiated l. an acute myeloproliferative disorder in which the cells involved cannot be identified.

leukemogen any substance that produces leukemia.

leukemogenesis the process of generation of myeloid cell lines in bone marrow and extramedullary sites; a critical feature in myeloproliferative disease; i.e. the induction or development of leukemia.

leukemoid exhibiting blood counts, particularly leukocytosis, and sometimes other clinical findings resembling those of leukemia, but not due to uncontrolled proliferation of leukocytes; it can be extremely difficult to differentiate from leukemia. Usually associated with severe inflammation such as pyometra, hepatic abscesses, etc.

leukergy nonspecific clumping of leukocytes.

leukin a lytic substance extractable from polymorphonuclear lymphocytes and that attacks spore-bearing aerobic bacteria, especially *Bacillus anthracis*.

leuk(o)- word element. [Gr.] *white, leukocyte*. For words beginning thus see also those beginning *leuc(o)-*.

leukoagglutinin an agglutinin that acts upon leukocytes.

leukoblast an immature granular leukocyte.
granular l. promyelocyte.

leukoblastosis a general term for proliferation of leukocytes.

leukocidin a substance produced by some pathogenic bacteria that is toxic to polymorphonuclear leukocytes (neutrophils).

leukocoria a white pupil.

leukocrit the volume percentage of leukocytes in whole blood.

leukocyte a white blood cell capable of ameboid movement, whose chief function is to protect the body against microorganisms causing disease and which comprise: granulocytes (basophils, eosinophils, neutrophils), nongranulocytes (lymphocytes, monocytes) and thrombocytes (platelets).
bovine l. adhesion deficiency lethal hematological defect inherited as a recessive trait in Holstein cattle; characterized by poor growth, recurrent infection and poor responsivity to standard treatments in calves from 2 to 8 weeks of age. Profound neutrophilia. Death supervenes before two years of age. Called also BLAD.
l. count tabulation of the numbers and kinds of leukocytes in a blood sample.
endothelial l. see ENDOTHELIOCYTE.
l. functional antigens a group of cell surface antigens involved in intracellular adhesion.
granular l's granulocytes; leukocytes containing abundant granules (lysosomes) in their cytoplasm, including neutrophils, eosinophils and basophils.
l. migration-inhibition factor a lymphokine elaborated by activated T or B lymphocytes that inhibits polymorphonuclear leukocyte migration.
polymorphonuclear l. any of the fully developed, segmented cells of the granulocyte series, especially a neutrophil, whose nuclei contain three or more lobes joined by filamentous connections.

leukocythemia leukemia.

leukocytic pertaining to or emanating from leukocytes.
l. pyrogen protein substances, e.g. interleukin-1, which stimulate the thermoregulator center of the hypothalamus via prostaglandins; produced by bone-marrow derived phagocytes.

leukocytoblast see LEUKOBLAST.

leukocytoclastic vasculitis see hypersensitivity angiitis.

leukocytogenesis the formation of leukocytes.

leukocytolysin a lysin that leads to disruption of leukocytes.

leukocytolysis disintegration of leukocytes.

leukocytoma a tumor-like mass of leukocytes.

leukocytopenia leukopenia.

leukocytoplania wandering of leukocytes; passage of leukocytes through a membrane.

leukocytopoiesis the production of leukocytes; leukopoiesis.

leukocytosis a transient increase in the number of leukocytes in the blood, due to various causes.

basophilic l. see BASOPHILIA (2).
eosinophilic l. see EOSINOPHILIA (2).
l.-inducing factor a factor which causes an increase in release of immature neutrophils into the circulation; an increased level of the factor in the circulation caused by endotoxin; called also neutrophil-releasing activity.
mononuclear l. mononucleosis.
pathological l. that due to some morbid reaction, e.g. infection or trauma.

leukocytotaxis see LEUKOTAXIS.

leukocytotoxin a toxin that destroys leukocytes.

leukocytozoonosis see LEUCOCYTOZOONOSIS.

leukocyturia leukocytes in the urine.

leukoderma loss of pigmentation of the skin.

leukodystrophic diseases diseases characterized by non-inflammatory degeneration and loss of myelin.

leukodystrophy disorders or metabolic defects in the system required for the maintenance and degradation of normally formed myelin in newborn and young animals. Clinical signs begin some time after birth. See also LEUKOENCEPHALOPATHY.
Afghan l. see hereditary MYELOPATHY of Afghan hounds.
cavitating l. a familial, probably inherited, disease of Dalmatian dogs in which there is blindness and progressive motor dysfunction from a few months of age.
fibrinoid l. a familial disease of astrocytes causing ataxia, paresis and behavioral changes from an early age; reported in Labrador retrievers. Similar to Alexander's disease in humans.
globoid cell l. an inherited lysosomal storage disease of polled Dorset sheep, cats, and dogs, particularly Cairn terriers and West Highland white terriers, caused by a deficiency of the enzyme beta-galactocerebrosidase. From a young age, there is weakness that progresses to paralysis. Called also galactocerebrosidosis and Krabbe's disease.
metachromatic l. a leukoencephalopathy reported in cats, caused by a deficiency of the enzyme arylsulfatase A. There is accumulation of a sphingolipid (sulfatide) in tissues, with diffuse loss of myelin in the central nervous system and progressive neurological dysfunction.

leuko-edema an abnormality of the buccal mucosa, consisting of an increase in thickness of the epithelium, with intracellular edema of the malpighian layer.

leukoencephalitis inflammation of the white substance of the brain.

leukoencephalomalacia ENCEPHALOMALACIA affecting especially the white matter. Occurs in carbon monoxide poisoning, mulberry heart disease of pigs and mycotoxic leukoencephalomalacia.
mycotoxic l. a syndrome of ataxia, tremor, circling, depressed consciousness, recumbency and death in horses and donkeys; caused by poisoning by fumonisins from the fungus *Fusarium moniliforme*, usually ingested with moldy corn.

leukoencephalomyelitis ENCEPHALOMYELITIS affecting particularly the white matter of the brain and spinal cord. See also CAPRINE arthritis–encephalitis.

leukoencephalomyelopathy a disease of white matter of the brain and spinal cord; a syndrome of progressive ataxia and weakness with dysmetria, quadriparesis, and conscious proprioceptive deficits, seen in adult Rottweiler dogs.

leukoencephalopathy any of a group of diseases affecting the white substance of the brain.

leukoerythroblastic pertaining to or emanating from the production of erythrocytes.
l. reaction a bone marrow response in which nucleated red blood cells and immature leukocytes are released. Seen in all species, most commonly in dogs and cats.

leukoerythroblastosis an anemic condition associated with space-occupying lesions of the bone marrow, marked by a variable number of immature erythroid and myeloid cells in the circulation.

leukogram a tabulation of the leukocytes present in a blood sample.

leukokinin see TUFTSIN.

leukolymphosarcoma lymphosarcoma cell leukemia.

leukolysin see LEUKOCYTOLYSIN.

leukolysis see LEUKOCYTOLYSIS.

leukoma a dense corneal opacity.
adherent l. one caused by adhesion of the iris.

leukomyelitis inflammation of the white matter of the spinal cord.

leukomyelopathy disease of the white matter of the spinal cord.

leukon the circulating leukocytes and the cells that produce them.

leukonecrosis gangrene with formation of a white slough.

leukonychia loss of pigmentation in a nail, claw or hoof.

leukopathia 1. leukoderma. 2. any disease of the leukocytes.
l. unguium leukonychia.

leukopedesis diapedesis of leukocytes through blood vessel walls.

leukopenia reduction of the number of leukocytes in the blood. It is a common manifestation of a number of diseases, especially those caused by viruses, by a severe inflammatory lesion that draws off large numbers of leukocytes, a consumption leukopenia, and by toxins which depress bone marrow function. See also RADIATION injury, PTERIDIUM AQUILINUM and STACHYBOTRIS ATRA.
malignant l., pernicious l. agranulocytosis.

leukophenothiazone one of the metabolic products of phenothiazine, which is excreted in the urine and produces the red color in the urine when it has been exposed to the air.

leukopoiesis the production of leukocytes; leukocytopoiesis.

leukopoietin a hypothetical substance presumed to be the humoral means of regulating leukopoiesis.

leukorrhagia profuse leukorrhea.

leukorrhea a whitish or yellowish, viscid discharge from the vagina or uterine cavity, which may be a sign of a disorder either in the reproductive organs or elsewhere in the body.

leukosarcoma the development of leukemia following a well-differentiated, lymphocytic type of malignant lymphoma.

leukosis proliferation of leukocyte-forming tissue; the basis of LEUKEMIA.
avian l. a complex of related diseases caused by retroviruses (oncornaviruses). LYMPHOID leukosis, ERYTHROBLASTOSIS, MYELOCYTOMATOSIS and MYELOBLASTOSIS are the principal component diseases. There are in addition a series of tumors of connective tissue, epithelium, endothelium and other miscellaneous related tumors.
cutaneous bovine l. see BOVINE viral leukosis.
enzootic bovine l. see BOVINE viral leukosis.
l.-sarcoma neoplastic diseases includes lymphoid leukosis, erythroblastosis, myeloblastosis, myelocytomatosis, connective tissue tumors, nephroma, nephroblastoma, miscellaneous epithelial and

endothelial tumors, osteopetrosis of birds caused by avian type C oncoviruses.

leukosis/sarcoma see avian LEUKOSIS, ROUS SARCOMA.

leukotaxine a polypeptide that appears in injured tissue and inflammatory exudates; it promotes leukocytosis and leukotaxis and increases capillary permeability.

leukotaxis cytotaxis of leukocytes; the tendency of leukocytes to collect in regions of injury and inflammation.

leukothionol one of the metabolic products of phenothiazine; is excreted in the urine and colors it red when the urine is exposed to the air.

leukotoxic destructive to leukocytes.

leukotoxin a toxin that destroys leukocytes.

leukotrichia whiteness of the hair.

hyperesthetic l. painful, crusted skin lesions on the dorsal midline of horses. White hairs emerge after several weeks.

periocular l. loss of pigmentation around the eyes; seen in Siamese cats, mainly females. It is usually transient and may be precipitated by estrus, pregnancy and systemic illness. Called also goggles.

reticulated l. seen in Quarter horses, Thoroughbreds and Standardbreds; linear crusts, which appear in a cross-hatched pattern over the back, are followed by loss of hair and regrowth of white hairs. Called also tiger stripe, variegated leukotrichia.

spotted l. seen mainly in Arabian horses; multiple white spots appear, most commonly over the rump and thorax.

variegated l. see reticulated leukotrichia (above).

leukotriene substance formed from arachidonic acid which participates in inflammatory reactions, probably as leukotoxin. May act as a slow-reacting substance in anaphylaxis.

leukovirus see ONCORNAVIRINAE.

levallorphan an analog of levorphanol, which acts as an antagonist to analgesic narcotics; used as tartrate in the treatment of respiratory depression produced by narcotic analgesics.

levamisole a broad-spectrum anthelmintic of proven efficiency against gastrointestinal and lung worms that can be administered orally, by injection and by pour-on in cattle. It has no effect on tapeworms or liver fluke; it has a secondary effect in enhancing depressed immune responsiveness by stimulation of T lymphocytes and phagocytosis.

l. poisoning causes a syndrome of lip licking, head shaking, salivation, tremor, excitement and increased frequency of urination and defecation.

levarterenol norepinephrine.

levator pl. *levatores* [L.] 1. a muscle that elevates an organ or structure, e.g. the levator labii muscle. 2. an instrument for raising depressed osseous fragments in fractures.

LeVeen shunt a peritoneal–venous shunt used in the control of ASCITES. It routes excess ascitic fluid out of the peritoneal cavity and into the superior vena cava or the jugular vein.

level of confidence see CONFIDENCE level.

leveret a young hare.

levigation the grinding to a powder of a moist or hard substance.

levo- word element. [L.] *left.*

levobunolol a β-adrenergic blocking agent, used as the hydrochloride in ophthalmic preparations to treat glaucoma.

levocardia a term denoting normal position of the heart associated with transposition of other viscera (situs inversus).

levodopa, L-DOPA the pharmaceutical name for DOPA.

levoduction movement of an eye to the left.

levogyration see LEVOROTATION.

levopropoxyphene the levo isomer of propoxyphene; the napsylate is used as a centrally acting cough suppressant.

levorotation a turning to the left; levogyration.

levorotatory turning the plane of polarization, or rays of light, to the left.

levorphanol a potent, synthetic, narcotic analgesic. The tartrate form is used.

levothyroxine the pharmaceutical name for the thyroid hormone thyroxine (T_4); used for replacement therapy in hypothyroidism.

levoversion a turning toward the left.

levulose a sugar from honey and many sweet fruits, used in solution as a fluid and nutrient replenisher; called also fructose and fruit sugar.

Lewis diagram a ladder diagram of cardiac impulse formation and conduction.

lewisite an arsenical mustard; used as a war gas. The possibility of arsenic poisoning in animals by this means now seems remote. The chief claim for the product in recent times is the production of an antidote which has come into general use for poisoning by metals; known as British antilewisite or BAL.

ley a highly productive pasture composed largely of annual grasses and clovers. It has a tremendous capacity to make milk but is susceptible to outbreaks of hypomagnesemia.

Leydig's cell interstitial cell of the testis, which secretes testosterone.

L. c. tumor a variant of ovarian sex cord-stromal tumurs which are composed of cells that resemble those of Leydig's cells in the testicle. Some of them secrete androgenic hormones, especially in the mare. See also INTERSTITIAL cell tumor.

Leyland cypress see CUPRESSOCYPARIS LEYLANDII.

LFA leukocyte functional antigen.

LH luteinizing hormone.

LH-RH luteinizing hormone-releasing hormone (gonadotropin releasing hormone).

Lhasa apso a small dog with a very long, straight haircoat in almost any color. The dark eyes are barely visible beneath the long coat; the tail is carried over the back with the long hair flowing onto the body. Called also the Bark lion sentinal dog, Tibetan apso. The breed is affected by an inherited renal cortical hypoplasia and lissencephaly.

Li chemical symbol, *lithium.*

liability financial or legal responsibility.

liberty cap see PSILOCYBE.

libido pl. *libidines* [L.] sexual drive, vigor, enthusiasm.

absent l. unwillingness to copulate on the part of a male.

Libyostrongylus a genus of nematodes in the family Trichostrongylidae.

L. douglassii causes proventriculitis in ostriches. Young birds are emaciated, poorly grown and anemic; death losses may be heavy.

lice plural of LOUSE.

bird l. see CHICKEN, TURKEY, DUCK, GOOSE, PIGEON lice.

licensing the award of a license.

poisons l. registration of dealers so that the sources of poisons can be determined and controlled. A veterinarian's right to trade in substances which are of pharmacological benefit but are poisonous is ensured by appropriate scheduling in the legislation.

professional l. see LICENSURE.
radioactive materials l. a license required in most countries for persons or institutions using radioactive materials of any sort. Granted only to persons who have had training in the subject.

licensure the granting of a permit to perform acts which, without it, would be illegal. The licensure of veterinarians has traditionally been the responsibility of the state licensing boards, governed by licensing statutes enacted by the state.
individual l. the granting of a legal permit that is personal and cannot be transferred to another. The individual seeking the licensure must meet standards for practice as established by the state licensing statutes. In most instances the initial license is granted upon successful completion of an examination administered by the state examining board of the specific profession or vocation, and annual re-registration is required to maintain the license.
institutional l. licensure of an agency providing a particular service to the public. In veterinary services this is usually limited to organizations that provide animal welfare services or which are teaching institutions.

licentiate a person holding a license from an authorized agency entitling him/her to practice a particular profession.

lichen 1. any of certain plants formed by the mutualistic combination of an alga and a fungus. 2. any of various papular skin diseases in which the lesions are typically small, firm papules set very close together, the specific kind being indicated by a modifying term.
l. tropicus see equine ALLERGIC dermatitis.

lichenification thickening and hardening of the skin, with exaggeration of its normal markings.

lichenoid resembling lichen.
l. infiltrate adopts a banded configuration parallel to the epidermis.
l. keratosis circumscribed, firm, scaling plaque. See also EAR plaque.
l.-psoriasiform dermatosis idiopathic, probably inherited skin disease of yearling Springer spaniels; lesions begin on the ear and groin and spread to all parts; lesions are symmetric, erythematous, hyperkeratotic, lichenoid papules and plaques.

Lichtenstern block a technique for a block anesthesia of the orbit of the horse.

lick 1. a stroke with the tongue, normally used in cleaning the coat or ingesting a substance from a flat surface. See also LICKING. 2. a mixture of salt plus other macro-elements, especially phosphorus, trace elements, vitamins and other feed additives, fed loosely in a box in the field or indoor housing. The objective is to get the animals to ingest small amounts daily by licking the mixture; salt hungry cattle may eat larger amounts. May be consolidated into a block which encourages licking. Called also mineral mix.
acral l. dermatitis see ACRAL lick dermatitis.
l. dermatitis see lick granuloma (below).
feline l. granuloma see feline EOSINOPHILIC granuloma complex.
l. granuloma called also lick dermatitis; see ACRAL lick dermatitis.

licked beef diffuse, often hemorrhagic, jelly-like edema along the back of a beef carcass, caused by warble fly larvae.

licking stroking with the tongue. There are three kinds of licking in animals: (1) licking of inanimate objects including soil and trees, i.e. pica, which is usually interpreted as an expression of malnutrition; (2) grooming licking of self; (3) abrasive licking of self, often at the same spot. Examples are the 'mad itch' of bovine pseudorabies and the production of acral lick dermatitis in dogs.
l. disease see licking sickness (below).
psychogenic l. see psychogenic DERMATOSIS.
l. sickness pica in cattle on a herd or area scale. Usually ascribed to nutritional deficiency of COPPER, but may also reflect inadequate salt intake.
l. syndrome usually refers to SODIUM chloride nutritional deficiency. See also licking sickness (above).

lid see EYELID.

Lidneria clavata South African plant in the family Liliaceae; contains a cardiac glycoside thought to cause cardiac irregularity, sudden death; called also *Pseudogaltonia clavata*, *P. pechuelli*, *P. subspicata*, cape hyacinth, Southwest African slangkop.

lidocaine a local anesthetic used as a cardiac antiarrhythmic and to produce infiltration anesthesia and epidural and peripheral nerve blocks. Called also lignocaine.

lien [L.] *spleen.*

lien(o)- word element. [L.] *spleen;* see also words beginning *splen(o)-*.

lienocele hernia of the spleen.

lienography radiography of the spleen; splenography.

lienomalacia abnormal softness of the spleen; splenomalacia.

lienomedullary pertaining to the spleen and bone marrow; splenomedullary.

lienomyelogenous formed in the spleen and bone marrow; splenomyelogenous.

lienomyelomalacia softening of the spleen and bone marrow; splenomyelomalacia.

lienotoxin splenotoxin.

lientery diarrhea with passage of undigested food.

lienunculus a detached mass of splenic tissue; an accessory spleen.

LIF leukocyte inhibitory factor.

life span average duration of life in animals of the species in average circumstances where special treatment to maintain life is not provided. Called also *characteristic life span*—commonest age of senile death.

Laboratory animals and small pets—gerbil 3–4 yrs; guinea pig 1–8 yrs; hamster 15 mths–2 yrs; mice 2–3 yrs; rabbit 5–6 yrs; rats 3–4 yrs.

Domestic pets—cat 18–20 yrs; dog small and medium size 15 yrs; large breeds 10 yrs.

Farm animals—cattle 9–11 yrs; sheep 5–6 yrs; goat 8–10 yrs; pig 8–10 yrs; domestic poultry 5–6 yrs; geese—no data but apparently much longer than other domestic birds; horse 25–30 yrs.

life table a tabulation of deaths occurring in age groups, often with other information; may be a current life table, when all of the animals in a population at one time are surveyed, or a cohort table, when all of the animals born in a particular time span are dealt with as a group.

lifetime for the duration of the animal's (usually productive) life.
average l. performance total of production data divided by the number of years of records.

ligament 1. a band of fibrous tissue connecting bones or cartilages, serving to support and strengthen joints. 2. a double layer of peritoneum extending from one visceral organ to another. 3. cordlike remnants of fetal tubular structures that are nonfunctional after birth.

The injury suffered when a joint is wrenched with sufficient violence to stretch or tear the ligaments is called a SPRAIN. For a complete list of named ligaments in the body, see Table 12. See also LIGAMENTUM.

accessory l. one that strengthens or supports another.

l. arteriosum fibrous remnant of the ductus arteriosus.

broad l. the peritoneal folds by which the uterus is suspended from the wall of the abdomen and pelvis.

capsular l. the fibrous layer of a joint capsule.

cruciate l. a pair of ligaments which cross over one another, as for example the cranial and caudal cruciate ligaments which tie the femur to the tibia.

median l. of the bladder a fold of peritoneum attaching the urinary bladder and urachus to the ventral abdominal wall.

pectinate l. a comb-like ligament at the iridocorneal angle.

phrenicocardial l. the continuation of the pericardial sac as a ligament attaching to the diaphragm; attaches to the sternum in species where the heart axis is less oblique.

round l. of the bladder remnants of the umbilical arteries and their mesenteries in the lateral ligaments of the urinary bladder.

round l. of the liver remnants of the umbilical veins found in the falciform ligament in young animals, and the adults of some species.

round l. of the uterus part of the gubernaculum of the female extending from the proper ligament of the ovary to the inguinal canal; in some species, e.g. dog, the ligament passes through the inguinal canal and is incriminated in the development of metrocele.

scrotal l. vestige of the gubernaculum testis of the fetus; connects the dartos surrounding the testicle to the vaginal tunic of the scrotum.

l. splitting a surgical procedure used in horses to stimulate vascularity of a diseased tendon. Through a single key-hole access incision, a series of fan-like incisions are made in the longitudinal axis of the tendon with a special knife.

sutural l. a band of fibrous tissue between the opposed bones of a suture or immovable joint.

l. of the tail of the epididymis a mesenchymal ligamentous caudal extension of the gubernaculum; a cord which binds the tail of the epididymis to the tunica vaginalis.

ligamentopexy fixation of the uterus by shortening the round ligament.

ligamentum pl. *ligamenta* [L.] ligament.

l. arteriosum remnants of the ductus arteriosus between the aorta and the pulmonary artery.

l. flavum connects the arches of adjacent vertebrae.

l. nuchae see NUCHAL ligament.

l. venosum remnants of the ductus venosus in the liver.

ligand an organic molecule that donates the necessary electrons to form coordinate covalent bonds with metallic ions. Also, an ion or part of a molecule that specifically binds to form a complex with another molecule.

ligandin an hepatic transport protein; measurement of it in serum and urine may be a means of estimating the severity of hepatocellular necrosis.

ligase an enzyme that repairs single-strand nicks in duplex DNA and covalently joins DNA fragments with complementary, overlapping (called also cohesive or sticky) ends or less efficiently, with blunt ends. Bacteriophage T4 ligase catalyzes the formation of a covalent phosphodiester bond between adjacent 5′-phosphate and 3′-hydroxyl groups in duplex DNA.

l. chain reaction a technique for detecting a specific nucleotide pair in a gene. Called also LCR.

ligate to apply a ligature.

ligation 1. application of a surgical ligature. 2. the joining of two DNA molecules by a phosphodiester bond. See also SPLICING.

rubber-band l. see RUBBER-BAND LIGATION.

ligature any material, such as a thread or wire, used in surgery to tie off blood vessels to prevent bleeding, or to treat abnormalities in other parts of the body by constricting the tissues.

light electromagnetic radiation with a range of wavelength between about 390 nm (violet) and 770 nm (red), capable of stimulating the subjective sensation of sight; sometimes considered to include ultraviolet and infrared radiation as well.

l. beam diaphragm adjustable lead shutters at the aperture of an x-ray tube. Usually includes a light bulb which delimits the area covered by the beam at the cassette level.

l. cattle store class cattle off range and destined for movement onto irrigated pasture or into feedlot for fattening.

l.–dark cycles an important environmental factor in proper housing of laboratory animals for optimal health and reproductive cycling. Most species do well on a 12 : 12 light–dark cycle but in rabbits more light for females and less for males is recommended.

l. pen a photosensor mounted in the tip of a pen-like instrument. The sensor is capable of reading the beam of a visual display unit (VDU) on a computer terminal and can be used to edit the characters displayed on the screen.

polarized l. light of which the vibrations are made over one plane or in circles or ellipses.

l. sensitization see PHOTOSENSITIZATION.

l. sheep sheep light in condition off subsistence range and destined to go to irrigated pasture or into a feedlot for fattening.

l. stimulus see ELECTRORETINOGRAPH.

Wood's l. see WOOD'S LIGHT.

Light Sussex a high-quality table poultry breed.

lightning visible discharge of electricity between storm clouds or between the clouds and an earthing point at ground level.

l. injury exposure to high voltage electric shock by means of a lightning strike, which causes sudden nervous shock and unconsciousness or permanent cessation of medullary vital centers, resulting in sudden death. Animals that recover may have residual signs. Called also lightning strike. Fish in enclosed waters, e.g. farmed fish, may have their backs broken by lightning striking the water.

l. strike when lightning finds an earthing point.

lights an abattoir term for lung as meat.

lignification the laying down of lignin in a plant; the last stage in maturation, representing a heavy loss in nutritional value.

lignin an almost completely indigestible plant polyphenol present in large quantities in wood, hulls and straw.

lignite pitch can cause poisoning. See PHENOL.

lignocaine see LIDOCAINE.

lignoceric acid a saturated fatty acid found in wood tar, various cerebrosides, and in small amounts in most natural fats.

lignosol a pellet binder known to cause black, sticky cecal contents which stick to the skin of broilers during processing.

Ligula a genus of tapeworms in the family Diphyllobothriidae.

L. intestinalis the plerocercoids are found in the body cavity of freshwater fish, where they cause infertility and loss of condition. The adults are found in the alimentary tract of piscivorous birds.

Ligularia amplexicaulis Asian plant in the family Asteraceae; contains pyrrolizidine alkaloids which cause hepatitis; called also *L. mortonii*, dola.

Ligustrum vulgare European plant in the family Oleaceae. Reputed to cause gastroenteritis, but this is an uncommon event in view of the widespread occurrence of the plant. No toxin has been identified. Called also privet.

likelihood probability.

l. function a method used to estimate unknown parameters, using a function constructed from a statistical model which gives the probability of the observed data for various values of the unknown parameter. The values which maximize the probability are the maximum likelihood estimates.

maximum l. estimates see likelihood function (above).

liksucht [Dutch] see COPPER nutritional deficiency.

lilac 1. a lilac-gray coat color of cats, most commonly seen as a variety of Siamese or Himalayan (Colorpoint). 2. breed of rabbits with a dove gray coat; originally called Cambridge blue.

Lilium longiflorum garden plant in the family Liliaceae; an unidentified toxin causes nephrosis in cats. Called also Easter or Christmas lily.

lily a common name for many plants in the family Liliaceae, many of them poisonous. In cases where such plants are suspected of causing poisoning it is probably safest to assume that they are. See also GLORIOSA, ARUM.

l.-of-the-valley see CONVALLARIA MAJALIS.

l.-of-the-valley tree see CLETHRA ARBOREA.

lima bean PHASEOLUS *lunatus*.

limb 1. one of the paired appendages of the body used in locomotion and grasping. 2. a structure or part resembling an arm.

l. absence may be an acquired characteristic, or a congenital defect caused by inheritance of a modifying factor, e.g. 'mole' calves, or the effect of an environmental noxious agent, e.g. beta-irradiation. Called also amputates.

anacrotic l. the ascending portion of an arterial pulse tracing.

catacrotic l. the descending portion of an arterial pulse tracing.

l. curvature medially or laterally as in rickets, *Trachymene* spp. poisoning.

l. deformity abnormal size, shape, position or composition of a limb, which may be congenital and inherited or an acquired defect.

l. drag the limb is insufficiently flexed and the toe is dragged; indicates weakness or paresis.

l.-hoof conformation the contours, angulation and relative size of the component parts of a limb, all of which are vital to a long and troublefree life of locomotion, the principal function of agricultural animals.

l. mange see CHORIOPTIC MANGE.

pectoral l. the frontlimb.

pelvic l. the hindlimb.

thoracic l. pectoral limb.

limb flexure see ARTHROGRYPOSIS.

limberleg flaccid paralysis or paresis. Used to describe cases of botulism or poisoning by *Karwinskia humboldtiana*.

limberneck flaccid paralysis or paresis of the neck, used principally in referring to poultry with botulism.

limbic pertaining to a limbus, or margin.

l. conjunctiva the mucous membrane at the place of transition from corneal to conjunctival epithelium.

l. system a system of brain structures common to the brains of all mammals, comprising the phylogenetically old cortex (archipallium and paleopallium) and its primarily related nuclei. It is associated with olfaction, autonomic functions and certain aspects of emotion and behavior.

limbus pl. *limbi* [L.] an edge, fringe or border; used in anatomical nomenclature to designate the edge of the cornea, where it joins the sclera (limbus corneae, scleral limbus), and other margins in the body.

eyelid l. the skin–conjunctival junction at the palpebral rim.

oval fossa l. edge of a fossa in the atrial wall, location of the original interatrial foramen in the fetus.

scleral l. see limbus (above).

lime 1. calcium oxide, a corrosively alkaline earth, used for absorbing carbon dioxide from air. 2. agricultural lime, feed lime and chalk, which are all calcium carbonate. Lime for building mortar is calcium hydroxide; quick lime is calcium oxyhydroxide. 3. the acid fruit of *Citrus aurantifolia*.

chlorinated l., chloride of l. a disinfectant and antiseptic with properties similar to chlorine. Contains at least 30% available chlorine which is quickly inactivated by organic material. Called also bleaching powder. In combination with sodium carbonate and sodium bicarbonate, it forms DAKIN'S SOLUTION which is used for wound disinfection.

sulfurated l. see LIME-SULFUR.

l. water a saturated aqueous solution of calcium hydroxide.

lime-sulfur used as an orchard spray and topically as an ectoparasiticide and antifungal in the treatment of skin diseases. Can cause skin irritation in some animals. Called also calcium sulfide, calcium polysulfide, sulfurated lime.

limen pl. *limina* [L.] a threshold or boundary.

insula l., l. insulae the point at which the cortex of the insula is continuous with the cortex of the frontal lobe.

l. pharyngoesphagaeum a mucosal ridge where the pharynx becomes the esophagus.

limestone rock which is largely calcium carbonate, used as a livestock feed when ground. Contains 38% calcium and is used as a calcium supplement. See also DOLOMITE.

Limey disease renal coccidiosis in birds.

liminal barely perceptible; pertaining to a threshold.

liming addition of lime to a pasture or crop field as a fertilizer and soil conditioner.

liminometer an instrument for measuring the strength of a stimulus that just induces a tendon reflex.

limit dextrinosis glycogenosis type III.

limitans [L.] *limiting*.

limitation avoidance of excessive size.

liability l. see LIABILITY.

statute of l. each state has a statute that limits the time after an event at which legal proceedings can be initiated based on the event. The time lapse varies with the subject of the action and between states.

limited feeding see restricted FEEDING.

limiting udder infection a mastitis control program aimed at limiting the rate of acquisition of new udder infections so that the quarter infection rate does not exceed 10%.

Limnaea see LYMNAEA.

Limnatis a genus of leeches in the class Hirudinea.

Live in water and infest animals that pass through or drink the water.

L. africana found in the nasal cavity, vagina and urethra of humans, dogs and monkeys.

L. nilotica found in the pharynx and nasal cavity in all species. Causes anemia and local edema and obstruction.

Limnotragus spekei see SITUTUNGA.

D-limonene extracted from the oil of citrus peel, used as an external parasiticide on dogs, but may be toxic to cats.

Limousin dark yellow, beef or draft breed of cattle.

limping syndrome joint pain, hyperesthesia and muscle soreness reported in cats infected with feline CALICIVIRUS.

***Limulus* test** a lysate of blood cells from the horseshoe crab (*Limulus polyphemus*) is used to test specimens for the presence of *Escherichia coli* endotoxin in blood or milk.

linalool a natural insecticidal compound found in oil extracted from citrus peel. Similar in activity to D-LIMONENE.

linamarase an enzyme in the plants *Linum* spp. which liberates hydrocyanic acid from a cyanogenetic glycoside in the same plant. Boiling for 10 minutes destroys the enzyme and renders the material, usually linseed, safe.

linamarin the toxic cyanogenetic glycoside in linseed and flax. See also LINATINE, LINUM.

Linaria vulgaris a European plant of the family Scrophulariaceae. Contains cardiac glycosides and is a potential cause of poisoning, manifested by diarrhea. Called also toad flax.

linatine a toxin found in linseed. Causes pyridoxine deficiency in fowls fed on linseed meal. See also LINAMARIN.

Lincoln an English longwool breed of polled, meat sheep, used as a base for new meat breeds.

Lincoln formula a formula used to estimate the number of animals in a wildlife population where the capture–release–recapture strategy is adopted. The formula is N/M = n/m, where N is the unknown population size, M is the number of marked animals released, n is the number of animals recaptured, and m is the number of recaptured animals that are marked.

Lincoln red a deep red breed of beef cattle, originating from Shorthorn cattle. A polled variety is also available.

lincomycin a lincosamide antibiotic produced by *Streptomyces lincolnensis*; used as the hydrochloride salt.

l.-associated colitis a disease of horses resembling colitis-X occurring in horses receiving therapy with lincomycin; an organism resembling *Clostridium cadaveris* has been suggested as a cause.

lincosamides bacteriostatic antibiotics that inhibit protein synthesis; includes lincomycin and clindamycin.

lindane the gamma isomer of benzene hexachloride used as a topical pediculicide and scabicide. Carries the same toxicity risks as all CHLORINATED hydrocarbons. Called also γ-HCH, γ-BHC, gamma benzene hexachloride.

line 1. a stripe, streak, mark, or narrow ridge; often an imaginary line connecting different landmarks. See also LINEA. 2. conversion of a broad beam of x-rays to a pencil beam. 3. a single consignment of livestock from one farm. Said of a group of cattle or sheep notable for their homogeneity.

absorption l's dark lines in the spectrum due to absorption of light by the substance through which the light has passed.

l. block a nerve block of local anesthesia produced by infiltrating the anesthetic along a line that the incision is to take.

blue l. lead line (below).

cell l. see CELL CULTURE.

cement l. a line visible in microscopic examination of bone in cross section, marking the boundary of an osteon (haversian system).

cervical l. see CEMENTO-ENAMEL JUNCTION.

cleavage l's linear clefts in the skin indicative of direction of the fibers.

l. dressing a system of handling carcasses in an abattoir. The carcasses move along an overhead chain line past a series of stations where the dressing and meat inspection is done.

l. feed the advance on a printer by one line.

l. focus utilization of a broad beam of electrons for the generation of x-rays by a rotating anode so that the area of the target on which the electrons fall is spread over a line instead of a point.

gingival l. 1. a line determined by the level to which the gingiva extends on a tooth; called also gum line. 2. any linear mark visible on the surface of the gingiva.

gum l. gingival line (1).

iliopectineal l. the ridge on the ilium and pubes showing the brim of the true pelvis.

incremental l's lines supposedly showing the successive layers deposited in a tissue, as in the tooth enamel.

intertrochanteric l. one running obliquely from the greater to the lesser trochanter.

lead l. a bluish line at the edge of the gums in lead poisoning. Rarely seen in animals.

median l. an imaginary vertical line dividing the body equally into right and left parts.

milk l. 1. the line of thickened epithelium in the embryo along which the mammary glands are developed. 2. the metal tube in a milking machine along which the milk, after extraction from the cow, passes to the storage vat.

mylohyoid l. a ridge on the inner surface of the lower jaw from the base of the symphysis to the ascending rami behind the last molar tooth.

pectinate l. one marking the junction of the zone of the anal canal lined with stratified squamous epithelium and the zone lined with columnar epithelium.

physeal l. one on the surface of an adult long bone, marking the junction of the epiphysis and diaphysis.

pleural reflection l. line of the junction between costal and diaphragmatic pleurae.

semilunar l. a curved line along the lateral border of each rectus abdominis muscle, marking the meeting of the aponeuroses of the internal oblique and transverse abdominal muscles.

temporal l. a curved ridge on the external surface of the cranium that marks the origin of the temporal muscle.

terminal l. one on the inner surface of each pelvic bone, from the sacroiliac joint to the iliopubic eminence cranially, separating the false from the true pelvis, and marking the pelvic inlet.

l. transects a technique for estimating the density of a population, e.g. the number of deer per hectare in a gamepark.

visual l. a line from the point of vision of the retina to the object of vision; called also visual axis.

linea pl. *lineae* [L.] a narrow ridge or streak on a surface, as of the body or a bone or other organ; a line.

l. alba white line; the tendinous median line on the ventral abdominal wall between the two rectus muscles.
l. albicantes see atrophic STRIA.
l. aspera one or two rough longitudinal lines on the back of the femur for muscle attachments.
lineae atrophicae see atrophic STRIA.

linear in a line.
l. assessment a method of expressing an assessment result as a score out of a possible perfect score of 10, or some other number. Used in body condition scoring, showring judging of conformation.
l. dodecyl benzene sulfonic acid teat dip see TEAT DIP.
l. energy transfer expresses the quality of electronic radiation. It is concerned with the spatial distributions of energy transfers which occur in the tracks of particles as they penetrate matter.
l. model see linear programming MODEL.
l. program a management program used to determine the best mix of ingredients or services to be used in a particular situation to maintain the highest level of productivity or profitability or other similar parameter.
l. regression statistical method used to study the relationship between independent and dependent variables when the dependent variable consists of continuous data.
l. scores numbers reduced to natural logarithms.

linearity the characteristic of being a straight line. If one variable is a linear function of another, a graph prepared by plotting one against the other will be a straight line.

linebreeding breeding to animals in the same family.

linen suture suture material made of flax fiber.

liner see TEAT CUP LINER.

lingua pl. *linguae* [L.] tongue.
l. nigra black tongue.

lingual pertaining to or near the tongue.
l. bone hyoid bone.
l. swellings primordia of the tongue, the median swelling and the distal and proximal swellings arise from the ventral aspect of the stomodeum.

Linguatula a genus of parasites in the class Pentastomida.
L. serrata adults occur in the nasal cavities of canines and larvae in mesenteric lymph nodes of the horse, goat, sheep and rabbit. Causes sneezing and a bloody nasal discharge. The larval stages may be confused with tuberculosis.

linguatulosis, linguatuliasis disease caused by infection with LINGUATULA.

linguitis inflammation of the tongue; the usual name is GLOSSITIS.

lingula pl. *lingulae* [L.] a small, tonguelike structure.

lingulectomy excision of a lingula.

linguo- word element. [L.] *tongue.*

linguo-occlusal angle where the lingual and the occlusal surfaces of a tooth meet.

linguofacial pertaining to the tongue and the face.

linguopapillitis inflammation or ulceration of the papillae of the edges of the tongue.

liniment a medicinal preparation in an oily, soapy or alcoholic vehicle, intended to be rubbed on the skin as a counterirritant or anodyne.

linitis inflammation of gastric cellular tissue.
l. plastica inelastic thickening and fibrosis of the gastric submucosa; called also leather bottle lesion.

link connecting one part or thing with another.
l. proteins stabilize the aggregates of proteoglycans in ground substance in supportive tissues forming large bottle-brush-like configurations.
l. relatives a method of analysis of series of values over time. The values for successive time periods are expressed as proportions of the values of the preceding time periods.

linkage 1. the connection between different atoms in a chemical compound, or the symbol representing it in structural formulae. See also BOND. 2. in genetics, the association of genes having located on the same chromosome, which results in the tendency of a group of such nonallelic genes to be associated in inheritance (linkage disequilibrium). Called also syntenic group.
disequilibrium l. the inheritance of two alleles together at a higher than expected frequency.
l. map see GENETIC map.

linnet small songbird in the family Fringillidae. Called also *Carduelis cannabina.*

Linognathus a genus of sucking lice of the family Linognathidae, mostly parasitic on ungulates. Includes *L. africanus* (goats), *L. ovillus* (sheep face or blue louse), *L. pedalis* (on hairless parts of limbs of sheep, called also foot louse), *L. setosus* (fox, dog), *L. stenopis* (goat), *L. vituli* (cattle—called also long-nosed cattle louse).

linoleate see LINOLEIC ACID.

linoleic acid an essential fatty acid; contains 18 carbons and 2 double bonds at carbons 9, 10 and 12,13; precursor of n-6 or omega 6 fatty acids; the major unsaturated fatty acid found in vegetable oils.
l. acid deficiency dry, scaling skin and alopecia have been reported in cats deficient in linoleic acid. Dietary deficiency occurs in cats fed diets low in fat, containing rancid fat, or with little or no animal-source fats.

linolenate see LINOLENIC ACID.

linolenic acid an essential fatty acid; *[alpha]-linolenic acid* is an 18 carbon fatty acid containing three double bonds at carbons 9, 12, and 15; found in plant leaves and some vegetable oils. *[gamma]-linolenic acid* is an 18 carbon fatty acid containing double bonds at carbons 6, 9 and 12; produced in animals by the desaturation of linoleic acid.

linoleum a floor-covering which contains lead; cows and dogs with pica may be poisoned when they eat it.

linseed LINUM *usitatissimum.*
l. cake the residue after the removal of the linseed oil by commercial processes. Contains cyanogenetic glycosides and may cause poisoning.
l. meal cake ground into meal.
l. oil used at one time as a lubricant laxative for horses in doses of 1 to 2 quarts as a drench. Has the unfortunate effect on unpredictable occasions of causing superpurgation and is generally supplanted by mineral oil.

Linstowia anoplocephalid cestode found in Australian marsupials.

lint an absorbent surgical dressing material.

Linton gag a gag in which two metal loops are hinged together at two sites so that they move inside each other. The closed loops are placed in the mouth and then opened by opening the other end of the loops. A good mouth speculum for sheep.

Linum a European plant genus containing LINSEED or flax, a member of the Linaceae family. Includes *L. catharticum* (purging flax), *L. usitatissimum* (common flax, linseed). Causes cyanide poisoning. Long-term ingestion can cause goiter.

linuron a methyl urea herbicide. Sprayed plants may contain higher than normal amounts of nitrate and cause nitrite poisoning.

lion the largest wild carnivore, yellow, tawny or gray in color; males have a distinctive mane. Called also *Panthera leo.*

l. jaw see CRANIOMANDIBULAR osteopathy.
mountain l. a lion-colored, maneless lion. Called also *Panthera concolor* (syn. *Felis concolor*), cougar, puma.
l.-tailed macaque *Macaca silenus*. See also MACAQUE.

liothyronine the pharmaceutical name for the thyroid hormone triiodothyronine (T_3); used in the treatment of hypothyroidism.

liotrix a mixture of liothyronine sodium and levothyroxine sodium in a ratio of 1 : 4 in terms of weight; used for replacement therapy in hypothyroidism.

lip 1. the upper or lower fleshy margin of the mouth. 2. any fleshy boundary; labium.
l. droop an unnatural hanging of the lower lip, which is not used during prehension and mastication; there is an accompanying lack of sensitivity of the part. Unilateral droop is usually an indication of facial paralysis; bilateral droop occurs in many conditions of general paralysis, e.g. botulism.
l. fold dermatitis see fold DERMATITIS.
l.–leg ulceration a disease of sheep. See ULCERATIVE dermatosis.
l. philtrum the vertical median groove or fissure in the upper lip of some mammals.
l. twitch see TWITCH.
l. ulcer see EOSINOPHILIC ulcer.

lip-curl see FLEHMEN.

lipacidemia an excess of fatty acids in the blood.

lipaciduria fatty acid in the urine.

lipase fat-splitting enzyme; abbreviated LPS. Any enzyme that catalyzes the splitting of fats into glycerol and fatty acids. The two important sources in the body are the pancreas and the intestinal mucosa. Measurement of the serum levels of lipase is an important diagnostic test for acute and chronic pancreatitis. See also PANCREATIC lipase.
triglyceride l. see TRIACYLGLYCEROL lipase.

lipectomy excision of a mass of subcutaneous adipose tissue.

lipedema an accumulation of excess fat and fluid in subcutaneous tissues.

lipemia an excess of lipids in the blood; hyperlipemia.
alimentary l. postprandial lipemia (below).
fasting l. that present when food has been withheld for at least 24 hours.
postprandial l. a physiological effect that occurs between 2 and 12 hours after the ingestion of food high in lipids.
l.-refrigeration test refrigeration of a lipemic blood sample may distinguish between triglyceride-rich lipoproteins, which persist in the turbid sample, and chylomicra, which rise to form a flocculent top layer while the sample clears.
l. retinalis that manifested by a milky appearance of the veins and arteries of the retina. Seen in hyperlipoproteinemia in dogs.

Lipeurus a genus of lice in the suborder Ischnocera.
L. caponis the wing louse of fowl and pheasants.

lipid a group of substances comprising fatty, greasy, oily and waxy compounds that are insoluble in water and soluble in nonpolar solvents, such as hexane, ether and chloroform.

Simple lipids are the triglycerides or neutral fats. Each triglyceride molecule is composed of one molecule of glycerol joined by ester linkages to three fatty acid molecules. They are an important source of oxidizable substrate to the body and have a greater caloric density (2.25 times) than carbohydrate.

Compound lipids are important structural components of cell membranes. Phospholipids include lecithin and the cephalins, which are composed of fatty acids linked to phosphatidic acid, and the sphingomyelins, which are composed of fatty acids linked to sphingosine. Glycolipids are composed of a carbohydrate chain and fatty acids linked to sphingosine or ceramide. Cholesterol is a steroid alcohol. Another important function of the phospholipids is as lung surfactants.
l. A a component of the cell wall of gram-negative bacteria, responsible for their toxic properties.
l. pneumonia see lipid PNEUMONIA.
protected l's fats treated to protect them against microbial degeneration in the rumen.
l. transport disease a group of diseases in which there is a disorder of lipid metabolism with abnormal levels or types of lipoproteins in the blood, e.g. HYPERLIPOPROTEINEMIA, HYPERLIPEMIA.

lipidosis see lipid STORAGE DISEASE.
idiopathic feline hepatic l. see FATTY liver syndrome (2).
sphingomyelin l. see SPHINGOMYELINOSIS.

lipiduria the presence of lipids in the urine.

lipiodol a radiopaque material at one time used as a contrast agent for salivary duct delineation and similar external tasks.

Lipitsa a famous breed of horses used at the Spanish Riding School in Vienna. Originated from Arab and Andalusian horses at Lipitsa stud in Yugoslavia. Light horses, usually gray, about 15.2 hands high. Foals are born black, gray or brown and change color gradually over a number of years. These horses are surprisingly small and muscular; one expects to see a much taller, more graceful animal. Called also Lipizzaner, Lippizaner and other similar spellings.

Lipizzaner see LIPITSA.

lip(o)- word element. [Gr.] *fat, lipid.*

lipoarthritis inflammation of the fatty tissue of a joint.

lipoatrophy atrophy of subcutaneous fatty tissues of the body.

lipoblast a connective tissue cell that develops into a fat cell.

lipocardiac pertaining to fatty degeneration of the heart.

lipochondrodystrophy mucopolysaccharidosis I.

lipochondroma a tumor composed of mature lipomatous and cartilaginous elements.

lipochrome any one of a group of fat-soluble hydrocarbon pigments, such as carotene, lutein, chromophane, and the natural yellow coloring material of butter, egg yolk, and yellow corn. They are also known as carotenoids.

lipocyte a fat cell.

lipodystrophy any disturbance of fat metabolism.
porcine cerebrospinal l. see GM_2 GANGLIOSIDOSIS.

lipofection using encapsulation in a phospholipid vesicle as a means of delivering RNA, DNA or other substances into a eukaryotic cell.

lipofibroma a lipoma containing fibrous elements.

lipofuscin any of a class of fatty pigments formed by the solution of a pigment in fat. They take the form of golden granular deposits derived from lipid components of membranous organelles, and commonly occur with advancing age or vitamin E deficiency. Called also abnutzen pigment.
l.-like pigment accumulates in the liver of patients, e.g. mutant Corriedale sheep, which lack enzymes necessary for bile salt conjugation and transport; the livers of affected sheep are black.

lipofuscinosis any disorder due to abnormal storage of lipofuscins.
ceroid l. an inherited disease in sheep, cattle, dogs

and cats, characterized by blindness, mental dullness and abnormal behavior. There is atrophy of the brain with extensive accumulation of lipopigments ('ceroid bodies') in nervous tissue and later viscera as well. The comparable, though possibly not identical, disease in humans is also called Batten disease.

hepatic l. a deposit of lipofuscin in partly oxidized form in the livers of sheep, which gives them a deep black color and makes them unsaleable. The condition is common in areas where the mulga tree (*Acacia aneura*) grows and the leaves are fed to sheep as fodder.

lipogenesis the formation of fat; the transformation of nonfat food materials into body fat.

lipogenic producing, forming or caused by fat.

lipogenous producing fatness.

lipogranuloma a nodule of lipoid material associated with granulomatous inflammation.

lipogranulomatosis a condition of faulty lipid metabolism in which yellow nodules of lipoid material are deposited in the skin and mucosae, giving rise to granulomatous reactions.

lipoic acid a vitamin prosthetic group in enzymes involved in oxidative decarboxylation of keto acids such as 2-oxoglutarate and pyruvate. Called also α-lipoic acid, thioctic acid.

lipoid pneumonia see lipid PNEUMONIA.

lipoidemia lipids in the blood; lipemia.

lipoidosis a disturbance of lipid metabolism with abnormal deposit of lipids in the cells.

lipoiduria lipids in the urine; lipiduria.

lipolysis the breakdown, splitting up or decomposition of fat.

lipoma a benign fatty tumor usually composed of mature fat cells. They have a special importance in horses, in which the pedunculated tumors in the abdominal cavity uncommonly twist themselves around a loop of small intestine, sometimes just below the pylorus or around the rectum. The occurrence of this particular form of colic is limited to horses 12 years or older. The clinical signs are not diagnostic except that the strangulation of the rectum causes a purse-string closure of the lumen just inside the anus and is easily detected at rectal examination.

infiltrating l. see LIPOSARCOMA.

skin l. localized nodules of normal looking fat in sucutaneous tissue in most species.

lipomatosis a condition characterized by abnormal localized, or tumor-like, accumulations of fat in the tissues. Large lipomatous masses occur in large numbers in the peritoneal cavity of cattle. They have importance in that they may be mistaken for calves on rectal examination. They may also cause chronic partial obstruction of the intestine with intermittent colic and indifferent appetite as the main signs. The common sites for the obstructions are the pylorus and the coiled colon. Called also massive fat necrosis.

lipomatous affected with, or of the nature of, lipoma.

lipomeningocele meningocele associated with an overlying lipoma, as in spina bifida.

lipomeria congenital absence of a limb.

lipometabolism metabolism of fat.

lipomyxoma a myxoma containing fatty elements.

liponeogenesis formation of fat, mostly in the liver and adipose tissue and lactating mammary gland, and principally from glucose and acetate in the ruminant.

Liponyssus see ORNITHONYSSUS.

lipopenia deficiency of lipids in the body.

lipophage a cell that absorbs or ingests fat.

lipophagia lipophagy.

lipophagy the absorption of fat; lipolysis.

lipophanerosis an outmoded concept relating to intracellular deposition of lipid.

lipophilia affinity for fat.

lipopolysaccharide a molecule in which lipids and polysaccharides are linked. See also ENDOTOXIN.

lipoprotein any of the macromolecular complexes that are the form in which lipids are transported in the blood. They consist of a core of hydrophobic lipids covered by a layer of phospholipids and apoproteins, which make the complex water-soluble. There are four main classes of lipoproteins: *chylomicrons*, in which lipids are transported after a meal from the intestine to tissues, where they are stored or used; *very low density lipoproteins* (VLDL); *low density lipoproteins* (LDL); and *high density lipoproteins* (HDL). VLDL and HDL are produced by both the liver and the intestine; LDL is produced by the metabolism of VLDL.

α-l. high density lipoproteins which migrate in the alpha position in paper chromatography. Inherited deficiency of these proteins is described in humans but there is no known animal model of the disease.

l. factor Xa inhibitor a blood coagulation inhibitor present in the low density lipoprotein fraction of plasma.

high density l. (HDL) a fraction of lipoproteins separable by ultracentrifugation.

intermediate density l. (IDL) intermediate in density between LDL and VLDL; migrate in electrophoresis with β-globulins.

l. lipase specific lipase hydrolyzing lipoproteins.

l. lipase deficiency see HYPERLIPOPROTEINEMIA.

γ-lipotropin a polypeptide hormone isolated from the hypophysis.

lipoproteinemia the presence of excessive lipoproteins in the blood. See also HYPERLIPOPROTEINEMIA.

lipoproteinosis accumulation of acidophilic, acellular material, e.g. within pulmonary alveoli.

Lipoptena a parasitic genus of flies in the family Hippoboscidae.

L. caprina a ked of goats.

L. cervi a parasite of deer, wild boar and badger.

liposarcoma a malignant tumor characterized by large anaplastic lipoblasts, sometimes with foci of normal fat cells.

liposis see LIPOMATOSIS.

liposoluble soluble in fats.

liposome a spherical structure, usually multilamelate, prepared from eukaryotic cell membranes which may be used as a carrier for glycoprotein antigens and drugs.

Lipotes vexillifer see DOLPHIN.

lipothymia see SYNCOPE.

lipotrope a lipotropic substance, e.g. choline, methionine.

γ-lipotropic hormone one of the products of a cleavage of a β-lipotrophic hormone.

β-lipotrophin see β-LIPOTROPIN.

lipotrophy increase of bodily fat.

lipotropic 1. acting on fat metabolism by hastening removal, or decreasing the deposit, of fat in the liver. 2. a lipotropic agent.

β-lipotropin a polypeptide which promotes the mobilization of fat; synthesized in the adenohypophysis.

lipotropism, lipotropy the condition of being lipotropic.

lipovaccine an inactivated vaccine in an oil adjuvant.

lipoxidase see LIPOXYGENASE.

lipoxygenase an enzyme that catalyzes the oxidation of polyunsaturated fatty acids to form a peroxide of the acid.

Lippia genus of South African plants in the family Verbenaceae; contain the triterpene lantadene which causes liver damage and photosensitization. Includes *L. javanica*, *L. pretoriensis*, *L. rehmanni* (*L. baziana*), *L. scaberrima*, *L. wilmsii*.
L. rehmanni a poisonous South African plant that contains icterogenin and rehmannic acid, both hepatotoxins that cause liver damage and a syndrome of depression, photosensitization and jaundice. Rehmannic acid is identical with lantadene A in *Lantana camara*.
lipuria lipids in the urine.
liquefacient 1. producing or pertaining to liquefaction. 2. an agent that produces liquefaction.
liquefaction conversion into a liquid form.
l. degeneration see HYDROPIC degeneration.
l. necrosis tissue undergoing liquefaction.
liquescent tending to become liquid or fluid.
liquid 1. a substance that flows readily in its natural state. 2. flowing readily; neither solid nor gaseous.
l. diet a diet limited to the intake of liquids or foods that can be changed to a liquid state.
l. nitrogen compressed nitrogen in liquid form; used as a supercoolant in freezing semen, and in cryosurgery.
l. paraffin, l. petrolatum see mineral OIL.
liquor 1. a liquid, especially an aqueous solution, containing medicinal substances. 2. a term applied to certain body fluids.
l. amnii amniotic fluid.
l. cerebrospinalis cerebrospinal fluid.
l. folliculi the fluid in the cavity of a developing graafian follicle.
l. pericardii pericardial fluid.
l. pleurae pleural fluid.
lisinopril an angiotensin-converting enzyme inhibitor, similar to captopril, but with longer duration of activity. Used in the treatment of heart disease in dogs.
lissencephaly a malformation in which the gyri of the cerebral cortex are not normally developed. In dogs it has been associated with behavioral abnormalities, visual deficits, ataxia and seizures. Called also agyria.
Lister scissors scissors designed for the crossways cutting of bandages that are in place on the patient. The blades take a 45° angle at the pivot so that they can be inserted under the bandage and leave the knuckles of the cutting hand clear of the patient. The lower blade has a rounded, blunt end to facilitate entry under the bandage without catching the blade.
listerellosis see LISTERIOSIS.
Listeria a genus of gram-positive bacteria in the form of small rods which frequently resemble diphtheroids. The most important species, *L. monocytogenes*, is found chiefly in ruminants. It causes a multi-syndrome disease referred to as LISTERIOSIS. *L. ivanovii* causes abortion in cattle and sheep.
listeriosis an infectious disease affecting all species and caused by *Listeria monocytogenes* and characterized by either meningoencephalitis and a syndrome of circling, facial paralysis, somnolence, endophthalmitis, head pressing, and abortion, or by septicemia in the newborn. Called also listerial meningoencephalitis.
listerism the principles and practice of antiseptic and aseptic surgery.
listlessness shows lack of interest in its surroundings.
Liston forceps standard bone-cutting scissor-type forceps; a heavy instrument with handles sprung to open and blades presenting opposing chisel faces.
Listrophorus a genus of mites in the family Listrophoridae.
L. gibbus may cause a mange-like condition in rabbits.
liter the unit of capacity of the metric system, being equal to 1 cubic decimeter; equivalent to 1.1365 Imperial quarts (1.0567 American quarts) liquid measure. See SI UNITS. Abbreviated l (or sometimes L).
lithagogue 1. expelling calculi. 2. an agent that promotes expulsion of calculi.
lithectasy extraction of calculi through a mechanically dilated urethra.
lithemia an excess of uric (lithic) acid in the blood.
lithiasis a condition marked by formation of calculi and concretions. See GALLSTONE, salivary CALCULUS, UROLITHIASIS, UROLITH, prostatic CALCULUS.
lithium a chemical element, atomic number 3, atomic weight 6.939, symbol Li. See Table 6.
l. carbonate used in the treatment of canine cyclic hematopoiesis to stabilize numbers of neutrophils.
lith(o)- word element. [Gr.] *stone, calculus.*
lithocholic acid the product of bacterial metabolism of bile acids in the intestine. Insoluble and not reabsorbed.
lithoclast see LITHOTRITE.
lithocystotomy incision of the bladder for removal of stone.
lithodialysis 1. the solution of calculi in the bladder by injected solvents. 2. litholapaxy.
lithogenesis formation of calculi, or stones.
litholapaxy the crushing of a stone in the bladder and washing out of the fragments. Called also lithotripsy.
litholysis dissolution of calculi.
lithonephritis inflammation of the kidney due to irritation by calculi.
lithonephrotomy excision of a renal calculus.
lithontriptic pertaining to LITHOLAPAXY.
lithopedion a fetus calcified in utero.
lithophagia ingestion of stones and rock.
lithophone a device for detecting calculi in the bladder by sound; a forerunner of ultrasound devices.
lithoscope an instrument for examining calculi in the bladder; a cystoscope.
Lithospermum arvense toxic plant genus in the family Boraginaceae; contains pyrrolizidine alkaloids; capable of causing liver damage. Called also *Buglossoides arvensis*, corn gromwell.
lithotomy incision of a duct or organ for removal of calculi.
lithotripsy see LITHOLAPAXY.
lithotrite an instrument for crushing calculi; lithoclast.
lithotrity see LITHOLAPAXY.
lithous pertaining to or of the nature of a calculus.
lithuresis passage of gravel in the urine.
litmus a blue pigment prepared from *Rocella tinctoria* and other lichens.
l. paper absorbent paper impregnated with a solution of litmus, dried and cut into strips. It is used to indicate the acidity or alkalinity of solutions. If dipped into alkaline solution, it remains blue; acid solution turns it red. It is used to test urine and other body fluids; it has a pH range of 4.5 to 8.3.
Litocranius walleri see GERENUK.
litre liter.
Littauer scissors scissors designed especially for cutting skin sutures; one blade is hook-shaped and designed to slip easily under a suture and to avoid the suture slipping off the end of the blade while it is being cut.
litter 1. the group of neonates, products of one gestation, provided the average number is in excess of two. 2. dry particulate material used for bedding or

as absorptive layer under animals or periodically by the animal to absorb urine and dry out feces. Dry litter system for poultry and litter for cats to use for urination and defecation while indoors.
l. size the number of young in a litter is an important statistic in pigs because of the need to maximize the output of piglets per sow per year.
l. tray the container, usually broad with low sides, that holds some absorbent material; used by indoor cats for urination and defecation.
little-leaf horsebrush see TETRADYMIA GLABRATA.
Little lion dog see LOWCHEN.
littoral pertaining to the shore.
live-leaf see BRYOPHYLLUM *pinnatum*.
live plant see BRYOPHYLLUM *pinnatum*.
liver 1. the large, dark-red organ located in the cranial portion of the abdomen, just behind the diaphragm. Its functions include storage and filtration of blood; secretion of bile; detoxication of noxious substances; conversion of sugars into glycogen; synthesis and breakdown of fats and temporary storage of fatty acids; and synthesis of serum proteins such as certain of the alpha and beta globulins, albumin, which helps regulate blood volume, and fibrinogen and prothrombin, which are essential blood clotting factors. See also HEPATIC. 2. a rich red-brown coat color in dogs that resembles the color of the organ.
l. abscess causes toxemia, possibly local signs of subacute abdominal pain, pain on percussion or palpation over the liver if peritoneal inflammation is present, when there may also be a positive paracentesis sample.
l. damage damage to the liver parenchyma causing some degree of hepatic insufficiency.
l. displacement may be because of a diaphragmatic hernia with the liver protruding into the thoracic cavity. Usually accompanied by dyspnea.
l. dullness dullness on percussion over the right rib cage, used to help in defining the size of the liver which must be grossly enlarged to register a recognizable change.
l. dysfunction the result of diffuse damage to the liver, e.g. in hepatitis. There may be clinical signs including photosensitization, jaundice, hepatic encephalopathy in the form of the dummy syndrome, dullness and anorexia, or there may be subclinical disease detectable by clinicopathological tests, e.g. hypoglycemia, hypoproteinemia, hyperammonemia. All of the functions of the liver will be affected at the one time.
l. enlargement may be caused by neoplasia, congestion (as with heart failure), and infiltration by fat or inflammatory cells.
l. enzyme when there is acute, diffuse damage to the liver some of its enzymes are liberated into the blood, where they can be measured. An indication of the severity of the damage can be obtained in this way. Different enzymes are used in each animal species.
l. failure when liver function is inadequate to sustain life; the end-stage of liver dysfunction.
fatty l. one affected with fatty infiltration.
fatty l. syndrome see FAT cow syndrome.
l. fluke FASCIOLA *hepatica*.
l. fluke disease see hepatic FASCIOLIASIS.
l. function summation of the functions of the liver.
l. function tests biochemical tests capable of demonstrating that the liver's functions are, or are not, at full capacity. The SULFOBROMOPHTHALEIN clearance test is the most commonly used in veterinary medicine.
l. inflammation see HEPATITIS.
inherited l. insufficiency occurs in several breeds of sheep and is characterized by the appearance of photosensitive dermatitis when the lambs begin to eat green feed. There is an accumulation of phylloerythrin in the blood and other biochemical indications of insufficiency, but the liver is histologically normal. Called also inherited photosensitization.
l. injury damage to the hepatic parenchyma, possibly by massive trauma, but usually by an hepatic toxin. A common cause of hepatic insufficiency.
l. insufficiency see liver dysfunction (above).
l. lobe torsion see liver torsion (below).
l. melanosis see hepatic LIPOFUSCINOSIS.
l. meridian points acupuncture points along the liver meridian.
l. necrobacillosis a disease characterized by multiple liver abscesses, usually containing *Fusobacterium necrophorum* and resulting from infection from a chemical rumenitis which originated from carbohydrate engorgement and lactic acid rumenitis.
l. protectant substance used for the treatment of liver failure. The important ones are choline, methionine, betaine, lecithin, vitamin B_{12} , selenium-vitamin E, essential phospholipids, glucose, fructose, vitamins E and B complex, and glucuronic acid.
l. rot see acute hepatic FASCIOLIASIS.
l. rupture is usually the result of severe trauma to the abdomen. In most cases there is massive hemorrhage into the peritoneal cavity, acute hemorrhagic anemia and mucosal pallor. Abdominal paracentesis recovers whole blood.
l. torsion is usually restricted to a single lobe. Causes severe abdominal pain and severe vomiting.
liverseed grass UROCHLOA *panicoides*.
livestock agricultural animals; animals kept for profit.
l. feed budget see FEED budget.
l. gross income total of income from sales of livestock or their produce.
l. insurance insurance against loss by death or production, recoupable in terms of loss of capital asset.
l. producer animal farmer, e.g. pig farmer.
l. production system management strategies, e.g. extensive grazing, zero-grazing, feedlotting, all-in–all-out system.
liveware people involved in computer utilization.
liveweight see body WEIGHT.
livid discolored, as from a contusion or bruise; black and blue.
lividity the quality of being livid; discoloration, as of dependent parts, by gravitation of blood.
lixiviation separation of soluble from insoluble material by use of an appropriate solvent, and drawing off the solution.
lizard member of the suborder Lacertilia. There are about 2500 species of true lizards and allied groups. None of them is poisonous.
l. poisoning infection with the fluke PLATYNOSOMUM *fastosum*.
Lizard canary a very old breed with distinctively colored feathers. The basic colors are gold or silver with black markings on the feathers' edges which makes them resemble scales. On the back this is called spangling, on the breast, rowing, and on the head, the cap.
llama together with camels, the South American camelids form the suborder Tylopoda. There are four species, the llama (*Lama glama*), the guanaco (*L. huanacos*, syn. *L. guanicoe*), the vicuña (*L. vicugna*, syn. *Vicugna vicugna*), and the alpaca (*L. pacos*). They are all long-legged, long-necked animals, like camels without humps. The alpaca is used for its wool, the others are used as pack animals.

Llewellin setter see ENGLISH SETTER.
LMF leukocyte mitogenic factor.
LMM light meromysin; produced by a digestion of myosin.
LMN lower motor neuron.
LNPF lymph node permeability factor.
Loa a genus of onchocercid worms in the superfamily Filarioidea.
L. loa causes subcutaneous nodules in humans and primates. Transmitted by *Chrysops* spp.
load 1. the quantity of a measurable form of work, e.g. metabolic or circulatory, borne by an organism, especially when it exceeds the normal amount of work for that process. Called also workload. 2. a computer command to load data or a program from a storage device into the memory of the computer.
loading administering sufficient quantities of a substance to test a subject's ability to metabolize or absorb it.
l. dose see loading DOSE.
loaiasis infection with nematodes of the genus *Loa*; loiasis.
lobar pertaining to a lobe.
congenital l. emphysema emphysema of one or more lung lobes usually the result of bronchial dysplasia or agenesis in the neonate.
l. pneumonia pneumonia affecting one or more lobes of the lungs. See also lobar PNEUMONIA.
lobate divided into lobes.
lobe 1. a more or less well-defined portion of an organ or gland. 2. one of the main divisions of a tooth crown.
caudate l. a small dorsally located lobe of the liver to the right of the caudal vena cava that frequently embraces the right kidney.
ear l. an elevated area of skin just below the external auditory meatus in birds.
frontal l. the anterior portion of the gray matter of the cerebral hemisphere.
hepatic l. one of the lobes of the liver.
occipital l. the most posterior portion of the cerebral hemisphere, forming a small part of its dorsolateral surface.
parietal l. the upper central portion of the gray matter of the cerebral hemisphere, between the frontal and occipital lobes, and above the temporal lobe. See also PARIETAL lobe.
prefrontal l. the part of the brain rostral to the ascending convolution.
quadrate l. 1. precuneus. 2. a small lobe of the liver, between the gallbladder on the right, and the left lobe.
temporal l. the lower lateral portion of the cerebral hemisphere.
lobectomy excision of a lobe, as of the lung, brain or liver.
Lobelia genus of toxic plants in the Campanulaceae family; toxins are pyridine alkaloids, e.g. lobeline; cause diarrhea, oral ulcers; include *L. berlandieri*, *L. inflata* (Indian tobacco), *L. pratioides*, *L. purpurascens*, *L. urens*.
lobeline a poisonous alkaloid found in plants of LOBELIA spp.
lobitis inflammation of a lobe, as of the lung.
loblolly pine see PINUS *taeda*.
Loboa loboi a unicellular organism, probably a yeast, that causes LOBOMYCOSIS in dolphins and keloidal blastomycosis in humans.
lobomycosis a skin disease of dolphins caused by the yeast LOBOA LOBOI and manifested by dermal granulomas or keloids, especially around the head. The disease is a debilitating one and may kill the dolphin.
lobotomy cutting of nerve fibers connecting a lobe of the brain with the thalamus. In most cases the affected parts are the prefrontal or frontal lobes; thus the operation is referred to as prefrontal, or frontal, lobotomy. Performed in humans as a form of psychosurgery. It has been applied in dogs for the treatment of aggressive behavior, but is of limited usefulness.
lobster see HOMARUS, NEPHROPS, PALINURUS.
lobulated made up of lobules.
lobulation the state of having lobules or of being lobulated.
lobule a small segment or lobe, especially one of the smaller divisions making up a lobe.
ansiform l. a lobule of the cerebellar hemispheres.
l's of epididymis the wedge-shaped parts of the head of the epididymis, each comprising an efferent ductule of the testis.
hepatic l. one of the small vascular units and associated parenchyme comprising the substance of the liver.
l. of lung one of the smaller subdivisions of the lobes of the lungs.
paracentral l. a lobe on the medial surface of the cerebral hemisphere, continuous with the pre- and postcentral gyri, limited below by the cingulate sulcus.
paramedian l. a lobule of the cerebellar hemispheres.
parietal l. one of two divisions, inferior and superior, of the parietal lobe of the brain.
portal l. a polygonal mass of liver tissue containing portions of three adjacent hepatic lobules, and having a portal vein at its center and a central vein peripherally at each corner.
primary l. of lung the functional unit of the lung, including a respiratory bronchiole, alveolar ducts and sacs, and alveoli. Called also respiratory lobule (below).
l. quadrangularis a lobule of the rostral lobe of the cerebellum.
respiratory l. see primary lobule of lung (above).
l. simplex a lobule of the cerebellar hemispheres.
testis l. a group of seminiferous tubules, connective tissue and smooth muscle, the basic unit of the testis.
lobulus pl. *lobuli* [L.] lobule.
lobus pl. *lobi* [L.] lobe.
local restricted to or pertaining to one spot or part; not general.
l. acupuncture points points which can be found only when a localized pathological process develops.
l. government government at substate level, i.e. at shire, municipality, city or county level. The ordinances of local government are the ones that are most constraining in terms of running a traditional urban veterinary practice.
l. infection fever fever associated with local infection such as abscess, empyema, cellulitis.
localization 1. restriction to a circumscribed or limited area. 2. the determination of a site or place of any process or lesion.
cerebral l. determination of areas of the cortex involved in performance of certain functions.
germinal l. the location on a blastoderm of prospective organs.
localized limited in area or volume.
l. infection see local INFECTION.
location a characteristic of data, for example those indicating central tendency, such as median, mean, mode.
lochia a vaginal discharge occurring during the first week or two after parturition.
l. alba the final vaginal discharge after parturition,

when the amount of blood is decreased and the leukocytes are increased.

l. cruenta lochia rubra.

l. purulenta lochia alba.

l. rubra that occurring immediately after parturition, consisting almost entirely of blood.

l. sanguinolenta the serous uterine discharge occurring four or five days after parturition. Called also lochia serosa.

l. serosa see lochia sanguinolenta (above).

lochiocolpos distension of the vagina by retained lochia.

lochiometra distension of the uterus by retained lochia.

lochiometritis puerperal metritis.

lochiopyra puerperal fever.

lochiorrhagia, lochiorrhea an abnormally profuse lochia.

lochioschesis retention of the lochia.

loci [L.] plural of *locus.*

lock-stitch suture pattern, locking-loop suture pattern a continuous suture pattern in which the needle is passed through the previous over-skin loop before taking the next bite.

Locke's solution an aqueous solution of sodium chloride, calcium chloride, potassium chloride, sodium bicarbonate and dextrose adjusted to pH 7.4; used in physiological experiments to keep the excised heart beating.

locking stifle see PATELLAR luxation.

lockjaw 1. tetanus. 2. trismus.

locks 1. inferior wool from the lower parts of the legs, under the forearm, inside the flank and the crutch. 2. normal fleece in longwool sheep. See STAPLE.

board l. locks of wool swept up from the shearing board after the fleece has been removed.

locky said of wool fleece that is open and of which the staples are thin, due to the absence of binder fibers to bind the staples together.

loco see LOCOISM.

locoism poisoning by some species of *Astragalus* and *Oxytropis.* Called also loco.

locomotion movement, or the ability to move, from one place to another. See also GAIT, AMBLE, GALLOP (2), RACK, TROT, WALK.

locomotor of or pertaining to locomotion.

l. area includes a mesencephalic locomotor area in the midbrain and a subthalamic locomotor area in the diencephalon.

l. dysfunction see INCOORDINATION, LAMENESS.

locoweed see ASTRAGALUS, OXYTROPIS.

loculus pl. *loculi* [L.] 1. a small space or cavity. 2. a local enlargement of the uterus in some mammals, containing an embryo.

locum tenens a replacement for an absent veterinarian whose responsibility is to provide exactly the same services and at the same standard as those provided by the absentee.

locus pl. *loci* [L.] place; site; in genetics, the specific site of a gene on a chromosome.

l. ceruleus a pigmented eminence in the superior angle of the floor of the fourth ventricle of the brain.

locust tree see ROBINIA PSEUDOACACIA.

Loefflerella mallei see BURKHOLDERIA *mallei.*

Löeffler's coagulated serum medium one used for the rapid presumptive identification of *Actinomyces pyogenes.*

log 1. logarithm of. 2. daily record of work. 3. large, friable, compacted mass of concentrate and roughage feed suitable for feeding to animals at pasture. Usually contains a total ration.

l. off procedure for terminating a session of using a terminal connected to a remote computer.

l. on procedure for commencing a session of using a terminal connected to a remote computer.

log-linear model a statistical model which models frequency counts in contingency tables by using an analysis of variance approach.

logadectomy excision of a portion of the conjunctiva.

logarithm a mathematical device.

common l. the value of the power when a number is expressed as to the power of 10 (has the base 10). Thus 100 expressed as to the power of 10 is 10^2 and the log of 100 is 2.

Napierian l. see natural logarithm (below).

natural l. as for common logarithm, except that the base is e or 2.178. Called also Napierian logarithm.

logarithmic pertaining to logarithm.

l. relationship when the logs of two variables plotted against each other create a straight line. A semilogarithmic relationship is when there is linearity when only one of the variables is scaled as a logarithm.

logic the principles of reasoning.

lognormal distribution see lognormal DISTRIBUTION.

logo- word element. [Gr.] *words, speech.*

-logy word element. [Gr.] *science, treatise, sum of knowledge in a particular subject.*

Lohmann's enzyme see CREATINE kinase.

loin the lumbar region of the back, between the thorax and pelvis.

l. disease see BOTULISM.

Loliginidae the family of octopus called calamary, e.g. *Loligo forbesi* (Northern European squid).

lolitrems complex indole tremorgenic mycotoxins found in *Lolium* spp. grasses infected with *Acremonium lolii*; includes lolitrems A and B.

Lolium grass genus of the family Poaceae; toxic when infested with ANGUINA LOLII, CLAVIBACTER TOXICUS, ACREMONIUM, *Pithomyces*, ENDOCONIDIUM TEMULENTUM or may contain toxic amounts of nitrate. Includes *L. multiflorum* (*L. italicum*, Italian rye grass), *L. perenne* (perennial rye), *L. rigidum* (Wimmera rye grass), *L. temulentum* (darnel, drake).

L. perenne a staple grass for permanent pastures. It is not in itself poisonous, except that it does contain high concentrations of alkaloids, e.g. perloline, at some times and may accumulate nitrate. There are doubts about the pathogenicity of these compounds. The diseases that do occur on perennial rye grass pastures are RYEGRASS staggers and FACIAL eczema. Called also perennial ryegrass.

L. rigidum an annual pasture grass of great productivity. Its seeds may be parasitized by a gall-inducing grass nematode *Anguina lolii*, and if it is accompanied by a *Clavibacter toxicus* which produces tunicaminyluracils (corynetoxins), it is very poisonous. Ataxia, convulsions and death are the common signs. Called also Wimmera rye grass.

L. temulentum varying reports on the toxicity of this grass may be because the poisoning is due to a fungal infection, e.g. *Endoconidium temulentum.* Called also darnel.

Lomandra longifolia Australian plant in the family Xanthorrhaceae; unidentified toxin causes myelomalacia and associated clinical signs of incoordination and paralysis. Called also iron grass, mat rush.

Lomatia silaifolia Australian plant in the Proteaceae family; may cause cyanide poisoning; called also crinkle bush.

lomustine cyclohexylchloroethylnitrosurea (CCNU); a nitrosourea used as an antineoplastic.

Lonchocarpus a plant genus, as well as *Derris* spp., that contains ROTENONE in its root.

London casting a complicated technique for casting a horse using two ropes and three hobbles. It is very easy on the horse and gives excellent exposure of the inguinal region.

London fancy a canary with a distinctive plumage pattern, consisting of a golden-yellow body with contrasting black wings and tail.

London rocket see SISYMBRIUM IRIO.

lone star tick see AMBLYOMMA *americanum.*

long-acting thyroid stimulator an autoantibody directed against thyroid-stimulating hormone receptors in the thyroid; abbreviated LATS. Its occurrence is associated with hyperthyroidism in humans.

long-keep said of animals in feedlots; groups kept in the lot to grow before entering an intensive fattening period; in cattle 9 months to a year.

long-necked bladder worm see CYSTICERCUS *tenuicollis.*

long-nosed louse LINOGNATHUS *vituli.*

long-spined thornapple DATURA *ferox.*

long-spurred thornapple DATURA *ferox.*

long terminal repeat (LTR) long, repeating sequences of genetic information located at the ends of genomes of retroviruses.

longeing lungeing.

longevity duration of life. In animal terms this frequently means productive life.

Longhorn see TEXAS LONGHORN.

longissimus [L.] *longest.* See also Table 13 for longissimus dorsi muscle.

Longistrongylus a genus of worms in the family Trichostrongylidae.

L. albifrontis, L. meyeri found in the abomasum of antelope, gazelle and African buffalo.

longitudinal study a chronologial study in epidemiology which attempts to establish a relationship between an antecedent cause and a subsequent effect. See also COHORT study.

longitudinalis lengthwise; a structure that is parallel to the long axis of the body or an organ.

longus [L.] *long.*

longwool-type sheep breeds with coarse wool which hangs down in locks or ringlets instead of a dense, upright fleece, e.g. Lincoln, Leicester, Border Leicester, Romney Marsh, Wensleydale.

loogbos see PSILOCAULON.

loop a turn or sharp curve in a cordlike structure.

capillary l's minute endothelial tubes that carry blood, as in the papillae of the skin.

closed l. a system in which the input to one or more of the subsystems is affected by its own output.

diuretic l. loop of Henle DIURETIC.

Henle's l. see HENLE's loop.

intestinal l. in most species the small intestine is arranged in a series of indefinite open loops. In ducks and geese the loops are closed, finite structures, five to eight in number, and are located more or less in fixed positions. The supraduodenal loop is one of them.

open l. a system in which an input alters the output, but the output has no effect on the input.

program l. in a computer program a sequence of commands which is repeated until a specified condition is reached.

loop twitch a twitch in which a rope loop is passed over the poll and through the mouth. For restraint purposes the rope is tightened. It may damage the mouth and is not a recommended method.

loose-box accommodation for a horse in which the animal is not tied up in any way. It needs to be big enough for the horse to be able to turn around and to lie down. 10 × 10 ft (3 × 3 m) is a minimum.

loose housing accommodation in which the animals, usually cattle, are not tied-in nor in pens but are free to roam between sleeping–loafing area and feed bunks and are driven to a parlor to be milked.

Lop a breed of rabbits, characterized by extremely large and long ears which cannot be carried erect.

Lop-eared Alpine a European group of sheep breeds with pendant ears and Roman nose, polled; the wool varies from carpet to medium-fine wool. The type breed is BERGAMO. Called also Alpine.

lop ears rigid, usually large, ears that fall at their base from the perpendicular. Seen in Nubian goats and occasionally in dogs.

lope a gait in a horse which is faster than a running walk; a relaxed, uncollected, slow canter.

loperamide a butyramide derivative; the hydrochloride is used as an antiperistaltic in the treatment of diarrhea.

lophodont having molar teeth with ridged surfaces. See also TEETH.

Lophophyton a genus of fungus which causes dermatitis in fowl; usually accompanies infestation with the mite EPIDERMOPTES BILOBATUS.

lophotrichous having two or more flagella at one end or both ends (of a bacterial cell).

Lophura nycthemera silver pheasant. See PHEASANT.

Lophyrotoma interrupta the Australian sawfly, whose host plant is *Eucalyptus melanophloia*, the silver-leaved ironbark; produces larvae which can cause poisoning if eaten, because of their content of lophyrotomin.

lophyrotomin toxic octapeptide in the larvae of sawfly (*Lophyrotoma interrupta*).

loquat see ERIOBOTRYA JAPONICA.

lorazepam a benzodiazepine derivative used as an antianxiety agent.

lorcainide an antiarrhythmic drug that blocks Na+ conduction; used in the treatment of ventricular arrhythmias.

lordoscoliosis lordosis complicated with scoliosis.

lordosis downward curvature of the lumbar spine.

lords-and-ladies ARUM *maculatum.*

lorikeet called also lories. See *Trichoglossus* spp.

loris primitive primate, nocturnal and arboreal, insectivorous and without a tail; very slow moving and related to lemurs. Includes slender loris (*Loris tardigradus*), slow loris (*Nycticebus coucang*).

Lorisidae a family of nonhuman primates that includes the LORIS.

Lorna towel clamp a non-penetrating clamp, useful for securing pieces of equipment to surgical drapes.

loss-of-form see POOR PERFORMANCE SYNDROME.

lot-fed cattle or sheep finished in a feedlot, usually on high density grain diets.

lotaustralin the cyanogenetic glycoside in white clover (*Trifolium repens*) and *Lotus australis.*

lotio [L.] *lotion.*

lotion a liquid suspension or dispersion for external application to the body.

calamine l. a mixture of calamine, zinc oxide, glycerin, bentonite magma and calcium hydroxide solution; used as a protectant.

Lotus a genus (family Fabaceae) of erect or semiprostrate leguminous plants for permanent pastures. They provide good feed, equal to alfalfa in nutritional quality, in many temperate regions, but some contain cyanogenetic glycosides, e.g. lotusin, or cause photosensitization. Includes *L. australis, L. cru-*

entus (*L. australis* var. *parviflorus*, *L. coccineus*), *L. corniculatus*, *L. major*; called also birdsfoot trefoils.
lotusin the cyanogenetic glycoside contained in trefoils.
Loudinia see GLISHROCARYON.
loup a bounding gait.
loupe a magnifying lens.
head l. a magnifying lens mounted on a headband, freeing both hands of the clinician. Used principally in ophthalmology.
louping ill an acute encephalomyelitis affecting mostly sheep, caused by a flavivirus and transmitted by ticks. Clinically it is notable as a syndrome of fever, a peculiar bounding (louping) gait, paralysis and convulsions. See also Russian spring–summer ENCEPHALITIS. Called also ovine encephalomyelitis.
louse pl. *lice;* a general name for various species-specific parasitic insects, the true lice, which infest mammals and belong to the order Phthiraptera. This is divided into two suborders, Mallophaga, the biting lice, and Anoplura, the sucking lice. They are grayish, wingless, dorsoventrally flattened, and vary in length from about 1.5 to 4 mm. They stimulate rubbing, scratching and restlessness, causing damage to fleece and loss of production. Heavy infestations with sucking lice may cause serious anemia. Louse infestation is also called pediculosis.
The term louse is also used loosely with respect to other external parasites, e.g. whale 'lice' are barnacles and small copepods.
lousewort see PEDICULARIS.
love bean see ABRUS *precatorius*.
love-in-a-mist PASSIFLORA *foetida*.
lovebird name often applied to the budgerigar (MELOPSITTACUS UNDULATUS), but more correctly to *Agapornis* spp.
l. eye disease a severe, often fatal disease of *Agapornis* spp., characterized by ocular discharge, blepharitis, depression and weight loss. The cause is unknown.
l. pox see POXVIRIDAE.
Loven reflex an ancient discovery that impulses within an organ can cause systemic vasoconstriction leading to hypertension and a localized vasodilation and increased blood flow.
low[1] a level lower than normal.
l.-calcium rickets see RICKETS.
l. contrast an x-ray film with a poorly defined image because of insufficient contrast between light and dark shadows.
l.-density lipoprotein see LIPOPROTEIN.
l. larkspur see DELPHINIUM.
l. lupin LUPINUS *pusillus*.
l. milk fat syndrome dramatic fall in butterfat content of milk (as low as 50%) while volume remains normal, due to low fiber content of ration.
l.-phosphorus rickets see RICKETS.
l. whorled milkweed ASCLEPIAS *pumila*.
l. withers a conformation defect in a horse.
low[2] the recognition call of cattle.
low-flow breathing system an anesthetic system, usually a circle, in which there is a low input of fresh gas and a high percentage of rebreathed air.
Lowchen a small (8–18 lb) lively dog with a long, wavy coat of any color which is traditionally clipped in the pattern of a lion, i.e. full coat over the head, shoulders, feet and end of the tail, but very short on the loin and hindquarters. Called also Little lion dog.
Lowenstein–Jensen medium one containing eggs for the cultivation of mycobacteria.
lower closer to ground surface.
l. airway the trachea from the entrance to the thorax, bronchi and bronchioles.
l. burner syndrome acupuncture term meaning chronic accumulation of fluid in the lungs because of failure of the kidneys to excrete the fluid.
l. motor neuron (LMN) the final common nervous path; the ventral horn cell in the spinal cord and the peripheral motor neuron. A lesion of a sufficient number of these neurons causes atrophy of the muscles supplied by the nerve, weak reflexes and flaccid paralysis.
l. nephron nephrosis see RENAL cortical necrosis.
l. respiratory tract the trachea, bronchial tree, lungs, pulmonary vessels and pleura.
l. urinary tract includes, ureters, bladder and urethra.
Lowman clamp a clamp designed to hold fractured ends of bone in position while plates are screwed into place, and so on. Consists of opposing sets of incurving claws which can be screwed into a tight position.
Lown–Ganong–Levine syndrome a pre-excitation syndrome, similar to Wolff–Parkinson–White syndrome.
Loxodonta africana see ELEPHANT.
Loxodontofilaria loxodontis see DIPETALONEMA *loxodontis*.
lozenge 1. a medicated tablet or disk; a troche. 2. a triangular area of tissue marked for excision in plastic surgery. 3. a name given to the chestnut-colored spot on the head of Blenheim type Cavalier King Charles and King Charles spaniels. Called also 'kissing spot'.
LPS lipopolysaccharide.
LRF luteinizing hormone releasing factor.
LSA lymphosarcoma.
LSD a hallucinogenic compound (lysergic acid diethylamide), derived from lysergic acid, a constituent of ergot alkaloids; called also lysergide.
LT lymphotoxin.
LTF lymphocyte transforming factor.
LTH luteotropic hormone (prolactin).
Lu chemical symbol, *lutetium*.
lubb a syllable used to represent, or mimic, the first sound of the heart in auscultation. See also HEART SOUNDS.
l.-dupp two syllables used to mimic the first (lubb) and second (dupp) sounds of the heart in auscultation.
Lubra plate a plastic plate use to support segments of the spinal column or to maintain reduction of a pelvic fracture. The plates are arranged on either side of the spinous processes and are bolted to each other between the processes.
lubricants preparations for the lubrication of passages to reduce frictional injury, e.g. oily preparations, including petroleum jelly, lanolin or water-soluble preparations such as methyl cellulose.
lubricin a polydisperse glycoprotein synthesized by synovial lining cells which provides boundary lubrication to articular cartilage.
lucerne MEDICAGO *sativa*.
lucifugal avoiding, or repelled by, bright light.
Lucilia a genus of blowflies in the family Calliphoridae.
L. caesar, L. illustris flies with bright metallic colors. Called copper-bottle or green-bottle flies.
L. cuprina, L. sericata important causes of blowfly strike in sheep. See also cutaneous MYIASIS.
Lucioperca see PIKE-PERCH.
lucipetal seeking, or attracted to, bright light.
lucky bean see ABRUS *precatorius*.
Ludwigia Australian plant in the family Onagraceae,

causes diarrhea and paralysis in all species. The toxin has not been identified.

Luebering–Rapoport pathway a biochemical pathway in mature erythrocytes involving the formation of 2,3-BISPHOSPHOGLYCERATE and which regulates oxygen release from hemoglobin and delivery to tissues. Called also Luebering–Rapoport shunt.

lufenuron a benzoylphenyl urea insecticide which acts as an insect development inhibitor. It blocks normal synthesis and deposition of chitin. Administered orally once a month to control fleas.

Lugol's iodine a 2 to 4% solution of LUGOL'S SOLUTION, used as a uterine irrigant in the treatment of bovine endometritis.

Lugol's solution strong iodine solution, each 100 ml containing 4.5 to 5.5 g of iodine and 9.5 to 10.5 g of potassium iodide; a source of iodine.

Luing a Scottish breed of beef cattle derived by crossbreeding Beef Shorthorn and Highland breeds.

lumbar pertaining to the loins.

l. epidural analgesia see EPIDURAL anesthesia.

l. paralysis paraplegia generally and specifically that due to CEREBROSPINAL nematodiasis.

l. plexus one formed by the ventral branches of the last four or five lumbar nerves in the psoas major muscle.

l. puncture insertion of a needle and stylet into the subarachnoid space between the seventh lumbar vertebra and sacrum in most species except the dog, where the space between the sixth and seventh lumbar vertebrae is usually used; called also SPINAL puncture. A lumbar puncture may be done to measure the pressure of CEREBROSPINAL fluid and obtain a specimen for examination, and to inject a contrast medium for special radiographic examinations such as myelography. As a therapeutic measure it is sometimes done to relieve intracranial pressure or to remove blood or pus from the subarachnoid space. A lumbar puncture also is necessary for injection of a spinal anesthetic.

l. spinal stenosis see LUMBOSACRAL stenosis.

l. tap see lumbar puncture (above).

l. vertebrae the vertebrae between the thoracic vertebrae and the sacrum, numbering seven in dogs and cats, six in horses and cattle, and six or seven in sheep and pigs.

lumbarization nonfusion of the first and second segments of the sacrum so that there is one additional articulated vertebra, the sacrum consisting of one fewer segment.

lumb(o)- word element. [L.] *loin*.

lumbocostal pertaining to the loin and ribs.

lumbodynia pain in the lumbar region.

lumbosacral pertaining to the lumbar and sacral region, or to the lumbar vertebrae and sacrum.

l. instability see lumbosacral stenosis (below).

l. intumescence the thicker portion of the spinal cord from which the roots of the lumbosacral plexus originate, corresponding to the caudal, cervical lumbar and the sacral spinal segments.

l. luxation may result from trauma; common in dogs and cats. Neurological deficits result from injury to spinal nerves, and parenchymal hemorrhage and edema in spinal cord segments distant from the site.

l. plexus a network made up of the caudal lumbar and sacral spinal nerves giving rise to the femoral, obturator, cranial gluteal, caudal gluteal, sciatic and pudendal nerves; innervates the perineum and muscles of the pelvic limb.

l. plexus injury severe trauma to the hindlimbs may cause injury to the lumbosacral plexus, causing femoral and sciatic nerve deficits (inability to bear weight, extend or flex the stifle, dropped hock, and knuckling onto the digits).

l. spondylopathy see lumbosacral stenosis (below).

l. stenosis a reduction in diameter of the spinal canal at the level of the lumbosacral articulation may be caused by congenital anomalies of the vertebrae or acquired lesions. Weakness, pain and paresthesia with self-mutilation of the pelvic limbs and tail are clinical signs in dogs. Occurs as a congenital anomaly in some smaller dog breeds, and as an acquired defect in larger breeds, particularly the German shepherd dog.

l. syndrome lesions involving the lumbosacral tumescence or the lumbosacral nerve roots. Signs include flaccid paresis or paralysis of pelvic limbs, paresthesia and sensory loss in the pelvic limbs, anal sphincter, tail, bladder and urethral sphincter, depressed or absent postural reactions in the pelvic limbs, and urine retention with passive incontinence. See also lumbosacral stenosis and lumbosacral plexus injury (above), CAUDA EQUINA NEURITIS.

lumbricoid resembling the earthworm; designating the ascaris, or intestinal roundworms.

Lumbriculus variegatus intermediate host of *Dioctophyme renale*. Called also mudworm.

lumbricus pl. *lumbrici* [L.] 1. the earthworm. 2. ascaris.

lumbus [L.] *loin*.

lumen pl. *lumina* [L.] 1. the cavity or channel within a tube or tubular organ, as a blood vessel or the intestine. 2. the SI unit of light flux.

luminescence the property of giving off light without a corresponding degree of heat.

luminophore a chemical group that gives the property of luminescence to organic compounds.

lumirhodopsin an intermediate product of exposure of rhodopsin to light.

lumpectomy excision of a 'lump', usually applied to lesions of the mammary gland, in contrast to a radical excision of the entire gland.

lumpy characterized by the presence of a lump or lumps.

l. disease see lumpy-skin disease (below).

l. jaw see ACTINOMYCOSIS. The etiology in captive macropods is unclear but is probably *Fusobacterium* spp.

l.-skin disease there are two distinct lumpy-skin diseases of cattle with a similar clinical syndrome, in which there is a sudden appearance of cutaneous nodules on all parts of the body. Some of the lesions may become necrotic and slough, but most just subside. The more acute and systemic of the two diseases is caused by the 'Neethling' poxvirus. The milder form is caused by the 'Allerton' herpesvirus, which appears to be identical to the virus of bovine ulcerative mammillitis (bovine herpesvirus 2). Called also knopvelsiekte.

l. wool see MYCOTIC dermatitis.

lunate 1. moon-shaped or crescentic. 2. the lunate bone. See Table 10.

Lundehund a small to medium-sized dog with large erect ears, curved tail and short, rough coat which is usually brown with black tipping and white markings. It is a Norwegian breed developed for hunting the puffin (*lunde*) on Arctic islands. It is has an extremely flexible body and has at least two dewclaws and up to eight digital footpads on each foot.

Lund's fly see CORDYLOBIA *rodhaini*.

lung either of the two main organs of respiration, lying on either side of the heart, within the chest cavity.

The lungs supply the blood with oxygen inhaled from the outside air, and they dispose of waste carbon dioxide in the exhaled air, as a part of the process of RESPIRATION. They are usually divided into lobes, the left lung has up to three (cranial, middle and caudal), while the right lung has up to four (cranial, middle, caudal and accessory). Horse lungs are least subdivided; cat and dog lungs are deeply fissured into lobes.

The lungs are made of elastic tissue filled with interlacing networks of tubes and sacs carrying air, and with blood vessels carrying blood. The bronchi, which bring air to the lungs, branch out within the lungs into many smaller tubes, the bronchioles, which culminate in clusters of tiny air sacs called alveoli, whose total runs into millions. The alveoli are surrounded by a network of capillaries. Through the thin membranes of the capillaries, the air and blood make their exchange of oxygen and carbon dioxide. See also PULMONARY, RESPIRATORY.

accessory l. develop from an embryonic lung bud in an abnormal site, e.g. neck, abdomen.

l. birth changes include dilation of the alveoli and the bronchial tree, marked pulmonary vasodilation, decreased resistance to blood flow through the lungs, constriction of the ductus arteriosus, removal of fluid from the fetal bronchial tree.

l. breath sounds see BREATH sounds.

l. bud blunt end of the respiratory diverticulum which grows ventrally out of the proximal end of the foregut, then extends caudally and divides into two, forming the origins of the bronchial tree.

l. consolidation see CONSOLIDATION, HEPATIZATION.

ectopic l. edematous, lobulated masses of lung tissue in the abdominal or thoracic cavities or in subcutaneous sites.

l. factor closely related ipomeanols produced in rotting sweet potatoes by the catabolic activities of the fungus *Perilla frutescens* and other fungi of phytoalexins in the tubers. The factor is not toxic until it is activated by pulmonary microsomal enzymes.

l. fluke see PARAGONIMUS.

l. hilus that part of the lung that is not covered by pleura and through which blood vessels, bronchi, nerves and lymphatics enter and leave the lung.

l. lobe torsion occurs uncommonly in dogs and cats, most often of the right middle lobe. May occur spontaneously, following trauma, or in association with pleural effusion. Impaired venous return causes engorgement and rapid necrosis. Clinical signs include coughing and hemoptysis.

l. meridian points acupuncture points on the lung meridian.

l. mites see PNEUMONYSSUS, HALARACHNE, ORTHOHALARACHNE.

l. perforation may cause lung hemorrhage, emphysema, hemothorax or pneumothorax, or any combination of these conditions.

l. puller appliance for pulling the pluck, the heart and lungs on the trachea, out of the thorax at the abattoir.

l. puncture see lung perforation (above).

l. *Qi* deficiency in acupuncture terminology is a deficiency of *Qi* or energy in the lungs manifested by recurrent illness, weak cough, rapid shallow respiration, dry cracked muzzle.

l. reflexes HERING–BREUER REFLEXES.

l. resonance resonant sound achieved on percussion of the chest wall over normal lung.

shock l. see SHOCK lung.

l. sounds absent breath sounds audible on auscultation over normal lung are absent over consolidated, neoplastic and collapsed lung.

stiff l. one with decreased compliance.

total l. capacity the sum of the potential air spaces in the bronchioles and the alveoli.

l. volume see total lung capacity (above), VOLUME.

lungeing exercising a horse by having it circle at the end of a long lead, encouraged if necessary by a lungeing whip.

lunger see ATYPICAL INTERSTITIAL PNEUMONIA.

lungfish see DIPNOI.

lungmotor an apparatus for forcing air, or air and oxygen, into the lungs.

lungworm any parasitic worm that invades the lungs, but generally refers to worms that preferentially invade the lungs, come to maturity there and either lay their eggs or produce viable larvae there.

l. disease is caused by species-specific lungworms.

The lungworm is *Dictyocaulus viviparus*, which causes a verminous pneumonia, a secondary bacterial pneumonia and an atypical interstitial pneumonia. The cardinal signs in all of them are chronic cough and respiratory distress.

The worms involved are *Dictyocaulus filaria*, *Muellerius capillaris* and *Protostrongylus rufescens*, and the clinical picture is one of persistent cough.

Metastrongylus apri, *M. salmi* and *M. pudendodectus* are the causative worms and chronic cough the outstanding clinical sign.

Horses and donkeys are parasitized by *Dictyocaulus arnfieldi* and may be affected by coughing.

Filaroides hirthi, *F. milksi* and *Oslerus osleri* parasitize the respiratory tract at various levels and may be the cause of chronic cough. *Angiostrongylus vasorum* is found in pulmonary arteries and causes respiratory signs.

Mild to severe pulmonary disease with chronic cough and weight loss may be caused by *Aelurostrongylus abstrusus*.

lunula pl. *lunulae* [L.] a small, crescentic or moon-shaped area or structure, e.g. the segments of the semilunar valves of the heart.

luo points in acupunctorial theory these connect meridians; called also connection points.

lupanine toxin in LUPINUS. At its greatest concentration in the seeds.

lupiform resembling lupus.

lupin see LUPINUS.

lupine see LUPINUS.

lupinosis the hepatic injury syndrome caused by poisoning with dead *Lupinus* spp. plants, as stubble, infested with the fungi *Phomopsis leptostromiformis* or *P. rossiana*. Depression, jaundice and photosensitization are the common signs. Called also mycotoxic lupinosis.

Lupinus temperate zone plant genus of the Fabaceae family of legumes; mature plants can cause several syndromes (the green plants are safe): (1) convulsions after exercise due to alkaloids in the seeds; (2) liver damage caused by fungal toxins (phomopsins) produced by *Phomopsis* spp. growing on the crop stubble or in the seeds, which also causes intermittent photosensitization (called also LUPINOSIS); (3) possibly precipitation of acute attacks of copper poisoning; (4) skeletal myopathy; and (5) pregnancy toxemia and acetonemia in cows. Includes *L. albus*, *L. albicaulis*, *L. alpestris*, *L. andersonii*, *L. angustifolius*, *L. arboreus*, *L. argenteus*, *L. burkei*, *L. cosentini* (*L. digitatus*), *L. cumulicola*, *L. cyaneus*, *L. erectus*, *L. evermannii*, *L. formosus*, *L. greenei*, *L. latifolius*, *L. leucophyllus*, *L. leucopsis*, *L. littoralis*, *L. luteus*, *L. mon-*

tigenus, L. nootkatensis, L. onustus, L. perennis, L. polyphyllus, L. pusillus, L. spathulatus, L. varius.

L. caudatus, L. laxiflorus, L. sericeus these plants, together with many other *Lupinus* spp., contain quinolizidine alkaloids (anagyrine), the cause of the crooked calf syndrome, in which calves are born with limbs in excessive flexion, rotated, generally malpositioned, and malaligned.

lupoid 1. pertaining to lupus vulgaris. 2. a variant of sarcoidosis marked by small papular lesions.

l. dermatosis an hereditary disease of German shorthaired pointers. Scaling and crusting starts on the face, then spreads over the body, particularly to the hocks and scrotum. The lesions may be painful and pruritic.

l. leishmaniasis cutaneous LEISHMANIASIS.

l. onychodystrophy symmetrical sloughing of claws occurs, followed by regrowth of misshapen, crumbling claws. Histological changes show a lichenoid interface dermatitis. German shepherd dogs appear to be predisposed.

lupus [L.] *wolf, pike.*

l. band the deposit of immunoglobulin or complement, or both, at the basement membrane zone that can be demonstrated by direct immunofluorescence testing in lupus erythematosus.

l. panniculitis, l. profundus circumscribed, subcutaneous nodules of panniculitis associated with lupus erythematosus.

lupus erythematosus (LE) the Latin word *lupus* means wolf and erythematosus refers to redness; abbreviated LE. The name lupus erythematosus has been used since the 13th century because human medicine physicians thought the shape and color of the skin lesions (butterfly rash) gave affected patients a wolf-like appearance. Currently, there are at least two recognized autoimmune disorders: discoid lupus erythematosus and systemic lupus erythematosus.

l. e. cell a mature neutrophilic polymorphonuclear leukocyte, which has phagocytized a spherical, homogeneous-appearing inclusion, itself derived from nuclear material of degenerating leukocytes and coated with antinuclear antibody; a characterisitic of lupus erythematosus, but also found in analogous connective tissue disorders or immune-mediated disorders.

l. e. cell test see lupus erythematosus phenomenon (below).

cutaneous l. e. see discoid lupus erythematosus (below).

discoid l. e. (DLE) an autoimmune skin disease of dogs, characterized by depigmentation, erythema, scaling, erosions, ulcerations and crusting, particularly on and spreading up the bridge of the nose, and sometimes the face and lips. Immunoglobulins and/or complement are deposited at the basement membrane zone in the skin. The disease is exacerbated by exposure to ultraviolet light (sunlight). The disorder called 'collie nose' or solar dermatitis has in the past included many cases of dogs with DLE.

l. e. phenomenon, LE test the formation of LE cells on incubation of the clotted blood or bone marrow of affected animals at 98.6°F (37°C). The clot is disrupted and centrifuged, the white cells are smeared on a glass slide and examined for LE cells.

systemic l. e. (SLE) a multisystem, autoimmune disease of dogs and cats. An extremely wide variety of clinical signs may occur, but immune-mediated polyarthritis, hemolytic anemia and skin disease are most common.

Lurcher a traditional dog of the Romany gypsies in the United Kingdom; not an officially recognized breed, but generally a smooth-haired dog of variable conformation. It resembles a cross between a Whippet and a Greyhound. The name comes from the habit of hanging around in the background, more as a camp follower than as a family pet.

lure the skin-covered object which runs on a monorail on a Greyhound racing track and which the dogs are schooled to chase. The lure must be kept 30 to 40 ft ahead of the leading dog so that the field is stretched out. Bunching of the field is likely to cause too many injuries by bumping and fighting.

Lusitano a Portuguese gray horse, 15 to 16 hands high, very similar to ANDALUSIAN. An excellent riding and parade horse.

LUTD lower urinary tract disease.

luteal pertaining to or having the properties of the corpus luteum or its active principle.

l. cyst includes cystic corpora lutea, which are not evidence of ovarian malfunction, and luteinized cysts, which are usually anovulatory. The former can be identified by the presence of a palpable ovulation papilla. See also luteal CYST.

l. phase the stage of the estrous cycle during which the effect of the corpus luteum dominates and the cow is anestrous because of the high levels of progesterone in the blood.

lutein 1. a lipochrome from the corpus luteum, fat cells, and egg yolk. 2. any lipochrome.

luteinic pertaining to the corpus luteum, to lutein, or to luteinization.

luteinization the process taking place in the follicle cells of graafian follicles that have matured and discharged their egg: the cells become hypertrophied and there is vascularization and lipid accumulation (the latter in some species giving a yellow color), the follicles becoming corpora lutea.

luteinized cyst a cyst that may develop when there is delayed or insufficient release of LH during estrus. Ovulation does not occur and the theca becomes luteinized. Commonly seen in cattle and pigs. See also CYSTIC corpus luteum.

luteinizing cell-stimulating hormone see LUTEINIZING HORMONE.

luteinizing hormone a gonadotropic hormone of the anterior pituitary gland, acting with follicle-stimulating hormone to cause ovulation of mature follicles and secretion of estrogen by thecal and granulosa cells of the ovary; it is also concerned with corpus luteum formation. In the male, it stimulates development of the interstitial cells of the testes and their secretion of testosterone. Abbreviated LH. Called also interstitial cell-stimulating hormone.

l. h. releasing hormone (LH-RH) a hormone secreted by the hypothalamus that, together with a release-inhibiting factor, controls the secretion of, for example, the luteinizing hormone of the adenohypophysis. Called also Gn-RH.

luteohormone see PROGESTERONE.

luteolysis regression of the corpus luteum.

premature l. results in nonseptic abortion in the bitch and queen.

luteolytic factor prostaglandin-$F_{2[alpha]}$ synthesized and secreted by the uterine epithelium.

luteoma 1. a luteinized granulosa–theca cell tumor. 2. nodular hyperplasia of ovarian lutein cells, sometimes occurring in the last trimester of pregnancy.

luteoskyrin mycotoxin produced by *Penicillium islandicum*; causes hepatic necrosis and its metabolites are carcinogenic.

luteotrope see LACTOTROPE.

luteotroph see LUTEOTROPIN.
luteotropic stimulating formation of the corpus luteum.
l. hormone (LTH) see LUTEOTROPIN.
luteotropin a hormone of the anterior pituitary which stimulates formation of the corpus luteum; identical with prolactin. Called also luteotropic hormone (LTH).
lutetium a chemical element, atomic number 71, atomic weight 174.97, symbol Lu. See Table 6.
Lutra see OTTER.
Lutzomyia a genus of sandflies, e.g. *L. trapidoi*, capable of transmitting *Leishmania* spp.
lux the SI unit of illumination, being 1 lumen per meter squared.
luxation see DISLOCATION.
luxus [L.] *excess*.
LVH left ventricular hypertrophy.
Lw chemical symbol, *lawrencium*.
ly-1 marker a T lymphocyte marker, present only on a small set of B lymphocytes responsible for most antibodies to self antigens.
lyase any of a class of enzymes that remove groups from their substrates (other than by hydrolysis), leaving double bonds, or that conversely add groups to double bonds.
Lycium halimifolium plant in family Solanaceae; may contain a glycoalkaloid and cause convulsions and sudden death; called also matrimony vine.
lycoctinine a diterpene alkaloid found in *Aconitum* spp.
Lycopersicum esculentum the tomato, SOLANUM *lycopersicum*.
lycorine a toxic alkaloid found commonly in the bulbs of plants of the family Amaryllidaceae. Causes salivation, vomiting and diarrhea; large doses cause collapse and death.
Lycosa tarentula the large tarantula spider which is not poisonous.
Lycra plastic, segmented, polyurethane fiber used in making a snapback fabric, stronger and lighter than rubber. Used in surgical garments and as an implant to restore function to atrophied muscles, e.g. in prostheses in the treatment of laryngeal hemiplegia in horses.
lye an alkaline percolate from wood ashes; household lye is a crude mixture of sodium hydroxide with some sodium carbonate.
Lyell's disease see toxic epidermal NECROLYSIS.
Lygodesmia juncea North American member of the Asteraceae plant family; causes nitrate–nitrite poisoning; called also skeleton weed.
lying down getting up a pattern of behavior in most large animal species indicative of acute abdominal pain; the patient appears apprehensive of further bouts of pain, then flops down heavily and may, especially in horses, roll violently and uncontrollably, before getting up and standing in a dejected attitude until the next bout of pain, usually within a few minutes.
lying on back a pattern of behavior characteristic only of the horse and indicative of subacute abdominal pain; the patient lies on its back, without struggling, for minutes at a time. Other signs, e.g. poor appetite and weight loss, usually present also.
Lyme disease an acute, often recurrent, polyarthritis of dogs and humans caused by the spirochete *Borrelia burgdorferi*, and transmitted by the tick *Ixodes dammini*. The disease is endemic in the northeast and certain other areas of the United States.
Lymnaea a genus of snails, some of which act as intermediate hosts of *Fasciola hepatica*. The snails are *L. truncatula*, *L. tomentosa*, *L. columella*, *L. viridis*.
lymph a transparent, usually slightly yellow, often opalescent liquid found within the lymphatic vessels, and collected from tissues in most parts of the body and returned to the blood via the lymphatic system. It is about 95% water; the remainder consists of plasma proteins and other chemical substances contained in the blood plasma, but in a slightly smaller percentage than in plasma. Its cellular component consists chiefly of lymphocytes.
l. duct large vessels carrying lymph from smaller collecting vessels. Include thoracic DUCT, right lymphatic DUCT.
l. heart a muscular dilatation in a lymph vessel, capable of contraction and moving lymph along the vessel. Seen in embryos and lower vertebrates.
l. node any of the accumulations of lymphoid tissue organized as definite lymphoid organs along the course of lymphatic vessels, consisting of an outer cortical and an inner medullary part; they are the main source of lymphocytes of the peripheral blood and, as part of the reticuloendothelial system, serve as a defense mechanism by removing noxious agents, e.g. bacteria and toxins, and play a critical role in antibody formation. Sometimes called, incorrectly, lymph glands.
l. node abscess hard, usually cold swellings containing pus; secondary to primary lesion in node's drainage area; a feature of some chronic infections, e.g. tuberculosis, caseous lymphadenitis of sheep; specific nodes may cause specific syndromes, e.g. retropharyngeal nodes.
l. node hyperplasia increase in size due to increase in number of normal cells but with preservation of natal architecture.
l. node hypoplasia occurs in cattle and causes antenatal edema of the fetus, leading to dystocia in many cases. The calves are not viable.
l. nodule germinal centers in lymph nodes which produce lymphocytes. Called also lymphatic or lymphoid nodule.
periarteriolar l. sheath (PALS) the white pulp, heavily populated with T lymphocytes, that surrounds arteries in the spleen.
l. tissue see LYMPHOID tissue.
lymph-vascular pertaining to lymphatic vessels.
lympha [L.] *lymph*.
lymphadenectasis enlargement of a lymph node.
lymphadenectomy excision of one or more lymph nodes.
lymphadenia hypertrophy of lymph nodes.
lymphadenitis inflammation of lymph nodes; a common finding as an incidental sign in diseases of animals. It is also a principal presenting sign in some others, especially STRANGLES in horses, CERVICAL ABSCESS OF PIGS, bovine TUBERCULOSIS, GASEOUS LYMPHADENITIS of sheep and goats, and LYMPHOSARCOMA in dogs and cats.
lymphadenocele a cyst of a lymph node.
lymphadenogram the film produced by lymphadenography.
lymphadenography radiography of lymph nodes after injection of a contrast medium in a lymphatic vessel.
lymphadenoid resembling the tissues of the lymph nodes. Lymphadenoid tissue includes the spleen, bone marrow, tonsils and the lymphoid tissues of the organs and mucous membranes.
lymphadenoma lymphoma.
lymphadenopathy disease of the lymph nodes.

algal l. enlargement and bright green coloration of lymph nodes caused by the presence of *Prototheca* spp.

hilar l. enlargement of the tracheobronchial and pulmonary lymph nodes.

lymphadenosis hypertrophy or proliferation of lymphoid tissue.

lymphadenotomy incision of a lymph node.

lymphagogue an agent promoting the production of lymph.

lymphangial pertaining to a lymphatic vessel.

lymphangiectasia, lymphangiectasis dilatation of the lymphatic vessels; may be congenital or acquired. See also LYMPHATIC vessel obstruction.

intestinal l. leakage of protein from dilated lacteals in intestinal villi caused by lymphatic obstruction. May result in a protein-losing enteropathy with hypoproteinemia, diarrhea, edema, ascites and weight loss.

lymphangiectasis see LYMPHANGIECTASIA.

lymphangiectomy excision of one or more lymphatic vessels.

lymphangioendothelioma lymphangioma in which endothelial cells are the main component. See also LYMPHANGIOSARCOMA.

lymphangiofibroma a fibrosing lymphangioma.

lymphangiogram the film produced by lymphangiography.

lymphangiography radiography of lymphatic channels after introduction of a contrast medium.

lymphangiology the scientific study of the lymphatic system.

lymphangioma a tumor composed of newly formed lymph spaces and channels.

cavernous l. dilatation of the lymphatic vessels, resulting in cavities filled with lymph.

cystic l., l. cysticum a cystic growth thought to originate from a developmental anomaly of the primitive lymphatic spaces.

lymphangiophlebitis inflammation of lymphatic vessels and veins.

lymphangioplasty surgical restoration of lymphatic channels.

lymphangiosarcoma a malignant tumor of lymphatic vessels.

lymphangiotomy incision of a lymphatic vessel.

lymphangitis inflammation of a lymphatic vessel. It is a common finding in diseases of animals, and is of particular importance in horses because of the need to differentiate causes from GLANDERS, and in cows because of the importance of this lesion in bovine TUBERCULOSIS.

epizootic l. see EPIZOOTIC lymphangitis.

mycotic l. see bovine FARCY.

sporadic l. a noninfectious disease of horses, characterized by an acute onset of severe swelling in a hindleg, with lymphangitis, three-legged lameness and great distress. Incomplete recovery leads to extensive fibrosis of the entire limb. The disease is thought to be an extension from a pre-existing lymphadenitis and lymphangitis.

streptococcal l. occurs in young foals and is caused by *Streptococcus zooepidemicus*. It presents as an ulcerative lymphangitis.

ulcerative l. a mildly contagious disease of horses and cattle caused principally by *Corynebacterium pseudotuberculosis*. It is a lymphangitis of the lower limbs, marked by the presence of ulcers which discharge green pus.

lymphapheresis lymphocytapheresis.

lymphatic, lymphoid 1. pertaining to lymph or to a lymphatic vessel. 2. a lymphatic vessel.

l. aplasia causes distension of other lymphatics where lymph flow is blocked and local edema.

l. ducts the two larger vessels into which all lymphatic vessels converge. The right lymphatic duct joins the venous system at the junction of the right jugular and subclavian veins and carries lymph from the cranial right side of the body. The left lymphatic duct, or thoracic duct, enters the circulatory system at the junction of the left jugular and subclavian veins; it returns lymph from the cranial left side of the body and caudal to the diaphragm.

l. enlargement includes distension with lymph as in lymphangiectasia, or thickened as in cutaneous tuberculosis.

l. flow obstruction by local compression, congenital, segmental aplasia, lymphangitis, lymphadenitis.

l. follicle see LYMPH nodule; may be primary or secondary.

inherited l. obstruction edema inherited as a single recessive in Ayrshire and Hereford cattle; calves are edematous, locally or generally at birth and do not improve; the defect is in aplasia of lymph vessels and nodes.

l. leukemia see lymphatic LEUKEMIA.

l. lumbar trunks a plexus of lymphatics on the abdominal roof that drain into the cisterna chyli.

l. nodule see LYMPH nodule.

primary l. organs see LYMPHOID organs.

secondary l. organs see LYMPHOID organs.

l. system the lymphatic vessels and lymphoid tissue, considered collectively. See also CIRCULATORY system.

l. tissue see LYMPHOID tissue.

l. vessel obstruction occurs as a result of pressure from nearby tumors or other space-occupying lesions, because of hypoplasia of lymph nodes in the fetus, in extensive calcinosis, e.g. in *Solanum malacoxylon* poisoning and in horses not getting sufficient exercise. Called also lymphangiectasia.

l. vessels the capillaries, collecting vessels, and trunks that collect lymph from the tissues and carry it to the bloodstream; called also lymphatics.

lymphaticostomy surgical creation of a permanent opening into a lymphatic duct, usually the thoracic duct.

lymphatolysis destruction of lymphoid tissue.

lymphectasia distension with lymph.

lymphedema acute or chronic aggregation of lymph fluid in local tissues caused by obstruction to flow in lymphatic vessels or through lymph nodes; common causes of obstruction are aplasia, hyperplasia or hypoplasia of lymphatics or nodes due to inflammation, trauma or neoplasia, or secondary due to compression of these by adjoining organ enlargement. Aplasia of lymph nodes is an inherited disorder in cattle, dogs and possibly pigs.

lymphemia the presence of an increased number of lymphocytes or their precursors in the blood.

lymphnoditis inflammation of a lymph node.

lymph(o)- word element. [L.] *lymph, lymphoid tissue, lymphatics, lymphocytes.*

lymphoblast the immature, nucleolated precursor of the mature lymphocyte. Called also large lymphocyte.

lymphoblastic pertaining to a lymphoblast; producing lymphocytes.

lymphocryptovirus Epstein–Barr virus.

lymphocystis viral (iridovirus) disease of marine finfish characterized by multiple creamy-white nodules on the skin and fins. Self-cure occurs. The nodules are benign external growths composed of hypertrophied dermal fibroblasts.

Lymphocystivirus a genus of viruses of fish in the family *Iridoviridae*. They cause tumor-like growths on the skin.

lymphocytapheresis the selective removal of lymphocytes from withdrawn blood, which is then retransfused into the donor.

lymphocyte a mononuclear, nongranular leukocyte having a deeply staining nucleus containing dense chromatin and a sparse, pale-blue-staining cytoplasm. It participates in IMMUNITY.

activated l. one that has reacted on exposure to antigen or to a mitogen.

l.-activating antigen see lymphocyte-defined antigen (below).

B l's thymus-independent lymphocytes, which develop from stem cells in hematopoietic tissue, including the blood islands of the fetal yolk sack, the fetal liver and spleen, and the bone marrow. The *B* in B lymphocyte refers to the bursa of Fabricius, an organ in birds where B cell differentiation occurs. No analogous organ has been found in mammals, though an equivalent is assumed to exist—probably bone marrow.

B lymphocytes are involved in humoral IMMUNITY, i.e. the production of ANTIBODIES. A small, mature B lymphocyte can be activated by the binding of an antigen to specific cell-surface receptors. This induces proliferation of the cell, resulting in an expanded clone of cells specific for that antigen. These cells can then differentiate and begin to secrete immunoglobulin (Ig) molecules. Antibody production for most antigens involves interaction with helper T lymphocytes. All of the cells of a single clone secrete Ig that binds specifically to the antigen that stimulated the production of antibody. Mature antibody-secreting cells are plasma cells. Following blastogenesis some of the cells produced by division revert to small lymphocytes and remain as a longlived clone of 'memory' cells.

l. blastogenesis increased DNA synthesis followed by cell division and differentiation of lymphocytes in response to antigens or mitogens; an in vitro test of lymphocyte function.

l.-defined antigen histocompatibility antigens found on lymphocytes, macrophages, epidermal cells and sperm, capable of stimulating division in allogeneic lymphocytes. Called also lymphocyte-activating antigen.

helper l's a subset of T lymphocytes that is itself comprised of Th1 and Th2 cells that cooperate with and regulate B lymphocytes in the antibody response and with themselves and other effector T lymphocytes.

histiocytic l. see PROLYMPHOCYTE.

intraepidermal l's cellular components of the cutaneous immune system.

intraepithelial l's cellular components of the mucosal immune system.

large l. lymphoblast.

large granular l. see natural killer CELL.

memory l. see MEMORY cell.

natural killer (NK) l. see natural killer CELL.

non-T, non-B l. see null CELL.

pre-B l. a progenitor B cell derived from bone marrow stem cells.

resting l. small lymphocytes in the G_0 stage of the cell cycle, prior to activation.

small l. unstimulated B and T lymphocytes.

l. stimulation test see lymphocyte blastogenesis (above).

suppressor (Ts) l. see T lymphocytes (below).

T l's lymphocytes produced from pluripotential bone marrow stem cells which migrate during late embryogenesis to the thymus. Enormous numbers of cells are produced in the thymus, most of which are destroyed there. Less than 10% of cells which are non-self reactive leave the thymus to populate the T lymphocyte areas of the secondary lymphoid tissues (lymph nodes, spleen, Peyer's patches, etc.). At least four subsets of T lymphocytes are defined by cell surface markers and more especially by function.

Three of the subsets are regulatory cells called T helper (Th) 1 and 2, and T suppressor (Ts) lymphocytes. The other subset is an effector cell called cytotoxic T (Tc) lymphocytes or CTLs. Following antigen binding to antigen-specific T cell receptor (TCR) molecules, T lymphocytes, like B lymphocytes, undergo blastogenesis, in which they enlarge and divide. Some daughter cells revert to form an expanded clone of memory T lymphocytes. For both regulatory and effector functions, T lymphocytes produce a number of substances generally referred to as LYMPHOKINES. Lymphokines, unlike antibody, do not bind specifically with antigen, but rather they direct cell functions.

thymus-derived l. see T lymphocytes (above).

l. transfer test injection of lymphocytes from a potential graft recipient into the skin of a potential donor can be a test of histocompatibility, primarily in humans at the LD loci. Noncompatibility is marked by an inflammatory skin reaction.

l. transformation test see lymphocyte blastogenesis (above).

l. transforming factor (LTF) an obsolete term for a lymphokine that causes transformation and clonal expansion of nonsensitized lymphocytes.

tumor-infiltrating l's (TILs) T lymphocyte preparations from surgically removed cancer tissue that may be activated in vitro and returned to the host as a basis for specific anticancer therapy.

lymphocytic pertaining to, characterized by or of the nature of lymphocytes. See also LYMPHOCYTIC–PLASMACYTIC.

l. choriomeningitis (LCM) a disease of mice caused by an arenavirus and characterized by the occurrence of immunological tolerance and the subsequent development of an immune complex disease. The lesions caused by the immune reaction vary very widely and include meningeal and perivascular infiltration with lymphoid cells in many organs. There are several similar naturally occurring diseases.

l. leukemia see lymphatic LEUKEMIA.

l. synovitis see lymphocytic–plasmacytic SYNOVITIS.

lymphocytic–plasmacytic pertaining to plasmacytes and lymphocytes. See also GINGIVITIS, ENTERITIS, RHINITIS, SYNOVITIS.

lymphocytoblast a lymphoblast.

lymphocytoma well-differentiated lymphocytic malignant lymphoma.

lymphocytopenia see LYMPHOPENIA.

lymphocytopheresis lymphocytapheresis.

lymphocytopoiesis the formation of lymphocytes.

lymphocytosis increase in the number of normal lymphocytes in the blood or in an effusion.

lymphocytotoxicity the quality or capability of lysing lymphocytes, as in procedures in which lymphocytes having a specific cell surface antigen are lysed when incubated with antiserums and complement.

lymphoduct a lymphatic vessel.

lymphoepithelial emanating from or pertaining to lymphocytic and epithelial tissue.

l. thymoma a type of thymoma composed of lymphocytes and spindle cells; seen most frequently in goats and sheep.

l. organ an organ containing or composed of epithelial and lymphocytic tissue, e.g. thymus.

lymphogenous 1. producing lymph. 2. produced from lymph or in the lymph vessels.

lymphoglandula pl. *lymphoglandulae* [L.] a lymph node.

lymphoglandular pertaining to or emanating from combined lymphoid and glandular tissues.

l. bodies see lymphoglandular complexes (below).

l. complexes submucosal aggregates of follicular lymphoid tissue, invaded by glands from the mucosa, in the cecum and colon of dogs and pigs. Called also lymphoglandular bodies.

lymphogonia large lymphocytes with a large nucleus, little chromatin and nongranular cytoplasm.

lymphogram a radiograph of the lymphatic channels and lymph nodes.

lymphography radiography of the lymphatic channels and lymph nodes, after injection of radiopaque material in a lymphatic vessel.

lymphohistiocytic involving lymphocytes and histiocytes.

lymphoid resembling or pertaining to lymph or to tissue of the lymphatic system.

bronchus-associated l. tissue (BALT) aggregations of B and T lymphocytes in the lower respiratory tract.

l. cells lymphocytes and plasma cells.

l. foci small foci of lymphoid tissue which occur in almost all parenchymatous organs in birds. The foci are not encapsulated and blend with the surrounding tissue.

l. follicles see LYMPH nodule.

l. granuloma one of the lesions in chronic follicular pharyngitis in the horse and a cause of persistent cough, difficulty in swallowing and a stertorous respiration.

gut-associated l. tissue (GALT) aggregations of mucosal-associated lymphoid tissue in the gastrointestinal tract, including adenoids, tonsils, Peyer's patches and lamina propria of the intestine; responsible for a local immune response to antigens.

l. leukemia see lymphatic LEUKEMIA.

l. leukosis a very rare primary tumor in mammals characterized by high blood lymphocyte counts. It is the most common form of the avian leukosis complex of diseases caused by avian retroviruses. Birds are affected between the ages of 14 to 30 weeks and show nonspecific signs of emaciation, inappetence and weakness, but many also have enlarged abdomens and a palpably enlarged liver. The primary lesion is the transformation of B lymphocytes in the lymphoid follicles of the bursa of Fabricius, but multiple metastatic lesions occur in the liver, spleen, etc.

mucosal-associated l. tissue (MALT) aggregations and organized lymphoid cells tissue found immediately beneath mucous membranes lining the respiratory, gastrointestinal and urogenital system.

l. organs primary lymphoid organs include the thymus and the bursa of Fabricius and its mammalian equivalent; secondary lymphoid organs include lymph nodes, spleen, Peyer's patches, etc.

skin-associated l. tissues include a group of nonactivated T lymphocytes and Langerhans cells derived from lymphatic or hematopoietic tissues which have antigen-presenting properties; enable the skin to maintain a functional immunological relationship with the immune system. Called also SALT.

l. system the lymphoid tissue of the body, collectively; it consists of the bone marrow, thymus, lymph nodes, spleen, and gut-associated lymphoid tissue (tonsils, Peyer's patches).

l. tissue a lattice work of reticular tissue, the interspaces of which contain lymphocytes.

l. tumor see LYMPHOMA, LYMPHOSARCOMA, thymic LYMPHOMA, LEUKEMIA.

lymphoidectomy excision of lymphoid tissue.

lymphokine soluble protein mediators released by lymphocytes undergoing blastogenesis following contact with antigen. Lymphokines influence the behavior of the cells that produce them (autocrine) and of other cells in the vicinity (paracrine) and cells at a distance (endocrine), including macrophages, neutrophils, lymphocytes and other cells; a subset of cytokines many of which are also defined as INTERLEUKINS.

l.-activated killer (LAK) cells cytotoxic T lymphocytes produced by incubation with interleukin 2. See also K CELLS.

lymphokinesis 1. movement of endolymph in the semicircular canals of the internal ear. 2. the circulation of lymph in the body.

lymphology the study of the lymphatic system.

lympholytic causing destruction of lymphocytes.

lymphoma any neoplastic disorder of lymphoid tissue. Often used to denote malignant lymphoma, classifications of which are based on predominant cell type and degree of differentiation; various categories may be subdivided into nodular and diffuse types, depending on the predominant pattern of cell arrangement. There is also a great deal of difference in the types of disease in the different animal species. There is a system of classification based on the histological characteristics of the lymphocytes.

African l. see BURKITT'S LYMPHOMA.

angiotropic large-cell l. an uncommon form of the disease seen rarely in dogs; lesions most commonly in the lungs producing a syndrome similar in many ways to congestive heart failure.

bovine malignant l. the tumor form of BOVINE viral leukosis.

Burkitt's l. see BURKITT'S LYMPHOMA.

canine malignant l. the commonest hemopoietic neoplasm of dogs. It is characterized by lymphoid tumors in multiple lymph nodes, spleen, liver or other organs. Lymphocytic leukemia with involvement of bone marrow is much less common.

cutaneous l. round, raised cutaneous nodules or plaques caused by the infiltration of neoplastic lymphocytes with a tropism for epithelial cells. Occurs in cattle, dogs and humans. See also MYCOSIS fungoides.

follicular l. a malignant lymphoma in which the lymphomatous cells are in clusters in the lymph node resembling follicles. Called also giant follicular lymphoma, nodular lymphoma.

giant follicular l. see follicular lymphoma (above).

Hodgkin's type l. rare, but reported most frequently in the dog. A diagnosis depends on the identification of the Reed–Sternberg cell in a mixed population of lymphocytes accompanied by sclerosis.

immunoblastic l. may be nonsecretory or may secrete immunoglobulins. See also MYELOMA.

large cell l. classified as diffuse, large cells, large cell immunoblastic or mixed tumors with large cells.

lymphoblastic l. tumors of medium-sized lymphocytes or small noncleaved lymphocytes.

malignant l. (histiocytic) a form in which the predominant cell is the prolymphocyte (reticulum cell).

malignant l. (mixed cell) a form containing proliferations of both prolymphocytes and lymphocytes.

malignant l. (poorly differentiated lymphocytic) a form in which the predominant cell is morphologically similar to the lymphoblast, containing a fine nuclear chromatin structure and one or more nucleoli.

malignant l. (small cell lymphocytic, small cleaved cell, well-differentiated lymphocytic) the form in which the predominant cell is the mature lymphocyte.

malignant l. (undifferentiated) a form in which relatively large stem cells with large nuclei, pale, scanty cytoplasm and indistinct borders predominate.

nodular l. see follicular lymphoma (above).

T cell l. a form in which the predominant cell is the mature lymphocyte.

thymic l. occurs most commonly in yearling cattle and cats. In cattle, it causes obstruction of the esophagus leading to ruminal tympany, engorgement of jugular veins and edema of brisket and submandibular space. In cats it is caused by feline leukemia virus infection and is usually associated with pleural effusion and accompanying dyspnea and regurgitation.

lymphomatoid granulomatosis a rare pulmonary neoplasm of dogs characterized by infiltration by atypical lymphoreticular cells.

lymphomatosis the formation of multiple lymphomas in the body. In cows the lesions are caused by the virus of BOVINE viral leukosis, in cats by the FELINE leukemia virus, in chickens by the avian LEUKOSIS, ROUS SARCOMA group of viruses. The canine disease is canine malignant LYMPHOMA.

l. carcinomatosa invasion of alveolar septa by metastatic neoplastic cells. Occurs most commonly in dogs with metastasis from anaplastic scirrhous mammary carcinomas. Called also diffuse alveolar septal metastasis.

lymphomatous pertaining to, or of the nature of, lymphoma.

lymphopathia lymphopathy.

lymphopathy any disease of the lymphatic system.

lymphopenia, lymphocytopenia decrease in the number of lymphocytes of the blood.

lymphopoiesis the development of lymphocytes or of lymphoid tissue.

lymphoproliferative pertaining to or characterized by proliferation of lymphoid tissue.

l. disease a general term applied to a group of diseases characterized by proliferation of lymphoid tissue and abnormal lymphoid elements in the peripheral blood, such as lymphocytic leukemia and lymphosarcoma.

turkey l. disease a disease of young turkeys probably caused by a retrovirus and with lymphoproliferative lesions.

lymphoreticular system consists of the lymphoid tissues and the tissues of the reticuloendothelial system. Therefore includes reticular supporting cells, lymphoid cells and cells of the monocyte–macrophage series.

lymphoreticulosis proliferation of the reticuloendothelial cells of the lymph nodes.

benign l. cat-scratch disease.

lymphorrhea, lymphorrhagia flow of lymph from cut or ruptured lymphatic vessels.

lymphorrhoid a localized dilatation of a perianal lymph channel, resembling a hemorrhoid.

lymphosarcoma a general term applied to malignant neoplastic disorders of lymphoid tissue—a diffuse lymphoma. The clinical signs of the disease depend largely on the location of the tumors and their effects on the invaded and adjoining organs, e.g. alimentary, extranodal, multicentric. Also may be composed of particular types of lymphoid cells, e.g. B-cell lymphosarcoma.

bovine l. see BOVINE viral leukosis.

cutaneous l. SKIN leukosis.

feline l. see FELINE leukemia virus.

transmissible l. see canine transmissible VENEREAL tumor.

lymphosarcomatosis a condition characterized by the presence of multiple lesions of lymphosarcoma.

lymphoscintigraphy use of a radionuclear agent to demonstrate a lymphatic drainage system, using SCINTIGRAPHY.

lymphostasis stoppage of lymph flow.

lymphotaxis the property of attracting lymphocytes via chemotactic cytokines.

lymphotomy the anatomy of the lymphatic system.

lymphotoxin a lymphokine released by antigen-stimulated lymphocytes, particularly cytotoxic T lymphocytes, and involved in target-cell lysis, as in virus-infected target cells. The killing requires cell-to-cell contact and is restricted by Class I major histocompatibility antigens. Called also tumor necrosis factor-*[beta]* (TNF-*[beta]*).

Lyngbya a genus of marine cyanobacteria including the toxic *L. majuscula* algae which is not poisonous to fish but causes poisoning in the animals that eat the fish that eat the algae. Cases in humans may end fatally.

lynx medium-sized wild cats in the family Felidae, with characteristically short tails and tufted ears. They are generally spotted and of a rufous hue, though there are plain and fawn (bay lynx) varieties. Well known species are *Lynx* (*Felis*) *canadensis*, *L.* (*Felis*) *lynx* and *L.* (*Felis*) *rufus*. A related species is *Caracal caracal* (syn. *Lynx caracal*).

Lynxacarus a genus of mites.

L. radovsky the cat fur mite; may cause pruritus and exudative, crusted skin lesions.

Lyon hypothesis the random and fixed inactivation (in the form of sex chromatin) of all X chromosomes in excess of one in mammalian cells at an early stage of embryogenesis, leading to mosaicism for X-linked genes in the female, since the paternal X chromosome is inactivated in some cells and the maternal one in the remainder.

Lyonia ligustrina member of the Ericaceae plant family; contains andromedotoxin and causes gastroenteritis, tenesmus, vomiting, diarrhea, abdominal pain, sudden death; called also stagger bush, maleberry.

lyonization the process by which or the condition in which all X chromosomes of the cells in excess of one are inactivated on a random basis.

lyophil a lyophilic substance.

lyophile 1. lyophil. 2. lyophilic.

lyophilic having an affinity for, or stable in, solution.

lyophilization the creation of a stable preparation of a biological substance by rapid freezing and dehydration of the frozen product under high vacuum. Called also freeze-drying.

lyophobe a lyophobic substance.

lyophobic not having an affinity for, or unstable in, solution.

lyotropic readily soluble.

Lyperosia see HAEMATOBIA.

lypressin a synthetic preparation of lysine vasopressin used as an antidiuretic and vasoconstrictor in the treatment of diabetes insipidus due to deficiency of endogenous posterior pituitary antidiuretic hormone (vasopressin).

lyrate lyre shaped; said of horns, e.g. some Ayrshires, indigenous African breeds.
Lys lysine.
lyse, lyze 1. to cause or produce disintegration of a compound, substance or cell. 2. to undergo lysis.
lysemia disintegration of the blood.
lysergic acid a psychomimetic compound. Occurs naturally in some plants, e.g. members of the family Convolvulaceae.
l. acid diethylamide a hallucinogenic drug. Called also lysergide, LSD.
lysergide LYSERGIC ACID diethylamide.
Lysichiton americanus plant in the Araceae family; toxin unidentified, causes congenital, including cranio-facial, deformity; called also skunk cabbage.
lysin 1. an ANTIBODY capable of causing dissolution of cells, including hemolysin, bacteriolysin, etc. 2. a product of bacterial cells causing lysis. See BACTERIOLYSIN.
lysine Lys; a naturally occurring, essential amino acid, important in the formation of collagen, fibrin and keratin. Often the first limiting essential amino acid in growth and production. Nutritional deficiency in Bronzewing turkeys causes deficient pigmentation in the feathers.
l. vasopressin see VASOPRESSIN.
lysinogen lysogen.
lysis 1. destruction or decomposition, as of a cell or other substance, under the influence of a specific agent. 2. mobilization of an organ by division of restraining adhesions. 3. gradual abatement of the clinical signs of a disease, e.g. lysis of a fever.
-lysis word element. [Gr.] *dissolution*.
lysogen an antigen causing the formation of lysin; called also lysinogen.
lysogenesis 1. the production of lysis or lysins. 2. lysogenicity.
lysogenic cycle see LYSOGENICITY.
lysogenicity, lysogeny 1. the ability to produce lysins or cause lysis. 2. the potentiality of a bacterium to produce bacteriophage. 3. the specific integration of the phage genome (prophage) into the bacterial genome in such a way that only a few, if any, phage genes are transcribed; the integrated phage DNA behaves much as any other bacterial gene, including being passed to each daughter cell following DNA replication and cell division.
lysokinase a general term for substances of the fibrinolytic system that activate plasma proactivators.
lysol one of the original disinfectants; contains phenol, cresols. Toxic if ingested.
lysolecithin a lecithin with strong hemolytic properties; metabolized from lecithin by removal of its terminal fatty acid radical by phospholipase A.
lysophosphatide a phosphatide from which one molecule of fatty acid has been split off.
lysosomal pertaining to or emanating from lysosomes.
l. enzymes enzymes located in the lysosomes.
l. phospholipidosis overloading of lysosomes with phospholipids as caused by the inhibition of phospholipidases by aminoglycosides.
l. storage diseases diseases in which there is a congenital or acquired deficiency of an enzyme so that one or more specific metabolic processes are not completed. As a result there is an accumulation of metabolic products in the cellular lysosomes. The histological lesion indicates the error in function but not the cause. Most of these diseases are inherited but swainsonine poisoning is caused by plant (*Swainsona, Astragalus, Trachyandra* spp.) poisoning. See also ceroid LIPOFUSCINOSIS, GLYCOGENOSIS, GLYCOPROTEINOSIS, lipid STORAGE DISEASE, MUCOPOLYSACCHARIDOSIS.
lysosome a small intracellular organelle occurring in the cytoplasm of most cells, containing various hydrolytic enzymes and normally involved in the process of localized intracellular digestion. Lysosomes are particularly prominent in certain cells such as granulocytes, in which they are the granules, and activated macrophages. They play a major role in intracellular killing of microorganisms, destruction of foreign or damaged tissues, and in embryogenesis.
lysotype phage type.
lysozyme *lyso*—lyses bacteria; *zyme*—an enzyme naturally present in body fluids but ordinarily obtained from egg white for in vitro work. It hydrolyzes a specific glycoside bond in the peptidoglycan that forms bacterial cell walls, yielding the disaccharide *N*-acetylglucosamine-*N*-acetylmuramate. An important component of innate resistance.
lysozymuria urinary excretion of elevated levels of lysozyme.
lyssa 1. rabies. 2. a fusiform structure in the tip of the dog's tongue, made of connective, muscular and fatty tissue. Thought at one time to be the cause of rabies.
Lyssavirus a genus in the family RHABDOVIRIDAE. It contains RABIES virus, MOKOLA VIRUS, LAGOS VIRUS, Australian flying fox virus, and DUVENHAGE VIRUS.
lyssoid resembling rabies.
lysyl oxidase a copper-containing enzyme responsible for the maintenance of collagen and elastin in tissues; its absence leads to aneurysm formation in and rupture of large blood vessels.
lysylhydroxylase an enzyme involved in modification of collagen precursors.
Lythrum hyssopifolia plant in family Lythraceae; an unidentified toxin causes liver necrosis and nephrosis; called also lesser loosestrife.
lytic pertaining to lysis or a lysin.
l. necrosis local products of tissue destruction are reduced to liquid form.
l. test a simple method of cross-matching blood for transfusion in species that show little tendency to agglutinate, e.g. cattle, sheep and horses. Incompatibility causes hemolysis of red cells from either donor or recipient in the serum of the other.
Lytta vesicatoria see CANTHARIS VESICATORIA.
lyze lyse.

M

M macerate; maximal; symbol, *mega;* member; meter; minim; [L.] *mil* or *mille* (thousand); *misce* (mix); *mistura* (mixture); symbol, *molar* (solution)—the expressions M/10, M/100, etc., denote the strength of a solution in comparison with the molar, as tenth molar, hundredth molar, etc.; muscle; myopia.
M99 see ETORPHINE.
m symbol, *meter;* symbol *milli-*.
µ symbol, *micro-;* micron (µm).
m- symbol, *meta-*.
M & B 693 sulfapyridine.
M cells special epithelial cells associated with Peyer's

patches and lymphoid follicles that actively take up particulate matter from the intestinal contents. They are probably the portal of entry for bacteria and viruses.

M component a homogeneous immunoglobulin produced by a single clone of cells in a monoclonal GAMMOPATHY. May consist of either whole immunoglobulin molecules or their subunits, e.g. light chains or heavy chains. Called also paraprotein, myeloma protein or M protein.

M-CSF macrophage colony-stimulating factor.

M line a histological structure in myofibrils in skeletal muscle. The line runs transversely to the length of the myofibrils and corresponds to the segment occupied by myosin myofilaments.

M-mode motion mode. See M-mode ULTRASONOGRAPHY.

M phase see cell CYCLE.

M-plasty a technique for suturing a fusiform incision.

M protein myeloma protein; membrane protein.

M substance a dense zone in each myofilament of a muscle fiber and contributing to the M band which runs across the fiber.

mA milliampere.

MA test microscopic agglutination test.

MAb monoclonal antibody.

MAC in anesthetics, minimum alveolar concentration; in immunology, membrane attack complex.

MAC Test Kit a field test that determines the adequacy of plasma globulin levels in foal plasma.

MacAllan clamps aluminum clamps used as templates for the cropping of the ears of various breeds of dogs.

McBurney incision see grid INCISION.

McCullough forceps thumb forceps with very narrow points with cross-grooved blade faces. Designed for general ophthalmic surgery.

McDonald operation a purse-string retention technique for correction of cervical incompetence in breeding mares.

McDowall reflex a reflex in which section of the vagi in cats subjected to severe hemorrhage causes a decrease in blood pressure.

McFadyean's reaction a special staining reaction, demonstrating a pink capsule around a blue cell, after staining with methylene blue, which is used as a presumptive diagnosis for anthrax in a blood smear.

McFarland turbidity standard stock solutions of barium sulfate with consistent turbidity used to compare suspensions of bacteria in the disk diffusion method of ANTIMICROBIAL sensitivity tests.

McGuire scissors small, fine-bladed scissors, with the blades offset below the plane of the handles, for corneal surgery.

Mackenzie brush technique a method of collecting samples from the haircoat, particularly of cats, for diagnosis of dermatophytosis. A sterile toothbrush is used to brush the hair thoroughly and is then pressed onto a plate or slant of Sabouraud's agar and incubated.

Mackenzie river disease Australian name for poisoning by TERMINALIA OBLONGATA.

McLean suture pattern a mattress-type corneoscleroconjunctival suture.

McMaster technique a rapid, simple, quantitative technique for counting parasite eggs in ruminant feces, based on flotation on concentrated salt solution (specific gravity of 1.1 to 1.3) in a counting chamber.

MacMillan technique a conjunctival flap technique for the treatment of conjunctival ulcer in horses.

McNemar's chi-square test see CHI-SQUARE TEST.

McPherson speculum a mouth speculum for use in the horse. Called also HAUSSMAN–DUNN GAG.

Macaca genus of Old World monkeys very popular in zoos and for some aspects of human laboratory medicine. See MACAQUE.

Macadamia Australian genus of trees in the family Proteaceae; grown commercially for their fruits (Macadamia, Australian bush or Bopple Nut). The leaves and seeds contain cyanogenetic glycosides and are a potential cause of cyanide poisoning. Includes *M. integrifolia*, *M. ternifolia*, *M. tetraphylla*, *M. whelanii*.

macaque members of the genus *Macaca*, of the family Cercopithecoidae, the Old World monkeys. There are a large number of species including the rhesus and bonnet monkeys and the Barbary ape. They are thick-set monkeys, which are able to withstand the cold and often live above the snowline. Includes rhesus monkey (*M. mulatta*), Celebes macaque (*Cynopethicus niger*), pig-tailed macaque (*M. nemestrina*), Barbary ape (*M. inua*), *M. arctoides*, *M. fascicularis*, *M. nigra*, *M. silensus*.

macaw one of the tropical parrots of the family Psittacidae. Macaws are very colorful, have long tails and bare cheek patches. They are big birds (up to 3 feet long) and are members of the *Ara* genus, e.g. *Ara macao*, the scarlet macaw.

m. wasting disease a progressive weight loss associated with atony of the crop and proventriculus and atrophy of the gizzard, a nonsuppurative encephalitis and visceral ganglioneuritis. Called also proventricular dilatation syndrome and infiltrative splanchnic neuropathy.

Macdonaldius a genus of filaroid worms found in the blood vessels of colubrid and viperine snakes. In aberrant host snakes they cause cutaneous ulceration.

macerate to soften by wetting or soaking.

maceration the softening of a solid by soaking. In histology, the softening of a tissue by soaking, especially in acids, until the connective tissue fibers are dissolved so that the tissue components can be teased apart. In obstetrics, the degenerative changes with discoloration and softening of tissues, and eventual disintegration, of a fetus retained in the uterus after its death.

mach effect an optical illusion in radiography. Wherever there is a boundary between two objects of different luminosity the retina enchances the image. It leads to the misdiagnosis of fractures in the metacarpal and metatarsal bones.

Machaeranthera ramosa North American plant in the family Asteraceae and a selenium accumulator capable of causing selenosis in grazing livestock.

machine clipping clipping of the hair with an electric hair clipper, an important art in preparing dogs for show.

machine language see COMPUTER language.

machine milking milking machine.

macies [L.] *wasting*.

Macracanthorhynchus a genus of large acanthocephalans in the family Oligacanthorhynchidae.

M. catalinum found in the small intestine of dogs, wolves, badgers and foxes.

M. hirudinaceus found in the small intestine of domestic and wild pigs, where they cause granulomatous lesions in the intestinal wall, sometimes perforation and peritonitis.

M. ingens found in the small intestine of wild mammals including skunk, mink, raccoon and mole.

macrencephalia hypertrophy of the brain.

macro 1. a collection of commands or keystrokes which may be replayed by a small number of keystrokes or by a mouse click. 2. see MACR(O)-.

macr(o)- word element. [Gr.] *large, long.*

macroamylase a complex in which normal serum amylase is bound to a variety of specific binding proteins, forming a complex too large for renal excretion. It is not correlated with any specific disease state; however, in hyperamylasemia or pancreatitis, it can result in urinary amylase levels not rising concomitantly with serum levels.

macroamylasemia the presence of macroamylase in the blood.

macroblast an abnormally large, nucleated erythrocyte; a large young normoblast with megaloblastic features.

macroblepharia abnormal largeness of the eyelid.

macrocardius a fetus with an extremely large heart.

macrocarpa CUPRESSUS *macrocarpa.*

macrocephalous having an abnormally large head.

macrocephaly abnormal enlargement of the cranium.

macrochromosomes a pair of normal chromosomes.

macroclimate the climate as described by standard meteorological information. Paints a broad picture of the weather as perceived by animals and humans, but has little relevance to pasture plants and pathogens.

macrocolon see MEGACOLON.

macroconidium pl. *macroconidia;* a large conidium produced by some fungi such as *Microsporum* spp.

macrocrania abnormal increase in size of the skull in relation to the face.

macrocyclic lactones potent nematicidal and insecticidal compounds derived from *Streptomyces* spp. See also AVERMECTINS, MILBEMYCINS.

macrocyte an abnormally large erythrocyte.

macrocythemia, macrocytosis the presence of macrocytes in the blood. Observed in miniature poodles without overt anemia.

macrocytic manifested by or pertaining to the presence of macrocytes.

macrocytosis see MACROCYTHEMIA.

Macrodactylus subspinosus the rose chafer beetle. The population of these beetles can be very high in some years and ingestion of large numbers of them can cause poisoning in birds. Signs include drowsiness, weakness and some deaths. Called also *Cetonia aurata.*

macrodactyly abnormal largeness of the digits.

macrodontia abnormal increase in size of one or more teeth.

macroeconomics study of an economy as a whole; includes the total or aggregate level of output of an economy and prices for the economy, viewed as a whole. See also MICROECONOMICS.

macroelement a chemical element which has a minimal daily requirement greater than 100 mg; calcium, phosphorus, magnesium, potassium, sodium and chloride are macroelements.

macrogamete the larger, less active female gamete in anisogamy, which is fertilized by the smaller male gamete (microgamete).

macrogametocyte 1. a cell that produces macrogametes. 2. the female gametocyte of ampicomplexan protozoa which matures into a macrogamete.

macroglia neuroglial cells of ectodermal origin, i.e. the astrocytes and oligodendrocytes considered together.

macroglobulin immunoglobulin M, an antibody protein (globulin) of molecular weight in the range of 1,000,000.

α_2-m. a glycoprotein that inhibits proteolytic enzymes. Increased levels are seen in diabetes mellitus and diseases of the liver and kidney.

macroglobulinemia increased levels of immunoglobulin M in the blood.

Waldenström's m. a monoclonal gammopathy in which there are increased levels of IgM as a result of leukemia affecting IgM-producing B lymphocytes.

macroglossia excessive size of the tongue.

macrognathia abnormal overgrowth of the jaw.

macrogols a polyethylene glycol used in the manufacure of drugs as solvents.

macrogyria moderate reduction in the number of sulci of the cerebrum, sometimes with increase in the brain substance, resulting in excessive size of the gyri.

macrohabitat the immediate, large-scale environment, as can be seen with the naked eye; flora, fauna, topography, climate in the broad sense, as an animal would experience it.

macrolide as in antibiotic; any antibiotic with molecules having many-membered lactone rings, e.g. erythromycin, spiramycin, tylosin.

macromastia excessive size of the mammary glands.

macromelanosomes large pigment granules; seen in color dilution alopecia.

macromelia enlargement of one or more limbs.

macromelus a fetus with abnormally large or long limbs.

macromere one of the larger cells (blastomeres) formed in unequal cleavage of the fertilized ovum (at the vegetal pole).

macrometeorology measurement of the macroclimate.

macromineral the major minerals in animal nutrition (as distinct from trace minerals). Includes calcium, phosphorus, sodium, chlorine, potassium, magnesium, sulfur.

macromolecule a very large molecule having a polymeric chain structure, as in proteins, polysaccharides, etc.

macromonocyte a giant monocyte.

macromyeloblast a large myeloblast.

macronormoblast a very large nucleated erythrocyte; macroblast.

macronucleus the larger nucleus when there are two in the cell.

macronutrient an essential nutrient that has a large minimal daily requirement (greater than 100 mg for a ruminant); calcium, phosphorus, magnesium, potassium, sodium and chloride are macronutrients.

macronychia abnormally enlarged claws or hooves.

macropalpebral fissure an abnormally large opening between the eyelids that, in animals, allows greater exposure of sclera. Commonly seen in the brachycephalic dog breeds, where it predisposes to proptosis, abnormal distribution of the tear film, and may be the cause of exposure keratitis because of an inability to close the lids completely.

macrophage any of the large, mononuclear, highly phagocytic cells derived from bone marrow cells, promonocytes, the progeny of which, the monocytes, enter the bloodstream, where they stay for a few days before entering the tissues and developing into macrophages. They are components of the monocyte–macrophage system. Macrophages are usually immobile but become actively mobile when stimulated by inflammation, immune cytokines and microbial products. They are an important class of antigen presenting cells (APCs). See also IMMUNITY.

activated m. under the influence of cytokines, particularly γ-interferon and interleukin 4, released by antigen-stimulated Th1 lymphocytes, resting macrophages are activated whereby they become larger, more motile, stickier, express more MHCII proteins on their surface, contain more lysosomes and lysosomal enzymes, and secrete a variety of substances including interleukin 1, tumor necrosis factors; they have increased phagocytic antivity and increased killing via reactive oxygen intermediates, collagenases and lysosomal enzymes. Called also angry macrophage.
m. activating factor (MAF) a lymphokine produced by T lymphocytes following in vitro, probably γ-interferon, antigenic stimulation that activates macrophages.
alveolar m's rounded, granular, mononuclear phagocytes within the alveoli of the lungs that ingest inhaled particulate matter.
angry m. see activated macrophage (above).
armed m's those capable of inducing cytotoxicity as a consequence of binding antibodies via Fc receptors on their surfaces or by factors derived from T lymphocytes (specific macrophage arming factor [SMAF]).
m. chemotactic factor (MCF) a lymphokine that attracts macrophages.
m. colony-stimulating factor see COLONY-stimulating factors.
m. inhibition factor (MIF) a lymphokine that inhibits macrophage migration, causing them to accumulate at the site of antigen.
specific m. arming factor (SMAF) a lymphokine that stimulates macrophage cytotoxic activity.

macrophthalmia abnormal enlargement of the eyeball.

macropinosomes large droplets filled with fluid formed when excess tissue fluid is engulfed by cells as part of a clean-up of tissue spaces.

macropod members of the family Macropodidae; includes kangaroo, wallaby.

macropodia excessive size of the feet.

macropodid a member of the family Macropodidae, the kangaroos.

macropolycyte a hypersegmented polymorphonuclear leukocyte of greater than normal size.

macroprosopia excessive size of the face.

Macropus a large jumping marsupial with a very large tail, which balances the animal while it is airborne. Members of the family Macropodidae. Includes *Macropus rufus*, the red kangaroo, *M. foliginosus*, the Western gray kangaroo and *M. giganteus*, the Eastern or great gray kangaroo. Large male kangaroos stand 6 ft tall and weigh up to 220 lb. Some of the wallabies (*M. dorsalis* the black-striped wallaby, *M. eugenii* the Tammar wallaby) also belong in this genus.

macroreticulocyte large reticulocytes released prematurely from bone marrow; they have a reduced life span.

macroscopic of large size; visible to the unaided eye.
m. anatomy see gross ANATOMY.

macroscopy examination with the unaided eye.

macrosigmoid excessive size of the sigmoid colon.

macrosmatic pertaining to a good sense of smell, e.g. macrosmatic animals such as dogs.

macrosomatia, macrosomia great bodily size.

macrotia abnormal enlargement of the pinna of the ear.

Macrozamia one of the Australian genera of the cycads; contain cycad glycosides (e.g. macrozamin) and cause hepatitis, gastroenteritis and ZAMIA STAGGERS. Includes *M. communis*, *M. diplomera*, *M. heteromera*, *M. lucida*, *M. miquelii*, *M. moorei*, *M. pauliguilielmi*, *M. riedlei.* Called also burrawang palm, zamia.

macrozamin a glycoside of MAM in *Macrozamia* spp. and other cycads.

macula pl. *maculae* [L.] 1. a stain, spot, or thickening; 2. an area distinguishable by color or otherwise from its surroundings. Often used alone to refer to the macula retinae. 3. a macule: a discolored spot on the skin that is not raised above the surface. 4. a corneal scar that can be seen without special optical aids; presenting as a gray spot intermediate between a nebula and a leukoma. 5. macula lutea.
m. acusticae terminations of the vestibulocochlear nerve in the utricle and saccule.
m. adherens see DESMOSOME.
m. atrophica a white atrophic patch on the skin.
m. corneae a circumscribed opacity of the cornea.
m. cribrosa a perforated spot or area; one of three perforated areas (inferior, medial and superior) in the wall of the vestibule of the ear through which branches of the vestibulocochlear nerve pass to the saccule, utricle and semicircular canals.
m. densa a zone of heavily nucleated cells in the distal renal tubule.
m. folliculi the point on the surface of a vesicular ovarian follicle where rupture occurs; follicular stigma.
m. germinativa germinal area; the part of the conceptus where the embryo is formed.
inner ear m. sensory receptor areas in the walls of the utriculus and sacculus which monitor the position of the head relative to gravity; see also macula sacculi, macula utriculi (below).
m. lutea an irregular yellowish depression on the retina, lateral to and slightly below the optic disk. Called also macula retinae.
m. retinae see macula lutea (above).
m. sacculi a thickening on the wall of the saccule where the epithelium contains hair cells that receive and transmit vestibular impulses.
m. utriculi a thickening in the wall of the utricle where the epithelium contains hair cells that are stimulated by linear acceleration and deceleration and by gravity.

maculate spotted or blotched.

macule see MACULA.

maculocerebral pertaining to the macula lutea and the brain.

maculopapular both macular and papular.

mad apple DATURA *stramonium*.

mad cow disease see BOVINE SPONGIFORM ENCEPHALOPATHY.

mad itch see AUJESZKY'S DISEASE.

mad mushroom see PSILOCYBE.

Madagascan periwinkle see CATHARANTHUS *roseus*.

madarosis loss of eyelashes.

madeira vine see ANREDERA CORDIFOLIA.

madeira winter cherry SOLANUM *pseudocapsicum*.

madness see MANIA.

Madura foot see MADUROMYCOSIS.

maduramicin a polyether ionophore used in poultry feed as a coccidiostat.

Madurella a genus of fungi associated with the lesions of maduromycosis in humans.

maduromycetoma maduromycotic mycetoma.

maduromycosis a chronic disease due to various fungi or actinomycetes, affecting various body tissues, particularly the feet; called also mycetoma. The most common form in humans affects the foot

(Madura foot) and is characterized by sinus formation, necrosis and swelling. The disease is recorded in the horse, in which there are nasal granulomas and similar lesions in the skin. The fungi *Helminthosporium* spp., *Allescheria* spp. and *Curvularia* spp. are present in the lesions. See also MYCETOMA.

maduromycotic pertaining to or emanating from maduromycosis.

m. mycetoma see MYCETOMA.

maedi a chronic pneumonia of sheep caused by a lentivirus, which also causes visna when it invades the brain of sheep. In maedi the characteristic features are a prolonged incubation period of more than 2 years, a progressive pneumonia which lasts for about 6 months, and, at the inevitable death, an abnormally high density and heaviness of the lungs. Called also maedi–visna, Graff–Reinert disease, la bouhite, ovine progressive pneumonia and lymphoid interstitial pneumonia.

maedi–visna see MAEDI.

Maesa lanceolata an African plant of the family Myrsinaceae that causes diarrhea, polyuria, emaciation and death in cattle. The principal necropsy lesion is nephrosis; the toxin has not been identified.

MAF macrophage activating factor.

mafenide a sulfonamide that is not inhibited by the presence of pus and necrotic tissue; used mostly for local application to infected wounds. Called also homosulfanilamide, sulfamylon.

MAFF Ministry of Agriculture, Fisheries and Food, in the UK.

maggot the soft-bodied larva of an insect, especially one living in decaying flesh or tissue debris.

wool m. see cutaneous MYIASIS.

cattle m. see HYPODERMA.

magic mushroom see PSILOCYBE.

Magill circuit see Magill CIRCUIT.

magma 1. a suspension of finely divided material in a small amount of water. 2. a thin, paste-like substance composed of organic material.

Magner war bridle a type of restraint used on horses, it is a rope with a loop around the lower jaw, then passed over the head and back through the jaw loop.

magnesia magnesium oxide; aperient and antacid.

magnesium a chemical element, atomic number 12, atomic weight 24.312, symbol Mg. See Table 6. Its salts are essential in nutrition, being required for the activity of many enzymes, especially those concerned with oxidative phosphorylation. It is found in the intra- and extracellular fluids and is excreted in urine and feces.

m. ammonium phosphate (MAP) a common constituent of urinary calculi. See UROLITHIASIS.

blood m. level of magnesium in the blood.

m. carbonate, m. hydroxide, m. oxide, m. phosphate, m. trisilicate compounds used as antacids.

m. chloride used as a source of magnesium in the treatment of hypomagnesemia in cattle, and as a chemical defibrillator in cardiopulmonary resuscitation.

m. citrate a mild cathartic.

m. gluconate a magnesium replenisher.

m. nutritional deficiency is most important in the part that it plays in lactation tetany in ruminants. It also causes deformities of the limbs and nervous signs of tremor and convulsions in pigs. See also LACTATION TETANY (1).

m. salicylate the magnesium salt of salicylic acid used as an antiarthritic.

m. silicate talcum powder; capable of causing starch granulomatous peritonitis if introduced into the peritoneal cavity, so it has been superseded by other compounds for use on surgeon's gloves.

m. sulfate Epsom salts; used as an electrolyte replenisher, cathartic and local anti-inflammatory.

m. sulfate–chloral hydrate mixture see CHLORAL hydrate and magnesium sulfate.

magnet an object having polarity and capable of attracting iron.

oral dose m. see reticular MAGNET.

reticular m. a magnet placed in the reticulum to attract and isolate sharp metal and help to prevent traumatic reticuloperitonitis in ruminants.

magnetic having the properties of a magnet.

m. resonance imaging (MRI) the patient is placed in a magnetic field and radiofrequency signals are transmitted and received by surrounding coils. A computer processes the information and constructs cross-sectional images which provide detailed information on soft tissues.

m. therapy includes static magnets (magnets of 500 to 1500 gauss embedded in bandage applied to the injured part) and pulsed electromagnetic devices by which the frequency and the strength of the magnet can be varied.

magnetic tape flexible tape coated with magnetic material and used for the bulk storage of computer data. Suffers from a lack of immediate access compared to disks but can provide a large volume of removable data storage space.

m. t. drive the device that reads data onto and off magnetic tape from and to a computer.

magnetism magnetic attraction or repulsion.

magnetropism a growth response in a nonmotile organism under the influence of a magnet.

magnification 1. apparent increase in size, as under the microscope. 2. the process of making something appear larger, as by use of lenses. 3. the ratio of apparent (image) size to real size. 4. radiological magnification; a factor of object to film distance.

magnum the large diameter, second zone of the hen's left oviduct. The albumen-secreting zone.

magpie black and white crow-sized bird with melodious bell-like call and strong territorial behavior. Many species, e.g. *Gymnorhina* spp., *Pica pica*.

Mahaim fibers short, direct connections from the AV node (or the bundle of His or bundle branches) to muscle fibers in the interventricular septum.

M. fiber conduction a type of accessory AV conduction with abnormal beats originating below the region of normal delay in the AV-conducting system; causes an arrhythmia.

maiden 1. a female, e.g. ewe, gilt, heifer, bitch, mare, of breeding age but not yet mated. 2. a racehorse that has not yet won a race on a recognized track.

Main Drain virus one of the California serotype bunyaviruses isolated in California from a horse with encephalitis.

Maine-Anjou red, red-and-white, or red-roan dual-purpose cattle originating in northern France.

Maine coon cat a breed of cats originating from shipboard cats that landed in the American state of Maine in the 19th century. Now recognized as a distinct breed, it is a very large, muscular, long-haired cat in a variety of colors, although originally tabby.

mainframe computer see COMPUTER.

maintenance requirement in terms of animal nutrition, the amount and quality of the diet required to maintain an adult animal without providing additional nutriment for production, reproduction or weight gain.

m. r. for energy see ENERGY requirements.

m. r. interval the interval between doses of a medication arranged so as to maintain an appropriate blood level of the drug.

Maireana brevifolia Australian plant in the family Chenopodiaceae; toxin is soluble oxalate and the clinical findings include nephrosis and urolithiasis; called also small-leaved bluebush.

maize a staple crop part of the food supply for humans and animals in many countries. One of its best uses is as a chopped green crop or as ensilage. Called also *Zea mays.* The grain is usually referred to as CORN (3) in the USA or as maize in other countries. A full range of maize grain products is available and includes HOMINY, GRITS, maize germ meal and maize gluten meal (a high protein feed).

m. crop poisoning a form of carbohydrate engorgement caused when cattle accidentally gain access to a standing crop or when confined animals are fed too much of it. See also CARBOHYDRATE ENGORGEMENT.

m. stalk disease caused by ingestion of maize stalks infected with *Diplodia maydis* fungus. Characterized by dullness, head pressing, compulsive walking. Called also cornstalk disease.

Majocchi's granuloma a form of dermatophytosis with a granulomatous, pyogranulomatous or suppurative reaction containing fungal grains or hyphae. Called also nodular granulomatous perifolliculitis.

major histocompatibility complex see major HISTOCOMPATIBILITY complex.

mal [Fr.] *illness.* disease.

m. de caderas see TRYPANOSOMA *equinum.*

m. du coit see DOURINE.

m. do eucalipto disease caused by poisoning with the fungus *Ramaria* spp.

grand m. a generalized convulsive seizure attended by loss of consciousness. See also SEIZURE.

m. des mains sales see HYDATID disease.

m. de mer seasickness.

petit m. momentary loss of consciousness without convulsive movements. See also SEIZURE.

m. de playa South American name for LANTANA poisoning.

mal seco [Span.] disease of horses in Argentine, Chile; resembles GRASS sickness.

mala the cheek or cheek bone.

malabsorption impaired intestinal absorption of nutrients.

fat m. see STEATORRHEA.

m. syndrome a group of disorders marked by subnormal intestinal absorption of dietary constituents, and thus excessive loss of nutrients in the stool, with chronic diarrhea and weight loss; it may be due to a digestive defect, a mucosal abnormality, or lymphatic obstruction. A common disease in dogs and a major part of some of the enteric diseases of food animals. It is the pathogenesis of the diarrheas of trichostrongylosis of sheep and cattle, of the viral diarrheas of pigs and the undifferentiated chronic diarrheas of horses.

malaccol an insecticidal substance present in the roots of *Derris* spp. plants.

malachite green a green dye used to stain bacteria and as an antibacterial and antifungal. Used, with great caution, as a treatment of cutaneous mycosis in aquarium fish.

m. g. test used to determine the completeness of bleedout in an abattoir carcass. Also used to detect the presence of the meat preservative, sodium metabisulfite.

malacia morbid softening or softness of a part or tissue; also used as a word termination, as in osteomalacia, encephalomalacia, myelomalacia.

malacoma a morbidly soft part or spot.

malacoplakia a circumscribed area of softening on the membrane lining a hollow organ, such as the ureter, urethra or renal pelvis.

m. vesicae a flat yellow growth on the mucosa of the bladder.

malacosis malacia.

malacosteon softening of the bones; osteomalacia.

malacotic soft.

maladie see MAL.

m. du jeune âge du chat feline panleukopenia.

maladjustment syndrome see NEONATAL maladjustment syndrome.

malady a disease or illness.

malalignment displacement, especially of the teeth from their normal relation to the line of the dental arch.

Malamute, malemute see ALASKAN MALAMUTE.

malar pertaining to mala. See also ZYGOMATIC, JUGAL.

m. abscess abscessation at the root of the carnassial tooth (upper fourth premolar in dogs and upper third in cats) may give rise to an inflammatory reaction, then a fistula on the face, below the eye. Called also carnassial abscess, facial abscess, facial sinus. Less often, abscessation of the roots of the lower carnassial tooth (first molar in dogs and in cats) can drain through the skin over the mandible or into the mouth.

m. rash dogs with systemic lupus erythematosus sometimes develop a symmetric scaling erythematous lesion over the nose which resembles the change seen in humans with SLE.

malaris muscle the cutaneous muscle which depresses the lower eyelid.

Malassez named after L.C. Malassez, a French physiologist.

M. disease cyst of the testis.

M. epithelial rests epithelial remnant in the peridontal membrane; sometimes develops into a dental cyst.

Malassezia a lipophilic yeast which is commonly found on the skin and particularly in normal and diseased ears of dogs and cats. Includes *M. pachydermatis, M. canis.* Called also *Pityrosporum canis.*

***M. furfur* (syn. *P. orbiculare, P. ovale*)** causes a TINEA versicolor, a fungal dermatomycosis on the teats of goats.

malasseziasis infection with the yeast, *Malassezia.*

malassimilation 1. imperfect, faulty or disordered assimilation. 2. the inability of the gastrointestinal tract to take up one or more ingested nutrients, whether due to faulty digestion (MALDIGESTION) or to impaired intestinal mucosal transport (MALABSORPTION).

malate a salt of malic acid.

m.–aspartate shuttle system for the transfer of reducing equivalents as NADH and H+ between the site of generation in glycolysis in the cytosol and the site of oxidation in the electron transport chain for production of ATP in the mitochondria. Reducing equivalents are transported into the mitochondria as malate, using oxaloacetate as the carbon carrier. The oxaloacetate is generated from transamination of aspartate. Oxaloacetate does not have a mitochondrial transport protein.

m. dehydrogenase, NAD-linked malate dehydrogenase an enzyme found in the mitochondria (as part of the TCA cycle) or cytosol that participates in the reversible conversion of malate to oxaloacetate.

malathion one of the least toxic and most widely used organophosphorus insecticides in companion animals. Toxicity when it occurs is usually due to gross overconcentration of the compound in the topical preparation used. See also ORGANOPHOSPHORUS COMPOUND.

malaxate to knead, as in making pills.

malaxation an act of kneading.

maldescent faulty descent of the testicle into the scrotum.

maldevelopment abnormal growth or development.

maldigestion incomplete digestion such as occurs in pancreatic exocrine or bile salt deficiency. In ruminants a defect in ruminal microflora could have the same effect. See also MALASSIMILATION.

maldronksiekte Afrikaans term for poisoning with SOLANUM *kwebense*. Literal translation is 'mad drunk disease'.

male an individual of the sex that produces spermatozoa.

m. castrate see BARROW, CAPON, GELDING, STEER, WETHER.

m. feminizing syndrome see FEMINIZING SYNDROME.

m. genital system is comprised essentially of penis, prepuce, scrotum, testicles, epididymis, vas deferens, prostate, seminal vesicles, bulbourethral glands and the male urethra.

m. sex hormones testosterone is the most important male hormone. Weaker androgens are androstenedione and dihydroepiandrosterone.

m. pseudohermaphrodite see PSEUDOHERMAPHRODITE.

male fern see DRYOPTERIS.

maleberry see LYONIA LIGUSTRINA.

maleic hydrazide used experimentally to control the growth of grass without killing it. May cause vomiting in dogs walking in the grass.

maleruption see TEETH maleruption.

malformation defective or abnormal formation; deformity; an anatomical aberration, especially one acquired during development.

malic acid a compound that is found in the juices of many fruits and plants, and is an intermediate in the tricarboxylic acid cycle.

malic enzyme an adaptive enzyme involved in lipogenesis. Catalyses the irreversible conversion of malate to pyruvate + CO_2 in the cytosol. Called also the NADP-linked malate dehydrogenase.

malicious an act done to inflict an injury, not to redress a wrong.

m. poisoning laying a bait to poison an animal without the owner's consent.

m. prosecution instigating a lawsuit for the purpose of punishing the other person without having a proper justification for the litigation.

malignancy a tendency to progress in virulence. In popular usage, any condition that, if uncorrected, tends to worsen so as to cause serious illness or death. Cancer is the best known example.

malignant tending to become progressively worse and to result in death; having the properties of anaplasia, invasiveness and metastasis; said of tumors.

m. aphtha see contagious ECTHYMA.

m. carbuncle a form of anthrax in humans.

m. catarrhal fever (MCF) see BOVINE malignant catarrh.

m. edema an acute infection of wounds by *Clostridium septicum*, *C. chauvoei*, *C. welchii*, *C. sordellii* or *C. novyi*. The inflammation causes severe swelling and discoloration of skin and exposed tissues. There may be local subcutaneous emphysema and a frothy exudate, depending on the identity of the invading organism. There is a high fever and a profound toxemia; death follows within a few hours if treatment is not provided. Special occurrences are when a large number of animals are affected at one time. These include involvement of the vulva in recently lambed ewes, of shearing or docking wounds, and of the umbilicus or eyes of recently born lambs.

m. fibrous histiocytoma a rare aggressive tumor of dogs and cats; composed of densely packed fibroblasts and histiocytes.

m. head catarrh see BOVINE malignant catarrh.

m. histiocytosis see malignant HISTIOCYTOSIS.

m. hyperthermia see malignant HYPERTHERMIA, PORCINE stress syndrome.

m. lymphoma see LYMPHOSARCOMA.

m. pustule see malignant carbuncle (above).

m. theileriasis THEILERIASIS caused by *Theileria hirci*.

malignin a protein fragment present in the serum of human patients with malignant glial tumors.

malingerer in human terms, an individual who feigns illness. The word cannot really be applied to animals but is sometimes used as a name for an assortment of otherwise difficult to classify cases, e.g. cows which 'sulk' and will not rise even though they probably can, or animals that practice attention–attraction behavior, e.g. dogs feigning lameness.

Malinois see BELGIAN shepherd dog.

malkop-ui DIPCADI *glaucum*.

mallard see ANAS PLATYRHYNCHOS.

malleable susceptible of being beaten out into a thin plate.

m. retractor a flat elongated piece of metal shaped like a tongue depressor, which can be bent into a desired shape and used as a retractor for soft tissue. See RIBBON MALLEABLE RETRACTOR.

mallein a substance prepared from *Malleomyces mallei* (*Pseudomonas mallei*, now called *Burkholderia mallei*) that elicits a delayed-type hypersensitivity reaction when injected intradermally as a test for glanders.

m. test the intradermal test for glanders.

mallenders a chronic dermatitis on the posterior aspect of the carpal joint; a disease of cart horses with thick legs and coarse feather.

malleoincudal pertaining to the malleus and incus.

malleolus pl. *malleoli* [L.] a rounded process, especially either of the two rounded prominences on either side of the distal end of the fibula (external, lateral or outer malleolus) or of the tibia (inner, internal or medial malleolus).

Malleomyces see PSEUDOMONAS.

mallet a heavy-headed surgical instrument used for driving a bone chisel.

Kirk m. a mallet with a solid bronze head.

malleus 1. the largest of the three ossicles of the ear; called also hammer. 2. glanders.

Mallophaga suborder of insects comprising the biting or bird lice. Also found on mammals. See also LOUSE.

malnutrition the term used to describe the condition caused by a diet that contains all of the essential nutrients but in suboptimal amounts—an intermediate stage to starvation. It is compatible with life and the same metabolic changes occur as in starvation but to a lesser degree. Ketosis, loss of body weight and muscular power accompany a lower metabolic rate. There is also a fall in body temperature, reduced heart and respiratory rates and sexual activity. Could also be used to describe gross over-nutrition. See also CACHEXIA, STARVATION.

milk replacer m. see MILK replacer.

malocclusion malposition of the teeth resulting in the

faulty meeting of the teeth or jaws. Malocclusion of the incisors is a common defect in all species and is treated as an inherited defect in many of them. See also BITE (3), PARROT mouth.

malonate utilization a biochemical test used for the identification of *Salmonella arizonae* based on the utilization of malonate in the broth as the sole carbon source.

malonyl CoA first committed intermediate in the synthesis of fatty acids. Inhibitor or carnitine palmitoyl transferase I.

Malpighian named after Marcello Malpighi, an Italian anatomist.

M. body lymphoid follicles in the spleen.

M. capsule see BOWMAN'S CAPSULE.

M. corpuscle see renal CORPUSCLE.

M. layer the stratum basale (basal layer) and the stratum spinosum (prickle-cell layer) of the epidermis considered together.

malposition abnormal placement.

fetal m. see PRESENTATION.

malpractice in human medical practice, malpractice means bad, wrong or injudicious treatment of a patient professionally; it results in injury, unnecessary suffering or death of the patient. The court may hold that malpractice has occurred even though the physician acted in good faith. Also, malpractice may occur through omission to act as well as commission of an unwise or negligent act.

In veterinary practice, a client may proceed against a veterinarian if loss has been incurred and damages are sought. Malpractice suits are much more common in American law than in English law, where negligence suits are more usual. Misconduct charges are usually brought by the professional registering body, whose objective it is to preserve the reputation of the profession against the excesses of nonconformists and incompetents.

malpresentation faulty fetal presentation.

malrotation abnormal or pathological rotation, as of the vertebral column; failure of normal rotation of an organ, such as the gut, during embryological development.

MALT mucosal-associated lymphoid tissue.

malt feeds by-products of the brewing industry. Include malt cleanings (18% protein), malt culms (24% protein) and malt hulls which have a high fiber content. See also CULMS.

malt worker's lung an immediate, immune complex (antibody–antigen) mediated hypersensitivity pneumonitis of humans caused by inhalation of *Aspergillus clavatus* in moldy barley.

Malta fever brucellosis in humans caused by *Brucella melitensis*. Called also Mediterranean fever.

maltase an enzyme that hydrolyzes α-glucosides to glucose; there are two maltases found at the brush border of the intestinal epithelium, where they hydrolyze maltose (a product of the digestion of starch) to glucose for absorption. Maltase is absent from the intestine at birth and calves are unable to properly digest starch as a result.

Maltese 1. pertaining to or emanating from Malta. 2. a very small (4–6 lb) dog with dark brown eyes and a long, silky, flowing, white haircoat that obscures the long, pendant ears and small, arched tail. Sometimes called Maltese terrier. The breed is affected by white shaker dog disease.

M. cockspur CENTAUREA *melitensis*.

M. cross characteristic formation within phagocytes in peritoneal granulomas caused by granules of starch; visible in polarized light.

m. thistle CENTAUREA *melitensis*.

maltose a sugar (disaccharide) formed when starch is hydrolyzed by amylase.

maltotriose a trisaccharide product of amylase digestion of starch.

malunion faulty union (i.e. incorrect anatomical alignment) of the fragments of a fractured bone.

Malus sylvestris the common apple. The fruit can be eaten in sufficient amounts to cause CARBOHYDRATE ENGORGEMENT. The pips contain sufficient cyanogenetic glycoside to cause cyanide poisoning if they were eaten in quantity. Called also *M. pumila*, *Pyrus malus*.

Malva parviflora plant in the family Malvaceae; toxin may be a thiaminase; causes incoordination in sheep if they are made to exercise. If pressed the sheep go down but are able to get up and walk away within a few minutes. Called also marshmallow, small-faced mallow.

MAM methyl azoxyemethanol.

mamba highly venomous African tree-snake in the family Elapidae. Called also *Dendroaspis*.

mamilla pl. *mamillae* [L.] a nipple-like prominence or rounded breast-like eminence.

mamillated having nipple-like or rounded, breast-like projections or prominences.

mamillation 1. the condition of being mamillated. 2. a nipple-like elevation or projection.

mamilliform shaped like a nipple or breast.

mamilliplasty theleplasty; plastic reconstruction of the nipples or teats.

mamillitis, mammillitis thelitis; inflammation of the nipple.

bovine ulcerative m. see bovine herpes MAMMILLITIS.

mamma pl. *mammae* [L.] the milk-secreting gland of the female; mammary gland; the breast, udder.

mammal an individual of the class Mammalia, a division of vertebrates, including all that possess hair and suckle their young.

eutherian m's true placental mammals which develop chorion, amnion, yolk sac and allantois, all of which contribute to the placenta. Called also placental mammals.

metatherian m's marsupials including kangaroos, opossums which are born after a brief period of development and spend a long time being nurtured by the mother, usually in a pouch or marsupium.

placental m. see eutherian mammals (above).

prototherian m's monotremes, the egg-laying mammals.

mammalgia pain in the mammary gland.

mammalian emanating from or pertaining to mammals.

mammaplasty mammoplasty.

mammary pertaining to the mammary gland.

m. abscess usually an abscess of connective and subcutaneous tissue with no abnormality of the milk. Large masses of necrotic debris may occur in infection of the udder by *Corynebacterium pyogenes* but these are usually classified as mastitis because they connect with the duct system and cause the discharge of pus in the milk.

m. agalactia the absence of milk secretion in an animal that has recently given birth and has normal mammary development. See also AGALACTIA.

m. bud produced along the length of the embryonic mammary ridge these buds represent the future locations of the mammary glands. Invagination of ectoderm at each bud leads to the development of epithelial diverticula, later maturing as lactiferous ducts.

m. cyst recorded in ewes; filled with milk.
m. ductal ectasia milk ducts are distended with proteinaceous fluid containing cell debris. Common in bitches and queens. May rupture to the exterior causing granulomas. Called also mammary ductal hyperplasia.
m. ductal hyperplasia see mammary ductal ectasia (above).
m. ectopic tissue bilateral swellings in vulvar tissue; enlarge at parturition; milk can be aspirated.
m. edema occurs in the few days before or immediately after calving. The udder and the teats, often the escutcheon and sometimes the ventral abdominal and even the ventral thoracic wall are obviously misshapen by pitting edema. The teats may be so swollen that milking is difficult.
feline m. hypertrophy a hormone-dependent, benign enlargement of one or more mammary glands, occurring spontaneously in young, intact female cats and in others treated with progestins. Called also fibroepithelial hyperplasia, fibroadenomatous hyperplasia and fibroadenomatosis.
m. fibrosis diffuse thickening or local lumps palpable through skin, mostly in ventral part; may be sufficient to cause asymmetrical enlargement of the gland; terminally leads to atrophy.
m. gangrene a lesion which includes skin, a well demarcated mass of tissue usually involving whole or part of teat; secretion is watery, red-tinged; gangrenous mass eventually sloughs leaving a slow-to-heal gaping cavity.
m. gland a gland of female mammals developed from specialized sweat glands, which secrete milk for nourishment of the young. The mammary glands are composed of alveolar tissue, with the alveoli lined by milk-secreting epithelium, and connecting to a collecting duct system which empties into the milk cistern (sinus) at the base of the teat and then into the teat cistern (sinus). They exist in a rudimentary state in the male. In food animal females and mares, called also udder.
m. gland caking appears as a hard plaque along the floor of the udder, usually in a first calf heifer immediately after calving. The milk is normal but the udder is sore and let-down is poor.
m. gland suspensory ligament see UDDER suspensory apparatus.
m. hypertrophy normal tissue on palpation but quarter enlarged compared to opposite one of pair.
m. hypoplasia failure of the glands to develop. It is also usually extended to include those udders or individual quarters that do not undergo reconstitution after regression during a dry period.
m. inflammation see MASTITIS.
m. involution regression of mammary tissue to a non-secreting state, with disappearance of much of the epithelial tissue. The process can be induced by the infusion of colchicine into the milk system.
m. mazoplasia an increase in the number of ducts per lobule of mammary gland.
m. neoplasia is rare in food animals and mares. It accounts for approximately 25% of all neoplasms in dogs but is less common in cats.
m. pustular dermatitis an infectious disease of lactating cows consisting of 2 mm diameter thin-walled pustules on the skin of the teats and the ventral udder. There may be similar lesions on the hands of the milkers. The cause is bovine herpesvirus 2. Called also udder impetigo, udder acne.
m. secretion just before parturition and for the first week afterwards the secretion is thick, sticky COLOSTRUM. This is followed by MILK for the duration of the lactation and superseded in the weeks after drying off by honey-dew, a clear, viscid secretion. The gland may be completely dry for a variable period between lactations.
m. suspensory ligament rupture a condition manifested by separation of the median ligaments (medial laminae) resulting in the glands dropping ventrally. The teats point almost laterally. It is a problem of recently calved cows. Called also dropped udder.
m. tumor Gilbertson classification used in the classification of human breast tumors as an aid to prognosis; five grades of severity based on morphological criteria, especially degree of local invasion and lymph node involvement.
m. underdevelopment congenital lack of development of all glands, possibly an inherited defect.

mammatrope see MAMMOTROPE.
mammectomy see MASTECTOMY.
mammilla see MAMILLA.
mammillary pertaining to or resembling a teat or breast.
mammillitis mamillitis.
bovine herpes m. an infectious ulcerative dermatitis of the teats and udder of cows, caused by bovine herpesvirus 2 (BHV-2). The same virus also causes the Allerton form of lumpy skin disease. Spread between herds may be by insect vector. The lesions are severe and include vesicles, papules, sloughing of skin, scab formation and ulceration.
mammiplasia see MAMMOPLASIA.
mammiplasty see MAMMOPLASTY.
mammitis see MASTITIS.
mamm(o)- word element. [L.] *breast, mammary gland.*
mammogenesis development of the mammary gland.
mammogram a radiograph of the mammary gland.
mammography radiography of the mammary gland with or without injection of an opaque contrast medium into its ducts.
Mammomonogamus a genus of nematodes in the family Syngamidae. They are parasites of the nasal sinuses and trachea of mammals.
M. auris found in the puma.
M. ierei found in cats, a cause of chronic nasopharyngitis.
M. indicus found in the pharynx of the Indian elephant.
M. laryngeus found in the larynx of cattle, goats, water buffalo and deer, and occasionally in humans.
M. loxodontus in the trachea of the African elephant.
M. mcgaughei found in cats.
M. nasicola found in the nasal cavities of cattle, sheep, goats and deer.
mammoplasia development of mammary tissue.
mammoplasty plastic surgery of the breast.
mammotomy see MASTOTOMY.
mammotrope one of the acidophils of the adenohypophysis that secretes prolactin.
mammotrophic see MAMMOTROPIC.
mammotropic having a stimulating effect on the mammary gland.
mammotropin see PROLACTIN.
mammotrops one of the five types of secretory cells found in the adrenohypophysis; secrete prolactin.
man masculine member (sole) of the genus *Homo*, i.e. *Homo sapiens*.
management technique, practice or science of managing or controlling; the skillful use of resources and time; the specific treatment of a disease or disorder.

m. factors parts of the management program that influence the occurrence and prevalence of disease. They include such things as feeding, breeding program, culling program, genetic selection, disease prevention, cash flow, capital accessibility and MANAGER FACTORS.

m. groups livestock grouped according to management parameters, usually age, sex, purpose.

m. history history of a herd or flock which includes all management operations.

manager factors the unassessable characters which make the difference between a good and a bad manager. They include thoroughness, dependability, numeracy, money-wisdom, empathy with animals and acceptance of responsibility.

manatee members of the genus *Trichechus* which with the dugongs make up the order Sirenia, of sea-cows. They are almost completely aquatic mammals with a large, fish-like body with flippers in front and horizontal tail flukes behind. They can be up to 13 ft long and weigh up to 2000 lb.

Manchester terrier a small (12–22 lb), compact dog with a very short, black coat and mahogany markings on specified areas of the body, but generally on the face and legs. The 'candle-flame' shaped ears are v-shaped and folded over the head, which is long and wedge-shaped, and the tail is short and tapered. Sometimes called the Rat terrier, Black and tan terrier.

A variety weighing less than 12 lb is recognized in the United States and called the Toy Manchester, the English version is called the Black and tan toy terrier; called also English Toy Terrier.

Manchester wasting disease see ENZOOTIC calcinosis.

manchette see CAUDAL sheath.

Mancini technique see radial IMMUNODIFFUSION.

Mandalong special cattle a beef breed of cattle produced in Australia by intercrossing Charolais, Chianina, British white, Shorthorn, Brahman.

mandarin duck see AIX GALERICULATA. Called also *Dendronessa galericulata*.

mandatory required by law.

m. continuing education participation in a continuing education program is a prerequisite for continued registration in some countries.

mandelic acid a keto-acid used as a urinary antiseptic in nephritis, pyelitis and cystitis. It must be excreted in the urinary tract unchanged in order to have a bacteriostatic effect; therefore, a strongly acid urine must be maintained during its administration.

mandible the horseshoe-shaped bone forming the lower jaw.

Consists of a central body, which forms the chin and supports the lower teeth, and two vertical or perpendicular rami, which point upward from the back of the chin on either side and articulate with the temporal bones by their condylar processes. The rami end as coronoid processes. In ruminants and carnivores the mandible is permanently divided into two halves by the mandibular symphysis, a joint that allows some rotation.

swollen m. generally enlarged due to osteodystrophia in horses and pigs; localized enlargement in actinomycosis of jaw in cattle, bone neoplasm.

mandibular emanating from or pertaining to the mandible.

m. arch cartilage an early skeletal element in the embryonic viscerocranium, the cartilage eventually becomes the mandible.

m. duct the duct of the mandibular salivary gland.

m. enlargement causes a characteristic lateral silhouette in animals similar to that of bottle jaw. It is a common sign in osteodystrophia fibrosa in horses and pigs, CRANIOMANDIBULAR osteopathy in dogs, and lymphoma and actinomycosis of cattle.

m. gland a salivary gland situated behind the angle of the jaw, sometimes partly covered by the parotid salivary gland and the mandible.

m. lymph node one of a cluster of nodes grouped around the facial vein at the angle of the jaw.

m. nerve block an anesthetic agent is injected around the mandibular alveolar nerve where it enters the mandibular foramen. Usually used in large animals for dental procedures on the lower jaw.

m. neurapraxia bilateral trigeminal motor paralysis causing a dropped jaw that cannot be voluntarily closed. Seen in dogs as a result of trauma or as an idiopathic neuritis. Recovery is usual, but occasionally the condition persists with atrophy of the temporal, masseter, pterygoid, rostral digastricus and mylohyoid muscles.

m. osteodystrophy one of the regions of the body where a generalized OSTEODYSTROPHY is most readily observable. The ventral edge of each ramus is thickened and the intermandibular space reduced.

m. prognathism an abnormal protrusion of the mandible so that there is difficulty in prehending and masticating food, especially in animals at pasture. The defect is inherited in some breeds of cattle and also occurs as part of a more general range of defects, e.g. in achondroplastic dwarf cattle. Called also undershot. See also MALOCCLUSION.

mandibulectomy excision of the mandible.

mandrel a farrier's tool used in fitting frost nails to shoes.

mandrill Old World monkeys in the genus *Mandrillus*. They are the ugliest and most brutal-looking of the monkeys, with brightly colored genital regions and buttocks. They are large, walk on all four limbs and are terrestrial in habit.

mandrin a metal guide for a flexible catheter.

mane the region of long coarse hair at the dorsal border of the neck and terminating at the poll in the forelock. Present in the horse and other Equidae. Similar gatherings of coarse hairs are present in the giraffe, gnu, various antelope, cheetah and lion. Called also juba.

buzzed-off m. broken or sheared hairs in the mane, causing it to be irregularly shortened; seen with self-trauma in response to pruritic skin disease such as *Culicoides* hypersensitivity.

m. and tail dystrophy short, brittle hair in the mane and tail of horses; the cause is unknown.

maneb an organic compound used in agriculture as a fungicide; appears to have minimal toxicity.

mangabeys dark-colored, long-snouted Old World monkeys with a wide distribution and common as zoo specimens, e.g. crested mangabey (*Cercocebus albigena*).

manganese a chemical element, atomic number 25, atomic weight 54.938, symbol Mn. See Table 6. Its salts occur in the body tissue in very small amounts and serve as activators of liver arginase and other enzymes.

m. nutritional deficiency in cattle, sheep and pigs is thought to cause infertility and skeletal deformities, including enlarged joints, pain, knuckling at the fetlocks and twisting of the legs. It is a rare deficiency in dogs and cats.

mange a skin disease of domestic animals, caused by a number of genera of mites and described under those headings. See CHORIOPTIC MANGE, DEMODECTIC MANGE, NOTOEDRIC MANGE, OTODECTIC MANGE, PSOROPTIC MANGE and SARCOPTIC MANGE.

auricular m. see ear mange (below).

body m. PSOROPTIC MANGE.

ear m. called also auricular mange; see OTODECTIC MANGE, PSOROPTIC MANGE.

follicular m. DEMODECTIC MANGE.

fox m. see SARCOPTIC MANGE.

head m. NOTOEDRIC MANGE.

incognito m. a form of sarcoptic mange in well-groomed dogs in which lesions are virtually absent, but there is still intense pruritus.

leg m. CHORIOPTIC MANGE.

otodectic m. see OTODECTIC MANGE.

red m. synonym for SARCOPTIC MANGE in farm animals and DEMODECTIC MANGE in dogs.

ursicoptic m. pruritus and alopecia caused by a sarcoptiform mite (*Ursicoptes americanus*) found in the follicular sinuses of bears.

mangel-wurzel see MANGELS.

mangels *Beta vulgaris*; called also mangel-wurzel.

manger a receptacle, usually of wood or iron, for the feeding of grain and chopped roughage to farm and racing animals.

mangolds see BETA *vulgaris*.

mangrove snake see BOIGA *dendrophila*.

mania a disordered mental state of excitement. Affected animals act in bizarre ways and appear to be unaware of their surroundings. Their actions include licking and chewing of foreign materials, abnormalities of voice, apparent blindness, aggression and lack of response to normal stimuli.

maniac one affected with mania.

manica flexoria a tubular sheath on the palmar aspect of the metacarpophalangeal region of the front paw of carnivores, through which the tendons of the deep digital flexor muscle pass.

Manihot esculenta the cassava plant, a member of the Euphorbiaceae family. The tuber is used for food but contains high levels of cyanogenetic glycosides and can cause poisoning in animals if fed to them raw. Called *M. dulcis*, *M. utilissima*, cassava, manioc, tapioca.

manioc see MANIHOT ESCULENTA.

manipulation skillful or dextrous treatment by the hands. In physical therapy, the forceful passive movement of a joint beyond its active limit of motion.

Manis see PANGOLIN.

Manley ventilator a ventilator suitable for anesthetizing small animals. Operated by the gas flow from the anesthetic apparatus.

manna gum EUCALYPTUS *vinimalis*.

mannagrass see GLYCERIA.

Manning eye shield a tent-like, miniature aluminum and canvas shield applied to an injured eye in a horse to prevent self-mutilation.

mannitol a sugar alcohol occurring widely in nature, especially in fungi; utilization of mannitol is used in identification of some bacteria; used in diagnostic tests of kidney function and as an osmotic diuretic, particularly in the treatment of cerebral edema and oliguric acute renal failure.

mannose an aldohexose, a monosaccharide produced from mannitol by oxidation.

mannosidase deficiency see MANNOSIDOSIS.

mannosidosis an inborn error of metabolism, in which inactivity or an inherited deficiency of mannosidase results in lysosomal accumulation of mannose-rich substrates. Deficiency of the α-isomer (α-mannosidosis) is inherited in Aberdeen Angus and Murray Grey cattle as an autosomal recessive trait, and the resulting disease is of economic importance. From several months of age, affected calves show ataxia, head tremor, aggression, and finally paralysis. A similar disease has been reported in cats.

Deficiency of the β-isomer is inherited, also as an autosomal recessive trait, in Nubian goats, causing neurological deficits and tremors from birth. There are also skeletal abnormalities.

acquired m. caused by ingestion of ASTRAGALUS, OXYTROPIS and SWAINSONA spp., which contain alkaloids that inhibit α-mannosidase activity. Called also locoweed poisoning.

manometer an instrument for ascertaining the pressure of liquids or gases.

manometry technique of using a manometer and interpreting the result.

esophageal m. a method of recording pressures within the esophagus, particularly during the passage of a food bolus.

Mansonella a genus of nematode parasites of the superfamily Filaroidea transmitted by *Culicoides* and *Simulium* spp.

M. ozzardi a species found in the mesentery and visceral fat of humans in Central and South America; suspected sightings also in domestic animals.

Mansonia a genus of mosquitoes in the family Culicidae and vectors of *Dirofilaria immitis* of dogs and the virus of Rift Valley fever in all species. Now called *Taeniorhynchus* spp.

Mansonia altissima a tree in the family *Sterculiaceae*. Animals kept on its shavings as litter may abort and develop oral and cutaneous ulcers, diarrhea and death. No toxin has been identified. Called also African redwood.

Manson's eyeworm see OXYSPIRURA *mansoni*.

Mantel–Haenszl technique an odds ratio named after N. Mantel and W. Haenszl, modern day epidemiologists who devised the method.

mantle 1. an enveloping structure or layer, especially the brain mantle, or pallium. 2. see FRILLED.

m. zone an outer region surrounding germinal centers in the cortex of lymph nodes.

Mantoux test a tuberculin skin test used in humans to detect prior exposure to *Mycobacterium* spp.

manubrium pl. *manubria* [L.] 1. the most cranial portion of the sternum. 2. the largest process of the malleus, giving attachment to the tendon of the tensor muscle of the tympanum.

manufacturing beef see HAMBURGER BEEF.

manure the dung of farm animals used as replenishment for the ground.

m. disposal has become a major problem to animal farming in urban areas. Methods have been devised to avoid labor involvement by the use of pits under animal accommodation, or by discharging onto pasture or into evaporative lagoons by use of a slurry pushed through a hose. Housing animals on litter and rapid composting of the litter has advantages.

m. management includes collection, storage, fly and odor control, environmental pollution, avoiding soiling of cow's hair and udder, bedding supply and distribution, maintaining good footage.

m. pit gas poisoning large quantities of hydrogen sulfide gas are produced in pits and tanks in which animal manure is undergoing biological degradation. If the contents of the pit are stirred violently to facilitate emptying, the gas may be released into the atmosphere in a high concentration, and if the area is enclosed, poisoning of animals and humans can occur.

manus pl. *manus* [L.] hand.
Manx a shorthaired, medium-sized cat with long hindlegs, prominent hindquarters and some degree of taillessness which can range from absolute, with only a hollow at the end of the spine ('rumpies'), to a short, immobile tail only a few coccygeal vertebrae long and not projecting above the back ('rumpyriser'), to one longer, mobile, but often kinked or otherwise deformed ('stumpy'). Occasionally a normal looking, but abnormally short, tail is produced ('longie'). The Manx gene which is dominant is often associated with other deformities of the lower gastrointestinal tract, such as atresia ani, or spine, such as spina bifida, and many Manx have unusual hindleg gaits as a result. All Manx are heterozygotes, as the trait is lethal, prenatally, in the homozygous state. The usual breeding is Manx to normal, to avoid such losses, but Manx litters are normally very small. The breed is also affected by a hereditary corneal edema.
M. virus a strain of calicivirus, isolated from and named after a Manx cat, at one time incriminated in the etiology of the feline urological syndrome; its significance is unclear.
manyplies omasum.
MAO monoamine oxidase.
MAP 1. magnesium-ammonium-phosphate; a type of UROLITH. 2. microtubule-associated protein.
map distance, map unit the amount of recombination between two genes expressed as a percentage. See also CENTIMORGAN.
maple syrup urine disease an inherited disease of polled Hereford cattle and humans, in which there is a deficient decarboxylation of branched-chain α-ketoacids derived from several amino acids. It is marked clinically by mental and physical retardation, feeding difficulties and a characteristic odor of the urine resembling burnt sugar.
Mapleson classification a scheme for categorizing anesthetic breathing circuits, based on the position of the breathing bag, the fresh gas flow and the patient. See also Mapleson CIRCUIT.
mapoon see MORINDA RETICULATA.
mapping see GENETIC map.
maps an important feature of epidemiological investigations. Maps with special features suited to data analysis are GRID, ISODEMIC, ISOPLETH and SPOT maps.
maranguey see ZAMIA.
marasmus a form of protein-calorie malnutrition characterized by growth retardation and wasting of subcutaneous fat and muscle, but usually with retention of appetite and mental alertness. See COBALT nutritional deficiency.
marathon races races for horses. See also ENDURANCE RIDES.
marble bone disease see OSTEOPETROSIS.
marble spleen disease a disease of pheasants and a similar disease of chickens and turkeys which is caused by group II avian adenovirus and characterized by the postmortem finding of a marble-like mottling and enlargement of the spleen.
marbling 1. the presence of different stages of congestion and necrosis in adjoining lobules of an organ, giving a gross effect of a pattern similar to that of marble. 2. the desirable intermixing of fat and muscle fibers in good beef produced by feeding a high energy diet when the animal is still young.
marbofloxacin a fluoroquinolone with wide antibacterial activity, registered for veterinary use.
Marburg disease a severe, often fatal, viral hemorrhagic fever of humans first reported in Marburg, Germany, among laboratory workers exposed to African green monkeys. The virus is a member of the family *Filoviridae*.
marc grape pulp used as animal feed. When dried, it is called pomace.
Marcenac incision a low flank grid incision for entry to the equine abdomen for ovariectomy or cesarean section.
march fly see TABANUS.
Marche a gray Italian breed of beef cattle. Called also Marchigiana.
Marchigiana see MARCHE.
mare 1. a female horse, 4 years or older. 2. in Great Britain, also applied to a female donkey (jenny).
Marek's disease a transmissible disease of chickens caused by an alphaherpesvirus that carries some retrovirus oncogenes; characterized by a tumorous, mononuclear infiltration of peripheral nerves, causing limb paralysis. Infiltration of other organs and tissues is common, especially of the iris, causing blindness, and of the ovaries. Vaccination is highly effective and without it serious outbreaks with heavy losses can occur. Called also neural lymphomatosis, neurolymphomatosis gallinarum.
Marek's tumor-specific antigen see Marek's tumor-specific ANTIGEN.
Maremma sheepdog a large (80–100 lb) sturdy dog with a thick, long white coat which forms a collar on the neck. The small, v-shaped ears are folded over and the tail is long and carried low.
mare's nest something thought to be an extraordinary discovery but proving to be a delusion or hoax.
marestail see EQUISETUM.
Marfan's syndrome congenital defect in calves comparable to an inherited human defect; enlargement of the aortic root associated with a loud systolic murmur on the left side, long, thin limbs, joint laxity, lenticular displacement and opacity.
Margaropus a genus of ticks in the family Ixodidae, similar physically to *Boophilus* spp.
M. reidi found on giraffes.
M. winthemi found on horses, sometimes cattle; called also Argentine tick.
margay a wild cat about the size of a domestic cat which preys on small domestic animals and birds. Called also *Panthera tigrina*, American tiger cat.
margin border, margin or edge.
antitragal m. caudal edge of the ear.
central m. the inner margin of the sole of the horse's hoof, occupied by the bars and the apex of the frog.
coronal m. proximal border of the hoof where the horn meets the skin.
epididymal m. the attached border of the testis where the epididymis is attached.
free m. (margo liber) the unattached border of the testis.
interalveolar m. the ridge along the alveolar process of the maxillae and mandibles between the teeth.
mesometric m. the border of the uterus to which the broad ligament is attached.
parietal m. outer margin of the sole of the hoof, connected to the wall of the hoof by the white line.
plicated m. the raised cuticular ridge that separates the esophageal part of the stomach in the horse from the glandular part.
pupillary m. the free edge of the iris, the edge of the pupil.
safety m. 1. the ratio between the lethal dose for 1% of the population and the effective dose for 99% of the population. Used to describe the toxicity of a pharmaceutical agent. 2. estimate of the ratio of the

'no-observed-effect' level (NOEL) to the level accepted in regulations relating to epidemiology and disease control. Called also margin of safety.
tragal m. (margo tragicus) anteromedial edge of the ear.

marginal pertaining to margin; the economist's version, in which marginal means added or extra.
m. auricular dermatosis see EAR margin dermatosis.
m. cost the added cost incurred by producing an additional unit of product.
m. folds folds of endothelium found in lymphatics which provide a valve-like effect, permitting ingress only of fluid.
neural tube m. layer on the external surface of the embryonal neural tube; houses axonal processes of developing neurons.
m. product the added amount of product produced by the application of an additional unit of a particular input.
m. product value the value of an extra unit of output.
m. revenue the extra net income obtained by selling or using internally one additional unit of product.
m. zone the rim of tissue surrounding lymph follicles in the spleen which contains many lymphocytes and macrophages.

margination accumulation and adhesion of leukocytes to the epithelial cells of blood vessel walls at the site of injury in the early stages of inflammation.

marginoplasty surgical restoration of a border, as of the eyelid.

margo pl. *margines* [L.] border; margin. See also MARGIN.
m. plicatus the conspicuous folded edge of the mucous membrane between the large non-glandular portion of the horse's stomach and the dorsally located glandular portion.

marguerite see CHRYSANTHEMUM.

mariculture marine aquaculture.

Marie–Bamberger disease see hypertrophic OSTEOPATHY.

Marie's disease see hypertrophic OSTEOPATHY.

marijuana, marihuana a preparation of the leaves and flowering tops of *Cannabis sativa*, the hemp plant, which contains a number of pharmacologically active principles (cannabinoids).

marine of or pertaining to the sea.

marine biologist specialist in the biology of marine life.

marine flexibacter disease erosive skin and gill disease of marine fish caused by *Flexibacter maritimus*.

marine mammals mammals inhabiting the sea; generally taken to include the cetaceans (whales, porpoise, dolphin), the sirenians (sea-cows, including manatees and dugong) and the pinnipeds (the carnivores of the group, seals, sealions, walruses). Other mammals that spend a great deal of time in the water but are not classified as marine mammals are the polar bear and the sea otter.

marine orders the laws governing the conduct of sea travel and transport on board ship. They are relevant to the sea transport of animals.

mark-sensing method of entering data into a computer without needing to transcribe it; can be performed by marking the collected data form at predetermined positions.

marker a visual or electronic signal that permits identification and therefore sorting of individual items from a group.
m. animals males or teasers wearing chin-ball or siresine harness so that females mounted are marked by crayon or paint.
m. genes genes with a known location on a chromosome and an obvious phenotype which are used as reference points when mapping other genes.
histochemical m. marking of cells or tissues based on a chemical identification of the contents; the location of specific chemical substances in particular locations is marked by the installation of an electronic or color signal.

marketing margin difference between the purchase and resale prices of a product.

markhor CAPRA *falconeri*.

marking 1. docking of tails in lambs and, where appropriate, castration. 2. a form of olfactory communication or territorial marking by dogs and cats with urine or feces. Dogs deliberately defecate against a vertical surface such as tree, post, or bush. Cats uncharacteristically leave their feces uncovered. See also urine SPRAYING. 3. a color marking on a horse's coat.

Markov chain, Markov model a mathematical model that makes it possible to study complex systems by establishing a state of the system and then effecting a transition to a new state, such a transition being dependent only on the values of the current state, and not dependent on the previous history of the system up to that point.

Marmite disease affected pigs look as if they have been smeared with meat extract (Marmite). See EXUDATIVE epidermitis.

marmoset a small (1 to 2 ft), yellow-green monkey; they are fruit-eaters, arboreal and diurnal. Called also *Callithrix* spp., *Leontideus* spp., *Saguinus* spp.
common m. South American monkey 9 inches long, soft fur, bushy tail, hair black at base, yellow in the middle, white at the tip. Called also *Callithrix jacchus*.

marmot a member of the squirrel family Sciuridae, but heavy-set, burrowing animals, about 2 ft long and weighing 12 lb. Herbivorous and diurnal, they are remarkably agile. Red-gray in color with fine fur and a short tail. Inhabit very cold or high-altitude areas. Related to GROUND-HOG. Called also *Marmota* spp., woodchuck.

Marmota see MARMOT.

Maroteaux–Lamy syndrome mucopolysaccharidosis VI.

Marree disease *Pimelea simplex* subsp. *simplex* poisoning in north-eastern South Australia. Called also St. George disease.

marrow see BONE MARROW.

marrowstem kale BRASSICA *oleraceae* var. *acephala*.

Marsdenia rostrata Australian plant in the family Asclepiadaceae; toxin is probably cynanchoside; liana-type vine with milky sap. The leaves are unpalatable but if eaten cause signs of unsteadiness, collapse, convulsions, dyspnea and, in pigs, vomiting. Death follows within a few hours. Called also milk vine.

Marseilles fever boutonneuse fever.

marsh pertaining to or emanating from swamplands, marshes and bogs. Archetypal denizens are leeches, mangroves, baying hounds and bunyips.
m. arrowgrass TRIGLOCHIN *maritima*.
m. buck see SITUTUNGA.
m. hawk medium-sized, 20 inches long, gray to brown raptor bird with a distinctive white rump during flight. Called also hen harrier, *Circus cyaneus*.
m. horsetail EQUISETUM *palustre*.
m. marigold see CALTHA PALUSTRIS.
m. ragwort SENECIO *aquaticus*.

Marshallagia a genus of intestinal worms in the family Trichostrongylidae; not known to have significant pathogenicity.

M. dentispicularis found in sheep.

M. marshalli found in the abomasum of sheep, goats, antelopes, bighorn sheep and the like.

M. mongolica found in the abomasum of sheep, goat and camel.

M. orientalis found in hillgoats (*Capra sibirica*).

M. schikhobalovi found in sheep.

marshmallow see MALVA PARVIFLORA, ALTHAEA OFFICINALIS.

Marsilea drummondiii Australian aquatic fern; contains a thiaminase and contributes to the etiology of POLIOENCEPHALOMALACIA in sheep, horses and occasionally cattle. Called also nardoo fern.

marsupial an animal member of the order Marsupiala, infraclass Metatheria, which produces viviparous young by hatching eggs internally. The bean-sized fetus is transferred to the characteristic marsupial pouch on the anterior abdomen with its mammary gland and reared there. Two monotremes, the platypus and the spiny anteater, lay and hatch eggs and rear the young, the latter in rudimentary marsupial pouches.

carnivorous m. see DASYURIDS.

marsupialization conversion of a closed cavity, such as an abscess or cyst, into an open pouch, by incising it and suturing the edges of its wall to the edges of the wound. The urinary bladder and prostatic cysts are treated similarly.

marsupium pl. *marsupia* [L.] pouch; the scrotum.

Marteilia parasitic protozoa in the order Occlusosporidia. Includes *M. refringens* (in European oysters), *M. sydnei* (in Sydney rock oysters).

marteiliosis disease of the digestive gland of molluscs, caused by protozoan parasite *Marteilia* spp.

Martina Franca ass an Italian black donkey with paler underline.

Martindale the Extra Pharmacopoeia; published in 30 editions over a period of 110 years by the Royal Pharmaceutical Society of Great Britain; contains over 5000 monographs on substances used in pharmacy and medicine.

Martinez dissector a corneal dissector designed to allow the surgeon to separate the superficial from the deep layers of the cornea.

martingale a leather strap running from the girth to the reins or the noseband for the purpose of restricting the movements of the horse's head. There are many designs. The common ones are the standing martingale, which is attached to the noseband, and the running martingale, which is divided in two, each of which has a ring through which one of the reins passes.

mA·s, mAs milliampere seconds.

Mascagnia genus of South American plants in the family Malpighiaceae; contains an unidentified toxin which causes sudden death, incoordination, recumbency, convulsions, dyspnea and cardiomyopathy. Includes *M. pubiflora*, *M. rigida* etc.

masculine pertaining to the male sex.

masculinity the possession of masculine qualities.

masculinization the normal induction or development of male sex characteristics in the male; also, the induction or development of male secondary sex characteristics in the female.

masculinize to produce masculine qualities in the female or in the sexually maturing male.

masculinized females see VIRILISM.

maser a device that produces an extremely intense, small and nearly nondivergent beam of monochromatic radiation in the microwave region, with all the waves in phase.

mash dry food moistened with a little water. See also BRAN mash.

mask 1. to cover or conceal, as the masking of the nature of a disorder by the presence of unassociated signs, organisms, etc.; in audiometry, to obscure or diminish a sound by the presence of another sound of different frequency. 2. an appliance for shading, protecting, or medicating the face, e.g. a surgical mask. 3. the dark shaded markings on the face of some breeds, e.g. Boxer, Great Dane, Alaskan malamute.

Schimmelbusch m. see SCHIMMELBUSCH MASK.

Venturi m. see VENTURI mask.

masking 1. using a mask for administering a gaseous anesthetic. 2. covering part of an x-ray film, usually with lead, while the other part is being exposed. 3. see BLINDING.

m. down the use of a mask for inducing general anesthesia, using a gaseous anesthetic, followed by intubation.

Mason-meta splint spoon-shaped aluminum splint, curved lengthwise so as to fit around bones and limbs; similar extensions can be added on to the main splint.

Mason–Pfizer monkey virus a type D retrovirus isolated from a mammary carcinoma in a macaque.

mass 1. a lump or collection of cohering particles. 2. that characteristic of matter which gives it inertia.

m.–action ratios the ratio of substrate to product, where the predominance of one, usually the substrate, over the other thermodynamically favors a particular direction for a reaction.

inner cell m. an internal cluster of cells at the embryonic pole of the blastocyst which develops into the body of the embryo.

lean body m. that part of the body including all its components except neutral storage lipid; in essence, the fat-free mass of the body.

m. medication (or immunization, or treatment, or prophylaxis, or testing, or screening) application of the procedure to all of the animals in the population, which may be as small as a herd or as large as a national herd. This sort of strategy has been used extensively and for many years in the control of diseases of animals, and has been the principal reason for the dramatic virtual eradication of the major plagues in many countries. The unintelligent extension of the strategy to the control of wastage caused by endemic disease has contributed most to the problem of residues of antibacterial drugs in the human food chain. See also mass MEDICATION.

m. number the number used to express the mass of a nucleus, being the total number of nucleons, protons and neutrons in the nucleus of an atom or nuclide; symbol A.

m. reflex reflex actions by all the body parts controlled by the part of the spinal cord which has been injured.

thalamic intermediate m. see INTERTHALAMIC ADHESION.

massa pl. *massae* [L.] mass (1).

massage systematic therapeutic stroking or kneading of the body or part.

cardiac m. intermittent compression of the heart by pressure applied through the chest wall (closed cardiac massage) or directly to the heart through an opening in the chest wall (open cardiac massage). See also CARDIAC massage.

genitalic m. of the seminal vesicles in bulls or the penis in male dogs for the purpose of collecting semen, of the clitoris in cows and goat does for the collection of urine.

vibratory m. massage by rapidly repeated light percussion with a vibrating hammer or sound.

masseter see masseter MUSCLE and Table 13.1H.

massotherapy treatment of disease by massage.

mast cell a cell that may be derived from an undifferentiated precursor, which may be of monocytic origin, in the perivascular connective tissue. It elaborates granules that contain histamine, heparin and, in the rat and mouse, serotonin. It plays an important role in acute hypersensitivity (type I) reactions such as atopy and anaphylaxis.

m. c. leukemia see mast cell LEUKEMIA.

m. c. tumor a benign, local aggregation of mast cells forming a nodular tumor that occurs in the skin of most species, but most commonly in dogs. The release of histamine or other vasoactive substances may be associated with gastroduodenal ulceration. These tumors may become malignant. See also MASTOCYTOSIS.

mastadenitis inflammation of a mammary gland; see also MASTITIS.

Mastadenovirus one of the two genera in the family ADENOVIRIDAE, the members of which infect mammals.

mastatrophy atrophy of the mammary gland.

mastectomy surgical removal of mammary gland tissue. In dogs and cats, usually performed to treat malignant tumors, while in cows, does and ewes it is most used as an amputation of a gangrenous quarter which will otherwise kill the animal.

master superior, overseer.

m. problem list see problem-oriented MEDICAL record.

masterate master's degree.

mastication the act of chewing. Abnormalities of this function commonly occur and often have diagnostic significance. Painful teeth may cause slow, intermittent or one-sided eating. Dropping of the food from the mouth during eating may have a similar cause. Periodic stopping eating for long periods when there is food in the mouth is a common sign in encephalitis and encephalopathy. See also CUD dropping, QUIDDING, TOBACCO-CHEWERS.

masticatory 1. pertaining to mastication. 2. a substance to be chewed, but not swallowed.

m. muscles include the masseter, temporal, pterygoids and digastric muscles.

Mastiff a massive, very large (175–190 lb) muscular dog with very short fawn, silver, apricot or brindle coat. The ears are small and folded over the broad head, the muzzle is blunt and dark colored, and the tail is tapered. Called also Old English mastiff.

French M. see DOGUE DE BORDEAUX.

German M. see GREAT DANE.

Mastigophora a subphylum of protozoa, including all those that have one or more flagella throughout most of their life cycle and a simple, centrally located nucleus; many are parasitic in both invertebrates and vertebrates. Included are the Kinetoplastida (e.g. *Trypanosoma*), Diplomonadina (e.g. *Hexamita*) and Trichomonadida (e.g. *Trichomonas*).

mastigote any member of the subphylum Mastigophora.

mastitic emanating from or pertaining to mastitis.

mastitis inflammation of the mammary gland. Although it may be caused by chemical or physical agents, the causes are almost entirely infectious, and mostly bacterial. Clinical signs vary with the severity of the disease, but include pain, heat and swelling of the affected quarter or half or gland, and abnormality of the milk, either as clots or flakes, and wateriness of the liquid phase. Subclinical mastitis is the most important form and is diagnosed on the basis of bacteriological examination or by indirect tests, principally based on the cell count of the milk. Called also mammitis, garget. See also blue BREAST.

For a summary of the infectious agents which cause mastitis in each of the animal species consult Table 16. See also CALIFORNIA MASTITIS TEST, WISCONSIN MASTITIS TEST.

acute m. acute swelling of the mammary gland accompanied by heat and pain, together with grossly abnormal milk. There may be a slight systemic reaction.

black m. severe, usually peracute clinical mastitis in which one or more quarters become gangrenous. Usually caused by *Staphylococcus aureus*.

botryomycotic m. persistent local infection, usually by *Staphylococcus aureus,* causes granulomas and the collection of pus within them to produce a botryomycotic effect. See also COLIFORM mastitis.

coliform m. caused by *Escherichia coli, Klebsiella* spp. or *Enterobacter aerogenes*. See COLIFORM mastitis.

contagious m. caused by those bacteria which are resident in bovine udders or on teat skin and are spread primarily during milking. *Staphylococcus aureus, Streptococcus agalactiae, S. dysgalactiae* are the common causes. Called also 'cow-associated' mastitis.

m. control aimed at reducing new infection rate and the static quarter infection rate; based on dry period treatment, culling or treating infected animals, teat disinfection, TEAT CUP LINER sanitization, and milking machine maintenance and correct use.

discarding m. milk milk from infected quarters flushed to waste, not fed to calves.

m. dry cow treatment intramammary infusion with a long-acting formulation, at the time of the last milking for the lactation; may be blanket (all cows) or selective (infected quarters only). See also DRY PERIOD treatment.

environmental m. caused by those bacteria which are usually resident in the environment of the cow, especially in the feces, bedding or water. *Escherichia coli, Streptococcus uberis* are the common infections. See also coliform MASTITIS.

gangrenous m. the teat and much of the quarter are black and cold, the secretion is thin blood-stained fluid and there is a severe systemic reaction. The quarter is lost, and the cow may very well die.

granulomatous m. see botryomycotic mastitis (above).

m. infection rate rate of quarters or cows infected with pathogenic bacteria or showing clinical mastitis or, a much more commonly used index nowadays, the percentage of cows with a milk cell count in excess of a stated norm.

NIRD m. control program the basis of all modern mastitis control programs. Named after the National Institute for Research in Dairying (now called the Animal Grassland Research Institute) at Reading, UK, which introduced dry period treatment and teat dipping into mastitis control. Highly effective in reducing the prevalence of contagious mastitis pathogens such as *Streptococcus agalactiae, Staphylococcus aureus*. Called also 'five point program'.

peracute m. as for acute mastitis, but there is also a severe systemic reaction and the cow may die of the attending septicemia.

pyogranulomatous m. a chronic disease in cattle caused by *Nocardia asteroides*, also occurs in sows caused by *Actinomyces suis*.
m. screening testing for evidence of inflammation of mammary epithelium, of individual cows or entire herd, by use of milk cell counts, biochemical tests which measure products of inflammation, e.g. NAG-ase test, electrical conductivity.
subclinical m. mastitis in which the only evidence of disease is an abnormality of cell count or other clinicopathological parameter.
summer m. a serious disease likely to cause the loss of the quarter and a severe clinical illness. Caused by *Actinomyces (Corynebacterium) pyogenes* and other unspecified cocci. See also Table 16.
suppurative m. mastitis in which the secretion of the quarter is largely pus.
m. treatment withholding times after intramammary infusion in lactating cow—withhold 72 hours; dry cow intramammary infusion—administered at least 4 weeks before calving, withhold for 96 hours after calving.
traumatic m. mastitis in which the infection is introduced through the skin into the teat canal or mammary tissue by a penetrating injury; it is usually a mixed infection and causes a suppurative or gangrenous mastitis, depending on the bacteria that are present. The quarter is ruined and the cow may die. See also Table 16.
m. vaccination not proven to exert beneficial effect. Only vaccination with an autogenous bacterin against *Staphylococcus aureus*, where the infecting organism is highly antigenic, appears to even reduce the severity of the disease.

mastitis–metritis–agalactia a syndrome which occurs in sows that have farrowed for 12 to 48 hours; abbreviated MMA. It is manifested by an indeterminate set of signs including anorexia, lethargy, fever, agalactia, swelling of mammary glands, constipation and a marked disinterest in the piglets. There is always a mastitis, most often caused by *Escherichia coli*, but a variety of gram-negative organisms can be involved. Metritis is a rare occurrence. Called also toxemic agalactia, farrowing fever.

masto- word element. [Gr.] *mammary gland.*

mastocyte a mast cell.

mastocytoma see MAST CELL tumor.

mastocytosis an accumulation, local or systemic, of mast cells in the tissues. Occurs in horses of all ages where the lesions disappear spontaneously from the skin but the nodules are present for about a year. See also MAST CELL tumor.
systemic m. see mast cell LEUKEMIA.

mastography radiography of the mammary gland; mammography.

mastology study of the mammary gland.

mastoncus a tumor or swelling of the mammary gland.

masto-occipital pertaining to the mastoid process and occipital bone.

mastoparietal pertaining to the mastoid process and parietal bone.

mastopathy any disease of the mammary gland.

mastopexy surgical fixation of a pendulous mammary gland.

Mastophorus a genus of worms in the family Spirocercidae.
M. muris found in the stomach of a wide range of rodents.

mastoplasia mammoplasia.

mastoplasty mammoplasty.

mastoptosis a pendulous condition of the mammary glands.

mastorrhagia hemorrhage from the mammary gland.

mastoscirrhus hardening of the mammary gland.

mastotomy incision of a mammary gland.

masturbation self-stimulation of the genitals, seen in stallions, and an annoying habit seen in pet dogs which mount inaminate objects or the arms or legs of people.

Masugi nephritis an experimentally produced, immune-mediated nephritis. Called also nephrotoxic nephritis.

MAT microscopic agglutination test.

mat a localized, tight tangle of hairs, often seen in poorly groomed longhaired dogs and cats. They occur most commonly around the ears and on the legs, but in extreme cases, large areas of the body may be encased in a continuous mat.
m. rush see LOMANDRA LONGIFOLIA.
m. spurge EUPHORBIA *drummondii.*

match head toxicity ingestion may lead to poisoning by chlorates, which are nephrotoxic, and potent oxidizing agents, which cause methemoglobinemia.

matched study, matched control a comparison between groups in which each subject animal is matched by a comparable animal in terms of age and all other measurable parameters. Called also matched or paired CONTROL.

matching comparison for the purpose of selecting objects having similar or identical characteristics.
blood m. see cross-matching (below).
control m. see MATCHED STUDY.
cross-m. determination of the compatibility of the blood or tissue of a donor and that of a recipient before transfusion by placing erythrocytes or leukocytes of the donor in the recipient's serum and erythrocytes or leukocytes of the recipient in the donor's serum. Absence of agglutination, hemolysis and cytotoxicity indicates that the two blood or tissue samples belong to the same group and are compatible.

materia pl. *materiae* [L.] material; substance.
m. alba material that accumulates on teeth; it is a conglomeration of salivary protein, desquamated epithelial cells, degenerating leukocytes and bacteria. See also PLAQUE.
m. medica the study of materials used as medicine. It used to be a subject in veterinary curricula and dealt mostly with the physical and chemical characteristics of the medicinal substances. As a science it has now been largely superseded by pharmacology.

maternal pertaining to the female parent.
m. antibodies see maternal ANTIBODY and passive IMMUNITY.
m. bond see DAM–offspring bond.
m. effect the transitory influence of the mother on the phenotype of her offspring, caused by factors such as milk yield and uterine environment.
m. neglect failure of the dam to stay with the neonate, failure to groom it, help it to feed, find it if separated. The extreme degree is desertion. Characteristic of some breeds, e.g. merino ewes. See also MISMOTHERING.
m. nutritional status body condition of a dam, pregnant or with a neonate at foot; important management feature as insurance for the survival of the offspring.
m. obstetric paralysis a common abnormality after a difficult calving, especially in a heifer. It is caused by pressure on peripheral nerves, and manifests itself as weakness, paresthesia in one hindleg, or difficulty or inability to rise. The ligaments, joints and muscles are normal. See also OBTURATOR paralysis.

m. pelvic inlet the size of the aperture leading from the peritoneal to the pelvic cavity.

maternity motherhood and the establishment of the maternal–neonatal bond.

m. pen accommodation provided to encourage the establishment of the maternal–neonatal bond, to maximize the chances of survival of both and the return to a breeding status for the dam, and a good start for the growth period in the young animal. Includes maternity box stall, maternity barn.

Mathevotaenia a genus of cestodes in the family Linstowiidae. Includes *M. oklahomensis*, *M. pedunculata*, *M. wallacei* in raccoons and skunks.

Mathieu needle holder the conventional needle driver with a scissor action but with palm-held handles that spring open when the ratchet is activated. The face of the blades is grooved to avoid the needle slipping.

Mathieu retractor a surgical instrument with three prongs at one end and a right-angled bent at the other, used to retract tissues.

mating sexual union by vagina between male and female. Called also breeding, covering, joining, serving.

m. ability see SERVING CAPACITY TEST.

artificial m. see ARTIFICIAL INSEMINATION.

m. behavior in the female consists mostly of evading male advances while in proestrus and until she is in estrus when she stands quietly and copulation occurs. In males early attempts at mating occur during the females' proestrus; copulation behavior is very variable between species but generally consists of seeking, intromission, thrusting and a period of ejaculation which is very brief in ruminants, brief in horses, prolonged in pigs and very prolonged due to the development of the copulatory tie in dogs. Mating behavior in cats is the most demonstrative of all the species; the queen actively seeks the tom; copulation is very quick and characterized by the tom grasping the queen's neck nape with his teeth. During the queen's estrus period copulation usually occurs many times.

double m. putting the female to the male twice at an interval of some hours or days to optimize the chances of conception.

m. failure incomplete mating for any one of several causes and at any one of the several stages of the mating act.

hand m. mating in which the female is detected to be in estrus and is then handheld while she is mated or is let into a paddock or pen with a male, where she is the only female. Mating is observed and can be guaranteed to have occurred.

m. harness hobbles and sidelines are often used on mares to prevent them from kicking the stallion.

paddock m. males and females are allowed to run uncontrolled at pasture. The percentage of males to females varies between 1% and 5% in sheep and cattle.

pen m. see hand mating (above).

seasonal m. the males are put in with the females only at particular times of the year in order to match good feed supplies with the arrival of lambs or with a need for maximum ovulation and fertilization.

m. tie see COPULATORY tie.

Matricaria nigellifolia South African plant in the family Asteraceae; unidentified toxin causes hepatic encephalopathy in cattle, manifested by syndrome called stootsiekte including incoordination, compulsive walking, convulsions and apparent blindness. Called also staggers weed.

matrimony vine see LYCIUM HALIMIFOLIUM.

matrix pl. *matrices* [L.] 1. the intercellular substance of a tissue, such as bone matrix. 2. the tissue from which a structure develops, such as hair or nail matrix. 3. a rectangular arrangement of quantities or symbols.

bone m. (1) see BONE matrix.

cartilage m. (1) the intercellular substance of cartilage, consisting of cells and extracellular fibers embedded in an amorphous ground substance.

claw m. (2) the claw bed. Called also matrix unguis.

correlation m. (3) a square table giving a correlation between each pair of a set of variables. The diagonal elements give the correlation of a variable with itself, namely 1.

covariance m. similar to the correlation matrix but gives the variances and covariances.

m. Gla protein part of the organic phase of bones; found tightly bound to the bone morphogenetic protein of Urist.

transition m. (3) a table of values used in a MARKOV CHAIN mathematical model, giving the probability of a transition from one state to another in a specified time interval.

m. unguis see claw matrix (above).

MATSA Marek's tumor-specific ANTIGEN.

Matson elevator a handheld instrument with a tool at each end. At one end is a two-pronged rib lifter, at right angles to the handle. At the other end is a curved elongated periosteal stripper.

matter 1. physical material having form and weight under ordinary conditions of gravity. 2. pus.

gray m. matter of the central nervous system, which represents the aggregations of the nerve cells.

white m. matter of the central nervous system, which comprises the axons of the nerve cells.

mattress suture pattern a surgical suturing procedure. The needle goes into the skin, across the incison and out through the skin on the other side; then a bite parallel to the incision and on top of the skin; then back through the skin, across the wound and out to the surface again. It is tied to the end of the suture if the pattern is to be an interrupted one. It may be interrupted or continuous, vertical or horizontal, and direct or crossed. The interrupted horizontal pattern is called also the automatic ridge suture, the four-stitch interrupted suture and the U-suture.

maturation 1. the stage or process of attaining maximal development. In biology, a process of cell division during which the number of chromosomes in the germ cell is reduced to one-half the number characteristic of the species. 2. the formation of pus.

m. arrest an interruption in the progressive development of erythrocytes, characterized by a bone marrow dominated by macrocytes and megaloblasts. Seen in anemias caused by deficiency of folic acid and vitamin B_{12}.

maverick an unbranded calf whose ownership is in doubt.

maw worm OXYURIS *equi*.

Max Joseph spaces subepidermal clefts formed by acantholysis or hydropic degeneration of basal cells.

Maxam–Gilbert method used in DNA sequencing; four samples of end-labeled DNA restriction fragments are chemically cleaved at different specific nucleotides. The resulting subfragments are separated by gel electrophoresis, and the labeled fragments are detected by autoradiography. The sequence of the original end-labeled restriction fragment can be determined directly from parallel electropherograms of the four samples.

maxilla pl. *maxillae, maxillas* [L.] one of two identical bones that form the upper jaw. The maxillae meet in the midline of the face and often are considered as one bone. Together the maxillae form the floor of the orbit for each eye, the sides and lower walls of the nasal cavities, and the hard palate. The lower border of the maxilla supports the upper teeth. In most species, each maxilla contains an air space called the maxillary sinus.

maxillary emanating from or pertaining to the maxilla.

m. collapse includes failure of the maxilla to grow, as in achondroplastic dwarfism, or atrophy due to turbinate atrophy, as in atrophic rhinitis. The result is a dishing or depression of the face.

m. cyst a cyst that occurs in young horses and causes sufficient distortion of the bone as to obstruct the nasal passage.

m. myositis a localized myositis of unknown origin which occurs in young horses. It causes inability to eat or to suck the mare. The muscles of the cheeks are hard.

m. process an embryonic fold which develops from the first visceral arch and expands to produce the rostral bones of the upper jaw.

m. sinusitis infection in the maxillary sinus, often from an infected tooth. Causes local facial swelling and nasal discharge. See also MALAR abscess.

m. swelling a unilateral swelling which is usually an indication of an osteomyelitis, as in ACTINOMYCOSIS of cattle, tooth-root abscess of dogs or sinusitis in horses. Bilateral swellings are characteristic of osteodystrophia fibrosa in dogs and horses.

maxillectomy surgical removal of the maxilla.

maxilloethmoidectomy excision of the portion of the maxilla surrounding the maxillary sinus and of the cribriform plate and anterior ethmoid cells.

maxillofacial pertaining to the maxilla and the face.

maxillomandibular pertaining to the upper and lower jaws.

maxillotomy surgical sectioning of the maxilla which allows movement of all or part of the maxilla into the desired position.

maximum the greatest quantity, effect or value possible or achieved under given circumstances.

m. permissible dose see DOSE equivalent limits.

tubular m. the highest rate in milligrams per minute at which the renal tubules can transfer artificially administered test substances; the maximal tubular excretory capacity. Abbreviated T_m.

mayapple see PODOPHYLLUM PELTATUM.

Mayer waves waves in arterial blood pressure; brought about by oscillations in baroreceptor and chemoreceptor reflex control systems.

Mayne's pest see VERBENA *tenuisecta*.

Mayo–Hegar needle holder lightweight needle driver with finger holes at the end of ratcheted handles and blades with cross-hatched faces.

Mayo scissors heavy-duty surgical sissors with narrowed but blunt pointed blades, which may be straight or curved.

mayweed see ANTHEMIS COTULA.

maze a complicated system of intersecting paths used in intelligence tests and in demonstrating learning in experimental animals.

Mazzotti reaction a skin reaction that occurs in humans when the microfilariae of *Onchocerca volvulus* in cutaneous sites are killed by the administration of diethylcarbamazine.

MBC minimal bactericidal concentration. See MINIMAL lethal concentration.

MBD methylene blue dye binding test. See SABIN–FELDMANN DYE TEST.

MBD test methylene blue dye test.

MbO_2 oxymyoglobin.

MBV mixed bacterial vaccine.

Mc- for words beginning thus see under *Mac-*.

MCC milk cell count.

MCF malignant catarrhal fever. See BOVINE malignant catarrh.

mcg microgram.

MCH mean corpuscular hemoglobin, an expression of the average hemoglobin content of a single cell in picograms, obtained by multiplying the hemoglobin in grams by 10 and dividing by the number of erythrocytes (in millions).

MCHC mean corpuscular hemoglobin concentration, an expression of the average percentage hemoglobin concentration obtained by multiplying the hemoglobin in grams by 100 and dividing by the hematocrit determination.

mCi millicurie; a non-SI unit now replaced by the BECQUEREL.

μCi microcurie; a non-SI unit now replaced by the BECQUEREL.

MCPA, MCP 2-methyl-4-chlorophenoxyacetic acid; a weedkiller reported to be nontoxic at the levels likely to be encountered on pasture, though it has killed cattle dosed experimentally with large single doses.

MCT 1. mean circulation time. 2. medium-chain triglyceride.

MCT oil see medium-chain TRIGLYCERIDE.

MCV 1. mean corpuscular volume, an expression of the average volume of individual red cells in cubic microns, obtained by multiplying the hematocrit determination by 10 and dividing by the number of erythrocytes (in millions). 2. mean clinical value, obtained by assigning a numerical value to the response noted in a number of patients receiving a specific treatment, adding these numbers and dividing by the number of patients treated. 3. minute canine virus.

Md chemical symbol, *mendelevium*.

MDF myocardial depressant factor.

MDV mucosal disease virus.

ME metabolizable energy.

M:E ratio myeloid:erythroid ratio.

meadow grassland, used for grazing and/or haying.

m. rue see THALICTRUM.

m. buttercup RANUNCULUS *acris*.

m. crowfoot RANUNCULUS *acris*.

m. saffron COLCHIUM *autumnale*.

m. sweet AMMI *majus*.

meal 1. a portion of food or foods taken at some particular, and usually stated or fixed, time. 2. a ground feed which may be a plain cereal, e.g. barley meal, or a ground up cake which is a residue from oil extraction, e.g. linseed meal. It has an undefined particle size greater than that of flour.

m. pattern feeding pattern which may be imposed by humans or be a natural behavior pattern in the species.

mealworm see ALPHITOBIUS DIAPERINUS.

yellow m. see TENEBRIO MOLITOR.

mean an average; a numerical value intermediate between two extremes. Called also arithmetic mean.

m. arterial pressure average pressure in artery for one heartbeat.

m. cell constants see ERYTHROCYTE indices.

m. corpuscular hemoglobin (MCH) see MCH.

m. corpuscular hemoglobin concentration (MCHC) see MCHC.

m. corpuscular volume (MCV) see MCV.

m. deviation the average value of a set of absolute deviations from the mean of a set of observations.

m. electrical axis (MEA) in electrocardiography, a calculation based on the relative amplitude of Q, R and S waves in the three bipolar limb leads. It is an aid to recognizing right ventricular enlargement and various intraventricular conduction defects.

geometric m. the antilog of the mean of the logarithm of the calculated values, the same as the nth root of the product of the values. It is often a more useful mean for growth curves.

harmonic m. the reciprocal of the arithmetic mean of values converted to their reciprocals (used in dealing with skewed data).

rolling m. see moving AVERAGE.

measles 1. a highly contagious disease of humans characterized by a maculopapular skin rash and caused by a morbillivirus; called also rubeola. 2. a term used in veterinary science to identify animal diseases that have a speckled appearance thought to resemble the skin rash of measles in humans. The resemblance in most diseases is superficial and highly speculative.

beef m. see CYSTICERCUS *bovis*.

pork m. see CYSTICERCUS *cellulosae*.

sheep m. see CYSTICERCUS *ovis*.

m. vaccine a preparation containing attenuated human measles virus that is used to immunize dogs against canine distemper virus, based on the close antigenic relationship between the two viruses. It is only administered to young puppies, in which the persistence of maternal antibodies against canine distemper virus is likely to interfere with an immune response to canine distemper vaccine. It must always be followed by the administration of canine distemper vaccine by 4 months of age.

measly said of beef, pork and mutton because infected meat has a speckled appearance thought to resemble MEASLES (1) in humans. See also CYSTICERCUS.

measurement ascertaining a dimension by the physical act of measurement.

discretizing m. see DISCRETIZING MEASUREMENTS.

meat 1. flesh and other tissues of farm animals for human consumption. 2. the edible parts of nuts or fruit seeds. Called also kernels.

m. and bone meal meat meal that contains more than 4.4% phosphorus because bones have been included; used as a protein feed supplement.

conditionally admissible m. see FREIBANK SYSTEM.

m. inspection examination of all meat sold for human consumption to ensure that it is wholesome and free from any disease that might be communicated from the animals to humans. Includes antemortem examination of the living animal, examination of the carcass, the head and the viscera.

m. intoxication hepatic encephalopathy.

knackers' m. meat from animals dead on arrival or of insufficient quality to go into the human food chain; killed at a separate establishment. It is not always possible to keep this meat separate from butcher's meat—illegal substitutions are serious offenses but the rewards are high.

m. meal a by-product of meat-packing or abattoir industries containing about 50% protein but varying depending on the material included and whether preparation is by a wet-cooking or tankage process, or a dry-cooking method. A popular protein supplement for all classes of livestock. Use for food-producing animals now restricted because of the risk of transmitting the agents causing spongiform encephalopathies.

mechanically recovered m. meat harvested by putting a carcass through an industrial process to separate it from the bones, instead of carving it off by hand knife.

m. packing plant abattoir.

meatorrhaphy suture of the cut end of the urethra to the glans penis after incision for enlarging the urinary meatus.

meatoscopy visual examination of any meatus, especially the urinary meatus or the ureteral orifices.

meatotomy incision of the urinary meatus in order to enlarge it.

meatus pl. *meatus* [L.] an opening or passage.

acoustic m., m. acusticus, m. auditorius, auditory m. a passage in the ear; see external acoustic meatus and internal acoustic meatus (below).

external acoustic m. the passageway within the ear between the ear flap and the eardrum.

internal acoustic m. the passageway on the medial surface of the petrous temporal bone; transmits the facial and vestibulocochlear nerves.

ethmoidal m. the spaces between the ethmoturbinal bones.

m. nasi, m. of nose one of the three main airways of the nasal cavity which are found on either side of the septum; they are the dorsal, middle and ventral meati.

nasopharyngeal m. the common space shared by the right and left nasal cavities just before they enter the nasopharynx.

m. urinarius, urinary m. the opening of the urethra on the body surface through which urine is discharged.

mebendazole a broad-spectrum anthelmintic efficient against all gastrointestinal nematodes, lungworms and *Moniezia* in ruminants. It is not effective against *Trichuris* spp. and has reduced activity against benzimidazole-resistant worm species. It is not very effective against larval forms of *Taenia* spp., not effective against *Draschia* or *Habronema* spp. in horses, nor against *Trichostrongylus axei.* It is effective against *Strongylus* spp., but not against migrating *Strongylus vulgaris* larvae nor against *Trichostrongylus axei, Strongyloides* spp. or *Anoplocephala perfoliata.* It is recommended for general use in horses and combined with metriphonate for use against bot fly larvae. It is useful in dogs but does not remove *Echinococcus granulosus* or *Dipylidium caninum.* The drug has very low toxicity but has caused severe acute hepatic necrosis in some dogs.

mechanical extraction exposure to heat and pressure as a means of extracting oil from seeds. See also SOLVENT extraction of oil seeds.

mechanical milking see MILKING MACHINE.

mechanics the science dealing with the motions of material bodies.

body m. the application of kinesiology to the use of the body in normal activities.

mechanism 1. a machine or machine-like structure. 2. the manner of combination of parts, processes, etc., which subserve a common function.

mechanobullous disease see EPIDERMOLYSIS bullosa.

mechanoreceptor a nerve-ending sensitive to mechanical pressures or distortions, such as those responding to touch and muscle contractions.

cutaneous m. touch, pain, temperature, pressure receptors are defined in human skin; also some touch sensors which are stimulated only by firm pressure over a long period.

mechanotherapy use of mechanical apparatus in treatment of disease or its results, especially in therapeutic exercises.

mechloretham see MUSTINE HYDROCHLORIDE.
mechlorethamine see MUSTINE HYDROCHLORIDE.
mecillinam see AMDINOCILLIN.
Mecistocirrus a genus of worms in the family Trichostrongylidae.
M. digitatus found in the abomasum of domestic ruminants and buffalo, and in the stomach of pigs. In endemic areas it is an important parasite, causing effects similar to those of *Haemonchus* spp.
Meckel named after J.F. Meckel Jr, a German anatomist.
M's cartilage ventral cartilage of the first branchial arch.
M's diverticulum a congenital sac or appendage occasionally found in the ileum; a relic of a fetal structure that connects the yolk sac with the intestinal cavity of the embryo. In horses persistence of this structure has caused acute intestinal obstruction by creating a torsion of the ileum.
meclizine a centrally acting antiemetic used as the hydrochloride to control motion sickness.
meclocycline a tetracycline antibiotic derived from oxytetracycline; used topically.
meclofenamate a nonsteroidal anti-inflammatory agent with analgesic and antipyretic activity; used as the sodium salt for treatment of arthritis and osteoarthritis, mainly in horses and cattle.
meclofenamic acid has the same properties as meclofenamate but is not as soluble and has to be used orally.
meconium yellow-orange mucilaginous material in the intestine of the full-term fetus; it constitutes the first stools passed by the newborn.
m. aspiration aspiration of fragments of meconium into the pulmonary airways occurs in the fetus in the terminal stages of many infections.
m. ileus intestinal obstruction in the newborn due to the blocking of the bowels with thick meconium. This is an important disease of newborn colt foals. The syndrome is usually one of subacute abdominal pain, restlessness and straining, and a positive finding on rectal examination. Occasional cases show severe pain and tympany of the large intestine. Called also meconium retention.
m. retention see meconium ileus (above). See also impaction COLIC.
MED minimal effective dose; minimal erythema dose.
medehas one of the unusual fish that carries its fertilized eggs in a membranous sac attached to the abdomen. Called also *Oryzias latipes*, Japanese killifish.
medetomidine a potent α_2 adrenoreceptor agonist used widely as a sedative, hypnotic and analgesic. Used in combination with ketamine in wild animals where it provides good immobilization and can be reversed with α_2 antagonists.
medi- prefix meaning middle.
media [L.] 1. plural of *medium.* 2. middle, especially the middle coat of a blood vessel, or tunica media. 3. materials used as substrates on which to culture microbiological agents. See also BROTH.
medial pertaining to or situated toward the midline.
m. nasal process one of the frontal processes derived from frontonasal mesenchyme and forming part of the border of the nasal pits, the future nostrils.
m. palatine process see PALATINE process.
m. patellar ligament in the species in which the tendon is trifurcated (horse, cattle), the largest and most medial of the three patellar ligaments.
medialis [L.] *medial.*
median 1. situated in the median plane or in the midline of a body or structure. 2. the perpendicular line that divides the area of a frequency curve into two equal halves.
m. calving date the number of days between the first calving in the herd and the 50th percentile calving; an excellent measure of fertility status of seasonally calving herds; in dairy herds the target is 18 days.
m. eminence part of the hypophysis.
m. nerve see Table 14.
m. nerve block the anesthetic agent is injected on the medial aspect of the forelimb, just distal to the elbow. An area encircling most of the fetlock and pastern is desensitized.
m. nerve injury results in overextension and dropping of the carpus.
mediastinal of or pertaining to the mediastinum.
m. abscess an abscess that causes systemic signs of toxemia and fever but also severe pain with each inspiration, causing grunting as in pleurisy but without the auscultatory findings of pleurisy.
m. cyst remnants of branchial pouches may be found in the anterior mediastinum, particularly in brachycephalic dogs; bronchogenic cysts are found in the posterior mediastinum.
m. emphysema see PNEUMOMEDIASTINUM.
m. flutter movement of the tissues and organs of the mediastinum back and forth with each movement of air in and out of an open sucking wound in the thoracic cavity. The condition can produce serious impairment of cardiopulmonary function and is fatal if not treated promptly. Signs are similar to those of mediastinal shift (see below).
m. lymph node enlargement a condition due to abscess formation or neoplastic growth which may cause obstruction to the esophagus and dysphagia, or to the bronchi, causing inspiratory dyspnea. If it is in the anterior chest and of considerable size, it may mimic congestive heart failure, with jugular vein engorgement and edema of the brisket.
m. neoplasm characterized by progressive weight loss, reduced exercise tolerance, dyspnea, hydrothorax, areas of dullness on auscultation or percussion over lungs, neoplastic cells in pleural fluid if lesion intrudes into pleural cavity.
m. shift a shifting or moving of the tissues and organs that comprise the mediastinum (heart, great vessels, trachea and esophagus) to one side of the chest cavity. The condition occurs when a severe injury to the chest causes the entrapment of air in the pleural space (tension PNEUMOTHORAX). As the volume of air increases on the affected side, the lung collapses and the organs and tissues of the mediastinum are crowded to the opposite side of the chest. This can produce compression of the other lung and kinking or twisting of one or more of the great blood vessels, which in turn seriously impairs blood flow to and from the heart.
m. testis a partial septum of the testis that contains the rete testis.
mediastinitis inflammation of the mediastinum.
mediastinography radiography of the structures of the mediastinum.
mediastinopericarditis inflammation of the mediastinum and pericardium.
mediastinoscope a specially designed endoscope used in mediastinoscopy.
mediastinoscopy examination of the mediastinum by means of an endoscope inserted through an anterior midline incision just above the thoracic inlet.
mediastinotomy incision of the mediastinum.

mediastinum pl. *mediastina* [L.] 1. a median septum or partition. 2. the mass of tissues and organs separating the two lungs, between the sternum ventrally and the vertebral column dorsally, containing the heart and its large vessels, trachea, esophagus, thymus, lymph nodes, and other structures and tissues. In the horse, the caudal part of the mediastinum is usually fenestrated and the two pleural cavities communicate with each other through it.

MEDIC minimum essential drug information checklist.

medicable subject to treatment with medicine with reasonable expectation of cure.

Medicago plant genus of the legume family Fabaceae; contains coumestans, the phytoestrogens, in certain circumstances, and cause hyperestrogenism; can also cause photosensitivity possibly through steroidal saponins; causative plants include *M. littoralis*, *M. minima* (burr medic), *M. polymorpha* (*M. denticulata*, *M. hispida*, burr medic or trefoil), *M. sativa* (lucerne, alfalfa), also a common cause of primary frothy bloat, *M. trombiculata* (barrel clover), *M. truncatula* (barrel medic).

medical 1. pertaining to or emanating from the study or discipline of medicine, in the context of veterinary science in veterinary medicine. 2. a class of diseases that are traditionally treated by medicines rather than by surgery.

m. ecology study of the environment and its relationship to a population of animals with respect to the effect of the environment on the diseases of the animals.

problem-oriented m. record a standardized format for keeping clinical records in a problem-oriented case management system. An early decision is made on what is the nature of the patient's problem or problems and from then on the patient's status with respect to each problem is assessed daily. This has the undeniable advantage that the clinician does not lose sight of the objective with respect to the individual patient. Without this approach there is always an inclination for the clinician to attack the disease and place the patient on a lower priority. The attitude adopted as a result of this approach is very similar to the herd health approach in herd medicine—the objective is the farmer's survival, not the eradication of some bacteria.

m. records the detailed records, made at the time, of the clinical, clinical pathology and pathology examinations and treatments of each patient, or patient group. The records have importance to the welfare of the patient, and to potential medical research and legal investigations, and to be worth their full value they must be made contemporaneously.

m. technologist a qualified worker in a paramedical field such as laboratory scientist, veterinary nurse or livestock inspector.

medicament a medicinal agent.

medicated contains a medicinal substance.

m. feed feed containing medicines for the purpose of treating or controlling disease in animals.

medication 1. administration of remedies. 2. a medicinal agent. 3. impregnation with a medicine.

m. delivery the routes used in medication. See DRUG administration.

mass m. the medicament may be administered in the drinking water or in the feed. Mixing with the feed is limited to prophylactic dosing because sick animals rarely eat their feed in adequate amounts. Sick animals are more inclined to keep up their water intake, but still need to be observed to ensure that they are doing this. Animals suspected of not drinking must be treated individually. Special techniques of mass treatment include the laying of palatable baits for wildlife, although this is limited to once-only medications, such as oral vaccines, and aerosol administration, limited to closely confined groups such as chickens.

teratogenic m. teratogenous effects produced by medication; known agents include methallibure, griseofulvin, cyclophosphamide, folic acid antagonists, parbendazole, corticosteroids, phenytoin, thalidomide, hydroxyzine, metrifonate, hydroxyurea.

m. tube 1. a short esophageal tube used in sheep, perorally, and horses, pernasally, for the administration of medicines. 2. an in situ tube used for the treatment of the eye in horses. See also subpalpebral LAVAGE.

medication pneumonia see lipid PNEUMONIA.

medicinal having healing qualities; pertaining to a medicine.

medicine 1. any drug or remedy. 2. the nonsurgical treatment of disease.

food animal m. the veterinary medicine of the domesticated farm animals, including cattle, sheep, goats, pigs, poultry and, with some flexibility, horses, that are used for and in the production of human food and of fiber used in human raiment. It includes the increasingly important segment of preventive and herd/flock medicine.

nuclear m. that branch of veterinary medicine devoted to the use of radionuclides in the diagnosis and treatment of animal diseases.

veterinary m. the science and art of diagnosis, treatment and prevention of the diseases of animals, and the maintenance of normal health. This classic definition is now expanded in many areas to include the promotion of financially optimal production. It consists mostly of prevention of wastage caused by disease, but also includes inputs from nutrition, genetics, housing, and other management disciplines. See also VETERINARY MEDICINE.

medicolegal pertaining to medicine and law, or to forensic medicine. See forensic VETERINARY MEDICINE.

medina worm see DRACUNCULUS *medinensis*.

medionecrosis focal areas of destruction of the elastic tissue and smooth muscle of the tunica media of a blood vessel, especially of the aorta or its major branches.

mediotarsal pertaining to the center of the tarsus.

Mediterranean named after the Mediterranean Sea or region.

M. coast fever see THEILERIA *annulata* infection in cattle.

M. fever see MALTA FEVER.

M. lymphoma a human disease resembling plasmacytoid lymphoma in horses.

M. squill URGINEA *maritima*.

medium pl. *media, mediums* [L.] 1. an agent by which something is accomplished or an impulse is transmitted. 2. a substance providing the proper nutritional environment for the growth of microorganisms; called also culture medium.

basic nutritive m. one adequate for the growth requirements of most bacteria.

contrast m. a radiopaque (positive) substance, or (negative) gases used in radiography to permit visualization of body structures.

culture m. a substance used to support the growth of microorganisms or other cells.

dioptric m. refracting medium (see below).

disperse m., dispersion m. the continuous phase of

a colloid system; the medium in which a colloid is dispersed, corresponding to the solvent in a true solution.
enriched m. modification of a basic medium for the growth of fastidious bacteria. Common additions are blood, serum or egg yolk.
indicator m. a type of bacteriological medium which may contain a fermentable sugar plus a pH indicator that gives a color change. It is used to identify bacteria on the basis of a characteristic biochemical reaction.
refracting m. the transparent tissues and fluid in the eye through which light rays pass and by which they are refracted and brought to a focus on the retina.
m. sausage a technique for examining meat for bacterial contamination. The solid medium is made up in the form of a sausage and slices are removed from it after application of the exposed end to the suspect meat.
selective m. formulated to facilitate the isolation of specific bacteria, they contain substances to inhibit growth of others.
transport m. formulated to preserve a specimen, usually tissue or microbiological swab, and minimize bacterial overgrowth for the time necessary to transport it to the laboratory.

medius [L.] *situated in the middle.*

medlar body see CHROMO BODY.

MEDLARS acronym for *Med*ical *L*iterature *A*nalysis and *R*etrieval *S*ystem, a computerized bibliographic system of the National Library of Medicine (USA), from which the Index Medicus is produced.

MEDLINE acronym for *MED*LARS on-*line*, a computerized bibliographical retrieval system, an on-line segment of MEDLARS.

medroxyprogesterone acetate a synthetic progestogen used for estrus control and the treatment of behavioral problems in dogs and cats; abbreviated MPA.

medrysone a synthetic glucocorticoid used in the treatment of inflammatory and allergic conditions of the conjunctiva; applied topically.

medulla pl. *medullae* [L.] the central or inner portion of an organ.
adrenal m. the inner portion of the ADRENAL GLAND, where epinephrine is produced.
m. of bone BONE MARROW, contained in the medullary canal of bone.
m. oblongata that part of the hindbrain continuous with the pons anteriorly and the spinal cord posteriorly; it houses nerve centers for both motor and sensory nerves, where such functions as breathing and the beating of the heart are controlled. Called also myelencephalon. In animals the principal clinical manifestations of local lesions in the medulla are those of head rotation and circling, and facial and tongue paralysis with resulting difficulty in prehension and swallowing. With diffuse lesions spastic paralysis or a stiff-legged incoordination occurs.
m. ossium bone marrow.
renal m. the inner part of the substance of the kidney, composed chiefly of collecting tubules, and in some species organized into a group of structures called the renal pyramids.
spinal m., m. spinalis spinal cord.
m. of thymus the central portion of each lobule of the thymus; it contains many more reticular cells and far fewer lymphocytes than does the surrounding cortex.

medullary emanating from or pertaining to a medulla. Used most frequently in relation to diseases of glands, e.g. thyroids, or gland-like structures, e.g. lymph nodes.
m. cavity cavity of the bone marrow.
m. cord cords of tissue in lymph nodes; may be hyperplastic in cases of chronic localized disease.
m. reticular formation the part of the medulla oblongata which controls the trigeminal, facial, vagal and hypoglossal nerve nuclei.
m. sinus part of the flow system for lymph through lymph nodes; drain into efferent lymphatic vessels at the node hilus.

medullated 1. said of nerve fibers; means myelinated, equipped with myelin sheaths. 2. said of hair; means having a core of air-filled cells. If the medulla is coarse, the fiber is hairy and has irregular dyeing properties. It is a blemish in a wool fiber.

medullization the enlargement of the haversian canals in rarefying osteitis, followed by their conversion into marrow channels; also the replacement of bone by marrow cells.

medulloadrenal pertaining to the adrenal medulla.

medulloblast an undifferentiated cell of the neural tube that may develop into either a neuroblast or spongioblast.

medulloblastoma a brain tumor composed of medulloblasts.

medulloepithelioma a brain tumor composed of primitive neuroepithelial cells lining the tubular spaces.

medusa jellyfish; a colony of animals comprising a bell from which hang a number of filaments and tentacles. Called also hydromedusa. Inflict painful stings and can cause death, even of humans. See also HYDROZOA.
m. head colonies colonies of *Bacillus anthracis* on agar have this appearance of being domes with a fringe of filaments.

meerkat species of mongoose. Called also *Suricata suricatta.*

mefenamic acid a nonsteroidal anti-inflammatory agent with analgesic and antipyretic activity, used for relief of mild to moderate pain.

MEFR maximal expiratory flow rate.

mega- word element. [Gr.] *large;* used in naming units of measurement to designate an amount 10^6 (one million) times the size of the unit to which it is joined, e.g. megacuries (10^6 curies); abbreviation M.

Megabacteria an organism of uncertain taxonomic status which causes megabacteriosis in caged birds.

megabacteriosis a disease of caged birds, caused by *Megabacteria*, which is characterized by inflammation of the proventriculus with vomiting and diarrhea.

megabladder permanent overdistension of the bladder.

megabyte one million bytes (approximately 1 million characters = 1000 KB).

megacalorie 1000 kilocalories; a therm.

megacalycosis nonobstructive dilatation of the renal calices due to malformation of the renal papillae.

megacaryocyte megakaryocyte.

megacolon dilatation and hypertrophy of the colon.
acquired m. colonic enlargement associated with chronic constipation, but with normal ganglion cell innervation. Most common in dogs and cats, the usual causes are dietary factors, lack of exercise, prostatic enlargement, anal disease and neurological deficits.
aganglionic m. due to congenital absence of myenteric ganglion cells and abnormal motor activity in a distal segment of the large bowel. There is continuous spasm in the aganglionic segment that causes a

stenosis, and a massive distension of the normal proximal colon develops secondarily. The disease in humans is called Hirschsprung's disease and a similar, but not identical, condition occurs in piebald mice and Overo horses. Congenital megacolon may occur in dogs and cats, but acquired disease is much more common. Called also congenital megacolon.

congenital m. see aganglionic megacolon (above).

idiopathic m. recurrent episodes of constipation in aging cats over a long period of time is believed to lead to the progressive development of a dilated colon.

inherited m. is presumed in fattening pigs in which there is abdominal distension and wasting without rectal stricture.

psychogenic m. seen in cats and dogs that will not defecate indoors. Prolonged fecal retention causes loss of the defecation reflex, especially in aged patients.

Megadyptes see PENGUIN.

megaesophagus chronic dilatation and atony of the body of the esophagus, usually associated with asynchronous function of the esophagus and the caudal esophageal sphincter. It occurs sporadically in cattle, horses and cats, but is most common in dogs. It is usually a congenital condition, causing accumulation of food and saliva and regurgitation and aspiration pneumonia from an early age but may also be secondary to systemic disease, particularly general neuromuscular disorders such as myesthenia gravis. An inherited basis is suspected in dogs. Vascular ring anomaly and a defective local neuromuscular plexus are listed pathogeneses.

megahertz one million (10^6) hertz; abbreviated MHz.

megajoule 1 million joules.

megakaryoblast the earliest cytologically identifiable precursor in the thrombocytic series, which matures to form the promegakaryocyte.

megakaryoblastic characterized by the presence of megakaryoblasts.

megakaryocyte the giant cell of bone marrow; it is a large cell with a greatly lobulated nucleus and gives rise to blood platelets.

megakaryocytic characterized by the presence of large numbers of megakaryocytes.

m. hypoplasia depressed thrombopoiesis; a common cause of thrombocytopenia.

m. leukemia, m. myelosis see megakaryocytic LEUKEMIA.

megakaryocytopoiesis the production of megakaryocytes.

megakaryocytosis the presence of megakaryocytes in the blood or of excessive numbers in the bone marrow.

megakaryophthisis deficiency of megakaryocytes in bone marrow.

megakaryopoiesis megakaryocytopoiesis.

megalencephaly macrencephalia; hypertrophy of the brain.

megalgia a severe pain.

megal(o)- word element. [Gr.] *large, abnormal enlargement.*

megaloblast a large, nucleated immature progenitor of an abnormal erythrocytic series; megaloblasts are present in the blood in certain anemias. These changes reflect asynchronism in maturation between cytoplasm and nucleus. Observed in folic acid responsive anemias.

megaloblastic pertaining to or emanating from a megaloblast.

megaloblastoid resembling a megaloblast.

megalocardia cardiomegaly; enlargement of the heart.

megalocephaly abnormally increased size of the head.

megalocornea an enlarged cornea on an otherwise normal globe.

megalocystis an abnormally enlarged bladder.

megalocyte an extremely large erythrocyte.

megalocytosis strictly speaking, MACROCYTHEMIA. The term is also used in relation to hepatic, renal and pulmonary disease where there is gross enlargement of hepatocytes, tubular epithelium and pulmonary epithelium.

megalodactyly excessive size of the digits.

megaloenteron enlargement of the intestine.

megalo-esophagus megaesophagus.

megalogastria enlargement of the stomach.

megaloglobus enlargement of the eyeball; sequel to glaucoma in species with thin sclera, e.g. cats.

megaloglossia macroglossia; hypertrophy of the tongue.

megalohepatia enlargement of the liver; hepatomegaly.

megaloileitis a disease of unknown etiology in young laboratory rats and characterized by distension of the abdomen, segmental distension of the ileum and a mortality rate of 50%.

megalomelia abnormal largeness of the limbs.

megalonychosis hypertrophy of the claws and their matrices.

megalopenis abnormal largeness of the penis.

megalophthalmos abnormally large size of the eyes; buphthalmos.

megalopodia abnormal largeness of the extremities of the limbs.

megalosplenia enlargement of the spleen; splenomegaly.

megalosyndactyly a condition in which the digits are large and more or less webbed together.

megaloureter congenital ureteral dilatation without demonstrable cause.

-megaly suffix meaning enlargement.

meganeurites neurons swollen with ganglioside in ganglioside storage disease may store the ganglioside in a swollen compartment between the axonal hillock and the first axonal segment; the swollen section is the meganeurite.

megarectum a greatly dilated rectum.

Megasphaera elsdenii one of the bacterial participants in ruminal digestion.

megathrombocyte an enlarged thrombocyte.

megaureter dilatation of the ureter.

megavolt one million volts.

megestrol acetate a synthetic progestational agent, commonly used for estrus control in dogs and cats and also in the treatment of behavioral abnormalities and a variety of inflammatory skin diseases, including miliary dermatitis and eosinophilic granuloma.

meglumine 1. a crystalline base used in preparing salts of certain acids for use as diagnostic radiopaque media. Meglumine diatrizoate is used in angiocardiography and excretory urography; meglumine iodipamide is used in cholecystography; and meglumine iothalamate is used in cerebral angiography, excretory urography and peripheral arteriography. Called also methylglucamine. 2. meglumine antimonate, a pentavalent antimonial used as an antiprotozoal, a preferred drug in the treatment of leishmaniasis.

Megninia a genus of feather mites in the family Analgesidae. Considered to be nonpathogenic but may cause depluming itch on rare occasions.

M. columbae found on pigeons.
M. cubitalis found on fowl.
M. ginglymura found on fowl.
M. phasiani found on pheasants and peacocks.
M. velata found on ducks.

megohm one million ohms.

megophthalmos abnormally large eyes.

megrims pigeon fanciers' name for salmonellosis caused by *Salmonella typhimurium.*

Mehelya see FILE SNAKE.

Mehlis gland part of the reproductive system of a trematode.

meibomian named after H. Meibom, a German anatomist.
m. adenoma commonest canine peri-ocular neoplasm.
m. cyst see CHALAZION.
m. gland see meibomian GLAND.

meibomianitis inflammation of the meibomian glands. See also CHALAZION, internal HORDEOLUM.

meiogenic promoting meiosis.

meiosis the process of cell division by which reproductive cells (gametes) are formed. There are two successive divisions, meiosis I and meiosis II, in which four daughter cells that have the haploid chromosome number are formed. As in MITOSIS (somatic cell division), meiosis I and II are each divided into four phases: *prophase, metaphase, anaphase* and *telophase.*

meiotic pertaining to meiosis.

Melampyrum arvense European plant of the family Scrophulariaceae, members of which contain cardiac glycosides and are therefore potentially poisonous, causing dyspnea, diarrhea, sudden death. Called also cow wheat.

mélangeur [Fr.] an instrument for drawing and diluting specimens of blood for examination.

melan(o)- word element. [Gr.] *black, melanin.*

melaniferous containing melanin or other black pigment.

melanin a dark, sulfur-containing pigment normally found in the hair, skin, ciliary body, choroid of the eye, pigment layer of the retina, and certain nerve cells. It occurs abnormally in certain tumors, known as melanomas, and is sometimes excreted in the urine when such tumors are present (melanuria).
m. deficiency hypopigmentation, leukoderma, hypomelanosis.
excess m. hyperpigmentation, hypermelanosis, melanism, melanoderma, melanotrichia.
m.-stimulating hormone see MELANOCYTE-stimulating hormone.

melanism excessive deposition of melanin in the skin.

melanoblast a cell that develops into a melanocyte.

melanocyte any of the dendritic clear cells of the epidermis that synthesize tyrosinase and, within their melanosomes, the pigment melanin; the melanosomes are then transferred from melanocytes to keratinocytes.
m.-stimulating hormone (MSH) a peptide from the anterior pituitary which influences the formation or deposition of melanin in the body, especially in amphibians and fish.

melanocytoma see MELANOMA.

melanoderma an abnormally increased amount of melanin in the skin due to either an increase in production of melanin by the melanocytes normally present or to an increase in the number of melanocytes, with production of hyperpigmented patches.

melanodermatitis dermatitis with a deposit of melanin in the skin.

melanoepithelioma see MELANOMA.

melanogen a colorless chromogen, convertible into melanin, which may occur in the urine in certain diseases.

melanogenesis the production of melanin.

melanoglossia blackening and elongation of the papillae of the tongue; black tongue.

melanoid 1. resembling melanin. 2. a substance resembling melanin.

melanoleukoderma a mottled appearance of the skin.

melanoma a tumor arising from melanocytes, dendritic cells of neuroectodermal origin, or melanoblasts. They are most common in the skin, eye and oral cavity of dogs and aged gray horses, but occur occasionally as congenital lesions in pigs, goats and cattle. An inherited, malignant melanoma is recorded in swordtail–platyfish hybrids.
amelanotic m. one containing little or no melanin.
benign m's usually pigmented plaques or nodules. Those with junctional activity are analogous to the human compound junctional nevus.
congenital m. of pigs a single or multiple pigmented tumor of the skin or viscera that grows slowly and may metastasize. Spontaneous regression is common. An inherited form seen in Sinclair miniature pigs.
dermal m. a tumor which arises from rests of melanocytes in the dermis, remnants of neural crest precursors. Pigmentation is variable. It is usually benign.
malignant m. a malignant, rapidly growing, frequently ulcerated mass, consisting of either spindle cells or epithelioid cells or a mixture of the two, with a marked tendency to metastasize. The tumor cells may or may not (amelanotic) be pigmented. Although melanomas in pigs and cattle are usually benign and are not treated, those in horses, dogs, cats and occasional cases in sheep, goats and pigs are malignant. Called also nevocarcinoma.

melanomatosis the formation of melanomas throughout the body.

melanonychia blackening of the claws by melanin pigmentation.

melanophage a histiocyte laden with phagocytosed melanin.

melanophore a pigment cell containing melanin, especially such a cell from fish, amphibians and reptiles.

melanoplakia pigmented patches on the mucous membrane of the mouth.

melanosarcoma malignant melanoma.

melanosis 1. a condition characterized by dark pigmentary deposits. 2. a disorder of pigment metabolism.
m. coli brown-black discoloration of the mucosa of the colon.
congenital m. patches of melanin in the capsule and stroma of the liver or lung in the neonate.
liver m. see hepatic LIPOFUSCINOSIS.

melanosome any of the granules that contain melanin. The melanin is synthesized within melanocytes, then the melanosomes are transferred to keratinocytes.

melanotic characterized by the presence of melanin; pertaining to melanosis.

melanotrichia abnormally increased pigmentation of the hair.

melanotroph a pituitary cell that elaborates melanocyte-stimulating hormone (MSH).

melanotropin melanocyte-stimulating hormone.

Melanthera biflora WEDELIA *biflora*.
Melanthrium hybridum, Melanthrium virginicum North American plant in the Liliaceae family; unidentified toxin causes dyspnea, incoordination, recumbency. Called also bunchflower.
melanuria the discharge of darkly stained urine.
melarsomine a trivalent arsenical with activity against adult *Dirofilaria immitis*.
melarsoprol an antiprotozoal effective against *Trypanosoma* spp.
melasma dark pigmentation of the skin. Called also chloasma.
melatonin an indoleamine hormone synthesized and released by the pineal body during the hours of darkness; it may have a role in the control of the regulation of gonadotropin release.
Meleagris gallopavo gallopavo the South Mexican Turkey, from which the domestic turkey originated.
melena, melaena darkening of the feces by blood pigments. Typically the feces have a black color with a red tinge at the edges and are soft and almost slimy.
melengestrol acetate an effective oral progestational agent used as a feed additive in cattle to promote growth.
Meles a genus of small (3 ft long, 35 lb weight) mammals in the family Mustelidae. It includes *Meles meles*, the common (Eurasian) badger, and *Meles anakuma*, the Japanese badger. They are omnivorous, walk on all fours, massively built, placid, live in a burrow, and are grayish in color with two black stripes starting on the face and running over the top of the head to the back. There are also badgers in other genera, e.g. *Taxidea taxus*, the American badger.
Melia genus in the family Meliaceae.
M. azederach, M. dubia much used as a shade tree. The seed causes severe diarrhea with dysentery. There may also be excitement and dyspnea. Called also white cedar, chinaberry, dhrek.
M. major MELIANTHUS *comosus*.
Melianthus South African plant genus in the family Melianthaceae; the root is more toxic than the leaves and causes salivation, vomiting, colic, diarrhea and dysentery. The toxin is a cardiac glycoside. Honey produced from the shrub's nectar is toxic. Includes *Melianthus major* (tall Cape honey flower), *M. comosus* (Cape honey flower).
meliatoxin toxic tetranortriterpene from *Melia azederach* fruits.
Melica decumbens South African grass from family Poaceae; unidentified agent causes incoordination and recumbency. Called also staggers grass, dronkgras.
melilot see MELILOTUS.
Melilotus a genus of the legume family Fabaceae; plants contain coumarol, converted by fungal infestation of the hay to toxin dicoumarol, which causes greatly prolonged clotting time, spontaneous hemorrhage and often fatal anemia. Includes *M. alba* (white sweet clover, Bokhara clover), *M. altissima* (tall melilot), *M. indica* (Hexham scent, King Island melilot), *M. officinalis* (yellow sweet clover).
melioidosis a glanders-like disease of rodents, transmissible to humans, and caused by *Burkholderia pseudomallei*. Minor outbreaks, some with heavy mortalities have been recorded in all animal species. The syndromes seen vary widely and may include lymphangitis, meningoencephalitis, ocular and nasal discharge and pneumonia.
melitoptyalism secretion of saliva containing glucose.
melitose see RAFFINOSE.
melittin one of the toxic peptides in bee sting.
melituria the presence of any sugar in the urine.
melkbos EUPHORBIA *mauritanica*.
melktou SARCOSTEMMA *viminale*.
Melochia pyramidata a South American shrub in the Sterculiaceae family, toxin unidentified, causes posterior paralysis in cattle.
melochinine toxic alkaloid in *Melochia pyramidata*.
Melogale moschata the ferret badger, a partly arboreal member of the Mustelidae family. See also MELES.
melomelus a fetus with supernumerary limbs.
Melophagus a genus of insects in the family Hippoboscidae.
M. ovinus a permanent ectoparasite, the wingless, brown, leathery ked of sheep. Heavy infestations cause anemia, loss of condition and wool damage.
meloplasty plastic surgery of the cheek.
Melopsittacus undulatus the budgerigar. A mostly green with some yellow, small (3 to 4 inches long) psittacine bird with very affectionate ways. The most popular cage bird, it can be taught to speak. Domesticated birds have been bred to produce a great variety of colors, especially a powder blue. Called also love bird, but other species, especially *Psittacula* spp., probably have first call on the name.
melorheostosis a form of osteosclerosis, with linear tracks extending through the long bones.
melphalan a cytotoxic nitrogen mustard alkylating agent used as an antineoplastic.
melt butcher's name for spleen.
member a distinct part of the body, especially a limb.
membra [L.] plural of *membrum*.
membrana pl. *membranae* [L.] membrane.
m. granulosa the layer of small, actively mitotic cells in the wall of the ovarian follicle.
m. nictitans a fold of conjunctiva supported by a T-shaped cartilage and attached at the medial canthus of the eye; the so-called third eyelid in animals. In most animal species, it moves across the cornea when the upper and lower eyelids are closed. Prolapse of the membrane so that it is held in position halfway across the eye when the eyelids are open is a nonspecific sign of ill health in cats. Spasm of the membrane so that it is drawn smartly across the eye with a slow return to a normal position is a diagnostic sign of tetanus in all species. See also NICTITATING MEMBRANE, THIRD EYELID.
membrane a thin layer of tissue that covers a surface, lines a cavity, or divides a space or organ.
alveolocapillary m. a thin tissue barrier through which gases are exchanged between the alveolar air and the blood in the pulmonary capillaries.
m.-attack complex complement components C5–C9 which form in terminal stage of either of the complement pathways and lead to cell lysis.
basilar m. the lower boundary of the scala media of the ear.
Bowman's m. a thin layer of basement membrane between the outer layer of stratified epithelium and the substantia propria of the cornea.
Bruch's m. the inner layer of the choroid, separating it from the pigmented layer of the retina.
m. carrier a mechanism in the cell membrane of epithelial cells in the intestinal mucosa which facilitates the rapid transport of for example glucose, into the cell and thus into the bloodstream.
cell m. plasma membrane (below).
m. channels see CHANNEL.
continuous m. the middle of the three membranes on the outside of the yolk of the hen egg.

cricothyroid m. the membrane connecting the thyroid cartilage to the cricoid cartilage. It is extensive in the horse and surgical incision through it allows access to the interior of the larynx.
Descemet's m. the posterior lining membrane of the cornea; it is a thin hyaline membrane between the substantia propria and the endothelial layer of the cornea.
drum m. tympanic membrane (below).
extraembryonic m's those that protect the embryo or fetus and provide for its nutrition, respiration and excretion; the yolk sac (umbilical vesicle), allantois, amnion, chorion, decidua and PLACENTA.
extravitelline m. the outermost of the three membranes on the outside of the yolk of the hen egg.
false m. a membrane similar to the pseudomembrane; fibrinous exudates readily loosened from underlying tissue, as in croupous or pseudomembranous inflammation.
fenestrated m. one of the perforated elastic sheets of the tunica intima and tunica media of arteries.
fetal m's see FETAL membranes. See also extraembryonic membranes (above).
fibrous m. the strong, fibrous support layer in a joint capsule.
Henle's m. see HENLE's membrane.
hyaline m. 1. a membrane between the outer root sheath and inner fibrous layer of a hair follicle. 2. BASEMENT MEMBRANE. 3. a homogeneous eosinophilic membrane lining alveolar ducts and alveoli, frequently found at necropsy in premature human infants. See also HYALINE membrane disease.
hyoglossal m. a fibrous lamina connecting the under-surface of the tongue with the hyoid bone.
interosseous m. the membrane connecting the shaft of the fibula to the tibia.
limiting m. one that constitutes the border of some tissue or structure.
mucous m. the membrane covered with epithelium that lines many tubular organs of the body.
nictitating m. see MEMBRANA nictitans.
nuclear m. 1. either of the membranes, inner and outer, comprising the nuclear envelope. 2. nuclear envelope.
olfactory m. the olfactory portion of the mucous membrane lining the nasal fossa.
periodontal m. see PERIODONTIUM.
perivitelline m. the innermost of the three layers on the outside of the yolk in the hen egg.
placental m. the membrane that separates the fetal from the maternal blood in the placenta.
plasma m. the membrane that encloses a cell; it is composed of phospholipids, glycolipids, cholesterol and proteins. The primary structure is a lipid bilayer. Phospholipid molecules have an electrically charged 'head' that attracts water and a hydrocarbon 'tail' that repels water; they line up side by side in two opposing layers, with their heads on the inner or outer surface of the membrane and their tails in the core, from which water is excluded. The other lipids affect the structural properties of the membrane. Proteins embedded in the membrane transport specific molecules across the membrane, act as hormone receptors, or perform other functions.
m. potential of a cell is the voltage difference across the cell membrane resulting from the differential concentrations of sodium and potassium on either side of the membrane. The resting potential, for example in a nerve cell, is altered by the temporary opening of the sodium channels in the membrane during an action potential, allowing a redistribution of the ions.
m. proteins the large number of proteins attached to a cell membrane. They include *integral* proteins, called also intrinsic, which are embedded in the phospholipid bi-layer of the cell membrane, and *peripheral* proteins, called also extrinsic, because they are loosely bound and can readily be extracted without damage to the cell membrane.
pupillary m. a vascular membrane which occupies the pupil in the embryo stage, completely covering the anterior surface of the lens but subsequently disappears. See also persistent PUPILLARY membrane.
Reissner's m. the thin anterior wall of the cochlear duct, separating it from the scala vestibuli.
Scarpa's m. tympanic membrane, secondary.
semipermeable m. one permitting passage through it of some but not all substances.
serosal m. see serous membrane (below).
serous m. the membrane lining the walls of the body cavities and enclosing the contained organs; it consists of mesothelium lying upon a connective tissue layer and it secretes a watery fluid.
shell m. the membrane on the outside of the soft contents of the hen egg and just inside the shell. It consists of two membranes close together, with an air cell in between.
synovial m. see SYNOVIAL membrane.
m. transport transport of electrolytes across semipermeable membranes with the aid of a transporter.
unit m. the trilaminar structure of all cellular membranes (such as the plasma membrane, nuclear membranes, mitochondrial membranes, endoplasmic reticulum, lysosomes) as they appear in electron micrographs. The biochemical structure is a lipid bilayer.
wing m. the membrane comprising the wing of the bat.
yolk m. the membrane investing the yolk of the hen egg; it includes (from the inside out) the perivitelline, the continuous and the extravitelline membranes.

membrane keyboard a touch-sensitive keyboard with no mechanical linkages.

membranella a membrane formed of a fused row of cilia.

membraniform resembling a membrane.

membranocartilaginous 1. developed in both membrane and cartilage. 2. partly cartilaginous and partly membranous.

membranoid resembling a membrane.

membranous pertaining to or emanating from a membrane.
m. glomerulonephritis see membranous GLOMERULONEPHRITIS.
m. pneumocyte see ALVEOLAR epithelial cells (type 1).

membrum pl. *membra* [L.] a limb or member of the body; an entire leg.

memory the capacity to recall previously experienced sensations, information, data and ideas.
brain m. the ability of the brain to use knowledge gained from past experience. This is essential for the process of learning by animals. The process is poorly understood, but its practical application is sophisticated, especially in dogs.
m. cell an expanded clone of small lymphocytes derived from stimulated antigen-sensitive B and T lymphocytes. They have antigen receptors of the same specificity as the parent cell. Important in the secondary immune response.
computer m. the part of the computer that stores information and instructions for instantaneous recall. A small part of the memory that contains critical

information may be in *read only memory* (ROM), but most of the memory is *random access memory* (RAM), which can be modified at will. Disk storage is sometimes also called memory; strictly speaking, this is incorrect.

immunological m. the ability of the immune system to respond to more strongly and rapidly to the second and subsequent exposures to an antigen.

suture m. a property of some synthetic fibers which encourages the spontaneous untying of knots—the 'memory' of the fiber is that it is a straight fiber.

Menacanthus a genus of lice in the superfamily Amblycera.

M. cornutus resembles *M. stramineus*.

M. pallidulus a body louse of chickens.

***M. stramineus* (syn. *Eomenacanthus stramineus*)** yellow body louse of poultry.

menace reflex a reflex that may be tested by stabbing the finger towards the eye, with all precautions to avoid setting up a wind current. A positive reflex is a closing of the eyelids. An absence of the reflex indicates defective vision, paralysis of the eyelids or serious depression of consciousness. Called also eye preservation reflex, menace test, menace response, opticofacial reflex.

menadiol a water-soluble synthetic derivative of menadione. The sodium diphosphate salt is used in the treatment and prevention of vitamin K deficiency.

menadione a fat-soluble synthetic derivative of vitamin K used in the treatment and prevention of deficiency. Called also vitamin K_3.

m. sodium bisulfite is soluble in water and can be given by injection for a rapid effect.

menaquinone any of a series of compounds having vitamin K activity, in which the phytyl side-chain of phytomenadione (vitamin K_1) is replaced by a side-chain of prenyl units. Called also vitamin K_2.

mendelevium a chemical element, atomic number 101, atomic weight 256, symbol Md. See Table 6.

Mendelian pertaining to MENDEL'S LAWS.

m. inheritance the patterns of INHERITANCE (1) as explained by Mendel's laws.

m. rate an expression of the numerical relations of the occurrence of distinctly contrasted mendelian characteristics in succeeding generations of hybrid offspring.

Mendel's laws Law 1 The Law of Segregation—refers to the separation into different gametes, and therefore into different offspring, of the two members of every pair of alleles possessed by a parent. **Law 2** The Law of Independent Assortment—refers to the members of different pairs of alleles which are assorted independently into gametes, and that pairing of male and female gametes is a random activity. See also INHERITANCE.

Ménétrier's disease see giant hypertrophic GASTRITIS.

Menghini needle a long needle used for percutaneous biopsy of the liver.

Mengo virus a virus strain in the genus *Cardiovirus* which causes encephalomyocarditis.

menhaden oil an oil from a fish of the herring family which is found off the Atlantic coast of North America.

meningeal pertaining to the meninges.

m. hemorrhage common in neonates which have suffered forced traction to relieve dystocia and after normal births from cows being fed moldy sweet clover hay; whether or not they cause clinical signs depends on their size and location.

m. metaplastic ossification ossifying pachymeningitis. See dural OSSIFICATION.

m. worm PARAELAPHOSTRONGYLUS *tenuis*.

meningeal dura see DURA MATER.

meningeorrhaphy suture of membranes, especially the meninges.

meninges the three membranes covering the brain and spinal cord: the dura mater, arachnoid and pia mater. Consists of cranial and spinal membranes and special sections of it in diaphragma sellae, falx cerebri, tentorium cerebelli.

meningioangiomatosis a rare benign lesion characterized by circumscribed plaques on the brain surface.

meningioma a common, well-defined, firm intracranial neoplasm of animals arising from leptomeningeal cells, which occurs in basal locations, over the cerebral, cerebellar convexities, and in the spinal cord. One subtype is characterized by psammoma bodies (central calcified material).

angioblastic m. angioblastoma.

epithelioid m. see meningotheliomatous meningioma (below).

meningotheliomatous m. a diffusely cellular mesodermal tumor with cells in sheets or in pseudoalveoli.

meningism the signs of meningitis associated with acute febrile illness or dehydration but without actual inflammation of the meninges.

meningitis inflammation of the meninges. When the inflammatory process affects the dura mater, the disease is termed *pachymeningitis*; when the arachnoid and pia mater are involved, it is called *leptomeningitis* or *meningitis proper*. It is also classified as fibrinous, hemorrhagic, purulent or eosinophilic, depending on the principal reaction of the tissues.

The term *meningitis* does not refer to a specific disease entity but rather to the pathological condition of inflammation of the tissues of the meninges. The etiological agent can be anything that activates the inflammatory process, including both pathogenic and nonpathogenic organisms, such as bacteria, viruses and fungi; chemical toxins such as lead and arsenic; contrast media used in myelography; and metastatic malignant cells.

In animals there are no specific meningitides, most cases of meningitis occurring as secondary complications to other diseases and having a bacterial etiology. Clinical signs seen commonly include fever, cutaneous hyperesthesia and rigidity of the muscles of the neck and forelimbs. A CSF tap should assist in the diagnosis.

Beagle m. see BEAGLE pain syndrome.

Bernese Mountain Dog m. an acute, aseptic nonsuppurative meningitis seen in young Bernese Mountain Dogs of unknown etiology.

cerebrospinal m. an inflammation of the brain and spinal cord; it may be caused by many different organisms.

Pug m. see Pug MENINGOENCEPHALITIS.

spinal m. inflammation of the meninges of the spinal cord.

mening(o)- word element. [Gr.] *meninges, membrane*.

meningocele hernial protrusion of meninges through a defect in the skull or vertebral column.

meningocerebritis inflammation of the brain and meninges.

meningocortical pertaining to the meninges and cortex of the brain.

meningocyte a histiocyte of the meninges.

meningoencephalitis encephalomeningitis; inflammation of the brain and its meninges. Most meningoencephalitides in animals are bacterial and combine the fever, pain and rigidity of a meningitis with the tremor, convulsions and paralysis of an encephalitis. Localizing signs such as circling, falling to one side, unilateral facial paralysis and Jacksonian type seizures are more common than in a viral encephalitis.

bovine infectious m. see HEMOPHILOSIS.

eosinophilic m. see SODIUM CHLORIDE poisoning (in pigs).

listerial m. see LISTERIOSIS.

pasteurella m. can be caused by *Pasteurella multocida* or *P. haemolytica* in calves and in horses, mules and donkeys. Clinical signs include tremor, opisthotonos, rotation of the eyeballs, blindness, collapse and coma.

Pug m. an acute or chronic neurologic disease of young or adult Pugs with predominantly cerebral signs which include depression, circling, head pressing and blindness. Cerebellar signs sometimes also occur. A viral etiology is suspected.

streptococcal m. a common complication of streptococcal septicemia of newborn pigs. The cause is usually *Streptococcus suis* type 1. The syndrome includes stiffness, tremor, blindness, recumbency and violent, paddling convulsions.

thromboembolic m. see HEMOPHILOSIS.

West Nile equine m. a mosquito is the vector for this flavivirus that infects principally horses but probably also other species, including humans. Clinically the disease resembles equine viral ENCEPHALOMYELITIS.

meningoencephalocele hernial protrusion of the meninges and brain substance through a defect in the skull.

congenital m. occurs in CRANIUM bifidum. An inherited form has been identified in Landrace pigs. The piglets are not viable. Called also cranioschisis.

inherited m. possibly an inherited defect in Landrace pigs.

meningoencephalomyelitis inflammation of the meninges, brain and spinal cord.

granulomatous m. an acute, progressive disease of dogs characterized by diffuse or focal perivascular accumulations of histiocytes, lymphocytes and plasma cells in the meninges, brain and spinal cord. The distribution and severity of lesions and, accordingly, clinical signs are extremely variable, e.g. optic nerve involvement may cause blindness. The cause is unknown, but viral infection and immunological mechanisms have been suspected. Called also inflammatory reticulosis.

meningoencephalopathy noninflammatory disease of the cerebral meninges and brain.

meningogenic arising in the meninges.

meningomalacia softening of a membrane.

meningomyelitis inflammation of the spinal cord and its meninges.

meningomyelocele hernial protrusion of the meninges and spinal cord through a defect in the vertebral column, often spina bifida.

meningomyeloradiculitis inflammation of the meninges, spinal cord and spinal nerve roots.

Meningonema peruzzi a filarial parasite of the central nervous system of a number of African monkeys including talopin monkeys and *Cereopithecus aethions.* Thought also to cause cerebral filariasis of humans.

meningopathy any disease of the meninges.

meningoradicular pertaining to the meninges and the cranial or spinal nerve roots.

meningoradiculitis inflammation of the meninges and spinal nerve roots.

meningorhachidian pertaining to the spinal cord and meninges.

meningorrhagia hemorrhage from cerebral or spinal membranes.

meningorrhea effusion of blood between or upon the meninges.

meninx pl. *meninges* [Gr.] a membrane, especially one of the membranes of the brain or spinal cord—the dura mater, arachnoid and pia mater.

meniscectomy excision of a meniscus, as of the stifle joint.

menisci plural form of *meniscus.*

meniscitis inflammation of a meniscus.

meniscosynovial pertaining to a meniscus and the synovial membrane.

meniscus pl. *menisci* [L.] 1. something of crescent shape, such as the concave or convex surface of a column of liquid in a pipette or burette. 2. one of a pair of crescent-shaped fibrocartilages (semilunar cartilages) in the stifle joint that provide stability while permitting both flexion and rotation of the joint.

m. tear a common injury in dogs with rupture of the cranial cruciate ligament and the accompanying instability of the stifle joint. Most tears occur in the caudal horn of the medial meniscus.

Menopon a genus of bird lice in the suborder Amblycera.

M. gallinae the 'shaft louse' of fowl, ducks and pigeons.

M. pallidum a chicken louse found to harbor the virus of equine ENCEPHALOMYELITIS.

M. phaeostomum found on peacocks.

menotropins a purified preparation of gonadotropins extracted from the urine of postmenopausal women, containing follicle-stimulating hormone (FSH) and luteinizing hormone (LH); used in the treatment of human infertility.

menstruum the end product of a process of extraction using a solvent—the combined extract plus solvent.

mental 1. pertaining to the mind. 2. pertaining to the chin.

m. nerves see Table 14.

m. organ an accumulation of apocrine tubular glands in the intermandibular space of swine.

m. state includes states of excitement, e.g. frenzy, mania and panic, and depression states, including somnolence, lassitude, narcolepsy, catalepsy, syncope and coma. Delirium is not diagnosable in animals but aimless wandering and headpressing are reminiscent of that mental state in humans.

m. status assessment of level of patient awareness or consciousness.

mentation mental activity, state of mind.

Mentha genus of herbs in family Lamiaceae; unidentified toxin; clinical signs include incoordination, diarrhea; with some plants abortion and photosensitization also recorded; includes *M. australis* (native mint), *M. longifolia* (horse mint), *M. pulegium* (penny royal), *M. satureioides* (native mint).

menthol an alcohol from various mint oils or produced synthetically, used locally to relieve pruritus.

mentoplasty plastic surgery of the chin; surgical correction of deformities and defects of the chin.

mentum [L.] *chin.*

menu a list of options which are displayed at each step in a computer program and from which the computer user can choose.

m. bar section at the top of a window on a computer screen which contains items available in pull-down menus.

m.-driven program a program which uses menus to advance to the next step by responding to a prompt from the user.

Menziesia ferruginea North American plant in family Ericaceae; toxin is andromedotoxin; causes sudden death, abdominal pain, vomiting, diarrhea; called also *M. glabella*, mock azalea.

meow see MEW.

mepacrine see QUINACRINE.

mepenzolate an anticholinergic used in the form of the bromide to relieve abdominal pain and diarrhea.

meperidine a centrally acting analgesic with spasmolytic properties equal to those of atropine. Has little hypnotic effect and relieves pain without reducing consciousness, muscular activity, coordination or responsiveness of the special senses. An addictive drug for humans. Called also pethidine.

mephenesin a centrally acting muscle relaxant. Once used in association with pentobarbital for anesthesia, but no longer used because of its many side-effects, including venous thrombosis and hemolysis.

mephenytoin, methoin a hydantoin anticonvulsant drug, similar to phenytoin, but more toxic.

mephitic noxious; foul smelling.

Mephitis mephitis see SKUNK.

mephobarbital see METHYLPHENOBARBITAL.

mepivacaine hydrochloride a compound used as a local anesthetic.

meprobamate a tranquilizer and skeletal muscle relaxant.

mepyramine see PYRILAMINE.

mEq milliequivalent.

merbromin organic, hydroxomercury disodium salt; used as a topical antiseptic. Called also mercurochrome, which in some countries is a trademark name.

mercaptans organic mercurial compounds, used as fungicides on plants and animals. See CAPTAN.

2-mercaptoethanol (2 ME) test differentiates between IgM and IgG antibodies and used to identify a recent immune response to an infectious agent.

2-mercaptopropionylglycine a drug with properties similar to penicillamine; used in the treatment of cystine urolithiasis; abbreviated MPG. Called also tiopronin.

mercaptopurine, 6-mercaptopurine an antimetabolite that acts by blocking purine synthesis; used as an antineoplastic agent, primarily in the treatment of leukemia and lymphosarcoma.

merchandising a fringe activity for rural veterinarians; the selling of nonethical medicines which are generally available to the public without prescription. It is extended by some veterinarians to include general items such as grooming kits and dog collars.

mercurial 1. pertaining to mercury. 2. a preparation containing mercury.

Mercurialis European plant genus in Euphorbiaceae family; unidentified toxin causes hemolytic anemia and gastritis when eaten; includes *M. annua*, *M. perennis* (dog's mercury, annual mercury).

mercurialism chronic mercury poisoning.

mercuric pertaining to mercury as a bivalent element; containing bivalent MERCURY.

m. chloride, m. bichloride used as a skin antiseptic and disinfectant and counterirritant; is limited by its toxicity and irritant properties.

m. iodide a counterirritant and vesicant; use of this compound in blisters for horses has been discontinued because of its renal and hepatic toxicity.

m. nitrate has antiseptic and miticidal properties; once used topically in the treatment of demodectic mange in dogs, but replaced by safer and more effective agents.

m. oxide a topical antiseptic, used in ointment form for eye disorders. Called also yellow oxide.

mercurochrome see MERBROMIN.

mercurous pertaining to mercury as a monovalent element; containing monovalent MERCURY.

m. chloride used mainly as a cathartic and irritant vermicide, but largely superseded by more reliable preparations. It increases peristalsis and glandular secretions, especially of bile. It is also used rarely as an intestinal antiseptic and to reduce edema, or in an ointment as a local antibacterial agent. Called also calomel.

mercury a chemical element, atomic number 80, atomic weight 200.59, symbol Hg. See Table 6.

Mercury forms two sets or classes of compounds: *mercurous*, in which a single atom of mercury combines with a monovalent radical, and *mercuric*, in which a single atom of mercury combines with a bivalent radical. Mercury and its salts have been employed therapeutically as purgatives; as alternatives in chronic inflammations; and as intestinal antiseptics, disinfectants and astringents. They are absorbed by the skin and mucous membranes, causing chronic mercurial poisoning, or hydrargyria. The mercuric salts are more soluble and irritant than the mercurous. See also MERCUROUS, MERCURIC.

m. plant MERCURIALIS *annua*.

ammoniated m. used as an antiseptic skin and ophthalmic ointment.

organic m. includes the fungistats phenylmercurials, ethyl and methyl mercurials, e.g. methoxyethylmercury silicate; poisonous to animals and cause unacceptable residues in animal products.

m. poisoning by inorganic compounds causes gastritis and kidney damage manifested by diarrhea and terminal uremia. Organic mercury compounds were until recently extensively used as fungistatic agents in stored grain. They cause poisoning manifested by nervous signs, including incoordination, blindness and recumbency. With larger doses there are convulsions.

mercury bichloride see CORROSIVE sublimate.

mercy killing the euthanasia of animals for humane reasons is regarded by the veterinary profession as one of its responsibilities to the animal population. When the animal is in a great deal of pain and there is no chance of a favorable outcome, it is thought that the veterinarian is required to carry out euthanasia. In most Western countries this is enshrined in legislation relating to the protection of animals against cruelty. In awkward situations, e.g. when the owner resists or is not available to give consent to euthanasia, it is prudent to get another veterinary opinion if that is possible.

merge in computer terms, the combining of two or more files into one, according to a previously specified order.

meridian 1. an imaginary line on the surface of a globe or sphere, connecting the opposite ends of its axis. 2. in Western acupuncture includes the system of channels and their collaterals which are thought to connect all body parts and most acupuncture points are located on them. There are 12 bilaterally distributed meridians—lung meridian of the hand (*Tai Yin*), heart m. of the hand (*Shao Yin*), pericardium m. of the hand (*Jue Yin*), large intestine m. of the hand (*Yang Ming*), small intestine m. of the hand (*Tai Yang*), triple heater m. of the hand (*Shao Yang*), stomach m. of the foot (*Yang Ming*), urinary bladder

m. of the foot (*Tia Yang*), gallbladder m. of the foot (*Shao Yang*), spleen m. of the foot (*Tao Yin*), kidney m. of the foot (*Shao Yin*), liver m. of the foot (*Jue Yin*).

m. points acupuncture points located on one of the meridians.

m. theory traditional Chinese medicine is based on the theory that all body parts are connected by a network of main and collateral channels along which are situated the bulk of the acupuncture points; there are also some meridians, the dorsally located Governing Vessel and the ventrally located Conception Vessel, which are not connected to specific anatomical organs.

Merino a fine-woolled sheep with unpigmented hooves used for fabric wool; males are usually horned (polled strains are available), females are polled. Originated in Spain, now many ethnic varieties. Classes of Australian merinos include Superfine (18 microns), Medium (20–22 microns), and Strongwoolled (23–25 microns). Other strains exist, e.g. Booroola, which has a much better fertility performance than average merinos.

Merinolandschaf sheep polled, meat and medium wool, German sheep. originsted from local breed mated with imported breed.

Meriones unguiculatus see Mongolian GERBIL.

Merkel cell, Merkel disk found in the basal layer of the epidermis; believed to act as slow-acting tactile endorgans.

M. c. tumor see NEUROENDOCRINE cell tumor.

merle a pattern of coat color pigmentation with dark, irregular blotches on a lighter background. Seen in some Collies and Welsh corgis. In shorthaired dogs, e.g. Great Danes and Dachshunds, the similar pattern is called DAPPLE. The trait is sometimes associated with congenital defects such as deafness and heterochromia iridis. In the homozygous state, there are severe ocular defects and deafness.

merlin FALCO *columbarius*.

Mermis subnigrescens a worm in the family Mermithidae which is parasitic in grasshoppers and earwigs. Called also rainworm.

mero- word element. [Gr.] 1. part. 2. thigh.

meroblastic partially dividing; undergoing cleavage in which only part of the egg participates.

merocele femoral hernia.

merocrine partly secreting; denoting that type of glandular secretion in which the secreting cell remains intact throughout the process of formation and discharge of the secretory products, as in the salivary and pancreatic glands; see also APOCRINE, HOLOCRINE.

merogenesis cleavage of an ovum.

merogony the development of only a portion of an ovum.

meromelia congenital absence of a part, but not all, of a limb.

meromicrosomia unusual smallness of some part of the body.

meromyarian nematode whose somatic musculature is composed of closely packed units of three or four flattened muscle cells. Includes *Ancylostoma* and *Necator* spp.

meromyosin a fragment of the myosin molecule isolated by treatment with proteolytic enzyme; there are two types, heavy (H-meromyosin) and light (L-meromyosin).

meropia partial blindness.

merorachischisis fissure of part of the spinal cord.

merotomy a cutting into segments.

merozoite one of the organisms formed by multiple fission (schizogony) of a sporozoite within the body of the host.

mersalyl mercurial diuretic usually used in combination with theophylline.

Merthiolate trademark for an alcohol, acetone and water preparation of THIMEROSAL.

M.-iodine-formalin perservative a preparation used for the preservation and staining of protozoa.

Merychippus a primitive stage in the evolution of the horse that existed in the Miocene era.

mesalazine, mesalamine the component of sulfasalazine utilized in the treatment of acute colitis. Used orally or rectally as suppositories or enemas.

mésalliance, misalliance [Fr.] see MISMATING.

mesamnion the longitudinal chorioamniotic raphe, formed by the fusion of the two chorioamniotic folds.

mesangial of the nature of or pertaining to mesangium.

m. cell connective tissue cells of the glomerulus; occur singly or in pairs in a thin matrix.

m. sclerosis increased mesangial matrix.

mes(o)- word element. [Gr.] *middle*.

mesangiocapillary pertaining to or affecting the mesangium and the associated capillaries.

m. glomerulitis apparently inherited disease in Finnish-Landrace lambs younger than 4 months old; most are asymptomatic and found dead; kidneys enlarged, severe proteinuria.

mesangium the thin membrane in the form of a central matrix supporting the capillary loops in renal glomeruli.

mesaortitis inflammation of the tunica media of the aorta.

mesarteritis inflammation of the tunica media of an artery.

mesatipellic having a round pelvis.

mesaxon the pair of longitudinal adjoining membranes that mark the edge-to-edge contact of the Schwann cell that encircles the axon.

mescal bean see SOPHORA SECUNDIFLORA.

mescaline a poisonous alkaloid derived from the flowering heads (mescal buttons) of a Mexican cactus which produces hallucinations of sound. See also PEYOTE.

mescalism intoxication due to mescal buttons or mescaline. See PEYOTE.

Mesembryanthemum African genus of succulent plants in family Aizoaceae; includes *M. nodiflorum*, *M. crystallinum*; toxin is soluble oxalates characterized by occurrence of nephrosis, urolithiasis; called also pigface.

mesems see MESEMBRYANTHEMUM.

mesencephalic aqueduct constricted portion of the lumen of the neural tube in the midbrain.

mesencephalitis inflammation of the mesencephalon, or midbrain.

mesencephalon 1. the midbrain, including the colliculi of the tectum, the cerebral crura, the Edinger–Westphal nucleus, internal capsule, lemniscal trigone, pallidum, putamen and substantia nigra. 2. the middle of the three primary brain vesicles of the embryo.

mesenchyma mesenchyme.

mesenchymal cell see MESENCHYME.

mesenchyme the meshwork of embryonic connective tissue in the mesoderm, from which are formed the muscular and connective tissues of the body and also the blood vessels and lymph vessels.

mesenchymoma a mixed mesenchymal tumor composed of two or more cellular elements that are not commonly associated, exclusive of fibrous tissue.

mesenterectomy resection of the mesentery.
mesenteric pertaining to or emanating from the mesentery.
m. abscess in horses causes a syndrome of subacute abdominal pain, due usually to the coexistence of thromboembolic colic, plus the toxemia of the abscess and a commonly concurrent peritonitis.
m. arteritis see VERMINOUS mesenteric arteritis.
m. hemorrhage spontaneous rupture of a blood vessel in the mesentery in horses, which causes severe colic, hemorrhagic anemia and shock. Blood is found in a paracentesis sample.
m. lymph node cranial and caudal groups of nodes clustered about the arteries of the same names.
m. receptors Pacinian corpuscle mechanoreceptors plus some less readily adaptive mechanoreceptors found near mesenteric blood vessels.
m. root origin of the mesentery from the parietal peritoneum.
m. stretch a tight bowstring-like edge of mesenteric fold in equine colic, where the large bowel is impacted and very heavy, or in acute intestinal obstruction, with loops of bowel very heavy with fluid. The stretching is a significant factor in causing pain and may be relieved by the horse lying on its back.
m. tear see mesenteric HERNIA.
m. torsion torsion of the mesenteric root, causing ischemia of the mesentery and intestine so that the tissue is devitalized and the animal dies quickly of shock and toxemia.
m. vessel thrombosis causes thromboembolic COLIC.
mesenteriopexy fixation or suspension of a torn mesentery.
mesenteriorrhaphy suture of the mesentery.
mesenteriplication the operation of taking a tuck in the mesentery to shorten it.
mesenteritis inflammation of the mesentery.
mesenterium mesentery.
mesenteron the midgut.
mesentery a membranous sheet attaching various organs to the body wall, especially the peritoneal fold attaching the intestine to the dorsal body wall.
ovarian m. see MESOVARIUM.
testicle m. see PROPER LIGAMENT of the testis.
mesh interlaced structure; a net.
nylon m. woven fiber in sheets used to repair gaps in tissue. Other less reactive and more easily worked materials are also available.
surgical m. made of stainless steel, polyester fiber or polypropylene. Used in hernia repair or when there is a tissue deficiency.
mesiad toward the middle or center.
mesial situated in the middle; median; nearer the middle line of the body or nearer the center of the dental arch.
mesially toward the median line.
mesiobuccal pertaining to or formed by the mesial and buccal surfaces of a tooth, or the mesial and buccal walls of a tooth cavity.
mesiocervical pertaining to the mesial surface of the neck of a tooth.
mesiodistal pertaining to the mesial and distal surfaces of a tooth.
mesiolabial pertaining to the mesial and labial surfaces of a tooth or a tooth cavity.
mesion the plane dividing the body into right and left symmetrical halves.
mesio-occlusion anteroocclusion; malrelation of the dental arches, with the mandibular arch anterior to the maxillary arch. Called also prognathism.
mesoblast the mesoderm, especially in the early stages.
mesobronchitis inflammation of middle coat of the bronchi.
mesocardia location of the apex of the heart in the midline of the thorax.
mesocardium the part of the embryonic mesentery which connects the embryonic heart with the body wall in front and the foregut behind.
mesocecum the occasionally occurring mesentery of the cecum.
mesocephalon mesencephalon, or midbrain.
Mesocestoides a genus of tapeworms in the family Mesocestoididae.
M. corti, M. lineatus, M. variabilis found in the intestines in a range of carnivores including dogs, foxes, cats and humans. They may cause enteritis in humans, but are innocuous in other species. The worm has an unusual life cycle and has a stage of tissue invasion which may cause peritonitis.
mesocolon the mesentery that attaches the colon to the dorsal abdominal wall; it is called ascending, descending or transverse, according to the portion of the colon to which it attaches.
ascending m. see mesocolon (above).
pelvic m. the peritoneum attaching the sigmoid colon to the dorsal abdominal wall. Called also sigmoid megacolon.
sigmoid m. see pelvic megacolon (above).
mesocolopexy suspension or fixation of the colon.
mesocoloplication plication of the mesocolon to limit its mobility.
mesocord an umbilical cord adherent to the placenta.
Mesocricetus auratus see CRICETUS.
mesoderm the middle of the three primary germ layers of the embryo, lying between the ectoderm and entoderm; from it are derived the connective tissue, bone, cartilage, muscle, blood and blood vessels, lymphatics, lymphoid organs, notochord, pleura, pericardium, peritoneum, kidneys and gonads.
extraembryonic m. located outside the developing embryo and forming its accessory organs.
paraxial m. adjacent to the mid line beneath the epiblast of the embryo which develop into somites.
somatic m. the outer layer of the developing mesoderm.
splanchnic m. the inner layer of the developing mesoderm.
mesodiastolic pertaining to the middle of the diastole.
mesodiverticular band an anomalous persistence of a vitelline artery appearing as a fold of mesentery stretching from the cranial mesenteric artery to the antimesenteric side of the intestine, the site of Meckel's diverticulum. The pouch that it forms with the normal mesentery may entrap a loop of intestine and cause obstruction of it.
mesoductus deferens the peritoneal web or 'mesentery' of the ductus deferens.
mesoduodenum the mesenteric fold that supports the duodenum.
mesoepididymis a fold of tunica vaginalis connecting the epididymis and testis.
mesogastrium the portion of the primitive mesentery that encloses the stomach; from its dorsal sheet, the greater omentum develops, and from its ventral sheet, the lesser omentum.
mesogenic 1. a host–parasite relationship in which the parasite dominates but the host usually survives. 2. of medium virulence; said of some strains of NEWCASTLE DISEASE virus.

Mesogyna a genus of tapeworms in the family Mesocestoididae.

M. hepatica found in the small bile ducts and blood vessels of the liver in a little known fox (*Vulpis macrotis*) in California.

Mesohippus a prehistoric, three-toed, horse-like creature; probably not in the direct line of ancestors of the modern horse.

mesoileum the mesentery of the ileum.

mesojejunum the mesentery of the jejunum.

mesolymphocyte a medium-sized lymphocyte.

mesomelic the middle parts of limbs.

m. dysplasia deformity of the middle parts of a limb.

mesomere 1. a blastomere of size intermediate between a macromere and a micromere. 2. a midzone of the mesoderm between the epimere and hypomere.

mesometrium the portion of the broad ligament below the mesovarium.

meson 1. mesion. 2. any elementary particle having a mass intermediate between the mass of the electron and that of the proton.

mesonephric emanating from or pertaining to the mesonephros.

m. duct embryonal structure that develops into the vas deferens and epididymis in males and remains vestigial in females. Called also wolffian duct. It is subject to a variety of manifestations of segmental aplasia and hypoplasia, especially in bulls. In mares remnants of the ducts may become cystic and produce PARAOVARIAN cyst.

m. tube excretory tube of the mesonephros; becomes the mesonephric duct and contributes in the adult to the vasa efferentia of the male.

m. tubules embryonic tubules which connect at one end with a blood vessel, at the other with the mesonephric duct.

mesonephroma a malignant tumor of the female genital tract, usually the ovary, formerly thought to arise from mesonephric rests. Two types are recognized: one of müllerian duct derivation, the other an embryonal tumor which may also arise in the testis.

mesonephron mesonephros.

mesonephros pl. *mesonephroi* [Gr.] the excretory organ of the embryo, arising caudal to the pronephros and using its duct. Displaced by the metanephros which becomes the kidney of the postnatal animal.

mesopexy repair of the mesentery; mesenteriopexy.

mesophile a microorganism that grows best at 68° to 131°F (20° to 55°C).

mesophlebitis inflammation of the tunica media of a vein.

mesoporphyrin III a crystalline, iron-free porphyrin derived from heme.

mesorchium the portion of the primitive mesentery enclosing the fetal testis, represented in the adult by a fold between the testis and epididymis.

mesorectum the fold of mesentery connecting the cranial portion of the rectum with the sacrum.

mesoropter the normal position of the eyes with their muscles at rest.

mesorrhaphy suture of the mesentery.

mesosalpinx the part of the broad ligament cranial to mesovarium, investing the uterine tube.

mesosigmoid the peritoneal fold by which the sigmoid flexure is attached to the abdominal wall.

mesosome an invagination of the bacterial cell membrane, seen in fixed cells; the significance is unknown.

mesosternum the middle piece or body of the sternum.

mesotendineum, mesotendon the connective tissue sheath attaching a tendon to its synovial sheath. It may persist, disappear altogether, or leave vestigial strands called vincula (see VINCULUM).

mesotendon the space-occupying web of tissue between the inner and outer layers of a tendon sheath.

mesothelial pertaining to the mesothelium.

m. cells cover all serous membranes and normally found in fluid samples aspirated from the pleural or peritoneal cavities.

mesothelioma a rare malignant tumor made up of cells derived from the mesothelium. Recorded in the pleural cavity of animals, causing massive effusion and dyspnea. Found most commonly as a congenital tumor of calves.

mesothelium the layer of flat cells, derived from the mesoderm, that lines the body cavity of the embryo. In the adult it forms the simple squamous epithelium that covers the surface of all true serous membranes (peritoneum, pericardium, pleura).

mesotocin a posterior pituitary hormone in birds; involved in producing uterine contractions.

mesotympanum the portion of the middle ear medial to the tympanic membrane.

mesovarium the portion of the broad ligament enclosing and holding the ovary in place.

mesoviductus the peritoneal sheet or 'mesentery' which suspends the avian oviduct.

mesquite see PROSOPIS JULIFLORA.

messenger RNA (mRNA) see RIBONUCLEIC ACID.

mesulfen a sulfur-containing scabicide and antipruritic.

Met methionine.

met-enkephalin methionine ENKEPHALIN; abbreviated Met-ENK.

met-tRNA$_i$ a single species of methionyl tRNA that forms a tertiary complex with eukaryotic initiation factor 2 (eIF2) which has bound to GTP as a first step in the initiation of protein synthesis.

meta- word element. [Gr.] 1. change, transformation, exchange. 2. after, next. 3. the 1,3-position in derivatives of benzene.

metabasis change in the manifestations or course of a disease.

metabiosis the dependence of one organism upon another for its existence; commensalism.

metabolic pertaining to internal metabolism.

m. acidemia acidemia due to metabolic error.

m. bone disease includes a range of bone diseases associated with metabolic diseases, e.g. secondary hyperparathyroidism, rickets and osteoporosis.

m. defect generally an inherited defect that is present at birth, but which is not necessarily evident clinically for several months afterwards. The defect creates a metabolic error, which leads to the accumulation of end products which cause clinical signs, e.g. mannosidosis, porphyria or an exaggerated response from an end-organ, e.g. inherited goiter. See also INBORN error of metabolism.

m. diseases diseases in which normal metabolic processes are disturbed and a resulting absence or shortfall of a normal metabolite causes disease, e.g. hypocalcemia in cows, or an accumulation of the end products of metabolism causes a clinical illness, e.g. acetonemia of dairy cows. Many diseases in this group really have their beginnings in a nutritional deficiency state. See also PRODUCTION diseases.

m. encephalopathy many disorders of metabolism can lead to neurologic abnormalities through alterations in electrolytes and acid–base balance, accumulation of endogenous toxins. See also ENCEPHALOPATHY.

m. error see metabolic defect (above).

m. inhibition technique a virus neutralization test in tissue culture in which phenol-red indicator is used to detect the acid metabolic products of actively metabolizing cells or the lack of metabolism when cells are infected and destroyed by the virus.

m. laminitis see LAMINITIS.

m. myopathies muscular dystrophies caused by metabolic defects; include systemic glycogenoses, deposits of a PAS-positive glycoprotein, the lipid storage disease of cats caused by carnitine deficiency.

m. pathways groupings of enzymic processes leading to the synthesis or breakdown of carbohydrates, amino acids and lipids.

m. polymyopathy a muscle disease associated with a metabolic disorder, e.g. hyperadrenocorticism.

m. polyneuropathy a disease of the nerves associated with a metabolic disorder, e.g. uremia, diabetes mellitus or hypothyroidism.

m. profile results of a spectrum of tests of metabolic functions.

m. profile test see COMPTON METABOLIC PROFILE TEST.

m. rate the rate of energy metabolism in the body. The basal metabolic rate (BMR) is the rate of energy consumption by the body when it is completely at rest.

m. toxins include histamine, other toxic amines, ketone bodies, phenols and cresols from the large intestine, which are normal end-products of metabolism and indigestion but if their normal excretion and detoxication are impeded, cause intoxication. See also TOXIN.

m. water the water produced in the body by oxidative metabolism of food; it represents 5 to 10% of the body's water utilization.

metabolism the sum of the physical and chemical processes by which living organized substance is built up and maintained (anabolism), and by which large molecules are broken down into smaller molecules to make energy available to the organism (catabolism).

Essentially these processes are concerned with the disposition of the nutrients absorbed into the blood following digestion.

inborn error of m. a genetically determined biochemical disorder in which a specific enzyme defect produces a metabolic block that may have pathological consequences at birth, as in maple syrup urine disease of calves, or in later life, e.g. in mannosidosis in calves. See also METABOLIC defect.

metabolite any substance produced during metabolism.

metabolizable capable of being converted by metabolism.

m. energy (ME) said of a feed or ration, the net energy available to an animal after the utilization of some energy in the processes of digestion and absorption and the loss of some of the material as being undigested or indigestible.

metabolize to subject to or be transformed by metabolism.

metacarpal 1. pertaining to the metacarpus. 2. a bone of the metacarpus.

m. pad see FOOTPAD.

small m. bone see SPLINT BONE and Table 10.

metacarpectomy excision or resection of a metacarpal bone.

metacarpophalangeal pertaining to the metacarpus and phalanges.

m. joint see Table 11. Called also fetlock.

metacarpus the segment of the limb housing the aggregate of metacarpal bones.

metacentric a replicating chromosome with the centromere midway between the ends.

metacercaria pl. *metacercariae;* the encysted resting or maturing stage of a trematode parasite in the tissues of a second intermediate host or on vegetation.

metacestode larval stage of cestodes.

metachromasia 1. failure to stain true with a given stain. 2. the different coloration of different tissues produced by the same stain. 3. change of color produced by staining.

metachromatic having the characteristics of metachromasia.

m. leukodystrophy see metachromatic LEUKODYSTROPHY.

metachromophil, metachromatophil not staining normally.

metacresylacetate see *m*-CRESYL ACETATE.

metacyclic produced in an intermediate host, and infective for the definitive host; said of the infective stages of trypanosomes.

metagenesis alternation of generations; there are alternate sexual and asexual cycles of reproduction in the one species.

Metagonimus a genus of digenetic trematodes in the family Heterophydiiae.

M. yokogawai found in the small intestine of the dog, cat, pig, pelican and humans. May cause enteritis in humans but considered to be nonpathogenic in animals.

metahypophyseal abnormal hypophyseal function.

m. diabetes diabetes mellitus which occurs as a result of active hyperplasia or tumor of the acidophil cells of the pituitary gland.

metal any chemical element marked by luster, malleability, ductility and conductivity of electricity and heat, and which will ionize positively in solution.

alkali m. one of a group of monovalent elements including lithium, sodium, potassium, rubidium and cesium.

m. detector a portable electronic device used to detect metal in the reticulum of cows. Most clinically normal cows fed on prepared rations give positive results.

m. implants see IMPLANT.

m. retriever a long, probang-like instrument, passed orally into the reticulum in cattle for the retrieval of metallic foreign bodies that might cause traumatic reticuloperitonitis.

metaldehyde a common molluscicide; its formulation in a bran base, especially pellets, makes it a positive risk for all animal species and a very serious threat to all urban dogs.

m. poisoning clinical signs include tremor, incoordination, salivation, dyspnea, unconsciousness and death due to respiratory failure.

metalkamate a carbamate pesticide.

metalloenzyme any enzyme containing tightly bound metal atoms, e.g. cytochrome oxidase.

metalloid 1. any element with both metallic and nonmetallic properties. 2. any metallic element that has not all the characteristics of a typical metal.

metalloporphyrin a combination of a metal with porphyrin, as in heme.

metalloprotein a protein molecule bound to a metal ion, e.g. hemoglobin.

metallurgy the science and art of using metals.

metalosis a nonsuppurative osteomyelitis that occurs around metal implants as a result of corrosion or hypersensitivity reaction.

metamere one of a series of homologous segments of the body of an animal.
metameric of or pertaining to metamerism.
metamerism a system of structures in which similar segments succeed each other craniocaudally.
metamorphosis change of structure or shape; particularly, transition from one developmental stage to another, as from larva to adult form.
fatty m. any normal or pathological transformation of fat, including fatty infiltration and fatty degeneration.
metamyelocyte a precursor in the granulocytic series, being a cell intermediate in development between a promyelocyte and the mature, segmented (polymorphonuclear) granular leukocyte, between the myelocyte and the band stage, and having a U-shaped nucleus.
metanephric pertaining to the metanephros.
m. diverticulum first stage in the development of the metanephros; an evagination from the caudal end of the mesonephric duct. Called also ureteric bud.
m. duct embryonic ureter.
metanephrine a urinary metabolite of epinephrine.
metanephros pl. *metanephroi* [Gr.] the third and final attempt to produce a permanent embryonic kidney, developing later than and caudal to the mesonephros.
metaphase the second stage of cell division (mitosis or meiosis), in which the chromosomes, each consisting of two chromatids, are arranged in the equatorial plane of the spindle prior to separation.
Metaphen a proprietary name for NITROMERSOL.
metaphyseal pertaining to or emanating from the metaphysis.
m. aclasis see multiple cartilaginous EXOSTOSIS.
m. dysplasia see OSTEOCHONDRITIS, OSTEOPETROSIS.
m. osseous replacement occurs within the primary spongiosa and carried out by the trabecular endosteal envelope.
m. osteopathy see hypertrophic OSTEODYSTROPHY.
m. reduction part of the bone modeling process is funnelization of the metaphysis to reduce its diameter to conform with the smaller diameter of the diaphysis.
metaphysis pl. *metaphyses* [Gr.] the wider part at the end of the shaft of a long bone, adjacent to the epiphyseal disk.
metaplasia the change in the type of adult cells in a tissue to a form abnormal for that tissue.
metaplastic characteristic of metaplasia.
metapneumonic succeeding or following pneumonia.
metapodium the segment of limb supported by metacarpal or metatarsal bones.
metaproterenol a bronchodilator indicated in treatment of bronchial asthma, reversible bronchospasm of bronchitis, and emphysema. It is closely related to isoprenaline but has a longer duration and fewer cardiovascular side-effects. Called also orciprenaline.
metaraminol a noncatecholamine symphathomimetic amine, active at peripheral α-receptors; used as the bitartrate for its pressor effects in the treatment of shock.
metarteriole a branch of an arteriole.
metarubricyte an orthochromatic NORMOBLAST; an immature red cell erythrocyte.
metarubricytosis see NORMOBLASTOSIS.
metastasis pl. *metastases* [Gr.] 1. the transfer of disease from one organ or part to another not directly connected with it. It may be due either to the transfer of pathogenic microorganisms (e.g. tubercle bacilli) or to the transfer of cells, as in malignant tumors. 2. *metastases,* growths of pathogenic microorganisms or of abnormal cells distant from the site primarily involved by the morbid process.
See also CANCER.
metastasize to form new foci of disease in a distant part by metastasis.
metastatic pertaining to or of the nature of a metastasis.
m. abscesses abscesses seeded down in tissues distant from a mother abscess.
m. calcification deposition of calcification in soft tissues, e.g. muscles and connective tissue.
metasternum the xiphoid process.
Metastrongylidae a family of nematode parasites, the adults of which invade the bronchi and lung parenchyma.
Metastrongyloidea a superfamily of nematodes whose members are found in the bronchi, parenchyma and blood vessels of the lungs; the lungworms.
Metastrongylus a genus of nematodes in the family Metastrongylidae.
M. apri see *M. elongatus* (below).
M. brevivaginatus see *M. pudendotectus* (below).
***M. elongatus* (syn. *M. apri*)** occurs in the bronchi and bronchioles of pigs, occasionally in ruminants and very rarely in humans. No significant pathogenic effect.
M. madagascariensis found in the bronchi of pigs, where it causes bronchitis, verminous pneumonia and loss of body weight.
***M. pudendotectus* (syn. *M. brevivaginatus*)** found in the lungs of pigs.
M. salmi a pig lungworm.
metatarsal 1. pertaining to the metatarsus. 2. a bone of the metatarsus.
m. pad see FOOTPAD.
m. spur see SPUR (3).
metatarsectomy excision or resection of a metatarsal bone.
metatarsophalangeal pertaining to the metatarsus and the phalanges of the hindlimb.
m. joint the joint formed by the metatarsus and phalanges. Called also fetlock.
metatarsus the part of the hindlimb between the tarsus and the first phalanx. In the cat and dog it contains five bones (metatarsals) extending from the tarsus to the phalanges. See also Table 10.
m. primus varus angulation of the first metatarsal bone toward the midline of the body, producing an angle sometimes of 20 degrees or more between its base and that of the second metatarsal bone.
metathalamus the part of the diencephalon composed of the medial and lateral geniculate bodies; often considered to be part of the thalamus.
Metathelazia a genus of nematode worms of the family Pneumospiruridae, found in the lungs.
M. ascaroides found in langur monkey.
M. californica found in various cats.
M. felis found in *Felis pardalis*, etc.
M. multipapillata found in hedgehogs.
Metatheria see MARSUPIAL.
metathesis 1. artificial transfer of a morbid process. 2. a chemical reaction in which an element or radical in one compound exchanges places with another element or radical in another compound.
metatrophic utilizing organic matter for food.
Metazoa the division of the animal kingdom that includes the multicellular animals, i.e. all animals except the Protozoa.

metazoan member of the zoological division of Metazoa.

metazoon pl. *metazoa* [Gr.] an individual organism of the Metazoa.

metazoonosis a zoonosis transmitted to vertebrate hosts by invertebrates. It depends on the invertebrate vectors or other intermediate hosts to complete the life cycle. Rift Valley fever, babesiosis and fascioliasis are examples.

metencephalon pl. *metencephala* [Gr.] 1. the part of the central nervous system comprising the pons and cerebellum. 2. the anterior of two brain vesicles formed by specialization of the rhombencephalon in the developing embryo.

meteorism tympanites; drum-like distension of the abdomen caused by the presence of gas in the abdomen or intestines.

meteorismus see METEORISM.

meteorotropism the possible response to influence by meteorological factors noted in certain biological events, such as sudden death, attacks of milk fever, joint pain, colic and traffic accidents.

meter the basic unit of linear measure of the metric system, being equivalent to 39.371 inches; abbreviated m. See also Table 3 and SI UNITS.

-meter word element. [Gr.] *instrument for measuring.*

metestrus the period of early corpus luteum development, commencing at the end of estrus and lasting until the beginning of dioestrus. Generally a period of 2 days, but in the bitch the term is usually taken to include the pseudopregnancy (40–90 days).

methacholine a synthetic choline ester with pharmacological effects similar to those of acetyl choline, but has little effect on alimentary tract and is little used in veterinary medicine.

methacycline a derivative of oxytetracycline with similar activity.

methadone a synthetic opioid agonist used for analgesia and sedation. Commonly used in horses.

methallibure an inhibitor of pituitary gonadotropin, used to control estrus in sows. It causes congenital defects of cranium and limbs in fetuses of sows fed the compound in early pregnancy.

methamphetamine, methylamphetamine a central nervous system stimulant and pressor drug; used as the hydrochloride salt. See also AMPHETAMINE.

methandienone, methandrostenolone an anabolic steroid with androgenic effects.

methane CH_4; an inflammable, explosive gas from decomposition of organic matter. Large amounts are produced in the rumen. Attempts have been made to use the output from slurry pits to heat the animal accommodation in the building overhead.

methanearsonate a preparation which includes two herbicides, monosodium methanearsonate (MSMA), disodium methanearsonate (DSMA). See also organic ARSENICAL.

methanethiol 1. a flammable gas used in the manufacture of pesticides and fungicides. Called also methyl mercaptan. 2. an inflammable gas with the odor of rotten cabbage. Produced in the intestine by the actions of anaerobic bacteria on albumin. 3. a toxic metabolite of methionine that induces hepatic coma and encephalopathy.

Methanobrewbacter ruminantium a bacterial resident of the rumen involved in its digestive processes.

methanol a mobile, colorless liquid widely used as a solvent; methyl alcohol. A potent poison causing death due to its toxic effect on cardiac muscle. A component of methylated spirit.

Methanosarcina barkeri one of the wide range of digestive bacteria in the ruminal population.

methantheline a quaternary amine with antimuscarinic activity similar to atropine; the bromide is used as a smooth muscle relaxant.

methaqualone a nonbarbiturate hypnotic similar to barbiturates in its effects.

metharbital a long-acting barbiturate used as a central nervous system depressant with anticonvulsant action.

methazolamide a carbonic anhydrase inhibitor used orally in the treatment of glaucoma.

MetHb methemoglobin.

metHb methemoglobin.

methemalbumin a brownish pigment formed in the blood by the binding of albumin with heme; indicative of intravascular hemolysis.

methemalbuminemia the presence of methemalbumin in the blood.

methemoglobin a compound formed from hemoglobin by oxidation of the iron atom from the ferrous to the ferric state. A small amount of methemoglobin is normally present in the blood, but injury or toxic agents convert a larger proportion of hemoglobin into methemoglobin, which does not function as an oxygen carrier. See also HEMOGLOBIN.

m. reductase pathway an intraerythrocyte enzyme system that maintains hemoglobin in a reduced state. A deficiency of the enzyme, resulting in the formation of methemoglobinemia with insufficient oxygenation of the blood, occurs in the dog.

methemoglobinemia methemoglobin in the blood, usually due to the toxic action of drugs or other agents, or to hemolytic processes. The common cause in food animals is nitrite poisoning. Clinically there is dyspnea and sometimes coffee colored mucosae.

congenital m. an inherited condition suspected in horses.

methemoglobinuria methemoglobin in the urine. Urine containing a high concentration of hemoglobin from an intravascular hemolysis may also contain large amounts of methemoglobin.

inherited m. congenital defect recorded in horses, characterized by pale mucosae, hemic heart murmur, decreased exercise tolerance, hemolytic anemia. Rare and unproven as an inherited defect.

methenamine a white crystalline powder used orally as a urinary antiseptic; in acidic urine it is hydrolyzed to formaldehyde and ammonia. Called also hexamine.

m. hippurate hexamine combined with hippuric acid.

m. mandelate a salt of hexamine and mandelic acid, used in infections of the urinary tract.

methenolone an anabolic steroid; used as the acetate or enanthate.

methetharimide see BEMEGRIDE.

methicillin a semisynthetic penicillin which is highly resistant to inactivation by penicillinase; its sodium salt is used parenterally.

methimazole a thiourea antithyroid drug used in the treatment of feline hyperthyroidism.

methiocarb an organophosphorus compound which is used as a molluscicide; it causes poisoning in many species, particularly dogs, with vomiting, diarrhea, salivation, pupillary constriction, bradycardia, muscular tremor and convulsions.

methionine Met; a sulfur-containing amino acid occurring in proteins, which is an essential component of the diet of animals.

m. deficiency exacerbates deficiencies of choline and vitamin B_{12}.

m. enkephalin met-enkephalin; see ENKEPHALIN.

m. sulfoximine the convulsant agent produced in flour by the agene process. Causes HYSTERIA in dogs, ferrets, rabbits and cats, but other species are not affected.

dl-methionine racemethionine. See METHIONINE.

methisazone a thiosemicarbazone derivative that inhibits RNA and protein synthesis. Used as an oral antiviral agent.

methocarbamol a compound used as a skeletal muscle relaxant, particularly in dogs with intervertebral disk disease.

method procedure for carrying out a particular task, e.g. investigating a hypothesis.

agreement m. when a particular factor is common to all occurrences of the disease, it may be that the common factor is the cause of the disease.

analogy m. when the circumstances of occurrence in one disease are similar to those in which another disease occurs, the diseases may come about in the same way even though the causes are different.

concomitant variation m. when variation in the frequency of the disease is mirrored by a similar variation in the strength of a particular agent which may be the cause.

difference m. when there are wide differences in the rate of occurrence of a disease and a high frequency is accompanied by the presence of the suspected cause and a low frequency by its absence.

nearest neighbor m. a method for establishing the population density of a particular species of animal or plant. One of the units is identified and the distance to its nearest neighbor of the same species measured. The number of units of that species in an area can then be established, the accuracy increasing with the number of measurements made.

methodology the science dealing with principles of procedure in research and study.

methohexital, methohexitone an ultra-short-acting barbiturate.

methomyl a carbamate insecticide capable of causing poisoning similar to oganophosphorus poisoning.

methoprene an insect growth regulator used to control ectoparasites on animals and in their environment. A common ingredient of household flea-bombs.

methotrexate a folic acid antagonist used as an antineoplastic agent.

methotrimeprazine a phenothiazine tranquilizer used as a sedative and antiemetic.

methoxamine a sympathomimetic amine used as the hydrochloride for its vasopressor effects.

5-methoxy-*N*-methyl-tryptamine toxic tryptamine found in *Phalaris* spp.

methoxy-pyridone (4-methoxy-) toxic pyridoxine analog found in *Albizia* spp.

methoxychlor one of the group of CHLORINATED HYDROCARBON insecticides which cause typical signs of that poisoning.

methoxycoumestrol, 4-methoxycoumestrol toxic coumestan, phytoestrogen, found in plants.

5-methoxydimethyltryptamine one of the toxic substances in the grass *Phalaris aquatica*.

methoxyethyl mercury silicate used as a fungistatic seed dressing. Feeding the grain to livestock can cause MERCURY poisoning.

methoxyflurane an ether derivative compound used as a general anesthetic administered by inhalation.

8-methoxypsoralen the photodynamic agent in AMMI *majus*.

methscopolamine see SCOPOLAMINE.

methyl the monovalent radical, $-CH_3$.

m. alcohol see methyl ALCOHOL.

m. bromide a soil and grain fumigant. Poisoning by this compound causes incoordination and somnolence. Called also bromoethane.

m. carbamate see PROPOXUR.

m. demeton an organophosphorus insecticide. Called also methyl systox, oxydemeton-methyl.

m. harmane (3-methyl) carboline toxin found in plants.

m. hydroxybenzoate see METHYLPARABEN.

m. *p*-hydroxybenzoate a sex pheromone in the vaginal secretions of the bitch in estrus; it stimulates mounting behavior in dogs.

m. orange an orange-yellow aniline dye, used as an indicator with a pH range of 3.2–4.4 and a color change from pink to yellow.

m. parathion a very toxic organophosphorus insecticide.

m. red test a biochemical test for identification of enterobacteria.

m. salicylate a natural or synthetic wintergreen oil, used as a topical analgesic and as a clearing agent when mounting parasites. Called also oil of sweet birch.

m. systox see methyl demeton (above).

methyl mercaptan see METHANETHIOL.

2-methyl,9-fluorocortisol synthetic adrenal corticoid.

methylases host cell enzymes that introduce methyl groups into bases of DNA. In prokaryotic cells two methyl groups are introduced into the palindromic sequences by the restriction endonucleases that recognize the palindrome; when methylated, the restriction enzyme does not cut the DNA so that methylation protects host cell DNA from cleavage.

methylate 1. a compound of methyl alcohol and a base. 2. to add a methyl group to a substance.

methylated spirit a mixture of methyl ALCOHOL (4%) and ethyl alcohol. Used as fuel, and as a skin disinfectant; poisonous if taken orally.

methylation the addition of methyl groups.

methylatropine see ATROPINE methobromide.

methylazoxymethanol the aglycone which is linked with a sugar to make the toxic glycosides cycasin and macrozamin in CYCADS. Called also MAM.

methylbenzene see TOLUENE.

methylbenzethonium chloride a quaternary ammonium compound used as a disinfectant and antiseptic.

methylcellulose a methyl ester of cellulose; used as a bulk laxative and applied topically to the cornea during certain ophthalmic procedures to protect and lubricate the cornea. Used also as an obstetrical lubricant and, in squeeze bottles, as a lubricant for rectal examinations in large animals.

methylcholanthrene a thyroid initiator, capable of initiating thyroid tumors.

methylconiine one of the toxic alkaloids in CONIUM MACULATUM.

***S*-methylcysteine sulfoxide** the naturally occurring substance in plants of family Brassicaceae which is metabolized in the rumen and converted to dimethyldisulfide, the hemolytic agent. Called also SMCO.

methylcytosine a pyrimidine occurring in deoxyribonucleic acid.

methylene blue a synthetic organic compound, in dark green crystals or lustrous crystalline powder, used in treatment of methemoglobinemia, as an antidote in cyanide poisoning, as a stain in pathology and bacteriology, and as an antiseptic.

m. b. dye binding test see SABIN–FELDMANN DYE TEST.

new m. b. stain see new methylene blue STAIN.

3,3′-methylene (4-hydroxycoumarin) the anticlotting agent in moldy sweet clover hay. Called also dicoumarol. See also MELILOTUS.

methylenebis (3, 4, 6-trichlorophenol) hexachlorophane.

methylergometrine maleate, methylergonovine maleate a compound used as an oxytocic.

methylergonovine see METHYLERGOMETRINE MALEATE.

methylestrenolene a compound used to suppress estrus in cats.

***N*-methylglucamine** see MEGLUMINE (1).

3-methylindole an ingested substance that causes damage to pulmonary tissue and the development of ATYPICAL INTERSTITIAL PNEUMONIA in cattle and horses.

methyllycaconitine diterpenoid alkaloid toxin found in plants.

methylmalonic acid a normal ruminant metabolite detoxified in animals receiving a diet adequate in cobalt. A high content in the urine suggests nutritional deficiency.

methylmalonyl CoA intermediate in the conversion of propionate into glucose.

m. CoA mutase vitamin B_{12} containing enzyme catalyzing the conversion of propionate into glucose.

methylmercurialism poisoning with organic mercurial compounds.

methylmercury compounds fungistatic agents used in stored feeds. They include methylmercury acetate, chloride, dicyandiamide and hydroxide. When treated grain is accidentally fed to livestock, poisoning may result. See MERCURY poisoning.

methylmethacrylate used in orthopedic surgery to construct protective structures, e.g. in laminectomy to protect the spinal meninges, in dentistry, and to cement prostheses.

methylmorphine see CODEINE.

***N*-methyl-*N*-nitrosourea** poisoning can cause a higher than normal incidence of thyroidal tumors.

methylparaben an antifungal and antibacterial agent used as a preservative in pharmaceutical preparations. Called also methyl hydroxybenzoate. See also HYDROXYBENZOATE.

***N*-methyl-β-phenethylamine** the toxin in the tree *Acacia berlandieri*.

methylphenidate a central nervous system stimulant used in the treatment of hyperkinesis and narcolepsy in dogs.

methylphenobarbital, mephobarbital, methylphenobarbitone related to phenobarbital, but produces less sedation; is used as an anticonvulsant in dogs.

methylprednisolone a glucocorticoid with anti-inflammatory action similar to that of prednisolone. The acetate is often prepared in long-acting forms while the water-soluble, rapid-acting succinate is suitable for intravenous administration and is used in the treatment of shock.

m.-21-dimethylaminoacetate a long-acting glucocorticoid, used in the treatment of dermatoses and allergic conditions.

4-methylpyrazole an inhibitor of alcohol dehydrogenase, used in the treatment of ethylene glycol poisoning.

methylrosaniline chloride see GENTIAN violet.

methylselenocysteine a selenium-containing amino acid found in the selenium converter plant ASTRAGALUS *bisulcatus*.

methyltestosterone an orally effective, synthetic form of testosterone.

methylthiouracil a thiourea antithyroid drug.

methyltransferase any enzyme that catalyzes transmethylation.

methyluracil compounds compounds used as herbicides which could cause poisoning at the levels used if animals are allowed access to treated pasture. Signs include bloat, incoordination and anorexia. Includes bromacil and isocil.

methylxanthine methylated derivatives of xanthine, including caffeine, theobromine and theophylline.

methysergide a potent serotonin antagonist.

metichlorpindol see CLOPIDOL.

metipranolol a β-blocker used to lower intraocular pressure in glaucoma.

metirosine, metyrosine L-tyrosine, an inhibitor of catecholamine synthesis used in the treatment of pheochromocytoma.

metmyoglobin a compound formed from myoglobin by oxidation of the ferrous to the ferric state with essentially ionic bonds.

metoclopramide a dopamine antagonist that stimulates motility of the upper gastrointestinal tract, relaxes the pyloric sphincter, and promotes gastric emptying. Used as an antiemetic.

metocurine iodide a nondepolarizing muscle relaxant, similar to *d*-tubocurarine.

metoestrus see METESTRUS.

Metol a common developing agent for use with x-ray films. Commonly used together with hydroquinone.

metolazone a diuretic and saluretic.

metomidate a nonbarbiturate hypnotic with minimal analgesia; used in pigs and birds, especially raptors. It is often used in combination with azaperone.

metopic pertaining to the forehead.

metoprolol a cardioselective BETA-blocker having a greater effect on β_1-adrenergic receptors of the heart than on β_2-adrenergic receptors of the bronchi and blood vessels. Used as the tartrate.

Metorchis a genus of flukes (digenetic trematodes) parasitic in the gallbladder and bile ducts, members of the family Opisthorchiidae.

M. albidis found in dogs, cats, fox, gray seal; also in birds and humans.

M. conjunctus found in cat, dog, mink, raccoon, fox.

metoserpate a rauwolfia derivative, administered as the hydrochloride in drinking water to fowls as a tranquilizer before handling.

metoxenous requiring two hosts for the entire life cycle.

metra the uterus.

metra-, metro- word element. [Gr.] *uterus*.

metratonia uterine atony.

metratrophia atrophy of the uterus.

metre see METER.

metrectasia dilatation of the nonpregnant uterus.

metreurynter an inflatable bag for dilating the cervical canal of the uterus.

metreurysis dilatation of the cervix uteri by means of the metreurynter.

metric 1. of or pertaining to the metric system. 2. pertaining to measures or measurement. 3. having the meter as a basis.

m. system the system of units of measurement that is based on the meter, gram and liter, and in which new units are formed by prefixes denoting multiplication by a power of ten. See also Tables 4.1 to 4.6.

metrifonate an organophosphorus insecticide. See TRICHLORFON.

metritis inflammation of the uterus.
contagious equine m. called also CEM. See CONTAGIOUS equine metritis.
m. dissecans metritis with necrosis of portions of the uterine wall.
mastitis–m.–agalactia see MASTITIS–METRITIS–AGALACTIA.
puerperal m. infection of the pregnant uterus.
purulent m. see PYOMETRA.
septic m. metritis with a severe systemic reaction, either as a toxemia or a septicemia.
metritis–mastitis–agalactia in sows see MASTITIS–METRITIS–AGALACTIA.
metrizamide a nonionic, water-soluble, iodinated radiographic contrast medium used in myelography and cisternography. Replaced by newer contrast media because of a high rate of side-effects.
metrocele hernia of the uterus.
metrocolpocele hernia of the uterus with vaginal prolapse.
metrocystosis formation of cysts in the uterus.
metrodynia pain in the uterus.
Metroliasthes a genus of tapeworms in the family Paruterinidae.
M. lucida found in the small intestine of fowl and turkeys.
metrology the study of weights and measures used in prescription writing.
metrolymphangitis inflammation of the uterine lymphatic vessels.
metromalacia, metromalacoma abnormal softening of the uterus.
metronidazole an antimicrobial compound effective against protozoa and anaerobic bacteria. Commonly used to treat trichomoniasis, amebiasis, giardiasis and balantidiasis.
metroparalysis paralysis of the uterus.
metropathia any disorder of the uterus.
metropathy any uterine disorder.
metroperitoneal pertaining to the uterus and peritoneum.
metroperitonitis inflammation of the peritoneum about the uterus.
metrophlebitis inflammation of the uterine veins.
metroplasty reconstructive surgery on the uterus.
metroptosis prolapse of the uterus.
metrorrhagia uterine bleeding, usually of normal amount. Occurs normally in cows.
metrorrhea abnormal uterine discharge.
metrorrhexis rupture of the uterus.
metrosalpingitis inflammation of the uterus and uterine tubes.
metrosalpingography hysterosalpingography; radiography of the uterus and uterine tubes.
metroscope an instrument for examining the uterus.
metrostaxis slight but persistent uterine bleeding.
metrostenosis stenosis of the uterus.
-metry word element. [Gr.] *measurement*.
metyrapone a compound that selectively inhibits adrenocortical 11β-dehydroxylase and the synthesis of cortisol.
m. test blood levels of cortisol and 11-desoxycortisol are measured, before and after administration of metapyrone. In pituitary dependent hyperadrenocorticism, there is a decrease in cortisol and increase in 11-deoxycortisol; both values decrease if there is an adrenal tumor.
Metzenbaum scissors lightly built curved scissors with blunt-pointed, narrow blades.
Meuse–Rhine–Yssel red pied, dual-purpose European cattle. Called also Dutch red and white.
MEV mink enteritis virus.
MeV megaelectron volt.
mevalonic acid a step in the synthesis of cholesterol in the body. It is the rate of synthesis limiting step and the site of dietary control.
mevinphos an organophosphorus insecticide. Light poisoning can cause pupillary constriction in the absence of other signs. Called also phosdrin.
mew, miaow the vocal sound characteristic of domestic cats; in various languages it is spelled in 31 different ways, which include ‘miaow’, ‘meow’, ‘myaus’, ‘mio’, and ‘mau’. See also VOCALIZATION.
Mexican named after or originating in Mexico.
M. axolotl see AMBYSTOMA *mexicanum*.
M. beaded lizard (*Heloderma horridum*) a venomous lizard of North America whose bite causes local tissue reaction, vomiting, shock and central nervous system depression.
M. blue eye see porcine PARAMYXOVIRUS encephalomyelitis.
M. fireweed see KOCHIA SCOPARIA.
M. hairless a small lively dog with smooth skin that is hairless except on the head, feet and tip of the tail. The breed, which is recognized in the USA, is very similar to the Chinese Crested dog, and other hairless breeds. The body temperature is higher, about 104°F (40°C) than the normal range for domestic dogs.
M. poppy ARGEMONE *mexicana*, *A. ochroleuca*.
M. walking fish see AMBYSTOMA *mexicanum*.
M. rue PEGANUM *mexicana*.
M. tea see CHENOPODIUM *ambrosioides*.
M. walking fish Mexican axolotl (above).
M. whorled milkweed ASCLEPIAS *mexicana*.
mexiletine a cardiac antiarrhythmic agent with action similar to lignocaine, used in the treatment of heart disease in dogs.
Meyerding retractors a handheld retractor with a thumb grip at one end and a curved, sharp-toothed blade at the other. It is used for retracting large muscles during orthopedic surgery.
mezerein, mezereum an intensely irritating resin whose action resembles that of cantharides. Signs include vomiting, colic, prostration. The seeds and bark of *Daphne mezereum* and *D. laureola* are the important sources of the poison.
mezereinic acid the anhydride of this acid is MEZEREIN.
mezereon DAPHNE *mezereum*.
mezereum see MEZEREIN.
mezlocillin a ureidopenicillin with a broad spectrum of activity.
MF mitogenic factor.
M'Fadyean's reaction see MCFADYEAN'S REACTION.
MFD minimum fatal dose.
Mg chemical symbol, *magnesium*.
mg milligram.
μg microgram.
Mg^2+ magnesium ion.
MH malignant hyperthermia.
MHA microangiopathic hemolytic ANEMIA.
MHC major histocompatibility complex.
mho see SIEMENS.
MHV mouse hepatitis virus.
miaow see MEW.
miasma noxious exhalations from putrescent organic matter; the basis for an early concept of the origin of epidemics.
mibolerone a synthetic androgenic, anabolic, antigonadotrophic steroid used to control estrus in dogs; contraindicated for use in cats. Called also dimethylnortestosterone.

MIC minimal inhibitory concentration.
mica a heat-resistant transparent mineral found in large glass-like sheets and used in windows of furnaces; may have a high content of fluorine but seems unlikely to affect animals.
mication a quick motion, such as winking.
mice plural form of MOUSE.
micelle a supermolecular colloid particle, most often a packet of chain molecules in parallel arrangement. A stage in the luminal phase of fat digestion; bile salts form spheres containing fatty acids, monoglycerides and the fat-soluble vitamins.
critical m. concentration the concentration of bile salts in solutions at which they aggregate into poymolecular aggregates called micelles.
Michaelis constant, Michaelis–Mentin constant see $K_{7/8}$ CONSTANT.
Michaelis–Menten rate law specific rate law governing enzymatic reactions in steady-state with the constants, V_{max} and K_M.
Michel named after Gaston Michel, a French surgeon (1875–1937).
M. clip metal skin sutures in various sizes from 8 to 16 mm long. Each clip is a 2 mm wide band of metal with a downturned sharp prong at each end. When the clip is bent double the points face each other and approximate. There is a special instrument for applying and removing the clips. They are excellent in design and concept but can be easily removed by rubbing.
M.'s trephine a heavy-duty trephine with an adjustable head for cutting holes in bone of 0.5 to 0.8 mm diameter.
Michel's fixative a tissue fixative used for preservation of skin biopsy specimens to be examined by direct immunofluorescent testing for demonstration of tissue-fixed immunoglobulins.
Michigan test an indirect test on milk carried out to determine whether mastitis is present in the gland. Is based on the formation of a gel when there are a large number of cells in the sample. Now largely superseded by milk cell counts.
miconazole an imidazole antifungal agent used topically as the nitrate in the treatment of fungal and yeast infections of the skin.
micrencephaly abnormal smallness and underdevelopment of the brain.
micr(o)- word element. [Gr.] *small;* used in naming units of measurement to designate an amount 10^{-6} (one-millionth) the size of the unit to which it is joined; symbol μ, e.g. microgram (μg).
microabscess abscess visible only under a microscope.
Munro m. a small collection of neutrophils within or under the stratum corneum.
Pautrier m. a collection of malignant lymphocytes in the epidermis occurring as solid intraepidermal nodules; seen in epitheliotropic lymphomas.
microadenoma an adenoma less than 0.5 inch diameter.
microaerophilic requiring oxygen for growth but at a lower concentration than is present in the atmosphere, in conjunction with an enhanced carbon dioxide concentration; said of bacteria.
microagglutination test see microscopic AGGLUTINATION test.
microaggregate a microscopic collection of particles, such as platelets, leukocytes or fibrin, that occurs in stored blood.
microalgae unicellular aquatic plants (phytoplankton), the starting point of the aquatic food chain. Include toxic microalgae which are important causes of marine fish mortalities, especially *Alexandrium*, *Chaltonella*, *Heterosigma* spp., and pathogenic microalgae, e.g. *Chaetoceros* spp., phytoplankton with long, sharp spines which penetrate the gills of fish.
microanalysis the chemical analysis of minute quantities of material.
microanatomy see HISTOLOGY.
microaneurysm a minute aneurysm occurring on a vessel of small size, such as one in the retina of the eye or as occurs in thrombotic purpura.
microangiopathic having the characteristics of microangiopathy.
m. hemolytic anemia see microangiopathic ANEMIA.
microangiopathy a disorder involving the small blood vessels.
cerebrospinal m. in pigs is manifested by depression, incoordination, aimless wandering, circling and wasting. The characteristic microangiopathy is not restricted to the nervous system. Thought to be a sequel to chronic EDEMA disease.
dietetic m. one of the less commonly occurring lesions that can be prevented by the dietary addition of selenium and vitamin E.
thrombotic m. formation of thrombi in the arterioles and capillaries.
microatelectasis lung collapse visible only by microscope.
microbe a microorganism, especially a pathogenic bacterium.
microbial pertaining to or emanating from a microbe.
m. digestion the breakdown of organic material, especially feedstuffs, by microbial organisms. It is the basis of the functioning of the rumen, the large intestine of the horse, and a significant part of the digestive process in the crop of birds. The function can be seriously damaged by the prolonged or heavy dosing of the animal with antibiotics or sulfonamides.
m. flora see MICROBIOTA.
microbicidal destroying microbes.
microbicide an agent that destroys microbes.
microbiologist a specialist in microbiology.
microbiology the study of microorganisms, including bacteria, fungi, viruses and pathogenic protoza, and the diseases they cause.
microbiota the microscopic living organisms of a region. Called also microbial flora.
microblast an erythroblast of 5 μm or less in diameter.
microblepharia abnormal shortness of the vertical dimensions of the eyelids.
microbody any of the cytoplasmic particles found in kidney and liver cells and in certain other cells, surrounded by a limiting membrane, and containing dense crystalline-like inclusions and oxidases.
microbrachius a fetus with abnormally small forelimbs.
Microcalliphora see CHRYSOMYA.
microcapillary a small capillary.
m. hematocrit see MICROHEMATOCRIT.
microcardia abnormal smallness of the heart.
Microcebus see LEMUR.
microcephalus an animal with a very small head.
microcephaly small size of the head in relation to the rest of the body.
microcheilia abnormal smallness of the lips.
microchromosomes very small chromosomes found only in avian karyotypes.
microcirculation the flow of blood through the fine vessels (arterioles, capillaries and venules).
microclimate the temperature, humidity, pH and air

movement at a particular level, usually an interface between two systems, e.g. ground and air, skin and air.

Micrococcaceae a family of gram-positive, catalase-positive, aerobic or facultatively anaerobic spherical bacteria, containing *Staphylococcus* and *Micrococcus.*

micrococci any bacteria belonging to the Micrococcaceae.

Micrococcus a genus of gram-positive coccoid bacteria of the family Micrococcaceae found in soil, water, etc.

micrococcus pl. *micrococci* [Gr.] any organism of the genus *Micrococcus.*

microcolon abnormal smallness of the colon.

microcomputer stand-alone computers with limited memory both as random access memory and as storage on linked floppy disks or hard disks. Single computers can be linked together to give access to a larger database storage; they can also be linked to other computers, especially a mainframe computer, by a modem and can utilize all the resources, especially speed and size of storage, that the large machines offer. See also COMPUTER.

microconidium pl. *microconidia;* small conidia, as produced by *Trichophyton.*

microcoria smallness of the pupil.

microcornea unusual smallness of the cornea, usually bilateral.

Microcotyle a monogenetic trematode of marine fish that attaches to the skin of the host.

microcotyledons a microscopic grouping together of villi in the equine placenta in a manner similar to that in ruminants.

microcryoepilation use of freezing to destroy hair follicles; used in distichiasis.

microcrystalline made up of minute crystals.

microcurie one-millionth (10^{-6}) curie; abbreviated μCi. A non-SI unit, now replaced by the BECQUEREL.

microcurie-hour a non-SI unit of dose equivalent to that obtained by exposure for one hour to radioactive material disintegrating at the rate of 3.7×10^4 atoms per second; abbreviated μCi-h.

microcyst a cyst visible only under a microscope.

microcystin a group of toxic cyclic decapeptides, the hepatotoxins in some cyanobacteria. See also MICROCYSTIS, ANABAENA, GLOEOTRICHIA, OSCILLATORIA, NOSTOC RIVULARE.

Microcystis a genus of the CYANOBACTERIA; produces a peptide toxin, microcystin, which causes acute liver necrosis. Includes *M. aeruginosa*, *M. flosaquae* (*M. toxica*, *Anacystis cyanea*), *M. viridis* (*Anacystis*). Called also *Anacystis*, *Gloeotrichia*.

microcystoid retinal degeneration common retinal abnormality in the dog but of no apparent functional significance; called also cystic retinal degeneration.

microcyte an erythrocyte that has a smaller diameter than is normal for the species in which it occurs.

microcythemia, microcytosis a condition in which the erythrocytes are smaller than normal.

microdactyly abnormal smallness of the digits.

microdissection dissection of tissue or cells under the microscope.

microdontia abnormal smallness of the teeth.

microeconomics study of the economic behavior of individual, decision-making units, e.g. individual consumers or businesses, and the operation of individual markets. See also MACROECONOMICS.

microembolus pl. *microemboli* [L.] an embolus of microscopic size.

microencapsulation a manufacturing process in which an active agent is contained in microcapsules, suspended in a liquid. As the vehicle dries, the capsules dry out and the contents become active. Used to apply insecticides in order to prolong their period of effectiveness, usually for several days, and to reduce the hazard of ingestion by dogs and cats.

microencephaly small size of the brain. Usually accompanied by MICROCEPHALY.

microerythrocyte microcyte.

microfarad one-millionth (10^{-6}) farad; abbreviated μF.

microfauna microscopic animals, e.g. protozoa.

microfibril an extremely small fibril.

microfilament any of the submicroscopic filaments composed chiefly of actin, found in the cytoplasmic matrix of almost all cells, often in close association with the microtubules.

microfilaremia the presence of microfilariae in the circulating blood.

microfilaria the larva of worms in the superfamily Filarioidea. They are produced by adult worms residing in the bloodstream, tissues or body cavities, from where they can be ingested by biting insects. There they pass through a developmental stage and are transmitted to another permanent host when it is bitten by the insect. The microfilariae of some species are nocturnal and are therefore available for transmission only at night.

microfilarial emanating from or pertaining to microfilariae.

m. pityriasis a name given to a seasonal skin lesion on the backs of horses, characterized by hair loss and severe pruritus. Some of the lesions contain microfilariae, hence the name; but many of the cases appear to be allergic dermatitis. See also equine ALLERGIC dermatitis.

microfilariasis any disease caused by microfilariae. Includes equine microfilarial pityriasis, heartworm in dogs, filarial dermatoses, cerebrospinal nematodiasis and miscellaneous localizations in individual organs, e.g. *Onchocerca* spp. invasions of the eye.

microflora living microorganisms that are so small that they can be seen only with a microscope and that maintain a more or less constant presence in a particular area, e.g. the pharynx or the rumen. Includes bacteria, viruses, protozoa, fungi.

microgamete the smaller, actively motile male gamete which fertilizes the macrogamete in anisogamy.

microgametocyte a cell that produces microgametes.

microgastria congenital smallness of the stomach.

microgenia abnormal smallness of the chin.

microgenitalism smallness of the external genitalia.

microglia non-neural cells forming part of the adventitial structure of the central nervous system. They are migratory and act as phagocytes of waste products of the nervous system.

microgliosis accumulation of microglial cells as a reaction to injury to the parenchyma of the central nervous system, a characteristic of nonsuppurative encephalomyelitis.

microglobulin any globulin, or any fragment of a globulin, of low molecular weight.

β_2 m. a polypeptide found free in serum and which also combines with the α (heavy) chain to form class I major histocompatibility heterodimer. See also major HISTOCOMPATIBILITY complex.

microglossia abnormal smallness of the tongue.

micrognathia abnormal smallness of the jaws, especially the lower jaw.

microgram one-millionth (10^{-6}) gram, or one-thousandth (10^{-3}) milligram; abbreviated μg.
micrograph 1. an instrument for recording very minute movements by making a greatly magnified photograph of the minute motions of a diaphragm. 2. a photograph of a minute object or specimen as seen through a microscope.
electron m. see ELECTRON micrographs.
microgyria the convolutions in the cerebral cortex are smaller and more numerous than usual and the normal gyral pattern may be lost.
microgyrus pl. *microgyria;* an abnormally small, malformed convolution of the brain.
microhabitat the normal environment, the natural home, of a microorganism.
microhematocrit a method for rapid determination of the packed cell volume by high-speed centrifugation of blood contained in capillary tubes.
Drummond m. a high speed centrifuge used for microhematocrit determinations. See also ADAMS AUTOCRIT.
microhepatia a small liver.
microinfarct a very small infarct due to obstruction of circulation in capillaries, arterioles or small arteries.
microingredient a ration ingredient, such as minerals, vitamins, antibiotics, estimated to be present in parts per million or milligrams or micrograms per ton of feed.
microinjection a method in which very finely drawn glass pipettes held in a finely adjustable mechanical device are used to introduce new materials (antibodies, organelles, DNA) into cells as they are visualized under a microscope.
microinjector an instrument for infusion of very small amounts of fluids or drugs.
microinvasion microscopic extension of malignant cells into adjacent tissue.
microlesion a minute lesion.
microliter one-millionth (10^{-6}) part of a liter, or one-thousandth (10^{-3}) of a milliliter; abbreviated μl.
microlith a minute concretion or calculus.
microlithiasis the formation of minute concretions in an organ.
m. alveolaris pulmonum a rare condition in dogs of unknown etiology. There is deposition of minute calculi in the alveoli of the lungs and progressively compromised pulmonary function so that the affected dog shows dyspnea, cough and fatigue. Called also pulmonary calcinosis, and pumice-stone lung. Called also pulmonary alveolar microlithiasis.
pulmonary alveolar m. see microlithiasis alveolaris pulmonum (above).
micromanipulation the performance of surgery, injections, dissections, etc., by means of micromanipulators.
micromanipulator an instrument for the moving, dissecting, etc., of minute specimens under the microscope.
micromastia abnormal smallness of the mammary gland.
micromelia abnormal smallness of one or more extremities.
micromelus an animal with abnormally small limbs.
micromere one of the small blastomeres formed by unequal cleavage of a fertilized ovum.
micrometeorology study of the climate of a microhabitat or a microclimate.
micrometer 1. instrument for making minute measurements. 2. micron; one thousandth (10^{-3}) of a millimeter or one millionth (10^{-6}) of a meter. Abbreviated μm. 3. see MICRON.
micromethod a technique dealing with exceedingly small quantities of material.
micrometry measurement of microscopic objects.
micromicro- word element designating 10^{-12} (one-million-millionth) part of the unit to which it is joined; now supplanted by the prefix pico-.
Micromonospora purpurea an organism, cultures of which produce the antibiotic gentamicin.
micromyelia abnormal smallness of spinal cord.
micromyeloblast a small, immature myelocyte.
Micromys a genus of rodents in the subfamily Murinae of Old World rats and mice.
M. minutus the small, 2 to 3 inch, red-brown Eurasian harvest mouse.
micron pl. *micra, microns* [Gr.] micrometer; one thousandth (10^{-3}) of a millimeter or one millionth (10^{-6}) of a meter; abbreviated μm.
microneedle a fine glass needle used in micromanipulation.
Micronema deletrix a saprophytic worm usually found in decaying organic matter but also found in lesions about the head and in internal organs of a horse, including the brain.
microneurosurgery surgery conducted under high magnification with miniaturized instruments on microscopic vessels and structures of the nervous system.
micronization a process for preparing medication in which the particle size is greatly reduced, thereby increasing absorption following oral administration.
micronize an industrial process of heating grain or pharmaceuticals with microwaves from infrared burners and then rolling to achieve a standard size. The purpose is to produce a dry, free-flowing product.
micronodular marked by the presence of small nodules.
micronucleus 1. in ciliate protozoa, the kinetoplast, the smaller of two types of nucleus in each cell, which functions in sexual reproduction. 2. a small nucleus. 3. nucleolus.
micronutrient a dietary element essential only in small quantities.
micronychia abnormal smallness of the claws.
microorchidia, microorchidism abnormal smallness of the testicle.
microorganism a microscopic organism; those of veterinary interest include bacteria, rickettsiae, viruses, fungi and protozoa.
micropalpebral fissure an abnormally narrow or small eyelid opening. Can be associated with other ocular abnormalities such as microphthalmos. Sometimes apparent rather than real, because of the size or position of the globe.
micropapilla a small optic disk without blindness.
micropathology 1. the sum of what is known about minute pathological change. 2. pathology of diseases caused by microorganisms.
microphage a small phagocyte; an actively motile neutrophilic leukocyte capable of phagocytosis.
microphakia abnormal smallness of the crystalline lens. Inherited as a congenital defect, together with other ocular defects, in cattle.
Microphallidae a family of intestinal digenetic trematodes that parasitize anserine and gallinaceous birds and may cause losses if the infestations are heavy.
microphallus abnormal smallness of the penis.
microphone a device to pick up sound for purposes of amplification or transmission.
microphonia marked weakness of voice.
microphonic 1. serving to amplify sound. 2. cochlear microphonic.

cochlear m. any of the electrical potentials generated in the hair cells of the organ of Corti in response to acoustic stimulation.

microphotograph a photograph of small size.

microphthalmia see MICROPHTHALMOS.

microphthalmos abnormal smallness in all dimensions of one or both eyes, sometimes in association with other ocular abnormalities. Recorded as occurring in piglets from sows on vitamin A-deficient diets in early pregnancy, and in dogs, where it is associated with collie eye anomaly and is an inherited defect in some breeds.

pure. m. see NANOPHTHALMOS.

micropinocytosis pinocytosis.

micropipette a pipette for handling small quantities of liquids (up to 1 ml).

microplethysmography the recording of minute changes in the size of a part as produced by circulation of blood.

micropodia abnormal smallness of the feet.

Micropolyspora faeni a thermophilic actinomycete which produces spores in moldy hay. The spores are inhaled by cattle eating the hay and cause granulomas and bronchitis, bronchiolitis, and a chronic interstitial pneumonia. It is also associated with chronic obstructive pulmonary disease in horses.

microprobe a minute probe, such as one used in microsurgery.

microprocessor the central processing unit of a COMPUTER.

Micropterus salmoides finfish in family Centrarchidae. Called also largemouth bass. See Table 23.

micropyle an opening through which a spermatozoon enters certain ova.

microradiography radiography under conditions that permit subsequent microscopic examination or enlargement of the radiograph up to several hundred linear magnifications.

microrespirometer an apparatus for investigating oxygen utilization in isolated tissues.

microscope an instrument used to obtain an enlarged image of small objects and reveal details of structure not otherwise distinguishable.

acoustic m. one using very high frequency ultrasound waves, which are focused on the object; the reflected beam is converted to an image by electronic processing.

binocular m. one with two eyepieces, permitting use of both eyes simultaneously.

bright-field m. the standard bench microscope used in histology and requiring stained tissue sections.

compound m. the standard laboratory microscope used in veterinary science; consists of a two lens system whereby the image formed by the system near the object (objective) is magnified by the one nearer the eye (eyepiece).

confocal scanning m. one that utilizes a focused laser beam to visualize fluorescent molecules in a single plane.

darkfield m. used for examining unstained, often living cells, in which light is only directed into the objective lens if it is deflected by an object in its path. The object is thus viewed as a white structure in an otherwise black (darkfield) background.

electron m. one using an electron beam of very short wavelength as the source of illumination. It has a resolving power of 2 nm (which is 100 times greater than with the light microscope). Includes the transmission electron microscope and the scanning electron microscope (below). See also immunoelectron MICROSCOPY.

fluorescence m. one used for the examination of specimens stained with fluorochromes or fluorochrome complexes, e.g. a fluorescein-labeled antibody, which fluoresces in ultraviolet light. See also FLUORESCENCE microscopy.

interference m. a microscope similar to the phase contrast microscope but delivers a three-dimensional image. Called also Nomarski interference phase microscope.

light m. used for examining unstained or stained particles or the cellular structure of tissues that have been cut into sections and stained. It has a resolving power of 0.2 μm. Modern light microscopes have an eyepiece and objective lenses which provide magnification, and a condenser beneath the stage which gathers and focuses light on the object being examined.

operating m. one designed for use in performance of delicate surgical procedures, e.g. on the middle ear, eye or small vessels of the heart.

phase m., phase-contrast m. a form of light microscope useful for examining living, unstained structures, including animal cells and bacteria, e.g. leptospira. The phase of the light wave passing through different structures in the cell, e.g. nucleus vs. thin part of the cytoplasm, is changed by different amounts and thereby provides contrast.

polarizing m. based on the phenomenon of birefringence; useful in the study of bone and muscle.

scanning electron m. (SEM) an electron microscope that produces a high-magnification image of the surface of a metal-coated specimen (shadow casting) by scanning an electron beam and building up an image from the electrons reflected at each point. Particularly useful for determining the three-dimensional structure of objects.

simple m. one that consists of a single lens.

specular m. one used in the examination of the corneal endothelium.

stereoscopic m. a binocular microscope modified to give a three-dimensional view of the specimen.

surgical m. see operating microscope (above).

transmission electron m., TEM one that resembles an inverted light microscope in that the beam of electrons generated from a heated filament at the top of the instrument passes down through a column where it is focused by magnetic coils (lenses) and is differentially scattered when it passes through the specimen. The image is recorded either on a photographic plate or on a phosphorescent screen.

ultraviolet m. uses an ultraviolet light source; useful in histochemical studies; only photographic images are available.

microscopic of extremely small size; visible only with the aid of a microscope.

m. agglutination test see microscopic AGGLUTINATION test.

microscopical pertaining to a microscope or to microscopy.

microscopist a person skilled in using a microscope.

microscopy examination with a microscope.

immunoelectron m. the mixing of antibody with an antigen such as a virus on a specimen grid so as to increase the probability of visualizing a virus and to identify (type) the kind of virus present in the specimen, or antibody may be conjugated with gold and used to visualize and determine the location of specific antigenic determinants on a specimen.

microsecond one-millionth (10^{-6}) of a second; abbreviated μs or μsec.

microsomal pertaining to or emanating from microsome.
microsomatic having a poor sense of smell, e.g. primates.
microsome any of the vesicular fragments of endoplasmic reticulum produced during disruption and centrifugation of cells.
microsomia abnormally small size of the body.
microspectroscope a spectroscope and microscope combined.
microspherocyte an erythrocyte whose diameter is less than normal, but whose thickness is increased.
microspherocytosis the presence in the blood of an excessive number of microspherocytes.
microsphygmia that condition of the pulse in which it is perceived with difficulty by the finger.
microsplenia smallness of the spleen.
microsporid a secondary skin eruption which is an expression of hypersensitivity to *Microsporum* infection.
Microsporidia an order of the subphylum Sporozoa characterized by having small spores and one polar capsule. Common occurrence is as parasites of arthropods and fish. Includes NOSEMA. In finfish may cause xenomas, in crustaceans cause 'cotton flesh'.
microsporidiosis infection by species of the genus *Microsporidia*; common infections in flounder and other marine fish and in ornamental fish; include *Thelohania* and *Pleistophora* spp.
Microsporum a genus of fungi that cause various diseases of the skin and hair, referred to as RINGWORM. The sexual state is known as *Nannizia*.
M. audouinii an anthropophilic species which may occasionally infect domestic animals.
M. canis causes ringworm in dogs, cats, humans and occasionally other animals.
M. distortum principally an infection of laboratory primates, but occurs also in dogs and cats.
M. fulvum occasionally infects pigs, goats, monkeys, jaguars and lions.
M. gallinae causes favus in chickens and turkeys.
M. gypseum a soil dermatophyte that causes ringworm in dogs, horses and sometimes other species.
M. nanum causes ringworm in pigs and rarely other animals and humans.
M. persicolor infects voles.
Microstix-3 trademark for a reagent strip with a chemical test area for recognition of nitrite in urine that turns pink on contact with nitrate, and two culture areas for semiquantification of bacterial growth after 18–24 hours of incubation; one culture area supports both gram-negative and gram-positive organisms; the other, only gram-negative organisms.
microstomia abnormally decreased size of the mouth.
microsurgery dissection of minute structures under the microscope, with the use of extremely small instruments.
microsyringe a syringe fitted with a screw-threaded micrometer for accurate measurement of minute quantities.
Microtetramere a genus of spirurid nematode found in the proventriculus of birds.
Microthoracius a genus of sucking lice in the family Linognathidae.
M. cameli found on camels and dromedaries.
M. mazzai, M. minor, M. praelongiceps found on the neck of the llama.
microtia abnormal smallness of the pinna of the ear.
microtine said of rodents which belong to the subfamily Microtinae, e.g. voles, lemmings and muskrats.
microtiter a titer determined using small volumes of reagents.
microtitration procedure for titrating substances such as antibiotics, antibodies or viruses in which small volumes are used, often 0.025 or 0.05 ml, using special delivery and transfer equipment referred to as diluters, droppers or micropipettes. Commonly performed in 96 well plastic plates.
microtome an instrument for making thin sections for microscopic study.
freezing m. one for cutting frozen tissues.
rotary m. one in which wheel action is translated into a back-and-forth movement of the specimen being sectioned.
sliding m. one in which the specimen being sectioned is made to slide on a track.
microtomy the cutting of thin sections.
microtrauma a microscopic lesion or injury.
microtubule any of the slender, tubular structures composed chiefly of tubulin, found in the cytoplasmic ground substance of nearly all cells; they are involved in maintenance of cell shape and in the movements of organelles and inclusions, and form the spindle fibers of mitosis.
m.-associated protein (MAP) any of the high molecular weight proteins that bind to microtubules, enhancing polymerization.
m. organizing center (MTOC) the location in a cell from which microtubules regrow after depolymerization. See also CENTROSOME.
Microtus see VOLE.
microurolith microscopic urolith.
microvasculature the finer vessels of the body, such as the arterioles, capillaries and venules.
microvent ventilator see MINIVENT VENTILATOR.
microvesicle microscopic vesicle.
microvillus pl. *microvilli;* a minute process of protrusion from the free surface of a cell, especially cells of the proximal convolution in renal tubules and of the intestinal epithelium.
microvolt one-millionth (10^{-6}) of a volt; abbreviated μV.
microwave a wave typical of electromagnetic radiation between far infrared and radiowaves.
m. acupuncture utilizes deeply penetrating heat, produced by a microwave generator and transmitted via acupuncture needles.
micrurgy manipulative technique in the field of a microscope.
micturate urinate.
micturition urination.
m. disorders includes neurogenic disorders controlling urination, urinary incontinence from several causes, and behavioral disorders. See also INCONTINENCE, URINARY BLADDER, elimination BEHAVIOR, ectopic URETER and inappropriate micturition (below).
inappropriate m. done at the wrong time or place, as dogs or cats urinating in the house or away from a litter tray. See also SPRAYING.
m. reflex the sequence of neurological impulses and muscular responses that controls the retention and release of urine.
mid-lactation in a ten month lactation in a cow, month 2 to month 8, the peak of the lactation.
midazolam maleate a potent, short-acting benzodiazepine, similar to diazepam, suitable for intravenous injection, for use as a taming agent and for induction of anesthesia.
midbrain the short part of the brainstem just rostral to the pons. It contains the nerve pathways between the

cerebral hemispheres and the medulla oblongata, and also contains nuclei of the third and fourth cranial nerves. The centers for visual and auditory reflexes, such as moving the head and eyes, are located in the midbrain. Called also mesencephalon.

m. lesion causes spastic paresis or paralysis, tremor, nystagmus, opisthotonos and depression or coma.

midcrop mortality syndrome cause of severe mortality of Australian cultured prawns. Multifactorial cause including a yellow-head-like virus.

midden dungheap.

middle burner syndrome chronic lung problems caused by the accumulation of fluid in the lungs due primarily to splenic and pancreatic dysfunction.

middle ear see EAR, OTITIS media.

m. e. cavity cavity of the middle ear made up of the tympanic bulla and the epitympanic recess.

m. e. ossicles see OSSICLE.

middlings a by-product of the milling industry used as a protein supplement in diets for ruminants and pigs. A finer grade of offal than bran and it approximates POLLARD or shorts. The nomenclature is poorly defined.

midges see CERATOPOGONIDAE and CULICOIDES.

midget ACACIA *osswaldii.*

midgut the region of the embryonic digestive tube into which the yolk sac opens; ahead of it is the foregut and caudal to it is the hindgut.

midline the imaginary line that divides the body into right and left halves.

midshaft midway between the epiphyses of a long bone.

Miescher's tubes cysts of SARCOCYSTIS. Called also Miescher's corpuscles, tubules and Rainey's corpuscles and tubules, all expressions used in human medicine.

MIF 1. melanocyte-stimulating hormone-inhibiting factor. 2. macrophage migration inhibition factor.

mifepristone a compound with antiprogesterone and antiglucocorticoid activity. Used as an abortifacient and in the management of hyperadrenocorticism.

migram a disease of sheep occurring in the UK on the Romney Marsh, of unknown cause and characterized by incoordination and collapse while being driven.

migrating motor complexes regularly occurring motor complexes are recorded in the intestine of turkeys and chickens.

migrating myoelectric complex mechanisms for sweeping large food particles and residues in starving animals into the terminal small intestine; reported only in the fasting period and in humans and dogs.

migration movement of living things from one place to another by their own volition. Also used to describe movement of nonliving biological material, e.g. migration of protein in electrophoretic media.

m. inhibition factor see LEUKOCYTE migration-inhibition factor, MACROPHAGE inhibition factor, migration inhibition test (below).

m. inhibition test an in vitro test for detection of cell-mediated immunity (or delayed hypersensitivity) in which peritoneal exudate cells (lymphocytes and macrophages) are packed in capillary tubes and placed in a medium; if the medium contains an antigen to which the lymphocytes are primed, macrophage migration from the tubes is inhibited by lymphokines, particularly macrophage inhibiting factor, released by the antigen stimulated lymphocytes.

migratory emanating from or pertaining to migration.

Mikrocytos minute protozoan parasites infecting the hemocytes of oysters. See MIKROCYTOSIS.

mikrocytosis disease caused by minute protozoans infecting the hemocytes of oysters. Includes *Mikrocytos mackini* (Denman island disease in Pacific oysters), *M. roughlei* (winter mortality in Sydney rock oysters).

milagaipoondu CATHARANTHUS *pusilla.*

Milan frill a frilled canary of solid color, either white, red-orange or blue.

milbemycin a macrolone lactone, derived from *Streptomyces cyanogeneus*, similar to the avermectins, effective as an anthelmintic and parasiticide. Milbemycin oxime is used for the prevention of heartworm in dogs and it has found a use in the treatment of generalized demodecosis.

milch giving milk or kept for milking.

mild as in disease; does not interfere with normal activities such as grazing, ambulation.

miliary 1. like millet seeds. 2. characterized by the formation of lesions resembling millet seeds.

m. bronchiolithiasis see MICROLITHIASIS.

m. dermatitis see feline miliary DERMATITIS.

m. tuberculosis an acute form of tuberculosis in which minute tubercles are formed in a number of organs of the body, owing to dissemination of the bacilli throughout the body by the bloodstream.

milieu [Fr.] *surroundings, environment.*

m. extérieur external environment.

m. intérieur internal environment; the interstitial tissue fluid and lymph in which the cells are bathed.

milium pl. *milia* [L.] spheroidal follicular cyst of lamellated keratin lying just under the epidermis, which appears as small white or yellow nodule. Popularly called *whitehead.*

milk 1. a nutrient fluid produced by the mammary gland of many mammals for the nourishment of their young. 2. a liquid (emulsion or suspension) resembling the secretion of the mammary gland. 3. to remove milk from the mammary gland.

absent m. see AGALACTIA.

acid m. reported as a cause of death in neonatal puppies and kittens, presumably resulting from bacterial mastitis or metritis which concurrently lowers the pH of the bitch's milk. See also toxic milk (below).

acidophilus m. milk fermented with cultures of *Lactobacillus acidophilus*; used in gastrointestinal disorders to modify the bacterial flora of the intestinal tract.

African m. bush see SYNADENIUM ARBORESCENS.

m. allergy see milk ALLERGY.

augmented m. culture system includes preculture incubation, followed by freezing, then use of a larger inoculum than usual.

blood in m. see BLOOD in milk.

m. bush EUPHORBIA *tirucalli.*

casein m. a prepared milk containing very little salts and sugars and a large amount of fat and casein.

m. chickens very young chickens weighing 0.5 to 1 lb (0.25 to 0.50 kg); birds up to 2 lb (1.0 kg) are accepted. Called also poussins.

m. coagulation coagulation of milk in the abomasum of the calf, precipitated by rennin, the enzyme produced by the abomasal mucosa, converts the dissolved casein into a rubbery clot. See also RENNIN.

condensed m. milk that has been partly evaporated and sweetened with sugar.

m. cow, milch cow cow used expressly for the production of milk for human consumption.

m. dentition the dentition of sucklings, the deciduous TEETH.

dialyzed m. milk from which the sugar has been removed by dialysis through a parchment membrane.

m. drinker's syndrome metastatic calcification in

young animals kept on high milk intakes for long periods.
m. drop syndrome a sudden and often unexplained fall in milk production in a dairy herd. It can occur when any disease or condition affects a significant proportion of a herd at one time; identified causes include poisoning by *Acremonium coeniophialum* or *Claviceps purpurea*, infection with *Leptospira hardjo*, severe combined nutritional and environmental stress.
m.-ejection reflex filling of the teat and udder cisterns with milk in response to teat stimulation, the response being effected via a release of oxytocin from the posterior pituitary; called also letdown.
evaporated m. milk prepared by evaporation of half of its water content.
m. fat see BUTTERFAT, MILK lipid (below).
m. fat depression see BUTTERFAT.
m.-fed neonate a neonate still being suckled by the dam or being reared on artificial milk replacer.
m. fever a metabolic disease of mature dairy cows occurring just before or soon after calving; signs are muscular weakness, peripheral circulatory failure with cool skin, small amplitude pulse, soft heart sounds, recumbency and drowsiness. Definitive clinical pathology is hypocalcemia. The same syndrome occurs in ewes; called also moss-ill.
m. flake fine, flat sheets of fibrin as part of the inflammatory process in the cow's udder, especially in cases of coliform mastitis.
m. flow sensor a sensor fitted in the long milk tube from the cluster to the milk line which is sensitive to the rate of flow; designed to trigger the automatic removal of the cluster when the rate of flow of milk in the milk tube falls below a predetermined level.
fortified m. milk made more nutritious by addition of cream, egg white or vitamins.
m. harvesting the process of producing, extracting and storing milk on the farm.
homogenized m. milk treated so that the fats form a permanent emulsion and the cream does not separate.
m. impacts drops of milk from other teat cups propelled vigorously against the teat ends of susceptible-to-mastitis quarters during, and as a result of TEAT CUP LINER slips.
inappropriate production of m. see GALACTORRHEA.
m. intolerance deficiency of intestinal LACTASE which results in diarrhea, abdominal distension and cramping. Occurs most commonly in puppies and kittens.
m. knots palpable, milk-containing dilations in the lactiferous ducts in the udder, especially of cows.
m. lameness see milk LEG.
m. leakage teats which drip milk between milkings have defective external sphincters and are susceptible to infection. Also occurs when the udder is very full, e.g. just before calving, or when letdown has occurred prior to milking when the intramammary pressure exceeds the closing forces of the normal teat end sphincter.
m. letdown see LETDOWN (1).
m. line the site for future location of mammary glands developing early as a ridge along the ventral abdomen of the embryo.
m. lipid butter fat globules in the milk; some is synthesized by mammary epithelium, some is secreted unchanged from the bloodstream.
low-fat m. normal milk but with the normal fat percentage greatly reduced, e.g. to below 50%; usually due to feeding finely ground grain or low-fiber roughage.
m. of magnesia a suspension containing 7 to 8.5% of magnesium hydroxide, used as an antacid and laxative.
m. meter flow meter at each unit in a milking machine designed to measure the yield of milk for each cow at each milking.
peak m. yield in cows the period during early lactation when the amount of milk produced per day is higher than at any other time. In bitches and queens, maximum lactation is achieved at 3–4 weeks postpartum.
m. persistency rate of decline of milk production from the peak. This is in effect the duration of the cow's production of an amount of milk which is worth harvesting; in commercial dairying cows are usually dried off when their daily yield falls to less than 4 liters. In good herds most cows are dried off because they have been in milk for the specified duration.
m. production 1. the secretion of milk by the mammary epithelium. 2. the volume of milk produced, usually quoted for a year or a lactation, sometimes quoted as kg of butterfat or of milk solids produced. Used as the benchmark of productivity of dairy cows.
m. production data records of volume and components of milk produced by individual cows or the whole herd, either actually measured, or aspirated from periodic samplings.
m. progesterone tests see PREGNANCY tests.
protein m. milk modified to have a relatively low content of carbohydrate and fat and a relatively high protein content.
m. protein casein.
m. replacer used as replacement for milk in calf, lamb and piglet diets to permit early weaning and to rear orphans. Milk replacers are manufactured from dried milk products but may contain large amounts of animal fats, nonmilk carbohydrates and proteins. The dried milk powder used may also have been denatured during heat treatment. Poor replacers cause dietary diarrhea. Should contain less than 0.1% plant fiber, 36–40% lactose, 30–40% fat, 28–32% milk protein.
m. replacer malnutrition malnutrition in calves fed on poorly formulated milk replacer.
m. ring test is used for surveillance of brucellosis prevalence in dairy cattle. It depends on the presence of agglutinable antibodies in the milk and the agglutination of added stained antigen by antibodies in the milk of positive reacting cows.
m. sample culturing from cows may be composite of all quarters in one sample or single quarter samples. Samples must be refrigerated until cultured. Culture on sheep blood agar is standard but many special media available for particular purposes.
m. scald alopecic dermatitis around the muzzle of bucket-fed calves caused by frequent immersion in milk.
m. sickness the disease of humans caused by the drinking of milk from cows which have been eating EUPATORIUM *rugosum*; the milk contains tremetol.
skim m. see SKIM MILK.
m. spots 1 mm diameter white spots in the capsule of the pig's liver caused by migration of *Ascaris suum* larvae.
m. solids combined yield of fat and protein in the milk.
m. stage the period of plant growth after blooming has finished when the seed is formed but still soft and milky when squeezed.
m. stone a calcareous deposit which accumulates in milking machinery and utensils over a long period if proper cleaning techniques are not practiced.

m. sugar lactose.
m. teeth see milk dentition (above).
m. tetany see calf HYPOMAGNESEMIC tetany.
m. thistle see SILYBUM MARIANUM, SONCHUS.
toxic m. bacterial toxins in the dam's milk are believed to be the cause of death in neonatal puppies and kittens.
uterine m. see UTERINE milk.
m. veins subcutaneous abdominal veins of lactating cows. See also Table 15.
m. vetch see ASTRAGALUS.
m. vine see MARSDENIA ROSTRATA.
m. well opening through the ventral abdominal wall to permit entry of milk vein.
whole m. milk as it is drawn from the udder, undiluted, not separated into skim milk, buttermilk, whey. See also WHOLE MILK FED.
m. yield see milk production (above).

milk cell counts the counting of cells in milk, which is now standard practice for the assessment of cows for the presence of mastitis. The techniques used nowadays are electronically based and set to count somatic cells as a group without differentiation. The popular methods are the individual cow cell count and the bulk milk cell count. For the individual cow test, milk that has been collected for butter fat testing can be used, and this greatly reduces the cost of the operation. Another innovative technique is the preservation of the milk samples so that counting can be delayed. Counting is carried out on three or four occasions during lactation and a decision is made about culling the cow or giving her dry-period treatment at the end of the lactation. For the bulk milk cell count, a count is done on samples collected at regular intervals from the bulk milk supplied by the herd.

milk clots slimy lumps in milk affected by mastitis; block filters and teat canals; usually accompanied by a watery fluid in visible amounts.

milk of sulfur see precipitated SULFUR.

milk shake a solution of sodium bicarbonate administered to racehorses by stomach tube 4 to 6 hours before racing to produce a metabolic acidosis. Promoted as a means of producing relief from tying-up and delaying the onset of fatigue by producing additional buffering to counteract the accumulation of lactic acid, induced by anaerobic muscular activity. Some commercial preparations include a mixture of vitamins and minerals. Legislated against by limiting the blood level of CO_2. See also SALINE DRENCH.

milker's nodule, milker's node see PSEUDOCOWPOX.

milkfish see CHANNOS CHANNOS.

milking the procedure of extracting the milk from the udder usually with a milking machine. The process and the machine play a large part in the transmission of mastitis, pseudocowpox, bovine ulcerative mamillitis, cowpox, udder impetigo, teat papillomatosis, and in the causation of black spot. It is a special portal of entry for infection in the cow, goat and rarely sheep.
m. bail the head lock or stock which restrains the cow while she is milked.
m. hygiene includes milking machine sanitation between milkings, TEAT CUP sanitation during milking, teat washing, teat dipping or spraying, hand disinfection, fly control, shed floor washing.
m. machine see MILKING MACHINE.
m. order the order in which groups of cattle in a milking herd pass through the milking parlor twice each day; for reasons of mastitis control the order should be heifers first followed by uninfected senior cows, followed by known infected but clinically normal individuals and then cows with clinical mastitis last.
m. parlor the room or shed used for milking cows. The milking stalls may be in line abreast (a walk-through), angled away from a central pit, and often not divided into stalls (herringbone), in-line behind each other on either side of a pit (tandem), or on a milking platform that rotates around a central point (carousel or rotary); there are a number of other variations on these styles.
m. ratio the duration of the milk flow within each pulsation cycle expressed as a percentage of the period when milk does not flow.
m. time 1. the time of day at which milking occurs. 2. total time taken to milk the entire herd or the average time taken to milk each cow.

milking herd see DAIRY herd.

milking machine a machine for the milking of cows, occasionally sheep and rarely goats. It includes a vacuum pump, a pulsation system, clusters of teat cups, a rigid milk line, some flexible rubber tubes which connect the clusters to the milk line and a number of other components. Many of the components are replicated in the usual machine so that a number of cows can be milked at the same time. The vacuum applied directly to the teat sphincter effects milk removal from the teat, and an intermittent vacuum between the teat cup and the liner relieves the tendency to edema of the teat by squeezing it intermittently. The pressure used in the machine is critical, too great causes damage to the teat, too little causes incomplete milking. The art of good milking technique is to balance one against the other.
m. m. claw the metal handpiece to which are attached the four cups that, with their inflations, are used to milk the cow.
m. m. clean-in-place cleaning system consisting of the circulation of cleaning and rinsing fluids through the milking machine without disassembling it.
m. m. cluster claw plus cups, plus connecting rubber tubes.
high level m. m. a machine in which the distance between the milk inlet to the milkline and the floor on which the cow is standing exceeds 4 feet.
m. m. liner slip see TEAT CUP LINER slip.
low level m. m. a machine in which the milk inlet to the milkline is below the level of the floor on which the cow is standing.
m. m. milking extracting milk from the udder with a milking machine.
m. m. pulsation rate number of pulsation cycles per minute; varies between machine manufacturers but average is 40 vacuum releases/minute.
m. m. pulsation ratio the ratio of the time during which the teat cup liner is more than half open to the time for which it is less than half open.
m. m. pulsation system the intermittent increase in vacuum pressure in a milking machine mimics the application of sucking pressure by a sucking neonate by cyclic opening and closing of the teat cup liner; the intermittency is provided by the pulsator which consists of a servodiaphragm. The pulsation to a cluster may be alternate, when two teat cups move alternately with the other two, or simultaneous, when all four cups move at the same time.
m. m. reverse milk flow excessive changes in machine vacuum pressure cause reverse flow of milk for very brief periods, which allows contact of milk from infected quarters with the teat ends of unin-

fected quarters. The impact of this milk on a relaxed teat sphincter can effect the entry of infected milk.

m. m. stripping see machine STRIPPING.

m. m. teat cup liner see TEAT CUP LINER.

m. m. pump capacity air-moving capacity of the vacuum pump in a milking machine.

m. m. vacuum pressure varies with design but average is 50 kPa (37.5 cm Hg).

m. m. vacuum reserve governs vacuum stability, the protection against random acute fluctuations in vacuum pressure, the cause of milk flow reversal and elevation of the new mastitis infection rate.

Milking shorthorn a red, red-and-white or red-roan dual-purpose breed of cattle.

milklame see OSTEOMALACIA.

milkleg see OSTEOMALACIA.

milkline pipeline in a milking machine which carries milk and air during milking, thus providing milking vacuum and a conduit for the passage of milk.

milkweed see ASCLEPIAS.

milky mangrove *Excoecaria agallocha.*

milky pine ALSTONIA *scolaris.*

Miller–Abbott tube a double-channel intestinal tube with an inflatable balloon at its distal end, used for diagnosing and treating obstructive lesions of the small intestine. The tube is inserted via a nostril and gently passed through the stomach and into the small intestine. Used in humans in the treatment of intestinal obstruction.

miller's disease see OSTEODYSTROPHIA FIBROSA.

Miller's suture tie used as a ligature around a soft tissue stump. It is a clove hitch.

millet a summer fodder crop that matures very quickly. See also ECHINOCHLOA, PANICUM and PENNISETUM *americanum.*

m. ergot see CLAVICEPS *fusiformis.*

milli- word element, *one-thousandth;* used in naming units of measurement to designate one-thousandth (10^{-3}) the size of the unit to which it is joined, symbol m; e.g. milligram (mg).

milliamperage in radiography, the x-ray tube current during an exposure, measured in milliamperes (mA).

milliampere one-thousandth (10^{-3}) of an ampere; abbreviated mA.

milliampere-second a unit of radiographic exposure equal to the product of the milliamperage and the exposure time in seconds. Abbreviated mAs, mA·s.

millicurie a non-SI unit of radioactivity; one-thousandth (10^{-3}) of a curie. The quantity of radioactive material in which the number of disintegrations of nuclei is 3.7×10^7 per second; abbreviated mCi. Now replaced by the BECQUEREL.

millicurie-hour a non-SI unit of dose equivalent to that obtained by exposure for one hour to radioactive material disintegrating at the rate of 3.7×10^7 atoms per second; abbreviated mCi-h.

milliequivalent one-thousandth of a chemical equivalent. Abbreviated mEq.

milligram one-thousandth (10^{-3}) of a gram; equivalent of 0.015432 grain avoirdupois or apothecaries' weight; abbreviated mg.

milliliter one-thousandth (10^{-3}) of a liter; abbreviated ml.

millimeter one-thousandth (10^{-3}) of a meter; equivalent to 0.039 inch; abbreviated mm.

millimicro- word element, formerly used to designate one-thousand-millionth (10^{-9}) part of the unit to which it is joined; now supplanted by the prefix nano-.

millimole one thousandth (10^{-3}) part of a mole; symbol mmol.

milling the grinding or cracking of grain, and the mixing and compounding of feeds. Could reasonably include pelleting.

m. error an error in which the miller has usually included a wrong ingredient or the correct ingredient at the wrong concentration. A common cause of poisoning in housed cattle.

milliosmole one-thousandth (10^{-3}) of an osmole. Abbreviated mOsm.

millipede nonpoisonous, multisegmented, circular in cross-section, arthropod with two legs per segment.

Millipore filter trademark for cellulose acetate filters with pore sizes of 8 μm to 10 nm; such membranes are widely used for sterilizing liquid media.

millirad a non-SI unit of dosage of absorbed radiation, 10^{-3} rad; abbreviated mrad. Now replaced by GRAY.

millivolt one-thousandth of a volt; abbreviated mV.

Millotia greevesii toxic plant in family Asteraceae; causes nitrate–nitrite poisoning; called also creeping millotia.

milo a variety of sorghum used for grain, with the same toxic potential as fodder sorghum. Called also SORGHUM *vulgare.*

milphae, milphosis the falling out of the eyelashes.

milrinone a synthetic phosphodiesterase inhibitor compound, used to provide inotropic support to the failing myocardium.

milt fish spermatozoa.

milzbrand anthrax.

Mima now classified as *Acinetobacter.*

-mimetic imitating; used as a word ending to indicate what it is that is being imitated, e.g. sympathomimetic.

MIMI multifactorial intramural myocardial infarction.

Mimosa plant genus in the legume family Mimosaceae; contain toxin mimosine; includes *M. invisa* (giant sensitive plant), *M. pudica* (sensitive plant).

mimosine the toxic amino acid in *Leucaena leucocephala, Mimosa* spp. Causes depilation, especially of the long hairs of the mane and tail.

min. minim; minimum; minute.

Minamata disease mercury poisoning in cats, birds and humans originating from industrial pollution of Minamata bay in Japan, and the poisoning of fish and shellfish which were then absorbed into the local food chains.

mindi see MELIA *azederach.*

mineral any naturally occurring nonorganic homogeneous solid substance. There are 19 or more minerals forming the mineral composition of the animal body; at least 13 are essential to health. These minerals must be supplied in the diet and are generally found in a varied or mixed diet of animal and vegetable products which meet the energy and protein needs. Nutritional deficiencies of individual minerals are listed under each of them.

m. deficiencies see under the appropriate mineral, e.g. phosphorus, iodine.

m. flux the excessive output of a mineral from the animal body, leading to a state of deficiency; a negative balance.

m. imbalances imbalances between minerals that need to be maintained in a proper balance with others as well as being present in appropriate absolute amounts, e.g. calcium : phosphorus, sodium : potassium.

mineral-salt mixtures mixtures of stock grade salt, with sterilized bonemeal, copper, cobalt, iodine and other trace minerals where required, in granular form or in a hard cake for licking. Set out in barns or at pasture for AD LIB access by cattle, sheep, goats. Called also lick.

m. supplements minerals added to the diet of animals to prevent or correct a nutritional deficiency.

trace m. see TRACE ELEMENT.

m. tolerance limits of dietary supplementation with minerals which animals can survive for a limited period without a decline in their production or performance, and without creating unsafe residues in the human food chain.

mineralization the addition of mineral matter to the body, especially the skeleton.

cutaneous m. see CALCINOSIS cutis.

dystrophic m. see DYSTROPHIC calcification.

ectopic m. the deposition of calcium salts in abnormal locations, e.g. in uremia, hypervitaminosis D.

m. front the interface between the unmineralized osteoid and the mineralized bone. Called also phosphate ridge.

heterotopic m. see ectopic mineralization (above).

metastatic m. calcification of unusual tissues leading to the development of metastatic bone.

mineralized ring see PERICHONDRAL ring.

mineralocorticoid any of a group of hormones elaborated by the cortex of the ADRENAL gland, so called because of their effects on sodium, chloride and potassium concentrations in the extracellular fluids. They are the adrenocortical hormones that are essential to the maintenance of adequate fluid volume in the interstitial and intravascular fluid compartments, normal cardiac output and adequate levels of blood pressure. Without sufficient supply of the mineralocorticoids, fatal shock from diminished cardiac output can occur very quickly.

The principal mineralocorticoid is *aldosterone*, which accounts for most of the activities of this group of hormones. The primary effects of the mineralocorticoids are increasing the reabsorption of sodium and the secretion of potassium in the renal tubules. Secondary effects are related to the reabsorption of water, serum levels of sodium and potassium, anion reabsorption and secretion of hydrogen ions. The net result of these activities is maintenance of fluid and electrolyte balance and, therefore, adequate cardiac output.

miners lettuce see MONTIA PERFOLIATA.

miniature much smaller in size than normal animals of the species, but with normal proportions. Animals born prematurely are miniatures but show evidence of prematurity in their haircoat, unerupted teeth and immature hooves. A nonviable form of miniaturism in calves with these characteristics is thought to be inherited. See also DWARFISM.

m. dog breeds several dog breeds or varieties which are specified as miniatures, usually in contrast to a larger variety with similar characteristics except for size. They include the Miniature SCHNAUZER, Miniature BULL TERRIER, Miniature POODLE, Miniature DACHSHUND and MINIATURE PINSCHER.

m. endplate potentials the steady release of acetylcholine from the nerve terminal, which results in subthreshold responses.

m. pig see miniature PIG.

Miniature pinscher a very small (10 lb), lively dog with very short coat in solid red, brown, blue, chocolate or black, with tan markings on the face, throat, chest and legs. The ears may be erect, dropped, or cropped where practiced. The tail is docked. Sometimes regarded as a miniature Doberman pinscher. Called also 'Minpin' and Roe terrier.

minilaparotomy a small abdominal incision for liver biopsy, open transhepatic cholangiography, or sterilization by ovariectomy.

minim a unit of volume (liquid measure) in the apothecaries' system, equivalent to 0.0616 ml.

minimal the smallest possible; the least.

m. bactericidal concentration (MBC) see minimal lethal concentration (below).

m. disease pigs a variant on SPECIFIC PATHOGEN FREE pigs.

m. inhibitory concentration (MIC) the lowest concentration of an antimicrobial that inhibits the growth of a bacterium; usually in reference to an antimicrobial sensitivity test.

m. lethal concentration (MLC) the lowest concentration of antimicrobial that kills a particular bacterium; usually in reference to an antimicrobial sensitivity test.

m. viable gestational age the minimal gestational age at which the fetus can survive independently (horse 300 days, cattle 240 days, 138 for sheep, 108 for pig).

minimum see also MINIMAL.

m. alveolar anesthetic concentration the concentration of an anesthetic in the alveoli that prevents a muscular response to a painful stimulus in 50% of the subjects; abbreviated MAC.

m. daily requirement (MDR) the minimum amount of a nutrient that is required daily for the maintenance of good health.

m. data set an accepted list of terms and definitions necessary for veterinary records aimed at creating useful animal disease records. Called also uniform basic data set.

m. effective concentration (MEC) the minimal blood level at which a systemic drug exerts the desired effect.

m. effective strain level of strain below which bone shows no adaptive reaction.

Minimum Essential Drug Information Checklist (MEDIC) a checklist to be used in a problem-solving approach to the understanding of pharmacology.

Minivent ventilator a small, simple unit that fits onto any continuous-flow anesthetic apparatus and acts as a minute volume divider. Used for anesthesia of small animals.

mink a small mammal of the family Mustelidae; an aquatic carnivore much prized for its fur. Called also *Mustela lutreola*, *M. vison*.

Aleutian m. disease see ALEUTIAN MINK DISEASE.

m. encephalopathy a prion spongiform encephalopathy; there is similarity between this disease and scrapie produced experimentally in mink. There is a very long incubation period, hyperirritability, biting, paralysis, coma and death. Called also transmissible encephalopathy of mink, TEM.

m. enteritis a condition caused by the mink enteritis virus, which is closely related to feline panleukopenia virus, and characterized by mucoid, sometimes blood-stained, diarrhea that may contain casts.

ranch m. mink cultivated artificially on a mink farm or 'ranch'.

Minnesota disease reporting system a surveillance system for diseases in farm animals, initiated by the Minnesota Veterinary Association, and based on periodic reporting and analysis of the diseases occurring on SENTINEL farms.

minnie-minnie see ABRUS *precatorius*.

minocycline a second-generation, highly lipid-soluble derivative of tetracycline.

Minorca a lightweight, black breed of egglaying fowl with a large, erect, single comb, and black legs; it lays a bright, white-shelled egg.

minoxidil a potent, long-acting vasodilator, which acts primarily on arterioles. Used as an antihypertensive agent in humans and also topically as a hair restorer in male baldness. Has been used in the treatment of alopecia in dogs.
minpin see MINIATURE PINSCHER.
mint MENTHA *longifolia*.
Mintchew's operation an operation for dorsal fixation of a prolapsing vagina in a cow. A heavy suture is placed from the skin beside the tailhead into the vagina.
mintweed see SALVIA *reflexa*.
minute very small.
m. canine virus (MCV) see canine PARVOVIRUS type 1.
m. mouse virus a parvovirus recovered from mice. Experimental infection of neonatal or fetal mice causes runting and cerebellar hypoplasia, but natural infection has not been associated with clinical disease. Sometimes referred to as the 'mini-mouse' virus.
mio mio BACCHARIS *cordifolia*.
miocardia the contraction of the heart; systole.
Miohippus one of the early evolutionary stages of the horse; existed during the Oligocene period.
miopus a monster with two fused heads, one face being rudimentary.
miosis, myosis excessive contraction of the pupil.
miotic 1. pertaining to, characterized by or causing miosis. 2. an agent that causes contraction of the pupil.
mipafox a cholinesterase inhibitor, organophosphorus insecticide which causes degeneration of the spinal cord tract in fowl.
miracidium pl. *miracidia* [Gr.] the free-swimming, ciliated larva of a trematode parasite which emerges from an egg and penetrates the body of a snail host.
mirex an effective organic pesticide used in ant control and as a fire retardant; it is, however, very persistent in tissue and now banned because of residue problems.
Mirounga angustirostris largest of all pinnipeds; residents of the Pacific coast of the USA. Called also Northern ELEPHANT seal.
mirror-image artifact in ultrasonography, highly reflective interfaces, such as lung–diaphragm, may result in multiple reverberations of sound waves causing some echoes to be delayed in returning to the transducer so that a more superficial structure may appear deeper.
misalliance see MISMATING; called also mésalliance.
misbeksiektebos see GEIGEREIA.
misbredie see AMARANTHUS.
miscible susceptible to being mixed.
misconduct conduct as a professional person which brings sufficient discredit to the profession to damage its reputation and decrease the trust that the public places in it. Personal morality, social behavior, language and dress are all criteria that need to be included in any assessment, but they must be judged in the light of the prevailing community standards of the day.
miserotoxin the β-glycoside of 3-nitro-1-propanol in *Astragalus miser* (timber milk vetch) which when converted to an aglycone causes the signs of poisoning by this plant—loss of condition, incoordination on driving and a roaring respiration.
mismatch 1. in blood transfusions and transplantation immunology, an incompatibility between potential donor and recipient. 2. one or more nucleotides in one of the double strands in a nucleic acid molecule without complementary nucleotides in the same position on the other strand. Called also incomplete base-pairing.
mismating female mated to the wrong male, often by failure of restraint of one or the other. The emphasis in most cases is to ensure that the mating does not proceed to conception or to parturition. Called also mésalliance, misalliance.
mismothering failure of the newborn to be matched up with its own mother, which is one of the hazards of raising animals in flocks and submitting them to intensive management with much human intervention. The problem can be a serious one in sheep flocks, especially with timid merino-type sheep, and many newborn lambs may be lost.
misoprostol a synthetic analog of prostaglandin E and inhibitor of gastric secretion; used in the treatment of gastrointestinal ulceration, particularly those associated with the use of nonsteroidal anti-inflammatory drugs.
mispickel arsenical pyrites, an iron-rich ore containing a high content of arsenic. Fumes from an industrial plant handling the ore can cause local chronic arsenic poisoning in livestock.
mission bells BRYOPHYLLUM *tubiflorum*.
mission grass PENNISETUM *polystachya*.
Missulena one of the genera of venomous trapdoor spiders.
mist flower EUPATORIUM *riparium*.
mistletoe (European) see VISCUM ALBUM.
mistura [L.] *mixture*.
MIT monoiodotyrosine.
mitchell grass see ASTREBLA.
Mitchell markers lead letters containing a mercury bubble to indicate orientation of the cassette when the x-ray is taken.
Mitchell needle a needle designed especially for intravenous anesthesia, with a device that keeps the needle in place and prevents reflux of blood up the needle.
mite any arthropod of the order Acarina except the ticks; they are characterized by minute size, usually transparent or semitransparent body, and other features distinguishing them from the ticks. They may be free living or parasitic on animals or plants, and may produce various irritations of the skin. See MANGE, CHIGGER, HARVEST mites, PSORERGATES *ovis*, DEMODECTIC, NOTEDRIC, OTODECTIC, and many locality names, e.g. cat fur mites, ear mites, nasal mites, and other special titles, e.g. harvest mites, housedust mites.
chigger m. see CHIGGER.
m. fever see scrub TYPHUS.
grain itch m. see PEDICULOIDES VENTRICOSUS.
mithramycin see PLICAMYCIN.
mithridate mustard see THLASPI ARVENSE.
mithridatism acquisition of immunity to a poison by ingestion of gradually increasing amounts of it.
miticide an agent destructive to mites.
mitis medical Latin term for mild—opposite of forte.
mitochondria [Gr.] plural of *mitochondrion;* small, spherical to rod-shaped, membrane-bounded cytoplasmic organelles that are the principal sites of ATP synthesis; they also contain enzymes of the citric acid cycle and for fatty acid oxidation, oxidative phosphorylation, and other biochemical pathways. Mitochondria also contain DNA, RNA and ribosomes; they replicate independently and synthesize some of their own proteins.
mitochondrial pertaining to mitochondria.
m. RNAs a unique set of tRNAs, mRNAs, rRNAs, transcribed from mitochondrial DNA by a mitochon-

drial-specific RNA polymerase, that account for about 4% of the total cell RNA that are transcribed.

m. targeting signal a not fully defined sequence of amino acids, rich in hydroxyl amino acids and normally lacking acidic residues, that is recognized by a mitochondrial receptor that permits mitochondrial-specific proteins synthesized in the cytoplasm to be imported into mitochondria.

mitochondrion singular of MITOCHONDRIA.

mitogen an agent that induces mitosis and lymphocyte blastogenesis.

pokeweed m. (PWM) a lectin from the plant, *Phytolacca americana*, that produces B and T lymphocyte blastogenesis.

mitogenesis the induction of mitosis in a cell.

mitogenic factor one of the lymphokines.

mitomycin, mitomycin C a group of highly toxic antineoplastics (mitomycin A, B and C) produced by *Streptomyces caespitosus*, indicated for palliative treatment of certain neoplasms that do not respond to surgery, radiation and other drugs.

mitosis the ordinary process of cell division which results in the formation of two daughter cells, and by which the body replaces dead cells. The two daughter cells receive identical diploid complements of chromosomes, which are characteristic of somatic cells. Cell division that results in haploid reproductive cells is known as MEIOSIS. The period between mitotic divisions is called *interphase*. Mitosis itself occurs in four phases: *prophase*, *metaphase*, *anaphase* and *telophase*.

Originally, the term *mitosis* referred only to the division of the nucleus, which can occur without cytokinesis in certain fungi and in the fertilized eggs of insects. As used now, it usually refers to mitotic cell division.

mitotane an oral chemotherapeutic agent that causes selective necrosis and atrophy of the adrenocortical zona fasciculata and zona reticularis. Used in the treatment of inoperable adrenal cortical carcinoma in humans and in canine Cushing's syndrome. Called also *o,p,-DDD*.

mitotic pertaining to mitosis.

m. activity degree to which a cell population is proliferating; used as an index of tumor aggression. Can be quantified by counting the percentage of cells showing mitotic figures, or by flow cytometry.

m. figure the condensed chromosomes by which a cell that is undergoing mitosis can be identified.

m. index the percentage of cells simultaneously in the process of division, normally calculated after counting 1000 cells. Used in morbid pathology as a measure of the malignancy of a tumor, and in clinical pathology as an index of survival time of a neoplasm.

m. metaphase chromosomes chromosomes in metaphase manifesting as mitotic figures.

m. nondisjunction failure of proper disjunction of the paired chromosomes during metaphase which results in the chromosomal abnormalities of monosomy or trisomy.

m. potential estimate of the cell's potential reproductive capacity.

mitoxantrone, mitozantrone an anthracene derivative, similar to doxorubicin, used as an antineoplastic agent.

mitral shaped like a miter; pertaining to the mitral valve.

m. area that area of the thoracic wall through which sounds of the mitral valve can best be auscultated; generally the lower one-third of the mid- to anterior left thorax.

m. atresia–hypoplastic left heart syndrome defects in the development of the mitral valve, left heart and aortic valve, which occur rarely in cats.

m. complex includes the leaflets, annulus, chordae tendineae and papillary muscles of the mitral valve, left atrium and left ventricular muscle wall.

m. insufficiency a functional incompetence resulting in regurgitation of blood from the left ventricle to the left atrium during systole or from the great vessels into the left atrium during diastole.

m. regurgitation see mitral insufficiency (above).

m. valve the left atrioventricular valve, the valve between the left atrium and the left ventricle of the heart; it is composed of two cusps, anterior and posterior. Called also the bicuspid valve.

m. valve prolapse (MVP) a condition in which some portion of the mitral valve is pushed back too far during ventricular contraction. Often a complication of mitral endocardiosis.

Mittendorf's dot a congenital anomaly of the eye, without an effect on vision, manifested as a small gray or white opacity just inferior and nasal to the posterior pole of the lens, representing the remains of the lenticular attachment of the hyaloid artery. Detectable in puppies and kittens at 6 to 8 weeks after birth.

mivacurium a nondepolarizing drug used to achieve neuromuscular blockade.

mixed 1. affecting various parts at the same time. 2. having two or more characteristics. 3. comprising several different ingredients.

m. bacterial vaccine an experimental preparation once investigated as a nonspecific immunostimulant in the treatment of different types of tumors in dogs. It contained *Streptococcus pyogenes* and *Serratia marcescens*.

m. infection infection with more than one agent at the same time.

m. lymphocyte reaction a test for histocompatibility between donor and recipient; lymphocytes from both are mixed in vitro and the responses quantitated by measuring the uptake of tritium-labeled thymidine (^{3}H-TdR). In the usual assay one of the two populations which will serve as the target is blocked from undergoing blastogenesis by the drug mitomycin. The degree of incompatibility is reflected in the amount of cell division as measured by the uptake of ^{3}H-TdR, incompatibility increasing the uptake of ^{3}H-TdR.

m. tumor canine mammary tumors are often mixtures of epithelial, myoepithelial or connective tissues. Mixed tumors also occur in the dog in the thyroid, sweat and salivary glands.

Mixter forceps lightweight, ratchet-handled hemostats with the blades curved sharply downwards near their tip.

mixture a combination of different drugs or ingredients, such as a fluid with other fluids or solids, or a solid with a liquid.

Miyagawanella an obsolete name for a genus of organisms, the species of which are now assigned to the genus *Chlamydia*. *M. bovis*, *M. felis*, *M. ornithosis*, *M. ovis*, *M. pecoris*, *M. pneumoniae* and *M. psittaci* were originally introduced as names for particular isolates, but these are now all included as *C. psittaci*.

mizoribine an oral immunosuppressant used in organ transplantation.

mjölkhälta [Scand.] see PHOSPHORUS nutritional deficiency.

ml milliliter.

MLD minimum lethal dose.

MLR mixed lymphocyte reaction.
MLV modified live virus. See attenuated VACCINE.
mm millimeter; muscles.
μm micrometer.
MM disease *Mycoplasma meleagridis* disease. See TURKEY syndrome.
MMA called also MMA sow syndrome; see also MASTITIS–METRITIS–AGALACTIA.
MMF maximal midexpiratory flow (rate).
MMFR maximal midexpiratory flow rate.
mmHg millimeters of mercury; a unit of pressure.
mmol millimole; see MOLE.
Mn chemical symbol, *manganese.*
Mn^2+ manganese ion.
mnemodermia skin memory; the existence of a state of hypersensitivity in a particular location on the skin long after the initial reaction has disappeared. Thought to occur but difficult to prove in animals.
mnemonics words in commands or computer dialog boxes containing letters highlighted by underlining, bolding or coloring to indicate single keystroke access to the particular option.
Mo chemical symbol, *molybdenum.*
mob Australian vernacular for a group of sheep which stay together for an extended period.
mobilization the rendering of a fixed part movable.
Mobitz block see HEART BLOCK.
mock azalea see MENZIESIA FERRUGINEA.
modality 1. a method of application of, or the employment of, any therapeutic agent; limited usually to physical agents. 2. a specific sensory entity, such as taste. 3. in homeopathy, a condition that modifies drug action; a condition under which clinical signs develop, becoming better or worse.
mode 1. in statistics, the value or item in a variations curve that shows the maximum frequency of occurrence; in a series of values, the value that occurs most frequently. 2. in computer usage, a particular state of the system or program, e.g. edit, or print, selected by the operator for a particular task.
amplitude m. see A-mode ULTRASONOGRAPHY.
brightness m. see B-mode ULTRASONOGRAPHY.
motion m. see M-mode ULTRASONOGRAPHY.
modeccin toxalbumin in ADENIA DIGITATA.
model a simulation, a copy, occurring naturally or manufactured. Models used in statistical and epidemiological studies may be deterministic, stochastic or random.
m. 1 the fixed version of the linear additive model used in linear regression analysis.
m. 2 the random version of the linear additive model used in linear regression analysis.
animal m. any condition in an animal that has enough similarities to a condition in humans that studies of the animal disease are will assist in understanding the human disorder.
causal m. a model used to determine the part played by multiple factors in the cause or causes of disease; a path model in which the variables are arranged temporally.
descriptive m. consist largely of diagrams and maps or charts designed to describe a real-world system.
deterministic m. see epidemiological model (below).
epidemiological m. a mathematical model, which may be a computer simulation model, of a disease for the purpose of studying the behavior of the disease in a variable animal population under variable conditions of climate, density of population, mix of population, and so on. It may be an *analytical* model, an *economic decision making* model, an *explanatory* model or a *predictive* model. It may also be a *causal* model, which allows the operator to vary the determinants of prevalence and observe the respective outcomes. It may permit only the use of fixed numbers so that it will always return the same answer to the same question, in which case it is a *deterministic* model, or it may introduce the element of chance into the selection of outcomes, in which case it is a *stochastic* model.

Specific computer simulation models have been prepared for the study of rinderpest, the costs of mastitis control, the cost-benefits of foot-and-mouth disease control, and the costs of mortality in dairy calves. For example see REED–FROST MODEL.
linear programming m. a statistical model of a dependent variable, e.g. Y, as a linear combination of other variables, e.g. X. The model is based on a series of linear equations with a linear equation, called the objective function, as the desired end. Such an end could, in the determination of lowest cost rations, be the total cost of each ration.
mathematical m. a representation of a system, process or relationship in a mathematical form; see also mathematical MODELING.
physical m. e.g. a model of a molecule utilizing colored balls connected by rigid wires.
probabilistic m. includes basic concepts of probability theory and may be deterministic or stochastic.
Reed–Frost m. a deterministic probability model of a theoretical epidemic.
stochastic m. see epidemiological MODEL.
symbolic m. mathematical symbols used to describe the status of variables at a given time and to define the manner in which they change and interact.
modeling the art and science of constructing models.
mathematical m. the use of a set of consequential mathematical formulae to create a numerical model of the possible events in a system. Introduction of a series of values for individual constants makes it possible to produce a series of results that mirror the outcome of practical experiments. See also COMPUTER simulation model.
modem acronym for *mod*ulator–*dem*odulator. Electronic equipment that translates digital signals from a computer into codes that can be transmitted between computers over telephone lines, television cables or radiotelephone. Called also data set.
moderate said of a disease or condition that interferes with normal activities, such as eating and ambulation, without completely blocking them out.
moderator band see septomarginal TRABECULA.
modified contemporary comparison a two-step method of comparing the productivity of herd mates to establish breeding values; sires are evaluated first, then the sire data is used in the evaluation of the cows.
Modiola toxic plant in family Malvaceae; unidentified toxin causes incoordination, recumbency, convulsions; includes *M. caroliniana* (creeping mallow, *M. multifida*).
modiolus the central pillar or columella of the cochlea.
MODS multiple organ dysfunction syndrome.
modulation the capacity to regulate; widely used in biology, e.g. modulation of immune responses, food intake, etc.
antigenic m. the alteration of antigenic determinants in a living cell surface membrane following interaction with an antibody.
covalent m. activation or inactivation of enzymes, either by phosphorylation/dephosphorylation or by

proteolytic cleavage. A major means of regulation of enzyme action by hormones.

module a discrete and identifiable unit that is repeatable with minor variations. In computer terminology, a part (e.g. accounts receivable) of a whole program (e.g. an accounting program for a practice).

modus mode of.

MOET multiple ovulation and embryo transfer.

moggy term of endearment addressed to a cat.

mohair goat hair, product of the Angora goat.

moiety any equal part; a half; also any part or portion, such as a portion of a molecule.

moist having a moderate moisture content, slightly wet to the touch.

m. dermatitis see moist DERMATITIS of rabbits.

m. grain storage grain stored at about 30% moisture in airtight silos. (Normally grain is stored at 10 to 15% moisture.) Care is needed to avoid errors in the ensiling process and the storage costs are much higher, but the grain is more digestible. To avoid the silo costs, the grain can be treated with propionic or acetic acid and stored in bins, but care needs to be given to the grain's vitamin E content, which may be diminished by this treatment.

m. lung sounds sounds heard on auscultation of the lungs that indicate the presence of inflammatory or edema fluid in the bronchi or alveoli.

moisture wetness due to any liquid; usually refers to water as a component, e.g. in feed.

m. free a substance heated at 220°F (105°C) to constant weight. Called also oven-dry or 100% dry matter.

moisturizers hydroscopic agents, applied to the skin and hair, as creams, rinses or shampoos, to increase hydration of the stratum corneum. Examples are propylene glycol, glycerine and lactate.

Mokola virus a rhabdovirus found in bats that has serological similarities to, but significant differences from, the rabies virus.

mol see MOLE (2).

mol. wt. molecular weight.

molal containing one mole of solute per kilogram of solvent. See also MOLAR (4).

molality the number of moles of a solute per kilogram of solvent.

molar 1. massive; pertaining to a mass; not molecular. 2. adapted for grinding. See also molar TEETH. 3. pertaining to an amount of substance specified in moles rather than mass units. 4. containing 1 mole of solute per liter of solution; symbol M.

NOTE: *molal* refers to the *mass* of *solvent*, *molar* to the *volume* of the *solution*.

m. extinction coefficient constant n the equation describng the Lambert–Beer law pertaining to light spectrophotometry. Usually given the symbol ε.

m. extractor the universal heavy-duty plier-type instrument with jaws offset to the plane of the handles.

m. gland see SALIVARY GLAND.

inherited displacement of m. teeth a deformity of the mandible with gross displacement of the teeth. Affected calves are not viable.

m. tooth see molar TEETH.

m. tooth cutter long-handled, heavily constructed cutter, usually with a double-action scissor system of closing. The chisel-edged blades face each other and are brought together in parallel. They are operated from outside the mouth of the anesthetized horse and are sufficiently powerful to remove a protruding piece of tooth.

molarity the number of moles of a solute per liter of solution.

molasses thick syrup obtainable as sugar cane, beet, citrus or wood molasses. All contain 50 to 55% sugar except citrus, which contains 42%. All are low in protein but high in minerals. The common form is black treacle, a biproduct of the cane sugar industry. Used as a feed supplement to supply additional energy. Because of its high carbohydrate content and palatability it is a common cause of carbohydrate engorgement in cattle. It is also a common cause of polioencephalomalacia in cattle in feedlots.

m. sugar-beet pulp a cattle feed made of sugar beet pulp, after sugar extraction, and molasses.

mold any of a group of parasitic and saprophytic fungi causing a cottony growth on organic substances; also, the deposit of growth produced by such fungi. See also FUNGI, FUNGAL.

m. nephrosis ochratoxin A and citrinin in moldy feed cause nephrosis in pigs.

moldy animal feed overgrown with fungus; the feed may be harvested and stored or be still in the ground.

m. corn disease see LEUKOENCEPHALOMALACIA, FUSARIUM *moniliforme*.

m. feed causes mycotoxic nephropathy in horses.

m. garden beans causes acute interstitial pneumonia in cattle.

m. hay see MICROPOLYSPORA FAENI.

m. sweet clover MELILOTUS *alba*.

m. sweet potato FUSARIUM *javanicum*.

mole 1. a fleshy mass formed in the uterus by abortive development of an ovum. 2. the amount of a substance that contains as many elementary entities (atoms, ions, molecules, or free radicals) as there are atoms in 0.4 oz (12 grams) of pure carbon-12, i.e. equivalent to Avogadro's number (6.023×10^{23}) of elementary entities; the amount of a chemical compound having a mass in grams equal to its molecular weight. 3. a fleshy growth caused by a defect in development of the skin; a NEVUS. The name is also sometimes incorrectly used to describe the tactile hairs and underlying tubercles which are sometimes distinctively pigmented, on either side of the face in dogs. 4. a highly efficient burrowing insectivorous, small mammal in the family Talpidae or Chrysochloridae, with black, velvety fur, and almost blind and deaf.

hydatid m., hydatidiform m. a condition in females characterized by an abnormal pregnancy resulting from a pathological ovum, with proliferation of the epithelial covering of the chorionic villi and dissolution and cystic cavitation of the avascular stroma of the villi. It results in a mass of cysts resembling a bunch of grapes.

pigmented m. see pigmented NEVUS.

molecular of, pertaining to, or composed of molecules.

m. activity see enzyme ACTIVITY.

m. biology study of the biochemical and biophysical aspects of the structure and function of genes and other subcellular entities, and of such specific proteins as hemoglobins, enzymes and hormones; it provides knowledge of cellular differentiation and metabolism and of comparative evolution.

m. layer layers of cells in both cerebellar and cerebral cortices.

m. mimicry see ANTIGENIC mimicry.

m. weight see molecular WEIGHT.

molecule a group of atoms joined by chemical bonds; the smallest amount of a substance that possesses its characteristic properties.

möle [Scand.] a deformity of calves which have short and malformed limbs, hydrocephalus, mandibular hypoplasia and facial tissue deficits. The body is edematous. An inherited defect in Danish cattle.

molera a term for the frontal fontanelle that persists in some dogs, particularly Chihuahuas.

Möller–Barlow's disease see hypertrophic OSTEODYSTROPHY.

mollies popular, all-black, viviparous aquarium fish, *Poecilia* spp. (syn. *Mollienesia sphenops*).

mollities abnormal softening.

m. ossium see OSTEOMALACIA.

Moll's glands sweat glands that have become arrested in their development, situated at the edges of the eyelids; called also ciliary glands, glands of Moll. See also external HORDEOLUM.

mollusc members of the phylum Mollusca, which comprises about 50,000 species. Includes snails, slugs and the aquatic molluscs—oysters, mussels, clams, cockles, arkshells, scallop, abalone, cuttlefish, squid. Also includes gastropods, whose main veterinary interest is as an intermediate host for animal flukes and lungworms.

molluscicide an agent used for killing molluscs (mainly snails and slugs), e.g. copper sulfate, METALDEHYDE, METHIOCARB.

molluscum any of various skin diseases in humans marked by the formation of soft rounded cutaneous tumors.

m. body intracytoplasmic inclusion body, containing poxvirus particles, seen in keratinocytes in molluscum contagiosum.

m. contagiosum a disease of the skin in humans and a similar condition in horses, macropods and chimpanzees caused by a virus in the genus *Molluscipoxvirus*. It is characterized by the formation of firm, rounded, translucent, crateriform papules containing caseous matter that occur mainly on the muzzle, penis, prepuce, and axillary and inguinal skin in horses. The lesions are usually an incidental finding. Two similar diseases occur in horses: viral PAPULAR dermatitis and UASIN GISHU DISEASE.

molly see mare HINNY.

molopo moth see GONOMETA.

molt the physiological shedding of the integument, usually annual, and at the beginning of the breeding season, including the shedding of the skin by reptiles, of hair by many species, and of feathers by birds; the phenomenon is gradual, has severe metabolic overtones and leaves the bird flightless and off lay for several weeks. It is assumed to be related to hormonal changes related to changes in the length of daylight hours.

Molteno disease a disease of cattle in South Africa caused by *Senecio burchellii*.

molting 1. the change of coat in animals at the change of season, most noticeable in animals kept outside in cold climates that stimulate a long winter coat. 2. the replacement in birds of all their feathers once each year in the autumn. Hens stop laying for 8 to 12 weeks at this time. Molting may occur at other times if there is a feed stress.

molybdenosis MOLYBDENUM poisoning.

molybdenum a hard, silvery-white, metallic element, atomic number 42, atomic weight 95.94, symbol Mo. See Table 6. It is an essential trace element, being a component of the enzymes xanthine oxidase, aldehyde oxidase and nitrate reductase.

Molybdenum poisoning causes a secondary hypocuprosis, and clinical signs including chronic diarrhea, illthrift and depigmentation of hair. It occurs most commonly on pastures growing on soils naturally rich in the element, but can be caused by excessive pasture supplementation in an attempt to stimulate the growth of *Rhizobium* spp., the nitrogen-fixing bacteria of legume roots.

moment 1. the force exerted by a lever about a fulcrum. 2. statistically, the mean. The first moment is the same as the mean, the second moment is the mean of the square of a variable, and so on.

momentum the quantity of motion; the product of mass and velocity.

mona grass PASPALUM *scrobiculatum*.

monad 1. a single-celled protozoon or coccus. 2. a univalent radical or element. 3. in meiosis, one member of a tetrad.

monarthric pertaining to a single joint.

monarthritis inflammation of a single joint.

monarticular pertaining to a single joint.

monathetosis athetosis of one limb.

monatomic 1. containing one atom. 2. univalent.

Monday morning disease diseases of horses which occur most frequently after a period of rest. See SPORADIC LYMPHANGITIS, PARALYTIC myoglobinuria.

monecious monoecious.

monensin used as a growth promotant in ruminants, produced by cultures of *Streptomyces cinnamonensis*. Not to be used in horses because of its toxicity in this species.

Large doses in cattle and normal doses in horses cause sudden death due to heart failure. Signs include jugular engorgement, edema and dyspnea. Monensin also increases chances of nitrite poisoning occurring in ruminants fed on high-nitrate rations.

m.-tiamulin poisoning simultaneous administration of both compounds can result in the development of monensin poisoning.

monestrous animals completing only one estrus cycle in each sexual season.

money plant *Epipremnum pinnatum* cv. *aureun*.

Mongolian pony Chinese multipurpose pony, including riding and draft, meat, milk, all coat colors,

Mongolian sheep fat-tailed, meat and carpetwool sheep; white with black or brown head, polled or horned.

Mongolian wild horse a primitive dun-colored pony with a dark dorsal stripe and zebra markings on the legs, 12.1 to 14 hands high. Called also Przewalski's horse, after the Russian explorer who discovered them.

mongoose small, cat-sized mammal in the family Viverridae. There are a number of varieties and genera including the Egyptian mongoose (*Herpestes ichneumon*) and the banded mongoose (*Mungos mungo*). A voracious eater of rodents and reptiles and a favorite house pet.

mongrel of mixed or uncertain breeding; said of dogs in particular but also used adjectivally to refer to any species.

Moniella suaveolens one of the fungi implicated in causing pheohyphomycosis in animals.

Moniezia a genus of tapeworms in the family Anoplocephalidae.

M. benedini, M. expansa common inhabitants of the small intestine in young ruminants up to the age of 6 months. Massive infestations may cause diarrhea and wasting.

Monilia former name of a genus of parasitic fungi, now called CANDIDA.

monilial pertaining to or caused by *Monilia* (CANDIDA).

moniliasis see CANDIDIASIS.

moniliform beaded; having the appearance of a string of beads.

Moniliformis moniliformis acanthocephalid (thorny

headed) worms found in the small intestine of rodents.

Monin technique a surgical procedure for urethroplasty as part of the repair of a rectovaginal fistula in a mare.

monitor 1. continuous observation and measurement of a variable; to check constantly on a given condition or phenomenon, e.g. blood pressure or heart or respiration rate. 2. an apparatus by which such conditions or phenomena can be constantly observed and recorded, e.g. the visual display unit of the computer. 3. very large lizard, up to 10 feet long. Aquatic or terrestrial, carnivorous and carrion-eating. Members of the family Varanidae, e.g. *Varanus griseus*, the desert monitor.

m. alarm devices used to monitor an anesthetized patient to alert the anesthetist and surgeon of abnormalities in the heart rate, respiration and blood pressure. Most are electrical and rely on a satisfactory connection to the patient.

monk-fish see SQUATINA SQUATINA.

monkey members of the families Cebidae (New World monkeys) and Cercopithecidae (Old World monkeys). Those families and the families Pongidae (anthropoid apes) and Callithricidae (marmosets) make up the suborder Anthropoidea (syn. Simiae). They are all diurnal animals with great anatomical similarity to humans, including orbital cavities that are closed laterally, digits that end in nails and pectoral mammary glands. There are minor differences between the New World and Old World monkeys and the total number of genera and species is very large. Individual species are dealt with under their individual titles.

m. dog see AFFENPINSCHER.

m. mouth common deformity in goats, especially the breeds selected for the Roman nose; the upper jaw is shorter than the lower.

m. muscle the triceps brachii muscle of the shoulder; a term used by Greyhound fanciers.

m. pox see MONKEYPOX.

m. rope CYNANCHUM *africanum*.

m. terrier see AFFENPINSCHER.

monkeypox a disease of monkeys caused by a poxvirus in the genus *Orthopoxvirus*. Typical pox lesions occur on the face, hands, feet and ears, and there is a systemic reaction with bronchitis. Healing of the umbilicated, pustular lesions is complete in about a month.

monkshood see ACONITUM.

mono- word element. [Gr.] *one, single, limited to one part, combined with one atom*.

monoacylglycerol hydrolase, lipase enzyme catalyzing the final hydrolytic removal of a fatty acid from monoacylglycerol releasing glycerol into the bloodstream; present in adipose tissue.

monoamine an amine containing only one amino group.

m. oxidase a cuproprotein enzyme that deaminates monoamines such as serotonin, epinephrine, norepinephrine, dopamine, tyramine and tryptamine. Called also MAO.

m. oxidase inhibitors substances that inhibit the activity of monoamine oxidase, increasing catecholamine and serotonin levels in the brain; they are used as antidepressants and antihypertensives. Called also MAO inhibitors.

monoaminergic of or pertaining to neurons that secrete the monoamine neurotransmitters dopamine, norepinephrine and serotonin.

monoamniotic having or developing within a single amniotic cavity; said of monozygotic twins.

monobactam a group of monocyclic β-lactamase resistant antibiotics which includes AZTREONAM and CARUMONAM SODIUM.

monobasic having but one atom of replaceable hydrogen.

monoblast the earliest precursor arising from a committed stem cell in the monocytic series, which develops into the promonocyte.

monobrachia see MONOBRACHIUS.

monobrachius a fetus with only one forelimb.

monocephalus a monster with two bodies and one head.

Monocercomonas a genus of protozoa of the family Monocercomonadidae. No pathogenic effect is associated with the following notable species: *M. caviae*, *M. minuta*, *M. pistillum* (guinea pig), *M. cuniculi* (rabbit), *M. gallinarum* (chicken), all in ceca, and *M. ruminantium* (cattle rumen).

monochloroacetate used in agriculture as a defoliant; nontoxic unless taken in large doses.

monochorial said of twins that have developed sharing a single chorion. Called also monochorionic.

monochorionic having or developing in a common chorionic sac; said of monozygotic twins.

monochromatic 1. existing in or having only one color. 2. staining with only one dye at a time.

monocistron an mRNA encoding a single polypeptide.

monocistronic mRNAs each eukaryotic mRNA contains information coding for only one protein, hence monocistronic, whereas prokaryotic mRNAs may encode more than one protein and are said to be POLYCISTRONIC.

monoclonal derived from a single cell; pertaining to a single clone.

m. antibodies identical immunoglobulin molecules formed by a single clone of plasma cells; may occur naturally in plasma cell myelomas or in vitro by the fusion of an antibody producing B lymphocyte with a non-antibody-producing myeloma B cell. The fused heterokaryon has the properties of immortality and production of a monoclonal antibody. For the most part, monoclonal antibodies are made in mouse systems.

m. gammopathy see monoclonal GAMMOPATHY.

monocontaminated infected by only one species of microorganism or a single contaminating agent.

monocotyledonous said of plants the seeds of which have only one cotyledon.

monocrotaline a pyrrolizidine alkaloid in CROTALARIA *spectabilis*.

monocrotophos an organophosphorus compound used as a pesticide and capable of poisoning raptor birds that eat the poisoned vermin.

monocular 1. pertaining to one eye. 2. having but one eyepiece, as in a microscope.

monoculus 1. a bandage for one eye. 2. a cyclops.

monocyte a mononuclear, phagocytic leukocyte, 13 to 25 μm in diameter, having an ovoid or kidney-shaped nucleus and azurophilic cytoplasmic granules. Monocytes are derived from promonocytes in the bone marrow. They circulate in the blood for about 24 hours before migrating to the tissues, as in the lung and liver, where they develop into macrophages.

m. leukemia see monocytic LEUKEMIA.

m.–macrophage system see RETICULOENDOTHELIAL SYSTEM.

monocytic leukemia see monocytic LEUKEMIA.

monocytopenia a deficiency of monocytes in the blood.

monocytopoiesis the production of monocytes.
monocytosis an excess of monocytes in the blood.
monodactyl a foot with one digit, as in the horse. See also SOLIPED.
monodactyly the presence of only one digit on a limb.
monodermoma a tumor developed from one germinal layer.
monodon baculovirus disease affects larval *Penaeus monodon*, *P. merguiensis*, *P. semisulcatus*, and to a lesser extent other penaeids under conditions of poor husbandry and stress.
monoecious having reproductive organs typical of both sexes in a single individual.
monofilament suture a suture made of a single filament. Causes less irritation than a braided suture.
monogastric referring to a stomach with a single chamber as in the dog, cat, horse or pig.
Monogenea a subclass of trematode parasites that infest cold-blooded aquatic or amphibious vertebrates. Includes the genera *Benedenia*, *Dactylogyrus*, *Diplozoon*, *Discocotyle*, *Gyrodactylus*.
monogenean pertaining to or emanating from Monogenea.
monogenic pertaining to or influenced by a single gene.
monogerminal developed from one ovum; said of identical twins.
monoglyceride a compound consisting of one molecule of fatty acid esterified to glycerol.
monohydric alcohols includes ethanol, benzyl alcohol, methanol.
monoiodotyrosine the first step in the production of thyroxine. Iodine trapped in the thyroid gland is conjugated with the tyrosine moiety of thyroglobulin; abbreviated MIT.
monokine a cytokine produced by macrophages that act on T lymphocytes to enhance cell-mediated immunity, e.g. interleukin 1.
monolayer pertaining to or consisting of a single layer of molecules or cells, as in a monolayer cell culture, as used for the isolation and assay of viruses.
monolocular having but one cavity, as in a cyst.
monomastest an indirect test for bovine mastitis based on the concentration of serum albumen in the milk.
monomelic affecting one limb.
monomer 1. a simple molecule of relatively low molecular weight, which is capable of reacting chemically with other molecules to form a polymer, in which the monomers are linked by covalent bonds. 2. a single protein molecule that combines with other monomers by hydrogen bonds to form a larger protein.
fibrin m. the material resulting from the action of thrombin on fibrinogen, which then polymerizes to form fibrin.
monomeric 1. pertaining to a single segment. 2. in genetics, determined by a gene or genes at a single locus. 3. consisting of monomers. 4. see also monomeric DIET.
monomolecular pertaining to a single molecule or to a layer one molecule thick.
monomorphic existing in only one form.
monomphalus a double monster joined at the navel.
monomyelocytic leukemia in horses causes ventral edema, weight loss, splenomegaly, some lymph node enlargement and susceptibility to infection.
monomyoplegia paralysis of a single muscle.
monomyositis inflammation of a single muscle.
Mononegavirales an order of RNA viruses containing four families, *Paramyxoviridae*, *Rhabdoviridae*, *Filoviridae* and *Bornaviridae*.
mononeural supplied by a single nerve.
mononeuritis inflammation of a single nerve.
m. multiplex simultaneous inflammation of several nerves remote from one another.
mononeuropathy a lesion or lesions affecting a single peripheral nerve.
m. multiplex neuropathy involving a number of peripheral nerves but in a random manner.
mononuclear having only one nucleus.
blockade of m.–phagocytic system results when large numbers of particles or bacteria absorb all available receptor sites or otherwise interfere with phagocytosis. May be a factor in reducing host defense mechanisms.
m. phagocytes macrophages.
m. phagocyte system the group of highly phagocytic cells that have a common origin from stem cells of the bone marrow and develop circulating monocytes and tissue macrophages, which develop from monocytes that have migrated to connective tissue of the liver (Kupffer's cells), lung, spleen and lymph nodes. The term has been proposed to replace *reticuloendothelial system*, which includes some cells of different origin.
mononucleosis excess of mononuclear leukocytes (monocytes) in the blood.
monooxygenase one of the microsomal enzyme systems; mixed function enzyme systems.
monoparesis paresis of a single part.
monopathy a disease affecting a single part.
monophthalmus, monops a fetus with one eye; a cyclops.
monophyletic descended from a common ancestor or stem cell.
monophyodont an animal in which permanent teeth do not have a temporary precursor.
monoplegia paralysis of a single limb.
monopodia agenesis of one limb.
monopoiesis the development of monocytes.
monopolar having a single pole.
monops see MONOPHTHALMUS.
monopus a fetus with only one foot.
monorchid an animal having only one testis in the scrotum.
monorchidism, monorchism the condition of having only one testis or one descended testis.
Monordotaenia taxidiensis a tapeworm of the family Taeniidae recorded in wild amimals, skunk, mink, ermine, marten and badger.
monosaccharide a simple sugar; a carbohydrate that cannot be broken down to simpler substances by hydrolysis, e.g. glucose, fructose and galactose.
m. absorption tests see oral GLUCOSE tolerance test; D-XYLOSE absorption test.
monosodium methyl arsenate a potent brushwood killer, toxic to animals by mouth or percutaneously, causing diarrhea and weight loss. See also organic ARSENIC poisoning.
monosomy existence in a cell of only one instead of the normal diploid pair of a particular chromosome.
monospace font see fixed-pitch FONT.
monospecific having an effect on only a particular kind of cell or tissue, or reacting with only a single antigen, as, for example, a monospecific antiserum.
Monosporium see SCEDOSPORIUM APIOSPERMUM.
monostotic affecting a single bone.
monosulfiram an ectoparasiticide, called also Tetmosol and sulfiram; used extensively against mites, but toxic if overused.

monosymptomatic manifested by only one clinical sign.
monosynaptic pertaining to or passing through a single synapse.
monothermia a condition in which the body temperature remains the same throughout the day.
monotocous having one offspring per gestation.
monotreme a member of the animal order of Momotremata, the egg-laying mammals. Includes only two species, the duck-billed platypus and the spiny anteater.
monotrichous having a single flagellum, usually at a polar position; applied to a bacterial cell.
monotypic said of a genus with only one species.
monovalent 1. having a valency of one. 2. capable of binding with only one antigenic or antibody specificity.
monovular twins twins developed from one fertilized ovum, i.e. identical twins.
monoxenous requiring only one host to complete the life cycle.
monozygotic pertaining to or derived from a single zygote (fertilized ovum); said of TWINS.
m. twins see monozygotic TWINS.
monozygous see MONOZYGOTIC.
mons pl. *montes* [L.] a prominence.
monster a fetus or neonate with such pronounced developmental anomalies as to be grotesque and usually nonviable. Classified in many ways, e.g. single or double.
Monstera deliciosa toxic plant in the Araceae family; contains raphide crystals of oxalate; causes oral erosions.
monstriparity the act of giving birth to a monster.
monstrosity 1. great congenital deformity. 2. a monster or teratism.
Montadale an American medium-woolled, meat sheep produced by crossing COLUMBIA and CHEVIOT breeds.
Montana progressive pneumonia a chronic pneumonia of sheep caused by a virus closely related antigenically to MAEDI virus.
Monte Carlo method a computer trial or study which uses random numbers in the simulation and analysis of complex relationships and events.
Monteggia's fracture a fracture in the proximal half of the shaft of the ulna, with dislocation of the head of the radius.
Montenegro test an immunodiagnostic test suitable for use in chronic cases of cutaneous LEISHMANIASIS.
Monterey cypress CUPRESSUS *macrocarpa*.
Montgomery T tube a T-shaped tube used in a tracheostomy to treat laryngeal and tracheal injuries. It serves as a stent and to provide an airway.
Montgomery's disease African swine fever.
monthly accounts receivable the accounts raised for the month for which statements are to be sent out.
Montia perfoliata plant in Portulacaceae family; causes nitrate–nitrite poisoning; called also miner's lettuce, winter purslane, *Claytonia perfoliata*.
monticulus pl. *monticuli* [L.] a small eminence.
m. cerebelli the projecting part of the superior vermis cerebelli.
monuron a selective urea-based herbicide. Can cause anemia and methemoglobinemia. Vomiting, ataxia and urticaria are also recorded.
moo the subdued talking voice of cattle.
moon blindness see periodic OPHTHALMIA.
Moore technique an imbrication technique for replacement of a prolapsed third eyelid, using a purse-string suture.
moose largest of the deer, 6 feet at the withers, 2000 pounds. Males have a prominent roman nose and overhanging upper lip, dark brown coat with white legs. Called also American moose, *Alces americana, Alces alces*.
m. disease/sickness see NEUROFILARIASIS. Called also moose sickness.
m. tick see DERMACENTOR *albipictus*.
MOPP a regimen of mechlorethamine (mustine), Oncovin (vincristine), procarbazine and prednisone, used in cancer chemotherapy.
Mopshond an early Dutch name for the Pug.
Moraea poisonous plants in the family Iridaceae; contain a bufadienolide which causes cardiac irregularity, diarrhea, abdominal pain and sudden death; includes *M. bellendini, M. bipartitia, M. graminicola, M. juncea, M. lilacina, M. polyanthos, M. polystachya, M. venenata*.
morantel a general purpose anthelmintic for horses and cattle, used as the tartrate. Can be used against worms that have benzimidazole resistance. Mode of action is similar to levamisole.
Moraxella a genus of short, rod-shaped bacteria that occur in pairs. *M. lacunata* and *M. phenylpyruvica* are of unknown pathogenicity in animals.
M. anatipestifer see PASTEURELLA *anatipestifer*.
M. bovis causes INFECTIOUS bovine keratoconjunctivitis.
morbid 1. pertaining to, affected with, or inducing disease; diseased. 2. unhealthy; unwholesome.
morbidity the condition of being diseased.
proportional m. the proportion of all of the diseased animals in the population that have the particular disease under discussion.
m. rate the ratio of diseased to healthy animals in the population. The ratio is said to be standardized when it is expressed as a proportion of the expected rate compared with a standard group. It is also expressed as a proportional rate when it is stated as a proportion of all of the cases of illness due to all causes in the group.
morbific causing or inducing disease.
Morbillivirus one of the three genera of viruses in the family PARAMYXOVIRIDAE. It includes the viruses of human measles, canine distemper, rinderpest, equine morbillivirus disease and peste des petits ruminants.
equine m. see EQUINE morbillivirus.
morbus [L.] *disease*.
morcellation division of solid tissue (as a tumor) into pieces, followed by piecemeal removal.
mordant 1. a substance capable of intensifying or deepening the reaction of a specimen to a stain. 2. to subject to the action of a mordant before staining.
Morellia a genus of flies in the family Muscidae. They are essentially flies of flowers and vegetation, but are attracted to sweat and mucus and can be a significant source of insect worry in summer. The common species are *M. aenescens, M. hortorum* and *M. simplex*. Called also sweat flies.
Morel's disease a disease of sheep characterized by abscesses containing green pus located near lymph nodes, and is caused by a gram-positive micrococcus.
Moreton Bay chestnut see CASTANOSPERMUM AUSTRALE.
morgagnian globule proteinaceous globule produced from the degeneration of optic lens fibers.
Morgagni's hydatid small cysts adjacent to the head of the epididymis in the horse, probably remnants of the Mullerian ducts. Called also 'appendix testis'.
morgan flower see MORGANIA FLORIBUNDA.
Morgan horse an American light horse, named after

a famous sire Justin Morgan. An all-round pleasure horse in harness or under saddle. Bay, black, brown or chestnut; 14.2 to 15.2 hands high.

M. h. cuneate nucleus neuraxonal dystrophy suspected inherited defect in Morgan horse foals less than 6 months old; characterized by hindlimb ataxia progressing gradually over a period of several years and dystrophic neuraxonal lesions only in the accessory cuneate nucleus.

Morganella morganii member of the bacterial family Enterobacteriaceae; may be associated with otitis externa and urinary tract infections in dogs and cats.

Morgania floribunda Australian plant in the Scrophulariaceae family; contains a cardiac glycoside causing vomiting, diarrhea; called also Morgan flower.

moribund in a dying state.

Morinda reticulata Australian plant in the Rubiaceae family; a converter plant which preferentially absorbs selenium and has a higher content of it than other plants; causes alopecia, laminitis in horses; called also mapoon.

morning glory IPOMOEA *muelleri*, *I. purpurea*.

Morocco leather the appearance of the abomasal mucosa, hyperplasia and covered with small, 2 to 3 mm diameter, circular nodules, in cattle with heavy infestations of *Ostertagia ostertagi*.

Morone genus of finfish in family Perichthyidae. Includes *M. chrysops* (white bass), *M. saxatilis* (striped bass). See Table 23.

morph- prefix meaning shape.

morphea see canine localized SCLERODERMA.

morphine the principal and most active opium alkaloid, a narcotic analgesic and respiratory depressant, usually used as morphine sulfate.

m. substitutes those used in veterinary medicine include MEPERIDINE, METHADONE, PENTAZOCINE LACTATE.

morphium see MORPHINE.

morphogenesis the developmental changes of growth and differentiation occurring in the organization of the body and its parts.

morphogeny morphogenesis.

morphology the science of the forms and structure of organisms; the form and structure of a particular organism, organ, tissue or cell.

morphometry the measurement of forms.

-morphous word element. [Gr.] *shape, form*.

mors [L.] *death*.

morsus [L.] *bite*.

m. diaboli the fimbriated end of a uterine tube.

mortal 1. destined to die. 2. causing or terminating in death; fatal.

mortality 1. the quality of being mortal. 2. death as a statistic.

embryonic m. see early EMBRYONIC mortality.

m. rate the death rate; the ratio of the total number of deaths to the total number of the population during a specified time period. Commonly used specific mortality rates include *disease*, *case fatality*, *neonatal*, *perinatal* and *preweaning* mortality rates.

The rate may also be expressed as a standardized rate, when it is stated as a ratio of the expected death rate in a standard group of animals. It may also be expressed as a proportional rate, when it is stated as a proportion of all of deaths due to all causes in the group.

mortar 1. wooden or ceramic vessel with a rounded internal surface, used with a pestle, for reducing a solid to a powder or producing a homogeneous mixture of solids. 2. a material used to cement bricks in place.

m. licking a form of pica usually ascribed to a nutritional deficiency of calcium.

Mortierella wolfii a mucoraceous fungus causing mycotic abortion in cattle. See also MORTIERELLOSIS.

mortierellosis a disease caused by infection with *Mortierella wolfii*. Abortion is the best known manifestation of the disease. There is in addition the uncommon finding of acute necrotizing pneumonia in the cow that has just aborted.

mortification gangrene.

morula 1. a solid mass of cells (blastomeres) resembling a mulberry, formed by cleavage of a fertilized ovum. 2. a cluster of organisms appearing as an inclusion in the cytoplasm of circulating leukocytes infected by *Ehrlichia* spp.

mosaic a pattern made of numerous small pieces fitted together; in genetics, the occurrence in an animal of two or more cell populations, each having a different chromosome complement, e.g. XY/XXY mosaic.

m. animals all the genotypes arise from a single zygotic genotype because of chromosomal loss or mitotic nondisjunction.

ecological m. a pattern of interspersed ecosystems of similar size and on a recurring basis.

mosaicism the presence in an individual animal of cells derived from the same zygote, but differing in chromosomal constitution.

Moskoff's islets islets of seminiferous tissue, supplied with blood from the tunic of the testis, which survive ligation of the spermatic artery in the prepubertal lamb and regenerate. However, recanalization does not occur and the tissue ultimately degenerates.

mOsm milliosmole.

mosquito blood-sucking insect of the genera *Aedes*, *Anopheles*, *Culex*, *Taeniorhynchus* (*Mansonia*) and *Psorophora*. Some species are concerned with the transmission of diseases, such as equine encephalomyelitis, filarial nematodes, avian malaria and Rift Valley fever.

m.-bite dermatitis pruritic papules and plaques develop on the face of cats with hypersensitivity reactions to mosquito bites.

m. forceps see HALSTED mosquito forceps.

moss-ill see MILK fever.

mossy passion flower PASSIFLORA *foetida*.

most common fee the average fee charged for a particular professional service, as a guide to what should be charged; the recommended fee.

mother maternal parent; in animals, usually called the dam.

m. hairs kemp hairs in the fleece of newborn lambs which are shed soon after birth and do not recur.

m. of millions see BRYOPHYLLUM.

m.-young relationship the bond established between the newborn and the mother—a critical factor in maintaining high survival rates; a matter of great importance in enhancing lamb survival.

mothering the instinct in a dam to provide the best protective care for the young. See also MATERNAL neglect, MISMOTHERING.

m. capability lack of this capacity can cause loss of the neonate, a characteristic of some individual dams and of merino ewes.

motherumbah ACACIA *cheelii*.

moths insects belonging to the order Lepidoptera; see ARCYOPHORA.

motif for proteins a three-dimensional structural unit formed by a particular sequence of amino acids, found in proteins and which is often linked with a particular function. For nucleic acids a particular, usually short, nucleotide sequence that forms a recognition site usually to which other proteins bind.

structural m's in proteins, certain specific orderings of secondary structure that may have a functional role and include β-α-β helix-turn-helix, leucine zippers, calcium binding EF hands, zinc fingers and longer orderings that take on a structural domain such as the β-barrel and the immunoglobulin fold.

motile having spontaneous but not conscious or volitional movement.

motilin a polypeptide hormone secreted by enterochromaffin cells of the gut; it causes increased motility of several portions of the gut and stimulates pepsin secretion. Its release is stimulated by the presence of acid and fat in the duodenum.

motility the ability to move spontaneously.

abomasal m. synchronized contractions and motility of the abomasal wall and the opening of the pyloric sphincter are dependent on the fullness of the abomasum, the degree of trituration and the pH of the contents and the integrity of the vagal and sympathetic nerve supplies.

intestinal m. is essential to onward movement of the digesta and excreta. Absence leads to lack of absorption, accumulation of fluid and gas, and development of paralytic ileus. Audible over the flank with a stethoscope.

m. modifiers a class of drugs used to regulate activity of gastrointestinal smooth muscle; includes cholinergics, anticholinergics, DOMPERIDONE, CISAPRIDE, opioids, LOPERAMIDE, METOCLOPRAMIDE and DIPHENOXYLATE hydrochloride.

ruminal m. audible and visible in the upper left flank. The best indicator of the state of activity of the alimentary tract in cattle.

m. tests carried out to characterize the motility of some bacteria. Methods include the direct microscopy of a hanging-drop, semisolid media with an indicator dye, and other specialized types of media.

motion mode see M-mode ULTRASONOGRAPHY.

motion sickness discomfort observed by some companion animals while being transported. It is caused by irregular and abnormal motion that disturbs the organs of balance located in the inner ear. There may be hypersalivation, restlessness and vomiting.

motivation see DRIVE.

motoceptor any muscle sense receptor.

motor 1. pertaining to motion. 2. a muscle, nerve or center that effects movements.

m. activity limb movement the most obvious of these forms of activity.

m. alpha-neuron ventral spinal cord neurons which innervate skeletal muscle. Called also final common pathway, lower motor neuron.

m. depressant anticonvulsant a drug that depresses motor activity and hence prevents convulsions, e.g. phenobarbital sodium, phenytoin sodium.

m. dysfunction abnormality of the motor system.

m. end-plate sites of neuraptic transmission of acetylcholine from nerve to muscle receptors.

m. fibers innervate the body effectors.

m. lubricating oil ingestion may cause lead poisoning.

m. nerve conduction the transmission of impulses along motor nerves to skeletal muscle.

m. unit includes the motor neuron, neuromuscular junction, and the myofibrils innervated by the neuron.

m. unit action potential the electrical activity of voluntary muscle contractions recorded by needle electromyography.

motor neuron a neuron having a motor function; an efferent neuron conveying motor impulses.

m. n. disease see ABIOTROPHY.

lower m. n's peripheral neurons whose cell bodies lie in the ventral gray columns of the spinal cord and whose terminations are in skeletal muscles. Called also LMN. See also LOWER motor neuron.

peripheral m. n's neurons in a peripheral reflex arc that receive impulses from interneurons and transmit them to voluntary muscles.

upper m. n's neurons in the cerebral cortex that conduct impulses from the motor cortex to the motor nuclei of the cerebral nerves or to the ventral gray columns of the spinal cord. Lesions of the upper motor neuron interrupt the inhibitory effect that upper motor neurons have on lower motor neurons, resulting in exaggerated or hyperactive reflexes. This is called also extensor rigidity. See also UPPER motor neuron. Called also UMN.

MOTT mycobacteria other than tuberculosis.

moufflon the European wild sheep, characterized by a reddish color, short wool and big curly horns, and an ability to survive in very tough conditions. Called also *Ovis musimon*.

moulage [Fr.] *a wax model of a structure or lesion.*

mould mold.

mount 1. to prepare specimens and slides for study. 2. a preparatory step to mating in animals.

Mount Rose lupine LUPINUS *montigenus*.

mountain related in some way to high altitude.

m. devil see LAMBERTIA *formosa*.

m. disease see ALTITUDE SICKNESS.

m. gorilla *Gorilla gorilla beringei*.

m. laurel see KALMIA.

m. lion see mountain LION.

m. mahogany see CERCOCARPUS.

m. pink CENTAURIUM *beyrichii*.

m. sickness see ALTITUDE SICKNESS.

m. silvery lupine LUPINUS *alpestris*.

m. thermopsis THERMOPSIS *montana*.

Mountain collie see BEARDED COLLIE.

mounting see MOUNT.

m. behavior the placement of the forequarters over the hindquarters of another animal, as occurs in mating. Seen particularly in pet dogs that mount other dogs, male or female, humans or sometimes objects. Usually considered unacceptable behavior by owners.

inappropriate m. commonly seen in puppies, but occasionally continues into adulthood. Commonly a displacement activity, in response to conflict or excitement.

mouse pl. *mice*. 1. small rodent, various species of which are used in laboratory experiments and kept as domestic pets. 2. a small loose body, e.g. in a joint. 3. a microcomputer peripheral device used to control cursor movement by means of a ball and a sensor.

athymic m. see NUDE MOUSE.

banana m. *Dendromus*.

common m. members of several subfamilies of the family Muridae which includes the mice, rats and Eurasian voles. Old World mice (subfamily Murinae) include many species such as house mouse (*Mus musculus*), harvest mouse and wood mouse. New World mice (subfamily Cricetinae) also include many species and varieties such as deer mice (*Peromyscus leucopus*). Banana mice (*Dendromus* spp.) live in banana trees and are related to the fat mice which live in sandy burrows.

m. deer see CHEVROTAIN.

m. ectromelia see ECTROMELIA (2).

field m. lives in fields, woods and gardens. Includes *Apodemus flavicollis* (yellow-necked field mouse) and *A. sylvaticus* (European long-tailed field mouse).
house m. see MUS *musculus*.
joint m. a movable fragment of synovial membrane, cartilage or other body within a joint; usually associated with degenerative osteoarthritis and osteochondritis dissecans.
laboratory m. similar in many ways to wild mice, but selectively bred to be of a consistent type for experimental work under laboratory conditions. Many lines are closely inbred to produce selected genetic characteristics that make them develop certain diseases or biochemical abnormalities. Most laboratory mice are white, but some colored varieties exist.
m. lactic dehydrogenase elevating virus an arterivirus, originally isolated as a contaminant of transplantable mouse tumor cells. Subsequently found to cause life-long virema associated with elevated blood levels of lactic dehydrogenase, but no clinical disease.
marsupial m. an insectivorous, mouse-like member of the subfamily Phascogalinae; the smallest of existing marsupials.
m. parvovirus see MINUTE mouse virus.
peritoneal m. a free body in the peritoneal cavity, probably a small detached mass or omentum, sometimes visible radiographically.
m. pneumonia virus a pneumovirus that causes chronic illness and emaciation in athymic mice, but subclinical infection in others.
m. pointer a symbol on the computer screen to indicate the position of the mouse and/or the state of the system.
m. poliomyelitis a picornavirus disease causing generalized paralysis in older mice (6 to 10 weeks) and encephalitis in younger mice (up to 30 days). Called also THEILER'S DISEASE.
m. pox see ECTROMELIA (2).
spiny pocket m. small rodent with large food pockets in its cheeks; called also *Perognathus spinatus*.
m. tick IXODES *muris*.
m. typhoid infection by *Salmonella enteritidis*.
white-footed m. see PEROMYSCUS LEUCOPUS.

mouse-tailed crumbleweed see DYSPHANIA RHADINOSTACHYA.

mouth an opening, especially the oral cavity, which forms the beginning of the DIGESTIVE system and in which the chewing of food takes place. It is also the site of the organs of taste and the teeth, tongue and lips, and the entrance to the body for food and sometimes air. In animals it is a part of the system of defense and attack. Called also oral cavity, buccal cavity. See also ORAL.
African m. breeders fish that breed in isolated pairs and the spawn of which are incubated in the mouth of the male. Called also *Tilapia macrocephala*.
m. carcinoma in food animals may occur in those eating bracken. It is usually a squamous cell carcinoma of gum epithelium.
m. dryness characteristic of dehydration, atropine poisoning.
m. erosions EROSIVE STOMATITIS.
full m. a mature animal with all teeth erupted and in wear.
m. gag see mouth speculum (below).
m. inflammation see STOMATITIS, GINGIVITIS, GLOSSITIS, etc.
monkey m. mandibular prognathism; undershot jaw.
m. mucosal lesions includes stomatitis, necrobacillosis, ulcer, foreign body lodgment, laceration.
m. necrobacillosis necrosis, ulceration caused usually by *Fusobacterium necrophorum*.
m. neoplasms see ORAL neoplasm.
parrot m. see BRACHYGNATHIA.
paw and m. disease a name for feline CALICIVIRUS or HERPESVIRUS infection because of the infrequent occurrence of ulcerations on the skin, usually of the front paws, as well as the usual location in the mouth; probably the result of transmission from grooming.
scabby m. see contagious ECTHYMA.
shear m. malocclusion producing marked pointing of the enamel. Seen particularly in horses.
m. shyness avoidance of handling around the mouth may be a sign of dental disease in animals.
sow m. mandibular prognathism; undershot jaw.
m. speculum a device for preventing the mouth from being closed which permits the passage of the hand or an easily damaged piece of equipment such as a rubber stomach tube. See also FRICK, MCPHERSON, SCHOUPE, DRINKWATER, BAYER specula. There are several unnamed pieces: a wooden one used in cows, which is inserted crossways between the teeth and a stomach tube passed through a hole in its middle; a metal one used in horses by placing its two dental plates over the tables of the incisor teeth and screwing them apart with a thumbscrew working inside the frame that supports the plates; and a similar, simpler device used in sheep and small pigs which has two horizontal bars running crossways between the two parallel prongs of a handheld, fork-like device. It is inserted horizontally between the molar teeth and then turned to a vertical position.
m. ulcers in large animals, ulcers of the oral mucosa usually caused by secondary bacterial infection of less severe mucosal lesions caused by a primary disease, e.g. mucosal disease. In cats, ulcerations are often associated with FELINE viral respiratory disease complex.
m. wart a common location for infection by papilloma virus.
wry m. a twisted mouth caused by unilateral malocclusion.

mouthing 1. familiarizing the unbroken horse with the novelty of having a bit in its mouth. A special mouthing bit with dangling players on the bit is used. 2. checking the teeth of a grazing animal, e.g. to identify sheep with a BROKEN MOUTH.

mouthrot necrotic stomatitis of reptiles caused by *Corynebacterium* spp. and *Staphylococcus aureus*.

mouton lamb pelt made to resemble seal or beaver.

Movar 33/63 herpesvirus a strain of bovine herpesvirus 4.

movement an act of moving; motion.
m. abnormality includes involuntary movement, lack of flexion or rigidity, hyper- or hypometric.
active m. movement produced by the animal's own muscles.
ameboid m. movement like that of an ameba, accomplished by protrusion of cytoplasm of the cell.
associated m. movement of parts that act together, such as the eyes.
brownian m. continuous movement of particles suspended within a liquid.
conjugate m. two parts moving synchronously in the same direction, e.g. the eyes.
disjunctive m. two parts moving synchronously but in opposite directions.
involuntary m. a movement which the animal is unable to prevent.

m. keys keys on a keyboard which control the movement of the cursor within a page or document; includes arrow keys, page up, page down, end, home keys.
molecular m. the peculiar, rapid, oscillatory movement of fine particles suspended in a fluid medium.
passive m. a movement of the body or of the extremities of an animal performed by a person without voluntary motion on the part of the animal.
vermicular m's the wormlike movements of the intestines in peristalsis.
voluntary m. performed out of the will of the animal; an intentional purposeful movement.
moving average see moving AVERAGE.
moxa a tuft of soft, combustible herb *Artemisia vulgaris* is burned upon the skin as a cautery. A procedure in Chinese traditional medicine.
moxalactam a third-generation cephalosporin antibiotic having an oxa-β-lactam ring and a broad spectrum of activity, effective against β-lactamase-producing strains of *Haemophilus influenzae* and gram-negative enteric bacilli, including multiple drug-resistant strains.
moxibustion cauterization by the burning of a moxa; a procedure in traditional Chinese medicine.
moxidectin a macrolide derived from *Streptomyces cyaneogriseus noncyanogenus* with activity against nematodes and arthropods.
MPA medroxyprogesterone acetate.
MPD maximum permissible dose.
MPF mitosis-promoting factor.
MPS mononuclear phagocytic system.
MR methemoglobin reductase.
mR milliroentgen.
mrad millirad. A non-SI unit now replaced by the GRAY.
MRI magnetic resonance imaging.
MRL maximum residue limit.
mRNA a unique set of tRNAs, mRNAs, rRNAs, transcribed from mitochondrial DNA by a mitochondrial-specific RNA polymerase, which account for about 4% of the total cell RNA which is transcribed.
MRT milk ring test.
MRV minute respiratory volume.
MS-DOS acronym for MicroSoft disk operating system; probably the commonest computer operating system used in microcomputers.
MSH melanocyte-stimulating hormone.
MSMA monosodium methanearsonate; an organic arsenical herbicide which can cause poisoning characterized by the signs of organic ARSENIC poisoning.
mtDNA mitochondrial DNA.
MTOC microtubule-organizing center.
mu the twelfth letter of the Greek alphabet, M or μ.
***mu* points** see ALARM POINTS.
mu tree ALEURITES *montana.*
muciferous secreting mucus.
muciform resembling mucus.
mucigen a substance present in mucous cells, convertible into mucin and mucus.
mucilage an aqueous solution of a gummy substance, used as a vehicle or demulcent.
mucilloid a preparation of a mucilaginous substance.
psyllium hydrophilic m. a powdered preparation of the mucilaginous portion of blond psyllium seeds, used in treatment of constipation. See also PSYLLIUM.
mucin a mucopolysaccharide or glycoprotein which is the chief constituent of mucus.
m. clot test the adding of acetic acid to normal synovial fluid, which causes clot formation. The compactness of the clot and the clarity of the supernatant fluid are the criteria on which the result is based.
mucinase an enzyme that acts upon mucin.
mucinogen a precursor of mucin.
mucinoid 1. resembling mucin. 2. mucoid (2).
mucinosis a state with abnormal deposits of mucin in the skin, often associated with hypothyroidism (myxedema).
follicular m. see ALOPECIA mucinosa.
idiopathic m. see Shar-Pei mucinosis (below).
Shar-Pei m. increased amounts of mucin in the dermis is associated with the greatly wrinkled skin which is characteristic of this breed. Called also idiopathic mucinosis.
mucinous relating to, resembling or containing mucin.
m. carcinoid see goblet-cell CARCINOID.
muciparous secreting mucin.
muck itch see SWEET itch.
mucking out removing manure and soiled straw from a horse's loose box.
mucoarteritis a degenerative disease in which glycosaminoglycan is deposited in the subendocardium of the left atrium and in the intima of the large arteries in dogs. Seen in uremic dogs, significant only in dogs on a high fat diet.
mucocele 1. dilatation of a cavity with accumulated mucous secretion. 2. a mucous polyp.
nasolacrimal m. see DACRYOPS.
orbital m. may be due to leakage from a salivary gland or lacrimal secretions. Causes exophthalmos and protrusion of the nictitating membrane.
salivary m. extravasation of saliva into subcutaneous tissue following injury to a salivary gland or duct. Most commonly seen in dogs as a fluctuant, sometimes large and pendulous, nonpainful mass in the intermandibular, cranial, cervical or sublingual area.
mucocervix a condition in cows in which the cervix is much enlarged (4 inches diameter × 5 to 6 inches long or 10 cm diameter × 12–15 cm) and has a tenacious and enlarged seal of mucus.
mucociliary pertaining to a combination of cilia and mucus.
m. blanket a blanket of mucus overlying cilia beating in a watery sol on the surface of the respiratory mucosa.
m. escalator the nonimmunological defense mechanism involving ciliary action and flow of mucus from bronchioles, through the bronchi and trachea to the larynx, by which particulate matter is removed from the respiratory tract. Called also mucociliary ladder.
m. ladder see mucociliary escalator (above).
m. transport the effect of the operation of the mucociliary escalator.
mucocutaneous pertaining to mucous membrane and skin.
m. margin the sites where skin and mucosae merge, e.g. at the anus, mouth, urethra. Called also mucocutaneous junction.
mucoenteritis see irritable COLON syndrome.
mucoepidermoid composed of mucus-producing epithelial cells, e.g. mucoepidermoid carcinoma.
mucogingival junction, mucogingival line the junction between gingiva attached to underlying bone and the flap overlying the tooth.
mucohemorrhagic characterized by hemorrhage and mucus, e.g. mucohemorrhagic diarrhea.
mucoid 1. resembling mucus. 2. a mucus-like conjugated protein of animal origin, differing from mucin in solubility.
m. degeneration see mucoid DEGENERATION.
m. enteritis see mucoid ENTEROPATHY, irritable COLON syndrome.
m. valvular degeneration see ENDOCARDIOSIS.

mucolipidosis a group of inherited lysosomal storage diseases in which mucopolysaccharides and lipids accumulate in tissues. Mucolipidosis I is also called sialosis.

m. II lysosomes contain large inclusions of undigested glycosaminoglycans and glycolipids. Called also I-cell disease.

mucolytic 1. destroying or dissolving mucus. 2. an agent that so acts.

mucomembranous pertaining to or composed of mucous membrane.

mucometra a uterus distended with a fluid containing much mucin. Occurs in segmental aplasia, imperforate hymen and cystic ovarian degeneration. See also HYDROMETRA.

mucoperiosteum periosteum having a mucous surface, as in parts of the auditory apparatus.

Mucophilus cyprini algae in tanks and ponds which may asphyxiate fish by blocking the gills.

mucopolysaccharide a group of polysaccharides that contain hexosamine, which may or may not be combined with protein; when dispersed in water, mucopolysaccharides form many of the mucins.

acid m. the amorphous, PAS-positive intercellular substance of most connective tissue. Formed by fibroblasts and osteoblasts.

mucopolysaccharidosis any of a group of genetically determined disorders due to a defect in glycosaminoglycan (GAG) metabolism, marked by skeletal changes, mental retardation and visceral involvement; abbreviated MPS. Achondroplastic dwarfism in cattle may be a defect of this type.

m. I caused by an inherited deficiency of α-L-iduronidase with increased urinary excretion of dermatan sulfate and heparan sulfate. Affected dogs and cats show facial dysmorphia, stunted growth, corneal clouding, lameness and granulation of leukocytes. Called also Hurler's syndrome.

m. VI caused by an inherited deficiency of arylsulfatase B with increased urinary excretion of dermatan sulfate. Affected Siamese cats show facial dysmorphia, corneal clouding, granulation of leukocytes, posterior paresis, and skin nodules. Called also Maroteaux–Lamy syndrome.

m. type VII caused by a deficiency of β glucaronidase. Affected dogs have facial dysmorphism and corneal edema.

mucopolysacchariduria an excess of mucopolysaccharides in the urine.

mucoprotein a compound present in all connective and supporting tissues, containing, as prosthetic groups, mucopolysaccharides; soluble in water and relatively resistant to denaturation. An important component of many uroliths.

Tamm–Horsfall m. locally secreted in Henle's loops, the distal tubules, and the collecting ducts of the kidney; the principal constituent of hyaline casts.

mucopurulent marked by an exudate containing both mucus and pus.

mucopus mucus blended with pus.

Mucor a genus of saprophytic mold fungi; some species cause MUCORMYCOSIS.

M. amphibiorum the cause of ulcerative dermatitis in platypus in Tasmania, Australia.

mucormycosis a fungal disease which may take the form of: (1) a necrotic placentitis which causes abortion; sometimes there are cutaneous lesions over much of the skin of the calf; (2) granulomatous lesions in various tissues and closely resembling lesions of tuberculosis; (3) gastroenteritis and ulceration of the alimentary tract mucosa at all levels; (4) a secondary invasion of rumenitis lesions, which leads to peritonitis and lesions in the liver. The causative fungi may be *Rhizopus*, *Absidia* and *Mucor* spp.

mucosa pl. *mucosae* [L.] mucous membrane.

m.-only rectal tears a tear in the rectal wall, usually along the length of the rectum, which penetrates only as far as the submucosa and is without clinical effect. Possibly caused by any rectal penetration by a rigid object but observed mostly during manual examination by a veterinarian.

mucosal pertaining to or emanating from mucosa.

m.-associated lymphoid tissue (MALT) see mucosal-associated LYMPHOID tissue.

m. block a concept relating to the prevention of absorption of more iron by the intestinal epithelium when the rate of absorption passes a certain limit.

m. crypts invaginations of mucosa; occur in many organs, e.g. biliary and intestinal mucosae.

m. disease see BOVINE virus diarrhea.

m. glands small glands which lie within the lamina propria of the mucosa.

m. transport a means of effecting absorption of materials from the intestinal lumen through the cell membrane of the epithelial cell. Much of this movement has to be in addition to passive diffusion based on osmotic, pH or electromagnetic gradient. It is carried out by membrane carriers, which provide an active transport system.

mucosanguineous composed of mucus and blood.

mucoserous composed of mucus and serum.

mucositis inflammation of a mucous membrane.

mucosocutaneous pertaining to a mucous membrane and the skin.

mucosubstances a superseded name for glycosaminoglycans.

mucous pertaining to or resembling mucus; secreting mucus.

m. cell a cell which secretes mucus.

m. colitis see irritable COLON syndrome.

m. membrane see mucous MEMBRANE.

m. thread accumulations of mucus at the conjunctival fornices.

m. tissue a jelly-like connective tissue, such as occurs in the umbilical cord.

mucus the free slime of the mucous membrane, composed of the secretion of its glands, various salts, desquamated cells and leukocytes. See also MUCOUS.

m. agglutination test an agglutination test carried out on mucus, e.g. the test for the presence of antibodies to *Campylobacter* spp. carried out on vaginal mucus.

gastric m. a protective gelatinous material coating gastric mucosal cells.

respiratory m. part of the protective MUCOCILIARY blanket of the upper respiratory tract.

vaginal m. the appearance of the mucus from the cow's vagina is a good indication that she is in estrus. Laboratory examination of the mucus for cell patterns and arborization is used to determine the stage of reproduction in bitches.

mud pertaining to or emanating from wet conditions underfoot.

m. fever said of horses affected by DERMATOPHILOSIS, LEPTOSPIROSIS, GREASY HEEL.

m. snail LYMNAEA *truncatula*.

mudworm see LUMBRICULUS VARIEGATUS.

mudworm 1. polychete worms, especially *Polydora websteri* which infect the shells of molluscs and can cause significant losses. 2. *Lumbriculus variegatus*.

Muellerius a genus of nematodes in the family Protostrongylidae.

M. capillaris the common lungworm of sheep; occurs also in goat and chamois. In sheep the worm causes little harm, but in goats it may cause dyspnea and cough and occasionally severe interstitial pneumonia.

mugwort ARTEMISIA *vulgaris*.

mulberry heart disease a common form of vitamin E/selenium deficiency in pigs, usually manifested by sudden death, or by dyspnea, cyanosis and recumbency. Extensive subepicardial hemorrhage gives the disease its name.

mule 1. sterile offspring of a mating between a jack (male donkey) and a mare. 2. a bird-fancier's term for a hybrid bird with one parent, usually the female, a canary, and the other a finch; they are usually sterile. Breeding and exhibiting of these birds is a popular hobby in the UK.

horse m. the male mule.

mare m. the female mule.

mule deer small, 3 ft deer with large, mule-like ears and tail tipped with black. Called also *Odocoileus hemionus* (syn. *Dama hemionus*).

Mules operation the removal of strips of skin from the perineal area of lambs so as to increase the area of woolless skin and confer a lower susceptibility to blowfly strike.

mulesing the performance of the MULES OPERATION.

mulga Australian vernacular for inland areas where mulga trees, several species of *Acacia*, especially *A. aneura*, grow. See also hepatic LIPOFUSCINOSIS.

m. fern see CHEILANTHES *sieberi*.

m. nettle see HALORAGIS *odontocarpa*.

m. snake see PSEUDECHIS *australis*.

mulgee ACACIA *osswaldii*.

mullein a plant in the genus *Verbascum* spp.

müllerian duct, Muellerian duct either of the paired embryonic paramesonephric ducts developing into the vagina, uterus and uterine tubes, and becoming largely obliterated in the male or retained as the uterus masculinus or prostatic utricle. Named after J.P. Müller, a German physiologist.

m. d. aplasia the ovaries cycle normally and the lumen of the tube oral to the obstruction distends with secreted fluids. The lumen may be obstructed at any location along its length, including only one horn; the commonest form is hymenal persistence. Called also 'white heifer disease'.

m. d. inhibitory factor produced by the Sertoli cells in the developing testis; causes müllerian duct regression, a key step in sexual differentiation.

multi- word element. [L.] *many*.

multiallelic pertaining to or occupied by many different genes affecting the same or different hereditary characters.

multiarticular pertaining to or affecting many joints.

multicapsular having many capsules.

multicellular composed of many cells.

multicentric the same pathological lesion occurring in many different sites at the same time, e.g. multicentric periarticular calcinosis.

Multiceps see TAENIA.

multicuspidate having numerous cusps; said of teeth.

multicystic polycystic.

multifactorial 1. of or pertaining to, or arising through the action of, many factors. 2. in genetics, arising as a result of the interaction of several genes, i.e. polygenic.

m. etiology see MULTIPLE causation.

multifocal arising from or pertaining to many foci.

m. cystic iris separation separation of the posterior iridal epithelium of aged dogs.

m. intramural myocardial infarction a result of hyalinization of small, intramural, coronary arteries in old dogs. Called also MIMI.

m. symmetrical myelinolytic encephalopathy a fatal disease of Limousin and Simmental calves, beginning at about a month of age with blindness and dysmetria (Limousins) or at 5–8 months of age with signs of ataxia and weight loss (Simmentals).

multiform occurring in many forms; polymorphic.

multiformat camera one used to record frozen ultrasound images on x-ray film.

multigene family see GENE cluster.

multiglandular affecting several glands.

multigravida a female pregnant for the third (or more) time.

multilobar having numerous lobes.

multilobular having many lobules.

m. chondroma and osteoma nodular masses involving membranous bones, as in the canine cranium, causing local disfigurement, and sometimes pressure on the brain.

multilocular having many compartments.

m. hematic bone cyst aneurysmal BONE cyst.

m. hydatid cysts see ECHINOCOCCUS *multilocularis*.

multimeric a protein containing two or more, same or different, polypeptide chains.

multinodular having many nodules.

multinuclear, multinucleate cells having more than one nucleus.

m. chondrone characteristic cell clusters which accompany the proliferation of chondrocytes. Called also brood capsules, clones.

multinucleated characterized by having more than one nucleus per cell.

m. giant cell see giant CELL.

multipara a female which has had two or more pregnancies resulting in viable offspring.

multiparity the condition of being a multipara.

multiple manifold; occurring in various parts of the body at once.

m. alleles see ALLELE.

m. birth more than one offspring in a gestation and parturition.

m. causation a disease in which a combination, or alternative combinations, of causes, are required to produce it. Called also multifactorial etiology.

m.-crush surgical instruments, e.g. heavy duty emasculators, ecraseurs in which each jaw has more than one crushing surface, mounted one behind the other, each successive surface coming into contact with its counterpart as increasing pressure is applied to the handles of the instrument.

m. endochondromas see ENDOCHROMATOSIS.

m. fission a method of reproduction in protozoa. See SCHIZOGONY.

m. infection simultaneous infection with more than one virus or a combination of virus and bacteria may be caused by one agent lowering resistance to the other. There may be synergism between the agents.

m. least squares regression the major method of analysis used to sort through a large number of potential risk factors permitting the examination of one factor while the other factors in the regression equation are held mathematically constant.

m. limb defects patients with more than one congenital limb defect.

m. myeloma see multiple MYELOMA.

m. organ dysfunction syndrome in critical care medicine, a state in which intervention is required to maintain homeostasis. Called also MODS.

m. ovulation an important feature in the technique of embryo transfer. See SUPEROVULATION.
m. pregnancies twins, triplets and more in usually uniparous species.
m. regression an analytical method which determines the relationship between a dependent variable and one or more independent variables.
m. risk situations in which more than one risk factor for a disease is present and their combined presence contributes to an increased risk.
m. suckling when a cow accepts more calves to suckle than her own; a system for foster-rearing of orphan or purchased calves.

multiplier second tier in the conventional structure of breed organizations; takes males and females from the nucleus herds and flocks and produces mostly males to supply commercial herds.

multipolar having more than two poles or processes.

multisynaptic pertaining to or relayed through two or more synapses.

multisystemic affecting more than one body system.
equine m. eosinophilic epitheliotropic syndrome includes chronic eosinophilic enteritis, eosinophilic granulomatous pancreatitis and eosinophilic dermatitis; there is no peripheral eosinophilia.
m. neuronal degeneration in red-haired Cocker spaniel dogs; signs commence at about 6 months of age with behavioral changes, gait and balance disorders, tremors, some seizures sufficient to warrant euthanasia.

multivalent 1. combining with several univalent atoms. 2. a vaccine that is active against several strains of an organism.

multivariate analysis see multivariate ANALYSIS.

multivesicular body a primary lysosome with engulfed vesicles.

mummification conversion to a dehydrated state; commonly said of a fetus. The soft tissues are very much reduced in volume, the skin is leathery and the tissues are deeply brown-stained.
corneal m. see CORNEAL sequestrum.

mumps a communicable paramyxovirus disease of humans that attacks one or both of the parotid salivary glands. Called also epidemic parotitis. There is some evidence that the infection also occurs rarely in dogs and cats.

Münchener 1. a dog breed, the Giant SCHNAUZER. 2. a breed of canaries, originating in Munich; similar to the Scotch Fancy, but without the exaggerated curvature of the body.

munga ergot the seed of the bullrush millet, *Pennisetum typhoides*, which may be infested with CLAVICEPS *fusiformis*.

Mungos mungo see MONGOOSE.

Munro microabscess spongiform microabscesses sometimes found in seborrheic skin disease.

Munsterlander see LARGE MUNSTERLANDER.

Muntiacus muntjak see MUNTJAC.

muntjac, muntjak Asian rib-faced deer with slit-like scent gland openings on the face and two-tined antlers. Called also *Muntiacus muntjak*.

munyeroo PORTULACA *oleracea*.

mupirocin a bacteriostatic antibiotic produced by *Pseudomonas fluorescens* and used topically, mainly against gram-positive bacteria.

mural pertaining to or occurring in a wall of an organ or cavity.

muramidase see LYSOZYME.

muramyl dipeptide a component of the cell wall of the mycobacteria that is active in Freund's complete adjuvant and in purified form also used as an adjuvant. In both instances, it enhances T cell mediated immune responses.

Murdock eye speculum a speculum in which two curved retractor blades are mounted back to back on a bar along which one of them can be moved to part the eyelids.

μ-receptors see OPIOID receptors.

murine pertaining to or affecting mice or rats. Strictly speaking refers to members of the subfamily Murinae, the Old World rats and mice. See also MOUSE.
chronic m. pneumonia see murine respiratory mycoplasmosis (above).
chronic m. respiratory disease see murine respiratory mycoplasmosis.
m. epizootic diarrhea occurs in young mice up to 3 weeks of age. Caused by a rotavirus and characterized by mucoid yellow diarrhea, a high morbidity but a low mortality. Called also epizootic diarrhea of infant mice (EDIM).
m. leukemia virus a number of viruses in the family *Retroviridae* which are associated with the naturally occurring and experimentally induced leukemia or lymphosarcoma in mice.
m. respiratory mycoplasmosis a disease of mice caused by *Mycoplasma pulmonis* and characterized by dyspnea, nasal discharge, head tilt and incoordination. In most mice, infection occurs without clinical signs. Called also chronic respiratory disease of rats and mice, chronic murine pneumonia.
m. typhus a disease of rats caused by *Rickettsia typhi*, transmitted by the rat flea *Xenopsylla cheopis* and the rat louse *Polyplax spinulosa*. It is an important disease of humans.

murmur an auscultatory sound, particularly a periodic sound of short duration of cardiac or vascular origin.
anemic m. see blood murmur (below).
aortic m. a sound indicative of disease of the aortic valve.
apex m. one heard over the apex of the heart.
arterial m. one in an artery, sometimes aneurysmal and sometimes constricted.
blood m. one due to an abnormal, commonly anemic, condition of the blood. Called also anemic murmur.
cardiac m. see heart murmur (below).
cardiopulmonary m. one produced by the impact of the heart against the lung.
continuous m. a humming murmur heard throughout systole and diastole.
crescendo m. one marked by progressively increasing loudness.
crescendo–decrescendo m. one with increasing intensity until mid- to late systole, then a decreasing intensity, giving a diamond-shaped tracing on phonocardiography. Characteristic of pulmonary stenosis.
decrescendo m. one with an intensity that gradually decreases. Heard during diastole in aortic or pulmonary valvular insufficiency.
diamond-shaped m. refers to the phonocardiographic tracing of a crescendo–decrescendo murmur.
diastolic m. one at diastole, due to mitral obstruction or to aortic or pulmonary regurgitation.
ejection m. systolic murmur heard predominantly in mid-systole, when ejection volume and velocity of blood flow are at their maximum.
friction m. friction rub.
functional m. a cardiac murmur occurring in the absence of structural changes in the heart.
heart m. any adventitious sound heard over the region of the heart. It may indicate a leaking or

stenotic valve, a congenital patency between the right and left sides of the heart, or be a functional murmur which does not indicate cardiac disease. These occur in young foals, some of them disappear before maturity.

hemic m. see blood murmur (above).

innocent m. one caused by increased velocity of blood rather than a cardiac lesion.

machinery m., machinery-like m. a long, rumbling sound occupying most of systole and diastole. Characteristic of patent ductus arteriosus and arteriovenous fistulas.

mitral m. one due to disease of the mitral valve.

musical m. a cardiac murmur having a periodic harmonic pattern.

organic m. one due to structural change in the heart.

pansystolic m. one heard throughout systole.

prediastolic m. one occurring just before and with diastole, due to mitral obstruction or to aortic or pulmonary regurgitation.

presystolic m. one occurring shortly before the onset of ventricular ejection, usually associated with a narrowed atrioventricular valve.

pulmonary m. one due to disease of the valves of the pulmonary artery.

radiating heart m. one which is heard over a wider area or over another area. The systolic murmur of subaortic stenosis radiates up the aortic arch and carotid arteries. It can be heard over the right, as well as left, heart base and occasionally over the head.

regurgitant m. one due to a dilated valvular orifice, with consequent regurgitation of blood through the valve.

seagull m. a raucous murmur resembling the call of a seagull, frequently heard in aortic insufficiency.

systolic m. one occurring at systole, usually due to mitral or tricuspid regurgitation, or to aortic or pulmonary obstruction.

tricuspid m. one caused by disease of the tricuspid valve.

vascular m. one heard over a blood vessel.

vesicular m. the normal breath sounds heard over the lungs.

Murocytomegalovirus a genus of betaherpesviruses. See CYTOMEGALOVIRUS.

Murphy eye the distal opening in the side or wall of an endotracheal tube which allows airflow in the event of the tube opening lying against the tracheal wall or being obstructed in other ways.

Murrah a group of breeds of Indian (or European) buffalo including the Kundi, Nili-Ravi and Murrah.

Murray Grey a gray to gray-dun, polled breed of beef cattle, which originated in Australia from gray calves produced by mating a nearly white Shorthorn cow with an Aberdeen Angus bull. The breed carries a number of inherited defects, including mannosidosis and Elso heel.

Murray Valley encephalitis see Murray Valley ENCEPHALITIS.

murrina [Span.] *Trypanosoma evansi* infection.

Murrurrundi disease probably the same disease as inherited ovine degenerative AXONOPATHY.

Mus a genus of rodents in the subfamily Murinae.

M. musculus small gray rodents. Called also house mouse, a variety of the common mouse.

Musca a genus of flies in the family Muscidae, including the common house fly, *M. domestica*, bush flies (*M. sorbens*, *M. fergusoni*, *M. terraereginae*, *M. hilli*) and face fly (*M. autumnalis*). *M. larvipara*, *M. convexifrons* and *M. amica* all act as intermediate hosts for *Thelazia* spp.

M. amica, M. convexifrans, M. larvipora are intermediate hosts for *Thelazia* spp. worms.

M. autumnalis congregates on the face of cattle and may spread infectious keratoconjunctivitis. Called also face fly.

M. bezzi, M. fasciata, M. lusoria, M. pattoni, M. vetustissima, M. vitripennis flies that follow the blood-sucking fly species and clean up the spilt blood.

M. conducens transmits *Stephanofilaria* spp.

M. domestica a mechanical carrier of a good many bacterial, viral and protozoan diseases and an intermediate host for the helminths *Habronema* and *Raillietina* spp. Called also house fly.

M. crassirostris is able to draw blood.

M. fergusoni, M. hilli, M. terraeregina bush flies.

M. sorbens a complex of bush flies.

M. vetustissima the Australian bush fly, an intermediate host for *Habronema* spp.

musca volitantes literally, gliding fly; a small opacity in the vitreous body, a vitreous floater.

muscarine a deadly alkaloid from various mushrooms, e.g. *Amanita muscaria* (the fly agaric), and also from rotten fish.

muscarinic pertaining to the transmission of nerve impulses mediated by muscarinic receptors; these may be adrenergic or cholinergic.

m. activity includes slowing and reduced stroke volume of the heart, bronchiolar constriction, arteriolar dilatation, increased tone, motility and secretion in the alimentary tract, and increases in salivation and lacrimation.

m. blocking agents block muscarinic receptors, e.g. atropine and the synthetic agents homatropine, methantheline, propantheline and methylatropine.

m. receptors cholinergic receptors of autonomic effector cells (and also on some autonomic ganglion cells and some central neurons) that are stimulated by muscarine and parasympathomimetic drugs and antagonized by atropine.

Muscina a genus of flies in the family Muscidae.

M. assimilis, M. pabulorum, M. stabulans denizens of rotting fruit and carrion.

muscle an organ composed of bundles of fibers that has the power to contract and hence to produce movement. Muscles are responsible for locomotion and help support the body, generate heat and perform a number of other functions. They are of two varieties: *striated* (or striped, voluntary or skeletal), which makes up most of the meat of a carcass, and *smooth* (unstriated), which includes all the involuntary muscle of the viscera, heart and blood vessels.

Skeletal muscle fibers range in length from a few millimeters to many centimeters. They also vary in color from white to deep red. Each muscle fiber receives its own nerve impulses, which trigger fine and varied motions. At the signal of an impulse traveling down the nerve, the muscle fiber changes chemical energy into mechanical energy, and the result is muscle contraction. At least two major types of muscle fibers have been identified by histochemical techniques: type I (red) fibers, which have a slow contraction; and type II (white) fibers, which have a fast contraction.

Some muscles are attached to bones by tendons. Others are attached to other muscles, and to skin, producing, for example, the skin twitch, the eye blink and hair erection. Parts of the walls of hollow internal organs, such as the heart, stomach and intestines and also blood vessels, are composed of muscles. See also MUSCULAR. For a complete list of named muscles see Table 13.

agonistic m. prime mover; a muscle opposed in action by another muscle, called the antagonist.
antagonistic m. one that counteracts the action of another muscle (the agonist).
appendicular m. one of the muscles of a limb.
arrector pili m. small, smooth muscle attached to the bulb of the hair which causes erection of the hair and compression of the attending sebaceous gland when it contracts.
arterial m. part of the tunica media; smooth muscle fibers arranged in a circular pattern around the lumen.
articular m. one that has one end attached to the capsule of a joint.
axial m. 1. muscles derived from the somites in the embryo. 2. the muscles around the vertebral column.
m. biopsy sample of living muscle obtained by excision or punch.
cardiac m. striated involuntary muscle with branched fibers and containing modified fibers which act as cardiac conducting cells.
congenital m. defects may be environmental, e.g. nutritional muscular dystrophy, or inherited, e.g. splayleg of piglets.
congenital type II m. fiber hypertrophy occurs in the hip joint musculature in German shepherd dogs but there is no detectable abnormality of gait.
cutaneous m. striated muscle that inserts into the skin.
double m. see MYOFIBER hyperplasia.
esophageal m. the tunica muscularis of the esophagus in most domestic animals is mostly striated; in pigs, horses and cats there are small segments of smooth muscle; in birds the entire tunic is smooth muscle.
extraocular m's the six or seven voluntary muscles that move the eyeball: dorsal, ventral, medial and lateral recti, dorsal and ventral oblique, and retractor bulbi muscles.
extrinsic m. one that originates in another part than that of its insertion, e.g. those originating outside the eye, which move the eyeball.
fast-twitch skeletal m. two of the three types of skeletal muscle are pale in color and fast-twitch—type IIa (fast-twitch oxidative–glycolytic), type IIb (fast-twitch glycolytic). Type IIa fibers are fatigue-resistant, type IIb fatigue easily.
m. fiber see muscle (above).
fixation m's, fixator m's accessory muscles that serve to steady a part.
hamstring m's the biceps, semimembranosus and semitendinosus muscles. See also HAMSTRING.
intraocular m's the intrinsic muscles of the eyeball.
intrinsic m. one whose origin and insertion are both in the same part or organ, such as those entirely within the eye.
involuntary m. see smooth muscle (below).
iridial m. layers of circular (sphincter) and radial (dilator) muscles. See also IRIS.
jaw m. see Table 13.1H muscles of mastication.
laryngeal m. see Table 13.1E muscles of the larynx.
limb m. see Table 13.3, 13.4 muscles of the fore- and hindlimbs.
masseter m. the principal muscle of mastication. See also Table 13.1H.
mylohyoid m. see Table 13.1D muscles of the hyoid apparatus.
m. neoplasms of striated muscle—rhabdomyoma, rhabdomyosarcoma; of plain muscle—leiomyoma, leiomyosarcoma.
m. nonstriated see smooth muscle (below).
orbicular m. one that encircles a body opening, e.g. the eye or mouth.
m.-paralyzing drugs drugs which produce neuromuscular blockade, used as muscle relaxants during surgical procedures. Include *d*-TUBOCURARINE, ALCURONIUM CHLORIDE, PANCURONIUM, VECURONIUM, ATRACURIUM BESYLATE, SUCCINYLCHOLINE.
red m. type 1 fibers predominate with slow contraction cycles and aerobic metabolism.
m. rupture the muscle may have torn away from its insertion, in which case the tendon will be slack, or it may be a complete or partial separation of the belly of the muscle, when the muscle will be swollen and hard. Structural and conformational changes may result, e.g. in rupture of the gastrocnemius muscle, and the hernias caused by rupture of the ventral abdominal muscles or the diaphragm.
skeletal m's striated muscles that are attached to bones and typically cross at least one joint. Called also voluntary or striated muscles.
slow-twitch skeletal m. type 1 skeletal muscle fibers are bright red and contain large amounts of myoglobin; not easily fatigued.
smooth m. plain or involuntary muscle which powers the internal organs and is controlled by the autonomic nervous system; slow contracting cycles and fatigue resistant. Two types listed, visceral and vascular.
sphincter m. a ringlike muscle that closes a natural orifice; called also sphincter.
m. spindle sensory end-organ attached to the perimysial connective tissue of the muscle.
m. strain soreness and stiffness in a muscle due to overexertion or contusion, especially in muscles that have not been conditioned for hard use; some of the muscle fibers may actually tear.
striated m. see skeletal muscles (above).
synergic m's those that assist one another in action.
temporal m. a significant muscle of mastication. See also Table 13.1H.
m.–tendon junction the union between connective tissue investing muscles and anchoring connective tissue.
type I m. fiber see slow-twitch skeletal muscle (above).
type II m. fiber see fast-twitch skeletal muscle (above).
type II m. fiber deficiency a relative deficiency of type II muscle fibers, with a predominance of type I fibers. An inherited defect in Labrador retrievers. Clinical signs include stunted growth, and muscle weakness and abnormal gait, which subside with rest, from an early age.
voluntary m. see skeletal muscle (above).
white m. consist of type II fibers; fast contraction fibers and aerobic metabolism are characteristic.
yoked m's those that normally act simultaneously and equally, as in moving the eyes.

muscle relaxant an agent that specifically aids in reducing muscle tone. Most such agents inhibit the transmission of nerve impulses at the somatic neuromuscular junctions. They include tubocurarine, gallamine, pancuronium, succinylcholine and decamethonium bromide.

Muscovy treated as a duck, but it is really a member of the goose family. A meat duck, white mostly but some varieties are black, or black with white wings. Poor egg producers. Called also *Cairina moschata*.

muscular 1. pertaining to a muscle. 2. having well developed muscles.
m. asymmetry due usually to neuronal or disuse atrophy on one side of the body.

m. atrophy wasting away of muscle or a muscle because of reduction in cross sectional area of muscle fibers; may be due to disease of the muscle or its nerve supply, or to disuse or nutritional inadequacy. See also hereditary spinal muscular atrophy of Brittany spaniels and of Rottweilers (below).

m. degeneration varies in severity from degeneration of only the myofibrils or degeneration of the myofibrils plus sarcoplasm, leaving satellite cells and myonuclei and sarcolemmal laminae unaffected, or further levels of increasing severity.

m. denervation destruction or congenital absence of the motor nerve supply to the muscle; manifested by paralysis and atrophy and absence of spinal reflexes.

m. denervation atrophy progressive shrinkage of muscle fibers when the nerve supply to the muscle is severed.

Duchenne m. dystrophy an X-linked inherited disease in humans, which is believed to be due to a deficiency of a membrane-associated protein, dystrophin. An analogous disease has been identified in Irish terriers, Golden retrievers and mice.

m. dystrophy any degenerative muscular disorder due to faulty nutrition of the muscles. Causes muscle weakness, liberation of myoglobin into the circulation from skeletal muscle and subsequent wasting and possible contracture. In humans there are a group of genetically determined, painless, degenerative myopathies that are progressively crippling because muscles are gradually weakened and eventually atrophy. In food animals the principal disease in this group is ENZOOTIC muscular dystrophy caused by a nutritional deficiency of selenium and/or vitamin E. Sporadic cases of muscular dystrophy of unknown etiology occur rarely in dogs.

m. fascicle see FASCICLE.

m. fasciculation see FASCICULATION.

m. fatigue during brief, intense exercise probably due in large part to the accumulation of lactate.

hereditary spinal m. atrophy progressive degeneration of the motor cells of the spinal cord. It is an inherited, slowly progressive flaccid tetraparesis from an early age, with muscular atrophy. Occurs as an autosomal recessive trait in Swedish lapland dogs, a dominant trait in Brittany spaniels. Also reported in German shepherd dogs, English pointers and Rottweilers. See also hereditary neuronal ABIOTROPHY of Swedish Lapland dogs.

m. hernia hernia through an enclosing muscle sheath.

m. hyperplasia an increase in the size of a muscle mass due to an increase in the number of muscle cells. See also MYOFIBER hyperplasia, ILEAL muscular hypertrophy.

m. hypertrophy an increase in the size of a muscle mass due to an increase in the length and thickness of each muscle cell without any increase in the number of cells.

m. ischemia short duration or temporary or partial cessation of blood supply causes loss of muscle power and possibly some muscle fiber necrosis; long duration or severe or complete cessation cause ischemic muscle necrosis and atrophy. See also COMPARTMENT syndrome, DOWNER COW SYNDROME.

m. ischemic necrosis see ISCHEMIC myonecrosis.

m. mineralization ectopic deposition of minerals in muscle. See MINERALIZATION.

myelopathic m. atrophy muscular atrophy due to a lesion of the spinal cord, as in spinal muscular atrophy.

nutritional m. dystrophy see muscular dystrophy (above).

m. parasitic diseases includes cysticercosis, hepatozoonosis, *Neosprum caninum* myositis, sarcocystosis, toxoplasmosis, trichenellosis.

m. receptors muscle spindles which respond to stretch.

m. steatosis excess fat deposits in muscle; a problem only at meat hygiene inspection.

m. vascular occlusive syndrome see ISCHEMIC myonecrosis.

X-linked m. dystrophy see Duchenne muscular dystrophy (above).

m. weakness see WEAKNESS.

muscularis [L.] relating to muscle, specifically a *muscular layer* or *coat*.

musculature the muscular system of the body, or the muscles of a particular region.

musculocutaneous pertaining to muscle and skin.

m. nerve notable because in the horse it is connected to the median nerve forming a sling in which the axillary artery is supported. See also Table 14.

musculomembranous pertaining to muscle and membrane.

musculophrenic pertaining to (chest) muscles and the diaphragm.

musculoskeletal pertaining to muscle and skeleton.

m. system the muscles and the skeleton.

musculotendinous pertaining to muscle and tendon.

musculotropic exerting its principal effect upon muscle.

musculus pl. *musculi* [L.] muscle.

mushroom the fruiting bodies of fungi of the class Basidiomycetes. See AMANITA, RAMARIA, CLAVARIA and CORTINARIUS.

m. worker's lung an immediate, immune complex-mediated hypersensitivity pneumonitis of humans caused by inhalation of thermophilic actinomycetes in compost.

mushy chick disease see avian OMPHALITIS.

musk ox a longhaired, shortnecked, thickset ruminant that survives well in the Arctic wastes. It averages 6 ft high and 800 lb when fullgrown, looks like a cross between a ram and an ox, has lowset droopy horns and a smell of musk—hence the name *Ovibos moschatus*.

muskrat a rabbit-sized aquatic rat that lives in a burrow and lives on vegetable matter, has thick, shiny, brown and gray fur and gives off a musky odor. Called also *Ondatra zibethica*.

musky storksbill ERODIUM *moschatum*.

Muslim slaughter Muhammadan ritual in which animals are slaughtered while conscious. Has much in common with the JEWISH SLAUGHTER method. The objective is to obtain an instant painless death, after food and water have been provided, and the slaughter does not take place in the sight of other animals. Death is achieved by drawing a very sharp knife across the throat and cutting both carotid arteries and both jugular veins with one stroke. Called also the Halal or Al-Dhabh method. See also SLAUGHTER.

Musophaga genus of wild subsaharan African birds including *M. rossae* (Lady Ross turaco), *M. violacea* (violet turaco).

musophagid members of the Musophagidae family of noisy cuckoo birds which inhabit African forests. Includes go-away birds (*Corythaixoides*, *Criniferoides* spp.), plantain eaters (*Crinifer* spp.), turacos (*Musophaga violacea*, *M. rossae*).

mussel there is a great variety of mussels; some of which are farmed commercially for human food, e.g. *Mytilus*, *Perna* spp. See Table 23.

mustang American for feral horse, also charitably

described as a scrub-type of light horse varying a good deal in conformation. Any color, 14 to 15 hands high. Descended from the horses brought into Central America by Spanish conquistadores.

mustard an irritant compound derived from the dried ripe seed of *Brassica (Sinapis) alba*, *B. nigra* or *B. juncea*. Contains toxic allyl isothiocyanate in nontoxic glycoside form, though the plant also contains myrosinase, an enzyme that converts the glycoside to the toxic form. Used as a carminative, emetic and counterirritant in poultices.

m. gas one of several gases used in military activities, e.g. dichlorodiethylsuphide. Causes vesication of skin, blindness due to corneal damage, and pulmonary edema if inhaled.

m. greens green foliage of several mustard-type plants, used in salads.

m. oil present in high concentrations in mustard plants and causes acute indigestion in animals.

m. oil glucosinolates toxic oil glucosinolates found in plants.

sulfur m. a synthetic compound with vesicant and other toxic properties.

tansy m. see DESCURAINIA PINNATA.

Mustela a genus of the family Mustelidae.

M. erminea see ERMINE.

M. lutreola see MINK.

M. nigripes black-footed ferret.

M. nivalis see WEASEL.

M. putorius furo see FERRET.

M. putorius putorius called also *Putorius putorius*; see POLECAT.

mustelid a member of the Mustelidae family.

Mustelidae a family of carnivores, both aquatic and terrestrial, and almost 70 species. The mustelids include weasel, ferret, mink, wolverine, American badger, skunk, otter, sea otter and European stoat (ermine).

muster to collect sheep or cattle into a herd (cattle) or flock or mob (sheep).

musth the period of great sexual activity in the male Asian elephant. The elephant is very aggressive at this time and the temple glands drain continuously. See also RUT.

mustine hydrochloride a nitrogen mustard compound used as a chemical warfare agent and as an antineoplastic agent.

musty taint an unpleasant odor in poultry meat from chickens raised on litter containing wood shavings. The odor is caused by chloroanisoles generated by bacterial action on wood preservatives in the shavings.

mutagen a physical agent or chemical reagent that causes mutation to occur, e.g. x-irradiation, nitrous acid, and thereby increases the mutation rate of a gene.

mutagenesis the process of inducing genetic mutation.

site directed m. the controlled alteration of a selected region of a DNA molecule which may involve the insertion or deletion of selected nucleotides or nucleotide substitution.

mutagenic inducing genetic mutation.

mutagenicity the property of being able to induce genetic mutation.

mutant 1. an organism with a mutant gene which expresses itself in the phenotype. 2. a normal organism that is genetically different in one or more characteristics from an arbitrarily defined, previously existing 'wild-type' organism. 3. produced by a change in the nucleotide sequence of the genome.

conditional lethal m. mutations that occur in viruses, rendering them unable to grow under certain conditions which can be controlled experimentally. See permissive TEMPERATURE.

defective interfering m. see DEFECTIVE INTERFERING VIRUS.

ts m. see TEMPERATURE-SENSITIVE.

mutase any of a group of enzymes (transferases) that catalyze the intramolecular shifting of a chemical group from one position to another.

mutation 1. a nucleotide change, including base substitutions, insertions or deletions in DNA, or RNA in the case of some viruses, that gives rise to the mutant phenotype. 2. an animal exhibiting such change. Called also a sport.

back m. see reverse mutation (below).

base substitution m. may be a *transition* in which a purine–pyrimidine pair is substituted by the other purine–pyrimidine pair, or *transversion* in which a purine–pyrimidine pair is replaced by one of the two pyrimidine pairs.

chain termination m. one in which the new base sequence introduces a stop codon and thereby prematurely terminates synthesis of the polypeptide; the three mutations are also called amber (UAG), ochre (UAA) and opal (UGA).

deletion m. one produced by loss of nucleotides from a DNA sequence.

frame shift m. occur as a result of either the insertion of a new base pair or the deletion of a base pair or a block of base pairs from the DNA base sequence; these, unless they occur in 3 or multiples of 3, are most serious in that the message to the right of the frame shift is garbled.

leaky m. one in which the amino acid substitution only partially disrupts the function of the protein; in bacteria this is usually manifested by reduced growth rate.

mis-sense m. one causing an amino acid substitution in the protein.

nonsense m. one in which a stop codon is substituted for a codon that specifies an amino acid.

operator constitutive m. one or more base changes in the operator region (originally defined for the lactose operon) which stop the repressor protein from tightly binding to sequence such that it is less effective in preventing RNA polymerase from inhibiting transcription.

point m. a single changed base pair in the DNA of an organism which may be a base substitution, base insertion or base deletion.

m. rate the frequency of mutations in the population over time.

repressor-constitutive m. in regulation of gene expression, a mutation in the repressor protein that decreases the binding affinity of the repressor protein for the operator which leaves the gene permanently turned on.

reverse m. one in which the wild-type phenotype is restored; such organisms are called revertants. Called also back mutation, reversion mutation.

second-site m. see suppressor MUTATION.

silent m. one in which there is a base change but because of the redundancy of the genetic code the same amino acid is coded, or one in which there is an amino acid substitution in the protein which has no detectable effect on the phenotype.

somatic m. a change in the DNA sequence that occurs in somatic cells, i.e. not gametes. The mechanism underlying the generation of diversity of antigen recognition by immunoglobulins and T cell receptor molecules. The fundamental cause of cancer, in which the mutation occurs spontaneously or is induced by carcinogens, such as sunlight, chemicals or viruses.

suppressor m. a particular type of reversion mutation in which a mutation at a second site restores the original phenotype; most simply a mutation produced by a base deletion may be restored to wild type by a proximate but independent base substitution. Called also second-site mutation.

temperature-sensitive (ts) m. one in which there is an altered protein that is active at one temperature, typically 86°F (30°C) and inactive at a higher temperature, usually 104° to 108°F (40 to 42°C), e.g. ts mutant virus and bacteria.

transdominant m. occur in genes producing diffusible products, in contrast to *cis*-dominant mutation in which mutations occur in regulatory sequences that are recognized by other proteins.

transition m. one in which the base change does not change the pyrimidine–purine orientation. See also base substitution mutation (above).

transposition m. one produced by the insertion of a transposable genetic element.

transversion m. one in which the purine–pyrimidine orientation is changed to pyrimidine–purine or vice versa. See also base substitution mutation (above).

mutilation the cutting off or otherwise depriving an animal of a limb or other essential part. Farming procedures, classified as mutilations by animal welfare organizations, include tail-docking of cows and horses, ear-cropping in dogs, mulesing of sheep, debarking of dogs, debeaking of birds.

acral m. syndrome see hereditary sensory NEUROPATHY.

muting removal of the capacity of an animal to make a loud call. In the dog this is done by removal of a small part of each vocal cord.

muton a gene when specified as the smallest hereditary element that can be altered by mutation.

mutt vernacular for dog.

mutton meat obtained from ewe, wether, hogget or ram and from lambs not finished to lamb quality.

mutualism the biological association of two animals or populations of different species, both of which are benefited by the relationship and sometimes unable to exist without it.

mutualist one of the organisms or species living in a state of mutualism.

muzzle 1. the part of the face supported by the maxillae and nasal bones; the part of a dog's head anterior to the stop and cheeks, containing the nasal passages and bearing the nosepad. Longer in dolichocephalics and practically nonexistent in brachycephalics. In farm animals it comprises the nasolabial plane, between the edge of the upper lip, the two nostrils and the junction between the nasolabial plane and the haired part of the face. It includes the skin and fascia and the muscles of the upper lip. 2. an appliance placed over the mouth of an animal, usually a dog, to prevent it biting. The simplest form is a clove-hitch made of bandage and wound around the two jaws.

m. bagging occluding the muzzle, usually of a horse, to cause temporary asphyxia and succeeding dyspnea, during an auscultatory examination of the lungs.

box m. a solid, box-like appliance, usually made of stiff leather over a frame. It prevents the animal sucking or feeding, but holes in the box allow it to drink.

calf-weaning m. a cavesson with spikes on the noseband.

tape m. a piece of tape or bandage tied in a half-hitch around the upper and lower jaws. A temporary measure only.

wire m. a muzzle made of strong wire mesh. Used to prevent dogs fighting or biting, especially Greyhounds during races. Companion animal appliances are more commonly made of leather.

MV [L.] *Medicus Veterinarius* (veterinary physician).

Mv chemical symbol, *mendelevium.*

mV millivolt.

μV microvolt.

MVC minute virus of canines.

MVV maximal voluntary ventilation.

MVY virus Yucaipa virus.

My 301 see GUAIFENESIN.

my(o)- word element. [Gr.] *muscle.*

myalgia pain in muscle.

myasthenia primary skeletal muscle weakness in the absence of nervous system lesions or myositis or myodystrophy. For the most part the weakness is reversible or temporary. Examples amongst animal diseases are myasthenia gravis, hypocalcemia, hypopotassemia, hypoglycemia, and many plant toxins that cause the so-called staggers syndromes in food animals.

angiosclerotic m. excessive muscular fatigue due to vascular changes; intermittent claudication.

m. gastrica weakness and loss of tone in the muscular coats of the stomach; atony of the stomach.

m. gravis a syndrome of muscular weakness that is aggravated by activity and relieved by rest. There is no muscular atrophy or loss of sensation. Affected dogs and cats show predominantly episodic weakness, but various other manifestations, such as laryngeal paralysis, dysphagia and megaesophagus, may also be seen. Clinical signs are rapidly reversed by anticholinesterase drugs and this is used as a diagnostic test for the disease. It may be congenital or acquired as an autoimmune disease, inherited in some breeds.

paraneoplastic m. gravis seen in association with neoplasms and other lesions of the thymus.

myatonia defective muscular tone. See MYOTONIA.

m. congenita amyotonia congenita.

myatrophy atrophy of a muscle.

mycelium pl. *mycelia;* the mass of threadlike processes (hyphae) constituting the fungal thallas.

mycetism mushroom poisoning.

mycetogenic caused by fungi.

mycetoma chronic granulomatous infection of the skin and underlying tissues, with edema, draining sinuses and grains, giving the appearance of a tumor. May be caused by bacteria (actinomycetoma) or fungi (eumycetoma).

actinomycotic m. containing filamentous bacteria of the order Actinomycetales.

blackgrain m. a mycetoma may contain small, dense masses of necrotic material, some of them calcified. They may be yellow or white or black—hence blackgrain mycetoma.

eumycotic m. mycetoma containing fungi.

maduromycotic m. a disease of humans, but with a similar disease in horses and dogs. The common findings in lesions are the fungi *Curvularia geniculata*, *Petriellidium boydii* (syn. *Allescheria boydii*, *Monosporium apiospermum*). In horses *Brachycladium spiciferum* has also been identified. Characterized by an extensive distribution of mycetomas. The name originated from a commonly associated fungus *Madurella* spp.

white-grain m. caused by non-pigmented fungi, such as *Acremonium* spp. and *Pseudallescheria* spp.

myc(o)- word element. [Gr.] *fungus*.
mycobacteria members of the genus *Mycobacterium*.
anonymous m. see opportunist (atypical) mycobacteria (below).
nontubercular m. see opportunist (atypical) mycobacteria (below).
opportunist (atypical) m. saprophytic mycobacteria which may cause disease in animals. Included are *M. chelonae*, *M. fortuitum*, *M. phlei*, *M. smegmatis*. Called also anonymous and nontuberculous. See also RUNYON CLASSIFICATION, opportunist MYCOBACTERIAL granuloma.
rapid growing m. a distinguishing characteristic used for classifying mycobacteria, based on growth rate in cultures. Rapid growth is defined as less than 7 days. This group includes the saprophytic or opportunist mycobacteria, only some of which are associated with disease.
slow growing m. these mycobacteria take more than 7 days for the appearance of colonies. This group includes the tubercle bacilli, *M. avium*, *M. bovis* and *M. tuberculosis*, and many of the others pathogenic for animals and humans.
mycobacterial emanating from or pertaining to MYCOBACTERIUM.
m. granuloma may be caused by *Mycobacterium tuberculosis* (see cutaneous TUBERCULOSIS), *Mycobacterium lepraemurium* (see FELINE leprosy) or opportunist mycobacteria (see opportunist mycobacterial granuloma, below).
opportunist m. granuloma a chronic infection of the skin and subcutaneous tissue, caused by saprophytic mycobacteria, usually as a result of wound contamination. Seen most commonly in cats, particularly in the inguinal region, the lesion may be extensive with ulceration and draining fistulas. Called also pyogranulomatous panniculitis.
mycobacteriosis infection by *Mycobacteria* spp. Includes JOHNE'S DISEASE, MYCOBACTERIAL granuloma, TUBERCULOSIS, FELINE leprosy. See also MASTITIS (Table 16).
atypical m. infection by one of the opportunistic or atypical species in the genus *Mycobacteria* which cause mild to moderate infections in most animals and fish and make them react positively to the tuberculin tests. The bacteria are *M. aquae*, *M. fortuitum*, *M. intracellulare*, *M. kansasii*, *M. scrofulaceum*. See also opportunist MYCOBACTERIAL granuloma, opportunist (atypical) MYCOBACTERIA.
cutaneous m. see skin TUBERCULOSIS, FELINE leprosy, opportunist MYCOBACTERIAL granuloma.
nontubercular m. infection by a species of bacteria in the genus *Mycobacteria*, other than *M. tuberculosis*.
tubercular m. tuberculosis.
Mycobacterium the only genus in the family Mycobacteriaceae of bacteria; slender acid-fast rods which may be straight or slightly curved. They may produce filaments or cocci. The most serious disease caused by members of this genus is TUBERCULOSIS. *M. fortuitum*, *M. chelonea*, *M. marinum* are listed as causes of piscine tuberculosis Other species, including *M. aquae*, *M. kansasii* and *M. scrofulaceum*, may occasionally cause disease in a number of different species.
M. avium found mostly in birds but occasionally also in other animals and in humans. The tubercle bacillus of birds, it causes avian TUBERCULOSIS.
***M. avium–intracellulare* complex** see *M. intracellulare* (below).
M. bovis the tubercle bacillus of the bovine, it causes TUBERCULOSIS in many animal species and humans.
M. chelonei, M. fortuitum, M. phlei, M. smegmatis, M. thermoresistible cause disease in a number of animal species, including mastitis in cattle and cutaneous MYCOBACTERIAL granuloma in cats and dogs. See also opportunist (atypical) MYCOBACTERIA.
M. farcinogenes, M. senegalense associated with BOVINE farcy.
M. intracellulare found in tuberculin-positive cattle and causes limited lymph node lesions in pigs. Closely related to *M. avium* and also described as *M. avium–intracellulare* complex.
M. kansasii causes tuberculosis-like disease in pigs, deer and cattle.
M. leprae the cause of leprosy in humans.
M. lepraemurium causes murine and FELINE leprosy.
M. marinum found in water, it causes tuberculosis in fish and skin ulcers in humans.
M. microti the vole bacillus; lesions sometimes occur in other species.
***M. paratuberculosis* (syn. *M. johnei*)** causes JOHNE'S DISEASE in cattle, sheep, goats, deer and camelids.
M. tuberculosis the tubercle bacillus of humans, but found also in monkeys and pigs, and rarely in cattle, dogs and parrots.
M. ulcerans causes skin ulcers in humans and cats.
M. xenopi causes MYCOBACTERIAL granuloma in cats and lymph node lesions in pigs.
mycobactin a substance in some mycobacteria capable of promoting the growth of other mycobacteria; it is capable of extracting ferric ion from the medium which some *Mycobacterium* spp. are unable to do.
mycodermatitis fungal infection of the skin.
mycolic acid the component of mycobacterial cell walls that confirms their acid-fast characteristic.
mycological pertaining to or arising from mycology.
mycologist a specialist in mycology.
mycology the study of fungi and fungal diseases.
mycomyringitis fungus inflammation of the eardrum.
mycophenolic acid an immunosuppressant used in organ transplantation.
Mycoplasma a genus of highly pleomorphic, aerobic or facultatively anaerobic bacteria that lack cell walls, including the pleuropneumonia-like organisms (PPLO).
***M. agalactiae, M. capricolum, M. conjunctivae, M. mycoides* subsp. *mycoides and* subsp. *capri, M. ovipneumoniae, M. putrefaciens, M.* strain F-38** cause disease in sheep and goats. See CONTAGIOUS agalactia, CONTAGIOUS caprine/ovine pleuropneumonia, ENZOOTIC pneumonia, KERATOCONJUNCTIVITIS, mycoplasmal POLYARTHRITIS and Table 16.
M. alkalescens, M. bovis, M. bovoculi, M. bovigenitalium, M. bovirhinis M. californicum, M. canadense, M. dispar* and *M. mycoides* subsp. *mycoides found in cattle and may cause disease, including pneumonia, mastitis, arthritis, ocular infection and mastitis. See CONTAGIOUS bovine pleuropneumonia, ENZOOTIC pneumonia, KERATOCONJUNCTIVITIS and Table 16.
M. anatis, M. gallinarum, M. gallisepticum, M. gallopavonis, M. iowae, M. meleagridis, M. synoviae cause disease in poultry. See CHRONIC respiratory disease, infectious avian SYNOVITIS, infectious SINUSITIS of turkeys, and TURKEY syndrome.
M. arthritidis, M. neurolyticum, M. pulmonis cause disease in rats and mice. See MURINE respiratory mycoplasmosis, ROLLING disease.
M. columbinasale, M. columborale found in pigeons, but pathogenicity is not known.

M. cynos, M. gateae, M. spumans found in dogs and cats and may be associated with disease. See also histiocytic ulcerative COLITIS, KENNEL COUGH.
M. felis found in the respiratory tract of horses and may cause pleuritis. It causes conjunctivitis in cats.
M. flocculare, M. hyorhinis, M. hyosynoviae, M. hyopneumoniae cause disease in pigs. See ATROPHIC rhinitis, mycoplasma ARTHRITIS and ENZOOTIC pneumonia.

mycoplasma microorganisms in the class Mollicutes; the genera of importance in animals are *Mycoplasma, Ureaplasma* and *Acholeplasma.*
t-strain m. UREAPLASMA *urealyticum.*

mycoplasmal emanating from or pertaining to infection with *Mycoplasma.*

mycoplasmosis any disease caused by infection with *Mycoplasma* spp., e.g. bovine mycoplasmosis; includes contagious bovine pleuropneumonia, enzootic calf pneumonia, mycoplasmal mastitis, murine respiratory mycoplasmosis and granular vulvovaginitis.

mycosis pl. *mycoses;* any disease caused by fungi.
dermal m. see RINGWORM, EPIZOOTIC lymphangitis, SPOROTRICHOSIS, SWAMP CANCER. Called also dermatophytosis.
m. fungoides a chronic, malignant, lymphoreticular neoplasm of the skin, and, in late stages, lymph nodes and viscera; a type of cutaneous lymphosarcoma involving T lymphocytes. It occurs in humans, dogs and cats.
guttural pouch m. see GUTTURAL POUCH mycosis.
opportunistic m. a fungal or fungus-like disease occurring in an animal with a compromised immune system. Opportunistic organisms are normal resident flora that become pathogenic only when the host's immune defenses are altered, as in immunosuppressive therapy, in a chronic disease, such as diabetes mellitus, or during steroid or antibacterial therapy that upsets the balance of bacterial flora in the body.
superficial m. those involving the superficial layers of the skin; typical of infections caused by DERMATOPHYTES.
systemic m. fungal infection spread via the bloodstream and characterized by multiple granulomatous lesions in many organs. See ASPERGILLOSIS, BLASTOMYCOSIS, COCCIDIOIDOMYCOSIS, CRYPTOCOCCOSIS, HISTOPLASMOSIS, MUCORMYCOSIS.

mycostasis prevention of growth and multiplication of fungi.

mycostat an agent that inhibits the growth of fungi.

mycota see FUNGUS.

mycotic pertaining to a mycosis; caused by fungi. Fungal infections occur in most organs of the body, e.g. mycotic mastitis, keratitis, hepatitis, rumenitis, colitis.
m. abortion is common only in cattle and is caused by *Mortierella wolfii, Mucor* and *Aspergillus* spp. *Petriellidium boydii* (*Allescheria boydii*) is also recorded as a cause.
m. dermatitis the name is a misnomer because it is caused by a bacterium *Dermatophilus dermatonomus.* It occurs in all species but is a disease of high prevalence only in cattle and sheep. Lesions are worst on the dorsal parts of the body. They are thick, tenacious scabs, difficult to remove, underrun by granulation tissue. Continual wetness is an exacerbant. In sheep the lesions are in the woolled parts and damage the fleece badly. There is often vivid discoloration.
m. granuloma see SWAMP CANCER.
m. lymphangitis see bovine FARCY.
m. nasal granuloma a disease of cows, characterized by noisy and distressed breathing and nasal discharge. There are large polyps containing yellow-green granulation tissue in the nasal cavities. Histologically the lesions are eosinophilic granulomas containing fungal elements. *Drechslera rostrata* has been isolated from the lesions. *Rhizobium* spp. fungus is also recorded as a cause in cattle.
m. stomatitis is regarded as a secondary lesion produced by the invasion of devitalized tissue or existing mucosal lesions by fungi, especially *Candida* spp. Characterized by a growth of soft, white, elevated patches, which are felted masses of mycelia on an inflamed or ulcerated mucosa. Occurs especially in very young animals still drinking milk. The lesions usually extend into the pharynx and in fatal cases further still down the alimentary tract.

mycotoxic pertaining to or emanating from a mycotoxin, e.g. mycotoxic lupinosis, mycotoxic nephropathy.
m. nephrotoxic tubular necrosis caused by OCHRATOXIN and CITRININ in pigs.

mycotoxicosis 1. poisoning due to a fungal toxin. 2. poisoning due to ingestion of fungi is poisoning caused by fungal toxins, resulting from the ingestion of moldy feeds or as toxins produced by fungi that parasitize living plants externally or live in the tissues of the plants as endophytes.
The common toxic fungi on standing crops are *Alternaria, Claviceps, Fusarium, Helminthosporium* and *Rhizopus* spp. On stored feeds the common ones are *Aspergillus, Fusarium* and *Penicillium.* There are a number of identified specific poisonous fungi, but it is probable that there are a great number of fungal toxic incidents that go unnoticed. Food animals are frequently exposed to fungi on moldy stored food and also on standing plants and on the litter lying at the ground surface in a pasture. See also FACIAL eczema, RYEGRASS STAGGERS, LUPINUS poisoning, STACHYBOTRYOTOXICOSIS.

mycotoxin poisonous substance produced by a fungus.
m. hyperthermia see ACREMONIUM *coenophialum,* CLAVICEPS *purpurea.*

mydriasis gross dilatation of the pupil. Common causes in animals are atropine poisoning, hypocalcemia and tiger snake envenomation. Permanent dilatation may be due to damage to the retina, as in toxoplasmosis, or to the optic nerve, as in avitaminosis A.

mydriatic 1. dilating the pupil. 2. a drug that dilates the pupil.
m. test measurement of intraocular pressure before and after the administration of a short-acting mydriatic; used in the diagnosis of narrow-angle glaucoma.

myectomy excision of a muscle or a portion of a muscle.
caudal m. see NICKING (2). Instead of severing the ventral sacrococcygeal muscle, a portion is removed.
pectineal m. see PECTINOTOMY.

myectopia displacement of a muscle.

myelapoplexy hematomyelia; hemorrhage in the spinal cord.

myelatelia imperfect development of the spinal cord.

myelatrophy atrophy of the spinal cord.

myelemia see MYELOCYTOSIS.

myelencephalon 1. the part of the central nervous system comprising the medulla oblongata and caudal of the fourth ventricle. 2. the posterior of the two brain vesicles formed by specialization of the rhombencephalon in the developing embryo.

myelin 1. the lipid substance forming a sheath around

the axons of certain nerve fibers; these nerve fibers are spoken of as myelinated or medullated fibers. 2. lipoid substance found in various normal and pathological tissues, which differs from fats in being doubly refractive.

Myelinated nerve fibers occur predominantly in the cranial and spinal nerves and compose the white matter of the brain and spinal cord. It is the myelin sheath that gives the whitish color to the areas of white matter. Unmyelinated fibers are abundant in the autonomic nervous system.

myelinated having a myelin sheath.

myelination, myelinization production of myelin around an axon.

myelinic edema disruption of the lamellar structure of peripheral and central myelin; caused by chemicals, e.g. hexachlorophene; leads to spongy degeneration of white matter.

myelinogenesis formation of myelin in the nervous system. Commences in the embryo at about the midpoint of gestation but is not complete until after parturition, later in those species in which neonates do not walk immediately after birth; myelinogenesis is not simultaneous in all parts of the nervous system so that clinical signs may appear temporarily and recover spontaneously, e.g. some types of neonatal tremor in pigs.

myelinolysis destruction of myelin; demyelination.

myelinolytic of the nature of or pertaining to myelin.

myelinopathy general term used to include any disease of myelin; includes hypomyelination, dysmyelination, leukodystrophies, myelinolytic diseases, spongiform myelinopathies, encephalomyelinopathies.

feline spinal m. an iodiopathic, adult-onset, progressive myelin loss in the spinal cord in Californian cats.

myelinosis fatty degeneration, with formation of myelin.

myelinotoxic having a deleterious effect on myelin; causing demyelination.

myelitis 1. inflammation of the spinal cord; there are no specific myelitides in animals but myelitis is a significant lesion in listeriosis, equine herpesvirus-1 infection in horses, caprine arthritis–encephalitis, equine protozoal myeloencephalitis. 2. inflammation of bone marrow (see also OSTEOMYELITIS).

bulbar m. that involving the medulla oblongata.

spinal cord m. is most commonly caused by a viral infection, though protozoa and helminth parasites are also significant causes. The signs are weakness through to complete flaccid paralysis, including paralysis of the anus and the tail. See also MYELOMALACIA, ENCEPHALOMYELITIS.

myel(o)- word element. [Gr.] *marrow* (often with specific reference to the spinal cord).

myeloblast an immature cell of bone marrow, not normally found in peripheral blood; it is the most primitive precursor in the granulocytic series, which develops into the promyelocyte and eventually into a granulocyte.

myeloblastemia myeloblasts in the peripheral blood.

myeloblastoma a focal malignant tumor composed of myeloblasts, observed in acute myelocytic leukemia.

myeloblastosis 1. an excess of myeloblasts in the blood. 2. one of the specific viral diseases in the leukosis–sarcoma group of diseases of fowl. It is characterized by a spectacular leukemia with a great preponderance of myelocytes. There are general signs of debility, anemia and spontaneous hemorrhage.

myelocele protrusion of the spinal cord through a defect in the vertebral column.

myelocyst a cyst developed from rudimentary medullary canals.

myelocystocele hernial protrusion of spinal cord through a defect in the vertebral column.

myelocystomeningocele protrusion of cystic spinal cord and meninges through a defect in the vertebral column.

myelocyte 1. a precursor in the granulocytic series intermediate between a promyelocyte and a metamyelocyte, normally occurring only in the bone marrow. In this stage, differentiation into specific cytoplasmic granules has begun. 2. any cell of the gray matter of the nervous system.

myelocythemia an excess of myelocytes in the circulating blood.

myelocytoma see MYELOMA.

myelocytomatosis one of the virus-induced diseases in the leukosis–sarcoma group of diseases of fowl. It is characterized by tumors of the skull, ribs and limb bones. There is emaciation, weakness, pallor of the comb and a course of several months. There are often bony protuberances at the head and on the thorax and shanks.

myelocytosis increase of myelocytes in the blood.

myelodysplasia 1. defective development of the spinal cord. 2. disorders of myeloid cells of the bone marrow, either in number or degree of maturity.

hemopoietic m. includes myeloid metaplasia and myelofibrosis, refractory anemia with excess blast cells, and myelomonocytic leukemia.

m. syndrome qualitative defect in stem cells characterized by dysplastic hematopoietic cells and the presence of abnormal blast cells in the blood. There is also anemia, leukopenia and sometimes thrombocytopenia. See also MYELOPROLIFERATIVE disease.

myeloencephalic pertaining to the spinal cord and brain.

myeloencephalitis see ENCEPHALOMYELITIS.

myeloencephalopathy any degenerative disease affecting the brain and the spinal cord. Usually used as a pathoanatomical diagnosis when the etiological diagnosis is elusive.

equine degenerative m. an irreversible disease of young horses characterized by hypermetria of all limbs causing ataxia and falling backwards. One of the causes of ENZOOTIC equine incoordination. Demyelination is present in the medulla and spinal cord, especially the cervical and midthoracic regions.

progressive degenerative m. inherited disease of Brown Swiss cattle characterized by appearance at 6–8 months of age, progressive, bilateral hindlimb weakness causing a weaving gait; euthanasia inevitable after a 12–18 month course: called also weaver syndrome.

myeloencephaly any disease of the brain and spinal cord.

myelofibrosis replacement of bone marrow by fibrous tissue, e.g. in the end-stage of myeloid metaplasia and myelofibrosis.

myelogenesis 1. development of the central nervous system. 2. the deposition of myelin around the axon.

myelogenic, myelogenous produced in the bone marrow.

m. leukemia see myelocytic LEUKEMIA.

myelogeny development of the myelin sheaths of nerve fibers.

myelogone a white blood cell of the myeloid series having a reticulate violaceous nucleus, well-stained nucleolus, and deep blue rim of cytoplasm.

myelogram 1. the film produced by myelography. 2. a graphic representation of the differential count of cells found in a stained representation of bone marrow.

myelography radiography of the spinal cord after injection of a contrast medium into the subarachnoid space.

cervical m. injection of a radiopaque contrast medium into the subarachnoid space before taking an x-ray to outline more clearly the structures in the vertebral canal.

myeloid 1. pertaining to, derived from or resembling bone marrow. 2. pertaining to the spinal cord. 3. having the appearance of myelocytes, but not derived from bone marrow.

m.:erythroid (M:E) ratio the ratio of myeloid to erythroid cells found in an examination of the bone marrow; provides an assessment of bone marrow activity.

m. leukemia see myelocytic LEUKEMIA.

m. leukosis see MYELOBLASTOSIS (2).

m. metaplasia hyperplasia of the bone marrow, with erythroid phthisis and compensatory splenomegaly and sometimes hepatomegaly. It is usually succeeded by bone marrow fibrosis and sclerosis. The initiating cause is usually not apparent.

m. tissue red bone marrow.

myeloidosis formation of myeloid tissue, especially hyperplastic development of such tissue.

myelokathexis neutropenia resulting from bone marrow retention in the face of adequate reserves.

myelolipoma a rare benign tumor of the adrenal gland composed of adipose tissue, lymphocytes and primitive myeloid cells.

myeloma 1. a B lymphocyte tumor. 2. multiple myeloma.

giant cell m. giant cell tumor (1).

multiple m. a malignant neoplasm of plasma cells, in which the plasma cells proliferate and invade the bone marrow, causing destruction of the bone and resulting in pathological fracture and bone pain. A secretory form of the disease is characterized by the presence of an immunoglobulin recognized as Bence Jones protein (monoclonal immunoglobulin), Bence Jones proteinuria, anemia, and lowered resistance to infection. It is the most common type of monoclonal GAMMOPATHY. A non-secretory form of the disease also occurs.

osteosclerotic m. multiple myeloma associated with osteosclerosis (rather than bone destruction) and often with peripheral neuropathy.

plasma cell m. see multiple myeloma (above).

m. protein the immunoglobulin molecules produced by myeloma cells. See GAMMOPATHY.

myelomalacia morbid softening (necrosis) of spinal cord. It is not commonly recorded as an entity separate from encephalomalacia. Poisonings by *Phalaris tuberosa* in sheep and sorghum in horses are two examples. There is a gradual onset of paresis or paralysis.

progressive hemorrhagic m. a progressive, ascending and descending, intramedullary hemorrhage of the spinal cord that sometimes follows trauma; the result of ischemic and hemorrhagic infarction of the parenchyma, but not nerve roots in the leptomeninges. Called also hematomyelia.

myelomatosis see multiple MYELOMA.

myelomeningitis inflammation of the spinal cord and meninges.

myelomeningocele hernial protrusion of the spinal cord and its meninges through a defect in the vertebral column.

myeloneuritis inflammation of the spinal cord and peripheral nerves.

myelopathy 1. any functional disturbance or pathological change in the spinal cord; often used to denote nonspecific lesions, as opposed to myelitis. Examples are ischemic encephalopathy, that due to intervertebral disk disease, in the wobbler syndrome in horses. 2. pathological change in bone marrow.

bovine spinal m. inherited disease of Murray Grey cattle conditioned by a recessive gene; congenital or appears at up to one year old; characterized by paresis progressing to recumbency and necropsy lesions of neuronal degeneration in midbrain, cerebellum and spinal cord.

degenerative m. of German shepherd dogs a slowly progressive ataxia and paresis of the hindlegs in older German shepherd dogs. Marked muscle atrophy is common and fecal and urinary incontinence often develops. The etiology is unknown, but an immune-mediated mechanism is suspected as a depression of T lymphocyte responsiveness has been demonstrated in affected dogs.

demyelinating m. of Miniature poodles a diffuse demyelination with sparing of spinal gray matter and dorsal and ventral nerve roots. There is a progressive weakness, then paralysis of hindlegs and later forelegs as well, beginning at a few months of age; believed to be inherited.

fibrocartilaginous embolic m. extrusion of degenerate intervertebral disk material into meningeal or intramedullary blood vessels, which results in an ischemic myelopathy. It occurs in horses and, most frequently, in large breeds of dogs, and is manifested by acute paresis or paralysis.

hereditary m. of Afghan hounds an autosomal recessive inherited degenerative myelopathy of young Afghan hounds, in which there is ataxia, paresis and eventually paralysis, first in the hindlimbs, then in the forelimbs as well. Called also a leukodystrophy.

spondylotic cervical m. myelopathy secondary to encroachment of cervical spondylosis upon a congenitally small cervical spinal canal.

myeloperoxidase a hemoprotein having peroxidase activity, occurring in the primary granules of promyelocytes, myelocytes and neutrophils, and which exhibits bactericidal, fungicidal and virucidal properties.

myelopetal moving toward the spinal cord.

myelophthisic pertaining to or emanating from myelophthisis.

m. anemia see myelopathic ANEMIA.

myelophthisis 1. wasting of the spinal cord. 2. reduction of the cell-forming functions of bone marrow.

myeloplast any leukocyte of the bone marrow.

myelopoiesis the formation of bone marrow or the cells arising from it.

ectopic m., extramedullary m. formation of myeloid tissue outside bone marrow.

myeloproliferative pertaining to or characterized by abnormal proliferation of bone marrow constituents.

m. disease a group of diseases related histogenetically and marked, at varying times in varying degrees, by medullary and extramedullary proliferation of one or more lines of bone marrow constituents, including myelocytic, erythroblastic and megakaryocytic forms, in addition to various cells derived from the reticulum and mesenchymal elements. It occurs most commonly in cats, often associated with feline leukemia virus infection, causing anemia, weight loss, fever and hepatosplenomegaly. Hematological findings usually include the presence of abnormal cells, corresponding to the proliferating cell type. The forms seen include erythremic myelosis, reticuloendothelosis, myeloid leukemia, erythroleukemia, monocytic leukemia, myelomonocytic leukemia, megakaryocytic myelosis and eosinophilic leukemia.

myeloradiculitis inflammation of the spinal cord and posterior nerve roots.

myeloradiculodysplasia abnormal development of the spinal cord and spinal nerve roots.

myeloradiculopathy disease of the spinal cord and spinal nerve roots.

myelorrhagia hematomyelia; spinal hemorrhage.

myelosarcoma a sarcomatous growth made up of myeloid tissue or bone marrow cells.

myeloschisis a cleft neural tube and an incompletely closed spinal cord.

myelosclerosis 1. sclerosis of the spinal cord. 2. obliteration of the marrow cavity by small spicules of bone. 3. myelofibrosis.

myelosis 1. proliferation of bone marrow tissue, producing the blood changes of myelocytic leukemia. 2. formation of a tumor of the spinal cord.

erythremic m. a malignant blood dyscrasia, one of the MYELOPROLIFERATIVE disorders, with progressive anemia, megaloblastic erythroid hyperplasia, myeloid dysplasia and hepatosplenomegaly. Seen most often in cats with feline leukemia virus infection.

megakaryocytic m. see megakaryocytic LEUKEMIA.

myelospongium a network developing into the neuroglia.

myelostimulation stimulation of the bone marrow to produce blood cells; an important therapeutic objective in treating conditions which involve bone marrow suppression, such as aplastic anemia and in cancer chemotherapy. Various hemopoietic growth factors are used, including the COLONY-stimulating factors.

myelosuppression depression of bone marrow activity.

myelosuppressive 1. inhibiting bone marrow activity, resulting in decreased production of blood cells and platelets. 2. an agent having such properties.

myelotomy severance of nerve fibers in the spinal cord.

myelotoxicity state of being toxic to myeloid tissue, i.e. bone marrow.

myelotoxin a toxin that destroys bone marrow cells.

myenteric pertaining to the myenteron.

absent m. ganglia congenital defect associated with colonic atresia.

m. ganglionitis lesion of unspecified origin in horses, probably inflammatory; causes malfunction of intestinal movement, ingesta and fluid accumulation and colic.

m. plexus see AUERBACH PLEXUS.

myenteron the muscular coat of the intestine.

myesthesia muscle sensibility.

myiasis invasion of the body by the larvae of flies, characterized as cutaneous (subdermal tissue), gastrointestinal, nasopharyngeal, ocular or urinary, depending on the region invaded.

blowfly m. see cutaneous myiasis (below).

cutaneous m. infestation of devitalized skin, skin covered by hair or wool fouled by feces or urine, or skin wounds by maggots of *Lucilia* spp., *Phormia* spp., *Calliphora* spp. Sheep are especially susceptible and large areas of skin may be destroyed and the sheep die as a result. Called also calliphorine myiasis, blowfly myiasis or strike and struck.

gastrointestinal m. see gastric HABRONEMIASIS, GASTEROPHILOSIS.

nasal m. OESTRUS *ovis* infestation.

ocular m. see ONCHOCERCIASIS, THELAZIASIS.

oculovascular m. GEDOELSTIA *hassleri* infection, in which the eye is invaded by larvae per medium of the vascular system.

oestrid m. includes invasion of tissues by larvae of *Oestrus* spp. and *Hypoderma* spp.

screw-worm m. see SCREW-WORM myiasis.

warble m. see HYPODERMA.

myko- for words beginning thus, see those beginning *myco-*.

Mylabris phalerata, Mylabris sidae a beetle containing CANTHARIDIN. Called also Chinese blistering beetle, Chinese blister fly, mylabris.

mylohyoid pertaining to the hyoid bone and molar teeth.

mynah bird probably the most accomplished talking bird. Black with yellow beak, feet and wattles, 12 to 18 inches long and 0.25 to 0.5 lb. Called also *Gracula religiosa*, *Acridotheres* and *Sturnus* spp.

myo- word element. [Gr.] *muscle*.

myoarteritis inflammation of the smooth muscle in the arterial wall.

myoatrophy muscular atrophy.

Myobia a genus of parasitic mites in the family Myobiidae.

M. musculi causes alopecia and dermatitis in laboratory mice.

myoblast an embryonic cell that becomes a cell of a muscle fiber.

myoblastoma a benign circumscribed tumor-like lesion of soft tissue.

granular cell m. see GRANULAR cell myoblastoma.

myobradia slow reaction of muscle to stimulation.

myocardial pertaining to the muscular tissue of the heart (the myocardium).

m. asthenia myocardial weakness and decrease in the power of the heart's contraction, leading to reduction in cardiac reserve and ultimately to congestive heart failure.

m. cells 1. being surrounded by an intact sarcolemma prevents the cells forming a true syncytium; but do form a functional syncytium because of presence of gap junctions with low electrical resistance which allow the passage of ions and small molecules. 2. myocardial cells are specialized smooth muscle cells with acquired features and properties similar to those of skeletal muscles.

m. contractility myocardium has an intrinsic periodic contractility which enables the denervated heart to continue beating; in the intact animal neurogenic control of contractility is paramount, inhibited by parasympathetic effects, stimulated by sympathetic effects.

m. damage any disease causing loss of muscular or nervous function of the heart. Includes myocarditis, ischemia, degeneration.

m. depressant factor substances liberated from the pancreas, intestine and liver during any type of circulatory shock. They reduce cardiac and reticuloendothelial activity and cause vasoconstriction. Called also MDF.

m. dystrophy degenerative change in heart muscle, e.g. that occurring as a result of nutritional deficiency of selenium or vitamin E. Death usually occurs suddenly, with blood-stained froth pouring from the nostrils.

m. fiber see myocardial cells (above).

m. heart failure heart failure due to myocardial inefficiency.

m. hypertrophy increase in size of myocardial mus-

cle due to increase in size of individual myocardial cells, usually in response to an added afterload.
m. infarction (MI) necrosis of the cells of an area of the heart muscle (myocardium) occurring as a result of oxygen deprivation, which in turn is caused by obstruction to the blood supply; commonly referred to in humans as a 'heart attack'. This is not a common disease in animals, but does occur, e.g. in horses, especially in the right atrium. It is a cause of myocardial weakness. See myocardial asthenia (above).
m. inflammation see MYOCARDITIS.
m. injury see myocardial damage (above).
ischemic m. necrosis localized or widespread necrosis due to interruption of the blood supply via the coronary arteries.
m. lipofuscinosis occurs in aged or cachectic cattle, also in healthy cattle; most common in Ayrshires; no apparent significance in terms of health; called also brown atrophy.
m. necrosis focal or massive and subsequent scarring caused by infection, e.g. *Haemophilus somnus*, the encephalomyocarditis virus, nutritional deficiency, e.g. vitamin E–selenium, poisoning by plants, e.g. *Acacia georgina,* farm chemicals, e.g. monensin, and ischemic necrosis due to general or local inadequacy of blood supply to the myocardium.
m. tension affects myocardial contractility but the importance of the effect in the living animal is obscure.
myocardiograph an instrument for making tracings of heart movements.
myocardiopathy any noninflammatory disease of the myocardium.
myocarditis inflammation of the muscular walls of the heart (the myocardium). The condition may result from bacterial or viral infections or it may be a toxic inflammation caused by drugs or toxins from infectious agents. A striking example is the myocarditis of foot-and-mouth disease. The effect is to reduce cardiac reserve, possibly to the point of precipitating heart failure. Focal lesions may cause cardiac arrhythmia.
fibrotic m. healed lesion with much myocardium replaced by scar tissue; cardiac function will be severely compromised.
infectious myocarditis see GOOSE hepatitis.
primary m. usually the result of a primary viral or protozoal infection of the myocardium.
secondary m. associated with an infectious or noninfectious systemic disease or associated with another cardiovascular disorder.
myocardium the middle and thickest layer of the heart wall, composed of cardiac MUSCLE.
myocardosis any degenerative, noninflammatory disease of the myocardium.
Myocastor coypus see COYPU.
myocele hernia of muscle through its sheath.
myocellulitis myositis with cellulitis.
myoceptor the motor end-plate of the muscle fiber.
myocerosis waxy degeneration of muscle.
myoclonia congenita see CONGENITAL TREMOR SYNDROME.
myoclonic pertaining to myoclonus.
m. epilepsy see GLYCOPROTEINOSIS.
m. jerk a generalized SEIZURE consisting of a jerk of most muscles in the body.
myoclonus repetitive, rhythmic contractions of a group of skeletal muscles, persisting in sleep. The result of encephalitis or myelitis caused by distemper virus in dogs. Called also canine chorea, flexor spasm and tremor syndrome.
familial reflex m. a familial disease seen in young Labrador retriever puppies; myoclonus is followed by a generalized extensor rigidity and opisthotonos.
inherited congenital m. inherited as a recessive trait in Polled Hereford cattle; at birth affected calves are unable to stand because of myoclonic jerks to skeletal muscles in response to external stimuli; affected calves are not viable. One of the diseases originally classified together as neuraxial edema.
palatal m. a condition characterized by a rapid rhythmic movement of one or both sides of the palate.
Myocoptes a genus of mites in the family Listrophoridae.
M. musculinus found on the hair of guinea pigs and laboratory mice.
M. romboutsi see TRICHOECIUS ROMBOUTSI.
myocyte a cell of muscular tissue.
myocytolysis dissolution of muscle cells.
myocytoma a tumor composed of myocytes.
myodemia fatty degeneration of muscle.
myodesmone a furanosesquiterpenoid plant poison found in *Lasiospermum*, *Myoporum* spp.
myodysplasia abnormal development of muscles. An inherited form of the disease occurs in calves, manifested by small, pale skeletal muscles and an inability to stand. Hydrocephalus is an additional lesion. See also MYODYSTROPHIA fetalis deformans.
myodystonia disorder of muscular tone.
myodystrophia see MUSCULAR dystrophy.
m. fetalis deformans muscular dystrophy with limb deformity in the newborn. Occurs as an inherited disease in lambs. See also inherited ARTHROGRYPOSIS.
myodystrophy see MUSCULAR dystrophy.
myoedema edema of a muscle.
myoelectric pertaining to the electric properties of muscle.
myoendocarditis combined myocarditis and endocarditis.
myoepithelioma a tumor composed of outgrowths of myoepithelial cells from a sweat gland.
myoepithelium tissue made up of contractile epithelial cells.
myofascitis inflammation of a muscle and its fascia.
myofiber MUSCLE fiber.
m. hyperplasia an inherited marked increase in the number of fibers in the muscle masses of affected cattle. There is a corresponding diminution in the amount of fat and connective tissue in the carcass. There is no deleterious effect on the animals except a higher prevalence of dystocia, and some other minor musculoskeletal defects, including elso-heel. Called also culard, doppellender, doppellendigkeit, double muscle.
myofibril a muscle fibril, one of the slender threads of a muscle fiber, composed of numerous myofilaments.
myofibrillar pertaining to a myofibril.
m. ATPase muscle enzyme which can be stained histochemically to aid in the differentiation between type I and type II muscle fibers.
m. hypoplasia see SPLAYLEG.
myofibroblast an atypical fibroblast combining the ultrastructural features of a fibroblast and a smooth muscle cell.
myofibroma a myoma combined with a fibroma.
myofibrosis replacement of muscle tissue by fibrous tissue.
myofibrositis inflammation of the sheath of muscle fibers.
myofilament any of the ultramicroscopic threadlike structures composing the myofibrils of striated muscle fibers.

myogenesis the formation of muscle fibers and muscles in embryonic development.
myogenic giving rise to or forming muscle tissue.
m. atrophy atrophy which is intrinsic to the muscle and not to its nerve, neurogenic atrophy, or to its blood supply, ischemic atrophy.
myogenous originating in muscular tissue.
myoglobin the oxygen-transporting pigment of muscle, a conjugated protein resembling a single subunit of hemoglobin, being composed of one globin polypeptide chain and one heme group.
myoglobinuria the presence of myoglobin in the urine. It is evidence of severe muscle degeneration, though all such degenerations do not necessarily lead to myoglobinuria; it depends on the content of the pigment in the muscle and the renal threshold for it. The urine is red to dark red-brown, but in severe cases may be almost black.
paralytic m. see PARALYTIC myoglobinuria.
myoglobinuric nephropathy accumulation of large quantities of myoglobin in renal convoluted tubules during an episode of severe muscle damage can result in damage by the myoglobin to the tubular epithelium and lead to nephrosis; renal ischemia may also contribute to the epithelial damage.
myoglobulin a globulin from muscle serum.
myogram a record produced by myography.
myograph an apparatus for recording the effects of muscular contraction.
myography 1. the use of a myograph. 2. description of muscles. 3. radiography of muscle tissue after injection of a radiopaque contrast medium.
myoid resembling muscle.
m. cell striated muscle cells found in thymus tissue; they contain acetylcholine receptors and may be a target in immune-mediated myasthenia gravis.
myointimal cell cells of the muscle layer of arterial wall that migrate to a subendothelial site and are responsible for organization of deposits on the vessel wall.
myoischemia local deficiency of blood supply in muscle.
myokinase see ADENYLATE kinase.
myokinesimeter an apparatus for measuring muscular contraction induced by electrical stimulation.
myokinetic pertaining to the motion or kinetic function of muscle, as contrasted with the myotonic or tonic function.
myokymia a benign condition in which there is persistent quivering of the muscles.
myolipoma myoma with fatty elements.
myology scientific study or description of the muscles and accessory structures (bursae and synovial sheaths).
myolysis degeneration of muscle tissue.
myoma a tumor formed of muscle tissue.
m. uteri, m. of uterus a benign tumor of the smooth muscle fibers of the uterus. See LEIOMYOMA uteri.
myomalacia morbid softening of a muscle.
myomatosis the formation of multiple myomas.
myomectomy 1. excision of a myoma. 2. myectomy.
myomelanosis melanosis of muscle.
myomere myotome; the muscle plate or portion of a somite that develops into voluntary muscle.
myometer an apparatus for measuring muscle contraction.
myometritis inflammation of the myometrium.
myometrium the smooth muscle coat of the uterus.
myonecrosis necrosis or death of individual muscle fibers.
ischemic m. see ISCHEMIC myonecrosis.
myoneural junction the junction of nerve and muscle fibers. Called also somatic myoneural junction; see also MOTOR end-plate.
myoneuralgia neuralgic pain in a muscle.
myopalmus muscle twitching.
myoparalysis paralysis of a muscle.
myoparesis slight muscle paralysis.
myopathic emanating from or pertaining to myopathy.
m. syndrome generalized muscle weakness with fatigue and reduced exercise tolerance.
myopathy strictly speaking, any disease of a muscle. Common usage is to restrict its use to describe the noninflammatory degenerations of skeletal muscle characterized by hyaline degeneration of muscle fibers, muscle weakness, myoglobinuria and a high serum level of muscle enzymes. This includes post-exertional rhabdomyolysis, enzootic nutritional muscular dystrophy, congenital myopathies, neurogenic atrophy and pale, soft, exudative pork. See also MUSCULAR.
capture m. an acute myopathy occurring most frequently in wild animals after a long chase or with a lot of struggling. The course is short and the death rate high. Affected animals are recumbent, dyspneic, hyperthermic and show muscle tremor. It is basically an exertional myopathy.
centronuclear m. myotubular myopathy.
congenital myotonic m. see MYOTONIA congenita.
exertional m. acute myopathy occurring as a result of intensive activity of large muscle masses. See PARALYTIC myglobinuria, TYING-UP SYNDROME, capture myopathy (above), PORCINE stress syndrome.
fibrotic m. fibrous adhesions between the muscle masses in the posterior thigh muscles in horses. A sequel to traumatic mysositis. See also ossifying myopathy (below).
Golden retriever m. a congenital disorder of muscles seen from a very young age in male Golden retrievers that show a stiff gait, abduction of thoracic limbs, bunny-hopping in the pelvic limbs, and enlargement of the tongue. The clinical signs worsen with exercise and as the dog matures. Now recognized as an X-linked inherited deficiency of dystrophin, analogous to the human disorder, Duchenne MUSCULAR dystrophy.
hereditary m's see X-linked MUSCULAR dystrophy, Golden retriever myopathy (above), NEMALINE BODY myopathy, type II MUSCLE fiber deficiency.
hypokalemic m. see feline HYPOKALEMIC polymyopathy.
lipid storage m. increased amounts of lipid accumulate in myofibers causing weakness, muscle pain and atrophy and rarely cardiomyopathy. Reported in dogs; the cause is unknown but abnormalities in levels of lactate, pyruvate and carnitine have been found.
mitochondrial m. caused by a deficiency of pyruvate dehydrogenase; reported in Clumber spaniels, Sussex spaniels and Old English sheepdogs.
myotubular m. a form marked by myofibers resembling those of early fetal muscle, i.e. myotubules.
ossifying m. calcification of the adhesions of fibrotic myopathy. A special occurrence is in the semimembranosus, semitendinosus and biceps femoris muscles of Western performance horses. See OSSIFYING fibrotic myopathy.
m. post-exercise see exertion myopathy (above).
postoperative m. after a period of recumbency with general anesthesia, affected horses are usually unable to rise. If they do rise, they show severe tremor, weakness and easy falling. Serum muscle enzyme

levels indicate gross muscle damage and both fore- and hindlimbs are affected.

myopericarditis inflammation of both the myocardium and pericardium.

myopia short sightedness; light rays focus in front of the retina. The opposite of hypermetropia.

axial m. results from the anteroposterior length of the eye being longer than normal.

myoplasm the contractile part of the muscle cell.

myoplasty plastic surgery on muscle in which portions of detached muscles are used, especially in the field of defects or deformities.

Myoporum Australian genus of plants in the Myoporaceae family; contain a number of poisonous substances, of which sesquiterpenes are the most significant; the most important is a hepatoxin, ngaione, which causes photosensitization, jaundice and death in animals eating them. Includes *M. acuminatum* (boobialla), *M. deserti* (Ellangowan poison bush), *M. laetum* (ngaio), *M. montanum*, *M. serratum* (boobialla), *M. tetrandrum*, *M. adscendens*, (boobialla), *M. insulare* (boobialla).

Myoprocta a small South American forest rodent. Called also acuchi.

Myoptes musculinus see MYOCOPTES *musculinus*.

myoreceptor a receptor situated in skeletal muscle that is stimulated by muscular contraction, providing information to higher centers regarding muscle position.

myorrhaphy suture of a muscle.

myorrhexis rupture of a muscle.

myosarcoma a malignant tumor derived from myogenic cells.

myosclerosis hardening of muscle tissue.

myosin one of the two main proteins of muscle. Myosin and actin are the proteins involved in contraction of muscle fibers.

m. ATPase catalyzes the physicochemical interactions of actin and myosin during muscle contraction.

m. light chains each molecule of smooth muscle cell myosin contains two pairs of light molecular weight chains (MLCs), one alkali MLC and one regulatory MLC.

myosis see MIOSIS.

myositis inflammation of a voluntary muscle. Causes heat, swelling, pain and lameness if a limb is affected. Trauma is the common cause, especially in racing and work horses. Blackleg is a specific myositis. See also POLYMYOSITIS.

atrophic m. a form of masticatory myositis in dogs. There is a chronic, progressive atrophy and fibrosis of the masticatory muscles of dogs which finally makes it impossible for the mouth to be opened wider than a few inches.

eosinophilic m. 1. a form of masticatory myositis seen in German shepherd dogs. It is acute, often recurrent, and there is painful, bilaterally symmetrical swelling of the masticatory muscles, mainly temporals and masseters. Often there is an eosinophilia found in the hemogram. Occasionally other muscles are also involved. There is a progressive atrophy and fibrosis of the muscles, frequently resulting in an inability to open the mouth. In the latter it may be confused clinically with atrophic myositis (above). 2. a lesion found at meat inspection. It reduces the value of the carcass. The cause is unknown.

familial m. see canine familial DERMATOMYOSITIS.

m. fibrosa a type in which there is formation of connective tissue in the muscle.

masticatory m. see atrophic myositis and eosinophilic myositis (above).

maxillary m. a slowly developing myogenic degeneration of the muscles of the jaw in horses.

multiple m. polymyositis.

m. ossificans a generalized myositis with dystrophic ossification in muscle. It occurs in pigs, in which it may be familial, and rarely in dogs and cats.

trichinous m. caused by the presence of *Trichinella spiralis*.

myospasm spasm of a muscle.

myospherulosis a granulomatous reaction containing saclike structures with spherules; associated with lipid medications being applied to open wounds or being injected. There are solid subcutaneous or dermal nodules.

myotactic pertaining to the proprioceptive sense of muscles.

m. reflex see tendon REFLEX.

myotasis stretching of muscle.

myotatic pertaining to the stretching of a muscle.

m. reflex spinal reflex elicited by the tapping (stretching) of a muscle tendon, which causes a response, usually seen as the flexion or extension of a joint. The patellar, biceps and triceps reflexes are examples.

myotendinous junction see MUSCLE–tendon junction.

myotenositis inflammation of a muscle and tendon.

myotenotomy surgical division of the tendon of a muscle.

myotic see MIOTIC.

Myotis genus of bats. Includes *M. thysanodes* (fringed myotis bat), *M. myotis* (European common mouse-eared bat), *M. lucifugus* (little brown bat).

myotome 1. an instrument for dividing muscles. 2. the muscle plate or portion of a somite that develops into voluntary muscle. 3. a group of muscles innervated from a single spinal nerve.

myotomy cutting or dissection of muscular tissue or of a muscle.

circumferential m. a means of relieving tension when attempting resection and anastomosis of the cervical or thoracic esophagus.

coccygeal m. transection of a dorsal sacrococcygeal muscle to correct a crooked tail in horses.

Heller's m. an esophagomyotomy at the esophagogastric junction, usually performed as a treatment for megaesophagus caused by achalasia. Called also CARDIOPLASTY.

ventral caudal m. see NICKING (2).

myotonia any disorder involving tonic spasm of muscle.

acquired m. see PSEUDOMYOTONIA.

m. congenita an inherited muscle stiffness with stilted gait that worsens with excitement is observed from a few months of age in Chow Chows, Labrador retrievers and Irish terriers.

inherited congenital m. a disease of goats, characterized by inability to move quickly. The limbs become rigid due to muscle contraction, but after a few minutes rest the animal is able to move normally. It is similar to myotonia congenita in humans.

myotonic pertaining to or emanating from myotonia.

m. dimple a depression or furrow that forms from a sudden local contraction of muscle in response to percussion and persists for up to a minute. It occurs in MYOTONIA and is used as a diagnostic test for the condition.

m. myopathy see MYOTONIA congenita.

myotonus tonic spasm of a muscle or a group of muscles.

myotoxin toxins affecting muscle fibers only.

myotrophic 1. increasing the weight of muscle. 2. pertaining to myotrophy.
myotrophy nutrition of muscle.
myotropic having a special affinity for muscle.
myotube, myotubule a developing skeletal muscle fiber with a centrally located nucleus.
myovascular pertaining to muscle and blood vessels.
Myriapoda originally a class of arthropods, including the millipedes and centipedes now superseded by two classes—Diplopoda (millipedes) and Chilopoda (centipedes).
myringa see TYMPANIC membrane.
myringectomy, myringodectomy excision of the tympanic membrane.
myringitis inflammation of the tympanic membrane.
myring(o)- word element. [L.] *tympanic membrane.*
myringodectomy myringectomy.
myringomycosis fungus disease of the tympanic membrane.
myringotomy tympanotomy; incision of the tympanic membrane.

The procedure is usually performed to relieve pressure and allow for drainage or irrigation of the middle ear behind the tympanic membrane.

Myrmecophaga a genus in the family of anteaters (Myrmecophagidae).
M. tetradactyla **(syn.** ***Tamandua tetradactyla*****)** the tamandua, an arboreal anteater with a prehensile tail and a yellow ochre color.
myrosinase the enzyme in mustard that releases the toxic allyl isothiocyanate from the nontoxic glycoside that occurs in the plant.
myrotheciotoxicosis poisoning due to ingestion of the fungi *Myrothecium roridum* and *M. verrucosum*, characterized by diarrhea, dysentery, abomasal hemorrhage, hepatitis, pulmonary congestion and a fatal outcome. The toxin is a trichothecene.
Myrothecium *Myrothecium roridum* and *M. verrucosum* (*M. verrucaria*) are fungi that grow on standing grasses or clover, and on stored feed. There is a special disposition to grow on kikuyu grass. See MYROTHECIOTOXICOSIS, PENNISETUM *clandestinum*.
Mystax see TAMARIN.
mystery pig disease see PORCINE reproductive and respiratory syndrome.
Mysticetes baleen whales; 11 species including the blue whale.
Mytilus genus of farmed mussels in the suborder Lamellibranchiae. Includes *M. edulis* (blue mussel), *M. galloprovincialis* (Mediterranean mussel), *M. smaragdinus* (green mussel), *M. crassitesta* (Korean mussel). See Table 23.
myxadenitis inflammation of a mucus-secreting gland.
myxadenoma an epithelial tumor with the structure of a mucous gland.
myxasthenia deficient secretion of mucus.
myxedema a mucinous degeneration with thickening of the skin that occurs in hypothyroidism. In animals it occurs mainly in newborn piglets and dogs.
myxedematoid resembling myxedema.
myx(o)- word element. [Gr.] *mucus, slime.*
Myxobolus cerebralis a myxosporean parasite which invades the cranial cartilages of juvenile rainbow trout, causing whirling disease.
myxochondroma chondroma with stroma resembling primitive mesenchymal tissue.
myxocyte one of the cells of mucous tissue.
myxofibroma a fibroma containing myxomatous tissue; called also fibroma myxomatodes and fibromyxoma.
myxofibrosarcoma fibrosarcoma with myxomatous areas.
myxoid resembling mucus.
myxolipoma lipoma with foci of myxomatous degeneration.
myxoma a tumor composed of primitive connective tissue cells and stroma resembling mesenchym.
heart valve m. developmental abnormality caused by persistence of embryonic myxomatous tissue in the endocardial cushions.
m. virus a poxvirus in the genus *Leporipoxvirus*; the cause of MYXOMATOSIS of rabbits.
myxomatosis 1. the development of multiple myxomas. 2. myxomatous degeneration.
infectious m. of rabbits a highly infectious, mosquito and rabbit flea or contact transmitted, generalized disease caused by myxoma virus which is very similar to the rabbit fibroma virus. It is characterized by swelling of the eyelids and a profuse, purulent ocular and nasal discharge, subcutaneous lumps 0.5 to 1 inch in diameter, especially on the head, and swelling of the genitalia. The case fatality rate with virulent virus strains is 100% and the morbidity in a closed rabbitry is usually more than 50%.
myxomatous characterized by the development of lesions resembling myxomas.
m. transformation see mucoid DEGENERATION.
myxomyoma a myoma with myxomatous degeneration.
myxopoiesis the formation of mucus.
myxorrhea a flow of mucus.
m. intestinalis excessive secretion of intestinal mucus.
myxosarcoma a sarcoma containing myxomatous tissue.
Myxosoma a genus of myxozoan parasites in the class Myxosporea. Cause serious disease losses in free-living fishes.
M. cartilaginis invades cartilage in the head of fish without causing deformity or nervous signs.
M. cerebralis causes whirling disease and twist disease characterized by tail chasing, black pigmentation of the tail and deformity, including sunken heads and twisted spines. The parasite invades and destroys skeletal discharge.
M. dujardini causes cysts in the gills, followed by dyspnea and death due to asphyxia.
myxosporean cyst-producing parasite found in many organs of fish. Previously regarded as protozoans, now believed to be metazoans.
myxovirus a synonym for influenza virus. See ORTHOMYXOVIRIDAE.
myxozoan member of the phylum Myxozoa, a phylum of parasitic protozoa found chiefly in fish, amphibians and reptiles.
Myzorhynchus one of the mosquito vectors of the canine heartworm, *Dirofilaria immitis.*
myzorhyncus the apical glandular region of the scolex of a cestode belonging to the order Tetraphyllidea, parasitic in sharks.

N

N 1. symbol, *newton*. 2. chemical symbol, *nitrogen*. 3. symbol, *normal* (solution); the expressions 2N (double normal), 0.5N (half-normal), 0.1N (tenth-normal), etc., denote the strength of a solution in comparison with the normal.

n 1. symbol, *refractive index*. 2. symbol, *nano-*. 3. statistically speaking, the number of individuals or values in a sample.

N-3-pyridyl methyl N^1-*p*-nitrophenyl urea see VALOR.

N banding a staining technique for karyotypes; performed with Giemsa or silver stains; called N band because it identifies nucleolus organizer regions.

N-CAMs nerve-cell adhesion molecules.

***n*-capric acid** see DECANOIC ACID.

***N*-methylconiine** plant toxin found in *Conium maculatum*.

***n*-propyl disulfide** see PROPYL disulfide.

N region a highly variable region on the H chain of immunoglobulins.

N^5,N^{10}-methylene H_4 folate form of tetrahydrolate essential to the synthesis of purines.

N5,N10A band the wide (1.5–2 μm) anisotropic central zone in the sarcomere or contractile unit of the myofibril, made of both actin and myosin filaments.

NA Nomina Anatomica.

Na chemical symbol, *sodium* (L. *natrium*).

Na+ sodium ion.

Na+ gradient the rate of increase or decrease of sodium ion concentration.

Na+ pump see sodium PUMP.

Na+-dependent transport voltage-sensitive protein 'gates' with complex subunit structure of large α-subunit and smaller β-subunits. Present in axonal fibers and involved in transmission of action potential along a nerve.

NAA Nomina Anatomica Avium.

naalehu [Hawaiian] see ENZOOTIC calcinosis.

Naboth's cyst see cervical CYST.

Naboth's cysts see cervical CYST.

NaCl sodium chloride.

nacreous having a pearl-like luster.

NAD+ the oxidized form of nicotinamide adenine dinucleotide.

NAD+ malate dehydrogenase see MALATE dehydrogenase.

NAD in medical records, an abbreviation for no abnormalities detected.

NADH the reduced form of nicotinamide-adenine dinucleotide.

NADH-methemoglobin reductase the enzyme in the erythrocyte that converts methemoglobin to hemoglobin, which is the form responsible for the transport of oxygen.

nadolol an adrenergic blocking agent that affects both β_1- and β_2-receptors.

NADP nicotinamide-adenine dinucleotide phosphate.

NADP diaphorase an enzyme system in the erythrocyte involved in the efficient transport of oxygen.

NADP-linked malic enzyme see MALIC ENZYME.

NADPH reduced form of nicotinamide adenine dinucleotide phosphate (NADP) used in a number of reductive synthesis such as fatty acids and steroids.

Naegleria a genus of protozoa in the family Vahlkampfiidae.

N. fowleri persists in thermally heated swimming pools and causes fatal meningoencephalitis in humans.

Naemorhedus see GORAL.

naevus see NEVUS.

nafcillin a semisynthetic, acid- and penicillinase-resistant penicillin that is effective against staphylococcal infections. Used as the sodium salt.

naftalofos see NAPHTHALOPHOS.

nag vernacular for horse; called also steed, cayuse, neddy.

nagana see TRYPANOSOMIASIS.

NAGase mastitis test an indirect test for mastitis based on the presence in the milk of mastitic quarters of high levels of a cell-associated enzyme *N*-acetyl-β-*D*-glucosaminidase.

Nagler's reaction a test for the identification of alpha toxin of *Clostridium perfringens*; the addition of antitoxin to cultures on egg yolk agar prevents visible opacity, due to lecithinase action which is normally observed around colonies.

Nagpuri breed of Indian buffalo; used for draft and milk production; long horns, usually black, sometimes white on face, legs and tail.

nail 1. a rod of metal, bone or other material used for fixation of the ends of fractured bones. 2. see horseshoe nail (below). 3. a horny cutaneous plate overlying the dorsal surface of the distal phalanx of the human fingers and toes; similar structures are found in other primates. 4. (loosely) one of the claws of dogs, cats, chickens, etc.

n. bed infection see PARONYCHIA.

n. bind usually used to indicate a nail prick of the horse's hoof caused by the blacksmith driving a nail too close to the soft tissues and causing pressure on the sensitive laminae without penetrating them. See also nail prick (below).

n.-hole curette a curette with a fine stem and a tiny, half-cup shaped end designed to be inserted in a nail-hole in the hoof to curette out damaged tissue and to provide drainage. Called also Hughes nail-hole curette.

n. dermatophytosis see ONYCHOMYCOSIS.

horseshoe n. a nail made of a special soft metal and with a specific shape that directs the point of the nail away from the soft tissues and out through the side wall of the hoof.

intramedullary n. one placed within the medullary cavity, bridging the fracture site and providing support and immobilization although rotation may be a problem. See INTERNAL fixation.

n. prick penetration of the sole of the horse's hoof by a nail or other sharp object to the depth of the sensitive laminae. Causes acute lameness and may lead to infection, HOOF abscess and tetanus. See also nail bind (above). Called also nail tread.

pulled n. an injury common in racing Greyhounds, in which the attachment of the nail to the nail bed is separated by trauma. Causes severe pain and lameness.

n. tread see NAIL prick.

n. trimmers see RESCO NAIL TRIMMER, toenail SCISSORS.

Nairobi bleeding disease see canine EHRLICHIOSIS.

Nairobi sheep disease an infectious disease of sheep caused by an arbovirus in the genus Nairovirus and transmitted by the tick *Rhipicephalus appendiculatus* and possibly other ticks. It is characterized by acute hemorrhagic gastroenteritis and blood-stained purulent nasal discharge.

Nairovirus a genus of viruses in the family BUNYAVIRIDAE; includes Nairobi sheep disease virus.

Naivasha star grass *Cynodon plectostachyus.*
naive in immunology, an individual that has not been exposed to a particular antigen.
Naja see COBRA.
Na+,K+-ATPase widely distributed enzyme consisting of two large α-subunits and two smaller β-subunits, whose function is to transport Na+ and K+ against their concentration gradients using hydrolysis of ATP as the thermodynamic couple. The stoichiometry of exchange is two K+ for every three Na+ pumped. Often called the sodium PUMP.
nakanuke a characteristic sign in avian reticuloendotheliosis. The barbs of the central portion of the wing and tail feathers of some affected birds remain adherent to the shaft.
naked ladies see COLCHICUM AUTUMNALE.
Nakuru grass CYNODON *aethiopicus.*
nalbuphine a potent synthetic narcotic agonist–antagonist used as the hydrochloride for relief of moderate-to-severe pain.
naled an organophosphorus insecticide.
nalidixic acid a naphthylidine derivative that inhibits DNA synthesis. Used for the treatment of urinary tract infections due to susceptible gram-negative bacteria. Side-effects in dogs include vomiting, diarrhea and seizures.
nalmefene, nalmetrene a narcotic antagonist, similar to naloxone, used to temporarily control obsessive behavior such as crib-biting in horses and self-mutilation in dogs.
nalorphine a semisynthetic congener of morphine used as the hydrochloride to antagonize morphine and related narcotics and as an analgesic.
naloxone a narcotic antagonist structurally related to oxymorphone used as the hydrochloride to reverse the effects of previously administered narcotics.
naltrexone an opiate antagonist similar to naloxone but with longer action and greater potency.
namaqua THESIUM *namaquense.*
name title; identifying word(s).
business n. a legal title for a veterinary hospital or practice, approved by the local veterinary registering authority and the registrar under the Companies Act or similar authority responsible for the registration of such names.
problem n. key name; key indicant. The name of the problem, which may be a clinical sign, a production average, or a performance figure. A critical identification in a problem-oriented system of record keeping.
Nandina domestica horticultural plant in family Berberidaceae; can cause cyanide poisoning; called also sacred or heavenly bamboo.
nandrolone an androgenic, anabolic steroid. The decanoate and phenpropionate esters are long-acting repository preparations.
nanism dwarfism or marked small size from any cause.
Nannizia see MICROSPORUM.
nanny mature goat doe.
nano- word element. [Gr.] *dwarf, small size;* used in naming units of measurement to designate an amount 10^{-9} (one-thousand-millionth) the size of the unit to which it is joined, e.g. nanogram (ng).
nanocephaly microcephaly.
nanocormia abnormal smallness of the body or trunk.
nanocurie a non-SI unit of radioactivity, being 10^{-9} curie, or the quantity of radioactive material in which the number of nuclear disintegrations is 3.7×10, or 37, per second; abbreviated nCi. Now replaced by the BECQUEREL.
nanogram one-thousand-millionth (10^{-9}) gram.
nanoid dwarfish.
nanomelus micromelus.
nanometer a unit of linear measure or wave length equal to one-thousand-millionth (10^{-9}) of a meter; nm; millimicron.
nanophthalmia nanophthalmos.
nanophthalmos abnormal smallness in all dimensions of one or both eyes in the absence of other ocular defects. Called also pure microphthalmos.
nanophthalmus 1. nanophthalmos. 2. an animal affected with nanophthalmos.
nanophyetiasis see SALMON poisoning.
Nanophyetus a genus of digenetic trematodes in the family Nanophyetidae, parasites in the intestines of mammals.
N. salmincola found in the small intestines of cats, dogs and many small, wild mammals, and occasionally in piscivorous birds and humans. The second intermediate host is fish. The fluke carries the rickettsia that causes SALMON poisoning and ELOKOMIN FLUKE FEVER in the terminal host.
nanosecond one-thousand-millionth (10^{-9}) second; abbreviated ns or nsec.
nanosomia dwarfism.
nanous dwarfed; stunted.
nanus a dwarf.
Nanyang cattle Chinese draft cattle, usually red with gray or white spots.
nape the back of the neck. Called also nucha.
naphthalene a hydrocarbon from coal tar oil; used as an antiseptic.
chlorinated n. see CHLORINATED NAPHTHALENES.
naphthalophos, naftalofos a species-specific anthelmintic against *Haemonchus contortus,* most useful in areas where benzimidazole resistance has developed in the worm population and where frequent treatment is necessary. It also has the advantage that it is used at a single dose level for sheep of all sizes. It is an organophosphate compound but is safe at the recommended dose rates. Higher dose rates are of moderate efficiency against most intestinal nematodes of sheep, but may be toxic. Called also phthalophos.
naphthlindandione an anticoagulant rodenticide, related to warfarin.
naphthol a phenol occurring in coal tar: α-naphthol (1-hydroxynaphthalene) or β-naphthol (2-hydroxynaphthalene). It has antiseptic properties and is used in compound form as a skin antiseptic.
2-naphthylamine an industrial chemical identified as a urinary bladder carcinogen.
[alpha]-naphthylthiourea a rodenticide. Causes fatal pericardial and pleural effusion and pulmonary edema in most domestic animal species if taken accidentally. Little used nowadays. Abbreviated ANTU.
Napier grass *Pennisetum purpureum.* Called also elephant grass.
napkin ring lesion a circumferential adenocarcinoma of the rectum, often a cause of rectal stricture.
naproxen a propionic acid derivative with analgesic, antipyretic and anti-inflammatory activity (a nonsteroidal anti-inflammatory agent); its use is associated with gastroduodenal ulceration in dogs.
napsylate USAN contraction for 2-naphthalenesulfonate.
narasin an ionophore used as an aid to gastrointestinal absorption and to improve weight gains as for monensin. Causes poisoning similar to monensin poisoning.
Narcissus European genus of plants in the family Liliaceae. Includes the daffodil and narcissus. Can be

poisonous if plant residues, especially bulbs, are ingested by animals because of the high content of lycorine, which causes salivation, vomiting and diarrhea.

narco- word element. [Gr.] *stupor, stuporous state.*

narcolepsy cataplectic episodes, often precipitated by exercise or excitement, with partial to complete flaccid paralysis. It occurs in dogs and is thought to be inherited in Shetland ponies.

narcosis a reversible state of central nervous system depression induced by a drug.

basal n., basis n. narcosis with complete unconsciousness, amnesia and analgesia.

narcotic 1. pertaining to or producing narcosis. 2. a drug that produces insensibility or stupor.

In veterinary medicine the term narcotic includes any drug that has this effect, but care is needed to avoid confusion with the more common usage of the word to mean the habit-forming drugs—for example, opiates such as morphine and heroin, and synthetic drugs such as meperidine. These can be legally obtained for use in animals only with a veterinarian's prescription. The sale or possession of narcotics for other than strictly therapeutic purposes is prohibited by law.

n. analgesics opiate derivatives such as morphine and etorphine.

n. antagonists substances used to reverse the effects of morphine derivatives. They include naloxone, and partial antagonists such as levallorphan and nalorphine.

n. antitussives cough suppressants, usually containing codeine.

narcotize to put under the influence of a narcotic.

nardoo fern see MARSILEA.

nares [L.] plural of *naris;* the openings of the nasal cavity. See also NOSTRIL, CHOANA.

caudal n. see CHOANA.

holorhinal n. the type of external nostrils found in many gallinaceous and anserine birds. The nostril does not reach beyond the nasal-frontal hinge.

schizorhinal n. a kind of nostril found in some birds. The external nares are long and slit-like and extend caudally beyond the nasal-frontal hinge.

stenotic n. a congenital anomaly found most commonly in brachycephalic dogs. There is inspiratory dyspnea, often forcing open-mouth breathing, and sometimes coughing or gagging. Associated anomalies, such as elongated soft palate and everted laryngeal saccules, are common, as are secondary changes in the respiratory tract, including laryngeal and tracheal collapse.

Narrawa burr SOLANUM *cinereum.*

narrow-leaved plants whose foliage consists of narrow, as opposed to round, leaves.

n.-l. sumpweed see IVA ANGUSTIFOLIA.

n.-l. vetch VICIA *sativa* var. *angustifolia.*

Narthecium toxic plant genus in the family Liliaceae; contain steroidal saponins which cause crystal-associated cholangiopathy and a resulting jaundice and photosensitive dermatitis; also cause nephrosis; includes *N. asiaticum*, *N. ossifragum* (bog asphodel).

narwhal an Arctic whale *Monodon monoceros* with an extraordinary dentition, no conventional teeth, two upper central teeth only, one of which develops into a long tusk in the male.

nasal pertaining to the nose.

n. acariasis characterized by mild nasal discharge and hyperemia, occasionally severe rhinitis. See also PNEUMONYSSUS *caninum.*

n. actinobacillosis a chronic granulomatous lesion in the nasal cavity of the sheep, causing nasal obstruction and discharge, usually unilaterally.

n. amyloidosis in horses analogous to AL-amyloidosis in humans; can occur independently of a generalized disease, affecting nasal vestibule and anterior septum and turbinates, with sufficient nodular or diffuse deposits to obstruct the nasal passage.

n. areae, n. plane the polygonal, raised, epidermal markings on the skin of the nasolabial plane of the dog. The pattern of marking is individual to each dog and can be used for identification, similar to the use of fingerprints in humans.

n. bot fly infestation causes sneezing and constant nasal discharge. The presence of the flies in the flock causes some insect worry. See also OESTRUS *ovis.*

n. breath flow of the breath from the nostrils as distinct from the breath from the mouth.

n. breath volume as determined by holding the palms of the hands in front of the nostrils; diminution or cessation of flow are readily appreciated.

n. catarrh chronic nasal discharge without obvious physical cause. A specific problem of unknown etiology in rabbits, although *Bordetella bronchiseptica* is thought to be implicated. Manifested by sneezing, constant nasal and ocular discharge and matting of the fur on the insides of the forelimbs. Called also snuffles.

n. cavity erectile tissue erectile tissue present only in some patients; usually collapsed.

n. cavity hemorrhage see EPISTAXIS.

n. cavity obstruction by mucosal inflammation, foreign body, neoplasm; detected by assessing the nasal breath flow.

n. cavity olfactory region located on ethmoturbinates, turbinates and nasal septum; covered by olfactory epithelium including sustentacular, basal and olfactory cells.

n. cavity respiratory region covers most of the cavities; covered by respiratory epithelium containing many, mainly serous, glands and carrying cilia.

n. cavity-sinuses see paranasal SINUSES.

n. cavity vestibular region place of transition from skin to respiratory epithelium.

n. conchae see Table 10.

n. cycling reciprocal change in degree of congestion between nostrils; when the mucosa of one nasal cavity becomes congested the mucosal congestion of the opposite nasal cavity diminishes.

n. discharge may be unilateral or bilateral, serous, purulent, hemorrhagic, or contain food material.

n. diverticulum see nasal DIVERTICULUM.

encapsulated n. hematoma persistent because of its size; blood is accumulated under respiratory mucosa so as to resemble a polyp. Like a polyp the hematoma obstructs the flow of breath through the nasal cavity.

enzootic n. adenocarcinoma of sheep and cattle may occur at a sufficiently high incidence to suggest an infectious cause. Usually unilateral in front of the ethmoid bone.

n. fold see facial FOLD[1].

n. foreign bodies take the form of grass seeds or sticks poked up while the animal is scratching its muzzle in allergic rhinitis, especially in cattle. Cause sneezing, nasal discharge, inspiratory dyspnea, snoring noise and rubbing of the nose. Foreign bodies may be viewable or palpable.

n. fossa see nasal FOSSA.

n. fundus the caudal part of the nasal cavity, close to the ethmoid bone.

n. granuloma see ENZOOTIC nasal granuloma, MYCOTIC nasal granuloma, SCHISTOSOMA nasalis.

n. hemorrhage see EPISTAXIS. Called also rhinorrhagia, nose bleed.
n. hematoma cause unilateral nasal obstruction; are usually the result of foreign body injury, rarely due to inept passage of a nasal tube or endoscope.
n. meatus see nasal CAVITY.
n. mites see nasal acariasis (above).
n. mucosal inflammation see RHINITIS.
n. obstruction causes respiratory stertor, mouth breathing, and small airstreams from the nostrils. It may be caused by a palpable foreign body.
n. odor smell of the nasal breath; may be necrotic, smell of ketones.
n. passage see nasal CAVITY.
n. plane see nasal PLANE.
n. polyp see nasal POLYP.
progressive n. hematoma see PROGRESSIVE nasal hematoma.
n. schistosomiasis infection with the blood fluke SCHISTOSOMA, which is largely asymptomatic but can cause dyspnea, snoring and profuse nasal discharge.
n. septum a vertical plate of bone and cartilage covered with mucous membrane that divides the cavity of the nose. See also SEPTUM.
n. sinus see paranasal SINUS.
n. swab cotton swab on a stick, passed up the nostril to obtain a sample of exudate and epithelial debris for microbiological or cellular examination.
n. tube see NASOGASTRIC tube.
n. turbinates see nasal conchae (above) and Table 10.
n. vestibule the part of the nasal cavity just inside the nostrils that is lined with skin.
n. wash flushing of the nasal cavity, usually with sterile saline, to recover cells or infectious agents for cytology or culture.

nascent 1. being born; just coming into existence. 2. just liberated from a chemical reaction, and hence more reactive.
n. DNA see OKAZAKI FRAGMENTS.

nasion a landmark found at the middle point of the frontonasal suture.

naso- word element. [L.] *nose.*

nasociliary pertaining to the eyes, brow, and root of the nose.

nasodigital pertaining to the specialized epidermal tissue of the planum nasale and footpads of carnivores.

nasofrontal pertaining to the nasal and frontal bones.

nasogastric pertaining to the nasal cavity and the stomach.
n. intubation the flexible tube with a rounded end is passed through the nasal cavity to the stomach; the technique requires expert knowledge and care to avoid damage to the nasal conchae and mucosa and to avoid passing medicines or feed into the lungs. The intubation may be therapeutic to relieve the stomach of a large volume of regurgitated fluid, or to pass a purgative fluid to the intestines, or the passing may be diagnostic in cases of colic to determine if there is fluid being recycled from the intestine back to the stomach. In small animals also used for enteral feeding.
n. tube a tube of soft rubber or plastic that is inserted through a nostril and into the stomach.

nasolabial pertaining to the nose and lip.
n. gland multilobular, tubuloalveolar, seromucoid glands in the muzzle and lips of cattle, sheep, goats.

nasolabiogram LABIOGRAM.

nasolacrimal pertaining to the nose and lacrimal apparatus.
n. apparatus see LACRIMAL duct.
n. duct see nasal DUCT.
n. duct obstruction may be a congenital defect or the result of infection or injury; causes tears to run down the affected side.
n. furrow formed in the embryo by the fusion of the two maxillary processes; develops eventually into the nasolacrimal duct.
n. groove nasolacrimal furrow.
n. radiography see DACRYOCYSTORHINOGRAPHY.
n. sac see LACRIMAL sac.
n. system includes the lacrimal ducts, lacrimal sac and nasolacrimal duct.
n. urticaria hay fever; an uncommon manifestation of atopy in dogs.

nasomaxillary pertaining to the maxilla and the nasal cavity.
n. aperture see nasomaxillary APERTURE.

naso-oral pertaining to the nose and mouth.

nasopalatine pertaining to the nose and palate.

nasopharyngeal pertaining to the nasal and pharyngeal cavities.
n. meatus see nasopharyngeal MEATUS.
n. spasm see reverse SNEEZE.
n. swab a sterile swab inside a plastic sleeve is passed up the nostril to the pharynx, the swab exteriorized, then withdrawn inside the sleeve and the appliance withdrawn.

nasopharyngitis inflammation of the nasopharynx.

nasopharyngolaryngoscope a flexible fiberoptic endoscope for examining the nasopharynx and larynx.

nasopharyngoscopy visual examination of the pharynx via a fiberscope passed up the nostril.

nasopharynx the part of the pharynx above the soft palate.

nasosinusitis inflammation of the paranasal sinuses.

nasty child syndrome constrictive foreign bodies, usually rubber bands or string, applied around the scrotum, muzzle, neck, tail or limbs of dogs or cats.

Nasua nasua see COATIMUNDI.

nasus [L.] *nose.*

natal 1. pertaining to birth. 2. pertaining to the nates (buttocks).

Natal gousiektebossie PACHYSTIGMA *thamnus.*

Natal yellow tulp HOMERIA *glauca* (*H. natalensis*).

natality the birth rate.

natamycin a polyene antibiotic used in topical treatment of fungal infections of the skin, eye and nasal cavity.

nates [L.] *the buttocks.*

natimortality the proportion of stillbirths to the general birth rate.

National cautery kit for electrocautery which includes a rheostat, pistol and appropriate cautery tips. The pistol is a handheld applicator with a finger operated on–off switch.

National Formulary see UNITED STATES NATIONAL FORMULARY.

National Institute for Research in Dairying at Reading, UK, this was for many years the world's leading institution for research into dairying, especially in the fields of mastitis and milking procedure. Called also NIRD. Now called Animal Grassland Research Institute.

National Research Council a body representing the (United States) National Academy of Sciences, National Academy of Engineering, and the Institute of Medicine, and established to further knowledge and advise the USA government; abbreviated NRC. It issues a series of publications on the nutrient requirements of each species of domestic animal, laboratory animals, primates and fish.

native 1. indigenous. 2. in the veterinary context, wild, unimproved, not cultivated. The listed plants were named native in their Australian context.

n. birdsfoot trefoil LOTUS *australis*.

n. candy tuft ZIERIA *laevigata*.

n. couch BRACHYACHNE *convergens*.

n. fuchsia EREMOPHILA *maculata*.

n. indigo INDIGOFERA *australis*.

n. leek BULBINE *semibarbata*.

n. lily DIPLARRENA *moraea*.

n. loquat see RHODOMYRTUS MACROCARPA.

n. millet see PANICUM *decompositum*.

n. mint MENTHA *australis*.

n. pennyroyal MENTHA *satureoides*.

n. thornapple DATURA *leichhardtii*.

n. tobacco NICOTIANA *debneyi*, *N. suaveolens*, *N. megalosiphon*.

n. tulip HOMERIA *flaccida*.

n. verbine PSORALEA *patens*.

n. willow see ACACIA *salicina*.

natremia see HYPERNATREMIA.

natrium [L.] *sodium* (symbol Na).

natriuresis the excretion of abnormal amounts of sodium in the urine.

natriuretic 1. pertaining to or promoting natriuresis. 2. an agent that promotes natriuresis.

n. factor see ATRIAL natriuretic factor.

natural occurs in nature, without the intervention of humans.

n. experiments occur by chance when all variables for a population are constant except one, which is different for one large part of the population compared with the other, e.g. when half of a flock comes from one climate and the other half is a local resident in another climate.

n. focus the ecology that is best suited to a biological system, e.g. an individual insect-borne disease; the area in which the disease naturally flourishes best; an ecological niche.

n. history history of a process or organism as it occurs in nature, e.g. course of a disease from infection to resolution.

n. killer (NK) cell see natural killer CELL.

n. selection selection occurring in nature, without any human intervention, direct or indirect.

n. ventilation ventilation without the use of artificially induced energy and the machines which it drives; the forces used are wind and the exchange of heat from within the barn and the external air, controlled by ventilation devices in the walls and the ceiling.

naturally bred see BULL-BRED HERD.

naturietic hormone a hypothetical humoral substance responsible for controlling many aspects of renal regulation of sodium homeostasis.

naturopath a practitioner of naturopathy.

naturopathy a drugless system of healing by the use of physical methods, such as light, air, water, etc.

nausea a subjective sensation in humans which probably occurs in animals. It is an unpleasant sensation, vaguely referred to the epigastrium and abdomen, with a tendency to vomit. Nausea may be a symptom of a variety of disorders, some minor and some more serious.

Nausea is usually felt when nerve endings in the stomach and other parts of the body are irritated, e.g in motion sickness. The irritated nerves send messages to the center in the brain that controls the vomiting reflex. When the nerve irritation becomes intense, vomiting results.

NAV Nomina Anatomica Veterinaria.

navel the umbilicus, the scar marking the site of entry of the umbilical cord into the fetal belly.

n. bleeding a problem in young piglets, up to 2 days old. Blood oozes from navel causing severe anemia, frequently death: prefarrowing vitamin C for more than 6 days before farrowing prevents it; called also umbilical hemorrhage.

n. ill see OMPHALITIS. Called also omphalophlebitis.

navelwort COTYLEDON *umbilicus*.

navicular boat-shaped; applied to certain bones, such as the navicular bones of the horse's foot and human ankle.

n. block a specially carved block of wood in which a horse's foot is lodged to enable a radiograph of the navicular bone to be taken at a suitable angle.

n. bone 1. the distal sesamoid bone of a horse's foot; it lies on the palmar side of the coffin joint and serves to change the direction of the deep digital flexor tendon as it inserts on the distal phalanx. Its palmar surface is covered with fibrocartilage, its dorsal surface with hyaline cartilage and its dorsal surface is pocked with a row of nutrient foramina. 2. (rare) the central tarsal bone.

n. bursa inflammation in the horse may contain *Brucella abortus*; a cause of intermittent lameness.

n. disease a chronic degeneration of the navicular bone in which there is damage to its flexor surface and the overlying flexor tendon in the front feet of horses. There may be an accompanying navicular bursitis and osteophyte formation. Characterized by intermittent lameness and pointing when the animal is standing. Called also podotrochlitis.

navy bean PHASEOLUS *lunatus*.

Nb chemical symbol, *niobium*.

nCi nanocurie; see BECQUEREL.

Nd chemical symbol, *neodymium*.

N'Dama a West African small, humpless type of beef cattle, fawn, dun or light red in color, with lyre or crescent horns. There are a large number of varieties.

NE Nomina Embryologica.

Ne chemical symbol, *neon*.

Neapolitan farcy see EPIZOOTIC lymphangitis.

near-drowning non-fatal water inhalation.

Near East fat-tailed a group of sheep breeds used for milk, meat or carpetwool; white, white with a colored face, black, brown or broken colored. Males are horned, females are polled; tails are fat, S-shaped and bi-lobed. Called also Semitic fat-tailed.

Near Eastern encephalomyelitis see Near Eastern equine ENCEPHALOMYELITIS.

near–far–far–near suture pattern an excellent tension suture. The first bite is made at right angles to the wound and close to it, under the wound, to emerge a long way from the wound, on the far side. The second bite begins closer to the wound, and crosses underneath it to emerge beyond the first point of entry. The two ends are tied there.

near-side a horse's left-hand side.

nearest neighbor the basis for the means of analyzing the spatial relations of free-living populations; consists of measuring distance between infected herds and their nearest neighbors.

nearthrosis a false or artificial joint.

neat an archaic word for cattle.

neatsfoot oil an oil manufactured by boiling cattle hooves. Used in leather maintenance.

Nebraska virus the calf diarrhea ROTAVIRUS.

nebula 1. a slight corneal opacity. 2. an oily preparation for use in an atomizer.

nebulization 1. conversion into a spray. 2. treatment by a spray.
nebulizer an atomizer; a device for creating an aerosol.
Necator a genus of HOOKWORM in the subfamily Necatorinae.
N. americanus the common hookworm of humans, found also in pigs and dogs.
N. suillus see *N. americanus* (above), found in pigs.
necatoriasis infection with organisms of the genus *Necator*; hookworm disease. Manifested by anemia and melena.
neck a constricted portion, such as the part connecting the head and trunk of the body, or the constricted part of an organ, as of the uterus (cervix uteri) or other structure.
n. band a band worn around the neck of a dairy cow, attached to which is a name or number plate or plaque.
n. chain used to tether dairy cows in standing stalls in enclosed barns; attached to the cow by a leather or webbing neck band.
n. collar a part of most horse draft harnesses, providing a point of attachment for plow chains or cart or buggy harness. Made of leather stuffed with straw and lined with felt, it closes over the top of the neck, just in front of the withers, lies on the front of the shoulder and is a support for the hames to which the traces or chains are actually attached. Pressure from a badly fitted collar can cause suprascapular nerve paralysis or sweeny.
ewe n. a concave neck; a fault in conformation in most species except sheep.
femoral n. the column of bone connecting the head of the femur and the shaft.
n. flexion abnormal presentation of the fetus, with the neck flexed and its dorsal flexure at the pelvis.
humeral n. the constriction of the humerus just distal to its head.
n. lesions resorption of tooth structure around the cemento-enamel junction. See also CERVICAL line lesions.
n. reining see neck REIN.
tooth n. the narrowed part of certain teeth, between the crown and the root.
n. twist injury see HEAD twist injury.
uterine n., n. of uterus cervix uteri.
wry n. see TORTICOLLIS.
n. yoke see HEADSTOCK.
neck stab see EVERNAZIONE.
neckbread butcher's term for the cervical segment of the thymus.
necklace fern see ASPLENIUM FLABELLIFOLIUM.
necrectomy excision of necrosed tissue.
necro- word element. [Gr.] *death*.
necrobacillosis tissue damage, especially in liver, caused by infection by *Fusobacterium necrophorum*. Manifested usually as areas of necrosis, occasionally as cellulitis or phlegmon. The pus has a characteristic rotting odor. See also HEPATIC abscess.
interdigital n. see bovine FOOTROT.
oral n. see ORAL necrobacillosis.
ruminal n. see RUMINAL necrobacillosis.
necrobiosis the physiological death of individual effete cells in any tissue; a normal mechanism in the constant turnover of many cell populations.
necrocytosis death and decay of cells.
necrogenic productive of necrosis or death.
necrogenous originating or arising from dead matter.
necrology statistics or records of death.
necrolysis separation or exfoliation of necrotic tissue.
toxic epidermal n. an acute exfoliative disease of skin and mucous membranes in dogs, cats and monkeys. Characterized by full thickness epidermal necrosis and accompanied by erythema, vesicles, bullae and ulcers, and systemic signs of fever, anorexia and lethargy. It is associated with concurrent infections or neoplasia, and drug reactions.
necroparasite an organism that lives in dead tissue.
necrophagous feeding upon dead flesh.
necrophilous showing a preference for dead tissue; said of microorganisms.
necropneumonia gangrene of lung.
necropsy examination of a body after death. See also AUTOPSY.
necroscopy see NECROPSY.
necrose to become necrotic or to undergo necrosis.
necrosis pl. *necroses* [Gr.] the morphological changes indicative of cell death caused by enzymatic degradation.
aseptic n. necrosis without infection or inflammation.
caseous n. necrosis in which the tissue is soft, dry and cheesy, occurring typically in tuberculosis.
central n. necrosis affecting the central portion of an affected bone, cell or lobule of the liver.
cheesy n. that in which the tissue resembles cottage cheese; most often seen in tuberculosis.
coagulation n. death of cells, the protoplasm of the cells becoming fixed and opaque by coagulation of the protein elements, the cellular outline persisting for a long time.
colliquative n. see liquefactive necrosis (below).
liquefactive n. necrosis in which the necrotic material becomes softened and liquefied.
moist n. necrosis in which the dead tissue is wet and soft.
Zenker's n. hyaline degeneration and necrosis of striated muscle; called also Zenker's degeneration.
necrospermia a condition in which the spermatozoa are dead or motionless.
necrotic of or pertaining to cell death and enzymatic degradation.
n. cervicovaginitis necrosis in cows and ewes, usually as a result of trauma during parturition.
n. colitis common in older cats as a cause of chronic, foul, bloody diarrhea.
n. dermatitis gangrene and necrosis of inflamed, wet skin caused by *Clostridium septicum*; characterized by a sudden onset of severe depression, a short course of a few hours and a high death rate; mostly in 4–16 week old chicks.
n. ear syndrome extensive necrosis of ear edges in baby pigs probably caused by biting by pen mates plus *Staphylococcus hyicus*.
n. enteritis a name used to refer to: (1) subacute or chronic enteritis in pigs, usually a sequel to an acute episode of enteritis caused by *Salmonella* spp. or *Campylobacter hyointestinalis* and other anaerobic flora. Characterized by unthriftiness, and intermittent or chronic diarrhea; (2) a hemorrhagic enteritis in young chickens caused by *Clostridium welchii* type C.
n. glossitis necrosis and loss of the tip of the tongue in feeder steers; cause unknown.
n. hepatitis see INFECTIOUS necrotic hepatitis.
n. laryngitis see calf DIPHTHERIA.
n. rhinitis a cellulitis of soft tissues of the face and nose of pigs. The face is swollen and the nasal cavity occluded. It causes dyspnea, stertor and difficult mastication. *Fusobacterium necrophorum* is the cause, usually entering through fight wounds. Called also bullnose.

n. stomatitis see ORAL necrobacillosis.
n. ulcer of swine see ULCERATIVE granuloma of swine.
n. vulvovaginitis usually the result of injury during dystocia.

necrotic tips see AVASCULAR chorion.

necrotizing causing necrosis; exuding a brown to green, putrid discharge containing tissue debris.
n. epithelioma, necrotizing calcifying epithelioma see PILOMATRIXOMA.
n. hepatopancreatitis disease of shrimps caused by a small obligate intracellular unidentified bacterium; subacute to chronic syndrome with cumulative mortality of up to 90%.
n. panniculitis multifocal, erythematous, nonpruritic cutaneous lesions which ulcerate in the center and discharge seropurulent exudate; identifiable on histopathological examination.
n. scleritis a rare eye lesion, inflammatory proliferation of the anterior sclera, in dogs.
n. ulcerative gingivitis see necrotizing ulcerative GINGIVITIS.
n. vasculitis important feature of the Arthus reaction; damage to the endothelium results from deposition of immune complexes in the vessel wall, usually on the basement membrane of the endothelium.

necrotomy 1. dissection of a dead body. 2. excision of a sequestrum.

necrotoxin a factor or substance produced by certain staphylococci that kills tissue cells.

neddy vernacular for horse; called also nag, cayuse, steed.

needle 1. a sharp instrument for suturing or puncturing. 2. to puncture or separate with a needle.
acupuncture n's stainless steel needles with silver-plated handles 0.5 to 1 inch long, which are inserted into tissues at those points on the skin surface which are considered relevant to the problem being treated.
aneurysm n. one with a handle used in ligating blood vessels.
aspirating n. a long, hollow needle for removing fluid from a cavity.
aspiration biopsy n. a needle to which suction can be applied in order to withdraw a core of tissue from a solid organ.
atraumatic n. surgical needles with suture material fused to the end, which is less traumatic to tissues then suture doubled back through the end of a needle. See SWAGE (2).
blunt-point n. a noncutting, blunt-pointed needle used in general surgery and for suturing liver and kidney. Needle pricks are less likely. This is an issue in modern surgery on humans.
n. burr AMARANTHUS *spinosus*.
n.-cannula a needle used as a cannula, as for introduction of an intravenous catheter or for passing a suture thread.
cataract n. one used in removing a cataract.
discission n. a two-way needle or cannula which permits flushing and aspiration of liquid cataract material. See also DISCISSION.
n. driver see needle holder (below).
n. feeling the sensation perceived by the operator when the insertion of an acupuncture needle reaches the acupuncture point.
n. grass *Stipa* spp. Called also spear grass.
Hagedorn's n. a form of flat suture needle.
n. holder a strong scissor-type instrument used to hold a suture needle while pushing it through tissue. The handles are ratcheted and have to be squeezed to release the needle. The face of each blade is grooved so that the needle will not twist or swivel while being driven. The natural action is for a right-handed surgeon.
hypodermic n. a hollow, sharp-pointed needle to be attached to a hypodermic syringe for injection of solutions.
knife n. a slender knife with a needle-like point, used in ophthalmic operations.
ligature n. a long-handled, slender steel needle, having an eye in its curved end, used for passing a ligature underneath an artery.
n. puncture puncture of a mass, tissue or fluid accumulation in order to relieve pressure or to collect sample for field or laboratory examination.
reverse cutting n. a curved cutting needle with the cutting edge on the back of the curve rather than on the concave surface.
Rosenthal n. used for aspiration of bone marrow.
round bodied n. a noncutting surgical needle used for suturing tissues that separate easily such as intestine, liver, lung and fascia. Called also taperpoints.
spatula n. a flat, rather than round, special cutting needle for ophthalmic work.
stop n. one with a shoulder that prevents too deep penetration.
tape n. a special, heavy duty needle with a palm-fitting handle, for sewing with tape.
tapercut n. a suture needle with a flattened shaft, so that it is three times as wide as it is thick, and a point which has a gradually diminishing triangular cross-section, a cutting point. Modern design has a circular cross-section and a short cutting tip.

needling includes introduction and withdrawal of needles, lifting and thrusting, twirling, and combinations of the three basic movements in acupunctorial technique.

NEEE Near Eastern equine encephalitis.

neem see AZADIRACHTA INDICA.

Neethling virus the poxvirus that causes the severe form of LUMPY skin disease.

neg negative.

negative 1. having a value of less than zero. 2. indicating lack or absence, as coagulase-negative or Brucella-negative. 3. characterized by denial or opposition.
n. feedback see FEEDBACK.
n. reinforcement in animal psychology the stimuli which produce withdrawal, immobility, aversion, escape.

negative sense in RNA viruses, the genomic RNA is of opposite polarity, 5′ to 3′, to messenger RNA so that after adsorption, penetration, uncoating and release of the viral RNA into the cytoplasm of the cell, the viral RNA must first be transcribed to produce messenger RNAs which is initially accomplished by a RNA dependent RNA polymerase that is a structural component of the virus and released along with the viral RNA.

negatron a negatively charged electron.

negligence in law, the failure to do something that a reasonable person of ordinary prudence would do in a certain situation or the doing of something that such a person would not do. Negligence may provide the basis for a lawsuit when there is a legal duty, as the duty of a veterinarian, to provide reasonable care to patients and when the negligence results in damage to the patient.
contributory n. a defense against a negligence suit, in which evidence is presented that the client contributed to the unsatisfactory outcome of a case by being negligent himself/herself, e.g. by not returning the animal for further treatment soon enough.

Negri bodies see Negri BODY.
Nei Ching the Yellow Emperors' Classic of Internal Medicine as part of the history of Chinese medicine.
Neisseria a genus of gram-negative bacteria in the family Neisseriaceae. Commonly found as normal flora in the oral cavity and respiratory tract of many species and only rarely associated with disease except in humans where *N. meningitidis* is the cause of meningococcal meningitis, and *N. gonorrheae* is the cause of gonorrhea.
nelia ACACIA *osswaldii*.
Nelson scissors blunt-pointed, curved or straight-bladed, long-handled scissors designed for thoracic surgery.
Nelson's syndrome the development of an ACTH-producing pituitary tumor after bilateral adrenalectomy in Cushing's syndrome.
nemaline body the name of the lesion arises from the electron microscopic image; an inclusion-like structure found in muscles but with no specific disease significance.
n. b. myopathy myopathy associated with the presence of nemaline bodies in the muscle fibers; recorded in cats and dogs, characterized by weakness, tremor, ataxia, fatigue.
nematocerans members of the suborder of insects Nematocera. It includes the gnats, mosquitoes, midges, black flies and gall flies.
nematocide 1. destroying nematodes. 2. an agent that destroys nematodes, including PHENOTHIAZINE, PIPERAZINE, BENZIMIDAZOLE, the IMIDAZOTHIAZOLES, the TETRAHYDROPYRIMIDINES, ORGANOPHOSPHORUS COMPOUNDS and a wide variety of miscellaneous compounds, including the AVERMECTINS.
nematocysts the stinging capsules of marine animals in the phylum Cnidaria. They are the characteristic feature of members of the phylum.
nematode a roundworm; any individual organism of the class Nematoda. Parasitism with any of the worms in this group represents a significant proportion of the diseases of animals. Includes: *Ancylostoma*, *Ascaris*, *Capillaris*, *Dictyocaulus*, *Dioctophyma*, *Dirofilaria*, *Habronema*, *Haemonchus*, *Metastrongylus*, *Muellerius*, *Onchocerca*, *Ostertagia*, *Oxyuris*, *Parafilaria*, *Parascaris*, *Protostrongylus*, *Rhabditis*, *Skrjabinema*, *Spirocerca*, *Strongyloides*, *Strongylus*, *Syngamus*, *Thelazia*, *Trichuris*, *Toxocara*, *Trichinella*, *Trichostrongylus*.
n. galls hard, fibrous excrescences produced in the seedheads of grasses by chronic inflammation created by an invasion by larvae of grass seed nematodes, e.g. *Anguina* spp.
grass-seed n. the grass seed nematode *Anguina lolii* infests Wimmera ryegrass and causes a fatal poisoning in animals eating the grass. Called also *A. fenesta*, *A. agrostis*. See also LOLIUM *rigidum*.
nematodiasis state of infestation with nematodes.
cerebral n. sporadic occurrence of chance invasion of brain by migrating nematode larvae, e.g. strongyles in horses. See also CEREBROSPINAL nematodiasis. Called also kumri.
Nematodirella a genus of worms in the trichostrongyloid family Molineidae.
N. cameli found in camel and reindeer.
N. dromedarii found in dromedary and sheep.
N. longispiculata found in the small intestine of sheep, goats and other ruminants.
nematodiriasis infestation in the small intestine with the nematode *Nematodirus* spp. Characterized clinically by persistent diarrhea and wasting. Usually found in mixed infestations.
Nematodirus a genus of roundworms in the trichostrongyloid family Molineidae, cause of NEMATODIRIASIS.
N. abnormalis found in sheep, goats and camels.
N. andrewi found in sheep.
N. aspinosus found in rabbits and hares.
N. battus a parasite of sheep; causes nematodiriasis.
N. filicollis found in sheep, cattle, goat and deer.
N. helvetianus found in cattle and occasionally sheep.
N. hsuei found in sheep.
N. lamae found in sheep.
N. leporis found in rabbits and hares.
N. odocoilei found in sheep.
N. oiratianus found in camels and wild ruminants.
N. spathiger found in the small intestine of sheep, cattle and other ruminants.
N. tarandi found in sheep.
Nembutal a proprietary name for pentobarbital sodium.
neo- word element. [Gr.] *new, recent.*
neoantigen a newly acquired and expressed antigen, e.g. a T antigen, present in cells infected by oncogenic viruses.
neoarsphenamine an organic arsenical antiprotozoal agent which used to be used extensively, particularly in the treatment of swine dysentery and blackhead of turkeys, but is now replaced by more effective compounds.
neoarthrosis see NEARTHROSIS.
Neoascaris vitulorum see TOXOCARA *vitulorum*.
Neobassia proceriflora toxic plant in family Chenopodiaceae; contains soluble oxalates causing nephrosis and urolithiasis; can cause heavy mortalities in sheep, characterized by hypocalcemia, paralysis, coma and death; called also soda bush, *Threlkeldia proceriflora*.
Neobenedinia cutaneous, ocular and oral flukes of marine fish; in order Capsalidae; characterized by being transparent. Called also *Benedinia*.
neoblastic originating in or of the nature of new tissue.
neocerebellum the cerebellar hemispheres. Phylogenetically, the newer parts of the cerebellum, especially those supplied by corticopontocerebellar fibers.
neocortex neopallium.
Neocuterebra a genus of flies in the family Oestridae, the larvae of which parasitize animals.
N. squamosa found in the African elephant.
Neodactylogyrus a genus of monogenetic flukes in the family Dactylogyridae, which parasitize marine and freshwater fish.
Neodiplostomum a genus of intestinal digenetic trematodes in the family Diplostomatidae. Includes *N. multicellulata* (in herons), *N. perlatum* (in piscivorous birds), *N. tamarini* (in New World primates).
neodymium a chemical element, atomic number 60, atomic weight 144.24, symbol Nd. See Table 6.
n.:yttrium-aluminum-garnet (Nd:YAG) laser a type of continuous wave laser used for hemostasis, coagulation and in ophthalmic surgery for ablation of specific structures.
Neofelis nebulosa see clouded LEOPARD.
neogenesis tissue regeneration.
neohemocyte experimental, artificial erythrocytes consisting of hemoglobin contained in liposomal membranes, capable of transporting and delivering oxygen to tissues.
neokinetic pertaining to the nervous motor mechanism regulating voluntary muscular control.

neomembrane a false membrane.

neomycin an aminoglycoside antibiotic produced by *Streptomyces fradiae*; the sulfate is used as an intestinal antiseptic and in treatment of systemic infections due to gram-negative bacteria. High doses and prolonged treatment can be nephrotoxic and ototoxic.

n. B see FRAMYCETIN.

neon a chemical element, atomic number 10, atomic weight 20.183, symbol Ne. See Table 6.

neon fish disease see PLISTOPHORA *hyphessobryconis*.

neonatal pertaining to the period immediately after birth; the duration varies between species; in humans refers to the first four weeks of life; in animals the first week seems appropriate. Some neonatal disorders are listed in entries below. Others are listed elsewhere under titles specific to their anatomic location, including HYALINE membrane disease, RESPIRATORY distress syndrome.

n. cardiac murmur is observed in foals and most disappear before the fifth day. Persistence after that time may suggest valvular dysfunction. Many congenital murmurs are functional and cause no signs of disease.

n. diarrhea see undifferentiated DIARRHEA of the newborn.

n. distress see neonatal maladjustment syndrome (below).

n. edema usually caused by obstruction to lymphatic flow by defective development of lymph drainage system.

n. hyaline membrane disease see HYALINE membrane disease.

n. hyperbilirubinemia see neonatal jaundice (below).

n. hypoglycemia a metabolic disease of newborn piglets caused by restriction of food intake. Clinical signs include weakness, shivering, hypothermia and terminal convulsions.

n. isoerythrolysis see ALLOIMMUNE hemolytic anemia of the newborn.

n. jaundice is an important clinical sign in foals because of the possibility of alloimmune hemolytic anemia. Some cases of benign, physiological jaundice also occur in foals. There is jaundice but no other clinical or pathological abnormality. Called also neonatal hyperbilirubinemia.

n. isoimmune purpura see neonatal thrombocytopenic purpura (below).

n. maladjustment syndrome a disease of newborn thoroughbred foals caused by premature severance of the umbilical cord in assisted foalings and by hypoxia due to other causes. The foals may be normal for some hours after birth. Clinical signs include aimless wandering, apparent blindness, and convulsions including a sound like a dog barking. Called also barkers and wanderers.

n. mortality death in the neonatal group.

n. neoplasm occurs rarely. Lymphosarcoma, benign and malignant melanoma and myeloid leukosis are recorded. Sporadic bovine leukosis, manifested by many subcutaneous tumors, is the most common form of the disease.

n. ophthalmia see OPHTHALMIA neonatorum.

n. septicemia many bacteria, which are not widely invasive in older animals, can cause septicemia in neonates because of their immunological immaturity; common examples are *Escherichia coli*, *Listeria monocytogenes*, *Salmonella* spp., streptococci, e.g. *S. suis*.

n. spasticity an inherited disease of calves which are normal at birth but soon develop a susceptibility to tetanic convulsions when stimulated. See also NEURAXIAL EDEMA.

n. streptococcal infection occurs in all species, but is especially important in piglets and foals. Bacteremia and septicemia may result in the animal's death or the development of arthritis, endocarditis, meningitis or ophthalmitis. Causative bacteria are: foals—*Streptococcus zooepidemicus* (*S. pyogenes equi*); piglets—*S. suis* types 1 and 2, *S. equisimilis*; calves—*S. pyogenes*; lambs—*S. faecalis* and group C streptococci.

n. thrombocytopenic purpura a severe bleeding disease in piglets a few days old which have drunk colostrum containing antiplatelet antibody from their alloimmune dam.

n. vigor amount of physical activity displayed by the newborn animal; an indication of the potential viability of the patient.

neonate a newborn animal. The duration of the state of neonaticity varies between 48 hours for a chicken to about 4 weeks for mammals, depending on the ability of the animal to survive without its dam.

n. abandonment abandoned newborn of any species due principally to poor maternal instincts in the dam. See also MISMOTHERING.

neonatologist a veterinarian who specializes in neonatology.

neonatology the branch of theriogenology dealing with disorders of the newborn animal.

neonicotine see ANABASINE.

Neonyssus a genus of mites in the family Rhinonyssidae.

N. columbae*, *N. melloi nasal mites of pigeons.

neopallium that part of the pallium (cerebral cortex) showing stratification and organization of the most highly evolved type; called also isocortex and neocortex.

neoplasia the formation of a neoplasm.

neoplasm 1. a TUMOR. 2. any new and abnormal growth, specifically one in which cell multiplication is uncontrolled and progressive. Neoplasms may be benign or malignant. Neoplasms of particular organs and of particular cell types are to be found under their individual headings, e.g. pharyngeal, adenocarcinoma.

benign n. a neoplasm having none of the characteristics of a malignant neoplasm (see below), i.e. it grows slowly, expands without metastasis, and usually does not recur.

n. fever due to extensive necrosis in rapidly growing tumors.

histoid n. a neoplasm whose cells and organization resemble those of the tissue from which it is growing.

malignant n. a neoplasm with the characteristics of anaplasia, invasiveness and metastasis.

organoid n. a neoplasm whose cellular architecture resembles that of some organ in the body.

transmissible n. a neoplasm capable of being transmitted between individuals. Includes BOVINE viral leukosis, avian LEUKOSIS, ROUS SARCOMA complex, MAREK'S DISEASE, canine transmissible VENEREAL tumor, squamous cell CARCINOMA of cattle, and canine viral PAPILLOMATOSIS.

neoplastic pertaining to neoplasia or a neoplasm.

n. disease see NEOPLASIA.

Neopolitan mastiff a very large (110–150 lb), heavy dog with loose-fitting skin over the body and the large, broad head. The tail may be docked by one-third. The coat is short and colored black, blue, gray or brown.

neoprene oil-resistant synthetic rubber.

neopulmo the functional division of the respiratory system of birds formed by the parabronchi from the laterodorsal and lateroventral bronchi.

neopulmon a part of the avian lung composed of an anastomotic system of parabronchi, ventral and lateral to the primary bronchus in some species of birds.
Neorickettsia helminthoeca the rickettsia-like agent that causes SALMON poisoning in dogs.
Neoschongastia a genus of mites in the family Trombiculidae.
N. americana infest chicken, quail and turkey, and may cause dermatitis.
Neospora recent assumption of important status; closely resembles *Toxoplasma*; the life cycle is unknown but transplacental transmission is known to occur; causes ascending paralysis in kittens, puppies, calves and abortion in cattle. Includes *N. caninum*.
neosporosis infection by the protozoa *Neospora caninum*. In dogs, there are clinical signs referable to the central nervous system and myositis. Young puppies are most commonly and severely affected, showing a characteristic ascending limb paralysis with hyperextension, cervical weakness and dysphagia. Infection is a significant cause of late abortion, and some defective live calves, in cattle in Australia and New Zealand. An infected carnivore is the likely source of infection.
neostigmine an anticholinesterase used in the treatment of myasthenia gravis and glaucoma and as an antidote for nondepolarizing muscle relaxants, such as tubocurarine.
n. test muscle weakness caused by myastenia gravis is temporarily reversed following the administration of neostigmine; used as a diagnostic test.
neostriatum the more recently developed part of the corpus striatum, comprising the caudate nucleus and the putamen.
Neostrongylus a genus of nematodes in the family Protostrongylidae.
N. linearis found in the lungs of sheep and goats.
neoteny prolongation of the larval form in a sexually mature organism.
neothalamus the part of the thalamus connected to the neopallium.
Neotoma see pack RAT.
Neotrombicula autumnalis an acarine mite in the family Trombiculidae that causes dermatitis, usually on the head and extremities, in most animal species. Called also *Trombicula autumnalis*.
neovascularization formation of new blood vessels.
Nepeta a genus of plants in the family Labiatae.
N. hederacea causes pulmonary edema and enteritis in horses. Called also *Glechoma hederacea*, ground ivy.
N. cataria see CATNIP.
nepetalactone the volatile terpenoid found in catnip (*Nepeta cataria*).
nephelometer an instrument for measuring the concentration of substances in suspension by the amount of light that is scattered by the suspended particles.
nephelometry measurement of the concentration of a suspension by means of a nephelometer.
nephralgia pain in a kidney.
nephrectomy surgical removal of a kidney. The procedure is indicated when chronic disease or severe injury produces irreparable damage to the renal cells. Tumors, multiple cysts and congenital anomalies may also necessitate removal of a kidney. A single healthy kidney can carry on the functions formerly performed by both kidneys.
nephric pertaining to the kidney.
nephridium pl. *nephridia* [L.] 1. either of the paired excretory organs in each body segment of certain invertebrates, having the inner end of the tubule opening into the coelomic cavity. 2. various excretory structures such as the nephron of the embryo.
nephritic 1. pertaining to or affected with nephritis. 2. pertaining to the kidneys; renal. 3. an agent useful in kidney disease.
nephritis inflammation of the kidney; a focal or diffuse proliferative or destructive disease that may involve the glomerulus, tubule or interstitial renal tissue. See also GLOMERULONEPHRITIS, interstitial nephritis (below), NEPHROSIS, PYELONEPHRITIS.
autoimmune n. see GLOMERULONEPHRITIS.
embolic n. caused by infected emboli lodging in renal vessels. One or more abscesses may develop, causing signs referable to toxemia. There may be intermittent pyuria. Renal dysfunction is likely only if most of the renal mass is destroyed.
glomerular n. see GLOMERULONEPHRITIS.
interstitial n. a diffuse lesion characterized by interstitial inflammation and fibrosis, sometimes attributed to hematogenous infection with *Leptospira* spp. There is a secondary glomerular and vascular injury. It is manifested by polyuria, urine of low specific gravity, and terminal uremia.
lupus n. glomerulonephritis associated with systemic lupus erythematosus.
parenchymatous n. nephritis affecting the parenchyma of the kidney.
suppurative n. a form accompanied by suppuration and abscessation of the kidney.
transfusion n. nephropathy following transfusion from an incompatible donor.
nephritogenic causing nephritis.
nephr(o)- word element. [Gr.] *kidney*.
nephroblastoma a rapidly developing malignant mixed tumor of the kidneys, made up of embryonal elements. It may reach an enormous size, even distending the abdomen, e.g. in pigs.
nephrocalcinosis deposition of calcium phosphate in the renal tubules, resulting in renal insufficiency. Occurs in association with HYPERCALCEMIA. in cultivated finfish can be caused by a high CO_2 content of the water or by a high calcium:magnesium ratio in the diet.
nephrocapsectomy excision of the renal capsule.
nephrocardiac pertaining to the kidney and the heart.
nephrocele hernia of a kidney.
nephrocolic 1. pertaining to the kidney and the colon. 2. renal colic.
nephrocystitis inflammation of the kidney and bladder.
nephrogenesis producing kidney tissue.
nephrogenic producing kidney tissue.
nephrogenous arising in a kidney.
nephrogram a contrast radiograph of the kidney.
nephrography radiography of the kidney. See also PYELOGRAPHY.
nephroid resembling a kidney.
nephrolith a calculus in a kidney.
nephrolithiasis a condition marked by the presence of renal calculi. See also UROLITHIASIS.
nephrolithotomy incision of kidney for removal of calculi.
nephrology the branch of medicine dealing with the kidneys.
nephrolysin nephrotoxin, a toxin destructive to kidney tissue.
nephrolysis 1. freeing of a kidney from adhesions. 2. destruction of kidney substance.
nephroma a tumor of kidney tissue.
congenital mesoblastic n. a mesenchymal tumor composed of fibromatous and myxomatous areas.

nephromegaly enlargement of the kidney.

nephron the structural and functional unit of the KIDNEY, each nephron being capable of forming urine by itself. The nephron consists of the renal corpuscle, the proximal convoluted tubule, the descending and ascending limbs of the loop of Henle, the distal convoluted tubule, and the collecting tubule. Each kidney is an aggregation of many nephrons. The specific function of the nephron is to remove from the blood plasma certain end-products of metabolism, such as urea, uric acid and creatinine, and to regulate excretion of sodium, chloride, potassium and other ions. By allowing for reabsorption of water and some electrolytes back into the blood, the nephron also plays a vital role in the maintenance of normal fluid balance in the body.

The nephron is a complex system of tubules. Blood is brought to the nephron via the afferent arteriole. As the blood flows through the glomerulus (a network of capillaries), about one-fifth of the plasma is filtered through the glomerular membrane and collects in the glomerular (Bowman's) capsule, which encases the glomerulus. The fluid then passes through the proximal tubule, from there into the loop of Henle, then into the distal tubule, and finally into the collecting tubule (collecting duct). As the fluid is making its tortuous journey through these various tubules, most of its water and some of the solutes are reabsorbed into the blood via the peritubular capillaries. The water and solutes remaining in the tubules become urine.

intact-n. hypothesis see INTACT-NEPHRON HYPOTHESIS.

n. loop see renal TUBULE.

nephronophthisis wasting disease of the kidney substance.

nephropathy any disease of the kidneys.

analgesic n. see ANALGESIC nephropathy.

familial n. different types of renal disease have been recorded as occurring on a familial basis in Finnish-Landrace sheep and several breeds of dogs, including Lhasa apsos, Shih tzus, Samoyeds, Bull terriers, Norwegian elkhounds, Cocker spaniels and Basenjis.

hypercalcemic n. see NEPHROCALCINOSIS.

juvenile n. suspected of being familial in many dog breeds especially Malamute, Miniature schnauzer, Keeshond, German shepherd; characterized by renal failure in immature or young adult dogs. The pathogenesis is poorly understood, hence the retention of the title nephropathy.

mycotoxic n. caused by mycotoxins, such as ochratoxin and citrinin, produced by *Penicillium* and *Aspergillus* spp.

pigment n. see HEMOGLOBINURIC nephrosis.

reflux n. pyelonephritis in which the renal scarring results from vesicoureteric reflux, with radiological appearance of intrarenal reflux.

nephropexy surgical fixation of a floating or hypermobile kidney (NEPHROPTOSIS).

Nephrops farmed lobsters in the family Nephropsidae; includes *N. norvegicus* (Norwegian lobster). See Table 23.

nephroptosis downward displacement of a kidney; called also floating kidney.

nephropyelitis inflammation of the kidney and its pelvis; pyelonephritis.

nephropyelography radiography of the kidney. See also PYELOGRAPHY.

nephropyelostomy a diversion of urine to the exterior by placement of a catheter into the renal pelvis.

nephropyleocentesis aspiration of urine from the renal pelvis.

nephropyosis suppuration of a kidney.

nephrorrhagia hemorrhage from the kidney.

nephrorrhaphy suture of the kidney.

nephrosclerosis hardening of the kidney associated with chronic glomerulonephritis and in humans especially with hypertension and disease of the renal arterioles.

nephroscope an instrument inserted into an incision in the renal pelvis for viewing the inside of the kidney; it is equipped with three channels, for telescope, fiberoptic light input and irrigation.

nephroscopy visualization of the kidney by means of the nephroscope.

nephrosis disease characterized by purely degenerative lesions of the renal tubules.

amyloid n. chronic nephrosis with amyloid deposition in glomerular capillaries, in basement membranes of tubules and eventually around tubules.

biliary n. the renal component of acute hepatic failure characterized by oliguria and azotemia.

infectious avian n. an acute, viral, highly contagious disease of young chickens, characterized by edema of the cloacal bursa, lymphoid necrosis, prostration and death. Called also Gumboro disease, infectious bursal disease.

lipid n. nephrosis marked by edema, albuminuria, and changes in the protein and lipids of the blood and accumulation of globules of cholesterol esters in the tubular epithelium of the kidney.

lower nephron n. now called acute renal tubular necrosis where tubular degeneration occurs as a consequence of ischemia and nephrotoxins. Complete urinary outflow obstruction follows, resulting in acute renal failure. Also seen after severe injuries, especially crushing injury to muscles. See also CRUSH SYNDROME.

mycotic n. caused by ingested toxins of *Aspergillus ochraceus*, *Penicillium viridicatum*. Characterized by enlarged, terminally fibrosed kidneys, polyuria and polydipsia. See also MYCOTOXICOSIS.

nephrosonephritis renal disease with nephrotic and nephritic components.

nephrosplenic entrapment see left COLON displacement colic.

nephrostoma one of the ciliated funnel-shaped orifices of the excretory tubules that open into the celom in the embryo; best seen in lower vertebrates.

nephrostomy creation of a permanent opening into the renal pelvis.

nephrotic syndrome a condition marked by edema, marked proteinuria, hypoalbuminemia and hypercholesterolemia.

nephrotome one of the segmented divisions of the embryonic mesoderm connecting the somite with the lateral plates of unsegmented mesoderm; the source of much of the urogenital system. Called also intermediate cell mass.

nephrotomogram a tomogram of the kidney obtained by nephrotomography.

nephrotomography radiological visualization of the kidney by tomography after introduction of a contrast medium.

nephrotomy incision of a kidney.

nephrotoxic destructive to kidney cells.

n. nephritis an experimental disease induced by the injection of anti-rat-kidney antibodies. Called also Masugi nephritis.

nephrotoxicity quality of being toxic for kidneys.

nephrotoxin a toxin having a specific destructive effect on kidney tissue.

nephrotropic having a special affinity for kidney tissue.

nephrotuberculosis renal disease due to *Mycobacterium tuberculosis*.

nephroureterectomy surgical removal of a kidney and ureter.

neps small (2 mm) aggregations of matted wool fibers created during processing.

Neptunia amplexicaulis Australian plant in the legume family Mimosaceae; selectively absorbs selenium and can cause selenium poisoning. A selenium-converter plant. Called also selenium weed. Also grows preferentially on selenium-rich soils and is therefore an indicator plant.

neptunium a chemical element, atomic number 93, atomic weight 237, symbol Np. See Table 6.

nequinate a quinolone cocciostat used in poultry.

Nerine a plant genus in the family Liliaceae which causes poisoning when eaten by cattle. The toxic agent is lycorine, which causes salivation, vomiting and diarrhea. Called also nerine.

nerioside a cardiac glycoside found in NERIUM *oleander* and one of the causes of poisoning by this plant.

Nerium widespread genus of plants in the family Apocynaceae; popular garden specimens in hot climates. Their leaves and branches are very poisonous, causing death due to ventricular fibrillation. The toxic agents are cardiac glycosides, especially nerioside and oleandroside. Signs include dyspnea, cardiac arrhythmia, diarrhea and convulsions. Lesions include cardiomyopthy. Includes *N. indicum*, *N. odorum*, *N. oleander*. Called also oleander.

Nernst equation gives the amplitude and sign of the electronic potential created when a semipermeable membrane separates charged ions.

nerve a macroscopic cordlike structure of the body, comprising a collection of nerve fibers that convey impulses between a part of the central nervous system and some other body region. For a complete list of the named nerves of the body, see Table 14.

Depending on their function, nerves are known as sensory, motor or mixed. Sensory nerves, or afferent nerves, carry information from the periphery of the body to the brain and spinal cord. Sensations of heat, cold, pressure and pain are conveyed by the sensory nerves. Motor nerves, or efferent nerves, transmit impulses from the brain and spinal cord to the periphery, especially the muscles. Mixed nerves are composed of both motor and sensory fibers, and transmit messages in both directions.

Together, the nerves make up the peripheral nervous system, as distinguished from the central nervous system, which consists of the brain and spinal cord. There are 12 pairs of CRANIAL nerves, which carry messages to and from the brain. Spinal nerves arise from the spinal cord and pass out between the vertebrae. The various nerve fibers and cells that make up the autonomic nervous system innervate the glands, heart, blood vessels and involuntary muscles of the internal organs. For a complete list of nerves, see Table 14.

accelerator n's the cardiac sympathetic nerves, which, when stimulated, accelerate the heart rate.

n. biopsy specimens taken from representative nerves by separation and removal of fascicles may provide useful information in the investigation of neuromuscular disorders or neuropathies. Consideration must be given to any resulting motor or sensory deficits that might result from the procedure. In dogs, the common peroneal, ulnar and tibial nerves are the usual sources.

n. cuff device used in the surgical repair of nerves to protect the site of anastomosis from an in-growth of connective tissue and to promote linear regeneration of neural elements.

depressor n. 1. an inhibitory nerve whose stimulation depresses a motor center. 2. a nerve that lessens activity of an organ.

dermal n. network the organization of sensory nerve fibers to the dorsal root ganglia found in the dermis.

n. endings comprise afferent and efferent endings. ***Afferent endings*** transform sensations into acceptable stimuli by the CNS; include diffuse-free endings, free, modified free or encapsulated (e.g. tactile corpuscles, Krause's endbulbs, Golgi–Mazzoni corpuscles, genital corpuscles, lamellated corpuscles, Herbst corpuscles, Uffini corpuscles). ***Efferent endings*** transform nerve impulses into stimuli delivered to effector end organs; they include neuromuscular spindles, Golgi tendon organs.

encapsulated n. endings see nerve endings (above).

excitor n. one that transmits impulses resulting in an increase in functional activity.

excitoreflex n. a visceral nerve that produces reflex action.

n. fiber a process of a neuron, especially the long slender axon which conducts nerve impulses away from the cell. It may be medullated or nonmedullated.

free n. endings see nerve endings (above).

fusimotor n's those that innervate the intrafusal fibers of the muscle spindle.

gangliated n. any nerve of the sympathetic nervous system. Called also ganglionated.

n. gas organophosphorus compounds specially selected for their toxicity to humans and used in chemical warfare.

n. growth factor a protein dimer composed of two identical polypeptide chains secreted by nerve cells and necessary for the growth and survival of certain classes of nerve cells during development.

n. impulses the physicochemical change in a nerve fiber's membrane which is caused by stimulation, e.g. from a stretch receptor, and which transmits a record of the sensation, or, in another case, of a motor instruction to an effector organ.

inhibitory n. one that transmits impulses resulting in a decrease in functional activity.

medullated n. myelinated nerve.

modified free n. endings see nerve endings (above).

myelinated n. one whose axons are encased in a myelin sheath.

pelvic n's nerves of the parasympathetic outflow. See Table 14.

peripheral n. any nerve outside the central nervous system. Injury to a nerve causes pain initially and if tissue is destroyed, loss of function follows; signs are weakness or paralysis, atrophy, lower temperature and depressed reflexes.

pilomotor n's those that supply the arrector muscles of hair.

pressor n. an afferent nerve whose impulses stimulate a vasomotor center and increases intravascular tension.

retinal n. fiber layer layer number 9 of the retina; axons of ganglion cells, make up bundles of nerve fibers and pass to the optic disk and lamina cribrosa; from there on they become the optic nerve.

secretory n. an efferent nerve whose stimulation increases glandular activity.

n. sheath see NEURILEMMA.

n. sheath tumor neurilemmoma or schwannoma.

somatic n's the sensory and motor nerves supplying skeletal muscle and somatic tissues.
somatic afferent n's sensory neurons whose cell bodies reside in spinal and cranial nerve ganglia.
somatic efferent n's motor neurons originating in ventral gray columns of the spinal cord and certain parts of the brain and are connected to striated muscles derived from embryonic somites.
spinal n. a segmental nerve which consists of afferent and efferent axons from its dorsal and ventral roots.
splanchnic n's those of the blood vessels and viscera, especially the visceral branches of the thoracic, lumbar and pelvic parts of the sympathetic trunks.
n. stimulator an electrical device used to deliver a short stimulus to a peripheral nerve as a test of its function. It can be used to assess the effects of a neuromuscular blocking agent during clinical anesthesia.
sudomotor n's those that innervate the sweat glands.
sympathetic n's 1. see SYMPATHETIC trunk. 2. any nerve of the sympathetic nervous system.
n. terminal nerve ending.
trophic n. one concerned with regulation of nutrition.
n. trunk the main body of a nerve; subsequently divides into branches.
unmyelinated n. one whose axons are not encased in a myelin sheath.
vasoconstrictor n. one whose stimulation causes narrowing of blood vessels.
vasodilator n. one whose stimulation causes dilatation of blood vessels.
vasomotor n. one concerned in controlling the caliber of vessels, whether as a vasoconstrictor or vasodilator.
vasosensory n. any nerve supplying sensory fibers to the vessels.
visceral afferent n's nerves with cell bodies in spinal and cranial ganglia and which provide sensory innervation to thoracic and abdominal tissues.
visceral efferent n's the parasympathetic component of the autonomic nervous system.

nervi erigentes nerves containing preganglionic, parasympathetic motor fibers to the genitalia that are involved in erection of the penis. Called also pelvic splanchnic nerves.

nervi vasorum nerve supply to the blood vessels.

nervimotor pertaining to a motor nerve.

nervone a cerebroside isolated from nerve tissue.

nervous 1. pertaining to a nerve or nerves. 2. unduly excitable.
n. acetonemia in contrast to the more common form of this disease of cattle, the wasting form, this one is manifested by delirious signs of circling, head pushing, leaning, straddling, forceful licking including themselves, salivation and incoordination. There is a strong acetonuria and odor on the breath.
autonomic n. system the branch of the nervous system that works without conscious control. The voluntary nervous system governs the striated or skeletal muscles, whereas the autonomic governs the glands, the cardiac muscle, and the smooth muscles, such as those of the digestive system, the respiratory system and the skin. The autonomic nervous system is divided into two subsidiary systems, the sympathetic system and the parasympathetic system.

It is also divided into central and peripheral sections. The core of the central section is the hypothalamus which receives afferent input from many other parts of the brain including the cerebral cortex. Its efferent output goes to many lower centers in the nervous system that have visceral control as their functions, e.g. the respiratory center in the medulla. The peripheral section consists of nonmedullated nerve fibers that leave the central nervous system in the craniosacral outflow (parasympathetic system) or the thoracolumbar outflow (sympathetic) system, and terminate in effector organs after passing through a ganglion, visible paravertebral ganglia in the sympathetic system, or ganglia embedded in the wall of the target organ in the parasympathetic system.
central n. system the portion of the nervous system consisting of the brain and spinal cord. See also NERVOUS, BRAIN, CEREBRAL.
n. dysfunction can occur in any of four ways: (1) Excitation or irritation, an increase in the number of electrical stimuli or facilitation in their passage. (2) Release phenomena, from the damping, modifying effects of higher centers; includes spasticity, exaggerated tendon jerks. (3) PARALYSIS, due to reduction or cessation of transmission of nerve impulses. (4) Nervous SHOCK, a temporary cessation of activity in the nervous system as a whole in response to an insult applied to a part of it.
n. excitation see nervous dysfunction (above).
n. paralysis see nervous dysfunction (above).
peripheral n. system the portion of the nervous system consisting of the nerves and ganglia outside the brain and spinal cord.
n. release phenomena see nervous dysfunction (above).
n. shock see nervous dysfunction (above).
n. system the organ system that along with the endocrine system, correlates the adjustments and reactions of an organism to internal and environmental conditions, comprising the central, peripheral and autonomic nervous systems.

nervousness a state of excitability, with great mental and physical unrest.

nervus pl. *nervi* [L.] nerve.

nesidiectomy excision of the islet cells of the pancreas.

nesidioblast any of the cells giving rise to islet cells of the pancreas.

nesidioblastosis pancreatic ductular and islet cell proliferation in children and in dogs with islet cell neoplasms.

nest 1. the bed or shelter constructed by a bird for deposition of its eggs and rearing of its young. 2. a bed prepared by an animal. 3. an accumulation of cells in a foreign location.
n. building a signal of oncoming broodiness in female birds and of imminent parturition in some mammals.

nesting see AVIAN nesting.

net, nett the correct amount; not subject to further deductions; the amount remaining after all deductions have been made.
n. calf crop calves surviving until weaning.
n. energy energy available to the ingester for metabolic purposes. See also METABOLIZABLE energy.
n. profit gross income less all costs incurred by the enterprise.
n. worth statement balance sheet.

Netherland dwarf small, cobby rabbit, weighing up to 2.5 lb.

netilmicin a semisynthetic aminoglycoside antibiotic.

netobimin a broad-spectrum pobenzimidazole anthelmintic.

nettle a common name used for a variety of plants including bull nettle (*Solanum carolinense*), white horsenettle (*S. elaeagnifolium*), dead nettle (*Lamium* *amplexicaule*), field nettle (*Stachys arvensis*), spurge nettle (*Jatropha stimulosa*), mulga nettle (*Haloragis odontocarpa*) and the stinging nettles (*Urtica incisa, U. urens* and *U. dioica*).

n. gases used in crowd control in humans. Cause a very painful irritation of the skin. Includes dichloroformoxime.

n. rash see URTICARIA. Called also hives.

nettlerash urticaria.

nettling mimicking the effect of a nettle. Causing irritation to the skin and eyes, and to the bronchi if inhaled and the oral mucosa if ingested.

network a mesh-like structure of interlocking fibers or strands.

computer n. 1. a group of computers linked together so that the user of one of them can access the data and programs of another one of them. 2. the physical equipment to connect the computers together.

immunological n. idiotypes produced in an immune response may in turn act as antigens, provoking anti-idiotype antibodies with idiotypes that also may act as antigens, leading to a network of interacting reactions. Considered to be the possible basis for the overall regulation of immune responses.

networking see computer NETWORK.

Neubauer ruling a specific pattern of precise markings on a hematocytometer slide that facilitates the counting of leukocytes, erythrocytes and platelets in blood and all cells in other fluids.

neurad toward the neural axis or aspect.

neural pertaining to a nerve or to the nerves.

n. crest cells a group of neuroepithelial cells which condenses dorsal to the neural tube in the embryo; they subsequently migrate and set up dorsal root ganglia, the ganglia of the autonomic nervous system, and the pigment cells of the integument (melanocytes).

n. folds in the embryo, the sides of the invaginated neural plate that meet and fuse over the neural groove to form the neural tube.

n. groove the longitudinal furrow in the neural plate of the embryo.

n. lymphomatosis see MAREK'S DISEASE.

n. plate the thickened ectoderm dorsal to the notochord in the embryo that gives rise to the neural tube.

n. retina separated from the outer layer of the optic retina by the intraretinal space; constitutes the *pars optica retinae*, with its neuroepithelial layer (contains rods and cones—the receptor cells), bipolar ganglion layer, multipolar ganglion layer, and a layer of axons of the latter layer. Light must pass through the latter three layers before reaching the receptor cells.

n. substrates functional units of the central nervous system, often composed of a series of structural units which may be widely separated anatomically but which interact to support or drive complex nervous system functions, such as hunger and sleepiness. They are the counterparts of simple centers, e.g. the respiratory center, which control simple physiological mechanisms.

n. tropic influence the tropic influence of nerves on, for example, muscle, demonstrated by the atrophy of muscle when it is denervated.

n. tube the precursor of the central nervous system in the embryo, formed by invagination and fusion of the neural plate.

neuralgia pain in a nerve or along the course of one or more nerves. Assumed to occur in animals.

neuraminic acid a nine-carbon sugar; parent of a family of amino sugars containing nine or more carbon atoms (the sialic acids or nonulosaminic acids).

neuraminidase 1. an enzyme that cleaves the terminal *N*-acetylneuraminic acid from mucoproteins. 2. a structural component occurring as a spike in the envelope of ortho- and paramyxoviruses.

neuranagenesis regeneration of nerve tissue.

neurapophysis the structure that forms either side of the neural arch; also, the part supposedly homologous with this structure in a so-called cranial vertebra.

neurapraxia failure of nerve conduction in the absence of structural changes, due to blunt injury, compression or ischemia.

mandibular n. see MANDIBULAR neurapraxia.

neurarthropathy neuroarthropathy.

neuratrophia impaired nutrition of the nervous system.

neuratrophic characterized by atrophy of the nerves.

neuraxial edema a disease complex of newborn calves, recorded only in polled Herefords and their crosses; characterized clinically by extreme extensor spasm if stimulated by touch or lifting to their feet. They appear normal while recumbent, are unable to stand but can suck normally. Two diseases have been identified, inherited, congenital MYOCLONUS and a poorly defined 'congenital brain edema'. See also MAPLE SYRUP URINE DISEASE.

neuraxis 1. axon. 2. central nervous system.

neuraxon axon.

neuraxonal dystrophy see inherited ovine degenerative AXONOPATHY.

neurectasia, neurectasis the surgical stretching of a nerve; neurotony.

neurectoderm ectoderm destined to be nervous tissue.

neurectomy excision of a part of a nerve.

posterior (low) digital n. used for relief of incurable lameness in horses, usually resulting from navicular disease or fractures of the navicular bone or wing of the third phalanx. The procedure is relatively simple and can be performed under local or general anesthesia, but the consequences for a neurectomized horse can be disastrous. Rules of racing in many places limit or exclude participation of neurectomized horses.

neurectopia displacement or abnormal situation of a nerve.

neurenteric pertaining to the neural tube and archenteron of the embryo.

neurepithelium see NEUROEPITHELIUM.

neurergic pertaining to or dependent on nerve action.

neurexeresis the operation of tearing out (avulsion) of a nerve.

neurilemma the plasma membrane of a Schwann cell, forming the sheath of Schwann of a myelinated or unmyelinated peripheral nerve.

neurilemmitis inflammation of the neurilemma.

neurilemmoma a tumor of a peripheral nerve sheath (neurilemma); called also schwannoma. Occur as small subcutaneous tumors on the head of goldfish.

neurinoma neurilemmoma.

neurite axon.

neuritis pl. *neuritides*; inflammation of a nerve; also used to denote noninflammatory lesions of the peripheral nervous system. See also NEUROPATHY.

There are many different forms of neuritis. Some increase or decrease the sensitivity of the body part served by the nerve; others produce paralysis; others cause pain and inflammation. The cases in which pain is the chief symptom are generally called NEURALGIA.

Neuritis and neuralgia affect the peripheral nerves,

the nerves that link the brain and spinal cord with the muscles, skin, organs, and all other parts of the body. These nerves usually carry both sensory and motor fibers; hence both pain and some paralysis may result.

allergic n. see experimental allergic neuritis (below).

autoimmune n. see experimental allergic neuritis (below).

cauda equina n. see CAUDA EQUINA NEURITIS.

equine exudative optic n. a cause of sudden blindness in old horses of unknown etiology but sometimes associated with trauma to the head. There are signs of acute inflammation with optic neuritis and later atrophy.

equine proliferative optic n. an incidental unilateral finding in old horses of cauliflower-like mass attached to the optic disk; vision is not impaired.

experimental allergic n. (EAN) an ascending polyneuritis produced experimentally by the administration of nerve tissue. The condition resembles GUILLAIN–BARRÉ SYNDROME, CAUDA EQUINA NEURITIS in horses, and COONHOUND paralysis. Called also allergic, autoimmune neuritis.

interstitial n. inflammation of the connective tissue of a nerve trunk.

multiple n. neuritis affecting several nerves at once; polyneuritis.

optic n. inflammation of the optic nerve, affecting the part of the nerve within the eyeball (neuropapillitis) or the part behind the eyeball (retrobulbar neuritis).

parenchymatous n. neuritis affecting primarily the axons and the myelin of the peripheral nerves.

retrobulbar n. optic neuritis affecting the part of the optic nerve behind the eyeball.

toxic n. neuritis due to some poison.

traumatic n. neuritis following and due to injury.

neur(o)- word element. [Gr.] *nerve, neurology, neurological.*

neuroaminidase see NEURAMINIDASE.

neuroanastomosis surgical anastomosis of one nerve to another.

neuroanatomy anatomy of the nervous system.

neuroanesthesia anesthesia in animals with neurological disease, particularly of the central nervous system.

neuroanesthesiology the study of neuroanesthesia.

neuroarthropathy any disease of joint structures associated with disease of the central or peripheral nervous system.

neuroaxial dystrophy see inherited ovine degenerative AXONOPATHY.

neuroaxonal dystrophy a degenerative disease believed to be inherited in several breeds of dogs and cats. Progressive signs of cerebellar dysfunction with ataxia, hypermetria, proprioceptive deficits, incoordination and tremors develop from an early age. It has been reported in Rottweilers, Collie sheepdogs and Bull mastiffs.

neurobehavioral relating to neurological status as assessed by observation of behavior.

neurobiologist a specialist in neurobiology.

neurobiology biology of the nervous system.

neuroblast an embryonic cell from which nervous tissue is formed.

neuroblastoma rare neoplasm arising from primitive neuroepithelial cells which differentiate toward neuroblasts (neuroblastoma) or neurons (ganglioneuroma). They usually arise in the central or autonomic nervous system or in the adrenal medulla (sympathicoblastoma).

neurocanal vertebral canal.

neurocardiac pertaining to the nervous system and the heart.

neurocentrum one of the embryonic vertebral elements from which the spinous processes of the vertebrae develop.

neurochemistry that branch of neurology dealing with the chemistry of the nervous system.

neurochorioretinitis inflammation of the optic nerve, choroid and retina.

neurochoroiditis inflammation of the optic nerve and choroid.

neurocirculatory pertaining to the nervous and circulatory systems.

neurocladism the formation of new branches by the process of a neuron; especially the force by which, in regeneration of divided nerves, the newly formed axons become attracted by the peripheral stump, so as to form a bridge between the two ends.

neuroclonic marked by nervous spasm.

neurocommunications the branch of neurology dealing with the transfer and integration of information within the nervous system.

neurocranium the part of the cranium enclosing the brain.

neurocrine 1. denoting an endocrine influence on or by the nerves. 2. pertaining to neurosecretion.

neurocristopathy any disease arising from maldevelopment of the neural crest.

neurocutaneous pertaining to nerves and skin, or the cutaneous nerves.

neurocyte a nerve cell of any kind.

neurocytoma a brain tumor of undifferentiated cells of nervous origin. Called also neuroepithelioma.

neurodegeneration selective degeneration of neurons; may be entire neuron (neuronopathy) or restricted to the axon (axonopathy); may also be central, or peripheral, or central and peripheral.

neurodegenerative diseases diseases characterized by NEURODEGENERATION. Lesions are microscopic only but in chronic disease with massive involvement there may be grossly visible atrophy of affected nervous tissue.

neurodendrite, neurodendron dendrite.

neurodermatitis a general term for a dermatosis presumed to result primarily from self trauma, usually scratching, from behavioral causes.

canine n. see ACRAL lick dermatitis.

feline n. see idiopathic HYPERESTHESIA syndrome.

neurodynamic pertaining to nervous energy.

neurodynia pain in a nerve.

neuroectoderm the portion of the ectoderm of the early embryo which gives rise to the central and peripheral nervous systems, including some glial cells.

neuroectodermal pertaining to or emanating from neurectoderm.

neuroeffector of or relating to the junction between a neuron and the effector organ it innervates.

neuroencephalomyelopathy disease involving the nerves, brain and spinal cord.

neuroendocrine pertaining to neural and endocrine influence, and particularly to the interaction between the nervous and endocrine systems.

n. cell present in skin and oral mucosae of some species; thought to act as pressure receptors.

n. cell tumor rare tumors of neuroendocrine cells in the skin and oral mucosa, where they are pedunculated and located on the lips and gums. In the skin, they occur on the lips, ears or digits, where they may grow rapidly and ulcerate. Called also Merkel cell tumor.

n. receptors receptors located on the membrane of the target cell.

n. system the nervous system plus the endocrine system and the interactions between them.

neuroendocrinology the study of the interactions of the nervous and endocrine systems.

neuroepithelial pertaining to the neuroepithelium.

n. body an APUD respiratory system cell occurring in the bronchiolar mucosa either singly or as small aggregates.

neuroepithelioma see NEUROCYTOMA.

neuroepithelium 1. epithelium made up of cells specialized to serve as sensory cells for reception of external stimuli. Called also sense, or sensory, epithelium. 2. the ectodermal epithelium, from which the central nervous system develops.

neurofibril one of the delicate threads running in every direction through the cytoplasm of a nerve cell, extending into the axon and dendrites.

neurofibroma a tumor of peripheral nerves due to abnormal proliferation of Schwann cells. In cattle neurofibromas appear as subcutaneous swellings. They seem to be transmitted from a cow to her calf. Called also fibroneuroma, schwannoma.

neurofibromatosis seen commonly as swellings on peripheral and intercostal nerves, and on the myocardium in old cows at the abattoir. Also occurs in very young calves and is passed from cow to calf. May be visible as subcutaneous swellings. See also NEUROFIBROMA.

neurofibrosarcoma a malignant tumor originating from Schwann cells of the peripheral nervous system and seen most commonly in cattle.

neurofilament any of the slender, fibrillar elements which, along with the neurotubules, forms a neurofibril.

Neurofilaria cornelliensis see PARELAPHOSTRONGYLUS *tenuis*.

neurofilariasis a disease caused by *Parelaphostrongylus tenuis*; principally a parasite of deer but also infests sheep in which the worms invade the spinal cord and cause a syndrome of lameness, incoordination and paralysis. Called also moose disease (sickness).

neurogenesis the development of nervous tissue.

neurogenic 1. forming nervous tissue, or stimulating nervous energy. 2. originating in the nervous system.

n. atrophy wasting of a muscle due to damage to its peripheral nerve supply.

n. colic colic in the horse, caused by stimulation of nerve supply to intestine by verminous aneurysm. Colic is spasmodic.

n. lung edema pulmonary edema as a consequence of acute brain injury.

n. hyperthermia elevation of body temperature due to a lesion, e.g. spontaneous hemorrhage, in the hypothalamus.

n. muscular atrophy see neurogenic atrophy (above).

n. myopathy the muscle lesions resulting from interruption of its nerve supply.

neurogenous arising from the nervous system, or from some lesion of the nervous system.

neuroglia the supporting cells of central nervous system, consisting of astrocytes, oligodendrocytes and microglia; called also glia.

neuroglial emanating from or pertaining to neuroglia.

neurogliocyte one of the cells composing the neuroglia.

neuroglioma a tumor composed of neuroglial tissue.

neurohemal organs organs in which intimate relationships between axons and terminal blood vessels are established.

neurohistology histology of the nervous system.

neurohormone a hormone stimulating the neural mechanism.

neurohumor a chemical substance formed in a neuron and able to activate or modify the function of a neighboring neuron, muscle or gland.

neurohumoral pertaining to or emanating from neurohumor.

n. substances include epinephrine, norepinephrine, acetylcholine, possibly histamine, serotonin and gamma-aminobutyric acid.

n. transmission the transmission of a nervous impulse from neuron to neuron or from neuron to effector organ by means of a neurohumoral substance.

neurohypophysis the posterior lobe of the pituitary gland. It stores and secretes two hormones, oxytocin and antidiuretic hormone (vasopressin), which are released in response to neural stimulation.

neuroid resembling a nerve.

neuroimmunology that branch of science which deals with the interaction of the nervous and immune systems in health and disease, as in the effect of autonomic nervous activity on the immune response and the role of antibodies in myasthenia gravis.

neurokeratin non-lipid component of the myelin sheath.

neurolathyrism the form of LATHYRISM manifested as irreversible paralysis of the legs.

neurolemma neurilemma.

neurolemmal pertaining to or emanating from the neurolemma.

neurolemmitis neurilemmitis.

neurolemmocytus see Schwann CELL.

neurolemmoma neurilemmoma, schwannoma.

neuroleptanalgesia a state of quiescence, reduced awareness and analgesia produced by the simultaneous administration of a neuroleptic agent, e.g. acepromazine, and a narcotic analgesic, e.g. meperidine. Fixed-dose combinations used extensively in veterinary science are droperidol–fentanyl citrate and etorphine–acepromazine.

neuroleptanalgesic a suitable combination of agents used to produce NEUROLEPTANALGESIA.

neuroleptanesthesia a state of neuroleptanalgesia and unconsciousness produced by the simultaneous administration of a narcotic analgesic agent and a neuroleptic agent, e.g. a mixture of methadone and acepromazine for dogs and a mixture of pethidine and acepromazine in horses, supplemented by the inhalation of nitrous oxide and oxygen.

neuroleptanesthetic an agent producing neuroleptanesthesia, such as the combinations droperidol–fentanyl, acepromazine–meperidine, acepromazine–oxymorphone and diazepam–oxymorphone.

neuroleptic 1. modifying psychotic behavior. 2. any drug that favorably modifies psychotic clinical signs; the main categories of neuroleptics include the phenothiazines, butyrophenones and thioxanthenes. Called also antipsychotic and major tranquilizer.

Drugs of this type stabilize mood and reduce anxiety, tension and hyperactivity. They are also effective in helping to control agitation and aggressiveness.

neurolipidoses a group of lysosomal storage diseases in which lipids accumulate in the central nervous system, e.g. gangliosidosis, galactocerebrosidosis, leukodystrophy, glucocerebrosidosis and sphingomyelinosis.

neurological, neurologic pertaining to or emanating from the nervous system or from neurology.

n. assessment evaluation of the health status of a patient with a nervous system disorder or dysfunction. The purposes of the assessment include establishing a diagnosis to guide the veterinarian in prescribing medical and surgical treatments and in planning and implementing nursing measures to help the patient cope effectively with daily living. Includes evaluation of CRANIAL nerves, GAIT, MENTAL state, muscle TONE (1), POSTURAL reactions, SENSORY perceptivity, spinal nerves and visceral function.

n. deficit any defect or absence of function of a peripheral nerve or a system; e.g. nystagmus is a vestibular deficit.

neurologist a specialist in neurology.

neurology that branch of veterinary science which deals with the nervous system, both normal and in disease.

clinical n. that especially concerned with the diagnosis and treatment of disorders of the nervous system.

neurolymphomatosis lymphoblastic infiltration of a nerve.

n. gallinarum see MAREK'S DISEASE.

neurolysin a cytolysin with a specific destructive action on neurons.

neurolysis 1. release of a nerve sheath by cutting it longitudinally. 2. operative breaking up of perineural adhesions. 3. relief of tension upon a nerve obtained by stretching. 4. exhaustion of nervous energy. 5. destruction or dissolution of nerve tissue.

neuroma a tumor or new growth largely made up of nerve cells and nerve fibers.

acoustic n. a benign tumor within the auditory canal arising from the eighth cranial (acoustic) nerve.

amputation n. traumatic neuroma occurring after amputation of an extremity or part.

traumatic n. an unorganized bulbous or nodular mass of nerve fibers and Schwann cells produced by hyperplasia of nerve fibers and their supporting tissues after accidental or purposeful sectioning of the nerve.

neuromalacia morbid softening of the nerves.

neuromere 1. any of a series of transitory segmental elevations in the wall of the neural tube in the developing embryo; also, such elevations in the wall of the mature rhombencephalon. 2. a part of the spinal cord to which a pair of dorsal roots and a pair of ventral roots are attached.

neuromuscular pertaining to nerve terminations in muscles.

n. blockade deliberate paralysis of the motor endplates; important in veterinary surgery for immobilization. It is effected by the use of competitive (non-depolarizing) agents such as *d*-tubocurarine, and depolarizing agents such as succinylcholine.

n. blocking agents drugs capable of producing neuromuscular blockade (above).

n. junction the point of junction of a nerve fiber with the muscle that it innervates. It includes an area of folded sarcolemma of the muscle fiber, and an axon terminal located in the folds and containing vesicles of the neurotransmitter acetylcholine. Called also MYONEURAL JUNCTION.

n. junction disease examples are TICK paralysis, BOTULISM, MYASTHENIA gravis.

n. paralysis paralysis caused by malfunction at the neuromuscular junction, e.g. after administration of a neuromuscular blocking agent. The paralysis may be flaccid or spastic.

phase-II n. block alteration of the end-plate threshold to depolarization by acetylcholine following prolonged use of a depolarization agent such as succinylcholine.

n. spindle consists of muscle fiber, afferent and efferent nerve endings and connective tissue; maintains muscle tone via stretch reflex mediated through two neurons at spinal cord level.

n. transmission release of acetylcholine from the nerve ending and activation of the receptors in the muscle end-plate.

neuromycotoxins fungal toxins which affect nervous functions, e.g. ergotamine, tunicamycin, lolitrems.

neuromyelitis inflammation of nervous and medullary substance; myelitis attended with neuritis.

neuromyopathy any disease of muscles and nerves combined.

neuromyositis neuritis with myositis.

neuron a nerve cell; any of the conducting cells of the nervous system, consisting of a cell body, containing the nucleus and its surrounding cytoplasm, and the axon and dendrites.

Neurons are highly specialized cells having two characteristic properties: irritability, which means that they are capable of responding to stimulation; and conductivity, which means that they are able to conduct impulses. They are composed of a cell body (the neurosome or perikaryon), containing the nucleus and its surrounding cytoplasm, and one or more processes (nerve fibers) extending from the cell body.

The processes are actually extensions of the cytoplasm surrounding the nucleus of the neuron. A nerve cell may have only one such slender fiber extending from its body, in which case it is classified as unipolar. A neuron having two processes is bipolar, and one with three or more processes is multipolar. Most neurons are multipolar, this type of neuron being widely distributed throughout the central nervous system and autonomic ganglia. The multipolar neurons have a long single process called an *axon* and several branched extensions called *dendrites*. The dendrites receive stimuli from other nerves or from a receptor organ, such as the skin or ear, and transmit them through the neuron to the axon. The axon conducts the impulses to the dendrite of another neuron or to an effector organ that is thereby stimulated into action.

Many processes are covered with a layer of lipid material called MYELIN. Peripheral nerve fibers have a thin outer covering called the neurilemma.

adrenergic n. nerve cells which secrete norepinephrine as a neurotransmitter; they are mostly sympathetic postganglionic nerves plus some within specific brainstem foci.

association n. see internuncial neuron (below).

cholinergic n. nerves which synthesize the neurotransmitter acetylcholine in their terminals; they include α-motor neurons of the spinal cord, cranial nerves innervating skeletal muscle, preganglionic sympathetic and postganglionic parasympathetic neurons.

internuncial n. neurons found in the brain and spinal cord that conduct impulses between neurons such as from afferent to efferent neurons. Called also association neurons or interneurons.

Golgi n's see GOLGI NEURONS.

lower motor n's see lower MOTOR NEURON.

motor n. see MOTOR NEURON.

neurosecretory n. neurons of the hypothalamus that receive nervous impulses from higher centers and translate them into the regulation of hormone secretion.

parvicellular n. in the hypothalamus; regulate the secretion of adenohypophyseal hormones via releasing and inhibiting factors.

postganglionic n's neurons whose cell bodies lie in the autonomic ganglia and which relay impulses beyond the ganglia to the effector organ.

preganglionic n's neurons whose cell bodies lie in the central nervous system and whose efferent fibers terminate in the autonomic ganglia.

n. transmission the transmission of impulses along axons by means of electrical impulses and across synapses by neurotransmitters, especially norepinephrine and acetylcholine.

upper motor n's see upper MOTOR NEURON.

neuronal pertaining to or emanating from a neuron.

n. abiotrophy see hereditary neuronal ABIOTROPHY of Swedish Lapland dogs.

n. ceroid-lipofuscinosis see ceroid LIPOFUSCINOSIS.

n. glycoproteinosis see GLYCOPROTEINOSIS.

n. heterotopia a collection of nerve cells at a site where they are normally absent.

n. inclusion-body disease an idiopathic disease of female Japanese Brown cattle; characterized by an acute onset of excitability, fever, sweating, sudden death plus cytoplasmic inclusion bodies in axons in the pons, medulla, midbrain.

n. lipodystrophy see GANGLIOSIDOSIS.

n. processes dendrites and axons.

n. vacuolar degeneration a probably inherited scrapie-like neuronopathy in young Australian Angora goats; ataxia commences at 3 months of age and progesses to severe paresis; characterized by vacuolation of large brain and spiral cord neurons.

neuronopathy any disease affecting nerve cells.

n. and pseudolipidosis see MANNOSIDOSIS.

neuronophage a phagocyte that destroys nerve cells.

neuronophagia phagocytic destruction of nerve cells.

neuronophagic pertaining to or emanating from neuronophagia.

n. nodule a focus of microglia formed around degenerating neurons.

neuro-ophthalmology that branch of ophthalmology dealing with portions of the nervous system related to the eye.

neuropapillitis optic NEURITIS affecting the part of the optic nerve within the eyeball.

neuroparalysis paralysis due to disease of a nerve or nerves.

neuropathic pertaining to disease of the nervous system.

neuropathogenicity the quality of producing or the ability to produce pathological changes in nerve tissue.

neuropathology pathology of the nervous system.

neuropathy a general term denoting functional disturbances and pathological changes in the peripheral nervous system. The etiology may be known (e.g. poidoning by arsenicals, ischemic or traumatic neuropathy) or unknown. Encephalopathy and myelopathy are corresponding terms relating to involvement of the brain and spinal cord, respectively. The term is also used to designate noninflammatory lesions in the peripheral nervous system, in contrast to inflammatory lesions (neuritis).

central peripheral n. see Boxer progressive AXONOPATHY.

diabetic n. a chronic symmetrical sensory polyneuropathy associated with diabetes mellitus in humans, which occurs uncommonly in dogs and cats.

entrapment n. a neuropathy due to mechanical pressure on a peripheral nerve.

giant axonal n. a familial disease of German shepherd dogs, characterized by ataxia, hypotonia, reduced pain sensation, and loss of reflexes and proprioception in the hindlegs, which develops from a young age. Vomiting, associated with esophageal dilatation, also occurs.

hereditary n. recorded in Tibetan mastiff as an inherited defect in myelin production. Weakness, loss of reflexes and quadriplegia develop quickly and at an early age.

hereditary sensory n. an inherited abnormality in which affected dogs have impaired perception of pain in the feet and lower limbs from a young age; causes extensive self-mutilation of toes and footpads. It occurs in German shorthaired pointers, English pointers and English springer spaniels. Called also acral mutilation syndrome.

infiltrative splanchnic n. see MACAW wasting disease.

progressive n. disease of young Cairn terriers with many similarities to globoid cell LEUKODYSTROPHY. Affected dogs show quadriparesis, ataxia and head tremors.

retrobulbar n. see DRYOPTERIS.

trigeminal n. see MANDIBULAR neurapraxia.

neuropeptide any of the molecules composed of short chains of amino acids (endorphins, enkephalins, vasopressin, etc.) found in brain tissue.

neuropharmacology the scientific study of the effects of drugs on the nervous system.

neurophthisis wasting of nerve tissue.

neurophysin any of a group of soluble proteins secreted in the hypothalamus that serve as binding proteins for vasopressin and oxytocin, playing a role in their transport in the neurohypophyseal tract and their storage in the posterior pituitary.

neurophysiology physiology of the nervous system.

neuropil, neuropile a dense feltwork of interwoven cytoplasmic processes of nerve cells (dendrites and axons) and of neuroglial cells in the central nervous system and some parts of the peripheral nervous system.

neuroplasm the protoplasm of a nerve cell.

neuroplasty plastic repair of a nerve.

neuropodium a bulbous termination of an axon in one type of synapse.

neuropore an opening in the cranial or caudal end of the neural tube of the developing embryo that closes eventually.

neuroradiology radiology of the nervous system.

neuroretinitis inflammation of the optic nerve and retina.

neuroretinopathy pathological involvement of the optic disk and retina.

neurorrhaphy suture of a divided nerve.

neurosarcoma a sarcoma with neuromatous elements.

neuroscience the embryology, anatomy, physiology, biochemistry and pharmacology of the nervous system.

neurosclerosis hardening of nerve tissue.

neurosecretion 1. the secretory activities of nerve cells. 2. a substance secreted by nerve cells.

neurosecretory pertaining to or emanating from the secretory activities of nerve cells.

n. bodies the form in which neurosecretions are passed along axons to release them into the blood.

n. neurons neurons capable of secreting neurosecretions.

n. substances substances secreted by neurosecretory neurons, e.g. oxytocin, antidiuretic hormone, releasing factors, inhibiting factors.

neurosis pl. *neuroses;* an emotional disorder that can interfere with an animal's ability to lead a normal life; sometimes called psychoneurosis. Examples are WEAVING, CRIB-biting and psychogenic DERMATOSIS.

neurosome 1. cell body of a neuron. 2. small particle in a neuron cell body.
neurospasm nervous twitching of a muscle.
neurosplanchnic pertaining to the cerebrospinal and sympathetic nervous systems.
neurospongioma neuroglioma.
neurospongium 1. the fibrillar component of neurons. 2. a meshwork of nerve fibrils, especially the inner reticular layer of the retina.
Neurospora a genus of fungi, comprising the bread molds, capable of converting tryptophan to niacin; used in genetic and enzyme research.
neurosurgeon a physician who specializes in neurosurgery.
neurosurgery surgery of the nervous system.
neurosuture neurorrhaphy.
neurotendinous pertaining to both nerve and tendon.
neurotensin a tridecapeptide which induces vasodilatation and hypotension; present in human brain tissue and postulated to be a neurotransmitter.
neurothekeoma benign tumors arising from Schwann cells; occur rarely in dogs.
neurotherapy the treatment of nervous disorders.
neurotization 1. regeneration of a nerve after its division. 2. the implantation of a nerve into a paralyzed muscle.
neurotmesis partial or complete severance of a nerve, with disruption of the axon and its myelin sheath and of the connective tissue elements.
neurotome 1. a needle-like knife for dissecting nerves. 2. neuromere.
neurotomy dissection or cutting of nerves.
neurotony the surgical stretching of a nerve; neurectasia; neurectasis.
neurotoxic pertaining to or emanating from a neurotoxin.
n. state a case of poisoning by a neurotoxin.
neurotoxicity the quality of exerting a destructive or poisonous effect upon nerve tissue.
neurotoxin a substance that is poisonous or destructive to nerve tissue.
neurotransmission see NERVE impulses.
neurotransmitter a substance (e.g. norepinephrine, acetylcholine, dopamine) that is released from the axon terminal of a presynaptic neuron on excitation, and which travels across the synaptic cleft to either excite or inhibit the target cell.
adrenergic n. see NOREPINEPHRINE.
n. receptor each neurotransmitter has its own receptor molecule; these show a high degree of structural homology.
neurotrauma mechanical injury to a nerve.
neurotrophy nutrition and maintenance of tissues as regulated by nervous influence.
neurotropic pertaining to or emanating from neurotrophy, e.g. neurotropic osteopathy.
neurotropism 1. the quality of having a special affinity for nervous tissue. 2. the alleged tendency of regenerating nerve fibers to grow toward specific portions of the periphery.
neurotubule any of the long, straight, parallel tubules within neurons, which together with neurofilaments form neurofibrils.
neurovaccine a vaccine virus, classically rabies, prepared by growing the virus in the brain and spinal cord of a rabbit.
neurovascular pertaining to both nervous and vascular elements, or to nerves controlling the caliber of blood vessels.
neurovisceral see NEUROSPLANCHNIC.
neurula the early embryonic stage following the gastrula, marked by the first appearance of the nervous system.
neurulation formation in the early embryo of the neural plate, followed by its development into the neural tube.
neuter 1. to desex an animal. This has assumed an important role in the management and control of companion animal populations. CASTRATION and OVARIOHYSTERECTOMY are the usual procedures. 2. a desexed animal. 3. a castrated male cat.
neutral neither basic nor acid.
n. endopeptidase synthesized by tracheobronchial epithelium, this is an important enzymatic regulator of airway neuropeptides which stimulate increased vascular permeability and smooth muscle contraction.
n. stress evokes responses which do not affect the comfort, well-being or reproduction of the patient.
neutralization the state of having been converted to neutrality from acid or base. Used also in microbiology to indicate neutralization of a toxin or of infectivity.
n. tests tests based on the ability of an antibody to neutralize the biological activity of an antigen. These may utilize antitoxins and toxins or immune serum and viruses or bacteria. The tests are often quantitative whereby antibody (serum) is serially diluted; the reciprocal of the highest dilution of serum neutralizing a standard amount of toxin or virus or bacteria is the neutralizing antibody titer of that serum.
neutralize to render neutral.
neutrino a subatomic particle with an extremely small mass (theoretically zero rest mass) and no electric charge.
neutroclusion class I malocclusion involving abnormalities of individual teeth.
neutrocyte neutrophil (2).
neutron an electrically neutral or uncharged particle of matter existing along with protons in the atoms of all elements except the mass 1 isotope of hydrogen.
neutropenia a diminished number of neutrophils in the blood.
cyclic n. periodic neutropenia. See also canine CYCLIC hematopoiesis.
malignant n. agranulocytosis.
periodic n. see canine CYCLIC hematopoiesis.
neutrophil 1. one of the three granular leukocytes having a nucleus with three to five lobes connected by threads of chromatin, and cytoplasm containing lysosomes that stain characteristically and enable neutrophils to be distinguished from basophils and eosinophils; called also a granulocyte or polymorphonuclear leukocyte. See also HETEROPHIL (1). 2. any cell, structure or histological element readily stainable with neutral dyes.
band n. see stab neutrophil (below).
n. chemotactic factor see CHEMOTACTIC FACTOR.
hypersegmented n. increased number of nuclear lobes; seen in hyperadrenocorticism or during treatment with corticosteroids, and in blood that has been in transit for long periods.
hyposegmented n. a lack of nuclear lobes; may occur in chronic infections and is a feature of PELGER–HUET ANOMALY.
n.:lymphocyte ratio correlates directly with the magnitude of the total leukocyte count in response to disease in domestic animals; it varies from 0.5 in cattle to 3.5 in dogs.
stab n. a neutrophilic leukocyte whose nucleus is not divided into segments.

toxic n. one with blue-black or large reddish cytoplasmic granules and diffuse cytoplasmic basophilia and vacuolation; caused by disruption of maturation.

neutrophil-releasing activity see LEUKOCYTOSIS-inducing factor.

neutrophilia an increase in the number of neutrophils in the blood.

inflammatory n. see true neutrophilia (below).

physiological n. see pseudo-neutrophilia (below).

pseudo-n. one caused by a shift of neutrophils from the marginal pool to the circulating pool; there is no real increase in the total number of neutrophils. It is seen with stress and exercise.

stress n. see pseudo-neutrophilia (above).

true n. one in which there is an increase in the total blood granulocyte pool. It is seen in chronic infection.

neutrophilic 1. pertaining to neutrophils. 2. stainable by neutral dyes.

nevi plural form of NEVUS.

nevocarcinoma see malignant MELANOMA.

nevoid resembling a nevus.

nevus pl. *nevi* [L.] a circumscribed stable malformation of the skin and occasionally of the oral mucosa, which is not due to external causes; the excess (or deficiency) of tissue may involve epidermal, connective tissue, adnexal, nervous, or vascular elements; called also mole.

blue n. a dark blue nodular lesion composed of closely grouped melanocytes and melanophages situated in the mid-dermis.

connective tissue n. any nevus occurring in the dermal connective tissue and characterized by nodules, papules or plaques, or by combinations of such lesions. Histologically, there is inconstant focal or diffuse thickening and abnormal staining of collagen.

epidermal n. congenital skin tumors that do not contain melanocytes, which vary widely in appearance, size and distribution, and which are commonly hyperkeratotic.

hair follicle n. occur on the proximal extremities and have thick, brushlike hairs protruding.

intradermal n. a nevocytic nevus in which the nevus cells occur in nests in the upper part of the dermis, with no evidence of the proliferative process by which they originated.

melanocytic n. any nevus, usually pigmented, composed of melanocytes. See also MELANOMA.

pigmented n., n. pigmentosus one containing melanin; the term is usually restricted to nevocytic nevi (moles), but may be applied to other pigmented nevi.

sebaceous n. an epidermal nevus containing an overgrowth of sebaceous glands, frequently growing larger during puberty or early adult life, and rarely giving rise to a variety of new growths, including basal cell carcinoma.

n. vascularis, n. vasculosus, vascular n. a reddish swelling or patch on the skin due to hypertrophy of the skin capillaries. Seen on the scrotum of old dogs, sometimes bleeding.

new duck disease see PASTEURELLA *anatipestifer*.

New Forest named after the New Forest in the UK.

N. F. disease see INFECTIOUS bovine keratoconjunctivitis.

N. F. fly see HIPPOBOSCA *equina*.

N. F. pony an English pony, any solid color, 12.2 to 14.2 hands high; an all-round riding pony.

New Hampshire red a deep red dual-purpose breed of chicken, probably derived from Rhode Island red. Used extensively for crossbreeding.

New Holland rattlepod CROTALARIA *novae-hollandiae*.

new methylene blue see new methylene blue STAIN.

new process said of oil cake or meal. See SOLVENT extraction of oil seeds.

New York dressed poultry a special poultry meat inspection technique in which the viscera are left in the carcass.

New Zealand named after the country, New Zealand.

N. Z. blue lupin LUPINUS *angustifolius*.

N. Z. cattle tick see HAEMAPHYSALIS *longicornis*.

N. Z. red a bright, red-buff fur rabbit, 7 to 9 lb, with a harsh 1 inch long coat.

N. Z. spinach TETRAGONIA *expansa*.

N. Z. white a white-coated, pink-eyed, 10 lb meat rabbit, also commonly used as a laboratory rabbit with medium length ears and a double chin.

Newberry knife see Newberry castrating KNIFE.

newborn animals recently born. See also NEONATAL, NEONATE.

Newbury virus a calicivirus associated causatively with diarrhea in calves.

Newcastle disease an infectious, highly contagious disease of chickens, turkeys and many wild birds, occasionally infecting humans, caused by a paramyxovirus. The disease causes very heavy losses in birds of all ages and frequently occurs as massive outbreaks. There are a number of clinical forms of the disease, including a nervous form characterized by tremor, opisthotonos and paralysis, and a mortality rate of 90%, an acute respiratory form with high mortality, up to 90% in chickens, an acute respiratory form without significant death losses, and a clinically inapparent form. The disease is also classified, on epidemiological grounds, into velogenic (peracute), mesogenic (acute) and lentogenic (subacute) forms, which are caused by viruses with a corresponding variation in virulence. Called also avian pneumoencephalitis.

Newfoundland a very large (100–150 lb), black or bronze, longhaired dog with massive head, small pendulous ears and bushy tail. A black and white version is known as Landseer. The breed is predisposed to subaortic stenosis, cardiomyopathy and hypothyroidism.

Newman's stain a defatting stain, useful for the examination of direct smears of milk.

Newmarket named after the famous racing center in the United Kingdom.

N. cough see EQUINE influenza.

N. itch see RINGWORM.

newspaper columns in computer printouts a format in which the text flows down the first column to the bottom of the page, then resumes at the top of the page in the next column.

newsprint low grade paper used for newspapers. Old newspapers are fed to cattle as an alternative roughage and may occasionally be ingested by dogs. Significant amounts of lead are accumulated in tissues; no cases of poisoning have been recorded in cattle, though it has been recorded in dogs.

newt newts and salamanders belong to the subclass Urodela (syn. Caudata) and comprise eight families and a very large number of species. The newts spend some of their lives on land, in a form called efts, and then metamorphose to aquatic newts. They are small, lizard-like creatures, which are becoming popular as house pets or decorations.

n. poisoning dogs and cats mouthing newts and salamanders may develop salivation, muscular weakness and motor incoordination leading to paralysis, vomiting and diarrhea, caused by a salivary toxin.

newton the SI unit of force; the force that, when acting continuously upon a mass of 1 kilogram, will impart to it an acceleration of 1 meter per second squared. Symbol N.

nexin the connecting link between microtubules in cilia and flagella.

nexus 1. a bond, as between members of a series or group. 2. a gap junction.

NF National Formulary.

NFE nitrogen free extract.

ng nanogram.

ngaio tree MYOPORUM *laetum*.

ngaione a hepatotoxic sesquiterpene ketone present in the poisonous tree MYOPORUM *laetum* and in a fungus growing on sweet potatoes. See also CERATOSTOMELLA FIMBRIATA.

NGF nerve growth factor.

NGL no gross lesions.

NH_3 ammonia.

Ni chemical symbol, *nickel*.

niacin a water-soluble vitamin of the B complex found in various animal and plant tissues. Essential for normal carbohydrate metabolism. Most natural animal feeds have high enough content to avoid need for supplementation, except for pigs fed a heavy corn diet. Called also nicotinic acid, vitamin PP. See also NICOTINAMIDE.

n. nutritional deficiency causes hemorrhagic diarrhea, dermatitis, anemia and a severe stomatitis with ulceration of the mouth and tongue ('black tongue'). In cats, the signs are diarrhea, emaciation and death. Called also pellagra.

n. production a test for differentiating *Mycobacteria tuberculosis* (positive) and *M. avium* (negative).

niacinamide see NICOTINAMIDE.

nibbling reaction seen in sheep with scrapie; the patient makes rapid, exaggerated, nibbling movements with the upper lip for the duration of a light stroking of the wool over the hindquarters.

Nicandra physalodes toxic plant in the family Solanaceae; contains an unidentified toxin which causes sudden death, ruminal tympany; called also apple of Peru.

nicarbazin an efficient coccidiostat but causes mottling of the egg yolk and lowered egg production in laying hens. Excessive dosing causes incoordination, inanition and loss of weight.

niche a small recess, depression or indentation, especially a recess in the wall of a hollow organ that tends to retain contrast media, as revealed by radiography.

ecological n. the geographical location in the physical environment which the particular organism occupies best, in which it thrives best. The boundaries are determined by the suitability of the climate and the feed provided and competition with predators and collaboration with synergists.

n. pericarditis an abattoir finding in normal cattle; small red velvety patches on the outside of the great vessels.

nick 1. said of a mating that is likely to produce superior offspring. 2. slang for body condition; an animal in good body condition is said to be in good nick. 3. a break in a strand of nucleic acid.

nickel a chemical element, atomic number 28, atomic weight 58.71, symbol Ni. See Table 6.

nicking 1. localized constriction of the retinal blood vessels. 2. making a small cut. A specific surgical procedure done on the underside of a horse's tail, which is then set so it is carried higher. Called also ventral caudal myotomy. Considered an unnecessary mutilation in most circles and may be illegal. 3. in animal breeding the phenomenon observed when the offspring are significantly better than either of the parents.

niclofolan a nitrosubstituted analog of hexachlorophane used as a fasciolicide and effective against mature liver flukes in sheep.

niclosamide a nitrosalicylanilide anthelmintic effective against tapeworms in all species except *Echinococcus granulosus* and *Dipylidium caninum* in dogs. Has some activity against paramphistomes in ruminants.

Nicotiana a genus of plants in the family Solanaceae; contain nicotine which causes dyspnea, incoordination, tremor and convulsions; includes *N. amplexicaulis*, *N. attenuata*, *N. debneyi*, *N. exigua*, *N. glauca* (tree tobacco), *N. gossei*, *N. megalosiphon*, *N. suaveolens*, *N. suaveolens* var. *parviflora* (*N. debneyi*), *N. trigonophylla*, *N. velutina*. Most of the species are also called wild or native tobacco.

N. tabacum ingestion of the leaves or stalks of this plant by sows in early pregnancy causes congenital arthrogryposis of their piglets. Cows may also be affected. The teratogen is the alkaloid anabasine. Called also tobacco—the commercial tobacco plant.

nicotinamide the amide of the B group vitamin, niacin, occurring naturally in the body and interconvertible with niacin; used in the prophylaxis and treatment of pellagra in humans. Called also niacinamide.

n. adenine dinucleotide (NAD) a coenzyme that is involved in many biochemical oxidation–reduction reactions. The symbols for the oxidized and reduced forms are NAD+ and NADH.

n. adenine dinucleotide phosphate (NADP) a coenzyme similar to nicotinamide adenine dinucleotide but involved in fewer reactions. The symbols for the oxidized and reduced forms are NADP+ and NADPH.

nicotine a very poisonous piperidine alkaloid that in its pure state is a colorless, pungent, oily liquid, having an acrid burning taste. It is a constituent of tobacco and is produced synthetically.

n. sulfate has been used as an anthelmintic but is very poisonous. Signs are dyspnea, tremor and convulsions. Death is due to respiratory paralysis. Has also been used as an insecticide and acaricide. It was once used against sheep scab and is still used against poultry lice.

nicotinic pertaining to the transmission of nerve impulses mediated by nicotinic receptors.

n. acid see NIACIN.

n. receptors cholinergic receptors of autonomic ganglion cells and motor end-plates of skeletal muscle that are stimulated by low doses of nicotine and blockaded by high doses, or by tubocurarine.

n. synapses synapses in which nicotinic transmitters effect the transmission of impulses.

nicotinism nicotine poisoning, marked by stimulation and subsequent depression of the central and autonomic nervous systems, with death due to respiratory paralysis.

nicoumalone see ACENOCOUMAROL.

nictitans pertaining to the nictitating membrane.

nictitating membrane see also MEMBRANA nictitans, THIRD EYELID.

n. m. flap using the membrana nictitans (third eyelid) as a flap in the treatment of corneal ulcer by sewing the eyelid across the cornea.

n. m. prolapse occurs when the globe of the eye is depressed in the orbit, as in dehydration and emaciation. It is also a diagnostic sign of tetanus in many species; the membrane flicks across the eye whenever the animal is startled.

nictitation the act of winking.

nidation implantation of the fertilized ovum in the endometrium of the uterus in pregnancy.

nidicolous said of a bird that does not leave the nest for a long time after it is hatched.

nidifugous said of birds that leave their nests soon after they are hatched.

nidogen an adhesive glycoprotein involved in the cell/basal lamina/matrix interface.

Nidorella foetida toxic plant, a member of the Asteraceae family; contains an unidentified toxin which causes hepatic insufficiency and photosensitization.

nidus pl. *nidi* [L.] 1. a nest; point of origin or focus of a morbid process, e.g. a urolith, a local infection. 2. nucleus (2).

NIEA negative inotropic effect of activation.

Niemann–Pick disease see SPHINGOMYELINOSIS.

Nierembergia veitchii toxic plant in the family Solanaceae; contains a calcinogenic glycoside which causes enzootic calcinosis.

nifedipine a calcium channel blocker used principally as a vasodilator.

nifuraldezone anitrofuran antibiotic used to treat enteritis in calves.

nifuratel an oral nitrofuran antibiotic with activity against *Candida* spp.

nifuroxime a topical nitrofuran with antifungal properties.

nifurtimox a nitrofuran derivative used as an antitrypanosomal agent.

night blindness inability or a reduced ability to see in dim light. In night blindness, the eyes not only see more poorly in dim light, but are slower to adjust from brightness to dimness. It is a sign of hypovitaminosis A and early progressive retinal atrophy. Testing for night blindness entails construction of an obstacle race and putting an animal through it at dusk. Difficult to interpret results.

congenital n. b. occurs in Appaloosa horses. There is a retinal defect which is detectable by electroretinography.

night-flowering cestrum CESTRUM *nocturnum*.

night lighting the management practice of exposing laying hens and brood mares to bright lights at night time to stimulate egg production in the hens and to stimulate the early appearance of estrus at the beginning of the mating season in the mares.

night monkey soft, curly-haired, nocturnal monkey; red to gray-brown with a long, nonprehensile tail. Good house pets. Called also douroucouli, owl monkey, *Aotus* spp.

night-scented cestrum CESTRUM *nocturnum*.

night stool cecotroph.

nightshade there are many plants with variants of this name. See SOLANUM, ATROPA BELLADONNA.

nigra [L.] *black;* see SUBSTANTIA nigra.

nigricans blackening.

nigroid bodies corpora nigra. See IRIDIAL granule.

nigropallidal encephalomalacia a condition caused by ingestion of *Centaurea solstitialis* or *C. repens*. In horses it causes somnolence, aimless wandering and difficulty in prehending and then eating feed.

nigrostriatal projecting from the substantia nigra to the corpus striatum; said of a bundle of nerve fibers.

nikethamide a central nervous system and respiratory stimulant.

Nikolsky's sign in pemphigus vulgaris and some other bullous diseases, the outer epidermis separates easily from the basal layer on exertion of firm sliding manual pressure.

nil fees provision of a service by a veterinarian for which no fee is charged. The procedure does not diminish in any way the responsibility of the veterinarian for the patient's welfare.

Nile tilapia TILAPIA *niloticus* (*Oreochromis niloticus*).

nilgai, nylghaie a large Asian antelope, 5 ft high, 6 ft long and weighing 400 to 500 lb. Gray or tan in color. Called also *Boselaphus tragocamelus*.

Nili-Ravi one of the Murrah type of breeds of Indian buffalo; usually black, sometimes brown; wall eyes and white marks on head, legs and tail are common.

nimorazole a 5-nitroimidazole derivative with antimicrobial activity similar to metronidazole. Used in the treatment of intestinal protozoal infections.

nine-mile fever see Q FEVER.

niobium a chemical element, atomic number 1, atomic weight 92.906, symbol Nb. See Table 6.

nipper a tool for clipping, e.g. for claws and beaks of small cagebirds.

hoof n. a pincer-like tool with the blades curved in to face each other at the ends which are composed of two chisel edges opposing one another. Used in horses and cattle to nip off the bottom edge of the wall of the hoof and the adjoining sole.

pig tooth n. the equivalent of an electrician's sidecutters. A single-handed, scissor type tool, the blades consisting of two chisel edges facing one another laterally. Used to nip off the needle teeth of baby pigs.

nipple fleshy projection on each mammary gland of the bitch, queen and other species; exit for milk produced by the gland. In ruminants called the TEAT.

n. drinkers nipple-shaped metal devices mounted on tanks of water or on mains pipes that have a ball in the point and from which animals can get a sufficient daily intake of water by licking or, in the case of birds, pecking the tip of the device.

Nippon Inu an ancient purebred Japanese dog. There are three types, each recognized as a separate breed. The AKITA is the largest, the SHIBA INU the smallest, and the Kari, a medium-sized dog.

Nippostrongylus braziliensis a nematode found in the intestine of rats.

NIRD abbreviation for National Institute for Research in Dairying, now called Animal Grassland Research Institute, Reading, UK.

NIRD mastitis control program see NIRD MASTITIS control program.

nisin an antibiotic substance isolated from cultures of lactic acid producing streptococci and reputed to have antibacterial activity against gram-positive bacteria.

Nissl named for Franz Nissl (1860–1919), German neurologist.

N. bodies large granular bodies that stain with basic dyes, forming the reticular substance of the cytoplasm of neurons, composed of rough endoplasmic reticulum and free polyribosomes.

N. granules location of synthesis of most nervous system proteins.

N. substance see CHROMAPHILIC SUBSTANCE.

nit louse egg.

nitarsone an arsenical compound used as a feed additive for the prevention and treatment of histomoniasis in turkeys. Called also 4-nitrophenylarsonic acid. See also organic ARSENICAL.

nithiazide drug used in the treatment of histomoniasis and hexamitiasis in turkeys.

nitralin a dinitroaniline compound used as a herbicide.

The toxicity is low and poisoning would occur only with serious error in usage; signs of poisoning are nervousness, diarrhea, anorexia and loss of weight.

nitrate any salt of nitric acid. High intakes by animals may occur when they eat large quantities of lush herbage that has been heavily fertilized with a nitrogen fertilizer such as potassium or ammonium nitrate. It can also occur after a long drought during which nitrification bacteria accumulate large amounts of nitrate in the soil and the first growth after the drought breaks may also be toxic.

Pigs fed on food residues may ingest potassium nitrate used in meat curing when their swill contains butcher's residues.

n. explosives nitroglycerine and others used to blast out water holes and left in the hole may cause subsequent nitrate poisoning.

n. poisoning unusual unless animals get access to unguarded fertilizer or butcher shop residue containing potassium nitrate. Causes gastroenteritis with diarrhea and vomiting. Long-term, low level intake thought to cause abortion in cattle. Chief importance is as a constituent of ruminant diet and its conversion in the rumen to nitrite causing NITRITE poisoning.

n. reduction test a biochemical reaction used in the identification of bacteria, particularly mycobacteria. It is based on the reduction of nitrate to nitrite and/or the release of nitrogen gas.

nitrazine yellow a dye used in a test for degree of composition of meat. If the dye stays yellow the meat is safe, gray-green is a doubtful result, and a purple color indicates that the meat is not suitable for human consumption.

nitremia excess of nitrogen in the blood, e.g. in uremia.

nitric pertaining to or containing nitrogen in one of its higher valences.

n. acid. a highly caustic, fuming acid that has a characteristic choking odor. It was used at one time in the immediate treatment of rabid animal bites to prevent rabies becoming established, and as a cauterizing agent in the eradication of various kinds of warts. It is also used in the form of its potassium and sodium salts. It can be fatal if swallowed, and large amounts of nitric acid applied to the skin can cause necrosis. The antidote for nitric acid poisoning is an alkali or sodium bicarbonate applied liberally.

n. oxide is produced during the ensiling process and animals in confined spaces and exposed to silo gas may develop severe respiratory disease due to irritation of the alveolar epithelium. Called also silo-filler's disease. See also ATYPICAL INTERSTITIAL PNEUMONIA.

nitride a binary compound of nitrogen with a metal.

nitrification the bacterial oxidation of ammonia and organic nitrogen to nitrites and nitrates in the soil.

nitrifying oxidizing ammonia into nitrites and then into nitrates; said of certain bacteria.

nitrile an organic compound containing trivalent nitrogen attached to one carbon atom, $-C{\equiv}N$.

nitrite any salt of nitrous acid; organic nitrites are used in the treatment of angina pectoris in humans.

n. poisoning causes methemoglobinemia and anemic anoxia. Signs are dyspnea and coffee color of mucosae and blood. Pregnant cows may abort several weeks later. Nitrite may come preformed in feed contaminated by a chemical agent, or in nitrate-rich food in which the nitrate is converted to nitrite during processing, e.g. low temperature cooking, heating of hay in a stack or moldering. Most cases are in ruminants which convert nitrate to nitrite in the rumen, the source being nitrate-rich plants. See also NITRATE.

n.-treated fish meal used as a preservative and color-preservation agent the nitrite is converted biologically to a toxic nitrosamine, dimethylnitrosamine.

nitrituria the presence of nitrites in the urine.

nitro abbreviation of nitrogen. Usually taken to indicate the presence of an $-NO_2$ radical.

n.-chalk a fertilizer in the form of lime or chalk mixed with ammonium nitrate.

n. compounds toxins in *Astragalus* spp. plants which are converted to nitrite in the rumen, and cause nitrite poisoning, and into other toxins causing weakness and paralysis. See also CARDUUS.

nitroblue tetrazolium a yellow dye converted to a blue color on reduction.

n. t. test used to measure the phagocytic activity of polymorphonuclear leukocytes by the amount of color change in the dye.

nitrocellulose pyroxylin, a base which is dissolved in alcohol or ether to form collodion.

nitrofuran a group of antibacterials, including nitrofurantoin, nitrofurazone, etc., that are widely used in food animals because of their effectiveness against gram-negative bacteria. They are used orally for mass medication in both feed and water. See also FURAZOLIDONE, NITROFURANTOIN, NITROFURAZONE, NIFUROXIME, NIFURATEL.

nitrofurantoin a nitrofuran derivative antibacterial agent used in the treatment of urinary tract infections.

nitrofurazone a nitrofuran derivative antibiotic used mostly for topical application, and orally for treatment of coccidiosis in poultry and in swine dysentery. Heavy or continuous dosing may cause paralysis or convulsions in calves. Called also Furacin.

nitrogen a chemical element, atomic number 7, atomic weight 14.007, symbol N. See Table 6. It is a gas constituting about four-fifths of common air; chemically it is almost inert. It is not poisonous but is fatal if breathed alone because of oxygen deprivation. Nitrogen occurs in proteins and amino acids and is thus present in all living cells.

n. balance the state of the body in regard to the rate of protein intake and protein utilization. When protein is metabolized, about 90% of the protein nitrogen is excreted in the urine in the form of urea, uric acid, creatinine and other nitrogen end products. The remaining 10% of the nitrogen is eliminated in the feces.

A *negative* nitrogen balance occurs when more protein is utilized by the body than is taken in. A *positive* nitrogen balance implies a net gain of protein in the body. Negative nitrogen balance can be caused by such factors as malnutrition, debilitating diseases, blood loss and glucocorticoids. A positive balance can be caused by exercise, growth hormone and testosterone.

blood urea n. (BUN) see UREA nitrogen.

n. dioxide see NITRIC oxide.

n. fixation conversion of atmospheric nitrogen into organic nitrogenous compounds by bacteria which may be symbiotic, e.g. *Rhizopus* spp., which grow on the roots of legumes and put those plants in an advantageous position with respect to nonlegumes.

n.-free extract the water-soluble, nitrogen-free contents of a feed. Consists of sugars, starches, pentoses and organic acids.

n. mustards a group of toxic, blistering alkylating agents homologous to dichlorodiethyl sulfide (mustard gas), some of which have been used as antineoplastics. The group includes mustine hydrochloride, cyclophosphamide, thiotepa, chlorambucil and melphalan.

nonprotein n. (NPN) 1. the nitrogenous constituents of the blood exclusive of the protein bodies, consisting of the nitrogen of urea, uric acid, creatine, creatinine, amino acids, polypeptides, and an undetermined part known as rest nitrogen.

Measurement of nonprotein nitrogen is used as a test of renal function, but has been largely replaced by measurement of specific substances, e.g. urea and creatinine. 2. also used in relation to feeds and refers to those nitrogen-containing constituents which are not proteins, e.g. nucleic acids, amino sugars, urea, etc.

n. trichloride see AGENE PROCESS.

n. washout test measures the rate at which the nitrogen concentration in the expired air is reduced when the horse is made to breathe pure oxygen. The rate is less in incompetent lungs, e.g. those affected by emphysema.

nitrogenous containing nitrogen.

nitroglycerin a chemical well known as an explosive but also a venodilator and used medically, principally in the treatment of angina pectoris in humans; called also glyceryl trinitrate.

3-nitro-4-hydroxyphenylarsonic acid a feed additive used as a growth promotant; is capable of causing organic arsenical poisoning.

nitroimidazoles antiprotozoal agents, the most common being metronidazole.

nitromersol an organic mercurial used as a disinfectant on the skin and for surgical instruments.

nitromide see 3,5-DINITROBENZAMIDE.

nitrophenide a coccidiostat with low usefulness because of its toxicity, manifested by paralysis, at relatively low dose rates.

nitrophenol a parasiticide which is applied to buildings and fixtures. Can cause poisoning manifested as high fever, dyspnea, stumbling gait, terminal convulsions, a short course of a few hours and a high mortality rate. A substituted nitrophenol (DISOPHENOL) is used as an anthelmintic against blood-sucking nematodes such as hookworms and *Haemonchus* spp.

4-nitrophenylarsonic acid see NITARSONE

nitropropanol one of the nitro compunds in *Astragalus* spp. from which neurotoxins, e.g. miserotoxin, are developed in the plant.

3-nitro-1-propanol the β-glycoside of this substance is miserotoxin, the toxic agent of ASTRAGALUS *miser*, the timber milk vetch.

3-nitropropionic acid one of the nitro compounds in *Astragalus* spp. which are precursors to neurotoxins in the plant.

nitroprusside sodium nitroferricyanide, a vasodilator used in the treatment of heart failure in dogs, and used as a reagent in Rothera's test for ketone bodies.

cyanide n. reaction detects sulfhydryl group compounds and is used to test urine in screening tests for the metabolic diseases, cystinuria and homocystinuria.

nitrosamines highly hepatotoxic compounds formed in the rumen by the combination of amines and nitrite. They do not appear to occur naturally in large quantities. Nitrosamine poisoning has also been caused by feeding nitrite- treated fishmeal and *Solanum incanum*.

nitroscanate an anthelmintic used in cats and dogs; effective against some cestodes.

nitrosohemochrome the compound responsible for the red color of cooked corned beef.

nitrosomyoglobin the compound formed in meat by the interaction of myoglobin and nitrite in the curing process; creates a rich red color which soon disappears because of oxidation of the compound.

nitrosourea any of a group of lipid-soluble biological alkylating agents, including carmustine and lomustine, which cross the blood–brain barrier and are used as antineoplastic agents.

nitrothiazoles a group of related compounds used in the treatment of histomoniasis in turkeys. Used excessively they can depress fertility and cause liver and kidney damage.

nitrotoxin includes miserotoxin, karakin.

nitrous pertaining to or containing nitrogen in its lowest valence.

n. oxide a gas used by inhalation as a general anesthetic; called also laughing gas.

nitrovin a nonantibiotic nitrofuran, used in some countries as a growth promotant in poultry, pigs and calves.

nitroxynil, nitroxinil an injectable fasciolicide with good efficiency against *Fasciola hepatica* in cattle and sheep and against *Haemonchus contortus* strains that are resistant to benzimidazoles.

nivalenol see DEOXYNIVALENOL.

nizatidine a histamine H_2-receptor antagonist, similar to cimetidine, used to reduce gastric acidity in the treatment of gastrointestinal ulceration.

NK cell natural killer CELL.

NMB new methylene blue.

No chemical symbol, *nobelium*.

no- absence of.

n.-effect level, n.-observed-effect level the maximum dose of a poison that can be given over a stated period without producing detectable ill effects.

n.-lesion pathology the clinical pathology of diseases in which no physical lesion is demonstrable.

n.-visible lesion (NVL) case a case in which no gross lesion is demonstrable by a routine postmortem examination.

no-see-ums slang for midges, sandflies.

nobbling illegal interference with a horse before a race to ensure that it does not race well.

nobelium a chemical element, atomic number 102, atomic weight 253, symbol No. See Table 6.

Nocardia a genus of gram-positive, modified acid-fast bacteria, with branching filaments that break into cocci or bacilli, in the family Nocardiaceae. Most are soil saprophytes which uncommonly may cause pyogranulomatous infections in a number of species.

N. asteroides, N. brasiliensis may cause MASTITIS in cattle, pneumonia, mastitis and lymphadenitis in pigs, sheep and goats, and cutaneous or systemic NOCARDIOSIS of dogs and cats.

N. farcinica there is some uncertainty about the taxonomic status of this species; causes BOVINE farcy.

N. otitidiscaviarum causes dermatitis on guinea pig ears.

nocardial pertaining to or caused by NOCARDIA.

nocardiosis infection with *Nocardia* spp. See also bovine FARCY.

cutaneous n. caused by *N. asteroides* and manifested by the formation of pyogranulomas and the drainage to the surface of pus which may contain sulfur granules.

systemic n. lesions may be in any organ; the disease rarely is disseminated, but most commonly causes pyogranulomatous pleurisy and pneumonia producing a voluminous effusion and a resulting dyspnea. In fish the most common lesion is a granulomatous disease. Nocardiosis of Pacific oysters is almost indistinguishable grossly from Denman Island disease caused by *Mikrocytos machini*.

noci- word element. [L.] *harm, injury*.

nociception perception of a painful stimulus.

nociceptor a receptor that is stimulated by injury; a receptor for pain.
noci-influence injurious or traumatic influence.
noctalbuminuria excess of albumin in the urine secreted at night.
nocturnal active by night.
n. mite see DERMANYSSUS GALLINAE.
nodding blue lily see STYPANDRA GLAUCA.
node pl. *nodi;* 1. a small mass of tissue in the form of a swelling, knot or protuberance, either normal or pathological. 2. in information management, the point where an information system tree branches, e.g. a computer or terminal in a computer network. See also decision tree.
n. of Aschoff and Tawara atrioventricular node.
cutaneous n. an elevated, solid lump, without a necrotic center, about 0.5 inch diameter, caused by acute or chronic inflammation, with an unbroken surface. Called also cutaneous nodule.
Flack's n. see SINOATRIAL node.
hemal n's see HEMAL node.
Keith's n., Keith–Flack n. see SINOATRIAL node.
lymph n. see LYMPH node.
n's of Ranvier constrictions of myelinated nerve fibers at regular intervals of about 1 mm at which the myelin sheath is absent and the axon is enclosed only by Schwann cell processes.
sinoatrial (S-A) n. see SINOATRIAL node.
n. of Tawara atrioventricular node.
nodose having nodes or projections.
nodosity 1. a node. 2. the quality of being nodose.
nodular marked with, or resembling, nodules.
n. dermatofibrosis see DERMATOFIBROSIS.
n. episcleritis see nodular fasciitis (below).
n. fasciitis a firm painless nodular swelling, 0.25 to 0.5 inch diameter, under the conjunctiva at the corneoscleral junction of the eye in dogs. Alternative sites for lesions are the nictitating membrane, and in the subcutis anywhere in the body and in deeper fascia and muscles of the head, face and eyelid. The lesion is an inflammation of fascia and not a neoplasm but acts in a similar manner and may require enucleation because of its size. Called also nodular episcleritis, collie granuloma and proliferative keratoconjunctivitis.
n. hyperplasia a characteristic lesion in nodular regeneration in the liver.
n. infiltrates cells aggregated in one site.
n. intestinal worm disease see ESOPHAGOSTOMIASIS.
n. liver regeneration nodules covering the surface of the liver in patients subjected to persistent or repetitive poisoning, usually by poisonous plants.
n. lungworm see MUELLERIUS *capillaris*.
n. necrobiosis multiple, cutaneous nodules of unknown etiology on the neck, withers and back of the horse. They are composed of degenerate collagen and an eosinophilic and granulomatous response. Called also equine nodular collagenolytic granuloma or eosinophilic granuloma.
n. necrosis see ROECKL'S GRANULOMA.
n. panniculitis see nodular PANNICULITIS.
n. scleritis see nodular fasciitis (above).
n. subepidermal fibrosis fibroma.
n. thyroid hyperplasia see nodular GOITER.
n. venereal disease see GRANULAR vaginitis.
n. worm OESOPHAGOSTOMUM *columbianum*.
n. worm disease see ESOPHAGOSTOMIASIS.
Nodularia spumigena a toxic cyanobacterium occurring in blooms in brackish or salt water and causing sudden death or acute hepatoxicity in animals drinking infested water. Toxin is NODULARIN.
nodularin hepatoxic cyclic pentapeptide from *Nodularia spumigena*.
nodulation the formation of or presence of nodules.
nodule a small boss or node that is solid and can be detected by touch.
acral pruritic n. see ACRAL lick dermatitis.
aggregated lymphatic n's groups of small masses of lymphoid tissue. In the intestinal mucosae they are PEYER'S PATCHES.
n. of Arantius see semilunar valve nodule (below).
cutaneous n. see cutaneous NODE.
milker's n's see PSEUDOCOWPOX.
semilunar valve n. a small mass of fibrous tissue in the center of the free edge of each semilunar valve. Called also nodule of Arantius.
n. of vermis the part of the vermis of the cerebellum, on the ventral surface, where the inferior medullary velum attaches.
nodulectomy see LUMPECTOMY.
nodulus pl. *noduli* [L.] nodule.
nodus pl. *nodi* [L.] node.
noils short and broken fibers combed out of the wool staple during processing.
noise 1. a loud, harsh and objectionable sound. 2. interference in an ecological or electronic system, but insufficient to stop the system. 3. in statistics when extraneous, uncontrolled variables cause errors in the distribution of data.
n. pollution noise in the environment that adversely affects, in our context, the animal inhabitants. No such ill effects have been demonstrated.
Nolina genus of North American plants in the family Agavaceae; contain a hepatotoxin, probably steroidal saponins, causing hepatogenous photosensitization. Includes *N. microcarpa*, *N. texana* (sacahuiste, bear grass).
Nolvasan a proprietary name for chlorhexidine.
noma an idiopathic disorder similar to oral necrobacillosis; a rapidly spreading pseudomembranous to gangrenous stomatitis.
Nomarski interference phase microscope see interference MICROSCOPE.
nomenclature terminology; a classified system of technical names, as of anatomical structures, organisms, etc.
binomial n. the system of designating plants and animals by two latinized words signifying the genus and species.
Nomina Anatomica a book that lists the internationally approved official body of human anatomical nomenclature; abbreviated NA. It now contains items in gross anatomy, histology and embryology.
N. A. Avium (NAA) the internationally approved list of terms used to describe the gross anatomy of birds.
N. A. Veterinaria (NAV) the veterinary counterpart of the NA, now in its third edition, and based largely on the NA.
nominal data a type of data in which there are limited categories but no order.
nominal interest rate the real rate of interest plus the anticipated rate of price inflation.
nomogram a graph with several scales arranged so that a straightedge laid on the graph intersects the scales at related values of the variables; the values of any two variables can be used to find the values of the others.
nomotopic occurring at a normal place.
non-acid-fast readily decolorized by acids after staining; said of bacteria.
non-infectious infections hypothetically viruses which produce no disease but may be capable of reducing resistance to other agents.

non-invasive 1. not penetrating the skin, e.g. a non-invasive test. 2. a neoplasm which spreads over a surface and does not invade and destroy healthy tissue.
non-perforating abomasum ulcer see ABOMASAL ulcer.
non-self see NOT-SELF.
non-sister chromatid chromatid from two different homolog chromosomes.
noncatecholamines adrenergic drugs which do not contain the catechol nucleus but still activate, directly or indirectly, the α- and β-receptors. They include ephedrine, amphetamine, phenylephrine, methoxamine and metaraminol.
nonchaser a Greyhound which will not chase the lure.
nonchromaffin lacking chromaffin characteristic.
n. paraganglia the chemoreceptor organs such as the aortic and carotid bodies.
n. paraganglionoma see CHEMODECTOMA.
nonchromogenic not producing colored pigments. Said of bacteria, e.g. nonchromogenic *Mycobacterium* spp.
nonciliated bronchiolar epithelial cell see CLARA CELL.
noncompetitive antagonist see noncompetitive ANTAGONISM.
noncompliance failure of the owner to follow instructions, particularly in administering medication as prescribed; a cause of a less than expected response to treatment.
nonconductor a substance that does not readily transmit electricity, light or heat.
noncytocidal infection one in which cells are not killed but continue to grow and divide. Characteristic of persistent virus infections.
nondepolarizing agents anticholinergic drugs that compete with acetylcholine at cholinergic receptors. Used as muscle relaxants. Called also competitive drugs. Examples are *d*-tubocurarine, gallamine, pancuronium.
nondisease a diagnosis reserved for cases in which abnormalities are observed in examinable functions but in which no disease can be demonstrated.
nondisjunction failure (1) of two homologous chromosomes to pass to separate cells during the first division of meiosis, or (2) of the two chromatids of a chromosome to pass to separate cells during mitosis or during the second meiotic division. As a result, one daughter cell has two chromosomes or two chromatids, and the other has none. Death of the fetus or chromosomal anomalies may result.
nonelectrolyte a compound which, dissolved in water, does not separate into charged particles and is incapable of conducting an electric current.
nonequilibrium reaction reaction in which the concentration of the substrates and products is much smaller than the value of the equilibrium constant so that the value of ΔG is large and negative. These reactions are important in providing directionality in pathways in that the flux through the reaction is usually controlled by allosteric factors.
nonheme iron proteins proteins containing iron usually in the form of iron-sulfur centers rather than iron in the heme configuration.
nonhuman primate see PRIMATE.
noninflammatory degenerative, neoplastic.
nonkeratinizing squamous cell tumor see TRANSITIONAL CELL tumors.
nonliving disease agents agents causing disease which are not infectious agents; includes chemicals, physical agents, allergens, genetic conditioning.
nonmilk feed ingredients used in milk replacers for calves but made from materials other than milk, principally as an economy measure.
n. carbohydrates carbohydrates other than lactose; very young animals have little intestinal disaccharidase other than lactase and the addition of nonmilk carbohydrate to milk replacers will lead to dietary problems.
n. proteins include proteins from legume seeds, especially soy beans, fish, potatoes, rapeseed.
nonmyelinic spongiform encephalomyelopathies a group of diseases that includes bovine citrullinemia, scrapie, bovine spongiform encephalopathy, the internationally infamous disease known as 'mad cow disease', Creutzfeld–Jakob disease, Gerstmann–Straussler disease (the last two are diseases of humans), and neuronal vacuolar degeneration of Angora goats and focal spongiform encephalopathy of dogs; in all of these diseases spongiform vacuolation of neurons and their processes is the characteristic lesion.
non-NAV terms anatomical terms not included on the official list of terms, the Nomina Anatomica Veterinaria.
Nonne–Apelt test a test for the presence of globulin in cerebrospinal fluid.
non-neuronal pertaining to or composed of nonconducting cells of the nervous system, e.g. neuroglial cells.
non-normality said of values of which the frequency distribution is markedly different from that of the NORMAL (3) probability distribution.
nonoxynol a group of compounds of the general composition, $C_{15}H_{24}O(C_2H_4O)_n$, which are assigned a number according to the value of *n*. Nonoxynol 4, 15 and 30 are nonionic surfactants; nonoxynol 9 is a spermaticide.
nonparametric said of statistical techniques which do not depend on the data having a normal or some other definable distribution.
nonphotochromogen Runyon's group III bacteria of the mycobacteria.
nonpolar not having poles; not exhibiting dipole characteristics.
nonproprietary names generic names; said of drugs.
nonprotein body constituents other than proteins.
n. calorie calories provided by carbohydrates or lipids.
n. nitrogen the nitrogenous constituents of the blood exclusive of the protein bodies; abbreviated NPN. Measurement of NPN is used as a test of renal function. See also nonprotein NITROGEN.
nonrandom selection some individuals or values have more chance of being selected than others.
nonrespiratory originating elsewhere than in the respiratory system.
n. acidosis results from loss of bicarbonate from the extracellular fluid, e.g. in diarrhea and paralytic ileus. Called also metabolic acidosis.
n. alkalosis results from loss of chloride ions, e.g. in gastric dilatation, vomiting, abomasal torsion.
nonreturn rate the proportion of cows not seen to come back into estrus within a specified period after breeding, and are thus considered to be pregnant. They can also be classified as 28, 35, 60 or 90 day nonreturns depending on the interval since mating that is specified.
nonruminant single stomached species, e.g. horse, pig.
nonscreen film see nonscreen FILM.
nonscutate tick see SOFT ticks.

nonsegregational methods those methods of statistical examination in epidemiological studies where disease etiologies are complex or multiple and in which it may not be appropriate to segregate animals into classes on the basis of whether they have been exposed to one or other of the suspected causes. Includes the use of studies of small isolated populations and of twins.

nonspecific 1. not due to any single known cause. 2. not directed against a particular agent, but rather having a general effect.

n. colitis diarrheic disease of growing pigs resembling a mild form of swine dysentery; associated with infection by *Serpulina innocens*. Called also grower pig scours.

nonsporting dog a group of dog breeds in registration and show ring classifications. Breeds included vary between countries and registration bodies, but often it includes, among others, the Boston terrier, Chow Chow, Dalmatian, French bulldog, German pinscher, Keeshond, Lhasa apso, Poodle and Schipperke. Generally, those other than the working, hunting, toy or terrier breeds.

nonsteroidal anti-inflammatory drugs a group of drugs having analgesic, antipyretic and anti-inflammatory activity due to their ability to inhibit the synthesis of prostaglandins; abbreviated NSAID, NSAIDs. Includes aspirin, acetaminophen, phenylbutazone, indomethacin, tolmetin, ibuprofen and related drugs. Excessive use in animals can lead to development of gastric and intestinal ulcers, especially in cats.

nonstick surfaces see POLYTETRAFLUOROETHYLENE.

nonsuppurative pertaining to inflammation without the production of pus, e.g. nonsuppurative polyarthritis of lambs and calves.

nonsweating disease see ANHIDROSIS.

nontapetal region the highly pigmented, non-reflective part of the retina in the optic fundus.

nontropical sprue see SPRUE.

nonunion failure of the ends of a fractured bone to unite.

nonviable not capable of living.

Noogoora burr XANTHIUM *pungens*, *X. occidentale*.

nootka lupine LUPINUS *nootkatensis*.

nor- chemical prefix denoting (1) a compound of normal structure (having an unbranched chain of carbon atoms) that is isomeric with one having a branched chain, or (2) a compound whose chain or ring contains one less methylene (CH_2) group than does that of its homolog.

noradrenaline see NOREPINEPHRINE.

noradrenergic activated by or secreting norepinephrine.

Norberg angle, Norberg's index the angle formed by a line connecting the centers of both femoral heads and one drawn between the center of a femoral head and the craniodorsal rim of the acetabulum on the same side. It is a means of assessing hip laxity and is used in the detection of hip dysplasia.

norbormide a selective rodenticide affecting only rats (*Rattus* spp.). Not toxic for domestic animals, primates, birds and fish.

Nordic goat from Norway, Sweden, Finland; long-haired, polled or horned, many colors, dairy goat.

nordihydroguaiaretic acid one of a group of chemicals which cause renal cysts when administered to experimental animals.

norepinephrine a catecholamine which is the neurotransmitter of most sympathetic postganglionic neurons and also of certain tracts in the central nervous system. It is also a neurohormone stored in the chromaffin granules of the adrenal medulla and released in response to sympathetic stimulation, primarily in response to hypotension. It produces vasoconstriction, an increase in heart rate, and elevation of blood pressure. It is used as a vasopressor, administered by intravenous infusion, to restore blood pressure in certain cases of acute hypotension and as an adjunct in the treatment of cardiac arrest. Called also norepinephrine.

norethandrolone a synthetic androgen having less androgenic activity than testosterone but equal anabolic activity. Used primarily as a growth promotant in poultry.

norethisterone, norethindrone a progestin.

norfloxacin a fluoroquinolone antibiotic, used particularly in urinary tract infection.

Norfolk terrier a small (11–12 lb) lively, compact dog with short legs, small turned over, v-shaped ears, and a medium length (optional) docked tail. The coat is hard and wiry in black and tan, shades of red or wheaten, or grizzle. See also NORWICH TERRIER, which is essentially identical, but has erect ears.

norharmane a β-carboline found in plant members of the family Zygophyllaceae.

Noric horse all colors, including spotted, Austrian draft horse. Called also Pinzgau, Pinzgauer.

norloline an alkaloid thought to provide some of the toxic effects of *Lolium temulentum*—darnel grass.

norm a fixed or ideal standard.

normal 1. agreeing with the regular and established type. When said of a solution, it denotes one containing one chemical equivalent of solute per liter of solution; e.g. a 0.5 normal (0.5 N) solution has a concentration of 0.5 Eq/l. The use of standard units (Eq/l) is now generally preferred in pharmacy and clinical medicine although elsewhere molarity (M) is used. 2. in the context of infectious diseases, not immunized or infected. 3. statistically speaking, the values of a variable which follow a bell-shaped or Gaussian distribution.

n. distribution see normal DISTRIBUTION.

n. limits limits of the classification of 'normal' in the results of a test.

n. saline contains 0.9% sodium chloride. Called also isotonic saline.

normalize to convert a set of data by, for example, converting them to logarithms or reciprocals so that their previous non-normal distribution is converted to a normal one.

Norman–Landing disease type 1, GM_1 gandliosidosis.

Normande cattle dual-purpose cattle, red brown and white, sometimes brindled, red spectacles, originated from local French breeds.

normetanephrine metabolite of norepinephrine excreted in the urine and found in certain tissues.

norm(o)- word element. [L.] *normal, usual, conforming to the rule.*

normoblast a nucleated precursor cell in the erythrocytic series; metarubricyte.

Four developmental stages are recognized: the PRONORMOBLAST (prorubricyte); the basophilic normoblast (basophilic rubricyte, erythroblast), in which the cytoplasm is basophilic, the nucleus is large with clumped chromatin, and the nuclei have disappeared; the polychromatic normoblast (polychromatic erythroblast, rubricyte), in which the nuclear chromatin shows increased clumping and the cytoplasm begins to acquire hemoglobin and takes on an acidophilic tint; and the orthochromatic normoblast (acidophilic normoblast, metarubricyte, orthochromatic erythroblast), the final stage before nuclear loss, in which the nucleus is small and ultimately becomes a blue-black homogeneous structureless mass.

normoblastosis excessive production of normoblasts (metarubricytes) by the bone marrow. Called also metarubricytosis.

normocalcemia a normal level of calcium in the blood.

normocapnemia see NORMOCAPNIA.

normocapnia normal level of carbon dioxide in the blood.

normochromia normal color of erythrocytes.

normocyte an erythrocyte that is normal in size, shape and color.

normocytosis a normal state of the blood in respect to erythrocytes.

normoglycemia normal glucose content of the blood.

normokalemia a normal level of potassium in the blood.

normonatremia a normal level of sodium in the blood.

normospermic producing spermatozoa normal in number and motility.

normotensive characterized by normal tension, tone, or pressure, as by normal blood pressure.

normothermia a normal state of temperature.

normotonia normal tone or tension.

normoventilation normal respiratory exchanges.

normovolemia normal blood volume.

normoxemia normal blood levels of oxygen.

North American named after North America.

N. A. blastomycosis see North American BLASTOMYCOSIS.

N. A. cattle tick see BOOPHILUS *annulatus*.

N. A. chigger see EUTROMBICULA *alfreddugesi*.

N. A. Dräger a mechanical ventilator, used in gaseous anesthesia in horses, which operates as a flow generator and controller. See also DRÄGER VAPORIZER.

N. A. equine encephalomyelitis western and eastern equine encephalomyelitis; see equine viral ENCEPHALOMYELITIS.

North Dutch frill a medium-sized canary with voluminous frills.

North Ronaldsay a breed of sheep kept on the island of North Ronaldsay, close to the Orkney Isles. It has an extraordinary susceptibility to primary copper poisoning. It ordinarily subsists on a diet of seaweed which has a low content of copper and molybdenum and a high content of zinc. Exposure to normal terrestrial herbage may cause fatal copper poisoning.

northern demonstrating a geographical predilection.

n. black bullhead a frog, called also *Ictalurus melas*, a paratenic host for the worm *Dioctophyma renale*.

n. forest grasstree XANTHORRHOEA *johnsonii*.

n. fowl mite see ORNITHONYSSUS *sylviarum*.

n. red oak QUERCUS *rubra* var. *borealis*.

Northern blot an immunologic technique for the detection of specific messenger RNAs using complementary DNA. Called also Northern transfer.

Northern short-tailed sheep a group of European breeds of horned, carpetwool sheep with short tails; black, gray or brown. It includes Icelandic, Orkney, Romanov and Shetland.

Northern transfer see NORTHERN BLOT.

nortryptyline a tricyclic antidepressant.

Norway rat see brown RAT.

Norwegian associated in some way with Norway.

N. buhund, N. sheepdog a medium-sized (26–40 lb), spitz-type dog with a short, dense coat in wheaten, black, red or sable, sometimes with black markings on the face, ears and tip of the curled tail. The ears are large, pointed and erect.

N. elkhound a medium-sized (40 lb) compact dog with a short body, very thick, medium length coat, pointed erect ears and a bushy tail tightly curled over the back. The hair is gray, tipped with black, and there is a thick, light-colored undercoat. The breed is predisposed to progressive retinal atrophy.

N. forest cat a medium- to large-sized, muscular cat with a woolly undercoat and long outer coat in any color combination. The breed is affected by glycogenosis IV.

N. red cattle red or red and white dairy cattle, may be polled, originated from two native Norwegian breeds.

N. scabies see Norwegian SCABIES.

N. tetany-paresis a special form of LACTATION TETANY (1) caused by feeding cows on a herring and cellulose, low-energy high-protein, diet which is very low in magnesium.

Norwich canary a very popular breed, it is short, cobby bird with silky plumage. It is sometimes crested with a saucer-shaped hat of feathers (called Crested Norwich or Gloucester).

Norwich terrier a small (11–12 lb) dog which is almost identical to the NORFOLK TERRIER, but has erect ears.

noscapine an alkaloid present in opium; used as a nonaddictive antitussive.

nose the specialized structure of the head that serves both as the organ of smell and as the first segment of the respiratory apparatus. Air breathed in through the nose is warmed, humidified and filtered by the richly vascular mucous membrane. On breathing out through the nose some of the heat gained is returned to the nasal mucous membrane. See also NASAL.

n. bleed see EPISTAXIS.

collie n. see solar DERMATITIS.

Dudley n. see nasal DEPIGMENTATION.

n. lead, n. tong, n. grip, bulldog a scissor-like instrument with the blades curved towards each other and fitted with a knob on each of their ends. The tool is inserted into the nostrils with the blades opened, positioned on either side of the septum, then closed tight. The end of the nasal septum is grasped between the ends of the tongs. Provides fair restraint for a cow having a minor interference, such as an intravenous injection. Comparable in effect to a twitch on a horse.

n. mite *Speleognathus australis*; occurs in wild ruminants and may cause bouts of sneezing. See also NASAL acariasis.

n. picking a vice in quail kept in overcrowded conditions. The birds pick at the soft tissue where the beak and skin join. Causes blood loss and subsequent beak deformity.

n. printing epidermal contours in the skin of the nose of dogs and the muzzle of ruminants are reflections of dermal structures; they are individually distinctive and can be replicated by applying ink to the part with an inking pad and imprinting on paper; provide a means of identification similar to fingerprints in humans. See also TRANSPONDER, NASAL areae.

snow n. see nasal DEPIGMENTATION.

nosebag canvas bucket with a poll strap to go over the horse's poll and to contain a small meal for the horse. A portable manger.

noseband a broad leather band worn across the nose between the eyes and the nostrils and connecting the two cheek straps. Usually part of a CAVESSON.

drop n. worn below the bit and around the muzzle. Used to prevent the horse opening its mouth too wide. Pressure on the band, produced by the reins, causes compression of the nasal cartilages.
sheepskin n. has the effect of obscuring forward shadows which might balk the horse. See also SHADOW ROLL.

nosebleed see EPISTAXIS.

Nosema a genus of protozoa in the class Microsporea. All are obligate intracellular parasites.
N. branchialis, N. lophi found in fish.
N. cuniculi see ENCEPHALITOZOON *cuniculi.*

nosematosis see ENCEPHALITOZOONOSIS.

nos(o)- word element. [Gr.] *disease.*

nosocomial pertaining to or originating in a hospital.
n. infections those acquired during hospitalization or during attendance at any veterinary medical facility.

nosogeny the development of a disease; pathogenesis.

nosography a nomenclature of disease entities.

nosology classification of patients into groups.

nosoparasite an organism found in a disease that it is able to modify, but not to produce.

nosopoietic causing disease.

Nosopsyllus fasciatus a flea that infests mice and rats. It maintains plague in rats but is reluctant to bite humans and is rarely involved in cases in them.

nosotaxy the classification of disease.

Nostoc rivulare cyanobacterium contains the toxic peptide microcystin, causing sudden death or hepatic necrosis.

nostril either of the two apertures (nares) of the nose that lead into the nasal cavity. See also nasal CAVITY.
n. dilatation accompanies dyspnea, is also present in tetanus as part of the generalized muscular tetany.
false n. a blind pouch of skin dorsal to the true nostril in the horse. Called also nasal DIVERTICULUM.
false n. cyst developmental abnormality in the false nostril of a horse.
n. fly see OESTRUS *ovis.*
hemorrhage from n. see EPISTAXIS.
regurgitation from n. a common finding in food animals as part of a syndrome of esophageal obstruction; also in horses with gastric dilatation and cows with severe rumen distension; also occurs in recumbent ruminants with motor paralysis as in milk fever or general anesthesia.
n. vibrissae the special tactile hairs around the nostrils.

nostrum a quack, patent or secret remedy.

not-self a term denoting antigenic constituents foreign to the organism (self), which are eliminated through antibody or cell-mediated IMMUNITY.

not(o)- word element. [Gr.] *the back.*

notarium the bony structure created by the fusion of two or more thoracic vertebrae as occurs in some birds. Called also os dorsale.

notch an indentation, especially one on the edge of a bone or other organ.
acetabular n. in the medial part of the rim of the acetabulum.
antitragohelicine n. in the caudal process of the cartilage of the pig's ear separating it from the tragus and antitragus.
aortic n. a small downward deflection in the arterial pulse or pressure contour immediately following the closure of the semilunar valves, sometimes used as a marker for the end of systole or the ejection period. Called also dicrotic notch.
cardiac n. an indentation in the ventral margin of the lungs that allows the heart in its coverings to lie against the chest wall. Useful for ultrasound examination, auscultation, pericardiac and cardiac puncture. The extent of the notch varies between species and enlarges during expiration.
costal n. indentations in the sternum with which the costal cartilages of the ribs articulate.
dicrotic n. see aortic notch (above).
glenoid n. in the cranial part of the rim of the glenoid cavity of the scapula.
greater sciatic n. indentation in the dorsal edge of the ilium over which the sciatic nerve passes.
intertragic n. the notch in the auricular cartilage between the tragus and antitragus.
lesser sciatic n. indentation in the lateral border of the ischium between the ischial spine and the ischial tuber.
mandibular n. separates the coronoid and condylar processes of the mandible.
mandibular vascular n. the notch on the lower edge of the mandible below which facial vessels cross to reach the face in some species such as the horse.
nasoincisive n. deep notch separating the pointed nasal bone and the incisive bone.
pretragic n. the palpable depression rostral to the tragus of the ear.
tragohelicine n. the slot in the auricular cartilage between the tragus and the medial border of the ear cartilage; a useful surgical landmark.
vertebral n. the notch in the pedicle of the vertebral arch, at the cranial and caudal ends of each vertebra which combines with its opposite number to create an intervertebral foramen.

notching pliers an instrument used to produce an EAR mark.

notchplasty an orthopedic procedure to remove osteophytes, which form on the inner margin of the lateral femoral condyle because of stifle instability resulting from cranial cruciate ligament rupture, and reshaping of the intercondylar notch to facilitate placement of the fascial graft during reconstruction of the joint.

Notechis scutatus see TIGER snake.

notedric mange a crusting, pruritic dermatitis on the ears and neck of cats caused by *Notoedres cati.* It may extend onto the face, paws and elsewhere on the body. Called also head mange. Occasionally occurs on rabbits.

notencephalocele hernial protrusion of brain at the back of the head.

notencephalus a fetus affected with notencephalocele.

Notesthes robusta a venomous scorpion or wasp fish. Called also bullrout.

Notholaena distans rockfern. See CHEILANTHES.

notifiable necessary to be reported to the relevant government authority. Said of individual diseases.

notochord a cylindrical cord of cells on the dorsal aspect of an embryo, marking its longitudinal axis; a defining characteristic of all chordates. It is the center of development of the axial skeleton. Its remnants in adult mammals are found in the pulpy centers of the intervertebral disks.

Notocotylus a genus of intestinal flukes (digenetic trematodes) in the family Notocotylidae.
N. attenuatus found in the ceca and rectum of fowl, duck, goose and wild aquatic birds. Can cause erosion, diarrhea and emaciation in young birds.
N. impricatus found in domestic poultry.
N. thienemanni found in domestic and wild ducks.

Notoedres a genus of mange mites in the family Sarcoptidae.

N. cati causes NOTEDRIC MANGE in cats and occasionally rabbits.
N. douglassi occurs in gray squirrels; causes severe dermatitis in koalas and bandicoots in captivity.
N. muris causes ear mange in rats.
N. oudemansi found on rats.

Nova Scotia duck tolling retriever a medium-sized, compact hunting dog with a dense, medium length coat of red or orange, and a well feathered tail. The breed is noted for its hunting activity in which it jumps and plays in the water to attract waterfowl.

November lily see LILIUM LONGIFLORUM.

novobiocin an antibacterial produced by *Streptomyces niveus*, used in the treatment of infections caused by staphylococci and other gram-positive organisms. Called also albamycin, cathomycin.

Novocain a proprietary name for procaine.

noxious hurtful; injurious; pernicious.
n. gases those encountered in nature include ammonia, hydrogen sulfide, methane, sulfur dioxide; industrial intoxicants include ammonia, carbon monoxide, cyanide, and a variety of toxic smokes and fumes.

Noyes forceps see alligator FORCEPS.

Np chemical symbol, *neptunium*.

NPH 3-nitropropionic acid.

NPN nonprotein nitrogen.

NPOH 3-nitropropanol.

NPY neuropeptide-Y.

NRA neutrophil-releasing activity.

NRC National Research Council.

ns nanosecond.

NSAIDs see NONSTEROIDAL ANTI-INFLAMMATORY DRUGS.

NSD Nairobi sheep disease.

nsec nanosecond.

NSH nutritional secondary hyperparathyroidism.

NSHP nutritional secondary hyperparathyroidism.

Nubian see ANGLO-NUBIAN.

nucha the nape, or top, of the neck.

nuchal pertaining to the top of the neck.
n. crest see nuchal CREST.
n. disease fistulous withers and poll evil.
n. ligament a powerful elastic apparatus that serves to support the head without muscular effort. It joins either the occipital bone or the axis to the dorsal thoracic spines (withers in the horse) and is continuous with the thoracolumbar part of the supraspinous ligament. The dorsal, rope-like funicular part is connected by the lamellar part to the spinous processes of the cervical vertebrae. In some species the lamellar part consists of two independent sheets closely applied to each other; in others it is absent.

nuclear pertaining to a nucleus.
n. bag fibers fibers found in neuromuscular spindles; have an extensive nerve supply.
n. chain fibers fibers, which like nuclear bag fibers, are found in neuromuscular spindles; shorter but more numerous than the bag variety.
n. ground substance, n. matrix the matrix substance in a nucleus, surrounded by the limiting membrane.
n. imaging see SCINTIGRAPHY.
n. index see SCHILLING COUNT.
n. medicine technologist see RADIOLOGICAL technologist.
n. sap soluble phase of the nuclear matrix.
n. veterinary medicine see nuclear VETERINARY MEDICINE.

nuclease any of a group of enzymes that cleave or digest nucleic acids into fragments or single nucleotides.
S1 n. a single-strand-specific endonuclease that degrades DNA and RNA to nucleoside 5′-monophosphates. The enzyme is a single polypeptide chain of molecular weight 32,000 and is isolated from 'takadiesterase', a digestive enzyme preparation from *Aspergillus oryzae*. Widely used in molecular biology to map the position of mRNA to its DNA, and also used to remove single-stranded tails from DNA fragments, to produce blunt ends to open up hairpin-loop structures.

nucleated having a nucleus or nuclei.
n. erythrocyte see NORMOBLAST, METARUBRICYTE.

nucleation sites the ends of microtubules in the cytoplasmic skeleton; contributes to the growth of protofilaments.

nuclei plural of *nucleus*.

nucleic acids threadlike, high-molecular-weight molecules that occur naturally in the cells of all living organisms. They form the genetic material of the cell and direct the synthesis of protein within the cell.

Nucleic acids are composed of repeating smaller units, called *nucleotides* or bases, which are made up of a pentose sugar, a nitrogenous base, and a phosphate group. There are two major classes of nucleic acids: DEOXYRIBONUCLEIC ACID (DNA) whose pentose sugar is deoxyribose, and RIBONUCLEIC ACID (RNA) whose pentose sugar is ribose. The major purine and pyrimidine bases in the nucleic acids are adenine (A), guanine (G) and cytosine (C), which occur in both, and thymine (T) in DNA and uracil (U) in RNA.

RNA is present in both the nucleus and the cytoplasm of many cells. Most of the cytoplasmic RNA is associated with ribosomes (called rRNA), which are the site of protein synthesis. RNA molecules perform several functions in the cell, depending on the type of RNA molecule and its specific properties. DNA is a major constituent of chromosomes in the nuclei of all cells. Its chief function is to provide a genetic message that is encoded in the sequence of bases.
n. acid sequencing see DNA sequencing.

nuclein an intermediate product in the decomposition pathway between nucleoprotein and nucleic acid.

nucleocapsid a minimum unit of viral structure, consisting of a protein capsid with the enclosed nucleic acid. For some viruses the nucleocapsid is enclosed within an envelope.

nucleofugal moving away from a nucleus.

nucleohistone the nucleoprotein complex made up of deoxyribonucleic acid (DNA) and histones. It is the principal constituent of chromatin.

nucleoid 1. resembling a nucleus. 2. a nucleus-like body sometimes seen in the center of an erythrocyte. 3. the genetic material (nucleic acid) of a rickettsia, chlamydia and some viruses, e.g. poxviruses, situated in the center of the microorganism.

nucleolar pertaining to or emanating from nucleolus.

nucleoli plural form of nucleolus.

nucleolonema a network of strands formed by organization of a finely granular substance, perhaps containing RNA, in the nucleolus of a cell.

nucleolus pl. *nucleoli* [L.] a rounded refractile body in the nucleus of most cells, which is the site of synthesis of ribosomal RNA, becoming enlarged during periods of synthesis and smaller during quiescent periods; multiple nucleoli occur in some cells.
n. organizer site chromosomal sites for attachment of nucleoli.

nucleon a particle of an atomic nucleus; a proton or neutron, the total number of which constitutes the mass number of the isotope.

nucleonics the study of nucleons or of atomic nuclei and their reactions; nuclear physics.
nucleopetal moving toward a nucleus.
nucleophile an electron donor in chemical reactions involving covalent catalysis in which the donated electrons bond other chemical groups (electrophiles).
nucleoplasm karyoplasm; the protoplasm of the nucleus of a cell.
nucleoprotein any of a class of conjugated proteins, consisting of nucleic acids and simple proteins, e.g. a histone.
nucleosidase an intracellular enzyme that is capable of causing the decomposition of nucleosides.
nucleoside any of a class of compounds produced by hydrolysis of nucleotides, consisting of a sugar (a pentose or a hexose) and a purine or pyrimidine base.
nucleosome any of the complexes of histone and DNA in eukaryotic cells, seen under the electron microscope as beadlike bodies on a string of DNA.
nucleotidase an enzyme that splits nucleotides into nucleosides and phosphoric acid.
5-n. elevated levels may be detected in liver disease.
nucleotide any of a group of compounds obtained by hydrolysis of nucleic acids, consisting of a purine or pyrimidine base linked to a sugar (ribose or deoxyribose), which in turn is esterified with phosphoric acid. See also NUCLEOSIDE, DEOXYRIBONUCLEIC ACID.
cyclic n's those in which the phosphate group bonds to two atoms of the sugar forming a ring, as in cyclic AMP and cyclic GMP, which act as intracellular second messengers.
n. sequences see DNA sequencing.
nucleotidyl a nucleotide residue.
nucleotoxin a toxin from cell nuclei, or one that affects cell nuclei.
nucleus pl. *nuclei* [L.] 1. cell nucleus; a spheroid body within a cell, contained in a double membrane, the nuclear envelope, and containing the CHROMOSOMES and one or more nucleoli. The contents are collectively referred to as *nucleoplasm.* The chromosomes contain DEOXYRIBONUCLEIC ACID (DNA), which is the genetic material that codes for the structure of all the proteins of the cell. 2. a mass of gray matter in the central nervous system, especially such a mass marking the central termination of a cranial nerve. 3. in organic chemistry, the combination of atoms forming the central element or basic framework of the molecule of a specific compound or class of compounds. 4. the dense core of an atom; called also atomic nucleus. It is made of protons and neutrons held together by the strong nuclear force. Traveling in orbit around the nucleus is a cloud of negatively charged particles called ELECTRONS. The number of protons in the atomic nucleus gives a substance its identity as a particular ELEMENT (2).
n. abducens located in the floor of the fourth ventricle; its axons constitute the abducent nerve.
n. ambiguus the nucleus of origin of motor fibers of the glossopharyngeal, vagus and accessory nerves that supply the striated muscle of the pharynx and larynx. Found in the medulla oblongata.
arcuate n., n. arcuati small irregular areas of gray substance on the ventromedial aspect of the pyramid of the medulla oblongata.
atomic n. nucleus (3).
basal n. large brain nuclei, the caudate and lentiform nuclei, which combine with the white matter to form the corpus striatum. Important in the regulation of motor function.
caudate n., n. caudatus an elongated, arched gray mass closely related to the lateral ventricle throughout its entire extent, which, together with the putamen, forms the neostriatum.
central nervous system n. aggregations of neurons within the brain.
cerebellar n. there are a number of them; they are surrounded by the medulla oblongata caudal to the cerebellum.
cochlear n. (dorsal and ventral) the nuclei of termination of sensory fibers of the cochlear part of the vestibulocochlear (eighth cranial) nerve, which partly encircle the inferior cerebellar peduncle at the junction of the medulla oblongata and pons.
cranial nerve n. aggregations of cell bodies associated with the cranial nerves, which in general are organized as continuations of the four gray matter components of the spinal cord plus three others which appear in the medulla oblongata developed for innervation of the organs in the head.
cuneate n. medial and lateral nuclei are situated in the medulla oblongata.
dentate n., n. dentatus the largest of the deep cerebellar nuclei lying in the white matter of the cerebellum.
Edinger–Westphal n. located in the midbrain and a center for coordination of oculomotor activity.
facial n. in the medulla oblongata and the origin of the facial nerve.
lateral geniculate n. concerned in the transmission of visual stimuli.
medial geniculate n. a nucleus within the thalamus; involved in transmission of auditory stimuli.
gracile n. located in the medulla oblongata.
habenular n. the gray matter of the habenula.
hypoglossal n. located in the medulla oblongata, the origin of the hypoglossal nerve.
lenticular n., lentiform n. the part of the corpus striatum just lateral to the internal capsule, comprising the putamen and globus pallidus.
motor n. any collection of cells in the central nervous system giving origin to a motor nerve.
oculomotor n. the cells of the midbrain which make up the origin of the oculomotor nerve.
olivary n., n. olivaris 1. a folded band of gray matter enclosing a white core and producing the elevation (olive) on the medulla oblongata. 2. olive (2).
n. of origin any collection of nerve cells giving origin to the fibers, or a part of the fibers, of a peripheral nerve.
paraventricular n., n. paraventricularis a band of cells in the wall of the third ventricle in the supraoptic part of the hypothalamus; many of its cells are neurosecretory in function and project to the neurohypophysis, where they secrete oxytocin (and, to a lesser extent, antidiuretic hormone).
pontine n., n. pontis groups of nerve cell bodies in the part of the pyramidal tract within the ventral part of the pons, upon which the fibers of the corticopontine tract synapse, and whose axons in turn cross to the opposite side and form the middle cerebellar peduncle.
pulpy n., n. pulposus a semifluid mass of fine white and elastic fibers forming the center of an intervertebral disk. It serves to distribute pressure over the vertebral body. It shows early age changes, may calcify and herniate through the fibrous rings that enclose it to cause disk disease.
red n. an oval mass of gray matter (pink in fresh specimens) in the anterior part of the tegmentum and extending into the posterior part of the hypothalamus; one of the important relay stations in the extrapyramidal motor pathway of the CNS; origin of

the rubrospinal tract in the cord; called also nucleus ruber.

n. ruber see red nucleus (above).

salivatory n. groups of preganglionic parasympathetic neurons concerned with salivary secretion organized into a rostral nucleus, of the facial nerve, and the caudal nucleus, of the glossopharyngeal nerve.

sensory n. the nucleus of termination of the afferent (sensory) fibers of a peripheral nerve.

supraoptic n., n. supraopticus one just above the lateral part of the optic chiasm; many of its cells are neurosecretory in function and project to the neurohypophysis, where they secrete antidiuretic hormone (ADH) and, to a lesser extent, oxytocin; other cells are osmoreceptors that stimulate ADH release in response to increased osmotic pressure.

tegmental n. several nuclear masses of the reticular formations of the pons and midbrain, especially of the latter, where they are in close approximation to the superior cerebellar peduncles.

thoracic n., n. thoracicus a column of cells in the dorsal gray column of the spinal cord, extending from the seventh or eighth cervical segments to the second or third lumbar level.

trapezoid body n. a relay station in the auditory pathways.

trigeminal n. there are three sensory nuclei and one motor nucleus of the trigeminal nerve found in the brainstem; the sensory nuclei comprise the mesencephalic nucleus, the nucleus of the descending tract, and the principal sensory nucleus, but none is exclusive to the trigeminal nerve, all of them receiving sensory inputs from other cranial nerves.

trochlear n. source of the trochlear nerve; located in the tegmentum of the midbrain.

vagus n. source of the vagus nerve.

vestibular n., n. vestibularis the four cellular masses (superior, lateral, medial and inferior) in the floor of the fourth ventricle, in which the branches of the eighth cranial (vestibulocochlear) nerve terminate.

nuclide a species of atom characterized by the charge, mass, number and quantum state of its nucleus, and capable of existing for a measurable lifetime (usually more than 10^{-10} s).

nude mouse inbred strain of laboratory mouse which is hairless and has no thymic tissue. Because it has no source of T lymphocytes, it suffers from a defect in cell-mediated immunity and is highly susceptible to infections. This trait is utilized for immunological studies. Called also athymic mouse.

Nugent forceps general purpose thumb forceps with fine points for ophthalmic work.

null an absence of information, as contrasted with zero or blank or nil, about a value.

n. cell called also null lymphocyte; see null CELL.

n. hypothesis a statistical hypothesis which states that one variable has no association with another variable, or set of variables. That is, the observed results can be explained by chance alone.

n. lymphocyte see null CELL.

nullipara a female who has not produced a viable offspring; PARA 0.

nulliparity the state of being a nullipara.

number a symbol, as a figure or word, expressive of a certain value or a specified quantity determined by count.

atomic n. a number expressive of the number of protons in an atomic nucleus, or the positive charge of the nucleus expressed in terms of the electronic charge; symbol A.

Avogadro's n. see AVOGADRO'S number.

n. crunching said of a program which performs much computation and manipulation of numerical data.

mass n. see MASS number.

Reynold's n. see REYNOLD'S NUMBER.

numerator the upper part of a fraction.

n. relationship see ADDITIVE genetic relationship.

numeric see NUMERICAL.

n. cluster see TEN-KEY PAD.

numerical expressed in numbers, i.e. Arabic numerals of 0 to 9 inclusive.

n. nomenclature a numerical code is used to indicate the words, or other alphabetical signals, intended.

Numidicola antennatus lice of guinea fowl.

Numidinae see GUINEA FOWL.

Numinbah horse sickness see EUPATORIUM *adenophorum*.

nummular 1. coin-sized and coin-shaped. 2. made up of round, flat disks. 3. arranged like a stack of coins.

numnah a thick felt pad cut to the shape of a saddle and worn under it as protection for the horse's back. Fitted with straps which fasten it to the saddle and prevent it moving.

nurse see ANIMAL nurses.

nursery a building or part of a building constructed especially for the rearing of animals on a largely milk diet. Requires special attention to mechanical services and the maintenance of a stable external environment. Hygiene, preferably an all-in, all-out management strategy, and strict microbial isolation are important parts of the management system.

n. diarrhea enteropathogenic bacterial or viral infections in young animals.

nursing see SUCKLING.

artificial n. feeding on milk replacer; implies by sucking a teat, on a bottle or a multiple sucking device usually described as a calfeteria.

n. sickness a disease of lactating mink characterized by aimless wandering, anorexia, emaciation and hepatic lipidosis. No specific cause has been identified.

nutation the act of nodding, especially involuntary nodding.

nutmeg liver the appearance given by a chronic passive congestion of the liver; a mosaic of red and gray caused by blood replacement of necrotic periacinar hepatocytes contrasted with areas of grayish, fatty, surviving hepatocytes in the periportal tissue.

nutraceutical a nutrient with drug-like properties but not legally recognized as a therapeutic agent.

nutria see COYPU.

nutrient 1. nourishing; aiding nutrition. 2. a nourishing substance, food or component of food. Includes minerals, vitamins, fats, protein, carbohydrate and water.

n. allowance the total feed provided to an animal for a day. Includes its basic nutritional requirements plus allowances for waste in the feeding process, special allowances for special states and activities, and for special qualities of the feed being used.

n. analysis chemical analysis of feedstuff with measurement of fiber, protein, fat, carbohydrate, individual minerals and vitamins.

n. artery one of the arterial blood supplies to a typical long bone; enters the bone via an oblique canal. Other blood supply routes to bone include metaphyseal, epiphyseal and periosteal arteries.

n. content the proportion of a feed or diet that is digestible and assimilable. See also TOTAL DIGESTIBLE NUTRIENTS.

n. profile a listing of the optimal level of each nutrient in dog and cat foods; published by the Association of American Feed Control Officials.

n. requirements daily requirement for each nutrient for each animal species at the recognized stages of life and production; usually presented in feeding tables.

n. veins mimics the nutrient artery.

nutriment nourishment; nutritious material; food.

nutrition 1. the sum of the processes involved in taking in nutriments and assimilating and utilizing them. 2. nutriment.

It includes all the processes by which the body uses food for energy, maintenance and growth. See also MALNUTRITION, INANITION, STARVATION, THIRST, NUTRITIONAL.

critical care n. provision of nutritional support for patients in critical care units; usually requires modification of normal nutritional requirements to meet the demands of stress, injury and disease, and to support recovery from these states.

enteral n. see ENTERAL feeding.

intravenous n. see parenteral nutrition (below).

N. Labeling and Education Act of 1990 an amendment to the (US) Federal Food, Drug, and Cosmetic Act which defines how foods, claimed to affect disease, are not regulated as drugs.

parenteral n. a technique for meeting a patient's nutritional needs by means of intravenous feeding; sometimes called *hyperalimentation*, even though it does not provide excessive amounts of nutrients. Nutrition by intravenous feeding may be total parenteral nutrition (TPN) or supplemental. TPN provides all of the carbohydrates, proteins, fats, water, electrolytes, vitamins and minerals needed for the building of tissue, expenditure of energy, and other physiological activities.

total parenteral n. called also TPN; see parenteral nutrition (above).

nutritional pertaining to or emanating from nutrition.

n. anemia see nutritional ANEMIA.

n. assessment chemical analysis of ration ingredients or, more commonly, consultation of a table of approximate composition of feedstuffs.

n. deficiency disease disease caused by a deficiency of a particular nutrient in the feed. Includes the micro- and macronutrients of minerals, vitamins, carbohydrates, fats and proteins. The specific diseases are described under their individual titles.

n. gill disease caused by a nutritional deficiency of pantothenic acid. The gills of affected fish hypertrophy, show clubbing and fuse together causing interference with gaseous exchange.

n. gout an excess of protein in the diet may cause visceral and even articular GOUT.

n. hyperparathyroidism see nutritional secondary OSTEODYSTROPHIA FIBROSA.

n. infertility infertility due to a nutritional deficiency, principally caloric.

n. muscular dystrophy see ENZOOTIC muscular dystrophy.

n. myodegeneration see ENZOOTIC muscular dystrophy.

n. myopathy see ENZOOTIC muscular dystrophy.

n. panniculitis disease of cats, mink, foals and pigs associated with the feeding of fish offal, fish meal or rations containing high levels of unsaturated fatty acids. Palpable thickening and solidity of subcutaneous fat; may be associated with myopathy, gastric ulcer or hepatosis dietetica.

n. secondary hypercalcitonism see nutritional secondary HYPERCALCITONISM.

n. secondary hyperparathyroidism see nutritional secondary HYPERPARATHYROIDISM.

n. status the state of the body with respect to each nutrient and to the overall state of the body weight and condition.

n. stress the stress of inadequate nutrition of total nutrients.

n. supplement addition of a nutrient to an existing diet to make good what might be only a temporary shortfall. May be made available in a salt or mineral mix or block, or may be mixed in with a feed or even in drinking water. For pastured animals other means are used but foliar dusting comes close to being a nutritional supplement.

nutritionally related disease disease caused by deficiencies or excesses of specific feed nutrients or of a total ration; also includes diseases in which susceptibility to a separate risk factor is increased by a nutritional aberration, e.g. enterotoxemia (*Clostridium welchii* type D) in lambs.

nutritious affording nourishment.

nutritive pertaining to or promoting nutrition.

n. ratio the ratio of digestible protein to other digestible components in the feed.

nutriture nourishment.

Nuttallia see BABESIA.

nuttalliosis see BABESIOSIS.

nux vomica powdered nut of the plant *Strychnos nux-vomica*. In earlier times was used as a stimulant to appetite. Also finds use in small animals as a herbal remedy, but the strychnine content presents the possibility of toxicity.

NVE see no visible ESTRUS.

NVL no visible lesion. Said of cows that react positively to a tuberculin test but no lesions can be found in them at autopsy.

NVO no visible oestrus (see no visible ESTRUS). Called also NVE.

nyala a bushbuck antelope, called also *Tragelaphus angasi*, especially susceptible to nutritional myopathy.

nyctalopia night blindness.

Nycteribiidae a family of flies similar to the hippoboscids and found on bats in the Old World.

nycterine occurring at night.

Nycticebus slow LORIS.

nyct(o)- word element. [Gr.] *night, darkness*.

nyctohemeral pertaining to both day and night.

nyctotyphlosis night blindness, or nyctalopia.

Nye tourniquet a strong rubber cord with a friction grip holder. Used also as a muzzle.

Nylander test a test for glucose in the urine using a solution containing bismuth subnitrate which forms a black precipitate in a positive reaction.

nylon a long-chain polymer available in monofilament and multiple filament forms.

nymph a developmental stage in certain arthropods (e.g. ticks, mites and lice) between the larval form and the adult, and resembling the latter in appearance.

nymphomania behavioral state in which the female is in estrus continually or for longer periods at shorter intervals than is normal. Rectal palpation may reveal cystic follicles or there may be no detectable abnormality.

nymphomaniac an individual patient habitually showing signs of nymphomania.

Nyquist limit the maximum frequency shift that can be accurately interpreted in a pulsed Doppler ultrasound unit.

nystagmiform, nystagmoid resembling nystagmus.

nystagmograph an instrument for recording the movements of the eyeball in nystagmus.

nystagmus a periodic, rhythmic, involuntary movement of both eyeballs in unison. There is a slow component in one direction and a quick return. The movement may be vertical, horizontal or rotary. Common causes are lesions of the cerebellum or the vestibular apparatus, or increased intracranial pressure.

aural n. labyrinthine nystagmus.

cerebellar n. one characterized by tremor, without fast and slow components.

Cheyne's n. a peculiar rhythmical eye movement resembling Cheyne–Stokes respiration in rhythm.

congenital n. may be a primary functional defect or secondary to lesions in the visual pathways, sometimes associated with albinism. Reported in cattle, cats (particularly Siamese), and dogs.

dissociated n. that in which the movements in the two eyes are dissimilar.

gaze n. nystagmus made apparent by looking to the right or to the left.

horizontal n. that in which the eyes move from side to side with the fast component opposite to the side of the lesion; seen with central or unilateral peripheral vestibular disease.

jerk n. vestibular nystagmus (see below).

labyrinthine n. vestibular nystagmus due to labyrinthine disturbance.

latent n. that occurring only when one eye is covered.

lateral n. involuntary horizontal movement of the eyes.

ocular n. wandering movement of the eyes as though searching for something. Associated with congenital blindness.

optokinetic n. nystagmus induced by looking at objects moving across the field of vision.

oscillatory n. pendular nystagmus.

pendular n. that which consists of to-and-fro movements of equal velocity.

positional n. that which occurs, or is altered in form or intensity, on assumption of certain positions of the head.

postrotatory n. a normal finding after the animal has been rotated, with the fast phase away from the direction of rotation.

resting n. that occurring while the head is stationary.

retraction n., n. retractorius a spasmodic backward movement of the eyeball occurring on attempts to move the eye; a sign of midbrain disease.

rotatory n. involuntary rotation of the eyes about the visual axis.

spontaneous n. that occurring without specific stimulation of the vestibular system.

vertical n. involuntary up-and-down movement of the eyes.

vestibular n. nystagmus due to disturbance of the labyrinth or of the vestibular nuclei; the movements are usually jerky.

undulatory n. an inherited disorder of Finnish Ayrshire cattle; there is a synchronous, tremor-like movement of the eyes but affected aninals are otherwise healthy.

nystatin a polyene antibiotic produced by *Streptomyces noursei*; used topically in treatment of infections due to *Candida albicans*, *Aspergillus* spp., yeasts and some dermatophytes.

nystaxis see NYSTAGMUS.

nyxis puncture, or paracentesis.

O

O-F test see OXIDATION-FERMENTATION TEST.

O chemical symbol, *oxygen;* [L.] *oculus* (eye); [L.] *octarius* (pint); opening.

O_2 oxygen.

o- symbol, *ortho-*.

O antigen see O ANTIGEN.

oak see QUERCUS.

o. buds see ACORN.

oak-leaved goosefoot CHENOPODIUM *glaucum*.

oat member of the plant genus *Avena* in the family Poaceae.

oats see AVENA *sativa*.

o. grain seed of *Avena sativa,* and as 'oats' the favored grain for the feeding of horses. Too light in energy concentration for the heavy feeding of ruminants.

o. grass *Avena pubescens*. See also OATGRASS.

o. hair calculi large, intestinal trichobezoars composed entirely of oat hairs and capable of causing intestinal obstruction.

o. hay made from cereal oat crop (*Avena sativa*) it is a popular feed for herbivores but it may have a high nitrate content if it has been well fertilized, and if it gets moldy and overheated, develops a high nitrite content and is poisonous. See also NITRITE poisoning.

o. hulls a high-fiber, low-protein, low-energy feed.

o. sickness stiffness and restriction of movement in horses soon after a heavy feed of grain; a vague syndrome thought to be due to sensitivity to grain of any sort in particular horses.

o. straw used as bedding and as feed when supplemented with a nitrogen-rich feed such as urea. Like oaten hay may cause nitrite poisoning if moldy.

oat-shaped cell inflammatory cells seen in pneumonic lung, and characterized by elongated or streaming nuclei.

oaten pertaining to or emanating from oats.

oatgrass *Arrhenatherum elatius* (tall oatgrass), *Danthonia* (California oatgrass).

OB obstetrics.

ob- word element. [L.] *against, in front of, towards*.

obcecation incomplete blindness.

obedience training a standardized program of training for dogs calculated to give owners mastery of their dogs at all times. The grades of increasing excellence vary between countries. A popular grading is Companion Dog, Companion Dog Excellent, Utility Dog and Tracking Dog.

Obeliscoides a genus of nematodes in the family Trichostrongylidae.

O. cuniculi found in the stomach of rabbits; in heavy infestations causes gastritis.

Obermayer's test a test for indican in the urine using a solution of ferric chloride and hydrochloric acid and added chloroform. A blue-violet color develops in a positive test.

obese characterized by OBESITY.

obesity excessive accumulation of fat in the body; increase in weight beyond that considered desirable with regard to age, height and bone structure.

o. fold pyoderma see fold DERMATITIS.

obex a small triangular membrane at the caudal end of the roof of the fourth ventricle of the brain.

object code a computer term. See object CODE.

object–film distance in the taking of a radiograph the distance between the object and the film; the shorter the distance the sharper the image and the less the magnification.

objective 1. perceptible by the external senses. 2. the lens or system of lenses of a microscope nearest the object that is being examined.

immersion o. one designed to have its tip and the coverglass over the specimen connected by a liquid instead of air.

obligate necessary, essential.

o. accumulators see ACCUMULATOR PLANTS.

o. carrier the subject is always available as a carrier of the infection.

obligatory unavoidable; something that is bound to occur.

o. water diuresis polyuria resulting from a decrease or inactivity of antidiuretic hormone on distal tubules and collecting ducts.

oblique slanting; inclined.

obliquity the state of being oblique or slanting.

obliteration complete removal, by disease, degeneration, surgical procedure, irradiation, etc.

obliterative cardiomyopathy see restrictive CARDIOMYOPATHY.

oblongata medulla oblongata. See also BRAIN.

Obodhiang virus a rhabdovirus closely related to RABIES virus.

O'Brien–Elschnig forceps thumb-operated fixation tissue forceps similar to O'Brien forceps except that there is a slide catch that keeps the teeth locked together.

O'Brien forceps thumb-operated tissue forceps with blades tipped by long rat-teeth, two on one side, one on the other.

observation something perceived by the senses of the clinician, e.g. pallor of mucosae, as distinct from an interpretation of what is sensed, e.g. anemic.

obsessive-compulsive behavior normal activities or behavior for the species, but repetitive or constant, even to the point of being damaging to the animal. Includes tail chasing, flank licking and licking.

obstacle test small objects such as hay bales, a drum, or furniture placed randomly in a hall or laneway that is unfamiliar to the patient which is then made to move through the test course in a dim light. The ability of the patient to pass without bumping into objects is accepted as freedom from night blindness. Because of the inability to communicate with the subject the results of such tests are usually impossible to interpret.

obstetrical, obstetric pertaining to or emanating from obstetrics.

o. anesthesia an anesthetic procedure designed especially for patients undergoing cesarean operation or intrauterine manipulation of the fetus. The particular additional responsibility in this kind of anesthesia is the survival of the fetus.

o. assistance assistance to the dam in the expulsion of the fetus varying from simple traction to episiotomy, fetal manipulation in the uterus, fetotomy and cesarean section.

o. chains see obstetric CHAIN.

o. instruments there is a large range including long-handled and finger-grip fetotomy knives; eyehooks, either long-handled or threaded onto obstetric rope; fetotome; obstetric wire; Kuhn's crutch for repelling or rotating the fetus; obstetric forceps; traction chains and handles; fetal extractor.

o. saw wire saw used in fetotomes. There are two types, Swedish and GIGLI WIRE SAW.

obstetrician a veterinarian who specializes in obstetrics.

obstetrics classically in human medicine the branch of medical science dealing with pregnancy, labor and the puerperium. In the veterinary context it is usually limited to the care of the dam and the unborn young during a parturition that cannot be completed, or has slowed to the point that the life of one or both patients is at risk.

obstipation intractable constipation.

obstruction the act of blocking or clogging; state of being clogged; refers usually to a tubular structure. See INTESTINAL, LARYNGEAL, NASOLACRIMAL duct obstruction, ESOPHAGEAL, OVIDUCTAL, URETHRAL, URETERAL obstruction.

ventricular outflow o. see VENTRICULAR outflow obstruction.

pseudo-o. functional, rather than physical, obstruction of the small intestine can occur with hypomotility and ileus.

obstructive having the characteristic of obstruction.

o. colic see equine COLIC.

o. constipation constipation of sufficient severity as to obstruct the rectum.

o. pulmonary disease see CHRONIC obstructive pulmonary disease.

o. shock circulatory failure caused by physical obstruction, e.g. cardiac tamponade or pulmonary embolism.

o. urolithiasis see URETERAL, URETHRAL obstruction.

o. uropathy any obstructive disease of the urinary tract.

obstruent 1. causing obstruction. 2. any agent or agency that causes obstruction.

obtund to render dull or blunt.

obtundent 1. having the power to dull sensibility or to soothe pain. 2. a soothing or partially anesthetic agent.

obturating pertaining to, having the characteristic of obturation.

obturation the act of closing off, as in intestinal obstruction; in orthodontics filling a root canal.

obturator a disk or plate that closes an opening, e.g. to close a cleft palate temporarily or permanently.

o. muscles the muscles that rotate the thigh laterally. See also Table 13.

o. nerve degeneration causes permanent obturator nerve paralysis (below).

o. paralysis commonly follows pressure on the obturator nerve during parturition; causes inability to adduct the thighs and the cow does the splits. When recumbent the legs are splayed with one on either side of the body.

Occam's razor a principle named after William of Occam, a 14th century philosopher. The generalization states that, if there are a number of explanations for observed phenomena, the simplest explanation is preferred. Called also scientific parsimony.

occipital pertaining to the occiput; located near the occipital bone, as the occipital lobe.

o. bone the unpaired bone constituting the back and part of the base of the skull. See also Table 10.

o. crest see external occipital CREST.

o. fracture see BASISPHENOID fracture.

o. lobe see occipital LOBE.

o. somites the most anterior of the embryo's somites; they are the origin of the occipital cartilages of the skull.

occipitalization synostosis of the atlas with the occipital bone.

occipitoatlantal of or relating to the occipital bone of the skull and the atlas cervical vertebrae.

occipitoatlantoaxial pertaining to the occiput, the atlas and the axis.

o. malformation see ATLANTO-OCCIPITAL malformation of Arab horses.
occipitocervical pertaining to the occiput and neck.
occipitofrontal pertaining to the occiput and the face.
occipitomastoid pertaining to the occipital bone and mastoid process.
occipitomental pertaining to the occiput and chin.
occipitoparietal pertaining to the occipital and parietal bones or lobes of the brain.
occipitotemporal pertaining to the occipital and temporal bones.
occipitothalamic pertaining to the occipital lobe and thalamus.
occiput the back of the skull. The external occipital protruberance and the occipital crests; may normally be very prominent in some dogs. Sometimes traumatized with hematoma formation resulting.
occlude to fit close together; to close tight; to obstruct or close off.
occlusal pertaining to closure; applied to the masticating surfaces of the teeth.
occlusio pupillae a complete fibrovascular membrane across the pupil.
occlusion 1. the act of closure or state of being closed; an obstruction or a closing off. 2. the relation of the teeth of both jaws when in functional contact during activity of the mandible.
abnormal o. malocclusion.
coronary o. see CORONARY occlusion.
functional o. contact of the maxillary and mandibular teeth that provides the highest efficiency in the centric position and during all exclusive movements of the jaw that are essential to mastication without producing trauma.
traumatic o. any abnormality of occlusion which causes injury to structures within the mouth.
occlusive pertaining to or effecting occlusion.
o. dressing 1. a surgical dressing applied to close off an aperture, e.g. a trephine opening into a maxillary sinus. 2. a dressing used on the skin that retains moisture and heat while increasing the concentration and absorption of medication being applied.
occult obscure or hidden from view.
o. blood test examination, microscopically or by a chemical test, of a specimen of feces, urine, gastric juice, etc., to determine the presence of blood not otherwise detectable. Feces are tested when intestinal bleeding is suspected but there is no visible evidence of blood in the stools.
o. heartworm infection infection by *Dirofilaria immitis* in which circulating microfilariae cannot be detected in the peripheral blood by the usual test methods.
o. spavin see occult SPAVIN.
o. virus the virus or infectious agent cannot be isolated but there is strong circumstantial evidence that it is present, e.g. scrapie prion.
occupation time parameter for usage of pens in a feedlot.
occupational therapy not a significant part of veterinary activity, but the term is applied to the teaching of tricks and activity patterns to big cats in captivity so that they escape boredom.
occurrence in epidemiological terms means frequency of a disease without defining incidence or prevalence.
OCD osteochondritis dissecans.
ocelli simple eyes of insects.
ocelot one of the nine species in the group of New World cats in the family Felidae. Called also *Panthera pardalis* and painted leopard. It has a small, 3 ft long body, golden to silver color with dark metallic spots on the body and stripes on the head and neck.
Ochotona see PIKA.
ochratoxicosis the nephropathy caused by poisoning by the mycotoxin OCHRATOXIN A. Characterized by degeneration of renal epithelium, polydipsia, polyuria, diarrhea and uremia. Pigs most affected. Resembles Balkan nephropathy in humans.
ochratoxin, ochratoxin A an isocoumarin derivative mycotoxin produced by the fungus *Acpergillus* spp. fungi. A nephrotoxin causing ochratoxicosis. Experimentally it has been shown to have teratogenic effects, especially in pigs, including eye malformation, hydrocephalus, short jaw, other skeletal and cardiac defects.
ochrometer an instrument for measuring capillary blood pressure.
ochronosis a yellow, brown or chocolate discoloration of cartilage, tendon sheaths and ligaments but not bone. Caused by deposit of alkapton bodies as the result of a metabolic disorder. Affected parts must be condemned as not suitable for human consumption.
ocular o. brown or gray discoloration of the sclera, sometimes involving also the conjunctivae and eyelids.
Ochsner forceps a strongly built, curved hemostat with rat-tooth tips to the blades.
Ocicat a new breed of cats, derived from crossing a chocolate point Siamese with a hybrid Abyssinian pointed Siamese. It is large with a long nose, large ears and a distinctive spotted coat in many different colors. Named because of its resemblence to an ocelot.
O'Connor program a breeding management system designed to ensure pregnancy in beef cows, based on a 63 day breeding season, having the cows in good body condition, the cows gaining weight during the breeding season, removal of sucking calves, and the use of fertile bulls.
OCR optical character recognition.
OCT ornithine carbamoyl transferase, a liver specific enzyme.
octa- word element. [Gr., L.] *eight.*
octachloronaphthalene one of the toxic highly CHLORINATED NAPHTHALENES.
octan occurring on the eighth day (every 7 days).
octatropine see ANISOTROPINE.
octavalent having a valency of 8.
Octodon degus see DEGU.
octopus a mollusc in the order Octopoda which has eight legs and eats crustaceans and shellfish.
blue-ringed o. see HAPALOCHLAENA MACULOSA.
Octopus maculatus see HAPALOCHLAENA MACULOSA.
ocular 1. pertaining to the EYE. 2. eyepiece (of a microscope).
o. albinism hypopigmentation of the iris.
o. carcinoma see CARCINOMA of skin.
extrinsic o. muscles see extraocular MUSCLES. See also Table 13.1F.
o. filariasis see THELAZIASIS, ONCHOCERCIASIS.
o. fornix the fold formed by the reflection of the conjunctiva from the eyelid to the globe of the eye.
o. globe see EYEBALL.
o. lymphomatosis see MAREK S DISEASE.
o. neurectoderm ECTODERM which gives rise to ocular tissues.
o. osteosarcoma see feline posttraumatic SARCOMA.
o. reflexes see MENACE REFLEX, PUPILLARY light reflex, CORNEAL reflex, CONSENSUAL light reflex.

o.-skeletal dysplasia combined ocular and skeletal defects found in Samoyeds and Labradors; ocular lesions include cataract and retinal detachment, the skeletal lesions include hip dysplasia, varus and valgus deformities, and many others.

o. ultrasound ultrasound examination of the eye is used to detect foreign bodies, intraocular masses, retinal detachment and asterid hyalitis. Especially useful when the cornea is opaque and ophthalmoscopic examination is impossible.

ocul(o)- word element. [L.] *eye*.

oculocardiac reflex bradycardia or cardiac arrest in the anesthetized animal as a result of manipulating the eyeball. A potential hazard of ophthalmic surgery.

oculocentesis paracentesis of the eyeball.

oculocephalic reflex see DOLL S EYE reflex.

oculocutaneous pertaining to or affecting both the eyes and the skin.

o. hypopigmentation affected Angus cattle are brown instead of black and have heterochromia; they are photophobic.

oculofacial pertaining to the eyes and face.

oculogyration the movement of the eyeball about the anteroposterior axis.

oculomotor pertaining to or affecting eye movements.

o. nerve the third cranial nerve; it contains motor and parasympathetic fibers. Various branches of the oculomotor nerve provide for muscle sense and movement in most of the muscles of the eye, for constriction of the pupil, and for accommodation of the eye. See also Table 14.

o. nerve paralysis causes pupillary dilatation, absence of pupillary light reflex, ventrolateral deviation of the eye, defective eye movement and palpebral ptosis.

oculomotorius the oculomotor nerve.

oculomycosis any fungal disease of the eye.

oculonasal pertaining to the eye and the nose.

oculoplastic denoting plastic surgery of the eye, eyelids, ocular muscles, lacrimal apparatus, or orbit.

oculopupillary pertaining to the pupil of the eye.

oculoskeletal dysplasia a syndrome of disproportionate dwarfism and retinal dysplasia with blindness reported in Labrador retrievers.

oculovestibulocephalic reflex see DOLL S EYE reflex.

oculozygomatic pertaining to the eye and the zygoma.

oculus pl. *oculi* [L.] eye.

OD 1. [L.] *oculus dexter* (right eye). 2. overdose.

oddi sphincter see SPHINCTER of Oddi.

oddments in wool marketing includes locks, bellies, crutchings, stained wool.

odds a method of expressing probability, e.g. at odds of 3 to 2 this can be converted to conventional terminology by using each number as the numerator and the sum of them as the denominator, i.e. 3/5, 2/5 or 60% or 40% or 0.6, 0.4. The odds are quoted as for or against. So that at odds of 3 to 2 the chances for an event happening are 3/5. The odds against it happening are 2/5.

posterior o. probability determined after consideration of the results of a study.

o. ratio the ratio, used particularly in case-control studies, estimates the chances of a particular event occurring in one population in relation to its rate of occurrence in another population.

Odland's bodies keratinosomes.

Odobenus rosmarus see WALRUS.

Odocoileostrongylus tenuis see PARELAPHOSTRONGYLUS *tenuis*.

Odocoileus a genus of North American deer. Includes *O. virginianus* (white-tailed deer; called also *Dama virginianus*), *O. hemionus* (mule deer), *O. hemionus columbiana* (black-tailed deer), *O. virginianus leucurus* (Columbian white-tailed deer).

odontalgia pain in a tooth.

odontectomy excision of a tooth.

odontic pertaining to the teeth.

odont(o)- word element. [Gr.] *tooth*.

odontoameloblastoma a tumor containing areas of ameloblastic epithelium and compound or complex odontoma.

odontoblast one of the connective tissue cells that deposit dentine and form the outer surface of the dental pulp adjacent to the dentine.

odontoblastic emanating from or pertaining to odontoblast.

o. layer the epithelioid layer of odontoblasts in contact with the dentine of teeth.

o. processes see DENTINAL fibers.

odontocetes members of the Odontoceti, a suborder of whales which have teeth, contrasted with the baleen whales which have plates of whalebone as their dental apparatus.

Odontoceti the suborder of toothed whales. Includes sperm whales, porpoises, grampuses, dolphins, beaked whales, bottle-nosed whales and narwhals.

odontoclast an osteoclast associated with absorption of the roots of deciduous teeth.

odontodysplasia cystica congenita a disease of calves recorded in Germany and thought to be due to environmental influences; characterized by abortion or stillbirth and congenital fibrous, cystic enlargement of mandibles and maxillae, and absence or deformity of some teeth.

odontodystrophy diseases of teeth caused by nutritional, metabolic or toxic errors and insults.

odontogenesis the origin and development of the teeth.

o. imperfecta dentinogenesis imperfecta.

odontogenic 1. forming teeth. 2. arising in tissues that give origin to the teeth.

o. cyst epithelium-lined cysts derived from cell rests or malformed enamel organs.

odontogeny odontogenesis.

odontoid like a tooth.

o. process see odontoid PROCESS.

odontology 1. scientific study of the teeth. 2. dentistry.

odontolysis the resorption of dental tissue.

odontoma a non-neoplastic malformation, a hamartoma, consisting of a mixture of enamel, dentine and cementum.

ameloblastic o. contains true neoplastic ameloblastic tissue. See AMELOBLASTIC odontoma.

complex o. all the dental tissues are represented but not in an organized form.

composite o. one consisting of both enamel and dentine in an abnormal pattern.

compound o. all the dental tissues are present and organized into denticles, tooth-like structures.

radicular o. one associated with a tooth root, or formed when the root was developing.

temporal o. most commonly in the mastoid process of the petrous temporal bone manifested as a discharging sinus at the base of the ear. Is a dentigerous cyst.

odontopathy any disease of the teeth.

odontoplasty the removal of enamel from teeth, but also applied to the remodeling of filling material or cast crowns.

odontoprisis see BRUXISM.
odontosis formation or eruption of the teeth.
odontotomy incision of a tooth.
odor a volatile emanation, usually unpleasant, perceived by the olfactory sense of the clinician. See also TAINT.
boar o. the rank male odor of the male pig, present in the meat of uncastrated male pigs more than 4 months old. Caused by androsterone. See also BOAR taint.
butyric acid o. odor of rancid butter.
irradiation o. meat sterilized by irradiation may develop a hydrogen sulfide odor.
sexual o. includes boar odor. Buck goat meat has a similar taint but in other ruminants the odor is much weaker. Female odors are not noteworthy with the possible exception of the meat from a sow in estrus at the time of slaughter.
odorant any substance capable of stimulating the sense of smell.
-odynia word element. [Gr.] *pain.*
odynometer an instrument for measuring pain.
odynophagia painful swallowing of food.
oe- for words beginning thus, see also those beginning *e-*.
Oeciacus vicarius the cliff swallow bug, possibly an overwintering vector for the western equine encephalomyelitis virus.
oedema see EDEMA.
Oedemagena a genus of flies similar to *Hypoderma* spp.
O. tarandi found in the caribou, musk-ox and reindeer. Causes significant damage to the skin and the lesions are conducive to blowfly strike. Called also reindeer warble fly.
Oenanthe a genus of the plant family Apiaceae; contain the toxin oenanthotoxin, a toxic alcohol which causes sudden death, convulsions and no lesions; includes *O. aquatica* (horsebane), *O. crocata* (hemlock water dropwort), *O. fistulosa* (water dropwort), *O. lachenalii* (parsley water dropwort), *O. palustris*, *O. pimpinelloides*, *O. sarmentosa*, *O. silaifolia*.
oenanthetol one of the poisonous alcohols in the plant *Oenanthe crocata.*
oenanthetone one of the poisonous alcohols in the plant *Oenanthe crocata.*
oenanthotoxin one of the poisonous alcohols in the plant *Oenanthe crocata.* Used loosely also to identify the group of three acetylenic alcohols, oenanthotoxin, oenanthetol, oenanthetone. Causes pupillary dilatation, salivation and convulsions in cattle, pigs and horses. Sheep are not as susceptible.
oesophageal see ESOPHAGEAL.
Oesophagodontus a blood-sucking nematode genus in the family Strongylidae.
O. robustus one of the blood-sucking strongyles of horses. Causes STRONGYLOSIS.
Oesophagostomum a genus of roundworms in the family Chabertiidae. Found in the large intestine. Cause the important disease ESOPHAGOSTOMOSIS (esophagostomiasis) in sheep. Includes *O. aculeatum*, syn. *O. apiosternum* (monkeys); *O. asperum*, syn. *O. indicum* (goats, sheep); *O. bifurcum* (monkeys); *O. brevicaudatum* (pig); *O. columbianum* (sheep, goats, camels and wild antelopes); *O. dentatum* (pig); *O. georgianum* (pig), *O. granatensis* (pig), *O. hsiungi* (pig), *O. indicum*, syn. *O. asperum* (goat, sheep), *O. longicaudatum*, syn. *O. quadrispinulatum* (pig), *O. maplestonei* (pig), *O. multifoliatum* (goat, sheep), *O. okapi* (okapi); *O. quadrispinulatum,* syn. *O. longicaudatum* (pig), *O. radiatum* (water buffalo, cattle); *O. rousseloti* (pig); *O. staphanostomum* (monkeys), *O. venulosum* (camel, deer, goat, sheep), *O. walkeri* (eland).
oesophagus see ESOPHAGUS.
oestrogen see ESTROGEN.
oestrogenism see ESTROGENISM.
Oestromyia leporina a fly similar to *Hypoderma* spp. which parasitizes moles and muskrats.
oestrone see ESTRONE.
Oestrus a genus of bot flies in the family Oestridae.
O. ovis a widespread species that deposits its larvae on the nostrils of sheep and goats. Invasion of the nasal cavity causes irritation manifested by sneezing, nose rubbing, noisy breathing and nasal discharge. It may cause ocular myiasis in humans. Called also sheep nasal bot fly.
oestrus see ESTRUS.
OFA Orthopedic Foundation for Animals; an organization dedicated to recording statistical data on orthopedic diseases, especially hip dysplasia in dogs.
off term used when talking of a horse's age, e.g. '6 off' for a horse which has just passed 6 years, as opposed to 'rising 7' for approaching 7 years.
off-center said of an x-ray beam which is not centered exactly over the part to be examined; the rays will be diverging as they pass it and the image will be distorted.
off feed the animal's food intake is less than normal.
off-flavor abnormal unappetizing flavor.
off-focus in radiography the radiation composed of x-rays produced by the interaction of electrons with objects, usually metal, other than the tube's target.
off-shears said of sheep which have been recently shorn.
off-side the off-side of a horse is the horse's right hand side. The horse is always mounted from the left or near side.
offal 1. nonmeat edible products from animal slaughter. Includes brains, thymus, pancreas, liver, heart, kidney, tripes, sausage casings, chitterlings, crackling rind. 2. by-product of milling, called also weatlings, middlings. A high-protein supplement for herbivores.
Office International des Epizooties a bureau in Paris established in 1924 for the accumulation and dissemination of information about animal diseases of international importance, particularly epidemiological information; abbreviated OIE. A voluntary organization that also publishes a valuable periodical on the subject.
office laboratory procedures clinical pathology tests suitable for use in a consulting room or from a country practitioner's vehicle.
official drugs medicines authorized by pharmacopeias and recognized formularies. Use of drugs other than these could be regarded by a court of law as being experimental.
offspring progeny generally; includes calf, lamb, kid, pig, foal, chicken, poult, duckling, puppy, kitten, cria. See also Table 20.
ofloxacin a fluoroquinolone antibiotic, similar to ciprofloxacin.
Ogmocotyle a genus of intestinal flukes (digenetic trematodes) in the family Notocotylidae.
O. indica a parasite of sheep, goats and cattle, infecting stomach and small and large intestines, but thought to be nonpathogenic.
Ohara's disease see TULAREMIA.
OHCS hydroxycorticosteroids.
OHE medical record abbreviation for ovariohysterectomy.
Ohio buckeye tree AESCULUS *glabra.*

ohm the SI unit of electrical resistance, being that of a resistor in which a current of 1 ampere is produced by a potential difference of 1 volt. Symbol Ω.

ohmmeter an instrument that measures electrical resistance in ohms.

Ohm's law the electric current flowing through a conductor is equal to the voltage divided by the resistance.

-oid suffix meaning resembling.

OIE Office International des Epizooties.

oil 1. an unctuous, combustible substance that is liquid, or easily liquefiable, on warming, and is not miscible with water, but is soluble in ether. Such substances, depending on their origin, are classified as animal, mineral or vegetable oils. 2. a fat that is liquid at room temperature.

automobile o. see SUMP OIL.

o. of chenopodium extracted from the plant *Chenopodium ambrosioides*. An old-time anthelmintic.

o.-contamination the coating of spilled crude oil on waterbirds that destroys the waterproofing and insulating properties of their feathers, predisposing them to hypothermia and impairing flight and swimming abilities. It also blocks nares, causes aspiration pneumonia, and has toxic effects on kidneys, reproduction and the gastrointestinal tract.

o. crop crops grown primarily for their oil production, e.g. linseed, safflower, sunflower, rapeseed.

crude petroleum o. crude oil and its several distillates are all relished by cattle and can cause poisoning. The oil as it is extracted from subterranean deposits varies widely in its additional contents. These may be salt or sulfur and cause poisoning by those substances. Oil causes vomiting and death from aspiration pneumonia. Animals do not do well and oil stays in the gut, appearing in the feces for long periods.

diesel and fuel o. see CRUDE OIL.

essential o. called also ethereal oil; see volatile oil (below).

ethereal o. see volatile oil (below).

fixed o. an oil that does not evaporate on warming and occurs as a solid, semisolid or liquid.

o. gland see UROPYGIAL GLANDS.

irritant o. occurs in plants; causes gastroenteritis; includes bryonin, croton and castor oils.

mineral o. a mixture of liquid hydrocarbons from petroleum. Mineral oil is available in both light (light liquid petrolatum) and heavy (liquid, or heavy liquid, petrolatum) grades. Light mineral oil is used chiefly as a vehicle for drugs, though it may also be used as a cathartic and to cleanse the skin. Heavy mineral oil is used as a cathartic, solvent and oleaginous vehicle. Excessive intake over a long period results in hypovitaminosis A.

o. pollution aquatic birds are worst affected because of pasting together of feathers, poisoning because of contamination of food source, blocking of nares and eyes and starvation because of unpalatability of food supply.

o. products includes kerosene (or kerosine, or paraffin), gasoline (or petrol), diesoline and additives to lubricating oils, e.g. highly chlorinated naphthalenes; any of them may cause poisoning.

o. spill accidental or negligent discharge of industrial oil on a body of water; effect is that the oil floats and pollutes the shore and covers aquatic birds and mammals with fatal results in most cases; salvage depends on capture of affected birds and animals and removing the oil.

sump o. see SUMP OIL.

sweet birch o. see METHYL salicylate.

turpentine o. see TURPENTINE oil.

volatile o. an oil that evaporates readily; such oils occur in aromatic plants, to which they give odor and other characteristics.

o. of Wintergreen see METHYL salicylate.

yew o. an irritant oil in *Taxus baccata*, but not the principal irritant in that plant—TAXINE is.

oilseed the seeds of the linseed plant, rapeseed or canola, peanut, safflower (*Carthamus tinctorius*); biproduct oils from seeds include corn, grapeseed, olive, sesame, sunflower.

ointment a semisolid preparation for external application to the body. Official ointments consist of medicinal substances incorporated in suitable vehicles (bases).

okapi a member of the giraffe family Giraffidae, but with short legs and neck. It has a similar head, face and lips to the giraffe, is about 5 ft tall at the withers and has horizontal stripes on its hindquarters and limbs. Called also *Okapia johnstoni*.

Okapia johnstoni see OKAPI.

Okazaki fragments DNA sequences, 100 to 200 nucleotides long, synthesized on the lagging strand of DNA in DNA replication. The fragments are subsequently ligated together to form a continuous strand. They are produced because of the need for DNA polymerase to always synthesize in a 5′ to 3′ direction.

Okie a system of grading of feeder calves purchased for feedlots and based on percentage of beef versus dairy blood in the breeding. The bulk of these cattle are yearling, baldy-faced, Hereford cross steers. The name is a contraction of Oklahoma.

OL [L.] *oculus laevus* (left eye).

-ol word termination indicating an alcohol or a phenol.

olamine USAN contraction for ethanolamine.

olaquindox a growth stimulant used as a feed additive for pigs.

Olax benthamiana Australian plant in the family Olacaceae; causes cyanide poisoning.

old dog encephalitis see old dog ENCEPHALITIS.

Old English mastiff see MASTIFF.

Old English sheepdog a large, compact dog distinguished by its profuse, shaggy, gray and white coat that covers the body, including the face, and obscures most of the body features. The tail is either naturally short or docked to a very short length. Called also the English bobtail. The breed is predisposed to congenital deafness, myelopoietic disorders, inherited cataracts and demodectic mange.

old man's beard CLEMATIS *vitalba*.

old tuberculin see TUBERCULIN.

Old World the Eastern Hemisphere; that part of the world (generally Europe, Asia, Africa) which was known before the discovery of America.

Oldenburgh, Oldenburgh whitehead polled, German, mutton and wool sheep. Called also German Whitehead.

-ole suffix meaning a small.

oleaginous oily; greasy.

oleander NERIUM *oleander*.

oleandomycin a macrolide antibiotic extracted from cultures of *Streptomyces antibioticus*, similar to, but less active and more toxic than erythromycin. Used as the phosphate salt.

oleandroside a digitoxin-like glycoside, one of the toxic substances in *Nerium oleander*.

oleate 1. a salt of oleic acid. 2. a solution of a substance in oleic acid.

olecranarthritis inflammation of the elbow joint.

olecranarthropathy disease of the elbow joint.
olecranoid resembling the olecranon.
olecranon the bony projection of the ulna at the elbow.
olefin oil-forming.
oleic acid a long-chain, 18-carbon, monounsaturated fatty acid found in animal and vegetable fats; the double bond is located at carbons 9,10; precursor of n-9 or omega 9 fatty acids.
olein 1. pertaining to oleic acid. 2. a principal constituent of nondrying fats and oils. Called also triolein, glyceryl trioleate. Animal fat containing a high proportion of olein has a greasy character.
oleo- word element. [L.] *oil.*
oleo oil the oily fraction of rendered animal fat.
oleoresin 1. a compound of a resin and a volatile oil, such as exudes from pines, etc. 2. a compound extracted from a drug by percolation with a volatile solvent, such as acetone, alcohol, or ether, and evaporation of the solvent.
oleostearin a firm fraction of rendered animal fat, used in margarine manufacture.
oleotherapy treatment by injections of oil.
oleothorax intrapleural injection of oil to compress and inactivate the lung.
oleovitamin a preparation of fat-soluble vitamins in fish liver or edible vegetable oil.
oleum pl. *olea* [L.] oil.
olfact a unit of odor, the minimal perceptible odor, being the minimal concentration of a substance in solution which can be perceived by a large number of normal individual animals, expressed in terms of grams per liter.
olfact- prefix meaning sense of smell.
olfaction 1. the act of smelling. 2. the sense of smell.
olfactology the science of the sense of smell.
olfactometer an instrument for testing the sense of smell.
olfactory pertaining to the sense of smell.

o. bulb the bulblike extremity of the olfactory tract on the rostral surface of the frontal lobe of each cerebral hemisphere; it is lodged against the cribriform plate through which the olfactory nerves pass.

o. glands in the mucosa of the nasal olfactory region; branched tubuloalveolar glands secreting serous fluid; cleanse the mucosal surface, dissolve odor-producing substances.

o. hair modified cilia projecting from olfactory cells in the mucosa of the nasal olfactory area.

o. mucosa specialized olfactory cells in a region of nasal mucosa covering ethmoturbinates, turbinates and nasal septum.

o. nerve the first cranial nerve made up of about 20 bundles and concerned with the sense of smell. The cell bodies are situated in the olfactory mucous membrane of the nose. Nerve fibers lead upward through openings in the cribriform plate of the ethmoid bone and connect with the cells of the olfactory bulb. From there the fibers pass inward to the cerebrum. See also Table 14.

o. neuroblastoma rare neoplasm, commonest in pups and kittens, characterized by local invasion of surrounding bone.

o. pit primordia of the nasal cavities commencing as pits in the olfactory placodes of the embryo. The pits deepen and finally open into the oral cavity as the choanae; the external orifices become the nostrils. Called also nasal pit.

o. system includes the olfactory part of the nasal mucosa, the olfactory nerves and the olfactory bulbs of the cerebrum.

o. tract a band of white nerve fibers visible on the ventral surface of the brain running caudally from the olfactory bulbs.

o. tractotomy surgical removal or transection of the olfactory tracts to produce an anosmia may be performed in cats as a means of controlling spraying and inappropriate urination.

olifantvel [Af.] the thickened, wrinkled, alopecic skin caused by BESNOITIA *besnoiti* in cattle.
oligemia deficiency in volume of the blood. Estimation of the degree of oligemia, the severity of dehydration, is a vital assessment in many diseases of animals. See PACKED CELL VOLUME, DEHYDRATION.
olig(o)- word element. [Gr.] *few, little, scanty.*
oligochromemia deficiency of hemoglobin in the blood.
oligochymia deficiency of chyme.
oligocythemia deficiency of the cellular elements of the blood.
oligodactyly congenital absence of one or more digits.
oligodendrocyte a cell of oligodendroglia.
oligodendroglia 1. the non-neural cells of ectodermal origin forming part of the adventitial structure of the central nervous system. 2. the tissue composed of such cells.
oligodendrogliocytes cells which form myelin in the nervous system; they are non-neuronal cells in nervous system adventitia.
oligodendroglioma a neoplasm derived from and composed of oligodendroglia.
oligodipsia abnormally diminished thirst.
oligodontia congenital absence of some of the teeth.
oligodynamic active in a small quantity.
oligogalactia deficient secretion of milk.
oligohemia oligemia.
oligohydramnios deficiency in the amount of amniotic fluid.
oligohydruria abnormally high concentration of urine.
oligomeganephronia congenital renal hypoplasia in which there is a reduction in the total number of nephrons, and hypertrophy of the nephrons.
oligomer a short polymer.
oligomucous cell a cell which develops into a goblet cell in the intestinal epithelium.
oligomycin inhibitor of oxidative phosphorylation, acting at the O-sensitivie subunit of F_0F_1-ATPase.
oligonucleotide a polymer made up of a few to a hundred or more nucleotides. Can be made synthetically to a specified sequence.

o. ligation assay a technique for detecting a specific nucleotide pair in a gene.

oligopeptides small peptides containing mixtures of amino acids.
oligophosphaturia deficiency of phosphates in the urine.
oligoplasmia deficiency of blood plasma.
oligopnea hypoventilation. Usually refers to reduced rate; apnea is complete cessation.
oligoptyalism diminished secretion of saliva.
oligosaccharide a carbohydrate which yields only a small number, usually 3 to 10, of monosaccharides on hydrolysis.
oligospermia deficiency of spermatozoa in the semen.
oligotrophia, oligotrophy a state of poor (insufficient) nutrition.
oligozoospermia see OLIGOSPERMIA.
oliguria reduced daily output of urine. This has veterinary significance if the net intake is normal or if water

is available ad lib; then it is a sign of renal insufficiency.

olingo a small, 14 to 20 inches high, yellow to brown bear. It is arboreal, nocturnal, omnivorous and forages in packs. Called also *Bassaricyon gabbii* (syn. *B. beddardi*).

olivary shaped like an olive.
o. body called also olivary nucleus; see OLIVE (2).
o. nucleus see OLIVE (2).

olive 1. the tree *Olea europaea* and its fruit. 2. olivary body; a rounded elevation lateral to the upper part of each pyramid of the medulla oblongata.
o. oil an emollient lubricant and mild laxative.

olivifugal moving or conducting away from the olive.

olivipetal moving or conducting toward the olive.

olivocerebellar tract nerve fibers passing from olive to contralateral cerebellum.

olivopontocerebellar pertaining to the olive, the middle peduncles and the cerebellar cortex.

Ollier's disease multiple enchondromatosis, dyschrondroplasia.

Ollulanus a genus of roundworms in the family Ollulanidae.
O. tricuspis found in the stomach of cats, foxes, wild cats and pigs. Causes chronic gastritis and emaciation in pigs and vomiting and wasting in cats.

olsalazine 5-amino-salicylate; used in the treatment of ulcerative colitis.

Olsen–Hegar needle holder a combination instrument constructed as a needle holder except that the half of each blade nearest to the pivot is shaped like a regular scissor blade. Used for driving the needle, then cutting the suture without changing instruments.

-olus suffix meaning a small.

-oma word element. [Gr.] *tumor, neoplasm.*

omarthritis inflammation of the shoulder joint.

omasal pertaining to or emanating from the omasum.
o. atony due to poorly digestible roughage in the diet; feed stagnates, leading to atony and eventually impaction.
o. functional stenosis achalasia of the reticulo-omasal sphincture as part of the syndrome of vagus indigestion of cows; causes accumulation of ingesta in the reticulorumen.
o. impaction usually identified at autopsy. Clinically there is recurrent indigestion with anorexia, scant, hard feces and possibly palpation of hard, distended omasum through the right flank or per rectum.
o. sulcus see omasal GROOVE.
o. transport failure see VAGUS indigestion.

omasitis usually accompanies rumenitis and, like it, is caused by infection with e.g. *Fusobacterium necrophorum* or with normal fungal inhabitants of the forestomachs, secondary to rumenoreticular acidosis as a sequel to grain engorgement; a necropsy finding rather than a clinical diagnosis.

omasoabomasal pertaining to the omasum and the abomasum.

omasum the third and smallest compartment of the forestomachs of the ruminant. Connects with the reticulum through the reticulo-omasal orifice and with the abomasum through the omasoabomasal orifice. Called also the bible because of its many, tightly packed leaves.

ombudsman a public official appointed to look into complaints by members of the public about mistreatment by officers of government instrumentalities.

omega the twenty-fourth and last letter of the Greek alphabet, Ω.
o. protein topoisomerase I of *Escherichia coli.*

3-omega fatty acids see omega-3 FATTY acids.

omental pertaining to or emanating from the omentum.
o. bursitis see intra-abdominal ABSCESS.
o. hernia passage of a loop of intestine through a tear in the omentum.
o. tear see omental hernia (above).
o. veil a lace-like omentum.

omentectomy excision of all or part of the omentum.

omentitis inflammation of the omentum.

omentofixation fixation of the omentum to the abdominal wall, especially to establish collateral circulation in portal obstruction or, in ruminants, to avoid recurrence of abomasal displacement. Called also omentopexy.
Hanover method o. in a right flank laparotomy the omentum is included in the suture line when the incision is closed.
Utrecht method o. through a left flank incision the omentum is sutured to the midline with a suture that passes through the abdominal wall and is tied on the outside of the skin.

omentopexy see OMENTOFIXATION.

omentorrhaphy suture or repair of the omentum.

omentum pl. *omenta* [L.] a fold of peritoneum extending from the stomach to adjacent abdominal organs. Lace-like in pigs, carnivores and the horse, sheetlike in ruminants.
gastrocolic o. the part of the greater omentum attached to the colon.
gastrohepatic o. the part of the lesser omentum attached to the liver.
greater o. the double fold of peritoneum derived from the dorsal mesogastrium that extends from the greater curvature of the stomach over the floor of the abdomen like an apron; poorly developed in the horse and well developed in ruminants.
lesser o. a peritoneal fold joining the lesser curvature of the stomach and the first part of the duodenum to the porta hepatis.
o. majus greater omentum.
o. minus lesser omentum.

omeprazole a substituted benzimidazole that is a long-acting inhibitor of gastric ATPase; used in the treatment of gastric ulcers.

omitis inflammation of the shoulder.

omnivore an OMNIVOROUS animal.

omnivorous eating both plant and animal foods.

omnopon see PAPAVERETUM.

omocervical artery see Table 9.

omohyoid pertaining to the shoulder and the hyoid bone.

OMP orotidine 5′ monophosphate.
OMP decarboxylase enzyme catalyzing the synthesis of uridine monophosphate, the first pyrimidine nucleotide essential for RNA structure.
OMP synthesis first nucelotide synthesized in the pathway of pyrimidine synthesis.

omphalectomy excision of the umbilicus.

omphalelcosis ulceration of the umbilicus.

omphalic pertaining to the umbilicus.

omphalitis inflammation, usually by infection, of the tissues of the umbilicus, usually involving the umbilical veins. See also JOINT-ILL.
avian o. caused by infection of the yolk by *Escherichia coli*, *Proteus* spp., bacilli and enterococci and manifested by embryonic and early chick mortality. The yolks are caseous or watery and the chickens edematous. Called also mushy chick disease.

omphal(o)- word element. [Gr.] *umbilicus.*

omphaloangiopagus twin fetuses, one of which

derives its blood supply from the umbilicus or placenta of the other.

omphaloarteritis inflammation of the umbilical arteries.

omphalocele protrusion, at birth, of part of the intestine through a defect in the abdominal wall at the umbilicus.

omphalomesenteric pertaining to the umbilicus and mesentery.

o. duct the duct which connects the yolk sac with the embryonal alimentary tract in vertebrates.

o. vessels arteries and veins carrying blood between the embryonal circulation and the yolk sac; destined to contribute to the blood supply to the gut and the portal venous drainage.

omphalopagus twins joined at the umbilicus.

omphalophlebitis inflammation of the umbilical veins. See also JOINT-ILL.

omphalorrhagia hemorrhage from the umbilicus.

omphalorrhea effusion of lymph at the umbilicus.

omphalorrhexis rupture of the umbilicus.

omphalosite the underdeveloped member of allantoidoangiopagous twins, joined to the more developed member (autosite) by the vessels of the umbilical cord.

omphalotomy the cutting of the umbilical cord.

Omsk hemorrhagic fever see ENCEPHALITIS.

on call see CALLING.

on-cost the supplementary costs, e.g. of a salary, include workers' compensation, leave loading, superannuation, payroll tax etc.

on-line the operation of computer terminals or peripherals in direct interactive telephonic communication with and under control of a central processing unit of a computer.

o. bibliographic database a database of reference material in the form of titles only or as abstracts which can be searched, usually by key words but possibly also by author or journal, and the selected data reproduced. The largest veterinary system is the program operated by the Commonwealth Agricultural Bureaux in the American Lockheed DIALOG system.

o. processing the interactive processing of data, e.g. by adding or deleting, while connected to a distant database. Contrast with BATCH PROCESSING.

on-the-rail dressing abattoir dressing of carcasses while they are still suspended from an overhead monorail and workers are stationed at key points along the chain.

***onc* genes** genetic elements that are causatively associated with cancer. Originally applied to genes found in rapidly transforming oncogenic retroviruses, particularly sarcoma viruses, which were designated v*onc* genes, most of which have a cellular homolog termed c*onc*. The term has been broadened to include genes found in other viruses and other cellular genes that are causatively associated with cancer.

Onchocerca a genus of nematode parasites in the family Onchocercidae. They are important as causes of ONCHOCERCOSIS. Their life cycles depend on the carriage of larval microfilariae by a variety of insects, chiefly mosquitoes, black flies and midges (families Simuliidae and Ceratopogonidae). The microfilariae are found in the lymph and connective tissue spaces of the skin. Called also *Wehrdikmansia*.

O. armillata the microfilariae are found in the skin of the hump, withers, neck, dewlap and umbilicus and the adults in the aorta of cattle, buffalo, sheep, goats and donkeys.

O. bohmi see ELAEOPHORA *bohmi*.

O. cebei found in nodules on the brisket and the lateral aspects of the hindlimbs of buffalo. Called also *O. sweetae*.

O. cervicalis found in the ligamentum nuchae of the horse and mule. The microfilariae are commonest in the area of the linea alba. Etiologically related to the occurrence of fistulous withers, poll evil, equine conjunctivitis and possibly equine recurrent ophthalmitis.

O. cervipedis found in the subcutaneous tissues of the neck and limbs of deer.

O. dukei adults are found in nodules in subcutaneous and perimuscular sites in cattle, mostly in the thorax, abdomen, diaphragm and thighs.

O. flexuosa occurs in deer.

O. garmsi parasites of deer.

O. gibsoni found in nodules under the skin of the brisket or the lateral aspect of the hindlimbs of *Bos taurus* and *Bos indicus* cattle.

O. gutturosa found in cattle and buffalo in the ligamentum nuchae, on the scapular cartilage and in the hip, shoulder and stifle areas.

O. lienalis found in the gastrosplenic ligament, on the capsule of the spleen and above the xiphisternum in cattle.

O. ochengi found in cattle, in nodules in cutaneous and subcutaneous sites on the udder, scrotum and flanks.

O. raillieti adult worms are found in the ligamentum nuchae, in subcutaneous cysts on the penis and in perimuscular connective tissue of donkeys.

O. reticulata a parasite of horses, mules and donkeys. Adult worms are found in the connective tissue of flexor tendons and suspensory ligament of the fetlock, mostly in the forelimb.

O. rugosicauda found in the subcutaneous fascia in the shoulders and back of roe deer.

O. sweetae see *O. cebei* (above).

O. synceri found in subcutaneous tissues in African buffalo.

O. tarsicola a parasite of deer.

O. tubingensis a parasite of deer.

O. volvulus causes dermatitis and ocular disease in humans.

onchocerciasis infestation by the filarioid worm *Onchocerca* spp.; can cause a variety of diseases listed generally under the heading of ONCHOCERCOSIS.

onchocercosis the diseases caused by infection with the nematodes *Onchocerca* spp. The presence of large numbers of microfilariae in the skin is associated with a severe, summer dermatitis called also wahi, kasen in cattle and summer mange or allergic dermatitis in horses. See also SWEET itch.

An association is suspected between periodic OPHTHALMIA in horses and onchocerciasis because of the finding of microfilariae in the eye and because *Onchocerca volvulus* is a known cause of blindness in humans.

The adult worms cause little problem to the animals but the hides and carcasses are damaged and reduced in value. The relationship between the worms and the occurrence of fistulous withers, poll evil and tendonitis is unproven. The lesions in the aorta caused by *O. armillata* are often extensive but appear to cause little clinical disease.

onchosphere see ONCOSPHERE.

Oncicola a genus of thorny-headed worms (acanthocephalans) in the family Macracanthorhynchidae.

O. campanulatus found in the intestine of dogs.

O. canis found in the intestine of dogs, coyotes, cats, lynx and bobcats. Chance infections can occur in young turkeys and cause cysts in the esophageal wall.

onco- word element. [Gr.] *tumor, swelling, mass.*
oncocyte oxyphil cells with acidophilic and granular cytoplasm, found in the endocrine glands and epithelial tissues.
oncocytoma a rare benign neoplasm arising from oncocytes.
oncofetal antigen a fetal antigen that is also produced by some types of cancer cells, such as carcinoembryonic antigen (CEA) or alpha-fetoprotein (AFP). See also oncofetal ANTIGEN.
oncogenes 1. genes carried by tumor viruses that are directly and solely responsible for the neoplastic transformation of host cells. Many oncogenes function after integration into the DNA of the host cell and some up-regulate normal downstream host cell genes to cause neoplasia. 2. any genetic element linked to cancer.
oncogenesis the production or causation of tumors.
multistep o. a theory of tumor induction involving several sequential stages including initiation, promotion and mutations.
viral o. a characteristic of some retroviruses, papovaviruses, adenoviruses, hepadnaviruses, herpesviruses and poxviruses.
oncogenic giving rise to tumors or causing tumor formation; said especially of tumor-inducing viruses.
oncogenous arising in or originating from a tumor.
oncology the sum of knowledge regarding tumors; the study of tumors.
oncolysate any agent that lyses or destroys tumor cells.
oncolysis destruction or dissolution of a neoplasm.
oncoma a swelling or tumor.
Oncorhynchus genus of finfish in family Salmonidae; include *O. clarki* (cutthroat trout), *O. gorbuscha* (pink salmon), *O. kisutch* (coho salmon), *O. mykiss* (rainbow trout), *O. tshawytscha* (chinook salmon). See Table 23.
Oncornavirinae a subfamily of viruses in the family RETROVIRIDAE, members of which cause leukosis in animals and include the viruses of avian LEUKOSIS, BOVINE viral leukosis, ROUS SARCOMA, MURINE leukemia virus, FELINE leukemia virus.
oncornavirus a member of the subfamily ONCORNAVIRINAE.
o.-associated cell membrane antigen see feline oncornavirus cell membrane ANTIGEN (FOCMA).
oncosis a morbid condition marked by the development of tumors.
oncosphere the larva of the tapeworm contained within the external embryonic envelope within the egg and armed with six hooks. Called also onchosphere.
oncotherapy the treatment of tumors.
oncotic pertaining to swelling.
o. pressure see oncotic PRESSURE.
oncotomy incision of a tumor or swelling.
oncotropic having special affinity for tumor cells.
oncovirus any virus that causes cancer. Includes the viruses of avian LEUKOSIS, ROUS SARCOMA complex, FELINE leukemia virus, FELINE sarcoma virus, BOVINE viral leukosis.
ondansetron a serotonergic antagonist, used as an antiemetic in chemotherapy.
Ondatra zibethica see MUSKRAT.
Ondiri disease a petechial fever caused by *Cytoecetes ondiri* in cattle and sheep. There is a pancytopenia, fever and petechiation of mucosae. See also BOVINE petechial fever.
one cell–one antibody rule the principle that any given B lymphocyte produces a specific antibody with a particular H chain isotype and one L chain isotype; because of class switching can be rephrased to imply one cell–one antibody specificity.
one-day event a contraction of the three-day event but like that contest is aimed at selecting the best all-round horse and rider. The events usually contested are show-jumping, dressage and cross-country.
one-hit theory lysis of an erythrocyte by complement can result from only one site of injury to the cell.
one-leafed cape tulip HOMERIA *flaccida.*
one-stage prothrombin time see PROTHROMBIN time test.
Ongole cattle draft, dairy, zebu type Indian cattle; gray-white with shorthorn horns.
onion *Allium cepa*; feeding of large quantities of bulbs causes hemolytic anemia, the hemolytic agent is *n*-propyl disulfide.
o. grass ROMULEA *rosea* (*R. australis*).
o. grass + ***Helminthosporium biseptatum*** causes incoordination and fall in fertility rate to very low level. Called also romulosis.
o. weed BULBINE *bulbosa.*
onion skinning said of blood vessels.
onlay a graft applied or laid on the surface of an organ or structure.
onomatology the science of names and nomenclature.
ONPG test *o*-nitrophenyl-β-D-galactopyranoside test, a test used to distinguish *Salmonella arizonae* from other *Salmonella* spp.
Ontario encephalitis, Ontario encephalomyelitis see hemagglutinating ENCEPHALOMYELITIS virus disease of pigs.
ontogeny the developmental history of an individual.
onychauxis overgrowth or thickening of nails.
onychectomy excision of a claw or nail or claw or nail bed. A surgical procedure carried out on single, damaged or diseased claws and at other times in domestic cats for social reasons and exotic cats, canines and ursids for the well-being of handlers and cage-mates.
onychia inflammation of the nail or claw bed, resulting in loss of the nail or claw.
Onychium contiguum Indian fern in the family Adiantaceae (ferns); contains the toxin ptaquiloside; causes neoplasm of the bladder wall and intermittent hematuria in cattle. Called also fuh.
onych(o)- word element. [Gr.] *the nails.*
onychodystrophy malformation of a nail or claw.
onychogenic producing or stimulating the formation of the substance of the claw, nail or hoof.
onychogryphosis, onychogryposis abnormal hypertrophy and curving of the nails or claws. In a racing Greyhound, a serious defect that reduces racing performance.
onychoid resembling a nail or claw.
onycholysis loosening or separation of a nail or claw from its bed; onychoschizia.
onychomadesis complete loss of the nails (claws).
onychomalacia softening of the nail or claw.
onychomycosis fungal disease of the nails or claws; the nails (claws) become misshapen, discolored, thickened and friable.
onychopathy any disease of the nails or claws.
onychorrhexis spontaneous splitting or breaking of the nails or claws.
onychoschisis fissures in the nails or claws.
onychosis disease or deformity of a nail or the nails.
onychotomy incision into a fingernail or toenail.
onyx 1. a variety of hypopyon. 2. a claw or nail.
oo- word element. [Gr.] *egg, ovum.*

ooblast a primitive cell from which an ovum ultimately develops.
Oochoristica a genus of tapeworms in the family Listowiidae. Primarily parasitic in reptiles.
O. megatoma found in squirrel monkeys.
oocyst the resistant stage of the life cycle of coccidial parasites. It contains a zygote and under appropriate conditions sporulates to become a mature infective oocyst. It may also remain infective for long periods in dry conditions.
o. patches see OOCYST plaques.
o. plaques raised patches up to 0.5 inch diameter in small intestinal epithelium in goats and sheep caused by heavy infestation by coccidial oocysts.
oocyte an immature ovum; it is derived from an oogonium, and is called a primary oocyte prior to completion of the first maturation division, and a secondary oocyte between the first and second maturation division.
Oodinium a protozoan parasite of fish affecting the skin and the gills. Called also *Piscinoodinium*, *Amyloodinium*, velvet disease.
O. limneticum causes a dermatitis in fish which gives them a varnished appearance. It may kill the fish within a few days.
O. pillularis a skin parasite of fish, tadpoles, axolotls and newts; causes a greenish appearance to the skin and kills by blocking the gills.
oogamous pertaining or relating to or produced by oogamy; heterogamous.
oogamy 1. fertilization of a large nonmotile egg by a small, motile male gamete or sperm, as seen in certain algae. 2. conjugation of two dissimilar gametes; heterogamy.
oogenesis the development of mature ova from oogonia. See also AVIAN oogenesis.
oogonium pl. *oogonia* [Gr.] an ovarian egg during fetal development; near the time of birth it becomes a primary oocyte.
ookinesis the mitotic movements of an ovum during maturation and fertilization.
oolemma see ZONA pellucida.
Oomycetes a class of fungi.
oomycosis infection with fungi of the class Oomycetes; a serious problem of aquarium fish.
Oonopsis North American plant genus in family Asteraceae; contains a selenocompound; causes alopecia, lameness, laminitis, hoof deformity, recumbency; includes *O. condensata*; called also golden weed.
oophorectomy excision of one or both ovaries; called also ovariectomy. The procedure is done for sterilization, tumors, severe infection, or other disorders of the ovary. Removal of the ovaries from a sexually immature animal prevents the development of secondary sex characters. If both ovaries are removed from an adult animal reproduction is not possible and the female sex hormones estrogen and progesterone are no longer produced.
oophoritis inflammation of an ovary; ovaritis.
oophor(o)- word element. [Gr.] *ovary*.
oophorocystectomy excision of an ovarian cyst.
oophorocystosis the formation of an ovarian cyst.
oophorohysterectomy excision of the ovaries and uterus.
oophoron an ovary.
oophoropexy see OVARIOPEXY.
oophoroplasty plastic repair of an ovary.
oophorostomy incision of an ovarian cyst for drainage purposes.
oophorotomy incision of an ovary.

ooplasm cytoplasm of an ovum.
oosperm a fertilized ovum.
oosporein a plant toxin which may produce nephritic gout in poultry.
ootid the cell produced by meiotic division of a secondary oocyte, which develops into the ovum. In mammals, this second maturation division is not completed unless fertilization occurs.
oozing exudation of fluid.
O/P oropharyngeal.
opacification the development of an opacity.
opacity 1. the condition of being opaque, e.g. corneal opacity, lenticular opacity. 2. an opaque area. 3. radiopacity is the capacity of a substance to absorb radiation, rather than permit its passage.
opalescent showing a milky iridescence, like an opal.
Opalina a common ciliated protozoon in the gut of fish and amphibians.
opaque impervious to light rays or, by extension, to x-rays or other electromagnetic radiation; neither translucent nor transparent.
o,p′-DDD see MITOTANE.
open 1. said of tissues, cavities and lesions which are normally enclosed when they are exposed to the environment. 2. not pregnant but capable of being pregnant. 3. a computer command which starts an application, inserts a document into a new document window or accesses a dialog box.
o. case lesions which carry a heavy load of infection are exposed to the air and represent a potent source of infection for other animals, e.g. an open case of bovine tuberculosis where the cow has extensive pulmonary lesions which are open to the bronchi.
o.-chest usually refers to thoracotomy or other procedure in which there is an opening in the chest wall.
o.-heart surgery in which the heart itself is exposed.
o. heels when the heels in the horse's feet are wide apart.
o. joint the joint capsule and synovial membrane have been punctured and the synovial lining of the joint is exposed to the air.
o. pen feedlot the animals in the lot are without shelter.
o. wound one without apposition of skin edges or left without sutures, usually to allow drainage and healing by granulation.
open nucleus breeding scheme a method of selecting and using breeding animals, consisting of a small number of elite breeding animals in a nucleus, or upper tier, and a large number of animals in a lower tier. In contrast to closed nucleus schemes, more flexible programs permit animals from the lower tiers to contribute progeny to the upper tiers.
A popular variation on this system is the GROUP breeding scheme.
opening an aperture, orifice or open space.
aortic o. 1. the aperture of the ventricle into the aorta. 2. the aperture in the diaphragm for passage of the descending aorta.
cardiac o. the opening from the esophagus into the stomach.
pyloric o. the opening between the stomach and duodenum.
operable subject to being operated upon with a reasonable degree of safety; appropriate for surgical removal.
operant see instrumental and operant CONDITIONING.
operate 1. to perform an operation. 2. the subject of an experiment which has undergone a specific surgical procedure.
operating 1. pertaining to operative surgery. 2. per-

taining to the operation of a computer. 3. pertaining to the operation of a business enterprise such as a farm or veterinary practice.

o. costs the total of variable and overhead costs.

o. profit gross income less the variable and operational overhead costs.

o. room a room set aside in which to perform surgical operations. Called also operating theater.

o. room emergency when a patient in the room is suddenly involved in a life threatening situation.

o. system a computer term; a collection of computer programs which control the operation of a computer as a whole. It is software often provided by the computer manufacturer. It controls input, output and management of files, the interaction of the central processing unit with the peripheral devices.

o. table designed for operative surgery with maximum flexibility to permit optimum positioning of the patient.

o. theater room devoted to the conduct of veterinary surgery.

operating theater a room in which surgical operations are conducted.

operation 1. any action performed with instruments or by the hands of a surgeon; a surgical procedure. 2. an agricultural, farming undertaking, e.g. cow–calf operation; an enterprise. 3. any effect produced by a therapeutic agent. For specific operations, see the specific name, such as Caslick operation.

o. code a computer term. See operation CODE.

cosmetic o. one intended to remove or correct a deformity in an esthetically acceptable manner.

covered o. one performed without exposing the part to the external air or to the possibility of confined tissues or organs escaping, e.g. covered CASTRATION.

exploratory o. incision into the body for determination of the cause of otherwise unexplainable symptoms.

flap o. any operation involving the raising of a flap of tissue.

radical o. one involving extensive resection of tissues for the complete extirpation of disease.

operations research mathematical or scientific analysis of a process.

operative 1. pertaining to an operation. 2. effective; not inert.

o. technique the actual step-by-step procedure of performing a specific surgical procedure.

operator 1. DNA sequence of 21 base pairs which is present within the promoter region of the *Escherichia coli* gene for β-galactosidase to which the regulatory protein called gene repressor protein binds. 2. sequences similar to (1), believed to be present in all genes.

opercular fold the fold formed by the second visceral arch in the embryo which expands caudoventrally and overgrows the caudal visceral arches of fish.

operculum pl. *opercula* [L.] 1. a lid or covering. 2. the folds of pallium from the frontal, parietal and temporal lobes of the cerebrum overlying the insula. 3. gill cover in a fish.

dental o. the hood of gingival tissue overlying the crown of an erupting tooth.

trophoblastic o. the plug of trophoblast that helps close the gap in the endometrium made by the implanting blastocyst.

operon a segment of a chromosome comprising an operator gene and closely linked structural genes having related functions, the activity of the latter being controlled by the operator gene through its interaction with a regulator gene.

Ophidascaris a genus of roundworms found in reptiles, including *O. morelia* in pythons and *O. robertsi*, *O. labiato-papillosa* in a variety of snakes.

Ophidia the suborder of reptiles which includes the snakes, as distinct from the lizards.

ophidian member of the suborder Ophidia; see SNAKE.

ophidism poisoning by snake venom. Called also envenomation—properly the injection of the poison rather than the effects of the poison on the patient.

Ophionyssus a genus of mites of the family Dermanyssidae.

O. natricis blood-sucking mite of captive snakes. May cause anemia or transmit bacterial disease.

ophthalmencephalon the retina, optic nerve and visual apparatus of the brain.

ophthalmia severe inflammation of the eye or of the conjunctiva or deeper structures of the eye.

albinistic o. occurs in the pseudo-albinistic fry of the Atlantic salmon; results from the bilateral exophthalmia which is inherited in the species.

contagious o. a disease of sheep and goats caused by RICKETTSIA (*Colesiota*) *conjunctivae*. Characterized by lacrimation, blepharospasm, keratitis and corneal opacity.

o. neonatorum a purulent conjunctivitis occurring during the first 10 days of life, before the eyelids separate in puppies and kittens. In kittens usually caused by feline herpesvirus (rhinotracheitis).

periodic o. a disease of horses with a causal relationship to infection wtih *Leptospira* spp. and possibly *Onchocerca cervicalis*. Manifested by recurrent attacks of photophobia, lacrimation, conjunctivitis, keratitis, hypopyon and iridocyclitis. Usually terminates in blindness.

sympathetic o. inflammation of the uveal tract of the originally unaffected eye following a wound or disease involving the uveal tract or lens of the other eye.

ophthalmic pertaining to the eye.

o. genetics the study of inherited eye diseases.

o. reaction ophthalmoreaction.

ophthalmitis inflammation of the eyeball.

follicular o. see CHERRY EYE.

ophthalm(o)- word element. [Gr.] *eye*.

ophthalmocele see EXOPHTHALMOS.

ophthalmodonesis trembling motion of the eyes.

ophthalmodynamometry determination of the blood pressure in the retinal artery.

ophthalmoeikonometer an instrument used to determine both the refraction of the eye and the relative size and shape of the ocular images.

ophthalmography description of the eye and its diseases.

ophthalmogyric see OCULOGYRATION.

ophthalmolith a lacrimal calculus.

ophthalmologist a veterinarian who specializes in diagnosing and prescribing treatment for defects, injuries and diseases of the EYE, and is skilled at delicate eye surgery, such as that required to remove cataracts. Called also eye specialist.

ophthalmology that branch of veterinary medicine dealing with the eye, its anatomy, physiology, pathology, etc.

ophthalmomalacia abnormal softness of the eyeball.

ophthalmometer an instrument used in ophthalmometry.

ophthalmometry determination of the refractive powers and defects of the eye.

ophthalmomycosis any disease of the eye caused by a fungus.

ophthalmomyiasis infection of the conjunctival sac by fly larvae. See GEDOELSTIA and OESTRUS *ovis*.

ophthalmomyotomy surgical division of the muscles of the eyes.
ophthalmoneuritis inflammation of the optic nerve.
ophthalmopathy any disease of the eye.
ophthalmoplasty plastic surgery of the eye or its appendages.
ophthalmoplegia paralysis of the eye muscles.
o. externa paralysis of the extraocular muscles.
o. interna paralysis of the iris and ciliary apparatus.
nuclear o. that due to a lesion of nuclei of motor nerves of the eye.
partial o. that affecting some of the eye muscles.
progressive o. gradual paralysis of all the eye muscles.
total o. paralysis of all the eye muscles, both intraocular and extraocular.
ophthalmoptosis see EXOPHTHALMOS.
ophthalmoreaction local immune hypersensitivity reaction of the conjunctiva after instillation into the eye of toxins or organisms causing glanders and tuberculosis, being more severe in those animals affected with these diseases. Called also ophthalmic reaction.
ophthalmorrhagia hemorrhage from the eye.
ophthalmorrhea oozing of blood from the eye.
ophthalmorrhexis rupture of an eyeball.
ophthalmoscope an instrument for examining the interior of the eye. It sends a bright, narrow beam of light through the lens of the eye, and contains a perforated mirror and lenses through which the veterinarian can examine interior parts of the eye. It is helpful in detecting possible disorders of the eyes, as well as disorders of other organs that are reflected in the condition of the eyes.
direct o. one that produces an upright, or unreversed, image of approximately 15 times magnification.
indirect o. one that produces an inverted, or reversed, direct image of two to five times magnification.
ophthalmoscopic pertaining to the ophthalmoscope.
o. examination see OPHTHALMOSCOPY.
ophthalmoscopy examination of the eye by means of the ophthalmoscope. In animals the procedure presents difficulties because of the need for restraint. For best results requires darkness, pupil dilatation, absence of distraction, minimum of restraint. See also OPHTHALMOSCOPE.
ophthalmostasis fixation of the eye with the ophthalmostat.
ophthalmostat an instrument for holding the eye steady during operation.
ophthalmosteresis loss of an eye.
ophthalmosynchysis effusion into the eye.
ophthalmotomy incision of the eye.
ophthalmoxerosis xerophthalmia; abnormal dryness and thickening of the conjunctiva and cornea due to vitamin A deficiency or to local disease.
Ophyra aenescens a muscid fly which is a predator for filth flies.
opiate any sedative narcotic containing opium or any of its derivatives. Used chiefly to induce sleep and to suppress cough. See also OPIOID.
endogenous o. naturally occurring substances with opiate effects.
Opiliones see HARVESTMEN.
opioid 1. any synthetic narcotic that has opiate-like activities but is not derived from opium. 2. denoting naturally occurring peptides, e.g. enkephalins, that exert opiate-like effects by interacting with opiate receptors of cell membranes.
endogenous o. see ENDORPHIN, ENKEPHALIN.
o. receptors specific receptor sites for opioids, named for the drugs which have a high binding affinity for them. The main ones are mu (morphine), kappa (opioid agonist-antagonists such as pentazocine) and delta (enkephalin endogenous opioids). Subtypes exist and others, such as sigma and epsilon, have been identified.
opisthorchiasis infection and obstruction of the biliary tract by the liver flukes *Opisthorchis* spp. Characterized by abdominal pain, diarrhea, jaundice and ascites.
Opisthorchis a genus of flukes (digenetic trematodes) parasitic in the liver and biliary tract of various reptiles, birds and mammals, including humans. Causes opisthorchiasis.
O. felineus see *Opisthorchis tenuicollis* (below).
O. sinensis see CLONORCHIS *sinensis*.
O. tenuicollis found in the bile ducts, rarely the pancreatic duct and intestine, of dogs, cats, foxes, pigs and the Cetacea and humans.
O. viverrini occurs in domestic and wild cats, civets, dogs and humans.
opisthotonos a form of spasm in which the head and tail are bent upward and the abdomen bowed downward. Indicates a lesion in the area of the medulla, pons and midbrain, or a general decrease in synaptic resistance, as in tetanus.
opium the air-dried milky exudation from unripe capsules of the opium poppy *Papaver somniferum* or its variety *P. somniferum album*. Opium contains some 25 alkaloids, the most important being morphine (from which heroin is derived), narcotine, codeine, papaverine, thebaine and narceine; the alkaloids are used for their narcotic and analgesic effect. It is poisonous in large doses. Because it is highly addictive, opium production and cultivation of opium poppies is prohibited by most nations by international agreement, and its sale or possession for other than medical or veterinary uses is strictly prohibited by law.
camphorated tincture of o. see PAREGORIC.
o. poppy see PAPAVER *somniferum*.
opocephalus a monster with ears fused to the head, one orbit, no mouth, and no nose.
opodidymus a monster with two fused heads and sense organs partly fused.
opossum a cat-sized, arboreal, insectivorous and carnivorous marsupial with dense, black through every shade to white, fur with a pointed snout, bare prehensile tail and a noted ability to play dead when in danger—hence playing 'possum. Called also American or Virginian opossum, *Didelphis virginiana*.
opportunistic 1. denoting a microorganism which does not ordinarily cause disease but becomes pathogenic under certain circumstances. 2. denoting a disease or infection caused by such an organism.
opportunity cost the amount of money that is alienated by choosing to use it for one project rather than another, i.e. the opportunity to make a profit by investing in another project is lost.
opsin the protein component of retinal pigments, e.g. rhodopsin.
opsinogen a substance (antigen) capable of stimulating the formation of opsonins.
opsiuria excretion of urine more rapidly during fasting than after a meal.
opsoclonia, opsoclonus involuntary, nonrhythmic horizontal and vertical oscillations of the eyes.
opsogen see OPSINOGEN.
α_2-opsonic protein see FIBRONECTIN.
opsonin a substance such as antibody, complement or

properdin that renders bacteria and other cells more susceptible to phagocytosis.

immune o. an antibody that, when bound to particulate antigen, enhances in vivo or in vitro phagocytosis; the Fc portion of the antibody binds to an Fc receptor on the surface of the phagocytic cell.

opsoninopathy a condition marked by reduced levels of serum opsonins, leading to increased susceptibility to infection.

opsonization the rendering of bacteria and other foreign substance subject to phagocytosis.

opsonize to subject to opsonization.

opsonocytophagic denoting the phagocytic activity of blood in the presence of serum opsonins and homologous leukocytes.

opsonotherapy treatment based on the administration of bacterial antibodies to increase the opsonic index.

optic of or pertaining to the eye.

o. chiasma see optic CHIASM.

o. cortex see VISUAL cortex.

o. cup activity see INTRARETINAL SPACE.

o. disk the disk in the fundus of the eye marking the point at which the optic nerve enters; it is accompanied by blood vessels, is oval, light in color and the blind spot of the retina.

o. nerve the second cranial nerve; it is purely sensory and is concerned with carrying impulses for the sense of sight. The rods and cones of the retina are connected with the optic nerve which leaves the eye slightly to the nasal side of the center of the retina. The point at which the optic nerve leaves the eye is called the blind spot because there are no rods and cones in this area. The optic nerve passes through the optic foramen of the skull and into the cranial cavity. It then passes backward and undergoes a division; those nerve fibers leading from the nasal side of the retina cross to the opposite side in the optic chiasma while those from the temporal side continue to the thalamus uncrossed. The nerve tracts proceeding backward from the optic chiasm, pass around the cerebral peduncle, and dividing into a lateral and medial root, which end in the superior colliculus and lateral geniculate body, respectively. After synapsing in the thalamus the neurons convey visual impulses to the occipital lobe of the brain.

Injury to the nerve leads to partial or complete loss of sight on the opposite side. Commonly bilateral.

o. nerve aplasia an uncommon congenital anomaly, most frequently seen in Collie dogs; affected animals are blind from birth. Hypovitaminosis A and prenatal infection with bovine virus diarrhea are possible causes.

o. nerve inflammation optic neuritis.

o. primordia the eyes begin in the embryo as a pair of shallow optic grooves on each side of the developing forebrain. The grooves form optic vesicles which invaginate to form a double-walled optic cup.

o. radiation fibers from the lateral geniculate body entering the occipital cortex.

o. stalk the evagination from the neural tube of the developing embryo which develops the optic cup at its extremity; the stalk persists as the optic nerve.

o. sulcus see optic GROOVE.

o. vesicle the initial evagination from the neural tube which gives rise to the optic cup and the optic stalk.

optical pertaining to vision.

opticele, opticoele in the embryonic eye, the potential space between the pigment epithelium and the neural retina.

opticociliary pertaining to the optic and ciliary nerves.

opticofacial reflex see MENACE REFLEX.

opticopupillary pertaining to the optic nerve and pupil.

optics the science of light and vision.

opto- word element. [Gr.] *visible, vision, sight.*

optochin susceptibility test a means of distinguishing *Streptococcus pneumoniae* from other alpha hemolytic streptococci.

optogram the visual image formed on the retina by bleaching of visual purple under the influence of light.

optokinetic pertaining to movement of the eyes, as in nystagmus.

optometer a device for measuring the power and range of vision.

optomyometer a device for measuring the power of ocular muscles.

Opuntia American plant genus in family Cactaceae; spines cause stomatitis; called also prickly pear.

OR operating room.

or- prefix meaning mouth.

ora[1] pl. *orae* [L.] an edge or margin.

o. ciliaris retinae the marginal zone between the sensitive retina and nonsensitive retina and the commencement of the ciliary body.

o. serrata retinae the zigzag margin of the human retina of the sensory part of the eye. Located near the ciliary body. In domestic mammals the margin is less obviously serrated.

ora[2] [L.] plural of *os*, mouth.

orache ATRIPLEX *patula.*

orad toward the mouth.

oral 1. pertaining to the mouth; taken through or applied in the mouth, as an oral medication. 2. denoting that aspect of the teeth which faces the oral cavity or tongue.

o. cavity see MOUTH.

o. contraceptive contraceptive agent taken by mouth.

o. dysphagia see oropharyngeal DYSPHAGIA.

o. necrobacillosis an infectious stomatitis of calves caused by *Fusobacterium necrophorum.* There are deep necrotic ulcers in the mouth, e.g. lateral to the molar teeth, foul breath, drooling saliva, fever and toxemia. See also calf DIPHTHERIA. Called also necrotic stomatitis.

o. neoplasm is usually squamous cell carcinoma of the gum epithelium. It impedes mastication.

o. plasmacytoma an unusual benign oral neoplasm of older dogs; appears as a red, lobulated, raised mass on the gingiva.

o. plate separates the stomodeum from the pharyngeal cavity; subsequently breaks down to become the palatoglossal arch; called also oropharyngeal membrane.

o. restraint the use of a mouth speculum, gag or wedge to permit examination and the carrying out of procedures in the mouth without danger of being bitten.

orang-utan a small anthropoid ape, 150 lb, 5 ft tall, covered with mahogany colored hair and with a striking facial similarity to humans. Herbivorous, not very agile and sleeps in trees. Called also *Pongo pygmaeus.*

orange[1] a composite color between yellow and red.

o. sneezeweed HELENIUM *hoopesii.*

o.-flowered cestrum CESTRUM *auranticum.*

orange[2] the tree *Citrus aurantium* and its edible yellow fruit; the peel of two varieties is used in making various pharmaceuticals.

orb-weavers spiders of the family Epeiridae; they

contain poisonous substances in their body fluids and eggs and may cause illness in animals that eat them accidentally.

orbicular circular; rounded.

orbicularis oculi muscle see Table 13.1F.

orbicularis oris muscle see Table 13.1A.

orbiculus ciliaris the posterior part of the ciliary body, the ciliary ring.

orbit 1. the bony cavity containing the eyeball and its associated muscles, vessels and nerves; the ethmoid, frontal, lacrimal, nasal, palatine, sphenoid and zygomatic bones and the maxilla contribute to its formation. 2. the path of an electron around the nucleus of an atom.

orbital pertaining to the eye socket.

o. abscess may be associated with orbital cellulitis. Can be caused by foreign bodies, wounds, tooth infection, or fractures. Clinical signs include protrusion of the globe, pain on opening of the mouth, and often edema of the eyelids.

o. arteries the external and internal ophthalmic arteries.

o. gland see HARDERIAN GLAND.

o. index the ratio of the height of the orbit to the width.

o. ligament the fibrous band which completes the lateral margin of the orbit in the cat, dog and other species which do not have a post-orbital bar; reaches from the frontal process of the zygomatic bone to the zygomatic process of the frontal bone.

o. neoplasm in dogs sarcoma and carcinoma common, multilobular osteoma occurs; in other species tumors uncommon except for metastatic lymphoma and cancer eye in cattle and to a lesser extent in horses.

o. sinus bleeding often the method of bleeding small rodents; the anesthetized rat or mouse is bled via a microhematocrit tube or pipette inserted through the medial canthus of the eye.

orbitography radiography of the orbit.

contrast o. the use of positive or negative contrast agents injected into the orbital cone to define space-occupying lesions.

orbitomeatal a line running from the external auditory meatus of the skull to the lower border of the orbit.

orbitonasal pertaining to the orbit and nose.

orbitonometer an instrument for measuring backward displacement of the eyeball produced by a given pressure on its anterior aspect.

orbitotomy incision into the orbit.

Orbivirus a genus of viruses in the the family REOVIRIDAE that includes African horse sickness, bluetongue, epizootic hemorrhagic disease of deer and Ibaraki disease viruses.

orcein a brownish-red coloring substance obtained from orcinol; used as a stain for elastic tissue.

orcein-Giemsa stain useful because of its capacity to stain elastic fibers, the metachromatic granules of mast cells, and differentiates smooth muscle from collagen.

orchard grass see DACTYLIS GLOMERATA.

orchard sorrel see RUMEX.

orchidectomy see ORCHIECTOMY.

orchidic pertaining to a testis.

orchidorrhaphy see ORCHIOPEXY.

orchiectomy excision of one or both testes. This procedure is common in animal husbandry as a promoter of growth. It may also be necessary when a testis is seriously diseased or injured. In farm parlance it is castration, caponizing for birds and gelding for horses. It is included in the term mark for lambs. The euphemism in dogs and cats is to 'have him fixed up', 'doctored' or 'dressed' (Scotland).

Removal of both testes before puberty prevents the development of secondary sex characters and behavior because of the deficiency of testosterone. If the procedure is performed after puberty, when the masculine characteristics are already developed, the changes that occur are much less extreme. The ability to reproduce is ended, there is a diminution of the production of testosterone and sexual activity disappears, for the most part.

orchiepididymitis inflammation of a testis and epididymis.

orchi(o)- word element. [Gr.] *testis*.

orchiocele 1. hernial protrusion of a testis. 2. scrotal hernia. 3. tumor of a testis.

orchiopathy any disease of the testes.

orchiopexy surgical fixation of an undescended testis in the scrotum; an unethical practice in veterinary medicine.

orchioplasty plastic surgery of a testis.

orchioscheocele scrotal tumor with scrotal hernia.

orchiotomy incision and drainage of a testis.

orchitis inflammation of a testis. *Brucella abortus* and *B. suis* are known causes in cattle and pigs respectively. In rams *Actinobacillus seminis* is cultured from some lesions. *Corynebacterium pseudotuberculosis* causes a suppurative orchitis. The lesions may be specified as interstitial, intertubular or intratubular.

The clinical signs of acute orchitis are swelling of one or both testes with pain and sensitivity to touch. In chronic orchitis there is no pain but the testes swell slowly and become hard.

Orchopeas howardii a flea that parasitizes squirrels but can be found on poultry.

Orcinus orca see killer WHALE.

orciprenaline see METAPROTERENOL.

order a taxonomic category subordinate to a class and superior to a family (or suborder).

o. statistic see RANK.

ordinate the vertical line in a graph along which is plotted one of the factors considered in the study, as temperature in a time–temperature study. The other line is called the abscissa.

Oregon disease DEEP PECTORAL MYOPATHY of turkeys and broilers.

Oreochromis niloticus see TILAPIA NILOTICUS.

orexigenic increasing or stimulating the appetite.

orf see contagious ECTHYMA.

organ a somewhat independent body part that performs a specific function or functions.

o. of Corti the organ lying against the basilar membrane in the cochlear duct, containing special sensory receptors for hearing, and consisting of neuroepithelial hair cells and several types of supporting cells.

effector o. a muscle or gland that contracts or secretes, respectively, in direct response to nerve impulses.

enamel o. see ENAMEL organ.

genital o. see PENIS, VULVA, etc.

Golgi tendon o. see GOLGI TENDON ORGAN.

gustatory o. TASTE bud.

gustus o. see TASTE bud.

o. of Jacobson see vomeronasal organ (below).

ocular o. see EYE.

olfactory o. the organ of smell in the nasal mucosa consisting of specialized cells with a tuft of very fine processes protruding into the nasal cavity. Internally they communicate with the olfactory nerves which pass through the cribriform plate of the ethmoid bone to synapse with cells in the glomeruli of the olfactory bulb of the brain.

reproductive o's those concerned with reproduction. See also PENIS, VULVA, etc.

female reproductive o. paired ovaries, uterine tubes, uterus, vagina and vulva.

male reproductive o. paired testes, gonadal duct systems (epididymis, ductus deferens), accessory glands, urethra, penis, prepuce and scrotum.

sense o's, sensory o's organs that receive stimuli that give rise to sensations, i.e. organs that translate certain forms of energy into nerve impulses which are perceived as special sensations.

solid o. any organ which does not contain a cavity or lumen and which is not gaseous; that is an organ which consists of parenchyma and stroma, the latter often arranged as trabeculae or surrounding groups of parenchymatous cells to provide support, e.g. liver, kidney.

spiral o. organ of Corti.

spiral o. of the inner ear the COCHLEA.

subfornical o. a small tubercle in the floor of the third ventricle.

target o. the organ affected by a particular hormone.

tubular o. an organ characterized by the presence of a lumen and four concentric tunics in its wall; centrifugally the layers are mucosal, submucosal, muscular and adventitia-serosal.

urinary o.'s see KIDNEY, URETER, URETHRA, URINARY BLADDER.

vascular o. of the lamina terminalis in the wall of the third ventricle of the brain.

vestibulocochlear o. the cochlear duct, semicircular canals, utricle and saccule that occupy the osseous labyrinth.

vestigial o. an undeveloped organ that, in the embryo or in some remote ancestor, was well developed and functional.

vomeronasal o. part of the olfactory sense system that consists of a pair of fleshy tubes found on the floor of the nasal cavity on either side of the nasal septum, supported by cartilage sleeve. Probably concerned with scenting and aftersmell of food.

organ grinder monkey see CAPUCHIN MONKEY.

organ-specific restricted to, or having an effect only on, a particular organ, as an organ-specific antigen or enzyme.

organelle a specialized structure of a cell, such as a mitochondrion, Golgi complex, lysosome, endoplasmic reticulum, ribosome, centriole, chloroplast, cilium or flagellum.

organic 1. pertaining to an organ or organs. 2. having an organized structure. 3. arising from an organism. 4. pertaining to substances derived from living organisms. 5. denoting chemical substances containing carbon. 6. pertaining to or cultivated by use of animal or vegetable fertilizers, rather than synthetic chemicals.

o. acids acids which contain carbon.

o. arsenic see ARSENIC.

o. chemistry see organic CHEMISTRY.

o. disease a disease due to or accompanied by structural changes.

o. fluoride see FLUORINE.

o. mercury see MERCURY.

organification conversion of glycoprotein in the thyroid gland resulting in the formation of thyroglobulin.

organism an individual animal or plant.

organization 1. the process of organizing or being organized. 2. the replacement of blood clots by fibrous tissue. 3. an organized body, group or structure.

organizer a special region of the embryo that is capable of determining the differentiation of other regions.

primary o. the dorsal lip region of the BLASTOPORE.

organo- word element. [Gr.] *organ*.

organoarsenicals see ARSENIC.

organobromine includes some toxic compounds, e.g. polybrominated biphenyls.

organochlorines see CHLORINATED HYDROCARBONS.

o. poisoning cause excitement and irritability, tremor, ataxia, weakness, paralysis, convulsions.

organogenesis, organogeny the development of organs.

organoid 1. resembling an organ. 2. a structure that resembles an organ.

organology the sum of what is known regarding the body organs.

organomegaly enlargement of a viscus; visceromegaly.

organomercurial any mercury-containing organic compound, e.g. the mercurial diuretics. See also MERCURY.

organometallic consisting of a metal combined with an organic radical, e.g. organical arsenical, organomercurial.

organon pl. *organa* [Gr.] organ.

organophosphate term commonly used to describe ORGANOPHOSPHORUS COMPOUNDS.

organophosphorus compound an organic ester of phosphoric or thiophosphoric acid; such compounds are powerful acetylcholinesterase inhibitors and are used as insecticides and anthelmintics. They are also used industrially as fire-resistant hydraulic fluids, coolants and lubricants and animals may be accidentally exposed to them. All organophosphorus compounds are poisonous, even those used pharmacologically, if given in large enough doses or in particular circumstances.

o. c.-induced delayed neurotoxicity paralysis occurring 3 weeks after exposure to organophosphorus compounds, especially industrial organophosphates; the degree of paralysis varies from weakness appearing as knuckling of the fetlocks to complete flaccid paralysis.

industrial o. c. see organophosphorus compound (above). Includes aryl-, cresyl-, and tolyl- phosphates used commercially as flame retardants and wood preservatives. Access to the substances or, more commonly, premises contaminated by them may cause poisoning, especially delayed neurotoxicity.

o. c. insecticide includes a very wide range of contact insecticides, systemic insecticides for animals and plants; all have significant toxic potential.

o. c. poisoning signs of poisoning differ between the species. (1) Cattle show salivation and diarrhea, tremor and stiffness and a pathognomonic constriction of the pupil. (2) Sheep and pigs show predominantly nervous signs. In sheep ataxia, posterior paralysis and spinal cord degeneration are indicators. In pigs nystagmus, tremor, recumbency, posterior paralysis and drowsiness occur. (3) Horses show abdominal pain, diarrhea, ataxia, dyspnea and in foals acute bilateral laryngeal paralysis. (4) Dogs and cats show salivation, tremors and muscle fasciculations, vomiting and diarrhea, constriction of the pupils, ataxia and convulsions.

organotherapy therapeutic administration of animal endocrine organs or their extracts.

organotrophic 1. relating to the nutrition of organs

of the body. 2. deriving energy from the oxidation of organic compounds; said of bacteria.

organotropism the special affinity of chemical compounds or pathogenic agents for particular tissues or organs of the body.

organum pl. *organa* [L.] an organ; a somewhat independent part of the body that performs a special function.

orgling the guttural sound made by the male camelid during mating.

orgotein a superoxide dismutase used as an anti-inflammatory agent.

oribatid mite freeliving, nonparasitic mites, intermediate hosts to tapeworms found in grazing animals, e.g. *Moniezia*, *Anoplocephala*, *Paranoplocephala*, *Avitellina* spp. Members of the superfamily Oribatoidea.

oriental having some connection with the Orient.

o. avian eye fluke see PHILOPHTHALMUS *gralli*.

o. blood fluke SCHISTOSOMA *japonicum*.

o. cattle plague see RINDERPEST.

o. liver fluke see CLONORCHIS *sinensis*.

o. lung fluke see PARAGONIMUS *westermani*.

o. mustard BRASSICA *juncea*.

o. sore see LEISHMANIASIS.

o. theileriosis a mild form of East Coast fever caused by *Theileria orientalis*.

Oriental longhair a new cat breed, derived from crossing a Balinese and an Oriental shorthair. It is basically a longhaired Siamese, without points. The coat can be any color.

Oriental shorthair a solid colored, long slim cat with very large, pointed ears, and green eyes.

oriental sore see cutaneous LEISHMANIASIS.

orienting reflex a component of the behavioral state of readiness or arousal.

Orientobilharzia see ORNITHOBILHARZIA.

orifice 1. the entrance or outlet of any body cavity. 2. any foramen, meatus or opening.

The names of most orifices are self-defining, e.g. atrioventricular, preputial. See also OSTIUM.

atrioventricular o. the opening between the atria and ventricles.

cecocolic o. aperture through which the cecum connects with the colon.

ileocolic o. the communicating orifice between the ileum and the colon.

infundibular o. slit-like orifice at the ovarian end of the avian oviduct; positioned near the ovary so that it can grasp the newly extruded oocyte.

intrapharyngeal o. the orifice between the nasopharynx and oropharynx which is bounded by the palatopharyngeal arches.

nasomaxillary o. the slit-like opening between the maxillary sinus and the middle meatus of the nasal cavity.

omasoabomasal o. large, oval opening at the end of the omasal canal which communicates with the abomasum.

oviductal o. a slit-like opening in the avian urodeum.

pyloric o. aperture between the stomach and duodenum; opens infrequently, solely for the passage of ingesta.

ureteric o. paired orifices in the neck of the bladder.

orificium pl. *orificia* [L.] orifice.

origin the source or beginning of anything before which there is nothing. In statistical terms expressed by the equation $x = y = 0$. In anatomy the more fixed end or attachment of a muscle or the end closer to the trunk (as distinguished from its insertion), or the site of emergence of a peripheral nerve from the central nervous system.

original antigenic sin the observation that a secondary immune response occurs when B lymphocytes are exposed to closely related, but not identical, antigens and that the antibodies formed react more strongly with the antigen that elicited the primary response. Called also the doctrine of original antigenic sin. Noted originally for influenza virus. See also MEMORY cells.

oris see MOUTH.

Orlov trotter horse Russian light horse, any color, bred from mating many light breeds together including Arab, Thoroughbred, Persian, Spanish saddle, Dutch draft, Mecklenberg, Hackney.

ormetoprim a close analog of diaveridine and a folic acid antagonist used in potentiated sulfonamide mixtures used as coccidiostats.

Ormskirk terrier see LANCASHIRE HEELER.

ornamental fowl any of several breeds of fowl used for ornamental purposes, e.g. bantams, game birds and many other breeds such as the Yokohama, Silver spangled Hamburgs, Bearded silver Polish.

ornidazole a nitroimidazole used to treat anaerobic enteric protozoa.

ornithic of or pertaining to birds.

ornithine an amino acid obtained from arginine by the action of the enzyme arginase which also splits off urea; it is an intermediate in urea biosynthesis.

o. carbamoyl transferase (OCT), o. transcarbamoylase see ornithine carbamoyl TRANSFERASE.

o. cycle alternative name for urea CYCLE since ornithine is the carrier of the nitrogens.

o. decarboxylase test a means of identifying different members of the Enterobacteriaceae as well as other gram-negative bacteria.

o.-δ aminotransferase deficiency see GYRATE atrophy.

Ornithobacterium rhinotracheale gram-negative, pleomorphic, rod-shaped bacteria associated with acute exudative pneumonia and airsacculitis in turkeys and broiler chickens.

Ornithobilharzia a genus of blood flukes (digenetic trematodes) in the family Schistosomatidae. Includes, as well as those listed below, *O. dattai*.

O. bomfordi occurs in the mesenteric veins of zebu cattle.

O. turkestanicum found in the mesenteric veins of most grazing herbivores and cats. Causes hepatic cirrhosis and nodules in the intestinal wall accompanied by loss of body weight in small ruminants.

Ornithobius mathisi louse of duck and geese.

Ornithocoris cimicid bug pest of poultry. Includes *O. toledoi* (Brazilian chicken bug), *O. pallidus*.

Ornithodorus a genus of soft-bodied ticks in the family Argasidae.

O. coriaceus found on cattle and deer. A vector of EPIZOOTIC bovine abortion.

O. erraticus a possible vector of African swine fever.

O. guerneyi the kangaroo tick, a vector of *Coxiella burnetii*. Its bite can cause severe local and systemic reactions in humans.

O. lahorensis causes tick paralysis.

O. moubata a parasite of mammals, including humans, birds and reptiles. A vector of African swine fever and Q fever and possibly of *Borrelia anserina* and *Aegyptianella pullorum* in fowls.

***O. moubata porcinus* (syn. *O. porcinus*)** infests wart hog burrows and transmits African swine fever.

O. puertoicensis a possible transmitter of the African swine fever virus.

O. savignyi occurs on most domestic animals and may bite humans.

O. turicata a vector of Q fever, *Theileria* and *Anaplasma* spp., and a cause of tick paralysis.

Ornithofilaria a roundworm genus in the family Onchocercidae. Called also *Splendido filaria.*

O. fallisensis found in the subcutaneous tissues in ducks, including domesticated species.

Ornithogalum a genus of African plants in the family Liliaceae; contain an unidentified toxin (possibly cardiac glycosides) which causes dyspnea due to pulmonary edema, diarrhea, dysentery, abdominal pain; *O. umbellatum* contains the alkaloid lycorine; includes *O. angustifolium* (snowdrop), *O. caudatum* (pregnant onion), *O. ceresianum*, *O. conicum* subsp. *conicum* (bulrush), *O. gilgianum*, *O. hermanii*, *O. lacteum* (bulrush), *O. longibracteum*, *O. ornithogaloides*, *O. prasinum*, *O. sundersiae*, *O. tenellum*, *O. thyrsoides*, *O. umbellatum* (daffodil), *O. virens*, *O. zeyheri.* Most of these plants are referred to as 'chincherinchee'.

Ornithoglossum viride African plant in the family Liliaceae; contains bufadienolide, which causes sudden death, abdominal pain; called also Cape poison onion.

Ornithonyssus a mite genus in the family Dermanyssidae.

O. bacoti* (syn. *Bdellonyssus, Liponyssus*) *bacoti parasitic in rats and humans, the intermediate host of the filarial nematode of rats, *Litomosoides sigmodontis*, vector of *Yersinia pestis* (human plague), murine typhus and Q fever. Called also tropical rat mite.

O. bursa parasitizes birds. Called also tropical fowl mite.

O. sylviarum a parasite of birds.

Ornithopus sativus African plant in legume family Fabaceae; indigestible fiber causes phytobezoars; called also seradella.

Ornithorhynchus anatinus see PLATYPUS.

ornithosis a systemic, contagious disease of nonpsittacine birds including domestic poultry, transmissible to humans, caused by a strain of *Chlamydia psittaci.* The avian disease is called also CHLAMYDIOSIS. In psittacine birds and humans the same disease is called PSITTACOSIS.

Ornithostrongylus a genus of worms in the superfamily Trichostrongyloidea.

O. quadriradiatus found in the crop, proventriculus and intestine of pigeons. Causes catarrhal and hemorrhagic enteritis and may cause heavy losses in young birds.

Orobanche minor parasitic plant in family Orobanchaceae; an unidentified toxin causes polydipsia, polyuria; called also broom rape.

orogastric pertaining to the mouth and stomach.

o. intubation passing a stomach tube via the mouth. The tube is of rubber or plastic. To avoid having the animal chew it there is a preference for a nasogastric tube. If it is passed per os, it is standard practice to use a mouth gag.

o. tube see orogastric intubation (above).

orogranulocyte any of the polymorphonuclear leukocytes suspended in the mucus layer on the free surfaces of oral tissues.

orolingual pertaining to the mouth and tongue.

oronasal pertaining to the mouth and nose.

o. membrane temporary partition replacing the nasal pit in the embryo; degenerates to open the passage from the nostril into the oronasal cavity.

oropharyngeal pertaining to the mouth and pharynx. Called also O/P.

o. membrane a transient embryonic membrane which separates the stomodeum from the pharyngeal cavity in the early fetus. Called also oral plate.

oropharynx the part of the pharynx between the soft palate, the tongue and the epiglottis.

orosomucoid a glycoprotein found in the blood.

orotic acid an intermediate in the biosynthesis of pyrimidine nucleotides.

orotracheal pertaining to the mouth and trachea.

Oroya fever see BARTONELLA.

orphan a newborn animal without a dam.

o. virus usually enteroviruses, that have no known disease attributed to them.

orphenadrine an anticholinergic agent and analgesic used as a skeletal muscle relaxant.

orpiment a sulfide ore containing arsenic.

Orpington two breeds, Black and Buff, of meat fowl. All black or buff in color.

orthesis pl. *ortheses* [Gr.] orthosis.

orth(o)- word element. [Gr.] *straight, normal, correct.* In chemistry, *ortho-* indicates an isomer; also, a cyclic derivative having two substitutes in adjacent positions.

ortho-aminophenol an industrial chemical exposure associated with a high incidence of urinary bladder neoplasms.

ortho para'DDD see MITOTANE.

orthochromatic staining normally.

orthodontic pertaining to orthodontia.

o. applicance intraoral devices used to carry out orthodontic procedures, e.g. to correct abnormalities of occlusion; may be fixed or removable.

orthodontics, orthodontia that branch of dentistry concerned with irregularities of teeth and malocclusion.

orthodromic conducting impulses in the normal direction; said of nerve fibers.

orthognathics the science dealing with the cause and treatment of malposition of the bones of the jaw.

orthograde carrying the body upright in walking.

Orthohalarachne mesostigmatid mites of the family Halarachnidae.

O. attenuata, O. diminuta found in the nostrils, trachea and bronchi of seals and sealions, causing sneezing and a nasal discharge.

Orthohepadnavirus a genus in the family *Hepadnaviridae.* It includes mammalian hepatitis B-like viruses.

orthometopic tending to have a vertical forehead as in some primates.

orthomolecular pertaining to the theory that certain diseases are associated with biochemical abnormalities resulting in increased needs for certain nutrients, e.g. vitamins, and can be treated by administration of large doses of these substances.

Orthomyxoviridae a family of viruses containing influenza viruses A, B and C of which only influenza A viruses cause disease in domestic animals. Virions are 100 nm diameter, enveloped and contain a single-stranded negative sense RNA genome in eight segments. The envelope carries two glycoprotein spikes, hemagglutination (H) and neuraminidase (N), each of which is coded for by a different genome segment and undergo continuous antigenic variation, either because of mutation (antigenic drift) or genetic recombination (antigenic shift).

Orthomyxovirus a genus of viruses in the family ORTHOMYXOVIRIDAE. They cause influenza in various species, including human influenza, SWINE influenza, EQUINE influenza and AVIAN influenza.

orthopedic pertaining to ORTHOPEDICS.

o. implant see IMPLANT.

Orthopedic Foundation of America an independent organization devoted to the evaluation of x-rays of orthopedic conditions in dogs, particularly hip dysplasia.
orthopedics that branch of surgery dealing with the preservation and restoration of the function of the skeletal system, its articulations, and associated structures; particularly associated with the correction of deformities of the musculoskeletal system.
orthopedist an orthopedic surgeon.
orthopercussion percussion with the distal phalanx of the finger held perpendicularly to the body wall.
orthophenylphenol see *o*-PHENYLPHENOL.
orthophoria normal equilibrium of the eye muscles, or muscular balance.
orthophosphoric acid used in ACID ETCH TECHNIQUE in dentistry.
orthopnea ability to breathe easily only while standing, seen in congestive heart failure.
orthopneic position dogs with congestive heart failure will resist lying down, preferring to stand or sit in order to relieve pulmonary congestion.
Orthopoxvirus a genus of viruses in the family POXVIRIDAE.
***O.* infections** see POX.
orthopraxy, orthopraxis mechanical correction of deformities.
Orthoptera an order of insects of little direct importance to veterinary science except that some act as the intermediate host for some worms. Includes grasshoppers, crickets, cockroaches.
Orthoreovirus a genus of viruses in the family *Reoviridae*. It includes the mammalian reoviruses of mammals and birds.
orthoscope an apparatus that neutralizes the corneal refraction by means of a layer of water; used in ocular examinations.
orthoscopic 1. affording a correct and undistorted view. 2. pertaining to orthoscopy.
orthoscopy examination by means of an orthoscope.
orthosis pl. *orthoses* [Gr.] an orthopedic appliance or apparatus used to support, align, prevent or correct deformities or to improve function of movable parts of the body.
orthostatic pertaining to or caused by standing.
orthotic serving to protect or to restore or improve function; pertaining to the use or application of an orthosis.
orthotics the field of knowledge relating to orthoses and their use.
orthotist a person skilled in orthotics and practicing its application in individual cases.
orthotoluidine see TOLUIDINE TEST.
orthotonos, orthotonus tetanic spasm that fixes the head, body, and limbs in a rigid straight line.
orthotopic occurring at the normal place.
orthotricresyl phosphate see TRICRESYL PHOSPHATE.
orthovoltage in radiation therapy, voltage in the range of 140 to 400 kV.
orthozoonosis a disease transmitted from birds to animals or humans.
Ortolani's sign a test of hip laxity, used in dogs to diagnose hip dysplasia. A positive sign is a snap as the head of the femur moves back into the acetabulum after being moved to the rim of the acetabulum.
orts leftover feed that the animals will not eat.
-ory suffix meaning pertaining to.
Orycteropus see AARDVARK.
Oryctolagus cuniculus European rabbit. See SYLVILAGUS.
Oryx a genus of antelopes.
O. algazel see ORYX.
O. gazella see GEMSBOK.
oryx a large, graceful antelope with curved horns. Called also *Oryx algazel*.
Oryx gazella see GEMSBOK.
Oryzias latipes see MEDEHAS.
OS [L.] *oculus sinister* (left eye).
Os chemical symbol, *osmium*.
os[1] pl. *ora* [L.] 1. any body orifice. 2. the mouth.
os[2] a bone. See Table 10.
o. acetabuli the cotyloid bone, one of the bones of the pelvis forming a portion of the floor of the acetabulum.
o. brevia short bones, e.g. tarsus, carpus bones.
o. compedale first phalanx of ungulates.
o. cordis the bone in the heart of some species such as the ox.
o. cornu, o. cornua the bony process of the frontal bone as a component of the horn.
o. coronae the pastern bone, the second or intermediate phalanx of ungulates.
o. costale bony part of the rib.
o. coxae hip bone.
o. dorsale formed by the fusion of two or three thoracic vertebrae in some birds. Called also notarium.
o. longa long bone.
o. malleolare a small separate bone representing the distal end of the fibula, found in ruminants.
o. membri pelvini bones of the pelvic limb.
o. metacarpalia metacarpal bones.
o. opticus a U-shaped bone around the optic nerve in adult game cocks.
o. pedis the coffin bone, the third phalanx of ungulates.
o. penis a bone in the penis of carnivores, and many other groups.
o. plana flat bone.
o. rostrale the bone in the nose of the pig at the rostral end of the cartilaginous nasal septum.
o. suffraginis (archaic term) the first or proximal phalanx of ungulates.
o. tarsi tarsal bone.
o. ungulare third phalanx of ungulates.
OS strain an obese strain of White Leghorn chickens which have a selective IgA deficiency and in which there is an inherited predisposition to autoimmune thyroditis.
oscar vernacular for fish *Artromotus ocellatus*. See Table 23.
OSCC ocular squamous cell carcinoma.
oscheitis inflammation of the scrotum.
osche(o)- word element. [Gr.] *scrotum*.
oscheocele a swelling or tumor of the scrotum.
oscheoma tumor of the scrotum.
oscheoplasty plastic surgery of the scrotum.
Oschmarenia see MATHEVOTAENIA.
oscillating saw the saw oscillates backwards and forwards instead of rotating in a full circular path as is conventional with power saws. Used for bone surgery. The Stryker is the model.
oscillation a backward and forward motion, like that of a pendulum; also vibration, fluctuation or variation.
Oscillatoria genus of benthic (bottom-dwelling) cyanobacteria or plankton (blue-green algae) occurring in blooms in fresh water; toxins include anatoxins and microcystin; causes hepatic necrosis, sudden death, photosensitization. Includes *O. aghardii*.
oscillatory characterized by oscillation.
o. nystagmus see pendular NYSTAGMUS.

oscillo- word element. [L.] *oscillation.*
oscillometer an instrument for measuring oscillations.
oscillometry the measurement of oscillations.
oscilloscope an instrument that displays a visual representation of electrical variations on the fluorescent screen of a cathode-ray tube.
oscitation the act of yawning.
osculum a small aperture or minute opening.
Osgood–Schlatter disease avulsion of the tuberosity of the tibia, usually seen in puppies. Similar, but not identical to the disease seen in humans. Called also Schlatter–Osgood disease.
-osis word element. [Gr.] *disease, morbid state, abnormal increase.*
Osleroides massinoi see VOGELOIDES *massinoi.*
Oslerus a genus of nematodes in the family Filaroididae and the superfamily Metastrongyloidea. Found in the respiratory tract of mammals.
O. osleri found in the trachea and bronchi of dogs.
osmatic pertaining to the sense of smell.
osmic acid a fixative used in the preparation of pathology slides, especially those to be examined by electron microscope. See also OSMIUM tetroxide.
osmics the science dealing with the sense of smell.
osmidrosis the secretion of foul-smelling sweat; bromhidrosis.
osmiophilia the state in which tissue stains readily with osmic acid.
osmiophobia the state in which tissue stains poorly with osmic acid.
osmium a chemical element, atomic number 76, atomic weight 190.2, symbol Os. See Table 6.
o. tetroxide a pathology stain and fixative; called also osmic acid.
osmolal adjectival form of mole, a one osmolal solution contains 1 mole of solute in 1 L of water.
o. gap difference between the measured plasma osmolality and the osmolality calculated from the plasma concentration of normally measured solutes.
osmolality the concentration of a solution in terms of osmoles of solutes per kilogram of solvent.
serum o. a measure of the number of dissolved particles per unit of water in serum. In a solution, the fewer the particles of solute in proportion to the number of units of water (solvent), the less concentrated the solution. A low serum osmolality would be indicative of a higher than usual amount of water in relation to the amount of particles dissolved in it. It would be expected, then, that a low serum osmolality would accompany overhydration, or EDEMA, and an increased serum osmolality would be present in a state of FLUID volume deficit.

Measurement of the serum osmolality gives information about the hydration status within the cells because of the osmotic equilibrium that is constantly being maintained on either side of the cell membrane (HOMEOSTASIS).

Water moves freely back and forth across the membrane in response to the osmotic pressure being exerted by the molecules of solute in the intracellular and extracellular fluids. Serum osmolality reflects the status of hydration of the intracellular as well as the extracellular compartments and thus describes total body hydration.
urine o. a measure of the number of dissolved particles per unit of water in the urine. A more accurate measure of urine concentration than specific gravity, urine osmolality is useful in diagnosing renal disorders of urinary concentration and dilution and in assessing status of hydration.
osmolar pertaining to the concentration of osmotically active particles in solution.
o. gap the difference between the calculated and measured osmolality of a solution. The gap is due to laboratory error or to disease states.
osmolarity the concentration of a solution in terms of osmoles of solutes per liter of solution. See also OSMOLALITY.
osmole a unit of osmotic pressure equivalent to the amount of solute substances that dissociates in solution to form one mole (Avogadro's number) of particles (molecules and ions). Abbreviated Osm.
osmometer 1. a device for testing the sense of smell. 2. an instrument for measuring osmotic pressure.
osmometry the technique of measuring osmolar concentrations. The definitive method of measuring solute:solvent ratios.
osmophiles bacteria and protozoa that can withstand high osmotic pressures.
osmophilic having an affinity for solutions of high osmotic pressure.
osmophore the group of atoms in a molecule of a compound that is responsible for its odor.
osmoreceptor 1. a specialized sensory nerve ending sensitive to stimulation giving rise to the sensation of odors. 2. any of a group of specialized neurons of the supraoptic nuclei of the thalamus that are stimulated by increased extracellular fluid osmolality to cause the release of antidiuretic hormone (ADH) from the posterior pituitary.
osmoregulation adjustment of internal osmotic pressure of a simple organism or body cell in relation to that of the surrounding medium.
osmose to diffuse by osmosis.
osmosis [Gr.] the passage of pure solvent from a solution of lesser to one of greater solute concentration when the two solutions are separated by a membrane which selectively prevents the passage of solute molecules, but is permeable to the solvent.

The process of osmosis and the factors that influence it are important clinically in the maintenance of adequate body fluids and in the proper balance between volumes of extracellular and intracellular fluids.

The term osmotic pressure refers to the amount of pressure necessary to stop the flow of water across the membrane. The hydrostatic pressure of the water exerts an opposite effect; that is, it exerts pressure in favor of the flow of water across the membrane. The osmotic pressure of the particles in a solute depends on the relative concentrations of the solutions on either side of the membrane, and on the area of the membrane. The osmotic pressure exerted by the nondiffusible particles in a solution is determined by the numbers of particles in a unit of fluid and not by the mass of the particles.
osmostat the regulatory centers that control the osmolality of the extracellular fluid.
osmotherapy the use of hypertonic solutions to produce dehydration.
osmotic emanating from or pertaining to the pressure of osmosis.
o. concentration concentration of osmotically active particles in solutions.
o. fragility the susceptibility of red blood cells to hemolyze in hypotonic saline solutions; may be used as a test of red cell fragility when a series of increasing concentrations is used. See also erythrocyte FRAGILITY.
Osphranter robustus see WALLAROO.
osphresiology the science of odors and sense of smell.

osphresis the sense of smell.
osprey a large brown bird of prey with white underparts and head. Called also *Pandion haliaetus*.
OSPT one stage prothrombin time.
ossa cordis see HEART bones.
ossein the collagen of bone.
osselets periosteal inflammation on the anterior aspect of the epiphysis of the large metacarpal bone, the proximal end of the first phalanx and the joint capsule of the fetlock. Caused by overtraining of young horses.
osseocartilaginous composed of bone and cartilage.
osseofibrous made up of fibrous tissue and bone.
osseoligamentous made of bone and ligament.
osseomucin the ground substance that binds together the collagen and elastin fibrils of bone.
osseous of the nature or quality of bone; bony.
o. cochlea see COCHLEA.
ossicle a small bone, especially one of those in the middle ear.
auditory o's the small bones of the middle ear: incus, malleus and stapes.
heart o. see HEART bones.
ossiculectomy excision of one or more of the ossicles of the middle ear.
ossiculotomy incision of the auditory ossicles.
ossiculum pl. *ossicula* [L.] ossicle.
ossiferous producing bone.
ossific forming or becoming bone.
ossification formation of or conversion into BONE or a bony substance.
biceps brachii o. causes a progressive lameness of the shoulder joint of the horse. The calcification of the tendon can be identified radiologically.
o. center a locus in an epiphysis or other part of a bone at which ossification commences and from which it spreads over the entire section. Radiological examination can detect the appearance of each ossification center and this is of assistance in aging.
dural o. occurs in large and giant breed dogs. Detected radiographically, most commonly in the lumbar and cranial and caudal cervical areas, but rarely produces clinical signs. Called also ossifying pachymeningitis.
ectopic o. see ECTOPIC mineralization.
enchondral o. ossification that occurs in and replaces cartilage.
o. groove located at the physeal end of the perichondrial ring of long bones. It supplies chondrocytes to the physis for the diametric growth of the bone. Called also groove of Ranvier.
intramembranous o. the formation of bone directly from fibrous tissue without the use of a cartilaginous model, e.g. as occurs in the parietal and frontal bones.
lateral cartilage o. see SIDEBONE.
retarded enchondral o. the ossification of cartilage in growing large dogs may be retarded and, at the distal ulnar growth plate, resembles premature closure of the plate; the characteristic lesion is a cone of uncalcified cartilage in the growth plate.
ossify to change or develop into bone.
ossifying changing or developing into bone.
o. fibrotic myopathy metaplastic ossification in the semitendinosus, semimembranosus and biceps femoris muscles of the horse in areas that have been subjected to fibrotic myopathy.
osslets see OSSELETS.
ostearthritis osteoarthritis.
ostearthrotomy excision of an articular end of a bone.
ostectomy excision of a bone or part of a bone.
oste-ectopia displacement of a bone.
ostein ossein.
osteitis inflammation of bone. The term is used to describe a number of conditions; for instance, advanced cases of brucellosis can lead to brucellar osteitis. See also OSTEOMYELITIS.
alveolar o. necrosis of alveolar bone at the site of a tooth extraction. Called also dry socket.
o. deformans osteitis causing deformity of bones.
o. fibrosa see OSTEODYSTROPHIA FIBROSA.
o. fibrosa cystica rarefying osteitis with fibrous degeneration and the formation of cysts and the presence of fibrous nodules on the affected bones, due to osteoclastic activity secondary to HYPERPARATHYROIDISM. See also OSTEODYSTROPHIA FIBROSA.
rarefying o. a bone disease in which the inorganic matter is diminished and the hard bone becomes cancellated.
sclerosing o. 1. sclerosing nonsuppurative osteomyelitis. 2. condensing osteitis.
ostempyesis suppuration within a bone.
oste(o)- word element. [Gr.] *bone*.
osteoarthritis a noninflammatory degenerative joint disease marked by degeneration of the articular cartilage, hypertrophy of bone at the margins, and changes in the synovial membrane; called also degenerative joint disease.
There is chronic lameness, bulls are reluctant to serve, the gait is stiff, the animals are reluctant to rise and have difficulty doing so. The affected limb shows atrophy, the joint is painful on passive movement and may show crepitus. In pigs epiphysiolysis may occur. See also OSTEOCHONDROSIS, LEG WEAKNESS of pigs.
chronic progressive o. result of repeated injury to joint surfaces, ligaments and cartilages of serving bulls.
inherited o. in cattle the coxofemoral joint is most affected in Herefords, the stifle in Holstein–Friesian and Angus. In horses the coxofemoral joint is affected.
osteoarthropathy any disease of the joints and bones.
osteoarthrosis chronic noninflammatory bone disease. See degenerative JOINT disease.
osteoarthrotomy ostearthrotomy.
osteoblast a cell arising from a fibroblast, which, as it matures, is associated with bone production.
inactive o. see surface OSTEOCYTE.
osteoblastic emanating from or pertaining to an osteoblast.
osteoblastoma a giant osteoid osteoma; a benign, painful, rather vascular enostotic tumor of bone characterized by trabeculae of osteoid produced by well-developed osteoblasts. It has not been described in animals.
osteocalcin a product of the resorption of bone.
osteocampsia curvature of a bone.
osteocartilaginous exostoses see multiple cartilaginous EXOSTOSIS.
osteochondral pertaining to bone and cartilage.
osteochondritis inflammation of bone and cartilage.
o. dissecans (OCD) osteochondritis resulting in the splitting off of a piece of articular cartilage due to fissure formation in an area of dysplastic subarticular cartilage so that it forms a flap or separates completely and falls into the joint space ('joint mouse'); occurs most commonly on the distal condyles of the humerus and femur in dogs and pigs. Is a manifestation of OSTEOCHONDROSIS.
osteochondrodysplasia any disorder of cartilage and bone growth.

osteochondroid resembling bone and cartilage.
osteochondrolysis see OSTEOCHONDRITIS dissecans.
osteochondroma a benign bone tumor consisting of projecting adult bone capped by cartilage which is proliferating and undergoing endochondral ossification; cartilaginous exostosis.
osteochondromatosis the occurrence of multiple osteochondromas. See multiple cartilaginous EXOSTOSIS.
osteochondrosis a disease characterized by abnormal differentiation of growth cartilage. Called also dyschondroplasia. It is a common disease in pigs and dogs and is also recognized in horses, turkeys and possibly in young bulls. The manifestations and sequelae vary with the species. In pigs osteochondrosis includes osteochondritis dissecans, epiphysiolysis deformities of bones and arthropathy. See also LEG WEAKNESS.
o. and arthrosis this disease of pigs causes severe degenerative lesions of the articular cartilage and underlying bone which are recognizable to autopsy but often without clinical signs. See also LEG WEAKNESS.
osteoclasia absorption and destruction of bony tissue.
osteoclasis surgical fracture or refracture of a bone.
osteoclast 1. a large, multinuclear cell frequently associated with resorption of bone. 2. a surgical instrument used for osteoclasis.
o.-activating factor (OAF) a product of activated T lymphocytes that takes part in local resorption of bone.
osteoclastoma giant cell tumor of bone.
osteoconduction the growth of bony tissue into the structure of an implant or graft.
osteocranium the fetal skull during the period of ossification.
osteocyte an osteoblast that has become embedded within the bone matrix, occupying a bone lacuna, and sending through canaliculi cytoplasmic processes that connect with other osteocytes in developing bone.
o.–osteoblast pump the interaction of osteocytes and osteoblasts, in response to parathyroid hormone, in moving calcium from the bone fluid to the extracellular fluid compartment.
surface o. a leaky barrier between cancellous and dense bone and lining the vascular channels in cortical bone. Called also resting osteoblast, inactive osteoblast.
osteocytic pertaining to osteocyte.
o. osteolysis one of the mechanisms involved in the resorption of bone by primary metastatic tumors.
osteodentin dentine that resembles bone.
osteodiastasis the separation of two adjacent bones.
osteodysplasia abnormal development of bone.
osteodystrophia fibrosa a lesion of bone in which fibro-osseous tissue replaces resorbed bone. The resorption is caused by HYPERPARATHYROIDISM which may be primary or, more commonly, secondary to nutritional error, or to renal insufficiency. Called also osteitis fibrosa, osteitis fibrosa cystica.
nutritional secondary o. f. see nutritional secondary HYPERPARATHYROIDISM.
renal secondary o. f. see renal secondary HYPERPARATHYROIDISM.
osteodystrophic pertaining to or emanating from osteodystrophy.
osteodystrophy diseases of bone in which there is failure of normal development or abnormal metabolism in bone which is already mature. Principal clinical signs are distortion and enlargement of bones, susceptibility to fracture, and abnormalities of gait and posture. See also OSTEODYSTROPHIA FIBROSA.
hypertrophic o. a disease of unknown etiology that occurs in young, rapidly growing dogs primarily of the large or giant breeds, in which there is pain and soft tissue swelling usually around the distal radius, ulna and tibia, lameness, and varying degrees of fever, lethargy and anorexia. Periosteal new bone is formed around the metaphyses and sometimes diaphyses, contributing to the enlargement of the limbs. The cause is unknown but hypovitaminosis C has at various times been suggested. Called also Möller–Barlow's disease (from a similar human disease), Barlow's disease, skeletal scurvy, infantile scurvy, osteodystrophy II, metaphyseal osteopathy, canine hypertrophic osteodystrophy.
renal o. see renal secondary HYPERPARATHYROIDISM.
osteoepiphysis any bony epiphysis.
osteofibroma ossifying fibroma; a benign, sometimes multiple, supraosseous ossifying spindle cell tumor.
osteofluorosis a generalized disturbance of bones caused by chronic fluorine poisoning and characterized by the development of multiple exostoses. There is lameness, ease of fracture of bones and mottling and pitting of the teeth.
osteogen the substance composing the inner layer of the periosteum, from which bone is formed.
osteogenesis the formation of bone; the development of the bones.
o. imperfecta an inherited condition marked by abnormally brittle bones that are subject to fracture. Affected lambs and calves are normal in appearance but are unable to stand. There is a defect in formation of bone matrix caused by a deficiency of PROCOLLAGEN *N*-peptidase. Called also paper-bone disease, juvenile osteoporosis.
osteogenic derived from or composed of any tissue concerned in bone growth or repair.
o. precursor cell see OSTEOPROGENITOR CELLS.
o. sarcoma see OSTEOSARCOMA.
osteogenin a morphogenetic bone matrix-derived protein which stimulates bone growth.
osteogeny osteogenesis.
osteography description of the bones.
osteohalisteresis deficiency in mineral elements of bone.
osteohematochromatosis see bovine congenital erythropoietic PORPHYRIA.
osteoid 1. resembling bone. 2. the organic matrix of bone; young bone that has not undergone calcification.
osteolathyrism an experimental form of lathyrism which occurs only in laboratory animals and characterized by skeletal deformities and aortic aneurysms.
osteolipochondroma osteochondroma with fatty elements.
osteoliposarcoma a malignant form of mesenchymoma in dogs; contains liposarcomatous and osteosarcomatous elements.
osteologist a specialist in osteology.
osteology scientific study of the bones.
osteolysis dissoluton of bone; applied especially to the removal or loss of calcium from the bone.
osteoma a benign tumor composed of bony tissue. In animals seen most commonly on jaws and in the nasal sinuses of horses and cattle. Histologically similar to ossifying fibroma, fibrous dysplasia, heterotopic ossification and exostosis.
osteoid o. a small, benign but painful, circumscribed tumor of spongy bone, occurring especially in

the bones of the extremities and vertebrae in humans. Similar lesions have been reported in cats.

o. spongiosum one containing cancellated bone.

osteomalacia softening of the bones of adult animals, resulting from impaired mineralization, with excess accumulation of osteoid, caused by a nutritional deficiency of vitamin D or phosphorus. The clinical signs are those of a painful condition of the bones and joints, including stiff gait, lameness, restlessness while standing, cracking sounds in the joints while walking, an abnormal posture including an arched back. Affected animals are disinclined to move and lie down for long periods. Fractures and tendon ruptures occur frequently and pelvic deformity may cause dystocia. Called also stifsiekte, stiffs, creeps, peglegs, cripples, bog-lame, milk-leg, milk-lame.

osteomatoid resembling an osteoma.

osteomere one of a series of similar bony structures, such as a vertebra.

osteometry measurement of the bones.

osteomycosis osteomyelitis caused by a fungus; fungal infection of bone, e.g. *Aspergillus* spp. in chickens.

osteomyelitis inflammation of bone, localized or generalized, due to a pyogenic infection. It may result in bone destruction, in stiffening of joints if the infection spreads to the joints, and, in extreme cases occurring before the end of the growth period, in the shortening of a limb if the growth center is destroyed.

Specific osteomyelitides in animals are actinomycosis and necrotic rhinitis of pigs. Clinical signs include persistent, severe pain, surrounding cellulitis sometimes with sinuses to the exterior. The affected bone is subject to pathological fracture and is readily recognizable radiographically. There are local signs related to the position and function of the affected bone, e.g. lameness, inability to eat.

cervical vertebral o. causes abnormal posture and motor difficulties including stumbling, then stiff and restricted gait, reluctance to bend neck, resulting in kneeling to graze.

juvenile o. see PANOSTEITIS.

osteomyelodysplasia a condition characterized by thinning of the osseous tissue of bones, increase in size of the marrow cavities, and associated leukopenia and fever.

osteon the basic unit of structure of compact bone, comprising a haversian canal and its concentrically arranged lamellae. Called also haversian system.

osteonal pertaining to the osteone.

o. canal canal around which the concentric laminae or sheets of osteonal bone are disposed.

osteone the microscopic unit of compact bone construction; consists of thin lamellae of bone arranged in a series of concentric tubules around a small central canal.

osteonecrosis necrosis of a bone.

osteonectin a glycoprotein found in bone but not cartilage or other connective tissues.

osteopath a practitioner of OSTEOPATHY.

osteopathia osteopathy (1).

osteopathology any disease of bone.

osteopathy 1. any disease of a bone. 2. a system of therapy utilizing generally accepted physical, medicinal and surgical methods of diagnosis and therapy, and emphasizing the importance of normal body mechanics and manipulative methods of detecting and correcting faulty structures.

hypertrophic o. (HOA) symmetrical periosteal proliferation of new bone on the four limbs, chiefly localized to the phalanges and terminal epiphyses of the long bones, almost always associated with a chronic intrathoracic, occasionally an intra-abdominal, disease particularly a neoplasm. Called also Marie–Bamberger's disease (osteopathy), hypertrophic pulmonary osteopathy, secondary hypertrophic osteopathy.

metaphyseal o. see hypertrophic OSTEODYSTROPHY.

nutritional o. includes rickets, osteomalacia, osteodystrophia fibrosa.

osteopenia reduced bone mass due to a decrease in the rate of osteoid synthesis to a level insufficient to compensate for normal bone lysis. The term is also used to refer to any decrease in bone mass below the normal.

osteoperiosteal pertaining to bone and its periosteum.

osteoperiostitis inflammation of a bone and its periosteum.

osteopetrosis in mammals, a hereditary disease marked by abnormally dense bone, and by the common occurrence of fractures of affected bone. It may lead to obliteration of the marrow spaces, causing anemia. Readily diagnosable radiographically. Occurs in rats, rabbits and cattle, in which it is usually associated with other inherited, congenital skeletal defects including shortness of long bones. In calves needs to be differentiated from similar lesions caused by infection in utero by the bovine virus diarrhea virus.

avian o. occurs as part of the avian LEUKOSIS, ROUS SARCOMA complex. All bones are affected but the long bones are most obviously deformed. Called also thick leg disease of poultry.

osteopetrotic having the characteristics of osteopetrosis.

o. lymphomatosis a disease of birds, possibly a part of the avian LEUKOSIS, ROUS SARCOMA complex.

osteophage osteoclast.

osteophagia chewing of debris bones found in pasture by herbivores. Indicative of nutritional deficiency of phosphorus. Sequelae include foreign body stuck in mouth, esophageal obstruction, botulism. See also PICA.

osteophlebitis inflammation of the veins of a bone.

osteophony bone conduction.

osteophore a bone-crushing forceps.

osteophyte, osteophyma a bony excrescence; a bony outgrowth. See also EXOSTOSIS, SPONDYLOSIS.

osteoplasty plastic surgery of the bones.

osteopoikilosis a mottled condition of bones, apparent radiographically, due to the presence of multiple sclerotic foci and scattered stippling.

osteopontin a sialopontin found in cells in bone tissue but its function is not understood.

osteoporosis a pathological loss of bone but the remaining bone is structurally normal. There is an imbalance in bone formation and resorption in favor of resorption. Bone becomes light and porous and fragile so that it fractures easily. It is associated with general undernutrition rather than specific nutritional deficiencies. Other causative factors are disuse, senility, lactation, weightlessness.

disuse o. that occurring when the normal laying down of bone is slowed because of lack of the normal stimulus of functional stress on the bone.

post-traumatic o. loss of bone substance after an injury in which there is nerve damage, sometimes due to decreased blood supply caused by the neurogenic insult, or to disuse secondary to pain.

osteoprogenitor cells the stem cells of the stromal system, the only cells capable of independent osteogenesis. Called also osteogenic precursor cells.

osteoradionecrosis necrosis of bone as a result of excessive exposure to radiation.

osteorrhagia hemorrhage from bone.

osteorrhaphy fixation of fragments of bone with sutures or wires; called also osteosuture.

osteosarcoma bone-producing malignant tumor; common in dogs and cats, but rare in other species. Dogs of large breeds are more frequently affected and the most common sites are distal humerus or femur and proximal radius or tibia. Lameness, swelling and rapid metastasis to the lungs are usual features.

osteosclerosis the hardening, or abnormal density, of bone.

o. congenita achondroplasia.

o. fragilis osteopetrosis; so called because of frequency of pathological fracture of affected bones.

o. fragilis generalisata osteopoikilosis.

osteosis degeneration and necrosis of osseous tissue.

Osteospermum toxic plant genus in family Asteraceae; causes cyanide poisoning; includes *O. cuneata* (*Arctotis glutinosa*), *O. ecklonis*, *O. jucundum* (*O. barbariae*), *O. spectabilis* (*Castelis spectabilis*); called also *Dimorphotheca* spp., South African daisy.

osteostixis surgical puncture of a bone.

osteosuture osteorrhaphy.

osteosynovitis synovitis with osteitis of neighboring bones.

osteosynthesis surgical fastening of the ends of a fractured bone.

osteothrombosis thrombosis of the veins of a bone.

osteotome a chisel-like knife for cutting bone.

US Army o. there are two versions of this heavy duty instrument, which resembles a standard cold chisel. In one the cutting edge is beveled on one side, in the other on both sides.

osteotomoclasis correction of bone curvature by partial division with the osteotome, followed by forcible fracture.

osteotomy incision or transection of a bone.

bulla o. a surgical procedure that drains the middle ear cavity, usually in the treatment of otitis media. Several different techniques may be used to penetrate the ventral or lateral portion of the tympanic bulla.

cuneiform o. removal of a wedge of bone.

displacement o. surgical division of a bone and shifting of the divided ends to change the alignment of the bone or to alter weight-bearing stresses.

linear o. the sawing or simple cutting of a bone.

pelvic o. a surgical technique used to reposition the acetabulum; used in the treatment of hip dysplasia in dogs. Involves an osteotomy of the ilium, ischium and pubis, that is, triple pelvic osteotomy.

wedge o. see cuneiform osteotomy (above).

Oster the archetypal hair clipper used worldwide. Has a range of interchangeable heads.

Ostertagia a genus of worms in the family Trichostrongylidae. They are found in the abomasum, rarely the intestine, of ruminants, are thin and brown and called brown stomach worms. They cause OSTERTAGIASIS. Includes *O. bisonis* (cattle, wild ruminants), *O. circumcincta* (goats, sheep), *O. crimensis* syn. *O. leptospicularis*, *O. hamata* (springbok), *O. leptospicularis* (cervid deer, cattle), *O. lyrata*, syn. *Skrjabinagia lyrata*, *Grosspiculagia lyrata* (cattle), *O. orloffi* (Barbary sheep, cattle, deer), *O. ostertagi* (cattle, goats, rarely sheep, horses), *O. podjapolskyi*, syn. *Grosspiculagia podjapolskyi* (cattle, sheep, moufflon), *O. trifurcata* (sheep, goats, also cattle).

ostertagiasis a disease of ruminants caused by invasion of the abomasum by *Ostertagia* spp. Two forms occur. Type I is in lambs or calves in their first summer at pasture and is characterized by the presence of large numbers of adult worms in the abomasum, profuse watery diarrhea, depressed appetite and a high morbidity rate. Type II occurs in cattle in the late winter after that first summer and sometimes in adults. It is characterized by emergence of large numbers of inhibited larvae from the abomasal mucosa, by chronic diarrhea, emaciation, a high death rate and a greatly thickened and edematous abomasal mucosa, subcutaneous edema and high plasma pepsinogen levels. The timing of the two forms varies between countries.

The disease is more properly referred to as ostertagiosis but common usage is ostertagiasis.

ostertagiosis see OSTERTAGIASIS.

ostia plural form of ostium.

ostitis see OSTEITIS.

ostium pl. *ostia* [L.] a mouth or orifice; a general term to designate an opening into a tubular organ, or between two distinct body cavities. The names of most ostia are self-defining.

o. abdominale the fimbriated end of the uterine tube.

o. cardiacum the opening of the esophagus into the stomach.

coronary o. either of the two openings in the aortic sinuses which mark the origin of the (left and right) coronary arteries.

o. ejaculatorium the common orifice of the ductus deferens and the excretory duct of the seminal vesicle into the urethra.

o. internum ostium uterinum tubae.

o. pharyngeum the nasopharyngeal end of the auditory tube.

o. primum an opening in the lower portion of the membrane dividing the embryonic atria into right and left sides. Called also foramen primum. See also ATRIAL septal defect.

o. pulmonary vein the opening of the pulmonary vein into the left atrium.

o. ruminoreticulare the opening between the rumen and the reticulum.

o. secundum an opening in the upper portion of the membrane dividing the embryonic atria into right and left sides, appearing later than the ostium primum. Called also foramen secundum. See also ATRIAL septal defect.

tympanic o., o. tympanicum the opening of the auditory tube on the carotid wall of the tympanic cavity.

o. uteri the external opening of the cervix of the uterus into the vagina.

o. uterinum tubae the point where the cavity of the uterine tube becomes continuous with that of the uterus.

o. vaginae the external orifice of the vagina.

ostomate an animal which has undergone enterostomy or ureterostomy.

ostomy general term for an operation in which an artificial opening is formed, as in colostomy, ureterostomy, tracheostomy, etc. See also STOMA (2).

Ostrea flat oysters; includes *O. angasi* (flat oyster), *O. edulis* (European oyster). See Table 23.

ostrich large, 9 ft high, weighing 400 lb, running birds with long necks and legs. They are gregarious herbivores. Called also *Struthio camelus*.

Oswaldocruzia a trichostrongyloid nematode genus found in amphibians and rarely in lizards.

OT old tuberculin.

otarid member of the Otariidae family of eared seals which includes the sealions (hair seals) and the fur seals (sea bears).

o. ataxia see otarid ATAXIA.

otectomy excision of tissues of the internal and middle ear.

othelcosis 1. ulceration of the auricle or external meatus of the ear. 2. suppuration of the middle ear.

othematoma see AURICULAR hematoma.

othemorrhea see OTORRHAGIA.

otic pertaining to the ear; aural.

o. capsule cartilaginous envelope which surrounds the nervous elements of the embryo's inner ear, and which subsequently ossifies.

o. cup the invagination of the otic placode, destined to form an otic vesicle and ultimately the inner ear.

otitis inflammation of the ear.

ceruminous o. that in which there is excessive cerumen and a characteristic rancid odor.

o. externa inflammation of the external ear characterized by frequent shaking of the head, pawing at the ear, intermittent rotation of the head with the affected ear down, pain on palpation of canal, bad odor and discharge.

furuncular o. the formation of furuncles in the external acoustic meatus.

o. interna labrynthitis; usually due to an extension of otitis media. Clinical signs include varying degrees of peripheral vestibular dysfunction. Deafness may also occur. Called also otitis labyrinthica.

o. labyrinthica see otitis interna (above).

o. media inflammation of the middle ear. It may occur in young animals by hematogenous spread of infection from omphalophlebitis, but it may also arise from extension of otitis externa or by infection ascending the eustachian tube. Clinical signs are usually referable to an associated otitis externa (odor, discharge, pain) or otitis interna which may cause vestibular signs such as rolling, ataxia and nystagmus. In addition, inflammation of the middle ear may cause facial paralysis, Horner's syndrome or keratitis sicca.

parasitic o. see OTOACARIASIS.

ot(o)- word element. [Gr.] *ear*.

otoacariasis infestation of the ear with mites, e.g. with *Otodectes cynotis*, *Raillietia auris*, *R. caprae*, causing shaking of the head and scratching at the ear. The ear canal contains a waxy exudate. Called also parasitic otitis.

Otobius a genus of soft-bodied ticks in the family Argasidae.

O. lagophilus found on rabbits.

O. megnini found in the ears of most mammals, but most commonly in dogs, sheep, horses and cattle. They cause irritation, head shaking and general debility. Mainly a problem in cattle and horses, but recorded from a wide range of hosts.

otoblennorrhea mucous discharge from the ear.

otocephalic pertaining to or emanating from otocephaly.

o. syndrome a complex of inherited abnormalities, recorded in Beagles, that include distortion of craniofacial structures, hydrocephalus, partial agnathia and neurological signs.

otocephalus an animal exhibiting otocephaly.

otocephaly a congenital malformation characterized by lack of a lower jaw and by ears that are united below the face.

otocleisis closure of the auditory passages.

otoconia see STATOCONIA.

otocranium 1. the chamber in the petrous bone lodging the internal ear. 2. the auditory portion of the cranium.

otocyst 1. the auditory vesicle of the embryo. 2. the organ of hearing in some lower animals.

Otodectes acarid mite genus in the family Psoroptidae.

O. cynotis the ear mite of dogs, foxes, cats, raccoons and ferrets and causes otodectic mange.

otodectic mange the ear and skin disease caused by infestation with *Otodectes cynotis*. Signs include those of OTITIS externa, with thick, brownish-red crusts in the ear canal, and occasionally a pruritic dermatitis.

otoencephalitis inflammation of brain extending from an inflamed middle ear.

otoganglion the otic ganglion.

otogenic, otogenous originating within the ear.

o. abscess usually part of a widespread abscessation; no specific syndrome associated with it.

otogenic precursor cells see OSTEOPROGENITOR CELLS.

otognathia a rudimentary, accessory mandible located at the base of the ear.

otography description of the ear.

otolaryngology, otorhinolaryngology that branch of veterinary medicine dealing with disease of the ear, nose and throat.

otolith an earstone; concretions of calcium carbonate and protein in the labyrinth of the inner ear and which move with every change in the posture of the head. Called also STATOLITH.

otolithic emanating from or pertaining to otolith.

o. membrane gelatinous matrix in the labyrinth of the ear; contains otoliths or otoconia.

o. organs utricle and saccule; detect the position of the head in a gravitational field.

otologist a specialist in otology.

otology the branch of veterinary medicine dealing with the ear and its anatomy, physiology and pathology.

otomucormycosis mucormycosis of the ear.

otomycosis a fungal infection of the external auditory meatus and ear canal. *Aspergillus* spp. and the yeasts *Pityrosporum* spp. are most commonly found in the ears of animals with otitis externa, sometimes as a result of prolonged antibiotic therapy rather than as primary pathogens.

otoneurology that branch of otology dealing especially with those portions of the nervous system related to the ear.

otopathy any disease of the ear.

otopharyngeal pertaining to the ear and pharynx.

otoplasty plastic sugery of the ear.

cosmetic o. see EAR CROPPING.

otopolypus a polyp in the ear.

otopyorrhea a copious purulent discharge from the ear.

otorhinolaryngology the branch of veterinary medicine dealing with disease of the ear, nose and throat; called also otolaryngology.

otorhinology the branch of veterinary medicine dealing with ear and nose.

otorrhagia hemorrhage from the ear.

otorrhea a discharge from the ear.

otosclerosis the formation of spongy bone in the capsule of the labyrinth of the ear, often causing the auditory ossicles to become fixed and less able to pass on vibrations when sound enters the ear. May be an inherited condition in humans.

otoscope an instrument for inspecting the ear.

otoscopy examination of the external acoustic meatus with an otoscope.

otospongiosis the formation of spongy bone in the bony labyrinth of the ear.

otosteal pertaining to the ossicles of the ear.

Otostrongylus a genus of lungworms in the family Crenosomatidae.

O. circumlitus found in the lungs or heart of true seals. Causes anorexia and coughing.
ototomy dissection of the ear.
ototoxic having a deleterious effect upon the eighth cranial (vestibulocochlear) nerve or on the organs of hearing and balance.
ototoxicity the property of being ototoxic.
otter an aquatic mustelid, closely related to polecat and marten. Has dark brown glossy, dense fur, webbed toes and a broad tail, short face whiskers and ears that can be closed off when diving. There are several species, *Lutra*, *Aonyx* spp. and the much bigger sea otter (*Enhydra lutis*).
Otter hound a large (approximately 65 to 115 lb), muscular dog with a large head and distinctive long, pendulous ears that curl inward on the leading edge, large feet and a long tail. The coat is long, dense and rough with an oily, waterproof topcoat in solid colors. The breed is affected by an inherited platelet disorder (thromboasthenic thrombocytopathia).
Otter sheep extinct achondroplastic mutant sheep. Similar to ANÇON sheep.
OU [L.] *oculi uterque* (each eye).
ouabain a cardiac glycoside obtained chiefly from the plant *Strophanthus gratus*; its effect is similar to that of digitalis, but digitalization is achieved more rapidly.
Ouchterloney technique see IMMUNODIFFUSION tests.
Oulou fato a form of nonfatal rabies described in dogs in Africa.
ounce 1. a measure of weight in both the avoirdupois and the apothecaries' system; abbreviation oz. The ounce avoirdupois is 28.3495 g, 1/16 lb, or 437.5 gr. The apothecaries' ounce is 31.103 g, 1/12 lb, or 480 gr.; symbol ℥. See also Tables 4.1 and 4.2. 2. see SNOW LEOPARD.
fluid o. a unit of liquid measure of the apothecaries' system, being 8 fluid drams, or the equivalent of 29.57 ml.
-ous suffix meaning pertaining to.
out-cross the mating of unrelated or only distantly related animals. Opposite to inbreeding or close-breeding.
out-of-court settlement a suit for damages listed for a court hearing which is settled out of court by mutual agreement between the parties.
out-of-hours before or after stated hours during which a clinic or hospital is fully staffed.
outbreak see EPIDEMIC.
outbreeding the mating of unrelated organisms. Called also crossbreeding.
outcome information data on result of treatment of disease, change in management, especially breeding and feeding, introduction of new genetic material or hygienic practice.
outdoor pen lambing see PEN lambing.
outflow tract the vascular structures associated with movement of blood from the ventricles. See also VENTRICULAR outflow obstruction.
outlet a means or route of exit or egress.
outlier an extremely high or low value lying beyond the range of the bulk of the data.
outpatient a patient who comes to the hospital, clinic or dispensary for diagnosis and/or treatment but does not occupy a cage or stall.
outpocketing evagination.
output the yield or total of anything produced by any functional system of the body.
computer o. the response to a command such as print, list, display. Usually taken to mean printed material but does include other materials, e.g. magnetic tape recordings put out on other output media by various output devices.
energy o. the energy a body is able to manifest in work or activity.
stroke o. the amount of blood ejected by each ventricle at each beat of the heart.
tube o. the output of an x-ray tube usually quoted in milliamps, the amount of current supplied to the cathode filament and the determining influence in the quantity of x-rays produced.
urinary o. the amount of urine secreted by the kidneys. See also FLUID balance.
ova plural of *ovum*.
ovalbumin principal protein in an egg white.
ovalocyte elliptocyte, an elliptical erythrocyte.
ovalocytosis elliptocytosis.
ovarian pertaining to an ovary.
o. agenesis one or both ovaries absent; usually accompanies defects of the tubular reproductive organs.
o. anomaly includes ovarian dysgenesis (see below), agenesis (above) or hypoplasia, as in Swedish Highland cattle.
o. bursa a pouch formed by the mesosalpinx and the mesovarium that encloses the infundibulum of the uterine tube and the ovary. It is shallow in the mare and does not enclose the ovary. It is capacious in sows and deep with a fat-filled wall in the bitch.
o. bursitis inlammation of the ovarian bursa; likely to affect the function of the ovary and ovulation.
o. cycle the cycle of follicle maturation and rupture, then luteinization and regression of the corpus luteum followed by recommencement of the cycle, unless pregnancy intervenes.
o. cyclicity the regular appearance of estrus as an indication of the regular occurrence of estrous cycles.
o. cyst see cystic ovarian disease (below).
cystic o. degeneration persistent cysts derived from ovarian follicles which do not ovulate. Follicular cysts are thin-walled and fluctuant, and often multiple. Luteal cysts have a thick wall of luteal tissue about the cyst, are firm to palpate and do not rupture easily. There is abnormal estral behavior, either anestrus or nymphomania, and diminished fertility.

Cystic corpora lutea form after ovulation has occurred and do not interfere with reproduction. They have a characteristic ovulation papilla.
cystic o. disease common disease of cows, less common in sows, characterized by gross abnormalities of estrus, either anestrus or more frequent and prolonged. In cows the cysts can be palpated per rectum.
o. dysgenesis small, inactive ovaries lacking germ cells such as occur in mares lacking a second X chromosome.
o. follicle see ovarian FOLLICLE.
follicular o. cyst see cystic FOLLICLE.
o. hormones estrogens, progesterone.
o. hypoplasia functional hypoplasia in immature females and undernourished females of all ages are common findings; in the absence of these risk factors hypoplasia is genetic in origin in Swedish Highland and possibly white Ayrshire cattle.
o. imbalance an alternative name of endocrine dermatoses caused by abnormalities of ovarian function in bitches. *Type I*, associated with cystic ovaries or functional ovarian tumors, consists of a bilaterally symmetrical alopecia, gynecomastia, enlargement of the vulva, and abnormalities of the estrous cycle. *Type II* is a bilaterally symmetrical alopecia, sometimes with seborrhea, in spayed bitches. It is respon-

sive to treatment with estrogen. Called also estrogen-responsive dermatosis.
o. inflammation see OOPHORITIS.
intrafollicular o. hemorrhage hemorrhage into an ovarian follicle occurs in all species during ovulation; also rarely in anovulatory follicles.
luteal o. cyst see LUTEAL cyst.
luteinized o. cyst see LUTEAL cyst.
o. neoplasms includes mostly granulosa cell tumors, but also rarely carcinomas, fibromas, thecomas, sarcomas.
o. pain a rare cause of colic in mares; identifiable by eliciting pain by rectal palpation of ovary.
premature o. failure defective differentiation of ovarian tissue and the patient shows no signs of pubertal estrus until long past the customary age.
o. rebound return of cyclical ovarian activity after a period of inactivity, usually pregnancy and parturition.
o. remnant syndrome the return of estral activity in a desexed female; due to failure to remove all of the ovarian tissue or to dropping, and allowing to implant, a piece of the ovary.
rete ovarii o. cyst a convoluted system of epithelial cell cords and tubules occupying part of the ovarian medulla; the cysts are found mostly in the hilar region of the ovary.
o. serous inclusion cyst similar in size and appearance to, but distinguishable from, ovarian cysts by their intraovarian position; lined by cuboidal epithelium thought to be pinched off from indentations of surface epithelium.
tubular epithelial o. cyst formed from epithelial cells from the surface of the ovary.

ovariectomy excision of an ovary. See also OOPHORECTOMY.

ovari(o)- word element. [L.] *ovary*. See also words beginning *oophor(o)-*.

ovariocele hernia of an ovary.

ovariocentesis surgical puncture of an ovary.

ovariocyesis ovarian pregnancy.

ovariohysterectomy surgical excision of the ovaries and the uterus, used as a means of preventing pregnancy and ovarian cyclicity, and for removal of a diseased uterus. The common 'spay' operation in dogs and cats.
o. hooks see spay HOOK.

ovariopexy the operation of elevating and fixing an ovary to the abdominal wall.

ovariorrhexis rupture of an ovary.

ovariosalpingectomy excision of an ovary and uterine tube.

ovariostomy incision of an ovary, with drainage; oophorostomy.

ovariotomy surgical removal of an ovary, or removal of an ovarian tumor.

ovariotubal pertaining to an ovary and uterine tube.

ovaritis inflammation of an ovary; oophoritis.

ovarium pl. *ovaria* [L.] ovary.

ovarobursal pertaining to or emanating from the ovary and the ovarian bursa, e.g. adhesions.

ovary pl. *ovaries;* the female gonad; either of the sex glands in the female in which the ova are formed and from which the sex hormones, estrogen and progesterone, are released. Small, round bodies varying in size with the species and the stage of the estral cycle, they are located one each at the end of the ovarian (fallopian) tubes, in the ovarian bursa. In birds two ovaries are present but usually the right one remains small and nonfunctional.
accessory o. very rare in domestic animals; usually located close to or attached to a normal ovary. See also supernumerary ovary (below).
cystic o. see cystic OVARIAN disease.
supernumerary o. occurs widely situated from normal ovary, formed presumably from a separate anlage in contradistinction to an accessory ovary which results from a splitting of the embryonic gonad and is usually attached to the normal gonad.

oven-dry see MOISTURE free.

over at the knees a conformation defect in horses in which the carpal joints are incompletely extended when the horse is standing normally.

over sticking see BACK BLEEDING.

over-the-counter medicines available to anyone, patent medicines, as opposed to ethical drugs which are available only to veterinarians.

over the hooks an abattoir term for meat purchased while still in the carcass stage and paid for by weight; contrast with 'on the hoof'.

overcheck a strap stretching from the pollstrap of the bridle to the saddle. It prevents the horse getting its head down to kick.

overconditioned said of beef cattle; means overfat.

overcrowding overcrowding of animal accommodation. Many countries now publish codes of practice which define what the appropriate volumetric allowances should be for each species of animal when they are housed indoors. Breaches of these codes is overcrowding. Pastoral conditions are too varied for similar guidelines to be drawn up for range animals. The consequences of overcrowding include the development of neuroses, inability to gain proper access to food and water and spread of contagious disease.

overdosage 1. the administration of an excessive dose. 2. the condition resulting from an excessive dose.

overdose 1. to administer an excessive dose. 2. an excessive dose.

overdrive suppression inhibitory effect of a fast cardiac pacemaker on a slow pacemaker.

overeating eating too much food too quickly; leads to acute gastric dilatation in dogs and horses, acute carbohydrate engorgement in ruminants, dietetic (dietary) diarrhea in young calves and foals, abomasal tympany in bottle fed lambs and calves.
o. disease 1. acute carbohydrate engorgement in ruminants. 2. enterotoxemia due to *Clostridium welchii* type D.

overexertion horses appear to be able to race beyond their real capacity when they are not properly fit and develop pulmonary edema as a result.

overexposure too long an exposure time or too high a milliamperage causing too black a picture, loss of detail and some anomalies of translucency.

overextension extension beyond the normal limit for a joint, commonly causing sprain of its ligaments.

overfeeding provision of more feed than necessary. Results in obesity, interference with normal parturition, fat cow syndrome, pregnancy toxemia in ewes, laminitis in ponies, diarrhea in puppies and kittens.

overflow in a computer operation, the generation of a quantity of output that is greater than the capacity of the register, buffer, field or record can accommodate.

overgrazing see OVERSTOCKING.

overgrown said of a part that has not been kept trimmed.
o. hoof overgrown hooves put unusual stresses on bones and tendons and allow for distortion of the wall and sole.
o. incisors occurs in guinea pigs, rabbits, rats, usually because malocclusion prevents wearing down by

opposing teeth, or the lack of hard surfaces in the environment for chewing. Excessively long teeth need to be clipped.

overhead costs see FIXED COSTS.

overhydration a state of excess fluids in the body. Usually the result of the excessive administration of fluids parenterally. Causes pulmonary edema with dyspnea, froth from airways, watery feces without unpleasant odor, usually for only a brief period, polyuria.

overlay a later component superimposed on a pre-existing state or condition.

overload a larger load than the system can comfortably bear.

tube o. when repeated exposures are made at high output. This may vaporize the target or damage the cathode.

veterinary o. the popular term for the knowledge explosion and the need to learn more by the veterinarian.

overlying suffocation of piglets by the sow. The piglets may be weak from illness or malnutrition, the sow may be clumsy or ill, the pen may be inadequate in size or poorly designed so that piglets cannot escape.

overmilking leaving the milking machine cups on a cow after the rate of milk flow has fallen to negligible levels.

overnutrition feeding, particularly calories, in excess of requirements; leads to obesity, rapid weight gain, and developmental skeletal abnormalities in dogs.

Overo Spanish-American name for a coat color in a horse. A broken colored horse in which white coat is continuous over the body but there is pigmented hair continuously from the ears to the tail. Matings between two of these horses produces a high ratio of foals with atresia of gut segments. Called also paint horses. See also TOBIANO.

Overo lethal white foal syndrome see LETHAL white.

overpopulation overcrowding of housing or pasturage.

overproduction jaundice see hemolytic JAUNDICE.

overreach the error in a fast gait when the toe of a hindhoof of a horse strikes and injures the back of the pastern of the leg on the same side.

o. boot a circular rubber boot worn on the front foot to protect against injury by an overreaching hindhoof.

overriding 1. the position of fracture fragments in which they overlap one another. 2. anomalous positioning of major blood vessels, e.g. aorta or pulmonary arteries. 3. a law or order which overrides, or takes precedence over, a law or order of a court or legislature of lower standing.

o. aorta a congenital anomaly occurring in tetralogy of Fallot, in which the aorta is displaced to the right so that it appears to arise from both ventricles and straddles the ventricular septal defect.

o. pulmonary artery a congenital cardiac defect in which the pulmonary artery straddles a defective interventricular septum and the aorta originates in the right ventricle.

overscald to scald chicken carcasses for too long in water that is too hot so that they have a cooked appearance and are not suitable for sale for human consumption.

overservicing carrying out more clinical or preventive work on an animal or herd than is needed or was requested by the owner with the express intention of raising a higher fee.

overshot protruding.

o. fetlock see KNUCKLING over.

o. jaw See BRACHYGNATHIA. Called also parrot mouth.

overstocking carrying more livestock on a particular area of pasture than it can support for any length of time. The pasture is killed, exposing the soil to erosion and the invasion of weeds. Called also overgrazing.

overtraining training horses or dogs too hard so that they lose spirit.

overventilation hyperventilation.

overwintering the ability of animals, plants or parasites to survive outdoors through a winter season.

overwork the condition produced by working a draft animal or working dog, an eventing or endurance horse too hard. See also EXHAUSTION.

overwrite in computer terms, to record new data over the top of existing data thus obliterating it.

ovi- word element. [L.] *egg, ovum.*

Ovibos moschatus see MUSK OX.

ovicide an agent destructive to the ova of certain organisms, usually helminths and arthropods.

oviduct a passage through which ova leave the maternal body or pass to an organ communicating with the exterior of the body. See also UTERINE tube. In birds generally only the left oviduct and ovary are functional. See INFUNDIBULUM of uterine tube, MAGNUM, ISTHMUS of uterine tube.

accessory o. see MÜLLERIAN DUCT.

o. hypoplasia failure of the tube to develop in the fetus; a rare cause of infertility.

o. impaction blockage of the oviduct in the hen by an inspissated mass of egg material.

o. inflammation see OVIDUCTITIS.

oviductal emanating from or pertaining to the oviduct.

o. obstruction may be a congenital defect or the result of infection or injury; adhesions prevent the passage of the ovum, causing infertility from the ipsilateral ovary.

oviductitis inflammation of the oviduct.

oviferous producing ova.

oviform egg-shaped.

ovigenesis oogenesis.

ovine pertaining to, characteristic of, or derived from sheep.

o. atopic dermatitis symmetrical erythema, alopecia, lichenification, excoriation on woolless areas; sporadic cases, recur each summer.

o. balanoposthitis see ENZOOTIC balanoposthitis.

o. encephalomyelitis see LOUPING ILL.

enzootic o. abortion see ENZOOTIC ovine abortion.

o. genital campylobacteriosis see VIBRIONIC abortion.

infectious o. keratoconjunctivitis see contagious OPHTHALMIA.

o. interdigital dermatitis see INTERDIGITAL dermatitis.

o. pneumonic complex involves one or more of the following pathogens: parainfluenza 3 virus, *Mycoplasma ovipneumoniae*, *Pasteurella haemolytica*, *P. multocida*, *Chlamydia psittaci.*

o. progressive pneumonia see MAEDI.

o. pulmonary adenomatosis see ovine PULMONARY adenomatosis.

o. respiratory syncytial virus a syncytium-forming virus; the cause of pneumonia lesions in sheep.

o. staphylococcal dermatitis see ovine staphylococcal DERMATITIS.

o. staphylococcal pyoderma see ovine staphylococcal DERMATITIS.

oviparity the characteristic of being OVIPAROUS.
oviparous producing eggs in which the embryo develops outside of the maternal body, as in birds.
oviposition the act of laying or depositing eggs.
ovipositor a specialized organ by which many female insects deposit their eggs.
Ovis a genus of ruminant animals in the subfamily Caprinae. Includes wild and domestic sheep, small ruminants with spirally curled horns which are ridged transversely.
O. ammon wild sheep.
O. aries see SHEEP.
O. canadensis see BIGHORN SHEEP.
Ovis canadensis californiana California Bighorn sheep.
Ovis canadensis canadensis Rocky Mountain bighorn sheep.
Ovis canadensis cremnobates desert wild sheep.
O. dalli see DALL SHEEP.
O. musimon see MOUFFLON.
ovisacs small sacs in the ovarian tissue that contain the immature ovocytes that develop into ova; a graafian follicle.
ovo- word element. [L.] *egg, ovum.*
ovocytes embryonic stages of ova.
ovoid having the oval shape of an egg.
o. body colloid body.
ovoplasm the cytoplasm of an unfertilized ovum.
ovotestis a gonad containing both testicular and ovarian tissue.
ovoviviparity the characteristic of being ovoviparous.
ovoviviparous bearing living young that hatch from eggs inside the maternal body, the embryo being nourished by food stored in the egg; said of lizards, etc.
ovular pertaining to an ovule or an ovum.
ovulate see OVULATION.
ovulation the discharge of the ovum from the GRAAFIAN FOLLICLE.
The discharged ovum enters the UTERINE tube adjoining the ovary and moves toward the uterus; if it encounters a spermatozoon while it is still alive (about 48 hours), the two merge. Fertilization usually takes place in the uterine tube. The fertilized ovum then makes its way to the uterus, where it becomes embedded in the prepared wall as the first stage of growth of the embryo. See also ESTRUS, ESTROUS cycle.
double o. simultaneous ovulation in both ovaries.
o. failure the ripe follicle does not rupture and discharge its ovum.
o. fossa site of rupture of mature follicles.
multiple o. see SUPEROVULATION.
noncopulatory o. standard procedure in species other than cats.
quiet o. see silent ESTRUS.
o. tags strands of fibrin, proliferating capillaries and leukocytes on the peritoneal serosa close to ovulation sites especially in mares and cows.
ovule 1. the ovum within the graafian follicle. 2. any small, egglike structure.
ovum pl. *ova* [L.] egg; the female reproductive or germ cell which, after fertilization, is capable of developing into a new member of the same species; sometimes applied to any stage of the fertilized germ cell during cleavage and even until hatching or birth of the new animal.
centrolecithal o. one with the yolk concentrated at the center of the egg, surrounded by a peripheral shell of cytoplasm, and with an island of cystoplasm surrounding the nucleus.
holoblastic o. one that undergoes total cleavage.
isolecithal o. one with a small amount of yolk evenly distributed throughout the cytoplasm.
meroblastic o. one that undergoes partial cleavage.
o. penetration assay a biological assay using hamster, or other, zona-free ova as the test medium for the penetrating ability of individual samples of semen.
primitive o., primordial o. any egg cell very early in its development.
telolecithal o. one with a comparatively large amount of yolk massed at one pole.
o. transplant an ovum that has been fertilized in utero is recovered from the dam by flushing from the uterus, inspected under the microscope to ensure viability and transferred to the uterus of an estral female. The donor female has usually been superovulated so that a number of ova can be salvaged in the one operation.
Owen contour lines accentuated incremental lines in dentin caused by sublethal systemic insults such as infectious disease which injure odontoblasts. Called also Owen's contour lines.
owl a bird of the order Strigiformes with very distinctive characteristics including nocturnal predation, soft feathers and silent flight, frontset eyes and ears that can be closed. There are a number of families including barn owls, nightjars, frogmouths, potoos, monkey owls and the tropical owls.
o. midge see SANDFLY.
owl monkey nocturnal, New World monkey with very large eyes, gray-brown to red in color. Make good pets; eat fruits, insects and birds. Called also *Aotus trivirgatus*, night ape, douroucouli.
owner proprietor.
absentee o. pays a manager to run the farm.
o.-manager the owner who also manages his own farm.
ox pl. *oxen;* mature, castrated male reared for meat production or draft purposes.
o. warbles see HYPODERMA.
oxacillin a semisynthetic penicillin used as the sodium salt.
oxalate any salt of oxalic acid.
o. calculi see oxalate UROLITH.
o. crystalluria associated with ethylene glycol poisoning in dogs and cats.
o.-induced equine nutritional secondary hyperparathyroidism see nutritional secondary HYPERPARATHYROIDISM.
insoluble forms (calcium) o. appear as raphide crystals in some plants; irritate oral mucosa causing severe stomatitis.
o. soluble forms sodium, magnesium and ammonium oxalates.
soluble o. poisoning in ruminants acute poisoning due to ingestion of large amounts causes hypocalcemia with muscle weakness and recumbency. Precipitation of oxalate crystals in renal tubules causes nephrosis. Long-term ingestion in horses can cause osteodystrophia fibrosa. Most cases are the result of eating large amounts of oxalate-bearing plants, e.g. *Oxalis* spp., *Setaria* spp., *Halogeton glomeratus*, *Portulaca oleracea*.
oxalemia excess of oxalates in the blood.
oxalic acid a poisonous, dibasic acid found in various fruits and vegetables, and formed in the metabolism of ascorbic acid. In plants the acid is present in the form of OXALATE.
The commercial acid is highly toxic and if ingested should be neutralized by the administration of lime

water (calcium hydroxide solution) or other convenient source of calcium, which reacts with the acid to form insoluble calcium oxalate.

o. a. test papers used to detect indole production in an INDOLE test.

Oxalis a plant genus of the family Oxalidaceae; poisonous to herbivora because of high soluble oxalate content causing nephrosis and urolithiasis. Includes *O. acetosella* (wood sorrel), *O. corniculata* (creeping oxalis), *O. latifolia*, *O. pes-caprae* (*O. cernua*, soursob, Bermuda buttercup).

oxalism poisoning by oxalic acid or by an oxalate.

oxaloacetate a salt or ester of oxaloacetic acid.

oxaloacetic acid a metabolic intermediate in the tricarboxylic acid cycle, which is also a substrate of aspartate aminotransferase.

Oxalobacter formigenes a resident ruminal digestive adjunctal bacteria.

oxalocetate plays a role in gluconeogenesis and the production of CO_2.

oxalosis generalized deposition of calcium oxalate, in renal and extrarenal tissues, as may occur in primary hyperoxaluria.

pulmonary o. results from infection with *Aspergillus niger*; the fungus produces oxalic acid which causes tissue necrosis in adjacent tissues.

oxaluria hyperoxaluria.

oxazepam a benzodiazepine tranquilizer. See also DIAZEPAM.

oxazolidinediones a group of anticonvulsants that includes troxidone (trimethadione) and paramethadione.

oxen adult castrated male of any breed of *Bos* spp.

oxethazaine a topical anesthetic.

oxfendazole a benzimidazole anthelmintic used extensively in ruminants against a wide spectrum of worms. A special formulation is available for intraruminal injection. Also effective against equine strongyles.

Oxford see OXFORD DOWN.

Oxford Down a short-woolled, Downs-type meat sheep with dark brown face and legs. Called also Oxford, Oxfordshire Down.

Oxford ragwort SENECIO *squalidus*.

Oxfordshire Down see OXFORD DOWN.

oxibendazole a benzimidazole anthelmintic similar to oxfendazole.

oxidant the electron acceptor in an oxidation–reduction (redox) reaction.

oxidase any of a class of enzymes that catalyze the reduction of molecular oxygen independently of hydrogen peroxide.

o. test used to identify bacteria that contain cytochrome *c* oxidase.

oxidation the act of oxidizing or state of being oxidized.

Chemically it consists in the increase of positive charges on an atom or the loss of negative charges. Univalent oxidation indicates loss of one electron; divalent oxidation, the loss of two electrons. The opposite reaction to oxidation is reduction.

alpha o. important in the metabolism of fatty acids.

beta o. major process for the oxidation of fatty acids in the body leading to the production of ATP. Occurs predominantly in the mitochondrial matrix, but can occur in peroxisomes. Oxidation of the fatty acid occurs at the beta-carbon, leading to the release of the preceding two carbon as acetyl CoA.

omega o. oxidation beginning at the last carbon (omega carbon) of an acyl chain, usually a fatty acid.

oxidation–fermentation test used to identify bacteria by their ability to ferment or oxidize glucose in the test media. Called also the O-F test.

oxidation–reduction potential measure of the capacity of an element or compound, usually contained in half-cells consisting of electron donor and its conjugate electron acceptor, to donate electrons in aqueous medium. Often called redox potential and given the symbol E_O or E'_O for pH 7.0. Electrons flow from the half-cell of lower to that of higher redox potential.

oxidation–reduction reactions reactions involving electron transfer; the electron donor is the reductant, which becomes oxidized while transferring electrons to the other substrate, the oxidant.

oxidative pertaining to or emanating from oxidation.

o. deamination oxidative breakdown of amino acids; specialized enzyme systems carry out the process, e.g. D-amino oxidase.

o. metabolism enzymic pathways leading to the addition of oxygen or removal of hydrogen from intermediates in the pathway.

o. phosphorylation the mitochondrial process by which the free energy from the oxidation of intracellular substrates is made available in the form of ATP for cellular endergonic processes.

oxide a compound of oxygen with an element or radical.

oxidize to cause to combine with oxygen or to remove hydrogen.

oxidized having been modified by the process of oxidation.

o. cellulose see absorbable CELLULOSE.

oxidized cellulose a specially treated form of surgical sponge which promotes clotting and is used as a temporary dressing.

oxidoreductase a class of enzymes that catalyze the reversible transfer of electrons from one substance to another (oxidation–reduction, or redox reaction).

oxime any of a series of compounds formed by action of hydroxylamine on an aldehyde or ketone.

oximeter a device for measuring oxygen concentration.

oximetry measurement of the oxygen content of arterial blood.

pulse o. use of a spectrophotoelectric instrument applied to the skin which measures pulse rate and the percentage of oxygenated and reduced hemoglobin.

oxirane see ETHYLENE oxide.

2-oxoglutaric acid a metabolic intermediate involved in the tricaboxylic acid cycle, in amino acid metabolism, and as an amino group acceptor in transamination reactions. Called also α-ketoglutaric acid.

oxolinic acid a long-acting antibacterial agent, derived from quinolone, used orally in the treatment of urinary tract infections caused by susceptible gram-negative organisms. Side-effects in dogs include vomiting, diarrhea and CNS signs.

5-oxoproline a modified amino acid occurring in several proteins. Called also pyroglutamic acid.

oxosteroids ketosteroids.

oxtriphylline see CHOLINE theophyllinate.

oxy- word element. [Gr.] *sharp, quick, sour, presence of oxygen in a compound.*

oxyblepsia unusual acuity of vision.

oxybutynin an anticholinergic having direct antispasmodic effect on smooth muscle; used in the treatment of uninhibited neurogenic bladder and reflex neurogenic bladder.

oxycephaly congenital condition in which the top of the head is pointed due to premature closure of the coronal and lambdoid sutures. Called also acrocephaly, acrocephalia.

oxychlorosene a stabilized organic complex of hypochlorous acid used as a topical antiseptic in the treatment of localized infections.

oxycinesia pain on motion.

oxyclozanide a useful treatment for adult liver fluke in dairy cattle. It has a short withholding period and is also effective against immature paramphistomes.

oxycodone a semisynthetic narcotic analgesic derived from morphine.

4-oxycoumarin a hypothrombinemic substance in *Ferula communis*.

oxydemeton-methyl see METHYL demeton.

oxygen a chemical element, atomic number 8, atomic weight 15.999, symbol O. See Table 6. It is a colorless and odorless gas that makes up about 20% of the atmosphere. In combination with hydrogen, it forms water; by weight, 90% of water is oxygen. It is the most abundant of all the elements of nature. Large quantities of it are distributed throughout the solid matter of the earth, because the gas combines readily with many other elements. With carbon and hydrogen, oxygen forms the chemical basis of much organic material. Oxygen is essential in sustaining all kinds of life.

o. analyzer an instrument that measures the concentration of oxygen in a gas mixture.

o. deficiency significant cause of losses in cultivated finfish in enclosed dams, but also in rivers and estuaries, caused by lack of natural aeration of the water or to heavy algal blooms, bushfire ash deposits and overcast conditions leading to respiration rather than photosynthesis or a high concentration of organic matter and leading to the development of a bacterial bloom; a high temperature exacerbates the development.

o. flux equation a calculation that determines the rate at which oxygen is made available to tissues, based on cardiac output and arterial oxygen content.

o.–hemoglobin dissociation curve a graphic explanation of the release and acquisition of oxygen from and to the hemoglobin in the blood in varying circumstances of oxygen partial pressure in the environment.

o. regulator see reducing VALVE.

o. saturation the amount of oxygen bound to hemoglobin in the blood expressed as a percentage of the maximal binding capacity.

o. saturation curve graphical representation describing the relationship (usually curvilinear) between fraction of oxygen-binding sites (of a protein) that have oxygen bound to them and the partial pressure (concentration) of free oxygen.

o. tension see TENSION (2).

o. tent an enclosed space or plastic canopy used for oxygen therapy, humidity therapy or aerosol therapy.

o. therapy supplemental oxygen administered for the purpose of relieving hypoxemia and preventing damage to the tissue cells as a result of oxygen lack (HYPOXIA). Companion animals are usually placed in a special cage with oxygen piped to it. A mask is used for short-term administration. Large animals can be supplied by a nasal tube taped in place to deliver oxygen into the pharynx.

o. toxicity tissue damage may occur with exposure to high concentrations of oxygen for long periods. See also RETROLENTAL fibroplasia.

o.-transfer chain a functional chain describing the transfer of oxygen from the external environment to the metabolizing tissue; includes uptake in the respiratory system, binding to hemoglobin, transport through the circulatory system, diffusion and dissociation in tissues and utilization in mitochondria, i.e. oxidatable substrates and enzymes.

o. transport process of transfer of oxygen around the body either attached to hemoglobin or myoglobin.

oxygenase any enzyme of the oxidoreductase class that catalyzes the incorporation of both atoms of molecular oxygen into the substrate.

oxygenation saturation with oxygen.

hyperbaric o. exposure to oxygen under conditions of greatly increased pressure See also HYPERBARIC oxygenation.

oxygenator an apparatus by which oxygen is introduced into the blood during circulation outside the body, as during open-heart surgery. See also EXTRACORPOREAL circulatory support unit.

bubble o. a device in which pure oxygen is bubbled through an extracorporeal reservoir of blood, either directly or through a filter.

film o. a device, encased in a container of oxygen, that makes possible reduction of a thin film of blood to facilitate the exchange of gases.

rotating disk o. a type of film oxygenator in which a series of parallel disks rotate through an extracorporeal pool of venous blood in a container of oxygen; gaseous exchange occurs between the thin film of blood on the exposed surface of the disks and the oxygen in the container.

screen o. a type of film oxygenator in which the venous blood is passed over a series of screens in a container of oxygen, gaseous exchange taking place in the thin film of blood produced on the screens.

oxyhemoglobin hemoglobin combined with molecular oxygen, the form in which oxygen is transported in the blood. See also HEMOGLOBIN.

o. dissociation curve see HEMOGLOBIN–oxygen dissociation curve.

Oxylipeurus a genus of lice that parasitize turkeys. Includes *O. polytrapezius*, *O. corpelentis*.

Oxylobium see GASTROLOBIUM.

oxymetazoline a vasoconstrictor used topically as the hydrochloride salt in nasal congestion.

oxymetholone a 17α-alkylated androgen used for its anabolic effects in the treatment of aplastic and other nonregenerative anemias.

oxymorphone hydrochloride a narcotic analgesic that is more potent and has longer duration than morphine.

oxymyoglobin MbO_2; myoglobin charged with oxygen.

oxyntic secreting acid, as the parietal (oxyntic) cells of the stomach.

o. cells gastric mucosal cells that secrete gastric acid.

o. glands glands in the gastric mucosa that contain oxyntic cells.

oxyphenbutazone, oxyphenylbutazone a nonsteroidal anti-inflammatory agent, similar to phenylbutazone.

oxyphil 1. Hürthle cell. 2. oxyphilic, i.e. stainable with an acid dye.

o. cell acidophilic cells found in parathyroid gland.

oxyphilic, oxyphilous stainable with an acid dye.

oxyquinoline see HYDROXYQUINOLINES.

Oxyspirura a genus of nematodes in the family Thelaziidae. They are parasites of the eyes of birds and cause ophthalmitis, with ocular discharge, and scratching at the eyes.

O. mansoni, O. parvorum found under the third eyelid of fowls, turkeys and peafowl.

***O. petrowi* and many others** found in the eyes of wild birds.

Oxysporum see FUSARIUM *solani*.

oxytalan a connective tissue fiber found in the periodontal membrane.
Oxytenia acerosa North American plant member of the family Asteraceae containing an unidentified hepatoxin. Syndrome includes depression, recumbency; necropsy lesions include hepatitis and nephrosis. Called also copperweed.
oxytetracycline a short-acting water-soluble tetracycline. Called also Terramycin.
oxytocia rapid labor.
oxytocic 1. pertaining to, marked by, or promoting oxytocia. 2. an agent that promotes rapid labor by stimulating contractions of the myometrium.
oxytocin a hypothalamic hormone stored in and released from the posterior pituitary, or prepared synthetically. Produced also by the corpus luteum of sheep, and perhaps other animals. Involved in the release of $PGF_{2[alpha]}$ which induces luteolysis. It acts as a powerful stimulant to the pregnant uterus, especially toward the end of gestation. The hormone also causes milk to be expressed from the alveoli into the lactiferous ducts during suckling.
Oxytropis a genus of plants in the legume family Fabaceae. Very closely related botanically to *Astragalus* spp. and with very similar characteristics as poison plants. Contain the indolizidine alkaloid swainsonine; causes excitability, paralysis, blindness. Includes *O. besseyi*, *O. condensata*, *O. deflexa*, *O. glabra*, *O. glabra* var. *drakana*, *O. kansuenis*, *O. lambertii*, *O. ochrocephala*, *O. puberula*, *O. saximontana*, *O. sericea*. Called also locoweeds.
Oxyuranus scutellatus see TAIPAN.
oxyuriasis the disease caused by infestation with OXYURIS nematodes. Manifested by intense irritation of the perianal region causing rubbing and biting at the tail.
oxyuricide an agent that kills oxyurids.
oxyurid an individual nematode of the family Oxyuridae.
Oxyuris a genus of nematodes in the family Oxyuridae. Occupants of the large intestine; the females have long, tapering tails. Includes *O. equi* (horse), *O. karamoja* (rhinoceros), *O. poculum* (horse), *O. tenuicorda* (Burchell's zebra—*Equus burchelli*).
oyster see CRASSOSTREA, SACCOSTREA COMMERCIALIS, OSTREA and Table 23.
oyster feet said of horses having flat feet with ridges in the wall giving a general appearance not unlike an oyster shell. Usually the result of chronic laminitis.
oyster velar disease caused by an iridovirus this disease causes severe losses in Pacific oyster hatcheries.
oz ounce.
ozena, ozoena an atrophic rhinitis marked by a thick mucopurulent discharge, mucosal crusting and fetor.
Ozobranchus branchiatus a leech found on green sea turtles in association with cutaneous fibroepitheliomas.
ozone a bluish explosive gas or blue liquid, being an allotropic form of oxygen, O_3; it is antiseptic and disinfectant, and irritating and toxic to the pulmonary system.
ozonization exposure of stored meat to ozone to preserve it and especially to reduce any taint in the meat.
ozostomia foulness of the breath.

P

P chemical symbol, *phosphorus*; symbol, *peta-;* position; presbyopia; [L.] *proximum* (near); pulse; [L.] *punctum* (point); pupil.
 P cells found in the sinoatrial and atrioventricular nodes. May be a source of electrical impulses.
P_1 parental generation.
P_2 pulmonic second sound. See HEART SOUNDS.
Pco_2 carbon dioxide partial pressure or tension; also written PCO_2, pCO_2 and pCO_2. See RESPIRATION and BLOOD GAS ANALYSIS.
Po_2 oxygen partial pressure (tension); also written PO_2, pO_2 and pO_2. See also BLOOD GAS ANALYSIS.
p symbol for (1) the short arm of a chromosome; or (2) the frequency of the more common allele of a pair; (3) pico-.
p- symbol, *para-*.
P-450 enzymes enzymes, which are at high levels in some fish-eating birds, e.g. Atlantic puffins, capable of metabolizing xenobiotic substrates including pesticides.
p-cresol see CRESOLS.
P-K reaction Prausnitz-Küstner reaction.
P mitrale an electrocardiographic abnormality in which the P wave is prolonged, in dogs more than 0.04 s. Associated with left atrial enlargement.
P pulmonale an electrocardiographic abnormality in which the P wave is tall and peaked. Indicative of right atrial enlargement which is often associated with chronic pulmonary disease.
P site see peptidyl-tRNA binding site (under TRNA).
Pa chemical symbol, *protactinium*; symbol, *pascal.*
P_aco_2 symbol for partial pressure of carbon dioxide in the arterial blood. See also BLOOD GAS ANALYSIS.
P_ao_2 symbol for partial pressure of oxygen in arterial blood. See also BLOOD GAS ANALYSIS.
PA inhibitor PLASMINOGEN activator inhibitor.
Paatsama technique a surgical method for reconstruction of a ruptured cranial cruciate ligament using a strip of fascia lata.
PAB, PABA para-aminobenzoic acid.
pabulum food or aliment.
paca a large, plump rodent, brown in color, with three to five lines of white spots down the sides of the body. Called also sooty paca, spotted cavy, *Cuniculus paca* (formerly *Coelogenys* spp.).
 sooty p. see paca (above).
pacchionian granulations enlargements of the arachnoid villi which protrude into the dorsal sagittal sinus, as seen in the horse.
pace an equine gait similar to a trot except that the front and rear limbs on each side are moved in unison instead of the diagonal limbs. A comfortable even gait for the rider, producing an even speed for the duration of a race. Similar to the AMBLE gait but at a fast speed. Many pacing horses are raced and trained in harness. Called also sidewheel.
pacemaker an object or substance that controls the rate at which a certain phenomenon occurs; often used alone to indicate an artificial cardiac pacemaker; however, there are other natural and artificial pacemakers. In biochemistry, a pacemaker is a substance whose rate of reaction sets the pace for a series of interrelated reactions.
 asynchronous p. an implanted cardiac pacemaker in which the induced ventricular rhythm is independent of the atrium; it is usually set at a fixed rate of ventricular stimulation.

p. cells cells within the heart capable of spontaneous discharge.
gastric p. a saddle-shaped area of the greater curvature of the stomach at the junction of its proximal and middle thirds, which regulates the frequency of gastric contractions.
phrenic p. a device designed to facilitate respiration by converting radiofrequency signals into electrical impulses that stimulate the phrenic nerve, resulting in contraction and flattening of the diaphragm and improved inspiration of air.
uterine p. either of the two regulating centers that control uterine contractions.
wandering p. a condition in which the site of origin of the impulses controlling the heart rate shifts from the head of the sinoatrial node to a lower part of the node or to another part of the atrium.

Pacheco's disease a disease of parrots caused by a species-specific herpesvirus and characterized by weakness, diarrhea and focal necrosis in the liver and spleen. Intranuclear inclusion bodies in hepatocytes suggest the diagnosis. The disease causes very heavy mortalities in zoo colonies.

pachy- word element. [Gr.] *thick*.

pachyacria enlargement of the soft parts of the extremities.

pachyblepharon thickening of the eyelids.

pachycephaly abnormal thickness of the bones of the skull.

pachycheilia thickening of the lips.

pachychromatic having the chromatin in thick strands.

pachycurares a group of neuromuscular blocking agents characterized by large, bulky molecules. Includes *d*-tubocurarine, gallamine, pancuronium; all of them are competitive blockers.

pachydactyly enlargement of the digits.

pachyderma abnormal thickening of the skin.
p. vesicae thickening of the mucous membrane of the bladder.

pachydermatocele plexiform neuroma attaining large size, producing an elephantiasis-like condition.

pachyglossia abnormal thickness of the tongue.

pachygyria see MACROGYRIA.

pachyhematous pertaining to or having thickened blood.

pachyleptomeningitis inflammation of the dura mater and pia mater.

pachymeninges dura mater.

pachymeningitis inflammation of the dura mater; perimeningitis.
ossifying p. see dural OSSIFICATION.

pachymeningopathy noninflammatory disease of the dura mater.

pachymeninx the dura mater.

pachynsis an abnormal thickening.

pachyonychia abnormal thickening of the nails or claws.

pachyperiostitis periostitis of long bones resulting in abnormal thickness of affected bones.

pachyperitonitis inflammation and thickening of the peritoneum.

pachypleuritis fibrothorax.

pachysalpingitis chronic interstitial inflammation of the muscular coat of the oviduct producing thickening; called also mural salpingitis and parenchymatous salpingitis.

pachysalpingo-ovaritis chronic inflammation of the ovary and oviduct, with thickening.

pachysomia thickening of parts of the body.

Pachystigma a genus of South African plants in the family Rubiaceae; the causative toxin is unidentified but causes myocardial problems resulting in congestive heart failure. The syndrome is called goosiekte. Includes *P. latifolium*, *P. pygmaeum*, *P. thamnus*. Called also *Vangueira* spp., goubos, gousiektebossie.

pachytene in prophase of meiosis, the stage following zygotene during which the chromosomes shorten, thicken and separate into two sister chromatids joined at their centromeres. Paired homologous chromosomes, which were joined by synapsis, now form a tetrad of four chromatids. Where crossing over has occurred between nonsister chromatids, they are joined by Y-shaped chiasmata.

pachyvaginalitis inflammation and thickening of the tunica vaginalis of the testis.

pachyvaginitis chronic vaginitis with thickening of the vaginal walls.

Pacifastacus leniusculus American crayfish. See Table 23.

Pacific Coast tick see DERMACENTOR *occidentalis*.

Pacific cupped oyster CRASSOSTREA *gigas*.

Pacific harbor porpoise see PHOCOENA SINUS.

Pacific labrador tea LEDUM *columbianum*.

pacific pond turtle CLEMMYS *marmorata*.

pacing 1. normal gait of some horses. See PACE. 2. stereotyped pacing; a habit in all caged animals, especially if they are active species and are confined in very small areas. May cause excessive wear in footpads, in snakes the damage is usually to the front of the head. 3. setting the pace or rate of movement. See CARDIAC pacing.

pacinian corpuscle cutaneous mechanoreceptors that sense pressure and stretch.

pack 1. see sterile SURGICAL pack. 2. jute container (1350 mm × 750 mm × 750 mm) into which wool is packed to make a bale; other similar containers in which wool is packed include butts and sacks.

packalacca PHYTOLACCA *dioica*.

packed cell volume the percentage of the volume of whole, unclotted blood occupied by the erythrocytes. Abbreviated PCV. A useful prognostic indicator in dehydration when the PCV rises markedly.

packer 1. an instrument for introducing a dressing into a cavity or a wound. 2. proprietor of a meat packing plant.

packet knot slip knot; useful for the beginning of a continuous suture.

packing 1. the filling of a wound or cavity with gauze, sponge or other material. 2. the material used for this purpose.

packing plant a complete meat production unit including facilities for slaughtering animals, processing of meat and offal, boning out, making up of blocks of carcasses, chilling, freezing, storing of the meat, preparation of by-products.

pad a cushion-like mass of soft material which may be (1) anatomical; (2) surgical.
abdominal p. a pad for the absorption of discharges from abdominal wounds, or for packing off abdominal viscera to improve exposure during surgery.
fat p. a pad of fat lying within a joint, covered with synovial membrane and thought to assist in the spreading of synovial lubricant, e.g. infrapatellar fat pad of stifle joint.
foot p's see FOOTPAD.
Mikulicz's p. a pad made of folded gauze, for packing off viscera in surgical procedures.
pressure p. in surgery, gauze sponges used to apply pressure in the control of minor hemorrhage.
stripped p. avulsion of the pad with exposure of the dermis. A common injury in Greyhounds which have

raced on asphalt or been over-exercised on a walking machine with a rough belt.

pad-saddle a thick pad of felt made like a saddle but without a tree. Can be made in leather with a minor arch. Used for riding horses in track work.

Padda oryzivora see Java SPARROW.

paddock a fenced field or enclosure.

joining p. used for mating.

Paecilomyces a genus of soil-inhabiting imperfect fungi which are sometimes found as contaminants of the skin and oral mucosa. See also HYALOHYPHOMYCOSIS.

P. fumosoroseus associated with cutaneous and disseminated infections in dogs and cats.

P. varioti an opportunistic fungal infection of the respiratory tract of birds.

PAF platelet activating factor.

Pagrus auratus finfish in family Sparidae. Called also snapper, red sea bream. See Table 23.

-pagus word element. [Gr.] *conjoined twins*.

PAHA para-aminohippuric acid.

Pahvant Valley fever see TULAREMIA.

pail-fed said of neonates reared on milk or replacer fed from a pail instead of a bottle. Called also bucket-fed.

pail-feeding a method of rearing calves by weaning them off the dam and feeding them on her or another cow's milk or milk replacer in a bucket without the use of a nipple. Because of the common practice of feeding at too long intervals with cold milk there is a higher prevalence of dietary diarrhea in pail-fed calves than in calves that are suckled. See also dietary DIARRHEA.

pain a feeling of distress, suffering or agony, caused by stimulation of specialized nerve endings. Its purpose is chiefly protective; it acts as a warning that tissues are being damaged and induces the sufferer to remove or withdraw from the source.

All receptors for pain stimuli are free nerve endings of groups of myelinated or unmyelinated neural fibers abundantly distributed in the superficial layers of the skin and in certain deeper tissues such as the periosteum, surfaces of the joints, arterial walls, and the falx and tentorium of the cranial cavity. The distribution of pain receptors in the gastrointestinal mucosa apparently is similar to that in the skin; thus, the mucosa is quite sensitive to irritation and other painful stimuli. Although the parenchyma of the liver and the alveoli of the lungs are almost entirely insensitive to pain, the liver as an organ and the bile ducts are extremely sensitive, as are the bronchi, ureters, parietal pleura and peritoneum.

Some pain receptors are selective in their response to stimuli, but most are sensitive to more than one of the following types of excitation: (1) mechanical stress of trauma; (2) extremes of heat and cold; and (3) chemical substances, such as histamine, potassium ions, acids, prostaglandins, bradykinin and acetylcholine.

The conscious perception of pain probably takes place in the thalamus and lower centers; interpretation of the quality of pain is probably the role of the cerebral cortex.

There are some naturally occurring internal systems in the body that are known to control pain but none of them has been completely verified. One of the best known is the GATE CONTROL system in which it is thought that pain impulses are mediated in the substantia gelatinosa of the spinal cord.

abdominal p. pain occurring in the area between the thorax and pelvis. Manifestations vary between species. Identifiable syndromes include: (1) horse—pawing, flank watching, rolling, straddling as though to urinate, lying on the back; (2) cattle—may depress back and paddle with hindfeet but mostly arched back, grunting, immobility; (3) dogs and cats—arched back, grunting, depression, reluctance to move. Sometimes there is elevation of the hindquarters, with the chest and forelegs on the ground (the so-called 'praying dog' attitude).

Beagle p. syndrome see BEAGLE pain syndrome.

projected p. pathology in one area can affect the nerve supply to a distant area in which pain is experienced.

p. receptors free nerve endings of tufts of fine points or buttons.

referred p. pain felt in an area distant from the site of pathology but not mediated through a common innervation. There is no evidence that referred pain occurs in animals but it seems likely on anatomical grounds.

p. threshold the lowest level at which a stimulus can be applied and cause perceptible pain.

p. tolerance the level of stimulation at which pain becomes intolerable.

painful defecation see DYSCHEZIA.

paint 1. commercial paint products are used in animal accommodation. Most contain some lead, even so-called lead-free paints. Therefore they are capable of causing lead poisoning in animals. 2. see PINTO.

paint horse see PINTO.

paintbrushes see CASTILLEJA.

painted turtle *Chrysemys picta*.

paired pertaining to data or animals that are matched as being very similar.

p. controls see paired CONTROL.

p. data values which fall normally into pairs and can therefore be expected to vary more between pairs than within pairs.

Pajaroello tick see ORNITHODORUS *coriaceus*.

pakoein a toxic cycad glycoside found in *Bowenia*, *Cycas* etc.

palae(o)- for words beginning thus see *pale(o)-*.

palatability pleasantness of taste of feed; willingness of animals to eat the feed in preference to others, which may be based on factors other than taste, e.g. smell, appearance, the sound of cows munching on ensilage.

palate the roof of the mouth.

The front portion braced by the upper jaw bones (maxillae) is known as the hard palate and forms the partition between the mouth and the nose. The fleshy part arching from the hard palate to the throat is called the soft palate and separates the oropharynx from the nasopharynx. When the animal swallows, the rear of the soft palate swings up against the back of the pharynx and blocks the passage of food and air to the nose. See also SOFT PALATE.

cleft p. see CLEFT lip.

displaced p. the soft palate of the horse, except during deglutition, rests below the epiglottis. It may be displaced and come to lie above the epiglottis, due either to hypoplasia of the epiglottis or paresis of the soft palate.

midline defect of p. see CLEFT lip.

p. reflexes swallowing caused by stimulation of the palate.

palatine, palatal pertaining to the palate. See also PALATE.

p. abscess commonly diagnosed in companion birds. Are often accumulations of keratinized cellular debris as a result of a dietary deficiency of vitamin A.

p. fissure narrow gap beside the palatine process of the incisive bone; covered by the vomeronasal organ and pierced by the naso-incisive duct.
p. process medial and lateral palatine processes contribute to the development of the palate and the separation of the oral and nasal cavities.
p. sinus one of the paranasal sinuses connecting with the nasal cavity that is particularly large in ruminants.
p. slit the caudal half of the palate in birds is divided by a median choanal slit.
p. tonsil tonsils found on the ventrolateral border of the soft palate, which are large and housed in a tonsillar sinus in dogs and cats, are absent from the pig and are follicular in ruminants and the horse.

palatitis inflammation of the palate.

palat(o)- word element. [L.] *palate.*

palatoglossal pertaining to the palate and tongue.
p. arch see palatoglossal ARCH.

palatognathous having a congenitally cleft palate.

palatomaxillary pertaining to the palate and maxilla.

palatopharyngeal pertaining to the palate and pharynx.
p. arch see palatopharyngeal ARCH.

palatoplasty plastic reconstruction of the palate.

palatoplegia paralysis of the palate.

palatorrhaphy surgical correction of a cleft palate.

palatoschisis see CLEFT lip.

palatum [L.] *palate.*

pale lacking the pink color of normal viable tissue that is perfused with blood.
p. laurel KALMIA *polifolia* var. *microphylla.*
p. willow weed PERSICARIA *lapathifolia.*

pale soft exudative pork see PORCINE stress syndrome.

pale-encephalon the (phylogenetically) old brain; all of the brain except the cerebral cortex and its dependences.

pale(o)- word element. [Gr.] *old.*

paleocerebellum originally, the phylogenetically older parts of the cerebellum; the term is now applied specifically to those parts whose afferent inflow is predominantly supplied by spinocerebellar fibers.

paleocortex paleopallium.

paleogenetic originated in the past; not newly acquired; said of traits, structures, etc., of species.

paleokinetic old kinetic; a term applied to the nervous motor mechanism concerned in automatic associated movements.

paleopallium that part of the pallium (cerebral cortex) developing with the archipallium in association with the olfactory system; it is phylogenetically older and less stratified than the neopallium, and composed chiefly of the piriform cortex and parahippocampal gyrus. Called also paleocortex.

paleopathology study of disease in bodies that have been preserved from ancient times.

paleopulmo the functional division of the avian respiratory tract formed by the parabronchi arising from the mediolateral and medioventral bronchi.

paleostriatum the phylogenetically older portion of the corpus striatum, represented by the globus pallidus.

paleothalamus the phylogenetically older part of the thalamus, i.e. the medial portion which lacks reciprocal connections with the neopallium.

Palicourea South American plant genus in the family Rubiaceae; contain fluoroacetate, a cause of myocardial damage and sudden death; includes *P. aeneofusca*, *P. grandiflora*, *P. juruana*, *P. marcgravii*, cafezinho, cafe bravo, erva cafe, erva de rato, roxa, roxinha, roxona, vick.

pali(n)- word element. [Gr.] *again, pathological repetition.*

palindrome literally, something that reads the same backwards as forwards. In nucleic acid biochemistry palindromic sequences of 4 to 10 or more base pairs occur not infrequently. These are of interest because they are recognition sites for cleavage by restriction endonuclease enzymes; responsible for secondary structures in nucleic acids such as the folding of RNA molecules or the hairpin structures found at the termini of the single-stranded DNA genome of parvoviruses.
interrupted p. restriction enzymes such as *Bgl*I recognize sequences which are interrupted palindromes, e.g. GCNNN↓NGGC where N is any nucleotide.

palindromia a recurrence or relapse.

palisade worms see STRONGYLUS.

palisading giving the appearance of palisades in a fence.
p. crust alternating horizontal layers of keratin and exudate in a crust or scab.
p. granuloma see palisading GRANULOMA.

palladium a chemical element, atomic number 46, atomic weight 106.4, symbol Pd. See Table 6.

palliate to relieve clinical signs.

palliative affording relief; also, a drug that so acts.

pallidum the globus pallidus of the brain.

pallium the cerebral cortex viewed in its entirety, i.e. the mantle of gray matter covering both cerebral hemispheres. Also, the cerebral cortex during its development.

pallor paleness, as of the skin or mucosae. Although it is commonly associated with anemia, many long-term cases show mucosae of normal color; pallor is also a common sign in shock.

Palma christi see RICINUS *communis.*

palmar descriptive of the palm of the human hand, or of the homologous surface or direction of the limbs of other animal species.
p. nerve block see PLANTAR nerve block.

Palmer's dental notation a scheme for charting the position and number of teeth. A horizontal line indicates the occlusal plane and a vertical line in the middle indicates the midline. The teeth in each quadrant are numbered, starting from the point closest to the midline.

palmitate ester of palmitic acid, a common dietary fatty acid.

palmitic acid a 16-carbon saturated fatty acid from animal and 16-carbon vegetable fats.

palmitin glycerol tripalmitate, one of the common fats in animal fat. A crystallizable and saponifiable substance.

palmitoleic acid a 16-carbon monounsaturated, with a double bond at carbons 7,8, endogenously synthesized nonessential fatty acid.

palmityl-CoA-carnitine transferase an enzyme involved in the transport of fatty acids across the mitochondrial membrane.

palmus 1. palpitation. 2. clonic spasm of limb muscles, producing a jumping motion.

palo santo tree see BULNESIA SARMIENTII.

palomino not a breed of horse but a color type of gold with white mane and tail.

palpable perceptible by touch.

palpate to perform palpation.

palpation the technique of examining parts of the body by touching and feeling them.
abdominal p. palpation of the contents of the abdomen and the state of the abdominal wall either through the wall or per rectum.

gastric p. internal palpation of the stomach via the esophagus is performed in dolphins and other cetaceans.
pharyngeal p. palpation via the external wall in small animals; can be performed per os in cattle but requires a mouth speculum for all but the most deft practitioners.
rectal p. palpation of the posterior abdomen and the organs in it by inserting the finger (in dogs) or hand and arm (in horses, cattle and pigs) in the rectum.

palpebra pl. *palpebrae* [L.] eyelid.

palpebra tertia third eyelid; MEMBRANA nictitans.

palpebral pertaining to the eyelid.
p. conjunctiva conjunctiva at the back of the eyelid.
p. fissure see palpebral FISSURE.
medial p. ligament the ligament which connects the medial ends of the tarsi to the orbit.
p. nerve a branch of the auriculopalpebral nerve which serves the muscles of the eyelid (see Table 14).
p. reflex the eyelids close when the eyelids are touched.

palpebritis blepharitis.

PALS periarteriolar lymphoid sheath. See white PULP.

palsy paralysis. A word used commonly in human medicine but rarely if ever in veterinary medicine.

palustrine a toxic alkaloid in *Equisetum* spp.

Palyam viruses a group of viruses in the genus *Orbivirus* which cause abortion and congenital abnormalities, including hydranencephaly and cerebellar hypoplasia, in cattle in Africa, Japan and Australia.

PAM, 2-PAM 2-pyridine aldoxime methchloride (pralidoxime chloride).

pampas grass see CORTADERIA SELLOANA.

pampiniform shaped like a tendril, e.g. pampiniform plexus, a plexus of veins which tangle around the tortuous testicular artery.

PAMS para-amino salicylic acid.

pan- word element. [Gr.] *all*.

Pan troglodytes see CHIMPANZEE.

panacea a remedy for all diseases.

Panacur a proprietary name for fenbendazole.

Panaeolina foenisecii see PSILOCYBE.

panagglutinin an agglutinin that agglutinates the erythrocytes of all human blood groups.

panangiitis inflammation involving all the coats of a vessel.

panaritium an obsolete expression for PARONYCHIA. Still used with reference to cattle and meaning bovine footrot.

panarteritis nodosa see PERIARTERITIS nodosa.

panarthritis inflammation of all the joints.

panatrophy atrophy of several parts; diffuse atrophy.

panautonomic pertaining to or affecting the entire autonomic (sympathetic and parasympathetic) nervous system.

pancarditis diffuse inflammation of the heart.

pancolectomy excision of the entire colon, with creation of an outlet from the ileum on the body surface.

pancreas a large, elongated, racemose gland located in the anterior abdomen between the liver, kidneys, stomach, spleen and duodenum.

The pancreas is composed of both exocrine and endocrine tissue. The *acini* secrete digestive enzymes, and small ductules leading from the acini secrete ions, mainly sodium and bicarbonate. The combined product, *pancreatic juice*, enters a long pancreatic duct and from there is transported duct to the duodenum. The pancreatic juice contains enzymes for the breakdown of proteins, carbohydrates and fats. The bicarbonate ions in the pancreatic secretion help neutralize the acidic chyme that is passed along from the stomach to the duodenum.

The endocrine functions of the pancreas are related to the islets of Langerhans which occur throughout the pancreas. These small islands contain three major types of cells: the *alpha*, *beta* and *delta* cells. The alpha cells secrete the hormone *glucagon*, which elevates blood sugar. The beta cells secrete *insulin*, which affects the metabolism of carbohydrates, proteins and fats. The delta cells secrete *somatostatin*, the functions of which are not fully understood, but it is known that it can inhibit the secretion of both glucagon and insulin and may act as a controller of metabolic processes. The somatostatin produced by the delta cells of the pancreas is the same as that produced by the hypothalamus as an inhibitor of the release of growth hormone from the pituitary gland.
p. disease pancreatic atrophy of post-smolt Atlantic salmon caused by a togavirus infection; clinical signs include anorexia, emaciation. Called also sleeping disease.
endocrine p. see pancreas (above).
exocrine p. see pancreas (above).

pancreatectomy excision of the pancreas.

pancreatic pertaining to the pancreas. See also PANCREATITIS, DIABETES MELLITUS, CYSTIC pancreatic duct.
p. abscess occurs as a complication of acute pancreatitis or subsequent to pancreatic surgery due to bacterial contamination but is most common as an extension from a leaking gastric ulcer.
p. acinar atrophy the islets of Langerhans remain normal but acinar tissue atrophies and exocrine function is compromised. Seen most commonly in large breeds of dogs, particularly German shepherd dogs. Clinical signs are related to the exocrine pancreatic insufficiency (see below).
acute p. necrosis see acute hemorrhagic PANCREATITIS.
p. α-cells cells in the islet of Langerhans which secrete glucagon.
p. anomaly includes acinar hypoplasia and congenital Islet of langerhans aplasia.
p. β-cells comprise the majority of pancreatic islet cell population; secrete insulin.
p. bladder a diverticulum in the pancreatic duct like a gallbladder in the bile duct. Seen in some cats.
p. C-cells cells in the islet of Langerhans with no known function.
p. calculus small concretions, 4 to 5 mm diameter, in the pancreatic ducts, caused by chronic inflammation. Seen, usually in large numbers, in cattle.
p. cysts anomalous obstructions of ducts, often associated with similar cysts in kidneys and bile ducts.
p. D-cells cells in the islet of Langerhans; known to secrete somatostatin, and vasoactive intestinal peptide.
p. duct one of the two excretory ducts of the pancreas. Depending on the species, it may unite with the common bile duct before entering the duodenum at the major duodenal papilla. Absent from the pig and ox which only have an accessory pancreatic duct (developed from the dorsal primordium) which opens on the minor duodenal papilla. See also BILE DUCT.
p. duct obstruction congenitally by agenesis of the duct, by pancreatic lithiasis or inflammation; causes initial distension followed by atrophy of acinar tissue.
p. ectopic tissue small masses of pancreatic exocrine or endocrine tissue found occasionally in the wall of the stomach or intestines and in the gallbladder; presumed to be functional.

p. enzymes the exocrine secretion into the intestine includes amylase, endo- and exopeptidases, and lipase. The endopeptidases include trypsin, chymotrypsin and elastase, the exopeptidases are the carboxypeptidases A and B.

exocrine p. insufficiency insufficient secretion of digestive enzymes, usually due to loss of acinar tissue from idiopathic atrophy or acute or chronic inflammation, causes maldigestion and malabsorption with diarrhea, steatorrhea and weight loss.

p. fibrosis a sequel to pancreatitis, pancreatic duct obstruction, zinc poisoning.

p. fluke see EURYTREMA.

p. gastrinoma a gastrin-producing tumor arising from the delta cells of the pancreatic islets that causes hypergastrinemia, hypersecretion of gastric acid and ulceration of the upper gastrointestinal tract. Occurs rarely in dogs. See also ZOLLINGER–ELLISON SYNDROME.

p. hypertrophy physiological response to diets high in protein and energy.

p. islets islets of cells scattered through the pancreas; contain α, β, C and D cells.

p. islet cell tumor see GASTRINOMA, INSULINOMA.

p. lipase enzyme released from the exocrine pancreas; catalyzes the hydrolysis of dietary lipids in the presence of bile salts. See also LIPASE.

p. lithiasis see pancreatic calculus (above).

p. nodular hyperplasia hard, pale elevations on the surface of the gland; involve only the exocrine tissue; common in old cats and dogs; cause unknown; no discernible effect on patient.

p. polypeptide secreted by the pancreas into the blood but has no apparent function.

p. trypsin inhibitor see TRYPSIN inhibitor.

pancreatico- word element. [Gr.] *pancreatic duct.*

pancreaticoduodenal pertaining to the pancreas and duodenum.

pancreaticoenterostomy anastomosis of the pancreatic duct to the intestine.

pancreaticomesojejunal ligament an anomalous structure that extends between the pancreaticoduodenal vein, under the ileum and colon, to the left side of the mesojejunum. Reported to be the cause of diarrhea in kittens.

pancreatin a substance from the pancreas of the hog or ox containing enzymes, principally amylase, protease and lipase; used in the treatment of pancreatic exocrine insufficiency.

pancreatitis inflammation of the PANCREAS.

acute hemorrhagic p. a condition due to autolysis of pancreatic tissue caused by escape of enzymes into the substance, resulting in hemorrhage into the parenchyma and surrounding tissues. Seen most commonly in dogs, rarely in horses and pigs. Clinical signs include abdominal pain that may be severe and associated with cardiovascular shock, vomiting and diarrhea. Fatalities are not uncommon. In the longer term, the process may be slowly progressive, appearing clinically to be relapsing, often with eventual destruction of the islets of Langerhans that leads to diabetes mellitus. Called also acute pancreatic necrosis.

chronic p. relapsing or continuing acute pancreatic necrosis. Called also relapsing pancreatitis.

focal p. focal lesions discovered incidentally in patients dying of other disease, e.g. canine distemper, foot and mouth disease.

interstitial p. inflammation of the interstitial tissue; may be acute or chronic.

necrotizing p. see acute hemorrhagic pancreatitis (above).

relapsing p. see chronic pancreatitis (see above).

pancreato- word element. [Gr.] *pancreas.*

pancreatoduodenectomy excision of the head of the pancreas along with the encircling loop of the duodenum.

pancreatogenous arising in the pancreas.

pancreatolithectomy excision of a calculus from the pancreas.

pancreatolithiasis the presence of calculi in the ductal system or parenchyma of the pancreas.

pancreatolithotomy incision of the pancreas for the removal of calculi.

pancreatolysis destruction of pancreatic tissue.

pancreatotomy incision of the pancreas.

pancreatotropic having a special affinity for the pancreas.

pancrelipase a preparation of hog pancreas containing enzymes, principally lipase with amylase and protease, having the same actions as pancreatic juice; used in the treatment of exocrine pancreatic insufficiency.

pancreolithotomy pancreatolithotomy.

pancreolysis pancreatolysis.

pancreozymin a hormone of the duodenal mucosa that stimulates the external secretory activity of the pancreas, especially its production of amylase; identical with CHOLECYSTOKININ.

pancuronium a non-depolarizing neuromuscular blocking agent, used as the bromide salt.

pancystitis cystitis involving the entire thickness of the wall of the urinary bladder, as occurs in interstitial cystitis.

pancytopenia abnormal depression of all the cellular elements of the blood. Results from the depression of activity of bone marrow, spleen and lymph nodes such as occurs in radiation injury and a number of poisonings, e.g. *Pteridium aquilinum*, trichlorethylene extracted soybean meal, nitrofurans and stachybotrytoxicosis.

myelophthisic p. resulting from loss of bone marrow function.

tropical canine p. see canine EHRLICHIOSIS.

pancytopenic relating to pancytopenia.

panda includes *Ailuropoda melanoleuca* (giant panda) and *Ailurus fulgens* (lesser panda). Arboreal, plantigrade animal, vegetarian for the most part but may be omnivorous in some circumstances. Black and white in color with a white face and a black patch around each eye. The lesser or red panda has glossy red fur on its back The genera vary in size from a large cat to a small bear.

pandemic a widespread epidemic, i.e the disease is clustered in time but not in space.

Pandion haliaetus see OSPREY.

Pandy test a screening test for globulin in the cerebrospinal fluid; a positive result is an indication of inflammation in the central nervous system.

panencephalitis encephalitis with parenchymatous lesions of both the gray and white matter of the brain.

sclerosing p. see old dog ENCEPHALITIS.

panendoscope a cystoscope that gives a wide-angle view of the bladder.

Paneth cell narrow, pyramidal or columnar epithelial cell with a nucleus close to its base. Found in the fundus of the mucosal crypts in the intestine.

pangenesis a now discarded hypothesis about heredity stating that the whole organism reproduces itself through all of its parts. The proposed mechanism is based on the supposed existence of gemmules in the blood each of them representing a cell of the body and each of them throws off an atom which is inherited by an offspring.

pangola grass DIGITARIA *decumbens*.

pangolin scaly anteater, of the genus *Manis* and the order Pholidota; covered with overlapping scales like roof tiles. Plantigrade, often arboreal and adapted for destroying anthills and eating the termites or ants that are exposed.

Pangonia a genus of flies in the family Tabanidae; some feed on blood and cause insect worry in horses and cattle. Called also deer fly. Do not suck blood but will mop up spilled blood.

panhypopituitarism generalized hypopituitarism due to absence or damage to the pituitary gland, which in its complete form, leads to absence of gonadal function and insufficiency of thyroid and adrenal function. When cachexia is a prominent feature, it is called SIMMONDS' DISEASE or pituitary CACHEXIA.

juvenile p. most frequent in German shepherd dogs but also in other breeds; puppy dwarfism not apparent until 2–3 months old; small stature, delayed dentition, alopecia, infantile genitalia and short life span are characteristic. See also German shepherd dog DWARFISM.

panhysterectomy total hysterectomy.

panhysterosalpingectomy excision of the uterus, cervix and oviducts.

panhysterosalpingo-oophorectomy excision of the uterus, cervix, oviducts and ovaries.

panic grasses grasses that are members of the genus *Panicum*, e.g. *P. antidotale*.

panicled amaranth AMARANTHUS *cruentus*.

panicled redshank AMARANTHUS *cruentus*.

Panicum a genus of grasses in the family Poaceae. May contain sufficient nitrate or oxalate to cause poisoning with these substances. They are highly productive and popular annual and perennial grasses and cereal crops but many of them cause hepatogenous photosensitization due probably to a high content of steroidal saponins in the plants. Edematous enlargement and icteric staining of the cranial tissues gives rise to the common names of yellow bighead and yellow thickhead.

P. anticum BRACHIARIA *mutica*.

P. antidotale may contain sufficient oxalate to cause oxalate poisoning in sheep or osteodystrophia in horses. Also reported as a cause of atypical interstitial pneumonia. Called also blue panic grass.

P. capillare causes nitrate–nitrite poisoning; called also witchgrass.

P. coloratum may contain high oxalate (see above) or cause hepatogenous photosensitization. Called also Coolah grass, kleingrass.

P. crus-galli reputed to cause photosensitization.

P. decompositum suspected high levels of steroidal saponins causing hepatogenous photosensitization. Called also native millet (Australia).

P. dichotomiflorum causes hepatogenous photosensitization due to steroidal saponins; called also smooth witchgrass.

P. effusum causes hepatogenous photosensitization due probably to steroidal saponins. Called also hairy millet.

P. maximum poisoning characterized by hepatogenous photosensitization due probably to steroidal saponins Called also pigeon grass, guinea grass.

P. maximum* var. *trichoglume causes equine osteodystrophia fibrosa, Called also green panic.

P. miliaceum an annual cereal crop. Causes hepatogenous photosensitization due probably to steroidal saponins. Called also French millet.

P. muticum BRACHIARIA *mutica*.

P. purpurascens a coarse, high-producing pasture grass. Called also para grass.

P. queenslandicum causes hepatogenous photosensitization due probably to steroidal saponins. Called also Yabila grass.

***P. schinzii* (syn. *P. laevifolium* var. *contractum*)** causes hepatogenous photosensitization due to steroidal saponins. Called also sweet grass.

P. virgatum causes hepatogenous photosensitization due probably to steroidal saponins.

P. whitei causes hepatogenous photosensitization due probably to steroidal saponins. Called also *P. laevinode*, pepper grass.

Panilurus spiny lobster, potentially farmable, members of the family Palinura; called also rock lobster, langouste.

panimmunity immunity to a wide range of bacterial and viral infections.

panleukopenia 1. abnormal depression in numbers of white blood cells. 2. the name of a disease caused by feline parvovirus; see FELINE panleukopenia.

feline p. virus feline parvovirus; the etiologic agent of FELINE panleukopenia.

p.-like syndrome is characterized by decreased numbers of leukocytes, often an anemia and thrombocytopenia, resembling clinically infection by the feline panleukopenia virus. Occurs in cats infected by feline leukemia virus.

panlife cycle life history; the series of stages in physical which an organism passes through from the primary stage to the germinal stage of adult demise.

panmyeloid pertaining to all elements of the bone marrow.

panmyelophthisis aplastic anemia.

panmyelosis proliferation of all the elements of the bone marrow.

feline p. a myeloproliferative disorder seen in cats; associated with infection by feline leukemia virus.

panniculitis a rare multifactorial inflammatory condition involving subcutaneous fat.

lobular p. the inflammatory process primarily involves the fat lobules rather than the interlobular connective tissue.

lupus p. see LUPUS ERYTHEMATOSUS.

necrotizing p. multifocal, non-pruritic cutaneous nodules which may ulcerate and discharge serous fluid; recorded in dogs. See also nodular PANNICULITIS (below).

nodular p. subcutaneous nodules that may become cystic or ulcerate or develop fistulous tracts that drain an oily material. They occur in dogs, cats and horses, and may be sterile or caused by infectious agents.

nodular nonsuppurative p. a disease marked by fever and the formation of tender, sterile nodules in the subcutaneous fatty tissues which drain oily, bloody material. Occurs in dogs, particularly Dachshunds. Similar to Weber–Christian or Christian–Weber disease in humans. Called also sterile panniculitis, or relapsing, febrile, nonsuppurative panniculitis.

postinjection p. occurs after a subcutaneous injection; a discrete nodule with a necrotic center.

pyogranulomatous p. see opportunist MYCOBACTERIAL granuloma.

relapsing, febrile, nonsuppurative p. see nodular nonsuppurative panniculitis (above).

septal p. the inflammatory process primarily involves the interlobular connective tissue septae rather than the fat lobules.

sterile p. see nodular nonsuppurative panniculitis (above).

Weber–Christian p. a subcutaneous panniculitis with systemic features. See nodular nonsuppurative panniculitis (above).

panniculus pl. *panniculi* [L.] a layer of membrane.

p. adiposus the subcutaneous fat; a layer of fat underlying the corium, well developed in pigs and marine mammals.

p. carnosus a muscular layer in the superficial fascia of most quadripedal mammals; it includes the cutaneous trunci.

p. muscle see panniculus carnosus (above).

p. reflex a quick twitch of the subcutaneous muscle along the back in response to a pinprick in the thoracolumbar area. Absence of the reflex is important in helping to localize the location of a lesion in the spinal cord.

pannus 1. superficial vascularization of the cornea with infiltration of granulation tissue. 2. an inflammatory exudate overlying synovial cells on the inside of a joint capsule, usually occurring in rheumatoid arthritis or related articular rheumatism. 3. panniculus adiposus.

degenerative p. see chronic superficial KERATITIS.

panophthalmitis inflammation of all the eye structures or tissues. May occur as a result of a penetrating injury but is of greatest importance as a part of a generalized infection, e.g. streptococcal septicemia of the newborn foal.

panosteitis 1. inflammation of every part of a bone. 2. a self-limiting disease of young, large breed dogs, particularly German shepherd dogs, characterized clinically by shifting lameness and radiographically by enosteal and subperiosteal new bone formation on long bones. Called also panosteitis eosinophilica because some cases are reported to have eosinophilia in peripheral blood.

p. eosinophilica see PANOSTEITIS.

panostosis see PANOSTEITIS.

panotitis inflammation of all the parts or structures of the ear.

pansinusitis inflammation involving all the paranasal sinuses.

pansteatitis 1. inflammation of body fat. 2. a disease of cats and aquarium fish fed on a diet high in polyunsaturated fats and low in vitamin E. In cats there is inflammation of all fat tissues; in fish there is also thickening of the swim bladder. See also YELLOW fat disease.

pansystolic the whole of systole; includes presystolic and systolic phases. See also heart MURMUR.

panters ATYPICAL INTERSTITIAL PNEUMONIA of cattle.

panthenol nonproprietary name for pantothenyl alcohol.

Panthera includes cougar (*P. concolor*), jaguar (*P. onca*), jaguarundi (*P. jaguarundi*), leopard (*P. pardus*), lion (*P. leo*), margay (*P. tigrina*), ocelot (*P. pardalis*), tiger (*P. tigris*), Siberian tiger (*P. tigris altaica*), snow leopard (*P. uncia*).

panting rapid, shallow breathing, a characteristic heat-losing reaction in dogs; represents an increase in dead-space ventilation resulting in heat loss without necessarily increasing oxygen uptake or carbon dioxide loss.

p. disease see ATYPICAL INTERSTITIAL PNEUMONIA, ZIERIA *arborescens*.

pant(o)- word element. [Gr.] *all, the whole.*

pantocaine see TETRACAINE.

Panton–Valentine leukocidin a nonhemolytic toxin produced by *Staphylococcus aureus* which kills segmented neutrophils and macrophages.

pantothenate any salt of pantothenic acid.

pantothenic acid a vitamin of the B complex group present in all living tissues as part of the coenzyme A (CoA) molecule or the acyl carrier protein.

p. a. nutritional deficiency a nutritional essential in all species other than ruminants which synthesize it in the rumen. Recorded as a natural occurrence only in poultry and pigs on heavy corn diets. Manifested in pigs by diarrhea, dermatitis, incoordination with a spastic gait and ulcerative colitis. Fowls show poor hatchability of eggs, poor feather development and dermatitis.

pantothenyl alcohol a compound that is oxidized in the body to pantothenic acid.

pantotropic, pantropic having affinity for tissues derived from all three of the germ layers (ectoderm, entoderm and mesoderm).

Panulirus potentially farmable spiny lobster; members of the family Palinura; called also rock lobster, langouste.

panuveitis inflammation of all parts of the uveal tract.

panzootic rarely used equivalent of pandemic when referring to animal diseases.

papain a proteolytic enzyme from the latex of pawpaw, *Carica papaya*, the active ingredient of meat tenderizers. In surgery it is used as a protein digestant and for enzymatic débridement and promotion of normal healing of surface lesions. Papain is also used in immunology to cleave immunoglobulin molecules into Fab and Fc fragments.

Papaver a plant genus of the family Papaveraceae which includes the poppies.

P. aculeatum may cause nitrate–nitrite poisoning.

P. nudicaule causes ataxia and muscle tremor. Called also Iceland poppy.

P. rhoeas a common weed in cultivation fields in Europe. Contains an isoquinoline alkaloid, e.g. rhoadine, and causes somnolence, abdominal pain, recumbency. Called also red poppy.

P. somniferum causes excitement and gastrointestinal disturbance. Called also opium poppy. See OPIUM.

papaveretum a mixture of all of the alkaloids of the opium poppy and is better tolerated by dogs than morphine. Called also omnopon.

papaverine an alkaloid obtained from opium and prepared synthetically; the hydrochloride salt is used as a smooth muscle relaxant.

paper see NEWSPRINT.

p. bark albizia ALBIZIA *tanganyicensis*.

p. bark thorn ACACIA *sieberana*.

p. bone disease see OSTEOGENESIS imperfecta, OSTEODYSTROPHIA FIBROSA.

p. flowers see PSILOSTROPHE.

papilla pl. *papillae* [L.] a small, nipple-shaped projection or elevation.

buccal p. see under dental, conical, lingual etc. papilla (below).

circumvallate p. vallate papilla.

conical p. one of the sparsely scattered fleshy elevations on the tongue or lining the cheeks of cattle.

p. of corium conical extensions of the fibers, capillary blood vessels, and sometimes nerves of the corium into corresponding spaces among downward- or inward-projecting rete ridges on the undersurface of the epidermis. Special papillae coriales occur on the sensitive corium of the frog of the horse's hoof.

dental p., dentinal p. the small mass of condensed mesenchyme capped by each of the enamel organs in a developing tooth.

dermal p. finger- and ridge-like projections of the

dermis which interdigitate with similar depressions in the epidermis.
duodenal p. either of the small elevations (major and minor) on the mucosa of the duodenum, the major at the entrance of the conjoined pancreatic and common bile ducts, the minor at the entrance of the accessory pancreatic duct.
filiform p. one of the short threadlike elevations covering most of the tongue surface. In cats and cattle they are heavily cornified to give a rasping tongue.
foliate p. one of the parallel mucosal folds on the tongue margin at the junction of its body and root, best developed in the horse and pig but rudimentary or absent from other domestic animals.
fungiform p. one of the knob-like projections of the tongue scattered among the filiform papillae.
gingival p. the triangular pad of the gingiva filling the space between the proximal surfaces of two adjacent teeth.
hair p. the fibrovascular mesodermal papilla enclosed within the hair bulb.
ileal p. papilla carrying the terminal orifice of the ileum and its entrance to the large bowel.
incisive p. an elevation at the anterior end of the raphe of the palate onto which the incisive ducts open.
lacrimal p. see LACRIMAL punctum.
lingual p. elevations on the surface of the tongue, containing the taste buds; the conical, filiform, foliate, fungiform and vallate papillae.
major duodenal p. the papilla in the duodenum for the common opening of the bile duct and the pancreatic duct.
mammary p. the teat or nipple of the mammary gland.
optic p. optic disk.
palatine p. incisive papilla.
parotid p. the oral opening of the duct of the parotid salivary gland located opposite the third upper molar.
p. pili hair papilla.
renal p. the blunted apex of a renal pyramid.
ruminal p. papillae up to 0.5 inch long, flat or filiform that cover most of the ruminal wall but are absent from the pillars and the dorsal part of the dorsal sac.
tactile p. tactile corpuscles.
p. unguiculiformes horny claw-shaped papillae at the reticulo-omasal orifice.
terminal hoof p. papillae on the distal ends of the sensitive laminae of the hoof.
tongue p. small projections from the mucous membrane of the tongue that include filiform, lenticular, fungiform, foliate and vallate papillae; most are to assist in grooming, food prehension and movement; some carry orifices for glands and others for taste.
marginal tongue p. temporary filiform papillae in puppies, piglets and kittens which are thought to facilitate sucking.
urethral p. a slight elevation in the vestibule of the vagina at the external orifice of the urethra.
vallate p. one of the eight to 12 large circular papillae arranged in a V near the base of the tongue.
p. of Vater, Vater's p. major duodenal papilla.
wool p. as for hair papilla (above).

papillary pertaining to a papilla; having the characteristics of a papilla.
p. duct urine passes from the collecting tubules into the papillary ducts as the last section of the renal tubular system.
p. necrosis necrosis of the renal papilla.
p. squirting a feature of seborrheic dermatitis, zinc-responsive dermatoses; the superficial papillae are edematous and contain dilated vessels, the overlying epidermis is edematous and parakeratototic.
p. sulcus gustatory glands open into a sulcus in the mouth.

papillectomy excision of a papilla.

papilledema edema and hyperemia of the optic disk, usually associated with increased intracranial pressure; called also choked disk.

papillitis inflammation of a papilla, especially of the optic disk.

papilloadenocystoma papillary cystadenoma.

papillocarcinoma papillary carcinoma.

papilloma the common wart. A benign tumor derived from epithelium, which may arise from skin, conjunctiva, mucous membranes or glandular ducts. Varies from keratinized, to fibrovascular, squamous. Caused by a species-specific papillomavirus. In cattle, papilloma occurring particularly in the bladder may become carcinoma where cattle are grazing bracken fern. Transmissible by intradermal injection. See also PAPILLOMATOSIS, FIBROPAPILLOMA, TRANSMISSIBLE porcine genital papillomatosis.
cutaneous p. the common form; distinguishable from papilloma of the esophageal groove and reticulum, bladder.
fibrovascular p. single or multiple, small, benign fibrovascular skin tumors, that occur occasionally on the extremities or ventral thorax of dogs. Called also skin tag, keratin tag, soft fibroma.
plexus p. a rare tumor of the choroid plexus, often causing an internal hydrocephalus.
transmissible p. see PAPILLOMA.

papillomatosis disease state characterized by the development of multiple papillomas. See also PAPILLOMA, FIBROPAPILLOMA.
canine viral p. multiple papillomas, caused by a papillomavirus, occur most commonly on the oral mucosa and lips of young dogs. Occasionally skin, cornea, conjunctiva and eyelids are also involved. The tumors may persist for several months, occasionally longer, but spontaneous regression is usual.
cottontail rabbit p. infection by a papilloma virus specific to *Sylvilagus floridanus*, causes cutaneous papillomas which may become malignant.
genital p. multiple fibropapillomas of the anogenital skin transmitted venereally in cattle, usually involving the vulva and penis. There is also a genital form of the disease in pigs affecting principally the boars.
oral p. see oral lapine papillomatosis (below), canine viral papillomatosis (above).
oral lapine p. small, gray, sessile or pedunculated tumors on the undersurface of the tongue and rarely at other sites in the mouth, caused by a papillomavirus. Seen in *Oryctolagus* and *Sylvilagus* spp.
teat p. there are five antigenically identified papillomaviruses which cause warts on the teats of cows. Lesions vary from ricegrain lesions to long tags of keratinized tissue.

Papillomavirus a genus in the family *Papovaviridae*. They are naked, icosahedral viruses with a circular, supercoiled DNA genome of ~8 kilobases and are specific to each animal species and in some cases to specific epithelial sites in that species. Virions are very stable and readily transmissible especially if there is abrasion such as by grooming with a curry comb. The type virus is the Shope papilloma virus of rabbits. See also SARCOID, PAPILLOMA, PAPILLOMATOSIS.

Papillon a small, dainty dog with an alert expression, rounded head and long, silky coat in white with colored patches. The large, rounded ears are distinctive with their flowing fringe of hair and may be erect, resembling a butterfly, hence the name of the breed, or they may be dropped, a type called Phalene (moth). Called also butterfly dog.

papilloretinitis inflammation of the optic nerve and disk.

papillotomy incision of a papilla, as of a duodenal papilla.

Papio see BABOON.

Papovaviridae a family of viruses containing two genera: *Papillomavirus*, which cause warts in various species, and *Polyomavirus*, which cause tumors in rodents (mice, hamsters) and have been extensively studied as models of viral oncogenesis. Virions are icosahedral, 45–55 nm in diameter, naked, ether-resistant and contain a supercoiled circular double-stranded DNA genome of ~8 kilobases.

papovavirus a virus in the family PAPOVAVIRIDAE.

Pappenheimer body see Pappenheimer BODY.

papple-shaped abdomen an abdomen pear-shaped on the right side and apple-shaped on the left.

PAPS 3′-phosphoadenosine 5-phosphosulfate.

Papuan black snake see PSEUDECHIS *papuanus*.

papular characterized by the development of epidermal or oral mucosal papules.

bovine p. stomatitis a benign stomatitis caused by a poxvirus in the genus *Parapoxvirus*. Lesions occur in young cattle and are characterized by round papules that develop a roughened center which expands and may merge with other adjacent lesions to give a network effect. The lesions are on the buccal mucosa and the adjoining skin of the muzzle and occasionally esophagus and forestomachs.

papulation the formation of papules.

papule a small circumscribed, solid, elevated lesion of the skin.

follicular p. one arising from a hair follicle; hair projects from the center.

lichenoid p. one that is elevated and flat-topped.

papulopustular marked by papules and pustules.

papulosis the presence of multiple papules.

papulosquamous both papular and scaly.

papulovesicular marked by papules and vesicles.

papyraceous like paper.

p. fetal mummification the commonest form of fetal mummification; fluids are resorbed, the placenta being reduced to paper-like sheets.

PAR post-anesthesia recovery.

par [L.] *pair*.

para [L.] used with numerals to designate the number of pregnancies that have resulted in the birth of viable offspring, as para 0 (none—nullipara), para I (one—unipara), para II (two—bipara), para III (three—tripara), para IV (four—quadripara). The number is not indicative of the number of offspring produced where multiple offspring occur with a pregnancy.

para- word element. [Gr.] *beside, beyond, accessory to, apart from, against.* In chemistry, a prefix indicating the substitution in a derivative of the benzene ring of two atoms linked to opposite carbon atoms in the ring; abbreviated *p*-.

para-aminobenzoic acid a compound that is a growth factor for certain bacteria that use it to synthesize folic acid. Sulfonamides act by blocking a step in this synthesis. Abbreviated PAB, PABA.

para-aminohippurate any salt of para-aminohippuric acid.

para-aminohippuric acid a derivative of para-aminobenzoic acid used to measure the effective renal plasma flow and to determine the functional capacity of the renal tubular excretory mechanism. Called also aminohippuric acid. Abbreviated PAH, PAHA.

para-aminophenol a substance used in the manufacture of dyes and drugs. May cause skin sensitization and methemoglobinemia.

p. derivative analgesics include acetanilid, acetophenetidin and acetaminophen.

para-aminophenylarsonic acid arsanilic acid. See also organic ARSENIC poisoning.

para-aminosalicylic acid see *p*-AMINOSALICYLIC ACID.

para-anesthesia 1. anesthesia of the lower part of the body. 2. anesthesia-related.

para-aortic beside the aorta.

p. bodies see para-aortic BODY.

para-aural surrounding the ear.

p. abscess infection in the external ear canal or middle ear that extends to the surrounding soft tissues and forms a draining sinus through the skin because of obstruction of the external ear canal by atresia, neoplasm or proliferative tissue.

para grass BRACHIARIA *mutica*, PANICUM *purpurascens*.

para-ureidobenzenearsonic acid used for the treatment of avian histomoniasis; fed in excessive amounts causes peripheral neuropathy with lameness in turkeys.

parabens see HYDROXYBENZOATE.

parabiosis 1. the union of two individuals, as conjoined twins, or of experimental animals by surgical operation. 2. temporary suppression of conductivity and excitability.

parablackleg bacillus see MALIGNANT edema.

parabronchi tertiary bronchi in the avian lung. The domestic fowl has some 500 parabronchi each 1 to 2 mm diameter with the wall of each containing the complex respiratory epithelium.

Parabronema a genus of alimentary tract nematodes found in wild animals Includes *P. africum*, *P. rhodesiense* (in African elephants), *P. rhinocerotis* (rhinoceros, elephant).

parabuxine one of the toxic alkaloids found in the plant BUXUS SEMPERVIRENS.

paracasein casein. The insoluble product of rennin acting on caseinogen. In American terminology the term for casein; not included in British nomenclature.

paracentesis surgical puncture of a cavity for the aspiration of fluid.

abdominal p. insertion of a trocar through a small incision or a needle into the abdominal cavity, to remove ascitic fluids, inject a therapeutic agent, or to collect a sample for cytological and chemical examination. It is an important technique in the examination of horses for colic and in investigation of causes of ascites in all species. Called also abdominocentesis.

anterior chamber p. aspiration of aqueous humor from the anterior chamber may be indicated as a diagnostic procedure in diseases such as hypopyon, hyphemia, glaucoma and iridocyclitis.

pericardial p. see PERICARDICENTESIS.

thoracic p. surgical puncture for drainage of the thoracic cavity and for collection of a sample of fluid for clinical pathology examination See also THORACENTESIS.

vitreous p. may be useful in the diagnosis of diseases of the posterior segment of the eye, e.g. endophthalmitis, panophthalmitis and neoplasms. Called also hyalocentesis.

paracephalus a fetus with a defective head and imperfect sense organs.

paracervical beside the neck, such as the uterine cervix.

paracetamol see ACETAMINOPHEN.

parachordal beside the notochord.

paraclinical pertaining to abnormalities (e.g. morphological or biochemical) underlying clinical manifestations (e.g. abdominal pain or fever). Used also as a collective term for the sciences that deal with pathology, including clinical pathology and immunology, and pathogenic agents including microbiology, parasitology and toxicology.

p. tests laboratory tests in the area of pathology, clinical pathology, immunology, microbiology, parasitology, toxicology.

Paracoccidioides a genus of fungi that proliferate by multiple budding yeast cells in the tissues.

P. brasiliensis the etiological agent of PARACOCCIDIOIDOMYCOSIS. Called also *Blastomyces brasiliensis*.

paracoccidioidomycosis an often fatal, chronic granulomatous disease of humans, dogs, cats and most mammals caused by *Paracoccidioides brasiliensis*. The disease is endemic in South America, particularly Brazil. Infection primarily involves the lungs, but spreads to the skin, mucous membranes, lymph nodes and internal organs. Called also South American blastomycosis.

paracolitis inflammation of the outer coat of the colon.

Paracolobactrum not a valid genus. These bacteria rightly belong in *Escherichia*, *Klebsiella*, *Salmonella*, *Edwardsiella* spp. For *P. arizonae*, see SALMONELLA *arizonae*.

paracolon bacteria see PARACOLOBACTRUM.

Paracooperia a genus of nematodes in the family Trichostrongylidae.

***P. nodulosa* (*P. matoffi*)** occurs in the intestines of buffalo and other wild animals and may cause nodules in the intestinal wall.

Paracoroptes allenopitheci a mange mite species in the family Psoroptidae. Found in the ears and on the body of primates.

paracortex the thymus-dependent part of the lymph node.

paracrine indicative of the action of the secretion of one kind of endocrine cell on another kind which is not the normal effector cell.

p. hormones in contrast to true endocrines these hormones are not released into the bloodstream but into the surrounding tissues and act in the immediate vicinity, e.g. intestinal mucosal hormones.

paracystic situated near the bladder.

paracystitis inflammation of tissues around the bladder.

paradental 1. having some association with dentistry. 2. periodontal.

paradidymis remnants of mesonephric tubules sometimes found as a small body near the head of the epididymis.

paradigm a pattern of thought, a similarity of conceptualization.

paradistemper an oldfashioned term for clinical syndromes which are now known to be manifestations of canine DISTEMPER, e.g. hardpad disease, or which have been shown to be separate diseases, e.g. infectious canine HEPATITIS.

paradoxical different from what is expected; at variance with the established laws.

p. motion see paradoxical respiration (below).

p. respiration a type of breathing in which all or part of a lung inflates during inspiration and balloons out during expiration; the opposite of normal chest motion. Called also paradoxical motion. The condition seriously inhibits the movement of gases during respiration and can produce severe and even fatal cardiovascular disturbances and respiratory insufficiency if not quickly relieved by emergency treatment.

Paradoxical respiration or paradoxical motion of the lung usually results from traumatic injury to the thorax (FLAIL chest) in which several ribs are fractured in two or more places and are no longer attached by bony cartilage to the rest of the rib cage. The condition can also be seen following surgical removal of several ribs and in paralysis of the diaphragm.

p. septal motion in echocardiography, the interventricular septum moves away from the left ventricular free wall during systole. Normally, it would move towards the wall. It is seen in right ventricular hypertrophy.

Paraelaphostrongylus see PNEUMOSTRONGYLUS.

paraesophageal beside the esophagus.

p. herniation see paraesophageal HERNIA.

Parafasciolopsis a genus of flukes (digenetic trematodes) in the family Fasciolidae.

P. fasciolaemorpha found in the digestive tract and gallbladder of the elk and deer.

paraffin 1. a purified hydrocarbon wax used for embedding histological specimens. 2. a saturated hydrocarbon used as a fuel oil. Poisoning causes gastroenteritis and aspiration pneumonia, the latter being secondary to vomiting. Called also alkane, kerosene, lamp oil. See also OIL. 3. petrolatum.

liquid p. liquid petrolatum. See mineral OIL.

p. embedding technique the most commonly used technique for the preparation of slides of tissue for light microscopic examination.

paraffinoma a chronic granuloma produced by prolonged exposure to paraffin.

Parafilaria a genus of nematodes in the filarioid family Filariidae.

P. antipini found in deer.

P. bovicola causes hemorrhagic nodules in the skin of cattle and buffalo.

***P. multipapillosa* (syn. *Filaria haemorrhagica*)** causes nodules in the subcutaneous and intermuscular tissues of horses. The nodules break open and discharge blood and then heal. They reappear each summer.

parafilariasis see PARAFILARIA *multipapillosa*.

Parafilaroides a genus of nematodes in the metastrongyloid family Filaroididae; cause lesions in the lungs of aquatic mammals. Includes *P. decorus* (sealions), *P. gymnurus* (harbor seals), *P. nanus* and *P. prolificus* (Stellar's sealion).

parafollicular close to a follicle.

p. cell a C CELL of the thyroid gland.

paraformaldehyde an additive fixative used in the preparation of histology and pathology slides of animal tissues.

paraganglioma a tumor of the tissue composing the paraganglia.

paraganglion pl. *paraganglia* [Gr.] a collection of chromaffin cells derived from neural ectoderm, occurring outside the adrenal medulla, usually near the sympathetic ganglia and in relation to the aorta and its branches. Most secrete epinephrine or norepinephrine.

paragle fly see PARAGLE REDICUM.

Paragle redicum an anthomyiid fly that lays its eggs in canine feces.

paraglossia inflammation of the oral tissues under the tongue.

paragonimiasis infection with lung flukes of the genus *Paragonimus*. Characterized by lethargy, cough, dyspnea. On autopsy there is an eosinophilic peritonitis, pleurisy and myositis, and a chronic bronchitis and granulomatous pneumonia.

Paragonimus a genus of trematode parasites in the family Paragonimidae. Causes PARAGONIMIASIS.

P. africanus, P. caliensis, P. iloktsuenensis, P. mexicanus, P. ohirai, P. peruvianus, P. uterobilateralis found in the lungs of a large number of animal species.

P. kellicotti found in the lungs of cat, dog and pig. Mink and muskrat are the probable primary hosts.

P. westermani found in the lungs and other organs of most animal species, and humans.

Parahistomonas a genus of protozoa in the family Monocercomadidae.

P. wenrichi some similarity to *Histomonas* spp. but is nonpathogenic in gallinaceous birds, especially pheasants.

parahormone a substance, not a true hormone, that has a hormone-like action in controlling the functioning of some distant organ.

Parainfluenzavirus one of the three genera of viruses in the family PARAMYXOVIRIDAE; abbreviated PI virus.

p. 1 causes bronchopneumonia in young pigs. Called also SENDAI VIRUS. Occurs also in humans.

p. 2 a group of viruses one of which causes infectious tracheobronchitis of dogs (SV-5 disease).

p. 3 involved in the complex etiology of shipping fever in cattle and similar respiratory tract infections in sheep and possibly horses.

p. SV-5 an earlier name for parainfluenza 2 (above).

parakeelia, parakeelya see CALANDRINIA.

parakeets one of the bird groups known as typical parrots in the family Psittacidae. Small parrots with long tails and include the BUDGERIGAR.

parakeratosis persistence of the nuclei of keratinocytes as they rise into the horny layer of the skin; it occurs normally in the epithelium of the true mucous membrane of the mouth and vagina. When it occurs on the external skin it constitutes a lesion. The appearance is of thickening of the skin with thick scale formation, cracking and fissuring, and an underlying raw red surface. Occurs as a specific disease in pigs fed on rations deficient in zinc; the effect is exacerbated on diets high in calcium.

inherited p. occurs in calves, which are normal at birth but develop parakeratosis all over the body, especially on the legs and die after a long illness. Responds to treatment with zinc given orally. See also THYMIC hypoplasia. Called also lethal trait A46, adema disease.

ruminal p. the ruminal papillae are enlarged, leathery and adhered in clumps. The lesion is most severe in the dorsal part of the sac. Occurs principally in animals fed pelleted feed.

parakeratotic pertaining to parakeratosis.

p. caps focal parakeratotic hyperkeratosis.

parakinesia perversion of motor powers causing strange and unnatural movements; in ophthalmology, irregular action of an individual ocular muscle.

parakinesis parakinesia.

paraldehyde a sedative and hypnotic that has an unpleasant taste and imparts an unpleasant odor to the breath. Because of its low therapeutic index, it is now little used.

parallagma displacement of a bone or of the fragments of broken bone.

parallel two or more lines which run continuously at exactly the same distance apart.

p. columns text is arranged across the page in rows; the next row commences just below the longest column of the previous row.

p. grid see parallel GRID.

parallergy a condition in which an allergic state, produced by specific sensitization, predisposes the body to react to other allergens with clinical manifestations that differ from the original reaction.

paralumbar next to the lumbar area.

p. fossa see paralumbar FOSSA.

paralysis loss or impairment of motor function in a part due to a lesion of the neural or muscular mechanism; also, by analogy, impairment of sensory function (sensory paralysis). Called also palsy. Motor paralysis may be expressed as flaccid, in the case of lower motor neuron lesion, or spastic, in the case of an upper motor neuron lesion. See also PARAPLEGIA, QUADRIPLEGIA, HEMIPLEGIA and paralyses of individual cranial and peripheral nerves.

p. of accommodation paralysis of the ciliary muscles of the eye so as to prevent accommodation.

anal p. manifested by flaccidity and lack of tone of the anal sphincter, and loss of house training restraint in companion animals.

antepartum p. pressure on sciatic nerves by a large fetus in late pregnancy in a cow can cause posterior paralysis that is cured by a cesarean section.

ascending p. spinal paralysis that progresses forwards involving first the hindlimbs then the forelimbs, then the intercostal muscles, then the diaphragm, and finally the muscles of the neck.

birth p. that due to injury received by the neonate at birth.

bladder p. manifested by fullness of the bladder and response to manual pressure. See also motor paralytic URINARY BLADDER.

cage p. see THIAMIN nutritional deficiency.

central p. any paralysis due to a lesion of the brain or spinal cord.

cerebral p. paralysis caused by some intracranial lesion.

Chastek p. see THIAMIN nutritional deficiency.

compression p. that caused by pressure on a nerve.

congenital p. paralysis of the newborn. Many cases are due to birth trauma especially when lay persons exert excessive traction. Other causes are enzootic ataxia, inherited congenital paraplegias in calves and pigs, spina bifida and spinal dysraphism and occipito-alanto-axial malformations in foals and puppies.

conjugate p. loss of ability to perform some parallel ocular movements.

coonhound p. see idiopathic POLYRADICULONEURITIS.

crossed p. paralysis affecting one side of the head and the other side of the body.

curled toe p. a disease of poultry caused by a nutritional deficiency of riboflavin. See also CURLED TOE PARALYSIS.

decubitus p. paralysis due to pressure on a nerve from lying for a long time in one position.

esophageal p. manifested by inability to swallow, and regurgitation.

facial p. weakening or paralysis of the facial nerve. See also FACIAL paralysis.

flaccid p. paralysis characterized by loss of voluntary movement, decreased tone of limb muscles, absence of tendon reflexes and neurogenic atrophy.

immunological p. the absence of immune response to a specific antigen. See also TOLERANCE.

infectious bulbar p. see AUJESZKY'S DISEASE.
ischemic p. local paralysis due to stoppage of circulation.
lambing p. MATERNAL obstetric paralysis in the ewe.
laryngeal p. see LARYNGEAL hemiplegia.
mixed p. combined motor and sensory paralysis.
motor p. paralysis of the voluntary muscles.
nerve p. paralysis caused by damage to the local motor nerve supply. See also peripheral nerve paralysis (below).
obstetric p. see MATERNAL obstetric paralysis.
partial p. see PARESIS.
peripheral nerve p. the part deprived of its peripheral nerve supply shows flaccid paralysis, absence of spinal reflexes, muscle atrophy and a subnormal temperature.
postcalving p. see MATERNAL obstetric paralysis.
posterior p. paralysis of the hindlimbs, tail and perineum. See also PARAPLEGIA.
range p. see MAREK'S DISEASE.
sensory p. loss of sensation resulting from a morbid process.
spastic p. paralysis with rigidity of the muscles and heightened deep muscle reflexes.
tongue p. see HYPOGLOSSAL nerve paralysis.

paralytic 1. pertaining to paralysis. 2. an animal affected with paralysis.
p. bladder see atonic neurogenic URINARY BLADDER.
p. ileus loss of all intestinal tone and motility as a result of reflex inhibition in acute peritonitis, from excessive handling during bowel surgery, prolonged and severe distension due to intestinal obstruction and in grass sickness of horses. The effect is the same as that of an acute intestinal obstruction. Called also ileus, adynamic ileus.
p. myoglobinuria a disease of horses characterized by red-brown urine due to myoglobinuria, and acute myopathy with muscle weakness, often to the point of being unable to get up. It occurs after exercise after several days of inaction while still being fed a high-energy ration. Called also azoturia and Monday morning disease.
p. rabies see RABIES.
p. shellfish poisoning syndrome of flaccid paralysis after ingestion of bivalve molluscs whose tissues have accumulated tetrahydroxypurine toxins from some marine DINOFLAGELLATES; syndrome identical with TETRODOTOXIN poisoning. See also SAXITOXIN. Called also PSP.

paralyzant 1. causing paralysis. 2. a drug that causes paralysis.

paramastitis inflammation of tissues around the mammary gland.

parameatal situated near or around a meatus.

Paramecium a genus of ciliate protozoa.

paramedian beside the midplane.

paramesonephric see MÜLLERIAN DUCT.
p. duct inhibiting factor secreted by the sustentacular cells of the testis; promotes the degeneration of the paramesonephric ducts.

parameter 1. in mathematics and statistics, an arbitrary constant, such as a population mean or standard deviation. It wholly or partly determines a probability distribution. 2. a property of a system that can be measured numerically.

paramethadione an anticonvulsant.

paramethasone a glucocorticoid used as the 21-acetate ester for its anti-inflammatory and antiallergic effects.

Parametorchis a genus of digenetic trematodes in the family Opisthorchidae.
P. complexus found in the bile ducts of dogs and cats. May cause abdominal pain, ascites, jaundice.

parametric 1. situated near the uterus; parametrial. 2. pertaining to or defined in terms of a parameter.
p. method a method of testing a hypothesis which requires the user to assume a particular model for the distribution of data, e.g. Poisson, normal.

parametritis inflammation of the parametrium.

parametrium the extension of the subserous coat of the uterus laterally between the layers of the broad ligament.

Paramoeba cause of AMEBIC gill disease in salmonids.

Paramonostomum intestinal flukes (digenetic trematodes); *P. alveatum* and *P. parvum* are found in ducks but appear to cause little injury.

paramphistomes members of the family Paramphistomatidae; belonging to genera such as *Paramphistomum*, *Calycophoron*, *Cotylophoron*, *Gigantocotyle*.

paramphistomiasis infestation with members of the family Paramphistomatidae.

paramphistomosis the disease caused by infestation of ruminants with stomach flukes. Adult flukes cause weight loss, loss of production and anemia. Immature flukes cause diarrhea also. Called also stomach fluke disease. See also PARAMPHISTOMUM, CALICOPHORON, CEYLONOCOTYLE and COTYLOPHORON.

Paramphistomum a genus of ruminal flukes (digenetic trematodes) in the family Paramphistomatidae.
P. cervi, P. ichikawai, P. microbothrium important parasites of cattle, sheep, goats and buffalo.
P. cotylophoron see PARAMPHISTOMOSIS.
P. explanatum, P. gotoi, P. hiberniae, P. liorchis, P. microbothrioides, P. scotiae other paramphistomes of cattle.

paramyloidosis accumulation of an atypical form of amyloid in tissues.

paramyoclonus a condition characterized by myoclonic contractions of various muscles.
p. multiplex a condition characterized by sudden shocklike contractions.

paramyotonia a disease marked by tonic spasms due to disorder of muscular tonicity, especially a hereditary and congenital affliction.
p. congenita myotonia congenita.

paramyotonic syndromes signs include stiffness and reluctance to walk, exacerbated by cold and by exercise; include congenital paramyotonia in King Charles spaniels, HYPERKALEMIC PERIODIC PARALYSIS in Quarter horses, feline HYPOKALEMIC polymyopathy.

Paramyxoviridae a family of viruses in the order *Mononegavirales* containing three genera: *Parainfluenzavirus*, which includes Newcastle disease virus, mumps virus and parainfluenza viruses 1 to 4; *Morbillivirus*, which includes measles, canine distemper, rinderpest and possibly equine morbillivirus; *Pneumovirus*, which includes the respiratory syncytial viruses of humans, cattle and turkeys. They are large (180 nm diameter) enveloped viruses containing a genome that is a single molecule of single-stranded negative sense RNA.

paramyxovirus a member of the family PARAMYXOVIRIDAE.
avian p. see NEWCASTLE DISEASE.
p. encephalomyelitis a disease of pigs in Mexico, believed to be caused by a paramyxovirus. In addition to encephalomyelitis, there is reproductive failure and corneal opacity. Called also porcine blue eye disease. Mexican blue eye. Paramyxovirus-like agents

have also been associated with encephalomyelitis in domestic and large exotic Felidae.

paranal sacs see ANAL SACS.

Paranaplasma a genus of organisms of uncertain validity in the family Anaplasmataceae, with a close resemblance to *Anaplasma* spp. They are often found in mixed infections with *A. marginale* in cattle. Includes *P. caudatum*, *P. discoides*.

paranasal beside the nasal cavity.

p. sinuses mucosa-lined air cavities in the bones of the skull, communicating with the nasal cavity. See also SINUS.

p. sinus polyps rare cause of nasal bleeding in horses.

paraneoplastic auxiliary to neoplasia.

p. syndrome a collective term for disorders arising from metabolic effects of cancer on tissues remote from the tumor; such disorders may, for example, appear as primary endocrine, hematological or neuromuscular disorders. See also PSEUDOHYPERPARATHYROIDISM.

paranephric 1. near the kidney. 2. pertaining to the adrenal gland.

paranephritis 1. inflammation of the adrenal gland. 2. inflammation of the connective tissue around the kidney.

paranephros pl. *paranephroi* [Gr.] an adrenal gland.

paranesthesia para-anesthesia.

paraneural alongside a nerve.

Paranoplocephala a genus of tapeworms in the family Anoplocephalidae. Parasitic in rodents. See also ANOPLOCEPHALOIDES.

P. mamillana see ANOPLOCEPHALOIDES.

paranucleus a body sometimes seen in cell protoplasm near the nucleus.

paraovarian beside the ovary.

p. cyst remnants of mesonephric or paramesonephric ducts and tubules.

paraparesis a partial paralysis of the lower extremities.

paraphimosis inability to retract the penis because of its swollen state, or because of constriction of the preputial orifice.

paraplasm 1. any abnormal growth. 2. hyaloplasm (1).

paraplastic exhibiting a perverted formative power; of the nature of a paraplasm (1).

paraplectic paraplegic.

paraplegia paralysis of the hindlimb and, in some cases, the posterior part of the body caudal to the last cervical vertebrae. The paralysis may be acute in onset as in fracture of a lumbar vertebra, or gradual; it may be spastic or flaccid.

Paraplegia is a form of central nervous system paralysis, in which the paralysis affects all the muscles of the parts involved. In the majority of cases, paraplegia results from disease or injury of the spinal cord that causes interference with nerve paths connecting the brain and the muscles.

inherited congenital p. is observed in cattle and pigs. The paralysis may be flaccid or spastic and there may or may not be degenerative lesions in the spinal cord.

paraplegiform resembling paraplegia.

Parapoxvirus a genus of viruses in the family POXVIRIDAE.

p. infection includes bovine papular stomatitis, contagious ecthyma.

paraprofessional 1. a person who is specially trained in a particular field or occupation to assist a veterinarian. 2. allied animal health professional. 3. pertaining to a paraprofessional.

paraprostatic beside the prostate.

p. cyst appears to result from anomalous development from vestiges of the müllerian duct.

paraprotein immunoglobulin produced by a clone of neoplastic plasma cells proliferating abnormally, e.g. myeloma proteins and cryoglobulins. See also monoclonal GAMMOPATHY.

paraproteinemia the presence in the blood of paraproteins.

paraproteinuria the presence in the urine of paraproteins.

parapsoriasis a disease resembling psoriasis of humans. There are erythematous, scaly plaques on the body, with hair loss and secondary bacterial infection.

paraquat a dipyridilium herbicide which initially causes stomatitis, colic, vomiting and diarrhea, then 2 to 10 days later causes pulmonary edema and hemorrhage which leads to a fibrosing pneumonitis and death in all species if given in sufficiently large doses.

parareflexia any disorder of the reflexes.

pararosaniline a basic dye; a triphenylmethane derivative, one of the components of basic fuchsin.

pararotaviruses atypical rotaviruses that have been isolated from pigs, cattle and lambs.

pararrhythmia parasystole.

parasacral situated near the sacrum.

Parascaris a genus of roundworms in the family Ascarididae.

***P. equorum* (syn. *Ascaris equorum*)** found in the small intestine of horses and zebras. In foals up to 9 months of age heavy infestation with migrating larvae causes coughing. Heavy burdens of adult worms may cause diarrhea, debility, potbelly in young animals.

parasinoidal situated along the course of a sinus.

parasite a plant or animal that lives upon or within another living organism at whose expense it obtains some advantage. See also SYMBIOSIS.

Among the many parasites in nature, some feed upon animal hosts, causing diseases ranging from the mildly annoying to the severe and often fatal. Parasites include multicelled and single-celled animals, fungi and bacteria. Viruses are sometimes considered to be parasites. However, the commonest use of the word refers to the multicellular helminth, arachnid, crustacean (copepod) and arthropod parasites.

accidental p. one that parasitizes an organism other than the usual host.

facultative p. one that may be parasitic upon another organism but can exist independently.

incidental p. accidental parasite.

obligate p., obligatory p. one that is entirely dependent upon a host for its survival.

periodic p. one that parasitizes a host for short periods.

temporary p. one that lives free of its host during part of its life cycle.

parasitemia the presence of parasites, including filariae and protozoa, in the blood.

parasitic pertaining to parasites. See also ARTERITIS, BRONCHITIS, GASTRITIS, GASTROENTERITIS, HYPERSENSITIVITY, PNEUMONIA, TRACHEOBRONCHITIS, HELMINTIC.

parasiticide destructive to parasites; also, an agent that is destructive to parasites.

parasitism 1. symbiosis in which one population (or individual) adversely affects another, but cannot live without it. 2. infection or infestation with internal or external parasites.

parasitize to live on or within a host as a parasite.

parasitogenic due to parasites.
parasitological pertaining to or emanating from parasitology.
p. examination includes examination of feces for protozoa, worm eggs or larvae and for tapeworm segments, skin scrapings for arthropod parasites, blood samples for protozoa, microfilariae, for plasma pepsinogen levels, and examination of gross specimens.
parasitologist a person skilled in parasitology.
parasitology the scientific study of parasites and parasitism.
parasitosis a disease caused by a parasitic infestation. See also HELMINTHIASIS.
parasitotropic having affinity for parasites.
paraspadias a congenital condition in which the urethra opens on one side of the penis.
Paraspidodera a genus of nematodes in the superfamily Heterakoidea.
P. uncinata occurs in the large intestine of guinea pigs and agouti and appears to be nonpathogenic.
parasternal beside the sternum.
Parastrigea intestinal digenetic trematodes in the family Strigeidae.
P. robusta found in the intestine of domestic ducks and may cause anemia and hemorrhagic enteritis.
parasympathetic pertaining to the parasympathetic nervous system.
p. cholinergic vasodilator fibers cause dilatation of blood vessels in tissues including cerebral vessels, tongue, salivary glands, external genitalia, bladder, rectum.
p. nervous system part of the AUTONOMIC nervous system, the preganglionic fibers of which leave the central nervous system with cranial nerves III, VII, IX and X and several sacral nerves (depending on species); postganglionic fibers are distributed to the heart, smooth muscles, and glands of the head and neck, and thoracic, abdominal and pelvic viscera. Almost three-quarters of all parasympathetic nerve fibers are in the VAGUS nerves, which serve both the thoracic and abdominal regions of the body.

The predominant secretion of the nerve endings of the parasympathetic nervous system is *acetylcholine*, which acts on the various organs of the body to either excite or inhibit certain activities. For example, stimulation of the parasympathetic system causes constriction of the pupil of the eye and contraction of the ciliary muscle; increase of the glandular secretion of enzymes, as in the case of the pancreas; increased peristalsis; and a slowed heart rate. Excitation of the sympathetic nervous system often results in an effect opposite to that of the parasympathetic system; however, most organs are predominantly under the control of either one or the other of the two nervous systems that compose the autonomic nervous system.
p. outflow the total of parasympathetic nerves which leave the central nervous system. Includes the cranial and sacral outflows.
parasympatholytic anticholinergic; producing effects resembling those of interruption of the parasympathetic nerve supply of a part; having a destructive effect on the parasympathetic nerve fibers or blocking the transmission of impulses by them. Also, an agent that produces such effects, e.g. atropine.
parasympathomimetic cholinergic; producing effects resembling those of stimulation of the parasympathetic nerve supply of a part. Also, an agent that produces such effects, e.g. physostigmine.
parasynapsis the union of chromosomes side by side during meiosis.
parasynovitis inflammation of the tissues about a synovial sac.
parasystole a cardiac irregularity attributed to the interaction of two foci independently initiating cardiac impulses at different rates. Called also pararrhythmia.
paratenic host an animal acting as a substitute intermediate host of a parasite, usually having acquired the parasite by ingestion of the original host; no development of the parasite takes place but the phenomenon aids in the transmission of infection. Called also transfer or transport host.
paratenon, paratendon loose connective tissue filling the interstices of the fascial compartment in which a tendon is situated and which allows it to move freely. Is not organized into discrete tendon sheaths.
parathion an agricultural insecticide highly toxic to humans and animals. See also ORGANOPHOSPHORUS COMPOUND.
p.-methyl a less toxic form of parathion.
parathormone parathyroid hormone.
parathyroid 1. situated beside the thyroid gland. 2. one of the parathyroid glands. 3. a preparation containing parathyroid hormone from animal parathyroid glands; used for diagnosis and treatment of hypoparathyroidism.
p. calcium-regulating hormone see parathyroid hormone (below).
p. cyst remnants of the embryonic duct that connects the parathyroid and the thymus during embryogenesis. Called also Kursteiner's cyst.
p. gland small body in the region of the thyroid gland, occurring in a variable number of pairs, commonly two.

The parathyroid contains two types of cells: chief cells and oxyphils. Chief cells are the major source of parathyroid hormone (PTH), the secretion of which is dependent on the serum calcium level. Through a closed-loop feedback mechanism a low serum calcium level stimulates secretion of PTH; conversely, a high serum calcium level inhibits its secretion. The essential role of PTH is maintenance of a normal serum calcium level in association with vitamin D and calcitonin.
p. gland hyperplasia may be focal and nodular or, more importantly diffuse. The latter occurs in cases suffering long-standing nutritional deficiency of calcium or renal insufficiency.
p. hormone (PTH) a simple, straight-chain polypeptide, synthesized in chief cells and stored in secretory granules. The hormone stimulates the formation and activity of resorptive osteocytes so that calcium is released into body fluids without extensive bone remodeling. This is its mineral homeostatic function and is a relatively quick, short duration response. It is also concerned in skeletal homeostasis by stimulating osteoclastic osteolysis, the slower acting process of bone remodeling.
p. hormone-related protein, p. hormone-like peptide associated with humoral hypercalcemia of malignancy (HHM); see PSEUDOHYPERPARATHYROIDISM.
p. hyperfunction see HYPERPARATHYROIDISM, OSTEODYSTROPHIA FIBROSA.
p. secretory protein stored in secretory granules with parathyroid hormone but has no known function. Called also chromogranin A.
p. tumors carcinomas occur rarely and adenomas more commonly, particularly in older dogs. Either type of tumor may be nonfunctional or functional, causing a primary hyperparathyroidism.

parathyroidectomy excision of a parathyroid gland. Complete removal of all parathyroid tissue results in severe hypocalcemia.

parathyroiditis usually a diffuse lymphocytic lesion, probably immune-mediated, and terminating in loss of most of the chief cells and replacement with fibrous tissue. Hypocalcemia may result.

lymphocytic p. a common cause of idiopathic hypoparathyroidism in dogs; the gland tissue may be almost completely replaced by lymphocytes. It may be an autoimmune disease.

parathyrotropic having an affinity for the parathyroid glands.

paratope the site in the variable region of an antibody or T cell receptor that binds to an epitope of an antigen.

paratrichial literally beside the hair or hair follicle; used to refer to the apocrine sweat glands.

p. cystic dilation cystic dilation of the apocrine sweat gland occurs with or without hyperplasia of the glandular tissue.

p. sweat gland see SWEAT glands.

paratrophy dystrophy.

paratuberculosis a tuberculosis-like disease not due to *Mycobacterium tuberculosis*, *M. bovis* or *M. avium*. Usually reserved as an alternative name for JOHNE'S DISEASE.

paratyphoid infection with any *Salmonella* sp. other than *S. typhi* in humans. See SALMONELLOSIS.

p. nodule very small, yellow, necrotic foci in the liver in calves and pigs with salmonellosis.

paraurethral near the urethra.

paravaccinia a synonym for PARAPOXVIRUS.

paravaginitis inflammation of the tissues alongside the vagina.

paravertebral near the vertebrae.

p. block a local anesthetic agent is injected close to emerging spinal nerves between the transverse lumbar processes to produce regional analgesia of the flank for the purpose of conducting a laparotomy. The approach to the nerves may be dorsal, the Cambridge or Farquharson method, or lateral, the Magda method. Called also the Cakala or Cornell technique.

p. ganglia postganglionic sympathetic neurons synapse in these ganglia close to the aorta.

paraveterinary allied to the veterinary profession.

p. technicians persons trained to assist veterinarians. Includes veterinary nurses, and also animal technicians who assist in laboratory animal care, animal welfare work and field testing of large numbers of agricultural animals. In developing countries these personnel are used more extensively in carrying out preventive and treatment work in the small groups of animals that are likely to be owned by small farm holders. A number of them usually work under the direction of a veterinarian.

parbendazole a broad-spectrum benzimidazole anthelmintic used with good effects against the common parasites of cattle, pigs and horses. It acts quickly reaching peak blood levels 6 to 8 hours after administration. Its use in pregnant animals is contraindicated because of its teratogenicity; the defects are largely skeletal. Like other benzimidazoles it suffers from the problem of resistance developing in the resident worm population if it is used persistently.

parboiled partly cooked.

paregoric a mixture of powdered opium, anise oil, benzoic acid, camphor and glycerin, in diluted alcohol, used as an antiperistaltic, especially in the treatment of diarrhea.

parelaphostrongylosis see PARELAPHOSTRONGYLUS *tenuis*.

Parelaphostrongylus a genus in the worm family Protostrongylidae.

P. andersoni found in the musculature, especially in the longissimus dorsi, in white-tailed deer.

P. odocoilei found in connective tissue around blood vessels and lymphatics of musculature below the vertebral column, abdomen and proximal parts of the limbs in mule and black-tailed deer and in moose.

***P. tenuis* (syn. *Pneumostrongylus tenuis*, *Odocoileostrongylus tenuis*, *Elaphostrongylus tenuis*, *Neurofilaria cornelliensis*)** found in the cranial venous sinuses of white-tailed deer but is nonpathogenic in this species. Infection also occurs in moose, elk, caribou, red deer, black-tailed deer, llama, sheep and goat. In these species the migrating larvae cause serious damage in the spinal cord and posterior paralysis, often in a number of animals at the one time. Called also moose sickness.

Some infected goats also develop a local, linear dermatosis over the shoulders, thorax and flanks, believed to be caused by migrating *P. tenuis* larvae irritating nerve roots which leads to pruritus and self-trauma along dermatomes.

parenchyma the essential or functional elements of an organ, as distinguished from its stroma or framework.

parenchymatitis inflammation of a parenchyma.

parent generation the immediate parents of the F_1 generation. Denoted by P_1.

parentage the animal's sire and dam. In animal circles the dam is usually evident, the sire is often a subject of conjecture.

p. determination see parentage testing (below).

p. exclusion testing see parentage testing (below).

p. testing a test originally based on red cell antigens but increasingly on restriction fragment length polymorphisms (RFLPs), also called DNA fingerprinting. The offspring can have only those blood group antigens possessed by one or both of its parents. Identification of the offspring's antigens makes it possible to exclude some possible sires because they carry antigens not possessed by the subject animal. Similarly, the inheritance of a particular RFLP is directly linked to that found in each parent. Called also parentage determination, parentage exclusion testing.

parental emanating from or pertaining to a parent.

p. aggression in agricultural animals observed only in sows. See FARROWING hysteria.

parenteral not through the alimentary canal, e.g. by subcutaneous, intramuscular, intrasternal or intravenous injection, e.g. parenteral fluid therapy.

p. alimentation see parenteral nutrition (below).

p. hyperalimentation see parenteral nutrition (below).

p. nutrition the provision of adequate carbohydrate, protein, vitamins, minerals and fluids parenterally to maintain the animal over a relatively long period of several weeks. Called also parenteral alimentation, parenteral hyperalimentation. See also parenteral NUTRITION.

p. therapy treatment by the parenteral route is limited to those substances that are soluble in a solvent that can be injected into tissues including the bloodstream. The choice of routes may depend on the nature of the vehicle used, e.g. oily preparations are injected into tissues, irritant substances are injected intravenously slowly.

parepididymis paradidymis.

parer see hoof KNIFE.

paresis slight or incomplete paralysis. Includes the animals that can make purposeful attempts to rise without being able to do so, those that are able to rise with assistance, those that are able to rise and walk with major difficulty including frequent falling, and those able to stand and walk without assistance but with slight errors, e.g. stumbling.

hypocalcemic p. a stage or form of hypocalcemia in which the patient remains ambulatory.

inherited spastic p. an inherited defect of cattle that appears several months after birth. A hindleg is stiff and straight on rising and the hoof does not reach the ground. After several minutes the gastrocnemius muscle relaxes and the animal walks normally although the leg is still abnormally straight. Gradually the stiffness worsens until the animal is unable to walk. Called also Elso heel.

parturient p. see periparturient HYPOCALCEMIA.

progressive canine p. see dural OSSIFICATION, degenerative MYELOPATHY of German shepherd dogs.

paresthesia morbid or perverted sensation; an abnormal sensation, as burning, prickling, formication, etc. Difficult to define in animals because of its subjectivity. Sensations which give rise to itching or rubbing in animals are probably best classified as pruritus.

pareto improvement any change in economic management that improves the situation of one or more members of the community without worsening the lot of anyone.

pargyline a monoamine oxidase inhibitor, used as the hydrochloride salt.

Parhadjelia neglecta a habronematid larva found in the proventricular submucosa of ducks in Brazil.

pari-mutuel, parimutuel betting on the totalizator. Literally means betting between ourselves. All of the money wagered is divided up equally between those who have backed the winning and placed horses.

paries pl. *parietes* [L.] wall of an organ (e.g. hoof) or cavity (e.g. abdomen).

p. labyrinthicus, p. mastoideus, etc. medial wall of the middle ear that separates it from the internal ear.

parietal 1. of or pertaining to the walls of an organ or cavity. 2. pertaining to or located near the parietal bone.

p. block abnormal electrical conduction through the left branch of the bundle of His.

p. bone one of two quadrilateral bones forming the sides and roof of the cranium. See Table 10.

p. cells cells of the proper gastric mucosa that secrete hydrochloric acid. Called also oxyntic cells.

p. decidua see parietal DECIDUA.

p. hernia when only the antimesenteric edge of the intestine is incarcerated in the defect of body wall or mesentery.

p. lobe the upper central portion of the cerebral hemisphere, between the frontal and occipital lobes, and above the temporal lobe. In the human brain, it is the receptive area for fine sensory stimuli, and the highest integration and coordination of sensory information is carried on in this area. Damage to the parietal lobe can produce defects in vision and aphasia.

p. peritoneum, p. pleura that part of the serous membrane that invests the wall of the cavity, as distinct from the visceral part.

parietofrontal pertaining to the parietal and frontal bones, gyri or fissures.

parietography radiographic visualization of the walls of an organ.

Parinaud's oculoglandular syndrome cat-scratch disease.

Paris green an oldfashioned green pigment used in plaster and still found in old buildings. Can cause inorganic ARSENIC poisoning.

Parisian frill a large canary characterized by a mass of frilled feathers which appear to completely cover the body.

parity 1. para; the condition of a breeding female with respect to her having borne viable offspring. 2. equality; close correspondence or similarity.

Parker casting a method of casting a horse using two ropes, one of which pulls the feet of two limbs on one side together, while the other pulls the horse over.

Parker–Kerr suture pattern one used to close the stump of a hollow viscus, e.g. in intestinal anastomosis. A Cushing suture pattern is put in first over the top of the bowel clamp which is then gradually withdrawn and the suture pulled tight. A layer of Lembert pattern is then used to oversew the first row.

Parker retractor a shaped piece of flat metal with rounded ends both of which are curved back against the main blade. Used for holding a laparotomy incision open.

Parkinsonia aculeata plant in the legume family Caesalpiniaceae; causes nitrate–nitrite poisoning; called also horse bean, Jerusalem thorn, retama.

paroccipital beside the occipital bone.

paromomycin a broad-spectrum antibiotic derived from *Streptomyces rimosus* var. *paromomycinus*; poorly absorbed after oral administration, it is used for intestinal infections. Called also aminosidine.

paromphalocele hernia near the navel.

paronychia inflammation involving the folds of tissue surrounding the nail or claw. Causes much pain and often results in loss of the nail or abnormalities in its growth such as grooves, discoloration or fragility. Called also perionychia, perionychitis.

paroophoron an inconstantly present, small group of coiled tubules between the layers of the mesosalpinx, being a remnant of the excretory part of the mesonephros.

parophthalmia inflammation of the connective tissue around the eye.

parorchidium displacement of a testis or testes.

parosteal pertaining to the outer surface of the periosteum, e.g. parosteal osteoma.

parostosis ossification of tissues outside of the periosteum.

parotid near the ear.

p. adenitis inflammation of the parotid gland characterized by regional swelling, pain and heat.

p. duct see parotid glands (below).

p. duct transposition a surgical procedure in which the parotid duct is redirected so that it discharges into the lower conjunctival cul-de-sac. Used in the treatment of keratoconjunctivitis sicca.

p. glands the largest of the main pairs of salivary glands, located on either side of the head, just behind the jaw and below the ears. From each gland a duct, the parotid duct, runs forward across the cheek (carnivores and small ruminants) or runs on the inside of the jaw to wind around the ventral border of the jaw to the cheek (pig, horse and ox) and opens on the inside surface of the cheek generally opposite the upper molars, the precise location depending on the species.

p. region the region below the ear.

parotidectomy excision of a parotid gland.

parotiditis, parotitis inflammation of the parotid gland.

contagious p., epidemic p. MUMPS; an acute, communicable viral disease of humans involving chiefly the parotid gland, but frequently affecting other oral glands or the pancreas or gonads. There are sporadic reports of the infection occurring in dogs.

parous having produced offspring.

parovarian 1. beside the ovary. 2. pertaining to the parovarium (epoophoron).

p. cyst developmental remnants of the mesonephric duct system; thin-walled sacs distended with clear fluid located in the mesosalpinx and the infundibulum of the oviduct. They appear to have no effect on fertility.

parovarium a vestigial structure associated with the ovary; consists of a group of mesonephric tubules with a corresponding section of mesonephric duct. Called also epoophoron.

paroxysm 1. a sudden recurrence or intensification of clinical signs. 2. a spasm or seizure.

paroxysmal having the characteristic of a paroxysm.

p. dysrhythmia a cardiac rhythm disturbance which occurs briefly and transiently.

parr a juvenile salmonid, especially *Salmo* spp., at a stage before it becomes a smolt; characterized by parallel transverse bands on its sides.

parrot any of a group of birds in the family Psittacidae which also includes cockatoos and lories. All are characterized by curved beaks with the lower one fitting inside the larger upper beak when they are closed. The typical parrots are the macaws, parakeets, lovebirds and budgerigars. They are characterized by their bright plumage, their gift of mimicry and their popularity as pets.

p. fever see PSITTACOSIS.

p. mouth serious malocclusion of the incisors with the upper arcade protruding beyond the lower. Called also overshot. See also BRACHYGNATHIA.

p. pox see PARROTPOX.

parrotpox a pox disease caused by a poxvirus in the genus *Avipoxvirus*. Occurs in South American and Australian psittacine birds as dry scabs around the mouth, eyelids, face and legs or as a 'wet' form with white plaques in the oral cavity and with blunting of the choanal papillae.

pars pl. *partes* [L.] a division or part.

p. ciliaris retinae see CILIARY body.

p. distalis the major part of the anterior lobe of the pituitary gland, the adenohypophysis. It is separated from the neurohypophysis by the intraglandular cleft, the residual lumen of Rathke's pouch.

p. disseminata the thin layer of the prostate that surrounds the urethra; as distinct from the body of the gland.

p. flaccida the small, triangular portion of the tympanic membrane lying between the lateral process of the malleus and the margins of the tympanic incisure.

p. infundibularis the neural stalk that connects the neurohypophysis with the hypothalamus.

p. intermedia the part of the adenohypophysis consisting of a layer of cells contiguous with the neurohypophysis. The source of melanocyte-stimulating hormone.

p. iridica retinae see IRIS[1].

p. longa glandis the long, cylindrical part of the dog glans; distinct from the bulbar part.

p. major uteri the section of the bird's oviduct in which the egg is held while the shell is formed.

p. mastoidea the mastoid portion of the temporal bone, being the irregular, posterior part.

p. nervosa of the pituitary gland. See NEUROHYPOPHYSIS.

p. optica retina the large, posterior part of the retina which contains the nervous elements of rods, cones and optic nerve fibers.

p. petrosa the petrous portion of the temporal bone, containing the inner ear.

p. pigmentosa the pigmented part of the retina.

p. plana the thin flat part of the ciliary body; the ciliary disk.

p. plicata the folded part of the ciliary body.

p. pylorica distal segment of the stomach or abomasum, curved behind the omasum.

p. pylorica ventriculi the distal (aboral) third of the stomach.

p. squamosa the flat, scalelike, anterior and superior portion of the temporal bone.

p. tensa the drumlike part of the tympanic membrane.

p. tuberalis a layer of cells surrounding the neural stalk of the pituitary gland and forming part of the adenohypophysis.

p. tympanica the tympanic portion of the temporal bone, forming the anterior and inferior walls and part of the posterior wall of the external acoustic meatus.

parsley PETROSELINUM *crispum*.

parsley water dropwort OENANTHE *lachenalii*.

parsnip see PASTINACA SATIVA.

Parson Jack Russell terrier similar to but larger (14 in or 36 cm tall) than the JACK RUSSELL TERRIER.

Parsonsia Australian genus of woody vines in the Apocynaceae family. *P. eucalyptophylla*, *P. lilacina* and *P. straminea* are the species that are most suspect. Firm evidence about their toxic effects is lacking but some can cause nitrate–nitrite poisoning. Cardiac glycosides or cyanogenic glucosides may also be present. Called also gargaloo.

part–film distance the distance between the part being x-rayed and the film; the greater the distance the less definition of the image. See OBJECT–FILM DISTANCE.

Parthenium hysterophorus plant member of Asteraceae family; contains a sesquiterpene lactone which causes hepatopathy, dermatitis, stomatitis, nephropathy. Called also parthenium weed.

parthenium weed see PARTHENIUM HYSTEROPHORUS.

parthenogenesis asexual reproduction in which an egg develops without being fertilized by a spermatozoon, as in certain lower animals, especially arthropods; it may occur as a natural phenomenon or be induced by chemical or mechanical stimulation (artificial parthenogenesis).

parti-color variegated in two or more colors; used to describe coat color in dogs.

partial pertaining to or having the characteristics of a part of something.

p. budget see partial BUDGET.

p. pressure the pressure exerted by a specific gas in a mixture of gases. Because the amount of the gas dissolved in a liquid is proportional to the pressure of the gas on the fluid the concentration of a gas in a fluid is expressed as its partial pressure.

p. thromboplastin time (PTT) see ACTIVATED partial thromboplastin time.

particle an extremely small mass of material. See also ALPHA particles and BETA particle.

elementary p. any of the subatomic particles, including electrons, protons, neutrons, positrons, neutrinos and muons.

particulate composed of separate particles.

parting of hair where hairstreams of hair diverge, exposing the skin.

partridge two genera of gallinaceous game birds (*Perdix*, *Alectoris*) in the pheasant family Phasianidae. They are ground feeders and tree perchers. They are poor flyers but can run quickly when disturbed. The common species are the red-legged and the common partridges.

parts per million mg/kg or ml/l; see PPM.

parturient giving birth or pertaining to birth.

p. disease disease related to parturition and which occurs during or in close relationship to parturition.

p. injury injury sustained during birth, to the neonate or to the dam, not necessarily restricted to the birth canal or even the reproductive system, e.g. hip dislocation.

p. paresis see periparturient HYPOCALCEMIA.

p. recumbency recumbency in a female that has just borne young. May be due to hypocalcemia, toxemia, physical injury or to being unable to find suitable footing.

parturiometer a device used in measuring the expulsive power of the uterus.

parturition the act or process of giving birth to a calf, foal, lamb, puppy, etc.

p. acceleration used most commonly in sows with uterine inertia; usual medication is oxytocin; carazolol a recent introduction to the list.

p. delaying attempted to give more time for relaxation of the cervix; clenbuterol the common medication.

difficult p. see DYSTOCIA.

p. induction is a common management practice in dairy herds in order to synchronize calvings and lactations. It is also used for therapeutic reasons when large fetuses are expected or in sows when mastitis–metritis–agalactia is a problem in the herd. The usual method is the injection of a suitable corticosteroid, oxytocin or $PGF_{2[alpha]}$. Undesirable side-effects include high calf mortality rate, retained placenta, photosensitive dermatitis and unusual metabolic diseases. Called also calving induction. Called also parturition initiation.

p. initiation see parturition induction (above).

p. injury includes laceration of the cervix, vaginal wall or vulva, uterine rupture, fat hernia through the vaginal wall, uterine prolapse, rupture of middle uterine artery, sciatic nerve injury, maternal obstetric paralysis.

prolonged p. prolongation of parturition beyond the normal for the species is attended by risks to the dam and the fetuses.

p. psychosis see FARROWING hysteria.

synchronized p. control of the date of parturition by controlling the date of estrus and of mating, or by the induction of parturition.

p. syndrome a loose diagnosis embracing many toxemias that occur about the time of calving. See ACETONEMIA, FAT cow syndrome, PREGNANCY toxemia, MASTITIS, METRITIS and PERITONITIS.

parulis a subperiosteal abscess of the gum.

parumbilical alongside the navel.

parvaquone an antiprotozoal agent.

parvicellular composed of small cells.

parvo slang for parvovirus infection.

parvoviral pertaining to a parvovirus.

Parvoviridae a family of small (20 nm diameter) icosahedral single-stranded DNA viruses that are nonenveloped. There are three genera: *Parvovirus*, which includes feline panleukopenia virus, mink enteritis virus, canine, bovine and porcine parvoviruses and Aleutian mink disease virus; *Densovirus*, which occur in insects; and *Dependovirus*, which are defective, requiring adenoviruses to complete their replication, and are nonpathogenic (called also adeno-associated viruses). Autonomously replicating parvoviruses replicate only during S phase of the cell cycle, i.e. they attack dividing cells.

parvovirus a virus of the family PARVOVIRIDAE.

bovine p. commonly infects the intestinal tract of cattle, but does not cause clinical disease; called also Hadenvirus for hemadsorbing enterovirus.

canine p. type 1 (CPV1) is not associated with clinical disease. Called also minute canine virus (MCV).

canine p. type 2 (CPV2) the cause of enteritis in dogs, particularly puppies. Clinical signs include vomiting and diarrhea, often with blood, high fever, dehydration and a leukopenia. Perinatal or in utero infection may result in generalized disease or acute myocarditis. There is a high mortality rate in young puppies, but vaccines are available for prevention of the disease.

porcine p. a cause of stillbirths, abortion, mummification, embryonic death and infertility in young sows (SMEDI) which become infected with a parvovirus in early gestation.

PAS 1. *p*-aminosalicylic acid, used at one time in the treatment of tuberculosis in humans; also abbreviated PASA. 2. periodic acid–Schiff reaction (stain).

pas-de-côte the sidestep in equine dressage.

Pascal a computer language which emphasizes structured programming. The name is not an acronym; the language was named after Pascal, the French mathematician.

pascal the SI unit of pressure, which corresponds to a force of one newton per square meter; symbol, Pa.

Paschen bodies, Paschen's corpuscles inclusion bodies in the cells of tissues infected with vaccinia or variola viruses.

paspalitrems tremorgens produced by *Claviceps paspali* which parasitize *Paspalum* spp. grasses.

Paspalum a grass genus of the Poaceae family, containing a number of valuable pasture grasses, all of which are capable of causing poisoning by *Claviceps paspali* which infests their seed heads; includes *P. commersonii*, *P. compressum*, *P. conjugatum*, *P. dilatatum* (paspalum, Dallas grass), *P. distichum* (*P. vaginatum*, salt water couch), *P. notatum* (Bahia grass), *P. orbiculare* (ditch millet), *P. paspalodes* (water couch), *P. scrobiculatum*, *P. urvillei* (water couch).

paspalum ergot the ergot fungus that grows on the seedheads of members of the *Paspalum* genus of grasses. See also PASPALUM STAGGERS. Called also *Claviceps paspali*, *C. cinerea*.

paspalum grass see PASPALUM.

paspalum staggers caused by the ingestion of *Claviceps paspali*, *C. cinerea*, the ergot of PASPALUM. Characterized by ataxia, gross muscular tremor, frequent falling, hypermetria, hyperesthesia. Recovery is spontaneous.

pasque flower ANEMONE *pulsatilla*.

passage introduction followed by recovery of an infectious agent in an experimental animal or culture medium.

blind p. passage of an infectious agent through an experimental animal or medium without there being any evidence, clinical or cultural, that the agent is present.

serial p. repeated passage through a series of experimental animals or media, often with the objective of altering the virulence of the agent or adapting it to grow better.

Passalurus a genus of nematodes in the family Oxyuridae.

P. ambiguus found in the cecum and colon of rabbits, hares and other lagomorphs. They appear to be harmless even in very large numbers.

Passer genus of small brown birds. Includes *P. montanus*, *P. domesticus*; see also SPARROW.

Passeriformes the order of birds including all of the 5000 or more perching birds, including the finches, sparrows, buntings, mynahs, canaries and serins.

passerines birds belonging to the order Passeriformes.

Passeromyia a genus of screw-worm flies of birds in Australia.

Passiflora a plant genus of vines in the family Passifloraceae. Includes passion fruit valued for their edible fruits. Most of the plants in the genus that have been tested have high concentrations of cyanogenetic glycosides and are potential causes of cyanide poisoning and there is good field evidence of poisoning of livestock by some of them.

Suspected species are *P. aurantia* (red passion flower), *P. cinnabarina* (vermilion passion flower), *P. foetida* (stinking or mossy passion flower), *P. herbertiana*, *P. suberosa* (small passion flower), *P. subpeltata* (white or wild passion flower).

passion flower see PASSIFLORA.

passivation the final stage in instrument manufacture, passing the finished instruments through a bath of nitric acid which removes foreign particles and promotes the formation of a protective coating of chromium oxide.

passive neither spontaneous on the part of the patient, nor active response by the patient, the stimulus having been applied externally.

p. cutaneous anaphylaxis (PCA) test see passive cutaneous ANAPHYLAXIS.

p. diffusion passage of electrolytes to all parts of a solution, including through a permeable membrane. Plays some part in intestinal absorption.

p. hemagglutination test see HEMAGGLUTINATION test.

p. immunization see passive IMMUNIZATION.

p. neonatal immunity see passive IMMUNITY.

p. transfer see passive diffusion (above).

p. venous congestion noninflammatory distension of vessels with blood. Caused by simple accumulation resulting from obstruction or failure of the heart to eject the full volume of blood returned to it.

Passulurus ambiguus an oxyurid nematode of rabbits, cottontails and hares.

paste highly viscous ointment containing a large amount of powder.

pastern in ungulates the segment of the limb between the fetlock and hoof, supported by proximal and middle phalanges; in dogs the metacarpal region.

equine p. dermatitis see GREASY HEEL.

congenital p. flexure a common neonatal deformity in all species. If it is the only deformity it commonly corrects itself spontaneously or with minimal interference. Occurs also as part of multiple deformities, e.g. Akabane virus disease.

p. folliculitis folliculitis of the posterior pastern in horses from which *Staphylococcus hyicus* has been isolated.

p. joint in ungulates, the articulation between the proximal and middle phalanges.

Pasteur named after Louis Pasteur, French microbiologist and biochemist.

P.–Chamberland filter see PASTEUR–CHAMBERLAND FILTER.

P. effect the decrease in the rate of glycolysis and the suppression of lactate accumulation by tissues or microorganisms in the presence of oxygen.

Pasteur–Chamberland filter a hollow column of unglazed porcelain through which liquids are forced by pressure or by vacuum exhaustion.

Pasteurella a genus of gram-negative facultatively anaerobic, rod-shaped bacteria.

P. anatipestifer causes an acute or chronic septicemic disease of ducks and other birds characterized by fibrinous pericarditis, perihepatitis and airsacculitis and caseous salpingitis and arthritis. Called also new duck disease, infectious serositis, goose influenza.

P. avium, P. gallinarum, P. langaa, P. volantium recovered from chickens. *P. gallinarium* may cause disease in poultry.

P. caballi causes respiratory infections in horses.

P. canis, P. dagmatis, P. pneumotropica, P. stomatis recovered from dogs, cats and rodents and may be involved in infected bite wounds. *P. pneumotropica* also causes pneumonia and abscesses in rodents.

P. granulomatis causes fibrogranulomatous disease in cattle in Brazil.

***P. haemolytica* (biotypes A and T)** cause septicemic and pneumonic PASTEURELLOSIS in cattle and sheep, usually in conjunction with a virus infection such as parainfluenza 3. Also recorded as a cause of acute mastitis in cattle.

***P. multocida* (syn. *P. septica*) types A, B, D, E, F** the cause of HEMORRHAGIC septicemia in cattle, sheep and pigs, FOWL cholera of birds, PASTEURELLOSIS of rabbits, and gangrenous mastitis of ewes. It is also commonly found in atrophic rhinitis of pigs.

P. pestis see YERSINIA *pestis*.

P. piscicida causes pasteurellosis in a range of marine warm water species especially in the Mediterranean and Japan.

P. salpingitidis see ACTINOBACILLUS *salpingitidis*.

P. testudinis causes abscesses in tortoises and turtles.

P. tularensis see FRANCISELLA *tularensis*.

pasteurellosis infection with organisms of the genus *Pasteurella*. In animals includes septicemic pasteurellosis, pneumonic pasteurellosis, both of cattle, SNUFFLES in rabbits and pasteurellosis of swine, sheep and goats. The causative bacteria include *Pasteurella multocida* types A, B, C and D, and *P. haemolytica*.

epidemic p. see HEMORRHAGIC septicemia.

ovine, porcine and caprine p. a pneumonic, sometimes septicemic, form of pasteurellosis. The pneumonic form is caused by *P. haemolyticum* type A, and the septicemia form by *P. haemolyticum* type T.

pneumonic p. the common pasteurellosis of cattle caused by *P. haemolytica*, sometimes *P. multocida* type A. Characterized by acute bronchopneumonia with fever, dyspnea, abnormal breath sounds, weak cough, severe toxemia and death in 24 to 48 hours.

septicemic p. see HEMORRHAGIC septicemia.

pasteurization heating of milk or other liquids to a temperature of 140°F (60°C) for 30 minutes, killing pathogenic bacteria and considerably delaying other bacterial development.

Pastinaca sativa the domestic parsnip; causes dermatitis, probably primary photosensitization, due to furanocoumarin produced in response to the fungus *Ceratocystis fimbriata* growing on the plant.

pastoral emanating from or pertaining to the use of land for pasture.

p. rearing raising of young, after weaning, on pasture where they are more susceptible to nutritional deficiencies and parasitic infestation than young reared indoors.

pasture fields or paddocks carrying a permanent or semipermanent growth of grasses and clovers or other legumes and usually some volunteer herbaceous plants. It is used as a complete or partial diet for herbivores and in some economies for omnivores. It may be permanent or temporary, even annual, irrigated or dry, native or improved.

p. bloat primary ruminal tympany characterized by frothing of the ruminal contents; occurs in cattle on legume-rich pastures.

p. breeding the males are turned into the pasture with a group of females. Called also paddock mating.

clean p. refers to the status of the pasture as a source of infective helminth larvae and implies relative freedom. The degree of freedom from parasite larvae is important as a factor in prevention of parasitoses.

p. diarrhea see COPPER nutritional deficiency.

p. ley see LEY.

p. meter device for measuring the amount of feed remaining; based on a design in which a flat metal plate traverses up a central spindle when the spindle is inserted through the plants so that it reaches the ground, the plate floating on top of the plants; measures in cow days.

native p. consists of the plants normally found growing wild in the area. Agriculturally speaking, this usually refers to areas with an annual rainfall of less than 20 in (500 mm). Areas with larger rainfalls usually carry improved pastures.

p. plants plants which occur naturally or are cultivated especially for growing in pasture to provide feed for grazing animals, with excess growth made into hay or ensilage.

p. rotation see rotational GRAZING.

pasturing the system of management based on the use of pasture as the principal source of dietary energy.

pasveer process the channel aeration method of sewage disposal in which the effluent is passed along deep channels 3 to 7 ft deep to undergo aeration.

patagiectomy excision of the wing membrane on one side of the bird to prevent flight. See also PROPATAGIUM.

patas monkey Old World monkey of the family Cercopithecidae. An orange terrestrial monkey with white underparts and a black face. Called also *Erythrocebus patas*.

patch a small area differing from the rest of a surface.

p. grafting see patch GRAFT.

serosal p. creation of an adhesion between serosal surfaces in order to cover a defect or perforation of bowel, often accomplished by suturing another section of bowel over the area.

p. test a test of delayed type hypersensitivity in the skin used in the diagnosis of allergic contact dermatitis. The substance suspected of being the cause is applied to the skin, either under a dressing (closed patch test) or without a covering (open patch test). The site is examined at regular intervals for up to 5 days to detect any inflammatory reaction of the skin.

patching antibody induced clustering of plasma membrane molecules, usually proteins or glycoproteins. Patching can also be induced by lectins.

patella pl. *patellae* [L.] a large sesamoid bone at the femorotibial joint. See also Table 10.

p. cubiti an anomalous sesamoid over the extensor aspect of the elbow.

patellar of or pertaining to the patella.

p. cartilage a cartilaginous process borne on the medial side of the patella of horses and cattle.

p. fossa the depression in the anterior face of the vitreous humor in which the lens sits.

p. ligament the continuation of the central portion of the tendon of the quadriceps femoris muscle distal to the patella, extending from the patella to the tuberosity of the tibia; it is single in carnivores, pigs and sheep and triple in horses and cattle; called also patellar tendon.

p. ligament desmotomy section of the medial patellar ligament for relief of upward luxation of the patella in horses (and rarely, cattle).

p. luxation, p. dislocation a common, congenital or acquired orthopedic abnormality in dogs, causing mild to severe, continuous or intermittent lameness. *Medial* luxation is more common in toy or miniature breeds, often as an inherited defect and frequently associated with structural abnormalities of the distal femur and proximal tibia. *Lateral* luxation is less frequent, and occurs more often in large breeds associated with genu valgum.

p. reflex involuntary contraction of the quadriceps muscle and jerky extension of the hindlimb when the patellar ligament is sharply tapped. It is often used as a test of nervous system function. Absence of the reflex, together with deficient muscle tone in the limb, suggests paralysis or paresis due to lower motor neuron lesion. Called also quadriceps reflex.

p. tendon see patellar ligament (above).

patellectomy excision of the patella.

patelliform shaped like a small plate.

patellofemoral pertaining to the patella and femur.

patency the condition of being open.

patent 1. open, unobstructed, or not closed. 2. apparent, evident.

p. ductus arteriosus (PDA) abnormal persistence of an open lumen in the ductus arteriosus, between the aorta and the pulmonary artery, after birth. The ductus arteriosus is open during prenatal life, allowing most of the blood of the fetus to bypass the lungs, but normally this channel closes shortly before birth. When the ductus arteriosus remains open, it places special burdens on the left ventricle and causes a diminished blood flow in the aorta. May remain open for up to 5 days in foals. One of the most common congenital heart defects in dogs, but less common in cats. Causes a continuous 'machinery' murmur loud in systole, soft in diastole, and 'bounding' pulse.

p. ductus venosus see DUCTUS venosus.

p. foramen ovale see FORAMEN ovale (1).

p. medicine a drug or remedy protected by a trademark, available without a prescription.

p. period the period during a disease in which the causative agent can be detected by clinicopathological tests, e.g. for helminth eggs.

p. urachus the urachus persists after birth and allows urine to drip out of the bladder through the umbilicus. See also URACHUS.

p. ventricular septum includes several entities characterized by incomplete closure of ventricular wall. Characterized by palpable cardiac thrill and audible pansystolic murmur on both sides of the chest at birth, accompanied by exercise intolerance and developing dyspnea at rest.

paternity testing see PARENTAGE testing.

Paternoster bean ABRUS *precatorius*.

Paterson's curse ECHIUM *plantagineum*.

path 1. a course for a procedure, especially in statistical matters. 2. in computers is the complete name of a file or directory on a disk or tape; the sequence of drive, root directory, subdirectory or sequence of subdirectories, as well as the file name and extension, all of which leads the user to the exact spot where the desired information is lodged.

p. analysis an analytical method suitable for the study of multiple variables. It has the advantage over the usual stepwise multiple regression analysis in that it allows the epidemiologist to decide the order in which the independent variables enter the regression equations, thus improving the chance that the modeled sequence of events will approximate the pattern in nature.

path(o)- word element. [Gr.] *disease*.

pathergasia mental malfunction, implying functional or structural damage, marked by abnormal behavior.

pathergy 1. a condition in which the application of a stimulus leaves the organism unduly susceptible to subsequent stimuli of a different kind. 2. a condition of being allergic to several antigens.

pathfinder 1. an instrument for locating urethral strictures. 2. a dental instrument for tracing the course of root canals.

pathoanatomical diagnosis a diagnosis which defines the type and location of the lesion without identifying the cause, e.g. polioencephalomalacia.

pathobiology pathology.

pathoclisis a specific sensitivity to specific toxins, or a specific affinity of certain toxins for certain systems or organs.

pathogen any disease-producing agent or microorganism.

p. risk factors risk factors dependent on the characteristics of the pathogen, e.g. virulence or persistence in the environment of a bacterium or virus.

pathogenesis the development of morbid conditions or of disease; more specifically the cellular events and reactions and other pathological mechanisms occurring in the development of disease. Includes the study of the relationship between the cause and the lesions, and that between the lesion and the clinical signs.

pathogenic capable of causing disease, e.g. bacteria, fungi, protozoa.

pathogenicity the ability of a pathogenic agent to produce disease in a host. See also VIRULENCE.

pathogeny pathogenesis.

pathognomonic specifically distinctive or characteristic of a disease or pathological condition; denoting a sign or other indicant on which a diagnosis can be made.

pathological, pathologic pertaining to or emanating from pathology.

p. anatomy see morbid ANATOMY.

pathologist a specialist in pathology.

pathology 1. the branch of veterinary science treating of the essential nature of disease, especially of the changes in body tissues and organs which cause or are caused by disease. 2. the structural and functional manifestations of a disease.

clinical p. see CLINICAL pathology.

comparative p. that which considers human disease processes in comparison with those of the lower animals.

experimental p. the study of artificially induced pathological processes.

oral p. that which treats of conditions causing or resulting from morbid anatomical or functional changes in the structures of the mouth.

surgical p. the pathology of disease processes that are surgically accessible for diagnosis or treatment.

pathomorphism perverted or abnormal morphology.

pathonomia the science of the laws of disease.

pathophysiology the physiology of disordered function.

pathosis a diseased condition.

pathway a course usually followed. In neurology, the nerve structures through which a sensory impression is conducted to the cerebral cortex (afferent pathway), or through which an impulse passes from the brain to the skeletal musculature (efferent pathway). Also used alone to indicate a sequence of reactions that convert one biological material to another (metabolic pathway).

biosynthetic p. the sequence of enzymatic steps in the synthesis of a specific end product in a living organism.

coagulation p's see COAGULATION pathways.

Embden–Meyerhof p. see EMBDEN–MEYERHOF PATHWAY.

final common p. 1. the motor neurons by which nerve impulses from many central sources pass to a muscle or gland in the periphery. 2. any mechanism by which several independent effects ultimately exert a common influence.

pentose phosphate p. a pathway of hexose oxidation in which glucose-6-phosphate undergoes two successive oxidations by NADP, each producing NADPH, the final forming a pentose phosphate.

properdin p. alternative complement pathway.

-pathy word element. [Gr.] *morbid condition* or *disease;* generally used to designate a noninflammatory condition.

patient an animal that is ill or is undergoing treatment for disease.

p. data name, initials, sex, address, postcode, phone number.

p. monitoring continuous or frequent periodic clinical assessment.

p. rights are adapted from the statement applicable to human medicine. They are really only applicable to the client in the veterinary situation. See CLIENT rights.

patrilineal descended through the male line.

Patterdale terrier a small (12–13 lb) hunting dog with a short, coarse coat in black, red, chocolate or black and tan. It has a broad head and ears that fold over; the tail is docked to a medium length. Called also Black fell terrier.

patterns the distribution of cases of disease, production maxima, population density or other measurable variable, in time or space. It may be random, or it may be in a pattern that is helpful in suggesting a diagnosis.

p. generators populations of neurons which generate a standard pattern of movements, e.g. respiratory basic rate and rhythm, rumination, mastication, eructation; they are not self-initiating but require stimulation from the brain or a sensory input.

Patterson milkvetch ASTRAGALUS *pattersonii*.

patulin an antibiotic substance derived from a group of fungi, including *Byssochlamys nivea*, *Penicillium* spp., which caused deaths when given to animals. The information suggests that patulin may also be a toxin.

patulous spread widely apart; open; distended.

paunch see RUMEN.

pause an interruption, or rest.

compensatory p. the pause after a premature ventricular systole, related to blockage of one beat of the basic pacemaker of the heart.

Pautrier microabscess see Pautrier MICROABSCESS.

Pavetta an African plant genus in the family Rubiaceae; plants contain an unidentified toxin which causes myocarditis and sudden death due to acute heart failure. The condition is also known as gousiekte. Includes *P. harbori*, *P. schumanniana*. Called also pavettabossie, tonnabossie, gousiekte tree, poisonous bride's bush.

pavettabossie see PAVETTA.

pavilionitis inflammation of the fimbriated end of the oviduct.
Pavlovian conditioning see classical CONDITIONING.
Pavo see PEAFOWL.
paw foot; especially of carnivores and other digitigrade animals.
p. and mouth disease see paw and MOUTH disease.
pawing a form of behavior characterized by persistent use of one forelimb to dig in the ground, or to thump it, or to scratch at a fixed object such as a door; stimulated by subacute pain, boredom.
pawpaw see CARICA PAPAYA.
payback method a method of assessing the potential profitability of two or more competing strategies; based on the assessment of the period of time required before the financial returns from the strategy recoup the original investment.
payoff table a table showing the financial returns minus costs for each of the strategies under consideration.
payroll a list of employees, their salary rates, tax deductions, amounts paid, payroll tax, long service leave entitlements.
PB *Pharmacopoeia Britannica* (British Pharmacopoeia).
Pb chemical symbol, *lead* (L. *plumbum*).
PBB polybrominated biphenyl.
PBG-D porphobilinogen diaminase.
PBI protein-bound iodine.
PBS phosphate buffered saline.
p.c. [L.] *post cibum* (after meals).
PCA passive cutaneous anaphylaxis.
PCB polychlorinated biphenyl.
PCD polycystic disease.
PCG phonocardiogram.
PCNB pentachloronitrobenzene.
PCP pentachlorophenol.
PCR[1] polymerase chain reaction. The amplification of a specific DNA sequence, termed target or template sequence, that is present in a complex mixture, by adding two or more short oligonucleotides, also called primers, that are specific for the terminal or outer limits of the template sequence. The template–primers mixture is subjected to repeated cycles of heating to separate (melt) the double-stranded DNA and cooling in the presence of nucleotides and DNA polymerase such that the template sequence is copied at each cycle. Thermostable polymerases such as those obtained from a hot springs bacterium *Thermus aquaticus*, commonly termed *Taq* polymerase, are used.

At the end of 20 to 30 such cycles, the amplified target sequence, which may have been present in as few as a single copy in the original mixture, can be readily detected, for example by electrophoresis and ethidium bromide staining in an argarose gel.

multiplex PCR the detection of more than one template in a mixture by addition of more than one set of oligonucleotide primers.
nested PCR the primers used in the first round of amplification are either both replaced (nested PCR) or only one is replaced (semi-nested PCR) for the second and subsequent cycles of amplification. Increases the sensitivity and specificity of the PCR.
quantitative PCR a means for quantifying the amount of template DNA present in the original mixture. Usually achieved by the addition of a known amount of a target sequence that is amplified by the same primer set but can be differentiated, usually by size, at the end of the reaction.
reverse-transcriptase PCR (RT-PCR) a reaction applied when the target sequence is RNA, such as viral RNA or messenger RNA. Reverse transcriptase that copies DNA from an RNA template is present in the first round.
PCR[2] protein–calorie ratio.
PCT prothrombin consumption time.
PCTA see percutaneous transluminal ANGIOPLASTY.
PCV packed-cell volume, the volume of packed red cells in milliliters per 100 ml of blood.
PD 1. pregnancy diagnosis. 2. predicted differences.
Pd chemical symbol, *palladium.*
pd potential difference; prism dioptre.
PD_{50} the dose of antiserum or vaccine that protects 50% of the animals challenged.
PDA patent ductus arteriosus.
PDGF platelet-derived growth factor; interacting with cell surface receptors and stimulating hydrolysis of inositol 1,4,5-triphosphate (IP_3).
PDS polydioxanone suture.
pe- for words beginning thus, see also those beginning *pae-*.
PE4 see CYCLONITE.
pea leguminous plants, members of the family Fabaceae. The plants may be used as green feed but are too succulent to make into hay. Silage is made from the crop residue after harvesting canning peas but is very subject to fungal infestation. Peas used for livestock feed include canning peas (*Pisum sativum*), field peas (*Pisum sativum*), chick peas (*Cicer arietinum*) and cow peas (*Vigna sinensis*, syn. *V. catjang*, *V. unguiculata*). See also LATHYRUS.
p. hulls a source of dietary fiber in manufactured pet foods.
p.-struck poisoning by Darling pea. See SWAINSONA.
p. vine ensilage is made from the commercial green pea plants after harvesting and removal of pods. It is now more common to harvest pods from the standing crop, which livestock then graze. Ensilage can be poisonous. Lambs show nervous signs soon after birth, an abnormal gait and intermittent recumbency with exercise, and there are degenerative lesions in the cerebral and cerebellar cortices at autopsy.
peach the fruiting tree of the genus *Prunus* and the family Rosaceae. The leaves and pips of this and other members of the family contain cyanogenetic glycosides and are potentially poisonous. Engorgement on the fruit may cause lactic acidosis and in occasional cases an entire fruit lodges in the esophagus and obstructs it. Called also *Prunus persica*.
peach-leaf poison bush see TREMA TOMENTOSA.
peacock see PEAFOWL.
peafowl members of the genus *Pavo* of which there are a number of species including the common and the Javan. With the argus pheasant they represent the largest, most dramatically colored and longest tailed birds of the pheasant family Phasianidae. The peacock is a popular zoological specimen but has a typically raucous voice and is frequently muted surgically.
Péan forceps compression foceps with ratchet handles and long, wide, slightly bowed blades with longitudinal grooves.
peanut seed kernels of the plant *Arachis hypogaea* cultivated as a commercial crop. Made into peanut meal after the oil is extracted. The kernels and meal are subject to fungal growth and may cause AFLATOXICOSIS. Called also groundnut.
p. hulls a source of supplementary fiber in manufactured pet foods; it is high in lignin.
p. meal residue after the extraction of peanut oil; a

high protein (40 to 50%) feed supplement; low in methionine, lysine and tryptophan. May be mixed with hulls when it becomes of less value because of the high (30%) of fiber.

p. oil a refined fixed oil extracted from peanuts; used as a solvent for drugs.

pearl 1. a small medicated granule, or a glass globule with a single dose of volatile medicine, as amyl nitrite. 2. a rounded mass of tough sputum, as seen in the early stages of an attack of bronchial asthma.

p. disease calcification of the nodular lesions of pleural tuberculosis in cattle.

enamel p. small rounded masses of enamel adherent to the dentine of a tooth.

epidermic p's rounded concentric masses of epithelial cells found in certain papillomas and epitheliomas and as epithelial remnants of the dental lamina in the gingiva and jaws where they may give rise to cysts and tumors. Called also epithelial pearls.

epithelial p's see epidermic pearls (above).

p. millet see PENNISETUM *americanum*.

squamous p. see HORN pearls.

pearled a method of processing grain feeds to increase digestibility; the grain is hulled and broken into small, smooth, pearl-like pieces. A process more suited to human nutrition where the appearance of the grain is more important.

PEARS porcine enzootic abortion and respiratory syndrome.

Pearson saw a chain saw used in large animal obstetrics. It is safe in operation but limited to making cuts in a longitudinal direction.

Pearson square a quick, simple method of calculating the amount of a supplement required to achieve the desired composition of a ration. Copies of tables of feed standards and feed compositions are necessary to carry out the sums involved.

Pearson's chi-square test see CHI-SQUARE TEST.

peat, peat moss used as bedding for housed cattle and horses and is very absorbent of water.

p. scours chronic diarrhea in ruminants grazing pasture on peat-derived soils low in copper and/or high in molybdenum. See also COPPER nutritional deficiency, MOLYBDENUM.

peavine 1. see LATHYRUS. 2. the haulms of pea vines after canning peas have been harvested. The ensilage made from these vines may be poisonous. See PEA.

pebulate a thiocarbamate herbicide of low toxicity. Heavy doses cause muscular weakness, recumbency and weight loss.

peccary a South American suiform animal, of the genus *Tayassu*. Gregarious, omnivorous, small in size, black in color, with a sacculated stomach like a ruminant. Resembles a miniature wild boar. Species include *Catagonus wagneri* (chacoan peccary), *Tayassu tajacu* (collared peccary), *Tayassu peccari* (white-lipped peccary).

p. flea PULEX *porcinus*.

pecilomycosis infection with PAECILOMYCES.

peck order the order of dominance established in a flock of birds and changed only by fighting. The concept is now transposed to all species and is of major importance where animals are kept in groups and have to compete for feed supplies and shelter.

pecten pl. *pectines* [L.] 1. a comb; comblike structures. 2. a narrow zone in the anal canal, bounded above by the pectinate line.

p. oculi a black trapezoidal structure attached to the optic disk of the fowl.

p. ossis pubis cranial edge of the two pubic bones.

pubic p. cranial edge of the pubis bone; provides attachment to the abdominal muscles.

retinal p. a black pleated outgrowth from the retina to cover the optic papilla in the avian eye.

Pecten yessoensis farmed scallop in the family Pectinidae; called also Japanese scallop. See Table 23.

pectenitis inflammation of the pecten of the anus.

pectenosis stenosis of the anal canal due to an inelastic ring of tissue between the anal groove and anal crypts.

pectin a homosaccharidic polymer of sugar acids of fruit, which forms gels with sugar at the proper pH; a purified form obtained from the acid extract of the rind of citrus fruits or from apple pomace is used as a protectant and in cooking. Has a gelatinizing capacity and may be important in stabilizing the foam in frothy bloat.

p. methyl esterase a plant enzyme thought to have significance in the cause of bloat in cattle because of its role in the digestion of pectin and liberation of frothing agents pectic and galacturonic acids.

pectinate comb-shaped.

p. ligament the comb-like trabeculae of the corneoiridial angle.

imperforate p. ligament a cause of primary glaucoma; considered to be an inherited defect in a number of breeds of dogs. See also pectinate ligament (above).

p. line see pectinate LINE.

pectineal pertaining to the pecten.

pectineus muscle see Table 13.4.

pectiniform comb-shaped.

pectinotomy surgical transection of the pectineal muscle is a method of treatment in canine hip dysplasia; it provides relief from the pain associated with the condition.

pectoral 1. of or pertaining to the chest. 2. relieving disorders of the respiratory tract, as an expectorant.

p. girdle in birds is the three pairs of bones that support the wings: the furculae (fused clavicles), coracoids and scapulae. In mammals the coracoids and clavicles are often reduced, making the girdle incomplete.

p. limb the forelimb.

p. muscles extrinsic muscles of the forelimb arising from the brisket (ventral chest). See also Table 13. Outbreaks of defective development of these muscles are recorded in cattle.

p. myopathy a meat hygiene term for the lesions found in turkey and meat chicken breasts causing rejection of the meat. Called also green muscle disease.

pectoralis [L.] pertaining to the chest or breast; pectoral.

pectus [L.] *breast, chest, thorax.*

p. excavatum a congenital deformity in which the sternum and caudal ribs are concave, reducing the thoracic cavity space. Seen in puppies and kittens.

pedal pertaining to the foot or feet.

p. arthritis seen most often in cattle with septic arthritis of the distal interphalangeal joint.

p. bone the distal phalanx of ungulates, especially the horse.

p. bone rotation causing penetration of the sole of the horse's foot; a characteristic of severe laminitis.

p. fracture fractures of the pedal bone occur most commonly in horses. They may involve a wing or extensor process. They are usually transverse in cattle.

p. osteitis a rarefying osteitis of the pedal bone in the foot of the horse. Causes local pain and lameness.

pediatrics a branch of human medicine that deals with the diseases of children; the name is also used in describing the medicine of young animals.
pedicellation the development of a pedicle.
Pedicinus a genus of lice that infests monkeys. Members of the family Pediculidae.
P. eurygaster found on macaques.
P. mjobergi found on howler monkeys.
P. obtusus found on leaf and green monkeys and baboons.
P. patas found on colobus monkeys.
pedicle a footlike, stemlike, or narrow basal part or structure, such as a narrow strip by which a graft of tissue remains attached to the donor site.
p. advancement technique a surgical technique, commonly used in the repair of skin defects and defects in eyelids, in which a pedicle of tissue, usually skin, is formed and moved forward to fill a defect, without lateral movement. Various forms include the single or sliding flap, bipedicle flap, and V-Y technique. See also FLAP (1).
p. flap see pedicle GRAFT.
omental p. flap a segment of omentum can be mobilized as a flap to aid in the reconstruction of the thoracic or body wall.
vertebral p. one of the paired parts of the vertebral arch that connect a lamina to the vertebral body.
Pedicularis a genus of plants in the family Scrophulariaceae that contain digitalis-like alkaloids and are potentially dangerous as poisons for animals. Called also lousewort.
pediculation 1. the process of forming a pedicle. 2. infestation with lice.
pediculicide 1. destroying lice. 2. an agent that destroys lice.
Pediculoides ventricosus the grain itch mite that infests cereal crops and stored hay and grain; parasitizes animals causing a mild dermatitis but a severe pruritus.
pediculosis LOUSE infestation.
pediculous infested with lice.
pedigree a table, chart, diagram, or list of an animal's ancestors, used in genetics in the analysis of mendelian inheritance, and in the prediction of productivity and breed quality in the offspring.
p. analysis a useful basis for planning a program to eliminate an inherited defect; the analysis determines the probability that each prospective parent is homozygous for the normal gene, i.e. is not a carrier for the anomaly gene; potential parents with a probability of >95% can be used with confidence.
p. herds herds or flocks composed of animals whose pedigrees are known. Not necessarily stud herds or registered herd but the terms are usually synonymous.
p. index the average of the PREDICTED DIFFERENCE of the sire and the cow index of the dam. The pedigree index is allotted to the offspring.
p. selection use of an individual's pedigree to select breeding animals.
p. verification verification via breed societies and production testing agencies, horse stud books and race records are all used; checks via coat color, blood cell antigens may assist.
Pedipalpi whip scorpions, nonpoisonous arachnids.
ped(o)- [L.] *foot.*
pedogenesis metamorphotic phenomenon of production of a number of separate individuals in an intermediate host, e.g. a snail, by a single larval form.
peduncle a stemlike connecting part, especially: (1) a collection of nerve fibers coursing between different regions in the central nervous system, or (2) the stalk by which a nonsessile tumor is attached to normal tissue.
cerebellar p's three pairs of thick, white fiber trunks that arise from the midbrain, pons and medulla and pass into the cerebellum.
cerebral p. the ventral half of the midbrain, divisible into a dorsal part (*tegmentum*) and a ventral part (*crus cerebri*), which are separated by the substantia nigra.
p. disease a disease of marine fish caused by the flexibacter *Cytophaga psychrophila.*
olfactory p. caudal continuation of the olfactory bulb of the brain.
pineal p. see HABENULA (2).
peduncle disease see COLDWATER DISEASE.
pedunculated having a peduncle or stalk.
pedunculus [L.] *peduncle.*
PEEP positive-end-expiratory pressure.
peer review judgments of other scientists who work in the same field on the merits of papers submitted for publication, applications for reseach funding,
pefloxacin a fluoroquinolone antibiotic, similar to ciprofloxacin. Used as the mesylate.
PEG polyethylene glycol; percutaneous endoscopic gastrostomy.
peg a projecting structure; usually a small diameter, pointed piece of wood or metal, driven into a solid object.
rete p's see RETE pegs.
p. sticking see TENT pegging.
peg-leg osteomalacia. See PHOSPHORUS nutritional deficiency.
Pega ass Brazilian roan or dark gray donkey.
Peganum a genus of plants in the family Zygophyllaceae. The plants contain β-carboline alkaloids, e.g. harmine, harmalol which cause incoordination and paralysis; includes *P. harmala* (African rue), *P. mexicana* (Mexican rue).
pegleg see OSTEOMALACIA.
PEGS polyethylene glycols used as drug solvents.
PEI pancreatic exocrine insufficiency.
Peke-faced a longhaired Persian cat with a very short, flattened face, resembling that of a Pekingese dog.
Pekin a deep-cream or buff canary meat duck with bright orange legs, which also has a fair egg output.
Pekingese a very small, thickset dog with a large head, very short nose, prominent eyes and pendulous ears. The coat is long, straight and profuse over the body, particularly around the neck where it forms a 'mane', and on the tail, which is carried over the back. The breed is predisposed to distichiasis, hemivertebrae, intervertebral disk disease, proptosis, central corneal ulceration, facial fold pyoderma and anomalies of the upper respiratory tract.
pelage [Fr.] the hairy coat of mammals; the hairs, fur or wool of the body, limb and head, collectively.
pelagic living in the middle or near the surface of large bodies of water such as lakes or oceans.
Pelecitus roemeri filaroid nematode found in subcutaneous tissues, especially around the stifle joints, of wallabies and kangaroos. Called also *Dirofilaria roemeri.*
Pelger–Huët anomaly an anomaly, probably inherited, of neutrophils and eosinophils in which there is hyposegmentation of the nuclei. Seen rarely in dogs and cats with no clinical significance.
pseudo-P.–H. a. a transient hyposegmentation in neutrophils and eosinophils, usually from unknown causes. May be mistaken as the congenital anomaly.
pelican large aquatic piscivorous birds with large bills

and commodious sub-bill pouches, and white or gray plumage. Belong to the genus *Pelecanus* in the family Pelecanidae.

peliosis purpura.

p. hepatis focal, blood-filled spaces in the liver. Occurs in poisoning by PIMELEA in cattle. See also TELANGIECTASIA.

pellagra a syndrome in humans caused by a diet seriously deficient in niacin (or by failure to convert tryptophan to niacin). In dogs called blacktongue. See also NIACIN nutritional deficiency.

feline p. ulcerative stomatitis, especially of the tongue, and conjunctivitis.

pellagroid resembling pellagra.

pellet a small pill or granule.

p. feeding see pelleted FEED.

pellicle 1. a thin scum forming on the surface of liquids. 2. a thin, nonliving outer covering.

dental p. see DENTAL pellicle.

pellucid translucent.

Pelodera a genus of nematodes in the family Rhabditida.

P. strongyloides a freeliving worm which invades broken skin, usually from damp and infected bedding. Causes pelodera DERMATITIS.

pelt the undressed, raw skin of a wild animal with the fur in place. If from a sheep or goat there is a short growth of wool or mohair on the skin.

Peltophryne lemur Puerto Rican crested toad.

pelves plural form of pelvis.

pelvic pertaining to the pelvis.

p. abscess commonest in horses as a result of a rectal tear during a manual examination. The tear is only mucosa deep and the infection is deposited in the pelvic fascia where an abscess develops. This has the potential to erode into the peritoneal cavity. The syndrome begins as a toxemia and fever caused by the local abscess but a common sequel is the abrupt appearance of severe abdominal pain and toxemic shock.

p. bone os coxae, comprising the ilium, ischium and pubis. See also Table 10.

p. canal the canal from the pelvic inlet to the pelvic outlet.

p. cavity the space bounded by the bones of the pelvis.

p. girdle the bony ring formed by the pair of hip bones fused at the symphysis and their firm articulation with the sacrum, and in some species one or two coccygeal vertebrae.

p. inlet the cranial opening of the pelvis.

p. intestinal hernia see pelvic HERNIA.

p. ligaments include the dorsal sacroiliac, the sacrotuberal and the iliolumbar ligaments.

p. limb the hindlimb.

p. nerve see Table 14.

p. organs includes reproductive organs, urinary bladder, ureter, rectum.

p. outlet the caudal opening of the pelvis, guarded by the pelvic diaphragm.

p. plexus the autonomic plexus that is distributed to the pelvic viscera that consists of the cranial vesical plexus, the middle genital plexus and the caudal hemorrhoidal plexus, located on the ventrolateral surface of the rectum. It innervates the urinary bladder, prostate, ductus deferens and cranial urethra. It is supplied by the hypogastric and pelvic splanchnic nerves.

p. splanchnic nerves see NERVI ERIGENTES.

p. symphysiotomy surgical separation of the symphysis in immature animals as an aid in dystocia due to maternal pelvic inadequacy.

p. urethra that part of the urethra that passes through the pelvis.

p. viscera includes urinary bladder and pelvic ureters and urethra, rectum, prostate, seminal vesicles, vas deferens and ampullae in males, and vagina cervix and uterus, possibly ovaries, in the female.

pelvicaliceal, pelvicalyceal pertaining to the renal pelves and calices.

pelvicephalometry measurement of the fetal head in relation to the maternal pelvis.

pelvifixation surgical fixation of a displaced pelvic organ.

pelvimeter an instrument for measuring the pelvis.

pelvimetry measurement of the capacity and diameter of the pelvis, either internally or externally or both, with the hands or with a pelvimeter.

pelviotomy 1. incision or transection of a pelvic (hip) bone. 2. pyelotomy; incision of the renal pelvis.

pelviperitonitis inflammation of the pelvic peritoneum.

pelvirectal pertaining to the pelvis and rectum.

pelvis pl. *pelves;* the caudal portion of the trunk of the body, forming a basin bounded ventrally and laterally by the hip bones and dorsally by the sacrum and coccygeal vertebrae. Also applied to any basin-like structure, e.g. the renal pelvis.

The bony pelvis is formed by the sacrum, coccyx, ilium, pubis and ischium, bones that form the hip and pubic and sciatic arches.

android p. one with a wedge-shaped inlet and narrow cranial segment typically found in the male.

extrarenal p. see renal pelvis (below).

rachitic p. one distorted as a result of rickets.

renal p. the funnel-shaped expansion of the cranial end of the ureter; it is usually within the renal sinus, but under certain conditions, a large part of it may be outside the kidney (extrarenal pelvis).

split p. one with a congenital separation at the symphysis pubis.

tipped p. a tilted pelvis as occurs in cows and causes the external urinary meatus to be higher than the anterior pelvic floor so that urine accumulates in the vagina. See also UROVAGINA.

pelviureteral relating to the renal pelvis and the ureter.

pelvospondylitis inflammation of the pelvic portion of the spine.

Pembroke Welsh corgi see WELSH CORGI.

pemmican, pemican dried raw beef. See also BILTONG.

pemoline a central nervous system stimulant, similar to dexamphetamine.

pemphigoid 1. resembling pemphigus. 2. a group of skin disorders similar to but clearly distinguishable from pemphigus.

bullous p. an autoimmune disease of skin and oral mucosa with vesicles, bullae and ulcerations; occurs rarely in dogs and humans.

cicatricial p. a form that involves the oral and ocular mucosa.

pemphigus [Gr.] *pemphix* (blister); a group of immune-mediated diseases of the skin and mucous membranes characterized by vesicles, bullae, erosions and ulcerations; occurs in dogs, cats and horses.

p. erythematosus a form with features of both pemphigus foliaceus and lupus erythematosus; occurs in dogs and cats. There are erythematous, pustular lesions, mainly on the nose, periorbital skin and pinnae, and hypopigmentation of the planum nasale.

p. foliaceus a generalized, exfoliative, scaling disease sometimes with the formation of heavy crusts, marked hyperkeratosis of footpads, and involvement of the nail beds that may lead to loss of the nails. Occurs in dogs, cats, horses and goats.

p. vegetans a benign variant of pemphigus vulgaris, occurring only rarely in animals, in which the bullae are replaced by verrucoid hypertrophic vegetative masses.

p. vulgaris consists of shallow ulcerations with a generalized distribution and frequently involving the mucocutaneous junctions and oral mucosa.

pen 1. a small enclosure in which animals are restrained for handling or on a long term basis for intensive feeding. Called also corral. 2. female swan.

p. check the daily or twice daily examination of cattle in a feedlot to detect any sick animal. More frequent checks are made in the early period of a feeding program.

p. checker the specially selected cowboys whose task it is to carry out intensive pen checks.

p. design includes materials for floor and walls, floor drainage and warmth, disposal of feces and urine, sleep area versus feeding area, troughage and drinking facilities, space and number of occupants proposed.

pen-fed fed in small, compatible groups in pens to optimize feed utilization.

p. lambing the ewes are brought in from the pastures and those close to lambing are brought into pens where they can be kept under close observation to ensure carefree lambing and maximum lamb survival. The pens may be indoors or outside.

p. mating cows on heat are cut out from the herd and put into the bullpen. Mating is observed and recorded. Provided heat detection is good the reproductive efficiency can be maximal.

p. space space allocation per head of livestock proposed to be accommodated.

p. sweeps wool swept up from pens, shearing board, races.

Penaeus genus of farmed crustaceans in suborder Penaeidae; includes *P. chinensis* (fleshy or white prawn), *P. monodon* (giant tiger prawn), *P. vannamei* (whiteleg shrimp), *P. merguiensis* (banana prawn). See Table 23.

pencil bush MYOPORUM *deserti*.

pencil caustic SARCOSTEMMA *australe*.

pendulous hanging loosely; dependent.

p. crop see pendulous CROP.

penectomy surgical removal of the penis.

penetrance the frequency with which a heritable trait is manifested by individuals carrying the principal gene or genes conditioning it.

incomplete p. when penetrance is less than 100%.

penetrating breaching the tissues of the body.

penguin completely marine, aquatic flightless bird inhabiting only the southern hemisphere. There are six genera, all of them gregarious, monogamous and piscivorous, including *Aptenodytes* and *Megadyptes* in the order Sphenisciformes. Varieties include black-footed, pigeon-toed.

-penia word element. [Gr.] *deficiency*.

penicillamine, D-penicillamine a product of penicillin which chelates copper and other metals; used in the treatment of copper accumulation associated with chronic hepatitis, copper-associated hepatopathy of Bedlington terriers, and lead poisoning.

penicilliary radicles arborizing arterioles of the spleen, the blood supply for the splenic germinal centers.

penicillic acid an antibiotic substance isolated from cultures of various species of *Penicillium* and *Aspergillus*.

penicillin any of a large group of natural or semisynthetic antibacterial antibiotics derived directly or indirectly from strains of fungi of the genus *Penicillium* and other soil-inhabiting fungi grown on special culture media. Penicillins exert a bactericidal as well as a bacteriostatic effect on susceptible bacteria by interfering with the final stages of the synthesis of peptidoglycan, a substance in the bacterial cell wall. Despite their relatively low toxicity for the host, they are active against many bacteria, especially gram-positive pathogens (streptococci, staphylococci); clostridia; certain gram-negative forms; certain spirochetes (*Treponema pallidum* and *T. pertenue*); and certain fungi. Certain strains of some target species, for example staphylococci, secrete the enzyme *penicillinase*, which inactivates penicillin and confers resistance to the antibiotic. Some of the newer penicillins, for example methicillin, are more effective against penicillinase-producing organisms. An additional class of extended-spectrum penicillins has been approved for use; it includes piperacillin and mezlocillin.

There are four groups of penicillins, the natural penicillins, penicillin G and penicillin V, with a narrow spectrum of activity, mainly against gram-positive bacteria; the aminopenicillins (amoxicillin, ampicillin and hetacillin) are semisynthetic derivatives and have a broad spectrum of activity against gram-positive and many gram-negative organisms, but are susceptible to penicillinase-producing *Staphylococcus* spp.; penicillinase-resistant penicillins, which include cloxacillin, methicillin, nafcillin and oxacillin; and the extended-spectrum penicillins (azlocillin, carbenicillin, mezlocillin, piperacillin and ticarcillin), which are effective against gram-positive and gram-negative organisms, including *Pseudomonas aeruginosa*.

Allergic reaction to penicillin occurs in some animals. The reaction may be slight—a stinging or burning sensation at the site of injection—or it can be more serious—severe dermatitis or even anaphylactic shock, which may be fatal.

p. allergy degradation products of the penicillins act as haptens, binding to proteins and stimulating an immune response.

p. G benzylpenicillin; the most widely used penicillin; used principally in the treatment of infections due to gram-positive bacteria. *Procaine* penicillin G is a parenteral preparation that gives extended action for up to 24 hours and *benzathine* penicillin G is a very slow-release, parenteral preparation that maintains blood levels for several days.

p.-induced hemolytic anemia rare problem in horses which develop IgG anti-penicillin antibodies.

phenoxymethyl p. a biosynthetically or semisynthetically produced antibiotic, similar to penicillin G, for oral administration; not affected by gastric acid and is suitable for oral administration. Its antibacterial spectrum is the same as for penicillin G. Called also penicillin V.

p. V see phenoxymethyl penicillin (above).

penicillinase an enzyme produced by bacteria that inactivates penicillin, thus increasing resistance to the antibiotic; a purified form from *Bacillus cereus* is used in the treatment of reactions to penicillin.

penicilliosis infection by the blue-green mold, *Penicillium*; causes a necrotic rhinitis and sinusitis that occasionally extends to the mouth or orbit. The disease is similar to aspergillosis.

Penicillium a genus of mold-forming fungi that grow on stored feed and in growing plants. Some produce antibiotics, some can be opportunistic pathogens and some produce mycotoxins, including patulin.

P. chrysogenum, P. notatum cultures of these fungi produce penicillin.

P. citreo-viride produces the neurotoxin citreoviridin which causes paralysis, convulsions and death in humans eating contaminated yellow rice. Resembles beriberi, thought originally to be due to thiamin deficiency.

P. citrinum produces ochratoxin, citrinin, causes growth retardation, hepatic necrosis and nephropathy.

***P. claviforme, P. cyclopium, P. divergens, P. equinum, P. expansum, P. griseofulvum, P. lapidosum, P. leucopus, P.melinii, P. novae-zeelandiae, P. patulum* (syn. *P. urticae*)** produce the antibiotic patulin.

P. crustosum produces tremorgens which cause incoordination and recumbency and was thought at one time to cause ryegrass staggers.

P. cyclopium, P. jantinellum, P. nigricans, P. palitans, P. piscarum, P. puberulum are soil fungi and produce tremorgens which cause tremor, ataxia and muscular rigidity in animals grazing infested pasture. The fungi were once thought to be involved in causing ryegrass staggers.

P. estinogenum produces tremorgens and causes incoordination and recumbency.

P. islandicum causes hepatic necrosis and has carcinogenic properties.

P. purpurogenum produces rubratoxin and causes anemia and widespread hemorrhages in chickens.

P. roqueforti grows on stored grain and ensilage; suspected of causing bovine abortion and retained placenta via an unidentified toxin. Produces roquefortine which causes tetanic convulsions in dogs.

P. rubrum contains rubratoxin which causes abdominal pain, jaundice, convulsions.

P. simplicissimus fungus which produces tremorgens, causing incoordination and recumbency.

P. viridicatum grows on stored grain and produces ochratoxin which causes nephrosis mostly in pigs. Also produces citrinin and viomellin.

penicilloyl-polylysine prepared from polylysine and a penicillic acid, it is used as a diagnostic agent; intradermal reaction elicits a wheal and erythema response in those sensitive to penicillin.

penicillus pl. *penicilli* [L.] any of the brushlike groups of arterial branches in the lobules of the spleen.

penile of or pertaining to the penis.

p. abscess causes apparent swelling of the ventral body line of affected bulls. The lesions are moderately painful to touch, are firm and hard and persist for long periods. Associated adhesions make it impossible for the bull to extrude the penis.

p. amputation carried out in horses for treatment of extensive neoplasms and granulomas and for paralysis of the penis.

p. bulb a swelling at the origin of the corpus spongiosum penis.

p. crura the origins of the corpus cavernosum penis at the ischial arch.

p. deviation a common defect only in bulls in which an abnormality of the apical ligament, present congenitally or caused by trauma, causes a spiral, lateral or ventral deviation of the penis, causing difficulty in mating. See also CORKSCREW penis.

p. erection see ERECTION.

p. eversion see penile prolapse (below).

p. frenulum see penile preputial FRENULUM.

p. glans see GLANS penis.

p. hair-ring long hairs from the preputial orifice pack up around the penis of the bull and cause pressure necrosis occasionally creating a hypospadias. Can occur in any species carrying preputial hairs.

p. hematoma in bulls, in which it is a common event, it is caused by trauma while the bull is mating a cow. It occurs halfway along the penis with an obvious swelling and an inability to breed cows. There is a tear in the tunica albuginea of the corpus cavernosum and a surrounding hematoma.

p. hypoplasia occurs as part of an intersex deformity or as a sequel to prepubertal castration.

inadequate p. protrusion due to congenital shortness of the penis, adhesions caused by injury and hematoma, and persistence of the penile frenulum.

p. ossification common radiological finding in aged dogs; ossification caudal to os penis.

p. paralysis common only in stallions, due to local neurological lesion, or as a rare occurrence after the administration of phenothiazine-derived tranquilizers or severe debility.

persistent p. frenulum see penile preputial FRENULUM.

p. prepuce see PREPUCE.

p. prolapse inability to withdraw the penis into the prepuce, other than a paraphimosis. Not to be confused with PHIMOSIS; paralysis does occur in disease of the spinal cord, e.g. in some cases of rabies.

p. protrusion failure caused by persistent frenulum, adhesions to prepuce, fibropapilloma.

p. sigmoid flexure the S-shaped bend in the penis of ruminants and pigs, present when the penis is not erect, and the principal mechanism for reducing the length of the organ in these species.

p. tiedown an adhesion of the penis to the prepuce created artificially to prepare the animal as a teaser.

p. translocation surgical operations to direct the penis so that the bull cannot serve a cow.

p. tunica albuginea the dense connective tissue covering of the corpus cavernosum penis.

penis the external male organ of urination and copulation. Its structure varies a great deal between the species. In carnivores and horses the bulk of the organ is erectile tissue; in cats and dogs there is a bone included in the glans. In cats the penis is directed backwards (retromingent). In ruminants and pigs the bulk of the penis is connective tissue and the organ is long and firm and has a large sigmoid flexure which disappears when the penis is in the erect state. In rams and goat bucks the penile urethra is continued beyond the glans as the urethral process. See also PENILE.

corkscrew p. see CORKSCREW penis.

corpus cavernosum p. one of the two bodies that make up the dorsal compartment of erectile tissue, grooved below to carry the corpus spongiosum penis (syn. corpus cavernosum urethrae). It arises from each side of the ischial arch as the crus penis and at its anterior end is enclosed by the glans which is an extension of the corpus spongiosum.

corpus spongiosum p. a column of erectile tissue around the urethra of the penis and extending into the glans penis.

short p. an uncommon, possibly inherited, defect in some breeds of cattle.

supernumerary p. a rare deformity, usually ectopic.

p. urethral process detached the free end of the penis has a bifid structure.

penitis inflammation of the penis.

penitrem-A a tremorgen toxin causing nervous signs and renal damage; isolated from the fungi *Penicillium cyclopium, P. palitans, P. puberulum, P. viridicatum*.

PennHIP Pennsylvania Hip Improvement Program. A system for standardized evaluation of radiographs in the diagnosis of canine hip dysplasia. It uses an adjustable hip distraction device in positioning dogs for the x-rays.
penniform shaped like a feather.
Pennisetum a genus of grasses in the family Poaceae.
P. americanum, P. typhoides, P. glaucum a large grass used as a fodder crop. Can be poisonous if infested with the fungus *Claviceps fusiformis*, known to cause agalactia in sows. Called also bulrush, Indian, horse or pearl millet.
P. clandestinum perennial, creeping grass with hairy leaves and inconspicuous seedheads. Has a rapid summer growth period; suitable for green chop, silage or grazing. May have a low fiber content and cause depression of fat content of milk. A very valuable grass producing an enormous bulk of feed in suitable climates. It can be poisonous, causing abdominal pain, paralysis of tongue and pharynx, and tremor. Probably caused by ingestion of fungi *Myrothecium* spp. and *Phoma herbarum* growing on plant debris after period of lush growth or infestation with army caterpillars. Can also cause oxalate and nitrite poisoning. Called also Kikuyu grass.
P. glaucum see *Pennisetum americanum* (above).
P. polystachyon *P. purpureum*. Called also mission grass.
P. purpureum its oxalate content is known and is associated with the occurrence of osteodystrophia fibrosa in horses. Called also elephant or Napier grass.
P. typhoides see *Pennisetum americanum* (above).
penny-cress see THLASPI ARVENSE.
pennyroyal MENTHA *palegium*.
pennyroyal oil an aromatic extract of several mint plants, particularly *Mentha pulegium* and *M. canadensis*. Sometimes used as an insecticide or insect repellent on dogs and cats, but can be a cause of poisoning, particularly in cats, with signs that include panting, dyspnea and abortion.
pennywort COTYLEDON *umbilicus*.
Penrose drain see Penrose DRAIN.
Penstemon a North American genus of plants in the family Scrophulariaceae which act as facultative selenium converters; the selenocompounds produced by the plant cause alopecia, lameness, laminitis; called also beard tongue.
pent(a)- word element. [Gr.] *five*.
pentachloronaphthalene see CHLORINATED NAPHTHALENES.
pentachloronitrobenzene a soil fungicide used extensively in agricultural crops and not known to cause illness but it is of environmental concern because of its capacity to enter the human food chain and cause tissue residues in all species; abbreviated PCNB.
pentachlorophenol a wood preservative with great capacity to enter the body by any route, including percutaneously; causes weight loss, low milk production and general debility.
pentadactyl having five digits.
pentadiene isomers compounds used as herbicides; can cause excitability, incoordination and prostration.
pentagastrin a synthetic pentapeptide consisting of β-alanine and C-terminal tetrapeptide of gastrin; used in a test of gastric secretory function.
pentamer a polymer formed from five molecules of a monomer.
pentamidine isethionate a diamidine derivative effective against protozoa. Used in the treatment of *Babesia*, *Leishmania* and *Pneumocystis* spp.
pentaploidy having a chromosome number which is five times the standard number.
pentasomy the presence of three additional chromosomes of one type (e.g. 5 X chromosomes) in an otherwise diploid cell (2n + 3).
pentastome aberrant arthropod parasite belonging to the class Pentastomida. Includes *Linguatula*, *Porocephalus* and *Armillifer* spp.
pentastomiasis infection by parasites of the phylum Pentastomida; found in the respiratory tract of reptiles.
Pentastomida see PENTASTOME.
pentastomidiasis infection with pentastomes.
Pentatrichomonas a genus of protozoan parasites with five flagella.
***P. hominis* (syn. *Trichomonas hominis, T. intestinalis*)** found in dogs, primates and humans but appears to be nonpathogenic.
pentavalent having a valence of five.
p. antimony compounds see ANTIMONY.
p. organic arsenicals includes the pharmaceuticals arsanilic acid, roxarsone, nitarsone. See also organic ARSENICAL.
pentazocine lactate a synthetic narcotic used as an analgesic.
pentetic acid diethylenetriamine penta-acetic acid, an iron-chelating agent.
Penthrane a proprietary name for methoxyflurane.
pentobarbital, pentobarbitone a short- to intermediate-acting barbiturate; used as a hypnotic and sedative in the form of the sodium salt. Nembutal—the sodium salt.
pentobarbitone see PENTOBARBITAL.
pentosans pentose polysaccharides found in fruits and other foods; form pentoses on hydrolysis.
pentose a monosaccharide containing five carbon atoms in a molecule.
p. cycle see pentose phosphate pathway (below).
p. phosphate pathway called also pentose cycle; see pentose phosphate PATHWAY.
pentoside a compound (glycoside) of pentose with another substance.
pentosuria high levels of pentose in the urine.
Pentothal a proprietary name for thiopental.
pentylenetetrazol see LEPTAZOL.
penumbra a blurred edge to an image, a halo effect, in an x-ray film caused usually by an overlarge focal spot exacerbated by a long object-to-film distance.
PEP phosphoenolpyruvate.
peplomer a glycoprotein structural unit found in the lipoprotein envelope of enveloped viruses, e.g. H and N spikes of influenza virus. Called also spikes.
peplos the lipoprotein envelope of some types of virions.
pepper grass PANICUM *whitei*.
Peppin famous strain of Australian merino sheep.
pepsin a proteolytic enzyme that is the principal digestive component of gastric juice. It acts as a catalyst in the chemical breakdown of protein to form a mixture of polypeptides; it is formed from pepsinogen in the presence of acid or, autocatalytically, in the presence of pepsin itself. Pepsin also has milk-clotting action similar to that of rennin and thereby facilitates the digestion of milk protein.
p. barrier the gastric mucosal mechanism which prevents rediffusion of hydrochloric acid back into gastric tissues; includes an electrical resistance, mucus, plus bicarbonate ions trapped in the mucus, endogenous prostaglandins.

pepsinogen a zymogen secreted by the chief cells of the gastric glands and converted into pepsin in the presence of gastric acid or of pepsin itself.

plasma p. high levels are indicative of extensive mucosal damage in the abomasum, as in ostertagiasis in ruminants.

peptic pertaining to pepsin or to digestion or to the action of gastric juices.

p. ulcer an ulceration of the mucous membrane of the esophagus, stomach or duodenum, caused by the action of the acid gastric juice. There are two kinds of peptic ulcers: *gastric* ulcers occur in the stomach; *duodenal* ulcers occur in the duodenum, the part of the small intestine nearest the stomach. Most common in cattle and dogs, but they do occur sporadically in other species. See also ZOLLINGER–ELLISON SYNDROME.

peptidase any of a subclass of proteolytic enzymes that catalyze the hydrolysis of peptide linkages.

peptide any of a class of compounds of low molecular weight which yield two or more amino acids on hydrolysis; known as di-, tri-, tetra- etc. peptides, depending on the number of amino acids in the molecule. Peptides form the constituent parts of proteins. See also POLYPEPTIDE.

leader p. a step in the signal hypothesis advanced to explain the mechanisms governing the fate of newly formed polypeptides or secretory proteins.

p. map a pattern of peptide fragments, characteristic of a particular protein. Produced by using either proteolytic enzymes such as trypsin or chemicals such as cyanogen bromide to cut proteins at a relatively small number of particular sites, the peptide fragments are then separated by chromatographic or electrophoretic procedures. Called also fingerprint.

p.-para-aminobenzoic acid test see BT-PABA TEST.

peptidergic of or pertaining to neurons that secrete peptide hormones.

p. neurons a group of enteric interneurons which contain peptides; the peptides include enkephalins and somatostatins.

peptidoglycan a glycan (polysaccharide) attached to short cross-linked peptides; found in bacterial cell walls and is responsible for their structural rigidity.

peptidolytic capable of splitting up peptide bonds.

peptidoma see APUDOMA.

peptidyl site see peptidyl-TRNA binding site.

Peptococcus a genus of non-spore-forming, gram-positive anaerobic cocci which have been recovered from infected dog bite wounds. The type species is *P. niger*.

peptogenic 1. producing pepsin or peptones. 2. promoting digestion.

peptolysis the splitting up of peptone.

peptone protein derivative formed by partial hydrolysis of a protein.

Peptostreptococcus gram-positive round or oval bacteria occurring singly or in long chains. Found as an normal flora in many species and humans.

P. anaerobius isolated from abscesses in dogs and cats.

P. heliotrinreductans a ruminal organism thought to detoxify pyrrolizidine alkaloids in the rumen of sheep.

P. indolicus implicated in the etiology of mastitis in cattle, especially in summer mastitis.

per- word element. [L.] 1. throughout, completely, extremely. 2. in chemistry, a large amount, combination of an element in its highest valency.

per anum [L.] *through the anus.*

per-head fees see FEES.

per oral peroral; per os.

per os [L.] *by mouth.*

per primam [L.] *by first intention;* see also HEALING.

per rectum [L.] *by way of the rectum.*

per secundam [L.] *by second intention;* see also HEALING.

per tertiam [L.] *by third intention;* see also HEALING.

per tubam [L.] *through a tube.*

per vaginam [L.] *through the vagina.*

peracetic acid a potent disinfectant used as a 3% concentration; suitable for the destruction of anthrax spores.

peracid an acid containing more than the usual quantity of oxygen.

peracute very acute; a duration of a few hours only.

Perameles see BANDICOOT.

peramine metabolite of the fungus *Acremonium lolii*; repellent to insects.

Perca see PIKE-PERCH.

P. pluviatilis European freshwater fish species used extensively as food; introduced into many countries. Variously regarded as a valuable sports species or as a pest. Called also redfin perch.

percentile 1. one of 100 equal parts of a series of measurements, each group being of equal size, and arranged in order of their magnitude; the 20th percentile is the value in the series below which 20% of the values fall. 2. the dividing points between such groups.

perception the conscious mental registration of a sensory stimulus. The ability of animals to perceive is apparent from their responses to the application of stimuli but the nature of the perceptivity is only surmised. The difficulty in examining an animal is to decide whether a failure to respond to a stimulus is due to lack of perception, inability to respond or disinclination to do so.

Percheron a French heavy draft horse, of graceful build and action. Gray, white or black, 15.2 to 17 hands high.

perching characteristic resting posture of birds on thin branches or perches; facilitated by anatomical arrangement of the digital flexor tendons—when the bird squats the knee and hock joints are flexed and the digital tendons flex passively, the digits grasping the perch.

perchlorate ion one of the competing ions which blocks the uptake and transport of iodine ions.

percolate 1. to strain; to submit to percolation. 2. a liquid that has been submitted to percolation. 3. to trickle slowly through a substance.

percolation the extraction of soluble parts of a drug by passing a solvent liquid through it.

percolator a vessel used in percolation.

percuss to perform percussion.

percussible detectable on percussion.

percussion in veterinary diagnosis, striking a part of the body with short, sharp blows of the fingers in order to determine the size, position and density of the underlying parts by the sound obtained. Percussion is most commonly used on the chest and back for examination of the heart and lungs. For example, since the heart is not resonant and the adjacent lungs are, when the examiner's fingers strike the chest over the heart the sound waves will change in pitch. This serves as a guide to the precise location and size of the heart. The value of percussion in animals is limited by their haircoat, their reluctance to cooperate and their anatomy. Radiology and ultrasonographic imaging have pretty much supplanted the percussionist.

auscultatory p. auscultation of the sound produced by percussion. See also AUSCULTATION with percussion.
immediate p. that in which the blow is struck directly against the body surface.
mediate p. that in which a pleximeter is used.
palpatory p. a combination of palpation and percussion, affording tactile rather than auditory impressions. See also BALLOTTEMENT.

percussor an instrument for performing percussion.

percutaneous performed through the skin, e.g. percutaneous cystocentesis.

Père David's deer Chinese deer found only in zoos. Called also *Elaphurus davidianus*.

perencephaly porencephaly.

Perendale a dual-purpose, polled, New Zealand sheep, produced by crossing the Romney Marsh and Cheviot breeds; wool 28 to 32 microns. It has a head clear of wool and a profile and stance like the Cheviot.

perennial a plant with a life cycle of more than one year.
p. broomweed GUTIERREZIA *microcephala*.
p. pea LATHYRUS *latifolius*.
p. ryegrass LOLIUM *perenne*.
p. snakeweed GUTIERRHEZIA *microcephala*.
p. urochloa grass UROCHLOA *mozambicensis*.

perfect state the sexual stage in the life cycle of fungi.

perforans [L.] *penetrating;* a term applied to various muscles and nerves.

perforating canals canals in bone through which blood vessels pass.

perforation a hole or break in the containing walls or membranes of an organ or structure of the body. Perforation occurs when erosion, infection or other factors create a weak spot in the organ and internal pressure causes a rupture. It also may result from a deep penetrating wound caused by trauma.
bladder p. usually the result of obstructive urolithiasis with eventual leakage of urine into the peritoneal cavity. See also congenital URINARY BLADDER rupture.
eardrum p. occurs when an infectious process erodes the tympanic membrane or leads to increased pressure in the middle ear.
esophageal p. causes local cellulitis and obstruction of the esophagus.
gallbladder p. sometimes occurs as a complication of CHOLECYSTITIS and GALLSTONES. When the gallbladder is infected, necrosis may progress to the point of destroying the wall so that the bile spills out into the abdominal cavity causing biliary peritonitis.
intestinal p. a complication of ulcerative colitis (see COLITIS), INTESTINAL obstruction, ulceration and other disorders in which there is inflammation of the intestinal wall or obstruction of the intestinal lumen.
ulcer p. a complication of duodenal and gastric ulcers. It requires immediate surgical correction to prevent hemorrhage, shock and peritonitis.
urethral p. is usually a result of obstructive urolithiasis; urine collects in a ventral subcutaneous site,

perforin a protein in cytotoxic T lymphocytes that creates transmembrane pores that act as ion channels in the target cell. Structurally and chemically related to C9 protein of complement which performs a similar function.

performance in the context of animals, a comprehensive term including productivity, racing performance, reproductive efficiency, and any other form of activity that contributes to the owner's financial and psychological welfare.
p. diet one formulated to be high in energy, fat and protein, and highly digestible. Used not only for performance animals, but also suitable for other above-maintenance requirements such as reproduction, lactation, growth, stress and after surgery or trauma.
p. testing a widely used technique in agricultural animals. Sample animals are tested in controlled surroundings and on controlled diets and ranked in the order of their productivity, e.g. bull test stations.

performing animals animals trained to perform unusual acts as an entertainment for humans. The practice could be subject to cruel procedures and the animals could be brutalized to perform painful movements. Of some importance is the imposition by humans of training in tricks that are demeaning to the animals and hold them up to ridicule.

perfusate a liquid that has been subjected to perfusion.

perfusion 1. the act of pouring through or over; especially the passage of a fluid through the vessels of a specific organ. 2. a liquid poured through or over an organ or tissue.
p. pressure the gradient between arterial blood pressure and venous pressure in a comparable location in the vascular tree.
pulmonary p. blood flow through the pulmonary capillaries.
renal p. the rate of perfusion in the kidney is much higher than in any other organ. The rate of formation of urine depends to a large extent on the perfusion rate.
p. scan using pulmonary scintigraphy, radionucleotide agents injected into a peripheral vein can be detected where it is trapped in the pulmonary capillary bed. Used to assess pulmonary blood flow.
p. technique maintenance of blood circulation to tissues during cardiopulmonary bypass.
p.:ventilation ratio see VENTILATION:perfusion ratio.

peri- word element. [Gr.] *around, near*. See also words beginning *para-*.

periacinal, periacinous around an acinus.

periacinar see PERIACINAL.
p. necrosis see CENTRILOBULAR necrosis.

periadenitis inflammation of tissues around a gland.

periampullary situated around an ampulla.

perianal around the anus.
p. abscess under the skin outside the anal canal. Causes sufficient pain to inhibit defecation.
p. fistula a syndrome of inflammation, ulceration, and draining sinuses and fistulae in the perianal region of dogs, particularly German shepherd dogs. The specific lesions include fistulae of the anal sinuses, anal sac rupture and fistulae, submucous fistulae and sinuses and fistulae of the rectum. Clinical signs include painful defecation and unpleasant odor. A variety of surgical techniques have been developed, but the condition is very resistant to treatment. Called also anal furunculosis.
p. gland modified sebaceous glands found in skin around the anus of dogs. Other regions also contain modified glands, e.g. the perineum, prepuce, thigh, dorsal lumbosacral area and tail base. Called also circumanal glands, hepatoid glands.
p. gland hyperplasia most perianal gland enlargements in male dogs are hormone-dependent hyperplasia and regress when the patient is castrated.
p. gland tumors nodular hyperplasia, adenomas and carcinomas are common in older male dogs, occurring occasionally in females.
p. pyoderma see perianal fistula (above).
p. sinus see perianal fistula (above).

p. warts papilloma around anus, virus possibly transmitted by veterinarian performing rectal examination.

periangiitis inflammation of the tissue around a blood or lymph vessel.

periangiocholitis inflammation of tissues around the bile ducts; pericholangitis.

periaortitis inflammation of tissues around the aorta.

periapical surrounding the apex of the root of a tooth.

periaqueductal gray a core of gray matter nervous tissue surrounding the cerebral aqueduct in the midbrain.

periarterial around an artery.

periarteriolar lymphoid sheath splenic white pulp, containing mainly T lymphocytes, surrounding arteries.

periarteritis inflammation of the outer coat of an artery and of the tissues surrounding it.

p. nodosa an inflammatory disease of the coats of small and medium-sized arteries, marked by a variety of systemic signs. Seen sporadically in domestic animals and in humans associated with hepatitis B antigen. See also COLLAGEN diseases. Called also Kussmaul's disease, polyarteritis, panarteritis nodosa.

periarthritis inflammation of the tissues around a joint.

periarticular situated around a joint.

p. osteophytes bony excrescences around the periphery of a joint.

periauricular cyst dentigerous cyst. See DENTAL cyst.

periaxial around an axis.

periaxillary around the axilla.

periblast the portion of the blastoderm of telolecithal eggs, the cells of which lack complete cell membranes.

peribronchial around a bronchus or bronchi.

peribronchiolar around the bronchioles.

peribronchiolitis inflammation of the tissues around the bronchioles.

peribronchitis a form of bronchitis consisting of inflammation and thickening of the tissues around the bronchi.

pericaliceal, pericalyceal situated near or around a renal calix.

pericallosal situated around the corpus callosum.

pericardectomy surgical excision of the pericardial sac. A form of treatment for pericardial effusion.

pericardiac pertaining to the pericardium; around the heart.

pericardial pertaining to the pericardium.

p. diaphragmatic hernia see PERITONEOPERICARDIAL hernia.

p. effusion the second stage of pericarditis when much inflammatory exudate accumulates, part of a general edematous state or in cases of neoplasia involving the epicardium or pericardium. Characterized by enlargement of the cardiac silhouette on radiography and outline on percussion, muffling of heart sounds and congestive heart failure due to compression of the heart by cardiac tamponade.

p. fibrosis a chronic change in pericarditis, leading to constriction that limits diastolic ventricular volume. See also constrictive PERICARDITIS.

p. friction rub see pericardial RUB.

p. inflammation see PERICARDITIS.

p. knock an early diastolic sound caused by loss of pericardial elasticity accompanying fibrosis that limits ventricular filling.

p. meridian points acupuncture points located along the pericardial meridian.

p. paracentesis see PERICARDICENTESIS.

p. tamponade see cardiac TAMPONADE.

pericardicentesis surgical puncture of the pericardial cavity with aspiration of fluid, usually for the purpose of obtaining fluid for cytological examination or to relieve cardiac tamponade.

pericardiectomy excision of a portion of the pericardium.

pericardiocentesis pericardicentesis.

pericardiolysis the operative freeing of adhesions between the visceral and parietal pericardium.

pericardiophrenic pertaining to the pericardium and diaphragm.

pericardiopleural pertaining to the pericardium and pleura.

pericardiorrhaphy suture of the pericardium.

pericardiostomy creation of an opening into the pericardium, usually for drainage of effusions.

pericardiotomy incision of pericardium.

pericarditis inflammation of the pericardium. Initially there is an audible friction rub on auscultation. Later as fluid accumulates there is a muffling of the heart sounds and sometimes a washing machine sound on auscultation. Congestive heart failure develops terminally. Classified according to exudate produced as fibrinous, fibrinohemorrhagic, hemorrhagic, purulent.

bread-and-butter p. see BREAD AND BUTTER PERICARDITIS.

constrictive p. adhesions between the epicardium and pericardium limit the movement of the heart sometimes sufficiently to cause congestive heart failure.

niche p. see NICHE pericarditis.

traumatic p. occurs in cattle and goats, rarely sheep, when a sharp foreign body is swallowed and lodges in the reticulum, subsequently perforating its wall. The perforation may go as far forward as the pericardial sac, especially if the animal is pregnant. The animal dies of a combination of congestive heart failure and toxemia due to the bacterial infection.

pericardium the fibroserous sac enclosing the heart and the roots of the great vessels, composed of external (fibrous) and internal (serous) layers. See also PERICARDIAL.

adherent p. one abnormally connected with the heart by dense fibrous tissue.

congenitally absent p. the heart lies free in the pleural sac; recorded in dogs.

fibrous p. the external layer of the pericardium, consisting of dense fibrous tissue.

parietal p. the parietal layer of the serous pericardium, which is in contact with the fibrous pericardium.

serous p. the inner, serous portion of pericardium, consisting of two layers, visceral and parietal; the space between the layers is the pericardial cavity.

visceral p. the inner layer of the serous pericardium, which is intimately attached to the heart and roots of the great vessels. Called also epicardium.

pericecal around the cecum.

pericecitis inflammation of the tissues around the cecum.

pericellular surrounding a cell.

pericementitis periodontitis.

pericervical around the cervix.

p. abscess caused by trauma during parturition or laceration during mating. Causes infertility.

pericholangitis inflammation of tissues surrounding the bile ducts; periangiocholitis.

pericholecystitis inflammation of tissues around the gallbladder.

perichondral, perichondrial pertaining to or composed of perichondrium.

p. mineralization aberrant deposits of calcium salts in the perichondrium.

p. ring surrounds and supports the growth plate at the end of each long bone.

perichondrial see PERICHONDRAL.

perichondritis inflammation of the perichondrium.

perichondrium the layer of fibrous connective tissue investing all cartilage except the articular cartilage of synovial joints.

perichordal surrounding the notochord.

perichoroidal surrounding the choroid coat of the eye.

pericolic around the colon.

pericolitis, pericolonitis inflammation around the colon, especially of its peritoneal coat.

pericolpitis inflammation of the tissues around the vagina; perivaginitis.

periconchal around the concha.

Periconia a fungus that grows on forage growing in the field and contains an unidentified hepatoxin. Livestock grazing the infected forage may develop hepatic injury and photosensitization.

pericorneal around the cornea.

pericoronal around the crown of a tooth.

pericoronitis inflammation of the gums around a crown, usually associated with eruption.

pericranitis inflammation of the pericranium.

pericranium the periosteum of the skull.

pericystitis inflammation of tissues about the bladder.

pericyte one of the peculiar elongated, contractile cells found wrapped about precapillary arterioles outside the basement membrane.

pericytial around a cell.

peridentitis periodontitis.

periderm the outer layer of the bilaminar fetal epidermis, generally disappearing before birth. Called also epitrichium.

peridesmitis inflammation of the peridesmium.

peridesmium the areolar membrane that covers the ligaments.

perididymis the tunica vaginalis testis, the membrane covering the front and sides of the testis and epididymis.

perididymitis inflammation of the tunica vaginalis testis.

peridiverticulitis inflammation around an intestinal diverticulum.

peridontal periodontal.

periductal around a duct.

periduodenitis inflammation around the duodenum.

peridural external to the dura mater.

p. anesthesia see EPIDURAL anesthesia.

periencephalitis inflammation of the surface of the brain.

periencephalomeningitis inflammation of the cerebral cortex and meninges.

perienteritis inflammation of the peritoneal coat of the intestines.

periesophageal around the esophagus.

p. hiatal hernia see paraesophageal HERNIA.

periesophagitis inflammation of the tissues around the esophagus.

perifistular around a fistula.

perifollicular surrounding a follicle.

perifolliculitis inflammation around the hair follicles.

nodular granular p. see MAJOCCHI'S GRANULOMA.

perigangliitis inflammation around a ganglion.

perigastric around the stomach; pertaining to the peritoneal coat of the stomach.

perigastritis inflammation of the peritoneal coat of the stomach.

periglandular infiltrates dermal cellular infiltrates around glands.

perihepatic around the liver.

perihepatitis inflammation of the peritoneal coat of the liver and the surrounding tissue.

peri-islet situated around the islets of Langerhans.

perijejunitis inflammation around the jejunum.

perikaryon the cell body of a neuron.

perilabyrinthitis inflammation of the tissues around the labyrinth.

perilacunar around the lacunae.

p. bone see perilacunar BONE.

perilaryngitis inflammation of the tissues around the larynx.

perilenticular around the optic lens.

perilesional located or occurring around a lesion.

perilimbic around the limbus of the eye.

Perilla frutescens North American plant, in the family Lamiaceae, containing ipomeanol-like toxins which cause acute bovine pulmonary emphysema (interstitial pneumonia). Called also purple mint plant, wild mint.

perilla mint ketone toxic ketone found in *Perilla frutescens* (mint bush) causes interstitial pneumonia in cattle.

perilymph, perilympha the fluid contained in the space separating the membranous and osseous labyrinths of the ear.

perilymphangitis inflammation around a lymphatic vessel.

perimeningitis pachymeningitis; inflammation of the dura mater.

perimetritis a localized inflammation of the tissues around the uterus.

perimetrium the serous membrane enveloping the uterus.

perimyelitis inflammation of (1) the pia of the spinal cord, or (2) the endosteum.

perimyositis inflammation of connective tissue around a muscle.

perimysiitis inflammation of the perimysium; myofibrositis.

perimysium connective tissue demarcating a fascicle of skeletal muscle fibers.

perinatal relating to the period shortly before and after birth; the actual time varies between species. The last 10 to 15% of the pregnancy before parturition to the end of a comparable period after birth would cover present usage of the term.

p. mortality the percentage of animals in the danger period which die, as a ratio of the total number exposed.

perinatologist a specialist in perinatology.

perinatology the branch of veterinary medicine (obstetrics and pediatrics) dealing with the fetus and the newborn during the perinatal period.

perineal pertaining to the perineum.

p. body central tendon of the perineum. The fibromuscular mass in the median plane of the perineum where the bulbospongiosus and external anal sphincter muscles, and the levator ani and transverse perineal muscles attach.

Gelpi p. retractor a small self-retaining tissue retractor.

p. hernia a defect in the pelvic diaphragm that permits deviation of the rectum and protrusion of pelvic fat and abdominal contents, particularly the prostate and urinary bladder. Clinical signs include a uni- or bilateral ventrolateral perianal swelling with constipation or straining. Seen most often in middle-aged, male dogs, but occurs rarely in females and in cats.

p. laceration laceration of the perineal area such as by the birth of a foal. Three degrees of severity are recognized. *First degree* laceration is when only the mucosa of the vulva and vagina are involved. *Second degree* is when the submucosa and muscularis layers of the vulva, the anal sphincter and the perineal body are involved. *Third degree* is when there is also tearing through the rectovaginal septum, the muscles of the vagina and rectum, and the perineal body.

p. reconstruction various surgical techniques are used to repair perineal lacerations. It is necessary to reconstruct the rectal floor and vaginal roof.

p. reflex stimulation of the perineum causes contraction of the anal sphincter and flexion of the tail. It is a test of the integrity of the caudal spinal segments and the pudendal nerve. Called also the anal reflex.

p. sling a surgical technique that uses a fascial strip under the urethra to increase resistance to urine flow in the treatment of urinary incontinence.

perineocele a hernia between the rectum and the prostate or between the rectum and the vagina.

perineomelia an ectopic limb which projects from the perineum.

perineoplasty plastic repair of the perineum.

perineorrhaphy suture of the perineum.

perineotomy incision of the perineum.

perineovaginal pertaining to or communicating with the perineum and vagina.

perinephric around the kidney.

perinephritis inflammation of the perinephrium.

perinephrium the peritoneal envelope and other tissues around the kidney.

perineum the region between the tail and the ischiatic arch, especially the region between the anus and genital organs made up of the pelvic diaphragm and associated structures occupying the pelvic outlet, bounded ventrally by the pelvic symphysis, laterally by the ischial tuberosities, and dorsally by the coccygeal vertebrae. During parturition the perineum may be torn, resulting in possible damage to the urinary meatus and anal sphincter. To avoid a perineal laceration the veterinarian may cut the perineum just before delivery and suture the incision after delivery. See also EPISIOTOMY, PERINEORRHAPHY.

perineural around a nerve.

p. block regional anesthesia produced by injection of the anesthetic agent close to the nerve.

perineuritis inflammation of the perineurium.

perineurium the connective tissue sheath surrounding each bundle (fascicle) of nerve fibers in a peripheral nerve.

perinuclear space the space between the inner and outer nuclear membranes as illustrated in electron microscope recordings.

periocular around the eye.

p. hemorrhage a sign of viral hemorrhagic septicemia and vitamin C deficiency in fish.

period prevalence see period PREVALENCE.

periodic repeated or recurring at intervals.

p. acid–Schiff stain (PAS) periodic acid followed by Schiff reagent stains polysaccharides, glycoproteins and glycolipids. It is used to demonstrate fungal elements.

p. breathing alternating periods of apnea and hyperventilation. See also BIOT'S RESPIRATIONS, CHEYNE–STOKES RESPIRATION.

inherited p. spasticity a defect in cattle which does not appear until they are adults. On rising from a recumbent position the hindlimbs are extended and the animal is unable to flex them. Spasticity may last for 15 minutes but the patient will eventually relax and walk normally. Causes inconvenience only. Called also stall-cramp, the stretches.

p. movement see CYCLICAL.

p. myelodysplasia see canine CYCLIC hematopoiesis.

p. ophthalmia see periodic OPHTHALMIA.

p. reassessment re-examination at intervals of registered veterinarians to ensure their continued educational refreshment. Adequate performance obligatory for reregistration.

periodicity recurrence at regular intervals of time.

circadian p. every 24 hours.

diurnal p. twice daily.

periodontal around a tooth; pertaining to the periodontium.

p. abscess a localized, acute infection that may drain into the gingival pocket or directly through the gum. There is often local bone destruction. See also MALAR abscess.

p. charting recording the periodontal indices in dental records.

p. disease any disease or disorder of the periodontium. See also PERIODONTITIS and PERIODONTOSIS.

p. fibrous hyperplasia see periodontal fibromatous EPULIS.

p. indices indicators of periodontal health; includes amount of plaque and calculus, changes in the gingiva, probing depth, evaluation of attachment, and grade of mobility.

p. ligament the connective tissue that occupies the space between each tooth and its socket and that suspends the tooth.

p. pocket a deep space between the gingiva and the crown or root of a tooth. It can be the result of hyperplasia of the gingiva (false pocket) or migration of the epithelial attachment toward the apex (true pocket).

p. probe a dental instrument used to measure the depth of the periodontal pocket.

periodontics the branch of dentistry dealing with the study and treatment of diseases of the periodontium.

periodontist a dentist who specializes in periodontics.

periodontitis inflammation of the periodontium. The condition is caused by residual food, bacteria and calcium deposits (tartar) that collect in the spaces between the gum and lower part of the tooth crown. If it continues unchecked the infection will spread to the bone in which the teeth are rooted. The bone then resorbs and the teeth are slowly detached from their supporting tissues. A common problem on some sheep farms causing premature loss of teeth and culling of the sheep. The specific cause is undetermined. Called also peridentitis.

periodontium pl. *periodontia* [L.] the tissues investing and supporting the teeth, including the periodontal ligament, alveolar bone and gingiva.

periodontoclasia any degenerative or destructive disease of the periodontium.

periodontosis a degenerative, noninflammatory condition of the periodontium, characterized by destruction of the tissues.

periomphalic situated around the umbilicus.

perionychia see PARONYCHIA.

perionychitis see PARONYCHIA.

perionychium the epidermis bordering a nail or claw.

perioophoritis inflammation of the tissues around the ovary.

perioophorosalpingitis inflammation of the tissues around the ovary and oviduct.

perioperative pertaining or relating to the period

immediately before and/or after an operation, as perioperative care. Usually relates to immediately before, as in perioperative antibiotics, extending to just after.

periophthalmic around the eye.

periople the layer of soft, light-colored horn which covers the coronary border of the hoof in ungulates and serves as a transition between soft skin and hard hoof wall.

perioplic pertaining to or emanating from periople.

perioral around the mouth.

periorbita the fascial sheet that encloses the eyeball and its muscles that is continuous medially with the periosteum of the bones forming the orbit.

periorbital around the eye socket.

p. eczema ovine staphylococcal DERMATITIS.

periorbitis inflammation of the periorbita.

periorchitis inflammation of the tunica vaginalis testis; vaginalitis.

periorchitis–orchitis inflammation of the investing membranes, the tunica vaginalis of the testis and the testicular parenchyma.

periosteal pertaining to or emanating from the periosteum.

p. bud a stage in the development of bone to replace existing cartilage; periosteal bud formation results in the removal of calcified cartilage.

p. elevator a heavy metal instrument, with a broad, flat thin end for prising between periosteum and bone and lifting the periosteum prior to working on the bone. See also SAYRE ELEVATOR, MATSON ELEVATOR.

p. reaction production of new bone by the periosteum in response to injury or irritation.

p. stripping may occur in association with fractures, damaging vascular supply and delaying callus formation.

periosteitis periostitis.

periosteoma a morbid bony growth surrounding a bone.

periosteomyelitis inflammation of the entire bone, including periosteum and marrow.

periosteophyte a bony growth on the periosteum.

periosteotomy incision of the periosteum.

periosteum a specialized connective tissue covering all bones of the body, and possessing bone-forming potentialities. It is made up of an outer tough fibrous layer and a deeper more succulent osteogenic layer. Periosteum also serves as a point of attachment for certain muscles, tendons and ligaments. The connective tissues fuse with the fibrous layers of periosteum.

periostitis inflammation of the periosteum.

dental p. periodontitis.

diffuse p. widespread periostitis of the long bones.

periostosis abnormal deposition of periosteal bone; the condition manifested by the growth of periosteomas.

periotic 1. situated about the ear, especially the internal ear. 2. the petrous and mastoid portions of the temporal bone, at one stage a distinct bone.

periovarian around the ovary, e.g. periovarian adhesions.

peripachymeningitis inflammation of the substance between the dura mater and the bony covering of the central nervous system.

peripancreatitis inflammation of tissues around the pancreas.

peripapillary around a papilla, such as the optic papilla.

p. conus small hyper-reflective zone of the canine retina immediately adjacent to the optic disk.

peripartum occurring during the last 10% of the gestation period or the first few weeks after delivery, with reference to the mother.

periparturient see PERIPARTUM.

p. rise the phenomenon of increase in number of nematode eggs produced by ewes and sows in the period 4 to 8 weeks after parturition. A reduction in the resistance of the dam permits greater establishment and fecundity of the worms.

periphacitis inflammation of the capsule of the eye lens.

peripharyngeal around the pharynx.

peripherad toward the periphery.

peripheral 1. pertaining to or situated at or near the periphery. 2. abbreviation for any of the equipment belonging to a computer; that is, peripheral to the central processing unit. Includes monitor, printer, disk drive.

p. circulatory failure see CIRCULATORY failure.

p. gangrenous ergotism gangrene of the tips pf the ears and tail and of the lower limbs caused by rye ergot poisoning; see also rye ERGOT.

p. giant cell granuloma see giant-cell EPULIS.

p. lymphatics see LYMPHATIC.

p. nerve see peripheral NERVE.

p. nerve degeneration see AXONAL degeneration, WALLERIAN DEGENERATION.

p. nerve paralysis see peripheral NERVE.

p. nervous system see peripheral NERVOUS system.

p. proteins see MEMBRANE proteins.

p. sinus the peripheral lymph space just beneath the capsule of a lymph node.

peripheralization colonization of other tissues by T lymphocytes from the thymus which populate specific regions of lymph nodes and the periarteriolar zone of splenic corpuscles.

periphery an outward structure or surface; the portion of a system outside the central region.

periphlebitis inflammation of the tissues around a vein, or the external coat of a vein.

periplantar shoe see CHARLIER SHOE.

periplasmic around the plasma membrane; between the plasma membrane and the cell wall of a bacterium.

periportal situated around the portal vein of the liver.

p. necrosis necrosis of hepatocytes localized around the portal vein. Usually associated with ingested toxins.

periproctitis inflammation of tissues around the rectum and anus.

periprostatic around the prostate.

periprostatitis inflammation of the tissues around the prostate.

peripylephlebitis inflammation of tissues around the portal vein.

peripyloric around the pylorus.

perirectal around the rectum in the tissues of the pelvic cavity.

p. abscess caused usually by minor perforation of vagina or rectum.

perirenal around the kidney.

p. edema an exaggeration around the kidney of generalized subserous edema; seen only in pigs and cattle.

feline p. cysts uni- or bilateral accumulations of fluid in cystlike masses (pseudocysts) between the renal parenchyma and capsule or entirely extracapsular occur in aged, male cats causing a progressive abdominal enlargement, but not usually renal dysfunction. Called also perinephritic pseudocyst, renal capsular cyst, capsulogenic renal cyst, perirenal hygroma, capsular hydronephrosis and retroperitoneal perirenal cyst.

perirhinal around the nose.
perisalpingitis inflammation of tissues around the uterine tube.
periscopic affording a wide range of vision.
perisigmoiditis inflammation of the peritoneum of the sigmoid flexure of the colon.
perisinusitis inflammation of the tissues around a sinus.
perisinusoidal space the space separating sinusoids from hepatocytes; it is occupied by cells, reticular fibers and hepatocytic microvilli.
perispermatitis inflammation of tissues around the spermatic cord.
perisplanchnic around a viscus or the viscera.
perisplanchnitis inflammation of tissues around the viscera.
perisplenic around the spleen.
perisplenitis inflammation of the peritoneal surface of the spleen.
perispondylitis inflammation of tissues around a vertebra.
perissodactyl, perissodactylids any member of the order Perissodactyla, animals which have an odd number of toes. Includes the pentadactyls, e.g. elephants, tridactyls, e.g. tapir (but only on the hindlimbs, the front limbs have four digits), and the monodactyls, e.g. horses.
peristalsis the wormlike movement by which the alimentary canal or other tubular organs with both longitudinal and circular muscle fibers propel their contents, consisting of a wave of contraction passing along the tube. Increased peristalsis means faster movement of ingesta through the gut and less absorption of fluid, both tending to diarrhea. Reduced peristalsis means a longer alimentary sojourn, greater inspissation of ingesta and a tendency to constipation. See also PERISTALTIC, PARALYTIC ileus.
reverse p. peristalsis directed orally is a result of intestinal obstruction and acute, significant distension of the intestinal lumen; it is a major contributing mechanism in vomiting.
peristaltic pertaining to or emanating from peristalsis.
p. reflex onward movement of a bolus of ingesta in the intestine is preceded by a reflex dilation of the intestine.
p. rush a rapid movement of intestinal contents that results in diarrhea caused by an absence of peristaltic rhythm and sphincter tone.
p. sounds made by the vigorous and rapid mixing of fluid and gas by peristaltic movement in the intestines and forestomachs. Are loudest and evocative in the rumen of the cow and the colon and cecum of the horse. Thoracic peristaltic sounds can be suggestive of intestines located in thorax via a diaphragmatic hernia and need to be differentiated from normal intestinal sounds transmitted via viscera from the peritoneal cavity.
perisynovial around a synovial structure.
peritectomy excision of a ring of conjunctiva around the cornea in treatment of pannus.
peritendineum connective tissue investing larger tendons and extending between the fibers composing them.
peritendinitis, peritenonitis inflammation of the sheath of a tendon; TENOSYNOVITIS.
peritenon the connective tissue structures attached to and surrounding a tendon.
perithelioma see HEMANGIOPERICYTOMA.
perithelium the connective tissue layer surrounding the capillaries and smaller vessels.
perithyroiditis inflammation of the capsule of the thyroid.
peritomy 1. surgical incision of the conjunctiva and subconjunctival tissue about the whole circumference of the cornea. 2. circumcision.
peritoneal pertaining to the peritoneum.
continuous ambulatory p. dialysis the use of an indwelling catheter with external tubing that is strapped to the body wall when not being used for infusion and drainage of the dialysate fluid.
p. cysts include vestigial remnants of primordial urogenital organs, cestode intermediate stages, inclusion cysts or lymphatic ectasia.
p. dialysis the employment of the peritoneum surrounding the abdominal cavity as a dialyzing membrane for the purpose of removing acumulated waste products or toxins. In veterinary medicine, the main indication is acute, reversible renal failure. Certain crystalloids such as urea, creatinine and electrolytes, and some drugs, such as the salicylates, bromides and barbiturates, can be removed.

Fluid equal in osmolarity and similar in chemical composition to normal body fluid is introduced into the peritoneal cavity via a catheter. After a period of time ('dwell time') determined by the molecular weight of the substance being used as the dialyzing solution, the fluid is drained and the cycle repeated.
p. implantation attachment and growth of other tissues to the peritoneum, e.g. a fetus escaped from the genital tract, direct metastasis of malignant tumors.
p. lavage see abdominal LAVAGE.
p. lymph the fluid normally present in very small amount in the peritoneal cavity.
p. membrane see PERITONEUM.
peritoneocentesis paracentesis of the abdominal (peritoneal) cavity.
peritoneoclysis injection of fluid into the peritoneal cavity.
peritoneography radiography of the peritoneal cavity.
peritoneopathy any disease of the peritoneum.
peritoneopericardial pertaining to the peritoneum and pericardium.
p. hernia anomalous development of the diaphragm and pleuropericardial membranes that allows herniation of variable amounts of abdominal contents into the pericardial sac. May cause dyspnea, tachypnea, vomiting, diarrhea, cardiac tamponade and congestive heart failure, but some cases are only detected incidentally at postmortem examination. Seen in dogs and cats.
peritoneoscope an endoscope for use in peritoneoscopy.
peritoneoscopy visual examination of the organs of the abdominal (peritoneal) cavity with a peritoneoscope.
peritoneotomy incision into the peritoneum.
peritoneovenous communicating with the peritoneal cavity and the venous system. See also LeVeen SHUNT.
peritoneum the serous membrane lining the walls of the abdominal and pelvic cavities (parietal peritoneum) and investing contained viscera (visceral peritoneum), the two layers enclosing a potential space, the peritoneal cavity. The diseases which are important in the peritoneum of animals are peritonitis, including a special group of rectal tear, retroperitoneal abscess, lipomatosis, neoplasia, ascites and peritoneal effusion.
peritonitis inflammation of the peritoneum. The cause may be infectious or chemical. Typical signs

are rigidity and pain on palpation of the abdominal wall, absence of feces, severe toxemia and fever. In horses there is a mild colic and in dogs and cats there is often effusion. Paracentesis may show evidence of inflammation.

acute diffuse p. in the early stages pain is evident all over the abdomen. There is soon a disappearance of pain, a profound toxemia develops and the disease may go undetected.

acute local p. added to the usual signs there is a sharp pain response over the site of the lesion.

adhesive p. peritonitis characterized by adhesions between adjacent serous structures.

aseptic p. see chemical peritonitis (below).

biliary p., bile p. that due to the presence of bile in the peritoneum; choleperitoneum. Is detected by the color of the fluid withdrawn by paracentesis. See also BILE peritonitis.

chemical p. may be caused by leakage of bile, urine, gastric juices or pancreatic enzymes in acute pancreatitis. Infusion of irritant materials can cause a similar chemical irritation.

chronic p. is manifested by chronic toxemia, bouts of colic due to adhesions and an accumulation of exudate which may cause a visible distension of the abdomen. See also RETROPERITONEAL abscess.

chylous p. an uncommon result of abdominal trauma or tumors, intestinal obstruction or lymphangiectasia.

egg p. peritonitis in birds due to release of an egg into the peritoneal cavity with subsequent infection by *Escherichia coli* which have ascended via the oviduct.

feline infectious p. (FIP) see FELINE infectious peritonitis.

idiopathic p. one caused by a primary infection of the peritoneal cavity, e.g. feline infectious peritonitis, or hematogenous spread from a noncontiguous site.

post-stripping p. fatal peritonitis occurring in cultured salmonid fish soon after stripping, sometimes before. Caused by a number of gram-positive cocci and coccobacilli; *Carnobacterium piscicola* considered to be the most important infection.

primary p. see idiopathic peritonitis (above).

septic p. secondary to disruption of the abdominal cavity or a hollow viscus, particularly leakage from the gastrointestinal tract.

silent p. asymptomatic peritonitis.

starch granulomatous p. talcum powder, and to a lesser extent, other powders used on surgical gloves can cause a granulomatous reaction on the peritoneum.

traumatic p. perforation of the gut wall or abdominal wall introducing infection into the peritoneal cavity. May result from stake or bite wound, inexpert passing of urinary or insemination catheter, sadistically by a broom handle in the vagina, or stabbing of the rumen as an emergency measure in acute ruminal tympany. See also TRAUMATIC reticuloperitonitis.

urine p. prolonged exposure of the peritoneum to urine, usually due to leakage from the bladder or a ureter, results in a peritonitis and the development of uremia. Bacterial infection may also be introduced.

peritonsillar around a tonsil.

p. abscess a localized accumulation of pus in peritonsillar tissue subsequent to suppurative inflammation of the tonsil. Called also quinsy.

peritonsillitis inflammation of peritonsillar tissues.

peritracheal around the trachea.

peritrichous 1. having flagella around the entire surface; said of bacteria. 2. having flagella around the cytostome only; said of Ciliophora.

peritubular investing the uriniferous tubules.

p. plexus a plexus of capillaries formed by the renal intertubular arterioles around cortical uriniferous tubules.

p. space water and electrolytes resorbed by tubular epithelium passes into this space.

periumbilical around the umbilicus.

periureteral around the ureter.

periureteritis inflammation of tissues around the ureter.

periurethral around the urethra.

periuterine around the uterus.

perivaginal around the vagina.

p. needle see GERLACH NEEDLE.

perivaginitis inflammation of tissues around the vagina; pericolpitis.

perivascular around a vessel.

p. cellulitis may be caused by the introduction of infection at the time of an injection or the injection of an irritant substance such as thiacetarsamide into tissues while attempting an intravenous injection.

p. cuffing the accumulation of lymphocytes or plasma cells in a dense mass around the vessel. An indication of inflammation or of an immune reaction.

p. dermatitis a classification of inflammatory dermatosis in which the reaction is centered around superficial or deep dermal blood vessels.

perivasculitis inflammation of a perivascular sheath and surrounding tissue.

periventricular gray a diffuse mass of neurons and fiber tracts which surrounds the spinal canal and the ventricular system cranial to the mid-cervical region in the medial part of the reticular formation.

perivenular around a vein; in the connective tissue about a vein.

perivesical around the bladder.

perivesiculitis inflammation of tissues around the seminal vesicles.

periwinkle see VINCA.

Perkinsus protozoan parasite genus of molluscan tissues. Includes *P. marinus* (major pathogen of the american oyster), *P. olseni* (pathogen of abalone in warm waters).

perlèche inflammation with exudation, maceration and fissuring at the labial commissures.

perloline photosensitizing agent in *Lolium perenne*.

permanganate salts of permanganic acid; the potassium salt is an oldfashioned, out-of-favor, weak disinfectant compound which used to be used topically. Its purple color in solution was an advantage. Called also Condy's crystals.

permeability the level or degree of the state of being permeable.

permeable not impassable; pervious; permitting passage of a substance.

permease any carrier protein involved in transporting substances across cell membranes.

permeate 1. to penetrate or pass through, as through a filter. 2. the constituents of a solution or suspension that pass through a filter.

permethrin a third-generation synthetic pyrethroid widely used in the control of ectoparasites. It is very stable and lasts for several weeks.

permissible dose see DOSE equivalent limits.

permissible medication treatments that are permitted of animals before racing or performing or just appearing at shows, race meetings and the like.

pernicious tending to a fatal issue.

p. anemia a form of anemia in humans caused by a genetically determined lack of the intrinsic factor, which normally is produced by the stomach mucosa.

The deficiency results in inadequate and abnormal formation of erythrocytes, and failure to absorb vitamin B_{12}. Not reported in animals.

pero- word element. [Gr.] *deformity, maimed.*

perobrachius a fetus with deformed forelimbs.

perocephalus a fetus with a deformed head.

perochirus a fetus with deformed forelimb extremities.

Perodicticus potto see POTTO.

perodontium see PERIODONTIUM.

Perognathus spinatus see spiny pocket MOUSE.

peromelia congenital deformity of the limbs.

peromelus a fetus with deformed limbs.

Peromyscus leucopus deermouse; called also white-footed mouse.

peroneal pertaining to the fibula or to the outer side of the leg or shank; fibular.

common p. nerve a nerve originating in the sciatic nerve; innervates parts of the calf and foot. See also Table 14.

p. muscles see Table 13.4.

p. nerve block achieved by injection of a local anesthetic into the groove between the tendons of long and lateral digital extensors on the hindlimb, usually in a horse. Anesthesia is obtained mainly over the craniolateral surface of the limb distal to this site and over the medial fetlock.

p. nerve paralysis causes a characteristic inability to flex the hock and extend the digits so the animal bears weight on the dorsum of the foot. There is anesthesia of the cranial leg and dorsal paw or foot. Occurs in recumbent cattle and from trauma to the lateral stifle in dogs.

Peronia rostrata a tertiary blowfly parasitizing carcasses which are tending to dry out.

peroral performed or administered through the mouth. Called also per os.

perosis a disease of young birds caused by a nutritional deficiency of manganese and characterized by a deformity of the leg bones. There is gross enlargement of the tibiotarsal joint and deformity of the bones above and below the joint, and slipping of the gastrocnemius tendon from the condyles. The birds are crippled and usually die of starvation.

perosomus elumbus a congenital skeletal defect commonest in calves and lambs. The vertebral column stops at the caudal thoracic region and the posterior part of the body is joined to the front half by soft tissue only.

Perostrongylus a subgenus of nematodes in the family Filaroididae. See AELUROSTRONGYLUS.

peroxidase any of a group of iron–porphyrin enzymes that catalyze the oxidation of some organic substrates in the presence of hydrogen peroxide.

p. stain a group of staining techniques that demonstrate peroxidases in tissue sections or smears.

peroxidation conversion of oxides to peroxides.

peroxide that oxide of any element containing more oxygen than any other; more correctly applied to compounds having such linkage as –O–O–.

hydrogen p. see HYDROGEN peroxide.

p. value said of a feed sample; an indication of the degree of rancidity of oils and fats in the feed.

peroxisome a membrane-bound body found in vertebrate animal cells, especially kidney and liver cells, that contains urate oxidase, amino acid oxidase, catalase and other enzymes.

perphenazine a phenothiazine compound used as a tranquilizer and antiemetic.

Perralderia coronopifolia North American plant in family Asteracea; causes cyanide poisoning, characterized by dyspnea, in camels. Called also tafes, lahiel el tis.

Perreyea lepida South American SAWFLY whose larvae cause severe liver necrosis when ingested; toxin is LOPHYROTOMIN.

Persea americana tree in the Lauraceae family; contains an unidentified cardiotoxin which causes cardiomyopathy manifested by heart failure; called also avocado; the leaves of the Guatemalan varieties are toxic, the Mexican varieties are not.

Persian cat the traditional longhaired cat with a broad head, short nose and cobby body, medium to large size, with short legs. A variety of colors are seen in the coat and eyes. Also known as Angora, although originally that was a type with finer, satiny coat, or simply as longhair.

Persian insect powder see PYRETHRUM.

Persicaria plant genus in the Polygonaceae family; contains an unidentified hepatotoxin which causes hepatitis and photosensitive dermatitis; includes *P. hydropiper* (willow weed), *P. lapathifolia*, *P. maculosa* (*P. vulgaris*), *P. orientalis*. Called also smart weeds.

persistent relative to embryological defects refers to persistence of an entity into external life in such a way as to cause some reduction of efficiency. The common defects are listed under the names of the compromised organs. See also persistent right AORTIC ARCH, DUCTUS arteriosus, penile preputial FRENULUM, imperforate HYMEN, persistent URACHUS, persistent hyperplastic VITREOUS, persistent PUPILLARY membrane.

p. corpus luteum see CORPUS luteum.

p. ductus arteriosus see PATENT ductus arteriosus.

p. ductus venosus see DUCTUS venosus.

p. omphalomesenteric duct see OMPHALOMESENTERIC duct.

p. posterior perilenticular vascular tunic the tunic is generated in the embryo but atrophies just before birth. Persistence of some part of the tunic into adult life is common but of no clinical significance.

p. recumbency the animal is normal in other respects but does not rise to its hooves for a period exceeding 24 hours.

p. right aorta arch see persistent right AORTIC ARCH.

p. truncus arteriosus may cause neonatal congestive heart failure and cyanosis; the interventricular septum is usually patent. See also TRUNCUS arteriosus.

personal limited in its accessibility to individual people.

p. advertising advertising of a particular practice or veterinarian. Formerly controlled in order to prevent individuals from unfairly attracting business; nowadays largely deregulated to permit more vigorous competition.

p. computer see COMPUTER.

personality that which constitutes, distinguishes and characterizes an animal as an entity over a period of time; the total reaction of an animal to its environment. Many factors that determine personality are inherited; they are shaped and modified by the animal's environment.

perspiration see SWEAT, SWEATING (1).

insensible p. sweat lost from skin and mucosal surfaces which is not secreted by sweat glands.

pertechnate ion a competitive agent in the uptake and transport of iodine in the thyroid gland.

perthane a CHLORINATED HYDROCARBON insecticide with conventional toxicity.

Perthes' disease see LEGG–CALVÉ–PERTHES DISEASE.

Peru balsam see BALSAM.

peruke bizarre collection of velveted antlers developed by male caribou and roe deer males castrated as adults. Called also wigged.
Peruvian bark tree see ALSTONIA *constricta*.
Peruvian guinea pig see GUINEA PIG.
perverted appetite see PICA.
pervious urachus see persistent URACHUS.
pes pl. *pedes* [L.] foot; the terminal organ of the lower limb; any footlike part; the tarsus, metatarsus and digits (the phalanges and sesamoid bones). See also DIPES.
pessary 1. an instrument placed in the vagina to support the uterus or rectum or as a contraceptive device. 2. a medicated vaginal suppository.
pessulus a wedge-shaped cartilage in the syrinx of the fowl, lying at the bifurcation of the trachea and dividing it into the two bronchi.
pest 1. an organism that injures, irritates or damages livestock or crops. 2. a highly fatal, rapidly spreading disease with an acute course. See also PLAGUE, PESTE DES PETITS RUMINANTS, PESTE DU PORC, PESTE SUINA.
fowl p. see AVIAN influenza. Newcastle disease was at one time known as new fowl pest and as pseudo fowl pest.
peste des petits ruminants [Fr.] a highly infectious and fatal disease of sheep and goats caused by a paramyxovirus in the genus *Morbillivirus* which is very closely related to the rinderpest virus. Typical signs are purulent nasal discharge, erosive stomatitis, diarrhea and bronchopneumonia. The spread is rapid and the mortality rate high. See also RINDERPEST. Called also contagious pustular stomatitis.
peste du porc [Fr.] HOG cholera.
peste suina [Span.] HOG cholera.
pesticide a poison used to destroy pests of any sort. See ARSENICAL, CARBAMATES, CHLORINATED HYDROCARBONS, ORGANOPHOSPHORUS COMPOUND, PYRETHROIDS.
p. poisoning pesticides are selective poisons chosen for use because of their relative safety for humans and animals. It is likely that they will poison these species if they are used in sufficient quantity or in special circumstances, for example when the water intake of the subject animals is limited.
p. resistance continued use of a single agent, or a group of closely allied agents, can cause selective survival of insects with innate tolerance of the agent and lead to the development of a resistant population.
p. tissue residues some pesticides have had to be withdrawn from use because of their persistence in the tissues of animals including humans. The passage of the agent in the milk of the animal is a comparable problem.
pestilence a virulent contagious epidemic or infectious epidemic disease.
pestis see PLAGUE.
pestis equorum see AFRICAN HORSE SICKNESS.
Pestivirus a genus in the family FLAVIVIRIDAE. Includes hog cholera, bovine virus diarrhea–mucosal disease and ovine border disease viruses. Not arthropod borne.
pestle an instrument with a rounded end, used in a mortar to reduce a solid to a powder or produce a homogeneous mixture of solids.
PET positron emission TOMOGRAPHY, a nuclear medicine technique that combines computed tomography and radioisotope brain scanning.
pet a nonfood animal included in a human household as a companion and on a status almost equivalent to that of a human being. They are used as instructional media for children about biological matters, as companions for lonely people of all sorts, as a guarding and watchdog presence, as psychological support for disturbed people and as a means of entrance into a different social group. Called also companion animals. Includes dogs, cats, cage birds, aquarium fish, and exotic species such as monkeys, alligators, tortoises, monkeys, big cats, axolotls, newts, yabbies, seahorses, snakes, gerbils, hamsters, mice, rats and spiders.
p.-assisted therapy, p. facilitated therapy the use of animals in a specific medical program as an adjunct to conventional therapy, especially for seriously ill and recuperating persons and persons with psychological problems. See also ANIMAL facilitated therapy.
children's p's those pets which can be properly cared for by children; usually taken to include the common companion pets, dogs, cats and cage birds, and the unusual species such as lizards, tortoises, terrapins, hamsters, guinea pigs, mice, rats, gerbils, rabbits, and even snakes and spiders.
exotic p's those other than the conventional dogs, cats, aquarium fish and cage birds.
peta- a word element used in naming units of measurement to designate a quantity 10^{15} (a thousand-million-million) times the unit to which it is joined. Symbol P.
-petal word element. [L.] *directed, moving toward.*
Petaurus see POSSUM.
petechia pl. *petechiae* [L.] a minute, pinpoint, nonraised, perfectly round, purplish red spot caused by intradermal or submucous hemorrhage, which later turns blue or yellow.
petechial fever see BOVINE petechial fever.
petechiation a state in which petechiae are present.
Peter's anomaly an abnormality of ocular development in which there is an absence of Descemet's membrane and corneal endothelium with an adherent corneal leukoma.
Peterson block a regional nerve block of the orbit to facilitate optic surgery, especially ablation, in cows.
petfood see pet FOOD.
pethidine see MEPERIDINE.
petiole a stem, stalk or pedicle.
epiglottic p. the pointed caudal end of the epiglottic cartilage, attached to the thyroid cartilage.
petiolus petiole.
Petit Basset Griffon Veneen a short-legged, compact hound with a slightly elongated body and head, pendulous, narrow ears and straight tail. The coat is long and harsh and can be any solid color, bicolored or tricolored. See also GRAND BASSET GRIFFON VENDEEN.
petit mal a relatively mild seizure contrasting with grand mal, a major seizure. Occurs in humans where the patient loses consciousness only momentarily and there are few motor signs. True petit mal seizures would be difficult to detect, but probably do occur occasionally in animals. See also SEIZURE.
petits poussins milk-fed chickens, 6 weeks old, approximately 1.5 lb (650 to 700 g) in weight, and fattened on a special diet. A gourmet delicacy.
Petiveria alliacea South American plant in the family Phytolaccaceae; causes digestive disturbance, muscular atrophy and glomerulonephritis. Contains an unidentified garlic-odored, carbamate-like toxin. Called also anamu.
Petri dish a shallow, circular, glass or disposable plastic dish used to grow bacteria on solid media such as agar.
Petriellidium boydii a saprophytic fungus which

causes abortion in cattle, eumycotic mycetoma (pseudoallescheriosis) in dogs and maduromycosis in humans. Previously called *Allescheria boydii*.

petrolatum a purified mixture of hydrocarbons obtained from petroleum; used as a base for ointments, protective dressings and soothing applications to the skin. Called also petroleum jelly. Two types of liquid petrolatum are recognized, light and heavy. See also mineral OIL.

petroleum a thick natural oil obtained from beneath the earth. It consists of a mixture of various hydrocarbons of the paraffin and olefin series. See crude petroleum OIL.

p. jelly petrolatum.

petromastoid 1. pertaining to the petrous portion of the temporal bone and its mastoid process. 2. OTOCRANIUM (2).

petrosal pertaining to the pars petrosa, or petrous portion of the temporal bone.

Petroselinum cultivated plant in family Apiaceum; contains furocoumarins which cause primary photosensitization. Includes *P. crispum*, *P. hortense*, *P. sativum*. Called also parsley.

petrositis inflammation of the pars petrosa or petrous portion of the temporal bone.

petrosphenoid pertaining to the petrous portion of the temporal bone and to the sphenoid bone.

petrosquamous pertaining to the petrous and squamous portions of the temporal bone.

petrous resembling rock or stone; stony.

p. bone the pars petrosa, or petrous portion of the temporal bone. See also Table 10.

petty spurge EUPHORBIA *peplus*.

pexis 1. the fixation of matter by a tissue. 2. surgical fixation, usually by suturing.

-pexy word element. [Gr.] *surgical fixation*.

Peyer's patches oval, elevated patches of closely packed lymph follicles in mucous and submucous layers of the small intestine. Called also aggregated lymphatic nodules.

continuous p. p. found in the terminal ileum in calves, lambs, piglets. Thought to be a primary site for B-cell generation; involute with age.

peyote a stimulant drug from mescal buttons, the flowering heads of the cactus *Lophophora williamsii*, whose active principle is mescaline; used by North American Indians in certain ceremonies to produce an intoxication marked by feelings of ecstasy. See also HALLUCINOGEN.

Peyronella glomerata a fungus isolated from hyperkatoses on the ears of wild goats.

Pezzer's catheter a self-retaining urinary catheter with a bulbous extremity.

PF-3 platelet factor-3.

Pfeifferella a bacterial name no longer in use.

P. anatipestifer see PASTEURELLA *anatipestifer*.

P. mallei see BURKHOLDERIA *mallei*.

Pfiesteria microalgae which produce water blooms which cause deaths in local fish. Only found in the presence of live fish, hence the term 'phantom dinoflagellate'. See also DINOFLAGELLATES.

PFK phosphofructokinase.

PFU plaque-forming unit; in virology, areas of cell lysis (CPE) in monolayer cell culture, under overlay conditions, initiated by infection with a single virus particle.

PG prostaglandin.

pg picogram.

PGA pteroylglutamic (folic) acid.

$PGF_{2[alpha]}$ prostaglandin $F_{2[alpha]}$.

PGK phosphoglycerate kinase.

PGM-2 phosphoglucomutase-2.

pH the negative logarithm of the hydrogen ion concentration [H+]; a measure of the degree to which a solution is acidic or alkaline. An acid is a substance that can give up a hydrogen ion (H+); a base is a substance that can accept H+. The more acidic a solution the greater the hydrogen ion concentration and the lower the pH; a pH of 7.0 indicates neutrality; a pH of less than 7 indicates acidity, and a pH of more than 7 indicates alkalinity.

p.–bicarbonate diagram an aid to the assessment of an acid–base problem; expresses the relationship between bicarbonate ions and the pH of the plasma.

blood p. normal blood pH varies a little between species but is of the order of 7.32 to 7.5. In moderate acidosis this falls to 7.25 to 7.30, severe acidosis 7.20 to 7.25 and grave acidosis to 7.00 to 7.10.

p. partition the partition that occurs in the degree of ionization of electrolytes, including soluble drugs, about semipermeable membranes depending on the pH of the medium.

skin p. in haired mammals, the pH of skin is usually acidic. In dogs it is from 5.5 to 7.2; in cats from 5.6 to 7.4; in cattle from 5.4 to 5.75; and in the horse from 4.8 to 6.8.

PHA phytohemagglutinin, a plant lectin.

phacitis inflammation of the crystalline lens of the eye.

phac(o)- word element. [Gr.] *lens*.

phacoanaphylaxis hypersensitivity to the protein of the crystalline lens of the eye, induced by escape of material from the lens capsule.

phacocele hernia of the eye lens.

Phacochoerus aethioicus see WART HOG.

phacoclastic uveitis inflammation of the iris, ciliary body and choroid due to release of lens material after penetration by a foreign body.

phacocystectomy excision of part of the lens capsule for cataract.

phacocystitis inflammation of the capsule of the eye lens.

phacoemulsification a technique of CATARACT extraction, utilizing high-frequency ultrasonic vibrations to fragment the lens combined with controlled irrigation to maintain normal pressure in the anterior chamber, and suction to remove lens fragments and irrigating fluid.

phacoerysis removal of the eye lens in cataract by suction.

phacofragmentation see PHACOEMULSIFICATION.

phacoid shaped like a lens.

phacoiditis phacitis.

phacolysis dissolution or discission of the crystalline lens.

phacoma a tumor of the lens of the eye.

phacomalacia softening of the eye lens; a soft cataract, that is, one without a hard nucleus.

phacometachoresis displacement of the eye lens.

phacosclerosis hardening of the eye lens; a hard cataract, that is, one with a hard nucleus.

phacoscope an instrument for viewing accommodative changes of the eye lens.

phacotoxic exerting a deleterious effect upon the crystalline lens.

Phaenicia see LUCILIA.

phaeo- for words beginning thus see words beginning *phe(o)-*.

phaeochromocytoma see PHEOCHROMOCYTOMA.

phaeohyphomycosis opportunistic infections caused by the pigmented (dematiaceous) fungi, including *Alternaria*, *Aureobasidium*, *Bipolaris*, *Cladosporium*,

Curvularia, Drechslera, Exophiala, Exserohilum rostratum, Moniliella and *Phialophora, Wangiella* spp.
subcutaneous p. subcutaneous nodules containing yellow-brown fungal hyphae, and which may ulcerate and produce a sinus tract. May cause mycetoma if the lesions develop to granuloma.
phage see BACTERIOPHAGE.
p. type an intraspecies type of bacterium demonstrated by phage typing; called also lysotype and phagotype.
p. typing characterization of bacteria, extending to strain differences, by demonstration of susceptibility to one or more (a spectrum) races of bacteriophage; widely applied to staphylococci, typhoid bacilli, etc., for epidemiological purposes.
phagedena rapidly spreading and sloughing ulceration.
phagedenic pertaining to or emanating from phagedena.
-phagia, -phagy word element. [Gr.] *eating, swallowing.*
phag(o)- word element. [Gr.] *eating, ingestion.*
phagocyte any cell that ingests microorganisms or other cells and foreign particles.
phagocytic emanating from or pertaining to phagocytes.
p. deficiency usually related to a deficiency in opsonization or a failure of intracellular killing.
p. system see RETICULOENDOTHELIAL SYSTEM.
p. vacuole see PHAGOSOME.
phagocytin a bactericidal substance from neutrophilic leukocytes.
phagocytize phagocytose.
phagocytoblast a cell giving rise to phagocytes.
phagocytolysis destruction of phagocytes.
phagocytose to envelop and destroy bacteria and other foreign material; phagocytize.
phagocytosis the engulfing of microorganisms or other cells and foreign particles by phagocytes.
phagodynamometer an apparatus for measuring the force exerted in chewing food.
phagokaryosis phagocytosis effected by the cell nucleus.
phagolysosome a phagocytosed substance is initially engulfed by the cell to form from an invagination of a small region of the cell membrane a phagocytic vacuole, which then fuses with a lysosome to form a phagolysosome within which the lysosomal enzymes are released and other killing mechanisms are activated and the phagocytosed material is degraded.
phagosome a membrane-bound vesicle in a phagocyte containing the phagocytized material. Called also a phagocytic vacuole.
phagotype phage type.
phak(o)- for words beginning thus see words beginning *phac(o)-*.
Phalacrocorax see CORMORANT.
phalangeal pertaining to a phalanx.
phalangectomy excision of a phalanx.
phalanger see POSSUM.
phalanges plural of *phalanx*.
Phalangida see HARVESTMEN.
phalangitis inflammation of one or more phalanges.
phalanx pl. *phalanges* [Gr.] any of the principal bones of a digit. See also Table 10.
inherited reduced p. a congenital absence of the first two phalanges on all limbs. The hoof and third phalanx are attached by skin. An inherited defect in cattle.
Phalaris a grass genus of the Poaceae family containing some of the best pasture grasses which can, on occasion, be poisonous. Cause two kinds of poisoning: (1) acute heart failure and sudden death in sheep—caused by *P. aquatica, P. arundinacea* and Rhompa grass (a hybrid variety); (2) incoordination with tremor and head nodding, finally recumbency and convulsions. (Called also phalaris staggers and caused by all species.) New cases occur for many weeks after removal from the pasture. There is a characteristic gray-green discoloration of the brainstem and midbrain. Includes *P. aquatica* (*P. tuberosa*, Toowoomba canary grass), *P. arundinacea* (reed canary grass), *P. minor* (canary grass), *P. angusta, P. brachystachys, P. canariensis, P. caroliniana* and Rhompa grass, a hybrid form. Toxins include β-carbolines, tryptamine and indole alkaloids.
phalaris staggers see PHALARIS.
phallectomy amputation of the penis.
phallic pertaining to the penis.
p. body see phallic BODY.
phallitis penitis.
phallocampsis curvature of the penis during erection.
phallocrypsis retraction of the penis.
phalloidin, phalloidine a hexapeptide toxin from the mushroom *Amanita phalloides*, which causes fatal liver necrosis.
phalloncus a pathological swelling, including a neoplasm, of the penis.
phallopexy surgical fixation of the penis, e.g. as performed to create a teaser bull, or to correct a chronically prolapsed penis in a horse.
phallus the penis.
phanerosis 1. the process of becoming visible. 2. the liberation of a substance previously undetectable because of being in a combined state.
phantom 1. a model of the body or of a specific part thereof. 2. a device for simulating the in vivo effect of radiation on tissues.
p. mare a dummy of a mare used to collect semen for artificial insemination. A padded, hollow device about the height and width that would suit the stallion to be used. Excellent for collecting from an insecure or lame stallion.
p. parturition see false PREGNANCY.
p. pregnancy see false PREGNANCY.
phar., pharm. pharmacy; pharmaceutical; pharmacopoeia.
Pharaoh hound a medium-sized, lean, graceful dog with broad-based, erect ears and a long, thin tail. The coat is very short and fine, colored tan with white markings with a white tip on the tail and spot on the chest ('star').
pharmaceutical 1. pertaining to pharmacy or drugs. 2. a medicinal drug.
p. incompatibility substances that react chemically with each other, e.g. acids and alkalis, and cannot both be included in the same formulation.
p. industry the manufacturers of pharmaceuticals. Also one of the biggest research contributors to human and veterinary medicine. This includes basic research into chemotherapy but includes also the otherwise neglected fields of formulations, packaging, dosing regimens and dispensing information. The industry also has access to the biggest database relating to chemicals and their uses.
pharmaceutics 1. pharmacy. 2. pharmaceutical preparations.
pharmacist an individual who is licensed to prepare, compound and dispense drugs upon written order (prescription) from a licensed veterinary, medical or dental practitioner. A pharmacist is a health care pro-

fessional who cooperates and consults with and sometimes advises the licensed practitioner concerning drugs.

pharmac(o)- word element. [Gr.] *drug, medicine.*

pharmacodiagnosis use of drugs in diagnosis.

pharmacodynamics the study of the mechanisms of action of drugs and other biochemical and physiological effects.

pharmacogenetics the study of the relationship between genetic factors and the nature of responses to drugs.

multifactorial p. the metabolism of many drugs is determined by the action of an unknown number of genes, besides an unknown number of non-genetic effects; as a result a continuous distribution of drug concentrations in patients, ranging from subtherapeutic to toxic, may ensue.

pharmacognosy the branch of pharmacology dealing with natural drugs and their constituents.

pharmacokinetics the study of the movement of drugs in the body, including the processes of absorption, distribution, localization in tissues, biotransformation and excretion.

pharmacological, pharmacologic pertaining to pharmacology.

p. antagonism the relationship between drugs in which an antagonist inhibits the activity of an agonist by reacting with the receptor or other part of the effector mechanism. The antagonist has no other pharmacological function. It may be a competitive or noncompetitive antagonist.

pharmacologist a specialist in pharmacology.

pharmacology the science that deals with the origin, nature, chemistry, effects and uses of drugs; it includes pharmacognosy, pharmacokinetics, pharmacodynamics, pharmacotherapeutics and toxicology.

pharmacopeia, pharmacopoeia an authoritative treatise on drugs and their preparations. For example the European Pharmacopoeia, United States Pharmacopeia, British Pharmacopoeia, British Pharmaceutical Codex, United States Dispensatory. See also MARTINDALE.

pharmacophore the group of atoms in the molecule of a drug responsible for the drug's action.

pharmacotherapy treatment of disease with medicines.

pharmacy 1. the branch of the health sciences dealing with the preparation, dispensing and proper utilization of drugs. 2. a place where drugs are compounded or dispensed.

pharyngeal pertaining to the pharynx.

p. abscess an abscess in the wall of the pharynx causing painful and difficult swallowing, pain on palpation, cough and if sufficiently large, the signs of pharyngeal obstruction.

p. cyst subepiglottic cysts (remnants of thyroglosssal duct) and cysts on dorsum of pharynx and soft palate (remnants of craniopharyngeal ducts) may cause obstruction of the pharynx in the horse.

p. diverticulum a small, 3–4 cm, midline diverticulum dorsal to the pharyngeal opening of the esophagus. Found only in pigs. It can become impacted with dried food and cause dysphagia.

p. dysphagia see oropharyngeal DYSPHAGIA.

p. hypophysis cyst a distended remnant of the pharyngeal anlage of the pituitary gland. It may protrude into the nasopharynx and obstruct respiration.

p. lymphadenopathy enlargement of the pharyngeal lymph nodes, due to abscess, neoplasia, e.g. bovine viral leukosis, or hyperplasia and granuloma in chronic pharyngitis, is a possible cause of pharyngeal obstruction.

p. lymphoid hyperplasia there is hyperplasia of lymphoid follicles on the roof of the pharynx thought to be a sequel of an upper respiratory tract virus infection. Clinically there is a chronic cough and a poor racing performance and the lesions can be observed via a fiberoptiscope.

p. neoplasia a high incidence of squamous cell carcinoma in the mouth, pharynx and rumen is recorded in several countries, some associated with grazing on bracken. Chronic dysphagia and tympany result.

p. obstruction characterized by noisy breathing, difficult swallowing, coughing and the coughing up of food. In dogs and cats pawing at the mouth is usual. There is no regurgitation through the nostrils. Manual or endoscopic examination of the interior of the pharynx is necessary. A common cause is foreign body impaction. See also THROAT abscess (1), pharyngeal cyst and pharyngeal lymphadenopathy (above), pharyngeal polyp (below) and impaction of the pharyngeal diverticulum (above) in pigs.

p. paralysis presents a syndrome similar to pharyngeal obstruction with coughing, inability to swallow, but with no signs of pain or respiratory obstruction. See also CUD dropping.

p. phlegmon a peracute peripharyngitis, most commonly of cattle, characterized by profound toxemia, respiratory distress, swelling and pain of the throat area, painful cough and high fever. *Fusobacterium necrophorum* is usually present in the lesion. Called also intermandibular cellulitis.

p. polyp a fibrous or mucoid, usually pedunculated mass that causes intermittent pharyngeal obstruction.

p. pouch one of the paired bilateral outpockets of the embryonic pharynx located opposite external branchial clefts and separated from each other by the developing visceral or branchial arches.

p. reflex gag reflex.

p. swab NASOPHARYNGEAL swab.

pharyngectomy excision of part of the pharynx.

pharyngemphraxis obstruction of the pharynx.

pharyngismus muscular spasm of the pharynx.

pharyngitis inflammation of the pharynx, characterized by coughing, painful swallowing and lack of appetite. The throat is sore on palpation. In severe cases food and saliva may be regurgitated through the nostrils.

chronic equine p. is relatively common after viral infections. There is persistent coughing and moderate dyspnea on exercise. Training cannot be done. Endoscopic examination shows lymphoid infiltration and follicular hyperplasia.

equine lymphoreticular p. see chronic equine pharyngitis (above).

plasma cell p. see feline plasma cell GINGIVITIS–pharyngitis.

pharyng(o)- word element. [Gr.] *pharynx.*

Pharyngobolus a genus of parasitic flies in the family Oestridae. The larval stages resemble those of *Oestrus ovis*.

P. africanus found in the pharynx of African elephants. Called also elephant throat bot fly.

pharyngocele a herniation or cystic deformity of the pharynx.

pharyngoesophageal pertaining to the pharynx and esophagus.

pharyngoglossal pertaining to the pharynx and tongue.

pharyngogram a radiograph of the pharynx aided by the administration of contrast agent.
pharyngokeratosis keratosis of the pharynx.
pharyngolaryngitis inflammation of the pharynx and larynx.
pharyngomycosis any fungal infection of the pharynx.
pharyngonasal pertaining to the pharynx and nose.
pharyngoparalysis paralysis of the pharyngeal muscles; pharyngoplegia.
pharyngoperistole pharyngostenosis.
pharyngoplasty plastic repair of the pharynx.
pharyngoplegia pharyngoparalysis.
pharyngorhinitis inflammation of the nasopharynx.
pharyngorrhea mucous discharge from the pharynx.
pharyngoscope an instrument for inspecting the pharynx.
pharyngoscopy direct visual examination of the pharynx.
pharyngospasm spasm of the pharyngeal muscles.
pharyngostenosis narrowing of the pharynx; pharyngoperistole.
pharyngostomy creation of an artificial opening into the pharynx.
p. intubation an opening created through the skin of the neck or throat can be used to insert (1) an esophagostomy tube for feeding when the oral cavity must be bypassed following injury or surgery, or (2) an endotracheal tube.
pharyngotomy incision of the pharynx.
pharyngotympanic tube the narrow channel that connects the middle ear with the nasopharynx; called also auditory tube, eustachian tube. The tube serves to equalize pressure on either side of the tympanic membrane (eardrum).
pharynx the throat; the musculomembranous crossroads of the digestive and respiratory systems, found behind the nasal cavities and mouth, and rostral to the larynx and esophagus.

The pharynx includes many individual structures and may be divided into three parts: the nasopharynx (above), oropharynx (below) and laryngopharynx (behind). The nasopharynx, connected with the nasal cavities, provides a passage for air during breathing; it also contains the openings of the auditory tubes through which air enters the middle ear. The oropharynx and laryngopharynx provide passageways for both air and food. The pharynx also functions as a resonating organ in vocalization.

The pharynx is subdivided by the soft palate. In swallowing, the palate lifts up, closing off the nasopharynx as food passes from the mouth to the esophagus.

Phascolarctos cinereus see KOALA.
phase 1. one of the aspects or stages through which a varying entity may pass. 2. In physical chemistry, a component that is homogeneous of itself, bounded by an interface, and mechanically separable from other phases of the system.
continuous p. in a heterogeneous system, the component in which the disperse phase is distributed, corresponding to the solvent in a true solution.
disperse p. the discontinuous portion of a heterogeneous system, corresponding to the solute in a true solution.
p. feeding a poultry feeding strategy based on varying the amount and kind of feed fed with varying egg production levels, body weight, age, environmental temperature and cost of feed ingredients.
p. plate a critical component of a phase microscope.
p. transition temperature temperature, usually between 30°C and 40°C, at which biological membranes change from a rigid gel phase to a thinner, more fluid phase.
phase variation a mechanism of differential gene regulation found in *Salmonella* whereby two alternative forms of the flagellin gene, H1 and H2, are expressed.
phaseolunatin a cyanogenetic glycoside found in PHASEOLUS *lunatus*—the Java bean.
Phaseolus a genus of bean plants in the family Fabaceae; contain a number of phytotoxins including phaseolus hemolytic agent, lunatin, a cyanogenetic glucoside, and a hemagglutinating lectin which causes vomiting, diarrhea. Includes garden kidney beans (*P. vulgaris*, e.g. French beans, scarlet runner climbing bean) and crop beans such as Lima and Java beans (*P. lunatus*).
phaseolus hemolytic agent hemolytic agent found in members of the genus *Phaseolus*.
Phasianus see PHEASANT.
phasmid either of the two caudal chemoreceptors occurring in certain nematodes (Phasmidia).
Phe phenylalanine.
pheasant gallinaceous birds which are members of the family Phasianidae, which also includes partridge, quail and peafowls. They are ground feeders and tree roosters, with profuse, brightly colored plumage and a long tail and are the best game bird. There very many species, the best known being *Phasianus colchicus*, the common ringneck pheasant. Others include blue-eared pheasant (*Crossoptilon auritum*), golden pheasant (*Chrysolophus pictus*), Reeves pheasant (*Syrmaticus reevesii*), silver pheasant (*Lophura nycthemera*).
pheasant eye ADONIS *annua*, *A. microcarpa*.
phemerol see BENZETHONIUM CHLORIDE.
phenacemide an anticonvulsant.
phenacetin see ACETOPHENETIDIN.
phenamidine isethionate an aromatic diamidine used as an antiprotozoal, particularly in the treatment of infections by *Babesia*, *Leishmania* and *Pneumocystis* spp.
phenanthrene a colorless, crystalline hydrocarbon used in industry. Has caused photosensitization.
phenanthridium, phenanthridine a group of chemotherapeutic agents used in the treatment of trypanosomiasis. Includes isometamidium, homidium, pyrithidium (Prothidium) and quinapyramine.
phenarsonic acid pharmaceutical aliphatic organic arsenical; see also organic ARSENICAL.
phenazone an analgesic and antipyretic. Poisoning is characterized by convulsions and collapse. Called also antipyrine.
phenazopyridine an azo dye, used as a urinary analgesic and antiseptic in humans. Causes hemolytic anemia and hepatic injury in cats.
phencyclidine a dissociative agent most used in nonhuman primates and other wild animals.
phenelzine a monoamine oxidase inhibitor, used as an antidepressant.
phenethicillin a semisynthetic acid-resistant penicillin, which is a methyl analog of phenoxymethyl penicillin.
phenethylamine a toxic substance in North American mistletoe, *Phoradendron villosum*.
phenidone 1-phenyl-3-pyrazolidone; a developer used with hydroquinone in the development of x-ray film.
pheniprazine one of the monoamine oxidase inhibitors used as an antidepressant but is toxic on continued use in dogs, causing irreversible cerebellar ataxia and hemolytic anemia.

pheniramine an antihistaminic, used as the maleate salt.

phenobarbital, phenobarbitone a hypnotic, anticonvulsant and sedative.

phenocopy 1. an environmentally induced phenotype mimicking one usually produced by a specific genotype. 2. an individual exhibiting such a phenotype; the simulated trait in a phenocopy. 3. experimentally produced phenocopies have been created in unfertilized rabbit eggs by the microinjection of the nuclei of embryonic rabbit cells.

phenodeviant an individual whose phenotype differs significantly from that of the typical phenotype in the population.

phenogroup alleles that are always inherited in groups of two or more.

phenol 1. an extremely poisonous compound obtained by distillation of coal tar or produced synthetically; used as a disinfectant and used extensively as a wood preservative. Called also carbolic acid. 2. any organic compound containing one or more hydroxyl groups attached to an aromatic or carbon ring.

p. coefficient a measure of the bactericidal activity of a chemical compound in relation to phenol. The activity of the compound is expressed as the ratio of dilution in which it kills in 10 minutes under specified conditions. It can be determined in the absence of organic matter, or in the presence of a standard amount of added organic matter.

p. Folin–Ciocalteau a sensitive, colorimetric method for estimating the protein content of cerebrospinal fluid.

plant p. includes gossypol, tannins.

p. poisoning animals can be exposed to phenol by skin contact with floors and housing which have been treated with the disinfectant, or other phenol-rich substance such as lignite pitch, or by nibbling at wood treated with it. Causes local tissue necrosis and hepatic injury. Cats are particularly susceptible.

p. red see PHENOLSULFONPHTHALEIN.

phenolphthalein 1. an acid–base indicator dye; it is colorless below pH 8.5, but turns red above pH 9.0. 2. in monogastric animals, a cathartic administered orally, usually with a bulk laxative such as agar. When ingested by ruminants causes the urine to change color to red on exposure to air.

phenolsulfonphthalein an acid–base indicator dye; abbreviated PSP.

p. (PSP) clearance test after an injection of the dye, urine samples are collected at timed intervals and the amount of excreted dye is determined and plotted against time as an indicator of renal function, particularly renal blood flow, tubular excretion, and to some extent glomerular filtration.

phenoltetrachlorphthalein a dye used intravenously as a liver function test.

phenomenon pl. *phenomena* [Gr.] any observable occurrence or fact of which the cause is not immediately evident. In veterinary science usually relates to laboratory findings but can relate to clinical signs. Typical examples are BERRY–DEDRICK PHENOMENON, CAMP PHENOMENON, KOCH phenomenon, RICKETTSIAL INTERFERENCE PHENOMENON, SATELLITISM, SWARMING (1).

phenothiazine the first broad-spectrum veterinary anthelmintic and the market leader in all agricultural animals for many years. Now largely superseded by more efficient compounds. Used now only in horses. Not recommended for use in pregnant mares because of the fear of causing abortion. Its principal use is in mixtures with piperazine and in small daily doses to inhibit egg-laying by resident worms. It must be supported by regular dosing at full dose rates. The name is also used to denote a group of major tranquilizers resembling phenothiazine in molecular structure.

phenotype 1. the outward appearance of the animal in all of its anatomical, physiological and behavioral characteristics as dictated by the genetic and environmental influences in its environment; in contradistinction to genotype in which only the inherited factors are taken into account. 2. an individual exhibiting a certain phenotype; a trait expressed in a phenotype.

phenoxyacids phenoxy derivatives of fatty acids used as herbicides; are largely innocuous to animals. They may make poisonous plants temporarily more palatable and increase their content of cyanide or nitrate. The common members of the group are 2,4-D, 2,4,5-T, MCPA, 2,4-DB, MCPB and fenoprop.

phenoxybenzamine an α-adrenergic blocking agent with prolonged action; the hydrochloride salt is used as a vasodilator and as a relaxant in functional urethral obstruction. Has proved useful in some cases of chronic diarrhea in horses.

phenoxymethylpenicillin see phenoxymethyl PENICILLIN.

phenpropionate USAN contraction for 3-phenylpropionate.

phensuximide an anticonvulsant. See SUCCINIMIDES.

phentanyl see FENTANYL.

phentolacin an indandione derivative used as an anticoagulant rodenticide.

phentolamine a potent α-adrenergic blocking agent; it blocks the hypertensive action of epinephrine and norepinephrine and most responses of smooth muscles that involve α-adrenergic cell receptors. Its hydrochloride and mesylate salts are used in the diagnosis of hypertension due to pheochromocytoma.

phenyl the monovalent radical, C_6H_5.

p. salicylate a salicylic acid ester used as an analgesic.

phenylalanine a naturally occurring amino acid essential for optimal growth in young animals and for nitrogen equilibrium in adults.

p. deaminase test a biochemical test used for the identification of enterobacteria, based on the formation of phenylpyruvic acid.

phenylbutazone a nonsteroidal anti-inflammatory drug resembling cortisone in its action; used in the treatment of painful conditions of joints and skeletal muscles. It has powerful analgesic and antipyretic effects, but causes bone marrow suppression with high doses or prolonged administration.

phenylephrine an α-adrenergic stimulant used as the hydrochloride salt as a nasal decongestant and in ophthalmology to produce mydriasis.

phenylhydrazine a chemical reagent for detection of reducing substances such as sugars, ketones and aldehydes.

phenylmercuric denoting a compound containing the radical $C_6H_5Hg–$, forming various antiseptic, antibacterial and fungicidal salts; compounds of the acetate and nitrate salts are used as bacteriostatics, and the former is also used as a herbicide.

p. acetate used as a bacteriostatic preservative in pharmaceutical preparations, as a topical fungistatic agent, and as a herbicide.

p. chloride used as a bacteriostat in pharmaceuticals.

p. nitrate used as a bacterial preservative in pharmaceutical preparations, and as a topical antiseptic.

***o*-phenylphenol** a preservative approved for use in foodstuffs.

phenylpropanolamine a β-adrenergic agent used chiefly as a nasal and sinus decongestant in the form of the hydrochloride salt and to increase urethral pressure in the treatment of urinary incontinence.

phenylpyruvic acid an intermediate product of the metabolism of phenylalanine in the body.

phenylurea a chemical compound on which relatively nontoxic herbicides are based. Very high intakes of these cause loss of appetite and weight and weakness of the hindquarters.

phenytoin an anticonvulsant used as the sodium salt. Occasionally used in the treatment of tonic–clonic and psychomotor seizures; also used for the control of cardiac arrhythmias, especially those caused by digitalis intoxication. Formerly called diphenylhydantoin.

pheo- a combining form meaning brown, dun or dusky.

pheochrome chromaffin.

pheochromoblast, phaeochromoblast any of the embryonic structures that develop into chromaffin (pheochrome) cells.

pheochromocyte a chromaffin cell.

pheochromocytoma, phaeochromocytoma a small chromaffin cell tumor, usually located in the adrenal medulla but occasionally occurring in chromaffin tissue of the sympathetic paraganglia. It occurs most often in dogs and cattle; in bulls it develops concurrently with C-cell tumors of the thyroid gland. Functional tumors secrete catecholamines, causing arteriolar sclerosis and medial hyperplasia and clinical signs of hypertension: tachycardia, edema and cardiac hypertrophy.

pheomelanin yellow to red-brown pigment produced by melanocytes. See also EUMELANIN.

pheomelanosome brown-colored MELANOSOME producing pheomelanin.

pheresis any procedure in which blood is withdrawn from a donor, a portion (plasma, leukocytes, etc.) is separated and retained, and the remainder is retransfused into the donor. It includes plasmapheresis, leukapheresis, etc.

pheromone a substance secreted to the outside of the body and perceived (as by smell) by other individuals of the same species, releasing specific behavior in the percipient.

phi the twenty-first letter of the Greek alphabet, Φ or ϕ.

phialide an open-ended, tubular or flask-like conidiophore that produces phialoconidia. Seen in *Aspergillus* and *Penicillium* spp.

phialoconidium pl. *phialoconidia;* a conidium that develops from a phialide.

Phialophora a dematiaceous fungus associated with phaeohyphomycosis and chromoblastomycosis.

Philadelphia chromosome the 9:22 chromosomal translocation characterisitic of human patients with inherited predilection for chronic myelogenous leukemia.

Philaemon grandidieri a leech that invades the dorsal lymph sac of New Guinea frogs.

-philia word element. [Gr.] *affinity for, morbid fondness of.*

Phillips technique a method of teat stripping of dairy cows before commencing milking. Aimed at reducing the rate of new quarter infections. The top of the teat is clamped off with one hand and the teat is stripped with the other, preventing reflux of infected milk into the udder cistern.

Philodendron plant genus in the family Araceae and a popular house plant. Toxin is insoluble calcium oxalate raphide crystals. Causes stomatitis and renal damage in cats.

Philometra genus of deep red-colored, large nematode of the Dracunculoid family Philometridae; found in the peritoneal cavity of fish.

Philophthalmus a genus of flukes (digenetic nematodes) in the family Philophthalmidae.

P. gralli found in the conjunctival sacs of birds causing congestion and erosion of the conjunctiva. Called also oriental avian eye fluke.

philtrum the junction between the left and right upper lips; not distinctive in many animal species. In some, such as dogs, the term also applies to the noticeable junction between the two sides of the nose pad.

Philydrum languinosum Australian plant in the family Philydraceae; contains an unidentified toxin which causes diarrhea; called also woolly water lily.

phimosis constriction of the orifice of the prepuce so that it cannot be drawn back over the glans.

phlebangioma a venous aneurysm.

phlebarteriectasia general dilatation of veins and arteries.

phlebectasia dilatation of a vein or veins; a varicosity.

phlebectomy excision of a vein, or a segment of a vein.

phlebedema edema resulting from venous insufficiency.

phlebemphraxis stoppage of a vein by a plug or clot.

phlebismus obstruction and consequent turgescence of veins.

phlebitis inflammation of a vein.

Phlebitis is not serious when the inflammation is located in a superficial vein since these veins are numerous enough to permit the flow of blood to be rechanneled, so that the inflamed vein is bypassed. When a deep vein is involved, however, phlebitis is potentially more dangerous. It can also have serious consequences if it leads to cerebral abscesses.

The common causes in animals are omphalophlebitis and injection phlebitis caused by the inadvertent injection of irritant substances or the prolonged use of intravenous catheters. The vein is swollen and painful and the blood flow obstructed.

phleb(o)- word element. [Gr.] *vein.*

phleboclysis injection of fluid into a vein; venoclysis. See also INTRAVENOUS infusion.

phlebogram 1. a radiograph of a vein filled with contrast medium. 2. a phlebographic or sphygmographic tracing of the venous pulse.

phlebograph an instrument for recording the venous pulse.

phlebography 1. radiography of a vein filled with contrast medium. 2. the graphic recording of the venous pulse. 3. a description of the veins.

phlebolith a venous calculus or concretion.

phlebolithiasis the development of phleboliths.

phlebomanometer an instrument for the direct measurement of venous blood pressure.

phlebophlebostomy operative anastomosis of one vein to another, as of the portal vein and inferior vena cava.

phleboplasty plastic repair of a vein.

phleborrhaphy suture of a vein.

phleborrhexis rupture of a vein.

phlebosclerosis fibrous thickening of the walls of veins.

phlebostasis 1. retardation of blood flow in veins. 2. temporary sequestration of a portion of blood from the general circulation by compressing the veins of an extremity.

phlebothrombosis the development of venous thrombi in the absence of associated inflammation of the vessel wall, as opposed to thrombophlebitis, in which there are inflammatory changes in the vessel wall. See also VENOUS thrombosis.

Phlebotomus a genus of biting flies, called sandflies, the females of which are blood-sucking. They are vectors of various human diseases, including kala-azar (*P. argentipes, P. chinensis, P. martini, P. perniciosus*), Carrion's disease (*P. noguchi, P. verrucarum, P. columbianum*), cutaneous leishmaniasis (*P. sergenti, P. papatasi, P. major, P. caucasicus*) and phlebotomus or sandfly fever (*P. papatasi, P. chinensis, P. mongolensis*).

phlebotomy incision of a vein. See VENISECTION.

Phlebovirus a genus of viruses in the family BUNYAVIRIDAE.

phlegm viscid mucus excreted in abnormally large quantities from the respiratory tract.

phlegmasia inflammation.

phlegmon diffuse inflammation of the soft or connective tissue due to infection.

throat p. see PHARYNGEAL phlegmon.

phlegmonous pertaining to or emanating from phlegmon.

Phleum pratense the oldfashioned but still popular pasture grass in the family Poaceae which can be infested with *Claviceps purpurea* and cause ergotism. Called also timothy grass.

phlogistic inflammatory.

phlog(o)- word element. [Gr.] *inflammation.*

phlogogenic producing inflammation.

phloridzin, phlorizin a dihydrochalcone extracted from the root bark of the apple tree. Thought at one time to be present in cherry, plum and pear. Blocks the renal tubular reabsorption of glucose hence promoting the development of glycosuria.

phlyctena 1. a small blister made by a burn. 2. a small vesicle containing lymph seen on the conjunctiva in certain conditions.

phlyctenoid resembling a phlyctena.

phlyctenular associated with the formation of phlyctenules, or of vesicle-like prominences.

phlyctenule a minute vesicle; an ulcerated nodule of the cornea or conjunctiva.

phlyctenulosis a condition marked by formation of phlyctenules.

phobia an excessive or unreasonable fear of something.

Phoca vitulina see HARBOR SEAL.

Phocaena see PORPOISE.

Phocanema a genus of nematodes in the family Anisakidae. This genus parasitizes codfish and may be transmitted to humans who eat the fish,

P. decipiens found in the South American sealion and fur seals.

phocine pertaining to or emanating from seals.

p. distemper see phocine DISTEMPER.

Phocitrema fusiforme a liver fluke found in fur seal, ringed seal and otter.

Phocoena sinus marine mammal in the family Delphinidae; called also Pacific harbor porpoise.

phocomelia congenital absence of the proximal portion of a limb or limbs, the distal parts being attached to the trunk by a small, irregularly shaped bone.

phocomelus an animal exhibiting phocomelia.

Phoebetria see ALBATROSS.

Phoenicopterus ruber flamingo; the long-legged, long-necked wading birds that live in very large colonies on lakes. They have the unusual ability to stand on one leg with the head laid on the back for hours at a stretch.

Pholcus phalangoides daddy-long-legs; crane fly; harvestman.

pholedrine an adrenergic vasopressor and cardiac stimulant used in cases of shock and toxemia.

Phoma herbarum a fungus growing on Kikuyu grass and possibly contributing to outbreaks of poisoning by that grass. See also PENNISETUM *clandestinum.*

phomopsins hepatoxic mycotoxins in the fungus PHOMOPSIS LEPTOSTROMIFORMIS.

Phomopsis leptostromiformis a toxic fungus growing on dead lupin plants (luypin stubble) and contributing to the toxicosis, lupinosis, caused by the plant. The toxins are PHOMOPSINS. See also LUPINOSIS. Called also *Diaporthe toxica.*

phonal pertaining to the voice.

phonasthenia weakness of the voice; difficult phonation from fatigue.

phonation the utterance of vocal sounds.

phonatory subserving or pertaining to phonation.

phonendoscope a stethoscopic device that intensifies auscultatory sounds. Consists of a flat chamber closed at its contact with the skin by a thin plastic diaphragm. It is most useful in picking up low pitched sounds from the respiratory tract. The classical bell stethoscope is more suited to picking up the higher pitched heart sounds.

phonic pertaining to the voice.

phon(o)- word element. [Gr.] *sound, voice.*

phonoangiography the recording and analysis of arterial bruits to estimate the extent of arterial stenosis.

phonocardiogram the record produced by phonocardiography.

phonocardiograph the instrument used in phonocardiography.

phonocardiography the graphic recording of heart sounds and murmurs; by extension, the term includes pulse tracings (carotid, apex and venous pulse).

Phonocardiography involves picking up, through a highly sensitive microphone, sonic vibrations from the heart which are then converted into electrical energy and fed into a galvanometer, where they are recorded on paper. The procedure is most useful when there is evidence of heart murmurs or unusual heart sounds, such as gallops, that are difficult to discern by the human ear. Most recordings are made through an externally applied microphone but intracardiac recordings, made through a phonocatheter, are possible.

phonocatheter a catheter with a device in its tip for picking up and transmitting sound.

phonoendoscope a stethoscope with a large diameter flat head sealed by a thin plastic or celluloid diaphragm. Most useful for picking up small sounds from lung.

phonogram a graphic record of a sound.

phonometer a device for measuring the intensity of sounds.

phonomyoclonus myoclonus in which a sound is heard on auscultation of an affected muscle, indicating fibrillar contractions.

phonomyogram a record produced by phonomyography.

phonomyography the recording of sounds produced by muscle contraction.

phonophotography photographic recording of the movements of a diaphragm set up by sound waves.

phonoreceptor a receptor for sound stimuli.

phonorenogram a record of the sounds produced by pulsation of the renal artery obtained by a phonocatheter passed through a ureter into the renal pelvis.

phonostethograph an instrument by which chest sounds are amplified, filtered and recorded.

Phoradendron villosum North American plant in the family Viscaceae; contains cardiotoxic amines β-phenylethylamine and tyramine and causes sudden death due to heart failure; called also mistletoe.

phorate an ORGANOPHOSPHORUS COMPOUND used as an insecticide and capable of causing poisoning.

phorazetim a very toxic ORGANOPHOSPHORUS COMPOUND used as a rodenticide.

-phore word element. [Gr.] *a carrier.*

-phoresis word element. [Gr.] *transmission.*

phoresy a method of dispersal, e.g. of insect pests, in which the insect clings to a moving animal or other insect. Includes transmission of a parasite by a parasite, e.g. *Histomonas meleagridis* by *Heterakis gallinarum.*

Phormia a genus of blowflies. *P. regina* and *P. terranovae* are involved in cutaneous MYIASIS in North America.

phosdrin see MEVINPHOS.

phosgene a suffocating and highly poisonous war gas, carbonyl chloride, $COCl_2$.

phosmet an organophosphorus insecticide used as a spray or pour-on to control ectoparasites.

phosphatase any of a group of enzymes capable of catalyzing the hydrolysis of esterified phosphoric acid, with liberation of inorganic phosphate, found in practically all tissues, body fluids and cells, including erythrocytes and leukocytes.

acid p. a lysosomal enzyme that hydrolyzes phosphate esters liberating phosphate, showing optimal activity at a pH between 3 and 6; found in erythrocytes, prostatic tissue, spleen, kidney and other tissues.

alkaline p. an isoenzyme showing optimal activity at a pH of about 10; found in bone, liver, kidney, leukocytes, adrenal cortex and other tissues, often used in clinical diagnosis of liver and/or bone damage. Called also AP; see also ALKALINE phosphatase.

p. inhibitor-1 inhibitor of phosphatase enzymes known to activate glycogen synthesis or inactivate glycogen breakdown. Need to themselves be phosphorylated by cAMP-dependent kinases before they are effective in their inhibitory activity.

phosphate any salt or ester of phosphoric acid.

1. Phosphates are widely distributed in the body, the largest amounts being in the bones and teeth. They are continually excreted in the urine and feces, and must be replaced in the diet. Inorganic phosphates function as buffer salts to maintain the ACID–BASE BALANCE in blood, saliva, urine and other body fluids. The principal phosphates in this buffer system are monosodium and disodium phosphate. Organic phosphates, in particular adenosine triphosphate (ATP), are used to store the chemical bond energy released during the oxidation of compounds such as glycogen or fatty acids, which may later be expended in muscle contraction. This is thought to occur through the hydrolysis of the so-called high-energy phosphate bond present in ATP, phosphocreatine and certain other body compounds. See also HYPOPHOSPHATEMIA, HYPERPHOSPHATEMIA. 2. used extensively in agricultural industry as fertilizers and organic compounds as cleaning agents.

p. binders usually aluminum carbonate or hydroxide preparations, used to bind phosphates and limit their absorption from the intestine. Used in the treatment of the hyperphosphatemia of renal failure.

p. buffer important phosphate-containing buffers.

p. buffered saline a special phosphate buffered saline used in tissue cultures and for the storage and transport of bovine embryos. Abbreviated PBS.

p. calculi see struvite UROLITH.

dietary p. supplementation of the diet with phosphate in some form is a very common practice in farm animals. Materials used include rock phosphate (defluorination may be necessary), sodium dihydrogen phosphate produced by the agricultural chemical industry, calcium triphosphate and bone meal or flour.

inorganic p. any salt of phosphoric acid.

p. retention a phenomenon resulting from reduced glomerular filtration; contributes to a chronic hypocalcemic state.

p. ridge see MINERALIZATION front.

p. rock see ROCK PHOSPHATE.

p. yielding endonucleases a class of ribonuclease involved in the usually fairly rapid turnover of RNA in the cell that degrades RNA by cleavage of the phosphodiester bonds within the molecule.

phosphatemia an excess of phosphates in the blood.

phosphatidic acid a precursor of triacylglycerols and some phospholipids. Its biologically important derivatives include cardiolipin and compounds consisting of a phosphate ester linked to ethanolamine, inositol, serine or choline, i.e. phosphatidylcholine, phosphatidylethanolamine, phosphatidylinositol, phosphatidylserine.

phosphatidyl any of several univalent groups derived from phosphatidic acid; includes phosphatidyl choline, phosphatidyl ethanolamine, phosphatidyl inositol, and phosphatidyl serine.

p. inositol 4,5-biphosphate activated form of sulfur for S transfer.

p. serine a phospholipid found in mammalian cells.

phosphatidylcholine one of the lipids concerned in the structure of cell membranes.

phosphatidylserine one of the lipids concerned in the structure of cell membranes.

phosphaturia an excess of phosphates in the urine.

phosphine 1. PH_3, a toxic war gas called hydrogen phosphide. 2. a coal tar dye; called Philadelphia yellow.

phosphoamidase an enzyme that catalyzes the conversion of phosphocreatine to creatine and orthophosphate.

phosphocreatine a compound of creatine and phosphoric acid occurring in muscle, being an important storage form of chemical bond energy, an energy source in muscle contraction.

phosphodiester group the bonds that join the 5′ phosphate of one nucleotide and the 3′-OH group of the adjacent nucleotide, i.e. the phosphate group esterified to both the 3′- and 5′-carbon atoms of the sugar.

phosphodiesterase a group of enzymes that catalyze the hydrolysis of a phosphodiester.

phosphoenolpyruvate an intermediary metabolite in the Embden–Myerhof glycolytic pathway; abbreviated PEP.

phosphoenolpyruvate–carboxykinase an enzyme in gluconeogenic metabolism; abbreviated PEP–CK. It assists in the conversion of oxaloacetate to phosphoenolpyruvate (PEP).

6-phosphofructokinase 1 an enzyme of the glycolytic (Embden–Meyerhof) pathway that catalyzes the conversion of fructose-6-phosphate to fructose-

1,6-bisphosphate using ATP as the source of the phosphate. Allosteric enzyme regulating glycolysis.
p. deficiency inherited disorder of glucose metabolism in English springer spaniel dogs. Affected dogs develop a chronic hemolytic anemia. Called also Type 7 glycogen storage disease.

6-phosphofructokinase 2 enzyme catalyzing the phosphorylation of fructose-6-phosphate to fructose 2,6-bisphosphate using ATP as the source of the phosphate. Fructose 2,6-bisphosphate is a key allosteric influence of the activity of 6-phosphofructokinase 1.

phosphoglucomutase a glycolytic pathway enzyme that catalyzes the conversion of glucose-1-phosphate to glucose-6-phosphate in a reversible reaction.
p.-2 a minor histocompatibility system in dogs; genetic polymorphism of this enzyme has been associated with graft-versus-host reactions.

6-phosphogluconate pathway see HEXOSE monophosphate shunt, pentose phosphate PATHWAY.

phosphoglycerate kinase an enzyme which catalyzes the transfer of high-energy phosphate to ADP.

phosphoglyceride a class of phospholipids, including lecithin and cephalin, consisting of a glycerol backbone, two fatty acids, and a phosphorylated alcohol, e.g. choline, ethanolamine, serine or inositol. They are a major component of cell membranes.

phosphoglyceromutase an enzyme which converts 3-glycerophosphate to 2-glycerophosphate in one of the steps in the Embden–Meyerhof pathway. There are two enzymes, one labeled PGM-1 and the other PGM-2.

phosphokinase see KINASE.

phospholine iodide see ECHOTHIOPHATE IODIDE.

phospholipase any of four enzymes (phospholipase A to D) which catalyze the hydrolysis of a phospholipid.

phospholipase A_2 enzyme catalyzing the hydrolysis of the fatty acyl group esterified in the 2-position of a phospholipid. Key enzyme in the release of arachidonic acid from this position for subsequent conversion to the eicosanoid group of humoral agents.

phospholipase C enzyme catalyzing the removal of polar head group such as choline from phospholipids.

phospholipid any lipid that contains phosphorus, including those with a glycerol backbone (phosphoglycerides and plasmalogens) or a backbone of sphingosine or a related substance (sphingomyelins). They are the major lipids in cell membranes.
p. bilayer a layer containing two phospholipid molecules which is the basic structural unit of all biological membranes.

phospholipidosis a generalized phospholipid disturbance with major deposits, derived from alveolar surfactant, in the pulmonary alveoli.

phosphoprotein a conjugated protein in which phosphoric acid is esterified with a hydroxy amino acid.

phosphorated charged or combined with phosphorus.

phosphorescence the emission of light without appreciable heat; it is characterized by the emission of absorbed light after a delay and at a considerably longer wavelength than that of the absorbed light. Caused by a number of bacteria, especially in seawater. One of them, *Pseudomonas phosphorescens*, may infect coldrooms via infected fish but does not constitute decomposition so that phosphorescent meat is still edible.

phosphoribulokinase an enzyme that catalyzes the conversion of ATP and D-ribulose 5-phosphate to ADP and D-ribulose 1,5-diphosphate.

phosphoric acid a crystalline acid formed by oxidation of phosphorus; its salts are called phosphates. See also PHOSPHATE.

phosphorolysis cleavage of a chemical bond with simultaneous addition of the elements of phosphoric acid to the residues.

phosphorus a chemical element, atomic number 15, atomic weight 30.974, symbol P. See Table 6. Phosphorus is an essential element in the diet. In the form of phosphates it is a major component of the mineral phase of bone and is involved in almost all metabolic processes. It also plays an important role in cell metabolism. It is obtained by the body from milk products, cereals, meat and fish, and its use by the body is controlled by vitamin D and calcium.
p.-32 a radioisotope of phosphorus having a half-life of 14.3 days and emitting only beta rays; used in the form of sodium phosphate P-32 for treatment of polycythemia vera, chronic myelocytic leukemia and chronic lymphocytic leukemia, and in localizing certain tumors during surgery. Symbol ^{32}P.
calcium:p. ratio see CALCIUM:phosphorus ratio.
inorganic p. any phosphorus-containing compound which does not also contain carbon.
p. nutritional deficiency causes rickets in the young and OSTEOMALACIA in adult ruminants. In less severe deficiency states there is pica, growth retardation, infertility and possibly retention of placenta. See also POSTPARTURIENT hemoglobinuria. An unlikely nutritional deficiency in carnivores.
p. poisoning is very rare because of the absence of elemental phosphorus from the environment. Causes severe gastroenteritis with vomiting and diarrhea. If the animal survives the gastroenteritis there is a subsequent acute hepatic insufficiency.
p. restriction indicated in the dietary management of chronic renal disease and secondary hyperaparathyroidism; in dogs and cats, usually accomplished by reducing the content of meat.
p. supplements supplementing the diets of animals exposed to phosphorus deficient feeds is usually achieved by feeding bone meal, or calcium or sodium phosphates. All are readily assimilable but none are palatable and special devices are often necessary to get animals to take required amounts. See also dietary PHOSPHATE.

phosphorylase a key regulatory enzyme that, in the presence of inorganic phosphate, catalyzes the removal of one glucose unit from glycogen to glucose-1-phosphate.
citrulline p. see ornithine carbamoyl TRANSFERASE.
p. kinase an enzyme that activates phosphorylase by catalyzing the phosphorylation of serine. See also KINASE.

phosphorylated glycerolipids chief constituents of the lipid bilayer of cell membranes in which apolar acyl chains face each other in the membrane interior.

phosphorylation the process of introducing a phosphate group into an organic molecule.
oxidative p. the final common oxidative pathway in which high-energy phosphate bonds are formed by phosphorylation of ADP to ATP by harnessing by F_0F_1-ATPase of the proton motive force generated from pumping of protons from the matrix of mitochondria across the inner mitochondrial membrane to the intermembrance space and is coupled with the transfer of electrons along a chain of carrier proteins with molecular oxygen as the final acceptor.

phosphosphingolipids a subset of sphingolipids; are membrane constituents of cells, constituents of plasma lipoproteins, blood group substances and act as receptors for bacterial toxins.

phosphotransacetylase an enzyme which catalyzes the transfer of an acetyl group between acetylphosphate and acetylcoenzyme A.

phosphotransferase any of a class of enzymes that catalyze the transfer of a phosphate group.

photic pertaining to light.

Photinia genus of garden plants in the family Rosaceae; can cause cyanide poisoning; called also Christmas berry, Chinese hawthorn.

phot(o)- word element. [Gr.] *light*.

photo timer an alarm device for use in a darkroom to advise the need to move to the next stage of the developing program. More commonly used to control x-ray exposure time automatically for spot filming or photofluorography connected with the output optical detector.

photoactivated see PHOTOAGGRAVATED.

photoactive reacting chemically to sunlight or ultraviolet radiation.

photoaggravated condition produced when a preexisting condition worsens on being exposed to sunlight. Called also photoactivated.

p. dermatoses term used in human medicine when referring to pemphigus, lupus erythematosus, bullus pemphigoid; may be applicable to the same diseases in dogs.

p. vasculitis a dermatosis of horses affecting only the white extremities of the limbs.

photoallergy a hypersensitivity that develops against the photoproduct of an exogenous chemical.

photobiology the branch of biology dealing with the effect of light on organisms.

photobiotic living only in the light.

photocatalysis promotion or stimulation of a chemical reaction by light.

photocatalyst a substance, e.g. chlorophyll, that brings about a chemical reaction on exposure to light.

photochemistry the branch of chemistry that deals with the chemical properties or effects of light rays or other radiation.

photochemotherapy treatment by means of drugs (e.g. methoxsalen) that react to ultraviolet radiation or sunlight.

photochromogen a microorganism whose pigmentation develops as a result of exposure to light. A characteristic of Runyon Group I mycobacteria.

photocoagulation condensation of protein material by the controlled use of an intense beam of light (e.g. argon laser); used especially in the treatment of retinal detachment and destruction of abnormal retinal vessels or intraocular tumor masses.

photodermatitis, photodermatosis an abnormal state of the skin in which light is an important causative factor, e.g. actinic DERMATITIS.

photodynamic activated or made more powerful by light.

p. agent a substance that is activated by light to cause damage to tissue. It may be exogenous and absorbed preformed from the environment, or endogenous in that it is formed within the body as an abnormal metabolite, e.g. porphyrins, or as a normal metabolite, e.g. phylloerythrin, and accumulate in tissues because of faulty excretion, e.g. in hepatic disease.

p. therapy the use of photodynamic agents in the treatment of disease.

photoelectric pertaining to the electrical effects of light or other radiation.

p. absorption the basis of diagnostic radiology. The difference in absorption of x-ray energy by different tissues causes differences in electromagnetic energy arriving at the film.

photofluorography the photographic recording of fluoroscopic images on small films, using a fast lens. Called also fluorography and fluororadiography.

photogenic 1. produced by light. 2. emitting or producing light.

photogrammetry a stereophotographic technique for estimating body weight and parts of the body by three-dimensional measurement.

photohemolysis lysis of red cells when the patient is exposed to sunlight. Occurs in erythropoietic protoporphyria.

photokinetic moving in response to the stimulus of light.

photolysis chemical decomposition by light.

photolyte a substance decomposed by light.

photometer a device for measuring the intensity of light.

photometry measurement of the intensity of light.

photomicrograph a photograph of an object as seen through an ordinary light microscope.

photomirex environmental pollutant capable of causing testicular degeneration in animals ingesting it.

photomyoclonic photomyogenic.

photomyogenic clonic spasm of muscles when the patient is exposed to flashes of light. Requires electoencephalographic recognition of response to be a valid result.

photon a particle (quantum) of radiant energy.

x-ray p. a particle of x-ray energy.

photoperiod the period of time per day that an organism is exposed to daylight (or to artificial light).

photoperiodicity the rhythm of certain biological phenomena such as hibernation and reproductive activity which are determined by the regularly recurring changes in light and dark caused by the annual passage of the earth about the sun.

photoperiodism the physiological and behavioral reactions brought about in organisms by changes in the duration of daylight and darkness, e.g. in reproductive activity, shedding of hair. Birds respond to longer daylight hours by increased sexual activity. Use is made of the phenomenon by using artificial light to stimulate egg production.

photophilic thriving in light.

photophobia abnormal visual intolerance to light. Expressed in animals by closing of the eyelids when exposed to light. Difficult to differentiate from blepharospasm due to conjunctivitis.

photophthalmia ophthalmia caused by exposure to intense light.

photopia day vision.

photoreactivation reversal of the biological effects of ultraviolet radiation on cells by subsequent exposure to visible light.

photoreception perception of light waves which are in the range of visible light.

photoreceptive sensitive to stimulation by light.

photoreceptor a nerve end organ or receptor sensitive to light. In the retina of the eye, the outer limbs of rods and cones make up the photoreceptor layer.

photorefractoriness the state of being refractory to the stimulus of light; an important feature of sexual non-receptivity in some species.

photoretinitis retinitis due to exposure to intense light.

photosensitive exhibiting abnormally heightened sensitivity to sunlight.

p. conjunctivitis conjunctivitis that begins on the lateral quadrant of the cornea and reduces in severity to the center of the cornea—the area exposed to the sun's rays. If left unattended progresses to keratitis.

p. dermatitis is confined to the dorsal parts of the body exposed to the sunlight, and to parts with little or no pigment and the least hair or wool covering. The dermatitis is diffuse and often sufficiently severe to kill the animal. Initially there is itching and rubbing, then edema, followed by weeping, then necrosis or gangrene. Additional lesions may be on the undersurface of the tongue, at the mucocutaneous junction at the lips and on the lateral aspects of the teats.

photosensitivity the state of being photosensitive.

photosensitization the development of abnormally heightened reactivity of the skin to sunlight. In food animals the principal photodynamic agents are porphyrins and phylloerythrin. The principal clinical manifestations are as dermatitis and conjunctivitis. There may be an accompanying hepatic insufficiency or porphyrinuria. See LIVER dysfunction, PHOTOSENSITIVE dermatitis. Called also light sensitization.

There is a long list of drugs that can cause photosensitization reactions. Antineoplastics, antimicrobials, diuretics, hypoglycemic agents, and even antihistamines are capable of triggering photosensitivity reactions in certain individuals.

inherited p. in Corriedale and Southdown sheep is caused by an inherited liver transport defect. The liver is histologically normal but phylloerythrin excretion is impeded. Photosensitive dermatitis appears as soon as the lambs begin to eat grass.

primary p. caused by the ingestion of exogenous photosensitizing agents such as dianthrone derivatives (e.g. hypericin, fagopyrin), furanocoumarins, perloline, phenothiazine, rose bengal.

secondary p. secondary to hepatic cell damage, biliary obstruction leading to the accumulation in the body of phylloerythrin, a metabolic end-product of chlorophyll.

photosensitizing causing photosensitivity.

p. plants. some plants carry primary photodynamic agents, e.g. *Hypericum perforatum.* Others are hepatotoxic or carry mycotoxin-producing fungi that are, and are indirectly photosensitizing in that they interfere with the excretion of phylloerythrin through the animal's biliary system.

photostable unchanged by the influence of light.

photostimulator a source of an intense flash of light of very short duration that serves as the light stimulus for electroretinography.

photosynthesis a chemical combination caused by the action of light; specifically the formation of carbohydrates from carbon dioxide and water in the chlorophyll tissue of plants under the influence of light.

phototaxis the movement of cells and microorganisms under the influence of light.

phototherapy treatment of disease by exposure to light. Malignant tumors are treated by using photosensitizing drugs and laser light.

phototoxic having a toxic effect triggered by exposure to light.

phototoxicity pertaining to phototoxic.

primary p. see solar DERMATITIS, SUNBURN.

phototrophic capable of deriving energy from light.

phototropism 1. the tendency of an organism to turn or move toward (positive phototropism) or away from (negative phototropism) light. 2. change of color produced in a substance by the action of light.

photuria excretion of urine having a luminous appearance.

PHPV persistent hyperplastic primary vitreous.

phrenetic maniacal.

phrenic pertaining to the diaphragm.

p. nerve one of the paired nerves to the diaphragm that arises from the caudal cervical nerves (4–7, the specific branches varying with species), passes through the thoracic inlet and in the mediastinum and adjacent structures to the diaphragm.

phrenicectomy resection of the phrenic nerve.

phrenicoexeresis avulsion of the phrenic nerve.

phrenicotomy surgical division of the phrenic nerve.

phrenicotripsy phrenemphraxis.

phrenitis 1. delirium or frenzy. 2. diaphragmitis.

phren(o)- word element. [Gr.] 1. diaphragm. 2. mind.

phrenocolic pertaining to the diaphragm and colon.

phrenogastric pertaining to the diaphragm and stomach.

phrenohepatic pertaining to the diaphragm and liver.

phrenoplegia paralysis of the diaphragm.

phrenosin a cerebroside containing cerebronic acid attached to the sphingosine.

phrynoderma a follicular hyperkeratosis probably due to deficiency of vitamin A or of essential fatty acids.

phthalamic acid an organic herbicide. Poisoning is manifested by bloat and incoordination.

alpha-pthalic-acid esters, *o*-phthalic acid plasticizers in polyvinyl products; cause testicular degeneration in rats.

phthalofyne an anthelmintic used specifically for the treatment of whipworm (*Trichuris vulpis*) in dogs.

phthalophos see NAPHTHALOPHOS.

phthalylsulfacetamide a sulfonamide with a high solubility and suited for systemic use for diseases of the eye. Used for topical application to the skin and the conjunctiva.

phthalylsulfathiazole the phthyl form of SULFATHIAZOLE which is poorly absorbed from the gastrointestinal tract. Administered orally it is hydrolyzed to sulfathiazole which is the effective antibacterial agent.

phthisis 1. a wasting of the body. 2. tuberculosis.

p. bulbi shrinkage of the eyeball.

phyco- word element. [Gr.] *seaweed, algae.*

phycology the scientific study of algae.

Phycomycetes a group of fungi comprising the common water, leaf and bread molds. Called also Zygomocota. Includes *Mucor* spp. and *Rhizopus* spp.

phycomycosis any of a group of acute fungal diseases caused by members of the Phycomycetes. See also ZYGOMYCOSIS.

equine p. see SWAMP CANCER.

Phyllanthus a genus in the plant family of Euphorbiaceae.

P. abnormis North American plant; contains an unidentified toxin which causes liver and kidney damage manifested by compulsive walking, tenesmus, rectal prolapse, petechiation and death. Called also spurge.

P. gasstroemii may cause cyanide poisoning.

P. lacunarius causes gastroenteritis.

phylloerythrin an end-product of chlorophyll metabolism normally excreted in the bile. It is a photodynamic agent and its accumulation in the tissues in animals on a diet of green feed and with liver insufficiency leads to the development of photosensitization.

phyllomenaquinone see PHYTOMENADIONE.

phylloquinone see PHYTOMENADIONE.

phylogeny the evolutionary history of a race or group of organisms.

phylum pl. *phyla* [L., Gr.] a primary division of the plant or animal kingdom, including organisms that are assumed to have a common ancestry.

phyma pl. *phymata* [Gr.] a skin tumor or tubercle.

Physalia physalis common blue-colored jellyfish in the genus *Physalia* with stinging filaments trailing from a central medusa. Records of poisoning in animals are very rare but deaths do occur in infested colonies of farmed fish. Called also Portuguese man-of-war, bluebottle.

Physalis genus of plants in the family Solanaceae; suspected of poisoning livestock. Includes *P. minima*, *P. peruviana*. Called also wild ground cherry.

Physaloptera a genus of spirurid worms in the family Physalopteridae. The gastric mucosa may become eroded, inflamed and produce much mucus. Clinically there may be vomiting, melena, anorexia and weight loss.

P. alata found in the gizzard and intestines of doves and other birds.

P. canis found in the stomach of cats and dogs.

P. caucasica found in the esophagus, stomach and intestines of simian primates.

P. clausa, P. dispar, P. erinacea found in hedgehogs.

P. dilitata found in the stomach of simian primates.

P. felidis found in the stomach and intestines of cats.

P. gemina found in fowl and cat.

P. maxillaris found in skunks and *Procyon* and *Mustela* spp.

P. poicilometra found in simian primates.

P. praeputialis found in the stomach of cats and wild cats.

P. pseudopraeputialis found in the stomach and larynx of cats and coyotes.

P. rara found in the stomach and duodenum of dogs and wild dogs and cats.

P. tumefasciens occurs in the stomach of simian primates.

Physconelloides zenaidurae a pigeon louse.

physeal pertaining to growth or to that part of a bone that is responsible for lengthening—the physis.

p. delayed closure occurs when there is inadequate growth hormone, as in hypopituitarism.

p. dysplasia essentially a disease of horses which consists of a self-limiting disturbance of endochondral ossification affecting the metaphyseal physes of young horses; called also physitis, epiphysitis.

p. focal closure occurs as a result of damage to or displacement of the growth plate; bony bridges develop uniting the epiphysis and the metaphysis, many leading to bone deformities.

p. premature closure usually the result of injury and seen most often in dogs. Causes abnormal development of the bone, the type and severity depending on the age of the animal and the particular location. The most vulnerable are the radius and ulna, mainly because closure of one physis results in unequal growth of the two parallel bones and angular deformity often results.

p. scar see EPIPHYSEAL scar.

Physeter macrocephalus sperm whale. See also WHALE.

physic 1. the art of medicine and therapeutics. 2. a medicine, especially a cathartic. See also PURGING ball.

p. nut JATROPHA *curcas*, *J. multifida*.

physic ball see PURGING ball.

physical pertaining to the body, to material things, or to physics.

p. agent the physical causes of disease. Includes altitude, radiation, wetness, exercise, fire, electricity including lightning.

p. diagnosis a preliminary diagnosis made solely on the basis of a physical examination. Often all that is possible in private practice.

p. examination examination of the bodily state of a patient by ordinary physical means, as inspection, palpation, percussion and auscultation.

p. exhaustion see physical EXHAUSTION.

p. findings results of a physical examination. Observations made visually, by auscultation, palpation, smell, percussion, succussion and ballottement.

p. fitness quality of being able to perform physically, to turn in a good physical performance. Best tested by performance but in horses can be vaguely predicted by a series of tests including hemoglobin content of blood, heart size, duration of the QRS interval on an ECG, and low levels of muscle enzymes in blood.

p. insults physical agencies that cause disease. These include trauma, stress (physical as in stress fracture of long bones in horses), hyperthermia (as a cause of congenital defects), persistent wetting, high altitude, lightning stroke, electrocution, bushfire and fire injury, volcanic eruption and exposure to radiation.

p. map in genetics, determination of the array of genes within a DNA segment of a chromosome.

p. restraint the use of halters, collars and chains, ropes, harness, twitches of various sorts, squeeze cages, hog holders, dog catchers and many more devices. As distinct from the use of analeptic agents—chemical restraint.

p. stress see STRESS.

p. therapist one who is skilled in the physical and therapeutic techniques of helping to alleviate suffering from muscle, nerve, joint and bone diseases and from injuries and to overcome or prevent disabilities. Among the procedures used by the physical therapist are exercise to increase strength, endurance, coordination, and range of motion; electrical stimulation to activate paralyzed muscles; massage, vibrators and many other patented devices to try to improve the circulation and condition of a part.

physician a veterinarian who devotes him or herself to work with medical rather than surgical or reproductive diseases.

physicochemical pertaining to both physics and chemistry.

physics the study of the laws and phenomena of nature, especially of forces and general properties of matter and energy.

physio- word element. [Gr.] *nature, physiology, physical.*

physiochemical pertaining to both physiology and chemistry.

physiological, physiologic 1. pertaining to physiology; 2. normal; not pathological. Conforming to the normal function of an organ or the body as a whole.

p. age age as measured by events rather than years. For example: first-calf heifer, fourth litter sow, stallion in his fourth season.

p. saline 0.9% solution of sodium chloride. See also NORMAL saline.

physiologist a specialist in physiology.

physiology 1. the science which deals with the functions of the living organism and its parts, and of the physical and chemical factors and processes involved. 2. the basic processes underlying the functioning of a species or class of organism, or any of its parts or processes.

cell p. the scientific study of phenomena involved in

cell growth and maintenance, self-regulation and division of cells, interactions between nucleus and cytoplasm, and general behavior of protoplasm.

morbid p., pathological p. the study of disordered functions or of function in diseased tissues.

physiopathological pertaining to pathological physiology.

physiotherapist physical therapist.

physiotherapy physical therapy.

physique the body organization, development and structure. In animals it is more customary to speak of conformation.

physis the segment of a bone that is responsible for lengthening. There are four zones within the physis, the resting cartilage zone, the proliferating cartilage zone, the zone of hypertrophy and the zone of calcification. Called also the growth plate. See also PHYSEAL.

-physis root meaning to grow, growth.

physitis see PHYSEAL dysplasia.

physo- word element. [Gr.] *air, gas.*

Physocephalus a spirurid nematode in the family Spirocercidae. Causes gastritis manifested by anorexia, increased thirst, loss of weight and rarely death.

P. cristatus found in the dromedary.

P. sexalatus found in the stomach of the pig.

physohematometra gas and blood in the uterine cavity.

physohydrometra gas and serum in the uterine cavity.

physometra gas in the uterine cavity.

Physopsis water snail intermediate host for *Schistosoma* spp.

physopyosalpinx gas and pus in the oviduct.

physostigmine an alkaloid usually obtained from the dried ripe seed of *Physostigma venenosum*; used as a topical miotic in the form of the base and of the salicylate and sulfate salts.

p. challenge test a test for the diagnosis of cataplexy; after increasing doses of physostigmine, affected dogs show a dose-related severity of reactions when offered food.

phytase a hydrolase enzyme found in plants; catalyzes the hydrolysis of phytic acid to inositol and phosphoric acid.

phytate inositolhexaphosphoric acid; a source of phosphorus for ruminants and horses but indigestible to carnivores. Present in large amounts in plants.

phytate-phosphorus relatively unavailable phosphorus combined with phytic acid, in feeds with a high fiber content. See also PHYTATE.

phytic acid used synonymously with PHYTATE. See also PHYTIN.

phytin the calcium and magnesium salt of phytic acid.

phyt(o)- word element. [Gr.] *plant, an organism of the vegetable kingdom.*

phytoagglutinin an agglutinin of plant origin.

phytoalexins substances in plants which destroy plant pathogens. They are released in response to a chemical substance released by the pathogen.

phytoallexin chemical produced by plants in response to tissue damage by microbes or herbivores, usually insects. Such chemicals may be toxic to animals the affected plants, e.g. furanocoumarins in fungus-infected parsnips may cause primary photosensitization in pigs.

phytobezoar a bezoar composed of vegetable fibers. Common in cattle as abomasal inclusions. Important as a cause of pyloric or intestinal obstruction. See INTESTINAL obstruction, ROMULEA, bovine COLIC.

phytoestrogens substances with activity as estrogens produced in plants. Includes isoflavones and coumestans. Most of these agents undergo major changes in the rumen, the agents becoming much more potent as a result of the change, e.g. formononetin, which has very little activity is converted to a potent estrogen.

phytogenous derived from plants, or caused by a vegetable growth.

p. chronic copper poisoning see TOXEMIC jaundice.

phytohemagglutinin a hemagglutinin of plant origin.

phytoid resembling a plant.

Phytolacca genus of plants in the family Phytolaccaceae; suspected to contain a toxic saponin which causes enteritis with vomiting, abdominal pain and diarrhea. The illness may be fatal. Includes *P. americana* (*P. decandra*, poke or pokeweed), *P. dioica*, *P. octandra* (ink weed), *P. dodecandra*.

phytomenadione, phytonadione vitamin K_1; a naturally occurring form of vitamin K obtained from plants; used as an antidote in poisoning by warfarin and other anticoagulant rodenticides.

Phytomonas a genus of protozoan parasites found in plants and insects.

phytonadione vitamin K.

phytoparasite any plant parasitic organism.

phytophagous plant-eating.

phytophotocontact dermatitis photosensitization following skin contact with plants which leads to absorption of psoralens.

phytophotodermatitis phototoxic dermatitis due to contact with certain plants and subsequent exposure to sunlight.

phytoplankton see PLANKTON.

phytoprecipitin a precipitin formed in response to vegetable antigen.

phytosis any disease caused by a phytoparasite.

phytosterol a sterol of vegetable origin.

phytotoxic 1. pertaining to phytotoxin. 2. poisonous to plants.

phytotoxin an exotoxin produced by certain species of higher plants; any toxin of plant origin.

phytotrichobezoars fiber balls found in the intestines. They are light compared with enteroliths, being composed of plant or animal fiber cemented by some phosphate salt. They are smooth and usually have a hairy surface. They are usually innocuous.

P_i inorganic orthophosphate.

pI isoelectric point.

pi the sixteenth letter of the Greek alphabet, Π or π.

PI-3 virus parainfluenzavirus 3.

Pi lines thin, black lines running longitudinally across the x-ray film caused by chemical deposits on the rollers in the automatic developer tank.

pia mater [L.] the innermost of the three meninges covering the brain and spinal cord.

pia-arachnitis leptomeningitis; inflammation of the leptomeninges, or pia mater and arachnoid.

pia-arachnoid the pia mater and arachnoid considered together as one functional unit; the leptomeninges.

piaffe [Fr.] *a strut;* a horse dressage gait in which the horse moves actively but stays in place. The action is high.

pial pertaining to the pia mater.

pialabatement decrease in severity of a pain or sign.

piarachnitis leptomeningitis; pia-arachnitis.

piarachnoid pia-arachnoid.

pica craving for unnatural articles of food; a depraved appetite. Expressed in animals by licking or eating foreign materials. Often caused by a nutritional deficiency of bulk, fiber or a specific nutrient, e.g. phosphorus, salt or copper. May lead to botulism, foreign body lodgement in mouth, pharynx, esophagus, in the reticulum to cause reticuloperitonitis, at the pylorus and, in the horse, in the small colon. Called also allotriophagia.

Pica pica see MAGPIE.

Pichia ohmeri a yeast that has caused bovine mastitis. See also Table 16.

pick a sharp-pointed instrument, of varying size and function, e.g. tooth pick, hoof pick.

hoof p. consists of a palm grip and a stem with a sharp point. Used for picking out debris, especially stones, from between the bars and the frog of horses' hooves.

picking out removing the accumulated dirt, manure and stones from the sole of the horse's feet with a hoof pick.

pickling a form of curing in which the meat is immersed in a solution of the curing agents instead of being rubbed with and packed in the dry agent (BACON CURING). The method is faster but does not provide the mouthwatering, smoky dryness of a York or Virginian ham.

Pick's cell see Pick's CELL.

pickwickian syndrome alveolar hypoventilation, somnolence and erythrocytosis associated with extreme obesity as seen in Charles Dickens' fat boy in the *Pickwick Papers*. A similar syndrome is observed rarely in dogs.

picloram a picolinic acid derivative used as a herbicide; causes weakness, anorexia and depression in poisoned animals.

pico- designating 10^{-12} (one-million-millionth) part of the unit to which it is joined. Symbol p.

picobirnaviruses a name provisionally applied to small (35 nm) double segment, double-stranded RNA viruses which may cause diarrhea in humans, pigs and rodents.

picogram one million-millionth (10^{-12}) gram. Abbreviated pg.

picolinic acid a base compound from which a number of derivatives are produced and used as herbicides.

picometer a unit of length, 10^{-12} meter. Abbreviated pm.

Picornaviridae a family of small (25 nm diameter), nonenveloped single-stranded, plus sense RNA viruses, the members of which cause a variety of diseases including poliomyelitis in pig and chickens (*Enterovirus*), respiratory disease in cattle and horses (*Rhinovirus*), encephalomyocarditis in pigs (*Cardiovirus*), foot-and-mouth disease (*Aphthovirus*), *Orphanovirus* and hepatitis A of humans (*Hepatovirus*); equine rhinovirus 1 which may be prototype of a new genus.

picornavirus a member of the virus family PICORNAVIRIDAE.

picrate any salt of picric acid.

p. test a field test for cyanogenetic compounds in plants and gut contents. Based on the conversion of yellow sodium picrate to a brick red color in contact with hydrocyanic acid. Called also Henrici test.

picric acid a substance used as dye, tissue fixative, antiseptic, astringent and stimulant of epithelialization; it can be detonated on percussion or by heating above 570°F (300°C). Called also trinitrophenol.

picrocarmine a histological stain consisting of a mixture of carmine, ammonia, distilled water and aqueous solution of picric acid.

picrotoxin a central nervous system and respiratory stimulant formerly used in barbiturate and other anesthetic poisonings; extracted from the seeds of the plant *Anamirta cocculus*.

Pictou disease Canadian term for pyrrolizidine alkaloidosis in cattle eating *Senecio jacobaea*.

picture frame theory a theory of wound healing and contraction stating that mitotically active cells migrate inward from the margin of the wound, pulling on the material within the margins of the defect. See also PULL THEORY.

PIE syndrome pulmonary infiltration with eosinophilia; a disease of dogs of unknown origin characterized by dyspnea, reduced exercise tolerance, diffuse pulmonary infiltration by eosinophils and an eosinophilia.

piebald a horse coat color of large, distinct patches of black and white. The patches are irregular in shape.

piebaldism a condition in which the skin is partly brown and partly white, as in partial albuminism and vitiligo. See also WAARDENBURG'S SYNDROME.

piecemeal patchy, e.g. necrosis of the liver in which groups of hepatocytes are separated by small groups of inflammatory cells and fine, fibrous septa following extension of the inflammatory process beyond the limiting plate.

pieces a wool-classer's term; when classing fleece wool preparatory to sale, these are the inferior pieces of wool, including skirtings from around the edge and broken wool.

pied a coat color in dogs that consists of uneven patches or spots of color on a white or cream background.

Piedmont, Piedmontese a breed of white or pale gray, with black points, dual-purpose cattle. They have short horns and a deep forehead, like other brachyceros-type cattle.

piedra a fungal disease of the hair in which white or black nodules of fungi form on the shafts.

piercing jaundice needle large wide pointed acupuncture needle, threaded with horse tail or hemp thread passed through the skin of the edematous region and the ends of the thread knotted together and a weight tied to them; used to maintain drainage through the holes.

Pieris[1] temperate zone garden plant genus in the family Ericaceae. Contains andromedotoxin. Includes *P. formosanum*, *P. japonicum* (*Andromeda japonica*, Japanese pieris), *P. ovalifolia*.

Pieris[2] an insect genus in the order Lepidoptera.

P. brassicae the cabbage butterfly of which the caterpillars are cryptoxic, causing colic, stomatitis and paraplegia.

-piesis word element. [Gr.] *pressure*.

Pietrain dirty white pig with black or red spots and semi-lop ears.

Pietrain creeper pigs inherited defect in the Pietrain breed of pigs; characterized by progressive muscular weakness in young pigs.

piezoelectric the generation of electricity in response to mechanical stimulation.

PIF prolactin inhibitory factor.

pig an even-toed nonruminant ungulate with a simple stomach. A member of the suborder Suiformes of the order Artiodactyla. Includes domestic pigs, which are very prolific, heavy, ponderous, rapid-growing, grunting creatures bred almost completely for the purpose of providing meat, but in some cultures are assuming importance as house pets. There are many breeds and colors, the ears may be erect or lop, there are a large number of mammary glands and they have a characteristic snout, thin skin and heavy bristles.

They are descendants of the wild boar, *Sus scrofa*. Preferred name swine. Called also hog.

There are many indigenous domesticated breeds. Popular commercial breeds include BERKSHIRE, CHESTER WHITE, DUROC (DUROC JERSEY), GLOUCESTER OLD SPOT, HAMPSHIRE, LACOMBE, LANDRACE, LARGE WHITE, PIETRAIN, POLAND CHINA, TAMWORTH, WESSEX SADDLEBACK, YORKSHIRE.

Wild genera include wild boar, wild pigs (both *Sus* spp.), bush pigs (*Potamochoerus* spp.), wart hog (*Phacochoerus aethiopicus*), forest hog (*Hylochoerus meinertzhageni*), babirussa (*Babirussa babyrussa*).

Pigs are becoming popular as companion animals, especially pot-bellied pigs. it seems reasonable to assume that this trend will increase because of the advent of 'Babe'.

miniature p. developed in the early 1960s as research animals by interbreeding local American feral pigs with natural dwarf pigs of Yucatan, Vietnamese, Taiwanese breed origin. Pet pigs called 'miniature pet pigs' may be purebred Vietnamese pot-bellied pigs (black, short-nosed, heavy-jowled, pot-bellied, with straight wagging tail), or Yucatan type (straight-bellied, long-snouted, coarse-haired and coarse-coated, without a pot belly and weighing 120–250 lb when mature—called also Mexican hairless), or African Pygmy—called also Guinea hog (with straight back, no pot belly, short to medium length hair, kinky tail, black, sometimes with white markings).

pot-bellied p. not a specific breed; originate from dwarf, pot-bellied indigenous Chinese and South East Asian pigs.

p. pox see SWINEPOX.

p. typhoid see SALMONELLOSIS.

pig-sticking the so-called sport of hunting wild pigs on horseback and stabbing them to death with spears.

pigCHAMP commercial swine database program produced by University of Minnesota.

pigeon a member of the family Columbidae which also includes the doves. The domestic pigeons are generally gray, medium-sized birds which exist in a large number of breeds and races including Romans, Jacobins, tumblers, fantails, pouters, carrier pigeons and turtle-doves.

p. berry PHYTOLACCA *americana*.

p. breast deep-seated abscesses in the pectoral muscles of horses. Called also pectoral abscess.

p.-breeder's lung see BIRD-fancier's lung.

carrier p. pigeon with strong homing instincts used to carry messages over relatively long distances. Produced by breeding and selection between races of domestic pigeons. See also homing pigeon (below).

p. fly a member of the parasitic fly family Hippoboscidae or louse fly and an important parasite of domestic pigeon. Called also *Pseudolynchia canariensis*.

p. grass PANICUM *whitei*, SETARIA spp.

p. herpesvirus the cause of respiratory disease (coryza) in domestic pigeons.

homing p. pigeon with strong homing instincts used in racing and as a carrier pigeon (above). Produced by breeding and selection between races of domestic pigeon.

p. pox see PIGEONPOX.

slender (small) p. louse COLUMBICOLA *columbae*.

p. strongyle ORNITHOSTRONGYLUS *quadriradiatus*.

p. toed a condition in which the toes are turned inwards.

pigeonpox a disease caused by a poxvirus in the genus *Avipoxvirus*; characterized by the presence of pox lesions in the mouth and serious involvement of the eyes which may be sufficiently serious as to cause blindness.

pigeonwood see HEDYCARYA ARBOREA.

pigface see MESEMBRYANTHEMUM.

piggery condensate the liquid or dried condensate which collects on walls of piggeries in very cold climates; may be toxic because of its high nitrate content.

piglet baby pig from birth to conventional weaning age, usually 8 weeks. Called also erroneously suckler.

p. anemia see IRON nutritional deficiency.

hysterectomy-derived p. see HYPAR.

pigment 1. any coloring matter of the body. 2. a stain or dyestuff. 3. a paintlike medicinal preparation applied to the skin.

abnutzen p. see LIPOFUSCIN.

bile p. any one of the coloring matters of the bile, derived from heme, including bilirubin, biliverdin, etc.

blood p. any one of the pigments derived from hemoglobin, including heme, hematoidin, etc.

p. cells see MELANOCYTE.

p.-enhancing media formulated to promote the production of pigment by some bacteria, such as *Pseudomonas aeruginosa* and *Rhodococcus equi*, to aid in identification.

p. genes genes for each of the coat colors, e.g. white gene, black gene, orange gene.

respiratory p's substances, e.g. hemoglobin, myoglobin or cytochromes, which take part in the oxidative processes of the animal body.

pigmentary pertaining to or emanating from pigment.

p. incontinence a histopathological lesion in which melanin granules are free in the dermis and within dermal macrophages; it is associated with damage to the stratum basale and basement membrane of the epidermis.

p. keratitis see CORNEAL pigmentation.

pigmentation the deposition of coloring matter; the coloration or discoloration of a part by a pigment. See also HYPERPIGMENTATION, HYPOPIGMENTATION.

bacterial p. production of pigment is a characteristic of some bacteria which may be useful in identification. Examples are *Pseudomonas aeruginosa*, *Chromobacterium violaceum* and *Serratia marcescens*.

p. disorders see HYPERPIGMENTATION, LEUKODERMA, LEUKOTRICHIA, HYPOPIGMENTATION.

hematogenous p. pigmentation produced by accumulation of hemoglobin derivatives, such as hematoidin or hemosiderin.

pigmented colored by deposit of pigment.

p. villonodular synovitis a disease of humans characterized by the development of nodular and villous synovial proliferations; similar lesions are reported in horses and dogs; pigmentation results from deposition of blood pigments.

pigmentolysin a lysin that destroys pigment.

pigmentophage any pigment-destroying cell, especially such a cell of the hair.

pigweed *Amaranthus* spp., *Portulaca oleracea*, *Trianthema portulacastrum*.

PIH prolactin-inhibitory hormone.

piitis inflammation of the pia mater.

pika a genus of animals in the family Ochotonidae. Guinea-pig-sized rabbits with short ears found only in rough, high mountain terrain of North America. Called also rock rabbits, mouse hares, calling hares, *Ochotona* spp.

pike see ESOX.

p. fry rhabdovirus the cause of disease similar to SPRING VIREMIA OF CARP.

pike-perch important food fish in Europe and the USSR, including *Lucioperca*, *Perca* and *Stizostedion* spp.

pil- prefix meaning hair.

pila pillar, e.g. pila coronaris dorsalis—one of the several pillars in the rumen that divides it into semiseparate sacs.

pilar, pilary pertaining to the hair.

p. cyst TRICHILEMMAL cyst.

pilary canal lumen of the hair follicle.

pilewort RANUNCULUS *ficaria*.

pili plural of *pilus*.

p. torti curvature of the hair follicle results in twisted, flattened hairs; may be caused by systemic disease or inflammation of the hair follicle. Reported in cats.

pill a small globular or oval medicated mass to be swallowed; a tablet.

enteric-coated p. one enclosed in a substance that dissolves only when it has reached the intestines.

pillar a supporting column.

p's of the fauces folds of mucous membrane at the sides of the throat.

p. reins short reins attached to each side of a horse's headstall and fixed to a pillar on each side of the horse, the ties at 5 ft above the ground and the pillars 3 ft apart; method of restraint while grooming or saddling a horse.

ruminal p. fleshy ridges which circle the rumen dividing it into dorsal and ventral sacs; lesser coronary pillars demarcate the caudal sacs.

pillory a contrivance of pipe or wood that fits around the neck of the cow and stops the head from getting loose, but allows it to move up and down. Called also yokebail.

pilo- word element. [L.] *hair, composed of hair.*

Pilobolus a fungus which grows prolifically on cow feces and facilitates the spread of lungworm larvae by projecting them up to 10 feet when the fungal sporangia explode, as they do when they ripen.

pilocarpine a cholinergic alkaloid from leaves of *Pilocarpus jaborandi* and *P. microphyllus*; used as an ophthalmic miotic in the form of its hydrochloride and nitrate salts.

pilocystic hollow or cystlike, and containing hair; said of dermoid tumors.

piloerection erection of hair.

pilojection introduction of one or more hairs into an aneurysmal sac, to promote formation of a blood clot.

pilomatricoma pilomatrixoma.

pilomatrixoma a benign, circumscribed, calcifying epithelial neoplasm derived from hair matrix cells, manifested as a small firm intracutaneous spheroid mass. Kerry blue terriers have a predisposition to develop these. Called also epithelioma of Malherbe, calcifying epithelioma.

pilomotor causing movement of the hairs, piloerection; pertaining to the arrector muscles.

p. nerves the nerves supplying the arrector muscles of the hair.

pilonidal having a nidus of hairs.

p. sinus see DERMOID cyst.

pilose hairy; covered with hair.

pilosebaceous pertaining to the hair follicles and sebaceous glands.

p. follicle sebaceous glands empty into the pilary canal.

pilot trials preliminary trial using a small number of animals to obtain general information without necessarily achieving statistical significance.

pilot whale see GLOBICEPHALA.

pilus pl. *pili* [L.] 1. a hair. 2. fine, filamentous appendage found on the surface of many gram-negative bacteria, shorter, thinner and straighter than flagella. There are two kinds of pili: (a) a larger form that is hollow and found on male bacterial cells only; it is used in bacterial cell conjugation, and (b) a smaller form which is of major significance in adherence of bacterial cells to epithelial surfaces such as the intestinal mucosa or mammary gland epithelium. Antipilus antibody can provide protection against disease. Called also fimbria.

p. cuniculatus pl. *pili cuniculati;* burrowing hair.

p. incarnatus pl. *pili incarnati;* ingrown hair.

p. lanei wool fiber.

p. tacti tactile hairs about the lips, nostrils and eyes.

p. tortus pl. *pili torti;* twisted hair; see also PILI torti.

Pimelea Australian genus of poisonous annual herbs and perennial shrubs in the family Thymelaeaceae; cause two major syndromes: (1) generalized edema, called also St. George or Moree disease, caused in cattle only by a diterpenoid ester, simplexin; the syndrome is one of chronic, right-sided heart failure leading to hydrothorax, massive anasarca and jugular vein distension plus profound anemia and persistent diarrhea; (2) in species other than cattle the only sign is severe diarrhea and a fatal outcome caused by dihydroxycoumarin glycosides; toxic species include *P. decora* (Flinders poppy), *P. elongata*, *P. flava*, *P. glauca*, *P. haematostachya* (pimelea or red poppy), *P. latifolia* (*P. altior*), *P. linifolia*, *P. microcephala*, *P. neoanglica*, *P. pauciflora*, *P. prostrata* (Strathmore weed), *P. simplex*, *P. trichostachya*. Called also many common names, mostly some variation on riceflower, flaxweed.

pimelitis inflammation of the adipose tissue.

pimelosis 1. conversion into fat. 2. obesity.

pimozide an antipsychotic agent in humans; used for its long-acting central antiemetic effect in dogs.

Pimpinella genus of plants in family Apiaceae; includes *P. anisum*. See ANISE.

pimple an elevated inflamed lesion about 0.5 inch diameter, raised above the skin surface, with a necrotic center which commonly points and bursts.

pimply gut see ESOPHAGOSTOMIASIS.

pin a slender, elongated piece of metal used for securing fixation of parts.

p. bone the triangular ischial tuber; a term used almost exclusively in cattle.

p. cutter a sophisticated, surgical version of a boltcutter, usually with multiple scissor joints.

p. drill a sterilizable drill chuck can be fitted to a surgical power drill and fitted with a surgical bit to match plating screws or orthopedic pins.

intramedullary p. see INTERNAL fixation.

Steinmann p. a metal rod for the internal fixation of fractures. See also STEINMANN pin.

p. teat inverted nipple, seen mostly in sows.

p. toes toes turned inwards. Called also pigeon toes.

p. vise a device for attaching to the end of an intramedullary pin to provide a grip for placement in bone. See also CHUCK.

Pin Yin one of the methods used to convert spoken Chinese into Roman alphabet and numbers.

pincement [Fr.] pinching of the flesh in massage.

Pincer emasculatome see BURDIZZO EMASCULATOME.

pinch biopsy a method for gastrointestinal biopsy using forceps, introduced by endoscopy, to grasp and cut small specimens of mucosa and lamina propria.

pinch technique a method of correcting entropion in which forceps are used to crush enough skin of the lower lid to correct the abnormal position; it is then cut away and the defect sutured.

pincherry PRUNUS *pennsylvanica.*

pindan poison VELLEIA *panduriformis.*

pindborg tumor see CALCIFYING epithelial odontogenic tumor.

pindone one of a series of 2-aryl-1,3-indandiones which have potent anticoagulant activity. Can cause fatal hemorrhage in animals.

pine 1. unthriftiness of calves due to nutritional deficiency of copper. There is a stiff gait, painful joints, graying of the haircoat and diarrhea in some. May also be used to describe the unthriftiness caused by nutritional deficiency of cobalt. 2. a tree; see PINUS. 3. many other trees are also called pine incorrectly, e.g. 'cypress pine'.

p. needle abortion see PINUS, ISOCUPRESSIC ACID.

p. lupine LUPINUS *albicaulis.*

p. oil an extract from pine trees which is used as an astringent, antiseptic, antitussive and in cattle as an antifoaming agent to treat bloat.

pineal 1. shaped like a pine cone. 2. pertaining to the pineal body.

p. body, p. gland a small, conical endocrine gland attached by a stalk to the dorsal wall of the third ventricle of the cerebrum. In certain amphibians and reptiles the gland functions as a light receptor. In most mammals, including humans, it appears to be the major or unique site of melatonin biosynthesis. The effect of melatonin on the body and the exact function of the pineal body remain uncertain. There is an increasing body of evidence that the pineal body is inhibitory to the gonads and that it is the principal mechanism in the known effect of environmental illumination on estrous cycles. It is proposed that the retina perceives the changes in light intensity and stimulates the pineal gland via the sympathetic nervous system.

p. extract see MELATONIN.

p. eye in lower vertebrates the pineal body is a third or pineal eye.

p. gland see pineal body (above).

pinealism the condition due to deranged secretion of the pineal body.

pinealoblastoma pinealoma in which the pineal cells are not well differentiated.

pinealocyte an epithelioid cell of the pineal body.

pinealoma a rare tumor of the pineal body composed of neoplastic nests of large epithelial cells; it may cause hydrocephalus, precocious puberty and gait disturbances.

pinene the principal component of turpentine oil.

ping clear, sharp, high-pitched, metallic, musical note created by a flicking percussion stroke over a viscus containing gas under moderate pressure and a small amount of fluid; used extensively in the physical examination of the abdomen in cattle and horses.

pingue HYMENOXYS *richardsonii.*

pinholing minute holes in a can that permit entry of air and spoilage of the contents. The pinholes may be selfsealing causing the cans to blow, often late in their shelf life.

piniform conical or cone-shaped.

pining the state of having PINE (1).

pinion rear section of a bird's wing; holds the flight feathers.

pinioning a permanent alteration of a bird to prevent its flying. The standard operation is amputation of the distal wing including the carpal, metacarpal and phalangeal bones of one wing. Alternative procedures are tenotomy and ankylosis of a joint.

pink disease pink color of tissues in broiler chickens dying of fatty liver and kidney disease which responds to dietary supplementation with biotin. Called also pinks.

pink dock RUMEX *vesicarius.*

pink-eyed coat color series the *p* allele series causes dilution mainly of dark colors, loss of retinal pigmentation and sometimes male sterility.

pink nose LANTANA poisoning.

pink rot see FLEECE rot.

pink rot fungus of celery *Sclerotinia* spp.; of parsnip *Ceratocystis* spp.

pink salmon ONCORHYNCHUS *gorbuscha.*

pink tooth see pink TEETH.

pinkeye see INFECTIOUS bovine keratoconjunctivitis, contagious OPHTHALMIA (sheep and goats).

pinks see PINK DISEASE.

pinky syndrome vitiligo. See also Arabian FADING syndrome.

pinna the projecting part of the ear lying outside the head; auricle.

pinnal pertaining to or emanating from the pinna, e.g. pinnal ALOPECIA. See also AURICULAR, EAR.

p. cartilage see auricular CARTILAGE.

p. fissure see ear FISSURE.

pinnate featherlike; said of a muscle in which the fibers lie at angles to its tendon. The fibers may be unipinnate, bipinnate, etc.

pinnation in a pinnate muscle, the way in which the muscle fibers are attached to its tendon.

pinning a method of bone fixation, usually for treatment of fractures, in which metal pins are placed within the medullary cavity or anchored in bone. Two types of pins in common use are Steinmann and Rush. See also INTERNAL fixation.

pinniped member of the mammal family of Pinnipedia, including seals, sealions, walruses. Their bodies are fishlike, covered with hair, have four limbs and can move around on land. Their tails are vestigial.

p. stranding the largely unexplained migrational phenomenon of cetaceans and pinnipeds in which the animals swim into shallow water and up onto land from where they are unable or unwilling to depart. Single strandings may be due to disease. Multiple strandings may similarly result from illness in the leader of the pod. They are also known to occur in specific locations where the local land appears to confuse the whales' direction-finding ability.

pinocyte a cell that exhibits pinocytosis.

pinocytosis a mechanism by which cells ingest extracellular fluid and its contents; it involves the formation of invaginations by the cell membrane, which close and break off to form fluid-filled vacuoles in the cytoplasm.

pinosome the intracellular vacuole formed by pinocytosis.

pinscher a medium-sized working dog with characteristic proportions; its head is approximately half the length of the back, from withers to the base of the tail. The coat is short in any solid color, with red or tan markings. See also DOBERMAN PINSCHER, MINIATURE PINSCHER.

pint a unit of liquid measure in the apothecaries' system, 16 fluid ounces. The Imperial pint is 568.26 milliliters and the American pint is 473.17 milliliters.

Pinta fever see ROCKY MOUNTAIN SPOTTED FEVER.

pinto a broken colored or paint horse used for riding. See also PIEBALD, SKEWBALD. Called also paint. Special pinto colorings are OVERO and TOBIANO.

Pinus a genus of coniferous trees in the family Pinaceae.

P. cubensis*, *P. ponderosa*, *P. radiata the leaves of the trees *P. ponderosa* (western yellow pine), *P. radiata* and *P. cubensis* contain isocupressic acid and are abortifacient when fed to cows.

P. taeda the leaves are reported to cause fatal indigestion in cows. Called also loblolly pine.

pinworm any oxyurid, especially *Oxyuris equi* and *Probstmayria vivipara* both in horses, *Passalurus ambiguus* in rabbits, *Syphacia obvelata* in hamster and mouse.

Pinzgau a multipurpose breed of central European cattle, red-brown color, colorsided, colored head. Called also Pinzgauer.

Pinzgauer 1. PINZGAU cattle. 2. NORIC HORSE.

Piophila casei the cheese or ham fly. The larvae are the skippers of neglected food. They leap around when they are looking for a dry spot to pupate.

pipecurium pipecuronium bromide.

pipecuronium bromide a long-acting, non-depolarizing neuromuscular blocking agent similar to tubocurarine.

pipemidic acid a quinolone antibiotic, similar to nalidixic acid.

piperacetazine a phenothiazine tranquilizer used as a sedative and antipruritic.

piperacillin an extended-spectrum semisynthetic penicillin active against a wide variety of gram-negative, gram-positive and anaerobic bacteria.

piperazine an anthelmintic; several of its salts are used, especially in horses and dogs. A useful agent especially against ascarids. Combined with a benzimidazole is effective against *Parascaris equorum* and benzimidazole-resistant small strongyles.

Piperazine is a very safe medicament but poisoning occurs on doses that are several times normal. Signs include incoordination, pupillary dilatation, hyperesthesia, somnolence, tremor, swaying at rest and recumbency. Spontaneous recovery usual.

piperidine alkaloids include CONIINE, CYNAPINE, LOBELINE, NICOTINE.

piperidolate hydrochloride a hydrochloric acid salt used to treat achlorhydria.

piperocaine a local anesthetic, used as the hydrochloride salt. Has the characteristic of being able to be autoclaved repeatedly without loss of potency.

piperonyl butoxide a synergist used with, and as an enhancer for, pyrethrum and rotenone in the control of ectoparasites.

pipestem long, thin and rounded like the stem of a pipe.

p. feces loose feces passed through a stenotic or undilated sphincter.

p. liver one marked by the calcified, fibrosed bile ducts of chronic FASCIOLIASIS.

pipette, pipet [Fr.] 1. a volumetrically accurate glass or transparent plastic tube used in measuring or transferring small quantities of liquid or gas. 2. to dispense by means of a pipette.

pipimedic acid an early quinolone antibiotic.

Pipturus argenteus toxic plant in the family Urticaceae; an unidentified toxin causes diarrhea, dyspnea, recumbency.

pirbuterol a synthetic β-receptor agonist, used as the acetate or hydrochloride salt in the treatment of bronchospasm.

pirenzepine a selective M_1 cholinergic antagonist; used as an antiemetic in dogs.

piriform pear-shaped.

piritrexin a folate antagonist used in the treatment of toxoplasmosis.

pirlimycin a lincosamide antibiotic, similar to lincomycin.

Piroplasma see BABESIA, THEILERIA.

piroplasmosis see BABESIOSIS.

piroxicam a nonsteroidal anti-inflammatory agent with antineoplastic activity; used in the treatment of transitional cell carcinoma in dogs.

Piry virus in the genus *Vesiculovirus*.

Piscinoodinium see OODINIUM.

Piscirickettsiosis rickettsial disease of salmonids caused by *Piscirickettsia salmonis*. Has caused huge losses of Coho salmon in Chile.

piscivorous fisheating; said of birds.

pisgoed [Af.] see ULCERATIVE dermatosis.

pisgras [Af.] see ULCERATIVE dermatosis.

pisiform 1. resembling a pea in size and shape. 2. the accessory carpal bone.

pistol a weapon for delivery of a missile; usually a weapon to fire a bullet, used in euthanasia.

balling p. a device shaped like a pistol but loaded with a medicinal bolus which is fired into the pharynx of a horse by the operation of a spring loaded piston.

Pisum a genus of plants in the legume family Fabaceae; an unidentified toxin causes lameness, incoordination, recumbency; includes *P. arvense* (field or Austrian pea), *P. sativum* (domestic pea, field pea), *P. sativum* var. *arvense* (field pea).

pit 1. a hollow fovea or indentation. 2. a pockmark. 3. to indent, or to become and remain for a few minutes indented, by pressure. 4. seed of a fruit, e.g. cherry. Strictly refers to the hard woody coating which surrounds the seed.

anal p. the proctodeum of the embryo.

auditory p. a distinct depression in each auditory placode, marking the beginning of the embryonic development of the internal ear.

p. bull a term used in describing various types of dogs used in past times for fighting in pits. Now, usually refers to the specific breed, AMERICAN PIT BULL TERRIER.

lens p. a pitlike depression in the fetal head where the lens develops.

nasal p. a depression appearing in the olfactory placodes in the early stages of development of the nose. Called also olfactory pit.

olfactory p. see nasal pit (above).

otic p. early stage in the development of the embryonic inner ear.

p. pony pony used in a mine to haul mined rock. Breed varies as long as it is small, e.g. Shetland pony.

p. of stomach the epigastric fossa or epigastric region.

p. viper see VIPER.

pitch 1. a dark, more or less viscous residue from distillation of tar and other substances. 2. natural asphalt of various kinds. 3. the quality of sound dependent on the frequency of vibration of the waves producing it. 4. horizontal spacing of characters in a computer printer.

coal tar p. see COAL TAR PITCH.

pitchblend a black mineral containing uranium oxide; from it are obtained radium, polonium and uranium.

pitchery DUBOISIA *hopwoodii*.

pith soft, spongy, plant tissue.

Pithecia see SAKI.

pithecoid apelike.

pithing 1. destruction of the brain and spinal cord by thrusting a blunt needle into the vertebral canal and cranium, done on animals to destroy sensibility preparatory to experimenting on their living tissue. 2. an abattoir method of euthanasia; the animal is stunned by a captive bolt pistol and a cane or coiled wire passed into the cranium through the hole. The brain is destroyed by moving the cane about.

Pithomyces chartarum called also *Sporidesmium bakeri.* See FACIAL eczema.

pithomycotoxicosis liver damage caused by the toxins of *Pithomyces chartarum.* See also FACIAL eczema.

Pitressin see VASOPRESSIN.

P. tannate test see ANTIDIURETIC hormone response test.

pitting 1. the formation, usually by scarring, of a small depression. 2. the removal from erythrocytes, by the spleen, of such structures as iron granules, without destruction of the cells. 3. remaining indented for a few minutes after removal of firm-finger-pressure, distinguishing fluid edema from myxedema.

pituicyte any of the distinctive fusiform cells comprising most of the neurohypophysis.

pituicytoma a neoplasm of the neurohypophysis.

pituitary 1. a neuroepithelial endocrine gland of dual origin at the base of the brain in the sella turcica, attached by a stalk to the hypothalamus; called also hypophysis. It is composed of two main lobes, the anterior lobe (anterior pituitary, ADENOHYPOPHYSIS), secreting several important hormones that regulate the proper functioning of the thyroids, gonads, adrenal cortex, and other endocrine glands, and the posterior lobe (posterior pituitary, NEUROHYPOPHYSIS) whose cells serve as a reservoir for hormones having antidiuretic and oxytocic action, releasing them as needed, and in response to signals from the hypothalamus, itself responding to incoming signals from the nervous system received by the thalamus. Called also hypophysis. See also PITUITRIN, VASOPRESSIN, OXYTOCIN, ANTIDIURETIC hormone, THYROTROPIN releasing hormone, ADRENOCORTICOTROPIC hormone, FOLLICLE-STIMULATING HORMONE, LUTEINIZING HORMONE, MELANOCYTE-stimulating hormone, PROLACTIN and GROWTH HORMONE. 2. pertaining to the pituitary gland. 3. a preparation of the pituitary glands of animals, used therapeutically.

p. abscess abscess in the rete mirabile of the pituitary is recognizable clinically in cattle. The syndrome begins with a characteristic inability to close the mouth. Saliva drools, the tongue is prolapsed slightly, and there may be blindness, opisthotonos, loss of balance and recumbency.

p.-adrenal axis the interactions between hypothalamus, pituitary and adrenal cortex, involving releasing factors, tropic hormones and negative feedback mechanisms.

p. alopecia see GROWTH HORMONE-responsive dermatosis.

p. cachexia see pituitary CACHEXIA.

p. dwarfism congenital dwarfism with all parts properly proportioned. Affected animals are miniatures of normals. There is delayed bone development and epiphyseal fusion is retarded. It is inherited in cattle and German shepherd dogs. See also German shepherd dog DWARFISM.

p. giantism acromegaly.

p. gonadotropins FOLLICLE-STIMULATING HORMONE, LUTEINIZING HORMONE.

fetal p. hormones in sheep, cows and goats fetal pituitary ACTH stimulates fetal adrenal cortisol production inducing in turn placental estrogen secretion. Hence fetal placental hormone is important in the induction of parturition.

p. hypoplasia congenital absence (aplasia) or incomplete growth (hypoplasia) of gland. Occurs in one form of inherited prolonged gestation in cattle and in poisoning by the weed *Salsola tuberculata* var. *tomentosa.* It is an inherited trait in German shepherd dogs.

posterior p. 1. the posterior lobe of the pituitary gland; the neurohypophysis. 2. a preparation of animal posterior pituitary having the pharmacological actions of its hormones, oxytocin and vasopressin; used mainly as an antidiuretic in the treatment of diabetes insipidus and as a vasoconstrictor.

p. rete mirabile abscess see PITUITARY abscess.

p. tumor includes adenoma, carcinoma and craniopharyngioma. All cause pressure on surrounding tissue and some cause endocrinological disturbances.

pituitrin an extract of bovine pituitary gland containing oxytocin and vasopressin, now displaced by preparations containing only one of the hormones.

pituri, pitury DUBOISIA *hopwoodii.*

pityriasis a group of skin diseases in humans characterized by branlike scales on the skin surface. The skin is not thickened and its surface is unbroken. Pityriasis rosea of pigs is the only diseases in animals that is similar.

p. rosea see porcine juvenile pustular psoriasiform DERMATITIS.

pityroid furfuraceous; branny; resembling pityriasis.

Pityrosporon see MALASSEZIA.

pivalate USAN contraction for trimethylacetate.

pivamdinocillin, pivmecillinam an ester of amdinocillin.

pivampicillin an ester of ampicillin with the same broad spectrum of antibiotic activity.

PIVKA proteins induced by vitamin K deficiency or antagonists; nonfunctional precursor forms of vitamin K-dependent coagulation factors, lacking carboxylation of glutamic acid residues, found in animals treated or poisoned with anticoagulants.

pivmecillinam pivamdinocillin.

pivoters a term used in the meat industry for animals that walk in circles.

pivoting said of the exercise demanded of a horse when testing a limb for weakness or lameness; the horse is forced to turn very tightly so that it actually pivots on the limb being examined.

pixel a *pic*ture *el*ement such as a dot on a video display screen. The greater the concentration of pixels the clearer the image.

A CT scan or PET scan is composed of an array of squares (pixels), each of which is colored a uniform shade of gray or another color. The corresponding region in the tissue slice that is imaged is called a *voxel* (volume element). See also computed TOMOGRAPHY.

pizzle 1. prepuce. 2. penis.

p. dropping a farm procedure used in male sheep to reduce local wetting of the wool as a prevention against pizzle rot. The anterior attachment of the prepuce to the abdominal wall is severed.

p. rot see ENZOOTIC balanoposthitis.

p. stain wool stained by urine; in belly wool from male sheep.

PK pyruvate kinase.

pK the negative logarithm of the ionization constant (K) of an acid, the pH of a solution in which half of the acid molecules are ionized.

PKU phenylketonuria.

placebo [L.] a substance given to a patient as medicine or a procedure performed on a patient that has no intrinsic therapeutic value but pleases the patient's owner who expects to have to give the animal some medicine. A placebo may be administered in the form of a sugar pill or an injection of sterile water.

Placebos are also used in controlled clinical trials of new drugs. While some patients selected at random are given the new drug, others are given a placebo. Often this is an active placebo that mimics the new drug's side-effects. Neither the patients nor the veterinarians know who is receiving the real drug. The patients taking the new drug must have significantly more relief of signs than the control group taking the placebo for the new drug to be considered to be effective. Placebos can produce an effect that is either positive, with improvement of signs, or negative, with worsening of signs or the appearance of adverse side-effects.

placenta pl. *placentae, placentas* [L.] an organ characteristic of true mammals during pregnancy, joining mother and offspring, providing endocrine secretion and selective exchange of soluble bloodborne substances through apposition of uterine and trophoblastic vascularized parts. Called also afterbirth. See also FETAL membranes, PLACENTATION.

Domestic animals have a chorioallantoic placenta in which the outer layer of the allantois is fused with the chorion and the fetal umbilical vessels are distributed in the connective tissue between the two. Placentae are classified in several ways; based on the tissues of the dam and the fetus that contact each other; based on the proportion of the surface area of the fetal membranes that is in fact placentacious; based on loss of tissue at birth, etc. Thus the bovine placenta is epitheliochorial, cotyledonary and nondeciduate.

The major function of the placenta is to allow diffusion of nutrients from the dam's blood into the fetus's blood and diffusion of waste products from the fetus back to the dam. This two-way exchange takes place across the placental membrane, which is semipermeable. The placenta also produces hormones such as progesterone and estrogen.

choriovitelline p. a placentation in which the yolk sac becomes involved in the fetal–maternal union.

cotyledonary p. distribution of the villi on the fetal chorion is localized in multiple circumscribed areas—the cotyledons.

diffuse p. the villi on the fetal chorion is diffuse over the entire placenta as in mares and sows.

discoid p. a placenta in which the chorionic villi are arranged in a circular plate as in human and rodent placentae.

endotheliochorial p. the maternal vessels in the endometrium are bared to their endothelium and these are in contact with the chorion of the fetal membranes. This occurs in the bitch and queen.

epitheliochorial p. the uterine epithelium of the uterus and the chorion are in contact in this placentation, and there is no erosion of the epithelium. Characteristic of cows, sows and mares. Called also adeciduate placenta.

hemochorial p. a type of placenta in which all maternal layers are lost so that fetal tissue is in contact with frank maternal blood, as occurs in insectivores, rodents, rabbits and most primates.

nondeciduate p. no maternal tissue is lost when the pregnancy terminates.

retained p. the placenta has not been passed within 12 hours after the fetus has been delivered. Represents a potential beginning for metritis and infertility. Often difficult to assess in carnivores which rapidly eat the placenta.

syndesmochorial p. a type of placentation characterized by an endometrial attachment to the chorion with a limited amount of destruction of the endometrial epithelium. Formerly thought to be characteristic of the ewe and goat doe, these species are now known to have epitheliochorial placentae.

zonary p. a placenta in which the chorionic villi are restricted to an equatorial girdle, as in the bitch and queen.

placental pertaining to or emanating from placenta.

p. barrier the placental separation of maternal and fetal blood which varies in its structure and permeability between the species. In general the more layers of cells between the two circulations the less permeable the membrane. In none of the domestic animals are significant amounts of immune globulins or erythrocyte antigens passed through the membranes unless the epithelium is damaged. See also PLACENTA.

p. calcification accumulations of mineral deposit especially around the vessels and in the allantois, a normal occurrence in most species.

p. edema edema of the placenta, without necessarily any involvement of the fetus.

p. hormones the placenta in all species produces estrogens and progesterone. In the cow it also produces lactogen, a hormone that influences structural and functional aspects of milk production. In the mare the ENDOMETRIAL cups produce PMSG (now called eCG) which assists in the maintenance of pregnancy. The equine, feline and primate placentae also produce RELAXIN which has a similar action.

p. implantation the placenta of a viable fetus, escaped from the genital tract, can implant successfully to the peritoneum.

p. inflammation see PLACENTITIS.

p. lactogen a placental hormone present in the cow's peripheral circulation at about 160 days of pregnancy; thought to have prolactin and growth-hormone capabilities.

p. mole see MOLE.

p. plaques are normal structures on the amnion in most species. They are foci of squamous epithelium.

p. removal manual removal per vagina, detaching the placenta from each caruncle in turn.

p. transfer of immunoglobulins see placental barrier (above) and passive IMMUNITY.

placentation 1. the series of events following implantation of the embryo and leading to development of the placenta. 2. the nature of the implantation. See also PLACENTA.

adventitial p. developmental of additional areas outside the normal areas, e.g. intercotyledonary in cattle.

cotyledonary p. the areas of placentation are limited to caruncles, approximately circular masses scattered over the placenta. Characteristic of the cow, ewe and goat doe.

diffuse p. the whole of the surface of the chorion is placental.

intercotyledonary p. abnormal placental attachments between the cotyledons, in cows.

zonal p. only some zones of the placenta have a vascular area involved in placentation. Characteristic of the bitch and the queen.

placentitis inflammation of the placenta; causes abortion or, by adhesions, retention of the placenta.

placentography radiological visualization of the placenta after injection of a contrast medium.

placentoid resembling the placenta.

placentome the cotyledon plus the caruncle.

placentopathy any placental disease.

placentophagia eating of placenta by the dam; common in carnivores.

placing the way in which an animal places its feet when moving.

p. reflex a postural reaction tested by supporting the animal and approaching a surface such as a table to see how the animal positions its feet; performed with and without a blindfold to test its tactile and visual responses.

Placobdella leeches found in the nasal cavities of aquatic anatid birds. Recorded species include *P. rugosa*, *P. catanigera*.

placode a platelike structure, especially a thickening of the ectoderm marking the site of future development in the early embryo of an organ of special sense, e.g. the *auditory placode* (ear), *lens placode* (eye) and *olfactory placode* (nose).

lens p. the ectodermal thickening which develops into the lens vesicle and later the lens.

nasal p. one of a pair of ectodermal thickenings which are the forerunners of the external nares and nasopharyngeal epithelium.

olfactory p. an ectodermal thickening of the embryo which ultimately provides the sensory nerves for the olfactory region of the nasal mucosa.

otic p. one of the pair of ectodermal thickenings in the vertebrate embryo which invaginates and is a major contributor to the internal ear.

placoid platelike or plaquelike.

Plagiobothrys genus of plants in family Boraginaceae; causes nitrate–nitrite poisoning; called also popcorn flower.

plagiocephaly bizarre distortion of the shape of the skull resulting from irregular closure of the cranial sutures.

Plagiorchis a genus of flukes (digenetic trematodes) in the family Plagiorchiidae.

P. arcuatus found in, and causes inflammation of, the oviduct of fowls.

P. lutrae found in otters.

***P. megalorchis* (syn. *P. laricola*)** found in turkey poults and in wild birds.

Plagiorhynchus formosus see PROSTHORHYNCUS FORMOSUS.

plague an epidemic of disease attended by great mortality.

bubonic p. an acute febrile, infectious, highly fatal disease caused by the bacillus *Yersinia pestis.* It is primarily a disease of rats and other rodents, dogs and cats, and is usually spread to humans by fleas. The more common form of plague is the bubonic. There is also a pneumonic type in humans, which can be spread directly from person to person by droplet infection. The clinical signs in all species are fever, vomiting and enlargement of lymph nodes, the buboes that give the disease its name.

cattle p. see RINDERPEST.

duck p. an acute infectious disease of ducks caused by a herpesvirus and characterized by tissue hemorrhages and blood free in body cavities, eruptions on the mucosae of the digestive tract, degeneration of parenchymatous organs and lesions in lymph nodes. Called also duck virus enteritis.

equine p. see AFRICAN HORSE SICKNESS.

fowl p. see AVIAN influenza.

pneumonic p. see bubonic plague (above).

septicemic p. hematogenous spread of infection to many organs may occur without the formation of buboes; occurs in the cat with pulmonary involvement, disseminated intravascular coagulopathy and death.

swine p. see SWINE plague.

sylvatic p. bubonic plague in wild animals in uninhabited areas. See also SYLVATIC plague.

plain lacking in style; unadorned.

p.-bodied said of a sheep with very few wrinkles.

p. quarters a horse with fat, rounded hindquarters resembling those of a pig.

p. wool when the crimp in the staple is barely visible.

plainhead in canaries, one with plain feathering on the head instead of a crest.

plains bahia see BAHIA OPPOSITIFOLIA.

plains milkweed ASCLEPIAS *pumila*.

plains plover-daisy see IXIOLAENA BREVICOMPTA.

plane 1. a flat surface determined by the position of three points in space. 2. a specified level, as the plane of anesthesia. 3. to rub away or abrade. See also PLANING and PLASTIC surgery. 4. a superficial incision in the wall of a cavity or between tissue layers, especially in plastic surgery, made so that the precise point of entry into the cavity or between the layers can be determined.

coronal p. frontal plane, an ambiguous term when applied to quadripeds and bipeds.

dorsal p. any plane passing longitudinally through the body from side to side, at right angles to the median plane and dividing the body into dorsal and ventral parts. Called also coronal plane, frontal plane.

horizontal p. one passing through the body at right angles to the median plane, and dividing the body into upper and lower parts.

inclined p. an intraoral acrylic or metal appliance used in orthodontics to guide a tooth into a new position by using pressure applied when the mouth is closed normally. Commonest use is to move canines laterally.

median p. one passing longitudinally through the body from front to back and dividing it into right and left halves.

nasal p. the space between the nostrils.

nasolabial p. the extension of the nasal plane between the nostrils into the upper lip in cattle.

nuchal p. the flat surface at the back of the occipital bone below the nuchal crest.

rostral p. the bare area on the dorsum of the snout of the pig.

sagittal p. a vertical plane through the body parallel to the median plane (or to the sagittal suture) and dividing the body into left and right portions.

transverse p. one passing through the body, at right angles to the sagittal and dorsal planes, and dividing the body into cranial and caudal portions.

vertical p. one perpendicular to a horizontal plane, dividing the body into left and right, or front and back portions.

planigraphy a method of body-section radiography that shows in detail structures lying in a predetermined plane of the body while blurring structures in other planes, produced by movement of the film and x-ray tube in certain specified directions. See also TOMOGRAPHY.

planing abrasion of disfigured skin to promote re-epithelization with minimal scarring; done by mechanical means (dermabrasion) or by application of a caustic (chemabrasion). See also plastic SURGERY.

dental p. the scraping or abrasion of the cemental surface of a tooth after the removal of calculus in order to remove bacterial endotoxins.

plank method a method of relieving a torsion of the uterus in a mare. The mare is cast and laid on her back. A plank with several people standing on it is used to put pressure on the abdomen while the mare is rolled on her back towards the plank.

plankton a collective name for small animal and plant

(phytoplankton) organisms that drift passively in all natural bodies of water. The starting point of the aquatic food chain. Called also microalgae.

planktonophagous eating or subsisting solely on plankton.

planned animal health/production program regular visits to farms by a veterinarian to monitor health parameters, especially fertility and mastitis in dairy herds, and check productivity indexes, e.g. weight gains in beef cattle, followed by reports on achievement relative to targets and the application or recommendation about treatment or preventive measures.

planoconcave flat on one side and concave on the other.

planoconvex flat on one side and convex on the other.

planography planigraphy.

Planorbis a water snail intermediate host to paramphistomes.

plant a member of the vegetable kingdom; living things characterized by absence of locomotion, absence of special senses, and feeding only on inorganic substances.

abortigenic p. plants that cause abortion include *Pinus*, *Cupressus* and *Astragalus* spp.

p. alkaloids see ALKALOID.

p. awns sharp, long processes attached to seed casings of plants, mostly grasses; important causes of skin and oral lesions in grazing animals, and to housed animals when fed hay containing the plants.

p. eating both dogs and cats may eat GRASS; indoor animals sometimes eat ornamental plants, some of which are poisonous.

p. edemagens plant substances that cause edema in animals, e.g. 3-methyl indole, produced in the rumen from tryptophan.

p. hormones organic substances produced by plants which are extracted and used as herbicides or plant growth stimulants. Some of them cause long-term ill health in animals if drunk in large quantities.

p. poisoning the list of poison plants is very large and it is necessary to know the suspect plant's botanical name to begin an effective search for information about it. In order to exert an effect on an animal the plant has, in most cases, to be eaten. There are a few plants that exert a toxic effect by inhalation or by skin contact.

p. protein the proteins in plants. Common, protein-rich plants include alfalfa, the oilseed meals, e.g. soyabean, cottonseed and linseed meals, clover, the legume seeds, e.g. peas, beans.

teratogenic p. plants that cause congenital defects include *Lupinus*, *Lathyrus*, *Leucaena*, *Nicotiana*, *Conium*, *Astragalus*, *Oxytropis*, *Veratrum*, *Vicia*, *Salsola* spp.

p. toxins phytotoxins, elaborated by plants, in some cases incorporating an inorganic element, e.g. selenocompounds, and in some cases present in the plant in an inert state, requiring an additional ingredient, e.g. ruminal fermentation to activate it.

Plantago a large genus of plants in the family Plantaginaceae.

P. psyllium a plant whose seeds resemble fleas. Used at one time as a flea repellent. See also PSYLLIUM.

P. varia a common weed of native pastures providing scant feed. Called also plaintain and sometimes lamb's tongue, a name best reserved for *Chenopodium* spp., which have a potential to cause oxalate poisoning.

plantain two plant species are called by this common name. See PLANTAGO *varia*.

plantain-eaters see MUSOPHAGID.

plantar pertaining to the sole or caudal aspect of the digit.

p. cushion see DIGITAL cushion.

p. ligament strong ligaments running down the backs of the hind paws, or the plantar surface of the hock in ungulates.

p. nerve block nerve block of the medial and lateral plantar nerves to desensitize the digit in the horse. May be done at a high or low site. Called also palmar nerve block.

plantaris [L.] 1. plantar. 2. the superficial digital flexor muscle of the hindlimb.

plantation flies see HYDROTOEA *irritans*.

plantation walk the four-beat, running walk gait characteristic of the Tennessee walking horse.

plantigrade a method of locomotion seen in bears, monkeys and humans, in which the animal walks on the phalanges, metacarpal and carpal bones, as distinct from digitigrade.

p. stance seen in dogs and cats with various neuropathies and myopathies, particularly in diabetic neuropathy and hypokalemic myopathy.

planula a larval coelenterate.

planum pl. *plana* [L.] plane.

p. nasale see nasal PLANE.

p. nasolabiale the plate of moist, highly cornified epidermis, completely hairless, containing tubular merocrine glands around the nostrils and upper lip which is characteristic of the muzzle of cattle.

p. rostrale the front plate of the muzzle of pigs; highly cornified epithelium, contains many tubular merocrine glands and a few fine hairs.

plaque 1. any patch or flat area. 2. a clear area of cell lysis caused by viral replication on a cell monolayer.

amniotic p. small, 1 to 2 inch diameter, poxlike lesion on the inside of the amnion. Constant on the bovine amnion during the middle trimester and causes no problems.

annular p. seen in equine lupus erythematosus panniculitis.

p. assay a method of quantifying the number of infectious units by inoculating serial dilutions of a viral suspension on a cell culture monolayer, overlaying with a medium containing agarose and after several days incubation, counting the number of plaques formed; recorded as plaque forming units/ml.

atheromatous p. a deposit of predominantly fatty material in the lining of blood vessels occurring in atherosclerosis.

bacterial p., dental p. a mass adhering to the enamel surface of a tooth, composed of a mixed colony of bacteria in an intercellular matrix of bacterial and salivary polymers and remnants of epithelial cells and leukocytes. It may cause caries, dental calculi and periodontal disease.

cutaneous p. an elevated, solid structure without a necrotic center, up to 1 to 2 inch diameter with an unbroken surface.

drug p. cutaneous, subcutaneous or subconjunctival deposits formed as a result of injection of some drugs, particularly repository steroid preparations. May be unsightly and a cause of conjunctivitis.

ear p. see EAR plaque.

eosinophilic p. see EOSINOPHILIC plaque.

p.-forming cells see plaque assay (above).

p.-forming count the number of plaques formed in the plaque assay.

senile p. described in the brain of old dogs.

siderotic p. nodules observed as dry, yellow encrustations on the splenic capsule of old dogs.

plasm 1. plasma. 2. formative substance (cytoplasm, hyaloplasm, etc.).

plasma the fluid portion of the blood in which corpuscles are suspended. Plasma is to be distinguished from serum, which is plasma from which the fibrinogen has been separated in the process of clotting.

p. bound many electrolytes exist in plasma in a form in which they are bound to protein which reduces their lability and liability to loss in the urine, e.g. protein-bound iodine.

p. cell gingitivitis–pharyngitis see feline plasma cell GINGIVITIS–pharyngitis.

p. cell myeloma see multiple MYELOMA.

p. cell pododermatitis a nonpainful swelling with ulceration and exuberant granulation tissue on the footpads of cats. The cause is unknown but believed to be immunological.

p. clearing factor a lipoprotein lipase which lipolyses the triglyceride in the chylomicrons of the plasma and hence clears it of cloudiness.

p. exchange the removal of plasma from withdrawn blood (plasmapheresis) and retransfusion of the formed elements and type-specific fresh-frozen plasma into the donor; done for removal of circulating antibodies or abnormal plasma components.

p. expanders see plasma volume EXPANDER.

p. protein the heterologous group of proteins in circulating blood that includes albumin, lipoproteins, glycoproteins, transcortin, haptoglobin, ceruloplasmin, cholinesterase, α_2-macroglobulin, erythropoietin, transferrin, hemopexin, fibrinogen, plasminogen and the immunoglobulins (γ-globulins).

p. protein:fibrinogen (PP:F) ratio an indicator of significant changes in fibrinogen levels, taking into account dehydration.

p. substitute a fluid suitable for use as a replacement for plasma in the animal body. Usually a solution of gelatin or dextran.

therapeutic p. concentration a therapy–response relationship determined only by experiment; the plasma level which is matched by the desired therapeutic response.

p. thromboplastin antecedent CLOTTING factor XI; see plasma THROMBOPLASTIN antecedent.

p. turbidity test a qualitative test for fat absorption, performed by comparing the turbidity of plasma before and 2, 3 and 4 hours after the oral administration of fats, usually vegetable oil. Results are greatly influenced by delays in gastric emptying, so normally this test can only be relied upon to rule out malabsorption or maldigestion when evidence of absorption is found.

p. volume the estimation of plasma volume is essential to a complete knowledge of a patient's fluid status. The common technique is by the intravenous injection of a known amount of a dye such as Evans blue and the subsequent measurement of the dilution that it has undergone in a set time period.

plasmablast the immature precursor of a plasmacyte, or plasma cell.

plasmacyte, plasmocyte see plasma CELL.

plasmacytic of the nature of or pertaining to plasmacyte.

p. stomatitis see feline plasma cell GINGIVITIS–pharyngitis.

plasmacytic–lymphocytic see LYMPHOCYTIC–PLASMACYTIC.

plasmacytoma any focal neoplasm of plasmacytes, including those of multiple myeloma (immunoblastic sarcoma). Isolated plasmacytomas may occur outside the bone marrow (extramedullary plasmacytomas), affecting such tissues as the nasal, oral, pharyngeal and gastrointestinal mucosa and other viscera; called also PLASMA cell tumor.

plasmacytosis 1. an excess of plasmacytes in the blood. 2. a synonym for ALEUTIAN MINK DISEASE.

plasmalemma plasma membrane.

plasmalogen one of a group of phospholipids found in platelets, cell membranes of muscle and myelin sheaths of nerve fibers. In platelets their hydrolysis produces aldehydes which appear to play a significant part in the coagulation function of those cells.

plasmapheresis the removal of plasma from withdrawn blood, with retransfusion of the formed elements into the donor; generally, type-specific fresh frozen plasma or albumin is used to replace the withdrawn plasma. The procedure may be done for purposes of collecting plasma components or for therapeutic purposes. See also PLASMA exchange.

plasmatic pertaining to plasma; of the nature of plasma.

plasmatorrhexis bursting of a cell from internal pressure.

plasmic plasmatic; pertaining to or of the nature of plasma.

plasmid an extrachromosomal self-replicating genetic element of a cell. In bacteria, plasmids are circular DNA molecules that reproduce themselves and are thus conserved, apart from the chromosome, through successive cell divisions; they include the F factor and R factor.

R factor p. see R FACTOR.

relaxed p. occurs in tens to several hundred copies per bacterium and are dependent solely on host enzymes for replication.

plasmin the active principle of the fibrinolytic or clot-lysing system, a proteolytic enzyme formed from plasminogen which hydrolyzes fibrin, fibrinogen, factor V and other proteins. It has the particular ability to dissolve formed fibrin clots. Called also fibrinolysin.

p. inhibitors include α_2-macroglobulin, α_1-antitrypsin, C1-inactivator, antithrombin III.

plasminogen the inactive precursor of plasmin, occurring in plasma and converted to plasmin by activators present in most tissues, blood, vessel walls and body fluids; called also profibrinolysin.

p. activator inhibitor can protect the fibrin clot from premature lysis; called also PA inhibitor.

plasmocyte plasmacyte.

plasmocytoma plasmacytoma.

plasmodesma pl. *plasmodesmata;* a bridge of cytoplasm connecting adjacent cells.

plasmodicidal destructive to plasmodia; malariacidal, antimalarial.

Plasmodium a genus of Apicomplexa in the family Plasmodiidae parasitic in the blood cells of animals and humans; the malarial parasite. See also AVIAN malaria.

P. berghei occurs naturally in tree rats; transmissible experimentally to other rodents.

P. brasilianum occurs in several monkey species, transmissible experimentally to humans and marmosets.

P. cathemerium occurs in passerine birds including sparrows, blackbirds.

P. chabaudi occurs in tree rats, transmissible to mice.

P. circumflexum parasitizes a wide range of birds including passerines, Canada goose.

P. coatneyi occurs in cynomolgus monkey; transmissible to other monkeys.

P. cynomolgi occurs in a wide range of monkeys; transmissible to humans causing tertian type malaria.
P. durae occurs in turkeys, transmissible to ducks.
P. elongatum transmissible experimentally to sparrow, canaries, ducks.
P. eylesi found in gibbon monkeys.
P. falciparum, P. malariae, P. ovale, P. vivax the causes of the four specific types of human malaria. They are transmitted to the bloodstream of humans by the bite of anopheline mosquitoes. The sporozoites migrate directly to the liver, where they develop and multiply within the parenchymal cells as merozoites, which then burst the liver cells and invade erythrocytes. Some of the merozoites develop into gametocytes, which are ingested by mosquitoes, beginning the sexual stage, which ends with the development of sporozoites.
P. fallax occurs in guinea fowl; transmissible to other birds.
P. gallinaceum occurs in fowls and transmissible to some other birds; many are resistant.
P. gonderi occurs in mandrills, mangabeys, rhesus monkeys.
P. griffithsi occurs in turkeys.
P. hexamerium found in passerine birds.
P. inui found in several species of monkeys.
P. juxtanucleare occurs in fowls; transmitted experimentally to turkeys.
P. knowlesi occurs in several species of monkeys.
P. lophurae occurs in pheasants; experimentally transmitted to chickens and ducklings.
P. reichenowi occurs in chimpanzee and gorilla.
P. relictum occurs in a variety of bird species.
P. rouxi found in sparrows and finches.
P. schwetzi occurs in chimpanzee and gorilla; transmissible experimentally to humans.
P. simium occurs in howler monkeys and humans.
P. vaughani found in many bird species.
P. vinckei occurs in a variety of rat species; transmissible to mice.

plasmodium pl. *plasmodia* [Gr.] 1. an ampicomplexan protozoon parasite of the genus *Plasmodium*; includes the avian malaria protozoa. 2. a multinucleate continuous mass of protoplasm.

plasmogen the more vital or essential part of the cytoplasm; called also bioplasm.

plasmolysis contraction of cell protoplasm due to loss of water by osmosis.

plasmoma plasmacytoma.

plasmon extrachromosomal hereditary factors.

plasmorrhexis see ERYTHROCYTORRHEXIS.

plasmoschisis the splitting up of cell protoplasm.

plasmotropism destruction of erythrocytes in the liver, spleen or marrow, as contrasted with their destruction in the circulation.

plaster 1. a mixture of materials that hardens; used for immobilizing or making impressions of body parts. 2. an adhesive substance spread on fabric or other suitable backing material, for application to the skin, often containing some medication, such as an anodyne or rubefacient.
p. cast see CAST (5).
p. of Paris calcium sulfate dihydrate, reduced to a fine powder; the addition of water produces a porous mass used in making casts and bandages to support or immobilize body parts.
p. rolls the dry material for constructing plaster casts is packaged as rolls of impregnated gauze which is thoroughly soaked in water before being applied by unrolling around the site of the fracture.
p. shears special shears to cut plaster of Paris casts. Designed to cut upwards away from the tissues to avoid injury. Called also plaster scissors, Esmarch plaster shears.
p. spreader a reverse pincer device with flat blades that are fitted down into a cut made in a plaster cast that is to be removed. Opening the handles forces the plaster apart.

plastic 1. tending to build up tissues to restore a lost part. 2. capable of being molded. 3. a substance produced by chemical condensation or by polymerization. 4. material that can be molded.
p. dish dermatitis an inflammatory skin reaction on the muzzle of dogs caused by a hypersensitivity to plastic feeding dishes.
p. toy poisoning nervous signs including ataxia, hyperexcitability and muscle twitching sometimes occur in cats after eating chidren's plastic toys made of rubber and polythene.
p. vinyl sheeting a surgical drape made of synthetic material with the advantage of not being capillary and not abrasive to exposed tissue.

plasticity the quality of being plastic, or capable of being molded.
nervous system p. the ability of the nervous system to change its capabilities by experience; plays a major role in compensating for the loss of neurons with age.

plasticizers mostly triaryl phosphates, such as tricresyl, triphenyl phosphates, which are poisonous. See also TRIORTHOCRESYL PHOSPHATE.

plastid 1. any elementary constructive unit, as a cell. 2. any specialized organ of the cell other than the nucleus and centrosome, such as chloroplast, mitochondria or amyloplast.

plastron skeletal structure protecting the abdomen of chelonians.

-plasty word element. [Gr.] *formation, plastic repair of.*

plate 1. a flat structure or layer, as a flat layer of bone. 2. used as a fracture repair medium, including compression plates. 3. to apply a culture medium to a glass plate. 4. to cultivate bacteria on such plates.
axial p. the primitive streak of the embryo.
basal p. primordial ventral horn of the spinal cord.
p. bender a strong crimping device for manually bending a plate for a tricky bit of orthopedic repair.
buttress p. (2) a metal plate used in fracture repair to bridge and support a diaphyseal gap filled with a cancellous bone graft.
cloacal p. blind ending of the hindgut in the embryo.
cribriform p. a sievelike partition between the cranial and nasal cavities. The posterior surface is divided by the vertical ethmoidal crest into two concave surfaces which contain the olfactory bulbs. It contains many small perforations through which the filaments of the olfactory nerves pass.
deck p. see roof PLATE.
dorsal p. see roof PLATE.
equatorial p. the collection of chromosomes at the equator of the spindle in mitosis.
floor p. the unpaired ventral longitudinal zone of the neural tube; called also ventral plate.
foot p. the flat portion of the stapes.
medullary p. neural plate.
muscle p. myotome (2).
nasal p. region of modified skin around the nostrils in the embryonic carnivore or small ruminant.
nasolabial p. region of modified skin around the nostrils in the embryo of cattle.
neural p. a thickened band of ectoderm in the midbody region of the developing embryo, which develops into the neural tube; called also medullary plate.

neutralization p. (2) a bone plate placed to protect against the forces acting on the fracture site.
orthopedic bone p. a metal plate screwed to the two fragments of a fractured bone to provide fixation and permit healing in correct alignment.
roof p. the unpaired dorsal longitudinal zone of the neural tube; called also dorsal plate and deck plate.
rostral p. region of modified skin around the nostrils in the porcine embryo.
sole p. a mass of protoplasm in which a motor nerve ending is embedded.
spinal p. metal or plastic plates may used to stabilize thoracolumbar or lumbar spinal fractures. With one plate on each side of a row of dorsal spinal processes, they are bolted together in the spaces between processes.
tarsal p. one of the plates of connective tissue forming the framework of either (upper or lower) eyelid.
tectorial p. the roof of the ethmoidal labyrinth of the internal ear.
tension band p. (2) a bone plate placed on the tension side of a fracture and which counteracts tensile forces, converting them into compression forces at the fracture site.
ventral p. floor plate.

platelet a small disk or platelike structure, the smallest of the formed elements in blood. Blood platelets (called also thrombocytes) are disk-shaped, non-nucleated blood elements with a very fragile membrane; they tend to adhere to uneven or damaged surfaces. They average about 250,000 per cubic millimeter of blood and are formed in the red bone marrow by fragmentation of megakaryocytes, the largest of the bone marrow cells. Platelet production is controlled by a hormone, thrombopoietin, and regulatory lymphocytes acting at the stem cell level. At any given time about one-third of the total blood platelets can be found in the spleen; the remaining two-thirds are in the circulating blood.

The functions of platelets are related to the clotting of blood. Because of their adhesion and aggregation capabilities platelets can occlude small breaks in blood vessels and prevent the escape of blood. Platelets which have adhered to exposed collagen in damaged vessels release ADP in milliseconds which in turn initiates the synthesis of thromboxane A_2, a very potent prostaglandin which causes platelet aggregation and localized vasoconstriction. Fibrinogen, factors V and VIII, calcium ions, platelet phospholipid (PF-3), associated with the platelet membrane are also released. Substances contained within the platelet granules such as thromboglobulin, heparin neutralizing activity (PF-4) mitogens such as platelet derived growth factor, thrombospondin, ADP, serotonin and calcium ions are also released by aggregated platelets.
p.-activating factor (PAF) see platelet-activating FACTOR.
p. adhesion the adherence of platelets to any area with damaged blood vessels; an important component of hemostasis.
p. aggregation the progressive accumulation of platelets, attracted by other platelets once adhesion begins. Thromboxane A_2 causes irreversible platelet aggregation.
p. aggregation test a known platelet aggregating factor such as collagen, ADP or thrombin is added to a suspension of the platelets under test and the degree of aggregation measured by decrease in turbidity of the suspension.
p. count may be performed directly (in a hemocytometer chamber) or indirectly (estimating from the stained blood smear by number per field or in comparison to the number of white blood cells), expressed as number of cells per liter of blood.
p.-derived growth factor one of three growth factors released by platelets which undergo the release reaction; the growth factors stimulate endothelial cell proliferation.
p. factor 3 (PF-3) test, p. release test test the antiplatelet activity of serum; used to detect circulating antiplatelet antibodies. Antibody–antigen reactions involving platelets cause the release of PF-3 from platelets which in turn shortens the contact-activated clotting time of platelet-rich plasma (PRP).
p. factors factors important in hemostasis which are contained in or attached to the platelets: platelet factor 1 is adsorbed CLOTTING factor V from the plasma; platelet factor 2 is an accelerator of the thrombin–fibrinogen reaction; platelet factor 3 is a phospholipid with potent procoagulant activity; platelet factor 4 is capable of inhibiting the activity of heparin (heparin neutralizing activity).
p. plug formation see platelet aggregation (above).
p. release reaction measured by the degree of secondary ADP-mediated aggregation that occurs. This is assessed by the amount of PF-4, PF-3 or serotonin, etc. released.
p. retention tested by testing the adhesiveness of a suspension of the subject platelets to a glass bead column or standard size filter.
p. storage-pool disease an inherited autosomal thrombopathia in American foxhounds and cats characterized by a deficiency of platelet storage granules.
p. transfusion transfusion of fresh, nonchilled whole blood is the usual method of transfusing platelets to an animal with thrombocytopenia.

plateletpheresis thrombocytapheresis.

Platemys platecephala Bolivian side-neck turtle.

platen a rubber cylinder in a typewriter or similar device such as a computer printer around which the paper passes while a printout is made.
pin feed p. a platen with sprockets at the sides, the pins of which move the continuous stationery past the printer head. Called also tractor feed.

platform scales a weighing machine which has a platform on which animals can stand to be weighed.

plating the process of using a PLATE as in orthopedic surgery and in bacteriology, the cultivation of bacteria on artificial media.
bone p. a method of fracture fixation in which one or more metal plates are applied across the fracture and anchored, usually by screws, in the fragments.
replication p. the transfer of cells from bacterial colonies on one plate to another plate, with a colony growing in the same position as in the original plate.

platinum a chemical element, atomic number 78, atomic weight 195.09, symbol Pt. See Table 6.
p. chemotherapy see platinum complexes (below).
p. complexes inhibit DNA synthesis and have some alkylating activity. They are sometimes used in cancer chemotherapy, but have marked side-effects of nausea, vomiting, nephrotoxicity and bone marrow suppression. See also CISPLATIN, CARBOPLATIN.

platy- word element. [Gr.] *broad, flat.*

platybasia malformation of the base of the skull, with forward displacement of the upper cervical vertebrae and bony impingement on the brainstem. It is accompanied by neurological signs referable to the medulla oblongata, cervical spinal cord and cranial nerves. Called also basilar impression.

platycephalic, platycephalous having a wide, flat head.

Platycobboldia loxodontis a stomach bot of the African elephant. The fly lays eggs around the nostrils and the larvae migrate to the stomach through the tissues.

platycoelous having one surface flat and the other concave, referring to vertebrae.

platycoria a dilated condition of the pupil of the eye.

platyfishes aquarium fish—*Platypoecilus maculatus*—one of those that gives birth to live young. Called also *Xiphophorus* spp. Malignant melanomas are inherited in these and hybrids with swordtails.

platyhelminth one of the Platyhelminthes; the flatworms. Includes cestodes and trematodes, the tapeworms and the flukes.

platyhieric having a wide sacrum.

platynosomiasis infection with trematodes in the genus *Platynosomum*.

Platynosomum a genus of digenetic trematodes in the family Dicrocoeliidae.

P. ariestis a nonpathogenic fluke found in the intestine of sheep.

P. fastosum occurs in the liver and bile ducts of cats; causes a mild disease characterized by vomiting, diarrhea and jaundice. Cats become infested by eating infected lizards. Called also lizard poisoning.

platypellic, platypelloid having a broad pelvis.

platypus an aquatic animal of the order Monotremata, found only in Australia. It resembles a beaver, being about 12 to 16 inches long, covered with fine red-brown to gray fur, with a broad, dorsally flattened tail, webbed and clawed paws, and a broad flat, duck-like beak. It lives in a burrow that has an underwater entrance. It lays eggs, hatches them and feeds the young from milk which is discharged through the skin in a skinfold. Called also duckbill, duckmole, *Ornithorhynchus anatinus*.

platyrrhine having a broad nose.

platys see PLATYFISHES.

platysma the superficial sheet of cutaneous muscle over the face and neck.

Playdo a child's modeling medium useful in obliterating air spaces in superficial sites, e.g. clefts in the sole of the normal horse hoof, and improving the quality of the radiographical image.

PLE protein losing enteropathy.

pledget a small compress or tuft, usually of cotton or cotton wool, cotton batting, used to apply disinfectant or medicament to the skin.

-plegia word element. [Gr.] *paralysis*.

pleiotropism, pleiotropy the production by a single gene of multiple phenotypic effects.

pleocytosis the presence of a greater than normal number of cells, as of more than the normal number of lymphocytes in cerebrospinal fluid.

pleomastia the presence of supernumerary mammary glands or nipples; polymastia.

pleomorphism having more than one shape or form.

pleonasm an excess of parts.

pleonectic characterized by having a higher than normal O_2 content at a given Po_2; said of blood.

pleonosteosis abnormally increased ossification.

plerocercoid the second larval stage of a pseudophyllidean cestode which follows the procercoid. This larva infects a wide range of vertebrate hosts including fish, amphibia, reptiles, mammals, birds. They are elongated, have a solid body and carry an adult scolex. As a migrating larva of a tapeworm, this is an infectious stage of importance in predation; the definitive host becomes infected by eating the tissues of the second intermediate host.

Plesiomonas facultatively anaerobic gram-negative rods which are mainly found in fish and reptiles. The only species is *P. shigelloids*.

plesiotherapy a form of very superficial radiotherapy; ^{90}Sr probes are used.

plessesthesia palpatory percussion.

plessimeter pleximeter.

plessor plexor.

PLET agar for growth of *Bacillis anthracis*.

plethora a general term denoting an overabundance, or specifically, an excessive amount of blood.

plethysmograph any device for measuring and recording variations in the volume of an organ, part or limb.

body p. a device used in PULMONARY function tests to measure parameters such as functional residual capacity (FRC) and lung–thorax compliance (C_{LT}). It consists of a large box in which the subject can be sealed so that volume of the thorax can be determined from pressure changes in the box while the lung volume and gas pressure in the lungs are measured by spirometry.

plethysmography the determination of changes in volume by means of a plethysmograph.

pleura pl. *pleurae* [Gr.] the serous membrane investing the lungs (pulmonary pleura) and lining the walls of the thoracic cavity (parietal pleura), the two layers enclosing a potential space, the pleural cavity.

pleuracotomy incision into the pleural cavity.

pleural emanating from or pertaining to the pleura.

p. effusion accumulation of fluid in the space between the membrane encasing the lung and that lining the thoracic cavity. The normal pleural space contains only a small amount of fluid to prevent friction as the lung expands and deflates. If, however, there is a disturbance in either the production of this fluid or its removal, the fluid accumulates and threatens collapse of the lung. In extreme cases there is total collapse of the lung and MEDIASTINAL shift.

p. friction rub the abrasive sound made by the rubbing together of two acutely inflamed serous surfaces, as in acute pleurisy. Later separation of the surfaces by accumulated exudate marks the disappearance of the rub. The sound is synchronous with the respiratory movements.

p. gas may be produced by gas-forming bacteria or be caused by leakage from thoracentesis or lesions of the airways.

p. hemorrhage see HEMOTHORAX.

p. infection see PYOTHORAX.

p. inflammation see PLEURITIS.

p. paracentesis see THORACENTESIS.

p. peel heavy fibrinous deposits on the pleura.

p. stripping 1. removal of the pleura at an abattoir when the tissue is discolored or superficially diseased and the remainder of the carcass is suitable for human consumption. 2. surgical removal of excessive pleural fibrin deposits via thoracotomy.

pleurapophysis a rib, or a vertebral process corresponding to a rib.

pleurectomy excision of a portion of the pleura.

pleuritic pertaining to or emanating from pleurisy. See also PLEURAL.

p. ridge thoracic immobility with the chest expanded combined with abdominal respiration causes the costochondral arches to be more visible than usual. Called pleuritic ridge because of its occurrence in pleurisy as a response to pain on chest movement.

p. thrill palpable counterpart of the pleural friction rub.

pleuritis, pleurisy inflammation of the pleura; it may be caused by infection, injury or tumor. It may be a

complication of lung diseases, particularly of pneumonia or lung abscess. Typical signs of acute pleurisy include painful respiratory movements causing grunting and rapid shallow breathing. Chronic pleurisy includes empyema with collapse of lung and dyspnea with toxemia, or interference with respiratory movements by adhesions.
bile p. see BILE pleuritis.
constrictive p. adhesions between the parietal and visceral pleura restrict movement of the lungs and the chest wall.
dry p. inflammation of the pleura without effusion. Painful, the cause of dry cough, shallow, rapid respiration and sounds of friction rubbing. Can be a stage in the development or healing of serous or purulent pleuritis.
restrictive p. development of fibrous tissue on pleura may restrict expansion of lungs.

pleur(o)- word element. [Gr.] *pleura, rib, side.*

pleurocele hernia of lung tissue or of pleura.

pleurocentesis thoracentesis; paracentesis of the pleural cavity.

pleurocentrum the lateral element of the vertebral column.

pleuroclysis injection of fluids into the pleural cavity.

pleurodesis the production of adhesions between the visceral and parietal pleurae. May be produced intentionally by the instillation of irritating drugs into the pleural cavity for the purpose of limiting space for pleural effusion.

pleurodont a tooth with no root, but attached to the jaws.

pleurodynia paroxysmal pain in the intercostal muscles due to muscular disease or irritation of the pleural surface.

pleurogenic, pleurogenous originating in the pleura.

pleurography radiography of the pleural cavity by coating the parietal and visceral pleura with a contrast agent.

pleurohepatitis hepatitis with inflammation of a portion of the pleura near the liver.

pleurolith a concretion in the pleura.

pleurolysis surgical separation of the pleura from its attachments.

pleuroparietopexy the operation of fixing the visceral pleura to the parietal pleura, thus binding the lung to the chest wall.

pleuropericardial pertaining to the pleura and pericardium.
p. celom, p. coelom that part of the original body cavity in the fetus which subsequently divides into the pericardial and pleural cavities.
p. fold the beginnings of the pleuropericardial septum in the developing embryo.
p. septum the septum produced by the fusion of the two pleuropericardial folds; it divides the original pleuropericardial coelom into the pleural and pericardial coeloms, later the cavities of the same names.

pleuropericarditis inflammation involving the pleura and the pericardium.

pleuroperitoneal pertaining to the pleura and peritoneum.
p. canal an embryonic, transient canal venting pleural and peritoneal cavities.
p. hernia herniation of abdominal viscera through a pleuroperitoneal hiatus defect.
p. hiatus defect faulty closure of the pleuroperitoneal canals by the embryonic diaphragm.
p. membrane folds of tissue which extend into the peritoneal cavity of the developing embryo and participate in the separation of the pleural and peritoneal cavities.

pleuropneumonia pneumonia accompanied by pleurisy.
contagious bovine p. see CONTAGIOUS bovine pleuropneumonia.
contagious caprine p. see CONTAGIOUS caprine/ovine pleuropneumonia.
porcine p. a highly contagious disease of pigs caused by *Actinobacillus (Haemophilus) pleuropneumoniae (parahaemolyticus)* and characterized by severe dyspnea, and a short course and high mortality rates.

pleuropneumonia-like organisms a term applied to a group of filtrable microorganisms similar to *Mycoplasma mycoides*, the cause of pleuropneumonia in cattle; abbreviated PPLO.

pleuroscopy visual examination of the pleural cavity via a pleuroscope introduced through an incision in the chest wall.

pleurothotonos, pleurothotonus tetanic bending of the body to one side.

pleurotomy incision of the pleura.

pleurovisceral pertaining to the pleura and viscera.

plexiform resembling a plexus or network.

pleximeter a plate to be struck in mediate percussion; preferably with a percussion hammer.

plexitis inflammation of a nerve plexus.

plexogenic giving rise to a plexus or plexiform growth.
p. pulmonary arteriopathy pulmonary vascular lesions caused by pulmonary hypertension and hyperfusion in congenital cardiac defects such as patent ductus arteriosus.

plexopathy any disorder of a plexus, especially of nerves.
lumbar p. neuropathy of the lumbar plexus.

plexor a hammer used in diagnostic percussion; plessor. See also PLEXIMETER.

plexus pl. *plexus, plexuses* [L.] a network or tangle, chiefly of veins or nerves.
brachial p. see BRACHIAL plexus.
cardiac p. the plexus around the base of the heart, chiefly in the epicardium, formed by cardiac branches from the vagus nerves and the sympathetic trunks and ganglia, and made up of sympathetic, parasympathetic and visceral afferent fibers that innervate the heart.
carotid p's nerve plexuses surrounding the common, external and internal carotid arteries.
celiac p. a plexus of autonomic fibers and sympathetic nerve ganglia which surround the origin of the celiac artery, and supply the abdominal viscera.
celiacomesenteric p. a plexus of autonomic nerve fibers and sympathetic ganglia around the origin of the celiac and cranial mesenteric arteries; called also solar plexus.
cervical p. a network of nerve fibers formed by the first four cervical nerves and supplying the structures in the region of the neck.
choroid p. infoldings of blood vessels of the pia mater covered by a thin coat of ependymal cells that form tufted projections into the third, fourth, and lateral ventricles of the brain; they secrete the cerebrospinal fluid.
coccygeal p. a nerve plexus formed by the ventral branches of the coccygeal and last sacral nerves.
coronary p. a venous plexus within the coronet of the hoof.
cutaneous p's superficial, middle and deep, intercommunicating plexuses of blood vessels are identified as supplying blood to haired skin.

cystic p. a nerve plexus near the gallbladder.
dental p. either of two plexuses (inferior and superior) of nerve fibers, one from the inferior alveolar nerve, situated around the roots of the lower teeth, and the other from the superior alveolar nerve, situated around the roots of the upper teeth.
gonadal p. the collection of parasympathetic and sympathetic nerves to the gonads.
hoof p. plexus of veins draining the hoof region in the horse.
lumbar p. see LUMBAR plexus.
lumbosacral p. see LUMBOSACRAL plexus.
mesenteric p. parasympathetic and sympathetic nerve supply to the abdominal organs.
myenteric p. see AUERBACH PLEXUS.
nerve p. a plexus composed of intermingled nerve fibers.
pampiniform p. 1. a plexus of veins from the testis and the epididymis, constituting part of the spermatic cord. 2. a plexus of ovarian veins in the broad ligament of the uterus.
parametrial p. the venous plexus within the broad ligament providing venous drainage to the uterus and vagina.
p. papilloma see plexus PAPILLOMA.
pulmonary p. the array of autonomic nerves which supply the lungs.
renal p. autonomic nerve supply to the kidney.
sacral p. a plexus arising from the ventral branches of the last few lumbar and first few sacral spinal nerves.
solar p. see celiacomesenteric plexus (above).
tympanic p. a network of nerve fibers supplying the mucous lining of the tympanum and auditory tube.

PLH PHARYNGEAL lymphoid hyperplasia.

plica pl. *plicae* [L.] a ridge or fold.
p. abomasi permanent folds in the abomasal mucosa.
p. circulares permanent folds in the mucosa of the small intestine.
p. glossoepiglottica a median fold in the pharyngeal mucosa that passes from the root of the tongue to the base of the epiglottis.
pterygomandibular p. passes from the lower jaw to the upper behind the last molar teeth on both sides of the mouth.
p. rumenoreticularis the fold that partly separates the rumen from the reticulum.
p. semilunaris conjunctivae the fold of conjunctiva that encloses the substance of the third eyelid.
p. venae cavae the pleural fold which extends from the mediastinum to the caudal vena cava.

plicamycin an antineoplastic antibiotic produced by *Streptomyces argillaceus* and *S. tanashiensis*; particularly effective in treating the hypercalcemia associated with canine lymphosarcoma. Called also mithramycin.

plicate plaited or folded.

plication the operation of taking tucks in a structure to shorten it.

plicotomy surgical incision of the posterior fold of the tympanic membrane.

Pliohippus the last three-toed horse in the evolution of Equidae; existed during the Pliocene era. The lateral toes were small and finally disappeared in this stage. The connecting link from the primitive horse to the modern day *Equus*.

Plistophora obligate, intracellular parasites, mostly of fish, belonging to the class Microsporidea.
P. anguillarum occurs in the muscles of eels and causes body deformities when muscles atrophy.
P. cepedianae produces large cysts that protrude from the body wall of affected fish.
P. hyphessobryconis found in the skeletal muscles of aquarium fish causing 'neon fish disease'. The muscles are patchily transparent and the fish lose their balance and the fins degenerate.
P. macrozoarcidis causes the development of cysts and tumors in the muscles of marine fish.
P. ovariae infects the ovaries of minnows causing infertility.
P. salmonae infects the gills of trout causing clubbing and fusion.

plombage [Fr.] the filling of a space or cavity in the body with inert material.

plooks colloquial term for 3 to 4 week old lamb.

Plott hound a medium-sized, sturdy dog with large, pendulous ears. The black and brindle coat is short and the tail is long and tapered. The breed is used in packs for hunting bear, wild boar, wolves and mountain lions, traditionally in the Great Smoky Mountains of the eastern United States.

plotter a computer device specialized for the production of high quality graphs, maps and drawings.

plow harness a harness which consists of a collar and hames, a backstrap and chains that run from the hames through the back strap to the swingle-bar of the plow.

plowman's spikenard see INULA *conyza*.

plowshare bone see PYGOSTYLE.

PLP pyridoxal phosphate.

PLR pupillary light reflex.

PLT *p*sittacosis-*l*ymphogranuloma venereum-*t*rachoma (group). See CHLAMYDIA.

pluck 1. an abattoir term for the thoracic viscera plus the liver, after separation from the esophagus and the diaphragm. Includes the larynx, trachea, lungs, heart and liver, plus the spleen in sheep. 2. removal of the feathers from birds during the preparation of the carcass for meat. Scalding for 2 minutes in water plus detergent at 134°F is a great aid. 3. removal of wool from the carcass of a sheep dead long enough for the wool to become loose.

plucking box restraint box used for feather harvesting of ostriches.

plug an obstructing mass.
epithelial p. mass of ectodermal cells that temporarily closes the external naris of the fetus.
mucous p. a plug formed by secretions of mucous glands, of the cervix uteri and closing the cervical canal during pregnancy.

plug-compatible said of devices from different manufacturers which may be connected to a computer, without the need to modify the computer.

plum PRUNUS *domestica*.

plum pudding dog see DALMATIAN.

'plum pudding' liver see TELANGIECTASIA.

plumage the feather coat of a bird for one molt.

plumas lupine LUPINUS *onustus*.

plumbic pertaining to lead.

plumbism a chronic form of poisoning caused by absorption of lead or lead salts. See also LEAD[1] poisoning.

plumbum [L.] *lead* (symbol Pb).

plumeless thistle see CARDUUS.

plumping forming up of the egg in the hen's oviduct before investing it with the shell.

pluri- word element. [L.] *many*.

pluriglandular pertaining to several glands or their secretions.

plurigravida multigravida; a female pregnant for the third (or more) time.

plurilocular multilocular; having many cells or compartments.
pluripara multipara; a female which has had two or more pregnancies that resulted in viable offspring.
pluriparity multiparity; the condition of being a pluripara (multipara).
pluripotent having the capacity to develop in one of several ways.
p. stem cell. see stem CELL.
pluripotential characterized by pluripotentiality.
pluripotentiality having the ability to develop in any one of several different ways, or to affect more than one organ or tissue.
pluronic detergent used as an oral prophylactic against bloat in ruminants; overdosing can have toxic effects.
plus sense in RNA viruses, the genomic RNA is of the same polarity 3′ to 5′ as messenger RNA so that after adsorption, penetration, uncoating and release of the viral RNA into the cytoplasm of the cell the viral RNA acts immediately as a messenger RNA for the synthesis of viral proteins, some of which are essential for the replication of the virus.
plutonium a chemical element, atomic number 94, atomic weight 242, symbol Pu. See Table 6.
Plymouth Rock a black-and-white barred colored fowl, with distinctive crossbands of black and white across the feathers, giving the bird a spangled look. A heavyweight meat bird with a single comb.
Pm chemical symbol, *promethium.*
PMI point of maximal intensity.
PMN polymorphonuclear neutrophil.
PMS pregnant mare's serum.
PMSG pregnant mare serum gonadotropin. Now equine chorionic gonadotropin (eCG).
-pnea, -pnoea word element. [Gr.] *respiration, breathing.*
pneo- word element. [Gr.] *breath, breathing.*
pneogram spirogram.
pneograph spirograph.
pneometer spirometer.
pneoscope pneograph.
pneumarthrograph a radiograph obtained by pneumarthrography.
pneumarthrography radiography of a joint after it has been injected with a gas as a contrast medium; pneumoarthrography.
pneumarthrosis gas or air in a joint.
pneumatic pertaining to air or respiration.
pneumatization the formation of air cavities in tissue, especially such formation in the temporal bone.
pneumat(o)- word element. [Gr.] *air* or *gas; lung.*
pneumatocele 1. hernia of lung tissue. 2. a usually benign, thin-walled, air-containing cyst of the lung. 3. a tumor or sac containing gas, especially a gaseous swelling of the scrotum.
pneumatogram spirogram.
pneumatograph spirograph.
pneumatometer spirometer.
pneumatometry measurement of the air inspired and expired.
pneumatonograph a pneumatic tonometer–tonographer.
pneumatorrhachis the presence of gas in the vertebral canal.
pneumatosis air or gas in an abnormal location in the body.
p. coli gas or air dissecting the tissues in the wall of the large intestine.
p. cystoides intestinalis a condition characterized by the presence of thin-walled, gas-containing cysts in the wall of the intestines in humans, a condition similar to intestinal emphysema in pigs.
pneumaturia gas or air in the urine.
pneumectomy pneumonectomy.
pneum(o)- word element. [Gr.] *air* or *gas; lung.*
pneumoangiography radiography of the blood vessels of the lungs.
pneumoarthrography roentgenography of a joint after injection of air or gas as a contrast medium; pneumarthrography.
pneumocephalus air in the intracranial cavity.
pneumococcus see STREPTOCOCCUS *pneumoniae.*
pneumocolon air in the colon; it may be placed there as an aid to diagnosis.
pneumocolonography radiography of the colon after air or gas has been introduced to aid in contrast.
pneumoconiosis any of a group of lung diseases resulting from inhalation of particles of industrial substances, such as the dust of iron ore or coal, and permanent deposition of substantial amounts of such particles in the lungs.

The disease is rare in animals unless there is an unusual exposure to a dusty environment. Horses are the ones most commonly exposed, usually in a mining operation (pit ponies). Exercise intolerance and chronic cough are the cardinal signs.
Pneumocystis a genus of organisms of uncertain status, but considered to be protozoa.
P. carinii the causative agent of interstitial plasma cell pneumonia in humans and immunocompromised Arab foals and dogs with combined immune deficiency.
pneumocystogram a radiograph obtained by pneumocystography.
pneumocystography radiography of the urinary bladder after injection of air or gas.
pneumocystosis 1. pneumonia characterized by interstitial accumulation of plasma cells. 2. pneumonia caused by *Pneumocystis carinii* infection; usually latent or sucbclinical except in immunocompromised humans, dogs, cats, pigs, horses, goats, primates, rabbits.
pneumocyte includes granular and alveolar pneumocytes; see ALVEOLAR² cell.
pneumoderma subcutaneous emphysema; air or gas in subcutaneous tissues.
pneumodynamics the dynamics of the respiratory process.
pneumoencephalitis see NEWCASTLE DISEASE.
pneumoencephalogram the radiograph produced by pneumoencephalography.
pneumoencephalography radiographic visualization of the fluid-containing structures of the brain after cerebrospinal fluid is withdrawn and replaced by air, oxygen or helium.
pneumoenteritis inflammation of the lungs and intestine as in stomatitis pneumoenteritis. See PESTE DES PETITS RUMINANTS.
pneumoextraperitoneography infiltration of the subperitoneal tissues with nitrogen or carbon dioxide to give a better visualization of the kidney.
pneumogastric nerve vagus nerve. See Table 14.
pneumogastrogram radiograph of an air-filled stomach, used to screen for gastric foreign bodies and assessment of stomach position, size and shape. Not useful for defining details of the mucosa.
pneumogastrography a radiographic technique which utilizes a gas-filled stomach to visualize the organ. See also GASTROGRAPHY.
pneumography 1. description of the lungs. 2. graphic recording of the respiratory movements. 3. radiography of a part after injection of a gas.

pneumohemopericardium air or gas and blood in the pericardium.
pneumohemothorax gas or air and blood in the pleural cavity.
pneumohydrometra gas and fluid in the uterus.
pneumohydropericardium air or gas with fluid in the pericardium.
pneumohydrothorax air or gas with fluid in the thoracic cavity.
pneumolith a pulmonary concretion.
pneumolithiasis the presence of concretions in the lungs.
pneumomediastinum the presence of air or gas in tissues of the mediastinum, occurring pathologically or introduced intentionally.
pneumometer spirometer.
pneumomycosis any fungal disease of the lungs.
pneumomyelography a generally unused technique of radiography of the spinal canal after withdrawal of cerebrospinal fluid and injection of air or gas.
pneumonectomy excision of lung tissue, of an entire lung (total pneumonectomy) or less (partial pneumonectomy), or of a single lobe (lobectomy).
pneumonia inflammation of the parenchyma of the lung. It is often accompanied by inflammation of the airways and sometimes of the adjoining pleura. Clinically it is manifested by an increase in the rate and depth of respiration at all degrees of severity up to dyspnea. There is also cough, and abnormality of the breath sounds on auscultation. In bacterial pneumonia there is usually a severe toxemia, in viral pneumonia it is usually minor. See also BRONCHOPNEUMONIA, PLEUROPNEUMONIA.
Arabian foal p. an inexorably progressive pneumonia of certain Arabian foals born with primary severe combined immunodeficiency in which adenovirus plays a dominant role but is complicated by other microorganisms, particularly *Pneumocystis carinii*.
aspiration p. see ASPIRATION pneumonia.
atypical p. histologically the pneumonia is atypical in that there are no signs of acute inflammation and it is characterized by an exudation of eosinophilic, protein-rich fluid in the alveoli which may become organized to form a hyaline membrane. In animals that survive for several days there is epithelialization of the alveolar walls. In humans there is a primary atypical pneumonia caused by *Mycoplasma pneumoniae*. In animals the best known example is ATYPICAL INTERSTITIAL PNEUMONIA of cattle.
bronchointerstitial p. the lesions are centered on the bronchioles and a prominent feature is the accumulation of lymphocytes in interstitial tissue; typical of pneumonias caused by aerogenous virus infections, especially myxoviruses.
brooder p. see BROODER pneumonia.
chronic undifferentiated p. of sheep see ENZOOTIC pneumonia.
corynebacterial p. of foals see CORYNEBACTERIAL pneumonia.
cuffing p. chronic undifferentiated pneumonia of sheep in which lymphofollicular sheaths around the bronchioles are a feature.
equine cryptococcal p. see EPIZOOTIC lymphangitis.
desquamative p. a chronic pneumonia associated with *Mycoplasma* spp. and characterized by organization of the exudate within bronchioles and bronchi, and proliferation of the interstitial tissue and epithelium.
desquamative interstitial p. chronic pneumonia with desquamation of large alveolar cells and thickening of the walls of distal air passages; marked by dyspnea and nonproductive cough.
embolic p. results from hematogenous spread from an intravascular lesion elsewhere in the body. The best known example is CAUDAL vena caval thrombosis.
endogenous-lipid p. focal alveolar accumulations of foamy, lipid-filled macrophages which may impede alveolar clearance. Usually an incidental postmortem finding in laboratory rodents, fur-bearing animals and uncommonly cats and dogs.
enzootic p. see ENZOOTIC pneumonia.
fibrinous p. an acute fulminating pneumonia, often lobar in distribution, characterized by a fibrinous exudate. Fibrinous describes the exudate, not the anatomical distribution so that the term fibrinous pneumonia should not be used interchangeably with lobar pneumonia.
foreign body p. see ASPIRATION pneumonia.
gangrenous p. usually an accompaniment of aspiration pneumonia.
giant-cell p. a secondary lesion in dermatosis vegetans in pigs; lesions marked by the presence of a proliferative giant-cell type of diffuse interstitial pneumonia.
granulomatous p. has a slow course characterized by granulomatous, not exudative, lesions. Sporadic cases occur in immunodeficient animals. It is a characteristic of tuberculosis and systemic fungal infections, e.g. coccidioidomycosis.
hypostatic p. caused by pooling of blood and some decrease in viability of the dependent lung in an old, sick or debilitated animal that is in lateral recumbency for a long period. The infection is secondary to hypostasis.
inhalation p. see ASPIRATION pneumonia.
interstitial p. pneumonia in which there is diffuse or patchy damage to alveolar septa widely distributed through the lungs. There is an early intra-alveolar exudative phase followed by significant proliferation and enlargement of the alveolar epithelial cells and a thickening of the interstitial tissue. Most interstitial pneumonias in animals are infectious including viral, bacterial, fungal and protozoal causes, but may be caused by chemical injury, acute pancreatitis or shock, as in acute respiratory distress syndrome.
lipid p. a specific type of aspiration pneumonia caused by the inhalation of oil droplets; most commonly associated with the forced administration of paraffin oil or cod-liver oil to cats. Called also medication pneumonia, lipoid pneumonia. See also ASPIRATION pneumonia.
lobar p. a fulminating bronchopneumonia in which entire pulmonary lobes are diffusively inflamed and then consolidated. Pneumonic pasteurellosis in cattle is the type disease. The animal is critically ill with anoxia and toxemia.
lobular p. an oldfashioned term for BRONCHOPNEUMONIA.
lymphoid interstitial p. see MAEDI.
ovine progressive p. see MAEDI.
parasitic p. see LUNGWORM disease.
stable p. see EQUINE influenza.
suppurative p. of foals see CORYNEBACTERIAL pneumonia.
uremic p. occurs in dogs with terminal uremia; lesions characterized by absence of inflammatory cells.
pneumonic pertaining to the lung or to pneumonia.
p. pasteurellosis see pneumonic PASTEURELLOSIS.
pneumonitis inflammation of lung tissue. See also PNEUMONIA.

feline p. see FELINE pneumonitis.
hypersensitivity p. a local type III hypersensitivity reaction resulting from inhalation of antigens, seen in cattle fed moldy hay and the group of diseases in humans that includes FARMER'S LUNG and BIRD-fancier's lung.
pneumono- word element. [Gr.] *lung*.
pneumonocentesis surgical puncture of a lung for aspiration.
pneumonocyte collective term for the alveolar epithelial cells (great alveolar cells and squamous alveolar cells) and alveolar phagocytes of the lungs.
pneumonolysis division of tissues attaching the lung to the wall of the chest cavity, to permit collapse of the lung.
pneumonomycosis pneumomycosis.
pneumonopathy any lung disease.
pneumonopexy fixation of the lung to the thoracic wall.
pneumonorrhaphy suture of the lung.
pneumonosis any lung disease.
pneumonotomy incision of the lung.
Pneumonyssoides see PNEUMONYSSUS.
P. stammeri a mite found in the lungs of New World primates.
Pneumonyssoides caninum see PNEUMONYSSUS *caninum*.
Pneumonyssus a genus of mites in the family Dermanyssidae.
P. caninum found in the nasal passages and sinuses of dogs causing irritation manifested by sneezing, and rubbing of the nose.
P. simicola found in the bronchi of the rhesus monkey where it may cause irritation with sneezing and coughing.
pneumopericardiography injection of air or carbon dioxide into the pericardial sac, usually after a comparable amount of fluid has been withdrawn.
pneumopericardium the presence of air or gas in the pericardial cavity.
pneumoperitoneography a radiograph taken of the abdomen after the intraperitoneal infusion of air or carbon dioxide to give better contrast.
pneumoperitoneoscopy the infusion of air into the peritoneal cavity in order to improve the view obtained through a laparoscope.
pneumoperitoneum the presence of air or gas in the peritoneal cavity, occurring pathologically or introduced intentionally.
pneumoperitonitis peritonitis with accumulation of air or gas in the peritoneal cavity.
pneumopleuritis inflammation of the lungs and pleura.
pneumopyopericardium air or gas and pus in the pericardium.
pneumopyothorax air or gas and pus in the pleural cavity.
pneumoradiography radiography of a part after injection of air or other gas as contrast material.
pneumoretroperitoneum the presence of air or gas in the retroperitoneal space.
pneumorrhagia hemorrhage from the lungs; severe hemoptysis.
Pneumospirura a genus of spiruroid nematodes in the family Pneumospiruridae.
P. bassarisci found in the bronchioles of the ringtail.
P. capsulata found in the common badger.
P. rodentium found in the lungs of gerbils and birds.
Pneumostrongylus a genus of nematodes in the family Protostrongylidae. Parasites of the lungs of African antelopes. Called also Paraelaphostrongylus.
pneumotachograph an instrument for recording the velocity of respired air.
pneumotachography the science of using a PNEUMOTACHOGRAPH.
pneumotachometer a transducer for measuring expired air flow.
pneumotaxic regulating the respiratory rate.
p. center one of the four respiratory centers; located in the upper, rostral part of the pons; rhythmically inhibits inspiration.
pneumotherapy treatment of disease of the lungs.
pneumothorax entry of air into the pleural cavity in sufficient quantity to cause collapse of the lung and consequent respiratory embarrassment. If it is unilateral there is a mediastinal shift with displacement of the heart to the other side of the chest. Breath sounds are absent from the affected side.
closed p. air leaks from a discontinuity in the lung into the pleural cavity.
iatrogenic p. may occur following intrathoracic surgery or in association with procedures which involve entry into the pleural cavity, such as thoracentesis or placement of a chest drain.
open p. caused by an open wound in the chest wall.
spontaneous p. due to an unknown cause.
tension p. a particularly dangerous form of pneumothorax that occurs when air escapes into the pleural cavity from a bronchus but cannot regain entry into the bronchus. As a result, continuously increasing air pressure in the pleural cavity causes progressive collapse of the lung tissue. If not relieved, it can lead to lung collapse and MEDIASTINAL shift.
pneumotomy pneumonotomy.
pneumovagina involuntary aspiration of air into the vagina so that the vagina is chronically distended. Usually incompatible with fertility. See also RECTOVAGINAL fistula.
pneumoventriculogram the radiograph produced by the use of VENTRICULOGRAPHY (1).
pneumoventriculography pneumoencephalography.
Pneumovirinae a subfamily of viruses in the family *Paramyxoviridae*. See PNEUMOVIRUS.
Pneumovirus one of the three genera of viruses in the family PARAMYXOVIRIDAE. Includes respiratory syncytial virus of humans, cattle, sheep and turkeys.
PNS peripheral nervous system.
PO, p.o. [L.] *per os* (by mouth; orally).
Po chemical symbol, *polonium*.
Poa genus of grasses in family Poaceae. Contains many very productive fodder grasses including the bluegrasses, e.g. Canadian, Kentucky.
P. aquatica GLYCERIA *maxima*.
P. hueca South American grass; contains an indole alkaloid which causes incoordination and convulsions.
poach damage caused to sodden pasture by the hooves of cattle and sheep. In clay soils and when the ground is sufficiently wet the damage caused by a heavy stocking rate of sheep may be very high. Said also of the take-off in front of a jump in an equitation course or a race. Called also pugging.
poaching 1. illegal, secret trapping or killing of game. 2. excessive traffic by animals, especially ungulates, on wet pasture fields causing rupture of pasture mat and loss of grass and clover carrying capacity.
pock a pustule typified by the cutaneous lesions of poxviruses.
pocket small enough to fit into a pocket, figuratively speaking.
p. gopher see GOPHER.

p. pet a general term, used to describe very small animals kept as pets; usually includes hamsters, guinea pigs, gerbils, rats and mice.
pockmark a depressed scar left by a pustule.
pod a small herd or school of seals or whales, etc.
podarthritis inflammation of the joints of the feet.
poddy 1. the act of artificial rearing. 2. an animal being reared in this way, e.g. a poddy calf.
poddying technique for artificial rearing of young, e.g. on a bottle, with an eyedropper, from a bucket. See also ARTIFICIAL rearing.
podencephalus a monster without a cranium, the brain hanging by a pedicle.
poditis see BUMBLEFOOT.
podium pl. *podia* [L.] a footlike process, such as an extension of the protoplasm of a cell.
pod(o)- word element. [Gr.] *foot.*
podocyte an epithelial cell of the visceral layer of a renal glomerulus, having a number of footlike radiating processes (pedicles).
pododemodicosis pododermatitis caused by *Demodex* spp.
pododerm the specially adapted part of the skin that provides nourishment to the hooves or claws. See also CORIUM.
pododermatitis inflammation of that portion of the skin which continues downward within the horny structure of the hoof. Most common use is with reference to cattle where it is used synonymously with FOOTROT, but also used increasingly to describe dermatitis or pyoderma of the feet in dogs.
p. circumscripta bruising and necrosis of the sole in the angle between the bar and the wall of the hoof in horses. See also CORN (2).
demodectic p. see DEMODECTIC MANGE.
plasma cell p. see PLASMA cell pododermatitis.
suppurative p. underrun sole with pus formation.
ulcerative p. a disease of rabbits, guinea pigs and other caged small mammals, caused by pressure from a cage floor on the backs of the metatarsal bones; it may progress to arthritis. *Staphylococcus aureus* is most commonly recovered. Called also sore hocks in rabbits, and bumblefoot in guinea pigs.
pododynamometer a device for determining the strength of the leg muscles.
podophyllin the pharmacologically active resin extracted from PODOPHYLLUM.
podophyllotoxin podophyllin resin.
podophyllum the dried rhizome and roots of *Podophyllum peltatum*.
p. resin a mixture of resins from podophyllum, used as a topical caustic in the treatment of certain papillomas. Was used at one time as a purgative but was capable of causing fatal superpurgation.
Podophyllum peltatum Northern American plant in the family Berberidaceae; contains podophyllum resin which causes diarrhea; called also American mandrake, mayapple.
podotrochlitis see NAVICULAR disease.
podotrochlosis podotrochlitis.
Poecilia see GUPPY, MOLLIES.
pogonion the anterior midpoint of the chin.
-poiesis word element. [Gr.] *formation.*
poikil- prefix meaning irregular.
poikiloblast an abnormally shaped erythroblast.
poikilocyte an abnormally shaped erythrocyte.
poikilocytosis the presence of poikilocytes in the blood.
poikiloderma a condition characterized by pigmentary and atrophic changes in the skin, giving it a mottled appearance.
poikilospherocyte small spheroidal erythrocytes caused by fragmentation.
poikilotherm an animal that exhibits poikilothermy; a cold-blooded animal.
poikilothermic characterized by poikilothermy.
poikilothermism the state induced by poikilothermy.
poikilothermy the physiological state of having body temperature that varies with that of the environment.
poinsettia see EUPHORBIA.
point 1. a small area or spot; the sharp end of an object. 2. to approach the surface, like the pus of an abscess, at a definite spot or place. 3. unit of measurement of the size of a print font; 72 points = 1 inch. 4. a single tine of an antler. 5. extremities of a sheep fleece which has been removed from the sheep and laid out on a classing table.
auricular p. the center of the opening of the external acoustic meatus.
boiling p. the temperature at which a liquid will boil: at sea level, 212°F (100°C).
p. of buttock the prominence caused by the ischial tuberosity.
p. of croup highest point of the croup; caused by the sacral tuberosity.
dew p. the temperature at which moisture in the atmosphere is deposited as dew.
p. of the elbow the summit of the olecranon process.
p. firing see FIRING.
freezing p. the temperature at which a liquid begins to freeze; for water, 32°F (0°C).
p. of the hip the most lateral point of the hip; caused by the coxal tuberosity.
p. of the hock the summit of the calcaneus.
ice p. the temperature of equilibrium between ice and air-saturated water under one atmosphere pressure.
isobestic p. the wavelength at which two substances have the same absorptivity.
isoelectric p. (pI) the pH of a solution in which molecules of a specific substance, such as a protein, have equal numbers of positively and negatively charged groups and therefore do not migrate in an electric field.
lacrimal p. lacrimal puncta.
p. of lay the age of sexual maturity in female fowls.
p. of maximal impulse (PMI) the point on the chest where the impulse of the left ventricle is felt most strongly. It is usually on the left chest wall, around the area of the 5th costochondral junction.
melting p. the minimum temperature at which a solid begins to liquefy.
nodal p's two points on the axis of an optical system situated so that a ray falling on one will produce a parallel ray emerging through the other.
p. outbreak see point EPIDEMIC.
paper p. very fine, tapered swabs used in endodontics to dry up the root canal.
p. prescriptions details of the exact needle procedures and locations of insertions for the treatment of specific diseases.
p. prevalence rate the proportion of the animals in a population at a point in time which are affected by the subject disease at that point. Called also instantaneous prevalence.
p. selection can be based on a table of prescriptions for specific diseases, or on the basis of which acupoints are tender, or on the basis of the innervation of the area of the lesion, and so on for a series of eleven, and possibly more, strategies.
p. of the shoulder the point over the greater tubercle of the humerus.

p. source epidemic see point EPIDEMIC.
p. of the sternum the most cranial point of the sternum, caused by the manubrium.
trigger p. a spot on the body at which pressure or other stimulus gives rise to specific sensations or clinical signs.
triple p. the temperature and pressure at which the solid, liquid, and gas phases of a substance are in equilibrium.

Pointer a medium-sized, lean gun dog with long neck, pendulous ears, and long pointed tail. The coat is short and fine in solid color or white with lemon, black, liver or orange patches or ticks. Called also English pointer.
Hungarian p. see VIZSLA.
Italian p. see SPINONI ITALIANI.

pointer an injury such as a contusion or avulsion of muscle attachments at a bony prominence.

pointfinder an electronic device used to detect the exact location of points for the insertion of acupuncture needles, based on variations in electrical impedance of the skin.

pointillage [Fr.] massage with the points of the fingers.

pointing 1. the posture adopted by a horse with one lame limb, lame with a weight-bearing lameness. The toe of the affected limb is rested on the ground in front of its normal position and less weight is taken on it than normal. 2. the posture adopted by a pointer type hunting dog when it detects the presence of a bird—looking straight at the location of the bird, perfectly still with the tail straight out behind and one front limb flexed with the carpus at right angles. 3. the coming to a head or maturation of an abscess.

points 1. specific parts of the conformation. 2. restricted areas of color. In dogs this refers to contrasting coloring over the eyes, on the face, legs and feet. In cats it is the face, ears, feet and tail and is used to describe the pigmentation pattern seen in Siamese, e.g. seal-point, blue-point, tabby-point, etc.
p. of the horse a list of the outstanding anatomical landmarks of the animal which are used as guiding points when judging the quality of the animal's conformation. This is used mostly in show judging. The list is usually expressed in lay terms such as muzzle, pastern, hock.

poise the unit of viscosity of a liquid; the number of grams per centimeter per second. Centipoise, 0.01 poise, is the standard unit used.

Poiseuille's law, Poiseuille's equation the law which expresses the relationship between the rate of flow of a liquid in a tube and the pressure gradient in the tube, the radius of the tube, the length of the tube and the viscosity of the liquid.

poison a substance that, on ingestion, inhalation, absorption, application, injection or development within the body, in relatively small amounts, may cause structural damage or functional disturbance.

Corrosives are poisons that destroy tissues directly. They include the mineral acids, such as nitric acid, sulfuric acid and hydrochloric acid, and the caustic alkalis, such as ammonia, sodium hydroxide (lye), sodium carbonate and sodium hypochlorite; and carbolic acid (phenol).

Irritants are poisons that inflame the mucous membranes by direct action. These include copper sulfate, salts of lead, cantharidin, oxalate raphides, and many plant and insect poisons.

Nerve toxins act on the nerves or affect some of the basic cell processes. This large group includes the narcotics, such as opium, heroin and cocaine, and the barbiturates, anesthetics and alcohols.

Blood toxins act on the blood and deprive it of oxygen. They include carbon monoxide, carbon dioxide, hydrocyanic acid and the gases used in chemical warfare. Some blood toxins destroy the blood cells or the platelets.

See also POISONING and names of individual poisons.
p. bean SESBANIA spp., THERMOPSIS *montana*.
berry p. GASTROLOBIUM *parvifolium*.
box p. GASTROLOBIUM *parviflorum*.
bullock p. GASTROLOBIUM *trilobum*.
p. bush THESIUM *namaquense*.
bushman's p. ACOKANTHERA spp.
p. buttercup RANUNCULUS *scleratus*.
camel p. ERYTHROPHLEUM *chlorostachys*.
candyup p. STYPANDRA GLAUCA.
Champion Bay p. GASTROLOBIUM *oxyloboides*.
clover-leaf p. GOODIA *lotifolia*.
cluster p. GASTROLOBIUM *bennettsianum*.
p. Control Center public facility set up to provide information around the clock to persons with poisoning problems.
crinkle-leaf p. GASTROLOBIUM *villosum*.
desert p. bush GASTROLOBIUM *grandiflorum*.
p. elder TOXICODENDRON *vernix*.
Gilbernene p. GASTROLOBIUM *rotundifolium*.
granite p. GASTROLOBIUM *graniticum*.
heart-leaf p. bush GASTROLOBIUM *bilobum* or *G. grandiflorum*.
p. hemlock CONIUM MACULATUM.
Hill River p. GASTROLOBIUM *polystachyum*.
hook-point p. GASTROLOBIUM *hamulosum*.
horned p. GASTROLOBIUM *polystachyum*.
Hutt River p. GASTROLOBIUM *propinquum*.
insect p. see BEE STING, EPICAUTA VITTATA, TICK paralysis.
p. ivy TOXICODENDRON *radicans*.
kite-leaf p. GASTROLOBIUM *laytonii*.
lamb p. ISOTROPIS *cuneifolia*.
p. leaf DICHAPETALUM *cymosum*.
p. lobelia LOBELIA *pratioides*.
mallet p. GASTROLOBIUM *densifolium*.
marlock p. GASTROLOBIUM *parviflorum*.
p. morning glory IPOMOEA *muelleri*.
narrow-leaf p. GASTROLOBIUM *stenophyllum*.
net-leaf p. GASTROLOBIUM *racemosum*.
p. oak TOXICODENDRON *diversilobum, T. quercifolium*.
p. onion DIPCADI *glaucum*.
pea-blossom p. ISOTROPIS spp.
p. peach TREMA *tomentosa*. Called also peach-leaf poison bush.
p. pimelea PIMELEA *pauciflora*.
p. pod albizia ALBIZIA *versicolor*.
prickly p. GASTROLOBIUM *spinosum*.
rigid-leaf p. GASTROLOBIUM *rigidum*.
river p. GASTROLOBIUM *forrestii*.
river p. tree EXCOECARIA *dallachyana*.
rock p. GASTROLOBIUM *callistachys*.
Roe's p. GASTROLOBIUM *spectabile*.
round-leaf p. GASTROLOBIUM *pycnostachyum*.
runner p. GASTROLOBIUM *ovalifolium*.
p. sage ISOTROPIS *atropurpurea*.
sandplain p. GASTROLOBIUM *microcarpum*.
scale-leaf p. GASTROLOBIUM *appressum*.
p. sedge SCHOENUS *asperocarpus*.
slender p. GASTROLOBIUM *heterophyllum*.
slender lamb p. ISOTROPIS *juncea*.
spike p. GASTROLOBIUM *glaucum*.
Stirling Range p. GASTROLOBIUM *velutinum*.

p. suckleya SUCKLEYA SUCKLEYANA.
p. sumac TOXICODENDRON *vernix*.
thick-leaf p. GASTROLOBIUM *crassifolium*.
p. vetch ASTRAGALUS spp., OXYTROPIS spp.
wallflower p. GASTROLOBIUM *grandiflorum*.
p. walnut CRYPTOCARYA PLEUROSPERMA.
wodjil p. GASTROLOBIUM *floribundum*.
woolly p. GASTROLOBIUM *tomentosum*.
York Road p. GASTROLOBIUM *calycinum*.

poisoning the morbid condition produced by a poison. The poison may be swallowed, inhaled (as in CARBON MONOXIDE poisoning), injected by a stinging insect as in a BEE STING, or spilled or otherwise brought into contact with the skin.
blood p. septicemia.
food p. a group of acute illnesses due to ingestion of contaminated food. See also FOOD poisoning.

poisonous having the properties of a poison.
p. bride's bush PAVETTA *schumanniana*.
p. plants plants which contain specific chemical poisons, although they may not be identified. They are a different group from plants which cause illness if eaten in very large amounts or have physical qualities that cause illness, e.g. clover in bloat, tree loppings in omasal impaction. There is a third group of plants, those that are only intermittently poisonous. These form a very large group known to have caused nitrite, cyanide or oxalate poisoning but are valuable plants and are safe if used with care. See also under the names of individual plants or the toxins that they contain.

Poisson distribution a statistical distribution which often describes the sampling frequency of individual, isolated counts in time and space.

Poitou ass a French, longhaired, black or dark brown donkey.

poke PHYTOLACCA *americana*.

pokeroot PHYTOLACCA *americana*.

pokeweed PHYTOLACCA *americana*.
p. mitogen (PWM) see pokeweed MITOGEN.

***pol* gene** a gene which encodes reverse transcriptase, found in the retroviral genome.

Poland China a black pig with white points produced in the USA.

polar 1. emanating from or pertaining to a pole. 2. being at opposite ends of a spectrum of values.
p. bodies 1. the small cells consisting of a tiny bit of cytoplasm and a nucleus that result from unequal division of the primary oocyte (*first polar body*) and, if fertilization occurs, of the secondary oocyte (*second polar body*). 2. metachromatic granules located at the ends of bacteria.
p. bond a covalent bond in which the electron pair is held unequally by two bonded atoms.
p. spongioblastoma an astrocytoma with a predilection for the optic nerve and pons.

polarimeter a device for measuring the rotation of plane polarized light.

polarimetry measurement of the rotation of plane polarized light.

polarine a glycoalkaloid found in plants of the family Solanaceae and thought to contribute to poisoning by them.

polariscope an instrument used to measure polarized light.

polarity the condition of having poles or of exhibiting opposite effects at the two extremities.
cell p. a feature of epithelial cells which defines an apical surface facing the outside which is separated by a tight junction from the basolateral surface.

polarization the production of that condition in light in which its vibrations are parallel to each other in one plane, or in circles and ellipses.

polarizer an appliance for polarizing light.

polarography an electrochemical technique for identifying and estimating the concentration of reducible elements in an electrochemical cell by means of the dual measurement of the current flowing through the cell and the electrical potential at which each element is reduced.

pole 1. either extremity of any axis, as of a body organ. 2. either one of two points that have opposite physical qualities (electric or other).
control p. a pole with a loop at one end for capturing wild or dangerous small animals. The loop is put over the animal's head and pulled tight. Good poles have a nonslip device so that the animal cannot slip free because of relaxation on the cord by the operator.
frontal p. the most prominent part of the anterior end of each hemisphere of the brain.
occipital p. the posterior end of the occipital lobe of the brain.
temporal p. the prominent anterior end of the temporal lobe of the human brain.

poleaxe a long-handled hammer, about 9 to 10 lb, originally with an axe blade at the front, used at one time for stunning cattle prior to bleeding out at slaughter.

polecat *Putorius putorius* (syn. *Mustela putorius putorius*), a member of the Mustelidae family of Carnivora. It has a long body, short legs, short furry tail and beady eyes and is about 2 ft long. Brown in color but some varieties, e.g. the ferret, have their own distinctive color. Can eject a foul smelling material from its anal glands when attacked. Its pelt is called fitch.

poley 1. a polled animal; one without horns. 2. a pad on an American saddle.

poli(o)- word element. [Gr.] *gray matter*.

polioclastic destroying the gray matter of the nervous system.

poliodystrophia poliodystrophy.

poliodystrophy atrophy of the cerebral gray matter.

polioencephalitis inflammatory disease of the gray matter of the brain.

polioencephalomalacia softening of the cerebrocortical gray matter distributed in a laminar pattern. Called also laminar cortical necrosis, cortical necrosis.
periventricular p. degenerative changes in periventricular nuclei in carnivores in thiamin deficiency. See THIAMIN nutritional deficiency.
ruminant p. a sporadic disease of unknown etiology occurring in cattle and sheep. The lesion is associated with thiamin deficiency or a disturbance in thiamin metabolism. It is characterized by a sudden onset of blindness, nystagmus, opisthotonos and tonic convulsions. Mild cases may remain standing, walk aimlessly and head press. At autopsy there is cerebral edema and laminar necrosis of the gray matter of the brain. Called also cerebrocortical necrosis.

polioencephalomeningomyelitis inflammation of the gray matter of the brain and spinal cord and of the meninges.

polioencephalomyelitis inflammation of the gray matter of the brain and spinal cord.
feline p. a slowly progressive disease of unknown etiology in cats, including large Felidae; clinical signs include ataxia, paresis and hyperesthesia.

polioencephalopathy any disease of the gray matter of the brain.

poliomalacia softening of the gray matter of the central nervous system.
focal symmetrical spinal p. a disease of young sheep and of unknown etiology observed only in Kenya and characterized by focal softening of the gray matter of the spinal cord, especially the cervical cord, and paralysis especially of the forelimbs. Similar lesions and clinical signs are also observed in pigs, except that the paralysis is posterior. It is associated with selenium toxicosis.

poliomyelitis inflammation of the gray matter of the brain; also the name applied to the viral disease of humans and also known as polio.
feline p. see feline POLIOENCEPHALOMYELITIS.
p. suum see porcine viral ENCEPHALOMYELITIS.

poliomyelopathy any disease of the gray matter of the spinal cord.

poliosis localized loss of pigment in the hair.
uveitis–p.–vitiligo syndrome see VOGT–KOYANAGI–HARADA-LIKE SYNDROME.

poliovirus the human poliomyelitis virus capable of infecting nonhuman primates. Causes paralysis due to encephalomyelitis in which motor neurons are selectively destroyed.

Polish lowland sheepdog a medium-sized, cobby dog with a long, thick, shaggy coat which covers the eyes. The tail is docked or the dog may be born tailless.

Polish rabbit a compact, sprightly breed with a white coat and red or blue eyes.

polishing the final step in dental prophylaxis which smooths the tooth surface and delays the rate of new plaque adhesion. Carried out with a mechanical polisher, prophy cup and paste.

polishings byproduct of the rice industry; the material removed from the rice grain. Its quality varies depending on whether hulls are included; without them it is a high-protein supplement. With them it is largely fiber.

poll top of the head; the occiput.
p. evil a condition of horses involving inflammation of the supra-atlantal bursa and infection with *Brucella abortus,* occasionally *Brucella suis* or *Actinomyces* spp. The bursa is swollen and painful initially and may rupture to discharge through a sinus.
p. Hereford cattle see HEREFORD.
p. pad worn on top of the bridle to protect a horse's poll while traveling.
p. presentation see poll PRESENTATION.
p. Shorthorn cattle see SHORTHORN.

Poll Dorset an Australian meat sheep produced by crossing the Dorset Horn with the Corriedale or Ryeland. A DOWNS SHEEP with all of their characteristics.

pollakiuria abnormally frequent passage of urine.

pollard fine protein-rich feed supplement for farm animals; a byproduct from the milling of wheat for flour. Called also shorts.

polled an individual animal of a normally horned breed, or a breed of a normally horned species, that does not grow horns. Selection for polledness amongst horned breeds has produced some remarkable breeds, e.g. polled Dorset, polled Hereford.

polledness the hornless characteristic.

pollen the male fertilizing element of flowering plants.
p. allergy see canine ATOPY.

Pollenia a genus of flies in the family Calliphoridae. Larvae occur in earthworms.
P. rudis messy and a nuisance in animal accommodation because of their habit of clustering in roof spaces. Called also cluster fly.

pollenosis pollinosis.

pollex [L.] *thumb.*

pollinosis an allergic reaction to pollen; hay fever.

pollutants see ENVIRONMENTAL pollution.

pollution defiling or making impure, especially contamination by noxious substances. See also ENVIRONMENTAL pollution.
anesthetic p. escape of inhalant anesthetic agents into the surgery environment has been linked to cases of spontaneous abortion, birth defects, cancer, liver disease, loss of cognitive and motor skills and drug dependence in operating room personnel. See also ANESTHETIC scavenging.

polo a game played between two teams of four mounted riders armed with polo sticks, consisting of wooden mallets on long sticks, and contesting the driving of a ball through a set of goals at either end of the ground which is 300 yd (274 m) long and 160 yd (146 m) wide. A match consists of six chukkas (eight in Argentina) each of 7 minutes.

polo pony not a breed but a type of horse adapted for playing polo. The majority are Argentinian thoroughbreds, and well over 15 hands high. They have a typical wiry quality, like Australian Stock horses and American and Canadian Cutting horses.

polocrosse a combination of polo and lacrosse played on horseback by teams of three players armed with polo-type sticks with nets attached on a field 146 m × 54 m. The ponies used must not be taller than 15 hands.

polonium a chemical element, atomic number 84, atomic weight 210, symbol Po. See Table 6.

poloxalene a block polymer of ethylene and propylene oxides; it is a surfactant and given daily in the feed or as a drench. An effective preventer of RUMINAL tympany.

Polwarth an Australian medium-woolled (22 to 25 microns) Merino (75%) crossed with a Lincoln (25%) sheep with at least five generations of inbreeding within the foundation stock.

poly- word element. [Gr.] *many, much.*

poly I–poly C POLYINOSINIC ACID–POLYCYTIDILIC ACID.

poly(A) synthesis see RIBONUCLEIC ACID.

poly(A) tail see POLYADENYLATION.

polyadenitis inflammation of several glands.

polyadenosis disorder of several glands, particularly endocrine glands.

polyadenylation the addition of up to 250 adenylate residues to the 3′ end of eukaryotic mRNAs to form a so-called poly(A) tail. The primary transcript is cleaved by a specific endonuclease that recognizes the sequence AAUAAA which is also referred to as a polyadenylation signal sequence. The poly(A) tail protects the mRNA from digestion with nuclease and greatly increases the efficiency of translation.

polyamide material used in the creation of nonabsorbable, synthetic, nylon sutures.

polyamines widely distributed cationic cell components especially abundant in rapidly proliferating cells. Major polyamines are spermidine and spermine but the diamine, putrescine is often grouped in this category. Multiple role in stabilizing intracellular negatively charged nucleic acids and membranes.

polyandry the mating of a female animal with more than one male.

polyanethol sulfonate an anticoagulant and inhibitor of complement and lysozymes, included in bacterial culture media.

polyangiitis inflammation involving multiple blood or lymph vessels.

polyarteritis inflammatory and degenerative lesions of the arterial walls in a number of isolated locations.
p. nodosa See PERIARTERITIS nodosa.
polyarthric polyarticular.
polyarthritis inflammation of several joints. More common in very young animals because of the frequency of navel infection and bacteremia and the immaturity of the arthrodial tissues. See also ARTHRITIS.
chlamydial p. caused by *Chlamydia psittaci* and characterized by joint enlargement, lameness, stiff gait, fever, conjunctivitis, a high morbidity and mortality in young animals. There are also lesions and signs of involvement of other organs, e.g. pneumonia, encephalomyelitis and interstitial focal nephritis. An important disease of feedlot lambs.
chronic villous p. chronic inflammation of the synovial membrane of several joints.
crystal-induced p. see GOUT, PSEUDOGOUT.
feline chronic progressive p. see periosteal proliferative polyarthritis (below).
Greyhound p. an erosive joint disease of unknown etiology occurring in young Greyhounds. See GREYHOUND polyarthritis.
immune-mediated p. see immune-mediated ARTHRITIS.
inherited p. a disease of young Akita dogs, in which there is sytemic illness with fever, lethargy and peripheral lymphadenopathy, as well as polyarthritis.
p.–meningitis syndrome an immune-mediated, nonerosive polyarthritis, seen in Weimaraners and several other breeds. There is fever and spinal pain.
mycoplasmal p. *Mycoplasma hyorhinis* and *M. hyosynoviae* cause polyarthritis in pigs, the first in suckling pigs in which there may also be a serositis, the latter more common in older growing pigs. *M. agalactiae bovis* causes polyarthritis in feedlot cattle, *M. mycoides* var. *capri* causes polyarthritis and serositis in goats and *M. capricolum* causes polyarthritis in goats and sheep.
periosteal proliferative p. occurs in young, adult male cats as an acute, febrile illness accompanied by severe joint pain and stiffness, followed by generalized stiffness, swollen joints and akylosis. The disease is believed to be immune-mediated and associated with infection by feline leukemia virus and feline syncytium-forming virus. In a variant form, the onset is insidious and the joint changes are erosive and deforming.
p.-polymyositis an immune-mediated, nonerosive polyarthritis seen in spaniels. There is a chronic myositis with muscle atrophy.
polyarticular affecting many joints; polyarthric.
polyatomic made up of several atoms.
polybasic having several replaceable hydrogen atoms.
polybrominated biphenyls see BIPHENYL.
polybutester a synthetic material used in suture materials. It has the advantage of being flexible, very strong and forms knots well.
polycarbophil see CALCIUM polycarbophil.
polychemotherapy simultaneous administration of several chemotherapeutic agents.
polychlorinated biphenyls see BIPHENYL.
polycholia excessive flow or secretion of bile.
polychondritis inflammation of many cartilages of the body.
relapsing p. affected cats have a history of swollen, painful ears which eventually become deformed; most cats are infected with feline leukemia or feline immunodeficiency viruses.
polychromasia 1. variation in the hemoglobin content of erythrocytes. 2. polychromatophilia.
polychromatic many-colored.
polychromatocyte a cell stainable with various kinds of stains.
polychromatophil a structure stainable with many kinds of stains.
polychromatophilia 1. the property of being stainable with various stains; affinity for all sorts of stains. 2. a condition in which the erythrocytes, on staining, show various shades of blue combined with tinges of pink.
polychromatophilic having the property of polychromatophilia.
p. erythrocyte see POLYCHROMATOPHILIA (2).
p. rubricyte see RUBRICYTE.
polychrome methylene blue the preferred stain for a smear when the presence of anthrax bacilli is suspected. A positive result is a McFadyean reaction of a purple capsule around a blue bacillus.
polychromemia increase in the coloring matter of the blood.
polycistronic a single mRNA encoding several different polypeptide chains.
p. mRNAs a mRNA found in prokaryotes that encodes more than one protein. See also MONOCISTRONIC MRNAS.
polyclinic a hospital and school where diseases and injuries of all kinds are studied and treated.
polyclonal derived from different cells; pertaining to several clones.
p. antiserum see polyclonal ANTIBODY.
p. gammopathy see polyclonal GAMMOPATHY.
polyclonia a disease marked by many clonic spasms; called also polymyoclonus.
polycloning site in recombinant DNA technology, an artificially synthesized nucleotide sequence incorporated in a plasmid that contains multiple cleavage sites for different restriction enzymes enabling a choice of the most appropriate restriction enzyme for cloning. Called also restriction site bank or polylinker site.
polycoria more than one pupil in an eye.
polycrotism the quality of having several secondary waves to each beat of the pulse.
polycyclic having two or more usually fused chemical ring structures in their molecule.
p. hydrocarbons thyroid initiators, i.e. they increase the incidence of thyroid tumors.
polycyesis multiple pregnancy.
polycystic containing many cysts.
p. kidney disease see polycystic KIDNEY disease.
p. liver congenital anomaly in which cystic remnants of the bile duct occur in the liver; the bile duct is patent; seen in kittens, pups, piglets.
p. ovarian disease multiple thin-walled cysts in one or both ovaries of the mature bitch; may cause hyperestrogenism.
p. pancreas cystic pancreatic and bile ducts and polycystic kidneys may occur in the same patient.
p. renal disease see polycystic KIDNEY disease.
polycythemia an increase in the circulating red blood cell mass.

There are two distinct forms:

Primary polycythemia is a myeloproliferative disorder of unknown etiology. It occurs as an inherited defect in cattle and is a rare disease in dogs and cats. There is hyperplasia of the cell-forming tissues of the bone marrow, with resultant elevation of the erythrocyte count and hemoglobin level, and an increase in the number of leukocytes and platelets. Called also polycythemia vera.

Secondary polycythemia is a physiological condition

resulting from a decreased oxygen supply to the tissues, caused by living at high altitudes, heart disease, circulatory insufficiency or severe pulmonary disease, or the production of erythropoietin or erythropoietin-like compounds, as in polycystic kidney disease, hydronephrosis or renal neoplasms.

absolute p. an increase in total hemoglobin and red cell mass with a normal plasma volume. May be a primary or secondary polycythemia.

compensatory p. a secondary polycythemia, occurring in response to impairment of oxygenation.

familial p. occurs as an autosomal recessive trait in Jersey cattle. See primary polycythemia (above).

inherited p. an inherited defect of cattle. Clinically there is dyspnea.

relative p. apparent polycythemia resulting from loss of plasma and the hemoconcentration that follows. Called also spurious polycythemia.

p. vera see primary polycythemia (above).

polydactylia polydactyly.

polydactylism, polydactyly the presence of supernumerary digits; occurs as an inherited defect in cattle, cats and some breeds of dogs; occurs not uncommonly also in horses.

Polydelphis an ascarid nematode parasitic in the esophagus, stomach and small intestine of reptiles.

polydioxanone a polymer of paradioxanone, used in a monofilament suture material.

polydipsia excessive thirst manifested by excessive water intake. The histories that accompany animal patients are often inaccurate on this point and should be qualified quantitatively.

compensatory p. one caused by an obligatory polyuria.

drug-induced p. diuretics, corticosteroids, salt, vitamin D, and megestrol acetate may cause a polyuria and, secondarily, a polydipsia.

primary p. excessive water drinking in hyperactive, stressed dogs. See also psychogenic DIABETES INSIPIDUS.

psychogenic p. horses confined in a stall and having little or no exercise may drink excessively from boredom, up to three times normal amounts. It may also occur in dogs, apparently from psychological causes, with large amounts of water a day being consumed and a corresponding polyuria with a large volume of dilute urine produced. Yet, when water intake is restricted normal tubular function with concentration of urine is possible. See also psychogenic DIABETES INSIPIDUS.

polydysplasia faulty development of several tissues, organs or systems.

polyembryony the production of two or more embryos from one ovum, e.g. monozygotic twins. Armadillos are the only consistently polyembryonic mammals.

It is a phenomenon in some helminths, e.g. *Gyrodactylus* spp., in which viviparous adults produce trematodes that are identical with themselves and as larvae they carry larvae within their uteri which contain larvae in their uteri. The rate of reproduction can be very high. Also occurs in some insects in which fertilized eggs give rise to a number of larvae.

polyemia excessive blood in the body.

polyendocrine pertaining to several endocrine glands.

p. gland failure see POLYGLANDULAR syndrome.

polyene chemical compound characterized by the presence of several conjugated double bonds.

p. antibiotics a group of agents, synthesized by *Streptomyces* spp., with antifungal activity; includes amphotericin B, nystatin and candicidin.

polyester a multifilament strand of synthetic polymer.

p. base the film on which the photographic emulsion is added to make an x-ray plate.

p. mesh see surgical MESH.

p. suture a multifilament strand, Dacron impregnated or coated with Teflon, silicone or polybutylate used as nonabsorbable sutures. Their virtue is their strength, their disadvantage the difficulty encountered in tying a knot that holds.

polyestrus having two or more estral cycles in each breeding season.

seasonally p. having estrous cycles only during part of the year. Increasing daylight hours stimulates cycling in spring and summer in mares and cats, but decreasing hours of daylight stimulates cyclicity in ewes and does in autumn.

polyethylene polymerized ethylene $(CH\text{–}CH_2)_n$, a synthetic plastic material, forms of which have been used in reparative surgery.

p. glycol a polymer of ethylene oxide and water, available in liquid form (polyethylene glycol 300 or 400) or as waxy solids (polyethylene glycol 1540 or 4000), used in various pharmaceutical preparations as a water-soluble ointment base.

p. glycol electrolyte solution an osmotic solution used as a cathartic to empty the bowel in preparation for endoscopy. Abbreviated PEG. Called also GoLYTLEY.

p. suture one of the better monofilament fibers because of its good handling, low capillarity, high tensile strength and longevity in tissue. It has only moderate knot-holding capacity.

Polygala klotzchii South American plant in the family Polygalaceae; an unidentified toxin causes heavy mortality in cattle. Manifested by diarrhea, tremor and incoordination.

polygalactia excessive secretion of milk.

polygamous as a male or female, having more than one mate.

polygene a group of nonallelic genes that interact to influence the same character with additive effect.

polygenic pertaining to or determined by several different genes.

polyglactin 910 a synthetic absorbable monofilament surgical suture material, an alternative to catgut.

polyglandular pertaining to or affecting several glands.

p. syndrome immune-mediated disease of more than one organ or endocrine gland in the animal, associated with the presence of autoantibodies. A heritable disorder in humans. In dogs, hypothyroidism and hypoadrenocorticism (Addison's disease) are the most frequent findings. Called also Schmidt's syndrome.

polyglycolic acid (PGA) a polymer of glycolic acid used as an absorbable suture material and capable of replacing catgut. Does not swell when wet and is nonantigenic. Is available coated in tissue lubricant which improves passage through tissue. See also POLYGLACTIN 910.

polyglyconate a monofilament synthetic absorbable suture material with good tensile strength.

polygnathus a double monster in which a parasitic twin is attached to the autosite's jaw.

Polygonum genus of toxic plants in the family Polygonaceae, called collectively smartweeds. Some cause nitrate–nitrite poisoning, some cause photosensitization; includes *P. aviculare* (wireweed), *P. convolvulus* (*Fallopia convolvulus*), *P. esculentum*, *P. fagopyrum* (*Fagopyrum sagittatum*), *P. hydropiper* (water pepper), *P. lapathifolium* (*Persicaria lapathi-*

folium), *P. orientale* (*Persicaria orientalis*), *P. pennsylvanicum* (willow weed), *P. persicaria* (spotted persicaria).

polygram a tracing made by a polygraph.

polygraph an apparatus for simultaneously recording several mechanical or electrical impulses, such as blood pressure, pulse and respiration, and variations in electrical resistance of the skin.

polygyny 1. union of two or more female pronuclei with one male pronucleus, resulting in polyploidy of the zygote. 2. as a male, having more than one mate.

polygyria a condition in which there is more than the normal number of convolutions in the brain.

polyhedral having many sides or surfaces.

polyhidrosis hyperhidrosis.

polyhydramnios hydramnios.

polyhydric a molecule containing more than two hydroxyl groups.

polyhydroxydine an iodine-containing skin and wound disinfectant.

polyinfection infection with more than one organism at the one time.

polyinosinic acid–polycytidylic acid synthetic double-stranded RNA polynucleotides, once considered for use as antiviral agents that act by inducing host interferon production. Abbreviated poly I–poly C.

polyionic containing a number of different ions, e.g. sodium, potassium, chloride, bicarbonate.

p. replacement solutions used in the treatment of patients with fluid and electrolyte deficit, the choice of solution to be used depending on the exact nature of the deficit. In the uncompromised patient undergoing elective surgery it is usual to use an alkalizing, isotonic solution such as lactated Ringer's.

polyleptic having many remissions and exacerbations.

polylinker site see POLYCLONING SITE.

polymastia the presence of supernumerary mammary glands or nipples; pleomastia.

polymelia the presence of supernumerary limbs.

polymelus an animal with supernumerary limbs.

polymer a compound, usually of high molecular weight, formed by combination of simpler molecules (monomers).

p.-fume fever see POLYTETRAFLUOROETHYLENE.

polymerase an enzyme that catalyzes polymerization, particularly of nucleic acids.

p. chain reaction see PCR[1].

RNA p. 1. an enzyme that synthesizes an RNA copy of the sequence in a limited region of DNA in a process known as DNA transcription. Called also DNA-dependent RNA polymerase. 2. a viral enzyme that synthesizes RNA from an RNA template during viral replication. Called also RNA-dependent RNA polymerase.

RNA-dependent RNA p. see RNA polymerase (above).

***Taq* p.** a DNA polymerase that functions at high temperature; derived from the bacterium *Thermus aquaticus* and used in the polymerase chain reaction.

polymeric exhibiting the character of a polymer.

p. biguanide see BIGUANIDES.

p. diet see polymeric DIET.

polymerization the combining of several simpler compounds to form a polymer.

polymerized caprolactam a braided synthetic fiber used as a nonabsorbable suture material but only in animals. It has high tensile strength, modest knot-holding capacity, reduced capillarity because of a coating over the twisted fibers, and low tissue reactivity. Called also Vetafil.

polymicrobial, polymicrobic marked by the presence of several species of microorganisms.

polymicrogyria a brain malformation marked by development of numerous microgyri.

polymorph a colloquial term for a polymorphonuclear leukocyte.

polymorphic occurring in several or many forms; appearing in different forms in different developmental stages.

polymorphism the quality of existing in several different forms.

balanced p. an equilibrium mixture of homozygotes and heterozygotes maintained by natural selection against both homozygotes.

polymorphocellular having cells of many forms.

polymorphonuclear 1. having a nucleus so deeply lobed or so divided as to appear to be multiple. 2. a polymorphonuclear leukocyte.

p. neutrophil (PMN) see NEUTROPHIL.

polymorphous polymorphic.

Polymorphus a genus of thorny-headed worms in the phylum Acanthocephala.

P. boschadis found in the posterior part of the small intestine of many domesticated and wild birds including ducks and fowls. Causes anemia, wasting and enteritis, and heavy infestations cause death losses in colonies of aquatic birds.

P. botulus causes death losses in eider duck colonies.

P. magnus found in the intestines of wild anseriform birds.

polymyarian the distinctive somatic musculature of *Ascaris*, *Dracunculus*, *Filaria*.

polymyoclonus 1. a fine or minute muscular tremor. 2. polyclonia.

polymyopathy any disease affecting a number of muscles simultaneously.

endocrine p. occurs in association with hyperadrenocorticism in dogs.

idiopathic p. a cause of acute pain, muscle weakness and lameness or, in a chronic form, muscle atrophy, in dogs. May be generalized or affecting only certain muscle groups, particularly of the head.

polymyositis inflammation of several or many muscles at once, along with degenerative and regenerative changes, and marked by muscle weakness. See also POLYMYOPATHY.

equine p. see TYING-UP SYNDROME.

polymyxin a generic term for antibiotics derived from various strains of *Bacillus polymyxa*, several closely related compounds being designated by letters.

p. B a bacteriostatic and bactericidal antibiotic, effective mainly against gram-negative organisms. It is used as the sulfate salt, and is especially effective against *Pseudomonas aeruginosa* and is also used against *Klebsiella* spp. It is used mostly in combinations with other antibiotics as a topical dressing including ophthalmic and aural preparations. It is not absorbed from the alimentary tract and is not recommended for systemic use because of its nephrotoxicity and neurotoxicity.

p. E see COLISTIN.

polynesic occurring in many foci.

polyneural pertaining to or supplied by many nerves.

polyneuralgia neuralgia of several nerves.

polyneuritis inflammation of many nerves simultaneously.

p. equi see CAUDA EQUINA NEURITIS.

idiopathic p. see GUILLAIN–BARRÉ SYNDROME, idiopathic POLYRADICULONEURITIS.

p. equi see CAUDA EQUINA NEURITIS.

postinfectious p. see GUILLAIN–BARRÉ SYNDROME.

polyneuromyositis inflammation involving the muscles and peripheral nerves, with loss of reflexes, sensory loss and paresthesias.

polyneuropathy a disease involving several nerves. See also NEUROPATHY.

acute idiopathic p. see idiopathic POLYRADICULONEURITIS.

distal p. of Birman cats a noninflammatory, diffuse loss of myelinated fibers in the distal portions of the central and peripheral nervous systems, resulting in progressive hindlimb ataxia and hypermetria in young Birman kittens. Believed to be inherited as an autosomal recessive trait.

familial p. see Boxer progressive AXONOPATHY, hereditary neuronal ABIOTROPHY of Swedish Lapland dogs, giant axonal NEUROPATHY.

hypoglycemic p. associated with hyperinsulinism of β-cell insulinomas; there is generalized muscle weakness, paraparesis and tetraparesis.

hypothyroid p. a progressive lower motor neuron disease associated with hypothyroidism.

idiopathic p. see idiopathic POLYRADICULONEURITIS.

immune-mediated p. may occur in association with systemic lupus erythematosus in dogs.

polyneuroradiculitis inflammation of spinal ganglia, nerve roots and peripheral nerves.

polynomial a relationship between two variables such that $y = a + bx + cx^2 + \dots qx^n$. A straight line is $y = a + bx$. Any curve can be approximated with a polynomial formula.

polynuclear 1. polynucleate. 2. polymorphonuclear.

polynucleate having many nuclei.

polynucleosomes a level of organization of nucleoprotein consisting of numerous nucleosomes joined by 'linker' DNA.

polynucleotide any polymer of mononucleotides.

polyodontia the presence of supernumerary teeth. See also PSEUDOPOLYODONTIA.

heterotopic p. see EAR cyst.

polyol dehydrogenase see L-iditol DEHYDROGENASE.

polyolefin synthetic material used for surgical sutures, e.g. in polyethylene and polypropylene sutures.

Polyomavirus a genus of viruses in the family *Papovaviridae* that includes simian virus 40 and polyomavirus, both of which cause tumors in rodents and have been extensively studied as models of oncogenic DNA viruses. A polyoma-like virus may cause an acute disease in psittacine birds.

polyonychia the presence of supernumerary nails or claws.

polyorchidism the presence of more than two testes.

polyorchis an animal exhibiting polyorchidism.

polyorchism polyorchidism.

polyosteomyelitis osteomyelitis at a number of sites in the one patient.

polyostotic affecting several bones.

polyotia the presence of more than two ears.

polyovular pertaining to or produced from more than one ovum, as polyovular twins.

polyovulatory discharging several ova in one ovarian cycle.

polyoxyethylenes alcohols used as emulsifiers in pharmaceuticals. They have low toxicity but may reduce growth rate.

polyp 1. any growth or mass protruding from a mucous membrane. Polyps may be attached to a membrane by a thin stalk, in which case they are known as pedunculated polyps, or may have a broad base (sessile polyps). They are usually an overgrowth of normal tissue, but sometimes polyps are true tumors or masses of new tissue separate from the supporting membrane. Usually benign, they may lead to complications or eventually become malignant.

Polyps may occur wherever there is mucous membrane: in the nose, ears, mouth, lungs, heart, stomach, intestines, urinary bladder, uterus and cervix. Terminology includes location and/or contents, e.g. adenomatous, fibrous, gastric, tracheal. 2. a sedentary form of hydrozoan, e.g. sea anemone.

nasal p. causes nasal obstruction in sporadic cases. Mycotic nasal granuloma of cattle is manifested by respiratory obstruction and polyps in the anterior part of the nasal cavity. They are eosinophilic granulomas containing spores and hyphae of the fungus *Drechslera rostrata*. In cats, inflammatory polyps arise from mucosa of the nasal cavity or auditory canal.

nasopharyngeal p. occur in cats of any age; inflammatory in origin, they may cause dyspnea, sometimes sneezing.

pharyngeal p. cause difficult swallowing and breathing. In cattle they are pedunculated and capable of much movement and erratic clinical signs.

polypathia the presence of several diseases at one time.

polypectomy excision of a polyp.

polypeptide a compound containing two or more amino acids linked by a peptide bond; called dipeptide, tripeptide, etc., depending on the number of amino acids present.

polypeptide-oma see APUDOMA.

polypeptidemia the presence of polypeptides in the blood.

polyphagia excessive ingestion of food. Polyphagia is a permanent objective with food animals in which carbohydrate engorgement and gastric dilatation are constant threats to health. In companion animals it may be a sign of metabolic disease in which the nutritional requirements of the subject are greater than normal. See also DIABETES MELLITUS, HYPERTHYROIDISM, CUSHING'S SYNDROME.

polyphalangia, polyphalangism excess of phalanges in a digit.

polypharmacy 1. the administration of many drugs together. 2. administration of excessive medication.

polyphosphate a chemical preservative used as a 2 to 4% solution in the treatment of meat.

polyphyodonty having many generations of teeth.

polyplastic 1. containing many structural or constituent elements. 2. undergoing many changes of form.

Polyplax a genus of sucking lice in the family Hoplopleuridae.

P. serrata common louse of laboratory mice. Transmits *Eperythrozoon* and *Francisella* spp.

P. spinulosa the common louse of the laboratory rat. Transmits *Haemobartonella* spp.

polyplegia paralysis of several muscles.

polyploid 1. characterized by polyploidy. 2. an individual or cell characterized by polyploidy.

polyploidy the state of having more than two sets of homologous chromosomes; that is a multiple of the normal diploid number. Results from replication within a nucleus without nuclear division.

polypnea increased rate of respiration. See also HYPERPNEA.

polypnoea see POLYPNEA.

polypodia the presence of supernumerary feet.

Polypogon monspeliensis Australian grass in family Poaceae; causes poisoning when the grass seed head is infested with *Anguina agrostis* nematodes carrying *Clavibacter toxicus* producing corynetoxins; causes incoordination, tremor, convulsions, sudden death. Grass called also annual beard grass, Steward Range syndrome.

polypoid resembling a polyp.

polyporous having many pores.

polyposia ingestion of abnormally increased amounts of fluids for long periods.

polyposis the formation of numerous polyps.

polypous polyp-like.

polypropylene a polyolefin available in monofilament form and used as a nonabsorbable surgical suture. Very popular as a vascular suture material. Like most synthetics it has poor knot security but it causes little tissue reaction and has very long life. It is also available in mesh form.

polyptychial arranged in several layers.

polypus pl. *polypi* [L.] polyp.

polyradiculitis inflammation of the nerve roots.

polyradiculoneuritis an acute polyneuritis that involves the peripheral nerves and spinal nerve roots.

ganglionic p. see GANGLIORADICULITIS.

idiopathic p. an acute, progressive ascending paralysis, usually leading to complete tetraplegia, that occurs in dogs and rarely cats. A slow recovery is usual but occasional cases are chronic or relapsing. The condition follows raccoon bites in some dogs, hence the name 'Coonhound paralysis', but the etiology is unclear; other cases occur sporadically with no known cause. Similar to GUILLAIN–BARRÉ SYNDROME in humans.

protozoan p. canine NEOSPOROSIS.

polyribonucleotide a RNA molecule.

polyribosome a cluster of ribosomes connected with messenger RNA; they are formed for the translation of mRNA to proteins. See also RIBOSOME.

polysaccharide a complex carbohydrate which, on acid hydrolysis, yields many monosaccharides.

polyscelia the presence of more than two hindlimbs.

polyserositis general inflammation of serous membranes, with effusion.

porcine p. see GLÄSSER'S DISEASE, mycoplasmal POLYARTHRITIS.

polysinusitis inflammation of several sinuses.

polysome polyribosome. See also RIBOSOME.

polysomia doubling or tripling of the fetal body.

polysomus a monster exhibiting polysomia.

polysomy an excess of the numbers of a particular chromosome present.

polyspermia 1. excessive secretion of semen. 2. polyspermy.

polyspermy fertilization of an ovum by more than one spermatozoon; occurring normally in certain species (physiological polyspermy) and sometimes abnormally in others (pathological polyspermy).

polystichia two or more rows of eyelashes on an eyelid.

polystyrene the resin produced by polymerization of styrol, a clear resin of the thermoplastic type.

sodium p. sulfonate a potassium exchange resin that may be administered orally or rectally in the treatment of hyperkalemia.

polysulfated glycosaminoglycan see GLYCOSAMINOGLYCAN polysulfate.

polysynaptic pertaining to or relayed through many synapses.

polysyndactyly hereditary association of polydactyly and syndactyly.

polysynovitis synovitis at a number of sites in the one patient.

polytef the pharmaceutical name for Teflon, a polymer of POLYTETRAFLUOROETHYLENE; used as a surgical implant material for many prostheses, such as artificial vessels and orbital floor implants, and for many applications in skeletal augmentation and skeletal fixation.

polytenosynovitis inflammation of several or many tendon sheaths at the same time.

polytetrafluoroethylene a synthetic material commonly used as a nonstick lining in domestic cooking utensils (frypans); abbreviated PTFE; called also Teflon. Overheating produces toxic fumes that cause an acute hemorrhagic pneumonitis and death in small caged birds, which are particularly susceptible. Called also polymer-fume fever, kitchen deaths. See also POLYTEF.

polythelia the presence of supernumerary nipples.

polythiazide a diuretic and antihypertensive.

polytocous giving birth to several offspring at one time.

polytomogram the record produced by polytomography.

polytomography tomography of tissue at several predetermined planes.

polytrichia hypertrichosis; excessive hairiness.

polyunsaturated denoting a fatty acid, e.g. linoleic acid, having more than one double bond in its hydrocarbon chain.

p. fatty acids see FATTY acids.

polyurethane a synthetic material used for nonwoven vascular grafts.

polyuria the formation and excretion of a large volume of urine. A history of polyuria in an animal is as unreliable as a history of polydipsia. A quantitative assurance that polydipsia is present suggests an error of renal tubular efficiency either as a result of toxic damage or an absence of the pituitary gland's antidiuretic hormone.

compensatory p. see physiological polyuria (below).

pathological p. that caused by a disease of the kidney or disorder elsewhere in the body, e.g. diabetes mellitus or liver failure.

pharmacological p. is caused by administered fluids or medication, such as glucocorticoids or diuretics.

physiological p. the result of increased fluid intake; called also compensatory polyuria (above).

polyvalent multivalent; having more than one valence.

p. vaccine see polyvalent VACCINE.

polyvinyl a polymer of a normally monomeric compound, e.g. vinyl chloride.

p. alcohol technique a method of fixation and preservation of feces for later examination.

polyvinylpyrrolidone see POVIDONE; called also PVP.

pomace the residue of fruits after juice is extracted and contains skins, pips and stalks; refers usually to grapes. Used as animal feed but useful only if dried. Called also pulp, marc.

Pomax umbellata Australian plant of the family Rubiaceae; causes cyanide poisoning.

Pomeranian a very small (3–7 lb), alert dog with prominent eyes, a foxy expression, erect ears and a tail carried over the back. The long, straight coat covers the body. The breed is predisposed to patent ductus arteriosus, patellar luxation and tracheal collapse.

pommel the high part at the front of the seat of the riding saddle.

Pompe's disease see bovine generalized GLYCOGENOSIS, GLYCOGENOSIS type I.

Pomphorhynchus an acanthocephalan or thorny-headed genus of worms.

P. laevis found in the intestine of freshwater and marine fish.

POMR Problem-Oriented Medical Record (see problem-oriented MEDICAL record).

ponderosa pine PINUS *ponderosa*.

Pongamia glabra Asian oil tree in plant legume family Fabaceae; toxicity is in cake made by expressing oil from seeds; contains an unidentified toxin which causes hepatitis and nephrosis; called also *Pongamia pinnata*, poonga oil tree, karanja, Indian beech.

Pongidae see APE.

Pongo pygmaeus see ORANG-UTAN.

pons 1. that part of the metencephalon lying between the medulla oblongata and the midbrain, ventral to the cerebellum. See also BRAINSTEM. 2. slip of tissue connecting two parts of an organ.

p. varolii PONS (1).

ponticulus pl. *ponticuli* [L.] delicate plates of white matter passing across the anterior end of the pyramid, just caudal to the pons.

pontine pertaining to the pons.

pontobulbar pertaining to the pons and the region of the medulla oblongata dorsad to it.

pontocerebellar pertaining to the pons and cerebellum.

pontomedullary pertaining to the pons and the medulla oblongata.

p. syndrome lesions in this area cause spastic, uni- or bilateral weakness to paralysis, depression of ipsilateral postural reactions, cranial nerve deficits, and sometimes alterations in consciousness.

pontomesencephalic pertaining to or involving the pons and the mesencephalon.

pony an equine animal of about 14 hands high. Breed definitions vary from 14 to 14.2 hands. The term is also used regardless of height, e.g. polo pony. The only safe procedure when writing a certicate for a pony, e.g. for sale, is to state the animal's actual height, preferably in cm.

p. hypertriglyceridemia see equine HYPERLIPEMIA.

pit p. see PIT pony.

Poodle a dog characterized by its thick curly coat and the intriguing, yet standardized, patterns created by clipping and grooming that usually leave isolated patches of profuse coat separated by areas that are closely clipped. Three varieties are recognized as separate breeds: *Standard*, which must be 15 inches or more tall; *Miniature*, 10–15 inches tall; and *Toy*, which is less than 10 inches (11 inches in the British Kennel Club standards). The breeds are predisposed to otitis externa, progressive retinal atrophy, epilepsy, patent ductus arteriosus, cystinuria, patellar luxation, cataracts, distichiasis and atlanto-axial luxation.

P. cat see REX (1).

Poole suction tube a tube with multiple holes at the end, which reduces plugging with fat and omentum.

poonga oil tree see PONGAMIA GLABRA.

pooper-scooper a flat-bottomed shovel and separate spatula of corresponding size and shape, each on a long handle; used to collect dog feces from the ground, usually for disposal.

poor performance syndrome said of horses which have performed well in the past but are now having a string of poor performances without any obvious disease. Called also loss-of-form.

poor quality roughage corn or sorghum plant tops, cut when very mature, grass hay where the grass has been allowed to seed and the leaves to dry out.

poorness a state of agricultural animals of being thin or emaciated.

popany vetch see VICIA *benghalensis*.

popcorn flower see PLAGIOBOTHRYS.

popliteal pertaining to the area behind the femorotibial joint, the stifle.

p. lymph node a node found behind the stifle joint, between the semimembranosus and semitendinous muscles; deep and superficial groups may occur, the latter being less frequent.

p. tendon transposition a surgical technique for reconstruction of the caudal cruciate ligament.

popped knee see CARPITIS. A term usually reserved for diseases of horses.

poppy member of the plant family Papaveraceae. Includes the genera *Papaver*, *Chelidonium* and *Argemone*.

poppy (horticultural) see PAPAVER *somniferum*.

poprosie HELICHRYSUM *argyrosphaerum*.

population all of the animals in a specifically defined area considered as a whole. The population may also be defined in modes other than geography, e.g. the cow population, a species specification, the nocturnal bird population.

binomial p. see BINOMIAL population.

p. cartogram a map of populations.

case p. see CASE population.

closed p. e.g. closed herd or flock; a population into which no introductions are permitted, including artificial insemination or embryo transfer; the population is genetically and/or hygienically isolated.

comparison p. see COMPARISON population.

contiguous p's the populations are separated but have a common border. Some diseases are very difficult to restrain from spreading from one population to the next.

control p. see CONTROL population.

p. density see population DENSITY.

experimental p. the population in which the experiment, or trial, is being conducted.

finite p. one capable of total examination by census.

genetic p. see DEME.

genetically defined p. one in which the ancestry of the animals in it is known.

p. genetics deals with the frequency of occurrence of inherited characteristics in a population.

infinite p. cannot be examined as a total population because they may never actually exist but are capable of statistical importance.

p. limitation restricting the growth of an animal population by desexing, by culling or by managemental means of interfering with reproduction.

p. mean the mean of the population.

p. numbers see population size (below).

open p. one in which immigration in and out is unrestrained.

parent p. the original population about which it is hoped to make some inferences by examination of a sample of its constituent members.

p. proportion the percentage of the population that has the subject characteristics.

p. pyramid a graphic presentation of the composition of a population with the largest group forming the baseline, the smallest at the apex.

p. at risk see risk population (below).

risk p. the population which is composed of animals that are exposed to the pathogenic agent under discussion and are inherently susceptible to it. Called also population at risk. High or special risk groups are those which have had more than average exposure to the pathogenic agent.

p. size actual counting of a total population, the *census* method, is not often possible in large animal populations. Alternatives are by various sampling techniques including *area trapping*, the trapping of all animals in an area, the *capture–release–recapture* method, the *nearest neighbor* and *line transect* methods,

The population size is expressed as the population present at a particular instant. Alternatively it can be expressed as an animal-duration expression when the population is a shifting one and it is desired to express the population size over a period (e.g. cow-day).

stable p. a population which has constant mortality and fertility rates, and no migration, therefore a fixed age distribution and constant growth rate.

target p. in epidemiological terms the population from which an experimenter wishes to draw an unbiased sample and make inferences about it.

POR Problem-Oriented Record.

poradenitis inflammation of lymph nodes with formation of small abscesses.

Poranthera plant genus in the family Euphorbiaceae; suspected of poisoning livestock. May contain high levels of cyanogenetic glycosides and some toxic alkaloids. Includes *P. corymbosa*, *P. microphylla* (small-leaf poranthera).

porcine pertaining to pig. See also HOG (1), SWINE.

p. circovirus a nonpathogenic virus.

p. contagious pleuropneumonia see porcine PLEUROPNEUMONIA.

p. epidemic abortion and respiratory syndrome (PEARS) see porcine reproductive and respiratory syndrome (below).

p. epidemic diarrhea see porcine epizootic diarrhea (below).

p. epidemic diarrhea virus coronavirus 777.

p. epizootic diarrhea outbreaks of diarrhea similar to TRANSMISSIBLE gastroenteritis caused by coronavirus 777.

p. hemagglutinating encephalomyelitis see hemagglutinating ENCEPHALOMYELITIS virus disease of pigs.

p. herpesvirus-1 see AUJESZKY'S DISEASE.

p. idiopathic chronic recurrent dermatitis a dermatitis observed only in sows and only in specific farrowing houses; affected sows recovered when moved from the houses; lesions consisted of annular macules and patches of erythema.

p. inclusion body rhinitis see INCLUSION BODY rhinitis.

p. intestinal adenomatosis see porcine intestinal ADENOMATOSIS.

p. juvenile pustular psoriasiform dermatitis see porcine juvenile pustular psoriasiform DERMATITIS.

p. lymphosarcoma a rare tumor in pigs but a high proportion of all porcine tumors. Caused by an oncovirus.

p. malignant hyperthermia see porcine stress syndrome (below).

p. necrotic ear syndrome see NECROTIC ear syndrome.

p. parvoviral abortion see porcine PARVOVIRUS.

p. polioencephalomyelitis see porcine viral ENCEPHALOMYELITIS.

p. poliomyelitis see porcine viral ENCEPHALOMYELITIS.

p. proliferative enteritis complex PROLIFERATIVE hemorrhagic enteropathy.

p. reproductive and respiratory syndrome (PRRS) a virus disease of pigs first recognized in the United States in 1987 and subsequently in many other countries; characterized by severe reproductive failure in sows and respiratory disease in young pigs and an influenza-like syndrome in grower finisher pigs. The prototype virus is Lelystad virus 60 nm diameter with an isometric nucleocapsid of 35 nm diameter, enveloped with a single-stranded, plus sense polyadeylated RNA genome coding for about 8 proteins with a genomic organization and strategy of replication similar to coronaviruses and tentatively classified in the family *Arteriviridae.* Prior to a consensus, called also mystery swine disease, swine infertility syndrome, porcine epidemic abortion and respiratory syndrome, blue ear disease, Heko-Heko.

p. respiratory coronavirus may be a minor primary respiratory pathogen causing mild bronchointerstitial pneumonia.

p. SMEDI viruses enteroviruses or parvoviruses causing stillbirths, mummification, embryonic deaths and infertility in sows.

p. streptococcal meningitis see STREPTOCOCCAL meningitis.

p. stress syndrome is an acute death syndrome in pigs occurring usually after transportation, fighting, exercise or even high environmental temperature. If signs are observed they include increasing dyspnea, tremor and stiffness, severe hyperthermia and a rapid onset of rigor mortis after death. Called also herztod, pale soft exudative pork, malignant hyperthermia.

p. ulcerative spirochetosis see ULCERATIVE granuloma of swine.

p. wattles see porcine WATTLES.

porcupine two families of rodents, the New World (Erethizontidae) and Old World (Hystricidae) porcupines have long, erectile spines or quills. All are nocturnal, some are arboreal, some live in burrows. The quills are a cause of major injury to individual dogs that attack the animals. Called also *Hystrix cristata* (common porcupine), *Erythizon dorsatum* (Canadian porcupine).

p. fish members of the family Diodontidae, the flesh of which is poisonous, causing hypotension, hypothermia, emesis and paralysis.

pore a small opening or empty space.

nuclear p. a group of proteins with a central hole through which molecules pass through a nuclear membrane.

dilated p. of Winer a benign follicular tumor that occurs on the head and neck of older cats; they resemble epidermal cysts with a keratin filled, wide opening (pore).

porencephalia porencephaly.

porencephalitis porencephaly with inflammation of the brain.

porencephalous characterized by porencephaly.

porencephaly development or presence of abnormal cysts or cavities in the brain tissue, usually communicating with a lateral ventricle.

porging the process of removing all blood vessels from meat to be sold for consumption in Jewish households. This is a religious requirement.

pork the fresh, uncured meat of the pig.

p. measles TAENIA *solium* and CYSTICERCUS *cellulosae*.

porker the class of pig judged to be most suitable for conversion to pork. The target age and weight vary too much between localities to make a general statement worthwhile.

porocele scrotal hernia with thickening of the coverings of the testes.

Porocephalus internal parasites in the class Pentastomida and the family Porocephalidae.

P. clavatus, P. crotali, P. subulifer the adults of these wormlike arthropods are found in the respiratory passages of large snakes. Heavy infestations may kill the snakes.

poroconidia conidia produced through a pore in the conidiophores. Seen in *Alternaria* spp.
poroporo SOLANUM *aviculare*.
porosis 1. formation of the callus in repair of a fractured bone. 2. cavity formation.
porosity the condition of being porous; a pore.
porotomy meatotomy.
porous penetrated by pores and open spaces.
porphin the fundamental ring structure of four linked pyrrole nuclei around which porphyrins, hemin, cytochromes and chlorophyll are built.
porphobilinogen an intermediary product in the biosynthesis of heme. Not detectable in normal animals.
p. deaminase an enzyme involved in the condensation of porphobilinogen. Now called uroporphyrinogen I synthetase.
porphobilinogen synthase see AMINOLEVULINATE DEHYDRATASE.
porphynuria see bovine congenital erythropoietic PORPHYRIA.
porphyria a group of inherited or acquired diseases in which there are abnormalities of porphyrin metabolism, with accumulation in the tissues and increased excretion of porphyrins.
bovine congenital erythropoietic p. inherited as an autosomal recessive trait in cattle; from birth, affected animals have varying degrees of reddish-brown discoloration of bones, teeth and urine, anemia and photosensitization, associated with a deficiency of the enzyme uroporphyrinogen III cosynthetase.
feline p. inherited as an autosomal dominant trait; affected cats have discolored teeth, urine and tissues, severe anemia and photosensitivity associated with a deficiency of uroporphyrinogen III cosynthetase.
inherited p. the disease is inherited in cattle and swine and is similar to erythropoietic porphyria of humans. There are excessive amounts of porphyrins in urine and deposits in the bones and teeth causing a dark red-brown discoloration. The animals are very photosensitive and cannot live outside. See also PROTOPORPHYRIA, HEMATOPORPHYRINURIA, OSTEOHEMATOCHROMATOSIS.
pig p. an erythropoietic porphyria, similar to bovine congenital erythropoietic porphoryia, but inherited as a dominant trait. Discoloration of the teeth, bones and tissues occurs, but not of the urine, except in severely affected cases. Photosensitization is not a feature. The enzymatic defect is unknown.
porphyrin any of a group of iron- or magnesium-free cyclic tetrapyrrole derivatives which forms the basis of the respiratory pigments of animals and plants. Porphyrins, in combination with iron, form hemes.
p. test the presence of porphyrin in cultures of *Hemophilus* spp. or *Tayorella equigenitalis* indicates that hemin is not required for growth.
porphyrinogen partly reduced precursor form of porphyrin rings which can then have metals such as iron introduced to produce heme or other porphyrin structures.
porphyrinuria an excess of porphyrin in the urine. The urine is of normal color on voiding but darkens to a red-brown after exposure to light.
porphyropsin a visual pigment.
porpoise the smallest cetacean, 6 ft long weighing 100 lb, black on top, white belly, piscivorous and an excellent swimmer. The common porpoise is *Phocaena phocaena*. There are other species, e.g. *P. sinus* (Pacific harbor porpoise).
Porrocaecum a genus of roundworms in the family Ascarididae.
P. angusticolle found in birds of prey.
P. aridae found in the heron.
P. crassum found in the intestine of ducks; causes nasal discharge, diarrhea, anemia and loss of weight.
P. decipiens found in the small intestine of the walrus.
P. depressum found in birds of prey.
port 1. the socket into which the peripherals are attached to a computer. The data for a *serial* port are sent along a single wire, bit by bit. The data for a *parallel* port are sent down several wires simultaneously, and at a faster speed than a serial port. 2. the upward curve in a bar bit on a horse's bridle.
porta pl. *portae* [L.] an entrance or gateway, especially the site where blood vessels and other supplying or draining structures enter an organ.
p. hepatis the fissure on the visceral surface of the liver, where the portal vein and hepatic artery enter and the bile duct leaves. Called also portal fissure and transverse fissure.
portacaval, portocaval pertaining to or connecting the portal vein and caudal vena cava.
p. anastomosis surgical, traumatic or congenital defect resulting in an anastomosis between the portal vein and the caudal vena cava including a portal–azygos anastomosis, or the portal vein and the hepatic artery resulting in portal hypertension. More commonly provides the physical basis for a portacaval shunt.
p. shunt single or multiple abnormalities, intrahepatic or extrahepatic in location, result in venous blood from the intestine bypassing the liver. Hyperammonemia results and leads to neurological dysfunction (hepatic encephalopathy). Other clinical signs include weight loss or poor growth from an early age, vomiting, diarrhea, voracious appetite and polydipsia.
portal 1. an avenue of entrance; porta. 2. pertaining to an entrance, especially the porta hepatis.
p.–azygos anastomosis a form of portacaval shunt with the portal vein bypassing the liver and emptying directly into the azygos vein.
p. biliary bacterial circulation a continuous normal circulation of bacteria brought to the liver in the portal vein from the gut and excreted back into the gut via the biliary system.
p. canal tissue space situated between three or more hepatic lobules; carries the blood and lymphatic vessels and connective tissue.
p.-caval see PORTACAVAL.
p. circulation circulation of blood from the capillaries of one organ to those of another; applied especially to the passage of blood from the gastrointestinal tract and spleen through the portal vein to the liver. See also CIRCULATORY system.
p. of entry the pathway by which bacteria or other pathogenic agents gain entry to the body.
p. fibrosis see BILIARY fibrosis.
p. hypertension see PORTAL obstruction.
p. obstruction obstruction of portal venous blood flow through external pressure on the portal vein, by abscess or tumor or by hepatic fibrosis constricting the hepatic vascular bed, causes interference with digestion and absorption and eventually venous return so that ascites and diarrhea develop.
p. system an arrangement by which blood collected from one set of capillaries passes through a large vessel or vessels and another set of capillaries before returning to the systemic circulation, as in the pituitary gland and liver.
Includes the hepatic portal system consisting of

portal vein and its tributaries from the stomach, intestine, pancreas and spleen, the vessels into which the portal vein divides in the liver and the hepatic veins that enter into the caudal vena cava.

p. systemic shunt see PORTACAVAL shunt.

p. triad anatomically close association of interlobular bile duct, branches of hepatic artery and portal vein.

p. vascular anomalies see PORTACAVAL anastomosis.

p. vein a short, thick trunk formed by the union of the caudal mesenteric and splenic veins; at the porta hepatis, it divides into successively smaller branches, following branches of the hepatic artery, until it forms a capillary system of sinusoids that permeates the entire substance of the liver.

p. vein obstruction acute, complete obstruction causes a syndrome similar to that of intestinal obstruction without signs suggesting liver involvement; partial occlusion causes shrinkage and eventual atrophy of the relevant section of the liver.

p. vein rupture rare complication of epiploic foraminal herniation; sudden death from internal hemorrhage results.

p. venule absence a congenital defect resulting in the development of multiple shunts within the liver, hepatoportal fibrosis and ascites, general immaturity and hepatic encephalopathy.

Porthesia chrysorrhoea the brown-tail moth; has body scales that have a NETTLING effect, causing irritation of skin and bronchi on contact. The caterpillars of the moth have similarly irritant hairs.

portio pl. *portiones* [L.] a part, division or portion.

p. dura (obsolete) the facial nerve.

p. intermedia intermediate nerve, a root of the facial nerve.

p. mollis (obsolete) vestibulocochlear nerve.

p. vaginalis the portion of the uterus that projects into the vagina.

portocaval see PORTACAVAL.

portoenterostomy surgical anastomosis of the jejunum to a decapsulated area of liver in the porta hepatis region, and to the duodenum; done to establish a conduit from the intrahepatic bile ducts to the intestine in biliary atresia.

portogram the film obtained by portography.

portography radiography of the portal vein after injection of opaque material.

portal p. portography after injection of opaque material into the superior mesenteric vein or one of its branches, the abdomen being opened.

splenic p. see SPLENOPORTOGRAPHY.

portosystemic pertaining to the portal vein and the systemic circulation.

p. anastomosis see PORTACAVAL anastomosis.

p. shunt persistence of an anastomosis between the vitelline veins, later the portal system, with any of the large systemic veins, e.g. the azygos vein or the caudal vena cava.

p. vascular anomaly see PORTOSYSTEMIC shunt.

portovascular dysplasia dysplasia of the liver caused by interference with the organ's blood supply; e.g. obstruction of radicles of the portal vein leads to rapid atrophy with condensation and scarification of the affected tissue.

portrait the position of a page when its longer border is vertical.

Portuguese fishing dog see PORTUGUESE WATER DOG.

Portuguese man-of-war, man-o'-war see PHYSALIA PHYSALIS.

Portuguese oyster *Crassostrea angulata*, *C. pipas*.

Portuguese sheepdog see ESTRELA MOUNTAIN DOG.

Portuguese water dog a medium-sized, well-muscled dog with characteristic swimming and fishing traits. The coat is profuse and may be either long, loosely waved, or short, harsh and curled. In addition, the dog may be shown with a lion clip, which involves short clipping of the mid-body, hindquarters, muzzle and tail, except the tip; or a working-retriever clip in which the coat is trimmed evenly to a length of about 1 inch over the whole body, except at the end of the tail where it is left full length. Called also Portuguese fishing dog.

Portulaca plant genus in the family Portulacaceae. Contains high concentrations of oxalic acid and sometimes nitrate, either of which can cause fatal poisoning in hungry stock. Manifested by recumbency and high mortality in sheep. Includes *P. australis*, *P. filifolia*, *P. oleracea* (pigweed, purslane), *P.* sp.aff. *oleracea* (munyeroo, inland pigweed).

porus pl. *pori* [L.] an opening or pore.

p. acusticus externus the outer end of the external acoustic meatus.

p. acusticus internus the opening of the internal acoustic meatus in the cranial cavity.

p. opticus the opening in the sclera for passage of the optic nerve.

-posia word element. [Gr.] *intake of fluids*.

position a bodily posture adopted by a patient to facilitate breathing or a distended viscus or cavity, or to relieve pain by moving pressure from an organ.

positional pertaining to position or posture.

p. nystagmus see positional NYSTAGMUS.

positioning passive arrangement of the head, trunk or limbs in order to obtain the optimum x-ray image, or to make a physical clinical examination, e.g. palpation of the abdomen.

p. equipment devices to hold limbs or head and neck in a predetermined position for radiographic or other examination.

positive having a value greater than zero; indicating existence or presence, as chromatin-positive or coagulase-positive; characterized by affirmation or cooperation.

p. end-expiratory pressure (PEEP) In mechanical ventilation, a positive airway pressure maintained until the end of expiration. A PEEP higher than the critical closing pressure holds alveoli open until the end of expiration and can markedly improve the arterial Po_2 in patients with a lowered functional residual capacity (FRC), as in acute respiratory failure.

positron the antiparticle of the electron. When a positron is emitted by a radionuclide it combines with an electron and both undergo annihilation, producing two 511 keV gamma rays traveling in opposite directions. This effect is used in positron emission TOMOGRAPHY (PET).

posological pertaining to posology.

posology the science of dosage or a system of dosage.

posological table one listing drugs and their dosages.

possum a member of the family Phalangeridae, of marsupials. Insectivorous and frugiferous these squirrel-like animals have a beautiful dense fur and a prehensile tail. There are a number of species including brush-tailed possum (*Trichosurus* spp.), ring-tailed possum (*Pseudochirus* spp.), phalangers or gliding possums (*Petaurus* spp.).

post- word element. [L.] *after, behind*.

post-anesthetic occurring after recumbency imposed by general anesthesia; any sequel may be the result of either.

p. compartment syndrome syndrome caused by

compression of an anatomical part of the body causing decreased blood flow, i.e. ischemia and loss of function and sensation, and eventually necrosis; see also DOWNER COW SYNDROME.
p. morbidity tissue damage resulting from hypoxia during anesthesia.
p. myonecrosis see post-anesthetic myopathy (below).
p. myopathy muscle ischemia sufficient to cause death of muscle fibers results from prolonged recumbency.

post-dipping lameness lameness in sheep due to laminitis caused by infection with *Erysipelothrix rhusiopathiae* after dipping in insecticidal solutions which do not contain a bactericidal agent.

post-milking teat disinfection see TEAT DIP.

post mortem see POSTMORTEM.

post oak QUERCUS *stellata*.

post-surgery starvation starving of horses after surgery can have the unfortunate sequel that the patient, intellectually incompetent, will gorge on bedding if not muzzled and develop gastric impaction.

post-transcriptional RNA processing a series of enzymatic reactions that convert the primary transcript to a mature functional molecule. Processing includes: base modification, sugar modification, pyrimidine ring rearrangements, formation of helices and tertiary conformations, additions to the 5′- and 3′-termini, specific exonucleolytic and endonucleolytic cleavages, complex cleavages with splicing and the formation of RNA–protein complexes. The number, type and order of the processing events varies with the RNA species.

post-traumatic occurring as a sequel to trauma.

post-traumatic sarcoma see feline post-traumatic SARCOMA.

post-weaning pertaining to the period of about 2 weeks after weaning. Relates to the dam or the offspring.
p. anestrus a problem in sows. See ANESTRUS.
p. diarrhea a cause of serious losses in young pigs during the first 2 weeks after weaning; a form of coliform gastroenteritis.
p. *Escherichia coli* diarrhea see COLIFORM gastroenteritis.
p. growth check the sudden slowing of weight gain in piglets when they change from sow's milk to prepared grain rations.

postalbumin a peak on the electrophoresis pattern of serum proteins producing a shoulder on the cathodal side of the albumin peak.

postantibiotic effect the period after antibiotic serum levels have dropped below the minimum inhibitory concentration when no bacterial growth occurs.

postauricular located or performed behind the auricle of the ear.

postaxial behind an axis; the ulnar aspect of the forelimb, and the fibular aspect of the hindlimb.

postbrachial on the posterior part of the upper arm.

postcapillary a venous capillary.
p. venule located in lymphoid tissue these are the site of recirculation of the lymphocytes from the blood to the lymphoid tissue.

postcardiotomy occurring after open-heart surgery.

postcava the caudal vena cava.

postcibal postprandial; after eating.

postcoital after coitus.

postcordial behind the heart.

postcornu the posterior horn of the lateral ventricle.

postdiastolic after diastole.

postdicrotic after the dicrotic elevation of the sphygmogram.

postdistemper after an attack of canine DISTEMPER.
p. convulsions convulsions due to encephalitis caused by the distemper virus.
p. encephalitis see old dog ENCEPHALITIS.

postduplication phase termination of DNA replication; histone and RNA synthesis occurs during this phase: called also postsynthesis or G_2 phase.

postencephalitic occurring after or as a consequence of encephalitis.

postepileptic following an epileptic attack.

posterior directed toward or situated at the back; opposite of anterior. In quadripeds usually applied only to parts of the head.
p.–anterior with the x-ray beam passing from the back to the front, especially to the limbs.
p. chamber luxation see LENS luxation.
p. (caudal) drawer sign instability of the stifle joint with caudal movement of the proximal tibia in relation to the distal femur; normally restricted by the intact posterior (caudal) cruciate ligament. This movement is used as a test in the diagnosis of rupture of the ligament in the dog.
p. functional stenosis failure of pyloric outflow from the abomasum, as part of the syndrome of vagus indigestion in cattle.
inherited p. paralysis congenital paraplegia recorded in cattle and pigs. There are other nervous signs, e.g. opisthotonos, in some forms.
p. limiting membrane see DESCEMET'S MEMBRANE.
p. pituitary see PITUITARY.
p. polar cataract see CATARACT.
p. segment the vitreous body, retina, choroid and optic disk.
p. station trypanosomes one of the two types of cyclical development of trypanosomes. In this form the metacyclic trypomastigotes accumulate in the hindgut of the arthropod vector and are passed out with its feces. Infection of the definitive vertebrate host occurs via the skin or skin wound. Called also stercoracic.
p. vena caval thrombosis see CAUDAL vena caval thrombosis.

postero- word element. [L.] *the back, posterior to.*

posteroanterior directed from the back toward the front.

posteroexternal situated on the outside of a posterior aspect.

posteroinferior behind and below.

posterolateral situated on the side and toward the posterior aspect.

posteromedian situated on the middle of a posterior aspect.

posterosuperior situated behind and above.

postesophageal dorsal to the esophagus; retroesophageal.

postextrasystolic potentiation occurs in mammalian ventricular muscle after a premature contraction which is weaker than preceding beats; for several regular beats after the premature beats, the contractions are greater than normal.

postganglionic distal to a ganglion.
p. axon an axon arising from a cell body within an autonomic ganglion, and distal to it.
p. fibers nerve fibers arising from cell bodies within an autonomic ganglion, and distal to it.

postgraduate after first degree graduation, the registerable degree in veterinary science.
p. degree may be a research degree, e.g. PhD, or a

course-work masterate with a vocational bias, or any combination of these. Oriented towards a research career, or a vocational one.

p. internships clinical posts in teaching hospitals, usually at university veterinary schools, which include a large segment of in-service training. An essential step for veterinarians contemplating academic careers in the clinical sciences or eventual registration as a specialist. Mostly of 2 years' duration; some have an incorporated diploma or course-work masterate achievable by examination at the end of the internship.

p. professional education continuing education, usually structured to provide a continuum of training in a particular segment of professional work, e.g. companion animal medicine and surgery.

Postharmastomum a genus of intestinal flukes (digenetic trematodes) in the family Brachylaemidae.

***P. commutatus* (syn. *P. gallinarum*)** found in the ceca of fowl and other birds and may cause typhlitis.

P. suis occurs in the small intestine of pigs but causes little apparent injury.

posthepatitic occurring after or as a consequence of hepatitis.

posthetomy circumcision.

posthioplasty plastic repair of the prepuce.

posthitis inflammation of the prepuce.

enzootic p. of sheep see ENZOOTIC balanoposthitis.

Posthodiplostomum a genus of flukes (digenetic trematodes) in the family Diplostomatidae.

P. cuticula the adults are found in the intestine of herons and kingfishers, but it is the second intermediate stage, the metacercariae, which occur in the skin, fin, cornea and superficial muscles of fish that are pathogenic. They cause black spot disease of cyprinid fish, especially carp, and may cause some deaths.

P. minimum the metacercaria cause 1 mm diameter white cysts in most internal organs of many freshwater fish. Called also white grub. Herons are the definitive host.

postholith a preputial concretion or calculus. See also preputial UROLITH.

postholithiasis see preputial UROLITHIASIS.

postictal following a seizure.

postiness the thickness and heaviness of the lower limbs of bulls and horses. The animal with thick, heavy legs is said to be posty.

posting the rising of the rider to the trot.

postmaturity the condition of a neonate after a prolonged gestation period.

postmitotic occurring after or pertaining to the time following mitosis.

postmortem performed or occurring after death.

p. decomposition changes that take place at a fairly predictable rate, depending on body temperature at the time of death, and environmental temperature once death has taken place. The size of the body and the presence or absence of bacterial infection also influence these changes.

Rigor mortis is the first of these changes after cessation of circulation and respiration. Within 2 to 4 hours after death depletion of glycogen stores prevents synthesis of adenosine triphosphate (ATP). Without ATP the muscle fibers do not relax, resulting in rigid contraction of the fibers and immobilization of the joints. The rigor first occurs in the involuntary muscles and then involves the voluntary musculature, starting with the head and neck and descending gradually to the trunk and lower extremities. The process usually takes about 45 hours and continues for about 96 hours.

Another noticeable change is cooling of the body, which occurs rather rapidly once circulation stops and the heat-regulating center in the brain no longer is functioning. This postmortem loss of body heat is called *algor mortis*.

Decomposition of the tissues begins almost as soon as blood supply stops. With the breakdown of hemoglobin, discoloration, or *livor mortis*, appears as mottled, reddened areas that can be mistaken for bruises, particularly in the extremities or other parts of the body where there is a pooling of blood. As deterioration of tissues continues and bacterial fermentation occurs the tissues soften and then liquefy. Refrigeration or some other method of cooling the body inhibits this process.

p. examination a careful dissection of a cadaver with the objective of deciding the cause of death. Called also autopsy or necropsy examination.

p. inspection that part of a meat inspection or food inspection at an abattoir that is conducted after the animal has been killed and dressed. Supplements the antemortem examination.

p. report a detailed report of a postmortem examination of a cadaver, including a complete identification of the animal, the body condition, age, sex, species, breed, parity and the changes observed.

postnatal relates to the newborn in the period immediately after birth. A suitable subdivision is: early postnatal—within 48 hours of birth; delayed postnatal—2 to 7 days; late postnatal—1 to 4 weeks. See also PERINATAL, PARTURIENT disease.

p. diseases diseases which are more prevalent at this time in the animal's life because of its small size, its immunological inadequacy and its dependence on the dam for nourishment, protection from predators and from inclement weather, especially protection from the cold.

postnecrotic scarring a reaction to primary parenchymal injury in organs such as liver and pancreas; after the primary injury the resulting connective tissue undergoes condensation and scarification.

postobstruction subsequent to relief of a uni- or bilateral obstruction of the urinary tract.

p. diuresis diuresis occurring after relief of the obstruction. Caused by the retention of natriuretic substances and extracellular fluid during the obstruction. May cause fluid and electrolyte imbalance.

postOp postoperative.

postoperative after a surgical operation.

p. care care of the patient following a surgical procedure. Includes correct positioning relative to the surgery performed and the application of minimum pressure and strain on the operation site, maintenance of an open airway, maintenance of body temperature, moving from side to side if the recovery period is prolonged, maintenance of fluid and electrolyte balance and monitoring for signs of developing shock.

postoral in the back part of the mouth.

postparalytic following an attack of paralysis.

postpartum [L.] *after parturition;* see also POSTPARTURIENT.

p. metritis *Actinomyces pyogenes* the common cause with *Fusobacterium necrophorum* and *Bacteroides melaninogenicus* as contaminants. End result can be pyometra or infertility due to endometritis.

p. septic metritis commonly associated with retained placenta and poor uterine involution. *Escherichia coli*, *Staphylococcus aureus*, *Actimomyces pyogenes*, *Streptococcus* spp., *Pseudomonas aeruginosa*, *Proteus* spp., rarely *Clostridium* spp. are common infections responsible for the putrid smell of the exudate and severe toxemia.

postparturient relates to the dam, in the period immediately after parturition.

p. debilitation the effects of pregnancy, parturition and the onset of heavy lactation especially in animals with multiple offspring, coupled with the high incidence of metabolic diseases and disease of the uterus and the mammary gland at this time can cause serious debilitation which requires intensive management to correct.

p. endometritis inflammation of the endometrium as a result of infection introduced usually at parturition; one of the principal causes of infertility.

p. fever of sows see MASTITIS–METRITIS–AGALACTIA.

p. hemoglobinuria a disease of high-producing dairy cows in the period of about a month after calving characterized by acute intravascular hemolysis, hemoglobinuria, pallor of mucosae and a heavy mortality rate. Predisposed by a nutritional deficiency of phosphorus or copper.

p. hemolytic anemia see postparturient hemoglobinuria (above).

p. hypocalcemia see MILK fever.

p. immunosuppression drain of antibodies in colostrum depletes maternal resources and reduces immune status.

p. paresis see periparturient HYPOCALCEMIA.

postprandial after eating. Called also postcibal.

p. alkaline tide see postprandial alkaline TIDE.

postpuberal, postpubertal after puberty.

postpubescent after puberty.

postradiation following exposure to radiation.

postrenal pertaining to those parts of the urinary system that, anatomically and physiologically, are distal to the kidney. Includes ureters, bladder and urethra.

postrotatory occurring after the patient has been spun around passively.

p. nystagmus see postrotatory NYSTAGMUS.

postshearing sheep in a state of susceptibility to cold stress immediately after shearing.

p. mortality death of sheep due to hypothermia, especially if they are thin and poorly fed, in the period immediately after shearing.

postsphygmic after the pulse wave.

p. interval, p. period the short period (0.08 second) of ventricular diastole, after the sphygmic period, and lasting until the atrioventricular valves open.

poststenotic located or occurring distal to or beyond a stenosed segment.

postsynaptic distal to or occurring beyond a synapse.

p. potentiation increased rate of discharge of a nerve cell that has been subjected to intensive stimulation. Appears to be related to the appearance of a greater number of dendritic spines.

postsynthesis phase see POSTDUPLICATION PHASE.

postulate anything assumed or taken for granted.

Koch's p's see KOCH'S postulates.

postural pertaining to posture or position.

p. reflexes, p. reactions reflexes which respond to changes of position of the body or head to maintain the eyes looking straight ahead and the poll–nose axis pointing similarly, e.g. hanging the animal by its hindlimbs should provoke a lifting of the nose, and if this is obstructed an upward rotation of the eyeball.

posture an attitude of the body. Good posture cannot be defined by any rigid formula. It is usually considered to be the natural and comfortable bearing of the body in normal, healthy animals. This generally means that in a standing position the body is naturally, but not rigidly, straight with the four legs evenly placed below the body, the back straight and the head held up so that the eyes look directly ahead. The position of the ears varies with the mental state of the animal. Continuous or frequent departure from this norm may indicate the need to look further for overt signs of disease.

p. abnormality includes sternal or lateral recumbency, head deviation or rotation, head-pressing, dog-sitting, arched back.

kangaroo p. one which mimics the characteristic pose of kangaroos, sitting upright on the hindquarters with front legs held against the chest. Adopted by some cats affected by the spinal exostoses of hypervitaminosis A.

praying p. one in which the forequarters are close to the ground while the hindquarters are elevated by extension of the hindlegs. Assumed in dogs and cats, often because of abdominal pain.

sawhorse p. one in which the feet are placed wider apart than would normally be required to remain standing. Seen in tetanus and neurological diseases in which there are proprioceptive deficits.

postvaccinal occurring after vaccination. Usually used in reference to an adverse reaction to the vaccine or occurrence of disease caused by the infectious agent contained in the vaccine because of an altered immune status in the recipient or a fault in the vaccine manufacture.

p. anaphylaxis see ANAPHYLAXIS.

p. hepatitis is most common after vaccination of horses against equine encephalomyelitis but also occurs after other vaccinations and in some cases at times unrelated to any vaccination. Clinically there is intense jaundice, gut stasis, oliguria and stupor or mania.

potable fit to drink.

Potamochoerus porcus see BUSH PIG.

potash, potassa chemically speaking, potassium hydrate, a strong caustic. In farming terms, potassium carbonate as it is mixed into fertilizers to redress a deficiency of potassium in the soil.

potassa see POTASH.

potassemia hyperkalemia, hyperpotassemia.

potassium a chemical element, atomic number 19, atomic weight 39.102, symbol K. See Table 6. In combination with other minerals, potassium forms alkaline salts that are important in body processes and play an essential role in maintenance of its acid–base and water balance. All body cells, especially muscle tissue, require a high content of potassium. A proper balance between sodium, calcium and potassium in the blood plasma is necessary for proper cardiac function. Alfalfa meal, molasses and soyabean meal are good sources for herbivores.

p. acetate, bicarbonate, bitartrate, citrate, gluconate electrolyte replenishers, weak diuretics and urinary alkalinizers. Some are also used as expectorants.

p. arsenite see FOWLER'S SOLUTION.

p. bromide used in the treatment of seizures in humans and dogs.

p. carbonate used commercially as a fertilizer.

p. channel see CHANNEL.

p. chloride a compound used orally or intravenously as an electrolyte replenisher.

p. cyanide may be present in industrial effluents. A potent cause of cyanide poisoning.

p. deficiency nutritional deficiency of potassium is very rare. In calves can cause poor growth, anemia and diarrhea. Experimental deficiency in piglets causes also incoordination and cardiac insufficiency.

p. exchange resins an oral preparation administered to limit the amount of potassium available for absorption; used in the management of hyperkalemia. See also ION-EXCHANGE RESIN; sodium POLYSTYRENE sulfonate.

p. guaiacolsulfonate an expectorant.

p. hydroxide (syn. potassium hydrate) used commercially as a caustic. In veterinary medicine used mostly for clearing skin scrapings in the diagnosis of ectoparasite infestation.

p. iodate used as a constituent of salt blocks and mixes to supplement the diet with iodine. Overdosing will cause IODISM.

p. iodide an expectorant and antithyroid agent.

p. nitrite a compound sometimes used in place of potassium nitrate. Overdosing causes methemoglobin formation and severe, sometimes fatal hypoxia.

p. nitrate used commercially as a fertilizer and a meat preservative. Can cause nitrate poisoning or nitrite poisoning in ruminants.

p. nutritional deficiency causes poor growth, anemia and diarrhea in pigs and calves. Electrocardiographic changes are also recorded. See also HYPOKALEMIA.

p. oxalate causes oxalate poisoning.

p. permanganate a topical anti-infective, oxidizing agent, and antidote for many poisons. See also PERMANGANATE.

p. phosphate a cathartic.

p. pump see sodium PUMP.

p. sodium tartrate a compound used as a saline cathartic and also in combination with sodium bicarbonate and tartaric acid (Seidlitz powders, a cathartic).

potato SOLANUM *tuberosum*.

p. bush SOLANUM *esuriale*.

p. dermatitis scabby dermatitis on the lower limbs in cattle on a diet heavily supplemented with potatoes over a period of some weeks.

p. poisoning see CARBOHYDRATE ENGORGEMENT.

p. weed HELIOTROPUM *europaeum*.

potbellied abnormal relative enlargement of the abdomen. May be caused by increased size of viscera and contents, or diminution in volume of skeletal muscle, fat and fascia due to malnutrition or wastage due to parasitism.

potency power; especially (1) the ability of the male to perform coitus; (2) the power of a medicinal agent to produce the desired effects; (3) the ability of an embryonic part to develop and complete its destiny.

potential 1. existing and ready for action, but not active. 2. electric tension or pressure.

action p. see ACTION POTENTIAL.

after-p. the period following termination of the spike potential.

membrane p. see MEMBRANE potential.

resting p. the potential difference across the membrane of a normal cell at rest.

spike p. the initial, very large change in potential of an excitable cell membrane during excitation.

zeta p. a net negative charge.

potentiation enhancement of one agent by another so that the combined effect is greater than the sum of the effects of each one alone.

Potentilla anserina member of the plant family Rosaceae, has a high tannic acid content. Reputed to poison horses. Called also silver weed.

Poteriostomum a genus of strongylid roundworms in the subfamily of Cyathostominae.

Poth-Gold suture pattern a simple interrupted suture pattern used in intestinal anastomosis which is tied very tightly so that it cuts through the serosa, mucosa and muscularis and remains holding the submucosa in apposition.

potion a large dose of liquid medicine.

Potomac horse fever see equine intestinal EHRLICHIOSIS.

potoroo a rat kangaroo in the genus *Potorous*. The most primitive and smallest of the kangaroos, they gallop instead of hopping, are the size of a rat, and one of the species has a long, pointed, ratlike snout. There is also a broad-faced species. Called also kangaroo rat.

Potos flavus see KINKAJOU.

Pott's technique a surgical technique for management of tetralogy of Fallot involving a side-to-side anastomosis of the aorta and pulmonary artery.

Potter–Bucky famous names in human radiology. See Potter–Bucky GRID, DIAPHRAGM.

Potter–Bucky tray see BUCKY TRAY.

potteries possible source of fluorine, used in glazes and art work, causing poisoning of livestock grazing on surrounding contaminated pasture.

potto African equivalent of a slow lemur, but really a loris, a slow moving primate intermediate between a monkey and an insectivore. Arboreal and nocturnal, insect-eating. Called also *Perodicticus potto*.

Potts anastomosis a method of joining the aorta and the pulmonary artery, side-by-side, in the surgical repair of tetralogy of Fallot.

Potts scissors 60° to 90° angled, fine-pointed scissors used in vascular surgery.

Potts–Smith forceps long, fine-pointed, serrated jaw, tissue forceps useful for cardiovascular work.

pouch a pocket-like space, cavity or sac, e.g. one formed by bending back of the peritoneum on the surfaces of adjoining organs. See also BURSA, PHARYNGEAL pouch.

abdominovesical p. the pouchlike reflection of the peritoneum from the abdominal wall to the ventral surface of the bladder.

adenohypophyseal p. see Rathke's pouch (below).

cutaneous p. an invagination of the skin, especially a glandular invagination such as the infraorbital, inguinal or interdigital pouch of sheep (see below).

guttural p. see GUTTURAL POUCH.

infraorbital p. a cutaneous pouch rostral to the medial canthus of the eye, 0.5 to 1 inch deep, in the sheep and many other ungulates. Called also lacrimal pouch.

inguinal p. an extensive cutaneous pouch in the inguinal region of male and female sheep. Called also mammary pouch.

interdigital p. occurs in the foot of the sheep and some other cloven-footed animals. Is a tubular invagination of the skin between the toes that anoints the hooves with its waxy secretion.

lacrimal p. see infraorbital pouch (above).

mammary p. see inguinal pouch (above).

pubovesical p. formed by a reflection of the peritoneum from the floor of the pelvis onto the neck of the bladder.

Rathke's p. a diverticulum from the embryonic buccal cavity from which the anterior lobe of the pituitary gland is developed.

rectogenital p. the pouch contained by the extension of the peritoneal cavity into the pelvic cavity between the rectum and the uterus or the uterus masculinus in the male.

rectouterine p. the pouch formed by the extension of the peritoneal cavity into the pelvic cavity between the uterus (or the uterus masculinus in the male) and the bladder.

Seesel's p. an outpouching of the embryonic pharynx rostrad to the pharyngeal membrane and caudal to Rathke's pouch.

vesicogenital p. the peritoneal pouch between the bladder and the genital fold in the male, or the uterus in the female.

poudrage [Fr.] application of a powder to a surface, as done to promote fusion of serous membranes (e.g. two layers of pericardium or pleura).

poult a young turkey.

poultice a soft, moist, mass about the consistency of cooked cereal, spread between layers of muslin, linen, gauze or towels and applied hot to a given area in order to create moist local heat or counterirritation.

poultry farmed, domestic birds including fowls, turkeys, ducks, geese. For other words relating to domestic birds, see under AVIAN.

p. flea see ECHIDNOPHAGA *gallinacea*.

p. hemorrhagic syndrome see HEMORRHAGIC syndrome.

p. mite see DERMANYSSUS GALLINAE.

p. waste spilled feed, dried litter and fecal residues from chicken houses can be used to provide a high-protein supplement feed for livestock. There are hazards, especially botulism and poisoning by feed additives such as copper and phosphorus. The material may also contain an unidentified hepatoxin. Called also dried poultry waste.

pound 1. a unit of weight in the avoirdupois (453.6 g, or 16 ounces) or apothecaries' (373.2 g, or 12 ounces) system. 2. said of the gait of a horse which strikes the ground hard with the front feet at the canter. 3. an enclosure or building maintained by a local government authority in which stray animals are kept until claimed by their owners. See also ANIMAL shelter.

Poupart's ligament inguinal ligament.

pour-on a technique for the application of insecticides, in which a small amount of liquid is poured onto the animal's back without any attempt to spread it over the surface. It is suited to systemic insecticides which are absorbed percutaneously.

Pouret technique a surgical procedure for the correction of pneumovagina and urovagina in mares.

poussin [Fr.] see MILK chickens.

pouters see PIGEON.

poverty weed PIMELEA *trichostachya*.

povidone polyvinylpyrrolidone, a synthetic polymer used as a dispersing and suspending agent; abbreviated PVP. It has also been used as a plasma volume expander.

povidone–iodine a complex produced by reacting iodine with the polymer POVIDONE; used as a topical anti-infective. Called also Betadine.

Powassan virus see FLAVIVIRIDAE.

powder an aggregation of particles obtained by grinding or triturating a solid.

dusting p. a fine powder used as a talc substitute.

glove p. sterile and special grind for powdering surgical gloves.

powderpuff a CHINESE CRESTED dog with a full haircoat.

power energy or force available to perform work.

p. down sequence of steps taken by a computer when power is shut off. The objective is to preserve the status of the computer and avoid damage to the peripheral appliances.

powered driven by explosive or electrical power.

p. missiles used in euthanasia of animals. Includes conventional weapons such as revolvers, rifles and shotguns, Greenough humane killers and captive bolt pistols.

p. surgical instruments include saws, drills.

pox a group of diseases caused by poxviruses and affecting primarily the skin and manifested by a characteristic progression of lesions from erythema to papule to vesicle to pustule to a round, reddish, raised scab about 0.5 inch diameter to a pock mark which remains at the site of lesions after healing. Includes BUFFALOPOX, CAMELPOX, CANARYPOX, CATPOX, COWPOX, ECTROMELIA (2), elephantpox, FOWLPOX, GOATPOX, HORSEPOX, MONKEYPOX, PARROTPOX, PSEUDOCOWPOX, RABBITPOX, SEALPOX, SHEEPPOX, SWINEPOX.

Poxviridae a family of viruses, the members of which are large, brick- or oval-shaped particles containing a double-strand DNA genome that replicate in the cytoplasm of cells. There are six genera in the family: (1) *Orthopoxvirus*, which includes alastrim, buffalopox, camelpox, cowpox, ectromelia (mousepox), horsepox, monkeypox, rabbitpox, vaccinia, variola; (2) *Avipoxvirus*, closely related viruses that include canarypox, fowlpox, juncopox, lovebirdpox, pigeonpox, quailpox, sparrowpox, starlingpox, turkeypox and others; (3) *Capripoxvirus*, which includes goatpox, lumpy skin disease, and sheeppox viruses; (4) *Leporipoxvirus*, which includes squirrel, hare, and rabbit (Shope) fibroma viruses and myxoma viruses; (5) *Suipoxvirus*, which includes swinepox virus; (6) *Parapoxvirus*, which includes contagious ecthyma, bovine papular stomatitis, sealionpox and pseudocowpox viruses. There are also unclassified poxviruses isolated from cats, elephants, lions, raccoons and gerbils.

poxvirus a virus in the family POXVIRIDAE.

p. officinalis vaccinia virus.

PPD purified protein derivative form of tuberculin.

PP_i inorganic pyrophosphate.

PPLO pleuropneumonia-like organisms. See also MYCOPLASMA.

ppm abbreviation for parts per million; a weight-for-weight (w/w) concentration equal to 1 mg/kg or 1 g/tonne. Used most commonly to express the concentration of toxicants or trace elements in water, feeds, solvents and tissues.

PPR peste des petitis ruminants.

PPV porcine parvovirus.

P–R in electrocardiography, refers to the P and R waves.

P–R interval the period from the beginning of the P wave to the beginning of the QRS complex.

P–R segment the isoelectric tracing that follows the P wave and ends with the deflection of the Q wave. It represents the delay of the electrical impulse at the atrioventricular node.

Pr chemical symbol, *praseodymium*.

PRA progressive retinal atrophy.

practice the exercise of a profession.

advisory p. practice limited to giving advice, usually to farmers on the subjects of breeding, feeding and housing in relation to maximum health maintenance and optimum production. Usually called a consultation practice.

association p. a group of individual practices contract to use common facilities, possibly franchised by a central practice. Similar to a group practice, having the benefits of a large group of veterinarians but maintaining independence of the individual practitioner.

branch p. a practice operated from another center, often with limited hours and facilities but clients can proceed to the main center of the practice at other times or for other purposes.

company p. where the law permits is practice by a company with all of the commercial and financial benefits that the arrangement permits. Has the unattractive appearance of an attempt to evade financial responsibilty to clients.

consultant p. practice as a specialist providing consultations and carrying out referrals for other veterinarians. Commonly used to refer to advisory practices (see above).

contract p. contracts are made with individual clients for work to be done for a flat fee or a sliding scale based on time spent, or per head in the risk population or a percentage of the profit.

corporate p. see company practice (above).

domiciliary p. house calls. The average country practice is mostly domiciliary in that the veterinarian visits the patient in its own surroundings.

emergency p. a practice set up specifically to attend to emergencies that arise at times when most other surgeries are not available, e.g. nights, weekends, public holidays.

fire engine p. the standard practice based on providing attention for sick and injured animals in the surrounding area. For small animals the service is available at the veterinarian's premises but large animals are seen at the owner's domicile.

group p. individual veterinarians use the same facilities and provide mutual support but each has his/her own clients and receives their fees after central costs are deducted.

illegal p. includes practice by veterinarians who are not registered and practice by persons who are not veterinarians.

partnership p. partners are co-owners of a practice, not necessarily by equal shares, and have consequential proportional entitlement to the profits.

principal–assistant p. the principal owns the practice and hires assistants who are paid salaries and allowances. Most veterinarians work as assistants for one or two years after graduation.

private p. practice by a self-employed veterinarian who is obliged by convention to be available to the public although it is accepted that such a veterinarian is entitled to limit the practice to a particular class of work, or to a geographical area or to a particular list of clients.

special interest p. a practice in which the veterinarian limits the species or the kind of work that will be done, e.g. 'practice limited to cagebirds'.

specialist p. see consultant practice (above).

subsidized p. the veterinarian does not subsist on fee income only but is subsidized, usually by an organization interested in having a veterinary presence in an area that is sparsely populated. The sponsor is usually a government but may be a dairy manufacturing company or a wool-selling agency.

practitioner a person who practices a profession. This may be in one of the many forms of PRACTICE.

practolol a β-adrenergic blocking agent with the same actions as PROPRANOLOL.

prae- for words beginning thus, see those beginning *pre-*.

prairie pertaining to or emanating from the prairie.

p. dog small, 12 inches, 2 lb, gray-brown, herbivorous, diurnal rodent, living in burrows, in colonies or towns. Called also *Cynomys ludovicianus*.

p. grass PASPALUM *urvillei.*

pralidoxime a cholinesterase reactivator, effective against the nicotinic cholinergic effects of organophosphorus compounds; it also has limited value in counteracting carbamate-type cholinesterase inhibitors; abbreviated 2-PAM.

prallethrin a pyrethroid insecticide used to control fleas and ticks on dogs and cats.

pramocaine a topical anesthetic.

pramoxine pramocaine.

prandial pertaining to a meal.

praseodymium a chemical element, atomic number 59, atomic weight 140.907, symbol Pr. See Table 6.

Pratt twitch a twitch which combines the LOOP TWITCH and GALVAYNE'S TWITCH.

Prausnitz–Küstner (PK) reaction a local hypersensitivity reaction induced by intradermal injection into a normal person of serum from a hypersensitive individual. Injection 24 hours later of the antigen to which the donor is allergic results in a wheal-and-flare response.

prawn see PENAEUS, METAPENAEUS, MACROBRANCHIUM; called also shrimp.

praxiology the science or study of conduct.

praying posture see praying POSTURE.

prazepam a benzodiazepine tranquilizer, similar to diazepam.

praziquantel a widely used cestocide in dogs and cats. Has a very high efficiency against *Echinococcus granulosus,* removing all of the worms with a single dose. Called also Droncit.

prazosin a postsynaptic α-adrenergic receptor blocker that acts as a peripheral vasodilator; used as the hydrochloride salt in the treatment of congestive heart failure.

PRD progressive retinal degeneration.

pre- word element. [L.] *before* (in time or space).

pre-ejection period the period between when the ventricular contraction occurs and the semilunar valves open and blood ejection into the aorta commences.

pre-mRNA precursor mRNA.

preagonal immediately before the death agony.

prealbumin an electrophoretically fast-migrating protein in human serum but not positively identified in animals. Concerned in thyroxine binding and transport.

preanesthesia preliminary anesthesia; sedation, light anesthesia or narcosis induced by medication as a preliminary to administration of a general anesthetic.

preanesthetic 1. pertaining to preanesthesia. 2. an agent that produces preanesthesia. Acepromazine, atropine, diazepam are examples. 3. occurring before the administration of an anesthetic.

preantiseptic pertaining to the time before the discovery of antisepsis.

preauricular in front of the auricle of the ear.

p. alopecia an area of sparse haircoat located between the eyes and base of the ears in cats; a normal variation, but sometimes incorrectly interpreted as alopecia.

preaxial situated before an axis; the lateral radial aspect of the forelimb, and the tibial aspect of the hindlimb.

prebetalipoprotein very low-density lipoprotein.

prebetalipoproteinemia hyperprebetalipoproteinemia.

prebloom the last stage of a plant's growth, just before it blooms. It is at maximum bulk and the nutriment is still largely in the foliage. Subsequently the nutritional mass moves out of the foliage and into the seeds and fruits.

precancer a condition that tends to become malignant but does not necessarily do so, e.g. precancerous eye lesions in cancer-eye of cattle (see SQUAMOUS cell carcinoma). See also CANCER.

precapillary a vessel lacking complete coats, intermediate between an arteriole and a capillary.

p. sphincters capillaries with a muscle layer which controls the flow of blood from the arterioles into the capillary bed.

precardial pertaining to the PRECARDIUM.

precardium the area of the chest wall ventral to the heart.

precatory bean see ABRUS *precatorius*.

precava the anterior vena cava.

preceptor an instructor. Common usage of the term is that of a skilled practitioner or veterinarian in other field of work who gives one-to-one in-service training to undergraduate students in their practices or other places of work.

preceptorships an appointment as a preceptor.

prechordal situated in front of the notochord in the developing embryo.

precipitant a substance that causes precipitation.

precipitate 1. to cause settling of a soluble substance in solution. 2. a deposit of solid particles settled out of a solution. 3. occurring with undue rapidity, as precipitate labor.

precipitation the act or process of precipitating.

p. test see PRECIPITIN reaction.

precipitin an antibody to soluble antigen that specifically aggregates the antigen in vivo or in vitro to give a visible precipitate.

p. curve a plot showing the amount of antibody precipitated with increasing amounts of antigen added in a precipitin reaction.

p. reaction, p. test a reaction involving the specific precipitation of an antigen in solution by mixing with a specific antiserum in the presence of electrolytes. See also LATTICE theory.

precipitinogen a soluble antigen that stimulates the formation of and reacts with a precipitin.

precision the quality of being sharply defined by virtue of exact detail, an important criteria of a diagnostic test. A precise test is free from random error. Precision is a requirement of ACCURACY.

preclinical before a disease becomes clinically recognizable.

precocial precocious.

p. birds birds which are well developed, have their eyes open and are active as soon as they are hatched.

precocity unusually early development of physical and sexual traits.

preconditioning preparation of 6 to 8 months old range-reared, recently weaned beef calves for entry into a feedlot and an intensive fattening program. Includes castration, dehorning and branding 3 weeks before and all vaccinations 2 weeks before weaning, and weaning 3 to 4 weeks before sale or entry to the feedlot. During this postweaning period the calf should become accustomed to feedlot feeds and conditions.

precordial pertaining to the precordium.

p. electric shock see CARDIOVERSION.

p. thump a sharp blow to the sternum to revive heart action is used in certain types of cardiac arrest in humans. It has not been of proven benefit in animals.

precordium area of the chest wall over which the heart contractions can be palpated and auscultated; typically it is found on the ventral third of the left chest wall behind the elbow, which may be advanced cranially for better access.

precorneal anterior to or outside the cornea.

p. tear film the thin layer of secretions from the conjunctival goblet cells and lacrimal, tarsal and nictitans glands that covers the outer surface of the cornea and conjunctiva.

precostal ventral to the ribs.

precuneus pl. *precunei* [L.] a small convolution on the medial surface of the parietal lobe of the cerebrum.

precursor something that precedes. In biological processes, a substance from which another, usually more active or mature substance is formed. In clinical medicine, a clinical sign or syndrome that heralds another.

p. fragments see OKAZAKI FRAGMENTS.

predation the characteristic of preying on other animals as a source of food. Can be a big cause of loss in animal flocks and herds, especially lambs. See also PREDATORY.

predator an animal that derives its life support by PREDATION.

predatory pertaining to PREDATOR.

p. behavior the hunting of birds, mice and small reptiles by cats and the hunting and herding behavior of dogs, often facilitated in a pack.

Wild predators kill mostly for prey, only one victim at a time. Urban dogs kill a lot of sheep in a flock, many more than they could eat.

p. lesions dog attacks cause massive hemorrhages, much tissue disruption, broken bones; attack mostly thighs, flanks, lambs have crushed skulls; foxes attack tongue, lower jaw, tail area, thigh; coyotes eat a part of the carcass, crushing and tearing of larynx, fang marks in skin, lambs crushed head and neck; crows attack eyes, tongue, anus, umbilicus of already immobilized victim.

predentin immature, uncalcified dentin, consists chiefly of fibrils.

prediabetes a state of latent impairment of carbohydrate metabolism in which the criteria for diabetes mellitus are not all satisfied.

prediastole the interval immediately preceding diastole.

predicrotic occurring before the dicrotic wave of the sphygmogram.

predicted difference predicting the improvement in production of the offspring as compared with that of the dam's which will result with the use of a particular sire. The estimate is based on the actual performance of the male in this regard, as measured on a sample of his offspring.

predictive value a measure used by clinicians to interpret diagnostic test results. See also SENSITIVITY, SPECIFICITY.

positive p. v. the probability that a patient with a positive test result really does have the condition for which the test was conducted.

negative p. v. the probability that a patient with a negative test result really is free of the condition for which the test was conducted.

predigestion partial artificial digestion of food before its ingestion into the body.

predisposition a latent susceptibility to disease which may be activated under certain conditions.

prediverticular denoting a condition of thickening of the muscular wall of the colon and increased intraluminal pressure without evidence of diverticulosis.

prednisolone a glucocorticoid; an analog of hydrocortisone with 3–5 times the potency. Used as the crystalline form for oral administration, as the acetate or butylacetate for soft tissue injection or the sodium phosphate or sodium succinate for intravenous administration.

prednisone a glucocorticoid; a synthetic analog of cortisone, used like prednisolone.

preen gland see uropygial GLAND.

pre-excitation premature excitation of a portion of the ventricle caused by stimuli passing along one of the auxiliary pathways of cardiac stimulation that are not subject to the same physiological delays as the A-V node. Characterized electrocardiographically by a short P–R interval and a wide QRS interval. See also accessory tract atrioventricular CONDUCTION, WOLFF–PARKINSON–WHITE SYNDROME, LOWN–GANONG–LEVINE SYNDROME.

preferred name the name amongst two or more which refer to a single disease, condition or clinical sign, which is recommended to be used generally.

preformation theory a defunct theory that each germ cell contains a complete microscopic replica of the organism.

prefrontal 1. situated in the anterior part of the frontal region or lobe of the brain. 2. the central part of the ethmoid bone.

preganglionic nerve fibers, usually autonomic ones located proximal to a ganglion.

PregChek a computer program which analyzes bovine reproductive performance.

pregnable capable of becoming pregnant.

pregnancy the condition of having a developing embryo or fetus in the body, after union of an ovum and spermatozoon. The duration of pregnancy in each animal species varies widely. See also GESTATION.

abdominal p. ectopic pregnancy within the peritoneal cavity.

p. diagnosis see pregnancy tests (below).

p. duration see GESTATION period.

ectopic p., extrauterine p. development of the fertilized ovum outside the cavity of the uterus. The site of implantation usually is one of the uterine tubes. Not recorded as occurring in animals.

p. edema see UDDER edema.

p. failure includes fetal resorption, fetal mummification, abortion, miscarriage.

false p., phantom p. development of all the signs of pregnancy without the presence of an embryo. Commonly seen in bitches, 40 to 60 days after estrus, associated with the persistence of corpora lutea. There may be all the signs of impending parturition with mammary development, milk and behavior changes including nest building and aggression. Tends to recur in the same bitch. Sometimes pyometra is a sequel. Called also pseudopregnancy, pseudocyesis.

p. prolonged see PROLONGED GESTATION.

p. rate (overall) the percentage of all services given to a group of females during a defined period which result in pregnancies (diagnosed at 42 days or more after service), or percentage of all females which become pregnant during a specified (usually seasonal) breeding period.

p. specific protein B a potential pregnancy diagnosis test; secreted by the trophoblastic ectoderm and present in the cow's peripheral circulation at day 24 of gestation; persists in the circulation for long periods after parturition.

p. termination in the early stages of pregnancy prostaglandins are used; in the later stages corticosteroids are used. The efficacy of the various treatments varies between the species. See also PARTURITION induction.

p. tests cover a wide range with different tests being most satisfactory in different species. *Mare*—ultrasound at 24 days, rectal palpation of the uterus 30 to 35 days, serum gonadotropin levels at day 40 to 100. *Cow*—rectal palpation from 35 days onwards; progesterone assay in milk at day 24 after breeding. *Ewes*—ultrasound after 60 days, rectal probe after 70 days. *Sow*—estrone sulfate content of the urine at 25 days, rectal examination at 30 days, ultrasound at 28 days. *Bitch, queen*—palpation through the abdominal wall in a cooperative patient at 21 days, radiographic examination at day 45, ultrasound at 35 days.

p. toxemia is recorded in ruminants. 1. Ewes. Pregancy toxemia occurs only in the last month of pregnancy, most commonly in fat ewes carrying twin lambs, and in circumstances in which the feed supply is declining. 2. Cows. Fat cows in the last 6 weeks of pregnancy and which suffer a sharp decrease in feed are subject. Dairy cows that calve in an excessively fat state and then are stressed nutritionally develop a syndrome very similar to pregnancy toxemia but called more commonly FAT cow syndrome. In all of the diseases there is blindness, recumbency and severe ketosis. In early cases there may be some excitation, even convulsions. 3. in guinea pig sows, particularly obese ones, uteroplacental ischemia caused by aortic compression and iliac arterial hypoplasia occurs in late pregancy, causing lethargy, anorexia and rapid death.

pregnane one of the two major types of steroid hormone involved in female reproductive processes; includes progesterone.

pregnanediol a crystalline, biologically inactive dihydroxy derivative of pregnane, formed by reduction of progesterone and found especially in urine of pregnant women.

pregnanediol-3-glucuronide a common urinary metabolite of progesterone used in assays of the hormone.

pregnanetriol a metabolite of 17-hydroxyprogesterone; its excretion in the urine is greatly increased in certain disorders of the adrenal cortex.

pregnant having one or more developing embryo or fetus within the uterus; gravid; in calf, in lamb, in pig, in foal, in pup.

p. mare serum gonadotropin (PMSG) originates in the endometrial cups and present in the blood during the period 40 to 140 days of pregnancy. Used pharmaceutically to stimulate growth of follicles in inactive ovaries in adult animals, and in combination with prostaglandin to induce superovulation in cows which are acting as donors for embryo transfers. Now called equine chorionic gonadotropin (eCG).

pregnenolone a precursor in the synthesis of steroid hormones, formed from cholesterol.

prehemiplegic preceding hemiplegia.

prehensile adapted for grasping or seizing.

prehension the act of grasping. Common usage is grasping with the mouth for food.

difficult p. needs to be classified into difficulty in approaching food, paralysis of the tongue or jaws, malapposition of incisor teeth, pain in the mouth, foreign body in the mouth, and defective development of the lips or tongue.

prehormone prohormone.

prehypophysis the anterior lobe of the hypophysis, or pituitary gland.

preictal occurring before a seizure.

preicteric preceding the appearance of jaundice.

preimmunization vaccination well in advance of the expected threat, e.g. 4 weeks before cattle go into a feedlot rather than the day of entry.

preinvasive not yet invading tissues outside the site of origin.

Preisz–Nocard bacillus see CORYNEBACTERIUM *pseudotuberculosis*.

prekallikrein FLETCHER FACTOR in blood coagulation. Precursor of plasma kallikrein which circulates in the blood. Acts in the initiation of intrinsic coagulation.
prekeratin a fibrous protein synthesized by basal cells of the epidermis.
preleukemia a stage of bone marrow dysfunction which may progress to the development of granulocytic leukemia. It occurs in cats which in most cases are infected by feline leukemia virus. The disease is also called subleukemic granulocytic leukemia.
prelimbic in front of a limbus; refers usually to the limbus fossae ovalis.
preload see CARDIAC preload.
premalignant precancerous.
premating uterus disinfection a routine practice in some herd health programs; includes uterine infusion in all or selected cows with antibiotic or other antibacterial material.
premature born or interrupted before the state of maturity; occurring before the proper time.
p. activation potentiation see POSTEXTRASYSTOLIC POTENTIATION.
p. heartbeats arise from irritable foci from within the myocardium in either the atrium or ventricle or close to the A-V node (junctional premature beats). They may cause irregularity of the heartbeat but they can be accurately identified only by the use of an electrocardiograph.
p. ventricular contraction (PVC) see premature heartbeats (above).
p. young a newborn animal born before the full term of its pregnancy but capable of maintaining an independent existence.
prematurity underdevelopment; the condition of being born prematurely.
premaxilla the incisive bone, the bone which bears the upper incisor teeth.
cleft p. see CLEFT lip.
premaxillary 1. situated in front of the maxilla proper. 2. incisive bone. 3. pertaining to the premaxilla.
premaxillectomy surgical removal of a premaxilla, usually performed for radical excision of an oral neoplasm.
premedication preliminary medication, particularly internal medication to produce sedation or narcosis prior to general anesthesia, e.g. acepromazine, diazepam, promethazine.
premilking in the period immediately before commencing to milk the cow, ewe or doe goat.
p. udder preparation includes cleaning of the teats and udder so as to provide milk of good quality, massage to encourage let-down and fast milking, and physical examination and rejection of the first few streams of milk which are most likely to contain transient bacterial infections.
premises a building or part of a building, including land and other appurtenances, especially mechanical services.
veterinary p. does not define whether the accommodation is classified as a hospital, or a clinic, or is less than those and does not fit any special criteria. Does indicate that the premises are used for veterinary purposes, e.g. branch premises indicates that the premises are used for veterinary work but is serviced from a main clinic at a distance and is not manned for sufficiently long periods each day to qualify as a branch practice.
premium pet food a commercially prepared dog or cat food, sold through selected outlets and at higher prices than other pet foods, suggesting a superior quality. The formula is generally constant, irrespective of variations in cost and availability of ingredients.
premix a finite mixture of nutritional supplements such as minerals and vitamins, usually combined with a carrier and ready for mixing with a total ration.
premolar in front of the molar teeth. See also TEETH.
premorbid occurring before the development of disease.
premucin mucin prior to its discharge from its goblet cell; gives the cell a foamy appearance.
premunition resistance to infection by the same or closely related pathogen established after an acute infection has become chronic, and lasting as long as the infecting organisms are in the body.
premyeloblast a precursor of a myeloblast.
premyelocyte promyelocyte; progranulocyte.
prenarcosis the induction of narcosis usually as a preliminary to general anesthesia or as an adjunct to local or regional anesthesia.
prenatal preceding birth.
p. care care of the pregnant female before delivery of the neonate.
p. cytogenetic studies cytogenetic studies carried out on amniotic fluid cultures, the fluid being collected by amniocentesis, is not much used in veterinary medicine because of lack of knowledge of congenital disease linked to chromosomal abnormality. Could be used as a means of early sex determination.
p. infection infection of the fetus via an intact placenta, in the case of viruses, or via a placentitis in the case of bacterial or metazoan infections.
p. loss see ABORTION, STILLBIRTH, early EMBRYONIC mortality, MUMMIFICATION.
preneoplastic before the formation of a tumor. See also PRECANCEROUS.
Prenia vygie PSILOCAULON *rogersiae*.
preOp preoperative.
preoperative preceding an operation.
p. care the preparation of a patient before operation. The preoperative period may be extremely short, as with an emergency operation, or it may encompass several days during which diagnostic tests, specific medications and treatments, and measures to improve the patient's general well-being are employed in preparation for surgery.
p. cleansing preparation of the patient and surgical personnel to minimize contamination of the wound. See also SCRUB (2).
p. scrub-up see surgical SCRUB.
preoptic nuclei nuclei in the anterior part of the hypothalamus.
preoral situated rostral to the mouth; in front of the mouth.
preparalytic preceding paralysis.
prepartum just before parturition.
p. milking milking of cows for a week or so before calving to reduce pressure in the udder and prevent development of udder edema, or to stimulate parathyroid activity and reduce chance of milk fever occurring. Has the disadvantage of reducing the colostral antibodies available for the calf.
prepatellar in front of the patella.
prepatent before it becomes manifest. Used with reference to infection with bacteria, viruses and particularly helminth parasites.
p. period the period between infection of the host and the earliest time at which the causative agent can be recovered from the patient or, in the case of para-

sites, eggs or larvae can be recovered from feces, urine or blood. It is usually shorter than the INCUBATION period but may be longer in some parasitic infestations, e.g. hookworm infestation in puppies.

prepotent having great power; of the two parents, the one with greater power to transmit heritable characteristics to the offspring.

preprandial before meals.

prepriming complex in DNA replication, an assembly of proteins that include dnaB–dnaC complex and proteins n, n′, n″ and i, formed at an intermediate time during DNA replication.

prepriming protein in the initiation of DNA replication, a group of proteins that bind to tetranucleotide motifs (T7 phage) prior to the synthesis of oligonucleotide primers by primase.

preprocessing controls in an ultrasound machine, controls which alter the character of the incident beam of ultrasound, thus enhancing the resultant image.

preprocollagen chain primary translational product in the production of collagen.

preproinsulin the precursor of proinsulin, containing an additional polypeptide sequence at the *N*-terminal.

preproparathyroid hormone a precursor of proparathyroid hormone, synthesized on the ribosomes of chief cells; abbreviated pre-proPTH.

preproprotein any precursor of a proprotein.

prepuberal, prepubertal before puberty; pertaining to the period preceding gonadal maturity.

prepubescent prepuberal.

prepubic in front of the pubis.

prepuce an invagination of skin which covers the free portion of the penis in the non-erect state. In horses the invagination is a double one. In cattle called also pizzle.

preputial emanating from or pertaining to the prepuce.

p. anastomosis a treatment for preputial prolapse in pigs involving resection of the prolapsed portion and joining of the skin and mucosal surfaces at the margin of the prolapsed tissue.

p. annulus the fibrous ring contained in the skin around the external orifice of the prepuce.

p. calculus top-shaped mass; may act as valve and obstruct preputial orifice.

p. diverticulitis inflammation of the preputial diverticulum in the pig.

p. diverticulum an evagination of the prepuce such as of the dorsal wall of the preputial cavity of the boar just inside the external preputial orifice. Called also preputial sac.

p. eversion because of injury or infection the skin lining the preputial cavity becomes swollen and edematous and prolapses through the preputial orifice where it is likely to undergo more injury. Commonest in cattle and amongst them in polled animals which are likely to have a higher incidence of weak preputial muscles and therefore the most dependent pizzles. Called also preputial prolapse.

p. hypoplasia with concurrent smallness of other genitalia occurs with early castration and in intersex specimens.

p. inflammation posthitis.

p. prolapse seen in pigs and may be treated by replacement and use of a purse-string suture, or in more severe cases by preputial anastomosis (above).

ring method of p. amputation a surgical method of treating prepucial prolapse in bulls, using a rigid plastic ring as a framework for ligation.

p. sac see preputial diverticulum (above).

p. varicosities distended veins that often cause local distension of the prepuce in stallions but do not appear to interfere with breeding.

preputiotomy incision of the prepuce of the penis to relieve phimosis.

preputium prepuce.

prepyloric just oral to the pylorus.

prerace testing a procedure for testing a horse's urine or saliva for drugs before the race is run with the objective of excluding the horse if the result is positive. This does not achieve the real objective of avoiding fraudulent betting coups and because the logistics are difficult and expensive, and because postrace testing is still necessary in the same animal, prerace testing is not a common strategy.

prerenal in front of the kidney, used usually in a physiological sense rather than an anatomical one. The most important prerenal mechanism is severe reduction in renal blood flow and therefore glomerular filtration in shock, dehydration and severe hemorrhage.

p. failure failure of the urinary mechanism due to inadequate perfusion of the kidney.

presacral cranial to the sacrum.

presby- word element. [Gr.] *old age*.

presbyacusia see PRESBYCUSIS.

presbyatrics geriatrics.

presbycardia impairment of cardiac function attributed to aging, with senescent changes in the body and no evidence of other cause of heart disease.

presbycusis, presbyacusia progressive, bilateral loss of hearing with advancing age; occurs in several animal species, especially old dogs.

presbyopia diminution of visual acuity due to old age; caused by loss of accommodation resulting from decreased elasticity of the lens.

prescription a written directive, as for the compounding or dispensing and administration of drugs, or for other service to a particular patient. Any prescription relating to restricted drugs must be directed to a qualified pharmacist and can be authorized only by a registered veterinarian, dentist or medical practitioner.

There are four parts to a drug prescription. The first is the symbol ▬ from the Latin *recipe*, meaning 'take'. This is the superscription. The second part is the inscription, specifying the ingredients and their quantities. The third part is the subscription, which tells the pharmacist how to compound the medicine. The signature is the last part, and it is usually preceded by an S or sig. to represent the Latin *signa*, meaning 'mark'. The signature is where the veterinarian indicates what instructions are to be put on the outside of the package to tell the patient when and how to take the medicine and in what quantities.

The pharmacist keeps a file of all the prescriptions he/she fills.

p. drugs drugs limited in their availability so that a prescription is needed to obtain them. Called also restricted substances.

presentation lie; the relationship of the long axis of the fetus to that of the dam. In foals and ruminants the normal presentation of a fetus during parturition is with the forelimbs extended forwards so that the hooves are presented first, followed by the head between the forearms, followed by the trunk, abdomen and lastly the hindlimbs extended backwards, i.e. anterior presentation.

In piglets the usual presentation is the nose first followed by the shoulders with the forelimbs beside the trunk, followed by the hindlimbs extended backwards. The nose of puppies and kittens is presented first with the front paws forward under the neck and chin.

anterior p. presentation of the front feet and limbs followed by the fetal head in labor.

breech p. presentation of the fetal buttocks and tail in labor.

funic p. presentation of the umbilical cord in labor.

poll p. the fetus is presented with the forelimbs retained and the neck flexed so that the poll is presented in the cervix.

posterior p. the hindfeet are presented followed by the hindlimbs and hindquarters and tail; a normal variation in dogs and pigs.

transverse p. at birth the fetus is presented at the pelvic inlet with its long axis running across the long axis of the pelvic canal in the dorsotransverse position. It is the back of the fetus that can be palpated. There are no fetal parts with which to effect a correction.

ventral head p. the fetus presents with the head and neck flexed beneath the body. Called also neck flexion.

preservation 1. of food by any means which will inhibit the growth of microorganisms. Includes salting, wet pickling, drying, cold storage, smoking, vacuum packing, heating, gamma-radiation. 2. preservation of specimens for teaching purposes.

preservative a substance added to a product to destroy or inhibit multiplication of microorganisms.

food p. substances added to food for humans; hence they are not poisonous.

wood p. chrome–copper–arsenic, chlorinated naphthalene, creosote; poisonous to most animals. See also WOOD PRESERVATIVE.

preslaughter tenderizing the intravenous injection of a tenderizing agent, usually a proteolytic enzyme, a few minutes before slaughter. The concept is a repugnant one to most people, the effects are dubious and some animals die of anaphylaxis immediately after the injection.

presomite referring to embryos before the appearance of somites.

presphenoid the anterior portion of the body of the sphenoid bone.

presphygmic preceding the pulse wave.

p. interval, p. period the first phase of ventricular systole, being the period immediately after closure of the atrioventricular valves and lasting until the semilunar valves open.

pressor tending to increase blood pressure.

pressor receptor pressoreceptor.

pressoreceptive sensitive to stimuli due to vasomotor activity; pressosensitive.

pressoreceptor a receptor or nerve ending sensitive to stimuli of vasomotor activity.

pressosensitive pressoreceptive.

pressure stress or strain, by compression, expansion, pull, thrust or shear.

arterial p. the blood pressure in the arteries.

atmospheric p. the pressure exerted by the atmosphere, about 15 lb per square inch (2.17 kPa) at sea level.

capillary p. the blood pressure in the capillaries.

central venous p. (CVP) see CENTRAL venous pressure.

cerebrospinal p. the pressure of the cerebrospinal fluid, normally 100 to 150 mmHg.

diastolic p. the lowest pressure recorded in the arterial blood pressure cycle. Represents the minimal pressure in the left ventricle which can maintain its ejection phase. See also BLOOD PRESSURE.

intracranial p. (ICP) see INTRACRANIAL pressure.

intraocular p. (IOP) the pressure exerted against the outer coats by the contents of the eyeball.

p. gradient the rate of increase (or decrease) in the magnitude of the pressure being measured.

p. load see FLOWLOAD.

mean circulatory filling p. a measure of the average (arterial and venous) pressure necessary to cause filling of the circulation with blood; it varies with blood volume and is directly proportional to the rate of venous return and thus to cardiac output.

p. natriuresis thought to participate in regulating the volume of extracellular fluid levels when the normal neurohumoral mediators are impaired; the increase in water and sodium ion excretions which occur when blood pressure is elevated because of an increase in the circulating blood volume.

p. necrosis necrosis of tissue caused by exclusion of circulation by external compression, e.g. in prolonged recumbency, or due to too-tight bandage, collar, harness.

negative p. pressure less than that of the atmosphere.

oncotic p. the osmotic pressure of a colloid in solution.

osmotic p. the potential pressure of a solution directly related to its solute osmolar concentration; it is the maximum pressure developed by osmosis in a solution separated from another by a semipermeable membrane, i.e. the pressure that will just prevent OSMOSIS between two such solutions.

p. point granuloma see pressure points (below).

p. point pyoderma see pressure points (below).

p. points parts of the body subject to pressure when the animal is recumbent, wearing harness or saddlery, or during restraint. Usually bony prominences such as the point of the hock, hip, shoulder, elbow and lateral aspects of limbs. These are predisposed to callus formation, infection pyoderma and granulomas.

positive p. pressure greater than that of the atmosphere.

pulse p. difference between systolic and diastolic pressures in arteries.

p. receptors e.g. the blood pressure receptors in the aortic arch and the carotid sinus.

p. sore decubitus ulcer.

systolic p. the highest reading in the arterial blood pressure cycle. A reflection of the ejection pressure of left ventricular systole, and the elasticity of the arterial system.

venous p. the blood pressure in the veins. See also CENTRAL venous pressure.

wedge p. intravascular pressure as measured by a SWAN–GANZ CATHETER introduced into the pulmonary artery; it permits indirect measurement of the mean left atrial pressure.

p. wrap bandages which apply pressure to underlying tissues; used after trauma to limit the development of edema, and in the management of lymphedema.

presternal ventral to the sternum.

p. calcification calcification of originally fat necrotic lesions in the brisket of cattle resulting from repeated trauma caused by lying down or by pressure by feed trough. Called also putty brisket.

presternum the manubrium; the cranial part of the sternum.

presuppurative preceding suppuration.

presuturing the suturing of skin over a lesion 12 to 24 hours before it is to be surgically removed. This allows for stretching of skin which assists in closure of the defect at the time of surgery.

presymptomatic existing before the appearance of clinical signs.

presynaptic situated or occurring proximal to a synapse.

presystole the interval in the cardiac cycle just before systole.

presystolic pertaining to PRESYSTOLE.

pretarsal dorsal to the tarsus.

pretibial cranial to the tibia.

prevalence the total number of cases of a specific disease in existence in a given population at a certain time, i.e. PREVALENCE. See also CROSS-SECTIONAL STUDY.

instantaneous p. the prevalence at a particular moment. Called also spot prevalence.

period p. the number of cases of a disease which occur during a specified period, e.g. annual, lifetime, as a percentage of the total or average total number of animals at risk during the same period.

point p. as for period prevalence (above) except that the assessment is made at a specific point in time rather than over a period, a rather impractical exercise.

p. rate the number of patients who have the disease at a particular time, divided by the population at risk of having the disease at that time.

spot p. see instantaneous prevalence (above).

prevalent widespread occurrence.

prevention in disease control terms includes measures designed to prevent the introduction of a disease into areas where it does not already exist, and improve the resistance of the population and reduce the chances of the infection spreading, when the disease already exists in the population.

preventive serving to avert the occurrence of; prophylactic.

veterinary p. medicine science aimed at preventing disease in animals. Preventive medicine has been a large part of general practices for many years and is currently expanding the sorts of services that it provides by the inclusion of such items as herd health programs, cytogenetic surveillance, embryo transfer.

veterinary p. screening see SCREENING test.

veterinary p. therapeutics the positive aspects of repair of nutritional deficiencies; the provision of therapeutic agents as part of a preventive medicine program. Daily administration of small doses of anthelmintics, treatment of the trypanosomiases are examples.

prevertebral ventral to a vertebra.

prevesical ventral to the bladder.

previable before the time at which the fetus is capable of maintaining a separate existence.

p. period the period of fetal life just prior to the time at which the fetus is capable of being viable.

Prevoltella ruminocola one of the digestive bacteria commonly found in rumens.

preweaning the period just before the young animal is weaned. This includes the neonatal period and is the period during which most deaths occur.

prezygotic before a zygote is formed; occurring before completion of fertilization.

priapism persistent abnormal erection of the penis, accompanied by pain and tenderness. It is seen in diseases and injuries of the spinal cord, and may be caused by vesical calculus and certain injuries to the penis.

Pribnow box the sequence of five to 10 bases in the promotor region of *Escherichia coli* genes. It is a variant of a basic sequence TATAATG. See also TATA BOX.

Pricetrema zalophi a liver fluke found in fur seals in large numbers without causing apparent clinical illness.

prick-eared in dogs, used to describe upright ears, usually with a pointed tip.

pricket a male deer with his first set of horns at 2 years of age.

prickle cell a cell with delicate radiating processes connecting with similar cells, being a dividing keratinocyte of the prickle-cell layer of the epidermis.

prickly many sharp spines protrude.

p. black rolypoly SCLEROLAENA *muricata*.

p. jack EMEX AUSTRALIS.

p. lettuce LACTUCA SERRIOLA.

p. paddymelon CUCUMIS *myriocarpus*.

p. pear OPUNTIA spp.

p. poppy ARGEMONE spp.

p. roly-poly SCLEROLAENA *muricata*.

prickly heat miliaria of humans; not a disease known to occur in animals.

PRID progesterone releasing intravaginal device.

pride of California LATHYRUS *splendens*.

prilocaine a local anesthetic, used as the hydrochloride salt.

primaquine an antiprotozoal agent used as the phosphate in the treatment of theileriosis, babesiosis, leishmaniasis and trypanosomiasis.

primary first; basic.

p. accession the first contact with the veterinarian by an animal for the particular condition or disease incident that is the cause of the visit.

p. accession practice a veterinary practice that does most of its work with primary accession cases—not a specialty practice.

p. bile acids see BILE acids.

p. carcinogens substances that react directly with a specific biological group in living tissue resulting in the development of a neoplasm. They are mostly synthetic compounds or metals.

p. case the patient which brings the disease into the population.

p. complex of Ranke in the pathogenesis of tuberculosis is the primary lesion with a similar lesion in the draining lymph node.

p. health care routine outpatient care.

p. immune response see humoral IMMUNITY.

p. intention healing see HEALING by first intention.

p. rumen cycle see RETICULORUMINAL CONTRACTIONS.

p. ruminal tympany intrinsic to reticuloruminal dysfunction; not secondary to traumatic reticulitis, esophageal obstruction.

p. ruminant gastrointestinal dysfunction dysfunction intrinsic to the gastrointestinal tract of the ruminant; not secondary to dysfunction in some other organ.

primase a specialized RNA polymerase that synthesizes short stretches of RNA used as primers.

primate an animal belonging to the highest order of mammals, Primates, which includes humans and the nonhuman primates, the apes, monkeys, lemurs, tree-shrews, lorises, aye-ayes, pottos, bush babies and tarsiers. They are characterized by being plantigrade, pentadactyl, by having clavicles, a complete dentition without specialized molars, a voluminous and complicated brain and a supple hand with a thumb that can be approximated to any of the fingers. They have excellent sight and are highly adapted to an arboreal existence, including the possession by some of a prehensile tail.

prime first grade or best quality.
primer oligonucleotide which is hydrogen-bonded to the template strand of DNA; required for the replication of DNA by polymerase.
random p. method a method of labeling DNA in vitro.
p. walking an orderly method for sequencing DNA which involves obtaining some sequence, then making an oligonucleotide primer to the end of the sequence obtained and using it as a primer for the next sequencing reaction and repeating this until the whole sequence is determined.
primidone an anticonvulsant related to phenobarbital. Used in dogs to control seizures of epilepsy and encephalitis.
primigravida an animal pregnant for the first time; gravida I.
primipara unipara; a female which has had one pregnancy that resulted in viable offspring, para I.
primiparity the state of being a primipara.
primitive first in point of time; existing in a simple or early form; showing little evolution.
p. groove longitudinal furrow in the primitive streak of the embryo.
p. knot see HENSEN'S NODE.
p. node enlarged cranial end of the primitive streak.
p. streak the thickened median area of the epiblast which sets out the future longitudinal axis of the early embryo.
primordial original or primitive; of the simplest and most undeveloped character.
p. germ cell cells which provide the origins of the spermatozoa and the ovum; they originate from the yolk sac endoderm and migrate to the developing gonad.
primordium the first beginnings of an organ or part in the developing embryo. Called also anlage.
Prince of Wales feather AMARANTHUS *reflexus*.
Prince's plume see STANLEYA PINNATA.
principle 1. a chemical component. 2. a substance on which certain of the properties of a drug depend. 3. a law of conduct.
active p. any constituent of a drug that helps to confer upon it a medicinal property.
reasonable person p. the basis for many decisions in cases alleging negligence. The court bases its judgment on what it considers a reasonable person, a reasonable veterinarian in our context, would have done in the circumstances. This is the evidence that most expert witnesses are asked to give, evidence about what should be expected of a member of their profession in terms of quality of performance. Called also principle of the reasonable person.
print 1. identifying mark left by part of an animal's anatomy. The print left by the nasolabial plane is sometimes used as an identification. 2. a medium of communicating by the printing of letter, numbers and other characters.
p. queue a list of print jobs waiting in line at a printer.
print-out the paper copy of the output of a computer program.
printed circuits the circuit of a computer. They are printed on cards, called boards, which can be used as add-ons to a basic unit and which can be replaced as a single unit. The elements of the computer including the diodes, transistors, resistors and capacitors are soldered to it.
printer a computer output device that produces a printed version or *hard copy* of the information in the computer by acting as an electric typewriter and printing out information provided by the computer.
daisy wheel p. provides letter quality printing at from 10 to 50 characters per second. The daisy wheel can be changed to alter the type font.
dot matrix p. uses a matrix of dots to form its letters and can print at speeds of 100 to 300 characters per second.
p. driver software connecting the computer to the printer.
impact p. a printhead strikes a carbon or cloth ribbon to produce an imprint. May be a *line* printer printing an entire line at a time or a *character* printer printing one character at a time across the page, usually bidirectionally. The printhead comes in a variety of forms presenting print of differing legibility.
laser p. uses xerographic methods to produce high quality output at 4 to 12 pages per minute.
line p. prints a line at a time, from 300 to 1200 lines per minute.
nonimpact p's include inkjet, thermal and laser printers which use other mechanisms to create a character on the paper.
prion a small protein which is believed capable of infecting cells and causing itself to be replicated, even though it contains no nucleic acid, i.e. it is believed to induce transcription of the gene that codes for the prion protein. In some way the horizontally acquired prion also alters the folding of the expressed protein and it is the altered protein that polymerizes to form fibrils within neurons and causes the spongiform encephalopathy. Aspects of this prion theory remain controversial. Prions cause spongiform encephalopathies of humans and animals, such as Creutzfeldt–Jakob disease, kuru, scrapie, transmissible mink encephalopathy and bovine spongiform encephalopathy.
prism needle has a prism-like or triangular head used for drawing blood.
pritchel a metal tool used to punch nailholes in horseshoes.
private owned by an individual person.
p. label pet food a product marketed under the label of the retailer; the house brand.
p. law the law relating to individual persons including contracts, property, torts, wills, matrimony and divorce.
p. practice see private PRACTICE.
p. practitioner a veterinarian who conducts a private practice.
p. sale sold by private agreement between buyer and seller; the alternative to sale by auction.
privet see LIGUSTRUM VULGARE.
privileged not generally available; can be used only by selected persons or substances.
p. information information about a client's animals or business to which the veterinarian has access because of his/her professional activities; it is a convention that such information is regarded as confidential. See also CONFIDENTIALITY.
p. sites areas of the body that escape immune surveillance, e.g. cornea.
p.r.n. [L.] *pro re nata* (according to circumstances).
Pro proline.
pro- word element. [L., Gr.] *before, in front of, favoring.*
pro-climax in ecological terms the stage reached in an ecosystem when humans intervene to prevent the natural climax or balance in the ecosystem from developing, e.g. vaccination of a large part of a canine population against distemper achieves a different climax serologically than the natural climax achieved by allowing the disease to develop unrestrained.

pro-drug a compound that, on administration, must undergo chemical conversion by metabolic processes before becoming an active pharmacological agent; a precursor of a drug.
pro-oestrus see PROESTRUS.
pro re nata [L.] *according to circumstances;* abbreviated p.r.n.
pro-time see PROTHROMBIN time test.
proaccelerin CLOTTING factor V.
proacrosomal granules precursors of the acrosomal vesicle in the Golgi complex of the spermatid.
proactinomyces see ACTINOMYCES.
proactivator a precursor of an activator; a factor that reacts with an enzyme to form an activator.
proatlas a rudimentary vertebra which in some animals lies in front of the atlas; sometimes seen in many as an anomaly.
probability the basis of statistics. The relative frequency of occurrence of a specific event as the outcome of an experiment when the experiment is conducted randomly on very many occasions. The probability of the event occurring is the number of times it did occur divided by the number of times that it could have occurred. Defined as:

$$p = \frac{x}{(x + y)}$$

where p = probability, x = positive outcomes, y = negative outcomes.
prior p. estimation of the probability that a particular phenomenon or character will appear before putting the patient to the test, e.g. testing the probable productivity of a patient by testing its forebears.
subjective p. the measure of the assessor's belief in the probability of a proposition being correct.
proband propositus.
probang a flexible rod with a ball, tuft or sponge at the end; used to apply medications to or remove matter from the esophagus or larynx. Instruments used in large animals consist of flexible tubes containing a flexible stilette.
p. gag a wooden rod which is placed across the mouth in cattle, and jammed between the molars and above the tongue. It has a hole transfixing its center through which the probang is passed.
probatocephaly an inherited, congenital deformity of the head in a calf giving the appearance of a sheep head. Called also sheepshead.
probe 1. a long, slender instrument for exploring wounds or body cavities or passages. 2. a radiolabeled DNA molecule such as a phage, viral or plasmid carrying a foreign DNA sequence used in hybridization to detect DNA homologous to the fragment.
cryosurgical p. see CRYOPROBE.
electroejaculation p. a probe containing electrodes which is inserted in the rectum of the male animal and connected to an electrical power source to stimulate the nerves controlling emission and ejaculation of the semen.
freezing p. see CRYOSURGERY.
probenecid used in the treatment of gout to promote excretion of uric acid; also used with certain antibiotics such as penicillin G and ampicillin to delay excretion and prolong their action.
probiotic hypothetical substances in the alimentary tract that aid in establishing the best balance of microorganisms.
problem a question to which there is no obvious, immediate answer; a question that requires some work done on it before a solution can be available.
p. herds herds which do not respond to the general control program for a particular disease and require special examination to elucidate the error and additional control measures to overcome it, e.g. a mastitis problem herd with a bacterially contaminated water supply.
p. knowledge coupler system computer-assisted diagnosis system designed for use in human medicine; based on a special matching algorithm known as pattern recognition.
p. list the list of problems to be overcome in a particular patient; in hospitals using a problem-oriented case management system.
p. name a generally accepted, preferred name for a clinical sign, syndrome or other indicant such as a positive laboratory test, poor work or production performance or poor reproductive result.
p.-oriented case management a system of managing patients based on the recognition of the patient's problems as targets for correction, planning the treatment program to achieve that, and assessing performance in terms of results with each of the problems and with the case overall. It is an excellent teaching procedure but is also helpful in maintaining the correct perspective in the patient's program.
p.-oriented diagnosis a system of diagnosis that starts off with the cardinal sign presented by the patient and proceeds in steps to identify the body system involved, the part of the system affected, the nature of the lesion and the cause of the lesion.
p.-oriented medical record see problem-oriented MEDICAL record.
p. solving the basis of clinical veterinary (and most other) education; learning diagnosis by practicing resolving clinical problems—the essential problem being 'which disease is most likely to be the cause of the syndrome presented by this patient'.
proboscis elongated, flexible feeding apparatus, formed of the fused mouthparts, in some insects.
Probstmayria a genus of roundworms in the family Kathlaniidae.
P. vivipara a minute worm found in the colon of horses, often in enormous numbers but without apparent pathogenic effect.
procainamide an antiarrhthymic agent, similar to quinidine, used as the hydrochloride salt in the treatment of cardiac arrhythmias.
procaine a local anesthetic; the hydrochloride salt is used in solution for infiltration, nerve block and spinal anesthesia.
p. penicillin see PENICILLIN G.
Procambarus clarkii farmed crustacean in family Astacidae; called also red swamp crawfish. See Table 23.
procarbazine an antineoplastic agent that acts by inhibiting the synthesis of DNA, RNA and protein.
procarboxypeptidase the inactive precursor of carboxypeptidase, which is converted to the active enzyme by the action of trypsin.
procarcinogen a chemical substance that becomes carcinogenic only after it is altered by metabolic processes.
procaryote prokaryote.
Procavia see HYRAX.
procedure-based fees see FEES.
procentriole the immediate precursor of centrioles and ciliary basal bodies.
procephalic pertaining to the anterior part of the head.
procercoid the first larval stage in the life cycle of a pseudophyllidean cestode, e.g. *Spirocerca erinacei.*

The procercoid is a solid bodied stage with oncospheral hooks carried on the cercomer in the posterior region.

process 1. a prominence or projection, as from a bone. 2. a series of operations or events leading to achievement of a specific result; also, to subject to such a series to produce desired changes.

accessory vertebral p. a process which protrudes backwards from the vertebral arch of the thoracic and lumbar vertebrae and overlap the succeeding vertebra in dogs and some other species.

acromial p. acromion.

alveolar p. the part of the bone in either the maxilla or mandible that surrounds and supports the teeth.

anconeal p. the point of the elbow; a prolongation vertically of the ulna.

articular p. one of the pair of processes at each end of a typical vertebrae which articulate with adjacent vertebral articular processes.

arytenoid cartilage corniculate p. a horn-like process which extends dorsomedially and forms one side of the caudal margin of the entrance to the larynx.

basihyoid lingual p. a median process which projects from the basihyoid bone into the root of the tongue in the horse and cow.

basilar p. a quadrilateral plate of the occipital bone projecting superiorly and anteriorly from the foramen magnum.

caudate p. the right of the two processes on the caudate lobe of the liver.

ciliary p's meridionally arranged ridges or folds projecting from the crown of the ciliary body.

clinoid p. any of the three (anterior, medial and posterior) processes of the sphenoid bone.

condylar p. carries the articular surface with which the mandible articulates with the temporal bone at the temporomandibular joint.

coracoid p. a small curved process arising from the glenoid rim and neck of the scapula; called also coracoid; large in humans and animals with large clavicles.

coronoid p. 1. the anterior part of the upper end of the ramus of the mandible. 2. a projection at the proximal end of the ulna.

See also CORONOID PROCESS.

distal phalangeal extensor p. the process on the dorsal border of the distal phalanx to which the common digital extensor tendon is attached.

ensiform p. xiphoid process.

ethmoid p. a bony projection above and behind the maxillary process of the inferior nasal concha of some species.

frontal p. 1. of the zygomatic bone forms the anterior part of the zygomatic process. 2. a cone-shaped mass of red vascular tissue that lies across the base of the turkey's beak. Called also snood, nasal comb.

frontal bone cornual p. the bony core of the horn which projects from the frontal bone.

frontonasal p. an expansive facial process in the embryo that develops into the forehead and upper part of the nose.

malar p. zygomatic process of the maxilla.

mamillary p. a tubercle on each cranial articular process of a lumbar vertebra.

mandibular angular p. a process which protrudes from the ventral caudal angle of the mandible, and acts as the attachment of the digastric muscle.

mastoid p. a conical projection at the base of mastoid portion of temporal bone.

odontoid p. a toothlike projection of the axis that articulates with the atlas. See also DENS.

paracondylar p. a prominent process lateral to the occipital condyle at the caudal extremity of the skull.

pterygoid p. one of the wing-shaped processes of the sphenoid bone.

retroarticular p. a flange of bone which protrudes ventrally from the caudal end of the zygomatic arch; carries part of the articular surface of the temporomandibular joint on its rostral edge.

spinous p. of vertebrae a dorsal median process of a vertebra giving attachment to muscles of the back.

styloid p. a long, pointed projection, particularly a long spine projecting downward from the inferior surface of the temporal bone.

suprahamate p. a flat, caudally directed process on the acromion of cats and some other species.

tail vertebral hemal p. paired ventral processes of the more cranial tail vertebrae; the coccygeal vessels run between them.

uncinate p. any hooklike process, as of vertebrae, the lacrimal bone, or the pancreas.

urethral p. an extension of the urethra beyond the end of the glans penis in the male horse, sheep and goat. In the horse it is buried in a deep recess. In the small ruminants it is a thin, loose, wormlike appendage.

xiphoid p. the caudal sternebra, consisting of a rod of bone that typically supports a xiphoid cartilage. Called also xiphoid.

zygomatic p. a projection from the frontal or temporal bone, or from the maxilla, by which they articulate with the zygoma.

processing exposure to a set of processes.

data p. conversion of crude data into usable and storable information by checking it for errors, incompatibilities, spelling, sorting it alphabetically or numerically or both, performing functions such as adding, dividing, storing, retrieving, deleting, packing, merging, all of which can be done manually but which can also be done automatically, in series and error-free by a computer program.

feed p. includes mechanical (crushing, crimping) thermal (boiling, exploding) chemical (acid or alkali treatment) and combinations of these.

meat p. meat being exposed to any one of a series of curing or preserving processes such as salting, wet pickling, drying, cooking and canning, sausage manufacture, ham curing.

x-ray film p. developing and fixing an exposed x-ray film. Some of this work is now done in automatic machines.

processor see COMPUTER.

processus pl. *processus* [L.] process.

p. anconeus non-union ununited anconeal process.

prochlorperazine a phenothiazine derivative; the edisylate is used as a tranquilizer and antiemetic.

prochondral occurring before the formation of cartilage in embryological development.

procidentia a state of prolapse, especially prolapse of the uterus.

procoagulant 1. tending to promote coagulation. 2. a precursor of a natural substance necessary to coagulation of the blood.

procoelous having the cranial surface concave; said of vertebrae.

procollagen the precursor of collagen, synthesized in osteoblasts and fibroblasts and subsequently converted to form collagen by procollagen peptidase.

p. *N*-peptidase one of the enzymes involved in the conversion of procollagen to collagen. There is inadequate activity of this enzyme in OSTEOGENESIS imperfecta, DERMATOSPARAXIS.

proconvertin clotting factor VII.

p. deficiency occurs in Beagle dogs and also Alaskan malamutes, causing no apparent bleeding tendency but may be associated with a predisposition to demodectic mange.

procreation the act of begetting or generating.

proctatresia imperforate anus.

proctectasia dilatation of the rectum or anus.

proctectomy excision of the rectum.

proctitis inflammation of the rectum.

ulcerative p. an early stage in the development of rectal stricture in pigs. See also RECTAL stricture.

proct(o)- word element. [Gr.] *rectum;* see also words beginning *rect(o)-*.

proctocele hernial protrusion of part of the rectum into the vagina; rectocele.

proctoclysis slow introduction of large quantities of liquid into the rectum.

proctocolonoscopy visual inspection of the interior of the rectum and lower colon with a proctoscope or sigmoidoscope.

proctocolpoplasty repair of a rectovaginal fistula.

proctocystotomy removal of a bladder calculus through the rectum.

proctodeum, proctodaeum the ectodermal depression of the caudal end of the embryo, which becomes the anal canal; called also anal pit, avian cloaca.

proctolitis proctitis.

proctology the branch of veterinary medicine concerned with disorders of the rectum and anus.

proctoparalysis paralysis of the anal and rectal muscles; proctoplegia.

proctopexy fixation of the rectum to adjacent tissue.

proctoplasty plastic repair of the rectum and anus.

proctoplegia proctoparalysis.

proctoptosis prolapse of the rectum.

proctorrhaphy suture of the rectum.

proctorrhea a mucous discharge from the anus.

proctoscope a speculum or tubular instrument with illumination for inspecting the rectum.

proctoscopy inspection of the rectum with a proctoscope. The examination is usually done prior to rectal surgery or as part of the physical examination of a patient with rectal bleeding, stricture or other signs of a rectal disorder.

proctosigmoiditis inflammation of the rectum and sigmoid colon.

proctospasm spasm of the rectum.

proctostenosis stricture of the rectum.

proctostomy surgical creation of a permanent artificial opening from the body surface into the rectum.

proctotomy incision of the rectum, usually for anal or rectal stricture.

proctovalvotomy incision of the rectal valves.

procumbent prone; lying on the abdomen. Called also ventral recumbency.

Procyon lotor see RACCOON.

procyonid a member of the family PROCYONIDAE.

Procyonidae a family of animals comprising the ring-tailed cat, cacomistle, raccoon, coatimundi, mountain coati, kinkajou, olingo, lesser panda and giant panda.

prod a prod to make animals move or move faster. Ranges from a pointed stick to an electric instrument. The electrically powered units may be battery-powered or operate off mains power, most suited to use in a fixed location such as an abattoir, or a portable model with a small generator which is operated by opening and clenching the hand. Invaluable when loading or encouraging downer animals to rise but are brutalizing and cruel if used unnecessarily.

prodromal the stage of premonitory signs presaging the onset of disease or of specific clinical signs such as seizures.

prodrome a premonitory clinical sign; a clinical sign indicating the onset of a disease.

product endorsement a public statement declaring the virtues and recommending the use of a product. Discouraged by codes of veterinary ethics other than by the publication of research results.

production 1. the act of producing. 2. the total of things produced.

animal p. see ANIMAL PRODUCTION.

p. diseases diseases caused by systems of management, especially feeding and the breeding of high-producing strains of animals and birds, in which production exceeds dietary and thermal input. Includes the group of diseases known in veterinary literature as 'metabolic diseases'. They differ from nutritional deficiencies in which it is the nutritional supply which falls short of normal production.

p. efficiency the efficiency of conversion of feedstuffs to animal product. The basis of the cost-efficiency of any animal production undertaking.

p. function the relationhip between the input of a single variable and the output of the product.

p. indices specific indices such as live pigs produced per sow per year, intercalving interval, rate of gain of body weight per day in beef cattle, used as benchmarks of productivity.

p. ketosis ketosis (acetonemia) as a production disease, one which is produced by animal management; failure of the dietary input to satisfy the demands of the energy output in milk.

p. losses product which is produced but not harvested or sold, e.g. mastitic milk from cows with mastitis.

p. medicine see production diseases (above).

p. program a schedule of activities relating to feeding, breeding and health maintenance aimed at maximizing the profitability of an animal enterprise. Includes the establishment of targets of production in the areas of specific indices of productivity and the monitoring of production. The programs may be computerized so that the entry of data is simplified and analysis of the data automatic and regularly periodic. The establishment of programs and their maintenance by way of modification of practices and strategies to match changes of production efficiency require the participation of SPECIES specialists. See also MANAGEMENT factors.

productive producing or forming. Said especially of (1) an inflammation that produces new tissue or of a cough that brings forth sputum or mucus, and (2) an animal or animal enterprise that has a net excess production which is available to the farmer and produced in a cost-effective operation.

p. life that part of an animal's life during which it is productive.

productivity the amount or quality or value of the output of a food animal. Best measured in terms of the percentage productivity compared with a target based on productivity of peers. It is customary nowadays to state productivity in terms of return on capital invested, or per head of livestock or per hectare or per unit of workforce, and may be for a period, e.g. annual, lifetime, for a specific unit, e.g. farm, the dairy herd on a mixed farm.

p. index includes such items as wool yield per hectare, wins per race starts.

p. marginal value see MARGINAL revenue.

proelastase the inert precursor of ELASTASE, found in the pancreas.

proencephalus a fetus with a protrusion of the brain through a frontal fissure.
proenzyme zymogen; an inactive precursor of an enzyme.
proerythroblast pronormoblast; rubriblast.
proestrogen a substance without estrogenic activity but which is metabolized in the body to active estrogen.
proestrus the period of heightened follicular activity preceding estrus.
profession 1. an avowed, public declaration or statement of intention or purpose. 2. a calling or vocation requiring specialized knowledge, methods and skills, as well as preparation, in an institution of higher learning, in the scholarly, scientific and historical principles underlying such methods and skills. A profession continuously enlarges its body of knowledge, functions autonomously in formulation of policy, and maintains by force of organization or concerted opinion high standards of achievement and conduct. Specifically in this regard it maintains and polices a code of ethics and conducts a professional organization of which a large majority of the profession are members. Members of a profession are committed to continuing study, placing service above personal gain, and are committed to providing practical services vital to human and social welfare.
professional 1. pertaining to one's profession or occupation. 2. one whose income is derived from the practice of his/her profession.
professionalism the upholding by individuals of the principles, laws, ethics and conventions of their profession.
profibrinolysin an old term for plasminogen; the precursor of plasmin, which is an active enzyme in the fibrinolytic system.
profilaggrin a structural protein synthesized by cells of the stratum granulosum and a precursor of filaggrin.
profile a simple outline, as of the side view of the body or head; by extension, a graph representing quantitatively a set of characteristics determined by tests. In animals the same purpose may be served by photographing it against a grid background. Profiles are used to determine an animal's conformational similarity to a standard set by a breed society and, especially in ruminants, as an aid to the diagnosis of diseases of the abdomen.
biochemical p. a panel of tests, usually selected for their ability in the particular species to evaluate the functional capacity of several critical organ systems and general health. The 'profile' may literally be the results plotted on individual, parallel numerical scales, producing a pattern similar to a bar graph.
cost–benefit p. a written or graphic description of the costs and production returns of an animal enterprise, set out according to a set of standard indices and parameters so that inter-herd comparisons are facilitated. A standard feature in modern animal health and production programs.
Profilicollis minutus see POLYMORPHUS *boschadis*.
profilometer a device for measuring the shape of a facial profile and expressing the results mathematically. Such an instrument was used extensively at one time as a means of detecting the heterozygotes for inherited achondroplastic dwarfism.
profilometry a system for studying disorders of micturition using electromyography and measurement of intraurethral pressures. See also URETHRAL pressure profile.
profit the amount by which income exceeds expenditure.
p. sharing profit sharing between a professional and a lay person is illegal in most countries because it is considered to be improper for a nonveterinarian to have any authority over the quality and style of the work of a professional person.
profitability the quality of making a profit; the extent of the profit-making of an enterprise.
proflavine a constituent of acriflavine, $C_{13}H_{11}N_3$, used as a topical and urinary antiseptic in the form of the hemisulfate salt.
profundus [L.] *deep*.
Progamotoenia anoplocephalid cestodes found in the bile ducts of kangaroos, wallabies, wombats.
progastrin an inactive precursor of gastrin.
progenesis the maturation of gametes within an organism before it has reached physical and sexual maturity.
progenitor ancestor, including parent.
p. cell stem cells.
progeny testing testing the potential productivity of an animal by measuring the production of some of its progeny under normal field conditions. The efficiency of the test will depend on the size of the sample of progeny.
progestagen progestogen.
progestational preceding gestation; referring to changes in the endometrium preparatory to implantation of the developing ovum should fertilization occur.
p. agent (hormone) a group of hormones secreted by the corpus luteum and placenta and, in small amounts, by the adrenal cortex, including progesterone, Δ^4-3-ketopregnen-20(α)-ol, and Δ^4-3-ketopregnene-20(β)-ol; agents having progestational activity are also produced synthetically.
progesterone a steroid sex hormone that is the principal progestational hormone. Used therapeutically in the treatment of threatened abortion in some species, in estrus control in dogs and cats, and occasionally in treatment of some types of skin diseases.

During the maturation of the ovum, estrogen, the principal female sex hormone, is produced at a high rate. At ovulation estrogen production is sharply reduced and the follicle is replaced by the corpus luteum of which the main function is to produce progesterone. Unless fertilization takes place, the corpus luteum disappears when it has performed its function.

The progesterone produced by the corpus luteum is promptly carried by the blood to the uterus, as was the estrogen that preceded it. Both hormones now work to prepare the uterus for possible conception.

In pregnancy, progesterone acts in a way that protects the embryo and fosters growth of the placenta. By decreasing the frequency of uterine contractions it helps to prevent expulsion of the implanted ovum. It also promotes secretory changes in the mucosa of the uterine tubes, thereby helping to provide nutrition for the fertilized ovum as it travels through the tube on its way to the uterus.

Another function of progesterone is promotion of the development of the mammary glands in preparation for lactation. Prolactin, from the anterior lobe of the PITUITARY gland, stimulates production of the milk, and progesterone prepares the glands for secretion.
p. assay the estimation of progesterone in milk is used as a PREGNANCY test.
p.-induced lactation see LACTATION induction.

p. milk test assay of progesterone in milk used as a pregnancy test.

p. plasma test the original pregnancy test which survives as the milk progesterone test; used in dogs as a guide in predicting the time of ovulation.

p. releasing intravaginal device used as a means of synchronizing estrus in cows and sheep as an aid to structured artificial insemination programs. Called also PRID.

progestin originally, the crude hormone of the corpus luteum; it has since been isolated in pure form and is now known as PROGESTERONE. Certain synthetic and natural progestational agents are called progestins.

progestogen any substance having progestational activity.

proglossis the tip of the tongue.

proglottid, proglottis one of the segments making up the body of a tapeworm.

prognathia prognathism.

prognathism abnormal protrusion of one or both jaws, especially the lower jaw.

prognathous having a projecting jaw.

prognose to give a prognosis.

prognosis a forecast of the probable course and outcome of an attack of disease and the prospects of recovery as indicated by the nature of the disease and the clinical signs of the case. In keeping with modern day usage of decision making on the basis of statistics it is now becoming commonplace to give a percentage probability of a successful outcome in terms of survival, and a similar figure for probability for return to full function.

progoitrin an antithyroid substance in the seeds, and to a lesser extent the foliage, of rape and other plants in the family Brassicae. It is a glycoside which is converted to an active oxazolidone by an enzyme also resident in the plant. This substance 1,5-vinyl-2-thiooxazolidone is goitrogenic and inhibits growth.

program, programme 1. a planned course of action, e.g. HERD health program, PRODUCTION program. 2. a sequence of encoded instructions for directing a computer to perform specified logical actions on data. 3. the writing of a computer program. See also COMPUTER.

application p. a computer program written for a particular function required by a user, e.g. HERD health program, inventory monitoring program, PRODUCTION program.

benchmark p. a computer program designed to assess efficiency of hardware or software.

computer p. a set of instructions, written in the appropriate language for the machine and the software, that directs a digital computer to perform a particular operation or series of operations. This could, for example, include adding up a series of figures, taking an average of them and adding the answer to each of the accounts on the database that are located in a particular postal district.

p. language see COMPUTER language.

proprietary p. a computer program owned by an individual or company. Usually sold on the understanding that the program will not be copied to other persons.

public p. a disease control program available to all members of the public, e.g. rabies control, tuberculosis eradication.

whole farm p. one which takes into account all of the enterprises on a farm and presents a financial accounting of the farm as a whole.

programmed cell death proposed system of cell death, often including poly(ADP)-ribosylation, ensures that a cell will not survive if it is so badly damaged that its recovery would harm the organism.

programmer in computer work a person who writes and tests programs but does not perform the more sophisticated task of designing the programs.

programming writing a computer program.

progranulocyte promyelocyte.

progravid denoting the phase of the endometrium in which it is prepared for pregnancy.

progress notes narrative records kept on changes in the animal's condition and treatment administered. In the problem-oriented MEDICAL record, it is written in the SOAP format.

progressive advancing, increasing in scope and severity.

p. ataxia an inherited disease of cattle in which stiffness and stumbling commence at about a year of age and worsen over 1 to 2 more years to the point of recumbency. Called also progressive sensory ataxia of Charolais cattle.

p. ethmoid hematoma see progressive nasal hematoma (below).

p. interstitial pneumonia in sheep see MAEDI.

p. motor neuron disease various forms of these diseases, all characterized by progressive paresis, paralysis and local muscle atrophy, progressive muscular dystrophy, are recorded in dogs (Brittany spaniel, Rottweiler, Swedish Lapland), horses, Brown Swiss calves, pigs (Yorkshire, Hampshire).

p. nasal hematoma a disease of horses characterized by epistaxis and nasal obstruction. The large hemorrhagic mass originates from the ethmoid region and has a high rate of recurrence after surgery. Called also hemorrhagic nasal polyp, progressive ethmoidal hematoma.

p. posterior paralysis see progressive ataxia (above).

prohemistomiasis disease caused by infection with *Prohemistomum vivax*; occurs in humans, dogs and cats in Israel, North Africa and Romania.

Prohemistomum vivax a digenetic trematode found in the intestines of cats and dogs.

prohormone a precursor of a hormone, such as a polypeptide that is cleaved to form a shorter polypeptide hormone, or a steroid that is converted to an active hormone by metabolism.

proinsulin a precursor of insulin, having low biological activity.

projectile something thrown forward.

p. syringe see BLOW DART.

p. vomiting forceful vomiting, usually without preceding retching, in which the vomitus is thrown well forward. In dogs and cats, a feature of gastric retention and particularly pyloric obstruction. Cattle do not vomit easily and when they do it is usually projectile and voluminous.

projection throwing forward, e.g. x-ray projection.

somatotopical p. an arrangement by which a picture of the body is represented on a surface, such as projection onto the cerebral cortex of the topography of the body from which the efferent nerve impulses depart or to which afferent impulses come.

prokaryocyte prokaryote.

prokaryon 1. nuclear material scattered in the cytoplasm of the cell, rather than bounded by a nuclear membrane; found in some unicellular organisms, such as bacteria. 2. prokaryote.

prokaryote a unicellular organism lacking a true nucleus and nuclear membrane, having genetic material composed of a single molecule of double-stranded DNA. Prokaryotes with the exception of mycoplasmas have a rigid cell wall. Includes the blue-green algae and bacteria—the Cyanophyceae.

prokinetics drugs which enhance the passage of intraluminal contents of the gastrointestinal tract.

prolactin a hormone secreted by the anterior pituitary that promotes the growth of mammary tissue and stimulates and sustains milk production in postpartum mammals, and shows luteotropic activity in certain mammals. Promotes the secretion of milk in the crop of pigeons and doves. Called also lactogenic hormone, luteotropic hormone, LTH and mammotropin. It is identical with luteotropin.

p. inhibitory factor (PIF) probably the catecholamine dopamine, released in the hypothalamus, carried to the anterior pituitary via the hypophyseal portal system, and inhibits the secretion of prolactin.

p. releasing factor (PRF) appears to be released from the hypothalamus in a pulsatile fashion and it is the fluctuation in PRF that regulates the circulating level of prolactin.

prolamine a globular protein, e.g. zein in maize grain.

prolan an outdated name for chorionic gonadotropin. Thought originally to be the hormone responsible for the uterine enlargement seen in the Ascheim–Zondek test.

prolapse 1. literally the falling down, or downward displacement, of a part or viscus. In many instances in animals the prolapse is lateral or even dorsal, e.g. in intervertebral disk prolapse. 2. to undergo such displacement.

cloacal p. caused in companion birds by parasitic enteritis.

eye p. the eyeball is displaced from the orbit and is lying on the lower eyelid.

fat p. see perivaginal FAT prolapse.

oviduct p. a minor prolapse of oviductal mucosa may stimulate cannibalism in others and the entire oviduct be removed via the cloaca.

parturient bladder p. see parturient URINARY BLADDER prolapse.

preputial p. see PREPUTIAL eversion.

rectal p., p. of rectum protrusion through the anus of the mucosa only or the complete wall of the rectum. Uncommon in most species but commonplace in the pig because of anatomical weakness in the area, especially in some breeds. The feeding of estrogens exacerbates the tendency.

p. retainer 1. a frame made of strong wire or thin metal rod and shaped like a lattice with obvious apertures for defecation and urination; strapped to the rear end of the cow so that the perineum will not bulge when the animal strains. 2. a bottle-shaped appliance sewn in to the vagina to prevent prolapse of the vagina.

third eyelid gland p. see CHERRY EYE.

uterine p. displacement of the uterus so that the cervix is within the vaginal orifice (first-degree prolapse), the cervix is outside the orifice (second-degree prolapse), or the entire uterus is outside the orifice (third-degree prolapse). May be related causally to hypocalcemia in cattle.

vaginal p. usually the prolapse contains only the mucosa of the ventral floor, but it may also contain the urinary bladder or the cervix. Kinking of the urethra may cause obstruction and eventual rupture of the bladder.

prolapsus [L.] *prolapse*.

prolepsis recurrence of a paroxysm before the expected time.

prolidase an enzyme that catalyzes the hydrolysis of the imide bond between an α-carboxyl group and proline or hydroxyproline.

proliferation the reproduction or multiplication of similar forms, especially of cells.

proliferative pertaining to or emanating from proliferation.

p. dermatitis see strawberry FOOTROT.

p. enteropathy see proliferative ILEITIS.

p. exudative pneumonia of lambs see ENZOOTIC pneumonia.

p. hemorrhagic enteropathy an acute or peracute disease of young pigs, characterized by anemia and dysentery, and a proliferative, hemorrhagic lesion in the terminal ileum and proximal colon, and a high death rate. The cause is obscure but the disease is related etiologically and pathologically to several other intestinal diseases from which *Campylobacter hyointestinalis* is isolated regularly. Part of the intestinal adenomatosis complex of pigs.

p. ileitis see porcine intestinal ADENOMATOSIS.

p. interstitial pneumonia see ENZOOTIC pneumonia.

p. kidney disease important disease of salmonids; caused by a pre-spore stage of a myxosporean species presumably carried by other fish inhabiting the same waters.

p. optic neuropathy a raised gray mass on the surface of the optic disk but there is no effect on vision.

p. phase in uterine activity; called also follicular phase. The lining epithelium of the uterus hypertrophies and becomes congested and edematous.

p. stomatitis see proliferative STOMATITIS.

proligerous producing offspring.

proligestone a long-acting progestin used in estrus control in bitches.

prolinase an enzyme that catalyzes the hydrolysis of dipeptides containing proline or hydroxyproline as *N*-terminal groups.

proline Pro; a cyclic amino acid occurring in proteins; it is a major constituent of collagen.

prolonged gestation may be inherited, caused by plant toxins or occur sporadically. In all forms of the disease there is absence or developmental abnormality of the fetal adrenal or pituitary glands.

inherited p. g. occurs in several forms in cattle. Pregnancy is prolonged for 3 weeks to 3 months; in one form the fetus is normal except that it is of very great size and can only be delivered by cesarean section. In another the fetus does not develop beyond the 6 month stage and is a cyclops monster with only one eye. In a third there are multiple skeletal deformities and cleft palate.

phytogenous p. g. poisoning by VERATRUM *californicum* or SALSOLA *tuberculata* causes prolonged gestation. Called also phytogenous prolonged gestation.

prolymphocyte a cell of the lymphocytic series intermediate between the lymphoblast and lymphocyte.

promastigote one of the morphological stages in the development of certain protozoa, characterized by a free anterior flagellum and the kinetoplast and axoneme at the anterior end of the body. There is no undulating membrane. They are found in arthropods and plants.

promazine a phenothiazine derivative used as a major tranquilizer in the form of the hydrochloride salt.

promecarb a carbamate pesticide.

promegakaryocyte a precursor in the thrombocytic series that is a developmental form intermediate between the megakaryoblast and the megakaryocyte.

promegaloblast the earliest form in the abnormal erythrocyte maturation sequence occurring in vitamin B_{12} and folic acid deficiencies in humans; it corresponds to the pronormoblast or rubriblast, and develops into a megaloblast.

promethazine a phenothiazine derivative used as an antihistaminic, antiemetic and tranquilizer in the form of the hydrochloride salt.

promethestrol a synthetic estrogenic agent; used as the dipropionate ester.

promethium a chemical element, atomic number 61, atomic weight 147, symbol Pm. See Table 6.

prometon, prometone a plant hormone herbicide; one of the triazine compounds and capable of causing anorexia, poor weight gain and muscle weakness if there is excessive contact with animals.

prometryne see PROMETON.

prominence a protrusion or projection.

promonocyte a cell of the monocytic series intermediate between the monoblast and monocyte, with coarse chromatin structure and one or two nucleoli.

promontory a projecting process or eminence.

middle ear p. a bulge in the medial wall of the middle ear overhanging the cochlea.

sacral p. in the midline of the ventral surface of the lumbosacral junction, a lip at the junction of the cranial extremity of the sacrum with its ventral surface, an easily recognized prominence of the roof of the pelvic cavity.

promotants see GROWTH promotants.

promoter a specific DNA sequence to which RNA polymerase binds and signals where RNA synthesis (transcription) should begin.

internal p. a class of enhancers which are gene-specific sequences that increase transcription.

p. region the non coding nucleotide sequence at the transcription start region that is characterized by the presence of a number of conserved or consequence sequences.

prompt a message which indicates that the computer requires further information from the user before it can proceed.

prompting a stimulus that gets an animal to perform a desired behavior.

promyelocyte a precursor in the granulocytic series, intermediate between myeloblast and myelocyte, containing a few, as yet undifferentiated, cytoplasmic granules.

promyelocytic pertaining to a promyelocyte.

pronate in humans, to turn the palm downwards or from the body to face the ground; not easily done in most animal species, except primates, dogs and cats; compare with SUPINATION.

pronation the plantar surface of the paw is turned to face backwards, the customary position in animals other than primates.

pronator a muscle that pronates an extremity.

prone lying face downward, or on the ventral surface.

p. sticking a method of slaughtering pigs in which the pigs are stunned, then conveyed in a prone position on a conveyor belt past the various stations including the sticking or jugular opening station.

pronephric see PRONEPHROS.

p. duct a duct reaching from the pronephros to the cloaca.

p. tubules transient tubules of the primitive kidney which are produced in embryos of the lower vertebrates but in the domestic animals are found only in the sheep; they are nonfunctional in other mammals. Connect the pronephros to the pronephric duct.

pronephros pl. *pronephroi* [Gr.] the primordial kidney; nonfunctional in mammals; functional only in amphioxuses and lampreys; an excretory structure or its rudiments developing in the embryo before the mesonephros; its duct is later used by the mesonephros, which arises caudal to it.

pronghorn antelope a fast-moving, wild North American ruminant with hollow core, branched horns which shed their outer sheath each year. Called also *Antilocapra americana*.

pronormoblast the earliest erythrocyte precursor, having a relatively large nucleus containing several nucleoli, surrounded by a small amount of cytoplasm (see also NORMOBLAST). Called also proerythroblast and rubriblast.

pronucleus pl. *pronuclei*; the haploid nucleus of a sex cell.

female p. the haploid nucleus of the fully mature ovum which loses its nuclear envelope and liberates its chromosomes to meet the synapsis with those from the male pronucleus.

male p. the nuclear material of the head of a spermatozoon, after it has penetrated the ovum and acquired a pronuclear membrane.

proof reading 3′→5′ exonuclease activity of DNA polymerase that results in the removal of erroneously incorporated nucleotides during DNA replication; responsible for the very high fidelity ($>10^6$) of polymerase.

p. r. site a distinct site of aminoacyl-tRNA synthetases that preferentially recognizes and hydrolyzes mis-acylated tRNA.

pro-otic in front of the ear.

propagation reproduction.

propagule an ecological term; the minimum number of individuals of a species required to colonize an island.

propanediol see PROPYLENE GLYCOL.

propanidid see EUGENOL.

propantheline a smooth muscle relaxant, used particularly in urethral spasm and irritable bowel syndrome.

proparacaine the preferred topical anesthetic for ophthalmic use. Called also proxymetacaine hydrochloride.

proparathyroid hormone an intermediate precursor of parathyroid hormone, formed from preproparathyroid hormone in the rough endoplasmic reticulum of chief cells; abbreviated proPTH.

propatagiectomy surgical removal of part of one of the wing membranes of a bird to prevent it from flying. See also DEFLIGHTING.

propatagium the web of skin that makes up the wing membrane of birds in front of the elbow and that stretches from shoulder to carpus.

propazine a triazine herbicide. Sprayed pastures may cause poisoning of livestock up to 7 days later. Causes anorexia, weight loss and muscle weakness.

propedeutics preliminary instruction; preparatory teaching.

propepsin pepsinogen; the inactive precursor of pepsin.

proper ligament a fold of peritoneum which unites the ovary to the uterus or the testis to the epididymis.

p. ligament of the ovary a fold of peritoneum in the free edge of the mesometrium between the ovary and the horn of the uterus.

p. ligament of the testis the ligament which binds the tail of the epididymis to the testis.

properdin a normal, relatively heat-labile, nonantibody serum protein (a euglobulin) that, in the presence of COMPLEMENT component C3 and magnesium ions, is involved in the alternative complement pathway, and acts nonspecifically against gram-negative bacteria and viruses and plays a role in lysis of erythrocytes. It may act in conjunction with complement-fixing ANTIBODY.

p. pathway alternative complement pathway.

prophage the latent stage of a BACTERIOPHAGE in a lysogenic bacterium, in which the viral genome becomes inserted usually at a specific location within the host chromosome and is duplicated into each cell generation.

propham a herbicide and fungicide used as a seed dressing; has little if any toxicity.

prophase the first stage of cell replication in either meiosis or mitosis.

prophy cup a deformable rubber cup which flares when applied to a tooth being polished.

prophylactic 1. tending to ward off disease; pertaining to prophylaxis. 2. an agent that tends to ward off disease.

p. antibiotic therapy treatment with antibiotics, beginning just before a surgical procedure, to minimize or prevent development of infection. See also PERIOPERATIVE.

p. vaccination vaccination carried out in expectation of the occurrence of the disease.

prophylaxis prevention of disease; preventive treatment.

dental p. scaling and polishing teeth carried out regularly to prevent and control peridontal disease.

propiocortin precursor protein to ACTH found in the adenohypophyseal pars distalis.

propiolactone a disinfectant with bactericidal, sporicidal, fungicidal and virucidal activities used as a vapor for sterilizing large enclosed spaces. Of limited usefulness because of toxicity and carcinogenic properties.

propiomazine see PROPIONYLPROMAZINE.

propionanilide a hormone weedkiller which is likely to be toxic only if massive doses are administered.

propionate any salt of propionic acid. A precursor for glucose in the ruminant.

sodium p. used as a prophylactic against acetonemia in cows.

Propionibacterium gram-positive pleomorphic rods which are common skin residents, found also in dairy products and the alimentary tract.

P. acnes activates macrophages, increases proliferation of lymphoblasts, and stimulates resistance to bacterial infection. Used as a bacterial immunostimulant.

propionic acid CH_3CH_2COOH, found in chyme and sweat, and one of the products of bacterial fermentation of wood pulp waste; also an important gluconeogenic volatile fatty acid synthesized by the ruminal microflora. Its salts (calcium and sodium propionate) are used as mold inhibitors in stock feeds and pharmaceuticals, and in topical antifungal preparations.

propionyl CoA activated intermediate in the utilization of the volatile fatty acid, propionic acid; or end product of the beta-oxidation of odd-carbon chain fatty acids.

propionylpromazine, propiopromazine a phenothiazine derivative used as a tranquilizer, usually in combination with methadone.

propiopromazine see PROPIONYLPROMAZINE.

proplatelets elongated strands of megakaryocyte cytoplasm which extend into the bone marrow sinuses; fragmentation produces platelets.

proplexus the choroid plexus of the lateral ventricle of the brain.

propofol a rapidly acting, short duration, intravenous hypnotic anesthetic induction agent, which has low excitatory effect. It is harmless when injected into tissues or intra-arterially. The active ingredient is 2,6-di-isopropylphenol.

proportion percentage or fraction of a whole. Often expressed also as a rate or ratio by comparison to a total or other population.

p. differences estimating the significance of differences between two proportional morbidities or mortalities.

proportional values expressed as a proportion of the total number of values in a series.

p. dwarf the patient is a miniature without disproportionate reductions or enlargements of body parts.

p. morbidity a percentage estimate of the morbidity of a disease in a group. See also proportional MORBIDITY.

p. mortality the mortality rate due to a specific disease in a group expressed as a proportion of all of the causes of death in the group. See also MORTALITY rate.

propositus pl. *propositi* [L.] the original animal presenting a disease or disorder which serves as the basis for a hereditary or genetic study; called also proband.

propoxur a carbamate insecticide used widely on companion animals to control ectoparasites.

propoxycaine a local anesthetic with longer action than procaine.

propoxyphene an analgesic used as the hydrochloride and napsylate salts. Called also dextropropoxyphene.

proppy a gait in which the animal's movements are stilted with a lack of flexion of the knees and pasterns; usually used in describing horses.

propranolol a β-adrenoceptor blocking agent, useful in the treatment of cardiac dysrhythmias including paroxysmal tachycardia, atrial flutter and fibrillation.

proprietary medicine any chemical, drug or similar preparation used in the treatment of diseases, if such article is protected against free competition as to name, product, composition or process of manufacture by secrecy, patent, trademark or copyright, or by other means.

proprioception perception mediated by proprioceptors or proprioceptive tissues.

proprioceptive pertaining to or emanating from proprioceptor.

p. deficit a defect of proprioception in which the animal acts as though it does not know where its feet are (in contrast to a cerebellar defect when the feet do not end up where the animal appears to intend that they should go).

p. positioning positioning of the limbs or head and neck in response to proprioceptive inputs. The basis of postural reflexes.

p. reflex a reflex that is initiated by stimuli arising from some function of the reflex mechanism itself.

proprioceptor any of the sensory nerve endings that give information concerning movements and position of the body; they occur chiefly in muscles, tendons and the labyrinth.

proprotein a protein which is cleaved to form a smaller protein, e.g. proinsulin, the precursor of insulin.

proptometer an instrument for measuring the degree of exophthalmos.

proptosis forward displacement or bulging, especially of the eye; exophthalmos.

propyl the univalent radical $CH_3CH_2CH_2$, from propane.

p. disulfide the toxic principle in ALLIUM *validum* and domestic onions and garlic. Called also *n*-propyl disulfide.

propylene glycol a chemical used industrially as an antifreeze, solvent stabilizer, as a preservative in liquid livestock feeds and pharmaceutically as a vehicle or solvent for medicinal preparations. It is used extensively in food animal medicine as an oral medicament to boost the blood glucose level, e.g. in bovine acetonemia. Doses that are innocuous to cows can cause ataxia, depression and death in horses. Called also propanediol.

propylene oxide a gas used to disinfect animal feeds.

propyliodone a radiopaque medium used in bronchography.

propylparaben an antifungal agent used as a preservative in pharmaceuticals. See also HYDROXYBENZOATE.

propylthiouracil a thyroid inhibitor used in the treatment of hyperthyroidism, but because of severe hematologic toxicity in cats other drugs are preferred.

prorennin the zymogen (proenzyme) in the gastric glands that is converted to rennin.

prorubricyte basophilic normoblast.

Prosarcoptes a genus of mange mites in the family Sarcoptidae.

P. faini, P. pitheci found on monkeys.

prosecretin the precursor of secretin.

prosection carefully programmed dissection for demonstration of structure.

prosector one who performs prosection.

p.'s wart infection of the skin of humans by *Mycobacterium tuberculosis* picked up while dissecting infected tissue.

prosencephalic pertaining to or emanating from prosencephalon.

p. hypoplasia a congenital malformation in calves; there is a small opening on the surface of the calvaria; the hole connects with a deformed diencephalon which may discharge cerebrospinal fluid.

prosencephalon the forebrain consisting of the diencephalon (thalamus, epithalamus, subthalamus, hypothalamus) and the telencephalon (cerebral hemispheres).

prosencephaly fusion of the cerebral hemispheres with a single lateral ventricle.

prosimian member of the suborder Prosimii of the order of Primates.

Prosimii a suborder of nonhuman primates that includes indirses, lemurs, treeshrews, lorises and tarsiers.

pros(o)- word element. [Gr.] *forward, anterior.*

proso millet see PANICUM *miliaceum.*

prosodemic passing directly from one animal to another instead of reaching a large number at once, through such means as water supply; said of a disease progressing in that way.

Prosopis juliflioria, Prosopis glandulosa American plant in the legume family Fabaceae; can cause chronic liver damage. Called also algarroba, mesquite, kioxa bean, kiowa bean.

prosoplasia 1. abnormal differentiation of tissue. 2. development into a higher state of organization or function.

prosop(o)- word element. [Gr.] *face.*

prosopoplegia facial paralysis.

prosoposchisis congenital fissure of the face.

prosopospasm spasm of the facial muscles.

prosoposternodymia a double monster joined face to face and sternum to sternum.

prosopothoracopagus twin fetuses fused from the face to the thorax.

prospective not yet done; in the future.

p. history maintaining a surveillance over a patient in order to accumulate a history of an illness after the initial attack.

p. surveillance an epidemiological strategy of maintaining a watch over a suspected population after an event.

p. trial in a field trial of a preventive or therapeutic regimen the trial can be conducted in a series of consequential or contingent steps with each step contingent on the results in the one preceding it.

prostacyclin a metabolite of arachidonic acid formed by prostaglandin endoperoxides in the walls of arteries and veins; it is a potent vasodilator and an inhibitor of platelet aggregation. The exogenous form is called EPOPROSTENOL.

prostaglandin a group of naturally occurring, chemically related, long-chain hydroxy fatty acids that stimulate contractility of the uterine and other smooth muscle and have the ability to lower blood pressure, regulate acid secretion of the stomach, regulate body temperature and platelet aggregation, and control inflammation and vascular permeability. They also affect the action of certain hormones. First found in semen, they have since been found in cells throughout the body. There are six types, A, B, C, D, E and F, the degree of saturation of the side chain of each being designated by subscripts 1, 2 and 3.

The main use of prostaglandins in veterinary medicine is in the treatment and regulation of activity of the female reproductive tract. The E and F series stimulate myometrial contraction. F_2 is luteolytic.

p. $F_{1[alpha]}$ promotes platelet aggregation; actively removed from the circulation by the vascular endothelium.

p. I_2 see PROSTACYCLIN.

p. synthase complex a central enzyme system in the synthesis of prostaglandins.

prostanoid having the form of a prostaglandin.

prostate a gland in the male which surrounds the neck of the bladder and the urethra. It is a diffuse gland in rams and goat bucks, a lobed gland in stallions and dogs and a combination of lobed and diffuse in bulls and boars. The prostate consists of glandular tissue, the ducts from which empty into the prostatic portion of the urethra, and partly of muscular fibers which encircle the urethra. It contributes to the seminal fluid a secretion containing acid phosphatase, citric acid and proteolytic enzymes, which account for the liquefaction of the coagulated semen. The rate of secretion increases greatly during sexual stimulation.

prostatectomy surgical removal of the PROSTATE.

prostatic pertaining to or emanating from the prostate.

p. abscess occurs in dogs, often as a complication of benign prostatic hypertrophy and squamous metaplasia. Clinical signs are variable, sometimes resembling those of acute prostatitis with fever and systemic illness, or they can be similar to those of chronic prostatitis with straining, dysuria and hematuria.

benign p. hyperplasia a diffuse glandular and stromal hyperplasia and hypertrophy of the prostate is commonly seen in dogs from middle age, increasing in frequency and degree with advancing age. Clinical effects are minimal or absent in the majority of dogs, but occasionally dysuria and constipation result. Infection can be a complication, causing an acute or chronic prostatitis.

p. calculi occur uncommonly in dogs. May originate in the urinary tract, becoming lodged in the prostate, or form within prostatic tissue.

p. cyst may occur in association with benign prostatic hyperplasia or as a separate entity, developing from vestiges of müllerian ducts.

p. fluid secretion of the prostate; the third, sperm-free, fraction in a dog semen collection.

p. inflammation see PROSTATITIS.

p. massage firm digital pressure and massage of the prostate, applied per rectum, may be performed to increase the amount of cellular material and secretions collected in a urine or prostatic wash sample.

p. neoplasms adenocarcinomas occur infrequently in older dogs, invading locally and metastasizing to sublumbar lymph nodes and lumbar vertebrae.

p. wash placement of a urinary catheter in the prostatic urethra and a flush followed by aspiration of fluid is used to obtain samples for culture and cytology in the diagnosis of prostatic disease.

prostatitis inflammation of the PROSTATE. Occurs mostly in dogs where it may be acute, causing fever, leukocytosis, pain and gait abnormalities, or chronic with dysuria, hematuria and constipation.

prostatocystitis inflammation of the neck of the bladder (prostatic urethra) and the bladder cavity. The clinical syndrome is a combination of those of cystitis and prostatitis.

prostatocystotomy incision of the bladder and prostate.

prostatolith see PROSTATIC calculi.

prostatolithotomy incision of the prostate for removal of a calculus.

prostatomegaly hypertrophy of the prostate.

prostatorrhea catarrhal discharge from the prostate.

prostatotomy surgical incision of the prostate.

prostatovesiculitis inflammation of the prostate and seminal vesicles.

Prosthenorchis a genus of parasites in the phylum Acanthocephala.

***P. elegans*, *P. spirula* (syn. *P. sigmoides*)** found in the terminal small intestine, colon and cecum of monkeys. Heavy infestations cause diarrhea, dehydration and death. There are yellow nodules on the serosal surface of the intestine which is swollen. There may be obstruction of the ileocecal valve and perforation of the intestinal wall.

prosthesis pl. *prostheses* [Gr.] 1. the replacement of an absent part by an artifical substitute. 2. an artificial substitute for a missing part, such as an eye, leg or tooth, used for functional or cosmetic reasons, or both.

femoral p. see total HIP replacement.

joint p. the principal example in veterinary surgery is total HIP replacement.

ocular p. is used infrequently in animals. It may be fitted in the orbit after enucleation (intraorbital), within the sclera after evisceration of the defective globe (intrascleral), or over the surface of a deformed globe (extrascleral).

skeletal p. not much used in animals, largely because of the great variability in the sizes needed and the small volume required. Human prostheses have been adapted for use in primates.

urethral p. metal or synthetic conduits may be implanted in the treatment of urethral stricture and obstruction in male cats.

prosthetic serving as a substitute; pertaining to prostheses or to prosthetics.

p. implants see PROSTHESIS, CARBON FIBER IMPLANTS.

prosthetics the field of knowledge relating to prostheses, their design, use, etc.

prosthetist a person skilled in prosthetics and practicing its application.

prosthodontics a specialty in dentristy concerned with the restoration of damaged or missing teeth.

Prosthogonimus a genus of flukes (digenetic trematodes) in the family Prosthogonimidae which parasitize birds but are found occasionally in mammals.

P. anatinus found in domestic ducks.

P. cuneatus found in swans.

P. macrorchis*, *P. ovatus found in the bursa of Fabricius and oviduct of domestic poultry and wild birds.

P. oviformis found in ducks.

P. pellucidus occurs in the bursa of Fabricius, oviduct and posterior intestine of fowl, ducks and wild birds.

prosthokeratoplasty surgical replacement of a damaged section of cornea by an inert graft.

Prosthorhyncus formosus an acanthocephalan parasite found in the small intestine of domestic fowl and some wild bird species. Has doubtful pathogenicity.

prostration extreme exhaustion, or lack of energy or power.

heat p. a condition caused by exposure to excessive heat. See also HEAT[1] exhaustion.

protactinium a chemical element, atomic number 91, atomic weight 231, symbol Pa. See Table 6.

protamine any of a class of simple proteins, soluble in water, not coagulated by heat, and precipitated from aqueous solution by addition of alcohol, found combined with nucleic acids in the sperm of certain fish, and having the property of neutralizing heparin. Protamine sulfate is used as an antidote to heparin overdosage.

p. paracoagulation used to examine a blood sample for fibrin monomers and fibrinogen-split products.

p. zinc insulin (PZI) see INSULIN.

protandry, protogyny a state of hermaphroditism in which the male gonad matures before the female gonad.

protean changing form or assuming different shapes.

protease any proteolytic enzyme.

p.-antiprotease imbalance thought to play a part in the pathogenesis of emphysema by permitting excessive proteolysis, especially of elastin.

fecal p. originate from the pancreas and include trypsin, chymotrypsin and carboxypeptidases. Proteolytic activity of the feces may be evaluated by tests that measure digestion of gelatin or casein-based substrates.

α_1-p. inhibitor α_1-antitrypsin.

protectant, protective 1. affording defense or immunity. 2. an agent affording defense against harmful influence.

intestinal p. a preparation that given orally provides a protective coating for the intestinal mucosa, and absorbs bacteria and toxins. Kaolin, pectin and activated charcoal are commonly used for this purpose.

protected not generally available; surrounded by some mechanism that prevents access.

p. fat see protected LIPID.

p. field information on the computer screen which cannot be overwritten.

protection prevention against injury.

p. tests neutralization tests using serial dilutions of antiserum to protect animals against challenge by a standard dose of microorganism.

x-ray p. includes taking x-rays only in designated areas, the use of portable warning signs when radiography is done elsewhere, the wearing of leadlined gloves and aprons by staff working near active apparatus, a red warning light which is switched on when the apparatus is being used. Personnel working near x-ray apparatus should wear dosimeter badges which are checked periodically.

protective 1. providing protection. 2. substances used to provide protection to tissues.

p. clothing varies with the risk prevailing, e.g. radiation (see x-ray PROTECTION), waterproof gear for highly infectious diseases, coveralls for normal large animal practice, metal studded gloves for catching aggressive companion animals.

p. isolation a type of ISOLATION designed to prevent contact between potentially pathogenic microorganisms and uninfected animals which have seriously impaired resistance. Called also reverse isolation. It is recommended for patients suffering from agranulocytosis, severe and extensive dermatitis, certain types of lymphomas and leukemias, and those who are receiving immunosuppressive therapy.

p. substances finely ground, absorbent, insoluble, inert substances that absorb toxins, cover sensitive and damaged tissues with a fine film. Includes starch, kaolin, talc, zinc oxide, zinc stearate. See also intestinal PROTECTANT.

protein any large organic compound made from one or more polypeptides, which are chains of AMINO acids joined in a genetically determined order by peptide linkages between the carboxyl group of one amino acid and the amino group of the next. They contain carbon, hydrogen, oxygen and nitrogen and usually sulfur, occasionally phosphorus.

Proteins form a large and essential part of the body mass, comprising especially cell membranes, connective tissue, muscles, enzymes, hormones, blood proteins. To maintain this mass the diet must contain a high proportion of protein, especially in growing animals and those recovering from debilitating diseases.

p. A a surface protein of *Staphylococus aureus* which binds to the Fc region of some IgG molecules. Fluorochrome labeled protein A is used in an indirect immunofluorescence test for detecting bound immunoglobulins.

authentic p. a recombinant protein with all its naturally occurring properties.

p. binding a property of many drugs which limits their distribution and availability in the blood, as well as affecting elimination from the body.

p. bumps see BUMPS.

p.-calories calories derived from proteins in the diet.

p. calorie malnutrition inadequate protein in the diet leads to impaired cell-mediated immunity, delayed wound healing and loss of lean body mass.

p.–calorie ratio the number of calories provided from protein sources, compared with the total caloric intake; an indication of the level of protein intake.

carrier p. one which, when coupled to a hapten, renders it capable of eliciting an immune response.

complete p. one containing the essential amino acids in the proportion required in the diet.

p. concentrates feeds containing a high concentration of protein, e.g. legume grains and forages, meat meal, fish meal, oil cakes, milling residues including bran, shorts, middlings, brewer's grains.

conjugated p's those in which the protein molecule is united with nonprotein molecules or prosthetic groups, e.g. glycoproteins, lipoproteins and metalloproteins.

p.–creatinine ratio in urine is valuable in correcting for variation in urine contents due to variable dilutions.

crude p. the total nitrogen content of a feed multiplied by 6.25. Includes several obvious errors but is still a close approximation of the protein content.

dietary p. is usually the most expensive part of the diet, except for animals at pasture, and the constituent most likely to be deficient. An excess of protein in the diet in ruminants can cause a sharp rise in alkalinity, due to the release of ammonia, of the ruminal contents causing ruminal atony and indigestion.

digestible p. the crude protein ingested less the protein excreted in the feces. The estimation requires a digestibility trial involving animals.

p. equivalent said of a feed. The total nitrogen content expressed as protein if it were all in that form. That is the percentage nitrogen in the feed multiplied by the average percentage of nitrogen in plant protein (6.25%).

p. excretion t. one that uses ^{51}Cr-labeled protein which measures protein excretion in the feces in cases of protein-losing enteropathy.

p.–fibrinogen ratio see PLASMA protein:fibrinogen ratio.

fibrous p's characterized by shape, structure and low water solubility; they have a structural role. Examples are COLLAGEN, KERATIN and TROPOMYOSIN.

fusion p. in recombinant DNA technology when a foreign gene is inserted into a plasmid vector to interrupt a gene, such as *lac*Z, the mRNA transcript of the recombinant plasmid contains the lacZ Shine–Dalgarno sequence and codons for the 3′ end of the lacZ gene protein followed by the codons of the foreign gene; the protein expressed is a fusion protein containing a few N-terminal *lac*Z amino acids and the contiguous foreign protein.

p. hydrolysates pharmaceutical preparations used in the treatment of severe, acute protein loss. Available for use orally or parenterally. They are partly digested proteins and contain a mixture of polypeptides, amino acids and other breakdown products.

myeloma p. see multiple MYELOMA.

p. nutritional deficiency causes lack of muscle development, and slow growth rate and maturation. In adults there is a low milk production and poor weight gain. In severe states tissue and blood levels fall, hypoproteinemic edema may occur, and a degree of immunosuppression could be expected.

partial p. one having a ratio of essential amino acids different from that of the average body protein.

peripheral p. any protein located in the membrane but not essential to the reconstitution of that protein.

plasma p's all the proteins present in the blood plasma, including the immunoglobulins. See PLASMA protein.

rec A p. an enzyme that binds to DNA and plays an important role in genetic recombination.

serum p. proteins in the blood serum, including immunoglobulins, albumin, complement, coagulation factors and enzymes.

p. shock ANAPHYLAXIS occurring after the intravenous injection of protein.

p.-sparing in times of energy deficiency the animal body may raid protein stores for glucogenic amino acids, thus depleting body stores of proteins. Substances such as acetic acid which can fill the energy deficiency and avoid the protein loss are known as protein-sparing.

p. supplements feeds which contain more than 20% protein.

urine p. see PROTEINURIA.

viral p. proteins encoded by the viral genome.

protein-bound said of a chemical bonding of calcium, iodine, iron, copper and other electrolyte ions in the blood to plasma proteins. The bound electrolyte is not immediately available biologically nor is it as vulnerable to sudden loss.

p.-bound iodine (PBI) test determination of thyroid function by measuring the amount of iodine contained in compounds bound to plasma proteins. It has been largely replaced by radioimmunoassay for the thyroid hormones thyroxine (T_4) and tri-iodothyronine (T_3).

proteinaceous pertaining to or of the nature of protein.

proteinase any enzyme that catalyzes the splitting of interior peptide bonds in a protein; an endopeptidase.

p. resistant protein (prp) a protein which resists digestion by proteinases; the amyloid fibrils in brain tissue of sheep affected with scrapie contain such a prp.

proteinemia excess of protein in the blood.

proteinosis the accumulation of excess protein in the tissues.

proteinuria an excess of serum proteins in the urine; an important indicator of renal disease. It is a constant finding in glomerulonephritis, renal infarction, amyloidosis and nephrosis, but is also common in congestive heart failure and renal ischemia of all kinds. The significance of proteinuria as an indicator of renal disease is greatly enhanced by the presence of renal casts in the urine.

Bence Jones p. see BENCE JONES PROTEIN.

neonatal p. occurs transiently during the period of intestinal absorption of proteins, some of which are small enough to pass the glomerular membrane.

Proteles cristatus see AARDWOLF.

Proteocephalus a genus of tapeworms in the order Proteocephalidea.

P. ambloplitis found in cultured fish, especially bass. The parasite affects the gonads and causes sterility. Called also bass tapeworm.

proteoglycan any of a group of glycoproteins found primarily in connective tissue and formed of subunits of glycosaminoglycans (long polysaccharide chains containing amino sugars) linked to a protein core like bristles on a bottle brush. Hydrated proteoglycans form the highly viscous fluid of mucus and the matrix of the intercellular ground substance of connective tissue. Called also mucopolysaccharide.

proteolipid a combination of a peptide or protein with a lipid, having the solubility characteristics of lipids.

proteolysis the splitting of proteins by hydrolysis of the peptide bonds, with formation of smaller polypeptides.

proteolytic 1. pertaining to, characterized by, or promoting proteolysis. 2. a proteolytic enzyme.

p. enzyme includes pepsin from the stomach; trypsin, chymotrypsin, elastase, carboxypeptidase A and B, ribonuclease and deoxyribonuclease—all from the exocrine pancreas; enteropeptidase, aminopeptidase, dipeptidase, nuclease, nucleotidases and nucleosidases—all from the intestinal mucosa.

proteometabolism the metabolism of protein.

proteopeptic digesting protein.

proteoses a mixture of split products formed by the hydrolysis of protein molecules short of the amino acid stage.

proteroglypha members of the Proteroglyphae group of snakes. Venomous but not aggressive and most are too small to be dangerous.

Proteromonas flagellate protozoa found in the intestines of all lizards; not thought to be pathogenic.

Proteus a genus of gram-negative, motile bacteria, members of the family Enterobacteriaceae, usually found in fecal and other putrefying matter. Also found associated with infections of the external ear and skin and in pyometra and pyelonephritis.

P. mirabilis a common inhabitant of animal fecal material found particularly in infections of the eye, skin, urinary and respiratory tract.

P. vulgaris found in canine epididymo-orchitis, prostatitis and cystitis.

prothrombin a glycoprotein present in the plasma that is converted into thrombin by extrinsic thromboplastin during the second stage of blood CLOTTING; called also clotting factor II.

p. consumption test determines thromboplastin generating capacity, which provides information about the first stage of coagulation. When clotting of a normal blood sample occurs, prothrombin is converted to thrombin, thus there should be little or no prothrombin in the serum after the clot is formed. If, however, there is deficiency of blood coagulation, some of the prothrombin will not be utilized (consumed). Abnormal results of the test are found in deficiencies of the first-stage factors of coagulation (factors VIII and IX), and in the presence of circulating anticoagulants, thrombocytopenia, and any other condition leading to inadequate generation of thromboplastin. Called also serum clot time.

p. converting activity the step in blood coagulation in which factor Xa, together with factor V react with phospholipid in the presence of calcium, activates prothrombin to form thrombin.

p. deficiency see HYPOPROTHROMBINEMIA.

p. time test a test to measure the activity of clotting factors V, VII and X, prothrombin and fibrinogen. Deficiency of any of these factors leads to a prolongation of the one-stage prothrombin times, as will circulating anticoagulants that are active against factors V, VII, or against thromboplastin. Called also protime.

The *one-stage* (OSPT) test is performed by measuring the time required for clot formation after tissue extract and calcium are added to citrated plasma. Called also Quick's prothrombin test. A *two-stage* test determines plasma levels of prothrombin by finding the dilution of plasma that clots a standard fibrinogen reagent in a set period of time.

prothrombinase thromboplastin; tissue factor, factor III.

prothrombinogenic promoting the production of prothrombin.

protirelin thyrotropin releasing hormone.

protist any member of the Protista.

Protista a kingdom comprising bacteria, algae, slime molds, fungi and protozoa; it includes all single-celled prokaryotic organisms.

protium the mass 1 isotope of hydrogen, symbol ^1H; ordinary, or light, hydrogen.

proto- word element. [Gr.] *first*.

protoanemonin pentadienoic lactone in all members of the plant family Ranunculaceae. In the living plant it is present as an inert glycoside ranunculin. When it is released enzymatically it is irritant, causing erythema and blistering of the skin and mucosae. See also RANUNCULUS.

protoblast 1. a cell with no cell wall; an embryonic cell. 2. a blastomere from which a particular organ or part develops.

protocol 1. the original notes made on a necropsy, an experiment, or on a case of disease. 2. a strict plan of formal procedure at a prestigious gathering. 3. a set of rules governing the format and chronology of message exchange in a communications system.

protocollagen an abnormal form of collagen when the hydroxylation stage of its formation is interrupted.

protodiastole the beginning of ventricular relaxation, terminating when the semilunar valves close.

protodiastolic pertaining to early diastole, i.e. immediately following the second heart sound.

protoduodenum the first or proximal portion of the duodenum, extending from the pylorus to the duodenal papilla.

protofibril the first elongated unit appearing in formation of any type of fiber.

protofilament a filament formed by the aggregation of tubulin in the form of microtubules; a stage in the development of the cytoplasmic skeleton.

protogaster archenteron.

protogyny see PROTANDRY.

protokylol hydrochloride a sympathomimetic agent with activity similar to isoproterenol. Used as a bronchodilator.

Protolepsis tesselata a species of leech that commonly parasitizes the nasal cavity of aquatic birds.

protolipids hyrophobic lipoproteins present in many membranes, particularly in myelin.

proton an elementary particle of mass number 1, with a positive charge equal to the negative charge of the electron; a constituent particle of every nucleus, the number of protons in the nucleus of each ATOM of a chemical element being indicated by its atomic number.

p. pump see sodium PUMP.

p. pump inhibitor a class of therapeutic agents which are used to counteract the effects of proton pumps in tissues and organs, particularly used in counteracting gastric hypersecretion and acidity.

protoneuron the first neuron in a peripheral reflex arc.

proto-oncogene a gene that is progenitor of an oncogene.

Protophormia terraenovae one of the primary flies in cutaneous MYIASIS.

protophyrinogen oxidase a mitochondrial enzyme.

protoplasm the viscid, translucent colloid material, the essential constituent of the living cell, including cytoplasm and nucleoplasm.

protoplast a bacterial or plant cell deprived of its rigid wall but with its plasma membrane intact; the cell is dependent for its integrity on an isotonic or hypertonic medium. In bacteria, specifically refers to gram-positive organisms. See also SPHEROPLAST.

protoplatelet a stage in the maturation and release of platelets by megakaryocytes consisting of a strip of platelets in the peripheral circulation, which will eventually separate into individual platelets. See also PROPLATELET.

protoporphyria porphyria marked by excessive protoporphyrin in the erythrocytes, plasma and feces. The excess is due to a deficiency of the enzyme ferrochelatase and an increased formation of the protoporphyrin. The disease occurs in cattle and is similar to congenital erythropoietic PORPHYRIA but less severe with the only clinical abnormality being photosensitive dermatitis. The defect is inherited as a dominant trait.

protoporphyrin a porphyrin whose iron complex united with protein occurs in hemoglobin, myoglobin and certain respiratory pigments.

p. III combines with 4 moles of iron to form the heme moiety of hemoglobin.

protoporphyrinogen III a two carboxyl porphyrinogen, precursor of protoporphyrin III.

protoporphyrinuria protoporphyrin in the urine.

Protospirura a genus of spirurid nematodes in the family Spiruridae.

P. bestianum, P. muricola, P. numidia found in the stomach of various felids and rodents.

Protostrongylus a genus of hairlike lungworms found in the bronchioles, alveoli and parenchyma of the lungs of some mammals.

P. boughtoni in cottontail rabbits and hares.

P. brevispiculum, P. davtiani, P. hobmaieri in bighorn sheep.

P. kochi in sheep and goats.

P. oryctolagi in rabbits.

P. pulmonalis in rabbit and hare.

P. rufescens found in sheep, goats and deer.

P. rushi in bighorn sheep.

P. skrjabini in sheep and goats.

P. stilesi in bighorn sheep.

P. sylvilagi in cottontail and jackrabbits.

P. tauricus found in hares.

Prototheca a genus of achloric algae, possibly a mutant form of *Chlorella*. They are saprophytic organisms that usually occupy freeliving niches in a great variety of places. Very rarely infection may occur in canine and feline skin, bovine mammary gland, canine eye and the canine colon. Identified species are *P. stagnora*, *P. trispora*, *P. wickerhami*, *P. zopfi*.

protothecal enterocolitis caused by oral infection with *Prototheca* spp. may cause chronic intractable diarrhea, with or without dysentery; necropsy lesions include ulcerative and hemorrhagic colitis.

protothecosis granulomatous panuveitis, enterocolitis, mastitis, dermatitis or a systemic spread of infection with the alga PROTOTHECA.

prototroph an organism with the same growth factor requirements as the ancestral strain; said of microbial mutants.

prototype the original type or form that is typical of later individuals or species.

protoveratrine one of the poisons found in the members of the plant genus *Veratrum*. Causes salivation, purgation, vomiting, diuresis, excitement, prostration, convulsions and cardiac arrhythmia.

Protozoa a phylum comprising the unicellular eukaryotic organisms; most are freeliving, but some lead commensalistic, mutualistic, saprophytic or parasitic existences. There are two subphylla of veterinary interest: (1) Sarcodina—including coccidia, cryptosporidia, *Toxoplasma*, *Babesia*, *Plasmodium* and others; (2) Mastigophora—including trypanosomes, *Histomonas*, *Trichomonas* spp.

Pathogenic protozoa for animals include: *Acanthamoeba*, *Babesia*, *Balantidium*, *Besnoitia*, *Chilomastix*, *Cochlosoma*, *Cryptobia*, *Cryptosporidium*, *Cystoisospora*, *Dientamoeba*, *Eimeria*, *Encephalitozoon*, *Endolimax*, *Entamoeba*, *Frenkelia*, *Giardia*, *Haemoproteus*, *Hammondia*, *Hartmannella*, *Hepatozoon*, *Hexamita*, *Histomonas*, *Iodamoeba*, *Isospora*, *Klossiella*, *Leishmania*, *Leucocytozoon*, *Naegleria*, *Parahistomonas*, *Pentatrichomonas*, *Plasmodium*, *Sarcocystis*, *Theileria*, *Toxoplasma*, *Trichomonas*, *Tritrichomonas*, *Trypanosoma*, *Tyzzeria* and *Wenyonella* spp.

protozoacide destructive to protozoa; an agent destructive to protozoa.

protozoal pertaining to or caused by protozoa.

p. encephalomyelitis probably the same disease as equine protozoal myeloencephalitis caused by *Sarcocystis neurona*.

p. hepatitis caused usually by *Toxoplasma*, *Neospora*, *Leishmania*. Rare cases of hepatic coccidiosis are observed but the causative organisms are not identified.

protozoan 1. of or pertaining to protozoa. 2. an organism belonging to the Protozoa.

protozoiasis any disease caused by protozoa.
protozoology the scientific study of protozoa.
protozoon pl. *protozoa* [Gr.] any member of the Protozoa.
protozoophage a cell having phagocytic action on protozoa.
protractor an instrument for extracting foreign bodies from wounds.
protransglutaminase the inactive precursor of transglutaminase; called also coagulation factor XIII (fibrin stabilizing factor) in the blood coagulation system.
protrusion extension beyond the usual limits, or above a plane surface.
protryptyline a tricyclic antidepressant.
protuberance a projecting part, or prominence.
external occipital p. on the occipital surface of the occipital bone, above the foramen magnum. The ligamentum nuchae is attached to it.
intercornual p. the prominence between the horns of cows.
protuberantia pl. *protuberantiae* [L.] protuberance.
protyrosinase precursor of tyrosinase, an enzyme critical in the formation of melanin.
proud exuberant.
p. cut see CUT proud.
p. flesh exuberant amounts of soft, edematous, granulation tissue developing during healing of large surface wounds.
proven sire a sire whose genetic credentials have been established by the production performances of his offspring in a properly conducted progeny test.
proventricular pertaining to or emanating from the PROVENTRICULUS.
p. dilatation syndrome see MACAW wasting disease.
proventriculotomy performed in large birds, usually for the removal of ingested foreign bodies.
proventriculus 1. the elongated, spindle-shaped, glandular stomach of birds. Supplemented by the muscular stomach just distal to it. 2. the ruminant FORESTOMACHS.
Providencia a genus of gram-negative, non-lactose-fermenting enterobacteria; occasionally isolated from diseased animals.
P. heimbachae isolated from penguin feces and an aborted bovine fetus.
P. stuartii identified as a cause of severe enteritis in newborn calves.
provirus the genome of an animal virus integrated into the chromosome of the host cell, and thus transferred to in all of its daughter cells.
provitamin a substance, e.g. ergosterol, from which the animal organism can form a vitamin.
p. A see CAROTENE.
provocative exposure see provocative EXPOSURE.
proximad in a proximal direction.
proximal nearest to a point of reference, as to a center or median line or to the point of attachment or origin.
proximalis [L.] *proximal.*
proximate immediate; nearest.
p. analysis a chemical method of assessing and expressing the nutritional value of a feed. It divides each feed into six categories and states the percentage of each that is present in the feed:
(1) water (or dry matter).
(2) total or crude protein (total nitrogen $\times$ 6.25).
(3) fat (or ether extract).
(4) ash (minerals).
(5) crude fiber (incompletely digested carbohydrates).
(6) nitrogen-free extract (readily digestible carbohydrate).
proximobuccal pertaining to the proximal and buccal surfaces of a posterior tooth.
proxymetacaine see PROPARACAINE.
Prozac see FLUOXETINE.
prozone the phenomenon exhibited by some sera, in which agglutination or precipitation occurs at higher dilution ranges, but is not visible at lower dilutions or when undiluted.
PRPP phosphoribosylpyrophosphate.
PRSL protein renal solute load.
prulaurasin a cyanogenetic glycoside found in the seeds, and to a less extent foliage, of plants in the family Rosaceae.
prunasin a cyanogenetic glycoside found in the seeds, and to a less extent in the foliage, of plants of the Rosaceae family.
Prunus a genus of trees in the family Rosaceae. The seeds of these trees contain cyanogenetic glycosides which are potentially poisonous. The fruit pulp appears to quite safe. The glycosides are amygdalin, prunasin, prulaurasin.

The following are the known toxic plants—*P. amygdalus* var. *amara* seeds (bitter almond), *P. armeniaca* (apricot), *P. brachybotrya*, *P. caroliniana*, *P. laurocerasus* (cherry laurel), *P. cerasus* (cherry), *P. domestica* (plum), *P. padus* (bird cherry), *P. pennsylvanica* (pincherry), *P. persica* (peach), *P. sellowii*, *P. serotina* (wild black cherry), *P. sphaerocarpa*, *P. virginiana* (chokecherry), *P. virginiana* var. *demissa* (western chokecherry), *P. virginiana* var. *melanocarpa* (western chokecherry).
pruritogenic causing pruritus, or itching.
pruritus itching; common in many types of skin disorders, especially allergic inflammation and parasitic infestations. Its presence in animals is inferred because of the presence of scratching, which would be a more accurate description. Pruritus is epidermal in origin and does not occur in deep ulcerations, although they may be painful. It is most intense at mucocutaneous junctions. See also PARESTHESIA, HYPERESTHESIA.
p. ani intense chronic itching in the anal region. May be caused by perianal dermatitis, intestinal parasitism and anal sac disease in dogs and cats.
cholinergic p. caused by stimulation of afferent cholinergic fibers at the neuroglandular junction of the sweat gland with release of acetylcholine and sweat. There is mast cell degranulation. Called also heat reflex urticaria.
essential p. that occurring without known cause.
symptomatic p. that which occurs secondarily to another condition.
Prussian blue ferric ferrocyanide; a dark blue dye, used to demonstrate ferric iron and in the treatment of chronic thallium poisoning.
prussic acid see CYANIDE.
PRV pseudorabies virus.
Przevalskiana a parasitic fly with a life cycle resembling that of *Hypoderma* spp. Parasitizes goats, sheep, gazelle.
Przewalski's horse see MONGOLIAN WILD HORSE.
psammomas bodies which occur in meningiomas. They are calcified material within the center of a laminated whorl of elongated fibroblastic cells. See also ACERVULI, CORPORA arenacea.
psammomatous pertaining to a psammoma.
p. meningioma a meningioma in which psammoma bodies occur.
Psammomys obesus an arid-zone sand rat which

develops diabetes when fed entirely on laboratory chow.

psammona bodies see CORPORA arenacea.

psammosarcoma a sarcoma containing granular material.

Psathyrotes annua North American plant in the family Asteraceae; a highly poisonous plant causing acute or chronic hepatic injury caused by an unidentified hepatoxin. Death may occur in as little as 24 hours. Chronic cases develop jaundice.

PSCID primary severe combined immunodeficiency disease. See COMBINED IMMUNE DEFICIENCY SYNDROME.

PSE 1. pale soft exudative pork. 2. portosystemic encephalopathy.

Pseudallescheria boydii (syn. *Petriellidium boydii, Allescheria boydi*) perfect state of SCEDOSPORIUM APIOSPERMUM.

pseudallescheriosis infection by *Pseudallescheria boydii* (syn. *Petriellidium boydii, Allescheria boydii*). See eumycotic MYCETOMA.

Pseudamphistomum a digenetic trematode, parasitic in the liver, of the family Opisthorchiidae.

P. truncatum occurs in carnivores and humans and has a life cycle and pathogenicity similar to those of *Opisthorchis* spp.

pseudarthrosis, pseudoarthrosis a pathological entity characterized by a nonosseous union of bone fragments of a fractured bone due to inadequate immobilization leading to existence of the 'false joint' that gives the condition its name.

Pseudaspidodera a genus of roundworms in the family Heterakidae.

P. jnanendre, P. pavonis found in the cecum of peafowl. Do not appear to be pathogenic.

Pseudechis a genus of venomous snakes.

P. australis the mulga or king brown snake with a highly poisonous neurotoxin. A brassy red-brown color with a cream and orange belly and up to 10 ft long.

P. papuanus Papuan black snake. A highly poisonous but unaggressive black snake with a blue-gray belly and gray underthroat and up to 8 ft long.

P. porphyriacus the red-bellied black snake. A purple-black snake with a pink-white belly up to 8 ft long. Not aggressive and has a poison of relatively low neurotoxicity but has a high content of hemolysin and hemorrhagic factor.

pseudencephalus a fetus with a tumor in place of the brain.

pseud(o)- word element. [Gr.] *false*.

pseudoachondroplastic dysplasia see EPIPHYSEAL dysplasia.

pseudoachrondoplastic dysplasia see EPIPHYSEAL dysplasia.

pseudoalbinism a defect of pigmentation similar to albinism. Most suspected cases of albinism in animals are of pseudoalbinism with pigment in some places, e.g. the eyes. Many equine pseudoalbinos die in utero or have a congenital absence of a gut segment. See also CHEDIAK–HIGASHI SYNDROME.

flatfish p. claimed to be due to too bright aquarium lights prior to hatching.

pseudoalbino see ALBINO.

pseudoallele one of two or more genes that are seemingly allelic, but which can be shown to have distinctive but closely linked loci.

pseudoanemia marked pallor with no evidence of anemia.

pseudoaneurysm false aneurysm; differs from a true aneurysm in that its wall does not contain the components of an artery, but consists of fibrous tissue, which usually continues to enlarge, creating a pulsating hematoma.

pseudoankylosis a false ankylosis.

pseudoanodontia failed eruption rather than absence of teeth. Occurs in gray lethal mice and in Lhasa apso and Shih tzu dogs. See also ANODONTIA.

Pseudobilharziella a genus of blood flukes in the family Schistosomatidae. Found in the blood vessels of some anatid birds.

pseudoblackleg a disease of cattle caused by *Clostridium septicum* and resembling blackleg clinically but occurring only when precipitated by trauma such as shearing wounds. The disease occurs also in pigs but is a systemic infection by *C. septicum* with a primary lesion in the stomach.

pseudobulbar apparently, but not really, due to a lesion of the medulla oblongata.

Pseudocalymma elegans South American plant in the family Bignoniaceae; an unidentified toxin causes staggering, tremor and convulsions followed by death all within a few hours.

Pseudocaranx dentex finfish in family Caragidae. Called also silver trevally or striped jack. See Table 23.

pseudocarcinomatous hyperplasia hyperkeratosis resembling carcinoma.

pseudocartilaginous resembling cartilage.

pseudocast an accidental formation of urinary sediment resembling a true cast.

pseudocele the 'fifth' ventricle of the brain, the space between the two halves of the septum pellucidum.

pseudocervix false or phantom cervix created during examination of the canine reproductive tract, when the dorsomedial fold of the vagina and the lateral walls of the vagina cause a temporary obstruction.

Pseudocheirus see POSSUM.

P. peregrinus ringtail POSSUM.

pseudocholinesterase see BUTYRYLCHOLINESTERASE.

pseudochorea a state of general incoordination resembling chorea.

pseudochromhidrosis discoloration of sweat by surface contaminants, such as pigment-producing bacteria or chemical substances on the skin.

pseudochylothorax see CHYLOID effusion.

pseudochylous effusion see CHYLOID effusion.

pseudocirrhosis a condition suggestive of, but not due to cirrhosis; often due to pericarditis (pericardial pseudocirrhosis).

pseudocoarctation a condition radiographically resembling coarctation but without compromise of the lumen, as occurs in a congenital anomaly of the aortic arch.

pseudocoele see PSEUDOCELE.

pseudocolloid a mucoid substance sometimes found in ovarian cysts.

pseudocoloboma a line or scar on the iris resembling a coloboma.

pseudocontinuity abnormal healing and regeneration of severed nerve fibers; the space between the cut ends becomes filled with fibrous tissues rather than nerve fibers.

pseudocoprostasis constipation caused by matting of haircoat around the anus that impedes passage of feces. Seen in longhaired dogs and cats.

pseudocowpox an infectious disease of the skin of teats of cows caused by a paravaccinia virus. Typical lesions commence as erythema, progress to a vesicle, pustule or scab which is shed leaving a horseshoe-shaped ring of small scabs. Persons milking the cows may develop lesions on their hands. Called also milker's nodule.

pseudocoxalgia osteochondrosis of the capitular epiphysis of the femur.

pseudocrisis sudden but temporary abatement of febrile signs.

pseudo-Cushing's syndrome see GROWTH-HORMONE-responsive dermatosis.

pseudocyesis see false PREGNANCY.

pseudocylindroid a shred of mucin in the urine resembling a cylindroid.

pseudocyst an abnormal dilated space resembling a cyst but not lined with epithelium, e.g. a retroperitoneal accumulation of urine from a leaking ureter.

perirenal p., perinephritic p. see feline PERIRENAL cysts.

salivary p. see salivary MUCOCELE.

pseudodiabetes early diabetes.

azotemic p. a glucose intolerance seen in association with azotemia, thought to be due to a peripheral resistance to insulin-mediated uptake of glucose by tissues. Severe hyperglycemia, glucosuria, ketonemia, ketonuria and metabolic acidosis are not features.

Pseudodiscus a genus of intestinal flukes (digenetic trematodes) in the family Paramphistomatidae.

P. collinsi found in the colon of horses.

pseudodistemper TYROSINEMIA in mink.

pseudodominant the phenotypic expression of a recessive allele as the reult of a deletion of the dominant allele.

pseudoedema a puffy state resembling edema.

pseudoemphysema a condition resembling emphysema, but due to temporary obstruction of the bronchi.

pseudoenophthalmos apparent enophthalmos, resulting from a small globe or swollen eyelids.

pseudo-eosinophil the heterophil of rabbits and guinea pigs with prominent granules.

pseudoephedrine one of the optical isomers of EPHEDRINE.

pseudoepitheliomatous hyperplasia hyperkeratosis resembling an epithelioma.

pseudoexstrophy a developmental anomaly marked by the characteristic musculoskeletal defects of exstrophy of the bladder, but with no major defect of the urinary tract.

pseudofarcy see EPIZOOTIC lymphangitis.

pseudofilling defects abnormalities of the outline of the urinary bladder as seen on radiographs. They result from external pressure on the wall by colonic fullness, and can be differentiated from filling defects by use of a retrograde cystogram.

pseudo-focused grid see GRID.

pseudo-fowl pest see NEWCASTLE DISEASE.

pseudofracture radiological appearance of a thickened periosteum and new bone formation over what looks like an incomplete fracture.

Pseudogaltonia see LIDNERIA.

pseudoganglion an enlargement on a nerve resembling a ganglion.

pseudogene a nonfunctional DNA sequence, nearly homologous to a functional gene.

pseudoglanders see EPIZOOTIC lymphangitis. See also MELIOIDOSIS.

pseudoglandular a stage in the growth of the embryonic lung before ciliated cells are differentiated.

pseudoglioma any condition mimicking retinoblastoma, e.g. retrolental fibroplasia or exudative retinopathy.

pseudoglottis 1. the aperture between the false vocal cords. 2. neoglottis.

pseudogout an apparently hereditary, arthritic condition of humans, associated with chondrocalcinosis. In dogs, deposition of calcium phosphate crystals has been described as a cause of arthritis.

pseudohematuria the presence in the urine of pigments that impart a pink or red color, but with no detectable hemoglobin or blood cells.

pseudohemophilia von Willebrand's disease.

pseudohepatorenal syndrome many disease states in which there are clinical indications of renal and hepatic disease but there is no relationship between the two, e.g. a systemic disease in which the agent causes both hepatic and renal damage.

pseudohermaphrodite an individual exhibiting pseudohermaphroditism.

pseudohermaphroditism a state in which the gonads are of one sex but one or more contradictions exist in the morphological criteria of sex. In female pseudohermaphroditism, the individual is a genetic and gonadal female with partial masculinization; in male pseudohermaphroditism, the individual is a genetic and gonadal male with incomplete masculinization. Pseudohermaphroditism is not to be confused with hermaphroditism, in which the individual possesses both ovarian and testicular tissue.

pseudohernia an inflamed sac or gland simulating strangulated hernia.

p. inguinalis a mass of cod fat distends the scrotum and dilates the inguinal canal.

pseudo-Horner's syndrome see HAW'S syndrome.

pseudohyperkalemia elevated levels of serum potassium resulting from an increased release from cells during clotting of the sample. Associated with thrombocytosis, extreme leukocytosis, or abnormal white or red blood cells.

pseudohyperparathyroidism persistent hypercalcemia and hypophosphatemia, due to ectopic secretion of parathyroid hormone (-like) polypeptides or other bone resorbing substances by neoplasms. Lymphosarcoma and apocrine adenocarcinoma of the anal sac in dogs are the most common source. Affected dogs show muscle weakness, anorexia, vomiting, bradycardia, polyuria and polydipsia. Nephrocalcinosis may also occur. The clinical and biochemical abnormalities are reversed if the tumor is removed. See also HYPERPARATHYROIDISM.

pseudohypertrophic muscular dystrophy see ERB'S DYSTROPHY.

pseudohypertrophy increase in size without true hypertrophy.

pseudohypha pl. *pseudohyphae*; a chain of blastoconidia.

pseudohypoaldosteronism an unresponsiveness of the distal renal tubule to aldosterone, resulting in severe loss of salt in the urine, despite elevated secretion and urinary excretion of aldosterone. An inherited disorder in humans.

pseudohyponatremia a condition in which marked increases in serum proteins or lipids decrease the percentage of serum water and therefore sodium.

pseudohypoparathyroidism a condition in which there are changes characteristic of HYPOPARATHYROIDISM (hypocalcemia and hyperphosphatemia) in association with hyperactive parathyroid glands and increased blood levels of parathyroid hormone. It is the result of nonresponsive target cells in bone and kidneys. Not reported in animals.

pseudojaundice yellowness of the skin due to blood changes and not to liver disease.

pseudojervine one of the toxic alkaloids in *Veratrum* spp. Causes vomiting, purgation, salivation, diuresis, convulsions and death.

pseudokidney in ultrasonography, a contracted stomach or an intussuscepted bowel can be mistaken as a kidney.

Pseudoletia separata caterpillars which appear in massive waves and completely devour crops and pasture. Plants such as kikuyu grass are reputed to be more toxic when they regrow after such decimation. Called also army caterpillars.

pseudoleukemia the condition in which there are excessive numbers of lymphocytes in tissues but not in blood. See also LEUKOSIS. Called also aleukemic leukemia.

pseudolipidosis the original name for MANNOSIDOSIS. Called also pseudolipidosis with neuronopathy.

pseudo-lumpy-skin disease the disease of cattle that resembles a mild form of lumpy skin disease but is caused by bovine herpesvirus 2, known as the Allerton virus, identical to the bovine herpes mammillitis virus.

pseudolymphoma lesions likely to be mistaken for lymphoma include nodular lymphocytic–plasmacytic lesions of panniculitis, vasculitis, perifolliculitis, nodules created by vaccinations, arthropod stings.

Pseudolynchia a genus of flies in the family Hippoboscidae.

P. canariensis, P. capensis, P. lividicolor found on domestic pigeons and some wild birds. Dark brown flies resembling a sheep ked. They transmit *Haemoproteus columbae* of pigeons and *H. lophortyx* of quail.

pseudomalleus see MELIOIDOSIS.

pseudomelanosis pigmentation of tissues after death by blood pigments.

pseudomembrane a layer of coagulated fibrin, leukocytes and bacteria overlying a badly damaged mucous membrane and giving the appearance of being a viable tissue. Called also false membrane.

pseudomembranous pertaining to or emanating from pseudomembrane.

p. colitis see pseudomembranous COLITIS.

Pseudomicrodochium suttonii a fungus associated with phaeohyphomycosis in dogs.

Pseudomonas a genus of gram-negative, strictly aerobic bacteria, some species of which are pathogenic for plants and vertebrates.

P. aeruginosa a common isolate from wounds, burns and urinary tract infections and from many other accumulations of pus in all species. Also commonly found in otitis externa, fleece rot in sheep, and some cases of bovine mastitis. Its presence may be indicated by a distinctive blue or green color of the pus or infected site.

P. fluorescens a common cause of food spoilage and a frequent isolate from wounds and other contaminated sites in animals.

P. mallei see BURKHOLDERIA *mallei*.

P. pseudomallei see BURKHOLDERIA *pseudomallei*.

P. putida causes septicemia in aquarium fish.

pseudomucin a mucin-like substance found in ovarian cysts.

pseudomucinous pertaining to pseudomucin.

p. cystadenoma an ovarian tumor originating from the celomic epithelium of the ovary. Most often seen in aged nulliparous bitches.

pseudomycetoma rare manifestation of infection in the dermis and subcutis with *Microsporum canis*; recorded only in Persian cats.

pseudomycosis cutaneous and subcutaneous lesions ranging from nodules to fungating growths, usually on the lower limbs and abdomen of horses and composed of connective tissue riddled with necrotic tracts containing thick pus and small yellow-white granules. Usually contain a variety of bacteria and a foreign body.

pseudomyotonia muscle weakness accompanying canine Cushing's syndrome and some primary muscle disorders which can resemble myotonia, clinically and on electromyography.

pseudomyxoma a mass of epithelial mucus resembling a myxoma.

p. peritonei the presence in the peritoneal cavity of mucoid material from a ruptured ovarian cyst or a ruptured mucocele.

Pseudonaja nuchalis see DEMANSIA *nuchalis nuchalis*.

pseudoneuritis a congenital hyperemic condition of the optic papilla.

pseudo-odontoma see PERIOSTITIS.

pseudo-oligodontia the appearance of having less than the correct number of teeth erupted; due to failure of eruption of formed teeth. See also OLIGODONTIA.

pseudopapilledema anomalous elevation of the optic disk.

pseudoparalysis apparent loss of muscular power without real paralysis.

pseudo-Pelger–Hüet anomaly see pseudo-PELGER–HÜET ANOMALY.

Pseudopezzia medicaginis a leaf-spotting organism which causes a manifold increase in the concentration of coumestrol in the leaves of alfalfa (lucerne).

pseudophyllidean pertaining to tapeworms (cestodes) of the order Pseudophyllidae. Members within this order usually have a three-host aquatic life cycle. Adult tapeworms are parasitic in the intestines of fish-eating mammals, birds, fish and humans. Lengths of the adults range from 10 to 100 feet.

pseudoplague see NEWCASTLE DISEASE.

pseudopodium a temporary protrusion of the cytoplasm of an ameba or other motile simple cell, serving for purposes of locomotion or to engulf food.

pseudopolycoria full-thickness colobomas of the iris which may appear to be multiple pupils.

pseudopolyodontia retention of the deciduous teeth until the permanent teeth have erupted, giving the impression of more than the normal number of teeth. See also POLYODONTIA.

pseudopolyp a hypertrophied tab of mucous membrane resembling a polyp, but caused by ulceration surrounding intact mucosa.

pseudopolyposis numerous pseudopolyps in the colon and rectum, due to longstanding inflammation.

pseudopregnancy see false PREGNANCY.

pseudoproptosis apparent exophthalmos, as when the globe is very prominent or the eyelids are retracted.

pseudopseudohypoparathyroidism an incomplete form of pseudohypoparathyroidism, marked by the same constitutional features but by normal levels of calcium and phosphorus in the blood serum.

pseudopterygium an adhesion of the conjunctiva to the cornea following inflammation or injury.

pseudoptosis decrease in the size of the palpebral aperture.

pseudoptyalism the dribbling of saliva caused by a difficulty in swallowing or paralysis of the lips.

pseudorabies see AUJESZKY'S DISEASE.

Pseudorca see false killer WHALE.

pseudoreaction a false or deceptive reaction; in intradermal skin tests, a reaction not due to the specific test substance but to protein in the medium employed in producing the toxin.

pseudorickets see renal secondary HYPERPARATHYROIDISM.
pseudorinderpest see PESTE DES PETITS RUMINANTS.
pseudoringworm see porcine juvenile pustular psoriasiform DERMATITIS.
pseudosarcomatous fasciitis see NODULAR fasciitis.
Pseudostertagia bullosa a roundworm in the family Trichostrongylidae found in the abomasum of sheep, bighorn and Barbary sheep and pronghorn antelope.
pseudotetanus persistent muscular contractions resembling tetanus but not associated with *Clostridium tetani.*
pseudotrismus inability to completely open the mouth due to causes other than muscular spasm, e.g. in eosinophilic myositis of dogs.
pseudotruncus arteriosus the most severe form of tetralogy of Fallot.
pseudotuberculosis resembles tuberculosis. See also YERSINIOSIS.
avian p. a contagious disease of birds, both domestic and wild, caused by *Yersinia pseudotuberculosis* and characterized by an initial, brief septicemia, followed by a bacteremic phase in which there is the development of multiple abscesses and granulomas as in avian tuberculosis.
The disease causes major epornithics in populations of canaries, finches, cockatoos, parakeets. Called also canary cholera.
bovine p. see JOHNE'S DISEASE.
pseudotumor phantom tumor.
p. cerebri cerebral edema and raised intracranial pressure without neurological signs except occasional sixth cranial nerve palsy.
pseudotype phenotypic mixing in retroviruses results in a genome from a parent with a defective envelope, contained within the envelope capsid from a helper retrovirus.
pseudoulcer ulcer-shaped defects seen in the mucosa of the duodenum on radiographs following contrast studies. A change of no significance.
pseudouremia see AZOTEMIA.
pseudourticaria see LUMPY-skin disease.
psi the twenty-third letter of the Greek alphabet, Ψ or ψ.
p.s.i. pounds per square inch, equivalent to one-seventh of a kilopascal (kPa), the metric measure of pressure.
Psilocaulon genus of South African plants in the family Aizoaceae; have high content of soluble oxalates; cause oxalate poisoning manifested by nephrosis, uremia and urolithiasis. Also contain toxin psilocauline; includes *P. absimile*, *P. rogersiae*. Called also asbos, loogbos, prena vygie, asbosvygie.
Psilocybe genus of toxic mushrooms; contain an indole alkaloid which causes incoordination, tremor, stumbling, recumbency and hypersensitivity. Includes *P. cubensis*, *P. semilanceata*. Called also mad or magic mushrooms.
psilocybin a HALLUCINOGEN having indole characteristics, isolated from the mushroom *Psilocybe mexicana*.
psilostomatid a member of the family Psilostomatidae of small, globose flukes.
Psilostrophe North American plant genus in the family Asteraceae; contains an unidentified toxin which causes incoordination, coughing, vomiting, emaciation and death. Includes *P. gnapholodes*, *P. sparsiflora*, *P. tagetinae*. Called also paper flowers.
psittaciform a bird member of the order *Psittaciformes*, the parrots and parakeets.
psittacine said of birds which are members of the order Psittaciformes, the parrots and parakeets.
p. beak and feather disease occurs predominantly in young birds with their first contour feathers, but sometimes adults with previously normal feathers. There is a loss of contour and down feathers over most of the body, often progressing to complete baldness. The upper and lower beak may also be involved with inflammation, abnormal elongation, uneven wearing and transverse fracture lines. The disease is believed to be caused by a circovirus.
psittacosis a disease of psittacine birds due to a strain of *Chlamydia psittaci*, first seen in parrots and later found in other birds and domestic fowl, in which it is called ORNITHOSIS. It is transmissible to humans. In birds psittacosis causes a systemic infection and signs including diarrhea and ocular and nasal discharge.
p.–lymphogranuloma venereum group the family Chlamydiaceae of organisms.
psoas a sublumbar muscle. See Table 13.
p. tubercle on the ventral border of the shaft of the ilium; attachment point for the psoas minor muscle.
psocid a member of the order Psocoptera of book lice.
Psocoptera an order of insects; book lice found in dust and debris in many situations. Inconspicuous, soft-bodied insects which live on vegetable matter of various sorts and have no veterinary importance other than their ubiquity so that they are constantly suspected of causing disease.
psoitis inflammation of a psoas muscle or its sheath.
Psoralea a genus of plants in the legume family Fabaceae; may cause primary photosensitization. Includes *P. argophylla*, *P. cinerea*, *P. patens*, *P. tenuiflora*. Called also scurf pea. See also PSORALEN.
psoralen a furanocoumarin, one of the constituents of certain plants (e.g. *Psoralea corylifolia*) that have the ability to produce phototoxic dermatitis in humans when an individual is first exposed to it and then to sunlight; certain perfumes and drugs (e.g. methoxsalen) contain psoralens.
Psorergates a genus of parasitic mites in the family Cheyletidae. Called also *Psorobia* spp.
P. bos found on cattle but there is no lesion.
***P. oettlei* (syn. *P. simplex*)** found on laboratory mice and rats.
***P. ovis* (syn. *Psorobia ovis*)** causes a mild pruritus and scaly dermatitis on the body of sheep with some damage to the wool. Called also itch mite.
P. simplex see *P. oettlei* (above).
psorergatic mange see PSORERGATES *ovis*.
psoriasiform a dermatosis resembling psoriasis.
p. exfoliative dermatosis an idiopathic disease of cats and dogs characterized by asymptomatic, large, erythematous, irregular, scaly plaques symmetrically disposed over the forelimbs and trunk. A similar disease is also recorded in goats but the lesions are on the face under the belly and on the perineum.
p.-lichenoid dermatosis multiple lichenoid, hyperkeratotic papules and plaques begin to appear in young adult English springer spaniel dogs, first on the pinnae, ear canal and inguinal skin and later other areas.
psoriasis a usually chronic, recurrent skin disease in humans marked by discrete macules, papules or patches covered with lamellated silvery scales resulting from an increased turnover of epidermal cells. The cause is multifactorial and poorly understood. There is no equivalent disease in animals.
Psorobia ovis see PSORERGATES *ovis*.
Psorophora a genus of mosquitoes; a cause of severe insect worry when in large numbers and may cause deaths of poultry.

Psoroptes a genus of mange mites in the family Psoroptidae. See PSOROPTIC MANGE.

P. cervinus found on bighorn sheep, wapiti.

P. communis see *Psoroptes ovis* (below).

P. cuniculi found on the ears of rabbit, goat, horse, donkey and mule.

P. equi the body louse of horses. Found also on the donkey and mule.

P. hippotis see *P. cuniculi* (above).

P. natalensis found on the body of cattle (*Bos taurus*, *B. indicus*), Indian water buffalo.

P. ovis causes sheep-scab; found also on cattle and goats.

psoroptic mange a parasitic dermatitis of many species caused by *Psoroptes* spp. mites. They are *P. cervinus* (deer), *P. equi*, *P. natalensis* (cattle and water buffalo) and *P. ovis* (sheep, goats and cattle). The common ear mange mites are *P. cuniculi*. The disease in sheep is serious with much damage to fleece and some deaths. Goats and horses show mostly ear mange with much head shaking but lesions can occur anywhere on the body. In cattle the lesions are widespread and itching is severe. Called also sheep-scab, body mange, ear mange.

PSP 1. phenolsulfonphthalein. 2. paralytic shellfish paralysis.

PSP toxins paralytic shellfish poisoning toxins.

PSS 1. porcine stress syndrome. 2. portosystemic shunt.

psychic pertaining to the mind or psyche. See also PSYCHOGENIC.

psych(o)- word element. [Gr.] *mind*.

psychoanaleptic exerting a stimulating effect on the mind.

psychodid a member of the family Psychodidae. The sandflies or owl midges. Includes PHLEBOTOMUS.

psychogenic having an emotional or psychological origin. Some diseases of animals are considered to have a psychogenic origin, e.g. esophagogastric ulcer of pigs, in spite of our limited knowledge of their psychological makeup.

p. alopecia anxiety and excessive grooming in cats can cause loss of hair from barbering and pulling. In a more severe form, injury to the skin occurs and eosinophilic plaques may appear.

p. dermatitis see ACRAL lick dermatitis, idiopathic HYPERESTHESIA syndrome, TAIL biting, TAIL sucking, FLANK sucking.

p. vomition in cats, may be caused by rapid, overeating as an attention-seeking or compulsive activity.

psychomimetic resembling a psychosis.

psychomotor pertaining to motor effects of cerebral or psychic activity.

p. epilepsy see psychomotor SEIZURE.

psychoneurosis a neurosis based on emotional conflict.

psychopathology the pathology of mental disease. There is no branch of veterinary medicine which deals with this subject.

psychosis pl. *psychoses;* any major mental disorder of organic or emotional origin, marked by derangement of the personality and loss of contact with reality, often with delusions, hallucinations or illusions.

There is no scientific study of animal psychiatry and no specific psychoses but some well-identified and traumatic vices, e.g. crib-biting, weaving, tail chasing and flank sucking in dogs, are often classified as such. FARROWING hysteria in sows seems to be the animal disease with the closest approximation to a derangement of personality.

parturient p. of sows see FARROWING hysteria.

psychosomatic pertaining to the interrelations of mind and body; having bodily clinical signs of psychic, emotional or mental origin.

p. disease there are no identified psychosomatic diseases in animals. Abomasal ulcer in bulls in artificial insemination centers, esophagogastric ulcer in pigs, ulcerative colitis in dogs are possible candidates for the classification. The suggested mechanism for the development of disease in this way is that the cerebral cortex (via the psyche) overrides the normal, adaptive, feedback mechanisms by which the pituitary gland regulates the secretion of corticosteroids in response to stress of any sort. For this reason the adrenal cortex is overstimulated, develops hyperadrenocorticism first and then exhaustion.

psychosurgery neurosurgery for the purpose of altering behavior. See OLFACTORY tractotomy.

psychotropic capable of modifying mental activity.

p. drugs the important groups in veterinary medicine are the phenothiazine, thioxanthene, butyrophenone and benzodiazepine derivatives.

psychr(o)- word element. [Gr.] *cold*.

psychrometer an instrument for measuring the moisture of the atmosphere.

psychrophile a psychrophilic organism.

psychrophilic fond of cold; said of bacteria that grow best in the cold (40–68°F; 5–20°C).

psychrophore a double catheter for applying cold, per medium of cold water, to e.g. the urethra.

psychrotherapy treatment of disease by applying cold. See also CRYOSURGERY.

psyllium a fecal softener made from the seeds of the plants *Plantago psyllium*, *P. indica* and *P. ovata*. The mucilloid portion of the seeds of *P. ovata* is used to make psyllium hydrophilic mucilloid which is a bulk aperient to relieve constipation caused by a low residue diet.

PT prothrombin time.

Pt chemical symbol, *platinum*.

pt pint.

PTA plasma thromboplastin antecedent, CLOTTING factor XI.

ptaquiloside a norsesquiterpene glucoside of the illudane type; a major toxic principle of bracken (*Pteridium aquilinum*) and rock fern (*Cheilanthes sieberi*); is retinotoxic, radiomimetic, carcinogenic and responsible for thrombocytopenia leading to generalized hemorrhages in acute poisoning of cattle, bovine enzootic hematuria and bright blindness.

ptarmic causing sneezing.

ptarmus spasmodic sneezing.

PTC plasma thromboplastin component, CLOTTING factor IX, Christmas factor.

Pteridium a fern in the family Dennstadiaceae.

The fern is classified by some authorities as more than one species including: *P. aquilinum*, *P. esculentum*, *P. revolutum*, *P. yarrabense*. Called also bracken. It causes poisoning in several unique ways: (1) Ingestion by cattle over a short period causes depression of bone marrow activity, leading to pancytopenia evidenced principally as ecchymotic hemorrhages in mucosae and terminal septicemia. Severe diarrhea and dysentery may be terminal events. Ingestion over a long period causes proliferative lesions in and bleeding from the urinary bladder mucosa. See ENZOOTIC hematuria. Bright BLINDNESS of sheep also occurs when intake of bracken is prolonged. There is also a relationship between access to bracken and a higher than normal occurrence of intestinal carcinoma in ruminants. (2) A thiaminase in bracken causes a clinical syndrome of THIAMIN deficiency in horses. Signs are muscle tremor, incoordination, frequent falling and bradycardia and cardiac irregularity.

pteridophyte a member of the fern community and their allies.

Pteris aquilina PTERIDIUM *aquilinum*.

Pteroglossus see TOUCAN.

Pterolichus a genus of mites in the family Dermoglyphidae.

P. bicaudatus found on the feathers of the South African ostrich.

P. obtusus found on the feathers of fowls.

Pteronia pallens South African plant in the family Asteraceae; contains an unidentified toxin which damages liver and kidneys. Called also Scholtz bush, witbossie, *P. geigeroides* (syn. *Asaemia axillaris*).

Pteronyssus striatus a feather mite found on sparrow, linnet and chaffinch.

Pterophagus a genus of mites in the family Proctophyllodidae.

P. strictus found on the feathers of pigeons.

Pterophyllum small, highly colored, laterally compressed aquarium fish with thin, trailing fins. Called also angelfish. Members of the family Chaetodontidae.

Pteropus see CHIROPTERA.

pteroside a sesquiterpenoid found in bracken (*Pteridium aquilinum*).

pterosin a sesquiterpenoid found in bracken (*Pteridium aquilinum*).

pteroylglutamic acid see FOLIC ACID.

pterygium a winglike structure, especially an abnormal triangular fold of membrane in the interpalpebral fissure, extending from the conjunctiva to the cornea.

pterygoid shaped like a wing.

p. bone see pterygoid BONE. See also Table 10.

p. process see pterygoid PROCESS.

pterygomandibular pertaining to the pterygoid process and the mandible.

pterygomaxillary pertaining to a pterygoid process and the maxilla.

pterygopalatine pertaining to a pterygoid process and the palatine bone.

pterylae tracts on the skin of birds into which feathers are implanted and which establish the pattern of the plumage of that bird for that molt.

pterylosis the distribution of feathers in the pterylae.

PTFE polytetrafluoroethylene.

PTH parathyroid hormone.

ptilopody feathering of the foot and toes of birds.

ptilosis 1. falling out of the eyelashes. 2. the feather coat, total feather covering, of birds.

ptomaine any of an indefinite class of toxic bases, usually considered to be formed by the action of bacterial metabolism on proteins.

p. poisoning a term commonly misapplied to FOOD poisoning. Contrary to popular belief, ptomaines are not injurious to the carnivorous or omnivorous digestive systems, which are quite capable of reducing them to harmless substances. Decomposed foods are often responsible for food poisoning, however, because they may harbor certain forms of poison-producing bacteria, especially *Clostridium botulinum*.

ptosed affected with ptosis.

ptosis 1. prolapse of an organ or part. 2. paralytic drooping of the upper eyelid.

-ptosis word element. [Gr.] *downward displacement*.

PTS put to sleep; a common euphemism for euthanasia, but also used to describe general anesthesia.

PTT partial thromboplastin time.

ptyalagogue see SIALAGOGUE.

ptyalectasis 1. a state of dilatation of a salivary duct. 2. surgical dilatation of a salivary duct.

ptyalin see AMYLASE.

ptyalism excessive secretion of saliva; seen in rabbits, guinea pigs with malocclusion or heat stress, ruminants poisoned by *Rhizoctonia leguminicola*.

ptyal(o)- word element. [Gr.] *saliva*.

ptyalocele a cystic tumor containing saliva.

ptyalogenic formed from or by the action of saliva.

ptyaloreaction a reaction occurring in or performed on the saliva.

ptyalorrhea ptyalism.

Pu chemical symbol, *plutonium*.

pubertal pertaining to or emanating from puberty.

p. period the period approaching puberty when gonadal function, accessory sex gland function and behavior develop to the point where reproduction is possible.

puberty the time at which reproduction by an individual animal becomes possible for the first time; a term used infrequently in veterinary medicine but there is no other word which can substitute for it.

delayed p. varies widely between species and between breeds; negatively influenced by undernutrition and obesity.

pubescent 1. arriving at the age of puberty. 2. covered with down or lanugo.

pubic pertaining to or lying near the pubis.

p. ligament see Table 12.

pubiotomy surgical separation of the pubis lateral to the symphysis.

pubis pl. *pubes* [L.] the bone beneath the human pubis (pubic hair) and its homolog in other animals; the cranioventral part of the pelvic girdle. See also Table 10. Called also pubic bone.

public health the field of human medicine that is concerned with safeguarding and improving the physical, mental and social well-being of the community as a whole. There are marginal roles for veterinarians in this service, especially in the area of zoonoses.

veterinary p. health the part played by veterinarians in human public health, relating chiefly to the recognition and control of zoonotic disease.

public programs see public PROGRAM.

pubocaudal muscles the more caudal of the two parts of the levator ani muscles; origin at the dorsal surface of the pubis; insertion at the ventral surface of the caudal vertebrae.

pubofemoral pertaining to the pubis and femur.

puboprostatic pertaining to the pubis and prostate.

pubovesical pertaining to the pubis and bladder.

Puccinia graminis a toxic fungus which contains an unidentified toxin and causes salivation and stomatitis and, in severe cases, death of horses.

pudding a food preparation with a farinaceous base and cooked by steaming or boiling.

black p. one containing whole blood.

pudendal pertaining to the pudendum.

p. block anesthesia produced by blocking the pudendal nerves, accomplished by injection of the local anesthetic into the tuberosity of the ischium.

p. fissure see RIMA pudendi.

internal p. block local nerve block used mostly for exteriorizing the bull's penis for examination or treatment. The hypodermic needle is introduced through the ischiorectal fossa and directed to the nerve by a hand in the rectum.

pudendum pl. *pudenda* [L.] the external genitalia, especially of the human female.

pudic pudendal.

Pueraria lobata a coarse, perennial leguminous vine.

Has woody stems but very palatable and nutritious foliage equal in value to alfalfa. Called also kudzu.

puerperal pertaining to a puerpera or to the puerperium.

p. fever see MASTITIS–METRITIS–AGALACTIA.

p. laminitis see LAMINITIS.

p. metritis infection of the uterus in a puerperal female.

p. psychosis 1. whelping bitches sometimes display frenzied, destructive behavior and aggression. 2. sows, see FARROWING hysteria.

p. tetanus see TETANUS.

p. tetany see puerperal TETANY.

puerperalism a morbid condition incident to parturition.

puerperium the period or state of confinement after parturition.

Puerto Rican crested toad *Peltophryne lemur*.

PUFA polyunsaturated fatty acids.

puff adder see puff ADDER.

puff disease see ANHIDROSIS.

puffer see TETRAODONTIDAE. Called also toadfish, a poisonous fish.

p. fish poison see TETRODOTOXIN.

puffin see FRATERCULA.

Puffinus tenuirostris short-tailed shearwater.

Pug a small (14–18 lb), cobby dog with a large rounded head, prominent eyes, very short nose, and large, deep wrinkles on the forehead and face. The small ears fold over, the tail is curled over the back, and the coat is fine and very short in black, silver, apricot or fawn with a black mask. Called also Mopshond. The breed is predisposed to pigmentary keratitis and proptosis.

pugging see POACH.

pukatea see LAURELIA NOVAE-ZEALANDIAE.

pulegone a toxic ketone found in pennyroyal oil. It causes hepatotoxicity in dogs and cats.

Pulex a genus of fleas, several species of which transmit the microorganism causing bubonic plague in humans.

P. irritans a widely distributed species, known as the human flea, which infests domestic animals as well as humans, and may act as an intermediate host of certain helminths.

P. porcinus the peccary flea.

Puli a medium-sized dog distinguished by its long, wiry haircoat, usually black, gray or white, that forms long, tightly coiled cords in adults which obscure the body features. In the United States, dogs may be shown either corded or brushed. The breed was developed for guarding and driving sheep.

pulicicide an agent destructive to fleas.

pull to remove a sick animal from a pen in a feedlot for treatment. See also DAILY PULL AND DEAD RECORDS.

pull rate a daily percentage of the cattle in a feedlot which are pulled out of the feeding pens and relegated to the hospital yards or sent for emergency slaughter.

pull-out suture pattern removable, nonabsorbable, interrupted sutures for apposition of deep tissues. The suture starts on one side of a wound, crosses it at right angles at the deep tissues. Having taken a bite of these tissues it returns to the entry side and emerges at the skin close to the entry. Individual sutures are inserted on both sides in an alternating pattern.

pull theory a theory of wound healing and contraction stating that material within the healing wound contracts and pulls the margins of the wound together.

pull-through a surgical technique for abdominoperineal resection of the rectum. After removal of a segment, the rectum is sutured to the perineal skin, forming a new mucocutaneous junction. Used in the treatment of rectal neoplasms and anal furunculosis.

pullet young, female fowl from heat-weaning at about 4 weeks of age, up to point of lay at about 5 months. In some circles the first laying season is referred to as the pullet year.

p. disease see visceral GOUT.

pullorum disease a disease of birds caused by infection with *Salmonella pullorum* and characterized by moribund and dead birds at hatching time, by dyspnea and diarrhea in older birds and a reduction in egg yield, and reduction in fertility of the eggs in adults. The disease has been largely eradicated.

pullulation development by sprouting, or budding.

pulmo pl. *pulmones* [L.] lung.

pulmo- word element. [L.] *lung*.

pulmoaortic pertaining to the lungs and aorta.

pulmonary pertaining to the lungs, or to the pulmonary artery. See also LUNG.

p. abscess causes a syndrome of chronic toxemia, cough, loss of body weight. Careful auscultation may elicit squeaky rales around the lesions. See also CAUDAL vena caval thrombosis, ASPIRATION pneumonia.

p. acinus basic structural unit of the lung parenchyma; the gas exchange unit, supplied by a single terminal bronchiole and includes branches of the terminal bronchiole, alveolar ducts, alveolar sacs, alveoli and associated blood vessels. A pulmonary lobule consists of many acini.

p. agenesis incompatible with life; found only in fetal or neonatal necropsy specimens.

p. alveolar microlithiasis see MICROLITHIASIS alveolaris pulmonum.

p. alveolar parenchyma include epithelial cells (pneumonocytes or pneumocytes), alveolar capillary endothelial cells, and interstitial cells (fibroblasts) and alveolar macrophages.

p. alveolar proteinosis a disease of unknown etiology marked by chronic filling of the alveoli with a proteinaceous, lipid-rich, granular material consisting of surfactant and the debris of necrotic cells.

p. arteriopathy see AELUROSTRONGYLUS.

p. artery wedge pressure see wedge PRESSURE.

p. atelectasis see ATELECTASIS.

p. bed the network of capillaries in lung tissue.

p. calcinosis see MICROLITHIASIS alveolaris pulmonum.

p. calculus see BRONCHIAL calculus.

p. carcinomatosis see ovine pulmonary adenomatosis (below).

p. circulation the circulation of blood to and from the lungs. Deoxygenated blood from the right ventricle flows through the right and left pulmonary arteries to the right and left lung. After entering the lungs, the branches subdivide, finally emerging as capillaries which surround the alveoli and release the carbon dioxide in exchange for oxygen. The capillaries unite gradually and assume the characteristics of veins. These veins join to form the pulmonary veins, which return the oxygenated blood to the left atrium. See also CIRCULATORY system.

p. compliance a measure of the ability of the lung to distend in response to pressure without disruption. Expressed as the unit volume of change in the lung per unit of pressure. Compliance or distensibility of the lung is increased in conditions such as emphysema in which the lung distends more readily, and is decreased in fibrotic conditions in which the lung distends with difficulty. See also COMPLIANCE.

p. congestion caused by engorgement of the pulmonary vascular bed and it may precede pulmonary edema when the intravascular fluid escapes into the parenchyma and the alveoli. There is a loss of air space and the development of respiratory embarrassment.
p. cysts may be congenital or acquired, caused by trauma, parasites (*Paragonimus* spp.), or associated with bronchiectasis. Rarely, metastatic tumors cavitate forming cysts.
p. defense mechanisms include aerodynamic filtration in nasal cavities, sneezing, local nasal antibody, laryngeal and cough reflexes, mucociliary transport mechanisms, alveolar macrophages, systemic and local antibody systems.
p. edema an effusion of serous fluid into the pulmonary interstitial tissues and alveoli. Preceded by pulmonary congestion (see above). If the extravascular exudation is sufficiently severe a critical level of hypoxia may be reached. The breathing will then be labored, the normal breath sounds on auscultation may be absent, and a frothy nasal discharge, often blood-tinged, may appear. At this stage the animal's life is about to terminate.
p. embolus obstruction of the pulmonary artery or one of its branches by an embolus. The embolus usually is a blood clot swept into circulation from a large peripheral vein.
Signs vary greatly, depending on the extent to which the lung is involved. Simple, uncomplicated embolism produces such cardiopulmonary signs as dyspnea, tachypnea, persistent cough, pleuritic pain and hemoptysis. On rare occasions the cardiopulmonary signs may be acute, occurring suddenly and quickly producing cyanosis and shock. A septic embolus can lead to local pulmonary abscess or an extension to pneumonia as in caudal vena caval syndrome. See also CAUDAL vena caval thrombosis, pulmonary abscess (above).
p. eosinophilic granulomatosis a lesion common in heartworm disease; eosinophiles and neutrophils surround trapped microfilariae causing nodules as large as 3 inches diameter. May be preceded by lesions of allergic pneumonitis.
exercise-induced p. hemorrhage traces of blood can be found in about 60% of horses after racing. Less than 1% of these bleed from the nostrils. See also EPISTAXIS.
p. function tests tests used to evaluate lung mechanics, gas exchange, pulmonary blood flow and blood acid–base balance. Pulmonary function testing is used to detect emphysema and chronic obstructive bronchitis at an early stage.
p. hemorrhage as distinct from hemothorax, is recognized because of a syndrome of dyspnea, increased lung density radiographically, and hemorrhagic anemia. If a large vessel ruptures into an abscess cavity there is usually a massive hemoptysis and instant death. Frothy blood-stained nasal discharge is an indication of pulmonary edema rather than of pulmonary hemorrhage. See also exercise-induced pulmonary hemorrhage (above).
p. horse sickness the predominantly pulmonary form of AFRICAN HORSE SICKNESS.
p. hypertrophic osteoarthropathy see hypertrophic OSTEOPATHY.
p. hypoplasia a congenital defect resulting in decreased lung development.
p. infarction see pulmonary INFARCTION, pulmonary embolus (above).
p. infiltration with eosinophilia (PIE) see PIE SYNDROME.
p. malformation includes accessory lungs, pulmonary hypoplasia, pulmonary agenesis, congenital pulmonary cysts, endodermal heteroplasia, respiratory distress syndrome, neonatal maladjustment syndrome, immotile cilia syndrome.
p. mycoses includes aspergillosis, mortierellosis, blastomycosis, cryptococcosis, coccidioidomycosis.
p. neoplasm many types are recorded in all species but the prevalence is very low in food animals. A common site for metastases in companion animals. Characterized clinically by decreased exercise tolerance, progressive dyspnea, chronic cough and emaciation. Most diagnoses result from radiographic examination of the thorax for secondary growths.
neurogenic p. edema results from head trauma, central nervous system lesions and toxins, which may cause increased pulmonary blood pressure and alteration to sympathetic innervation leading to fluid leakage from vessels.
overriding p. artery see OVERRIDING pulmonary artery.
ovine p. adenomatosis a very chronic progressive pneumonia of sheep and goats caused by a retrovirus. Dyspnea, emaciation and a profuse nasal discharge are the cardinal signs, but coughing is not evident. The disease is always fatal. It is of great importance if it occurs in flocks that are housed for long periods. Characteristically the extensive lung involvement includes large areas of neoplastic tissue. Called also jaagsiekte, pulmonary carcinomatosis.
p. patterns see ALVEOLOGRAM PATTERN, BRONCHIAL pattern.
re-expansion p. edema edema, emphysematous bullae and serosanguinous fluid in the airways with generalized pulmonary capillary endothelial damage; associated with chronic pulmonary collapse and removal of pleural effusions or pneumothorax with rapid re-expansion.
p. rupture traumatic, especially when there is rib fracture, or spontaneous due to coughing and a weak parenchyma. The most common cause of pneumothorax.
p. thromboembolic disease thromboembolism causing blockage of large sections of the pulmonary vascular bed will result in at least temporary severe dyspnea. It may also lead to right heart congestive failure, i.e. cor pulmonale.
p. thrombosis see THROMBOEMBOLISM.
p. valve the pocket-like structure that guards the orifice between the right ventricle and the pulmonary artery.
p. valve stenosis causes right ventricular hypertrophy and a poststenotic dilatation of the pulmonary artery. There is a systolic murmur and thrill on the left side of the chest. A common congenital defect in dogs.
p. vein the large vein (right and left branches) that carries oxygenated blood from the lungs to the left atrium of the heart.
p. wedge pressure see wedge PRESSURE.

pulmonic pulmonary.
p. stenosis a common anomaly in dogs; rare in other species. Inherited in beagles, probably in Chihuahuas, English bulldog and terrier breeds. Includes supravalvular, valvular and subvalvular (infundibular) stenosis.

pulmonitis inflammation of the lung; pneumonitis; pneumonia.

pulmotor an apparatus for forcing oxygen into the lungs, and inducing artificial respiration.

pulp any soft, juicy animal or vegetable tissues, e.g. citrus pulp.

p. canal root canal.
p. cap pulp of the feather produced inside the calamus by the follicular tissue. The pulp protrudes through the aperture in the wall of the shaft and forms the external pulp caps. Internal pulp caps are formed within the calamus.
p. cavity the pulp chamber and the root canal in a tooth.
p. chamber the cavity at the center of the tooth which contains most of the pulp.
dental p. see DENTAL pulp.
p. polyp superficial hyperplasia of dental pulp, usually after exposure due to injury such as fracture of a tooth.
red p., splenic p. the dark reddish brown substance filling the interspaces of the splenic sinuses.
tooth p. dental pulp.
white p. sheaths of lymphatic tissue surrounding the arteries of the spleen.

pulpa pl. *pulpae* [L.] pulp.

pulpal pertaining to pulp, usually dental.
p. axis the direction in which pulp is distributed in a tooth, generally from the apex to the occlusal surface.
p. stones calcified deposits in the pulp cavity.

pulpectomy removal of dental pulp.
partial coronal p. a procedure in which some exposed pulp is amputated and the remainder is covered. Sometimes called pulpotomy.

pulpefaction conversion into pulp.

pulpitis pl. *pulpitides* [L.] inflammation of dental pulp; endodontitis.

pulpotomy surgical excision of a vital pulp.

pulpy soft; having the consistency of pulp.
p. kidney disease *Clostridium welchii* (type D) ENTEROTOXEMIA.

pulsatile characterized by a rhythmic pulsation.

Pulsatilla vulgaris ANEMONE *pulsatilla*.

pulsation chamber space between the TEAT CUP shell and the liner of a milking machine teat cup.

pulsator mechanism in a milking machine which governs the cyclic pressure changes necessary to the function of the machine.

pulse 1. a rhythmic wave. 2. any leguminous seed used in animal feed or human food. Contain about 20% protein. 3. the beat of the heart as felt through the walls of arteries. What is felt is not the blood pulsing through the arteries but a shock wave, generated by the abrupt ejection of blood from the heart, that travels along the arteries. The arterial pulse wave can be measured by a sphygmograph. The resulting tracing shows ascending and descending limbs.
abdominal p. that over the abdominal aorta.
p. abnormality includes irregularity of timing and amplitude, large or small amplitude, waterhammer pulse, Corrigan's pulse, dropped pulse, pulse deficit, alternating pulse and many others.
alternating p. pulsus alternans; one with regular alteration of weak and strong beats without changes in cycle length.
p. amplitude indicative of arterial blood pressure; estimated on the difference of pressure exerted by the fingers to occlude and then reopen the arterial pulse.
anacrotic p. one in which the ascending limb of the tracing shows a transient drop in amplitude, or a notch.
anadicrotic p. one in which the ascending limb of the tracing shows two small additional waves or notches.
anatricrotic p. one in which the ascending limb of the tracing shows three small additional waves or notches.
arterial p. the wave of pressure generated by the ejection of blood from the left ventricle into the aorta. Although the size (amplitude) of the pulse depends on the volume ejected it is not the blood passing the finger that is palpated, it is only the pressure wave. The pulse is a good indicator of the heart's activity with respect to amplitude, rate and regularity. It may also provide information on the state of the vessel walls and the efficiency of the aortic semilunar valves. It may be palpated in the median, facial, femoral or coccygeal arteries, the preferred site varying with the species and the occasion.
atrial venous p. atriovenous pulse, a cervical pulse having an accentuated 'a' wave during atrial systole, owing to increased force of contraction of the right atrium; a characteristic of tricuspid stenosis.
B-B shot p. see water-hammer pulse (below).
bigeminal p. one in which two beats occur in rapid succession, the groups of two being separated by a longer interval, usually related to regularly occurring ventricular premature beats.
catadicrotic p. see CATADICROTISM.
catatricrotic p. see CATATRICROTISM.
p.-chase experiment to study the movement of macromolecules, cells are incubated with a radiolabeled precursor (pulse) and then replaced with unlabeled precursor (chase). The label can be followed as it is incorporated into newly synthesized compounds and through different cellular compartments.
Corrigan's p. see CORRIGAN'S PULSE.
p. deficit the difference between the apical pulse and the radial pulse. Obtained by counting apical beats as heard through a stethoscope over the heart and counting the arterial pulse at the same time. A characteristic of several arrhythmias.
dicrotic p. a pulse characterized by two peaks, the second peak occurring in diastole and being an exaggeration of the dicrotic wave.
p. dosing the administration of drugs, usually antibiotics or corticosteroids, in a single, large dose which might be repeated after an interval of days. Thought to have the advantage of high tissue levels and fewer of the undesirable side-effects associated with more frequent dosing.
dropped p. arrhythmic pulse.
femoral p. that which is located at the site where the femoral artery passes through the groin in the femoral triangle; the usual site for palpating the pulse in dogs and cats.
fetal p. detector an ultrasound detector based on the Doppler principle used to detect the presence of a living fetus in utero.
funic p. the arterial tide in the umbilical cord.
p. generator the power source for a cardiac pacemaker system, usually powered by a lithium battery. It supplies electrical impulses to the implanted electrodes. See also PACEMAKER.
hard p. one characterized by high tension.
jerky p. see water-hammer pulse (below).
jugular p. comprises the movements of the wall of the jugular vein in response to pressure changes in the right atrium. Much more visible if the vein is distended. A reflection of increased pressure in the right atrium or insufficiency of the right A-V valve. A small pulse is normal in most food animals. A large pulse which goes high up the neck when the head is in the normal position, and which is synchronous with the heart cycle and is systolic in time, indicates insufficiency of the right atrioventricular valve.
p. monitor a pulse detector which uses the Doppler principle.

paradoxical p. one that markedly decreases in amplitude during inspiration.
peripheral p. that palpable in the extremities, e.g. legs, neck and head; the usual sites for measuring the pulse rate.
pistol-shot p. one in which the arteries are subject to sudden distension and collapse.
p. pressure the difference between the systolic and diastolic pressures.
radial p. that felt over the radial artery.
p. rate the number of pulsations per minute palpable in an artery, usually of a limb. The normal rates per minute for the common domestic animal species are: horses, 30 to 40; young horses up to one year of age, 70 to 80; cattle, 60 to 80; young calves, 100 to 120; sheep and goats, 70 to 120; pigs (heart rate), 60 to 70; dogs, 100 to 130; cats, 110 to 140; adult fowls 250 to 300.
p. rhythm regularity of the pulse in time and amplitude.
thready p. one that is very fine and barely perceptible.
p. tracing see SPHYGMOGRAM.
tricrotic p. see TRICROTISM.
trigeminal p. one with a pause after every third beat.
undulating p. one giving the sensation of successive waves.
vagus p. a slow pulse.
venous p. the pulsation over a vein.
wiry p. a small, tense pulse.
water-hammer p. one in which the artery is suddenly and markedly distended and relaxed. Characteristic of patent ductus arteriosus. Called also Corrigan's, jerky and B-B shot pulse.

pulse-diagnosis the technique of locating the points for acupuncture to be used in an individual human case. No application to animal patients.

pulsion a pushing outward.

pulsus [L.] *pulse.*
p. alternans see alternating PULSE.
p. bigeminus bigeminal pulse.
p. bisferiens a pulse characterized by two strong systolic peaks separated by a midsystolic dip, most commonly occurring in pure aortic regurgitation and in aortic regurgitation with stenosis.
p. celer a swift, abrupt pulse.
p. differens inequality of the pulse obervable at corresponding sites on either side of the body.
p. paradoxus an abnormal inspiratory decrease in arterial blood pressure, seen in cardiac tamponade and caused by a decreased pulmonary venous return.
p. parvus et tardus a small hard pulse that rises and falls slowly.
p. tardus an abnormally slow pulse.

pultaceous like a poultice; pulpy.

pulverization in dentistry, high-speed burs may be used to remove root fragments that cannot be extracted or are ankylosed.

pulverulent powdery; dusty.

pulvinar the posterior medial part of the posterior end of the thalamus.

pulvinus cushion, pad.
p. dentalis the dental pad which replaces the upper incisors in the mouth of ruminants.
p. digitalis the digital cushion, a pad of fat, white fibrous and elastic tissue located between the distal phalanx and the sole and frog of the hoof of the horse.

puma see mountain LION.

pumice a substance consisting of silicates of aluminum, potassium and sodium; used in dentistry as an abrasive.

p.-stone lung MICROLITHIASIS alveolaris pulmonum.

pumiced hoof a rough, porous appearance of the hoof in a horse with chronic coronitis.

pump 1. an apparatus for drawing or forcing liquid or gas. 2. to draw or force liquids or gases. 3. a mechanism or structure that mediates ACTIVE transport of ions or molecules across a biological membrane.
blood p. a machine used to propel blood through the tubing of extracorporeal circulation devices.
calcium p. the mechanism of active transport of calcium (Ca^2+) across a membrane, as of the sarcoplasmic reticulum of muscle cells, against a concentration gradient; the mechanism is driven by hydrolysis of ATP.
infusion p. an electronic device used to control the administration of intravenous fluids in very small amounts and at a carefully regulated rate over long periods.
p. oxygenator heart–lung machine. See EXTRACORPOREAL circulatory support unit.
sodium p., sodium–potassium p. the mechanism of active transport driven by hydrolysis of ATP, by which sodium (Na+) is extruded from a cell and potassium (K+) is brought in, so as to maintain the low concentration of Na+ and the high concentration of K+ within the cell with respect to the surrounding medium. See also NA+,K+-ATPASE.
stomach p. an apparatus used to remove material from the stomach. It consists of a rubber stomach tube to which a bulb syringe is attached. The tube is inserted into the mouth or nose and passed down the esophagus into the stomach. Suction from the syringe brings the contents of the stomach up through the tube. For cattle and horses a reversible metal pump adapted from a yachting bilge pump is most suitable. In small animals, gravity is the usual method of moving fluid into and out of the stomach during lavage.

pumpkin large edible fruit, used extensively as cattle feed and for human consumption, *Cucurbita maxima.*

punch a metal, rodlike instrument with one pointed or cavitied end and one propulsion end to be pushed hard with the palm of the hand or driven with a hammer in order to drive a hole or to excise a small round piece of tissue.
p. biopsy a circular piece of skin excised by a hand driven biopsy punch. See also KEYES PUNCH.
dental p. has a slight cavity at the end so that the tooth to be driven will seat into the end and not slip off.
p. graft see punch GRAFT.

punched cards see CARD FILES.

puncta plural form of PUNCTUM.
p. maxima points on the chest wall where heart sounds are heard best.

punctate spotted; marked with points or punctures.

punctiform like a point.

punctograph an instrument for radiographic localization of foreign bodies.

punctum pl. *puncta* [L.] a point or small spot.
imperforate p. congenital absence of an opening in the lacrimal punctum, usually the lower, occurs most often in toy and miniature poodles. Commonly absent also in pigs.
misplaced p. variations in the position of the lacrimal puncta, seen most commonly in brachycephalic dogs, may interfere with tear drainage.
p. nasolacrimal see LACRIMAL punctum.
obstructed p. may result from foreign bodies, inflammation, or swelling of the lower eyelid.

puncture 1. the act of piercing or penetrating with a

pointed object or instrument; a wound so made. Wounds of special interest because of their potential seriousness are to the cornea, the sole of the horse's foot and the synovial cavity. 2. Surgical puncture of an anatomical tissue to obtain material for clinicopathological examination. Includes CISTERNAL puncture, LUMBAR puncture, SPINAL puncture, STERNAL puncture.

puncture vine see TRIBULUS *terrestris*.

punishment the use of an undesirable stimulus to modify or prevent an undesirable behavior.

punitive damages damages awarded by the court, in addition to damages awarded as compensation for loss, as a punishment to the guilty party and an assuagement to the suffering party.

punkies see BITING midge.

puntilla a short, double-edged, stabbing knife which is plunged into the occipitoatlantal space to sever the medulla oblongata in the EVERNAZIONE method of slaughter.

Puntius javanicus farmed finfish in the family Cyprinidae; called also Java barb. See Table 23.

PUO pyrexia of unknown origin.

pupa pl. *pupae* [L.] the second stage in the development of an insect, between the larva and the imago. Usually an inactive stage such as a coccoon.

puparium the hard pupal case of the insect pupa.

pupate to proceed to the stage of pupa in an insect life cycle.

pupil the aperture in the center of the iris which regulates the amount of light that reaches the retina.

Adie's p. dilated pupil due to parasympathetic denervation.

Argyll Robertson p. one that is miotic and responds to accommodation effort, but not to light.

fixed p. a pupil that does not react either to light or on convergence, or in accommodation.

multiple p's polycoria.

occluded p. a congenital or acquired pupillary membrane that obstructs the pupil.

secluded p. a complete posterior synechia that separates the anterior and posterior chambers of the anterior compartment.

spastic p. syndrome anisocoria with pupils that fail to dilate in darkness. Seen in cats infected with feline leukemia virus. The virus has been observed in the short ciliary nerves and ciliary ganglia of some affected cats.

tonic p. see PUPILLOPLEGIA.

pupilla [L.] *pupil.*

pupillary pertaining to or emanating from the pupil.

p. aperture the pupil.

p. block an obstruction to the flow of aqueous between the border of the pupil and the anterior capsule of the lens.

p. consensual light reflex constriction of the pupil in the eye opposite to the one receiving an intensified beam of light, and reversal when the light is removed. The reflex is clearcut in humans and dogs but little used in food animals. Presence of the reflex is a guarantee of integrity of the optic pathways.

p. constriction see MIOSIS.

p. cyst see IRIS cyst.

p. dilatation see MYDRIASIS.

p. light reflex constriction of a dilated pupil in response to an increase in light intensity and a dilatation of a constricted pupil in response to a decrease in the intensity. Activity of the reflex indicates the efficiency of the retina, the optic and oculomotor nerves and the musculature of the iris.

p. membranectomy a surgical technique for resection of an iridocapsular membrane, formed as a sequela to cataract surgery.

persistent p. membrane nonvascular remnants of the tunica vasculosa lentis may extend across the iris or from the iris to the cornea, often producing a corneal opacity at the site. A common defect in dogs, particularly in Basenjis.

p. zone the portion of iris closest to the pupillary border.

pupillatonia dilated pupil due to parasympathetic denervation.

pupillodilator 1. a mechanism responsible for dilatation of the pupil. 2. a substance having the effect of dilating the pupil.

pupillometer an instrument for measuring the width or diameter of the pupil.

pupillometry measurement of the diameter or width of the pupil of the eye.

pupillomotor pertaining to the movement of the pupil. Includes pupilloconstrictor, pupillodilator.

p. pathways the nerves and mediators involved in regulating the size of the pupil.

pupilloplegia a pupil that responds in a slow delayed fashion to accommodation and convergence stimuli. Called also tonic pupil.

pupilloscopy skiametry; retinoscopy.

pupillostatometer an instrument for measuring the distance between the pupils.

puppy the young of the canine species; usually used up to the age of 12 months.

fading p. syndrome see FADING kitten/puppy syndrome.

p. pyoderma see IMPETIGO.

p. strangles see juvenile PYODERMA.

p. walker a person who cares for a puppy during its formative stage, from weaning to about a year of age. A practice with dogs destined for the hunt or as guide dogs for the blind.

purebred progeny derived from at least several generations of animals of the same breed.

p. herds herds (or flocks) composed of purebred animals. Not necessarily registered animals. Distinct from crossbred herds.

p. pedigree pedigree of a purebred animal.

puréed pet foods foods of a gruel-like consistency; designed for enteral feeding.

purgation the effect of a purge; catharsis; purging effected by a cathartic medicine.

purgative 1. a purge or CATHARTIC (1); causing bowel evacuation. 2. a cathartic, particularly one stimulating peristaltic action. See also LAXATIVE.

purge 1. a purgative medicine or dose. 2. to cause free evacuation of feces. 3. to remove outdated data from a file or other store of data.

p. nut JATROPHA *curcas*.

purging pertaining to purge.

p. ball a bolus given periodically to horses by owners and trainers in the belief that a good clean-out is good for a horse, especially if it is racing poorly. Usually contains aloes; 7 to 14 g (2 to 4 drachms) is the usual dose. Anthraquinone purgatives are more reliable in their action but the procedure is basically empirical and is not recommended by veterinarians. Called also physic ball.

p. buckthorn RHAMNUS *cathartica*.

p. facility part of a computer program for data storage which automatically selects data of a particular kind, usually aged data, and purges it either from the records altogether or to an archive storage where it is not readily accessible.

p. flax LINUM *catharticum*.

p. nut JATROPHA *curcas*.

purified protein derivative see purified protein derivative of TUBERCULIN.

purine a heterocyclic compound that is the nucleus of the purine bases (or purines) such as adenine and guanine, which occur in DNA and RNA, and xanthine and hypoxanthine. All living cells contain purines as purine nucleotides. They can be synthesized using amino acids, or by salvage of dietary or endogenous nucleotides derived from cell wastage.

A p. adenine.

low p. diet one with a low content of organ meats, seafood, beans, lentils, peas and spinach; used in the dietary management of xanthine or urate uroliths in dogs.

p. nucleoside phosphorylase a transferase enzyme that acts in the degradation of nucelotides and nucleic acids.

Purkinje named after J.E. Purkinje, Bohemian anatomist (1787–1869).

P. cell neuronal cell bodies in the middle layer of the cerebellar cortex; characterized by a large, globose body and massive, branching dendrites but a single, slender axon.

P. fiber modified cardiac muscle fibers in the subendothelial tissue, concerned with conducting impulses through the heart.

P's image, P.–Sanson images in a normal eye, reflections of light off the surface of the cornea, anterior lens capsule, and posterior lens capsule. When viewed from different angles, can be used to localize intraocular opacities.

P. network a reticulum of modified muscle fibers in the subendocardial tissue of the cardiac ventricles.

P. neuron see Purkinje cell (above).

puromycin an antibiotic that inhibits protein synthesis. Used in the treatment of protozoal infections and as an antineoplastic agent.

purple 1. a color between blue and red. 2. a substance of this color used as a dye or indicator.

p. cudweed GNAPHALIUM PURPUREUM.

p.-flowered bell vine IPOMOEA *purpurea*.

p.-flowered morning glory IPOMOEA *purpurea*.

p.-leafed goosefoot SCLEROBLITUM ATRIPLICINUM.

p. loco ASTRAGALUS *mollisimus*.

p. mint PERILLA FRUTESCENS.

p. pigeon grass SETARIA *incrassata*.

p. plume grass TRIRAPHIS MOLLIS.

p. rattlebox SESBANIA *punicea*.

p. top VERBENA *bonariensis*.

p. sesbane SESBANIA *punicea*.

p. viper's bugloss ECHIUM *plantagineum*.

visual p. rhodopsin.

purpura a hemorrhagic disease characterized by extravasation of blood into the tissues, under the skin and through the mucous membranes, and producing spontaneous ecchymoses and petechiae on the skin. Similar lesions are produced in many specific diseases, e.g. epizootic hemorrhagic disease of deer, bracken poisoning in cattle, and leptospirosis in calves. In immune-mediated purpura there is a defect in the integrity of the vessel wall due to immunological mechanisms, which may also cause a THROMBOCYTOPENIA.

anaphylactoid p. immune-mediated purpura; see also PURPURA.

fibrinolytic p. purpura associated with increased fibrinolytic activity of the blood.

p. hemorrhagica a well-defined disease of horses, occurring sporadically, usually associated with a respiratory tract infection. Clinical signs include cold, subcutaneous, edematous swellings, usually about the head and not always symmetrical, mucosal petechiation and high heart rate; affected horses commonly die within a few days. Nonthrombocytopenic.

neonatal p. ALLOIMMUNE hemolytic anemia of the newborn in pigs is sometimes accompanied by a thrombocytopenic purpura, caused by antiplatelet antibodies. See also alloimmune THROMBOCYTOPENIA.

nonthrombocytopenic p. purpura without any decrease in the platelet count of the blood. In such cases the cause of purpura is either abnormal capillary fragility or a clotting factor deficiency.

thrombocytopenic p. purpura associated with a decrease in the number of platelets in the blood. See also immune-mediated THROMBOCYTOPENIA.

vascular p. that caused by loss of vascular integrity or function, as seen in vitamin C deficiency (scurvy), diabetes mellitus and hyperadrenocorticism.

purring a physiologically very complicated, semi-automatic, cyclic, controlled respiration involving alternating activity of the diaphragm and intrinsic laryngeal muscles in cats. The frequency of the alternation is about 25 times per second. Each cycle includes three phases of glottal closing, glottal opening with sound produced, further glottal opening with rapid airflow and low resistance at the glottis.

Purring occurs when cats are contented, sick or sleeping. It also provides the equivalent of complementary breaths during periods of shallow breathing.

purse-string suture a suture pattern adapted to closing of the end of a hollow viscus or fixing tissue around a tube such as a catheter. Stitches are made into the wall completely surrounding the orifice but without entering the lumen of the viscus. The suture is tightened and tied with the free end of the viscus returned back inside the purse-string.

purslane PORTULACA *oleracea*.

pursuit space the amount of space in a wild animal enclosure which is necessary to provide sufficient space for pursued animals to outrun their aggressors. The amount of space will vary widely depending on the species and on the individuals.

purulence the formation or presence of pus.

purulent containing or forming pus.

poultry p. synovitis swellings on the feet and in the limb joints causing lameness and spondylitis in fowls and turkeys. Caused by *Staphylococcus aureus*.

puruloid resembling pus.

pus a protein-rich liquid inflammation product made up of cells (leukocytes), a thin fluid (liquor puris) and cellular debris.

blue p. pus with a bluish tint, seen in certain suppurative infections, the color occurring as a result of the presence of an antibiotic pigment (pyocyanin) produced by *Pseudomonas aeruginosa*.

p. in milk indicates complete destruction of the mammary secretory tissue.

pushing disease a syndrome of compulsive walking and head pressing in cattle in southern Africa, caused by a number of hepatotoxic agents, especially *Matricaria nigellaefolia*. Called also stootsiekte.

pusly PORTULACA *oleracea*.

puss, pussy term of endearment addressed to a cat. Called also moggy.

pustula pl. *pustulae* [L.] pustule.

pustular pertaining to or of the nature of a pustule; consisting of pustules.

contagious viral p. dermatitis see contagious ECTHYMA.

infantile p. dermatosis see infantile pustular DERMATOSIS.

ovine p. dermatitis see contagious ECTHYMA.

subcorneal p. dermatosis see subcorneal pustular DERMATOSIS.

superficial p. dermatitis see superficial pustular DERMATITIS.

p. vulvovaginitis see infectious pustular VULVOVAGINITIS.

pustulation the formation of pustules.

pustule a small, elevated, circumscribed, pus-containing lesion of the skin or cornea; usually thin-walled and ruptures easily. Cutaneous pustules may be epidermal, intraepidermal or subepidermal. The corneal lesions may be superficial or subcorneal.

pustulosis a condition marked by an eruption of pustules.

sterile eosinophilic p. an acute, pruritic pustular dermatitis of dogs. Numerous eosinophils are found in the sterile lesions. The cause is unknown.

put down see EUTHANASIA.

put-to-sleep see EUTHANASIA.

putamen the larger and more lateral part of the lenticular nucleus.

Putorius putorius called also *Mustela putorius;* see POLECAT, FERRET.

putrefaction enzymatic decomposition, especially of proteins, with the production of foul-smelling compounds, such as hydrogen sulfide, ammonia and mercaptans. Called also decomposition.

putrefy to undergo putrefaction.

putrescence the condition of undergoing putrefaction.

putrescine a polyamine first found in decaying meat; small quantities occur in most cells.

putrid rotten; putrified.

Putti rasp a bone rasp with a curved, pointed rasp surface at both ends of this handheld metal instrument.

putty a malleable carpenter's material consisting of white lead and linseed oil. It is palatable to cattle and causes lead poisoning.

p. brisket see PRESTERNAL calcification.

PVA polyvinyl alcohol.

PVC premature ventricular contraction.

PVCT posterior vena caval thrombosis.

PVNT predictive value of a negative test.

PVP polyvinylpyrrolidone. Called also povidone.

PVP–I povidone–iodine.

PVPT predictive value of a positive test; the proportion of disease-positive animals amongst those which test positive.

Px abbreviation for prognosis; used in medical records.

py- prefix meaning pus.

pyarthrosis suppuration within a joint cavity; acute suppurative arthritis.

Pycnomonas a subgenus of trypanosomes. Includes *Trypanosoma suis.*

Pycnosorus chrysanthus see CRASPEDIA CHRYSANTHA.

pye-dog any mongrel dog.

pyelectasis dilatation of the renal pelvis.

pyelitis inflammation of the renal pelvis, the outer basin-like portion of the kidney at the attachment of the ureter.

cystic p. pyelitis with formation of multiple submucosal cysts.

p. glandularis the pelvic mucosa is modified to cylindrical epithelium and the formation of glandular acini.

pyel(o)- word element. [Gr.] *renal pelvis.*

pyelocaliectases dilatation of the renal pelvis and calices.

pyelocentesis aspiration of fluid from the renal pelvis, usually for diagnostic purposes.

pyelocystitis inflammation of the renal pelvis and bladder.

pyelogram the film produced by pyelography.

pyelography radiography of the kidney and ureter after injection of a contrast medium, introduced by the intravenous or retrograde method. Preparation of the animal for pyelography includes clearing the intestinal tract of as much fecal material and gas as possible so that there can be adequate visualization of the urinary tract structures. Called also intravenous pyelography (IVP).

intravenous p. see pyelography (above).

retrograde p. see RETROGRADE pyelography.

pyelointerstitial pertaining to the interstitial tissue of the renal pelvis.

pyelolithotomy incision of the renal pelvis for removal of calculi.

pyelonephritis inflammation of the kidney and renal pelvis (see also PYELITIS and NEPHRITIS). Clinical signs include pyuria, pain on palpation of the kidney, ureteritis, cystitis and passage of blood-stained urine. Called also nephropyelitis.

contagious bovine p. see CONTAGIOUS bovine pyelonephritis.

porcine p. pyelonephritis caused by *Eubacterium suis.* The infection is transmitted by the boar. Signs include dysuria, bloody urine and a short course and a high mortality rate.

pyelonephrosis any disease of the kidney and its pelvis.

pyelopathy any disease of the renal pelvis.

pyeloplasty plastic repair of the renal pelvis.

pyeloplication reduction in size of a dilated renal pelvis by surgical infolding of its walls.

pyelostomy the operation of forming an opening in the renal pelvis for the purpose of temporarily diverting the urine from the ureter.

pyelotomy incision of the renal pelvis.

pyelovenous pertaining to the renal pelvis and renal veins.

pyemesis the vomiting of pus.

pyemia septicemia in which secondary foci of suppuration occur and multiple abscesses are formed.

arterial p. a form due to the dissemination of septic emboli from the heart.

cryptogenic p. that in which the source of infection is in an unidentified tissue.

pyemic pertaining to or emanating from pyemia.

p. hepatitis disease caused by *Yersinia pseudotuberculosis* in sheep. Characterized by septicaemia and necrotic foci in liver, spleen and lymph nodes and fibrinohemorrhagic enteritis.

Pyemotes a genus of mites; *P. tritici* (straw-itch mite) and *P. ventricosus* (harvest mite) can cause transitory dermatitis on animals eating infested feeds.

pyencephalus abscess of the brain.

pygal pertaining to the buttocks.

pygmy hippopotamus *Choeropsis liberiensis*; see HIPPOPOTAMUS.

pygmy hog SUS *sylvanius.*

pygoamorphus asymmetrical conjoined twins, in which the parasite is an amorphous mass attached to the sacral region of the autosite.

pygodidymus a fetus with double hips and pelvis.

pygomelus a fetus with a supernumerary limb or limbs attached to or near the buttocks.

pygopagus conjoined twins fused in the sacral region.

pygostyle a bony termination of the vertebral column in birds formed by fusion of the last four to eight spinal vertebrae. Called also plowshare bone or rump post. The tail feathers are attached to its fascia so that it is very important in flight.
pyknic having a short, thick, stocky build.
pykn(o)- word element. [Gr.] *thick, compact, frequent.*
pyknocyte a distorted and contracted, occasionally spiculed erythrocyte.
pyknocytosis conspicuous increase in the number of pyknocytes.
pyknometer an instrument for determining the specific gravity of fluids.
pyknomorphous having the stained portions of the cell body compactly arranged.
pyknosis a thickening, especially degeneration of a cell in which the nucleus shrinks in size and the chromatin condenses to a solid, structureless mass or masses.
pyle- word element. [Gr.] *portal vein.*
pylephlebectasis dilatation of the portal vein.
pylephlebitis inflammation of the portal vein.
pylethrombophlebitis thrombosis and inflammation of the portal vein.
pylethrombosis thrombosis of the portal vein.
pylorectomy excision of the pylorus.
pyloric pertaining to the pylorus or to the pyloric part of the stomach.
antral p. hypertrophy syndrome a narrowing of the pyloric antrum caused by hypertrophy of the circular smooth muscle and mucosa; occurs most commonly in dogs of small breeds. Obstruction to gastric emptying causes chronic vomiting.
p. antrum the part of the stomach cavity just cranial to the pylorus.
p. dysfunction the usual effect is to delay gastric emptying. See pyloric ACHALASIA, pyloric obstruction (below).
p. gastropathy chronic hypertrophic pyloric GASTROPATHY.
p. gland situated in the pyloric region of the stomach and secreting gastrin and mucus. The secretion is slightly alkaline.
p. obstruction may be functional due to spasm or achalasia, or physical due to foreign body, e.g. phytobezoar, or external compression by, e.g. lipoma or fat necrosis or tumor or cicatrical contraction. Clinical signs are vomiting, distress due to gastric dilatation, possibly visible abdominal enlargement. In ruminants gross distension of abdomen, rumen contents running from nose, scant feces. In dogs and cats delayed gastric emptying usually causes vomiting, sometimes characteristically projectile, of undigested food.
p. outflow failure achalasia of the pylorus with obstruction to the flow of ingesta into the intestine; impaction of material in the abomasum follows; pyloric ulcer a common sequel.
p. spasm see pyloric achalasia (above).
p. stenosis, congenital p. hypertrophy usually a congenital lesion in dogs, particularly the brachycephalic breeds, that causes vomiting and poor growth from weaning age. Occasionally hypertrophy of the pyloric sphincter may be acquired.
pylor(o)- word element. [Gr.] *pylorus.*
pylorodiosis dilatation of a pyloric stricture with the fingers during a surgical operation.
pyloroduodenitis inflammation of the pyloric and duodenal mucosa.
pylorogastrectomy excision of the pylorus and adjacent portion of the stomach.
pyloromyotomy incision of the longitudinal and circular muscles of the pylorus.
Fredet–Ramstedt p. see RAMSTEDT OPERATION.
pyloroplasty plastic surgery of the pylorus, especially for pyloric stricture, to provide a larger communication between the stomach and duodenum.
Finney p. enlargement of the pyloric canal by establishment of an inverted U-shaped anastomosis between the stomach and duodenum after longitudinal incision.
Fredet–Ramstedt p. see RAMSTEDT OPERATION.
Heineke–Mikulicz p. enlargement of a pyloric stricture by incising the pylorus longitudinally and suturing the incision transversely.
Y-U antral advancement flap p. an antral flap is created and advanced over the incision through the pylorus.
pyloroscopy endoscopic inspection of the pylorus.
pylorospasm spasm of the pylorus or of the pyloric portion of the stomach.
pylorostenosis pyloric stenosis.
pylorostomy surgical formation of an opening through the abdominal wall into the stomach near the pylorus.
pylorotomy incision of the pylorus.
pylorus the distal aperture of the stomach or abomasum, opening into the duodenum. The term pylorus is variously used to mean the pyloric part of the stomach, and the pyloric antrum, canal, opening or sphincter. A ring of muscles, the pyloric sphincter, serves as a 'gate', closing the opening from the stomach to the intestine. It opens periodically, allowing the contents of the stomach to move into the duodenum. See also PYLORIC.
pyo- word element. [Gr.] *pus.*
pyoarthritis pyarthrosis.
pyocele a collection of pus, as in the scrotum.
pyocephalus the presence of purulent fluid in the cerebral ventricles.
pyochezia the presence of pus in the feces.
pyococcus a pus-forming coccus.
pyocolpocele a vaginal tumor containing pus.
pyocolpos pus in the vagina.
pyocyanic pertaining to blue pus, or to *Pseudomonas aeruginosa.*
pyocyanin a blue-green antibiotic pigment produced by *Pseudomonas aeruginosa*; it gives the color to 'blue pus'.
pyocyins antibacterial proteins produced by strains of *Pseudomonas aeruginosa*; used in strain typing.
pyocyst a cyst containing pus.
pyoderma any purulent skin disease. Includes pustule, pimple, acne, impetigo and furunculosis.
callus p. see CALLUS pyoderma.
contagious porcine p. see CONTAGIOUS porcine pyoderma.
deep p. bacterial infections involving the dermis and often subcutaneous tissues. There may be systemic illness.
dry p. see zinc-responsive DERMATOSIS.
fold p. see fold DERMATITIS.
p. gangrenosum a rapidly evolving cutaneous ulcer or ulcers, with undermining of the border.
interdigital p. infection of the interdigital skin in dogs; may be associated with trauma, *Demodex canis* infestation, or foreign bodies such as grass seeds.
juvenile p. a sterile, pustular skin disease on the face and head and sometimes ears, anus and prepuce, in one or more puppies of a litter, usually around weaning age. Dachshunds, Golden retrievers and Gordon setters appear to be predisposed. There is often fever, anorexia and lymphadenopathy, particularly of sub-

mandibular lymph nodes which may form abscesses and drain, hence the alternative name of puppy strangles. *Staphylococcus* spp. are frequently cultured from affected skin, but the etiology of the disease is unclear. Called also juvenile cellulitis, and juvenile sterile granulomatous dermatitis and lymphadenitis.

mucocutaneous p. occurs on the lip margins and perioral skin of dogs; German shepherd dogs are predisposed.

nasal p. a deep bacterial folliculitis and furunculosis on the dorsum of the nose in dogs, particularly German shepherd dogs, Bull terriers, Collies and Pointers. Trauma may be a factor in the etiology.

perianal p. see PERIANAL fistula.

pressure point p. see PRESSURE points.

skin-fold p. see fold DERMATITIS.

superficial pustular p. see IMPETIGO.

surface p. see acute moist DERMATITIS.

tail fold p. see fold DERMATITIS.

pyodermatitis pyoderma.

pyodermia pyoderma.

pyogenesis the formation of pus.

pyogenic producing pus.

p. dermatitis pyoderma.

p. gingival granuloma a bright red or blue mass on the gum, caused by chronic inflammation. Composed of vascular granulation tissue.

p. spondylitis vertebral osteomyelitis.

pyogranuloma an inflammatory process in which there is infiltration of polymorphonuclear cells into a more chronic area of inflammation characterized by mononuclear cells, macrophages, lymphocytes and possibly plasma cells.

pyogranuloma idiopathic see idiopathic sterile GRANULOMA.

pyohemia pyemia.

pyohemothorax pus and blood in the pleural cavity.

pyohydronephrosis the accumulation of pus and urine in the kidney.

pyoid resembling or like pus.

pyolabyrinthitis inflammation with suppuration of the labyrinth of the ear.

pyometra an accumulation of pus within the uterus. In the bitch, it is a distinct disease syndrome associated with cystic endometrial hyperplasia and usually infection by a variety of bacteria, especially *Escherichia coli*, occurring during diestrus. Clinical signs may include abdominal enlargement, purulent vaginal discharge if the cervix is open, polyuria, polydipsia, and a systemic response, which is more severe if the cervix is closed. An immune-mediated glomerulonephritis may also occur.

stump p. infection in the remaining portion of uterus after ovariohysterectomy.

pyometritis purulent inflammation of the uterus. See also PYOMETRA.

pyomyositis purulent myositis characterized by suppurating masses in the muscle.

pyonephritis purulent inflammation of the kidney.

pyonephrolithiasis pus and calculi in the kidney.

pyonephrosis suppurative destruction of the renal parenchyma, with total or almost complete loss of kidney function.

pyo-ovarium an abscess of the ovary.

pyopagus twin fetuses joined together at the sacrum.

pyopericarditis purulent pericarditis.

pyopericardium pus in the pericardium.

pyoperitoneum pus in the peritoneal cavity.

pyoperitonitis purulent inflammation of the peritoneum.

pyophthalmitis purulent inflammation of the eye.

pyophysometra pus and gas in the uterus.

pyopneumocholecystitis distension of the gallbladder, with the presence of pus and gas.

pyopneumohepatitis abscess of the liver with pus and gas in the abscess cavity.

pyopneumopericardium pus and gas in the pericardium.

pyopneumoperitonitis peritonitis with the presence of pus and gas.

pyopneumothorax pus and air or gas within the pleural cavity.

pyopyelectasis dilatation of the renal pelvis with pus.

pyorrhea a copious discharge of pus.

p. alveolaris a purulent inflammation of the dental periosteum, with progressive necrosis of the alveoli and looseness of the teeth. See also PERIODONTITIS.

pyosalpingitis purulent salpingitis.

pyosalpingo-oophoritis purulent inflammation of the uterine tube and ovary.

pyosalpinx an accumulation of pus in a uterine tube.

pyosepticemia pyemia and septicemia in the one patient; most common in neonates (pyosepticemia neonatorum).

pyostatic arresting suppuration; an agent that arrests suppuration.

pyothorax an accumulation of pus in the thorax. Commonly seen in cats, caused by a variety of bacteria, especially *Pasteurella*, *Staphylococcus*, *Nocardia* and *Bacteroides* spp. Large amounts of pleural fluid accumulate. Affected cats frequently show a rapid development of dyspnea and cyanosis, and often die suddenly. See also EMPYEMA.

pyotraumatic dermatitis see acute moist DERMATITIS.

pyoureter pus in the ureter.

pyr- prefix meaning heat.

Pyramicocephalus phocarus a cestode parasite found in seals.

pyramid a pointed or cone-shaped structure or part.

p. breed structure a standard format for a multiple herd system comprising a breed structure; headed by an open or closed nucleus, a second tier of multiplier herds and a terminal tier of commercial herds which produce the end-product to be marketed. The nucleus, perhaps one herd, produces all of the basic genetic material and supplies breeding stock to the multiplier herds which have the prime role of multiplying the progeny for supply to commercial herds who produce the end product. The entire system is under the control of one organization. Ideally suited to the pig industry.

p. of cerebellum pyramid of vermis.

p. of light a triangular reflection seen upon the tympanic membrane.

malpighian p's renal pyramids.

p's of the medulla oblongata either of two rounded masses, one on either side of the median fissure of the medulla oblongata.

renal p's the conical masses constituting the medulla of certain kidneys, the base toward the cortex and culminating at the summit in the renal papilla.

p. of tympanum the hollow elevation in the inner wall of the middle ear that contains the stapedius muscle.

p. of vermis the part of the vermis cerebelli between the tuber vermis and the uvula.

pyramidal shaped like a pyramid.

p. disease abnormal growth of the wall of the hoof in the horse in which the vertical midline of the front of the hoof bulges, causing lameness. Caused by fracture of the extensor process of the third phalanx or by low ringbone.

p. nervous system pyramidal-shaped nerve cells in the cerebral cortex and their efferent neurons to skeletal muscles.
p. tracts collections of motor nerve fibers arising in the brain and passing down through the spinal cord to motor cells in the ventral horns.
pyramis pl. *pyramides* [Gr.] pyramid.
pyran a cyclic compound in which the ring consists of five carbon atoms and one oxygen atom.
pyranose a six-membered ring structure formed by the reaction of the carbonyl group and a hydroxy group of a sugar to form a hemiacetal.
pyrantel a broad-spectrum anthelmintic of low toxicity, used as the pamoate and tartrate salts; has extensive use in dogs and cats.
pyrazinamide, pyrazinecarboxamide an antibacterial agent used for the oral treatment of tuberculosis in humans. Also used in a biochemical test for the identification of mycobacteria.
pyrazines volatile compounds with a strong odor; contribute part of the odor of meat.
pyrazolone derivatives a group of agents which have analgesic and antipyretic actions. They include phenylbutazone and dipyrone.
pyrectic 1. pertaining to fever; feverish. 2. a fever-inducing agent.
Pyrenean associated with the Pyrenean region in northern Spain.
P. goat France and Spain, dark brown or black with pale belly and feet, dual-purpose goat, longhaired, horned or polled.
P. mountain dog see GREAT PYRENEES.
P. sheepdog a small (16–18 inches tall) sheepdog with a haircoat which may be long, with long hair on the legs, or semi-long, with short hair on the legs, in shades of fawn, gray, blue merle, blue or brindle.
pyrethrins the active insecticidal ingredients of the flowers of the PYRETHRUM plant. Can cause systemic or cutaneous allergic reactions. Are esters of PYRETHROLONE and CINEROLONE with chrysanthemum mono- and dicarboxylic acids.
pyrethroids synthetic substances with activity similar to the naturally occurring pyrethrins. They include cypermethrin, cyhalothrin, deltamethrin, flumethrin, permethrin.
pyrethrolone one of the insecticidal agents in the PYRETHRINS.
pyrethrum flowers of the plants *Chrysanthemum cinerariaefolium* (syn. *Pyrethrum cinerariaefolium*) and *C. coccineum* (syn. *C. roseum*). Called also Dalmatian or Persian insect powder. The insecticidal agents are the PYRETHRINS.
pyretic pertaining to fever.
pyretogenesis the origin and causation of fever.
pyretogenous 1. caused by high fever. 2. pyrogenic.
pyretotherapy 1. treatment by artificially increasing the patient's body temperature. 2. the treatment of fever.
pyrexia a fever, or febrile condition. Can be said to be present if body temperature exceeds the normal range for the particular age and species: horse 102.0°F (39.0°C), cattle 103.0°F (39.5°C), pig 103.5°F (40.0°C), sheep 104.0°F (40.0°C), goat 105.0°F (40.5°C), dog and cat 102.0°F (39.0°C). Called also fever. See also HYPERTHERMIA.
p.-pruritus-hemorrhage syndrome a syndrome in dairy cattle thought to be due to use of a chemical aid in the making of ensilage, possibly via the intervention of a mycotoxin. Clinically characterized by widespread pruritic dermatitis, fever and mucosal petechiation.
pyridine 1. a substance derived from coal tar and also from tobacco and various organic materials. Used in industry as a solvent and in the synthesis of organic compounds. 2. any of a group of substances homologous with normal pyridine. The pyridines are serious poisons causing damage to most organs especially nervous and respiratory systems and skin.
pyridostigmine a cholinesterase inhibitor; used as the bromide in the treatment of myasthenia gravis and as an antidote to nondepolarizing muscle relaxants, e.g. tubocurarine.
pyridoxal, pyridoxaldehyde a form of vitamin B_6.
p. phosphate PLP; a major coenzyme involved in amino acid metabolism.
pyridoxamine one of the three active forms of vitamin B_6.
p. phosphate a coenzyme involved in amino acid metabolism.
pyridoxine one of the forms of vitamin B_6, chiefly used, as the hydrochloride salt, in the prophylaxis and treatment of vitamin B_6 deficiency. Nutritional deficiency is not known to occur under natural conditions in animals. Called also pyridoxal, adermin.
pyriform pear-shaped.
p. apparatus pair of triangular structures in the eggs of anoplocephalid tapeworms surrounding the oncosphere.
p. lobe a swelling on the ventral surface of the brain, made up of the combined lateral olfactory gyrus and the hippocampal gyrus.
pyrilamine an ethylenediamine histamine H_1-receptor antagonist, used topically and systemically in the treatment of allergic disorders. Called also mepyramine.
pyrimethamine a folic acid antagonist used in combination with sulfonamides in the treatment of toxoplasmosis and avian coccidiosis.
pyrimidine an organic compound that is the fundamental form of the pyrimidine bases, including uracil, cytosine and thymine.
A p. cytosine.
pyriminil see VACOR.
pyro- word element. [Gr.] *fire, heat;* (in chemistry) *produced by heating.*
pyrocatechol a metabolite of tannic acid used as a topical antiseptic. Prepared synthetically or extracted from powdered catechu. Called also catechol.
pyrogen an agent that causes fever.
endogenous p. (EP) the mediator of fever, produced by polymorphonuclear leukocytes, monocytes and macrophages.
exogenous p. lipopolysaccharides and other substances produced by pathogenic microorganisms.
pyrogenic reaction one causing fever.
pyroglobulinemia the presence in the blood of an abnormal globulin constituent that is precipitated by heat.
pyroglutamic acid see 5-oxoproline.
pyrolysis decomposition by heating; said of organic materials.
pyrometer instrument for measuring the intensity of heat when this is beyond the range of the mercury thermometer.
pyronine a red aniline histological stain.
pyroninophilic having an affinity for pyronine.
p. cell contains large quantities of RNA stainable with pyronine. Called also immunoblast.
pyrophosphatase any enzyme that catalyzes the hydrolysis of central pyrophosphate linkages.
pyrophosphate any salt of pyrophosphoric (diphosphoric) acid.

pyrophosphoric acid a dimer of phosphoric acid, $H_4P_2O_7$. Called also diphosphoric acid.
pyrotic caustic; burning.
pyroxylin a product of the action of a mixture of nitric and sulfuric acids on cotton, consisting chiefly of cellulose tetranitrate; a necessary ingredient of collodion.
pyrrole a basic, cyclic substance, obtained by destructive distillation of various animal substances. Critical components in the synthesis of porphyrins.
pyrrolidine a simple base obtained from tobacco or prepared from pyrrole.
pyrrolizidine a specific chemical configuration which is common to a number of naturally occurring compounds called the pyrrolizidine alkaloids. Common plant sources are in the genera *Crotalaria*, *Echium*, *Heliotropium*, *Senecio*.
p. alkaloidosis the disease caused by poisoning with pyrrolizidine alkaloids. The hepatic lesion tends to be chronic and is characterized by necrosis, megalocytosis of hepatocytes due to inhibition of mitosis, biliary ductule, proliferation, vasculitis and perivenous fibrosis. Lesions are most severe in the liver and result in the syndrome of jaundice, photosensitization and hepatic encephalopathy. Some alkaloids cause lung damage characterized by edema, fibrosis, alveolar epithelialization and emphysema, e.g. jaagsiekte. Megalocytosis also occurs in the kidney and there may be extensive nephrosis. There may also be ulceration of the mucosa of the esophagus, stomach and intestines and carcinogenesis is a feature in some animals. An incidental pathogenesis is a concurrent chronic copper poisoning causing the disease TOXEMIC jaundice.
p. alkaloids toxic alkaloids, esters of retronecine, heliotridine, including senecionine, jacobine, monocrotaline, spectabiline, heliotrine and lasiocarpine. All cause pyrrolizidine alkaloidosis (see above). Common plant sources are in the genera CROTALARIA, ECHIUM, HELIOTROPIUM, SENECIO.
Pyrus malus see MALUS SYLVESTRIS.
pyruvate a salt, ester or anion of pyruvic acid. The term is used interchangeably with pyruvic acid. Pyruvate is the end product of glycolysis and may be metabolized in the body to lactate or to acetyl CoA. In yeast it is metabolized to ethanol.
p. carboxylase an enzyme concerned in the conversion of pyruvate to oxaloacetic acid.
p. dehydrogenase actively concerned in the decarboxylation of pyruvate to acetyl CoA and CO_2.
p. kinase a glycolytic pathway enzyme (called also PK) which catalyzes the formation of pyruvate from phosphoenolpyruvate (PEP). A deficiency of the enzyme is a hereditary defect in humans and occurs also in Beagle and Basenji dogs, causing a familial nonspherocytic ANEMIA.
p. transaminase see ALANINE AMINOTRANSFERASE.
pyruvic acid a compound formed in the body in metabolism of carbohydrate; also formed by dry distillation of tartaric acid. Used synonymously with pyruvate.
pyruvic kinase see PYRUVATE kinase.
pythiosis see OOMYCOSIS.
equine p. see SWAMP CANCER.
Pythium insidiosum*, *Pythium destruens previously called *Hyphomyces destruens*; the cause of pythiosis in dogs, cattle and horses.
python large snake, up to 26 ft long, with big, square head, prominent jaws and a distinct neck. Awesome but not venomous. Includes carpet snakes often kept as housepets because of their appetite for rodents which they swallow whole.
pyuria pus in the urine. The pus may be obvious or be detectable only on microscopic examination and be in the form of leukocytes in casts or rafts. Usually accompanied by bacteria.
PZI protamine zinc insulin.

Q

Q abbreviation for ubiquinone (CoQ).
Q. quadrant.
q symbol for (1) the long arm of a chromosome or (2) the frequency of the rarer allele of a pair.
Q banding a laboratory technique for staining a karyotype with quinacrine dye.
Q fever (query fever) a rickettsial infection of most animal species, including humans, and some birds. It is caused by *Coxiella burnetii* and spread by inhalation, especially of inspissated reproductive exudates, and by ticks, and by the ingestion of raw infected milk. The disease is inapparent in most infected animals but can cause abortion in sheep and goats, and probably cattle. Called also Queensland fever.
q.d. [L.] *quaque die* (every day).
q.h. [L.] *quaque hora* (every hour).
Qi in acupuncture terms this is the 'life force'; it is the source of all movement within the body, the protection against invasion of the body, the source of all metabolic activity, provides for the holding of tissues and components in place, maintaining body temperature and for the circulation of nourishment in the bloodstream.
q.i.d. [L.] *quater in die* (four times a day).
Qinchuan cattle red or yellow Chinese draft cattle with a cervical hump.
q.q.h. [L.] *quaque quarta hora* (every 4 hours).
QRS complex, QRS wave a group of waves depicted on an electrocardiogram; it actually consists of three distinct waves created by the passage of the cardiac electrical impulse through the ventricles and occurs at the beginning of each contraction of the ventricles. In a normal ELECTROCARDIOGRAM the R wave is the most prominent of the three; the Q and S waves may be extremely weak and sometimes are absent.
q.s. [L.] *quantum satis* (a sufficient amount).
qt quart.
QT interval the portion of an electrocardiogram between the onset of the Q wave and the end of the T wave, representing the total time for ventricular depolarization and repolarization.
quack slang for a person who misrepresents his/her qualifications as a veterinarian, and therefore ability and experience in diagnosis and treatment of animal disease or the effects to be achieved by the treatment. Refers usually to a person without any qualifications who practices in breach of the local veterinary regulations and is liable to a heavy fine as a result.
quackery the practice or methods of a QUACK.
quadrangular having four angles.
quadrant 1. one-quarter of the circumference of a circle. 2. one of four corresponding parts, or quarters, as of the surface of the abdomen or of the field of vision.
quadrate square or squared.

quadr(i)- word element. [L.] *four.*
quadriceps having four heads; refers to quadriceps muscle. See also Table 13.
q. reflex see PATELLAR reflex.
quadrigemina the corpora quadrigemina.
quadrigeminal fourfold; in four parts; forming a group of four.
quadrilateral having four sides.
quadrilocular having four cavities.
quadripartite divided into four.
quadriplegia paralysis of all four limbs; tetraplegia. Indicative of spinal cord injury in the upper cervical area. May be acute or gradual in onset depending on the nature of the lesion.
hereditary amblyopia with q. see hereditary AMBLYOPIA with quadriplegia.
quadrisect to cut into four parts.
quadritubercular having four tubercles or cusps.
quadrivalent having a valence of four.
quadruped 1. four-footed. 2. an animal having four feet.
quadruplet one of four offspring produced at one birth. Said of species that normally have single births.
quagga an extinct member of the family Equidae which was characterized by stripes like a zebra but only on the head and neck.
quail a small, gallinaceous, insectivorous game bird, gray-brown with black, white and yellow spots. They are poor flyers but migrate long distances annually and reproduce at a high rate. The common species is the common quail, *Coturnix coturnix*. In North America the native quail is the bobwhite (*Colinus virginianus*).
q. bronchitis caused by an adenovirus in captive or freeliving bobwhite quail, manifested by coughing, sneezing, lacrimation and conjunctivitis but usually without nasal discharge. Morbidity is usually 100% in young birds where the mortality may also be high.
q. disease see ulcerative ENTERITIS.
qualimeter an early instrument for measuring the penetrating power of x-rays; penetrometer.
qualitative pertaining to observations of a categorical nature, e.g. breed, sex.
q. data data measured on a categorical scale.
q. trait see qualitative TRAIT.
quality purity of contents, care in presentation and finish of a product.
q. assurance planned and systematic action necessary to provide adequate confidence that a product or service will satisfy given requirements for quality. Quality is built into the product or service, rather than 'inspected in'.
q. control the use of operational techniques, particularly end-product testing or inspection to ensure that a product or service satisfies its stated or implied role.
protein q. relates to the content and balance of amino acids in the protein. A good quality protein contains the amino acids in the correct proportions required by the specific animal species.
radiographic q. depends on the correct positioning of the subject part, good contrast, clear image due to good detail and absence of artefacts.
quantal pertaining to specific quantities; used usually in reference to drugs and their dose rates.
q. drug–receptor relationship the variation in effect observed with increasing doses of a drug.
quantile division of a total into equal subgroups; includes terciles, quartiles, quintiles, deciles, percentiles.
quantimeter an instrument for measuring the quantity of x-rays generated by a Coolidge tube. The first hot-cathode tube.
quantitative pertaining to observations of a numerical kind, e.g. 50 kg, 2 m, 24 hands.
q. characters features of animal productivity or performance which can be measured quantitatively.
q. data numerical data.
q. inheritance genetic transmission of phenotypes which are quantitative and continuous.
q. trait see quantitative TRAIT.
quantity 1. a characteristic, as of energy or mass, susceptible of precise physical measurement. 2. a measurable amount.
quantivalence valence (1).
quantum pl. *quanta* [L.] an elemental unit of energy; the amount emitted or absorbed at each step when energy is emitted or absorbed by atoms or molecules.
q. theory radiation and absorption of energy occur in quantities (quanta) which vary in size with the frequency of the radiation.
quarantine 1. a place or period of detention of ships or aircraft coming from infected or suspected ports. 2. restrictions placed on entering or leaving premises or regions where a case of communicable disease exists or is suspected.
q. station a government institution which houses animals or people that have to serve out a mandatory period of quarantine because they have come from an infected port or been exposed to, or affected by, one or more exotic diseases.
quarrian see COCKATIEL.
quart one-quarter of a gallon or 2 pints. The Imperial quart is 1136.5 milliliters (1.1365 liters) and the American quart is 946 ml (0.946 liters); abbreviated qt.
quartan 1. recurring in 4-day cycles (every third day). 2. a variety of intermittent fever of which the paroxysms recur on every third day.
quarter 1. hindquarter. 2. lateral or medial sides of the wall of the hoof of the horse. 3. one of the four individual glands in the udder of a cow.
black q. see BLACKLEG.
blind q. a quarter in the udder of a lactating cow that does not produce any milk when the other quarters are doing so. Caused usually by a prior attack of mastitis.
q. crack crack in the lateral or medial wall of the hoof, beginning at the coronet. Usually cause no lameness.
hoof q. side of the hoof.
q. infection rate percentage of udder quarters at risk in a herd found to be infected with mastitis-causing bacteria by bacteriological examination of quarter samples of milk. May be as low as 10% in herds utilizing a full mastitis control program. See also MASTITIS infection rate.
q. marks designs made in the haircoat of a horse by grooming the hair in a direction the reverse of its normal growth pattern.
q. sheet an item of horse clothing; a lightweight half blanket covering the horse from the girth to the tail.
Quarter horse an American light horse of compact build and muscular hindquarters, about 15.2 hands high, often chestnut but any solid color. It originated from THOROUGHBRED and CRIOLLO. Primarily a cattle horse but also used in short sprint races.
quartile one of the values establishing the division of a series of variables into fourths, or the range of items included in such a segment.
quartipara quadripara; a female which has had four pregnancies that resulted in viable offspring; para IV.
QUAT quaternary ammonium compound.
quater in die [L.] *four times a day;* abbreviated q.i.d.

quaternary 1. fourth in a series. 2. made up of four elements or groups.

q. ammonium compounds synthetic cationic detergents commonly used as disinfectants. They act against cell wall lipids in bacteria. An example is benzalkonium chloride. Effective in teat dips for mastitis control. Called also QUATs.

q. structure the arrangement of separate polypeptide subunits in the structure of a multimeric protein.

Quebec Jersey see CANADIAN.

Queckenstedt's test when the veins in the neck are compressed on one or both sides there is a rapid rise in the pressure of the cerebrospinal fluid of healthy animals, and this rise quickly disappears when pressure is taken off the neck. But when there is a block in the spinal canal the pressure of the cerebrospinal fluid is affected little or not at all by the maneuver.

queen a mature, entire female cat used for breeding.

Queen Anne legs valgus deformity (inward bowing) of the forelegs, seen most commonly in dogs.

Queen Anne's lace DAUCUS CAROTA, AMMI *majus*.

Queen's delight see STILLINGIA DENDATA.

queen-of-the-bush PIMELIA *linifolia*.

queening parturition in the female cat.

Queensland having some geographical relationship to the state of Queensland, Australia.

Q. fever see Q FEVER.

Q. blue heeler see AUSTRALIAN cattle dog.

q. nut tree see MACADAMIA.

Queensland itch see SWEET itch.

Queensland tick typhus a tickborne fever of humans, similar to Rocky Mountain spotted fever, caused by *Rickettsia australis* and transmitted by ixodid ticks. Dogs and cats may be unusual hosts.

quena SOLANUM *esuriale*.

quench to put out, extinguish, or suppress; to cool (as hot metal) by immersing in water. In liquid scintillation counting, any process taking place within the sample container which results in a decrease in number or intensity of the light flashes produced, thus lowering the amount of energy recorded.

Quercus plants of the northern temperate zone in the family Fagaceae; oaks; vary from shrubs to great trees. Leaves and acorns are poisonous because of their content of gallotannins. Poisoning is manifested by abdominal pain, thirst, frequent urination, ventral edema and lesions of gastritis and nephritis. Toxic species include *Q. aliena*, *Q. breviloba* (*Q. durandii*), *Q. coccinea*, *Q. cutissima*, *Q. dentata*, *Q. douglesii*, *Q. gambelii*, *Q. garyanna*, *Q. glandulifera* var. *acuteserrata*, *Q. havardii* (shin oak), *Q. incana*, *Q. lobata*, *Q. marilandica*, *Q. petraea*, *Q. prinus*, *Q. robur* (*Q. pedunculata*), *Q. rubra* var. *borealis*, *Q. stellata* (post oak), *Q. variabilis*, *Q. velutina*.

query fever see Q FEVER.

questionnaire a planned set of questions used to collect data. It can be sent to the respondents by mail (when the response rate is poor and the sample of respondees is often biased) or used as the basis of a personal interview. The latter procedure has the advantage of quickly detecting questions that are ambiguous or are couched in terms that will elicit information on the wrong subject. The biggest problem is to keep the size of the questionnaire small enough to avoid exasperating the subjects. It is also desirable to couch the questions so that the responses can be easily categorized and the results computerized.

queue dynamic storage area in a computer in which items, e.g. print files for a printer, wait to be processed.

quick disease sudden death due to cardiac arrest in poisoning by *Urechites lutea*, *Albizia* spp., *Fadogia* spp., *Galena africana*, *Pavetta* spp. Called also gousiekte.

quick freezing very quick freezing of carcasses of meat by passage through a freezing tunnel beneath jets of liquid nitrogen.

quick of hoof the area of the sensitive laminae; penetrated by a misguided farrier nail to draw blood.

Quick prothrombin test see PROTHROMBIN time test.

quicklime calcium oxide, called also unslaked lime.

quidding the disability in horses of dropping food from the mouth while in the process of masticating it. Due usually to stomatitis caused by bad teeth. Paralysis of the tongue has the same effect. See also CUD dropping.

quiddor a horse affected by QUIDDING.

quiescent at rest; latent; the G_0 stage of the cell cycle.

quiet ovulation see silent ESTRUS.

quill the shaft of a bird's FEATHER (1).

q. suture technique a secure, external method of closing the vulva against prolapse; now obsolete. A vertically placed piece of rubber tubing on either side of the vulva is encircled in a row of four or five horizontal mattress sutures.

Quilonia a genus of roundworms in the subfamily Cyathostominae.

Q. africana*, *Q. ethiopica*, *Q. uganda found in the African elephant.

Q. renniei*, *Q. travancra found in the Indian elephant.

quilt suture pattern see HALSTED suture pattern.

quinacrine an antimalarial, antiprotozoal and anthelmintic used especially for suppressive therapy of malaria in humans and also in the treatment of giardiasis in dogs. Called also mepacrine.

quinalbarbitone see SECOBARBITAL.

quinaldine used as a fish anesthetic agent.

quinapyramine a drug used in the treatment of trypanosomiasis. A toxic reaction can occur within 2 hours after the administration of a therapeutic dose to cattle; signs include salivation, tremor, dyspnea, incoordination, tachycardia.

quince see CYDONIA OBLONGA.

quinestrol a long-acting estrogen.

quinidine the dextrorotatory isomer of quinine, used in treatment of cardiac arrhythmias. Several salts are used, including the gluconate, sulfate and bisulfate.

quinine an alkaloid from *Cinchona* spp. plants of South America used in some forms of malaria in humans. Quinine also has analgesic, antipyretic, mild oxytocic, cardiac depressant, and sclerosing properties, and it decreases the excitability of the motor end-plate. It may be the cause of an immune-mediated hemolytic anemia.

q. tree see ALSTONIA *constricta*.

quininism cinchonism; poisoning from cinchona bark or its alkaloids. See also ALSTONIA *constricta*.

quinoline a drug used originally as an antimalarial. Some of its derivatives are used as antiprotozoal and topical antifungal agents, e.g. quinuronium sulfate, 4-aminoquinoline, di-iodohydroxyquinoline and clioquinol (iodochlorhydroxyquin).

quinolizidine alkaloid includes plant-origin alkaloids causing nervous dysfunction (e.g. sparteine, lupinine, lupanine, hydroxylupanine, spathulatine, thermopsine), and those causing congenital defects (e.g. anagyrine).

quinolones drugs that have good effect against all species of chicken coccidia but have a bad tendency to generate resistant strains and are now rarely used for that purpose; newer derivatives are used as antibacterials.

quinquevalent pentavalent; having a valence of five.
quinsy peritonsillar abscess.
quint- word element. [L.] *five*.
quintan recurring every 5 days (every fourth day).
quintuplet one of five offspring produced at one birth. Used in species that normally have single births.
quinuronium an antiprotozoal agent effective against *Babesia* spp. Has a low margin of safety because of its marked parasympathomimetic effects.
Quiscalus quiscala see GRACKLE.
quittor a chronic, suppurative inflammation of the lateral cartilage of the third phalanx of the foot of the horse. Causes lameness and usually the appearance of a discharging sinus at the coronet.
quokka a small, nocturnal wallaby (*Setonyx brachyurus*) which is especially sensitive to nutritional myopathy. Called also Rottnest quokka.
quota the portion of a whole that belongs to one person. In agriculture it usually refers to a share of a market, e.g. Australia's quota of the USA's beef market.
q. sampling see quota SAMPLING.
quotid. [L.] *quotidie* (every day); abbreviated q.d.
quotidian recurring every day.
quotient a number obtained by division.
caloric q. the heat evolved (in calories) divided by the oxygen consumed (in milligrams) in a metabolic process.
respiratory q. see RESPIRATORY quotient.

R

R symbol, *roentgen*; a symbol used in general chemical formulae to represent an organic radical; Rankine (scale); Réaumur (scale); [L.] *remotum* (far); respiration; *Rickettsia;* right.
r symbol for ring chromosome.
R 1929 see AZAPERONE.
R 2028 see FLUANISONE.
R 4749 see DROPERIDOL.
R banding a technique for staining a karyotype using Giemsa stain; produces effects the reverse of G banding.
R conformational state oxyhemoglobin ('relaxed') conformational form of hemoglobin.
R-on-T phenomenon a form of ventricular arrhythmia in which the electrocardiographic tracing shows premature ventricular complexes occurring in early diastole. It is believed to lead to ventricular fibrillation in most cases.
RA see rheumatoid ARTHRITIS, RAGOCYTE.
Ra chemical symbol, *radium*.
rabbit see SYLVILAGUS.
brush r. SYLVILAGUS *bachmani*.
r. calicivirus disease see RABBIT HEMORRHAGIC DISEASE.
r. fever see TULAREMIA.
r. fibroma virus see LEPORIPOXVIRUS, Shope rabbit FIBROMA.
r. fur mite CHEYLETIELLA *parasitivorax*.
laboratory r. some specialized strains have been developed to provide a consistent type of rabbit for experimental work in laboratories. The International Index of Laboratory Animals is a reference source for these strains. The most commonly used variety is the NEW ZEALAND White.
r. pasteurellosis see rabbit septicemia (below).
r. pox see RABBITPOX.
pygmy r. *Brachylagus idahoensis*; a native of North America.
rock r. *Ochotona princeps*; see PIKA.
r. septicemia a disease of rabbits caused by *Pasteurella multocida* and characterized by sudden death preceded by fever, dyspnea and nasal discharge. In mild cases there is nasal catarrh and conjunctivitis. Called also SNUFFLES (1).
r. syphilis see SPIROCHETOSIS (2).
r. tick HAEMAPHYSALIS *leporispalustris*.
volcano r. *Romerolagus diazi*; a native of Mexico.
rabbit hemorrhagic disease a highly fatal, contagious disease of European rabbits (*Oryctolagus cuniculus*) but other rabbit species and other wildlife are not susceptible. Caused by rabbit calicivirus; the virus while typical of caliciviruses has not been cultivated. The disease is related to European Brown Hare syndrome but cross-transmission between hares and rabbits of either virus does not occur; spread is by contact, possibly by infected feces, fomites, possibly by spread of carrion by birds, and by recently contaminated insects such as bush flies. After infection rabbits show few clinical signs other than depression and immobility and die after an illness of about 18 hours. Characteristic gross necropsy lesions are enlargement of the liver and spleen and small, focal, pulmonary hemorrhages. There is massive liver necrosis which is believed to be the trigger for disseminated intravascular coagulation. Rabbits less than 6 weeks of age are curiously not susceptible to fatal disease. An effective vaccine is available. Called also rabbit calicivirus disease.
rabbitbrush see TETRADYMIA GLABRATA.
rabbitpox a disease of rabbits caused by a poxvirus in the genus *Orthopoxvirus*. There are typical skin lesions with a systemic illness, ocular and nasal discharge, and a high mortality rate.
rabiate, rabid affected with rabies; pertaining to rabies.
rabid affected by rabies.
rabies a highly fatal viral infection of the nervous system which affects all warm-blooded animal species. The causative rhabdovirus is transmitted in the saliva and the principal method of infection in animals is by a bite. Separate furious and dumb (paralytic) forms are described but both commonly occur in the one animal. The syndrome includes an ascending paralysis which may be preceded by a period of mania and aggression. Rabies is one of the most important of the zoonoses because of the inevitably fatal outcome for the infected human.
bat r. an infection which is endemic in bats and may be caused by the rabies virus or by other similar rhabdoviruses such as Lagos, Mokola and Australian flying fox bat viruses.
fixed r. virus see fixed VIRUS.
r. inhibiting substance present in the salivary glands and brain tissue of infected animals and may make the tissue nonlethal for mice by the intracerebral route. It does not interfere with detection of rabies antigen by immunofluorescent staining.
rabies-like viruses Mokola, Lagos bat, Duvenhage, European and Australian bat viruses. So called because they cause rabies-like disease in humans and animals.
rabiform resembling rabies.
raccoon a gray-brown animal with a long, furry tail

ringed with black, a sharp, pointed face, and about as big as a medium-sized dog. It is terrestrial, arboreal and aquatic, omnivorous and nocturnal. Called also coon, *Procyon lotor*.

r. dog see COONHOUND.

r. poxvirus a poxvirus that causes typical POX lesions in the raccoon.

r. rabies a major wildlife reservoir and source of human exposure in the southeastern United States.

r. roundworm BAYLISASCARIS *procyonis*.

race 1. a class or breed of animals subordinate to species, i.e. a subspecies; a group of animals having certain characteristics in common, because of a common inheritance. 2. a fenced lane just one animal wide leading to a dipping tank, spray dip, branding chute, drafting gate, etc. 3. see STRIPE.

racehorse refers usually to THOROUGHBRED but may also include STANDARDBRED, TROTTER.

racemase an enzyme that catalyzes the racemization of an optically active substance, such as L-lactic acid.

racemate a racemic compound.

racemethionine a racemic mixture of D- and L-methionine used as a dietary supplement with lipotropic action.

racemic optically inactive, being composed of equal amounts of dextrorotatory and levorotatory isomers.

racemization the transformation of one-half of the molecules of an optically active compound into molecules that possess exactly the opposite (mirror-image) configuration, with complete loss of rotatory power because of the statistical balance between equal numbers of dextrorotatory and levorotatory molecules.

racemose shaped like a bunch of grapes.

rachianesthesia loss of sensation produced by injection of an anesthetic into the spinal canal.

rachicentesis puncture into the lumbar spinal canal. See also SPINAL puncture.

rachidial, rachidian pertaining to the spine.

rachigraph an instrument for recording the outlines of the spine and back.

rachi(o)- word element. [Gr.] *spine*.

rachiocampsis spinal curvature.

rachiomyelitis inflammation of the spinal cord.

rachiotomy incision of a vertebra or the vertebral column.

rachipagus twin fetuses joined at the vertebral column.

rachis 1. the vertebral column. 2. the shaft of a feather.

rachischisis congenital fissure of the vertebral column.

rachitic pertaining to rickets.

r. rosary the visible enlargements of the costochondral junctions in rickets.

rachitis 1. rickets. 2. inflammatory disease of the vertebral column.

rachitogenic causing rickets.

rachitomy the surgical or anatomical opening of the spinal canal.

racing contests of speed and endurance with serious biochemical and physiological consequences lessened by adequate training beforehand. See also PHYSICAL fitness, EXERTIONAL rhabdomyolysis, HEAT exhaustion, PULMONARY hemorrhage, EPISTAXIS, EXHAUSTION.

r. dogs usually refers to Greyhounds and Whippets, but in some instances may be used to describe the dogs used for endurance sledge racing.

r. pigeons a variety of pigeons, bred and selected to fly long distances back to their own homes. Races are conducted as time trials with groups of birds being released at specific times and their arrival clocked in.

r. plates lightweight, single-use, horseshoes made of aluminum and with a fullered contact surface; see also HORSESHOEING.

rack a fast, four beat artifical (taught) gait of horses, similar to the running walk and slow gait, but with more up and down movement. Performed by the five-gaited American saddle horse.

Racosperma melanoxylon see ACACIA *melanoxylon*.

Racosperma salicinum see ACACIA *salicina*.

rad 1. acronym for *r*adiation *a*bsorbed *d*ose; a superseded, non-SI unit of measurement of the absorbed dose of ionizing radiation. It corresponds to an energy transfer of 100 ergs per gram of any absorbing material (including tissue). The biological effect of 1 rad of radiation varies with the type of radiation. When the dose is in REM, all types have the same biological effect. Now replaced by the GRAY. 2. abbreviation for radiograph; used in medical records.

rad. [L.] *radix* (root).

radar tracking an electronic technique used to follow the flight of birds.

raddle color marker in crayon or cake form used to temporarily identify sheep by marking them on the tip of the fleece.

radectomy excision of a portion of the root of a tooth.

Radfordia a genus of mites in the family Myobiidae.

R. affinis found on mice.

R. ensifera found on wild and laboratory rats. May cause sufficient pruritus to result in self-trauma.

radiability the property of being readily penetrated by x- or other rays.

radiad toward the radius or radial side.

radial 1. pertaining to the radius of the forelimb or to the radial aspect of the forelimb as opposed to the ulnar aspect; pertaining to a radius. 2. radiating; spreading outward from a common center.

r. agenesis a common congenital deformity in animals, particularly in cats. The defect may be uni- or bilateral, causing a marked medial deviation of the lower forelimb.

r. dysplasia a developmental disorder of the radius and ulna in which growth rates differ and deformities of the limb result.

r. hemimelia absence of the radius.

r. paralysis caused by loss of function of the radial nerve. See Table 14. Manifested by loss of function of extensor muscles and impaired sensory perception in the thoracic limb especially over the dorsum of the paw. Lesions at or distal to the level of the elbow result in difficulty in extending the carpus and foot so that weight may be carried on the dorsum of the foot. Lesions above that level, usually associated with injury to the brachial plexus, also cause an inability to actively extend the elbow (dropped elbow) and the animal cannot bear weight on the limb.

radialis [L.] *radial*.

radiant 1. diverging from a center. 2. emitting rays, as of light or heat.

radiata pine see PINUS *radiata*.

radiate 1. to diverge or spread from a common point. 2. arranged in a radiating manner.

radiathermy short wave diathermy.

radiatio pl. *radiationes* [L.] a radiating structure; a collection of nerve fibers connecting different portions of the brain.

r. acoustica auditory radiation of the internal capsule in the brain.

radiation 1. divergence from a common center. 2. a structure made up of diverging elements, especially a tract of the central nervous system made up of diverging fibers. 3. energy carried by waves or a stream of particles. One type is *electromagnetic radiation*, which consists of wave motion of electric and magnetic fields. The *quantum theory* is based on the fact that electromagnetic waves consist of discrete particles, called *photons*, that have an energy inversely proportional to the wavelength of the wave. In order of increasing photon energy and decreasing wavelength, the electromagnetic spectrum is divided into radio waves, infrared light, visible light, ultraviolet light and x-rays.

Another type is the radiation emitted by radioactive materials. *Alpha particles* are high-energy helium-4 nuclei consisting of two protons and two neutrons, which are emitted by radioisotopes of heavy elements, such as uranium. *Beta particles* are high-energy electrons, which are emitted by radioisotopes of lighter elements. *Gamma rays* are high-energy photons, which are emitted along with alpha and beta particles and are also emitted alone by metastable radionuclides, such as technetium-99m. Gamma rays have energies in the x-ray region of the spectrum and differ from x-rays only in that they are produced by radioactive decay rather than by x-ray machines.

Radiation with enough energy to knock electrons out of atoms and produce ions is called *ionizing radiation*. This includes alpha and beta particles and x-rays and gamma rays.

r. biology study of the effects of ionizing radiation on living tissues.

corpuscular r. particles emitted in nuclear disintegration, including alpha and beta particles, protons, neutrons, positrons and deuterons.

r. detection special equipment, including Geiger–Müller tubes and a scintillation crystal, is available to detect radiation which may be accidental, or detect small amounts where this is expected but it needs to be measured in terms of accumulated dose.

electromagnetic r. energy, unassociated with matter, that is transmitted through space by means of waves (electromagnetic waves) traveling in all instances at 3×10^{10} cm or 186,284 miles per second, but ranging in length from 10^{11} cm (electrical waves) to 10^{-12} cm (cosmic rays) and including radio waves, infrared, visible light and ultraviolet, x-rays and gamma rays.

r. exposure means more than the patient being exposed intentionally to an x-ray beam. Technical persons in the vicinity will also be exposed to a much less dangerous but perniciously cumulative load of radiation.

infrared r. the portion of the spectrum of electromagnetic radiation of wavelengths ranging between 0.75 and 1000 μm. See also INFRARED.

r. injury is caused by exposure to radioactive material. High doses cause intense diarrhea and dehydration and extensive skin necrosis. Median doses cause initial anorexia, lethargy and vomiting then normality for several weeks followed by vomiting, nasal discharge, dysentery, recumbency, septicemia and a profound pancytopenia. Death is the most common outcome. Chronic doses cause cataract in a few. Congenital defects occur rarely.

interstitial r. energy emitted by radium or radon inserted directly into the tissue.

ionizing r. corpuscular or electromagnetic radiation that is capable of producing ions, directly or indirectly, in its passage through matter. Used in treatment of radiosensitive cancer, in sterilization of animal products and food for experimental use.

r. necrosis see RADIONECROSIS.

r. physicist the person responsible for the administration of radiation therapy including estimating the dose required for a treatment, arranging for the dose to be delivered and making arrangements for safety of the patient and staff, and disposing of any residual radioactive material. Technical aspects of the work include computer estimations, preparation of isodose curves, preparation of wedge and compensating filters, and calibration of teletherapy equipment.

primary r. radiation emanating from the x-ray tube which is absorbed by the subject or passes on through the subject without any change in photon energy.

r. protection includes proper control of emissions from the x-ray machines, proper protective clothing for staff, keeping unnecessary people out of the way while the tube is actually generating its beam, the wearing and regular examination of a dosimeter and the proper storage of radioactive materials or residues.

pyramidal r. fibers extending from the pyramidal tract to the cortex.

r. sensitivity tissues vary in their sensitivity to the damaging effects of irradiation. The rapidly growing tissues are most susceptible, e.g. the embryo, rapidly growing cancer, gonads, alimentary tract, skin and blood-forming organs.

r. sickness see radiation injury (above).

solar r. see SOLAR.

r. striothalamica a fiber system joining the thalamus and the hypothalamic region.

tegmental r. fibers radiating laterally from the nucleus ruber.

thalamic r. fibers streaming out through the lateral surface of the thalamus, through the internal capsule to the cerebral cortex.

r. therapist a person skilled in RADIOTHERAPY. See also radiation therapy (below).

r. therapy see RADIOTHERAPY.

ultraviolet r. the portion of the spectrum of electromagnetic radiation of wavelengths ranging between 0.39 and 0.18 μm. See also ULTRAVIOLET rays.

radiative pertaining to or emanating from radiation.

radical 1. directed to the cause; going to the root or source of a morbid process. 2. a group of atoms that enters into and goes out of chemical combination without change and that forms one of the fundamental constituents of a molecule.

free r. a radical, extremely reactive, and having a very short half-life (10^{-5} s or less in an aqueous solution), which carries an unpaired electron.

radicle one of the smaller branches of a vessel or nerve.

radicotomy rhizotomy; division or transection of a nerve root.

radicular pertaining to a root or radicle.

radiculitis inflammation of a spinal nerve root, especially of the portion of the root that lies between the spinal cord and the spinal canal.

radiculoganglionitis inflammation of the posterior spinal nerve roots and their ganglia.

radiculomedullary affecting the nerve roots and spinal cord.

radiculomeningomyelitis inflammation of the nerve roots, meninges and spinal cord.

radiculomyelopathy disease of the nerve roots and spinal cord.

degenerative r. slowly progressive in adult German shepherd and other breeds of dogs; cause unknown; characterized clinically by paraparesis and truncal ataxia.

radiculoneuritis inflammation of nerve roots and their attendant peripheral nerves.

radiculoneuropathy disease of the nerve roots and spinal nerves.

radiculopathy disease of the nerve roots.

spondylotic caudal r. compression of the cauda equina due to encroachment upon a congenitally small spinal canal by spondylosis, resulting in neural disorders of the lower limbs. See also LUMBOSACRAL stenosis.

radiectomy excision of the root of a tooth.

radii lentis the sutures formed by the union of the ends of the lens fibers create a three-pointed star formation.

radio- word element. [L.] *ray, radiation, emission of radiant energy, radium, radius* (bone of the forearm); affixed to the name of a chemical element to designate a radioactive isotope of that element.

radio-pulse transmitters small electronic devices which give off a small electronic pulse which is reiterated for very long periods, sufficient for a search to be conducted for the beeper. A valuable tool in wildlife studies.

radioactivation analysis see ACTIVATION analysis.

radioactive characterized by radioactivity.

r. decay spontaneous decomposition of the nuclei of the atoms of radioactive substances. Measured as the proportion of the atoms in a radionuclide that decompose per unit of time, usually stated as the half-life of that particular isotope.

r. fallout dissemination of radioactive substances through the atmosphere and deposition on the environment generally; causes radiation injury.

r. isotope radionuclide. A radioactive NUCLIDE, e.g. radioactive iodine or strontium.

r. tracer see radioactive TRACER.

radioactivity the quality of emitting or the emission of particulate or electromagnetic radiation as a consequence of the decay of the nuclei of unstable elements, a property of all chemical elements of atomic number above 83, and possible of induction in all other known elements.

The chemical elements are made up of atoms, each of which consists of a nucleus around which orbits a cloud of negatively charged electrons. The nucleus itself is made up of two kinds of particles: *neutrons*, which have no electrical charge; and *protons*, each of which has a single positive charge. A neutral atom has an equal number of protons and electrons and no electric charge. The *atomic number* of an element is the number of protons in the nucleus of each of its atoms. The *mass number* of an element is the sum of the number of protons and neutrons in the nucleus.

All of the atoms of a particular element have the same atomic number, but can have different numbers of neutrons. An *isotope* of a chemical element consists of atoms having the same number of protons, but a different number of neutrons. When an atomic nucleus is unstable it decomposes or decays spontaneously, emitting high-energy particles. The emissions from radioactive decay can consist of electrons (beta particles), or electromagnetic energy in the form of photons, or helium ions (alpha particles). (See also RADIATION.) The process of decay can produce a product that is itself unstable, in which case it too will decay. The process continues until a stable nuclide is finally formed.

The radioactivity of a substance can be measured by determining the rate at which atoms decay in a given period of time. The basic unit of measurement of radioactivity is the *becquerel* (Bq), which is equal to 1 disintegration per second. The now outdated but possibly still used unit is the *curie* (Ci), which equals 37 thousand-million disintegrations per second. One-thousandth of a curie is a *millicurie;* one-millionth is a *microcurie.* These units of measure are used to calculate the dosage of radioactivity administered for various therapeutic procedures in much the same way that units of measure such as the gram and milligram are used to measure dosages of medications.

The *half-life* of an element is the time necessary for one-half of a given amount of the isotope to decay. Half-lives can range from thousands of millions of years to fractions of a second. The rate at which atomic decay occurs in a particular isotope cannot be altered by any outside force such as temperature, pressure or chemical reaction. The knowledge of the half-life of a particular isotope is essential to the proper handling of the substance for the protection of the medical staff and the animal receiving some form of radiation therapy.

radioallergosorbent test (RAST) a radioimmunoassay for the detection and measurement of specific IgE antibody to a variety of allergens, using antigen fixed in a solid-phase matrix and radiolabeled anti-IgE antibody.

radioautograph autoradiograph.

radioautography autoradiography.

radiobicipital pertaining to the radius and biceps muscle of the forelimb.

radiobiologist an expert in radiobiology.

radiobiology the branch of science concerned with effects of light and of ultraviolet and ionizing radiations on living tissue or organisms. See also RADIOTHERAPY.

radiocardiogram the graphic record produced by radiocardiography.

radiocardiography graphic recording of variation with time of the concentration, in a selected chamber of the heart, of a radioactive isotope, usually injected intravenously.

radiocarpal pertaining to the radius and carpus.

radiochemicals radioactive chemicals such as the isotopes [^{125}I] iodohippurate.

radiochemistry the branch of chemistry dealing with radioactive materials.

radiocinematograph see PHOTOFLUOROGRAPHY.

radiocurability responsiveness to treatment with radiotherapy.

radiocurable curable by radiation.

radiocystitis inflammatory tissue changes in the urinary bladder caused by irradiation. Best called radiation cystitis.

radiodense radiopaque.

radiodensity the property of being relatively resistant to the passage of radiant energy.

radiodermatitis a cutaneous inflammatory reaction to exposure to biologically effective levels of ionizing radiation; x-ray dermatitis.

radiodiagnosis diagnosis by means of x-rays or gamma rays.

radioelectrocardiogram the tracing obtained by radioelectrocardiography.

radioelectrocardiograph the apparatus used in radioelectrocardiography.

radioelectrocardiography the recording of alterations in the electric potential of the heart, with impulses beamed by radio waves from the subject to the recording device by means of a small transmitter attached to the patient.

radioencephalogram a curve showing the passage of an injected tracer through the cerebral blood vessels as revealed by an external scintillation counter.

radioencephalography the recording of changes in the electric potential of the brain without direct attachment between the recording apparatus and the subject, the impulses being beamed by radio waves from the subject to the receiver.

radiofrequency current heating a form of heat therapy in which low-frequency electrical current is passed directly through the tissue being treated, usually skin tumors.

radiogold a radioisotope of gold, especially ^{198}Au, which has a half-life of 2.7 days and emits gamma and beta radiation. See GOLD-198.

radiogram radiograph.

radiograph the film produced by radiography.

scout r. see SURVEY radiograph.

radiographer a RADIOLOGICAL technologist whose work is the making of diagnostic radiographs. Duties depend on legislative constraints but may include positioning animals for radiological examinations; determining the proper voltage, current and exposure time for each radiograph and adjusting the x-ray equipment; the production of radiographs requested by the veterinarian; developing the x-ray film; and assisting the radiologist in special procedures and in the preparation of radiopaque contrast media.

radiographic pertaining to or emanating from radiography.

r. contrast agent see CONTRAST medium.

r. film digestion test a quantitative test for fecal trypsin in which a strip of x-ray film is incubated in an alkaline suspension of feces. Clearing of the film's gel indicates the prescence of trypsin. Used in the diagnosis of exocrine pancreatic insufficiency.

r. geometry relates to the loss of clarity of the radiographic image as the subject moves further away from the film.

r. interpretation translation of the radiographic image into an explanation of the pathology underlying the abnormalities that are observed.

radiography the making of film records (radiographs) of internal structures of the body by exposure of film specially sensitized to x-rays or gamma rays.

body-section r. a special technique to show in detail images and structures lying in a predetermined plane of tissue, while blurring or eliminating detail in images in other planes; various mechanisms and methods for such radiography have been given various names, e.g. laminagraphy, tomography, etc.

contrast r. the use of means of exaggerating the differences in density of tissues or organs or intraluminal filling defects, usually by the introduction of contrast agents.

double contrast r. see double CONTRAST.

intraoral r. small non-screen film is placed in the mouth and x-rays are directed from outside the mouth. Used to assess alveolar bone and roots of teeth.

mucosal relief r. a technique for revealing any abnormality of the intestinal mucosa, involving injection and evacuation of a barium enema, followed by inflation of the intestine with air under light pressure. The light coating of barium on the inflated intestine in the radiograph reveals clearly even small abnormalities.

neutron r. that in which a narrow beam of neutrons from a nuclear reactor is passed through tissues; especially useful in visualizing bony tissue.

scout r. see SURVEY radiograph, STRAIGHT (2).

serial r. the making of several exposures of a particular area at arbitrary intervals.

spot-film r. the making of localized instantaneous radiographic exposures during fluoroscopy.

radiohumeral pertaining to the radius and humerus.

radioimaging see IMAGING.

radioimmunity diminished sensitivity to radiation.

radioimmunoassay a sensitive assay method used for the measurement of minute quantities of specific antibodies or any antigen, such as hormones or drugs, against which specific antibodies can be raised; abbreviated RIA. An assay for a specific hormone uses antihormone antibody produced by injecting the human hormone into an animal, such as a rabbit. In the assay either the antigen or antibody is labeled with radioisotope.

radioimmunodiffusion immunodiffusion conducted with radioisotope-labeled antibodies or antigens.

radioimmunoelectrophoresis electrophoresis in which a particular antigen is identified by adding the corresponding radioactive-labeled antibody and subjecting the gel to autoradiography.

radioimmunosorbent test (RIST) a radioimmunoassay technique for measuring IgE immunoglobulins in serum, using radiolabeled IgE and anti-IgE bound to an insoluble matrix.

radioiodine any radioactive isotope of IODINE.

r. therapy see IODINE-131.

r. uptake t. ^{131}I or ^{125}I are used by oral or intravenous administration as a test of thyroidal function.

radioisotope a radioactive form of an element. A radioisotope consists of unstable atoms that undergo radioactive decay emitting alpha, beta or gamma radiation. Radioisotopes occur naturally, as in the cases of radium and uranium, or may be created artificially. See also RADIONUCLIDE.

Artificial radioisotopes are created by bombarding stable atoms of an element with subatomic particles in a nuclear reactor or in an atom smasher, or cyclotron. When the nucleus of a stable atom is charged by bombarding particles, the atom usually becomes unstable, or radioactive, and is said to be 'labeled' or 'tagged'.

r. organ scanning injection of an isotope and scanning of organs in which the isotope is planned to locate, e.g. radioactive iodine in the thyroid gland.

radiolabeling incorporation of a radioactive element into a compound in order to investigate its metabolism, fate and utilization.

radioligand a radioisotope-labeled substance, e.g. an antigen, used in the quantitative measurement of an unlabelled substance by its binding reaction to a specific antibody or other receptor site.

radiological pertaining to radiology.

r. diagnosis see radiological DIAGNOSIS.

mobile r. apparatus x-ray machines that can be moved but are not portable because of their weight. This is imposed because of the large transformer required to achieve the desired output.

portable r. apparatus can be carried because of the small transformer used. However, the exposure time is prolonged and the image is less clear. The machine is easily dismantled.

r. technologist a health care worker who is skilled in the theory and practice of the technical aspects of the use of x-rays and radioisotopes in the diagnosis and treatment of disease. Radiological technologists can specialize in radiography, radiation therapy or nuclear medicine. See also RADIOGRAPHER, RADIATION therapist. Called also nuclear medicine technologist.

radiologist a specialist in radiology.

radiology the branch of science dealing with use of x-rays, radioactive substances, and other forms of radiant energy in diagnosis and treatment of disease.
veterinary r. dealing with the diseases of animals by radiological methods.
radiolucency the quality of being radiolucent.
radiolucent permitting the passage of radiant energy, such as x-rays, yet offering some resistance to it, the representative areas appearing dark on the exposed film.
radiometer 1. an instrument for estimating x-ray quantity. 2. an instrument in which radiant heat and light may be directly converted into mechanical energy. 3. an instrument for measuring the penetrating power of radiant energy.
radiomimetic producing effects similar to those of ionizing radiations.
radionecrosis, radiation necrosis tissue destruction due to radiant energy.
radioneuritis neuritis from exposure to radiant energy.
radionuclide a radioactive nuclide; one that disintegrates with the emission of corpuscular or electromagnetic radiations. Used in diagnosis for whole body or individual organ scanning. See also RADIOACTIVE isotope, NUCLIDE.
radiopacity the quality or property of obstructing the passage of radiant energy, such as x-rays, the representative areas appearing light or white on the exposed film.
radiopaque not permitting the passage of x-rays, such areas appearing light in color on the x-ray film.
radiopathology the pathology of radiation effects on tissues.
radiopharmaceutical a radioactive pharmaceutical used for diagnostic or therapeutic purposes. See also RADIONUCLIDE.
radiophosphorus either of two radioactive isotopes of phosphorus, ^{32}P and ^{33}P; the former, a pure beta emitter, has a half-life of 14.3 days and is used in solution or colloidal form in erythrocyte studies and in the treatment of polycythemia vera and chronic leukemia in humans.
radiopotentiation the action of a drug in enhancing the effects of irradiation.
radioprotective agents chemicals that reduce the effects of radiation on tissues; may be useful in radiotherapy because of the differential concentration between normal and target (tumor) tissues following parenteral administration.
radioreceptor a receptor for the stimuli that are excited by radiant energy, such as light and heat.
radioresistance resisting the effects of radiation, especially in reference to the treatment of malignancy.
radioresponsive reacting favorably to irradiation.
radioresponsiveness quality of being radioresponsive.
radioscopy fluoroscopy.
radiosensitivity sensitivity, as of the skin, tumor tissue, etc., to radiant energy, such as x-ray or other radiations.
radiosensitization the application of heat therapy as an adjunct to radiotherapy to increase the radiosensitivity of target cells.
radiotelemetry measurement based on data transmitted by radio waves from the subject to the recording apparatus.
radiotherapist a specialist in radiotherapy.
radiotherapy the treatment of disease by ionizing radiation. The purpose of radiation therapy is to deliver an optimal dose of either particulate or electromagnetic radiation to a particular area of the body with minimal damage to normal tissues. The source of radiation may be outside the body of the patient (external radiation therapy) or it may be an isotope that has been implanted or instilled into abnormal tissue or a body cavity. Called also radiation therapy.

Modern radiation therapy primarily uses high-energy x-rays or gamma rays with peak photon energies above 1 MeV. This is called 'supervoltage' or 'megavoltage' therapy. These high voltages are produced by linear accelerators or by cobalt-60 teletherapy units. Megavoltage radiation is more penetrating than lower energy radiation. It produces less damage to the skin at the entry port, is absorbed less in bone, and is scattered less, thus reducing the exposure to tissues outside the x-ray beam. Low-energy x-rays that do not penetrate are used for treatment of superficial skin lesions.

Internal radiation therapy can involve the implantation of sealed radiation sources in or near cancerous tissue. Isotopes, such as radium-226, cesium-137, iridium-192 and iodine-125, are introduced either temporarily or permanently into body tissues (interstitial application) or body cavities (intercavitary application). Permanent sources have a short half-life so that the dose received by the patient is limited. Another form of internal radiation therapy is the administration of radioactive materials into the bloodstream or a body cavity.

See also RADIATION, external BEAM therapy, ORTHOVOLTAGE, BRACHYTHERAPY.
external beam r. see TELETHERAPY.
fractionated r. the full dose is divided and given as a number of separate small treatments.
intraoperative r. the use of radiotherapy during a surgical procedure, usually in the treatment of diffuse neoplasia that cannot be totally removed by surgical methods alone.
supervoltage r., megavoltage r. the use of energy in excess of 500 keV.
radiothermy short-wave diathermy.
radiotoxemia toxemia produced by a radioactive substance, or resulting from radiotherapy.
radiotracer a radioactive tracer.
radiotranslucent radiolucent.
radiotransparent permitting the passage of x-rays or other forms of radiation. See also RADIOLUCENT.
radiotropic influenced by radiation.
radioulnar pertaining to the radius and ulna.
radish see RAPHANUS *sativus*.
radium a chemical element, atomic number 88, atomic weight, 226, symbol Ra. See Table 6. Radium is highly radioactive and is found in uranium minerals. Radium-226 has a half-life of 1622 years. It and its short-lived decay products emit alpha particles, beta particles and gamma rays. One of the decay products, radon-222, is a radioactive gas. In clinical use, radium is contained in a metal container that stops alpha and beta particles and traps radon.

Radium is used in the treatment of malignant diseases, particularly those that are readily accessible, for example, tumors of the eye. In the form of needles or pellets, it can be inserted in the tumorous tissue (interstitial implantation) and left in place until its rays penetrate and destroy malignant cells. It can also be used in the form of plaques applied to the diseased tissue. Large amounts of radium are used as a source of GAMMA rays, which are capable of deep penetration of matter. See also RADIOTHERAPY.
radius pl. *radii* [L.] 1. a line radiating from a center, or

a circular limit defined by a fixed distance from an established point or center. 2. one of the two long bones of the forearm that extends from the lateral side of the elbow to the medial side of the wrist or carpus. See also Table 10.

r. curvus syndrome see CURVUS.

radix pl. *radices* [L.] root.

radon a chemical element, atomic number 86, atomic weight 222, symbol Rn. See Table 6. Radon is a colorless, gaseous, radioactive element produced by the disintegration of radium.

raffinose a crystalline, trisaccharide obtained from cottonseed meal and Australian manna, a substance obtained from a number of eucalypts. Contains dextrose, fructose and galactose. Called also melitose.

Rafinesquia californica toxic plant in the family Asteraceae; causes nitrate–nitrite poisoning; called also California chicory.

rafoxanide a very efficient flukicide which is also effective against *Haemonchus contortus* and *Oestrus ovis*. Available for both oral and injectable administration. There is a good safety margin but poisoning can occur in sheep with heavy doses. There is blindness, with degeneration of the optic nerve, recumbency, polypnea, clonic convulsions and death.

Ragdoll a recently developed breed of cats, derived from Persians, Birmans and Burmese. It is a very large cat with medium to long hair and blue eyes. When held, it relaxes completely, hence the name.

rage 1. a state of violent anger. 2. [Fr.] *rabies*.

sham r. an outburst of motor activity resembling the outward manifestations of fear and anger, occurring in decorticated animals and in certain pathological conditions in humans.

r. syndrome possibly a type of psychomotor seizure, of uncertain etiology; reported in Springer spaniels. Because of the unpredictable and dangerous nature of the episodes or rage, euthanasia is usually advised.

ragged hips defective conformation in a horse characterized by asymmetry, irregularity or ugly prominence of the ilial tuberosities; caused mostly by fractures of the ilium caused by falling.

ragocyte a cell found in the joints in rheumatoid arthritis; RA cell. Such cells are produced when polymorphonuclear leukocytes ingest aggregated IgG immunoglobulin, rheumatoid factor, fibrin and complement. Rare in dogs.

ragpicker's disease anthrax.

ragweed see ARTEMISIA, a name sometimes used for SENECIO but more commonly AMBROSIA ELATIR, or *Franseria discolor* (white ragweed).

ragwort SENECIO *jacobea*, *S. latifolius*, *S. tetrotsus*.

tansy r. see AMBROSIA ELATIR.

Raillietia a genus of mites in the family Gamasidae.

R. auris found on the ears of cattle.

R. australis found in the ears of wombats.

R. caprae found in the ears of goats.

R. hopkinsi found on the ears of antelopes.

Raillietiella a genus of pentastomid internal parasites in the class Pentastomida found in ophidians, lacertilians and birds.

Raillietina a genus of cyclophyllidean tapeworms containing a very large number of species, many of them uncommon. In the family Davaineidae.

R. cesticillus common in domestic poultry.

R. echinobothrida a common finding in the small intestine of chickens and turkeys.

R. georgiensis found in domestic and wild turkeys.

R. magninumida found in guinea fowl.

R. ransomi found in domestic and wild turkey.

R. tetragona found in the posterior small intestine of many birds including domestic fowls.

R. williamsi found in wild turkey.

railroad disease, railroad sickness see TRANSIT tetany.

rain rot see DERMATOPHILOSIS.

rain scald a patchy alopecia and pityriasis on the back and croup of horses without any obvious involvement of the epidermis. Caused by persistent heavy rain in summer months and disappears spontaneously when the weather turns dry. DERMATOPHILOSIS is a much more serious disease with a significant dermatitis.

rainbow lorikeet TRICHOGLOSSUS *haematodus*.

rainbow trout ONCORHYNCHUS *mykiss*.

r. t. fry syndrome severe septicemic condition of rainbow trout fry caused by *Cytophaga psychrophila*.

Rainey's corpuscles cysts of SARCOCYSTIS.

rainworm see MERMIS SUBNIGRESCENS.

rake a grooming instrument, used to comb through thick mats in the haircoat of dogs.

rake marks lacerations which leave parallel scars on the skin.

rakefisk fermented trout, a Scandinavian delicacy, a potent source of botulism in humans.

raking of an elephant—see BACK raking.

rakta karabi NERIUM *indicum*.

rale an abnormal respiratory sound heard in auscultation and indicating some pathological condition. Rales are distinguished as *dry* or *moist*, according to the absence or presence of fluid in the air passages, and are classified according to their site of origin as *bronchial*, *cavernous*, *laryngeal*, *pleural*, *tracheal* and *vesicular* (*crepitant*).

amphoric r. a coarse, musical and tinkling rale due to the splashing of fluid in a cavity connected with a bronchus.

atelectatic r. a nonpathological rale which is dissipated by deep breathing or coughing. Such rales are frequently heard in those who breathe feebly and superficially, when on deep inspiration the moist walls of the unexpanded alveoli are suddenly forced apart by the entering air; after a few deep inspirations such rales become lost.

bubbling r. a moist rale, finer than a subcrepitant rale, heard in bronchitis, in the resolving stage of pneumonia, and over small cavities.

cavernous r. a hollow and metallic rale caused by the alternate expansion and contraction of a pulmonary cavity during respiration.

cellophane r. a dry, crackling chest sound, as heard in interstitial pulmonary emphysema.

clicking r. a small sticky sound heard on inspiration, due to the passage of air through secretions in the smaller bronchi.

consonating r. a clear, ringing sound produced in bronchial tubes that are surrounded by consolidation tissue.

crepitant r. a very fine crackling rale.

dry r. a rale produced by the presence of viscid secretion in the bronchial tubes, or by spastic contraction of the walls of the tubes; it has a whistling, musical or squeaking quality.

gurgling r. a very coarse rale resembling the bursting of large bubbles; in pulmonary edema, heard over large cavities that contain fluid, and in the trachea in the 'death rattle'.

sibilant r. a hissing sound resembling that produced by suddenly separating two oiled surfaces. It is produced by the presence of a viscid secretion in the bronchial tubes or by thickening of the walls of the tubes; heard in asthma and bronchitis.

subcrepitant r. a fine, moist rale associated with fluid in the bronchioles.
ralgro synthetic zearalenol, an estrogen, used commercially as a growth promotant, capable of causing hyperestrogenism.
RAM random access memory.
ram male, entire sheep which has attained sexual maturity at about the age of 6 months.
r. effect introduction of a ram into a flock of nonpregnant ewes in the period between deep anestrus and the commencement of the breeding season tends to advance the onset of estrus and enhances its synchronization.
r. epididymitis ovine BRUCELLOSIS.
r. mating harness leather or webbing harness worn around the forequarters and carrying a marking crayon or paint pad on the brisket to mark the rumps of ewes that have been mated.
stud r. pedigree ram used to mate with purebred ewes.
teaser r. vasectomized ram. See also TEASER.
ramal pertaining to a ramus.
Ramaria a genus of macrofungi of the class Basidiomycetes (Clavariaceae). Their fruiting bodies contain an unidentified toxin which causes death in cattle. Signs include salivation, mucosal erosions, ocular lesions and abortion. See also MAL do eucalipto. Called also fairy clubs, coral fungus.
Rambouillet French fine-woolled, merino sheep; males are horned, females polled.
rami [L.] plural of *ramus*.
r. communicantes bundles of nerve fibers connecting a sympathetic ganglion to spinal nerve; categorized as gray rami (unmyelinated postganglionic fibers) or white rami (myelinated preganglionic fibers).
ramification 1. distribution in branches. 2. a branch or set of branches.
ramify 1. to branch; to diverge in different directions. 2. to traverse in branches.
ramisection section of the appropriate rami communicantes of the sympathetic nervous system.
ramitis inflammation of a ramus.
ramose branching; having many branches.
Ramphastos see TOUCAN.
Rampley forceps obstetrical forceps for use in dogs and cats. Scissors type with ratchet handles and blades which end in loops suitable for grasping a fetal head.
ram's horn tree see ACACIA *osswaldii*.
Ramstedt operation longitudinal incision through the serosa and sphincter muscles at the pyolorus in order to relax a stenotic or closed-by-spasm sphincter. Called also Fredet–Ramstedt operation. See also PYLOROMYOTOMY.
ramulus pl. *ramuli* [L.] a small branch or terminal division.
ramus pl. *rami* [L.] a branch, as of a nerve, vein or artery.
r. communicans pl. *rami communicantes;* a branch connecting two nerves or two arteries.
mandibular r. the vertical extension of each half of the mandible that ends at the coronoid process.
RANA abbreviation for Registered Animal Nursing Auxiliary in the UK. Used as a qualification by persons admitted to its membership.
Rana a genus of amphibians in the family Ranidae. The genus of frogs.
R. catesbeiana American bullfrog; farmed commercially to produce frog meat for human consumption.
R. clamitans green frog.
R. pipiens leopard frog.
Ranavirus a genus of viruses in the family *Iridoviridae* that cause disease in amphibians. In frogs, it causes death in tadpoles.
ranch extensive grazing or pastoral farm or holding. See also RANGE (2). Called also station, run, selection.
r. cattle brood cows, commercial cattle used for producing young cattle for fattening.
rancid having a musty, rank taste or smell; applied to fats that have undergone decomposition, with the liberation of fatty acids.
rancidity the state of being rancid.
random unplanned, without direction or purpose.
r. assignment see RANDOMIZATION.
r. mating where each member of the population has an equal opportunity of mating with every member of the opposite sex.
r. numbers a list of numbers obtained by a standard randomization procedure; used commonly to select individual animals from a pack.
r. sample see random SAMPLE.
r. sampling a procedure for selecting units from a group in such a way that each unit has an equal chance of being selected in the sample.
r. selection selection in such a way as to produce a random SAMPLE.
r. variable a group or quantity that takes various values, each with varying probabilities.
random access memory see computer MEMORY; abbreviated RAM.
randomization the performance of a function, e.g. selection, in a random manner.
randy budgie syndrome mating behavior seen in caged budgerigars; it includes courtship feeding and regurgitation, attempts to copulate with inanimate objects or humans.
range 1. the difference between the upper and lower limits of a variable or of a series of values. 2. extensive grazing land which provides seasonal feed supply of pasture comprising grasses and clovers and other legumes supplemented by forbs and browse. 3. a husbandry system where animals are permitted to roam free, within reasonable limits, i.e. they are not confined in corrals, lots, yards, houses, barns, byres and the like. Called also free range. 4. animals maintained as in 3 above, e.g. range cattle. Called also range-reared.
r. of audibility the range between the extreme frequencies of sound waves beyond which the ear of each species perceives no sound.
r. cubes large pellets of compacted feed, between a pellet and a log, approximately 1 inch cubed, used to feed animals at pasture. Can be fed on the ground with very little loss.
free r. see (3) (above).
r. goldenrod SOLIDAGO *mollis*.
r. of motion the range, measured in degrees of a circle, through which a joint can be extended and flexed. See also range of motion exercises (below).
r. of motion exercises exercises calculated to extend the range of extension and flexion of an impaired joint.
r. paralysis see MAREK'S DISEASE.
r.-reared see range (3 above).
r. stiffness a disease of lambs. See BLUETONGUE.
Rangifer tarandus see REINDEER.
rangiora see BRACHYGLOTTIS *repanda*.
rangy a term describing conformation; generally a light frame with long body and legs.
ranikhet disease see NEWCASTLE DISEASE.
ranine pertaining to (1) a frog; (2) a ranula, or to the lower surface of the tongue; (3) the sublingual vein.

ranitidine a histamine H_2-blocking agent used in the treatment of gastric ulceration and chronic hypertrophic gastritis.

rank the place in a series occupied by a value when the series has been set in order according to a particular trait, usually size. Called also order statistic.

r. sum test nonparametrical statistical test used to compare two methods by seeing if one method contributes more to the higher ranked values.

Ranke primary complex the initial lesion plus the lesion in the regional lymph node in a case of tuberculosis.

ranking arranging units, e.g. cows, in order according to a predetermined criterion e.g. milk production, with the superior unit first in the list.

ransoms ALLIUM *ursinum*.

ranula a cystic enlargement beneath the tongue due to obstruction and dilatation of the sublingual or submaxillary gland.

pancreatic r. a retention cyst of the pancreatic duct.

ranunculin glycosidic precursor for PROTOANEMONIN; found in *Anemone* spp.

Ranunculus a very large plant genus of family Ranunculaceae; the buttercups. All of them should be regarded as potentially poisonous. The species listed below have been reported as causing poisoning in animals. They contain protoanemonin glycosides which cause abdominal pain, convulsions, stomatitis, diarrhea. See also PROTOANEMONIN.

R. abortivus (small-flowered buttercup), *R. acris* (tall buttercup), *R. bulbosus* (bulbous buttercup), *R. colonorum*, *R. cymbalaria*, *R. ficaria* (lesser celandine), *R. flammula* (spearwort), *R. inundatus*, *R. lingua* (greater spearwort), *R. multifidus*, *R. parviflorus* (small-flowered buttercup), *R. pentandrus*, *R. pumilio*, *R. repens* (creeping buttercup), *R. rivularis* (*R. amphitrichus*, river buttercup), *R. sceleratus* (celery buttercup, cursed crowfoot, poison buttercup), *R. sessiliflorus*, *R. testiculatus* (burr buttercup), *R. undosus*.

Ranvier node see NODE of Ranvier.

rapamycin a macrolide compound obtained from *Streptomyces hygroscopicus* used as an immunosuppressant in tissue transplantation.

rape see BRASSICA *napus*.

r. blindness a manifestation of polioencephalomalacia in ruminants caused by ingestion of *Brassica napus*; characterized by compulsive walking, head pressing, behavior indicating impaired vision.

rapeseed the seed of Target rape grown specifically for the seed and its oil.

r. meal as oil cake or meal after rapeseed oil is removed this is a high-protein feed supplement used in cattle. It can be goitrogenic because of its content of isothiocyanate but can be detoxified.

Raphanus a plant genus in the family Brassicaceae; contains the poisonous principle *S*-methylcysteine sulfoxide and causes poisoning characterized by hemoglobinuria, jaundice, diarrhea and liver damage.

R. raphanistrum called also jointed charlock, wild radish.

R. sativus may contain toxic amounts of nitrate. The culinary radish.

raphe a seam; line of union of the halves of various symmetrical parts.

abdominal r. linea alba.

r. nuclei small group of serotenergic cells in the midline of the brainstem; may be involved in the initiation of sleep.

raphide needle-like microscopic crystals of calcium oxalate found in plants (*Dieffenbachia*, *Philodendron*, *Zantedescgia*, *Colocasia*, *Alocasia* spp.); reputedly capable of causing painful laceration of the tongue.

Rapistrum rugosum member of the plant family Brassicaceae; contains goitrogenic glucosinolates which cause goiter; may also cause polioencephalomalacia; called also wild turnip, turnip weed.

Rapoport–Luebering cycle see 2,3-BISPHOSPHOGLYCERATE pathway.

Rappaport's acinus the modern and current concept of structural function in the liver is based on this description of the hepatic acinus.

raptor a predator; an animal or bird adapted for capturing prey. Usually limited in its application to birds of prey.

rare-earth intensifying screen see rare-earth INTENSIFYING SCREEN.

rarefaction the condition of being or becoming less dense.

rash a temporary eruption on the skin.

drug r. dermatitis medicamentosa.

rasp a flat, round-toothed instrument used to débride the surface of hard materials such as teeth, bones, hooves.

bone r. for trimming rough ends of bone prior to repair of a fracture. See also PUTTI RASP.

hoof r. for fine trimming of hoof while shoeing a horse.

tooth r. used for smoothing teeth in horses. See FILING TEETH.

raspweed, raspwort see HALORAGIS *heterophylla*.

RAST radioallergosorbent test.

rat small, furred mammal; members of the family Murinae (Old World rats) and the family Cricetinae (New World rats) both of the order Rodentia. They are omnivorous, nocturnal, do not hibernate and live commensally with humans. They have pointed snouts, a long, thin, almost hairless tail. Only some of the members of the rat and allied groups are listed below.

r. bite fever STREPTOBACILLUS *moniliformis*.

black r. Old World rat with long tail and ears. Called also *Rattus rattus*.

brown r. Old World rat with short tail and ears. Called also *Rattus norvegicus*.

r. flea see LEPTOPSYLLA SEGNIS.

kangaroo r. a solitary rodent with long legs with which it progresses in leaps like a kangaroo and uses its large tail as a balancer. Called also *Dipodomys deserti*.

r. leprosy a chronic, largely cutaneous disease of rats caused by *Mycobacterium lepraemurium* and characterized by subcutaneous granuloma and similar involvement of superficial lymph nodes, containing large numbers of acid-fast organisms. The disease has little similarity to nor any relationship with human leprosy. See also FELINE leprosy.

Long–Evans r. laboratory rat with brown or black head and shoulders.

musk r. properly called muskrat and is really a water vole. Called also *Ondatra zibethica*.

pack r. New World rat-like creature. Called also *Neotoma* spp., wood rat.

sand r. see GERBIL.

Sprague–Dawley r. albino laboratory rat.

water r. properly called water vole; in Australia, water rat is a native rodent *Hydromys chrysogaster*.

white r. common laboratory rat.

Wistar r. a white laboratory rat.

rat-tail syndrome see SARCOCYSTOSIS.

rat-tailed maggot larva of *Eristalis* spp., a hover fly of no veterinary importance other than in confusing an identification. Called also filth fly. The maggots are found in areas with high concentrations of organic matter, e.g. stable drains.

rat terrier see MANCHESTER TERRIER.

rat-tooth pointed projections (teeth) on the tips of some surgical instruments, particularly forceps, which intermesh when brought together, for grasping tissue with a minimum of trauma or crushing.

ratchet a steplocking device on surgical instruments. As the handles are closed the jaws are also closed and the ratchet holds them in a locked position. The ratchet consists of a notched bar on each handle, the notches facing and overriding when the handles are closed.

rate the frequency with which an event or circumstance occurs per unit of time.

attack r. the proportion of a population affected by a specific condition during a prescribed, usually short, period of time.

attribute-specific r. the rate of occurrence of a specific attribute.

basal metabolic r. (BMR) an expression of the rate at which oxygen is utilized in a fasting subject at complete rest as a percentage of a value established as normal for such a subject.

birth r. the number of births during one year for the total population (crude birth rate), for the female population (refined birth rate), or for the female population of reproductive age (true birth rate).

case r. morbidity rate.

case fatality r. the number of deaths due to a specific disease as compared with the total number of cases of the disease.

cohort r. the rate of occurrence of e.g. disease in cohorts.

death r. the number of deaths per stated number of animals (1000 or 10,000 or 100,000) in a certain region in a certain time period.

erythrocyte sedimentation r. (ESR) see ERYTHROCYTE sedimentation rate.

fatality r. the number of deaths caused by a specific circumstance or disease, expressed as the absolute or relative number among individuals encountering the circumstance or having the disease.

five-year survival r. an expression of the number of survivors with no trace of disease 5 years after each has been diagnosed or treated for the same disease.

forced expiratory flow r. (FEF) see maximal expiratory flow rate (below).

glomerular filtration r. an expression of the quantity of glomerular filtrate formed each minute in the nephrons of both kidneys, calculated by measuring the clearance of specific substances, e.g. inulin or creatinine.

growth r. an expression of the increase in size of an organic object per unit of time.

heart r. the number of contractions of the cardiac ventricles per unit of time.

incidence r. describes the probability of a new case occurring during a stated time interval.

infection r. percentage of the population from which a specific infectious pathogen is isolated.

r.-limiting enzymes rate controlling enzymic steps in metabolic pathways. Often allosteric enzymes with allosteric effector sites but can be controlled through substrate availability, product removal or enzyme concentration.

maximal expiratory flow r. (MEFR) the slope of the line connecting the points 200 ml and 1200 ml on the forced expiratory volume curve. See also PULMONARY function tests. Called also $FEF_{200-1200}$.

metabolic r. an expression of the amount of oxygen consumed by the body cells.

morbidity r. the number of cases of a given disease occurring in a specified period per unit of population.

mortality r. death rate; the mortality rate of a disease is the ratio of the number of deaths from a given disease to the total number of cases of that disease.

reactor r. percentage of reactors in a tested population.

respiration r. the number of movements of the chest wall per unit of time, indicative of inspiration and expiration.

response r. see RESPONSE.

risk r. see RELATIVE risk.

sedimentation r. the rate at which a sediment is deposited in a given volume of solution, especially when subjected to the action of a centrifuge. See also SEDIMENTATION rate.

specific r. expresses the frequency of a characteristic per unit of the population.

r. standardization adaptation of a rate so that the conditions under which it occurred are comparable with those in which other rates have been estimated. There are several methods, e.g. the equivalent average death rate.

Rathke's pouch, cleft, pocket a diverticulum from the embryonic buccal cavity from which the anterior pituitary is developed.

R. pouch cyst failure of the ectoderm of Rathke's pouch to differentiate into adenohypophyseal tissue. A cyst fills the space normally occupied by the pituitary gland and the animal is a dwarf with panhypopituitarism.

ratio [L.] an expression of the quantity of one substance or entity in relation to that of another; the relationship between two quantities expressed as the quotient of one divided by the other. It differs from a proportion in that the numerator is not included in the denominator. Thus $x/(x + y)$ is a proportion, $x:y$ is a ratio.

A–G r. ALBUMIN–globulin ratio.

area–incidence r. the number of new cases of a specific disease in a population during a specified time period, divided by the geographic area size in which the observations are made, multiplied by the time elapsed, e.g. cases per hectare per month.

arm r. a figure expressing the relation of the length of the longer arm of a mitotic chromosome to that of the shorter arm.

A/S r. the diameter of the ascending aorta divided by the diameter of the aorta at the sinus of Valsalva; less than 1 in a normal dog. In subaortic stenosis it becomes greater than 1.

cardiothoracic r. the ratio of the transverse diameter of the heart to the internal diameter of the chest at its widest point just anterior to the dome of the diaphragm.

cross r. see ODDS ratio.

fetal death r. the number of fetal deaths divided by the number of live births.

gain r. individual animal's gain/average gain in group × 100.

lecithin–sphingomyelin r. the ratio of lecithin to sphingomyelin in amniotic fluid. See also LECITHIN, SPHINGOMYELIN.

odds r. see ODDS ratio.

rates r. the ratio between two rates. See ODDS ratio and relative risk ratio (below).

relative risk r. the ratio between the rate (of mortality or some such parameter) in one group of animals and the rate in another group, used as a standard and the comparison expressed as a ratio. See also RELATIVE risk.

sex r. the number of males in a population per number of females, usually stated as the number of males per 100 females.

S/P ratio secondary-to-primary ratio. An indicator of fleece type in sheep, the greater the ratio the finer the fleece. Coarse-wool sheep have ratios of 3:1 to 4:1; merinos have a ratio of 20:1.

stillbirth r. the ratio of stillbirths to total births in the population.

urea excretion r. the ratio of the amount of urea in the urine excreted in one hour to the amount in 100 ml of blood. The normal ratio is 50.

ration a fixed allowance of total feed for an animal for one day. Usually specifies the individual ingredients and their amounts and the amounts of the specific nutriments such as carbohydrate, fiber, individual minerals and vitamins. See also BLENDED RATIONS, CREEP ration, CUT-AND-FIT RATION BALANCING.

r. analysis chemical analysis to determine the proportions of principal nutrients in the feed; no tests of digestibility are included.

balanced r. a ration which has been balanced so that it contains appropriate proportions of the principal nutritional components, that is carbohydrates, protein, fat, minerals and vitamins, for the specific class, including especially age and lactational status, of livestock for which the ration is formulated.

complete r. all of the constituents of a ration fed to a confined animal are mixed together and fed at the one time. It does not require supplementation other than drinking water.

r. formulation the recipe; list and amounts of feed ingredients to be included in a ration.

rational based upon reason.

r. deductive diagnosis a diagnosis based on rationalization of the signs with pathological and epidemiological principles, as distinct from empirical diagnosis.

ratite a running bird with flat, raft-like sternum and strong muscular legs, e.g. ostrich.

ratsbane DICHAPETALUM *toxicarium.*

rattle bush CROTALARIA *burkeana.*

rattlebox SESBANIA *punicea, S. drummondii.*

rattlebrush SESBANIA *drummondii.*

rattlepod see CROTALARIA.

rattles vernacular for purulent bronchopneumonia in foals with pneumonia caused by *Rhodococcus equi*; name derived from the moist, loud crackles heard on auscultation of the lungs.

rattlesnake a snake of the genera *Crotalus* or *Sisustrus,* both members of the family Crotalidae and of the series Splenoglypha which have movable fangs. Rattlesnakes are characterized by the retention of dried skin segments at the end of the tail which give them their ominous rattle. The bites of these snakes cause severe local inflammation with much tissue destruction. See also SNAKEBITE.

rattleweed ASTRAGALUS *diphysus.*

Rattus see RAT.

R. norwegicus see brown RAT.

R. rattus see black RAT.

rauwolfia, *Rauvolfia* any member of the genus *Rauwolfia* in the plant family Apocynaceae; the dried root, or extract of the dried root, of *Rauwolfia*; contains reserpine; causes abdominal pain, diarrhea, jaundice, hepatitis; includes *R. serpentina, R. tetraphylla* (*R. canescens*), *R. vomitoria.*

RAVC Royal Army Veterinary Corps.

raven's beak the coracoid bone in the bird.

raw in its natural state; uncooked; unaltered.

r. data see raw DATA.

r. fiber see FIBER[2].

rawhide untanned cattle hide. Used in manufacture of stiff lariats, hackamores. Stretches and becomes malleable when soaked.

ray a line emanating from a center, as a more or less distinct portion of radiant energy (light or heat), proceeding in a specific direction.

alpha r's, α-r's high-speed helium nuclei ejected from radioactive substances; they have less penetrating power than beta rays. See also ALPHA particles.

beta r's, β-r's, beta particles electrons ejected from radioactive substances with velocities as high as 0.98 of the velocity of light; they have more penetrating power than alpha rays, but less than gamma rays.

digital r. a digit of the hand or foot and corresponding metacarpal or metatarsal bone, regarded as a continuous unit.

r. fungus branched filamentous appearance of *Actinomyces bovis* in granules in pus.

gamma r's, γ-r's electromagnetic radiation of short wavelengths emitted by an atomic nucleus during a nuclear reaction, consisting of high-energy photons, having no mass and no electric charge, and traveling with the speed of light and with great penetrating power.

They have very great range in penetrating tissues and cytotoxic effects, especially on nuclei and on tissues which are replicating rapidly. The fetus, bone marrow, blood, liver and gonads are particularly susceptible. See also RADIATION injury, RADIATION therapy.

medullary r. a cortical extension of a bundle of tubules from a renal pyramid.

roentgen r's x-rays.

x-r's see X-RAY.

rayless goldenrod HAPLOPAPPUS *heterophyllus.*

razor back a fault in conformation of any modern farm animal; a sharp-ridged backbone produced by long spinous processes of the vertebrae and scant longissimus dorsi muscles.

razor-billed Auk see ALCA TORDA.

razorbill see ALCA TORDA.

Rb chemical symbol, *rubidium.*

RBC red blood cells; red blood (cell) count (see BLOOD COUNT).

RBE relative biological effectiveness; effectiveness of absorbed doses of radiation delivered by different types of radiation. The unit RBE is the SIEVERT which has replaced the REM.

RCVS Royal College of Veterinary Surgeons of the United Kingdom.

Rd see RUTHERFORD.

RD114 virus an endogenous retrovirus of cats, not associated with disease.

RDA recommended daily (nutritional) allowance.

RDS respiratory distress syndrome.

RE reticuloendothelial.

Re chemical symbol, *rhenium.*

reabsorb to absorb again; to undergo or to subject to reabsorption; to resorb.

reabsorption 1. the act or process of absorbing again, as the absorption by the kidneys of substances (glucose, proteins, sodium, etc.) already secreted into the renal tubules. 2. resorption.

reach the distance covered with each stride.

react 1. to respond to a stimulus. 2. to enter into chemical action.

reactant a substance which takes part in a reaction and is altered by it.

reaction 1. opposite action or counteraction; the response of a part to stimulation. 2. the phenomena caused by the action of chemical agents; a chemical process in which one substance is transformed into another substance or substances.
chain r. one which is self-propagating; a chemical process in which each time a free radical is destroyed a new one is formed.
coupled r. one in which the free energy released by one chemical reaction drives the other reaction.
dark r. photosynthetic reaction which fixes CO_2 into sugar and which occurs without exposure to light. Called also Calvin cycle.
r. of degeneration the reaction to electrical stimulation of muscles whose nerves have degenerated, consisting of loss of response to a faradic stimulation in a muscle, and to galvanic and faradic stimulation in the nerve.
delayed r. a reaction, such as an allergic reaction, occurring hours to days after exposure to an inducer.
false negative r. an erroneously negative reaction to a test.
false positive r. an erroneously positive reaction to a test.
first set r. see REJECTION.
immune r. 1. IMMUNE response; see also IMMUNITY. 2. formation of a papule and areola without development of a vesicle following smallpox vaccination.
lengthening r. reflex elongation of extensor muscles that permits flexion of a limb.
leukemic r., leukemoid r. a peripheral blood picture resembling leukemia or indistinguishable from it on the basis of morphological appearance alone, characterized by immature leukocytes in the blood.
r. pattern analysis designed to replace archaic, nonspecific descriptions of the reactions of the skin to noxious influences; recommended categories are (1) perivascular dermatitis, (2) interface dermatitis, (3) vasculitis, (4) nodular and diffuse dermatitis, (5) intradermal vesicular and pustular dermatitis, (6) subepidermal vesicular and pustular dermatitis, (7) perifolliculitis, folliculitis and furunculosis, (8) fibrosing dermatitis, (9) panniculitis, (10) atrophic dermatosis, (11) mixed reaction patterns.
second set r. see REJECTION.
r. specificity lack of production of by-products in enzymatic reactions with yields of products being nearly 100%.
Strauss r. development of suppurative peritonitis, localized to the scrotal sac, in the guinea pig after the intraperitoneal injection of material containing *Burkholderia mallei.*
stress r. 1. alarm reaction. 2. gross stress reaction.
r. time the time elapsing between the application of a stimulus and the resulting reaction.
wheal–flare r. a cutaneous sensitivity rection to skin injury or administration of antigen, due to histamine production and marked by edematous elevation and erythematous flare.

reactivation to become active after a period of quiescence or, as in bacterial and viral infections, latency.
cross r. in immunology, the capacity of an antibody made in response to one antigen including microorganisms to recognize other, different antigens; the two antigens share common antigenic sites (epitopes).
multiplicity r. in virology, a population of viruses that has been inactivated, say by irradiation, may when introduced into a cell at high multiplicity of infection, replicate because of complementation between different member viruses in the inactivated population.

reactor an animal that reacts positively to a particular test.
false positive r. an animal that does not have the subject disease but reacts positively to a test for it.

read only memory see computer MEMORY; abbreviated ROM.

read-through transcription DNA or translation of RNA that proceeds past the point of termination because of the absence of a terminal signal.

read–write head the part of the disk drive of a computer that actually reads or writes down to or from the disk.

readiness response see AROUSAL.

reading frame the actual codons that are translated (read) during mRNA synthesis. In principle a DNA sequence can be transcribed in any one of three different reading frames, each of which will specify a completely different polypeptide. Usually only one of the three reading frames is transcribed.
open r. f. (ORF) an extended sequence in mRNA that is free of stop codons.

reagent a substance used to produce a chemical reaction so as to detect, measure, produce, etc., other substances.

reagin an old term for immunoglobulin E antibody (IgE).
atopic r. the antibody responsible for hypersensitivity reactions to specific substances with signs of atopy resulting.

reaginic pertaining to reagin.
r. antibody immunoglobulin E.

real prevalence a technique of measuring prevalence. It is needed because of the significant errors in estimation of prevalence when the definitive test has high sensitivity but low specificity. When S_e = selectivity, S_p = specificity, the real prevalence (RP) can be estimated from the apparent prevalence (AP) by the formula:

$$RP = \frac{(AP + S_p - 1)}{(S_p + S_e - 1)}$$

real time a term used to describe the making of electronic observations and the processing of them while the data is being collected rather than later.
r. t. computer program a program in which the analyses and computation are made while the user is using the computer; an interactive program.

real-time scanning see real-time ULTRASONOGRAPHY.

realgar a naturally occurring deposit of arsenic disulfide, used as a pigment and a potential source of poisoning in animals.

reamer an instrument used to enlarge the diameter of a pulp cavity in the practice of endodontics.

reannealing see RENATURATION.

rear[1] hind, as in limb.

rear[2] 1. feeding of a sucking animal that is not able to survive without milk or milk replacer. Called also hand-rearing. See also ARTIFICIAL rearing. 2. in a horse, to stand up on its hindlimbs with the spine almost vertical.

reasonable person see reasonable person PRINCIPLE.

reasonable veterinarian see reasonable person PRINCIPLE.

reassortment see RECOMBINATION.

reata [Span.] *lasso.*

reboot restarting the computer after it hangs.

rebreathing bag conductive rubber, reservoir bag in a circle system gas anesthesia machine. It can be used to assist ventilation manually or to completely control respiration in open-chest surgery.

rebreeding the practice of mating the female two or

more times during the one estrous period; applicable only to controlled breeding systems, especially artificial insemination of dairy cows. Called also double MATING.

recapitulation theory ontogeny recapitulates phylogeny, e.g. an organism, in the course of its development goes through the same successive stages (in abbreviated form) as did the species in its evolutionary development.

receiver operating characteristic curve see ROC CURVE.

receptacle of the deferent duct slight terminal enlargement of the avian deferent duct.

receptaculum pl. *receptacula* [L.] a vessel or receptacle.

r. chyli cisterna chyli.

receptive field an area of the body surface over which a single sensory receptor, or its afferent nerve fiber, is capable of sensing stimuli. In some body area, e.g. face, ears, front paws, the sensitive areas are small; over the back they are larger.

receptor 1. a molecule on the surface or within a cell that recognizes and binds with specific molecules, producing some effect in the cell, e.g. the cell-surface receptors of immunocompetent cells that recognize antigens, complement components or lymphokines, or those of neurons and target organs that recognize neurotransmitters or hormones; see also OPIOID receptors. 2. a sensory nerve ending that responds to various stimuli, e.g. arterial stretch, baroreceptors, cold, Golgi tendon organs, joint, muscle and tendon, olfactory, retinal, taste and warmth.

r. activation the cell of a sensory receptor responds to a specific energy change in its environment and initiates a corresponding sensory input.

adrenergic r's receptors for epinephrine or norepinephrine, such as those on effector organs innervated by postganglionic adrenergic fibers of the sympathetic nervous system. Classified as α-adrenergic receptors, which are stimulated by norepinephrine, and β-adrenergic receptors, which are stimulated by epinephrine. See also ADRENERGIC receptors.

autonomic r's. includes adrenergic and muscarinic receptors.

cholinergic r's receptor sites on effector organs innervated by cholinergic nerve fibers and which respond to the acetylcholine secreted by these fibers. There are two types: MUSCARINIC receptors and NICOTINIC receptors.

complement r. a cell-surface receptor capable of binding activated complement components. For example, component C3b is bound to neutrophils, B lymphocytes and macrophages.

dopamine r's. there are dopamine-inhibitory and dopamine-excitatory receptors.

drug r. a component of tissue with which a drug reacts. Classified according to the type of drugs that react with them.

Fc r. bind immunoglobulins via Fc part of the molecule.

histamine r's receptors for histamine, classified as *H_1-receptors*, which produce bronchoconstriction and contraction of the gut and are blocked by antihistamines, such as mepyramine or chlorpheniramine, and *H_2-receptors*, which produce gastric acid secretion and are blocked by H_2-receptor blockers, such as cimetidine.

muscarinic r. see MUSCARINIC receptors.

nicotinic r. see NICOTINIC receptors.

peripheral r. sensory receptors including cutaneous warm and cold, dermoreceptors touch and pain plus receptors in the mucosae.

sensory r. an endorgan at the end of an afferent neuron which is capable of stimulation by a specific change, physical or chemical, in the internal or external environment of the patient.

r. tyrosine kinases a large class of cell-surface receptors with tyrosine-specific protein kinase activity.

receptor adaptation see receptor ADAPTATION.

recess a small, empty space or cavity.

costodiaphragmatic r. the largest of the pleural recesses, lying between the diaphragm and the thoracic wall into which the basal border of the lung encroaches during inspiration.

costomediastinal r. a pleural recess between the mediastinum and costal wall into which the ventral border of the lung encroaches during inspiration.

hepatomesenteric r. the part of the celomic cavity confined between the stomach and the right lobe of the liver, the vestibule of the omental bursa.

maxillary r. a modified form of maxillary sinus in the dog. It communicates with the ventral nasal meatus.

mesenterico-enteric r. a pouch of the omental bursa.

neurohypophyseal r. the pouch of the third ventricle that protrudes into the stalk of the pituitary gland.

pharyngeal r. dorsal and caudal to the orifice of the auditory tube in the pharynx of the ruminant.

pleural r. one of the potential spaces within the thorax where two layers of parietal pleura lie in close apposition. The borders of the lung extend into the pleural recesses during inspiration; pleural effusions fill them.

pyriform r. paired gutters which run beside the anterior projection of the larynx and below the epiglottis, into the pharynx.

supraomental r. formed by the caudal suspensions of the omentum to the rumen and dorsal abdominal walls in the ruminant abdomen.

terminal r. of the kidney tubular extensions of the renal pelvis of horses which receive collecting ducts.

recessive gene a gene which expresses itself in the homozygous state, but not in the presence of the dominant allele.

recessus pl. *recessus* [L.] a recess.

recidiva leishmaniasis cutaneous LEISHMANIASIS.

recidivation the relapse or recurrence of a disease.

recipe [L.] 1. take; used at the head of a prescription, indicated by the symbol ℞. 2. a formula for the preparation of a combination of ingredients.

recipient an animal which receives a blood transfusion, or a tissue or organ graft.

reciprocal mathematically the reciprocal of x is 1/x. See also TRANSLOCATION.

r. crosses matings of two phenotypes in which both the male and the female of both phenotypes are crossed, usually to detect sex linkage.

reciprocating grid see reciprocating GRID.

reciprocity in terms of international registration of veterinarians refers to the agreement between countries for reciprocal acceptance of each other's qualifications for registration. The members of the European Economic Community have such an agreement.

reclamation disease a disease of oat cereal plants which indicates a deficiency of copper in the soil.

recognin any of a group of protein fragments produced from cancer cells that are capable of recognizing specific cells; they include astrocytin and malignin.

recognition 1. the act of recognizing or state of being recognized. 2. in immunology, a term used to describe the functional changes occurring in immunologically competent cells on contact with antigen, involving antigen binding with a receptor on the cell surface. Called also antigen recognition.
r. sequence most recognition sequences used by restriction enzymes are palindromes, some enzymes have more than one recognition sequence and some have nonpalindrome recognition sequences and may cut several nucleotides away from the recognition sequence. See also PALINDROME.
r. site see RESTRICTION SITE.

recombinant 1. the new cell or individual that derives some of its genetic material from one parent and some from another, genetically different parent. 2. pertaining or relating to such cells or individuals.
r. DNA technology a mixture of technologies developed in the 1970s that include (a) specific cleavage of DNA by restriction endonucleases; (b) nucleic acid hybridization which makes it possible to identify specific sequences of DNA or RNA; (c) DNA cloning whereby a specific DNA fragment is integrated (spliced) into a rapidly replicating, high yielding genetic element (plasmid or virus) so that it can be amplified in bacteria or yeast; (d) DNA sequencing of the nucleotides in a cloned DNA fragment.

recombinase a function of the recA protein in *Escherichia coli* that catalyzes the binding and unwinding of the double strands of DNA that form a synapse during DNA recombination.

recombination the reunion, in the same or different arrangement, of formerly united elements that have been separated; in genetics, the formation of new gene combinations due to crossing over by homologous chromosomes. Recombination occurs between viruses such as influenza or bluetongue which have segmented genomes. Called also reassortment.
r. frequency the frequency of exchange between two genes on the same chromosome.

recommended daily allowance the amount of each nutrient that provides for the animal's nutritional requirements; abbreviated RDA. It is greater than the minimum daily requirement (MDR), allowing for individual variation.

recompression return to normal environmental pressure after exposure to greatly diminished pressure.

recon the smallest unit of genetic material capable of recombination.

reconstruction to reassemble or re-form from constituent parts, such as the mathematical process by which an image is assembled from a series of projections in computed TOMOGRAPHY.

reconstructive surgery surgery to rebuild damaged or lost structure, e.g. rectovaginal fistula.

record 1. a permanent or long-lasting account of something (as on film, in writing, etc.); see also MEDICAL records. 2. in computer terminology, a group of fields of information that relate to a particular client or animal; a row in a database TABLE.
fixed-length r. a common fixed length for all records in a program is predetermined and that space is consumed by a record whether it fills it or not. The length of the record must be based on the maximum possible length of the record. The system can be a very wasteful of space if the maximum length is overestimated.

recorder jar graduated measuring jar at each unit on a milking machine designed to measure the milk yield of each cow during milking.

recovery return to normal after illness or period of devitalization, e.g. anesthesia, surgery.
r. period period after surgery when the patient needs to be closely monitored to ensure that its return to normal is uneventful.
r. room a special room with special monitoring and resuscitation equipment used for monitoring the patient recovering from surgery.
surgical r. the process of healing of a surgical wound and restoration to normal of body functions and systems, e.g. fluid and acid–base balance, that have been disturbed by the original disease or by the surgical procedure.

recrement saliva, or other secretion, that is reabsorbed into the blood.

recrudescence recurrence of clinical signs after temporary abatement; a recrudescence occurs after some days or weeks, a relapse after weeks or months.

recruitment the gradual increase to a maximum in a reflex when a stimulus of unaltered intensity is prolonged.
collateral r. dilatation of collateral capillaries in the lungs with exercise.

recrystallization in cryosurgery, the conversion of small crystals, produced during the freezing process, to larger ones which are more damaging to cells. Occurs during a slow rewarming phase.

rectal pertaining to the rectum.
r. examination digital (in small animals) or manual examination of the visceral contents of the posterior abdomen for the purposes of diagnosis, in cattle and horses especially of pregnancy. See also RECTUM, PROCTOSCOPY.
r. fistula see RECTOVAGINAL fistula.
r. impaction see fecal IMPACTION.
r. inflammation see PROCTITIS, RECTITIS.
r. massage massage of the accessory sex glands, a method of semen collection in dogs.
r. paralysis occurs especially in cows and mares in late pregnancy. No feces are passed and the rectum is distended with feces, and there is no peristalsis during their manual removal. Dogs may show posterior paresis.
r. polyp see COLORECTAL polyp.
r. probe used in pregnancy diagnosis in ewes and in electroejaculation.
r. rupture the wall is perforated into the peritoneal cavity. Death occurs quickly as a result of endotoxic shock because of the absorption of enteric toxins through the peritoneum.
r. stricture stenosis of the rectum occurs in dogs, presumably resulting from trauma and anorectal disease, and in pigs following local ulceration caused by infection with *Salmonella* spp. Abnormal abdominal distension, small diameter feces and straining result.
r. tear most common in mares in association with manual rectal examinations. The mucosa is damaged but the wall is not ruptured. Leads to perirectal abscessation and subsequent peritonitis.
r. temperature see rectal TEMPERATURE.

rectectomy excision of the rectum.

rectification 1. the act of making straight, pure, or correct. 2. redistillation of a liquid to purify it.
radiological r. changing the flow of electrical current from alternating to direct.
surgical r. reconstructive surgery.

rectified refined; made straight.

rectilinear scanner a scintillation crystal probe on an arm that traverses the area to be scanned in a rectilinear pattern. Used to measure the distribution of radionuclide in organs. The output is recorded photographically.

rectitis proctitis; inflammation of the rectum.

rect(o)- word element. [L.] *rectum*. See also words beginning *proct(o)-*.

rectoabdominal pertaining to the rectum and abdomen.

rectoanal junction the division between rectum and anus marked by the transition of the mucous membrane from one bearing a columnar epithelium to one bearing a stratified squamous epithelium.

rectocele hernial protrusion of part of the rectum into the vagina.

rectocolitis coloproctitis; inflammation of the rectum and colon.

rectocutaneous pertaining to the rectum and the skin.

r. fistula communication between the rectum and the perirectal skin; may be the result of trauma, pelvic fracture, rectal foreign body, pararectal abscess or surgery. Fecal material is discharged through the skin wound.

rectopexy proctopexy.

rectoplasty proctoplasty.

rectoscope proctoscope.

rectosigmoid the lower portion of the sigmoid colon and the upper portion of the rectum.

rectostomy the operation of forming a permanent opening into the rectum for the relief of stricture of the rectum.

rectourethral pertaining to or communicating with the rectum and urethra.

rectouterine pertaining to the rectum and uterus.

rectovaginal pertaining to the rectum and vagina.

r. constriction inherited defect in Jersey cattle; fibrous bands cause dystocia and difficulty performing a rectal examination.

r. fistula a common event in mares because of the precipitate nature of the equine birth process. Perforation of the rectovaginal shelf occurs at foaling. The lesion does not extend to include the perineum. Feces accumulate in the rectum and there is a chronic vaginitis. Called also wind-sucking, gill-flirter.

r. tear see PERINEAL laceration.

rectovesical pertaining to or communicating with the rectum and bladder.

rectovestibular pertaining to or communicating with the rectum and the vestibule of the vagina.

rectovulvar pertaining to or communicating with the rectum and vulva.

rectum the distal portion of the large intestine, beginning at the pelvic inlet and ending at the anal canal. The feces, the solid waste products of digestion, are formed in the large intestine and are gradually pushed into the rectum by the muscular action of the intestine. Distension of the rectum by the accumulating feces sets up nerve impulses that indicate to the brain the need to empty the bowels; defecation follows. See also RECTAL.

rectus [L.] *straight*.

r. abdominis muscle see Table 13.2.

ocular r. muscle see Table 13.1F.

r. sheath the sleeve of fascia which surrounds the rectus abdominis muscle and which is derived from the aponeurotic tendons of the other abdominal muscles.

recumbency a clinical term is used to describe an animal that is lying down and unable to rise. See also PARALYSIS, DOWNER COW SYNDROME.

dorsal r. lying on the back.

lateral r. lying on side.

sternal r. see ventral recumbency (below).

ventral r. sitting up on the brisket with the legs tucked under the body.

recumbent pertaining to RECUMBENCY.

recuperation recovery of health and strength.

recurrence the return of clinical signs soon after a remission.

r. risk in genetics the probability of a particular defect occurring again if the type of mating which produced it is repeated.

recurrent characterized by recurrence at intervals of weeks or months.

r. airway obstruction chronic obstructive pulmonary disease of horses when the disease recurs after remimissions when the patient is in a dust-free environment.

r. fever relapsing fever.

r. impaction colic form of the disease likely to occur in equine patients which are overfed by indulgent owners; a common problem in American miniature horses.

r. iridocyclitis see periodic OPHTHALMIA.

r. laryngeal nerve paralysis see ROARING, LARYNGEAL hemiplegia.

r. mastitis clinical mastitis recurring in the same quarter due usually to residual foci of infection in tissue where udder infusion therapy does not penetrate; caused usually by infection with coagulase-positive *Staphylococcus aureus*.

r. tetany see Scottie CRAMP.

recurvation an upward bending or curvature.

recycled animal wastes poultry manure, litter, feathers and spilt feed processed and fed to cattle; other animal wastes are also used. The dangers are relatively low except that there are occasional devastating outbreaks of botulism, and there may be a gradual accumulation of residues of substances used as feed supplements in the original species.

red the color at the lowest end of the visible spectrum; the color of blood.

r. dye used in food coloring, reputed to reduce fertility.

red amaranth see AMARANTHUS *retroflexus*.

Red Angus a breed of beef cattle similar to the Aberdeen Angus in all respects except for its gold-red color.

red-bellied black snake see PSEUDECHIS *porphyriacus*.

red blood cell erythrocyte.

r. b. c. count see BLOOD COUNT.

nucleated r. b. c. see NORMOBLAST, METARUBRICYTE.

red bone marrow see BONE MARROW.

red buckeye AESCULUS *pavia*.

red bug see EUTROMBICULA *alfreddugesi*.

red burr BASSIA *hyssopifolia*, SCLEROLAENA *calcarata*.

Red canary one carrying the RED FACTOR gene.

red cell erythrocyte.

r. c. count (RCC) see BLOOD COUNT.

r. c. pit see PITTING (2).

red cestrum CESTRUM *fasciculatum*.

red clover TRIFOLIUM *pratense*.

red cotton bush ASCLEPIAS *curassavica*.

red crumbweed see DYSPHANIA.

red deer the principal hunting deer; golden red-brown, large, 5 ft tall, and up to 650 lb; males have very large antlers. Called also *Cervus elaphus*.

red dock RUMEX *vesicarius*.

red-eared sliders see SLIDERS.

red factor a gene responsible for red coloring in canaries, but strong red color is produced by a combination of several interacting genes, plus essential food substances in the diet. Canthaxanthin is fed to obtain the best results.

red-flowered birdsfoot trefoil LOTUS *cruentus*.

red-flowered mallow MODIOLA *caroliniana*.

red-flowering summer pheasants eye ADONIS *aestivalis*.

red foot disease lethal defect, similar to epidermolysis bullosa; seen in Scottish blackface and Welsh mountain sheep. Characterized by sloughing of hooves, limb and ear skin, conjunctiva, oral mucosa skin in lambs at 2 to 4 days of age, affects limbs, ears, tongue dorsum and conjunctiva. Separation of hoof horn exposing sensitive laminae is basis for name. Probably inherited.

red gums gingivitis.

red gut syndrome cecal torsion in lambs grazing lush legume pasture in New Zealand characterized by a very short illness, high mortality and a distinctive bright red distended cecum.

red hair syndrome red-brown discoloration of the hair of the paws, flanks and ventral abdomen of dogs receiving low-protein diets.

red-heart bullock bush ALECTRYON *oleifolius*.

red-ink plant PHYTOLACCA *octandra*.

red leg a disease of amphibians caused by *Aeromonas hydrophila* characterized by hemorrhages of the legs and abdomen. There are also hemorrhages elsewhere and ulceration of the skin and septicemia.

red-legged tick see RHIPICEPHALUS *evertsi*.

red maple see ACER *rubrum*.

red mite see DERMANYSSUS GALLINAE.

red mouth septicemic disease of young rainbow trout infected by *Yersinia ruckeri*; manifested by hyperemia and hemorrhagic ulceration of perioral tissues.

red nose see INFECTIOUS bovine rhinotracheitis.

red paper bark ALBIZIA *tanganyicensis*.

red passion flower PASSIFLORA *aurantia*.

red plague cutaneous vesicles, focal mecrosis of muscle, widespread hemorrhage in salmonids caused by *Aeromonas salmonicida*.

Red poll a breed of red, polled dual-purpose cattle.

red poppy see PAPAVER *rhoeas*.

red rock cod one of the Scorpaenidae family of venomous fish. Called also *Ruboralga jacksoniensis*.

red-root amaranth AMARANTHUS *retroflexus*.

red salvia see SALVIA *coccinea*.

red sea bream see PAGRAS AURATUS.

red sesbania, purple sesbania SESBANIA *punicea*.

Red setter see IRISH SETTER.

red shank AMARANTHUS *cruentus*.

Red Sindhi a red zebu breed of dairy cattle.

red sore disease focal hemorrhagic necrosis accompanied by deep ulceration of the perioral epidermis of some freshwater fish; caused by *Aeromonas hydrophila*.

red spinach TRIANTHEMA *triquetra*.

red spot disease see EPIZOOTIC ulcerative syndrome.

red squill a cardiac glycoside (scilliroside) extracted from the dried bulbs of *Urginea maritima*. Was used therapeutically as a cardiac stimulant at one time, now used as a rodenticide. Poisoning, with signs of bradycardia and convulsions, occurs with very large doses.

red staining inocybe INOCYBE *patouillardii*.

red-stemmed peavine ASTRAGALUS *emoryanus*.

Red Steppe red breed of dairy cattle derived from Red Friesian. Called also Red Ukranian.

red stomach worm see HAEMONCHUS.

red swamp crawfish see PROCAMBARUS CLARKII.

Red Ukrainian see RED STEPPE.

red wattle bird see ANTHOCHAERA CARUNCULATA.

red wings see COMBRETUM PLATYPETALUM.

redback spider see LATRODECTUS.

Redbone coonhound a medium-sized, sturdy dog, with a short, rich red coat, large, pendulous ears and a long, tapered tail. The dog is derived from bloodhounds and foxhounds and originated in the Ozark Mountains of central USA. It is used for tracking bear, mountain lions and raccoons.

redfin perch see PERCA *pluviatilis*.

redia pl. *rediae* [L.] a larval stage of certain trematode parasites, which develops in the body of a snail host and gives rise to daughter rediae, or to the cercariae.

redintegration the restoration or repair of a lost or damaged part.

redleg see LACHNANTHES TINCTORIA.

rednose see INFECTIOUS bovine rhinotracheitis.

redox oxidation–reduction.

redroot see AMARANTHUS, LACHNANTHES TINCTORIA.

reduce 1. to restore to the normal place or relation of parts, as to reduce a fracture. 2. to undergo reduction. 3. to decrease in weight or size.

reduced said of a fracture which has been exposed to reduction.

reducible permitting of reduction.

reducing agents substances that act as electron contributors in a reduction reaction, e.g. glucose, creatinine, uric acid.

reductant the electron donor in an oxidation–reduction (redox) reaction.

reductase an enzyme that catalyzes a chemical reduction.

5α-r. an enzyme that catalyzes the irreversible reduction of testosterone to dihydrotestosterone.

reduction 1. the correction of a fracture, luxation or hernia. 2. the addition of hydrogen to a substance, or more generally, the gain of electrons; the opposite of oxidation.

closed r. the manipulative reduction of a fracture without incision.

open r. reduction of a fracture after incision into the fracture site.

reductionism policy of reducing subjects to its parts in an attempt to simplfy the understanding of the whole. The opposite of holism.

reduplication 1. a doubling back. 2. the recurrence of paroxysms of a double type. 3. a developmental anomaly resulting in the doubling of an organ or part, with a connection between them at some point and the excess part usually a mirror image of the other.

heart sound r. see gallop RHYTHM.

reduviid bug a member of the family Reduviidae. Called also cone-nose bug, assassin bug or kissing bug. One of the TRIATOMA species is involved in the transmission of CHAGAS' DISEASE.

redwater red urine; see HEMOGLOBINURIA, HEMATURIA, MYOGLOBINURIA, PHENOTHIAZINE, PHENOLPHTHALEIN, XANTHORRHOEA.

r. fever see BABESIOSIS.

redwood see ENTANDROPHRAGMA CYLINDRICUM.

redworm see STRONGYLUS.

r. infestation see STRONGYLOSIS.

reed abomasum.

reed canary grass PHALARIS *arundinacea*.

Reed–Frost model a simple mathematical model of an outbreak of hypothetical disease; a chain-binomial model, based on the development of an outbreak of disease occurring as a chain of events, each of which is assessable in terms of a binomial equation, suitable for class-room use. See also epidemiological MODEL.

Reed–Sternberg cell see Reed–Sternberg CELL.

reed sweet grass GLYCERIA *maxima*.
reef an infolding or tuck of tissue, as a tuck made in plication.
reef knot see SQUARE KNOT.
reefing surgery involving taking in a reef of tissue, e.g. in reducing a prolapse of the preputial lining in a bull.
re-entry in cardiology, a postulated mechanism by which a premature beat can be coupled to the normal beat.
r. tachyarrhythmia see re-entrant TACHYARRHYTHMIA.
Rees–Ecker fluid a diluting fluid for use in direct thrombocyte counts; contains sodium citrate, formaldehyde and brilliant cresyl blue.
REF renal erythropoietic factor.
refection recovery; repair. A special use of the word is the function of the cecal and colonic flora to synthesize B vitamins.
refeeding the process of restoring nutrition to a previously starved animal. This should initially consist of a diet of predominantly protein and fat, gradually becoming more complex.
r. syndrome excessive dietary carbohydrate intake after a period of starvation leads to potentially fatal insulin-induced transport of phosphorus and potassium into cells.
reference group the group against which a comparison is being made, e.g. reference sires.
referral the professional etiquette by which a primary accession clinican refers a case to a specialist for further diagnosis and treatment. The case passes out of the care of the first veterinarian for the time being. It is usually returned to him/her when the specialist has concluded with the problem at hand. See also CONSULTATION (2).
referred pain see referred PAIN.
referring the act of referral.
refine to purify or free from foreign matter.
reflection a turning or bending back, such as the folds produced when a membrane passes over the surface of an organ and then passes back to the body wall that it lines.
reflector a device for reflecting light or sound waves.
reflex a reflected involuntary action or movement; the sum total of any particular automatic response mediated by the nervous system.

A reflex is built into the nervous system and does not need the intervention of conscious thought to take effect.

For reflexes used in clinical examination of a patient see under individual titles including anal, blink, corneal, conjunctival, crossed extensor, extensor thrust, eyelid, gastrocnemius, hopping, palpebral, panniculus, patellar, perineal, placing, pupillary, withdrawal.

accommodation r. the coordinated changes that occur when the eye adapts itself for near vision; they are constriction of the pupil, convergence of the eyes and increased convexity of the lens.
r. action an involuntary response to a stimulus conveyed to the nervous system and reflected to the periphery (see also REFLEX).
r. bradycardia bradycardia occurring as a reflex initiated by severe atrial or ventricular stretch.
chain r. a series of reflexes, each serving as a stimulus to the next, making a complete activity.
conditioned r. see CONDITIONED response.
cutaneous trunci r. see PANNICULUS reflex.
dazzle r. a test of the retina, optic nerve, and central retinal pathways. Shining a bright light into the eye should cause squinting.
r. dyssynergia see detrusor-urethral DYSSYNERGIA.
gastroileal r. increase in ileal motility and opening of the ileocecal valve when food enters the empty stomach.
light r. see PUPILLARY light reflex.
nociceptive r. reflexes initiated by painful stimuli.
palatal r. see SWALLOWING reflex.
rectosphincteric r. relaxation of the anal sphincter which occurs with distension of the rectum and during defecation.
stepping r. movements of progression elicited when the animal is held upright and inclined forward with the feet touching a flat surface.
stretch r. reflex contraction of a muscle in response to passive longitudinal stretching.
superficial r. any withdrawal reflex elicited by noxious or tactile stimulation of the skin, cornea or mucous membrane, including the corneal and pharyngeal reflexes.
tapetal r. tapetal reflection of light.
tendon r. a method of testing the patency of reflex arc. The tendon is stretched sharply by tapping it close to its insertion. A positive reaction is a sharp contraction of the muscle of which the tendon is part. The patellar reflex is the best known of these reflexes. Absence indicates a defect in the reflex arc, an exaggerated response suggests an upper motor neuron lesion. Called also myotactic reflex.
tonic r. see TONIC neck response.
triceps surae r. Achilles reflex.
trigemino-abducens r. a test of the ophthalmic and mandibular divisions of the trigeminal nerve, and the abducens nerve. Light touching of the cornea should result in retraction of the globe and protrusion of the nictitating membrane.
r. walking spinal reflexes can provide support and uncoordinated use of the hindlegs that resembles walking, in dogs with transection of the spinal cord between T13 and L4.
reflexogenic, reflexogenous producing or increasing reflex action.
reflexograph an instrument for recording a reflex.
reflexometer an instrument for measuring the force required to produce myotactic contraction.
reflux a backward or return flow.
esophageal r. reflux of the stomach contents into the esophagus; likely to occur during anesthesia and may be a cause of esophageal strictures. Called also gastroesophageal reflux. See also peptic ESOPHAGITIS.
gastroduodenal r. reflux of duodenal contents, especially bile salts into the stomach; a cause of injury to the gastric mucosa and a possible factor in the genesis of gastric ulceration.
gastroesophageal r. see esophageal reflux (above).
intrarenal urine r. reflux of urine into the renal parenchymal tissue.
vesicoureteral r., vesicoureteric r. backward flow of urine from the bladder into a ureter.
refractile bodies see ERYTHROCYTE refractile bodies.
refractive capacity to refract light.
r. error a difference between the focal length of the cornea and lens, and the length of the eye, resulting in myopia or hyperopia.
r. media of the eye include the vitreous humor and the lens.
refractometer 1. an instrument for measuring the refractive power of the eye. 2. an instrument for determining the indexes of refraction of various substances. 3. an instrument for measuring the concentration of solutes, e.g. protein in solutions, immunoglobulins in serum.

refractometry the science of measuring by refractometer.

refractory not readily yielding to treatment.

r. period the period of depolarization and repolarization of the cell membrane after excitation; during the first portion (absolute refractory period), the nerve or muscle fiber cannot respond to a second stimulus, whereas during the relative refractory period, it can respond only to a strong stimulus.

myocardial r. state the myocardium is refractory to stimulation during the action potential period, excitability returning in the repolarization phase; initially there is a period of supernormality.

refracture the process of breaking a bone which has previously been fractured, but healed in an unsatisfactory manner, usually with a deformity.

refresh to freshen or make raw again; to denude a wound of epithelium to enhance tissue repair.

refrigerant 1. relieving fever and thirst. 2. a cooling remedy.

refrigeration 1. therapeutic application of low temperature. See also induced HYPOTHERMIA. 2. a major part of the preservation of perishable food, biologicals and other materials by chilling or freezing.

r. test see CHYLOMICRON test.

refusion the temporary removal and subsequent return of blood to the circulation. See also EXTRACORPOREAL circulatory support unit.

regeneration the natural renewal of a structure, as of a lost tissue or part.

regenerative left shift see SHIFT to the left.

regimen a strictly regulated scheme of diet, exercise, or other activity designed to achieve certain ends.

regio pl. *regiones* [L.] region.

region a general term to designate certain areas on the surface of the body within certain defined boundaries.

abdominal r's nine arbitrary areas into which the ventral surface of the abdomen is divided, including the epigastric, right and left hypochondriac, umbilical, right and left lateral, pubic, right and left inguinal.

I r. that part of the major histocompatibility complex where immune response genes are present.

lumbar r. the region of the back lying lateral to the lumbar vertebrae.

perineal r. the region over the pelvic outlet, including the anal and urogenital regions.

precordial r. the part of the chest covering the heart.

pubic r. the middle portion of the most caudal region of the abdomen, located caudal to the umbilical region and between the inguinal regions.

regional pertaining to a certain region or regions.

r. acceleratory phenomenon permits a number of mineralization foci to commence repair or modeling simultaneously.

r. enteritis inflammation of the terminal portion of the ileum. See also terminal ILEITIS, CROHN'S DISEASE and porcine intestinal ADENOMATOSIS.

r. hypotrichosis a congenital hypotrichosis over particular areas, usually symmetrical, of skin recorded in many dog and some dog breeds; hair follicles may be absent.

register 1. in law, a list of names of persons registered as veterinary surgeons under local or national legislation. May be in two categories, practitioners and specialists. 2. in computer terms, a part of a computer's random access memory that is used specifically for temporary storage of a small amount of data until the program can deal with it.

registrant a veterinarian listed on the register as available for consultation by virtue of registration.

registrar 1. an official keeper of records. 2. in large veterinary teaching hospitals, a staff specialist who acts as head of the relevant clinical unit, e.g. the surgical or medical unit.

registration the act of registering.

registry 1. an office for the maintenance of a register. 2. a central agency for collection of pathological material and related data in a specified field of pathology, so organized that the data can be properly processed and made available for study.

Registry of Comparative Pathology a national resource center for comparative pathology and animal models of human disease, at the (US) Armed Forces Institute of Pathology.

regression 1. return to a former or earlier state. 2. subsidence of clinical signs or of a disease process. 3. in biology, the tendency in successive generations toward the mean. 4. the relationship between pairs of random variables; the mean of one variable and its location is influenced by another variable.

r. analysis see regression ANALYSIS.

r. coefficient is the factor which determines the slope of a regression line; the greater the coefficient the steeper the line.

curvilinear r. when the relationship between two variables is not linear.

linear r. the relationship between two variables is a straight line.

regular crossing the same cross is made on a regular basis as a breeding program; the object is usually to produce a standard offspring and to benefit from heterosis.

regulated system regulation of a substance in the body; requires a receptor, a regulator and an effector.

regulation 1. the act of adjusting or state of being adjusted to a certain standard. 2. in biology, the adaptation of form or behavior of an organism to changed conditions. 3. the power of a pregastrula stage to form a whole embryo from a part. 4. the biochemical mechanisms that control the expression of genes. 5. in law the lesser rules promulgated under the authority of an Act of Parliament, and which can be altered by consultation short of presenting a bill to the Parliament.

feedback r. a mechanism for regulating metabolic processes involving the active and regulatory sites of allosteric enzyme proteins.

regulator see reducing VALVE.

regulatory proteins 1. proteins which regulate the contraction of muscle by controlling the interaction of myosin and actin. Calcium is an essential component of this reaction. The two proteins are TROPONIN and TROPOMYOSIN. 2. special proteins that bind to specific regulatory sequences of DNA and act to switch genes on and off and thereby regulate the transcription of genes.

regulatory site that portion of a protein, usually an enzyme, to which the product of the enzyme–substrate interaction binds and down-regulates the active site of the enzyme by altering in conformation so as to prevent further binding to the substrate. A basis for feedback regulation.

regulatory veterinary authorities governmental authorities of city, county, shire, province, state, national administrations which apply and enforce laws and regulations which control all matters relating to animal health and to animal diseases which are communicable to humans.

regurgitant flowing back.

regurgitation a backward flowing, as the casting up of undigested food, or the backflow of blood through a defective heart valve. In the alimentary canal the regurgitation of food comes from the esophagus, as distinct from vomiting in which the food comes from the stomach. A sign of pyloric obstruction or megaesophagus.

r. cycle see RETICULAR cycle.

neurotic r. regurgitation by budgerigars is a common phenomenon with no physiological explanation and is considered to be an expression of affection.

valvular r. backflow of blood through the orifices of the heart valves owing to imperfect closing of the valves (valvular insufficiency); named, according to the valve affected, aortic, mitral, pulmonic or tricuspid regurgitation.

regurgitus the material voided in a regurgitation. Includes saliva, ingesta from the esophagus (plus forestomachs in ruminants).

Rehfuss tube a single-lumen oral tube used in humans to obtain specimens of biliary secretions for diagnostic study. The tube is weighted on one end so that it can be passed orally and positioned at the point where the bile duct empties into the duodenum. Done with a flexible endoscope to position a catheter to do the sampling.

rehmannic acid LANTADENE A.

rehydration the restoration of water or fluid content to a body or to a substance that has become dehydrated.

Reich–Nechtow curette a long slim handheld instrument with a slim neck and an upturned, sharp-edged oval cup, 8 mm × 4 mm with a complete bottom, used to collect biopsy samples from the uterine cervical canal.

Reichert's cartilage the dorsal cartilage of the second branchial arch.

Reighardia a genus of pentastomes in the family Porocephalidae and found in the air sacs of gulls and terns.

Reimer emasculator a complicated, multiple-crush emasculator for horses. A scissor type with the main pair of handles ratcheted. The crushing jaws are multiple and there is a secondary crushing jaw operated by a third handle or lever. There are two blades on either side; these interlock and it is important that the instrument is applied in the correct way so that the last crushing action is applied to the cord that remains in the horse.

reimplantation replacement of tissue or a structure in the site from which it was previously lost or removed.

rein narrow strip of thin leather or other fabric attached to both ends of a bit in a horse's bridle making a loop which passes through the hands of the driver/rider. Used to direct the horse's head and so change its direction.

bearing r. a fixed rein attached to the saddle or backpad and to the bridle to prevent the horse from lowering its head too far.

check r. runs from the bit or the crown of the bridle to the saddle in vehicle harness. Limits the range of movements that the horse can make. Is a fixed but adjustable check and is not under the control of the rider/driver.

neck r. not a piece of harness; is the technique in which the rider moves his/her hands to one side of the horse's neck thus touching the horse with the rein on one side of the neck. The well-schooled horse will move in the other direction.

running r. runs from the rider, through the rings of the bit and back to the girth. For horses in harness is a very powerful restrainer.

side r. extends on either side from the bit, through rings on a saddle or pad and ends with the driver walking beside the horse. Used in training a horse to cart harness.

reindeer *Rangifer tarandus*, the large, wild ruminant of Christmas mythology, a mirror image of the North American caribou except that the latter cannot be domesticated whereas reindeer adapt easily. Large brown animals with a white buttock patch and lower parts, large antlers in both male and female.

r. warble fly see OEDEMAGENA *tarandi*.

reinfection a second infection by the same agent.

reinforcement the use of a stimulus to modify an existing form of response. The stimulus may be a reward or a punishment and the reinforcement may correspondingly be positive or negative.

reinforcer the stimulus that provides reinforcement.

second-order r. a conditioned reinforcer; a neutral stimulus is paired with a natural reinforcer thereby acquiring reinforcing properties.

reinfusate fluid for reinfusion into the body, usually after being subjected to a treatment process.

reinfusion infusion of body fluid that has previously been withdrawn from the same individual, e.g. reinfusion of ascitic fluid after ultrafiltration.

reinnervation the operation of grafting a viable nerve to restore the nerve supply of an organ or paralyzed muscle.

Reinsch test a test for heavy metals in urine, using copper wire or foil in heated hydrochloric acid. If metals are present, they form visible deposits on the copper.

reiteration in eukaryotes, mulitple copies of certain relatively short nucleotide sequences that are repeated from a few times to milliions of times; three classes are defined, single copy, moderately reiterated and highly reiterated; some occur as inverted repeats.

rejection the immune reaction of a recipient to a graft, usually an allograph, after transplantation. The recipient recognizes antigens, particularly major histocompatibility complex antigens that are different from self antigens. The rapidity and severity of the graft rejection parallels the degree of antigenic difference between donor and recipient. The primary rejection of a graft, called *first set reaction*, typically begins 6 to 10 days after engraftment and in the case of skin is characterized by an erythematous zone around the graft which subsequently shrinks and is rejected. Rejection is predominantly a cell-mediated immune response, particularly Th1 lymphocytes and activated macrophages. If the same recipient receives a second graft from the same donor the graft is rejected more rapidly and the response is more severe, called a *second set reaction* which is also a cell-mediated response. Lymphocytes from the recipient can be adoptively transferred to a naive recipient which if also given a graft from the same donor responds with a second set reaction.

r. factors antibodies, particularly IgM but also IgG, directed against antigenic determinants on the Fc region of other immunoglobulins. When the immunoglobulin binds to antigen, changes occur in the folding of the protein of the Fc region such that new, nonself antigenic determinants are exposed and it is to these that rheumatoid factors, i.e. other antibodies, are directed.

reksiekte disease see STRETCHING DISEASE.

relapse the return of a disease weeks or months after its apparent cessation.

relationship the state that exists when one variable is related to another variable in some way.

direct r. when changes in the value of one of the variables is mirrored by a change in the same direction in the other variable.

relative relates to the condition of one animal when it is considered in connection with another.
r. biological effectiveness (RBE) see RBE.
r. frequency the proportion of the total number of observations of a variable which are observations of a particular value.
r. odds see ODDS ratio.
r. population index a measure of a population based on a sampling technique such as LINE transects which determine the number of animals in a given ecological niche relative to a period of examination, or other parameter.
r. risk the ratio of the disease incidence rate in animals exposed to an hypothesized cause to the incidence rate in animals not exposed. A measure of association commonly used in epidemiological studies. Called also risk ratio.
relatives animals which share common ancestors.
first-degree r. parents, offspring, full-sibs.
second-degree r. grandparents, half-sibs, grandchildren.
relaxant 1. causing relaxation. 2. an agent that causes relaxation.
muscle r. an agent that specifically aids in reducing muscle tension.
relaxation a lessening of tension.
relaxin a factor that produces relaxation of the symphysis pubis and dilatation of the cervix uteri in certain animal species including pigs, cattle, dogs and cats. Produced in the corpus luteum of pregnancy.
relaxing factor sarcoplasmic reticulum, a protein synthesized by and contained in the platelets.
release reaction a reaction which occurs when platelets react with exposed collagen fibers due to injury of a blood vessel; the release reaction causes the release of constituents from the platelets, including histamine, fibrinogen, serotonin, adenine nucleotides and other substances.
release signs in neurological terms, the signs evident when the lower motor neuron is released from the damping effects of the upper motor neuron, e.g. tetany, exaggerated tendon reflexes.
releaser device in the milking machine which discharges milk from the vacuum pressure system to atmospheric pressure.
releasing factors hypothalamic hormones that stimulate the secretion of effector hormones in the pituitary, e.g. follicle-stimulating hormone releasing hormone.
relocation syndrome the moderation of inappropriate behavior that occurs when the animal is placed in a different situation or environment. Can be used to provide an opportunity to reinforce appropriate behavior.
REM rapid eye movement. See also SLEEP.
rem acronym for *r*oentgen *e*quivalent *m*an; the amount of any ionizing radiation which has the same biological effect as 1 rad of x-rays; 1 rem = 1 rad × RBE (relative biological effectiveness). Now replaced by the SIEVERT (Sv) SI unit. 1 Sv = 100 rem.
remedy anything that cures or palliates disease.
specific r. one that is invariably effective in treatment of a certain condition.
remex pl. *remiges;* one of the large flight feathers of the wing. There are primary and secondary remiges.
remiges see REMEX.
remineralization restoration of mineral elements, as of calcium salts to bone.
remission diminution or abatement of the clinical signs of a disease; the period during which such diminution occurs.
remittence temporary abatement, without actual cessation, of clinical signs.
remittent having periods of abatement and of exacerbation.
remodeling a constant, normal process in bone comprising removal–replacement of minute sections of bone without alteration to the visible skeletal volume; may be periosteal or endosteal.
remote at a distance.
r. access in computer terms means being able to access a computer by a telephone and a modem.
r. cause predisposing cause.
r. sensing perceiving or measuring change in physical or chemical parameters from a distance.
r. treatment see INJECTION collar.
remounts all horses owned by the army to be used for army service.
removal trapping a means of measuring a wild animal population by the change in the population resulting from the trapping of a known number of animals and their removal to a distant site.
remuda the group of saddle horses kept on a beef cattle ranch, or station, or run.
ren pl. *renes* [L.] kidney.
r. mobilis hypermobile kidney; nephroptosis.
renal pertaining to the kidney. See also KIDNEY.
r. abscess results from infected emboli and infarcts. Usually without localizing signs unless they are very large and palpable, or when they extend into the renal pelvis and cause pyelonephritis.
r. adenoma rare, incidental necropsy finding.
r. agenesis failure of the renal tissue to develop; unilateral agenesis causes compensatory hypertrophy in the single kidney; bilateral is fatal. Commonly accompanies genital tract malformation.
r. artery see Table 9.
avian r. hemorrhage sporadic unexplained disease of turkeys; sudden death is common.
r. biopsy is conducted usually with a biopsy needle introduced percutaneously through the flank. In food animals it is possible to fix the left kidney via a rectal manipulation, but the right kidney can be impossible to reach.
r. calculus see UROLITHIASIS.
r. capsular cyst see feline PERIRENAL cysts.
r. carcinoma commonest in old male dogs. They are very large, spread locally and metastasize widely.
r. casts see urinary CAST.
r. clearance tests laboratory tests that determine the ability of the kidney to remove certain substances from the blood. See also PHENOLSULFONPHTHALEIN clearance test, INULIN clearance.
r. cortical fissures external fissures created by the lobar structure of the large ruminant kidney.
r. cortical hypoplasia see renal dysplasia (below).
r. cortical necrosis results from patchy or complete renal ischemia and is part of the terminal state of many diseases, e.g. severe metritis, grain overload in cattle, azoturia in horses.
r. countercurrent system see COUNTERCURRENT.
r. cyst incidental necropsy finding except for polycystic KIDNEY disease. See also feline PERIRENAL cysts.
r. cystadenoma inherited as an autosomal dominant trait in middle-aged German shepherd bitches with generalized nodular dermatofibrosis.
r. diabetes insipidus see nephrogenic DIABETES INSIPIDUS.
r. dialysis the application of the principles of dialysis for treatment of renal failure (below). See also HEMODIALYSIS and PERITONEAL dialysis.
r. diverticuli diverticuli of the renal pelvis.

r. dysfunction reduced capacity to excrete metabolic products which accumulate systemically and are detectable clinicopathologically by renal function tests. The early stage of uremia.

r. dysplasia small, misshapen kidneys at birth. May be caused by intrauterine infection of the fetus by virus, but numerous inherited renal dysplasias occur in dogs. They occur in several breeds and are manifested by signs of chronic renal insufficiency, e.g. polyuria, polydypsia, poor growth and weight gain, pale mucous membranes, and renal secondary osteodystrophia fibrosa, from an early age.

r. ectopia see pelvic KIDNEY, horseshoe KIDNEY.

r. erythropoietic factor erythropoietin.

r. failure inability of the kidney to maintain normal function. Impairment of kidney function affects most of the body's systems because of its important role in maintaining fluid balance, regulating the electrochemical composition of body fluids, providing constant protection against acid–base imbalance, and controlling blood pressure. See also KIDNEY.

r. function tests include blood urea nitrogen and serum creatinine estimations, tests of concentrating ability, tests of ability to excrete test substances, e.g. phenolsulfonphthalein (PSP) clearance test. Of the urine tests, only specific gravity (SG) has any significance in terms of a function test but abnormalities of urine should lead to a function test being conducted.

r. hypophosphatemic rickets inherited as an X-linked dominant trait in children and mice; characterized by hypophosphatemia and normocalcemia due to failure of phosphate resorption in renal tubules, and skeletal deformities. Called also vitamin-resistant rickets.

r. infarct results from embolic or thrombotic occlusion of renal arteries or branches. Clinical signs are those of renal colic initially followed by toxemia if the infarct is infected.

r. insufficiency see renal dysfunction (above).

r. ischemia a significant cause of renal dysfunction and cortical and medullary necrosis. Is usually part of a general state of shock, dehydration and severe toxemia.

r. lobe a large mass of a kidney, comprising the tissue contributing to each pyramid; kidneys may be unilobar (unipyramidal), e.g. cats, dogs, small ruminants, horses, or multilobar (multipyramidal), e.g. cattle, pigs.

r. lobule small masses of kidney tissue comprising a medullary ray and its associated nephrons.

r. medullary necrosis necrosis of the renal medulla due to restriction of blood flow in medullary vessels, usually due to venous occlusion.

r. medullary washout see medullary solute WASHOUT.

r. mineralization see NEPHROCALCINOSIS.

r. osteodystrophy, r. osteitis fibrosa, r. osteitis fibrosa cystica see renal secondary HYPERPARATHYROIDISM.

r. oxalosis deposition of oxalate crystals in renal tubules of patients poisoned by dietary oxalate, usually in poisonous plants.

r. papillae see renal PAPILLA.

r. papillary necrosis necrosis of renal papillae due usually to obstruction to urinary flow or poisoning or dehydration.

r. pelvis the chamber in the kidney into which the collecting tubules discharge urine and from which urine is voided into the ureter.

r. plasma flow the effective rate of blood flow through the kidneys; the determining factor relative to the rate of glomerular filtration.

r. portal system a system unique to birds; half to two thirds of the blood supply to the kidney comes from the hindlimbs via veins and terminates in peritubular capillaries where it is mixed with arteriolar blood coming from the glomeruli.

r. rickets see renal secondary HYPERPARATHYROIDISM.

r. shutdown cessation of the excretory function of the kidney; oliguria.

r. spongiform encephalopathy spongiform encephalopathy associated with renal failure.

r. tubular casts see urinary CAST.

r. vein thrombosis commonly associated with renal amyloidosis in dogs.

renaturation the reassembly of a protein or nucleic acid molecule after denaturation.

rendering of fat, the melting of the tissue material and collection and solidification of the molten fat.

dry r. separation of edible fat from abattoir residues by dry steam heat and the driving off of water.

renguerra [Span.] secondary nutritional deficiency of copper. Called also renguerra.

Renibacterium salmoninarum see BACTERIAL kidney disease of fish.

Renicola a genus of renal flukes (digenetic trematodes) in the family Renicolidae.

R. hayesanniae found in turkeys and eider ducks and may cause sufficient damage to lead to renal failure.

renicolid a member of the family Renicolidae of flukes.

reniform kidney-shaped.

renin a proteolytic enzyme synthesized, stored and secreted by the juxtaglomerular cells of the kidney; it plays a role in regulation of blood pressure by catalyzing the conversion of the plasma glycoprotein angiotensinogen to angiotensin I. This, in turn, is converted to angiotensin II by an enzyme that is present in relatively high concentrations in the lung. Angiotensin II is one of the most potent vasoconstrictors known, and also is a powerful stimulus of aldosterone secretion.

r.–angiotensin system renin, secreted by the juxtaglomerular apparatus, activates the precursor angiotensinogen. This liberates angiotensin I, then angiotensin II, a vasoconstrictor and stimulant to the secretion of aldosterone.

big r. a relatively inactive protein with a higher molecular weight than normal renin, which is activated after exposure to low pH or to proteolytic enzymes.

renin–angiotensin–aldosterone system see RENIN–angiotensin system.

reninism a condition marked by overproduction of renin.

primary r. a syndrome of hypertension, hypokalemia, hyperaldosteronism and elevated plasma renin activity, due to proliferation of juxtaglomerular cells.

renipelvic pertaining to the pelvis of the kidney.

reniportal pertaining to the portal system of the kidney.

renipuncture surgical incision of the capsule of the kidney.

rennet extract of the abomasal mucosa of the unweaned calf used in curdling milk in the preparation of cheese.

rennin an outdated term. See CHYMOSIN.

renninogen prorennin; the proenzyme in the gastric glands which is converted into rennin.

renogastric pertaining to the kidney and stomach.

renogram a graphic record of kidney function produced by externally monitoring the level of radioactivity in the bladder as a radiopharmaceutical agent enters it from the kidney via the ureters.

renography radiography of the kidney.

renointestinal pertaining to the kidney and intestine.

renolith see renal UROLITH.

renomegaly enlargement of the kidney.

renopathy any disease of the kidneys; nephropathy.

renoprival pertaining to or caused by lack of kidney function.

renotropic having a special affinity for kidney tissue.

Renshaw cells interneurons in the central nervous system that provide a regulatory feedback system to control the excitability of motor neurons.

renule an area of the kidney supplied by a branch of the renal artery, usually consisting of three or four medullary pyramids and their corresponding cortical substance.

Reoviridae a family of nonenveloped, medium-sized viruses that have a double capsid structure and a segmented double-strand RNA genome. There are three genera of importance in veterinary medicine: *Reovirus*, *Orbivirus* and *Rotavirus*.

Reovirus a genus of viruses in the family *Reoviridae*. They are widespread in nature but have little known pathogenicity and are not identified as causing any specific animal diseases. Reoviruses isolated from cattle and dogs appear to cause clinically inapparent infections; in cats they uncommonly cause conjunctivitis and gingivitis, in horses coughing and ocular discharge without fever, and in poultry respiratory disease and arthritis.

reoxygenation in radiobiology, the phenomenon in which hypoxic (and thus radioresistant) tumor cells become more exposed to oxygen (and thus more radiosensitive) by coming into closer proximity to capillaries after death and loss of other tumor cells due to previous irradiation.

rep acronym for *r*oentgen *e*quivalent *p*hysical, an unofficial unit of radiation equivalent to the absorption of 93 ergs per gram of water or soft tissue. An equivalent dose of ionizing radiation as that delivered to tissues by 1 roentgen of x-radiation.

repair the physical or mechanical restoration of damaged tissues, especially the replacement of dead or damaged cells in a body tissue or organ by healthy new cells.

plastic r. restoration of anatomical structure by means of tissue transferred from other sites or derived from other individuals, or by other substance.

repeat breeder said of cows that have no apparent physical abnormality of the reproductive tract and have normal estral cycles but fail to conceive to matings at two or more successive estral periods. Called also FTC.

repeat units see repeat DNA.

repeat visit reminders reminders to clients that their animals should be revaccinated, treated for worms or returned for routine repeat examination.

repeatability 1. the ability to get similar results at a series of examinations. 2. in genetics a measure of the extent to which an animal's superiority (or inferiority), based on aninitial measurement, will be seen in future measurements. Denoted by R. 3. in diagnostic tests, the ability of the test to give consistent results in repeated measurements. See also PRECISION.

repeated periodic health care periodic preventive medical measures such as testing for heartworm infection in dogs, brucellosis testing in rams, drenching of young sheep for worms, vaccination of poultry against infectious laryngotracheitis (ILT).

repellent able to repel or drive off; also, an agent that repels. Refers usually to insect repellent.

repeller an obstetrical instrument used in large animal obstetrics to repel a fetus during correction of a dystocia, e.g. KÜHN'S CRUTCH. See also REPULSION (3).

repensol estrogenic coumestan compound found in plants.

reperfusion injury damage to renal blood vessels during periods of hypotension does not become apparent until reperfusion occurs in the recovery stage of the vascular incident.

reperitonealization the regeneration of mesothelium lining the peritoneal cavity, following injury.

replacement alternative or back-up groups of animals.

r. flocks flocks of poultry dedicated to the production of eggs for production of day-old chicks, requiring particular attention to the prevention of diseases transmitted vertically through the egg.

r. heifers heifers retained in a herd, or sold to other herds, to replace cows culled for age, low production or disease.

replacement proteins the dietary proteins in milk replacer which need to be of good biological value, contain the essential amino acids and not be denatured in the heat preparation of the feed.

replantation restoration of an organ or other body structure to its original site.

replenishment the addition of an appropriate quantity of properly prepared solution containing the correct concentration of chemicals to the developer solutions used in radiography.

replicate to repeat an experiment or an object a number of times.

replication 1. a turning back of a part so as to form a duplication. 2. repetition of an experiment to ensure accuracy. 3. the process of duplicating or reproducing, as replication of an exact copy of a polynucleotide strand of DNA or RNA. See also DEOXYRIBONUCLEIC ACID.

r. bubble seen in electron micrographs of DNA in replicating eukaryotic cells, suggesting bidirectional growth.

conservative r. an invalid hypothetical model for DNA replication in which both strands of the double helix remain together after replication. DNA replicationoccurs via semiconservative mechanisn in which one parental and one nascent strand are produced.

dispersive r. in DNA replication, a hypothetical model in which nucleotides of the parental DNA strand would be randomly scattered along the strands of the newly synthesized DNA, as compared with semiconservative and conservative DNA replication.

r. fork a 'y' shaped structure in replicating DNA, the arms of which are the newly synthesized DNA molecules composed of one parental and one nascent strand and the stem of which is the parental DNA that is progressively unwinding as it is copied.

semiconservative r. a reference to the preservation of one of the original parental DNA strands in each of the two nascent DNA molecules produced following DNA replication.

replicative form a double-stranded intermediate in the replication of DNA or RNA viruses.

replisomes in DNA replication, the final and complete assembly of proteins and enzymes at the replication origin necessary to carry out replication.

repolarization the re-establishment of polarity, especially the return of cell membrane potential to resting potential after depolarization.
repopulation 1. introduction of new animals to a farm or part of it after it has been depopulated for health or production reasons. 2. the additional growth of normal cells around a tumor that is being destroyed by irradiation.
Reporyje virus a strain of porcine enterovirus isolated in Czechoslovakia from pigs with procine viral ENCEPHALOMYELITIS (Teschen disease).
repositol medicine in a formulation suitable for a depot injection which will deliver the medication to the vascular system over a prolonged period, e.g. repositol diethylstilbestrol.
repositor an instrument used in returning displaced organs to the normal position.
representative representative of the population as a whole; e.g. erythrocyte counts of randomly selected samples of a population. See also RANDOM.
repression 1. the act of restraining, inhibiting or suppressing. 2. in molecular genetics, inhibition of gene transcription by a repressor.
enzyme r. interference, usually by the end product of a pathway, with synthesis of the enzymes of that pathway.
repressor that which restrains or inhibits; a specific protein molecule coded for by a regulatory gene, which acts to repress the synthesis of a specific protein.
***lac* r.** interacts specifically with the *lac* operator.
repressor-constitutive mutation see repressor-constitutive MUTATION.
reproduction 1. the process by which a living entity or organism produces a new individual of the same kind. It may be asexual or sexual. 2. the creation of a similar object or situation; duplication; replication.
In sexual reproduction the gonads, or sex glands—the ovaries in the female and the testes in the male—produce the germ cells that unite and grow into a new individual. Reproduction begins when the germ cells unite, the process called fertilization.
asexual r. reproduction without the fusion of germ cells; usually by budding or fission.
cytogenic r. production of a new individual from a single germ cell or zygote.
sexual r. reproduction by the fusion of a female germ cell with a male sexual cell or by the development of an unfertilized egg.
somatic r. production of a new individual from a multicellular fragment by fission or budding.
reproductive subserving or pertaining to reproduction.
r. behavior see SEXUAL behavior.
r. cycle in all mammalian species other than humans the reproductive cycle is an ESTROUS cycle.
r. efficiency fertility or efficiency in terms of input, e.g. services per conception, bull serving capacity estimates.
r. failure infertility; failure to produce viable offspring; the end-stage of reproductive inefficiency.
r. fitness a pre-mating examination of cows in an intensive herd health program; includes manual examination of genitalia per rectum, cervical sample for microbiological examination, blood sample for locally relevant abortogenic diseases, manual examination of udder, milk cell count and composite bacteriological examination of milk.
r. history computerized or card-based record of individual cow's complete breeding record including all services and identity of donor or naturally mated bull.
r. organs (female) the ovaries, which produce the ova, or eggs; the uterine tubes; the uterus; the vagina, or birth canal; and the vulva, comprising the external genitalia. The udder is a secondary sex character, enclosing the mammary glands.
r. organs (male) the testes, external genitalia and accessory glands that secrete special fluids and the ducts through which these organs and glands are connected to each other and through which the spermatozoa are ejaculated during coitus.
r. performance the productivity of the animal or herd or flock in terms of offspring produced, can be expressed in many ways, e.g. live piglets per litter or per year or per sow-year or per cubic meter of shed space.
r. rate viable, full-term offspring produced per female per year.
r. senescence the end of cyclic reproductive activity in primates; not recognized in domestic animals.
r. system the genital tract plus the endocrinal control systems, especially the hypothalamus, pituitary, gonads and placenta, the products of pregnancy and the mammary glands.
r. tract see reproductive organs (above).
reptilase an enzyme from Russell's viper venom used in determining blood clotting time.
reptiles terrestrial or aquatic vertebrates which breathe air through lungs and have a skin covering of horny scales. They are poikilothermic, oviparous or ovoviviparous, and, if they have legs they are short and constructed solely for crawling. Includes snakes, reptiles, crocodilians and the chelonians. Members of the class Reptilia.
repulsion 1. the act of driving apart or away; a force that tends to drive two bodies apart. 2. in genetics, the occurrence on opposite chromosomes in a double heterozygote of the two mutant alleles of interest. 3. in obstetrics the forcible displacement of the fetus back into the uterus so that limbs or head and neck can be brought into a proper position and a dystocia be relieved. 4. in dentistry, especially in the horse, involves gaining access to the root of the tooth by an external approach and repelling it into the mouth by hammering at its root.
RES reticuloendothelial system.
Resco nail trimmer a pincer-like instrument in which closing of the handles pushes a sharp blade through a guillotine fitting, clipping off a claw or beak that has been placed in the guillotine loop.
rescue grass BROMUS *catharticus*.
research careful study of a subject with the object of establishing one or more facts.
animal r. the use of animals in a careful study of a subject, which may be related to the health or other welfare of animals of the same or other species, including humans.
comparative medical r. the use of animals in research projects directed at establishing facts of direct value to human health and welfare.
holistic r. see HOLISTIC MEDICINE.
reductionistic r. see REDUCTIONISM.
resect to excise part of an organ or other structure.
resection excision of a portion of an organ or other structure.
en bloc r. radical resection or amputation.
gastric r. partial gastrectomy.
lateral ear r. a surgical procedure, usually performed in dogs with otitis externa, in which the lateral cartilaginous plate of the vertical portion of the external ear canal is removed, thereby exposing the horizontal canal for drainage and easier application of topical

medications. See also FORMSTON–MCCUNN METHOD, LACROIX OPERATION, ZEPP OPERATION.
submucosal r. a procedure in which the mucosa, e.g. of a prolapsed vagina, is stripped from a circumferential segment and the opposing edges sutured so as to take a tuck in the length of the wall of the viscus.
vertical ear canal r. total removal of the vertical portion of the external ear canal. Performed in dogs with chronic otitis externa with severe hyperplasia of the meatal epithelium without involvement of the horizontal canal.
wedge r. removal of a triangular mass of tissue.

resectoscope an endoscope with a wide-angle telescope and an electrically activated wire loop for transurethral removal or biopsy of lesions of the bladder, prostate or urethra.

resectoscopy resection or biopsy of lesions by means of the resectoscope.

reserpine an active alkaloid from various species of *Rauwolfia*, used as an antihypertensive, tranquilizer and sedative. Little used in veterinary medicine.

reserve 1. to hold back for future use. 2. a supply, beyond that ordinarily used, that may be utilized in emergency.
alkali r., alkaline r. the amount of buffer compounds in the blood that are capable of neutralizing acids, such as sodium bicarbonate and proteins. See also ALKALI reserve.
cardiac r. the potential ability of the heart to perform work beyond that necessary under basal conditions. See also CARDIAC reserve.

reservoir 1. a storage place or cavity. 2. an alternative host or passive carrier of a pathogenic organism.
r. control control of infection in animal, bird or insect populations which act as reservoirs for infection of domesticated animals.

resident a graduate and licensed veterinarian receiving training in a specialty in a hospital.

residual remaining or left behind.
r. body an amorphous body formed by the separation of the original tail of the spermatid during its metamorphosis to spermatozoon.
r. spray insecticide spray for surfaces. Has a residual effect either because of the ingredient or the vehicle. Aimed at killing the larvae that are still to hatch.
r. urine urine remaining in the bladder after voiding; seen with bladder outlet obstruction and disorders affecting nerves controlling bladder function.

residue a remainder; that which remains after the removal of other substances; in organic chemistry a portion of a molecule that is incorporated into another molecule, e.g. an amino acid residue of a polypeptide. See also UNINTENTIONAL RESIDUE.
r. avoidance procedures in the handling of chemicals adopted on the farm and in food processing facilities to ensure that human food is not contaminated.
cannery r. cannery wastes used as supplementary feed for cattle in feedlots. Tomato and onion wastes have caused poisoning incidents. Damaged materials, especially those infected with fungi, may cause mycotoxicoses.
chemical food r. chemicals used in agriculture present a real threat to the saleability of animal products if they are contaminated with chemical residues. The residues are often harmful to human health and are also the target of some very stringent pure foods legislation. Mercury in fish, sulfonamides in pig products, iodine in milk and chlorinated hydrocarbons in beef have been some of the celebrated examples of environmental and human food chain pollution.
drug r. see DRUG residue.
maximum r. limits maximum concentrations of individual chemicals, or groups of chemicals, especially metabolites, and including pharmaceutical and industrial chemicals, in commodities or tissues to be used as human or animal feeds, and as defined by the food standard codes of a particular country or state; permissible levels vary with local legislation. Called also MRL.

resin 1. a solid or semisolid, amorphous organic substance of vegetable origin or produced synthetically. True resins are insoluble in water, but are readily dissolved in alcohol, ether and volatile oils. 2. rosin.
acrylic r's products of the polymerization of acrylic or methacrylic acid or their derivatives and used in the fabrication of surgical prostheses and equipment.
anion-exchange r. see ION-EXCHANGE RESIN.
cation-exchange r. see ION-EXCHANGE RESIN.
cholestyramine r. a synthetic, strongly basic anion-exchange resin in the chloride form which chelates bile salts in the intestine, thus preventing their reabsorption.
composite r. usually a mixture of organic matrix and inorganic filler, used in restorative dentistry.
ipomoea r., jalap r., scammony r. severe cathartics and irritants; little used because of their disastrous effects.

resistance 1. opposition, or counteracting force, as opposition of a conductor to passage of electricity or other energy or substance. 2. the natural ability of a normal organism to remain unaffected by noxious agents in its environment. See also IMMUNITY. 3. acquired ability of a bacterium or helminth or arthropod parasite to survive in the presence of concentrations of a chemical which are normally lethal to the organisms of that species. Occurs usually as a result of prolonged growth of the organism in sublethal concentrations of the agent and the survival of the organisms which have the least innate susceptibility to the agent. Has serious implications for animals which may find themselves without a suitable remedy for a disease, and for humans who may experience transfer of a resistant organism from the food supply. 4. in studies of respiration, an expression of the opposition to flow of air produced by the tissues of the air passages, in terms of pressure per amount of air per unit of time.
drug r. the ability of a microorganism to withstand doses of a drug that are lethal to most members of its species.
peripheral r. resistance to the passage of blood through the small blood vessels, especially the arterioles.
transferable r. antimicrobial resistance genes carried by bacteria on plasmids or transposons can often be readily acquired by other strains of the same species, by different species, and sometimes by organisms in different genera. Of considerable import in consideration of the implications of antimicrobial therapy in animal populations and in public health. The full significance is difficult to ascertain.

resistance-determinant segment an accumulation of transposons or resistance genes into one large transposon or resistance-determinant segment.

resistance inducing factor test a test used to detect viruses; based on the increased resistance to a test virus by a tissue culture which has been previously infected with a known virus.

resistive index an indicator of resistance of an organ to perfusion. In ultrasonography, it can be calculated from the peak systolic velocity and the end diastolic velocity of blood flow.

resmethrin a synthetic pyrethroid insecticide used to control fleas and ticks on dogs and cats.

resolution 1. subsidence of a pathological state, as the subsidence of an inflammation, or the softening and disappearance of a swelling. 2. perception as separate of two adjacent points; in microscopy, the smallest distance at which two adjacent objects can be distinguished as separate.

resolvent 1. promoting resolution or the dissipation of a pathological growth. 2. an agent that promotes resolution.

resolving power the ability of the eye or of a lens to make small objects that are close together separately visible, thus revealing the structure of an object.

resonance 1. the prolongation and intensification of sound produced by transmission of its vibrations to a cavity, especially such a sound elicited by percussion. Decrease of resonance is called *dullness;* its increase, *flatness.* 2. a vocal sound heard on auscultation.

amphoric r. a sound resembling that produced by blowing over the mouth of an empty bottle.

skodaic r. increased percussion resonance at the upper part of the chest, with flatness below it.

tympanic r. drumlike reverberation of a cavity filled with air.

tympanitic r. the peculiar sound elicited by percussing a tympanitic abdomen.

vesicular r. normal pulmonary resonance.

vocal r. the sound of ordinary speech as heard through the chest wall.

resonant giving an intense, rich sound on percussion; exhibiting resonance.

resonator 1. an instrument used to intensify sounds. 2. an electric circuit in which oscillations of a certain frequency are set up by oscillations of the same frequency in another circuit.

resorantel a safe, hydroxybenzanilide cestocide highly effective against *Moniezia* and *Thysaniezia* spp. and moderately effective against *Paramphistomum* spp.

resorb to take up or absorb again; to undergo resorption.

resorcinism chronic poisoning by resorcinol, resulting in methemoglobinemia, paralysis and damage to the capillaries, kidneys, heart and nervous system.

resorcinol a phenol with bactericidal, fungicidal, keratolytic, exfoliative and antipruritic activity; used especially as a topical keratolytic in the treatment of dermatoses.

resorcylic acid lactones found in plants, e.g. zearalenone, an estrogenic substance found in fungi.

resorption 1. the lysis and assimilation of a substance, as of bone or fetus. 2. reabsorption.

r.-formation sequence while bones are being formed for the first time the sequence is formation followed by resorption and modeling; in remodeling of an existing bone resorption occurs first and is then followed by bone formation.

r. lacuna concavities in bone created by osteoclasts.

r. space a continuous series of resoption lacunae.

respirable suitable for respiration.

respiration 1. the exchange of oxygen and carbon dioxide between the atmosphere and the body cells, including inspiration and expiration, diffusion of oxygen from the pulmonary alveoli to the blood and of carbon dioxide from the blood to the alveoli, and the transport of oxygen to and carbon dioxide from the body cells. 2. cellular respiration, the metabolic processes by which living cells break down carbohydrates, amino acids and fats to produce energy in the form of ATP (adenosine triphosphate).

abdominal r. inspiration and expiration accomplished mainly by the abdominal muscles and diaphragm. Occurs in acute pleurisy because of pain in the chest and fixation of the thorax, and tick paralysis due to paralysis of the intercostal muscles.

aerobic r. oxidative transformation of certain substrates into secretory products, the released energy being used in the process of assimilation.

anaerobic r. respiration in which energy is released by chemical reactions in which free oxygen takes no part.

artificial r. that maintained by force applied to the body. Called also artificially assisted respiration.

artificially assisted r. see artificial respiration (above).

Biot's r's rapid, deep respirations with abrupt pauses in breathing. See also BIOT'S RESPIRATIONS.

cell r. the processes in the living cell by which organic substances are oxidized and chemical energy is released.

Cheyne–Stokes r. breathing characterized by rhythmic waxing and waning of respiration depth, with regularly recurring apneic periods. See also CHEYNE–STOKES RESPIRATION.

cogwheel r. breathing with jerky inspiration.

controlled r. during general anesthesia using an endotracheal tube with an inflated cuff, the animal's respiration can be controlled completely by compression alternating with relaxation on the rebreathing bag of the breathing circuit. See also intermittent positive-pressure VENTILATION.

costal r. the respiratory movements are mostly carried out by the chest wall.

diaphragmatic r. that performed mainly by the diaphragm.

electrophrenic r. induction of respiration by electric stimulation of the phrenic nerve.

external r. the exchange of gases between the lungs and the blood.

internal r. the exchange of gases between the body cells and the blood.

Kussmaul's r. see KUSSMAUL'S RESPIRATION.

labored r. see DYSPNEA.

r. monitors machines that monitor respiratory movement and efficiency are most desirable during anesthesia. They include rate monitors, apnea alarms, tidal and minute volume monitoring respirometers, infrared gas analyzers to measure carbon dioxide content of end-tidal air,

paradoxical r. that in which a lung, or a portion of a lung, is deflated during inspiration and inflated during expiration. See also PARADOXICAL respiration.

tissue r. internal respiration.

respirator a device for giving artificial respiration or to assist in pulmonary ventilation. See also VENTILATOR.

r. shock circulatory SHOCK due to interference with the flow of blood through the great vessels and chambers of the heart, causing pooling of blood in the veins and the abdominal organs and a resultant vascular collapse. The condition sometimes occurs as a result of increased intrathoracic pressure in patients who are being maintained on a mechanical VENTILATOR.

respiratory pertaining to respiration. See also PULMONARY.

acute r. disease of turkeys see turkey CORYZA.

acute r. distress syndrome a noncardiogenic pulmonary edema characterized by disruption of pulmonary capillary endothelium and accumulation of high-protein edema fluid in the lungs. See also SHOCK lung, ATYPICAL INTERSTITIAL PNEUMONIA, NEONATAL maladjustment syndrome.

r. arrest sudden complete cessation of respiratory movement.

r. burst of neutrophils the series of biochemical reactions that take place within a neutrophil when a particle is phagocytosed. Important in the host defense mechanisms.

r. centers see respiratory CENTERS.

chronic r. disease see CHRONIC respiratory disease.

r. cilia see CILIA.

r. clearance clearance of inhaled particles from the respiratory system by absorption of finally solubilized material through the respiratory epithelium, passage through the alveolar epithelium at special sites near the alveolar ducts, or to the exterior by a flow of alveolar fluid to the bronchi, a moving sheet of mucus into the bronchioles, up the bronchioles, bronchi and trachea with the assistance of repiratory cilia to the pharynx.

r. control quantitative relationship between oxidative phosphorylation and electron transfer. Traditionally presented as a P/O ratio indicating the number of ATP molecules synthesized per atom of oxygen consumed.

r. control ratio ratio of oxygen uptake in the presence of ADP to that in the absence of ADP. Used as an index of the functional integrity of prepared mitochondria since it is above 10 in good preparation and unity in aged or damaged mitochondria.

r. cycle the cycle of inspiration, expiration, pause of the normal resting cycle depends on sensors in the respiratory system which provide stimuli to initiate the next part of the cycle.

r. dead space see dead SPACE (2).

r. depression the rate and/or depth of respiration are insufficient to maintain adequate gas exchange in the lungs; a subjective judgment tending to be superseded, at least during anesthesia, by instrumentation. See RESPIRATION monitors.

r. depth amplitude of each respiratory movement.

r. difficulty see DYSPNEA.

r. disease pattern may be aerogenous when the pathogen is inhaled or hematogenous when the pathogen is delivered to the lungs in the blood supply.

r. distress syndrome of newborn (RDS) see HYALINE membrane disease.

r. exchange ratio the carbon dioxide output divided by the oxygen uptake; see also respiratory quotient (below).

r. failure a life-threatening condition in which respiratory function is inadequate to maintain the body's need for oxygen supply and carbon dioxide removal while at rest; called also acute ventilatory failure. The type of failure varies with the CO_2 content of the blood and may be asphyxial, when there is gasping, dyspneic when there is dyspnea, paralytic when the respiratory movements gradually fade away, tachypneic when the movements are fast and shallow.

r. grunting grunting at the peak of each inspiration, or on percussion of the chest wall; indicates pain in the pleura.

r. insufficiency a condition in which respiratory function is inadequate to meet the body's needs when increased physical activity places extra demands on it. Insufficiency occurs as a result of progressive degenerative changes in the alveolar structure and the capillary tissues in the pulmonary bed.

r. noises includes sneezing, snorting, stridor, stertor (snoring), wheezing, roaring, grunting.

r. paralysis see respiratory failure (above).

r. quotient (RQ) the ratio of the volume of expired carbon dioxide to the volume of oxygen absorbed by the lungs per unit of time. Called also respiratory exchange ratio (above).

r. rate the number of respirations per minute. Normal rates per minute are: horses 8 to 10; cattle 10 to 30; sheep and pigs 10 to 20; goats 25 to 35; dogs 10 to 30; cats 20 to 30.

r. rhythm normally consists of three phase cycles of inspiration, expiration, pause; prolongation of inspiration suggests obstruction of the upper respiratory tract, prolongation of expiration, or a double respiratory effort suggests loss of recoil elasticity of the lungs. See also BIOT'S RESPIRATIONS, CHEYNE–STOKES RESPIRATION.

r. secretion includes samples collected by nasal swab, nasopharyngeal swab, percutaneous tracheobronchial lavage and fiberoptic endoscopic sampling. Assessment is by laboratory examination for cellular content, bacteria, viruses, helminth parasites, fungi.

r. system the group of specialized organs whose specific function is to provide for the transfer of oxygen from the air to the blood and of waste carbon dioxide from the blood to the air. These functions are performed by the tubular and cavernous organs which allow atmospheric air to reach the membranes across which gases are exchanged with the blood. The system includes the organs of the respiratory tract (below) plus the respiratory centers in the medulla. The supportive roles of the nervous system, the muscular, cardiovascular and hemopoietic systems are also essential.

r. tract the organs of the tract include the UPPER respiratory tract of the nasal cavities, the pharynx, larynx, trachea and bronchi, and the LOWER respiratory tract comprising the bronchioles and alveoli of the lungs.

r. viruses see Table 8.2.

respirometer an instrument for determining the nature of the respiration, including the rate, the volume and the rhythmicity.

RESPITE an interactive computer-based guide to demonstrate the effect of specific management practices on the expected prevalence of swine pneumonia.

respondent an animal that responds to a particular stimulus.

r. behavior reflex responses elicited by stimuli; generally not under voluntary control.

r. conditioning see classical CONDITIONING.

response any action or change of condition evoked by a stimulus.

autoimmune r. the immune response in which antibodies or immune lymphoid cells are produced against the body's own tissues.

conditioned r. see also CONDITIONED response, CONDITIONING.

galvanic skin r. the alteration in the electrical resistance of the skin associated with sympathetic nerve discharge.

immune r. specifically altered reactivity of the animal body after exposure to antigen, manifested as antibody-production, cell-mediated immunity, development of hypersensitivity, or as immunological tolerance. Called also immune reaction. See also IMMUNE response.

maze r. a test of vision for animals.

placing r. see PLACING reflex.

r. rate in surveys, the number of completed survey instruments (questionnaires, interview records) divided by the total number of persons approached.

r. trial a field trial conducted to test a hypothesis, often about the cause of a disease but can encompass therapeutics or control of a disease. The hypothesis is tested by observing the response to an alteration in the system, e.g. in feeding or in management.

triple r. (of Lewis) a physiological reaction of the skin to stroking with a blunt instrument: first a red line develops at the site of stroking, owing to the release of histamine or a histamine-like substance, then a flare develops around the red line, and lastly a wheal is formed as a result of local edema.

unconditioned r. an unlearned response, i.e. one that occurs naturally. See also CONDITIONING.

responsible ownership the motto for the companion animal owner of this decade. Includes avoidance of cruelty and discomfort, preservation of the animal's dignity, prevention of disease, optimum nutrition and shelter and some consideration for what are the animal's pleasures. It also includes the avoidance of nuisance to other animals and people.

responsive diagnoses a diagnosis couched in terms of what the disease responds to, implying the at least partial involvement of the risk factor in the causation, e.g. copper-responsive achromotrichia.

rest 1. repose after exertion. 2. a fragment of embryonic tissue retained within the adult organism.

restenosis recurrent stenosis, especially of a cardiac valve after surgical correction of the primary condition.

restibrachium the inferior peduncle of the cerebellum.

restiform shaped like a rope.

resting pertaining to or having the characteristics of a REST (1).

limb r. posture adopted when the standing animal rests its weight on three limbs and allows the other to relax. The relaxed limb is said to be being rested.

r. line basophilic lines in the cement in bones. The lines are smooth and level and indicate that the previous activity in the bone was formative.

r. membrane potential see resting POTENTIAL.

r. osteoblast see surface OSTEOCYTE.

restis the caudal peduncle of the cerebellum.

restlessness a state manifested by increased motor activity, constant walking, vocalizing, lying down and getting up. May be caused by psychological factors, e.g. separation from young, or by pain, or deprivation of water.

Reston virus an Ebola-like virus isolated in Reston, Virginia from monkeys imported from Asia. It has not been shown to be pathogenic for humans.

restoration 1. induction of a return to a previous state, as a return to health or replacement of a part to normal position. 2. partial or complete reconstruction of a body part, or the device used in its place.

dental r. see restorative DENTISTRY.

restorative 1. promoting a return to health or to consciousness. 2. a remedy that aids in restoring health, vigor or consciousness.

r. dentistry see restorative DENTISTRY.

restraining chute a chute used for restraining cattle and to a limited extent horses that are not sufficiently tame to be handled in the normal manner. Of metal or wood with a head stock for restraining cattle by the head, a gate behind to prevent the animal from backing out but providing access over a rail so that a rectal examination can be performed, quick-release side gates with access ports to enable the operator to reach the animal's sides, and bars over the top to prevent escape by that route.

restraint control of an animal so that it can be examined or treated.

r. bag see FELINE restraint bag.

r. cage see squeeze CAGE.

chemical r. tranquilizers, sedatives and anesthetics are used depending on the wildness of the animal. See also BLOW DART.

diversionary r. use of various techniques to distract the animal and permit minimal physical restraint, usually used on horses. Examples are tapping or rubbing the head, using a blindfold, pressure on a skin fold, holding an ear, applying a chain shank over the bridge of the nose and use of a war bridle.

physical r. includes everything from halters to casting harness for horses, from hog-holders to dog-catchers.

restricted substances substances which because of the danger that would arise if the substances were released for uncontrolled use are available to the public only on the order of a veterinarian, or a medical or dental practitioner.

restriction digest a unique family of DNA fragments produced by digestion of a given DNA molecule by a particular restriction enzyme; usually visualized by agarose gel electrophoresis and ethidium bromide or other fluorescent procedures.

restriction endonuclease one of over 200 enzymes isolated from bacteria that cleave any DNA molecule at specific sites which are usually palindromes of 4 to 10 or so nucleotides to yield a collection of restriction DNA fragments that can be separated, usually by electrophoresis in agarose or polyacrylamide gels, and which are highly characteristic for a particular DNA. They evolved as a defense mechanism for bacteria in that they modify the bacteria's own DNA by methylation which blocks the restriction fragmentation function but allows restriction of any foreign DNA that enters the cell. Called also restriction-modification enzyme. See also RESTRICTION MAP.

restriction fragment length polymorphism (RFLP) when the restriction endonuclease DNA fragment patterns of organisms of the same type or species are compared minor differences in the patterns are observed which are produced by gain or loss of restriction sites or by insertion or deletion of DNA to make a particular fragment larger or smaller. Where a large amount of DNA, such as all the chromosomal DNA from a cell, is digested with a restriction enzyme and separated on an agarose gel, the fragments can be transferred to a nylon membrane (Southern blot) and probed with a particular probe, usually directed at repetitive DNA sequences. The pattern so obtained is unique to a particular individual. Called also restriction endonuclease DNA fingerprints. See also PARENTAGE testing.

restriction map for a DNA molecule, is constructed for a particular restriction endonuclease by ordering the fragments left to right in the DNA molecule. By convention, there are six fragments which are labeled in order of decreasing size, ABCDEF, but the order left to right in the genome may be DCBAFE.

restriction mapping the ordering, left to right, of the set of DNA fragments of a DNA molecule produced by a particular restriction enzyme.

restriction site the specific nucleotide site recognized by restriction endonuclease. Called also restriction endonuclease site.

r. s. bank see POLYCLONING SITE.

restrictive cardiomyopathy see restrictive CARDIOMYOPATHY.

resurrection plant see BRYOPHYLLUM *pinnatum*.

resuscitation restoration to life or consciousness of

an animal apparently dead or dying, or whose respirations have ceased. See also artificial RESPIRATION.
cardiopulmonary r. an emergency technique used in cardiac arrest to re-establish heart and lung function until more advanced life support is available. See also CARDIOPULMONARY resuscitation.
cerebral r. treatment to counteract the cerebral edema resulting from low cerebral blood flow and hypoxia that occurs during cardiopulmonary resuscitation.
r. equipment inludes cardiac defibrillator, laryngoscope, endotracheal tubes, tracheotomy tubes, plus the stimulants and the administration sets needed in an emergency.

resuscitator an apparatus for initiating respiration in animals whose breathing has stopped.

retained kept in an original position when dehiscence or movement to another location is more appropriate.
r. cartilage core see retained enchondral CARTILAGE cores.
r. corpus luteum the corpus luteum is not resorbed at the appropriate time in the reproductive cycle and the animal remains anestral.
r. meconium see MECONIUM ileus.
r. placenta see retained PLACENTA.
r. testicle failure of the testicle(s) to migrate out of the peritoneal cavity, through the inguinal ring and into the scrotum before the animal reaches puberty. The retention may be uni- or bilateral.

retainer a regular periodic payment made to a veterinarian in order to ensure that his/her services will be available if a particular need arises.

retama see PARKINSONIA ACULEATA.

Retama retam North African plant in family Fabaceae; contains alkaloids anagyrine, cytisine; cause abortion, incoordination, tremor, milk taint in camels. Called also r'tem.

retch vomiting movements without the production of regurgitus.

retching an unproductive effort to vomit.

rete pl. *retia* [L.] a network or meshwork, especially of blood vessels.
arterial r., r. arteriosum an anastomotic network of minute arteries, just before they become capillaries.
articular r. a network of anastomosing blood vessels in or around a joint.
blood vessel r. visible networks of vessels; see also rete mirabile (below).
r. carpi dorsale a network of small vessels over the dorsal aspect of the carpus in the horse.
r. malpighii the innermost stratum of epidermis.
r. mirabile a vascular network formed by division of an artery or vein into many smaller vessels that reunite into a single vessel, such as the carotid rete mirabile (epidural rete) at the base of the brain of ruminants.
r. mirabile ophthalmicum a small arterial network in the orbit of ruminants.
r. pegs inward projections of the epidermis into the dermis, as seen histologically in vertical sections.
r. ridge marked undulations of the dermoepidermal junction; not a feature of normal skin in animals except in certain areas such as the footpads and planum nasale of carnivores.
r. testis the network of channels formed in the mediastinum of the testis by the seminiferous tubules.
r. tubules a network composed of tubules, e.g. seminiferous tubules.
r. vasculosa networks of vessels as in the lungs.
r. venosum an anastomotic network of small veins.

retention the process of holding back or keeping in a position, such as persistence in the body of material normally excreted. See also RETAINED.
renal r. cysts these are acquired and result from scarring and obstruction of tubules in chronic renal disease.
urine r. accumulation of urine within the bladder because of inability to urinate.

reticular[1] resembling a net.
r. activating system the system of cells of the reticular formation of the medulla oblongata that receive collaterals from the ascending sensory pathways and project to higher centers; they control the overall degree of central nervous system activity, including wakefulness, attentiveness and sleep; abbreviated RAS. Called also ascending reticular formation.
ascending r. formation see reticular activating system (above).
r. cells stellate cells that form the reticular fibers of connective tissue; they form the supporting framework of bone marrow, lymph nodes, lymphatic nodules, spleen and tonsils.
r. colliquation, epidermal r. degeneration severe intracellular edema of epidermal cells, characterized by the degeneration of cells to form reticulated septa separating lobules of fluid.
descending r. system a diffuse motor control mechanism which descends from the midbrain to lower motor neurons in the brainstem and spinal cord.
r. dysgenesis a congenital error in stem cell numbers in the bone marrow; a rare cause of anemia.
r. formation see ascending reticular formation, reticular activating system (above).
medullary r. formation see ascending reticular formation (above).
r. tissue, reticulated tissue connective tissue composed predominantly of reticulum cells and reticular fibers.

reticular[2] pertaining to or emanating from the reticulum of the fore-stomachs.
r. cycle the reticular contraction which terminates in regurgitation. Called also regurgitation cycle.
r. foreign body sharp, ferrous objects causing traumatic reticuloperitonitis, flakes of lead paint.
r. groove the first part of the gastric GROOVE extending from the cardia to the reticulo-omasal orifice.
r. groove malfunction damage to the ruminal branches of the vagus nerve, or a foreign body lodged in the groove, causes a variety of malfunctions including vomiting when an eructation cycle occurs in the rumen, and failure of the reticulo-omasal orifice to open and allow onward movement of ruminal contents during a ruminal mixing cycle.
r. grunt a grunt audible on tracheal auscultation which occurs at each reticular contraction; an uncommon observation because the inflammation caused by reticular penetration, and therefore theoretically the grunt, is a potent cause of complete reticuloruminal atony.
r. papillomas not uncommon, especially in the esophageal groove where they interfere with normal ruminal cycles and may cause chronic bloat or vagus indigestion.
r. retention pellet dense, heavy pellet designed to be taken orally and to lodge, by virtue of its weight, in the reticulum.

reticulate body a stage in the development of elementary bodies in *Chlamydia*.

reticulated reticular.

reticulation the formation or presence of a network.

radiographic r. network appearance of the film; caused, for example, by hot developer and cold fixer, sometimes by weak fixer solution.

reticulemia the presence in the blood of increased numbers of immature erythrocytes.

reticulin a scleroprotein present in the connective fibers of reticular tissue, closely related to collagen in composition.

reticulitis inflammation of reticulum. Is rare except in specific disease entities. See also TRAUMATIC reticuloperitonitis.

reticulocerebellar tract one of the tracts in the reticular formation.

reticulocyte a stage of erythrocyte maturation, between normoblast (metarubricyte) and mature erythrocyte, showing a basophilic reticulum (residual RNA) under vital staining.

r. count performed on blood mixed with a supravital stain such as new methylene blue or brilliant cresyl blue. An increased count indicates active erythropoiesis.

r. production index (RPI) corrects the reticulocyte count, taking into account the presence of anemia and the presence of shift reticulocytes producing a more accurate indicator of red cell production.

r. response the release of reticulocytes in response to erythropoietin or administration of specific therapy for anemia, e.g. a deficiency of iron or folic acid. A reticulocyte response does not develop until the anemia is marked in cattle and not at all in horses.

shift r., stimulated r. with intense stimulation of erythropoiesis there is premature release of reticulocytes from the bone marrow into peripheral blood. These are larger and contain more reticulum than normal reticulocytes.

reticulocytopenia a deficiency of reticulocytes in the peripheral blood.

reticulocytosis an excess of reticulocytes in the peripheral blood. See also RETICULOCYTE response.

reticuloendothelial system a term that encompasses the monocyte–macrophage or mononuclear phagocytic system and also includes reticulum cells. It consists of a population of cells called macrophages, which are of bone marrow origin and are widely distributed throughout the body. Immature macrophages or monocytes make up about 5% of peripheral blood leukocytes. Mature macrophages are found in connective tissue (histiocytes), lining hepatic sinusoids (Kupffer cells), in the lung (alveolar macrophages), brain (microglia) and skin (Langerhans cells). They are also found in the spleen, lymph nodes and bone marrow. The major roles of these cells include: phagocytosis, antigen-processing and trapping, regulation of immune responses and the secretion of several biologically important factors such as interleukin 1, lysozyme, plasminogen activator and complement components.

The macrophages of the SPLEEN possess the ability to dispose of disintegrated erythrocytes. They do not, however, destroy hemoglobin, which is liberated in the process.

Kupffer cells, together with the cells of the general connective tissue and bone marrow, are capable of transforming into bile pigment the hemoglobin released by disintegrated erythrocytes.

reticuloendotheliosis a superseded term for neoplasia of hemopoietic precursors. See also blast form of ERYTHREMIC MYELOSIS.

avian r. a group of diseases of poultry caused by the REV group of retroviruses, and includes a chronic neoplastic disease of turkeys and chickens, a runting disease in chickens accidentally injected with the virus, and possibly an acute reticulum cell neoplasia. The chronic neoplasia is manifested by nodular tumors in visceral organs.

feline r. see ERYTHREMIC MYELOSIS, MYELOPROLIFERATIVE disease.

leukemic r. leukemia marked by splenomegaly and by an abundance of large, mononuclear abnormal cells with numerous, irregular cytoplasmic projections that give them a flagellated or hairy appearance in the bone marrow, spleen, liver and peripheral blood; called also hairy-cell leukemia.

reticuloendothelium the tissue of the reticuloendothelial system.

reticulohistiocytoma a granulomatous aggregation of lipid-laden histiocytes and multinucleated giant cells.

reticulo-omasal orifice aperture in the gastric groove as it passes from the reticulum into the omasum. Obstruction by a foreign body causes ruminal distension and hypermotility and the passage of small amounts of feces. See also VAGUS indigestion.

r.-o. sphincter achalasia part of the vagus indigestion pathogenesis; causes accumulation of ingesta in the reticulorumen. Called also anterior functional stenosis.

reticulopenia reticulocytopenia.

reticuloperitonitis see TRAUMATIC reticuloperitonitis.

reticulopodium a threadlike, branching pseudopodium.

reticuloruminal contractions contractions occur in two types, primary and secondary. Primary contraction cycles commence with a double reticular contraction, the second accompanied by a contraction of the anterior dorsal sac of the rumen; next comes a contraction of the ventral sac of the rumen which completes the cycle. The frequency of the cycle in the normal animal depends on the volume and physical characteristics of the contents of the reticulorumen.

Secondary cycles follow primary cycles mostly when the patient is feeding; usually they commence in the caudal sacs and terminate in eructation.

reticulosarcoma malignant lymphoma, histiocytic or undifferentiated.

reticulosis an abnormal increase in cells derived from or related to the monocyte macrophage.

familial histiocytic r., histiocytic medullary r. see malignant HISTIOCYTOSIS.

inflammatory r. see granulomatous MENINGOENCEPHALOMYELITIS.

pagetoid r. a lymphoproliferative disease of the skin in dogs; it may be a variant of mycosis fungoides. There are erythematous plaques, ulcers and vesicles on the oral mucosa and footpads.

reticulospinal tract spinal cord tract originating in the reticular formation in the brainstem and impinging on motor fibers arising in the spinal cord.

reticulum pl. *reticula* [L.] 1. a small network, especially a protoplasmic network in cells. 2. reticular tissue. 3. the smallest, most cranial section of the compound stomach of ruminants, lined with mucous membrane folded into a hexagonal pattern. Called also honeycomb. It communicates cranially with the esophagus and caudally with the rumen.

r. (1) cell see RETICULAR[1] cells.

r. (1) cell leukemia see malignant HISTIOCYTOSIS.

r. (1) cell sarcoma see cutaneous LYMPHOSARCOMA.

endoplasmic r. (1) an ultramicroscopic organelle of nearly all higher plant and animal cells, consisting of a system of membrane-bound cavities in the cytoplasm, occurring in two types: granular or rough-surfaced, bearing large numbers of ribosomes on its outer surface, and concerned mainly with protein production, and agranular or smooth-surfaced, concerned with lipid and glycogen synthesis and cholesterol metabolism. See also ROUGH ENDOPLASMIC RETICULUM.

sarcoplasmic r. (1) a form of agranular reticulum in the sarcoplasm of striated muscle, comprising a system of smooth-surfaced tubules surrounding each myofibril.

transmissible r. (1) cell tumor see canine transmissible VENEREAL tumor.

transmissible venereal r. (1) cell tumor see canine transmissible VENEREAL tumor.

retiform reticular.

retina the innermost of the three tunics of the eyeball, surrounding the vitreous body and continuous posteriorly with the OPTIC nerve. The retina is composed of two parts: an optical part in the fundus of the eye that is sensitive to light, and a nonsensitive pigmented part that lines the ciliary body and iris. The light-sensitive neurons are arranged in three layers; the first layer is made up of rods and cones and the other two transmit impulses from the rods and cones to the optic nerve The rods are sensitive to dim light of a variety of wavelengths, and the cones are sensitive to bright light of more restricted wavelengths and are responsible for color vision. Visual acuity is greatest in the central part of the retina. See also EYE.

silent r. syndrome see sudden acquired RETINAL degeneration.

retinaculum pl. *retinacula* [L.] 1. a structure that retains an organ or tissue in place. 2. an instrument for retracting tissues during surgery.

carpal r. a superficial transverse ligament passing obliquely across the palmar aspect of the carpus, completing the carpal tunnel.

hock r. one of three transverse ligamentous bands across the dorsal aspect of the hock, holding the digital extensor tendons in place.

r. morgagni a ridge formed by the coming together of segments of the ileocecal valve. Called also frenulum of ileocecal valve.

patellar r. medial and lateral patellar ligaments.

r. tendinum a tendinous restraining structure, such as an annular ligament.

retinal 1. pertaining to the retina. 2. the aldehyde of retinol, having vitamin A activity. One isomer(11-*cis*-retinal) combines with opsin in the retinal rods (scotopsin) to form rhodopsin (visual purple); another, all-*trans*-retinal, or visual yellow, results from the bleaching of rhodopsin by light, in which the 11-*cis*-form is converted to the all-*trans*-form. Retinal also combines with opsins in the retinal cones to form the three pigments responsible for color vision.

r. absence inherited as a recessive character in foals.

central progressive r. atrophy a disease of the retinal pigmented epithelium, generally in middle-aged Labrador retrievers, Border collies, Golden retrievers, Irish setters, and English springer spaniels. There are pigmentary changes in the tapetal fundus, with attenuation of retinal vasculature, and atrophy of the optic disk. Day vision is affected first, followed by impairment, but not always blindness, in any situation. Called also CPRA.

r. degeneration see progressive retinal atrophy (below), bright BLINDNESS, TAURINE nutritional deficiency, RETINOPATHY.

r. detachment see retinal DETACHMENT.

r. dialysis, r. disinsertion separation of the sensory retinal layer from the pigment layer at the ora ciliaris retinae.

r. dysplasia a congenital anomaly in many species, consisting of an abnormal differentiation of retinal cells and proliferation of photoreceptors, forming rosettes. May be caused by viral infections such as feline panleukopenia, bluetongue, bovine virus diarrhea and canine herpesvirus; an inherited defect in some breeds of dogs and cattle.

r. ganglionic cell layer the layer of the retina which contains ganglion cell bodies.

r. hemorrhages occur in association with many systemic diseases and intoxications in most species, including ethylene glycol poisoning, ehrlichiosis, severe anemia and thromboembolic meningoencephalitis in cattle.

light-induced r. degeneration a phototoxic degeneration in rats and mice caused by exposure to continuous light and high temperatures.

r. nuclear layer the layer of the retina which includes inner and outer nuclear layers of the retina.

inner r. nuclear layer the layer of the retina which contains the cell bodies of bipolar neurons and association neurons.

outer r. nuclear layer the layer of the retina which contains the cell nuclei of the photoreceptor cells.

r. optic nerve fiber layer retinal layer of axonal processes of the ganglion cells as they approach the optic papilla and emerge as the optic nerve.

r. photoreceptor layer the retinal layer which contains rods and cones, modified neuronal processes of the photoreceptor rod and cone cells.

r. pigment epithelial layer retinal layer just beneath the choroidal basal complex of the eye; probably serves as a store of vitamin A. Long cellular processes extend to and between the photoreceptor cells in the next layer.

r. plexiform layer the retinal layer which includes inner and outer plexiform layers; both consist of a network of cell processes of adjacent nerve cells, especially photoreceptor and ganglion cells.

progressive r. atrophy a group of inherited, degenerative diseases of the retina, occurring most commonly in dogs and consisting of a progressive, noninflammatory degeneration or dysplasia of rods and cones or purely cones, leading to blindness. Specific features, such as age of onset, pattern of degeneration, and ultrastructural and biochemical changes vary between the many breeds in which the disease is found. Night blindness followed by a loss of day vision are clinical signs common to most. There may also be an associated cataract formation. See also central progressive retinal atrophy (above), CONE dysplasia, ROD–cone dysplasia. Called also PRA.

progressive r. degeneration in one system of classification, a term encompassing a range of retinal disorders otherwise referred to as various types of retinal atrophy, retinal dysplasias or retinal degenerations. The inherited rod–cone dysplasias of dogs and cats are included in Type I; pigment epithelial dystrophy (central progressive atrophy) is Type II; and hemeralopia of Alaskan malamutes and miniature poodles is Type III. Called also PRD.

sudden acquired r. degeneration a nonspecific degeneration of rods and cones that progresses to complete retinal atrophy and blindness in mature dogs. The cause is unknown. Called also silent retina syndrome, metabolic toxic retinopathy, SARD.

retinene an ocular pigment derived from vitamin A

and formed by the bleaching action of light on rhodopsin. It occurs in two forms: retinene$_1$ is RETINAL (2), and retinene$_2$ is DEHYDRORETINAL.

retinitis inflammation of the retina. Occurs in association with many viral infections, particularly canine distemper, scrapie, hog cholera and rabies.

neurotrophic r. caused by infection such as canine distemper virus.

r. pigmentosa a group of diseases in humans, frequently hereditary, marked by progressive retinal atrophy, attenuation of retinal vessels, and clumping of the pigment, with contraction of the field of vision. See progressive RETINAL atrophy.

retinoblastoma a tumor arising from retinal cells.

retinochoroiditis inflammation of the retina and choroid.

retinoic acid form of vitamin A, derived from retinal. See TRETINOIN.

retinoid 1. resembling the retina. 2. any derivative of retinal.

retinol vitamin A_1; the form of vitamin A found in mammals, which is reversibly dehydrogenated by enzymatic action into its aldehyde, RETINAL (2).

retinomalacia softening of the retina.

retinopapillitis inflammation of retina and optic disk (papilla).

retinopathy any noninflammatory disease of the retina; occurs in systemic disorders, e.g. nephritis, diabetes mellitus and in a number of poisonings in agricultural animals. Examples are poisoning by *Astragalus*, *Oxytropis*, *Pteridium* spp.

diabetic r. retinal manifestations of diabetes mellitus, including microaneurysms and punctate exudates, occur in dogs but are often obscured by cataract formation.

hypertensive r. that associated with hypertension; seen in dogs and cats. There is sudden loss of vision, retinal hemorrhages and detachment, and sometimes glaucoma.

nutritional r. may occur with deficiency of vitamin A or E, or TAURINE.

senile r. retinal thinning, cyst formation, atrophy and fibrosis occur in aged dogs and horses.

toxic r. see bright BLINDNESS.

retinoschisis splitting of the retina.

retinoscope skiascope; an instrument used in retinoscopy.

retinoscopy an objective method of investigating, diagnosing and evaluating refractive errors of the eye, by projection of a beam of light into the eye and observation of the movement of the illuminated area on the retina surface and of the refraction by the eye of the emergent rays. Called also pupilloscopy, shadow test, skiametry and skiascopy.

retinosis any degenerative, noninflammatory condition of the retina.

retinotopic relating to the organization of the visual pathways and visual area of the brain.

retinyl esters of retinol, the alcohol form of vitamin A.

retort a globular, long-necked vessel used in distillation.

Retortamonas a genus of nonpathogenic, pyriform, protozoan parasites in the family Retortamonadidae.

R. caviae found in the cecum of guinea pigs.

R. cuniculi found in the cecum of rabbits.

R. intestinalis found in humans and nondomesticated primates.

R. ovis found in sheep.

retothelium the layer of cells covering a reticular tissue.

retractile capable of being drawn back.

retraction the act of drawing back, or condition of being drawn back.

clot r. see CLOT retraction.

retractor 1. an instrument for holding open the edges of a wound or edges of a fissure such as the eyelids. 2. a muscle that retracts.

flexible r. a simple surgical instrument made of metal, usually copper, and shaped like a simple spatula or tongue-depressor. It can be bent into any shape so as to get into tricky sites to hold back tissues. Usually bent into a hook shape.

Weitlaner r. see WEITLANER RETRACTOR.

retrices the very long contour feathers coming from the side of the tail. These are the longest feathers of all in the domestic fowl.

retrieval obtaining access to and bringing information out, usually a specific record, of a storage medium, e.g. into the memory of a computer.

r. basket an instrument used with endoscopy which permits removal of small, round and smooth foreign bodies, usually from the gastrointestinal tract.

retriever a type of hunting dog used for recovering the shot bird, often from water; includes the specific breeds, Chesapeake Bay, Curly-coated, Flat-coated, Golden and Labrador retrievers, and Wire-haired pointing griffon, but various spaniels may also perform retrieving duties in the field.

retrix pl. *retrices* a large tail feather at the pelvic inlet.

retro- word element. [L.] *behind, backward.*

retroaction action in a reversed direction; reaction.

retroauricular behind the auricle of the ear.

retrobulbar 1. behind the pons. 2. behind the eyeball.

r. block regional anesthesia of the eyeball by blocking the nerve supply as it emerges from the orbital fissure. There are two techniques, a four-point injection and the Peterson technique, used in cattle for enucleation of the eyeball.

r. neuropathy see DRYOPTERIS.

retrocecal behind the cecum.

retrocervical behind the cervix uteri.

retrocession a going backward; backward displacement.

retrocochlear 1. behind the cochlea. 2. denoting the eighth cranial nerve and cerebellopontine angle as opposed to the cochlea.

retrocolic behind the colon.

retrocollic pertaining to the dorsum of the neck; nuchal.

retrocursive marked by stepping backward.

retrodeviation a general term including retroversion, retroflexion, retroposition, etc.

retrodisplacement backward or posterior displacement.

retroesophageal behind the esophagus.

r. right subclavian artery a vascular anomaly resulting in constriction of the esophagus in the newborn. See also vascular RING.

retroflexion the bending of an organ so that its top is turned backward.

retrogasserian pertaining to the sensory (dorsal) root of the trigeminal (gasserian) ganglion.

retrognathia underdevelopment of the maxilla and/or mandible.

retrognathism a state of being affected by retrognathia.

retrograde going backward; retracting a former course; catabolic.

r. pyelography radiography of the kidney after introduction of contrast medium through the ureter.

retrogression degeneration; deterioration; regression; return to an earlier, less complex condition.

retroinsular behind the insula of the cerebral cortex.
retrolective data harvested from records already collected, usually for another purpose.
retrolental behind the lens of the eye.
r. fibroplasia a retinopathy caused by exposure to high concentrations of oxygen at a young age; reported in kittens.
retrolingual behind the tongue.
retromammary behind the mammary gland.
retromandibular behind the lower jaw.
retromastoid behind the mastoid process.
retromingent urinating backwards, e.g. cats, other Felidae, elephants. Such an undignified posture for these kings of beasts, perhaps accounting for their nocturnal proclivities.
retromorphosis retrograde metamorphosis.
retronasal pertaining to the back part of the nose.
retro-ocular behind the eye.
retroparotid behind the parotid gland.
retroperistalsis reverse peristalsis.
retroperitoneal behind the peritoneum.
r. abscess characterized by fever and toxemia, chronic or intermittent colic in horses, weight loss and a positive paracentesis sample. See also PELVIC abscess and MESENTERIC abscess.
r. perirenal cyst see feline PERIRENAL cysts.
r. space see RETROPERITONEUM.
retroperitoneum the retroperitoneal space; the space between the peritoneum and the abdominal wall.
retroperitonitis inflammation in the retroperitoneal space. In animals, occurs most often in association with migrating foreign bodies, particularly grass awns, and in bitches following spaying.
retropharyngeal behind the pharynx.
r. abscess see PHARYNGEAL abscess.
r. lymphadenopathy see PHARYNGEAL lymphadenopathy.
r. lymph nodes lymph nodes in the tissues in the dorsum of the pharynx.
r. lymph node abscess see PHARYNGEAL abscess.
r. lymph node enlargement enlargement causes interference with respiration and swallowing. The principal sign is snoring. In large animals the glands are palpable via the oral cavity or inspected by fiberoptoscopic viewing. See also PHARYNGEAL lymphadenopathy.
retropharyngitis inflammation of posterior part of the pharynx.
retroplasia retrograde metaplasia; degeneration of a tissue or cell into a more primitive type.
retropneumoperitoneography a radiograph taken of the abdomen after the injection of air or carbon dioxide into the retroperitoneal space to give better contrast.
retroposed displaced backward.
retroposition backward displacement.
retropulsion a driving back, as of the fetal head during correction of a dystocia; performed manually or with a crutch during pauses between contractions and straining efforts.
retrorsine a pyrrolizidine alkaloid in *Crotalaria* spp.
retrospective said of data already collected or of events that have already occurred. Hence a retrospective study is a study of past events, in contradistinction to a prospective study.
retrotarsal behind the tarsus of the eye.
retrotransposon, retroposon a mobile sequence of DNA that transposes via a RNA intermediate.
retrouterine behind the uterus.
retroversion a turning backwards; as in surgically created deviation of the penis in the creation of a teaser bull.
retrovesical behind the urinary bladder.
Retroviridae a family of medium-sized (about 100 nm diameter) enveloped viruses with an icosahedral capsid enclosing the single-strand RNA genome which is diploid, i.e. two copies per virion. There are three subfamilies: *Oncornavirinae*, which includes avian, bovine, feline and murine leukemia/sarcoma viruses; *Lentivirinae*, which includes maedi/visna virus of sheep, caprine arthritis encephalitis and equine infectious anemia viruses and human immunodeficiency virus 1 and 2; *Spumavirinae*, which includes nonpathogenic viruses of monkey, cattle and cats, recognized only in cell culture where they produce syncytia (bovine and feline syncytia-forming viruses) which have a vacuolated cytoplasm, hence also called foamy viruses.
retrovirus a member of the family RETROVIRIDAE.
defective r. a virus unable to replicate independently; commonly the result of loss of part of the envelope gene when leukosis viruses acquire an oncogene. Propagation is achieved by coinfection with a leukosis virus able to provide the envelope for the defective virus.
endogenous r. one transmitted in germ-line DNA from an infected parent to offspring.
exogenous r. one transmitted horizontally.
rapidly transforming r. characterized by rapid oncogenesis attributable to the v-*onc* gene which they carry.
slowly transforming r. weakly oncogencic after a long incubation period. They do not carry the v-*onc* gene.
return 1. income earned. 2. the key on the keyboard of a computer terminal which carries out the commands previously typed in.
r. to assets the annual operational profit expressed as a percentage of the total assets of the farm.
r. to capital the annual operational profit expressed as a percentage of the capital invested in the enterprise.
internal r. rate the rate of discount at which the present value of a future income from a project equals the present value of the total expenditure (capital and running) on the project.
retzius enamel incremental lines incremental lines in normal enamel.
REU recurrent equine uveitis.
Reuff casting a casting in which, using a single rope, a loop is passed around the horns, followed by three halfhitches, one around the neck, one around the chest behind the elbows and one just in front of the udder.
revascularization the restoration of an adequate blood supply to a part by means of a blood vessel graft, as in aortocoronary bypass.
reverberation an artifact in ultrasound imaging resulting from the production of spurious echoes which are caused by reflections at the skin–transducer interface or by bone or gas. See also COMET-TAIL.
Reverchonia arenaria North American plant in the family Euphorbiaceae; contains an unidentified toxin which causes chronic liver damage.
Reverdin pertaining to the Swiss surgeon, Jacques Louis Reverdin.
R's needle a surgical needle with an eye that can be opened by means of a slide.
R's continuous suture see LOCK-STITCH SUTURE PATTERN.
reversal a turning or change in the opposite direction.

r. band band separating the osteoid seam in developing bone from the remaining osteoid tissue.
r. line basophilic cement lines in bone that are wavy rather than smooth and are an indication that the previous cellular activity at the site was resorptive. See also RESTING line.
reverse genetics methods such as antisense nucleic acids and site-directed mutagenesis that are used to selectively study gene function. Contrasts with classical genetics which depends on the isolation and analysis of cells (animals) with random mutations that can be identified.
reverse isolation see PROTECTIVE isolation.
reverse T_3 3,3′,5′-tri-iodothyronine.
reverse transcriptase see reverse TRANSCRIPTASE.
reverse zoonosis infections transmitted from humans to animals.
reversed marker mirror images of letters and numbers for marking x-ray films that are to be viewed from the reverse.
reversed title for purposes of sorting data the titles of items are often set out in reversed form, e.g. brucellosis, bovine for bovine brucellosis.
reversion 1. a returning to a previous condition; regression. 2. in genetics, inheritance from some remote ancestor of a character that has not been manifest for several generations.
Revivon a proprietary name for DIPRENORPHINE.
revulsant revulsive.
revulsion the drawing of blood from one part to another, as in counterirritation; the diminution of morbid action in any part of the body by irritation in another.
revulsive 1. causing revulsion. 2. an agent causing revulsion; a counterirritant.
reward a specific, intuitive drive in all animals; utilized in most animal training systems.
rewarming the restoration of normal body temperature in the management of cases of hypothermia. Several methods are used: (1) passive, which relies on retention of basal heat, (2) active, which employs a heat source externally or internally ('core') with lavage, irrigation, dialysis or extracorporeal blood heating.
Rex 1. a breed of cats derived from several mutants with a short, wavy or curly haircoat, including the whiskers. Many colors are recognized and there are several strains, each named after the origin of one of founding mutants, e.g. Cornish rex, Devon rex. The Cornish rex has curly hair, the Devon rex has wavy hair. The unusual coat has been linked with a specific genetic trait and virtually any variety of cat can be 'rexed'. Sometimes called 'Poodle cats'. The breed is affected by hereditary hypotrichosis. 2. a type of rabbit with short guard hairs in their coats which do not protrude above the level of their undercoat, producing a short, plush coat. As in cats, this characteristic can be produced in many different colored varieties or breeds. The Castor Rex was the original variety introduced into the United States. It was a chestnut-brown agouti color. Other varieties are 'rexed' versions of the normal breeds. Variation can also be found in the character of the coat. The rough-coated varieties are the Astrex, which have a wavy coat, and the Oppossum coat, which have curly guard hairs.
Reynaud body nodular proliferations of Schwann cells; common finding in normal horses.
Reynold's number a dimensionless number allotted empirically to the circumstances in which turbulence occurs in fluids flowing through vessels. It takes into account the velocity of the flow, the diameter of the vessel, and the density and viscosity of the fluid. Used to explain the development of heart murmurs.

$$\text{Reynold's number} = \frac{\text{radius} \times \text{velocity} \times \text{density}}{\text{viscosity}}$$

Rf chemical symbol, *rutherfordium;* rheumatoid factor.
RFFIT rapid fluorescent focus inhibition test for rabies.
RFLP restriction fragment length polymorphism.
RH releasing hormone.
Rh chemical symbol, *rhodium.*
Rhabdias a genus of nematodes which cause verminous pneumonia in reptiles and amphibians; they may also be found in their body cavities. Includes *R. fuscovenosa*.
rhabditic dermatitis see pelodera DERMATITIS.
rhabditiform esophagus an anterior esophagus shaped like a club connecting through a narrow neck (isthmus) to a bulbous posterior part (corpus); all free-living nematodes have an esophagus of this type.
Rhabditis a genus of minute nematodes found mostly in damp earth but they may temporarily invade damaged skin; members of the family Rhabditidae.
R. axei not recorded as pathogenic.
R. bovis causes bovine parasitic otitis and secondary myiasis.
R. clavopapillata, R. macrocerca found as a contaminant on the hair of dogs and monkeys.
R. gingivalis found in a granuloma of the gum in a horse.
R. strongyloides see PELODERA *strongyloides*.
rhabd(o)- word element. [Gr.] *rod, rod-shaped.*
rhabdocyte metamyelocyte.
rhabdoid resembling a rod; rod-shaped.
rhabdomyoblastoma rhabdomyosarcoma.
rhabdomyolysis disintegration of striated muscle fibers with excretion of myoglobin in the urine.
equine r. see PARALYTIC myoglobinuria.
exertional r. see EXERTIONAL rhabdomyolysis.
transient exertional r. see TYING-UP SYNDROME.
rhabdomyoma a tumor containing striated muscle fibers.
rhabdomyomatosis a non-neoplastic, nodular glycogenic infiltration of myocardial cells, seen in guinea pigs.
rhabdomyosarcoma a highly malignant tumor arising in striated muscle or in embryonal mesenchymal cells, and exhibiting differentiation along rhabdomyoblastic lines, including but not limited to the presence of cells with recognizable cross striations.
rhabdosarcoma rhabdomyosarcoma.
Rhabdoviridae a family in the order *Mononegavirales*, of bullet-shaped, enveloped viruses with a single-strand negative sense RNA genome and a helical nucleocapsid. Two genera cause disease in animals: *Vesiculovirus*, which contains vesicular stomatitis virus, and *Lyssavirus*, which contains rabies. There are two unnamed subgroups which include bovine ephemeral fever virus and the fish rhabdoviruses that cause viral hemorrhagic septicemia, infectious hemopoietic necrosis, spring viremia of carp. Lagos bat virus, Mokola virus and Australian flying fox lyssavirus are examples of bat rabies-like viruses that cause rabies-like illness in humans and animals. See also EEL rhabdovirus.
rhabdovirus a member of the family RHABDOVIRIDAE.
rhachi- for words beginning thus, see those beginning *rachi-*.
Rhadinovirus a genus of gammaherpesviruses. They cause disease in chimpanzees and baboons.
rhagades fissures, cracks or fine scars in the skin, especially such lesions around the mouth or other regions subjected to frequent movement.

Rhamnus a genus of small trees in the family Rhamnaceae all of which contain glycosides from which anthraquinone, a purgative, can be prepared. Includes *R. cathartica* (buckthorn), *R. frangula* (*Frangula alnus*, alder buckthorn), *R. purshiana* (buckthorn).

rhamphotheca beak, as in birds; made of hard keratinized epidermis.

rhaphe raphe.

-rhaphy, -rrhaphy word element. [Gr.] *seam, suture;* surgical repair of.

RHDV rabbit hemorrhagic disease virus.

rhea a large, flightless, ostrich-like bird, with a black head and yellow to white body. Includes *Rhea americana* and *Pterocnemia pennata.*

rhegma a rupture, rent or fracture.

rhegmatogenous arising from a rhegma, as rhegmatogenous detachment of the retina.

rhenium a chemical element, atomic number 75, atomic weight 186.2, symbol Re. See Table 6.

rheo- word element. [Gr.] *electric current, flow* (as of fluids).

rheobase the minimum electric current necessary to produce stimulation.

rheology the science of the deformation and flow of matter, such as the flow of blood through the heart and blood vessels.

rheostat an apparatus for regulating resistance in an electric circuit.

rheostosis a condition of hyperostosis marked by the presence of streaks in the bones; melorheostosis.

rheotaxis orientation of an organism in a stream of liquid, with its long axis parallel with the direction of flow, designated negative (moving in the same direction) or positive (moving in the opposite direction).

rhestocythemia the occurrence of broken-down erythrocytes in the blood.

rhesus monkey a gray, longhaired monkey with red ischial callosities. They are very agile, strong and curious. They learn easily and are used extensively in research work. Called also *Macaca mulatta.*

rheum any watery or catarrhal discharge.

Rheum rhaponticum culinary rhubarb, member of plant family Polygonaceae; the leaves can cause oxalate poisoning if fed in large amounts.

rheumarthritis rheumatoid arthritis.

rheumatic pertaining to or affected with rheumatism.

rheumatoid resembling rheumatism.

r. arthritis see rheumatoid ARTHRITIS.

r. factor antibodies, particularly IgM but also IgG, that are directed against antigenic determinants on the Fc region of other immunoglobulins. When the immunoglobulin binds to antigen, changes occur in the folding of the protein of the Fc region such that new, 'non self' antigenic determinants are exposed and it is to these that rheumatoid factors, i.e. other antibodies, are directed.

rheumatoid-like arthritis rare disease in mostly toy and small breeds of dogs characterized by episodes of anorexia, depression, fever, generalized or shifting lameness and periarticular swelling.

rhexis the rupture of a blood vessel or of an organ.

rhinal pertaining to the nose.

rhinalgia pain in the nose.

Rhinanthus a northern hemisphere plant genus in the family Scrophulariaceae, the members of which contain sufficient toxic cardiac glycosides to cause poisoning but are not recorded as having caused clinical illness in animals. Called also yellow rattle.

rhinencephalon 1. the part of the brain once thought to be concerned entirely with olfactory mechanisms, including olfactory nerves, bulbs, tracts and subsequent connections (all olfactory in function) and the limbic system (not primarily olfactory in function); homologous with olfactory portions of the brain in lower animals. 2. one of the parts of the embryonic telencephalon.

rhinesthesia the sense of smell.

rhinion the lower end of the suture between the nasal bones.

rhinitis inflammation of the mucous membrane of the nose. It may be mild and chronic, or acute. There are signs of wheezing, sneezing and respiratory stertor at all levels. There is a strong nasal discharge which may be serous to purulent.

allergic r., anaphylactic r. any allergic reaction of the nasal mucosa, occurring perennially (nonseasonal allergic rhinitis) or seasonally.

atrophic r. see ATROPHIC rhinitis.

bovine atopic r. see ENZOOTIC nasal granuloma.

catarrhal r. the common form of rhinitis with a transitory catarrhal discharge.

familial allergic r. a rarely recorded disease of cattle.

fibrinous r. rhinitis with development of a false membrane.

hypertrophic r. that with thickening and swelling of the mucous membrane.

inclusion body r. see INCLUSION BODY rhinitis.

membranous r. chronic rhinitis with a membranous exudate.

necrotic r. see NECROTIC rhinitis.

parasitic r. see PNEUMONYSSUS *caninum.*

polypous r. chronic rhinitis associated with polyps in the nasal cavity.

pseudomembranous r. coagulated discharge clings to the mucosa like a membrane but can be peeled off without leaving a mucosal lesion.

purulent r. chronic rhinitis with formation of pus.

vasomotor r. 1. nonallergic rhinitis in which transient changes in vascular tone and permeability (with the same symptoms of allergic rhinitis). 2. any condition of allergic or nonallergic rhinitis, as opposed to infectious rhinitis.

rhin(o)- word element. [Gr.] *nose, noselike structure.*

rhinoantritis inflammation of the nasal cavity and maxillary sinus.

rhinocanthectomy rhinommectomy; excision of the medial canthus of the eye.

rhinocephalus a fetus exhibiting rhinocephaly.

rhinocephaly a developmental anomaly characterized by the presence of a proboscis-like nose above eyes partially or completely fused into one.

rhinoceros an odd-toed ungulate in the family Rhinocerotidae of the order Perissodactyla, with a massive size, thick, armourplate-like skin and one or two horns low down in the middle of the face. They are herbivorous, partly nocturnal, unpredictable and aggressive. There are several genera including *Diceros* (white and black rhinos), *Ceratotherium simum* (white rhino), *Dicerorhinus* (Sumatran rhino) and *Rhinoceros* (Indian rhino).

rhinocheiloplasty plastic surgery of the nose and lip.

Rhinocladiella a genus of fungi responsible for chromomycosis.

rhinocleisis obstruction of the nasal passage.

rhinodacryolith a lacrimal concretion in the nasal duct.

Rhinoestrus a genus of flies, resembling *Oestrus* spp., and obligate parasites of *Equus* spp.

R. purpureus larvae parasitize larynx and nasal sinuses of Equidae. Called also Russian gad fly.

rhinogenous arising in the nose.

rhinograph a contrast radiograph of the nasal cavity.

rhinokyphosis an abnormal hump on the ridge of the nose.
rhinolaryngitis inflammation of the mucosa of the nose and larynx.
rhinolaryngoscope a long, rigid instrument with a lamp at the tip and a built-in optical system enabling the operator to view the interior of the upper respiratory tract. Largely replaced by the fiber-endoscope.
rhinolaryngoscopy the technique of use of the rhinolaryngoscope.
rhinolith a nasal calculus.
rhinolithiasis a condition associated with formation of rhinoliths.
rhinologist a specialist in rhinology.
rhinology the sum of knowledge about the nose and its diseases.
rhinomanometer a manometer used in rhinomanometry.
rhinomanometry measurement of the air flow and pressure within the nose during respiration; nasal resistance or obstruction can be calculated from the figures obtained.
rhinometer an instrument for measuring the nose or its cavities.
rhinommectomy excision of the medial canthus of the eye.
rhinomycosis fungal infection of the nasal mucosa.
rhinonecrosis necrosis of the nasal bones.
Rhinonyssus a genus of mites which parasitize birds without being important pests.
R. rhinolethrum found in ducks and geese.
rhinopathy any disease of the nose.
rhinopharyngitis inflammation of the nasopharynx.
rhinophore a nasal cannula to facilitate breathing.
rhinophycomycosis a fungal disease of humans caused by *Entomophora coronata*, marked by formation of large polyps in the subcutaneous tissues of the nose and paranasal sinuses; orbital involvement and unilateral blindness may follow. Cerebral involvement is common.
rhinoplasty plastic surgery of the nose.
rhinopneumonitis inflammation of the mucosae of the nasal cavities and the lungs.
equine viral r. see EQUINE viral rhinopneumonitis.
rhinopolypus a nasal polyp.
rhinorrhagia nosebleed; see EPISTAXIS.
rhinorrhea the free discharge of a thin nasal mucus.
cerebrospinal r. discharge of cerebrospinal fluid through the nose, usually due to skull fracture.
rhinosalpingitis inflammation of the mucosa of the nose and eustachian tube.
rhinoscope a speculum for use in nasal examination.
rhinoscopy examination of the nose with a speculum, through either the anterior nares or the nasopharynx.
rhinosinusitis inflammation of the nasal cavity and sinuses.
rhinosporidiosis a fungal disease caused by *Rhinosporidium seeberi*, marked by large polyps on the mucosa of the posterior nares of horses and cattle. The fungi can be found in the polyps. They cause interference with respiration and noisy breathing.
Rhinosporidium a genus of fungi in the phylum Deuteromycota (Fungi Imperfecti).
R. seeberi causes RHINOSPORIDIOSIS.
rhinotomy incision into the nose.
rhinotracheitis a combined inflammation of the mucosae of the nasal cavities and the trachea, the sort of lesion encountered in viral infections of the upper respiratory tract or in cattle maintained in a dusty environment such as a feedlot.
canine viral r. see KENNEL COUGH.
dust r. steers in a feedlot fed on a finely chopped ration develop a syndrome of cough, nasal and ocular discharge but without signs of fever or toxemia.
feline viral r. (FVR) an acute upper respiratory infection of cats, caused by feline herpesvirus. Sneezing, coughing, ocular and nasal discharges, and often chemosis, keratitis and corneal ulceration are the main signs. Occasionally there is fatal pneumonia or generalized infection in young kittens. Most cats recovered from infection become lifelong carriers of the virus, with shedding precipitated by stress. See also FELINE viral respiratory disease complex.
infectious bovine r. see INFECTIOUS bovine rhinotracheitis.
turkey r. see TURKEY rhinotracheitis.
rhinotracheitis virus see feline viral RHINOTRACHEITIS, INFECTIOUS bovine rhinotracheitis.
Rhinovirus a genus of single-stranded positive sense RNA viruses in the family PICORNAVIRIDAE. They cause common colds in humans and similar diseases in cattle.
rhinovirus a member of the genus *Rhinovirus*.
bovine r. some isolates cause nasal discharge, cough, dyspnea and fever. Others are innocuous.
equine r. see EQUINE rhinovirus 1; not a member of the *Rhinovirus* genus.
Rhipicentor a genus of ticks in the family Ixodidae that resemble *Dermacentor* spp.
R. bicorinis, R. nuttalli found on a wide range of wild and domesticated animals.
Rhipicephalus a genus of ticks in the family Ixodidae.
R. appendiculatus a three-host tick found on most animal species. Called also brown ear tick. Transmits *Theileria parva*, *Babesia* spp. and other protozoan and viral diseases including Nairobi sheep disease and louping ill. It is the principal vector of East Coast fever.
R. ayrei transmits *Theileria parva*.
R. bursa transmits *Babesia*, *Theileria*, *Anaplasma*, *Rickettsia*, *Anaplasma*, *Coxiella* spp.
R. capensis a three-host tick, parasitic on cattle; transmits East Coast fever.
R. evertsi a two-host tick; transmits *Theileria*, *Babesia*, *Borrelia*, *Rickettsia* spp. Called also red-legged tick.
R. jeanelli transmits *Theileria parva*.
R. neavei transmits *Theileria parva*.
R. pulchellus transmits Nairobi sheep disease virus and *Theileria parva*.
R. sanguineus a three-host tick, mainly a parasite of dogs but occurs on all species of mammals and birds. It transmits *Babesia*, *Borrelia*, *Coxiella*, *Rickettsia*, *Anaplasma* and *Pasteurella* spp. Also causes tick paralysis.
R. simus a three-host tick that transmits *Theileria parva*.
rhizo- word element. [Gr.] *root*.
Rhizoctonia leguminicola a fungus of clover hay which causes profuse salivation, lacrimation, lameness, frequent urination, bloat and diarrhea. The toxic agent is slaframine, an indolizidine alkaloid. Also produces swainsonine.
rhizoid resembling a root; said of hyphae produced by fungi which infiltrate the substrate.
rhizolysis interruption of spinal nerve roots by coagulation with radiofrequency waves.
rhizome an underground plant stem that develops roots and leaves at nodes along its length, e.g. in bracken, *Sorghum halepense*.
rhizomelic pertaining to the hips and shoulders (the roots of the limbs).

rhizomeningomyelitis radiculomeningomyelitis; inflammation of the nerve roots, meninges and spinal cord.

Rhizomucor a genus of fungi in the order Mucorales. See MUCORMYCOSIS.

rhizoneure a nerve cell forming a nerve root.

Rhizopoda a class of protozoa of the subphylum Sarcodina, having pseudopodia, and including the amebae.

rhizopodium pl. *rhizopodia* [Gr.] a filamentous pseudopodium, characterized by branching and anastomosis of the branches.

Rhizopus a genus of fungi involved in opportunistic infections. Members of order Mucorales of the class Zygomycetes. One of its species *R. microspora* is commonly found in gastric ulcers of pigs but it is thought that there is no etiological relationship. It also acts as a secondary invader in lesions of rumenitis initiated by lactic acid in carbohydrate engorgement in cattle. It is thought to cause bovine abortion.

rhizotomy division or transection of a nerve root, either within the spinal canal or outside it.

rhodamine a dye used in fluorescent staining techniques and FLUORESCENCE microscopy. It emits red light.

Rhode Island red a deep red-brown, dual-purpose poultry breed which lays a deep brown egg. It has a single comb, with clean yellow legs.

Rhodes grass CHLORIS *gayana*.

Rhodesian ridgeback a large, very muscular dog with a short, light to red wheaten coat. The distinctive feature of the breed is a band (ridge) of hair over the spine, between the neck and hips, in which the hairs grow in the reverse direction. Called also African lion hound. The breed is predisposed to the occurrence of dermoid sinuses associated with the ridge.

Rhodesian sleeping sickness see TRYPANOSOMA *rhodesiense*.

Rhodesian star grass CYNODON *nlemfuensis*.

Rhodesian tick fever East Coast fever.

rhodium a chemical element, atomic number 45, atomic weight 102.905, symbol Rh. See Table 6.

Rhodnius prolixus a triatomine bug, vector of trypanosomiasis. Member of the insect family Reduviidae of assassin or kissing bugs.

rhod(o)- word element. [Gr.] *red*.

rhodococcal pneumonia a disease of foals. See CORYNEBACTERIAL pneumonia.

Rhodococcus equi gram-positive rods of varying length; causes CORYNEBACTERIAL pneumonia and abscesses in foals and cervical lymphadenitis in pigs. It has also been associated with suppurative infections in cats. Previously called *Corynebacterium equi*. See also RATTLES.

Rhododendron plant genus in the family Ericaceae; contains andromedotoxin which causes a syndrome of repeated swallowing, bloat, vomiting, abdominal pain and frequent defecation. The course is short and the outcome may be death from aspiration pneumonia or complete recovery. Called also azalea.

The list of toxic plants includes *R. albiflorum*, *R. arboreum*, *R. campanulatum*, *R. cinnabarinum*, *R. indicum*, *R. macrophyllum* (*R. californicum*, California rose bay), *R. maximum* (great laurel), *R. molle*, *R. occidentale* (western azalea), *R. ponticum* (horticultural rhododendron).

rhodogenesis regeneration of retinal rhodopsin after its bleaching by light.

Rhodomyrtus macrocarpa northern Australian plant in the family Myrtaceae; fruit causes permanent blindness and paralysis; called also finger cherry.

rhodophylaxis the property of the retinal epithelium of facilitating rhodogenesis.

rhodopsin visual purple: a photosensitive purple-red chromoprotein in the retinal rods that is bleached to visual yellow (all-*trans*-retinal) by light, thereby stimulating retinal sensory endings. Lack of rhodopsin results in NIGHT BLINDNESS. Vitamin A is the primary source of rhodopsin.

Rhodotorula an imperfect yeast, a skin contaminant and occasional secondary infection of skin lesions, and occasional cause of bovine mastitis.

rhoeadine an alkaloid in the red poppy (*Papaver rhoeas*) which can cause signs similar to those of opium poisoning.

rhombencephalon 1. the hindbrain, including the medulla oblongata, pons and cerebellum. 2. the most caudal of the three primary vesicles formed in embryonic development of the brain, which later divides into the metencephalon and the myelencephalon.

rhombic lip one of a pair of folds which develops to form the roof of the fourth ventricle.

rhombocoele the terminal expansion of the canal of the spinal cord.

rhomboid shaped like a rectangle that has been skewed to one side so that the angles are oblique.

Rhombosolea tapirina finfish in the family Pleuronectidae. Called also greenback flounder. Not yet a species used in aquaculture.

rhompa grass a *Phalaris* spp. hybrid grass.

rhonchus pl. *rhonchi* [L.] a rattling in the throat; also, a dry, coarse rale in the bronchial tubes, due to a partial obstruction. Suggests the presence of chronic inflammation accompanied by presence of small amounts of tenacious exudate.

rhubarb see RHEUM RHAPONTICUM.

Rhus plant genus in family Anacardiaceae. Includes *Toxicodendron* spp.

rhythm a measured movement; the recurrence of an action or function at regular intervals.

alpha r. a uniform rhythm of waves in the normal electroencephalogram.

beta r. a rhythm in the electroencephalogram consisting of waves smaller than those of the alpha rhythm, having an average frequency of 25 per second, typical during periods of intense activity of the nervous system. See also ELECTROENCEPHALOGRAPHY.

biological r's the cyclic changes that occur in physiological processes of living organisms; called also biorhythms. These rhythms are so persistent throughout the living kingdom that they probably should be considered a fundamental characteristic of life, as are growth, reproduction, metabolism and irritability. Many of the physiological rhythms occur in animals about every 24 hours (circadian rhythm). Examples include the peaks and troughs that are manifested in body temperature, vital signs, brain function and muscular activity. Biochemical analyses of urine, blood enzymes and plasma serum also have demonstrated rhythmic fluctuations in a 24-hour period.

It has long been believed that the cyclic changes observed in plants and animals were totally in response to environmental changes and, as such, were exogenous or of external origin. This hypothesis is now being rejected by some chronobiologists who hold that the biological rhythms are intrinsic to the organisms, and that the organisms possess their own physiological mechanism for keeping time. This mechanism has been called the 'biological clock'.

circadian r. see CIRCADIAN rhythm.

circamensual r. that which occurs in cycles of about one month (30 days).

circannual r. the recurrence of a phenomenon in cycles of about one year.
circaseptan r. that which occurs in cycles of about 7 days (one week).
coupled r. heartbeats occurring in pairs, the second beat of the pair usually being a ventricular premature beat.
escape r. a heart rhythm initiated by lower centers when the sinoatrial node fails to initiate impulses, its rhythmicity is depressed, or its impulses are completely blocked.
gallop r. an auscultatory finding of three or four heart sounds, the extra sounds by convention being in diastole and related to atrial contraction (fourth sound, presystolic gallop), to early rapid filling of a ventricle with an altered ventricular compliance (protodiastolic gallop), or to concurrence of atrial contraction and ventricular early rapid filling (summation gallop).
idioventricular r. a series of ventricular escape complexes occuring at a regular rate.
infradian r. the regular recurrence in cycles of more than 24 hours, as certain biological activities which occur at such intervals, regardless of conditions of illumination.
nodal r. heart rhythm initiated in the specialized junctional tissue, i.e. the atrioventricular node and the main (His) bundle.
nyctohemeral r. a day and night rhythm.
pendulum r. alternation in the rhythm of the heart sounds in which the diastolic sound is equal in time, character and loudness to the systolic sound, the beat of the heart resembling the tick of a watch.
sinus r. normal heart rhythm originating in the sinoatrial node.
ultradian r. the regular recurrence in cycles of less than 24 hours, as certain biological activities which occur at such intervals, regardless of conditions of illumination.
ventricular r. the ventricular contractions which occur in cases of complete heart block.

rhythmic cycling hormone release pulsatile release of hormones like cortisol.

rhythmicity in cardiology, the ability to beat, or the state of beating, rhythmically without external stimuli.

rhytidectomy excision of skin for elimination of wrinkles.

rhytidoplasty plastic surgery for the elimination of wrinkles or skin folds, as around the face or vulva of some dogs.

rhytidosis a wrinkling, as of the cornea.

RIA radioimmunoassay.

rib any one of the paired, curved, cylindrical bones, extending from the thoracic vertebrae to the ventral aspect of the trunk, forming the major part of the thoracic skeleton, and consisting of a dorsal bony part and a ventral cartilaginous part that may or may not articulate with the sternum. Typically 13 pairs in the dog, cat and ruminants, 18 pairs in horses and 14 or 15 pairs in the pig. Called also costa. See Table 10.
abdominal r's, asternal r's a rib whose ventral end does not meet the sternum. See also false ribs (below).
cervical r. a supernumerary rib arising from a cervical vertebra.
r. contractor a strongly built device for pulling ribs together following retraction for surgical access to the thoracic cavity.
false r's the caudal ribs, not attached directly to the sternum but are attached too each others sternal cartilage to form the costal arch.
floating r. a rib whose distal extremity is unattached to an adjacent rib or the sternum.
r. retractor heavy duty surgical instrument for separating ribs to allow surgeon better access to thoracic contents. See FINOCHIETTO RIB SPREADER.
slipping r. one whose attaching cartilage is repeatedly dislocated.
sternal r. true ribs articulating with the sternum.
true r's the ribs attached to both vertebrae and sternum.
vertebral r's floating ribs.
vertebrocostal r's the false ribs that contribute to the costal arch.
vertebrosternal r's true ribs.

ribavirin a broad-spectrum, non-interferon inducing, antiviral nucleoside.

ribbed melilot MELILOTUS *officinalis*.

ribbed-up see WELL RIBBED-UP.

ribbon gum EUCALYPTUS *viminalis*.

ribbon malleable retractor a surgical instrument made of malleable metal which can be molded to different shapes to assist in holding back tissues.

ribbons in harness horse terminology, reins.

ribbonwood see IDIOSPERMUM AUSTRALIENSE.

Ribeiroia a genus of alimentary tract flukes (digenetic trematodes) in the family Cathaemasiidae; found in fowl, domestic ducks and geese in which they cause proventricular inflammation and ulceration.
R. ondatrae found in fish-eating birds, chicken and geese.

riboflavin, riboflavine vitamin B_2, a component of FAD and FMN, which are coenzymes or prosthetic groups for certain enzymes (flavoproteins) that catalyze many oxidation–reduction reactions. Called also vitamin G, lactoflavin.
r. kinase an enzyme (a phosphotransferase) that catalyzes the conversion of free riboflavin and ATP to flavin mononucleotide (FMN) and ADP. Called also flavokinase.
r. nutritional deficiency causes conjunctivitis with corneal vascularization, dermatitis, glossitis and muscular weakness. Occurs rarely in dogs, but not a natural deficiency in farm mammals. In birds it causes a fall in egg production, decreased hatchability, CURLED TOE PARALYSIS and poor growth.

ribonuclease an enzyme that catalyzes the breakdown of ribonucleic acid.

ribonucleic acid NUCLEIC ACIDS present in all living cells which are particularly involved in cellular protein synthesis and replace DNA as a carrier of genetic information in some viruses; abbreviated RNA. RNA is similar in composition to DNA with two exceptions: the sugar in RNA is ribose (in DNA it is deoxyribose) and in RNA the pyrimidine uracil replaces the thymidine of DNA.

The structure of RNA varies from helical to uncoiled linear strands of varying lengths, depending on the number of nucleotides forming the strand. This variance in structure is evident in the different types of RNA. For example, *transfer RNA* (tRNA) contains only about 75 nucleotides, while some mRNAs may contain thousands of nucleotides.

Messenger RNA (mRNA) receives its name from its function of carrying the genetic code from DNA in the nucleus of the cell to the cytoplasm, where proteins are synthesized. The transfer of the genetic code from DNA to mRNA is called transcription. Molecules of mRNA migrate to the cytoplasm and bind to ribosomes, to form polyribosomes. RNA moves along the ribosomes and its information content as codons (three nucleotides) is translated into a particular sequence of amino acids, i.e. a protein or polypeptide. Stop codons, UAA, UAG and UGA, terminate translation of mRNA.

Transfer RNA (tRNA) called also soluble RNA, brings about the transfer of specific amino acid molecules to the growing protein molecules during the synthesis of proteins. Each of the 20 common amino acids found in protein molecules has a corresponding type of tRNA. Thus, a specific tRNA carries the appropriate amino acid to its appropriate place in the nascent chain of the protein molecule being synthesized. tRNA has a triplet of nucleotides called the anticodon which is able, by base pairing to the codon triplet in mRNA as it moves along the ribosomes, to place the amino acids in the specific order characteristic of the particular protein. See also TRNA.

Ribosomal RNA (rRNA) is so called because it is found as a major structural component of ribosomes are the cytoplasmic organelle required for linking of amino acids into protein molecules.

Large amounts of RNA are also found in the nucleus of cells. One class of nuclear RNA, called *heterogeneous RNA* (hnRNA), represents primary RNA transcripts, i.e. before processing including splicing of introns, to form mRNA. A second class of nuclear RNA is called *small nuclear RNA* (snRNA) one species of which, called *small nuclear ribonucleoprotein* (snRNP), is believed to play an important role in the processing of hnRNA to mRNA. In the splicing reaction RNA itself acts as an 'enzyme' in that it is able to cut and religate other RNA molecules.

ribonucleoprotein particles small stable RNA species found in the nucleus, cytoplasm and mitochondria with one or more protein subunits attached; implicated in a variety of functions including: RNA trimming, splicing, transport, translation control and protein export.

ribonucleoside a nucleoside in which the purine or pyrimidine base is combined with ribose.

ribonucleotide a nucleotide in which the purine or pyrimidine base is combined with ribose.

ribose 5-carbon sugar present in ribonucleic acid (RNA).

60S ribosomal particle the largest of the two (40S and 60S) ribosome RNA structures that is itself composed of one copy of the 28S, 5.8S, and 55 rRNA; the entire complex ribosome structure is called 80S ribosome. Also includes 70 to 80 proteins.

ribosome ribonucleoprotein particles concerned with protein synthesis; they consist of two, one large and one small, reversibly dissociable units (called also 50S and 30S subunits) that are found either bound to cell membranes, particularly rough endoplasmic reticulum, or free in the cytoplasm. They may occur singly or in clusters, called polyribosomes or polysomes, which are ribosomes linked by mRNA and are actively engaged in protein synthesis.

r. binding site a nucleotide sequence near the 5′ terminus of mRNA required for binding of mRNA to the small ribosomal subunit. Called also Shine–Dalgarno sequence.

ribostamycin an aminoglycoside antibiotic with activity similar to gentimicin. It is effective against *Prototheca* spp.

ribosyl a glycosyl radical formed from ribose.

ribozyme enzyme whose catalytic function is carried out by an RNA subunit; of the four known classes, three carry out self processing reactions while the fourth, ribonuclease P (RNase P), is a true catalyst; discovered in the context of RNA splicing.

rice a cereal not used much for animal feed for socio-economic reasons. The grain also has a low protein content but is otherwise suitable for animal use. Milling by-products are available. Called also *Oryza sativa*.

r. flower see PIMELEA.

Richards bone holding forceps a surgical instrument with curved jaws designed to grasp bones during orthopedic surgery.

Richards bone plating kit a kit which contains a wide range of plates, plate bender, compression device, screws, wrench, screwdriver, bone clamp, hammer, power drill, drills, drill guide and rack, and pin cutter.

Richter's syndrome an aggressive large cell lymphoma of humans, suggested to occur in animals.

richweed see EUPATORIUM *rugosum*.

ricin phytotoxin (combining lectin, toxalbumin, hemagglutinin) in the seeds of the castor oil plant (*Ricinus communis*), inhalation or ingestion of which causes intoxication, producing superficial inflammation of the respiratory mucosa with hemorrhages into the lungs, or edema of the gastrointestinal tract with hemorrhages.

Ricinus communis toxic plant in the Euphorbiaceae family; contains ricin which causes diarrhea and convulsions when eaten. Called also castor oil plant, castor bean, palma christi.

rickets a disease of young growing animals caused by a nutritional deficiency of phosphorus or vitamin D. There is a failure of calcification of osteoid and cartilage of the bones which become bowed and a persistence with enlargement of the epiphyses so that the joints appear swollen. The animals are lame and dentition is delayed. Radiological examination shows a wider and thicker growth plate.

adult r. osteomalacia; a rickets-like disease affecting adults.

fetal r. see ACHONDROPLASIA.

hypervitaminosis D r. deposition of large amounts of osteoid matrix in the metaphyses with a delay in its mineralization occurs in feeding excessive amounts of vitamin D.

inherited r. affected piglets are normal at birth but develop rickets indistinguishable from classical rickets. There is a defect in calcium absorption.

renal r. see renal secondary HYPERPARATHYROIDISM.

vitamin D-resistant r. a condition almost indistinguishable from ordinary rickets clinically but resistant to unusually large doses of vitamin D; it is often familial but may occur sporadically. In hypophosphatemic vitamin D-resistant rickets, hypophosphatemia is the main characteristic, while in hypocalcemic vitamin D-resistant rickets, the serum concentration of phosphate is within normal limits or nearly so, and the concentration of calcium is abnormally low.

Rickettsia a genus of small, rod-shaped, round to pleomorphic microorganisms in the family Rickettsiaceae. They are true bacteria, gram-negative, and cultivable only in living tissues. They cause disease in humans and domestic animals but are also found in the cytoplasm of tissue cells of lice, fleas, ticks and mites, which may act as reservoirs and vectors. See also EHRLICHIA and COXIELLA.

R. akari causes rickettsial pox in humans, mice and rats.

R. australis causes QUEENSLAND TICK TYPHUS in humans, small marsupials, rats.

R. bovina see TICKBORNE FEVER.
R. canada causes new typhus in humans and rabbits.
R. conjunctivae causes contagious OPHTHALMIA of sheep. See also COLESIOTA CONJUNCTIVAE.
R. conorii causes BOUTONNEUSE FEVER in humans and dogs and small feral mammals.
R. equina, R. ovina, R. phagocytophilia see EHRLICHIA.
R. melophagi a nonpathogenic organism found in the sheep ked.
R. phagocytophila see CYTOECETES *bovis*.
R. prowazeki causes epidemic typhus in humans and possibly cattle, sheep and goats.
R. rickettsii causes spotted fever in humans and many feral animals, especially rodents and in dogs and birds. See also ROCKY MOUNTAIN SPOTTED FEVER.
R. ruminantium see COWDRIA RUMINANTIUM.
R. rupricapae has been isolated from keratoconjunctivitis in chamois.
R. siberica causes Siberian tick typhus in humans and many feral mammals, especially rodents.
R. tsutsugamushi causes scrub typhus in humans and many small feral mammals, especially rodents and occasionally dogs.
R. typhi causes murine typhus in humans and the brown rat.

rickettsia pl. *rickettsiae*; an individual organism of the family Rickettsiaceae.

rickettsial pertaining to or caused by rickettsiae.
r. fish disease caused by rickettsia-like organisms; most often asymptomatic in teleosts; characterized by granular, blue inclusions in epithelial cells of the gills. Similar bodies are found in the digestive glands of molluscs and crustaceans. More generalized infections sometimes cause ill-defined syndromes in crustaceans. Called sometimes epitheliocystis. See also PISCIRICKETTSIOSIS.

rickettsial interference phenomenon the protection of an experimental animal against an injection of virulent rickettsiae by a large dose of a low virulence strain. Abbreviated RIP.

Rickettsiales the order of bacteria containing the families Rickettsiaceae and Anaplasmataceae.

rickettsialpox a febrile disease of humans marked by a vesiculopapular eruption, clinically resembling chickenpox, caused by *Rickettsia akari* and transmitted from mice by mites. Called also Kew Gardens spotted fever.

rickettsicidal destructive to rickettsiae.

rickettsiosis any disease caused by infection with rickettsiae.
canine r. see canine EHRLICHIOSIS.

rida see SCRAPIE.

Riddell's groundsel SENECIO *riddellii*.

ride 1. control and direct a horse while mounted on it. 2. lane cut through a wood.
r. work to ride a horse for the purpose of training it for a race.

Rideal–Walker coefficient a measure of the efficiency of a disinfectant compared with that of phenol. Called also phenol coefficient.

ridge a linear projection or projecting structure; a crest.
dental r. any linear elevation on the crown of a tooth.
healing r. an indurated ridge that normally forms deep to the skin along the length of a healing wound.
interureteric r. a fold of mucous membrane extending across the bladder between the ureteric orifices.
mammary r. milk line; an ectodermal thickening in early embryos, along which the mammary glands subsequently develop.
mesonephric r. the more lateral portion of the urogenital ridge of the embryo, giving rise to the mesonephros.
palatine r. a number of transverse ridges across the hard palate in some animals.
urogenital r. a longitudinal ridge in the embryo, lateral to the mesentery.

ridgling cryptorchid; usually said of a horse.

riding school covers a wide range of establishments catering to the pleasure horse trade. Includes schools for the training of dressage horses, schools for dressage riders and more importantly, schools for training horse and rider units, and establishments of all degrees of quality including those that rent horses to people for an hour's pleasure.

Riedelliella graciliflora South American plant in the legume family Fabaceae; contains an unidentified toxin which causes generalized hemorrhages and liver and kidney damage.

Riegel's pulse a pulse that is smaller during respiration.

Riesenschnauzer Giant schnauzer.

RIF resistance-inducing factor.
R. test resistance-inducing factor test for the assay of avian leukosis viruses.
R. virus a virus that has the effect of increasing the resistance of an experimental animal or tissue culture against infection by another related virus.

rifabutin a rifamycin antibiotic with activity against mycobacteria.

rifampin, rifampicin a derivative of rifamycin; an antibacterial and antifungal agent used in the treatment of mycobacterial infections, actinomycosis and histoplasmosis.

rifamycin a family of antibiotics produced in cultures of *Streptomyces mediterranei*. Effective against gram-positive cocci and gram-negative bacilli and mycobacteria including *Mycobacterium tuberculosis*.

Rift Valley fever an acute infectious febrile disease of humans, cattle and sheep caused by a *Phlebovirus* and spread by biting insects, especially mosquitoes. Clinically there is high fever, incoordination and sudden death. Abortion is a common accompaniment. The autopsy findings include extensive hepatic necrosis. The disease is an important zoonosis.

rig see CRYPTORCHID.

right abomasal displacement see right ABOMASAL displacement.

right aortic arch a condition in which the fourth aortic arch on the right hand side may persist from the embryonic state instead of the left, causing a syndrome of persistent right AORTIC arch.

right colon displacement causes colic in horses; the right colon is displaced anteriorly between the cecum and the right body wall so that the pelvic flexure reaches the diaphragm.

rightangle forceps surgical tissue forceps or hemostats with a rightangle turn at the tip which permits an alternative approach to some sites that are inaccessible with the more common straight or gently curved forceps.

righting reflex a postural reaction that turns a falling animal's body in space so that its paws or feet are pointed at the ground or, less traumatically, returns the animal to sternal recumbency after being placed on its back or side; the animal may be blindfolded or in a darkened room to remove visual responses. A normal reaction is dependent on normal vestibular, visual and proprioceptive functions. Called also righting response.

righting response see RIGHTING REFLEX.

rights of animals see ANIMAL rights.
rigid lamb disease see ENZOOTIC muscular dystrophy, AKABANE VIRUS disease.
rigidity inflexibility or stiffness.
clasp-knife r. increased tension in the extensor of a joint when it is passively flexed, giving way suddenly on exertion of further pressure; seen especially in upper motor neuron disease.
cogwheel r. tension in a muscle that gives way in little jerks when the muscle is passively stretched.
lead-pipe r. posture adopted when the rigidity of the limb is maintained equally throughout the passive flexion.
r. reflex the state of immobility generated in female animals, especially those in estrus, when they make physical contact with a male.
rigor a subjective sensation of feeling cold, accompanied by muscle tremor, characteristic of the increment stage of fever. Because of its subjectivity it is not a term that can be used in animal medicine.
r. complexes formed when actin and myosin bond together strongly in the absence of ATP; occurs in rigor mortis.
r. mortis the stiffening of a dead body accompanying depletion of adenosine triphosphate in the muscle fibers.
rima pl. *rimae* [L.] a cleft or crack.
r. cornealis the groove in the scleral margin into which the rim of the cornea fits.
r. glottidis the kite-shaped opening between the true vocal folds and between the vocal processes of the arytenoid cartilages.
r. oris the opening of the mouth.
r. palpebrarum palpebral fissure.
r. pudendi the space between the labia of the vulva; called also pudendal fissure, rima vulvae.
r. vestibuli the entrance to a cavity from a vestibule, especially that of the larynx.
r. vulvae r. pudendi (above).
rimula pl. *rimulae* [L.] a minute fissure, as of the spinal cord or brain.
rinderpest a highly contagious disease of ruminants caused by paramyxovirus (genus *Morbillivirus*). It is characterized by high fever, focal erosive lesions in the mouth and throughout the alimentary tract, by severe diarrhea and a high fatality rate. Called also cattle plague. See also PESTE DES PETITS RUMINANTS, JEMBRANA DISEASE.
ring 1. any annular or circular organ, structure or area. 2. in chemistry, a collection of atoms united in a continuous or closed chain.
abdominal r. (external) an opening in the aponeurosis of the external oblique muscle for the spermatic cord or round ligament. Called also external inguinal ring.
abdominal r. (internal) an aperture in the transverse fascia for the spermatic cord or round ligament. Called also internal inguinal ring.
Bandl's r. see BANDL'S RINGS.
r. cell an immature granulocyte, intermediate between the myelocyte and metamyelocyte, found in the bone marrow of rats. There is a 'hole' in the nucleus.
ciliary r. the posterior part of the ciliary body of the eye, a continuation of the choroid.
conjunctival r. a ring at the junction of the conjunctiva and cornea.
constriction r. a contracted area of the uterus, where the resistance of the uterine contents is slight, as over a depression in the contour of the fetus, or below the presenting part.
deep inguinal r. an aperture in the transverse fascia for the spermatic cord or the round ligament.
docking r. see ELASTRATOR.
femoral r. the abdominal opening of the femoral canal through which the femoral nerve and blood vessels pass from the peritoneal cavity to the limb.
inguinal r. see abdominal ring (above).
pancreatic r. the ring in the pancreas that accommodates the portal vein.
preputial r. the rim of the external orifice of the prepuce proper, the internal prepuce, on the penis of the horse.
retraction r. (pathological) a complication of prolonged labor marked by failure of relaxation of the circular fibers at the internal opening of the cervix, obstructing delivery of the fetus.
retraction r. the demarcation between the upper, contracting portion of the uterus in normal parturition and the lower, dilating part.
r. precipitin test see PRECIPITIN reaction.
Schwalbe's r. see SCHWALBE'S RING.
scleral r. see RING OF OSSICLES.
stallion r. a rubber ring fitted over the glans penis of the stallion which discourages erection and masturbation.
superficial inguinal r. a fissure-like opening in the aponeurosis of the external abdominal oblique muscle for the spermatic cord or the round ligament.
r. test see ASCOLI TEST.
tympanic r. the bony ring forming part of the temporal bone at birth and developing into the tympanic plate.
umbilical r. the orifice in the abdominal wall of the fetus for transmission of the umbilical vein and arteries.
r. vaccination vaccination of all animals in a zone around an area in which the subject disease occurs. A preventive strategy that contains the infected population so that the eradication team has a finite target.
vascular r. any of a number of congenital anomalies of the aortic arch and its branches, the vessels forming a ring about the trachea and esophagus that cause varying degrees of compression, vomiting and esophageal dilatation. See also persistent right AORTIC ARCH.
ring-dove wood-pigeon.
ring-eyes see WALLEYE (4).
ring-in said of a racehorse; means not the horse referred to but one criminally substituted for it with the intention of defrauding the punters.
ring of ossicles a circlet of bony overlapping plates which serve as reinforcement in the sclera, near the cornea, in the eyes of birds. Called also scleral ring.
ring-tailed characterized by a tail that is banded with black rings.
r. cat an arboreal, nocturnal, squirrel-like animal, *Bassariscus astutus*, in the family Procyonidae. Has a banded black and white tail. Called also cacomistle.
r. lemur see LEMUR.
ringbinden aberrant myofibrils that wrap themselves around an existing muscle fiber in a tight spiral. Occur most commonly in muscles affected by neurogenic atrophy.
ringbone osteoarthritis or periostitis of the first or second phalanx of a limb of a horse. Causes lameness and in the later stages swelling of the pastern due to the development of exostoses.
ringed octopus a venomous mollusc of the order Octopoda with eight tentacles, blue rings around them and a beak which inflicts a bite and provides for the injection of a potent neurotoxin from the salivary

glands. Death is due to respiratory failure. Called also *Hapalochlaena maculosa*.

Ringer's solution a sterile solution of sodium chloride, potassium chloride and calcium chloride in purified water, a physiological salt solution for topical use. See also LACTATED RINGER'S SOLUTION.

ringing removal of a circle of wool from around the prepuce at crutching time to reduce the chance of soiling with urine and subsequent cutaneous myiasis.

ringtail a disease of mice, rats and hamsters; caused by low humidity and high temperatures in the environment. The tail swells and becomes annulated as a result of constrictions along its length. It eventually becomes gangrenous and drops off. The feet may also be swollen and reddened.

ringtail monkey see CAPUCHIN MONKEY.

ringwomb a disease of the ewe characterized by failure of the cervix to relax so that there is no evidence of impending parturition. Many full-term fetuses die in utero.

ringworm an infection of the superficial layers of the skin and the hair fibers with one of a group of dermatophytic fungi. Some of the fungi are obligate parasites of animals, others have the same relationship with humans, and some are freeliving in the soil and only invade animal skins in unusual circumstances. See also TINEA. The common species are TRICHOPHYTON *verrucosum* in cattle, *T. equinum* in horses; in dogs and cats the infections are MICROSPORUM *canis*, *M. gypseum* and *T. mentagrophytes*. In sheep and goats the infection is usually *T. verrucosum* and in pigs *M. nanum*.

The infection is very superficial and does almost no injury to animals but efforts are usually made to prevent its spread because it is highly infectious, including for humans. In companion animals this zoonotic aspect is very important in management of cases. Called also dermatophytosis.

honeycomb r. see FAVUS.

rinsing wash the brief washing stage between developing an x-ray film and fixing it.

RIP rickettsial interference phenomenon.

ripening said of meat. See CURING.

RIS rabies inhibiting substance.

Risdon wiring technique use of a wire twisted around teeth to support rostral jaw fractures.

rising said of age, means just before, e.g. rising 7 years means 6 years nearly 7 years old.

difficulty r. having to make a number of attempts, or requiring assistance or improvement in the footing before being able to rise; a stage in the development of spinal cord compression, or a sequel to injury to peripheral, e.g. sciatic or obturator, nerves.

risk the chance of an unfavorable event occurring.

acceptable r. risk for which the benefits rank larger than the potential hazards.

at r. that part of a total population which is subject to the disease being reviewed, e.g. only milking cows are at risk to milk fever, only grazing cows to enzootic nasal granuloma.

r. aversion reluctance to take risks.

r. factor an attribute or exposure which increases the probability of occurrence of a disease or other outcome.

r. premium the amount of money required to convince a person to take a specific risk.

r. ratio the ratio of two risks.

relative r. see RELATIVE risk.

surgical r. an animal that has poor general health and must be assessed as a poor survival risk to undergo major surgery or anesthesia.

RIST radioimmunosorbent test.

ristocetin an antibiotic produced by cultures of the actinomycete *Nocardia lurida*. Used also in the assessment of platelet function.

r. cofactor inolved in platelet aggregation. Called also von Willebrand factor.

risus [L.] *laughter*.

r. sardonicus a grinning expression produced by spasm of the facial muscles, typical of tetanus in humans. The term is also applied to dogs with tetanus in which the lips are drawn back by muscle spasms.

Rivanol precipitation test a serological test for the differentiation of antibodies to *Brucella* spp.

river blindness infection with ONCHOCERCA *volvulus*.

river buttercup RANUNCULUS *inundatus*.

river poison EXCOECARIA *agallocha*, GASTROLOBIUM *forrestii*.

riverine tsetse GLOSSINA *pallidipes*, *G. palpalis*.

Rivina humilis toxic plant in the family Phytolaccaceae; an unidentified toxin causes milk taint; called also coral or turkey berry.

Rivinus' incisure a defect in the upper tympanic part of the temporal bone, filled by the upper portion of the tympanic membrane.

riziform resembling grains of rice.

Rn chemical symbol, *radon*.

RNA ribonucleic acid.

RNA primer a sequence of about 10 nucleotides long copied from DNA by RNA primase and required for the priming of the synthesis of each Okazaki fragment during DNA replication.

RNA viruses viruses distinguished by having a ribonucleic acid genome, usually as a single strand which may be positive or negative sense, a single molecule or a segmented; in at least two families the genome is a double-strand segmented form.

secondary structure RNA folding of single-stranded RNA molecules which arises from intramolecular base pairing.

small cytoplasmic RNA small (7S; 129 nucleotides) RNA molecules found in the cytosol and rough endoplasmic reticulum associated with proteins that are involved in specific selection and transport of other proteins. Abbreviated scRNA.

RNase ribonuclease.

RNP see RIBONUCLEOPROTEIN.

R/O abbreviation for rule out; used in medical records.

roach back a defect in conformation, most commonly in the horse, which does not affect performance but is unattractive esthetically. The dorsal spinous processes of the caudal thoracic and lumbar vertebrae protrude excessively giving the animal a convex topline. Called also kyphosis.

roached mane the mane is clipped but a central narrow fringe of erect short hairs is left, like the plume on a Roman soldier's helmet.

road related to animals on roadways.

r. accidents results in traumatic injuries because of collisions with vehicles, falling on uneven or slippery surfaces.

r. founder traumatic LAMINITIS.

r. transportation motor transport.

roan a coat color consisting of a relatively uniform mixture of white and colored hairs, giving a 'silvered' hue; self-describing colors are red-roan, blue-roan, chestnut roan.

roaring the stertor in respiration caused by air passing through a stenosed larynx. The commonest cause is laryngeal hemiplegia in the horse. The disease is incompatible with fast exercise. The cause of the basic lesion, degeneration of fibers in the left recurrent laryngeal nerve, is unknown. See also LARYNGEAL hemiplegia.

r. burr surgical instrument used to evert the mucosal lining of the lateral ventricle in the horse in the operation for laryngeal hemiplegia—ventriculectomy; the lining is then excised. Strawberry type has a rough surface reminiscent of the surface of that fruit. French type has a surface covered with small hooks.

roast beef plant IRIS *foetidissima.*

roaster a young fowl for eating; weighs 5 to 7 lb at 6 months of age.

robenidine a guanidine derivative used at one time as an anticoccidial in poultry. Little used now because of the rapid development of resistance to it by the protozoa.

Robert–Jones bandage see Robert–Jones BANDAGE.

Robertsonian translocation see Robertsonian TRANSLOCATION.

robin 1. a bird. 2. a phytotoxin in the plant ROBINIA PSEUDOACACIA.

Robinia pseudoacacia toxic tree in the legume family Fabaceae; the bark contains a toxalbumin which causes purging and paralysis. Called also black locust, black acacia, false acacia, locust tree.

Robinson sling see pelvic limb SLING.

Robson–Heggers biopsy see Robson–Heggers BIOPSY.

robust 1. strong and healthy. 2. in statistical terminology said of methods of analysis that are insensitive to nonnormality of data distribution.

robust star grass CYNODON *nlemfuensis.*

ROC curve acronym for receiver operating characteristic curve. A graphical method of assessing the characteristic of a diagnostic test.

Rochalimaea a genus of the family Rickettsiaceae resembling the genus *Rickettsia*, but usually found extracellularly in the arthropod host, including *R. quintana*, the etiological agent of trench fever of humans and voles, transmitted by the body louse *Pediculus humanus.*

Rochester–Carmalt forceps scissor-type, ratchet handle, hemostatic forceps with longitudinal grooves on the blade faces with cross-hatching at the tip.

Rochester–Pean forceps scissor-action hemostat forceps with ratcheted handles, long blades with deep transverse grooves, straight or curved.

rock centaury CENTAURIUM *beyrichii.*

rock fern see CHEILANTHES *sieberi.*

rock lobster see PANULIRUS.

rock phosphate a mined mineral used as a fertilizer and as a dietary phosphorus supplement for animals. Some deposits of the mineral contain high levels of fluorine and its use as a feed supplement leads to poisoning in the livestock. See also FLUOROSIS.

rock salt salt in large crystalline masses, mined from extensive underground deposits. Used commonly as salt licks on pasture.

rocket electrophoresis see rocket IMMUNOELECTROPHORESIS.

Rocky mountain bee plant see CLEOME SERRULATA.

Rocky Mountain Bighorn sheep *Ovis canadensis canadensis.*

Rocky Mountain spotted fever an infectious disease of small mammals, dogs and humans. It occurs mainly in certain areas within the USA. Called also tick fever, and it is also known by various names according to the geographic area.

Rocky Mountain spotted fever belongs to a group of insect-borne fevers caused by rickettsiae, which attack endothelium. The species, *Rickettsia rickettsii*, responsible for Rocky Mountain spotted fever is transmitted from rodent by various ticks. The clinical signs associated with infection in dogs are lethargy, anorexia, ocular and nasal discharge, lymphadenopathy and splenomegaly. A thrombocytopenia also occurs. Kennel epizootics have been recorded.

Rocky Mountain wood tick see DERMACENTOR *andersoni.*

rod a straight, slim mass of substance; specifically, one of the retinal rods; are highly specialized cylindrical segments of the neuroepithelial visual cells containing rhodopsin and modified to receive, transduce and transmit visual stimuli; together with the retinal cones, they form the light-sensitive elements of the retina. See also CONE (1).

r.–cone dysplasia an inherited defect in dogs, particularly Irish setters, Elkhounds and Miniature poodles, causing a progressive retinal atrophy with impairment of night vision, then day vision starting at an early age. There are differences in the ultrastructural and biochemical features in each breed, but generally rods are more severely affected than cones. See also progressive RETINAL atrophy.

olfactory r. the slender apical portion of an olfactory bipolar neuron, a modified dendrite extending to the surface of the epithelium.

rodent a member of the order Rodentia. Includes rats and mice and allied species, the squirrels and beavers, the porcupines and their related species, and the African mole rat in four separate suborders.

r. bot see CUTEREBRA.

r. ulcer see EOSINOPHILIC ulcer.

rodenticide 1. destructive to rodents. 2. an agent destructive to rodents. They are all toxic to animals and are a common cause of poisoning. The common ones are warfarin and its related compounds and sodium fluoroacetate, called also compound 1080. Other agents are cyanide, alphanaphthylthiourea (ANTU), thallium salts and zinc phosphide. Although these substances are selected because of their relatively low toxicity for domestic animals, they can all cause severe losses in them if used carelessly.

rodeo a sporting event in which riders compete for points in contests related to buckjump riding, bull riding, calf roping.

Rodontocaulus ondatrae a nematode parasite in the family Angiostrongylidae, found in the pulmonary artery of rodents.

roe eggs of fish, still in the fish.

roe deer red-gold to black with white buttock patch. Lives in small family groups. Called also *Capreolus capreolus.*

Roe terrier see MINIATURE PINSCHER.

Roeckl's granuloma nodular lesion of unknown cause occurring principally in skeletal muscles but also in other organs in European cattle. There are usually multiple lesions which are up to 5 cm in diameter. Called also nodular necrosis.

Roeder forceps see BACKHAUS TOWEL CLAMP.

roentgen a superseded international unit of x- or γ-radiation; it is the quantity of x- or γ-radiation such that the associated corpuscular emission per 0.001293 g of air produces, in air, ions carrying 1 electrostatic unit of electrical charge of either sign. Abbreviated R. Now replaced by coulomb/kg (C/kg); see COULOMB. 1 R = 2.58×10^{-4} C/kg; 1 C/kg = 3876 R.

r. equivalent man (rem) see REM.

r. equivalent physical (rep) see REP.

r. ray x-ray.

roentgenkymogram the film obtained by roentgenkymography.

roentgenkymography a technique of graphically recording the movements of an organ on a single x-ray film.
roentgenogram see RADIOGRAPH.
roentgenograph see RADIOGRAPH.
roentgenography see RADIOGRAPHY.
roentgenologist radiologist.
roentgenology see RADIOLOGY.
roentgenoscope a term not now used; a fluoroscope; an apparatus for examining the body by means of the fluorescent screen excited by x-rays.
roentgenoscopy see FLUOROSCOPY.
roentgenotherapy see RADIOTHERAPY.
Rolando's fissure see Rolando's FISSURE.
rolitetracycline a semisynthetic, broad-spectrum, tetracycline antibiotic administered intravenously or intramuscularly.
rolled said of grain rolled into flat plates by passing through flat rollers, e.g. rolled oats. Improves digestibility at the cost of the processing. See also CRACKED.
Roller a breed of canaries bred solely for their distinctive voice. It is soft with long, intricate rolls or tours. Color is variable. A number of different song passages are recognized; in exhibitions are judged on their songs.
roller harness of a wide leather band that encircles the horse at the girth place, behind the elbows. Good models have stuffed pads that fit on either side of the dorsal spine and keep pressure off it. Can be used for decoration, for anchoring check-reins when breaking in to harness and for keeping a rug, quarter sheet and other horse garments in place.
rolling involuntary rolling in animals; an important sign of abdominal pain or of disease of the vestibular apparatus. In the latter it is accompanied by persistent head rotation. Passive rolling is a therapeutic manipulation for the correction of torsion of the uterus in mares and cows. The animal is cast, laid on its back and swung sharply from side to side, sometimes with one hand in the rectum attempting to retard any movement of the fetus. The objective is to rotate the dam's body around an immobilized fetus and uterus.
r. average see moving AVERAGE.
r. disease a nervous system disease of mice caused by *Mycoplasma neurolyticum*.
r. mean see moving AVERAGE.
r. skin syndrome see idiopathic HYPERESTHESIA syndrome.
rolling circle replication a description of the replication of circular DNA molecules in which linear daughter DNA molecules that contain repeated DNA sequences called concatemers are produced from the parent; the concatemers are cleaved to form unit length genomes which themselves circularize.
ROM 1. read only memory. 2. range of motion.
Romagna a gray to white breed of beef cattle originating in Italy. Called also Romagnola.
Romagnola see ROMAGNA.
roman-nosed the lateral view of the face of a horse that has a convex silhouette.
Romanizing conversion of the spoken sounds of the Chinese language to the Roman alphabet and numbers.
Romanov a breed of sheep maintained for their carpetwool and pelt. Gray with black head and legs, white face stripe and feet. May be horned or polled.
Romanowsky stains a group of eosin–methylene blue stains generally used for blood smears, protozoa and bacteria. Includes Giemsa, Wright and Leishman stains.
romerillo BACCHARIS *cordifolia*.
Romney Marsh English longwool-type meat sheep; polled, 33 micron wool, prized as fat lamb mother, used extensively in development of carpetwool breeds. Called also Kent Marsh.
R. M. disease see STRUCK.
Romney sheep see ROMNEY MARSH.
Rompun a proprietary name for XYLAZINE.
Romulea toxic genus of plants in the family Iridaceae; small, onion-like plant with a mauve flower, pineapple-like fruit and a deeply situated bulb. A very persistent weed causing much loss of productivity in the pasture. Is also a common cause of intestinal obstruction with phytobezoars produced from the fibrous leaves. Causes infertility and incoordination in sheep if infested with the leaf fungus *Helminthosporium biseptatum*. Called also onion grass. Includes *R. bulbocodium*, *R. longifolia* (syn. *R. bulbocordium*, *R. rosea*), *R. rosea* var. *australis*.
romulosis poisoning by ROMULEA.
rongeur [Fr.] an instrument for cutting tissue, particularly bone; also for cracking gross deposits of dental calculus.
bone r. a multijointed, springloaded, plier-like instrument used to break off pieces of bone. The opposing surfaces of the blades have sharp-edged, scooped out surfaces like a curette.
ronidazole a nitroimidazole derivative, similar to metronidazole. Used in the treatment of histomoniasis and swine dysentery.
ronnel see FENCHLORPHOS.
roofing felt contains lead compounds and may be a cause of poisoning.
room a place in a building enclosed and set apart for occupancy or for the performance of certain procedures.
operating r. one especially equipped for the performance of surgical operations. Called also operating theater.
recovery r. a hospital unit adjoining operating rooms, with special provisions for the care of animals recovering from surgery. For large animals, it must be designed and equipped to minimize the risk of injury to the animal as it regains consciousness and returns to its feet, while permitting close, but safe, supervision by nursing staff. Closed circuit television is commonly utilized for this purpose.
roost mite see DERMANYSSUS GALLINAE.
rooster entire, sexually mature, male fowl, more than about 5 months old.
root 1. the descending and subterranean part of a plant. 2. that portion of an organ, such as a tooth, hair or nail, that is buried in the tissues, or by which it arises from another structure, or the part of a nerve that is adjacent to the center to which it is connected, e.g. root of neck, root of tail.
calcified r. canal restriction of the diameter of the root canal due to calicification; seen in older animals.
r. canal that part of the dental pulp cavity extending from the pulp chamber to the apical foramen. Called also pulp canal.
r. canal therapy see ENDODONTICS.
dental r. elevator screwdriver-shaped instrument with a grooved and beveled blade. By pushing the tip of the blade between the tooth root and the alveolar wall the periodontal membrane is broken and the root is elevated and removed.
r. directory the top of a hierarchical directory structure for a computer disk.
dorsal r. the sensory division of each spinal nerve, attached centrally to the spinal cord and joining

peripherally with the ventral root to form the nerve before it emerges from the intervertebral foramen.
hair r. the part of the hair buried in the hair follicle.
mesenteric r. the small area of attachment of the mesentery to the dorsal abdominal wall at about the level of the first lumbar vertebrae. It encloses the vessels and nerves that supply the intestine.
motor r. ventral root.
nerve r's the series of paired bundles of nerve fibers which emerge at each side of the spinal cord, termed dorsal (or posterior) or ventral (or anterior) according to their position. A series of dorsal and ventral roots join to form a spinal nerve. Certain cranial nerves, e.g. the trigeminal, also have nerve roots.
penis r. the attachment of the penis by two crura to the lateral parts of the ischial arch.
r. perforation an accidental occurrence when filing a root canal.
r. planing see dental PLANING.
sensory r. dorsal root.
r. signature referred pain down a limb, causing lameness or elevation of the limb, resulting from entrapment of the spinal nerve, usually by an extruded intervertebral disk.
r. sheath cuticle single layer of cornified cells of the hair follicle interdigitating with the cornified cells of the hair cuticle.
tongue r. caudal part of the tongue attached to the hyoid bone, soft palate and pharynx.
ventral r. the motor division of each spinal nerve, attached centrally to the spinal cord and joining peripherally with the dorsal root to form the nerve before it emerges from the intervertebral foramen.

rootlets attachments of the basal bodies of cells to their cytoplasm.

roots inclusive term for underground parts of plants used as animal feed. Includes turnips, swedes, beets, mangels.

ROP record of performance, a series of programs for recording milk yield in cows, egg production in fowls and rate of gain in meat producing animals.

rope burn skin abrasion caused by the heat of friction by a rope on the skin; caused by entanglement in a rope or poor casting technique.

roped poultry see NEW YORK DRESSED POULTRY.

roping lassooing with a rope. See also LASSO.

roquefortine tremorgenic mycotoxin produced by *Penicillium roqueforti*.

roridin a macrocyclic trichothecene mycotoxin produced by *Stachybotrys atra*. Includes roridin A(1), roridin E(2).

rosaniline a substance from coal tar, the basis of various dyes and stains, including gentian violet, crystal violet and fuchsin.

rosaramicin a macrolide antibiotic produced in cultures of *Micomonospora rosaria* and effective against gram-positive and some gram-negative bacteria.

rosary a structure resembling a string of beads.
r. pea see ABRUS *precatorius*.
rachitic r. a succession of beadlike prominences along the costal cartilages, in rickets; caused by compression of metaphyses under pressure.

rosaxoacin a quinolone antibiotic, similar to naladixic acid. Called also acrosoxacin.

rose bengal a fluorescein compound used as a pink dye, in a liver function test, and as a coloring agent in feed. It is also used in the eye to stain necrotic tissue and devitalized cells of the cornea in keratitoconjunctivitis sicca. Animals injected with the dye are temporarily photosensitive.
r. b. test an oldfashioned field plate test for brucellosis in serum. The dye was used to mark the antigen and make its clumping visible. Suitable only as a screening test.

rose chafer see MACRODACTYLUS SUBSPINOSUS.

rose grower's disease sporotrichosis.

Rose–Waaler test a passive hemagglutination test for rheumatoid factor in the serum.

roseate cockatoo see GALAH.

Roseneath terrier an early name for the West Highland white terrier.

Rosenthal fiber irregularly shaped, hyaline, eosinophilic structures formed within astrocytes; a feature of Alexander's disease of dogs.

Roseolovirus a proposed genus of betaherpesvirus. It contains human herpesvirus 6.

rosette any structure or formation resembling a rose, such as (1) the clusters of polymorphonuclear leukocytes around a globule of lipid nuclear material, as observed in the test for disseminated lupus erythematosus, or (2) a figure formed by the chromosomes in an early stage of mitosis.
r. of Furstenberg the white ridges of mucous membrane that radiate from the internal orifice of the teat of ruminants.
r. inhibition test used to detect the presence of 'early pregnancy factor' but has problems of application and limited usefulness.

rosewood ALECTRYON *oleifolius*.

rosin the solid resin obtained from species of *Pinus*, a genus of trees; used in preparation of ointments and plasters.

Ross River encephalitis see Ross River ENCEPHALITIS.

Ross test a test which uses sodium nitroprusside in the detection of ketone bodies in urine and milk.

rostellum apical projection of the scolex of a tapeworm, which may or may not bear hooks.

rostr- prefix meaning nose.

rostrad 1. toward a rostrum; nearer the rostrum in relation to a specific point of reference. 2. cephalad.

rostral 1. pertaining to or resembling a rostrum; having a rostrum or beak. 2. situated toward a rostrum or toward the beak, i.e. toward the front of the head.
r. colliculus see midbrain COLLICULUS.
r. salivatory nucleus see salivatory NUCLEUS.

rostrate beaked.

rostrum pl. *rostra* [L.] 1. a beak-shaped process. 2. the most anterior part of the body.
nasal r. snout; apex of the nostrils and upper lip.

rot decay.
r. fungus *Ceratocystis* spp. on parsnip (*Pastinaca* spp.).

rotameter see FLOWMETER.

rotated turned around; pivoted.
r. tibia see rotated TIBIA.

rotation a state of having been pivoted around an axis. See also TORSION, ROTATIONAL.
r. flap graft see pedicle GRAFT.
r. fork an obstetrical instrument used in mares and cows. A 3 ft long rod with a crossbar handle and a two-pronged fork at the other end. The prongs have eyelets to which cord or canvas hobbles are attached. Two presenting limbs are threaded through these and the instrument pushed into the uterus to the body. Rotation of the bar handle helps to rotate the calf or foal, or uterus if it is closely applied. See also CAMMERER ROTATION FORK.
pedal r. see PEDAL bone rotation.
r. programs alternation of crops (crop rotation), of grazing of pastures (paddock or field rotation), of bulls or rams running with breeding females (bull

rotation), of anticoccidial agents to poultry or anthelmintics to sheep to avoid the development of resistance to the medication by the target organism. Rotational GRAZING of pastures is beneficial to pasture growth when livestock concentration is high, and aids in the control of helminth parasites by interrupting their life cycles.

rotational characterized by ROTATION.

r. crossbreeding system a program in which the sire for the terminal cross of lamb or calf is changed each year so that the state of heterosis is maintained at a high level.

r. grazing see rotational GRAZING.

rotator an obstetrical instrument used in cows and mares. See ROTATION fork.

Rotavirus a genus of viruses in the family REOVIRIDAE which cause diarrhea in the young of many species, including avian, but particularly calves, foals, piglets and lambs, particularly in conditions of poor hygiene, crowding and failure of maternal antibody transfer. The morbidity rate is usually very high but death losses are not heavy provided the hydration of the animals is maintained. There is some species specialization but interspecies transmission is common.

rotenone a compound derived from the root and rhizomes of derris (*Derris elliptica*) and lonchocarpus (*Lonchocarpus utilis*). Used as an insecticide and as an acaricide, mainly on dogs, cats, cattle, birds and fish. Toxic to pigs, causing incoordination, tremor, recumbency and terminal respiratory paralysis.

Rothera's test a test for the presence of ketone bodies, diacetic acid and acetone in urine. May also be applied to milk.

rotifer see BRACHIONUS PLICATILIS.

Rotterdam tuberculin a bovine purified protein derivative tuberculin used in testing cattle for tuberculosis. Contains 1 mg/ml of tuberculoprotein.

Rottnest quokka see QUOKKA.

Rottweiler a large, very powerfully built dog with massive, broad head, small pendant ears and short docked tail. The short coat is black with tan markings on the face, chest and legs. The breed is predisposed to osteochondrosis, diabetes mellitus, sesamoiditis, leukoencephalomyelopathy and neuroaxonal dystrophy.

rotula 1. the patella. 2. any disklike bony process. 3. a lozenge or troche.

rotular patellar.

rotund tick see IXODES *kingi*.

Rouen a beautifully colored and marked duck used for eating, but has dark flesh which is unpopular. Head and upper neck green (drake) or brown (female), then a white band, followed by a rich brown breast; the rest of the body feathers are green to black.

rough-bearded grass see ECHINOPOGON.

rough chervil CHAEROPHYLLUM *temulentum*.

rough comfrey SYMPHYTUM *asperum*.

rough endoplasmic reticulum parts of the endoplasmic reticulum to which ribosomes are attached on the cytoplasmic side; involved in the biosynthesis of proteins for export to the outside of the cell and enzymes to be incorporated into cellular organelles such as lysosomes. See also endoplasmic RETICULUM.

rough-scaled snake an olive green to brown snake with rough scales, dark bands and a pale belly which secretes a powerful neurotoxin. Called also *Tropidechis carinatus*.

roughage coarse, bulky feeds, largely indigestible, fed to species other than ruminants and horses. High in fiber, low in digestible carbohydrates and proteins. Includes hay, pasture, ensilage, which promote peristalsis by their bulk. Material that is too indigestible, e.g. straw, may cause impaction of the rumen or the cecum and colon in horses.

rouleau pl. *rouleaux* [Fr.] a roll of red blood cells resembling a pile of coins.

r. formation occurs when there is increased fibrinogen concentration or other changes in plasma proteins. It will disappear when blood is diluted with saline.

round heart disease a familial disease of turkeys characterized by sudden death due to cardiac arrest, associated with a deficiency of of the plasma protein, alpha$_1$-antitrypsin. Most common in inbred, broad-breasted, white turkeys.

round ligament 1. the ligament of the head of the femur which attaches to the acetabular fossa. Rupture usually accompanies dislocation of the hip. 2. the remnant of the fetal umbilical vein in the adult. 3. the remnant of the umbilical artery as it forms the cranial boundary to the lateral ligament of the bladder of the adult.

round-up see MUSTER.

roundworm any of the parasitic, unsegmented, cylindrical in cross-section, elongated in shape, nematode worms which invade principally the gastrointestinal tract. Almost any organ can be involved. Comprises the class Nematoda and its large number of genera.

roup any disease of poultry manifested by signs of coryza and involvement of the nasal chambers. See also avian TRICHOMONIASIS.

Rous sarcoma a spindle-cell sarcoma of fowls which is transplantable, metastasizes freely and usually destroys the host bird within a short time. It is caused by the Rous sarcoma virus, a retrovirus, which occurs in several serotypes and is transferable to rabbits, mice, rats, hamsters and primates as well as chickens.

roxa PALICOUREA *marcgravii*.

roxarsone an organic arsenical compound used as a growth promotant and coccidiostat in swine and poultry. Called also 4-hydroxy-3-nitrophenylarsonic acid. See also organic ARSENICAL.

roxinha PALICOUREA *marcgravii*.

roxithromycin a macrolide antibiotic.

roxona PALICOUREA *marcgravii*.

Royal Society for the Prevention of Cruelty to Animals an international organization, originating in the UK, and dedicated to the promotion of the humane use of animals by humans; abbreviated RSPCA. Although its principal target is the prevention of cruelty by the institution of deterrent litigation it also provides animal shelters and ambulances, conducts education programs and in general promotes the positive aspects of animal welfare.

RPF renal plasma flow.

r.p.m. revolutions per minute.

RQ respiratory quotient.

-rrhage, -rrhagia word element. [Gr.] *excessive flow*.

-rrhaphy see -RHAPHY

-rrhexis word element. [Gr.] *rupture of a vessel or organ*.

-rrhea word element. [Gr.] *profuse flow*.

rRNA ribosomal RNA. See RIBONUCLEIC ACID.

RSHP renal secondary hyperparathyroidism.

RSPCA Royal Society for the Prevention of Cruelty to Animals.

rT$_3$ reverse tri-iodothyronine.

RTA renal tubular acidosis.

r'tem see RETAMA RETAM.

RTG abbreviation for ready to go; used in medical records.

Ru chemical symbol, *ruthenium*.

rub friction rub, an auscultatory sound caused by the rubbing together of two serous surfaces.

pericardial r. a scraping or grating noise heard with the heartbeat, usually a to-and-fro sound, associated with an inflamed pericardium.

pleural r., pleuritic r. a rub produced by friction between the visceral and costal pleurae.

rub sore a sore found between the toes of Greyhounds and caused by pressure from a joint of a lesser digit on the side of a greater digit.

Rubarth's disease infectious canine hepatitis.

rubber-band ligation surgical removal of horns, tails, scrotums and contents by the application of rubber ligatures so that the ligated portion sloughs away after several days. Called also Barron ligation, elastration. The same technique is sometimes applied maliciously to a noisy or annoying animal without the owner's knowledge. This is a serious trespass and therefore actionable. The animal usually shows no evidence of pain and the sadism is unsuspected until the ligated part is gangrenous. When the ligature is placed around the neck attention is drawn to the area by a weeping discharge down the neck. Accidental ligation can happen to captive animals in zoos and the like when they are thrown feed parcels fastened with rubber bands.

rubber jaw, rubber nose see renal secondary HYPERPARATHYROIDISM.

rubber puppy syndrome, rubber kitten syndrome see EHLERS–DANLOS SYNDROME.

rubber ring castration see ELASTRATOR.

rubber tree see CALOTROPIS PROCERA.

rubber vine see CRYPTOSTEGIA GRANDIFLORA.

rubberweed HYMENOXYS *odorata.*

rubefacient 1. reddening the skin. 2. an agent that reddens the skin.

rubella see RUBIVIRUS.

rubeola human measles; can assume epidemic proportions in primate colonies with a syndrome of exanthematous rash on the body, rhinitis, conjunctivitis and in some interstitial giant-cell pneumonia.

rubeosis redness.

r. iridis a condition characterized by a new formation of vessels and connective tissue on the surface of the iris.

ruber [L.] *red.*

rubescent growing red; reddish.

rubidium a chemical element, atomic number 37, atomic weight 85.47, symbol Rb. See Table 6.

rubidomycin see DAUNORUBICIN.

rubijervine one of the toxic principles in the plant *Veratrum album.*

Rubin nerve block a technique for regional anesthesia of the equine orbital cavity.

Rubivirus a genus in the family *Togaviridae* that includes rubella (German measles) virus of humans which also infects nonhuman primates. Not arthropod borne.

rubor [L.] *redness;* one of the cardinal signs of inflammation.

Ruboralga jacksoniensis a venomous fish called the twelve-spined red rock cod. A sting from a spine causes intense local pain and rapid hyperthermia followed by hypothermia and prostration.

rubratoxin a series of two mycotoxins produced by the fungus *Penicillium rubrum.* Chronic exposure to these toxins causes extensive liver damage with much of the organ being completely destroyed. *P. pururogenum* produces similar toxins.

rubriblast pronormoblast; proerythroblast.

rubric red; specifically, pertaining to the red nucleus.

rubricyte polychromatic normoblast.

rubrospinal pertaining to the red nucleus and the spinal cord.

r. tract spinal cord motor tract emanating from the red nucleus.

rubrothalamic pertaining to the red nucleus and the thalamus.

rubrum [L.] red.

rubruria red urine.

ruby dock RUMEX *vesicarius.*

ruby saltbush see ENCHYLAENA TOMENTOSA.

Ruby spaniel see CAVALIER KING CHARLES SPANIEL.

Rudbeckia genus of North American plants in family Asteraceae; contain an unidentified toxin which causes incoordination, abdominal pain, diarrhea; includes *R. hirta* (black-eyed Susan), *R. laciniata* (golden glow, thimble weed, cone flower), *R. occidentalis* (western cone flower).

ruddy cyanosis mucosal congestion combined with cyanosis.

rudiment 1. primordium. 2. an organ or part that has failed to realize its potential function.

rudimentary 1. imperfectly developed. 2. vestigial.

rudimentum rudiment; the first indication of a structure in the course of its embryonic development.

ruffed grouse a forest species of game birds; called also *Bonasa umbellus.*

ruffled border see brush BORDER.

rufous red.

rufus red.

rug horse gear used to cover and protect from the weather from the root of the neck to the tail.

New Zealand r. canvas, waterproof rug with breast strap and leg straps that pass inside the thighs and anchor the rug behind.

ruga pl. *rugae* [L.] a ridge or fold.

rugae palatal transverse ridges of hard palate mucosa shaped so as facilitate the movement of food backwards towards the pharynx.

Rugopharynx gastrointestinal nematode found in free-living macropods.

R. australis found in free-living macropods.

R. rosemariae gastrointestinal nematodes found embedded in nodules in the saccular stomachs of kangaroos.

rugosa wrinkled.

rugoscopy the study of the patterns of the grooves and ridges (rugae) of the palate to identify individual patterns.

rugose marked by ridges; wrinkled.

rugosity 1. the condition of being rugose. 2. a fold, wrinkle or ruga.

rule of 20 a checklist of twenty parameters important in the care of critically ill patients.

rule of six a mnemonic for aging horses: in each arcade, a foal has two incisors from 6 days to 6 weeks of age, four incisors from 6 weeks to 6 months of age, and six incisors over 6 months of age.

rumen pl. *rumens, rumina;* the largest of the compartments of the forestomach of ruminant animals that serves as a fermentating vat. It is lined by a keratinized epithelium bearing numerous absorptive papillae; it is partly subdivided by folds (pillars). These include dorsal and ventral sacs and a caudodorsal blind sac and a caudoventral blind sac. It communicates directly with the reticulum cranially and has no other exit. It covers most of the floor of the adomen on the left in the nonpregnant animal and in animals not affected by left displacement of the abomasum. Caudally it may reach the brim of the pelvis and is palpable rectally.

r. transplant see CUD transfer.

rumen-degradable proteins those digested by ruminal microflora; there is no other simple way of categorizing them with respect to digestibility; some are digestible, some are not.

rumen-undegradable proteins only about half of the dietary protein of ruminants is digested in the rumen; some, e.g. those in maize, or those treated to pass though to the abomasum by heating or the addition of formaldehyde, are readily digestible by intestinal digestion systems.

rumenitis inflammation of the rumen commonly caused by carbohydrate engorgement. Also a result of ingestion of irritating substances such as crude oil or oil products. The lesions can be classified as necrobacillary, necrotizing.

rumenoreticular contractions combining the names of the rumen and reticulum has become an increasingly popular convention, acknowledging the preeminence of functionality over structure; the movements of the combined organs include a biphasic reticular contraction followed by a contraction of the dorsal ruminal sac, followed by a contraction of the ventral sac, then a repetition of the cycle.

rumenostomy creation of a permanent or semipermanent ruminal fistula. Suturing the ruminal wall to the skin and incising the rumen is the most permanent. Insertion of a bloatwhistle or a screw device that approximates the skin and ruminal mucosa are sufficient for temporary relief of persistent bloat or distension due to other causes.

rumenotomy surgical opening of the rumen through the left upper flank for the purpose of examining the reticulum, rumen or esophageal groove or for emptying the rumen.

r. shroud a large DRAPE used to cover exposed skin around a rumenotomy incision.

rumensin see MONENSIN.

Rumex plant genus of the Polygonaceae family; dock and sorrel plants which contain oxalate but are unpalatable and are rarely recorded as causes of poisoning. Includes *R. acetosa* (sorrel), *R. acetosella* (*R. angiocarpus*, dock sorrel), *R. brownii* (swamp dock), *R. conglomeratus* (clustered dock), *R. crispus* (curly dock), *R. venosus* (veined dock), *R. vesicarius* (red or ruby dock). See also soluble OXALATE poisoning.

ruminal, rumenal pertaining to the RUMEN.

r. acidosis see ruminal pH (below).

r. atony cessation of normal rhythmic contractions for more than 2 minutes. Caused by many factors including peritonitis, ruminal acidity or alkalinity. Recognized by palpation or auscultation in the left flank. Called also ruminal stasis.

r. collapse collapse of ruminal function, e.g. resulting from complete anorexia, severe toxemia for several days; complete atony, shrunken, collapsed rumen, little content other than fluid.

r. contractions see RETICULORUMINAL CONTRACTIONS.

r. cycles see RETICULORUMINAL CONTRACTIONS.

r. distension due to froth, free gas, fluid or feed. In the early stages rumen cycles are increased in rate and intensity. In the very last stages there is ruminal atony. See also ruminal tympany (below), VAGUS indigestion, PYLORIC obstruction, CARBOHYDRATE ENGORGEMENT.

r. drinkers calves fed milk or milk replacer in which reticular groove closure is incomplete so that much milk leaks into the rumen where it ferments causing a disabling indigestion.

r. fill dry matter capacity; the limitation on intake of the animal.

r. flora see rumen FLORA.

r. flora reconstitution see CUD transfer.

r. flukes see PARAMPHISTOMIASIS.

foul smelling r. contents putrefaction of ruminal contents, especially protein, in an atonic and defaunated rumen.

r. hyperkeratosis occurs in calves nutritionally deficient in vitamin A.

r. hypermotility rumen cycles occur almost continuously, at least faster than the normal high level of two cycles per minute. See VAGUS indigestion.

r. impaction dense packing of rumen with indigestible roughage, accompanied by ruminal hypomotility. Dietary error causing slight increase in ruminal acidity or alkalinity. Called also indigestion.

r. indigestion the clinical syndrome associated with ruminal atony. Includes low food intake, rumen atony, reduced fecal output.

r. inflammation see RUMENITIS.

r. necrobacillosis infection of the rumen wall by *Fusobacterium necrophorum*, usually secondarily to rumenitis after carbohydrate engorgement. Commonly a precursor of liver necrobacillosis.

r. overload see CARBOHYDRATE ENGORGEMENT.

r. parakeratosis significant lesion in ruminants fed high concentrate rations; characterized by black, club- or tongue-like papillae which tend to stick together in clumps.

r. pH the normal pH of 7.0 can fall as low as 5.5 to 6.5 in moderate acidosis caused by carbohydrate engorgement, 5 to 6 in acute engorgement, and 4 to 5 in the peracute disease.

r. protozoa absent see DEFAUNATE.

r. rotation partial rotation about the long anteroposterior axis has caused chronic tympany.

r. sounds the sounds which accompany normal ruminal movements in normal cows and are audible over the left upper flank. The sounds referable to the first movement in the cycle resembles water gurgling over a gravel bed, the second sound has a booming quality like distant thunder.

r. squamous-cell carcinoma rarely occurs in the rumen and may obstruct the esophageal cardia causing chronic ruminal tympany.

r. stasis complete absence of ruminal movement indicated by no audible sounds and no palpable ruminal movements during a two minute auscultation.

r. tympany distension of the rumen with gas. In cattle affected by eating too much wet legume—so-called clover bloat—the gas may be mixed with fluid phase to cause stable froth and the animal is unable to eructate and dies of asphyxia. Free gas bloat is due to physical obstruction of the esophagus by a foreign body, or by pressure from outside, or failure of the esophageal groove reflex, or acute atony of ruminal musculature as in anaphylaxis. Called also bloat.

r. ulceration an uncommon lesion due usually to bacterial or fungal infection of a primary erosive lesion or chemical rumenitis; clinically inapparent unless leakage or rupture causes peritonitis.

r. villous atrophy encountered in weanling ruminants on low fiber diets, e.g. pelleted feed. Causes no apparent impairment of digestion.

r. zoospores motile fungal bodies, chemotactically attracted to soluble carbohydrate and may represent 8% of the total ruminal biomass in animals on high fiber diets. Their role in digestion is unsure but they do form rhizoids which penetrate plant tissue.

ruminant 1. member of the mammalian suborder Ruminantia. 2. an animal that has a stomach with four complete cavities, and that characteristically regurgitates undigested food from the rumen and masticates it when at rest.

r. forestomach see FORESTOMACHS.

r. ketosis see PREGNANCY toxemia, ACETONEMIA.

r. stomachs include the forestomach (reticulum, rumen, omasum) and abomasum.

rumination includes regurgitation, remastication, ensalivation and reswallowing. The regurgitation of fluid reticular contents occurs as a result of a positive lowering of intrathoracic pressure, the arrival of a ruminal contraction at the cardial sphincter at the appropriate time, relaxation of the cardia and reverse peristalsis in the lower esophagus. The regurgitus is compressed at the back of the tongue and the fluid immediately reswallowed. The solid material is chewed for about a minute and reswallowed. The cycle is then ready to recommence. Rumination requires a positive approach by the cow and it is easily dissuaded by fright or food. Called also chewing the cud, cudding.

Ruminobacter amylophilus a standard ruminal bacterial denizen useful in bacterial fermentation of plant ingesta.

Ruminococcus ruminal bacteria which participate in bacterial fermentation of ingested plant material; includes *R. albus*, *R. flavefaciens*.

ruminoreticulum the rumen and reticulum as a unit.

rump the gluteal region; the region around the pelvis, hindquarters, buttocks.

goose r. a very steep slope to the back over the pelvis.

rump post see PYGOSTYLE.

rumpy 1. overendowed with buttocks. 2. a variety of MANX cat without any coccygeal vertebrae.

rumpyriser a variety of MANX cat with a few coccygeal vertebrae.

runch poisoning by SINAPIS *arvensis*.

runners a defective gait in foxhounds in which affected animals are unable to gallop or jump fences.

running fits see canine HYSTERIA, psychomotor SEIZURE.

running out said of a horse that is not stabled but running at pasture.

running walk a four-beat horse gait faster than a walk and slower than a rack. Said to be a trot in front and a walk behind.

runt small, stunted, weak; an undersized offspring. See also INTRAUTERINE growth retardation.

r. disease disease produced by immunologically competent cells in a foreign host that is unable to reject them, resulting in gross retardation of host development and in death. Classically observed in neonatal mice given bone marrow or leukocytes from an adult, genetically different strain of mice; a form of GRAFT VERSUS HOST DISEASE.

runting syndrome a condition which occurs in newborn pigs infected often with porcine parvovirus during gestation. The piglets do not thrive, suffer thymic atrophy and die at the age of 2 to 12 months.

Runyon classification an older system of classification of MYCOBACTERIA, based on growth rate, morphology of colonies and pigmentation.

Rupicapra a genus of European wild goats; includes *R. rupicapra*, *R. tragis*; see CHAMOIS (2).

RUPs rumen undegradable proteins.

rupture 1. tearing or disruption of tissue. 2. hernia.

For details of individual diseases see under each organ, e.g. abomasal, aortic, atrial, cecal, intestinal, rectal, gastric, ventricular, vesical, esophageal, ligamentous, individual ligaments (e.g. cruciate, round, Achilles) urethral, hepatic, splenic, egg yolk.

Rusa unicolor see SAMBAR DEER.

rush peristaltic rush; a powerful wave of contractile activity that travels very long distances down the small intestine, caused by intense irritation or unusual distension.

Rush pin internal splinting pin of stainless steel and vitallium that is semicircular in cross-section and has a pointed tip with a bevel edge. When properly placed in the intramedullary cavity of a long bone, it provides three-point fixation under spring-loaded tension.

rushes aquatic plants; called also bulrush. See JUNCUS.

Ruskin forceps heavy duty, double action, spring-loaded handle with two chisel-shaped blades approximating each other. The standard bone forcep.

Ruskin rongeur similar to RUSKIN FORCEPS except that the blades are excavated spoon-shaped, classical rongeur blades.

Russell bodies globular plasma cell inclusions composed of aggregates of immunoglobulin. Called also cancer body.

Russell's viper venom the venom of Russell's viper (*Vipera russelli*), which acts in vitro as an instrinsic thromboplastin and is useful in defining deficiencies of blood clotting factor X.

R. viper venom time (RVVT) a one-stage prothrombin time test, used to distinguish between deficiency of factor VII and factor X. Called also Stypven time.

Russian associated in some way with Russia.

R. blue a breed of cats with short, dense, silver-tipped blue-colored coat and vivid green eyes.

R. heavy draft heavy draft or milk Russian horse, usually chestnut, also brown or bay.

R. rabbit a breed of white domestic rabbit with black extremities.

R. trotter light horse bred by mating Orlov horse and American trotters; all coat colors.

R. wolfhound see BORZOI.

Russian comfrey SYMPHYTUM.

Russian forceps tissue handling forceps with broad, spoon-shaped tips, serrated around the edge.

Russian gad fly see RHINOESTRUS *purpureus*.

Russian knapweed *Acroptilon repens*. See also CENTAUREA.

Russian spring–summer encephalitis see Russian spring–summer ENCEPHALITIS.

Russian thistle SALSOLA *kali*.

rust 1. a disease of tropical fish in aquariums caused by the protozoa *Oodinium limneticum* and characterized by loss of luster of the skin surface. Causes heavy mortality. 2. a bacterial disease of the shell in turtles. See also SHELL ROT.

rusty male fern DRYOPTERIS *borreri*.

rut the period of increased sexual activity occurring in the autumn (fall) in some male mammals, especially deer and elephants. It is accompanied by increased testicular activity, especially spermatogenesis, and in deer by shedding of the antlers and a marked increase in vocalizing and aggression. The vocalizing is a distinctive deep roar known as 'the rut'. The aggressive actions have the effect of keeping attending females close and competing males at a distance.

rutabaga BRASSICA *napobrassica*.

ruthenium a chemical element, atomic number 44, atomic weight 101.07, symbol Ru. See Table 6.

rutherford a unit of radioactive disintegration, representing one million disintegrations per second. Called also Rd. The term is no longer used having been replaced by CURIE which is also now superseded by BECQUEREL.

rutherfordium a chemical element, atomic number 104, atomic weight 261, symbol Rf. See Table 6.

ruttling a rough wheezing sound made by guinea pigs; sometimes it is associated with pneumonia, but may occur in normal animals.

RV residual volume.
RVH right ventricular hypertrophy.
RVVT Russell's viper venom time.
Rx, ℞ recipe; used as a heading for a prescription.
rye the cereal plant *Secale cereale*, and its nutritious seed. May be infected with CLAVICEPS *purpurea* and cause poisoning.
r. ergot see rye ERGOT.
ryegrass highly productive pasture grasses including Wimmera or annual ryegrass (*Lolium rigidum*), Italian ryegrass (*L. multiflorum*) and perennial ryegrass (*L. perenne*).
r. staggers ruminants and horses grazing pastures dominated by *Lolium perenne* (perennial ryegrass) may be affected with a severe incoordination which appears with forced exercise but disappears if the animals are left to their own devices. Caused by tremorgen lolitrems from the endophyte *Acremonium lolii* which infests the grass.
Ryeland a breed of English polled, short-woolled, meat sheep.
ryodoraku a specific form of acupuncture developed by the Japanese; ryodo points are very close to or at the site of acupuncture points. Ryodoraku lines are comparable to acupuncture meridians.

S

S chemical symbol, *sulfur;* symbol for *siemens* and *svedberg;* [L.] *semis* (half); sight; [L.] *signa* (mark); [L.] *sinister* (left).
S phase see cell CYCLE.
S-A, SA sinoatrial.
S-T segment the portion of an electrocardiogram between the end of the QRS complex and the beginning of the T wave. It represents the period of slow repolarization of the ventricles.
S1-mapping a method for mapping precursor or mature mRNA to particular DNA sequences using the enzyme S1-nuclease.
SA node see SINOATRIAL.
Saanen a breed of all-white, although cream is acceptable, dairy goat with prick ears and always polled.
Sabin–Feldmann dye test a test which detects serum antibody against *Toxoplasma gondii*. In the presence of antibodies, live organisms are not stained with methylene blue. Called also methylene blue dye binding test.
sable 1. a coat color pattern with black-tipped hairs on a light background. Seen in the German shepherd dog. 2. breed of fur rabbit that is dark sepia with paler underside in a dense, soft coat. There are two varieties, Siamese and Marten, the latter having white markings on the belly and legs.
Sabouraud's dextrose agar see Sabouraud's dextrose AGAR.
sabulous gritty or sandy.
saburra sordes; foulness of the mouth or stomach.
saburral pertaining to saburra.
sac a pouch; a baglike organ or structure. See also CONJUNCTIVAL sac.
air s. 1. alveolar sac. 2. one of the large air-filled diverticula of the respiratory system of birds. See also AIR SACS.
allantoic s. see ALLANTOIS.
alveolar s's the spaces into which the alveolar ducts open distally, and with which the alveoli communicate.
anal s. see ANAL SACS.
endolymphatic s. the blind, flattened cerebral end of the endolymphatic duct.
heart s. the pericardium.
hernial s. the peritoneal pouch that encloses a herniated viscus or mesentery.
lacrimal s. see LACRIMAL sac.
paranal s. see ANAL SACS.
pleural s. the pleura-lined cavity which contains the lung.
ruminal s. one of the dorsal and ventral sacs of the rumen which are themselves further subdivided to create a caudodorsal sac and a caudoventral sac.
yolk s. the extraembryonic membrane connected with the midgut; in vertebrates other than true mammals, it contains a yolk mass. See also YOLK SAC.
sacahuiste, sacahuista NOLINA *texana*, *N. microcarpa*.
saccade the series of involuntary, abrupt, rapid, small movements or jerks of both eyes simultaneously in changing the point of fixation.
saccadic said of the eye; small, rapid, jerky movements of the orbit, such as occur in humans while reading.
saccadic movement a quick return movement of the eyeball in order to establish a new image on the retina.
saccate 1. shaped like a sac. 2. contained in a sac.
saccharated iron, saccharated ferric oxide a brown powder, soluble in water, used as a hematinic. Given by intramuscular injection to newborn piglets. See also IRON poisoning.
saccharide one of a series of carbohydrates, including the sugars; they are divided into monosaccharides, disaccharides, trisaccharides and polysaccharides according to the number of saccharide groups present.
sacchariferous containing sugar.
saccharogalactorrhea secretion of milk containing an excess of sugar.
saccharogenic capable of producing a sugar.
saccharolytic capable of splitting up sugar.
saccharometabolic pertaining to the metabolism of sugar.
saccharometabolism the metabolism of sugar.
Saccharomyces farciminosum see HISTOPLASMA *farciminosum*.
Saccharomycopsis guttulatus a fungus associated with enteritis in young animals.
saccharum [L.] *sugar* (especially sucrose).
sacciform shaped like a bag or sac.
Saccostrea commercialis farmed bivalve; called also Sydney rock oyster. See Table 23.
saccular pertaining to or resembling a sac.
s. stage lung growth about the midpoint of fetal development when the lung volume increases markedly due to saccule development; subdivision of the saccules into alveoli commences.
sacculated containing saccules.
sacculation 1. a saccule, or pouch. 2. the quality of being sacculated. 3. the formation of pouches.
large intestinal s. see HAUSTRUM.
saccule 1. a little bag or sac; a small, pouchlike cavity. 2. the smaller of the two divisions of the membranous labyrinth of the vestibule, which communicates with the cochlear duct by way of the ductus reuniens.
laryngeal s. sacculus laryngis.

sacculectomy surgical removal of saccular structures.
anal s. performed in dogs with anal sac disease. It is also the basis for descenting of skunks and ferrets. There are number of different procedures described, many of which are modifications intended to enable the surgeon to more easily visualize and handle the structures.
sacculitis inflammation of a saccule, e.g. AIRSACCULITIS, ANAL sacculitis.
sacculus pl. *sacculi* [L.] a saccule.
s. laryngis the lateral ventricle of the larynx, especially when of large size; its entrance in most species lies between the vocal and the vestibular folds. In pigs the ventricle lies between the two parts of the vocal ligament and there is no sac in the cat nor in ruminants.
saccus pl. *sacci* [L.] a sac.
s. cecus fundus of the stomach in the horse.
s. hypophysialis an outgrowth of ectoderm coming directly from the roof of the stomodeum in the embryo; it comes into contact with a downgrowth from the forebrain and is later transformed into the anterior lobe of the pituitary.
sacrad toward the sacrum.
sacral pertaining to the sacrum.
s. dysgensis defective development of sacral vertebrae as in Manx cats.
s. paralysis see AZOTURIA.
sacralgia pain in the sacrum.
sacralization anomalous fusion of the last lumbar vertebra with the first segment of the sacrum.
sacrectomy excision or resection of the sacrum.
sacred bamboo see NANDINA DOMESTICA.
Sacred cat of Burma see BIRMAN.
sacr(o)- word element. [L.] *sacrum*.
sacrocaudal pertaining to the sacrum and the tail.
s. agenesis, s. dysgenesis abnormal development of the vertebrae in the area; seen most commonly in Manx cats and dogs naturally tailless, e.g. Old English sheepdogs, British bulldogs and others. It is often associated with abnormalities of innervation to the anus, urinary bladder and sometimes hindlegs and tail.
s. fusion an anomalous union between the sacrum and coccygeal vertebrae.
s. joint the joint between the sacrum and the tail.
s. luxation a relatively common traumatic injury in dogs and cats, caused by traction on the tail. Neurological deficits result from hemorrhage, edema and avulsion of nerve roots in the terminal spinal cord. There may be urinary and fecal incontinence, posterior paresis and paralysis of the tail.
sacrococcygeal see SACROCAUDAL.
sacroiliac pertaining to the sacrum and the ilium, or the joint between these two bones, or to the part of the back where these bones meet on both sides of the back.
s. joint see Table 11.
sacroiliitis inflammation of the sacroiliac joint.
sacrolumbar pertaining to the sacrum and lumbar vertebra; the loins.
sacropelvic pertaining to the pelvis and sacrum.
sacrosciatic pertaining to the sacrum and ischium.
sacrospinal pertaining to the sacrum and vertebral column.
sacrotuberous ligament see Table 12.
sacrouterine pertaining to the sacrum and uterus.
sacrovertebral pertaining to the sacrum and vertebrae.
sacrum the triangular-shaped bone between the lumbar and coccygeal vertebrae; formed usually by five fused vertebrae (four in pigs, three in dogs) that are wedged dorsally between the two hip bones. See also Table 10.
SAD rabies vaccine Street–Alabama–Dufferin strain of attenuated rabies vaccine.
saddle 1. the back region over the thoracic vertebrae. 2. a coat color marking in dogs, usually black, located over the back. Seen in Beagles. 3. a piece of harness for either riding or draft.
basket s. an oldfashioned saddle with a basket in place of the seat into which a child could be strapped and taken for a ride.
s. cloth worn between the saddle and the horse it provides a little extra protection for the horse but mainly keeps the saddle lining clean.
draft s. has the same basic structure as a riding saddle but has ornaments in the place of the rider's seat. It is attached to the horse by the girth and supports two leather loops or tugs at about elbow height which carry the shafts and support the weight of the vehicle being drawn.
riding s. has a metal tree and bars as a skeleton, the tree providing a structure to keep pressure off the dorsal processes of the spinal vertebrae and the bars to spread the pressure of the rider's weight evenly over the muscles on either side. Covered with leather, lined with serge and stuffed with wool flock. There are many styles, the simplest being the English army saddle which has no adornments, no comfort index but never wears out.
s. scab see EQUINE staphylococcal dermatitis.
s. sore, s. gall a pressure sore caused by bad riding technique or more commonly a badly fitting or poorly stuffed saddle.
saddlepatch disease see COLUMNARIS DISEASE.
safe light red, yellow or orange light for use in photographic darkroom used for developing x-ray film; should comply with the specifications of the type of filter being used and the screen-film combination.
safety avoidance of occupational, iatrogenic or personal injury.
drug s. freedom from undesirable side-effects; increases with specificity and selectivity of a drug. See also safety index (below).
s. index maximum tolerated dose/recommended dose, the doses being expressed in similar terms, e.g. mg/lb, mg/kg.
radiological s. routine the specific routine to be followed in an x-ray room to ensure minimal risk to all parties.
restraint s. proper use of appropriate restraint procedure when dealing with any animal.
s. specifications specifications laid down by a local government authority about the construction and equipment to be used in a radiological facility.
safety pin appearance the appearance of *Clostridium perfringens* spores in fecal examinations; the open end represents the remains of the vegetative cell.
Saffan a steroidal preparation containing two pregnanediones (ALPHAXALONE and ALPHADOLONE acetate) and used for the induction of anesthesia. Induces short-term anesthesia immediately when administered intravenously. Called also CT 1341.
safflower meal ground cake made of decorticated residue of seeds of *Carthamus tinctorius*, rich in linoleic acid. A modest protein dietary supplement deficient in methionine and lysine. Called also kurdee.
saffron see COLCHICUM AUTUMNALE.

Sagatal a proprietary name for PENTOBARTITAL.
sage ARTEMISIA *filifolia*, *A. spinescens*.
s. sickness unspecified poisoning by *Artemisia* spp.
sagebrush sage.
sagging crop see pendulous CROP.
sagging posture comprises drooping ears, head hung low, tail down (unkinked in the case of pigs), lackluster facial expression.
sagittal 1. shaped like an arrow. 2. situated in the direction of the sagittal suture; said of a plane or section parallel to the median plane of the body.
sago palm CYCAS *revoluta*.
sago spleen the white pulp of the spleen is enlarged and protrudes through the capsule like grains of sago. Occurs in amyloidosis.
Saguinus see MARMOSET.
saharan pertaining to or emanating from the Sahara desert.
Sahelian emanating from or pertaining to Sahel, the region south of the Sahara desert in Central Africa.
S. goat many varieties of this dual-purpose breed in North West Africa.
Sahiwal a reddish-dun zebu type breed of dairy cattle. Usually has white markings.
SAIDS simian acquired immune deficiency syndrome.
sail sign the thymus, seen as a triangular structure in the left, cranial mediastinum on ventrodorsal radiographs of the thorax in young dogs.
Saimiri sciureis see SQUIRREL monkey.
St. Anthony's turnip RANUNCULUS *bulbosus*.
St. Barnaby's thistle CENTAUREA *solstitialis*.
St. Bernard a very large (110–200 lb) dog with massive, broad head, medium-sized ears lying close to the head, and a long tail. There are two varieties, the most familiar (rough) has a long, thick coat, while the smooth variety has a shorter coat, lying close to the body. The breed is predisposed to osteogenic sarcoma, ectropion, entropion, hip dysplasia, osteochondrosis, hemophilia and congestive cardiomyopathy.
St. George disease see PIMELEA.
St. Hubert hound see BLOODHOUND.
St. John's wort HYPERICUM *aethiopicum*, *H. perforatum*.
St. Louis encephalitis see St. Louis ENCEPHALITIS.
St. Lucia grass BRACHIARIA *brizantha*.
St. Mary's thistle see SILYBUM MARIANUM.
saki a longhaired, bushy-tailed, New World monkey, about 1.5 ft long and weighing 2 lb. They are diurnal, arboreal and gregarious and in two genera *Pithecia* and *Chiropotes*.
sal [L.] *salt*.
salamander a suborder of amphibians that includes three families and a wide variety of genera. They are all characterized by their unique life history which they pass partly on land in a terrestrial form (efts) and partly in water as an aquatic form (newt). Both forms are lizard-like and some of them have bright and distinctive coloring. Reproduction usually occurs in the aquatic phase. Neoteny, the maintenance of larval characteristics throughout life, is a common phenomenon in these animals.
s. poisoning dogs and cats mouthing salamanders may become distressed with excessive salivation, muscular weakness and incoordination and rarely convulsions.
Sala's cells star-shaped cells of connective tissue in the fibers that form the sensory nerve endings situated in the pericardium.
salbutamol see ALBUTEROL.
Salers mahogany red, dual-purpose French cattle.
salicyl-sulfonic acid test precipitation of protein in a urine sample by a 20% aqueous solution of salicylsulfonic acid. Placing the urine over a layer of reagent in a test tube results in the formation of a white ring where the two solutions meet, indicating that protein is present.
salicylamide an amide of salicylic acid; used as an analgesic; toxic in cats.
salicylanilides a group of anthelmintics which exert their action by uncoupling mitochondrial reactions which are critical to electron transport and associated phosphorylation in the metabolic system of the parasite. They are effective against cestodes and trematodes but not nematodes. Some are active against *Haemonchus contortus*, e.g. rafoxanide and closantel.
salicylate any salt or ester of salicylic acid. The salicylates used as drugs for their analgesic, antipyretic and anti-inflammatory effects include aspirin (acetylsalicylic acid, ASA), methyl salicylate and sodium salicylate. Low dosages of salicylates are used primarily for the relief of mild-to-moderate pain or fever.

The mechanism of most of the effects of aspirin and other salicylates is inhibition of prostaglandin synthesis, thus blocking pyretic and inflammatory processes that are mediated by prostaglandins.

Aspirin also prolongs the bleeding time through its effects on platelets owing to both inhibition of prostaglandin synthesis and acetylation of platelet structures. Salicylates also cause ulceration and hemorrhagic lesions of the gastric mucosa; the same mechanisms involved in the anti-inflammatory effects increase the production of stomach acid, decrease the secretion of protective mucus and increase bleeding. See also ASPIRIN poisoning.
salicylazosulfapyridine see SULFASALAZINE.
salicylic acid *o*-hydroxybenzoic acid; used as a keratolytic. See also SALICYLATE.
salicylism toxic signs caused by salicylic acid.
saline salty; of the nature of a salt.
s. cathartic see saline CATHARTIC.
s. drench an orally administered preparation of electrolytes in water used in racehorses but more particularly in endurance and event horses in which heavy electrolyte losses in sweat are likely. A variety of formulations is used but all contain sodium, potassium, calcium and magnesium ions; some also contain glucose.
s. solution a solution of salt (sodium chloride) in purified water. Physiological saline solution is a 0.9% solution of sodium chloride and water and is isotonic, i.e. of the same osmotic pressure as blood serum.
s. water poisoning see SODIUM chloride poisoning.
s. waters waters from surface running mineral springs, water obtained from natural underground storages in artesian and subartesian bores.
salinomycin an ionophore coccidiostat with a broad spectrum of efficiency and closely related to monensin.
s.–tiamulin poisoning fed concurrently or close together to pigs enhances the myonecrotic effect of salinomycin.
saliuresis diuresis due to high electrolyte excretion; e.g. the feeding of additional salt as a prevention against urolithiasis in sheep and cattle acts in this way. Some useful salt or osmotic diuretics may have to be administered parenterally because of poor absorption.
saliva the enzyme-containing secretion of the salivary glands.
s. tests tests conducted on the saliva of horses com-

peting in races or show events to detect the presence of drugs used to affect the horse's performance.

salivant causing flow of saliva.

Salivaria the ANTERIOR station group or Group B trypanosomes which transmit the protozoa with their mouthparts.

salivarian said of trypanosomes which belong to the subgenera of *Duttonella*, *Trypanozoon*, *Pycnomonas* and *Nannomonas*. These trypanosomes are passed to the recipient in the saliva of the tsetse fly (*Glossina* spp.). See also SALIVARIA.

salivary pertaining to the saliva.

s. amylase an α-amylase, ptyalin, initiates digestion of starch and glycogen in the mouth. Dogs, cats and horses appear not to secrete the enzyme.

s. calculus see SIALOLITH.

s. duct atresia a congenital absence of lumen in the duct; causes distension then atrophy of the gland.

s. duct dilatation see RANULA.

s. ducts excretory ducts that carry the saliva from the glands to the mouth cavity.

salivary gland any of the glands around the mouth that secrete saliva. The major ones are the three pairs known as the parotid, mandibular or submandibular and sublingual glands. There are other smaller salivary glands within the cheeks, e.g. zygomatic gland, and in the tongue.

s. g. inflammation see SIALOADENITIS, PAROTIDITIS.

s. g. squamous metaplasia of the interlobular duct of the salivary gland is a feature of hypovitaminosis A.

salivation 1. the secretion of saliva. 2. ptyalism.

excessive s. may be caused by slaframine toxicosis from the fungus *Rhizoctonia leguminocola*, by foreign bodies or painful lesions in the mouth. To be distinguished from drooling of saliva because of failure to swallow.

s. inhibitor antisialagogue; examples are atropine and glycopyrrolate.

salivon a functional salivary unit consisting of several acini and their related ducts and tubules.

sallenders a localized chronic dermatitis in front of the hock of heavy draft horses. The cause is unknown. The lesion is scabby, alopecic, with thick, hardened skin.

sally wattle ACACIA *glaucescens*.

Salmincola parasitic crustaceans which attach to the gills of salmonid fish and cause obstruction of respiration and blood loss resulting in delayed sexual maturity, reduced growth rate and some mortality.

Salmo genus of finfish in the family Salmonidae, many of them farmed. Includes *S. trutta* (brown trout), *S. salar* (Atlantic salmon). See Table 23.

salmon farmed finfish; many species in the genera *Salmo* and *Oncorhyncus*.

s. louse *Lepeophtherius salmonis*.

s. poisoning, salmon disease a disease of dogs and other canids which eat salmon from streams in the Pacific Northwest of the USA, and caused by NEORICKETTSIA HELMINTHOECA. The infection is transmitted by the fluke, *Nanophyetus salmincola*, parasitic in the salmon. The disease in dogs is characterized by fever, ocular discharge and edema of the eyelids, followed by vomiting, then diarrhea and later severe dysentery and death in untreated cases. See also ELOKOMIN FLUKE FEVER.

Salmonella a genus of gram-negative, non-lactose fermenting, medium-sized, rod-shaped, bacteria, members of the family Enterobacteriaceae, most species having flagella and pili. The genus contains one species which has been divided into seven subgroups and a very large number of serotypes. Most species pathogenic for warm-blooded animals are in subgroup I (*S. enterica*). Subgroups IIIa (*S. salamae*) and IIIb (*S. arizonae*) include some species occasionally pathogenic for animals and birds. The salmonella include the typhoid–paratyphoid bacilli and bacteria usually pathogenic for lower animals but which are often transmitted to humans. They cause SALMONELLOSIS which has a number of manifestations and some are specific causes of abortion.

S. abortusequi causes abortion in horses.

S. abortusovis, S. montevideo cause abortion in sheep.

S. arizonae the name now applied to subgroup IIIa, these organisms cause severe enteritis and septicemia in chicks and turkey poults.

S. bovismorbificans causes enteritis in cattle and horses.

***S. choleraesuis* biotype Kunzendorf** causes septicemic and enteric salmonellosis of swine. Called the hog cholera bacillus because of the similarity of the clinical diseases.

S. dublin causes septicemia, meningitis, enteritis and abortion in cattle and abortion in sheep.

S. enteriditis a common cause of gastroenteritis in humans. Recorded also in most domestic animal species and fowl.

S. gallinarum causes FOWL typhoid.

S. heidelberg an occasional isolate in horses.

S. pullorum causes PULLORUM DISEASE.

S. typhimurium the causative agent of mouse typhoid and of food poisoning in humans. Causes outbreaks of enteritis in most species, often related to rodent infestation. The cause of fowl paratyphoid.

S. typhisuis an uncommon isolate in pigs.

salmonellosis a highly contagious disease of all animal species caused by SALMONELLA. It may cause septicemia, and acute or chronic enteritis. Abortion is a common accompaniment, particularly in food animals and horses. Localization may occur in almost any organ. It is a rare occurrence in companion animals. Called also paratyphoid. The disease is transmissible to humans and is an important zoonosis, with special implications for veterinarians involved in food hygiene.

salmonid a member of the fish family Salmonidae. Includes salmon, trout, char.

salpingectomy excision of a uterine tube.

salpingemphraxis obstruction of a eustachian tube.

salpingian pertaining to the auditory or the uterine tube.

salpingion a point at the apex of the petrous bone on the lower surface.

salpingitis 1. inflammation of a uterine tube. 2. inflammation of the eustachian tube.

mural s. pachysalpingitis.

parenchymatous s. pachysalpingitis.

salping(o)- word element. [Gr.] *tube* (eustachian tube or uterine tube).

salpingocele hernial protrusion of a uterine tube.

salpingocyesis development of the embryo within a uterine tube; tubal pregnancy.

salpingography radiography of the uterine tubes after intrauterine injection of a radiopaque medium.

salpingolithiasis the presence of calcareous deposits in the wall of the uterine tubes.

salpingolysis surgical separation of adhesions involving the uterine tubes.

salpingo-oophorectomy excision of a uterine tube and ovary.

salpingo-oophoritis inflammation of a uterine tube and ovary.

salpingo-oophorocele hernia of a uterine tube and ovary.
salpingopexy fixation of a uterine tube.
salpingopharyngeal pertaining to the auditory tube and the pharynx.
salpingoplasty plastic repair of a uterine tube.
salpingostomy 1. formation of an opening or fistula into a uterine tube for the purpose of drainage. 2. surgical restoration of the patency of a uterine tube.
salpingotomy surgical incision of a uterine tube.
salpinx 1. a uterine tube. 2. an auditory tube.
salsa IPOMOEA *asarifolia*.
Salsola plant genus in the family Chenopodiaceae; contains soluble oxalates and causes oxalate poisoning characterized by nephrosis, urolithiasis; includes *S. barbata*, *S. kali* (tumbleweed, soft roly-poly, Russian thistle).
S. tuberculatiformis, S. tuberculata* var. *tomentosa poisoning of sheep with this South African plant causes prolongation of gestation, enlargement of the fetus and dystocia. Syndrome called grootlamsiekte.
SALT see skin-associated LYMPHOID tissues.
salt 1. any compound of a base and an acid. 2. *salts*, a saline purgative. See also SODIUM chloride.
bile s's glycine or taurine conjugates of bile acids, which are formed in the liver and secreted in the bile. They are powerful detergents which break down fat globules, enabling them to be digested.
s. brine strong solution of common salt used to pickle meat and other human foods. Sodium chloride is the biggest component but large quantities of nitrate are usually present and represent a greater toxicity hazard than does the salt.
buffer s. a salt in the blood that is able to absorb slight excesses of acid or alkali with little or no change in the hydrogen ion concentration.
common s. see SODIUM chloride.
s. gland nasal gland in birds.
s. hunger common in circumstances in which animals are derived of any salt; manifested by leather chewing, earth eating, coat licking and urine drinking.
s. lick 1. naturally occurring deposit of salt in the form of a shallow pan that wild and domestic animals can share by licking. 2. a prepared mixture of salt with other minerals added, the composition varying with the local nutritional deficiency but the common additive is one containing phosphorus. The cattle or sheep are encouraged to lick by the taste of the salt and serendipitously acquire the other minerals. May be loose and put out in containers covered against the weather or formed into blocks that resist rain erosion and are fitted into holders fixed to buildings or free-standing in the pasture. See also MINERAL–salt mixture.
Rochelle s. potassium sodium tartrate, a cathartic.
s. sick see COPPER nutritional deficiency.
smelling s's aromatic ammonium carbonate, a stimulant and restorative.
s. tolerant capable of surviving in a high concentration of salt, e.g. some bacteria, including staphylococci.
salt-losing crisis vomiting, dehydration, hypotension and sudden death due to very large sodium losses from the body. It may be seen in abnormal losses of sodium into the urine (as in adrenocortical insufficiency or one of the forms of salt-losing NEPHRITIS) or in large extrarenal sodium losses, usually from the gastrointestinal tract.
salt sickness dual copper and cobalt deficiency.
salt-stored ovum penetration assay a test of the ability of spermatozoa in a semen sample to attach to and penetrate the zona pellucida of ova. Salt storage in NH_4SO_4 enables eggs from abattoir-collected ovaries to be used for several months.
salt water couch PASPALUM *distichum*.
saltation 1. the action of leaping, as in louping ill or the dancing of porcine myotonia congenita. 2. conduction along myelinated nerves. 3. in genetics, an abrupt variation in species; a mutation.
saltatory pertaining to or emanating from saltation.
s. conduction the leaping action transfer of electric potential from node of Ranvier to node of Ranvier along a medullated nerve fiber instead of a steady flow along the length of the nerve.
saltbush a widespread forage or browse plant on extensive range in Australian arid zones. Called also ATRIPLEX spp. Strictly a maintenance feed.
salted meats meats cured for preservation by the addition of salt to the external surface. The salt draws out water by osmosis. Plain salting is not a very sophisticated procedure and most commercial curing has at least nitrate in the curing mixture. See also BACON CURING.
Salter classification a system for classifying fractures, fracture-separations, and separations of the physis into five types. They are: *Salter type I*—a separation line through the epiphyseal plate only; *Salter type II*—a partial separation of the epiphyseal plate and fracture into the metaphyseal bone; *Salter type III*—a partial separation of the epiphyseal plate and a fracture through the epiphysis; *Salter type IV*—a fracture through the metaphysis, across the epiphyseal plate and through the epiphysis; *Salter type V*—a crushing or compression injury to the epiphyseal plate. Called also Salter–Harris classification.
Salter–Harris classification see SALTER CLASSIFICATION.
salting the mustering of cattle in wild country by training them to come for salt when called. The practice of putting out the salt is called salting.
salting out the separation of protein fractions in the serum or plasma by precipitation in increasing concentrations of neutral salts.
saltpeter, saltpetre potassium nitrate.
salubrious conducive to health; wholesome.
Saluki a medium-sized, very fine, graceful dog with a fine, silky coat of white, cream or shades of tan or red, sometimes with black and tan, that is flat on the body, but forms slight 'feathers' on the legs, ears, tail, and sometimes thighs and shoulders. There is also a smooth variety, which has no feathering. The entire dog is long and supple, suggesting its origins as a sight-hunting, desert dog. Believed to be the oldest known breed of domesticated dog. Called also Gazelle hound, Persian greyhound.
saluresis excretion of sodium and chloride in the urine.
saluretic 1. pertaining to saluresis. 2. an agent that promotes saluresis.
salutary healthful.
salvage pathways energy-saving re-utilization of preformed constituents, often purine and pyrimidine compounds that would otherwise be lost to degradation.
salvage statistics see salvage STATISTICS.
Salvation Jane ECHIUM *plantagineum*.
salve ointment.
Salvelinus genus of farmed finfish in family Salmonidae. Includes *S. fontinalis* (brook trout, splake), *S. namaycush* (splake, lake trout). See Table 23.

Salvia a genus of the plant family Lamiaceae.
S. coccinea an unidentified toxin causes abortion, diarrhea, recumbency. Called also *S. lineata*, red salvia.
S. reflexa has a high nitrate content and causes nitrate–nitrite poisoning in ruminants. Called also mintweed.

SAM *S*-adenosylmethionine.

samarium a chemical element, atomic number 62, atomic weight 150.35, symbol Sm. See Table 6.

sambar deer Indian deer with three-tined antlers. Called also *Rusa unicolor.*

Sambucus coarse bushes, members of the family Sambucaceae; contains toxic oil which causes diarrhea; sometimes also causes cyanide poisoning. Includes *S. canadensis*, *S. ebulus* (danewort, dwarf elder), *S. nigra* (common elder), *S. pubens*.

samore trypanosomiasis; called also nagana.

Samoyed a medium-sized dog characterized by a very thick, straight, white or cream-colored coat that stands out from the body, with brown eyes and black-rimmed eyelids and lip margins. It is said to have a 'smiling expression'. The ears are erect and the tail, with profuse haircoat, is curled over the back. The breed is predisposed to hemophilia, congenital heart defects and familial renal disease.

sample 1. a specimen of fluid, blood or tissue collected for analysis on the assumption that it represents the composition of the whole. 2. for statistical purposes a small collection of individual units taken from the population which is under investigation on the assumption that they represent the characteristics of the entire population.
EPSEM s. acronym for 'equal opportunity of selection method'.
grab s. sample of greasy wool taken at random by a special machine from each bale on the sale floor. Buyers price the bale on the basis of the appearance of the grab sample and the objective measurements.
multi-stage random s. with very large populations it may be desirable to arrange the data into groups on one criterion, e.g. address by area of postcode, and to select randomly from within this group, then select from within this sample to obtain randomly a representative number of specimens, such as dogs of each age group.
random s. the selection from a population of the units which are to constitute the sample of that population is made in such a way that each unit of the population has an equal chance of being selected. Called also simple random sample.
simple random s. see random sample (above).
stratified random s. the data is arranged into subsets or strata based on the possession of certain characteristics which are common to the members of the subset. The selection of units to comprise the sample of the parent population is arranged so that the proportional representation of each subset in the final sample fits a prearranged schedule.
volunteer s. sample donated by interested parties; a biased sample because it does not represent all sections of the population. Called also self-selection.

sampling the process of selecting a sample.
area s. dividing the population into equal areas and randomly selecting from among the areas.
cluster s. when the population to be sampled exists in clusters, e.g. herds, sampling can be done by random selection between the herds. This assumes that each cluster is a homogeneous group.
s. fraction ratio of the number of units in the population to the number of units in the population.
s. frame the names of the component parts of the population from which the sample is to be collected.
quota s. the sections of the population, e.g. milking cows, dry cows, yearlings, calves are represented in the sample in the same proportion as they exist in the population.
stratified s. a simple random selection is performed in each stratum of those created in order to permit a different sampling percentage to be used in each stratum.
systematic s. the sampling is random but the samples are drawn systematically, say every third unit, the first unit also being chosen randomly.
two-stage s. an example of multi-stage sampling. The first sampling is of large groups, e.g. herds, then a second-stage sampling is carried out within herds, e.g. sire families, with possibly a third stage, of individual cows within the sire families.
s. units individual members of a population. It is often difficult to define exactly what is a unit because of the design of the study.
s. variation the variation that occurs between samples of the one population. A measure of the random error of the sampling technique used.

San Joaquin Valley fever the primary form of COCCIDIOIDOMYCOSIS.

San Miguel sealion virus disease a disease of sealions, caused by a calicivirus that is transmissible to swine in which it causes a disease indistinguishable from vesicular exanthema of swine. Vesicular lesions of the skin and mucosae, abortion, pneumonia and encephalitis are associated with the infection in sealions. Related viruses have been recovered from other pinniped species.

sanative curative; healing. Said of trypanocidal drugs used between long courses of more popular drugs to avoid the development of resistance to those drugs by the trypanosomes.

sanatory conducive to health.

Sancassania berlessei a mite of stored products occasionally infests sheep.

sand 1. material occurring in fine, gritty particles loose in the body. 2. geological sand is ingested by animals, especially horses, grazing on very sandy soil. The animals may take in large amounts and this accumulates in the large sacs of the alimentary tract, the reticulum of the cow and the cecum and colon in horses. Sand or dust storms, or volcanic dust fallout may produce a similar, acute situation.
s. colic see sand COLIC.
s. enteritis acute sand ingestion may cause enteritis with severe, sometimes fatal diarrhea. See also ENTERITIS.
s. flea see TUNGA *penetrans*.
s. rash irritation and weeping of the toe webbing in racing Greyhounds causing lameness. Caused usually by racing in sand.
s. shin oak QUERCUS *havardii*.
s. toe Greyhounds racing in sand suffer impaction of sand under the coronary band, causing lameness, mostly in the inner and outer toes of the hind paws.
uterine s. see UTERINE sand.

sand rat see GERBIL.

sand sagebrush ARTEMISIA *filifolia*.

sand twin leaf ZYGOPHYLLUM *ammophilum*.

sandbags small sacks containing sand used to support an anesthetized animal in dorsal recumbency and prevent it from rolling sideways during anesthesia or surgery.

sandbath, sand roll a stall covered with deep sand used for horses to roll in after exercise.

sandcrack vertical cracks in the hoof that commence at the coronet and run parallel to the horn tubules and towards the toe. Are serious defects because they indicate an injury to the coronet and a possible extension to the sole.

sandfly *Phlebotomus* spp. *Culicoides*, *Simulium* and *Austrosimulium* spp. are also called called sandflies in some countries. Called also owl midges.

s. zieria ZIERIA *smithii*.

sandhill crane GRUS *canadensis*.

Sandhoff's disease see GM_2 GANGLIOSIDOSIS.

sandplain lupin LUPINUS *cosentinii*.

sandplain woody pear XYLOMELUM *angustifolium*.

sandwort see ARENARIA SERPYLLIFOLIA.

Sanfilippo's III-D syndrome a human disease similar to *N*-ACETYL-GLUCOSAMINE-6-SULFATASE deficiency in Nubian goats.

Sanga a type of draft cattle with a small cervicothoracic hump and long horns, originating in eastern and southern Africa. It includes many varieties.

Sanga Nguni cattle a breed of *Bos indicus* cattle in which testicular hypoplasia is recognized as being inherited.

Sanger–Coulson method a method of sequencing DNA; called also dideoxy or chain termination method. It involves the use of 2′3′ dideoxynucleoside triphosphates (dd NTPs) which lack a 3′-hydroxyl group.

sangui- word element. [L.] *blood*.

sanguifacient forming blood.

sanguinarine one of the isoquinoline alkaloids found in CHELIDONIUM MAJUS.

sanguine 1. abounding in blood. 2. ardent; hopeful.

sanguineous bloody; abounding in blood.

Sanguinicola a genus of the family Sanguinicolidae, digenetic flukes of the vascular system of freshwater and marine fish.

S. inermis*, *S. klamanthensis found in cyprinid and salmonid fish in which it is a serious pathogen, especially in cultured carp and trout. The gills and kidneys are affected most and mortality may be high.

sanguinolent of a bloody tinge.

sanguinopurulent containing both blood and pus.

sanguis [L.] *blood*.

sanguivorous blood-eating; said of female mosquitoes that prefer blood to other nutrients.

Sanhe named after Mongolian district.

S. cattle Chinese meat and draft cattle, red and white or black and white; originated from local breeds plus Simmental or Friesian.

S. horse riding and draft light horse, all coat colors.

sanies a fetid ichorous discharge containing serum, pus and blood.

saniopurulent partly sanious and partly purulent.

sanioserous partly sanious and partly serous.

sanitarian one skilled in sanitation and public health science.

sanitary promoting or pertaining to health.

s. trap container located between the air system and the milk system in a milking machine designed to trap fluids which would otherwise pass from one to the other.

sanitation the establishment of conditions favorable to health, especially with respect to infectious diseases. Includes disposal of infective materials, especially carcasses, discharges and excrement, application of disinfectants and general cleaning to make disinfection effective, isolation of infective animals and improvement in ventilation of buildings, improving feeding and watering arrangements to avoid fecal and urinary contamination of food and water.

sanitization the process of making or the quality of being made sanitary.

sanitize to clean and sterilize.

sanitizer a sanitizing product capable of cleaning and disinfecting; usually a formulation containing a disinfectant and a detergent.

Santa Gertrudis a red, beef breed, originated in southern USA by crossbreeding Shorthorn and Brahman cattle.

Santorini's duct, duct of Santorini see accessory pancreatic DUCT.

Sao_2 symbol for percentage of available hemoglobin that is saturated with oxygen. See BLOOD GAS ANALYSIS.

SAP serum alkaline phosphatase.

saperconazole a triazole antifungal agent.

saphena the small saphenous or the great saphenous vein.

saphenous pertaining to or associated with a saphenous vein; applied to certain arteries, nerves, etc. See also Tables 9, 14 and 15.

s. nerve block achieved by injection of a local anesthetic onto the saphenous vein, proximal to the hock. Anesthesia is obtained mainly over the medial thigh and metatarsal region. Usually performed in the horse.

Sapium sebiferum member of plant family Euphorbiaceae; contains an unidentified toxin which causes nephrosis and diarrhea. Called also Chinese tallow tree.

sapo [L.] *soap;* a compound of fatty acids with an alkali.

saponaceous soapy; of soaplike feel or quality.

Saponaria genus of the plant family Caryophyllaceae; contain toxic saponins which cause diarrhea. Includes *S. officinalis*, *S. vaccaria*. Called also cow cockle, soapwort, hedge pink, bouncing bet.

saponifiable capable of being made into soap.

saponification conversion of an oil or fat into a soap by combination with an alkali. In chemistry, the term now denotes the hydrolysis of an ester by an alkali, resulting in the production of a free alcohol and an alkali salt of the ester acid.

saponin a group of glycosides widely distributed in the plant world and characterized by (1) their property of forming durable foam when their watery solutions are shaken; this property may have importance in some plants in the development of frothy bloat in ruminants; (2) their ability to lyse erythrocytes even in high dilutions; and (3) their having the compound sapogenin as their aglycones.

lithogenic s's saponins in panicoid grasses (*Panicum*, *Brachiaria*) *Agave lecheguilla*, *Narthecium ossifragum*, *Tribulus terrestris* are probably responsible for causing crystal-associated cholangiohepatopathy and subsequent secondary photosensitization; this is suspected as the cause of photosensitization associated with other plants. Called also steroidal saponin.

steroidal s. see lithogenic saponins (above).

sapophore the group of atoms in the molecule of a compound that gives the substance its characteristic taste.

sapremia septicemia caused by a saprophytic organism.

sapr(o)- word element. [Gr.] *rotten, putrid, decay, decayed material*.

saprocyclozoonoses a disease with features of both the SAPROZOONOSES and CYCLOZOONOSES, e.g. tick paralysis.

Saprolegnia common cause of fungal dermatitis in fish and fungal infection of fish eggs. There are white/gray, cotton-type growths on the skin and in some internal organs.

saprolegniasis infection of fish with the fungus *Saprolegnia* spp. Causes typical 'cotton wool' mat type lesions on the skin. All ages including eggs are affected.

saprophagous feeding on dead or decaying organic matter.

saprophyte any organism, such as a bacterium, capable of living in inanimate media.

saprophytic pertaining to saprophyte.

saprozoic living on decayed organic matter; said of animals, especially protozoa.

saprozoonosis zoonosis which uses soil, water or decaying organic matter as a reservoir, e.g. coccidioidomycosis, tetanus.

saralasin a competitive angiotensin II antagonist.

sarc(o)- word element. [Gr.] *flesh*.

sarcoarthrosis a joint without bone to bone contact, e.g. between scapula and thorax in quadripeds. Called also fleshy joint, synsarcosis.

Sarcobatus vermiculatus North American member of the plant family Polygonaceae; contains soluble oxalates which can cause oxalate poisoning. Called also greasewood.

sarcoblast a primitive cell that develops into a muscle cell.

sarcocele any fleshy swelling or tumor of the testis.

sarcocyst any member of, or any cyst formed by, *Sarcocystis* spp.

Sarcocystis a genus of parasitic protozoa in the family Sarcocystidae. The definitive hosts are domestic and wild carnivores in which they appear as a form of COCCIDIOSIS. Birds and reptiles are also infected. It appears to be part of any prey–predator system, e.g. snake, rat, owl, mice, etc. The effects of their intermediate stages are manifested as the disease SARCOCYSTOSIS.

***S. bertrami* (syn. *S. equicanis*)** has a dog–horse cycle and produces cysts in muscles but without clinical disease.

S. bovifelis see *S. hirsuta* (below).

S. capracanis has a dog–goat cycle; not pathogenic.

S. cervi cysts found in deer.

S. cruzi has a dog (and other feral canids)–cattle cycle; causes fever, anorexia, anemia and weight loss in cattle but the microscopic cysts found in dogs are not pathogenic. See also SARCOCYSTOSIS.

S. cuniculi cysts found in wild and domesticated rabbits but without apparent pathogenicity in rabbits. It has a cat–rabbit cycle and the macroscopic cysts in cats are pathogenic.

S. equicanis see *S. bertrami* (above).

S. fayeri has a dog–horse cycle but appears not to be pathogenic to the horse.

S. fusiformis has a cat–buffalo cycle but appears not to be pathogenic in the water buffalo.

***S. gigantea* (syn. *S. ovifelis*)** has a cat–sheep cycle; the cysts in sheep are very large and visible with the naked eye but are not pathogenic.

S. hemionilatrantis has dog or coyote–mule deer cycle and the disease in young deer may be fatal.

***S. hirsuta* (syn. *S. bovifelis*)** has a cat–cattle cycle and is not pathogenic in cattle.

S. hominis has a human–cattle cycle, the enteric infection in humans causing diarrhea, and the cysts in the muscles of cattle having no observable effect.

S. kortei the definitive host is unknown, the intermediate host is the rhesus monkey but the cysts in its muscles appear to cause no disability.

S. levinei has a dog–buffalo cycle but causes no illness.

S. lindemanni humans are the intermediate host but the final host is unknown.

S. miescheriana has a dog–pig cycle but no pathogenicity.

S. muris has a cat–mouse, rat, vole, etc., cycle but the cysts are not pathogenic.

S. nesbitti rhesus monkeys are the intermediate hosts but the muscle cysts are clinically silent. The final host has not been identified.

S. neurona causes equine protozoal encephalomyelitis.

S. orientalis goats are the intermediate host but are unaffected. Dogs are probably the final host.

S. ovicanis see *S. tenella* (below).

S. ovifelis see *S. gigantea* (above).

S. porcifelis has a cat–pig cycle and is pathogenic for pigs, causing diarrhea, myositis and lameness.

S. porcihominis see *S. suihominis* (below).

S. rileyi cysts occur in the muscles of many species of domestic and wild birds without appearing to cause any ill-effects.

S. suihominis has a human–pig cycle without pathogenic effects.

***S. tenella* (syn. *S. ovicanis*)** has a dog–sheep cycle and causes mortality in lambs if the infection is a heavy one.

sarcocystosis a rare clinical disease in all food animal species caused by the intermediate stage of the protozoan parasite *Sarcocystis* spp. The terminal stages are passed in the dog or cat. Clinically the disease is manifested by emaciation, lameness, hypersalivation, loss of tail switch, anemia and abortion. The subclinical infection with the intermediate stage of cysts in muscles is very common in all species. The common sites are the esophageal, cardiac and lingual muscles. Abnormally there are localizations in brain, uterus and lungs. Called also rat-tail syndrome, Dalmeny disease. See also SARCOSPORIDIOSIS.

Sarcodina a subphylum of Protozoa, including all the amebae, both freeliving and parasitic, characterized by the ability to produce pseudopodia during most of the life cycle; flagella, when present, develop only during the early stages.

sarcoid 1. tuberculoid; characterized by noncaseating epithelioid cell tubercles. 2. pertaining to or resembling sarcoidosis. 3. sarcoidosis. See also EQUINE sarcoid.

sarcoidal pertaining to or of the nature of sarcoid.

s. granulomatous disease a sterile, sarcoidal granulomatous dermatitis in dogs characterized by multiple cutaneous plaques, nodules or papules, non-pruritic, not painful, mostly on the neck and trunk.

sarcoidosis a disease of horses characterized by scaly, crusting dermatitis with alopecia extending to a generalized exfoliative dermatitis, followed by wasting, anorexia and exercise intolerance.

sarcolemma the delicate plasma membrane covering every striated muscle fiber.

Sarcolobus globosus a plant of Asian origin in the family Asclepiadaceae. Its fruits are recorded as causing incoordination, tremor, paralysis and death in a cat.

sarcoma a tumor, often highly malignant, composed of cells derived from connective tissue such as bone and cartilage, muscle, blood vessel or lymphoid tissue. These tumors usually develop rapidly and metastasize through the lymph vessels.

The different types of sarcomas are named after the specific tissue they affect: fibrosarcoma—in fibrous connective tissue; lymphosarcoma—in lymphoid tissues; osteosarcoma—in bone; chondrosarcoma—in cartilage; rhabdosarcoma—in muscle; liposarcoma—in fat cells.

feline post-traumatic s. seen in cats, usually following injury from a penetrating injury to the eye. An orbit-destructive and sometimes metastasizing spindle-cell sarcoma develops months or years later.

giant cell s. a malignant form of giant cell tumor of bone.

infectious s. see canine transmissible VENEREAL tumor.

mast cell s. see MAST CELL tumor.

melanocytic s. melanoma.

osteogenic s. see OSTEOSARCOMA.

post-traumatic s. see feline post-traumatic sarcoma (above).

reticulum cell s. an old term for a form of malignant lymphoma, histiocytic lymphosarcoma, in which the dominant cell type is thought to be derived from histiocytic or macrophage origin. There is increasing evidence, however, that this neoplasm arises from transformed lymphocytes or immunoblasts.

Rous s. see ROUS SARCOMA.

spindle-cell s. see HEMANGIOPERICYTOMA.

Sticker's s. see canine transmissible VENEREAL tumor.

transmissible venereal s. see canine transmissible VENEREAL tumor.

s. virus see FELINE sarcoma virus.

sarcomatoid resembling a sarcoma.

sarcomatosis a condition characterized by development of many sarcomas.

sarcomatous pertaining to or of the nature of a sarcoma.

sarcomere the contractile unit of a myofibril; sarcomeres are repeating units, delimited by the Z bands along the length of the myofibril.

sarcomphalocele a fleshy tumor of the umbilicus.

Sarcophaga a genus of flesh flies in the family Sarcophagidae that deposit their larvae in wounds or sores.

S. carnaria, S. dux, S. fuscicauda, S. haemorrhoidalis the only clinical difference between these species appears to be their geographical distribution.

sarcophagid pertaining to *Sarcophaga* spp.

sarcoplasm the interfibrillary matter of striated muscle.

sarcoplasmic pertaining to or emanating from sarcoplasm.

s. organelles include a number of organelles associated with sarcoplasm.

sarcoplast an interstitial cell of a muscle, itself capable of being transformed into a muscle.

sarcopoietic forming muscle.

Sarcopterinus a genus of mites in the family Myobiidae.

S. nidulans found in the feather follicles of pigeons and other birds.

S. pilirostris found in the skin on the head of the sparrow.

Sarcoptes a widely distributed genus of mites in the family Sarcoptidae which causes SARCOPTIC MANGE. Their nomenclature is confused but the most widely used system of nomenclature is *Sarcoptes scabiei* var. *canis*, var. *suis*, var. *equi*, var. *ovis*, var. *bovis*, etc.

S. tapiri potentially pathogenic for tapirs.

sarcoptic mange an intensely pruritic dermatitis caused by the acarid mite *Sarcoptes scabiei*. Although there is some species specificity with subspecies of the mite this is not complete. Lesions commence as erythema and small red papules. Extensive self-trauma leads to loss of hair and secondary infection. In long-standing cases, debilitation is also common. The lesions are usually widespread but are most easily seen on the abdominal skin and inside the thighs. In dogs, the elbows, hocks and pinnae are most commonly affected. Besides the common infections in domestic species the disease occurs frequently in captive and freeliving primates, monkeys, rodents, canids and ungulates. Called also red mange, fox mange. See also SCABIES.

sarcosis abnormal increase of flesh.

Sarcosporidia see SARCOCYSTIS.

sarcosporidiasis see SARCOCYSTOSIS.

sarcosporidiosis the condition observed at meat inspection in which lesions caused by *Sarcocystis* spp. are observed. See also SARCOCYSTOSIS.

Sarcostemma a South African and Australian genus of the plant family Asclepiadaceae; suspected to contain cynachoside, which causes incoordination, tremor, recumbency and convulsions in sheep. Includes *S. australe*, *S. brevipedicellatum*, *S. viminale*. Called also, caustic vine, caustic creeper or caustic bush.

sarcostosis ossification of fleshy tissue.

sarcotubules the membrane-limited structures of the sarcoplasm, forming a canalicular network around each myofibril.

sarcous pertaining to flesh or muscle tissue.

Sarot needle holder long-handled, standard type needle holder with diamond-shaped grooving on blade faces.

Sarothamnos see HALOGETON GLOMERATUS.

Sartwellia flaveriae North American plant in the Asteraceae family; contains an unidentified toxin which causes nephrosis, liver damage, ascites, hydrothorax.

Saskatoon serviceberry see AMELANCHIER ALNIFOLIA.

sassafras an extract from the roots of *Sassafras albidum* or certain species of *Ocotea*. the oil is used topically as a rubifacient and may be toxic if ingested.

sassy bark bark of the African tree *Erythrophleum guineense* which contains cassaine; used as an arrow poison.

SAT serum agglutination test.

sat. saturated.

satellite 1. in genetics, a knob of chromatin connected by a stalk to the short arm of certain chromosomes. 2. a minor, or attendant, lesion situated near a large one. 3. a vein that closely accompanies an artery. 4. exhibiting satellitism.

s. cell cells present in nervous and muscle tissue, whose numbers diminish with age, which are involved in repair when damage occurs. They are capable of migration, reorientation, can proliferate, form myoblasts and myotubes, and form long cytoplasmic tails that act as tethers when they migrate.

s. DNA see DEOXYRIBONUCLEIC ACID.

satellitism the phenomenon in which certain bacterial species grow much better in the immediate vicinity of colonies of other unrelated species, owing to the production of an essential metabolite by the latter species.

satellitosis accumulation of neuroglial cells about neurons; seen whenever neurons are damaged.

satiation full satisfaction of desire to eat and drink.

satiety being in a state of satiation; in experimental animals used with reference to eating and drinking.

s. center located in the ventromedial hypothalamic nucleus. Lesions may cause hyperphagia with obesity or anorexia with cachexia. See also ADIPOSOGENITAL DYSTROPHY.

Satin rabbit small fur rabbit with a satin-like texture and sheen to the coat. The numerous varieties differ only in color.

Satinsky vena cava clamp scissor-action, ratchet handles, long, thin double-curved blades. Tangential occlusion clamp.

satratoxins the toxins produced by STACHYBOTRYS ALTRA. Classified as C, D, F, G, H depending on their chromatographic mobility.

saturated 1. denoting an organic compound that has only single bonds between carbon atoms and is therefore less reactive than one with double bonds, e.g. saturated fatty acids. 2. holding all of a solute that can be held in solution by the solvent (saturated solution).

s. fatty acids see FATTY acids.

saturation the state of being saturated, or the act of saturating.

s. kinetics point of high initial concentration of substrate after which the rate of reaction is independent of further increases in initial substrate concentration, and the enzyme is saturated with substrate.

saturnine pertaining to lead, the poisonous metal.

saturnism lead poisoning; plumbism.

saucerization 1. the excavation of tissue to form a shallow shelving depression, usually performed to facilitate drainage from infected areas of bone. 2. the shallow saucer-like depression on the anterior surface of a vertebra which has suffered a compression fracture.

Sauerbruch retractor simple handheld retractor with a broad blade turned down at right angles at the end. Used for short-term exposure of abdominal cavity.

sausage boot a stuffed leather roll worn above the coronet by a horse. Used to prevent pressure by the shoe on the elbow when the horse is lying down, which may cause a shoe boil.

sausage casing the tube used to stuff with sausage meat; some are synthetic. Small intestine is used as edible casing.

savaging severe trauma by biting. Said of horses savaging people, sows and bitches savaging litters.

savannah tsetses GLOSSINA *longipalpis*, *G. morsitans*.

savin a neurotoxic war gas similar to organophosphorus insecticides but considerably more toxic, as demonstrated in the Tokyo subway massacre in 1995.

Savlon a proprietary name for preparations of chlorhexidine gluconate.

saw multi-toothed cutting instrument.

chain s. see PEARSON SAW.

Stryker s. see STRYKER SAW.

surgical s. modeled on carpentry tools but made of sterilizable materials; used for cutting cartilage and bone.

wire s. see WIRE saw, GIGLI WIRE SAW.

sawdust used as litter for chickens and bedding for horses. Sawdust made from treated timber may cause pentachlorophenol and other wood preservative poisoning. Fungi growing in sawdust litter in poultry houses may cause poisoning in the birds. See also ENTANDROPHRAGMA CYLINDRICUM, JUGLANS NIGRA.

sawdust liver an abattoir term used to identify livers in which the external surface has the appearance of having been dusted with sawdust; multiple foci of nonsuppurative necrosis with leukocytic infiltration. The cause is not known.

sawfly member of the insect family Pergidae. Includes *Arge pullata* (Denmark), *Lophyrotoma interrupta* (Australia), *Perreyea lepida* (South America). The larvae of these leaf-eating insects collect in piles under the trees they parasitize; cattle eat them avidly and develop acute hepatitis due to the ingestion of LOPHYROTOMIN in the larvae.

sawhorse stance see sawhorse POSTURE.

saxitoxin neurotoxic tetrahydropurine of the PARALYTIC shellfish poisoning (PSP) toxin group from poisonous mussels, clams and plankton; a sodium channel blocker with the same mode of action as TETRODOTOXIN; originates in some toxic DINOFLAGELLATES and in some ANABAENA spp.

Saxon, Saxony popular strain of Australian merino fine or superfine woolled sheep.

Sayre elevator double-ended, handheld instrument with one rongeur type end and one curved blade; designed for lifting periosteum off bone during surgery.

Sb chemical symbol, *antimony* (L. *stibium*).

SBE sporadic bovine ENCEPHALOMYELITIS.

Sc chemical symbol, *scandium*.

sc subcutaneously.

s.c. in medical records, an abbreviation for subcutaneous.

scab 1. a crust composed of coagulated serum, blood, pus and skin debris covering a skin lesion. 2. used colloquially to mean PSOROPTIC MANGE.

s. mites see CHORIOPTES, PSOROPTES, SARCOPTES.

scabbard trachea congenital lateral compression of the trachea; seen in horses.

scabby cat disease see feline miliary DERMATITIS.

scabby mouth see contagious ECTHYMA.

scabicide 1. lethal to *Sarcoptes scabiei*. 2. an agent lethal to *Sarcoptes scabiei*.

scabies infestation by mites of the genus *Sarcoptes*. See also SARCOPTIC MANGE.

feline s. see NOTOEDRES *cati*.

s. incognito a variant of sarcoptic mange in dogs in which mites are difficult or impossible to recover in skin scrapings, presumably because of the extensive grooming and generally high level of skin hygiene that lacks only the use of a scabicide. Also there are usually only a few mites present once an immunity develops. Further infection may cause a hypersensitivity but the mites present will still be in small numbers.

Norwegian s. a variety characterized by immense numbers of mites and marked scaling of the skin. Seen in immunocompromised patients.

scabietic pertaining to scabies.

Scabiosa succisa European plant in the family Dipsaceae. Contains an unidentified toxin which has caused severe irritation of the oral mucosa in cattle. Called also *Succisa pratensis*, devil's bit.

scad transitory lameness in sheep, reputed to follow frosty conditions and to be a dermatitis caused by cold injury.

scala pl. *scalae* [L.] a ladder-like structure, applied especially to various passages of the cochlea.

s. media the cochlear duct: a space in the ear between Reissner's membrane and the basilar membrane.

s. tympani the part of the cochlea below the spiral lamina.

s. vestibuli the part of the cochlea above the spiral lamina.

scalar in electrocardiography, a single magnitude value of a recorded electrical potential, expressed in millivolts.

scald 1. a burn caused by a hot liquid or a hot, moist vapor; to burn in such fashion. 2. see BENIGN footrot. 3. alopecia, pityriasis and hair loss over the rump of the horse without dermatitis; occurs in warm wet weather when the skin is wet continuously for long periods.

sheep s. see INTERDIGITAL dermatitis.

scalded skin syndrome a disease of human skin mirrored closely by a lesion in Greyhounds from which pure cultures of *Staphylococcus aureus* can be isolated. The lesions commence as large, thin-walled bullae along the dorsum of the neck and trunk which cause erection of a patch of hair. Rupture of the bullae leads to loss of hair and scab formation. See also SORE.

scalding plunging of pig or poultry carcasses into very hot water to facilitate scraping and dehairing and plucking. Chicken scalding water is 130°F for broilers (larger birds higher) applied for 1 to 2 minutes. Modern pig abattoirs use steam at 144 to 147°F for about 3 minutes. This avoids overheating the carcasses.

scale 1. a thin flake or compacted platelike body, as of cornified epithelial cells. 2. a scheme or device by which some property may be measured (as hardness, weight, linear dimension). See also CELSIUS SCALE, CENTIGRADE, FARENHEIT SCALE, KELVIN SCALE. 3. to remove incrustations or other material from a surface, as from the enamel of teeth.

absolute s. a temperature scale with zero at the absolute zero of temperature.

contrast s. the range of densities or contrasts on a radiograph.

French s. see FRENCH GAUGE.

s. rot a disease of snakes with no specific cause, characterized by ulceration of the skin at multiple sites. Death is the usual sequel.

scalene muscle see Table 13.1I.

scalenectomy resection of a scalene muscle. See Table 13.1I.

scaler a manual or mechanical instrument used to remove deposits from the surface of teeth. See also TARTAR scraper.

rotosonic s. an air-driven scaler with a rotating bur.

subsonic s. one with a tip that vibrates less than 20,000 cycles per minute.

ultrasonic s. the scaling tip, which vibrates at high frequency, is cooled by water. There are several types, including magnetostrictive and piezoelectric, which differ in the mechanisms producing the vibrations. Cleaning occurs by cavitation. See also ULTRASONIC cleaning.

scales dry, flaky exfoliations of the skin without any discontinuity of its surface.

scaling 1. removal of tartar from teeth. See also ULTRASONIC tooth scaling, TARTAR scraper. 2. in statistical terms the changing of the scale on which a variable is measured, usually to match the scaling of another lot of data and simplify comparison.

scallop see PECTEN YESSOENSIS.

scalpel small surgical knife. The traditional fixed blade model usually has a convex edge. Modern instruments have detachable blades in a great variety of shapes. There are other more sophisticated cutting instruments such as the argon plasma scalpel, the carbon dioxide laser scalpel, the electrosurgical scalpel and the high-energy scalpel.

scaly skin condition characterized by scales; scalelike.

s. face, s. leg see CNEMIDOCOPTES *pilae*.

s. leg mite see CNEMIDOCOPTES.

scan an image produced using a moving detector or a sweeping beam of radiation, as in scintiscanning, B-mode ultrasonography or computed tomography.

s. generator the basic mechanism in a scanning electron microscope, moving the beam across the specimen.

static s. in ultrasonography, a static image built up by movement of the transducer sequentially over the body. Now largely replaced by real-time ULTRASONOGRAPHY.

scandium a chemical element, atomic number 21, atomic weight 44.956, symbol Sc. See Table 6.

scanning close visual, electronic or radiographical examination of a small area or of different isolated areas of the body.

radioisotope s. production of a two-dimensional record of the gamma rays emitted by a radioactive isotope concentrated in a specific organ or tissue of the body, such as brain, kidney or thyroid gland.

total body s. utilization of computed TOMOGRAPHY (CT) to examine a cross-section of the entire body. The CT scanner produces an image of tissue density in a complete cross-section of the part of the body being scanned.

For the most part total body scanning does not require the injection of a radiopaque substance, nor is there a need for use of a radioactive material to produce a record of the findings. However, contrast is used in some areas, particularly the skull, as it enhances the image.

The total body scanner is particularly useful in visualizing organs in the retroperitoneal space, for example, the pancreas, liver, spleen and ovaries, the abdominal section of the aorta, and in viewing the spine and skull.

scanography a method of making radiographs by the use of a narrow slit beneath the tube, so that, as the x-ray tube moves over the target, all the rays of the central beam pass through the part being radiographed at the same angle.

scansorial of or pertaining to climbing.

scant feces small, hard feces are passed infrequently; occur in dehydration, reduced feed intake, alimentary tract stasis.

scanty rice-flower PIMELEA *pauciflora*.

scapha pl. *scaphae* [L.] the hollow inside the peripheral part of the ear flap that leads into the tubular concha.

scaphoid 1. shaped like a boat. 2. radial carpal bone. See Table 10.

scaphoiditis inflammation of the scaphoid bone.

scapula pl. *scapulae* [L.] the flat triangular bone at the top of the shoulder; the shoulder blade. See also Table 10.

winged s. see ANGEL WINGS.

scapular pertaining to the scapula.

scapulectomy excision or resection of the scapula.

scapulohumeral pertaining to the scapula and humerus.

s. joint shoulder joint.

scapulopexy surgical fixation of the scapula.

scapulothoracic pertaining to the scapula and thorax.

scar cicatrix; a mark remaining after the healing of a wound, such as one caused by injury, illness or surgery.

constricting s. contraction of scar tissue causing constriction of vascular channel or hollow viscus.

honorable s. in judging dogs, scars resulting from injuries suffered as a result of work are permissible and do not detract from the dog's features.

hypertrophic s. an overabundance of connective tissue in a wound, identified by history of traumatized wound, infection and histological examination reveals hairs, foreign body, pockets of infection.

s. tissue a dense mass of granulation tissue.

scarification production in the skin of many small superficial scratches or punctures, as for introduction of vaccine. Erroneously used to mean scarring.
scarificator scarifier.
scarifier an instrument with many sharp points, used in scarification.
scarlet oak QUERCUS *coccinea*.
scarlet pimpernel ANAGALLIS *arvensis*.
scarlet red an azo dye used for demonstrating sex chromatin, basic protein and connective tissue in histology, and as a stimulant to healing in wounds. Called also Biebrich scarlet.
scarlet runner PHASEOLUS *vulgaris*.
Scarpa's membrane see TYMPANIC membrane (secondary).
Scatchard equation describes the irreversible binding of a univalent ligand by antibody.
scatemia alimentary toxemia in which the chemical poisons are absorbed through the intestine.
scatology study and analysis of feces, as for diagnostic purposes.
scatoscopy examination of the feces.
scatter 1. the diffusion or deviation of x-rays produced by a medium through which the rays pass. 2. the distribution of two variables in relation to each other, e.g. the numbers of a population in terms of time, place or any other variable.
back s. backward diffusion of x-rays.
s. diagram a graphic representation of a scatter of two variables.
s. radiation the scattering of radiation in all directions as a result of interaction between the beam of the x-ray and the patient. See also COMPTON EFFECT.
scattergram a graph in which the values found in a statistical study are represented by disconnected, individual symbols.
scattering a change in the direction of motion of a photon or subatomic particle as the result of a collision or interaction.
scavenger cell see GITTER CELLS.
scavenging of anesthetic. See ANESTHETIC scavenging.
SCCS self-contained-cleaning-system in an abattoir.
Scedosporium apiospermum the imperfect state of *Pseudallescheria boydii*; a fungus associated with bovine and equine abortion, bovine mastitis and nasal infections in horses.
Sceletium African plant genus in the family Aizoaceae; contain soluble oxalates which cause nephrosis, uremia and urolithiasis.
scenario building predicting the future by assuming a series of alternative possibilities, as opposed to predicting the future solely on the basis of extrapolated mathematical data.
scent a distinctive, agreeable odor. Animals secrete them from sweat and sebaceous glands and special scent glands. See also PHEROMONE.
s. gland impaction the secretion in the gland becomes inspissated and forms an irritating foreign body.
scented thorn ACACIA *nilotica* subsp. *kraussiana*.
Schalm classification a morphological classification system for anemias based on the erythrocyte indexes of MCV and MCHC.
schechita see SHECHITA.
scheduled diseases diseases listed in the schedules of the regulations of the local Stock Diseases Act or similar Act. The diseases are listed as contagious and the Act specifies that they are to be reported to the appropriate government authority with appropriate penalties for default. The schedules are included in the regulations rather than in the main body of the Act so that they can be changed without opening the Act to the Parliament.
Schefflera actinophylla Australian tree in Araliaceae family; leaves contain calcium oxalate raphide crystals causing stomatitis, salivation, vomiting, diarrhea in dogs which ingest them. Called also umbrella tree.
schema a plan, outline or arrangement.
Schiff–Sherrington syndrome extensor hypertonia of the thoracic limbs and paraplegia resulting from acute, severe, compressive lesions of the thoracolumbar spinal cord that remove the inhibitory effects of neurons in the lumbar spinal cord. Seen in dogs, usually caused by trauma or herniated intervertebral disk.
Schilling count a differential leukocyte count in which the neutrophils are divided into blasts, progranulocytes, myelocytes, metamyelocytes, bands, and mature segmented cells. Called also nuclear index. The terms 'left shift', and 'right shift' are based on this classification of neutrophils by age.
Schilling test see VITAMIN B_{12} absorption test.
Schimmelbusch mask a wire frame over which a cloth is spread and an inhalant anesthetic added.
schindylesis an articulation in which a thin plate of one bone is received into a cleft in another, as in the articulation of the perpendicular plate of the ethmoid bone with the vomer.
Schiotz tonometer see indentation TONOMETER.
Schipperke a small, lively dog with cobby build and thick, medium-length coat, usually black but may be another whole color, that forms a ruff around the neck and 'coulottes' on the back of the thighs. The head has a foxy appearance with pointed, erect ears. The tail is docked to a short length. Called also Belgian barge dog.
Schirmer tear test a measure of lacrimal secretory capacity and used in the diagnosis of keratoconjunctivitis sicca. A standardized strip of filter paper is inserted into the conjunctival sac, projecting over the lower eyelid. The length of paper wet after a specified period of time is measured and compared with normals for the species being tested.
schist(o)- word element. [Gr.] *cleft, split*.
schistocelia, schistocoelia congenital fissure of the abdomen.
Schistocephalus a genus of tapeworms in the family Diphyllobothriidae.
S. solidus adults found in the intestine of birds and can cause mortality in ducks. Intermediate stages in cyprinid fishes cause marked swelling of the abdomen.
schistocephalus a fetus with a cleft head.
schistocormus a fetus with a cleft trunk.
schistocyte a fragment of an erythrocyte, commonly observed in the blood in hemolytic anemia.
schistocytosis an accumulation of schistocytes in the blood.
schistoglossia cleft (bifid) tongue. See also BIRD tongue.
schistomelus a fetus with a cleft limb.
schistometer an instrument for measuring the aperture between the vocal cords.
schistoprosopus a fetus with a cleft face.
Schistosoma a genus of elongated dioecious trematodes which inhabit blood vessels of the host. The eggs are found in the wall of the bladder, uterus and urethra. Includes *S. bovis* (ruminants), *S. curassoni* (ruminants), *S. haematobium* (humans), *S. incognitum* (pigs, dogs), *S. indicum* (ruminants, horses), *S. inter-*

calatum (humans, ruminants, horses), *S. japonicum* (humans, many other species), *S. magrebowiei* (ruminants, zebra), *S. lieperi* (wild artiodactyls), *S. mansoni* (humans, wild animals), *S. mattheei* (most species), *S. mekongi* (humans, dogs), *S. nasalis* (ruminants, horses), *S. rodhaini* (dogs, rodents), *S. spindale* (ruminants, dogs), *S. suis* (see *S. incognitum*, above).

schistosoma reflexus a common fetal monster and cause of dystocia requiring a cesarean delivery. Characterized by acute angulation of the spine so that the tail lies close to the head, the thoracic and abdominal cavities have no ventral wall and the viscera are uncontained.

Schistosomatium a genus of flukes in the family Schistosomatidae. Found in rodents.

S. douthitti occurs in mesenteric veins and may cause dermatitis.

schistosome a member of the family Schistosomatidae. Includes the genera *Austrobilharzia*, *Bilharziella*, *Bivitellobilharzia*, *Dendritobilharzia*, *Gigantobilharzia*, *Heterobilharzia*, *Ornithobilharzia*, *Pseudobilharziella*, *Schistosoma*, *Schistosomatium*, *Trichobilharzia*.

s. dermatitis a disease of humans caused by invasion of the skin by the cercariae of nonhuman schistosomes, especially avian ones. Called also clam-digger's itch, swimmer's itch, rice-paddy itch, swamp itch.

schistosomiasis the disease caused by the trematode *Schistosoma* spp. The commonest syndrome is one of hemorrhagic enteritis, anemia and emaciation with many affected animals dying after an illness of several months. Necropsy lesions include distended mesenteric vessels filled with flukes, hemorrhagic enteritis with granuloma formation in some cases. Granulomatous lesions occur in the liver in an hepatic form of the disease. Nasal schistosomiasis, caused by *Schistosoma nasalis,* is characterized by nasal discharge, snoring and dyspnea. *S. haematobium* causes hematuria. Human infestation with cercariae causes swimmer's itch, swamp itch.

schistosomicide an agent that destroys schistosomes.

schistosomus a fetus with a cleft abdomen.

s. reflexus the lateral edges of the somatic disk in the developing embryo curve upwards instead of downwards. The viscera float free in the amnion, the head and tail are curved up towards each other. The fetus creates a dystocia with the free-floating viscera, or the four limbs and the head all together, presenting in the cervical canal.

schistothorax congenital fissure of the chest or sternum.

schizaxon an axon that divides into two nearly equal branches.

schiz(o)- word element. [Gr.] *divided, division.*

schizocyte schistocyte.

schizodemes parasites with mitochondrial DNA of similar characteristics.

schizogenesis reproduction by fission.

schizogony an asexual reproductive stage of an apicomplexan parasite by multiple fission within the body of the host, giving rise to merozoites.

schizogyria a condition in which the cerebral convolutions have wedge-shaped cracks.

schizomycete an organism of the class Schizomycetes.

Schizomycetes a taxonomic class comprising the bacteria; they are typically unicellular organisms, considered plants which commonly multiply by cell division, and which may be freeliving, saprophytic, parasitic, or even pathogenic, the last causing disease in plants or animals.

schizont the asexual reproductive stage in the development of the *Eimeria* spp. and in many other coccidians, e.g. *Toxoplasma* spp. in the cat, *Cystoisospora*, *Hammondia*, *Frenkelia* and *Isospora* spp., following the trophozoite whose nucleus divides into many smaller nuclei.

schizonychia splitting of the nails or claws.

schizotrichia splitting of the hairs at the ends.

Schizotrypanum see TRYPANOSOMA.

Schlatter–Osgood disease see OSGOOD–SCHLATTER DISEASE.

Schlemm's canal a circular canal at the junction of the sclera and cornea that receives aqueous humor draining from the anterior chamber. Called also scleral venous sinus.

Schlesinger's test a test for the presence of urobilinogen in urine, determined by a color change after the addition of zinc sulfate.

Schmauch bodies see Heinz BODY.

Schmidt's syndrome see POLYGLANDULAR syndrome.

Schmidt's test a test for the detection of bilirubin in feces based on the development of a pink color in a fecal sample after the addition of mercuric chloride.

Schmidt–Waldmann vaccine the widely used foot-and-mouth disease vaccine composed of inactivated virus and adjuvant.

Schmieden's suture a technique for closing incisions of the intestinal wall, it is a continuous inverting suture through all three layers of the wall and which is then buried by a second layer of sutures.

Schmorl's disease herniation of the nucleus pulposus of the intervertebral disk.

Schmorl's node an irregular or hemispherical bone defect in the upper or lower margin of the body of a vertebra into which the nucleus pulposus of the intervertebral disk herniates.

Schnauzer a dog with hard, wiry, black or salt-and-pepper colored coat that is short on the body but longer on the legs and face, where it forms the characteristic eyebrows, moustache and chin whiskers. The small, v-shaped ears are set high and fold over except in countries where ear-cropping is practiced. The tail is docked to a short length. There are three varieties of Schnauzers, each regarded as a separate breed, similar in appearance but varying in size. The *miniature* (12–14 inches tall) is classed as a terrier while the *standard* (17–20 inches tall) and *giant* (23–27 inches tall) are classed as working dogs in the United States. The miniature Schnauzer is predisposed to congenital cataracts, progressive retinal atrophy and Schnauzer COMEDO syndrome.

schochet see SHOCHET.

Schoengastia see HARVEST mites.

Schoenocaulon officinalis a member of the Liliaceae family; the plant source of veratrine for pharmaceutical use.

Schoenus genus of the plant family Cyperaceae; two Australian species contain the toxin galegine; causes fatal pulmonary edema and hydrothorax in sheep when eaten in quantity. Includes *S. asperocarpus*, *S. rigens*. Called also poison sedge.

Scholtz bush see PTERONIA PALLENS.

schomer see SHOMER.

school to train a horse in dressage or Greyhounds to perform on the racetrack. See also RIDING SCHOOL.

schooling see SCHOOL.

Schoupe speculum used in equine dentistry to keep the mouth open. Consists of a long metal rod with a cross handle. The other end returns on itself and has at its end a coiled springlike structure which is placed between the molars on the side opposite to where work is to be done.

schrock SORGHUM *vulgare*.

Schroeder–Thomas splint see Schroeder–Thomas SPLINT.

Schroeder vulsellum forceps long, scissor type forceps with ratchet handles and long, thin, sideways curved blades that have inward facing, double-pointed claws. Designed for grasping the uterus.

Schubert forceps designed for collecting a biopsy of uterine wall. Scissor type instrument with blades designed to pick up and punch out a piece of mucosa when the handles are closed.

Schultz–Dale reaction, test an experimental in vitro test for hypersensitivity in which a strip of smooth muscle is removed from a sensitized animal and exposed to specific antigen, resulting in contraction.

Schwalbe's ring a circular ridge composed of collagenous fibers surrounding the outer margin of Descemet's membrane.

Schwann cells see Schwann CELL.

schwannoma a neoplasm originating from Schwann cells (of the myelin sheath). Most occur in the skin, but they are also found in nerve trunks and roots. The Schwann cell is also a component of neurofibromas. Called also neurilemmoma.

cardiac s. single or multiple round or nodular masses on the epicardial surface or within the myocardium.

granular cell s. see GRANULAR cell tumor.

Schweinepest [Ger.] *hog cholera*.

Schweinsberger disease pyrrolizidine alkalosis caused by the ingestion of *Senecio* spp.

schwitzkrankheit *Hyalomma* toxicosis. See SWEATING sickness.

sciage [Fr.] a sawing movement in massage.

sciascopy see RETINOSCOPY.

sciatic pertaining to the ischium.

s. nerve a large nerve extending from the lumbosacral plexus down the thigh, with branches throughout the lower leg and foot. It is the widest nerve of the body and one of the longest. See also Table 14.

s. nerve degeneration occurs during parturition in cows due to passage of a large fetus through the pelvic canal causing pressure and subsequent degeneration of one or both sciatic nerves leading to posterior paresis or paralysis.

s. nerve paralysis injury to the sciatic nerve, commonly during difficult parturition in heifers, causes weakness or paralysis of one hindleg and the animal is recumbent. See also MATERNAL obstetric paralysis.

SCID severe combined immunodeficiency disease. See COMBINED IMMUNE DEFICIENCY SYNDROME DISEASE.

scientific method the process of extending knowledge by forming a hypothesis based on observations and epidemiological patterns, which is then tested on a subset of the total population, then generalizing the results to the appropriate population through the process of inductive logic. Before implementation of the hypotheses they should be tested by studies planned on the basis that the hyopothesis will be proved or denied.

scientific parsimony see OCCAM'S RAZOR.

Scilla African plant genus in the family Liliaceae; includes *S. maritima* (*Urginea maritima*, source of commercial red, white squills), *S. natalensis*, *S. non-scripta* (bluebell), *S. rigidifolia*; contains bufadienolide cardiac glycoside.

scillerin A cardiac glycoside found in *Urginea* (syn. *Scilla*) *maritima*.

scilliroside cardiac glucoside in *Urginea maritima*.

scintigram an image produced by scintigraphy.

scintigraphy the production of two-dimensional images of the distribution of radioactivity in tissues after the internal administration of a radiopharmaceutical imaging agent, the images being obtained by a scintillation camera.

scintillation 1. the emission of sparks. 2. a particle emitted in disintegration of a radioactive element.

s. camera a stationary device that records a photographic image of the distribution of radioactivity of an organ after the administration of a radionuclide. A sequence of photographs records the uptake and the distribution of the radionuclide.

s. counter see scintillation COUNTER.

scintiphotography scintigraphy.

scintiscan a two-dimensional representation (map) of the gamma rays emitted by a radioisotope, revealing its concentration in a specific organ or tissue.

scintiscanner the system of equipment used to make a scintiscan.

scirrho- word element. [Gr.] *hard*.

scirrhoid resembling scirrhous carcinoma.

scirrhous hard or indurated.

s. carcinoma carcinoma with a hard structure owing to the formation of dense connective tissue in the stroma.

s. cord see scirrhous CORD.

scirrhus scirrhous carcinoma.

scissor pertaining to scissors; like scissors in effect.

s. bite see scissor BITE.

s. mouth a narrow space between the rami of the mandible so that the molar arcades do not meet.

scissors cutting instruments consisting of two blades pivoted centrally. The blades are closed and material cut by closing the handles. In cutting tissue the preferred technique is to hold the blades in a firmly half-closed position and to push the instrument along the grain of the tissues.

bandage s. designed for cutting tight bandages on patients without cutting the patient. Have one blade with a knob at the point for slipping under the bandage. Varieties are Knowles and Lister.

blunt-sharp s. see standard surgical scissors (below).

corneal s. small, with angled blades. See CASTROVIEJO OPHTHALMIC INSTRUMENTS, MCGUIRE SCISSORS.

dissection s. used for separating tissues. See MAYO SCISSORS, METZENBAUM SCISSORS.

iris s. small, 3-4 inches long with sharp points, for ophthalmic surgery.

plaster s. robust for the cutting of plaster casts. See PLASTER shears, SEUTIN SHEARS.

standard surgical s. have one narrow sharp-pointed and one wide, blunt-pointed blade. Called also blunt-sharp scissors.

stitch s., suture s. for stitch removal; have a hook-shaped point on one blade to hook under the stitch before cutting it with the opposing blade.

tenotomy s. small, 4 inches long, very narrow blades, with large finger rings, for ophthalmic surgery. Called also Stevens scissors.

thoracic s. very long, up to 14 inches, scissors for reaching deeply located tissues. See NELSON SCISSORS.

toenail s. for trimming claws and beaks. May be guillotine style, see RESCO NAIL TRIMMER, or with curved blades, see WHITE SCISSORS.

uterine s. 9 inches long with long handles and short jaws. See MAYO SCISSORS.

wire suture s. short, strong construction with very short, sharp-pointed, angled blades.
scissura pl. *scissurae* [L.] an incisure; a splitting.
Sciurus see SQUIRREL.
sclera pl. *sclerae* [L.] the tough, usually white, outer coat of the eyeball, covering all the posterior surface and continuous anteriorly with the cornea. The stroma is banded by loose connective tissue, the lamina fusca internally and episclera externally.
s. inflammation see SCLERITIS.
scleradenitis inflammation and hardening of a gland.
scleral pertaining to sclera.
s. annulus a thickened roll of sclera at the junction with the cornea.
s. ectasia see SCLERECTASIA.
s. fixation sutures the placement of suture material around an extraocular muscle or partially through the sclera for purposes of immobilizing and controlling the position of the globe during ocular surgery.
sclerectasia, scleral ectasia a bulging state of the sclera; see also COLLIE eye anomaly.
sclerectoiridectomy excision of part of the sclera and of the iris.
sclerectoiridodialysis sclerectomy and iridodialysis.
sclerectomy 1. excision of part of the sclera. 2. removal of sclerosed parts of the middle ear after otitis media.
sclerema induration of the subcutaneous fat.
scleriritomy incision of the sclera and iris in anterior staphyloma.
scleritis inflammation of the sclera. It may be superficial (episcleritis) or deep.
anterior s. inflammation of the sclera adjoining the limbus of the cornea.
posterior s. scleritis involving the retina and choroid.
scler(o)- word element. [Gr.] *hard, sclera.*
scleroblastema the embryonic tissue from which bone is formed.
Scleroblitum atriplicinum toxic plant in the family Chenopodiaceae; causes oxalate poisoning manifested by nephrosis, uremia, urolithiasis. Called also *Chenopodium atriplicinum*, lamb's tongue.
sclerochoroiditis inflammation of the sclera and choroid.
sclerocornea the sclera and cornea regarded as one.
Scleroderma genus of toxic macrofungi; toadstools containing an unidentified toxin causing vomiting, tenesmus. Includes *S. aurantium*, *S. citrinum*, *S. flavidum*.
scleroderma chronic hardening and shrinking of the connective tissues of any organ of the body, including the skin, heart, esophagus, kidney and lung. The skin may be thickened, hard and rigid, and pigmented patches may occur.
canine localized s. sclerotic linear plaques on the trunk and limbs of dogs. Called also morphea.
sclerogenous producing sclerosis or a hard tissue or material.
scleroiritis inflammation of the sclera and iris.
sclerokeratectomy excision of a portion of cornea and sclera.
sclerokeratitis inflammation of the sclera and cornea.
Sclerolaena Australian genus of plants in family Chenopodiaceae; contain soluble oxalates which cause nephrosis, uremia, urolithiasis. Include *S. anisacanthoides* (yellow burr), *S. calcarata* (red or copper burr), *S. muricata* (prickly rolypoly).
scleroma a hardened patch or induration of skin or mucous membrane.
scleromalacia degeneration (softening) of the sclera.
scleronyxis surgical puncture of the sclera.
sclero-oophoritis sclerosing inflammation of the ovary.
sclerophthalmia encroachment of the sclera upon the cornea so that only a portion of the central part remains clear.
scleroplasty plastic repair of the sclera.
scleroprotein a simple protein characterized by its insolubility and its fibrous structure; it usually serves a supportive or protective function in the body.
sclerosant see SCLEROSING AGENTS.
sclerose to become, or cause to become, hardened.
sclerosing agents used to create scar tissue and obliterate a lumen or fix a moving part. Called also internal blister, e.g. ethanolamine oleate, sodium iodide.
sclerosis an induration or hardening, especially hardening of a part from inflammation and in disease of the interstitial substance. The term is used chiefly for such a hardening of the intestine in the dog, hardening of the nervous system due to hyperplasia of the connective tissue or for hardening of the blood vessels.
arteriolar s. arteriolosclerosis.
nuclear s. increased density of the lens causing a gray-blue haze; seen as a normal feature of aging in dogs. This is often mistaken as cataract formation, but seldom is a cause of blindness.
scleroskeleton the part of the bony skeleton formed by ossification in ligaments, fasciae and tendons.
sclerostenosis induration or hardening combined with contraction.
sclerostomy surgical creation of an opening through the sclera for the relief of glaucoma.
sclerotherapy the injection of sclerosing agents.
sclerothrix abnormal hardness and dryness of the haircoat.
sclerotica [L.] *sclera.*
Sclerotinia sclerotiorum fungal pathogen of commercial celery which is toxic when infested with the fungus.
sclerotitis scleritis.
sclerotium pl. *sclerotia*; a hard blackish mass of mycelia formed during the resting phase by certain fungi, as *Claviceps purpurea*.
sclerotome 1. an instrument used in incision of the sclera. 2. the area of a bone innervated from a single spinal segment. 3. one of the paired segmented masses of mesenchymal tissue, separated from the ventromedial part of a somite, which develop into vertebrae and ribs.
sclerotomy incision of the sclera.
anterior s. the opening of the anterior chamber of the eye, chiefly done for the relief of glaucoma.
posterior s. an opening made into the vitreous through the sclera, as for detachment of the retina or the removal of a foreign body.
sclerous hard; indurated.
s. tissues the cartilaginous, fibrous and osseous tissues.
scoke *Portulaca americana.*
Scolebasidium genus of fungi in the family Dematiaceae which are a cause of phaeohyphomycosis.
S. humicola, S. tshawytschae have been recovered from cats and fish.
scolex pl. *scoleces* [Gr.] the attachment organ of a tapeworm, generally considered the anterior, or cephalic, end.
scoli(o)- word element. [Gr.] *crooked, twisted.*

scoliokyphosis combined lateral (scoliosis) and posterior (kyphosis) curvature of the spine.
sclorachitic affected with scoliosis and rickets.
scoliosiometry measurement of spinal curvature.
scoliosis lateral deviation in the normally straight vertical line of the spine; it may or may not include rotation or deformity of the vertebrae.
Scolopendra a genus of arthropods in the class Myriapoda. Called also centipede (Chilopoda). They have poison claws used to stun prey and can cause a painful bite to an animal.
S. gigantea a large tropical centipede credited as being able to kill a human.
scooting a form of behavior limited largely to dogs. Sliding along on the ground while sitting on the perineal area and with the hindlimbs extended forwards. Caused usually by irritation in the perineal area, chiefly anal sac irritation.
scopolamine an anticholinergic alkaloid derived from various plants, used as the hydrobromide in parasympathetic blockade and as a central nervous system depressant.
Scopulariopsis a fungus causing hyalohyphomycosis.
S. brevicaulis an uncommon cause of ringworm in cattle.
-scopy word element. [Gr.] *examination of.*
scoracratia fecal incontinence.
scorbutic pertaining to scurvy.
scorbutigenic causing scurvy.
scorbutus [L.] *scurvy.*
score a rating, usually expressed numerically, based on specific achievement or the degree to which certain qualities are manifest.
scoring determining a SCORE.
s. system systematic awarding of points for each performance or appearance.
scorpenid scorpion fish.
scorpion eight-legged, venomous arthropod of varying sizes but all possessing massive claws at the head and a flexible, segmented tail, which is carried in a characteristic forward curve over the back and has a sting in it. The neurotoxin produced causes severe pain and numbing at the site but there is not usually sufficient to cause paralysis of a human. There are several species, including *Tityus*, *Centruroides*, *Androctonus*.
scorpion fish members of the family Scorpaenidae including bullrout, twelve-spined red rock cod, sixteen-spined fortescue, goblin fish and South Australian cobbler, all capable of administering a very painful sting from their spines. There may be a precipitate rise then fall in temperature and finally a fatal cardiovascular collapse.
scorpionid a member of the order Scorpionida, the true SCORPION.
Scotch collie see COLLIE.
Scotch cramp see Scottie CRAMP.
Scotchcast see FIBERGLASS CAST.
scoto- word element. [Gr.] *darkness.*
scotochromogen a microorganism whose pigmentation develops in the dark, used particularly in the classification of mycobacteria.
scotochromogenic pertaining to scotochromogen.
scotopsin the protein moiety in the retinal rods that combines with 11-*cis*-retinal to form rhodopsin.
Scottish blackface a breed of carpetwool and meat sheep with a black or pied face. From northern England and Scotland.
Scottish deerhound a very large (75–110 lb; 28–32 inches tall) dog with medium length, ragged, usually dark gray hair, long neck and quite long tail. The coat forms a 'mane' on the neck. The head is relatively small and elongated with small, pendant ears. Said to resemble a very large, thick boned, rough-coated Greyhound.
Scottish fancy an old, ornamental breed of canaries, popular in Victorian times. It is a long, slim bird, with a characteristic posture. The body is curved, head thrust forward and tail carried under the perch, forming the shape of a crescent moon.
Scottish fold a breed of cats all of which trace their parentage to a mutant Scottish farm cat. Their distinctive feature is the forward and downward folding of ear cartilages that becomes apparent as kittens mature. This is inherited as a dominant trait which when homozygous is associated with multiple cartilaginous and bony malformations. To avoid these defects, Scottish fold cats are bred to normal eared cats and about half the offspring are otherwise normal cats with the fold.
Scottish osteodystrophy the cartilaginous and bony malformations associated with the SCOTTISH FOLD trait in cats.
Scottish terrier, Scottie a small (19–23 lb) thickset dog with short legs. The coat is hard and wiry, trimmed to a short length on the body but allowed to be full and longer on the legs, under the body, and over the eyes and around the muzzle where it forms a beard. It may be black, wheaten or brindled. The head is long and the ears sharply pointed and erect. The tail is docked to a medium length and carried upright. Called also 'diehard'. The breed is affected by Scottie cramp, craniomandibular osteopathy, cystinuria, von Willebrand's disease and atopic dermatitis.
Scotty cramp see Scottie CRAMP.
scour, scours 1. the chemical and physical cleaning of fleece wool. 2. diarrhea.
dietetic s. see dietary DIARRHEA.
peat s. see secondary nutritional COPPER deficiency.
s. weed see SISYRINCHIUM.
s. worm includes the genera *Trichostrongylus*, *Ostertagia*, *Cooperia* and *Nematodirus* spp.
scouring characterized by SCOUR.
s. disease a colloquial name for secondary nutritional COPPER deficiency.
SCPK serum creatine kinase.
scr. scruple.
scraper see TARTAR scraper.
scrapie an infectious, fatal, chronic disease of sheep and goats with clinical signs of pruritus, abnormalities of gait, recumbency and a long illness of about 6 months. The incubation period is about 2 years.
s. agent scrapie is caused by an agent that acts like a virus but does not have the physical characteristics of one. Despite intensive study the true nature of the scrapie agent has not been defined; it is not a conventional virus or a viroid and current studies suggest that it may be a small-molecular-weight, 'self-replicating' basic protein for which the term prion has been proposed. The scrapie agent is of interest beyond its role as a rare pathogen for sheep in that it is a prototype of a new class of infectious agents responsible for a number of slow degenerative central nervous system diseases of humans and other animal species. See SCRAPIE, PRION, BOVINE SPONGIFORM ENCEPHALOPATHY.
s.-associated fibrils characteristic proteinaceous fibrils in the neurons of sheep with scrapie; the fibrils consist of membrane glycoprotein the DNA of which exists in the patient's brain cells. The glycoprotein accumulates because horizontally acquired scrapie

agent induces transcription of the related host chromosomal gene and converts it to a polymerized proteinase-resistant fibrillar form.

scraping 1. a scraping of the superficial elements of the skin for laboratory examination for parasitic and fungal elements. 2. removal of superficial layers of skin after scalding of pig carcasses.

scratch test a test for hypersensitivity in which a minute amount of the substance in question is inserted in small scratches made in the skin. A positive reaction is swelling and reddening at the site within 30 minutes. Used in allergy testing and in testing for tuberculosis. In animals, intradermal testing is used more commonly. See also SKIN test.

scratches 1. excoriations caused accidentally or during rubbing to ease pruritus. 2. excoriations across the back of the pastern in a horse with the early stages of GREASY HEEL. These are very painful and are the cause of the severe lameness evident at this stage of the disease.

scratching 1. the common motor response to pruritus in dogs and cats. It frequently causes more severe injury and secondary infection to the skin. 2. withdrawing a horse or Greyhound from a race after it has finally accepted. 3. a rodeo term for when a horse's sides are raked with spurs.

screen 1. a framework or agent used as a shield or protector. 2. to examine.

fast s. permits big reduction in exposure to x-ray beam.

s. film prepared to be used with intensifying screens. The standard film and marketed as being of standard, fast or ultrafast speeds.

rare-earth s. see rare-earth INTENSIFYING SCREEN.

screening 1. examination of a large sample of animals in a population in order to detect the presence of disease or to ascertain the prevalence of certain diseases, such as tuberculosis or diabetes mellitus. 2. in diagnostic tests the use of a test which has a high sensitivity but often only a moderate specificity. Usually this is a quick and cheap test which is followed by a more expensive but more accurate test carried out on the positive reactors to the screening test. 3. fluoroscopy or image intensification (Great Britain).

biochemical s. using biochemical tests for purposes of detecting the presence of a disease.

multiphasic s., multiple s. simultaneous examination of a population for several different diseases.

preventive s. screening of a population with a preventive medical program in prospect.

s. test any test, e.g. tuberculin, brucellosis tests, used to screen a population.

screw 1. a mechanical device for fixing one object to another, characterized by a spiral ridge cut on the external surface of a cylindrical rod of decreasing diameter towards its point. This is a male screw. In a female screw the screw is cut on the inside of a cylindrical cavity. 2. a colloquial term for a worn out or inferior horse.

AISF bone s. see buttress thread bone SCREW.

buttress thread bone s. the thread is not a simple V as in the standard thread but has one side of the groove at right angles to the direction of the screw and the other side at a 45° angle. Called also AISF, Howmett compression, Richards–Bechtol.

cancellous bone s. has a coarse thread; threaded to only the first third of the length of the screw.

cortical s. threaded the full length of the screw; fine thread to hold in dense bone.

Howmett compression bone s. see buttress thread bone SCREW.

lag bone s. used as a compressing unit between two fragments with the first half of the screw near the point threaded, with the diameter of the ridges greater than that of the unthreaded half near the head. As the ridged part of the screw bites in the walls of the drill hole in the distal fragment, the unthreaded part is free to move within the drill hole in the proximal fragment, thus compressing the two pieces of bone together.

Richards–Bechtol bone s. see buttress thread bone screw (above).

standard bone s. with a V thread the full length of the screw, with a single slot, cruciate or Phillips head.

transfixation s. orthopedic screw used to reattach bone fragments to a solid skeletal part. The proximal part near the head is not threaded and needs to be of a smaller diameter than the threaded portion nearer the tip.

screw-neck twisting of the neck causing rotation of the head. Called also torticollis.

screw-tail inherited tail formation in some breeds of dogs with naturally short tails, e.g. British bulldog, in which there are usually multiple malformations of the coccygeal vertebrae producing a curled or otherwise distorted, stumpy tail. Called also ingrown tail.

s. dermatitis irritation and sometimes significant secondary infection occurring in the skin fold surrounding the base of a screw-tail. See also fold DERMATITIS.

screw twitch a twitch in which a ring encloses a bar moved by a screw. A fold of lip is caught between the bar and the ring and screwed tight.

screw-worm the larvae of CALLITROGA, CHRYSOMYA *bezziana* and PASSEROMYIA.

s. flies the flies that produce screw-worms.

s. myiasis invasion of normal skin wounds by maggots of CALLITROGA, CHRYSOMYA *bezziana* and PASSEROMYIA flies. Large masses of tissue may be destroyed and the case fatality rate approximates 100%. All animal species including humans are susceptible.

script file see BATCH FILE.

scRNA small cytoplasmic RNA.

scrobic *Paspalum scrobiculatum*, toxic when infested with *Claviceps paspali*.

scrobiculate marked with pits.

scroll moving the cursor on a computer screen through information which may extend beyond the window being viewed.

s. bar bars on the side and bottom of the window which are used to move the cursor horizontally or vertically through a document around a computer screen by clicking on the directional arrows in the scroll bar.

Scrophularia aquatica European member of plant family Scrophulariaceae. Probably contain toxic cardiac glycosides; causes excitement, tachypnea, pupillary dilatation, oral mucosal congestion and ulceration, dysuria and profuse diarrhea. Called also water figwort, water betony.

scrotal pertaining to SCROTUM.

s. abscess usually the result of infection at the time of castration and absence of drainage from the site. May be accompanied by extensive local cellulitis.

s. anomalies include aplasia, congenital cleft and bifurcation.

s. circumference an essential part of the examination of a ruminant male for breeding soundness. A special tape is used and the measurement taken at the point of greatest diameter of the scrotum and contents—usually within the range of 13.5 to 16 inches is considered normal for adult bulls.

s. fat fat accumulates in the scrotum of most fat males; it is most obvious in castrates.
s. mange chorioptic mange.
s. myiasis blowfly strike of a recently castrated ram lamb.
scrotectomy excision of part of the scrotum.
scrotitis inflammation of the scrotum.
scrotocele scrotal hernia.
scrotoplasty plastic reconstruction of the scrotum.
scrotum the pouch that contains the testes and their accessory organs. It is composed of skin, the dartos, fascia and the parietal layer of tunica vaginalis.
scrub 1. low trees and bushes. Called also browse. Edible enough for livestock to graze them especially when more conventional feed is short. Lopping of this material for feeding is a husbandry practice in some arid zones. Lends itself to indigestion in ruminants because of its indigestibility, especially if it is the main article of diet. 2. to cleanse by vigorous scrubbing with a brush. See also surgical scrub (below).
s. ironbark BRIDELIA *exalta, B. leichhardtii.*
s.-itch mite see ACOMATACARUS, TROMBICULA *minor.*
s. kurrajong PIMELEA *microcephala, P. pauciflora.*
s.-up see scrub (2).
s. suit the outer, protective clothing worn by operating room personnel. Usually specially prepared within the hospital's sterilizing facility to minimize contamination in the surgical suite.
surgical s. the ritualistic presurgical preparation of hands and arms by surgeons and their assistants. Includes thorough, vigorous and systematic cleaning with a brush of all skin surfaces. Persons prepared in this manner are then considered 'scrubbed-up', ready to take part in the surgical procedure, and are not allowed to touch any nonsterile surfaces.
s. tick see IXODES *holocyclus.*
s. typhus a disease of humans transmitted by *Trombicula akamushi* and resident in rodents which serve as reservoirs. Called also Japanese river fever, tsutsugamushi disease.
scrubbed-up see surgical SCRUB.
scruple a unit of weight of the apothecaries' system, equal to 20 grains; the equivalent of 1.296 g.
scur vestigial frontal horn at the normal site in an animal expected to be polled. It is not attached to the skull and there may or may not be an associated bony protuberance beneath it. The animal is not acceptable as being genetically polled.
scurf loose, dry scales on the haircoat and skin. May be a sign of dry skin or associated with a variety of skin diseases. See also PITYRIASIS.
scurf pea see PSORALEA.
scurvy the disease caused by a nutritional deficiency of ascorbic acid (vitamin C). See also ASCORBIC ACID nutritional deficiency.
s. rickets see hypertrophic OSTEODYSTROPHY.
scute any squama or scalelike structure, especially one of the thick epidermal plates on the head of snakes, or the shell of a tortoise.
scutiform shaped like a shield.
Scutigera see JOHNNY HAIRY-LEGS.
scutulum pl. *scutula* [L.] one of the disk- or saucer-like crusts characteristic of FAVUS.
scutum 1. scute. 2. a protective covering or shield, e.g. a chitin plate in the exoskeleton of hard-bodied ticks. 3. a pressure pad that serves as a bearing surface for tendons as they bend around a prominence. The horse digit bears three scuta over the fetlock, pastern and coffin joints for the passage of the deep digital flexor tendon.
scybalous of the nature of a scybalum.
scybalum pl. *scybala* [Gr.] a hard mass of fecal matter in the intestine.
scyphoid shaped like a cup or goblet.
scyphozoa true jellyfish.
SD 1. streptodornase. 2. sorbitol dehydrogenase. 3. skin dose. 4. standard deviation.
SDA specific dynamic action.
SDH sorbitol dehydrogenase.
SDS–PAGE sodium dodecyl sulfate–polyacrylamide gel electrophoresis.
SE standard error.
Se chemical symbol, *selenium.*
SEA sheltie eye anomaly; see COLLIE eye anomaly.
sea said of denizens of the ocean. Called also marine.
s. cage netting enclosure anchored to the sea bed or to buoys in which cultivated fish for human consumption are kept captive and fed special diets.
s. canary see DELPHINAPTERUS LEUCAS.
s. horse bizarre aquarium fish with a snout, a skin covered with bony rings and a prehensile tail; the male has a brood pouch on the belly into which the female deposits her eggs. Called also *Hippocampus.*
s. onion URGINEA *maritima.*
s. otter see OTTER.
s. snakes members of the family Hydrophiidae, venomous snakes, inhabiting the sea, with paddle-shaped tails. Unlikely to bite unless pressed.
s. squill URGINEA *maritima.*
s. wasp see CUBOMEDUSAE.
s. water if natural sea water is not available a substitute can be used: sodium chloride—27.2; magnesium chloride—3.8; magnesium sulfate—1.6; calcium sulfate—1.3; potassium sulfate—0.9; calcium carbonate and magnesium bromide—each 0.1, all in g/l.
seagull a noisy, gregarious bird that frequents the seashore. Web-footed, hook-billed, white with gray wings. Member of the family Laridae and of the genus *Larus.*
seal 1. a marine mammal; member of the suborder Pinnipedia. There are two major groups, the earless seals (family Phocidae) including many species, and the eared seals (family Otariidae) including sealions and fur seals. They are carnivorous and have four paddles which enable them to move on land and to swim. 2. a very dark brown coat color of cats, seen in brown (or sable) Burmese and on the extremities of seal-point Siamese and Colorpoint cats.
s. pox see SEALPOX.
seal-point see POINTS.
sealant see BONE sealant.
sealer in meat hygiene terms, see SHOMER.
sealion member of the family Otariidae, identifiable by having external ears. There are several genera including *Otaria*, the southern sealion, *Zalophus*, the Californian sealion and *Eumetopius*, Steller's sealion. They are large seals with a hairy coat and lacking the fur of the fur seals.
s. virus see SAN MIGUEL SEALION VIRUS DISEASE.
sealpox multiple raised nodules on the head and neck of harbor seals and sealions; caused by a virus in the genus *Parapoxvirus.*
Sealyham terrier a small (22–25 lb), stocky dog with short legs and a harsh, wiry coat that is predominantly white, but may have lemon, brown, blue or badger pied markings on the head and ears. The coat is trimmed to a short length on the body but forms thick feathers on the legs and body and a beard with bushy 'eyebrows'. The breed is predisposed to atopic dermatitis, lens luxation and retinal dysplasia.
searcher 1. an instrument (a sound) used in examin-

ing the bladder for calculi; called also stone searcher. 2. a farrier's tool for excavating a small hole in the sole of the hoof in a search for a puncture site. Has a slightly curved blade with a sharp cutting hook at the end. Resembles a hoof knife but the blade is much narrower.

Searcy trephine miniature trephine like a skin biopsy punch for removal of chalazions.

seashore lupine LUPINUS *littoralis*.

seaside arrowgrass TRIGLOCHIN *maritima*.

season see ESTRUS.

seasonal pertaining to season of the year.

s. air flow patterns the changes in the patterns of air flow which occur in animal housing which are ventilated by natural means, according to the seasonal variation in the environmental temperature.

s. anestrus see ANESTRUS.

s. calvers cattle herds in which the mating is arranged so that the cows calve at a particular season of the year.

s. herds see seasonal calvers (above).

seaweed sea plants harvested for livestock feed; claimed to be a rich source of minerals and vitamins. When fed to laying hens may discolor yolks.

sebaceous pertaining to or secreting sebum.

s. adenitis inflammation of the sebaceous gland; includes granulomatous lesions.

s. adenoma particularly common in the skin of aged dogs. On the eyelids they arise from the meibomian glands.

s. cyst a benign retention cyst containing sebum.

s. epithelioma basal cell tumor with sebaceous differentiation.

s. gland holocrine glands in the skin that secrete sebum usually through the hair follicles. They vary in size and activity between species and location. In dogs, large sebaceous glands are located on the dorsum of the tail (see TAIL gland) and at mucocutaneous junctions. In cats, large glands are located also on the dorsum of the tail, on the lip margins and under the chin (see SUBMENTAL organ).

s. gland secretion abnormality includes sebolith, seborrhea.

s. secretion see SEBUM.

supracaudal s. gland see SUPRACAUDAL ORGAN.

Sebecia a pentastome, the larvae of which occur in fish and the adults in crocodiles.

sebiferous, sebiparous secreting or producing a fatty substance.

sebolith a calculus in a sebaceous gland.

seborrhea an abnormal secretion from the sebaceous glands, often associated with abnormalities of keratinization. The clinical features vary from dandruff to the formation of greasy scales and crusts with accompanying inflammation. See also FLEXURAL seborrhea, EAR margin dermatosis.

congenital s. occurs in several dog breeds as scaling skin at birth and progressively worsening seborrhea oleosa with advancing age. Called also dirty-puppy syndrome.

idiopathic s., primary s. that caused by endocrine- or lipid-related metabolic abnormalities; may have an inherited basis.

s. oleosa moist, oily seborrhea with the formation of yellow-brown crusts. See also EXUDATIVE epidermitis.

primary s. an inherited disorder of keratinization recognized in several breeds, particularly Cocker spaniels, English springer spaniel, West Highland white terrier and Chinese shar pei. Clinical signs may appear at a young age and worsen with advancing age. There is often ceruminous otitis externa and secondary bacterial and *Malassezia* infections are common. Reported occasionally in Persian cats. In horses, it usually occurs as seborrhea of the mane and tail, rarely as a generalized disease.

secondary s. that associated with a wide variety of unrelated diseases including parasitism, pyoderma, hypersensitivity reactions and autoimmune skin disease.

s. sicca dry, scaly seborrheic dermatitis.

seborrheic affected with or of the nature of seborrhoea.

s. dermatitis see seborrheic DERMATITIS.

s. disease see SEBORRHEA.

s. keratosis see seborrheic KERATOSIS.

s. plaque chronic, erythematous, scaly skin plaque which is associated with staphylococcal hypersensitivity.

seborrheid a seborrheic eruption.

sebotropic having an affinity for or a stimulating effect on sebaceous glands; promoting the excretion of sebum.

sebum the oily secretion of the sebaceous glands, whose ducts open into the hair follicles. It is composed of fat and epithelial debris from the cells of the malpighian layer, and it lubricates the skin. It is also secreted by the tarsal glands of the eyelids.

Secale cereale cereal rye. Grown mainly as a grain crop for animal feed, production of rye bread and rye whisky. The crop may be infected with CLAVICEPS *purpurea*.

secobarbital a short- to intermediate-acting oxybarbiturate, used for sedation and anesthesia. Called also quinalbarbitone.

secodont teeth with sharp cutting edges that produce a shearing action. Seen in the feline and canine.

second the SI unit of time. Symbol s. Abbreviated sec.

second cross progeny of a mating between a half-bred and a purebred of one of the parents.

second cuts short pieces of fleece wool resulting from the shearer cutting over the same area twice.

second cutting said of hay made from a field which has already been cut for hay in the current summer. Does not have the weeds and old growth of the first cutting hay.

second-order reactions the rate of product formation either depends directly on the concentrations of two substrates (as in condensation reactions) or the square of the concentration of a single substrate (as in dimerization reactions).

second-set reaction, phenomenon see REJECTION.

secondary derived from another condition, the primary condition.

s. attack rate number of cases in the outbreak divided by the total number of susceptible animals in the population.

s. carcinogens relatively inert substances that are converted by a host-mediated reaction to an active carcinogen, e.g. nitrosamines, pyrrolizidine alkaloids.

s. health care the level of care in the HEALTH CARE SYSTEM that consists of emergency treatment and critical care. Called also acute care.

s. hypertrophic osteopathy see hypertrophic OSTEOPATHY.

s. immune response see ANAMNESTIC response.

s. pregnancy toxemia pregnancy toxemia secondary to another condition which reduces the ewe's or cow's feed intake.

s. radiation see SCATTER radiation, COMPTON EFFECT.

s. ruminal contraction occurs after the primary ruminal cycles during feeding and terminate with eructation. See also RETICULORUMINAL CONTRACTIONS.

s. spongiosa see secondary SPONGIOSA.

secrecy see CONFIDENTIALITY.

secreta [L.] *secretion products.*

secretagogue 1. causing a flow of secretion. 2. an agent that stimulates secretion.

secrete to synthesize and release a substance.

secretin a hormone secreted by the mucosa of the duodenum and jejunum when acid chyme enters the intestine; carried by the blood, it stimulates the secretion of pancreatic juice and, to a lesser extent, bile and intestinal secretion.

s. test an examination of the gastric and duodenal contents after intravenous administration of exogenous secretin; useful in the diagnosis of disorders affecting pancreatic exocrine function, for example, pancreatitis and neoplastic disease.

secretinase a substance in the serum that inactivates secretin.

secretion 1. the cellular process of elaborating a specific product. This activity may range from separating a specific substance of the blood to the elaboration of a new chemical substance. 2. any substance produced by secretion. One example is the fatty substance produced by the sebaceous glands to lubricate the skin. Saliva, produced by the salivary glands, and gastric juice, secreted by specialized glands of the stomach, are both used in digestion. The secretions of the endocrine glands include various hormones and are important in the overall regulation of body processes. Secretion of milk is an essential physiological activity in all mammals. Secretion of tears in animals has a simple protectory function and has no overriding emotional involvement. 3. categories of secretion include APOCRINE, HOLOCRINE, MEROCRINE, SEBACEOUS, SEROUS.

secretoinhibitory inhibiting secretion; antisecretory.

secretomotor stimulating secretion; said of nerves.

secretory pertaining to secretion.

s. cells the specialized cells in a secretory gland that perform the secretory function.

s. component a polypeptide synthesized by epithelial cells that binds to IgA to form secretory IgA (SIgA).

s. diarrhea see secretory DIARRHEA.

s. endpieces see ADENOMERE.

s. granules intracellular granules composed of secretory proteins after their conversion by the Golgi apparatus.

s. IgA (SIgA) a class of immunoglobulin found in some body secretions, e.g. saliva, respiratory secretions, milk and colostrum, that is responsible for local immunity. See also IMMUNOGLOBULIN.

sectio pl. *sectiones* [L.] section.

section 1. an act of cutting. 2. a cut surface. 3. a segment or subdivision of an organ.

abdominal s. laparotomy; incision of the abdominal wall.

cesarean s. delivery of a fetus by incision through the abdominal wall and uterus; see also CESAREAN SECTION.

frontal s. a section through the body passing at right angles to the median plane, dividing the body into dorsal and ventral parts.

frozen s. a specimen cut by microtome from tissue that has been frozen; see also FROZEN section.

perineal s. external urethrotomy.

sagittal s. a section through the body coinciding with the sagittal suture, thus dividing the body into right and left halves.

serial s's histological sections of a specimen made in consecutive order and so arranged for the purpose of microscopic examination.

trial s. the gradual transverse cutting of a tissue or structure, usually to ascertain its composition or to limit the incision to only one component, e.g. scar tissue surrounding a nerve.

sectioning preparation of sections from fixed and embedded blocks of tissue by thin shaving with a microtome.

sections thin shavings of fixed and embedded blocks of tissue, collected by biopsy or at necropsy examination, for histological or pathological microscopy.

-sectomy surgical removal of.

sector an arc-shaped section of the magnetized surface of a computer disk; the smallest amount of information that can be read from or written to a disk. The disk drive read–write head can locate any sector quickly and without having to read all the information before the desired location. The sectoring may be *hard* or *soft*. In the latter the program determines the size of the sector. Which one is used is determined by the physical characteristics of the disk. Nowadays disks are standardized so that a knowledge of sectoring characteristics is unnecessary.

sectorial cutting; said of TEETH.

secular 1. not religious. 2. over long periods of time; gradual.

s. changes, trends changes that occur over long periods, as long as decades.

secundigravida a female pregnant the second time; gravida II.

secundines afterbirth; the placenta and the membranes expelled after parturition.

secundipara a female which has had two pregnancies that resulted in viable offspring; para II.

security security of information, especially that on computer disks, needing to have access limited to specified persons. Provided usually by passwords.

sedamine a poisonous alkaloid in the plant *Sedum acre*.

sedation 1. the allaying of irritability or excitement, especially by administration of a sedative. 2. the state so induced.

sedative 1. allaying irritabiliy and excitement. 2. an agent that calms nervousness, irritability and excitement. In general, sedatives depress the central nervous system and tend to cause lassitude and reduced mental activity. They may be classified, according to the organ most affected, as cardiac, gastric, etc.

The degree of relaxation produced varies with the kind of sedative, the dose, the means of administration, and the mental state of the patient. By causing relaxation, a sedative may help an animal go to sleep, but it does not 'put it to sleep', a dangerous lay euphemism for euthanasia. Medicines that induce sleep are known as hypnotics. A drug may act as a sedative in small amounts and as a hypnotic in large amounts.

The barbiturates such as phenobarbital are the best-known sedatives. They are also widely used as hypnotics. Other effective sedatives are the bromides, paraldehyde and chloral hydrate.

sedentary of inactive habits; pertaining to a fat, castrated or confined animal.

sedge numerous aquatic plants including *Carex vulpina*, *Schoenus* spp.

sediment a deposit, often a precipitate, that develops spontaneously.

s. activity test a test of ruminal function based on the speed with which the sediment in a sample of rumen fluid floats to the top, an indication that it has been digested.

sedimentation the settling out of sediment.

s. coefficient the ratio of molecular velocity to centrifugal force usually expressed in Svedberg (S) units.

s. rate the rate at which a sediment is deposited in a given volume of solution, especially when subjected to the action of a centrifuge. The ERYTHROCYTE sedimentation rate is the rate at which erythrocytes settle out of unclotted blood. Abbreviated sed. rate or ESR. The test is based on the fact that inflammatory processes cause an alteration in blood proteins, resulting in aggregation of the red cells, which makes them heavier and more likely to fall rapidly when placed in a special vertical test tube. Normal ranges vary according to the type of tube used, each type being of a different size, and with the species, horse erythrocytes falling faster than those of other species.

sedridine a toxic alkaloid in the plant *Sedum acre*.

Sedum acre a plant in the family Crassulaceae. Contains the toxic alkaloids sedamine and sedredine but there is no record of poisoning in animals by the plant.

seed 1. the mature ovule of a flowering plant. 2. semen. 3. a small cylindrical shell of gold or other suitable material, used in application of radiation therapy. 4. to inoculate a culture medium with microorganisms.

s. dressing chemicals mixed with seed grain to prevent infestion with insects and rodents and infection by fungi. Most are poisonous to animals and deaths may occur if the grain is not used as seed and is put back into the animal feed chain. The amount of feed in a collection of seed is usually very large and the probability is that it would be fed without dilution which would reduce its toxicity. Grain or grain products are also used as bait for birds, or to repel birds and to poison snails and other garden pests and all of them may be accessible to animals.

s. grain cereal grain intended to be used as seed for a crop.

s. mixtures mixtures of small grass and cereal seeds used as feed for companion birds. Some of the seeds used are the millets, chopped oat groats, canary grass (*Phalaris* spp.) seed, sunflower seed, hemp seed, rape seed.

plantago s., plantain s., psyllium s. cleaned, dried ripe seed of species of *Plantago*; used as a cathartic.

radon s. a small sealed container for radon, for insertion into the tissues of the body in radiotherapy.

s. tick larval form, the stage prior to the nymph.

seeding the plaques of hard tissue in the subcutaneous tissue in the floor of the udder of some recently calved cows. The milk is normal and the plaques disappear within a few days, sooner if they are massaged and hot fomented. Called also caking.

seedy cut belly tissue in a pig carcass, including mammary gland, which is streaked with melanin.

seedy toe a defect in the wall of the hoof of the horse, seen best from the sole. The inner part of the wall is crumbly and soft and is easily picked out. The defect extends up behind the wall sometimes as far as the coronet. Called also hollow wall, dystrophia ungulae.

seedy wool wool heavily contaminated with plant seeds.

seeing practice the activity in which an undergraduate veterinary student accompanies a practicing veterinarian and receives in-service training. In some countries this is a formal arrangement in which the practitioners are Academic Associates of the University Veterinary School.

seeker a probe or sound; a long thin rod used to probe the opening or a tract or a cavity in order to determine its direction, source or depth.

seeterwort HELLEBORUS *foetidus*.

segment a demarcated portion of a whole.

bronchopulmonary s. one of the subdivisions of the lobe of a lung, sometimes separated from others by a connective tissue septum and supplied by its own branch of the bronchus leading to the particular lobe.

hepatic s's subdivisions of the hepatic lobes based on arterial and biliary supply and venous drainage.

segmental pertaining to a segment or to segmentation. See also segmental APLASIA, AXONOPATHY, CEREBELLAR atrophy, MYELITIS.

segmentation 1. division into similar parts. 2. cleavage.

intestinal s. periodic constriction of segments of intestine without movement backwards or forwards; a mixing rather than a propulsive movement; the movements are reflex and can be initiated by intrinsic nerves in the wall of the small intestine.

segmenter neutrophil see NEUTROPHIL.

segregation the separation of allelic genes during meiosis as homologous chromosomes begin to migrate toward opposite poles of the cell, so that eventually the members of each pair of allelic genes go to separate gametes.

adjacent s. during meiosis adjacent centromeres segregate together.

alternate s. when diagonally opposite centromeres segregate together.

segregator an instrument for obtaining the urine from the ureter of each kidney separately.

Segugio Italiano a medium-size, lightly built hunting dog with an elongated, narrow head, deep chest and thin tail which is carried high. The coat is black and tan of any shade, with white markings. There are two varieties: coarsehaired and shorthaired.

seismotherapy treatment of disease by mechanical vibration.

Seitz filter a filter made of compressed asbestos fibers used in microbiological work to sterilize fluids such as serum and to filter off bacteria but permit the passage of viruses.

seizure 1. the sudden attack or recurrence of a disease. 2. a CONVULSION or attack of EPILEPSY.

audiogenic s. a seizure brought on by sound.

cerebral s. an attack of EPILEPSY.

epileptiform s. see EPILEPTIFORM.

focal s. see partial seizure (below).

generalized s. see grand mal seizure (below).

grand mal s. one with no localizing signs. After a brief period of restlessness, there is unconsciousness, generalized muscular activity, excessive salivation, chewing activity, opisthotonos, running movements, and often urination and defecation. The most common type of seizure in dogs and cats.

partial s. one restricted to a focus in the brain; signs correspond to the area affected, e.g. motor activity of an isolated area or limb, hallucinations such as fly catching, apparent blindness, behavioral abnormalities, etc. Called also focal seizures.

petit mal s. a mild, very brief generalized seizure. See also PETIT MAL.

photogenic s. a seizure brought on by light.

psychomotor s. motor seizures accompanied by a psychic stage. There are hallucinations, salivation, pupillary dilatation, mastication, fecal and urinary excretion, and wild running. Seen in dogs with lesions in the pyriform lobe or hippocampus and from poisoning with agenized flour (canine HYSTERIA). Called also running fits.

tetanic s. see TETANY.

s. threshold the level of stimulation at which a seizure is precipitated.

tonic s. one in which the muscles are rigid.

tonic–clonic s. alternating tonic (rigid muscles) and clonic (jerking of muscles) phases; a grand mal seizure.

selectins carbohydrate-binding proteins that mediate selective leukocyte adhesion.

selection 1. choosing the individual units to be included in a sample. See also RANDOM selection. 2. choosing the animals to be retained for breeding purposes; genetic selection.

artificial s. selection based on human decisions.

s. coefficient proportionate reduction in the average genetic contribution made by a specific genotype, relative to the contribution made by another genotype. Denoted by **s**.

s. criteria the animal characteristic which is used in a selection program.

s. differential a measure of the gain achieved by selection; the phenotypic superiority of selected individuals, compared to the population from which they were selected.

s. index a single overall estimate of the patient's true breeding value obtained from as many sources of information as are available.

individual s. selection on the results of performance testing of the subject.

s. intensity the superiority of the individuals selected for breeding, relative to the population from which they were selected.

s. limit the situation in which the entire population is homozygous for the same set of favorable genes; called also selection plateau.

s./mutation balance when the rate of removal of a gene from the population by selection equals the rate at which mutations occur.

s. plateau see SELECTION limit.

s. program the method used to select individuals from a population to be used for breeding. Usually includes nomination of the characters to be selected, the optimum size of the population in which the program is to operate, the intensity of selection available, the accuracy of the selection procedures, lengths of the generations in the species, the target rate of response.

selective the use of procedures on selected animals contrasted with blanket application to all members of the group.

s. slaughter slaughter of positive reactors or clinical cases during a disease control program.

s. dry-period mastitis therapy application of dry period intramammary therapy only to those cows known or suspected of being infected with organisms which cause mastitis; contrasts with blanket therapy in which all cows in the group are treated.

selectivity 1. the accuracy of a test in identifying animals that have the disease which is under investigation; the number of false positives to the test will be low in a selective test. 2. in pharmacology, the degree to which a dose of a drug produces the desired effect in relation to adverse effects.

selector plant see INDICATOR plants.

selegiline hydrochloride see L-DEPRENYL.

seleniferous rich in selenium.

selenite broth an enrichment broth for the growth of salmonellae.

selenium a chemical element, atomic number 34, atomic weight 78.96, symbol Se. See Table 6. It is an essential mineral nutrient and a very potent poison.

s.-75 a radioisotope of selenium having a half-life of 120 days and a principal gamma ray photon energy of 265 keV; used in the radiopharmaceutical selenomethionine. Symbol ^{75}Se.

s. accumulator plants see ACCUMULATOR plants.

s. converter plants see CONVERTER PLANTS.

s. indicator plants see INDICATOR PLANTS.

s.-induced infection resistance selenium deficiency in the diet may increase the patient's susceptibility to infection.

s. nutritional deficiency there are well-defined deficiency and poorly defined selenium responsive diseases. A nutritional deficiency of vitamin E has many of the same effects of selenium deficiency and it is often difficult to separate the two. See also ENZOOTIC muscular dystrophy, MULBERRY HEART DISEASE, HEPATOSIS dietetica, IRON poisoning, WEANER illthrift.

s. poisoning can occur on pasture growing on selenium rich soil, especially if there are selenium indicator plants growing in it. Also when selenium supplementation is carried out carelessly and there is accidental access to poisonous amounts. Acute poisoning features diarrhea, dyspnea and death. Subacute poisoning is hallmarked by blind staggers (see DUMMY). Chronic poisoning produces a syndrome of stiff gait, loss of haircoat and separation, perhaps sloughing, of the hooves. Called also alkali disease.

s.-responsive diseases diseases such as reproductive inefficiency and illthrift in sheep and cattle respond in some situations to dietary supplementation with selenium but the diseases are not proven to be caused by nutritional deficiency of the element.

s. sulfide, s. disulfide a commonly used keratolytic in medicated shampoos employed in the treatment of skin disease in dogs and cats.

s. weed see NEPTUNIA AMPLEXICAULIS.

seleno-DL-methionine sulfur-containing amino acid.

selenocompounds organic compounds containing selenium; found in plants and providing the medium by which selenium poisoning occurs via the ingestion of unpolluted plants.

selenodont said of the occlusive surfaces of cheek teeth which have crescent shapes, a characteristic of even-toed ungulates.

Selenomonas ruminantium bacterial resident of the rumen; participates in fermentation, and hence digestion, of plant ingesta.

selenosis see SELENIUM poisoning.

self a term used to denote an animal's own antigenic constituents, in contrast to 'not-self', denoting foreign antigenic constituents. The 'self' constituents do not normally elicit an immune response, i.e. there is self-tolerance, whereas the antigens which are 'not-self' do elicit an immune response. Self reactive lymphocytes, particularly T lymphocytes within the thymus, are eliminated. The breakdown of self-tolerance by a number of mechanisms is the basis for autoimmune diseases. See also IMMUNITY.

self-antigen any constituent of the body's own tissues capable of stimulating autoimmunity. See also IMMUNITY.

self-colored whole-colored.

self-contained cleaning system an abattoir cleaning unit containing all of the necessary functions including cleaning, application of live steam or a disinfectant.

self-cure a phenomenon in sheep in which a hypersensitivity to an adult worm load develops and the worms are discharged. The hypersensitivity is induced by a second larval infestation. The apparent cure of the sheep is misleading in the assessment of a control program.

self-feeder a feed container from which animals can take feed at will, but which is protected against weather, and wastage by scattering is minimal. Carbohydrate engorgement can occur if the livestock are not used to the system and eat too much grain. Dogs on such a system may overeat and become obese.

self-limited limited by its own peculiarities, and not by outside influence; said of a disease that runs a definite limited course and resolves itself without intervention.

self-mutilation the animal damages itself by biting or by violent and persistent scratching or rubbing, e.g. cattle with pseudorabies, sheep with pseudorabies. A degree of injury beyond self-trauma.

self-nursing see SELF-SUCKING.

self-recognition see SELF.

self-rectification property of an x-ray tube which means that it acts as a valve permitting the flow of current in only one direction, from the cathode to the anode.

self-replicating elements include plasmids, epizomes and transposons.

self-selection a circumstance in which the allocation of units of a population to one or other of two groups which are to be compared is done by the units, e.g. the sick animals in one group, the not-sick in the other. See also volunteer SAMPLE.

self-sucking a vice in which a female animal sucks her own milk. Seen in cows, bitches and queens.

self-tolerance immunological tolerance to self-antigens.

self-trauma self-inflicted injury, usually to the skin caused by an animal's response to pruritus. Depending on the species, this may be scratching, biting, rubbing or rolling. See also SCRATCHING (1).

sella pl. *sellae* [L.] a saddle-shaped depression.

empty s. see EMPTY-SELLA SYNDROME.

s. turcica a depression on the upper surface of the sphenoid bone, lodging the pituitary gland.

selodont teeth that have crescent-shaped cusps.

SEM 1. scanning electron microscope. 2. standard error of the mean.

semeiography a description of the clinical signs of a disease.

semeiology symptoms or signs of disease.

semeiotic 1. pertaining to clinical signs. 2. pathognomonic.

semelincident affecting an animal only once.

semen fluid discharged at ejaculation in the male, consisting of spermatozoa in their nutrient plasma, secretions from the prostate, seminal vesicles and various other glands, epithelial cells and minor constituents.

s. collection for artificial insemination or laboratory evaluation or examination in a clinicopathological sense. Done by artificial vagina, electroejaculation, genital massage.

s. concentration the number of spermatozoa per ml in the ejaculate.

s. diluent there are a number of suitable diluents with some preference being given to one or other of them in each species. There are also different diluters for chilled liquid semen as distinct from frozen semen. Most diluters are based on biological fluids such as whole or skim milk, buttermilk, cream and egg yolk. The general cryoprotectant for freezing is glycerol. Called also semen extender.

s. extender see semen diluent (above).

frozen s. semen stored in liquid nitrogen at −196°C (-321°F).

s. non-sperm portion see SEMEN pre-sperm fraction (below).

s. pre-sperm fraction the accessory gland fluid emitted at the beginning of ejaculation.

s. samples part of an ejaculate collected for laboratory examination.

s. sperm-rich fraction the portion of the ejaculate containing most of the spermatozoa.

s. stones concretions of amorphous cellular debris and clumps of nuclear material found in seminal vesicles of bulls.

s. storage chilled bull semen stored at 5°C can be stored and used for 5 days; frozen bull semen (−79°C using dry ice or −196°C using liquid nitrogen) can be stored and used successfully for up to 10 years, with only a small drop in fertility after 40 years.

semi- word element. [L.] *half.*

semiarid said of regions of the earth which have dry climates but not as dry as those of arid climates.

semicanal a trench or furrow open at one side.

semicircular shaped like a half-circle.

s. canals the passages in the inner ear, in the bony labyrinth concerned with the sense of balance, especially the detection of movement. Each ear has three semicircular canals (anterior, lateral and posterior) situated approximately at right angles to each other. They contain the semicircular ducts.

s. ducts the membranous tubes housed within the semicircular canals.They have enlarged portions at one end, called ampullae, which contain nerve endings, and which are filled with fluid.

The semicircular ducts respond to movement of the head. When the head changes position, the fluid in the duct that lies in the plane of movement also moves but, because of its inertia, the fluid flow lags behind the head movement. Thus the fluid presses against the delicate hairs of the nerves in the ampulla, and these nerves then register the fact that the head is turning in such a direction.

It is the fluid movement in the semicircular ducts that causes the feeling of dizziness or vertigo after spinning. When the spinning stops, the fluid in the horizontal canal continues to move for a moment in the direction of the spin, giving a temporary false reading that the head is turning in the other direction. Motion sickness is caused by the unusual and erratic motions of the head in an airplane, car or ship, and the resulting stimulation of the semicircular ducts. Many animals, even fish, can experience motion sickness.

semicoma a stupor from which the animal may be aroused.

semiconsciousness see SEMICOMA.

semiflexion the position of a limb midway between flexion and extension; the act of bringing to such a position.

semihairlessness an autosomal recessive trait in Hereford and polled Hereford cattle; affected calves are born with a thin, curly haircoat and some fail to thrive.

semilunar shaped like a half-moon or crescent.

s. valve valve guarding the entrances into the aorta and pulmonary trunk from the cardiac ventricles.

s. valve anomaly abnormal development causes an irregular central perforation of the valve and the signs of valvular stenosis.

seminal emanating from or pertaining to SEMEN.

s. colliculus see seminal COLLICULUS.

s. fluid some of the fluid originates in the testis but most is contributed by the various sex glands, the amount and the composition from each gland varying between species.

s. glands see seminal VESICLE.

s. peritonitis peritonitis caused by rupture of the vagina by the stallion during mating, or of the cow's uterus by the inseminator; causes a low-grade, chronic peritonitis in the caudal abdomen.

s. plasma the liquid supernatant after sedimentation or centrifugation of semen.

s. vesicle see seminal VESICLE.

s. vesiculitis inflammation of the seminal vesicles.

semination insemination.

seminiferous producing or carrying semen.

s. tubule develop as hollow tubes in the testis after birth, from solid gonadal cores.

seminin a proteolytic enzyme of human semen.

seminoma tumor of the testis thought to arise from basal spermatogonia. They are common in older dogs and occur often in cryptorchid testes. Seminomas also occur in the male of other domestic species.

seminoperitoneum see SEMINAL peritonitis.

seminuria discharge of semen in the urine.

semipermeable permitting passage only of certain molecules; said of a membrane.

semiplacenta diffusa see adventitial PLACENTATION.

semiquantitative yielding an approximation of the quantity or amount of a substance; falling short of a quantitative result.

semis [L.] *half;* abbreviated *ss.*

semisulcus a depression that, with an adjoining one, forms a sulcus.

semisupination a position halfway toward supination.

semisynthetic produced by chemical manipulation of naturally occurring substances.

semitendinosus muscle see Table 13.4.

Semitic fat-tailed sheep see NEAR EAST FAT-TAILED.

Semkin forceps thumb-operated, very fine-pointed, tissue forceps for pediatric work.

Semliki forest virus an alphavirus associated with illness in horses in Africa.

Sendai virus a paramyxovirus that causes a highly contagious disease of the respiratory tract of mice. It also affects rats but is usually subclinical in that species. The syndrome is one of pneumonia with dyspnea and a high mortality rate in young mice.

Senecio a widespread genus of the Asteraceae family. The genus contains more than 1200 species of which at least 25 are known to be poisonous. Some of them are listed here; the toxins are a group of pyrrolizidine alkaloids which cause seneciosis hepatic injury, and the dummy syndrome, jaundice, emaciation and photosensitization; includes *S. abyssinicus*, *S. alpinus*, *S. biligulatus*, *S. bipinnatisectus* (Australian fireweed), *S. braziliensis*, *S. burchelii*, *S. cineraria* (dusty miller), *S. cisplatinus*, *S. cunninghamii*, *S. desfontainei*, *S. desiderabilis*, *S. erraticus*, *S. glabellus*, *S. harvieanus*, *S. heterotrichus*, *S. integerrimus*, *S. integrifolius* (fleawort), *S. isatideus* (Dan's cabbage), *S. jacobaea* (ragwort, tansy ragwort), *S. latifolius*, *S. lautus*, *S. linearifolius* (*S. australis*, fireweed), *S. longilobus* (woolly groundsel), *S. madagascariensis* (fireweed), *S. magnificus* (tall yellowtop), *S. moorei*, *S. oxyphyllus*, *S. plattensis*, *S. pterophorus* (African daisy), *S. quadridentatus* (cotton fireweed), *S. raphanifolius* (gantho metho), *S. retrorsus* (ragwort), *S. riddellii* (Riddell's groundsel), *S. ruwenzoriensis*, *S. scleratus*, *S. selloi*, *S. spartioides* (broom groundsel), *S. spathulatus*, *S. squalidus* (Oxford ragwort), *S. tweediei*, *S. vernalis*, *S. vulgaris* (groundsel).

senecionine hepatoxic pyrrolizidine alkaloid found in *Senecio* spp. and *Crotalaria* spp.

seneciosis acute or chronic hepatic insufficiency caused by the ingestion of pyrrolizidine alkaloids in SENECIO. Characterized by a syndrome of jaundice and central nervous system derangement and possible photosensitization. Most outbreaks occur in animals on pasture but housed animals fed hay that is contaminated by the foliage or seeds can be affected. Called also Molteno disease, Pictou disease, Schweinsberger disease, Winton disease.

senescence depression of body functions as part of the process of growing old.

senile pertaining to old age; manifesting senility.

s. deafness due probably to degeneration of the hair cells in the organ of Corti, and to loss of neurons in the spinal ganglion; called also presbycusis.

s. osteoporosis reduced mineralization of bone due to advanced age.

s. retinopathy see senile RETINOPATHY.

Senkobo disease see MYCOTIC dermatitis.

Senn retractor a handheld instrument with a curled, three-pronged claw at one end and a right-angled, single blade at the other. Suitable for short-term displacement of soft tissue.

Senna plant genus in the legume family Caesalpiniaceae; contain anthraquinone glycosides which cause diarrhea; an unidentified toxin causes muscle necrosis. Includes *S. floribunda*, *S. obtusifolia*, *S. occidentale*, *S. roemeriana.* All also called *Cassia* spp., e.g. *C. floribunda.*

senna the dried leaflets of *Cassia acutiflora*; used in a syrup, fluid extract or compound powder as a cathartic.

s. bean see CASSIA *occidentalis.*

coffee s. see CASSIA *occidentalis.*

sensation an impression produced by impulses conveyed by an afferent nerve to the sensorium. Includes cold, distension, hunger, itch, pain, taste of various kinds, thermal, thirst, tickle, touch, warmth and some psychological and emotional experiences which animals obviously experience but cannot describe. See also SENSE.

s. disturbance cutaneous sensation errors include paresthesia, hyperesthesia, anesthesia. See also BLINDNESS, DEAFNESS.

sense a faculty by which the conditions or properties of things are perceived. Hunger, thirst, malaise and pain are varieties of sense; a sense of equilibrium or of well-being (euphoria) and other senses are also distinguished. The five major senses comprise VISION, HEARING, SMELL (2), TASTE and TOUCH (1).

The operation of all senses involves the reception of stimuli by sense organs. Each sense organ is sensitive to a particular kind of stimulus. The eyes are sensitive to light; the ears, to sound; the olfactory organs of the nose, to odor; and the taste buds of the tongue, to taste. Various sense organs of the skin and other tissues are sensitive to touch, pain, temperature and other sensations.

On receiving stimuli, the sense organ translates them into nerve impulses that are transmitted along the sensory nerves to the brain. In the cerebral cortex, the impulses are interpreted, or perceived, as sensations. The brain associates them with other information, acts upon them, and stores them as memory. See also SENSATION.

cutaneous s. skin senses including touch, pressure, pain, heat and cold.

s. organs 1. the organs of special sense including eye, olfactory organ, gustatory organs. 2. all organs containing sensory receptors.
special s's the five senses including feeling, hearing, seeing, smelling, tasting.
s. strand see CODING STRAND.
sensibility susceptibility of feeling; ability to feel or perceive.
deep s. the sensibility of deep tissue (muscle, tendon, etc.) to pressure, pain and movement.
epicritic s. the sensibility to gentle stimulations permitting fine discriminations of touch and temperature, localized in the skin.
proprioceptive s. the sensibility afforded by receptors in muscles, joints and other parts, by which one is made aware of their position and state.
protopathic s. the sensibility to strong stimulations of pain and temperature; it is low in degree and poorly localized, existing in the skin and in the viscera, and acting as a defensive agency against pathological changes in the tissues.
somatesthetic s. proprioceptive sensibility.
splanchnesthetic s. the sensibility to stimuli received by splanchnic receptors.
sensible perceptible to the senses; capable of sensation.
sensitive 1. able to receive or respond to stimuli. 2. unusually responsive to stimulation, or responding quickly and acutely.
s. vessel syndrome temporary engorgement of conjunctival blood vessels in the absence of disease. Seen most commonly in small dogs and cats.
sensitive plant MIMOSA *pudica*.
sensitivity the state or quality of being sensitive.
antibiotic s., antimicrobial s. the degree of susceptibility of a bacterial isolate to individual antibiotics. Measured by growth in liquid culture media with serial dilutions of the antimicrobial, or on agar plates as measured by the width of the zone of growth inhibition around a special disk impregnated with the antimicrobial.
bacterial s. see antibiotic sensitivity (above).
contact s. see contact HYPERSENSITIVITY.
diagnostic test s. the probability that a test will correctly identify the patients which are infected or have a specified non-infectious condition. A fundamental parameter for all diagnostic tests. A sensitive test will pick up the minutest quantity of antibody or other agent in a biological fluid. There are times when this is a desirable characteristic but the loss of specificity that usually accompanies the high sensitivity, needs to be taken into account. See also SPECIFICITY.
radioimmunoassay s. the smallest amount of hormone which the assay can accurately detect above a zero amount.
sensitization a state in which the body is sensitized to particular stimuli, e.g. (1) certain individuals exposed to some antigens by a particular route elicit an immune response which may be antibody-mediated, particularly IgE, or cell-mediated which sensitizes them such that subsequent exposure to the same antigen elicits an allergic response; said especially of such exposure resulting in a hypersensitivity reaction. (2) The coating of cells with antibody as a preparatory step to some detectable reaction such as their lysis if complement is added. (3) The preparation of a tissue or organ by one hormone so that it will respond functionally to the action of another.
active s. the sensitization that results from the injection, ingestion or inhalation, of antigen into the animal. See also active IMMUNITY, active IMMUNIZATION.
passive s. that which results when blood serum from a sensitized animal is injected into a normal animal. See also passive IMMUNITY, passive IMMUNIZATION.
protein s. that bodily state in which the individual is sensitive or hypersusceptible to some foreign protein, so that when there is absorption of that protein a typical reaction is set up.
sensitized rendered sensitive.
s. cells see sensitization (2).
sensitizer see ANTIGEN.
sensitogen allogen.
sensomobile moving in response to a stimulus.
sensomotor sensorimotor.
sensor a device, usually electronic, which detects a variable quantity and measures and converts the measurement into a signal to be recorded elsewhere.
sensorial pertaining to the sensorium.
sensorimotor both sensory and motor.
s. plegia loss of sensory and motor function caudal to the level of a spinal cord injury.
sensorineural of or pertaining to a sensory nerve or sensory mechanism, as sensorineural deafness.
sensorium 1. the part of the cerebral cortex that receives and coordinates all the impulses sent to individual nerve centers. 2. the state of an individual as regards consciousness or mental awareness.
s. commune the part of the cerebral cortex that receives and coordinates all the impulses sent to individual nerve centers. Includes auditory, gustatory, olfactory, somatosensory and visual centers.
sensory pertaining to sensation.
equine s. ataxia see ENZOOTIC equine incoordination.
s. input produced by sensory organs and transmitted by afferent nerve fibers to the central nervous system. See also SENSE.
s. nerve a peripheral nerve that conducts impulses from a sense organ to the spinal cord or brain; called also afferent nerve. See also NERVE.
s. neuropathy see hereditary sensory NEUROPATHY.
s. paralytic urinary bladder see atonic neurogenic URINARY BLADDER.
s. perceptivity the ability to perceive, to feel. Tests for this in animals are based on the assumption that the observer can differentiate between a reflex response and a central perception.
s. receptor see sensory RECEPTOR.
sentient able to feel; sensitive.
sentinel a recording mechanism, such as an animal, a farm or a veterinarian, posted explicitly to record a possible occurrence or series of occurrences in a prospective surveillance program.
sentry dog one trained for guard duty, particularly as used by the military for patrolling perimeter fences.
separation anxiety see separation ANXIETY.
separation from group sick animals, frightened animals may separate themselves from the group.
sepsis the presence in the blood or other tissues of pathogenic microorganisms or their toxins; the condition associated with such presence. See also TOXEMIA, BACTEREMIA.
puerperal s. sepsis occurring after parturition. See also MASTITIS–METRITIS–AGALACTIA.
septa plural of *septum*.
septal pertaining to a septum.
s. defect see VENTRICULAR septal defect, AORTIC septal defect, ATRIAL septal defect.
septan recurring on the seventh day (every 6 days).
septate divided by a septum or septa.
septectomy excision of part of the nasal septum.

septic pertaining to sepsis.
s. fever is fever associated with infection either as local abscess or cellulitis or as a septicemia or bacteremia. The infective agent may be a bacteria, virus, fungus, protozoa or even algae.
s. mastitis mastitis characterized by the presence of bacteria in the milk.
s. shock see TOXEMIC shock.
septicaemic see SEPTICEMIC.
septicemia systemic disease associated with the presence and persistence of pathogenic microorganisms and their toxins in the blood. The resulting syndrome is a combination of the signs of toxemia and hyperthermia, i.e. fever, mucosal and conjunctival petechiation and evidence of localization in joints, eyes, meninges, heart valves. Proof is by positive blood culture or smear. See also specific infections, e.g. ANTHRAX, PASTEURELLOSIS, COLIBACILLOSIS. Called also blood poisoning.
bacterial hemorrhagic s. includes many bacterial diseases of fish, e.g. vibriosis, but usually restricted to systemic infection by opportunists such as *Aeromonas hydrophila*, *Pseudomonas* spp.
cryptogenic s. septicemia in which the focus of infection is not evident during life.
foal s. rapidly fatal septicemia of the newborn foal caused by *Actinobacillus equuli*, *Escherichia coli*, *Klebsiella pneumoniae*, *Pseudomonas aeruginosa*, *Staphylococcus aureus*, *[beta]-hemolytic streptococcus*.
hemorrhagic s. septicemia characterized by marked petechiation on mucosae and serosae. Also used as a specific name for septicemic pasteurellosis in cattle; see HEMORRHAGIC septicemia.
puerperal s. that in which the focus of infection is a lesion of the mucous membrane received during parturition.
puppy s. puppies normal at birth, weaken and die after the first 24 hours. The usual causes are infection by hemolytic streptococci, *Escherichia coli* and *Brucella canis*.
septicemic emanating from or pertaining to septicemia. See also septicemic COLIBACILLOSIS, LEPTOSPIROSIS, LISTERIOSIS, PASTEURELLOSIS, SALMONELLOSIS.
s. cutaneous ulcerative disease (SCUD) disease of reptiles and amphibians caused by *Citrobacter freundii*. Characterized by cutaneous ulceration, paralysis, flaccidity and positive cultures in lesions and blood.
septicophlebitis septicemic inflammation of veins.
septicopyemia septicemia with pyemia.
septomarginal pertaining to the margin of a septum.
s. trabeculae the moderator bands that stretch from the ventricular septum to the opposite wall of the ventricle. They are partly muscular and partly tendinous.
septonasal pertaining to the nasal septum.
septoplasty surgical reconstruction of the nasal septum.
septostomy surgical creation of an opening in a septum.
septotomy incision of the nasal septum.
septula testis septa of connective tissue and plain muscle in the testis, subdividing it into lobules.
septulum pl. *septula* [L.] a small separating wall or partition.
septum pl. *septa* [L.] a wall or partition dividing a body space or cavity.

Some septa are membranous, some are composed of bone, and some of cartilage. The wall separating the atria of the heart, for instance, is called the interatrial septum.

atrioventricular s. the part of the membranous portion of the interventricular septum between the left ventricle and the right atrium.
bulbar s. a septum, formed by merging of the bulbar cushions, divides the bulbus cordis into aortic and pulmonary outflows.
cystic s. pellucidum an embryonic malformation resulting in the formation of a fluid-filled cavity in the septum between the two lateral ventricles, instead of the normal glial raphe.
horizontal s. in the avian body cavity there is no diaphragm but the cavity is divided into three compartments; this is one of the divider organs; thin and membranous for the most part, the septum forms the ventral boundary of paired cavities containing the lungs.
interalveolar s. the bony partition between adjacent tooth sockets.
interatrial s. the partition separating the right and left atria of the heart.
interlobar s. a septum that converts an organ into lobes.
intermuscular s. fascial septum separating muscle masses.
interorbital s. bony partition between the large orbital cavities of birds.
interventricular s. the partition separating the right and left ventricles of the heart. See also VENTRICULAR septum.
s. lucidum septum pellucidum (below).
median s. membranous partition in the ventral median fissure of the spinal cord.
oblique s. a partition which divides the lower part of the bird's body cavity; the part of the cavity cranial to this septum contains the thoracic air sacs and the thoracic parts of the cervical and clavicular air sacs. The part of the body cavity caudal to this septum contains heart, liver, spleen, gastrointestinal, urinary and reproductive tracts and abdominal air sacs.
orbital s. a fold which detaches from the periorbital fascia at the orbital rim, and which leads into the tarsi, the thickened margins of the eyelids.
s. pellucidum, pellucid s. the triangular double membrane separating the anterior horns of the lateral ventricles of the brain. Called also septum lucidum, telencephalic septum.
pharyngeal s. a transitory partition between the mouth and pharynx in the embryo.
s. primum a septum in the embryonic heart, dividing the primitive atrium into right and left chambers.
rectovaginal s. the membranous partition between the rectum and vagina.
rectovesical s. a membranous partition separating the rectum from the prostate and urinary bladder.
s. secundum develops during embryonic life to contribute to the formation of the foramen ovale between the cardiac atria.
telencephalic s. see septum pellucidum (above).
s. transversum a major contributor to the development of the diaphragm and the liver.
truncal s. a partition which develops from truncal cushions within the truncus arteriosus and contributes to the separation of cardiac outflow into pulmonary and systemic circulations.
urorectal s. a septum which divides the urinary passages from the hindgut in the embryo by horizontally partitioning the cloaca.
septuplet one of seven offspring produced at one birth.
sequel sequela.
sequela pl. *sequelae* [L.] a morbid condition following or occurring as a consequence of another condition or event.

sequence the order in which monomers occur in polymeric molecules; the order of amino acids in a polypeptide chain or of nucleotides in nucleic acid.

autonomously replicating s. usually plasmids that replicate independently of chromosomal DNA.

coding s's sections of DNA which code for the amino acids of a protein.

consensus s. a sequence of nucleotides that is always present in a large set of independently determined sequences. See also BOX.

enhancer s. in DNA transcription, an upstream *cis*-acting DNA sequence that enhances expression of a particular gene and forms part of a complex array of upstream sequences that control gene expression.

expressed s's in eukaryotic pre-messenger RNA the noncoding sequences, also called intervening sequences or introns, are removed in the nucleus; the mRNA is transported to the cytoplasm where the exons are translated to a protein.

intervening s. see INTRON.

palindromic s. see PALINDROME.

signal s. a collection of hydrophobic amino acid residues at the amino terminus of secretory or integrated membrane proteins that direct the protein to cell membranes, particularly endoplasmic reticulum where the proteins are modified, e.g. glycosylated, and the signal sequence is removed prior to secretion or integration of the protein into the lumen of the endoplasmic reticulum.

temporal s. in protein synthesis, is from the amino to the carboxyl end.

sequencing see DNA sequencing.

sequential characterized by a regular sequence of additions or modifications.

s. analgesia the use of a partial opioid agonist after a pure agonist to reverse respiratory depression but maintain analgesia. Called also agonist/antagonist analgesia.

s. analysis data are analyzed as they become available so that the experiment or survey can be terminated as soon as the required result is available at the desired rate of statistical significance.

s. trials see sequential analysis (above).

sequester to detach or separate abnormally a small portion from the whole.

sequestrant a sequestering agent, as, for example, cholestyramine resin which binds bile acids in the intestine, thus preventing their absorption.

sequestration 1. abnormal separation of a part from a whole, as a portion of a bone by a pathological process, or a portion of the circulating blood in a specific part occurring naturally or produced by application of a tourniquet. 2. isolation of a patient.

feline corneal s. see CORNEAL sequestrum.

pulmonary s. loss of connection of lung tissue with the bronchial tree and the pulmonary veins.

sequestrectomy excision of a sequestrum.

sequestrum pl. *sequestra* [L.] a piece of dead tissue that has become separated during the process of necrosis from sound tissue; refers usually to bone, but occurs also in cornea and lung.

feline corneal s. see CORNEAL sequestrum.

lung s. a critical feature in the epidemiology of contagious bovine pleuropneumonia; the sequestrum provides a long-term source of the causative bacteria.

sequoiosis a hypersensitivity pneumonitis of humans caused by inhalation of *Corphium* and *Pullularia* species in moldy redwood bark.

SER smooth endoplasmic reticulum.

Ser serine.

sera plural of *serum*.

seradella see ORNITHOPUS SATIVUS.

serendipity happy finding of an unexpected object or solution while searching for something else.

Sereny test a test of the invasiveness of bacterium. The organism is inoculated into the conjunctival sac of a guinea pig; invasiveness is measured by the occurrence of a keratoconjunctivitis within 24 hours. Used particularly for strains of *Escherichia coli* and *Listeria monocytogenes*.

serial part of a series.

s. homology see serial HOMOLOGY.

s. interface the device that transmits data from a processor to a peripheral device such as a printer, one bit at a time. The alternative method is to use a parallel interface in which transmission is one bit at a time, but simultaneously down several wires.

Seridon mexicanum see AMBYSTOMA *mexicanum*. Called also Mexican axolotl.

series a group or succession of events, objects or substances arranged in regular order or forming a kind of chain; in electricity, parts of a circuit connected successively end to end to form a single path for the current.

erythrocytic s. the succession of developing cells that ultimately culminates in the erythrocyte. The morphologically distinguishable forms are pronormoblast (rubriblast), basophilic normoblast (prorubricyte), polychromatophilic normoblast (rubricyte), orthochromatic normoblast (metarubricyte), reticulocyte and erythrocyte.

granulocytic s. the succession of developing cells that ultimately culminates in mature granulocytes (neutrophils, eosinophils, or basophils). The morphologically distinguishable forms are myeloblast, promyelocyte (progranulocyte), myelocyte, metamyelocyte, band granulocyte and segmented granulocyte. Stem cells are committed to become either neutrophils or eosinophils before the myelocyte stage. This may also be true for basophils.

lymphocytic s. the succession of developing cells that ultimately culminates in mature lymphocytes. The morphologically distinguishable forms are lymphoblast, prolymphocyte and lymphocyte.

monocytic s. the succession of developing cells that ultimately culminates in the monocyte. The morphologically distinguishable forms are monoblast, promonoblast and monocyte.

thrombocytic s. the succession of developing cells that ultimately culminates in platelets (thrombocytes). The morphologically distinct cell types are megakaryoblast, promegakaryocyte and megakaryocyte, which fragment to form platelets.

Serin finch small passeriform bird, the origin of the domestic canary. Called also *Serinus canaria*.

serine Ser; a naturally occurring amino acid.

Serinus a genus of the bird family Fringillidae.

S. canaria a small, stocky, seed-eating cage bird with a short conical bill. Called also canary, SERIN FINCH. Popular breeds are GLOSTER FANCY, YORKSHIRE, NORWICH, BORDER FANCY, LIZARD, BELGIAN fancy and ROLLER. They are noted for their crisp, bell-like tone combined with warbles and trills.

Seriola farmed finfish genus in the family Carangidae. Includes *S. lalandi* (yellowtail kingfish), *S. quinqueradiata* (Japanese amberjack). See Table 23.

serocolitis inflammation of the serous coat of the colon.

seroconversion the development of antibodies to an infectious organism in response to natural infection or to the administration of a vaccine.

seroculture a bacterial culture on blood serum.

serodiagnosis diagnosis of disease based on serum reactions.
seroenteritis inflammation of the serous coat of the intestine.
seroepidemiology a system of epidemiological surveillance and examination based on mass and serial testing of sera of samples of the animal populations.
serofibrinous marked by both a serous exudate and precipitation of fibrin.
serological pertaining to or emanating from SEROLOGY.
s. test one involving examination of blood serum usually for antibody.
serologist a specialist in serology. An old term for immunologist.
serology the conduct of antigen–antibody reactions in vitro.
serolysin a lysin of the blood serum.
seroma a collection of serum in the body, producing a tumor-like mass.
seromembranous pertaining to or composed of serous membrane.
seromucoid glands glands which secrete mucus and serous fluid; these glands occur in the skin of the muzzle and lip of ruminants and the skin of the snout and lip, and the caudomedial aspects of the carpus, of the pig.
seromucous both serous and mucous.
seromuscular pertaining to the serous and muscular coats of the intestine.
s. suture a suture placed across the serosa and muscular layers, but not the mucosa, of the bowel. Used in the closure of enterotomy incisions.
seronegative showing a negative serum reaction; i.e. an animal with no detectable serum antibodies to a specified microorganism.
seropositive showing positive results on serological examination, i.e. an animal with detectable serum antibodies to a particular microorganism.
seroprognosis prognosis of disease based on serum reactions.
seroprophylaxis the injection of immune serum for protective purposes.
seropurulent both serous and purulent.
seropus serum mingled with pus.
seroreaction any reaction taking place in serum, or as a result of the action of a serum.
seroresistant showing a seropositive reaction to a pathogen after treatment.
serosa any serous membrane.
serosanguineous composed of serum and blood.
seroserous pertaining to two serous surfaces.
serositis inflammation of a serous membrane.
s.-arthritis of sheep and goats see CAPRINE arthritis–encephalitis.
transmissible s. see sporadic bovine ENCEPHALOMYELITIS.
serosity the quality of serous fluids.
serosurvey a screening test of the serum of animals at risk to provide data about specific diseases.
serosynovitis synovitis with effusion of serum.
serotherapy the treatment of infectious disease by the injection of serum from immune animals.
serotonergic containing or activated by serotonin.
serotonin a hormone and neurotransmitter, 5-hydroxytryptamine (5-HT), found in many tissues, including blood platelets, intestinal mucosa, pineal body and central nervous system; it has many physiological properties, including inhibition of gastric secretion, stimulation of smooth muscles and production of vasoconstriction.
serotoninergic pertaining to neurons that release serotonin as a neurotransmitter, as those of the raphe nuclei of the brainstem, or that secrete serotonin as a hormone.
serotype the type of a microorganism determined by its constituent antigens based on one of several different antibody–antigen reactions, or a taxonomic subdivision based thereon.
serous 1. pertaining to serum; thin and watery, like serum. 2. producing or containing serum.
s. atrophy see serous ATROPHY.
s. cells one of the two kinds of cells in the acinar portions of salivary glands. Contain secretory granules the precursors of salivary amylase. Their secretion is serous and of low specific gravity.
s. membrane see serous MEMBRANE.
s. membrane inflammation see SEROSITIS.
s. ovarian inclusion cysts may be mistaken for cystic follicles but play no part in ovarian activity.
serovaccination injection of serum combined with bacterial vaccination to produce passive and active immunity.
serow goat antelope, genus *Capricornis*, in eastern Asia.
serpiginous creeping from part to part; having a wavy border like a snake.
Serpulina a genus of bacteria in the order Spirochaetaceae. Several species were previously in the genus *Treponema*.
S. hyodysenteriae the cause of swine dysentery. Previously called *Treponema hyodysenteriae*.
S. innocens may contribute to swine dysentery in association with *S. hyodysenteriae*.
Serra emasculator single action emasculator with a ratchet on the handle so that the jaws can be clamped shut. One of the jaws is a single, curved blade that closes between two blades on the other side. Designed for use in horses.
serrated having a sawlike edge or border.
Serratia gram-negative, flagellated rods, members of the family Enterobacteriaceae, found commonly in water, soil and food and only occasionally in pathological specimens. *S. marcescens* and *S. liquefaciens* are rare causes of bovine mastitis. See Table 16.
S. rubidaea a nonpathogen sometimes used as a marker because of the red colonies it produces.
serration 1. the state of being serrated. 2. a serrated structure or formation.
Serratospiculum amaculatum an air sac nematode infecting falcons.
Sertoli cell any of the elongated cells in the tubules of the testes to which the spermatids become attached; they provide support, protection and, apparently, nutrition until the spermatids are transformed into mature spermatozoa.
ovarian S. c. tumor Sertoli–Leydig tumor of an atopic ovary in a bitch, commonly associated with cystic endometrial hyperplasia.
testicular S. c. tumor occurs most commonly in dogs, particularly in retained testicles. Production of estrogen may cause feminization in which the dog is attractive to other males with reduced libido, feminine distribution of body fat, symmetrical alopecia, atrophy of the penis, increased size of the mammary glands and prepuce, and prostatic enlargement. Rarely there is depression of bone marrow activity with anemia, thrombocytopenia and granulocytopenia.
serum pl. *sera*, *serums* [L.] the clear portion of any animal or plant fluid that remains after the solid elements have been separated out. The term usually

refers to blood serum, the clear, straw-colored, liquid portion of the plasma that does not contain fibrinogen or blood cells, and remains fluid after clotting of blood.

Blood serum from animals whose bodies have built up antibodies is called antiserum or immune serum. Inoculation with such an antiserum provides temporary, or passive, immunity against the disease.

s. albumin mastitis test a high concentration of serum albumin in milk indicates the presence of mastitis in the quarter.

antilymphocyte s. see ANTILYMPHOCYTE SERUM.

s. breaks in hog cholera (swine fever) vaccination when a serum-simultaneous vaccination program is not effective and it is assumed that the hyperimmune serum was ineffective.

s. clot time see PROTHROMBIN consumption test.

s. enzymes enzymes of individual tissues are released into the blood when the tissue is damaged or when there is much activity in it. The levels are used as a measure of activity or injury.

s.-fast resistant to the effects of serum.

s. glutamic–oxaloacetic transaminase (SGOT) see ASPARTATE AMINOTRANSFERASE.

s. glutamic–pyruvic transaminase (SGPT) see ALANINE AMINOTRANSFERASE.

immune s. serum from an immunized animal, containing specific antibody or antibodies.

s. osmolality a measure of the number of dissolved particles per unit of water in serum. See also serum OSMOLALITY.

pooled s. the mixed serum from a number of animals.

s. protein see serum PROTEIN.

s. sickness a group of immediate or antibody-mediated hypersensitivity reactions (also referred to as type III hypersensitivities) that includes Arthus reaction, serum sickness and immune complex diseases. The pathogenesis involves formation of bulky antibody–antigen complexes in the walls of small blood vessels; the complexes fix complement and cause necrosis and thrombus formation. There is infiltration of polymorphonuclear cells from which lysosomal enzymes are released.

s.-simultaneous immunization an outdated method of vaccination, most popular at one time in the vaccination of pigs against hog cholera. Live virus and antiserum to the virus were injected into the patient simultaneously; breakdowns in the system were frequent, leading to severe outbreaks of the target disease.

s. thymic factor a humoral factor enhancing T lymphocyte responsiveness.

serumal pertaining to or formed from serum.

server a computer which can be accessed by other computers in a network and is dedicated to that task. Used widely by providers of network services. It is the critical feature, supported by imaginative software, which makes the Internet possible.

service 1. mating; the physical act of natural mating. 2. in terms of the delivery of services to animals includes surgical, pathological, clinicopathological, dispensary, radiological, anesthesiology services.

s. boots padded boots worn by mares during mating to prevent them injuring the stallion by kicking.

s. collar a broad leather pad worn over the withers by mares during mating to prevent the stallion injuring them by biting.

s. hobbles worn by mares during mating to prevent them kicking the stallion.

s. period in a controlled mating program the period during which the males are left in with the breeding females, or during which inseminations are carried out.

services per conception a measure of the fertility of a herd; the number of services required to effect a pregnancy.

serving see MATING.

serving capacity test supplementary to a physical examination of a male's genitalia and of semen, the testing of a male's capacity to mate with several females during a set test period.

sesamoid 1. denoting a small nodular bone embedded in a tendon or joint capsule. 2. a sesamoid bone. See Table 10.

carpal s. bone a small sesamoid in the tendon of the abductor pollicis longus muscle of the dog.

ectopic s. bone an anatomically inexact, and no longer used, name for ununited anconeal process.

metacarpal s. proximal sesamoid bone. See Table 10.

sesamoiditis ischemic disease of the proximal sesamoid bones in horses. Characterized by lameness, pain on deep pressure, heat and pain of the suspensory ligament.

Sesbania plant genus in the legume family Fabaceae. Annual herbaceous plants with a confused terminology but similar in their toxicity. Contain galactomannan, a toxic gum which causes diarrhea. Includes *S. cannabina*, *S. drummondii* (*S. cavanillesi*), *S. longifolia*, *S. punicea* (red or purple sesbania), *S. vesicaria* (*S. platycarpa*). Called also *Glottidium* spp., *Daubentonia* spp., rattlepod, bagpod, coffee bean, rattlebox, rattlebrush, poison bean, and many others.

sesqui- word element. [L.] *one and one-half.*

sesquiterpene common group of plant poisons, e.g. ipomeanols, ngaiones, sporidesmin, furanoid sesquiterpenes, sesquiterpene lactones.

s. lactones plant poisons found in *Geigeria*, *Hymenoxys*, *Helenium* spp., *Iphenia aucheri*, *Parthenium hysterophorus*.

Sessea brasiliensis South American plant in the family Solanaceae; causes serious losses in livestock. Poisoning characterized by hypothermia, bradycardia, incoordination, convulsions and severe liver injury. The toxic agent is thought to be a polypeptide.

sessile not pedunculated; attached by a broad base.

s. oak QUERCUS *petraea*.

s. wart without pedicle.

set-fast 1. see TYING-UP SYNDROME. 2. the area of superficial skin gangrene that develops on an acute saddle pressure sore on a horse's back.

seta a bristle. Called also chaeta.

setaceous bristle-like.

Setaria[1] a genus of filarioid worms in the family Onchocercidae found usually in the peritoneal cavity of ungulates. They cause no apparent clinical illness unless they invade abnormal tissues such as the central nervous system.

S. altaica found in the deer *Cervus canadensis asiaticus*.

S. cervi found in deer and possibly buffalo. Possibly also in the spinal cord of deer causing spinal nematodiasis.

S. congolensis found in pigs.

S. cornuta found in antelope.

S. digitata found in cattle, buffalo. May also occur in the urinary bladder in these species and in the central nervous system of sheep, goats and horses. Causes CEREBROSPINAL nematodiasis.

S. equina found in horses and in the eyes, scrotum,

pleural cavity and lungs as well as the peritoneal cavity. Found also in the eyes of cattle.

S. labiato-papillosa found in cattle, deer, giraffe, antelope.

S. marshalli found in sheep.

S. tundrae found in reindeer.

S. yehi found in deer, moose, caribou, bison.

Setaria[2] genus in the grass family Poaceae. Several cultivars are used commercially as pasture grasses; some have a high oxalate content. Acute intoxication in cattle causes hyocalcemia and nephrosis subsequently. Long-term ingestion in horses causes osteodystrophia. Includes *S. glauca, S. incrassata* (*S. porphyrantha*), *S. sphacelata* (*S. anceps, S. trinervia*).

S. lutescens is a grass with bristly seedheads and causes a traumatic stomatitis in cattle and horses. The lesions contain obvious plant fibers. Called also yellow bristle grass.

seton 1. a thin woven fabric wick, 6 in × 0.25 in, used as a primitive vaccination technique by dipping the seton in a bowl of 'vaccine', e.g. pleural exudate from a case of contagious bovine pneumonia. 2. a thread of gauze or other suture material threaded through tissue and used to keep a wound open.

Setonyx brachyurus see QUOKKA.

Setosphaeria rostrata the telomorph of the fungus *Exserohilum rostratum*.

setterwort HELLEBORUS *foetidus*.

setting 1. said of meat while it is cooling after slaughter and the processes of rigor mortis are precipitating the protein in the muscle fibers. 2. a clutch of eggs to set under a broody hen—usually 13 eggs.

'setting sun' phenomenon ventrolateral strabismus, seen in associated with lesions of the midbrain.

settlement legal term for a claim for damages resolved out of court by the defendant by making a settlement.

Seutin shears heavy duty shears for cutting plaster cast. Blades are angled to one side so that bottom, bulb-pointed blade can be inserted under plaster without the handles getting in the way.

severe a clinical qualifier that describes a disease that is so severe that it dominates all other activities.

s. combined immune deficiency disease (SCID) (syndrome) see COMBINED IMMUNE DEFICIENCY SYNDROME (DISEASE).

severity-of-disease scoring system a modification of the APACHE SYSTEM, for use in dogs.

sevoflurane a halogenated ether inhalation anesthetic.

sewage human sewage is utilized for animal husbandry purposes as a fertilizer for pastures. It may be in the form of crude sewage or as the sediment in settling tanks. It may cause cadmium or lead poisoning, or spread infectious disease, e.g. salmonellosis.

crude s. has caused goiter in the calves of cows grazing the pasture.

s. sludge the sediment of sewage collected in settling tanks.

sewejaartjie [Af.] HELICHRYSUM *argyrosphaerum*.

sex 1. the fundamental distinction, found in most species of animals and plants, based on the type of gametes produced by the individual or the category to which the individual fits on the basis of that criterion. Ova, or macrogametes, are produced by the female, and spermatozoa, or microgametes, are produced by the male. The union of these distinctive germ cells results in the production of a new individual in sexual reproduction. 2. to determine the sex of an animal.

s. cell see GERM cell, GAMETE.

s. chromatin the persistent mass of chromatin situated at the periphery of the nucleus in cells of normal females; it is the material of the inactivated sex chromosome. Called also Barr body.

chromosomal s. sex as determined by the presence of the XX (female) or the XY (male) genotype in somatic cells, without regard to phenotypic manifestations. Called also genetic sex.

s. chromosomes see sex CHROMOSOMES.

s. determination 1. the change in the fetus to a male or female configuration; the process by which the sex of an organism is fixed, associated, in animals, with the presence or absence of the Y chromosome. 2. diagnosis of the sex of the fetus before birth performed by examination of fetal fluids obtained by amniocentesis.

s. determining region of Y a single gene responsible for determining the sex of an animal.

s. drive see LIBIDO.

endocrinological s. the phenotypic manifestations of sex determined by endocrine influences, such as mammary development, etc.

genetic s. chromosomal sex.

s. glands in the male includes the prostate, seminal vesicles, ampullae and bulbourethral glands; in the female includes ovaries.

gonadal s. the sex as determined on the basis of the gonadal tissue present (ovarian or testicular).

s. hormones glandular secretions involved in the regulation of sexual functions. The principal sex hormone in the male is TESTOSTERONE, produced by the testes. In the female the principal sex hormones are the ESTROGENS and PROGESTERONE, produced by the ovaries.

These hormones influence the secondary sex characters, such as the shape and contour of the body and head, mammary development and the pitch of the voice. The male hormones stimulate production of spermatozoa, and the female hormones control ovulation, pregnancy and the estral cycle.

sex-linkage includes X-linked (much the most common) and Y-linked loci.

sex-linked inheritance see sex-linkage (above).

morphological s. sex determined on the basis of the morphology of the external genitals.

neutrophil s. lobe see DRUMSTICK lobe.

nuclear s. the sex as determined on the basis of the presence or absence of sex chromatin in somatic cells, its presence normally indicating the XX (female) genotype, and its absence the XY (male) genotype.

s. parity see sex ratio (below).

s. pheromone see PHEROMONE.

s. ratio proportion of female to male births.

s. reversal the sexual condition of animals in which gonadal sex and chromosomal sex are dissimilar.

s. steroids steroidal compounds acting as hormones in reproductive processes; the principal ones are estrogen, progesterone, testosterone.

sex-associated said of diseases that are predisposed to or affected in their severity by the sex of the patient.

sex-conditioned sex-influenced.

sex-cord stromal tumor ovarian tumors of granulosa and thecal cells and their luteinized forms.

sex-influenced denoting an autosomal trait that is expressed differently, either in frequency or degree, in males and females.

sex-limited affecting individuals of one sex only.

sex-linked determined by a gene located on a sex chromosome. Although a trait may be X-linked or Y-linked, virtually all clinically significant sex-linked traits are transmitted by genes located on the X chromosome; therefore, the terms sex-linked and X-linked are used synonymously. See also sex-linked GENE.

sexing see CHICKEN sexing.

sextan recurring on the sixth day (every 5 days).

sexual pertaining to sex.

s. behavior includes masturbation, courtship, mating, estral display.

s. cycle estral cycle.

s. differentiation identification of the sex of a patient is done usually by an examination of external genitalia; preparation and examination of a karyotype is the preferred laboratory method.

s. dimorphism differences in structure or physical characteristics between males and females of the same species, e.g. horns in some breeds of sheep, feather coat color in many species of birds.

s. intercourse see MATING.

s. maturity capable of mating. Occurs at different ages in different species and in different races and even breeds.

s. receptivity behavioral changes in female animals at the time of estrus; involves acceptance of male efforts at copulation and, in some species, actively seeking the male.

s. rest circumstances in which no sexual intercourse takes place.

Seymour Jones disinfection method a method used in the disinfection of hides. Consists of immersion in a solution of 1:5000 solution of bichloride of mercury plus 1% formic acid for 24 hours.

Sézary syndrome an exfoliative erythroderma due to cutaneous infiltration of reticular lymphocytes, with alopecia, edema and hyperkeratosis; believed to be a variant of MYCOSIS fungoides. This condition of humans is similar to the epidermotropic form of cutaneous lymphoma which occurs in dogs. The Sézary cell is a characteristic cerebriform lymphocyte which occurs in the dermis and blood of patients with Sézary syndrome. It has a distinctive markedly convoluted nuclear membrane.

SG specific gravity.

SGOT serum glutamic–oxaloacetic transaminase; see ASPARTATE AMINOTRANSFERASE.

SGPT serum glutamic–pyruvic transaminase; see ALANINE AMINOTRANSFERASE.

SGPV sheep and goat pox virus.

SH sulfhydryl.

shackle a bar 2.5 ft long with an iron loop at either end, used in restraint of large pigs. A chain is threaded through the loops and around the lower hindlimbs of the pig. When the chain is pulled the pig is stretched and is cast with the limbs held wide apart.

A similar device is used in the abattoir to lift the live pig before it is slaughtered and scalded.

shackling see SHACKLE.

shadow-casting application of a coating of gold, chromium, or other metal for the purpose of increasing contrast and thereby the visibility of ultramicroscopic specimens under the electron microscope. The heavy metal is evaporated under vacuum and deposited on the surface of the specimen.

shadow cell one that appears in a section only as an outline. Called also ghost cell.

shadow roll a thick roll of material, usually sheepskin, worn on the nose band of a bridle while racing to avoid having the horse shy at a shadow on the ground.

shadow test see RETINOSCOPY.

shadowgram the shades of gray at the edge of an image on a radiograph. They are the features that the expert can interpret; they define the silhouette of the object being imaged.

shaft a long slender part, such as the portion of a long bone between the wider ends or extremities, the shaft of a hair and the central shaft of a feather.

s. louse see MENOPON *gallinae*.

shafty said of wool in which the staples are long, wide and thick.

shag see CORMORANT.

shaggy heart see COR villosum.

shaker calf syndrome inherited degenerative disease of spinal cord in Hereford and Holstein–Friesian cattle characterized by neonatal tremor, paresis, spastic gait, aphonia, terminal spastic paraplegia.

shaker dogs a syndrome of generalized muscle tremors, aggravated by excitement or handling, seen most often in young, mature dogs of the West Highland White and Maltese breeds. The cause is unknown but an acquired immunological disease involving cells that metabolize tyrosine to produce neurotransmitting substances is suspected. Called also generalized tremor syndrome.

shaker foals a disease of young foals characterized by inability to stand up and gross muscle tremor if lifted. The foal is bright and alert but dies in about 72 hours. The cause is unknown.

shaker pigs see CONGENITAL TREMOR SYNDROME.

shaking pup a term used to describe the severe tremors observed in very young English springer spaniel puppies affected with X-linked hypomyelinogenesis.

sham drinking the phenomenon of an animal constantly playing with its drinking water but drinking little. A common sign in a horse with colic.

sham feeding intake of food by an animal with a surgically created esophageal fistula that prevents the ingested food from reaching the stomach. Used in studies of physiological and psychological mechanisms of hunger and feeding behavior.

sham urination most apparent in horses which stretch out to urinate, males relax the penis but urine is not passed; common sign in subacute colic. There is no grunting or straining to pass urine as there is in urethral obstruction.

shampoo a cleaning agent, usually liquid, for hair; usually consists of a detergent and perfume. Some, usually referred to as medicated shampoos, contain therapeutic substances such as parasiticides, antimicrobials, ketatolytic agents, and antiseborrheic compounds such as selenium sulfide.

shank 1. the tibia or shin; a leglike part. In the dog fancy, shank refers to the hindlimb between the hip and stifle. 2. the lead part of a halter.

shankings wool, usually containing hair fibers, from below the knees and hocks.

Shar pei a medium-sized, compact dog with distinctive, loose skin that forms many deep wrinkles over the entire body, particularly on the large head. The ears are small and the small eyes are almost hidden in the skin folds. There are two types of coat; one is very short and harsh, the other is slighty longer and brushy. The breed is predisposed to a variety of skin disorders and entropion, all associated with the skin folds.

share-farm a common form of farm lease arrangement; the land-owner leases the grazing and cropping rights to his land, natural resources and usually facilities including house, hay shed, milking parlor, in return for a share in the income of the enterprise.

Sharlea a type of sheep, called after a locality in Australia where they were developed by the Sharlea Sheep Society. The sheep are superfine Merinos with an average fiber diameter of less than 17 microns. The sheep are kept indoors at all times and are usually clad in nylon coats to minimize contamination of the wool that is used in the manufacture of superior garment fabrics.

sharp freezers freezing chambers for meat preservation which operate at lower temperatures than the average freezer, i.e. at 0°F (−18°C).

Sharpey's fibers see Sharpey's FIBERS.

sharps 1. needles, scalpel blades, broken ampoules; anything in a hospital or clinic which has been used on patients, and which may be contaminated with infectious material; to be discarded into special containers for disposal without any risk to disposal personnel. 2. see CALKINS.

Shattenfroh method a method for disinfecting hides; the hides are soaked in a solution of 2% hydrochloric acid and 10% sodium chloride for 48 hours.

shavings curly wafers of wood produced when trimming wood with a plane; used as bedding for horses. See also SAWDUST.

SHBG sex hormone-binding globulin.

shear 1. to remove the fleece of a sheep. 2. pressure on a mass in such a way that planes within it are pressured to move in a direction parallel to the pressure. Any movement is proportional to the distance from the plane at which movement occurs.

s. injury injury to tissues caused by shear pressure. See SHEARING injuries (2).

s. stress the stress to which a tissue is subjected by a shear force without injury actually occurring.

shearer person whose occupation is shearing sheep.

shearing 1. mechanical removal of the sheep's fleece. A traumatic event in the sheep's annual calendar. A time for the transmission of diseases between sheep, e.g. mycotic dermatitis, caseous lymphadenitis, infection with environmental infections, e.g. gas gangrene, tetanus, and for exposure to inclement weather without the protection of a fleece.

CHEMICAL shearing, the shedding of the fleece after administration of a chemical agent, is in the very early stages of exploration. Automatic shearing done by robots is perhaps a little closer. Breeding of sheep which shed their fleece annually is always a good cause for a research program. The Wiltshire horned breed does this to a varying degree. 2. a type of injury. See shearing injuries (below).

s. board open area in a shearing shed on which the sheep are restrained while they are shorn.

s. hypothermia see HYPOTHERMIA.

s. injuries 1. injuries inflicted to a sheep during shearing and by the shearing machine. Lacerations are frequent but cause little damage if they do not become infected. They appear to cause no discomfort and heal very quickly. The serious injuries are the removal of teats in ewes, damage to the prepuce and removal of the tip of the vulva. The last two lead to deviation of the stream of urine, fouling of the nearby fleece and increased risk of blowfly strike. 2. injuries in which there is the application of a shearing force tending to cause local deformity or diplacement; usually involve the carpus or tarsus in small animals hit by motor vehicles. There is extensive loss of soft tissues and bone, with exposure of the joint.

shearmouth the state of the molar teeth when occlusion is poor leading to wear in such a way that the teeth pass each other like the blades of a pair of shears. Most common in horses.

shears cutting instruments for the removal of wool—sheep shears, or for trimming the hooves of sheep and goats—hoof shears.

hoof s. a rugged pair of shears like secateurs but with sharp-pointed blades. The spring in the handle keeps the blades open and pressing the handles shut operates the shears.

plaster s. see PLASTER shears.

sheep s. 1. hand shears are sharp-pointed, with wide blades and have a spring at the handle which opens the blades. They have to be closed to cut the wool. 2. mechanical or power shears are driven by a rotating, flexible shaft converting to a reciprocating movement of a cutter in a comb at right angles to the shearer's hand; the cutter and comb comprise the handpiece.

sheath 1. a tubular case or envelope. 2. vernacular for prepuce.

adrenal pericapsular s. contains a plexus of large nerve trunks with numerous ganglion cells.

arachnoid s. the delicate membrane between the pial sheath and the dural sheath of the optic nerve.

carotid s. a portion of the cervical fascia enclosing the carotid artery, internal jugular vein, and vagus or vagosympathetic nerve.

carpal tendon s's sheaths to the tendons of the muscles which course over the carpus.

crural s. femoral sheath.

dural s. the external investment of the optic nerve.

femoral s. the fascial sheath of the femoral vessels.

Henle's s. the endoneurium, especially the delicate continuation around the terminal branches of nerve fibers.

lamellar s. the perineurium.

medullary s., myelin s. the sheath surrounding the axon of myelinated nerve cells, consisting of concentric layers of myelin formed in the peripheral nervous system by the plasma membrane of Schwann cells, and in the central nervous system by the plasma membrane of oligodendrocytes. It is interrupted at intervals along the length of the axon by gaps known as *nodes of Ranvier.* Myelin is an electrical insulator that serves to speed the conduction of nerve impulses.

pial s. the innermost of the three sheaths of the optic nerve.

root s. the epidermal layer of a hair follicle.

s. of Schwann neurilemma.

synovial s. a synovial membrane sleeve through which a tendon moves; found commonly where a tendon passes over a joint.

sheath rot see ENZOOTIC balanoposthitis.

Sheather's flotation method a method for examining feces for the presence of worm eggs or larvae by mixing with a saturated solution of sodium chloride or sugar and collecting a sample from the top of a column for microscopic examination.

shechita, shehita the Jewish method of ritual slaughter in which the animal is killed by one stroke of a very sharp knife across the throat, completely severing the trachea, carotid arteries and jugular veins. Called also schechita.

shed rural building used for agricultural pursuits.

s. hands miscellaneous workers in a shearing shed at shearing time, i.e. persons other than the shearers, wool classers.

s. lambing a system of indoor lambing for ewes which normally run at pasture so that the lambs have protection against the inclemency of the weather and where close observation can be maintained over every ewe. The ewes are brought in when they are individually on the point of lambing and moved out as soon as the ewe–lamb bond is established and the lamb is vigorous, usually 24 hours.

shearing s. contains a shearing 'board' supplied with a number of 'stands' which are locations for shearing machines. The sheep are shorn on the 'board' and are pushed out through small doors down chutes into counting pens where they are held until a sufficient group is accumulated. In the shed the sheep to be shorn are held in catching pens. The shed is usually large enough to hold several hundred sheep overnight so that there will be some dry sheep for the morning. The shorn wool is classed and packed into bales in the shed which is usually high off the ground; the droppings fall through the slatted floor.

s. sheet standard recording medium for dairy cow reproductive data—a structured cardboard poster pinned on the wall of the milking shed. Replaced in some sheds by a computer terminal.

shedding 1. exfoliation of entire skin, called also ecdysis, exuviate. 2. falling out of haircoat. 3. putting animals into a shed. 4. excretion of an infectious agent from the body of an infected host.

s. agent an agent, e.g. a wild animal, shedding an infectious agent.

sheep member of the species *Ovis aries*. They are classified into several types including merino, shortwool meat breeds, longwool, carpetwool, fat-tail, wool-shedding, Karakul. All domesticated types are characterized by a wool fleece.

Bighorn s. see BIGHORN SHEEP.

carpetwool s. includes BLACKFACED MOUNTAIN, CARPETMASTER, DRYSDALE, ELLIOTTDALE and TUKIDALE.

Dall s. see DALL SHEEP.

s. dog see SHEPHERD DOGS.

s. dip see DIP.

dual-purpose s. breeds generated to provide meat and wool. Include CHAROLLAISE, CORRIEDALE, CORMO, DORMER, GROMARK, PERENDALE, POLWARTH, ZENITH.

easy-care s. see EASY-CARE SHEEP.

fat-tailed s. see FAT-TAILED SHEEP.

s.–goat hybrid mating and fertilization can be achieved but the fetus dies early or is aborted.

s. itch mite see PSORERGATES *ovis*.

s. ked see MELOPHAGUS *ovinus*.

s. loco ASTRAGALUS *nothoxys*.

s. measles see ovine CYSTICERCOSIS.

meat s. includes English Longwool breeds (see under wool sheep below) and shortwool or Downs sheep, e.g. SOUTHDOWN, SUFFOLK, HAMPSHIRE, OXFORD DOWN, DORSET HORN, POLL DORSET, RYELAND, SHROPSHIRE and CHAROLLAISE, CHEVIOT, CLUN FOREST, COLBRED, COLUMBIA, COOPWORTH, DORMER, DORPER, many indigenous fat-tailed and fat-rumped breeds, FINNISH-LANDRACE, NORTH RONALDSAY, WENSLEYDALE.

s. nasal bot OESTRUS *ovis*.

s. pox see SHEEPPOX.

s.-scab see PSOROPTIC MANGE.

s. sorrel RUMEX *acetosella*.

s. tick sheep ked. See MELOPHAGUS *ovinus*.

wool s. includes AUSTRALIAN merino (including a wide range of strains and types especially BOOROOLA and COMEBACK), CORMO, CORRIEDALE, POLWARTH, SHARLEA, AMERICAN RAMBOUILLET and English Longwools such as LINCOLN, LEICESTER, BORDER LEICESTER, CHEVIOT, COOPWORTH, ROMNEY MARSH.

sheep-associated bovine malignant catarrah virus see BOVINE malignant catarrah.

sheep-head fly see HYDROTOEA *irritans*.

sheepdog any of various breeds of dogs produced to help manage sheep flocks. Three general types, the herding breeds that bring sheep to the operator, e.g. Border collie, the huntaway breeds that move sheep ahead, e.g. kelpie, and the guarding types that protect the flock from predators, e.g. Komondor.

sheepkill KALMIA *angustifolia*.

sheeppox a highly contagious, generalized disease of sheep caused by a poxvirus in the genus *Capripoxvirus* and characterized by the presence of typical pox lesions on the unwoolled skin, especially under the tail. Most recover. A much more lethal, generalized disease that resembles smallpox in its pathogenicity occurs in lambs with many dying and showing lesions in the bowel and respiratory system. A number of isolates have distinctive geographic distribution, but are indistinguishable serologically. These include Kenya and Middle East strains.

sheepshead see PROBATOCEPHALY.

sheet feeder a device fitted to a printer which feeds single sheets or envelopes into the printer one at a time.

shell disease 1. pitting of the shell of crustaceans initially due to a chitinoclastic *Vibrio* spp. 2. proliferative disease of oysters caused by an uncharacterized fungus.

shell rot softening and ulceration of the carapace and plastron of softshell turtles caused by the bacteria *Beneckea chitinovora*. Called also rust, ulcerative shell disease.

shellfish an aquatic animal having a shell; includes molluscs, e.g. oyster, and crustaceans, e.g. shrimp, lobster.

paralytic s. poisoning see PARALYTIC shellfish poisoning.

shellgrit crushed shells of marine crustaceans; mined on ocean beaches where the animals are prolific. Used in rations for birds, especially domesticated cage birds.

shelly thin, hollow, brittle.

s. hoof extensive separation of the hoof wall from underlying tissue in contagious footrot in sheep.

sheltie, shelty a common name for the Shetland sheepdog.

s. eye anomaly (SEA) see COLLIE eye anomaly.

s. syndrome see EPIDERMOLYSIS bullosa.

shepherd dogs any of several dog breeds used in working sheep (sheepdogs), but most commonly applied to the German shepherd dog. See also SHEEPDOG.

Shepherd's crook explorer a handheld instrument used to detect subgingival cavities and calculus, and to detect erosive lesions of the tooth surface.

Sherman bone plate the plate is narrowed in the spaces between the screw holes so that it has approximately the same strength at every point.

Shetland pony miniature or dwarf Scottish pony, most commonly black and dark brown, but can be any color, including broken colors; 9.2 to 10.2 hands high. Its most common use is as a child's pony, as depicted in Thelwell's fabulous cartoons.

Shetland sheepdog a small (13–16 inches tall), alert dog with abundant, medium-length haircoat that forms a thick 'mane' around the neck. It may be black and while, black and tan, blue merle, sable or tricolor (black, tan and white). The head is long, narrow and flat in profile with small ears that fold over at the tips. The dog looks like a collie in miniature. The breed is predisposed to collie eye anomaly, retinal atrophy, hemophilia, nasal solar dermatitis and iris heterochromia. Called also sheltie, shelty.

Shiba Inu the smallest (20–30 lb) of the Japanese

native dogs, it was bred as a hunting dog. A medium-sized, muscular dog with a thick coat in all solid colors but often red. See also NIPPON INU.

shift a change or deviation.

antigenic s. see ANTIGENIC shift.

chloride s. see CHLORIDE shift.

s. to the left an alteration in the distribution of leukocytes in the peripheral blood in which there is an increase in the numbers of immature neutrophils, primarily band forms but metamyelocytes or more immature cells may also be present; usually in response to an infection.

s. red cell see MACRORETICULOCYTE.

s. to the right an alteration in the distribution of leukocytes in the peripheral blood in which there is an increased number of mature neutrophils but no immature cells are present.

shiga-like toxins toxins produced by certain strains of *Escherichia coli* which disrupt the function of the ribosome. Responsible for the lesions seen in edema disease in pigs, hemolytic uremic syndrome in humans and dogs. Called also verotoxin and vero cytotoxin.

Shigella a genus of gram-negative rods in the family Enterobacteriaceae. There are four subgroups or species. The type species, *S. dysenteriae*, causes bacillary dysentery in humans and nonhuman primates. Other animals are resistant to infection, but organisms have been isolated from dogs without clinical signs.

shigella pl. *shigellae;* any individual organism of the genus *Shigella.*

shigellosis an acute highly fatal septicemia of very young foals, caused by *Actinobacillus equuli* and characterized by fever, prostration, diarrhea and dyspnea. The presence of minute abscesses in the renal cortex is confirmatory.

Shih tzu a small (9–16 lb), lively dog with a very short muzzle, broad, round head, large, prominent eyes and short eyes. The coat is long, straight and flowing in a variety of colors with a white blaze on the face and a white tip on the tail. Called also Chrysanthemum-faced dog. The breed is predisposed to cleft palate and a familial renal cortical hypoplasia.

shin in horses, the large metacarpal and metatarsal bones, especially the dorsal surface.

bucked s's see sore shins (below).

sore s's periostitis of the shins seen most commonly in 2- and 3-year-old thoroughbreds in hard training, mostly in the forelimbs. The horse is lame and worsens with work. In severe cases an enlargement is visible.

shin oak QUERCUS *havardii.*

Shine–Dalgarno sequence part of the leader sequence preceding the start codon of mRNA that is AGGAGGU or a variant thereof that binds the mRNA to a complementary sequence in the 16S component of rRNA so that translation of the mRNA can proceed.

shingle tick see DERMACENTOR *albipictus.*

shinnery oak QUERCUS *havardii.*

shipping 1. movement of any livestock to packing plant or feedlot; usually refers to long distance transport by rail. 2. slang phrase for sale to market or packing plant for immediate slaughter. The choice for the outcome in a damaged animal may be to treat or ship.

s. fever see BOVINE respiratory disease; EQUINE influenza.

shippon a stable used for the housing of farm animals.

Shire a massive English draft-horse, 17 to 18 hands high, bay, brown, black, gray, white markings commonly with dark colors; long feather on legs.

Shirley drain surgical drain; see DRAIN.

Shirodkar technique a surgical procedure for the correction of cervical incompetence in the mare. Uses a strap of fascia lata buried under the mucosa.

shiver involuntary shaking of the body, as with cold. It is caused by contraction or twitching of the muscles, and is a physiological method of heat production in all animals.

shivering see SHIVER, STRINGHALT.

shochet the operant slaughterer in the Jewish method.

shock a condition of acute peripheral circulatory failure due to derangement of circulatory control or loss of circulating fluid. It is marked by hypotension, coldness of the skin and tachycardia.

allergic s. see ANAPHYLACTIC shock.

s. bodies hyaline globules composed of fibrin degradation products which act as microthrombi and cause hemorrhage and necrosis.

burn s. the loss and redistribution of fluid, electrolytes and plasma protein, increased blood viscosity and increased peripheral resistance that follow a severe burn contribute to shock.

cardiogenic s. classically associated with acute myocardial infarction in humans; in animals may be caused by intrinsic congestive heart failure, cardiac depression caused by anesthetic overdosage or other drugs with negative inotropism, rarely, thromboembolism.

colloidoclastic s. shock due to breakdown of the physical equilibrium of the body colloids. Thought to cause anaphylactic shock due to the absorption of the colloids into the bloodstream.

distributive s. see vasogenic shock (below).

electric s. see ELECTRICAL injuries.

electroplectic s. electric shock. See also ELECTRICAL stunning.

endotoxic s. caused by endotoxins, especially *Escherichia coli.* See also TOXEMIC shock.

s. gut animals in shock develop changes in the gut including congestion and hemorrhage into the lumen.

hypovolemic s. shock due to reduced blood volume as a result of water deprivation, fluid loss due to diarrhea, vomiting, extensive burns, intestinal obstruction, whole blood loss.

insulin s. a condition of circulatory insufficiency resulting from overdosage with insulin, which causes too sudden reduction of blood sugar. It is marked by tremor, weakness, convulsions and collapse.

irreversible s. shock which has reached the stage where irreparable damage has been done to tissues, e.g. liver, kidneys and treatment will not salvage the patient although it might prolong life for a long time.

s. lung animals in shock due to massive burns, septicemia, disseminated intravascular coagulation (DIC), acute viral or bacterial pneumonias or trauma develop an acute respiratory distress syndrome. The pulmonary lesion is a nonspecific acute or subacute interstitial pneumonia.

nervous s. a temporary cessation of function in nervous tissue caused by an acute insult such as trauma without the part having been directly or detectably damaged. The loss of function is only temporary, usually for a few minutes but it may last for several hours. There may be residual signs due to direct damage when the shock passes. Stunning by a lightning stroke is an example.

s. organs those organs, specific to each animal

species, which respond to allergens circulating in the blood.

septic s. see TOXEMIC shock.

spinal s. flaccid paralysis up and down the body from the site of the spinal cord lesion. Accompanied by a fall in skin temperature, vasodilatation and sweating. Signs disappear within an hour or two. There may be residual signs due to physical injury to tissue.

toxic s. see TOXEMIC shock.

vasogenic s., vasculogenic s. shock exists because of the severe reduction in effective circulating blood volume caused by sequestration of blood and other fluids in the vascular system and their withdrawal from the circulating blood. Is the classical shock of traumatic injury, burns, uterine prolapse, extensive surgery.

shoe a foot covering; see HORSESHOEING.

s. covers protective coverings for shoes worn by surgical personnel working in a sterile environment in order to minimize contamination.

shoeing the application of metal shoes; a universal practice in horses. Hot shoeing with shoes made by the local blacksmith has been superseded by machine made shoes fitted cold—cold shoeing. In draft cattle small shoes are applied to each claw. See also HORSESHOEING.

Shohl's solution a solution containing 140 g citric acid and 98 g hydrated crystalline salt of sodium citrate, distilled water to make 1000 ml; used to correct electrolyte imbalance in the treatment of renal tubular acidosis.

shomer slaughterer's assistant and stamper of the carcass in the Jewish ritual slaughter procedure.

Shope named after R. E. Shope, American virologist.

S. fibroma see Shope rabbit FIBROMA.

S. papilloma caused by a papilloma virus and manifested by gray to black, tall, thin, horny structures on the skin of wild rabbits. The lesions may be on the head, neck, shoulders, abdomen and inside the thighs. The disease is transmissible.

shore thistle see CARDUUS.

short-bowel syndrome any of the malabsorption conditions resulting from massive resection of the small bowel, the degree and kind of malabsorption depending on the site and extent of the resection; it is characterized by diarrhea, steatorrhea and malnutrition.

short-coupled the animal has a short coupling and therefore a compact, usually well-muscled trunk; a prized conformation in a working horse.

short-crowned milkweed ASCLEPIAS *brachystephana*.

short feed see SHORT KEEP.

short hair syndrome a disease of Yorkshire and Australian silky terriers in which the normal, long coat is replaced by a shorter coat with no abnormality in the appearance of the skin. The cause is unknown.

short keep said of steers in a feedlot when they are expected to be fattened for 140 days or less. Called also short feed.

short-nosed cattle lice see HAEMATOPINUS *eurysternus*.

short rotation rye grass SECALE *cereale* var. *rosen*.

short-tailed a group of breeds of sheep characterized by naturally short tails. It includes the Heath and Marsh breeds of Europe, many Indian and Pakistani breeds, and others of the Indian subcontinent.

short-tailed shearwater *Puffinus tenuirostris*.

short-term behavior patterns behavior patterns which occur for short periods only, e.g. sunset and sunrise eating times, nocturnal estrus display, evening running in feedlot steers and other daily, or at shorter time intervals, activities have a considerable effect on productivity and disease wastage.

short thermal test subcutaneous injection of tuberculin in an animal with tuberculosis results in an abrupt hyperthermia 6 to 8 hours later. Occasional cows die of what appears to be an anaphylactic reaction.

short-woolled a class of sheep with short fleece wool, e.g. Southdown, Ryeland, Dorset Horn, the Downs breeds.

Shorthorn a breed of red, red-roan, white, red and white, roan and white dual-purpose cattle. Polled varieties exist. Also Dairy Shorthorn, Australian Illawarra Shorthorn, Beef Shorthorn, Milking Shorthorn.

shortnosed louse see HAEMATOPINUS *eurysternus*.

shorts see POLLARD.

shot 1. lead shot may be eaten by aquatic birds in sufficient amounts to cause lead poisoning. 2. vernacular for injection.

shotgun hunting firearm discharging mostly round lead shot over a wide area. Associated with lead poisoning in ducks that eat the failed shot, pitch poisoning in animals that eat the residues of clay pigeons at shooting ranges, and sometimes wounds in dogs that have the misfortune to be in the line of fire.

s. injuries typically occur in hunting dogs. Depending on the distance from the gun, the wounds range from extensive with much tissue damage to minor, almost undetectable, with the shot becoming imbedded in soft tissue.

s. pharmacy using a number of medicines to treat an animal because of uncertainty in the diagnosis. Called also polypharmacy.

s. procedure cloning DNA fragments in a random manner for a clone library from which fragments can later be selected.

shotty eruption round, cystic papules around the tailhead and buttocks of pigs. The lesions are in sweat glands and are thought to be caused by *Eimeria fusca*, a protozoan parasite.

shoulder the region around the large joint between the humerus and the scapula. The shoulder is a shallow ball-and-socket joint, similar to the hip joint.

s. blade scapula.

s. flexion a fetal postural cause of dystokia; flexion of the shoulder joint results in the affected forelimb, it may be bilateral, is lying back beside the sternum; the shoulder joint prevents entry of the fetus into the pelvic canal.

s. joint scapulohumeral joint.

s. luxation uncommon in most species. Occurs most frequently in dogs and cats associated with trauma.

slipped s. see SUPRASCAPULAR paralysis.

s. tick see IXODES *scapularis*.

shovel beak a disease of young chickens up to 8 weeks old characterized by deformity of the beak and caused by feeding on dry mash. There may be secondary infection with *Fusobacterium necrophorum*.

showy milkweed ASCLEPIAS *speciosa*.

shrew a small, 2 to 3 inches long, pointed-nosed, insectivorous mammal which has a moderately long tail and a very savage disposition. They are members of the family Soricidae and there are a large number of species including the common shrew (*Sorex araneus*).

s. virus a rhabdovirus with some antigenic relationship to rabies virus.

shrimp *Artemia*, *Penaeus* spp. See Table 23.

shrink in carcasses loss of weight of carcass, due to loss of fluids, from time of slaughter to sale.

shrinkage 1. a characteristic of freshly killed meat. Weight loss occurs because of evaporation of moisture from cut surfaces. Humidity of the chilling chamber determines how much shrinkage there is. 2. loss of body weight when live animals are exposed to bad weather, deprivation of feed and water, transportation or mixing with another group.

Shropshire an type of English DOWNS SHEEP. It has short wool, and is used mainly for meat; it has a black-brown face and legs.

***shu* points** see ASSOCIATION points.

shuffling gait short, uncertain steps, with minimal flexion and toes dragging.

shunt 1. to turn to one side; to divert; to bypass. 2. a passage or anastomosis between two natural channels, especially between blood vessels. Such structures may be formed physiologically (e.g. to bypass a thrombosis), or they may be structural anomalies. 3. a surgical anastomosis.

arteriovenous (A-V) s. a U-shaped or straight tube inserted between an artery and a vein (usually between the radial artery and cephalic vein), bypassing the capillary network; commonly done to allow repeated access to the arterial system for the purpose of HEMODIALYSIS.

cardiovascular s. an abnormality of the blood flow between the sides of the heart or between the systemic and pulmonary circulation; see left-to-right shunt (below) and right-to-left shunt (below).

left-to-right s. diversion of blood from the left side of the heart to the right side, or from the systemic to the pulmonary circulation through an anomalous opening such as a septal defect or patent ductus arteriosus.

LeVeen s. a device whose purpose is to remove excess ascitic fluid from the peritoneal cavity and return it to the venous system. Called also peritoneal-venous shunt.

peritoneal-venous s. see LeVeen shunt (above).

portacaval s., postcaval s. see PORTACAVAL shunt.

reversed s. right-to-left shunt.

right-to-left s. diversion of blood from the right side of the heart to the left side or from the pulmonary to the systemic circulation through an anomalous opening such as septal defect or patent ductus arteriosus.

ventriculovenous s. a surgical procedure used in the treatment of hydrocephalus.

shunted blood blood that has not been fully exposed to the oxygenation and carbon dioxide removal systems.

shuttle the transport of electrons or organic groups across biological membranes.

s. system means of transfer of reducing equivalents as NADH and H+ from the cytosol to mitochondria. The two main systems are: α-glycerophosphate shuttle and malate-aspartate shuttle.

shuttle pin a pin for internal fixation of a fractured long bone. See also LEIGHTON PIN.

shuttle programs programs for providing coccidiostats to poultry and avoiding breakdowns as a consequence because of the development of resistance to the agent. The coccidiostat is changed during the course of a feeding program to one batch of chickens.

Shwartzman phenomenon, Shwartzman reaction, Shwartzman–Sanarelli reaction a reaction to a second dose of bacterial endotoxin. It may be a local tissue reaction characterized by thrombosis, infarction and hemorrhagic necrosis, or generalized with disseminated intravascular coagulation and bilateral renal cortical necrosis.

shy timid.

s. breeder difficult to get pregnant because of timid disposition and disinclination to copulate.

s. feeder fussy, finicky eater; difficult to get to eat a full feed.

shying taking fright easily; said of horses that are startled easily and inclined to take a great leap sideways or to bolt with little provocation.

Si chemical symbol, *silicon.*

SI units the units of measurement generally accepted for all scientific and technical uses. Together they make up the International System of Units. The abbreviation SI, from the French *Système International d'Unités*, is used in all languages. There are seven base SI units, defined by specified physical measurements and two supplementary units. Units are derived for any other physical quantities by multiplication and division of the base and supplementary units. The derived units with special names are shown in Table 3.

SI is a *coherent* system. This means that units are always combined without conversion factors. The derived unit of velocity is the meter per second (m/s); the derived unit of volume is the cubic meter (m^3). If you know that pressure is force per unit area, then you know that the SI unit of pressure (the pascal) is the unit of force divided by the unit of area and is therefore equal to 1 newton per square meter.

The metric prefixes can be attached to any unit in order to make a unit of a more convenient size. The symbol for the prefix is attached to the symbol for the unit, e.g. nanometer (nm) = 10^{-9} m. The units of mass are specified in terms of the gram, e.g. microgram (μg) = 10^{-9} kg.

Only one prefix is used with a unit. The use of units such as the millimicrometer is no longer acceptable. When a unit is raised to a power, the power applies to the prefix as well, e.g. a cubic millimeter (mm^3) = 10^{-9} m^3. When a prefix is used with a ratio unit, it should be in the numerator rather than in the denominator, e.g. kilometers/second (km/s) rather than meters/millisecond (m/ms). Only prefixes denoting powers of 10^3 are normally used. Hecto-, deka-, deci- and centi- are usually attached only to the metric system units, gram, meter and liter.

Owing to the force of tradition, one noncoherent unit, the liter, equal to 10^{-3} m^3 or 1 dm^3, is generally accepted for use with SI. The internationally accepted abbreviation for liter is the letter l; however, this can be confused with the numeral 1 in typescript. For this reason, the capital letter L is also sometimes used as a symbol for liter. The lower case letter is generally used with prefixes, e.g. dl, ml, fl. The symbols for all other SI units begin with a capital letter if the unit is named after a person and with a lower case letter otherwise. The name of a unit is never capitalized.

SIADH syndrome of inappropriate secretion of antidiuretic hormone.

sialadenitis inflammation of a salivary gland.

sialadenosis noninflammatory swelling of the salivary glands.

sialagogue, sialogogue an agent that stimulates the flow of saliva.

sialectasia dilatation of a salivary duct.

sialic sialagogue.

sialic acid acetylated derivative of neuraminic acid.

sialine pertaining to the saliva.

sialismus ptyalism.

sialisosis see MUCOLIPIDOSIS.

sialitis inflammation of a salivary gland or duct; in guinea pigs may be caused by a cytomegalovirus.

sial(o)- word element. [Gr.] *saliva, salivary glands.*
sialoadenectomy excision of a salivary gland.
sialoadenitis inflammation of a salivary gland.
sialoadenotomy incision of a salivary gland.
sialoaerophagia the swallowing of saliva and air.
sialoangiectasis dilatation of a salivary duct.
sialoangiitis inflammation of a salivary duct.
sialoangiography radiography of the ducts of the salivary glands after injection of radiopaque material.
sialocele a salivary cyst.
sialodacryoadenitis severe, transient inflammation of the salivary and ophthalmic glands in suckling rats caused by a coronavirus. Affected animals have exophthalmos, swelling of the face and neck and red pigmentation around the eyes. There may be a secondary conjunctivitis and keratitis.
sialodentitis inflammation of salivary glands.
sialodochitis inflammation of a salivary duct.
sialodochoplasty plastic repair of a salivary duct.
sialoductitis sialoangiitis.
sialogen an agent that induces salivation.
sialogenous producing saliva.
sialogram a film obtained by sialography.
sialography radiographic demonstration of the salivary ducts by means of the injection of substances opaque to x-rays.
sialolith a salivary calculus.
sialolithiasis the formation of salivary calculi.
sialolithotomy excision of a salivary calculus.
sialomucin an acid mucopolysaccharide containing sialic acid, a component of airway secretions of the lungs.
sialoprotein glycoproteins containing sialic acid.
sialorrhea ptyalism.
sialoschesis suppression of secretion of saliva.
sialosis 1. the flow of saliva. 2. ptyalism.
sialostenosis stenosis of a salivary duct.
sialosyrinx 1. salivary fistula. 2. a syringe for washing out the salivary ducts, or a drainage tube for the salivary ducts.
siamang an anthropoid ape of the genus *Hylobates;* one of the heavier gibbons.
Siamese cat a medium-sized, svelte breed of domestic cats with blue eyes, and short hair with a distinctive pattern of pigmentation. Due to the presence of a color-limiting gene, the body is lightly pigmented while the face, ears, tail and legs are more intensely colored. The distribution corresponds to differences in skin temperature so that only in cooler areas is pigmentation fully developed. Several color varieties exist including seal-point (dark brown), blue, lilac, chocolate, red, tabby, cream and tortie. Siamese are also renowned for their loud, often demanding, manner of vocalizing. The breed is affected by mucopolysaccharidosis and sphingomyelinosis.
  S. c. disease sometimes used to refer to nutritional secondary HYPERPARATHYROIDISM because of the prevalence of that disease in this breed; breed predisposition, however, has not been proven.
Siamese fighting fish see BETTA SPLENDENS.
Siamese twins identical (monozygotic) twins joined together at birth. The connection may be slight or extensive. It involves skin and usually muscles or cartilage of a limited region, such as the head, chest, hip or buttock. The twins may share a single organ, such as an intestine, or occasionally may have parts of the spine in common. A rare congenital malformation in animals. Called also conjoined twins.
sib 1. a blood relative; one of a group of animals all descended from a common ancestor. 2. sibling.
  half-s. see half SIBLING.
  s. mating brother mated to sister.
Siberian a handsome breed of rabbits with distinctive rollback or blanket fur which looks as though it has been shorn. Its color can be black, blue or brown; its weight is about 6 lb.
Siberian husky a medium-sized (45–60 lb), muscular dog with a medium length, thick, double coat in a variety of colors and often dark markings on the head. The prominent ears are erect and the eyes are blue or brown, often not the same, and frequently show iris heterochromia. The tail is fox brush shape and usually carried over the back. Called also Arctic husky. The breed is predisposed to corneal dystrophy, cataracts and congenital laryngeal paralysis.
Siberian tick typhus a disease of humans and many species of feral mammals, especially rodents, caused by *Rickettsia siberica* and transmitted by the ticks *Dermacentor* and *Haemaphysalis.*
sibilant shrill, whistling or hissing.
sibling any of two or more offspring of the same parents; a brother or sister.
  half s. animals with only one parent in common, i.e. the same sire or dam.
sibship a group of animals born of the same parents.
sic [L.] *thus;* a parenthetical insertion in text to call attention to something anomalous which exactly reproduces the original.
siccative 1. drying; removing moisture. 2. an agent that produces drying.
siccus [L.] *dry.*
Sicilian ass an Italian donkey, almost black, with pale muzzle and belly. Can be gray.
sick not in good health; ill; afflicted with disease.
  s. sinus syndrome a complex cardiac arrhythmia manifested as severe sinus bradycardia alone, sinus bradycardia alternating with tachycardia, or sinus bradycardia with atrioventricular block.
sickle cell a crescentic or sickle-shaped erythrocyte. In humans, the abnormal shape is caused by a structural hemoglobinopathy. Sickle cells are found in normal members of the family Cervidae (deer).
sickle hocks the hock joint has too acute an angle and the foot is carried too far forward and the metatarsus is not vertical but is inclined forward distally. It is a serious defect because of the likelihood of arthrosis in the joint.
sickle shin deformity of the tibia and fibula in osteoporotic primates, accompanied by pathological fractures, paraplegia and kyphosis.
sickled erythrocyte see SICKLE CELL.
sicklepod SENNA *obtusifolia.*
sickling the development of sickle cells in the blood.
sickness the role assumed by ill humans; not a term applicable to animals.
SID single intradermal test for tuberculosis.
side to one side.
  s. bar see SIDEROD.
  s. effect a consequence other than that for which an agent is used, especially an adverse effect on another organ system.
  s. lines a means of restraining a horse which can also be used for casting. A 60 ft cotton rope is knotted so that there is a fixed loop in the center. This is placed over the head and seated on the shoulder and the two ends passed between the forelimbs. Each rope end is passed around a hind pastern and brought back to the shoulder loop. Pulling one of the legs up so that the hoof just reaches the ground is used as restraint to prevent the horse rearing. Pulling both legs forward causes the horse to fall.
  s. reins see side REIN.

side chain commonly referred to as –R; group that confers specific identity to compounds, particularly amino acids.
side-to-side anastomosis a method for establishing continuity between two blood vessels or segments of gut, whose ends have been closed. The resultant opening is wider than an end-to-end anastomosis.
sidebone ossification of the alar cartilages of the third phalanx of the foot of horses. Attention is usually drawn to the disease by lameness but it is possible for the lesion to be far-advanced and the gait to be normal. There may be obvious enlargement at the site and the cartilages can be felt to have lost their flexibility.
Sideranthus North American plants in the family Asteraceae; includes *S. grindeloides*; facultative accumulators of selenium and can cause poisoning by selenocompounds which cause alopecia, lameness, laminitis, hoof deformity, diarrhea. Called also ironweed.
sidero- word element. [Gr.] *iron.*
sideroblast a nucleated erythrocyte containing iron granules in its cytoplasm.
siderocalcinosis deposition of iron salts with calcium in tissues, principally blood vessels.
siderochrome siderophore.
siderocyte a red blood cell containing nonhemoglobin iron.
siderod rod attached at one end to the headstall and at the other end to a roller or surcingle; it prevents a horse from biting at a hindlimb.
siderofibrosis fibrosis associated with deposits of iron.
sideroleukocyte a leukocyte containing iron; associated with intracellular hemolytic anemia.
s. test staining a smear of concentrated leukocytes with potassium ferrocyanide to demonstrate hemosiderin and ferritin. Used as a general test for equine infectious anemia.
sideropenia deficiency of iron in the body or blood.
siderophil 1. siderophilous. 2. a siderophilous cell or tissue.
siderophilin transferrin.
siderophilous tending to absorb iron.
siderophore a macrophage containing hemosiderin.
siderosis 1. a form of PNEUMOCONIOSIS due to the inhalation of iron or other metallic particles. 2. excess of iron in the blood. 3. the deposit of iron in the tissues.
hepatic s. the deposit of an abnormal quantity of iron in the liver.
urinary s. the presence of hemosiderin granules in the urine.
siderotic emanating from or pertaining to siderosis.
s. nodule see GAMMA–GANDY BODY.
s. pigmentation of neurons situated close to contusions and hemorrhages; caused by encrustation of the cells by basophilic complexes of iron, calcium and phosphorus.
sidewheel see PACE.
siemens the SI unit of conductivity, equal to one reciprocal ohm (Ω^{-1}); symbol S. Called also mho.
sierra laurel LEUCOTHOE *davisiae.*
Sievert the SI unit of radiation absorbed dose equivalent, defined as that producing the same biological effect in a specified tissue as 1 gray of high-energy x-rays; symbol Sv. 1 sievert equals 100 rem.
sig., Sig. [L.] *signa* (mark); see SIGNA.
Sigesbeckia orientalis plant member of family Asteraceae; can cause nitrate–nitrite poisoning.
Siggaard-Andersen nomogram a nomogram used to determine the base excess level of a blood sample from its pH and $P\text{co}_2$ values.
sigh complementary breathing cycles characterized by a quick, deep inspiration followed by a slower expiration; probably a compensatory mechanism to counter poor ventilation.
sight 1. the act or faculty of VISION, involving the EYE itself, the visual center in the brain, and the optic nerve and nerve fibers in the brain that connect the two. 2. a thing seen.
sigma the Greek letter σ or Σ; the former frequently denotes a standard deviation, the latter is used in mathematics for the sum of the values of the term nominated.
sigmoid shaped like the letter C or S.
s. colon the distal part of the colon of some species, such as humans, shaped like an S, from the level of the iliac crest to the rectum.
s. curve an S-shaped curve of the relationship between two variables.
s. flexure of the penis situated in the bull's penis dorsal and caudal to the scrotal neck.
sigmoidal kinetics property of allosteric enzymes which are usually multisubunit enzymes with multiple active sites. Exhibit cooperativity in substrate binding and regulation of their activity by other effector molecules.
sign any objective evidence of disease or dysfunction recognizable by the veterinarian. Symptoms, the subjective sensations experienced by human patients, are not definable in veterinary medicine and the term has no application to veterinarians.
cardinal s's of greatest significance to the veterinarian; establishing the identity of the illness. Shown in abnormalities of the temperature, pulse and respiration. **Key sign** is a more appropriate expression for the important signs in a particular case on which the clinician will base his or her diagnosis.
presenting s's the signs or group of signs about which the client complains or from which relief is sought.
withdrawal s's those following sudden abstinence from a drug on which a patient is dependent.
sign test a nonparametric statistical test based on the comparison of the signs of the differences between paired values.
signa [L.] *mark, write;* abbreviated S, Sig. or sig. in prescriptions, followed by the SIGNATURE.
signal 1. audible or visible indications to animals in behavioral conditioning. Many signals have had long-term use in the animal world and are used worldwide. Whoa and Getup, Heel and Sit are common examples. Getawayback is perhaps more colloquial. Many sheepdogs are trained to react to whistles and performing animals are usually trained to react to gestures with the hand. 2. in biochemical terminology relates to staging in reactions; see signal SEQUENCE.
s. peptidase an integral membrane protein located on the luminal surface of the endoplasmic reticulum that cleaves the signal peptide and frees the protein for folding and export.
s. recognition particle (SRP) a particle composed of six different proteins and one small (7S) RNA that binds to the signal peptide as it emerges from the ribosome, temporarily halting the synthesis of the protein while the complex is transported to the endoplasmic reticulum where the SRP recognizes and docks to a docking protein located on the cytoplasmic surface followed by the transfer of the ribosome to a ribosome receptor on the membrane; the SRP

and its docking protein are released from the ribosome and translation resumes.

s. transduction proteins proteins which may be a protein kinase, an ion channel forming protein (as in nerve cells), or a protein that undergoes some energy dependent change in which the energy is supplied by the hydrolysis of a higher energy compound such as guanosine triphosphate.

signal grass BRACHIARIA *brizantha*, *B. decumbens*.

signal sequence see signal SEQUENCE.

signal-to-noise ratio the ratio of a specific response, e.g. counts per minutes (cpm) from a radiolabeled substance, to the background cpm; the latter is substracted from the former to give the value of the specific response.

signaling molecules substances synthesized by cells for purposes of extracellular communication between cells.

signalment that part of the veterinary medical history dealing with the animal's age, sex and breed.

signature that part of a drug prescription that gives directions to be followed by the patient in its use.

root s. see ROOT signature.

significance the quality of an assessment about the relationship between two or more values of a variable. Significance is achieved if the relationship is more common than would be achieved by a random selection.

significant said of an experimental result when it is greater than would be expected by chance. The degree of the significance can be expressed as a percentage, given the likely probability of the results occurring.

s. digit the number of decimal places for which the result is accurate.

Sigurdsson vaccine a vaccine composed of killed *Mycobacterium paratuberculosis* organisms used in the prevention of Johne's disease in sheep.

Sikh slaughter a method in which conscious sheep and goats are decapitated by a single blow of a special sword; used in India. Provided a special sword is used buffalo can be dealt with in the same way. Called also Jakta method.

silage see ENSILAGE.

s. disease see LISTERIOSIS.

s. poisoning. 1. overfeeding on silage may cause indigestion. Usually the result of a heavy feeding program and a shortage of hay so that the roughage supply is entirely silage. 2. a silage containing more than the usual proportion of butyric acid may predispose to acetonemia. 3. silage containing a thriving population of *Listeria monocytogenes* may cause that disease when fed out.

Silastic trademark for polymeric silicone substances having the properties of rubber; it is biologically inert and used in surgical prostheses, and Silastic tubing is used for temporary implants in tissue, e.g. for supra-palpebral irrigation of the conjunctival sac.

silent produces no audible sound.

s. atria see ATRIAL standstill.

s. estrus see silent heat (below).

s. heat the behavior pattern in which the animal gives no behavioral signals that an ovarian follicle is maturing and rupturing although it is doing so or has just done so. Called also silent estrus.

s. lung breath sounds absent on auscultation; occurs over collapsed lung or lung shielded by fluid, pus, solid tissue.

Siley tracheostomy tube a cuffed tube with removable inner cannula.

silhouette outline of a figure. The sharpness of the silhouette is a function of the shape, size and density of the object. This is most marked in radiography.

basketball-shaped s. the enlarged cardiac outline seen in the dorsal–ventral view of the thorax in a dog with chronic pericardial effusion.

s. sign produced when two fluid densities are contiguous and the individual outline of each is lost. Commonly used in the evaluation of chest problems.

silica silicon dioxide, a compound occurring naturally as quartz and in other forms. A common constituent of urinary calculi in agricultural animals, a rare occurrence in dogs.

s. calculi see silica UROLITH.

s. gel commonly used in the laboratory as a desiccant; has been used topically on dogs and cats for flea control.

silicate a salt of any of the silicic acids.

siliceous relating to or made of silica or a silicate.

silicon a chemical element, atomic number 14, atomic weight 28.086, symbol Si. See Table 6. See also SILICA.

silicone any organic compound in which all or part of the carbon has been replaced by silicon. Silicones are applied to glassware used for administering blood transfusions or for collecting blood for laboratory tests based on whole blood, and are important industrial lubricants.

silicosis deposits of inert dust in the lungs of animals; very rare because of lack of exposure of animals to such a polluted environment.

silk continuous, protein filament produced by the larvae of *Bombyx mori*, the white silkworm moth. Used as a SUTURE material.

Silkie a bantam with white, curly feathers, a prominent crest of feathers, rose comb and a black skin and legs.

silky lupin LUPINUS *sericeus*.

silky oak GREVILLEA *robusta*.

Silky terrier a small (8–10 lb), blue or gray with tan, silky-haired dog, larger but resembling a Yorkshire terrier. Called also Australian silky terrier, Sydney silky terrier.

silo an airtight and insect-proof container used to store agricultural products and to make ensilage. May be made of concrete, rarely of brick, or of glass-lined steel or be a hole dug in the ground, or two parallel barricades lined with plastic. Those used for grain storage need only to be insect-proof and airtight. Those used for ensilage making need also to be resistant to the corrosive effect of the acids produced during anaerobic fermentation. See also ENSILAGE.

s. gas nitrogen dioxide.

silo-filler's disease pulmonary inflammation of humans, often with acute pulmonary edema, due to inhalation of the irritant gases (especially oxides of nitrogen) which collect in recently filled silos. Often quoted as a disease similar to atypical interstitial pneumonia of cattle.

Silpha genus of the family of Silphidae of carrion beetles which infest pigeon droppings. Their larval maggots may invade the skin of live squabs.

silver 1. a chemical element, atomic number 47, atomic weight 107.870, symbol Ag. See Table 6. It is used in medicine for its caustic, astringent and antiseptic effects. Experimental poisoning with silver salts causes myopathy. 2. a coat color in dogs, foxes.

s. amalgam see AMALGAM.

s. collie syndrome see canine CYCLIC hematopoiesis.

s. grass ARISTIDA *contorta*.

s. halide any of the silver salts with halogens including bromine, chlorine, iodine used in photographic emulsion.

s. iodide soluble silver salt used in cloud seeding but presents no toxicological risk to local grazing cattle.

s.-leaf ironbark EUCALYPTUS *melanophloia*.

s.-leafed nightshade SOLANUM *elaeagnifolium*.

s. nitrate colorless or white crystals, used as a caustic and local anti-infective.

s. nitrate (toughened) a mixture of silver nitrate with hydrochloric acid, sodium chloride or potassium nitrate, occurring as white crystalline masses molded into pencils or cones, called caustic pencils; a convenient means of applying silver nitrate locally. Called also lunar caustic.

s. protein silver made colloidal by the presence of, or combination with, protein; an active germicide with a local irritant and astringent effect.

s. stain a method of demonstrating flagella on bacteria, or for visualizing very thin bacteria, such as leptospires.

s. sulfadiazine the silver salt of sulfadiazine, having bactericidal activity against many gram-positive and gram-negative organisms, as well as being effective against yeasts; used as a topical anti-infective for the prevention and treatment of wound sepsis in patients with second and third degree burns.

s. weed see POTENTILLA ANSERINA.

silver carp HYPOPHTHALMICHTHYS *molitrix*.

Silver Fox a very attractive and unusual breed of rabbit. They are 4 to 7 lb in weight and black, blue, chocolate or lilac in color, with profuse white ticking on the chest, flanks and feet. The insides of the ears, line of the jaw and tail underside are white, with white 'spectacles' around the eyes.

Silver rabbit small, well-fleshed, fur rabbit, gray brown or fawn in color with silvering of the tips of the hair.

silver trevally see PSEUDOCARANX DENTEX.

silverling see BACCHARIS.

Silverman's needle an instrument for taking tissue specimens. See also FRANKLIN–SILVERMAN BIOPSY NEEDLE.

silvery lupin LUPINUS *argenteus*.

silvex a weedkiller, warranted to be safe for animals at the concentrations used to spray plants. Poisoning can be produced experimentally. Characterized by depression, anorexia, weakness especially of the hindquarters. May cause an increase in nitrate content of plants and lead to nitrite poisoning in ruminants. Use of this compound has been discontinued.

Silybum marianum plant member of the family Asteraceae; has a very high feed value but a high nitrate content. May cause nitrate–nitrite poisoning in ruminants. Called also *Carduus marianus*, variegated thistle, milk thistle, bull thistle, St. Mary's thistle.

simazine a triazine weedkiller that is toxic if livestock are allowed access shortly after the plants have been sprayed. Signs of toxicity include staggering in sheep and colic in horses.

Simbu virus group antigenically related viruses in the Bunyamwera virus group in the *Bunyavirus* genus; includes Akabane virus.

simethicone an antiflatulent substance consisting of a mixture of dimethyl polysiloxanes and silica gel. Called also activated dimethicone.

Simford an Australian breed of beef cattle produced by crossing animals of Hereford and Simmental breeds.

simian 1. member of the suborder *Anthropoidea* or *Simiae*; includes the monkeys and apes. 2. ape-like.

s. acquired immune deficiency syndrome (SAIDS) a retrovirus-induced immune deficiency, similar to human acquired immune deficiency syndrome (AIDS).

s. exogenous type D retrovirus see simian acquired immune deficiency syndrome (above).

s. hemorrhagic fever a highly fatal disease of macaques, caused by an arterivirus. It is characterized by edema, hemorrhages and diarrhea.

Simmental dual-purpose Swiss cattle, reddish dun or yellow and white in color. There are many varieties throughout Europe. Black Simmental is a black variant.

Simmonds' disease panhypopituitarism in which cachexia is a prominent feature; called also pituitary cachexia. It follows the destruction of the pituitary gland by surgery, infection, injury or tumor.

Simondsia paradoxa member of the nematode family Thelaziidae. A thick white stomach worm of pigs. Causes chronic gastritis but unlikely to have any effect except perhaps to reduce growth rate.

Simonsiella gram-negative bacteria that form flat filaments. Common, nonpathogenic inhabitant of mouths of animals.

simplexin diterpenoid daphnane ester responsible for toxic effects of *Pimelea* spp.

Simplexvirus one of the two genera in the subfamily *Alphaherpesvirus* which includes bovine herpesvirus 2.

simuland characteristic of a real life system.

simular characteristic of a simulation model.

simulation 1. imitation of a system such as an ecological or farming system by a series of mathematical formulae. See also COMPUTER simulation model. 2. the act of running a model. 3. the imitation of one disease by another.

s. model mathematical models of dynamic processes which include combinations of mathematical and logical processes. They are generally used to compare several solutions to a problem.

simulator something that simulates, such as an apparatus that simulates conditions that will be encountered in real life.

simulid see SIMULIUM.

Simulium a genus of insects in the family Simuliidae causing insect worry with livestock. Cutaneous lesions may include vesicles and wart-like papules, and edema and petechiation of thin-skinned, ventral areas. Poultry may be affected by anemia. The species also transmits a number of animal diseases including the viruses of vesicular stomatitis and eastern equine encephalomyelitis, the protozoa, *Leucocytozoon* and *Haemoproteus* spp., and are intermediate parasites for some *Onchocerca* spp. Called also black fly, buffalo gnat.

There are a large number of species distinguished largely by their geographic distribution: *Simulium arcticum*, *S. callidum*, *S. columbaczense*, *S. damnosum*, *S. erythrocephalum*, *S. indicum*, *S. metallicum*, *S. neavei*, *S. ochraceum*, *S. ornatum*, *S. pecuarum*, *S. rugglesi*, *S. venustum*.

simultaneous serum–virus vaccination simultaneous administration of live virus and hyperimmune serum. Used at one time in the control of several diseases, including canine distemper and hog cholera.

SIMV synchronized intermittent mandatory ventilation.

sinalbin the glycoside in the seeds of white mustard (*Sinapis alba*) which is converted to isopropyl isothiocyanate and sinapine sulfate which can cause gastroenteritis manifested by abdominal pain and diarrhea.

sinapine sulfate one of the toxic agents produced by the metabolism of sinalbin, a glycoside in mustard seed.

Sinapis plant genus in the family Brassicaceae. The mustards. Cause poisoning due to sinalbin, sinigrin, mustard oil glucosinolates concentrated in the seeds, poisoning manifested by abdominal pain and diarrhea. Foliage can also cause nitrate–nitrite poisoning. Includes *S. alba* (white mustard, commercial mustard *Brassica alba, B. hirta*), *S. arvensis* (*Brassica sinapis, B. arvensis, B. kaber*, wild mustard, charlock—a common weed of cultivation), *S. nigra* (black mustard).

sinciput the upper and front part of the head.

Sinclair miniature swine developed in Minnesota, USA, specifically for the purpose of research.

sinew a tendon.

Singapura a native cat of Singapore; a small cat with a short sepia-colored coat with dark brown ticking. The eyes are hazel, green or yellow.

singeing flash application of flame to remove residual, esthetically unattractive hairs from poultry and pig carcasses.

Singer–Nicolson membrane model major current model of membrane structure. Incorporates a fluid mosaic structure whose major features include a discontinuous lipid bilayer composed predominantly of phospholipids, and proteins (often glycoproteins) that are integral to the structure, and peripheral proteins that are not essential to reassembly of a functional membrane.

Singhfilaria hayesi a tissue-dwelling nematode found in tissues around the crop and trachea of quail, turkeys in USA.

single-blind study see BLINDING.

single enterprise practice a veterinary practice in which the veterinarian has only one client, usually a large industrial enterprise such as a feedlot.

single-foot a fast, four-beat walking gait, short of a trot. Only one foot is on the ground at a time. See also broken AMBLE.

singletary pea LATHYRUS *pusillus, L. hirsutus.*

singultus hiccup.

sinigrin a toxic glycoside in the seed of *Sinapis nigra* (black mustard). Converted by the enzyme myrosin to allylisothiocyanate, the volatile oil of mustard.

sinister [L.] *left;* on the left side.

sinistrad to or toward the left.

sinistral pertaining to the left side.

sinistr(o)- word element. [L.] *left, left side.*

sinistrocardia levocardia.

sinistrocerebral situated in the left hemisphere of the brain.

sinistrogyration a turning to the left.

sinistrotorsion a twisting toward the left, as of the eye.

sinoatrial pertaining to the sinus venosus and the atrium of the heart or to the sinoatrial node; abbreviated S-A, SA.

s. block an absence of a discharge from the sinoatrial node. The heart is regular unless there is an underlying atrial arrhythmia. Considered to be within the limits of normality provided it disappears with exercise.

s. node a collection of atypical muscle fibers and nerve endings in the wall of the right atrium, adjacent to the sulcus terminalis, where the rhythm of cardiac contraction is usually established; therefore also referred to as the pacemaker of the heart. Called also sinoatrial bundle, Keith's node, Keith–Flack node.

Sinostrongylus see CABALLONEMA.

sinuotomy sinusotomy.

sinuous bending in and out; winding.

sinus 1. a recess, cavity, or channel, as (a) one in bone or (b) a dilated, valveless channel for venous blood. 2. an abnormal channel or fistula, permitting escape of pus. In common, unqualified usage, the word sinus refers to any of the cavities in the skull that are connected with the nasal cavity—the paranasal sinuses.

anal s's furrows, with pouchlike recesses at their distal ends, separating the rectal columns; called also anal crypts.

basilar s. a dural venous sinus which runs on the floor of the cranial cavity and out through the foramen magnum.

cavernous s. an irregularly shaped venous channel between the layers of dura mater of the brain, one on either side of the body of the sphenoid bone and communicating across the midline. Several cranial nerves and, when present, the rete mirabile, course through this sinus.

cavernous s. syndrome lesions of the cavernous syndrome, caused by neoplasia or infectious agents, result in a dilated pupil and paralysis of the globe; vision is usually spared.

cerebral s. one of the ventricles of the brain.

cervical s. a temporary depression in the neck of the embryo containing the branchial arches.

circular s. the venous channel encircling the pituitary gland, formed by the two cavernous sinuses and the anterior and posterior intercavernous sinuses.

conchal s. cavity of the conchal bone.

coronary s. the terminal portion of the great cardiac vein, which lies in the cardiac sulcus between the left atrium and ventricle, and empties into the right atrium.

dermoid s., dermal s. see DERMOID sinus.

dorsal sagittal s. a large dural venous sinus located within the falx cerebri.

dura mater venous s. large channels for venous blood forming an anastomosing system between the layers of the dura mater of the brain.

ethmoidal s. that paranasal sinus consisting of the ethmoidal cells collectively, and communicating with the nasal meatuses.

facial s. see MALAR abscess.

frontal s. one of the paired paranasal sinuses in the frontal bone, each communicating with the middle meatus of the ipsilateral nasal cavity.

hair s. see sinus HAIR.

infraorbital s. an air-filled recess in the head of birds which lies lateral to the nasal cavity into which it opens.

intercavernous s. channels connecting the two cavernous sinuses, one passing anterior and the other posterior to the stalk of the pituitary gland.

interdigitalis s. the cutaneous pouch, which lies between the claws of sheep and some other ruminants and whose wall contains apocrine glands, and whose duct surfaces on the skin just above the coronets; it serves as a trail gland.

lymphatic s. irregular, tortuous spaces within lymphoid tissues through which lymph flows.

maxillary s. one of the paired paranasal sinuses in the body of the maxilla on either side, opening into the middle meatus of the ipsilateral nasal cavity. In the horse it is divided into two compartments that communicate independently with the nasal chambers. All other sinuses of the horse communicate with the nasal chambers via the caudal maxillary sinus.

nasal s. see paranasal sinuses (below).

s. nerve a branch of the glossopharyngeal nerve; carries the afferent fibers of the stretch receptors in the wall of the carotid sinus.

s. node see SINOATRIAL node.

occipital s. a venous sinus between the layers of dura mater, passing along the midline of the cerebellum.

paranasal s's mucosa-lined air cavities in bones of the skull, communicating with the nasal cavity and including ethmoidal, frontal, maxillary and sphenoidal sinuses.

petrosal s. (inferior) a venous channel arising from the cavernous sinus and draining into the internal jugular vein.

petrosal s. (superior) one arising from the cavernous sinus and draining into the transverse sinus of the dura mater.

prostatic s. the dorsolateral recess between the seminal colliculus and the wall of the urethra.

pulmonary trunk s. spaces between the wall of the pulmonary trunk and cusps of the pulmonary valve at its opening from the right ventricle.

red pulp s. vascular storage in the spleen into which capillaries empty.

s. reflex arc afferent fibers are in the sinus nerve; these connect with the cardioinhibitory and vasomotor centers which control blood pressure and heart rate via sympathetic fibers to blood vessels; provides a route for the sinus reflex which relates pressure in the carotid sinus to the performance of the circulatory system.

renal s. a recess in the substance of the kidney, occupied by the renal pelvis, calices, vessels, nerves and fat.

sagittal s. (inferior) a small venous sinus of the dura mater of large animals found between the cerebral hemispheres and opening into the straight sinus.

sagittal s. (superior) a venous sinus of the dura mater that courses between the cerebral hemispheres and ends in the confluence of sinuses.

scleral venous s. see SCHLEMM'S CANAL.

sigmoid s. a venous sinus of the dura mater on either side, continuous with the straight sinus and draining into the internal jugular vein of the same side.

sphenoidal s. one of the paired paranasal sinuses in the body of the sphenoid bone of some species. In the horse it communicates with the nasal cavity via the frontal and caudal maxillary sinuses.

sphenoparietal s. one of the venous sinuses of the dura mater, emptying into the cavernous sinus.

splenic s. dilated venous channels in the substance of the spleen. See also red pulp sinus (above).

straight s. a venous sinus of the dura mater formed by junction of the great cerebral vein and inferior sagittal sinus, and ending in the confluence of sinuses.

tarsal s. a space between the calcaneus and talus.

tentorial s. straight sinus.

transverse dura mater s. a large venous sinus that runs in the attached border of the cerebellar tentorium on either side of the skull.

transverse pericardial s. a passage within the pericardial sac, between the aorta and pulmonary trunk cranioventrally, and the left atrium and cranial vena cava dorsally.

tympanic s. a deep recess on the medial wall of the middle ear.

urachal s. an anomalous closure of the urachal canal in the newborn in which the opening at the umbilicus remains open. The bladder is normal. It is the cause of persistent infection and swelling at the umbilicus in the young animal and may lead to cystitis and pyelonephritis.

urethral s a small cavity in the glans penis of the horse, above the urethral process; as a recess of the fossa glandis it is usually filled with a small mass (bean) of inspissated smegma.

urogenital s. an elongated sac formed by division of the cloaca in the early embryo, which ultimately forms most of the vestibule, urethra and vagina in the female, and some of the urethra in the male.

uterine s. venous channels in the wall of the uterus in pregnancy.

uteroplacental s. blood spaces between the placenta and uterine sinuses.

venae caval s. the posterior portion of the right atrium into which the inferior and the superior vena cava open.

s. venarum a chamber which is the greater part of the right atrium into which the great veins discharge.

venous s., s. venosus 1. the common venous receptacle in the heart of the early embryo that receives blood from the umbilical and vitelline veins and from the body via the ducts of Cuvier. 2. sinus of venae cavae.

vertebral s. a continuation of part of the common occipital vein in birds; it emerges from the foramen magnum and accompanies the vertebral vein.

sinusitis inflammation of one or more of the paranasal sinuses, often occurring during an upper respiratory infection, by extension from the nasal cavity. Sinusitis also may be a complication of tooth infection, allergy or certain infectious diseases. It is commonest in horses and cats, in cattle it is usually a complication of dehorning, and in dogs it often results from intranasal foreign bodies. In its chronic form it is characterized by a continuous or intermittent discharge of pus through the nostril on the affected side or through a sinus to the exterior. The face may be swollen and painful. See also SINUS.

infectious s. of turkeys caused by *Mycoplasma gallisepticum* and characterized by swelling of the infraorbital sinuses which are filled with thick pus. Some cases also have airsacculitis and conjunctivitis.

sinusoid 1. resembling a sinus. 2. a form of terminal blood channel consisting of a large, irregular, anastomosing vessel, having a lining of reticuloendothelium but little or no adventitia. Sinusoids are found in the liver, adrenal glands, heart, parathyroid glands, carotid bodies, spleen, hemolymph glands and pancreas.

sinusotomy incision of a sinus.

sipauba see THILOA GLAUCOCARPA.

siphon 1. a bent tube with arms of unequal length, for drawing liquid from a higher to a lower level by force of atmospheric pressure. 2. to draw liquid by means of a siphon.

Siphona see HAEMATOBIA.

siphonage the use of the siphon, as in gastric lavage or in draining the bladder.

Siphonaptera the order of fleas.

SIR systemic inflammatory response.

sire male parent.

s. evaluation in farm animals, the estimation of the breeding value of a male by PROGENY TESTING.

s.-family average the average performance of the half-sib family of which the individual is a member.

s. line characteristics contributed to the offspring of a cross mating by the sire.

s. verification verifying that a stated sire is indeed a parent by the use of a paternity testing technique.

sirenian aquatic mammal member of the order Sirenia; includes the sea-cow, manatee and dugong.

sirenomelus a fetus with fused legs and no feet.

sires of dams pathway breeding pattern for selecting sires who will be expected to produce good dams.

sires of sires pathway breeding pattern for selecting sires who will be expected to produce good sires.
siresine a type of harness worn over the forequarters by rams and as a headstall in bulls in mating groups. The harness carries a crayon on the brisket or under the chin in bulls so that females which are mounted by the male are marked by the crayon. Different colored crayons are used to identify females mated over a particular period of time or by individual males. This identifies the sire when more than one male is in the group.
SIRM see STERILE insect release method.
-sis word element. [Gr.] *state, condition.*
sisomicin, sissomicin an aminoglycoside antibiotic similar to gentamicin produced by cultures of *Micromonospora inyoensis.* Used as the sulfate.
Sistrunk scissors short dissecting scissors.
Sisymbrium irio a plant in the family Brassicaceae capable of causing severe gastroenteritis in cattle. Called also London rocket.
Sisyrinchium plant genus in the Iridaceae family, suspected to contain a cardiac glucoside which causes violent diarrhea in livestock. Includes *S. iridifolium*, *S. micranthum*, sisyrinchium species A. Called also scour weed, yellow rush lily.
sit-fast see SET-FAST.
sitiology, sitology the science of food and nourishment.
β-sitosterolemia high blood levels of β-sitosterol.
sitotherapy treatment by food; dietotherapy.
sitotropism tropism in response to the influence of food.
situs pl. *situs* [L.] site or position.
s. inversus total or partial transposition of the body organs to the side opposite the normal.
situtunga an antelope with spreading feet adapted to marshy ground. Called also marsh-buck, *Limnotragus spekei.*
Sium plant genus in the family Apiaceae; contain an unidentified toxin which causes several syndromes: (1) abdominal pain and diarrhea, (2) tremor, convulsions, bloat, bradycardia, (3) taints milk; includes *S. angustifolium* (cow-cress, fool's watercress), *S. latifolium* (water parsnip), *S. suave* (*S. cicutaefolium*).
six tooth in sheep, a 3 year old with all six permanent incisor teeth erupted.
size a criterion of growth other than height and weight; a combination of height, depth, width and weight. A large animal is tall but deep and wide in proportion; all of its dimensions are large.
Sjögren's syndrome a symptom complex marked by keratoconjunctivitis sicca and xerostomia often occurring in association with other inflammatory disorders such as immune-mediated arthritis and systemic lupus erythematosus. Reported in dogs.
SK streptokinase.
skatole a derivative of tryptophan formed in the putrefaction of proteins which contributes to the characteristic odor of the feces.
skatoxyl an oxidation product of skatole formed in the large intestine in certain diseases and excreted in the urine.
skeletal pertaining to the skeleton. See also skeletal MUSCLE.
s. remodeling the continuous dynamic process of resorption of some parts of the bony skeleton and mineralization of others.
s. scurvy see hypertrophic OSTEODYSTROPHY.
s. system the body's framework of bones and associated cartilages; see also SKELETON.
s. tissue the bony, ligamentous, fibrous and cartilaginous tissue forming the skeleton and its attachments.
skeletal patterning development of the limb primordia, pairs of limb buds, or other skeletal primordia, in the correct relationship to each other and to surrounding structures.
skeletization 1. extreme emaciation. 2. removal of soft parts from the skeleton.
skeletogenous producing skeletal structures or tissues.
skeleton the stiff, hardened tissues forming the supporting framework of an animal body.
appendicular s. the bones of the limbs.
axial s. the skull, spine, ribs and sternum.
visceral s. 1. the skeleton that forms part of an organ such as the os penis or os cordis. 2. the bony framework that protects the viscera, such as the sternum, ribs or pelvis.
s. weed see LYGODESMIA JUNCEA.
skeocytosis the presence of immature forms of leukocytes in the blood; shift to the left.
skeptophylaxis 1. a condition in which a minute dose of a substance poisonous to animals will produce immediate temporary immunity to the action of the poison, although the blood of the animal may be highly toxic during that period of immunity. 2. the method of allergic desensitization by the preliminary injection of a small amount of the allergen, as is commonly done before the injection of an antiserum.
skewbald a horse coat color of mostly white with some large, irregular patches of any other color than black.
skewed curve of a usually unimodal distribution with one tail drawn out more than the other and the median will lie above or below the mean.
skewer wood see EUONYMUS EUROPAEUS.
skia- word element. [Gr.] *shadow* (especially as produced by x-rays).
skiagraph radiograph.
skiametry see RETINOSCOPY.
skiascope an instrument which measures the refractive status of the eye.
skim milk the residue from whole milk after the cream has been skimmed off. In today's usage it is the residue after the butterfat is removed.
s. m. extender skim milk used as a diluent for semen. See also semen EXTENDER.
s. m. powder dehydrated skim milk used extensively as a milk replacer provided it is not too expensive. A high-protein supplement but deficient in vitamins A and D both of which will have been extracted with the butterfat.
skin the outer covering and largest organ of the body. It serves as a protective barrier against microorganisms, helps shield delicate tissues underneath from mechanical and other injuries, insulates against heat and cold, and helps eliminate body wastes. It guards against ultraviolet radiation by producing a protective pigment and it helps produce vitamin D. Its sense receptors detect pain, cold, heat, touch and pressure.

The skin consists of an outer cellular, avascular epidermis, and an inner fibrous corium (dermis, true skin) resting upon a hypodermis of fat and panniculus muscle.

See also CUTANEOUS, EPIDERMAL, EPIDERMIS.
s. appendages see HAIR, CLAW, HOOF, HORN, CHESTNUT (1), ERGOT[2], DEWCLAW, COMB, WATTLE, SPUR (3), PAD, FOOTPAD, BEAK, FEATHER (1), CERE, SCALE, FIN, ANTLER, BRISTLE (1), WOOL, MOHAIR, CASHMERE, ANGORA.

s.-associated lymphoid tissues (SALT) see skin-associated LYMPHOID tissue.
autoimmune s. disease see AUTOIMMUNE, PEMPHIGUS, LUPUS ERYTHEMATOSUS.
s. biopsy removal of a small section of skin for histopathological examination. See also KEYES PUNCH.
s. cancer include squamous cell carcinoma, papilloma and fibropapilloma, intracutaneous cornifying epithelioma (keratoacanthoma), basal cell tumors and tumors of the adnexa, perianal gland and hair follicles.
congenital absence of s. see EPITHELIOGENESIS imperfecta.
s. depigmentation see HYPOPIGMENTATION.
s. emphysema see subcutaneous EMPHYSEMA.
s. fold thickness a measure of obesity in humans but not a valid indicator in dogs or cats as the skin lifts off the subcutaneous tissue.
s. fungal infection see DERMATOMYCOSIS, DERMATOPHYTOSIS.
s. gangrene death of tissue and usually involves dermis, epidermis and subcutaneous tissue, e.g. severe saddle galls, heat burns, chemical burns, *Claviceps purpurea* poisoning. The affected area is cold and bluish in color. This changes to black and the area begins to lift at the edges and to dry out.
s. inflammation see DERMATITIS.
s. leukosis occurs in MAREK'S DISEASE. Called also cutaneous LYMPHOSARCOMA.
s.-maggot fly see CORDYLOBIA *anthropophaga*.
s. memory see MNEMODERMIA.
s. receptor cutaneous sensory endorgans.
s. resiliency test see skin tenting test (below).
s. tag see fibrovascular PAPILLOMA.
s. tension lines see TENSION line.
s. tenting test a fold of skin is picked up and then quickly let go. The amount that it will stretch is an indication of its extensibility. The speed with which it returns to a normal position is determined by the degree of hydration of the skin and subcutaneous tissue and the amount of fat in the subcutaneous tissue, e.g. in an animal that is 10 to 12% dehydrated the skin fold will not disappear until 20 to 45 seconds have elapsed.
s. test application or intradermal injection of a substance to the skin to test the body's reaction to it. Such a test detects an animal's sensitivity to such allergens as dust and pollen, or to preparations of microorganisms believed to be the cause of a disorder.

There are several types of skin tests, including the patch test, the scratch test, and the intradermal test.
s. wool scoured wool from a fellmonger.

skink the commonest lizards in the world with over 600 species, all of them in the family Scincidae.

Skinner box an experimental enclosure for testing animal conditioning, in which the subject animal performs (e.g. presses a bar or lever) to obtain a reward. See also instrumental CONDITIONING.

skippers larvae of *Piophila casei*, the cheese or ham fly. The larvae skip around on the cheese that they inhabit in a quite repulsive way.

Skirrow's medium a blood agar base suitable for growing *Campylobacter fetus* and *Brucella* spp.

skirt abattoir term for diaphragm.

skirted fleece a fleece from which the skirtings have been removed.

skirtings untidy pieces of inferior quality wool from the edges of a fleece. They are removed and sold separately.

Sklar forceps rack a flat plate with stand-up pins. The hemostats are laid on the plate with the finger grips over two of the pins and the blades positioned between two others. Suitable for compact, tidy transport and storage of large numbers of hemostats.

skler(o)- for words beginning thus, see those beginning *scler(o)-*.

skot(o)- for words beginning thus, see those beginning *scot(o)-*.

Skrjabinagia a genus of worms in the subfamily Ostertaginae and the family Trichostrongylidae.
S. boevi found in the large and small intestines of water buffalo.
S. dagestanica found in the small intestine of sheep.
S. kolchida found in the abomasum of deer.
S. lyrata OSTERTAGIA *lyrata*.
S. popovi found in the small intestine of sheep.

Skrjabinema a genus of worms in the family Oxyuridae. They inhabit the ceca of ruminants.
S. africana found in steinbock in Africa.
S. alata found in sheep.
S. caprae found in goats.
S. ovis found in sheep, goat and antelope.
S. tarandi found in reindeer and caribou.

Skrjabingylus a genus of worms in the metastrongyloid family Skrjabingylidae found in the nasal sinuses of their hosts.
S. chitwoodorum found in skunks.
S. magnus found in skunks.
S. nasicola found in nasal sinuses of mink, polecat and fox.
S. petrowi found in pine marten.

Skrjabinoptera phrynosome a physalopterid roundworm found in the stomach of lizards.

Skrjabinotrema ovis a digenetic trematode in the family Hasstilesiidae, found in the small intestine of sheep.

skull the bony framework of the head consisting of two parts, the cranium and the facial section.

The cranium is the domed top, back and sides of the skull that protects the brain. It is made up mostly of a roof of flat membrane bones united by sutures in the young, plus a series of cartilage bones at the base (occipital, sphenoid). Paranasal sinuses variably excavate the membrane bones.

The facial bones are mostly membrane bones and serve to support the dental arcades and the respiratory passages of the head.
s. bones the bones of the skull are the basisphenoid, ethmoid, frontal, hyoid, incisive, interparietal, lacrimal, nasal, occipital, nasal conchal, palatine, parietal, presphenoid, pterygoid, sphenoid, temporal, vomer and zygomatic.
brachycephalic s. short, broad skull.
dolicocephalic s. long, narrow skull.
mesaticephalic s. a medium skull in terms of width and length.
s. symmetry asymmetry common only in foals in which the lower part of the face is deviated to one side, involving mandibles, maxillae and nasal bones.

skunk a musteline mammal of the subfamily Mephitinae. The best-known animal in this group is the striped skunk *Mephitis mephitis*, a cat-size, mostly nocturnal, burrowing animal with a beautiful black coat and two longitudinal white stripes that run into the tail. It can also eject a powerfully pungent foul-smelling liquid up to 10 feet through the air.
s. cabbage see LYSICHITON AMERICANUS, SYMPLOCARPUS FOETIDUS, VERATRUM *californicum*.
s. descenting see DESCENTING.

s. rabies skunks are an important reservoir host of rabies in North America where they are the most common cause of rabies in cattle.

skunkweed CROTON *texensis*.

sky blue shrimp disease see BLUE SHELL SYNDROME.

Skye terrier a small (25 lb) dog with a distinctive appearance—the body is very long (the total length is specified in the breed standard as 41 in) and the legs are very short (height 10 in). The long, gray, fawn, cream or black coat is flat and straight, covering the face. The breed is affected by an inherited laryngeal hypoplasia.

skyline view tangential radiographic view of any structure; taken to provide more information than the standard projections. Used to examine the trochlear groove of the stifle in dogs and carpal slab fractures in horses.

slack loose; not taut.

s. cap a can of meat with one of the ends bulging slightly indicating the beginnings of a blown can.

s. loin hollow-flanked with too much room between the last rib and the thigh.

s. pastern too much slope in the pastern.

slaframine the sialagogic toxin in the fungus *Rhizoctonia leguminicola*.

slag vitreous residue after removal of metal in a smelting process.

basic s. a by-product of the smelting industry, basic slag is used as a fertilizer. Animals pastured on recently heavily dressed fields may be affected by colic, diarrhea and posterior paresis. The specific cause of the poisoning is not known.

slaked lime unslaked lime (calcium oxide) to which water has been added. Called also calcium hydroxide. See also LIME water.

slangkop [Af.] URGINEA *rubella*.

slap test see LARYNGEAL adductory reflex.

slatted floor wooden or metal floors with narrow gaps between slats to permit discharge of feces and urine to the external environment, e.g. in a shearing shed, or into a cesspit, the common construction on farms in the northern hemisphere. They are labor-saving but can cause serious damage to feet and limbs if not constructed carefully.

slaughter 1. the killing of animals for the preparation of meat for human consumption. Many methods are used. See also EMERGENCY slaughter, CAPTIVE BOLT PISTOL, CARBON DIOXIDE anesthesia, JEWISH SLAUGHTER, MUSLIM SLAUGHTER, PITHING, PUNTILLA, SHECHITA, SIKH SLAUGHTER. 2. destruction of animals because they are diseased, e.g. in test-and-slaughter programs.

casualty s. see EMERGENCY slaughter.

Danish s. data system a detailed system for keeping data on slaughter and meat inspection of pigs in Denmark. Based on tattooing of all pigs and a code for meat inspection findings with all information stored on a computer system.

s. hall, s. floor the part of an abattoir in which the slaughtering is conducted.

selective s. slaughter and disposal of infected animals as a tool in the eradication of disease. Those slaughtered may be infected or be positive reactors or in-contact animals.

s. spleen enlargement and congestion of the spleen with hemorrhages under the capsule which occur in some slaughter methods.

stunning–bleeding s. stunning either with a hammer or by electric shock followed by shackling and lifting, then by opening of the jugular vein.

slaughterhouse abattoir.

s. data data on lesions found in carcasses at abattoir; a biased sample because of the natural selection of animals for salvage as meat.

SLE systemic lupus erythematosus.

sleep a period of rest during which volition and consciousness are in partial or complete abeyance and the bodily functions partially suspended; a behavioral state marked by characteristic immobile posture and diminished but readily reversible sensitivity to external stimuli.

s. deprivation caused in animals by constant stimulation, e.g. preventing them from lying down, is followed by a compensatory period of prolonged sleep whenever the opportunity arises.

s. disorders see NARCOLEPSY, CATAPLEXY.

put to s. a common euphemism for euthanasia.

rapid eye movement s. that type of sleep characterized by low voltage but fast electroencephalographic activity and little muscular activity except of the ocular muscles. Believed to be the critical or necessary component of sleep. Called also 'sleep of the body' and paradoxical sleep. Called also REM.

sleeper foal syndrome newborn foals with severe toxemia or dehydration or anemia characterized by recumbency, sagging posture, lack of interest in food or the dam, listlessness to the point of coma.

sleeper syndrome see HEMOPHILOSIS.

sleeping beauty OXALIS *acetosella*.

sleeping disease narcolepsy.

s. d. syndrome disease affecting freshwater rainbow trout; characterized by lethargy and immobility; caused by a togavirus probably identical to the pancreatic disease virus.

sleeping sickness any disease characterized by drowsiness or somnolence. See also PREGNANCY toxemia (1) of ewes, equine viral ENCEPHALOMYELITIS, CRYPTOBIA *cyprini*, TRYPANOSOMIASIS.

sleepy characterized bY SLEEP.

s. foal disease see SHIGELLOSIS.

s. staggers see hepatic ENCEPHALOPATHY.

sleepygrass see STIPA *robusta*.

sleeve dog another name for the Pekingese dog.

slender ice plant MESEMBRYANTHEMUM *nodiflorum*.

slender lamb poison ISOTROPIS *juncea*.

slender native couch grass BRACHYACHNE *tenella*.

slender thistle see CARDUUS.

slender wild pea LATHYRUS *angulatus*.

slicker brush see CARDER.

slide a piece of glass or other transparent substance on which material is placed for examination under the microscope.

acetate tape s. see ACETATE tape slide.

s. culture technique a rapid method of preparing fungal colonies for examination and identification.

sliders a species of tortoise kept as pets. They have a black shell and a red stripe behind the eye. Called also *Chrysemys scripta elegans*, red-eared sliders.

sliding filament model mechanism proposed for muscle contraction where myosin head groups of the thick filaments move along the interdigitated actin of the thin filaments, sliding past them and thereby shortening the sarcomere.

slim amaranth AMARANTHUS *hybridus*.

slime balls form in which the cercariae of *Dicrocoelium dendriticum* are discharged from the intermediate host snail's lung; cercariae become infective only if the next intermediate stage, the ant, ingests the slime ball.

Slims BELGIAN fancy canary.

slimy skin disease a disease of aquarium fish caused by the flagellated protozoan *Costia necatrix* and characterized by a copious exudate on the skin of mucous and epithelial debris.

sling suspensory for supporting a part.

body s. canvas and metal sling for support of the abdomen with breastplate and breeching to prevent the horse slipping out forwards or backwards, and lifted from the ground by a block and tackle carried on an overhead beam or similar support. Used in horses; not a practicable proposition in cattle.

leg s. for the support of a limb in a cattle beast. For a front leg the rope is looped around the pastern, thrown over an overhead beam, back under the sternum behind the elbow on the same side, then back over the beam. For a hindleg the rope begins as a loop around the pastern, goes over an overhead support, back inside the thigh on the same side, half-hitched around the tibia and held by a helper. In both the leg is lifted off the ground to the required position and the rope tightened to create the sling.

pelvic limb s. the metatarsus is suspended by tape from a band of gauze and tape around the animal's abdomen. Used in small animals to prevent weight bearing on the limb, but not primarily for stabilization. Called also Robinson sling.

preputial s. a many-tailed bandage around the body with an aperture for the preputial orifice.

s. procedure a strip of fascia lata or synthetic material passed around the base of the tail or implanted in perianal tissue have been used in the treatment of fecal incontinence.

tail s. a half-hitch is applied to the tail hairs, ensuring that the tissue part is omitted. The rope can be used to support the hindquarters of a horse but not a cattle beast. The technique can be used in cattle as an aid, e.g. to keep the tail out of the way while correcting a dystocia; the rope is tied around the cow's neck.

udder s. a canvas bag with four strategically placed holes for the teats and supported by a harness over the hindquarters anchored to a neck collar to prevent it falling off the back. Not a particularly helpful device because of variation in the size of the vessel to be accommodated.

Velpeau s. a gauze wrapping around the thorax and forelimb with the elbow fully flexed and the carpus touching the opposite shoulder. Used in dogs to prevent weight-bearing following surgery, luxation of the shoulder or fracture of the scapula.

slink calves, slinks unborn calves retrieved at the abattoir. Their meat, slink veal, is not authorized for consumption in most countries. Their skins are valuable because they are so fine and clean.

slinkweed see GUTIERREZIA *microcephala*.

slip knot one in which the second and subsequent throws can still be snugged down to the surface. The knot is secured with a square knot for the last two throws.

slipe unscoured fell-mongered wool.

slipped 1. aborted. 2. dislocated or out of place in a more general sense.

s. claw flexion of the posterior claw in canaries so the dorsal surface becomes weight-bearing. May be caused by riboflavin deficiency.

s. disk see slipped DISK.

s. epiphysis see EPIPHYSIOLYSIS.

s. shoulder see SUPRASCAPULAR paralysis.

s. stifle see PATELLAR luxation.

s. tendon see PEROSIS.

slipper foot see LAMINITIS.

slit lamp biomicroscopy see slit LAMP.

slitter see TEAT slitter.

sliver in wool processing a continuous band of carded and combed wool which has not yet been twisted into yarn.

slobbering see DROOLING.

slobbers 1. moist dermatitis, or wet dewlap of rabbits; caused by continuous wetting of the dewlap due to poorly placed watering devices. 2. RHIZOCTONIA LEGUMINICOLA poisoning in cattle.

slope in statistical terms the slope of a line depicting the relationship of two variables is the gradient of the line or the regression coefficient of the relationship. A positive slope implies that increasing one variable will increase the other.

slope culture see slant CULTURE.

sloth member of the order Edentata of anteaters. A shaggy-haired, multicolored arboreal animal remarkable for its immobility and slowness of movement when it does move. It spends much time hanging by its paws in a belly-up, face-up position. There are several genera including the three-toed sloth (*Bradypus tridactylus*) and the two-toed sloth (*Choloepus didactylus*).

slough 1. a mass of dead tissue in, or cast out from, living tissue. 2. to shed or cast off.

anesthetic s. the iatrogenic slough caused by the injection of a necrotizing anesthetic solution subcutaneously in mistake for an intravenous injection. The common sites are over the anterior aspect of the forearm in small animals and over the jugular furrow in large animals.

epidermal s. occurs in captive cetaceans when the salinity of the pool water is insufficient.

Sloughi, Sloughui a medium-sized, lean, racy dog with a long, flat head, flat ears, a long, thin tail and a short, fine coat in sable or fawn. Called also Arabian greyhound.

slow reduced speed of action or reaction.

s. death factor see ALGAL poisoning.

s.-milking cows cows that require more than 6 minutes to milk right out; the average is 4 minutes. Caused by a too-small sphincter orifice at the tip of the teat.

s. muscles red (type I, slow twitch) muscles as distinct from white (type II, fast twitch) muscles. This is not a completely accurate definition but it serves as a generalization. Fast fibers require more stimulation to contract, develop greater tensions and fatigue more quickly than red fibers. See also MUSCLE.

s. release bolus formulation of drugs into a dense solid bolus, administered by balling gun, designed to dissolve slowly so as to provide a continuous intake of the medication over a period of 3 or 4 days.

s. virus infections somewhat imprecise term for persistent virus infections characterized by a very prolonged incubation period and a prolonged, slowly progressive clinical course. Originally applied to infection with lentiviruses and the subacute spongiform encephalopathies, now believed to be caused by prions.

slow-reacting substance a substance released in the anaphylactic reaction that induces slow, prolonged contraction of certain smooth muscles. So called because its effect is detected after the release and action of histamine; thought to be important in, for example, asthma. Symbol SRS or SRS-A. Called also leukotriene.

sludge a suspension of solid or semisolid particles in a fluid.

activated s. a means of encouraging biodegradation. See also ACTIVATED sludge.

sludging settling out of solid particles from solution.

s. of blood intravascular agglutination of erythrocytes into irregular masses, interfering with circulation of blood.

slug the garden pest *Agriolimax meticulatus*; may attract snail poison to a hitherto carefree garden and lead to metaldehyde poisoning in companion animals and may also harbor encysted larvae of *Syngamus trachea*.

slundhru KALANCHOE *integra*.

slurry solids in suspension. Used as a method of feeding pigs—slurry is pumped through fixed lines and delivered to troughs by hoses equipped with gasoline pump fittings. Used also as a means of disposing of feces and urine from cesspits under animal accommodation or trap tanks attached to milking sheds. Disposal is usually onto pasture. This creates poisoning hazards with respect to heavy metals and transmission of disease such as salmonellosis or Johne's disease.

sly syndrome human mucopolysaccharidosis, analogous to β-glucuronidase deficiency mucopolysaccharidosis in experimental dogs.

Sm chemical symbol, *samarium*.

SMAF specific macrophage arming factor.

small a lesser dimension.

s. buffalo grass PANICUM *coloratum*.

s. burr medic MEDICAGO *minima*.

s. colon the terminal colon in the horse between the right dorsal colon and the rectum. Because of its small diameter it is a common site for obstruction by phytobezoars and similar bodies.

s. colon impaction subacute colic in horses characterized by a palpable mass in the midlevel right abdomen.

s.-faced mallow see MALVA PARVIFLORA.

s.-flowered buttercup RANUNCULUS *parviflorus*.

s.-flowered Darling pea SWAINSONA *brachycarpa*.

s.-flowered mallow see MALVA PARVIFLORA.

s.-flowered melilot MELILOTUS *indica*.

s. golden tip GOODIA *medicagenea*.

s.-headed rice-flower PIMELEA *microcephala*.

s. intestine includes all of the intestine between the pylorus and the ileocecal valve; composed of the duodenum, jejunum and ileum. See also INTESTINE, INTESTINAL.

s. intestine meridian points acupuncture points on the small intestine meridian.

s.-leaf poranthera PORANTHERA *microphylla*.

s.-leaved bluebush see MAIREANA BREVIFOLIA.

s. liver fluke DICROCOELIUM *dendriticum*.

s. nuclear ribonucleoproteins see RIBONUCLEIC ACID.

s. passion flower PASSIFLORA *suberosa*.

s. stomach worm TRICHOSTRONGYLUS *axei*.

s. strongyles include *Caballonema*, *Cyathostomum*, *Cylicocyclus*, *Cylicodontophorus*, *Cylicostephanus*, *Cylindropharynx*, *Gyalocephalus*, *Poteriostomum* spp.

s. yellow foxglove LATHYRUS *splendens*.

smallhead sneezeweed HELENIUM *microcephalum*.

smallpox see VARIOLA.

smartweed see PERSICARIA, POLYGONUM.

SMCA monochloracetate.

SMCO *S*-methylcysteine sulfoxide.

smear a specimen for microscopic study, the material being spread thinly and unevenly across the slide with a swab or loop, or with the edge of another slide, e.g. blood smear, for differential white cell count, or trypanosome sighting, fecal for the presence of worm eggs or coccidial oocysts.

impression s. one made by pressing the slide against tissue, usually the surface of a neoplasm or the cut surface of a tissue specimen.

SMEDI group enteroviruses in three subgroups A, B and C. Found in pigs and cause a shortfall in live pigs, a high incidence of stillbirth and mummification and a high rate of piglet mortality. SMEDI group of diseases are also causatively linked to porcine parvovirus.

smegma the secretion of sebaceous glands, especially the cheesy secretion, consisting principally of desquamated epithelial cells, found chiefly within the prepuce.

smell 1. an odor. 2. the sense that enables an animal to perceive odors. The sense of smell depends on the stimulation of sense organs in the nose by small particles carried in inhaled air. It is important not only for the detection of odors, but also for the enjoyment of food. Flavor is a blend of taste and smell. Taste registers only four qualities: salt, sour, bitter and sweet; other qualities of flavor depend on smell. The organs of smell are small patches of special (olfactory) cells in the nasal mucosa. One patch is located in each of the two main compartments of the back of the nose. The olfactory cells are connected to the brain by the first cranial (olfactory) nerve.

abnormal s. see ODOR, TAINT.

organ of s. includes the olfactory sense organs, olfactory nerves, and the nerve cells of the olfactory bulb of the brain.

smelt small marine finfish *Osmerus eparlanus*, *O. mordax*.

Smith–Baskerville medium a selective medium for the growth of *Bordetella bronchiseptica*.

Smith–Petersen nail a flanged nail for fixing the head of the femur in fracture of the femoral neck.

smog smoke-laden fog, a form of environmental pollution.

smoke 1. a coat color of cats that consists of white hairs with black or blue tips. The intensity of the tip color varies on different parts of the body so that the face and back are very strongly colored. 2. a color variety of longhaired cats with orange or copper-colored eyes and a blue or black smoke coat color.

s. bombs after ignition may contaminate pasture with phosphorus.

s. inhalation animals confined in buildings, especially horses, suffer pulmonary congestion and edema after inhaling smoke from a building fire.

smoke injury injury caused by exposure to a fire where there is a great deal of smoke, especially one confined in a building. Animals are likely to suffer smoke injury to the respiratory system. The worst result is pulmonary edema and death due to asphyxia.

smoking a method of preserving meat or fish (most commonly bacon) which preserves the food's natural color and flavour. The food is pickled in salt first and then smoked in a smoke house, using special woods for special flavours, for about 3 days.

smoldering leukemia occult myeloproliferative neoplasia.

smolt young salmon on its way downriver en route to the sea; covered with distinctive silvery scales.

smoltification an internal metabolic process which enables a fish to adapt from fresh to sea water with a minimum of stress; characteristic of salmonid fish.

smooth absence of roughness.

s. Darling pea SWAINSONA *galegifolia*.

s. endoplasmic reticulum see endoplasmic RETICULUM.

s. gousiektebossie [Af.] PACHYSTIGMA *thamnus*.

s. mouth said of a horse's dentition when the molars are worn so that dentine and enamel are evenly worn and the tables are completely smooth and have lost their triturating capacity.

s. rice-flower PIMELEA *glauca*.
s. senna SENNA *floribunda*.
s. tongue a congenital defect in cattle characterized by the absence of papillae on the dorsum of the tongue, hypersalivation, poor haircoat and illthrift. Called also epitheliogenesis imperfecta lingua bovis.
s. witch grass PANICUM *dichotomiflorum*.
smothering death by asphyxiation. Occurs where poultry are carelessly herded into a corner where they cannot escape and where they are piled four or five birds deep; they will die of asphyxia very quickly. See also CROWDING.
SMSV San Miguel sealion virus.
smudge cell a ruptured leukocyte, seen in a blood smear.
smudge patterns the pattern of feces smeared on the buttocks of calves with diarrhea; thought to have diagnostic significance.
smut a group of fungal infections of the seedheads of cereals. Infected grain fed to livestock may be poisonous.
barley s. *Ustilago hordei* thought to cause infertility and stillbirths.
wheat s. *Tilletia tritici* thought to cause glomerulonephritis in pigs.
Sn chemical symbol, *tin* (L. *stannum*).
snail gastropod mollusc with a spiral, coiled shell. Some species of snails act as intermediate hosts for flukes and are thus of veterinary importance.
s. bait see METALDEHYDE, METHIOCARB.
snake a limbless reptile; many species are poisonous. See under the names of individual species. See also Table 22.
s. venom see SNAKEBITE.
snakebite injury caused by the mouthparts of a snake. (1) Cobra-type snakes inject a neurotoxin in their venom causing pupillary dilatation, excitement, convulsions and death due to asphyxia. (2) Adder-type snake venom contains also an agent that causes local swelling and necrosis. If the animal survives the neurotoxin, the part sloughs. (3) Other fractions in some venoms include hemolytic, cardiotoxic, coagulant and anticoagulant fractions. See also DEMANSIA *textilis*, TIGER snake, Table 22.
snakeroot see EUPATORIUM *rugosum*.
snake's head see FRITILLARIA MELEAGRIS.
snakeweed see GUTIERREZIA *microcephala*.
snap a short, sharp sound.
s. joint capable of moving abruptly from a stable, in the sense of having great stability than the sense of its domicile, to a more mobile position, e.g. the equine elbow joint.
opening s. a short, sharp, high-pitched click occurring in early diastole caused by opening of the mitral cusps, a characteristic sound in mitral stenosis.
snapper see PAGRUS AURATUS.
snare an entrapping loop.
cable s. see HOG holder.
obstetrical s. a looped cord for slipping over the head of a fetus to provide traction on the neck. Applied over the nape and through the mouth, not around the neck.
pig s. see HOG holder.
surgical s. a wire loop for removing polyps and other pedunculated growths by cutting them off at the base.
snatch removal of a newborn animal from the dam before it has an opportunity to suck. The objective is to rear it independently and free of colostrum-borne infection or of colostral antibodies.
SND standardized normal deviation.
sneeze 1. an involuntary, sudden, violent, and audible expulsion of air through the mouth and nose. 2. to expel air in such a manner. Sneezing is usually caused by the irritation of sensitive nerve endings in the mucous membrane that lines the nose. Allergies, drafts of cold air, and even bright light can produce sneezing. It is a predominant sign in inclusion body rhinitis in piglets, atrophic rhinitis in older pigs, and feline rhinotracheitis.
s. counts number of sneezes per pig per minute. Used as an indicator of the presence or absence of upper respiratory disease in a piggery—greater than 0.33 sneezes per pig per minute accepted as an indication of rhinitis in pigs.
reverse s. sporadic, brief periods of noisy, labored inspiratory effort seen in dogs that are otherwise normal. Postnasal drip, nasopharyngeal spasm, and entrapment of the epiglottis have been suggested as causes.
sneezeweed see HELENIUM.
sneezing sudden, reflex, noisy expiration through the nasal cavities; prominent sign in cases of rhinitis.
SNF solids-not-fat; a comment on the composition of milk.
sniffer dog one trained to detect the presence of specified materials, usually drugs or explosives, by smell. The dogs can be of any breed.
snip a white mark on the muzzle extending into one nostril.
SNOMED Standard Nomenclature of Medical Diseases and Operations.
snood see frontal PROCESS (2).
Snook hook a surgical instrument with a curved, button tip used to retrieve a horn of the uterus when performing ovariohysterectomy in dogs and cats.
snoring an involuntary, deep guttural sound emanating from the pharynx and soft palate on inspiration or expiration; often intermittent depending on posture of the head. May indicate a chronic, obstructive lesion of pharynx.
s. disease is an enzootic rhinitis of cattle caused by *Helminthosporium* spp.
snort a forceful expulsion of air through the nostrils as in a sneeze, but a snort is a voluntary act, sneezing is involuntary. Used by horses and cattle as a device to intimidate potential predators.
snorter dwarf an achondroplastic dwarf with stertorous respiration due to distortion of nasal passages. See achondroplastic DWARFISM.
snotsiekte [Af.] see BOVINE malignant catarrh.
snout the upper lip and the apex of the nose, especially of the pig. Called also rostrum. Has a specialized skin to survive the rigours of rooting, is supported by a separate bone (the os rostri), and also has a few sensory hairs.
s. rubbing a vice of pigs characterized by rubbing the snout into the flank until a friction sore develops.
s. twitch see HOG holder.
SNOVET Standard Nomenclature of Veterinary Diseases and Operations.
snow a freezing or frozen mixture consisting of discrete particles or crystals.
carbon dioxide s. the solid formed by rapid evaporation of liquid carbon dioxide, giving a temperature of about −110°F (−79°C); used locally in various skin conditions. See also CARBON DIOXIDE snow.
s. leopard see SNOW LEOPARD.
s. nose see nasal DEPIGMENTATION.
snow-on-the-mountain EUPHORBIA *marginata*.
snowflakes small patches of gray or white hair acquired after birth. Skin color is unchanged. See also ACHROMOTRICHIA, VITILIGO.

Snowshoe a recently recognized cat breed; it is a medium- to large-sized cat with blue eyes, and coat color similar to a sealpoint or bluepoint Siamese, but with a white nose, chin, and ventral midline, and white boots on all feet.

snowshoe hare virus one of the California serotype bunyaviruses isolated in Canada from the snowshoe hare. It is a cause of equine viral encephalomyelitis.

snRNA small nuclear RIBONUCLEIC ACID.

snRNP small nuclear ribonucleoprotein. See also RIBONUCLEIC ACID.

snuffles 1. a disease of the upper respiratory tract of rabbits caused by infection with *Pasteurella multocida* and characterized by serous and then purulent discharge from the nostrils and eyes which cakes the insides of the forepaws. The rabbit also sneezes and coughs. Pneumonia is a common sequel. 2. chronic rhinitis and sinusitis in cats. Sometimes called chronic snuffles syndrome.

snuffling a bubbling sound from the nasal cavities; an indication of inflammation and the presence of fluid exudate.

SNVDO Standard Nomenclature of Veterinary Diseases and Operations.

SOAP acronym for *s*ubjective data, *o*bjective data, *a*ssessment, *p*lan, the way the progress notes are organized in problem-oriented MEDICAL record keeping.

soap any compound of one or more fatty acids, or their equivalents, with an alkali. Soap is a detergent and is employed in liniments and enemas and in making pills. It is also a mild aperient, antacid and antiseptic.

green s. a potassium soap made by saponification of vegetable oils, excluding coconut oil and palm kernel oil, without the removal of glycerin; it is the chief ingredient of green soap tincture.

medicated s. those containing additional ingredients, usually for the treatment of skin disorders, e.g. insecticides, keratolytics, antiseptics, antipruritics.

s. poisoning common dishwashing and laundry soaps can be a source of poisoning for dogs and cats. There can be gastrointestinal and neurologic signs.

soft s. (medicinal) green soap.

s. substitute detergents or cleansing creams for cleaning the skin, especially removing greasy films or glandular exudates.

soapwort SAPONARIA *officinalis*.

Soboliphyme baturini a nematode in the family Soboliphymatidae; found in the intestines of foxes, sables and cats.

social pertaining to living in a community.

s. behavior behavior of an animal to others in its social group of herd, flock, neighbors. See also social BEHAVIOR.

s. benefits the benefits to a community that cannot be measured by material values, better social justice, freedom from fear, improvement in educational facilities. The fundamental parameter in a cost–benefit analysis.

s. costs the costs incurred by society as a whole rather than by individuals. Used in the estimation of benefit–cost analysis.

s. distance average distance between animals in a community. An expression of the concentration of the animals in the environment.

s. dominance heirarchy social order.

s. order the ranking in which a group of animals establishes itself with the most dominant one in the number one position and the most retiring one in the last position. The order is maintained unless new animals are introduced.

s. organization an aggregation of individual animals into an integrated group based on the interdependence of the animals and their responses to each other.

s. stress thought to be a common cause of illness in domestic pets and to a less extent in pigs, e.g. in ESOPHAGOGASTRIC ulcer.

socialization the process of familiarization between animals in a group and, in companion animals, between the animal and humans.

s. period the critical age when the young animal is most likely to establish social relationships, forming the basis for its personality, particularly toward humans, and trainability. In puppies, this is from approximately 3 to 12 weeks of age and approximately 2 to 7 weeks for kittens.

sociosexual behavior pertaining to sexual relationships between animals in groups; behavior such as dominance of one bull over another can have very important effects on the offspring of the groups of cows run with a group of bulls.

sock white mark on the feet. In horses this means from the coronet to halfway up the cannon. In dogs and cats, it is white from the paws up to the carpus or hock.

socket a hollow into which a corresponding part fits.

dry s. alveolar OSTEITIS.

tooth s. see ALVEOLUS.

sod-seeding resowing a pasture without ripping it up. Carried out with a special implement that places seed and fertilizer in a sliced furrow with minimum disturbance of existing sward.

soda sodium carbonate.

baking s. sodium bicarbonate.

s. bush see NEOBASSIA PROCERIFLORA.

s. lime a mixture of 90% calcium hydroxide, 5% sodium hydroxide, 5% silica and water, used to absorb carbon dioxide from the exhaled air in a closed circuit anesthetic system. See also BARALIME.

sodium a chemical element, atomic number 11, atomic weight 22.990, symbol Na. See Table 6. Sodium is the major cation of the extracellular fluid (ECF), constituting 90 to 95% of all cations in the blood plasma and interstitial fluid; it thus determines the osmolality of the ECF.

s. acetate a systemic and urinary alkalizer.

s. acetylsalicylate aspirin.

s. acid phosphate, s. biphosphate used as a dietary supplement of phosphorus for ruminants when only phosphorus is required and in small animals as a urinary acidifier.

s. aminoarsonate used as a feed additive to chickens and may cause arsenic poisoning if the dose rate is exceeded.

s. antimony gluconate, s. stibogluconate a pentavalent antimonial used in the treatment of leishmaniasis.

s. arsanilate used as a feed additive in the treatment of swine dysentery and in poultry and causes arsenic poisoning when dose rates are excessive.

s. arsenite used as a topical acaricide. See inorganic ARSENIC poisoning.

s. arsenate like the arsenite, a toxic compound used as an acaricide. Less toxic and less effective than the arsenite. See also inorganic ARSENIC poisoning.

s. ascorbate a form of ascorbic acid; vitamin C.

s. azide used in weed control and the prevention of rot in fruit; used in serum samples to prevent bacterial overgrowth.

s. bentonite see BENTONITE.

s. benzoate used topically as an antifungal agent in

companion animals, with caffeine as a CNS stimulant and as a diagnostic aid in a liver function test.
s. bicarbonate a white powder found in most households in the form of baking soda; called also bicarbonate of soda. Used as a gastric antacid and as a systemic and urinary alkalinizer. See also MILK SHAKE. Used locally to remove mucus and to remove exudates and scabs.
s. cacodylate an organic compound yielding trivalent inorganic arsenic on metabolism in the body, similar in effects and toxicity to arsenic trioxide. Formerly used as a systemic treatment for chronic skin disease and capable of causing arsenic poisoning if used to excess.
s.-calcium channels see CHANNEL.
s. carbonate $Na_2CO_3 \cdot H_2O$, used as an alkalizing agent in pharmaceuticals, and has been used as a lotion or bath in the treatment of scaly skin, and as a detergent in companion animals.
s. channels see CHANNEL.
s. chlorate an oldfashioned herbicide which is quite palatable to farm animals and toxic in moderate amounts. Large doses cause abdominal pain, staggering and purging. Lower doses cause methemoglobinemia and dyspnea.
s. chloride salt; a necessary constituent of the body and therefore of the diet; sometimes used parenterally in solution to replenish electrolytes in the body.
s. chloride nutritional deficiency not a common occurrence but is seen in grazing animals on sodium deficient pastures, where heavy potash fertilizer has been applied in animals that are milking heavily, growing rapidly or losing a lot of sweat. Signs include pica, e.g. drinking urine, polydipsia, polyuria and decrease in appetite, milk yield, body weight, and urinary sodium and chloride.
s. chloride poisoning (salt poisoning) can occur via the diet due to accidental inclusion of too much salt; is usually too unpalatable. Most common is drinking of natural saline water from bore or deep well. Causes gastroenteritis, diarrhea and dehydration most noticeable in lactating animals. Animals are restless and play with water, looking for fresh water. Water contains also magnesium, sulfate and carbonate ions. If water intake restricted and salt intake normal a relative poisoning occurs. If combined with water deprivation causes POLIOENCEPHALOMALACIA when the water intake returns to normal. In pigs the brain lesion is similar but because of the extensive infiltrations of eosinophils, characteristic of pigs, it is called eosinophilic meningoencephalitis.
s. chloroacetate a herbicide with very low toxicity potential.
s. citrate an alkalinizing agent; used also as an in vitro anticoagulant in blood stored for transfusion or diagnostic use.
s. cyanide a highly toxic industrial chemical and unlikely to enter the animal food chain unless as a result of a spill of reagents or industrial waste.
s. diethyldithiocarbamate a chelating agent used in the treatment for thallium poisoning; also used as an immunomodulator in the treatment of human immunodeficiency virus infection in humans.
s. fluoride a white, odorless powder used at one time for the treatment of ascariasis in pigs. Has no use in veterinary medicine comparable to its use as a prophylactic against dental caries in humans. See also FLUOROSIS.
s. fluoroacetamide 1081; causes poisoning similar to sodium fluoroacetate (below).
s. fluoroacetate occurs naturally in some plants and used in agriculture as a rodenticide known as 1080. The latter is a restricted substance and is only sold on license. Two forms of poisoning occur: (1) myocardial failure resulting in sudden death in herbivora; signs are dyspnea, cardiac irregularity; (2) excitement and convulsions in pigs and dogs. Both poisonings are highly fatal. Plants containing fluoroacetate are *Gastrolobium* spp., *Acacia georgina* (gidgee), *Dichapetalum* spp., *Palicourea* spp.
s. fluorosilicate is used as an insecticide in bait form for crickets and grasshoppers and as an insecticide dust for poultry. It is as toxic as sodium fluoride.
s. glutamate the monosodium salt of L-glutamic acid; used in treatment of encephalopathies associated with liver diseases. Also used to enhance the flavor of foods.
s. homeostasis maintenance of the body's sodium status at an appropriate level; effected principally by aldosterone increasing tubular resorption of sodium from the glomerular filtrate.
s. hyaluronate used in the treatment of degenerative joint disease in horses. See also HYALURONIC ACID.
s. hydroxide an all-purpose caustic. Its biggest use in veterinary science is to clean down fat-laden surfaces in abattoirs prior to disinfection.
s. hypochlorite a compound having germicidal, deodorizing and bleaching properties; used in solution to disinfect utensils, and in diluted form (Dakin's solution) as a local antibacterial and to irrigate wounds. A common disinfectant for a wide variety of uses in veterinary medicine, including application to cow's teats in mastitis control programs. Called also bleach.
s. iodide a compound used as a source of iodine and as an expectorant. At times used parenterally in the treatment of extensive ringworm, actinobacillosis and actinomycosis. Overuse causes IODISM.
s. lactate a compound used in solution to replenish body fluids and electrolytes.
s. lauryl sulfate an anionic surface-active agent used in shampoos as a detergent and wetting agent to increase skin penetration of active ingredients.
s. metabisulfite used as an antioxidant and as an aid in the making of ensilage. Also used as a preservative on meat, as a source of SULFUR dioxide.
s. methanearsonate a herbicide—monosodium acid methanearsonate—causes arsenic poisoning.
s. molybdate used in salt mixture and as pasture topdressing as a prophylaxis against chronic copper poisoning in ruminants.
s. monofluoroacetate see sodium fluoroacetate (above).
s. nitrate used in food preservation especially meat pickling and as a fertilizer. Can cause nitrate–nitrite poisoning or nitrite poisoning in ruminants.
s. nitrite a vasodilator; used in the treatment of cyanide poisoning. Can cause methemoglobinemia and death from anoxia.
s. oleate used by local injection in horses to cause inflammation and aid healing of chronic injuries such as splints and bucked shins.
s. oxalate see soluble OXALATE poisoning.
s. pentachlorophenate used as a fungicide in wood preservatives. Acute poisoning after heavy dosing causes dyspnea and death due to respiratory failure.
s. perborate an oxidizing agent; used as a topical antiseptic and mouthwash.
s. phosphate an osmotic cathartic.
s.-potassium-ATPase pump see PUMP.
s.-potassium channels see CHANNEL.

s./potassium ratio a low ratio, indicating hyponatremia and hyperkalemia, is characteristic of hypoadrenocorticism.
s. propionate used in the prophylaxis and treatment of acetonemia in cows, and as a fungistat both topically and in preparations for animal medication.
s. pump see sodium PUMP.
s.-restricted diets used in the dietary management of heart disease and hypertension in dogs and cats.
s. salicylate an analgesic, antipyretic compound. See SALICYLATE.
s. selenite used as treatment for severe nutritional deficiency of selenium. Overdose will cause poisoning by SELENIUM.
s. sulfanilate rate of excretion is used as a sensitive test of urinary function. See also SULFANILATE.
s. sulfate an osmotic cathartic; also used as a diuretic and sometimes applied topically in solution to relieve edema and pain of infected wounds. Called also Glauber's salts.
s. sulfite test 1. precipitates protein out of solution; a dramatic test for protein in urine. 2. a turbidity test on serum for proximate estimation of gamma globulin content and immunological status of newborn calf.
s. tetraborate called also borax; used as a weak disinfectant.
s. thiosulfate a compound used in the treatment of cyanide poisoning, and used in measuring the volume of extracellular body fluid and the renal glomerular filtration rate.
s. trichloroacetate a nontoxic herbicide.
s. versenate see EDETATE.

sodoku a relapsing type of infection in humans, dogs and cats due to *Spirillum minus*, an organism transmitted by the bite of an infected rat.

soft lacking in firmness.
s. copy in computer terms is the text displayed on the computer monitor—the opposite of hard copy.
s. fat unpleasant soft fat occurs in pigs fed for too long on kitchen swill.
s. font fonts which are generated by computer software rather than by the printer's firmware. They are located in a file on a disk; when the printer is switched on preparatory to printing a job the fonts must be loaded from the disk to the printer's memory.
s. khaki weed see GOMPHRENA CELOSIOIDES.
s. palate myositis a cause of dorsal displacement of the soft palate in horses, resulting in chronic obstruction of the airway during exercise.
s. rolypoly SALSOLA *kali*.
s. rush JUNCUS *effusus*.
s. shell disease fish eggs lose their turgidity and become flat and wrinkled; the cause is unknown.
s. shelled eggs hen eggs with soft shells occur in birds affected by avian infectious bronchitis and can persist for a long time into the recovery period.
s. ticks ticks lacking a dorsal shield or scutum; members of the family Argasidae, e.g. *Argas persicus*. Called also nonscutate.
s. tissue tissue other than bone and cartilage.
s. x-ray beam made at low kVp output. The beam has low energy and weak penetration.

Soft-coated wheaten terrier a medium-sized, compact dog with a soft, silky, wavy, wheaten-colored coat that covers the face and body. The tail is docked. The breed is affected by a familial nephropathy.

soft khaki weed see GOMPHRENA CELOSIOIDES.

soft palate the fleshy partition at the back of the mouth which separates the nasopharynx from the oropharynx and which, together with the hard palate, forms the roof of the mouth.
cleft s. p. commonly the posterior part is defective but may be part of a defect involving both soft and hard palates. Manifested by difficulties in sucking or nasal regurgitation of milk and food from a young age. Often associated with entrapment of the palate by the aryepiglottic fold. See also CLEFT lip.
s. p. dislocation see dorsal soft palate displacement (below).
dorsal s. p. displacement the free edge of the soft palate is displaced from its normal position under the epiglottis to lie over the opening of the larynx causing reduction in airflow. Common only in horses.
elongated s. p., overlong s. p. a common abnormality in brachycephalic dogs in which it causes inspiratory respiratory distress, gagging and coughing. The soft palate interferes with the epiglottis and glottis, particularly after it becomes inflamed and edematous. Other anomalies of the respiratory tract commonly are also present. Affected horses appear to choke, then continue to breathe through their mouth with a characteristic rattling sound. The cause and pathogenesis are unclear.
s. p. myositis may contribute to soft palate paresis.
s. p. paresis causes a functional pharyngeal paresis and the affected horse chokes up during exercise; often accompanies laryngeal hemiplegia.

softening a change of consistency, with loss of firmness or hardness.

software see COMPUTER software.

Sogdianella moshkovskii the identity of this rickettsia has not been fully established. Reported to occur in a number of wild and domestic birds.

soil the earth, origin of all plant growth and the basis of all animal agriculture. Its characteristics of chemical composition, physical structure, especially porosity and water retaining capacity, its humus content, pH and salinity exert enormous effects on its productivity.
s. analysis an essential activity in densely farmed farms. Measures the soil content of total and available amounts of each of the important soil minerals.
s. contaminated herbage either from dust storms or in loose soil by hoof movement may contribute to dental attrition in sheep, or sand colic in horses.
s. eating a form of pica; caused by salt deficiency.
s. fumigants are used to prepare fields for planting and may cause poisoning in animals grazing them or eating crops harvested from them. See METHYL BROMIDE.
s. type includes clay, sand, loam.

soilage see zero GRAZING.

soiling see zero GRAZING.

sol a liquid colloid solution.

sol. solution.

solanaceous pertaining to or emanating from SOLANUM.

solanidine a toxic steroid alkaloid in plants of SOLANUM.

solanine a toxic glycoalkaloid in plants of SOLANUM. Solanine is metabolized to the sugar solanose.
s. group the plants in *Solanum* spp. which contain solanine. Includes, e.g. *S. dulcamara*, *S. nigrum*, *S. tuberosum*, *S. lycopersicum*, *S. melongena* and *S. pseudocapsicum*.

Solanum a widespread plant genus of the family Solanaceae which contains a number of valuable crop plants but also some poisonous ones. Poisoning may be due to (1) the presence in the plant of toxic glycoalkaloids which cause diarrhea, (2) alkamines, e.g. nitrosamines, which cause neuromuscular signs of incoordination, and the 'crazy cow' syndrome, or (3) calcinogenic glycosides which cause excessive deposition of calcium in tissues.

Solanaceous plants which may cause diarrhea syndrome include *Solanum aculeastrum*, *S. americanum*, *S. aviculare*, *S. capsiciforme*, *S. capsicoides*, *S. carolinense*, *S. cinereum*, *S. dulcamara*, *S. elaeagnifolium*, *S. incanum*, *S. laciniatum*, *S. mauritianum*, *S. melongena*, *S. nigrum*, *S. panduriforme*, *S. pseudocapsicum*, *S. quadriloculatum*, *S. rostratum*, *S. seaforthianum*, *S. simile*, *S. sturtianum*, *S. symonii*, *S. triflorum*, *S. vescum*.

Solanaceous plants which cause nervous syndromes include *Solanum bonariensis*, *S. dimidiatum*, *S. fastigiatum*, *S. kwebense*, *S. luederitzii*, *S. lycopersicum*, *S. tenuiramosum*, *S. upingtoniae*.

Solanaceous plants causing calcinosis include *S. linneanum* (*S. hermanii*, *S. sodomaeum*), *S. malocoxylon* (*S. glaucophyllum*), *S. torvum*.

Solanaceous plants causing miscellaneous syndromes include *S. carolinense* (inflammation of the mouth and esophagus), *S. tuberosum* (the common potato), which can cause carbohydrate engorgement. Eating of large quantities over a long period causes dermatitis of the lower limbs. Greened and sprouted potato tubers contain solanine and cause poisoning if fed without cooking or paring.

solar emanating from or pertaining to the sun's rays.

s. burn see SUNBURN.

s. dermatitis see solar DERMATITIS.

s. elastosis degenerative changes in the dermis caused by excessive solar radiation.

s. keratosis see actinic KERATOSIS.

nasal s. dermatitis see solar DERMATITIS, COLLIE nose.

solar-induced squamous cell carcinoma see SQUAMOUS cell carcinoma.

solar plexus a network of ganglia and nerves in the center of the abdomen composed principally of the celiac and cranial mesenteric ganglia; it is part of the autonomic nervous system. It is important in the control of the function of the liver, stomach, kidneys and adrenal glands.

solarization exposure to sunlight and the effects produced thereby.

solation the liquefaction of a gel.

sole the bottom of the foot or HOOF.

s. abrasion traumatic injury to the sole of the hoof; more common and more serious in soft hooves caused by constant standing in wet footing.

s. abscess occurs in all ungulates but most common as a nonspecific disease in horses resulting from nail pricks. Causes pain and lameness, and tetanus in horses, and may extend up behind the wall of the hoof and discharge as a sinus at the coronet.

s. corium see solear CORIUM.

dropped s. see DROPPED sole.

s. puncture penetration of the sole by a sharp foreign body, e.g. nail.

soft s. syndrome soft, crumbly horn in the sole of the hoof, usually all four hooves of the patient are affected, caused usually by failure of wear of the hoof, exacerbated by continued wetness and failure to trim overgrown hooves.

s. trauma bruising from excessive walking or walking on rough surfaces occur in horses and cattle. In horses, CORNS (2) may develop.

solenoglyphid a snake with mobile fangs that can be moved to give the best position for envenomation of the prey. Includes the vipers, puff adders and rattlesnakes.

Solenopotes capillatus a sucking louse of cattle in the family Linognathidae.

Solenopsis invicta fire ant; capable of causing damage to the conjunctiva in recumbent newborn animals.

solicitation a personal approach by a veterinarian to a person who is not a client and soliciting for any veterinary work that the person may have is unprofessional, unethical and, in most countries, illegal under the law governing veterinary practice.

solid 1. not fluid or gaseous; not hollow. 2. a substance or tissue not fluid or gaseous.

s. color said of animal haircoats; the same color all over the animal.

Solidago North American plant genus in the family Asteraceae; contain an unidentified toxin. In some outbreaks there is suspicion that the poisoning is caused by a fungus growing on the plant but tests with the plant alone have proved its toxicity. Clinical signs include vomiting, dyspnea and death in most cases. Identified species include *S. chinensis*, *S. mollis* (*S. concinna*, range goldenrod), *S. odora*, *S. specios*, *S. spectabilis* (western goldenrod).

solids-not-fat the substances in milk other than butterfat and water; abbreviated SNF. They include casein, lactose, vitamins and minerals which contribute significantly to the nutritive value of milk.

soliped single-toed ungulate; an animal with a single uncloven hoof. Includes Equidae only. See also MONODACTYL.

solitary being the only one or ones.

s. cyst UNICAMERAL cyst.

s. tract nucleus the brainstem nucleus of the solitary tract, the tract carrying afferent parasympathetic nerve fibers.

solubility the quality of being soluble.

s. coefficient in anesthetics, a measure of the distribution of anesthetic agent between blood and gas and between blood and tissue. The greater the solubility, the greater the uptake of anesthetic agent by blood and the slower the period of induction and recovery.

soluble susceptible of being dissolved.

s. glass see soluble GLASS.

solubles liquid containing soluble and very fine suspended particles in water or solvent. Mostly by-products of fermentation for the manufacture of alcohol. A good dietary protein supplement.

solute the substance that is dissolved in a liquid (solvent) to form a solution.

s. diuresis increase in the volume of urine excreted as a result of an increase in the glomerular filtrate of any osmotically active solute.

solution 1. a liquid preparation of one or more soluble chemical substances usually dissolved in water. 2. the process of dissolving or disrupting.

aqueous s. one in which water is used as the solvent.

buffer s. one that resists appreciable change in its hydrogen ion concentration (pH) when acid or alkali is added to it.

colloid s., colloidal s. a preparation consisting of minute particles of matter suspended in a solvent.

hyperbaric s. one having a greater specific gravity than a standard of reference.

hypertonic s. one having an osmotic pressure greater than that of a standard of reference.

hypobaric s. one having a specific gravity less than that of a standard of reference.

hypotonic s. one having an osmotic pressure less than that of a standard of reference.

iodine s. a transparent, reddish brown liquid, each 100 ml of which contains 1.8 to 2.2 g of iodine and 2.1 to 2.6 g of sodium iodide; a local anti-infective.
iodine s. (strong) Lugol's solution.
isobaric s. a solution having the same specific gravity as a standard of reference.
isotonic s. one having an osmotic pressure the same as that of a standard of reference.
molar s. a solution each liter of which contains 1 mole of the dissolved substance; designated 1 M. The concentration of other solutions may be expressed in relation to that of molar solutions as tenth-molar (0.1 M), etc.
normal s. a solution each liter of which contains 1 chemical equivalent of the dissolved substance; designated 1 N.
ophthalmic s. a sterile solution, free from foreign particles, for instillation into the eye.
physiological saline s., physiological salt s., physiological sodium chloride s. an aqueous solution of sodium chloride and other components, having an osmotic pressure identical to that of blood serum.
priming s. the fluid used to fill tubing and the reservoir of a cardiac bypass unit before use.
saline s. a solution of sodium chloride, or common salt, in purified water.
saturated s. a solution in which the solvent has taken up all of the dissolved substance that it can hold in solution.
sclerosing s. one containing an irritant substance that will cause obliteration of a space, such as the lumen of a varicose vein or the cavity of a hernial sac.
standard s. one containing a fixed amount of solute.
supersaturated s. one containing a greater quantity of the solute than the solvent can hold in solution under ordinary conditions.
volumetric s. one that contains a specific quantity of solvent per stated unit of volume.

solvent 1. capable of dissolving other material. 2. the liquid in which another substance (the solute) is dissolved to form a solution.
s. drag transfer of solutes across the intestinal wall by being carried along with the water flow driven by osmotic gradients across cell membranes.
s. extraction of oil seeds the oil is extracted by organic solvents, a modern process largely displacing extraction by pressure. The resulting cake or meal may be toxic, e.g. trichloroethylene extracted soybean meal.
s. poisoning cases of poisoning may be due to the solvent used in a medication, especially when these are petroleum products, as they are in many insecticide preparations.

som- prefix meaning the body.

soma 1. the body as distinguished from the mind. 2. the body tissue as distinguished from the germ cells. 3. the cell body.

Somali a medium to large breed of cat, recently recognized in some countries. It is similar in appearance to the Abyssinian but with a medium length haircoat, bushy tail and ruff around the neck. Also like the Abyssinian, the coat colors are red ticked with chocolate-brown, orange-brown (ruddy) with black tips, or blue.

Somaphantus lusius a louse of guinea fowl.

somasthenia bodily weakness with poor appetite and poor sleep.

somatic 1. pertaining to or characteristic of the body or soma. 2. pertaining to the body wall, not the viscera.
s. afferent system the system of sensory neurons scattered around the body and responding to pain, touch, temperature and other external stimuli.
s. cell see somatic CELL.
s. cell hybridization fusion in the laboratory of two different populations of somatic cells.
s. mutation see somatic MUTATION.
s. myoneural junction see MYONEURAL JUNCTION.
s. nerves nerves supplying the body wall and limbs.
s. pain pain emanating from muscles, skeleton, skin; pain in the parts of the body other than the viscera.
s. sensation central perceptions of sensory stimuli from the body wall and limbs include touch, temperature, tickle, itch, pain, conscious proprioception.
s. theory this postulates that very few immunoglobulins are inherited but there is great diversification in differentiating somatic cells.

somation variations in somatic structure that are not hereditary.

somat(o)- word element. [Gr.] *body*.

somatochrome any neuron which has a well-marked cell body completely surrounding the nucleus, its colorable protoplasm having a distinct contour; used also adjectively.

somatocrinin see GROWTH HORMONE releasing hormone.

somatogenic originating in the body.

somatology the sum of what is known about the body.

somatome 1. an appliance for cutting the body of a fetus. 2. a somite.

somatomedin any of a group of peptides found in the liver and in plasma which mediate the effect of growth hormone (somatotropin) on cartilage; they are responsible for uptake of sulfate and increased synthesis of collagen and other proteins by cartilage.
s. C participates in the limitation of secretion of growth hormone by the pituitary; produced in various tissues, especially liver; called also IGF-1 or insulin-like growth factor.

somatometry measurement of the dimensions of the entire body.

somatopagus a double fetus united at the trunks.

somatopathy a bodily disorder rather than a mental one.

somatoplasm the protoplasm of the body cells exclusive of the germ cells.

somatopleure the part of the embryo which forms the lateral and ventral walls of the fetus. Consists of somatic mesoderm and ectoderm.

somatoschisis 1. splitting of the bodies of the vertebrae. 2. a fissure of the trunk.

somatoscopy examination of the body.

somatostatin a cyclic tetradecapeptide hormone and neurotransmitter that inhibits the release of peptide hormones in many tissues. It is released by the hypothalamus to inhibit the release of growth hormone (GH, somatotropin) and thyroid-stimulating hormone (TSH) from the anterior pituitary; it is also released by the delta cells of the islets of Langerhans in the pancreas to inhibit the release of glucagon and insulin and by the similar D cells in the gastrointestinal tract.

somatotherapy treatment aimed at relieving or curing ills of the body.

somatotopic related to particular areas of the body; a correspondence between the form of the body and its representation on an organ such as the brain. The motor and sensory cortices of the brain are arranged somatotopically, specific regions of the cortex being responsible for different areas of the body. See also somatotopical PROJECTION.

somatotopy see SOMATOTOPIC.
somatotrope somatotroph.
somatotroph any of the cells of the adenohypophysis that secrete growth hormone.
somatotrophin growth hormone. See also PITUITARY.
somatotropin somatotrophin.
somatotype a particular type of body build.
somatotyping objective classification of animals according to type of body build.
somatropin nonproprietary drug name for somatotropin (growth hormone).
somite one of the paired block-like masses of mesoderm beside the neural tube of a vertebrate embryo, formed by transverse subdivision, that develop into the vertebral column, skin and muscles of the body.
somitomere a segment of paraxial mesoderm.
somnifacient causing sleep.
somniferous producing sleep.
somnolence sleepiness; also, unnatural drowsiness. A depressive mental state commonly caused by encephalitis, encephalomalacia, hepatic encephalopathy, hypoxia and some poisonings, e.g. *Filix mas*, the male fern.
Somogyi effect a rebound phenomenon occurring in diabetes mellitus; overtreatment with insulin induces hypoglycemia, which initiates the release of epinephrine, ACTH, glucagon and growth hormone, which stimulate lipolysis, gluconeogenesis and glycogenolysis, which, in turn, result in rebound hyperglycemia and ketosis.
Sonchus genus of the plant family Asteraceae; can cause nitrate–nitrite poisoning; called also sow thistles.
songbird fever an acute, febrile illness with vomiting and hemorrhagic diarrhea, observed in cats in the Northeastern United States during periods of seasonal bird migration; believed to be caused by *Salmonella typhimurium*.
sonic bang loud sound made by a flying projectile when it passes through the sound barrier, that is by flying faster than the speed of sound.
sonicate 1. to expose to sound waves; to disrupt bacteria by exposure to high-frequency sound waves. 2. the products of such disruption.
sonication exposure to sound waves; disruption of bacteria by exposure to high-frequency sound waves.
sonitus tinnitus.
sonogram a record or display obtained by ultrasonic scanning.
sonography ultrasonography.
sonolucent in ultrasonography, permitting the passage of ultrasound waves without reflecting them back to their source (without giving off echoes).
sonopuncture ultrasonic stimulation of acupuncture points for 10 to 39 seconds using small sound heads 5 mm diameter.
sonorous resonant; sounding.
Sophora secundiflora North American plant in legume family Fabaceae; toxin is assumed to be an unidentified quinolizidine alkaloid which causes a staggers syndrome in range sheep. When driven affected sheep tremble, stiffen and fall but recover quickly. Most recover if access to the plant is denied. Called also mescal bean, frijolito.
sopor [L.] *deep or profound sleep.*
soporific 1. producing deep sleep. 2. an agent that induces sleep.
soporous associated with coma or deep sleep.
sorb to attract and retain substances by absorption or adsorption.
sorbate see SORBIC ACID.
sorbefacient 1. promoting absorption. 2. an agent that promotes absorption.
sorbent an agent that sorbs.
sorbic acid a fungistatic preservative used as a food preservative.
sorbitol a sugar alcohol found in various berries and fruits; in mammals, sorbitol is an intermediate in the conversion of glucose to fructose. It is found in lens deposits in diabetes mellitus. A 50% solution is used as an osmotic diuretic. Sorbitol is used as a sweetener in some dietetic foods; it has the same caloric value as other sugars.
  s. dehydrogenase called also SDH; see L-iditol DEHYDROGENASE (ID).
sorbose a sugar, a ketohexose, with properties similar to levulose; oral administration causes hemolytic anemia in dogs. Called also L-sorbose.
sordes foul matter collected on the lips and teeth in low fevers, consisting of food, microorganisms and epithelial elements.
sore a popular term for any lesion of the skin or mucous membrane.
  bed s. decubitus ulcer.
  foam s. see SCALDED SKIN SYNDROME.
  s. foot syndrome erosion of the pads in recently captured large cats. Caused by ceaseless walking and pivoting on a concrete floor.
  s. head see ELAEOPHORIASIS.
  s. hocks see ulcerative PODODERMATITIS.
  s. knee see CARPITIS.
  s. mouth see contagious ECTHYMA, vesicular STOMATITIS.
  s. muzzle in sheep, see BLUETONGUE.
  s. nose common name for facial dermatitis in gerbils. There is hypersecretion of the Harderian gland with accumulation of porphyrin pigment in the skin, causing irritation, self-trauma and secondary infection. Caused by overcrowding and excessive humidity.
  pressure s. decubitus ulcer.
  pus s. see SCALDED SKIN SYNDROME.
  summer s. see SWAMP CANCER.
  sweat s. see SCALDED SKIN SYNDROME.
Sorex see SHREW.
Sorghastrum nutans toxic plant in family Poaceae; causes cyanide poisoning.
Sorghum grass genus in the plant family Poaceae; can cause cyanide and nitrate–nitrite poisoning; the cyanide poisoning may be in the peracute, lethal, anoxia form or a chronic form manifested by spinal cord degeneration, ataxia, urinary incontinence and consequential pyelonephritis, or as congenital deformities including arthrogryposis. Includes *Sorghum almum*, *S. bicolor* (*S. vulgare*, grain sorghum), *S. halepense* (Johnson grass), *S. sudanense*, *S. verticilliflorum*. Includes very valuable fodder crops used extensively as ensilage or green chop, and a grain sorghum used for lot feeding. Fodder sorghum is the more dangerous but both should be considered as potentially poisonous.
sorption the process or state of being sorbed; absorption or adsorption.
sorrel 1. a weed and poisonous plant. See RUMEX. 2. a horse coat color, light or golden chestnut.
sort in computer terms to rearrange data, e.g. into alphabetical or numerical order.
sos [L.] *si opus sit* (if necessary); a pharmaceutical directive in a prescription.
souffle a soft, blowing auscultatory sound.
  cardiac s. any heart murmur of a blowing quality.
  fetal s. a murmur sometimes heard over the pregnant uterus, supposed to be due to compression of the umbilical cord.

funic s., funicular s. a hissing souffle synchronous with fetal heart sounds, probably from the umbilical cord.

placental s. a souffle supposed to be produced by the blood current in the placenta; called also placental bruit.

uterine s. a sound made by the blood within the arteries of the gravid uterus.

sound 1. percept resulting from stimulation of the ear by mechanical radiant energy, the frequency depending on the species. 2. a slender instrument to be introduced into body passages or cavities, especially for the dilatation of strictures or detection of foreign bodies. 3. a noise, normal or abnormal, emanating from within the body. 4. strong, in good condition and without significant defects, e.g. said of wool which has sufficient tensile strength to resist the rigors of processing; said also of teeth as *sound mouth*.

ejection s's high-pitched clicking sounds heard very shortly after the first heart sound, attributed to sudden distension of a dilated pulmonary artery or aorta or to forceful opening of the pulmonic or aortic cusps.

friction s. one produced by rubbing of two surfaces.

heart s's the sounds produced by the functioning of the heart. See HEART SOUNDS.

Korotkoff's s's those heard during auscultatory blood pressure determination.

percussion s. any sound obtained by percussion.

respiratory s. any sound heard on ausculation over the respiratory tract.

succussion s's splashing sounds heard on succussion over a distended stomach or in hydropneumothorax.

to-and-fro s. a peculiar friction sound or murmur heard in pericarditis and pleurisy.

urethral s. a long, slender instrument for exploring and dilating the urethra.

s. waves sound, the stimulus for hearing, consists of patterns of pressure waves generated in and passed through the air.

white s. that produced by a mixture of all frequencies of mechanical vibration perceptible as sound.

s. wool wool with no breaks in it that will stand up to the pressures of scouring, spinning and weaving.

soundness having the capacity to perform the function for which the animal is about to be purchased or about to be accepted as an entrant in a contest. The expression is usually used with reference to horses. See also BREEDING soundness.

s. certificate a certificate setting out the identity of the animal, the client and the veterinarian, the date of the examination, the parts and functions examined, the abnormalities noted and the conclusion of the examining veterinarian as to the ability of the subject animal to perform the tasks expected of it.

s. examination a clinical, (including clinicopathological and radiological segments if appropriate) examination of an animal with a view to providing a certificate of soundness or suitability for sale.

sour crop see pendulous CROP.

sour dock RUMEX *acetosa*.

sour side putrefaction on the sides of carcasses which have been hung too closely together in the chilling room and which have not cooled quickly enough at the points of contact.

source code the 'English-like' instructions of the program written by the programmer. It is converted to the machine code of the object program by a compiler or assembler, or an interpreter.

source points powerful acupuncture points in the carpal and tarsal areas, used additionally to tonification and sedation points, in the treatment of organ disease or dysfunction.

sourgrass RUMEX *acetosella*.

souring said of ham. See TAINT.

soursob OXALIS *pes-caprae*.

soutgannabos [Af.] SALSOLA *barbata*.

South African buffalo see SYNCERUS CAFFER.

South African daisy see OSTEOSPERMUM.

South African Merino sheep South African version of merino sheep, originated chiefly from Australian merino.

South American burr XANTHIUM *cavanillesii*.

South American camelids include alpaca, guanaco, llama, vicuna.

South Australian cobbler see GYMNOPISTES MARMORATUS, COBBLERFISH.

South Devon a red, dual-purpose breed of cattle. Called also Devon.

South Suffolk a breed of meat DOWNS-type sheep produced by crossing SOUTHDOWN and SUFFOLK sheep.

Southdown an English DOWNS type of short-woolled, meat sheep; polled, gray-brown face and legs. The origin of many crossbred flocks and popular sire of terminal fat-lamb cross. Dystocia is a problem in purebred flocks.

Southern blot a technique for detecting specific DNA sequences following agar gel electrophoresis of a set of DNA restriction enzyme digestion fragments. The fragments after electrophoresis are transferred to a nitrocellulose or nylon membrane by applying the membrane to the gel; the membrane is probed with a radioprobe that hybridizes to one or more of the separated fragments and used to produce an autoradiogram. Named for Edward Southern.

southern mock orange PRUNUS *caroliniana*.

Southern transfer a method for performing nucleic acid hybridizations in which fragments of DNA separated usually in agarose gels are transferred (blotted) from the gel to nitrocellulose or nylon membranes. The transferred fragments are then probed with a radiolabeled fragment of DNA. Called also Southern blot.

southwest Africa slangkop *Lidneria clavata*.

sow a female pig that has had a litter.

s. mouth the maxilla is foreshortened and the lower jaw protrudes beyond it.

s. stall a farrowing stall with limited room for movement but maximum protection for the suckers.

s. thistles SONCHUS.

soybean the leguminous plant *Glycine max* (syn. *G. soja*) used for the production of soya beans. The greatest use of the bean is the extraction of oil for industrial use. The beans are unsuitable for feeding in their raw state unless they are roasted because they contain growth-inhibiting factors.

s. meal the material left after extraction of soybean oil. It is poisonous if the oil is extracted by elution with trichloroethylene.

trichloroethylene-extracted s. meal causes a radiomimetic syndrome of anemia, leukopenia and submucosal petechiation.

sp. gr. specific gravity.

SPA staphylococcal protein A.

space 1. a delimited area. 2. an actual or potential cavity of the body. 3. the areas of the universe beyond the earth and its atmosphere.

dead s. 1. space remaining in tissues as a result of failure of proper closure of surgical or other wounds, permitting accumulation of blood or serum. 2. the portions of the respiratory tract (passages and space in the alveoli) occupied by gas not concurrently participating in oxygen–carbon dioxide exchange.

Disse s's small spaces between liver sinusoids and liver cells; conduits for liver lymph. Called also perisinusoidal space.

epidural s. the space between the dura mater and the lining of the spinal canal.

s's of Fontana fluid spaces separating solid trabeculae in the iridial angle meshwork.

interalveolar s. the part of the dental arch where there are no teeth.

intercostal s. the space between two adjacent ribs.

interpleural s. mediastinum.

intervillous s. the space of the human and some other placentae into which the chorionic villi project and through which the maternal blood circulates.

lumbosacral s. the intervertebral space between the last lambar and the first sacral vertebrae; suitable site for epidural injection.

lymph s's open spaces filled with lymph in connective or other tissue, especially in the brain and meninges.

Meckel's s. a recess in the dura mater that lodges the trigeminal ganglion.

mediastinal s. mediastinum.

medullary s. the central cavity and the intervals between the trabeculae of bone that contain the marrow.

parasinoidal s's spaces in the dura mater along the superior sagittal sinus which receive the venous blood.

perisinusoidal s. see Disse spaces (above).

perivascular s. a lymph space within the walls of an artery.

plantar s. a fascial space on the sole of the foot of primates, divided by septa into the lateral, middle and median plantar spaces.

pneumatic s. a portion of bone occupied by air-containing cells, especially the spaces constituting the paranasal sinuses.

retroperitoneal s. the space between the peritoneum and the dorsal abdominal wall.

retropharyngeal s. the space behind the pharynx, containing areolar tissue.

subarachnoid s. the space between the arachnoid and the pia mater, containing cerebrospinal fluid.

subdural s. the space between the dura mater and the arachnoid.

subphrenic s. the space between the diaphragm and subjacent organs of bipeds.

subumbilical s. somewhat triangular space in the body cavity cranial to the umbilicus.

Tenon's s. a lymph space between the sclera and Tenon's capsule.

space-occupying lesions substantial physical lesions, e.g. neoplasm, hemorrhage, granuloma, which occupy space; the effect is more significant if the lesion is within a space confined by bone, e.g. thorax, cranium, bone marrow cavity.

Spalding's sign in radiographs, overlapping of fetal cranial bones; a late sign of fetal death.

spaniel any of several breeds of bird dogs, used in hunting to 'flush' or 'spring' the game by following the scent. See AMERICAN WATER SPANIEL, BOYKIN SPANIEL, BRITTANY SPANIEL, CAVALIER KING CHARLES SPANIEL, CLUMBER SPANIEL, COCKER SPANIEL, CONTINENTAL TOY SPANIELS, ENGLISH SPRINGER SPANIEL, FIELD SPANIEL, IRISH WATER SPANIEL, KING CHARLES SPANIEL, SUSSEX SPANIEL, TIBETAN SPANIEL, WELSH SPRINGER SPANIEL.

Spaniopsis a genus of biting flies in the family Rhagionidae. They are blood-suckers but do not appear to transmit disease.

Spanish pertaining to or emanating from Spain.

S. blister fly see EPICAUTA VITTATA.

S. broom SPARTIUM JUNCEUM.

S. brown cattle Spanish version of Brown Swiss.

S. Merino sheep original Spanish merino finewool sheep, ewes mostly polled, rams mostly horned.

S. vetch LATHYRUS *clymenum*.

Spanish fly contains CANTHARIDES. Called also *Cantharis vesicatoria* (syn. *Lytta vesicatoria*).

spansules capsules containing medicines, coated with materials having slow dissolving rates so that the medicine is delivered at a time after the capsule is taken.

spanthoumelkbos SARCOSTEMMA *viminale*.

sparganosis infection with *Spirometra mansoni* (syn. *S. erinacei*), which invades the subcutaneous tissues of pigs causing inflammation and fibrosis. If the lymphatics are involved, there is edematous enlargement of the part. Transmissible to humans who eat infected meat.

sparganum pl. *spargana* [Gr.] a migrating plerocercoid of a tapeworm. Usually refers specifically to larvae of SPIROMETRA. Causes SPARGANOSIS in humans and pigs.

sparrow small gray-brown bird with a universal distribution.

Eurasian tree s. a denizen of rural areas, in copses and spinneys. Called also *Passer montanus*.

house s. the town bird. Called also *Passer domesticus*.

Java s. a large gray or white finch (up to 6 inches and 30 g) used as a companion bird; called also *Padda oryzivora*.

sparteine a toxic alkaloid found in Spanish broom and lupins. It causes paralysis of sympathetic ganglia and motor nerve endings.

Spartium junceum shrub in the family Fabaceae. Contains the quinolizidine alkaloid cytisine which causes convulsions and fatal respiratory failure. Called also Spanish broom.

Spartothamnella juncea Australian plant in the family Verbenaceae; causes nitrate–nitrite poisoning.

spasm 1. a sudden involuntary contraction of a muscle or group of muscles. 2. a sudden but transitory constriction of a passage, canal or orifice. Spasms usually occur when the nerves supplying muscles are irritated, and are commonly accompanied by pain. Occasionally a spasm may occur in a blood vessel, and is then called vasospasm.

Spasms vary from mild twitches to severe SEIZURES and may be the signs of any number of disorders.

bronchial s. bronchospasm; spasmodic contraction of the muscular coat of the smaller divisions of the bronchi.

esophageal s. occurs mostly in young horses, the cause is unknown and the clinical syndrome is one of esophageal obstruction.

inherited congenital s.'s in Jersey calves at birth; lethal within a few weeks; characterized by intermittent, vertical tremor of the head, neck and limbs, making progression and standing impossible; conditioned by a recessive gene.

muscle mass s. the basic functional defect in such diseases as Elso heel, inherited periodic spasticity.

nodding s. clonic spasm of the sternomastoid muscles, causing a nodding motion of the head.

spasmodic of the nature of a spasm; occurring in spasms.

s. colic see spasmodic COLIC.

spasmolysis the arrest of spasm.
spasmolytic 1. arresting or checking spasms. 2. an agent that arrests spasms, especially of smooth muscle.
spasmophilia abnormal tendency to convulsions; abnormal sensitivity of motor nerves to stimulation with a resultant tendency to spasm.
spasmus [L.] *spasm.*
s. nutans nodding spasm.
spastic characterized by spasms, or tightening of the muscles, causing stiff and awkward movements and in some cases a scissors-like gait.
s. colon see irritable COLON syndrome.
inherited s. paresis of cattle see ELSO HEEL.
spasticity the state of being spastic.
inherited neonatal s. signs appear in calves at 2 to 5 days of age. Unable to stand; if lifted rigidity of all muscles with extension of limbs.
inherited periodic s. see inherited PERIODIC spasticity.
inherited progressive s. possibly inherited disease of Angora goats; characterized by development of lethargy and ataxia at about 2 months of age, followed by paresis, recumbency and euthanasia and necropsy lesions of vacuolation in neurons of the brain and spinal cord.
spat juvenile aquatic shellfish, especially oysters ready for settlement on solid surfaces—'spat fall'.
spatial pertaining to space.
s. clustering in geographical terms the cases in an outbreak of disease are clustered in groups and not spread randomly.
s. distribution the distribution of a population within an area.
spatium pl. *spatia* [L.] space.
s. interarticulare spaces between the arches of the vertebrae, e.g. in pigs or young animals in which the body is longer than the arch.
s. zonularia the many spaces between the fibers of the suspensory ligament of the lens.
spatula a wide, flat, blunt, usually flexible instrument of little thickness, used for spreading material on a smooth surface or mixing.
obstetric s. Keller's spatula is a long-handled, 3 ft, rod with a blunt spatulate tip, introduced into the uterus and manipulated from outside the cow or mare. Used to remove the skin of the fetus by blunt dissection. De Bruin's spatula is similar and used for a similar purpose but is short-handled and is manipulated from inside the uterus.
spatulate 1. having a flat blunt end. 2. to mix or manipulate with a spatula.
spatulation the combining of materials into a homogeneous mixture by continuously heaping them together and smoothing the mass out on a smooth surface with a spatula.
spavin diseases of the hock joint.
bone s. osteoarthritis or osteitis of the distal intertarsal and tarsometatarsal joints of the horse. The lesions are those of a degenerative bone disease terminating in the formation of exostoses and in ankylosis of the joint. Lameness is a constant finding. There may or may not be a local bony swelling.
s. knife see Warmberg spavin KNIFE.
occult s. a spavin in which the clinical signs are evident but there is no external bony enlargement.
s. test the horse's hindlimb is held in a flexed position, with the metatarsus parallel to the ground for several minutes. Increased lameness afterwards is considered a positive test for spavin. Called also hock flexion test.
spawn fish eggs.
spawners see BROODFISH.
spay, spey to remove the ovaries. See also OVARIOHYSTERECTOMY.
s. hook see spay HOOK.
s. spreader a device with a spring loop, like a safety pin, at one end and an outcurving blade at the end of each arm. The blades are inserted into the spay incision and the arms released.
vaginal s. ovaries are removed through a colpotomy incision; sometimes performed on mares.
spaying pertaining to SPAY.
s. device see KIMBERLING–RUPP SPAYING DEVICE.
SPCA 1. serum prothrombin conversion accelerator (clotting factor VII). See also CLOTTING factors. 2. Society for the Prevention of Cruelty to Animals; the counterpart in the USA and Canada of the RSPCA in British Commonwealth countries.
SPD salmon poisoning disease.
spear grass see STIPA, STIPAGROSTIS.
spearwort RANUNCULUS *flammula.*
special out of the ordinary.
s. diagnostic strategies includes all techniques which are not provided in the ordinary course of the services available at veterinary clinics and hospital, e.g. Compton metabolic profile, field response trial, retrospective mating analysis.
s. incidence ratios ratios done specially for indexes that are not part of a regular surveillance system, e.g. a zoonosis incidence ratio which is the ratio of the number of new cases of the disease in the animal reservoir related to the number of people in the human population for the same period.
s. protocol a hospital case chart created specially to record observations in cases of a disease that is under examination by members of the staff.
s. risk population a population of animals that is especially likely to contract a disease because of some peculiarity of genetics or husbandry or because of geographic or climatic factors.
s. senses see special SENSE.
specialist a veterinarian whose practice is limited to a particular branch of medicine or surgery, especially one who, by virtue of advanced training, is certified by a specialty board as being qualified to so limit his/her practice.
specialty a legally recognized field of practice of a specialist.
species a taxonomic category subordinate to a genus (or subgenus) and superior to a subspecies or variety; composed of individuals similar in certain morphological and physiological characteristics, the important one of which is that they are capable of interbreeding to produce fertile and viable offspring.
s. difference the difference between species in their response to therapeutic agents, poisons and infections due to physical, biochemical, immunological differences.
s. specialist a veterinarian who specializes in the diseases and management of an individual animal species.
type s. the original species from which the description of the genus is formulated.
species-specific characteristic of a particular species; having a characteristic effect on, or interaction with, cells or tissues of members of a particular species; said of an antigen, drug or infective agent.
specific 1. pertaining to a species. 2. produced by a single kind of microorganism. 3. restricted in application, effect, etc., to a particular structure, function, etc. 4. a remedy specially indicated for a particular

disease. 5. in immunology, pertaining to the special affinity of antibody for the corresponding antigen.

s. acquired immunity see acquired IMMUNITY.

s. activity enzymes enzyme activity as V_{max}, measured as μmoles of substrate utilized or product produced per minute, expressed on a specific unit of comparison such as per mg protein or g of tissue weight or ml or L of solution such as plasma.

s. drug one that acts at only one type of receptor but may produce several pharmacological effects depending on which organs carry the operant receptor.

s. dynamic action heat produced by the metabolism of food and unavoidably lost to the animal. In cold environments it will be contributed to the maintenance of body temperature but in a hot environment it must be dispersed by the normal heat-dissipating mechanisms. Called also heat increment.

s. gravity (sp. gr.) the weight of a substance compared with the weight of an equal amount of some other substance taken as a standard. For liquids the usual standard is water. The specific gravity of water is 1; if a sample of urine shows a specific gravity of 1.025, this means that the urine is 1.025 times heavier than water. Specific gravity is measured by means of a hydrometer.

s. seasonals clusters of cases occurring at specific seasons.

specific pathogen free a term applied to animals reared for experimentation or to commence new herds or flocks of disease-free animals; abbreviated SPF. Animals usually obtained as for AXENIC animals but are then placed into a nonsterile environment in which they become infected with a range of microorganisms, many colonizing as so-called normal flora. Certain defined specific pathogenic microorganisms are not present in the environment so that SPF animals can be stated to be free of infection or previous infection with the specified microorganism. See also GNOTOBIOTIC animal.

specificity the quality of having a certain action, as of affecting only certain organisms or tissues, or reacting only with certain substances, as antibodies with certain antigens (antigen specificity).

drug s. the degree to which the effects of a drug are due to the one pharmacological action.

host s. the restricted infectivity of a particular parasite to a certain species or group of hosts.

test s. the probability of a test correctly identifying those patients which are not infected or which do not have the specified condition. A fundamental parameter of any diagnostic test. See also SENSITIVITY.

specimen a small sample or part taken to show the nature of the whole, such as a small quantity of urine for urinalysis, or a small fragment of tissue for microscopic study.

s. artifacts changes in tissues or other samples for laboratory examination, caused by the collection, transport, fixing, section cutting, staining or other procedural manipulations.

forensic s. specimen collected in the knowledge that there will probably be litigation relating to the case. Requires complete, accurate identification of the specimen and the patient and client, and that a separate reserve specimen be kept for any further testing required by the court. All containers should be sealed so that they cannot be tampered with, and preferably in the presence of witnesses.

speckled loco ASTRAGALUS *lentiginosus*.

speckling see TICKING.

spectacle a round lens. Snakes lack movable eyelids and their corneas are protected by a transparent spectacle which is shed and renewed at each ecdysis. See also SUBSPECTACLE.

s. retention a common problem in snakes; caused by lack of abrasive materials for the snake to rub against during the molting period.

spectinomycin an aminocyclitol antibiotic derived from *Streptomyces spectabili*; the hydrochloride is used as a feed additive for swine and chickens.

spectra plural of *spectrum*.

spectrin a contractile protein attached to glycophorin at the cytoplasmic surface of the cell membrane of erythrocytes, considered to be important in the determination of red cell shape.

spectrometry determination of the place of lines or absorption bands in a spectrum.

spectrophotometer an apparatus for determining the ability of a solution to absorb light of a specific wavelength by measuring the transmitted light.

spectrophotometry the use of the spectrophotometer.

spectroscope an instrument for developing and analyzing the spectrum of a substance.

spectroscopy examination by means of a spectroscope.

nuclear magnetic resonance s. technique depending on measurements of specific radiofrequency emissions produced in a strong magnetic field from molecules containing nuclei with magnetic properties, e.g. ^{31}P, the most prevalent isotope of phosphorus.

spectrum pl. *spectra, spectrums* [L.] 1. the series of images resulting from the refraction of electromagnetic radiation (e.g. light, x-rays) and their arrangement according to frequency or wavelength. 2. range of activity, as of an antibiotic, or of manifestations, as of a disease.

absorption s. one obtained by passing radiation with a continuous spectrum through a selectively absorbing medium.

antibacterial s. the range of bacteria susceptible to a particular antimicrobial or class of antimicrobials.

broad-s. effective against a wide range of microorganisms.

visible s. that portion of the range of wavelengths of electromagnetic vibrations (from 770 to 390 nanometers) which is capable of stimulating specialized sense organs and is perceptible as light.

speculum an instrument for opening or distending a body orifice or cavity to permit visual inspection.

mouth s. see MOUTH speculum, SCHOUPE SPECULUM, FRICK SPECULUM.

ophthalmic s. small, lightweight speculum consisting of two arms which are opened by a screw at one end. Called also Castroviejo eye speculum.

vaginal s. see GRAVES SPECULUM, THOROUGHBRED SPECULUM.

speedy-cutting when the medial aspect of the carpus or metacarpus of the horse is struck by the hoof on the opposite forelimb when moving at a fast speed and when turned sharply.

s. boot a boot worn over the wall of the hoof to prevent this injury.

Speleognathus respiratory tract mites found in commercial poultry and pigeons but not a significant pathogen.

spelt a low-grade variant of wheat with similar feed quality but lower yield. Used only as stock feed. Called also *Triticum spelta*.

Spencer hemoglobinometer see Spencer HEMOGLOBINOMETER.

Spencer scissors delicate stitch scissors for ophthalmic work. One of the blades has an indentation in its cutting edge near to the tip so that the suture will not slip out from between the blades.

sperm the male germ cell. See also SPERMATOZOON.

s. agglutinins anti-sperm antibodies of the IgG class occur as autoantibodies in dogs infected with *Brucella canis*.

s. capacitation acquisition of the capacity to penetrate an ovum, not present at the time of delivery of the spermatozoon, and which requires a period of incubation in the female tract. It involves increased metabolic activity and motility and the removal of a chemical decapacitation factor from the spermatozoon. Capacitation must take place for the acrosome reaction to occur.

s. concentration a sperm count as measured in a hemocytometer; an indication of the health of the relevant testicles and a guide to the prospective fertility of the ejaculate and the donor.

s. live–dead ratio an indicator of the viability of the ejaculate as expressed in a slide count of a specially stained smear of the semen in which the dead and live sperm can be distinguished because of their differential staining.

s. morphology the normal anatomical structure of the SPERMATOZOON. Abnormality of the structure of individual spermatozoa is used as a guide to the location and nature of the disease causing reduced reproductive efficiency.

s. motility the percentage of spermatozoa moving actively forward. Assessed under the microscope (400 × magnification) or by computerized imaging. See also WAVE motion; used to predict the probable fertility of the ejaculate.

s. motility index half the sum of the sample's sperm percentage motility + sperm progressive motility.

s. penetration assay see OVUM penetration assay.

s. stone hard bodies composed of inspissated masses of spermatozoa found in dilated remnants of epididymal ducts and produced by chronic epididymitis.

s. transport within both male and female reproductive tracts some movement forward results from the movements of the spermatozoa but most progress is the result of peristaltic movements by the tubular organs in which the spermatozoa find themselves at the time.

spermatheca accessory organ opening into the common oviduct in female insects; stores spermatozoa delivered by the male during copulation; the sperm may remain viable for the life of the female.

spermatic pertaining to the spermatozoa or to semen.

s. cord the structure extending from the deep inguinal ring to the testis, comprising the ductus deferens, testicular artery and vein including the pampiniform plexus, lymphatic ducts, autonomic nerves as a testicular plexus, smooth muscle tissue around the vessels, called also internal cremaster muscle, and the visceral layer of the vaginal tunic. Clinicians are likely to include the external cremaster muscle, and the parietal layer of the vaginal tunic as parts of the cord, although, strictly, these structures simply surround the cord. Called also funiculus spermaticus.

s. cord torsion torsion of the cord to the point where circulation in the blood vessels of the cord ceases; rare but occasional occurrence in dogs, particularly where the testicle is retained and enlarged by tumor. Causes acute abdominal pain and death due to shock.

spermaticide spermicide.

spermatid a cell produced by meiotic division of a secondary spermatocyte; it develops into the spermatozoon.

spermatitis inflammation of a vas deferens; deferentitis.

spermato- word element. [Gr.] *seed;* specifically used to refer to the male germinal element.

spermatoblast spermatid.

spermatocele a cystic distension of the epididymis or rete testis, containing spermatozoa.

spermatocelectomy excision of a spermatocele.

spermatocidal destructive to spermatozoa.

spermatocyst 1. a seminal vesicle. 2. spermatocele.

spermatocystectomy excision of a seminal vesicle.

spermatocystitis inflammation of a seminal vesicle.

spermatocystotomy incision of a seminal vesicle, for the purpose of drainage.

spermatocyte the mother cell of a spermatid.

primary s. daughter cell of a spermatogonium (an incongruous nomenclature in such an intensely masculine context). It undergoes the first meiotic division.

secondary s. a cell produced by meiotic division of the primary spermatocyte, and which gives rise to the spermatid.

spermatocytogenesis the first stage of formation of spermatozoa, in which the spermatogonia develop into spermatocytes and then into spermatids.

spermatogenesis the development of mature spermatozoa from spermatogonia; it includes spermatocytogenesis and spermiogenesis.

spermatogenic giving rise to spermatozoa.

s. cycle duration of the cycle which separates consecutive cell divisions of spermatogonia (pig is 8 days, sheep 10, cattle 14) to produce spermatocytes.

s. wave spermatogenesis occurs in sequential waves along the length of the seminiferous tubules so that spermatozoa are produced in waves; the phenomenon which ensures that spermatozoa are produced continuously, except for seasonal pauses when spermatogenesis is initiated and terminated each year.

spermatogonium pl. *spermatogonia* [Gr.] an undifferentiated male germ cell, originating in a seminal tubule and dividing into a new generation of spermatogonia or into two spermatocytes.

spermatoid resembling semen.

spermatolysin a lysin destructive to spermatozoa.

spermatolysis dissolution of spermatozoa.

spermatopathia abnormality of the semen.

spermatorrhea involuntary escape of semen, without orgasm.

spermatoschesis suppression of the semen.

spermatoxin a toxin that destroys spermatozoa.

spermatozoa see SPERMATOZOON.

spermatozoal pertaining to spermatozoa.

s. motility a guide to viability and potency of a semen sample; a highly motile sample shows wave movement under low power and individual sperm movement under high power.

spermatozoicide an agent that destroys spermatozoa; spermicide.

spermatozoon pl. *spermatozoa;* a mature male germ cell, the specific output of the testes, which impregnates the ovum in sexual reproduction.

The mature sperm cell is microscopic in size. It looks like a translucent tadpole, and has a flat, elliptical head containing a spherical center section, and a long tail by which it propels itself with a vigorous lashing movement.

spermaturia semen in the urine.

spermectomy excision of part of the spermatic cord.

spermicide an agent destructive to spermatozoa.

spermidine a polyamine first found in human semen but now known to occur in almost all tissues, in association with nucleic acids.
spermiduct the ejaculatory duct and vas deferens together.
spermine a polyamine first found in human semen but now known to occur in almost all tissues, in association with nucleic acids.
spermiogenesis the second stage in the formation of spermatozoa, in which the spermatids transform into spermatozoa.
spermioteleosis progressive development of the spermatogonium through various stages to the mature spermatozoon.
sperm(o)- word element. [Gr.] *seed;* specifically used to refer to the male germinal element.
spermolith a calculus in the vas deferens.
spermophlebectasia varicose state of the spermatic veins.
spermotoxin a toxin lethal to spermatozoa; especially an antibody produced by injection of an animal with spermatozoa.
spewing sickness *Helenium* spp., *Hymenoxys* spp. poisonings.
spey see SPAY.
SPF specific pathogen free.
sphacelate to become gangrenous.
sphacelation the formation of sphacelus; mortification.
Sphacelia typhina see ACREMONIUM *coenophialum.*
sphacelism sphacelation or necrosis; sloughing.
sphaceloderma gangrene of the skin.
sphacelous gangrenous; sloughing.
sphacelus a slough; a mass of gangrenous tissue.
Sphaeridiotrema a genus of small, globular digenetic trematodes in the family Psilostomatidae.
S. globulosus found in the intestine of wild and domestic ducks and in swans and causes severe enteritis. It has caused severe mortalities in swans.
S. spinoacetabulum inhibits the ceca and causes severe typhlitis.
Sphaerophorus necrophorus see FUSOBACTERIUM *necrophorum.*
sphenion the point at the sphenoid angle of the parietal bone.
spheno- word element. [Gr.] *wedge-shaped, sphenoid bone.*
sphenoid 1. wedge-shaped. 2. an irregular wedge-shaped bone at the base of the skull. See also Table 10.
s. bone fracture fracture of the basisphenoid bone occurs when the horse rears over backwards. Causes rotation of head, facial paralysis, occasionally hemorrhage into guttural pouch.
sphenoidal pertaining to the sphenoid bone.
sphenoiditis inflammation of the sphenoidal sinus.
sphenoidotomy incision of a sphenoid sinus.
sphenomaxillary pertaining to the sphenoid bone and the maxilla.
sphenopalatine pertaining to the sphenoid and palatine bones.
s. sinus in horses the sphenoid sinus is extended into the palatine bone.
Sphenosciadium capitellatum North American alpine plant in the family Apiaceae; contains an unidentified toxin which causes pulmonary edema and photosensitization. Called also whiteheads.
sphenotresia perforation of the base of the fetal skull in craniotomy.
sphenotribe an instrument used for crushing the base of the fetal skull.
sphere a ball or globe.
attraction s. centrosome.
segmentation s. 1. the morula. 2. a blastomere.
sphero- word element. [Gr.] *round, a sphere.*
spherocyte a small, globular, completely hemoglobinated erythrocyte without the usual central pallor; characteristically found in some types of acquired hemolytic anemia, particularly immune-mediated.
spherocytosis the presence of spherocytes in the blood.
spheroid a sphere-like body.
axonal s's these appear in axons in the early stages of development of progressive axonopathy; the spheroids are eosinophilic, round or oval swellings containing degenerate organelles.
spheroidal resembling a sphere.
spheroma a globular tumor.
spherophakia a spherical deformation of the lens.
spheroplast gram-negative bacterial cell deprived of its cell wall, but retaining an intact plasma membrrane. See also PROTOPLAST.
spherules double-contoured, highly refractile bodies in which the fungus *Coccidioides immitis* occurs in animal tissues. Called also sporangia.
sphincter a circular muscle that constricts a passage or closes a natural orifice. When relaxed, a sphincter allows materials to pass through the opening. When contracted, it closes the opening. The principal abnormalities relate to function. Failure to open may be because of spasm or achalasia, due usually to failure of parasympathetic nerve supply. Failure to close usually due to absence of sympathetic nerve supply. The important sphincters are the anal, ileal, pharyngoesophageal, pupillary, pyloric, reticulo-omasal, teat, urethral, vaginal and vesical.
cardiac s. the functional sphincter at the gastric end of the esophagus.
s. control is by the autonomic nervous system.
esophageal s. see cardiac SPHINCTER.
s. of Oddi bile duct sphincter.
pupillary s. a ring of smooth muscle around the pupillary border of the iris.
sphincterectomy excision of a sphincter.
sphincterismus spasm of a sphincter.
sphincteritis inflammation of a sphincter, particularly the sphincter of Oddi.
sphincterolysis surgical separation of the iris from the cornea in anterior synechia.
sphincteroplasty plastic reconstruction of a sphincter.
sphincterotomy incision of a sphincter.
sphingolipid one of the two dominant 'families' of lipids; a range of phospholipids containing sphingosine (e.g. ceramides, sphingomyelins, gangliosides and cerebrosides), occurring in high concentrations in the brain and other nerve tissue.
sphingolipidosis pl. *sphingolipidoses* [Gr.] a general designation applied to diseases characterized by abnormal storage of sphingolipids, such as GANGLIOSIDOSIS, GAUCHER'S DISEASE, GLUCOCEREBROSIDE, globoid cell LEUKODYSTROPHY and SPHINGOMYELINOSIS.
sphingolipodystrophy any of a group of disorders of sphingolipid metabolism. See also SPHINGOLIPIDOSIS.
sphingomyelin a group of phospholipids that on hydrolysis yield phosphoric acid, choline, sphingosine and a fatty acid.
s. lipidosis see SPHINGOMYELINOSIS.
sphingomyelinosis an inherited deficiency of sphingomyelinase in cats, dogs and mice that results in abnormal accumulation of sphingomyelin in nervous

tissue, liver and spleen. Clinical signs include retarded growth and neurological abnormalities from an early age. The disease in cats and miniature poodles closely resembles Niemann–Pick disease of humans. Called also sphingomyelin lipidosis.

sphingosine a basic amino alcohol present in sphingomyelin.

Sphinx cat see CANADIAN HAIRLESS CAT.

sphygm- prefix meaning pulse.

sphygmic pertaining to the pulse.

s. period the second phase of ventricular systole, between the opening and closing of the semilunar valves, while the blood is discharged into the aorta and pulmonary artery.

sphygmo- word element. [Gr.] *the pulse.*

sphygmobolometer an instrument for recording the energy of the pulse wave, and so, indirectly, the strength of the systole.

sphygmochronograph a self-registering sphygmograph.

sphygmodynamometer an instrument for measuring the force of the pulse.

sphygmogram the record or tracing made by a sphygmograph; called also pulse tracing.

sphygmograph an apparatus for registering the movements of the arterial pulse.

sphygmoid resembling the pulse.

sphygmomanometer an instrument for measuring arterial blood pressure.

sphygmometer an instrument for measuring the force and frequency of the pulse.

sphygmoscope a device for rendering the pulse beat visible.

sphygmotonometer an instrument for measuring the elasticity of arterial walls.

sphyrectomy excision of the malleus, or hammer, of the ear.

spica bandage figure-of-eight bandage which is applied around a joint or trunk.

spicule 1. a sharp, needle-like body or spike. 2. part of the male genital apparatus in nematodes; they engage the female genital orifice during copulation.

Spiculocaulus a genus of nematodes in the family Protostrongylidae and found in the lungs of small ruminants.

S. austriacus found in goats and ibex.

S. kwongi found in sheep and goats.

S. leuckarti found in sheep and ibex.

S. orloffi found in sheep, goats and ibex.

Spiculopteragia a genus of worms in the family Trichostrongylidae, found in the abomasum.

S. boehmi found in moufflon and deer.

S. peruviana found in llama, alpaca and vicuna.

S. spiculoptera found in sheep and deer.

spider an arthropod of the class Arachnida.

black widow s. see LATRODECTUS *mactans.*

brown recluse s. a poisonous spider, *Loxoceles reclusa*, whose bite causes severe poisoning in humans.

s. lily see CRINUM.

trapdoor s. *Atrax robustus.* Called also funnel-web spider.

s. grass BRACHYACHNE *convergens.*

s. lamb syndrome inherited ARACHNOMELIA.

spider cell cells in rhabdomyosarcoma that have extensively vacuolated cytoplasm.

spider monkey slim New World monkeys with long limbs and prehensile tails. There are several species in the genera *Ateles* and *Lagothrix.* They vary in color from black to red-brown and are very agile tree climbers.

spike 1. a sharp upward deflection in a curve or tracing, as on the encephalogram. 2. a sharp power surge in the electrical supply to a computer which may corrupt data and interrupt communication. 3. prepare samples with a known amount of substance for testing laboratory proficiency.

spiked rice-flower PIMELEA *trichostachya.*

spikes see PEPLOMER.

Spilopsyllus cuniculi a flea in the order Siphonaptera. A parasite of rabbits and hares and occasionally their predators; transmits myxomatosis. A cause of severe irritation on the pinnae of domestic cats. Called also European rabbit flea.

spina pl. *spinae* [L.] spine; a slender process such as occurs on many bones.

s. bifida a developmental anomaly characterized by defective closure of the two halves of the vertebral arch through which the spinal cord and meninges may or may not protrude.

s. bifida cystica spina bifida in which there is protrusion through the defect of a cystic swelling involving the meninges (meningocele), spinal cord (myelocele) or both (meningomyelocele).

s. bifida occulta spina bifida in which there is a defect of the bony spinal canal without protrusion of the cord or meninges.

s. bifida ventralis a defect of closure on the ventral surface of the bony spinal canal, often associated with defective development of the abdominal and thoracic viscera.

spinach *Spinacia oleracea.*

Spinacia oleracea plant in the family Chenopodiaceae; can cause soluble oxalate poisoning comprising nephrosis, urolithiasis. Called also spinach.

spinal pertaining to a spine or to the vertebral column and in many instances to the spinal cord.

s. abscess infection may be introduced hematologically from navel infection to a vertebral body or up the vertebral canal from an infected docking wound. Clinically there is a development of paresis over a few days then paraplegia when the abscess is in the lumbar region or quadriplegia when it is located in the cervical area.

s. accessory nerve see accessory nerve, Table 14.

congenital s. stenosis stenosis of the vertebral canal present at birth; recorded in calves.

s. fibrocartilaginous emboli see fibrocartilaginous embolic MYELOPATHY.

focal symmetrical s. poliomalacia see focal symmetrical spinal POLIOMALACIA.

s. fusion surgical creation of ankylosis of contiguous vertebrae.

s. meninges see MENINGES.

s. meningitis usually part of cerebrospinal meningitis. May be local related to spinal cord abscess and cause localized pain and muscle rigidity.

s. muscular atrophy see hereditary spinal MUSCULAR, hereditary neuronal ABIOTROPHY of Swedish Lapland dogs.

s. myelitis see MYELITIS.

s. myelopathy see MYELOPATHY.

s. nerve any of the paired nerves arising from the spinal cord and passing out between the vertebrae.

s. puncture introduction of a hollow needle into the subarachnoid space of the spinal canal, usually for the purpose of collecting a sample of cerebrospinal fluid, to introduce radiopaque material for myelography, or the injection of an anesthetic.

s. reflex any reflex action mediated through a center at the spinal cord.

s. stenosis see spinal cord compression (above).
s. tap see spinal puncture (above).
s. trauma temporary or permanent dislocation of one or more spinal vertebrae; or fracture; causes immediate flaccid paralysis caudal to injury due to spinal shock, followed by residual signs due to damage to spinal cord tissue.
s. walking see REFLEX walking.

spinal cord that part of the central nervous system lodged in the spinal canal, extending from the foramen magnum to a point in the lumbar or sacral vertebrae, depending on the species.
s. c. abscess see SPINAL abscess.
s. c. atrophy diminution in mass of the entire cord, is usually the hallmark of undernutrition or old age, or both.
s. c. compression may be gradual due to space-occupying lesion of vertebral canal, such as abscess, callus of a fracture, or a tumor, or acute due to fracture dislocation or thrombosis. In general, clinical signs include paresis or paralysis, but depending on the level of the spinal cord involved and the type of lesion present there may also be urinary incontinence, loss of sensation, Horner's syndrome, and in acute lesions, spinal shock.
s. c. degeneration see MYELOMALACIA.
s. c. hemorrhage see HEMATOMYELIA.
s. c. hypoplasia usually segmental, especially in the lumbar area.
s. c. local ischemia caused by embolus of a spinal artery; has the same effect as traumatic injury (see below).
s. c. tracts more or less distinct bundles of fibers within the white matter of the spinal cord. There are three funiculi on each side of the cord—dorsal, lateral and ventral; subdivisions within the funiculi include eleven major tracts—gracile and cuneate fasciculi, lateral and ventral corticospinal tracts, rubrospinal tract, dorsal and ventral spinocerebellar tracts, lateral and ventral spinothalamic tracts, elementary apparatus fibers, ventral corticospinal tract, vestibulospinal tract.
s. c. traumatic injury fracture or dislocation of one or more vertebrae; causes a syndrome of acute flaccid paralysis in the area supplied with nerves from the injured segment and spastic paralysis in the parts supplied by the cord segments caudal to the injury.

spinate thorn-shaped; having thorns.

spindle 1. mitotic spindle; the fusiform figure occurring during metaphase of cell division, composed of microtubules radiating from the centrioles and connecting to the chromosomes at their centromeres. 2. muscle spindle.
muscle s. a mechanoreceptor found within a skeletal muscle; the muscle spindles are arranged in parallel with muscle fibers. They contain three to 10 small, striated muscle fibers (intrafusal fibers) contained within a capsule and supplied with specialized motor and sensory nerves. They respond to passive stretch of the muscle but cease to discharge if the muscle contracts isotonically, thus signalling muscle length. The muscle spindle is the receptor responsible for the stretch or myotatic reflex.
s. wood, s. tree EUONYMUS *europaea*.

spindle-cell tumors, spindle-cell carcinoma tumors that arise from spindle-shaped cells of the dermis and subcutis.
cutaneous s.-c. tumors include fibroma, fibrous histiocytoma, schwannoma, hemangiopericytoma and their corresponding malignant counterparts, equine sarcoid, collagen nevi, papilloma-virus-induced fibropapillomas and spindle-cell dermal melanomas.

spindle-shaped shaped like a round stick tapered at both ends.

spindly leg syndrome a suspected nutritional myopathy seen in frogs and toads; after metamorphosis, the forelimbs are underdeveloped.

spine, spina 1. a thornlike process or projection. 2. the backbone, or vertebral column. See also SPINAL.
cuneal s. the axial ridge of the upper surface of the frog in the hoof of the horse that projects into the digital cushion.
iliac s. small salients along the dorsal and ventral borders of the ilium, divided into cranial and caudal, dorsal and ventral, in cats and dogs, contrasted to the single sacral and coxal tubers in large animals;
ischial s. the crest of bone to which the sacrosciatic ligament attaches and which provides the origin of the gluteus profundus muscle.
plant s's cause cutaneous laceration and subcutaneous abscess, oral mucosal laceration and ulceration, conjunctival injury.
scapular s. the ridge that divides the lateral surface of the scapula into the supraspinous and infraspinous fossae.

spineless horsebrush TETRADYMIA *canescens*.

spinifugal conducting or moving away from the spinal cord.

spinipetal conducting or moving toward the spinal cord.

spinners type said of wool which is attractive to makers of yarns.

spinning top a device used to assess the accuracy of the timer on the x-ray machine.

spinobulbar pertaining to the spinal cord and medulla oblongata.

spinocellular pertaining to prickle cells.

spinocerebellar pertaining to the spinal cord and cerebellum.
s. tract spinal cord tract carrying proprioceptive impulses from muscles, bones and joints to the cerebellum.

Spinoni Italiani a medium- to large-sized, strongly built, all-purpose gun dog with docked tail and a thick, medium-length wiry coat which forms a moustache and beard. The color is white with orange or brown markings, and the nose, lips and eyelids are fleshy red. Called also Italian pointer.

spinose ear tick see OTOBIUS *megnini*.

spinothalamic tract two spinal cord tracts carrying afferent nerve fibers to the thalamus; includes two principal tracts, the LEMNISCAL and the EXTRALEMNISCAL SYSTEMS.

spinous pertaining to or like a spine.
dorsal s. processes processes of the vertebrae that underlie the backline of the animal.
s. ear tick see OTOBIUS *megnini*.
s. layer see STRATUM spinosum.

spiny sharp spines protrude.
s. amaranth AMARANTHUS *spinosum*.
s. anteater see ECHIDNA.
s. clotburr XANTHIUM *spinosum*.
s. emex see EMEX AUSTRALIS.

spiracle small, circular openings in the exoskeleton of insects are the portal of entry for air into the insect body.

spiradenoma adenoma of the sweat glands.

spiral 1. winding like the thread of a screw. 2. a structure curving around a central point or axis.
Curschmann's s's see CURSCHMANN'S SPIRALS.
s. organ of Corti see ORGAN of Corti.

s. penile deviation a defect in bulls. See CORKSCREW penis.

s. septum the arterial partition between aorta and pulmonary trunk, formed by the fusion of the truncal, bulbar and aorticopulmonary septa of the great vessels attached to the embryonic heart.

s. worm *Dispharynx nasuta*. See SYNHIMANTUS *spiralis*.

spiramycin a macrolide antibiotic used primarily against penicillin-resistant staphylococci and for mycoplasmal diseases of swine and for swine dysentery. Administered by injection as the adipate ester.

spireme the threadlike continuous or segmented figure formed by the chromosome material during prophase.

spirilla plural of *spirillum*.

spirillicidal destroying spirilla.

spirillicide an agent that destroys spirilla.

spirillosis a disease caused by presence of spirilla, such as avian stomatitis.

Spirillum a genus of gram-negative, motile, helical bacteria isolated from fresh water. Neither of the animal pathogens bearing the genus name belong in this genus.

S. minus, S. minor pathogenic for guinea pigs, rats, mice and monkeys and is the cause of ratbite fever (Sodoku).

S. pulli recorded as causing a diphtheritic stomatitis in chickens.

spirillum pl. *spirilla* [L.] 1. a spiral-shaped bacterium. 2. a member of the genus *Spirillum*.

spirit 1. a volatile or distilled liquid. 2. a solution of a volatile material in alcohol.

ammonia s's, aromatic s's of ammonia a mixture of ammonia, ammonium carbonate, and other agents for use as a stimulant or alterative for a languishing horse.

rectified s. alcohol.

spir(o)- 1. [Gr.] a combining form denoting relationship to a coil or spiral. 2. [L.] a combining form denoting relation to the breath or to breathing.

Spirocerca a genus of spiruroid nematodes in the family Spirocercidae.

S. arctica found in dog, fox and wolf.

S. lupi found in domestic and wild Canidae and wild Felidae. The worms are located in the walls of the esophagus, the aorta and the stomach, and sometimes in other organs, persisting in nodules. The nodules may be large enough to cause obstruction of the esophagus and the aorta. The esophageal lesion converts to a fibrosarcoma or an osteosarcoma in a number of cases.

S. sanguinolenta see *S. lupi* (above).

spirocercosis see SPIROCERCA *lupi*.

Spirochaeta a genus of the family Spirochaetaceae of bacteria. Gram-negative, coiled bacteria, facultative or obligate anaerobes.

S. anserina now called *Borrelia anserina*; causes fowl SPIROCHETOSIS.

S. penortha of uncertain taxonomic status; described as a cofactor in ovine footrot.

spirochaetosis see SPIROCHETOSIS.

spirochete 1. a highly coiled bacterium; a general term applied to any organism of the order Spirochaetales, which includes the causative organisms of human syphilis (*Treponema pallidum*), of avian spirochetosis (*Borrelia anserina*) and rabbit spirochetosis (*Serpulina paraluiscuniculi*), and associated with swine dysentery (*T. hyodysenteriae*) and footrot of sheep. 2. an organism of the genus *Spirochaeta*.

spirocheticide an agent that destroys spirochetes.

spirochetolysis the destruction of spirochetes by lysis.

spirochetosis 1. an infectious disease of many species of fowl caused by *Borrelia anserina* and characterized by fever, cyanosis of the head and diarrhea. It is transmitted by the fowl ticks *Argas persicus, A. miniatus* and *A. reflexus*. Morbidity and mortality are very variable but may reach 100%. 2. a benign venereal disease of rabbits caused by *Treponema paraluiscuniculi*, characterized by small vesicles, scabs or ulcers which heal in 10 to 14 days. The lesions are confined to the genitalia, with a few animals also having lesions on the eyelids and lips. Called also rabbit syphilis, treponematosis, vent disease.

spirogram a graph of respiratory movements made by the spirometer.

spirograph an apparatus for measuring and recording respiratory movements.

spiroid resembling a spiral.

spirometer an instrument for measuring air taken into and expelled from the lungs. The spirometer provides a relatively simple method for determining most of the lung volumes and capacities that are measured in PULMONARY function tests.

Spirometra a pseudophyllidean tapeworm similar to *Diphyllobothrium* spp. that occurs in the intestines of wild carnivores and domestic cats and dogs. The larvae (plerocercoids) infest amphibians but humans can also be infected, the resulting disease being known as SPARGANOSIS. Includes *S. erinacei* (cats, dogs), *S. felis* (big zoo cats), *S. mansoni* (cats, dogs), *S. mansonoides* (cats, dogs, raccoons), *S. reptans* (New World primates).

spirometry measurement of the breathing capacity by means of a spirometer.

spironolactone a competitive antagonist of aldosterone, used as a diuretic. It increases resorption of sodium in the distal renal tubules.

Spironucleus one of the protozoan causes of 'hole-in-the-head disease' of ornamental fish.

S. muris a protozoon of mice. It causes weight loss, diarrhea and sometimes death.

Spiroptera incerta see HABRONEMA *incertum*.

Spirura a genus of nematodes in the family Spiruridae found in the alimentary tract of carnivores, rodents and insectivores.

S. rytipleurites there are two varieties, one found in the stomach of the cat and fox and one in the hedgehog.

S. talpae found in the European common mole (*Talpa europea*) and the black rat *Rattus rattus*.

spiruroid roundworms of the order Spirurida. Includes the genera of *Cyrnea, Draschia, Habronema, Hartertia, Mastophorus, Protospirura, Spirura, Streptopharagus*.

spitz a general description of so-called 'Northern' or Nordic dog breeds with conformational characteristics resembling wolves. They have bushy tails carried upright or over the back, thick short stand-off coat with a ruff around the neck, a wedge-shaped head and small pricked ears.

splake SALVELINUS *fontinalis, S. namaycush*.

splanchnapophysis a bony process, such as a ventral process on certain vertebrae, that is associated with the viscera.

splanchnectopia displacement of a viscus or of the viscera.

splanchnesthesia visceral sensation.

splanchnic pertaining to the viscera.

s. circulation includes the mesenteric, splenic and

hepatic beds, the first two comprising the major part of the inflow to the third.

s. nerves a group of sympathetic nerves serving the blood vessels and viscera of the abdomen.

splanchnicotomy transection of a splanchnic nerve.

splanchn(o)- word element. [Gr.] *viscus* (viscera), *splanchnic nerve*.

splanchnocele hernial protrusion of a viscus. The portion of the embryonic body cavity from which the abdominal, pericardial and pleural cavities are formed.

splanchnocoele see SPLANCHNOCELE.

splanchnodiastasis displacement of a viscus or viscera.

splanchnolith intestinal calculus.

splanchnology science of the organs of the body, as of the digestive, respiratory and genitourinary systems.

splanchnomegaly enlargement of the viscera; visceromegaly.

splanchnopathy any disease of the viscera.

splanchnopleure the embryonic layer formed by union of the splanchnic mesoderm with entoderm; the digestive tube develops from it.

splanchnoptosis prolapse or backward displacement of the viscera.

splanchnosclerosis hardening of the viscera.

splanchnoskeleton skeletal structures connected with viscera.

splanchnotomy anatomy or dissection of the viscera.

splanchnotribe an instrument for crushing the intestine to obliterate its lumen.

splashing an abattoir term for large areas of hemorrhage in the form of brush marks or groups of spots, usually evident in muscles and under serous membranes.

splayed digits an inherited defect in cattle in which the tendons and ligaments that hold the claws of the foot together are relaxed so that the digits splay. There is difficulty in standing and walking and affected animals lie down most of the time.

splayleg a congenital defect of the hindlimbs of piglets that prevents standing. The piglet is in sternal recumbency with the hindlimbs splayed and can only make swimming movements in attempts to rise. Some are crushed by the sow. Called also myofibril hypoplasia. Occurs also in rabbits.

spleen a large lymphoid organ usually situated in the cranial part of the abdominal cavity on the left of the stomach. The spleen contains the largest collection of reticuloendothelial cells in the body. In ruminants the spleen is located on the left lateral wall of the reticulum and under the last two ribs on the left side. Called also lien.

accessory s. a small mass of tissue, histologically and functionally identical with that composing the normal spleen but found elsewhere in the body.

slaughter s. see SLAUGHTER spleen.

splenadenoma hyperplasia of the spleen pulp.

Splendido filaria see ORNITHOFILARIA.

Splendore–Hoeppli material homogeneous, eosinophilic material that coats the grains that are characteristic of the exudate in lesions of BOTRYOMYCOSIS.

splenectasis splenomegaly.

splenectomy excision of the SPLEEN. Most commonly performed in dogs and cats because of trauma or neoplasia.

splenectopia, splenectopy see SPLENIC displacement.

splenial pertaining to a splenium (anatomical).

splenic pertaining to the spleen.

s. abscess caused by hematogenous spread of an infection elsewhere, by penetration by a foreign body from the reticulum in cattle, by ulceration from the stomach in the horse. Manifested by fever and toxemia, pain on palpation over the spleen and by a positive paracentesis sample.

s. artery see Table 9.

s. corpuscle lymph nodules in the splenic matrix.

s. displacement may be detectable on palpation. Usually caused by displacement of the stomach or intestine to which the spleen is attached.

s. enlargement see SPLENOMEGALY.

s. fever anthrax.

s. hyperfunction see HYPERSPLENISM.

s. meridian points acupuncture points situated along the splenic meridian.

s. phosphodiesterase a ribonuclease that is a $5'{\rightarrow}3'$ exonuclease.

s. rupture only likely in a grossly enlarged spleen, e.g. in bovine viral leukosis.

s. torsion a twisting or rotation of the spleen on its vascular pedicle, often in association with gastric dilatation–volvulus in large breed dogs, results in primarily venous congestion and possibly thrombosis and infarction. Clinical signs include abdominal distension and pain, vomiting, and in acute cases cardiovascular collapse and shock.

splenitis inflammation of the spleen, a condition that is attended by enlargement of the organ and severe local pain. Is usually a diffuse suppurative infection.

splenium 1. a compress or bandage. 2. bandlike structure.

s. corporis callosi the posterior, rounded end of the corpus callosum.

splenization the conversion of a tissue, as of the lung, into tissue resembling that of the spleen, due to engorgement and consolidation.

splen(o)- word element. [Gr.] *spleen*.

splenocele hernia of the spleen.

splenocolic pertaining to the spleen and colon.

splenocyte the monocyte characteristic of splenic tissue.

splenography 1. radiography of the spleen. 2. a description of the spleen.

splenohepatomegaly enlargement of the spleen and liver.

splenoid resembling the spleen.

splenolysin a lysin that destroys spleen tissue.

splenolysis destruction of splenic tissue by a lysin.

splenoma a splenic tumor.

splenomalacia abnormal softness of the spleen; lienomalacia.

splenomedullary of or pertaining to the spleen and bone marrow; lienomedullary.

splenomegaly enlargement of the spleen. Is largely without clinical signs but it may be palpated during an examination through the abdominal wall in dogs and cats, rectally in horses and not at all in ruminants. The enlargements may be caused by abscess or neoplasm or there may be a diffuse enlargement caused by accumulation of hemolyzed red cells.

asymmetrical s. usually the result of trauma or neoplasia.

congestive s. in animals, most often caused by splenic torsion.

hemolytic s. that associated with hemolytic anemia.

siderotic s. splenomegaly with deposit of iron and calcium.

symmetrical s. usually caused by congestion or infiltration of the splenic tissue.

splenometry determination of the size of the spleen.
splenomyelogenous formed in the spleen and bone marrow; lienomyelogenous.
splenomyelomalacia softening of the spleen and bone marrow; lienomyelomalacia.
splenoncus splenoma.
splenopancreatic pertaining to the spleen and pancreas.
splenopathy any disease of the spleen.
splenopexy surgical fixation of the spleen.
splenopneumonia pneumonia attended with splenization of the lung.
splenoportography radiography using a contrast agent injected into the pulp of the spleen to demonstrate portosystemic vascular anomalies.
splenoptosis backward displacement of the spleen.
splenorenal pertaining to the spleen and kidney, or to splenic and renal veins.
splenorrhagia hemorrhage from the spleen.
splenorrhaphy suture of the spleen.
splenosis widespread seeding of splenic implants on the serosal surfaces in the abdominal cavity; follows rupture of spleen, commonly after trauma.
splenotomy incision of the spleen.
splenotoxin a toxin produced by or acting on the spleen; lienotoxin.
spliceosome a ribonucleoprotein complex involved in the splicing of RNA.
splicing of RNA, the excision of introns from the primary transcript and the joining together of exons to make their finished mRNA. See also RIBONUCLEIC ACID.
splint 1. a rigid or flexible appliance for fixation of displaced or fractured bones. 2. see also SPLINTS.
biphase s. an external mandibular splint used to stabilize fractures. It consists of fixation bolts placed in the mandible with an acrylic bar placed across the protruding ends, parallel to the mandible.
gutter s. one with a central channel into which the well padded limb is placed for support of a fracture.
half-pin s. open reduction fracture repair based on placing Steinmann pins through the cortex and at an acute angle to the bone, in both sides of the fracture. The pins are connected to each other with rods which are then locked together with a Kirschner clamp, the fracture reduced and the pin-clamp assembly readjusted. Half-pin systems include Jonas and Kirschner.
Kirschner–Ehmer s. see KIRSCHNER–Ehmer splint.
lateral s. rigid splinting material such as plaster is applied to the lateral surface of a limb covered in a soft padded bandage to provide support and protection from angular or bending forces.
metal rod s. aluminum rods, bent to conform to the angles of the limb, are incoorporated into the outer layers of a soft padded bandage to provide support and protection from angular or bending forces.
modified spica s. similar to a lateral splint, but the bandaging and splinting is more extensive, being carried over the shoulder or hip and across the dorsal midline. Used to immobilize the humerus or femur, temporarily or as an adjunct to internal fixation.
Robert-Jones s. see Robert-Jones BANDAGE.
Schroeder–Thomas s. a traction splint, made of aluminum rods and consisting of a padded ring with extended bars bent to a shape determined by the size of animal and type of fracture. The limb is suspended and traction applied to the joints proximal and distal to the fracture site by wrapping with padded bandages. Modified versions are used for radial and tibial fractures in large animals.
snowshoe s. molded to fit the bottom of an avian foot, it is suitable for supporting fractures of the digits in those species.
spoon s. concave channel splints of metal or plastic, commonly used over soft padding for fractures of the lower limb in dogs and cats.
Stader s. the original half-pin splint now largely superseded by the KIRSCHNER splint. The pins have to be placed in the bone fragments in the position dictated by the configuration of the blocks into which the pins are fastened.
tape s. support with tape can be used on leg fractures in birds.
Thomas s. see Schroeder–Thomas splint (above).
traction s. see Schroeder–Thomas splint (above).
splint bone the second and fourth metacarpals or metatarsals of the horse that are greatly reduced in size and do not extend as far as the distal end of the third metacarpal.
splinting 1. the application of a splint to reduce a fracture or to restrict movement. 2. tensing of muscles, especially ventral abdominal muscles, as a response to pain and as a protection against further injury.
s. materials used in splinting fractures. Includes plaster, fiberglass, wood, balsa wood, aluminum rod, steel pins, nails, plates, screws.
splints inflammation of the interosseous ligament between the small and large metacarpal bones of horses and an accompanying periostitis and exostosis production on the small metacarpal bone. The metatarsal bones are similarly but less frequently involved. Lameness is apparent during the development of the splints and is most noticeable after working. Subsequently the soreness disappears but the enlargement can be palpated, and seen in the worst cases.
split divided.
s. estrus occurs in bitches, especially during the first heat. Early signs do not proceed and the bitch is not mated but comes on heat 6 weeks later but is likely to be infertile. Occurs sporadically also in most other species.
s. fats fats which have been split into fatty acids and glycerol by digestion. A preponderance of split fats over neutral fats in the feces suggests that the supply of lipase is adequate and that any steatorrhea that is present is probably due to malabsorption rather than maldigestion.
s. genes genes which contain coding segments (exons) interrupted by non-coding segments (introns); found in eukaryotes but not in prokaryotes.
s. hand deformity see ECTRODACTYLIA.
s. screen the screen of the computer is divided into several areas each of which is capable of displaying information from several processes independently of each other but simultaneously. A precursor to windows.
s. tongue may be congenital or the result of injury to the tongue.
spodo- word element. [Gr.] *waste material.*
spodogenous caused by accumulation of waste material in an organ.
spoilage decomposition; said of meat, milk, animal feeds especially ensilage.
spondylarthritis arthritis of the spine.
spondylitic pertaining to or marked by spondylitis.
spondylitis osteomyelitis of the vertebrae. See also SPONDYLOSIS, DISKOSPONDYLITIS.
spondyl(o)- word element. [Gr.] *vertebra, vertebral column.*
spondyloarthropathy disease of the joints of the spine.

spondylodymus twin fetuses united by the vertebrae.
spondylodynia pain in a vertebra.
spondyloepiphyseal dysplasia see EPIPHYSEAL dysplasia.
spondylolisthesis forward displacement of a vertebra over a posterior segment due to a congenital defect or fracture in the pars interarticularis. Occurs in the giant breeds of dogs as WOBBLER SYNDROME and as a developmental defect called kinky back in broiler chickens. Affected birds are unable to stand normally and may be completely paralyzed. The causative lesion is a deformity of the sixth thoracic vertebra but the cause of the defect is unknown.
spondylolysis the breaking down of a vertebra.
spondylopathy any disease of the vertebrae. Associated with compression of peripheral nerve roots and spinal cord, causing pain and stiffness of the part. See also SPONDYLITIS, SPINAL abscess, SPONDYLOSIS.
cervical s. see WOBBLER SYNDROME.
spondylopyosis suppuration of a vertebra.
spondyloschisis congenital fissure of a vertebral arch; spina bifida.
spondylosis ankylosis of a vertebral joint; also, a general term for degenerative changes in the spine. Commonly seen in dogs. In aged bulls spondylosis can cause pain in the back. There is difficulty rising, weakness, unsteadiness, knuckling and toe-dragging with the hind hooves.
s. deformans a chronic disease of the vertebrae, especially in the lumbar area, in old bulls, especially those in artificial insemination centers, and old dogs. There is degenerative arthropathy at the articular processes and osteophyte development along the ventral edge of the vertebrae. The lesions are visible radiographically but there may be no clinical signs unless the new bone is injured. When this happens the affected animals are reluctant to rise or move their backs because of the pain that movement causes.
spondylosyndesis surgical creation of ankylosis between contiguous vertebrae; spinal fusion.
sponge a porous, absorbent mass, as a pad of gauze or cotton surrounded by gauze, or the elastic fibrous skeleton of certain species of marine animals.
s. forceps see FOERSTER SPONGE FORCEPS.
gelatin s. (absorbable) a spongy form of denatured gelatin, soaked with thrombin and used for topical hemostasis.
spongiform resembling a sponge.
s. encephalopathy having the physical appearance of a sponge; includes scrapie, transmissible mink encephalopathy, and kuru and Creutzfeldt–Jacob disease of humans. See also BOVINE SPONGIFORM ENCEPHALOPATHY.
feline s. encephalopathy the counterpart of bovine spongiform encephalopathy in cats and presumed to be caused by the same agent as the bovine disease; characterized clinically by a progressive worsening of ataxia in mature cats. Other signs include a crouched stance, temperament change to timid or aggressive, hyperesthesia, head nodding, fine tremor and hypersalivation.
focal s. encephalopathy familial in Bull mastiffs; ataxia and blindness commence at 4–9 weeks; bilaterally symmetrical spongiform vacuolation of gray matter, especially in the cerebellum. Similar lesions recorded in Salukis.
s. myelinopathy very visible vacuolation of myelin without general signs of myelin degeneration. Includes idiopathic forms in Hereford calves and Samoyed, Labrador and Sydney silkie pups, Egyptian mau kittens, toxic and metabolic myelinopathies, including maple syrup urine disease, and non-myelinic encephalomyelopathies, e.g. scrapie, bovine citrullinemia,
s. pustule of Kogoj an aggregation of neutrophils within a bunch of loci, situated between and inside keratinocytes especially in the stratum granulosum and the stratum spinosum.
spongi(o)- word element. [L., Gr.] *sponge, spongelike.*
spongioblast any of the embryonic epithelial cells developed about the neural tube, which become transformed, some into neuroglial and some into ependymal cells.
spongioblastoma a tumor containing spongioblasts; a type of astrocytoma.
spongiocyte 1. a neuroglia cell. 2. one of the cells with spongy vacuolated protoplasm in the adrenal cortex.
spongioform spongiform.
spongioid resembling a sponge.
spongioplasm 1. a substance forming the network of fibrils pervading the cell substance and forming the reticulum of the fixed cell. 2. the granular material of an axon.
spongiosa spongy; sometimes used alone to mean the spongy substance of bone (substantia spongiosa ossium).
primary s. the mineralized cartilage in the developing metaphysis.
secondary s. second stage in the mineralization of bony trabeculae; comprises the enlarged, mineralized bony trabeculae of the primary spongiosa.
spongiosaplasty autoplasty of the spongy substance of bone (substantia spongiosa ossium) to potentiate formation of new bone or to cover bone defects; cancellous bone graft.
spongiosis intercellular edema within the epidermis.
spongiositis inflammation of the corpus spongiosum of the penis.
spongy of spongelike appearance or texture.
s. degeneration see spongy DEGENERATION.
spontaneous having no apparent external cause.
s. abortion most animal abortions are spontaneous in contradistinction to the surgically and medically procured abortions of humans. See also MISMATING, PARTURITION induction.
avian s. cardiomyopathy an idiopathic disease of 1 to 4 week old turkey poults causing sudden death or a brief period of dyspnea; the heart is visibly dilated.
s. internal hemorrhage causes sudden death in most cases; causes include cardiac tamponade, aortic or atrial rupture, splenic rupture.
s. pulmonary arteriopathy see AELUROSTRONGYLUS.
s. regression when diseases resolve themselves without outside assistance.
s. virus encephalitis so called because the disease appears without the subject animal coming in contact with a known encephalitogenic agent. In most instances the occurrence is eventually explained by the presence of a hitherto unknown virus.
sporadic occurring irregularly, usually infrequently.
sporadic leukosis leukosis of cattle which is other than bovine viral leukosis.
bovine s. l. occurs sporadically in animals less than 3 years old. There is a cutaneous form with temporary skin plaques which ultimately becomes systemic, a juvenile or calf form with multiple lymph node enlargement and a thymic form with compression of the jugular veins and brisket and submandibular edema.

equine s. l. characterized by subcutaneous and lymph node enlargements, jugular vein engorgement, cardiac irregularity, exophthalmos and anasarca or with diffuse involvement of the small intestine.
ovine s. l. characterized by lymph node enlargement, jugular vein engorgement, and hepatosplenomegaly; caused by bovine leukemia virus.
porcine s. l. characterized by emaciation, weakness, anorexia, bone marrow involvement and hepatosplenomegaly.

sporadic lymphangitis a noncontagious disease of horses characterized by a sudden onset of severe swelling and pain in one hindleg. There is a high fever. Associated with infection of minor wounds on the leg, a lymphangitis and lymphadenitis and spread of infection to surrounding tissues. Called also bigleg. sporadic equine lymphangitis.

sporangia see SPHERULES.

sporangiophore a specialized hypha which gives rise to a sporangium.

sporangium any cyst which contains spores or sporelike bodies.

spore 1. a refractile, oval or spherical body formed within bacteria, especially *Bacillus* and *Clostridium* spp., usually under adverse conditions such as nutritional deprivation, and which is regarded as a fully infectious, resting stage during the life cycle of the cell. Spores are inactive metabolically, highly resistant to environmental changes and may survive, for example in soil, for many years. Bacterial spores come in various shapes and are given illustrative names such as drumstick, terminal and subterminal. 2. the reproductive element, produced sexually or asexually, of organisms, such as protozoa, fungi or algae.
s. former a bacteria or other small life form that forms spores.

sporicide an agent that kills spores.

sporidesmin the toxin in the fungus *Pithomyces chartarum*; the cause of FACIAL eczema.

Sporidesmium bakeri *Pithomyces chartarum*. See FACIAL eczema.

sporoblast an asexual reproductive phase in the development of coccidial parasites. See also SPOROGONY.

sporocyst 1. any cyst or sac containing spores or reproductive cells; contained in the oocyst of coccidia in which sporozoites develop. 2. the larval stages of flukes in snails.

sporogenic producing spores.

sporogony an asexual stage in the life cycle of an apicomplexan parasite, with development of sporocysts and sporozoites within the oocysts. The oocysts are extraintestinal (e.g. *Eimeria*, *Isospora*), or intraintestinal (*Sarcocystis*, *Cryptosporidium*).

sporont a mature protozoon in its sexual cycle.

sporoplasm the protoplasm of a spore.

Sporothrix a genus of fungi.
S. carnis causes white mold on meat in storage.
***S. schenckii* (syn. *Sporotrichum schenckii, S. beurmonsis, S. beurmanii, S. equi, Ceratocystis stenoceras*)** causes SPOROTRICHOSIS.

sporotrichin a substance present in old fluid cultures of *Sporothrix schenckii* and capable of eliciting a specific delayed type hypersensitivity reaction in infected animals.

sporotrichosis a contagious disease in many species, including humans, caused by *Sporothrix schenckii*. It may occur in a cutaneous form, as localized, ulcerated nodules; a cutaneous–lymphatic form, seen particularly in horses as cutaneous nodules on the lower limbs, which may be connected by corded lymphatics and which discharge pus and then heal; or a disseminated form with infection of deep tissues, bone and viscera.

Sporotrichum see SPOROTHRIX.

Sporozoa a subphylum of endoparasitic protozoa in the Phylum Apicomplexa; marked by the lack of locomotor organs in adult stages and a complex life cycle including schizogony, gametogony and sporogony.

sporozoa plural of *sporozoon.*

sporozoan 1. pertaining to the Sporozoa. 2. an individual of the Sporozoa.

sporozoite a spore formed after fertilization; a sickle-shaped nucleated germ formed by division of the protoplasm of a spore of an apicomplexan organism during sporogony.

sporozoon pl. *sporozoa* [Gr.] an individual organism of the Sporozoa.

sport see MUTATION.

sport hunting hunting without collection of a food or other commercial product; hunting for trophy or prize.

sporting dog see GUN dog.

sporulation formation of spores.

spot a small, roundish part of a surface which differs from the surrounding surface.
s. disease of turtles. See SHELL ROT.
s. map a map with dots on it. Each dot marks where a case or some other incident of epidemiological interest occurred.

spot film see spot FILM.
s. film device a device attached to the x-ray machine which moves an x-ray cassette into position for exposure during a fluoroscopic examination.

spot-on a means of delivering medication topically, usually in a small area of the skin, where the active ingredient is absorbed percutaneously. A method used for flea control agents.

spot price price of a product available for immediate delivery.

spotted characterized by spots.
s. brown snake see DEMANSIA *nuchalis affinis*.
s. dick see DALMATIAN.
s. emu bush EREMOPHILA *maculata*.
s. fever a febrile disease characterized by a skin eruption, such as Rocky Mountain spotted fever, boutonneuse fever, and other human infections due to tickborne rickettsiae.
s. fever tick DERMACENTOR *andersoni*.
s. fuschia EREMOPHILA *maculata*.
s. gar the fish *Lepisosteus occulatus*.
s.-headed snake DEMANSIA *olivaceae*.
s. hemlock CONIUM MACULATUM.
s. horse Appaloosa.
s. locoweed ASTRAGALUS *lentiginosus*.
s. persicaria POLYGONUM *persicaria*.

spraddleleg, spraddle limb see SPLAYLEG.

sprain wrenching or twisting of a joint, with partial rupture of its ligaments. There may also be damage to the associated blood vessels, muscles, tendons and nerves.

A sprain is more serious than a strain, which is simply the overstretching of a muscle, without swelling. Severe sprains are so painful that the joint cannot be used. There is much swelling owing to hemorrhage from ruptured blood vessels.

sprained tendon see bowed TENDON, TENDON strain.

spray material applied in liquid form by pressure through a fine orifice creating a mist of fine droplets, e.g. insecticidal spray in a spray dip, pressure pack spray of insecticide or wound treatment.

s.-dehydrated a substance which has been dried by spraying onto a revolving heated drum and retrieved by scraping it from the drum.
s. drift chemical spray being applied to an agricultural crop may be toxic to animals and be carried from its target by wind. Poisoning by organophosphates and arsenic has been caused in this way.
s. freezing direct application of freezing agent, e.g. liquid nitrogen, by fine spray or stream.
s. race a lane with high fences, see RACE (2), used to restrain animals while they are being sprayed, usually with insecticide.

spraydip device for applying insecticide or other solution to the coat of animals, replacing the plunge dip. The animal walks through a compartment which carries spray nozzles on the sides, below and above. Excess spray drains into a sump and is reused.

spraying the pattern of urination typical of male cats but occasionally seen in females; after backing up to a vertical surface and while holding their tail erect, they void urine in a stream posteriorly onto the object. A form of olfactory communication, especially territorial marking. Called also urine marking.
inappropriate s. spraying on household objects. A common behavioral problem in domestic cats that may be related to stress or overcrowding, but sometimes it is caused by urinary tract disease.

spreading dogbane APOCYNUM *androsaemifolium*.

spreading factor said of biological fluids, used in pharmaceutical preparations. See HYALURONIDASE.

spreadsheet a computer software consisting of a program used for quick analysis of figures based on a grid of cells created by the intersection of vertical columns and horizontal rows, each cell containing data or formulae; much used in financial assessments and planning; also used to assess the effects of a number of changes to a system, e.g varying the feed supply and the average age of a sheep flock, a change in the price of wool and observing the profitability.

spring gag a gag used in dogs to keep the mouth open during treatment of teeth. It consists of two bars which run up and down a curved pillar. The bars have perforated disks at their ends, into which a canine tooth can be positioned. Pressure on the disks jams the sliding action of the bars.

spring parsley CYMOPTERUS *watsonii*.

spring rabbitbrush see TETRADYMIA GLABRATA.

spring rise a phenomenon in some nematode infestations, e.g. *Haemonchus* spp., in ruminants in which there is an increase in the number of eggs excreted in the feces during the spring months.

spring round-up traditional round-up (muster) each spring on beef cattle ranches to brand, dehorn, castrate the new calf crop and to draft off the yearlings into the group to be marketed.

spring viremia of carp an infection of European carp caused by a rhabdovirus which occurs when water temperature rises in the spring. It is characterized by edema and hemorrhage in viscera. Important in European carp culture. Suggested as a biological agent for the control of carp populations in Australia.

springbok the antelope *Antidorcas marsupialis*.

springbokbush see HERTIA PALLENS.

Springer spaniel see ENGLISH SPRINGER SPANIEL, WELSH SPRINGER SPANIEL.

sprouted grain used as feed; see HYDROPONICS.

sprue a chronic form of malabsorption syndrome in humans occurring in two forms, tropical, which is associated with ingestion of gluten-containing foods (called also CELIAC disease), and nontropical. Malabsorption syndromes in dogs are sometimes compared with, but are not identical with, sprue.

Spumavirinae a subfamily of viruses in the family *Retroviridae*.

spumavirus a member of the subfamily SPUMAVIRINAE.

spur 1. an abnormal projecting body, as from a bone. 2. a piece of riding gear worn on the heel of a horserider's boot and used to urge on a horse to a faster speed by digging the spur into the flank. 3. a sharp, horn-covered, bony projection from the shank of male birds of some species. Used as a weapon. Called also metatarsal spur. 4. tracheal spur, the ridge of tracheal cartilage that separates the beginning of the right bronchus from the beginnings of the left one.
s. veins subcutaneous veins visible over the ventral part of the chest of a horse (superficial thoracic vein). Subject to laceration by indiscriminate use of sharp spurs by the vigorous rider.

spurge see EUPHORBIA, PHYLLANTHUS *abnormis*.
s. flax DAPHNE *mezereum*.
s. laurel DAPHNE spp.
s. olive DAPHNE *mezereum*.

spurious simulated; not genuine; false.

sputum mucous secretion from the lungs, bronchi and trachea which is ejected through the mouth by humans but not so in animals and it is assumed that it is swallowed.
s. cup a small—1 inch diameter—cup on a long handle for the collection of sputum from the pharynx of a large animal.
s. specimen a sample of mucous secretion from the bronchi and lungs. The specimen may be examined microscopically for the presence of malignant cells (*cytological examination*) or tested to identify pathogenic bacteria (*bacteriological examination*).

SPV sheeppox virus.

SQ subcutaneous.

squab baby or fledgling pigeon.

squalene an unsaturated terpene, which is an intermediate in cholesterol synthesis, and occurs normally at low levels in blood plasma and at elevated levels in viral influenza; used as a vehicle for pharmaceuticals.

squama pl. *squamae* [L.] a scale, or thin, platelike structure.

Squamata an order of animals, the scaly-bodied reptiles, including snakes and lizards.

squamatization flattened, eosinophilic keratinocytes replace basophilic, cuboidal basal cells.

squame a scale or scalelike mass.

squamoparietal, squamosoparietal pertaining to the pars squamosa, or squamous portion of the temporal bone, and the parietal bone.

squamous scaly or platelike.
s. bone the pars squamosa, or squamous portion of the temporal bone.
s. cell carcinoma a carcinoma arising from squamous epithelium; relatively common, locally invasive and occasionally metastatic. In animals they occur on the conjunctiva, the mouth, salivary duct, stomach, trachea and bronchi, prostate, penis, prepuce, vulva, urinary bladder and skin. See also specific organ locations.
s. eddy a common histological pattern in neoplastic and hyperplastic epidermal disorders. They are whorl-like patterns of squamoid cells.
s. metaplasia affected cells are converted to a squamous stratified type from the surface of which squames are shed.
ocular s. cell carcinoma that arising from squamous epithelium and having cuboid cells.

Squamous cell carcinoma around the eye, also known as cancer eye, is a common neoplasm in cattle, especially those breeds with little pigment in the eyelids. Sunlight, viruses, skin pigmentation and heredity are all thought to be involved in causing the disease. Lesions begin on the third eyelid, unpigmented eyelid or vascular cornea. They are fungating masses of tissue, usually ulcerated, necrotic and apparently painful. They grow rapidly and commonly invade the local lymph nodes. Similar lesions occur on the eyeball and eyelid of the horse. What makes the cattle disease so remarkable is the high prevalence rate.

Squamous cell carcinomas are among the most common skin tumors in dogs and cats. They are particularly common in sun-exposed areas of skin such as the pinnae, eyelids or noses of white cats. Tumors are locally invasive and slow to metastasize.

s. papilloma the common papilloma in all species except cattle and deer. Composed largely of epithelial tissue in contrast to fibropapillomas but many lesions are intermediate in type.

s. pearl see HORN pearls.

square knot a secure knot made by a single throw of one of the two ends over the other, then a return and another single throw with both ends coming out on the same side of the loop, either both over or both under it. Called also reef knot.

squash CUCURBITA *maxima*.

Squatina squatina, S. angelus, S. laevis farmed finfish in family Squatinidae; called also angel-fish, monk-fish.

squeejit MENTHA *satureioides*.

squeeze compression.

s. cage see squeeze CAGE.

s. chute see CHUTE.

squid large marine invertebrate with eight arms with suckers, and two supplementary tentacles, almost suckerless, used for catching prey. Are members of the family Teuthoidea and there are a number of genera including *Loligo* spp. with many species and *Architeuthis* spp. the giant squids.

squill the fleshy inner scales of the bulb of the white variety of URGINEA *maritima*; it contains several cardioactive glycosides. The red variety is used as a rat poison. See also SCILLA.

squint convergent STRABISMUS; cross-eye.

squirrel small, arboreal, mostly herbivorous rodents varying in color from gray to shiny black, red and cream, and in size from mouse to large cat. Some are insectivorous, and many are terrestrial, e.g. the chipmunks. Some glide although they are called flying squirrels. Most squirrels are diurnal but the flying genera are nocturnal. They are all members of the family Sciuridae, which includes a very large number of species, and are distinguished by their fine, dense fur and their bushy, plume-like tails and ears that are often surmounted by tufts of hair.

s. corn DICENTRA *canadensis*.

s. fibroma a poxvirus disease caused by a member of the genus *Leporipoxvirus* in which there are typical subcutaneous fibroma lesions. The virus isolated from the lesions has been used to produce fibroma lesions in rabbits.

fox s. this species has a characteristic of inherited porphyria manifested by fluorescence of bones and teeth when viewed under ultraviolet light, and a pink coloration of these and other tissues. There is no photosensitization. Called also *Sciurus* spp.

s. monkey a dramatically colored, e.g. yellow-green with red lower limbs, squirrel-sized, carnivorous monkey distinguished by its large brain. Called also *Saimiri sciureus*.

squirreltail grass see HORDEUM.

squirting cucumber see ECBALLIUM ELATERIUM.

SR sedimentation rate.

Sr chemical symbol, *strontium*.

SRC Science Research Council (UK).

SRH somatotropin releasing hormone (growth hormone releasing hormone).

SRP signal recognition particle.

SRS, SRS-A see SLOW-REACTING SUBSTANCE.

ss. [L.] *semis* (one half).

SSA special somatic afferent system of dendritic zones of neurons associated with the eye and ear.

SSPE subacute sclerosing panencephalitis.

$S_1S_2S_3$ pattern an electrocardiographic abnormality in which S waves are present in leads I, II and III. It is associated with right ventricular enlargement involving the base of the heart or the ventricular outflow tract.

stabilate a mixture of blood and tick tissues, expected to contain infective elements of rickettsia or protozoa, in a stable state suitable for storage.

stabilization the process of making firm and steady.

stable 1. animal accommodation, usually for horses. 2. to accommodate an animal in a stable as distinct from running at pasture. 3. steady; not easily swayed.

s. blackleg caused by the germination of latent spores of *Clostridium septicum* in tissues. The clinical disease is similar to blackleg.

s. cough any of the viral diseases of the upper respiratory tract of horses, but most commonly equine influenza.

s. fly see STOMOXYS CALCITRANS.

s. footrot see stable FOOTROT.

stachybotryotoxicosis the disease caused by poisoning by STACHYBOTRYS ATRA.

Stachybotrys atra, S. alternans, S. chartarum a fungus that grows on stored feed and produces trichothecene mycotoxins. Poisoning is characterized by diarrhea, necrotic ulcers in the mouth, mucosal petechiation and agranulocytosis. See also SATRATOXINS. Poisoning called alimentary toxic aleucia.

Stachys arvensis European plant in the family Lamiaceae; contains an unidentified toxin which causes tremor, incoordination and recumbency if exercised. There is no permanent damage. Called also stagger weed.

stack work area in a computer's memory that expands and contracts dynamically as required to store temporary data.

stactometer a device for measuring drops.

Stader splint see Stader SPLINT.

staff 1. a wooden rod or rodlike structure. 2. the professional personnel of a hospital.

Staffordshire bull terrier a small (24–38 lb), very muscular and solidly built dog with broad head, moderately short muzzle, half-pricked ears and medium length tail. The coat is smooth and short and comes in many colors. See also AMERICAN STAFFORDSHIRE TERRIER.

stag 1. in abattoir terminology a male animal castrated after it has matured sexually, i.e. more than a year old. Used mostly about cattle beasts or pigs. In rams the age limit is 6 months. In some areas also applied to an unbroken colt more than a year old. 2. to the game hunter an adult male of any of the large deer species.

stage 1. a definite period or distinct phase, as of development of a disease or of an organism. 2. the platform of a microscope on which the slide containing the object to be studied is placed.

stagger bush SENECIO *latifolius*, *S. retrorsus*, LYONIA LIGUSTRINA.

stagger weed see STACHYS ARVENSIS.

staggergrass see AMIANTHIUM MUSCAETOXICUM, MELICA DECUMBENS.

staggers incoordination of any kind, including a tendency to fall, and recumbency if harassed.

blind s. incoordination, aimless wandering as in liver encephalopathy, carbohydrate engorgement.

grass s. see LACTATION TETANY (2).

paspalum s. see PASPALUM ERGOT.

ryegrass s. see RYEGRASS staggers.

staging 1. the determination of distinct phases or periods in the course of a disease, the life history of an organism, or any biological process. 2. the classification of neoplasms according to the extent of the tumor.

TNM s. staging of tumors according to three basic components: primary tumor (T), regional nodes (N) and metastasis (M). Subscripts are used to denote size and degree of involvement; for example, 0 indicates undetectable, and 1, 2, 3 and 4 a progressive increase in size or involvement. Thus, a tumor may be described as $T_1N_2M_0$.

stagnant loop syndrome the syndrome of toxemia and dehydration caused by a loop or loops of atonic small intestine caused by partial obstruction, paralytic ileus or radiation injury. The stasis has the effect of encouraging growth of anaerobic bacteria and damage to enterocytes causing diarrhea.

staib agar see birdseed AGAR.

stain 1. a substance used to impart color to tissues or cells, to facilitate microscopic study and identification. 2. an area of discoloration of the skin.

acid s. a stain in which the coloring agent is in the acid radical.

basic s. a stain in which the coloring agent is in the basic radical.

carbol fuschin s. used to stain some gram-negative bacteria, including *Campylobacter fetus*.

Castaneda's s. a technique for demonstrating chlamydial elementary bodies, using formol blue and safranine.

Diene's s. one containing methylene blue, maltose and azure II, used for staining mycoplasmal microcolonies.

differential s. one which facilitates differentiation of various elements in a specimen.

hematoxylin and eosin s. a staining method employed universally for routine histological examination of tissue sections.

India ink s. used to demonstrate capsules on *Cryptococcus neoformans* and some bacterial species.

lambing s. staining of the breech and back of the udder of a ewe caused by the passage of the fetal fluids and then the lochia. Used as a guide to whether or not the ewe has lambed and perhaps lost her lamb.

Macchiavello s. a basic fuscin solution for staining chlamydial elementary bodies.

metachromatic s. one that produces in certain elements color different from that of the stain itself.

methanamine silver s. stains fungal elements in tissue a dark brown.

new methylene blue s. a metachromatic dye used for staining blood, vaginal smears, and tissue samples for cytological examination. Particularly useful in demonstrating reticulocytes.

Newman's s. used on smears of milk for demonstrating organisms in mastitis.

nigrosin s. an aniline dye used in wet mounts to demonstrate capusules, especially with CRYPTOCOCCUS *neoformans*.

nuclear s. one that selectively stains cell nuclei, generally a basic stain.

ophthalmic s. used in the diagnosis of diseases of the eye, e.g. fluorescein and rose bengal dyes.

supravital s. a stain introduced in living tissue or cells that have been removed from the body.

tumor s. an area of increased density in a radiograph, due to collection of contrast material in distorted and abnormal vessels, prominent in the capillary and venous phases of arteriography, and presumed to indicate neoplasm.

vital s. a stain introduced into the living organism, and taken up selectively by various tissue or cellular elements. Often used to determine the live/dead cell ratio in a cell population.

Wright's s. a mixture of eosin and methylene blue, used for demonstrating blood cells.

Ziehl–Neelsen s. one of carbol fuchsin counterstained with methylene blue; used to demonstrate acid-fast organisms, especially *Mycobacterium* spp., in smears and tissues. A modified method using mild acid to decolorize is used for staining *Brucella* spp., *Nocardia asteroides* and *Chlamydia psittaci*. See also ACID-FAST.

stainable iron a method of staining a bone marrow smear to determine the amount of body storage of iron.

staining 1. artificial coloration of a substance to facilitate examination of tissues, microorganisms or other cells under the microscope. For various techniques, see under STAIN. 2. marring the appearance.

chromosomal s. blood is collected in a highly aseptic manner and placed in tissue culture medium containing a stimulant to cell division. The leukocytes are collected, killed with a cytotoxic agent, enlarged by osmosis in a hypotonic liquid, placed on slides, fixed and stained.

negative s. a procedure visualizing specimens by either light or electron microscopy. In light microscopy, India ink which blocks the transmission of light is used as a negative stain to detect bacterial capsules. In electron microscopy, electron-dense salts such as sodium phosphotungstate are used in the examination of particles particularly viruses.

radiograph s. may be yellow or brown stains due to inadequate rinsing, or doubly refracting exhibiting different colors depending on angle of viewing.

stainless steel see STEEL.

staircase phenomenon a characteristic of cardiac muscle, the strength of the contraction increases as the interval between contractions increases, up to a point.

stalagmometer an instrument for measuring surface tension by determining the exact number of drops in a given quantity of a liquid.

stale horseman's term for the act of urination by a horse.

stalkage residue of a maize crop after the cobs have been picked by a mechanical harvester. The feed is mature and dry. It may be fed standing or cut and chopped. See also STOVER.

stall a small compartment to house one animal, usually a horse, cow or pig. Calves may also be housed in stalls for reasons of hygiene or in veal fattening units. A stall is usually just large enough for an animal to stand and lie in but insufficient to turn around in; in fact they may be designed specifically so that the animal cannot turn around. There may be a chain across the back, which is always open, or the animal is tied in with a neck chain or a headstall. In open access housing in modern cow barns no attempt is made to keep the cows in their stalls. See also BOX (2).

s. bed the floor of a stall. Most commonly concrete covered with straw, sawdust or other bedding but earth floors or sand on concrete are probably more comfortable for cows. Pigs manage all right on concrete without bedding.

s. fed cattle confined and fed in individual stalls. Contrast with pen-fed or lot-fed.

s. kicking a vice in horses which are kept in stalls for too long without exercise.

s.-related injury injuries incurred by being restrained in stalls, e.g. teat treads, broken tail.

stall-cramp see inherited PERIODIC spasticity.

stallion 1. an entire male horse aged 4 years and over. 2. in UK, applied to a male donkey (jack).

s. ring see stallion RING.

teaser s. stallion used to detect those mares which are in estrus. During the breeding season those mares to be bred are brought into a crush and the teaser brought alongside. The mares that show estral signs are kept back, usually palpated per rectum to determine the state of their ovaries, and may be bred. The teaser is not used for breeding and is usually a pony or an infertile cryptorchid.

stance the posture or position.

sawhorse s. see sawhorse POSTURE.

stanchion cows are tied in for the winter in headlocks of wood or metal and have a confined space in which to lie but feed troughs and water bowls are at the front of the stall and a gutter, nowadays fitted with a mechanical dung remover, for the collection of manure and urine.

stand a standing crop of fodder plants or weeds, e.g. a stand of variegated thistle.

stand-alone computer see COMPUTER.

stand-off in ultrasonography, a device used to increase the distance between the transducer and skin in order to bring the area of investigation into the focal zone.

standard something established as a measure or model to which other similar things should conform.

bacteriological s. of meat the standard bacterial count of meat beyond which local legislation forbids the sale or use of meat. The international standard is for <107/g of meat and that *Salmonella* spp. should not be present in more than one of five 25 g samples, all held at 95°F (35°C) or 68°F (20°C) for chilled meat.

s. bicarbonate in blood gas analysis this is the plasma level of bicarbonate, under specified conditions, which eliminates the influence of respiration on the values obtained.

s. deviation a measure of the dispersal of a random variable; the square root of the average squared deviation from the mean. For data that have a normal distribution about 68% of the data points fall within one standard deviation from the mean and 95% fall within two standard deviations. Symbol is σ.

s. error the standard deviation of an estimate.

s. error of mean the sampling variability of the mean.

s. international (SI) units see Table 3.

s. population a population not yet divided into classes; the population against which each of its constituent classes can be compared.

s. *Salmonella pullorum* strains strains that contain only small amounts of 12_2 antigen.

Standard Nomenclature of Veterinary Diseases and Operations published by the US Department of Health, Education and Welfare in 1966. An eight digit code divided into two sections of four digits each, one section devoted to topography or anatomical location and the other to etiology. It is capable of enormous expansion. Its main problem is the difficulty of memorizing codes, an important feature for a practice which cannot afford to be consulting the code file every time it wants to make an entry. With increases in computer technology since 1966 a much more user-friendly code is required.

Standard Pinscher see GERMAN PINSCHER.

Standardbred a group of breeds of horses used in trotting races. See AMERICAN TROTTER. Called also Trotter.

standardization weighted averaging of a characteristic. It is usually specific to a standard distribution of age or other characteristic.

exposure factor s. in radiology is the elimination of variation as much as possible in as many as possible factors which affect the optimum exposure time. Includes using a standard anode-film distance, use of the same chemicals and preparation technique, eliminating surges and drops in input voltage, and use of the same screen-film combination.

standardized pertaining to data that have been submitted to standardization procedures.

s. morbidity rate see MORBIDITY rate.

s. mortality rate see MORTALITY rate.

standing heat the stage of estrus in which the cow stands to be mounted by other cows or by the bull.

standing lateral the positioning technique for a lateral projection of the x-ray beam through a standing animal to a vertically positioned cassette; useful for the assessment of fluid levels.

standstill cessation of motion, as of the heart (cardiac standstill) or chest (respiratory standstill).

Stangeria a genus of the family Stangeriaceae of cycads, restricted to southern Africa.

Stanleya pinnata North American selenium indicator plant in the family Brassicaceae; contains large amounts of selenium on soils rich in the element and can cause selenium poisoning characterized by lameness, hoof deformity, alopecia. Called also Prince's plume.

stannous containing tin as a bivalent element.

stannum [L.] *tin* (symbol Sn).

stanozolol, stanazol an androgenic anabolic steroid used in the treatment of weight loss, debility and nonregenerative anemias.

Stanton's disease melioidosis.

stapedial pertaining to the stapes.

stapediovestibular pertaining to the stapes and vestibule.

stapedius innermost auditory ossicle; shaped like a stirrup.

s. muscle a striated muscle which aids in the dampening of the effects of high-frequency vibrations on the auditory apparatus.

stapes the innermost of the three ossicles of the ear; called also stirrup.

staphage lysate staphylococcus phage lysate; a preparation of *Staphylococcus aureus* and polyvalent staphylococcus bacteriophage used as an immunomodulator in the treatment of refractory pyodermas.

staphylectomy uvulectomy in humans. In animals the term is used to describe resection of the posterior part of the soft palate.

staphyline 1. pertaining to the uvula. 2. shaped like a bunch of grapes.

staphylitis inflammation of the uvula or soft palate.

staphyl(o)- word element. [Gr.] *uvula, resembling a bunch of grapes, staphylococci.*

staphylococcal pertaining to *Staphylococcus* spp.
s. clumping test used as a means of measuring the quantity of fibrinogen-split products in a sample of blood.
equine s. dermatitis see EQUINE staphylococcal dermatitis.
s. food poisoning a disease of humans caused by enterotoxins elaborated by coagulase-positive *Staphylococcus aureus* of human origin. Dangerous foods for this disease are ham, dried milk and cold meats generally. Domestic animals appear not to be susceptible to the toxins but the disease is important to veterinarians because animal products, especially milk and chicken meat from animals in their care, may be the origin of this severe, often epidemic, gastroenteritis.
s. granuloma persistent, low-grade infection of connective tissue or muscle by *Staphylococcus aureus* causing the development of granulomas which can become very large, most commonly in the chest of the horse and the mammary gland of the sow. The granuloma is a dense mass of fibrous tissue containing a large number of small abscesses containing thick yellow pus containing granules of club colonies. Called also botryomycosis.
s. hypersensitivity see bacterial HYPERSENSITIVITY.
s. mastitis of cows caused by *S. aureus* may be chronic, acute or peracute with gangrene of the quarter and sometimes death of the cow.
s. phage lysate products see STAPHAGE LYSATE.
s. protein A a cell-bound protein expressed by most strains of *Staphyloccus intermedius* recovered from dogs and cats.
s. pyemia see TICK pyemia.
s. septicemia of lambs and less commonly other neonates; high mortality rate; umbilical infection the likely entry portal.

staphylococcemia septicemia with staphylococci in the blood.

staphylococcin see BACTERIOCIN (1).

staphylococcosis see ENZOOTIC staphylococcosis. Called also tick pyemia.

Staphylococcus a genus of spherical, gram-positive bacteria tending to occur in grapelike clusters; they are normal flora on the skin and in the upper respiratory tract and are the most common cause of localized suppurating infections. Pathogenic species are characterized by positive reactions to the COAGULASE test.
S. aureus a common and important cause of disease in animals including bovine MASTITIS, TICK pyemia (enzootic staphylococcosis), abscesses, dermatitis, furunculosis, meningitis, osteomyelitis, food poisoning, wound suppuration, and BUMBLEFOOT in poultry. *S. aureus* subsp. *anaerobius* causes lesions similar to caseous lymphadenitis in sheep.
S. epidermidis a common skin and mucosal inhabitant in humans and occasionally in animals living in association with humans.
***S. hyicus* (*S. hyos*)** causes EXUDATIVE epidermitis and occasionally septic arthritis in pigs.
S. intermedius the major isolate from pyoderma and occasionally other pyogenic infections in dogs and cats and a rare cause of infection in other species.
S. xylosus a rare cause of mastitis in cattle.

staphylococcus pl. *staphylococci* [Gr.] any organism of the genus *Staphylococcus*.
coagulase-positive s. see COAGULASE test.

staphylodemodicosis demodectic mange complicated by infection with *Staphylococcus* spp.

staphyloderma pyogenic skin infection by staphylococci.

staphylokinase a bacterial kinase produced by certain strains of staphylococci; it induces fibrinolysis by converting plasminogen to plasmin.

staphylolysin a substance produced by staphylococci that causes hemolysis.

staphyloma protrusion of the sclera or cornea, usually lined with uveal tissue, due to inflammation.
anterior s. staphyloma in the anterior part of the eye.
corneal s. 1. bulging of the cornea with adherent uveal tissue. 2. one formed by protrusion of the iris through a corneal wound.
posterior s., s. posticum backward bulging of sclera at posterior pole of eye.
scleral s. protrusion of the contents of the eyeball where the sclera has become thinned.

staphyloplasty plastic repair of the soft palate.

staphyloptosis elongation of the soft palate.

staphylorrhaphy surgical correction of a midline cleft in the soft palate.

staphyloschisis fissure of the soft palate.

staphylotomy 1. incision of the soft palate. 2. excision of a staphyloma.

staple a number of wool fibers naturally formed into a cluster about as thick as a human thumb but varying widely in size. Used with reference to fleeces of fine-wool sheep. Similar structures in longwool fleeces are called locks.
s. measurements includes staple length, staple strength, staple length variability, and the position of any break in the wool.
s. strength force required to break a staple of wool of a given thickness.

staples U-shaped stainless steel or vitallium units with sharp points used for surgical fixation.
epiphyseal s. used to staple epiphysis to metaphysis; have metal bracing at the corners. Are driven in to the bone while held in a special holder and are removed with a similar special instrument.
soft tissue s. come in a special appliance suitable for animal use. Are expensive but very saving of time. Used especially for skin closure, bowel anastomoses, ligation of pedicle, wherever conventional suturing is very consumptive of time or difficult because of awkward access.

stapling the use of staples as surgical sutures and fixation.

STAR see CORNELL STAR accelerated lambing system.

star a color marking in a horse's coat consisting of a white spot in the center of the forehead; just a few white hairs is sometimes called a flame.

star burr ACANTHOSPERMUM *hispidum*.

star of Bethlehem see ORNITHOGALUM.

starch 1. any of a group of polysaccharides of the general formula, $(C_6H_{10}O_5)_n$; it is the chief storage form of CARBOHYDRATES in plants. 2. granular material separated from mature grain of *Zea mays* (Indian corn, or maize); used as a dusting powder and tablet disintegrant in pharmaceuticals.
s. blockers inhibitors of alpha-amylase, used to decrease starch digestion and limit energy intake from starch.
s. digestion test, s. tolerance test a test to assess the ability of the intestine to digest and absorb a polysaccharide. Efficiency measured by the rise in blood glucose after oral administration of starch to an animal that has been fasted.
s. equivalent an outmoded way of estimating and expressing the energy value of a feed. Replaced now by METABOLIZABLE energy.
s. inhalation can occur in pigs in a poorly ventilated

environment and when the feed is fed dry. Causes foreign body pneumonia.

s.–iodine complex is a deep blue color and this is used as an indicator of the amount of starch in a solution.

s. tolerance test see starch digestion test (above).

stargrass CYNODON *plectostachys*.

staring coat a dry haircoat lacking in luster, usually carrying dandruff or scurf. May be caused by poor cutaneous circulation and lack of sebaceous secretion resulting from a general state of ill health such as in any toxemia.

Starling curves graphic curves that relate cardiac function to venous inflow. Called also cardiac function curve. See also FRANK–STARLING MECHANISM.

Starling's hypothesis, law the law relating to the passage of fluid out of a capillary depending on the hydrostatic and osmotic pressures of the blood and the same pressures of tissue fluid, the net effect of the opposing pressures determining the direction and rate of flow.

starry-sky effect the cytological effect created in a histological slide of a lymphosarcoma by the presence of a large number of tingible-body macrophages, usually associated with a high turnover of the tumor cells.

stars of Winslow prominent choroidal capillaries, seen as red or dark dots and lines in the tapetal area of equine, bovine and ovine eyes.

starter Welsh springer spaniel.

startle reaction the mental state of suddenly aroused awareness; manifested by a flight or fight or submit pattern of behavior and posture.

starvation long-continued deprival of food and its morbid effects. Hunger, loss of body weight and decreased muscle power and endurance occur early. Late stages include signs of milk yield drop, cessation of defecation and drinking, emaciation, loss of skin turgor without dehydration, weakness, slow heart rate and hypothermia.

preoperative s. see preoperative FASTING.

starve–feed cycle metabolic response to feeding usually involving an increased sensitivity to glucose resulting in markedly increased rates of insulin secretion after varying periods of starvation, such as an overnight fast in humans or a prolonged fast, or during winter in hibernating animals.

stasis a stoppage or diminution of flow, as of blood or other body fluid, or of intestinal contents.

gastric s. reduced motility, without primary organic disease, leading to retention of gastric contents; may be a cause of vomiting. Can be caused by stress, trauma, ulcers, peritonitis and gastritis.

urine s. may be caused by abnormalities in structure or innervation of the urinary outflow tract that result in incomplete emptying of the bladder or pooling of urine in diverticula. Important in the etiology of cystitis.

-stasis word element. [Gr.] maintenance of (or maintaining) a constant level; preventing increase or multiplication.

stat. [L.] *statim* (at once).

state condition or situation.

excited s. the condition of a nucleus, atom or molecule produced by the addition of energy to the system as the result of absorption of photons or of inelastic collisions with other particles or systems.

ground s. the condition of lowest energy of a nucleus, atom or molecule.

refractory s. a condition of subnormal excitability of muscle and nerve following excitation.

resting s. the physiological condition achieved by complete rest for at least 1 hour.

steady s. dynamic equilibrium.

static 1. stable with opposing forces in balance. 2. minor electric disturbance.

s. fetal cadaver see MUMMIFICATION.

s. reaction reflexes which maintain a steady posture; they may be local, segmental or general.

statim [L.] *at once;* abbreviated stat.

station stance.

statistic a numerical value calculated from a number of observations in order to summarize them.

statistical pertaining to or emanating from statistics.

s. efficiency between-test comparisons are based on the ratio of sample sizes required for the tests to have equal probabilities of detecting the same false null hypothesis; the more efficient test will have the smaller sample size.

s. methods procedures for collecting, classifying, summarizing, analyzing and making conclusions about, data. See also REGRESSION (4), PATH analysis, FACTOR, discriminant ANALYSIS.

s. significance see SIGNIFICANCE.

statistics 1. numerical facts pertaining to a particular subject or body of objects. 2. the science dealing with the collection, tabulation and analysis of numerical facts.

inferential s. conclusions, usually quantitative, drawn from an analysis of data.

salvage s. statistical technique used in an attempt to derive some useful information from a poorly designed or poorly executed experiment.

vital s. see VITAL statistics.

statoacoustic pertaining to balance and hearing.

statoconia [Gr.] plural of *statoconium*; minute calcareous particles in the gelatinous membrane surmounting the macula in the inner ear. Called also otoconia.

statoconial membrane part of each otolithic organ; the hair cells in the organ carry stereocilia which project from the hairs and into the statoconial membrane which is covered with otoliths.

statolith 1. a granule of the statoconia. 2. see OTOLITH.

stature the height of an animal in the standing position.

status [L.] *condition, state.*

s. asthmaticus asthmatic crisis; a sudden, intense and continuous asthmatic attack with dyspnea, gagging and cyanosis. May be seen in feline bronchial asthma.

s. epilepticus rapid succession of epileptic spasms without intervals of consciousness; brain damage may result.

s. line a portion of the computer screen which gives details of the computer's status.

s. spongiosum see spongy DEGENERATION.

Statute of Limitations the law which limits the time after an event during which a court action related to a claim for damages arising out of the event can be initiated.

stay apparatus the anatomical mechanism in both the fore- and hindlimbs of horses which enable the animal to stand with little or no muscular effort. Efficiency of the apparatus is based on the judicious location of fibrous tissue. Many muscles, ligaments and tendons participate, especially the suspensory ligament, the flexor tendons and their check ligaments, and in the hindlimb, the peroneus tertius and the patellar-locking mechanism.

stayer a horse that can gallop at racing speed for at least 1.5 miles (2.4 km).

steady-state level said of a medication regimen; a plateau.
steam the vapor created by heating water to 212°F (100°C).
s. sterilization see STERILIZATION (2).
steaming up the practice of commencing to feed extra rations, especially of grain and concentrates, to late pregnant cows in an attempt to promote maximum milk production from the very beginning of the lactation. Feeding usually commences about 4 weeks before the due date.
steapsin the fat-splitting enzyme (lipase) of the pancreatic juice.
steapsinogen the precursor metabolically of steapsin.
stearate any compound of stearic acid.
stearic acid an 18 carbon saturated fatty acid from animal and vegetable fats.
stearin a substance common in mammalian fat. Formed from the reaction of stearic acid with glycerol. See also OLEIN, PALMITIN.
stear(o)- word element. [Gr.] *fat.*
steatitis inflammation of fatty tissue. See also YELLOW FAT DISEASE.
steat(o)- word element. [Gr.] *fat, oil.*
steatocystoma a human term for an epithelial cyst.
steatogenous producing fat; lipogenic.
steatolysis the emulsification of fats preparatory to absorption.
steatoma pl. *steatomata, steatomas.* 1. lipoma. 2. a fatty mass retained within a sebaceous gland.
steatomatosis the presence of numerous sebaceous cysts.
steatonecrosis fat necrosis.
steatopathy disease of the sebaceous glands.
steatopygia excessive fatness of the buttocks; a normal state in FAT-TAILED SHEEP.
steatorrhea excess fat in the feces due to a malabsorption syndrome caused by disease of the intestinal mucosa or pancreatic enzyme deficiency. The feces are bulky, greasy, malodorous and pale in color.
pancreatic s. see exocrine PANCREATIC insufficiency.
steatosis fatty degeneration. See also MUSCULAR steatosis.
steed see NAG.
steel an industrial metal.
s. mesh see surgical MESH.
steely wool the appearance of wool of sheep which are suffering from a nutritional deficiency of copper. The wool loses its crimp and becomes straight and stringy and the fibers have reduced strength, elasticity and stainability. Caused by a defect of keratin metabolism.
steenboksuring RUMEX *acetosella.*
steeplechase a horse race conducted over fences, open ditches and water jumps.
steeplechaser a horse schooled in and used for steeplechase racing.
steer castrated male cattle beast over a year of age. See also BULLOCK, BULLER STEER.
s. bulling see BULLING.
steg stag.
stegnosis constriction; stenosis.
Stegomyia fasciata a mosquito vector of the virus of fowl pox.
Steinmann name given to specific designs of orthopedic hardware.
S. extension extension exerted on the distal fragment of a fractured bone by means of a nail or pin (Steinmann pin) driven into the fragment. Called also nail extension.
S. pin intramedullary pin with a choice of ends, either screw, chisel or trocar. Can be plain at one end or have one of the selected points at each end. Pin drills to drill the holes for the pins, and a chuck to grasp the end of the pin and drive or rotate it are available.
stell circular stone or metal corral providing shelter for sheep in windswept, snow-susceptible areas. Has lean-to, inward-facing roof around the wall.
stella pl. *stellae* [L.] star.
Stellaria media the widespread weed called chickweed, member of the family Caryophyllaceae, which may cause nitrate–nitrite poisoning.
stellate star-shaped; arranged in rosettes.
s. ganglion cervicothoracic and middle cervical ganglion.
s. reticulum center of the enamel organ of the embryonic tooth.
stem stalk; a stalklike supporting structure.
brain s. see BRAINSTEM.
stem line-template a process of development of new muscle fibers, evident in the fetal and newborn pig and important in the development of splayleg in that species. A centrally located muscle fiber in a sublobule of muscle divides longitudinally or acts as a template for myoblasts to form a new fiber. The process is repeated until a whole new sublobule is formed.
stemless loco OXYTROPIS *lambertii.*
Stemodia kingii plant in family Scrophulariaceae; causes cardiac glycoside poisoning.
sten- prefix meaning narrow.
steno- word element. [Gr.] *narrow, contracted, constriction.*
Stenocarpella naydis see DIPLODIA MAYDIS.
stenochoria stenosis.
stenocoriasis contraction of the pupil.
stenohaline species of fish capable of osmoregulation only in fresh water.
stenopeic having a narrow opening or slit.
stenosed narrowed; constricted.
stenosis narrowing or contraction of a body passage or opening. See also specific anatomical sites.
aortic s. obstruction to the outflow of blood from the left ventricle into the aorta. May be due to an anomaly of the valves (valvular), an obstruction in the ascending aorta (supravalvular), or an obstruction in the left ventricular outflow tract (subvalvular). See also AORTIC subvalvular stenosis, AORTIC valvular disease.
esophageal s. a common cause of esophageal obstruction, caused commonly by esophageal trauma; congenital stenosis often associated with TRACHEOESOPHAGEAL fistula.
left atrioventricular s. see mitral stenosis (below), VALVULAR stenosis.
mesonephric duct s. occurs as stenosis of the ductus deferens or epididymis; may be associated with renal aplasia.
mitral s. a narrowing of the left atrioventricular orifice. See also mitral COMMISSUROTOMY.
nasopharyngeal s. an acquired disorder in cats, usually following chronic upper respiratory infection, which causes upper airway obstruction with mucopurulent nasal discharge and a wheezing respiration, which is relieved with open mouth breathing.
paramesonephric duct s. focal defects in the duct lead to segmental aplasia or stenosis of the uterine tube or horn.
pulmonary artery s. the commonest cardiac defect in dogs; it is a narrowing of the pulmonary outflow tract and may occur in any one of a number of common sites including infundibular, valvular and subvalvular.

rectovaginal s. see RECTOVAGINAL constriction.
right atrioventricular s. see tricuspid STENOSIS (below).
subepiglottic s. has the effect of reducing air flow into and out of the lungs.
tricuspid s. narrowing or stricture of the tricuspid orifice of the heart.
valvular s. see AORTIC, PULMONARY, ATRIOVENTRICULAR.

stenostomia narrowing of the mouth.

stenothermal, stenothermic pertaining to or characterized by tolerance of only a narrow range of temperature.

stenothorax abnormal narrowness of the chest.

stenotic marked by abnormal narrowing or constriction.

Stenson's duct duct of the parotid salivary gland.

stent a mold for keeping a skin graft in place, made of Stent's mass or some acrylic or dental compound; by extension, a device or mold of a suitable material used to hold a skin graft in place or to provide support for tubular structures that are being anastomosed.

step cycle the sum of the movements made during locomotion by a limb from the time it leaves the ground until it leaves the ground on the next occasion.

step mouth sudden variation in the height of adjoining molars causing difficulty, possibly pain or discomfort, during mastication. Due usually to loss of opposing tooth.

Stephania japonica*, *S. hernandifolia plant member of the family Menispermaceae; contains an unidentified toxin which causes incoordination, recumbency, convulsions, paralysis.

Stephanofilaria a genus of nematodes in the family Filariidae; cause chronic dermatitis of cattle called cascado.
S. assamensis causes chronic dermatitis in buffaloes, goats and cattle. In cattle the disease is called humpsore.
S. dedoesi found in the skin of cattle.
S. dinniki causes filarioid dermatitis in black rhinoceros.
S. kaeli found on the legs of cattle.
S. okinawaensis causes dermatitis of the muzzle and teats of cattle.
S. stilesi causes dermatitis on the ventral abdominal wall of cattle.
S. zaheeri found on the inner side of the ear pinna of buffaloes.

stephanofilariasis see STEPHANOFILAROSIS.

stephanofilarosis infestation with filariid worms.
cutaneous s. infestation with *Parafilaria multipapillosa* causes subcutaneous nodules in horses, *P. bovicola* causes similar lesions in cattle, *Suifilaria suis* does the same in pigs, *Stephanofilaria dedoesi* causes dermatitis in cattle (cascado). *S. kaeli* and *S. assamensis* cause dermatitis in cattle (humpsore), *S. zaheeri* causes contagious otorrhea (earsore), a dermatitis around the ear in buffalo, *S. stilesi* and *S. okinawaensis* also cause dermatitis in cattle.
The dermatitis is manifested by small papules that enlarge to form itchy, scabby lesions that suffer much rubbing. The lesions occur at various sites on the body depending on the species of worm. See PARAFILARIA, STEPHANOFILARIA, ELAEOPHORA *schneideri*.

Stephanorossia palustris OENANTHE *palustris*.

Stephanostomum a genus of intestinal flukes in the family Acanthocolpidae.
S. baccatum found in the intestines of marine fish but thought to be not pathogenic.

stephanuriasis the disease of pigs caused by the kidney worm *Stephanurus dentatus*. Characterized by poor feed utilization and growth, and later emaciation, paralysis and ascites.

Stephanurus the only genus of importance in the nematode family of Stephanuridae.
S. dentatus found in the kidneys of pigs and rarely as aberrant parasites in cattle and horses. It may also be found in the liver, pancreas and other organs of pigs.

Steppe several Russian breeds of cattle, e.g. Red Steppe, Grey Steppe.

stepwedge a block of aluminum shaped like a series of steps. Used to test the characteristics of the x-ray beam, film, filters and to standardize exposure factors.

stepwise incremental; additional information is added at each step.
s. multiple regression used when a large number of possible explanatory variables are available and there is difficulty interpreting the partial regression coefficients. There are a number of computer programs available which select the 'best' subset of predictors. These are used first, then all of the predictors are used in succession and added stepwise to the set of predictors already selected.
s. prospective trial see PROSPECTIVE trial.

sterco- word element. [L.] *feces*.

stercobilin a bile pigment derivative formed by air oxidation of stercobilinogen; it is a brown-orange-red pigmentation contributing to the color of feces and urine.

stercobilinogen a bilirubin metabolite and precursor of stercobilin, formed by reduction of urobilinogen.

stercoracic see POSTERIOR station trypanosomes.

Stercoraria the posterior station group of trypanosomes transmitted by contamination through the feces of the insect vector. Includes *Trypanosoma cruzi*, *T. lewisi*, *T. melophagium*, *T. nabiasi*, *T. rangeli*, *T. theileri*, *T. theodori*.

stercorarian, stercoral, stercoraceous, stercoracic of fecal origin; said of trypanosomes in the subgenus *Schizotrypanum*. These trypanosomes are passed to the recipient in the feces of the tsetse fly (*Glossina* spp.). See also STERCORARIA.

stercorolith fecalith; an intestinal concretion formed around a center of fecal matter.

stercoroma a tumor-like mass of fecal matter in the rectum; fecaloma.

sterculia gum karaya gum.

stercus [L.] *dung, feces*.

stereo- word element. [Gr.] *solid, firm, three-dimensional*.

stereoarthrolysis surgical formation of a movable new joint in cases of bony ankylosis.

stereoauscultation auscultation with two stethoscopes, on different parts of the chest.

stereocampimeter an instrument for studying unilateral central scotomas and central retinal defects.

stereochemistry the branch of chemistry treating of the space relations of atoms in molecules.

stereocilium nonmotile, branched, long cellular processes of the nature of long microvilli.

stereocinefluorography recording by motion picture camera of images observed by steroscopic fluoroscopy, affording three-dimensional visualization.

stereoencephalotomy stereotaxic surgery.

stereognosis the sense by which the form of objects is perceived.

stereoisomer see ISOMER.

stereoisomerism isomerism in which the compounds have the same structural formulae, but the atoms are distributed differently in space.
stereoradiography, stereoroentenography paired radiographs of a part, taken from slightly different angles, and viewed with a stereoscopic device, giving a three-dimensional effect.
stereoscope an instrument for producing the appearance of solidity and relief by combining the images of two similar pictures of an object.
stereoscopic three-dimensional; having depth, as well as height and width.
stereospecific pertaining to enzymes that interact only with substrates of very specific structure.
stereotactic stereotaxic.
stereotaxic 1. pertaining to or characterized by precise positioning in space; said especially of discrete areas of the brain that control specific functions. 2. pertaining to or exhibiting stereotaxis.
s. surgery the production of sharply localized lesions in the brain after precise localization of the target tissue by use of three-dimensional coordinates.
stereotaxis, stereotropism movement or growth in response to contact with a solid or rigid surface.
stereotypy see OBSESSIVE-COMPULSIVE BEHAVIOR.
steric pertaining to the spatial arrangement of atoms.
sterigmatocystin a mycotoxin produced by *Aspergillus nidulans* and *A. versicolor.* In monkeys and rats causes nephritis and hepatitis and is hepatocarcinogenic in rats.
sterilant a sterilizing agent, i.e. an agent that destroys microorganisms.
sterile 1. not fertile; barren; not producing young. See also FERTILITY. 2. aseptic; not producing microorganisms; free from living microorganisms.
s. insect release method a method of insect control of particular use in insects in which mating occurs only once, e.g. screw-worm fly; artificially bred flies are sterilized by irradiation and released; if sufficient sterile flies are released most of the wild flies mate with a sterile fly and the population is sufficiently diminished to lead to a control situation. Called also SIRM.
s. pack see sterile SURGICAL pack.
sterility the state of being sterile. See also INFERTILITY.
cryptorchidism s. see CRYPTORCHIDISM.
hybrids s. offspring of parents of different species, these animals are usually sterile due to differences between the chromosomes of the two parents.
intersex s. sterility due to chromosomal differences within the patient.
nondisjunction s. sterility due to chromosomal errors.
polled goats s. a small percentage of all genetically female polled goats are sterile due to masculinization.
XX male dogs s. a Y chromosome-dependent character is an obligatory primary component in transforming the indifferent gonad into a testis.
sterilization 1. the process of rendering an animal incapable of reproduction, by castration, vasectomy, ovariohysterectomy or other procedure. 2. the process of destroying all microorganisms and their pathogenic products. It is accomplished by heat (wet steam under pressure at 120°C for at least 45 minutes, or dry heat at 160–180°C for 3 hours) or by bactericidal chemical compounds.
skin s. not a practical possibility, but a marked temporary reduction in the bacterial population of the skin, as in presurgical preparation of the surgical site and the hands of operating personnel, is achieved with thorough scrubbing, soaking or repeated applications of antiseptics.
sterilize to subject to sterilization.
sterilizer an apparatus used in ridding instruments, dressings, etc., of all microorganisms and their pathogenic products. See also AUTOCLAVE.
Stern anthrax vaccine avirulent spore vaccine producing 2 year immunity with no risk of causing the disease.
sternal pertaining to the sternum.
s. puncture insertion of a hollow needle into the manubrium of the sternum for the purpose of obtaining a sample of bone marrow. The sternum is chosen because of its accessibility and because it is a flat bone in many species.
s. recumbency the animal lies down on its ventral thoracic and abdominal walls, usually with the legs tucked underneath the body; the sagittal plane is vertical and the head is in a vertical plane. Called also dorsal recumbency.
Sternberg's giant cells see Reed–Sternberg CELL.
Sternberg–Reed cell see Reed–Sternberg CELL.
sternebra pl. *sternebrae;* one of the bony segments of the STERNUM.
stern(o)- word element. [L., Gr.] *sternum.*
sternocephalic muscle see Table 13.1I.
sternocostal pertaining to the sternum and ribs.
sternodymia union of two fetuses by the anterior chest wall.
sternodymus conjoined twins united at the anterior chest wall.
sternohyoid pertaining to the sternum and hyoid bone.
sternoid resembling the sternum.
sternomastoid pertaining to the sternum and the mastoid process of the temporal bone.
sternopericardial pertaining to the sternum and pericardium.
sternoschisis congenital fissure of the sternum.
Sternostoma a genus of mites of the family Rhinonyssidae. Found in the trachea, they cause respiratory difficulty in companion birds.
Sternostomum tracheacolum a tracheal mite in free-living finches.
sternothyroid pertaining to the sternum and thyroid cartilage or gland.
sternotomy incision of the sternum as an approach for a thoracotomy. The incision may be median, through the midline, or transverse, most commonly as an extension of an intercostal thoracotomy incision, across the sternum and up the other side.
sternum the breastbone, a median segmented skeletal structure made up of several elements or sternebrae, often with a considerable portion remaining cartilaginous into adulthood. It articulates with the cartilages of the sternal ribs and clavicles when large. It has three parts, the manubrium, the body and the xiphoid process, and consists of vascular, spongy bone covered with a thin layer of compact bone. In ruminants it has a flat ventral surface, while in horses it bears a keel (carina). It is especially well developed, as a nonsegmented keeled bone, in flying birds.
inherited short s. in the North Country Cheviot breed; characterized by a heavy mortality in newborn lambs resulting from rupture of the liver; the latter thought to occur because of the exposed position of the liver as a result of the absence of the sternum.
sternutator a substance that causes sneezing, vomiting, malaise, e.g. Adamsite. Used in chemical warfare.
sternutatory 1. causing sneezing. 2. an agent that causes sneezing.
steroid a complex molecule containing carbon atoms

in four interlocking rings forming a hydrogenated cyclopentophenanthrene-ring system; three of the rings contain six carbon atoms each and the fourth contains five.

Steroid derivatives are important in body chemistry. Among them are the male and female sex hormones, such as testosterone and estrogen, and the hormones of the cortices of the adrenal glands, including cortisone. Vitamins of the D group are steroids involved in calcium metabolism. The cardiac glycosides, a group of compounds derived from certain plants, are partly steroids. Sterols, including cholesterol, are steroids. Cholesterol is the main building block of steroid hormones in the body; it is also converted into bile salts by the liver.

s. I see ALPHAXALONE.

s. II see ALPHADOLONE.

s. diabetes see steroid DIABETES MELLITUS.

s. hormones see ANDROGENIC STEROIDS, CORTICOSTEROID, GLUCOCORTICOID, MINERALOCORTICOID, ANABOLIC steroid.

steroidal emanating from or pertaining to steroid.

s. saponins see lithogenic SAPONINS.

s. (*Solanum* spp.) alkaloid toxins including solanidine, soladulcidine, solasidine, tomatidine found in solanaceous plants.

steroidogenesis production of steroids, as by the adrenal glands.

sterol any steroid, e.g. cholesterol and ergosterol, having long (8–10 carbons) aliphatic side-chains at position 17 and at least one alcoholic hydroxyl group; the sterols have lipid-like solubility.

stertor snoring; sonorous respiration, usually due to partial obstruction of the upper airway. May be possible by careful auscultation to determine the site of the stertor, e.g. laryngeal stenosis, pharyngeal obstruction, nasal obstruction.

steth(o)- word element. [Gr.] *chest.*

stethogoniometer an apparatus for measuring the curvature of the chest.

stethoscope an instrument used to hear and amplify the sounds produced by the heart, lungs and other internal organs.

The modern stethoscope is binaural, with two earpieces and flexible rubber leading to them from the two-branched opening of the bell or cone. In this way, sound travels simultaneously through both of the branches to the earpieces. See also PHONENDOSCOPE.

electronic s. audible sounds are magnified through an amplifier to earphones, of which there may be more than one set, and may be broadcast through loudspeakers, but in both instances the results are mediocre.

esophageal s. one passed into the esophagus with the tip positioned at the level of the heart. It provides an excellent means of monitoring heart sounds and respiration while the animal is anesthetized.

stethospasm spasm of the chest muscles.

Stevens power law attempts to quantitate sensory inputs; the law holds that the perceived intensity of the sensation equals the actual intensity of the stimulus raised to a specified power, the value of the power varying with the type of receptor.

Stevens scissors see tenotomy SCISSORS.

stewardship the occupation of being a steward or custodian. Referring to animals it implies the caring sort of relationship based on an acceptance of the need to include the rights of animals in overall plans to maintain financial viability.

Stewart Range syndrome TUNICAMINYLURACIL poisoning of sheep in south-eastern Australia associated with *Clavibacter toxicus* in the seedheads of *Polypogon monspeliensis.*

STH somatotropic (growth) hormone.

sthenic active; strong.

stibialism antimony poisoning.

stibium [L.] *antimony* (symbol Sb).

stibogluconate an antimony compound used in the treatment of leishmaniasis.

stibophen a compound used at one time as a treatment for heartworm in dogs but now discarded because of toxicity.

stichochrome any neuron having the stainable substance arranged in more or less regular layers.

Sticker's sarcoma see canine transmissible VENEREAL tumor.

stickfast flea see ECHIDNOPHAGA *gallinacea.*

sticking the abattoir technique of bleeding the animal out at slaughter. There are many techniques used including those used in ritual slaughter. The traditional methods are the slash across the throat cutting arteries, veins, trachea and esophagus and even the spinal cord, and the stab method with the knife being thrust into the jugular vein at the base of the neck. The latter is used in cattle and pigs, the former in sheep. See also JEWISH SLAUGHTER, MUSLIM SLAUGHTER.

sticky ends see COHESIVE END.

sticky kid syndrome a defect of newborn kids of the golden Guernsey breed of goats; they have sticky, matted coats which remain sticky and harsh. Thought to be an inherited defect.

stiff lamb disease see ENZOOTIC muscular dystrophy.

stiff lung decreased lung compliance.

stiff sickness ephemeral fever.

stiffness half way to rigidity, tetany; result of insufficient use of the part.

stiffs one of the very large number of colloquial names given to the disease of cattle caused by a nutritional deficiency of phosphorus. See also OSTEOMALACIA.

stifle joint the homolog of the human knee in the quadriped, made up of the femorotibial and femoropatellar joints. It is subject to the problems associated with dislocation of the patella, rupture of the cruciate ligaments, injury to the cartilaginous menisci, and several other common disorders.

stifsiekte see OSTEOMALACIA.

stigma pl. *stigmas, stigmata* [Gr.] any physical mark or peculiarity that aids in identification or diagnosis of a condition.

follicular s. a 2 mm wide band around the meridian of all follicles greater than 4 mm diameter in the left ovary of the domestic fowl.

stigmatization the formation of stigmas.

stilbamidine see HYDROXYSTILBAMIDINE ISETHIONATE.

stilbestrol a synthetic estrogen used in the treatment of female animals for infertility and bitches for urinary incontinence. Its use as a growth promotant, especially in cattle, has been discontinued because of fears that it is a carcinogen. Its use is also not without toxicity hazards.

Overfeeding of stilbestrol as a growth promotant causes poisoning characterized by relaxation of pelvic ligaments, elevation of the tailhead, susceptibility to pelvic fracture and hip dislocation and prolapse of rectum and vagina. In castrated males there is a tendency for obstructive urolithiasis to occur. Pigs also show anuria, kidney enlargement and thickening of the ureters.

See also DIETHYLSTILBESTROL, ESTROGEN.

Stilesia a genus of tapeworms in the family Thyanosomatidae.

S. globipunctata found in the small intestine of ruminants and causes sufficient injury to kill some animals.
S. hepatica found in the bile ducts in all ruminant species and causes thickening of the duct walls but there is no clinical disease.
stilet stylet.
Still–Luer rongeur double-action, scissor type instrument with spoon-shaped, sharp-edged blades facing each other. The blades in different individual instruments are bent at different angles from the line of cutting so that inaccessible sites can be reached with the appropriate instrument.
stillbirth delivery of a fully formed dead neonate.
stillborn born dead.
Stille shears plaster shears with a powerful double action with angled blades that allow cutting while the handles are well away from the patient.
Stillingia dendata, S. treculeana an American plant in the family Euphorbiaceae. It contains cyanogenetic glucosides and may cause poisoning. Called also Queen's delight.
stimulant 1. producing stimulation. 2. an agent that stimulates.
stimulate to excite functional activity in a part.
stimulation the act or process of stimulating; the condition of being stimulated.
s. index the ratio of the number of proliferating T lymphocytes present in a lymphocyte culture after exposure to antigen or mitogen to the total number of cells. It is determined by adding tritiated thymidine to the culture usually 3 to 5 days after stimulation. The radiolabel is incorporated into DNA of those cells that are stimulated to divide.
stimulus pl. *stimuli* [L.] any agent, act, or influence that produces functional or trophic reaction in a receptor or an irritable tissue.
conditioned s. a neutral object or event that is psychologically related to a naturally stimulating object or event and which causes a conditioned response. See also CONDITIONING.
discriminative s. a stimulus associated with reinforcement, which exerts control over a particular form of behavior; the subject discriminates between closely related stimuli and responds positively only in the presence of that stimulus.
eliciting s. any stimulus, conditioned or unconditioned, which elicits a response.
s. generalization in learning by animals stimuli tend to be grouped together, the reactions lacking the discrimination of the higher mammals.
s. response coupling coupling of the neural or endocrine stimulus to the cellular response.
structured s. a well-organized and unambiguous stimulus, the perception of which is influenced to a greater extent by the characteristics of the stimulus than by those of the perceiver.
threshold s. a stimulus that is just strong enough to elicit a response.
unconditioned s. any stimulus that is capable of eliciting an unconditioned response. See also CONDITIONING.
unstructured s. an unclear or ambiguous stimulus, the perception of which is influenced to a greater extent by the characteristics of the perceiver than by those of the stimulus.
stimulus-response the key mechanism within the animal which permits it to adapt as perfectly as possible to its environment.
s.-r. apparatus a receptor region responding directly to a stimulus, e.g. sound, touch, smell, vision, an afferent neuron which conveys the stimulus towards the central nervous system, a synapse where the afferent path meets the efferent path, an efferent neuron conveying stimuli from the CNS, and an effector (a muscle, gland or neurosecretory cell).
sting 1. injury caused by a poisonous substance produced by an animal or plant (biotoxin) and introduced into a patient which it contacts, together with mechanical trauma incident to its introduction. See also INSECT bites and stings. 2. the organ used to inflict such injury. 3. the illicit prerace administration of a stimulant to a horse with the object of improving its performance.
stinger tree DENDROCNIDE *moroides*.
stinging nettle see URTICA.
stink fish fish member of the family Callionymidae. Cause immediate, forceful vomiting.
stinking having an intrinsic fetid smell.
s. elder SAMBUCUS *pubens*.
s. hellebore HELLEBORUS *foetidus*.
s. iris IRIS *foetidissima*.
s. milkvetch ASTRAGALUS *praelongus*.
s. passion flowers PASSIFLORA *foetida*.
s. willie SENECIO *jacobaea*.
stinkpeul ACACIA *nilotica* subsp. *Kreussiana*.
stinkweed see THLASPI ARVENSE.
stinkwood see ZIERIA *arborescens*.
stinkwort see DITTRICHIA GRAVEOLENS.
Stipa grass in the family Poaceae; the seed awns are found in great abundance in subcutaneous tissue of sheep grazing pasture containing these grasses when they are ripe. Called also spear grass. Includes *Stipa obtusa* (*Stipagrostis* spp.).
S. robusta* + *Acremonium* spp. endophyte, *S. vaseyi in North America causes stumbling, recumbency, saliva drooling but recovery if moved to new pasture; caused by ergot alkaloids generated by the fungus. In China has a similar endophyte and causes a similar sydrome. Called also sleepygrass.
Stipagrostis grass member of the family Poaceae; awns on the plant become entangled in the forestomachs forming phytobezoars; also cause grass seed abscess. Include *S. obtusa* (*Aristida obtusa*), *S. ciliata* var. *capensis* (*Aristida ciliata*).
stippled covered with many small dots.
s. cells see BASOPHILIC stippling.
stippling a spotted condition or appearance, such as an appearance of the retina as if dotted with light and dark points, or the spotted appearance of the erythrocytes in basophilic stippling.
basophilic s. see BASOPHILIC stippling.
stirk a heifer or bullock 6 to 12 months of age.
stirofos an organophosphorus insecticide.
stirrup 1. the stapes, the innermost of the three ossicles of the ear. 2. device usually made of metal, although some are wooden or laminated hard leather, attached by stirrup leathers to the saddle and providing support for the feet of the rider.
stitch a loop made in sewing or suturing.
s. abscess see stitch ABSCESS.
Stizostedion see PIKE-PERCH.
stochastic arrived at by skilful conjecturing; allowing the opportunity for variation.
stock livestock.
s. equivalents units of livestock measurement used when budgeting feed or assessing productive capacity. All forms of livestock are expressed in terms of one of them, e.g. dry sheep equivalents.
s. guard used in lieu of a gate; consists of a pit fitted with steel rollers close enough together to make a satisfactory crossing for a motor vehicle but sufficient to deter livestock. Called also cattle grid.

s. horse a riding horse used to work cattle, sheep or other horses. Small stature, light weight, wiry, fast for a short distance, agile, mostly bay. Called also cow pony, cutting horse.
s. and station agent person conducting a rural store dealing in implements, supplies and livestock pertaining to agricultural pursuits of all kinds.
Stockard's paralysis a progressive flaccid posterior paresis and paralysis in young Great Danes and crossbreds, believed to be a hereditary abiotrophy. There have been no reported cases since 1936.
stocker see STORE.
Stockholm tar a substance derived from certain species of *Pinus* spp. by destructive distillation of the wood. Called also wood tar and used extensively as a hoof dressing and general wound protectant by country people.
stockinet closely woven cotton material used extensively by surgeons mostly in the form of cylinders (e.g. Tubegauze) as a draping technique for surgery, as an undercoat for a plaster cast and as a means of keeping dressings in place on a limb.
stocking 1. white markings on the lower legs; in horses from the coronet to the carpus or hock and in dogs most of the leg up to the elbow or stifle. 2. populating a farm with animals.
set s. the livestock are left on the same pasture, in the same fields or paddocks for long periods, under range conditions often indefinitely. Compare with rotational grazing.
s. rate the number of livestock carried per unit of area of pasture. In order to make comparison more rational the procedure is to equate each animal in terms of a standard for the species. See also DRY SHEEP EQUIVALENT.
stocking-up accumulation of edema fluid in the lower limbs of horses which are not getting sufficient exercise.
stocks vertical metal or wooden pillars, arranged in a rectangular shape and connected by horizontal bars, designed to restrain a horse or bovine standing within.
stockwhip a whip used by a mounted horseman to help drive cattle; has a short, 3 foot long, handle and a long, 10 foot, thong. The best effect is gained by cracking the thong in the air making a sound like a pistol shot. This is achieved by a special snapper at the end of the thong.
stockyard 1. public saleyard where livestock are sold, usually by auction. 2. yards for working cattle or sheep on private property.
stoichiology the science of elements, especially the physiology of the cellular elements of tissues.
stoichiometry the determination of the relative proportions of the compounds involved in a chemical reaction.
stoke a unit of kinematic viscosity, that of a fluid with a dynamic viscosity of 1 poise and a density of 1 gram per cubic centimeter. Abbreviated St.
Stokes–Adams disease a condition due to cerebral ischemia, marked by sudden attacks of unconsciousness, with or without convulsions; associated with heart block or ventricular tachycardias. Called also Stokes–Adams attack, syndrome or syncope or Adams–Stokes syndrome.
Stoll's method a technique for counting nematode and trematode eggs in a fecal sample. The diluting fluid used is 0.1 M caustic soda solution.
stolon an above-ground prostrate stem that develops roots and leaves at nodes along its length, e.g. couch grass.
stoma pl. *stomas, stomata* [Gr.] 1. a mouthlike opening. 2. an incised opening that is kept open for drainage or other purposes, such as the opening in the abdominal wall for COLOSTOMY, URETEROSTOMY and ILEAL conduit.
stomach the curved, muscular, saclike structure that is an enlargement of the alimentary canal between the esophagus and the small intestine. See also ABOMASUM, RETICULUM (3), FORESTOMACHS, GASTRIC.
avian glandular s. see PROVENTRICULUS.
s. bot see GASTEROPHILUS.
compound s. a stomach made up of several compartments, e.g. ruminant stomach comprising forestomachs (reticulum, rumen, omasum) and abomasum.
s. fluke see PARAMPHISTOMUM.
glandular s. found in horses; includes cardiac, proper gastric and pyloric glandular zones.
hourglass s. one shaped like an hourglass.
s. meridian points acupoints situated along the stomach meridian.
s. mesenteries includes mesogastrium, lesser omentum, greater omentum and omental bursa.
muscular s. in birds the gizzard or ventriculus.
s. tube speculum see FRICK SPECULUM, HAUPTNER MOUTH GAG. For cattle there is also an instrument made out of a wooden rod with a hole through the center. This is placed between the cow's molars like a bit and held in position with a poll strap. It works adequately for a probang but is much inferior to the Frick speculum for a stomach tube.
s. worm see GNATHOSTOMA *spinigerum*, HAEMONCHUS, OSTERTAGIA.
stomachal pertaining to the stomach; stomachic.
stomachic 1. pertaining to the stomach. 2. a stimulant of gastric activity.
stomatitis inflammation of the mucosa of the mouth. It may be caused by one of many diseases of the mouth or it may accompany another disease. Both gingivitis (inflammation of the gums) and glossitis (inflammation of the tongue) are forms of stomatitis as are palatitis (or lampas in horses) and cheilitis (inflammation of lips). The specific identification of stomatitis is an important part of a clinical examination in a food animal because of the need to identify the highly infectious vesicular diseases and bluetongue.
angular s. superficial erosions and fissuring at the angles (commissures) of the mouth.
catarrhal s. diffuse erythema of lips, tongue, cheeks; causes some discomfort and unwillingness to eat.
contagious pustular s. see HORSEPOX.
erosive s. see EROSIVE STOMATITIS.
erosive–ulcerative s. advanced stage of stomatitis characterized by multiple erosions and deeper ulcers; complete anorexia results.
mycotic s. see MYCOTIC stomatitis.
necrotic s. of calves see ORAL necrobacillosis.
papular s. see bovine PAPULAR stomatitis.
s.-pneumoenteritis complex see PESTE DES PETITS RUMINANTS.
proliferative s. a very rare disease of cattle said to be caused by a filterable agent and recorded only in association with such conditions as chlorinated naphthalene poisoning. The lesions are papular and may also occur on the teats.
vesicular s. stomatitis characterized by vesicular lesions which soon rupture to leave denuded areas which become infected, necrotic, even ulcerative. See also VESICULAR stomatitis, VESICULAR exanthema of swine, SWINE vesicular disease, FOOT-AND-MOUTH DISEASE.

stomat(o)- word element. [Gr.] *mouth.*
stomatocyte erythrocyte with oval-shaped central area of pallor.
stomatocytosis anemia characterized by the presence of stomatocytes in the blood.
hereditary s. occurs in chondrodysplastic dwarf Alaskan malamute dogs.
stomatodeum see STOMODEUM.
stomatogastric pertaining to the stomach and mouth.
stomatognathic denoting the mouth and jaws collectively.
stomatology the study of the mouth and its diseases.
stomatomalacia softening of the structures of the mouth.
stomatomycosis any fungal disease of the mouth.
stomatonecrosis gangrene of the mouth.
stomatopapilloma papilloma on the oral mucosa.
eel s. a disease of eels thought to be caused by a virus.
stomatopathy any disorder of the mouth.
stomatoplasty plastic reconstruction of the mouth.
stomatorrhagia hemorrhage from the mouth.
stomocephalus a fetus with rudimentary jaws and mouth.
stomodeum, stomodaeum, stomatodaeum, stomatodeum the ectodermal depression at the head end of the embryo, which becomes the front part of the mouth.
Stomoxys calcitrans the ubiquitous stable fly, about house fly size, and a pest wherever horses are. It is a blood-sucker and transmits a number of trypanosomes including *Trypanosoma evansi* (Surra), *T. equinum* (Mal de Caderas), *T. brucei* and *T. vivax* (Nagana of cattle) and is an intermediate host for *Habronema majus.* It is probably also involved in the transmission of *Dermatophilus congolensis* (mycotic dermatitis).
-stomy word element. [Gr.] creation of an opening into or a communication between.
stone 1. a calculus. 2. a unit of weight, equivalent in the English system to 14 lb avoirdupois.
milk s. see MILK stone.
s. searcher see SEARCHER (2).
Stonebrinks medium an egg-based medium for the growth of *Mycobacteria bovis.*
stonefish fish member of the family Synancejidae which inhabits coral reefs and has an external appearance similar to a lump of coral. They have a number of spines along the back and if trodden on or bitten eject a very potent poison, which causes terrific pain, followed by local swelling and general paralysis ending in fatal respiratory paralysis. Includes *Synanceja trachynis, Synanceichthys verrucosa.*
stones commonly used to describe CALCULI.
stool the fecal discharge from the bowels. Normally, only used with reference to the cat and dog. See also FECES.
lienteric s. feces containing much undigested food.
night s. soft, moist fecal pellets ingested by rabbits, directly ftom the anus, usually in the early morning.
s. softeners agents such as bulk or lubricant laxatives which result in soft, but formed feces, without causing purgation.
stootsiekte [Af.] 'pushing disease' caused by *Matricaria nigellifolia* poisoning.
stop the steplike change in lateral profile of the face of dogs at the eyes, where the frontal bones meet the maxilla and nasal bones. It varies greatly between species, being most marked in brachycephalic breeds and barely detectable in Collies and Bull terriers.
stopcock a valve that regulates the flow of fluid through a tube.
stopper pad the normally non-weight-bearing footpad located at the posterior aspect of the forelegs, over the accessory carpal bone, in dogs and cats. Called also carpal pad, stoppers.
stoppers see STOPPER PAD.
storage disease any metabolic disorder in which some substance (e.g. fats, proteins or carbohydrates) accumulates in certain cells in abnormal amounts; called also thesaurismosis, thesaurosis.
lipid s. d. any disorder of cellular metabolism that results in accumulation of lipids in tissues, e.g. GANGLIOSIDOSIS, SPHINGOMYELINOSIS, GAUCHER'S DISEASE, globoid cell LEUKODYSTROPHY, metachromatic LEUKODYSTROPHY. Called also lipidosis.
lysosomal s. d. any inborn error of metabolism in which the deficiency of a lysosomal enzyme results in the accumulation of the substance normally degraded by that enzyme in the lysosomes of certain cells. These diseases are further classified, depending on the nature of the stored substance, as glycogen storage diseases (glycogenoses), sphingolipidoses, mucopolysaccharidoses and mucolipidoses.
storage fungi fungi that are particularly adapted to grow on stored feeds, e.g. *Stachybotrys, Aspergillus, Fusarium* and *Penicillium* spp.
storage mites many species, e.g. *Acarus siro,* in stored cereals.
storage pool disease a blood coagulation disorder due to an abnormality in the constituents of platelet storage granules. Characterized by mild to moderate bleeding. See also THROMBOPATHIA.
store used with reference to any species. Indicates that the animal is in a lean, lightweight condition, usually young and in most cases recently weaned. They are in a growing in stature phase and ready for good pasture so that in 2 to 5 months they have grown well and are ready for sale as replacement heifers or to go into lots as feeders.
forward s. meat sheep in good enough condition to go to the butcher but in need of topping off to be classified as prime.
storiform denoting a matted, irregularly whorled pattern, somewhat resembling that of a straw mat; said of the microscopic appearance of fibrous histiocytomas.
storksbill see ERODIUM.
Stormont test a more sensitive test for tuberculosis in cattle. The test is begun as a single INTRADERMAL test by an intradermal injection, usually into a caudal tail fold. The test is read at 72 or 96 hours and if it is inconclusive a second injection is made at the same site at 7 days after the first injection and the test read 24 hours later. A positive reaction is a 5 mm increase in the thickness of the skin.
stosstherapy treatment of a disease by a single massive dose of therapeutic agent or short-term administration of unphysiologically large doses.
stot steer.
Stout loop technique a method of wiring between teeth to provide support for fractures of the upper or lower jaws.
stoutly bred horseman's expression for a horse bred to stay; bred to run long distance races.
stover stalks of maize plants from which mature corn cobs have been harvested as grain, or grain sorghum plants from which heads have also been removed. The stover is usually fed by turning the cattle into the field and is subject to fungal infection, sometimes causing mycotoxicosis.

STPD standard temperature and pressure, dry; denoting a volume of dry gas at 32°F (0°C) and a pressure of 760 mmHg.

strabismus deviation of the eye that the patient cannot overcome; the visual axes assume a position relative to each other different from that required by the physiological conditions. Called also squint.

comitant s. extraocular muscles are not paralyzed and the degree of deviation is the same in all directions.

congenital s. medial strabismus is seen in Siamese cats. See convergent strabismus (below).

convergent s. that in which the visual axes converge; esotropia, or cross-eye. A frequent finding in Siamese cats, related to an anomaly of neuronal pathways between the retina and lateral geniculate nucleus in which more neurons project contralaterally rather than ipsilaterally as in other cats.

divergent s. that in which the visual axes diverge; called also exotropia and walleye.

inherited s. see inherited EXOPHTHALMOS.

noncomitant s. deviation due to paralysis of one or more muscles.

traumatic s. a complication of traumatic prolapse of the eye, due to rupture of extraocular muscles.

strabotomy cutting of an ocular tendon in treatment of strabismus.

straight 1. insufficient angulation of a joint or slope of a bone to give a horse a good conformation, e.g. straight hock, pastern, withers. 2. uncomplicated, e.g. a straight radiograph; one taken before the administration of contrast reagent so that any preexisting opacities can be identified. Called also scout radiography.

distal s. tubule last segment of the nephron loop.

proximal s. tubule first segment of the nephron loop.

straightbred purebred.

straights animal feeds that are plain feeds without additions of any sort, e.g oats, alfalfa hay, although they may have been processed in some way, e.g. cracked or chaffed.

strain 1. to overexercise. 2. to filter. 3. an overstretching or overexertion of some part of the musculature. 4. excessive effort. 5. one or more organisms within a species or variety, characterized by some particular quality, as rough or smooth strains of bacteria.

s. 19 *Brucella abortus* see STRAIN 19.

s. 45/20 *Brucella abortus* the strain of reduced virulence used as a living vaccine for adult cattle against bovine brucellosis.

s. 51 *Salmonella dublin* a rough strain with reduced virulence used in Europe to immunize young calves.

cell s. see CELL CULTURE.

compressive s. physical stress which tends to structural compaction.

tensile s. physical strain which tends toward structural elongation.

strain 19 naturally occurring mutant, low-virulence strain of *Brucella abortus*.

s. 19 vaccine living vaccine of strain 19 *Brucella abortus*, the vaccine which made virtual eradication of bovine brucellosis possible.

straining see TENESMUS.

s. to defecate tenesmus.

stramonium DATURA *stramonium*.

strand a term commonly used to describe one of the two complementary polynucleotide chains found in double-stranded DNA.

lagging s. in DNA replication, the strand in which the nascent strand is synthesized in discontinuous segments after the other or leading strand. See also OKAZAKI FRAGMENTS.

leading s. in DNA replication, the strand that is copied continuously.

stranding see PINNIPED stranding.

strangles an acute disease of horses caused by infection with *Streptococcus equi* subsp. *equi*, and characterized by fever, purulent rhinitis, pharyngitis, laryngitis, abscessation of the draining lymph nodes and cough.

puppy s., juvenile s. see juvenile PYODERMA.

strangulated congested by reason of constriction or hernial restriction, as strangulated HERNIA.

strangulation 1. arrest of respiration by occlusion of the air passages. 2. impairment of the blood supply to a part by mechanical constriction of the vessels. See also COLIC (2), INTESTINAL obstruction, INTESTINAL strangulation.

stranguria strangury.

strangury slow and painful discharge of urine.

strap cell long, flat cells found in some rhabdomyosarcomas.

strapper stable assistant engaged in the preparation of horses for racing.

strategic treatment prophylactic treatment, applied particularly in the prevention of parasitic and protozoal diseases, applied at strategic times in the life cycle of the causative agent, rather than on a strictly temporal basis.

Strathmore weed PIMELEA *prostrata*.

stratification 1. arrangement in layers. 2. in statistical terms the division of a population into subpopulations on the basis of specified criteria such as age, breed, parity. See stratified random SAMPLE.

stratiform occurring in layers.

stratigraphy a method of bodysection radiography.

stratum pl. *strata* [L.] a sheetlike mass of tissue of fairly uniform thickness; distinct layers making up various tissues or organs, as of the skin, brain, retina.

s. avasculosum the avascular stratum in the margin of the iris.

s. basale the mitotically active, basal layer of the epidermis, consisting of columnar to cuboidal keratinocytes on a basement membrane.

s. corneum the outer horny layer of the epidermis, consisting of cells that are non-nucleated, keratinized and desquamating.

s. germinativum in the epidermis, located between the stratum basale and the stratum granulosum. Together with the basal layer, called the malpighian layer. Called also germinative layer.

s. granulosum 1. the layer of cells between the stratum lucidum and the stratum spinosum of the skin, very thin and not always present. Called also the granular layer. 2. the deep layer of the cortex of the cerebellum. 3. the layer of follicle cells lining the theca of the vesicular ovarian follicle. Called also granular layer.

s. lamellatum laminae of the hoof corium.

s. lucidum the translucent layer of the skin just beneath the stratum corneum. Called also clear layer. Present in the epidermis of the planum nasale of several species and footpads of carnivores.

s. spinosum the layer of the epidermis between the stratum granulosum and the stratum basale, marked by the presence of prickle cells; called also spinous layer and prickle-cell layer.

s. tectorium the layer of horny scales claimed to exist on the surface of the horse's hoof that gives it the smooth glossy appearance.

Strauss reaction see Strauss REACTION.

straw 1. mature, dry foliage of a cereal crop after the grain has been harvested by a header or by threshing. Has very low digestibility, energy and protein content. Used principally as bedding but in some economies is used as feed. Causes impaction of the rumen in cattle and ileocecal valve in horses. Is more digestible if chopped and fed with a protein supplement or urea. If left standing in the field is referred to as stubble. When fed in this way there is a variable amount of spilt grain available also. 2. a hollow, plastic tube used for the storage of frozen semen. See also FRENCH STRAWS.

s. eating a vice in stabled horses which may require muzzling to avoid the occurrence of impaction colic.

straw-itch mite PYEMOTES *tritici*.

strawberry clover TRIFOLIUM *fragiferum*.

strawberry footrot see strawberry FOOTROT.

strawberry lymph nodes deeply congested lymph nodes such as seen in any septicemia.

strawberry mark a local granulomatous nodule in the intestinal wall of pigs caused by the deep penetration of the proboscis of *Macrocanthorynchus hirudinaceus*.

stray voltage accumulation of low voltages in the metalwork of a milking parlor due either to leakage from poor wiring or to poor earthing (grounding) with no outlet for static electricity. Very small voltages cause restlessness and a fall in milk yield. Stronger currents can cause stunning or even electrocution.

streak a line or stripe.

angioid s's red to black irregular bands in the ocular fundus running outward from the optic disk.

s. canal the papillary duct, the canal between the exterior and the lactiferous sinus within the teat of a ruminant.

primitive s. a faint white trace at the caudal end of the embryonic disk, formed by movement of cells at the onset of mesoderm formation, providing the first evidence of the embryonic axis.

streaked hairlessness, hypotrichosis irregular, narrow streaks of hairlessness, occurring only in females is recorded in Holstein cattle.

streaked rattlepod CROTALARIA *pallida*.

streaking 1. a fault in radiographs caused by inadequate rinsing or dirty hangers. 2. the process of inoculating microorganisms onto agar media with a loop such that the inoculum is seeded at decreasing concentration across the media, resulting in isolated colonies of the miroorganism.

focused grid s. a focused grid placed on the cassette upside down will cause streaking around the edges of the film.

streamlining physiological phenomenon of blood flow which passes through a vessel without complete mixing so that blood from two different sources and with different composition can flow side by side within the one vessel. May occur in the portal vein and be the possible explanation for the occasional limitation of lesions of toxopathic hepatitis to one lobe of the liver.

s. portal blood flow LAMINAR flow applied to the blood flowing through the portal vein to the liver.

Streblidae a family of flies similar to the hipposcids and which are found on bats in the tropics and subtropics.

Strepera graculina pied currawong.

Strepsiceros strepsiceros see KUDU.

streptavidin a protein found in *Streptomyces griseus* which has a high affinity for biotin and is used in immunofluorescent studies.

strepto- word element. [Gr.] *twisted*.

Streptobacillus a genus of gram-negative bacteria which sometimes forms filaments. The only species is *S. moniliformis*, which is found in the nasopharynx of rats. It is the cause of Haverhill fever, a form of ratbite fever, in humans and possibly dogs and cats. It may cause acute septicemia or chronic disease characterised by arthritis in mice. Previously called *Bacillus actinoides* and *Streptobacillus actinoides*.

streptobacillus pl. *streptobacilli* 1. a group of rod-shaped bacteria that remain loosely attached end-to-end in long chains as a result of failure of daughter cells to separate after cell division. 2. an organism of the genus *Streptobacillus*.

streptococcal pertaining to or caused by a streptococcus.

s. adenitis a specific disease of pigs; see CERVICAL ABSCESS OF PIGS. A similar disease occurs in epidemics in dogs in kennels caused by Lancefield Group C *Streptococcus*. It is characterized by fever, pharyngitis, submaxillary lymph node enlargement and conjunctival discharge.

s. dermatitis on the face of piglets in lesions made by unclipped needle teeth.

s. endocarditis see bacterial ENDOCARDITIS.

s. enteritis a rare disease in neonatal piglets and foals, characterized by mild enteritis and diarrhea.

s. lympadenitis see streptococcal adenitis (above).

s. mastitis bovine mastitis is caused by *Streptococcus agalactiae, S. dysgalactiae, S. uberis*.

s. meningitis a disease of young pigs caused by *Streptococcus suis* types I and II, type I in sucking pigs and type II in weaner pigs. Commonly the pigs are about 2 weeks old, and show signs of rigidity, hypersensitivity to touch and tetanic convulsions. There is a dramatic response to penicillin. Most pigs in a litter will be affected and successive litters will have the disease. There is also a suppurative arthritis.

neonatal s. septicemia streptococcal infection in newborn calves, piglets, lambs and puppies causes a syndrome of polyarthritis, meningitis, choroiditis and in calves an endophthalmitis.

s. pneumonia bacterial pneumonia of lambs, calves and in horses either primary or as secondary infections in viral disease. Infection is usually *Streptococcus pneumoniae* or *S. zooepidemicus*.

s. polyarthritis common in neonates of all species especially piglets; characterized by pain, heat and swellings of a number of joints.

s. septicemia is part of streptococcal infections in neonates and occurs also in calves caused by *Streptococcus pneumoniae*. Affected calves show a peracute illness with fever and petechiation of mucosae.

streptococcemia the presence of streptococci in the blood.

streptococci bacterial members of the genus *Streptococcus*.

streptococcosis a disease of domestic poultry caused by *Streptococcus zooepidemicus* (syn. *S. gallinarum*), *S. faecalis, S. faecium* and *S. durans*. The disease is characterized by bacteremia with localization of suppurative infection in many body sites and a variety of clinical pictures of fever, anorexia and pale comb.

In fish occurs in rainbow trout, yellowtail and eels; caused by *Enterococcus seriolicida*; manifested by exophthalmos, sometimes resulting in orbital rupture.

Streptococcus a genus of gram-positive, predominantly facultatively anaerobic cocci in the family Streptococcaceae occurring in pairs or chains. It is classifiable in several ways, none of them completely satisfactory in terms of species designation. Sherman's classification was based on tolerance tests. The system used most widely in veterinary bacteriology is Lancefield's grouping based on serological tests.

Another means of differentiating streptococci is on the basis of type of hemolysis produced around colonies grown on sheep blood agar. Alpha (α) is partial hemolysis or greening of the agar. Beta (β) hemolysis is seen as a clear zone and gamma (γ) is no hemolysis. Most of the pathogenic species are β hemolytic.

S. agalactiae causes mastitis in cattle, goats and sheep, neonatal septicemia and urogenital infections in dogs and cats.

S. avium, S. durans, S. faecalis, S. faecium* and *S. gallinarum reclassified in the genus ENTEROCOCCUS. Now called *Enterococcus avium* etc.

S. bovis an important organism in the development of lactic acidosis in cattle following carbohydrate engorgement because of its capacity to ferment starch to lactic acid.

***S. canis* (*canus*)** isolated from cases of septicemia and adenitis in puppies and kittens.

S. dysgalactiae causes mastitis in cows, ewes and goat does and polyarthritis in lambs.

S. dysgalactiae* subsp. *equisimilis causes suppurative arthritis in piglets and abscesses in lymph nodes of the head and neck of horses. Also a cause of cervicitis in mares. Previously called *S. equisimilis*.

S. equi* subsp. *equi causes STRANGLES in horses.

S. equi* subsp. *zooepidemicus occurs as a secondary infection in most species, particularly in horses in wounds, as a cause of cervicitis and a secondary infection associated with the viral infections of the upper respiratory tract. A cause of metritis and mastitis in cattle and septicemia in lambs, pigs and poultry. Previously called *S. zooepidemicus*.

S. equinus causes opportunist infections in many species.

S. parauberis, S. uberis, S. viridans may cause mastitis in cows.

S. pneumoniae formerly called *Diplococcus pneumoniae*; pneumococcus, causes pneumonia in humans, nonhuman primates, guinea pigs and calves and mastitis in cattle, and septicemia and arthritis in cats.

S. porcinus causes CERVICAL ABSCESS OF PIGS.

S. pyogenes a cause of lymphangitis in foals and an uncommon cause of bovine mastitis. An important pathogen of humans.

***S.* spp. biovar 1** causes disease in cultured finfish.

S. suis types I and II cause STREPTOCOCCAL meningitis and arthritis in pigs.

streptodornase an enzyme produced by hemolytic streptococci that catalyzes the depolymerization of deoxyribonucleic acid (DNA).

streptokinase an enzyme produced by streptococci that catalyzes the conversion of plasminogen to plasmin; abbreviated SK. Streptokinase, when administered as a thrombolytic, requires detailed and skilled control to avoid hemorrhage. It also is capable of producing severe antigenic reactions upon readministration. See also ANTICOAGULANT (2).

s.-streptodornase a mixture of enzymes elaborated by hemolytic streptococci; used as a proteolytic and fibrinolytic agent.

streptolysin the hemolysin of hemolytic streptococci.

Streptomyces a genus of nonpathogenic soil bacteria, but occasionally parasitic on plants and animals. Notable as the source of various antibiotics, e.g. the tetracyclines, erythromycin (*S. erythreus*), lincomycin (*S. lincolnensis*), tylosin (*S. fradiae*), rifampin (*S. mediterranei*), amphotericin B (*S. nodosus*) and monensin (*S. cinnamonensis*).

streptomycin one of the oldest of the aminoglycoside antibiotics. Because of its widespread use many previously susceptible gram-negative bacteria have developed a resistance to it and it has lost a great deal of its effectiveness and popularity. It is most effective against leptospira and *haemophilus*-associated infections. Like all other members of the group, streptomycin is absorbed poorly from the alimentary tract and must be given parenterally, usually by intramuscular injection for systemic effect. The group has moderate toxicity but this is of minor importance in food animals. Even in companion animals the risk is small but deafness and vestibular disturbances can occur, particularly in cats. Dihydrostreptomycin is a derivative and is used as an alternative to the parent antibiotic.

Streptopharagus a genus of roundworms in the family Spirocercidae.

S. armatus, S. pigmentatus found in the stomach of apes and monkeys.

streptosepticemia septicemia due to streptococci.

streptothricosis see MYCOTIC dermatitis.

Streptothrix bovis see DERMATOPHILUS *congolensis*.

streptotrichosis see DERMATOPHILOSIS.

streptozocin, streptozotocin a nitrosurea compound with antineoplastic activity, derived from *Streptomyces achromogenes*; used principally in the treatment of islet-cell tumors of the pancreas.

stress 1. forcibly exerted influence; pressure, e.g. compression, tension. 2. the sum of the biological reactions to any adverse stimulus, physical, mental, or emotional, internal or external, that tends to disturb the homeostasis of an organism. Should these reactions be inappropriate, they may lead to disease states. The term is also used to refer to the stimuli that elicit the reactions, e.g. heat, nutritional, lactational, confinement, transportation. See also PSYCHOSOMATIC disease.

s. induced diarrhea of the horse see acute undifferentiated and chronic undifferentiated DIARRHEA of the horse.

porcine s. syndrome see PORCINE stress syndrome.

s. reaction see ALARM REACTION.

s.-starvation syndrome said of sheep. See PREGNANCY toxemia.

s. testing a test for evaluating circulatory response to physical stress produced by exercise. See also EXERCISE testing.

stress-induced bone lesions found in horses doing heavy training but only by highly developed imaging techniques. Include sclerosis of the radial fossa of the third carpal bone, remodeling of the distal epiphysis of the third metacarpal or metatarsal bones.

stressor any factor that disturbs homeostasis producing stress. In animals there is a long list including nutritional, lactational and pregnancy stress, physical stressors including inclement climate, hard physical work such as endurance rides, racing, capture of wild animals, psychological including weaning, overcrowding, boredom, harassment by humans or other animals, absence of bedding or protection from drafts and poor ventilation.

stretch severe passive or active extension of a limb or the trunk.

s. injury commonly involves tendons and soft tissues surrounding a joint, particularly of the lower limbs. See dropped CARPUS.

s. receptor see RECEPTOR (2).

s. relaxation a not universally accepted characteristic of the smooth muscle of the gastrointestinal tract; if the muscle tension is being maintained by regular neural discharge, a distension of the organ which stretches the wall may temporarily inhibit the nervous impulses so that the muscle relaxes and accommodates the new length of the muscle.

stretcher a contrivance for carrying the sick or wounded.

stretches 'the stretches'; colloquial name for inherited periodic SPASTICITY.

stretching disease a description of the clinical signs shown by sheep with intussusception. Called also reksiekte.

Stretocara a genus of spiruroid worms found in the gizzard of many bird species; intermediate host is a crustacean.

stria pl. *striae* [L.] 1. a streak or line. 2. a narrow, bandlike structure; longitudinal collections of nerve fibers in the brain.

atrophic s., striae atrophicae atrophic, pinkish or purplish, scarlike lesions in the skin, later becoming white, due to weakening of elastic tissues. Seen in association with canine Cushing's syndrome.

habenular s. a bundle of nerve fibers connecting the olfactory centers with the habenular nuclei.

s. mallearis a light band visible through the tympanic membrane when it is examined with an otoscope; is the handle of the malleolus.

s. medullares bundles of white fibers across the floor of the fourth ventricle.

striate, striated having streaks or striae, e.g. striate retinopathy.

s. border see BRUSH BORDER.

s. duct the intralobular duct of major salivary glands.

striation 1. the quality of being streaked. 2. a streak or scratch, or a series of streaks.

striatonigral projecting from the corpus striatum to the substantia nigra.

s. degeneration the basic lesion in hereditary striatonigral and cerebello-olivary degeneration in Kerry blue terriers. See also CEREBELLAR abiotrophy.

striatonigral-cerebello-olivary degeneration hereditary see STRIATONIGRAL degeneration.

stricture an abnormal narrowing of a duct or passage, e.g. cervix, esophagus. See also STENOSIS and specific anatomic sites.

rectal s. of pigs see RECTAL stricture.

stricturization the process of decreasing in caliber or of becoming narrowed or constricted.

stridor a shrill, harsh sound, especially the respiratory sound heard during inspiration in laryngeal obstruction.

laryngeal s. that due to laryngeal obstruction. See also ROARING.

stridulation creation of a sound by rubbing two parts of the body together, e.g. cicada.

strigeids intestinal trematodes of birds in the family Strigeidae.

strike cutaneous MYIASIS.

striking a vigorous forward pounding action with a front limb. It is an instinctive defense or attack action by a horse which can be very dangerous to an inattentive handler.

string 1. twine, very thin rope. 2. in computer terminology, a sequence of alphanumeric characters.

s. foreign body see linear FOREIGN BODY.

s. sign seen in radiographs of the stenosed gastric pylorus as contrast medium is forced into the limited canal.

s. variable a sequence of characters, numerical or alphabetical which are treated by a computer program as a single entity.

stringent response in bacterial cells, a response to stress when the cell wall does not have a sufficient pool of amino acids to maintain protein synthesis in which the synthesis of rRNAs and tRNAs is reduced by 20-fold, which suspends many of the cell's activities until conditions improve.

stringhalt a sporadic disease of horses due to unknown cause. Characterized by involuntary repetitive exaggerated flexion of a hock. The horse is unable to move; there is wasting of thigh muscles.

Australian s. occurs as extensive outbreaks, often following a drought and associated with the abundance of herbaceous plants, particularly *Hypochoeris radicata* (called also flatweed, catsear).

classical s. the sporadic irreversible, severe form of the disease as it occurs in the northern hemisphere.

stringy wool see STEELY WOOL.

striocerebellar pertaining to the corpus striatum and cerebellum.

striola a curvilinear landmark in the middle ear to which the hairs (hair cells) in the macula are oriented.

strip 1. to press the contents from a canal, such as the urethra, teat canal or a blood vessel, by running the finger along it. 2. to excise lengths of large veins and incompetent tributaries by subcutaneous dissection and the use of a stripper.

s. cup a metal cup with a recessed black lid with a hole covered by wire mesh. To test the first milk of a cow for clots a few streams are squirted onto the lid so that watery milk can be recognized and some is squirted through the mesh so that any clots present can be detected.

s. grazing see strip GRAZING.

s. technique used in the treatment of deviated or corkscrew penis in the bull. Depends on the use of strips of the dorsal ligament of the penis to anchor the ligament to the dorsum and preventing it from slipping off during an erection.

stripe a white mark, narrower than the nasal bones, down the face of a horse. Called also race.

striped bass MORONE *saxatilis*.

striped jack see PSEUDOCARANX DENTEX.

striped wild cucumber CUCUMIS *africanus*.

stripper surgical instrument for stripping the periosteum from bone. See MATSON ELEVATOR.

stripping 1. abattoir technique for removal of esthetically unattractive pleura or peritoneum from a carcass of meat so rendering the meat saleable. 2. a technique for grooming dogs of the terrier type in which dead hairs are pulled out or cut with a razor blade incorporated into the 'stripping comb' or knife. The procedure may be a cause of mild folliculitis. 3. see also TEAT stripping. 4. referring to fish culture is the process of removing eggs or sperm from 'ripe' broodfish.

hand s. stripping the last of the milk from the udder by milking the teat manually.

machine s. stripping the last of the milk from the udder by pulling down on the teat cup cluster when milk flow has almost ceased; a common but deplored practice is to put a heavy weight on the handpiece at this time.

strobila pl. *strobilae* [L.] the chain of proglottides constituting the bulk of the body of an adult tapeworm.

strobilocercus larval stage of a tenid cestode; a fluid-filled cyst containing a scolex with a pseudosegmented elongated region connecting to the bladder, e.g. *Taenia taeniae* forms.

stroke 1. a sudden and severe attack. 2. in humans, rupture or blockage of a blood vessel in the brain, depriving parts of the brain of blood supply, resulting in loss of consciousness, paralysis or other symptoms depending on the site and extent of brain damage; see also CEREBRAL vascular accident. A very uncommon occurrence in animals.
canine s. see canine idiopathic VESTIBULAR syndrome.
lightning s. see LIGHTNING injury.
sun s. see HEAT stroke.
s. volume the volume of blood ejected by the left ventricle during a single ejection.

stroma pl. *stromata* [Gr.] the tissue forming the ground substance, framework, or matrix of an organ, as opposed to the functioning part or parenchyma, e.g. stroma iridis, stroma vitreum.

stromuhr an instrument for measuring the velocity of the blood flow.

strong wool wool with a comparatively wide fiber diameter, a classification now being superseded by stating the actual microns of diameter.

strongyle any roundworm in the superfamily Strongyloidea.
large s. includes *Craterostomum*, *Oesophagodontus*, *Strongylus asini*, *S. edentatus*, *S. equinus*, *S. vulgaris* and *Triodontophorus* spp.
small s. includes *Caballonema*, *Cyathostomum*, *Cylicocyclus*, *Cylicodontophorus*, *Cylicostephanus*, *Cylindropharynx*, *Gyalocephalus*, *Poteriostomum* and *Sinostrongylus*.

Strongyloides a genus of nematode parasites in the family Strongyloididae, the larvae of which are able to penetrate the intact skin of the host then migrate to the intestine via the bloodstream, lung, trachea and pharynx. Many species are passed from the dam to the young via the milk. See also STRONGYLOIDOSIS.
S. avium found in the ceca and small intestine of fowl, turkey and wild birds.
S. cati found in the small intestine of the cat.
S. felis in cats.
S. fuelleborni found in the small intestine of primates.
S. papillosus found in the small intestine of ruminants and rabbits.
S. planiceps in cats.
S. procyonis found in raccoons.
S. ransomi found in the small intestine of pigs.
S. ratti found in rats.
S. simiae see *S. fuelleborni* (above).
S. stercoralis a species found in the intestine of humans and other mammals, primarily in the tropics and subtropics, usually causing diarrhea and intestinal ulceration.
S. tumefaciens associated with tumors of the large intestine of cats.
S. venezuelensis found in rats.
S. westeri found in the small intestine of horse, pig and zebra.

strongyloidiasis infection with *Strongyloides* spp. See also STRONGYLOIDOSIS.

strongyloidosis, strongyloidiasis infestation with the nematode STRONGYLOIDES, a parasite of the small intestine. Can cause dermatitis and balanoposthitis due to percutaneous entry, or diarrhea when the intestinal infection is very heavy. In kangaroos it is a stomach parasite causing gastritis. *Strongyloides papillosus* may be associated with the introduction of organisms into the skin of the feet, causing footrot.

strongylosis infestation of horses with large strongyles (*Strongylus edentatus*, *S. equinus* and *S. vulgaris*), *Triodontophorus* spp., *Oesophagodontus* spp. and some members of the genera *Cyclostephanus*, *Cyathostomum*, *Cylicocyclus*, and the genera *Cylicodontophorus*, *Cylindropharynx*, *Gyalocephalus* and *Poteriostomum*. *S. vulgaris* sucks blood and also causes verminous arteritis and thromboembolic colic. The other *Strongylus* spp. and the *Triodontophorus* spp. cause anemia and debility. The small strongyles can cause severe enteritis and diarrhea. Called also redworm infestation.

Strongylus a genus of roundworms in the family Strongylidae. Called also redworm. See also STRONGYLOSIS.
S. asini found in the large intestine of the ass and wild equids.
S. edentatus found in the large intestine of horses.
S. equinus found in the cecum and colon of equids.
S. tremletti found in the rhinoceros.
S. vulgaris found in the large intestine of equids; larval stages are found in the anterior mesenteric and other arteries.

strontium a chemical element, atomic number 38, atomic weight 87.62, symbol Sr. See Table 6.
s.-90 is deposited in bones and removed with great difficulty. It has a very long half-life (28.1 years) and if sufficient is ingested it will have the same toxic and teratogenic effects as external irradiation. S-90 plates are used in the treatment of superficial squamous cell carcinomas involving the eye.
s. chloride experimental feeding to pigs causes gross bone abnormality and weakness and paralysis.

strophanthin, K-strophanthin a cardiac glycoside, obtained from the plant *Strophanthus kombé*. Has actions similar to ouabain, which is obtained from *S. gratus*, and scillerin A, obtained from *Urginea maritima*.

Strophanthus an African plant genus in the family Apocynaceae; contain cardiac glycosides, e.g. ouabain, strophanthin; are highly poisonous. Includes *S. gratus*, *S. kombé*.

struck an acute, highly fatal enterotoxemia of sheep caused by type C *Clostridium welchii*. At post mortem there is peritonitis and myositis. Called also Romney Marsh disease.

structural pertaining to structure, the components and their arrangement in constituting a whole unit.

struma enlargement of the thyroid gland; goiter.

strumectomy excision of a goiter.

strumitis thyroiditis.

Struthio camelus see OSTRICH.

struvite magnesium–ammonium–phosphate hexahydrate. See also UROLITH.
s. calculi see struvite UROLITHS.
s. crystalluria a normal finding in cats but large numbers of crystals and, rarely, calculi are found in FELINE urological syndrome, contributing to obstruction of the urinary tract.

strychnine a very poisonous alkaloid from seeds of the plant *Strychnos nux-vomica* and other species of *Strychnos*. A commonly used compound in malicious poisoning of dogs and used as a feral animal bait to which domestic dogs find access. The dogs may also be poisoned by eating the vermin. Clinical findings include tetanic convulsions especially in response to external stimuli.

strychnine bush STRYCHNOS *lucida*.

Strychnos a genus of tropical plant species in the family Loganiaceae; they contain strychnine or strychnine-like alkaloids including brucine, strychninine and lucidine and are therefore potentially poisonous. Includes *S. lucida*, *S. nux-vomica*, *S. psilospermia*, *S. toxifera* (a source of curare).

Stryker saw a power saw designed to cut plaster casts without cutting the patient. Has a unique oscillating action.

Stryphnodendron South American plant genus in the family Mimosaceae; probably contains tannins which cause hepatitis, nephrosis, diarrhea, photosensitivity. Includes *S. barbatimao*, *S. coriaceum*.

Stuart's carrier medium a special transport medium for bacteria, especially *Campylobacter* spp.

Stuart factor, Stuart–Prower factor factor X, one of the blood CLOTTING factors. Deficiency occurs in humans and Cocker spaniels, causing bleeding tendencies severe in neonatal puppies and mild in adults.

Stuart–Schwan cocci gram-positive cocci, one of the bacteria found in bovine summer mastitis.

stud 1. purebred. 2. a place, usually a farm, at which purebred animals are maintained and reproduced.
s. animal an animal registered in a stud book.
s. book the register in which the names and parentage of all of the animals that constitute the breed are kept.
s. breeder person conducting a business of a stud herd, flock, kennel, cattery etc.
s. crud see CANNON KERATOSIS.
double s. term used in the sheep industry; said of the best lines of rams.
s. farm a farm maintained for the purpose of breeding more stud animals.
s. herd a herd composed of purebred animals and used for producing more purebred animals.
s. tail hyperplasia of the sebaceous glands of the dorsum of the tail in sexually active male cats complicated by inflammation and orthokeratotic hyperkeratosis.

study a scholarly examination. Specific types of study are also detailed under BLIND, CASE-control, COHORT, CROSS-SECTIONAL.
analytical s. one in which a phenomenon is described and an attempt made to analyze the effects of variables on the phenomenon.
descriptive s. one in which a phenomenon is described but no attempt is made to analyze the effects of variables on the phenomenon.
follow-up s. one carried out to find out whether there has been change in the situation since the initial study.
longitudinal s. one carried out over a period of time so that chronological time has an opportunity to exert an effect as a variable.
observational s. see descriptive study (above).
prospective s. one in which the data to be studied are yet to be generated, the events having not yet occurred.
retrospective s. one based on examination of existing data, on events that have already occurred.
simulation s. one in which the real circumstances are simulated, either in fact, or by means of a set of mathematical formulae each of which expresses the probability of each outcome in a series of consequential events that mirror the possible pathways in a real-life situation.

stumbling an abnormal gait in which the animal does not fully extend the limb, the plantar surface is not properly placed with respect to the ground surface at the time of impact so that the limb is likely to collapse and the animal to fall.

stump the distal end of a limb left after amputation.

stump sucker see CRIB-biting.

stumped-up toe the toe of a horse's hoof that has been severely rasped back to make it coincide with a shoe that has been set too far back. A major fault in shoeing.

stumpy generally refers to a very short tail, as found in STUMPY-TAIL CATTLE DOG; also a variety of MANX cat with a mobile, often deformed, tail.

Stumpy-tail cattle dog a medium-sized dog with pricked ears and short coat, except around the neck where it forms a ruff. It can be blue, blue mottled, or red speckled with solid colored patches. The tail is naturally short.

stunner device used in abattoirs to stun an animal so that it is unconscious when it is bled out.
concussion s. a captive-bolt, nonpenetrating device, activated by a standard bullet. The explosion drives a mushroom-shaped head out of the handheld pistol which has been placed against the animal's forehead. Has the same effect as a hammer blow but is less subject to error or danger.
electrical s. see ELECTRICAL stunning.
penetrating captive-bolt s. the bolt that is driven out of the pistol (see concussion stunner above) is a 0.5 inch diameter rod which penetrates the skull bones and lacerates the brain.
pneumatic s. a penetrating captive-bolt unit (see above) in which the power is compressed air. Has problems when the compressor is not functioning.

stunning producing unconsciousness by a blow. See STUNNER. Various methods are used including a hammer blow, free bullet using a number of different projectiles, immersion of the head in carbon dioxide gas, electric shock, all of them aiming to allow the animal to bleed out while it is still alive. An animal that is dead before it has bled out will be unsuitable for marketing.

stunted chick disease see INFECTIOUS stunting syndrome.

stunting/runting syndrome see INFECTIOUS stunting syndrome.

stupe a hot, wet cloth or sponge, charged with a medication for external application.

stupefacient 1. inducing stupor. 2. an agent that induces stupor.

stupefactive producing narcosis or stupor.

stupor partial or nearly complete unconsciousness; a state of lethargy and immobility with diminished responsiveness to stimulation.

sturdy neurological disease in sheep caused by the pressure of a *Taenia multiceps* metacestode. Called also gid.

Sturges' rule a guide as to the number of categories into which a set of data should be divided for analysis or presentation:

$$\text{number of categories} = 1 + 3.3 \log N$$

where N = number of individuals in collected data.

Sturt's nightshade SOLANUM *sturtianum*.

Stuttgart casting a complicated technique for casting a horse which utilizes three ropes, a surcingle and two hobbles.

Stuttgart disease canine LEPTOSPIROSIS.

sty, stye see external HORDEOLUM.

styfziekte [Af.] another of the many colloquial names used to describe OSTEOMALACIA due to aphosphorosis.

style a term used in subjective appraisal of wool; combines brightness, density, character, dust penetration and tip shape.

stylet 1. a wire run through a catheter or cannula to render it stiff or to remove debris from its lumen. 2. a slender probe.

stylo a perennial legume adapted to grow in many

environments. An alternative to alfalfa in tough environments. Called also *Stylosanths gracilis*, Brazilian lucerne.

styl(o)- word element. [L., Gr.] *stake, pole, styloid process of the temporal bone.*

stylohyoid pertaining to the styloid process and hyoid bone.

styloid long and pointed, like a pen or stylus.

s. process 1. a pen-like process, as found at the distal end of the radius and the ulna, or of the auricular cartilage. 2. a small blunt cartilaginous process at the base of the petrous temporal bone.

styloiditis inflammation of tissues around the styloid process.

stylomastoid pertaining to the styloid and mastoid processes of the temporal bone.

stylomaxillary pertaining to the styloid process of the temporal bone and the maxilla.

stylopodium segment of a limb corresponding to the arm or thigh.

Stylosanthis gracilis see STYLO.

stylus 1. a stylet. 2. a pencil or stick, as of caustic.

Stypandra glauca, S. grandiflora, S. imbricata Australian member of the plant family Liliaceae; contains stypandrol which causes retinal degeneration, degeneration of optic nerves followed by blindness, incoordination, posterior paresis. Called also blind grass or candyup poison.

stypandrol neurotoxic naphthaquinone plant toxin found in *Stypandra, Dianella, Hemerocallis* spp.

stype a tampon or pledget of cotton.

stypsis 1. astringency; astringent action. 2. use of styptics.

styptic 1. arresting hemorrhage by means of an astringent quality. 2. a markedly astringent remedy. A chemical styptic works by causing the formation of a blood clot by chemical action. A vascular styptic checks bleeding by causing the blood vessels to contract. A mechanical styptic assists clotting by mechanical means—for example, when one applies a piece of paper or cotton to a slight razor cut.

Stypven time see RUSSELL'S VIPER VENOM time.

stywesiekte [Af.] 'stiff sickness', a pyrrolizidine toxicosis in livestock caused by *Crotalaria burkeana, C. barkae, C. steudneri*; characterized by painful hoof lesions.

sub [L.] preposition, *under.*

sub- word element. [L.] *under, less than.*

subacromial below the acromion.

subacute somewhat acute; between acute and chronic; of the order of a week's duration.

subalimentation insufficient nourishment.

subaortic, subaortal below the aorta.

s. septal defect ventricular septal defect in the pars membranaceae of, and high up in, the septum.

s. stenosis see AORTIC subvalvular stenosis.

subaponeurotic below an aponeurosis.

subarachnoid between the arachnoid and the pia mater.

s. block anesthesia produced by the injection of a local anesthetic into the subarachnoid space around the spinal cord. See also spinal ANESTHESIA.

subareolar beneath the areola of the nipple.

subastragalar below the astragalus (talus).

subastringent moderately astringent.

subaural below the ear.

subcapsular below a capsule.

subcartilaginous 1. below a cartilage. 2. partly cartilaginous.

subcellular organelles discrete, functioning structures within cells, e.g. mitochondria, nucleus, golgi apparatus and lysosomes.

subcephalic pocket a transverse furrow beneath the rostral margin of the forebrain.

subchondral below the cartilage.

s. bone providing support for the cartilage of the articular surface.

s. cysts cysts in the subchondral bone, usually an indication of osteochondrosis.

subclass a taxonomic category subordinate to a class and superior to an order.

subclavian literally means under the clavicle.

subclinical without clinical manifestations; said of the early stages or a very mild form of a disease, e.g. subclinical disease, infection, parasitism, or when a disease is detectable by clinicopathological tests but not by a clinical examination.

subcloning a restriction fragment of an original DNA that has been cloned may be further digested with another restriction enzyme and the smaller fragments cloned.

subconjunctival pertaining to the zone beneath the conjunctiva, e.g. subconjunctival hemorrhage, subconjunctival infection.

subcoracoid situated under the coracoid process.

subcorneal beneath the stratum corneum.

subcortex the brain substance underlying the cortex.

subcostal below a rib or ribs.

subcranial below the cranium.

subcrepitant somewhat crepitant in nature; said of a rale.

subculture a culture of microorganisms derived from another culture.

subcutaneous beneath the layers of the skin.

s. abscess the commonest site of an abscess; causes local pain and swelling and a positive indication is obtained by needle puncture.

s. edema accumulation of edema in subcutaneous tissues, usually of the dependent parts. If extensive referred to as anasarca. See also EDEMA.

s. fat necrosis manifested by many inert, painless lumps in the subcutis, is inherited in cattle.

s. hemorrhage the accumulation of blood in a subcutaneous site such as occurs in purpura hemorrhagica.

s. mite see LAMINOSIOPTES *cysticola*.

s. tissue the layer of loose connective tissue directly under the skin.

subcuticular below the epidermis.

subcutis the subcutaneous tissue, the panniculus adiposus.

hoof s. the connective tissue layer which attaches the dermis to the deeper structures of the hoof. Is thin in most places but thick in the coronary and digital cushions.

subdiaphragmatic below the diaphragm.

subduct to draw down.

subdural between the dura mater and the arachnoid.

s. abscess usually extensions from paranasal sinuses, e.g. in cattle after dehorning; localizing signs, head rotation, depending on location and volume of space occupied.

subendocardial beneath the endocardium.

s. coat layer of loose connective tissue beneath the endocarium.

s. fibrosis may be present at birth or acquired as a result of prolonged dilatation or as a result of persistent local turbulence as in the jet lesions caused by leaking cardiac valves.

s. mineralization may accompany subendocardial fibrosis or muscular degeneration or in association with persistent hypercalcemia or uremia.

subendothelial beneath an endothelial layer.

s. coat a layer of connective tissue and fibroblasts beneath the endothelium of blood vessels and the heart.

s. space potential connective tissue space beneath the endothelium of blood vessels and the heart.

subepidermal beneath the epidermis.

subepiglottic see PHARYNGEAL.

s. cyst in adult horses cause decreased exercise tolerance, respiratory stridor, choking.

subepithelial beneath the epithelium.

subestrus a very weak display of estral signs. See also silent ESTRUS.

subfamily a taxonomic division sometimes established, subordinate to a family and superior to a tribe.

subfascial beneath a fascia.

subfebrile marginally febrile.

subfertility marginal fertility.

subgallate a reduced salt of gallic acid, which is a hydrolysis product of tannins extracted from nutgalls or the spent broths of some antibiotic-producing fungal cultures. It is used as a styptic, intestinal astringent, and as a topical astringent in diseases of the skin. See also BISMUTH subgallate.

subgenus a taxonomic category sometimes established where the number of specimens is large, but not generally used; subordinate to a genus and superior to a species.

subgingival beneath the free margin of gingival tissue.

s. resorptive lesion commonly occur in cats, these may involve the pulp cavity. Affected teeth may become weak and fracture.

subglenoid beneath the glenoid (mandibular) fossa.

subglossal below the tongue.

subglottic below the glottis.

s. stenosis see LARYNGEAL stenosis.

subgrondation depression of one fragment of bone beneath another.

subhepatic below the liver.

subhyoid below the hyoid bone.

subiculum an underlying or supporting structure.

subiliac below the ilium.

subilium the lowest portion of the ilium.

subinfertility reduced fertility.

subinvolution incomplete involution; failure of a part to return to its normal size and condition after enlargement from functional activity.

s. of placental sites failure of involution of the sites of placental attachment in a postpartum bitch causes persistent intrauterine bleeding and may result in death due to blood loss or uterine perforation.

subjacent located below.

subject an animal subjected to treatment, observation or experiment.

s. contrast the difference in relative densities within the subject as distinct from the differences between the subject and the surroundings.

subjective perceived only by one examiner and not necessarily by any other examiner.

s. probability see subjective PROBABILITY.

subjugal below the zygomatic bone.

sublatio retinae detachment of the retina of the eye. See retinal DETACHMENT.

sublesional performed or situated beneath a lesion.

sublethal insufficient to cause death.

sublimate 1. a substance obtained by sublimation. 2. to accomplish sublimation.

sublimation the conversion of a solid directly into the gaseous state.

sublingual beneath the tongue.

s. gland a salivary gland on either side under the tongue.

sublinguitis inflammation of the sublingual gland.

sublobular veins veins which merge to form hepatic veins which receive tributaries from the central veins of liver lobules.

subluxate to partially dislocate.

subluxation a partial dislocation.

submandibular below the mandible.

s. salivary glands see SALIVARY GLAND.

s. swelling the swelling may be soft as in edema or hard and painful as in grass seed abscess, or lymphadenitis or inflammation of salivary glands. The accumulation of edema fluid is characteristic of grazing animals or those eating off the ground. Cows eating from a manger will not be affected. Called also bottle jaw.

submaxilla the mandible.

submaxillaritis inflammation of the submaxillary gland.

submaxillary below the maxilla.

s. gland the mandibular salivary gland.

submental below the chin.

s. organ a collection of large sebaceous glands located on the chin of cats.

submersion the act of placing, or the condition of being under, the surface of a liquid.

submetacentric having the centromere almost, but not quite, at the metacentric position.

submicroscopic too small to be visible with the microscope.

submission rate percentage of cows in a herd which come on heat and which are mated during a specified period, usually a month; the difference, i.e. those which come on heat and are not mated, are the deferred mating group.

submucosa connective tissue situated beneath a mucous membrane.

submucosal glands glands of the lamina epithelialis mucosae which perforate the lamina muscularis, with their adenomeres located in the submucosal connective tissue.

submucous beneath a mucous membrane.

subnarcotic moderately narcotic.

subneural beneath a nerve.

subnormal below or less than normal.

subnormality a state less than normal or that usually encountered.

suboccipital below the occiput.

suborbital beneath the orbit.

suborder a taxonomic category sometimes established, subordinate to an order and superior to a family.

subordinance see DOMINANCE aggression.

subordinate legislation legislation that depends on the delegation of authority from other, superior, legislation.

subpalpebral underneath the eyelid.

s. lavage see subpalpebral LAVAGE.

subpapillary plexus of skin a superficial plexus, one of three, of blood vessels in haired skin.

subpapular indistinctly papular.

subpatellar below the patella.

subpericardial beneath the pericardium.

subperiosteal beneath the periosteum.

subperitoneal beneath the peritoneum.

subpharyngeal beneath the pharynx.

subphrenic beneath the diaphragm.

subphylum pl. *subphyla* [L.] a taxonomic category sometimes established, subordinate to a phylum and superior to a class.

subpineal below the pineal body.

subplacenta below the placenta.

subpleural beneath the pleura.
subpreputial beneath the prepuce.
subpubic beneath the pubic bone.
subpulmonary beneath the lung.
subretinal beneath the retina.
subretrofacial nucleus located in the rostral, ventrolateral part of the medulla oblongata this nucleus is largely responsible for the tone of all blood vessels.
subroutine in computer usage a self-contained subsidiary program that is called upon by one program to carry out a specific task.
subscapular below the scapula.
subscription the third chief part of a drug prescription, comprising directions to be followed by the pharmacist in its preparation.
subserous beneath a serous membrane.
subsidized practice a system of private practice in which some organization, local government, cooperative dairy company, a farmers' club, subsidizes the veterinarian. The method of subsidy varies from a salary with the right to private practice to a guaranteed total income with the subsidy making up any shortfall. A novel and successful method has been to provide the professional premises for the veterinarian at a minuscule rental.
subsolar beneath the sole of the horse's hoof.
s. abscess usually a consequence of a nail prick causing lameness. See FOOT abscess.
subspecies a subdivision of a species; a variety or race.
subspectacle underneath the spectacles of a snake.
s. abscess an abscess between the spectacle and the cornea.
substage the part of the microscope underneath the stage.
substance the material constituting an organ or body.
black s. substantia nigra.
controlled s. see CONTROLLED SUBSTANCES ACT.
depressor s. a substance that tends to decrease activity or blood pressure.
gray s. nerve tissue composed of predominantly nerve cell bodies, unmyelinated nerve fibers, and supporting tissue. See also GRAY MATTER.
ground s. the gel-like material in which connective tissue cells and fibers are embedded.
medullary s. 1. the white matter of the central nervous system, consisting of axons and their myelin sheaths. 2. the soft, marrow-like substance of the interior of such structures as bone, kidney and adrenal gland.
s. P an undecapeptide present in the intestine, where it induces contraction of the intestine and dilatation of blood vessels; it is also present in a number of neuronal pathways in the brain and in primary sensory fibers of peripheral nerves, and may be a neurotransmitter associated with transmission of pain impulses.
perforated s. 1. *anterior perforated substance*, an area anterolateral to each optic tract, pierced by branches of the anterior and middle cerebral arteries. 2. *posterior perforated substance*, an area between the cerebral peduncles, pierced by branches of the posterior cerebral arteries.
pressor s. a substance that raises blood pressure.
reticular s. the netlike mass of threads seen in erythrocytes after vital staining.
slow-reacting s. see SLOW-REACTING SUBSTANCE.
threshold s's those substances (e.g. glucose) excreted into the urine only when their concentration in plasma exceeds a certain value.
white s. tissue consisting mostly of myelinated nerve fibers and constituting the conducting portion of the brain and spinal cord; see also WHITE MATTER.

substantia pl. *substantiae* [L.] substance.
s. alba the white matter of the spinal cord and the brain.
s. compacta compact bone.
s. gelatinosa the substance sheathing the posterior horn of the spinal cord and lining its central canal.
s. grisea the gray matter of the spinal cord and brain.
s. grisea centralis the central gray matter that surrounds the cerebral aqueduct.
s. nigra the layer of gray substance separating the tegmentum of the midbrain from the crus cerebri.
s. propria corneae layer of transparent lamellated fibrous connective tissue which constitutes the bulk of the cornea; composed of collagen fibers disposed in platelike formations, fibroblasts and ground substance with many nerve fibers but no blood vessels.
s. propria choroid loose connective tissue of the choroid.
substernal behind the sternum.
substituent 1. a substitute; especially an atom, radical, or group substituted for another in a compound. 2. of or pertaining to such an atom, radical or group.
substitution the act of putting one thing in the place of another, especially the chemical replacement of one atom or substituent group by another.
conservative s. in protein chemistry, one amino acid is substituted by another which has a similar polarity.
meat s. a common fraud in the meat industry in which uninspected meat is substituted for meat that has undergone inspection and been branded as satisfactory. The other not infrequent fraud is the substitution of meat of another species, e.g. horse for beef, cat for chicken or rabbit.
non-conservative s. in protein chemistry, one amino acid is substituted by another which has a markedly different polarity.
substrate any substance upon which an enzyme acts.
s. binding site part of the active site of an enzyme which includes the amino acid residues that come into contact with the substrate.
s. specificity range of substrates that can be catalytically converted to product by an enzyme.
suicide s. see SUICIDE SUBSTRATE.
substructure the underlying or supporting portion of an organ or appliance.
subsylvian situated deep in the lateral sulcus (sylvian fissure).
subsynaptic web the web of filaments in the postsynaptic membrane, i.e. on the effector organ.
subtarsal below the tarsus.
subtentorial beneath the tentorium of the cerebellum.
subterranean clover TRIFOLIUM *subterraneum*.
subthalamus the ventral thalamus or subthalamic tegmental region: a transitional region of the diencephalon interposed between the (dorsal) thalamus, the hypothalamus, and the tegmentum of the mesencephalon (midbrain); it includes the subthalamic nucleus and the zona incerta, all with unknown functions.
subtle 1. very fine, as a subtle powder. 2. very acute, as a subtle pain.
subtraction radiography highlighting the differences between two radiographs by covering one film of a part with a diapositive film of the same part. A photograph of this compilation will produce one which has grayed out the background but reinforced the differences. The method removes distracting material in the ordinary film. Used in angiography where the vessels are difficult to see, e.g. in the skull.

subtribe a taxonomic category sometimes established, subordinate to a tribe and superior to a genus.
Subtriquetra a genus of pentastomes in the family Porocephalidae found in fish (the nymphs) and crocodiles (the adults).
subtrochanteric below the trochanter of the femur.
subtympanic somewhat tympanic in quality.
Subulura a genus of roundworms in the family Subuluridae.
S. brumpti occurs in the ceca of fowls, turkey, guinea fowl and related wild birds and has low pathogenicity.
S. differens occurs in fowls and guinea fowl.
S. minetti occurs in chickens.
S. strongylina found in chickens, guinea fowl and wild birds.
S. suctoria found in the ceca of chickens and wild birds.
subungual beneath a nail or claw.
subunit vaccine see subunit VACCINE.
suburethral beneath the urethra.
subvaginal under a sheath, or below the vagina.
subvalvular below the heart valves.
s. aortic stenosis see AORTIC subvalvular stenosis.
subvertebral on the ventral side of the vertebrae.
subvirile having deficient virility.
subvolution the operation of turning over a flap to prevent adhesions.
succenturiate accessory; serving as a substitute.
Succinamonas amylolytica a common finding amongst the digestive bacteria in the rumen.
succinate any salt of succinic acid.
s. dehydrogenase an enzyme of the TCA cycle, located in the inner mitochondrial membrane that splits off hydrogen from succinic acid.
succinic acid an intermediate in the tricarboxylic acid cycle.
succinimides a group of anticonvulsant drugs that includes phensuximide, methsuximide and ethosuximide. Not widely used in animals.
Succinivibrio dextrinosolvens a bacterial digester of ruminal contents.
succinyl-CoA a high energy intermediate metabolite formed in the Krebs cycle by the oxidation of α-ketoglutaric acid.
succinylcholine a short-acting depolarizing neuromuscular blocking agent used as a muscle relaxant. Called also suxamethonium.
s. bromide the pharmaceutical form of succinylcholine; can cause death by cardiac arrest in even healthy horses.
succinylsulfathiazole a sulfonamide drug used for treatment of enteric infections because it is poorly absorbed and maintains high concentrations in the gut. Called also sulfasuxidine.
Succisa pratensis see SCABIOSA SUCCISA.
succorrhea excessive flow of a natural secretion.
succus pl. *succi* [L.] any fluid derived from living tissue; bodily secretion; juice.
s. entericus the secretion of the intestinal glands.
succussion shaking of the body or part of it to elicit a sound.
s. sound a splashing sound elicited when a patient is shaken, indicative of fluid and air in a body cavity.
suck reflex see SUCKING reflex.
sucker lamb a lamb still sucking the ewe and ready for slaughter. The most succulent lamb of all.
sucking the application of suction to an object by the mouth.
s. drive instinctive enthusiasm of the neonate to suck on a teat, or any object which even remotely resembles a teat.
s. lice lice in the order Anoplura. Includes the families Echinophthiriidae, Haematopinidae, Hoplopleuridae, Lignognathidae and Pediculidae.
s. reflex sucking movements of the lips of newborn and unweaned animals elicited by placing a warm, fleshy mass in the animal's mouth.
suckler a young animal that is still drawing milk from its dam; a nursing female animal, usually a cow.
s. herd a herd of cattle composed of dams and their young calves up to the point of weaning.
Suckleya suckleyana North American member of the plant family Chenopodiaceae; can cause cyanide poisoning. Called also poison suckleya.
suckling the nursing of the young by the dam; the young animal so nursed.
sucralfate a complex of aluminum hydroxide and sulfated sucrose used for short-term treatment of peptic ulcer; it forms a complex with proteins that resists digestion by acid and pepsin thereby making a protective coating for the ulcer.
sucrase an intestinal enzyme that hydrolyzes sucrose. It is not present in newborn animals so that they are unable to digest sucrose and feeding of the sugar will cause severe, osmotic diarrhea. Sucrase activity in the intestine increases as the need for, and secretion of, lactase decreases with age.
sucrose a sugar obtained from sugar cane, sugar beet, or other sources; used as a food and sweetening agent. Digestion is by sucrase secreted in the succus entericus. The feeding of large amounts to newborn and very young animals will cause osmotic diarrhea because of failure to hydrolyze the sugar. Overfeeding of ruminants with sucrose, or molasses, its crude form, causes carbohydrate engorgement.
suction aspiration of gas or fluid by mechanical means.
post-tussive s. a sucking sound heard over a lung cavity just after a cough.
s. tip sterilizable metal, handheld instrument, used for suction by inserting into the end of a suction tube. Has an angled neck for reaching into difficult pockets and a small bulb on the end with many holes in it it to permit placing it on tissue without obstructing the suction. Called also Yankauer tip.
suctioning removal of material through the use of negative pressure, as in suctioning an operative wound during and after surgery to remove exudates.
suctorial adapted for sucking.
sudamen pl. *sudamina* [L.] a small whitish vesicle caused by retention of sweat in the layers of the epidermis.
Sudan a group of lipophilic azo compounds used as biological stains for fats, e.g. Sudan III, Sudan IV.
S. stain test a useful screening test for steatorrhea. Feces mixed with Sudan III or Sudan IV stain are examined microscopically for detection of undigested (direct test) or digested (indirect test) fats that appear as red-stained globules.
Sudan grass SORGHUM *sudanense*.
Sudanese Fulani cattle West African, lyre-horned, milking cattle, usually light gray.
sudanophilia 1. affinity for a Sudan stain. 2. a condition in which the leukocytes contain particles staining readily with Sudan red III.
sudanophilic staining readily with Sudan III.
s. granules see SUDANOPHILIA (2).
sudation the process of sweating.
Sudax a Sudan grass hybrid with substantially less cyanogenetic glycoside content than the parent plant but still capable, in extreme circumstances, of causing cyanide poisoning.

sudden death a category of illness in which animals which are under frequent observation die either with no obvious illness or after a period of illness lasting only a few hours. Typical causes are spontaneous internal hemorrhage, trauma causing shock or blood loss, rupture of the gut, cardiac tamponade, trauma to brain or spinal cord at the occipitoatlantal joint, intravenous injection of inappropriate solution or given too rapidly causing cardiac arrest or pulmonary edema, anaphylactic shock.

In large animals, group deaths can be due to electrocution, lightning injury, many poisons especially cyanide, algal fast death factor, so-called Wimmera ryegrass poisoning, fluoroacetate and oleander. Monensin causes acute heart failure in horses. Septicemia due to anthrax, toxemia due to *Clostridium welchii* type D and colibacillosis can cause peracute deaths but signs are evident in animals kept under surveillance.

Animals that are 'found dead' are in a different category to sudden death and have a much wider range of possible causes.

s. d. factors see ANATOXIN.

sudomotor stimulating the sweat glands.

sudor sweat; perspiration.

sudoral characterized by profuse sweating.

sudoresis profuse sweating.

sudoriferous 1. conveying sweat. 2. sudoriparous.

s. glands sweat glands.

sudorific 1. promoting sweating; diaphoretic. 2. an agent that causes sweating.

sudoriparous secreting or producing sweat.

suet hard, raw fat from a beef carcass sold for cooking.

sufentanil an opioid analgesic, related to fentanyl.

suffocation the stoppage of breathing, or the asphyxia that results from it. If suffocation is complete—that is, no air at all reaches the lungs—the lack of oxygen and excess of carbon dioxide in the blood will cause almost immediate loss of consciousness. Though the heart continues to beat briefly, death will follow in a matter of minutes unless emergency measures are taken to get breathing started again.

Suffocation can be caused by drowning, electric shock, gas or smoke poisoning, strangulation, or choking on a foreign body in the trachea. That suffocation is occurring in an animal may not be obvious. Signs that suggest obstruction to the air passage, e.g. in acute pulmonary edema, are gasping dyspnea with mouth breathing, frantic demented activity including aggression, especially in horses, terminally violent convulsions and asphyxial respiratory failure.

Suffolk horse a compact, neat, heavy English drafthorse. Chestnut only, 16 to 16.2 hands high, limbs almost devoid of feather. Called also Suffolk Punch.

Suffolk Punch see SUFFOLK HORSE.

Suffolk sheep an English DOWNS-type breed of shortwoolled, meat sheep with a black, woolless head and distinctive Roman nose; polled, black legs. Scrapie is more common in this breed than in other breeds. Origin of WHITE SUFFOLK, SOUTH SUFFOLK.

suffusion 1. the process of overspreading, or diffusion. 2. the condition of being moistened or permeated through.

sugar a sweet carbohydrate of both animal and vegetable origin, the two principal groups of which are the disaccharides and the monosaccharides. Unless qualified, e.g. fruit sugar, milk sugar, usually refers to sucrose.

s. beet see BETA *vulgaris*.

s. beet pulp see BEET pulp.

s. beet tops see BETA *vulgaris*.

s. cane as such is not fed but molasses and the pith, bagasse, are fed (Camola is a feed composed of 4 parts pith and 10 parts molasses). Sugar cane may contain sufficient cyanogenetic glycoside to cause poisoning if the appropriate enzyme is also supplied.

s. fecal centrifugation using Sheather's solution; standard procedure for examination of feces for parasite eggs.

s. gum EUCALYPTUS *cladoclyx*.

invert s. a sugar obtained by hydrolyzing sucrose; a mixture of glucose and fructose. Called invert sugar because sucrose is dextrorotary—the mixture is levorotary. Used as a parenteral nutrient. Called also invertose.

s. of lead lead acetate, used in the preparation of white lotion. Occurs naturally on weathered paintwork and is attractive and poisonous to animals.

s. of milk see LACTOSE.

sugillation an ecchymosis.

suicide substrate a compound that is not of itself toxic to a cell, but which resembles a normal metabolite closely enough that it undergoes metabolic transformation to a product that does inhibit a crucial enzyme, e.g. fluoroacetate. A substrate-analog that binds irreversibly to amino acids, usually the catalytic amino acid, thereby blocking the active site of the enzyme to other molecules and effectively 'killing' the enzyme.

suid wild pig, e.g. wart hog, babirusa, bush pigs.

Suidasia nesbitti a grain mite in the family Acaridae which causes wheat pollard itch.

Suifilaria a genus of filarioid worms in the family Filariidae.

S. suis found in the intermuscular and subcutaneous connective tissue of pigs and cause no problems other than the physical presence of the worms in the meat.

suiform pig-like.

suint the water-soluble fraction of wool yolk.

Suipoxvirus a genus of viruses in the family POXVIRIDAE. The cause of SWINEPOX.

suipoxvirus a poxvirus in the genus *Suipoxvirus*, family *Poxviridae*.

sulbactam an irreversible β-lactamase inhibitor which increases the activity of β-lactam antibiotics. Commonly used in combination with ampicillin and occasionally with cephalosporins.

sulcate furrowed; marked with sulci.

sulcular pertaining to a sulcus.

s. epithelium the lining of the gingival sulcus.

s. lavage flushing of debris from the gingival crevice. Usually part of dental prophylaxis.

sulcus pl. *sulci* [L.] a groove or furrow; a linear depression, especially one separating the gyri of the brain.

abomasal s. the third or abomasal part of the gastric GROOVE.

alar s. lies between the dorsolateral cartilage at the nostril and the lateral accessory cartilage.

calcarine s. see CALCARINE sulcus.

central s. fissure of Rolando.

collateral s. see COLLATERAL fissure.

coronal s. a groove at the top of the hoof wall that houses the coronal matrix.

coronary s. an external groove which indicates the division of the ventricles of the heart and the atria. Houses the circumflex coronary blood vessels of the heart.

cruciate s. a deep groove which runs transversely across the rostro-dorsal surface of the cerebrum and which is one of the landmarks on the cerebral cortex.

s. cutis fine depressions of the skin between the ridges of the skin.
dorsal median s. see dorsal median FISSURE.
gingival s. the groove between the surface of the tooth and the epithelium lining the free gingiva.
hippocampal s. hippocampal fissure.
jugular s. see JUGULAR furrow.
lateral cerebral s. see sylvian FISSURE.
s. limitans a longitudinal groove in the neural tube wall of the embryo; stretches from the mesencephalon caudad.
omasal s. the second part of the gastric GROOVE in ruminants.
reticular s. the first part of the gastric groove in ruminants.
rhinal s. a deep groove which separates the neopallium from the paleopallium on the lateral surface of the brain.
rumenoreticular s. a groove on the external surface of the forestomachs that marks the division between the rumen and reticulum.
scleral s. the groove between the sclera and cornea.
sylvian s. a landmark groove on the lateral side of the cerebral cortex.
urethral s. the furrow in the ventral aspect of the corpus cavernosum of the penis that accommodates the corpus cavernosum urethrae and the urethra.

sulfa drugs a group of chemical compounds used as antibacterial agents; called also sulfonamides.

sulfabenzamide a sulfonamide antibiotic, similar to sulfamethoxazole.

sulfabrom, sulfabromomethazine a derivative of sulfamezathine which maintains blood levels for long periods, up to 48 hours in cattle.

sulfacetamide an antibacterial sulfonamide used mainly in ophthalmic preparations.

sulfachlorpyrazine an intermediate-acting sulfonamide, used as the soluble sodium salt in drinking water as a systemic antibacterial in chickens. It is absorbed rapidly from the gut.

sulfachlorpyridazine a sulfonamide antibacterial remedy used in pigs and calves. It is most effective against gram-negative bacteria including *Escherichia coli* and *Salmonella* spp., but is limited in its usefulness because of its rapid absorption and excretion.

sulfadiazine a rapidly absorbed and readily excreted sulfonamide antibacterial agent. Used commonly in triple-sulfa preparations. The sodium salt is used intravenously.
silver s. see SILVER sulfadiazine.
sodium s. an antibacterial compound used intravenously.
s.-trimethoprim a very popular combination of a potentiated sulfonamide because of its broad antibacterial spectrum and its small dose rate.

sulfadimethoxine a long-acting derivative of sulfadiazine.

sulfadimidine see SULFAMETHAZINE.

sulfadoxine a long-acting sulfonamide. Called also sulformethoxine.

sulfafurazole a sulfonamide antibacterial compound used orally, topically and parenterally, in infections of the urinary and respiratory tracts and of soft tissues. Called also sulfisoxazole.

sulfaguanidine the first sulfonamide designed to treat enteric infections. It is poorly absorbed and retains high levels in the gut but a number of similar but superior drugs are now available.

sulfallate a thiocarbamate herbicide which is poisonous if taken in large amounts. Not poisonous if used according to instructions. Causes muscle spasms, ataxia, depression and, in chronic cases, alopecia. Called also CDEC.

sulfamerazine a short-acting sulfonamide.

sulfameter see SULFAMETHOXYDIAZINE.

sulfamethazine a sulfonamide which is rapidly absorbed from the alimentary tract, slowly excreted and minimal precipitation in renal tubules. Used as an antibacterial and coccidiostat. Available also as a soluble sodium salt for injection. Called also sulfadimidine, sulfamezathine.

sulfamethizole a short-acting sulfonamide used in urinary tract infections.

sulfamethoxazole an antibacterial sulfonamide, especially useful in acute urinary tract infections and in infections of wounds and soft tissues. Commonly combined with trimethoprim.

sulfamethoxydiazine a long-acting sulfonamide, used in urinary tract infections. Called also sulfameter.

sulfamethoxypyridazine a long-acting sulfonamide that is rapidly absorbed but slowly excreted.

sulfamezathine see SULFAMETHAZINE.

sulfamylon see MAFENIDE.

sulfanilamide a potent antibacterial compound, the first of the sulfonamides, the first real antibacterial and the drug that opened the door into the antibiotic era.

sulfanilate used in clinical pathology, determination of clearance from the blood with blood samples collected at timed intervals after the intravenous injection of sodium sulfanilate is a sensitive test of renal insufficiency, particularly reduced glomerular filtration.

sulfanitran a coccidiostat used in fowls.

sulfapyridine one of the very early sulfonamides with significant toxicity. Now replaced by safer and more effective drugs.

sulfaquinoxaline a cocciodistat which was used extensively in chickens but has been superseded.

sulfarsphenamine an organic arsenical which was once used as a systemic antibacterial agent but is now largely discarded.

sulfasalazine a combination of sulfapyridine and salicylic acid, used in the treatment and prophylaxis of ulcerative colitis. Previously called salicylazosulfapyridine.

sulfasuxidine see SUCCINYLSULFATHIAZOLE.

sulfatase an enzyme that catalyzes the hydrolysis of sulfate esters.

sulfatases one of the more than 50 groups of hydrolases responsible for the digestive properties and defensive functions of lysosomes.

sulfate a salt of sulfuric acid.
s. conjugation an important in vivo mechanism for the detoxication mechanism for phenols and aliphatic alcohols.
high s. diets associated with increased prevalence of polioencephalomalacia in ruminants.

sulfathiazole a short-acting sulfonamide used as the phthalyl and succinyl forms for enteric infections. See also PHTHALYLSULFATHIAZOLE and SUCCINYLSULFATHIAZOLE.

sulfatide any of a class of cerebroside sulfuric esters.

sulfhemoglobin a step in the pathway of degeneration of hemoglobin and the formation of Heinz bodies.

sulfhemoglobinemia high levels of sulfhemoglobin in the blood.

sulfhydryl the univalent radical, –SH.
s. compounds compounds which contain sulfhydryl groups, principally the sulfur-containing amino acids. Used as radioprotective agents.

sulfide any binary compound of sulfur; a compound of sulfur with another element or base.

hydrogen s. see HYDROGEN sulfide.

sulfiding superficial black pigmentation in meat carcasses, especially pigs, in which, either because of hot weather or a long period between slaughtering and dressing, there is time for interaction between hydrogen sulfide formed in the gut and hemoglobin in the blood vessels of the kidney and liver.

sulfiram see MONOSULFIRAM.

sulfisoxazole see SULFAFURAZOLE.

sulfmethemoglobin a compound of hemoglobin and hydrogen sulfide.

sulfobromophthalein a sulfur- and bromine-containing compound used in liver function tests. The commercial name for the test reagent is Bromsulphalein.

s. clearance test used as a test of liver function. The compound is injected intravenously and measurement made at intervals of its serum concentration. Too slow a clearance is an indication of hepatic insufficiency. Called also BSP test.

sulfonamide 1. any compound containing the $-SO_2NH_2$ group. 2. any of a group of drugs that are derivatives of sulfanilamide, which competitively inhibit folic acid synthesis in microorganisms, and are bacteriostatic against gram-positive cocci (streptococci and pneumococci), gram-negative cocci (meningococci and gonococci), gram-negative bacilli (*Escherichia coli* and shigellae), and a wide variety of other bacteria. Sulfonamides have been supplanted by more effective and less toxic antibiotics in most uses. Called also sulfa drugs.

sulfone a compound containing two hydrocarbon radicals attached to the $-SO_2-$ group, especially dapsone (4,4′-sulfonylbisbenzenamine) and its derivatives, which are potent antibacterials effective against many gram-positive and gram-negative organisms, and are widely used in humans as leprostatics.

sulfonylurea a class of chemical compounds that includes the oral HYPOGLYCEMIC agents acetohexamide, chlorpropamide, tolazamide and tolbutamide.

sulformethoxine sulfadoxine.

sulfosalicylic acid test a turbidometric test for protein in the urine.

sulfoxide 1. the divalent radical =SO. 2. an organic compound intermediate between a sulfide and a sulfone.

sulfur a chemical element, atomic number 16, atomic weight 32.064, symbol S. See Table 6. Elemental sulfur is fed to animals to reduce their volume of feed intake, for example in a feedlot using self-feeders. It is also fed as an oldfashioned worm prophylaxis and coccidiostat.

Overfeeding of elemental sulfur causes enteritis characterized by black, evil smelling diarrhea. See also HYDROGEN sulfide poisoning.

s. dioxide a poisonous gas liberated by some industrial enterprises, e.g. copper smelting, from silage to which sodium metabisulfite has been added as a preservative and in oldfashioned treatments for mange. The gas causes irritation of the upper respiratory tract and pneumonia in severe cases. Commonly used as a meat preservative where it selectively destroys thiamin and has been incriminated as a cause of thiamin deficiency, particularly in dogs and cats.

s. granule small, soft to mineralized bodies in the pus of lesions of ACTINOMYCOSIS. Called also drusen.

lime-s. see LIME-SULFUR.

s. myopathy skeletal and myocardial degeneration caused by the feeding of toxic levels of sulfur.

s. nutritional deficiency ruminants may need supplemental inorganic sulfur if the bulk of their nitrogen is not in the form of protein but as urea or ammonium phosphate. A deficiency in these circumstances causes anorexia, weight loss, poor digestion and fall in milk yield.

precipitated s. a scabicide, antiparasitic, antifungal and keratolytic. Called also milk of sulfur.

s. stinker a can of preserved meat contaminated by *Clostridium nigrificans* causing the formation of hydrogen sulfide, and black or purple staining of the inside of the can.

s. sublimatum, sublimed s. a parasiticide and scabicide. Called also flowers of sulfur.

technetium coated s. colloid used in scintigraphy of the liver and reticuloendothelial systems. Called also ^{99m}Tc sulfur colloid.

sulfurated combined with sulfur.

sulfurated lime see LIME-SULFUR.

sulfuric acid an oily, highly caustic, poisonous compound, H_2SO_4.

Sulkowitch test an outmoded test of calcium concentration in urine. Used at one time as a diagnostic aid in milk fever diagnosis in cows.

sulky horse-drawn, ultra-lightweight, single-seater, two-wheeled vehicle used by Standardbreds in races. Called also bike, gig.

sulph- for words beginning thus, see those beginning *sulf-*.

sulphur see SULFUR.

sumac *Rhus* spp. trees and shrubs.

poison s. TOXICODENDRON *vernix*.

sumatrol one of the insecticidal substances, with rotenone, in DERRIS.

sumicidin synthetic, pyrethroid anthelmintic; poisonous causing a non-fatal syndrome of nervous signs, dyspnea, bloat and regurgitation of ruminal contents.

summation accumulate, add up, aggregate a series of numbers or quantities or events.

s. of effects a theory explaining clinical pruritus as the additive effects of pruritus from several causes which may raise the individual above the threshold, but pruritus from any single cause would be unlikely to do so.

s. gallop see gallop RHYTHM.

neurological s. physiological summation in synapses is a characteristic of the mammalian nervous system. It may be spatial, with additional synaptic junctions participating, or temporal, when succeeding stimuli catch up with the as-yet undischarged neurotransmitter. Seen in the retina of the cat, as an example of a nocturnal animal, where many millions of photoreceptors are connected to only one million axons, resulting in maximal sensitivity to light.

weighted s. the sum obtained by adding the numerical value for individual clinical signs, each weighted to express their importance, when making a diagnosis. The total, as a fraction or a percentage, provides an estimate of the probability of each diagnosis being the correct one.

summer said of diseases that are most prevalent during summer months.

s. bleeding see PARAFILARIA *multipapillosa*.

s. conjunctivitis see equine seasonal CONJUNCTIVITIS.

s. cypress see KOCHIA SCOPARIA.

s. dermatitis, s. eczema see SWEET itch.

s. flower see HELIANTHUS ANNUUS.

s. grass DIGITARIA *sanguinalis*.

s. itch see SWEET itch.

s. mange see ONCHOCERCOSIS.

s. mastitis bovine mastitis caused by *Corynebacterium pyogenes*. See also summer MASTITIS, Table 16.

s. slump chronic form of poisoning by FESTUCA *arundinacea* manifested by severe weight loss and severe abdominal fat necrosis.

s. snuffles is an acute rhinitis of cows characterized by sneezing, purulent nasal discharge, dyspnea. It occurs when pasture is in flower and is thought to be allergic. May be the initial stage of enzootic nasal granuloma.

s. sores see SWEET itch, SWAMP CANCER.

summer kill deaths amongst cultivated finfish caused by a higher temperature of the water in the water body than the particular species can tolerate, and/or the reduction in dissolved oxygen resulting from the elevated temperature.

summit metabolism when heat losses from the patient's body exceed the patient's ability to produce heat.

sump oil waste oil from engines: palatable to cattle. Cattle with access to rubbish dumps may lick large quantities. The oil causes lead poisoning as well as poisoning due to the oil if it is taken in large enough amounts. See also LEAD[I] poisoning, OIL.

sump–Penrose drain a Shirley wound drain (sump drain) enclosed within a Penrose drain.

sun conures a parrot in the family Psittacidae.

sun spurge EUPHORBIA *helioscopia*.

sunburn inflammation—an actual burn—of the skin caused by exposure to ultraviolet rays of the sun as it occurs in humans does not occur in animals. White pigs suffer most and may develop a chronic dermatitis along the back, some may lose the tips of the ears by sloughing. Called also primary phototoxicity. Dogs and cats, particularly those with unpigmented skin on the dorsum of the nose, eyelids, ears or groin, may develop a chronic actinic dermatitis. Fish in cultivation ponds show white patches on the top of the head and corneal cataracts. See also solar DERMATITIS.

s. cells dyskeratotic keratinocytes, either scattered or in a continuous band in the outer stratum spinosum, are characteristic of a sunburn lesion.

sunburst appearance, effect calcified streaks which appear on radiographs to radiate from a primary lesion at the surface of a bone. One possible feature of osteogenic sarcoma but can also occur in cases of osteomyelitis.

sunchillo WEDELIA *glauca*.

sundews see DROSERA.

sundry debtors the persons who have accounts with the practice and who are at present in debt to it. The accounts are kept in a sundry debtor's ledger.

sunflower a plant whose seed is used for oil for human food. The residual cake is a high-protein supplement but lacking in lysine. Decorticated seed cake contains 44% protein, undecorticated seed cake, suitable only for ruminants because it contains the seed hulls, contains 28% protein.

sunflower daisy WEDELIA *asperrima*.

sunlight the actinic rays of direct sunlight are known to have disinfectant properties, to be instrumental in the production of vitamin D in the skin and to be the trigger mechanism in photosensitive dermatitis, squamous cell carcinoma of the eye in cattle and of the vulva in sheep and solar dermatitis.

sunn hemp CROTALARIA *juncea*.

sunscreen a topical agent that filters ultraviolet rays reaching the skin; used to prevent sunburn, actinic dermatitis, and in the control of discoid lupus erythematosus.

sunstroke causing damage to the central nervous system by penetration of tissues by actinic rays is thought not to be an important physical pathogen. See also HEAT[I] exhaustion, HEAT[I] stroke.

super- word element. [L.] *above, excessive*.

superalimentation excessive feeding; sometimes used in the treatment of wasting diseases.

superalkalinity excessive alkalinity.

superantigen molecules that are potent T lymphocyte mitogens and simultaneously bind to class II MHC molecules. They are often associated with staphylococcal products and are involved in enterotoxemias and toxic shock syndrome in humans.

superbug a colloquial referrence to a bacterium that carries resistance genes to many antibiotics or to a bacterium or virus of greatly enhanced virulence.

superfamily a group of proteins related in structure but different in function, e.g. immunoglobulin superfamily which includes immunoglobulins, T cell receptor, major histocompatibility class I and II, β_2-microglobulin, α/β glycoprotein, neuronal cell-adhesive molecule (N-CAM) and neurocytoplasmic protein 3 (NP3).

superfecundation fertilization of two or more ova during the same ovulatory cycle, by separate coital acts.

superfetation the fertilization and subsequent development of an ovum when a fetus is already present in the uterus, a result of fertilization of ova during different ovulatory cycles and yielding fetuses of different ages.

superficial situated on or near the surface.

s. necrolytic dermatitis frequently associated with glucagon-secreting tumors of the pancreas and with cases of diabetes mellitus or chronic hepatitis; called also hepatocutaneous syndrome; lesions are erythematous, erosive, ulcerative and crusted with marked hyperkeratosis of the footpads.

s. plexus skin see SUBPAPILLARY PLEXUS OF SKIN.

s. pustular dermatitis see superficial pustular DERMATITIS.

superficialis superficial.

superficies an outer surface.

superfine a class of merino sheep with wool finer than that of FINE-WOOL. Usual limit is wool of 18.5 microns or less fiber diameter.

superinduce to bring on in addition to an already existing condition.

superinfection a new infection complicating the course of antimicrobial therapy of an existing infection, due to proliferation of bacteria or fungi resistant to the drug(s) in use.

superinvolution prolonged involution of the uterus after delivery, to a size much smaller than the normal, occurring in females that are still suckling their young.

superior situated above, or directed upward.

superjacent located just above.

superjuice Australian farmers' remedy for almost everything; saturated solution of superphosphate prepared by soaking enough of the fertilizer in a large drum of water to ensure that there is always a residue. A cupful per cow per day wards off nutritional deficiency of phosphorus.

superlactation oversecretion of milk; hyperlactation.

superlethal more than sufficient to cause death.

supermotility excessive motility.

supernatant the liquid lying above a layer of precipitated insoluble material.

supernumerary in excess of the regular number.
s. kidney an additional kidney which may be fused with or separate from a normal kidney; caused by the formation of an extra ureteric bud in the embryo.
s. teats in cows may be accompanied by a supernumerary mammary gland. May also be an adjunct to an existing teat and also share its teat cistern.
supernutrition see SUPERALIMENTATION.
superolateral above and to the side.
superovulation production of more than one ovum at ovulation. 1. Planned production of a number of ova from the one cow at the same ovulation period is an essential part of the technique of bovine embryo transfer. Can be effected with a single injection of PMSG or for better results, with FSH and LH in a 5:1 ratio, twice daily for 5 days. Called also multiple ovulation. 2. Can occur accidentally when cows are treated with large doses of FSH as a treatment for no visible estrus.
superoxide any compound containing the highly reactive superoxide ion O_2^-, a common intermediate in numerous biological oxidations and an important killing mechanism generated in lysosomes of phagocytes after they have phagocytosed microorganisms.
s. dismutase an enzyme that converts peroxides to two kinds of molecules in different states of oxidation. Present in aerobic bacteria.
superphosphate the common fertilizer for the application of phosphorus to a deficient soil. Used also to provide a direct nutritional supplement, as superjuice, the supernatant from a settled mixture of superphosphate and water. Fluorine poisoning may occur in animals with access to superphosphate made from rock phosphate with a high fluorine content.
superpurgation violent, watery diarrhea; life-threatening because of the imminence of irreversible dehydration.
supersaturate to add more of an ingredient than can be held in solution permanently.
superscription something written above; the first of four chief parts of a drug prescription, the ▪ prescription sign ('Take thou').
superseding taking over a case of a patient under treatment by another veterinarian. In general terms this is poor professional etiquette unless the other veterinarian has been consulted and agrees to the change. However, there are many situations in which professional etiquette is overridden by the need to provide the best treatment for the animal.
supersession see SUPERSEDING.
supertension extreme tension.
supervascularization in radiotherapy, the relative increase in vascularity that occurs when tumor cells are destroyed so that the remaining tumor cells are better supplied by the (uninjured) capillary stroma.
supervoltage in radiation therapy, pertaining to x-rays produced by a tube voltage in the range of 500–1000 kilovolts.
supination in humans, rotation of the forearm to bring the palm to face upward; in animals, the action is best in primates but is still significant in laboratory animals, cats and dogs.
supplejack see VENTILAGO VIMINALIS.
supplementary in addition to the already supplied basics.
s. feeding supplied to animals at pasture to supplement a shortfall due to inadequate supply of feed. In housed or lotted animals refers to supplements for special needs such as growth, pregnancy, lactation, flushing for fertility.
s. register when there is a register of accredited herds, registered veterinarians, studbooks, it is common practice to have a supplementary register of persons or animals who do not quite have the required qualifications but are trying to enter the list.
supplementation the provision of supplementary materials.
supplements materials used in a supplementary way. See also FEED supplements.
suppository an easily fusible medicated mass for introduction into the rectum, urethra or vagina.
suppressant 1. inducing suppression. 2. an agent that stops secretion, excretion or normal discharge.
suppression 1. sudden stoppage of a secretion, excretion or normal discharge. 2. in genetics, restoration of a lost function by a second mutation either in a gene other than that involved in the primary mutation, or within the same gene.
suppressor cells see T LYMPHOCYTE.
suppurant 1. promoting suppuration. 2. an agent causing suppuration.
suppurate produce pus.
suppuration formation or discharge of pus.
lamellar s. see LAMELLAR suppuration.
suppurative pertaining to or emanating from suppuration; pus in e.g. suppurative arthritis, bronchopneumonia.
supra- word element. [L.] *above*.
supra-acromial above the acromion.
supra-auricular above the auricle of the ear.
supracaudal organ, gland a collection of large sebaceous glands in the skin of the dorsum of the tail in cats. Excessive sebaceous secretion with inflammation gives rise to the condition known as STUD tail.
suprachiasmatic nucleus anatomic nucleus which innervates the pineal gland; thought to play a part in the management of circadian rhythms.
suprachoroid above or upon the choroid.
s. layer most superficial of the five laminae constituting the choroid; the layer is avascular and composed of collagen fibers, chromatophores, macrophages, fibroblasts.
suprachoroidea the outermost layer of the choroid.
supracondylar above a condyle.
supracostal above or outside the ribs.
supracotyloid above the acetabulum.
supradiaphragmatic above the diaphragm.
supraduction, sursumduction the turning upward of a part, especially the eyes.
supraepicondylar above the epicondyle.
supragingival a position on the side of the gingival margin towards the dental crown.
supraglenoid above the glenoid cavity.
suprahyoid above the hyoid bone.
supraliminal above the threshold of sensation.
supralumbar above the loin.
supramaxillary pertaining to the upper jaw.
supraorbital above the orbit.
s. foramen see supraorbital FORAMEN.
s. nerve block the anesthetic agent is injected into the supraorbital foramen. Anesthesia is obtained in the middle of the upper eyelid and the palpebral nerve supply is blocked.
suprapelvic above the pelvis.
suprapharmacological much greater than the usual therapeutic dose or pharmacological concentration of a drug.
suprapharyngeal diverticulum impaction impaction of the sac in pigs fed indigestible roughage causes pharyngeal obstruction and difficulty in swallowing.
suprapontine above or in the upper part of the pons.

suprapubic above the pubes.
suprarenal above a kidney; adrenal.
s. gland adrenal gland.
suprarenalectomy adrenalectomy; excision of one or both adrenal glands.
suprascapular above the scapula.
s. neuropathy suprascapular paralysis.
s. paralysis paralysis of the suprascapular nerve that leads to atrophy of the supraspinatus and infraspinatus muscles; usually due to trauma. Called also slipped shoulder, sweeney, equine suprascapular neuropathy.
suprascleral on the outer surface of the sclera.
suprasellar above the sella turcica.
supraspinal above the spine.
supraspinatus above the spine of the scapula.
suprasternal above the sternum.
supratrochlear above the trochlea.
supravaginal outside or above a sheath, specifically, above the vagina.
supravalvular above the heart valves.
s. aortic stenosis see aortic STENOSIS.
s. stenosis one of the forms of congenital constriction of the pulmonary trunk, which is dilated and thin-walled on the ventricular side of the lesion. There is a compensatory hypertrophy of the right ventricular wall.
supraventricular situated or occurring above the ventricles, especially in an atrium or atrioventricular node.
supraversion 1. abnormal elongation of a tooth from its socket. 2. sursumversion.
sura [L.] *gastrocnemius muscles.*
suramin a trypanocidal agent that is also toxic, causing degeneration of the liver, kidney and adrenal glands. It is also an inhibitor of reverse transcriptase, some types of growth factors, and causes suppression of the adrenal cortex, leading to investigations of its usefulness in the treatment of immunodeficiency infection in humans and cats, cancer and hyperadrenocorticism.
surcingle a separate, wide, thin strap or webbing passed around the horse and including the saddle and buckled tight underneath.
surditas deafness.
surface the outer part or external aspect of a body.
s.-active agent any substance capable of altering the physicochemical nature of surfaces and interfaces; an example is a detergent. Called also surfactant.
s. area conversion chart see Table 21.
s. body weight see BODY surface area.
s. catalysis in the intrinsic coagulation pathway, conversion of factor XII into its active state, factor XIIa, is catalyzed by contact with glass or a similar surface.
s. contact plates a bacteriological preparation in which the agar surface is slightly higher than the rim of the plate and inoculation is by inversion and direct contact with the surface being sampled.
surfactant a surface-active agent, such as soap or a synthetic detergent. In pulmonary physiology, a mixture of phospholipids (mainly dipalmitoylphosphatidylcholine) secreted by the great, or type II, alveolar cells into the alveoli and respiratory air passages, which reduces the surface tension of pulmonary fluids and thus contributes to the elastic properties of pulmonary tissue. See also HYALINE membrane disease.
surgeon a veterinarian who specializes in surgery. In many countries it is still the practice to continue the British tradition of having all veterinarians call themselves veterinary surgeon and for the registering legislation to be the Veterinary Surgeon's Act.
surgeon's knot same as a square knot except that the first throw is a double one. It is more secure than a square and holds its position better for the second throw. It is often reinforced by a third single throw.
surgery 1. that branch of veterinary science which treats diseases, injuries and deformities by manual or operative methods. 2. the place in a hospital, or doctor's or dentist's office where surgery is performed. 3. in some countries a room or office where a veterinarian sees and treats patients. 4. the work performed by a surgeon.
basic s. kit the collection of instruments, wrapped, sterilized and ready for use in the majority of uncomplicated surgical procedures. The choice of instruments may vary from one surgeon to another, but generally there are tissue forceps, thumb forceps, sponge forceps, hemostats, towel clamps, scalpel handle and needle holder. Scissors and needles may be added after cold sterilization.
bench s. surgery performed on an organ that has been removed from the body, after which it is reimplanted.
cold steel s. that performed with traditional cutting instruments; to distinguish from cryosurgical and electrosurgical methods.
cosmetic s. performed to improve the appearance, or change the appearance, of the animal; surgery that is not necessary for the health of the animal. Other than ear cropping and tail docking, where performed, generally discouraged or considered unethical for animals as it is usually done for purposes of improving their appearance in the show ring or to disguise traits that might be heritable.
elective s. surgery carried out at a time convenient to client and surgeon. The opposite of emergency surgery. Distinctly different to cosmetic surgery.
experimental s. that carried out as part of a planned experimental protocol, usually on animals selected specifically for the purpose and which are often sacrificed afterwards. Increasingly, use of animals in this way is under the control of institutional or governmental authorities.
plastic s. that concerned with the restoration, reconstruction, correction or improvement in the shape and appearance of body structures that are defective, damaged or misshapen by injury, disease or anomalous growth and development.
replacement s. transplanting of tissues or organs from another host. Not commonly undertaken in veterinary surgery.
veterinary s. see VETERINARY surgery.
surgical emanating from or pertaining to surgery.
s. abdomen see acute ABDOMEN.
s. cap an accompaniment to the surgical gown (below) which covers the head, and sometimes facial hair, of members of the surgical team; the object is to avoid contamination of the wound.
s. fever resulting from extensive tissue damage in major surgery.
s. gut see CATGUT.
s. insemination carried out by gaining access to the uterus by surgical means including per vaginam and via laparotomy.
s. instruments a group of instruments used in the performance of surgical operations. Nowadays there are subdivisions including ophthalmic, orthopedic, vascular, gut, thoracic and obstetric surgery.
s. mask a protective covering over the mouth and

nostrils of members of a surgical team, usually held in place by tapes tied over or behind the head, intended to minimize wound contamination.

s. needle see NEEDLE.

s. pins see PINNING.

s. scissors see standard surgical SCISSORS.

s. shock shock occurring as a result of massive or traumatic surgery. To a large extent the term is a contradiction because one of the principal objectives of surgery is the avoidance of shock but there are occasions, e.g. in a major resection of the gut in a horse or a cesarean in a mare, when extensive handling of heavy viscera is unavoidable and shock must be considered as inevitable unless preventive therapy is provided.

sterile s. pack all of the instruments and other equipment such as drapes, gloves, etc. required for a particular operation, or part of an operation, specially arranged, wrapped and sterilized by autoclaving then stored for future use.

s. suite a group of rooms designed to provide all surgical services to patients. Includes surgery, preparation and anesthesia for the patient, sterile preparation of the surgeon, instrument and materials sterilization and storage, instrument cleaning, and recovery room.

Suricata suricatta see MEERKAT.

suring RUMEX *acetosa*.

Surital a proprietary name for sodium thiamylal.

surra the disease occurring principally in camels and horses, caused by *Trypanosoma evansi* and transmitted by biting flies. The clinical syndrome, which has no diagnostic highlights, includes intermittent fever, anemia and weight loss and a high mortality rate.

surreptitious independent practice carrying on a private practice whilst supposedly fully employed by another veterinarian. This includes government or university employment. Conducting the practice in the same geographical area as that serviced by the employer is implied in the charge.

surrogate a substitute; a thing or animal that takes the place of something or some animal, as a drug used in place of another, or, in animal husbandry, an animal which takes the place of another in the family or herd environment.

sursumduction the turning upward of a part, especially the eyes.

Surti an Indian black or brown buffalo with two white collars; used for dairying.

surveillance keeping a watch over.

active s. sampling, including necropsy examination, of clinically normal samples of the population; important in the surveillance of diseases in which subclinical cases and carriers predominate.

epidemiological s. watching over a population and recording data likely to have epidemiological significance, usually with the aim of early detection of disease. Essentially an interventionist exercise compared with monitoring, which is passive.

passive s. examination of only clinically affected cases of specified diseases in the population.

survey a comprehensive examination of an area or population for a particular purpose. The survey may be of a part, e.g. cross-sectional survey, or for a particular end-result, e.g. a prevalence survey, or by the use of a particular method, e.g. aerial survey, or a combination of these, e.g. seroepidemiological.

s. radiograph a plain radiograph of a large area before embarking on a special radiographic technique for achieving special results. Called also scout radiography.

survivorship rate proportion of the population that are still alive at successive annual ages.

Sus a genus of wild pigs typified by the wild boar (*Sus scrofa*). Other species are *S. barbatus* (bearded pig), *S. salvanius* (pygmy hog), *S. verrucosus* (Javan warty pig); occurs on most continents.

susceptibility the state of being susceptible. Refers usually to infectious disease but may be to physical factors such as wetting or to psychological factors such as harassment. Signs which suggest a state of increased susceptibility to infection are: infections in the first few weeks of life, repeated bouts of infection, infections with nonvirulent pathogens, attacks of illness after vaccination with attenuated vaccines, and low leukocyte counts. See also IMMUNE deficiency disease.

susceptible readily affected or acted upon; lacking immunity or resistance.

suscitate to arouse to greater activity.

suscitation an arousal to greater activity.

suspension 1. temporary cessation, as of pain or a vital process. 2. a supporting from above, as in treatment of spinal disorders. 3. a preparation of a finely divided, undissolved substance dispersed in a liquid vehicle.

colloid s. one in which the suspended particles are very small.

suspensoid a colloid system in which the disperse phase consists of particles of any insoluble substance, such as a metal, and the dispersion medium may be gaseous, liquid or solid.

suspensory 1. serving to hold up a part. 2. a ligament, bone, muscle, bandage or sling for supporting a part.

s. ligament 1. the modified interosseous muscle of the horse that arises from the palmar carpal ligament behind the knee (or the hock in the hindlimb) and suspends the pair of sesamoid bones behind the fetlock. The distal continuation of the ligament is composed of the cruciate, oblique and straight sesamoidian ligaments and the pair of extensor branches that unite with the common digital extensor tendon. 2. various other supporting ligaments.

s. ligament of the lens delicate ligament suspending the lens from the ciliary body of the eye.

ovarian s. ligament a peritoneal fold which forms the cranial limit to the mesovarium.

rupture of udder s. ligament the medial attachment separates, the udder floor drops down and outwards so that the teats point laterally. The cow is difficult to milk, especially with a machine.

Sussex a solid red breed of beef cattle similar to the Devon. There are horned and polled breeds.

Sussex spaniel a massive, strongly built dog with short, well-boned legs. It has a broad head, deep chest, pendulous ears and an abundant, flat, golden liver-colored coat with feathering on the legs, ears and lower body. The tail is docked to a medium length. The breed has a characteristic rolling gait.

sustained-release preparations formulations of medicines which limit their solubility so that they are delivered at a slow but steady rate into the blood supply. Includes oral preparations in the form of reticular bullets of metal or ceramic and slow-release granules, intramuscular injection of slowly soluble substances, e.g. procaine penicillin, or drugs suspended in oil or in tablets, usually deposited under the skin. Microsyringes, described as osmotic pumps, are also being used for the pulsatile delivery of hormones over a long period.

s.-r. p. for bloat control capsules containing antifoaming agents or ionophores are administered by mouth.

sustentacular supporting; sustaining.
s. cell a supporting epithelial cell which lacks a specialist function.
sustentaculum pl. *sustentaculi* [L.] a support.
s. tali a medial process of the calcaneus, extending over the plantar aspect of the talus.
susurrus [L.] *murmur*.
sutilains proteolytic enzymes derived from a strain of *Bacillus subtilis* used for wound débridement.
sutura pl. *suturae* [L.] suture; used in anatomical nomenclature to designate a type of joint in which the apposed bony surfaces are united by fibrous tissue, permitting little or no movement; found only between bones of the skull.
s. lambdoides see lambdoid SUTURE.
s. sagittalis see sagittal SUTURE.
suturation the process or act of suturing.
suture 1. the line of union of adjoining bones of the skull. See also SUTURA. 2. the linear union of fibers from the equator of the lens, meeting on the anterior and posterior surfaces. May be the location of metabolic cataracts. 3. a stitch or series of stitches made to secure apposition of the edges of a surgical or traumatic wound (see suture pattern below); used also as a verb to indicate application of such stitches. 4. material used in closing a wound with stitches.
absorbable s. (4) a strand of organic or synthetic material used for closing wounds, which becomes dissolved in the body fluids and disappears, such as catgut and tendon or polydioxanone.
apposition s. (3) a superficial suture used for exact approximation of the cutaneous edges of a wound.
approximation s. (3) a deep suture for securing apposition of the deep tissue of a wound.
automatic ridge suture see MATTRESS SUTURE PATTERN.
braided s. (4) thin filaments braided into a single suture; has the virtues of strength, flexibility, ease of handling and good knot security.
Bunnell s. (3) see BUNNELL SUTURE PATTERN.
buried s. (3) one placed deep in the tissues and concealed by the skin.
Caslick s. (3) see CASLICK operation.
catgut s. (4) see CATGUT.
Chinese finger cuff s. (3) a method of securing a thoracostomy tube to the thoracic wall in which the suture is placed deeply into the skin and underlying tissue and the ends are wrapped around the protruding tube in a spiral pattern ('Chinese finger cuff') and tied.
circular s. (3) one applied around the cicumference of a hollow viscus to close it, or to a portion of the wall to bring about inversion of the wall.
cobbler's s. (3) one made with suture material threaded through a needle at each end.
Connell s. (3) see CONNELL SUTURE PATTERN.
continuous s. (3) one in which a continuous, uninterrupted length of material is used. Called also whip stitch.
continuous lock s. (3) see LOCK-STITCH SUTURE PATTERN.
coronal s. (1) the line of union between the frontal bone and the parietal bones.
cotton s. (4) a multifilament suture used mainly for closure of skin.
cranial s. (1) the lines of junction between the bones of the skull.
cruciate s. (3) see CRUCIATE suture pattern.
Cushing s. (3) see CUSHING SUTURE PATTERN.
Czerny s. (3) see CZERNY SUTURE.
Czerny–Lembert s. (3) see CZERNY–LEMBERT SUTURE.
false s. (1) a line of junction between apposed surfaces without a serrated union of the bones.
far–near–far s. (3) see NEAR–FAR–FAR–NEAR SUTURE PATTERN.
figure-eight s. (3) a row of surgical pins are placed through both edges of the wound and suture material is wound back and forth around each pin, as with a shoelace.
four stitch interrupted s. (3) see MATTRESS SUTURE PATTERN.
furrier's s. (3) simple continuous suture.
Gambee s. (3) see GAMBEE SUTURE PATTERN.
Gély's s. (3) see GÉLY'S SUTURE PATTERN.
Goetze's s. (3) see GOETZE'S SUTURE PATTERN.
Halsted s. (3) see HALSTED suture pattern.
interrupted s. (3) one in which each stitch is made with a separate piece of material.
intradermal s. (3) one placed in the lower dermis; a buried suture. May be interrupted or continuous.
intracutaneous s. (3) one totally within the substance of the skin, not emerging externally and not into the subcutaneous tissues. See also intradermal suture (above).
inverting s. (3) one that turns the edges of the incision inward so the exposed surfaces, usually serosa, contact each other and the edges of the incision are buried. Used in closure of hollow viscera such as the stomach, uterus, intestine or visceral stumps. Includes the Connell, Cushing, Halsted, Lembert and Parker–Kerr suture patterns.
lambdoid s. (1) the line of union between the upper borders of the occipital and parietal bones, shaped like the Greek letter lambda; called also sutura lambdoides.
Lembert s. (3) see LEMBERT SUTURE PATTERN.
McLean s. (3) see MCLEAN SUTURE PATTERN.
mattress s. (3) see MATTRESS SUTURE PATTERN.
Mersilene s. (4) an uncoated polyester suture material.
metal s. (4) stainless steel is used universally. There are also special metal devices including Michel clips and skin staples and staples for intestinal repair.
near–far–far–near s. (3) see NEAR–FAR–FAR–NEAR SUTURE PATTERN.
non-absorbable s. (4) includes silk, steel, polyester, polymerized caprolactam, polypropylene, polyethylene, nylon and cotton.
nylon s. (4) may be braided or monofilament.
Parker–Kerr s. (3) see PARKER–KERR SUTURE PATTERN.
s. pattern (3) the placement of suture material, usually designed to achieve a particular purpose in relation to the tissue, organ or surgical procedure being performed, e.g. inversion or eversion of wound edges, relief of tension on the wound, or cosmetic results.
s. pin (4) sharp-pointed pins that can be pushed through tissue, e.g. vulval lips, and secured at both ends by knobs so that they stay in situ.
pull-out s. (3) see PULL-OUT SUTURE PATTERN.
purse-string s. (3) a type of suture commonly used to bury the stump of the appendix, a continuous running suture being placed about the opening, and then drawn tight.
relaxation s. (3) any suture so formed that it may be loosened to relieve tension as necessary.
retention s. (3) used in the replacement of vaginal and uterine prolapse in cattle. Usually thick, heavy suture material, sometimes tape, is placed through adjacent tissues.

round-wound s. (3) used for tension relief, it consists of surgical pins placed through both sides of the wound and suture material wound around the protruding ends and across the incision.
safety s. (3) used in the surgical correction of patent ductus arteriosus, particularly in small dogs, to ensure that any slippage of ligatures or tissue will not result in excessive blood loss before being controlled by other means.
sagittal s. (1) the line of union of the two parietal bones, dividing the skull anteroposteriorly into two symmetrical halves; called also sutura sagittalis.
silk s. (4) braided silk is used as a nonabsorbable suture. It may be coated with wax or silicone to reduce its absorption of fluids. Its great advantages are its ease of handling and good knot-holding quality.
squamous s. (1) a suture where the uniting bones overlap such as the suture between the pars squamosa of the temporal bone and parietal bone.
stainless steel s. (4) see wire suture (below).
stent s. (3) a tension suture for closing wounds created by placing a roll of bandage along the line of incision and tying the sutures over the top of it.
subcuticular s. (3), subcutaneous s. a method of skin closure involving placement of stitches in the subcuticular tissues parallel with the line of the wound.
tension s. (3) one placed to relieve tension on the incision; may be the same suture pattern that closes the incision or a separate suture or line of sutures of a different pattern.
U-s. see MATTRESS SUTURE PATTERN.
vest-over-pants s. (3) see VEST-OVER-PANTS SUTURE PATTERN.
walking s. (3) a pattern of interrupted sutures used in closing large skin wounds. Each suture is placed first in the deep dermis and then into the deeper tissues, usually fascia, at a point closer to the center of the wound. The effect is to move the skin closer to the closing position with each suture, obliterate dead space, and relieve tension on the sutures eventually placed to close the wound edges.
wire s. (4) stainless steel wire used as suture material as monofilament or braided. Problems are kinking, bulk knots, tearing of tissues and the need for special cutting instruments.
Zimmerman's aluminum wire s. (3) a technique used for tension support. The stitches are placed with a cannula and ends are rolled instead of being tied.

suture knot may be tied manually or by instrument in several patterns. See also SQUARE KNOT, SURGEON'S KNOT.

suture pattern see SUTURE pattern.

suxamethonium see SUCCINYLCHOLINE.

Sv sievert.

SV-5 virus simian virus type 5; see PARAINFLUENZA-VIRUS 2.

SVD swine vesicular disease.

SVE special visceral efferent.

Svedberg a unit used to express sedimentation coefficients. Symbol S.

swab 1. a small pledget of cotton or gauze wrapped around the end of a slender wooden stick or wire for applying medications or obtaining specimens of secretions, etc., from body surfaces or orifices. 2. use of a swab to collect a specimen, e.g. collection of a sample of saliva for testing horses for doping.

swage 1. to shape metal by hammering or by adapting it to a die. 2. to fuse, as suture material to the end of a suture needle.

Swainsona Australian genus of plants in the legume family Fabaceae, closely related to *Astragalus*; contain the toxic indolizidine alkaloid swainsonine which causes tremor, incoordination, mania and death from an acquired lysosomal storage disease through inhibition of α-mannosidase so that mannose accumulates in nervous and other tissues. Toxic species include *S. brachycarpa* (small-flowered Darling pea), *S. canescens* (gray Swainson pea), *S. galegifolia* (smooth Darling pea), *S. greyana* (Darling pea), *S. luteola* (dwarf Darling pea), *S. procumbens* (Broughton pea), *S. swainsonioides*. See also MANNOSIDOSIS, ASTRAGALUS, SWAINSONINE, LYSOSOMAL storage diseases.

swainsonine a trihydroxylated indolizidine alkaloid found in *Swainsona* spp., *Schizoctonia leguminicola* and *Astragalus* spp. It is a potent α-mannosidase inhibitor and poisoning by it leads to accumulation of mannosidose in tissues.

Swale gag see BAYER GAG.

Swaledale sheep English carpetwool, meat sheep, black face, gray muzzle; similar to Black-faced mountain sheep.

swallow 1. the amount of ingesta that can be swallowed at one time. 2. to perform the act of swallowing.
barium s. see BARIUM swallow.

swallowing the taking in of a substance through the mouth and pharynx and into the esophagus. It is a combination of a voluntary act and a series of reflex actions. Once begun, the process operates automatically. Called also deglutition.
s. disorders difficulty in swallowing may be caused by foreign body obstruction, by inflammation of the lining or by a defect in nervous control. The nerves involved are the sensory and motor branches of the trigeminal nerve, the hypoglossal, the facial and the glossopharyngeal nerves. Called also dysphagia.
s. reflex begins as soon as the bolus of ingesta approaches the entry to the pharynx. In a series of reflex actions: breathing is halted, the soft palate elevates and closes the entrance to the nasal cavities, the tongue is clamped into the fauces, closing the exit from the pharynx back into the mouth, the epiglottis closes off the larynx, the pharynx contracts and forces the bolus into the esophagus, peristalsis-like movements in the esophagus carry the food to the cardia which relaxes and the food is propelled into the stomach. Called also palatal reflex.
repeated s. a sign of partial esophageal obstruction.

swamp pertaining to low-lying, marshy ground.
s. beaver see COYPU.
s. dock RUMEX *brownii*.
s. grass-tree XANTHORRHEA *fulva*.
s. maple ACER *rubrum*.
s. wilkweed ASCLEPIAS *incarnata*.

swamp cancer a common lesion of the skin and mucosae of horses in tropical and subtropical regions. The lesions are dense granulation tissue in the form of an ulcer which may rapidly extend to 8 inches diameter. The tissue may contain cores of necrotic yellow or black, sometimes calcified, material referred to colloquially as leeches, grains or kunkurs. Distribution of the lesions varies with the etiology, but is concentrated mostly on the legs and ventral abdomen, below the medial canthus of the eye and on the muzzle and nearby mucosae. The cause may be any one of the following: *Habronema megastoma* larvae, or one of the fungi *Hyphomyces destruens*, *Basidiobolus haptosporus* or *Entomophthora coronata*. Called also hyphomycosis, bursatti, cutaneous habronemiasis, summer sore, equine phycomycosis, equine pythiosis, Florida horse leech.

swamp fever see EQUINE infectious anemia.
swamp itch see SCHISTOSOME dermatitis.
swampy back said of sheep and cattle; an exaggerated depression of the back between the withers and the loin.
swan a member of the genera *Coscoroba* or *Cygnus* in the tribe Anserini (geese and swans) in the family Anatidae (ducks, geese and swans). The swans are the largest birds, they have long flexible necks, paddle and swim but they do not dive.
Swan–Ganz catheter a soft, flow-directed catheter with a balloon at the tip for measuring pulmonary arterial pressures, right atrial pressures, left atrial pressure, and reflected left ventricular end-diastolic pressure.

The catheter permits evaluation of cardiac function by assessing the effectiveness of right and left pumping action of the heart and providing a quantitative measurement of cardiac output, and by allowing for sampling of mixed arterial–venous oxygen levels and calculation of differences between the two.
swan plant GOMPHOCARPUS *physocarpus*.
Swann Report a report by the Swann Committee on Veterinary Education which made, among other matters, a strong recommendation that preventive veterinary medicine should be better taught in UK veterinary schools.
swarming 1. a phenomenon observed in cultures of *Proteus* spp. on solid media in which there is progressive surface spreading from the parent colony. 2. the periodic bee migration of the old queen and accompanying workers and drones from a full original hive which is left to be fought over by the new young queens.
Swartzia madagascariensis African plant in the legume family Fabaceae; ripe pods contain an unidentified toxin which causes red discoloration of the urine.
sway-backed a marked lordosis in the back of a horse.
sway response clinical test in which the animal is pulled laterally by the tail or pushed sideways on the rump while it is walking. Absence of the normal response, a resistance to being swayed or a smart sidestep to save from falling, is taken as indicating that normal balancing reflexes are not functioning.
swayback one of the syndromes caused by a primary nutritional deficiency of copper. It may be congenital with lambs unable to stand or suck, spastic paralysis, sometimes blindness, or delayed, appearing at 3 to 6 weeks of age. There is incoordination and spasticity. See also ENZOOTIC ataxia.
sweat the excretion of the sweat (sudoriparous) glands of the skin; perspiration. Sweating produces an evaporative cooling of the body, the importance varying between species, and also serves an excretory function. Substances eliminated in sweat include water, sodium chloride and small amounts of urea, lactic acid and potassium ions. In humans the ability to lose heat by sweating is much greater than that in domestic animals. Cattle have a high sweat rate (150 $g/m^2/h$ at 40°C), sheep lose less (32 $g/m^2/h$) and dogs lose an insignificant amount. Horses probably have the highest sweat rate of all.

Excessive sweating is called diaphoresis, hyperhidrosis.

atrichial s. gland see sweat glands (below).

eccrine s. gland called also atrichial sweat gland; see sweat glands (below).

s. fly *Morrelia aenescens*, *M. hortorum*, *M. simplex*.

s. glands the glands that secrete sweat, situated in the corium or subcutaneous tissue, and opening by a duct on the surface of the body. They are of two types: (1) the ordinary or eccrine sweat glands are unbranched, coiled, tubular glands that promote cooling by evaporation of their secretion. They are innervated by cholinergic nerve fibers; (2) the APOCRINE sweat glands are large, branched, specialized glands that empty into the upper portion of a hair follicle instead of directly onto the skin surface, and have no secretory innervation but are sensitive to epinephrine in the bloodstream. Called also sudoriferous, or sudoriparous, glands.

paratrichial s. gland see APOCRINE sweat gland.

s. scraper a semicircular band of metal with a handle to be dragged over a horse's skin like a squeegee to remove excess moisture quickly.
sweating 1. the production of sweat. Its importance as a cooling mechanism varies between species, being important in cows but not so in dogs. See also SWEAT. 2. meat that has been in cold store condenses air moisture onto it when it comes out into room temperature and is said to sweat. 3. see FELLMONGERING.

s. pens pens in which sheep are held before shearing.

s. sickness a tick toxicosis of young cattle caused by the bites of *Hyalomma truncatum* (syn. *H. transiens*) characterized by hyperemia of the mucosae and an extensive moist eczema which may lead to sloughing. Called also dyshidrosis tropicale.
swede BRASSICA *napobrassica*.

s. rape *B. napus*.

s. turnip *B. napobrassica*.
Swedish cattle indigenous to Sweden.

S. Friesian cattle Swedish version of Friesian.

S. red-and-white cattle red with small white markings, Swedish dairy cattle, originated from local breed plus Ayrshire.
Swedish cattledog see SWEDISH VALLHUND.
Swedish clover TRIFOLIUM *hybridum* (Alsike clover).
Swedish Lapland dog a medium-sized, spitz-type dog with a thick, standing haircoat in black, brown or other solid colors, sometimes with white marks on the chest, feet and tip of tail. Very similar to, but larger than, the Finnish Lapphund. The breed is affected with an hereditary neuronal abiotrophy. Called also Swedish lapphund.
Swedish lapphund see SWEDISH LAPLAND DOG.
Swedish red spotted cattle a breed of red cattle with small white markings, a white-spotted red cow; used for dairying. Called also Swedish red and white cattle.
Swedish Vallhund a small (20–32 lb), powerfully built working dog with a long body, long head, pointed erect ears and moderately short legs. (The breed standards call for a height to body length ratio of 2:5.) The coat is medium length, abundant and woolly in shades of gray, brown, red or yellow. The tail is naturally short or docked to a medium length. Called also Vasgotaspets, Swedish cattledog.
sweeney see SUPRASCAPULAR paralysis.
sweet opposite of sour.

s. birch oil see METHYL salicylate.

s. buckeye tree AESCULUS *octandra*.

s. clover MELILOTUS *alba*.

s. feed a mixture of rolled grain and molasses used to tempt convalescent horses and cattle.

s. grass PANICUM *schinzii*.

s. itch an intensely itchy dermatitis of horses caused by hypersensitivity to the bites of *Culicoides* spp. The lesions are worst in the summer months and most evident along the middle of the back. The skin is thickened and the hair is missing. Called also Queensland itch. See equine ALLERGIC dermatitis.

s. oil olive oil.

s. pea LATHYRUS *odoratus*.

s. potato IPOMOEA *batatas*.

s. vernal grass ANTHOXANTHUM ODORATUM.

sweetbread an abattoir expression for calf thymus.

gut s. pancreas.

true s. thymus.

sweetsiekte HYALOMMA toxicosis.

swell body the alar fold in the nostril of dogs.

swell can see BLOWER CAN.

swelled head a disease of rams, a form of malignant edema caused by *Clostridium septicum* or other *Clostridia* spp. The swelling and emphysema are present only on the head and neck. The disease is thought to occur as a result of fighting. Called also ovine bighead.

swellhead a disease of sheep caused by photosensitization. See also SWELLED HEAD.

swelling 1. transient abnormal enlargement of a body part of area not due to cell proliferation. 2. an eminence, or elevation.

cloudy s. a term which has been discarded. It was used to describe an early stage of toxic degenerative changes, especially in protein constituents of organs in infectious diseases, in which the tissues appear swollen, parboiled and opaque but revert to normal when the cause is removed. Called also albuminoid, or albuminous, degeneration.

genital s., labioscrotal s. in the male embryo overlie the inguinal canal development; in the female shift anteriorly and, in most species, disappear before birth.

laryngeal s. eminences which develop lateral to the laryngotracheal groove in the embryo.

scrotal s. primordial scrotum.

swept gain controls see TIME gain compensation.

swill cooked edible garbage fed to pigs.

swimmer see FLAT PUPPY SYNDROME.

swimmer's itch see SCHISTOSOMIASIS.

swimming exercise therapy a form of physical therapy employed in animals, usually horses or dogs.

swine pertaining to or emanating from swine (pigs, hogs). See also PORCINE.

African s. fever see AFRICAN SWINE FEVER.

s. dysentery a contagious disease of young pigs caused by *Serpulina hyodysenteriae*, characterized by severe porridge-like diarrhea, sometimes dysentery, dehydration and heavy morbidity and mortality rates.

s. erysipelas see ERYSIPELAS.

s. fever see HOG cholera.

s. influenza a highly contagious upper respiratory disease of pigs caused by swine influenza virus and a concurrent infection with *Haemophilus influenzae*. Clinical signs include fever, stiffness, recumbency, labored breathing, sneezing, paroxysmal cough and nasal and ocular discharge. Called also ferkelgrippe.

s. paramyxovirus see PARAMYXOVIRUS encephalomyelitis.

s. paratyphoid see SALMONELLOSIS.

s. plague fibrinous pneumonia caused by *Pasteurella multocida*. May occur in outbreak form with a number of litters of young pigs being affected within a short time.

s. vesicular disease is a highly infectious disease of pigs caused by an enterovirus related to human coxsackie B5 virus. It is clinically indistinguishable from foot-and-mouth disease in pigs. Vesicular lesions occur at the coronet, causing severe lameness, and in the mouth and on the snout.

vesicular exanthema of s. see VESICULAR exanthema of swine.

swine infertility and respiratory syndrome see PORCINE reproductive and respiratory syndrome.

swineherd's disease see LEPTOSPIROSIS.

swinepox a disease caused by either of two pox viruses, true swine poxvirus (suipoxvirus) or vaccinia virus. There are typical pox lesions, most commonly on the abdominal skin, and, in adult pigs, not much else. Piglets may have lesions on the face and have a concurrent conjunctivitis and some may die. *Haematopinus suis* is thought to transmit the disease in older pigs whereas suckers probably are infected by contact with the sow's udder.

swinge coat a haircoat that is short, sparse and curly.

swingle-bar wooden spreader used to keep trace chains apart behind draft animals.

swinney see SUPRASCAPULAR paralysis.

Swiss frill a breed of canary characterized by a curved body and voluminous, frilled breast feathers and a mantle with feathers falling symmetrically over the shoulders.

Swiss mountain dog see BERNESE MOUNTAIN DOG.

switch 1. in an x-ray machine, the on–off switch controls the input of electricity to the x-ray machine. 2. the hairy part of the tail of a cow. 3. in immunology refers to the change from the production of one form or class of antibody by a B lymphocyte to another; the differentiiation occurs only in the C region of their heavy chain.

s. sites repetitive nucleotide sequences located between most of the C genes.

switchgrass see PANICUM *virgatum*.

swollen head syndrome a disease of domestic poultry caused by a combination of a pneumovirus and adventitious bacteria, usually *Escherichia coli*. Often associated with outbreaks of rhinotracheitis in turkeys, thought to be caused by the same virus. Clinically the disease occurs in broiler breeders causing swelling of the periorbital and infraorbital sinuses and submandibular edema. Young birds also show signs of severe respiratory disease.

swordtail an aquarium fish, *Xiphophorus* spp., a member of the suborder Cyprinodontei.

Sx abbreviation for surgery; used in medical records.

sycosiform resembling sycosis.

sycosis a papulopustular inflammation of the hair follicles in humans. The term is not used in veterinary medicine but the animal diseases that fit this definition best are equine staphylococcal dermatitis, Canadian horsepox and demodectic mange.

Sydney golden wattle ACACIA *longifolia*.

Sydney rock oyster see SACCOSTREA COMMERCIALIS.

Sydney silky see SILKY TERRIER.

sylade a chemical additive used in the making of ensilage. A strong suspect at one time to be related in some way to the etiology of the pyrexia–pruritus–hemorrhage syndrome of cattle.

sylvan emanating from or pertaining to woods. See also SYLVATIC.

sylvatic found in the woods; occurring in animals of the forest.

s. plague the disease of wild rats, ground squirrels, mice, marmots, owls, gophers, badgers, rabbits, prairie dogs and chipmunks caused by *Yersinia pestis*, and which serves as a reservoir for urban rats which are the origin, via the oriental rat flea (*Xenopsylla cheopis*), of bubonic plague in humans.

s. rabies that form of the disease transmitted by forest-dwelling animals, particularly foxes and wolves.

s. ringworm ringworm in domestic animals transmitted from wild animals.
sylvian aqueduct cerebral aqueduct.
sylvian fissure a fissure extending laterally between the temporal and frontal lobes, and turning posteriorly between the temporal and parietal lobes. Called also fissure of Sylvius, lateral cerebral sulcus.
Sylvicapra see DUIKER.
Sylvicapra grimmia see DUIKER.
Sylvilagus the rabbit genus of lagomorphs in the family Leporidae. The wild rabbit lives in burrows, is herbivorous and feeds mostly at dawn and dusk. They have great powers of reproduction and have been a serious agricultural pest in some countries. The domestic variety is extensively used in laboratories and there are special varieties for the commercial production of rabbitmeat and for pelt and fur production. Common species are *Sylvilagus bachmani* (brush rabbit) the reservoir of the myxomatosis virus in USA, *Sylvilagus floridanus* (Eastern cottontail) and *Oryctolagus cuniculus* (European domestic and wild rabbit). See also ANGORA rabbit, ARGENTÉ, BELGIAN hare, BEVEREN, CALIFORNIAN, DUTCH, ENGLISH, FLEMISH GIANT, HAVANA, HIMALAYAN (2), LOP, NETHERLAND DWARF, NEW ZEALAND red, NEW ZEALAND white, POLISH, REX (2), RUSSIAN, SABLE (2), SATIN, SIBERIAN, SILVER FOX. Other colors include fox, harlequin, lilac, silver, smoke pearl, tan.
sym- prefix meaning together.
symballophone a stethoscope with two chest pieces, making possible the comparison and localization of sounds.
symbiont an organism or species living in a state of symbiosis.
symbiosis the biological association of two individuals or populations of different species, classified as mutualism, commensalism, parasitism, amensalism or synnecrosis, depending on the advantage or disadvantage derived from the relationship.
symbiote symbiont.
symbiotic mange chorioptic mange.
symblepharon adhesion of an eyelid(s) to the eyeball.
symblepharopterygium symblepharon in which the adhesion is a cicatricial band resembling a pterygium.
symmelus a fetus with fused legs.
symmetrical equally on both sides.
s. multifocal encephalopathy inherited disease in two forms: Limousin form appears at about a month old with blindness, forelimb hypermetria, hyperesthesia, nystagmus, aggression, weight loss; Simmental form does not appear until 5–8 months, no blindness, hindquarters affected instead of forelimbs. Euthanasia inevitable in both forms.
s. poliomalalacia see focal symmetrical spinal POLIOMALACIA.
symmetry correspondence in size, form and arrangement of parts on opposite sides of a plane, or around an axis. Often used to describe conformation.
bilateral s. the configuration of an irregularly shaped body (such as the body of a higher animal) that can be divided by a longitudinal plane into halves that are mirror images of each other.
radial s. that in which the body parts are arranged regularly around a central axis.
sympathectomize to deprive of sympathetic innervation.
sympathectomy excision or interruption of some portion of the sympathetic nervous pathway. The operation produces temporary vasodilatation leading to improved nutrition of the part supplied by the vessel.
chemical s. the interruption of the transmission of impulses through a sympathetic nerve by chemical agents.
periarterial s. surgical removal of the sheath of an artery containing the sympathetic nerve fibers; it produces temporary vasodilatation.
sympathetic pertaining to the sympathetic nervous system.
s. chain the sympathetic trunk whose ganglia suggest a chain of beads.
s. cholinergic vasodilator fibers a system of efferent dilator nerves distributed only to skeletal muscles; the existence of the system has been verified only in cats and dogs; in other species where it is not present vasodilation is achieved only by relaxation of vasoconstrictor tone.
s. nerves 1. see sympathetic trunk (below). 2. any nerve of the sympathetic nervous system.
s. nervous system the part of the AUTONOMIC nervous system whose preganglionic fibers arise from cell bodies in the thoracic and lumbar segments of the spinal cord; postganglionic fibers are distributed to the heart, smooth muscle, and glands of the entire body.
s. outflow the preganglionic fibers from the nerve cells in the thoracolumbar cord.
s. regurgitation see neurotic REGURGITATION.
s. trunk two long ganglionated nerve strands, one on each side of the vertebral column, extending from the base of the skull to the coccyx.
s. trunk ganglia ganglia situated segmentally along the paired sympathetic trunks beside the vertebral bodies.
sympathicoblast an embryonic cell that develops into a sympathetic nerve cell. See also SYMPATHOGONIUM.
sympathicoblastoma a malignant tumor containing sympathicoblasts.
sympathicolytic sympatholytic.
sympathicomimetic sympathomimetic.
sympathicotonia a stimulated condition of the sympathetic nervous system marked by vascular spasm, heightened blood pressure, and the dominance of other sympathetic functions.
sympathicotripsy surgical crushing of a nerve, ganglion or plexus of the sympathetic nervous system.
sympathicotropic 1. having affinity for or exerting its principal effect on the sympathetic nervous system. 2. an agent with such properties.
sympathicus the sympathetic nervous system.
sympathin a neurohormonal mediator of nerve impulses at sympathetic nerve synapses; the term is used only when the nature of the mediator is unknown.
sympathoadrenal 1. pertaining to the sympathetic nervous system and the adrenal medulla. 2. involving the sympathetic nervous system and the adrenal glands, especially increased sympathetic activity that causes increased secretion of epinephrine by the adrenal medulla and norepinephrine by the postganglionic sympathetic nerve endings.
s. discharge the sympathoadrenal system can discharge as one unit and prepare the animal in all systems for immediate fight or flight. There is an increase in heart rate, ventricular contractile strength, cardiac output, blood pressure plus pupillary dilatation, increased respiratory rate, bronchiolar dilatation, diversion of blood flow from the splanchnic to skeletal muscle circulation and elevation of the blood sugar.
sympathoblast sympathicoblast.

sympathoblastoma sympathicoblastoma.
sympathogonioma a tumor composed of sympathogonia.
sympathogonium pl. *sympathogonia* [Gr.] an embryonic cell that develops into a sympathetic cell.
sympatholytic antiadrenergic: blocking transmission of impulses from the adrenergic (sympathetic) postganglionic fibers to effector organs or tissues, inhibiting such sympathetic functions as smooth muscle contraction and glandular secretion. Also, an agent that produces such an effect.
sympathomimetic adrenergic: producing effects resembling those of impulses transmitted by the postganglionic fibers of the sympathetic nervous system. Also, an agent that produces such an effect.
sympathy an influence produced in any organ by disease or disorder in another part. See also sympathetic OPHTHALMIA.
symphalangism congenital ankylosis of the proximal phalangeal joints.
Symphoromyia a genus of flies which is ordinarily predatory on other flies but which are blood-suckers and do inflict a painful bite. They are members of the family Rhagionidae.
symphyseal, symphysial pertaining to a symphysis.
symphysiorrhaphy suture of a divided symphysis.
symphysiotomy surgical division of a symphysis.
mandibular s. performed in order to achieve better access to the pharynx and posterior buccal cavity.
pubic s. performed to facilitate delivery, most commonly in under-age or overfat heifers. In the management of chronic obstipation in cats, the pelvic diameter is enlarged by symphysiotomy and maintained with an iliac bone graft.
symphysis pl. *symphyses* [Gr.] a type of joint in which the apposed bony surfaces are firmly united by a plate of fibrocartilage or cartilage; e.g. intermandibular joint, pelvic symphysis. There is usually cartilage against each bone and fibrous tissue or fibrocartilage in the middle.
ischiatic s. the line of fusion between the bodies of the ischia.
mandibular s. the joint between the two halves of the mandible which allows each half to rotate, as in the jaws of the dog, cat, ruminants and many other species, is a cartilaginous symphysis. In the jaws of horses and pigs the mandibles are fused together.
pelvic s. the combined pubic and ischiatic symphyses, a cartilaginous symphysis.
pubic s., s. pubis the line of union of the bodies of the pubic bones in the median plane.
Symphytum genus in plant family Boraginaceae; contain pyrrolizidine alkaloids and can cause poisoning if eaten in large quantities. Include *S. asperum* (rough comfrey), *S. officinale* (comfrey), *S. uplandicum* (Russian comfrey).
Symplocarpus foetidus North American member of the plant family Araceae; contains calcium oxalate raphide crystals which cause stomatitis; called also skunk cabbage.
sympodia fusion of the lower extremities.
symport a structure that transports two compounds simultaneously across a cell membrane in the same direction, one compound being transported down a concentration gradient, the other against a gradient.
symptom any indication of disease perceived by the patient and a term therefore not applicable to animals. The expression used instead is 'clinical signs'.
symptomatic 1. pertaining to or of the nature of a symptom. The word symptom is not used in veterinary medicine because the subjective sensations of our patients are not known to us. However, because there is no comparable word relating to clinical sign, the principal means by which veterinarians arrive at diagnoses, it is customary to use the word symptomatic in this context, that is as pertaining to or in the nature of a clinical sign. 2. indicative (of a particular disease or disorder). 3. exhibiting the symptoms of a particular disease but having a different cause. 4. directed at the allaying of symptoms, as symptomatic treatment.
s. anthrax see BLACKLEG.
symptomatology 1. the study of the science of clinical signs. 2. the combined clinical signs of a disease.
symptomatolytic causing the disappearance of clinical signs.
sympus a fetus with feet and legs fused.
syn- word element. [Gr.] *union, association.*
Synadenium arborescens South African plant in the family Euphorbiaceae; used as a tropical garden shrub; contains a milky sap (latex) which irritates mucosae, causes diarrhea, but the toxin has not been identified. Called also African milk bush.
Synalar see FLUOCINOLONE ACETONIDE.
Synanceichthys verrucosa see STONEFISH.
Synanceja trachynis see STONEFISH.
synancejid see STONEFISH.
synanthropic ecologically associated with humans.
Synapis see SINAPIS.
synapse the junction between the processes of two neurons or between a neuron and an effector organ, where neural impulses are transmitted by chemical means. The impulse causes the release of a neurotransmitter (e.g. acetylcholine or norepinephrine) from the presynaptic membrane of the axon terminal. The neurotransmitter molecules diffuse across the synaptic cleft, bind with specific receptors on the postsynaptic membrane, causing depolarization or hyperpolarization of the postsynaptic cell. See also NEURON.
adrenergic s. the neurotransmitter is norepinephrine. See also ADRENERGIC (1).
axoaxonic s. see AXOAXONIC.
axodendritic s. see AXODENTRITIC.
axodendrosomatic s. one between the axon of one neuron and the dendrites and body of another.
axosomatic s. see AXOSOMATIC.
cholinergic s. the neurotransmitter is acetylcholine. See also CHOLINERGIC.
dendrodendritic s. one from a dendrite of one cell to a dendrite of another.
excitatory s. a synapse in which the transmission of impulses is electrical not chemical. Found only in fish and invertebrates.
inhibitory s. hyperpolarizing electrical current is used to raise the threshold for the stimulation of a discharge of an impulse from the particular kind of nerve cell, found only in fish.
synapsis the pairing off and union of homologous chromosomes from male and female pronuclei at the start of meiosis.
synaptic pertaining to a synapse.
s. cleft a narrow space between the plasma membranes of the presynaptic and postsynaptic cells.
s. junction see SYNAPSE.
s. vesicle one located in the axon terminal of a presynaptic cell, containing neurotransmitter substances.
synaptosomes discrete units of pre- and postsynaptic membranes.
synarthrodia synarthrosis.
synarthrodial pertaining to a synarthrosis.

synarthrophysis any ankylosing process.
synarthrosis pl. *synarthroses* [Gr.] a form of joint in which the bony elements are united by continuous intervening fibrous or cartilaginous tissue to make them immobile. Called also fixed joint.
syncanthus adhesion of the eyeball to the orbital structures.
syncephalus a twin monster with heads fused into one, there being a single face, with four ears.
Syncerus caffer a wild black ruminant, up to 6 ft high, with horns that drop down beside the head then wave out and up. There are a number of subspecies; the most common is the Cape buffalo of southeastern Africa. Called also South African buffalo.
synchilia congenital adhesion of the lips.
synchiria reference of sensation to the opposite side on application of a stimulus.
synchondrosis pl. *synchondroses* [Gr.] a type of cartilaginous joint in which the cartilage is usually converted into bone before or during early adult life and that serves to allow growth, e.g. intermandibular, intersternebrales (syn. sternales), spheno-occipitales.
synchondrotomy division of a synchondrosis.
synchronism occurrence at the same time.
synchronization arranging that events shall occur at the same time.
estrus s. see ESTRUS synchronization.
synchronous occurring at the same time.
s. diaphragmatic flutter see synchronous DIAPHRAGMATIC flutter.
s. timer an oldfashioned timer on an x-ray machine that permits of very short exposure times but has to be reset after each exposure. Use of this kind of timer is no longer legal in most countries.
synchysis a softening or fluid condition of the vitreous body of the eye.
s. scintillans floating cholesterol crystals in the vitreous, developing as a secondary degenerative change.
synclonus muscular tremor or successive clonic contraction of various muscles together.
syncope a temporary suspension of consciousness due to cerebral anemia; fainting.
cardiac s. sudden loss of consciousness due to cerebral anemia caused by ventricular asystole, extreme bradycardia or ventricular fibrillation.
drug-induced s. may result from abnormalities of cardiac rhythm, caused by treatment with digitalis, and hypotension caused by drugs such as diuretics, promazine and phenothiazine tranquilizers, and peripheral vasodilating agents.
laryngeal s. tussive syncope.
Stokes–Adams s. see STOKES–ADAMS DISEASE.
swallow s. syncope associated with swallowing, a disorder of atrioventricular conduction mediated by the vagus nerve.
tussive s. brief loss of consciousness associated with paroxysms of coughing.
vasovagal s. see VASOVAGAL attack.
syncytial pertaining to or producing a syncytium.
bovine s. virus see RETROVIRIDAE.
feline s. virus see RETROVIRIDAE.
s. giant cell multinucleated mass of protoplasm formed by the fusion of a number of cells; a stage in the formation of a syncytium.
syncytiotrophoblast the outer syncytial layer of the trophoblast.
syncytium a multinucleate cellular mass produced by the fusing of cells.
s.-forming virus members of the family *Retroviridae*, genus *Spumavirus*. The best known of these viruses are found in cats and cattle. It should be noted, however, that viruses of several families, including herpesviruses, paramyxoviruses, coronaviruses and retroviruses, produce syncytia.
syndactylia syndactylism.
syndactylism, syndactyly fusion of the claws or digits. An inherited defect in several breeds of cattle. Some affected animals are also susceptible to hyperthermia.
syndectomy peritectomy.
syndesis 1. arthrodesis. 2. synapsis.
syndesmectomy excision of a portion of ligament.
syndesmitis 1. inflammation of a ligament. 2. conjunctivitis.
syndesm(o)- word element. [Gr.] *connective tissue, ligament.*
syndesmochorial see syndesmochorial PLACENTA.
syndesmography a description of the ligaments.
syndesmology scientific study of the ligaments and joints.
syndesmoma a tumor of connective tissue.
syndesmoplasty plastic repair of a ligament.
syndesmosis pl. *syndesmoses* [Gr.] a joint in which the bones are united by fibrous connective tissue forming an interosseous membrane or ligament that allows a modest amount of movement.
syndesmotomy incision of a ligament.
syndrome a combination of clinical signs resulting from a single cause or so commonly occurring together as to constitute a distinct clinical picture. For specific syndromes, see under the specific name, as FLAT PUPPY SYNDROME, CUSHING'S SYNDROME.
s. recognition a preliminary stage in the making of a diagnosis based on the recognition of a particular combination of clinical signs.
s. search a computer search of a database of diseases using a syndrome as the string to be located.
testicular feminizing s. see TESTICULAR feminization syndrome.
triple XXX s. see XXX.
Turner's s. in humans; characterized by a small uterus and underdeveloped external genitalia; deafness and lowered mentality may be present.
syndrome of inappropriate secretion of antidiuretic hormone a syndrome in which the secretion of antidiuretic hormone (ADH) is not inhibited by hypotonicity of extracellular fluid and hyponatremia is produced; abbreviated SIADH.
syndromic occurring as a syndrome.
syndromology the field concerned with the taxonomy, etiology and patterns of congenital malformations.
synechia pl. *synechiae* [Gr.] adhesion, as of the iris to the cornea or the lens.
annular s. adhesion of the whole rim of the iris to the lens.
anterior s. adhesion of the iris to the cornea.
peripheral anterior s. adhesion of the peripheral iris to the cornea.
posterior s. adhesion of the iris to the capsule of the lens or to the surface of the vitreous body.
total s. adhesion of the whole surface of the iris to the lens.
s. vulvae a congenital condition in which the labia are sealed in the midline, with only a small opening below the clitoris through which urination may occur.
synechotomy incision of a synechia.
synencephalocele encephalocele with adhesions to adjoining parts.
syneresis a drawing together of the particles of the disperse phase of a gel, with separation of some of the

disperse medium and shrinkage of the gel. Occurs in the shrinkage of the gel of the vitreous with release of fluid.

synergism the joint action of agents so that their combined effect is greater than the algebraic sum of their individual parts, e.g. antibiotic synergism.

synergist an agent that acts with or enhances the action of another, e.g. parainfluenza 3 virus and *Pasteurella haemolytica* in cattle.

synergy correlated action or cooperation by two or more structures or drugs.

syngamiasis infestation with *Syngamus trachea* in fowl, turkey, pheasant, guinea fowl, goose and wild birds. Causes pneumonia while migrating through the lungs. In the trachea causes tracheitis and anemia because of heavy blood-sucking. The predominant clinical signs are dyspnea, head shaking and spasmodic gaping.

Syngamus a genus of nematodes in the family Syngamidae.

S. ierei a cause of chronic nasopharyngitis in cats in Puerto Rico.

S. laryngeus found in the larynx of cattle.

S. nasicola found in the nasal cavities of ruminants.

S. skrjabinomorpha found in the domestic goose and in chickens.

S. trachea found in fowl, turkey, pheasant, guinea fowl, goose and wild birds. Causes pneumonia while migrating through the lungs. In the trachea causes tracheitis and anemia because of heavy blood-sucking. The predominant clinical signs are dyspnea, head shaking and spasmodic gaping.

syngamy a method of reproduction in which two individuals (gametes) unite permanently and their nuclei fuse; sexual reproduction. A common form of reproduction in protozoa.

syngeneic in transplantation biology, denoting individuals or tissues having almost identical genotypes, i.e. animals of the same inbred strain, or their tissues. Grafts can be as readily exchanged between syngeneic animals as between identical twins which are called isogeneic.

syngenesis 1. the origin of an individual from a germ derived from both parents and not from either one alone. 2. the state of having descended from a common ancestor.

Synhimantus a genus of nematodes that infect birds; members of the family Acuariidae.

S. spiralis, S. nasula found in the walls of the proventriculus, esophagus, and sometimes intestine of most domestic and wild bird species, mainly in water birds, e.g. pelicans, but also in hawks and owls. It causes severe lesions in the proventriculus and affected birds waste away and die. Losses may be heavy.

synkaryon a nucleus formed by fusion of two pronuclei, the fertilization nucleus.

synkinesis an associated movement; an unintentional movement accompanying a volitional movement.

synnecrosis symbiosis in which the relationship between populations (or individuals) is mutually detrimental.

synonym an alternative name for the same disease, sign, bacteria, etc. A key word or sign may have a number of synonyms.

synophthalmus, synophthalmos, synophthalmia cyclops.

synorchidism synorchism.

synorchism congenital fusion of the testes into one mass.

synosteotomy dissection of the joints.

synostosis pl. *synostoses* [Gr.] normal or abnormal union of two bones by osseous material.

radioulnar s. occurs between the radius and ulna as a result of unsatisfactory reduction of fractures.

synotia a developmental anomaly with fusion of the ears, or their location near the midventral line in the upper part of the neck.

synotus a fetus exhibiting synotia.

synovectomy excision of a synovial membrane, as of that lining the capsule of the knee joint.

synovia synovial fluid; the yellow-white transparent viscid fluid secreted by the synovial membrane and found in joint cavities, bursae and tendon sheaths that serves to lubricate moving parts and nourish articular cartilage.

synovial of, pertaining to, or secreting synovia.

s. fluid a protein-free dialysate of plasma with added hyaluronate, glycoproteins and other unidentified substances added by the synovial membrane. Called also synovia.

s. folds pleats of synovial membrane infoldings into joint cavities.

s. fossa nonarticulating areas in synovial joint articular surfaces found in the larger joints of larger animals. They are recessed below the surface of the cartilage and are unevenly sculpted.

s. gout see articular GOUT.

s. joint a specialized form of articulation permitting more or less free movement, the union of the bony elements being surrounded by an articular capsule enclosing a cavity lined by synovial membrane. Called also diarthrosis.

s. membrane the inner of the two layers of the articular capsule of a synovial joint; composed of loose connective tissue and having a free smooth surface that lines the joint cavity; it secretes the synovia.

s. mucin the lubricant in synovial joints; an acidoglycoprotein, the acid polysaccharide portion of which is hyaluronic acid.

s. villus see synovial VILLUS.

synovialis synovial.

synovialoma, synovioma a tumor of synovial membrane origin.

synoviocytes cells of the synovial membrane are of two types: type A are mainly phagocytic and pinocytic; type B are chiefly synthesizers.

synovioma synovialoma.

synoviorthese irradiation of the synovium by intra-articular injection of radiocolloids to destroy inflamed synovial tissue.

synovitis inflammation of a synovial membrane, usually painful, particularly on motion, and characterized by fluctuating swelling, due to effusion in a synovial sac.

dry s. synovitis with little effusion.

granulomatous s. see GRANULOMATOUS synovitis/arthritis.

infectious avian s. an infectious disease of broiler chickens and young turkeys caused by *Mycoplasma synoviae* and manifested by acute or chronic exudative synovitis, tenosynovitis or bursitis. The birds are lame, the joints are often swollen and there is difficulty in moving and in maintaining a standing posture.

lymphocytic s. see lymphocytic–plasmacytic synovitis (below).

lymphocytic–plasmacytic s. an immune-mediated inflammatory joint disease seen most often in the stifle of dogs, with signs of joint laxity and instability resembling rupture of the cranial cruciate ligament. The synovial membrane is greatly thickened.

purulent s. synovitis with effusion of pus in a synovial sac.

serous s. synovitis with copious nonpurulent, serous effusion.

s. sicca dry synovitis.

simple s. synovitis with clear or slightly turbid effusion.

tendinous s. inflammation of a tendon sheath.

villonodular s. proliferation of synovial tissue, especially of the knee joint, composed of synovial villi and fibrous nodules infiltrated by giant cells and macrophages.

synovium a synovial membrane.

synsacrum the fused lumbar and sacral vertebra and pelvic girdle of birds.

synsarcosis union of parts of the skeleton by muscles, e.g. attachment of the thoracic limb to the trunk in the cow.

syntax the rules of a language. In computer languages, if the commands to a program are wrongly worded or the punctuation or capitalization is wrong the program may give the helpful message 'syntax error'.

syntenic groups see LINKAGE (2).

synteny the presence together on the same chromosome of two or more gene loci whether or not in such proximity that they may be subject to linkage.

synthase any enzyme, especially a lyase, which catalyzes a synthesis that does not involve the breakdown of a pyrophosphate bond, as opposed to *ligase*.

synthesis creation of a compound by union of elements composing it, done artificially or as a result of natural processes.

synthesize to produce by synthesis.

synthetase ligase; any of a class of enzymes that catalyze the joining together of two molecules coupled with the breakdown of a pyrophosphate bond in ATP or a similar triphosphate.

aminoacyl-tRNA s's see TRNA.

synthetic artificially produced.

s. fibers fibers such as nylon, Dacron and Teflon compete with the natural fibers in the weaving of fabrics. The rise in oil prices in the late 1970s made them less competitive. Synthetic fibers have revolutionized the manufacture and use of sutures in surgery.

s. milk see MILK replacer.

s. organic dyes includes azo, acridine and rosaniline dyes. Used topically as weak antimicrobial agents.

s. reaction a metabolic reaction in which two substances are synthesized into one, e.g. detoxication in the liver.

s. rubber may contain tricresyl phosphate and cause intoxication of animal having access to litter made of it.

syntopy the position of an organ relative to other organs.

syntrophoblast syncytiotrophoblast.

Syphacia obvelata the pinworm found in mice and hamsters, a common parasite in laboratory colonies.

syphilis see TREPONEMATOSIS (1).

syringe an instrument for introducing fluids into or withdrawing them from the body.

bulb s. a compressible rubber bulb with a pierced, pointed end that allows suction and expulsion of fluids. Useful in irrigating ears or small cavities as in abscesses.

s. driver an electronically controlled syringe used for delivering small volumes of fluid at a constant rate.

hypodermic s. one for introduction of liquids through a hollow needle into subcutaneous tissues.

pole s. a syringe on a long pole so that the syringe can be operated from a distance, e.g. through the bars of a cage.

projectile s. see BLOW DART.

syringectomy excision of a fistula.

syringitis inflammation of the eustachian tube.

syring(o)- word element. [Gr.] *tube, fistula.*

syringoadenoma syringocystadenoma.

syringobulbia the presence of fluid-filled cavities in the medulla oblongata and pons.

syringocarcinoma neoplasm of a sweat gland.

syringocele a cavity-containing herniation of the spinal cord through the bony defect in spina bifida.

syringocystadenoma adenoma of the sweat glands; called also hidradenoma.

syringocystoma a cystic tumor of a sweat gland.

syringomeningocele meningocele resembling syringomyelocele.

syringomyelia the presence of fluid-filled cavities in the substance of the spinal cord, with destruction of nervous tissue. Clinical signs are posterior paralysis, or if the animal is able to stand the posture is a wide spacing of the feet and overextension of the legs when walking. An inherited trait in Weimaraner dogs. See also spinal DYSRAPHISM.

syringomyelitis inflammation of the spinal cord with the formation of cavities.

syringomyelocele hernial protrusion of the spinal cord through the bony defect in spina bifida, the mass containing a cavity connected with the central canal of the spinal cord.

Syringophilus a genus of trombidiform mites found inside the quills of feathers of birds.

S. bipectinatus found in fowl feather quills.

S. columbae found in pigeon feather quills.

***S. uncinatus* (syn. *Cheyletoides uncinata*)** found in peacock feather quills.

syringotomy incision of a fistula.

syrinx 1. a tube or pipe; a fistula. 2. the principal voice organ of birds; a laterally compressed cartilaginous box at the end of the trachea and the beginning of the bronchi.

s. membrane one that creates the voice of birds; comprises two pairs of vibrating membranes, the internal and external tympanic membranes.

syrinxitis a condition seen in companion birds; inflammation of the trachea and syrinx, characterized by snoring, coughing, gagging, cyanosis and a threat of asphyxiation.

Syrmaticus reevesii Reeves PHEASANT.

syrup a viscous concentrated solution of a sugar, such as sucrose, in water or other aqueous liquid; combined with other ingredients, such a solution is used as a flavored vehicle for medications.

systaltic alternately contracting and dilating; pulsating.

system 1. a set or series of interconnected or interdependent parts or entities (objects, organs or organisms) that act together in a common purpose or produce results impossible by action of one alone. 2. an organized set of principles or ideas.

The parts of a system can be referred to as its elements or components; the environment of the system is defined as all of the factors that affect the system and are affected by it. A living system is capable of taking in matter, energy and information from its environment (input), processing them in some way, and returning matter, energy and information to its environment as output.

An *open* system is one in which there is an exchange of matter, energy and information with the environment; in a *closed* system there is no such exchange. A living system cannot survive without this exchange, but in order to survive it must maintain pattern and organization in the midst of constant change. Control of self-regulation of an open system is achieved by dynamic interactions among its elements or components. The result of self-regulation is referred to as the steady state; that is, a state of equilibrium. HOMEOSTASIS is an assemblage of organic regulations that act to maintain steady states of a living organism.

Definitions of individual systems are to be found under those titles, e.g. ALIMENTARY system.

general s's theory a theory of organization proposed by Ludwig von Bertalanffy in the 1950s as a means by which various disciplines could communicate with one another and duplication of efforts among scientists could be avoided. The theory sought universally applicable principles and laws that would hold true regardless of the kind of system under study, the nature of its components, or the interrelationships among its components. Since the introduction of the general systems theory, theoretical models, principles and laws have been developed that are of great value to scientists in all fields, including those of medicine, nursing, other health-related professions, and in veterinary medicine.

heterogeneous s. a system or structure made up of mechanically separable parts, as an emulsion or suspension.

homogeneous s. a system or structure made up of parts that cannot be mechanically separated, such as a solution.

systema [Gr.] *system.*

systematic in an organized manner; according to some system.

Système International d'Unités the International System of Units; introduced in 1977, a universally accepted system of units of measure and providing units for the health professions; abbreviated SI. See Table 3.

systemic pertaining to or affecting the body as a whole.

s. inflammatory response (SIR) a specific condition recognized in critical care medicine, characterized by febrile response, increased heart and respiratory rates, and leukocytosis.

s. lupus erythematosus see LUPUS ERYTHEMATOSUS.

s. neuroaxial dystrophy see NEUROAXIAL DYSTROPHY.

s. therapy treatment with a drug that is absorbed into the bloodstream and distributed to all parts of the body except where there is a specific BARRIER.

systole the contraction, or period of contraction, of the heart, especially of the ventricles, during which blood is forced into the aorta and pulmonary artery.

atrial s. contraction of the atria by which blood is forced into the ventricles; it precedes the true or ventricular systole.

extra s. see EXTRASYSTOLE.

ventricular s. contraction of the ventricles, forcing blood into the aorta and pulmonary artery.

systolic pertaining to or emanating from systole.

syzygy 1. the fusion of organs without the loss of identity by either. 2. temporary adherence of male and female protozoa of the subclass Gregarinomorpha before numerical increase occurs by sporogony.

T

2,4,5-T (2,4,5-trichlorophenoxy) acetic acid, a herbicide considered to be without toxicity hazard provided it is clear of the toxic contaminant dioxin.

t in genetics, symbol for translocation.

T antigen tumor antigen.

T banding a staining technique with Giemsa stain used in the preparation of karyotypes; stains the telomeres (ends) and the centromeres.

T-butylaminoethanol a coccidiostat which may induce a choline deficiency leading to depressed growth in chickens.

T conformational state deoxy ('tense') conformational form of hemoglobin.

T helper cell see helper LYMPHOCYTE.

t-PA tissue plasminogen activator.

T symbol, *tesla; tera-;* (absolute) temperature; intraocular TENSION; THYMINE.

T_{12} a value derived by multiplying the value for T_4 by the value for T_3 expressed as RT_3U (resin T_3 uptake).

T-1824 Evans blue dye.

T_m tubular maximum (of the kidneys); used in reporting kidney function studies, with inferior letters representing the substance used in the test, as T_{mPAH} (tubular maximum for para-aminohippuric acid).

T_2 toxin a trichothecene toxin (a secondary toxic metabolite) produced by a number of *Fusarium* spp. fungi including *F. tricinctum* growing on stored grain usually maize corn. The toxin affects rapidly dividing cells, thereby causing necrosis of skin and of cells lining the alimentary tract, lymphoid and hemopoietic tissues. This may result in panleukopenia and defective blood clotting. The toxin is also a teratogen and causes stillbirth, abortion and fetal abnormalities. Clinical signs include feed refusal and vomiting in species that can vomit. Called also moldy corn disease. See also TRICHOTHECENE.

T_3 tri-iodothyronine.

T_3 uptake see TRI-IODOTHYRONINE uptake.

T_4 thyroxine.

T_7 a value derived by dividing the T_4 value by the value for T_3 as expressed by RT_3U (resin T_3 uptake).

T cell see T LYMPHOCYTE.

T c. receptor antigen specific heterodimeric proteins, either αβ or γδ, present on the surface of T lymphocytes, the specificity of which is generated by somatic mutation and somatic recombination of a relatively small number of genes and is similar to that responsible for the generation of antibody diversity.

t-distribution see T STATISTIC.

T effector cell includes large granular lymphocyte, called also natural killer CELL and cytotoxic T lymphocytes.

T lymphocyte see T LYMPHOCYTE.

T wave see T WAVE.

***t* statistic, *t* distribution** the statistical distribution of the ratio of the sample mean to its sample standard deviation for a normal random variable with zero mean. It is the basis of various *t*-tests used to make inferences about the mean of a normal variable.

t-strain mycoplasma see UREAPLASMA.

***t*-test** a test of statistical significance which uses a formula from which a *t* value is derived. The value is then compared with a set of *t*-distribution tables to see whether the null hypothesis should be rejected or not.

T tubule see TRANSVERSE tubules.

TA toxin–antitoxin.
Ta chemical symbol, *tantalum.*
TAA tumor-associated antigen.
TAB a vaccine prepared from killed typhoid, paratyphoid A and paratyphoid B bacilli.
tabanid a fly of the family Tabanidae, including the genera *Chrysops*, *Haematopota*, *Pangonia* and *Tabanus.*
Tabanus a genus of blood-sucking biting flies (horse flies, deer flies or march flies) in the family Tabanidae which transmit trypanosomes and anthrax to various animals and have a painful bite.
tabby-point see POINTS.
tabes any wasting of the body; progressive atrophy of the body or a part of it.
tabescent growing emaciated; wasting away.
tabetiform resembling tabes.
tablature separation of the chief cranial bones into inner and outer tables, separated by a diploë.
table 1. a flat layer or surface, e.g. smooth surface on top of teeth especially on the incisors of the horse, used in telling the age of the horse. 2. a collection of related records in a data base.
t. food sometimes used to describe food from the owner's dining table that is fed to dogs and cats.
hydraulic t. used for surgery of large animals so it can be adjusted to the appropriate height and in some cases starting from floor level to accommodate animals anesthetized on the floor, then raised.
inner t. the inner compact layer of the bones covering the brain.
instrument t. used to arrange instruments for ready access by the surgeon and assistants. It often overhangs the surgery table.
outer t. the outer compact layer of the bones covering the brain.
statistical t. tables of values used in statistics, e.g. *t*-tables.
t. ties sterilizable nylon or cotton ropes that can be used to tie a recumbent, anesthetized dog or cat firmly to an operating table.
vitreous t. inner table.
table top technique a technique of radiography in which the use of a grid is unnecessary and the cassette can be moved about on the table top so that it is just below the part to be radiographed.
tablespoon a household unit of volume or capacity; equivalent to three teaspoons or approximately 15 milliliters; in metric measurement, equal to 20 milliliters.
tablet a solid dosage form containing a medicinal substance with or without a suitable diluent.
enteric-coated t. one coated with material that delays release of the medication until after it leaves the stomach.
tablet triturate a small, loosely packed tablet to be dissolved in water immediately before injection, e.g. apomorphine.
tabula vitrea inner layer of very dense bone in the bones of the cranium.
tabular resembling a table.
tabun an organophosphorus compound used as a war gas.
Tacazzea yototacolla African member of the plant family Asclepiadaceae; may contain cardiac glycoside which causes abdominal pain, vomiting, diarrhea, hepatitis.
tachogram the graphic record produced by tachography.
tachography the recording of the movement and speed of the blood current.
tachy- word element. [Gr.] *rapid, swift.*
tachyarrhythmia tachycardia associated with an irregularity in the normal heart rhythm. Includes atrial TACHYCARDIA, sinus TACHYCARDIA, PREMATURE ventricular contractions, atrial FLUTTER, atrial FIBRILLATION and VENTRICULAR tachycardia.
re-entrant t. one caused by a depolarization wave crossing areas of nonuniform conduction and excitability.
tachycardia abnormally rapid heart rate.
atrial t. rapid contraction of the atrium arising from an ectopic focus in the atrium. The heart rate remains normal.
ectopic t. rapid heart action in response to impulses arising outside the sinoatrial node.
idioventricular t. one occurring as a compensation for a sinus bradycardia and A-V block.
junctional t. that arising in response to impulses originating in the atrioventricular junction, i.e. the atrioventricular node.
orthostatic t. disproportionate rapidity of the heart rate on arising from a recumbent to a standing position.
paroxysmal t. episodes of an abrupt and marked increase in heart rate in a resting patient, with an equally sudden return to normal.
sinus t., simple t. an increase in heart rate from heightened activity of the sinoatrial node, such as occurs with excitement or pain.
supraventricular t. a combination of junctional tachycardia and atrial tachycardia.
ventricular t. see VENTRICULAR tachycardia.
Tachyglossus see ECHIDNA.
Tachygonetria a genus of oxyurid worms, in the superfamily Oxyuroidea, found in the large intestine of tortoises.
tachymeter an instrument for measuring rapidity of motion.
tachyphagia rapid eating.
tachyphylaxis 1. rapid immunization against the effect of toxic doses of an extract by previous injection of small doses of it. 2. rapidly decreasing response to a drug or physiologically active agent after administration of a few doses.
tachypnea very rapid respirations. The rate is fast and the depth shallow, as in heat stroke, because the initiating mechanism is hyperthermia and there is no hypercapnia.
tachypneic respiratory failure see RESPIRATORY failure.
tachysterol an isomer of ergosterol, an antirachitic substance, produced by irradiaton of ergosterol.
tachyzoite a fast multiplication stage of zoites in the life cycle of *Toxoplasma gondii* or *Neospora caninum*; found in tissues.
tack abbreviation for tackle; a horseman's word for saddlery and gear generally.
tactical treatment treatment at times when the activities of a disease are at their worst, e.g. when diarrhea caused by *Ostertagia* spp. in cattle is most severe.
tactile pertaining to touch.
t. hair hairs sensitive to touch. See also HAIR (1).
t. hair organ a group of vibrissae, such as the carpal organ of cats, made up of four vibrissae on the medial surface of the forelegs, sensitive to vibrations.
t. percussion a combination of touch and tap as in ballottement. The objective is to delineate the boundaries of a fetus or organ by a tap or thrust and allow the repelled organ to bounce back onto the fingers.
t. placing reaction, t. reflex see PLACING reflex.
t. receptors located in the skin most are connected to very fast, myelinated nerve fibers.

tactus [L.] *touch.*
tadpole edema virus see RANAVIRUS.
Taenia a genus of cyclophyllidean tapeworms of the family Taeniidae. The adult tapeworm inhabits the intestine of carnivores, the larval stage (metacestode) invades the tissues of a variety of animals, in some cases humans. They cause some economic loss due to condemnation of offal, but their greatest importance is their zoogenetic potential, and the preoccupation of humans with the danger of becoming infected.

Tapeworms and their hosts are listed below, but species whose intermediate hosts are unknown are: *T. bubesi* (lion), *T. crocutae* (spotted hyena), *T. erythraea* (black-backed jackal), *T. gongamai* and *T. hlosei* (lion and cheetah), *T. lycaontis* (hunting dog), *T. regis* (lion).

T. brauni adults tapeworms in dogs and jackals and the larval stage (coenurus) in rats, mice and porcupines. It is probably a subspecies of *T. serialis.*

T. crassiceps adult tapeworms in foxes and coyotes, the larval stage (cysticercus) in rodents.

T. hydatigena tapeworms in small intestine of dogs, wolves and wild Carnivora, and the larval stage, *Cysticercus tenuicollis*, found in the sheep and other ruminants, and in pigs and occasionally primates.

T. hyenae tapeworms are in hyenas and the cysticerci in antelopes.

T. krabbei adult tapeworms are found in the dog and in wild carnivores and the larval cestode, *Cysticercus tarandi*, in the muscles of wild ruminants, especially deer.

T. laticollis tapeworms found in carnivores and larval forms in rodents. possibly a synonym for *T. pisiformis.*

T. macrocystis adult tapeworms in lynx and coyote, and the intermediate stage in snowshoe lagomorphs.

T. martis the adult tapeworms in the marten and the cysticercus in the vole.

***T. multiceps* (syn. *Multiceps multiceps*)** the adult tapeworms are found in the dog and wild canids, the larvae, *Coenurus cerebralis*, in the brain and spinal cord of sheep and goat.

T. mustelae adult tapeworms in martens, weasels, otters, skunks, badgers and larval stages in voles and other rodents.

T. omissa adult tapeworms in the cougar and larvae in deer.

T. ovis adult tapeworms are found in dogs and wild carnivores and the larval stage, *Cysticercus ovis*, in the skeletal and cardiac muscles of sheep and goats.

T. parva adult tapeworms in genets, larval stage in rodents.

T. pisiformis adult tapeworms found in small intestine of dog, fox, some wild carnivores, and very rarely in cats. The metacestode stage (*Cysticercus pisiformis*) found in lagomorphs, in the liver and peritoneal cavity.

T. polyacantha adults are in the intestine of foxes and the metacestodes in microtine rodents.

T. rileyi adult tapeworms found in lynx, larvae in rodents.

T. saginata adult tapeworms are intestinal parasites of humans, and the metacestode (*Cysticercus bovis*) in cattle and some wild ruminants.

T. serialis the adult tapeworm is found in dogs and foxes and the metacestode, *Coenurus serialis*, in the subcutaneous and intramuscular tissues of lagomorphs.

T. serrata see *T. pisiformis* (above).

T. solium the adults are found in the small intestine of humans and some apes, the metacestode (*Cysticercus cellulosae*) in the skeletal and cardiac muscle of pigs and in the brain of humans.

T. taeniaeformis the adult is found in the small intestine of cats and other related carnivores and the metacestode (*Cysticercus fasciolaris*) in the livers of rodents.

T. twitchelli adult tapeworms found in wolverines, larvae in lungs and pleural cavity of porcupines.

taenia see TENIA.
taeniacide teniacide.
taeniafuge teniafuge.
Taeniorhyncus the modern genus for MANSONIA mosquitoes.
tafes see PERRALDERIA CORONOPIFOLIA.
tag 1. a small appendage, flap or polyp. 2. label. See EAR tag, TAIL tag.

cutaneous t. fibrovascular papilloma.

radioactive t. a radioisotope that has been incorporated in a chemical compound.

Tagetes minuta African grass in the family Poaceae; its sharp awns cause subcutaneous abscesses, dermatitis especially of the lower limbs. Called also kakiebos.
tahr short-horned, goat-like wild antelope. Called also *Hemitragus* spp.
Tahyna virus a virus of the California group of the genus *Bunyavirus*, family *Bunyaviridae*, associated with the occurrence of encephalitis in humans and for which many domestic and wild animals act as reservoirs.
tail the caudal terminal appendage of the vertebral column made up of the coccygeal vertebrae and their attendant tissues. See also CAUDA.

t. absence an inherited defect in cattle, cats and pigs, sometimes associated with other deformities of the vertebral column, atresia of the anus and urogenital system defects. See also MANX.

t. amputation may be required for removal of a diseased tail; also a common husbandry practice in pastoral dairy herds where tails full of sloppy feces are unwelcome industrial hazards to farmhands working in pit type milking parlors, especially on cold mornings. Standard practice is to amputate with a guillotine type dehorner.

banged t. see BANGTAIL.

t. biting a vice in pigs which bite each other's tail because of boredom initially and then as a habit, causing blood loss and frequently local abscess formation or spinal cord abscess. In dogs, seen as a vice in association with tail chasing (see below). In caged mice may be attributable to crowding.

t. bleeding collection of blood from the ventral median coccygeal vein, e.g. in cattle; laboratory rodents are also bled from the ventral coccygeal artery or by amputation of the end of the tail.

bob t., bobbed t. see BOBTAIL.

t. boot a leather sleeve that is wrapped around the butt of a horse's tail, laced up, and secured to a harness by a retaining strap. Designed to protect the tail from wear while traveling. Nowadays bandaging is a more common method of protection.

t. brace a device for supporting the tail in an elevated position for extended periods of time, usually as an adjunct to a surgical procedure on the tail or in the perineal region, e.g. dogs after surgery for perianal fistulae and horses after ventral myotomy ('nicking').

t. carriage the way in which the tail is carried relative to the body. A high carriage of the butt of the tail with the hair streaming in the wind is the objective in show horses. See also NICKING (2).

caudal t. fold see CAUDAL tailfold.
t. cellulitis at the tail tip, a common sequel to unsanitary vaccination against pleuropneumonia; at the butt incidental to injury.
t. chasing an obsessive-compulsive behavior seen occasionally in dogs, particularly Bull terriers. The dog periodically lapses into episodes of chasing its tail. Most deliberately do not catch it, but those that do can cause serious self-trauma.
t. deformity most cases are sporadic but it is inherited as part of the inherited tail-absent syndrome in cattle and pigs.
t. docking see DOCK (1).
t. elevation posture indicative of irritation in the vagina, e.g. after irrigation of cervix and uterus with Lugol's iodine; tail held out from the body, plus rigidity, a sure indication of the presence of tetanus.
t. fold dermatitis see fold DERMATITIS.
frozen t., limber t., rudder t. a painful condition of the tailbase recognized in gundogs, mainly Labrador retrievers. Usually seen the day after hunting, and believed to be a tendonitis or myositis associated with vigorous swimming or hyperextension of the tail when leaping into water. The affected dog holds the tail horizontally, away from the rump, and is reluctant to sit.
t. gland an oval area of skin on the dorsal aspect of the tail in dogs centered at the level of the eighth coccygeal vertebrae which contains a large number of sebaceous and apocrine glands.
t. gland hyperplasia in dogs, a spongy enlargement with alopecia and scaling of the area, usually associated with hormonal disturbances, in which the apocrine gland segment is especially hyperplastic.
ingrown t. dogs with naturally short, kinked tails (corkscrew tails), e.g. British bulldogs and Pugs, may have deep skin folds surrounding the tail that are subject to moist dermatitis and secondary infection.
t. jack see TAILING.
t. louse see HAEMATOPINUS *quadripertusus*.
t. and mane dystrophy see MANE and tail dystrophy.
t. mange see CHORIOPTIC MANGE.
t. paint special paint applied to the tailhead of cows as a heat mount detection aid. When cows stand to be mounted the paint is rubbed off.
t. paralysis is characterized by a flaccid, anesthetized tail. Occurs with injury, myelitis or myelomalacia of caudal segments of the spinal cord.
t. pulse the pulse as felt in the ventral coccygeal artery in cattle. Best felt at the level of the tip of the vulva.
t. pyoderma equine staphylococcal folliculitis.
t. restraint in cattle, holding the tail strongly over the back provides some control. See also TAIL-HITCH, TAILING.
t. rigidity tail is stiff instead of its usual, whip-like in cattle, flexibility. Indicative of the presence of tetanus.
t. root where the tail joins the body.
t. setting see NICKING (2).
t. skin dehiscence skin at the tip of the gerbil's tail is easily pulled off; never catch or lift a gerbil by the tail other than at its base.
t. sore the early or mild lesions in a tail-biting problem of pigs.
t. stock first part of the tail, of a whale or dolphin, before it divides into the flukes.
t. sucking a vice of cats, particularly Siamese, in which the tip of the tail is usually wet and becomes discolored.
t. switch louse see HAEMATOPINUS *quadripertusus*.
t. tag used extensively for the identification of cattle. Made of metal or plastic in sharply contrasting colors and with identifying marks or numbers and letters on them so that animals, owners and veterinarians can be easily identified. The tag is wrapped around the thinner, meaty part of the tail, just above the brush and fixed with one of several patented attachments. See also BACKTAG.
t. tip necrosis disease of confined cattle on slatted floors; caused by treading injury.
t. tone complete absence indicative of good outcome of epidural anesthesia; occurrence spontaneously indicative of lesion to cauda equine, in cattle usually due to mounting injury caused by a heavy bull or cow.
t. worm EQUINE staphylococcal dermatitis.

tail-hitch a half-hitch applied to a horse's tail, used in restraint for standing castration by pulling horse up on its toes to an overhead beam. Useful also in tying a cow's tail out of the way and in applying traction to a calf in posterior presentation at a dystocia.

tail root eczema itching, scaling, crusting, twitching of the tailhead in cows; responds to supplementary zinc in diet.

tailcup lupine LUPINUS *caudatus*.

tailhead dorsal aspect of the root of the tail.

tailing 1. the restraint technique used in cattle; the butt of the tail is grasped with both hands and raised vertically as far as it will go without breaking. While the tail is in this position the animal is unlikely to kick and then only lightly. Called also tail jack, tail restraint, tail-hitch. 2. the addition in vitro of the same nucleotide by terminal transferase to the 3′-hydroxyl terminus of a double-stranded DNA molecule. Called also homopolymeric tailing.

taillessness see TAIL absence.

taint an unpleasant odor and flavor in a human foodstuff of animal origin. Caused by the ingestion of the substance, commonly a plant such as Hexham scent, or while in storage, e.g. milk stored with pineapples, or as a result of animal metabolism, e.g. boar taint.

taipan a very venomous snake because of its large output of highly poisonous venom; dark brown on the dorsum with creamy yellow belly. Called also *Oxyuranus scutellatus*.

take-off part of the horse's jumping gait, the lifting of the forequarters off the ground and the thrust from the hindlegs at the beginning of the jump.

takin see GOAT-ANTELOPES.

talampicillin an antibiotic derived from ampicillin.

talapoin monkey a small yellow-green Old World monkey included among the guenons. Called also *Cercopithecus talapoin*.

talc a naturally occurring hydrous magnesium silicate, sometimes with a small amount of aluminum silicate; used as a dusting powder. Called also talcum.
t. granulomatous peritonitis talc, or starch, spilled in the peritoneal cavity provokes the development of granuloma by e.g. the serous membrane.

talcosis a condition due to inhalation or implantation in the body of talc.

talcum talc, talcum powder.

Talfan disease see porcine viral ENCEPHALOMYELITIS.

talipes see DACTYLOMEGALY.

tall higher than average.
t. fescue FESTUCA *arundinacea*.
t. Cape honeyflower MELIANTHUS *major*.
t. chloris CHLORIS *ventricosa*.
t. delphinium DELPHINIUM *trolliifolium*.
t. field buttercup RANUNCULUS *acris*.
t. larkspur DELPHINIUM *barbeyi*, *D. brownii*, *D. occidentale*.

t. melilot MELILOTUS *altissima*.

t silvery lupine LUPINUS *erectus*.

t. yellowtop SENECIO *magnificus*.

Tallebudgera horse disease see EUPATORIUM *adenophorum*.

tallow natural, hard fat taken from cattle or sheep. It is used in prepared animal feeds to act as a binder and reduce dust. It has a high calorific value and is palatable to pigs and poultry.

tallow tree see SAPIUM SEBIFERUM.

Tallqvist method a very old method for estimation of the hemoglobin content of blood in which a drop of blood is absorbed onto white paper and compared with a color chart.

talocalcaneal joint see tarsal joints, Table 11.

talocalcanean pertaining to the talus and calcaneus.

talocalcaneocentral joint the joint between the talus and central tarsal bone; see also tarsal joints, Table 11.

talocrural tarsocrural.

talofibular pertaining to the talus and fibula.

talonavicular pertaining to the talus and navicular bone.

talus the most proximal of the tarsal bones. Called also the tibial tarsal bone. See also Table 10.

Tamagotchi [Japanese; *cute little egg*] space-age cyberpet; a solely electronic state; indigenous to Japan, appearing as an egg on a liquid-crystal screen. Life history, consisting of hatching, feeding, beeping when not fed, sleeping in 12 hour snatches, growing, dying prematurely if neglected, flying away, is completed usually in 2 weeks with maximum recorded life span 4 weeks. The low maintenance costs and brief life span appear to have been designed to suit society's average desired investment level and affection span for a house pet. An unfriendly addition to the veterinary profession's list of exotic companion animals.

Tamandua small, 20 to 24 inches, nocturnal, arboreal anteater, cream, tan or black with a brown to black collar. Includes *Tamandua tetradactyla* (syn. *Myrmecophaga tamandua*). Called also tamandua.

tamandua see TAMANDUA.

tamarin one of the New World monkeys in the family Callithricidae. Called also *Mystax* spp. Similar to marmosets.

tamboril da campo see ENTEROLOBIUM.

Tamias striatus see CHIPMUNK.

Tamm–Horsfall mucoprotein a normal product of the ascending limb of the loop of Henle and the distal renal tubules; may appear in many cortical tubules.

tamoxifen an antiestrogen used as the citrate in the treatment of disseminated mammary cancer.

tampan a tick; see ORNITHODORUS.

tampon a pack, pad, or plug made of cotton, sponge or other material, variously used in surgery to plug the nose, vagina, etc., for the control of hemorrhage or the absorption of secretions.

tamponade 1. surgical use of a tampon. 2. pathological compression of a part.

cardiac t. compression of the heart due to collection of fluid or blood in the pericardial sac. Causes interference with heart action and subsequent sudden death or congestive heart failure. The heart shadow on radiography is enlarged, the heart sounds on auscultation are muffled.

Tamus communis European member of the plant family Dioscoreaceae; contains an unidentified toxin which causes vomiting, colic, paralysis and death. Called also black bryony.

Tamworth a golden-red, long faced, prick-eared bacon pig produced in the UK.

tan TANBARK.

Tanacetum member of the plant family Asteraceae; reported to be associated with abortion in cattle; includes *T. axillare* (ASAEMIA AXILLARIS), *T. parthenium* (feverfew), *T. vulgare* (tansy).

Tanaecium exitosium South American member of the plant family Bignoniaceae; contains an unidentified toxin which causes cardiomyopathy, enteritis, frequent micturition in cattle.

Tanaisia a genus of flukes in the family Eucotylidae.

T. bragai found in the kidneys and ureters of chickens, turkeys and pigeons but is apparently without much pathogenic effect.

T. zarudnyi found in ruffed grouse.

tanapox a poxvirus that infects African nonhuman primates, but may also cause disease in humans. Named after the Tana River Valley in Kenya.

tanbark dry shredded residue of the tree bark used in tanning leather. Springy and absorbent and is in demand as a surface for horses to work and exercise on or to stand on if they are sorefooted.

Tangier pea LATHYRUS *tingitatus*.

tangled hypericum HYPERICUM *triquetrifolium*.

tank an artificial receptacle for liquids.

horse flotation t. used to suspend horses with limb-bone injuries during repair phase. Water is warmed and filtered and the horse may be kept in the tank for periods of up to 3 months but if suspension has been almost complete and is ceased suddenly the osteoporosis due to weightlessness may cause bone fractures.

x-ray processing t. usually in four compartments, one for developing, one for wash water, one for fixing and one for rinsing.

tankage made from heat-digested animal abattoir residues without gut contents, hide, horn, hoof. Concentrated and dried and possessing a high biological value protein content of 60%. See also MEAT meal.

tannate any of the salts of tannic acid, all of which are astringent.

tanner grass BRACHIARIA *radicans*.

tannia see XANTHOSOMA.

tannic acid a substance obtained from bark and fruit of many plants, used as an astringent.

tanning the process of tanning hides to make leather; tanning is by a tanning bark process or a chemical process called chrome tanning.

tannins secondary plant metabolites, probably important in anti-herbivore defense; divisible into the common condensed tannins, and less common and more toxic hydrolyzable tannins, e.g. gallotannins in oak trees, punicalagin in *Terminalia oblongata,* capable of damaging the kidneys; condensed tannins bind to protein, interfere with the availability of proteins from feeds, and are pooly absorbed from the gut.

tansy TANACETUM *vulgare*.

tansy mustard see DESCURAINIA PINNATA.

tansy ragwort SENECIO *jacobea*.

tantalum a chemical element, atomic number 73, atomic weight 180.948, symbol Ta. See Table 6. It is a noncorrosive and malleable metal used for plates or disks to repair cranial defects, for wire sutures, and for making prosthetic appliances.

tanycyte special cell in the ependyma lining the third ventricle in the brain; the function is unknown.

tap 1. a quick, light blow. 2. to drain off fluid by paracentesis.

bone t. an instrument for cutting a screw thread inside a drill hole in bone. May have a fixed handle or come in bit form so that the bit size can be interchanged in a handle fitted with a chuck.

spinal t. lumbar puncture.

tape a long, narrow strip of fabric or other flexible material.

adhesive t. a strip of fabric or other material evenly coated on one side with a pressure-sensitive adhesive material.

t. closure application of tape strips across the incision can be used to hold wound edges in apposition.

magnetic t. inexpensive data storage medium but has the disadvantage of inaccessibility. It has to be dumped onto a disk before it can be accessed randomly. On the tape it can only be accessed by reading all of the data until the required sector is located.

vaginal t. special tape for use in closing the vulva to retain a prolapsed cervix or uterus. See also BUHNER METHOD.

tapeinocephaly flattening or depression of the skull.

taperpoint needle see round bodied NEEDLE.

tapetal emanating from or pertaining to the tapetum.

t. aplasia occurs in dogs, particularly Dalmations, and pigs.

t. degeneration occurs as an inherited defect in beagles and in cats with Chediak–Higashi syndrome.

t. hyperreflectivity a feature of retinal degeneration when less light is absorbed by the atophic retina.

t. rods crystalline structures containing zinc found in the cellular tapetum in carnivores.

t. stars nonreflective dots in the tapetum lucidum of certain species (such as the horse) caused by piercing blood vessels. Called also stars of Winslow.

tapetum pl. *tapeta* [L.] 1. a covering structure or layer of cells. 2. a stratum in the human brain composed of fibers from the body and splenium of the corpus callosum sweeping around the lateral ventricle.

t. cellulosum a type of tapetum lucidum made of cells called iridocytes, as found in carnivores.

choroidal t. see tapetum lucidum (below).

t. fibrosum a type of tapetum lucidum composed predominantly of organized bundles of collagen as found in ungulates.

t. lucidum the iridescent reflecting tissue layer of the choroid of some species of animals that gives their eyes the property of shining in the dark. It is characteristic of nocturnal animals and allows incident light two opportunities to stimulate the retinal receptors. Called also choroidal tapetum.

tapeworm members of the genera *Taenia*, *Diphyllobothrium*, *Dipylidium* and *Echinococcus*; includes infestation with members of the tapeworm class Eucestoda. Most tapeworm infestations have little apparent effect on the health of farm livestock and are mostly esthetic problems in companion animals.

armed t. TAENIA *solium*.

beef t. TAENIA *saginata*.

broad t. DIPHYLLOBOTHRIUM *latum*.

dog t. DIPYLIDIUM *caninum*.

fish t. DIPHYLLOBOTHRIUM *latum*.

hydatid t. ECHINOCOCCUS *granulosus*.

pork t. TAENIA *solium*.

unarmed t. TAENIA *saginata*.

tapioca MANIHOT *esculenta*.

tapir an odd-toed ungulate in the family Tapiridae, with four digits on the forelimbs and three on each of the hindlimbs. It has a short mobile trunk and simple, lophodont molars. It resembles a very large pig, has short woolly, dark brown fur, is 3 ft high and 6 ft long, nocturnal, shy and herbivorous. Called also *Tapir* spp.

tar a dark-brown or black, viscid liquid obtained from various species of pine or from bituminous coal. See also WOOD TAR DERIVATIVES.

coal t. see COAL TAR.

coal t. pitch see COAL TAR PITCH.

t. derivatives include phenol (carbolic acid), cresols, creosote, all potent poisons. See also WOOD TAR DERIVATIVES.

hot t. a cause of burns in dogs and cats, usually made more severe because it sticks to the skin.

juniper t. a volatile oil obtained from wood of *Juniperus oxycedrus*; used topically in the treatment of skin disease.

pine t. a product of destructive distillation of the wood of various pine trees; used as a rubefacient and treatment for skin disease.

t. pitch see COAL TAR PITCH.

Stockholm t. see STOCKHOLM TAR.

Tarai buffalo a black Indian dairy buffalo; occasionally brown in color; it has a white tail.

tarantula see LYCOSA TARENTULA.

Taraxacum officinale despite a widely held view, NOT the cause of Australian stringhalt in horses; called also dandelion. See HYPOCHOERIS RADICATA.

tarbush see FLOURENSIA CERNUA.

tardive late; applied to a disease in which the characteristic lesion is late in appearing.

tare 1. the weight of the vessel in which a substance is weighed. 2. to weigh a vessel which is to contain a substance in order to allow for it when the vessel and substance are weighed together.

Tarentaise cattle fawn to yellow, dual-purpose cattle from the French Alps.

target 1. an object or area toward which something is directed, e.g. target animal, population, level or nucleotide sequence. 2. the area of the anode of an x-ray tube where the electron beam collides causing the emission of x-rays. 3. a cell or organ that is affected by a particular agent, e.g. a hormone or drug.

t. cell see target CELL.

t.–film distance the distance from the target of the x-ray tube and the plane of the x-ray film.

t. lesion skin lesion consisting of annular or arciform areas of erythema with central pigmentation. Associated with bacterial hypersensitivity and seborrheic dermatitis. Called also bull's eye lesion.

performance t. in herd health programs target performances are set up in a number of production and health functions in order to provide an incentive and give some measure of performance other than an absolute one. This enables farmers to be rated on their effective performance in spite of the great variations that can occur between them in basic resources.

targetting of proteins mechanisms whereby proteins are sorted and transported to particular sites in the cell required for their synthesis or function.

Targhee an American medium-woolled, polled, meat sheep produced by crossing sheep of Lincoln and Rambouillet breeds.

tarichatoxin a neurotoxin from the newt (*Taricha*), identical with tetrodotoxin.

taro COLOCASIA *esculenta*, XANTHOSOMA spp.

tarry said of feces that are black and glutinous. See also MELENA.

tarsadenitis inflammation of the tarsus of the eyelid and the meibomian glands.

tarsal pertaining to the tarsus of an eyelid or of the foot. See also Table 10.

t. gland see meibomian GLAND.

t. hobbles tape applied around the hindlimbs, just above the tarsus, is used in dogs to provide support in walking after pelvic fractures.

t. hydrarthrosis see BOG SPAVIN.

t. joint see TARSUS.

t. pad see tarsal TORUS.
t. sheath the synovial sheath around the deep flexor tendon in the horse.
t. tunnel the osseofibrous passage for the tibial nerve, and flexor tendons, formed by the flexor retinaculum and the tarsal bones.

tarsalia the bones of the tarsus.

tarsalis [L.] *tarsal.*

tarsectomy 1. excision of one or more bones of the tarsus. 2. excision of the cartilage of the eyelid.

tarsier small, arboreal, almost hairless, South East Asian monkey, thought to be the ancestor of humans.

Tarsiidae a family of nonhuman primates that includes the TARSIER.

tarsitis inflammation of the cartilaginous portion of the eyelid; blepharitis.

tars(o)- word element. [Gr.] *edge of eyelid, tarsus of the foot.*

tarsoclasis surgical fracture of the tarsus.

tarsoconjunctiva the TARSUS (2) and palpebral conjunctiva.
t. graft, t. transposition transposition of the tarsus and palpebral conjunctiva by a sliding graft technique; used in reconstruction of the eyelid.

tarsocrural pertaining to the tarsal bones and the tibia and fibula.
t. joint the articulation between the tibial tarsal bone (talus) and the tibia and fibula.

tarsomalacia softening of the tarsal cartilage of an eyelid.

tarsometatarsal pertaining to the tarsus and metatarsus.

tarsometatarsus the bone of the lower shank of birds made up of fused tarsal and metatarsal bones.

tarsophyma any tumor of the tarsus.

tarsoplasty plastic repair of the tarsus of the eyelid.

tarsorrhaphy suture of a portion of or the entire upper and lower eyelids for the purpose of shortening or closing the palpebral fissure.

tarsotomy surgical incision of a tarsus, or an eyelid.

tarsus 1. the hock or ankle made up of up to seven bones—talus, calcaneus, navicular, medial, intermediate and lateral cuneiform, and cuboid—comprising the articulation between the cannon bone and the tibia. 2. the fibrous or cartilaginous plate forming the framework of either (upper or lower) eyelid.

tartar 1. the recrystallized sediment of wine casks; crude potassium bitartrate. 2. a yellowish film formed of calcium phosphate and carbonate, food particles, and other organic matter, deposited on the teeth by the saliva. See also DENTAL calculus.
t. emetic antimony potassium tartrate; used at one time as an emetic and as a treatment for trypanosomiasis but is very poisonous and is no longer used as an animal medicine.
t. scraper manual or mechanical, handheld instruments used to scrape tartar (dental calculus) from the teeth of dogs. There is a variety of tips including triangle, hoe (right and left) and claw. They may be single or double ended.

tartaric acid a compound used in preparing effervescent powders.

tartrate a salt of tartaric acid.

tarweed see AMSINCKIA.

Tasmanian ngaio MYOPORUM *insulare.*

Tasmanian white lily DIPLARRENA *moraea.*

tassel see caprine WATTLE.

tastant any substance, e.g. salt, capable of eliciting gustatory excitation, i.e. stimulating the sense of taste.

taste the peculiar sensation caused by the contact of soluble substances with the tongue; the sense effected by the tongue, the gustatory and other nerves, and the gustatory center.

There are four basic tastes: sweet, salt, sour and bitter. Sometimes alkaline and metallic are also included as basic tastes. All other tastes are combinations of these. The taste buds are specialized, and each responds only to the kind of basic taste that is its specialty. The location of and the number of taste buds varies between animal species.

Other senses, including smell and touch, also play an important role in tasting.
t. bud, t. organ the organ of taste; spherical nests of cells embedded in the mucosa of the mouth and tongue are composed of supporting and gustatory cells. The gustatory cells have a delicate, hairlike process which protrudes from the peripheral surface of the cell. Substances must be in solution to be tasted, solids must be chewed and mixed with saliva.
conditioned t. aversion animals have been shown to develop aversions to foods associated with illness or other adverse experiences.
conditioned t. preference theoretically, the reverse of conditioned taste aversion, which is a naturally occurring phenomenon; it is not widely accepted that animals will associate recovery from illness with a specific taste or food.
t. pore opening from the exterior to a taste bud.
t. receptor one of the three types of cell in a taste bud; called also gustatory cells.

TAT 1. tube agglutination test. 2. tetanus antitoxin.

TATA box a eukaryotic DNA sequence usually TATAAATA, similar to the Pribnow box of *Escherichia coli,* occurring in the promoter region 25 to 35 bases upstream from the transcriptional start site that binds the general transcription factor TFIID which begins the formation of the transcription initiation complex which includes RNA polymerase.

Tatera see GERBIL.

tattoo see TATTOOING.

tattooing the introduction, by punctures, of permanent colors in the skin. Used in animals as a means of permanent identification, the number code being placed inside the ear pinna in all species except the horse in which it is placed on the inside of the upper lip. In some schemes, dogs may be tattooed inside the hindleg.

Taura syndrome virus cause of severe losses in juvenile prawns *Penaeus vanammei.*

taurindicus breeds of cattle produced by crossing *Bos taurus* and *B. indicus* cattle. Examples are Santa Gertrudis, Chinese Yellow, Sanga.

taurine a sulfur-containing amino acid found in mammalian tissues. Because of obligatory excretion and only limited ability to synthesize taurine, it is a dietary essential amino acid for cats. Called also 2-aminoethanesulfonic acid.
t. nutritional deficiency taurine is the predominant free amino acid in the retina and in cats a dietary deficiency of the acid may result from diets low in animal protein, causing generalized retinal atrophy. Dilated cardiomyopathy has also been associated with taurine deficiency in cats.

taurocholate a salt of taurocholic acid, one of the bile acids.

taurocholic acid a bile acid; when hydrolyzed it splits into taurine and cholic acid.

tauroconjugates secondary bile acids linked to taurine in the liver and secreted into bile.

Taurotragus oryx see ELAND.

tautomer a chemical compound exhibiting, or capable of exhibiting, tautomerism.

tautomeral pertaining to the same part; said especially of neurons and neuroblasts sending processes to aid in formation of the white matter in the same side of the spinal cord.
tautomerase an enzyme that catalyzes tautomeric reactions.
tautomeric exhibiting, or capable of exhibiting, tautomerism.
tautomerism stereoisomerism in which the compounds are mutually interconvertible, under normal conditions, forming a mixture that is in dynamic equilibration.
taxel see BADGER.
Taxidea taxus see BADGER.
taxine a toxic alkaloid found in *Taxus baccata*. Causes depression of conduction in the myocardium and consequent heart failure and anoxia. It also causes depression of smooth muscle activity and possibly of activity of the respiratory center.
taxis 1. an orientation movement of a motile organism in response to a stimulus; it may be either toward (positive) or away from (negative) the source of the stimulus; used also as a word ending, affixed to a stem denoting the nature of the stimulus. 2. exertion of force in manual replacement of a displaced organ or part.
taxon pl. *taxa* [Gr.] 1. a particular taxonomic grouping, e.g. a particular species, genus, family, order, class, phylum or kingdom. 2. the name applied to a taxonomic grouping.
taxonomist a specialist in taxonomy.
taxonomy the orderly classification of organisms into appropriate categories (taxa), with application of suitable and correct names.
numerical t. a method of classifying organisms solely on the basis of the number of shared phenotypic characters, each character usually being given equal weight; used primarily in bacteriology.
Taxus genus of the Taxaceae family of trees and shrubs; contain the toxic alkaloid taxine which causes abdominal pain, convulsions, vomiting, dyspnea, diarrhea in most patients and acute heart failure and sudden death in a few cases. Includes *Taxus baccata*, *T. baccata* var. *fastigiata* (Irish or churchyard yew), *T. brevifolia* (western yew), *T. canadensis* (ground hemlock), *T. cuspitata* (Japanese yew).
Tay–Sachs disease a sphingolipidosis of humans in which the inborn error of metabolism is a deficiency of the enzyme hexosaminidase A that results in accumulation of GM_2 ganglioside in the brain. Similar to GM_2 GANGLIOSIDOSIS in German shorthaired pointer dogs.
Tayassu the peccary, a wild species of what look like small pigs with very thin legs but which have a compartmented stomach like a ruminant. They are omnivorous and gregarious. Includes *T. ajacu* (collared peccary).
tayassuids see PECCARY.
Taylorella equigenitalis a facultatively anaerobic, gram-negative rod. It is the cause of CONTAGIOUS equine metritis. Previously called *Haemophilus equigenitalis*.
tazi see AFGHAN HOUND.
tazobactam a penicillanic acid sulfone derivative, similar to sulbactam; often combined with other antibiotics to extend their spectrum of activity.
TB 1. tuberculosis. 2. thoroughbred horse.
Tb chemical symbol, *terbium*.
tb tuberculosis; tubercle bacillus.
TBA trichlorobenzoic acid.
TBG thyroxine-binding globulin.
TBZ thiabendazole.
Tc chemical symbol, *technetium*.
Tc cell cytotoxic T LYMPHOCYTE; CTL.
TCA 1. trichloroacetic acid. 2. tricarboxylic acid cycle (Krebs cycle).
TCA cycle tricarboxylic acid cycle.
TCDD tetrachlorodibenzodioxin.
TCE trichloroethylene.
TCID tissue culture infective dose; that amount of a pathogenic agent that will produce pathological change when inoculated on tissue cultures.
$TCID_{50}$ median tissue culture infective dose; that amount of a pathogenic agent that will produce pathological change in 50% of cell cultures inoculated. Expressed as $TCID_{50}$/ml.
T_{CO_2} total carbon dioxide content of a plasma sample; equivalent to bicarbonate plus carbonic acid.
TCR T cell receptor.
T.D. Tracking Dog; the first level degree or title awarded to dogs in scent tracking tests.
Td cell delayed hypersensitivity T lymphocyte. Called also T_{DTH} cell. This cell type is not individually well characterized and is probably a Th1 cell that is functioning to produce a delayed type hypersensitivity reaction.
TDE 1. tetrachlorodiphenylethane—a CHLORINATED hydrocarbon insecticide. 2. ethoglucid, an antineoplastic agent.
TDN total digestible nutrients.
TDS total dissolved solids.
t.d.s. [L.] *ter die sumendum* (three times a day).
TDTH cell see TD CELL.
T.D.X. Tracking Dog Excellent; the highest level degree or title, after T.D., awarded to dogs in scent tracking competition.
Te chemical symbol, *tellurium*.
te ch'i the state in the body created by successful needle therapy.
tea plant see THEA CHINENSIS.
Teale–Knapp technique a surgical procedure for the repair of symblepharon in which conjunctival flaps from each side of the cornea are used to reconstruct the fornix.
tear[1] the watery, slightly alkaline and saline secretion of the lacrimal glands that moistens the conjunctiva. See also LACRIMAL apparatus.
artificial t's ophthalmic solutions formulated to replace tear secretion when it is reduced, as in keratoconjunctivitis sicca, by stabilizing the precorneal tear film. The most common preparations contain polyvinylpyrrolidone or methylcellulose.
t. film, precorneal t. film the thin layer of lacrimal secretions covering the outer surface of the cornea; in conjunction with secretions from the meibomian glands and conjunctival goblet cells forms the preocular film. Deficiency of these secretions results in drying of the cornea and keratoconjunctivitis sicca.
t. film breakup time an indicator of normal tear film function; premature breakup results in less protection of the cornea.
t. gas see LACRIMATOR.
t. gland lacrimal gland.
Schirmer t. test see SCHIRMER TEAR TEST.
t. staining syndrome abnormal drainage with overflow of tears results in constant wetness and staining of facial hairs, usually in small breeds of dogs and brachycephalic cats.
tear[2] a rent in membranes, e.g. in omentum and mesentery, or mucosae, e.g. rectal tear.
tears see lacrimal FLUID.
teart a term describing pastures in the UK which have

a high molybdenum content, because of the high levels of the mineral in the underlying soil. The pastures cause molybdenosis and secondary hypocuprosis in the ruminants that graze on them.

t. scours see COPPER nutritional deficiency.

tease 1. to pull apart gently with fine needles to permit microscopic examination. 2. to tantalize, e.g. sexually by parading a male in front of a female, or the opposite, in the mating capacity test.

teaser an animal used to sexually tease but not to impregnate the members of the opposite sex. Usually males and they may be surgically prepared to ensure that they cannot mate or are not fertile. In cattle and sheep vasectomized animals or castrates injected with testosterone are used; in horses an entire or cryptorchid is used but at a distance so that no act of mating can take place.

t. buck male goat used as a teaser.

t. bull a bull that is used to make sexual advances to cows and detect those that are on heat without being able to fertilize them; this usually means that physical mating cannot occur but vasectomized bulls are able to do so. More commonly the bull has been altered surgically so that the penis is diverted or the bull wears an interfering harness.

t. male male animal used as a teaser.

teasing the act of parading a male before a female to see if she displays estrus, and is therefore in a state where mating is likely to be fertile.

teaspoon a household unit of volume or capacity approximately equal to 5 milliliters.

teat nipple, especially the large nipples of ruminants; the cistern of the mammary gland opens into the teat cistern (lactiferous sinus) which communicates with the exterior through the teat canal(s) or lactiferous duct(s), of which there may be one (cow), two (mare), or several (sow, bitch). The openings of these ducts are kept closed by a sphincter muscle. When the lactating female is stimulated to let down her milk the teat cistern fills with milk under pressure. At other times the teat is limp. See also TEAT CUP, TEAT CUP LINER, TEAT DIP, TEAT SINUS.

accessory t. a supernumerary teat, especially a small one; very common in cows; may be attached to secreting mammary tissue; may have separate ductal systems or be offshoots from an existing, major duct.

t. angulation teats which stick out at an angle instead of straight down are an inconvenience in a modern milking parlor especially if automatic cup placers are in use. Considered to be an inherited defect.

t. blackpox see BLACK SPOT (1).

blind t. characterized by the obvious presence of milk in the mammary gland but no milk can be gained through the teat orifice, nor can a teat cannula or sound be passed into the mammary gland cistern. The defect may be congenital with all or any part of the teat cistern and canal not present, or the defect may be at the junction of the teat and gland cisterns. Acquired permanent blockage of the duct system is usually due to trauma, occasionally infection, and can similarly be at any point in the teat cistern or duct. See also blind QUARTER.

bottle t. a cow's teat with a very distended base tapering down to a narrow neck at the tip; resembles an inverted bottle. They are a defect because of the difficulty in putting on the teat cups.

t. calculus mineralized concretions in the mammary ductal system; called also lactolith, MILK stone.

t. cannula short, narrow, 1 inch diameter round-pointed metal or plastic tube used to pass from the exterior, through the teat canal and into the teat cistern. Used to relieve pressure in the gland when the teat canal is obstructed. Well-designed ones have a bulge followed by a constriction near the hub so that the tube is self-retaining. Called also teat tube.

t. chap superficial erythema, soreness due usually to continued wetting; a sequel to use of a too concentrated or otherwise irritant teat dip.

t. cistern the cavity inside the teat. Called also teat sinus.

congenital t. defect includes supernumerary teats, fused teats, absence of the mammary gland and teat, absence of a teat canal or cistern, imperforate udder cistern orifice, teat angulation in cows; in sows insufficient teats, teats too far posteriorly, inverted or vestigial teats.

t. dipping the dipping of teats of dairy cows in a long-acting disinfectant at the end of each milking. It is an essential part of the NIRD mastitis control program. See also TEAT DIP.

t. fibroma rare tumor of heifer teats.

t. fibrosarcoma rare tumor of heifer teats or udder.

t. fistula laceration of the teat wall in a lactating cow results in a permanent leaker so that milk drains out continuously and the quarter is at great risk from infection.

t. flora considered to be normal, i.e. without pathogenetic significance, in dairy cows—*Staphylococcus hyicus*, *S. epidermidis*, *Corynebacterium bovis*, coagulase negative staphylococci.

fused t.'s two teats joined together along their length, with a common teat cistern.

imperforate t. a congenitally obstructed teat due to failure of formation of the teat canal (lactiferous duct).

insufficient t.'s 12 is minimal in sows.

t. inversion the tip of the teat is inverted so that the meatus of the teat canal is in a hollow. The end of the teat may close over the sphincter and obstruct it during sucking; an inherited defect in sows.

t. leak see teat fistula (above).

t. lesions common site for lesions caused by epitheliotropic viruses, e.g. cowpox, mammillitis; trauma common cause, tread lesions in housed cows, barbed wire cuts in cows at pasture; infections, e.g. udder acne transmitted by teat cup liners or milker's hands.

milking machine t. injuries see BLACK SPOT.

misplaced t. e.g. too far back in sows so that piglets cannot get access when the sow is lying down.

t. necrosis in piglets born onto rough, abrasive floors; may not be apparent until mature.

t. occlusion due usually to tread trauma; rarely a congenital defect in which case all teats are usually affected.

t. orifice the opening to the papillary duct; normally held closed by the sphincter muscle in the wall of the teat and elastic tissue around the orifice. Invasion through the orifice is the primary route in the causation of most cases of mastitis.

t. papillomas are better described as fibropapillomas of the bovine teat. May be long tag-like structures, or white sessile nodules 0.5 inch diameter or ricegrain nodules all caused by different strains of a papovavirus.

t. photosensitive dermatitis part of a generalized dermatitis (except in poisoning by corticosteroid); characterized by localization of inflammation to lateral teat surface.

t. polyp in teat cistern causes intermittent obstruction requiring surgical removal.

rudimentary t. standard equipment in males; inherited defect in cows.

t. sanitization cleaning and disinfection before milking; most farmers reduce this to a wash with running cold water followed, in meticulous parlors, by drying with a paper towel.

t. sealers, t. sealant are materials used to aid in bovine mastitis control. 1. a polyvinylpyrrolidone preparation used to put on teat skin to seal milk orifice and protect skin against infection for long periods. 2. an inert preparation to be infused into the teat at drying off to protect against new infections during the dry period.

t. siphon see teat tube (below).

t. slitter a surgical instrument in the form of 2 mm diameter tube containing a sharp cutting blade concealed in its tip. The slitter is introduced into the teat cistern in the closed position, opened so that the blade protrudes and then withdrawn so as to slit the stenosed sphincter.

t. slough as part of gangrene of the gland.

t. sphincter the muscle in the teat wall around the external orifice of the teat; its relaxation is necessary for the rapid expulsion of milk during 'let-down'.

t. sphincter contracted due usually to injury; milking is uneven with much milk left in the affected quarter; requires surgical dilation.

t. spider membranous obstruction of the teat canal.

t. stenosis partial obstruction of the teat canal or cistern as a result of injury or inflammation.

t. stripping removing the last of the milk in the teat after machine milking by occluding the teat at the top between the thumb and forefinger and then pulling downwards so as to express all the milk from the teat. See also machine STRIPPING, hand STRIPPING, HAND-MILKING.

supernumerary t. see SUPERNUMERARY teats; see also accessory teat (above).

t. tube a 1.5 mm diameter metal or plastic tube with a tapered end for insertion in the external orifice of the cow's teat. Exit from the lumen is via holes in the side wall of the tube. Vary in length from 1.5 to 4 inches depending on purpose. Used mostly for the infusion of medicament into the teat and udder, but also for clearing the teat canal and cistern of debris and for evacuating milk from a quarter with a blocked teat. Called also teat siphon, teat cannula.

t. tuberculoid granulomas granulomas in the teat wall and lower udder contain *Mycobacterium terrae*. See also ENZOOTIC nodular thelitis.

t. ulcerative dermatitis deep ulcers in cows bedded on infected straw.

vestigial t. rudimentary non-functional teats.

t. wart see teat PAPILLOMATOSIS.

teat canal the short, small caliber duct(s) at the tip of the teat and communicating to the exterior. Called also streak canal.

t. c. absent considered to be an inherited defect.

teat cup the solid metal cups which house the flexible teat cup liners at the end of the milk line on a milking machine. Called also teat cup shell.

t. c. cluster four cups and a manifold, called a claw, which connects them to make a cluster; designed to milk one cow.

t. c. crawl movement of the teat cup up the teat as internal pressure in the udder drops during milking. May pinch off the opening of the teat cistern and stop milk flow.

t. c. disinfection the principal objective of the disinfection procedure is the TEAT CUP LINER.

t. cup removal removal of the teat cups at the end of the milking process; performed manually or mechanically by the teat cup remover (see below).

t. c. remover an automatic device that turns off the vacuum pressure and pulls off the teat cups when the flow of milk from the quarter falls below a critical point.

teat cup liner the rubber inflation in the cup of a milking machine. Made of neoprene or silicone rubber, molded to approximate the shape of a teat or made of a simple extruded tube, consisting of a mouthpiece, a tube and a short milk tube which passes out the hole at the end of the teat cup and is connected to the milk line of the milking machine. Forced to alternately constrict and relax by variation of the vacuum pressure in the milking cup.

t. c. l. deflector shield a small disk in the bottom of the liner which prevents a jet of milk entering at the end of the milk line and impinging on the end of the teat; experiments show a significant reduction in mastitis new infection rates when they are installed.

t. c. l. disinfection disinfection of the liners between cows; performed manually, especially in barns where cows are milked in their stalls, or automatically, in some parlors as part of a complete cycle of backflush, disinfect, rinse.

t. c. l. slip the firm adhesion between the milking machine cup liner and the teat skin is lost and the cup drops down the teat, does not milk and squeaks or squawks as air leaks past the incomplete barrier; may cause milk droplets from the affected cup to impact on the ends of the other teats of the cow and result in the spread of mastitis infection.

teat dip for teat dipping or spraying in mastitis control. Suitable dips are Hibitane 1 in 5000, iodine preparations containing 100 ppm free iodine or chlorine solutions containing 800–1200 ppm of free chlorine, linear dodecyl benzene sulfonic acid.

barrier t. d. application of materials, latex or rubber-based, which physically protect the teat sphincter against infection; the common disadvantage is the difficulty in removing the material when milking commences.

teat sinus the cavity which occupies most of the volume of the teat; dorsally it is continuous with the mammary gland sinus; ventrally it leads into the papillary duct (teat canal) and to the exterior; its confines consist of the distensible teat wall. Called also teat cistern.

t. s. absent congenital defect immediately branding the animal as a cull.

technetium a chemical element, atomic number 43, atomic weight 99, symbol Tc. See Table 6.

t.-99m the most frequently used radioisotope in nuclear medicine, a gamma emitter having a half-life of 6.04 hours and a primary photon energy of 140 keV; symbol ^{99m}Tc.

^{99m}Tc sulfur coated scintiscan see SCINTISCAN.

technic technique.

technician a person skilled in the performance of the technical or procedural aspects of a profession. Generally, the minimum preparation for this role is a course of training of 2 years full time or the equivalent. The technician carries out the routine work of the profession under the supervision of a veterinarian. Includes animal technician, veterinary nurse.

animal t. after a basic training there is specialization into laboratory or agricultural animals, possibly zoo and wild animals.

technique the method of procedure and details of a mechanical or chemical process or surgical operation.

t. chart set of rules for an x-ray machine with the objective of obtaining the same quality of performance at each operation. Includes the coordination of the variables, kilovolt peak (kVp), milliamperage and time (milliamp-seconds, mA·s), and tube-to-table distance, screen-film combination and processing.

technologist a person skilled in the theory and practice of a technical profession; requires a minimum training of 2 years and the award of a diploma or associate degree.

tectorial pertaining to tectorium; of the nature of a roof or covering.

t. membrane a gelatinous, fibrous, tongue-like structure resting on the tactile hairs in the spiral organ of the inner ear.

tectorium Corti's membrane.

tectospinal extending from the tectum of the midbrain to the spinal cord.

tectum a rooflike structure.

t. of mesencephalon, t. of midbrain the dorsal portion of the midbrain.

TED threshold erythema dose.

teeth small, bonelike structures of the jaws for the biting and mastication of food. Plural of *tooth*. See also DENTAL, TOOTH.

t. abscess see ALVEOLAR[1] abscess, MALAR abscess.

accessional t. the permanent molars, so called because they have no deciduous predecessors in the dental arch.

anelodont t. teeth with a limited period of growth.

anterior t. usually taken to include incisors and canines.

t. attrition see DENTAL attrition.

baby t. see deciduous teeth (below).

brachyodont t. a type of dentition as seen in humans and pigs; the teeth have short crowns, well developed roots and a narrow root canal. See also HYPSODONT, BUNODONT.

bunodont t. see BUNODONT.

canine t. the long, pointed tooth in the interdental space between incisors and cheek teeth; there is one in each jaw on both sides.

carnassial t. see CARNASSIAL TOOTH.

t. cavity see dental CAVITY, pulp CAVITY.

deciduous t. the temporary set of teeth that erupt in the young and are shed before or near maturity. They have smaller crowns and root systems and are fewer in number than the permanent teeth that replace them. Called also milk teeth, temporary teeth, baby teeth. Occasionally, particularly in small breeds of dogs, shedding of the deciduous tooth may not occur when the permanent replacement has erupted, necessitating veterinary intervention.

diphyodont t. see DIPHYODONT.

displaced molar t. see inherited displacement of MOLAR teeth.

ectopic t. see DENTAL cyst.

embedded t. unerupted.

congenital t. enamel deficiency see inherited ENAMEL defect.

t. eruption time see Table 19.

t. excessive wear occurs in animals on high fluorine intake or on diets low in calcium.

geminous t. see GEMINATION.

t. grinding 1. grinding of the incisors to improve foraging ability. Has been done to sheep with an industrial angle grinder with indifferent results. 2. see BRUXISM.

heterodont t. see HETERODONT.

homodont t. see HOMODONT.

hypsodont t. a form of dentition, seen in horses and many ruminants; the crown is high (deep), the root is short.

impacted t. one so placed in the jaw that it is unable to erupt or to attain its normal position in occlusion.

incisor t. the front teeth used for cropping grass or rending flesh. From two to four in each quadrant, depending on the species, except that they are missing in the upper jaw of ruminants.

inherited molar t. displacement see inherited displacement of MOLAR teeth.

lophodont t. cheek teeth with ridged occlusal surfaces. See also LOPHODONT.

t. maleruption defective eruption; includes delayed eruption and more usually eruption out of its normal position.

milk t. see deciduous teeth (above).

molar t. the permanent, primary cheek teeth that are not preceded by premolars. They are typically big teeth used for grinding and with ridges on their occlusal surfaces (lophodont) in horses, worn rounded cusps (bunodont) in pigs, or including crescents (selenodont) in cattle, and either cutting edges or flattened areas in carnivores.

monophyodont t. see MONOPHYODONT.

needle t. any small sharp teeth in piglets but principally the canine teeth.

permanent t. see permanent DENTITION.

t. pigmentation see TETRACYCLINE stain.

pink t. caused by staining with porphyrin, or by deficiency of dentine and enamel, a congenital defect.

premature t. loss a problem in New Zealand sheep. Characterized by acute then chronic gingivitis, then periodontitis and loss of teeth. Cause unknown.

premolar t. cheek teeth present in both generations, found between the molars and canines. The first premolar is exceptional in humans because it erupts late and is never replaced. In domestic species, there are up to three or four deciduous, followed by up to four permanent premolars in both jaws and on both sides.

t. rasp see tooth RASP.

retained t. deciduous premolars or incisors may be retained even though the permanent teeth have erupted. The deciduous crowns are likely to protrude at odd angles and cause difficult mastication.

secodont t. see SECODONT.

sectorial t. a cutting tooth. See CARNASSIAL TOOTH.

selenodont t. teeth with crescents in their grinding surfaces, as in the cheek teeth of ruminants.

sharp t. the edges of molar teeth in the horse which require frequent rasping because of the injury that they might cause to the oral mucosa.

stained t. red-brown in inherited porphyrinuria in cattle, frequent dosing with tetracyclines, heavy staining with brown tartar in ruminants with a rumination and prehension problem, usually due to loss of anterior part of tongue.

supernumerary t. teeth in excess of the normal complement, e.g. double row of incisors. Called also polyodontia, heterotopic polydontia.

temporary t. see deciduous teeth (above).

wolf t. see WOLF TOOTH.

teething eruption of deciduous teeth may cause gingivitis, fever, diarrhea in infant primates.

Teflon see POLYTEF, POLYTETRAFLUOROETHYLENE.

tegmen pl. *tegmina* [L.] a covering structure or roof.

t. tympani 1. the thin layer of bone separating the tympanic antrum from the cranial cavity. 2. the roof of the tympanic cavity, related to part of the petrous portion of the temporal bone.

tegmentum pl. *tegmenta* [L.] a covering.

mesencephalic t. part of the mesencephalon, the midbrain; contains the motor nuclei of the oculomotor and trochlear nerves, the red nucleus and the reticular formation.

tegu skink-like lizards of the Americas; many genera and species including *Tupinambis teguexin*.

teichoic acids antigenic polymers of glycerol or ribitol phosphates found attached to the cell walls or in association with membranes of gram-positive bacteria; they determine group specificity of some species, e.g. the staphylococci.

teicoplanin a glycopeptide antibiotic, similar to vancomycin, used in the treatment of serious gram-positive infections.

tela pl. *telae* [L.] a thin weblike tissue or structure.

t. choroidea a thin, web-like layer of connective tissue; a component of the choroid plexus.

t. conjunctivae connective tissue.

t. elastica elastic tissue.

subcutaneous t. the deepest layer of the skin, between the dermis and the fascia of the muscles. Called also hypodermis.

submucosal t. the connective tissue that supports a mucous membrane and that lines the deep surface of the tunica muscularis of viscera. The tissue serves as a framework that adapts to the changes in shape and size of the organ.

subserosal t. the connective tissue beneath the serous layer of a viscus.

Teladorsagia genus of nematodes in the family Trichostrongylidae. Includes *T. circumcincta* (*T. davtiani*, *T. trifurcata*), found in sheep, goats. Considered sometimes as a synonym of *Ostertagia*.

telangiectasia a vascular lesion formed by dilatation of a group of small blood vessels. It occurs in all species but is most common in the liver of cattle. See also PELIOSIS hepatis.

telangiectasis pl. *telangiectases;* telangiectasia.

telangiectatic pertaining to or emanating from telangiectasis.

telangiosis any disease of the capillaries.

tele- word element. [Gr.] *far away, operating at a distance, an end.*

teleauction auction, usually of livestock, over the telephone using a conference call mode so that a number of buyers can bid after hearing a description of the produce. The animals are often on the producer's farm. Avoids shipping and commingling.

telecanthus abnormally increased distance between the medial canthi of the eyelids.

telecardiography the recording of an electrocardiogram by transmission of impulses to a site at a distance from the patient; now commonly done via a telephone to a referral center or consultant's office.

telecardiophone an apparatus for making heart sounds audible at a distance from the patient.

teleceptor a nerve terminal that is sensitive to stimuli originating at a distance. Such nerve endings exist in the eyes and ears.

telecommunication sending data over telephone communication lines.

telecopier a facsimile device that can send a letter-sized document over standard telephone lines to a similar device. Commonly called 'fax'.

telediagnosis determination of the nature of a disease at a site remote from the patient on the basis of transmitted telemonitoring data or closed-circuit television consultation.

telefluoroscopy television transmission of fluoroscopic images for study at a distant location.

telegony a discredited, superstitious belief that offspring bred from one sire may also inherit characteristics from another sire to which the dam had been successfully bred on a previous occasion.

Telemark cattle rare Norwegian breed of dairy cattle subject to an inherited lethal chondrodysplastic dwarfism; red or brindle with lyre horns.

telemedicine the provision of consultant services by off-site veterinarians to other veterinarians on the scene, as by means of closed-circuit television.

telemetry the making of measurements at a distance from the subject, the measurable evidence of phenomena under investigation being transmitted by radio signals.

telencephalon [Gr.] *endbrain.* 1. the paired brain vesicles, which are the anterolateral outpouchings of the forebrain, together with the median, unpaired portion, the terminal lamina of the hypothalamus; from it the cerebral hemispheres are derived. 2. the anterior of the two vesicles formed by specialization of the forebrain in embryonic development.

teleneurite an end expansion of an axon.

teleneuron a nerve ending.

teleomitosis completed mitosis.

teleomorph an end-stage e.g. of a fungus.

teleorganic necessary to life.

teleost fish of the class Osteichthyes, having the skeleton completely ossified.

teleradiography radiography with the x-ray tube located approximately 6 ft away from the plate in order to more nearly secure parallelism of the rays.

teleradiotherapy treatment with ionizing radiation from an x-ray source located at a distance from the body.

teletherapy treatment in which the source of the therapeutic agent, e.g. radiation, is at a distance from the body. Called also external beam radiotherapy.

telluric 1. pertaining to tellurium. 2. pertaining to or originating from the earth.

tellurium a chemical element, atomic number 52, atomic weight 127.60, symbol Te. See Table 6.

telo- word element. [Gr.] *end.*

telocentric chromosome having the centromere at one end of the chromosome (terminal centromere) so that the chromosome has only one arm.

telodendritic zones one of the three functionally significant zones of neurons and their transmission of impulses; includes terminal modifications which permit transfer of information to the next element in the path.

telodendron, telodendrion any of the fine terminal branches of an axon.

telogen the quiescent or resting phase of the hair cycle, following catagen, the hair having become a club hair and not growing further.

t. effluvium, t. defluxion, t. defluvium widespread loss of hair due to large numbers of hair follicles being in synchronized telogen. In animals, may be associated with stress, severe malnutrition and drug therapy. In bitches, and less frequently queens, it is a common postpartum change.

t. hair follicle one in a resting stage.

telognosis diagnosis based on interpretation of radiographs transmitted by radio or telephonic communication.

telolemma the covering of a motor end-plate, made up of sarcolemma and an extension of Henle's sheath.

telomere an extremity of a chromosome, which has specific properties, one of which is a polarity that prevents reunion with any fragment after a chromosome has been broken.

telomorph the sexual form of a fungus.

telophase the last of the four stages of mitosis and of the two divisions of meiosis.

telotherapy the use of x-rays or radioactive compounds applied from a distance away from the body, as compared with BRACHYTHERAPY, which delivers radiotherapy by being placed onto or into tissue.

TEM 1. transmission electron microscope. 2. triethylenemelamine. 3. transmissible encephalopathy of mink.

temazepam a benzodiazepine tranquilizer.

TEME thromboembolic meningoencephalitis.

temephos an organophosphorus insecticide.

temocillin a semisynthetic penicillin, very resistant to β-lactamase.

temperament the peculiar behavioral character and mental cast of an animal.

t. change can be important in animal management or indicative of disease, e.g. vicious change in mare with ovarian adenocarcinoma, assumption of male characters in cow with ovarian tumor, disengagement in dogs with brain tumor. In food animals, castration of male livestock and spaying of females is practiced to aid management with limited restraint. In companion animals desexing practiced for population control also has marked effect on temperament.

temperateness said of climate; includes consideration of temperature, humidity and wind speed, especially an absence of extremes of them. See also effective TEMPERATURE.

t. index comparable to comfort index in human meteorology.

temperature the degree of sensible heat or cold, expressed in terms of a specific scale. See also HYPOTHERMIA, HYPERTHERMIA.

absolute t. that reckoned from absolute zero (−459.67°F or −273.15°C).

air t. the temperature of the surrounding air as measured by a dry-bulb thermometer.

ambient t. temperature of the immediate environment.

body t. a prime technique for assessing health status of a patient. Always a rectal temperature. Average temperatures above which hyperthermia, pyrexia or fever can be said to occur are listed under PYREXIA.

critical t. 1. that below which a gas may be converted to a liquid by pressure. 2. the environmental temperature at which the body is unable to maintain a constant body temperature and at which heat production must be increased (cold temperatures) or at which heat loss must be increased (high temperatures).

effective t. the combination of air temperature, humidity and wind speed. See also TEMPERATENESS index.

environmental t. air temperature.

nonpermissive t. one at which a conditional gene mutation is nonfunctional. See also temperature-sensitive MUTATION.

normal body t. that usually registered by a healthy animal. See PYREXIA.

permissive t. one at which a conditional gene mutation can express its normal function. See also temperature-sensitive MUTATION.

premortal t. fall the sudden fall in body temperature of a previously fevered animal just before death.

rectal t. the body temperature as measured by a rectal thermometer which has been in situ and in contact with the mucosa of the rectum with the anal sphincter tightly closed for at least 30 seconds. Alternative equipment is a dipolar electrode in a rectal probe.

t. stress exposure to excessively high or low environmental temperature.

windchill t. a combination of wind velocity and air temperature. See also effective temperature (above).

temperature–humidity index air temperature as measured by a wet-bulb thermometer and an expression of apparent temperature and comfort of animals in it.

temperature-sensitive living organisms that are sensitive to air temperatures outside of a narrow range, e.g. virus vaccine that does not replicate at deep body temperature, but does replicate in the respiratory tract.

t.-s. (ts) mutants strains of viruses or other microorganisms that are able to grow at certain low temperatures, say 90°F (32°C), which is referred to as the permissive temperature, but are unable to grow at higher temperatures, say 102°F (39°C), which is referred to as the nonpermissive temperature. Such conditionally lethal mutants have been much used in the genetic analysis, i.e. gene mapping, of microorganisms. At the nonpermissive temperature the protein product of a particular gene is unstable and hence nonfunctional, whereas the protein function is normal at the permissive temperature. These mutants have also been selected for use in vaccines because of their growth requirements for lower temperatures and lower pathogenicity, e.g. ts strains of bovine herpesvirus 1 which, when administered intranasally, grow on nasal mucosa but do not cause systemic illness.

t.-s. proteins proteins that are functional at higher temperatures, but not at others. See temperature-sensitive mutants (above).

template the macromolecule that serves as a pattern for the synthesis of another macromolecule. In nucleic acid synthesis, the DNA from which a new strand is copied. See also DEOXYRIBONUCLEIC ACID, PCR.

temple the lateral region on either side of the head, above the zygomatic arch; a term commonly used in humans, but not in animals.

tempolabile subject to change with the passage of time.

temporal 1. pertaining to the temple. Said of bones and muscles—see Tables 10 and 13. 2. pertaining to time; limited as to time; temporary.

t. distribution distribution of events or population in chronological time; a suitable scatter graph may reveal clusters that have epidemiological significance.

t. lobe a long, tongue-shaped process constituting the lower lateral portion of the cerebral hemisphere.

t. summation occurs in the transmission of nerve impulses when a volley of impulses arrives at a synapse so that the duration of the impulses is briefer than the postsynaptic potential and their deliveries of transmitter are combined to create a larger than normal response.

temporary interim; for a short time only.

t. dentition the temporary or first set of teeth in animals with diphyodont dentition. See also deciduous TEETH.

t. environment factors e.g. rain, drought, heat.

t. registration registration to practice under local legislation but for a limited period only. A procedure used to permit a candidate for full registration to obtain some practice experience.

temporomandibular pertaining to the temporal bone and mandible.

t. dysplasia subluxation with open-mouth jaw locking occurs in Irish setters and Basset hounds, caused by developmental abnormalities in the condyloid process of the mandible and the mandibular fossa of the temporal bone. Called also temporomandibular joint (TMJ) syndrome.

t. joint syndrome see temporomandibular dysplasia (above).

temporomaxillary pertaining to the temporal bone and maxilla.

temporo-occipital pertaining to the temporal and occipital bones.

temporosphenoid pertaining to the temporal and sphenoid bones.

tempostabile not subject to change with time.

TEN toxic epidermal necrolysis.

ten eighty, 1080 see SODIUM fluoroacetate.

ten-key pad a key pad of numbers found on most computer keyboards in addition to the usual row of numbers to facilitate the touch typing of large volumes of numerical data. Universally referred to as a numeric cluster.

tenacious viscid; adhesive.

tenaculum a hooklike surgical instrument for grasping and holding parts.

tenascin adhesive glycoprotein contributing to the cell-to-basal lamina-to-matrix interface.

tender said of wool whose fibers break easily because of a weakness caused by an illness or feed stress.

tenderizing natural tenderizing is caused by the action of enzymes already in tissues. This effect can be enhanced by quick freezing before rigor mortis sets in, and by hanging the meat at the proper temperature for the proper time, especially just before cooking. Called also conditioning. Artificial tenderizing is carried out by stretching or pounding the meat with a proper hammer with a hobnail hammer face, by electrical stimulation or by application of one of the commercial enzyme preparations of papain (from pawpaw) or bromelin (from pineapple).

tenderness a state of unusual sensitivity to touch or pressure.

rebound t. a state in which pain is felt on the release of pressure over a part.

tenderstretch tenderizing see TENDERIZING.

tendinitis inflammation of tendons and of tendon–muscle attachments. It is one of the commonest causes of lameness. Tendinitis may be associated with a calcium deposit (calcific tendinitis), which may also involve the bursa around the tendon or near the joint, causing bursitis.

tendinoplasty tenoplasty.

tendinosuture tenorrhaphy.

tendinous pertaining to, resembling, or of the nature of a tendon.

tendo [L.] *tendon.*

t. Achillis, t. calcaneus ACHILLES TENDON.

tendolysis tenolysis; the freeing of a tendon from adhesions.

tendon a sheet, cord or band of strong white fibrous tissue that connects a muscle to a bone or other structure. When the muscle contracts, or shortens, it pulls on the tendon. Tendons serve to convey an action to a remote site, change the direction of pull and focus the force. Sheetlike tendons (aponeuroses) serve to support and squeeze, cordlike ones to act on joints. See also CUNEAN tendon.

t. aponeuroses see APONEUROSIS.

bowed t. chronic tendinitis of the superficial flexor tendons, usually of the front limbs, of a horse. The horse is lame or inclined to lameness, the tendon is thickened and is visibly enlarged. It may be painful on palpation in the early, acute stages.

calcaneal t. see ACHILLES TENDON.

t. cartilaginous metaplasia focal metaplasia with the formation of cartilage in tendons causes no apparent harm and is considered to be normal.

common calcanean t. see ACHILLES TENDON.

congenital t. contracture an inherited contracture of multiple tendons is identified in cattle. The joints are fixed in extension or flexion and cause serious dystocia. See also AKABANE VIRUS disease.

contracted t's see tendon contracture (below).

t. contracture permanent contraction of a tendon caused by chronic tendinitis. Most commonly of the flexor tendons of the digit in the horse. The action of the affected limb is restricted and the limb is not fully extended at rest causing the animal to stand up on its toe. Called also contracted tendons.

flexor t's tendons of the superficial and deep flexor muscles of the digit. Commonly strained, lacerated and separated in the racing horse.

t. graft done in horses with badly torn or ruptured flexor tendons. Autologous grafts are taken from the lateral digital extensor tendon.

hamstring t. see HAMSTRING.

t. implants see CARBON FIBER IMPLANTS.

internal biceps t. a core of fibrous tissue within the biceps muscle of horses which serves a significant role in the stay apparatus.

interosseous t. SUSPENSORY ligament (1).

t. luxation slipping of the superficial flexor tendon of the hindlimb of the horse off the tuber calcis, usually in the medial direction; also occurs rarely in dogs and ostriches. See also PEROSIS.

t. osseous metaplasia a pathological abnormality and usually attended by abnormality of movement. See also tendon ossification (below).

t. ossification occurs extensively in gallinaceous birds in the tendons of the legs and feet, the wings and the epaxial musculature. Although the ossification may be extensive the birds are normal and the reasons for the changes are unknown.

prepubic t. the tendon of insertion of the two abdominal recti muscles on to the pubis.

t. sheath a fluid-filled sleeve that resembles a synovial bursa wrapped around the tendon so as to form a continuous sheath, except for the MESOTENDON.

t. splitting performed by slitting the superficial flexor tendon (or the suspensory ligament) along its long axis and from lateral to medial sides as a treatment for tendinitis. The objective is to stimulate vascularization and hasten repair.

t. sprain see SPRAIN.

sprained t. see tendon strain (below).

t. strain the injury caused to flexor tendons in the horse during racing. Most commonly affected is the superficial flexor tendon in the front limb. See also bowed tendon (above). Called also sprained tendon.

symphysial t. a vertical median sheet which hangs from the pubic symphysis and provides an origin for the medial thigh muscles.

tendonectomy surgical severance of a tendon. Called also tenotomy.

tendonitis tendinitis.

tendovaginal pertaining to a tendon and its sheath.

tendovaginitis inflammation of a tendon and its tendon sheath.

Tenebrio molitor a pest of stored grain which may attack the claws of setting hens and tissues of newly hatched birds. Other mealworm species are known to have the same effect. Called also yellow mealworm.

tenectomy excision of a lesion of a tendon or of a tendon sheath.

tenesmus ineffectual and painful straining at defecation or in urinating. Called also straining. See also STRANGURY.

tenia pl. *teniae* [L.] a flat band or strip of soft tissue. A concentration of external longitudinal muscle and elastic fibers, e.g. on the large intestine of horses, pigs and some other species, dividing it into two to five longitudinal segments which are divided further into transient haustra or pockets. See tenia ceci (below).

t. ceci one of the four longitudinal muscular bands on the external surface of the cecum of some species, such as the horse, pig and rabbit, that puckers the tract into haustra.

t. coli the bands on the surface of the colon of some species. In the horse the thickened bands (tenia libera, tenia mesocolica and tenia omentalis) formed by longitudinal fibers in the tunica muscularis of the colon, the number varying from one to four.

teniacide, taeniacide 1. lethal to tapeworms. 2. an agent lethal to tapeworms.

teniafuge, taeniafuge a medicine for expelling tapeworms.

teniamyotomy an operation involving a series of transverse incisions of the teniae coli.

teniasis infection with tapeworms of the genus *Taenia*. The adult tapeworms do not cause a clinically recognizable disease. The larval stages may cause clinical signs described under COENUROSIS or CYSTICERCOSIS.

teniid pertaining to or emanating from cestodes in the family Taeniidae.

Tennessee walking horse a horse, originating in a Standardbred stallion, and bred for show and pleasure; the breed is characterized by its showy fast walk which can lapse into a pacing gait unless care is taken. It is a fast, four-beat gliding walk reputed to be the most comfortable of all of the gaits for the rider. A robust, less elegant version of the AMERICAN SADDLE HORSE, about 15 to 15.2 hands high, usually black or chestnut with white markings.

tennis racket spore classical shape of *Clostridium tetani* bacterium containing a terminal spore. Called also drumstick spore.

teno- word element. [Gr.] *tendon*.

tenodesis suture of the end of a tendon to a bone.

tenolysis the operation of freeing a tendon from adhesions.

tenomyoplasty plastic repair of a tendon and muscle, applied especially to an operation for inguinal hernia.

tenomyotomy excision of a portion of a tendon and muscle.

tenonectomy excision of part of a tendon to shorten it.

tenonitis 1. tendinitis. 2. inflammation of Tenon's capsule, the connective tissue enclosing the eyeball.

tenonometer an apparatus for measuring intraocular pressure.

Tenon's capsule the connective tissue enveloping the posterior eyeball.

tenontitis tendinitis.

tenonto- word element. [Gr.] *tendon*.

tenontography a written description or delineation of the tendons.

tenontology the sum of what is known about the tendons.

tenontothecitis tenosynovitis.

tenophyte a growth or concretion in a tendon.

tenoplasty plastic repair of a tendon.

tenoreceptor a nerve receptor in a tendon.

tenorrhaphy suture of a tendon.

three-loop t. a technique used for the repair of avulsion injuries of tendons, particularly the gastrocnemius tendon. It involves multiple throws of suture material through the tendon and the site of attachment. Its advantages are better closure of gaps with minimal distortion of tendon ends and disruption of blood flow.

tenositis tendinitis.

tenostosis conversion of a tendon into bone.

tenosuspension surgical attachment of the head of the humerus to the acromion by a strip of tendon; carried out as a treatment for habitual dislocation of the shoulder.

tenosuture tenorrhaphy.

tenosynovectomy excision or resection of a tendon sheath.

tenosynovitis inflammation of a tendon and its sheath, the lubricated layer of tissue in which the tendon is housed and through which it moves. It is painful, and may temporarily disable the affected part.

Arthritis frequently involves tendon sheaths. A less common cause of tenosynovitis is injury to the tendon sheath and subsequent infection.

villonodular t. a condition marked by exaggerated proliferation of synovial membrane cells, producing a solid tumor-like mass, may occur in periarticular soft tissues and less frequently in joints.

tenotome knife see tenotomy KNIFE.

tenotomy transection of a tendon.

graduated t. partial transection of a tendon.

tenovaginitis tenosynovitis.

tenrec an insect-eating mammal related to the hedgehogs and shrews belonging to the family Tenrecidae. Nocturnal eaters of earthworms, 8 to 12 inches long with a coat of hairs, bristles and spines and a long pointed nose.

Tenrecidae the otter shrews. Shrews are insectivorous mammals in many orders and genera. Include elephant, otter and tree shrews.

TENS transcutaneous electrical nerve stimulator.

Tensilon trademark for EDROPHONIUM chloride; used in the diagnosis of myasthenia gravis, known as the Tensilon test.

tension 1. the act of stretching or the condition of being stretched or strained. 2. the partial pressure of a component of a gas mixture or of a gas dissolved in a fluid, e.g. of oxygen in blood. 3. voltage.

arterial t. blood pressure within an artery.

t. band wires heavy gauge wire is inserted in fracture fragments and around pins placed in the fragments in order and adjusted to create compression on the fracture site. Suited for treatment of apophyseal or epiphyseal avulsion fractures. See also tension band PLATE.

intraocular t. intraocular pressure; intraocular tension, normal intraocular tension being indicated by Tn, while T + 1, T + 2, etc. indicate increased tension, and T − 1, T − 2, etc. indicate decreased tension.

t. line the direction of pull on the skin in any given region. A map of the body, drawn to show the various lines of pull, or tension, is useful in planning surgical closure of skin incisions, particularly ones with defects, in order to minimize forces that might cause dehiscence.

surface t. tension or resistance that acts to preserve the integrity of a surface.

tissue t. a state of equilibrium between tissues and cells that prevents overaction of any part.

tension–time index developed as a measure of the total tension of, for example, the left ventricle and is a product of the mean systolic pressure, times the duration of systole, times the heart rate.

tensor any muscle that stretches or makes tense.
t. veli palatini see Table 13.1C.
tent a conical, expansible plug of soft material for dilating an orifice or for keeping a wound open, so as to prevent its healing except at the bottom.
t. pegging equine sport invented in India. The horse is ridden at a canter and the rider attempts to uproot a tent peg from the ground with a sharp-pointed lance.
sponge t. a conical plug made of compressed sponge used to dilate the os uteri.
tentacle a slender, whiplike appendage in animals that may function in prehension and feeding or as a sense organ.
tenting see SKIN tenting test.
tentorial pertaining to the tentorium of the cerebellum.
t. hernia see BRAIN herniation.
tentorium pl. *tentoria* [L.] a part resembling a tent or covering.
t. cerebelli the sheet of dura mater separating the cerebrum from the cerebellum.
tenuazonic acid a metabolic product of *Alternaria* spp. fungus.
tephromyelitis inflammation of the gray matter of the spinal cord.
tephrosis incineration or cremation.
tepor [L.] *gentle heat.*
TEPP tetraethyl pyrophosphate.
ter- word element. [L.] *three, three-fold.*
ter in die [L.] three times a day; abbreviation is t.i.d.
tera- word element. [Gr.] *monster;* used in naming units of measurement to designate an amount 10^{12} (a million million) times the unit specified by the root to which it is joined, as teracurie; symbol T.
teras pl. *terata* [L., Gr.] a monster.
terat- prefix meaning congenital anomaly.
teratism an anomaly of formation or development; the condition of a monster.
terato- word element. [Gr.] *monster, monstrosity.*
teratoblastoma a neoplasm containing embryonic elements, differing from a teratoma in that its tissue does not represent all germinal layers.
teratocarcinoma a malignant neoplasm consisting of elements of teratoma with those of embryonal carcinoma or choriocarcinoma, or both; occurring most often in the testis, occasionally in uterus.
teratogen an agent or influence that causes physical defects in the developing embryo.
teratogenesis the production of deformity in the developing embryo, or of a monster.
teratogenic pertaining to or emanating from teratogen.
teratogenicity the capacity to act as a teratogen.
teratogenous developed from fetal remains.
teratogeny teratogenesis.
teratoid resembling a monster.
t. medulloepithelioma contains elements of cartilage, skeletal muscle and brain tissue.
teratology that division of embryology and pathology dealing with abnormal development and congenital deformations.
teratoma a true neoplasm made up of a number of different types of tissue, none of which is native to the area in which it occurs; usually found in the ovary or testis. See also DERMOID cyst.
malignant t. a solid, malignant ovarian tumor resembling a dermoid cyst but composed of immature embryonal or extraembryonal elements derived from all three germ layers.
teratomatous pertaining to or of the nature of teratoma.
teratosis the condition of a monster.
teratospermia malformed spermatozoa in the semen.
teratozoospermia the ejaculate contains a high percentage of morphologically abnormal spermatozoa.
terba *Chrozophora plicata.*
terbinafine an antifungal agent used as the hydrochloride in the treatment of fungal skin infections and particularly those involving the nails.
terbium a chemical element, atomic number 65, atomic weight 158.924, symbol Tb. See Table 6.
terbutaline a β-adrenergic receptor antagonist used as a bronchodilator.
terebration an act of boring or trephining.
terefa, terepha Jewish classification of meat meaning unsuitable for human food.
teres [L.] *long and round.*
t. ligament a round ligament; those of the bladder and liver are vestiges of umbilical vessels; that of the uterus is a rounded band from the broad ligament containing some smooth muscle.
terfenadine a nonsedating antihistamine used in the treatment of allergies.
term a definite period, especially the period of gestation, or pregnancy.
terminal 1. forming or pertaining to an end. 2. a termination, end or extremity, especially a nerve ending. 3. an input–output station of a COMPUTER. The terminal may be distant from the computer and be connected to it by an acoustic coupler or a modem attached to a telephone line. The terminal may have the sole function of entering and receiving data—a dumb terminal, or it may be capable of carrying out computing functions itself—an intelligent terminal. 4. the end-stages of a fatal illness.
t. cisterns the SER (smooth endoplasmic reticulum) in skeletal muscle fibers is a network of cisterns and tubules; the cisterns are attachments to the tubules and two tubules and a terminal cistern make up a triad.
t. crossbreeding a breeding program in which crossbreds are produced by mating two sets of purebreds but without further breeding among the crossbreds; a continuing F_1 generation.
efferent t. nerve endings transmitting nerve stimuli to effector organs; include neuromuscular spindles and Golgi apparatus.
t. ileitis see terminal ILEITIS.
t. pathway see terminal COMPLEMENT pathway.
terminal redundancy a stretch of several hundred nucleotides that is repeated at each end of the DNA molecule.
Terminalia oblongata Australian tree in the Combretaceae family of plants. Contains toxic hydrolyzable tannins (punicalagin) which causes nephrosis, hepatic necrosis. Clinically there is diarrhea and edema. Chronic cases show frequent straining and dribbling of urine. Causes Mackenzie river disease. Called also yellow-wood.
terminatio pl. *terminationes* [L.] an ending; the site of discontinuation of a structure, as the free nerve endings (terminationes nervorum liberae), in which the peripheral fiber divides into fine branches that terminate freely in connective tissue or epithelium.
termination signal a specific sequence in DNA at which the RNA polymerase and the newly made RNA transcript are released from their DNA association.
terminology 1. the vocabulary of an art or science. 2. the science that deals with the investigation, arrangement and construction of terms.
accurate t. essential for proper data storage and retrieval and requires an internationally recognized

nomenclature of diseases, pathology, clinical indicants, treatments and surgical operations.

terminus pl. *termini* [L.] an ending.

tern a large, marine bird in the family Laridae, together with gulls. They are effortless fliers, great divers and poor walkers. Can be infected with avian influenza virus.

ternary 1. third in order. 2. made up of three elements or radicals.

Ternidens a genus of strongylid worms in the family Chabertiidae.

T. deminatus found in the large intestine of primates and occasionally humans. They cause anemia and the development of nodules in the intestinal wall similar to those of *Oesophagostomum* spp.

terpene any hydrocarbon of the formula $C_{10}H_{16}$. A principal component of toxic oleoresins extracted from conifer trees and of TURPENTINE and CAMPHOR.

terpin a product obtained by the action of nitric acid on oil of turpentine and alcohol, used as an expectorant in the form of the hydrate.

Terramycin a proprietary name for oxytetracycline.

Terranova a genus of nematodes in the family Anisakidae that parasitize elasmobranch fish.

terrapin see TURTLE.

terrarium a closed glass container in which plants or small animals are cultivated.

terriers a group of dog breeds, developed as farm dogs in the British Isles for the hunting of vermin and ground dwelling mammals, e.g. rats, badgers, foxes and rabbits. The name is derived from the Latin *terra* because the dogs commonly pursue their quarry into burrows. Most have a harsh, wiry coat for the purpose. Includes such breeds as the AIREDALE, AUSTRALIAN, BEDLINGTON, BOSTON, BULL, CAIRN, DANDIE DINMONT, ENGLISH TOY, FOX, GLEN OF IMAAL, IRISH, JACK RUSSELL, KERRY BLUE, LAKELAND, MANCHESTER, NORFOLK, NORWICH, SCOTTISH, SEALYHAM, SILKY, SKYE, SOFT-COATED WHEATEN, STAFFORDSHIRE, TIBETAN, WELSH, WEST HIGHLAND WHITE and YORKSHIRE.

territoriality see territorial AGGRESSION.

tertian recurring in 3-day cycles (every second day).

tertiary third in order.

t. structure proteins unique structure made up of secondary structure elements (such as helices, β-sheets) folded in a specific way to determine the three-dimensional, biologically-active conformation of a protein.

tertigravida a female pregnant for the third time; gravida III.

tertipara tripara; a female which has had three pregnancies that resulted in viable offspring; para III.

Tervuren, Tervueren see BELGIAN shepherd dog.

Teschen disease see porcine viral ENCEPHALOMYELITIS.

tesla the SI unit of magnetic flux density, equal to one weber per square meter. Symbol T.

tessellated divided into squares, like a checker board.

test 1. an examination or trial. 2. a significant chemical reaction. 3. a reagent. See also under specific names of tests.

***cis-trans* t.** used in microbial genetics to determine whether two mutations that have the phenotypic effect, in a haploid cell or a cell with single phage infection, are located in the same gene or in different genes; the test depends on the independent behavior of two alleles of a gene in a diploid cell or in a cell infected with two phages carrying different alleles.

critical titer t. the titer of a test at which the patient is judged to have reacted positively to the test.

diazo t. a group of tests for bilirubin conjugates in urine and therefore suitable for the detection of biliary and hepatic disease. Based on the combination of bilirubin with a stable diazonium compound.

exact t. a statistical test based on the exact distribution of the data under the null hypothesis, rather than on a normal approximation.

hypothesis t. the method by which a hypothesis is judged.

sodium sulfanilate clearance t. see SULFANILATE.

t. station set up by the government or a cooperative organization for the purpose of testing individual livestock provided by farmers for productivity in terms of egg production, milk yield, weight gain. The feeding and measurement are under the control of the station.

statistical t. used to decide between two hypotheses.

surrogate t. an indirect test, e.g. milk cell count.

tolerance t. 1. an exercise test to determine the efficiency of the circulation. 2. determines the body's ability to metabolize a substance or to endure administration of a drug, e.g. insulin tolerance test.

triglyceride absorption t. see FAT absorption test.

urine concentration t. see WATER deprivation test.

V-t. a dexamethasone suppression test followed by an ACTH response test; the name refers to the change in plasma cortisone levels, first depressed then elevated, which if plotted on a graph would form a V.

test and slaughter a disease control program based on selective slaughter of animals, for diagnosis by necropsy, chosen by an immunological test.

test mating the technique of mating a suspected heterozygote with a group of known heterozygotes to test whether the suspect is in fact a carrier of the subject gene. The test needs an adequate number of test animals to achieve statistical significance.

test meal a portion of food or foods given for the purpose of determining the functioning of the digestive tract.

barium t. m. a meal containing barium sulfate as the opaque constituent. See also BARIUM study.

motor t. m. food or drink whose progress through the stomach, pylorus and intestinal tract is observed fluoroscopically.

opaque t. m. a meal containing some substance opaque to x-rays, permitting visualization of the gastrointestinal tract.

test tube a tube of thin glass, closed at one end; used in chemical tests and other laboratory procedures.

testectomy the removal of a testis. Called also orchiectomy.

tester population in breeding programs it is often necessary to evaluate a strain or breed; the evaluation is carried out by mating the population to be tested with a tester herd.

testes [L.] plural of *testis.*

testicle testis.

testicular pertaining to the testis.

t. agenesis absence of one or both testes, usually part of a wider range of defects.

t. anomaly includes hypoplasia, cryptorchidism, agenesis, heterotopia, polyorchidism, cystic rete testis and heterotopic Leydig cells and accessory adrenal cortical tissue.

t. biopsy percutaneous sampling of tissue for laboratory examination; disruption of normal spermatogenesis can be expected.

t. calcinosis common as a sequel to chronic inflammation and concurrent with fibrosis.

t. degeneration the most frequent cause of male infertility; many causes; regeneration and return to normal function possible provided some spermatogonia survive the insult and the basement membrane of the tubules is undamaged.

t. descent includes a long-distance, passive descent from the roof of the abdomen to near the inguinal canal followed by a short-distance, also passive, descent through the inguinal canal into the scrotum.

t. feminization syndrome an extreme form of male pseudohermaphroditism, with female external development, including secondary sex characteristics, but with the presence of testes and absence of uterus and tubes; it is due to end-organ resistance to the action of testosterone.

t. fibrosis a sequel to inflammation or degeneration; common in old bulls.

t. foreign body constriction malicious application of a constricting foreign body, usually an elastic band, around the base of the scrotum in dogs is an occasional cause of orchitis and often necessitates castration with scrotal ablation. Called also the 'nasty child syndrome', although 'bull terrier bite' would probably be more common.

t. hypoplasia occurs as an uncomplicated state, or as part of cryptorchidism or intersex anomaly; an inherited defect in Swedish Highland cattle.

t. inflammation see ORCHITIS.

t. lobuli lobules created in the testis by connective tissue septa.

t. mediastinum the central dividing plane of tissue which divides the testis and is continuous with its tunica albuginea.

t. septuli loose connective tissue septa which divide testis into lobules.

t. torsion causes pain and swelling of the scrotum, abdominal pain and vomiting. In dogs, testicles with neoplasms are predisposed to torsion. Occurs occasionally in stallions (180° torsion), with no apparent detrimental consequences on health or fertility.

t. tumors includes interstitial cell and Sertoli cell tumors and seminomas.

testis pl. *testes* [L.] the male gonad; either of the paired, egg-shaped glands normally situated in the scrotum; called also testicle. The testes produce the spermatozoa, the male reproductive cells, which are ejaculated into the female vagina during coitus, and the male sex hormone, testosterone, which is responsible for the secondary sex characters of the male.

ectopic t. the testis is in an abnormal position away from the normal descent pathway.

nonscrotal t. includes ectopic and cryptorchid testis.

retained t. see CRYPTORCHID.

supernumerary t. polyorchidism.

t. tubuli contorti seminiferous TUBULE.

undescended t. see CRYPTORCHID. Called also retained testicle.

testis-determining factor a single gene on the short arm of the Y chromosome.

testitis inflammation of a testis; called also ORCHITIS.

testoid a term applied to testicular hormones and other natural or synthetic compounds having a similar effect.

testosterone the most important male sex hormone (ANDROGEN) produced by the Leydig cells of the testes in response to luteinizing hormone (LH) secreted by the pituitary. Its chief function is to stimulate the development of the male reproductive organs and the secondary sex characters, such as the crest. It is necessary for the appearance of normal male sexual behavior. It encourages growth of bone and muscle, and helps maintain muscle strength. It is occasionally secreted in large amounts also by granulosa–theca cell tumors of the ovary, especially in mares.

t. cyclopentylpropionate, t. cypionate, t. propionate esters with a long period of activity.

t.-responsive dermatosis a bilaterally symmetrical alopecia, primarily affecting the flanks, ventral abdomen and caudomedial aspect of the thighs of male dogs. The cause is believed to be hypotestosteronism.

Testudo genus of land tortoises in the family Testudinidae. Includes *T. graeca* (spur-thighed tortoise), *T. hermannii* (Hermann's tortoise). See also TURTLE.

tetanic 1. tonic. 2. pertaining to tetanus.

t. convulsions convulsions characterized by prolonged muscle spasm without intervening periods of relaxation. The legs are extended, the neck is dorsiflexed. Seen in strychnine poisoning and tetanus.

tetaniform resembling tetanus.

tetanigenous producing tetanic spasms.

tetanism persistent muscular hypertonicity, as in the newborn.

tetanization the induction of tetanic convulsions or muscular spasms.

tetanize to induce tetanic convulsions or muscular spasms.

tetanode the unexcited stage of tetany.

tetanoid resembling tetanus.

tetanolepsin a toxin produced by *Clostridium tetani* which causes red cell hemolysis; it is not clinically significant.

tetanolysin the hemolytic fraction of the exotoxin formed by *Clostridium tetani*, the causative organism of tetanus; not known to play role in pathogenesis.

tetanospasmin the neurotoxic exotoxin produced by *Clostridium tetani*, which inhibits release of gamma amino butyric acid by inhibitory neurons, resulting in tetanic spasms.

tetanus a highly fatal disease of all animal species caused by the neurotoxin of *Clostridium tetani*. The bacterial spores are deposited in tissue, usually by traumatic injury, retained placenta or endometrial injury and under anaerobic conditions vegetate. Clinical features of the disease are remarkably similar in all species but there are differences in susceptibility to the disease. The muscle spasms cause a stiff gait, rigid posture (sometimes called 'sawhorse stance'), extension or elevation of the tail, protrusion of the third eyelid and trismus (lockjaw). Horses show flaring of the nostrils. In dogs, spasms of facial muscles cause abnormally erect ears and retraction of the lips that resembles the 'risus sardonicus' seen in humans with tetanus. Stimulation precipitates generalized muscle contractions and tetanic spasms or convulsions. The disease can be prevented by immunization with tetanus toxoid or the use of antitoxin, but this is done routinely only in humans and horses.

t. antitoxin see tetanus ANTITOXIN.

idiopathic t. a loosely defined syndrome of outbreaks of tetanus in young cattle without a wound being found; current practice is to refer to such outbreaks as being caused by the ingestion of preformed tetanus toxin.

localized t. tetany occurs predominantly in one limb, closest to the site of entry of the organism, but then usually spreads to the opposite limb and then the whole body. Seen in dogs and particularly cats.

t. toxin see tetanus TOXIN.

t. toxoid see TOXOID.

tetany continuous tonic spasm of a muscle; steady contraction of a muscle without distinct twitching. It is manifested clinically by rigidity of limbs, pricking of ears, flaring of nostrils. In extreme tetany as in tetanus, the rigidity is lead-pipe in nature in that the resistance to bending is constant. In less severe tetany, e.g. an upper motor neuron lesion, there is resistance at first but as soon as this is overcome the limb flexes easily.

grass t. see LACTATION TETANY (2).

hyperventilation t. tetany produced by forced inspiration and expiration continued for a considerable time.

hypocalcemic t. see puerperal tetany (below).

hypomagnesemic t. see calf HYPOMAGNESEMIC tetany, LACTATION TETANY (2).

lactation t. see LACTATION TETANY.

latent t. tetany elicited by the application of electrical and mechanical stimulation.

magnesium-deficiency t. a product of experimental nutrition but see also LACTATION TETANY.

milk t. see calf HYPOMAGNESEMIC tetany.

parathyroid t., parathyroprival t. tetany due to removal or hypofunctioning of the parathyroid glands.

t. pastures lush grass or cereal crop pastures, in the early spring when they have grown rapidly and their magnesium content is low. The weather is also inclined to be inclement with a high wind-chill factor and there is little or no shelter for the recently calved cows.

puerperal t. a syndrome of hypocalcemia in bitches, usually of small breeds, typically 2 to 3 weeks after whelping, caused by the loss of extracellular calcium in lactation. Affected bitchs show restlessness, panting and severe muscular spasms, all of which are relieved by the administration of intravenous calcium. Also occurs infrequently in queens. Called also lactational or puerperal tetany.

recurrent t. see Scottie CRAMP.

transit t. of cows, see TRANSIT tetany; of mares, see LACTATION TETANY.

tether to tie an animal up by the head or neck so that it can graze but not move away. See also BARTON TETHER.

tetmosol acaricide toxic to birds if used to excess. Called also monosulfiram.

tetra any one of a number of brightly colored tropical fish in the family Characinidae, much favored for home aquariums. Includes neon tetra (*Hyphessobrycon innesi*).

tetra- word element. [Gr.] *four.*

tetrabrachius a double monster having four forelimbs.

tetrabromophenol test an impregnated paper dip test for protein in urine. A change of color from yellow to green or even blue is a positive reaction and the concentration of protein can be estimated by the degree of color change.

tetracaine a member of the procaine series of compounds. It is a local and spinal anesthetic used in the form of the hydrochloride salt. Can be administered by local injection but is also useful by topical application to conjunctiva, mucosae and skin. Called also amethocaine.

tetrachlorodibenzodioxin a by-product in the manufacture of trichlorophenol which causes fatal centrilobular fibrosis and veno-occlusive disease in animals and humans.

tetrachlorodifluorethane a fasciolicide, some samples of which cause interference with blood clotting and the development of extensive hemorrhages, myocarditis and congestive heart failure. It is not recommended for general use. Called also Freon-112, difluorotetrachloroethane.

tetrachlorodiphenylethane non-degradable insecticide; relatively nontoxic; overuse in dogs causes adrenal cortical atrophy.

tetrachloroethane has had some usage as an anthelmintic and has a similar activity as carbon tetrachloride with less, but still significant risk of toxicity.

tetrachloroethylene a clear, colorless liquid used extensively at one time as an anthelmintic but now superseded in all species by safer and more effective drugs. Overdosing causes incoordination immediately, hepatic insufficiency later.

tetrachlorvinphos an organophosphorus insecticide used for ectoparasites.

tetracosactrin see COSYNTROPIN.

tetracrotic having four sphygmographic waves or elevations to one beat of the pulse.

tetracycline an antibiotic produced by cultures of *Streptomyces aureofaciens* and *S. rimosus*. It is effective against many different microorganisms, including rickettsiae, certain viruses, and both gram-negative and gram-positive microorganisms. Preparations include CHLORTETRACYCLINE hydrochloride (Aureomycin), OXYTETRACYCLINE hydrochloride (Terramycin), tetracycline hydrochloride (Achromycin), and demethylchlortetracycline (Declomycin). Administration of these compounds is associated with pigmentation of developing teeth and bones, and in horses with a severe colitis.

t. stain discoloration of dentine and enamel caused by systemic treatment with tetracycline during dental development; usually yellow to brown or green to gray.

tetrad a group of four similar or related entities, as (1) any element or radical having a valence, or combining power, of four; (2) a group of four chromosomal elements formed in the pachytene stage of the first meiotic prophase; (3) a square of cells produced by division into two planes of certain cocci (sarcina).

tetradactyly the presence of four digits on the hand or foot.

tetradifon an acaricide used in horticulture; minimally toxic and only if taken in over a long period. The liver is the principal target.

Tetradymia North American genus in plant family Asteraceae; contain an unidentified hepatoxin which causes secondary photosensitization. Includes *T. canescens* (spineless horsebrush), *T. glabrata* (spring rabbitbush, little leaf horsebrush, coal oil bush).

tetraethyl lead the additive in leaded petrol. See also LEAD^{I} poisoning.

tetraethyl pyrophosphate an insecticide used industrially and in agriculture and not to be used on animals. Accidental administration can cause death within an hour. Called also TEPP.

Tetragonia, Tetragonioides genus in the plant family of Aizoaceae; contains soluble oxalates capable of causing oxalate poisoning; includes *T. expansa* (New Zealand spinach).

tetragonum [L.] *a four-sided figure.*

tetrahydrobiopterin pterin cofactor in the mixed-function oxygenase, phenylalanine hydroxylase which catalyzes the conversion of phenylalanine to tyrosine. Hereditary deficiency of this enzyme is responsible for phenylketonuria (PKU).

tetrahydrocannabinol the active principle of cannabis, occurring in two isomeric forms, both considered psychomimetically active; abbreviated THC.

tetrahydrofolate H_4 folate; a coenzyme derived from the reduction of folic acid through dihydrofolate; an important cofactor in the synthesis of purines.

tetrahydronorharmane toxic carboline found in *Peganum* spp. plants.
tetrahydropteroylglutamate see TETRAHYDROFOLATE.
tetrahydropyrimidines a group of broad-spectrum anthelmintics including pyrantel and morantel.
tetrahymena free-living, freshwater ciliate sometimes capable of infecting and causing disease in fish.
tetraiodophenolphthalein a contrast agent used in radiography of the gallbladder and bile duct. Called also iodophthalein.
tetraiodothyronine thyroxine; see THYROID hormones. Called also T_4.
tetralogy a group or series of four.
t. of Fallot a congenital defect of the heart that combines four structural anomalies: pulmonary stenosis (narrowing of the pulmonary artery); ventricular septal defect, or abnormal opening between the right and left ventricles; dextroposition of the aorta, in which the aortic opening overrides the septum and receives blood from both the right and left ventricles; and right ventricular hypertrophy, or increase of volume of the myocardium of the right ventricle.
This is almost always a lethal defect. There is poor exercise tolerance, dyspnea, often cyanosis. A loud murmur and a strong thrill are palpable on the left side.
tetramastigote 1. having four flagella. 2. an organism having four flagella.
Tetrameres a genus of roundworms in the family Tetrameridae. They show marked sexual dimorphism, the female being globular and the male slender and filiform. They inhabit the proventriculus of birds and may kill young birds.
T. americana found in fowl and turkey.
T. confusa found in the fowl and pigeon.
T. crami found in domestic and wild ducks.
T. fissispina found in fowl, duck, turkey, pigeon and wild aquatic birds.
T. mohtedai found in fowl.
T. pattersoni found in quail.
tetrameres spiruroid nematodes in the family Tetrameridae.
tetrameriasis infestation with TETRAMERES.
tetrameric having four parts.
tetramethylthiuram disulfide relatively nontoxic acaricide. Experimentally rams show testicular degeneration, hen birds lay soft-shelled eggs and eggs with other abnormalities. Called also thiram.
tetramine 2,2,2,-tetramine (TRIENTINE) and 2,3,2-tetramine are copper chelating agents used to remove copper in chronic hepatobiliary disease, particularly Bedlington terrier copper-associated hepatopathy.
tetramisole a mixture of dextro- and levo isomers used as an anthelmintic. It is effective with a broad spectrum but a narrow safety margin; it has been superseded by the isomer LEVAMISOLE. Signs of toxicity include lip-licking, salivation, head shaking, tremor, excitement.
L-tetramisole levamisole.
Tetramitus rostratus a coprophilic, flagellate protozoan found in stagnant water and human and rat feces but no pathogenic effect is ascribed to it. A member of the family Tetramitidae.
tetranortriterpenes a class of plant toxins, e.g. the meliatoxins found in the plant *Melia azaderach* var. *australasica*.
Tetraodontidae the family of marine fish known as toadfish. They are extremely poisonous and ingestion of them causes severe illness and often death. The toxic agent is TETRODOTOXIN.
tetraparesis muscular weakness affecting all four extremities.
tetrapeptide a peptide which, on hydrolysis, yields four amino acids.
Tetrapetalonema a filarioid nematode found in the peritoneal cavity of primates and insectivores but even in very large numbers appear not to exert any damaging effect.
tetraplegia paralysis of all four extremities; QUADRIPLEGIA.
tetraploid 1. characterized by tetraploidy. 2. an individual or cell having four sets of chromosomes.
tetraploidy the state of having four sets of chromosomes (4n).
tetrapod a four-limbed, vertebrate animal, i.e. all vertebrates except fish. Compare with quadruped.
Tetrapteris tropical American plant genus in family Malpighiaceae; contains unidentified cardiotoxin which causes cardiac irregularity, congestive heart failure. Includes *T. acutifolia*, *T. multiglandulosa*.
tetrapus a monster with four hindfeet.
tetrascelus a monster with four hindlimbs.
tetrasomy the presence of two extra chromosomes of one type in an otherwise diploid cell.
tetraster a figure in mitosis produced by quadruple division of the nucleus.
tetrathyridium one of the forms of metacestodes in the life cycles of the cestodes of domestic animals, e.g. *Mesocestoides* spp.
Tetratrichomonas a genus of protozoa with four anterior flagella in the family Trichomonadidae.
T. anatis found in ducks but not pathogenic.
T. anseri found in the cecum of geese; not pathogenic.
T. bovis see *T. pavlovi* (below).
T. buttreyi found in the cecum and colon of pigs; no evidence of pathogenicity.
T. gallinarum found in fowl, duck, guinea fowl, quail, pheasant, partridge, and probably Canada goose. Causes hepatic lesions similar to those caused by *Histomonas meleagridis*.
T. microti found in the cecum of rodents.
T. ovis found in the cecum of sheep; not pathogenic.
***T. pavlovi* (syn. *T. bovis*)** found in the cecum of calves with diarrhea.
tetravalent having a valence of four.
tetrodotoxin a highly lethal neurotoxin present in numerous species of puffer and toadfish (suborder Tetraodontoidea) and in newts of the genus *Taricha* (tarichatoxin); ingestion results, within minutes, in malaise, dizziness and tingling about the mouth, which may be followed by ataxia, convulsions, respiratory paralysis and death.
teuthophagous feeding or subsisting solely on cephalopods.
Texas desert rue see THAMNOSMA TEXANA, T. OERTLI.
Texas fever see BABESIOSIS.
Texas longhorn a breed of beef cattle, of all colors but mostly red, and any pattern of marking; accoutred with a formidable spread of horns.
Texas sage SALVIA *coccinea*.
Texas thistle SOLANUM *rostratum*.
Texel a Dutch marsh type of long-woolled, polled, meat sheep.
textiform formed like a network.
textoblastic forming adult tissue; regenerative; said of cells.
textual–numeric said of databases that contain text accessed through a numeric code.
texture the structure or constitution of tissues.
TF transfer factor.

TG 1. thyroglobulins. 2. triacylglycerol.
TGE transmissible gastroenteritis.
TGEV transmissible gastroenteritis virus.
TGF-beta transforming growth factor beta; a growth factor synthesized by skeletal cells; found in most species.
TGH abbreviation for to go home; used in medical records.
Th chemical symbol, *thorium*.
Th cell helper T LYMPHOCYTE.
thalamencephalon that part of the diencephalon including the thalamus, metathalamus and epithalamus.
thalamocoele the third ventricle of the brain.
thalamocortical pertaining to the thalamus and cerebral cortex.
thalamolenticular pertaining to the thalamus and lenticular nucleus.
thalamus pl. *thalami* [L.] either of two large ovoid structures composed of gray matter and situated at the base of the cerebrum.

The thalamus functions as a relay station in which sensory pathways of the spinal cord and brainstem form synapses on their way to the cerebral cortex. Specific locations in the thalamus are related to specific areas on the body surface and in the cerebral cortex. A sensory impulse from the body surface travels upward to the thalamus, where it is received as a primitive sensation and then is sent on to the cerebral cortex for interpretation as to location, character and duration.

The thalamus has numerous connections to other areas of the brain as well, and these are thought to be important in the integration of cerebral, cerebellar and brainstem activity.

thalassoposia the drinking of sea water.
Thalictrum flavum European member of the plant family Ranunculaceae; contains the toxin protoanemonin; causes abdominal pain, diarrhea, salivation. Called also meadow rue.
thalidomide a sedative and hypnotic compound whose use during early pregnancy in women was frequently followed by the birth of infants with phocomelia.
thallium a chemical element, atomic number 81, atomic weight 204.37, symbol Tl. See Table 6. Its salts are active poisons. See THALLOTOXICOSIS.
t.-201 a radioactive isotope of thallium having a half-life of 73.5 hours; the principal emission is 71 keV x-rays.
t. poisoning see THALLOTOXICOSIS.
t. scan a scintillation scan involving the use of thallium-201 which localizes in the myocardium after intravenous injection. Areas of inadequate perfusion pinpoint the site of coronary artery occlusions.
thallotoxicosis thallium salts, especially the acetate and sulfate which have been used as rat baits, are very poisonous. Acute poisoning is manifested by severe abdominal pain, vomiting and hemorrhagic gastritis. Chronic poisoning causes characteristic hyperkeratosis and alopecia, plus tremors and convulsions, vomiting, diarrhea and respiratory difficulty.
thallous pertaining to thallium.
t. acetate a rodenticide. See THALLOTOXICOSIS.
t. chloride (Tl-201) the form in which thallium-201 is injected intravenously for myocardial perfusion imaging.
t. sulfate a rodenticide. See THALLOTOXICOSIS.
thallus 1. a simple plant body not differentiated into root, stem and leaf, characteristic of mycelial fungi and some algae. 2. the actively growing vegetative organism as distinguished from reproductive or resting portions, as in fungi.
THAM salt tromethamine, an alkalizing agent used in the manufacture of pharmaceuticals.
Thamnidium one of the fungi responsible for the growth of white whiskers on stored raw meat.
Thamnosma texana, T. oertli North American plant of the family Rutaceae; contains a toxic furocoumarin; causes primary photosensitization. Called also Dutchman's breeches, Texas desert rue, blisterweed.
thanato- word element. [Gr.] *death*.
thanatobiological pertaining to life and death.
thanatognomonic indicating the approach of death.
thanatoid resembling death.
thanatology the medicolegal study of death and conditions affecting human bodies.
Thargomindah nightshade SOLANUM *sturtianum*.
THC tetrahydrocannabinol.
Thea chinensis one of the few plants that absorbs fluorine in amounts that could be toxic. Called also tea plant. See also CAMELLIA, which is much more toxic.
thebesian foramina minute openings in the walls of the heart, especially the right atrium, through which the smallest cardiac veins empty into the heart.
thebesian valve the valve of the coronary sinus as it enters the right atrium.
thebesian veins smallest cardiac veins: numerous small veins arising in the muscular walls and draining independently into the cavities of the heart, and most readily seen in the atria.
theca pl. *thecae* [L.] a case or sheath.
t. cell an epithelioid cell of the corpus luteum.
t. cordis pericardium.
t. folliculi an envelope of condensed connective tissue surrounding a vesicular ovarian follicle, comprising an internal vascular layer (*theca interna*) and an external fibrous layer (*theca externa*).
granulosa t. cell tumor may secrete estrogen and progesterone in dogs and cause persistent or irregular estrus, alopecia, enlargement of nipples and vulva. Uterine changes range from cystic endometrial hyperplasia to pyometra.
thecal pertaining to a theca.
t. abscess abscess in a tendon sheath.
t. cone thecal cells in the ovarian stroma arrange themselves into a cone and may displace superficially situated follicles to make way for a deeper situated follicle which is undergoing enlargement.
thecitis tenosynovitis.
thecoma theca cell tumor.
thecostegnosis contraction of a tendon sheath.
Theileria a genus of protozoan parasites in the family Theileriidae. They are transmitted by ticks, multiply in leukocytes and then invade erythrocytes.
***T. annulata* (syn. *T. dispar*)** found in cattle and water buffalo, transmitted by *Hyalomma* spp. ticks and causes a clinical disease similar to EAST COAST FEVER.
T. buffali found in cattle and buffalo in Australia and transmitted by *Haemaphysalis longicornis* and *H. bancrofti*. Similar to *T. mutans*. Only sporadic cases of clinical disease and is seen mostly in splenectomized calves.
T. camalensis found in camels, transmission thought to be by *Hyalomma* spp. ticks.
T. cervi nonpathogenic, found in splenectomized deer.
T. dispar see *Theileria annulata* (above).

T. hirci found in sheep and goats. Vector uncertain but probably the tick *Rhipicephalus bursa*. Causes a disease similar to EAST COAST FEVER in cattle.

T. lawrenci found in cattle, buffalo and water buffalo. Transmitted by the tick, *Rhipicephalus appendiculatus;* causes fatal CORRIDOR DISEASE.

T. mutans found in cattle, transmitted by ticks including *Rhipicephalus* and *Haemaphysalis* spp. and causes a benign bovine THEILERIASIS.

T. orientalis usually benign but can cause severe anemia in imported cattle.

T. ornithorhynci found in platypus.

T. ovis found in sheep and goats, transmitted by ticks of the genera *Rhipicephalus*, *Dermacentor*, *Haemaphysalis* and *Ornithodoros* spp. It causes a mild form of THEILERIASIS.

T. parva found in cattle, African buffalo and Indian water buffalo; transmitted by *Rhipicephalus appendiculatus* and possibly other ticks. It causes the widespread and serious disease EAST COAST FEVER.

T. sergenti doubtful identity; mostly benign in cattle.

T. tarandi found in reindeer, transmitted by *Ixodes persulcatus* and causes an acute disease.

T. taurotragi mildly pathogenic; found in cattle in Africa, Asia.

T. velifera mildly pathogenic; found in cattle.

theileriasis in general the diseases may be acute and severe or mild. The severe disease is characterized by high fever, nasal discharge, jaundice, petechiation of mucosae, enlargement of the spleen and lymph nodes, enlargement of the kidneys and transient hemoglobinuria. Diagnosis is based on finding protozoa in the blood or in the lymph nodes. A feature, considered to be diagnostic is the presence of Koch's blue bodies or spots, lymphocytes containing macroschizonts, and detectable in smears stained with common blood-stain. See also EAST COAST FEVER, CORRIDOR DISEASE.

theileriosis THEILERIASIS.

benign t. caused by *Theileria orientalis*.

Theiler's disease murine encephalomyelitis caused by a picornavirus which is a normal inhabitant of the intestine.

Thelazia a genus of spiruroid worms in the family Thelaziidae. They are all parasites of the lacrimal duct or conjunctival sac of mammals and birds. The larvae are deposited in the conjunctival sac by the intermediate host, *Musca* spp. flies. Causes THELAZIASIS.

T. alfortensis found in cattle.

T. bubalis found in water buffalo.

T. californiensis occurs in cat, dog, humans, sheep and deer.

T. callipaeda occurs in dog, rabbit and humans.

T. erschowi found in pig.

T. gulosa found in cattle.

T. lacrymalis found in horses.

T. leesi found in dromedary.

T. rhodesii found in cattle, but also sheep, goat, buffalo.

T. skrjabini found in cattle.

thelaziasis infestation of the conjunctival sac with *Thelazia* spp. Causes conjunctivitis, lacrimation, blepharospasm and keratitis.

theleplasty a plastic operation on the nipple or teat.

thelitis inflammation of a nipple or teat.

thelium 1. a papilla. 2. a nipple.

Thelohanellus a genus of myxosporid protozoa in the class Myxosporea; parasites of freshwater fish.

T. piriformis causes cutaneous abscesses in cyprinid and coregonid fish.

Thelohania a genus of parasitic protozoa in the phylum Microspora.

T. apodemi found in the brain of field mice.

T. baueri found in the ovary of the stickleback fish.

thelorrhagia hemorrhage from the nipple.

thelygenic producing only female offspring.

Thelypodium lasiophyllum North American plant of the family Brassicaceae; can cause nitrate–nitrite poisoning. Called also mustard.

thenium closylate a very effective anthelmintic against hookworms in dogs, commonly teamed with piperazine to include control of ascarids.

Theobaldia one of the genera of mosquitoes which are the definitive hosts for *Plasmodium* spp., the cause of avian malaria.

Theobroma cacao tree of South American origin of the family Sterculiaceae; source of cocoa, chocolate; contains the toxin theobromine; causes diarrhea, sudden death. Commercial waste products from the plant may be fed to animals and cause THEOBROMINE poisoning.

theobromine an alkaloid prepared from dried ripe seed of the tropical American tree *Theobroma cacao*; or made synthetically from xanthine; used as a diuretic, myocardial stimulant, vasodilator and smooth muscle relaxant; available as theobromine calcium salicylate, sodium formate, sodium salicylate and salicylate.

theophylline an alkaloid derived from tea or produced synthetically; it is a smooth muscle relaxant used chiefly for its bronchodilator effect in the treatment of chronic obstructive pulmonary emphysema, bronchial asthma, chronic bronchitis and bronchospastic distress. It also has myocardial stimulant, coronary vasodilator, diuretic and respiratory center stimulant effects.

t. cholinate oxtriphylline, a smooth muscle relaxant, myocardial stimulant and diuretic.

t. ethylenediamine a smooth muscle relaxant, myocardial stimulant and diuretic. Called also aminophylline.

theory 1. the doctrine or the principles underlying an art as distinguished from the practice of that particular art. 2. a formulated hypothesis or, loosely speaking, any hypothesis or opinion not based upon actual knowledge.

cell t. all organic matter consists of cells, and cell activity is the essential process of life.

information t. a mathematical theory dealing with messages or signals, the distortion produced by statistical noise, and methods of coding that reduce distortion to the irreducible minimum.

recapitulation t. see RECAPITULATION THEORY.

theque [Fr.] a round or oval collection, or nest, of melanin-containing nevus cells occurring at the dermoepidermal junction of the skin or in the dermis proper.

therapeutic pertaining to therapeutics, or treatment of disease; curative.

t. decision making the use of decision theory in making decisions about treatment of individual cases.

t. incompatibility is the result of antagonistic pharmacological effects of several drugs in the one patient.

t. plasma concentration the blood concentration of a drug at which the desired therapeutic effect is obtained.

t. substances medicines with an identifiable value in the treatment of diseases of animals.

therapeutics 1. the science and art of healing. 2. a scientific account of the treatment of disease.

therapy the treatment of disease; therapeutics. See also TREATMENT.

animal-assisted t. the treatment of humans, usually for mental or psychological illness, which incorporates familiarization with a companion or pleasure animal. Called also pet-facilitated or pet-assisted therapy. See also ANIMAL facilitated therapy.

anticoagulant t. the use of drugs to render the blood sufficiently incoagulable to discourage thrombosis.

heat t. see HYPERTHERMIA (2).

immunosuppressive t. treatment with agents, such as x-rays, corticosteroids and cytotoxic chemicals, which suppress the immune response to antigen(s); used in organ transplantation, autoimmune disease, allergy, multiple myeloma, etc.

inhalation t. see AEROSOL.

oxygen t. the administration of supplemental oxygen to relieve hypoxemia and prevent damage to the tissue cells as a result of oxygen lack (hypoxia). See also OXYGEN therapy.

physical t. use of physical agents and methods in rehabilitation and restoration of normal bodily function after illness or injury; it includes massage and manipulation, therapeutic exercises, hydrotherapy, and various forms of energy (electrotherapy, actinotherapy and ultrasound). See also PHYSICAL therapist.

radiation t. treatment of disease by means of ionizing radiation. See also RADIOTHERAPY.

replacement t. treatment to replace deficient formation or loss of body products by administration of the natural body products or synthetic substitutes.

serum t. serotherapy; treatment of disease by injection of serum from immune animals.

substitution t. the administration of a hormone to compensate for glandular deficiency.

vaporization t. see AEROSOL.

theriogenological, theriogenologic pertaining to or emanating from theriogenology.

theriogenologist a veterinarian skilled in theriogenology.

theriogenology the discipline of animal reproduction; that branch of veterinary science which comprises the study of the normal physiology and anatomy and the pathology and diseases of the male and female reproductive tracts of animals. It includes the subjects of obstetrics and gynecology, as dealt with in human medicine, reproduction on a herd and flock basis, and with artificial insemination and embryo transfer and, in some countries, with neonatology.

theriotherapy treatment of all diseases of animals.

therm the amount of heat input required to raise the temperature of 1000 kg of water by 1°C. One therm = 1000 kilocalories = 1 megacalorie (Mcal) = 106 megajoule.

thermaburn thermal burn.

thermal pertaining to heat.

t. death point the state of heat content, as measured by temperature, at which the life of an organism ceases. Important in a consideration of sterilization procedures for certain organisms, especially those that produce spores.

t. energy the energy of heat.

t. injury see BURN.

t. processing the preservation of food by the application of heat either in boiling water, by live steam, in an autoclave or by flame.

t. sensation the sense of temperature.

t. stress see HYPERTHERMIA (1), HEAT stroke, FEVER.

thermelometer an electric thermometer for measuring small temperature changes.

thermic pertaining to heat.

thermistor a thermometer whose impedance varies with ambient temperature and so is able to measure extremely small temperature changes.

therm(o)- word element. [Gr.] *heat.*

Thermoactinomyces vulgaris thermophilic antigens of this and other fungi are thought to cause extrinsic allergic alveolitis (bovine farmer's lung); serum precipitins of the antigens have been found in cattle affected by the disease.

thermocautery cauterization by a heated wire or point.

thermochemistry the aspect of physical chemistry dealing with temperature changes that accompany chemical reactions.

thermocoagulation coagulation of tissue with high-frequency currents.

thermocouple a pair of dissimilar electric conductors so joined that with the application of heat an electromotive force is established; used for measuring small temperature differences.

thermodiffusion diffusion influenced by a temperature gradient.

thermodilution a technique for measuring size of a fluid-filled cavity by injecting a very cold sample of known volume and by measuring the change in temperature of the whole, assessing the degree of thermodilution, and hence the total volume of the cavity.

thermoduric able to endure high temperatures.

thermodynamics the branch of science dealing with heat and energy, their interconversion, and problems related thereto.

thermoexcitory stimulating production of bodily heat.

thermogenesis the production of heat, especially within the animal body.

diet-induced t. a portion of dietary calories in excess of those required for immediate energy requirements are converted to heat rather than stored as fat. Some types of obesity may be related to a defect in this mechanism.

neonatal t. thermogenesis is relatively inefficient in neonates, especially piglets, so that it becomes very important to protect them from cold stress. Most of their heat gain comes from the metabolism of their stores of brown fat.

nonshivering t. increased heat production due to enhancement of normal calorigenic metabolic processes.

shivering t. much the fastest thermogenic process which the static body can use. Shivering is an involuntary function with a tremor rate of about 10 per second.

thermogenin a thermogenic protein involved in the lipolysis of brown adipose tissue.

thermogram 1. a graphic record of temperature variations. 2. the visual record obtained by thermography.

thermograph 1. an instrument for recording temperature variations. 2. thermogram (2). 3. the apparatus used in thermography.

thermography a technique wherein an infrared camera photographically portrays the body's surface temperature, based on self-emanating infrared radiations; used as a diagnostic aid in the detection of superficial tumors and the assessment of joint and tendon disease; also used in the study of pain.

thermohygrograph an instrument which measures the environmental temperature and humidity at the same time, usually both continually.

thermoinhibitory retarding generation of bodily heat.

thermolabile easily affected by heat.

thermolysis 1. chemical dissociation by means of heat. 2. dissipation of bodily heat by radiation, evaporation, etc.

thermometer an instrument for determining temperatures, in principle making use of a substance (such as alcohol or mercury) with a physical property that varies with temperature and is susceptible of measurement on some defined scale.

Celsius t. one employing the Celsius scale, that is, with the ice point at 0 (0°C) and the normal boiling point of water at 100 degrees (100°C).

centigrade t. one having the interval between two established reference points divided into 100 equal units, as the Celsius thermometer.

clinical t. one used to determine the temperature of the patient in clinical situations.

electronic t. a clinical thermometer using a sensor based on thermistors, solid-state electronic devices whose electrical characteristics change with temperature. The reading is recorded within seconds, some having a red light or other device to indicate when maximum temperature is reached. Available models include handheld, desk-top and wall-mounted units, all having probes that are inserted orally or rectally. It is expected that electronic thermometers worn by the patient will have some use.

Fahrenheit t. one employing the Fahrenheit scale, that is, with the ice point at 32 and the normal boiling point of water at 212 degrees (212°F).

Kelvin t. one employing the KELVIN scale.

recording t. a temperature-sensitive instrument by which the temperature to which it is exposed is continuously recorded.

rectal t. a clinical thermometer that is inserted in the rectum for determining body temperature.

resistance t. one that uses the electric resistance of metals for determining temperature (thermocouple).

self-registering t. recording thermometer.

thermometry measurement of temperature.

thermophile a microorganism that grows best at elevated temperatures.

thermophore 1. a device or apparatus for retaining heat. 2. an instrument for estimating heat sensibility.

thermopile a number of thermocouples in series, used to increase sensitivity to change in temperature or for direct conversion of heat into electric energy.

thermoplacentography use of thermography for determination of the site of placental attachment.

Thermoplasma a genus of archebacteria which lack a cell wall; found in coal refuse piles.

thermoplastic materials materials used in making casts for broken limbs. Malleable when warmed in hot water or heated with a hairdrier, very quick setting and very strong, e.g. Hexcelite.

thermoplegia heat stroke.

thermopolypnea quickened breathing due to high body temperature or great environmental heat.

Thermopolyspora polyspora a fungus growing on stored forage thought at one time to be involved in the etiology of atypical interstitial pneumonia of cattle.

Thermopsis North American plant genus of the legume family Fabaceae; contain toxic quinolizidine alkaloid; causes myopathy, stiff gait, recumbency; includes *T. montana* (poison bean), *T. rhombifolia* (yellow bean). Called also false lupin, mountain thermopsis, golden banner.

thermoreceptor a nerve ending sensitive to stimulation by heat.

cutaneous t's come in two varieties, cold receptors and warm receptors. Called also peripheral receptors although the latter include, besides cutaneous receptors, those in the mucosae.

thermoregulation the physiological process controlling the balance between heat production and heat loss in the body so as to maintain body temperature; a function of a center in the hypothalamus. A lesion in that location can produce a central hyperthermia or hypothermia.

thermoregulatory mechanism the anatomical system that controls the body temperature; includes the temperature end-organs in the skin, the afferent nerves, the thalamus and hypothalamus, vasodilatation, respiratory center, the sweat glands, the muscular system and the hormonal and enzymic systems involved in the calorigenic metabolism of, stored fat and protein.

thermosensitivity the central perception of temperature is located in the anterior hypothalamus (preoptic region) and in the spinal cord. The preoptic sensitivity is the more important in mammals, the spinal cord center in birds.

thermostabile not affected by heat.

thermostasis maintenance of temperature, as in warm-blooded animals.

thermostat a device interposed in a heating system by which temperature is automatically maintained between certain levels.

thermostatic control a control system for the maintenance of a fixed temperature.

thermosteresis deprivation of heat.

thermosystaltic contracting under the stimulus of heat.

thermotaxis 1. normal adjustment of bodily temperature. 2. movement of an organism in response to the stimulation of a temperature gradient.

thermotherapy therapeutic use of heat.

thermotolerance the state of being relatively unaffected by hot conditions.

thermotonometer an instrument for measuring the amount of muscular contraction produced by heat.

thermotropism the orientation of a living cell in response to a heat stimulus.

Theromyzon tessulatum a small leech that normally parasitizes the nasal sinuses of geese, but which may migrate to the conjunctival sacs and cause keratoconjunctivitis.

thesaurismosis see STORAGE DISEASE.

thesaurosis a condition due to the storing up in the body of unusual amounts of normal or foreign substance.

Thesium genus of South African plants in family Santalaceae; contains bufadienolide cardiac glycosides; causes cardiomyopathy, sudden death; includes *T. lineatum* (vaalstorm, witstorm), *T. namaquense* (namaqua, gifbossie).

theta rhythm a rhythmic hippocampal electrical discharge correlated with movement and locomotion.

Thevetia shrub in the plant family Apocynaceae. Contains cardiac glycosides, e.g. thevetin. Causes sudden death in animals eating any part of the plant. Includes *T. peruviana*, *T. nereifolia* (yellow oleander, cook tree, daffodil tree, be-still tree).

thevetin a cardiac glycoside which occurs in *Thevetia peruviana*.

THF tetrahydrofolic acid.

thiabendazole a very safe and effective, broad-spectrum anthelmintic used widely in sheep. Also used extensively in horses in combination with piperazine. Poisoning with thiabendazole has been recorded but it is a very unusual occurrence requiring a massive overdose. It is capable of causing incoordination and collapse initially, and subsequently toxic nephrosis with terminal uremia.

thiacetarsamide sodium a parenteral anthelmintic used against adult heartworms in dogs with significant hepatic and renal toxicity. Commonly known as Caparasolate.

thialbarbital sodium, thialbarbitone a short-acting, intravenous anesthetic agent used in all species.

thiambutene hydrochloride see DIETHYLTHIAMBUTENE HYDROCHLORIDE.

thiamin, thiamine vitamin B_1; a component of the B complex group of vitamins, found in various foodstuffs and present in the free state in blood plasma and cerebrospinal fluid. The pharmaceutical products are thiamin hydrochloride and thiamin pyrophosphate.

t. nutritional deficiency an unlikely event in food animals with two exceptions: the secondary deficiency caused in horses and pigs by thiaminase in bracken and the primary deficiency in horses fed a diet almost entirely of turnips. In companion animals, the deficiency is much more common. Dogs, and particularly cats, fed diets in which thiamin has been destroyed, usually by excessive heat in processing but also by the inclusion of raw fish of certain marine species or sulfur dioxide as a food preservative, will develop signs of deficiency which include ataxia, mydriasis and convulsions.

thiaminase an enzyme that catalyzes the splitting of thiamin into a pyrimidine and a thiazole derivative. Is present in some ferns, e.g. bracken, and in some species of fish so that diets containing these materials are likely to be deficient in thiamin.

thiamphenicol an analog of chloramphenicol with similar activity, but reportedly a lower incidence of aplastic anemia in humans.

thiamylal an ultrashort-acting thiobarbiturate used as an intravenous anesthetic. The pharmaceutical product is thiamylal sodium.

thiazide any of a group of benzothiadiazinesulfonamide derivatives, typified by chlorothiazide, that act as diuretics by inhibiting the reabsorption of sodium in the proximal renal tubule and stimulating chloride excretion, with resultant increase in excretion of water.

thick forelegs see juvenile HYPEROSTOSIS.

thick leg disease of poultry, see OSTEOPETROSIS.

thick stomach worms see ASCAROPS *strongylina*, PHYSOCEPHALUS *sexalatus*.

thidiazuron a defoliant in cotton crops. It is not actually poisonous for animals but it may enter the human food chain via eggs and milk.

thiemia sulfur in the blood.

thienamycin see IMIPENEM.

thiethylperazine a phenothiazine derivative useful as an antiemetic.

thigh the portion of the leg above the stifle; the femur.

t. bone femur.

second t. in dogs, refers to the area from stifle to hock. Called also gaskin, calf.

thigmotaxis movement of an organism in response to contact.

thigmotropism the orientation of an organism in response to the stimulus of contact.

Thiloa glaucocarpa South American plant in the family Combretaceae; contains nephrotoxic tannin; called also sipauba, vaqueta.

thimble weed see RUDBECKIA.

thimbling the condition produced by the partial shedding of the horn on a claw of a pig. The horn separates from its laminae and a new claw's horn grows, gradually pushing the old horn off giving the effect that the pig is wearing a thimble. A good indication that the pigs have had a recent attack of foot-and-mouth disease.

thimerosal, thiomersal, thiomersalate a mercury-containing compound used as a local antibacterial agent in the form of the tincture. Used also as a preservative in pharmaceutical preparations. Known as Merthiolate.

thin 1. the body state in which the animal's weight is below normal but the eyes are bright and the coat good and the animal is physiologically and clinically normal. 2. the state of tissue in which the volume of connective tissue is diminished and other tissues lacking in size.

t. tubules renal tubules; includes thin ascending and thin descending tubules.

thin ewe syndrome a debilitating disease of adult ewes probably of mixed etiology but often associated with multiple internal abscesses containing *Corynebacterium pseudotuberculosis*, sometimes *Moraxella* spp.

thin-shelled egg thin egg shells can be caused by a nutritional deficiency of calcium, phosphorus, vitamin D, copper or manganese. Other causes are sulfonamides in the diet, end of the laying season, a diet contaminated by DDT and diseases at a chronic or subclinical level, e.g. infectious bronchitis. See also thin-shelled EGG.

thin sow syndrome the sow loses weight during pregnancy and after farrowing and does not return to feed or weight gain. There are no identifiable clinical signs. *Oesophagostomum* spp. and *Hyostrongylus* spp. infestations play a part in some cases but a bad environment and bullying of timid sows are also important.

thinness the state of being THIN. Called also light condition.

thi(o)- word element. [Gr.] *sulfur*.

thioarsenites salts of the hypothetical orthothioarsenious acid, e.g. arsenamide (caparsolate), used as anthelmintics, herbicides, insecticides, wood preservatives. They are organic arsenicals and potentially toxic.

thiobarbiturate a salt or derivative of thiobarbituric acid. Some are used as general anesthetics, some of them unstable in solution. Thiobarbital is used as a thyroid inhibitor.

thiocarbamates herbicides (allate, diallate, ETPC) which are poisonous causing clinical signs including tremor, dyspnea, salivation, vomiting and bloat.

thioctic acid see LIPOIC ACID.

thiocyanate a salt analogous in composition to a cyanate, but containing sulfur instead of oxygen and relatively nontoxic. It is one of the compounds produced in the body as a detoxicating mechanism. Continued ingestion can cause goiter.

thioesterase enzyme that catalyzes the hydrolytic cleavage of energy-rich thioester bonds as in acetyl CoA.

thioglucoside glucosinolate.

thioglycollate medium one used for culturing anaerobic bacteria.

thioglycoside a goitrogen found in plants, acts by inhibiting thyroidal hormonogenesis; its effects are only marginally reversible, if at all.

thioguanine an antineoplastic (2-aminopurine-6-thiol) used in the treatment of leukemia.

thiomolybdate forms insoluble complexes in the rumen with copper, contributing to the development of nutritional deficiency of copper.

thiones goitrogens produced by the hydrolysis of glucosinolates present in the seeds of cruciferous plants.

thionine a dark green powder, purple in solution, used as a metachromatic stain in microscopy.

thiopental, thiopentone, thiopentone a thiobarbiturate used extensively as a short-acting general anesthetic, administered by intravenous injection. Used as the sodium salt.

thiophanate a benzimidazole anthelmintic which was withdrawn from sale.

thioridazine a phenothiazine tranquilizer used in the treatment of stereotypic and aggressive behavior in dogs.

thiosemicarbazide a rodenticide with the capacity to cause pulmonary edema. Has an action similar to α-NAPHTHYLTHIOUREA (ANTU).

thiostrepton a polypeptide antibiotic produced in cultures of *Streptomyces aureus*. Is not absorbed from the alimentary tract and is used for topical application.

thiosulfate any salt of thiosulfuric acid. See also SODIUM thiosulfate.

thiotepa triethylenethiophosphoramide; a cytotoxic alkylating agent used as an antineoplastic agent.

thiouracil a thyrotoxic agent that inhibits the oxidation of iodine thus preventing the formation of thyroxine. Used to treat hyperthyroidism, and has been used as a fattening agent in cattle.

thiourea a goitrogenic agent used in industry as a photographic fixative. Mode of action is as for THIOURACIL.

thioureylenes a group of antithyroid agents used in the treatment of hyperthyroiditis; includes METHIMAZOLE, CARBIMAZOLE and PROPYLTHIOURACIL.

thioxanthene a class of structurally related neuroleptic drugs, including chlorprothixene and thiothixene.

thiram see TETRAMETHYLTHIURAM DISULFIDE.

third eye pineal eye, a photoreceptor organ, in lower vertebrates.

third eyelid see MEMBRANA nictitans, NICTITATING MEMBRANE.

t. e. eversion the free margin of the third eyelid is rolled outwards because of a curvature of the cartilage. More prevalent in large breeds of dogs and may be an inherited defect in St. Bernards and German shorthaired pointers.

t. e. protrusion syndrome see CHERRY EYE.

third phalanx fracture important, and most common in horses; pasture soundness may be achieved but degenerative joint disease is a common sequel.

thirst a sensation, often referred to the mouth and throat, associated with a craving for drink; ordinarily interpreted as a desire for water. Cellular dehydration also influences thirst and therefore water intake. Other factors may influence the role of the hypothalamus in maintaining water balance. See also POLYDIPSIA.

psychogenic t. see psychogenic POLYDIPSIA.

thistle any of a large number of plants in the family Asteraceae. Some poisonous ones are variegated thistle (*Silybum marianum*), yellow star thistle (*Centaurea solstitialis*).

thixotropism, thixotropy the property of certain gels of becoming fluid when shaken and then becoming solid again.

Thlaspi arvense North American annual weed of cultivation in the plant family Brassicaceae. It contains allyl isothiocyanate and causes hemolysis and gastric distress. Called also mithridate mustard, field penny-cress, fanweed, stinkweed.

thlipsencephalus a monster with a defective skull.

Thoma pipette a pipette used in the dilution of a blood specimen for counting of cells in a hemocytometer.

Thomas splint see Schroeder–Thomas SPLINT.

Thomomys see GOPHER.

thoracectomy thoracotomy with resection of part of a rib.

thoracentesis surgical puncture and drainage of the thoracic cavity. The procedure may be done as an aid to the diagnosis of inflammatory or neoplastic diseases of the lung or pleura, or it may be used as a therapeutic measure to remove accumulations of fluid from the thoracic cavity.

thoracic pertaining to the chest. See also THORACOLUMBAR.

t. asymmetry if obviously distorted can mean that the flatter side has a collapsed lung. Not a helpful sign in cattle because of the normal asymmetry caused by the rumen.

t. breath sounds breath sounds produced in the bronchi, bronchioles and alveoli by the passage of air; contrast with tracheal breath sounds.

t. cage the bony structure enclosing the thorax, consisting of the ribs, vertebral column and sternum.

t. cavity see THORAX; called also chest.

t. duct ligation a surgical procedure used in the treatment of chylothorax where medical management is unsuccessful.

t. girdle the incomplete ring of bones that support the thoracic limb, made up of the scapula, clavicle, coracoid and occasionally other elements. Mammals have no coracoids (except in monotremes) and nongrasping animals have no clavicle so that the girdle consists only of the scapula. Grasping or climbing animals have a clavicle. Birds have a complete bony girdle. Called also pectoral girdle.

t. inlet the entrance of the chest between the two first ribs, the manubrium, and the first thoracic vertebra.

t. limb forelimb.

t. pain such as that caused by broken ribs, torn intercostal muscles, pleurisy can cause a grunt at the end of each inspiration.

t. peristaltic sounds can be of assistance in diagnosing diaphragmatic hernia in a dog or cat but they occur commonly in normal horses and cattle.

t. positioner a sterilizable M-shaped metal trough which can be laid on an operating table and an animal propped up in it for surgery.

t. respiration the diaphragm and abdominal muscles remain immobilized and play little part in respiration, as in peritonitis with diaphragmatic hernia.

t. segmental spinal cord degeneration characteristic lesion in the inherited disease merino degenerative AXONOPATHY.

t. surgery surgical procedures involving entrance into the chest cavity. Until techniques for endotracheal anesthesia were perfected, this type of surgery was extremely dangerous because of the possibility of lung collapse. By administering anesthesia under pressure through an endotracheal tube it is now possible to keep one or both lungs expanded, even when they are subjected to atmospheric pressure.

t. symmetry lack of symmetry between the two sides, viewed from above, can suggest lung collapse or a space-occupying lesion on the smaller side; in ruminants the presence of the rumen always enhances the size of the left side.

t. tube see chest TUBE.

t. vertebrae the vertebrae between the cervical and lumbar vertebrae, giving attachment to the ribs and forming part of the dorsal wall of the thorax.

t. wall includes the ribs, sternum and thoracic vertebrae, the intercostal, superficial and deep, muscles, and the external respiratory muscles (transverse thoracic, rectus thoracic, serratus dorsalis and scalenus), and the costal pleura.

t. wall flap a surgical approach to the thoracic cavity that combines an intercostal incision and sternotomy. It allows great exposure to structures of the cranial mediastinum and caudal cervical region.

t. wall wound penetration through to the pleural cavity results in pneumothorax and collapse of the lung on that side.

thorac(o)- word element. [Gr.] *chest.*

thoracoacromial pertaining to the thorax and acromion.

thoracoceloschisis congenital fissure of the thorax and abdomen.

thoracocentesis thoracentesis.

thoracocyllosis deformity of the thorax.

thoracocyrtosis abnormal curvature of the chest wall.

thoracodelphus a double monster with one head, two forelimbs, and four hindlimbs, the bodies being joined above the navel.

thoracodidymus thoracopagus.

thoracodynia pain in the thorax.

thoracogastroschisis a developmental anomaly resulting from faulty closure of the body wall along the midventral line, involving both thorax and abdomen, i.e. fissure of the thorax and abdomen.

thoracolumbar pertaining to the thoracic and lumbar vertebrae.

t. disk intervertebral disk between vertebrae in the thoracolumbar segment of the vertebral column.

t. outflow symphathetic nervous system.

t. spinal cord lesion associated with a nerve deficit in the hindlimbs but no abnormality in the front limbs.

t. syndrome spinal cord lesions between T3 and L3 cause spastic paresis to paralysis in the hindlegs and sensory loss caudal to the level of the lesion. Most commonly seen in dogs with intervertebral disk protrusions.

thoracolysis the freeing of adhesions of the chest wall.

thoracomelus a monster with a supernumerary limb attached to the thorax.

thoracometer stethometer.

thoracopagus conjoined twins united at the thorax, facing each other, often with partly fused or compromised hearts.

thoracopathy any disease of the thoracic organs or tissues.

thoracoplasty surgical removal of ribs, allowing the chest wall to collapse a diseased lung.

thoracoschisis congenital fissure of the chest wall.

thoracoscope an endoscope for examining the pleural cavity through an intercostal space.

thoracoscopy examination of the pleural space with a thoracoscope.

thoracostenosis abnormal contraction of the thorax.

thoracostomy incision of the chest wall, with maintenance of the opening for drainage.

thoracotomy incision of the chest wall; may be intercostal, by rib resection or trans-sternal.

thorax the part of the body between the neck and abdomen; the chest. It is separated from the abdomen by the diaphragm. The walls of the thorax are formed by pairs of ribs, attached to the sides of the spine and curving toward the sternum. The cranial pairs of ribs are attached to the sternum, the next few connect with cartilage connected to the sternum and often the last one or two (the floating ribs) are unattached distally. The cavity of the thorax is divided by a thick partition, the mediastinum. The principal organs in the thoracic cavity are the heart with its major blood vessels, and the lungs with the bronchi. The trachea enters the thorax to connect with the lungs, and the esophagus travels through it to connect with the stomach caudal to the diaphragm. See also THORACIC.

thorium a chemical element, atomic number 90, atomic weight 232.038, symbol Th. See Table 6. Formerly used as a radiographic contrast medium.

thorn apple see DATURA.

thorn-headed worm see THORNY-HEADED WORM.

Thorn test a test of adrenal cortical function which originally measured the glands' response to ACTH by the change in the eosinophil count of blood samples taken before and after the injection. The modern version of the test measures the response by estimating plasma cortisol levels.

thorny-headed worm, thorn-headed worm member of the phylum Acanthocephala, a group of parasitic worms related to the nematodes. See CORYNOSOMA, FILICOLLIS, MACRACANTHORHYNCHUS, ONCICOLA and POLYMORPHUS.

Thoroughbred an English lightweight racing horse, incorporated into many breeds to improve speed and elegance. Black, brown, bay, chestnut or gray, usually 16 to 16.2 hands high.

thoroughbred speculum a speculum used for vaginal inspection in mares. There are three slightly curved plates which lie close together when the instrument is closed and can be inserted easily into the vagina. They are opened by a screw mechanism externally causing the plates to separate radially and dilating the vagina.

thoroughfare channel central channel in the arteriolar system; flow through the channel is controlled by the sphincter effect of the branch of the arteriole, the metarteriole.

thoroughpin tenosynovitis of the deep flexor tendon sheath of the hindlimb of the horse manifested by soft, nonpainful swellings just above the point of the hock and on the medial and lateral aspects of the hock. There is no lameness.

Thr threonine.

thread iris see GYNANDRIRIS SETIFOLIA.

threadleaf groundsel SENECIO *longilobus.*

threadworm any nematode worm.

abdominal t. SETARIA *equina.*

three-cornered garlic ALLIUM *triquetrum.*

three-day event a competition in the pleasure horse sport comprising usually one day each for dressage, cross country and show jumping.

three-day sickness see EPHEMERAL FEVER.

three-flowered nightshade SOLANUM *triflorum.*

three-way cross one in which a crossbred animal is mated with an animal from another population, e.g. AB × C.

Threlkeldia see NEOBASSIA PROCERIFLORA.

threonine Thr; a naturally occurring, hydroxy amino acid.

threpsology the scientific study of nutrition.

threshold the level that must be reached for an effect to be produced, as the degree of intensity of stimulus which just produces a sensation.

t. phenomenon a theory explaining pruritus which states that some degree of pruritus is tolerated by a patient, but a small increase from an additional source raises the patient above their threshold and causes clinical signs.

renal t. that concentration of a substance in plasma at which it begins to be excreted in the urine.

t. traits heritable traits which have specific thresholds, e.g. four rather than three toes on a guinea pig's hindfeet, alive or dead at a specific age.

t. unit the distance between two thresholds when an inherited abnormality can occur at a number of levels, e.g. completely patent ductus arteriosus, through partial closure (ductus diverticulum) and complete closure. See also threshold traits (above).

thrifty said of livestock that put on body weight or produce in other ways with a minimum of feed. The opposite of illthrift.

thrill a vibration caused by the movement of fluid felt by the examiner on palpation. Created by turbulence in a fluid column passing through an incompetent valve, or from a vessel of smaller caliber to a larger. The larger the orifice the bigger the thrill. Also by sharp firm percussion on one part of the abdomen and feeling a shock wave over a distant part of the abdomen—the so-called fluid wave.

diastolic t. one felt over the precordium during diastole in advanced aortic insufficiency.

presystolic t. one felt just before the systole over the apex of the heart.

systolic t. one felt over the precordium during systole in aortic stenosis, pulmonary stenosis and ventricular septal defect.

thyroid t. palpable over a colloid goiter with a large blood supply.

thrix hair.

t. annulata a condition in which a hair appears to be marked by alternating bands of white; called also ringed hair.

-thrix word element. [Gr.] *hair.*

throat the part of the body that includes the LARYNX and PHARYNX, where the passageways that link the nose and mouth with the respiratory and digestive systems of the body cross over. Called also the fauces.

t. abscess 1. one in the retropharyngeal lymph node causing partial obstruction to swallowing, dysphagia, and palpable through the pharynx and mouth in cattle. 2. an abscess in the parotid area just below the ear and behind the mandible. Usually ascribed to grass seed penetration.

t. cellulitis see PHARYNGEAL phlegmon.

t. lash, t. latch 1. the strap on a horse's bridle that goes under the throat and buckles just below the left ear. 2. the area under the throat where the head and neck are joined and where the harness throat latch fits.

throb a pulsating movement or sensation.

thrombapheresis thrombocytapheresis.

thrombasthenia a platelet abnormality characterized by defective clot retraction and impaired ADP-induced platelet aggregation. There are mild bleeding tendencies. Inherited as an autosomal recessive disorder in Otterhounds. Called also Glanzmann's disease, Glanzmann–Naegeli syndrome.

thrombectomy surgical removal of a clot from a blood vessel.

medical t. enzymatic dissolution of a blood clot in situ.

thrombin an enzyme resulting from activation of prothrombin, which catalyzes the conversion of fibrinogen to fibrin. It is also a potent stimulus to the aggregation of platelets. A preparation from prothrombin of bovine origin is used as a topical hemostatic.

t.–thrombomodulin complex thrombomodulin, a specific endothelial cell surface receptor, converts thrombin, a very weak activator of protein C in the anticoagulant pathway, to the status of a very active protein C activator.

t. time the time required for a standardized solution of thrombin to clot plasma. It is a measure of the rate of conversion of fibrinogen to fibrin.

thromb(o)- word element. [Gr.] *clot, thrombus.*

thromboangiitis inflammation of a blood vessel, with thrombosis.

thromboarteritis thrombosis associated with arteritis.

thromboasthenia thrombasthenia.

thromboclasis the dissolution of a thrombus.

thrombocyst, thrombocystis a sac formed around a clot or thrombus.

thrombocytapheresis the selective separation and removal of thrombocytes (platelets) from withdrawn blood, the remainder of the blood then being retransfused into the donor. Called also plateletpheresis and thrombapheresis.

thrombocyte a blood PLATELET.

thrombocythemia a fixed increase in the number of circulating blood platelets.

essential t., hemorrhagic t. a clinical syndrome with repeated spontaneous hemorrhages, either external or into the tissues, and greatly increased number of circulating platelets.

thrombocytocrit the volume of packed blood platelets in a given quantity of blood; also, the instrument used to measure platelet volume.

thrombocytolysis destruction of blood platelets (thrombocytes).

thrombocytopathy any qualitative disorder of blood platelets.

thrombocytopenia decrease in number of platelets in circulating blood. See also PURPURA.

alloimmune t. due to alloantibodies generated in response to blood transfusions or to maternal alloimmunization. Caused by the exposure of the platelets of a newborn animal to platelet alloantibodies which are present in the colostrum of the dam. Occurs in piglets as a syndrome of spontaneous hemorrhage at a few days of age. See also immune-mediated thrombocytopenia (below).

consumption t. excessive utilization of thrombocytes at hemorrhage sites causes significant reduction in circulating platelets.

drug-induced t. that associated with a drug being administered. Some drugs named as causing thrombocytopenia are phenylbutazone, diphenylhydantoin, sulfonamides, digitoxin and phenothiazine tranquilizers.

essential t. see megakaryocytic LEUKEMIA.

idiopathic t. see immune-mediated thrombocytopenia (below).

immune-mediated t. a loss of platelets caused by the presence of antiplatelet antibodies which can be demonstrated by the platelet factor-3 (PF-3) release test and immunofluorescence of megakaryocytes. Platelet production may be normal or impaired, also caused by antibodies directed against megakaryocytes. Includes alloimmune, autoimmune and some drug-induced thrombocytopenias.

infectious cyclic t. recurring cycles of parasitemia and reduced numbers of thombocytes in the peripheral blood are seen in dogs infected with *Ehrlichia platys*. Clinical signs are rarely observed, but coinfection may potentiate clinical disease caused by *E. canis*.

isoimmune t. see alloimmune thrombocytopenia (above).

myelophthisic t. that due to neoplastic invasion of the bone marrow.
surface-induced t. a form of nonimmune-mediated platelet destruction caused by exposure of platelets to a damaged or artificial surface.
thrombin-induced t. thrombin stimulates platelet aggregation and reduces circulating numbers.
vaccine-induced t. live-virus vaccines may be associated with a transient, nonimmunogenic aggregation and reduction in numbers of platelets.

thrombocytopenic of the nature of or pertaining to thrombocytopenia.

thrombocytopoiesis the production of blood platelets (thrombocytes).

thrombocytosis increase in the number of platelets in the circulating blood. See also THROMBOCYTHEMIA.
autonomous t. one resulting from a myeloproliferative disorder.
reactive t. one occurring in association with acute hemorrhage, trauma, neoplasia, etc.

thromboembolic pertaining to or emanating from THROMBOEMBOLISM.
t. meningoencephalitis see HEMOPHILOSIS.
t. parasitism see thromboembolic COLIC.

thromboembolism the lesion created by a THROMBOEMBOLUS. The exact form of the disease depends on the location of the thromboembolism, e.g. aortic, iliac, intestinal, pulmonary.

thromboembolus thrombotic material transported in the bloodstream to another site to form an embolus.
t. colic see thromboembolic COLIC.
t. meningoencephalitis see HEMOPHILOSIS.

thromboendarterectomy excision of an obstructing thrombus together with a portion of the inner lining of the obstructed artery.

thromboendarteritis inflammation of the innermost coat of an artery, with thrombus formation.

thromboendocarditis formation of a thrombus on a heart valve which has previously been eroded.

thrombogenesis clot formation.

thrombohemorrhagic the state of being hemorrhagic due to thrombocyte deficiency or malfunction.
consumption t. disorder hemorrhagic state due to excessive consumption of platelets.

thromboid resembling a thrombus.

thrombokinase activated clotting factor X.

thrombokinetics the dynamics of blood coagulation.

thrombolymphangitis inflammation of a lymph vessel due to a thrombus.

thrombolysis dissolution of a thrombus.

thrombolytic 1. dissolving or splitting up a thrombus. 2. an agent that dissolves or splits up a thrombus.

thrombomodulin an antithrombotic substance contained in the apical membrane of endothelial cells.

thrombon the circulating blood platelets and their precursors.

thrombopathia a disorder of blood coagulation resulting from a failure of ADP release from platelets on stimulation by aggregating factors, e.g. thromboplastin. See also STORAGE POOL DISEASE.

thrombopathy thrombocytopathy.

thrombopenia thrombocytopenia.

thrombophilia a tendency to the occurrence of thrombosis.

thrombophlebitis inflammation of a vein associated with thrombus formation. See also THROMBOSIS.

thromboplastic causing or accelerating clot formation in the blood.

thromboplastid a blood platelet.

thromboplastin a substance in blood and tissues which, in the presence of ionized calcium, aids in the conversion of prothrombin to thrombin. Extrinsic and intrinsic thromboplastin are formed as the result of the interaction of different clotting factors; the factors that combine to form extrinsic thromboplastin are not all derived from intravascular sources, whereas those that form intrinsic thromboplastin are.
activated partial t. time see ACTIVATED partial thromboplastin time.
extrinsic t. the prothrombin activator formed as a result of interaction of coagulation factors III, VII, and X which, with factor IV, aids in the formation of thrombin.
t. generation time (TGT) evaluates the first stage in blood coagulation by measuring the efficiency of prothrombinase formation.
intrinsic t. the prothrombin activator formed as a result of interaction of coagulation factors V, VII, IX, X, XI and XII and platelet factor 3 (PF-3), which, with factor IV, aids in the conversion of prothrombin to thrombin.
plasma t. antecedent (PTA) CLOTTING factor XI; deficiency occurs in cattle and dogs, causing mild to severe bleeding tendencies called hemophilia C.
plasma t. component (PTC) CLOTTING factor IX; deficiency causes CHRISTMAS DISEASE. Called also Christmas factor, antihemophilic factor B, autoprothrombin II.
t. time see ACTIVATED partial thromboplastin time.
tissue t. factor III, a material derived from several sources in the body (e.g. brain, lung), and is important in the formation of extrinsic prothrombin converting principle in the extrinsic pathway of blood coagulation. Called also tissue factor.

thrombopoiesis 1. thrombogenesis. 2. thrombocytopoiesis.

thrombopoietic cell cells in the normal hemopoietic production line; are in two classes proliferative phase and maturation phase.

thrombopoietin an α_2-globulin, a hormone involved in the differentiation and maturation of platelets but thought to be responsible for regulating the supply of platelets.

thromboresistance a function of intact endothelium contributed to by the production of a prostaglandin, prostacyclin, a potent inhibitor of platelet aggregation.

thrombosis formation, development, or presence of a thrombus.

A thrombus may form whenever the flow of blood in the arteries or the veins is impeded. If the thrombus detaches itself from the wall and is carried along by the bloodstream, the clot is called an embolus. The condition is known as EMBOLISM. Because blood normally flows more slowly through the veins than through the arteries, thrombosis is more common in the veins than in the arteries.

The effect of a thrombosis is engorgement of the obstructed vein, usually further aggravation of the thrombus formation, and edema of the local area drained by the vein. The clinical signs will depend on the location of the vessel, e.g. cerebrovascular, pulmonary.
caudal vena cava t. see CAUDAL vena caval thrombosis.
iliac t. see ILIAC artery thrombosis.

thrombospondin an osteoblast product which binds to connective tissues and serum proteins and binds calcium to hydroxyapatite and to osteonectin.

thrombostasis stasis of blood in a part with formation of thrombus.

thrombosthenin a contractile protein present in

platelets and instrumental in producing retraction of a blood clot.

thrombotic pertaining to or emanating from THROMBOSIS.

t. meningoencephalitis see HEMOPHILOSIS.

thromboxane an intermediate in the metabolic pathway of arachidonic acid, formed from prostaglandin endoperoxides, and released from suitably stimulated platelets; the unstable form, thromboxane A_2, is a potent inducer of platelet aggregation and constrictor of arterial smooth muscle.

thrombus an aggregation of blood factors, primarily platelets and fibrin with entrapment of cellular elements, frequently causing vascular obstruction at the point of its formation. The lesion and the syndrome produced by the thrombus depend on its location, e.g. pulmonary artery.

mural t. one attached to the wall of the endocardium in a diseased area.

obturating t. one which continues to grow distal to its site of attachment and the free end trails downstream with the current of blood.

occluding t. one that occupies the entire lumen of a vessel and obstructs blood flow.

parietal t. one attached to a vessel or heart wall.

saddle t. one formed at the terminal aorta and extending into the iliac arteries. Occurs most commonly in cats with arterial thromboembolism.

throw 1. in the restraint of horses and cows, to CAST (2) them. 2. when tying a knot, the action of making a loop and passing it (as if throwing a lariat) around an object, which may be a cow's tail or, more commonly, the suture material which has already been placed to commence a knot.

throw nets nets used in the capture and restraint of wild and zoo animals. A strong net which is flat when open but has a drawstring around its edge. It can be thrown over an otherwise unmanageable animal such as a seal, the drawstring pulled tight and the apex of the net and the drawstring end pulled tight in opposite directions.

throwback see ATAVISM.

thrush chronic, superficial, necrotic lesion of mucosa or epithelium. 1. stomatitis of the newborn caused usually by *Monilia* spp. See also CANDIDIASIS. 2. alimentary tract mycosis in birds usually associated with infection by *Monilia, Candida* spp. 3. a chronic disease of the horn of the sole of a horse's foot. *Fusobacterium necrophorum* is usually present and the smell is offensive.

t.-breast heart alternating strips of myocardium in cases of myocardial degeneration in which some of the strips appear more yellow than the others.

crop t. see thrush (2) (above).

frog t. see thrush (3) (above).

thrypsis a comminuted fracture.

thulium a chemical element, atomic number 69, atomic weight 168.934, symbol Tm. See Table 6.

thumb the radial or first digit of the hand; it has only two phalanges and is apposable to the four fingers of the hand. It is present in primates and a few other arborial (scansorial) animals.

thumps exaggerated expiratory movement and effort without necessarily any increase in respiratory rate nor evidence of dyspnea.

diaphragmatic t. see synchronous DIAPHRAGMATIC flutter.

thoracic t. pumping respiration of pigs with pneumonic pasteurellosis, due possibly to pleuritis.

thunarphobia fear of thunder; a common behavior problem in companion animals.

thunder lily see COOPERIA PEDUNCULATA.

thunderstorms a storm characterized by thunder and lightning caused by strong rising air currents; identified as agents of animal disease because of their involvement causing (1) spasmodic colic; (2) lightning strike; (3) injuries of cattle acquired in stampedes initiated by storms.

fear of t. see THUNARPHOBIA.

Thurber loco ASTRAGALUS *thurberi.*

Thy thymine.

Thy-1 antigen a cell membrane molecule of thymus lymphocytes.

Thygesen embryotome see FETOTOME.

thyme-leaved sandwort see ARENARIA SERPYLLIFOLIA.

thym(o)- word element. [Gr.] *thymus; mind, soul, emotions.*

thymectomize to excise the thymus.

thymectomy excision of the thymus.

thymelcosis ulceration of the thymus.

-thymia word element. [Gr.] *condition of mind.*

thymic pertaining to the thymus.

t. bovine leukosis see thymic LYMPHOMA.

t. corpuscles acidophilic bodies in the thymic medulla containing high concentrations of IgA.

t. humoral factor see THYMOSIN.

t. hypoplasia is the central lesion in COMBINED IMMUNE DEFICIENCY SYNDROME of Arab foals and inherited PARAKERATOSIS of cattle, both inherited diseases.

t. inflammation see THYMITIS.

inherited t. deficiency see thymic hyoplasia (above).

t. lymphocyte see T LYMPHOCYTE.

thymicolymphatic pertaining to the thymus and lymphatic nodes.

thymidine a nucleoside of DNA.

thymidine kinase (tk) gene a gene coding for thymidine kinase that is expressed in most mammalian cells and some viruses (herpes-, pox-viruses). Used as a selectable marker in that tk minus (tk^-) cells and viruses do not survive in medium containing hypoxanthine, aminopterin and thymidine (HAT medium); such cells cotransfected with a vector carrying a tk gene (tk+) can be rescued.

thymin former name for thymopoietin.

thymine a pyrimidine base in DEOXYRIBONUCLEIC ACID (DNA).

thymitis inflammation of the thymus.

thymocyte a lymphocyte arising in the thymus; a T lymphocyte.

thymokinetic tending to stimulate the thymus.

thymol a phenol obtained from thyme oil and other volatile oils or produced synthetically; used as a topical antifungal and antibacterial, and as an antimicrobial agent in trichloroethylene.

t. iodide a mixture of iodine derivatives of thymol, containing not less than 43% of iodine; mild antiseptic and fungicide.

thymoma thymic LYMPHOMA.

thymopathy any disease of the thymus.

thymopoietin a polypeptide hormone secreted by the thymus, which induces the proliferation of lymphocyte precursors and their differentiation into T lymphocytes.

thymoprivic, thymoprivous pertaining to or resulting from removal or atrophy of the thymus.

thymosin a humoral factor secreted by the thymus, which promotes the maturation of T lymphocytes. See also THYMUS.

thymus a primary lymphoid organ lying in the cranial

mediastinum or in the neck or throat, (depending on the species), which reaches its maximum development during puberty and continues to play an immunological role throughout life, even though its function declines with age. Called also sweetbread.

During the last stages of fetal life and the early neonatal period, the reticular structure of the thymus entraps immature 'stem' cells arising from the bone marrow and circulating in the blood. The thymus preprocesses these cells, causing them to become antigen-specific and therefore capable of maturing into a type of lymphocyte that is essential to the regulation of immune responses generally and the development of cell-mediated IMMUNITY. More than 90% of T lymphocytes produced in the thymus are destroyed there in a process sometimes referred to as clonal purging, which is conceptually associated with the removal of self-reactive cells, i.e. only nonself-reactive cells leave the thymus. After development in the thymus, these lymphocytes re-enter the blood and are transported to developing secondary lymphoid tissues, such as lymph nodes and spleen, where they seed the cells that eventually become thymus-dependent or T lymphocytes. If the thymus is removed or becomes nonfunctional during fetal life, the secondary lymphoid tissue and blood fail to become seeded with the T lymphocytes and the body's cell-mediated arm of immunity fails to develop. It is this arm of immunity that is mainly responsible for rejection of organ transplants and resistance to microbial infection, and plays a role in the elimination of cells potentially able to give rise to cancer.

t. atrophy leads to filure of the cell-mediated arm of the body's immunity.

thymus-derived originating in the thymus.

t.-d. lymphocytes see T LYMPHOCYTE.

Thynnascaris a genus of nematodes in the family Anasakidae. The adults parasitize fish.

T. aduncum occurs in fish.

thyratron switch a gas-filled triode used as a switch on an x-ray machine.

thyro- word element. [Gr.] *thyroid.*

thyroadenitis inflammation of the thyroid.

thyroaplasia defective development of the thyroid with deficient activity of its secretion.

thyroarytenoid pertaining to the thyroid and arytenoid cartilages.

thyrocalcitonin calcitonin.

thyrocardiac pertaining to the thyroid and heart.

thyrocardiac disease see THYROTOXIC heart disease.

thyrocele tumor of the thyroid gland; goiter.

thyrochondrotomy surgical incision of the thyroid cartilage.

thyrocricotomy incision of the cricothyroid membrane, the lower part of the fibroelastic membrane of the larynx.

thyroepiglottic pertaining to the thyroid and epiglottis.

t. ligament connects the epiglottis to the thyroid cartilage of the larynx.

thyrogenic, thyrogenous originating in the thyroid.

thyroglobulin 1. an iodine-containing glycoprotein of high molecular weight, occurring in the colloid of the follicles of the thyroid gland; the iodinated tyrosine moieties of thyroglobulin form the active hormones thyroxine and tri-iodothyronine. 2. a substance obtained by fractionation of thyroid glands from the pig, administered orally as a thyroid supplement in the treatment of hypothyroidism.

thyroglossal pertaining to the thyroid and tongue.

t. cyst developmental abnormality near the site of the thyroid diverticulum; may exist as a subepiglottic cyst, surrounded by thyroid follicular cells, embedded in the root of tongue; may cause inspiratory dyspnea and exercise intolerance.

t. duct vestigial canal of the epithelial outgrowth from the floor of the pharynx that develops into the thyroid gland. Parts of the duct and accessory thyroid tissue derived from it may become cystic or undergo neoplastic transformation.

thyrohyal 1. pertaining to the thyroid cartilage and the hyoid bone. 2. the thyrohyoid bone.

thyrohyoid 1. pertaining to the thyroid gland or cartilage and the hyoid bone. 2. one of the chain of hyoid bones, one that articulates with the thyroid cartilage and the basihyoid.

t. membrane the membrane connecting the thyroid cartilage to the hyoid bone.

thyroid 1. resembling a shield. 2. the thyroid gland (see below) secreting thyroid hormones (see below). 3. a pharmaceutical preparation of cleaned, dried, powdered thyroid gland, obtained from those domesticated animals used for food by humans.

accessory t. an additional thyroid located anywhere from the larynx to diaphragm, e.g. intrapericordial aorta; may be sufficient to supply the patient's need of thyroid hormone. Most common in dogs.

t. C cell see C CELL.

t. cartilage the shield-shaped cartilage of the larynx.

t. diverticulum primordium of the thyroid gland; appears as an outgrowth of the foregut between the first two pharyngeal pouches. This tube of epithelial cells grows ventrally into mesenchyme; the tube becomes the thyroglossal duct, the tip divides into two lobes, the thyroid glands.

t. dysfunction see HYPOTHYROIDISM, HYPERTHYROIDISM.

ectopic t. migration of thyroid diverticulum tissue to aberrant sites occurs, e.g. thyroid tissue in the thymus. These cause no apparent abnormality.

t. extract a pharmaceutical substance derived from thyroid glands, used in the treatment of hypothyroidism. See thyroid (3) (above).

t. function tests used to assess the functional capacity of the thyroid glands; most commonly employed in dogs and cats. Include plasma T_4, plasma T_3, free T_4, radioiodine uptake, and TSH response tests.

t. gland the largest of the ENDOCRINE glands, situated in the neck caudal to the larynx. It produces hormones (see below) that are vital in maintaining normal growth and metabolism. It also serves as a storehouse for iodine.

t. hormones iodothyronines secreted by the thyroid gland, principally THYROXINE (tetraiodothyronine, T_4) and TRI-IODOTHYRONINE (T_3); derived from iodination of tyrosyl residues in thyroglobulin. The pharmaceutical names for T_4 and T_3 are levothyroxine and liothyronine, respectively. Regulate basal metablic rate.

t. parafollicular cell see C CELL.

t. radioiodine uptake used as a thyroid function test but superseded these days by estimates of T_4 (thyroxine).

t.-stimulating hormone (TSH) see THYROTROPIN.

t. tumor mostly follicular adenomas in old-aged dogs, cats and horses; papillary adenomas are rare.

thyroidectomize to subject to thyroidectomy.

thyroidectomy surgical excision of the thyroid gland; indicated in the treatment of neoplasia or hyperfunction of the gland.

thyroidism hyperthyroidism; also, a morbid condition due to excess doses of thyroid.

thyroiditis inflammation of the thyroid gland.
autoimmune t. see lymphocytic thyroiditis (below).
Hashimoto's t. see also HASHIMOTO'S DISEASE, lymphocytic thyroiditis (below).
immune-mediated t. see lymphocytic thyroiditis (below).
lymphocytic t. progressive cellular infiltration of the thyroid gland, predominantly by lymphocytes, and replacement by fibrous tissue, resulting in hypothyroidism, associated with the presence of autoantibodies against thyroglobulin, follicular cell microsomes, and a second colloid antigen. It occurs in dogs, particularly Beagles, obese (OS) chickens, buffalo rats and primates. The disease has some similarity to Hashimoto's disease of humans.
thyroidization in renal amyloidosis the tubules may contain pink hyaline casts in such numbers as to obscure the normal histological cytotexture, the so-called thyroidization of the kidney.
thyroidotomy incision of the thyroid.
thyromegaly goiter.
thyromimetic producing effects similar to those of thyroid hormones or the thyroid gland.
thyroparathyroidectomy excision of the thyroid and parathyroids.
thyroprival, thyroprivic pertaining to, marked by, or due to deprivation or loss of thyroid function.
thyroprotein see IODINATED casein.
thyroptosis caudal displacement of a goitrous thyroid.
thyrosis any disease based on disordered thyroid action.
thyrotherapy treatment with preparations of thyroid.
thyrotomy 1. surgical division of the thyroid cartilage. 2. the operation of cutting the thyroid gland.
thyrotoxic marked by toxic activity of the thyroid.
t. crisis a fulminating increase in all the clinical signs of thyrotoxicosis.
t. heart disease heart disease associated with hyperthyroidism, marked by atrial fibrillation, cardiac enlargement and congestive heart failure. Most commonly seen in association with hyperthyroidism in aged cats. Called also thyrocardiac disease.
t. storm thyrotoxic crisis.
thyrotoxicosis a morbid condition due to overactivity of the thyroid gland.
thyrotrope one of the basophils (beta cells) of the adenohypophysis, the granules of which secrete thyrotropin.
thyrotroph thyrotrope.
thyrotrophic hormone thyroid-stimulating hormone, secreted from the pars distalis of the adenohypophysis.
thyrotrophin thyrotropin.
thyrotropic 1. pertaining to or marked by thyrotropism. 2. having an influence on the thyroid gland.
thyrotropin a hormone secreted by the anterior lobe of the pituitary gland that has an affinity for and specifically stimulates the thyroid gland. Called also thyroid-stimulating hormone (TSH).
t. releasing hormone (TRH) a tripeptide produced in the hypothalamus and released into the hypothalamohypophyseal portal circulation to reach the adenohypophysis where it triggers the release of thyroid-stimulating hormone. Called also TSH releasing factor, TSH releasing hormone.
t. releasing hormone stimulation test, response test measures serum levels of thyrotropin-stimulating hormone (TSH) before and after administration of TRH.
t.-stimulating hormone (TSH) stimulation test, response test measurement of serum levels of thyroid hormone(s) (T_3 and/or T_4) before and after the administration of TSH is a more reliable indicator of the functional capacity of the thyroid glands than single determinations and may distinguish between primary and secondary hypothyroidism.
thyrotropism affinity for the thyroid gland.
thyrotrops one of the five types of secretory cell found in the adenohypophysis; secrete thyroid-stimulating hormone.
thyroxine, thyroxin a hormone of the THYROID gland that contains iodine and is a derivative of the amino acid tyrosine. The chemical name for thyroxine is tetraiodothyronine (symbol, T_4); it is formed and stored in the thyroid follicles as thyroglobulin, the storage form. Thyroxine is released from the gland by the action of a proteolytic enzyme. T_4 is deiodinated in peripheral tissues to form tri-iodothyronine (T_3), which has a greater biological activity.

Thyroxine acts as a catalyst in the body and influences a great variety of effects, including metabolic rate (oxygen consumption); growth and development; metabolism of carbohydrates, fats, proteins, electrolytes and water; vitamin requirements; reproduction; and resistance to infection.

Thyroxine can be extracted from animals or made synthetically; it is used in the treatment of hypothyroidism and some types of goiter.
free t. the metabolically active fraction of thyroxine; abbreviated FT_4, T_f. $T_4 = T_f + TBG$. The amount is very small and difficult to estimate so that the amount present in serum is not used as a more accurate indicator of thyroxine status than T_4.
t.-binding globulin (TBG) most (99.95%) of the thyroxine in plasma is bound to globulin and a small amount bound to prealbumin.
t.-binding prealbumin bound to a small fraction of circulating T_4. This is the only known function of prealbumins.
L-t. see LEVOTHYROXINE.
Thysaniezia a genus of cyclophyllidean cestodes in the family Thysanosomatidae.
T. giardi occurs in the small intestine of sheep, goat and cattle. Appears to be of little pathogenic significance. Called also *Helictometra giardi*.
Thysanosoma actinioides a cyclophyllidean cestode in the family Thysanosomatidae found in the small intestine and biliary and pancreatic ducts of sheep, cattle and deer. Causes condemnation of livers and may cause unthriftiness. Called also fringed tapeworm.
Ti chemical symbol, *titanium*.
tiamulin a carboxypenicillin antibiotic effective against *Mycoplasma*, *Treponema* and *Hemophilus*. Used as a feed additive and growth promotant in pigs. The fumarate is water-soluble and can be administered in drinking water.
Tibetan apso see LHASA APSO.
Tibetan mastiff a very large (180 lb), powerful dog with pendulous ears, thick, medium length coat that forms a ruff around the neck and shoulders and is profuse on the long tail. The breed is affected by an inherited hypertrophic neuropathy.
Tibetan spaniel a small (9–15 lb), active dog with slightly short legs and a thick, silky coat that is short on the face but flat and of medium length on the body with feathering on the legs, tail and buttocks. The tail is carried over the back.
Tibetan terrier a medium-sized (18–30 lb), muscular dog with a profuse, medium length coat that covers the face and body. The ears are pendulous and the

thickly haired tail is carried over the back. The breed is affected by ceroid lipofuscinosis.

tibia the inner and larger bone of the hindlimb below the stifle; it articulates with the femur and head of the fibula above and with the talus below. See also Table 10.

rotated t. a disease of young turkeys characterized by rotation of the shaft of the tibiotarsus of one leg causing the metatarsus to point laterally and the bird to assume a spraddle leg posture. Up to 15% of a flock may be affected.

t. valga a bowing of the leg in which the angulation is away from the midline of the body.

t. vara a bowing of the leg in which the angulation is toward the midline of the body; bowleg.

tibia sours taint in a ham around the tibia, a much commoner site for taint than the femur.

tibial pertaining to the tibia.

t. crest a longitudinal prominence on the cranial border of the proximal tibia. Its proximal end (tibial tubercle) has a growth plate separate from the proximal tibia; hyperflexion injuries to the stifle may result in avulsion of this growth plate in dogs, seen in radiographs as a dorsal displacement of the tibial tubercle and patella.

t. dyschondroplasia a disease of broiler chickens and turkeys caused by a combination of dietary and genetic factors and characterized by dyschondroplasia in the proximal end of the tibiotarsal bone. In badly affected birds the leg is bowed and pathological fractures occur.

t. hemimelia see inherited tibial HEMIMELIA.

t. nerve block injection of an anesthetic agent above the tarsus, in the groove between the gastrocnemius tendon and the deep digital flexor tendon, produces anesthesia of the caudal, lateral and medial surfaces of the tarsus and metatarsus.

t. nerve injury results in overflexion of the hock (dropped hock).

t. rotation see rotated TIBIA.

t. tarsal bone see TALUS.

tibialis [L.] *tibial.*

tibiofemoral pertaining to the tibia and femur.

tibiofibular pertaining to the tibia and fibula.

t. joint see Table 11.

tibiotarsal pertaining to the tibia and tarsus.

tic a spasmodic twitching movement made involuntarily by muscles that are ordinarily under voluntary control. In dogs, the MYOCLONUS associated with infection by distemper virus is sometimes called a tic or chorea.

-tic suffix meaning pertaining to.

ticarcillin a semisynthetic penicillin with an extended spectrum of activity.

tick a blood-sucking arachnid parasite. There are two types, hard and soft. Includes American dog (DERMACENTOR *variabilis*), ARGASID TICK, bont (AMBLYOMMA *hebraeum*), British dog (IXODES *canisuga*), brown dog (RHIPICEPHALUS *sanguineus*), brown ear (RHIPICEPHALUS *appendiculatus*), brown winter (DERMACENTOR *nigrolineatus*), castor bean (RICINUS COMMUNIS), cayenne (AMBLYOMMA *cajennense*), Gulf Coast (AMBLYOMMA *maculatum*), IXODID, lone star (AMBLYOMMA *americanum*), pajaroello (ORNITHODORUS *coriaceus*), red-legged (RHIPICEPHALUS *evertsi*), Rocky Mountain wood (DERMACENTOR *andersoni*), shingle (syn. moose, DERMACENTOR *albipictus*), spinose ear (OTOBIUS *megnini*), tropical bont (AMBLYOMMA *variegatum*), yellow dog (HAEMAPHYSALIS *leachi leachi*) tick.

canine t. typhus see canine EHRLICHIOSIS.

t. collar a neck collar made of a PVC resin which releases particles of insecticide over a period of several months and aids in the control of tick infestations in companion animals.

t. fever see BABESIOSIS, ANAPLASMOSIS.

hard t. ticks of the family Ixodidae and members of *Ixodes*, *Boophilus*, *Margaropus*, *Hyalomma*, *Rhipicephalus*, *Haemaphysalis*, *Aponomma*, *Dermacentor*, *Amblyomma*, *Rhipicentor* spp. They have a hard chitinous shield on the dorsal surface of the body, on the entire back of the male but only the anterior portion of the female.

t. paralysis the female of several species of ticks but most commonly *Ixodes* or *Dermacentor* spp. elaborates a neurotoxin that typically causes an ascending flaccid paralysis in many animal species and humans but particularly in companion animals and young food animals. Affected dogs first develop weakness and paralysis of the hindlimbs, then forelimbs and ultimately respiratory paralysis unless the tick is removed and, in some cases, treatment with hyperimmune serum is given.

t. pyemia an infection of lambs caused by *Staphylococcus aureus* and transmitted by the bites of ticks. Newborn lambs die of septicemia or develop signs of arthritis, meningitis or dermatitis. Called also staphylococcal pyemia.

seed t. see SEED tick.

soft t. ticks of the family Argasidae including *Argas*, *Otobius*, *Ornithodorus* spp. These ticks have no dorsal protective shield.

t.-stained said of wool or fleece that is heavily discolored by the feces of sheep ked (*Melophagus ovinus*).

t. toxicosis see SWEATING sickness.

t. vectors ticks act as vectors of protozoa, bacteria, viruses, rickettsia.

t. worry an all-embracing term to describe the debilitating effects of heavy tick infestations. Includes anemia, irritation by the ticks, local infection as a result of bites, secondary blowfly and screw-worm infestation.

tick berry LANTANA *camara.*

tick-bite fever RICKETTSIA *conori.*

tickborne fever an infectious disease of cattle and sheep caused by *Ehrlichia phagocytophila* (called also *Rickettsia bovina* and *R. ovina* or *Cytoectes phagocytophila*). The organism is a parasite of white blood cells and the disease is characterized by fever, polypnea and abortion. Called also ehrlichosis, Ondiri disease, bovine petechial fever.

central European t. fever a meningoencephalitis of humans caused by a flavivirus which is present in the milk of ruminants although the principal reservoir is the tick *Ixodes ricinus.*

ticking a coat color pigmentation pattern in which hairs of one color are distributed in small groups throughout the background color, e.g. Australian cattle dog. Called also speckling.

tickling sensation no evidence exists that animals experience a tickling sensation but it is assumed that they do.

ticrynafen USAN name for TIENILIC ACID.

t.i.d. [L.] *ter in die* (three times a day).

tidal volume the amount of gas passing into and out of the lungs in each respiratory cycle.

tide a physiological variation or increase of a certain constituent in body fluids.

acid t. a temporary increase in the acidity of the urine that sometimes follows fasting.

fat t. the increase of fat in the lymph and blood following a meal.

postprandial alkaline t. the metabolic alkalosis that accompanies the active secretion of gastric acid following a meal.

tidemark undulating line that forms in the deep layer of the articular plate when growth of the bone ceases. It mineralizes but does not ossify. Called also blue line.

tie see GENITAL lock.

tie-bush see WIKSTROEMIA INDICA.

tie-stall a stall just large enough to accommodate one animal which is usually tied in by a neckchain if it is a cow, or by a halter if it is a horse. See also STALL.

tied-in a conformation defect in an animal in which a limb is perceptibly thinner at one point, e.g. tied-in below the knee, or below the hock.

Tiedmann's glands see BARTHOLIN'S GLANDS.

tienilic acid a diuretic, similar to the thiazide diuretics, but with greater uricosuric activity in humans.

Tiffany, Tiffanie (UK) a semi-longhaired version of the Burmese cat. It has a fine, silky coat in many colors.

tigemonam a monobactam antibiotic used orally.

tiger the large, 3 ft (1 m) high, 10 ft (3 m) long, yellow and black vertically striped cat. Called also *Panthera tigris*.

t. heart the striped and mottled myocardium of young cattle affected by a malignant form of foot-and-mouth disease.

t. snake tan to olive, with creamy yellow cross bands, venomous Australian snake. Envenomation is characterized by muscular weakness, flaccid paralysis, pupillary dilatation, restlessness, myoglobinuria, and a high serum creatine phosphokinase. Called also *Notechis scutatus*. Western tiger snake is called *Notechis scutatus occidentalis*.

t. stripe see reticulated LEUKOTRICHIA.

t. stripe colon the striking lesion of parallel lines of hemorrhages and congestion in the colon of cattle with rinderpest, acute mucosal disease and bovine malignant catarrh. Called also zebra marks.

Tiger River disease listeriosis.

tight junction a cell junction in which there is no intercellular space between cell membranes and so is impermeable. See also cell JUNCTION.

TIL tumor-infiltrating lymphocytes.

Tilapia niloticus freshwater, tropical fish of the family Cichlidae.

T. macrocephala see AFRICAN MOUTH BREEDER.

T. nilotica farmed finfish; called also Nile tilapia, *Oreochromis niloticus*. Table 23.

tile a display format for open windows in windows-type programs; the windows are displayed side by side, with no overlapping of some windows by others.

tiletamine a dissociative anesthetic agent, most commonly used in combination with zolazepam which provides better muscle relaxation and reduces the incidence of convulsions and muscle tremors.

Tilletia tritici the fungus of wheat grain, called also wheat smut; the smut is thought to contain an unidentified toxin which causes glomerulonephritis and poor weight gain in cattle.

tilmicosin a macrolide with antibacterial and antimycoplasma activity.

timber milk vetch see ASTRAGALUS.

timber tongue wooden tongue.

timbo de Palmeira see ATELEIA GLAZIOVIANA.

time a measure of duration. See under adjectives for specific times, e.g. BLEEDING time.

t. chart a graph on which the values of a variable are plotted on one axis and time on the other.

t. cluster a cluster of cases at particular points along a time axis.

developing t. for an x-ray film is about 3 to 5 minutes, but automatic processors complete the task in 90 seconds.

t. gain compensation (TGC) in ultrasonography, electronic amplification of returning sound waves, which are weaker because they come through deeper structures, is necessary so there is an even image density through the field. This is usually represented graphically by a TGC curve on most machines.

t. graph see time chart (above).

t. horizon the period until which the economic analysis under consideration applies.

t. series a distribution of data according to occurrence.

t.-space series a distribution of data according to the time and the place of occurrence.

t. value said of money; money now is more valuable than money later.

timer the device on the x-ray machine that controls the period of exposure to the beam. It may be a simple clockwork, wind-back timer, or one of two electronic timers which are capable of fast and repeated exposures. Only electronic timers are allowed on modern machines.

timolol a β-adrenergic blocking agent with antihypertensive and antiarrhythmic properties. Also used to decrease aqueous production in the management of glaucoma.

Timor pony dark-colored pony, about 12 hands high, tough, wiry, agile. Originated in the island of Timor.

timothy grass see PHLEUM PRATENSE.

tin a chemical element, atomic number 50, atomic weight 118.69, symbol Sn. See Table 6.

dibutyl t. dilaurate a cesticide used in poultry and cage birds. It is fed to chickens and is toxic if fed accidentally to calves. Causes tremor, diarrhea and convulsions.

tinct. tincture.

tincture an alcoholic or hydroalcoholic solution prepared from an animal or vegetable drug or a chemical substance.

benzoin t., compound a mixture of benzoin, aloes, storax and tolu balsam in alcohol; used as a topical protectant.

iodine t. a mixture of iodine and sodium iodide in a menstruum of alcohol and water; used as an anti-infective for the skin.

tinea RINGWORM; a name applied to many different kinds of fungal infection of the skin, the specific type (depending on characteristic appearance, etiological agent and site) usually being designated by a modifying term. Often used in humans but uncommonly in animals.

t. nigra superficial phaeohyphomycosis.

t. versicolor a skin disease of humans in which infection by *Malassezia furfur* (*Pityrosporum orbiculare*) causes skin lesions which differ in color from surrounding, noninfected skin. A similar disease has been described on the udder of goats.

ting point therapy a modern variant of classic acupuncture, based on symptomatic point selection plus classic meridian concepts of traditional Chinese medicine, and used in the treatment of diseases of the lower limbs of horses.

tingible stainable.

tinidazole an analog of metronidazole with a longer half-life but similar activity and uses.

tinnitus a noise in the ears, as ringing, buzzing or roaring.

objective t. one heard by others than the patient; reported in dogs and horses.

subjective t. one heard only by the patient; difficult to determine in animals.
-tion suffix meaning act or state of.
tiopronin see 2-MERCAPTOPROPIONYLGLYCINE.
TIP translation-inhibitory protein.
tip 1. a half horseshoe used to protect the toe from excessive wear but allows the frog and heels to stay free and not become contracted. 2. removal of the terminal 1 to 2 inches of horns in rams or cattle where they represent a risk to the animal from being caught in fences and the like, or to the people handling them. The horn at this point is insensitive and the operation can be performed without anesthetic. 3. outer extremity of a staple of wool.
hairy t. long, hairy fibers protrude beyond the tip of the wool staple; usually an example of non-selective breeding programs.
t. spraying spraying of an insecticide on the tip of the fleece anticipating its migration to deeper layers.
tipped pelvis see tipped PELVIS.
tipping an orthodontic procedure which forcibly pivots a tooth so that its crown is moved labially or lingually. Animals so treated should not be used for breeding.
tippy said of wool that has an open loose tip so that weather stain goes a long way down the staple. May be a natural defect or be the result of a long period of heavy rain.
tirefond [Fr.] an instrument like a corkscrew for raising depressed portions of bone.
tissue a group or layer of similarly specialized cells that together perform certain special functions. For anatomically specific tissues see under their identifying titles, e.g. adipose, connective.
t. death see NECROSIS.
t. density the penetrability of tissue by x-rays, bone and tooth being most dense, blood and soft tissue the next, fat the next, and gas and air least.
t. edema an abnormal accumulation of tissue fluid.
t. factor see tissue THROMBOPLASTIN.
t. fluid the extracellular fluid that constitutes the environment of the body cells. It is low in protein, is formed by filtration through the capillaries, and the excess drains away as lymph. See also INTERSTITIAL fluid.
t. inhibitors inhibitors of fibrinolysis; present in placenta.
indifferent t. undifferentiated embryonic tissue.
t. necrosis fever fever caused by pyrogens released by necrotic pyrogens.
t. plasminogen activator see plasminogen ACTIVATOR.
t. reacting agent substances that have a poorly defined but advantageous local effect on tissues.
t. receptor site a cell receptor common to cells of a particular tissue.
t. residue residues of chemical substances that are unacceptable to local pure food legislation especially sulfonamides, estrogens, chlorinated hydrocarbons, heavy metals. These are thought or known to have a deleterious effect on people eating or drinking the relevant animal product. See also chemical food RESIDUE.
t. sensitivity the susceptibility of individual tissues to injury by x-ray. The injury may be by way of inflammation, necrosis or cessation of cell growth. Fast-growing tissues in which the cells have a high mitotic index are the most sensitive, especially gonads, germinative layer of skin and erythropoietic tissues.
supportive t's cartilage and bone.
t. typing identification of tissue types for purposes of predicting acceptance or rejection of grafts and organ transplants. The process and purposes of tissue typing are essentially the same as for blood typing. The major difference lies in the kinds of antigens being evaluated. White blood cells, particularly lymphocytes, are used for tissue typing. The acceptance of allografts depends particularly on the matching of MHC antigens. If the donor and recipient are not MHC identical, the allograft is rejected. See also TYPING.
tit sign a small projection on the lesser curvature of the stomach seen on radiographs of dogs with pyloric stenosis due to accentuation of a haustral pouch.
titanium a chemical element, atomic number 22, atomic weight 47.90, symbol Ti. See Table 6.
t. dioxide used in ointment or lotion to protect the skin from the rays of the sun.
t. implant used for orthopedic implants, often in alloys, because of its good mechanical properties and resistance to corrosion.
titer the quantity of a substance required to react with or to correspond to a given amount of another substance.
agglutination t. the highest dilution of a serum which causes clumping of microorganisms or other particulate antigens.
titi monkey one of the many small New World monkeys, about the size of a squirrel with dense, short fur and a long, nonprehensile tail. It comes in several colors including black with white face, collar and hands. Called also *Callicebus* spp.
titoki ALECTRYON *excelsus*.
titrate to analyze by titration, to neutralize.
titration 1. in chemistry, the determination of a given component in solution by addition of a liquid reagent of known strength until a given end point, e.g. change in color, is reached indicating that the component has been consumed by reaction with the reagent. 2. in serology, the serial dilution of serum, often in two- or 10-fold steps to determine the highest dilution that still contains detectable amounts of antibody. The reciprocal of that dilution is referred to as the antibody titer of that serum. 3. in microbiology, the serial dilution of a suspension of microorganisms; each dilution, usually in replicas of 4 or 5, is then inoculated onto a substrate such as agar plate (bacteria) or cell culture (viruses) such that the number of organisms present in one or more of the higher dilutions can be accurately counted and used to infer the number of organisms in the original undiluted suspension.
Dean and Webb t. a test for measuring antibody in which varying dilutions of antibody are mixed with a constant quantity of antigen; antibody activity is determined by the dilution in which flocculation occurs most rapidly, i.e. the end point.
titre titer.
titrimetry analysis by titration.
titubation the act of staggering or reeling; a staggering gait with shaking of the trunk and head, commonly seen in cerebellar disease.
Tityus see SCORPION.
Tl chemical symbol, *thallium*.
TLC tender loving care; thin-layer chromatography; total lung capacity.
TLI trypsin-like immunoreactivity.
Tm 1. chemical symbol, *thulium*. 2. tubular maximum (in renal excretion). See also T_m.
TME transmissible mink encephalopathy.
TMJ syndrome temporomandibular joint syndrome.
TMTD tetramethylthiuram disulfide.

TNF tumor necrosis factor.
TNM tumor, nodes and metastases; a system of cancer staging (see TNM STAGING).
TNS transcutaneous neural stimulation.
TNT trinitrotoluene.
to-and-fro system a closed-circuit, rebreathing system used in inhalation anesthesia. A canister of soda lime is interposed between the animal and the rebreathing bag. Fresh gas is fed into the system as close as possible to the animal.
toad see BUFO.
toad flax see LINARIA VULGARIS.
toadfish see DIODONTIDAE, TETRAODONTIDAE.
toados colloquial for toadfish.
toadstool name may derive from German *todstuhl* (for death seat); for poisonous toadstools see RAMARIA and CLAVARIA.
Toano milkvetch ASTRAGALUS *toano*.
tobacco the dried prepared leaves of NICOTIANA *tabacum*, an annual plant widely cultivated which is the source of various alkaloids, the principal one being NICOTINE, a potent poison. Small animals ingesting cigarettes can be poisoned.
tobacco-chewers sheep that have had their tongues bitten off or pulled out by foxes or crows when they were lambs. Difficulty in controlling the regurgitated cud causes the juices to run out through the commissures of the lips and stain the chin. They resemble humans who chew tobacco.
Tobiano not a breed but a color type of spotted horse in which white extends from the dorsal midline in a ventral direction; the limbs are usually white and the distal half of the tail black. Most of the head, and always the poll and ears, are black. See also OVERO.
tobosa grass *Hilaria mutica*, may cause poisoning when it is infested with *Claviceps cinerea*. Called also tobo grass.
tobramycin an aminoglycoside antibiotic, similar to kanamycin and neomycin, produced by cultures of *Streptomyces tenebrarius*. Used as the sulfate.
tocainide an antiarrhythmic agent, similar to lidocaine, used in treating ventricular arrhythmias.
toco- word element. [Gr.] *parturition, labor*. See also words beginning *toko-*.
tocology the science of reproduction and the art of obstetrics.
tocolysis relaxation of the contracting pregnant uterus or undilated cervix to facilitate delivery in a dystocia or to briefly postpone parturition to ensure that surveillance is available.
tocolytic pertaining to tocolysis.
tocometer tokodynamometer.
tocopherol an alcohol isolated from wheat germ oil or produced synthetically; it has the properties of VITAMIN E.
α-t. vitamin E.
tocotrienol one of the eight structurally related compounds which are grouped together as vitamin E; tocotrienol indicates a compound with an unsaturated side chain.
toe a digit of the foot.
t. abscess see FOOT abscess.
t. crack see SANDCRACK.
curled t. see CURLED TOE PARALYSIS.
kicked-up t. a common injury in dogs, particularly racing Greyhounds, in which the deep flexor tendon is ruptured causing the affected claw to be elevated above others on the foot. Called also knocked-up toe.
t. out the limb is rotated slightly so that the toe points a little outward.
t. picking a vice of very young chickens that are hungry because feed supplies are inaccessible or inadequate. They pick each other's toes and start an outbreak of cannibalism.
sand t. see SAND toe.
seedy t. see SEEDY TOE.
splayed t. see SPLAYED DIGITS.
sprung t. a problem of racing Greyhounds characterized by dislocation of the proximal interphalangeal joint through rupture of the medial collateral ligament. The toe is displaced laterally, usually overriding the next toe.
toe-dragging stiff or tired gait in which unadequate flexing of the limbs causes dragging of the toes.
toe-pieces bars welded across the sole of a horseshoe behind the toe to give a draft horse grip on icy ground.
toenail occur in some animals, e.g. elephants, instead of the more conventional claws.
Togaviridae a large family of viruses; presently two genera are defined: *Alphavirus*, which contains arthropod-borne viruses that cause eastern, western and Venezuelan encephalitis, and *Rubivirus*, which contains rubella virus of humans and is not arthropod-borne. Members of both genera have similar physicochemical properties. They are enveloped (toga = cloak) about 60 nm diameter, contain a single-stranded, plus sense RNA genome, replicate in the cytoplasm of cells and mature by budding through cytoplasmic membranes. Flaviviruses, which are also arthropod-borne, were once included in the family, but are now a separate family, *Flaviviridae*.
togavirus a virus in the family TOGAVIRIDAE.
Toggenburg a polled dairy goat, brown to mouse-gray in color, with white facial stripes and extremities.
toggle the act of turning a feature for on to off and *vice versa* with the same keystroke.
toilet the cleansing and dressing of a wound.
toko- word element. [Gr.] *parturition, labor*. See also words beginning *toco-*.
tokodynagraph a tracing obtained by the tokodynamometer.
tokodynamometer an instrument for measuring and recording the expulsive force of uterine contractions.
tolazamide a first generation sulfonylurea derivative, used as a hypoglycemic agent in the treatment of diabetes mellitus.
tolazoline a smooth muscle relaxant and peripheral vasodilator; used as the hydrochloride salt.
tolbutamide a first generation sulfonylurea derivative, used as an oral hypoglycemic agent in the treatment of diabetes mellitus.
t. tolerance test the blood sugar curve after an intravenous injection of the hypoglycemic agent tolbutamide parallels the curve in a glucose tolerance test.
tolerance the ability to endure without effect or injury.
drug t. 1. decreased susceptibility to the effects of a drug due to its continued administration. 2. the maximum permissible level of a drug in or on animal feed or food at any particular time relative to slaughter.
high-dose t. in immunology, that induced by the intravenous administration of high doses of aqueous proteins.
immunological t. specific nonreactivity of the immune system to a particular antigen, which is capable under other conditions of inducing an immune response. There is, under normal circumstances, tolerance to self-antigens; identical (monozygotic) twins and dizygotic cattle or sheep twins where there has

been placental fusion and exchange of bone marrow stem cells are also tolerant of each other's tissues. Allophenic mice, that is mice produced by fusion of blastocysts from different mice are also tolerant of both 'parents'. The administration of antigens either at high or low dose and infection with certain viruses during critical early stages of immunological development may also induce tolerance.

t. level the concentration of a drug or chemical permitted by law to be present in human food.

t. limits the numerical limits within which a previously identified proportion of values of a variable, or observations in a population, can be expected to occur.

low-dose t. that induced by repeated administration of low doses of the antigen.

oral t. that induced by oral administration of the antigen.

self-t. the non-reactivity of the immune system to self-antigens.

t. test see tolerance TEST.

zero t. when no detectable amount of a chemical substance is permitted in human food.

tolerization the induction of tolerance, including the use of allergens, rendered nonimmunogenic, to stimulate formation of allergen-specific suppressor T lymphocytes that will suppress IgE synthesis; used in the treatment of atopy.

tolerogen an antigen that induces a state of specific immunological unresponsiveness to subsequent challenging doses of the antigen.

tolerogenesis induction of immunological tolerance.

Tollen's test a test for the presence of glycuronic acid in urine as an indicator of liver function.

Tollwut [Ger.] *rabies*. rabies. Called also *Wut*.

tolmetin a nonsteroidal anti-inflammatory analgesic, and antipyretic that causes gastrointestinal ulceration and hemorrhage in dogs.

tolnaftate a topical antifungal agent.

tolonium chloride see TOLUIDINE BLUE.

toltrazuril a triazinon drug with anticoccidial and antiprotozoal activity.

toluene the hydrocarbon C_7H_8 used as an anthelmintic against roundworms and hookworms in dogs. Vomiting occurs in some animals at even therapeutic dose rates. Overdosing causes incoordination and tremor soon after treatment, followed by diarrhea.

toluidine blue an antiheparin compound, used also as a biological stain. Called also tolonium chloride.

t. b. test a screening test for mucopolysaccharidosis, e.g. Hurler's syndrome; filter paper impregnated with toluidine blue turns blue when moistened with urine containing excessive amounts of chondroitin sulfuric acid.

***o*-toluidine test** a test for the presence of hemoglobin in feces or urine. The toluidine can be in solution, in a tablet or impregnated onto absorbent paper. A positive test is the development of a green to blue color.

tolyl any of three univalent radicals $CH_3C_6H_4$ derived from toluene.

tom 1. entire male feline. 2. male turkey.

tomato LYCOPERSICUM ESCULENTUM.

t. pomace residual pulp after extraction of juice from tomato fruit.

tombstones a cellular phenomenon in pemphigus vulgaris; rows of basal cells of the epidermis remain attached to the basal membrane, reminiscent of rows of tombstones.

-tome word element. [Gr.] *an instrument for cutting, a segment.*

tomia the sharp ventral edges of the upper beak of birds.

tomo- word element. [Gr.] *a section, a cutting.*

tomogram an image of a tissue plane or slice produced by tomography.

tomograph an apparatus in which the x-ray tube and film are moved in opposite directions during an exposure so that only a single plane of tissue remains in focus during the exposure. Other planes above and below are blurred by the motion.

tomography any method that produces images of single tissue planes. In conventional radiology, tomographic images (body-section radiographs) are produced by motion of the x-ray tube and film or by motion of the patient that blurs the image except in a single plane. In reconstruction tomography (CT and PET) the image is produced by a computer program. Called also laminagraphy, planigraphy, body-section technique.

computerized axial t. see computed tomography (below).

computed t. (CT) a revolutionary radiological imaging modality that uses computer processing to generate an image (CT scan) of the tissue density in a 'slice' about 0.5 inch thick through the patient's body. Called also computerized axial tomography (CAT) and computerized transaxial tomography (CTAT).

Because CT is noninvasive and has high contrast resolution, it has replaced some radiographic procedures using contrast media. However, in some areas the injection of contrast further enhances the image. CT also has a better spatial resolution than scintillation imaging (about 1 mm for CT compared with 15 mm for a scintillation camera).

positron emission t. (PET) a combination of computed tomography and scintillation scanning. Natural biochemical substances or drugs tagged with a positron-emitting radioisotope are administered to the subject. After injection, the tagged substance (tracer) is localized in specific tissues like its natural analog. When the isotope decays, it emits a positron, which then annihilates with an electron of a nearby atom, producing two 511 keV gamma rays traveling in opposite directions 180° apart. When the gamma rays trigger a ring of detectors around the subject, the line between the detectors on which the decay occurred is stored in the computer. A computer program (reconstruction algorithm), like those used in computed tomography, produces an image of the distribution of the tracer in the plane of the detector ring.

Most of the isotopes used in PET scanning have a half-life of only 2 to 10 minutes. Therefore, they must be produced by an on-site cyclotron and attached chemically to the tracer and used within minutes. Because of the expense of the scanner and cyclotron, PET is used only in research centers.

ultrasonic t. the ultrasonographic visualization of a cross-section of a predetermined plane of the body; see B-mode ULTRASONOGRAPHY.

-tomy word element. [Gr.] *incision, cutting.*

ton a measure of weight or mass. Includes short (or USA) 1 ton = 2000 lb and long (or UK) 1 ton = 2240 lb. See also TONNE.

tone 1. normal degree of vigor and tension; in muscle, the resistance to passive elongation or stretch. 2. a healthy state of a part; tonus. 3. a particular quality of sound or voice.

tongs long-handled, about 3 feet, shaped like pincers with knobs on the ends of the grasping blades.

Applied by standing behind the subject in a confined space and closing the jaws to grasp the animal's head just below the ears. Used for restraint of pigs and similarly built animals up to about 100 lb body weight.

tongue a muscular organ on the floor of the mouth; it aids in chewing, swallowing and speech, and is the location of organs of TASTE. The taste buds are located in the papillae, which are projections on the upper surface of the tongue.

t. abscess as well as true abscesses there are pseudoabscesses, common in companion birds, which are accumulations of inspissated, keratinized, epithelial debris, caused usually by a nutritional deficiency of vitamin A.

bifid t. a tongue with a lengthwise cleft.

bird t. see BIRD tongue.

black t. see BLACKTONGUE.

cleft t. bifid tongue.

coated t. one covered with a whitish or yellowish layer consisting of desquamated epithelium, debris, bacteria, fungi, etc.

t. cyst see THYROGLOSSAL cyst.

t. deformity the tongue may be shrunken because of prior inflammation, the tip may have been torn off, e.g. in lambs by predators. There is difficulty in prehending food and in managing in the mouth so that saliva and ruminal juices drool down the chin staining skin. Called tobacco chewers.

t. edema caused by local obstruction to venous blood flow, most dramatically displayed in a fetus presented anteriorly but delayed in parturition because of incompatibility in size between it and the birth canal, or bee or other hymenoptera sting.

t. frenulum see lingual FRENULUM.

furrowed t. a tongue with numerous furrows or grooves on the dorsal surface, often radiating from a groove on the midline.

geographic t. a tongue with denuded patches, surrounded by thickened epithelium.

hairy t. one with the papillae elongated and hairlike.

t. hypertrophy an occasional congenital anomaly in pigs.

t. inflammation see GLOSSITIS.

inherited smooth t. see SMOOTH tongue.

lolling t. one that protrudes from the mouth, usually to one side. Seen in some short-nosed dogs and as a vice in horses.

t. lyssa see LYSSA (2).

t. paralysis see GLOSSOPLEGIA.

t. protrusion caused by paralysis (hypoglossal nerve dysfunction), *Phalaris* spp. poisoning, swelling, e.g. edema, laceration.

t. rolling a vice in housed cattle. The animal rolls its tongue around in its half-opened mouth and may partially swallow it.

scrotal t. fissured tongue.

t. vice see tongue rolling (above).

wooden t. see ACTINOBACILLOSIS.

t. worm see LINGUATULA *serrata*.

tongue-tie abnormal shortness of the frenulum of the tongue, resulting in limitation of its motion; called also ankyloglossia. Occurs in dogs.

tonic 1. producing and restoring normal tone. 2. characterized by continuous tension. 3. a patent medicine dedicated to the restoration of normal 'tone' to bodily functions generally. Usually a pharmaceutical ragbag of stimulants, aromatics and alcohol, the paramount example of polypharmacy.

t.–clonic see CLONIC–tonic.

t. convulsion see tonic SEIZURE.

t. neck response a postural reaction in which extension of the head and neck causes extension of the forelimbs in a normal dog or cat.

t. seizure see tonic SEIZURE.

tonicity the state of tissue tone or tension; in body fluid physiology, the effective osmotic pressure equivalent.

tonification gentle stimulation of the acupuncture point; compare with sedation of it.

t. points acupuncture points used to increase or stimulate energy flow along a meridian or to stimulate an organ.

tonin an enzyme found in many tissues; can generate angiotensin II and bradykinin from their precursors; it appears to sustain blood pressure.

Tonkinese a cat breed derived from crossing the Burmese and Siamese; the build is intermediate between the two. They have the points of Siamese and coat color of Burmese. The eyes are aqua color.

tonnabossie see PAVETTA.

tonne measure of weight or mass; 1 tonne = 1000 kg. See also TON.

tono- word element. [Gr.] *tone, tension*.

tonoclonic both tonic and clonic; said of muscular spasms. See also tonic–clonic SEIZURE.

tonofibril one of the fine fibrils in epithelial cells, thought to give a supporting framework to the cell.

tonogram the record produced by tonography.

tonograph a recording tonometer.

tonography the recording of changes in intraocular pressure due to sustained pressure on the eyeball.

carotid compression t. a test for occlusion of the carotid artery by measuring ocular pressure and pulse before, during, and after the proximal portion of the carotid artery is compressed by the fingers.

tonometer an instrument for measuring tension or pressure, especially intraocular pressure.

applanation t. measures the force required to flatten or applanate an area of cornea. Includes the MacKay–Marg, Halberg, Dräger and Goldmann tonometers.

indentation t. measures the pressure required to indent the cornea; includes the Schiotz and pneumatonograph.

tonometry measurement of tension or pressure, e.g. intraocular pressure. See also TONOMETER.

digital t. estimation of the degree of intraocular pressure by pressure exerted on the eyeball by the finger of the examiner.

tonoplast the limiting membrane of an intracellular vacuole, the vacuole membrane.

tonoscope 1. an apparatus for rendering sound visible by registering the vibrations on a screen. 2. a device for examining the head or brain by means of sound. 3. tonometer.

tonsil 1. a small mass of lymphoid tissue, especially that found in close association with the mucous membrane of the throat; generally used alone to designate the palatine tonsil. Other structures referred to as tonsils are the cecal, lingual, esophageal, paraepiglottic, pharyngeal and tubal lymphoid aggregations. 2. a small mass of tissue.

cecal t. the accumulated mass of lymphoid tissue in the wall of cecum especially the proximal segment of the avian cecum.

cerebellar t. a rounded mass forming part of the cerebellum on its inferior surface.

esophageal t. large volume of lymphoid tissue in the caudal segment of the duck's esophagus.

follicular t. a tonsil bearing numerous invaginations of its surface epithelium (fossulae) each surrounded

by lymphoid tissue to form a follicle, as in the palatine tonsils of cattle or the lingual tonsils of the horse.
lingual t. diffuse collection of lymphoid tissue near the tongue root of most mammals.
palatine t. see PALATINE tonsil.
paraepiglottic t. a collection of lymphoid tissue craniolateral to the epiglottic base.
pharyngeal t. a collection of lymphoid tissue in the roof of the nasopharynx in pigs.
soft palate t. lymphoid tissue within the soft palate; principal tonsils in pigs in which it forms twin smooth patches of mucosa.
tubal t. the lymphoid tissue clustered close to the pharyngeal orifice of the auditory tube.
tonsillar pertaining to or emanating from TONSIL (1).
t. fossa the recess that houses a tonsil such as that which partly conceals the palatine tonsils of the dog.
t. inflammation see TONSILLITIS.
t. sinus the single opening of a compound follicle of a tonsil, as occurs in the palatine tonsil of cattle.
tonsillectomy excision of tonsils, most commonly performed in dogs.
tonsillitis inflammation and enlargement of a tonsil, especially the palatine tonsils.
follicular t. tonsillitis especially affecting the crypts.
parenchymatous t. that affecting the whole substance of the tonsil.
pustular t. a variety characterized by formation of pustules.
tonsillolith a calculus in a tonsil.
tonsillotomy incision of a tonsil.
tonus tone or tonicity; the slight, continuous contraction of a muscle, which in skeletal muscles aids in the maintenance of posture and in the return of blood to the heart.
tooth pl. *teeth;* one of the small, bonelike structures of the jaws for the biting and mastication of food. See also DENTAL, TEETH.
toothbrush technique see MACKENZIE BRUSH TECHNIQUE.
Toowoomba canary grass PHALARIS *aquatica.*
top continuous band of combed parallel wool fibers which have not yet been twisted.
top stud the best sheep in the stud.
tophaceous gritty or sandy; pertaining to tophi.
tophus pl. *tophi* [L.] 1. a chalky deposit of sodium urate occurring in GOUT; tophi form most often around the joints in cartilage, bone, bursae and subcutaneous tissue. 2. dental calculus.
topi see DAMALISCUS LUNATUS.
topical pertaining to a particular area, as a topical anti-infective applied to a certain area of the skin and affecting only the area to which it is applied.
t. agent a pharmaceutical preparation for topical application.
topline the top line of the animal as seen from the side at a distance of 10 feet or more. The general predilection is for the neat and tidy, straight topline.
top(o)- word element. [Gr.] *particular place or area.*
topmaker a commercial wool processor specializing in the manufacture of tops for sale to spinners.
topographic describing or pertaining to special regions.
topography a description of a region or a special part of the body, especially of the mutual relationships of adjacent structures.
topoisomerase an enzyme involved in DNA replication that introduces a single-strand nick in the DNA enabling it to swivel and thereby relieve the accumulated winding strain generated during unwinding of the double helix.
toponarcosis local anesthesia.
topping mowing the top, rank growth on an overgrown pasture to provide a more palatable and nutritious supply of feed.
toris pl. *tori;* footpad.
toro de lidia [Span.] FIGHTING BULL breed of beef cattle.
Torovirus a genus in the *Coronaviridae* family that includes Berne virus, recovered from horses in Switzerland, and Breda virus, recovered from diarrheic calf feces in the United States. Virions are enveloped and contain an elongated helical nucleocapsid with a single-stranded negative sense RNA genome. The capsid is bent into an open torus or doughnut-shaped structure.
torpedo fusiform swellings of proximal axonal segments of cerebellar Purkinje cells in cases of perennial rye grass mycotoxicosis and some forms of storage disease.
torpid not acting with normal vigor and accuracy.
torpor [L.] *sluggishness.*
torque a rotatory force.
Torrymeter an instrument for estimating freshness of meat. The estimates are based on changes in the dielectric properties of the meat as it ages.
torsalo grub larvae of *Dermatobia hominis.*
torsion 1. the act of twisting, e.g. of an artery in hemostasis. 2. the state of being twisted. For specific torsions see ABOMASAL, CECAL, COLONIC, GASTRIC, LIVER, MESENTERIC, SPLENIC, TESTICULAR, UTERINE.
torsiversion turning of a tooth on its long axis out of normal position.
torso the body, exclusive of the head and limbs.
torticollis wryneck, a contracted state of the cervical muscles, producing torsion of the neck. The deformity may be congenital, or secondary to pressure on the accessory nerve, to inflammation of tissues in the neck, or to muscle spasm.
tortipelvis distortions of the spine and hip produced by a disorder marked by irregular muscular contractions of the trunk and extremities.
tortoise see TURTLE.
tortoiseshell a coat color in cats consisting of a mixture of black and shades of red to yellow, usually broken into large patches. The color can be found in a variety of cats, both long- and shorthaired, and specific breeds, such as Burmese. Tortoiseshell-and-white is another variety, called calico in the USA and chintz in the United Kingdom. Because the genes for black and orange (including shades from red to yellow) are carried on an X chromosome, but not the same one, only females can carry both colors. Males from similar breeding are either orange or black. There are isolated examples of tortoiseshell or tortoiseshell-and-white male cats, but almost all are sterile due to the chromosomal abnormality of XXY. These are considered models of the human condition, KLINEFELTER'S SYNDROME. Rarely, the phenomenon may be attributed to somatic mutations, crossing over of chromosomes or mosaicism.
torts in law a wrong other than a criminal wrong, e.g. defamation, negligence.
Torula former name for CRYPTOCOCCUS.
toruli small elevations, papillae.
t. digitales digital pads on the feet of dogs, cats and other species with paws.
t. tactiles small tactile elevations associated with special guard hairs scattered on the skin of cats and dogs.
toruloid knotted or beaded, like a yeast cell.
Torulopsis a genus of imperfect fungi, similar to

Cryptococcus but without a capsule. Includes *T. neoformans*, *T. glabrata*. A normal inhabitant in the respiratory and gastrointestinal tract of many animals, but *T. glabrata* has been reported to be an uncommon cause of bovine mastitis.

torulopsosis infection by TORULOPSIS.

torulosis see CRYPTOCOCCOSIS.

torulus [L.] *pl. toruli a small elevation.*

torus pl. *tori* [L.] a swelling or bulging projection; a pad.

carpal t. chestnut on the leg of a horse; the stopper pad of a dog. Called also carpal pad.

t. corneus bulb of the heel in ungulates.

t. linguae the eminence on the dorsum of the tongue in ruminants.

t. metacarpal, t. metatarsal metacarpal pads, metatarsal pads.

t. pyloricus a fleshy protuberance at the pylorus of some species such as ruminants and pigs, that projects into the lumen of the pyloric canal.

tarsal t. chestnut on the leg of a horse. Called also tarsal pad.

tosylate USAN contraction for *p*-toluenesulfonate.

total body water includes the intracellular water and the extracellular water, the latter consisting of the interstitial or tissue fluid and the intravascular fluid or plasma. The extracellular fluids also contain the transcellular fluids that are formed by active transport processes and include saliva, cerebrospinal fluid, and the fluids of the eye and the secretory glands and so on. It may be ingested water or water produced by the body's metabolic processes (metabolic water).

total CO_2 content the CO_2 gas liberated from a sample of blood after the addition of acid.

total digestible nutrients an outmoded method of expressing the energy value of a feed; abbreviated TDN. Estimated as follows:

$$\%\text{TDN} = \frac{\text{DCP} + \text{DCF} + \text{DNFE} + (\text{DEE} \times 2.25)}{\text{feed consumed} \times 100}$$

where DCP = digestible crude protein, DCF = digestible crude fat, DNFE = digestible nitrogen-free extract, DEE = digestible ether extract.

One pound of TDN = 2000 kcal of digestible energy.

total frequency the number of observations in a set of data.

total intravenous feeding the only sustenance the patient gets is in solution via an intravenous device.

total milk solids butter fat, casein, lactose, minerals.

total parenteral nutrition see parenteral NUTRITION.

total peripheral resistance a measure of the total resistance to blood flow provided by the entire vascular system.

total plasma protein includes plasma prealbumin, albumin and globulin, fibrinogen.

total regional flow flow rate for a local area, e.g. a specific organ; depends largely on the resistance provided by the organ's vasculature, itself dependent on the lengths of the vessels and their diameters.

total solids meter refractometer.

total worm count see worm COUNT.

totalizator, totalisator a computer-driven, machine-operated betting system which eliminates the bookmaker in the betting industry which surrounds horse and dog racing. Called also parimutuel.

totipotential exhibiting totipotency; characterized by the ability to develop in any direction; said of cells that can give rise to cells of all types.

toucan a bizarre bird with an enormous brightly colored beak. It is insectivorous and a member of the woodpecker group. There are several genera, e.g. *Ramphastos* and *Pteroglossus* in the order Piciformes.

touch 1. the sense by which contact of an object with the skin is recognized. 2. palpation with the finger.

Touch is actually not a single sense, but several. There are separate nerves in the skin to register heat, cold, pressure, pain and touch. These thousands of nerves are distributed unevenly over the body, so that some areas are more responsive to cold, others to pain, and others to heat or pressure.

Each of these types of nerves has a different structure at the receiving end. A touch nerve has an elongated bulb-shaped end, and a nerve responsive to cold a squat bulb; the nerve that registers warmth has what looks like twisted threads, and the nerve for deep pressure has an egg-shaped end. Pain receptors have no protective sheath.

t. receptors see SENSE.

Toulouse a gray goose, with white underparts and orange legs and beak.

tourniquet a device for compression of an artery or vein, most commonly used in companion animals to facilitate obtaining blood samples or giving intravenous injections.

Rumel t. one constructed of ligature doubled back through a tube, with the exposed loop used to temporarily occlude large vascular structures.

touting the making of personal representations by a veterinarian to persons who are not clients in an attempt to solicit their business.

Touton giant cell large multinucleated cells characteristic of xanthomatous lesions. The cells are usually filled with lipid.

towel sterilizable piece of cloth with good water absorbing capacity used to mop up, as a temporary instrument store at a surgical site, as a local drape.

t. clamps see towel FORCEPS.

toxaemia see TOXEMIA.

toxalbumin a class of directly cytotoxic substances of a protein nature found in plants and snakes; plant toxalbumins, concentrated in seeds, occur in *Abrus precatorius* (abrin), *Adenia digitata*, *Ricinus communis* (ricin), *Robinia pseudoacacia*.

toxaphene an insecticide. See CHLORINATED HYDROCARBONS.

toxascariasis disease caused by infestation with *Toxascaris* spp.

Toxascaris a genus of roundworms in the family Ascarididae.

T. leonina found in the small intestine of dog, cat, fox and wild carnivora. Causes toxascariasis.

toxemia 1. the condition resulting from the spread of bacterial products (toxins) by the bloodstream. 2. a condition resulting from metabolic disturbances.

Clinically there is depression, lethargy, separation from the group, reduced appetite, slow growth, poor production, low fecal output, weak pulse of normal rate, hemic murmur, weakness, albuminuria. There may be localizing signs such as pressure by an abscess. See also TOXEMIC shock.

alimentary t. toxemia due to absorption from the alimentary canal of chemical poisons generated therein; a form of autointoxication.

pregnancy t. see PREGNANCY toxemia.

toxemic emanating from or pertaining to TOXEMIA.

t. agalactia see MASTITIS–METRITIS–AGALACTIA.

t. jaundice a complex of diseases in sheep including phytogenous chronic copper poisoning in which copper accumulation is fostered by copper converter plants such as subterranean clover, hepatogenous chronic copper poisoning, a combination of copper and plant poisoning, and simple poisoning by the same plants without any copper component. The clinical signs include jaundice, toxemia, possibly severe anemia.

t. shock caused by the presence of large quantities of potent toxins in the bloodstream. They cause peripheral vasodilatation and a precipitate fall in blood pressure accompanied by mucosal pallor, hypothermia, tachycardia and muscle weakness, e.g. in coliform toxicosis.

toxic poisonous; pertaining to poisoning.

t. algae see ALGAL poisoning.

t. biotransformations enzymatic changes of nontoxic to toxic substances, usually in the liver.

t. epidermal necrolysis see toxic epidermal NECROLYSIS.

t. fat syndrome see CHICKEN edema disease.

t. granulation see toxic GRANULES.

t. hepatitis, t. liver disease caused by a very large number of poisons including inorganic, organic, plant.

t. myopathy uncommon but is caused by e.g. gossypol, *Cassia* spp., monensin and the other ionophore coccidiostats.

t. nephrosis caused by many toxins, e.g. mercury, arsenic, copper, aminoglycoside antibiotics.

t. shock see TOXEMIC shock.

t. shock syndrome see TOXEMIC shock.

toxicant 1. poisonous. 2. a poison.

toxicity the characteristic or quality of being poisonous, especially the degree of virulence of a toxic microbe or of a poison. See also TOXICOSIS.

t. rating includes slightly toxic (with an oral LD_{50} in rats of 5000 to 15,000 mg/kg) up to supertoxic (with an LD_{50} of less than 5 mg/kg).

toxic(o)- word element. [Gr.] *poison, poisonous.*

Toxicodendron plant genus in the family Anacardiaceae; plants cause a serious contact dermatitis in humans and dogs; includes *T. diversilobum* (*Rhus toxicodendron, R. diversiloba*, western poison oak), *T. quercifolium* (*Rhus quercifolia*, eastern poison oak), *T. radicans* (*Rhus toxicodendron, Rhus radicans*, poison ivy), *T. vernix* (*Rhus vernix*, poison sumac, poison elder).

toxicodynamics the physiological mechanisms by which toxins are absorbed, distributed, metabolized and excreted.

toxicogenic producing or elaborating toxins.

toxicoid resembling a poison.

toxicoinfectious botulism see wound BOTULISM.

toxicologist a specialist in toxicology.

toxicology the science or study of poisons.

developmental t. abnormalities of development caused by exposure to deleterious agents; embryotoxicity.

genetic t. errors in the transmission of genetic information induced by a toxic agent; mutagenesis.

toxicopathy toxicosis.

toxicopexy the fixation or neutralization of a poison in the body.

toxicophidia venomous serpents collectively.

Toxicophloea spectabilis see ACOKANTHERA *spectabilis*.

toxicosis any disease condition due to poisoning. See also POISONING and under the titles of individual toxins. Compare with TOXICITY.

toxiferous conveying or producing a poison.

toxigenic caused by or producing toxins.

t. diarrhea see secretory DIARRHEA.

toxigenicity the capacity to produce toxins.

toxin a poison, especially a protein or conjugated protein produced by certain animals, some higher plants, and pathogenic bacteria. *Antigenic toxins*, produced by bacteria or helminths, stimulate production of antitoxins. Exotoxins are produced by bacteria and diffuse into surroundings, e.g. tetanus toxin, or can be ingested preformed, e.g. botulinum toxin. Endotoxins are released into the surrounding tissue only when the bacteria break down. They are lipopolysaccharides and form part of the cell wall, e.g. coliform endotoxins. *Metabolic toxins*, e.g. toxic amines absorbed from damaged intestine, ketones, lactic acid from carbohydrate engorgement, ammonia in liver damage, creatinine in renal dysfunction. See also METABOLIC toxins.

dermonecrotic t. an exotoxin produced by certain bacteria that causes extensive local necrosis on intradermal inoculation.

extracellular t. exotoxin.

intracellular t. endotoxin.

tetanus t. the potent neurotoxic exotoxin produced by *Clostridium tetani*. Called also tetanospasmin.

toxinology the science dealing with the toxins produced by certain higher plants, animals and humans and by pathogenic bacteria.

toxipathic pertaining to or caused by the pathogenic action of toxins, of whatever origin.

toxipathy toxicosis.

tox(o)- word element. [Gr., L.] *toxin, poison.*

Toxocara a genus of nematode parasites in the family Ascarididae.

T. canis the adults are found in the small intestine of the dog and fox; infection is via oral, transmammary and transplacental routes; the larvae migrate through tissues, including to the fetus where they establish a prenatal infection, eventually passing through the lungs and then to the alimentary tract. In hosts other than the dog and fox migration in abnormal tissues occurs and the life cycle is not completed. Is the cause of ocular and visceral LARVA migrans in humans.

T. cati the adults are found in the small intestine of domestic and wild cats. Larvae pursue a migratory course through tissues but intrauterine infection of the fetus does not occur.

T. pteropodis found in flying fox bats.

T. vitulorum occurs in the small intestine of cattle, buffalo and in sheep and goats. Calves are infected via the milk of the dam.

toxocariasis infection by worms of the genus *Toxocara*. Heavy infestations in young puppies and kittens may be responsible for abdominal distension, signs of colic, diarrhea and poor growth. Somatic tissue migration of larvae in neonatal puppies may cause respiratory and nervous signs.

toxoid a toxin treated by heat or chemical agent to destroy its deleterious properties without destroying its antigenicity. Most of the clostridial diseases, e.g. tetanus, are controlled by vaccination with toxoids.

toxophilic easily susceptible to poison; having affinity for toxins.

toxophore the group of atoms in a toxin molecule that produces the toxic effect.

toxophorous bearing poison; producing the toxic effect.

Toxoplasma a genus of sporozoan parasites in the family Sarcocystidae.

T. gondii a coccidian parasite of the intestine of all felids, including especially the domestic cat, jaguarundi, ocelot, mountain lion, leopard cat, and bobcat, which are definitive hosts. Most vertebrates, including humans and birds, can be infected with the intermediate stages and experience one or other forms of the disease TOXOPLASMOSIS.

T. hammondi see HAMMONDIA *hammondi*.

toxoplasmin an antigen prepared from mouse peritoneal fluids rich with *Toxoplasma gondii*; injected intracutaneously as a test for toxoplasmosis.

toxoplasmosis a contagious disease of all species caused by the sporozoan parasite *Toxoplasma gondii*. The principal manifestation in animals is as abortion in ewes. It is also a cause of sporadic cases of pneumonia, central nervous system disease, and less often retinochoroiditis, and hepatitis in dogs and cats. Clinical signs include fever, malaise, lymphadenitis, abortion, fetal malformation.

toy breeds the very small, decorative breeds of dogs, generally less than 20 lb weight, developed mainly for companionship and as novelties. Includes AFFENPINSCHER, BICHON FRISE, CAVALIER KING CHARLES SPANIEL, CHIHUAHUA, CHINESE CRESTED, ENGLISH TOY TERRIER, BRUSSELS GRIFFON, ITALIAN GREYHOUND, JAPANESE CHIN, KING CHARLES SPANIEL, LOWCHEN, MALTESE, MINIATURE PINSCHER, PAPILLON, PEKINGESE, POMERANIAN, PUG, SILKY TERRIER, Toy POODLE.

t. b. hypoglycemia see juvenile HYPOGLYCEMIA.

TPA total parenteral alimentation; see parenteral NUTRITION.

TPN total parenteral nutrition; see parenteral NUTRITION.

TPP 1. total plasma protein. 2. thiamin pyrophosphate.

TPR 1. temperature, pulse, respiration. 2. total peripheral resistance.

tr. tincture.

trabecula pl. *trabeculae* [L.] a small beam or supporting structure; various fibromuscular bands or cords providing support in various organs, such as heart, penis and spleen.

bone t. anastomosing bony spicules in cancellous bone which form a meshwork of intercommunicating spaces that are filled with bone marrow.

septomarginal t., t. septomarginalis the moderator bands passing from the interventricular septum to the peripheral ventricular wall of the heart.

trabeculate marked with crossbars or trabeculae.

trabeculation the formation of trabeculae in a part.

traberkrankheit scrapie.

trace element essential ingredients of the diet of a particular species of animals but the amount required is very small. Includes copper, cobalt, iron, iodine, manganese, molybdenum, selenium and zinc. Chromium, fluorine and silicon are also necessary in some experimental diets but their addition to livestock diets is not considered to be essential. See also MACROELEMENT. Called also trace minerals.

traceback an epidemiological strategy of locating the origin of an outbreak. The usual tactic is to enforce the use of identifying markers such as tailtags with codes identifying the vendors.

tracer a means by which something may be followed, as (1) a mechanical device by which the outline or movements of an object can be graphically recorded, or (2) a material by which the progress of a compound through the body may be observed.

radioactive t. a radioactive isotope replacing a stable chemical element in a compound introduced into the body, enabling its metabolism, distribution and elimination to be followed in the living animal.

traces long leather straps that run from the collar of a cart harness to the cart and provide the traction for moving it.

trachea the air passage extending from the larynx to the main bronchi; called also the windpipe.

This tube is reinforced by a series of C-shaped rings of cartilage that keep the passage uniformly open. The gaps between the rings are bridged by strong fibroelastic membranes. The arms of the C are bridged by the tracheal muscle which can vary the luminal diameter.

The trachea is lined with mucous membrane bearing cilia that continously sweep foreign material out of the breathing passages toward the mouth.

tracheal pertaining to or emanating from TRACHEA.

t. aspiration see TRANSTRACHEAL ASPIRATION.

t. band sign on contrast radiography of a dilated esophagus, the impression made ventrally by the trachea.

t. collapse, collapsing trachea a disorder of the tracheal membrane (trachealis muscle) or tracheal rings that results in a functional tracheal stenosis. Affected dogs, usually of miniature or toy breeds, have a cough and reduced exercise intolerance. See also goose honk COUGH.

t. compression pressure on the trachea sufficient to cause displacement and reduction in caliber, usually inside the thorax; most readily detected radiographically.

t. cough a nonproductive, or only slightly productive, resonant cough, often occurring in paroxysms and easily elicited by pressure on the cervical trachea. Typically associated with tracheitis.

t. duct paired lymphatic ducts running down the side of the trachea, commencing at the retropharyngeal lymph nodes, receiving tributaries from other nodes of the head and neck and terminating in either the thoracic duct or the jugular or other vein at the entrance to the chest.

t. hypoplasia a congenital defect in brachycephalic dogs in which the tracheal lumen is greatly reduced in size. Bronchopneumonia commonly occurs.

t. inflammation see TRACHEITIS.

t. intubation refers usually to the passage of an endotracheal tube for the purposes of anesthesia, resuscitation or external control of respiration for any other reason. See also tracheal tube (below).

t. lavage, t. wash introduction of a tracheal catheter via a cutaneous incision between two tracheal rings, passage of the catheter to the bronchi, introduction of normal saline, aspiration of the saline, retrieval of the catheter.

t. percussion a sharp percussion stroke on the trachea creates a sound which can be auscultated over the lung area.

t. rupture due usually to blunt trauma; there is escape of air into surrounding tissues which results in subcutaneous and mediastinal emphysema.

t. stenosis may be congenital or acquired, resulting from trauma or surgical procedures on the trachea. Causes respiratory distress, coughing, and secondary infections of the upper respiratory tract.

t. transection occurs as a result of trauma, in cats particularly from hyperextension of the head and neck, causing dyspnea.

t. tube a metal tube used in horses that have a long-term obstruction of the upper respiratory system. Different to a tracheotomy tube it is a flattened tube fixed to a broad flange with suture holes at its edge and a bend of 90° at 0.5 inch from the flange. See also ENDOTRACHEAL tube.

tracheitis inflammation of the trachea; characterized by cough, pain and coughing on compression of the trachea and, in severe cases with obstruction of the airway, dyspnea.

trachelectomy excision of the uterine cervix.

trachelematoma a hematoma on the sternocleidomastoid muscle.

trachelism, trachelismus spasm of the neck muscles; spasmodic reaction of the head in epilepsy.
trachelitis cervicitis; inflammation of the uterine cervix.
trachel(o)- word element. [Gr.] *neck, necklike structure,* especially the cervix uteri.
trachelocystitis inflammation of the neck of the bladder.
trachelomyitis inflammation of the muscles of the neck.
trachelopexy fixation of the uterine cervix.
tracheloplasty plastic repair of the uterine cervix.
trachelorrhaphy suture of the uterine cervix.
trachelotomy incision of the uterine cervix.
tracheo- word element. [Gr.] *trachea.*
tracheo-esophageal see TRACHEOESOPHAGEAL.
tracheoaerocele tracheal hernia containing air.
tracheobronchial pertaining to the trachea and bronchi.
t. aspiration see TRACHEAL lavage.
tracheobronchitis inflammation of the trachea and bronchi.
canine infectious t. see KENNEL COUGH.
parasitic t. see AELUROSTRONGYLUS, CAPILLARIA, CRENOSOMA, FILAROIDES, PARAGONIMUS, STRONGYLOIDES.
tracheobronchoscopy inspection of the interior of the trachea and bronchus.
tracheocele hernial protrusion of the tracheal mucous membrane.
tracheoesophageal pertaining to or arising from the trachea and the esophagus.
t. fistula a communication between the trachea and the esophagus; can occur during fetal life due to faulty separation of the laryngotracheal groove from the foregut; often associated with esophageal stenosis or atresia, aspiration pneumonia.
t. ridge primordium of the embryonic tracheoesophageal septum.
t. septum the partition which develops by fusion of the tracheoesophageal ridges; completes the separation of the trachea and esophagus in the developing embryo.
tracheography radiography of the trachea preferably after the intratracheal injection of an oily contrast agent.
tracheolaryngeal pertaining to the trachea and larynx.
tracheolaryngotomy incision of the larynx and trachea.
tracheomalacia softening of the tracheal cartilages.
tracheopathy disease of the trachea.
tracheopharyngeal pertaining to the trachea and pharynx.
Tracheophilus a genus of trematodes in the family Cyclocoelidae, parasites of aquatic birds.
T. cucumerinum found in the trachea, air sacs and esophagus of domestic and wild ducks; causes obstruction leading to dyspnea and asphyxia.
***T. cymbius* (syn. *T. sisowi*)** found in the trachea and bronchi of domestic and wild ducks; cause tracheal obstruction and asphyxia.
tracheophony a sound heard in auscultation over the trachea.
tracheoplasty plastic repair of the trachea.
tracheopyosis purulent tracheitis.
tracheorrhagia hemorrhage from the trachea.
tracheoschisis fissure of the trachea.
tracheoscopy inspection of the interior of the trachea.
tracheostenosis constriction of the trachea.
tracheostoma an opening through the neck and into the trachea.
tracheostomize to perform tracheostomy upon.
tracheostomy creation of an opening into the trachea through the neck, with insertion of an indwelling tube to facilitate passage of air or evacuation of secretions. The procedure may be an emergency measure or an elective one.
t. tube two identical down-curving, semicircular tubes are fitted one inside the other. They both have wide flanges which fit against the skin when the tubes are inserted in and down through the tracheostomy incision. When the tubes are snugly in position the inner tube is rotated through 180° making the tube self-retaining.
tracheotome an instrument for incising the trachea.
tracheotomy incision of the trachea through the skin and muscles of the neck for exploration, for removal of a foreign body, or for obtaining a biopsy specimen or removing a local lesion.
t. tube see TRACHEOSTOMY tube.
Trachyandra plant genus of South African origin, in family Liliaceae; contains an unidentified toxin; causes an acquired lipofuscinosis storage disease with exercise intolerance, incoordination, recumbency, tremor, paralysis; includes *T. divaricata* (branched onion weed), *T. laxa*.
Trachymene Australian plant genus of the Apiaceae family; contains an unidentified toxin; thought to cause bowie (bentleg), a congenital limb deformity, and sudden death of sheep; includes *T. cyanantha*, *T. glaucifolia*, *T. ochracea*. Called also wild parsnip.
trachyphonia roughness of the voice.
tracing a graphic record produced by copying another, or scribed by an instrument capable of making a visual record of movements.
track one of the many concentric circles of information recorded magnetically onto a computer disk. Each track is divided into sectors, and a sector is the smallest amount of information that can be read from or written to the disk at one time.
track leg severe sprain of the triceps or semitendinosus muscle in the racing Greyhound caused by injury while racing or training. There is severe lameness and the affected muscle is tense, swollen and painful.
tracker dog disease see canine EHRLICHIOSIS.
tract a longitudinal assemblage of tissues or organs, especially a bundle of nerve fibers having a common origin, function and termination, or a number of anatomical structures arranged in series and serving a common function. For anatomically specific tracts see under their identifying titles, e.g. alimentary, respiratory.
tractable easy to manage; tolerable.
traction the exertion of a pulling force, as that applied to a fractured bone or dislocated joint to maintain proper position and facilitate healing, or, in obstetrics, that along the axis of the pelvis to assist in delivery of a fetal part.
t. hook see KREY–SCHOTTLER HOOK.
t. splint see Schroeder–Thomas SPLINT.
tractor feed small nipples in a circle around each end of a printer platen on which computer paper is hooked to ensure even, slip-free progress of the paper.
tractor vaporizing oil English farmer's term for tractor fuel widely used during the second world war; approximates kerosene or paraffin.
tractotomy see OLFACTORY tractotomy.
tractus pl. *tractus* [L.] tract; certain collections of nerve fibers in the central nervous system.

Tradescanlia fluminens ubiquitous urban weed (wandering Jew) capable of causing allergic dermatitis in dogs.

trafficking see HOMING.

tragacanth the dried gummy exudation from *Astragalus gummifer* or other species of *Astragalus*; used as a suspending agent for drugs. Called also gum tragacanth.

Tragelaphus African bushbuck antelopes in the subfamily Antelopinae; includes *T. angasi*, *T. scriptus*, *T. spekei*, *T. strepciceros*.

T. angasi a very handsome antelope with lyrate horns. Very susceptible to capture myopathy. Called also nyala.

tragi plural of *tragus*.

tragulid a member of the family Tragulidae, the mouse-deer or chevrotain. The smallest ruminant, being 6 inches high.

tragus pl. *tragi* [L., Gr.] the knob-like projection at the base of the external ear supported by a plate of cartilage, part of the auricular cartilage.

trail a well-defined information pathway that leads from data point to data point and sequentially from analysis to conclusion.

audit t. as for accounting trail but designed for audit purposes.

diagnostic t. a diagnostic decision tree.

trail-ride a cross-country, noncompetitive, group saunter on horseback, principally with a view to seeing the sights.

trailer shoe a horseshoe in which the sidebars are carried well back beyond the heel. Useful when the flexor tendons have been damaged.

trailer-table a mobile operating table for large animals, moved from farm to farm behind a vehicle.

train of four a method of monitoring neuromuscular blockade in which four twitch responses are used to demonstrate depletion of acetylcholine.

trained-off pertaining to Greyhounds or racehorses which lose racing form during training or a racing program in the absence of any apparent physical or metabolic disease.

training 1. in racing horses and Greyhounds, a program of exercise to improve the animal's physical performance in a particular task. The effects of training include enlargement of spleen with greater erythrocyte storage and mobilization, increased heart size and stroke volume, and increased hemoglobin content of blood. A performance trial is the only satisfactory way of measuring the gains achieved. 2. in behavior includes BREAKING-IN and OBEDIENCE TRAINING in dogs.

trait 1. any genetically determined condition; also, the condition prevailing in the heterozygous state of a recessive disorder. 2. a distinctive behavior pattern.

t. A-46 see inherited PARAKERATOSIS.

qualitative t. a characteristic that is expressed only in descriptive terms, e.g. fine bone, deep chest.

quantitative t. a characteristic that is expressed mathematically, e.g. an annual yield of milk of 15,000 lb.

sex-linked t. the gene for the trait is located on the chromosomes which determine the sex of the individual.

Trakehner horse Russian and German light horse produced by crossing Thoroughbred and Arab; chestnut, bay or gray.

tranexamic acid an antifibrinolytic agent, used orally or intravenously to control hemorrhage. Called also Vasolamin.

tranquilizer any of a group of compounds that calm or quiet an anxious patient. There are two types: the *major tranquilizers* called also NEUROLEPTICS (2) or antipsychotic agents, such as acepromazine, and the *minor tranquilizers* called also antianxiety agents, such as diazepam (Valium). See also PSYCHOTROPIC drugs.

t. gun see BLOW DART.

trans 1. in organic chemistry, having certain atoms or radicals on opposite sides of a nonrotatable parent structure. 2. in genetics, having unlike members of a pseudoallelic, or closely linked, gene pair on the same member of a pair of homologous chromosomes. Compare *cis*.

t. acting in molecular biology a sequence or regulatory protein that is produced on one DNA molecule and acts on another, e.g. a sequence on one chromosome produces a regulatory protein that regulates expression of a gene on another chromosome. See also CIS acting.

trans- word element. [L.] *through, across, beyond*.

transabdominal across the abdominal wall or through the abdominal cavity.

t. needle biopsy insertion of a biopsy needle, such as Menghini or Tru-Cut, through the abdominal wall, for the purpose of obtaining a tissue sample from an organ, most commonly liver or kidney.

transacylase an enzyme that catalyzes the transfer of acyl groups.

transaldolase key enzyme of the non-oxidative pentose phosphate pathway.

transamidase an enzyme that catalyzes the transfer of an amide group from one molecule to another.

transamidation the process of transferring an amide group from one molecule to another.

transaminase an enzyme that catalyzes the transfer of an amino group from one molecule to another.

glutamic–oxaloacetic t. (GOT) see ASPARTATE AMINOTRANSFERASE (AST).

glutamic–pyruvic t. (GPT) see ALANINE AMINOTRANSFERASE (ALT).

transamination the reversible exchange of amino groups between different amino acids.

transanimation resuscitation of an asphyxiated person or animal by mouth-to-mouth breathing. See also artificial RESPIRATION.

transaortic performed through the aorta.

transarticular across an articulation.

t. stabilization placement of external skeletal fixation devices above and below a joint and connected by rigid bars. Useful where supporting soft tissues are damaged, requiring immobilization of the joint.

transatrial performed through the atrium.

transaudient penetrable by sound waves.

transaxial directed at right angles to the long axis of the body or a part.

transbasal through the base, as a surgical approach through the base of the skull.

transcalent penetrable by heat rays.

transcalvarial through or across the calvaria.

transcatheter performed through the lumen of a catheter.

transcellular fluids cerebrospinal fluid, aqueous humor of the eye, synovial fluids, urine, bile, pancreatic juice and so on.

transcervical 1. performed through the cervical opening of the uterus. 2. across or through the neck of a structure.

transcobalamin a group of proteins (of intestinal cells) that bind to cyanocobalamin (vitamin B_{12}) and transport it to other tissues.

transcortical connecting two parts of the cerebral cortex.

transcortin an α-globulin that binds and transports biologically active, unconjugated cortisol in plasma.

transcript an RNA molecule, formed during TRANSCRIPTION, from a DNA template.

primary t. the RNA molecule produced by TRANSCRIPTION prior to processing, including splicing.

transcriptase RNA polymerase; an enzyme that catalyzes the synthesis (polymerization) of RNA from ribonucleoside triphosphates, with DNA serving as a template.

reverse t. RNA-directed DNA polymerase; an enzyme of retroviruses and hepadnaviruses that catalyzes the transcription of RNA to DNA.

viral t. see reverse transcriptase above.

transcription the synthesis of an RNA copy from a nucleotide sequence in a limited region of DNA. See also DEOXYRIBONUCLEIC ACID and TRANSCRIPTASE.

t.-control region the *cis*-acting DNA sequences regulating transcription of a specific gene.

reverse t. the synthesis of a DNA copy from a RNA template, catalyzed by reverse transcriptase.

t. unit see OPERON.

transdifferentiation see ALVEOLAR². Metaplasia.

transducer a device that translates one physical quantity to another, e.g. pressure or temperature to an electrical signal. In ultrasonography, the device that emits sound waves.

annular array t. an ultrasound transducer with crystals arranged in concentric rings with different frequencies of sound produced. It allows for a greater depth of focus.

linear array t. an ultrasound transducer with crystals arranged in a line. It gives a rectangular field of view.

neuroendocrine t. a neuron, such as a neurohypophyseal neuron, that on stimulation secretes a hormone, thereby translating neural information into hormonal information.

sector t. an ultrasound transducer which produces a fan-shaped field of view.

transducin GDP/GTP-regulated protein, composed of three subunits designated α, β and γ, involved in the visual process. Photoactivated rhodopsin activates transducin to bind GTP, the transducin-GTP complex activates G-phosphodiesterase (G-PDE) by removing the inhibitory γ-subunit of G-PDE. The activated G-phosphodiesterase catalyzes the conversion of cGMP to GMP. Since the major action of cGMP is to open Na+-channels, the decrease in cGMP closes the Na+-channels leading to hyperpolarization of the nerve.

transductant a bacterium which has undergone transduction.

transduction the transfer of a genetic fragment from one bacterium to another by bacteriophage.

transdural through or across the dura mater.

transection a cross-section; division by cutting transversely.

transepidermal elimination a mechanism for the elimination of foreign constituents from the dermis.

transepithelial occurring through or across an epithelium.

transfaunation see CUD transfer.

transfection an introduction of free DNA into a cell.

transfer factor a factor extractable from sensitized lymphocytes of some species that has the capacity to transfer delayed hypersensitivity to a normal (nonreactive) individual; abbreviated TF. It confers cell-mediated IMMUNITY and therefore has been found to be useful in treating conditions in which there is a disorder of immune response. As an adjunct to antibiotic therapy it has been used in the treatment of such antibiotic-resistant diseases as candidiasis and coccidioidomycosis.

transfer RNA tRNA; see RIBONUCLEIC ACID.

transferase an enzyme that catalyzes the transfer, from one molecule to another, of a chemical group that does not exist in free state during the transfer.

gamma glutamyl t. (GGT) found in the cell membrane in most tissues, but particularly high levels are present in liver (bile duct cells, hepatocytes) and kidney (renal convoluted tubular cells). Increased serum levels occur primarily with cholestasis.

glucuronyl t. enzyme which converts bilirubin to a soluble glucuronide.

glutathione *S*-t's widely distributed enzymes catalyzing the detoxification of many compounds but particularly xenobiotics by linkage of the cysteine moiety of glutathione with the compound.

ornithine carbamoyl t. (OCT) catalyzes the transfer of carbamoyl, as from carbamoylphosphate to L-ornithine to form orthophosphate and citrulline in the synthesis of urea. Found almost exclusively in the liver. Determination of serum levels is used as an indicator of hepatocellular damage, particularly in cattle, sheep and pigs.

peptidyl t. a ribosomal enzyme that transfers the growing peptide from its carrier tRNA to the α-amino group of the amino acid residue of the aminoacyl-tRNA specified by the next codon of the mRNA.

transferation an introduction of free DNA into a cell.

transferrin a serum globulin that binds and transports iron.

transfix to pierce through or impale.

transfixation the process of transfixing.

t. ligature the suture material is passed through the stump to be ligatured, tied around a half of the stump, then around the entire stump.

t. pin used in orthopedic surgery in young animals, or where a medullary pin or plates are not applicable. The pin passes completely through the bone and is fixed by attachment to external bar splints. A series of them enable the surgeon to immobilize a number of fragments of a comminuted fracture.

transfixion a method of amputation in which the knife is passed directly through the soft parts, the cutting being done from within outward.

transforation perforation of the fetal skull.

transformation change of form or structure; conversion from one form to another. In oncology, the change that a normal cell undergoes as it becomes malignant. In statistics a functional change to the variable.

bacterial t. the process of intercellular transfer of genetic information in which a small portion of the total DNA of a lysed bacterium enters a related bacterium and is incorporated into the DNA genome of the recipient.

cell t. the changes in types of proteins expressed and growth characteristics that take place in cells infected by some viruses, including tumor formation by retroviruses.

transformer an induction apparatus for changing electrical energy at one voltage and current to electrical energy at another voltage and current, through the medium of magnetic energy, without mechanical motion.

t. fluid may cause poisoning due to its polychlorinated biphenyl content.

step-down t. one for lowering the voltage of the original current.

step-up t. one for raising the voltage of the original current.

transforming growth factor one of the three growth factors released by platelets when they undergo the release reaction; plays a part in stimulating endothelial proliferation and repair of vascular smooth muscle.

transfusion the introduction of whole blood or blood components directly into the bloodstream. Among the elements transfused, in addition to whole blood, are packed red blood cells, plasma, platelets, granulocytes and cryoprecipitate, a plasma protein rich in antihemophilic factor VIII. See also AUTOTRANSFUSION.

autologous blood t. transfusion of the animal's own blood.

blood t. whole blood is most often indicated to maintain or replace blood volume, to provide deficient blood elements and improve coagulation, to maintain or improve transport of oxygen, and in liver failure in which toxins accumulate in the blood, or in some other types of toxemia.

direct t. transfer of whole blood from the donor through a tube, directly to the recipient.

exchange t. blood is removed from the recipient at the same time and in the same amount as blood is being administered from the donor.

incompatible t. see transfusion reaction (below).

t. reaction a group of clinical signs due to antibody in the recipient's blood reacting with the transfused red blood cells when blood for transfusion is incorrectly matched, or when the recipient has an adverse reaction to some element of the donor blood. Most commonly, there is an immune-mediated hemolysis involving alloantibodies, which may be naturally occurring or the result of an earlier transfusion, in the recipient's serum and the donor's erythrocytes. In ruminants, signs appear during the transfusion, beginning with hiccough, then tremor, dyspnea, lacrimation, fever, ruminal tympany, hemoglobinuria and subsequent abortion. If death occurs, it is because of pulmonary edema. Similar signs are seen in other species. Urticaria and erythema sometimes occur in dogs and cats.

Nonimmunological transfusion reactions include cardiovascular overload, hypocalcemic tetany from citrate (used as the anticoagulant) overload, and disease transmission.

t. therapy the administration of whole blood or blood components, usually in the treatment of bleeding disorders.

transgene a gene that has been incorporated into the genome of another organism.

transgenesis transfer of genes from one individual into the genome of another who transmits it to successive generations.

transgenic the product of transgenesis.

t. animal one produced by transgenesis.

transglutaminase the activated form of protransglutaminase, which forms stabilizing covalent bonds within fibrin strands; called also coagulation factor XIIIa.

transhumance a husbandry procedure in which livestock are moved to another climatic region at particular seasons, e.g. mountain grazing in summer. It is a system which encourages the spread of some diseases such as pneumonic pasteurellosis.

transient paralysis syndrome a syndrome in birds affected with Marek's disease. Ataxia and paralysis last for several days followed by recovery and subsequently, after a lapse of several months, a fatal outcome from MD.

transiliac across the two ilia.

transillumination the passage of strong light through a body structure, to permit inspection by an observer on the opposite side.

ocular t. intense light placed on the sclera behind the ciliary body is transmitted to the interior of the eye, producing a tapetal reflex. Useful in identifying the presence of intraocular masses and demonstrating atrophy of the iris.

transit being conveyed from one place to another; in animal husbandry parlance used to mean being transported, usually with the qualification that the journey is undertaken over long distances without adequate preparation. Untoward sequels are heat stroke and transit tetany, especially in overweight and late pregnant animals.

t. erythema the carcasses of pigs which have been transported long distances before slaughter develop large patches of superficial erythema where they have lain for long periods. The stained areas have to be trimmed.

t. fever see BOVINE respiratory disease.

t. tetany, t. recumbency of mares, see LACTATION TETANY. Of ruminants it is a syndrome of recumbency, complete anorexia, rumen stasis and a gradual onset of coma and death after a course of 2 to 3 days. There may be tetany and excitement in the early stages. Occurs in ruminants transported long distances or forced to take too much exercise when in advanced pregnancy. Called also railroad disease, railroad sickness.

transit animals animals in sale yards, staging on a long move, e.g. to agistment, on dealer's premises, in veterinary hospital, holding yards at abattoirs.

transit time the time required for ingesta to pass through the gastrointestinal tract; a shorter transit time is seen in conditions associated with gut hypermotility, such as diarrhea. Delayed passage from any cause results in a longer transit time.

transition matrix see transition MATRIX (3).

transition state intermediate, higher free energy stage than initial stage in the reaction, often one in which the reacting molecule is strained or distorted or has an unfavorable electronic structure.

transitional cell cells which make up an epithelium, e.g. in the urinary bladder, consisting of several layers of soft cuboidal cells which flatten out when stretched.

t. c. tumors 1. adenomas, papillomas and carcinomas of transitional epithelium in the urinary tract; they are the most common tumors of the urinary bladder in dogs. 2. carcinoma of the upper respiratory tract.

transitional vertebra at the junction of two regions, e.g. lumbar and sacral, which take on the characteristics of the arch and articular processes of the next section.

transketolase an enzyme that participates in the transfer of ketol groups. Determination of activity in the red blood cell is an indirect indicator of thiamin deficiency.

translation the synthesis of a polypeptide using messenger RNA as a template, a complex process involving ribosomes and transfer RNAs; every three bases (a codon) along the mRNA beginning with the start codon specifies one amino acid in the polypeptide chain. See also DEOXYRIBONUCLEIC ACID.

t.-inhibitory protein (TIP) produced by cells with depression of DNA synthesis caused by the action of interferons. It inhibits viral replication by binding viral RNA on cell ribosomes.

nick t. an in vitro procedure for introducing radiolabeled nucleotides into DNA. A method for preparing highly radioactive probes for use in a wide variety of hydridization techniques both in vitro and in vivo. The DNA fragment to be labeled and used as a probe is mixed with DNA polymerase I and the 4 α NTPs, one of which is labeled; the polymerase nicks the DNA fragment and by strand displacement (exonuclease action) displaces and recopies, incorporating the labeled α NTP.

translocation the attachment of a fragment of one chromosome to a nonhomologous chromosome. See also CHROMOSOMAL abnormality. The translocations recorded include adjacent section, alternate segregation, centric fusion, distal segment, eye color, heterozygote, interstitial segment, reciprocal, Robertsonian.

Robertsonian t. that in which the breaks occur at the centromeres and entire chromosome arms are exchanged, usually involving two acrocentric chromosomes.

translucent slightly penetrable by light rays.

transmembrane across a membrane; usually referring to a cell membrane.

transmethylase an enzyme that catalyzes transmethylation.

transmethylation the transfer of a methyl group (CH_3^-) from the molecules of one compound to those of another.

transmigration 1. diapedesis. 2. change of place from one side of the body to the other.

transmissible said of a disease capable of being transmitted from one animal to another. There are very many such diseases but most are not included below because the word 'transmissible' is not a part of the disease's name in common usage.

canine t. venereal tumor see canine transmissible VENEREAL tumor.

t. gastroenteritis 1. a highly infectious disease of baby pigs caused by a coronavirus. It is manifested by vomiting and diarrhea, severe dehydration and a high mortality rate. In older pigs the syndrome is similar but less severe and many pigs survive—others are infected but show no clinical signs. Called also TGE. 2. a disease of turkeys caused by a coronavirus. It affects birds of all ages and is characterized by wet droppings and weight loss. Called also coronaviral enteritis, bluecomb.

t. lymphosarcoma, t. reticulum cell tumor see canine transmissible VENEREAL tumor.

t. murine colonic hyperplasia caused by *Citrobacter freundii* in suckling mice; characterized by diarrhea, weight loss, rectal prolapse, high mortality rate.

t. porcine genital papillomatosis in the prepuce of the boar as papular 0.5 to 1 inch diameter lesions; spontaneous disappearance and persistent subsequent immunity.

t. serositis see sporadic bovine ENCEPHALOMYELITIS.

transmission 1. transfer, as of an infection from one patient to another. 2. of nervous impulses. See NEUROMUSCULAR transmission. 3. heredity.

airborne t. spread of infection by droplet nuclei or dust through the air. Without the intervention of winds or drafts the distance over which airborne infection takes place is short, say 10 to 20 feet.

arthropod t. by insect, either mechanically via a contaminated proboscis or feet, or biologically when there is growth or replication of the organism in the arthropod. See also TRANS-STADIAL.

biological t. involving a biological process, e.g. passing a stage of development of the infecting agent in an intermediate host. Opposite to mechanical transmission.

colostral t. a form of vertical transmission via successive generations.

contact t. the disease agent is transferred directly by biting, sucking, chewing or indirectly by inhalation of droplets, drinking of contaminated water, traveling in contaminated vehicles.

cyclopropagative t. the agent undergoes both development and multiplication in the transmitting vehicle.

developmental t. the agent undergoes some development in the transmission vehicle.

horizontal t. lateral spread to others in the same group and at the same time; spread to contemporaries.

mechanical t. the transmittor is not infected in that tissues are not invaded and the agent does not multiply.

propagative t. the agent multiplies in the transmission vehicle.

vector t. see VECTOR.

vertical t. from one generation to the next, perhaps transovarially or by intrauterine infection of the fetus. Some retroviruses are transmitted in the germ line, i.e. their genetic material is integrated into the DNA of either the ovum or sperm.

transmural through the wall of an organ; extending through or affecting the entire thickness of the wall of an organ or cavity.

t. pressure gradient pressure difference across a wall, as of a capillary. See also STARLING'S HYPOTHESIS.

transmutation 1. evolutionary change of one species into another. 2. the change of one chemical element into another.

transonic in ultrasonography, the complete transmission of sound so the image appears black; anechoic; echolucent.

transorbital performed through the bony socket of the eye.

transovarial via the ovary. The infectious agent, often a virus, is passed to the fetus in the ovum, having been infected from the dam's circulation. A common occurrence in ticks and other arthropods, e.g. babesiosis in ticks.

transparent permitting the passage of rays of light so that objects may be seen through the substance.

t. overlay technique imposing different sets of data on a basic map by a succession of transparent acetate overlays.

transpeptidase an enzyme that catalyzes the transfer of an amino or peptide group from one molecule to another.

transperitoneal rectal tear see RECTAL tear.

transphosphorylase an enzyme that catalyzes the transfer of a phosphate group from one molecule to another.

transphosphorylation the exchange of phosphate groups between organic phosphates, without their going through the stage of inorganic phosphates.

transpiration discharge of air, vapor or sweat through the skin.

transplacental through the placenta.

transplant 1. an organ or tissue taken from the body and grafted into another area of the same individual or another individual. 2. to transfer tissue from one part to another or from one individual to another.

ovum t. see OVUM transplant.

t. rejection see REJECTION.

transplantation the transfer of living organs and tissue from one part of the body to another or from one individual to another. Transplantation and grafting mean the same thing, though the term grafting is more commonly used to refer to the transfer of skin. See GRAFTING (1).

Occasionally an organ is transplanted from one place to another within the body (autotransplants). Kidneys, for example, have been relocated to enable them to continue functioning after the ureters have been damaged. See also graft REJECTION.

t. antigen see HISTOCOMPATIBILITY antigen.

bone marrow t. has been used in the treatment of a variety of hematopoietic and immunological disorders, e.g. in dogs with aplastic anemia.

corneal t. full-depth and part-depth (lamellar) transplants are performed in animals when there is scarring of the cornea in the visual axis but the operation is difficult, the aftercare intensive and the failure rate high.

t. immunology the study of immune responses that distinguish between self and nonself and the rejection of transplanted tissue or organs.

tendon t. the procedure is not favored in horses where it was at one time used as a treatment for tendonitis. The success rate for return to racing performance is poor.

transponder implantable microchips used in animal identification; enclosed in inert glass; generate an alphanumeric code when stimulated by an external scanner's low-frequency radio signal.

transport 1. movement of materials in biological systems, particularly into and out of cells and across epithelial layers. 2. transport of animals, see TRANSIT, TRANSPORTATION.

active t. see ACTIVE transport.

t. death death during transportation, e.g. porcine stress syndrome.

t. host see PARATENIC HOST.

t. media see transport MEDIUM.

membrane t. proteins specific proteins associated with the plasma membrane of cells that are responsible for transferring solutes including ions, sugars, amino acids, nucleotides and many metabolites across cell membranes.

t. myopathy see EXERTIONAL rhabdomyolysis.

t. stress stress imposed by lack of access to water and feed, physical exhaustion caused by standing for long periods, heat stress, aggression by other animals.

t. tetany see TRANSIT tetany.

transportation an essential part of the livestock industries. It is an expensive on-cost to a farming enterprise. It also represents a source of contact infection and of stress and reduced resistance to infection, and of shrinkage in animals, from 4% to 9% in cattle transported long distances over 3 to 4 days.

Codes of ethics and guidelines for structure and use of transportation facilities are enforced in many countries.

transposase an enzyme that acts on transposable elements in DNA mutagenesis.

transposition displacement to the opposite side; in genetics, the nonreciprocal insertion of material deleted from one chromosome into another, nonhomologous chromosome.

t. of arterial trunks see transposition of great vessels (below).

t. of great vessels a congenital heart defect, in which the position of the chief blood vessels of the heart is reversed. Called also transposition of arterial trunks.

ulnar styloid t. a surgical procedure for correction of growth deformity resulting from premature closure of the distal ulnar physis. The distal tip of the ulna is fused to the distal radial epiphysis.

transposon see transposable GENETIC elements.

transpubic performed through the pubic bone after removal of a segment of the bone.

trans-segmental extending across segments.

trans-septal extending or performed through or across a septum.

trans-stadial across or between stages of a process or disease.

t. vector transmission when an infection is picked up by one stage in the vector's life cycle and transmitted to succeeding stages in its metamorphosis.

transthalamic across the thalamus.

transthoracic through the thoracic cavity or across the chest wall.

t. needle biopsy insertion of a fine needle through the thoracic wall for the purpose of obtaining a sample of lung tissue for cytological, microbiological or histopathological examination.

transtracheal aspiration, transtracheal wash a technique for collecting a sample of bronchial exudate for histological and microbiological examination. A needle is inserted through the skin overlying the trachea and through the cricothyroid ligament. A catheter is introduced into the trachea and passed to the level of the tracheal bifurcation, some saline introduced and then withdrawn.

transtympanic across the tympanic membrane or the cavity of the middle ear.

transudate a fluid substance that has passed through a membrane or has been extruded from a tissue; in contrast to an exudate, a transudate is characterized by high fluidity and a low content of protein, cells or solid matter derived from cells.

modified t. one with additional protein and/or cells. It may be a transitional stage, progressing to an exudate.

transudation 1. passage of serum or other body fluid through a membrane or tissue surface. 2. transudate.

transudative diathesis see EXUDATIVE diathesis.

transureteroureterostomy a method of urinary diversion consisting of anastomosis of one ureter to the other but maintaining the patency of the proximal and distal parts of the transplanted ureter.

transurethral performed through the urethra.

Transvaal having some relationship to the South African province of that name.

T. bietou see CASTALIS SPECTABILIS.

T. chincherinchee ORNITHOGALUM *saundersiae*.

T. gousiektebossie PACHYSTIGMA *pygmaeum*.

T. slangkop URGINEA *sanguinea*.

transvaginal through the vagina.

transversalis [L.] *transverse*.

t. fascia the fascia between the peritoneum and the abdominal muscles.

transverse extending from side to side; situated at right angles to the long axis.

t. ligaments see Table 12.

t. trabeculae see GROWTH arrest line.

t. tubules structures in myofibers which run transversely to the long axis of the myofibrils in skeletal and cardiac muscle. They are filled with basal lamina material and are part of the communication system of muscle fibers and provide a means for the passage of action potentials into the depths of the fibers. The tubules are invaginations of the sarcolemma.

transversectomy excision of a transverse process of a vertebra.

transversus [L.] *transverse*.

transvesical through the bladder.

trap-death syndrome deaths in small wild mammals subjected to close confinement in cages; includes gastric hemorrhage and ulceration.

trapdoor spider a very venomous spider that lives in a funnel-shaped web built into a horizontal crack or existing burrow. A bite causes intense pain at the site and then generally, sweating, dehydration and paralysis, and is often fatal. Called also *Atrax formidabilis*.

trapezium an irregular, four-sided figure.

trapnest a laying box in which the hen releases a spring when she enters. When it is released the egg that she has laid is recorded. A device for measuring eggs laid by each bird.

trapping an essential technique for sampling wildlife populations in surveys of their diseases or in order to establish the size and variety of the population, especially if carried out systematically with the traps set out in a grid formation. See also CAPTURE–RECAPTURE METHOD.

traps devices for the trapping of wild animals. Mostly used with an attractant, varying with the target species. Once in the target area the trap is sprung. The trap may be a limb snare, frowned on in many circles now, a cage with a dropdown door, a net dropped from above or fired from a gun, a sticky surface, a funneled entrance to a cage and so on.

Traube–Hering waves radiations of impulses from the respiratory center to the vasomotor center in the medulla oblongata during inspiration can increase arterial pressure.

trauma a wound or injury, especially damage produced by external force, e.g. surgical operation, impact, blunt instrument.

birth t. an injury to the fetus during the process of being born.

t. score a numerical assessment of injuries suffered as a result of trauma. Several systems are used, including the Glasgow Coma Scale and the Revised Trauma Score.

self-inflicted t. see SELF-TRAUMA.

traumatic 1. pertaining to, resulting from, or causing trauma. 2. in cattle, and in all ruminants, a special meaning is perforation of the reticular wall by a swallowed foreign body.

t. hepatitis penetration by a foreign body from externally via the skin or internally from the reticulum.

t. laminitis see LAMINITIS.

t. liver abscess caused usually by perforation of the stomach wall by a foreign body. Causes toxemia, leukocytosis, fever and pain on percussion over the posterior right ribs.

t. mastitis see traumatic MASTITIS.

t. peritonitis see traumatic PERITONITIS.

t. reticulopericarditis caused by an extension of reticuloperitonitis, especially in cows in late pregnancy; characterized by congestive heart failure with marked edema of the brisket and jowl, 'washing machine' heart sounds and disappearance of the normal sounds. There is a marked leukocytosis, fever and toxemia.

t. reticuloperitonitis caused by perforation of the reticular wall by a sharp foreign body in any ruminant but most common in adult dairy cows being fed processed feeds. Manifested by an acute fall in milk yield and appetite, a humped back and disinclination to move, pain on percussion over the xiphisternum, ruminal stasis, fever and a leukocytosis. Called also TRP, hardware disease, reticulitis, traumatic peritonitis.

t. reticulopleurisy inflammation of the wall of the reticulum and nearby pleura of cattle caused by the penetration of a foreign body from the reticulum into the pleural cavity. Characterized by toxemia, fever, leukocytosis, pain on percussion over the ribs, fast shallow grunting respiration, elbows abducted.

t. reticulosplenitis inflammation of the wall of the reticulum and nearby spleen of cattle caused by penetration of a foreign body into the spleen. Characterized by toxemia, leukocytosis, fever and pain on percussion over the upper posterior right ribs.

t. shock see vasogenic SHOCK.

t. splenitis see traumatic reticulosplenitis (above).

t. wet lung see SHOCK lung.

traumatism 1. the physical state resulting from an injury or wound. See also SHOCK. 2. a wound.

traumat(o)- word element. [Gr.] *trauma*.

traumatology the branch of surgery dealing with wounds and disability from injuries.

traumatopnea passage of air through a wound in the chest wall; a sucking injury.

travel edema wateriness of lamb carcasses, especially in the shoulders, when the lambs are transported long distances just before slaughter.

travel sickness see MOTION SICKNESS.

traveller's joy CLEMATIS *vitalba*.

tread injury to the coronet of the horse's hoof by treading on it by the opposite hoof, or by another horse when they are being worked in a team. If the coronary matrix is injured there may be a subsequent crack or deformity.

treading a part of a restlessness syndrome or a neurosis in ruminants or horses; the patient repeatedly changes weight from one limb to the opposite of the pair, lifting the hoof slightly at each change; the action looks as though the patient is treading grapes to make wine. The action is restricted largely to the hindlimbs and usually indicates subacute abdominal pain.

treatment management and care of a patient or the combating of disease or disorder.

active t. treatment directed immediately to the cure of the disease or injury.

causal t. treatment directed against the cause of a disease.

conservative t. treatment designed to avoid radical medical therapeutic measures or operative procedures.

empirical t. treatment by means that experience has proved to be beneficial.

expectant t. treatment directed toward relief of untoward clinical signs, leaving the cure of the disease to natural forces.

palliative t. treatment that is designed to relieve pain and distress, but does not attempt a cure.

preventive t., prophylactic t. that in which the aim is to prevent the occurrence of the disease.

rational t. that based upon knowledge of disease and the action of the remedies given.

specific t. treatment particularly adapted to the special disease being treated.

supporting t. that which is mainly directed to sustaining the strength of the patient.

treats see FOOD rewards.

tree 1. an anatomical structure with branches resembling a tree. 2. in information science, a decision tree.

bronchial t. the trachea, bronchi and successive branching generations of the respiratory passages.

t. daffodil THEVETIA *peruviana*.

decision t. see DECISION tree.

t. diagram see DECISION tree.

t. lupin LUPINUS *arboreus*.

t. nettle see URTICA.
t. shrew primitive arboreal mammal that some taxonomists place with the primates. Like squirrels in shape and size. Called also *Tupaia* spp.
t. snake a number of colubrid snakes that lead an arboreal existence and practice falling from trees with their body spread out, earning the name of flying snake.
t. tobacco NICOTIANA *glauca*.
tracheobronchial t. the trachea, bronchi and their branching structures.
t. zamia CYCAS *armstrongii, C. media*.
Treeing Walker coonhound a medium-sized hound with a short, smooth tricolor coat.
trefoil includes the *Medicago* and *Lotus* genera of the family Fabaceae.
t. dermatitis photosensitization caused by ingestion of MEDICAGO *polymorpha* (*M. denticulata*).
t. rattlepod CROTALARIA *medicaginea*.
Trema tomentosa Australian plant in the family Ulmaceae; causes acute liver necrosis in cattle. Called also *T. aspera, T. aspera* var. *viridis*, poison peach, peach-leaf poison bush.
trematocides drugs effective in the treatment of immature and adult flukes, e.g. rafoxanide, closantel, triclabendazole, diamphenethide. Bromsalans, oxyclozanide, nitroxynil and carbon tetrachloride are effective only against mature fluke.
trematode parasitic worm; member of the class Trematoda. There are three subclasses, Monogenea, containing parasites of fish, amphibians and mammals, Digenea, containing the flukes of domestic animals, called also digenetic trematodes. These cause parasitic disease of most systems, including the blood, eye, liver, reproductive tract, respiratory system, skin and urinary system. The third subclass is the Aspidogastrea, parasitic in molluscs, fish and reptiles.
trematodiasis infestation by trematodes.
trematoxin toxic glycoside in TREMA TOMENTOSA.
tremblante du mouton [Fr.] *scrapie*.
trembler pup hypomyelinogenesis in young puppies, particularly Bernese mountain dogs.
trembles porcine CONGENITAL TREMOR SYNDROME.
trembling visible muscle tremor caused by fever, fear, weakness, electrolyte imbalance, especially hypocalcemia and hypomagnesemia, and neuromuscular disease.
t. disease of sheep, scrapie; of piglets, congenital tremor syndrome.
tremetol toxic alcohol in EUPATORIUM *rugosum*.
tremor a continuous repetitive twitching of skeletal muscle, usually palpable and visible. The diseases characterized by tremor only, the tremor syndromes, may be caused by degenerative disease of the nervous system, e.g. hypomyelinogenesis, and by many toxins, especially plant ones. Tremor is also a sign in many other diseases of the nervous system.
action t. rhythmic, oscillatory, involuntary movements of the limbs.
coarse t. that involving large groups of muscle fibers contracting slowly.
congenital t. syndrome of piglets see CONGENITAL TREMOR SYNDROME.
epidemic t. see avian ENCEPHALOMYELITIS.
fibrillary t. rapidly alternating contraction of small bundles of muscle fibers.
fine t. one in which the vibrations are rapid.
intention t. one occurring when voluntary movement is attempted. See also volitional tremor (below).
rest t. tremor occurring in a relaxed and supported limb.
t. syndrome see SHAKER DOGS. Called also white dog shaker syndrome.
volitional t. trembling of the entire body during voluntary effort.
tremorgen group of toxins produced by fungi, e.g. *Penicillium* spp., which cause serious muscle tremor.
tremorgen staggers incoordination caused by tremorgens, usually mycotoxins.
tremorgenic pertaining to or emanating from tremorgen.
tremortin-A see PENITREM-A.
tremulous shaking, trembling or quivering.
trench mouth fusospirochetal stomatitis. See also VINCENT'S ANGINA.
trend a generally consistent movement in the same direction over a long period in a time series.
trendscriber the apparatus used in trendscription.
trendscription a programmed method of continuous electrocardiographic monitoring, wherein the tracing is condensed on a rotating drum recorder and the program permits selective sampling of rhythm data.
trepan trephine.
trepanation, trephination use of the trephine for creating an opening in the skull or in the sclera.
trephine 1. a crown saw for removing a circular disk of bone, chiefly from the skull. See also GALT TREPHINE, MICHEL'S trephine, SEARCY TREPHINE. 2. an instrument for removing a circular area of cornea, e.g. Castroviejo trephine. 3. to remove with a trephine.
trephocyte a cell which provides nourishment for another cell, e.g. Sertoli cell, avian thrombocytes.
Treponema a genus of spirochetes (family Spirochaetaceae), motile gram-negative, spiral-shaped rods. The species *T. hyodysenteriae* and *T. innocens* have been reclassified to the genus *Serpulina*.
T. paraluiscuniculi causes benign venereal SPIROCHETOSIS of rabbits called rabbit syphilis.
***T. penortha* (syn. *Spirochaeta penortha*)** see SPIROCHETE (1).
treponemata, treponemas members of the genus *Treponema* of bacteria.
treponematosis 1. see SPIROCHETOSIS (2). 2. infection by *Treponema* spp.; see also SWINE dysentery.
treponemicidal destroying treponemas.
treppe phenomenon the gradual increase in muscular contraction following rapidly repeated stimulation. Called also staircase phenomenon.
tresis perforation.
tretamine an alkylating agent used as an antineoplastic agent; a cause of testicular degeneration. Called also triethylenemelamine.
tretinoin the all-*trans* stereoisomer of retinoic acid, used in dermatology for the treatment of disorders of keratinization. It is a potent teratogen and must be used with great caution.
TRF thyrotropin releasing factor.
TRH thyrotropin releasing hormone.
tri- word element. [Gr., L.] *three*.
tri-allate a herbicide; large doses cause salivation, bradycardia, vomiting, weakness, tremor, dyspnea and convulsions.
triacetin glyceryl triacetate; used as a topical antifungal.
triacetyloleandomycin see TROLEANDOMYCIN.
triacylglycerol TG; most fat in excess of requirements is stored in adipose tissue in this form; the systematic chemical name for TRIGLYCERIDE.
t. lipase (LPS) produced primarily by the pancreas and in smaller quantities by the gastric and intestinal

mucosa. Determination of serum levels is used to detect acute necrosis of pancreatic acinar cells. Called also steapsin, lipase, triglyceride lipase.

triad 1. an element with a valence of three. 2. a group of three similar bodies, or a complex composed of three items or units.

t's of the tarsus the various combinations of (usually three) injuries that occur in trauma to the hock joint, based first on injury to the central tarsal bone.

Virchow's t. see VIRCHOW'S TRIAD.

Whipple's t. see WHIPPLE'S TRIAD.

Triadan system a system of identifying teeth in dental records. Each tooth has a three-digit number which identifies the quadrant, position and whether it is a primary or permanent tooth.

Triaenophorus a genus of tapeworms in the family Triaenophoridae.

T. nodulosus adults occur in pike and other predatory fish; intermediate hosts are first copepods, and second fish, especially trout. The plerocercoids in the trout tissues cause loss of value and liver damage may cause deaths.

triage sorting of patients from a disaster to establish priorities and allocation to special services.

t. nurse a nurse trained in triage procedures.

trial experiment; refers usually to the trying out of a substance or a material in order to determine its effect. The trial may be a BLIND experiment, a CLINICAL trial, a double BLIND trial or a PILOT TRIAL.

clinical t., therapeutic t. a test which uses patients as test objects for a drug regimen, a physical procedure, the results being compared with those in patients receiving a placebo or an alternative treatment.

trialling the running of Greyhounds and horses in practice races.

triamcinolone a prednisolone derivative used as an anti-inflammatory glucocorticoid in the form of the acetonide derivative and the diacetate ester.

triamterene a weak diuretic which increases sodium and chloride excretion, but not potassium.

triangle a three-cornered object, figure or area, as such an area on the surface of the body capable of fairly precise definition. Called also trigone.

facial t. a triangular area whose points are the basion and the alveolar and nasal points.

femoral t. the triangle bounded cranially by the sartorius, caudally by the pectineus and deeply by the iliopsoas muscles in the dog. The pulse of the femoral artery can be taken at this site.

vesical t. the area of the bladder wall within the triangle demarcated by the ureteral and urethral orifices. The bladder mucosa is firmly attached at this point and does not form folds.

Viborg's t. a surgical site on the side of the throat of the horse bounded by the caudal border of the mandible, the linguofacial vein and the tendon of the sternocephalic muscle.

triangularis [L.] *triangular*.

Trianthema genus of the Aizoaceae family of plants; have a high oxalate content and may cause acute oxalate poisoning. Includes *T. portulacastrum* (black or giant pigweed), *T. triquetra* (red spinach).

triaryl phosphates industrial chemicals used as plasticizers, lubricant additives and the like. Poisoning of animals has occurred and includes paralysis of the extremities and fetid diarrhea.

Triatoma a genus of bugs (order Hemiptera), the cone-nosed bugs, important in human medicine as vectors of *Trypanosoma cruzi* from its natural vectors, dogs, cats, foxes, monkeys and others. Includes *Triatoma dimidiata*, *T. infestans*, *T. protracta*, *T. sanguisuga* (vector for equine encephalomyelitis).

triatome a member of the genus TRIATOMA of true bugs.

triatomine pertaining to the genus TRIATOMA.

triazines selective herbicides including atrazine, propazine, simazine, prometone, prometryne. They are poisonous if given in sufficient quantity but the syndrome, weight loss, anorexia and weakness, is too nonspecific to be valuable diagnostically.

triazole antifungals azole derivatives with broad-spectrum antifungal activity; includes FLUCONAZOLE and ITRACONAZOLE.

tribe a taxonomic category subordinate to a family (or subfamily) and superior to a genus (or subtribe).

triboluminescence luminescence produced by mechanical energy, as by the grinding, rubbing, or breaking of certain crystals.

tribrachius a monster with three forelimbs.

Tribrissen a proprietary name for a mixture of trimethoprim and sulfadiazine.

tribromsalan see BROMSALANS.

tribulosis the disease caused by poisoning by TRIBULUS *terrestris*.

Tribulus a genus of the Zygophyllaceae family of plants.

T. micrococcus Australian species contains an unidentified toxin, which causes incoordination, recumbency, paralysis in sheep; called also yellow vine.

T. terrestris 1. this weed contains the toxic steroidal saponin which causes hepatic injury when eaten. The clinical syndrome consists of photosensitization, jaundice and hepatic encephalopathy. The disease is known also as 'geeldikkop' [Afrikaans] and yellow bighead. Called also caltrop, puncture vine, devil's thorn. 2. causes Coonabarabran disease of sheep in Australia; an ataxia syndrome thought to be caused by β-carboline alkaloids.

tributyl tin one of the constituents in defouling paint used on the exterior of boats.

tributyl triphosphorotrithioite an organophosphorus defoliant which causes typical signs of ORGANOPHOSPHORUS COMPOUND poisoning.

TRIC *tr*achoma and *i*nclusion *c*onjunctivitis.

tricaine methanesulfonate the most commonly used anesthetic for fish. It is dissolved in water and enters into the systemic circulation via the gills, producing a general anesthesia.

tricarboxylic acid cycle the cyclic metabolic mechanism by which the complete oxidation of the acetyl moiety of acetyl-coenzyme A is effected; abbreviated TCA cycle. It is the chief source of mammalian energy, during which acetyl groups derived from the metabolism of sugars, fatty acids and amino acid are oxidized to yield carbon dioxide, water and reduced coenzymes. Called also Krebs cycle and citric acid cycle.

Tricephalobus gingivalis see RHABDITIS *gingivalis*.

tricephalus a monster with three heads.

triceps a muscle having three heads; the triceps muscle of the forearm extends the forearm.

t. reflex contraction of the belly of the triceps muscle and slight extension of the forelimb when the tendon of the muscle is tapped directly, with the forelimb flexed and fully supported and relaxed.

trichiasis 1. a condition of ingrowing hairs about an orifice, or ingrowing eyelashes. 2. the appearance of hairlike filaments in the urine.

trichilemmal pertaining to the outer root sheath of a hair.

t. cyst greatly enlarged hair follicles, filled with keratin. They resemble epidermoid cysts. Called also pilar cysts.

trichilemmoma a rare, benign neoplasm of the lower outer root sheath of the hair; resembles trichoepithelioma.

trichina pl. *trichinae* [Gr.] a single larval stage worm of those in the genus *Trichinella.*

Trichinella a genus of nematode parasites in the family Trichinellidae.

***T. spiralis spiralis* (T1), *T. pseudospiralis* (T4), *T. spiralis domestica* (*T. spiralis*), *T. britovi* (T3), *T. nativa* (T2) and *T. nelsoni* (T7)** adult worms of the species listed above, together with their internationally recognized code numbers, are found in the intestines and the encapsulated, first stage larvae in the striated muscle of various animals. Three other species of uncertain taxonomy, T5, T6, T8, are also encountered. *T. spiralis* is a common cause of infection in humans as a result of ingestion of poorly cooked pork.

trichinellosis trichinosis.

trichinoscope a compression apparatus to squash a small sample of pork muscle and a projector to display the image of the tissue on a screen so that *Trichinella* spp. larvae can be identified.

trichinosis infection with the parasitic roundworm *Trichinella spiralis*, which enters the human body in infected meat eaten raw or insufficiently cooked. Found in most parts of the world with the exception of Australia and the Pacific Islands.

The larvae, or early forms, of *T. spiralis* live embedded in tiny capsule-like cysts of muscle tissue of infected pork. When the meat is properly cooked, the larvae are killed by the high temperature. If, however, the pork is undercooked, they survive; when the meat is eaten, digestive juices dissolve the cyst capsules and free the larvae in the intestines, where they grow to maturity.

trichinous affected with or containing trichinae.

trichlorfon an organophosphorus insecticide and anthelmintic, used in horses, often in combination with other anthelmintics, for treatment of endoparasites and cutaneous habronemiasis. Also used in dogs against whipworms and as a pour-on in cattle for control of warble flies. It is used in fishponds and commercial fish farms to control anchorworms, gill flukes and lice. Called also metrifonate.

trichloroacetate a relatively nontoxic herbicide.

trichloroacetic acid an extremely caustic acid, CCl_3COOH, used as a topical caustic for local destruction of lesions and as a protein precipitating agent.

trichlorobenzoic acid a nonselective weedkiller of very low toxicity.

trichlorocarbanilide a bacteriostat and disinfectant used in soaps and other cleansing compounds.

trichloroethanol a metabolic product of chloral and an hypnotic and analgesic in its own right.

trichloroethylene, trichlorethylene a volatile, nonflammable solvent with a similar odor to chloroform. Used in the extraction of oils and fats from plant and animal materials for the purpose of using the oil. The residue is available as animal feed. Has anesthetic and analgesic properties but is not recommended for use as either in animals.

t.-extracted soybean meal see trichloroethylene-extracted SOYBEAN meal.

trichloronaphthalene a CHLORINATED NAPHTHALENE used in industry and sometimes a cause of poisoning in cattle.

trichloronitromethane see CHLOROPICRIN.

trichlorophenol a wood preservative with fungistatic activity. Causes poisoning as with PENTACHLOROPHENOL.

trichlorphon, trichlorfon an organophosphorus compound used as an anthelmintic. It is toxic for sheep at recommended dose rates and is also hazardous for cattle. In pregnant sows it causes congenital cerebellar agenesis in the piglets and has been associated with left laryngeal hypoplasia in young horses. A solution of the compound is unstable and should be discarded if not used on the same day as the metabolite is toxic.

trich(o)- word element. [Gr.] *hair.*

trichoanesthesia loss of hair sensibility.

trichobezoar rounded masses of felted hairs caused by animals licking themselves. Common in cats ('hairballs'), particularly the longhaired varieties, in rabbits and in shaggy cattle wintered outdoors. Can cause pyloric or intestinal obstruction and in cats, occasional vomiting. A common finding in the abomasum of normal ruminants during abattoir slaughter.

Trichobilharzia a genus of blood flukes (digenetic trematodes) in the family Schistosomatidae.

T. ocellata*, *T. physellae*, *T. stagnicolae found in the portal veins of birds, especially waterfowl.

trichocardia a hairy appearance of the heart due to exudative pericarditis. See also BREAD AND BUTTER PERICARDITIS. Called also cor villosum, shaggy heart.

Trichocephalus see TRICHURIS.

trichoclasia brittleness of the hair.

trichoclasis TRICHORRHEXIS nodosa.

Trichodectes a genus of biting lice in the subfamily of Ischnocera.

T. canis found on dogs.

T. equi found on zebra and wild equids.

T. pinquis euarctidos found on wild black bear.

Trichodesma plant genus in the family Boraginaceae; contain pyrrolizidine alkaloids; cause hepatitis, dummy syndrome, photosensitization, death due to hepatic insufficiency; includes *T. ehrenbergii*, *T. incanum*, *T. zeylanicum* (camel bush).

Trichodina a genus of protozoa in the subclass Peritricha which parasitizes the skin and gills of fish and causes local irritation. They have a characteristic disklike appearance and are in constant revolving motion. Only pathogenic when in large numbers and/or in stressed fish.

Trichodinella a protozoan parasite of fish similar to and having similar effects to TRICHODINA.

Trichoecius romboutsi a mite that causes hair loss and dermatitis in mice. Called also *Myocoptes romboutsi.*

trichoepithelioma a benign skin tumor originating in the keratinocytes of the hair follicle outer sheath or the hair matrix. It occurs as single or sometimes multiple, firm, rounded skin nodules that may ulcerate. They are common in dogs, particularly Cocker spaniels. Called also epithelioma adenoides cysticum.

trichofolliculoma a benign neoplasm of the hair follicle with a large central follicle and numerous smaller follicle-like structures radiating from it; occur in dogs where they appear as firm nodules which may have tufts of hair protruding.

Trichoglossus genus of lorikeets. Includes *T. haematodus* (rainbow lorikeet).

trichogram the findings in TRICHOGRAPHY.

trichogranuloma a pyogranulomatous dermal reaction to the traumatic implantation of pieces of hair, often seen in dermatophytosis.

trichography examination of plucked hairs under the microscope; useful in assessing the status of hair follicle activity by examination of the hair bulbs, and in determining whether hair loss is due to self-trauma. See also ANAGEN–telogen ratio, BARBERING.

trichohyalin granules granules, like keratohyalin; found in cells of hair follicles.

trichoid resembling hair.

tricholemmoma a rare tumor of hair follicles in dogs; resembles TRICHOEPITHELIOMA.

trichology the sum of knowledge about the hair.

trichome a filamentous or hairlike structure.

trichomegaly excessively large eyelashes.

Trichomitus a genus of trichomonads in the family Trichomonadidae.

T. fecalis found in human feces.

T. rotunda found in the cecum and colon of pigs. Not thought to be pathogenic.

T. wenyoni found in the cecum and colon of rodents and rhesus monkeys.

trichomonacide an agent destructive to trichomonads.

trichomonad a parasite of the genera *Trichomonas*, *Tritrichomonas*, *Tetratrichomonas*.

trichomonal pertaining to trichomonads.

t. enteritis the cause-and-effect relationship between the numbers of trichomonads found in association with enteric disease, especially colitis in horses, is doubtful. The organisms may be opportunistic pathogens only.

Trichomonas a genus of flagellate protozoa parasitic in animals, birds, and in humans. Member of the family Trichomonadidae and characterized usually by the presence of a single flagellum.

T. caballi found in the colon of horses.

T. canistomae found in the mouth of dogs.

***T. equi* (syn. *T. faecalis*)** see TRITRICHOMONAS *equi*.

T. equibuccalis found in the mouth of horses.

T. felistomae found in the mouth of cats.

T. foetus see TRITRICHOMONAS *foetus*.

T. gallinae found in the upper digestive tract of many birds but mostly in pigeon squabs where it causes avian TRICHOMONIASIS.

T. gallinarum see TETRATRICHOMONAS *gallinarum*.

T. hominis see PENTATRICHOMONAS *hominis*.

T. intestinalis see PENTATRICHOMONAS *hominis*.

T. macacovaginae found in the vagina of the rhesus monkey.

T. phasioni causes diarrhea and dehydration of pheasant poults.

T. tenax found in the mouth of monkeys and humans but has no pathogenic effect.

trichomoniasis disease caused by infection with the protozoan parasite *Trichomonas* spp.

avian t. a disease of the upper digestive tract of young birds, especially pigeon squabs, caused by *Trichomonas gallinae*. Necrotic lesions are present in the mouth, pharynx, esophagus, crop and sometimes proventriculus and conjunctival sac. Called also canker, frounce, roup.

bovine t. a contagious venereal disease of cattle caused by *Tritrichomonas foetus* and characterized by infertility, abortion and pyometra.

trichomycosis any disease of the hair caused by fungi.

Trichonema a now discarded genus name of strongylid worms; replaced by the genera CYATHOSTOMUM, CYLICOCYCLUS, CYLICODONTOPHORUS, CYLICOSTEPHANUS.

trichonodosis a condition characterized by apparent or actual knotting of the hair.

trichopathy disease of the hair.

Trichophora a protozoan parasite of fish.

trichophytid a DERMATOPHYTID reaction to infection by *Trichophyton* spp.

trichophytin a filtrate from cultures of *Trichophyton* spp. used in testing for trichophytosis.

trichophytobezoar a bezoar composed of animal hair and vegetable fiber.

Trichophyton a genus of fungi that may cause various infections of the skin, hair and nails. It utilizes keratin as a source of nourishment and is therefore localized in its pathogenicity to the skin and its appendages. The perfect state is in the genus *Arthroderma*. Called also *Achorion*.

T. cutaneum an occasional cause of bovine mastitis.

T. equinum causes RINGWORM in horses.

T. erinacei occasionally causes RINGWORM in dogs and other species; the reservoir is the European hedgehog.

T. gallinae now called *Microsporum gallinae*; the cause of favus in fowl.

T. megninii, T. rubrum, T. shoenleinii, T. tonsurans, T. violaceum anthropophilic species which occasionally infect animals.

***T. mentagrophytes* (*T. gypseum*)** causes RINGWORM in horses, dogs and many other species.

T. mentagrophytes* var. *granulare causes RINGWORM in rabbits.

T. simii causes RINGWORM in monkeys and poultry.

T. verrucosum causes RINGWORM in cattle, sheep and goats.

trichophytosis infection with fungi of the genus *Trichophyton*.

trichoptilosis splitting of hairs at the end.

trichorrhexis the condition in which the hairs are split and feather-like.

t. nodosa structural abnormalities of the hair shaft result in breakage and hypotrichosis; seen in horses, dogs and humans. Physical or chemical damage to the hair is usually responsible.

trichoschisis trichoptilosis.

trichoscopy examination of the hair.

trichosis any disease or abnormal growth of the hair.

Trichosomoides crassicauda a nematode in the family Trichuridae; found in the urinary bladder of Norway and black rats and may cause granulomatous lesions.

Trichosporon a genus of yeast-like fungi that are soil saprophytes but may occasionally be pathogenic, especially as a cause of mastitis in cattle.

***T. beigelii* (syn *T. cutaneum*)** may be associated with disseminated infections in cats and cutaneous mycosis in horses.

T. capitatum has been incriminated in abortions in cattle and horses, and mastitis in cattle.

trichosporonosis infection with fungi of the genus *Trichosporon*; occurs rarely in immunosuppressed cats as papular or nodular skin lesions around the nostril or at the site of bite wounds on the legs.

trichosporosis infection with *Trichosporon* spp.

trichostrongyliasis, trichostrongylosis the disease caused by the infestation of the intestine and abomasum of ruminants by *Trichostrongylus* spp. Manifested by poor growth, wasting and persistent diarrhea. *T. axei* infestation is also seen in horses.

trichostrongylid a worm of the family Trichostrongylidae.

Trichostrongylus a genus of nematode parasites belonging to the family Trichostrongylidae, which infects animals and humans.

T. affinis found in the small intestine of rabbits, occasionally in sheep.

T. axei found in the abomasum of cattle, sheep, goats, deer, antelope and in the stomach of pigs, horses, donkeys and rarely humans.
T. capricola found in the small intestine of sheep and goats.
T. colubriformis found in the small intestine, sometimes abomasum also, in cattle, sheep, goat, antelope, camel. Also recorded in pig, human, dog and rabbit.
T. drepanoformis found in the small intestine of sheep.
T. falculatus found in the small intestine of sheep, goat and antelopes.
T. hamatus found in the intestine of sheep and steinbok.
T. longispicularis found in sheep and cattle.
T. orientalis found in the small intestine of humans and rarely sheep.
T. probolurus found in the small intestine of sheep, goats, camels and rarely humans.
T. retortaeformis found in the small intestines of rabbits, hares.
T. rugatus found in the small intestines of sheep and goats.
T. skrjabini found in sheep, moufflon, roe deer.
T. tenuis found in the small intestine and ceca of domestic and wild birds.
T. vitrinus found in the small intestine of sheep, goats, deer, and occasionally in pigs, rabbits, camels and humans.

Trichosurus vulpecula brush-tailed possum, an Australian marsupial; see POSSUM.

trichothecene a complex group of about 40 biologically active metabolites formed by *Fusarium* spp. fungi. Naturally occurring members of this group of mycotoxins are T-2 toxin, deoxynivalenol and nivalenol. They cause FUSARIOTOXICOSIS in animals and toxic aleukia in humans.

Trichothecium roseum a toxic fungus causing nervous signs.

trichotillomania a psychogenic dermatosis in which the animal pulls out its own hair; seen in cats.

trichotomous divided into three parts.

trichuriasis the disease caused by the infestation of the cecum by *Trichuris* spp. The most obvious clinical feature is diarrhea sometimes with mucus and blood.

Trichuris a genus of nematodes in the family Trichuridae, found in the large intestine of most species. Called also whipworms. Includes *T. cameli* (camels), *T. campanula* (cats), *T. discolor* (cattle, sheep. goat, buffalo, zebra), *T. globulosa* (ruminants), *T. leporis* (rabbits, hares, coypu), *T. ovis* (ruminants), *T. raoi* (dromedaries), *T. serrata* (cats), *T. skrjabini* (sheep, goats, camels), *T. suis* (pigs), *T. sylvilagi* (rabbits, hares, coypu), *T. tenuis* (dromedary), *T. trichiura* (humans, simian primates), *T. vulpis* (dogs, foxes).

trichurosis infection with the worm TRICHURIS.

tricipital 1. three-headed. 2. relating to the triceps muscle.

triclabendazole a highly effective fasciolicide against liver flukes.

tricolor describes a coat color of dogs and cats which has orange and black patches (similar to the tortoiseshell) but has in addition patches of white hair; see TORTOISESHELL.

tricornute having three horns, cornua or processes.

tricresol a mixture of *o*-, *m*- and *p*-cresols.

tricrotism the quality of having three sphygmographic waves or elevations to one beat of the pulse.

tricuspid having three points or cusps, as a valve of the heart.
t. dysplasia a congenital defect of the tricuspid heart valve commonest in cats. There is a variety of forms of the defect which causes enlargement of the right atrium and ventricle. See also EBSTEIN'S ANOMALY.
t. insufficiency a functional incompetence that may be caused by rupture of the chordae tendineae of the tricuspid valve, bacterial endocarditis, heartworms, endocardiosis or congenital anomalies, resulting in regurgitation of blood from the right ventricle into the right atrium during systole.
t. regurgitation see tricuspid insufficiency (above).
t. valve the valve located between the right atrium and right ventricle. Called also right atrioventricular valve.

tricyclic containing three fused rings in the molecular structure.

tridactylism the presence of three digits on each limb.

tridentate having three prongs.

tridermic derived from the ectoderm, entoderm and mesoderm.

tridihexethyl chloride an anticholinergic quaternary ammonium compound.

trientine triethylenetetramine dihydrochloride; a copper-chelating agent used in the treatment of chronic hepatopathies in which copper accumulates.

trier a meat inspector who inspects the viscera in an uneviscerated chicken carcass through a small incision in the abdominal wall. The prime target is the liver and if this appears to be unaffected by disease the carcass is passed. Called also abdominal trier.

triethanolamine see TROLAMINE.

triethylenemelamine tretamine.

triethylenethiophosphoramide see THIOTEPA.

trifenmorph see 4-TRITYLMORPHOLINE.

trifid split into three parts.

trifluomeprazine maleate a phenothiazine tranquilizer.

trifluorothymidine a synthetic nucleoside that blocks DNA synthesis. Once used as an antiviral agent in the treatment of ocular herpesvirus infections.

triflupromazine a phenothizine tranquilizer used as a sedative and antiemetic.

trifluralin a dinitroaniline compound used as a weedicide. Excessive, accidental access causes diarrhea, anorexia, nervousness.

trifluridine an antiviral agent used topically in the treatment of herpesvirus infections of the eye.

triflurothymidine see TRIFLURIDINE.

trifoliol one of the coumestan group of phytoestrogens.

trifoliosis photosensitive dermatitis caused by the ingestion of burr trefoil (*Medicago polymorpha*).

Trifolium the clover genus of the legume family Fabaceae. They are plants of the greatest importance in high-producing pastures but can have disadvantages in some circumstances, e.g. they are common causes of bloat in cattle. Major syndromes include hyperestrogenism (*T. alpestre*, *T. fragiferum*, *T. pratense*, *T. subterraneum*), neonatal goiter due to low-level cyanide poisoning (*T. repens*), slobbers (*T. pratense*), putative hepatopathy with encephalopathy and photosensitizaion (*T. hybridum*), molybdenum poisoning (*T. hybridum*), obstructive urolithiasis (*T. subterraneum*).
Useful pasture plants are alpestrine clover (*T. alpestre*), alsike clover (*T. hybridum*), red clover (*T. pratense*), strawberry clover (*T. fragiferum*), white clover (*T. repens*).

trifurcation division or the site of separation into three branches.

trigeminal 1. triple. 2. pertaining to the fifth cranial (trigeminal) nerve.

t. nerve paralysis causes an inability to close the mouth (dropped jaw), difficulty in mastication and atrophy of the masticatory muscles. See also MANDIBULAR neurapraxia.

t. neuropraxia see MANDIBULAR neurapraxia.

trigeminy the condition of occurring in threes, especially the occurrence of three pulse beats in rapid succession.

trigger zone the initial segment of a neuron; the first segment of the axon after it leaves the cell body.

Triglochin genus of marsh plants in the family Juncaginaceae; can cause cyanide poisoning. Includes *T. maritima*, *T. palustris*. Called also seaside or marsh arrowgrass.

triglyceride a compound consisting of three molecules of fatty acids bound with one molecule of glycerol; a neutral fat that is the usual storage form of lipids in animals.

t. absorption test see FAT absorption test.

t. lipase see TRIACYLGLYCEROL.

medium-chain t. (MCT) short and medium length chain fatty acids (containing four to 12 carbon atoms) are much more rapidly digested than those with long chains. Coconut oil contains a high proportion of medium-chain triglycerides and may be used in the diet of dogs with malabsorption syndrome.

trigonal 1. triangular. 2. pertaining to a trigone.

t.-colonic anastomosis a method of diverting urine flow by surgically joining the trigone of the bladder to the colon.

trigone 1. a triangular area. See also TRIANGLE. 2. the primary three cusps of an upper cheek tooth.

olfactory t. the triangular area of gray matter between the roots of the olfactory tract.

vesical t. a triangular region of the wall of the urinary bladder, the three angles corresponding with the orifices of the ureters and urethra; it is an area in which the muscle fibers are closely adherent to the mucosa.

trigonectomy excision of the vesical trigone.

Trigonella foenum-graecum member of the plant family Fabaceae; the source of pharmaceutical fenugreek. Has caused poisoning in grazing livestock.

trigonitis inflammation or localized hyperemia of the vesical trigone.

trigonocephalus an animal exhibiting trigonocephaly.

trigonum pl. *trigona* [L.] *trigone* or *triangle*.

tri-iodothyronine one of the thyroid hormones; an organic iodine-containing compound liberated from thyroglobulin by hydrolysis. It has several times the biological activity of thyroxine. Called also T_3.

t. (T_3) suppression test the difference between the serum levels of T_3 and T_4 before and after oral administration of tri-iodothyronine for two days. With normal thyroid function, there is a marked decrease in T_3 levels, but in hyperthyroidism there is little change. Used in cats when other laboratory indicators are ambiguous.

t. uptake the uptake of the compound by red blood cells is used as a measure of thyroid function. Called also T_3 uptake.

trilabe a three-pronged lithotrite.

trilaminar three-layered.

trilobate having three lobes.

trilocular having three loculi or cells.

trilogy a group or series of three.

t. of Fallot a term sometimes applied to concurrent pulmonic stenosis, atrial septal defect and right ventricular hypertrophy. See also TETRALOGY of Fallot.

trilostane an inhibitor of adrenal, ovarian and placental steroids. Used in the treatment of hyperadrenocorticism.

Trimenopon hispidum an amblycerid louse found on guinea pigs.

trimensual occurring every 3 months.

trimeprazine a drug with mild central nervous depressant, moderate antiemetic and anticonvulsant, and powerful antihistaminic action; used as an antipruritic in the form of the tartrate salt.

trimercaptopropane an impurity in dimercaptopropanol which may cause poisoning.

trimester a period of 3 months.

trimetaphan, trimethaphan a compound used in ganglionic blockade and as a vasodilator.

trimethobenzamide an ethanolamine derivative; a strong antidopaminergic antagonist which is used as a central antiemetic.

trimethoprim an antibacterial closely related to pyrimethamine; administered in combination with a sulfonamide because these drugs blockade two consecutive steps in the synthesis of tetrahydrofolate by microorganisms. See also SULFADIAZINE–trimethoprim.

trimethylamine a smelly substance that taints milk. Formed in sugar beet residues by the fermentation of betaine.

trimethylene glycol an alcohol that causes marked growth rate depression in chickens.

trimethyllysine component of histone proteins; precursor of carnitine, the coenzyme of fatty acid oxidation.

trimetrexate an antifolate and an antineoplastic agent, similar to methotrexate. Also used in the treatment of toxoplasmosis and *Pneumocystis* infections.

trimipramine a tricyclic antidepressant.

trimmer see RESCO NAIL TRIMMER, toenail SCISSORS.

trimorphous existing in three different forms.

trinitrophenol see PICRIC ACID.

Trinoton anserinum, T. anseris an amblycerid mite that is found on ducks and swans.

triocephalus a monster with no organs of sight, hearing or smell, the head being a nearly shapeless mass.

Triodontophorus one of the genera of large strongyles of horses in the family Strongylidae. They are all parasites of the large intestine of equids.

T. brevicauda in the horse and ass.

T. minor in donkey.

T. serratus in horse, ass, mule, zebra.

T. tenuicollis found in the right dorsal colon of horses where it causes deep, hemorrhagic ulcers.

triol an organic compound containing three hydroxy groups, a trihydric alcohol, e.g. glycerol.

triolein see OLEIN.

triorchidism the presence of three testes.

triorthocresyl phosphate, triorthotolyl phosphate the ortho isomer of cresyl phosphate; used in industry and very toxic to animals, causing degeneration of nerves, leading to stiffness, incoordination and paraplegia.

triorthotolyl phosphate see TRIORTHOCRESYL PHOSPHATE.

triose a monosaccharide containing three carbon atoms in a molecule.

triosephosphate isomerase an enzyme in the Embden–Meyerhof pathway which catalyzes the reversible conversion of dihydroxyacetone phosphate to glyceraldehyde-3-phosphate.

trioxymethylanthraquinone emodin; yielded by the glycosides in the bark and seeds of elder and buckthorn. Ingestion of the bark causes colic, diarrhea and some deaths.

tripara tertipara; a female which has had three pregnancies that resulted in viable offspring; para III.
tripe the scalded and cleaned rumen and reticulum. The omasum is discarded because of the difficulty in cleaning between the leaves.
tripelennamine an antihistamine used in treating allergic disorders and also as a stimulant in downer cows.
tripeptide a peptide formed from three amino acids.
tripery and guttery room at an abattoir set aside for salvaging, trimming and cleaning the rumen and reticulum for tripe, and the intestines for sausage casings.
triphalangism three phalanges in a digit normally having only two.
triphasic having three phases.
triphenylmethane a substance from coal tar, the basis of various dyes and stains, including aurin, rosaniline, basic fuchsine and gentian violet.
triphosphatase see ADENOSINE triphosphatase.
triple-burner in acupuncture a non-existent organ which is the seat of specific physiological functions, e.g. it facilitates the flow of fluid, promotes the circulation and aids secretion, excretion and all of the vital functions.
Triple Crown the three main events in the USA racing calendar for 3-year-old thoroughbreds, the Kentucky Derby, the Preakness Stakes and the Belmont Stakes.
triple-heater see TRIPLE-BURNER.
t.-h. meridian points acupuncture points located along the triple-heater meridian.
triple phosphate urolith see struvite UROLITH.
triple sugar iron (TSI) agar an indicator medium containing glucose, lactose and sucrose and ferrous sulfate or ferric ammonium to identify *Salmonella* spp. and other Enterobacteriaceae.
triple sulfa various combinations of sulfonamides used therapeutically to reduce the occurrence of crystalluria. The therapeutic efficiency of the compound is additive but the solubilities are independent of each other.
triplegia paralysis of three extremities.
triplet 1. one of three offspring produced at one birth. 2. a combination of three objects or entities acting together, as three lenses or three nucleotides. See also CODON.
triplex triple or threefold.
triploid having triple the haploid number of chromosomes (3n).
t. lower jaw deformity defect of Atlantic salmon comprising a short, curved lower jaw with misaligned symphyses in the jaw. Cause uncertain, possibly genetic.
triploidy state of being TRIPLOID.
triplokoria the presence of three pupils in an eye.
triplumbic tetroxide red lead.
triprolidine used as an antihistamine.
-tripsy word element. [Gr.] *crushing;* used to designate a surgical procedure in which a structure is intentionally crushed.
tripus a conjoined twin monster having three feet.
Triraphis mollis Australian grass of the Poaceae plant family; can cause cyanide poisoning; called also purple plume grass.
trisaccharide a sugar each molecule of which yields three molecules of monosaccharides on hydrolysis.
Trisetum flavescens European grass in the family Poaceae; contains a calcinogenic agent; causes ENZOOTIC calcinosis. Called also yellow (golden) oatgrass.
trismus motor disturbance of the trigeminal nerve, especially spasm of the masticatory muscles, with difficulty in opening the mouth (lockjaw); a characteristic early sign of tetanus.
trisomy the presence of an additional (third) CHROMOSOME of one type in an otherwise diploid cell (2n + 1); associated with many congenital deformities in humans.
trisplanchnic pertaining to the three great visceral cavities, the skull, thorax and abdomen.
tristichia the presence of three rows of eyelashes.
trisulcate having three furrows.
trisulfapyrimidine one of the commercially available triple sulfa mixtures; contains a mixture of the sulfonamides, sulfadiazine, sulfamerazine and sulfamethazine. See also TRIPLE SULFA.
trisulfide a sulfur compound containing three atoms of sulfur.
triterpene plant toxins, e.g. lantadenes A, B, found in *Lantana camara*, icterogenins A, B, C, found in *Lippia* spp. Called also triterpene acids.
t. acids see triterpene (above).
tetracyclic t. plant toxins found in *Cucumis* spp.
tritiated thymidine thymidine linked to the radioisotope tritium; abbreviated ^{3}HTdR. Used to label DNA in the study of cellular and viral DNA synthesis.
triticale a cereal crop plant, a hybrid of wheat and rye, used only for livestock feed. Has the same energy content as wheat but a higher content of better quality protein. Yield of grain per hectare is much less than that of wheat.
Triticum genus of cultivated cereals in the family Poaceae; grazing young green crop can contribute to hypomagnesemic tetany; includes *T. aestivum* (*T. vulgare*, wheat), *T. dicoccum* (emmer, close relative of wheat and similar quality to it but lower yield), *T. spelta* (spelt), *T. vulgare* (*T. aestivum*).
tritium the mass 3 isotope of hydrogen, symbol ^{3}H, obtained by bombardment of beryllium in the cyclotron with deuterium ions. It has a half-life of about 31 years, and is used as an indicator or tracer in metabolic studies. See also TRITIATED THYMIDINE.
Tritrichomonas a genus of protozoan parasites with three anterior flagella in the family Trichomonadidae.
T. caviae found in the cecum and colon of guinea pigs but is not pathogenic.
T. eberthi found in the ceca of the chicken, turkey and duck.
T. enteris found in the cecum and colon of *Bos indicus* and *Bos taurus*, but has no pathogenic effects.
T. equi thought at one time to be the cause of acute and chronic undifferentiated diarrhea in horses but thought now to have no pathogenic effect.
T. foetus found in cattle, pig, horse and deer but causes TRICHOMONIASIS only in cattle.
T. minuta found in the cecum and colon of rat, mouse and hamster.
T. muris found in the cecum and colon of mouse, rat, hamster and wild rodent.
T. suis found in the stomach, small intestine, cecum and nasal passages of pigs.
triturable susceptible of being triturated.
triturate 1. to reduce to powder by rubbing. 2. a substance powdered fine by rubbing.
trituration 1. reduction to powder by friction or grinding. 2. a finely powdered substance.
triturator an apparatus in which substances can be continuously rubbed.
4-tritylmorpholine a molluscicide used in the control of bilharziasis. Called also trifenmorph, Frescon.

trivalent having a valence of three.

t. phenylorganic arsenicals includes the pharmaceuticals thiacetarsamide, arsphencomplexamine. See also organic ARSENICAL.

Trixacarus a genus of mange mites in the family Sarcoptidae.

***T. caviae* (syn. *Caviacoptes caviae*)** causes mange in guinea pigs characterized by alopecia, pruritus and keratinization.

T. diversus causes mange in rats, mice and hamsters.

trixylenyl phosphate one of the compounds used in the manufacture of TRIARYL PHOSPHATES.

trixylyl phosphate an industrial aryl phosphate capable of causing organic phosphate poisoning in cattle.

tRNA transfer RNA (RIBONUCLEIC ACID).

aminoacyl-tRNA transfer RNA to which its specific amino acid has been coupled by its specific aminoacyl-tRNA synthetase.

aminoacyl-tRNA binding site one of two tRNA binding sites on a ribosome that holds the incoming tRNA molecule charged with an amino acid. Called also A site.

aminoacyl-tRNA synthetases a set of enzymes that couple each of the 20 amino acids to its appropriate tRNA molecule.

initiator tRNA a special methionine tRNA that binds to the initiation codon AUG that forms part of the initiation complex at the start of mRNA translation.

peptidyl-tRNA binding site one of two tRNA binding sites on a ribosome that holds the tRNA that is normally linked to the polypeptide chain. Called also P site.

trocar a sharp-pointed, needle-like instrument equipped with a cannula; used to puncture the wall of a body cavity and withdraw fluid or gas. An especially large bore trocar and cannula, 1.0 to 1.5 cm diameter, is used in the treatment of bloat in cattle.

bleeding t. a large bore, about 10 gauge, needle with a ferruled hub for the attachment of rubber tubing.

Duchenne's t. a trocar for obtaining specimens of deep-seated tissues.

trocarization the action of using a trocar to penetrate an organ or tissue.

trochanter one of three tuberosities on the femur, at the upper end of its lateral surface (greater trochanter), towards the upper end on its medial surface (lesser trochanter) and more distally on the lateral surface (third trochanter). The third trochanter is prominent in horses and rabbits.

trochlea pl. *trochleae* [L.] a pulley-shaped part or structure; various bony or fibrous structures through or over which tendons pass or with which other structures articulate, e.g. femoral, humeral, radial.

femoral t. the articular surface on the cranial aspect of the distal femur upon which the patella glides.

humeral t. grooved articular surface at the distal end of the humerus; articulates with the radius and ulna.

trochlear 1. pertaining to a trochlea. 2. pertaining to the fourth cranial (trochlear) nerve.

t. nerve see Table 14.

t. notch semicircular notch in the proximal extremity of the ulna, articulates with the trochlea of the humerus, overhung by the 'beak' of the ulna's anconeal process.

t. orbit a flat piece of cartilage, or loop of fibrous tissue, embedded in the dorso-medial wall of the orbit close to the edge of the orbit; acts as a pulley for the dorsal oblique muscle.

t. talus the proximal articular surface on the talus, articulates with the tibia.

trochoid pivot-like, or pulley-shaped.

trochoides a pivot joint.

Troglodytella ciliated protozoa isolated from cases of diarrhea in recently captured great apes, chimpanzees, gorillas. Includes *T. abrassarti*, *T. gorillae*.

Troglostrongylus a genus of nematodes in the family Crenosomatidae found in the lungs of members of the family Felidae.

T. brevior found in the respiratory tract of cats.

T. subcrenatus found in the lungs of domestic and wild cats.

Troglotrema a genus of trematodes in the family Troglotrematidae.

T. acutum found in the frontal and ethmoidal sinuses of fox, mink and polecat and may destroy the walls of the sinuses.

T. salmincola see NANOPHYETUS *salmincola*.

trohoc study see CASE-control study.

trolamine a mixture of alkanolamines consisting largely of triethanolamine and containing some di- and monoethanolamine; used as an alkalizing agent in pharmaceutical preparations.

troleandomycin the triacetyl ester of oleandomycin; a macrolide antibiotic, similar to erythromycin. Called also triacetyloleandomycin.

Trollius europaeus European plant member of Ranunculaceae family; contains protoanemonin; causes abdominal pain, stomatitis, diarrhea. Called also globeflower.

Trombicula a genus of mites (family Trombiculidae), whose larvae are parasitic on all animal species and cause dermatitis. Some also transmit diseases from their natural hosts rodents to humans, e.g. scrub typhus. The larvae are also called chiggers.

T. akamushi transmits scrub typhus of humans.

T. alfreddugesi see EUTROMBICULA *alfreddugesi*.

T. autumnalis distinctively red mite found on all domestic animal species including poultry. Attacks humans. It causes dermatitis, e.g. between dog's claws and on the heels of horses. Called also harvest mite, aoutat, lepte automnale.

T. batatas causes dermatitis.

T. delhiensis transmits scrub typhus of humans from rodents.

T. minor the scrub-itch mite.

T. sarcina see EUTROMBICULA *sarcina*.

T. spendens causes dermatitis.

trombiculiasis see TROMBICULIDIASIS.

trombiculid a member of the Trombiculidae family of mites whose parasitic larvae (CHIGGERS) infest vertebrates causing TROMBICULIDIASIS.

trombiculidiasis dermatitis in all pastoral animal species and birds caused by mites of the family Trombiculidae. The bites produce wheals and intense pruritus followed by the development of moderate to severe dermatitis. This is mostly on the lower part of the face and the distal extremities. The disease is most likely to occur in autumn when the parasites are active and is often confined to particular fields that provide the best ecological niche for the mite.

trombiculosis infestation with TROMBICULA.

trombidiform mite see TROMBICULA.

trop- prefix meaning changing.

tropane alkaloid plant toxins, e.g. atropine, hyoscyamine, scopolamine (hyoscine) found in solanaceous plants.

trophectoderm the earliest trophoblast.

trophesy defective nutrition due to disorder of the trophic nerves.

trophic pertaining to nutrition.

-trophic, -trophin word element. [Gr.] *nourishing, stimulating.*
troph(o)- word element. [Gr.] *food, nourishment.*
trophoblast the peripheral cells of the blastocyst, which attach the fertilized ovum to the uterine wall and contribute to the placenta and the membranes that nourish and protect the developing organism. The inner cellular layer is the cytotrophoblast and the outer layer is the syntrophoblast.
trophocyte a cell that provides nourishment for other cells.
trophology the science of nutrition of the body.
trophoneurosis any functional nervous disease due to failure of nutrition from defective nerve influence.
trophonosis any disease due to nutritional causes.
trophont sperm of the protozoon *Oodinium* spp. (called also *Piscinoodinium*, *Amyloodinium*) found attached to the skin or gills of fish.
trophonucleus macronucleus.
trophopathic pertaining to or emanating from TROPHOPATHY.
t. hepatitis hepatic injury caused by nutritional deficiency. In many cases the injury is not caused directly by the deficiency but the removal of the nutrient from the diet makes the animal susceptible to a constantly present but usually ineffective agent. Although it occurs it has limited importance in contrast to toxipathic hepatitis. Examples are the white liver disease of cobalt deficient sheep, and dietary hepatic necrosis in pigs which is preventable by selenium and alpha tocopherol.
trophopathy disease due to derangement of nutrition.
trophoplast a granular protoplasmic body, a plastid.
trophotaxis taxis in relation to nutritive materials.
trophotherapy treatment of disease by dietary measures.
trophozoite the active, motile feeding stage of an apicomplexan parasite, and the motile stage of flagellate protozoa, e.g. *Giardia* spp.
-trophy suffix meaning growth or development.
tropia a manifest deviation of an eye from the normal position when both eyes are open and uncovered. See also STRABISMUS.
-tropic word element. [Gr.] *turning toward, changing, tending to turn or change.*
tropical pertaining to the tropics, the regions of the earth lying between the tropic of Cancer above the equator and the tropic of Capricorn below.
t. anhidrotic asthenia a condition due to generalized absence of sweating in conditions of high temperature. See also ANHIDROSIS.
t. bont tick AMBLYOMMA *variegatum.*
t. canine pancytopenia (TCP) see canine EHRLICHIOSIS.
t. cattle tick BOOPHILUS *microplus.*
t. Dairy Criollo cattle Central American dairy cattle, light dun to deep red, often with black points and spectacles.
t. fish includes 400 species suitable for home aquariums. The common ones are GOLDFISH, MOLLIES, GUPPY, angelfish (PTEROPHYLLUM), SWORDTAIL and SEA horse.
t. fowl mite ORNITHONYSSUS *bursa.*
t. horse tick DERMACENTOR *nitens.*
t. rat mite ORNITHONYSSUS *bacoti.*
t. theileriosis Mediterranean coast fever.
tropicamide a rapid-acting parasympatholytic agent used topically as a mydriatic for ophthalmoscopic examination.
Tropidechis carinatus a banded, olive green snake with a yellow belly and rough scales. Has a very powerful neurotoxic venom. Called also rough-scaled snake.
tropillo SOLANUM *elaeagnifolium.*
tropine a crystalline alkaloid from atropine and various plants.
tropinin a protein aggregate in thin muscle filaments.
tropism a growth response in a nonmotile organism elicited by an external stimulus, and either toward (positive tropism) or away from (negative tropism) the stimulus; used as a word element combined with a stem indicating nature of the stimulus (e.g. phototropism) or material or entity for which an organism (or substance) shows a special affinity (e.g. neurotropism).
tropocollagen the molecular unit of all forms of collagen; it is a helical structure of three polypeptides.
tropomyosin a muscle protein of the I band that inhibits contraction by blocking the interaction of actin and myosin, except when influenced by troponin.
troponin a complex of muscle proteins which, when combined with $Ca^{2}+$, influence tropomyosin to initiate contraction.
trospectomycin a derivative of spectinomycin with greater activity against gram-positive bacteria.
trot one of the natural gaits of the horse; a two-beat gait on alternating diagonals.
collected t. the head is held well in and the horse is not permitted to fully extend its limbs. The gait can be very showy but not fast nor a great coverer of distance.
extended t. not a racing trot in that the rhythm is not fast but the horse takes long strides and covers a lot of distance; the head and neck are extended.
Trotter trotting racehorse; includes American, Baltic, Cuban, French, German, Russian, etc. Trotters. See AMERICAN TROTTER.
trotting gait see TROT.
trough 1. standard equipment for feeding and watering animals. 2. an M-shaped false top to be placed on a surgical table. A small patient laid in it is propped up in the groove. Made of sterilizable material. Useful also in radiology if made of radiolucent materials.
troughing collective term for water or feed troughs.
trout sport and food finfish. Includes brown, brook, cutthroat, rainbow, sea trout and Great Lakes trout, members of the family Salmonidae. Some are freshwater, some anadromous. See Table 23.
TRP traumatic reticuloperitonitis.
Trp tryptophan.
Tru-Cut biopsy needle a disposable needle with outer cannula and inner, notched rod in which a tissue specimen is cut, trapped and withdrawn. The needle is commonly used for percutaneous biopsy of lymph nodes, liver, kidney, etc.
true actual.
t. digestibility the endogenous source of a fecal content of a feed moiety under examination is taken into account when assessing the input–output relationship of the moiety.
t. glucose reducing substances in the blood less aldose sugars, galactose, mannose.
t. rosette a clustering of cells, e.g. neuroblasts, around a hollow central lumen, as in human retinoblastomas.
truncal of the nature of or pertaining to the trunk.
truncal endocardial cushions the first ingrowths of endocardium in the truncus arteriosus which begin the development of the truncal septum and the separation of the cardiac outflow into left and right channels.

truncate 1. to amputate; to deprive of limbs. 2. having the end cut squarely off.

truncus pl. *trunci* [L.] trunk; individual trunci are listed as trunks in Table 9 (arteries) and Table 14 (nerves).

t. arteriosus an artery connected with the fetal heart, developing into the aortic and pulmonary arches. The trunk may persist into extrauterine life. The single arterial trunk from the heart supplies blood to both aortic and pulmonary circuits.

t. brachiocephalicus a vessel arising from the arch of the aorta and giving origin to one or both of the common carotid and one or both right subclavian arteries.

t. celiacus celiac trunk.

t. pulmonalis pulmonary trunk.

trunk 1. the main part, as the part of the body to which the head and limbs are attached, or a larger structure (e.g. vessel or nerve) from which smaller divisions or branches arise, or which is created by their union. 2. the extended nose of the elephant, containing many muscles giving it extraordinary strength and mobility. Anatomically it includes the nose and upper lip. There is a single finger-like papilla on the dorsal part of the tip in the Asian elephant and two papillae on the African elephant.

bicarotid t. a short artery which is the origin of the common carotid arteries in ungulates.

brachiocephalic t. see Table 9.

celiac t. the arterial trunk arising from the abdominal aorta and giving origin to the left gastric, common hepatic, and splenic arteries; see Table 9.

costocervical t. a branch of the subclavian artery; see Table 9.

lumbar lymph t. a plexus of lymph vessels on the roof of the abdomen; drain into the cisterna chyli.

lumbosacral t. a nerve trunk formed by union of the ventral branches of the lumbar and sacral nerves; see also Table 9.

pudendoepigastric t. see Table 9.

pulmonary t. a vessel arising from the conus arteriosus of the right ventricle and bifurcating into the right and left pulmonary arteries; see also Table 9.

sympathetic t. see SYMPATHETIC trunk.

vagal t. see dorsal, ventral vagal trunks in Table 14.

trypan blue a supravital stain and a stain for amyloid. Also, a largely superseded trypanocide; causes tissue sloughs if injected around the vein, and stains tissues blue, an inconvenience in meat animals.

trypanocidal destructive to trypanosomes. The common drugs used are DIMINAZENE aceturate, HOMIDIUM bromide, QUINAPYRAMINE, SURAMIN.

trypanocide a TRYPANOCIDAL drug.

trypanolysis the destruction of trypanosomes.

Trypanoplasma cyprini a fusiform protozoan parasite with a flagellum at each pole. A member of the Cryptobiidae family. May invade the vascular system and cause depression and emaciation. See also CRYPTOBIA *cyprini*.

trypanoplasmiasis disease of finfish caused by *Trypanoplasma* spp.

Trypanosoma a multispecies genus of protozoa in the family Trypanosomatidae, parasitic in the blood, lymph and tissues of invertebrates and vertebrates, including humans; most species live part of their life cycle in the intestines of insects and other invertebrates, the flagellate stage being found only in the vertebrate host. The species which cause serious diseases of domestic animals are listed individually below. Species of minor pathogenicity include *T. avium* (birds), *T. binneyi* (platypus), *T. calmetti* (ducklings), *T. diazi* (capuchin monkeys), *T. dimorphon* (domestic animals generally), *T. gallinarum* (fowls), *T. melophagium* (sheep), *T. minasense* (monkeys, e.g. marmosets), *T. nabiasi* (rabbits), *T. primatum* (chimpanzees, gorillas), *T. rangeli* (humans, dogs, cats). Called also *T. ariarii*, *T. guatamalense*, *T. saimiriae* (squirrel monkeys), *T. sanmartini* (squirrel monkeys), *T. theodori* (pigs).

***T. brucei* (syn. *T. pecaudi*)** causes a severe disease in all species including horse, cattle, sheep, dogs and cats.

***T. congolense* (syn. *T. pecorum*, *T. nanum*, *T. montgomeryi*)** causes diseases in all domestic animals but most serious in humans (sleeping sickness), cattle (nagana); reservoir hosts are wild ruminants.

***T. cruzi* (syn. *T. escomeli*)** a disease of humans (Chagas' disease, American trypanosomiasis) which has reservoirs in pigs, dogs and cats and many wild animals. It causes disease in these hosts and may be fatal to dogs.

T. equinum occurs in all species but is most serious in equids, in which it is characterized by posterior paralysis; called Mal de Caderas.

T. equiperdum occurs in all species but a common infection and a serious disease only in equids in which it is transmitted venereally and is known as DOURINE.

T. evansi causes infection in many species especially in camels, horses and dogs. The disease in horses is SURRA. In cattle and buffalo the disease is subclinical but these species act as reservoirs.

***T. gambiense* (syn. *T. hominis*, *T. nigeriense*, *T. ugandense*)** a chronic disease of humans which can occur also in cattle, goats, sheep, horses, dogs and cats.

T. lewisi occurs in rats and may cause death in ratlings.

T. rhodesiense causes a serious disease in humans but only a mild one in ruminants and other domestic animals and monkeys.

T. suis found in pigs in which it causes a fatal disease.

T. theileri considered to be nonpathogenic in cattle, in which it occurs almost universally but may cause illness in stressed animals.

T. uniforme found in most ruminants. Similar to *T. vivax* in pathogenicity.

***T. vivax* (syn. *T. caprae*, *T. angolense*)** found in ruminants and horses but not pigs, dogs, cats. Causes a serious and fatal disease in cattle and goats, especially in animals under stress.

trypanosome a protozoan of the genus *Trypanosoma*.

trypanosomiasis clinically a nondescript disease which may be peracute, acute or chronic. Called also nagana, mal de caderas and others. See also DOURINE, SURRA. The diagnosis is based on a positive blood smear and the presence of an insect vector, often a tsetse fly, or a history of mating in the case of dourine.

American t. a disease of humans caused by infection with *Trypanosoma cruzi*.

trypanosomicide 1. lethal to trypanosomes. 2. an agent lethal to trypanosomes.

trypanosomid a skin eruption occurring in trypanosomiasis.

trypanotolerance resistance to infection with trypanosomes, inherent in some breeds of cattle, e.g. the N'dama, Nigerian shorthorn, Lagune and others.

trypomastigote developmental stage of trypanosomes, usually in the vertebrate host but may be in the invertebrate. A leaf-like form with an undulating membrane and often a free flagellum.

trypsin a proteolytic enzyme formed in the intestine by the cleavage of trypsinogen by enterokinase. Trypsinogen enters the intestine as part of the intestinal juice It is an endopeptidase that hydrolyzes peptides of arginine or lysine.

t. fecal tests see FECAL trypsin.

t. inhibitor small protein synthesized in the exocrine pancreas which prevents conversion of trypsinogen to trypsin, so protecting itself against trypsin digestion. Pancreatic trypsin inhibitor competitively binds to the active site of trypsin and inactivates it at a very low concentration. The binding is amongst the strongest noncovalent associations, but only a fraction of the potential trypsin is so inhibited.

t.-like immunoreactivity (TLI) serum proteins, particularly trypsinogen, react immunologically as trypsin and a normal level is dependent upon a normally functional pancreas. This is used in the diagnosis of exocrine pancreatic insufficiency.

trypsinogen the inactive precursor of trypsin, secreted by the pancreas and activated to trypsin by contact with enterokinase.

tryptamines poisonous compounds that occur in plants. Three tryptamine alkaloids in *Phalaris aquatica* are thought to be the cause of both nervous and cardiac forms of poisoning by this plant.

tryptase a protease that is active in inflammation and a mediator of anaphylaxis.

tryptic relating to or resulting from digestion by trypsin.

tryptophan, tryptophane Trp; a naturally occurring amino acid, existing in proteins. High levels of intake of D,L-tryptophan are thought to be a significant cause of atypical interstitial pneumonia in cattle. The actual toxic agent is 3-methylindole, a metabolic product of D,L-tryptophan in the rumen.

D,L-t. component of some roughages; high levels can cause acute bovine pulmonary emphysema and edema.

t. oxygenase first enzyme in the catabolic pathway for tryptophan. Essential step in the pathway to synthesis of nicotinamide nucleotides NAD+ and NADP+. Approximately 30% of the nicotinamide nucleotide requirement of some animals can be supplied through this enzyme. The cat is notably lacking in the latter capacity.

tryptophanase an enzyme that catalyzes the cleavage of tryptophan into indole, pyruvic acid and ammonia.

tryptophanuria excessive urinary excretion of tryptophan.

Ts cell suppressor T LYMPHOCYTE.

***tsang* organs** the body organs which have *yin*, a negative, passive quality; compare with *fu* organs.

tsetse an African fly of the genus GLOSSINA, which transmits trypanosomiasis.

t. fly disease nagana.

TSH thyroid-stimulating hormone (THYROTROPIN, thyrotropic hormone).

TSH releasing factor see THYROTROPIN releasing hormone.

TSST-1 toxic shock syndrome toxin.

TSTA tumor-specific transplantation antigen.

tsun the acupuncture basic unit of measurement, in the horse equals the width of the 16th rib at the level of the tuber coxae.

tsutsugamushi fever scrub typhus.

TTP thymidine triphosphate.

TU tuberculin unit.

tuba pl. *tubae* [L.] tube.

tube a hollow cylindrical organ or instrument.

chest t. one or more tubes inserted into the pleural space to provide relief from either PNEUMOTHORAX or accumulations of fluid within the thoracic cavity and to allow for re-expansion of the lung.

drainage t. a tube used in surgery to facilitate escape of fluids. See also DRAIN (2).

endobronchial t. a double-lumen tube inserted into the bronchus of one lung, permitting complete deflation of the other lung; used in anesthesia and thoracic surgery.

eustachian t. see PHARYNGOTYMPANIC TUBE.

feeding t. one for administering food into the alimentary tract. See also ENTEROSTOMY tube, JEJUNOSTOMY tube, tube GASTROSTOMY, nasoesophageal tube (below).

fermentation t. a U-shaped tube with one end closed, for determining gas production by bacteria. Called also Durham tube.

Levin t. a gastroduodenal catheter of sufficiently small caliber to permit transnasal passage.

nasoesophageal t. a feeding tube introduced through the nares and nasal cavity, then into the esophagus. Used in enteral feeding of dogs and cats.

otopharyngeal t. auditory tube.

pharyngostomy t. see PHARYNGOSTOMY intubation.

photomultiplier t. a vacuum tube that produces an electric current proportional to the intensity of light falling on its photocathode; it is sensitive enough to detect single photons.

t. rating chart provided by the manufacturer and containing the specifications for the safe operating limits of the x-ray tube in terms of kilovolt peak, milliamps and time.

stomach t. a flexible tube used for introducing food, medication, or other material directly into the stomach, or for removal of undesirable contents from the stomach. It can be passed into the stomach via the nose or mouth. Passage via the mouth requires the protection of a mouth speculum.

suction drainage t. see suction DRAINAGE.

test t. a tube of thin glass, closed at one end; used in chemical tests and other laboratory procedures.

thoracostomy t. one inserted through an opening in the chest wall for application of suction to the pleural cavity to facilitate re-expansion of the lung in spontaneous pneumothorax. See also chest tube (above).

tubectomy excision of a portion of the uterine tube.

tuber 1. a swelling or protuberance, especially on a bone. 2. a short, thick, fleshy, underground stem carrying a number of buds each capable of growing into a new plant, e.g. potato. A storage phase of plant growth.

t. calcaneus, t. calcis the point of the hock that serves as the attachment for the gastrocnemius tendon.

t. cinereum a mound on the undersurface of the forebrain to which the stalk of the pituitary gland is attached.

t. coxae, coxal t. the point of the hip; the most lateral point of the ilium.

facial t. the anterior point on the facial crest, just above the third and fourth cheek teeth of the horse. A homologous point in the cow.

t. ischii the caudal point on the floor of the pubis, the tuber ischium or pin bone.

sacral t. the most medial prominence on the ilium; above the sacroiliac joint.

t. scapulae supraglenoid tubercle.

tubercle 1. a small, rounded nodule produced by the bacillus of tuberculosis (*Mycobacterium bovis*). It is made up of small spherical masses that contain giant cells and are surrounded by spindle-shaped epithelioid cells. 2. a nodule or small eminence, especially one on a bone, for attachment of a tendon. See also CUNEATE tubercle.

dysgonic t. (1) one from which it is difficult to culture mycobacteria, typical of *Mycobacterium bovis*.

eugonic t. (1) one from which mycobacteria can be isolated with ease. Typical of *Mycobacterium avium*.

fibrous t. (1) a tubercle of bacillary origin that contains connective tissue elements.

genital t. see phallic tubercle (below).

gracile t. a small swelling; used as an anatomical landmark; also an attachment for the gracilis nucleus in the medulla oblongata.

humerus t. the point of the shoulder; the greater tubercle on the head of the humerus.

intercondylar t's situated on the intercondylar eminence on the head of the tibia, there are medial and lateral tubercles. Called also intercondylar eminences.

intermediate humerus t. a small ridge between the greater and lesser tubercles of the horse's humerus; it serves to restrain the bicipital tendon.

intervenous t. a fold on the inner wall of the right atrium, directing the flow of blood from the venae cavae to the atrioventricular opening.

miliary t. one of the many minute tubercles formed in many organs in acute miliary tuberculosis.

phallic t. primordia of the penis; called also genital tubercle.

pubic t. a prominent tubercle at the lateral end of the pubic crest.

supraglenoid t. a tubercle on the scapula for attachment of the biceps muscle.

tubercular tuberculous.

tuberculate, tuberculated covered or affected with tubercles.

tuberculid a papular skin eruption usually attributed to allergy to tuberculosis.

papulonecrotic t. an eruption of crops of deep-seated papules or nodules, with central necrosis or ulceration.

tuberculigenous causing tuberculosis.

tuberculin a sterile liquid containing the growth products of, or specific substances extracted from the tubercule bacillus; used in various forms in the diagnosis of tuberculosis.

heat concentrated synthetic medium (HCSM) t. similar to old tuberculin, but grown on synthetic medium.

new t. a suspension of the fragments of tubercle bacilli, freed from all soluble materials and with glycerine added.

old t. a sterile solution of concentrated, soluble products of the growth of the tubercle bacillus, adjusted to standard potency by addition of glycerin and isotonic sodium chloride solution, final glycerin content being about 50%.

purified protein derivative (PPD) of t. a form of tuberculin used in the testing of animals for tuberculosis; abbreviated PPD. It is a soluble protein fraction prepared from a synthetic medium on which the *Mycobacterium bovis* has been cultured. It has the advantage of reducing the number and severity of the reactions caused by nonspecific sensitizing materials in the culture medium in old tuberculin.

t. reaction the prototype delayed or type IV hypersensitivity; typified by swelling and redness at the site of inoculation of tuberculin.

t. tests a number of tests for tuberculosis, based on the use of tuberculin as a test agent, are used in animals. A short thermal test using a large volume of tuberculin injected subcutaneously is used in special circumstances. Most of the tests use an intradermal injection and a local swelling as a positive reaction.

tuberculitis inflammation of or near a tubercle.

tuberculocele tuberculous disease of a testis.

tuberculofibroid characterized by a tubercle that has undergone fibroid degeneration.

tuberculoid resembling a tubercle or tuberculosis.

tuberculoma a tumor-like mass resulting from enlargement of a caseated tubercle.

tuberculoprotein protein fraction isolatable from a culture of *Mycobacterium* spp. See also purified protein derivative of TUBERCULIN.

tuberculosis applied generally to diseases caused by tuberculous group of bacteria in the genus *Mycobacteria*, which includes *Mycobacteria tuberculosis*, *M. bovis* and *M. avium*. See also FISH tuberculosis, MYCOBACTERIOSIS.

atypical mycobacterial t. see atypical MYCOBACTERIOSIS.

avian t. see *Mycobacterium avium* tuberculosis (below).

bovine t. see *Mycobacterium bovis* tuberculosis (below).

cutaneous t. infection with *Mycobacterium tuberculosis* uncommonly involves the skin; in dogs and cats it can occur as cutaneous ulcers, abscesses, plaques and nodules. More often, the term is used to described infection with atypical mycobacteria.

fish t. see FISH tuberculosis.

***Mycobacterium avium* t.** causes a significant disease only in birds. In birds it is a chronic disease characterized by loss of body weight, poor egg production and eventual death. There are characteristic large gray, yellow or white tubercles in liver, spleen and intestinal wall. The disease is very persistent in a flock. In mammals it causes nonprogressive lesions, especially in lymph nodes, causing the animals to be positive to the tuberculin test.

***Mycobacterium bovis* t.** a chronic disease characterized by the development of tubercles or discrete nodular lesions in any organ. These may develop a necrotic center containing yellow-orange pus, often caseous. Diffuse involvement of lungs causing bronchopneumonia, and of uterus causing metritis, and of the udder also occur. The common clinical syndrome is wasting with localizing signs dependent on the organs involved. A common lesion in horses is osteomyelitis of a cervical vertebra.

***Mycobacterium tuberculosis* t.** infection with the human mycobacteria causes transient, usually lesionless infections in animals.

open t. 1. that in which there are lesions from which tubercle bacilli are being discharged out of the body. 2. tuberculosis of the lungs with cavitation.

skin t. is characterized by chronic indurated lesions on the skin of the lower limbs of cattle. There are nodules on the path of corded lymphatics. Nonpathogenic acid-fast bacteria are present in the lesions and affected cattle are positive to the tuberculin test. Also occurs uncommonly in dogs and cats as single or multiple nodules, ulcers, abscesses or plaques in the skin. See also MYCOBACTERIOSIS.

t. testing tuberculin testing.

tuberculostatic 1. inhibiting the growth of *Mycobacterium tuberculosis*. 2. a tuberculostatic agent.

tuberculotic pertaining to or affected with tuberculosis.

tuberculous pertaining to or affected with tuberculosis; caused by *Mycobacterium tuberculosis*, e.g. tuberculous adenitis.

t. mastitis chronic mastitis but with fibrosis commencing at the base of the udder, not around the milk cistern; abnormality of the milk is in the form of fine floccules in watery liquid, settling out on standing, and appearing at the end of milking instead of in the first few streams.

tuberculum pl. *tubercula* [L.] see TUBERCLE.

tuberosis a condition characterized by the presence of nodules.

tuberositas pl. *tuberositates* [L.] tuberosity; elevations on bones to which muscles are attached.

tuberosity an elevation or protuberance.

deltoid t. a prominence on the lateral aspect of the humerus; the point of attachment of the deltoid muscle.

facial t. a discrete elevation on the maxilla of cows which serves as an attachment for the rostral part of the masseter muscle.

ischial t. the pin bone; the most caudal process of the ischium.

olecranon t. the free end of the ulna; point of attachment of the triceps brachii muscle.

radial t. a rough patch on the cranial aspect of the proximal end of the radius.

tibial t. prominent tuberosity protruding from the cranial aspect of the proximal end of the tibia onto which the patellar ligament inserts.

tuberous covered with tubers; knobby.

tubo- word element. [L.] *tube.*

tubocurarine an alkaloid from the bark and stems of *Chondrodendron tomentosum*. *d*-tubocurarine chloride is used as a skeletal muscle relaxant.

tuboligamentous pertaining to the uterine tube and broad ligament.

tubo-ovarian pertaining to the uterine tube and ovary.

tuboperitoneal pertaining to the uterine tube and the peritoneum.

tuboplasty 1. salpingoplasty. 2. plastic repair of a tube, such as the eustachian tube.

tubouterine pertaining to the uterine tube and uterus.

tubular 1. pertaining to renal tubules. 2. pertaining to fallopian tube.

t. backleak leakage of tubular fluid into the interstitium of the kidney is one of the factors in the pathogenesis of acute renal failure.

t. maxima the concentrations of solutes at which the renal tubules are working at full capacity and further increases in concentration will not increase the function. Called also T_m.

t. necrosis acute necrosis of the tubular epithelium caused usually by ischemia or exposure to a nephrotoxin; in most cases the patient succumbs to uremia in a few days. See also NEPHROSIS.

t. proteinuria failure of the tubules to resorb small molecule proteins excreted by the glomerulus.

t. reabsorption reabsorption of solutes from the glomerular filtrate by the tubules, the conservation of protein, glucose and bicarbonate, and the conservation of the water that accompanies them.

t. transport refers to all processes which occur with renal tubular fluid during its transport from glomerular space to renal pelvis.

t. transport maximum when the tubular transport maximum for a renal tubular solute is exceeded the solute appears in the urine.

tubulation the mechanism and principle of development in the form of tubes such as the neural tube, and the visceral tube.

tubule a small tube; a minute canal found in various structures or organs of the body.

collecting t's the terminal channels of the nephrons which open on the summits of the renal papillae or renal crests.

convoluted t's channels which follow a tortuous course. See also renal tubules (below) and TUBULI contorti.

dentinal t's minute channels in the dentine of a tooth that extend from the pulp cavity to the cement or the enamel. Called also dentinal canaliculi.

galactophorous t's small channels for the passage of milk from the secreting cells in the mammary gland. Called also lactiferous ducts.

Henle's t's see HENLE'S tubules.

lactiferous t's see LACTIFEROUS ducts.

mesonephric t's the tubules comprising the mesonephros, or temporary kidney, of amniotes.

metanephric t's the tubules comprising the permanent kidney of amniotes.

proximal t. intrarenal site for the reabsorption of most of the protein in the tubular fluid.

proximal convoluted t. the portion of the nephron immediately succeeding the glomerulus; susceptible to disease because of its early exposure to toxins in the glomerular filtrate.

renal t's the minute canals made up of basement membrane and lined with epithelium, composing the substance of the kidney and secreting, reabsorbing, collecting and conducting the urine. Include proximal convoluted, the nephron loop (containing the proximal straight tubule, descending and ascending thin, and the distal straight tubules) and the distal convoluted tubules.

seminiferous t's the tubules of the testis, in which spermatozoa develop and through which they leave the gland.

uriniferous t's renal tubules; channels for the passage of urine.

tubuli [L.] plural of *tubulus*.

t. contorti convoluted seminiferous tubules.

t. recti straight seminiferous tubules.

tubulin the constituent protein of microtubules of cells which provide a skeleton for maintaining cell shape and is thought to be involved in cell motility.

α-t. with β-tubulins contributes to the heterodimer tubulin, the building blocks of the electron microscopically visible cell components, the microtubules.

β-t. one of the monomeric globular proteins which associate to form the dimer, α,β-tubulin, the basis of microfilaments.

tubuloalveolar glands glands that secrete from both alveoli (acini) and tubules as those secreting mucous onto the tracheal mucosa.

tubuloglomerular feedback an essential ingredient of the juxtaglomerular theory of renal autoregulation; TGF is the proposed mechanisms whereby the glomerular flow rate is modified by changes in the tubular flow rate.

tubulointerstitial nephropathy a familial renal disease in Norwegian elkhounds; the disease is caused by a nonspecific renal lesion, by an unknown pathogenesis and obviously inherited but the inheritance mode is unknown.

tubulorrhexis rupture of the tubules of the kidney.

tubulus pl. *tubuli* [L.] tubule.

tubus tube.

tucked-up describes an abdomen of small circumference as compared to the thorax or to the normal outline for the individual animal. Normally seen in some breeds of dogs, e.g. Whippet, Greyhound.

tuco-tuco see CTENOMYS TALARUM.

tuft a small clump or cluster; a coil.

t. cell see CAVEOLATED CELL.
malpighian t. renal glomerulus.
tufted burr daisy see CALOTIS SCAPIGERA.
tuftsin a basic tetrapeptide produced in the spleen that stimulates phagocytosis in polymorphonuclear leukocytes and in macrophages.
tugs stout leather loops, connected to the backband or saddle, into which vehicle shafts fit.
tui nar active stimulation of acupuncture points.
Tukidale a specialized, New Zealand carpetwool sheep, a mutant ROMNEY MARSH with a large percentage of medullated fibers in its high yielding fleece; the fiber diameter is 35 to 45 microns. It has a white face and dark skin.
Tula ixtle see AGAVE *lecheguilla*.
tularemia a highly contagious disease of rodents caused by *Francisella* (*Pasteurella*) *tularensis* which may infect farm animals and humans. In animals spread is by ticks. The clinical disease is very variable, depending on where the infection localizes.
tularin an extract of the organism *Francisella tularensis* used as an antigen in an intradermal test for tularemia in pigs.
tule elk see CERVUS.
tulip the horticultural tulip—see TULIPA. For Cape and Natal tulip see HOMERIA.
Tulipa the commercial tulip; member of the family Liliaceae; its bulbs have caused poisoning in cattle.
tullidora see KARWINSKIA HUMBOLDTIANA.
tulp [Af.] a form of poisoning caused by MORAEA and HOMERIA spp. plants.
tumbleweed SALSOLA kali.
tumbu fly see CORDYLOBIA *anthropophaga*.
tumefacient producing tumefaction.
tumefaction a swelling; the state of being swollen, or the act of swelling; puffiness; edema.
tumescence 1. the condition of being swollen. 2. a swelling.
tumid swollen; edematous.
tumor 1. swelling, one of the cardinal signs of inflammation; morbid enlargement. 2. neoplasm; a new growth of tissue in which cell multiplication is uncontrolled and progressive. A cancer.

Tumors are called also cancers or neoplasms, which means that they are composed of new and actively growing tissue. Their growth is faster than that of normal tissue, continuing after cessation of the stimuli that evoked the growth, and serving no useful physiological purpose.

Tumors are classified in a number of ways, one of the simplest being according to their origin and whether they are malignant or benign. Tumors of mesenchymal origin include fibroelastic tumors and those of bone, fat, blood vessels and lymphoid tissue. They may be benign or malignant (sarcoma). Tumors of epithelial origin may be benign or malignant (carcinoma); they are found in glandular tissue or such organs as the mammary gland, stomach, uterus or skin. Mixed tumors contain different types of cells derived from the same primary germ layer, and teratomas contain cells derived from more than one germ layer; both kinds may be benign or malignant.

ACTH secreting t. see CORTICOTROPH ADENOMA.
benign t. grows slowly, pushing aside normal tissue but not invading it. They are usually encapsulated, well-demarcated growths. They are not metastatic; that is, they do not form secondary tumors in other organs. Benign tumors usually respond favorably to surgical treatment and some forms of RADIATION therapy.
t. blush in cerebral arteriography, the pooling of contrast material where the blood–brain barrier has been interrupted.
brown t. a giant-cell granuloma produced in and replacing bone, occurring in osteitis fibrosa cystica and due to hyperparathyroidism.
Burkitt's t. see BURKITT'S LYMPHOMA.
button t. histiocytoma.
carotid body t. see CAROTID body tumors.
β cell t. see INSULINOMA.
t. clinical staging see STAGING (2).
connective tissue t. any tumor arising from a connective tissue structure, e.g. a fibroma or fibrosarcoma.
desmoid t. see DESMOID (2).
t. enhancement see tumor ENHANCEMENT.
erectile t. cavernous hemangioma.
false t. structural enlargement due to extravasation, exudation, echinococcus or retained sebaceous matter.
gastrin-secreting t. see GASTRINOMA, ZOLLINGER–ELLISON SYNDROME.
giant cell t. see GIANT CELL TUMOR.
granulosa t., granulosa cell t. a sex chord-stromal tumor, often referred to as granulosa–theca cell tumor, of the ovary originating in the cells of the cumulus oophorus. See also GRANULOSA CELL TUMOR.
granulosa–theca cell t. an ovarian tumor composed of granulosa (follicular) cells and theca cells; either form may predominate. See also GRANULOSA–THECA CELL TUMOR.
heterologous t. one made up of tissue differing from that in which it grows.
homoiotypic t., homologous t. one made up of tissue resembling that in which it grows.
Hürthle cell t. a new growth of the thyroid gland composed wholly or predominantly of Hürthle cells. See also HÜRTHLE CELL tumor.
t. immunology see tumor-specific ANTIGEN.
t. immunotherapy see IMMUNOTHERAPY.
islet cell t. a tumor of the islets of Langerhans, which may result in hyperinsulinism. See also INSULINOMA.
t. lysis syndrome a possible sequel to chemotherapy in which very rapid destruction of highly sensitive tumor cells results in release of large amounts of nucleic acid purines, lactate and uric acid which exceed renal and hepatic excretory mechanisms. Characterized by hyperkalemia, hyperphosphatemia, hypocalcemia, hyperuricemia and renal failure.
malignant t. composed of embryonic, primitive, or poorly differentiated cells. They grow in a disorganized manner and so rapidly that nutrition of the cells becomes a problem. For this reason necrosis and ulceration are characteristic of malignant tumors. They also invade surrounding tissues and are metastatic, initiating the growth of similar tumors in distant organs. See also CANCER.
mast cell t. a benign, but occasionally malignant, local aggregation of mast cells forming a nodulous tumor. Mast cell tumors with diffuse visceral involvement are called systemic mastocytosis. See also MAST CELL tumor.
mixed t. one composed of more than one type of neoplastic tissue, as in mammary tumors.
t. necrosis factor (TNF) two related cytokines produced by macrophages (TNF-α) and some T cells (TNF-β) that are cytotoxic for tumor cells but not for normal cells and which exert a variety of other inflammatory effects. See also LYMPHOTOXIN.
t.-node-metastases (TNM) classification see TNM STAGING.

non-neoplastic t. tumor (1).
organoid t. teratoma.
phantom t. abdominal or other swelling not due to structural change.
sand t. psammoma.
t.-specific antigen (TSA) see tumor-specific ANTIGEN.
true t. neoplasm.

tumoral calcinosis see CALCINOSIS circumscripta.
tumoricidal destructive to cancer cells.
tumorigenesis the production of tumors.
tumultus excessive organic action or motility.
tung oil tree ALEURITES *fordii.*
Tunga a genus of fleas native to tropical and subtropical America and Africa.
T. penetrans the chigoe or jigger flea, which attacks humans, dogs, pigs and other animals, as well as poultry, and causes intense skin irritation. See also CHIGOE.

tungiasis infestation with TUNGA fleas.
tungsten a chemical element, atomic number 74, atomic weight 183.85, symbol W. See Table 6.
tunic a covering or coat. See also TUNICA.
abdominal t. see TUNICA flava abdominis.
Bichat's t. tunica intima.

tunica pl. *tunicae* [L.] a covering or coat; a membranous covering of an organ or a distinct layer of the wall of a hollow structure, as a blood vessel. See also TUNIC.
t. adventitia the outer coat of various organs, blood vessels and other structures, usually made up of loose connective tissue.
t. albuginea a dense, white, fibrous sheath enclosing a part or organ, such as is present on the testis.
t. albuginea ovarii see tunica ovarii (below).
t. conjunctiva the conjunctiva.
t. dartos dartos.
t. externa an outer coat, especially the fibroelastic coat of a blood vessel.
t. flava abdominis an extensive sheet of elastic tissue that helps to support the abdomen. It is conspicuous in large animals as a yellow corset over the ventral abdomen and is a modified part of the deep fascia and aponeurosis of the external abdominal oblique muscle. It contributes to the deep fascia for the mammary gland or the scrotum.
t. intima the innermost coat of blood vessels; called also Bichat's tunic.
t. media the middle coat of blood vessels.
t. mucosa the mucous membrane lining of various tubular structures.
t. muscularis the muscular coat or layer surrounding the tela submucosa in most portions of the digestive, respiratory, urinary and genital tracts.
t. ovarii capsule of dense collagenous tissue, underlying the covering epithelium, covers each ovary. Called also tunica albuginea ovarii.
t. propria the proper coat or layer of a part, as distinguished from an investing membrane.
t. serosa the membrane lining the external walls of the body cavities and coating the surfaces of intruding organs; it secretes a watery exudate.
t. vaginalis the double-layered sleeve of peritoneum that lines the scrotum and inguinal canal (parietal layer) and invests the testis, epididymis and spermatic cord (visceral layer).
t. vasculosa a vascular coat, or a layer well supplied with blood vessels, e.g. of the eye.
t. vasculosa lentis vascular envelope of the lens in the developing fetus.

tunicaminyluracils mycotoxins and antibiotics, e.g. tunicamycin, produced by *Streptomyces* spp.; include corynetoxin produced by CLAVIBACTER TOXICUS.
tunicamycin 1. an antibiotic which inhibits the synthesis of all *N*-linked glycoproteins by blocking the transfer of acetylgalactosmaine from UDP-*N*-acetylgalactosamine to dolicholphosphate. 2. bacterial toxin produced by *Clavibacter rathayi* which infects galls on grass caused by the nematode *Anguina funesta.* Called also corynetoxin.
tuning fork auscultation see tuning fork AUSCULTATION.
Tunisian Barbary sheep white or red-brown head, carpetwool and meat sheep, male horned, female polled.
tunnel a passageway of varying length through a solid body, completely enclosed except for the open ends, permitting entrance and exit.
carpal t. see CARPAL tunnel, CARPAL tunnel syndrome.
t. of Corti spiral passage in the organ of Corti.
t. graft see rope FLAP.
tarsal t. see TARSAL tunnel.

tup ram.
Tupaia see TREE shrew.
Tupaiidae a family of nonhuman primates that includes tree shrews.
Tupinambis teguexin see TEGU.
tupping mating with a ram.
t. crayon a raddle crayon worn on the brisket in a harness by a ram running with ewes. Ewes that are mated are branded with the crayon. See also CRAYON-marking.

turacin crimson pigment in the feathers of turacos.
turacos see MUSOPHAGID.
turacoverdin the green pigment in the feathers of turacos.
turbid cloudy.
turbidimeter an apparatus for measuring turbidity of a solution.
turbidimetry the measurement of the turbidity of a liquid.
turbidity cloudiness; disturbance of solids (sediment) in a solution, so that it is not clear.
turbidometric emanating from or pertaining to turbidimetry.
turbinal, turbinate 1. shaped like a top. 2. turbinate bone (concha nasalis ossea).
turbinate atrophy see ATROPHIC rhinitis.
turbinate bones see Table 10.
turbinectomy excision of a turbinate bone (nasal concha).
turbinotomy incision of a turbinate bone.
turbulence filter the effect of the structure of the turbinates, trachea and bronchi in directing air flow against mucous membranes, serving to remove particulate matter from inspired air.
turbulent flow occurs in blood vessels where there is a stenosis or aneurysm or where there is a sudden increase in velocity; the laminar flow of normal tubes is disrupted and the fluid is randomly and completely mixed; turbulent flows have a greater apparent viscosity than laminar flows.
turgescence distension or swelling of a part.
turgescent becoming swollen.
turgid swollen and congested.
turgor the condition of being turgid; normal or other fullness.
Turino cattle Portuguese and Brazilian dairy cattle originated from Dutch Black Pied.
Türk cell see Türk's CELL.
turkey a bird in the family Meleagridae. The common

turkey is *Meleagris gallopavo*. There are two breeds, the American BRONZEWING and the WHITE HOLLAND. Bred entirely for meat mostly for human consumption on festive occasions.

t. berry see RIVINA HUMILIS.

t. bluecomb disease see turkey coronaviral ENTERITIS.

t. bordetellosis see turkey CORYZA.

t. bush MYOPORUM *deserti*.

t. coryza see turkey CORYZA.

t.-egg kidney a pale kidney covered with a large number of petechiae to give it the appearance of a turkey's egg; occurs in many septicemic diseases, particularly hog cholera, African swine fever and salmonellosis.

t. hemorrhagic enteritis an acute, infectious disease of turkeys 4 weeks old and older caused by a Group II avian adenovirus. Clinically there is illness for only 24 hours, bloody droppings and a mortality rate of up to 60%.

t. hepatitis a highly contagious disease of turkeys caused by an enterovirus. The disease is characterized by a high level of subclinical infection and sudden death in stressed birds. There is focal necrosis in the liver and pancreas.

t. herpesvirus antigenically related to Marek's disease virus (MDV) but not pathogenic in any species. Used to vaccinate chickens against Marek's disease. The infection is universal in domestic and wild turkey populations and is now widespread in chicken populations.

t. leg edema see leg EDEMA.

t. louse includes *Chelopistes meleagridis* (large turkey louse), *Colpocephalum tausi*, *Oxylipeurus polytrapezius* (slender turkey louse), *O. corpelentus*.

t. meningoencephalitis see Israeli turkey ENCEPHALOMYELITIS.

t. mullein see EREMOCARPUS SETIGERUS.

t. rhinotracheitis a catarrhal infection of the upper respiratory tract in young poults. In chickens, a similar disease is called swollen head syndrome. It is caused by a pneumovirus.

t. syndrome a common accompaniment of infection in 6-week-old turkey poults infected with *Mycoplasma meleagridis* and with airsacculitis as a result. The syndrome is characterized by deformity and shortening of the tarsometatarsal bone, hock joint swelling and deformity of cervical vertebrae. There may also be stunting of growth and abnormal feathering.

t. X disease the original name given to AFLATOXICOSIS.

Turkish Angora a small- to medium-sized cat originating in Turkey. It has a long, slender body with a flat, silky, wavy coat in any color.

turkish rue PEGANUM *harmala*.

Turkish Van an uncommon breed of domestic cats with a medium-length haircoat that is chalk white except where it is colored on the tail and in a few spots on the head. The breed is characterized by its attraction to water. Called also the swimming cat.

turnaround time in computer terminology, the time elapsed between submission of data to a computer bureau and the receipt of the result.

turned-in ears a defect in which the top part of the pinna is bent at an angle of 90° towards the animal's midline. A sporadic defect but also accompanies baldy calf disease (see also INHERITED EPIDERMAL DYSPLASIA).

turned-in toes a conformation defect in horses. May cause the gait to be abnormal and the horse to be subject to brushing or similar injury.

turned-out toes a conformation defect in horses because it may cause the gait to be very wide in front and therefore marginally inefficient.

Turner's (XO) syndrome see Turner's SYNDROME.

turning an obstetrical term for alteration of the presentation of a fetus in a dystocia. Called also version.

turning sickness an aberrant form of theileriasis in which parasitized lymphocytes cause emboli and hemorrhagic infarcts in central nervous tissue. *Theileria parva* is credited with causing the disease which is characterized by convulsive attacks of spinning followed by collapse and unconsciousness, or by a more chronic syndrome of circling, head pressing, incoordination and blindness.

turnip BRASSICA *rapa*.

t. rape BRASSICA *rapa* subsp. *campestris*.

t. stubble green top regrowth after the roots have been harvested. Used for grazing by ruminants but toxicity (nitrate–nitrite, hemolytic agent, goitrogen).

t. weed see RAPISTRUM RUGOSUM.

turnkey system a computer hardware–software package in which literally all that the user has to do is to switch on the computer and start typing. The seller of the program guarantees the validity of the program and its freedom from bugs, and the program prompts the user on what is the next step and the appropriate commands to use to effect it.

turnover the total of movement of an element or other body constituent in a given time, regardless of the gain or loss of the component.

iron t. much of the body's iron store is fixed in intracellular sites and is not available metabolically. The portion of the iron store that is available for mobilization into new sites is called the labile iron pool and may undergo a good deal of metabolic activity.

t. number see CATALYTIC CONSTANT.

turnsick see COENUROSIS.

turpentine a sticky oleoresin which exudes from *Pinus* spp. trees.

t. oil commercial extract from turpentine used as a solvent for waxes and varnishes. The active constituents are terpenes, α-pinene being the important one. In veterinary medicine has been used as a treatment for bloat in cattle and tympanitic colic in horses and as a constituent of general tonic drenches for cattle. Also has some use in stimulant ointments and liniments. Absorbed readily from the gut and the skin and is a significant poison for the kidney and intestine. Clinical signs of acute poisoning include colic, vomiting, diarrhea, incoordination and excitement followed by coma.

t. weed see GUTIERREZIA *microcephala*.

Turraea robusta an African tree in the plant family Meliaceae; the juice of the leaves is used as a treatment for diarrhea and as an anthelmintic, but the effective agent has not been identified. Overdosing causes dyspnea, ruminal stasis, diarrhea and apathy.

Tursiops truncatus bottle-nosed DOLPHIN.

turtle a reptile, member of the order Chelonia; most are aquatic or semiaquatic, fresh water or marine, but lay eggs on land. They have webbed feet or flippers and their body is covered by a horny shell from which only the legs, head and neck, and tail protrude when needed. The upper shell is called the carapace and the undershell the plastron.

There are inconsistencies in terminology. In the USA 'turtle' is used broadly for all reptiles with a shell, 'terrapin' applies to a large family, Emydidae, and 'tortoise' refers to the slow moving terrestial species (the land turtles) that enter water only to drink or soak. In Great Britain and Australia 'tortoise' is applied generally to all members of the group except the marine species with paddle-shaped limbs which are called 'turtles'. 'Terrapin' is often used to describe the young tortoises commonly sold as aquarium pets.

Includes genera *Chelonia*, e.g. *C. mydas* (green turtle), *Testudo*, e.g. *T. graeca* (spur-thighed tortoise), *T. hermanni* (Hermann's tortoise), *Gopherus*, e.g. *G. agassizi* (desert tortoise), *Clemmys*, e.g. *C. marmorata* (Pacific pond turtle), *Chrysemys*, e.g. *C. picta* (painted turtle), *Platemys*, e.g. *P. platycephala* (Bolivian side-neck turtle).

tush canine tooth in a horse.

tusk the well-developed canine tooth in the male pig and similar large projecting teeth in some wild species. They are open-rooted so that they continue to grow. The upper and lower ones in the pig have growth directions that brings them together in such a way that they sharpen each other as the jaws move. Elephant tusks are modified incisor teeth, with the ivory being dentine.

tussigenic causing cough.

tussis [L.] *cough.*

tussive pertaining to or due to a cough.

tutamen pl. *tutamina* [L.] a protective covering or structure.

tutamina oculi the protecting appendages of the eye, as the eyelids, eyelashes, etc.

tutin the toxic principle in the tree CORIARIA *arborea.*

Tuttle forceps thumb-type tissue forceps with the tips of the blades formed as loops lying at right angles to the line of closure.

tutu CORIARIA *arborea.*

TV tidal volume.

TVO tractor vaporizing oil.

TVT transmissible venereal tumor.

Tween-80 a proprietary name for a non-ionic surfactant use as an emusifier.

T.-80 hydrolysis a test used to differentiate *Corynebacterium cystitidis* from other corynebacteria.

twiggy midge bush see ZIERIA *laevigata.*

twin one of the two same-age fetuses in the one pregnancy. See also TWINS, TWINNING.

twin-lamb disease see PREGNANCY TOXEMIA.

twin leaf see ZYGOPHYLLUM.

twin-leaf senna CASSIA *roemeriana.*

twinning 1. the production of symmetrical structures or parts by division. 2. the simultaneous intrauterine production of two or more embryos. Twinning is a desirable feature in animals that depend for their profitability on the production of young, e.g. lambs of the meat-producing breeds, and selection for the characteristic is a standard husbandry strategy. In animals that are essentially uniparous, e.g. mares, twins represent a danger to the foals and to the mare. Twins in which one is a female and one a male have the added risk of the female being a FREEMARTIN.

twins two offspring produced in the same pregnancy. See also dizygotic and monozygotic twins (below).

conjoined t's fused, symmetrical twins formed by incomplete division of one embryo into two components. See also SIAMESE TWINS.

discordant t's a particular trait is present in only one of the twins.

dissimilar t. dizygotic twins (below).

dizygotic t's those that develop from two separate ova fertilized at the same time. They may be of the same sex or of opposite sexes, and are no more similar than any other two offspring of the same parents. Called also fraternal, binovular, dichorial, dissimilar and unlike twins.

fraternal t's dizygotic twins.

free symmetrical monozygotic t's see identical twins (below).

identical t's derived initially from a single zygote; placentas may be shared or separate.

impacted t's twins so situated during delivery that pressure of one against the other produces simultaneous engagement in the birth canal of both.

induced t. produced experimentally in ruminants using PMSG or FSH, or by immunization against androstenedione.

monovular t. see monozygotic twins (below).

monozygotic t's those which develop from a single ovum that divides after fertilization. Because they share the same set of chromosomes, they are always of the same sex, and are remarkably similar in haircoat color and pattern, teeth, and other respects. Monozygotic twins have exactly the same blood type and can accept tissue or organ transplants from each other. May be free and symmetrical, free and asymmetrical, cojoined and symmetrical or cojoined and asymmetrical. Called also identical, enzygotic, monochorial, mono-ovular, similar, or true twins.

Siamese t's cojoined twins. See also SIAMESE TWINS.

similar t. see monozygotic twins (above).

symmetrical t's twins of equal size, age and stage of development.

true t. see monozygotic twins (above).

unequal t's twins of which one is incompletely developed, called also asymmetric twins.

unlike t. see dizygotic twins (above).

twist disease a disease of salmonid fish, especially rainbow trout, caused by infection with the protozoan parasite MYXOSOMA *cerebralis* which erodes the skeleton especially the cranium. Affected fish lose their balance and chase their tails when startled. Survivors are usually badly deformed.

twisted leg a sporadic disease of fowls and turkeys of unknown etiology and low incidence in many flocks. There is deformity of the small tarsal bones and a resulting inward bending and twisting usually of only one leg.

twitch 1. a brief, contractile response of a skeletal muscle elicited by a single maximal volley of impulses in the neurons supplying it. 2. a device used in the restraint of horses; there are a great many designs. The standard twitch consists of a loop of cord or chain at the end of a short, 2 ft (0.6 m), wooden handle. A fold of muzzle is enclosed in the loop which is then screwed tight. The handle may be held by an assistant or tied to the halter.

Galvayne's t. a loop of soft rope is passed over the poll and through the mouth, below the upper lip but in front of and above the incisor teeth.

halter t. the shank of the halter is passed over the poll and back to the near side through the mouth and then through the halter again.

human t. for restraining horses, it consists of a hinged metal device which is placed over the upper lip and clipped to the halter.

leg t. a tourniquet applied above the carpal joint.

loop t. a loop in a soft rope is passed over the poll and through the mouth above the tongue and pulled tight.

Martingale t. see HUMANE twitch.

screw t. has the same effect as the standard twitch but the loop is of rigid metal and it is closed by screwing a bar up to clamp the fold of muzzle skin.

twitching the occurrence of a single contraction or a series of contractions of a muscle.

two-grooved milk vetch ASATRAGALUS *bisulcatus.*

two-leaf cape tulip HOMERIA *miniata*.
two-stage prothrombin test see PROTHROMBIN time test.
two-tailed test a test in which both 'large' and 'small' values of the test statistic indicate that the null hypothesis is not correct.
two tooth sheep with only the two central incisors erupted; average just over one year old.
two-way cross the male parent-to-be comes from one population, the female from another.
two-year-old a horse aged between 2 and 3 years, the age dating from the horse's date of birth. In racehorses the birth date of the horse is as determined by the local racing authority as the birthday of all horses.
Tx treatment.
TXA_2 thromboxane.
tying-up syndrome a disease in which horses become stiff in their limbs while performing exercise, or soon afterwards. The stiffness and soreness may be so severe that the horse cannot move. The creatine–phosphokinase and other relevant serum enzyme levels are very high. The disability is likely to be a permanent characteristic of an individual horse. Called also transient exertional rhabdomyolysis, polymyositis.
Tylecodon southern African genus in plant family Crassulaceae; contains bufadienolide cardiac glycosides; causes KRIMPSIEKTE (cotyledonosis); includes *T. cacalioides*, *T. grandiflorus*, *T. paniculatus*, *T. ventricosus*, *T. wallichii*. Previously COTYLEDON spp.
tylenol see ACETAMINOPHEN.
tyloma a callus or callosity.
interdigital t. see INTERDIGITAL fibroma.
tylosin an antibiotic produced by cultures of *Streptomyces fradiae*, with a structure similar to erythromycin. It is effective against gram-positive bacteria generally and especially those susceptible to members of the macrolide group.
tylosis formation of callosities.
tyloxapol a nonionic liquid polymer used as a surfactant to aid liquefaction and removal of mucopurulent bronchopulmonary secretions; administered by inhalation.
tympanal pertaining to the tympanum or to the tympanic membrane.
tympanectomy excision of the tympanic membrane.
tympanic 1. of or pertaining to the tympanum. 2. bell-like; resonant.
t. cavity middle ear.
t. membrane a thin, semitransparent membrane, nearly oval in shape, that stretches across the ear canal separating the middle ear from the external acoustic meatus (outer ear); called also the eardrum. It is composed of fibrous tissue, covered with skin on the outside and mucous membrane on the inside. It is constructed so that it can vibrate freely with audible sound waves that travel inward from outside. The manubrium (handle) of the malleus (hammer) of the middle ear is attached to the center of the tympanic membrane and receives the vibrations collected by the membrane, transmitting them to other bones of the middle ear (the incus and stapes) and eventually to the fluid of the inner ear.
t. membrane (secondary) the membrane enclosing the fenestra cochlearis; called also Scarpa's membrane.
t. nerve see Table 14.
t. plexus see tympanic PLEXUS.
t. ossicles see auditory OSSICLES.
tympanism, tympanites drumlike distension of the abdomen due to air or gas in the intestine or peritoneal cavity.
tympanites tympanism.
tympanitic 1. pertaining to or affected with tympanites. 2. bell-like; tympanic.
tympanitis otitis media.
tympanocentesis surgical puncture of the tympanic membrane or tympanum.
tympanogenic arising from the tympanum or middle ear.
tympanogram a graphic representation of the relative compliance and impedance of the tympanic membrane and ossicles of the middle ear obtained by tympanometry.
tympanohyoid the terminal segment in the chain of skeletal elements of the hyoid apparatus. One of a pair of rods of cartilage that connect the hyoid bone to the styloid process of the petrous part of the temporal bone.
tympanometry indirect measurement of the compliance (mobility) and impedance of the tympanic membrane and ossicles of the middle ear; it is done by subjecting the external acoustic meatus to positive, normal and negative air pressure and monitoring the resultant sound energy flow.
tympanosclerosis a condition characterized by the presence of masses of hard, dense connective tissue around the auditory ossicles in the middle ear.
tympanotomy myringotomy.
tympanous distended with gas.
tympanum 1. the part of the cavity of the middle ear, in the temporal bone, just medial to the tympanic membrane. 2. the tympanic membrane itself.
tympany 1. tympanitis. 2. a tympanic, or bell-like, percussion note. 3. distension of a hollow viscus with gas.
crop t. see pendulous CROP.
gastric t. see gastric dilatation COLIC.
intestinal t. see INTESTINAL tympany, INTESTINAL dilatation.
ruminal t. see RUMINAL tympany.
secondary t. ruminal tympany secondary to some other condition, e.g. traumatic reticulitis, vagus indigestion, esophageal obstruction.
Tyndall effect the light reflected by particles suspended in a gas or liquid. Called also Tyndall light phenomenon.
Tyndall light phenomenon see TYNDALL EFFECT.
type 1. the general or prevailing character of any particular case of disease, microorganism, person, substance, etc. 2. to determine or assign a character or category.
blood t's see BLOOD GROUP.
t. I to t. IV hypersensitivity see HYPERSENSITIVITY.
t. 1 muscle fiber slow twitch MUSCLE fiber.
t. 2 muscle fiber fast twitch MUSCLE fiber.
wild t. the normal or naturally occurring phenotype of an organism.
type 1 error an error which occurs when using data from a sample which demonstrates a statistically significant association when no such association is present in the population.
type 2 error an error which occurs when using data from a sample that fails to demonstrate a specific association when such association is present in the population.
typhlectasis distension of the cecum.
typhlectomy ablation of the cecum.
typhlitis cecitis.
typhl(o)- word element. [Gr.] *cecum, blindness.*
Typhlocoelium see TRACHEOPHILUS.
typhlocolitis inflammation of the cecum and colon.
typhlodicliditis inflammation of the ileocecal valve.

typhlolithiasis the presence of calculi in the cecum.
typhlopid a blind snake that burrows; about 10 inches long and looking like a polished, scaly worm; nonvenomous. Member of the family Typhlopidae. Called also worm snake.
typhloproctostomy a fistula between the rectum and the cecum.
typhlotomy incision of the cecum.
typhoid 1. resembling typhus. 2. typhoid fever, an infectious disease of humans caused by *Salmonella typhi*.
mouse t. salmonellosis.
typhus acute infectious diseases caused by *Rickettsia* which are usually transmitted from infected rats and other rodents to humans by lice, fleas, ticks and mites.
Abyssinian tick t. see BOUTONNEUSE FEVER.
canine t., canine tick t. see canine EHRLICHIOSIS.
epidemic t. see RICKETTSIA *prowazeki*.
Kenya t. see BOUTONNEUSE FEVER.
murine t. a disease of humans caused by *Rickettsia typhae*; rats and cats are the mammalian reservoir.
Queensland tick t. caused by *Rickettsia australis*. See QUEENSLAND TICK TYPHUS.
Sao Paulo t. see ROCKY MOUNTAIN SPOTTED FEVER.
scrub t. caused by *Rickettsia tsutsugamushi*. Wild rodents and occasionally dogs may be hosts.
typing in transplantation and transfusion immunology, a method of measuring the degree of organ, solid tissue, or blood compatibility between two individuals, in which specific histocompatibility antigens (e.g. those present on leukocytes) or other cell surface antigens, e.g. red blood cell antigens, are detected by means of suitable immune serum.
blood t. determining the antigenic determinants present on the surface of red blood cells by using specific antibodies (typing serums). See also BLOOD GROUP.
phage t. see PHAGE typing.
tissue t. see TISSUE typing.
typology the study of types; the science of classifying, as bacteria according to type.
Tyr tyrosine.
tyramine 1. a decarboxylation product of tyrosine, which may be converted to cresol and phenol, found in decayed animal tissue, ripe cheese, and ergot. Closely related structurally to epinephrine and norepinephrine, it has a similar but weaker action. 2. *N*-methyl-β-phenylethyamine, a toxic amine found in *Acacia berlandieri* and mistletoes.
Tyrell hook a very small, blunt-pointed, handheld instrument for moving the iris during ophthalmic surgery.
tyrocidin a bactericidal polypeptide antibiotic used in topical preparations.
tyrogenous originating in cheese.
Tyroglyphus a genus of mites in the family Acaridae. Parasites of grain and other vegetable matter and only parasitize animals accidentally. They cause itching and occasionally a mild dermatitis. The infestation is usually self-limiting.
***T. farinae* (syn. *Acarus farinae*)** lives in cheeses and grain.
***T. siro* (syn. *Acarus siro*)** the cheese mite; also infests grain and may cause diarrhea.
tyroid of cheesy consistency; caseous.
Tyrol Grey cattle silver-gray, multiple purpose cattle, from Austrian Tyrol.
tyroma a caseous tumor.
tyromatosis a condition characterized by caseous degeneration.
tyropanoate a radiopaque contrast medium for use in oral cholecystography.
Tyrophagus a genus of mites in the family Acaridae.
T. farinae housedust mites; common in stored cereal; thought to be associated with allergic dermatitis.
T. longior found in grains and copra. The cause of copra itch in humans.
T. palmarum a pasture mite found in the nostrils of cattle, especially those with nasal granuloma.
tyrosinase an enzyme important in the production of melanin from tyrosine. Deficiency has been reported in Chow Chows where it is transient and is associated with hypopigmentation of the oral mucosa and hair.
tyrosine, tyrosin Tyr; a naturally occurring amino acid present in most proteins; it is a product of phenylalanine metabolism and a precursor of melanin, catecholamines and thyroid hormones.
t. hydroxylase an oxidase which converts tyrosine to DOPA.
t. tolerance test used as a test of liver function but about 85% of liver parenchyma must be lost before the test gives a positive reaction.
tyrosine-specific kinases enzymes that phosphorylate specific tyrosine residues in proteins. Part of the insulin–receptor complex as well as several other growth factor receptors. Binding of the hormones leads to stimulation of the kinase activity. Associated with certain oncogene and proto-oncogene products.
tyrosinemia an excess of tyrosine in the blood. Several different types with varying clinical features occur in humans. A syndrome of dermatitis and keratoconjunctivitis resembling tyrosinemia type II of humans (Richner–Hanhart syndrome) occurs in rats fed a diet high in tyrosine, in mink as an inherited disorder (called also pseudodistemper) and it has been reported in a dog.
tyrosinosis a condition characterized by a faulty metabolism of tyrosine in which an intermediate product, parahydroxyphenyl pyruvic acid, appears in the urine and gives it an abnormal reducing power.
tyrosinuria the presence of tyrosine in the urine.
tyrosis CASEATION (2).
tyrosyluria increased urinary secretion of parahydroxyphenyl compounds derived from tyrosine, as in tyrosinuria.
tyrothricin a mixture of tyrocidins and gramicidins used for topical or intramammary application.
tyrotoxism poisoning from a toxin present in milk or cheese.
Tyzzeria a genus of protozoa in the family Eimeriidae. They are intracellular parasites in the intestinal epithelium.
T. alleni found in teal.
T. anseris found in domestic and wild geese.
T. pellerdyi found in wild birds.
T. perniciosa found in domestic duck.
Tyzzer's disease a fatal necrotizing hepatitis caused by *Clostridium piliforme*. Sporadic cases only. Recorded in foals and cats. Signs are severe diarrhea, jaundice and high serum levels of liver enzymes. Probably the commonest disease of gerbils, in which it is usually subclinical, but it can cause an acute disease characterized by death in young or stressed individuals.
tzaneen disease a mild disease of cattle without apparent clinical signs, caused by *Theileria mutans*.
tzetze tsetse.

U

U chemical symbol, *uranium*; unit; uracil.
U-suture interrupted horizontal mattress suture.
U wave seen in the human electrocardiogram; represents repolarization of Purkinje cells.
UAA ochre CODON, one of the three stop codons.
UAG amber CODON, one of the three stop codons.
uakari small, 2 ft, short, bushy-tailed, bald-faced New World monkey; brightly colored. Called also *Cacajao* spp.
Uasin gishu disease a viral disease of horses in Kenya. Highly contagious, large lesions and a generalized cutaneous eruption with a pathology similar to that of molluscum contagiosum of humans. There is a poxvirus similar to vaccinia associated with the disease.
Uberreiter's syndrome see chronic superficial KERATITIS.
ubiquinol the form of ubiquinone when reduced by two electrons.
ubiquinone coenzyme Q; component of the electron-transfer chain of oxidative phosphorylation.
ubiquitin heat shock (cell stress) protein present in mammalian cytosol; attaches to other cytosolic proteins and marks them for degradation either by specific proteases or by lysosomal enzymes.
U.D. Utility Dog; the highest level degree or title, after C.D. and C.D.X., awarded in obedience trial competition.
udder mammary gland of farm animals. The cow has four quarters and four teats. The rest of the ruminants and the mare have two. The sow may have as many as 18. See also MAMMARY gland, MASTITIS, TEAT.
u. abscesses these form at the base of the teat and are usually associated with summer mastitis.
u. acne see udder impetigo (below).
u. amputation done in cows with severe mastitis or rupture of the suspensory apparatus (below).
u. caking a plaque of hard tissue in the floor of the udder in a cow just calved. Makes milking difficult but frequent handmilking and hot water fomentation reduces the swelling. See also BLUE BREAST.
u. dermatitis see INTERTRIGO; FLEXURAL seborrhea.
u. development failure congenital defect of no mammary development in a female.
u. edema late and recent calving are often accompanied by edema of the udder and the subcutaneous tissue immediately in front of the udder. The swelling may be great enough to prevent the cow being milked or suckled and it may interfere with the cow moving about. Compression of the vascular drainage from the area probably contributes to the condition but there are obviously other unidentified factors which cause a very serious disability in only a few cows in a herd, all of which are being treated in exactly the same way.
u. impetigo staphylococcal dermatitis of the skin of the teats and lower udder. Transmissible between cows and to human attendants at milking.
u. inflation useful but no longer used farmer treatment for milk fever in cows; air, filtered through a layer of sterile gauze, was pumped into each of the four quarters of the patient by a hand-operated pump through a rubber tube attached to a teat siphon. Pumping ceased when air began to leak out past the teat siphon. If the teats were tied off with tape the ties were removed after 20 minutes. The back pressure of the air stopped further loss of calcium from the patient's blood which then regained a safe level of calcium.
u. infusion antibiotic or other antibacterial in water or, almost exclusively, an ointment base used to convey the medication, from the individual container, via the teat canal into the mammary tissue.
u. infusion tube see TEAT tube.
u. kinch a form of restraint by twitch. A loop of rope is made around the cow's abdomen just in front of the udder but the belly of the rope is passed around the udder base before the noose is tightened.
u. suspensory apparatus in the cow consists of two median sheets of yellow elastic tissue attached to the pelvic symphysis by its symphysial tendon and two less substantial lateral sheets of white fibrous tissue; all four sheets serve to suspend the udder from the pelvic skeleton.
u. symmetry the front pair and the mammary glands in the two hind quarters are very similar in shape and size; asymmetry usually indicates mastitis in an early hypertrophic stage, or a later atrophic stage.
u.-thigh dermatitis see FLEXURAL seborrhea.
u. washing see TEAT sanitization.
UDP uridine diphosphate.
UDP-G-pyrophosphorylase an enzyme that synthesizes uridine diphosphoglucose as part of glycogenesis.
UDP-galactose urinary diphosphate-galactose participates in the modification of procollagen.
UDP-glucose activated form of glucose required for glycosyltransferase reactions.
UGA opal CODON, one of the three stop codons.
Uhl's anomaly congenital hypoplasia of the myocardium of the right ventricle.
uitpeuloog a contagious disease of the eyes in ruminants and horses caused by the larvae of the fly GEDOELSTIA.
Ukrainian whiteheaded cattle red or black dairy cattle with white head, feet and belly; originated from Dutch Groningen whitehead plus local Ukrainian cattle.
Ulcardo melon CUCUMIS *melo* subsp. *agrestis*.
ulcer a local defect, or excavation of the surface of an organ or tissue, produced by sloughing of necrotic inflammatory tissue. They occur in all organs and tissues and are to be found under those headings, e.g. ABOMASAL, CORNEAL, GASTRIC.
button u. see BUTTON ulcer.
callous u. see SET-FAST (2).
collagenase u. a rapidly expanding, erosive ('melting') corneal ulcer, seen particularly in brachycephalic breeds of dogs.
Curling's u. acute ulceration of the stomach or duodenum seen after severe burns of the body in humans.
decubitus u. see DECUBITUS ulcer.
dendritic u. linear, branching pattern of ulceration on the cornea; characteristic of herpesvirus infections. See also herpetic KERATITIS.
eosinophilic u. see EOSINOPHILIC ulcer.
gastroduodenal u. common in foals 1–3 months old. Many are asymptomatic. Clinical cases manifest by mild, intermittent colic. See also GASTRIC ulcer, DUODENAL ulcer.
geographic u. a large, superficial, irregularly shaped corneal ulcer, typically formed by the coalescence of several dendritic ulcers.
indolent u. see EOSINOPHILIC ulcer, refractory ulcer (below).

infectious dermal u. a systemic, fatal bacteremia of snakes manifested by multiple, small cutaneous ulcers. Called also scale rot.

intestinal u. is rare in all species. When they do occur, intestinal ulcers usually cause signs of chronic enteritis. It is a common lesion in adenocarcinoma of the intestine. See also PEPTIC ulcer.

lip u. see EOSINOPHILIC ulcer.

lip and leg u. see ULCERATIVE dermatosis.

melting u. see collagenase ulcer (above).

u. mound a gastric ulcer viewed tangentially radiographically creates a mound in the otherwise smooth outline of radiopaque material in the stomach.

necrotic u. of swine see ULCERATIVE granuloma of swine.

perforating u. one that involves the entire thickness of an organ, creating an opening on both surfaces. See also ulcer PERFORATION.

phagedenic u. a necrotizing lesion in which tissue destruction is prominent.

refractory u. a chronic, superficial corneal ulceration in dogs, particularly common in Boxers, that extends into the superfical stroma, often undermining epithelium at the edges. The cause is unknown but abnormalities of the basal epithelial cells and anterior stroma have been noted. Response to the usual methods of treatment for corneal ulceration is characteristically very slow; superficial keratectomy is the treatment of choice. Called also superficial corneal erosion syndrome, Boxer ulcer.

rodent u. see EOSINOPHILIC ulcer.

stress u. superficial ulcerations or erosions of mucosa in the stomach, duodenum or colon. The possible predisposing factors include changes in the microcirculation of the gastric mucosa, increased permeability of the gastric mucosa barrier to H+, and impaired cell proliferation.

stromal u. a corneal ulcer involving the stroma.

trophic u. one due to imperfect nutrition of the part.

ulcerate to undergo ulceration.

ulceration 1. formation or development of an ulcer. 2. an ulcer.

ulcerative pertaining to or characterized by ulceration.

u. balanitis see ENZOOTIC balanoposthitis.

u. cellulitis see ulcerative LYMPHANGITIS.

u. colitis see eosinophilic ulcerative COLITIS, histiocytic ulcerative COLITIS.

u. dermal necrosis a skin disease of the head of Atlantic salmon and sea trout as they enter fresh water from the sea. The cause is unknown.

u. dermatitis disease of Belgian Landrace sows; lesions occur on the ear margins, anterior aspects of the limbs and around the teats; the cause is unknown.

u. dermatosis an infectious ulceration of the skin of the lips, feet, legs and external genitalia of sheep, of uncertain etiology, caused possibly by a paravaccinia virus. The lesions are ulcerative and destructive but the disease is not fatal and the morbidity rate is not high.

u. enteritis see ulcerative ENTERITIS.

u. gingivitis see necrotizing ulcerative GINGIVITIS.

u. glossitis, stomatitis in cats, a proliferative inflammation and ulceration of the oral cavity, particularly gum margins and mucosa at the fauces, a common disease of old cats characterized by painful ulcers at the fauces and surrounding tissues including the tongue. The cause is not known.

u. granuloma of swine an infectious disease of pigs caused by *Borrelia suilla* (unofficial nomenclature), and manifested by large, deep, ulcerative lesions on any part of the body. On the face they may cause destruction of the cheeks. The portal of infection is skin wounds and spread of the disease is enhanced by fighting in the group. Called also necrotic ulcer.

infectious bovine u. stomatitis an innocuous stomatitis of calves occurring in outbreak form but recorded rarely and not in recent years. Its existence separate from bovine virus diarrhea is not proven.

u. keratitis see CORNEAL ulcer.

u. lymphangitis see ulcerative LYMPHANGITIS.

u. mammilitis see bovine herpes MAMMILLITIS.

u. pododermatosis see ulcerative PODODERMATITIS.

u. posthitis occurs sporadically in rams and bulls and as part of ulcerative dermatosis in rams.

u. shell disease see SHELL ROT.

u. stomatitis 1. several virus infections cause oral ulcers in calves without any other clinical illness unless the calves are stressed, especially with hyperkeratosis caused by secondary nutritional deficiency of vitamin A. 2. outbreaks in horses are caused by grass with bristly seedheads and pasture infested with bristly caterpillars.

u. typhlocolitis one of the causes of idiopathic chronic diarrhea in horses; salmonellosis and intoxication with nonsteroidal anti-inflammatory drugs are possible culprits.

u. vulvitis of ewes, see ulcerative dermatosis (above).

ulcerogangrenous characterized by both ulceration and gangrene.

ulcerogenic causing ulceration; leading to the production of ulcers.

ulceromembranous characterized by ulceration and a membranous exudation.

u. stomatitis the gums are inflamed and bleed easily, ulcers develop and there are pseudomembranes over necrotic areas of gingival mucosa. Slimy brown, smelly saliva drools from the mouth and stains the forelimbs.

ulcerous 1. of the nature of an ulcer. 2. affected with ulceration.

ulcus pl. *ulcera* [L.] ulcer.

-ule suffix meaning a small.

ulectomy 1. excision of scar tissue. 2. excision of the gingiva; gingivectomy.

ulegyria a wrinkled appearance of the cerebral cortex resulting from scarring and atrophy.

Ulex europaeus a weedy shrub; member of the family Fabaceae; sometimes used as feed in times of shortage; contains ulexine a nerve and muscle poison but seldom causes poisoning. Called also furze, gorse.

ulitis inflammation of the gums.

ulna together with the radius, forms the skeleton of the forearm. See Table 10.

ulnad toward the ulna.

ulnar pertaining to the ulna; the medial aspect of the upper forelimb, as opposed to the radial or lateral aspect.

congenital lateral rotation of the u. seen in puppies from one to five months of age; they stand with the elbow flexed and the forearm markedly pronated.

u. nerve block injection of a local anesthetic in the caudal aspect of the forelimb, proximal to the carpus, produces anesthesia on the anterolateral aspect of the metacarpus.

u. nerve injury results in extension of the carpus, a 'dropped' carpus.

ulnaris [L.] *ulnar*.

ulnocarpal pertaining to the ulna and carpus.

ulnoradial pertaining to the ulna and radius.
ulocace ulceration of the gums.
ulocarcinoma carcinoma of the gums.
uloglossitis inflammation of the gums and tongue; gingivoglossitis.
uloncus swelling of the gums.
ulorrhagia a sudden discharge of blood from the gums.
ulotomy 1. incision of scar tissue. 2. incision of the gums.
ultimobranchial pertaining to the tissue originating from the fifth pharyngeal pouch of the embryo.
u. body the glandular tissue originating from the fifth branchial pouch which combines with the buccal cavity outgrowth to form the thyroid and contributes calcitonin-secreting cells to the gland.
u. duct cysts derived from remnants of the ultimobranchial body and found in the thyroid gland.
u. tumor a neoplasm containing thyroid C cells.
ultra- word element. [L.] *beyond, excess*.
ultracentrifugation subjection of material to an exceedingly high centrifugal force, which will separate and sediment the molecules of a substance or subcellular components.
ultracentrifuge the centrifuge used in ultracentrifugation.
ultradian pertaining to a period of less than 24 hours; applied to the rhythmic repetition of certain phenomena in living organisms occurring in cycles of less than a day (ultradian rhythm).
ultrafilter the filter used in ultrafiltration.
ultrafiltrate substances which pass through an ultrafilter, i.e. a semipermeable membrane through which the filtrate passes under pressure.
ultrafiltration filtration through a filter capable of removing colloidal particles from a dispersion medium, as in the filtration of plasma at the capillary membrane.
ultraheat heating to a very high temperature for a very brief period.
u. treated milk milk heated at 175° to 200°F (79° to 93°C) for a few seconds.
ultramicroscopic too small to be seen with the ordinary light microscope.
ultrasonic beyond the audible range; relating to sound waves having a frequency of more than 20,000 cycles per second.
u. cleaning surgical instruments can be thoroughly cleaned by the use of ultrasonic waves which cause the formation of minute gas bubbles which, when they collapse, form shock waves.
u. heating the use of ultrasound for producing localized hyperthermia.
u. pregnancy diagnosis see ULTRASONOGRAPHY.
u. probe used to disintegrate masses internally, e.g. the optic lens.
u. tooth scaling the use of vibrations to remove supragingival calculus. See ultrasonic SCALER.
ultrasonics that part of the science of acoustics dealing with the frequency range beyond the upper limit of perception by the human ear (above 20,000 cycles per second), but usually restricted to frequencies above 50,000 hertz. Ultrasonic radiation is injurious to tissues because of its thermal effects when absorbed by living matter, but in controlled doses it is used therapeutically to selectively break down pathological tissues, as in treatment of arthritis and lesions of the nervous system, and also as a diagnostic aid by visually displaying echoes received from irradiated tissues, as in ECHOCARDIOGRAPHY and echoencephalography. See also ULTRASONOGRAPHY.
ultrasonogram the record obtained by ultrasonography.
ultrasonography an imaging technique in which deep structures of the body are visualized by recording the reflections (echoes) of ultrasonic waves directed into the tissues.

Frequencies in the range of 1 million to 10 million hertz are used in diagnostic ultrasonography. The lower frequencies provide a greater depth of penetration and are used to examine abdominal organs; those in the upper range provide less penetration and are used predominantly to examine more superficial structures such as the eye.

The basic principle of ultrasonography is the same as that of depth-sounding in oceanographic studies of the ocean floor. The ultrasonic waves are confined to a narrow beam that may be transmitted through, refracted, absorbed, or reflected by the medium toward which they are directed, depending on the nature of the surface they strike.

In diagnostic ultrasonography the ultrasonic waves are produced by electrically stimulating a piezoelectric crystal called a *transducer*. As the beam strikes an interface or boundary between tissues of varying acoustic impedance (e.g. muscle and blood) some of the sound waves are reflected back to the transducer as echoes. The echoes are then converted into electrical impulses that are displayed on an oscilloscope, presenting a 'picture' of the tissues under examination.

Ultrasonography can be utilized in examination of the heart (echocardiography) and in identifying size and structural changes in organs in the abdominopelvic cavity. It is, therefore, of value in identifying and distinguishing cancers and benign cysts. The technique also may be used to evaluate tumors and foreign bodies of the eye, and to demonstrate retinal detachment. Ultrasonography is not, however, of much value in examination of the lungs because ultrasound waves do not pass through structures that contain air.

A particularly important use of ultrasonography is in the field of obstetrics and gynecology. It is a fast, relatively safe, and reliable technique for diagnosing pregnancy, and for detecting some typical fetal anomalies.
A-mode u. (amplitude modulation) that in which on the cathode-ray tube (CRT) display one axis represents the time required for the return of the echo and the other corresponds to the strength of the echo, as in echoencephalography.
B-mode u. (brightness modulation) that in which the position of a spot on the CRT display corresponds to the time elapsed (and thus to the position of the echogenic surface) and the brightness of the spot to the strength of the echo; movement of the transducer produces a sweep of the ultrasound beam and a tomographic scan of a cross-section of the body.
Doppler u. see DOPPLER ULTRASOUND.
endoscopic u. a high resolution ultrasound transducer, mounted on a flexible endoscope, can be used to gain images from within a hollow organ, such as the gastrointestinal tract. This overcomes some of the problems ingesta and fecal material cause in other methods of ultrasound examination.
gray-scale u. B-mode ultrasonography in which the strength of echoes is indicated by a proportional brightness of the displayed dots.
M-mode u. (motion mode) a type of B-mode ultrasonography in which spots on the CRT display pro-

duce a tracing of the motion of echogenic objects. Used in echocardiography.

real-time u. B-mode ultrasonography using an array of detectors so that scans can be made electronically at a rate of 30 frames a second, thus giving a true display of motion, such as that of the heart.

ultrasound mechanical radiant energy of a frequency greater than 20,000 cycles per second; used in veterinary medicine in the technique of ULTRASONOGRAPHY.

u. artifacts see ARTIFACT.

ultrastructure the structure visible under the electron microscope.

ultraviolet denoting electromagnetic radiation of wavelength shorter than that of the violet end of the spectrum, having wavelengths of 4–400 nanometers.

u. antisepsis because ultraviolet rays are capable of killing bacteria and other microorganisms, they are sometimes utilized in specially designed cabinets to sterilize objects, and may also be used to sterilize the air in operating rooms and other areas where destruction of bacteria is necessary.

u. irradiation the projection of ultraviolet light from a generator is used for the treatment of skin disease and for sterilization of materials.

u. rays electromagnetic radiation beyond the violet end of the visible spectrum (at 0.39 to 0.18 μm wavelength) and therefore not visible to humans. They are produced by the sun but are absorbed to a large extent by particles of dust and smoke in the earth's atmosphere. They are also produced by the so-called sun lamps.

Ultraviolet rays can produce sun-burning and affect skin pigmentation. When they strike the skin surface, these rays transform provitamin D, secreted by the glands of the skin, into vitamin D, which is then absorbed into the body.

u. therapy the employment of ultraviolet radiation in the treatment of various diseases, particularly those affecting the skin, is used in humans, but not commonly employed in veterinary medicine.

-um, -us suffix which creates a noun (indicates the presence of).

umbilical pertaining to the umbilicus.

u. abscess see URACHAL abscess.

u. clamp used in calves and foals for the closed method of herniorrhaphy. Consists of two lightweight bars that can be screwed together very tightly. The herniated gut is evacuated from the hernia and the clamp applied to as much of the hernial pouch as can be included. The tissue beyond the clamp sloughs and the clamp can be removed.

u. cord see umbilical CORD.

u. cord infection see OMPHALITIS.

u. diverticulum an evagination of the bowel wall at the vestigial point of attachment of the yolk sac. Called also Meckel's diverticulum.

u. gas gangrene umbilicus infected with *Clostridium septicum*, *C. oedematiens*.

u. hemorrhage a specific syndrome in newborn piglets. Bleeding from fleshy navel, also from ear notching, causes fatal anemia. The cause is unknown.

u. hernia protrusion of abdominal contents through the abdominal wall at the umbilicus, the defect in the abdominal wall and protruding intestine being covered with skin and subcutaneous tissue. Occurs sporadically in all species and inherited in cattle and some breeds of dogs. Soft swelling at umbilicus is reducible into the abdomen through a palpable ring. May accompany omphalitis.

u. hernia strangulation the intestinal loop in the hernia becomes incarcerated with its lumen occluded and its blood supply compromised.

u. inflammation see OMPHALITIS.

u. occlusion as when the umbilical cord is trapped between the fetus and the wall of the birth canal, causing loss of the fetal blood supply.

u. sinus created by persistence of only the distal end of the intraembryonic allantoic stalk at the umbilicus.

u. tape cotton tape, about 0.5 inch, with two selvedge edges. Used to tie off an umbilicus in calves and foals.

u. vein one of a pair of veins which return oxygenated blood from the placenta through the umbilical cord to the ductus venosus and thence to the heart.

u. vein infection see OMPHALOPHLEBITIS.

u. vein abscess residual after subsidence of acute omphalophlebitis.

umbilicated marked by depressed spots resembling the umbilicus.

umbilication a depression resembling the umbilicus.

umbilicus the scar marking the site of entry of the umbilical cord in the fetus; called also navel. It is usually only depressed in the human abdomen and is inconspicuous in most domestic species. In dogs it is a palpable knot advertised by a convergent whorl of hair.

feather u. see FEATHER (1).

Umbilicus rupestris COTYLEDON *umbilicus*.

umbo pl. *umbones* [L.] a round projection.

u. membrana tympanae the slight projection at the center of the outer surface of the tympanic membrane.

umbrella tree JATROPHA *multifida*, SCHEFFLERA ACTINOPHYLLA.

umbu PHYTOLACCA *dioica*.

UMN upper motor neuron.

UMP uridine 5′-monophosphate, a pyrimidine nucleotide.

UMP synthase deficiency an inherited absence of the enzyme, which assists in the conversion of orotate to UMP, results in the accumulation of orotate and its excretion in large amounts in the milk. Bovine homozygotes for the condition die at fetal age of about 40 days.

unapparent trauma trauma to a patient which could be fatal but is inapparent because it leaves no external mark.

unbound said of electrolytes, e.g. iron and calcium, and other substances which are circulating in the bloodstream and are not bound to plasma proteins so that they are available immediately for metabolic processes. See also CALCIUM, IRON.

Uncia uncia see snow LEOPARD.

unciform hooked or shaped like a hook.

Uncinaria a genus of canine hookworms in the order Strongylida.

U. criniformis occurs in the badger and fox.

U. lucasi found in the fur seal.

U. stenocephala the common species in the dog, cat and fox.

U. yukonensis found in all ursids.

uncinariasis the disease caused by UNCINARIA in cats and dogs. Similar to, but less severe than ANCYLOSTOMIASIS, with only mild blood loss and enteritis.

uncinate 1. unciform. 2. relating to or affecting the uncinate gyrus.

uncipressure pressure with a hook to stop hemorrhage.

unclassified viruses a diminishingly small number of viruses remain unclassified.

uncoating the removal of protein coat or envelope from a virus, one of the first steps in replication which releases the viral genome and enables viral genes to become available for transcription.
uncompetitive inhibition type of enzyme inhibition characterized by both increased K_M and decreased V_{max}.
unconscious insensible; incapable of responding to sensory stimuli and of having subjective experiences.
unconsciousness an abnormal state of lack of response to sensory stimuli, resulting from injury, illness, shock or some other bodily disorder. A brief loss of unconsciousness from which the animal recovers spontaneously or with slight aid is called fainting. Deep, prolonged unconsciousness is known as COMA. See also levels of CONSCIOUSNESS.
uncoupler an agent that inhibits ATP synthesis by dissociating it from the electron transport system at one or more of the phosphorylation sites.
uncovertebral pertaining to the uncinate processes of a vertebra.
unction 1. an ointment. 2. application of an ointment or salve; inunction.
unctuous greasy or oily.
uncus the medially curved anterior part of the hippocampal gyrus.
undecylenate see UNDECYLENIC ACID.
undecylenic acid, undecanoic acid, undecenoic acid an unsaturated fatty acid, used topically, in ointment or powder form, as an antifungal agent; toxic reactions are rare.
undercoat the fine hairs of an animal's coat which are usually shorter and more numerous than the coarse guard hairs. In some breeds of dogs and cats, however, these may predominate.
undercut in the preparation of a tooth cavity for restoration, a cavity under the edges of the opening which is intended to aid in retention of a filling.
underdevelopment an error in x-ray film developing procedure. Causes the production of a flat film with poor contrast; the unexposed background is gray instead of black.
underfeeding see MALNUTRITION, STARVATION.
underflue the soft, fluffy part of a feather, next to the skin. Called also flue.
underline an animal's ventral profile; the shape of the belly when viewed from the side, e.g. pendulous, potbelly, tucked up, gaunt.
undermilking removal of the teat cups before all the milk has been taken from an udder. In a dairy cow which is milked twice daily no more than 500 ml of milk should be left in the udder at the end of milking. Undermilking predisposes to mastitis.
undernutrition see MALNUTRITION, STARVATION.
underreach a gait defect at the trot; the toe of the foreshoe strikes and wears away the front of the hind hoof on the same side.
undershot the mandible is longer than the maxilla so that the lower incisors are forward of the upper incisors and there is no contact between them when the mouth is closed. A common abnormality in dogs and a normal feature in some breeds such as British bulldog.
undersized see DWARFISM, RUNT.
undescended testis see CRYPTORCHIDISM.
undifferentiated not differentiated; primitive. 1. in neoplasia refers to a primitive cell type and likely to be malignant. 2. In clinical medicine refers to a group diagnosis in which there is no differentiation from the pathoanatomical diagnosis, e.g. failure to take the additional step of differentiating between a diagnosis of diarrhea and the etiologically specific diagnosis, e.g. *Escherichia coli*. See also undifferentiated DIARRHEA of the newborn.
u. chronic diarrhea chronic diarrhea in horses which does not satisfy the diagnostic criteria for any of the known causes of that condition; most cases are irreversible and euthanasia is a common outcome.
u. chronic pneumonia see ENZOOTIC pneumonia.
undulant fever brucellosis of humans.
undulating membrane a fold of the protozoa's cell membrane formed when the flagellum of the protozoa beats and pulls up the membrane along the full length of the parasite's body.
undulation a wavelike motion in any medium; a vibration.
unethical said of conduct not conforming with professional ETHICS.
uneviscerated a term used to describe poultry and small game which are sold or hung without having the viscera removed, e.g. New York dressed poultry. The movement of bacteria and enzymes from the gut aids in the tenderizing of the meat and adds a new dimension to the flavor. Not suited to tropical climates nor uneducated palates.
unfavorable therapeutic response see adverse response.
unfit not properly prepared, e.g. physically incapable of performing hard work as in racing, because of lack of training. Said also of food prepared unhygienically.
u. for human consumption meat or other food considered by a qualified food inspector to be unsuited for entry into the human food chain because of the presence of disease, immaturity, physical damage, emaciation, edema, contamination by gut contents or unauthorized additives or being meat of another, unauthorized species, or meat that has not undergone approved inspection by health authorities.
ung. [L.] *unguentum* (ointment).
ungual pertaining to the nails, claws or hooves.
u. crest a crescent-shaped process on the distal phalanx, encircling the corium of the nail or claw, best developed in cats.
unguent an ointment.
unguentum pl. *unguenta* [L.] ointment.
unguicula claw or nail.
unguiculate having claws; clawlike.
unguilysis necrosis and dissolution of the claw or hoof as in equine CANKER.
unguinal pertaining to a nail.
unguis pl. *ungues* [L.] a nail. See also CLAW, NAIL.
ungula hoof.
ungulates, ungulata animals with hooves; cattle, sheep, goat, pig, horse and many wild and other domesticated species.
unguligrade the stance of an ungulate; the disposition of standing on hooves. The ultimate running gait.
uni- word element. [L.] *one*.
uniaxial 1. having only one axis. 2. developed in an axial direction only.
unicameral having only one cavity or compartment, e.g. unicameral cyst.
unicellular made up of a single cell, as the bacteria or protozoa.
uniform basic data set see MINIMUM data set.
uniglandular affecting only one gland.
unigravida a female pregnant for the first time; primigravida; gravida I.
unilocular having only one loculus or compartment; monolocular.
unintentional residue in terms of food hygiene, a

residue of a substance given to an animal for purposes other than improving, modifying or preserving its meat. An intentional residue is a legally authorized additive to the food.

uninucleated mononuclear.

uniocular monocular.

union the growing together of tissues separated by injury, as of the ends of a fractured bone, or of the edges of a wound.

uniovular monovular, monozygotic.

unipara a female which has had one pregnancy that resulted in a viable infant; primipara; para I.

uniparous 1. producing only one ovum or offspring at a time. 2. primiparous.

unipolar having a single pole or process, as a nerve cell.

unipotent, unipotential having only one power, as giving rise to cells of one order only.

unit 1. a single thing; one segment of a whole that is made up of identical or similar segments. 2. a specifically defined amount of anything subject to measurement, as of activity, dimension, velocity, volume, or the like.

Angstrom u. see ANGSTROM.

atomic mass u. see DALTON.

International u. 1. see SI UNITS. 2. a unit of enzyme activity equal to the amount of enzyme that catalyzes the conversion of one micromole of substrate or coenzyme per minute under specified conditions (temperature, pH and substrate concentration) of the assay method. Abbreviated U. 3. any of several arbitrary units that have been adopted by international bodies to express the quantities of certain vitamins (A, C, D and thiamin hydrochloride), hormones (androgen, chorionic gonadotropin, estradiol benzoate, estrone, insulin, progesterone and prolactin), and drugs (digitalis and penicillin).

SI u. any unit of the International System of units (the metric system). See SI UNITS.

unitary pertaining to a single object or individual.

United Kennel Club a privately owned, all-breed registry for purebred dogs in the United States.

United States Dispensatory an unofficial publication providing an international listing of existing and discontinued drugs.

United States National Formulary a book of standards for certain pharmaceuticals and preparations not included in the *United States Pharmacopeia*; revised every 5 years and recognized as a book of official standards by the United States Pure Food and Drug Act of 1906. Abbreviated USNF, NF.

United States Pharmacopeia a legally recognized compendium of standards for drugs, published by the United States Pharmacopeial Convention, Inc., and revised periodically; abbreviated USP. It also includes assays and tests for determination of strength, quality and purity.

United States straws see FRENCH STRAWS.

unitocous giving birth to a single young at one time.

univalent having a valence of one.

University of Illinois needle a rugged needle assembly for aspiration of a sample of bone marrow. The needle is advanced into the sternum by a screw device into which the needle and its lock-in stylus is fitted. The needle hub has a syringe fitting to which a syringe can be fitted to aspirate the marrow.

Unix a computer operating system which features multiprogramming and a hierarchial file structure and many useful but unforgiving utilities.

unmeasured anions see ANION gap.

unmyelinated not having a myelin sheath.

Unopette system a method for diluting blood in preparation for counting blood cells. It utilizes a premeasured volume of diluent in a chamber into which a specified amount of blood is drawn.

unphysiological not in harmony with the laws of physiology.

unsaturated 1. not having all affinities of its elements satisfied (unsaturated compound). 2. not holding all of a solute which can be held in solution by the solvent (unsaturated solution). 3. denoting compounds in which two or more atoms are united by double or triple bonds.

u. fatty acids see FATTY acids.

unsex to deprive of the gonads.

unsharpness lack of detail in an x-ray picture.

unslaked lime see QUICKLIME.

unsound said of an animal, usually a horse, which has been examined for SOUNDNESS and found to be unsatisfactory.

unstable having a tendency to disrupt, e.g. unstable chemicals.

u. fracture the principal fragments in a reduced fracture are overriding. Slow union or nonunion results.

unstriated having no striations, as smooth muscle.

unthriftiness failure to grow or to put on weight as well as expected in the presence of adequate quantity and quality of feed, and in the absence of overt clinical signs of illness. Called also illthrift. See also WEANER illthrift.

post-weaning u. occurs in young animals that are weaned at too young an age or without being weaned onto a suitable transitional diet.

selenium-responsive u. a condition seen in marginally deficient areas; affected ewes respond well in terms of body weight and milk yield to supplemental selenium although their clinicopathological indicants are in the normal range.

unthrifty weaner sheep see WEANER illthrift.

ununited a failure of union or closure, said of the union that occurs between an epiphysis and diaphysis.

u. medial coronoid process see fragmented CORONOID PROCESS.

update in computer terminology to modify a master file by replacing old information by new.

upper cranial; oral; rostral.

u. airway upper respiratory tract. See also AIRWAY.

u. burner syndrome in acupuncture terminology a chronic lung condition caused by an attack by a pathogen.

u. motor neuron motor nerve pathway originating in the brain and terminating at a peripheral motor neuron. Damage to this pathway releases the peripheral nerve from central control. See also upper MOTOR NEURON.

u. respiratory tract (URT) comprises the nasal cavities, pharynx and larynx. Some anatomists also include the upper segments of the bronchial tree. Inflammation of the URT is common to all species. It is usually caused by infection, most commonly viral, producing a syndrome of frequent, dry cough, serous or mucoid nasal discharge and pain on manual compression of the laynx, pharynx and trachea. It is a common precursor to more serious disease involving the lower respirtory tract.

u. respiratory tract virus disease see Table 8.2.

upright said of limb joints and bones, especially in the horse. Indicates a lack of angulation in the joint, e.g. upright hock, or slope in a bone, e.g. upright pastern. In horses, often associated with a bumpy ride and a tendency to joint injury and lameness.

upstream a term used in molecular biology to describe nucleotides of a nucleic acid molecule which lie in the 5′ direction from a particular reference point such as the site of initiation of transcription. See also DOWNSTREAM.

u. activating site DNA sequences that are upstream from the promoter and have a regulatory role in transcription.

Ura uracil.

urachal pertaining to URACHUS.

u. abscess a mass palpable in the abdomen dorsal to the umbilicus to which it is usually connected by a fistula that drips pus continually.

u. cyst symptomless fluid-filled cavities in the urachal ligament.

u. diverticulum visible with contrast radiography as an extension of the bladder at the vertex. See also VESICOURACHAL diverticulum.

u. inflammation usually results from an extensive infection of the umbilicus. The urachus may or may not be pervious. Cystitis or urachal abscess may follow.

persistent u. ligament maintains tension on the bladder leading to incomplete filling and emptying. The elongated bladder with a pointed vertex is readily visible radiologically.

urachitis inflammation of the urachus; often complicated by extension of the inflammation to the bladder.

urachus a fetal canal connecting the bladder with the allantois via the navel. It mostly disappears in the neonatal period although a nipple-like projection may remain on the bladder and in some species a cord may persist along the cranial border of the median ligament of the bladder.

persistent u. failure of the urachus to obliterate at birth so that urine dribbles from it continuously. The urine may also be passed from the urethra. Retrograde infection from an omphalitis is common, resulting in cystitis. Called also pervious urachus.

uracil U; Ura; a pyrimidine base found in nucleic acids.

uracrasia disordered composition of urine.

uraemia see UREMIA.

uragogue diuretic.

uraniscus the palate.

uranium a chemical element, atomic number 92, atomic weight 238.03, symbol U. See Table 6.

uran(o)- word element. [Gr.] *palate*.

uranoplasty plastic repair of the palate; palatoplasty.

uranorrhaphy suture of the palate; staphylorrhaphy.

uranoschisis cleft palate.

uranostaphyloschisis fissure of the soft and hard palates.

uranyl pertaining to uranium; the $UO^{22}+$ ion, as in uranyl sulfate.

u. nitrate causes depression, anorexia, hyperuricemia, nephrosis and visceral deposits of urates.

urate a salt of uric acid. Accumulates in tissues in large quantities in chickens fed excessive amounts of protein. See also visceral GOUT.

u. calculi see urate UROLITHS.

uratemia urates in the blood.

uratic pertaining to urates or to gout.

uratoma a concretion made up of urates; tophus.

uratosis the deposit of urates in the tissues.

uraturia urates in the urine.

urceiform pitcher-shaped.

urea 1. the diamide of carbonic acid found in urine, blood and lymph, the chief nitrogenous constituent of urine, and the chief nitrogenous end product of protein metabolism; it is formed in the liver from amino acids and from ammonia compounds. 2. a pharmaceutical preparation of urea occasionally used to lower intracranial pressure. 3. industrial urea is used as a fertilizer and feed additive for ruminants. Overfeeding or accidental access to large amounts can cause fatal poisoning.

u. cycle see urea CYCLE.

u. cycle enzyme deficiency see ARGINOSUCCINATE SYNTHETASE, CITRULLINEMIA.

u. hydrogen peroxide see CARBAMIDE peroxide.

u. nitrogen the urea concentration of serum or plasma, conventionally specified in terms of nitrogen content and called *blood urea nitrogen* (BUN), an important indicator of renal function.

u. poisoning causes tremor, dyspnea, abdominal pain, incoordination, bellowing, convulsions and death in 2 to 4 hours. Due to hyperammonemia.

urealytic bacteria those producing urease.

Ureaplasma a genus in the family Mycoplasmataceae. There are two species, *U. urealyticum*, found in humans, and *U. diversum*, which is associated with genital disease in cattle. See UREAPLASMOSIS. Called also t-strain mycoplasma.

ureaplasmosis infection with *Ureaplasma* spp.; occurs in the vagina and vulva of cows and ewes and there is speculation that they are causally associated with granular vaginitis and possibly with transitory endometritis. They are also mentioned in discussions about seminal vesiculitis in bulls, and in pneumonia in calves.

ureapoiesis formation of urea.

urease an enzyme that catalyzes the decomposition of urea to ammonia and carbon dioxide, present in high activity in ruminal microflora.

u. inhibitors compounds that inhibit or block the activity of urease, most commonly used in the management of struvite urolithiasis. See also ACETOHYDROXAMIC ACID.

u. tests a biochemical test used in the identification of some bacteria such as *Proteus* spp. Using urea agar or broth, bacteria producing urease will cause the formation of ammonia, which is detected by phenol red in the medium.

urecchysis an effusion of urine into cellular tissue.

Urechites lutea Central American plant in family Apocynaceae; causes sudden death, generalized hemorrhage and cardiomyopathy in cattle. Called also *Bejuro marrullero*.

uredema swelling from extravasated urine.

uredofos a broad-spectrum anthelmintic introduced for the treatment of canine and feline hookworms, ascarids, tapeworms and whipworms but withdrawn because of a large number of adverse reactions with many deaths.

ureidopenicillins a group of penicillins, susceptible to gastric acidity and β-lactamase, but with a greater range of activity against gram-negative bacteria, especially *Pseudomonas aeruginosa*. Includes AZLOCILLIN, MEZLOCILLIN and PIPERACILLIN.

urelcosis ulceration in the urinary tract.

uremia 1. an excess in the blood of urea, creatinine, and other nitrogenous end products of protein and amino acid metabolism; more correctly referred to as *azotemia*. 2. in current usage, the syndrome of chronic RENAL failure. As the glomerular filtration rate falls in either acute tubular necrosis or chronic renal failure, serum urea (usually expressed as blood urea nitrogen content, BUN) and creatinine rise to very high levels. However, BUN and creatinine measurements are only roughly correlated with the clinical signs of uremia. Other nitrogenous compounds present in small amounts may produce most of the toxic effects. Some uremic signs are due to losses of kidney function that do not involve azotemia.

Uremia is a syndrome that occurs as the end-stage in renal insufficiency. The pathology includes stomatitis, pneumonopathy, endocarditis and gastritis. In the dog and cat there is vomiting, diarrhea, anemia and sometimes ulcerative stomatitis. In horses there is depression and chronic diarrhea. Cattle show somnolence, depression and recumbency. Chickens develop visceral gout. Called also kidney failure.

prerenal u. see AZOTEMIA.

uremic pertaining to or emanating from UREMIA.

u. poisoning see UREMIA, visceral GOUT.

u. toxins a name given to the many products of metabolism that accumulate in the body with renal failure, and in association with uremia, because of impaired renal degradation and/or excretory capacity.

uremigenic 1. caused by uremia. 2. causing uremia.

ureogenesis hepatic synthesis of urea.

ureotelic having urea as the chief excretory product of nitrogen metabolism.

u. mammals humans, dogs, rat, sheep, cattle and pigs. These animals have high liver levels of arginase.

uresis the passage of urine; urination.

ureter the fibromuscular tube through which the urine passes from the kidney to the bladder.

ectopic u. an abnormally placed opening of the ureter, either into the urinary bladder or at another site in the lower urinary or genital tract. There is usually constant dribbling of urine and commonly an associated pyuria.

ureteral pertaining to or emanating from the URETER.

u. calculus ureterolith.

u. distension ureterectasis.

u. duplication a rare anomaly in animals in which there is more than one ureter from a kidney.

u. hypoplasia usually segmental underdevelopment of the ureter causing stenosis and hydronephrosis.

u. obstruction may be caused by intraluminal lesions, e.g. urolithiasis, or as part of pyelonephritis or by external compression of the ureter or as a congenital defect. Sudden blockage causes acute abdominal pain that lasts for several hours. Subsequently or if obstruction develops slowly the kidney on the affected side becomes hydronephrotic; if bilateral, renal failure follows.

u. reflux see vesicoureteral REFLUX.

u. rupture rupture usually results from trauma; leads to urinoma or peritoneal accumulation of urine.

u. stasis synonymous with obstruction.

u. valves a rare anomaly that may be a cause of urinary incontinence.

ureterectasis distension of the ureter.

ureterectomy excision of a ureter.

ureteric bud, ureteral bud see METANEPHRIC diverticulum.

ureteritis inflammation of a ureter. The epithelial reaction may be cystic, if the reaction is liquefaction, or glandular, if the epithelial reaction is by metaplasia.

ureter(o)- word element. [Gr.] *ureter*.

ureterocele ballooning of the submucosal segment of the ureter into the bladder.

ureterocelectomy excision of a ureterocele.

ureterocolostomy anastomosis of a ureter to the colon. May be carried out for permanent urinary diversion when cystectomy is required.

ureterocystoscope a cystoscope with a catheter for insertion into the ureter.

ureterocystostomy ureteroneocystostomy.

ureterodialysis rupture of a ureter; ureterolysis.

ureteroectasis megaureter.

ureteroenterostomy anastomosis of one or both ureters to the wall of the intestine.

ureterography radiography of the ureter, after injection of a contrast medium.

antegrade u. the contrast medium is injected through a catheter placed percutaneously into renal parenchyma and into the pelvis or ureter.

ureteroheminephrectomy excision of the diseased portion of a reduplicated kidney and its ureter.

ureteroileostomy anastomosis of the ureters to an isolated loop of the ileum, drained through a stoma on the abdominal wall.

ureterolith a calculus in the ureter.

ureterolithiasis formation of a calculus in the ureter.

ureterolithotomy incision of a ureter for removal of calculus.

ureterolysis 1. rupture of the ureter; ureterodialysis. 2. paralysis of the ureter. 3. the operation of freeing the ureter from adhesions.

ureteroneocystostomy surgical transplantation of a ureter to a different site in the bladder; ureterocystostomy.

ureteroneopyelostomy ureteropyeloneostomy.

ureteronephrectomy excision of a kidney and ureter.

ureteropathy any disease of the ureter.

ureteropelvic pertaining to the ureter and the renal pelvis.

u. junction junction of the renal pelvis and the ureter; strictly speaking the renal pelvis is the dilated proximal portion of the ureter.

ureteropelvioplasty surgical reconstruction of the junction of the ureter and renal pelvis; ureteropyelostomy.

ureteroplasty plastic repair of a ureter.

ureteropyelitis inflammation of a ureter and renal pelvis.

ureteropyelography radiography of the ureter and renal pelvis.

ureteropyeloneostomy surgical creation of a new communication between a ureter and the renal pelvis; ureteroneopyelostomy; ureteropyelostomy.

ureteropyelonephritis inflammation of the ureter, renal pelvis and kidney.

ureteropyeloplasty plastic repair of the ureter and renal pelvis.

ureteropyelostomy ureteropelvioplasty.

ureteropyosis suppurative inflammation of the ureter.

ureterorenoscope a fiberoptic endoscope used in ureterorenoscopy.

ureterorenoscopy visual inspection of the interior of the ureter and kidney by means of a fiberoptic endoscope for such purposes as biopsy, removal or crushing of stones, or other procedures.

ureterorrhagia discharge of blood from the ureter.

ureterorrhaphy suture of the ureter.

ureterostomy creation of a new outlet for a ureter.

ureterotomy incision of a ureter.

ureteroureterostomy end-to-end anastomosis of the two portions of a transected ureter.

ureterovaginal pertaining to or communicating with a ureter and the vagina.

u. fistula a complication of ovariohysterectomy in bitches and queens; causes urinary incontinence.

ureterovesical pertaining to a ureter and the bladder.

u. junction junction of the ureter with the urinary bladder; the ureter runs for a short distance in the wall of the bladder, providing a valvular action preventing reflux of urine up the ureter.

urethane a compound with limited use as an anesthetic in nonrecovery experiments with laboratory animals because it causes pulmonary edema and is carcinogenic.

urethra the tubular passage through which urine is discharged from the bladder to the exterior via the external urinary meatus. In males the urethra also conveys the secretions of the reproductive organs.

female u. runs ventrally to the reproductive tract, opening in its ventral wall at the junction of the vagina and the vestibule; at its entrance it may be joined with a diverticulum (cow, sow) or a hummock (bitch).

incomplete u. see URETHRAL atresia.

male u. consists of pelvic (bladder to entrance to penis) and penile or spongy part; the deferent and vesicular ducts enter the pelvic urethra soon after it leaves the bladder.

penile u. that part of the male urethra which passes through the penis; called also spongy urethra.

prosthetic u. limited use in male cats with urethral obstruction or stricture; some serious disadvantages and surgical perineal urethrostomy the preferred treatment.

spongy u. that part of the urethra surrounded by erectile tisssue; called also penile urethra.

urethra imperforate see URETHRAL agenesis.

urethral pertaining to or emanating from URETHRA.

u. agenesis, u. atresia failure of development of all or part of the urethra: characterized by complete urine retention. A rare cause of neonatal uremia.

u. calculus causes a syndrome of acute urethral obstruction (below).

u. diverticulum see URACHAL diverticulum.

u. fistula due to trauma; occurs in bulls in which the urethra lies superficially near its end. A fistula may affect the discharge of semen from the normal meatus sufficiently to cause infertility.

u. groove a median groove along the ventral surface of the genital tubercle providing an eventual location for the penile urethra in the male.

u. hydropulsion see HYDROPROPULSION.

u. hypoplasia a cause of urinary incontinence in female dogs and rarely cats.

u. muscle striated muscle in the wall of the male pelvic urethra.

u. obstruction causes acute abdominal pain with grunting and straining to urinate, tail switching, distension of the bladder, dripping of blood-stained urine, protrusion of the penis. Eventually the bladder ruptures or the urethra perforates. Caused usually by calculus. See also UROLITHIASIS.

u. perforation occurs usually at the site of urethral obstruction by a calculus. Causes urinary infiltration of the ventral abdominal wall and terminal uremia. Called also waterbelly. Rarely the accumulation occurs retroperitoneally and is palpable rectally. See also HYPOSPADIAS.

u. plate a solid cord of endodermal cells which arise from the floor of the urogenital sinus, contributing to the formation of the urethral groove.

u. plug occurs in male cats causing urethral obstruction; associated with feline urological syndrome. The plug is composed of proteinaceous material with cellular debris and struvite crystals.

u. pressure profile a study of the intraurethral pressure as a means of identifying the cause of urinary incontinence in dogs and cats.

u. pressure profilometry a measure of intraurethral pressures; used in the investigation of urinary incompetence in dogs and cats. Usually carried out with a pressure-measuring device in the tip of a catheter placed in the urethra and bladder.

u. process the extension of the urethra beyond the end of the glans penis. In the horse it is mostly concealed in the urethral fossa. In small ruminants it is in the form of a 1 to 2 inch long filiform appendage and is easily injured during shearing, interfering with the animal's subsequent fertility.

u. prolapse protrusion of urethral mucosa at the end of the penis.

u. prosthesis a synthetic conduit used in the treatment of urethral stricture or obstruction in cats, particularly following an unsuccessful urethrostomy.

proximal u. ulceration causes hematuria at the end of urination in horses.

u. rupture see urethral perforation (above).

u. sling see COLPOSUSPENSION.

u. sphincter mechanism incompetence a cause of urinary INCONTINENCE in female dogs and occasionally cats.

u. stricture caused by trauma, particularly injury associated with urethral calculi or urethral surgery. Clinically similar to obstruction except that the condition is subacute or chronic and characterized by a persistently distended bladder, dribbling of urine and the passage of a thin stream, usually accompanied by straining.

urethratresia imperforation of the urethra.

urethrectomy excision of the urethra.

urethremphraxis obstruction of the urethra.

urethrism irritability or chronic spasm of the urethra.

urethritis inflammation of the urethra due to injury or infection. The urethra swells and narrows, and the flow of urine is impeded. Both urination and the urgency to urinate increase. There may be a purulent discharge.

granulomatous u. occurs in female dogs, often complicated by bacterial infection. May cause partial obstruction and stranguria.

urethr(o)- word element. [Gr.] *urethra*.

urethrobulbar pertaining to the urethra and the bulb of the penis.

urethrocele prolapse of the female urethra through the urinary meatus.

urethrocolostomy anastomosis of the urethra to the colon.

urethrocystitis inflammation of the urethra and bladder.

urethrocystograph radiographic visualization of the urethra and urinary bladder utilizing contrast techniques.

urethrography radiography of the urethra.

prostatic u. the contrast material is delivered by catheter to the area of the prostate.

retrograde u. the contrast medium is injected into the terminal part of the urethra which has been occluded by a Foley catheter.

voiding u. contrast medium is injected into the urinary bladder and radiographs are taken as it is forced into the urethra.

urethrometry 1. determination of the resistance of various segments of the urethra to retrograde flow of fluid. 2. measurement of the urethra.

urethropenile pertaining to the urethra and penis.

urethroperineal pertaining to the urethra and perineum.

urethroperineoscrotal pertaining to the urethra, perineum and scrotum.

urethrophraxis obstruction of the urethra.

urethrophyma a tumor or growth in the urethra.
urethroplasty plastic repair of the urethra.
Brown u. technique a surgical treatment for urine reflux and accompanying chronic urogenital disease in mares. By using layers of the vestibular floor, the urethral lumen is extended caudally to open at the vulvar cleft.
sling u. a surgical technique for increasing proximal urethral resistance in the management of urinary incontinence. Seromuscular flaps, dissected from the midtrigone area, are reflected around the bladder neck and proximal urethra and sutured together, creating a constricting band.
urethroprostatic pertaining to the urethra and prostate.
urethrorectal pertaining to the urethra and rectum.
u. fistula may be a congenital defect. The male dog urinates into the rectum. Females usually have an opening into the vagina and sometimes an associated imperforate anus. Cystitis and urethritis are common sequels.
urethrorrhagia a flow of blood from the urethra.
urethrorrhaphy suture of a urethral fistula.
urethrorrhea abnormal discharge from the urethra.
urethroscope an instrument for viewing the interior of the urethra.
urethroscopy visual inspection of the urethra.
urethrospasm spasm of the urethral muscular tissue.
urethrostaxis oozing of blood from the urethra.
urethrostenosis constriction of the urethra.
urethrostomy creation of a permanent opening for the urethra in the perineum.
antepubic u. anastomosis of the urethra to skin of the abdominal wall. May be performed in the male or female, usually because of trauma to the urethra.
ischial u. see perineal urethrostomy (below).
perineal u. one performed in male cats in the perineal region, between the anus and scrotum. Called also ischial urethrostomy, Wilson–Harrison technique.
prepubic u. the opening is created on the ventral surface of the abdomen, cranial to the pubis.
scrotal u. one performed in dogs at the level of the scrotum, usually for chronic cystic calculi, penile amputation or traumatic strictures. After removal of the scrotum and testicles, the urethra is opened and sutured to the skin, creating a permanent opening.
Wilson–Harrison u. see perineal urethrostomy (above).
urethrotome an instrument for cutting a urethral stricture.
urethrotomy incision of the urethra.
ischial u. see perineal URETHROSTOMY.
urethrotrigonitis inflammation of the urethra and trigone of the bladder (vesical trigone).
urethrovaginal pertaining to the urethra and vagina.
urethrovesical pertaining to the urethra and bladder.
Urginea African-Mediterranean plant genus in the family Liliaceae; contains bufadienolide cardiac glycosides; causes abdominal pain, cardiac irregularity, diarrhea, dyspnea, sudden death; includes *U. altissima*, *U. capitata*, *U. lydenburgensis*, *U. macrocentra*, *U. maritima* (*Scilla maritima*, red squill), *U. physodes*, *U. pusilla*, *U. rubella* (snakehead), *U. sanguinea* (*U. burkei*). Called also slangkop, jeukbol, sea onion, red squill.
urhidrosis the presence in the sweat of urinous materials, chiefly uric acid and urea.
-uria word element. [Gr.] condition of the urine.
uric pertaining to the urine.
u. acid the end product of purine metabolism or oxidation in the body in species other than dogs which metabolize uric acid to allantoin (except Dalmatians). Amounts of more than 1 mg/100 ml of uric acid in the blood are an indication of hepatic insufficiency. In birds excess amounts of uric acid and urates in tissue occur in visceral GOUT.
u. acid calculi see urate UROLITH.
uricacidemia uric acid in the blood.
uricaciduria excess of uric acid in the urine.
uricase an enzyme that catalyzes the conversion of uric acid to allantoin.
uricemia uricacidemia.
uricolysis the cleavage of uric acid or urates.
uricosuria excretion of uric acid in the urine.
uricosuric 1. pertaining to, characterized by, or promoting uricosuria. 2. an agent that promotes uricosuria.
uridine a ribonucleoside containing uracil.
u. diphosphate (UDP) a nucleotide that participates in glycogen metabolism and in some processes of nucleic acid synthesis.
u. diphosphoglucuronic acid one of the incidental products in the glucuronate pathway and an important participant in detoxication processes in the body.
u. 5′-triphosphate (UTP) main activated form of pyrimidine bases, involved in the activation of sugars for synthesis and polymerization.
urina [L.] *urine*.
urinalysis analysis of the urine as an aid in the diagnosis of disease. Many types of tests are used in analyzing the urine in order to determine whether it contains abnormal substances indicative of disease. The most significant substances normally absent from urine and detected by urinalysis are protein, glucose, acetone, blood, pus and casts. Some renal function tests are based on clearance of metabolites into the urine. Urea clearance test is the most efficient.
urinary pertaining to the urine; containing or secreting urine.
u. bile pigment bilirubin and urobilinogen are found in the urine of normal animals.
u. calculi see UROLITH, UROLITHIASIS.
u. diversion various surgical procedures involving the ureters, bladder or urethra may be used to alter the usual route of urine flow, thereby bypassing portions of the urinary tract, usually the bladder and/or urethra. Ureters, bladder or urethra are transplanted or anastomosed to the bowel or placed so urine exits at an orifice created through the skin. See also URETEROILEOSTOMY, TRIGONAL–colonic anastomosis, URETEROCOLOSTOMY, TRANSURETEROURETEROSTOMY.
u. flow monitor periodic measurement of the amount of urine secreted. In an anesthetized animal a catheter draining into a calibrated container is used. In a conscious animal a clamped-off, self-retaining catheter is inserted and drained at intervals. A metabolism cage is an alternative.
u. flowmetry the measure of urinary flow rates.
u. incontinence an inability to control urination with the involuntary passage of urine. Most commonly occurs in dogs due to congenital abnormalities of the ureters or urethra. Other causes include congenital or acquired defects in nervous control of micturition, neoplastic or inflammatory disease of the lower urinary tract, and prostate gland and endocrine abnormalities.
u. obstruction urethral or ureteral obstruction often caused by lodgement of a urinary calculus in the narrow lumen. Constriction of urethra due to hyperplastic prostate in male dogs.

u. pole the point on the glomerulus where the proximal convoluted tubule exits.
u. pooling see UROVAGINA.
u. system, u. tract the system formed in the body by the KIDNEYS, the URINARY BLADDER (2), the URETERS and the URETHRA, the organs concerned in the production and excretion of urine.
u. territorial marking see SPRAYING.
u. tract see URINARY system.

urinary bladder a distensible reservoir with muscular walls and a lining mucous membrane that lies in the ventral part of the pelvic cavity or abdomen (especially far forwards in the cat). It receives urine from the kidneys via the ureters and discharges urine to the exterior of the body via the urethra. Urine trickles into the bladder from the kidneys every few seconds, where it remains until voided. There is no anatomical sphincter of circular muscle at the bladder neck, urine retention being maintained by the elastic tissues of the urethra—a physiological sphincter. Voiding occurs when the detrusor muscle contracts forcing the urine out. In the housetrained companion animal urination is resisted even when the bladder is uncomfortably full.
atonic u. b. a condition marked by a dilated, poorly contracting urinary bladder without evidence of a lesion of the central nervous system.
atonic neurogenic u. b. neurogenic bladder caused by destruction of the sensory nerve fibers from the bladder to the spinal cord (lateral spinal tracts), marked by the absence of awareness of bladder filling and of the desire to void. This leads to overdistension of the bladder, and an abnormal amount of residual urine with a tendency toward overflow incontinence. Seen in degenerative and traumatic injury to the spinal cord, especially intervertebral disk herniation, in dogs and cats. Called also retention and overflow incontinence, paralytic bladder and sensory paralytic bladder.
automatic u. b. neurogenic bladder due to complete resection of the spinal cord above the sacral segments, marked by complete loss of micturition reflexes and bladder sensation, violent involuntary voiding, and an abnormal amount of residual urine. Called also reflex neurogenic bladder.
autonomous u. b. neurogenic bladder due to a lesion in the sacral portion of the spinal cord that interrupts the reflex arc that controls the bladder. The lesion may be in the cauda equina, conus medullaris, sacral roots or pelvic nerve. It is marked by loss of normal bladder sensation and reflex activity, inability to initiate urination normally, and stress incontinence.
u. b. calculi can cause cystitis arising from the traumatic injury to the bladder epithelium. The initial stage may be hematuria and greatly increased frequency of urination. Dysuria may also be evident. Secondary bacterial infection is a common sequel. See also UROLITHIASIS.
congenital u. b. rupture there is gradually increasing abdominal distension soon after birth in the affected foal, which is almost always a male. Paracentesis reveals free urine in the peritoneal cavity. The tear is usually in the dorsal wall of the bladder.
u. b. duplication observed in dogs; the second bladder originates between the uterus and the urinary tract, or between the urinary tract and the rectum.
u. b. ectropion see urinary bladder eversion (below).
u. b. eversion turning inside out of the bladder; occurs in the mare, usually during labor.
u. b. extroversion failure of development of ventral abdominal wall so that the bladder and pelvic urethra are exposed.
u. b. hypertrophy due usually to long-standing partial obstruction of urinary flow.
u. b. inflammation see CYSTITIS.
irritable u. b. a state of the bladder marked by increased frequency of contraction with associated desire to urinate.
u. b. motility degree of motor activity of the bladder muscle as determined by the spinal sympathetic nerve supplies.
motor paralytic u. b. neurogenic bladder due to impairment of the motor neurons or nerves controlling the bladder. The *acute* form is marked by painful distension and inability to initiate micturition; the *chronic* form is marked by difficulty in initiating micturition, straining, a decrease in the size and force of the stream, interrupted stream, and recurrent infection of the urinary tract.
u. b. neck sling a surgical procedure that increases proximal urethral pressure; used to treat some forms of urinary incontinence.
u. b. neoplasia see urinary bladder tumors (below).
neurogenic u. b. any condition of dysfunction of the urinary bladder caused by a lesion of the central or peripheral nervous system.
u. b. papillary hyperplasia resembles papillomatosis in cattle bladders; may cause obstruction.
u. b. papilloma warts attached to the inner wall of the urinary bladder.
u. b. paralysis is caused by a lesion, usually a space-occupying one or due to trauma, in the lumbosacral region of the cord. In the early stages the bladder remains distended and urine dribbles from it. A good flow of urine can be obtained by firm pressure on the bladder. There may be some return to an emptying function later, but the evacuation is seldom complete. Cystitis is the almost certain outcome.
parturient u. b. prolapse may follow rupture of the floor of the vagina during parturition in the mare; it can protrude from the vulva.
u. b. reconstruction a surgical procedure performed to correct urinary incontinence caused by urethral hypoplasia in female dogs and cats. The caudal bladder is reshaped to form ventral bladder tubal flaps as a cranial extension of the urethra.
reflex neurogenic u. b. automatic bladder.
u. b. reflux see vesicoureteral REFLUX.
u. b. retroflexion seen in male dogs with tenesmus, due usually to prostatic hyperplasia or constipation; resumes normal position after voiding unless retained in a perineal hernia with a kinked urethra.
u. b. rupture failure to relieve an obstruction of the urethra may result in distension of the bladder to the point that its circulation is impaired and rupture of the organ follows. The pain of distension disappears, to be followed by a gradual distension of the abdomen, and somnolence and depression of developing uremia. In dogs and cats, trauma is also a common cause. See also URETHRAL perforation.
sensory paralytic u. b. atonic neurogenic bladder.
u. b. torsion a rare cause of complete anuria, bladder distension and eventual rupture.
u. b. trigone area of the bladder wall defined by imaginary lines joining the urethral orifice with the orifices of the ureters.
u. b. tumors rare in food animals except in cattle grazing bracken (see also ENZOOTIC hematuria). In dogs and cats they are usually carcinomas, or rarely adenomas, papillomas, leiomyomas or fibromas.

Botryoid rhabdomyosarcomas characteristically occur in young St. Bernards and may arise from mesenchymal cells.

u. b. uroliths see UROLITHIASIS.

u. b.-vaginal prolapse occurs occasionally in the cow as a complication of vaginal prolapse. The bladder is retrodeviated and the urethra kinked so that urine flow is obstructed.

u. b. warts see urinary bladder papilloma (above).

urinate to void urine.

urination the discharge of urine from the bladder; called also voiding of urine and micturition. Urine from the kidneys is passed every few seconds along the ureters to the bladder, where it collects until voided. During the act of urination the urine passes from the bladder to the outside via the urethra.

difficult u. the bladder is continually full; the animal is straining to urinate, often grunting, but producing only a thin stream, often under great pressure. Called also dysuria, strangury.

dribbling u. a steady, intermittent passage of small volumes of urine, sometimes precipitated by a change in posture or increase in intra-abdominal pressure, reflecting inadequate or lack of sphincter control. Seen with ectopic ureters and in paralysis of bladder. See also DRIBBLERS.

inappropriate u. see inappropriate MICTURITION.

increased u. frequency if output of urine per urination is reduced the increased frequency is probably related to irritation in the tract due to cystitis or urethritis.

painful u. dysuria; frequent passage of small amounts of urine with grunting and maintaining posture for some time afterwards.

submissive u. an expression of behavioral submission by dogs.

urine the fluid containing water and waste products which are secreted by the KIDNEYS, stored in the bladder and discharged by way of the urethra. See also URINARY.

u. albumin see ALBUMINURIA.

u. alkalinization increasing the pH of urine by the administration of alkalinizing agents such as sodium bicarbonate; used to increase the solubility of cystine in the management of cystine urolithiasis in dogs.

blood in u. see HEMATURIA.

u. burn see urine scald (below).

u. calculi see UROLITH, UROLITHIASIS.

u. casts see urinary CASTS.

u. cells see urine sediment (below).

u. chromogens see CHROMOGEN.

u. concentration test see WATER deprivation test.

u. creatine see CREATINURIA.

u. crystals see CRYSTALLURIA.

u. drinking in farm animals is observed in nutritional deficiency of sodium chloride.

u. flow the rate of flow may be reduced—OLIGURIA, absent—ANURIA, or increased—POLYURIA.

u. flowmetry measure of urine flow rates.

u. glucose see GLUCOSURIA.

u. hemoglobin see HEMOGLOBINURIA.

u. immunoglobulins may be found in small amounts in normal animals. Increased amounts occur in renal disease due to disruption of glomeruli and defects in tubular reabsorption.

u. indican see INDICANURIA.

u. ketones see KETONURIA.

u. marking see SPRAYING.

u. methemoglobin see METHEMOGLOBINURIA.

u. myoglobin see MYOGLOBINURIA.

u. osmolality a measure of the number of dissolved particles per unit of water in urine. See also OSMOLALITY.

u. peritonitis caused by the presence of urine in the peritoneal cavity as in rupture of the bladder.

u. pH the normal range varies with the animal species. Herbivores have a higher pH than carnivores because of differences in the diet. Alterations occur with changes in acid–base balance and infection in the urinary tract.

u. protein see PROTEINURIA.

pus in u. see PYURIA.

red u. see HEMATURIA, HEMOGLOBINURIA.

residual u. urine remaining in the bladder after urination; seen in bladder outlet obstruction (as by prostatic hypertrophy) and disorders affecting nerves controlling bladder function.

u. sample collection midstream collection is standard; for culture the sample should be collected by catheter or suprapubic, percutaneous needle insertion into the bladder.

u. scald scalding of the perineal area, and sometimes the hindlegs, by urine. It may be the result of urinary incontinence or the animal's inability to assume normal posture when urinating, i.e. paresis or paralysis of the hindlimbs. In rabbits it is caused by poor cage accommodation and frequent wetting of the area with urine. Secondary infection of the dermatitis is common.

u. sediment a centrifuged deposit suitable for microscopic examination for the presence of cells, casts, bacteria, crystals, etc.

u. specific gravity see SPECIFIC gravity.

subcutaneous u. aggregation urine leaking from a damaged urethra collects in a subcutaneous site.

urinemia uremia.

uriniferous transporting or conveying urine.

uriniparous excreting urine.

urin(o)- word element. [Gr., L.] *urine.*

urinogenital urogenital.

urinogenous of urinary origin.

urinology urology.

urinoma a subperitoneal accumulation or a cyst containing urine.

urinometer an instrument for determining the specific gravity of urine.

urinous pertaining to or of the nature of urine.

uriposia the drinking of urine.

uro- word element. [Gr.] *urine* (urinary tract, urination).

urobilin a brownish pigment formed by oxidation of urobilinogen; found in the feces and sometimes in the urine after standing in the air.

urobilinemia urobilin in the blood.

urobilinogen a colorless compound formed in the intestines by the reduction of BILIRUBIN. Small amounts of the bilirubin produced in the body by the breakdown of hemoglobin are excreted in the urine as urobilinogen. Increased amounts of urobilinogen in the urine indicate an excessive amount of bilirubin in the blood. Determination of the amount of urobilinogen excreted in a given period makes it possible to evaluate certain types of hemolytic anemia and also is of help in diagnosing liver dysfunction such as hepatocellular damage.

fecal u. a group of urobilinoid substances which react with Ehrlich's reagent. Presence indicates an open bile duct and a functional enterohepatic circulation of bile pigments.

urobilinoids resemble bilirubin.

urobilinuria excess quantities of bilirubin in the urine.

urocele distension of the scrotum with extravasated urine.

urochezia discharge of urine in the feces.

Urochloa genus of grasses in the family Poaceae; can cause nitrate–nitrite or oxalate poisoning; includes *U. mozambicensis*, *U. panicoides* (liverseed grass).

urochrome a breakdown product of hemoglobin related to the bile pigments, found in the urine and responsible for its yellow color.

uroclepsia the involuntary escape of urine.

urocrisia diagnosis by examining the urine.

urocyst the urinary bladder.

urocystitis inflammation of the urinary bladder.

urodeum, urodaeum see avian CLOACA.

urodynamics the dynamics of the propulsion and flow of urine in the urinary tract.

urogastrone a polypeptide secreted by the salivary glands and by Brunner's glands, which is a potent inhibitor of gastric acid secretion.

urogenital pertaining to the urinary system and genitalia; urinogenital; genitourinary.

u. folds elongated, ventral portion of the cloacal folds; contribute to the formation of the urethral groove on the ventral aspect of the genital tubercle.

u. membrane ventral part of the cloacal membrane separating the gut from the fetus's external environment.

u. orifice opening between the fetal urogenital sinus and the amniotic cavity.

u. sinus see urogenital SINUS.

u. system GENITOURINARY system.

u. tract, u. system genitourinary system.

urogenous 1. producing urine. 2. produced from or in the urine.

urogram a radiograph obtained by urography.

urography radiography of any part of the urinary tract.

ascending u., cystoscopic u. retrograde urography.

descending u., excretion u., excretory u., intravenous u. urography after intravenous injection of an opaque medium which is rapidly excreted in the urine.

retrograde u. urography after injection of contrast medium into the bladder through the urethra.

urokinase an enzyme found in the urine of humans and other mammals which is secreted by kidney parenchymal cells and converts plasminogen to plasmin and activates the fibrinolytic system; used as a fibrinolytic agent.

urolith a calculus in the urine or the urinary tract. See also UROLITHIASIS.

apatite u's consist of calcium phosphate in several forms, the most common being hydroxyapatite and carbonate-apatite. They may be only a component of uroliths of other mineral composition or occur in association with primary hyperparathyroidism, excessive intake of calcium and phosphorus or renal tubular acidosis. They are smooth and radiopaque.

ammonium acid urate u's the common form of urate uroliths in dogs. Occur particularly in Dalmation dogs because of their unique urate metabolism which results in high urinary levels of uric acid.

barium u's rare, iatrogenic curiosities.

brushite u. calcium hydrogen phosphate dihydrate.

calcium phosphate u's apatite uroliths.

carbonate u's found in ruminants with alkaline urine that ingest high-oxalate plants or pasture that is dominated by clover.

clover u's occurs in wethers grazing estrogen-rich clover pasture. May be a soft yellow body composed of benzocoumarin, a metabolite of estrogens in the subterranean clover, and desquamated epithelial cells or a pasty white material consisting largely of calcium carbonate and organic matter derived from isoflavones. Called also clover stone.

cystine u's occur in dogs excreting high levels of cystine in their urine due to an inherited transport defect in the proximal renal tubules.

u. dissolution may be part of the management of struvite and cystine uroliths in dogs. It involves increasing the solubility and reducing the quantity of crystalloids in the urine and increasing the volume of urine by the use of urinary acidifiers, dietary changes and promoting diuresis. See also calculolytic DIET, ACETOHYDROXAMIC ACID.

jackstone u's see silica uroliths (below).

magnesium ammonium phosphate u's see struvite uroliths (below).

oxalate u. hard, dense, white or yellow calculi with rough surfaces which may originate from ingested oxalate but in many cases is the endogenous product of liver metabolism.

preputial u. top-shaped calculi found rarely in the prepuce of steers. They have a valve-like effect and cause obstruction of the orifice, distension and sometimes local infiltration of subcutaneous tissues with urine.

purine u's includes ammonium acid urate, sodium acid urate and xanthine uroliths.

renal u. one formed in the renal pelvis and often of corresponding shape.

silica u's consist largely of silica. Are white to brown in color, may be laminated and measure up to 0.5 inch in diameter They may reach a high level of prevalence in groups of wethers from particular areas and from particular farms where the silicon level in the pasture is high. In dogs, they occur with low frequency except in certain areas, particularly Kenya. They often have a characteristic appearance with numerous spiked projections from the surface. Called also 'jackstones'.

struvite u's white, crumbly, smooth bodies composed of magnesium ammonium phosphate hexahydrate (triple phosphate). The most common type of urolith in dogs and cats; they are commonly associated with infection of the urinary tract. Obstruction of the urethra by crystals of struvite is common in cats. Called also triple phosphate uroliths. See also FELINE urological syndrome.

urate u's small (less than 2 inches diameter) yellow or brown calculi seen in dogs, especially Dalmatians, Bulldogs and pigs.

urease u's see struvite uroliths (above).

whitlockite u. tricalcium phosphate.

xanthine u's yellow to red, friable, irregularly shaped calculi in sheep and young cattle.

urolithiasis formation of calculi in the urinary tract, or the condition associated with urinary calculi. In many food animals the condition goes unnoticed. Castrated males are a special case because of the high risk of urethral obstruction. There is a high prevalence of urolithiasis in male cats. Recorded also in marine fish larvae. See also FELINE urological syndrome, UROLITH.

obstructive u. one or more uroliths obstructs the passage of urine. Obstruction of a ureter causes a period of acute abdominal pain followed by dilatation of the obstructed ureter and renal pelvis and later by HYDRONEPHROSIS. Obstruction of the urethra occurs almost exclusively in males and at a much higher prevalence in castrated males. It causes a syndrome of acute abdominal pain manifested by restlessness, swishing of the tail, groaning and grunting while straining to urinate but passing only a few drops of blood-stained urine. The penis is often protruded. There is pain on palpation of the urethra per rectum and distension of the bladder is also apparent during this examination or by palpation through the abdominal wall in small animals. Rupture of the bladder is inevitable unless the obstruction is relieved. No significant amount of urine is passed, an observation that may require that the animal be confined.

preputial u. in steers can cause obstruction of the preputial orifice and infiltration of the belly wall with urine. Called also postholithiasis.

urological syndrome see FELINE urological syndrome.

urologist a specialist in urology.

urology the branch of veterinary medicine dealing with the urinary system.

uromelus a monster with fused hindlimbs and a single foot.

urometry the measurement and recording of pressure changes caused by contraction of the ureter during ureteral peristalsis.

uronate pathway see GLUCURONATE PATHWAY.

uroncus a swelling caused by retention or extravasation of urine.

Uronema ciliated protozoa within the order Scuticociliatida. These or closely related genera cause severe losses in marine aquacultured finfish and in ornamental species.

uronephrosis distension of the renal pelvis and tubules with urine.

uronic acid one of the monosaccharide unit in the repeating disaccharide units involved in the formation of glycosaminoglycans.

uropathogen pathogenic organisms in the urinary tract.

uropathy any disease in the urinary tract.

uroperitoneum urine free in the peritoneal cavity.

urophanic appearing in the urine.

uroplania the presence of urine in, or its discharge from, organs not of the genitourinary system.

Uropodidae a family of scavenger mites which frequent poultry litter but do not infest birds.

uropoiesis the formation of urine.

uroporphyria porphyria with excessive excretion of uroporphyrin.

uroporphyrin one of a group of porphyrins produced during biosynthesis of natural porphyrins and excreted in urine. There are two isomers I and III.

uroporphyrinogen a precursor of uroporphyrin and coproporphyrinogen.

u. III first tetrapyrrole compound in the pathway of porphyrin synthesis from combination of four porphobilinogen compounds via the action of uroporphyrinogen I synthetase and uroporphyrinogen III cosynthetase.

u. III cosynthetase an enzyme involved in the synthesis of uroporphyrinogen.

u. isomerase see uroporphyrinogen III cosynthetase (above).

u. I synthetase an enzyme involved in the synthesis of uroporphyrinogen.

uropsammus urinary gravel.

uropygial glands bilobed oil glands on either side of the pygostyle of many birds which aid in waterproofing feathers. Some species, e.g pigeons and parrots, lack them.

uroradiology radiology of the urinary tract.

urorectal pertaining to or arising from the rectum and the urogenital sinus of the embryo.

u. fistula congenital defect in the urorectal septum resulting in passage of urine thro the rectum.

u. septal defects principally urorectal fistula.

u. septum divides the primitive fetal cloaca into dorsal rectum and ventral urogenital sinus.

urorrhagia excessive secretion of urine.

urorrhea involuntary flow of urine.

uroscheocele urocele.

uroschesis retention or suppression of the urine.

uroscopy diagnostic examination of the urine.

urosepsis bacteremia resulting from urinary tract infection.

urostealith a urinary calculus having fatty constituents.

urothelium the special epithelium of the urinary bladder.

urotoxia 1. the toxicity of the urine. 2. the toxic substances of the urine. 3. the unit of toxicity of the urine or a quantity sufficient to kill 1 kg of living substance.

urotropine see METHENAMINE.

uroureter distension of the ureter with urine.

urovagina pooling of urine in the anterior vagina due to upward tipping of the pelvis in old cows and mares, caused by forward and downward tension on the vagina and vestibule. Leads to vaginitis and infertility. See also tipped PELVIS.

Ursicoptes americanus American sarcoptiform mange mite which causes pruritus and alopecia in bears.

ursicoptic emanating from or pertaining to *Ursicoptes americanus*.

ursid a member of the family Ursidae, including the polar, brown, American brown, black, grizzly and Kodiak bears, the Himalayan black, Malayan and sloth bears. They are all very large, plantigrade carnivores.

Ursidae family of bears.

ursodeoxycholate a hydrophilic bile acid, used in the treatment of chronic hepatic disease.

ursodeoxycholic acid a natural bile acid; a degradation product of chenodeoxycholic acid, used therapeutically in the treatment of cholestatic liver disease.

Ursus a genus of bears in the family Ursidae. Includes black, brown, American black, grizzly, big brown and *U. theodorus*. See also BRUNUS EDWARDII.

Ursus theodorus see BRUNUS EDWARDII.

URT upper respiratory tract.

URTI upper respiratory tract infection.

Urtica plant genus in the family Urticaceae; called also stinging nettle. They have stinging leaves and stems which plague humans but appear to be harmless to animals; can cause nitrate–nitrite poisoning; includes *U. dioica*, *U. incisa*, *U. procera*, *U. urens*, *U. ferox*.

urticant producing urticaria.

urticaria a vascular reaction of the skin that is commonly immunologically based or may be due to direct exposure to a chemical. Marked by transient appearance of slightly elevated patches (wheals) which are redder or paler than the surrounding skin and often attended by severe itching; called also hives. The wheals may be in very large numbers, mostly over the body, 0.5 to 2 inches in diameter and there is no discontinuity of the epithelium. Called also nettle rash.

giant u., u. gigantea angioneurotic edema.

heat reflex u. see cholinergic PRURITUS.

u. hemorrhagica purpura with urticaria.

u. medicamentosa that due to use of a drug.

nasolacrimal u. conjunctivitis and rhinitis caused by hypersensitivity to inhaled allergens (atopy).

papular u., u. papulosa an allergic reaction to the bite of various insects, with appearance of lesions that evolve into inflammatory, increasingly hard, red or brownish, persistent papules. See also LICHEN.

u. pigmentosa a proliferative disorder of mast cells in humans; a similar disease has been reported in young cats. There is erythema and hyperpigmentation of the mouth, chin, neck and eyes.

urticarium hives.

urtication the development or formation of urticaria.

urushiol the toxic irritant principle of poison ivy and various related plants.

US Army a term applied to surgical instruments designed by members of the United States Army.

US Army chisel a heavyweight bone chisel with a bevel on one side of the cutting edge.

US Army osteotome like a chisel (above), but with a bevel on both sides.

US Army retractor handheld retractors, in pairs, flat metal with a right angle bend at both ends, both in the same direction. one long return, one short. Designed for short-term retraction of wound edges so as to view abdominal or thoracic contents.

USAN United States Accepted Nomenclature.

USDA United States Department of Agriculture.

user in computer terminology a person who uses either a computer or the information generated by one. A derogatory term used by information technology staff for their clients.

u. friendly a computer program or system which is easy to understand, to learn and to use.

USG urine specific gravity.

USNF see UNITED STATES NATIONAL FORMULARY.

USP United States Pharmacopeia.

USP unit one used in the United States Pharmacopeia in expressing potency of drugs and other preparations.

ustilaginism a condition resembling ergotism due to ingestion of maize containing *Ustilago maydis*.

Ustilago zeae a mold which grows commonly on the foliage and ears of the maize plant. Possibly related to CORNSTALK POISONING of cattle. The related smut on barley (*Ustilago hordei*) is suspected to cause abortion in ruminants.

uta see LEISHMANIASIS.

uterine pertaining to the UTERUS; see also ENDOMETRIUM, ENDOMETRIAL.

u. abscess most common in cattle and in dorsal wall due to injury during insemination or intrauterine therapy for infertility or instrumental obstetric manipulation.

u. accommodation limited may contribute to flexural deformities of limbs especially in foals; obesity of the dam may contribute to the limitation.

u. artery rupture occurs during parturition, and often accompanies uterine prolapse in cows. There is marked mucosal pallor and death occurs quickly due to hemorrhagic anemia. In mares, rupture of the middle uterine artery causes hemorrhage, colic, and often, death.

u. caruncle see uterine CARUNCLE.

u. cervix see CERVIX uteri.

u. discharge copious, foul-smelling discharge in postpartum septic metritis in cows; thick, white, small volume discharge in endometritis.

u. displacement includes torsion, downward deviation in sows, inguinal and ventral hernia, prolapse.

u. distension palpable per rectum in cows, mares, through the abdominal wall in cats and dogs; pregnancy the common cause, pyometra, accumulation of secretions in imperforate hymen rarely. Pregnancy distinguishable in cows and mares by presence of membranes, or cotyledons in cows or fetus or fremitus in middle uterine artery.

u. downward displacement occurs in deep-bodied, pregnant sows with large litters and dystocia results.

u. expulsive deficiency see uterine inertia (below).

u. gland simple or branched, tubular glands extending into the lamina propria–submucosa; secrete mucus, lipids, glycogen, protein.

u. horn one of the pair of tubular extensions from the uterine body. Amongst the domestic species the horns are largest in those that bear many young (polytocous), e.g. sows, bitches, and shorter in those that bear single young (unitocous). Birds have two but only the left one is well developed or functional.

u. inertia primary, due to overstretching of the uterus or toxemia or obesity, or secondary, due to exhaustion, lack of myometrial contractions.

u. infection see METRITIS.

u. involution return to normal size after the delivery of the fetus.

u. involution failure common sequel to normal parturition in aged, high-producing cows, especially those suffering from milk fever or ketosis; metritis is a common sequel.

u. lochia see LOCHIA.

u. malformation includes uterus didelphys, uterus unicornis and segmental aplasia of any part of the tubular organ.

u. milk secretions of the uterine endometrium in the early part of pregnancy; sustains the fetus until placental attachments are fully functional.

u. mucosa endometrium.

u. neoplasm uncommon but fibroleiomyoma occurs in bitches, leiomyoma and lymphosarcoma in cows.

u. prolapse see uterine PROLAPSE.

u. rupture occurs usually during parturition and due to human intervention. Reparable if recognized but may lead to peritonitis.

u. sand dry, inspissated granules, yellow in color, found occasionally on the exterior of the bovine placenta. Probably derived from blood leaked into the lumen of the uterus in early pregnancy.

u. stump granuloma chronic inflammation due to infection or nonabsorbable sutures used in closing the stump after ovariohysterectomy.

u. swab swab of the uterus for bacteriological and virological examination for pathogens likely to adversely affect fertility. Used in fertility maintenance of mares.

u. torsion torsion of the body of the uterus in cows and mares and of a horn of the uterus in the sow. Causes dystocia characterized by the nonappearance of any part of the fetus in the vulva. Occurs rarely in dogs and cats.

u. tube a slender tube extending from the uterus to the ovary on the same side, conveying ova to the cavity of the uterus and permitting passage of spermatozoa in the opposite direction. It is mostly suspended in a fold of peritoneum (mesosalpinx) that may enclose a cavity (ovarian bursa). It terminates at the ovarian end in a dilated funnel (infundibulum). Called also fallopian tube and oviduct.

When the mature ovum leaves the ovary it enters the fringed opening of the uterine tube, through which it travels slowly to the uterus. When conception takes place, the tube is usually the site of fertilization.

u. tube occlusion may be congenital, or constricted by scar tissue in chronic peritonitis; a rare cause of infertility.

uter(o)- word element. [L.] *uterus.*
uteroabdominal pertaining to the uterus and abdomen.
uterocervical pertaining to the uterus and cervix uteri.
uterofixation hysteropexy; surgical fixation of the uterus.
uterogenic formed in the uterus.
uterogestation uterine gestation; normal pregnancy.
uterography radiographic examination of the uterus; hysterography.
uterolith a uterine calculus; hysterolith.
uterometer an instrument for measuring the uterus; hysterometer.
utero-ovarian pertaining to the uterus and ovary.
uteropexy hysteropexy.
uteroplacental pertaining to the placenta and uterus.
uteroplasty plastic repair of the uterus.
uterorectal pertaining to or communicating with the uterus and rectum.
uterosacral pertaining to the uterus and sacrum.
uterosalpingography radiography of the uterus and uterine tubes, usually done with contrast in the non-gravid uterus. Called also hysterosalpingography.
uteroscope an instrument for viewing the interior of the uterus; hysteroscope.
uterotomy hysterotomy; incision of the uterus.
uterotonic 1. increasing the tone of uterine muscle. 2. a uterotonic agent.
uterotubal pertaining to the uterus and uterine tubes.
uterovaginal pertaining to the uterus and vagina.
uteroverdin the green lochia seen in postparturient bitches.
uterovesical pertaining to the uterus and bladder.
uterus the hollow muscular organ in female mammals in which the fertilized ovum normally becomes embedded and in which the developing embryo and fetus is nourished. It is composed of two horns, a body and a cervix; the cervix opens caudally into the vagina. Two UTERINE tubes enter the uterus at the upper end, one on each side. The walls of the uterus are composed of muscle; its lining is mucous membrane. The muscular substance of the uterus is called the myometrium; the inner lining is called endometrium.
  u. didelphys, duplex u. complete duplication of the cervix and uterus.
  u. masculinus see MÜLLERIAN DUCT.
  simple u. a uterus with a single large body, two small horns, and a single cervix as found in primates.
  u. unicornis one horn, except usually for its apex, is completely missing because of a developmental defect.
UTI urinary tract infection.
utility dogs those used for some tasks that are helpful to man; sometimes called WORKING DOGS. In some classification systems used for competitions, this is a separate group that includes the Alaskan malamute, Bull mastiff, Doberman pinscher, Newfoundland, Rottweiler and St. Bernard.
utilization coefficient in terms of oxygen transport in the blood this coefficient expresses the proportion of oxygen in the blood which diffuses into tissues as it passes through the capillaries.
UTP uridine triphosphate.
Utrecht technique see OMENTOFIXATION.
utricle 1. any small sac. 2. the larger of the two divisions of the membranous labyrinth of the inner ear. Called also utriculus.
  prostatic u., urethral u. a small blind pouch in the substance of the prostate.
utricular 1. bladder-like. 2. pertaining to the utricle.
utriculitis inflammation of the prostatic utricle or of the utricle of the ear.
utriculosaccular pertaining to the utricle and saccule of the membranous labyrinth of the inner ear.
  u. duct leads from the utricle of the internal ear to the endolymphatic duct.
utriculus see UTRICLE (2).
Utstein reporting scheme a system used in human medicine for uniform reporting of cardiac arrest and resuscitation data.
Uukuvirus a genus of viruses in the family BUNYAVIRIDAE.
U/V rays see ULTRAVIOLET rays.
uvea [L.] the iris, ciliary body, and choroid together.
  anterior u. see anterior UVEAL tract.
uveal pertaining to or emanating from the UVEA.
  anterior u. tract the iris and ciliary body.
  u. tract the vascular tunic of the eye, comprising choroid, ciliary body and iris.
uveitis inflammation of the uvea.
  anterior u. inflammation of the anterior uveal tract, i.e. iridocyclitis. Signs include pain, blepharospasm, tearing, conjunctivitis, constricted pupil, reduced intraocular pressure, aqueous flare, and sometimes keratic precipitates and hypopyon.
  endogenous u. arising from causes within the body.
  equine recurrent u. see periodic OPHTHALMIA.
  exogenous u. arising from causes external to the body.
  granulomatous u. associated with toxoplasmosis and systemic mycotic infections such as cryptococcosis, blastomycosis, coccidioidomycosis and candidiasis.
  heterochromic u. see heterochromic IRIDOCYCLITIS.
  lens-induced u. caused by escape of lens protein into the aqueous, initiating an immune response.
  phacolytic u. associated with resorption of hypermature cataracts in which there is rupture of the lens capsule and release of lens proteins.
  phacoclastic u. caused by disruption of the anterior lens capsule and leakage of lens proteins.
  posterior u. inflammation of the ciliary body and choroid.
  recurrent equine u. see periodic OPHTHALMIA.
  sympathetic u. see sympathetic OPHTHALMIA.
uve(o)- word element. [L.] *uvea.*
uveodermatologic syndrome see VOGT–KOYANAGI–HARADA-LIKE SYNDROME.
uveoneuraxitis uveitis associated with involvement of the optic nerve.
uveoscleral drainage an alternate route of aqueous drainage from the anterior chamber, through the ciliary body and choroid.
uveoscleritis scleritis due to extension of uveitis.
uviform shaped like a grape.
uvula pl. *uvulae* [L.] a small median prolongation of the soft palate occurring in humans and pigs.
  u. of bladder a rounded elevation at the neck of the bladder, formed by convergence of muscle fibers terminating in the urethra. Called also uvula vesicae.
  u. cerebelli a lobule that is the posterior limit of the fourth ventricle of the brain. Called also uvula vermis.
  palatine u., u. palatina the small, fleshy mass hanging from the soft palate above the root of the tongue.
  u. vermis the part of the vermis of the cerebellum between the pyramid and nodule.
  u. vesicae uvula of bladder.
uvulectomy excision of the uvula.

V

V chemical symbol, *vanadium;* symbol, *volt;* vision; visual acuity.
V_T tidal volume.
v. [L.] *vena* (vein).
V–D–J joining see ANTIBODY.
V domain the variable region or DOMAIN of immunoglobulins.
V factor see DIPHOSPHOPYRIDINE NUCLEOTIDE.
V–J joining see ANTIBODY.
V region variable region of immunoglobulins.
v tach ventricular tachycardia.
V to Y plasty a tension-relieving technique for closure of a skin incision in which a V-shaped incision is made alongside the primary incision and then closed in a Y shape.
vaalstorm THESIUM *lineatum.*
VAC vincristine, doxorubicin and cyclophosphamide; a cancer chemotherapy regime.
vaccigenous producing vaccine.
vaccina vaccinia virus.
vaccinable susceptible of being successfully vaccinated.
vaccinal 1. pertaining to vaccinia, to vaccine, or to vaccination. 2. having protective qualities when used by way of inoculation.
vaccinate to inoculate with vaccine to produce immunity.
vaccination the introduction of vaccine into the body to produce immunity to a specific disease. The vaccine may be administered by subcutaneous or intradermal injection, by infusion into the mammary gland, by mouth or by inhalation of an aerosol. The term vaccination comes from the Latin *vacca,* cow, and was coined when the first inoculations were given with organisms that caused the mild disease cowpox to produce immunity against smallpox. Today the word has the same meaning as IMMUNIZATION.
v. failure following administration of a vaccine, the animal develops the disease. The cause is often related to faulty inactivation of the vaccine due to improper handling or inappropriate administration, or the animal was incubating the disease at the time of vaccination.
v. schedules specified ages and intervals for administration of vaccines to ensure the best immunological response.
simultaneous serum-virus v. simultaneous administration of live virus and hyperimmune serum. Used at one time in the control of several diseases, including canine distemper and hog cholera.
vaccine a suspension of attenuated or killed microorganisms (viruses, bacteria or rickettsiae), administered for prevention, amelioration or treatment of infectious diseases.
anti-idiotype v. antibody made to antigenic determinants located in the variable domains of immunoglobulin molecules. Proposed as a means of regulating antibody responses and also as a substitute antigen for vaccination.
attenuated v. a vaccine prepared from live microorganisms that have lost their virulence but retained their ability to induce protective immunity. Attenuated microorganisms including particularly bacteria and viruses may be found naturally or they may be produced in the laboratory, for example by adaptation to a new medium or cell culture or they may be produced by recombinant DNA technology.
autogenous v. a vaccine prepared from cultures of material derived from a lesion of the animal to be vaccinated, e.g. wart vaccine.
bacterial v. a preparation of attenuated or killed bacteria, used to immunize against organisms injected, or sometimes for pyrogenetic effects in treatment of certain noninfectious diseases.
biosynthetic v. a formulation containing a protective, noninfectious, immunogenic subunit produced in or by a biological system.
caprinized v. a vaccine, usually a virus, attenuated by serial passage through goats, e.g. caprinized rinderpest vaccine. In highly susceptible cattle this vaccine may cause significant reactions and lapinized vaccines are preferred.
dead v. inactivated vaccine; one with organisms that have been killed.
DNA v. DNA sequences that code for immunogenic proteins located in appropriately constructed plasmids which include strong promoters, which when injected into an animal are taken up by cells and the immunogenic proteins are expressed and elicit an immune response. No vaccines of this type are licensed and concerns about safety have not been resolved.
heterotypic v. one developed from a virus that is antigenically distinct but related to that causing the disease for which the animal is being immunized, e.g. measles vaccine used to protect dogs from canine distemper.
homotypic v. one developed from the same virus as that causing the disease the animal is being immunized against.
human diploid cell v. an inactivated rabies vaccine made from rabies virus grown on human embryo lung fibroblast cells.
inactivated v. see dead vaccine (above).
killed virus (KV) v. see dead vaccine (above).
live v. a vaccine prepared from live, usually attenuated, microorganisms.
v. lymph material containing vaccinia virus collected from vaccinial vesicles of inoculated calves; used for active immunization against smallpox.
mixed v. see MIXED bacterial vaccine.
modified live virus (MLV) v. see attenuated vaccine (above).
polyvalent v. one prepared from more than one strain or species of microorganisms.
recombinant v. one created by recombinant DNA technology.
subunit v. one containing only specific antigenic proteins of the infectious agent.
synthetic peptide v. using synthetic short peptides which correspond with major epitopes of viral proteins to elicit a protective antibody response.
virus-vectored v. use of viruses as vectors to carry selected genes from another virus for immunization.
vaccinia the vaccinia virus; a laboratory generated virus, antigenically related to the cowpox virus, that causes a lesion on the teat skin of affected cows. It is indistinguishable from cowpox lesions and used to be used to vaccinate humans against smallpox.
vaccinial pertaining to or characteristic of vaccinia.
vacciniform resembling vaccinia.
vacciniola generalized vaccinia.
vaccinotherapy therapeutic use of vaccines.
Vacor a single dose rodenticide that acts as an antagonist of B vitamins, particularly nicotinamide; useful against warfarin-resistant rodents. Poisoning causes

vomiting, abdominal pain and weakness. Called also pyriminil.

vacuolar containing, or of the nature of, vacuoles.

vacuolated containing vacuoles.

vacuolation the process of forming vacuoles; the condition of being vacuolated.

vacuole a space or cavity in the cytoplasm of a cell.

contractile v. a small fluid-filled cavity in the cytoplasm of certain unicellular organisms; it gradually increases in size and then collapses; its function is thought to be respiratory and excretory.

vacuolization vacuolation.

vacuum a space devoid of air or other gas.

v. collection use of a handheld vacuum to recover ectoparasites from the coat of animals.

v.-dehydrated freed of moisture while in a vacuum. Used in the packaging of food.

v. gauge pressure gauge in a milking machine which indicates the level of vacuum in the system.

v. pack meat or other perishable food is packed in a tightly sealed bag made of copolymers with polyvinyldene chloride and a low vacuum created. A bag made of nylon–polythene laminate is used for bags that are heat-sealed and a high vacuum created. The pack is then frozen for storage or shipment.

v. pressure used as the basis of the modern milking machine; the negative pressure is generated by a vacuum pump and transmitted through metal and rubber pipes to the teat cups and thence to the teats; the continuous basic pressure is what keeps the teat cups on the teats; the periodic fluctuations is what causes the squezzing of the teat walls and the expulsion of the milk from the teats.

v. tube many clinical pathology specimens are now collected in evacuated test tubes. A needle connected to the tube through a rubber stopper is passed into a vein. The needle is then connected to the vacuum and the blood or other fluid withdrawn.

vagal pertaining to the vagus nerve.

v. attack see VASOVAGAL attack.

v. maneuver pressure on the carotid sinus or eyeball to terminate supraventricular tachycardia.

vagina 1. any sheath or sheathlike structure. 2. the canal in the female from the external genitalia (vulva) to the cervix uteri.

v. bulbi see TENON'S CAPSULE.

v. carotica the fascial sheath surrounding the carotid artery and also containing the internal jugular vein and vagus nerves. Called also carotid sheath.

double v. secondary vaginal pouch.

external v. of the optic nerve fascial sheath around the optic nerve and continuous with that of the eyeball.

pneumo-v. see PNEUMOVAGINA.

sunken v. a condition seen in older mares in which the vagina falls forward, resulting in pooling of urine and vaginal secretions and pneumovagina.

vaginal pertaining to the vagina, the tunica vaginalis testis, or to any sheath.

v. annulus see ANNULUS vaginalis.

v. aplasia manifested by imperforate hymen or residual strands of hymen. See imperforate HYMEN.

v. aspiration use of a suction apparatus to collect a sample of vaginal fluid for culture, cytological or immunological examination.

v. biopsy collection of a sample of mucosa by a pinch biopsy instrument for histopathogical examination.

v. constriction inherited defect in Jersy cows combined with anal constriction, sometimes with rectovaginal fistula.

v. cyclic changes see vaginal cytology (below).

v. cysts see GARTNER'S DUCTS, BARTHOLIN'S GLANDS.

v. cystocele the urinary bladder is lying on the floor of the vagina; the displacement has been via the urethra by eversion or via a tear in the floor of the vagina.

v. cytology cyclic changes in the exfoliated epithelial cells of the vaginal mucosa occurring synchronously with the stages of the estrous cycle; collection of samples by the use of a swab and laboratory examination of a smear is a useful aid in determining the most appropriate time to mate a bitch.

v. fornix see vaginal FORNIX.

v. hypoplasia segmental see MÜLLERIAN DUCT aplasia.

v. inflammation see VAGINITIS (1).

v. neoplasm include papilloma, sarcoma, myxofibroma.

v. process an outpocketing of the peritoneum into the gubernaculum at the site of the future inguinal canal in the male fetus; becomes the tunica vagina of the adult.

v. prolapse see vaginal PROLAPSE.

v. retainer see BEARING retainer.

v. ring see ANNULUS vaginalis.

v. rupture occurs during mating, dystocia, insemination, or by sadistic or malicious trauma. Results in peritonitis or cellulitis of the pelvic fascia.

v. smear examination of the cells in a smear is used as an aid in predicting the time of ovulation, which may be useful in selecting the optimal date for breeding.

v. speculum see GRAVES SPECULUM, THOROUGHBRED SPECULUM.

v. stricture cicatricial contraction after traumatic injury.

v. tunic the double peritoneal fold which encloses the spermatic cord and the testis; made up of a visceral layer which is adherent to the testis and cord, and a parietal layer which lines the scrotum and the inguinal canal.

v. vestibule entrance to the vagina enclosed between the lips of the vulva, the labia minor. Connects the vagina at the external urethral orifice to the external genital opening; develops from the embryonic urogenital sinus.

v. wash irrigation of the vagina with sterile saline can be used to recover cells, which are stained and examined microscopically to monitor estrus.

vaginalectomy vaginectomy.

vaginalitis inflammation of the tunica vaginalis testis; periorchitis.

vaginate enclosed in a sheath.

vaginectomy 1. resection of the tunica vaginalis testis. 2. excision of the vagina.

vaginismus painful spasms of the muscles of the vagina.

vaginitis 1. inflammation of the vagina; colpitis. 2. inflammation of a sheath.

adhesive v. that in which ulceration and exfoliation of the mucosa result in adhesions of the membranes.

contagious v. see infectious pustular VULVOVAGINITIS, EPIVAG.

granular v. see GRANULAR vaginitis.

pustular v. see infectious pustular VULVOVAGINITIS.

vaginoabdominal pertaining to the vagina and abdomen.

vaginocele colpocele; vaginal hernia.

vaginofixation vaginopexy; colpopexy.

vaginography radiography of the vagina using a contrast agent. Retrograde passage of the contrast agent can be used to demonstrate ectopic ureters in bitches.

vaginolabial pertaining to the vagina and labia.

vaginomycosis any fungal disease of the vagina.

vaginopathy any disease of the vagina.

vaginoperineal pertaining to the vagina and perineum.

vaginoperineorrhaphy suture of the vagina and perineum; colpoperineorrhaphy.

vaginoperineotomy incision of the vagina and perineum.

vaginoperitoneal pertaining to the vagina and peritoneum.

vaginopexy colpopexy; vaginofixation; suturing of the vagina to the abdominal wall in cases of vaginal relaxation.

vaginoplasty colpoplasty; plastic repair of the vagina.

vaginoscope illuminated tubular instrument designed for examining the interior of the vagina. A common alternative is to use a vaginal speculum and a flashlight.

vaginoscopy viewing of the vaginal lining with a vaginoscope.

vaginotomy colpotomy; incision of the vagina.

vaginourethrography radiography of the vagina and urethra. Contrast medium is introduced through a catheter into the vagina until it overflows into the urethra. Used in the diagnosis of lower urinary tract disease in bitches.

vaginovesical pertaining to the vagina and bladder.

vagolysis surgical destruction of the vagus nerve.

vagolytic having an effect resembling that produced by interruption of impulses transmitted by the vagus nerve; parasympatholytic.

v. agents includes atropine sulfate, glycopyrrolate, propantheline, isopropamide.

vagomimetic having an effect resembling that produced by stimulation of the vagus nerve.

vagosympathetic trunk the combined vagus nerve and the sympathetic trunk, invested in a common fascial sheath in the neck. In cats the two nerves remain separate.

vagotomy interruption of the impulses carried by the vagus nerve or nerves;

vagotonia irritability of the vagus nerve.

vagotonin a preparation of hormone from the pancreas that increases vagal tone, slows the heart, and increases the store of glycogen in the liver.

vagotropic having an effect on the vagus nerve.

vagovagal arising as a result of afferent and efferent impulses mediated through the vagus nerve.

vagus the tenth cranial nerve. For vagus nerve, see Table 14.

v. indigestion of cattle is the result of damage to branches of the vagus nerve which supply the rumenoreticulum, or to tension receptors in the wall of the reticulum. The two identified malfunctions are pyloric achalasia and reticulo-omasal achalasia (omasal transport failure). The clinical picture includes distension of the rumen or abomasum causing visible distension of the abdomen, emaciation and the passage of small amounts of pasty feces. Ruminal motility may be increased or decreased.

v. nerve signs dysfunction manifested by paralysis of pharynx, larynx, causing dysphagia, regurgitation through the nose, dyspnea, hypomotility of gastrointestinal tract.

v. nucleus any of four nuclei within the medulla oblongata; comprises the dorsal nucleus, the nucleus ambiguus, the nucleus of the tractus solitarius and the spinal nucleus of the trigeminal nerve.

Val valine.

valency, valence 1. the numerical measure of the capacity to combine; in chemistry, an expression of the number of atoms of hydrogen (or its equivalent) that one atom of a chemical element can hold in combination, if negative, or displace in a reaction, if positive. 2. in immunology, an expression of the number of antigenic determinants with which one molecule of a given antibody can combine.

valerian see VALERIANA.

Valeriana a genus of herbaceous plants providing second class forage for livestock. Has a fleshy root containing valeric acid. *V. officinalis* is used for extraction of commercial valeric acid.

valgus [L.] bent outward; twisted; denoting a deformity in which the angulation is away from the midline of the body, as in coxa valga.

valine Val; a naturally occurring amino acid.

valinemia hypervalinemia; elevated levels of valine in the blood and urine.

valinomycin ionophore consisting of a cyclic trimer of tetrapeptides. Specifically transports potassium ions across cell membranes. Inhibitor of oxidative phosphorylation due to its action in antagonizing the proton motive force.

Valium trademark for a preparation of diazepam, an anxiolytic and skeletal muscle relaxant. Also used as an appetite stimulant, particularly in cats.

vallate having a wall or rim; rim-shaped.

vallecula pl. *valleculae* [L.] a depression or furrow.

v. cerebelli a longitudinal fissure on the caudal cerebellum, in which the medulla oblongata rests.

v. epiglottica the depressions on either side of the median glossoepiglottic fold.

v. sylvii a depression made by the fissure of Sylvius at the base of the brain. Called also lateral cerebral fossa.

v. unguis the sulcus of the matrix of the nail.

Vallée's vaccine a vaccine composed of living *Mycobacterium paratuberculosis* organisms in a paraffin oil–pumice stone vehicle; used as a prophylactic against Johne's disease in cattle.

valley fever see COCCIDIOIDOMYCOSIS.

Valone an insecticide and rodenticide. One of the indandione compounds with actions similar to that of warfarin.

valor a rodenticide no longer marketed because of toxicity in horses causing dehydration, abdominal pain, hindlimb weakness, inappetence, fishy smell in urine. Called also N-3-pyridyl methyl N^1-*p*-nitrophenyl urea.

valproic acid an anticonvulsant.

Valsalva maneuver a forcible expiratory effort in combination with a closed glottis as occurs in coughing.

valsiekte [Af.] 'falling disease', characterized by myelomalacia, ataxia caused by *Chrysocoma tenuifolia.*

value a measure of worth or efficiency; a quantitative measurement of the activity, concentration, etc., of specific substances.

absolute v. the size of an observation or measurement regardless of its sign.

expected v. an estimate of the value of a population parameter, which would be achieved by sampling an infinite number of times.

normal v's the range in concentration of specific substances found in normal healthy tissues, secretions, etc.

valva pl. *valvae* [L.] a valve.

valve 1. a membranous fold in a canal or passage that prevents backward flow of material passing through it. 2. a mechanical device to regulate the flow of liquid or gas from an area of higher pressure to one of lower pressure. 3. automatic valve which maintains a steady vacuum in the system of a mechanical milking machine.

Adam's pressure reducing v. see reducing valve (below).

aortic v. see AORTIC valve.

atrioventricular v's the valves between the right atrium and right ventricle (tricuspid valve) and the left atrium and left ventricle (mitral valve).

bicuspid v. mitral valve.

cardiac v's valves that control flow of blood through and from the heart. See also AORTIC valve, MITRAL valve, PULMONARY valve, TRICUSPID valve.

coronary v. a valve at entrance of the coronary sinus into right atrium.

flair v. a cardiac valve having a cusp that has lost its normal support (as in ruptured chordae tendineae) and flutters in the bloodstream.

ileocecal v., ileocolic v. see ILEOCECAL valve.

nonreturn v. in anesthetic circuits, it prevents exhaled gas from returning to the patient.

portal v. regulates the amount of venous blood entering the kidney.

pressure reducing v. see reducing valve (below).

pyloric v. a prominent fold of mucous membrane at the pyloric orifice of the stomach.

reducing v. a special valve used on anesthetic machines and which reduces the pressure of the gas reaching the exit valve so that control of the flow is made easier. Called also regulator.

semilunar v's valves made up of semilunar segments or cusps (valvulae semilunares), guarding the entrances into the aorta and pulmonary artery.

thebesian v. coronary valve.

v. tube a thermionic diode that permits the flow of electric current in an x-ray machine in only one direction.

valvotomy incision of a valve.

valvula pl. *valvulae* [L.] a small valve; a single cusp of one of the semilunar valves of the heart.

valvular pertaining to, affecting or of the nature of a valve.

v. disease interferes with the normal rate and smoothness of blood flow through the cardiac orifices. The creation of turbulence results in the appearance of palpable thrills and audible murmurs, stenosis and insufficiency causing congestive heart failure. See also names of cardiac valves.

v. incompetence the valves do not close completely and when pressure is exerted on them blood leaks back through causing inefficient forward movement of the blood and turbulent flow leading to the development of cardiac murmurs.

v. stenosis narrowing of the lumen of the aperture through which the blood passes causing back pressure in the venous or pulmonary circuits. The clinical manifestations include cardiac murmurs and thrills and congestive heart failure. See also STENOSIS.

valvulitis inflammation of a valve, especially of a valve of the heart.

valvuloplasty plastic repair of a valve, especially a valve of the heart.

balloon v. use of a intracardiac catheter with an inflatable balloon to dilate stenotic cardiac valves.

valvulotome an instrument for cutting a valve.

valvulotomy valvotomy.

balloon v. see balloon VALVULOPLASTY.

vampire bat vector for rabies in animals, humans. See DESMODUS ROTUNDUS MURINUS.

van den Bergh test, reaction a test which differentiates between conjugated and unconjugated bilirubin in serum and assists in the differentiation between biliary or regurgitation hyperbilirubinemia, retention or hemolytic hyperbilirubinemia, or combined hyperbilirubinemia or jaundice. There are many variants of the basic test and the interpretation of them differs markedly between the species.

Van der Waals forces the relatively weak, short-range forces of attraction existing between atoms and molecules, which results in the attraction of nonpolar organic compounds to each other (hydrophobic bonding).

vanadium a chemical element, atomic number 23, atomic weight 50.942, symbol V. See Table 6. Its salts have been used in treating various diseases.

v. poisoning in humans poisoning is usually by inhalation causing respiratory irritation and pneumonia. In livestock poisoning is by ingestion of contaminated pasture and manifested by diarrhea, incoordination and oliguria.

vanadiumism poisoning by vanadium.

vancomycin a narrow-spectrum antibiotic produced by *Streptomyces orientalis*, highly effective against gram-positive bacteria; it is commonly reserved for use against serious infections caused by penicillinase-resistant *Staphylococci*. The toxic effects are quite severe and include damage to the eighth cranial (vestibulocochlear) nerve and renal disorders.

v. resistant enterococcus a group of multi-drug resistant bacteria associated with high mortality in humans.

vane the membranous or main part of the contour feather in birds as distinct from the shaft. It consists of the barbs held together by the interlocking barbules. Called also vexillum.

Vangueira PACHYSTIGMA *pygmaeum*.

vanillylmandelic acid an excretory product of the catecholamines found in the urine; used as a test in the diagnosis of phaeochromocytoma.

van't Hoff's law the velocity of chemical reactions is increased twofold or more for each rise of 10°C in temperature.

vapor steam, gas or exhalation.

Vapor vaporizer a type of temperature- and flow-compensating precision vaporizers for specific inhalation anesthetic agents.

vaporization 1. the conversion of a solid or liquid into a vapor without chemical change; distillation. 2. treatment by vapors; vapotherapy.

vaporize to convert into vapor or to be transformed into vapor.

vaporizer part of the apparatus used to deliver volatile anesthetic agents to patients. It is the vessel that vaporizes the liquid anesthetic and adds it to the flow of gas to the patient. The objective of them all is to deliver a suitable, accurately calibrated, quantity of anesthetic at all times and under all conditions. See also EMO VAPORIZER, DRÄGER VAPORIZER, VAPOR VAPORIZER.

bubble v., bubble through v. the carrier gas is dispersed through the anesthetic agent, usually through a diffuser, to form the anesthetic mixture to be inhaled. An example is the copper kettle vaporizer.

calibrated v. one with graduations to measure accurately the concentration of anesthetic vapor delivered.

wick v. carrier gas moves over the surface of the liquid anesthetic. Sheets of pliable material are used as wicks to increase the surface area. Examples are Vapor and 'tec' (Fluotec, Fortec) vaporizors.

vapotherapy therapeutic use of steam, vapor or spray.
VA/Q see VENTILATION:perfusion ratio.
Vaqueta see THILOA GLAUCOCARPA.
Vaquez–Osler disease primary polycythemia.
var. variety.
Varanus see MONITOR (3).
Varestrongylus see BICAULUS.
variability the state of being variable.
variable 1. any type of measurement, quantitative or qualitative, of which a series of individual observations is made so that it has, as a principal characteristic, the potential for variability. 2. has the quality of variability.
v. agent an agent in the cause of a disease which is capable of variation in intensity, e.g. weather, as contrasted to one that is not variable, e.g. *Salmonella dublin.*
concomitant v's in experimental design these refer to factors that affect the dependent variable, but are not themselves influenced by the treatment (e.g. age of animal). The effect of concomitant variables can be removed by suitable experimental design or by including them in the model.
continuous v. one in which all values within a given range are possible, e.g. birth weights of calves.
v. costs costs which vary with the dimensions of the activity. Includes seed, fertilizer, teat dip, worm drench. Called also direct costs. See also FIXED COSTS.
dependent v. 1. in statistics the variable predicted by a regression equation. 2. a variable which depends on other variables for its value.
discontinuous v. see discrete variable (below).
discrete v. one in which the possible values are not on a continuous scale, e.g. the number of sheep in a flock.
endogenous v. dependent variable.
exogenous v. independent or predetermined variable.
independent v. one not dependent on other variables but capable of affecting dependent variables, thus an input variable.
v. length record a computer record whose length is only as long as it needs to be. Many data storage programs have fixed length records which can waste much disk space especially if most of the records are likely to be short.
v. pitch font see proportionally spaced FONT.
spatial v. a measurement relating to area or location.
temporal v. one relating to chronological time.
variable formula pet food manufactured pet foods in which the ingredients vary according to their availability and cost; the type most commonly marketed.
variable groundsel SENECIO *lautus*.
variable region the *N*-terminal portion of heavy and light chains of immunoglobulin molecules in which the amino acid sequence varies as a consequence of somatic mutation and recombination during ontogeny of B lymphocytes and also occurring after antigen exposure. The variable amino acid sequence which provides more than 107 different antibody molecules is responsible for the antigen-binding specificity.
variance one of the measures of the dispersion of data; the mean squared deviation of a set of values from the mean.
additive genetic v. that portion of phenotypic variance which is due to the additive effect of genes (V_A).
analysis of v. a statistical method for comparing values, expressed in terms of means or variance, of one or more variables in several subgroups of a population. Called also anova.
non-additive genetic v. that portion of phenotypic variance which is due to epistatic interactions (V_I) and dominance deviations (V_D).
non-genetic v. that portion of phenotypic variance which is due to non-genetic effects such as environment (V_E).
phenotypic v. a measure of the extent to which individuals vary in their phenotype (V_P) – $V_P = V_A + V_D + V_I + V_E$.
v. ratio distribution see F DISTRIBUTION.
variant an organism or tissue that is different from the majority of the population but is still sufficiently similar to the common mode to be considered to be one of them, e.g. a variant strain of hog cholera (swine fever) virus.
variation divergence among individual animals of a group. The differences in the morphology or function of an organ or organism, are small enough to stay within the variability of the type organism or organ.
varicella-zoster virus causes chicken pox in humans and also infects gorillas, orang-utans and chimpanzees.
Varicellovirus one of two genera in the *Alphaherpesvirinae* subfamily of herpesviruses.
varices [L.] plural of *varix.*
variciform resembling a varix; varicose.
varicoblepharon a varicose swelling of the eyelid.
varicocele varicosity of the pampiniform plexus of the spermatic cord, forming a swelling in the scrotal neck that feels like a 'bag of worms'.
varicocelectomy excision of a varicocele.
varicomphalos a varicose tumor of the umbilicus.
varicose of the nature of or pertaining to a varix; unnaturally and permanently distended (said of a vein); variciform.
v. scrotal tumor benign vascular proliferation in dogs; resembles cavernous hemangioma.
v. veins are uncommonly found in animals except on the scrotum of old bulls, in the dorsal wall of the vagina in mares and on the prepuce in stallions. May also be associated with arteriovenous fistulae.
varicosity 1. a varicose condition; the quality or fact of being varicose. 2. a varix, or varicose vein.
varicotomy excision of a varix or of a varicose vein.
varicula a varix of the conjunctiva.
variegated thistle see SILYBUM MARIANUM.
variegated tick see AMBLYOMMA *variegatum*.
variety a taxonomic subcategory of a species.
variola a viral disease of humans and primates characterized by fever, rash and scab formation. Called also smallpox.
varix pl. *varices* [L.] an enlarged, tortuous vein, artery or lymphatic vessel.
aneurysmal v. a markedly dilated tortuous vessel; sometimes used to denote a form of arteriovenous aneurysm in which the blood flows directly into a neighboring vein without the intervention of a connecting sac.
arterial v. a racemose aneurysm or varicose artery.
lymph v., v. lymphaticus a soft, lobulated swelling of a lymph node, due to obstruction of lymphatic vessels.
varization a surgical procedure that decreases the angle of inclination of a part.
v. femoral osteotomy a surgical procedure involving an intertrochanteric osteotomy and removal of a bone wedge to create a varus deviation of the femoral head and neck. Used to increase hip stability in dogs with hip dysplasia.
varkoor see ZANTEDESCHIA AETHIOPICA.

Varnell gag a gag similar to the HITCHING GAG, except that the crossbars are rounded, and usually covered with leather or rubber, and fit into the interdental space.

varnish tree ALEURITES *moluccana*.

varolian pertaining to the pons varolii.

varus [L.] bent inward; denoting a deformity in which the angulation of the part is toward the midline of the body, as in coxa vara, genu varum.

vas pl. *vasa* [L.] a vessel.

v. aberrans 1. a blind tube sometimes connected with the epididymis; a vestigial mesonephric tube. 2. any anomalous or unusual vessel.

v. afferentia vessels that convey fluid to a structure or part.

v. brevia short vessels such as the gastric arteries.

v. deferens the excretory duct of the testis which conveys spermatozoa from the tail of the epididymis to the pelvic urethra and which sometimes unites with the excretory duct of the seminal vesicle to form the ejaculatory duct; called also ductus deferens.

v. efferentia vessels that convey fluid away from a structure or part.

v. lymphatica lymphatic vessels.

v. recta straight vessels, such as the long U-shaped vessels arising from the efferent glomerular arterioles of juxtamedullary nephrons and supplying the renal medulla.

v. vasorum the small nutrient arteries and veins in the walls of the larger blood vessels.

vasa [L.] plural of *vas*.

vascular pertaining to blood vessels or indicative of a copious blood supply.

v. clamps see hemostatic FORCEPS.

v. clip see CLIP (1).

v. disease see ARTERITIS, PHLEBITIS, LYMPHANGITIS, THROMBOSIS, ANEURYSM, capillary FRAGILITY.

v. grafts see vascular CONDUIT.

v. hemophilia von Willebrand's disease.

v. malformation includes HAMARTOMA, ARTERIOVENOUS fistula, TELANGIECTASIA.

v. neoplasm listed elsewhere; these include HEMANGIOMA, HEMANGIOENDOTHELIOMA, HAMARTOMA, TELANGIECTASIA, ANGIOKERATOMA, juvenile bovine ANGIOMATOSIS, bovine cutaneous ANGIOMATOSIS, VARICOSE scrotal tumor, MENINGIOANGIOMA, LYMPHOMATOID GRANULOMATOSIS, LYMPHANGIOMA, GLOMANGIOMA, HEMANGIOSARCOMA, LYMPANGIOSARCOMA.

v. nevus irregular shaped, cutaneous mass, congenital, hair-covered initially, subsequently hairless, usually 1–2 inches diameter in foals, may be inflamed, ulcerated; composed of densely packed blood vessels and bleed easily: most located on lower limbs; see also NEVUS.

v. occlusive syndrome complete occlusion of the vessel supplying blood to a part of the body causes temporary loss of function or death of the part, fall in temperature and change in color.

v. plaque a minor lesion in animals; manifested by slight thickening and wrinkling of the intima of the vessel over oval or elongated elevations.

v. pole the point on the renal glomerulus where the blood vessels enter and exit.

v. prosthesis see vascular CONDUIT.

v. ring anomaly see vascular RING.

v. sinus transformation marked dilation of sinuses in lymph nodes because of blockage of drainage from the node.

v. stasis serious slowing, or complete cessation, of blood or lymph flow through vessels.

v. system the vessels of the body including aorta, arteries, arterioles, capillaries, venules, sinusoids, sinuses, veins, lymphatics.

v. tone the state of contractile tension in the vessel walls.

v. tumor see vascular neoplasm (above).

v. tunic of the eye; consists of the choroid coat, the ciliary body and the iris.

vascularity the condition of being vascular.

vascularization the formation of new blood vessels in tissues.

vascularize to supply with vessels.

vasculature 1. the vascular system of the body, or any part of it. 2. the supply of vessels to a specific region.

vasculitis inflammation of a vessel; common causes include allergic, immune-mediated. Histopathologically differentiable types include eosinophilic, lymphocytic. Called also angiitis.

vasculopathy any disorder of blood vessels.

vasectomized subjected to VASECTOMY.

vasectomy excision of the vas (ductus) deferens, or a portion of it; bilateral vasectomy results in sterility.

Vaseline trademark for white petrolatum (USP), petroleum jelly.

vasey grass PASPALUM *urvillei*.

Vasgotaspets see SWEDISH VALLHUND.

vasifactive vasoformative.

vasiform resembling a vessel.

vasitis inflammation of the vas (ductus) deferens.

vas(o)- word element. [L.] *vessel, duct*.

vasoactive exerting an effect on the caliber of blood vessels.

v. intestinal peptide (VIP), v. intestinal polypeptide a peptide hormone that, in addition to its vasoactive properties, stimulates intestinal secretion of water and electrolytes, inhibits gastric secretion, promotes glycogenesis, causes hyperglycemia and stimulates secretion of pancreatic juice.

v. substances substances which cause constriction of blood vessels; substances which actively dilate vessels, rather than relax an existing vasoconstriction, should be included. See VASOCONSTRICTOR agents and VASODILATOR agents.

v. substances, endothelium-derived includes nitrous oxide, prostacyclin and other prostanoids, unnamed relaxing or constricting factors released as a result of a tissue insult, e.g. hypoxia or excessive stretch.

vasoconstriction decrease in the caliber of blood vessels; may be general or local, e.g. pulmonary, peripheral.

vasoconstrictor 1. causing constriction of the blood vessels. 2. a vasoconstrictive agent.

v. agents includes some prostaglandins, thromboxane A_2, leukotriene D_4, angiotensin II, vasopressin, neuropeptide Y, endothelin.

v. fibers adrenergic nerve fibers in the walls of all blood vessels except capillaries.

vasodepression decrease in vascular resistance with hypotension.

vasodepressor 1. having the effect of lowering the blood pressure through reduction in peripheral resistance. 2. an agent that causes vasodepression.

vasodilatation, vasodilation a state of increased caliber of blood vessels.

vasodilator 1. causing dilatation of blood vessels. 2. a nerve or agent that causes dilatation of blood vessels.

v. agents include prostaglandin E_2, prostacyclin, bradykinin, histamine, serotonin, vasoactive intestinal peptide, substance P, adenosine triphosphate, endothelium-derived relaxing factor.

vasoepididymography radiography of the vas deferens and epididymis after injection of a contrast medium.
vasoepididymostomy anastomosis of the vas (ductus) deferens and the epididymis.
vasoformative pertaining to or promoting the formation of blood vessels.
vasoganglion a vascular ganglion or rete.
vasogenic emanating from or pertaining to blood vessels.
v. circulatory failure see vasogenic SHOCK.
vasography radiography of the blood vessels.
vasohypertonic vasoconstrictor.
vasohypotonic vasodilator.
vasoinhibitor an agent that inhibits vasomotor nerves.
vasolamin see TRANEXAMIC ACID.
vasoligation ligation of the vas (ductus) deferens.
vasomotion change in caliber of blood vessels.
vasomotor 1. having an effect on the caliber of blood vessels. 2. a vasomotor agent or nerve.
v. system the part of the nervous system that controls the caliber of the blood vessels.
vasoneuropathy a condition caused by combined vascular and neurological defect, resulting from simultaneous action or interaction of the vascular and nervous systems.
vasoneurosis angioneurosis.
vaso-orchidostomy anastomosis of the epididymis to the severed end of the vas (ductus) deferens.
vasoparesis paralysis of vasomotor nerves.
vasopermeability the permeability of a blood vessel; the extent to which a blood vessel is permeable.
vasopressin a hormone secreted by cells of the hypothalamic nuclei and stored in the posterior pituitary for release as necessary; it stimulates contraction of the muscular tissues of the capillaries and arterioles, raising the blood pressure, and increases peristalsis, exerts some influence on the uterus, and influences resorption of water by the kidney tubules, resulting in concentration of urine. Its rate of secretion is regulated chiefly by the osmolarity of the plasma. Also prepared synthetically or obtained from the posterior pituitary of domestic animals; used as an antidiuretic. Called also antidiuretic hormone (ADH).
v. test see ANTIDIURETIC hormone response test.
vasopressor 1. stimulating contraction of the muscular tissue of the capillaries and arteries. 2. a vasopressor agent.
vasopuncture surgical puncture of the vas (ductus) deferens.
vasoreflex a reflex of blood vessels.
vasorelaxation decrease of vascular pressure.
vasorrhaphy suture of the vas (ductus) deferens.
vasosection the severing of a vessel or vessels, especially of the vasa deferentia (ductus deferentes).
vasosensory supplying sensory filaments to the vessels.
vasospasm spasm of blood vessels, decreasing their caliber.
vasostimulant stimulating vasomotor action.
vasostomy surgical formation of an opening into the ductus (vas) deferens.
vasotocin the normal antidiuretic hormone in birds. One of the hormones released by the avian posterior pituitary gland. Called also arginine vasotocin, AVT. Is also active in stimulating uterine contraction.
vasotomy incision of the vas (ductus) deferens.
vasotonia tone or tension of the vessels.
vasotonic pertaining to, characterized by, or increasing vasotonia.
vasotrophic affecting nutrition through alterations of the caliber of the blood vessels.
vasotropic exerting an influence on the blood vessels, causing either constriction or dilatation.
vasovagal vascular and vagal.
v. attack, v. syncope a transient vascular and neurogenic reaction in humans marked by pallor, nausea, sweating, bradycardia, and rapid fall in arterial blood pressure which, when below a critical level, results in loss of consciousness and characteristic electroencephalographic changes.
vasovasostomy anastomosis of the ends of the severed vas (ductus) deferens.
vasovesiculectomy excision of the vas (ductus) deferens and seminal vesicle.
vastus [L.] *great*.
VC vital capacity.
VCG vectorcardiogram.
V_d volume of distribution.
VDH valvular disease of the heart.
VDT visual display terminal of a computer.
VDU visual display unit of a computer.
veal in general terms means meat from young calves but there is no internationally acceptable definition of veal. The commonest starting point is 2 weeks of age. Any calves younger than that are considered to be too tasteless and uneconomical. White veal is from calves fed only on milk which necessarily limits their oldest permissible age. Most veal calves marketed at older than 8 weeks are fattened on grain. No roughage is fed and the calves are muzzled if they are allowed onto pasture. This kind of veal calf is grown out to produce a dressed carcass of 250 to 300 lb. In some countries veal carcasses are allowed to cool down with their skins still on to prevent dehydration. It also causes a distinct and desirable souring of the meat.
v. calves see VEAL.
vealer young calf destined to be marketed as veal.
v. feedlot calves are confined for a short period and fed intensively in a lot, usually under shelter.
vection the carrying of disease germs from an infected animal to a well animal.
vectis short metal rod with a loop at each end used in canine and feline obstetrics. The loops are of a size that they will engage the cranium or the front of the head in long-nosed breeds and permit traction or rotation of the fetus.
vector 1. a carrier, especially the animal (usually an arthropod) which transfers an infective agent from one host to another, e.g the tsetse fly, which carries trypanosomes from animals to humans, dogs, bats and other animals that transmit the rabies virus. In molecular biology, a DNA molecule which serves to transfer DNA into a host cell. 2. a quantity possessing magnitude, direction and sense (positivity or negativity).
biological v. an arthropod vector in whose body the infecting organism develops or multiplies before becoming infective to the recipient individual.
cloning v. a DNA molecule used to transfer an inserted DNA segment into a host cell. Includes other viruses, phages and bacterial plasmids. Called also cloning vehicle.
mechanical v. an arthropod vector that transmits the infective organisms from one host to another but is not essential to the life cycle of the parasite.
shuttle v's vectors which contain both prokaryotic and eukaryotic replication signals, thus allowing replication of the vector in both kinds of cells.
targeting v. a vector carrying a DNA sequence that

is able to take part in a specified chromosomal crossover in the host.

vectorcardiogram the record, usually a photograph, of the loop formed on the oscilloscope in vectorcardiography.

vectorcardiography the registration, usually by formation of a loop on an oscilloscope, of the direction and magnitude (vector) of the moment-to-moment electromotive forces of the heart during one complete cycle.

vecuronium a derivative of pancuronium, used as a short-acting neuromuscular blocking agent.

VEE Venezuelan equine encephalomyelitis.

vegetable 1. pertaining to or derived from plants. 2. any plant or species of plant, especially one cultivated as a source of food.

v. drugs derived from plants; includes alkaloids, glycosides, resins, gums and oils.

v. matter base residue after dissolving wool in a sample; a measure of the contamination of the wool.

v. oil oil derived from plants. Commercially used oils include peanut, linseed, sesame, cottonseed and castor. A separate group is the volatile oils including oil of turpentine, eucalyptus, peppermint and oil of cloves (eugenol). Animal oils are irritating to tissue and their accidental inhalation almost always causes a serious aspiration pneumonia. Vegetable oils are virtually nonpathogenic.

vegetal 1. pertaining to plants or a plant. 2. vegetative.

vegetation 1. any plant-like fungoid neoplasm or growth; a luxuriant fungus-like growth of pathological tissue. 2. plant growth.

vegetative 1. concerned with growth and nutrition. 2. functioning involuntarily or unconsciously. 3. resting; denoting the portion of a cell cycle during which the cell is not replicating. 4. pertaining to plants. 5. asexual reproduction.

inherited v. dermatosis see DERMATOSIS vegetans.

v. nervous system autonomic nervous system.

vehicle 1. a transporting agent, especially the component of a medication (prescription) serving as a solvent or to increase the bulk or decrease the concentration of the mixture. 2. any medium through which an impulse is propagated.

cloning v. see cloning VECTOR.

veil 1. a covering structure. 2. a caul or piece of amniotic sac occasionally covering the face of a newborn animal.

v. cell fibroblast-like cells which surround small vessels in the dermis.

Veillonella small, gram-negative anaerobic cocci that are part of the normal microflora in the mouth, intestine, respiratory system of animals.

vein a vessel through which blood passes from various organs or parts back towards the heart, in the systemic circulation carrying blood that has given up most of its oxygen. Veins, like arteries, have three coats, an inner, middle and outer, but the coats are not so thick and they collapse when the vessel is cut. Many veins, especially the superficial, have valves formed of reduplication of their lining membrane. For a complete list of the named veins of the body, see Table 15.

afferent v's veins that carry blood to an organ.

allantoic v's paired vessels that accompany the allantois, growing out from the primitive hindgut and entering the body stalk of the early embryo.

cardinal v's the major veins within the early embryo that include the pre- and postcardinal veins and the ducts of Cuvier (common cardinal veins).

emissary v. a vein escaping from a chamber or organ such as one passing through a foramen of the skull and draining blood from a cerebral sinus into a vessel outside the skull.

postcardinal v's paired vessels in the early embryo that return blood from regions caudal to the heart.

precardinal v's paired venous trunks in the embryo cranial to the heart.

pulp v's vessels draining the venous sinuses of the spleen.

subcardinal v's paired vessels in the embryo, replacing the postcardinal veins and persisting to some degree as definitive vessels.

sublobular v's tributaries of the hepatic veins that receive the central veins of hepatic lobules.

supracardinal v's paired vessels in the embryo developing later than the subcardinal veins and persisting chiefly as the lower segment of the inferior vena cava.

thebesian v's smallest cardiac veins: numerous small veins arising in the muscular walls and draining independently into the cavities of the heart, and most readily seen in the atria.

trabecular v's vessels coursing in splenic trabeculae, formed by tributary pulp veins.

varicose v's permanently dilated, tortuous veins. The milk vein of a lactating cow is a normal varicose vein. See VARICOSE veins.

vitelline v's veins that return the blood from the yolk sac to the primitive heart of the early embryo.

veined dock RUMEX *venosus*.

veined verbena see VERBENA *rigida*.

vela plural of velum.

velamen pl. *velamina* [L.] a membrane, meninx or velum.

velamentous membranous and pendent; like a veil.

veldt sickness see HEARTWATER.

vell abattoir term for abomasum of milk-fed calf used for the preparation of rennet for junket tablets.

Velleia Australian plant genus in the family Goodeniaceae; contains an unidentified toxin; causes dyspnea, depression in sheep. Includes *V. connata*, *V. discophora* (cabbage poison), *V. panduriformis* (pindan poison), *V. paradoxa*.

vellein coumarin glycoside of uncertain toxicity in *Velleia discora*.

vellus 1. fine hairs that appear on human skin after the lanugo hairs are cast off. 2. any fine, downy hair.

velogenic 1. a host–parasite relationship in which the parasite dominates and the host frequently dies. 2. highly virulent, e.g. velogenic Newcastle disease virus, as opposed to lentigenic which are low virulence strains.

velometer an instrument that measures air movement velocity in meat storage facilities. A variation on the anemometer.

velopharyngeal pertaining to the velum palatinum (soft palate) and pharynx.

Velpeau sling see Velpeau SLING.

velum pl. *vela* [L.] a covering structure or veil.

v. abomasicum two folds on either side of the omasoabomasal orifice.

v. interpositum the membranous roof of the third ventricle of the brain.

medullary v. one of the two portions (superior medullary velum and inferior medullary velum) of the white matter of the hindbrain that form the roof of the fourth ventricle.

palatine v., v. palatinum soft palate.

v. uteri see INTRACORNUAL frenulum.

velvet see ANTLER.

v. disease of fish, see OODINIUM, AMYLOODINIUM.
v. grass see HOLCUS LANATUS.
v. lupine LUPINUS *leucophyllus*.
v. mite see TROMBICULA.

ven-, vene-, veni-, veno- word element. [L.] *vein*.

vena pl. *venae* [L.] vein. See also Table 15.
caudal v. caval syndrome see CAUDAL vena caval thrombosis.
v. cava one of the the large vessels emptying venous blood into the right atrium; includes cranial and caudal venae cavae.
v. cava spontaneous rupture recorded as a cause of sudden death in horses.
v. cava thrombophlebitis due usually to spread from a hepatic abscess; a common precursor to vena caval syndrome.
v. caval hiatus see vena cava FORAMEN.
v. caval syndrome see CAVAL SYNDROME.
persistent left cranial v. cava an uncommon anomaly in dogs, often associated with other vascular anomalies such as persistent right aortic arch and tetralogy of Fallot.
posterior v. cava caudal vena cava.
cranial v. caval venipuncture a technique for blood sample collection in pigs; a needle is inserted into the cranial vena cava near the thoracic inlet.

venectasia phlebectasia.

venectomy phlebectomy.

venenation poisoning; a poisoned condition.

venenous venomous.

venereal due to or propagated by sexual intercourse. In human medicine now called sexually transmitted disease (STD).
v. balanoposthitis and vulvitis of sheep, see ULCERATIVE dermatosis.
canine transmissible v. tumor (TVT) occurs mainly on the genitalia, but sometimes other cutaneous sites, of dogs and bitches. The tumor, which is most common in certain geographic areas, especially where dogs roam freely, is transmitted by coitus and may regress spontaneously. The tumor cells contain only 59 chromosomes, compared with the normal complement of 78 in dogs. Called by a variety of names including Sticker's tumor or sarcoma, contagious venereal tumor, venereal granuloma, transmissible lymphosarcoma, transmissible reticulum cell tumor, and infectious sarcoma.
v. disease a contagious disease usually acquired by sexual intercourse or other genital contact. See also ULCERATIVE dermatosis.
v. epididymitis and vaginitis of cattle, see EPIVAG.
v. spirochetosis see SPIROCHETOSIS (2).
v. vulvitis/balanitis of horses, see equine COITAL EXANTHEMA.

Venerupis farmed bivalve mollusc in family Veneridae; includes *V. japonica* (Japanese or Manila clam).

Venezuelan equine encephalomyelitis an encephalomyelitis with clinical signs similar to those of western and eastern encephalomyelitis; abbreviated VEE. See also equine viral ENCEPHALOMYELITIS.

venipuncture, venepuncture surgical puncture of a vein.

venisection, venesection a vein is opened and a large volume of blood collected and discarded. Called also phlebotomy.

venison meat of the deer.

venisuture, venesuture phleborrhaphy.

Venn diagram a pictorial representation, usually in the form of two or more overlapping circles, of the extent to which two or more quantities or concepts have comparable or disparate characteristics.

venoclysis injection of fluid into a vein; phleboclysis. See also INTRAVENOUS infusion.

venoconstriction a venoconstrictive response can be elicited in the small and large cutaneous veins in cats and dogs.

venodilator an agent acting to increase the caliber of veins. See also VASODILATOR.

venogram 1. phlebogram. 2. venous-pulse tracing.

venography phlebography.
cavernous sinus v. injection of a contrast medium into the angularis oculi vein while the jugular vein is compressed permits radiographic visualization of the ophthalmic plexus and the cavernous sinus and may outline space-occupying lesions in the vicinity of the pituitary gland and cranial nerves II, III, IV and VI.
orbital v. radiopaque media can be used to outline veins around the orbit and retrobulbar veins.
vertebral v. injection of radiocontrast medium into the saphenous vein while the caudal vena cava is compressed causes the vertebral veins to be outlined; used to demonstrate cord compression.

venom poison, especially a toxic substance normally secreted by a serpent, insect or other animal.
Russell's viper v. the venom of the Russell viper (*Vipera russelli*), which acts in vitro as an intrinsic thromboplastin and is useful in defining deficiencies of clotting factor X. See also RUSSELL'S VIPER VENOM.

venomotor controlling dilatation or constriction of the veins.

venomous secreting poison; poisonous.

veno-occlusive pertaining to or characterized by obstruction of the veins.
v. disease of liver acute or chronic, partial or complete, occlusion of the branches of the hepatic veins by endophlebitis and thrombosis, leading to centrilobular necrosis, fibrosis and ascites; occurs at a higher than normal prevalence in cheetahs and snow leopards.

venoperitoneostomy anastomosis of the saphenous vein with the peritoneum for drainage of ascites.

venosclerosis sclerosis of veins; phlebosclerosis.

venosity 1. excess of venous blood in a part. 2. a plentiful supply of blood vessels or of venous blood.

venostasis retardation of the venous outflow in a part. See also PHLEBOSTASIS.

venotomy phlebotomy.

venous pertaining to the veins.
v. dilatation persistent dilatation of the vein but without necessarily any weakening of the wall or varicosity.
hepatic portal v. system includes the veins from the alimentary tract, the portal vein, the sinusoids in the liver, the hepatic veins and then the entry into the caudal vena cava.
v. infarct see venous INFARCT.
obstructed v. drainage may be generalized or local; manifested by dilation, local edema.
orbital v. plexus a plexus for venous drainage from the ophthalmic veins at the apex of the orbit; drains into the cavernous venous sinus within the cranium.
v. return the flow of blood into the heart from the peripheral vessels.
v. return curves relate venous return to atrial pressure; the inverse of the Starling relationship; an increase in atrial pressure decreases the venous return.
scleral v. plexus a ring of small vessels around the corneal limbus which forms a link in the chain of vessels which drain the aqueous humor. Called also canal of Schlemm.
v. sinuses see venous SINUS.

v. system the bodily system of veins commencing with the venae cavae, thence through the large veins and their tributaries, and immediately subsequent to the capillaries, the venules.

v. thrombosis the presence of a thrombus in a vein. Originates in phlebitis in most cases. It is a major problem in horses because of the high incidence of jugular phlebitis and periphlebitis as a result of injection of irritating materials. See also CAUDAL vena caval thrombosis.

venovenostomy phlebophlebostomy.

vent an opening or outlet, such as an opening that discharges pus, or the anus. In dogs, used to describe the area around the anus and in bitches also the vulva. Most appropriate use is the cloaca of birds.

cloacal v. the external opening to the cloaca. Comparable to the anus in mammals.

v. disease see spirochetosis (2).

v. gleet a chronic disease of the cloaca of domestic birds. Characterized by fouling of the feathers around the vent with exudate, and the presence of a diphtheritic membrane on the cloacal mucosa at the external orifice and a copious evil-smelling discharge.

v. picking the commonest and most severe of the cannibalistic vices of housed birds; most common in high producing pullet flocks probably related to the passage of large eggs causing some tearing of tissues at the vent. Other birds may cause fatal injury by picking at the part.

venter pl. *ventres* [L.] 1. any belly-shaped part; a fleshy contractible part of a muscle. 2. the abdomen or stomach. 3. a hollowed part or cavity.

Ventilago viminalis Australian plant in the family Rhamnaceae; a tree used as a fodder for sheep but causes poisoning if it is fed for a long period. Brown urine, stiff gait and convulsions are the prominent signs. The poison in the plant is tannin. Called also supple jack.

ventilation renewal or exchange of gas in an enclosed space. 1. the process or act of supplying a building or part of it continuously with fresh air. 2. in respiratory physiology, the process of exchange of air between the lungs and the ambient air. *Pulmonary ventilation* (usually measured in liters per minute) refers to the total exchange, whereas *alveolar ventilation* refers to the effective ventilation of the alveoli, where gas exchange with the blood takes place. See also AIR movement.

alveolar v. the amount of gas expelled from the alveoli to the outside of the body per minute.

artificial v. see artificial RESPIRATION.

assisted v. the depth of spontaneous ventilation is augmented by the anesthetist, as by squeezing the rebreathing bag.

controlled v. breathing is done entirely by a mechanical device or the anesthetist squeezing the rebreathing bag.

dead space v. see dead SPACE.

high frequency v. mechanical ventilation that delivers gas at more than four times the normal rate of breathing.

intermittent mandatory v. (IMV) a type of mechanical ventilation in which the VENTILATOR is set to deliver a prescribed tidal volume at specified intervals and a high-flow gas system permits the patient to breathe spontaneously between cycles. The ventilator rate is set to maintain the patient's P_aCO_2 at normal levels and is reduced gradually to zero as the patient's condition improves.

intermittent positive-pressure v. (IPPV) the provision of mechanical ventilation by a machine designed to deliver breathing gas until equilibrium is established between the patient's lungs and the VENTILATOR. IPPV machines are positive-pressure, pressure-cycled, assister-controller (pneumatic) devices.

Because of their compact size and capability of operating independently of an electrical current, the IPPV machines have the most widespread applicability in the employment of a form of treatment called INTERMITTENT positive-pressure breathing.

maximal voluntary v. (MVV) the maximal volume that can be exhaled per minute by the patient breathing as rapidly and deeply as possible.

mechanical v. that accomplished by extrinsic means.

minute v. the total amount of gas (in liters) expelled from the lungs per minute.

v. mismatch mismatches of ventilation and blood flow, as in chronic obstructive lung disease, are a common cause of hypoxemia.

v.:perfusion ratio the ratio of air ventilation to the blood perfused. Called also V_A/Q. The degree of oxygenation of the blood and the proportional excretion of CO_2 are both dependent on both variables being optimal.

positive pressure v. administration of oxygen under pressure, usually by use of an anesthetic bag or mechanical ventilator. See also CONTINUOUS POSITIVE AIRWAY PRESSURE, POSITIVE end-expiratory pressure.

spontaneous v. breathing without the assistance of any ventilator or mechanical device.

total v. the amount of air moved out of (or into) the airways and alveoli over a specified time period.

ventilator an apparatus designed to control air that is breathed through it or to either intermittently or continuously assist or control pulmonary ventilation; called also respirator. Use of a mechanical ventilator is indicated as a supportive measure in patients suffering from respiratory paralysis and in those with ventilatory failure manifested by either alveolar hypoventilation or distributive HYPOXIA, or both. It is a major activity in human nursing but of almost no importance in animals except for anesthetic purposes. See BIRD VENTILATOR, CAMBRIDGE VENTILATOR, FLOMASTA VENTILATOR, MANLEY VENTILATOR, MINIVENT VENTILATOR, NORTH AMERICAN Dräger.

ventilatory pertaining to or emanating from pulmonary ventilation.

v. failure respiratory acidosis.

ventilometry measurement of the volume of tidal volume; used in critical care.

ventrad toward a belly, venter or ventral aspect.

ventral 1. pertaining to the abdomen or to any venter. 2. directed toward or situated on the belly surface; opposite of dorsal.

v. coccygeal myotomy tail setting operation in horses. See also NICKING (2).

v. cord syndrome localized injury to the ventral portion of the spinal cord, characterized by complete paralysis and hypalgesia and hypesthesia up to the level of the lesion, but with relative preservation of dorsal column sensations of touch, position and vibration.

v. edema obvious swelling along ventral belly wall, may reach from brisket to pelvic brim, pits on pressure, so does urine from a leaking urethra. Manifestation of general edema due to congestive heart failure, hypoproteinemia, or to late pregnancy with compression on venous return by uterus and fetus.

v. funiculus nervous tissue white matter lying between the ventral columns of gray matter in the spinal cord.

v. respiratory group that part of the respiratory center which is located in the ventral medulla oblongata.

ventralis [L.] *ventral.*

ventr(i)-, ventr(o)- word element. [L.] *belly, front (anterior) aspect of the body, ventral aspect.*

ventricle a small cavity or chamber, as in the brain or heart.

cardiac v. the single fetal cardiac ventricle, formed by the looping of the bulboventricle; divided later by the growth of the interventricular septum as a projection from the wall of the bulboventricle.

fifth v. the median cleft between the two laminae of the brain's septum lucidum.

fourth v. a median, horizontally disposed, rhomboid cavity in the hindbrain, between the cerebellum and medulla, containing cerebrospinal fluid.

gastric v. stomach.

laryngeal v. a variably developed cavity of the larynx that opens into the laryngeal vestibule by a cleft between the vestibular and vocal folds; well developed in dogs and horses and especially certain apes.

lateral v. the cavity in each cerebral hemisphere, derived from the cavity of the embryonic tube, containing cerebrospinal fluid and communicating with the third ventricle.

left v. the lower chamber of the left side of the heart, which pumps oxygenated blood out through the aorta to all the tissues of the body.

pineal v. an extension of the third ventricle into the stalk of the pineal body.

right v. the lower chamber of the right side of the heart, which pumps venous blood through the pulmonary trunk and arteries to the capillaries of the lung.

third v. a vertically disposed, ring-shaped space that contains cerebrospinal fluid and that communicates anteriorly with the lateral ventricles and caudally with the cerebral aqueduct within the diencephalon between the two thalami.

ventricornu the ventral horn of gray matter in the spinal cord.

ventricular pertaining to a ventricle.

v. assist device a circulatory support device consisting of a pump with afferent and efferent conduits attached to the left ventricular apex and the ascending aorta, respectively, each conduit containing a porcine valve to ensure unidirectional blood flow; the pump rests on the external chest wall and is connected to an external pneumatic power source and control circuit.

v. asystole see ASYSTOLE.

v. bands folds of mucosa, parallel and craniolateral to the vocal cords. Called also false vocal cords, vestibular folds.

double right v. outlet a cardiac anomaly rarely seen in animals in which both the aorta and pulmonary artery arise from the right ventricle and there is a defect in the ventricular septum.

excessive v. moderator bands a rare syndrome of cardiomyopathy in cats caused by an excessive number of moderator bands in the left ventricle, extending from the papillary muscles to the ventricular septum.

v. extrasystoles see ventricular EXTRASYSTOLE.

v. fibrillation see ventricular FIBRILLATION.

v. function curve see STARLING CURVES.

v. hypertrophy see ventricular HYPERTROPHY.

v. outflow obstruction flow of blood from the ventricles is impaired by lesions or congenital abnormalities in the outflow tract. This is usually associated with hypertrophy of the ventricle and can be demonstrated with echocardiography or contract radiography. *Left outflow obstruction* occurs with stenosis and other anomalies of the aorta; *right outflow obstruction* occurs with pulmonic stenosis, pulmonic insufficiency, tetralogy of Fallot, and double-chambered right ventricle.

v. premature contraction (VPC) see PREMATURE heartbeats.

v. rupture due to focal weakness causes sudden death due to cardiac tamponade.

v. septal defect a congenital heart defect in which there is persistent patency of the ventricular septum in either the muscular or fibrous portion most often due to failure of the bulbar septum to completely close the interventricular foramen. The defect permits flow of blood directly from one ventricle to the other, bypassing the pulmonary circulation and producing varying degrees of cyanosis because of oxygen deficiency. Its clinical characteristics also include a systolic murmur and a palpable thrill on both sides of the chest, dyspnea and poor exercise tolerance. The occurrence is sporadic except that it is inherited in goats and dogs.

v. septum the muscular wall between the ventricles. A small section, between the aortic vestibule and the right atrium, is membranous. Failure of the septum to close completely during fetal growth causes a septal or subaortic defect.

v. shortening fraction in echocardiography, the percentage change in diameter from diastole to systole. Calculated from the internal systolic and diastolic dimensions. It is a measure of mycocardial function.

v. slice method a method for examination of fixed heart by cutting it into 0.5 inch thick slices, perpendicular to the plane of the ventricular septum, from apex to base. Useful in examination of myocardial lesions and cardiomyopathy.

v. tachycardia is manifested by a high heart rate with or without arrhythmia. In both cases there is severe cardiac disease and often acute heart failure.

ventriculectomy removal of the mucosa lining the lateral ventricles of the larynx for the relief of laryngeal hemiplegia in horses. The operation is performed through a laryngotomy incision in the cricothyroid membrane. It may be supplemented by the insertion of a laryngeal prosthesis.

ventriculitis inflammation of a ventricle, especially a cerebral ventricle.

ventriculoatriostomy introduction of a catheter with a one-way valve to drain cerebrospinal fluid from a cerebral ventricle to the right atrium via the jugular vein, for relief of hydrocephalus.

ventriculocisternostomy surgical creation of a communication between the third ventricle and the interpeduncular cistern, for drainage of cerebrospinal fluid.

ventriculocordectomy punch resection of the vocal cords. See also DEBARKING, DEVOCALIZATION.

ventriculogram a radiograph of the cerebral ventricles.

ventriculography 1. radiography of the cerebral ventricles after introduction of air or other contrast medium. Called also pneumoventriculogram. 2. radiography of a ventricle of the heart after injection of a contrast medium.

ventriculometry measurement of intracranial pressure.

ventriculonector the bundle of His.

ventriculopuncture surgical puncture of a lateral ventricle of the brain.

ventriculoscopy endoscopic examination of the cerebral ventricles.

ventriculostomy surgical creation of a free communication between the third ventricle and the interpeduncular cistern for relief of hydrocephalus.
ventriculosubarachnoid pertaining to the cerebral ventricles and subarachnoid space.
ventriculotomy incision of a ventricle of the heart.
ventriculus pl. *ventriculi* [L.] 1. a ventricle. 2. the stomach.
ventricumbent prone; lying on the belly.
ventriduct to bring or carry ventrad.
ventriflexion ventral flexion of the neck so that the head is carried near the knees.
ventrimeson the median line on the ventral surface.
ventrodorsal view the x-ray beam enters the animal ventrally and exits dorsally; usually taken with the animal lying on its back.
ventrofixation fixation of a viscus, e.g. the uterus, to the abdominal wall; ventrosuspension.
ventroflexion flexion of the cervical spine with movement of the head towards the ventrum; a clinical feature of THIAMIN deficiency in cats.
ventrohysteropexy ventral fixation of the uterus.
ventrolateral both ventral and lateral.
ventromedial pertaining to the ventral aspect and the midline.
ventroscopy illumination of the abdominal cavity for purposes of examination.
ventrose having a belly-like expansion.
ventrosuspension ventrofixation.
ventrotomy celiotomy.
venturi a tube with a decrease in the inside diameter that is used to increase the flow velocity of the fluid and thereby cause a pressure drop; used to measure the flow velocity (a *venturimeter*) or to draw another fluid into the stream.
v. mask a type of disposable mask used to deliver a controlled oxygen concentration to a patient. The flow of 100% oxygen through the venturi draws in a controlled amount of room air (21% oxygen). Commonly available masks deliver 24, 28, 31, 35 or 40% oxygen.
v. nebulizer a type of nebulizer used in AEROSOL therapy. The pressure drop of gas flowing through the venturi draws liquid from a capillary tube. As the liquid enters the gas stream it breaks up into a spray of small droplets.
venula pl. *venulae* [L.] venule.
venule any of the small vessels that collect blood from the capillary plexuses and join to form veins.
VEP visual evoked potential.
verapamil a calcium channel blocking agent used as a vasodilator and in the treatment of cardiac arrhythmias.
veratralbine a poisonous substance in plants of the genus *Veratrum*.
veratramine a potentially teratogenic alkaloid in the plant *Veratrum californicum*.
veratrine a commercial product obtained from the seeds of *Schoenocaulon officinalis*.
veratroidine one of the poisonous substances in the plant *Veratrum album*.
veratrosine teratogenic steroidal alkaloid found in *Veratrum* spp.
Veratrum a genus of the Liliaceae family of plants.
V. album contain alkaloids including protoveratrine, jervine, rubijervine, pseudojervine, veratroidine, veratralbine. Several alkaloids are extracted and used in therapeutic preparations. Poisoning by these plants causes salivation, purgation, vomiting, diuresis, excitability followed by paralysis and recumbency, then convulsions and death. Called also white hellebore, white veratrum, European veratrum.
V. californicum a poisonous weed which causes a number of congenital abnormalities especially congenital cyclopean deformity, prolonged gestation and absence of the pituitary gland in ruminants. The teratogen is cyclopamine. Called also skunk cabbage, western hellebore, false hellebore, corn-lily.
V. viride several alkaloid extracts are combined in the preparation alkavir, used as a rumenatoric and a hypotensive agent. Called also green veratrum, green hellebore, American hellebore.
verbal contract an agreement made verbally for the provision of goods or services in return for a consideration, in veterinary practice usually in the form of money.
Verbascum a potentially poisonous genus of plants in the family Scrophulariaceae. The plants contain cardiac glycosides similar to digitalis but poisoning is not recorded. Called also mullein.
Verbena a genus of plants in the family Verbenaceae.
V. bonariensis called also purple top; suspected of causing sickness and abortion in cattle.
V. officinalis contains a glycoside verbenalin reputed to cause contraction of the uterus and photosensitization. Called also common vervain.
V. rigida thought to cause photosensitization. Called also *Verbena venosa*, wild verbena.
V. tenuisecta suspected of causing deaths in chickens and photosensitization in sheep. Called also Mayne's pest.
verbenalin toxic glycoside found in *Verbena officinalis*.
Verbesina encelioides a plant of North American origin in the family Asteraceae known to contain toxic amounts of galegine. Death is sudden, often without clinical signs, but there may be a brief period of dyspnea, bloat, mouth-breathing, frothing at the mouth and cyanosis. Necropsy lesions include pulmonary edema and hydrothorax. Called also crown beard.
Verbrugge clamp a strongly built, scissortype bone clamp with ratcheted handles and sideways curving blades that have horizontal, semicircular, deeply ridged attachments to the end suited to grasping a long bone.
verge a circumference or ring.
anal v. the opening of the anus on the surface of the body.
vergence disjunctive movement of the eyes in opposite directions in adjusting to near or far vision; convergence or divergence.
vermeerbos [Af.] see GEIGERIA.
vermeeric acid the poisonous substance in the plant *Geigeria* spp.
vermeersiekte [Af.] poisoning by *Geigeria* spp. Called also vomiting sickness.
vermicide an agent lethal to worms or intestinal animal parasites.
vermicular wormlike in shape or appearance.
vermiculation peristaltic motion; peristalsis.
vermiculous 1. wormlike. 2. infected with worms.
vermiform worm-shaped.
vermifugal expelling worms or intestinal animal parasites.
vermifuge any agent that expels the worms or intestinal animal parasites; an anthelmintic.
vermin any vertebrate or invertebrate animals of an objectional kind.
vermination infestation with vermin or infection with worms.
verminous pertaining to, due to, or abounding in worms or in vermin.

v. aneurysm see verminous mesenteric arteritis (below).

v. bronchitis see LUNGWORM.

v. encephalitis is caused by migration of *Strongylus vulgaris* or larvae. The effect is one of paralysis due to destruction of nervous tissue. See also BRAIN trauma, NEUROFILARIASIS.

v. mesenteric arteritis is caused by migrating *Strongylus vulgaris* larvae. Defective blood supply to the intestine results and causes intermittent colic, sometimes terminal infarction. See also thromboembolic COLIC.

v. pneumonia see LUNGWORM.

Vermipsylla a genus of fleas in the order Siphonaptera.

V. alacurt, V. dorcadia, V. ioffi, V. perplexa found on sheep, goats, other ruminants and horses.

vermis [L.] a worm, or wormlike structure.

v. cerebelli the median part of the cerebellum, between the two hemispheres.

nodule of v. the part of the vermis of the cerebellum, on the ventral surface, where the inferior medullary velum attaches.

Vermont strain of merino sheep introduced into Australia from the United States of America.

vernix [L.] *varnish.*

v. caseosa the unctuous substance composed of sebum and desquamated epithelial cells, covering the skin of the fetus.

vernolate a thiocarbamate herbicide which may cause poisoning if there is accidental access to it. Causes anorexia, weight loss, muscle weakness and hairlessness.

Vernonia plant genus of the Asteraceae family; probably contains a toxic sesquiterpene; causes liver damage, incoordination, recumbency, convulsions. Includes *V. mollisima*, *V. rubricaulis*, *V. squarrosa*.

Verocay body a group of uniform, fusiform cells arranged in whorls, herringbones or palisades. Found in Schwann-cell tumors.

verocytotoxin see SHIGA-LIKE TOXINS.

verotoxin see SHIGA-LIKE TOXINS.

verruca pl. *verrucae* [L.] 1. a wart. See also PAPILLOMA, FIBROPAPILLOMA. 2. one of the wart-like elevations on the endocardium in various types of endocarditis.

v. plana flat warts.

verrucarin a toxic metabolite produced by the fungus STACHYBOTRYS ATRA.

verruciform wart-like.

verrucose, verrucous rough, warty.

v. dermatitis a proliferative inflammatory lesion on the back of the pastern from the bulb of the heel to fetlock of cattle. Caused by *Fusobacterium necrophorum*. Occurs in muddy overcrowded conditions. See also strawberry FOOTROT.

v. pododermatitis verrucose dermatitis extending onto the bulbs of the heel.

verruculogen tremorgenic mycotoxin produced by *Penicillium* spp. fungus.

verruga wart. Called also verruca.

Versa clip see Versa CLIP.

version the act of turning; especially the manual turning of the fetus in delivery.

vertebra pl. *vertebrae* [L.] any of the separate segments comprising the spine (vertebral column). See also SPINE, VERTEBRAL.

The vertebrae support the body and provide the protective bony corridor through which the spinal cord passes. The number of bones in the vertebral column varies with the animal species and even within each species. Average numbers are given in Table 10.

The compression-resisting portion of a typical vertebra is the vertebral body, the most ventral portion. This is a cylindrical structure that is separated from the vertebral bodies in front and behind by disks of cartilage and fibrous tissue. These intervertebral disks act as cushions to spread and absorb the mechanical shock during body movements. See also slipped DISK.

A semicircular arch of bone protrudes from the dorsum of each vertebral body, surrounding the spinal cord. Directly in its midline a bony projection, the spinous process, grows upward from the arch. Three pairs of outgrowths project from the arch. One of these protrudes horizontally on each side and in the thorax connects with the ribs. The remaining two form joints with the vertebrae in front and behind. The joints permit the spine to bend flexibly. The vertebrae are held firmly in place by a series of strong ligaments.

anticlinal v. 1. the vertebra whose spinous process is directed vertically at which point the backward slope of the cranial vertebrae changes to a forward inclination. Is usually the sixteenth thoracic vertebra in the horse. 2. (improperly) the diaphragmatic vertebra.

block v. anomalous development in which two or more vertebrae are fused.

butterfly v. anomalous development of a vertebra that is nearly divided in half by a longitudinal defect; caused by the persistence of the sagittal membrane remnant of the notochord. The vertebral body resembles a butterfly on ventrodorsal radiographs.

caudal v. coccygeal vertebrae.

cranial v. the segments of the skull and facial bones, regarded by some as modified vertebrae.

v. dentata the second cervical vertebra, or axis.

diaphragmatic v. the vertebra which marks the transition between those located cranially with a thoracic type of articular facet to those located caudally with a lumbar type. It is often the same vertebra as the anticlinal vertebra (above).

false v. those vertebrae which normally fuse with adjoining segments such as the sacral vertebrae or the human coccygeal vertebrae.

v. magnum the sacrum.

odontoid v. the second cervical vertebra, or axis.

opisthocoelus v. a vertebra with a concave caudal surface to the body.

v. plana a condition of spondylitis in which the body of the vertebra is reduced to a sclerotic disk.

transitional v. see TRANSITIONAL VERTEBRA.

true v. those segments of the vertebral column that normally remain unfused throughout life: the cervical, thoracic, lumbar and coccygeal vertebrae.

wedge-shaped v. hemivertebra.

vertebral of or pertaining to a vertebra.

v. abscess commonly associated with navel infection in the young. Usually infection delivered by the hematogenous route to the cervical or lumbar vertebral bodies or to meninges. Compression of the spinal cord by the abscess or a pathological fracture causes paraplegia or quadriplegia depending on location. See also vertebral osteomyelitis (below).

v. asymmetry a contributing factor in ENZOOTIC equine incoordination.

v. body see VERTEBRA.

v. body osteosclerosis occurs together with vertebral osteophyte development in old bulls with thyroid C-cell tumors.

v. canal see spinal CANAL.

v. column see spinal COLUMN.
v. curves the cervical, thoracic and lumbar curves.
v. exostosis may be the result of fractures, and in pigs, hypovitaminosis A. May cause compression of spinal cord and paralysis.
v. fracture often due to minor trauma in bone weakened by osteoporosis or osteomyelitis. In neonates may be dystocia-related. Usually causes acute onset of flaccid paralysis.
v. instability see canine WOBBLER SYNDROME.
v. joints are of two types, symphyseal between the vertebral bodies, and synovial between the facets of the neural arch.
v. malformation includes block vertebra and defective alignment such as scoliosis, kyphosis, torticollis.
v. osteomyelitis results in pathological fracture causing acute paralysis, or spinal cord abscess causing slower onset paralysis. Hematogenesis spread from omphalophlebitis is common so that disease is most often seen in young patients.
v. osteophytes see SPONDYLOSIS deformans.
v. stenosis compression of the spinal cord by a vertebral canal which has too small a diameter.
v. subluxation largely restricted to the cervical vertebrae where looser ligaments permit more intervertebral movement.

vertebrarium the spine, or vertebral column.
Vertebrata a subphylum of the Chordata, comprising all animals having a vertebral column, including mammals, birds, reptiles, amphibians and fish.
vertebrate 1. having a vertebral column. 2. an animal with a vertebral column; any member of the subphylum Vertebrata.
vertebrectomy excision of a vertebra.
vertebr(o)- word element. [L.] *vertebra, spine.*
vertebrobasilar pertaining to or affecting the vertebral and basilar arteries.
vertebrochondral pertaining to a vertebra and a costal cartilage.
vertebrocostal pertaining to a vertebra and a rib.
vertebrogenic arising in a vertebra or in the vertebral column.
vertebrosternal pertaining to a vertebra and the sternum.
vertex the summit or top, especially the top of the head.
v. corneae central part of the cornea.
vertical 1. perpendicular to the plane of the horizon. 2. relating to the vertex.
v. beam the radiographic technique in which the x-ray beam enters the surface of the recumbent animal at right angles.
v. scrolling in word processing the ability to move up or down through a page of script so that it can be accessed for editing.
verticalis [L.] *vertical.*
verticillate arranged in whorls.
Verticillium a genus of fungi which are normally plant, insect, nematode or arachnid pathogens. Opportunistic infection in mammals have been reported.
vertigraphy body-section radiography.
verumontanitis inflammation of the verumontanum.
verumontanum see seminal COLLICULUS.
vervain any member of the family Verbenaceae, e.g. VERBENA *officinalis.*
vervet monkey a species of Old World monkeys found in Africa. One of a large group known as guenons and members of the genus *Cercopithecus.* Called also *C. pygerythrus, C. lalandii.*
very low density lipoprotein see LIPOPROTEIN.
vesalianum a sesamoid bone in the tendon of origin of the gastrocnemius muscle, or in the angle between the cuboid and fifth metatarsal bones.
vesica pl. *vesicae* [L.] bladder.
v. fellea see GALLBLADDER.
v. urinaria see URINARY BLADDER.
vesical pertaining to or emanating from the urinary bladder.
vesicant 1. producing blisters. 2. an agent that produces blisters.
vesication 1. the process of blistering. 2. a blistered spot or surface.
vesicle 1. a small bladder or sac containing liquid. 2. a small circumscribed elevation of the epidermis containing a serous fluid; a small blister. See also VESICULAR disease.
auditory v. a detached ovoid sac formed by closure of the auditory pit in the early embryo, from which the percipient parts of the inner ear develop.
brain v's the five divisions of the closed neural tube in the developing embryo, including the telencephalon, diencephalon, mesencephalon, metencephalon and myelencephalon.
chorionic v. see CHORIONIC vesicle.
clear v. neuronal vesicles which occur in neuronal terminals in which acetylcholine is the transmitter.
coated v. see COATED PITS.
compound v. multilocular vesicle.
dense core v. neuronal vesicles which occur in neuronal terminals in which norepinephrine or other catecholamine is the transmitter. Called also granular vesicle.
encephalic v's brain vesicles.
germinal v. the fluid-filled nucleus of an oocyte toward the end of prophase of its meiotic division.
granular v. see dense core vesicle (above).
lens v. a vesicle formed from the lens pit of the embryo, developing into the crystalline lens.
matrix v's vesicles found in hyaline cartilage; are starting points for growth plate mineralization.
multilocular v. a vesicle with multiple chambers or compartments.
olfactory v. 1. the vesicle in the embryo which later develops into the olfactory bulb and tract. 2. a bulbous expansion at the distal end of an olfactory cell, from which the olfactory hairs project.
otic v. auditory vesicle.
pinocytotic v's vesicles which appear in vascular endothelium; may participate in transcapillary movement of macromolecules.
primary brain v's the three earlier subdivisions of the embryonic neural tube, including the forebrain, midbrain and hindbrain.
secondary brain v's the four brain vesicles formed by specialization of the forebrain and of the hindbrain in later embryonic development.
secretory v's vesicles found in rough excretory endoplasm of cells.
seminal v's paired sacculated pouches that overlie the urinary bladder in the males of some species; in some the pouch is a simple sac, in others a compound acinous gland, and in some the duct of each joins the ipsilateral ductus deferens to form the ejaculatory duct. In the boar and stallion it produces a bulky ejaculate. See also VESICULAR gland.
transfer v's vesicles found in rough endoplasmic reticulum of cells.
transport v. membrane bound vesicle, pinched off from endoplasmic reticulum, containing macromolecules to be transported to other parts of the cell.
umbilical v. the pear-shaped expansion of the yolk

sac growing out into the cavity of the chorion, joined to the midgut by the yolk stalk.

vesic(o)- word element. [L.] *blister, bladder.*

vesicocele hernia of the bladder.

vesicocervical pertaining to the bladder and cervix uteri.

vesicoclysis introduction of fluid into the bladder.

vesicoenteric, vesicointestinal pertaining to or communicating with the urinary bladder and intestine.

vesicoprostatic pertaining to the bladder and prostate.

vesicopubic pertaining to the bladder and the pubic area.

vesicopuncture cystocentesis.

vesicopustular involving vesicles and pustules.

vesicopustule a lesion of the epidermis consisting of a vesicle containing inflammatory cells.

vesicospinal pertaining to the bladder and spine.

vesicostomy the formation of an opening into the bladder; cystostomy.

cutaneous v. surgical anastomosis of the bladder mucosa to an opening in the abdominal skin, creating a stoma for bladder drainage.

vesicotomy incision into the bladder. In most cases the procedure is done to divert the flow of urine when the bladder can no longer function as a reservoir. After incising the bladder the surgeon moves it forward and sutures the bladder opening to the skin, forming a STOMA.

vesicourachal pertaining to the urinary bladder and the urachus.

v. diverticulum persistence of a segment of the urachus, present as a protrusion at the vertex of the bladder. It may predispose to urolith formation.

vesicoureteral, vesicoureteric pertaining to the bladder and ureter.

v. valve in the wall of the bladder where the ureter enters; prevents reflux of the urine from bladder to ureter.

vesicouterine pertaining to the bladder and uterus.

vesicovaginal pertaining to the bladder and vagina.

vesicula pl. *vesiculae* [L.] vesicle.

vesicular 1. composed of or relating to small, saclike bodies. 2. pertaining to or made up of vesicles on the skin.

avian v. dermatitis vesicles on the skin of the feet and toes and occasionally on the head, on all birds; caused usually by photosensitization.

v. disease a group of diseases of cloven-footed animals of major importance because of their high infectivity. See FOOT-AND-MOUTH DISEASE, vesicular stomatitis and vesicular exanthema of swine (below), SWINE vesicular disease, poisoning by the mushroom AMANITA.

v. emphysema see ALVEOLAR emphysema.

v. exanthema of swine an acute febrile disease caused by a calicivirus. The clinical syndrome is one of vesicular stomatitis, with lesions occurring also on the coronets. The disease only ever appeared in the USA and was eradicated from that country in 1959.

v. gland an accessory sex gland in ruminants, the counterpart of the seminal vesicle in the stallion but glandular instead of cystic. Consists of a much-coiled tube that exits at the seminal colliculus in the urethra.

v. murmur, v. sounds the soft, sibilant sounds heard by stethoscopic auscultation over the lung parenchyma. They are caused by air moving in and out of the alveoli and terminal bronchioles and are an expression of normality of the lung tissue. Called also vesicular murmur.

porcine idiopathic v. disease see porcine PARVOVIRUS.

v. stomatitis (VS) an infectious disease of horses, cattle and pigs caused by a vesiculovirus transmitted by mosquitoes and biting flies. The clinical syndrome is one of vesicular stomatitis but lesions can occur on the udder and coronets.

swine v. disease see SWINE vesicular disease.

v. vaginitis see infectious pustular VULVOVAGINITIS.

v. venereal disease see infectious pustular VULVOVAGINITIS.

vesicular-ulcerative dermatitis–glossitis of pigs a parvovirus has been suspected as causing outbreaks of dermatitis and glossitis in piglets; a more serious disease is thought due to a secondary infection with *Staphylococcus hyicus* or swinepox virus.

vesiculation formation of vesicles.

vesiculectomy excision of a vesicle, especially the seminal vesicle.

vesiculiform shaped like a vesicle.

vesiculitis inflammation of a vesicle, especially a seminal vesicle. See SEMINAL vesiculitis.

vesiculocavernous both vesicular and cavernous.

vesiculogram a radiograph of the seminal vesicles.

vesiculography radiography of the seminal vesicles.

vesiculopapular marked by or having the characteristics of vesicles and papules.

vesiculopustular marked by or having the characteristics of vesicles and pustules.

vesiculotomy incision into a vesicle, especially the seminal vesicles.

vesiculotympanic having both a vesicular and tympanic quality; said of percussion sounds.

Vesiculovirus a genus in the family RHABDOVIRIDAE; includes the vesicular stomatitis virus.

vessel any channel for carrying a fluid, such as blood or lymph. See also VAS.

absorbent v's lymphatic vessels.

blood v. any of the vessels conveying the blood; an artery, arteriole, vein, venule or capillary.

collateral v. 1. a vessel that parallels another vessel, a nerve, or other structure. 2. a vessel important in establishing and maintaining a collateral circulation.

great v's the large vessels entering the heart, including the aorta, the pulmonary arteries and veins, and the venae cavae.

lacteal v's those that take up chyle from the intestinal wall during digestion.

lymphatic v's the capillaries, collecting vessels, and trunks that collect lymph from the tissues and carry it to lymph nodes or the bloodstream.

nutrient v's vessels supplying nutritive elements to special tissues, e.g. arteries entering the substance of bone or the walls of large blood vessels.

vest-over-pants suture pattern an interrupted horizontal mattress pattern. Tissues to be sutured are overlapped instead of meeting end to end. Interrupted sutures pass through both layers at both edges.

vestibular 1. pertaining to any vestibule. 2. pertaining to the vestibular organ.

v. apparatus includes the vestibular organ and the vestibular branch of the vestibulocochlear nerve.

canine idiopathic v. syndrome seen in aged dogs, characterized by the sudden onset of head tilt, nystagmus, rolling, falling and circling, often with considerable distress. The cause is unknown, but a peripheral vestibular lesion is suspected. Signs usually regress within a few days. Called also geriatric vestibular syndrome, 'stroke'.

feline v. syndrome an acute onset of head tilt,

rolling and nystagmus in cats of all ages. There is usually rapid improvement over a few days. The cause is unknown.

geriatric v. syndrome see canine idiopathic vestibular syndrome (above).

v. gland see BARTHOLIN'S GLANDS.

v. membrane one of the membranes subdividing the osseous labyrinth into three compartments.

v. organ consists of a bony labyrinth containing a membranous labyrinth in the inner ear. Part of the membranous labyrinth is the nonacoustic labyrinth or vestibular organ. The vestibular organ consists of the membranous saccule and utricle and semicircular canals. The semicircular canals contain balance end organs called cristae and the saccule and utricle contain similar end organs called maculae. The organ is essential in the maintenance of the animal's balance.

paradoxical v. syndrome vestibular signs of head tilt and ataxia to the side opposite the lesion. Reported in dogs with tumors of the choroid plexus.

v. syndrome see vestibular ATAXIA, canine idiopathic vestibular syndrome (above), feline vestibular syndrome (above).

v. system see vestibular apparatus (above).

v. window see oval WINDOW.

vestibule a space or cavity at the entrance to another structure.

aortic v. a small space at the root of the aorta.

auricular v. an oval cavity in the middle of the bony labyrinth.

ear v. see VESTIBULAR apparatus.

laryngeal v. the part of the larynx between the entrance (aditus laryngis) and the vocal folds (rima glottidis).

mouth v. see oral vestibule (below).

nasal v. the anterior part of the nasal cavity.

oral v. the portion of the oral cavity bounded on the one side by teeth and gingivae, or the residual alveolar ridges, and on the other by the lips (labial vestibule) and cheeks (buccal vestibule).

pharyngeal v. 1. the fauces. 2. oropharynx.

vaginal v. see VAGINAL vestibule.

vestibulocerebellar tract one of the afferent sets of fibers passing to the cerebellum.

vestibulocochlear pertaining to the eighth cranial nerve. See also Table 14. The vestibular division serves the vestibule of the ear and the semicircular canals, carrying impulses for equilibrium. The cochlear division serves the cochlea and carries impulses for the sense of hearing. Called also acoustic nerve and auditory nerve.

v. nerve see Table 14.

v. nerve paralysis manifested by defective hearing if the cochlear nerve is damaged, or rotation, loss of balance and falling to one side if the cochlear branch is the affected one.

v. nerve root granuloma in calves a chronic inflammatory lesion causing facial paralysis and loss of balance.

v. nucleus a series of at least five nuclei on each side of the brainstem, three vestibular and two cochlear.

vestibulogenic arising in a vestibule, as that of the ear.

vestibulo-ocular pertaining to the vestibular and oculomotor nerves; or to the maintenance of visual stability during head movements.

vestibuloplasty surgical modification of gingiva–mucous membrane relationships in the vestibule of the mouth.

vestibulospinal tract a system of descending nerve fibers in the ventral funiculus of the spinal cord.

vestibulotomy incision into the vestibule of the inner ear.

vestibulourethral pertaining to vestibule of the vagina and the urethra.

vestibulovaginitis inflammation of the vaginal vestibule.

vestibulovaginoplasty plastic surgery of the vaginal vestibule. Used to correct hypoplasia of the vagina.

vestibulum pl. *vestibula* [L.] vestibule.

vestige the remnant of a structure that functioned in a previous stage of species or individual development.

vestigial reproductive tissue includes in the male—paradidymis, epididymal appendage, appendix testis, prostatic utricle, uterus masculinus; in the female—epoophoron, aberrant ductules, paroophoron, vesicular appendage, Gartner's duct.

vestigium pl. *vestigia* [L.] vestige.

vet common idiomatic version of veterinarian.

Vetafil trade name for polymerized caprolactam, a synthetic, white, plastic-coated, nonabsorbable suture material which is very popular in veterinary surgery. Designed for external use but is also used as a buried nonabsorbable suture.

vetch legumes in the genera *Lathyrus*, *Vicia*, *Astragalus*.

veterinarian a person trained and authorized to practice veterinary medicine and surgery; a doctor of veterinary medicine.

veterinary 1. pertaining to domestic animals and their diseases. 2. vernacular for veterinarian.

v. assistant 1. a veterinarian employed in a practice on a salary. 2. paraveterinary personnel with a variety of trainings including veterinary nurses, laboratory technicians, laboratory animal technicians, animal attendants. Usually with a minimum of 2 years' full-time training or its equivalent.

V. Board in countries with government services modeled on the British system is the registering authority for veterinarians who wish to conduct a practice.

v. certificate a certificate by a veterinarian relating to matters within the scope of veterinary medicine. Include certificates of soundness, more commonly these days a presale certificate, of freedom of products from diseased tissue, of vaccination or surgical alteration.

v. clinic 1. the title indicates that the establishment has the necessary facilities for the examination and treatment of animals but not necessarily ward accommodation and 24 hour surveillance. 2. the study of disease by direct examination of the living patient.

v. degree awarded by a university at the completion of a degree course in veterinary science and accepted in many countries as sufficient evidence of competence to practice, in others as sufficient to entitle the person to sit for the qualifying or board examination. The important degree, and the one on which registration to practice is based, is the first or primary degree. A postgraduate degree has no relevance to the registration procedure.

v. dermatology the study of the diseases of the skin of animals.

v. drugs medicines used in the treatment of animals. It is an important point in law that medicines used to treat animals should be registered by the relevant local authority, e.g. the Food and Drug Administration, for use in animals. The use of unregistered medicines could disadvantage the veterinarian if the outcome of the particular case was unfavorable and the client resorted to law to recoup any losses.

v. emergency service veterinary services provided at the patient's domicile or the veterinarian's premises for sick and injured patients when the emergency arises; the traditional and preponderant form of service provided by veterinarians everywhere.
v. facilities buildings and fixtures used to catch and restrain animals for veterinary examination and treatment. The use of faulty or incorrectly constructed races, chutes, operating tables may put the veterinarian in legal as well as physical jeopardy unless he/she warns the client beforehand that risk is involved.
v. farm visits veterinary services provided to patients on their home farm, the traditional and preponderant form of veterinary service to farm livestock.
v. hospital the title indicates that the establishment has all of the facilities available including surgery, radiology, clinical pathology, dispensary and ward accommodation and provision for 24 hour surveillance of patients.
v. internal medicine the study of the diseases of the internal organs of animals.
v. investigation centers the system in the UK of regional veterinary laboratories dedicated to the study and diagnosis of the diseases of animals in the region.
v. license the license to practice awarded by the country's registering authority on the basis of the applicant's university degree. Usually awarded annually to provide an opportunity for a periodic review of the candidate's capability.
v. literature includes textbooks, periodicals, proceedings of conferences, reports of institutions and computerized databases.
v. medical education includes undergraduate courses at universities, postgraduate courses either degree or diploma courses at universities or continuing professional education courses run by professional organizations such as associations and colleges.
v. nurse see ANIMAL nurses. Called also VN.
v. pharmacology the study of medicines used in the treatment of animals.
v. pharmacology industry the private companies and corporations which operate for the purpose of developing, manufacturing and selling medicines for use in animals. In some countries all of this work is done by government corporations and commissions rather than privately owned organizations.
v. physician a veterinarian who practices medicine as distinct from surgery; one who deals with medical diseases and not surgical diseases. This is not a common form of practice amongst veterinarians.
v. practice see PRACTICE.
v. practitioner 1. a registered veterinarian in practice on his/her own account and earning income as fees for service rendered, or a veterinarian employed by another veterinarian who is so employed. 2. in the UK refers to veterinarians on the supplementary register of the RCVS.
v. profession all of the veterinarians. Usually qualified in terms of area, e.g. country or international. See also PROFESSION (2).
v. science the study of the diseases and health maintenance of animals. This can only be a generalization because veterinary science is really what veterinarians do and are trained to do as well as it can be done. In some countries this includes what in other countries is classified as animal husbandry, especially the nutrition and breeding of farm animals and in the context of production efficiency unrelated to the health of the animals.
v. services includes veterinary practice, further subdivided into primary accession, consultant or specialist, advisory, contract, species specialist, government veterinary services in a preventive veterinary context, trouble-shooting services to back up services such as artificial insemination, drug and feed sales and domiciliary or house-call practice.
v. specialists veterinarians who provide services to other veterinarians in special areas, e.g. surgery, ophthalmology, radiology, anesthesiology, pathology, theriogenology and internal medicine, and at a higher level of expertise than the general practitioner could attempt to provide.
V. State Board set up under the registering Act to administer it. The constitution varies from elected veterinarians to veterinarians appointed by government, to a mixture of appointed and elected veterinarians and nonveterinarians. The function of the Board is to ensure that the level of veterinary professional service to the community is at the level that the public desires and the government authorizes.
v. surgeon 1. any qualified veterinarian. 2. a veterinarian providing specialist surgical services to other veterinarians.
V. Surgeon's Act legislation to empower a Veterinary Board to regulate the provision of veterinary services to the community.
v. surgery the study of the surgical diseases (those dealt with principally by surgical means) of animals.
v. technicians see veterinary assistant (above). A term used commonly in the USA.
v. toxicology the study of the poisons and poisonings affecting animals.

veterinary medicine the study of the diseases of animals including their diagnosis, prevention and treatment. Nowadays this is supplemented by the study of the medicine of herds and flocks as units.
clinical v. m. the study of disease by direct examination of the living patient.
emergency v. m. that specialty which deals with the acutely ill or injured animal which requires immediate veterinary treatment.
experimental v. m. study of the science of healing diseases based on experimentation in animals.
forensic v. m. the application of veterinary knowledge to questions of law; in human medicine this is an important subject, called also medical jurisprudence, legal medicine. There is no real counterpart in veterinary science or veterinary medical education, except that most veterinary colleges teach a small segment of a course on the subject.
group v. m. the practice of veterinary medicine by a group of veterinarians, usually representing various specialties, who are associated together for the cooperative diagnosis, treatment and prevention of disease.
internal v. m. that dealing especially with diagnosis and medical treatment of diseases and disorders of internal structures of the body.
legal v. m. see forensic veterinary medicine (above).
nuclear v. m. that branch of veterinary medicine concerned with the use of radionuclides in the diagnosis and treatment of disease.
patent v. m. a drug or remedy protected by a trademark, available without a prescription.
physical v. m. that branch of veterinary medicine using physical agents in the diagnosis and treatment of disease. It includes the use of heat, cold, light, water, electricity, manipulation, massage, exercise and mechanical devices.
preclinical v. m. the subjects studied in veterinary

medicine before the student observes actual diseases in patients.

preventive v. m. science aimed at preventing disease.

proprietary v. m. any chemical, drug, or similar preparation used in the treatment of diseases, if such article is protected against free competition as to name, product, composition or process of manufacture by secrecy, patent, trademark, or copyright or by other means.

space v. m. that branch of aviation medicine concerned with conditions to be encountered by animals in space.

sports v. m. the field of veterinary medicine concerned with injuries sustained in athletic endeavors, including their prevention, diagnosis and treatment.

state v. m. veterinary medical services supplied by the government.

tropical v. m. veterinary medical science as applied to diseases occurring primarily in the tropics and subtropics.

vexillum see VANE.

VFA volatile fatty acids.

via pl. *viae* [L.] way; channel.

viability the state or quality of being viable.

viable able to maintain an independent existence; able to live after birth.

vial a small bottle.

vibesate a modified polyvinyl plastic applied topically as a spray to form an occlusive dressing for surgical wounds and other surface lesions.

vibex pl. *vibices* [L.] a narrow linear mark or streak; a linear subcutaneous effusion of blood.

Viborg's triangle an area bounded rostrally by the vertical border of the mandibular ramus, dorsally by the tendinous insertion of the sternomandibularis muscle and ventrally by the linguofacial vein. One of the approaches to the guttural pouch for surgical intervention.

vibratile swaying or moving to and fro; vibratory.

vibration 1. a rapid movement to and fro; oscillation. 2. the shaking of the body as a therapeutic measure. 3. a form of massage.

vibrator an apparatus used in vibratory treatment.

vibratory vibrating or causing vibration; vibritile.

Vibrio a genus of gram-negative, short, motile, curved or straight rods in the family Vibrionaceae of bacteria. Microaerophilic species are now classified as *Campylobacter* spp.

V. anguillarum causes disease in freshwater and marine fish and eels.

V. coli, V. fetus see CAMPYLOBACTER.

V. meleagridis isolated from sinuses of turkeys with sinusitis. Not a recognized bacterial species.

V. metchnikovii found in the intestine of humans and birds; causes a cholera-like enteritis.

V. parahaemolyticus found in sea foods; causes enteritis in humans.

vibrio an organism of the genus *Vibrio*, or other spiral motile organism.

vibriocidal destructive to organisms of the genus *Vibrio*.

vibrion septique [Fr.] see MALIGNANT edema.

vibrionic an etiological qualification used in disease names and relating to bacteria which were at one time classified as *Vibrio* spp. but are now classified as CAMPYLOBACTER.

v. abortion a disease of sheep caused by *Campylobacter fetus jejuni* and characterized by abortion and by necrotic foci in the livers of the fetuses.

v. dysentery see SWINE dysentery, WINTER DYSENTERY.

vibriosis disease caused by infection with *Vibrio* or *Campylobacter* spp.

bovine v. a venereal disease of cattle caused by *Campylobacter fetus* subspp. *venerealis* and characterized by early embryonic death and its consequential infertility and by a low incidence of abortion. See also VIBRIONIC abortion.

canine v. caused by *Campylobacter fetus jejuni* and characterized by vomiting and bloody diarrhea. May be a source of infection for humans.

fish v. a variety of infections in fish, of especial importance in the aquaculture industry. Includes infections by *Vibrio anguillarum*, *V. ordalii*, *V. damsela*, *V. salmonicida*.

vibrissa pl. *vibrissae* [L.] 1. one of the hairs growing on the skin that is reflected into nostrils and on the skin about the nose (muzzle) of an animal. 2. any large tactile hair.

vibrocardiogram the record produced by vibrocardiography.

vibrocardiography graphic recording of vibrations of the chest wall of relatively high frequency that are produced by the action of the heart.

vibrotherapeutics the therapeutic use of vibrating appliances.

vice habitual abnormal behavior of a destructive kind. It is most common in horses, pigs and chickens but may occur in any species if the animals are kept in confined spaces. See CRIB-biting, WEAVING, PICA, TAIL biting, EAR sucking, TOE picking.

Vicia plant genus of the legume family Fabaceae; contains fodder plants that can be poisonous in a variety of ways. Called also vetch.

V. angustifolia contains the lathyrogenic agent β-cyano-L-alanine; also causes cyanide poisoning manifested by incoordination, recumbency, tremor, convulsions.

V. benghalensis unidentified toxin causes diarrhea, dermatitis, dyspnea and widespread eosinophilic granulomas; called also popany vetch.

V. dasycarpa unidentified toxin causes muscle wasting, jaundice, alopecia, diarrhea, pruritus and widespread eosinophilic granulomas. Called also woolly pod vetch.

V. faba reports of illness are confined to humans and are characterized by a toxic hepatitis. Called also broad bean.

V. nigricans reported to cause liver damage and photosensitization in horses.

V. sativa contains a cyanogenetic glycoside and also causes liver damage and photosensitization.

V. villosa reported to cause a syndrome of dermatis, conjunctivitis and diarrhea, with widespread eosinophilic granulomas in cattle. Called also hairy vetch.

viciousness a vice in animals, most commonly mentioned about stallions; AGGRESSION directed at people.

vick PALICOUREA *marcgravii*.

vicryl synthetic, slowly absorbed surgical suture material made of copolymer of lactide and glycolide, available as a braided suture.

Victoria blue stain a stain to demonstrate *Serpulina hyodysenteriae*.

Vicugna vicugna see VICUNA.

vicuna a species of wild LLAMA. A small compact form, fast disappearing because of uncontrolled hunting. Their fur is much in demand for heavy fabrics. Called also *Lama vicugna* (syn. *Vicugna vicugna*).

vidarabine a purine analog, adenine arabinoside (ara-A), that inhibits DNA synthesis; used as an antiviral agent to treat herpesvirus infection.

video auction an auction in which the livestock remain on the farm. The buyers and auctioneer are in one place and bid on the basis of a display on a video tape and screen.

videognosis diagnosis based on the interpretation of radiograms transmitted by television techniques to a radiological center.

videoradiography an x-ray system in which the image obtained by intensification fluoroscopy is displayed on a television screen or recorded on videotape.

videotext an obsolete interactive system for database examination utilizing a telephone, a television set and a converter. Called also dial-up information system.

vidian canal see pterygoid CANAL.

Vietnamese pot-bellied pig originated from the small Chinese pigs with swayed backs and pendulous abdomens and have similar physical characteristics. See also miniature PIG.

viewer a bright light in a box covered by glass on which radiographs are laid for reading.

viewing box the appliance used for examining radiographs; consists of a box and two fluorescent tubes under a sheet of white glass.

Vigna unguiculata plant in the legume family Fabaceae; high-protein legume; used as hay or the seed is used as a concentrate feed. Can cause nitrate–nitrite poisoning. Called also *V. catjang*, *V. sesquipedalis*, *V. sinensis*, cowpea.

vignetting a grid fault in x-ray technology causing areas of peripheral underexposure.

Viguiera annua North American plant in the family Asteraceae; contains an unidentified toxin; causes convulsions, dyspnea, sudden death; called also annual goldeneye.

villi [L.] plural of *villus*.

villin a protein binding the actin filaments of microvillar cores.

villitis coronitis.

villonodular characterized by a villous and nodular thickening.

v. synovitis see villonodular SYNOVITIS.

villose shaggy with soft hairs; covered with villi.

villositis a bacterial disease with alterations in the villi of the placenta.

villosity 1. condition of being covered with villi. 2. a villus.

villous pertaining to or emanating from villi.

v. atrophy reduction in size of the villi of the intestinal mucosa caused for example by invasion by enteric viruses such as rotavirus and coronavirus. The atrophy is the result of loss of the epithelial cells of the villus. Digestion is impaired leading to a syndrome of diarrhea and bulky feces.

villus pl. *villi* [L.] a small process or protrusion, as from the free surface of a membrane.

arachnoid v. microscopic projections of the arachnoid into some of the venous sinuses. Called also arachnoid granulations.

chorionic v. threadlike projections originally occurring uniformly over the external surface of the chorion.

intestinal v. multitudinous threadlike projections covering the surface of the mucous membrane lining the small intestine, serving as the sites of absorption of fluids and nutrients.

synovial v. slender projections from the surface of the synovial membrane into the cavity of a joint; called also haversian glands.

villusectomy synovectomy; excision of a synovial villus.

vimentin one of the Type II 1F proteins in the cytoskeleton; enmeshes the cell nucleus.

vinblastine a vinca alkaloid; the sulfate is used as an antineoplastic usually in combination with other, similar agents.

Vinca plant genus of Apocynaceae family; contains cardiac glycoside; causes diarrhea; includes *V. major* (blue periwinkle), *V. minor*, *V. rosea* (*Catharanthus roseus*).

vinca alkaloids a group of alkaloids, including vinblastine and vincristine, extracted from the periwinkle plant (*Vinca rosea*), which arrest cell division in metaphase by disrupting the microtubules that form the spindle apparatus; used as antineoplastic agents.

vincamine an alkaloid found in *Vinca* spp.

Vincent's angina gingivostomatitis caused by extension to the oral mucosa of necrotizing ulcerative gingivitis (TRENCH MOUTH), characterized by ulceration, pseudomembrane formation and odor, with lesions involving the palate or pharynx as well as the oral mucosa. Called also Vincent's disease, Vincent's gingivitis, necrotizing ulcerative gingivostomatitis.

Vincent's disease see VINCENT'S ANGINA.

vincristine a vinca alkaloid; the sulfate is used as an antineoplastic usually in combination with other antineoplastic agents.

vinculum pl. *vincula* [L.] a band or bandlike structure.

v. lingulae one of the lobules of the rostral lobe of the cerebellum.

v. tendinum filaments that connect the outer and inner sleeves of a synovial sheath.

vine tree see VENTILAGO VIMINALIS.

vinyl the univalent group, CH_2CH, from vinyl alcohol. A common radical in the production of plastic materials such as polyvinyl chloride (PVC).

1,5-vinyl-2-thioxazolidone an antithyroid substance found in the seeds of rape, kale, cabbage, turnips and other members of the *Brassica* spp.

violet the reddish blue color produced by the shortest rays of the visible spectrum.

crystal v., gentian v., methyl v. see GENTIAN violet.

viomellin nephrotoxin produced by several strains of *Penicillium* spp. fungus.

VIP vasoactive intestinal peptide.

viper any venomous snake, especially any member of the families Viperidae (true vipers) and Crotalidae (pit vipers).

viperine a snake of the family Viperidae. Their venom is mainly hemotoxic, causing intense local damage as well as general effects of paralysis. Includes the pit vipers (rattlesnake, moccasin) and the true vipers (puff adder, Russell's viper, English adder).

viper's bugloss ECHIUM *vulgare*.

viral pertaining to or caused by a virus.

v. abortion see equine viral abortion (below). See also EQUINE viral rhinopneumonitis, EQUINE viral arteritis, INFECTIOUS bovine rhinotracheitis.

v. arteritis see EQUINE viral arteritis.

v. arthritis a contagious disease of chickens and turkeys caused by a reovirus and characterized by a high incidence of inapparent infection and some cases of joint swelling and lameness.

v. assembly final steps in the replication of viruses in which virions are assembled from their separately synthesized components. The final steps of viral maturation prior to release from the cell.

v. cultivation viruses grow only in living cells which in the laboratory are provided by embryonated hen eggs, cell culture, or laboratory animals (rabbits, mice, etc.).

v. diarrhea occurs in most species, especially in the newborn. In cattle, rotavirus and coronavirus are the common agents but bovine herpesvirus 1 and others may also be the cause in this age group. In older cattle BOVINE virus diarrhea (mucosal disease) is the major cause. Some other diseases may have diarrhea as an incidental sign, e.g. rinderpest, bovine malignant catarrh.

equine v. abortion caused by equine herpesvirus 1, sometimes equine herpesvirus 4. Abortion occurs in the last trimester and often involves a majority of mares in a group (abortion storm). See also EQUINE viral rhinopneumonitis, EQUINE viral arteritis.

v. hemorrhagic septicemia important rhabdoviral infection of rainbow trout. Also causes infection, and sometimes disease, in other salmonids, pike, turbot, Pacific cod and Pacific herring. Acute infection is characterized by hemorrhages and a high mortality. Chronic infection may be inapparent.

v. hepatitis see DUCK hepatitis.

v. interstitial pneumonia bovine syncytial virus, a common cause of interstitial pneumonia in all age cattle, especially calves.

v. ligand a receptor binding molecule on the surface of a virus. See also LIGAND.

v. papular dermatitis see EQUINE papular dermatitis.

v. pneumonia see ENZOOTIC pneumonia.

v. pneumonia calf caused by parainfluenza-3 virus, bovine respiratory syncytial virus; infection with *Mycoplasma*, *Ureaplasma*, *Pasteurella* spp. may also accompany the viral infection.

v. recombination see RECOMBINATION.

v. replication see REPLICATION.

v. teratogen see AKABANE VIRUS disease, AINO VIRUS disease, BOVINE virus diarrhea, RIFT VALLEY FEVER, WESSELSBRON DISEASE, BLUETONGUE, BORDER DISEASE, HOG cholera, FELINE panleukopenia.

v. transcription see TRANSCRIPTION.

Virales obsolete term for the taxonomic order comprising the viruses.

Virchow–Robin space the potential perivascular space around the veins and arteries of the central nervous system.

Virchow's triad three factors leading to thrombosis: stasis, hypercoagulability and intimal change.

viremia the presence of viruses in the blood either as free virus or a cell associated viremia. In generalized virus infections there may be local invasion, proliferation in regional lymph nodes, followed by primary viremia with dissemination to other tissues. For some infections there may be a secondary viremia followed by increasing tissue damage and severe clinical disease sometimes including spread of virus to the central nervous system.

persistent v. virus can be isolated from the blood for periods longer than a few days.

virgin 1. a female who has not had coitus. 2. in immunology, a NAIVE lymphocyte.

virgin-soil epidemic one that occurs in a population that is largely susceptible.

virginiamycin an antibiotic mixture of virginiamycin M_1 and virginiamycin S_1, produced in cultures of *Streptomyces virginiae*; active against gram-positive cocci. Used mostly as a feed additive for pigs to promote growth.

Virginian opossum see OPOSSUM.

viridicatum a nephrotoxic mycotoxin produced by *Aspergillus* and *Penicillium* spp.

viridin antibiotic substance obtained from *Gliocladium virens*; used as an antifungal agent.

virile 1. peculiar to men or the male sex. 2. possessing masculine traits, especially copulative power.

virilescence the development of male secondary sex characters in the female.

virilism the presence of male characteristics in the female. See also VIRILIZATION.

adrenal v. virilism caused by a tumor of the zona reticularis of the adrenal gland.

virility possession of normal primary sex characters in a male.

virilization induction or development of male secondary sex characters, especially the appearance of such changes in the female. Called also masculinization.

virino hypothesis an explanation for the etio-pathogenesis of scrapie; a small nucleic acid genome is thought to be associated with a host membrane protein.

virion a complete virus particle, found extracellularly and capable of surviving in metabolically inert form and able to infect other living cells. Minimally viruses are composed of a core of genetic material which may be either RNA or DNA, single- or double-stranded surrounded by a protein coat (capsid) which together constitute a nucleocapsid. Additionally some viruses have a lipoprotein envelope that surrounds the nucleocapsid.

virogene viral antigen found in tumors from which infective virus cannot be isolated.

viroid the smallest known infectious agent consisting of a small circular RNA molecule of only 300 to 400 nucleotides that replicates entirely by means of host enzymes since the viroid RNA codes for nothing. It causes a number of important diseases in plants but has not been identified in animals.

virokine a protein encoded by viruses which influence the host's response to infection.

virolactia secretion of viruses in the milk.

virological pertaining to viruses.

virologist microbiologist specializing in virology.

virology the study of viruses and viral diseases.

virucidal, viricidal capable of neutralizing or destroying a virus.

virucide an agent that neutralizes or destroys a virus.

virulence the degree of pathogenicity of a microorganism as indicated by case fatality rates and/or its ability to invade the tissues of the host; the competence of any infectious agent to produce pathological effects.

v. alteration ATTENUATION (2).

viruliferous conveying or producing a virus or other noxious agent.

virulin see AGGRESSIN.

viruria the presence of viruses in the urine.

virus any member of a unique class of infectious agents, which were originally distinguished by their smallness (hence, they were described as 'filtrable' because of their ability to pass through bacteria-retaining filters) and their inability to replicate outside of a living host cell; because these properties are shared by certain bacteria (rickettsiae, chlamydiae), viruses are further characterized by their simple organization and their unique mode of replication. A virus consists of genetic material, which may be either DNA or RNA, and is surrounded by a protein coat and, in some viruses, by a membranous envelope.

For a list of animal viruses and their classification see Table 8.1.

Unlike cellular organisms, viruses do not contain all the biochemical mechanisms for their own replication; viruses replicate by using the biochemical mechanisms of a host cell to synthesize and assemble their separate components. When a complete virus particle (virion) comes in contact with a host cell, the viral nucleic acid and, in some viruses, a few enzymes are introduced into the host cell.

Viruses vary in their stability; some such as poxviruses, parvoviruses and rotaviruses are very stable and survive well outside the body while others, particularly those viruses that are enveloped, such as herpesvirus, influenza virus, do not survive well and therefore usually require close contact for transmission and are readily destroyed by disinfectants, particularly those with a detergent action. Some viruses produce acute disease while others, sometimes referred to as slow viruses, such as retroviruses and lentiviruses and the scrapie agent, produce diseases which progress often to death over many years. Viruses in several families are transmitted by arthropod vectors.

v. amplification see REPLICATION.

arbor v. an incorrect, obsolete term for arbovirus.

attenuated v. one whose pathogenicity has been reduced by serial animal passage or other means. See also ATTENUATION (2).

avianized v. see AVIANIZED.

bacterial v. one that is capable of producing transmissible lysis of bacteria. See also BACTERIOPHAGE.

C-type v. see C-TYPE VIRUS.

Coxsackie v. coxsackievirus.

defective v. one that cannot be completely replicated or cannot form a protein coat or envelope; in some cases replication can proceed if missing gene functions are supplied by other viruses, termed helper virus (see below).

ECHO v. see ECHOVIRUS.

enteric v. see ENTEROVIRUS.

enteric orphan v's orphan viruses isolated from the intestinal tract but not known to cause disease, hence *orphan*.

feline sarcoma v. see FELINE sarcoma virus.

filterable v., filtrable v. a pathogenic agent capable of passing through fine filters able to exclude bacteria; outdated terminology.

fixed v., v. fixé rabies virus whose virulence and incubation period have been stabilized by serial passage and have remained fixed during further transmission; used for inoculating animals from which rabies vaccine is prepared.

foaming v. feline syncytia-forming virus (FeSFV). So called because it causes foamy degeneration in feline cell cultures.

helper v. one that aids in the development of a defective virus by supplying or restoring the activity of the viral gene such as that forming the protein coat.

herpes v. herpesvirus.

human hepatitis v. infection of chimpanzees with some of the human hepatitis viruses can result in infection of human workers.

influenza v. any of a group of orthomyxoviruses that causes influenza. See INFLUENZA.

latent v. a noninfective state and is demonstrable by indirect methods that activate it.

lytic v. one that is replicated in the host cell and causes death and lysis of the cell.

masked v. latent virus.

v. N a type A influenza virus found in birds.

v. neutralization see NEUTRALIZATION tests.

occult v. see OCCULT virus.

orphan v. see ORPHAN virus.

parainfluenza v. see PARAINFLUENZAVIRUS.

pox v. see POX.

rabies v. an RNA virus of the rhabdovirus group that causes RABIES.

respiratory syncytial v. see PARAMYXOVIRIDAE.

slow v. the name given to certain viruses that cause diseases characterized by a long incubation period and a very prolonged clinical course, e.g. the lentiviruses of sheep, maedi and visna.

street v. rabies virus from a naturally infected animal, as opposed to a laboratory-adapted, fixed virus.

vis pl. *vires* [L.] force, energy.

viscera [L.] plural of *viscus*.

viscerad toward the viscera.

visceral pertaining to a viscus.

v. arch mesenchymal structures in the region of the embryonic pharynx and visible on the ventrolateral aspect of the head; give rise to skeletal elements, larynx and other structures of the head.

v. cleft temporary depressions between the visceral arches of the embryo.

v. efferent system that part of the AUTONOMIC nervous system which provides motor innervation to the viscera.

v. gout see GOUT.

v. granulomatosis a disease of farmed and freeliving freshwater and marine fish caused by the fungus *Ichthyophonus* spp. There are granuloma-like lesions in all organs.

v. larva migrans see visceral LARVA migrans.

v. lymphomatosis see LYMPHOID leukosis.

v. nervous system see autonomic NERVOUS system, visceral efferent system (above).

v. pain caused by inflammation of serous surfaces, distension of viscera and inflammation or compression of peripheral nerves. The pain caused by stretching of the wall of a hollow viscus is often intermittent because of its alternating relaxation and spasm in response to distension.

v. patterning the property in tissues of locating themselves in particular sites and with the appropriate three-dimensional shape.

v. receptors receptors in mucosae are sensitive to pH, slight touch, in ruminants there are sensors which recognize distension with or without gas.

visceralgia pain in any viscus.

viscer(o)- word element. [L.] *viscera*.

visceroinhibitory inhibiting the essential movements of any viscus.

visceromegaly splanchnomegaly.

visceromotor concerned in the essential movements of the viscera.

visceroparietal pertaining to the viscera and the abdominal wall.

visceroperitoneal pertaining to the viscera and peritoneum.

visceropleural pertaining to the viscera and the pleura.

visceroptosis splanchnoptosis; prolapse or downward displacement of the viscera.

viscerosensory pertaining to sensation in the viscera.

visceroskeletal pertaining to the visceral skeleton.

viscerosomatic pertaining to the viscera and the body.

viscerotropic acting primarily on the viscera; having a predilection for the abdominal or thoracic viscera.

v. velogenic Newcastle disease see NEWCASTLE DISEASE.

viscid glutinous or sticky.

viscidity the property of being viscid.

viscoelastic retardation a low shear viscometric method for the determination of the molecular weight of large ($>10^{10}$) DNA molecules based on mildly stretching long DNA molecules by hydrodynamic shear forces and then removing the force so that the molecule relaxes back to its normal conformation; the relaxation time is related to, and can be used to determine with accuracy, the molecular weight of DNA molecules of the size found in eukaryotic chromosomes.

viscoelastic substance a hyaluronate substance is used during intraocular surgery to protect structures and prevent adhesions.

viscosimeter an apparatus used in measuring viscosity of a substance.

viscosity resistance to flow; a physical property of a substance that is dependent on the friction of its component molecules as they slide by one another.

viscosum disease see SHIGELLOSIS.

viscotoxin A toxic polypeptide found in *Viscum album*.

viscous sticky or gummy; having a high degree of viscosity.

v. metamorphosis the swelling and fusion of platelet aggregates that occurs as part of a coagulation reaction and in response to thrombin.

viscousness viscosity.

Viscum album a plant in the family Loranthaceae. Called also European mistletoe. Contains tyramine and causes incoordination, salivation and pupillary dilatation followed by paralysis and death.

viscus pl. *viscera* [L.] any large interior organ in any of the great body cavities, especially those in the abdomen.

hollow v. tubular as distinct from solid, e.g. intestine.

Visicalc one of the first spreadsheet computer programs.

vision the faculty of seeing; sight.

The basic components of vision are the eye itself, the visual center in the brain, and the optic nerve, which connects the two. Abnormalities of vision in animals can only be inferred by an assessment of the animal's response to a variety of visual stimuli. The commonly used tests of vision are the MENACE REFLEX test, the watching of a moving object and the obstacle test. These can all be performed in subdued light as a test for night blindness.

achromatic v. vision characterized by lack of color vision.

aphakic v. vision after lens removal.

binocular v. the use of both eyes together, without diplopia.

central v. that produced by stimulation of receptors in the fovea centralis.

day v. visual perception in the daylight or under conditions of bright illumination.

double v. diplopia.

half v. hemianopia.

monocular v. vision with one eye.

night v. visual perception in the darkness of night or under conditions of reduced illumination.

panoramic v. 360° vision conferred on grazing herbivora by the lateral placement of their eyes.

peripheral v. that produced by stimulation of receptors in the retina outside the macula lutea.

photopic v. vision in bright illumination.

scotopic v. vision in low illumination.

v. test see VISUAL acuity test.

visna a meningoencephalitis of sheep caused by a lentivirus identical with the virus of maedi—hence the commonly used name of maedi–visna. The disease is characterized by a long incubation period, up to 2 years, followed by a prolonged clinical disease in which there is a demyelinating encephalomyelitis resulting in incoordination, tremor and wasting for a period of up to 2 years.

visnaga AMMI *visnaga*.

visual pertaining to vision.

v. acuity test performed by walking the animal through an obstacle course. A room full of unfamiliar furniture, or a stairway is usually used for companion animals. Farm animals are led or driven through a passage with drums or boxes strewn across it.

v. cortex the part of the cerebral cortex which deals with images received by the visual apparatu.

v. display the television screen attached to a computer which allows data to be viewed and editing to be performed on screen. Includes visual display unit, VDU, visual display terminal, VDT.

v. evoked potentials (VEPs) see visual EVOKED RESPONSE.

v. following movement of the eyes in watching a moving object.

v. pathway the bulk of the retinal ganglion cells have axons in the optic nerve which synapse with cells in the lateral geniculate nucleus in the thalamus, which project to the visual cortex in the occipital lobe of the cerebrum; in a secondary visual pathway the axons of the remainder of the retinal ganglion cells terminate in the anterior rostral colliculus (pretectal region).

v. system includes the eye, the optic nerve and the optic cortex in the cerebrum. The oculomotor, trochlear, abducent, trigeminal and facial nerves are all involved in reflexes which are part of the animal's responses to visual stimuli.

v. yellow all-*trans* retinal; see RETINAL (2).

visualization the act of viewing or of achieving a complete visual impression of an object.

visuoauditory pertaining to sight and hearing.

visuognosis recognition and interpretation of visual impressions.

visuosensory pertaining to perception of visual impressions.

vital pertaining to life; necessary to life.

v. capacity the greatest volume of gas that, following maximum inspiration, can be expelled during a complete, slow, unforced expiratory maneuver; equal to inspiratory capacity plus expiratory reserve volume. This is a commonly made and practicable measurement in humans but is not so in animals.

v. red dye injected into the circulation to estimate blood volume by calculating the concentration of the dye in the plasma.

v. signs the signs of life, namely pulse, respiration and temperature.

v. statistics that branch of biometry dealing with the data and laws of animal mortality, morbidity, natality and demography.

v. statistic rate vital statistics presented as a proportion of a population, e.g. fetal deaths as a percentage of total births. Includes case fatality rate, nonreturn rate at 60 days.

Vitallium trademark for a cobalt–chromium alloy used for surgical appliances.

vitamer a substance or compound that has vitamin activity.

vitamin an organic substance found in foods and essential in small quantities for growth, health and survival. The body needs vitamins as well as other food constituents such as proteins, fats, carbohydrates, minerals and water. The absence of one or more vitamins from the diet, or poor absorption of vitamins, can cause deficiency diseases such as rickets, enzootic muscular dystrophy and polioencephalomalacia.

Vitamins serve as coenzymes or cofactors in enzymatic reactions. They are required only in trace quantities because they are not consumed in the reactions.

fat-soluble v. one soluble in and absorbed from the intestine in fat. Includes vitamins A, D, E and K.

water-soluble v. one soluble in water. Includes vitamins B and C.

vitamin A a fat-soluble, organic alcohol formed in animal tissues from carotenoids found in plants. Called also retinol. It is formed from carotenoids, principally carotene, in the intestinal epithelium, except by cats, and stored in the liver. It is essential for the proper growth and maintenance of surface epithelium, for the accurate sculpting and proper growth of bones, and for the maintenance of light-sensitive pigments in the eye.

Nutritional deficiency due to lack of carotene in the diet in herbivores and to lack of carotene and preformed vitamin A in the diet in omnivores and carnivores causes hypovitaminosis A. The resulting clinical syndrome varies with species and age. In young animals there is compression of the brain and spinal cord caused by faulty bone growth and characterized by convulsions, blindness and posterior paralysis. In other animals there is night blindness, corneal keratinization, pityriasis, hoof defects, infertility and possibly congenital defects.

Hypovitaminosis in birds is manifested by poor egg production, ocular discharge at first watery then thick and caseous, a nasal discharge and pustular lesions and accumulations of caseous material in the mouth, pharynx, esophagus and trachea.

v. A_2 called also dehydroretinol and found in fish livers. Has the same effects and efficiency as retinol; it is absorbed unchanged and is immediately metabolically active.

v. A excess see HYPERVITAMINOSIS A.

v. A poisoning see HYPERVITAMINOSIS A.

v. A-responsive dermatosis seborrhea, particularly in Cocker spaniels, is sometimes found to be responsive to vitamin A.

teratogenic v. A causes abnormalities in closure of the neural tube in the developing fetus causing defects in the brain, eye and heart.

vitamin B, vitamin B complex a group of water-soluble substances described separately. Includes BIOTIN, CHOLINE, FOLIC ACID, NIACIN, PANTOTHENIC ACID, PYRIDOXINE, RIBOFLAVIN, THIAMIN and vitamin B_{12} (below). Most domestic animals do not require dietary supplementation if they are fed natural feeds. Artificially prepared feeds are usually supplemented because losses may occur during storage and preparation.

v. B_1 thiamin.

v. B_2 riboflavin.

v. B_3 the niacin group of B-vitamins, nicotinic acid and nicotinamide.

v. B_6 a group of methylpyridine derivatives that includes PYRIDOXINE, PYRIDOXAMINE, PYRIDOXAL.

v. B_7 an uncharacterized promoter of digestion in pigeons, possibly a mixture of compounds; called also vitamin I.

v. B_{12} a generic term describing all corrinoids with biological activity of cyanocobalamin. Required by all cells for nuclear maturation and cell division but required particularly for erythropoiesis. The vitamin is produced by ruminants who require only cobalt in sufficient quantities in their diet. A nutritional deficiency of the vitamin causes a maturation failure anemia, anorexia and failure to thrive. An inherited defect in absorption of vitamin B_{12} has been described in Miniature schnauzers. Called also cyanocobalamin. See also HYDROXOCOBALAMIN.

v. B_{12} absorption test measurement of radiolabeled cyanocobalamin excreted in the urine after oral administration (with parenteral administration to saturate the vitamin B_{12} binding sites). Used as a measure of intestinal absorption and, in humans, the presence of intrinsic factor. Called also Schilling test.

v. B_c folic acid.

v. B_T see CARNITINE.

vitamin C see ASCORBIC ACID.

v. C-responsive dermatosis scaling and hair loss occur in calves and piglets fed diets low in vitamin C. Serum levels of the vitamin are low and recovery follows supplementation.

vitamin D a group of closely related steroids that have antirachitic properties. They commence as provitamins in both plants and animals and are converted by exposure to ultraviolet light. In plants ergosterol is converted to vitamin D_2 (the provitamin ergocalciferol) by exposure to sunlight. In animals the provitamin 7-dehydrocalciferol (formed from cholesterol) is irradiated to form vitamin D_3. Pharmaceutical vitamin D is manufactured by the ultraviolet irradiation of ergosterol.

A deficiency of vitamin D, from a nutritional deficiency of vitamin D_2 and a deficiency of exposure to sunlight so that little vitamin D_3 is formed, is characterized by the development of RICKETS in young animals or OSTEOMALACIA in adults.

Poisoning due to overdosing with vitamin D causes demineralization of bones and mineralization of soft tissues. The same effect is achieved by feeding on some plants. See ENZOOTIC calcinosis.

v. D_2 ergocalciferol.

v. D_3 cholecalciferol.

vitamin E α-tocopherol, one of the three tocopherols found in wheat germ. Acts as an antioxidant in the prevention of enzootic muscle dystrophy, mulberry heart disease, hepatosis dietetica and exudative diathesis and yellow fat disease, and deficiency of the vitamin is a major cause of these diseases.

v. E-responsive dermatosis goats on selenium-deficient diets develop alopecia and seborrhea which responds to vitamin E supplementation; similar skin changes occured in calves fed a milk substitute deficient in vitamin E.

vitamin F thiamin.

vitamin G riboflavin.

vitamin H biotin.

vitamin I see VITAMIN B_7.

vitamin K a group of fat-soluble compounds which are required for the formation of prothrombin and therefore play a role in blood clotting. They are present in most green feeds and are not likely to be absent from natural diets. Failure to absorb the vitamin is a real risk in diseases in which fat absorption is defective, such as obstructive jaundice.

v. K deficiency most commonly due to anticoagulant rodenticide poisoning in dogs, and less often cats.

v. K_1 phylloquinone.

v. K_2 menaquinone.

v. K_3 menadione.

vitamin M folic acid.

vitamin PP niacin.

vitellarium a gland which forms yolk.

vitelline resembling or pertaining to the yolk of an egg or ovum.

v. diverticulum small outgrowth from the avian jejunum marking the previous connection to the yolk sac. See also MECKEL's diverticulum.

persistent v. artery creates an anomaly, a mesodiverticular band, stretching from the cranial mesenteric artery to the site of a Meckel's diverticulum, that may entrap a loop of intestine and cause its strangulation.

persistent v. duct creates an anomalous fibrous attachment between the site of a Meckel's diverticulum and the umbilicus. A partial band, reaching only part way to the intestine, may also be formed. Either development may result in an intestinal strangulation.

v. membrane the external envelope of the ovum.

v. vessel omphalomesenteric arteries and veins through which blood passes to and from the primitive heart, and the yolk sac and midgut of the embryo.

vitellochorion an intermediate stage in the development of a yolk sac type of placentation. The outer chorion of the embryo must be vascularized by an extraembryonic circulatory system in order to establish an organ of interchange between the dam and the fetus. If this is provided by the yolk sac vessels a vitellochorion is established. If the vascularization is by allantoic vessels the placentation is an ALLANTOCHORION.

vitellogenesis yolk formation in the liver, transport to ovaries, incorporation into ova.

vitellus the yolk of egg.

vitiligines depigmented areas of the skin.

vitiligo a condition of the skin in which destruction of melanocytes in small or large circumscribed areas results in patches of depigmentation, often having a hyperpigmented border, and often enlarging slowly. The condition is common in horses and cattle, often occurring after injury or surgery. Called also 'snowflakes', pinky syndrome. See also ACHROMOTRICHIA, Arabian FADING syndrome, FREEZE BRANDING.

vitrectomy surgical removal of a diseased vitreous of the eye.

anterior v. removal of vitreous present in the anterior chamber.

pars plana v. removal of vitreous by aspiration through a needle inserted over the pars plana ciliaris.

vitreocentesis see vitreous PARACENTESIS, HYALOCENTESIS.

vitreodentine an unusually hard and glasslike form of dentine.

vitreophage an instrument used in vitrectomy. It combines suction, cutting of vitreous strands with a rotary cutting blade within a needle, and delivery of a physiological solution to replace the vitreous removed.

vitreous 1. glasslike or hyaline. 2. the vitreous body.

v. body see vitreous BODY.

v. flare an opacity of the vitreous which occurs with uveitis.

v. floater a small opacity in the vitreous which may stimulate the retina and cause abnormal behavior patterns such as 'fly-biting'.

v. humor 1. vitreous body. 2. the watery substance contained within the interstices of the stroma in the vitreous body.

peripapillary v. that adjacent to the optic disk.

persistent hyperplastic v. a congenital anomaly, usually unilateral, due to persistence of embryonic remnants of the fibromuscular tunic of the eye and part of the hyaloid vascular system. Clinically, there is a white pupil, elongated ciliary processes, and often microphthalmia; the lens, although clear initially, may become completely opaque.

v. membrane 1. Descemet's membrane. 2. hyaline membrane (1). 3. Bruch's membrane. 4. a delicate boundary layer investing the vitreous body.

primary v. the first stage in development of the vitreous; it persists in the adult as Cloquet's canal.

v. removal vitrectomy.

secondary v. the secondary stage in development of the vitreous; an avascular mass secreted by the retinal ectoderm.

tertiary v. the third and final stage of development of the vitreous; it is secreted by the ciliary epithelium and persists in the adult as the suspensory ligament of the lens.

v. veils curtain-like opacities seen in a normal vitreous.

vitropression exertion of pressure on the skin with a slip of glass, forcing blood from the area.

vitrum [L.] *glass*.

viverrid a member of the family Viverridae. Includes civets, genets, mongoose.

Viverridae the family of civets, genets and mongoose; see MONGOOSE.

vivi- word element. [L.] *alive, life*.

vividialysis dialysis through a living membrane. See also PERITONEAL dialysis.

vividiffusion circulation of the blood through a closed apparatus in which it is passed through a membrane for removal of substances ordinarily removed by the kidneys. See also artificial KIDNEY.

vivification conversion of lifeless into living protein matter by assimilation.

viviparity the state of being viviparous.

viviparous giving birth to living young which develop within the maternal body.

viviperine viviparous.

vivisection surgical procedures performed upon a living animal for purpose of physiological or pathological investigation. It is illegal in most countries to perform such experiments without a license, without proper anesthesia or without all measures necessary to prevent cruelty to the experimental animal.

vivisectionist one who practices or defends vivisection.

vixen female fox.

Vizsla a medium-sized, muscular dog with pendulous ears, docked tail and short, russett gold coat. Called also Yellow pointer, Hungarian pointer, Hungarian vizsla. The breed is affected by hemophilia A.

VLDL very low-density lipoprotein.

vlei chinkerinchee ORNITHOGALUM *ornithogaloides*.

vlei poisoning plant cyanide poisoning caused by *Juncus* spp. in South Africa.

vleibossie HYPERICUM *aethiopicum*.

VMC vincristine, methotrexate, and cyclophosphamide; a cancer chemotherapy regime.

VMD Veterinary Medical Doctor.

VN veterinary nurse, see ANIMAL nurses.

VNO vomeronasal organ.

vocal pertaining to the voice.

v. cord acute bilateral paralysis manifestation of organophosphate poisoning in foals characterized by irreversible severe inspiratory dyspnea and stridor.

v. cord paralysis due to paralysis of the recurrent laryngeal nerve, e.g. in rabies. See also LARYNGEAL hemiplegia.

v. cord resection see VENTRICULOCORDECTOMY, DEBARKING.

v. cordectomy see DEBARKING.

v. cords the folds of mucous membrane in the LARYNX, the superior pair being called the false, and the inferior pair the true, vocal cords. These thin, reedlike bands vibrate to make vocal sounds and are capable of producing a vast range of sounds.

false v. cords ventricular bands.

vocalization to make a vocal sound; a form of communication. Studies of feline vocalization have identified murmur, vowel and strained intensity patterns.

excessive v. a behavioral problem of dogs and cats; may be a displacement activity or caused by separation anxiety.

Vogeloides a genus of nematodes in the family Pneumospiruridae. They are parasites of carnivores and primates.

V. massinoi, V. ramanujacharii found in the lungs of cats.

Voges–Proskauer (VP) test a biochemical test for the identification of members of the Enterobacteriaceae, as well as some other genera, including *Staphylococcus*.

Vogt–Koyanagi–Harada-like syndrome a disease occuring in humans that is believed to be immune-mediated; there is meningoencephalitis, uveitis and depigmentation of skin and hair. A similar disorder with uveitis and depigmentation of the nose, lips, eyelids, footpads and anus occurs in dogs.

voice the sound produced by the voice organs of the vocal cords, the soft palate and the nasal cavities. In birds it is the syrinx that plays the major part in what passes for voice.

v. abnormalities the normal voice patterns of barking, yelping, whining, whimpering, howling, baying, purring, meowing, bleating, mooing, bellowing, lowing, neighing, squealing, whinnying, whickering, nickering or grunting may be abnormal in that they are repeated ad nauseam, or are hoarse or altered in some other way. The myriad voices of birds and exotic species may be similarly affected. They may also be absent altogether so that the animal goes through the motions of making a call but no sound ensues.

v.-activated relay a device in a recording system which switches the recorder on whenever voice is audible and switches off when it disappears.

v. box see LARYNX.

v. response unit a device, usually attached to a computer, that can receive and interpret commands in the human voice and deliver output in synthesized speech. The unit is trained beforehand to the voice of each user.

void to cast out as waste matter, especially the urine.

voiding euphemism for urination, defecation.

vol. volume.

vola a concave or hollow surface.

v. manus the palm, as in primates.

v. pedis the sole, as in primates.

volar pertaining to the sole or palm of primates, the paw in many species and the hoof in ungulates; indicating the flexor surface of the forearm, wrist or hand or their counterparts.

volaris volar; palmar.

volatile evaporating rapidly.

v. anesthetic see inhalation ANESTHETIC.

v. fatty acids short-chain, soluble in water and steam-distillable; acetic, butyric, propionic acids. See also FATTY acids.

volatilization conversion into a vapor or gas without chemical change.

volcanic eruptions discharging of fumes, dust and lava from volcanoes. They have damaging potential in addition to those of being physically overpowering by the lava flow or the ash or dust fallout. However, the only recorded poisoning by contamination of water and pasture has been by fluorine.

vole free-living, small rodent often described as a country rat because of its resemblance to a rat and its disinclination to associate with humans. They are hoarders, live in burrows and eat plant material. Like lemmings, also members of the subfamily Microtinae, they experience massive surges in population, followed by mass migrations and very heavy mortalities. There are several genera including *Arvicola, Clethrionomys* and *Microtus*.

v. bacillus see MYCOBACTERIUM *microti*.

volition the act or power of willing.

Volkmann's canals see Volkmann's CANALS.

Volkmann curette has an oval cup at each end.

Volkmann retractor a handheld instrument shaped like a kitchen fork except that the prongs are curled back on themselves halfway through their length; two- to six-pronged.

volley a rhythmical succession of muscular twitches artificially induced; the aggregate of nerve impulses set up by a single stimulus.

volt the unit of electromotive force; 1 ampere of current against 1 ohm of resistance.

electron v. (eV) a unit of energy equal to the energy acquired by an electron in being accelerated through a potential difference of 1 volt; equal to 1.602×10^{-19} joule.

gigaelectron v. (GeV) one thousand million electron volts (10^9 eV).

kiloelectron v. (keV) one thousand electron volts (10^3 eV).

megaelectron v. (MeV) one million electron volts (10^6 eV).

voltage electromotive force measured in volts. In radiographic equipment it is important that there be no variation in the voltage supplied to the x-ray tube. The voltage supplied to the x-ray tube is controlled by a kilovoltage selector.

voltmeter an instrument for measuring electromotive force in volts, e.g. the one on the x-ray machine that registers the voltage being supplied to the machine.

volume the space occupied by a substance or a three-dimensional region; the capacity of such a region or of a container.

closing v. (CV) the volume of gas in the lungs in excess of the residual volume at the time when small airways in the dependent portions close during maximal exhalation. See also CLOSING VOLUME.

v. of distribution the calculated body space available for distribution of a drug. Abbreviated V_d.

minute v. the volume of air expelled from the lungs per minute.

v. overload see HEART FAILURE.

packed-cell v. (PCV) the volume of packed red cells in milliliters per 100 ml of centrifuged blood. See also PACKED CELL VOLUME.

volumetric pertaining to or accompanied by measurement in volumes.

v. pump a device for administration of intravenous fluids with great accuracy. See also infusion PUMP.

voluntary accomplished in accordance with the will.

v. culling culling by decision of the farmer to accommodate the farm's management plan. See also CULLING.

v. muscle skeletal muscle; controlled by cerebral cortical centers.

volute rolled up.

volvulus [L.] torsion of a loop of intestine, causing obstruction with or without compromising the blood supply to the part by strangulation.

gastric v. see GASTRIC dilatation–volvulus.

intestinal v. a common finding in horses because of the weight of the contents, the power and the duration of the peristaltic movements, and the long mesentery of some parts of the intestines.

Vombatus ursinus see WOMBAT.

vomer a bone forming part of the nasal septum. See also Table 10.

vomeronasal organ an organ thought to supplement the olfactory system in receiving pheromonic communication. The sensory part of the organ is in two long, thin sacs, situated on either side of the nasal septum at its base. The entrances to the sacs are from the incisive ducts which communicate with the nasal cavity and a pit in the roof of the mouth, just behind the dental pad or upper incisor teeth in horses. The function of the organ is probably related to the estrus-seeking action of FLEHMEN. Called also organ of Jacobson.

vomica pl. *vomicae* [L.] 1. the profuse and sudden expectoration of pus and putrescent matter. 2. an abnormal cavity in an organ, especially in the lung, caused by suppuration and the breaking down of tissue.

vomit 1. matter expelled from the stomach by the mouth. In horses the ejection must be via the nostrils and is always a terminal event. 2. to eject stomach contents through the mouth.

coffee-ground v., black v. dark granular material ejected from the stomach, produced by mixture of blood with gastric contents; it is a sign of bleeding in the upper alimentary canal. See also HEMATEMESIS.

vomiting forcible ejection of contents of stomach through the mouth. Called also emesis.

bilious v. the vomit contains bile which has been regurgitated from the duodenum.

v. budgerigar syndrome see neurotic REGURGITATION.

cyclic v. recurring attacks of vomiting.

dry v. attempts at vomiting, with the ejection of nothing but gas.

projectile v. vomiting with the material ejected with great force; seen commonly in congenital pyloric obstruction. See also PROJECTILE vomiting.

stercoraceous v. vomiting of fecal matter.

vomiting and feed refusal syndrome a disease of pigs caused by the ingestion of mycotoxins of *Fusarium roseum*, *Gibberella zeae*. Low concentrations cause vomiting and diarrhea, higher concentrations cause feed refusal.

vomiting and wasting disease see hemagglutinating ENCEPHALOMYELITIS virus disease of pigs.

vomiting sickness see VERMEERSIEKTE.

vomition the act of vomiting.

vomitory an emetic.

vomitoxin a trichothecene mycotoxin which causes emesis in pigs eating contaminated grain. Thought to be the cause of food refusal syndrome. Called also deoxynivalenol.

vomiturition repeated ineffectual attempts to vomit; retching.

vomitus 1. vomiting. 2. vomited material.

von Brunn's nests groups of proliferating urinary tract mucosal cells isolated in the urinary tract submucosa.

von Ebner's glands specialized lingual glands that secrete a serous product. Are associated with the large gustatory lingual papillae.

von Ebner's lines incremental lines in the dentin of normal teeth.

von Gierke's disease see GLYCOGENOSIS type I.

von Willebrand antigen factor VIII-related antigen.

von Willebrand's disease a congenital hemorrhagic diathesis, inherited as an autosomal dominant trait in dogs, pigs and rabbits; abbreviated VWD. It is characterized by a prolonged bleeding time, deficiency of coagulation factor VIII and factor VIII-related antigen, and often impairment of platelet adhesion and usually associated with mild bleeding tendencies. Called also angiohemophilia, pseudohemophilia and vascular hemophilia.

von Willebrand factor the property of factor VIII necessary for normal platelet function; abbreviated VWF. Called also factor VIII_{vwf}.

voorsiektebossie [Af.] see ASAEMIA AXILLARIS.

voracious said of appetite. See POLYPHAGIA.

vortex pl. *vortices* [L.] a whorled or spiral arrangement or pattern, as of muscle fibers, or of the ridges or hairs of the skin.

v. cordis the spiral pattern of the loops of muscle fibers at the apex of the heart.

v. pilorum the meeting place of hair streams to form whorls.

votheysveiki [Icelandic] *listeriosis*.

vox [L.] *voice*.

voxel a volume element; the region in a tissue slice that corresponds to a *pixel* (picture element) in an image. See also computed TOMOGRAPHY.

VPC ventricular premature contraction.

VRE vancomycin-resistant enterococcus.

VS volumetric solution.

v.s. vibration seconds (the unit of measurement of sound waves).

VSD ventricular septal defect.

VTEC verotoxigenic *Escherichia coli*.

vulgaris [L.] *ordinary, common*.

vulnerary 1. pertaining to wounds or the healing of wounds. 2. an agent that promotes the healing of wounds.

vulnus pl. *vulnera* [L.] a wound.

Vulpes velox, V. inacrotis see kit FOX.

Vulpes vulpes see red FOX.

vulsella, vulsellum a forceps with clawlike hooks at the end of each blade, usually with ratcheted handles.

vulture a large bird of prey in the order Falconiformes. In two major groups, the Old World vultures (family Accipitridae, subfamily Aegypiinae) and the New World vultures (family Cathartidae). The former include the Egyptian black (*Aegypius monachus*) and griffon (*Gypius fulvus*) vultures. The New World group include the condors and the black (*Coragyps atratus*) and turkey (*Cathartes aura*) vultures.

vulva the external genital organs in the female.

In primates two pairs of skin folds protect the vaginal opening, one on each side. The larger outer folds are the labia majora, and the more delicate inner folds are the labia minora. In carnivora and ungulates only one pair of labia is present. There is no hymen in the human sense in most domestic animal species but young fillies may have a thin membrane partially covering the opening of the vagina. Maiden bitches may also have a constriction of the vagina which interferes with intromission. A state of imperforate HYMEN in heifers and unmated bitches may cause accumulation of uterine exudates.

The clitoris, a small projection that is composed of erectile tissue like the male penis, is concealed deep in the vestibule of domestic animals. The opening of the urethra lies between the clitoris and the vagina and marks off the deepest portion of the vestibule. See also female REPRODUCTIVE ORGANS.

rosebud v. small, infantile vulva in an adult. Most common in sows. Usually accompanies infantile uterine horns and nonfunctional ovaries.

skyhooked v. tipped vulva (below).

tipped v. the dorsal commissure is almost as low as the ventral commissure because the whole vulva is tipped forward at the top. Difficulty may be encountered by the boar attempting to mate a sow with this defect.

vulvar pertaining to or emanating from the VULVA.

v. atresia failure of the orifice to open may occur with imperforate anus as a congenital defect.

v. bleeding occurs as part of any hemorrhagic diathesis; chronic local bleeding occurs in mares with varicose veins in the dorsal wall of the vulva; voluminous arterial bleeding can occur in cows after a difficult calving.

v. cyst see BARTHOLIN'S GLANDS, GARTNER'S DUCTS.

v. episioplasty surgery for repair of the vulvar orifice and its sphincter muscles most commonly for the correction of wind-sucking in the mare.

v. fibropapilloma a wart growing on the vulvar mucosa; caused by bovine papilloma virus; most cases recover spontaneously as do similar lesions on the prepuce and penis.

v. fold dermatitis see fold DERMATITIS.

v. inflammation see VULVITIS.

v. neoplasms includes papilloma, sarcoma and submucous fibroma.

v. parturient hematoma these can be dramatic in mares because of their size and the speed with which they develop.

v. rupture tears including the musculature are not uncommon in heifers and mares as a result of a difficult parturition.

v. squamous cell carcinoma may occur at a high level of incidence in ewes whose tails have been docked too short as part of a radical Mules operation, exposing the vulva to direct sunlight.

vulvectomy excision of the vulva.

vulvismus vaginismus.

vulvitis inflammation of the vulva.

enzootic v. in an outbreak of enzootic balanoposthitis in wethers some of the ewes will be observed to have vulvitis. The lesions are confined to the lips of the vulva and may predispose to blowfly infestation.

vulvocrural pertaining to the vulva and thigh.

vulvopexy see CASLICK operation.

vulvouterine pertaining to the vulva and uterus.

vulvovaginal pertaining to the vulva and vagina.

v. cleft see ANOGENITAL cleft.

v. glands see BARTHOLIN'S GLANDS.

vulvovaginitis inflammation of the vulva and vagina. In cows and mares this causes a high carriage and frequent switching of the tail in some species, a sticky discharge from the vulva and soiling of the perineum. It may interfere with breeding plans and can cause infertility.

infectious pustular v. a disease of cattle caused by bovine herpesvirus 1 and characterized by venereal transmission of multiple pustular eruptions 0.25 to 0.5 inch diameter on the vaginal mucosa. There is a moderate vaginal discharge. There may be similar lesions on the bull's penis.

vuursiekte [Af.] poisoning by *Asaemia axillaris*.

vv. pl. *venae* [L.] veins.

v/v volume (of solute) per volume (of solvent).

VWD von Willebrand's disease.

VX a nerve gas, the escape of which caused the 'Utah Sheep Kill' in Skull Valley, Utah, USA in 1968.

Vx in medical records, the abbreviation for vaccination.

vygies [Af.] *fire sickness*. See also MESEMBRYANTHEMUM.

W

W chemical symbol, *tungsten* (*wolfram*).

W/ with.

w symbol for *watt*.

W-plasty a technique in tension-relieving plastic surgery used mostly for the excision of unsightly scars. The edges of the excised part are left in the form of a zigzag and the triangles are interdigitated for suturing.

Waardenburg's syndrome, Waardenburg–Klein syndrome a hereditary disorder of humans characterized by pigmentary disturbances, including white forelock, heterochromia iridis, white eyelashes, leukoderma and sometimes cochlear deafness. Blue-eyed, white cats with congenital deafness are considered similar to this syndrome. See also COCHLEOSACCULAR degeneration.

Wachstumsprobe [Ger.] growth-agglutination test used in the identification of bacteria.

Wade-Giles one of the techniques used in romanizing the Chinese spoken word. Used extensively in the preparation of veterinary acupuncture literature.

wafers compressed roughage in flat plates useful for feeding to animals in transit.

Waheap milkvetch ASTRAGALUS *lentiginosus*.

wahi dermatitis caused by *Onchocerca gutturosa*.

waivers of responsibility documents signed by clients at the time of admission of their animals to hospital and which set out to absolve the veterinarian from any responsibility for an unfavorable outcome to the case. The documents have little value because they appear to deny the client the natural right to sue for damages.

wakefulness believed to occur when the tonic flow of impulses from the reticular activating system exceeds the critical level for sustaining consciousness; reduction of reticular activating system activity is the basis of the pharmacological induction of sedation.

Walchia americana one of the harvest mites that cause TROMBICULIDIASIS in domestic animals.

Waldenström's macroglobulinemia see Waldenström's MACROGLOBULINEMIA.

Waler an Australian saddle horse of great endurance, ideal for police horses and army remounts (name derives from New South Wales where the horse originated). Bay, brown, black or chestnut; averaging 16 hands high. Called also Australian Waler.

walk a slow, four-beat gait of horses in the sequence of near hind, near fore, off hind, off fore.

collected w. the horse is held in but is encouraged to walk vigorously by the rider.

extended w. fast, with long strides and the head carried well out in front. The horse is on a long but not loose rein and must not be hurried nor out of control.

free w. a walk on a loose rein with the head free.

walkabout a dummy syndrome in horses; usually pyrrolizidine alkaloses caused by CROTALARIA poisoning. Affected horses walk compulsively, head press, appear blind and walk into objects. They do not respond to usual external stimuli or commands. Called also walkabout, Kimberley horse disease.

Walker hound see TREEING WALKER COONHOUND.

walking a normal slow gait in all species.

aimless w. a similar but less severe sign to compulsive walking and part of the dummy syndrome characteristic of hepatic encephalopathy or chronic brain disease.

w. backwards a prodromal sign in pigs before opisthotonos and tetanic convulsions; some horses with colonic impaction will walk backwards, before sitting on their haunches, then lapsing into lateral recumbency.
w. in circles see CIRCLING.
w. dandruff cheyletiellosis.
w. disease see WALKABOUT.
wall a structure bounding or limiting a space or a definitive mass of material.
abdominal w. see ABDOMINAL wall.
cell w. a rigid structure that lies just outside of and is joined to the plasma membrane of plant cells and most prokaryotic cells, which protects the cell and maintains its shape.
w. chart see CALENDAR CHARTS, SHED sheet.
intestinal w. composed of serosa, muscular tunic, the submucosa containing intestinal submucosal glands, and the mucosa of lining cells, goblet and enterochromaffin cells.
wall-eyed see WALLEYE.
Wallabia the genus of wallabies; includes *W. bicolor* (swamp wallaby), *W. elegans* (pretty face wallaby).
wallaby kangaroo-like creatures of small size, some of them in the same genus (*Macropus*) as the kangaroos, others in related genera *Dendrolagus*, *Petrogale*, *Onychogalea*, *Lagorchestes*, *Lagostrophus*. There are many types including rock, swamp, Tammar, hare and nail-tailed wallabies.
wallaby tick see HAEMAPHYSALIS *bancrofti*.
wallaroo a small macropod marsupial similar to the kangaroo and wallaby but with an untidy appearance due to its sombre, brown-black color, shaggy haircoat and straggly facial hairs. Called also *Osphranter robustus*.
Wallerian degeneration degeneration of a nerve fiber and its myelin sheath that has been severed from its nutritive source.
walleye 1. leukoma; the eye appears white at first glance because of a white opacity of the cornea. Possible causes include inflammation of the cornea and corneal ulcer. 2. STRABISMUS in which there is permanent deviation of the visual axis of one eye away from the other eye, resulting in diplopia; called also exotropia and divergent strabismus. 3. heterochromia iridis; partial or complete lack of iridal pigment so that the iris is bluish-white or pinkish-white. Commonest in horses. Called also ring-eyes, watch eye. See also wall EYE. 4. one of the pike-perch fish; lives in fresh water and is a good source of human food.
wallow mud bath frequented by pigs, elephants, red deer, hippopotami as a cooling aid.
Walpole's solution an acetic acid and acetate buffer solution at pH 4.5, used to dissolve small struvite crystals and break down gritty plugs in the urethra of cats with feline urological syndrome.
walrus very large, up to 3500 lb, 15 to 20 ft long, pinniped similar to true seals. They are hairless, although furred at birth, fish-eaters with hindlimbs used for walking on land and the males have large, down-pointed tusks up to 20 inches long. Called also *Odobenus rosmarus* subspp., e.g. *O. rosmarus divergens*.
Walton–Liston forceps bone forceps with sharp-pointed blades which do not meet when the jaws are closed; double-actioned, blades straight or angled.
Wamberg's knife see Wamberg spavin KNIFE.
wamps farmers' name for cattle falling to one side while ataxic. Their explanation is that the cow falls over 'wamp'. Usually refers specifically to *Xanthorrhea* spp. poisoning.
wanderers see NEONATAL maladjustment syndrome.
wandering slow, purposeless walking.
w. Jew see TRADESCANTIA FLUMINENS, COMMELINA CYANEA.
Wangensteen clamp ratcheted, scissor type forceps with deep longitudinal grooves on the blade faces. Designed for use in closure of ductus arteriosus.
Wangensteen tube a small nasogastric tube connected with a special suction apparatus to maintain gastric and duodenal decompression.
Wangiella a fungus associated with animal diseases, especially phaeohyphomycosis.
wannakai see RHODOMYRTUS MACROCARPA.
waoriki RANUNCULUS *rivularis*.
wapiti large deer from North America. Called also American elk, *Cervus canadensis*.
war bridle see YANKEE WAR BRIDLE, MAGNER WAR BRIDLE.
warble fly see HYPODERMA. See also WARBLES.
warbles the disease caused by HYPODERMA. Includes damage to the hides where the larvae emerge, some cases of choke caused by periesophagitis, posterior paresis or paralysis in a small percentage of infested cattle due to a reaction to dead *H. bovis* in the spinal canal, and some deaths due to invasion of the brain or to anaphylaxis.
Warburg–Dickens scheme see pentose phosphate PATHWAY.
warfarin a coumarin compound used as an anticoagulant in humans and as a rodenticide, with serious toxicity implications for all species. It is readily absorbed from the intestinal tract and acts to inhibit the reduction of oxidized vitamin K, resulting in a depletion of active vitamin K that is required for carboxylation of coagulation factors VII, IX, X and II.
Accidental poisoning in all species causes massive, spontaneous hemorrhage and death due to anemia. Less severe cases often show pulmonary hemorrhage. In pigs it is the legs that are affected preferentially and in dogs hemorrhage into the anterior mediastinum and lungs is common. Vitamin K is the specific antidote.
Waring blender syndrome the shearing of erythrocytes by obstructions of the vascular bed, such as heartworms and disseminated intravascular coagulation, resulting in the formation of schistocytes. See also microangiopathic ANEMIA.
warm providing a sensation of approximately body heat.
w. water blanket a device containing circulating warm water; used to apply heat in the prevention or treatment of hypothermia.
w. receptors are not specifically identifiable but a given temperature receptor will respond to warm or cold stimuli but not both.
warm-up pre-race exercise by a horse.
Warmblood thoroughbreds, arabs and halfbreds (Hanoverian, Holsteiner etc.) in the German classification of horses. Called also Warmblut.
warmblut see WARMBLOOD.
warranty certification that particular animals or chattels are of a particular quality or quantity. Includes warranty of freedom from specifically nominated diseases, warranty of pregnancy, of vaccination or surgical procedure having been performed, of death of an animal. The warranty implies that the vendor will refund the purchase price or replace the item with a comparable one if the first falls short of the warranty.
wart see FIBROPAPILLOMA.
wart hog a grotesquely ugly member of the family Suidae, or wild pigs. They have large wart-like struc-

tures on the face, enormous sickle-shaped tusks, a misshapen head and run with their long tail held rigidly erect. Called also *Phacochoerus aethiopicus*.

w. h. disease see AFRICAN SWINE FEVER.

warty caltrop KALLSTROEMIA *parviflora*.

Wasatch milk vetch ASTRAGALUS *miser* var. *oblongifolius*.

wash a solution used for cleansing or bathing a part, such as an eye or the mouth. See also LAVAGE and specific sites.

washing a technique in the preparation of x-ray films to remove fixative; an important part of producing a good film that will keep for a long time without discoloring.

Washington lupine LUPINUS *polyphyllus*.

washout to disperse or empty by flooding with water or other solvent.

medullary solute w. a syndrome in which the relative hyperosmolarity of the renal medulla is reduced due to an excessive loss of sodium and chloride from the medullary interstitium, usually by diuresis. There is an inability to concentrate urine with polyuria and a compensatory polydipsia. Called also renal medullary washout.

w. period in drug trials, the period allowed for all of the administered drug to be eliminated from the body.

wasp stinging insect of the order Hymenoptera. There is local irritation at the site of the sting. Animals may be seriously affected if they eat fruit that is infested with wasps at the time. Wasp stings contain histamine, serotonin and 'wasp kinin' plus hyaluronidase and phospholipase. Unlike bees, wasps may sting several times.

w. fish see SCORPION FISH.

wastage a loss of product or productivity; in terms of animal production includes losses due to deaths of animals, lowered production from survivors, including reproduction, and lost opportunity income.

waste 1. gradual loss, decay, or diminution of bulk. 2. useless and effete material, unfit for further use within the organism. 3. to pine away or dwindle.

w. disposal techniques for disposing of a veterinary practice's, or abattoir or feedlot or milking shed wastes. By incineration, deep burial, washed away in a sewer as any other effluent or reclamation for industrial or agricultural use. Disposal of wastes from a veterinary practice or service has additional problems. There is a need for disposal of animal cadavers, kennel and pen wastes, tissue specimens, blood and milk and other samples. Much of the material is infected, some of it dangerous to humans, and therefore needs to be disposed of legally and systematically.

w. management system planned, economic and conservationist program for the recycling and conservation of waste.

recycled w. includes chicken litter, newsprint, sugar cane bagasse, fruit pomace, crude sewage, sewage sludge used as pasture topdressing and feed for farm animals, newsprint used as bedding for horses. See also RECYCLED ANIMAL WASTES.

wasting used in a general sense to indicate serious loss of body weight, or locally to indicate atrophy.

w. acetonemia see ACETONEMIA.

w. disease of deer and elk a disease with histopathologic features similar to scrapie.

w. syndrome used to describe terminal stages of feline immunodeficiency virus infection; similar to the cachexia associated with neoplasia.

watch eye heterochromia iridis; walleye.

water 1. a clear, colorless, odorless, tasteless liquid, H_2O. 2. an aqueous solution of a medicinal substance.

w. bag see WATERS.

body w. see TOTAL BODY WATER.

body w. loss is principally through the urine, supplemented by sweating, fecal water and evaporation in expired air.

w.-damaged grain recorded as toxic due to tunicamycin in mixture produced probably by fungi.

w. deprivation the animals are cut off from any source of water. May be by accident or neglect.

w. deprivation syndrome the animals become frenzied and begin to destroy their surroundings in an attempt to find water. There is abdominal gauntness, sunken eyes and weakness, and abortion may occur later.

w. deprivation test a test of the concentrating ability of renal tubules and their responsiveness to endogenous antidiuretic hormone. Urine specific gravity and/or osmolality is measured before water is withheld, at intervals during, and after an average time period of 12 to 24 hours. The normal animal should produce urine that is progressively more concentrated, with an osmolality becoming greater than that of the plasma.

distilled w. water that has been purified by distillation.

w. drowning a primitive method of euthanasia, especially for unwanted, newborn animals.

w.–electrolyte balance the concentration of individual electrolytes and of groups of, e.g. monovalent electrolytes, in serum, in tissue fluids and in intracellular fluid is critical to normal bodily function and is maintained by variation in the renal excretory rate of each electrolyte.

w. homeostasis conservation of body water during times of deprivation or excessive loss due to diarrhea or heavy sweating is effected by an increase in the concentration of the urine by the renal tubules.

w. immersion prolonged head-out water immersion has been used in the treatment of skeletal injuries in horses because of the weightlessness induced but there are serious implications of osteoporosis.

w. intoxication can occur if very thirsty animals, on limited salt intake, are allowed unlimited access to water. There is tremor, incoordination and convulsions and there may be polioencephalomalacia. Hemoglobinuria and hypothermia may also occur.

w. loading test measures the concentrating power of the kidney by combining the water deprivation and ADH tests.

w. marker a substance injected into the body that will diffuse through all of the body water compartments. The reduction in its concentration after injection can be used as a measure of body water. Tritiated water is used for the purpose.

w. marker decay curve the curve of declining concentration of a water marker in intravascular fluid.

w. medication administration of medication in drinking water is used particularly in birds and also in swine.

w. provocative test measurement of intraocular pressure before and after the administration of a large volume of water by stomach tube. A marked increase occurs in glaucomatous eyes.

w. salinity see SODIUM chloride.

w. seed see HYDROCELE.

w. vapor partial pressure in humans is the same in venous and arterial blood, in pulmonary alveolar air and in tissues; it is assumed that the same generalization applies to animals.

water betony see SCROPHULARIA AQUATICA.
water bloom see ALGAE, ALGAL poisoning, CYANOBACTERIA.
water buffalo see BUBALUS BUBALIS.
water bush MYOPORUM *acuminatum*.
water couch PASPALUM *paspalodes*.
water cowslip see CALTHA PALUSTRIS.
water dropwort see OENANTHE.
water figwort see SCROPHULARIA AQUATICA.
water flea see CYCLOPS, DIAPTOMUS GRACILIS.
water hemlock see CICUTA.
water hemlock dropwort see OENANTHE.
water horsetail EQUISETUM *limosum*.
water-jet lavage débridement of necrotic tissue and discharge by the use of a jet of water. A pulsating jet is recommended and the use of excessive pressure (optimum is 60 p.s.i.) must be avoided.
water parsnip SIUM *latifolium*, BERULA ERECTA.
water pepper POLYGONUM *hydropiper*.
water primrose see LUDWIGIA.
water rot see FLEECE rot.
water-soluble vitamin see water-soluble VITAMIN.
waterbelly anasarca and ascites in cattle, usually that caused by rupture of the bladder or perforation of the urethra in males as a result of obstructive urolithiasis.
waterbuck medium to large, semiaquatic antelope, called also *Kobus* spp.
waterfowl a loose term for anseriform birds especially ducks.
watering the giving of water to animals.
w. devices includes, troughs, ball-cock float valves, hydraulic rams, windmills, drinking nipples.
preslaughter w. ad. lib. water facilitates electrical stunning and hide removal and reduces danger of fecal contamination.
waterline disease a disease of black Labrador retrievers; there is pruritus, seborrhea and alopecia of the ventrum and legs. The cause is unknown.
waterpens [Af.] *Galenia africana* poisoning.
waters popular name for amniotic fluid. Called also waterbag.
watershed effect ischemic lesions, caused by slow flow of blood because of poor arterial perfusion, which occur at the periphery of a circulatory field where there is an inadequate collateral circulation.
Waterside terrier an early name for the Airedale terrier.
watery milk an important observation in the recognition of chronic bovine mastitis; the wateriness can be detected by squirting milk from the suspect quarter into a pool of normal milk from an unaffected quarter, the wateriness is immediately apparent, especially if the test is carried out on a shiny black surface; ingenuity is required if all four quarters are affected.
watery mouth 1. a prominent sign in toxemic newborn calves with colibacillosis. The calf is in a state of toxic shock, is hypothermic, recumbent and wet around the mouth to the point that fluid is dripping from it. 2. a disease of newborn lambs in which this sign is prominent. The cause is obscure but a bacterial cause, possibly *Escherichia coli*, seems likely.
watery pork the pale, soft exudative pork of pigs affected by PORCINE stress syndrome.
Watsonius watsoni a digenetic trematode found in the intestinal wall of some primates and causes mucohemorrhagic diarrhea, hepatomegaly, ascites and urinary tract disease.
Watson's test a test which measures urobilinogen and urobilin in urine using ferrous hydroxide to reduce the urobilin to urobilinogen.
watt a unit of electric power, being the work done at the rate of 1 joule per second. It is equivalent to 1 ampere under pressure of 1 volt. Abbreviated W.
wattage the output or consumption of an electric device expressed in watts.
wattle one of the fleshy appendages suspended from the head, spectacularly in turkeys, less so in other domestic birds, rarely in goats, and sheep and pigs.
avian w. a double fold of skin, similar anatomically to the tissue of the bird's comb, suspended from the mandible of domestic fowls. They are bilateral, without feathers and have a red, meaty appearance.
caprine w's variable in their location and their occurrence. Thought to be inherited as a single dominant gene. They are fusiform, 1.5 to 2 inches long, fleshy masses covered with normal skin and suspended usually from the mandibular area but may occur below the ear. Called also tassel.
w. cholera a localized form of FOWL cholera characterized by inflammation and necrosis of the wattles.
w. cyst fluid-filled cystic structure in the wattle of goats, most commonly Nubians; believed to be developmental abnormalities arising from the branchial cleft.
ovine w's identical to caprine but much less common.
porcine w's similar to caprine wattles in location and appearance but have a cartilaginous core and thought to be inherited.
wattle bird see ANTHOCHAERA CARUNCULATA.
wattle trees small trees and bushes in the plant genus *Acacia* in the family Mimosaceae.
wattmeter an instrument for measuring WATTAGE.
wave a uniformly advancing disturbance in which the parts undergo a double oscillation, as a progressing disturbance on the surface of a liquid or the rhythmic variation occurring in the transmission of electromagnetic energy.
brain w's changes in electric potential of different areas of the brain, as recorded by electroencephalography.
electromagnetic w's the entire series of ethereal waves which are similar in character, and which move with the velocity of light, but which vary enormously in wavelength. The unbroken series is known from the hertzian waves used in radio transmission, which may be miles in length (one mile equals 1.6×10^5 cm), through heat and light, the ultraviolet, x-rays, and gamma rays of radium to the cosmic rays, the wavelength of which may be as short as 40 femtometers (4×10^{-14} nm).
w. F 1. a muscle action potential seen on electromyographs; attributed to antidromically conducted motor nerve action potentials. 2. bidirectional, sawtoothed waves on an electrocardiographic tracing characteristic of atrial flutter.
light w's the electromagnetic waves that produce sensations on the retina. See also VISION.
w. motion swirling motion in a drop of dense semen when viewed microscopically (100 × magnification). The intensity and rapidity of the swirling is a reflection of the concentration of the spermatozoa and their level of motility. Called also mass activity.
P w. a deflection in the normal electrocardiogram produced by the wave of excitation passing over the atria.
positive sharp w. an electromyographic tracing associated with denervation and some types of primary muscle disease.
pulse w. the elevation of the pulse felt by the finger or shown graphically in a recording of pulse pressure.

Q w. in the QRS complex, the initial electrocardiographic downward (negative) deflection, related to the initial phase of depolarization.
R w. the initial upward deflection of the QRS complex, following the Q wave in the normal electrocardiogram.
S w. a downward deflection of the QRS complex following the R wave in the normal electrocardiogram.
T w. the second major deflection of the normal electrocardiogram, reflecting the potential variations occurring with repolarization of the ventricles.
T w. abnormalities a common finding in horses whose racing performance worsens. The cause is not identified but may be related to overtraining and the racing of unfit horses. Most animals recover spontaneously with rest. The validity of these abnormalities is now widely doubted.

wave mouth the tables of the molar teeth have a wavelike appearance due to uneven wear.

wavelength the distance between the top of one wave and the identical phase of the succeeding one in the advance of waves of radiant energy.

wavy-leaf St. Johns wort HYPERICUM *triquetrifolium*.

wax a plastic solid of plant or animal origin or produced synthetically, used as a vehicle in skin dressings.
bone w. see BONE sealant.
ear w. cerumen.

wax flower HOYA *australis*.

waxing covering with wax.
poultry w. a technique for removing final hairs and feathers from incompletely plucked birds. They are dipped in hot wax which is removed when it is set.
teat w. a phenomenon in mares which indicates that foaling is imminent. The teats which are already distended suddenly exude a soft waxy covering, probably derived from the thick first colostrum, from the teat orifice. Not a completely reliable guide to an imminent foaling.

waxy casts see urinary CASTS.

Wb weber.

WBC white blood cell (leukocyte); white blood (cell) count.

weak-at-birth due to early parturition, nutritional deficiency, especially of iodine, in the dam, injury during or prolonged birth, intra-uterine infection.

weak calf syndrome a group of undifferentiated diseases of newborn calves characterized by weakness, apathy, reluctance to stand, failure to suck and a humpbacked appearance.

weak lamb syndrome a group of undifferentiated diseases in which the lambs are weak, do not suck well and die of exposure or dehydration and starvation. Among the causes may be poor nutrition of the ewe before lambing, poor lamb–ewe bonding, poor milk supply in the ewe. It is common to find a combination of factors.

weak limb an important concept in the diagnosis of lameness in horses. The affected limb is dragged during progression, and has a low arc in the swing phase of the movement, the limb trembles, knuckles or collapses when weight is put on it, and knuckles or stumbles on it while walking.

weakness a weak bodily state as expressed by reluctance to and difficulty in rising, a shuffling, disinclination to move and then only slowly, eating slowly and a drooping posture. Can be the result of a general toxemia, of a mild form of paralysis, of anemia and other debilitating diseases.
episodic w. one that waxes and wanes, varying from mild or inapparent to severe in the same animal. A characteristic of certain neuromuscular, cardiovascular and metabolic disorders such as myasthenia gravis, polymyositis, hypoglycemia, abnormalities in blood potassium levels, and cardiac arrhythmias and conduction blocks.

wean to discontinue suckling by the dam and substitute other feeding procedures which may include the provision of milk substitutes or replacers.

weaner a young food animal in the period immediately after weaning and up to 6 to 8 months of age. Called also weanling.
w. colitis in 6 month old weaner lambs 1–2 months after weaning; characterized by diarrhea and a low case fatality rate. A *Campylobacter*-like organism can be isolated.
w. illthrift loss of weight at weaning and failure to gain weight subsequently in lambs which appear to have adequate feed and worm control programs. In most cases the problem is multifactorial.

weaning the act of separating the young from the dam that it has been sucking, or receiving a milk diet provided by the dam or from artificial sources.
w. age the average age at which groups of lambs, calves or piglets are weaned off milk, which may be provided by the dam or by artificial means. In pastured animals the age is that at which the young animals are judged to be able to survive on their own by grazing, say 4 to 6 months. In intensive farming systems where good quality, well-balanced diets can be fed, and the young kept under close surveillance, early weaning is practiced successfully. Also modern farming methods demand early weaning so that the dams are again available for mating. Dairy calves, sucking pigs and some lambs are now weaned at 2 to 7 days after birth. Under natural conditions more normal weaning ages, though still subject to a great deal of variation are: calves—4 to 6 months; lambs, goat kids—8 to 10 weeks; piglets—30 to 60 days; foals—5 to 6 months; puppies—6 to 8 weeks; kittens—7 to 8 weeks.
early w. weaning before the young have begun to take significant amounts of alternative diets, e.g. piglets at 3 weeks of age. Usually because of a shortage of feed for the dam, or because of the need to increase the number of young produced per female per year.
w. weight the weight of the young at weaning. Used as a target for young food animals raised for commercial purposes and is an expression of the size at which the young are capable of leading an independent existence. In calves, in particular, the age is related to the development of adequate rumen function.

weanling see WEANER.
w. enteritis see COLIFORM gastroenteritis.

wear and tear pigment lipofuscin. See also XANTHOSIS.

weasel small, short-legged, serpentine-bodied carnivore of great agility and voracity. Tawny colored, some turning white in winter. Members of the family Mustelidae. Called also *Mustela* spp., e.g. *M. nivalis* (common weasel).

weather climate, climatic conditions.
w. stain said of wool. See FLEECE rot.
w. stress cold, heat, wet stress.

weatlings see MIDDLINGS.

weavemouth uneven wear of teeth associated with accelerated attrition. See also WAVE MOUTH.

weaver syndrome see progressive degenerative MYELOENCEPHALOPATHY.

weaving a vice of stabled horses manifested by continuous and vigorous rocking from side to side with the head and neck, and to a less extent the trunk.

web 1. network of tissue, reasoning or electronic. 2. a tissue or membrane. See also WEBBED.

causation w. a network of interacting risk factors.

glottic w. the formation of granulation tissue across the lumen of the larynx, a complication of laryngeal surgery.

split w. a problem of racing Greyhounds. A split develops in the anterior edge of the interdigital web and causes lameness. If it is sufficiently deep it permits excessive spreading of the claws while racing, causing severe injury.

webbed connected by a membrane or strand of tissue.

weber the SI unit of magnetic flux which, linking a circuit of one turn, produces in it an electromotive force of one volt as it is reduced to zero at a uniform rate in one second; abbreviated Wb.

Weber–Christian disease see nodular nonsuppurative PANNICULITIS.

Weber–Fechner law in stimulus–response relations the ratio of changes in stimulus strength which are perceptible to a basic strength of the same stimulus is constant.

Weber spatula an ophthalmic spatula consisting of a handle and a spatulate blade which may be flat or halfround.

weddellite a form of calcium oxalate (calcium oxalate dihydrate). Found in oxalate UROLITHS.

wedder wether.

Wedelia genus of plants in America and Australia in the family Asteraceae; contain a carboxyatractyloside, wedeloside; causes acute hepatic necrosis, nephrosis and sometimes cardiomyopathy, congestive heart failure, death; includes *W. asperrima* (yellow daisy, sunflower daisy), *W. biflora* (*Melanthera biflora*), *W. glauca* (sunchillo).

wedeloside carboxyatractyloside found in *Wedelia asperrima*.

wedge a solid rectangular object, thin at one end, thick at the other.

mouth w. made of metal; used to force open the molar arcades of the anesthetized horse or cow. The planes on which the molars ride are roughened to prevent slippage. Called also Bayer gag.

w. osteotomy see cuneiform OSTEOTOMY.

w. vertebra see HEMIVERTEBRA.

wedge-leaved rattlepod CROTALARIA *retusa*.

WEE western equine encephalomyelitis.

weed 1. a plant growing out of place. 2. of horses, see sporadic LYMPHANGITIS.

Weed method PROBLEM knowledge coupler system.

WEED system problem-oriented medical recording of medical data.

weedfish where a fish, e.g. carp, escapes from a fish farming habitat and populates a natural environment where it destroys natural breeding habitats of native fish.

weedkiller see HERBICIDE.

Weeksella a genus of gram-negative, glucose-non-fermenting bacteria which are normal flora of dogs and cats.

weeping said of frozen meat on thawing; the fluid that runs away as thawing proceeds. It contains myoglobin, salts and protein and is fluid leaked from muscle fibers ruptured by the formation of crystals during the freezing stage. The amount of weeping, and it can represent 2.5% of the weight of a carcass, is greater if the freezing was done slowly and if the carcass is of poor quality. Beef is affected more than the other meats. Called also carcass drip.

weepy eye 1. a lay term for ocular discharge. 2. specifically, a conjunctivitis of rabbits caused mostly by *Pasteurella* spp. and characterized by ocular discharge which is soon spread over the face by the rabbit rubbing the eyes with its paws.

Wehrdikmansia see ONCHOCERCA.

Weibel–Palade body ultrastructural markers of endothelial cells in primates and horses.

weight heaviness; the degree to which a body is drawn toward the earth by gravity. See also Tables 4.1 and 4.2.

apothecaries' w. an outmoded system of weight used in compounding prescriptions based on the grain (equivalent 64.8 mg). Its units are the scruple (20 grains), dram (3 scruples), ounce (8 drams) and pound (12 ounces). See also Tables 4.2 and 4.3.

atomic w. the weight of an atom of a chemical element, compared with the weight of an atom of carbon-12, which is taken as 12.00000.

avoirdupois w. the system of weight still used for ordinary commodities in some English-speaking countries. Its units are the dram (27.344 grains), ounce (16 drams) and pound (16 ounces).

birth w. weight of the newborn at the time of birth.

body w. the animal's weight. In herbivores this is often debatable because of the variation in 'gut-fill' depending on the availability of palatable food. In the absence of scales the weights of large animals are often estimated on the basis of their age and their girth just behind the elbow. Called also liveweight. See also BODY CONDITION SCORE.

body w.-to-surface area determination of many drug dosages is physiologically more accurate when based on body surface area rather than body weight; used particularly in cancer chemotherapy. For conversion table for use in dogs see Table 21.

equivalent w. the weight in grams of a substance that is equivalent in a chemical reaction to 1.008 g of hydrogen. See also chemical EQUIVALENT.

w. gain increase in body weight for specific periods; the principal measure of productivity in meat animals.

w. loss the loss of body weight from that previously measured. This estimate must take into account the difference in 'gut-fill' and the effects of developing pregnancy and recent parturition.

metric w. see Tables 4.1 and 4.2.

molecular w. the weight of a molecule of a chemical compound as compared with the weight of an atom of carbon-12; it is equal to the sum of the weights of its constituent atoms. Abbreviated mol. wt. See also Table 6.

shifting w. limb to limb sign indicative of lameness especially in horses; while standing the horse is continually shifting its weight from one limb to the opposite one of the pair.

weightlessness in horses induces osteoporosis if the period of weightlessness is long enough; in dogs the effects of weightlessness are confused with those of head-out immersion in water.

weight/volume measurement the system in which the solids are weighed and the fluids measured volumetrically.

Weil's disease human leptospirosis caused by *Leptospira icterohaemorragiae* and transmissible from rats to humans.

Weimaraner a medium- to large-sized dog with a distinctive short, silver-gray coat and amber or blue-gray eyes, used for pointing and retrieving game. The ears are long and pendulous, the neck is long, and the tail is docked to a medium length. A longhaired variety is recognized in Europe. The breed is predisposed to spinal dysraphism, hemophilia A and an immunodeficiency syndrome. Called also gray ghost.

Weinberg pen a pen for restraining adult ruminants which are to be slaughtered by the Jewish or Muslim methods.
weir vine IPOMOEA sp. aff. *calobra*.
Weitlaner retractor a self-retaining instrument, shaped like a scissors but the blades open when the ratcheted handles are closed. The blades each have four downward-pointing, curved prongs which retain their position in a spread wound.
Welch bacillus see CLOSTRIDIUM *perfringens*.
welding fumes inhalation causes acute chemical irritation and bronchitis; severe cases develop pulmonary emphysema.
well ribbed-up a good spring of ribs with a short, well-muscled flank or coupling to the hindquarter.
well waters can be poisonous; see NITRATE, SODIUM chloride poisoning.
Wellingtons see GUM-BOOTS.
Welsh black dual-purpose black cattle breed originating in Wales, UK.
Welsh corgi a medium-sized, long, muscular dog with very short legs. Two types are recognized as separate breeds: *Cardigan* Welsh corgi, which is larger, has large, rounded, erect ears, a short, hard-textured coat, and a long, bushy tail. *Pembroke* Welsh corgi, which is more common, has a shorter body, smaller, pointed, erect ears, a medium length coat, and a very short, natural or docked, tail. The breed is predisposed to cystinuria, intervertebral disk disease and progressive retinal atrophy.
Welsh mountain a white or tan-faced wool and meat sheep; males are horned, females polled.
Welsh pig a long-faced, lop-eared, white pig, originating in Wales, UK.
Welsh Pony 1. Welsh Mountain pony, a riding pony of any color but not broken colors, up to 12 hands high. 2. Welsh pony, similar to the Welsh Mountain pony but larger, up to 13.2 hands high. 3. Welsh cob.
Welsh springer spaniel a medium-sized dog of the spaniel type, midway in size between the Cocker spaniel and English springer spaniel. It is compact with pendulous ears, docked tail, and a red and white, thick, silky coat that is flat on the body but forms feathering on the legs, ears and under the body. Called also Starter.
Welsh terrier a small (20 lb) dog with a wiry, black and tan coat that is shorter on the body and longer on the legs and muzzle. The ears are folded over, and the medium length tail is carried upright.
wen 1. a sebaceous or epidermal inclusion cyst. 2. pilar cyst.
Wenckebach's phenonemon a usually repetitive sequence seen in partial heart block, marked by progressive lengthening of the P–R interval until ventricular response occurs.
Wendener's disease chlorinated naphthalene poisoning.
Wensleydale an English longwool meat sheep, polled, with blue face and legs.
Wenyonella a genus of coccidia of the family Eimeriidae.
W. anatis found in domestic ducks.
W. gagari found in domestic ducks.
W. philiplevinei found in domestic ducks and causes severe inflammation of the mucosa of the ileum and rectum.
Werdnig–Hoffmann disease a human disease which has a possible model in hereditary spinal muscular atrophy of Brittany spaniels.
Wernicke encephalopathy Wernicke–Korsakoff syndrome.
Wernicke–Korsakoff syndrome an inflammatory hemorrhagic encephalopathy in humans due to thiamin deficiency. Called also Wernicke's encephalopathy (disease, syndrome).
Wesselsbron disease a disease of cattle and sheep in southern Africa caused by flavivirus transmitted by mosquitoes and characterized by abortion and heavy mortality in newborn lambs and jaundice in adult sheep. The disease is similar to Rift Valley fever but there is no antigenic or taxonomic relationship between the viruses. Serological evidence indicates that the infection is very widespread and occurs as an asymptomatic or mild infection in many other species including humans.
Wessex saddleback a black pig with a white saddle right around its thorax, including the forelimbs. The ears are pitched forward.
West African dwarf a southwest African breed of horned, hairy (woolless) sheep; white with red or black spots, may be all black.
West Australian blue lupin LUPINUS *cosentini*.
West dissector–elevator a handle with a long neck and a small curved, blunt end suitable for fine blunt dissection in ophthalmic sites.
West Highland see HIGHLAND cattle.
West Highland white terrier a small (15–22 lb), muscular, very alert dog with short legs and a distinctive, white, medium length, double coat made up outer, hard hairs and soft, fur underneath. The eyes and nose are dark, the ears erect and pointed, and the tail, which is naturally a medium length is carried upright or over the back. The breed is predisposed to atopic dermatitis, craniomandibular osteopathy and globoid cell leukodystrophy. Called also 'Westie'.
West Nile meningoencephalitis a disease caused by a flavivirus and occurs in horses on the south coast of France.
West Nile virus a flavivirus associated with bovine abortion and stillbirths in Africa.
Westermark's sign decreased filling of the pulmonary vasculature due to thromboembolism.
western azalea RHODODENDRON *occidentale*.
western bleeding heart DICENTRA *formosa*.
Western blot an immunologic technique for the detection of proteins using a radioactive probe. Called also Western transfer.
western brown snake see DEMANSIA NUCHALIS NUCHALIS.
western chicken flea CERATOPHYLLUS *niger*.
western chokecherry PRUNUS *virginiana* var. *melanocarpa*.
western duck disease, western duck sickness see BOTULISM.
western equine encephalitis see equine viral ENCEPHALOMYELITIS; abbreviated WEE.
western goldenrod SOLIDAGO *spectabilis*.
western hellebore see VERATRUM *californicum*.
western hen flea CERATOPHYLLUS *niger*.
western labrador tea LEDUM *glandulosum*.
western tiger snake a variety of TIGER snake.
Western transfer Western blot.
Western veal calves see HEAVY veal calves.
western yellow pine PINUS *ponderosa*.
western yew TAXUS *brevifolia*.
Westie West Highland white terrier.
wet-belly disease a disease of farmed, male mink characterized by urinary incontinence and staining of the pelt along the belly. The cause is unknown. It is not associated with illness nor fatality but the skin is damaged.

wet bench the facility in an x-ray dark room where the films are developed, fixed and washed.
wet brain brain edema.
wet calf disease HYALOMMA toxicosis.
wet dewlap a moist dermatitis of the dewlap in rabbits, often precipitated by drooling from malocclusion, moisture from drinking pans or bowls, and damp cages.
wet-drying a husbandry practice of classifying ewes according to whether they have had a lamb in the current lambing season. Ewes that have a dry udder and no lambing stain by fetal fluids on the perineum are classified as dry-dry and did not lamb. Those with a lambing stain and milk in the udder are wet-wet and have lambed and it has sucked. Wet-dry ewes, with a lambing stain and some milk but the teats are dirty, have had a lamb but lost it.
wet preparations a method of preparing specimens for examination in which they are kept in their liquid state or suspended in a liquid, rather than being dried and then examined. Used in the diagnosis of trichomoniasis, leptospirosis and fungal infections.
wet rendering abattoir offal is cooked in vats, the fat skimmed off and the residue dehydrated to meat meal. The alternative is DRY rendering.
wet tail proliferative ileitis, regional enteritis. A disease of hamsters of unknown etiology, thought to be associated with *Campylobacter jejuni*, characterized by diarrhea causing constant wetness of the tail, and dehydration. At necropsy there is marked hyperplasia of the ileal epithelium and a generalized enteritis. The disease is endemic in many commercial and laboratory colonies.
wether male sheep castrated at an early age before secondary sex characters have developed.
wetness constant wetness of the wool fleece or haircoat along the backs of animals, and caused by heavy rainfall over a long period, causes fleece rot in sheep and rain scald in horses. Constant wetness of the underparts caused by poor drainage in indoor housing, or too little bedding or a defect of urinary control by the animal causes local dermatitis referred to as wet, e.g. wet belly of mink, wet tail of hamsters, wet dewlap of rabbits.
wetting creating and maintenance of a wet surface. See also WETNESS.
w. agent substance that enhances wetting; detergents have been used internally as medicine, e.g. DIOCTYL SODIUM SULFOSUCCINATE in mineral oil for bloat in cows and impaction in horses as a fecal softener but has proved to be toxic to horses.
whale large mammal, member of the order Cetacea, well adapted to aquatic life.
false killer w. *Pseudorca crassidens;* much smaller than the killer whale and lacking its fiercely predatory behavior.
killer w. the greatest predator of the whales eating all kinds of fish life including other whales. Called also grampus, *Orcinus orca*.
w. lice see ISOCYAMUS DELPINI.
w. stranding see PINNIPED stranding.
Wharton's jelly the soft, jelly-like intercellular substance of the umbilical cord; rich in hyaluronic acid.
wheal a localized area of edema on the body surface, often attended with severe itching and usually evanescent. It is the typical lesion of urticaria.
w. and flare reaction a central blanching surrounded by an erythematous zone of varying diameter, sometimes with pseudopodia, observed on the skin in response to intradermal exposure to allergen (antigen). A basis for detecting particular immediate hypersensitivites in an individual. Produced following release of histamine from mast cells bearing IgE bound to Fc receptor.
wheal erythema response see WHEAL and flare reaction.
wheal–flare see wheal–flare REACTION.
wheat a plant used principally for its grain as human food and livestock feed. Wheat by-products of bran pollard, middlings, shorts are a major source of protein supplements for ruminants. Used also to a limited extent as a fodder by grazing the green crop or as green chop. Called also *Triticum vulgare*.
w. engorgement see CARBOHYDRATE ENGORGEMENT.
w. enteropathy see wheat-sensitive ENTEROPATHY.
w. germ the embryo of wheat salvaged during the milling process. A rich source of tocopherol, thiamin, riboflavin and other vitamins.
w. pasture poisoning a form of hypocalcemic and hypomagnesemic tetany which occurs in cattle and sheep grazed on a green cereal crop. This may be done in a time of feed shortage or as a measure to control excessive growth of the crop. It can also occur when animals are grazed on a cereal crop which has been used as a cover crop to help establish a pasture. See also LACTATION TETANY.
w. pollard itch dermatitis caused by the acarid mite SUIDASIA NESBITTI.
w. smut see TILLETIA TRITICI.
w. weevil disease an immediate immune complex-mediated hypersensitivity pneumonitis of humans caused by inhalation of flour infested with *Sitophilus granarius*.
wheaten a pale yellow or fawn coat color.
w. terrier see SOFT-COATED WHEATEN TERRIER.
wheelbarrowing a test for postural reactions in which the animal's hindquarters are supported and walking on the forelimbs is forced. Symmetry of movement, position of the head, neck and limbs, and abnormal movements are observed. Necessarily, only used in neurological examination of small animals.
wheeze a whistling respiratory sound.
wheezing breathing with a rasp or whistling sound. It results from constriction or obstruction of the throat, pharynx, trachea or bronchi.
whelping parturition in bitches.
w. box a low-sided, open-topped box designed to accommodate a whelping bitch and her newborn puppies. The bottom may have provision for heating.
whewellite a form of calcium oxalate (calcium oxalate monohydrate) found in uroliths.
whey liquid residue from milk after the removal of cheese curds in the manufacture of cheese. An excellent protein supplement but difficult to handle in the liquid form, except to pigs maintained close to the cheese factory. Dried whey is easy to handle but processing costs are high.
whinny the horse's call that expresses pleasure and expectancy.
whip muscle the sartorius muscle; a term used in Greyhounds.
whip stitch see continuous SUTURE.
Whippet a small (28 lb), very sleek, fine-boned dog with a short coat in any color or mixture of colors. The ears are small and folded over, the head long and flat, and the tail long and tapered. The dog resembles a miniature Greyhound and is often used for coursing. In earlier times, it was known as 'snap-dog'.
Whipple's operation a technique for repair of a prolapsed vagina in the bitch based on submucous resection and suturing of the cut ends.

Whipple's triad the three criteria on which hyperinsulinism due to pancreatic islet-cell disease (most commonly insulinoma) is diagnosed: (1) neuromuscular signs with fasting or exercise, (2) low blood glucose levels associated with clinical signs, and (3) reversal of clinical signs with the administration of glucose.
whipworm see TRICHURIS.
whirlbone lameness see trochanteric BURSITIS.
whirling disease important disease of juvenile rainbow trout. Caused by the myxosporean MYXOBOLUS CEREBRALIS which parasitizes the cartilage of the head.
whirlpool bath see whirlpool BATH.
whiskers 1. the coarse, long, widely spaced sensory hairs located around the muzzle of most animal species. See also sinus HAIR. 2. superficial fungal growth found on chilled meat carcasses and caused by infection with *Mucor* and *Thamnidium* spp. fungi. Cause no significant damage to the meat but may cause a musty smell.
whistling high-pitched respiratory sound made by forced breathing through a very narrow opening; usually indicative of stenosis of a passage.
white 1. a color lacking any hue; the color of fresh snow. 2. a coat color.
white bass MORONE *chrysops*.
white bile see white BILE.
w. bile syndrome fluid and mucus, lacking bile pigments, found in the gallbladder of cats with cholangiohepatitis and severe intrahepatic bile sludging.
white blood cell leukocyte.
w. b. c. count see BLOOD COUNT.
white bryony BRYONIA *dioica*.
white cedar see MELIA AZEDERACH.
white cell leukocyte.
white cloud disease infectious disease of carp causing copious mucus secretion so that the patient looks to be enclosed in a cloud. The causative infection is *Pseudomonas fluorescens*.
white clover TRIFOLIUM *repens*.
white comb disease of fowls. See FAVUS.
white dog shaker syndrome see SHAKER DOGS.
White emasculator a triple crush emasculator for use on horses. The central pivot is a thumb screw so that the joint can be tightened or the instrument dismantled.
white eye calf syndrome stillborn or weak calves with congenital cataract. Cause unknown, outcome fatal.
white face see BALDY.
white-flowered rhododendron RHODODENDRON *albiflorum*.
white foal syndrome see LETHAL white.
White forceps forceps with ratcheted handles, a scissor type construction, long, down-curved blades with inturning opposed rat-tooth ends. Designed for tonsillectomy.
White Fulani a white with black points multipurpose breed of Nigerian cattle, which has lyre horns. See also FULANI.
white goosefoot CHENOPODIUM *album*.
white grub see POSTHODIPLOSTOMUM *minimum*.
white gum EUCALYPTUS *viminalis*.
white heifer disease see imperforate HYMEN.
white hellebore see VERATRUM *album*.
White Holland a pure white turkey with pink shanks. Called also Australian white.
white horsenettle SOLANUM *elaeagnifolium*.
white iris DIPLARRENA *moraea*.
white lead basic lead carbonate.
White leghorn a pure white, egg-laying breed of poultry with bright yellow legs and bill. The comb, face and wattles are red, the earlobes are white.
white line 1. the fusion between the wall and the sole of the hoof as seen in the horse. 2. the linea alba.
w. l. disease a disease in sheep in which the wall of the hoof separates from the sole at the white line over a short part of its length. The cavity that is formed becomes packed with dirt causing pressure on the sensitive laminae and lameness. Eventually the cavity penetrates to the coronet and develops a sinus there.
white liniment a traditional, mildly stimulant proprietary embrocation containing oleic acid, turpentine oil and ammonium chloride; rubbed into sore and strained muscles and tendons.
white liver disease a specific hepatic dysfunction characterized by extensive hepatic lipidosis and seen only in cobalt deficient sheep. Clinically there is either photosensitization or anemia with emaciation. It is probably a toxic hepatopathy against which cobalt is protective.
white loco OXYTROPIS *lambertii*.
white lotion traditional astringent application for the treatment of superficial abrasions such as girth and saddle galls in horses. Contains lead acetate and zinc sulfate and is poisonous if licked over a long period.
white lupin LUPINUS *albus*.
white-margined spurge EUPHORBIA *marginata*.
white matter, white substance the white nervous tissue, constituting the conducting portion of the brain and spinal cord, composed mostly of myelinated nerve fibers. Gray matter or substance is the term used to describe the tissues composed of unmyelinated fibers.
white moth plant see ARAUJIA HORTORUM.
white muscle disease see ENZOOTIC muscular dystrophy.
white muscle fibers see MUSCLE.
white mustard SINAPIS *alba*.
white myofibers see MUSCLE.
white passion fruit PASSIFLORA *subpeltata*.
white petrolatum Vaseline.
white phosphorus pure phosphorus, used at one time as a rodenticide.
white point loco OXYTROPIS *sericea*, *O. lambertii*.
white poppy see PAPAVER *somniferum*.
white pulp see white PULP.
white ragweed see FRANSERIA DISCOLOR.
White scissors scissors designed for clipping tubular rather than flat nails, or claws. The cutting edges of the blades form a circle when open so that the claw cannot escape when they are closed.
white scours diarrhea in newborn animals on a milk diet. The name is usually used with reference to dietary diarrhea in which no bacteria or virus is etiologically involved.
white shaker disease see SHAKER DOGS.
white snakeroot see EUPATORIUM *rugosum*.
white spirit a petroleum distillate fraction used as an alternative to turpentine. The poisonous effects caused by ingestion are the same as for kerosene.
white spot 1. a fungal infection of the surface of chilled meat carcasses caused by *Sporotrichum carnis*. Appears as white, woolly spots that do no damage, can be wiped away easily but may give the meat a musty smell. 2. artefactual white spots on x-ray films are caused by dirt, specks of barium or iodine or medicines containing them on the animal or on the cassette or by dust or dirt on the screens.
white spot disease a disease of freshwater fish caused by the protozoan ICHTHYOPHTHIRIUS *multifiliis*

and manifested by white pustules on the skin and gills and in bad cases sloughing of extensive affected areas. Common in aquariums but occurs also in cultured fish in large groups in hatcheries and on fish farms.

white spot syndrome a baculovirus complex with probably three baculoviruses involved; clinical signs include a loose cuticle with white or reddish-brown spots; 100% mortality in 3–10 days not uncommon in *Penaeus monodon*, *P. japonicus*, *P. chinensis*, *P. indicus*, *P. merguiensis*, *P. setiferus*.

white-spotted kidney focal, nonsuppurative, interstitial nephritis in calves caused probably by bacteremia of undetermined origin. The lesion appears to exert little effect and is subsequently obliterated by changes in the kidney due to progressive fibrosis resulting from further increments of age.

white squill a cardiac glycoside called scillerin A obtained from the plant *Urginea maritima*.

White Suffolk a breed of Downs-type meat sheep produced by crossing SUFFOLK SHEEP and DORSET DOWN and selecting against colored points and fibers in the fleece.

white sweet clover MELILOTUS *alba*.

white sweet melilot MELILOTUS *alba*.

white-tailed deer called also *Odocoileus virginianus* (syn. *Dama virginianus*). A small, 3 ft high at the withers, graceful red to gray true deer with a distinctive white tail.

white veratrum see VERATRUM *album*.

white whale see DELPHINAPTERUS LEUCAS.

white zone horn of the hoof separating the wall horn from the sole horn; more common name is white line.

whitebrush ALOYSIA *lycioides*.

whiteheads see SPHENOSCIADIUM CAPITELLATUM.

Whitehouse technique surgery of the equine guttural pouch through a ventral midline or paramedian approach. A modification of the original technique is a paramedian approach immediately below the linguofacial vein.

whites see LEUKORRHEA.

whiteside test a precursor of the CALIFORNIA MASTITIS TEST and replaced by it; based on the development of viscosity in the milk when sodium hydroxide is added.

whitewood see ATALAYA HEMIGLAUCA.

Whitfield's ointment a mixture containing 6% benzoic acid and 3% salicylic acid; used on the skin as a fungistatic and keratolytic agent.

Whitmore's disease melioidosis.

Whitten effect the introduction of a male into a large group of females results in a synchronization of the estrous cycles of the females. Phenomenon observed in mice.

Whittingham's saline a phosphate-buffered saline used to store fertilized embryos.

WHO World Health Organization.

WHO juice an oral, hypertonic electrolyte solution, formulated by the World Health Organization for treatment of cholera in humans, but suitable for the treatment of gastroenteritis in many species; used particularly in dogs and cats. It contains dextrose, potassium chloride, sodium chloride and sodium bicarbonate.

whole blood blood as it comes from the artery or, more commonly, the vein, but usually assumed to be combined with an anticoagulant. Contains the cellular and plasma components of blood.

whole-colored there are no hairs of any color in the animal's coat other than those of the main color. Called also self-colored.

whole farm approach a method of assessing such parameters as the productivity or profitability, the freedom from disease and the mortality rate of a farm as a whole and not for a single enterprise or part of it.

whole farm budget one setting out the expected outcome of the whole farm's production plan in terms of profitability.

whole milk fed neonates fed on whole milk rather than diluted milk or milk replacer.

whole milk tetany of calves see calf HYPOMAGNESEMIC tetany.

whoop a sonorous and convulsive inspiration; suggestive of the sound associated with whooping cough in humans.

whorl a spiral arrangement, as in the hairs that go to make up a cowlick.

whorled milkweed ASCLEPIAS *subverticillata*.

wide behind said of a horse's gait in which the hindlimbs are moved wide apart.

wigged see PERUKE.

wiggings wool removed from around the eyes and face of the sheep.

Wikstroemia indica plant in the Thymelaceae family; contains toxic dihydroxycoumarin glycosides; has caused clotting defect, spontaneous hemorrhage in deer, dysentery in cattle; called also tie-bush.

Wilcoxon test a test used in statistics to compare paired data. Has the advantage of incorporating the size of the difference between the two sets of data in the comparison.

wild growing uncontrolled away from a domesticated environment. See under the name of the species, e.g. equid, sheep, swine, pig, turkey.

w. amaranth AMARANTHUS *cruentus*.

w. arum ARUM *maculatum*.

w. barley see HORDEUM.

w. black cherry, w. cherry PRUNUS *serotina*.

w. bleeding heart DICENTRA *eximia*.

w. boar the commonest wild pig. Shaped like a domestic pig but lean, long-legged and mean. They can move very quickly and have formidable tusks in their bottom jaws. Their long, pointed snout enables the pigs to get through undergrowth better than any other animal. Called also *Sus scrofa*.

w. carrot see DAUCUS CAROTA.

w. chervil CHAEROPHYLLUM *sylvestre*.

w. coffee see CASSIA *occidentalis*.

w. cotton see ASCLEPIAS.

w. cotton bush GOMPHOCARPUS *physocarpus*.

w. cucumber CUCUMIS *trigonus*.

w. date see FADOGIA HOMBLEI.

w. everlasting daisy HELICHRYSUM *argyrosphaerum*.

w. flax PIMELEA *trichostachya*.

w. garlic ALLIUM *ursinum*, *A. vineale*.

w. gooseberry see NICANDRA PHYSALODES.

w. grackle see GRACKLE.

w. ground cherry see PHYSALIS.

w. heliotrope HELIOTROPIUM *europaeum*.

w. hop RUMEX *vesicarius*.

w. hyacinth SCILLA *nonscripta*.

w. indigo see BAPTISIA LEUCANTHA.

w. iris see IRIS.

w. jasmine CESTRUM *diurnum*.

w. lettuce see LACTUCA SERRIOLA.

w. lucerne CROTALARIA *globifera*, *C. dura*.

w. lupin LUPINUS *laxiflorus*.

w. mint see PERILLA FRUTESCENS.

w. mustard SINAPIS *arvensis*.

w. onion ALLIUM *validum*, DIPCADI *glaucum*.

w. parsley CYMOPTERUS *longipes*.

w. parsnip any of several plant species including TRACHYMENE, CICUTA and a plant with the name *Pastinaca sativa* which is quite edible.
w. passion fruit PASSIFLORA *subpeltata*.
w. pea LATHYRUS *incanus*, *L. sylvestris*.
w. pepper DAPHNE *mezereum*.
w. pineapple see MACROZAMIA.
w. potato bush SOLANUM *esuriale*.
w. radish see RAPHANUS *raphanistrum*.
w. red cherry PRUNUS *pennsylvanica*.
w. sorghum SORGHUM *verticilliflorum*.
w. sunflower see DORONICUM HUNGARICUM, VERBESINA ENCELIOIDES.
w. tobacco see NICOTIANA.
w. tomato SOLANUM *esuriale*.
w. tree tobacco SOLANUM *mauritianum*.
w. turnip see RAPISTRUM RUGOSUM.
w. verbena see VERBENA *rigida*.
w. watermelon CITRULLUS *lanatus*.
w. winter pea see LATHYRUS *hirsutus*.

wild card characters (usually * or ?) used to replace one or a number of characters in a search string.

wildebeest an ungainly antelope with a head and horns like a buffalo; a carrier of the wildebeest-associated form of bovine malignant catarrh. Called also *Connochaetes gnou*, blue wildebeest (*Connochaetes taurinus*).
w.-associated bovine malignant catarrhal fever virus African malignant catarrhal fever.

wildedadel see FADOGIA HOMBLEI.

wilderoosmaryn LANTANA *camara*.

wildlife animals running unrestrained in a natural environment.

Willis circle see CIRCULUS arteriosus cerebri.

Willis technique a flotation method, utilizing saturated common salt solution to float helminth eggs, and hence separate eggs from fecal debris. The eggs can then be counted in a fecal sample. Suitable for most nematodes but not for cestodes or trematodes.

willow-leaved with long, lanceolate leaves, like those of the willow.
w.-l. cestrum CESTRUM *parqui*.
w.-l. jessamine CESTRUM *parqui*.

willow primrose LUDWIGIA.

willow weed PERSICARIA, POLYGONUM *pennsylvanicum*.

Wilms' tumor a rapidly developing malignant mixed tumor of the kidneys, made up of embryonal elements, and occurring chiefly in young pigs and chickens; called also embryonal nephroma, nephroblastoma.

Wilson–Harrison technique see perineal URETHROSTOMY.

Wilson's disease proposed as a model for chronic copper toxicosis in Bedlington and West Highland white terriers but there are significant differences. Called also hepatolenticular degeneration.

wilting dehydration of plants to the point where the leaves lose their turgor and hang limply. Can happen in living plants which later return to normal, or to cut plants before they are fed out. Thought to be a factor in increasing toxicity.

Wiltshire cure a special English method of curing bacon which includes a period of maturation in a dry cool environment after a 3 to 4 day soak in brine.

Wiltshire horn an English, horned, meat sheep with a characteristic short fleece which is shed spontaneously each year.

Wimmera ryegrass see LOLIUM *rigidum*.

wind 1. climatic expression of rate of air movement. 2. colloquial expression for ability to run a race without stopping for lack of respiratory reserve.
broken w. see CHRONIC obstructive pulmonary disease.
w. direction has an effect on the speed of spread of an airborne disease, as determined by the population density in different directions, and the temperature which can be expected with winds from each weather quarter.
w. dispersal refers to the direction and distance of spread and the area contaminated by radioactive fallout, fungal spores and other dangerous agents.
w. roses starburst effect given by a graphic representation of the direction and frequency of wind at a given spot over a period of time. Is a reflection of the prevailing wind.
w. speed for epidemiological purposes the height above ground level that wind speed is measured needs to be quoted.
vaginal w. sucking noisy ingress and egress of air from the vulva, especially when moving; usually accompanies pneumovagina and a result of rectovaginal laceration, sometimes fistulation.

wind-borne disease particles of infective material are carried through the air by wind. How far the material travels and how infective it remains is determined by a number of environmental factors, especially moisture, temperature and wind velocity.

wind chill because strong winds magnify convective heat loss from the body, a climatic hazard is not exposed simply by quoting the temperature. A combination of air temperature and mean wind speed gives the important wind chill index.
w. c. index derived from the equation:

$$W_{CI} = (10 \times W^{-2} + 10.45 - W)\ (33 - T)$$

where W_{CI} = wind chill index; W = mean wind speed in meters/sec; T = air temperature in degrees Celsius.
w. c. temperature special thermometers are available to express the effect of wind on the sensation of temperature. Based on the estimation of what the air temperature feels like to a human when the particular temperature is accompanied by a wind of a certain speed.

wind galls distensions of tendon sheaths and joint capsule at the fetlock of the horse. They can be quite obvious and esthetically unattractive but they appear to cause no interference to normal movement.

wind-sucking 1. see CRIB-biting. 2. see RECTOVAGINAL fistula. See also PNEUMOVAGINA.

windbreak a physical obstruction to the passage of the wind, usually in the form of a line or copse of tall bushes or low trees or a porous fence. Of very great importance in temperate climates and periods of cold, wet, windy weather. Neonatal lamb mortality, off-shears hypothermia of sheep and hypomagnesemia and lactation tetany are some of the risk diseases in these circumstances.

During sheep weather alerts it may be necessary to improvise shelter. Some methods are: rows of bales of hay, mowing swathes of tall vegetation in a cereal crop or overgrown pasture being kept for hay. The sheep lie down in the alleys and keep out of the wind.

windkessel circulation winkessel (air chamber) vessels convert pulsatile inflow into a smoother outflow; a laboratory model used to explain the steady rate of flow of blood though the vessels.

windmill grass see CHLORIS.

window 1. a circumscribed opening in a plane surface. 2. portion of a computer screen which is an entity in its own right. The size of the window can often be changed. Each application running on the computer has one or more windows in which to communicate to the user.

cochlear w., fenestra cochleae an aperture between the tympanic cavity of the middle ear and the cochlea of the internal ear; covered by the secondary tympanic membrane. Called also round window.

document w. the space on the computer screen where one's documents are typed.

oval w. an oval opening in the inner wall of the middle ear, which is closed by the stapes; called also fenestra vestibuli.

round w. see cochlear window (above).

Windows the first Microsoft software for IBM computers to be icon- and dialog box-driven and to feature split screen technology so that several applications could be run simultaneously; introduced in 1990. Macintosh computers had introduced the same technology years before.

windpipe the trachea.

windsucking equine neurosis manifested by arching the neck, swallowing air and grunting; there is no grasping of objects.

Winer's pore dilation see dilated PORE of Winer.

wing a modified limb suitable for generating aerodynamic lift. Wing membranes or patagia are stretched between bony elements. In birds the wing surface is increased by large flight feathers (remiges) borne on the hand (primaries) or ulna (secondaries). In bats the patagia are more extensive than in birds through enlargement of the bones of the hand.

w. amputation the extreme form of deflighting.

dropped w. a name for *Salmonella typhimurium* infection in young pigeons which causes arthritis in the wing.

w. louse LIPEURUS *caponis*.

w. vein cutaneous ulnar vein; on the under surface of the extended wing, the favored location for venepuncture in most avian species.

winged thistle see CARDUUS.

winkers see BLINKERS.

winking quick opening and closing of the eyelids. Called also eyelid snapping; usually done with much force.

jaw w. involuntary closing of the eyelids associated with jaw movements.

w. mares big feature during the daily search for mares in heat in the breeding season; see vulvar winking (below).

vulvar w. uncontrolled movement of the vulva in a mare on heat. Usually accompanied by protrusion of the clitoris.

Winkler's operation suture of the floor of the vagina to the prepubic tendon, performed as a prevention against prolapse of the ventral wall of the vagina and cervix in cows.

winter anestrus failure of mares to come into estrus during the months when daylight hours are below the minimal level. Can be overcome to some extent by exposing the mares to strong artificial light at night.

winter cherry SOLANUM *pseudocapsicum*.

winter cress see BARBAREA VULGARIS.

winter diet the daily ration of feed for animals in winter; in animals maintained outdoors there needs to be a dietary supplement in winter to compensate for the additional convection heat loss.

winter dysentery a highly contagious disease of cattle characterized by a short-lived attack of profuse diarrhea, sometimes accompanied by dysentery. The cause is uncertain but *Campylobacter fetus* var. *jejuni* appears to play a significant role.

winter infertility infertility caused by reduction in or absence of estrous periods during winter months in females of all species.

winter kill deaths in culivated finfish in water bodies where the temperature of the water is below the range of tolerance for the particular species.

winter mortality disease of Sydney rock oysters caused by *Mikrocytos roughlei*.

winter purslane see MONTIA PERFOLIATA.

winter Rhodes grass CHLORIS *distichophylla*.

winter tetany see LACTATION TETANY.

winter tick see DERMACENTOR *albipictus*.

winter vetch see VICIA *villosa*.

wintergreen oil methyl salicylate.

wintering ground a corral or other enclosure in which pastured animals are maintained during the snow season and fed on stored feed.

wintersweet ACOKANTHERA *spectabilis*.

Winton disease see SENECIOSIS.

Wintrobe method 1. a macromethod of hematocrit determination, centrifuging blood in a flat-bottomed glass tube with thick, parallel sides that are marked with calibrations. See also HEMATOCRIT. 2. for erythrocyte sedimentation; measures the rate of settling in a Wintrobe hematocrit tube placed in a vertical position. See also erythrocyte SEDIMENTATION rate.

wire very thin metal rod or thread.

Kirschner w. see KIRSCHNER wire.

w. loop lesion thickening of the glomerular basement membrane in glomerular tufts by deposition of immune complexes; seen in membranous glomerulonephritis.

w. saw very tough, braided steel wire used in obstetrics to cut through muscles and bone. Tends to clog up in skin and with viscera. Needs to be used with a protective fetotome to avoid injury to the vagina and uterus.

w. saw introducer 1. may be a long, 3 feet, blunt needle with an eye at the introduced end. Used to thread wire saw through the tube of an embryotome. 2. a heavy metal bean-shaped plaque, size of a hand palm, with two holes; used to carry the end of the wire saw through the uterus, around the object to be removed, and out again through the vagina. The two ends of the saw are then threaded into the tubes of the embryotome.

wire worm of cattle, see HAEMONCHUS *placei*.

wirehair a coarse, crimped and springy haircoat texture seen in some breeds of dogs, such as Dachshunds and German wirehaired pointers, and the American wirehaired cat.

Wirehaired pointing griffon a medium-sized (50–60 lb) hunting dog with a distinctive short, harsh dry coat which is steel gray, gray with or dirty white, mixed with chestnut.

wireweed see POLYGONUM.

wiring electrical installation within a building. Faults in the installation or subsequently due to age or wear may cause injury. See ELECTROCUTION, FREE electricity.

w. memory used in orthodontics, the wires return to their original shape after any distortion.

wirsung's duct see pancreatic DUCT.

Wisconsin mastitis test cowside test based on the development of a gel when a reagent is added if the number of inflammatory cells in the sample is high.

wishbone see FURCULA.

wisp a large, sponge-like piece of grooming apparatus home-made of woven straw.

Wisteria plant genus in legume family Fabaceae; contains glycoside wistarin, plus a lectin; causes diarrhea, abdominal pain, vomiting. Called also wisteria, a popular garden plant. Includes *W. sinensis*.

witch hazel an extract from the leaves of *Hamamelis*

virginiana, containing gallic acid and tannins, used topically as an astringent. Called also hamemelis.

witchgrass see PANICUM *capillare*.

witch's milk colloquial expression for milk secreted by newborn animals.

withdrawal pharmaceutically speaking, cessation of treatment with a particular drug.

w. reflex see FLEXOR reflex.

w. time time interval after cessation of treatment before the animal or any of its products can be used as human food. Based on determination of the time interval required for tissue levels of the substance to fall below critical levels as decreed by legislation. Called also withholding period.

withdrawal reflex see FLEXOR reflex.

withers the region over the backline where the neck joins the thorax and where the dorsal margins of the scapulae lie just below the skin.

fistulous w. see FISTULOUS withers.

high w. low pelvis see HYENA disease.

withholding period the time interval after the withdrawal of a drug from the treatment of an animal before the animal or its products can be used for human food.

witstorm THESIUM *lineatum*.

WMD white muscle disease.

wobble hypothesis proposed by Francis Crick to observations that the 5,-base of the anticodon was capable of 'wobble' in its position during translation, allowing it to make alternative hydrogen bonding arrangements with several different codon bases.

wobbler syndrome incoordination in horses and dogs.

canine w. s. compression of the cervical spinal cord caused by caudal cervical vertebral malformation–malarticulation or instability. Seen most commonly in large and giant breed dogs, particularly Great Danes and Dobermans. Affected dogs show an ataxia of the hindlimbs and occasionally the forelimbs. There is a base-wide stance with proprioceptive deficits and possibly neck pain.

equine w. s. see ENZOOTIC equine incoordination.

Wohlfahrtia a genus of flesh flies in the family Sarcophagidae.

W. magnifica, W. meigini, W. nuba, W. vigil deposit their larvae anywhere on the bodies of animals and cause tissue loss and some disfigurement.

wolf a wild member of the family Canidae. A brownish-gray dog which resembles a German Shepherd dog with a long nose and a bushy tail, noted for its ferocity as a hunter of game. Called also *Canis lupus*, other species *Canis rufus* (red wolf).

w. teeth see WOLF TOOTH.

wolf tooth small, rudimentary teeth in front of the first large cheek teeth in horses and if present counted as the first premolar. Usually only present in the upper jaw and usually shed in early maturity.

w. t. elevator special tool for extraction of equine wolf teeth.

Wolff–Chaikoff effect increased blood levels of thyroglobulin bound iodide inhibit further binding of iodide by the thyroid gland.

Wolff's law the law that skeletal transformation is dependent on the exertion of pressures from outside the animal.

Wolff–Parkinson–White syndrome the association of paroxysmal tachycardia (or atrial fibrillation) and pre-excitation, in which the electrocardiogram displays a short P–R interval and a wide QRS complex which characteristically shows an early QRS vector (delta wave). Called also anomalous atrioventricular excitation. Occurs occasionally in dogs, horses and cats.

wolffian named for Kaspar Friedrich Wolff, German anatomist and embryologist 1733–1794.

w. body mesonephros.

w. duct see MESONEPHRIC duct.

wolfhound see BORZOI, IRISH WOLFHOUND.

wolfram tungsten (symbol W).

wolf's bane see ACONITUM *napellus*.

wolfsmelk SARCOSTEMMA *viminale*.

Wolinella succinogenes one of the common bacterial residents of the rumen which participates in fermentative digestion of organic material.

wolverine a large, 4 ft long, dark brown furry, voracious carnivore with a long bushy tail. Called also *Gulo luscus*.

womb uterus.

wombat a thickset, nocturnal, herbivorous, burrowing marsupial with short legs and no tail. It is solitary and long-lived and peculiar to Australia. Called also *Vombatus ursinus*.

wood alcohol methyl alcohol.

wood anemone see ANEMONE.

wood bison BISON *bison athabascae*.

wood-eating a pica observed in sheep and horses kept in close confinement on diets low in roughage.

Wood's filter see WOOD S LIGHT.

wood garlic ALLIUM *ursinum*.

wood horsetail EQUISETUM *laevigatum*.

wood laurel DAPHNE *laureola*.

Wood's light, lamp ultraviolet radiation from a mercury vapor source, transmitted through a nickel oxide filter (Wood's filter), which holds back all but a few violet rays and passes ultraviolet wavelengths of about 365 nm; used in diagnosis of fungal infections of the skin and to reveal the presence of porphyrins and fluorescent minerals.

wood-pigeon a large gray pigeon with a red breast and a white collar. Called also ring-dove, *Columba palumbus*.

wood preservative substances used as dressing for lumber to protect it against mold, insects, pests, fire, etc. Animals housed in pens made of wood which has been treated with wood preservatives may be poisoned by these compounds if they chew the wood. Chlorinated phenols, chlorinated naphthalenes, copper–chrome–arsenate mixture, coal tar creosote and other coal tar preparations are some of the compounds used which are potentially toxic.

wood sorrel OXALIS *acetosella*.

wood tar derivatives substances obtained by the destructive distillation of pine, sometimes juniper, wood. Includes pine oil, turpentine and pine tar. Pine oil yields phenol, creosol, toluene, methyl alcohol and acetone. See also pine TAR, juniper TAR.

wood tick see DERMACENTOR *andersoni*.

woodchuck see MARMOT.

wooden tongue see ACTINOBACILLOSIS.

woody aster see XYLORRHIZA.

woody chest syndrome a syndrome caused by the thoracic musculature becomes rigid and interferes with respiration. Caused by rapid intravenous injection of droperidol-fentanyl and is reversible with naloxone hydrochloride.

woody nightshade SOLANUM *dulcamara*.

woody pear see XYLOMELUM.

wool the natural fiber produced by the skin of domesticated sheep, characterized by its quality of felting together by virtue of its imbricated surface.

w. ball see TRICHOBEZOAR.

black w. inherited coat color in sheep.

w. blind the state of having excess wool growth around the eyes to the point where the sheep is unable to see.
break in w. see wool BREAK.
carding w. wool suitable for the woollen trade.
carpet w. coarse low-grade wool, used in the manufacture of carpets.
w. classing see wool CLASSING.
clean w. the basis on which the price of wool is set; scoured wool less charges and loss incurred in scouring.
combing w. long-fibered wool suitable for processing in a combing machine. Used in textile manufacture, especially worsted.
colored w. fibers naturally colored fibers in a fleece.
dead w. wool plucked from a sheep which has been dead for some time; usually heavily contaminated and of little value.
dense w. staples carrying many fibers per unit area of skin surface.
w. depigmentation see ACHROMOTRICHIA.
w. discoloration see FLEECE rot, MYCOTIC dermatitis.
doggy w. unevenly or poorly crimped wool; found in old sheep.
w. eating eating of rabbits' wool by other rabbits, or wool from garments by cats causes intestinal wool balls and obstruction of the gut. May be a manifestation of pica due to boredom.
w. fat see LANOLIN.
w. fiber abnormalities includes straight, steely wool, wool break, pigmentation, achromotrichia in black sheep.
w. fiber diameter thickness of the fiber; wool is sold on the basis of the average fiber diameter of the wool in the lot as determined by a machine and quoted in microns (micrometers); a more sophisticated classification is made on the basis of the average fiber diameter and the variability of the diameter.
greasy w. wool in its natural state, after removal from the sheep and before any commercial processing; contains yolk, suint, moisture, extraneous soil and vegetable matter.
w. hairs the soft undercoat fibers in most cats and dogs, interspersed with the longer guard HAIR; the predominant fiber type in sheep.
hogget w. first fleece from a 10 to 14 month old sheep which has not been previously shorn.
hunger fine w. wool with a finer fiber diameter than expected for the sheep's age; caused usually by poor nutrition.
w. industry includes sheep farming, shearing, wool sales, wool processing and fiber and fabric manufacture.
w. maggots see cutaneous MYIASIS.
w. picking pulling at the wool of another sheep. It may be a vice due to over-confinement, or to an unspecified nutritional deficiency. Biting of another sheep as occurs in rabies may be confused with wool picking but not for long.
plain w. straight wool lacking crimp and character.
w. processing effluent liquid effluent from wool processing; has been a source of infection with anthrax.
w. pulling pulling by the sheep of its own wool, usually an indication of itchiness. See also PSORERGATES *ovis*.
w. rot see FLEECE rot.
w. rubbing the sheep rubs its fleece against a hard object. Usually an indication of itching caused by external parasites or to a systemic disease with manifestations in the skin. See also SCRAPIE.
w. slip alopecia of housed ewes that are shorn in winter. The wool is lost over a large area of the back. There is no systemic illness and the wool regrows normally. The cause is unknown but the condition appears to be related to a high level of serum corticosteroids.
straight-steely w. STEELY WOOL.
w. sucking a vice of cats, particularly Siamese and Siamese crosses, in which they suck or chew woollen objects. Believed to be an extension of sucking behavior.
tender w. wool which will break during the combing process in manufacturing.
w. wax see LANOLIN.
w. weight see FLEECE weight.
w. yield the percentage of raw wool that can be retrieved from processing in a state suitable for the particular type of production which is in hand, e.g. carpet making.

Wooley's solution a buffered-EDTA (ethylenediamine tetra-acetate) solution, pH 8.0, with bactericidal activity against gram-negative bacteria. Used topically, either alone or in combination with other antimicrobical agents, to treat resistant bacterial infections, particularly those involving *Pseudomonas* spp.

woollen fabrics such as tweeds, felts, flannels, blankets, knitwear made of wool with a shorter fiber length than that used for WORSTED.

woolly burr medic MEDICAGO *minima*.

woolly everlasting daisy see ARGENTIPALLIUM BLANDOWSKIANUM.

woolly foxglove DIGITALIS *lanata*.

woolly groundsel SENECIO *longilobus*.

woolly haircoat syndrome in horned and polled Herefords; the haircoat is abnormally short and curly; this sort of coat is also a marker for lethal inherited CARDIOMYOPATHY.

woolly-leaved lupine LUPINUS *leucophyllus*.

woolly loco ASTRAGALUS *mollissimus*.

woolly monkey a New World monkey with a gray woolly coat and a long prehensile tail in the genus *Lagothrix*.

woolly nightshade SOLANUM *mauritianum*.

woolly-pod milkweed ASCLEPIAS *eriocarpa*.

woolly-pod vetch see VICIA *dasycarpa*.

woolly syndrome haircoat of dogs with castration-responsive dermatosis may change in texture, becoming fluffy and crimped, resembling wool.

woolly water lily see PHILYDRUM LANUGINOSUM.

woolsorter's disease pulmonary anthrax.

Wooton loco ASTRAGALUS *wootonii*.

word processor a computer application created for the purpose of writing a document into memory, editing and amending it on screen, saving it, printing it, merging it with other documents, transmitting it by fax or E-mail or transmitting it to a printing press.

work in the context of farm animals work includes, besides the force times distance produced by the working or racing horse or dog, the caloric equivalent of such work measured as egg, milk, wool or meat production.
breathing w. breathing requires an energy utilization to overcome the resistance of the airway to air flow, repositioning of organs, the elasticity and surface tension forces in the respiratory system.
w. efficiency gross efficiency is the ratio of the caloric equivalent of work accomplished to the total energy metabolism. The gross work efficiency of muscular work by horses is about 25%, of milk production about 30%.

w. potential estimation estimation of the ability of a racehorse to perform work is an exercise in applied physiology but a satisfactory set of techniques has not yet been enunciated.

work-up the procedures done to arrive at a diagnosis, including history taking, laboratory tests, x-rays, and so on.

working capital see working CAPITAL.

working dogs breeds or individuals that are bred for or trained to do specific tasks that help humans in some way, such as guide dogs for the blind, sledge or cart dogs, police or guard dogs, and livestock tending dogs. In some dog classification systems used for competition, this group includes only those breeds that work livestock, e.g. Collie, Australian cattle dog, Australian kelpie, German Shepherd dog, Shetland sheepdog, Old English sheepdog, Hungarian puli and Welsh corgi, while other 'working dog' breeds, such as the Rottweiler and St. Bernard, are UTILITY DOGS.

Working terrier see AIREDALE terrier.

World Health Organization the specialized agency of the United Nations that is concerned with human health on an international level; abbreviated WHO. The agency was founded in 1948 and in its constitution are listed the following objectives.

'Health is a state of complete physical and social well being, and not merely the absence of disease or infirmity. The enjoyment of the highest attainable standards of health is one of the fundamental rights of every human being without distinction of race, religion, political belief, economic or social condition. The health of all peoples is fundamental to the attainment of peace and security and is dependent upon the fullest cooperation of individuals and States. The achievement of any State in the promotion and protection of health is of value to all'.

The major specific aims of the WHO are as follows:
(1) To strengthen the health services of member nations, improving the teaching standards in medicine and allied professions, and advising and helping generally in the field of health.
(2) To promote better standards for nutrition, housing, recreation, sanitation, economic and working conditions.
(3) To improve maternal and child health and welfare.
(4) To advance progress in the field of mental health.
(5) To encourage and conduct research on problems of public health.

In carrying out these aims and objectives the WHO functions as a directing and coordinating authority on international health. It serves as a center for all types of global and health information, promotes uniform quarantine standards and international sanitary regulations, provides advisory services through public health experts in control of disease and sets up international standards for the manufacture of all important drugs. Through its teams of physicians, nurses and other health personnel it provides modern medical skills and knowledge to communities throughout the world.

world scourge schistosomiasis.

world wide web a group of Internet servers using protocols such as HTTP which provides ready access to documents which contain text, sound, video.

worm egg count see EGG count.

worm nodule disease esophagostomiasis.

worm resistance a significant increase in the ability of worms to tolerate doses of individual drugs which have previously been lethal to the worms.

worm snake typhlopid.

worms in the context of veterinary science, endoparasitic helminths.

wormseed see CHENOPODIUM *ambrosioides*.

w. mustard see ERYSIMUM CHEIRANTHOIDES.

wormwood see ARTEMISIA *absinthium*.

worsted fabric made of combed wool with a longer fiber length than that used for WOOLLEN fabrics.

wound a bodily injury caused by physical means, with disruption of the normal continuity of structures.

avulsive w. see AVULSION.

blowing w. open pneumothorax.

w. contracture see CONTRACTURE.

contused w. one in which the skin is unbroken.

w. débridement see DÉBRIDEMENT.

w. dehiscence see DEHISCENCE.

w. drain any device by which a channel or open area may be established for the exit of material from a wound or cavity. See also DRAIN, DRAINAGE, wound healing (below).

w. healing the restoration of integrity to injured tissues by replacement of dead tissue with viable tissue. The process starts immediately after an injury and may continue for months or years, and is essentially the same for all types of wounds. Variations in wound healing are the result of differences in location, severity of the wound, and the extent of injury to the tissues. Other factors affecting wound healing are the age, nutritional status and general state of health of the animal and its body reserves and resources for the regeneration of tissue.

In *healing by first intention* (primary union), restoration of tissue continuity occurs directly, without granulation; in *healing by second intention* (secondary union), wound repair following tissue loss (as in ulceration or an open wound), is accomplished by closure of the wound with granulation tissue. This tissue is formed by proliferation of fibroblasts and extensive capillary budding at the outer edges and base of the wound cavity. *Healing by third intention* (delayed primary closure) occurs when a wound is initially too contaminated to close and is closed surgically 4 or 5 days after the injury.

The insertion of drains can facilitate healing by providing an outlet for removing accumulations of serosanguineous fluid and purulent material, and obliterating dead space.

w. healing agents topical agents which stimulate healing; includes preparations containing zinc, trypsin, neomycin, dyes and iodine.

incised w. one caused by a cutting instrument.

lacerated w. one in which the tissues are torn.

w. nonhealing failure to heal despite appropriate treatment being given.

open w. one that communicates directly with the atmosphere.

penetrating w. one caused by a sharp, usually slender object, which passes through the skin into the underlying tissues.

perforating w. a penetrating wound which extends into a viscus or bodily cavity.

puncture w. penetrating wound.

sucking w. a penetrating wound of the chest through which air is drawn in and out.

surgical w. one deliberately produced during a surgical procedure, e.g. the original incision.

tangential w. an oblique, glancing wound which results in one edge being undercut.

traumatopneic w. sucking wound.

woven bone see woven BONE.

wraparound a feature of most word-processing programs which automatically places a word that will not fit on a line or page onto the next line or page.

wraparound arthrogryposis the limb joints are rigid but in addition the limbs are held close to the body and appear to be wrapped around it.

Wright's stain see Wright's STAIN.

wrinkles small folds of skin in sheep, especially merino, that are susceptible to staining and wetness and therefore to blowfly strike.

wrist the carpus; this human term is sometimes applied to animals.

write-protect a physical method of preventing anyone from over-writing information on computer disk, or other computer media which has valuable data or systems on it.

wry bite see wry MOUTH.

wryneck hereditary condition in guinea pigs; the young are born with varying degrees of torticollis; less severely affected animals may appear normal after a few days.

wrytail a crooked tail as a result of malformation of coccygeal vertebrae; often an inherited defect and is desirable in some breeds of dogs, e.g. Bulldog, Boston terrier. In dogs, called also screw-tail.

wt weight.

Wuchereria see BRUGIA.

wut see TOLLWUT.

w/v weight (of solute) per volume (of solvent).

Wyandotte medium-sized, dual-purpose breed of poultry; white, buff, blue, black, blue-laced or barred plumage. Legs and beak yellow.

Wyman cantoplasty a procedure for correction of combined entropion–ectropion in dogs.

Wyoming strangles *Corynebacterium pseudotuberculosis* abscesses in horses.

Wyominia tetoni a cestode of the family Thysanosomatidae found in bighorn sheep.

X

X symbol, *Kienböck's unit* (of x-ray exposure).

X-deletion X ovarian dysgenesis a chromosomal defect identified in mares; causes failure of germ cells to survive and the ovaries become inactive.

X disease see CHLORINATED NAPHTHALENES.

X factor see HEMIN.

X-inactivation see the LYON HYPOTHESIS, DOSAGE compensation.

X-linked traits transmitted by genes on the X chromosome; sex-linked; the categories are X-linked dominant, X-linked recessive.

X-linked agammaglobinemia see Bruton's AGAMMAGLOBULINEMIA.

X-linked trait sex-linked, e.g. coat color in cats, hemophilia.

x radiation see RADIATION, X-RAY.

x-ray electromagnetic radiation of wavelengths ranging between 5.0×10^{-6} and 5.0×10^{-4} μm (including grenz rays).

X-rays are produced by the collision of a beam of electrons with a metal target in an x-ray tube. Called also roentgen rays. The penetrability and hardness of the x-rays increases with the voltage applied to the x-ray tube, which controls the speed with which the electrons strike the target. For diagnostic radiography, tube voltages in the range 50 to 120 kilovolts peak (kVp) are normally used. For radiation therapy, voltages in the 1 to 2 megavolt range are used for most treatment. Accelerating electrons to speeds high enough to produce megavoltage x-rays requires a linear accelerator (lineac).

The x-ray exposure is proportional to the tube current (milliamperage) and also to the exposure time. In diagnostic radiography, the tube voltage and current and exposure time are selected to produce a high-quality radiograph with the correct contrast and film density. In radiation therapy, these exposure factors are selected to deliver a precisely calculated radiation dose to the tumor. The total dose is usually fractionated so that tumor cells can be oxygenated as surrounding cells die; this increases the sensitivity of the cells to radiation.

Body tissues and other substances are classified according to the degree to which they allow the passage of x-rays (*radiolucency*) or absorb x-rays (*radiopacity*). Gases are very radiolucent; fatty tissue is moderately radiolucent. Compounds containing high-atomic-weight elements, such as barium and iodine, are very radiopaque; bone and deposits of calcium salts are moderately radiopaque. Water; muscle, skin, blood and cartilage and other connective tissue; and cholesterol and uric acid stones have intermediate density. See also RADIATION and RADIATION therapy.

A double contrast study uses both a radiopaque and a radiolucent contrast medium; for example, the walls of the stomach or intestine are coated with barium and the lumen is filled with air. The resulting radiographs clearly show the pattern of mucosal ridges.

x. tube a glass vessel with a high vacuum and two electrodes. A very high voltage electrical current is passed across the tube and drives a stream of electrons produced by a tungsten filament set in the face of the cathode to collide with the anode and generate x-rays.

xanthemia the presence of yellow coloring matter in the blood; carotenemia.

xanthic 1. yellow. 2. pertaining to xanthine.

xanthine a purine compound found in most bodily tissues and fluids; it is a precursor of uric acid. Xanthine compounds such as theophylline have diuretic properties.

x. calculi see xanthine UROLITH.

dimethyl x. theobromine.

x. oxidase key enzyme in the pathway for purine breakdown. Catalyzes the conversion of hypoxanthine to xanthine and then to uric acid. Generates hydrogen peroxide, which can be a generator of free radicals in biological systems through reactions with superoxide ions.

trimethyl x. caffeine.

xanthinuria excess of xanthine in the urine.

Xanthium plant genus in the family Asteraceae; the seeds contain a potent toxin, carboxyatractyloside, which causes acute hepatic necrosis. Poisoning results from eating the seeds, or the cotyledons of the young seedlings that grow in profusion after rain falls. Includes *X. ambrosioides*, *X. californicum*, *X. cavanillesii* (South American cockleburr), *X. chinense*, *X. italicum* (Italian cockleburr), *X. orientale*, *X. occidentale* (*X. pungens*, Noogoora burr), *X. spinosum* (Bathurst burr), *X. strumarium*. Called also cockleburr.

***X. strumarium* complex** includes, as a group, all of the above species except *X. spinosum*.

xanth(o)- word element. [Gr.] *yellow*.
Xanthocephalum lucidum GUTIERREZIA *sarothrae*.
Xanthocephalum sarothrae GUTIERREZIA *sarothrae*.
xanthochromatic yellow-colored.
xanthochromia yellowish discoloration of the skin or spinal fluid. Xanthochromic spinal fluid usually indicates hemorrhage into the central nervous system and is due to the presence of xanthematin.
xanthochromic yellow-colored.
xanthogranuloma a tumor having histological characteristics of both granuloma and xanthoma.
xanthoma a papule, nodule or plaque in the skin due to lipid deposits; the color of a xanthoma is usually yellow, but may be brown, reddish, or cream. Microscopically, the lesions show light cells with foamy protoplasm (foam cells, xanthoma cells). They occur most commonly in White Leghorn chickens and rarely in other species.
The formation of xanthomas may indicate an underlying disease, usually related to abnormal metabolism of lipids, including cholesterol. In reptiles they are associated with high cholesterol diets.
xanthomatosis an accumulation of excess lipids in the body due to disturbance of lipid metabolism and marked by the formation of foam cells and Touton giant cells in skin lesions. Occurs in association with diabetes mellitus in the dog and is common in humans and chickens. See also XANTHOMA.
xanthomatous pertaining to xanthoma.
xanthomegrin nephrotoxin produced by *Penicillium* spp. fungi.
xanthophyll yellow pigment in plants.
Xanthorrhoea Australian plant genus in the family Xanthorrhoeaceae; contains an unidentified toxin which causes posterior incoordination (wamps) with urinary incontinence in cattle; have also caused red coloration of urine; flower spikes most toxic. Includes *X. australis*, *X. fulva* (*X. hastile*, *X. hastilis*), *X. johnsonii*, *X. minor* subsp. *lutea*. All called also grasstree, blackboy.
xanthosine a nucleoside composed of xanthine and ribose.
x.-5′-monophosphate purine nucleotide found in many animals; intermediate ion pathway to synthesis of guanosine 5′-monophosphate.
xanthosis yellowish discoloration; degeneration with yellowish pigmentation.
Xanthosoma American plant genus in the family Araceae; probably contains calcium oxalate raphide crystals; causes stomatitis, salivation. Called also taro, tannia.
xanthurenic acid a metabolite of L-tryptophan, present in normal urine and in increased amounts in vitamin B_6 deficiency.
Xe chemical symbol, *xenon*.
xenobiothomochelidonine one of the toxic alkaloids found in the plant *Chelidonium majus*.
xenobiotic any substance, harmful or not, that is foreign to the animal's biological system.
x. transformation the principal mechanism for maintaining homeostasis during exposure to small foreign molecules such as drugs and toxins; the process deals with foreign chemicals which are too small for processing by the immune system; composed of enzyme systems evolved to render xenobiotics easily excreted, mainly in the liver; enzymic reactions classified as Phase I (add to or expose functional chemical groups; includes cytochrome P-450 monooxygenases) and Phase II (glucuronidation, conjugation and other reactions producing a large increase in water solubility to promote excretion). Cats lack the capacity for glucuronidation, making them more susceptible to certain poisonings, e.g. acetaminophen (paracetamol).
xenobiotics foreign organic compounds not produced in metabolism.
xenodiagnosis 1. diagnosis by means of finding, in the feces of clean laboratory-reared, parasite-free arthropod vectors allowed to feed on the host suspected of being infected by a protozoan, the infective forms of the organism causing the disease; used in diagnosis of trypanosomiasis. 2. diagnosis of trichinosis by means of feeding laboratory-bred rats or mice on meat suspected of being infected with *Trichinella*, and then examining the animals for the parasite.
xenogeneic in transplantation biology, denoting individuals or tissues from individuals of different species and hence of disparate cell type.
xenogenesis 1. heterogenesis (1). 2. production of offspring unlike either parent.
xenogenous caused by a foreign body, or originating outside the organism.
xenograft a graft of tissue or organ transplanted between animals of different species; a heterograft.
xenoimmunization development of antibodies in response to antigens derived from an individual of a different species.
xenoma a massive hypertrophic lesion caused in fish by the microsporidian protozoan parasites *Nosema* and *Pleistophora* spp.
xenon a chemical element, atomic number 54, atomic weight 131.30, symbol Xe. See Table 6.
x.-133 a radioisotope of xenon having a half-life of 5.3 days and a principal gamma ray photon energy of 81 keV; used for pulmonary ventilation imaging. Symbol ^{113}Xe.
xenoparasite an organism not usually parasitic on a particular species, but becomes so because of a weakened condition of the host.
xenophthalmia inflammation caused by a foreign body in the eye; called also ophthalmoxerosis.
Xenopsylla a genus of fleas, including more than 30 species, many of which transmit disease-producing microorganisms.
X. cheopis the rat flea, which transmits *Pasteurella pestis*, the causative organism of plague and *Rickettsia typhi*, the causative organism of murine typhus.
Xenopus laevis a toad used in the test of pregnancy in women. Called also African clawed toad.
xenoreactivity the reaction of lymphocytes or antibodies with xenoantigens.
xenotransplantation the transplantation of an organ or tissue from an animal of one species to an animal of a different species.
xer(o)- word element. [Gr.] *dry, dryness*.
xeroderma a mild form of ichthyosis; excessive dryness of the skin.
xerography xeroradiography.
xeroma abnormal dryness of the conjunctiva; xerophthalmia.
xeromammography xeroradiography of the mammary gland.
xerophagia the eating of dry food.
xerophthalmia abnormal dryness and thickening of the surface of the conjunctiva and cornea due to a deficiency of vitamin A or to local disease.
xeroradiography the making of radiographs by a dry, totally photoelectric process, using metal plates coated with a semiconductor, such as selenium.
The image produced by this process differs from conventional x-ray in that margins between tissues of

varying densities are more enhanced. Hence, xeroradiography is especially beneficial in the diagnosis of mammary tumors. Structures such as tendons are also visually enhanced. It does, however, require higher doses of radiation. Called also xerography.

xerosialography sialography in which the images are recorded by xerography.

xerosis abnormal dryness, as of the eye (xerophthalmia), skin (xeroderma) or mouth (xerostomia).

xerostomia dryness of the mouth from lack of the normal secretion.

xerotomography tomography in which the images are recorded by xeroradiography.

xi-cleft point accumulation points in acupuncture.

Ximenia americana plant in family Olacaceae; foliage of tree can cause cyanide poisoning; called also yellow plum.

xiphisternum xiphoid process.

xiph(o)- word element. [Gr.] *xiphoid process.*

xiphocostal pertaining to the xiphoid process and ribs.

xiphoid 1. sword-shaped; ensiform. 2. xiphoid process.

x. process the pointed process of cartilage, supported by a core of bone, connected with the posterior end of the body of the sternum.

xiphoiditis inflammation of the xiphoid process.

xiphopagus symmetrical conjoined twins united in the region of the xiphoid process.

Xiphophorus see PLATYFISHES, SWORDTAIL.

XLD medium one used for isolation of salmonellae and *Yersinia* spp.

XO symbol for the karyotype in which there is only one sex chromosome, an X chromosome.

XO genotype in horses, pigs and cats causes infertile, usually anestrous, females; the uterus and external genitalia may be small and undeveloped.

XO ovarian dysgenesis the second female X chromosome is missing, hence the XO of the title, and the animal, most commonly a mare, has small inactive ovaries which lack germ cells, and small uteri and external genitalia.

XX sex reversal inherited defect of sexuality occurring in goats and American Cocker spaniel puppies with an XX karyotype. They may be hermaphrodites if they also carry a Y-effect gene, e.g. the gene for polledness in goats.

XXX symbol for a chromosomal aberration found in mares and cows in which there is infertility because of ovarian hypoplasia.

XXX ovarian hypoplasia a chromosomal aberration found in mares and cows resulting in infertility caused by ovarian hypoplasia; estral cycles are long and irregular.

XX/XY chimaerism see CHIMERA.

XXXY males a cytogenetic chromosomal abnormality in bulls resembling human Klinefelter's syndrome and causing testicular hypoplasia.

XXY symbol for a karyotype associated with hypoplasia of the testes and hermaphroditism. It is seen in male TORTOISESHELL cats and has also been observed in sexually normal rams. See also Y CHROMOSOME.

XY sex reversal mares chromosomal abnormality in which affected mares vary from phenotypically normal, sterile mares with normal tubular reproductive organs but inactive ovaries to mares with ovotestes and aplastic tubular organs.

xylazine an analgesic and sedative which has become very popular for the immobilization of adult ruminants and is also registered for use in dogs, cats, horses, deer and elk. Often used in combination with ketamine. Care is needed with its use in cattle because of the very low dose required in that species. Xylazine also causes a marked increase in plasma growth hormone levels. Called also Rompun.

x. stimulation test used in the diagnosis of abnormalities of pituitary function, e.g. pituitary dwarfism, and specifically deficiency of growth hormone. Plasma levels of growth hormone are measured before and after the intravenous administration of xylazine. In normal dogs, there is a marked increase but hypopituitary dogs fail to respond.

xylene an organic solvent used industrially and as a cleaning agent and fat solvent in microscopy. Narcotic if inhaled in high concentration.

xylidine a compound used in blending gasoline; a potent hepatoxin.

xylitol an alcohol formed by the reduction of L-xylulose.

Xylocaine trademark for preparations of lidocaine, a topical and injectable anesthetic.

Xylohypha see CLADOSPORIUM.

xyloketosuria xylose and ketones present in the urine.

Xylomelum a genus of Australian shrubs and trees in the family Proteaceae. They contain cyanogenetic glycosides and have potential for causing cyanide poisoning. Includes *X. angustifolium* (sandplain woody pear), *X. pyriforme* (woody pear).

Xylorrhiza North American plant genus in the family Asteraceae. All of its members are selenium indicators and usually contain sufficient selenium, in the form of selenocompounds, to cause poisoning manifested by alopecia, lameness, laminitis, hoof deformity.

The recorded species are *X. glabriuscula*, *X. parryi*, *X. tortifolia*, *X. venusta*, *X. villosa*. All called also woody aster. Formerly classified in genus *Aster*.

xylose a pentose occurring in mucopolysaccharides of connective tissue and sometimes in the urine; also obtained from vegetable gum.

x. absorption test, D-x. absorption test D-xylose absorbed primarily in the duodenum and cranial jejunum; after oral administration, urine or plasma determination at timed intervals can be used as an indication of intestinal absorption.

xylulose a pentose sugar occurring as D-xylulose and as L-xylulose, one of the few L-sugars found in nature; it is sometimes excreted in the urine. See also PENTOSURIA.

xysma material resembling bits of membrane in stools of diarrhea.

xyster a filelike instrument used in surgery.

XY/XXY mosaic see MOSAIC.

Y

Y chemical symbol, *yttrium.*

Y-autosome chromosomal aberration created artificially by irradiation in the process of producing sterile flies by the STERILE insect release method.

Y chromosome the chromosome which causes the medulla of the embryonic gonad to form a testis. If there is one other chromosome present and it is X the newborn animal will be a fertile male. If there are two other X chromosomes, giving an XXY configuration, it will be a phenotypic male but sterile. Autosomal genes can have the same effect, creating an intersex newborn in an animal with XX chromosomes.

Y-linked inheritance inheritance determined by loci on the Y chromosome.

Y piece a leakproof connecting piece between the endotracheal tube and the anesthetic machine, the inspiratory and expiratory hoses of the machine each occupying an arm of the Y piece.

Y-plasty a technique for suturing V-shaped wounds in which part of the flap may be lost or destroyed, when the opposite end is extended and the flap is closed as the top of a Y. Also used for suturing circular wounds.

Y sutures anatomical structures connecting the concentric lamellae of the lens. The anterior one is erect, the posterior one is inverted.

yabapoxvirus a poxvirus of African nonhuman primates.

yabby, yabbie Australian term for *Cherax destructor* (freshwater crayfish).

Yabila grass see PANICUM *queenslandicum*.

YAC yeast artificial chromosome.

yak a large, up to 6 ft high at the shoulder, very long-haired ruminant with a round forehead, widely separated horns, a shoulder hump and a grunting call instead of a lowing one. Hunted for its meat and hair, it is also an excellent draft animal and can survive well at altitudes above 13,000 ft (4000 m). Called also *Bos mutus*.

yam see DIOSCOREA.

Yang organs the hollow organs in the acupuncture catalog including stomach, intestines, biliary system, ureter, bladder, urethra, triple heater.

Yangtze River fever schistosomiasis.

Yankauer tip see SUCTION tip.

Yankee war bridle a type of restraint used on horses; consists of a rope loop, passed around the horse's upper gum and over the head.

yard 1. a unit of linear measure, 3 feet, or 36 inches, equivalent to 86.44 cm. See also Table 4.5. 2. a small fenced enclosure called also corral. 3. in the UK is synonymous with feedlot. 4. to enclose animals in a small enclosure.

yarded enclosed within a fenced area. In the UK yarded cattle is synonymous with feedlotted cattle; the animals are enclosed in a yard for a brief period and fed fattening rations.

Yatapoxvirus a genus in the family *Poxviridae* that contains two viruses of African animals, yabapoxvirus and tanapoxvirus.

yawning a deep, involuntary inspiration with the mouth open, often accompanied by the act of stretching. Repeated yawning in the presence of other signs, may accompany signs of chronic abdominal pain or hepatic disease.

Yb chemical symbol, *ytterbium*.

yearling an animal in its second year of age, e.g. yearling cattle, yearling filly, yearling colt.

y. disease rinderpest in wildebeeste in the Serengheti.

yeast a general term including unicellular, nucleated, usually rounded fungi that reproduce by budding; some are fermenters of carbohydrates, and a few are pathogenic for animals. See also MASTITIS.

y. artificial chromosome cloning vectors developed for the cloning of large (200–500 kbp) DNA fragments; YAC libraries permit the cloning of large genes with their flanking regulatory sequences as well as families of contiguous genes. They are difficult to work with and have the further disadvantage that the cloned sequences are unstably retained.

brewer's y. *Saccharomyces cerevisiae* used in brewing beer, making alcoholic liquors, and baking bread. See also dried yeast (below).

dried y. dried cells of any suitable strain of *Saccharomyces cerevisiae*, usually a by-product of the brewing industry; used as a natural source of protein and B-complex vitamins.

yellow 1. the primary color produced by stimulation by light waves of wavelength of 571.5 to 578.5 nm. 2. a dye or stain that produces a yellow color.

yellow-barked oak QUERCUS *velutina*.

yellow bean THERMOPSIS *rhombifolia*.

yellow bighead see PANICUM.

yellow body see CORPUS luteum.

yellow bristle grass see SETARIA[2] *lutescens*.

yellow burr CENTAUREA *solstitialis*.

yellow burweed see AMSINCKIA.

yellow calf see COPPER nutritional deficiency.

yellow daisy WEDELIA *asperrima*.

yellow dog tick see HAEMAPHYSALIS *leachi leachi*.

yellow drumsticks see CRASPEDIA CHRYSANTHA.

yellow fat recessive trait in rabbits resulting in an inability to metabolize xanthophylls, plant pigments which are precursors of vitamin A. The accumulation is unsightly but not harmful.

yellow fat disease a disease of many species, but particularly cats and mink, characterized by inflammation of adipose tissue and deposition of lipofuscin pigment in the adipose cells. Caused by a diet high in unsaturated fatty acids and low in vitamin E. In cats, it has been associated with feeding canned red tuna. Affected animals usually show anorexia, fever and a generalized hypersensitivity that is due to painful fat depots. Especially in cats, subcutaneous fat may be palpably hard, lumpy and painful. Called also pansteatitis and steatitis.

yellow flag IRIS *pseudacorus*.

yellow grub see CLINOSTOMUM.

y. g. disease metacercariae of *Clinostomum marginatum* cause cyst development of the skin and viscera of freshwater fish.

yellow head disease rhabdovirus infection of cultured black tiger shrimp characterized by yellowish discoloration of gills and cephalothorax and general tissue necrosis.

yellow iris IRIS *pseudacorus*.

yellow jessamine see GELSEMIUM SEMPERVIRENS.

yellow lamb disease characterized by anemia, hemoglobinuria and jaundice caused by absorption of *Clostridium welchii* type A toxin from the intestine.

yellow lotion a devilishly ingenious way of marketing WHITE LOTION by including a yellow pigment.

yellow milkbush EUPHORBIA *mauritanica*.

yellow oat grass see TRISETUM FLAVESCENS.

yellow oleander THEVETIA *peruviana*.

yellow oxide see MERCURIC oxide.

yellow pheasant's eye ADONIS *vernalis*.

yellow pine tree PINUS *ponderosa*.

yellow plum see XIMENIA AMERICANA.

yellow pop flower see GLISHROCARYON.

yellow rattle see RHINANTHUS.

yellow rice discolored grain caused by contamination with the fungus *Penicillium citreo-viride*.

yellow rocket see BARBAREA VULGARIS.

yellow rush lily SISYRINCHIUM *micranthum*.

yellow star thistle CENTAUREA *solstitialis*.

yellow sweet clover MELILOTUS *officinalis*.

yellow thickhead see PANICUM.

yellow tulip HOMERIA *pallida.*
yellow vetchling LATHYRUS *aphaca.*
yellow vine see TRIBULUS *micrococcus.*
yellow weed see AMSINCKIA.
yellow-wood see TERMINALIA OBLONGATA.
yellowhead disease caused by an uncharacterized, rod-shaped, RNA virus. Causes massive mortality in juvenile and subadult *Penaeus monodon.* The characteristic lesion is a light yellow coloration of the cephalothorax.
yellowness average yellowness is now a required sale classification of scoured wool measured colorimetrically.
yellows enterotoxemic jaundice in lambs, caused by *Clostridium perfringens,* type A.
yellowses hepatic injury caused by poisoning by NARTHECIUM *ossifragum.*
yellow wood-sorrel OXALIS *corniculata.*
yelt gilt.
yerba-de-pasmo BACCHARIS *pteronioides.*
Yersinia a genus of ovoid or rod-shaped, nonencapsulated, gram-negative bacteria in the family Enterobacteriaceae.
Y. enterocolitica often carried by many animal species, especially pigs, and associated with sporadic diarrhea in humans and animals. Farmed deer are highly susceptible.
Y. pestis causes bubonic plague in humans and SYLVATIC plague in rodents and cats.
Y. pseudotuberculosis causes YERSINIOSIS in laboratory animals, wild rodents and domestic species, including cattle, sheep and cats. See also PYEMIC hepatitis.
Y. ruckeri causes enteric redmouth and salmonid blood spot disease especially of Atlantic salmon fry and parr.
Y. tularensis see FRANCISELLA *tularensis.*
yersiniosis septicemia often with signs of gastroenteritis, caused by *Yersinia pseudotuberculosis,* occurring in wild rodents, birds, and, uncommonly, most domestic species, particularly cats. There is fever, severe toxemia and a high fatality rate. At postmortem there are large numbers of embolic abscesses in most organs. Called also pseudotuberculosis.
Occurs also in many species of fish as a septicemia, caused by *Yersinia ruckeri.*
yesterday today and tomorrow see BRUNSFELSIA.
yew see TAXUS.
yield amount produced.
y. grade the amount of meat which will be harvested from a carcass; expressed in a code 1 to 5 with 1 being best. The assessment is based on weight of the carcass, the size of the longissimus dorsi muscle at the 12th rib, the thickness of fat at the same location and the percentage of kidney, heart and pelvic fat.
yin organs anatomical organs in the acupuncture catalog including the liver, pancreas, spleen, kidney, heart, pericardium, lungs.
Yin/Yang the balance between deficiency and excess in functional activity of the organs which is the basis of Chinese medicine's view of health versus dysfunction. The Yang organs are the hollow organs, stomach, intestines, biliary system, urinary bladder plus urethra and ureter. The Yin organs include the solid ones, the liver, spleen, pancreas, kidney, heart, pericardium, lungs.
yogurt, yoghurt a form of curdled milk produced by fermentation with organisms of the genus *Lactobacillus.* Used in the treatment of convalescing calves and other young animals after attacks of diarrhea.
yohimbine an $\alpha 2$ adrenoceptor antagonist used to reverse sedation produced by $\alpha 2$ adrenoceptor agonists such as xylazine.
y. challenge test used as a test for cataplexy in dogs; after administration, there is a marked reduction in the number and severity of clinical signs.
yoke 1. an anatomical connecting structure; a depression or ridge connecting two structures. 2. a primitive device for coupling two or more animals to one vehicle or implement. Usually a wooden bar that sits on the top of the neck with a metal loop to go around the neck of each animal.
y. muscles a pair of extraocular muscles.
yokebail see PILLORY.
yolk 1. the stored nutrient of the ovum; it is also rich in antibody which is absorbed into the circulation of the embryo in the last third of incubation and is the mechanism by which maternal antibody is transferred to the young bird. See also YOLK SAC, EGG. 2. the combined secretion of the sebaceous and sudoriferous glands of the sheep's skin and extractable from the fleece.
y. sacculitis see avian OMPHALITIS.
y. stalk the connection, passing through the umbilicus, between the yolk sac and the fetus.
y. stain a stain of wool originating from the yolk.
yolk sac one of the extraembryonic fetal membranes that balloons out from the fetal midgut. It helps to form a primitive placenta and promotes the development of the vitelline circulation. The vestigial yolk sac can be found about halfway along the small intestine of birds. The yolk sac membrane produces lymphoid stem cells that subsequently colonize the thymus and bursa of Fabricius. The stalk of the yolk sac is sometimes retained as Meckel's diverticulum of the small intestine.
y. s. infection see avian OMPHALITIS.
inverted y. s. a form of placentation in which fetal splanchnic mesoderm in direct contact with maternal uterine tissue; occurs in laboratory rodents. Called also yolk sac placenta.
y. s. placenta see inverted yolk sac (above).
y. s. tumor shows varying stages of differentiation into tissues of multiple germ layers. Called also endodermal sinus tumor.
York ham a special curing method based on a pickle injection followed by a long storage in dry salt.
Yorkshire boarding vertical wooden planks not butted together used as exterior cladding on buildings used as animal accommodation. Provides a wind break and is well ventilated.
Yorkshire boot a piece of Kersey horse cloth (felt) with a tape attached at the middle of its width and along its length. It is wrapped around a horse's fetlock and the tape tied around the felt above the joint. The top part of the felt is now folded down over the bottom part. Designed to protect the fetlock against injury while working.
Yorkshire canary a breed of long, slim, elegant canaries with upright posture.
Yorkshire fog see HOLCUS LANATUS.
Yorkshire pig see LARGE WHITE.
Yorkshire terrier a very small (up to 7 lb) dog with long, flowing, silky coat in dark steel blue and tan. The ears are erect and the tail is docked to a medium length. The breed is predisposed to retinal dysplasia and hypoplasia of the dens (atlantoaxial subluxation).
Young forceps scissor type forceps with ratcheted handles and a sideways curve. The blades end in opposing loops that are fitted with grooved rubber stoppers. Used for grasping the tongue.

Young gag see BAYER GAG.
ytterbium a chemical element, atomic number 70, atomic weight 173.04, symbol Yb. See Table 6.
yttrium a chemical element, atomic number 39, atomic weight 88.905, symbol Y. See Table 6.
Yucaipa virus a paramyxovirus which causes a mild respiratory disease in chickens. Called also MVY virus.
Yucatan pig see miniature PIG.
Yugoslavian hounds several breeds of scent hounds, most of which are not known outside Europe or the Balkan countries. They are medium-sized, have drop ears and long tails. Several coat types and colors are seen.

Z

Z band, Z line a band of electrodense, noncontractile protein which runs across the muscle fiber and to which the myofibrils are attached.
Z-inactivation occurs in birds because dosage compensation for Z-linked genes does not occur in birds.
Z-linkage genes with loci on the Z chromosome.
Z-linked sexing use of alleles at Z-linked loci to determine sex of chicks at an early age. See FAST feathering.
Z-myoplasty a technique for surgical correction of quadriceps muscle contracture.
Z-plasty repair of a skin defect by the transposition of two triangular flaps of adjacent skin, for relaxation of scar contractures. Called also zigzagplasty.
Z-tenectomy a technique for tendon shortening.
Z-tenotomy a technique for tendon lengthening.
Zackel sheep a group of horned breeds of sheep widely dispersed through Europe and Asia. Used for carpet-wool, meat and milk. Mostly white, some are brown, black or pied. Males have long spiral horns, females may be polled. Most breeds have long, thin tails.
Zaglossus see ECHIDNA.
Zalaphotrema a genus of digenetic trematodes which includes *Z. hepaticum* found in the liver of the sealion.
Zaleya galericulata member of the Aizoaceae plant family; suspected to cause soluble oxalate poisoning, causing nephrosis, urolithiasis. Called also hogweed.
Zalophus one of the sealion genera; see SEAL.
Zamia American genus of CYCAD; causes incoordination, due to degeneration of the spinal cord, and hepatic necrosis. The toxin is identified as a cycad glycoside. Includes *Z. integrifolia* (*Z. floridana*), *Z. portoricensis*, *Z. pujilla*, *Z. pumila* (*Z. debilis*, *Z. latifoliata*, *Z. silvicola*, *Z. umbrosa*). Called also coonties, Florida arrowroots, marangvey, derriengue, guayiga.
zamia CYCAD.
z. fern BOWENIA *spectabilis*.
z. staggers irreversible posterior paralysis in cattle in Australia; caused by poisoning by CYCADS; lesions present in the proprioceptive pathways in the white matter of the spinal cord.
zang-fu organs in acupuncture the collective Yin and Yang organs.
Zantedeschia aethiopica member of the plant family Araceae; toxin is calcium oxalate raphide crystals; causes stomatitis, salivation. Called also arum lily, calla lily, varkoor.
Zea mays a grass in plant family Poaceae. A staple part of human and animal diet in many countries as corn or maize meal. The standing green crop, up to 10 ft high, makes excellent ensilage and green chop. May be infested with poisonous fungi in the field or as stored grain. May cause nitrate–nitrite poisoning. Called also maize, corn.
zearalanol see ZERANOL.
zearalenone an estrogenic substance produced during the fermentation of stored grain by the fungus *Fusarium graminearum*. The effects of the toxin are enlargement of the external somatic addenda, infertility and death of the newborn. See also ZERANOL.
zeboid a class of cattle intermediate between zebu and humpless British breed cattle, e.g. Chinese yellow, Sanga, Santa Gertrudis, Droughtmaster. Called also taurindicus.
zebra ass-like animals with a distinctive black and white striped coat, large ears, tufted tail and stiff mane. Called also *Equus burchelli* (common zebra), *E. zebra* (mountain zebra), *E. grevyi* (Grevy's zebra) and some recognized subspecies.
z. diagnosis arriving at an unlikely diagnosis instead of a more common one.
z. marks faint striping in coats of horses, usually on the legs, also the neck and withers.
zebronkey a cross between zebra and donkey.
zebu a group of breeds of humped cattle, including Indian, East and West African, and most breeds of South-East Asian cattle. Origin of the Chinese Yellow, Sanga and Brahman. Includes Africander, Sahiwal, Sindhi and many others.
zein the principal protein in maize. Has low nutritive value, being deficient in lysine and tryptophan.
Zeis glands see GLANDS of Zeis.
Zenith an Australian medium-woolled (21.5 to 23 microns), dual-purpose, polled sheep, produced by crossing sheep of Merino and Lincoln breeds.
Zenker's necrosis, degeneration see Zenker's NECROSIS.
zeony progeny of a zebra and a pony.
Zephiran one of the early cationic detergents, used as the chloride. Proprietary preparation of benzalkonium chloride, a topical antiseptic.
Zephyranthes see COOPERIA PEDUNCULATA.
Zepp operation a modification of the lateral ear resection in dogs in which a cartilaginous flap is turned downward and sutured in place as a 'drainboard' at the bottom of the opening created. It serves to reduce the possibility of stricture of the horizontal canal and minimize growth of haircoat at the opening which might impede aeration and drainage.
zeranol a synthetic ZEARALENONE (6′-reduced zearalenone) marketed as Ralgro used as a growth promotant in cattle. Called also zearalanol.
zernike condenser special condenser used in phase contrast microscope.
zero the point on a thermometer scale from which the graduations begin. The zero of the Celsius (centigrade) scale is the ice point; on the Fahrenheit scale it is 32° below the ice point.
absolute z. the lowest possible temperature, designated 0 on the Kelvin or Rankine scale, the equivalent of −273.15°C or −459.67°F.
zero-order reactions generally pertaining to enzyme reactions where the rate of product formation is independent of substrate concentration.
zeta potential see zeta POTENTIAL.
zeugopodium the segment of the limb corresponding to either the forearm or the leg.
zho, zo see DZO.

zidovudine see AZIDOTHYMIDINE.
Ziegler knife needle an instrument used for opening the capsule of the lens of the eye and disrupting the lens material before aspirating it.
Ziehl–Neelsen stain a carbol-fuchsin stain most used for the detection of *Mycobcterium* spp.
Zieria an Australian genus of shrubs and trees of the Rutaceae family.
Z. arborescens causes atypical interstitial pneumonia in cattle. There is a grunting dyspnea and a nasal discharge. Called also stinkwood.
Z. laevigata, Z. smithii suspected of causing cyanide poisoning.
Zieve's syndrome a human disease characterized by hemolytic anemia related to a low lipid content of erythrocyte cell membranes; some clinical similarity to hemoglobinuria which occurs in event horses after prolonged exercise.
zigadenine, zigadine, zygadenine plant toxin found in *Zigadenus* spp.
Zigadenus, Zygadenus North American and African genus of the Liliaceae family. There are many species, some of them toxic some not. The toxins in the plants are steroid alkaloids of the veratrum group. Poisoning is characterized by salivation, vomiting, tachycardia, weakness, prostration and dyspnea. Death may occur within a few hours or not for a number of days. The list of toxic plants includes *Z. chlorantus*, *Z. densus*, *Z. elegans*, *Z. fremontii*, *Z. glaberimus*, *Z. glaucus*, *Z. gramineus*, *Z. leimanthoides*, *Z. nuttallii*, *Z. paniculatus*, *Z. venenosus*. Called also death camus.
zigzagplasty see Z-PLASTY.
Zimmerman's aluminum wire suture see Zimmerman's aluminum wire SUTURE.
zinc a chemical element, atomic number 30, atomic weight 65.37, symbol Zn. See Table 6.

Zinc is a trace element that is a component of several enzymes, including DNA and RNA polymerases, and carbonic anhydrase. Zinc salts are used in skin lotions, eye washes, the treatment and prevention of footrot of sheep and facial eczema of sheep and cattle.

z. acetate a salt used as an astringent and styptic.
z. cadmium sulfide used in the preparation of fluoroscopic screens; is fluorescent and emits yellow-green light when excited by x-rays.
z. carbonate a mild astringent; used mainly as CALAMINE.
z. chromate an industrial compound used in cold galvanizing of metal. Accidental access causes diarrhea and fatal enteritis.
z. finger motif sequence of approximately 30 amino acids, forming a helix-turn-helix, believed to form a structure that includes tetrahedrally coordinated zinc (II) ions. Found in many eukaryotic, prokaryotic and viral DNA-binding proteins.
z. finger protein DNA-binding proteins that contain zinc-finger motifs.
z. gelatin a mixture of zinc oxide, gelatin, glycerin and purified water; used topically as a protectant.
z. gluconate a source of supplementary zinc.
hereditary z. deficiency lethal trait A46; see inherited PARAKERATOSIS.
z. nutritional deficiency causes PARAKERATOSIS in pigs, a chronic, afebrile, noninflammatory disease of the epidermis characterized by crusty proliferation and cracking of the skin. Dogs fed diets with high levels of calcium or cereals may have poor absorption of zinc and develop signs of deficiency, primarily in the skin. See also zinc-responsive DERMATOSIS.
z. ointment a preparation of zinc oxide and mineral oil in white ointment; used topically as an astringent and protectant.
z. oversupplementation causes hemolytic anemia, anorexia and vomiting.
z. oxide a compound used as a topical astringent and protectant. Inhalation of fumes causes interstitial emphysema and atalectasis.
z. phosphate used as a phosphate-bonded cement in restorative dentistry.
z. phosphide used at one time as a rodenticide. When ingested the poisonous gas phosphine is liberated and kills the animal without diagnostic signs or lesions.
z. poisoning is usually chronic and causes stiffness and lameness with particular involvement of the shoulder joint in which there is a degenerative arthritis. In acute poisoning there is gastroenteritis with vomiting.
z.-responsive dermatoses see PARAKERATOSIS, zinc-responsive DERMATOSIS.
z. stearate a compound of zinc with stearic and palmitic acids; used as a water-repellent protective powder in dermatoses.
z. sulfate a compound used as an ophthalmic astringent, in skin lotions (see WHITE LOTION), for sheep footrot, and the treatment of facial eczema. It is the common form of zinc for oral supplementation and treatment of zinc-responsive diseases.
z. sulfate flotation test used to demonstrate nematode eggs, protozoan cysts, and larvae in feces and bronchial secretions.
z. sulfate turbidity test 1. serum globulins are precipitated by zinc sulfate. The test is used for the semiquantitative assessment of the immunological status of foals and calves when there is a question of whether they have suckled to receive immunoglobulins. 2. an outdated liver function test.
z. undecylenate a compound used topically in 20% ointment as an antifungal agent. See also UNDECYLENIC ACID.
zineb an antifungal preparation used extensively agriculturally but without any apparent toxicity hazard.
Zinn nodule see ciliary ZONULE.
zipper structure leucine see LEUCINE zipper.
zipper worm SPIROMETRA *erinacei*.
zirconium a chemical element, atomic number 40, atomic weight 91.22, symbol Zr. See Table 6.
Zn chemical symbol, *zinc*.
zoacanthosis a dermatitis caused by penetration into the skin, of bristles, hairs, etc., of lower animals.
zoetic pertaining to life.
zolazepam a benzodiazepine tranquilizer most commonly used in a fixed-ratio combination with tiletamine.
Zoletil a fixed-ratio combination of the tranquilizer, zolazepam, with the dissociative anesthetic, tiletamine; used for injection anesthesia in dogs, cats, wild and zoo animals. It produces dose-dependent sedation to general anesthesia.
Zollinger–Ellison syndrome a triad comprising intractable, sometimes fulminating, upper gastrointestinal ulceration, extreme gastric hyperacidity, and nonbeta cell, gastrin-secreting, islet cell tumors (gastrinomas) of the pancreas. Clinical signs in affected dogs include vomiting, often with blood, anemia, diarrhea, weight loss, and sometimes signs of peritonitis.
zona pl. *zonae* [L.] zone.
z. alba the white line in the horse's hoof.
z. arcuata see zona glomerulosa (see below).

z. fasciculata the thick middle layer of the adrenal gland.
z. glomerulosa the outermost layer of the adrenal cortex. Called also zona multiformis.
z. multiformis see zona glomerulosa (above).
z. pellucida 1. the transparent, noncellular, secreted layer surrounding an ovum. 2. area pellucida.
z. radiata a zona pellucida exhibiting conspicuous radial striations.
z. reaction caused by the penetration of the zona pellucida by the spermatozoa.
z. reticularis the innermost layer of the adrenal cortex.
z. striata a zona pellucida exhibiting conspicuous striations.

zona-free hamster ovum penetration ability assay a test of sperm function; the zona pellucida penetration assay is preferred.

zona pellucida penetration assay a test of sperm function preferred to the simpler zona-free hamster ovum penetration assay.

zone an encircling region or area; by extension, any area with specific characteristics or boundary. See also ZONA.
autonomous innervation z. areas of innervation supplied by a single nerve, as for example the patch of skin on the medial side of the horse fore pastern which is supplied solely by the median nerve; used to assess the integrity of individual nerves.
ciliary z. the outer of the two regions into which the anterior surface of the iris is divided by the angular line.
comfort z. an environmental temperature between 55° and 70°F (13° and 21°C) with a humidity of 30 to 55%.
epileptogenic z. an area, stimulation of which may provoke an epileptic seizure.
z. of inhibition the area without bacterial growth surrounding an antimicrobial-impregnated disk in an ANTIMICROBIAL sensitivity test.
provisional calcification z. in developing bone longitudinal tubes of mineralized matrix which surround hypertrophic chondrocytes.
transitional z. the circle in the equator of the lens of the eye in which epithelial fibers are developed into lens fibers.

zonifugal passing outward from a zone or region.

zonipetal passing toward a zone or region.

zonula pl. *zonulae* [L.] zonule.
z. adherens common component of junctional complexes between epithelial cells; forms an effective barrier between the lumen and connective tissue. Called also tight junction.
z. ciliaris suspensory ligament of the lens.
z. occludens part of the junctional complex of columnar epithelium.

zonule a small zone.
ciliary z. a series of fibers connecting the ciliary body and lens of the eye, holding the lens in place. Called also Zinn nodule.

zonulitis inflammation of the ciliary zonule.

zonulolysis, zonulysis dissolution of the ciliary zonule by use of enzymes, to permit surgical removal of the lens.

zonulotomy incision of the ciliary zonule.

zoo a collection of wild animals kept in close or open confinement, usually for public viewing. There are strict licensing provisions for such places to ensure that the welfare of the animals is taken care of, and the safety of the public, and that the possibility of an exotic disease being introduced with additions of animal specimens from foreign countries is avoided. See also GAME farm.

zoo- word element. [Gr.] *animal.*

zo(o)- word element. [Gr.] *animal.*

zoodermic performed with the skin of another species of animal, especially in reference to skin grafts.

zoogenous 1. acquired from animals. 2. viviparous.

zoogeny the development and evolution of animals.

zoogeography defining the location and numbers of animal populations, and their variability with time.

zoogony the production of living young from within the body.

zoografting the grafting of animal tissue.

zooid 1. animal-like. 2. an animal-like object or form. 3. an individual in a united colony of animals.

zoology the biology of animals.

zoom control in ultrasonography, a means of magnifying part of the image.

Zoomastigophora a class of protozoa (subphylum Mastigophora), including all the flagellates that parasitize higher animals.

zoonosis pl. *zoonoses;* disease of animals transmissible to humans.
direct z. one transmitted by contact or via an inanimate vehicle and which requires only one reservoir vertebrate (passing directly from animal to humans without the involvement of a vector or intermediate host) to maintain the cycle of infection, e.g. rabies. See also CYCLOZOONOSIS, METAZOONOSIS, SAPROZOONOSIS.

zooparasite any parasitic animal organism or species.

zoopathology the science of the diseases of animals.

zoophagous carnivorous.

zoophilic preferring animals to humans; said of certain fungi.

zoophobia abnormal fear of animals.

zoospore a motile mitospore; a motile, flagellated, asexual spore, as produced by certain algae and fungi, and *Dermatophilus congolensis.*

zoospores see RUMINAL zoospores.

zootechny animal management as distinct from animal husbandry which includes the science, economics and biometry of the care of farm animals.

zootoxicosis disease caused by a zootoxin.

zootoxin a toxic substance of animal origin, e.g. venom of snakes, spiders and scorpions.

Zr chemical symbol, *zirconium.*

zwitterion an ion that has both positive and negative regions of charge. Called also dipolar ion.

zwoegersiekte [Dutch] see MAEDI.

zygacine one of the toxic alkaloids in ZIGADENUS.

Zygadenus see ZIGADENUS.

zygadine one of the toxic alkaloids in ZIGADENUS.

zygal shaped like a yoke.

zygapophysis the articular process of a vertebra.

zygion the most lateral point on the zygomatic arch.

zyg(o)- word element. [Gr.] *yoked, joined, a junction.*

zygodactylous having two toes directed forwards and two backwards as in some birds, e.g. parrots.

zygodactyly union of digits by soft tissues (skin), without bony fusion of the phalanges involved.

zygoma 1. the zygomatic process of the temporal bone. 2. zygomatic arch. 3. a term sometimes applied to the zygomatic bone.

zygomatic pertaining to zygomatic bone.
z. arch the arch formed by the processes of the zygomatic and temporal bones.
z. bone the bone forming the hard part of the cheek and the lower, lateral portion of the rim of the orbit. See also Table 10.
z. gland a salivary gland, formerly known as the orbital or upper molar gland, best developed in carni-

vores; located above the zygomatic arch and below the eye. Enlargement or mucocele of the gland causes exophthalmos.

z. mucocoele accumulation of salivary secretions from the zygomatic gland. It appears as a protruding mass under the conjunctiva of the lower eyelid.

z. process a projection from the frontal or temporal bone, or from the maxilla, by which they articulate with the zygomatic bone.

zygomaticofacial pertaining to the zygoma and face.

zygomaticotemporal pertaining to the zygoma and temporal bone.

zygomorphism the anatomical principle of bilaterality of antimeres (right and left halves of the body).

Zygomycetes see PHYCOMYCETES.

zygomycetes members of the taxonomic class of fungi which includes two orders, Mucorales and Entomophthorales.

zygomycosis rare infection by fungi in the class, Zygomycetes, causes granulomatous lesions in many species, most often in the gastrointestinal tract. A rare example is *Conidiobolus incongruus* infection causing cutaneous granulomata and invasion of the lungs as in nasal zygomycosis in sheep. Immune suppression is believed to be a predisposing factor. See also MUCORMYCOSIS, ENTOMOPHTHOROMYCOSIS. Most infections previously called phycomycosis were believed to have been caused by zygomycetes.

zygomycotes members of the Zygomycota phylum of fungi. Includes *Mucor*, *Rhizopus* spp.

zygon the stem connecting the two branches of a zygal fissure.

Zygophyllum plant genus in the family Zygophyllaceae; can cause nitrate–nitrite poisoning; suspected of causing mortality in sheep and cattle. Called also twin leaf. Includes *Z. ammophilum*, *Z. apiculatum*.

zygosity the condition relating to conjugation, or to the zygote, as (1) the state of a cell or individual in regard to the alleles determining a specific character, whether identical (homozygosity) or different (heterozygosity); or (2) in the case of twins, whether developing from one zygote (monozygosity) or two (dizygosity).

zygospore a thick-walled sexual spore produced by fungi in the class Zygomycetes.

zygote the cell resulting from union of a male and female gamete; the fertilized ovum. More precisely, the cell after synapsis at the completion of fertilization until first cleavage.

zygotene the synaptic stage of the first meiotic prophase in which the two leptotene chromosomes undergo pairing by the formation of synaptonemal complexes to form a bivalent.

zymase enzyme.

zymic pertaining to enzymes or fermentation.

zym(o)- word element. [Gr.] *enzyme, fermentation.*

zymodemes populations of parasites with identical isoenzymes.

zymogen an inactive precursor that is converted into an active enzyme by action of an acid or another enzyme or by other means; a proenzyme.

z. cells the secretory cells that secrete the zymogens.

z. granules contained in the cytoplasm of the secretory cells in the relevant gland. Contain the zymogen.

Zymonema farciminosum see HISTOPLASMA *farciminosum.*

Appendix

Laboratory Services

1.1 Biochemical reference values:* conventional units

	Ox	Sheep	Goat	Swine	Horse	Dog	Cat
Alanine aminotransferase (ALT; SGPT) (U/l)	–	–	–	–	–	17–69	34–55
Alkaline phosphatase (AP; SAP) (U/l)	41–94	0–140	42–775	–	83–283	5–73	14–25
Amylase (U/l)	–	–	–	–	9–34	700–1700	1000–1700
Aspartate aminotransferase (AST; SGOT) (U/l)	42–98	31–111	67–117	–	153–411	12–37	11–29
Bile acids (μg/ml)	–	–	–	–	0–5	0–5	0–5
Bilirubin—total (mg/dl)	0–1.9	0–0.4	0–0.1	0–0.2	0.2–6.0	0–0.4	0–0.5
—direct (mg/dl)	0–0.4	0–0.3	–	–	0–0.4	0–0.1	0–0.1
Calcium (mg/dl)	8.0–10.5	11.5–13.0	8.5–10.2	11.0–11.3	11.2–13.8	8.7–11.8	9.2–11.9
Chloride (mEq/l)	95–110	98–110	99–110	100–105	98–110	99–110	117–123
Cholesterol (mg/dl)	39–177	40–58	80–130	117–119	46–177	117–345	100–165
Creatine phosphokinase (CPK; CK) (U/l)	66–220	0–330	108–211	–	92–307	12–292	0–540
Creatinine (mg/dl)	1.0–2.7	1.2–1.9	–	1.0–2.7	1.2–1.9	0.7–1.6	1.2–2.1
Gamma glutamyltransferase (GGT) (U/l)	13–32	35–67	43–71	–	11–44	0–11	0–1
Glucose (mg/dl)	35–55	30–65	58–76	65–95	60–100	55–102	55–114
Iron (μg/dl)	57–162	166–222	–	91–199	73–140	94–122	68–215
Lipase (U/l)	–	–	–	–	40–78	52–305	–
Magnesium (mg/dl)	1.2–3.5	1.9–2.5	2.8–3.6	1.9–3.9	1.8–2.5	1.5–2.4	1.9–2.7
Phosphorus (mg/dl)	4.0–7.0	4.0–7.0	7.5–12.3	4.0–11.0	3.1–5.6	2.8–7.6	4.6–7.1
Potassium (mEq/l)	3.9–5.8	4.8–5.9	3.5–6.7	4.7–7.1	3.0–5.0	3.7–5.6	4.0–4.5
Sodium (mEq/l)	132–152	145–160	142–155	140–150	132–150	137–149	147–156
Sorbitol dehydrogenase (SDH) (U/l)	18–46	14–41	35–80	–	0–15	–	–
Triglycerides (mg/dl)	–	–	–	–	5–55	10–140	30–100
Urea nitrogen (mg/dl)	6–27	8–20	15–33	8–24	10–20	7–21	18–34
Acid–base							
Bicarbonate (mmol/l)	20–30	21–28	26–30	18–27	23–32	17–24	17–24
pH	7.35–7.50	7.32–7.50	–	–	7.32–7.55	7.31–7.42	7.24–7.40
P_{CO_2} (mmHg)	34–45	–	–	–	38–46	–	–
Proteins							
Total protein (g/dl)	5.7–8.1	6.0–7.9	5.9–7.4	7.9–8.9	6.0–7.7	5.4–7.1	5.4–7.8
Albumin (g/dl)	2.1–3.6	2.4–3.0	2.7–3.9	1.8–3.3	2.9–3.8	2.6–3.3	2.1–3.3
α_1 globulin (g/dl)	0.7–1.2	0.3–0.6	0.5–0.7	0.3–0.4	0.7–1.3	0.2–0.5	0.2–1.1
α_2 globulin (g/dl)	–	0.3–0.6	–	1.3–1.5	0.7–1.3	0.3–1.1	0.4–0.9
β_1 globulin (g/dl)	0.6–1.2	1.1–2.6	0.7–1.2	0.1–0.3	0.4–1.2	0.7–1.3	0.3–0.9
β_2 globulin (g/dl)	–	–	0.3–0.6	1.3–1.7	–	0.6–1.4	0.6–1.0
γ_1 globulin (g/dl)	1.6–3.2	0.9–3.3	0.9–3.0	2.2–2.5	0.9–1.5	0.5–1.3	0.3–2.5
γ_2 globulin (g/dl)	–	–	–	–	–	0.4–0.9	1.4–1.9

All enzymes measured at 37°C.

* N.B. Reference values may be influenced by the method of measurement and by the animal's breed, sex, age and environment. Hence these values are guidelines only.

Updated from first edition by B.W. Parry, University of Melbourne, Werribee, Vic. Australia.

1.2 Biochemical reference values:* SI units

	Ox	Sheep	Goat	Swine	Horse	Dog	Cat
Alanine aminotransferase (ALT; SGPT) (U/l)	–	–	–	–	–	17–69	34–55
Alkaline phosphatase (AP; SAP) (U/l)	41–94	0–140	42–775	–	83–283	5–73	14–25
Amylase (U/l)	–	–	–	–	9–34	700–1700	1000–1700
Aspartate aminotransferase (AST; SGOT) (U/l)	42–98	31–111	67–117	–	153–411	12–37	11–29
Bile acids (μmol/l)	–	–	–	–	0–10	0–10	0–10
Bilirubin—total (μmol/l)	0–32	0–7	0–2	0–3	3–103	0–7	0–9
—direct (μmol/l)	0–7	0–5	–	–	0–7	0–2	0–2
Calcium (mmol/l)	2.00–2.63	2.88–3.25	2.13–2.55	2.75–2.83	2.80–3.45	2.18–2.95	2.30–2.98
Chloride (mmol/l)	95–110	98–110	99–110	100–105	98–110	99–110	117–123
Cholesterol (mmol/l)	1.01–4.58	1.03–1.50	2.07–3.36	3.03–3.08	1.19–4.58	3.03–8.92	2.59–4.27
Creatine phosphokinase (CPK; CR) (U/l)	66–220	0–330	108–211	–	92–307	12–292	0–540
Creatinine (μmol/l)	88–239	106–168	–	88–239	106–168	62–141	106–186
Gamma glutamyltransferase (GGT) (U/l)	13–32	35–67	43–71	–	11–44	0–11	0–1
Glucose (mmol/l)	1.9–3.1	1.7–3.6	3.2–4.2	3.6–5.3	3.3–5.6	3.1–5.7	3.1–6.3
Iron (μmol/l)	10–29	30–40	–	16–36	13–25	17–22	12–39
Lipase (U/l)	–	–	–	–	40–78	52–305	–
Magnesium (mmol/l)	0.49–1.44	0.78–1.03	1.15–1.48	0.78–1.60	0.74–1.03	0.62–0.99	0.78–1.11
Phosphorus (mmol/l)	1.29–2.26	1.29–2.26	2.42–3.97	1.29–3.55	1.00–1.81	0.90–2.45	1.49–2.29
Potassium (mmol/l)	3.9–5.8	4.8–5.9	3.5–6.7	4.7–7.1	3.0–5.0	3.7–5.6	4.0–4.5
Sodium (mmol/l)	132–152	145–160	142–155	140–150	132–150	137–149	147–156
Sorbitol dehydrogenase (SDH) (U/l)	18–46	14–41	35–80	–	0–15	–	–
Triglycerides (mmol/l)	–	–	–	–	0.05–0.60	–0.15–1.60	0.35–1.15
Urea (mmol/l)	2.1–9.6	2.9–7.1	5.4–11.8	2.9–8.6	3.6–7.1	2.5–7.5	6.4–12.1
Acid–base							
Bicarbonate (mmol/l)	20–30	21–28	26–30	18–27	23–32	17–24	17–24
pH	7.35–7.50	7.32–7.50	–	–	7.32–7.55	7.31–7.42	7.24–7.40
P_{CO_2} (kPa)	4.5–6.0	–	–	–	5.1–6.1	–	–
Proteins							
Total protein (g/l)	57–81	60–79	59–74	79–89	60–77	54–71	54–78
Albumin (g/l)	21–36	24–30	27–39	18–33	29–38	26–33	21–33
α_1 globulin (g/l)	7–12	3–6	5–7	3–4	7–13	2–5	2–11
α_2 globulin (g/l)	–	3–6	–	13–15	7–13	3–11	4–9
β_1 globulin (g/l)	6–12	11–26	7–12	1–3	4–12	7–13	3–9
β_2 globulin (g/l)	–	–	3–6	13–17	–	6–14	6–10
γ_1 globulin (g/l)	16–32	9–33	9–30	22–25	9–15	5–13	3–25
γ_2 globulin (g/l)	–	–	–	–	–	4–9	14–19

All enzymes measured at 37°C.

* N.B. Reference values may be influenced by the method of measurement and by the animal's breed, sex, age and environment. Hence these values are guidelines only.

Updated from first edition by B.W. Parry, University of Melbourne, Werribee, Vic 3030 Australia.

1.3 Conversion factors for biochemistry data

Analyte	Conventional unit	Multiplication factor	SI unit	Multiplication factor	Conventional unit
Alanine aminotransferase	U/l	1	U/l	1	U/l
Albumin	g/dl	10	g/l	0.10	g/dl
Alkaline phosphatase	U/l	1	U/l	1	U/l
Amylase	U/l	1	U/l	1	U/l
Aspartate aminotransferase	U/l	1	U/l	1	U/l
Bicarbonate	mEq/l	1	mmol/l	1	mEq/l
Bile acids	μg/ml	2.547	μmol/l	0.3926	μg/ml
Bilirubin	mg/dl	17.10	μmol/l	0.058	mg/dl
Calcium	mg/dl	0.2495	mmol/l	4.008	mg/dl
Chloride	mEq/l	1	mmol/l	1	mEq/l
Cholesterol	mg/dl	0.02586	mmol/l	38.67	mg/dl
Creatine (phospho)kinase	U/l	1	U/l	1	U/l
Creatinine	mg/dl	88.4	μmol/l	0.011	mg/dl
Gamma glutamyltransferase	U/l	1	U/l	1	U/l
Glucose	mg/dl	0.0555	mmol/l	18.0	mg/dl
Iron	μg/dl	0.1791	μmol/l	5.583	μg/dl
Lipase	U/l	1	U/l	1	U/l
Magnesium	mg/dl	0.4114	mmol/l	2.431	mg/dl
$P\text{CO}_2$	mm Hg	0.1333	kPa	7.502	mm Hg
Phosphorus	mg/dl	0.3229	mmol/l	3.097	mg/dl
Potassium	mEq/l	1	mmol/l	1	mEq/l
Proteins	g/dl	10	g/l	0.10	g/dl
Sodium	mEq/l	1	mmol/l	1	mEq/l
Sorbitol dehydrogenase	U/l	1	U/l	1	U/l
Triglycerides	mg/dl	0.01129	mmol/l	88.6	mg/dl
Urea (nitrogen)	mg/dl	0.3570	mmol/l	2.80	mg/dl

2.1 Hematological reference values:* conventional units

	Ox	Sheep	Goat	Swine	Horse	Dog	Cat
Haemoglobin (g/dl)	8.0–15.0	9.0–15.0	8.0–12.0	10.0–16.0	11.0–19.0	12.0–18.0	8.0–15.0
PCV (%)	24–46	27–45	22–38	32–50	32–53	37–55	24–45
RBC ($\times 10^6$/µl)	5–10	9–15	8–18	5–8	7–13	6–9	5–10
MCV (fl)	40–60	28–40	16–25	50–68	37–59	60–77	39–55
MCH (pg)	11–17	8–12	5–8	17–21	12–20	20–25	13–18
MCHC (g/dl)	30–36	31–34	30–36	30–34	31–39	32–36	30–36
Reticulocytes (% of RBC)	0	0	0	0–1.0	0	0–1.5	0–0.4†
WBC (/µl)	4000–12000	4000–12000	4000–13000	11000–22000	5400–14300	6000–17000	5500–19500
Neutrophils (mature) (/µl)	600–4000	700–6000	1200–7200	3080–10450	2260–8580	3000–115000	2500–12500
Neutrophils (bands) (/µl)	0–120	rare	rare	0–880	0–100	0–300	0–300
Lymphocytes (/µl)	2500–7500	2000–9000	2000–9000	4290–13640	1500–7700	1000–4800	1500–7000
Monocytes (/µl)	25–840	0–750	0–550	200–2200	0–1000	150–1350	0–850
Eosinophils (/µl)	0–2400	0–1000	50–650	55–2420	0–1000	100–1250	0–1500
Basophils (/µl)	0–200	0–300	0–120	0–440	0–290	rare	rare
Platelets ($\times 10^5$/µl)	1.0–8.0	2.5–7.5	3.0–6.0	3.2–7.2	1.0–3.5	2.0–5.0	3.0–8.0
Plasma proteins (g/dl)	6.0–8.5	6.0–7.5	6.0–7.5	6.0–8.0	5.8–8.7	6.0–8.0	6.0–8.0
Fibrinogen (mg/dl)	300–700	100–500	100–400	100–500	100–400	100–500	50–300

* N.B. Reference values may be influenced by the method of measurement and by the animal's breed, sex, age and environment. Hence these values are guidelines only.

† Aggregate reticulocytes derived from: Fan, L.C., Dorner, J.L. & Hoffman, W.E. (1978) *J. Am. Anim. Hosp. Assoc.*, **14**, 219.

Updated by B.W. Parry from first edition.

2.2 Hematological reference values:* SI units

	Ox	Sheep	Goat	Swine	Horse	Dog	Cat
Hemoglobin (g/l)	80–150	90–150	80–120	100–160	110–190	120–180	80–150
Hemogram (μmol/l)	5.0–9.3	5.6–9.3	5.0–7.4	6.2–9.9	6.8–11.8	7.4–11.2	5.0–9.3
PCV (l/l)	0.24–0.46	0.27–0.45	0.22–0.38	0.32–0.50	0.32–0.53	0.37–0.55	0.24–0.45
RBC ($\times 10^{12}$/l)	5–10	9–15	8–18	5–8	7–13	6–9	5–10
MCV (fl)	40–60	28–40	16–25	50–68	37–58	60–77	39–55
MCH (pg)	11–17	8–12	5–8	17–21	12–20	20–25	13–18
MCHC (g/l)	300–360	310–340	300–360	300–340	310–390	320–360	300–360
Reticulocytes ($\times 10^9$/l)	0	0	0	0–80	0	0–128	0–0.5†
WBC ($\times 10^9$/l)	4.0–12.0	4.0–12.0	4.0–13.0	11.0–22.0	5.4–14.3	6.0–17.0	5.5–19.5
Neutrophils (mature) ($\times 10^9$/l)	0.6–4.0	0.7–6.0	1.2–7.2	3.1–10.5	2.3–8.6	3.0–11.5	2.5–12.5
Neutrophils (bands) ($\times 10^9$/l)	0–0.1	rare	rare	0–0.9	0–0.1	0–0.3	0–0.3
Lymphocytes ($\times 10^9$/l)	2.5–7.5	2.0–9.0	2.0–9.0	4.3–13.6	1.5–7.7	1.0–4.8	1.5–7.0
Monocytes ($\times 10^9$/l)	0–0.8	0–0.8	0–0.6	0.2–2.2	0–1.0	0.2–1.4	0–0.9
Eosinophils ($\times 10^9$/l)	0–2.4	0–1.0	0.1–0.7	0.1–2.4	0–1.0	0.1–1.3	0–1.5
Basophils ($\times 10^9$/l)	0–0.2	0–0.3	0–0.1	0–0.4	0–0.3	rare	rare
Platelets ($\times 10^9$/l)	100–800	250–750	300–600	320–720	100–350	200–500	300–800
Plasma proteins (g/l)	60–85	60–75	60–75	60–80	58–87	60–80	60–80
Fibrinogen (g/l)	3–7	1–5	1–4	1–5	1–4	1–5	0.5–3.0

* N.B. Reference values may be influenced by the method of measurement and by the animal's breed, sex, age and environment. Hence these values are guidelines only.

† Aggregate reticulocytes derived from: Fan, L.C., Dorner, J.L. & Hoffman, W.E. (1978) *J. Am. Anim. Hosp. Assoc.*, **14**, 219.

Updated by B.W. Parry from first edition.

2.3 Conversion factors for hematology data

Analyte	Conventional unit	Multiplication factor	SI unit	Multiplication factor	Conventional unit
Hemoglobin	g/dl	10	g/l	0.10	g/dl
Hemoglobin	g/dl	0.6206	mmol/l	1.6113	g/dl
PCV	%	0.01	1/1	100	%
RBC	$\times 10^6$/μl	1	$\times 10^{12}$/l	1	$\times 10^6$/μl
MCHC	g/dl	10	g/l	0.10	g/dl
Leukocytes (all types)	/μl	0.001	$\times 10^9$/l	1000	/μ/l
Plasma proteins	g/dl	10	g/1	0.10	g/dl
Fibrinogen	mg/dl	0.01	g/l	100	mg/dl

3 The International System of Units: SI units

SI units

Quantity	Unit	Symbol	Derivation
Base units			
length	meter	m	–
mass	kilogram	kg	–
time	second	s	–
electric current	ampere	A	–
temperature	kelvin	K	–
luminous intensity	candela	cd	–
amount of substance	mole	mol	–
Supplementary units			
plane angle	radian	rad	–
solid angle	steradian	sr	–
Derived units			
force	newton	N	$kg \cdot m/s^2$
pressure	pascal	Pa	N/m^2
energy, work	joule	J	$N \cdot m$
power	watt	W	J/s
electric charge	coulomb	C	$A \cdot s$
electric potential	volt	V	J/C
electric capacitance	farad	F	C/V
electric resistance	ohm	Ω	V/A
electric conductance	siemens	S	Ω^{-1}
magnetic flux	weber	Wb	$V \cdot s$
magnetic flux density	tesla	T	Wb/m^2
inductance	henry	H	Wb/A
frequency	hertz	Hz	s^{-1}
luminous flux	lumen	lm	$cd \cdot sr$
illumination	lux	lx	lm/m^2
temperature	degree Celsius	°C	K – 273.15
radioactivity	becquerel	Bq	s^{-1}
absorbed dose	gray	Gy	J/kg
absorbed dose equivalent	sievert	Sv	J/kg

Prefixes for SI units

Multiplication factor	Prefix	Symbol
1 000 000 000 000 000 000 = 10^{18}	exa	E
1 000 000 000 000 000 = 10^{15}	peta	P
1 000 000 000 000 = 10^{12}	tera	T
1 000 000 000 = 10^{9}	giga	G
1 000 000 = 10^{6}	mega	M
1 000 = 10^{3}	kilo	k
100 = 10^{2}	hecto	h
10 = 10	deka	dk
0.1 = 10^{-1}	deci	d
0.01 = 10^{-2}	centi	c
0.001 = 10^{-3}	milli	m
0.000 001 = 10^{-6}	micro	μ
0.000 000 001 = 10^{-9}	nano	n
0.000 000 000 001 = 10^{-12}	pico	p
0.000 000 000 000 001 = 10^{-15}	femto	f
0.000 000 000 000 000 001 = 10^{-18}	atto	a

4.1 Weights and measures conversion: avoirdupois/metric weight

Avoirdupois to metric weight

Ounces (oz)	Grams (g)
1/16	1.772
1/8	3.544
1/4	7.088
1/2	14.175
1	28.350
2	56.699
3	85.049
4	113.398
5	141.748
6	170.097
7	198.447
8	226.796
9	255.146
10	283.495
11	311.845
12	340.194
13	368.544
14	396.893
15	425.243
16 (1 lb)	453.592

Pounds (lb)	Grams (g)	Kilograms (kg)
1 (16 oz)	453.59	
2	907.18	
3	1360.78	1.36
4	1814.37	1.81
5	2267.96	2.27
6	2721.55	2.72
7	3175.15	3.18
8	3628.74	3.63
9	4082.33	4.08
10	4535.92	4.54
14 (1 stone, UK)		6.35
100 (1 hwt, US)*		50.80
2000 (1 ton, US)*		1016.00

Metric to avoirdupois weight

Grams (g)	Ounces (oz)
0.001 (1 mg)	0.000035274
1	0.035274
1000 (1 kg)	35.274 (2.2046 1b)

* UK equivalents are 1 cwt = 112 lb, 1 ton = 2240 lb.

The 2000 lb ton also referred to as 'short ton', 2240 lb ton also referred to as 'long ton'.

The European tonne = 1000 kg.

4.2 Weights and measures conversion: apothecaries'/metric weight

Apothecaries' to metric weight

Grains	Grams (g)
1/150	0.0004
1/120	0.0005
1/100	0.0006
1/80	0.0008
1/64	0.001
1/50	0.0013
1/48	0.0014
1/30	0.0022
1/25	0.0026
1/16	0.004
1/12	0.005
1/10	0.006
1/9	0.007
1/8	0.008
1/7	0.009
1/6	0.01
1/5	0.013
1/4	0.016
1/3	0.02
1/2	0.032
1	0.065
1½	0.097 (0.1)
2	0.12
3	0.20
4	0.24
5	0.30
6	0.40
7	0.45
8	0.50
9	0.60
10	0.65
15	1.00
20(1)	1.30
30	2.00

Scruples	Grams (g)
1	1.296(1.3)
2	2.592(2.6)
3	3.888 (3.9)

Drams	Grams (g)
1	3.888
2	7.776
3	11.664
4	15.552
5	19.440
6	23.328
7	27.216
8	31.103

Ounces	Grams (g)
1	31.103
2	62.207
3	93.310
4	124.414
5	155.517
6	186.621
7	217.724
8	248.828
9	279.931
10	311.035
11	342.138
12	373.242

Metric to apothecaries' weight

Milligrams (mg)	Grains
1	0.015432
2	0.030864
3	0.046296
4	0.061728
5	0.077160
6	0.092592
7	0.108024
8	0.123456
9	0.138888
10	0.154320
15	0.231480
20	0.308640
25	0.385800
30	0.462960
35	0.540120
40	0.617280
45	0.694440
50	0.771600
100	1.543240

Grams (g)	Grains
0.1	1.5432
0.2	3.0864
0.3	4.6296
0.4	6.1728
0.5	7.7160
0.6	9.2592
0.7	10.8024
0.8	12.3456
0.9	13.8888
1.0	15.4320
1.5	23.1480
2.0	30.8640
2.5	38.5800
3.0	46.2960
3.5	54.0120
4.0	61.728
4.5	69.444
5.0	77.162
10.0	154.324

Grams (g)	Equivalents
10	2.572 drams
15	3.858 drams
20	5.144 drams
25	6.430 drams
30	7.716 drams
40	1.286 oz
45	1.447 oz
50	1.607 oz
100	3.215 oz
200	6.430 oz
300	9.644 oz
400	12.859 oz
500	1.34 lb
600	1.61 lb
700	1.88 lb
800	2.14 lb
900	2.41 lb
1000	2.68 lb

4.3 Weights and measures conversion: fluid measure

Apothecaries' to metric fluid measure

Minims	Milliliters (ml)
1	0.06
2	0.12
3	0.19
4	0.25
5	0.31
10	0.62
15	0.92
20	1.23
25	1.54
30	1.85
35	2.16
40	2.46
45	2.77
50	3.08
55	3.39
60 (1 fl dr)	3.70

Fluid drams (fl dr)	Milliliters (ml)
1	3.70
2	7.39
3	11.09
4	14.79
5	18.48
6	22.18
7	25.88
8 (1 fl oz)	29.57

Fluid ounces (fl oz)	Milliliters (ml)
1	29.57
2	59.15
3	88.72
4	118.29
5	147.87
6	177.44
7	207.01
8	236.58
9	266.16
10	295.73
11	325.30
12	354.88
13	384.45
14	414.02
15	443.59
16 (1 pt, US)	473.18
20 (1 pt, imp.)	591.48
32 (1 qt, US)	946.36
40 (1 qt, imp.)	1182.95
128 (1 gal, US)	3785.43
160 (1 gal, imp.)	4731.79

Metric to apothecaries' fluid measure

Milliliters (ml)	Minims
1	16.231
2	32.5
3	48.7
4	64.9
5	81.1

Milliliters (ml)	Fluid drams (fl dr)
5	1.35
10	2.71
15	4.06
20	5.4
25	6.76
30	7.1

Milliliters (ml)	Fluid ounces (fl oz)
30	1.01
40	1.35
50	1.69
500	16.91
1000 (1l)	33.815

4.4 Weights and measures conversion: capacity

Non-metric	to metric
1 cu. inch	= 16.387 milliliter (cu. cm)
1 cu. foot	= 0.028317 cu. meter
1 cu. yard	= 0.7646 cu. meter
1 gallon, imp. (1.2 gal, US)	= 4.546 liter
1 gallon, US (0.83 gal. imp.)	= 3.788 liter

* See also Table 4.3.

Metric	to non-metric
1 cu. centimeter	= 0.061 cu. inch
1 cu. meter	= 1.308 cu. yard
1 liter	= 0.220 gallon, imp.
1 liter	= 0.264 gallon US

4.5 Weights and measures conversion: length

Non-metric	to metric
1 inch	= 2.54 centimeters
1 foot	= 0.3048 meter
1 yard	= 0.9144 meter
1 rod (pole or perch)	= 5.0292 meters
1 chain	= 0.0201 kilometers
1 mile	= 1.609 kilometers

Metric	to non-metric
1 millimeter	= 0.03937 inch
1 centimeter	= 0.3937 inch
1 meter	= 1.0936 yards
1 kilometer	= 0.6215 mile

5 Temperature equivalents: Celsius/Fahrenheit

Celsius to Fahrenheit
(°F = (°C × $\frac{9}{5}$) + 32)

°C	°F	°C	°F
−50	−58.0	49	120.2
−40	−40.0	50	122.0
−35	−31.0	51	123.8
−30	−22.0	52	125.6
−25	−13.0	53	127.4
−20	−4.0	54	129.2
−15	−5.0	55	131.0
−10	14.0	56	132.8
−5	23.0	57	134.6
0	32.0	58	136.4
1	33.8	59	138.2
2	35.6	60	140.0
3	37.4	61	141.8
4	39.2	62	143.6
5	41.0	63	145.4
6	42.8	64	147.2
7	44.6	65	149.0
8	46.4	66	150.8
9	48.2	67	152.6
10	50.0	68	154.4
11	51.8	69	156.2
12	53.6	70	158.0
13	55.4	71	159.8
14	57.2	72	161.6
15	59.0	73	163.4
16	60.8	74	165.2
17	62.6	75	167.0
18	64.4	76	168.8
19	66.2	77	170.6
20	68.0	78	172.4
21	69.8	79	174.2
22	71.6	80	176.0
23	73.4	81	177.8
24	75.2	82	179.6
25	77.0	83	181.4
26	78.8	84	183.2
27	80.6	85	185.0
28	82.4	86	186.8
29	84.2	87	188.6
30	86.0	88	190.4
31	87.8	89	192.2
32	89.6	90	194.0
33	91.4	91	195.8
34	93.2	92	197.6
35	95.0	93	199.4
36	96.8	94	201.2
37	98.6	95	203.0
38	100.4	96	204.8
39	102.2	97	206.6
40	104.0	98	208.4
41	105.8	99	210.2
42	107.6	100	212.0
43	109.4	101	213.8
44	111.2	102	215.6
45	113.0	103	217.4
46	114.8	104	219.2
47	116.6	105	221.0
48	118.4	106	222.8

Fahrenheit to Celsius
(°C = (°F − 32) × $\frac{5}{9}$)

°F	°C	°F	°C	°F	°C
−50	−46.7	99	37.2	157	69.4
−40	−40.0	100	37.7	158	70.0
−35	−37.2	101	38.3	159	70.5
−30	−34.4	102	38.8	160	71.1
−25	−31.7	103	39.4	161	71.6
−20	−28.9	104	40.0	162	72.2
−15	−26.6	105	40.5	163	72.7
−10	−23.3	106	41.1	164	73.3
−5	−20.6	107	41.6	165	73.8
0	−17.7	108	42.2	166	74.4
1	−17.2	109	42.7	167	75.0
5	−15.0	110	43.3	168	75.5
10	−12.2	111	43.8	169	76.1
15	−9.4	112	44.4	170	76.6
20	−6.6	113	45.0	171	77.2
25	−3.8	114	45.5	172	77.7
30	−1.1	115	46.1	173	78.3
31	−0.5	116	46.6	174	78.8
32	0	117	47.2	175	79.4
33	0.5	118	47.7	176	80.0
34	1.1	119	48.3	177	80.5
35	1.6	120	48.8	178	81.1
36	2.2	121	49.4	179	81.6
37	2.7	122	50.0	180	82.2
38	3.3	123	50.5	181	82.7
39	3.8	124	51.1	182	83.3
40	4.4	125	51.6	183	83.8
41	5.0	126	52.2	184	84.4
42	5.5	127	52.7	185	85.0
43	6.1	128	53.3	186	85.5
44	6.6	129	53.8	187	86.1
45	7.2	130	54.4	188	86.6
46	7.7	131	55.0	189	87.2
47	8.3	132	55.5	190	87.7
48	8.8	133	56.1	191	88.3
49	9.4	134	56.6	192	88.8
50	10.0	135	57.2	193	89.4
55	12.7	136	57.7	194	90.0
60	15.5	137	53.3	195	90.5
65	18.3	138	58.8	196	91.1
70	21.1	139	59.4	197	91.6
75	23.8	140	60.0	198	92.2
80	26.6	141	60.5	199	92.7
85	29.4	142	61.1	200	93.3
86	30.0	143	61.6	201	93.8
87	30.5	144	62.2	202	94.4
88	31.0	145	62.7	203	95.0
89	31.6	146	63.3	204	95.5
90	32.2	147	63.8	205	96.1
91	32.7	148	64.4	206	96.6
92	33.3	149	65.0	207	97.2
93	33.8	150	65.5	208	97.7
94	34.4	151	66.1	209	98.3
95	35.0	152	66.6	210	98.8
96	35.5	153	67.2	211	99.4
97	36.1	154	67.7	212	100.0
98	36.6	155	68.3	213	100.5
98.6	37.0	156	68.8	214	101.1

6 Chemical elements

Element (date of discovery)	Symbol	Atomic number	Atomic weight	Valency	Specific gravity or density (g/l)	Comments
Actinium (1899)	Ac	89	[227]*	3	10.07	radioactive element associated with uranium
Aluminum (1827)	Al	13	26.9815	3	2.6989	silvery-white metal, abundant in earth's crust, but not in free form
Americium (1944)	Am	95	[243]	3, 4, 5, 6	13.67	fourth transuranium element discovered
Antimony (prehistoric)	Sb	51	121.75	3, 5	6.691	exists in four allotropic forms
Argon (1894)	Ar	18	39.948	0?	1.7837 g/l	colorless, odorless gas
Arsenic (1250)	As	33	74.9216	3, 5	5.73	(gray) semimetallic solid
					4.73	(black)
					1.97	(yellow)
Astatine (1940)	At	85	[210]	1, 3, 5, 7		radioactive halogen
Barium (1808)	Ba	56	137.34	2	3.5	silvery-white, alkaline earth metal
Berkelium (1949)	Bk	97	[247]	3, 4		fifth transuranium element discovered
Beryllium (1798)	Be	4	9.0122	2	1.848	light, steel-gray metal
Bismuth (1753)	Bi	83	208.980	3, 5	9.747	pinkish-white, crystalline, brittle metal
Boron (1808)	B	5	10.811	3	2.34, 2.37	crystalline or amorphous element, not occurring free in nature
Bromine (1826)	Br	35	79.909	1, 3, 5, 7	3.12	mobile, reddish-brown liquid, volatilizing readily
					7.59 g/l	red vapor with disagreeable odour
Cadmium (1817)	Cd	48	112.40	2	8.65	soft, bluish-white metal
Calcium (1808)	Ca	20	40.08	2	1.55	metallic element, forming more than 3% of earth's crust
Californium (1950)	Cf	98	[251]	2, 3		sixth transuranium element discovered
Carbon (prehistoric)	C	6	12.01115	2, 3, 4	1.8–2.1	(amorphous) element widely distributed in nature
					1.9–2.3	(graphite)
					3.15–3.53	(diamond)
Cerium (1803)	Ce	58	140.12	3, 4	6.67–8.23	most abundant rare earth metal
Caesium (1869)	Cs	55	132.905	1	1.873	silvery-white, soft, alkaline metal
Chlorine (1774)	Cl	17	35.453	1, 3, 5, 7	3.214 g/l	greenish-yellow gas of the halogen group
Chromium (1797)	Cr	24	51.996	2, 3, 6	7.18–7.20	steel-gray, lustrous, hard metal
Cobalt (1735)	Co	27	58.9332	2, 3	8.9	brittle, hard metal
Copper (prehistoric)	Cu	29	63.54	1, 2	8.96	reddish, lustrous, malleable metal
Curium (1944)	Cm	96	[247]	3, 4	13.51	third transuranium element discovered
Dysprosium (1886)	Dy	66	162.50	3	8.536	rare earth metal with metallic, bright silver luster
Einsteinium (1952)	Es	99	[252]	2, 3		seventh transuranium element discovered
Element 108 (1984)	–	–	[265]			sixteenth transuranium element discovered; no name yet proposed
Element 109 (1982)	–	–	[266]			fifteenth transuranium element discovered; no name yet proposed
Erbium (1843)	Er	68	167.26	3	9.051	soft, malleable rare earth metal
Europium (1896)	Eu	63	151.96	2, 3	5.259	lustrous, silvery-white rare earth metal
Fermium (1953)	Fm	100	[257]	2, 3		eighth transuranium element discovered
Fluorine (1771)	F	9	18.9984	1	1.696 g/l	pale yellow, corrosive gas of the halogen group
Francium (1939)	Fr	87	[223]	1		product of alpha distintegration of actinium
Gadolinium (1880)	Gd	64	157.25	3	7.8, 7.895	lustrous, silvery-white rare earth metal
Gallium (1875)	Ga	31	69.72	2, 3	5.907	silvery-appearing metal

Germanium (1886)	Ge	32	72.59	2, 4	5.323	grayish-white, brittle metal
Gold (prehistoric)	Au	79	196.967	1, 3	19.32	malleable yellow metal
Hafnium (1923)	Hf	72	178.49	4	13.29	gray metal associated with zirconium
Helium (1895)	He	2	4.0026	0	0.177 g/l	inert gas
Holmium (1879)	Ho	67	164.930	3	8.803	relatively soft and malleable rare earth metal
Hydrogen (1766)	H	1	1.00797	1	0.08988 g/l	(gas) most abundant element in the universe
					0.070	(liquid)
Indium (1863)	In	49	114.82	1, 2?, 3	7.31	soft, silvery-white metal
Iodine (1811)	I	53	126.9044	1, 3, 5, 7	4.93, 11.27 g/1	grayish-black, lustrous solid or violet-blue gas
Iridium (1803)	Ir	77	192.2	3, 4	22.42	white, brittle metal of platinum family
Iron (prehistoric)	Fe	26	55.847	2, 3, 4, 6	7.874	fourth most abundant element in earth's crust
Krypton (1898)	Kr	36	83.80	0	3.733 g/l	inert gas
Lanthanum (1839)	La	57	138.91	3	5.98–6.186	silvery-white, ductile, rare earth metal
Lawrencium (1961)	Lr	103	[260]	3		tenth transuranium element discovered
Lead (prehistoric)	Pb	82	207.19	2, 4	11.35	bluish-white, lustrous, malleable metal
Lithium (1817)	Li	3	6.939	1	0.534	lightest of all metals
Lutetium (1907)	Lu	71	174.97	3	9.872	rare earth metal
Magnesium (1808)	Mg	12	24.312	2	1.738	silvery-white metallic element, eighth in abundance in earth's crust
Manganese (1774)	Mn	25	54.9380	1, 2, 3, 4, 6, 7	7.21–7.44	exists in four allotropic forms
Mendelevium (1955)	Md	101	[258]	2, 3		ninth transuranium element discovered
Mercury (prehistoric)	Hg	80	200.59	1, 2	13.546	heavy, silvery-white metal, liquid at ordinary temperatures
Molybdenum (1782)	Mo	42	95.94	2, 3, 4?, 5?, 6	10.22	silvery-white, very hard metal
Neodymium (1885)	Nd	60	144.24	3	6.80, 7.004	exists in two allotropic forms
Neon (1898)	Ne	10	20.183	0?	0.89990 g/l	inert gas
Neptunium (1940)	Np	93	237.0482	3, 4, 5, 6	20.45	first transuranium element discovered
Nickel (1751)	Ni	28	58.71	0, 1, 2, 3	8.902	silvery-white, malleable metal
Niobium (1801)	Nb	41	92.906	2, 3, 4?, 5	8.57	shiny, white, soft ductile metal
Nitrogen (1772)	N	7	14.0067	3, 5	1.2506 g/l	colourless, odourless, inert element, making up 78% of the air
Nobelium (1958)	No	102	[259]	2, 3		
Osmium (1803)	Os	76	190.2	2, 3, 4, 8	22.57	bluish-white, hard metal of platinum family
Oxygen (1774)	O	8	15.9994	2	1.429 g/l	colourless, odourless gas, third most abundant element in the universe
Palladium (1803)	Pd	46	106.4	2, 3, 4	12.02	steel-white metal of the platinum family
Phosphorus (1669)	P	15	30.9738	3, 5	1.82	(white) waxy solid, transparent when pure
					2.20	(red)
					2.25–2.69	(black)
Platinum (1735)	Pt	78	195.09	1?, 2, 3, 4	21.45	silvery-white, malleable metal
Plutonium (1940)	Pu	94	[244]	3, 4, 5, 6, 7	19.84	second transuranium element discovered
Polonium (1898)	Po	84	[210]	2, 4, 6	9.32	very rare natural element
Potassium (1807)	K	19	39.102	1	0.862	soft, silvery, alkali metal, seventh in abundance in earth's crust
Praseodymium (1885)	Pr	59	140.907	3, 4	6.782, 6.64	soft, silvery rare earth metal
Promethium (1941)	Pm	61	[145]	3	7.22±0.02	produced by irradiation of neodymium and praseodymium; identity established in 1945
Protactinium (1917)	Pa	91	231.0359	4, 5	15.37	bright lustrous metal
Radium (1898)	Ra	88	226.0254	2	5.5	brilliant white, radioactive metal
Radon (1900)	Rn	86	[222]	0	9.73 g/l	heaviest known gas

Table continued over page

6 Chemical elements (*Continued*)

Element (date of discovery)	Symbol	Atomic number	Atomic weight	Valency	Specific gravity or density (g/l)	Comments
Rhenium (1925)	Re	75	186.2	–1, 2, 3, 4, 5, 6, 7	21.02	silvery-white lustrous metal
Rhodium (1803)	Rh	45	102.905	–2, 3, 4, 5	12.41	silvery-white metal of platinum family
Rubidium (1861)	Rb	37	85.47	1, 2, 3, 4	1.532	soft, silvery-white, alkali metal
Ruthenium (1844)	Ru	44	101.07	0, 1, 2, 3, 4, 5, 6, 7, 8	12.41	hard, white metal of platinum family
Rutherfordium (1969)	Rf	104	[261]			eleventh transuranium element discovered
Samarium (1879)	Sm	62	150.35	2, 3	7.536–740	bright silver lustrous metal
Scandium (1879)	Sc	21	44.956	3	2.992	soft, silvery-white metal
Selenium (1817)	Se	34	78.96	2, 4, 6	4.79, 4.28	exists in several allotropic forms
Silicon (1823)	Si	14	28.086	4	2.23	a relatively inert element, second in abundance in earth's crust
Silver (prehistoric)	Ag	47	107.870	1, 2	10.50	malleable, ductile metal with brilliant white lustre
Sodium (1807)	Na	11	22.9898	1	0.971	most abundant of alkali metals, sixth in abundance in earth's crust
Strontium (1808)	Sr	38	87.62	2	2.54	exists in three allotropic forms
Sulfur (prehistoric)	S	16	32.064	2, 4, 6	1.957, 2.07	exists in several isotopic and many allotropic forms
Tantalum (1802)	Ta	73	180.948	2?, 3, 4?, 5	16.6	gray, heavy, very hard metal
Technetium (1937)	Tc	43	98.9062	3?, 4, 6, 7	11.50	first element produced artificially
Tellurium (1782)	Te	52	127.60	2, 4, 6	6.24	silvery-white, lustrous element
Terbium (1843)	Tb	65	158.924	3, 4	8.272	silvery-grey, malleable, ductile rare earth metal
Thallium (1861)	Tl	81	204.37	1, 3	11.85	very soft, malleable metal
Thorium (1828)	Th	90	232.038	4	11.66	silvery-white, lustrous metal
Thulium (1879)	Tm	69	168.934	2, 3		least abundant rare earth metal
Tin (prehistoric)	Sn	50	118.69	2, 4	5.75 7.31	(gray) malleable metal existing in two or three allotropic forms, changing from white to gray on cooling and back to white on warming (white)
Titanium (1791)	Ti	22	47.90	2, 3, 4	4.54	lustrous white metal
Tungsten (1783)	W	74	183.85	2, 3, 4, 5, 6	19.3	steel-gray to tin-white metal
Unnilhexium (1974)	Unh	106	[263]			thirteenth transuranium element discovered
Unnilpentium (1970)	Unp	105	[262]			twelth transuranium element discovered
Unnilquadium (1969)	Unq	104	[261]			eleventh transuranium element discovered
Unnilseptium (1981)	Uns	107	[262]			fourteenth transuranium element discovered
Uranium (1789)	U	92	238.03	3, 4, 5, 6	18.95	heavy, silvery-white metal
Vanadium (1801)	V	23	50.942	2, 3, 4, 5	6.11	bright, white metal
Xenon (1898)	Xe	54	131.30	0?	5.887 g/l	one of the so-called rare or inert gases
Ytterbium (1878)	Yb	70	173.04	2, 3	6.977, 6.54	exists in two allotropic forms
Yttrium (1794)	Y	39	88.905	3	4.45	rare earth metal with silvery metallic lustre
Zinc (1746)	Zn	30	65.37	2	7.133	bluish-white, lustrous metal, malleable at 100–150°C
Zirconium (1789)	Zr	40	91.22	4	6.4	grayish-white, lustrous metal

* Figures in brackets represent the mass number of the most stable isotope.

7 Blood groups of domestic animals*

Species	Systems (number of factors)
Cattle	A (5), B (39), C (12), F (5), J (1), L (1), M (3), S (8), Z (1), T′ (1)
Sheep	A (2), B (9), C (2), D (2), M (3), R (2), X (2)
Pigs	A (2), B (2), C (1), D (2), E (16), F (4), G (3), H (5), I (2), J (2), K (7), L (12), M (11), N (3), O (2)
Horses	A (7), C (1), D (11), K (1), P (2), O (3), U (1)
Dogs	†DEA-1.1 (A_1), DEA-1.2 (A_2), DEA-3 (B), DEA-4 (C), DEA-5 (D), DEA-6 (F), and DEA-7 (Tr).
Cats	A-B (2)

* Adapted from Bell, T.K. (1983) In Agar, N.S. & Broad, P.G. (Eds) *Red Blood Cells of Domestic Mammals*, Amsterdam: Elsevier Science Publishers.

† Called also A (2), B (1), C (1), D (1), F (1), Tr (1), J (1), K (1), L (1), M (1), N (1)

8.1 A system of animal viruses

	DNA*			RNA†		
Size (nm)	**Enveloped cubical**	**Non-enveloped cubical**	**Complex**	**Enveloped helical**	**Enveloped cubical**	**Non-enveloped cubical**
300 × 200 × 200			*Poxviridae*‡ Orthopoxvirus§ Suipoxvirus Avipoxivirus Capripoxvirus Leporipoxvirus Parapoxvirus			
200	*Asfarviridae* Asfarvirus			*Paramyxoviridae* Paramyxovirus Morbillivirus Pneumovirus		
150	*Herpesviridae* *Alphaherpesvirinae*¶ *Betaherpesvirinae* *Gammaherpesvirinae*					
100				*Orthomyxoviridae* Influenza A Influenza B Influenza C		
130 × 300 × 70				*Rhabdoviridae* Vesiculovirus Lyssavirus Ephemerovirus		
2000				*Filoviridae* Filovirus		
90				*Bornaviridae* Bornavirus		
100				*Coronaviridae* Coronavirus Torovirus		
100					*Retroviridae* Oncovirinae Lentivirinae Spumavirinae	
100				*Bunyaviridae* Bunyavirus Phlebovirus		

		Nairovirus		
		Uukuvirus		
50–300			*Arenaviridae*	
			Arenavirus	
70	*Adenoviridae*			
	Mastadenovirus			
	Aviadenovirus			
60–80				*Reoviridae*
				Reovirus
				Orbivirus
				Rotavirus
60				*Birnaviridae*
45–55	*Papovaviridae*			
	Papillomavirus			
	Polyomavirus			
42	*Hepadnaviridae*			
60–70	Orthohepadnavirus		*Togaviridae*	
	Arihepadnavirus		Alphavirus	
40–50			*Flaviviridae*	
			Pestivirus	
			Arteriviridae	
			Arteriovirus	
35				*Caliciviridae*
20–30				*Picornaviridae*
				Enterovirus
				Cardiovirus
				Rhinovirus
				Aphthovirus
20	*Parvoviridae*			
15–23	Parvovirus			
	Dependovirus			
	Circoviridae			
	Circovirus			

* All DNA viruses are double-stranded, except those in the families *Parvoviridae* and *Circoviridae*, which are single-stranded, and *Hepadnaviridae*, which are partially single-stranded.
† All RNA viruses are single-stranded, except those in the families *Reoviridae* and *Birnaviridae*, which are double-stranded.
‡ Family name.
§ Genus name.
¶ Subfamily name.

8.2 Tropism of animal viruses

	Animal species						
Tropism	**Bovine**	**Ovine/caprine**	**Porcine**	**Equine**	**Canine**	**Feline**	**Avian**
Generalized	ephemeral fever* (Rhabdo-)† foot and mouth disease (Picorna-)	caprine herpesvirus (Herpes-) Rift Valley fever (Bunya-) foot and mouth disease (Picorna-)	African swine fever (Asfar-) pseudorabies (Herpes-) hog cholera (Flavi-) foot and mouth disease (Picorna-) reproductive – respiratory disease (Arteri-)	African horse sickness (Reo-) Getah (Toga-) equine infectious anemia (Retro-)	herpesvirus (Herpes-) infectious canine hepatitis (Adeno-) distemper (Paramyxo-)	feline infectious peritonitis (Corona-)	advenovirus infection (Adeno-) chicken anemia (circo-) Newcastle disease (Paramyxo-) infectious bursal disease (Birna-)
Respiratory	infectious bovine rhinotracheitis (Herpes-) adenovirus (Adeno-) parainfluenza 3 (Paramyxo-) respiratory syncytial (Paramyxo-) reovirus (Reo-) rhinovirus (Picorna-)	adeno (Adeno-) parainfluenza 3 (Paramyxo-) respiratory syncytial (Paramyxo-) reovirus (Reo-)	inclusion body rhinitis (Herpes-) adenovirus (Adeno-) influenza (Orthomyxo-)	rhinopneumonitis (Herpes-) Gammaherpesvirus (Herpes-) adenovirus (Adeno-) influenza (Orthomyxo-) Pneumonia (Morbilli-) reovirus (Reo-) rhinovirus (Picorna-)	tracheobronchitis (Adeno-) parainfluenza 2 (Paramyxo-) reovirus (Reo-)	rhinotracheitis (Herpes-) reovirus (Reo-) calicivirus (Calici-)	laryngotracheitis (Herpes-) influenza (Orthomyxo-) infectious bronchitis (Corona-) reovirus (Reo-)

Gastrointestinal tract	papular stomatitis (Pox-) malignant catarrhal fever (Herpes-) parvovirus (Parvo-) rinderpest (Paramyxo-) vesicular stomatitis (Rhabdo-) coronavirus (Corona-) torovirus (Corona -) reovirus (Reo-) rotavirus (Reo-) virus diarrhea (Toga-) calicivirus (Calici-) astrovirus (Astro-)‡ enterovirus (Picorna-)	adenovirus (Adeno-) peste des petits ruminants (Paramyxo-) bluetongue (Reo-) Wesselsbron (Flavi-) Nairobi sheep disease (Bunya-) reovirus (Reo-) rotavirus (Reo-) astrovirus (Astro-)‡ enterovirus (Picorna-)	transmissible gastroenteritis (Corona-) vesicular stomatitis (Rhabdo-) rotavirus (Reo-) vesicular exanthema (Calici-) swine vesicular disease (Picorna-) foot and mouth disease (Picorna-) enterovirus (Picorna-)	adenovirus (Adeno-) coronavirus (Corona-) vesicular stomatitis (Rhabdo-) torovirus (Corona-) reovirus (Reo-) rotavirus (Reo-) enterovirus (Picorna-)	parvovirus (Parvo-) coronavirus (Corona-) rotavirus (Reo-) calicivirus (Calici-) enterovirus (Picorna-)	panleukopenia (enteritis) (Parvo-) rotavirus (Reo-)	duck plague (Herpes-) duck hepatitis B (Hepadna-) rotavirus (Reo-) duck hepatitis A (Picorna-) enterovirus (Picorna-) turkey enteritis (Picorna-)
Genital tract	infectious pustular vulvovaginitis (Herpes-)			coital exanthema (Herpes-)			

Table continued over page

8.2 Tropism of animal viruses *(Continued)*

Tropism	Animal species						
	Bovine	**Ovine/caprine**	**Porcine**	**Equine**	**Canine**	**Feline**	**Avian**
Central nervous system	encephalitis (Herpes-) pseudorabies (Herpes-) rabies (Rhabdo-) Bovine spongiform encephalopathy (Prion*)	rabies (Rhabdo-) louping ill (Flavi-) visna (sheep) arthritis/encephalitis (goats) (Retro-) scrapie (Prion*)	rabies (Rhabdo-) haemagglutinating encephalitis virus (Corona-) encephalomyocarditis virus (Picorna-) polioencephalo-myelitis (Picorna-)	rabies (Rhabdo-) encephalosis (Reo-) Eastern and Western encephalitis (Toga-) Venezuelan encephalitis (Toga-) Japanese B encephalitis (Flavi-) Borna disease (Borna-)	pseudorabies (Herpes-) rabies (Rhabdo-)	pseudorabies (Herpes-) rabies (Rhabdo-)	turkey meningoencephalitis (Flavi-) avian encephalomyelitis (Picorna-)
Skin	cowpox/vaccinia (Pox-) Pseudocowpox (Pox) pseudo-lumpyskindisease/mammillitis (Herpes-)	sheep and goat pox (Pox-) contagious ecthyma (Pox-)	swinepox (Pox-) vaccinia (Pox-)	horsepox (Pox-)		poxvirus (Pox-)	fowlpox (Pox-)
Fetus (a) teratogenic	Akabane virus (Bunya-) virus diarrhea (Flavi-)	bluetongue (Reo-) Akabane virus (Bunya-) border disease (Flavi-)	hog cholera (Toga-)			panleukopenia virus (Parvo-)	

(b) abortion	bovine herpesvirus 1 (Herpes-)		pseudorabies (Herpes-) parvovirus (Parvo-) Japanese B virus (Flavi-)	equine herpesvirus 1 (Herpes-)			
Tumor	papilloma (Papova-) leukosis (Retro-)	Pulmonary adenomatosis/maedi (Retro-)	papilloma (Papova-)	papilloma (Papova-) sarcoid§	papilloma (Papova-)	leukemia/sarcoma (Retro-)	Marek's disease (Herpes-) papilloma (Papova-) leukosis (Retro-)

* Disease or virus name.
† Family name (add-viridae).
‡ Unconfirmed as a family or genus.
§ Unclassified.

Table prepared by M.J. Studdert.

Anatomy

9 Arteries

Artery	Other names	Origin	Comments
abdominal aa.	*see* cranial and caudal abdominal aa.		
abdominal aorta	aorta abdominalis (NAV)	from the thoracic aorta at its entrance into the aortic hiatus	the abdominal aorta runs in the midline, to the left of the vena cava, and terminates by bifurcation into the internal iliac aa. just cranial to the sacral promontory; it typically but not universally gives off paired lumbar, deep circumflex, external and internal iliac aa., renal aa., ovarian or testicular aa., caudal phrenic, cranial abdominal and suprarenal aa, the unpaired celiac a., and cranial and caudal mesenteric aa.
adrenal aa.	aa. adrenales mediae (NAV—pigs), a. adrenalis media (NAV—carnivores), suprarenal aa.	from the abdominal aorta	the adrenal glands are supplied by various aa. in different species; all receive blood from the caudal adrenal branches of the renal a.; the middle adrenal a. is only found in carnivores and pigs; cranial adrenal branches come from either the caudal phrenic, cranial abdominal, celiac or cranial mesenteric aa.
angularis oculi a.	a. angularis oculi (NAV)	from the terminal branch of the facial a. (in most species) or the buccal a. (pigs)	the vessel typically courses caudodorsally to reach the medial angle of the eye
angularis oris a.	a. angularis oris (NAV)	from the inferior labial a. (horse), the superior labial a. (ruminants) or the facial a. (dog)	a small a. to the corner of the mouth that has a variable origin
anterior ciliary aa.	aa. ciliares anteriores (NAV)	from the external ophthalmic a. (pigs) or from its muscular branches (others)	these vessels perforate the sclera near the corneoscleral junction and unite with the posterior ciliary vessels to supply the iris and ciliary body
anterior conjunctival aa.	aa. conjunctivales anteriores (NAV)	from the malar a. (pigs) or the supraorbital a. (ruminants)	these are vessels to the bulbar conjunctiva adjacent to the corneoscleral junction
aorta (NAV)		the base of the left ventricle	this, the largest artery in the body, is the parent to all others except the pulmonary aa.; its elasticity dampens the pulsatile flow from the left ventricle; see also its divisions: the ascending aorta, aortic arch and descending aorta
aortic arch	arcus aortae (NAV)	the ascending aorta	this is the communication between the ascending and descending aorta, derived embryologically in mammals from the left fourth aortic arch of the embryo and in birds from the right fourth arch; it gives off the brachiocephalic trunk, and in the dog and cat, the left subclavian a.
aortic arches 1–6	arcus aorticus I–VI	the ventral aorta of the embryo	the series of six paired embryonic aa. that connect the ventral and dorsal aortae; the first disappears totally, the second largely disappears, the third contributes to the internal carotids; the left (mammals) and right (birds) fourth arch forms the definitive aortic arch of the adult; the fifth only appears in lower vertebrates; the sixth contributes to the pulmonary aa. and the ductus arteriosus; anomalous forms may cause vascular rings around the structures passing through the mediastinum

aortic isthmus	isthmus aortae (NAV)	the aortic arch	this is a narrowing of the aortic arch that occurs in the fetus at or just proximal to the union of the aorta with the ductus arteriosus; it sometimes persists in the adult
arcuate a.	a. arcuata (NAV)	from the dorsal pedal a.	this short a. of carnivores crosses the hock transversely giving off the dorsal metatarsal aa.
arterial circle of the brain	*see* cerebral arterial circle		
a. of the clitoris	a. clitoridis (NAV)	a terminal branch of the internal pudendal a.	a homologue of the a. of the penis in the male; it gives off the a. of the vestibular bulb
a. of the ductus deferens	a. ductus deferentis (NAV)	from the prostatic a. (carnivores) or the umbilical a. (others)	this a., the homologue of the uterine a., supplies the deferent duct and forms an anastomotic loop with a branch of the testicular or prostatic a.
a. of the penile bulb	a. bulbi penis (NAV)	from the dorsal a. of the penis	this vessel supplies the corpus spongiosum of the penis near the sciatic arch
a. of the penis	a. penis (NAV)	a terminal branch of the internal pudendal a.	this a. to the penis arises at the sciatic arch and gives off the a. to the penile bulb, and the dorsal and deep aa. of the penis; in the horse it is augmented by a supply from the middle and cranial penile aa.
a. of the vestibular bulb	a. bulbi vestibuli (NAV)	from the a. of the clitoris	this is the homologue of the a. of the penile bulb in males; it passes to the ventral surface of the vulva
ascending aorta	aorta ascendens (NAV)	from the left ventricle	this is the initial segment of the aorta; at its origin it is expanded by the aortic sinuses to form the aortic bulb from which the left and right coronary aa. arise; it continues as the aortic arch
ascending palatine a.	a. palatina ascendens (NAV)	from the common carotid a. (sheep), the lingual a. (dogs, pigs), the linguofacial trunk (horses) or the occipital a. (cattle)	a. small a. to the muscles and mucosa of the soft palate
ascending pharyngeal a.	a. pharyngea ascendens (NAV)	from the common carotid a. (ruminants), the cranial thyroid a. (most horses) or the external carotid a. (dogs)	a vessel that runs in the roof of the pharynx where it supplies the local tissues and often gives off palatine, pharyngeal and, in cattle, tonsillar branches
auricular aa.	*see* caudal and rostral auricular aa.		
axillary a.	a. axillaris (NAV)	the continuation of the subclavian a.	this a. is arbitrarily named the axillary as the subclavian passes round the first rib; it provides the main supply to the forelimb and gives off the external and lateral thoracic, subscapular and cranial circumflex humeral aa. before it continues down the arm as the brachial a.
basilar a.	a. basilaris (NAV)	from the fusion of the two vertebral aa. and the rostral continuation of the ventral spinal a.	this a. is typically unpaired and runs forwards onto the ventral aspect of the medulla to end on the cerebral arterial circle; it gives off the caudal cerebellar and labyrinthine aa. plus branches to the medulla and pons
bicarotid trunk	truncus bicaroticus (NAV)	from the brachiocephalic trunk	in pigs, horses and ruminants the brachiocephalic trunk terminates by dividing into a right subclavian a. and a short bicarotid trunk; this then divides into the two common carotid aa.; these usually arise independently in dogs

Table continued over page

9 Arteries (*Continued*)

Artery	Other names	Origin	Comments
brachial a.	a. brachialis (NAV)	this a. is the continuation of the axillary a.	this largest a. of the forelimb begins just distal to the shoulder and runs along the medial aspect of the arm to the elbow, navigating the supracondyloid foramen in the cat; its main branches typically include the deep and superficial brachial, bicipital, collateral ulnar, transverse cubital and common interosseous aa.; it continues as the median a.
brachiocephalic trunk	truncus brachiocephalicus (NAV), brachiocephalic a.; common brachiocephalic trunk	the aortic arch	this is the largest branch of the aorta; it runs forwards from the aortic arch and typically supplies the head by giving off a bicarotid trunk or two independent common carotid aa.; it also supplies the right forelimb by giving off the right subclavian a.; in ruminants and horses it also supplies the left forelimb by giving off the left subclavian a.
broncho-esophageal a.	a. bronchoesophagea (NAV)	from the thoracic aorta, or from one of the dorsal intercostal aa.	this a., like many to the alimentary tract, is usually unpaired; it gives off one or more bronchial branches that provide oxygenated blood to the lung, especially the bronchial tree, and esophageal branches
buccal a.	a. buccalis (NAV)	the maxillary a.	in most species the a. supplies the pterygoids and muscles and glands of the cheek; it sends a branch to the zygomatic gland in dogs and an additional rostral deep temporal a. in pigs and cattle
carotid aa.	*see* common, external and internal carotid aa.		
caudal abdominal a.	a. abdominalis caudalis (NAV)	from the external iliac a. (carnivores) or the deep femoral or pudendoepigastric trunk (ruminants)	this a. is found in carnivores and ruminants; it is relatively small and runs cranially parallel to the rectus abdominis muscle
caudal auricular a.	a. auricularis caudalis (NAV)	from the external carotid a.	the a. runs dorsally to reach the back of the ear where it variably gives off lateral, medical and intermediate auricular branches, parotid and occipital branches, and a deep auricular a.
caudal cerebellar a.	a. cerebelli caudalis (NAV)	from the basilar a.	the a. runs under the trapezoid body, wraps around the medulla and reaches the cerebellar hemispheres; it gives branches to these structures plus ones to the choroid plexus
caudal cerebral a.	a. cerebri caudalis (NAV), deep cerebral a.	from the caudal communicating branch of the cerebral arterial circle	this large a. of the brain wraps around the cerebral peduncle and is distributed mainly to the midbrain; it is mostly concealed by the overlying cerebral hemispheres; it gives off central (perforating), cortical and choroidal branches and a rostral cerebellar a.
caudal circumflex humeral a.	a. circumflexa humeri caudalis (NAV)	from the subscapular a.	this a. runs with the axillary nerve on the flexor surface of the shoulder; it gives off the collateral radial a. and anastomoses with the cranial circumflex humeral a.; it supplies the shoulder region
caudal communicating a.	a. communicans caudalis (NAV)	from the internal carotid and basilar aa.	this vessel forms the caudal quadrant of the cerebral arterial circle; its major branch is the caudal cerebral a.

caudal deep epigastric a.	*see* caudal epigastric a.		
caudal epigastric a.	a. epigastrica caudalis (NAV), caudal deep epigastric a.	from the pudendoepigastric trunk, or occasionally, the deep femoral a.	the a. runs forwards and penetrates the deep surface of the rectus abdominis muscle and, near the umbilicus, anastomoses with its cranial epigastric counterpart
caudal femoral aa.	*see* proximal, middle and distal caudal femoral aa.	from the femoral a.	these three aa. are directed caudally into the medial muscles of the thigh including the adductors and the semimembranosus
caudal gluteal a.	a. glutea caudalis (NAV)	a terminal branch of the internal iliac a.	a large a. that arises at widely different sites in different species—from near the lumbosacral junction in horses and dogs, to the lesser sciatic notch in pigs and ruminants; it supplies the hamstrings and tail and may give off the iliolumbar, cranial gluteal, obturator, dorsal perineal and caudal rectal aa. and various aa. to the tail
caudal interosseous a.	a. interossea caudalis (NAV)	from the continuation of the common interosseous a.	this large a. of the carnivore forearm runs on the interosseous membrane to the carpus where it is called the palmar branch; there it supplies the deep palmar arch; in cats it gives off the ulnar a.
caudal mammary a.	a. mammaria caudalis (NAV)	from the external pudental a.	this a. to the mammary gland is found in the mare, ewe and cow; it is the homologue of the male cranial a. of the penis
caudal meningeal a.	a. meningea caudalis (NAV)	from the occipital a.	this a. passes through the mastoid foramen to supply the dura; before entering the foramen it supplies the atlanto-occipital joint and adjacent tissues; it is absent from the cat
caudal mesenteric a.	a. mesenterica caudalis (NAV)	from the abdominal aorta	this is the smallest and most caudal of the three unpaired aa. that supply the abdominal parts of the alimentary canal; it arises beneath the fourth to the sixth lumbar vertebra, runs in the mesocolon and supplies the terminal parts of the large intestine; it divides into the left colic and cranial rectal aa.; in ruminants it gives off the sigmoidal aa. too
caudal pancreaticoduodenal a.	a. pancreaticoduodenalis caudalis (NAV)	from the cranial mesenteric a.	this a. runs in the mesentery of the ascending limb of the duodenum; it divides to give branches that anastomose with the jejunal aa. near the duodenojejunal flexure and with the cranial pancreaticoduodenal a. at the caudal flexure of the duodenum
caudal phrenic a.	a. phrenica caudalis (NAV)	from the abdominal aorta; in carnivores by a common trunk with the cranial abdominal a.	this a. may have a variable origin from the aorta or its branches near the aortic hiatus; it ramifies in the crura of the diaphragm
caudal rectal a.	a. rectalis caudalis (NAV)	from the internal pudendal a. or one of its branches	this is one of the three rectal aa.; it divides into dorsal and ventral branches which supply the anus, its sphincters and the overlying skin and cutaneous glands
caudal superficial epigastric a.	a. epigastrica caudalis superficialis (NAV)	from the external pudendal a.	this a. lies superficially on the ventral surface of the rectus abdominis muscle and runs forwards to anastomose with the cranial superficial epigastric a.; in ruminants and mares its initial part is called the cranial mammary a.
caudal thyroid a.	a. thyroidea caudalis (NAV)	of variable origin from the brachiocephalic trunk or nearby branches	this small vessel runs cranially by the trachea to join the cranial thyroid a. by the thyroid gland, which it supplies; it also supplies the esophagus and the trachea
caudal tibial a.	a. tibialis caudalis (NAV)	from the popliteal a.	this a. supplies the muscles of the calf, especially the digital flexors

Table continued over page

9 Arteries *(Continued)*

Artery	Other names	Origin	Comments
caudal vesical a.	a. vesicalis caudalis (NAV)	from the prostatic or vaginal a., or one of their branches	this a. supplies the neck of the bladder over the caudolateral surface, and provides the main blood supply to the bladder; it gives off ureteric and urethral branches
celiac a.	a. celiaca (NAV)	from the abdominal aorta	this is the most cranial of the three unpaired aa. from the abdominal aorta that supply the alimentary tract; it supplies the stomach, spleen liver, and parts of the pancreas and small intestine; it usually has three branches—the splenic, left gastric and hepatic aa. (and in some, the caudal phrenic a.)
celiacomesenteric a.		from the abdominal aorta	this a. is a common variant in which the celiac and cranial mesenteric aa. share a common origin
central a. of retina	a. centralis retinae (NAV)	it arises from the union of a branch of the external with the internal ophthalmic a.	an a. that runs within the terminal portion of the optic nerve to enter the eye at the optic papilla; its branches spread out over the retina and were long thought to be true anatomical end-arteria, but are now considered to be physiological end-arteria only; this a. is significant because it nourishes the retina and individual vessels are visible with an ophthalmoscope
cerebral aa.	*see* cerebral arterial circle; rostral, middle and caudal cerebral aa.		
cerebral arterial circle	circulus arteriosus cerebri (NAV), circle of Willis, arterial circle of the brain	from the paired internal carotid aa., and the median basilar a.	this main source of blood to the brain is typically hour-glass shaped and encircles the optic chiasma and the hypophysis on the ventral surface of the brain; its formation from an anastomosis of three major aa. guarantees a constant supply along its branches; its four quadrants are made up of the paired rostral cerebral and caudal communicating aa.
ciliary aa.	*see* long and short posterior ciliary aa., and anterior ciliary aa.		
circle of Willis	*see* cerebral arterial circle		
circumflex humeral aa.	*see* cranial and caudal circumflex humeral aa.		
circumflex scapular a.	a. circumflexa scapulae (NAV)	from the subscapular a.	this a. gives off the nutrient a. of the scapula and supplies the adjacent region of the caudal part of the scapula
collateral radial a.	a. collateralis radialis (NAV)	from the caudal circumflex humeral a. (most species) or the deep brachial a. (horses)	this a. runs with the radial nerve in the brachial groove to the craniolateral aspect of the forearm supplying muscles on its course; it gives off a medial collateral a. and in pigs and ruminants a superficial antebrachial a.
collateral ulnar a.	a. collateralis ulnaris (NAV)	from the brachial a. (most species) or the superficial brachial a. (cats)	this a. curves around the inside of the elbow with the ulnar nerve and courses down to the carpus; it supplies parts of the triceps and the flexors of the carpus and digits

common carotid a.	a. carotis communis (NAV), the carotid	from the bicarotid trunk (pigs, horses and ruminants) or the brachiocephalic trunk (dogs)	this is the largest of the paired arteries that run to the head; it usually ascends the neck in a sleeve of connective tissue, the carotid sheath, in company with the vagosympathetic trunk and the internal jugular vein on either side of the trachea; its main branches are the cranial and caudal thyroid aa.; it terminates by dividing into the external and internal carotid aa.
common interosseous a.	a. interossea communis (NAV)	this is the terminal branch of the brachial a.	this short a. runs across to the space between the radius and ulna just distal to the elbow where it soon divides into the cranial and caudal interosseous aa.; in dogs it gives off the ulnar a.
communicating aa.	*see* rostral and caudal communicating aa.		these vessels unite the left and right halves of the cerebral arterial circle
condylar a.	a. condylaris (NAV)	from the occipital a. (dogs, ruminants and horses) or the internal carotid a. (pigs)	a variably developed vessel that enters the cranium through foramina near the occipital condyles and supplies the local dura; it also sends twigs to the inner and middle ear
conjunctival aa.	*see* anterior and posterior conjunctival aa.		
cornual a.	a. cornualis (NAV)	the superficial temporal a.	this a. supplies the horn of ruminants; because the adventitia of its branches is firmly applied to grooves in the bony cornual process, the a. tends not to retract when an animal is dehorned, thus encouraging extensive hemorrhage
coronary aa.	*see* right and left coronary aa.		these vessels supply the myocardium; in all species their main branches run subepicardially where they cannot be compressed by ventricular systole; they receive about 10% of the cardiac output; the left is larger in dogs and ruminants, the right in pigs and horses
costoabdominal a.	*see* dorsal costoabdominal a.		
costocervical trunk	truncus costocervicalis (NAV)	from the subclavian a.	this a. forms a common trunk for two to five of the branches of the subclavian, namely the deep cervical, dorsal scapular and thoracic vertebral aa. (dogs), plus the supreme intercostal and vertebral aa. (ruminants); in pigs and horses it is a common trunk to only the supreme intercostal and dorsal scapular aa.
cranial abdominal a.	a. abdominalis cranialis (NAV)	from the abdominal aorta (pigs) or by a common trunk with the caudal phrenic a. (carnivores)	this a. arises at about the level of the third lumbar vertebra and ramifies in the cranial part of the abdominal wall, mostly between the transverse abdomnis and the internal abdominal oblique muscles; it is absent from horses and ruminants
cranial a. of the penis	a. penis cranialis (NAV)	from the external pudendal a.	this a. passes forwards on the body of the penis to the glans; it is only large in the stallion; in the mare it is represented as the caudal mammary a.
cranial circumflex humeral a.	a. circumflexa humeric cranialis (NAV)	the last branch of the axillary a.; occasionally from neighboring aa.	an a. that supplies some of the muscles on the cranial aspect of the shoulder and arm
cranial epigastric a.	a. epigastrica cranialis (NAV)	from the internal thoracic a.	this a. pierces the diaphragm then runs first on and then in the rectus abdominis muscle until it anastomoses with the caudal epigastric a.; in dogs and ruminants it gives off a superficial branch
cranial gluteal a.	a. glutea cranialis (NAV)	from the internal iliac a. (ruminants, cats and pigs) or the caudal gluteal a. (dogs and horses)	this a. supplies the musculature over the wing of the ilium including the gluteal muscles themselves, and in some species sends twigs to the longissimus; its branches in some species include the obturator and iliolumbar aa.

Table continued over page

9 Arteries *(Continued)*

Artery	Other names	Origin	Comments
cranial interosseous a.	a. interossea cranialis (NAV)	from the terminal division of the common interosseous a.	this a., which arises on the medial side just below, pierces the interosseous membrane between the radius and ulna to gain the lateral side; it gives off a recurrent interosseous a. and supplies local muscles as it runs down the forearm
cranial laryngeal a.	a. laryngea cranialis (NAV)	from the common carotid a. (pigs and ruminants), cranial thyroid a. (horses) or the external carotid a. (dogs)	this vessel arises near the termination of the common carotid and supplies the muscles and mucosa of the larynx
cranial mammary a.	a. mammaria cranialis (NAV)	from the external pudendal a.	this a. of cows, ewes and mares is the highly developed proximal part of the caudal superficial epigastric a. of others
cranial mesenteric a.	a. mesenterica cranialis (NAV)	from the abdominal aorta just caudal to the celiac a.; sometimes from a combined celiacomesenteric a.	this is the middle of the three unpaired aa. that supply the abdominal part of alimentary canal; it nourishes most of the intestines and arises under the first or second lumbar vertebra; it serves as an axis about which the developing gut rotates and passes caudal to the transverse colon; it gives off the caudal pancreaticoduodenal, jejunal, ileal, ileocolic, right and middle colic aa., and in ruminants a large collateral branch
cranial pancreaticoduodenal a.	a. pancreaticoduodenalis cranialis (NAV)	from the gastroduodenal branch of the right gastric a.	this a. often runs partly within the pancreas; it typically anastomoses with the caudal pancreaticoduodenal a. near the caudal flexure of the duodenum
cranial phrenic a.	a. phrenica cranialis (NAV)	from the thoracic aorta	this a. is found only in the horse and supplies the right or left crus of the diaphragm (in the horse the caudal phrenic a. is absent)
cranial rectal a.	a. rectalis cranialis (NAV)	from the caudal mesenteric a.	this a. begins in the mesentery usually supplying the terminal parts of the colon before passing to the rectum where it anastomoses with the middle and caudal rectal aa.
cranial superficial antebrachial a.	a. antebrachialis superficialis (NAV)	from the superficial brachial a. (dogs and cats)	this small vessel rapidly divides into lateral and medial branches which run with the superficial branches of the radial nerve down the forearm; these branches may interfere with cephalic vein venipuncture
cranial thyroid a.	a. thyroidea cranialis (NAV)	from the common carotid a.	this large a. arises near the termination of the common carotid; it supplies the thyroid gland and typically gives off pharyngeal, cricothyroid and caudal laryngeal branches to the laryngeal muscles and pharynx
cranial tibial a.	a. tibialis cranialis (NAV)	a. terminal branch of the popliteal a.	the largest a. of the shank that runs between the muscle groups on its craniolateral side; it gives off the recurrent cranial tibial a. and others and terminates as the dorsal pedal a. over the flexor aspect of the hock
cranial vesical a.	a. vesicalis cranialis	the umbilical a.	this a. is small in dogs and cattle and best developed in sheep; it supplies the cranial aspect of the bladder
crural interosseous a.	a. interossea cruris (NAV)	from the caudal tibial a.	an a. of the shank of pigs and cattle that supplies the digital flexors of the hindlimb
deep antebrachial a.	a. profunda antebrachii (NAV)	from either the common interosseous or the brachial a.	this a. and its branches supply the deep heads of the flexors of the carpus and digits

deep a. of the clitoris	a. profunda clitoridis (NAV)	from the dorsal a. of the clitoris	this a. supplies the erectile tissue of the clitoris
deep a. of the penis	a. profunda penis (NAV)	from the dorsal a. of the penis	this a. penetrates the corpus cavernosum of the penis
deep auricular a.	a. auricularis profunda (NAV)	from the caudal auricular a.	a vessel derived from the caudal auricular, or one of its branches, that gains the inner surface of the ear cartilage and which supplies the skin of the external acoustic meatus
deep brachial a.	a. profunda brachii (NAV)	from the brachial a.	this a. is given off near the middle of the arm and mainly supplies the triceps muscles; in the horse it gives off the collateral radial a.
deep cerebral a.	*see* caudal cerebral a.		
deep cervical a.	a. cervicalis profunda (NAV)	mostly from the costocervical trunk, but in horses from the brachiocephalic and left subclavian aa.	the a. leaves the thorax through the first or second intercostal space and runs up to the nape, supplying the epaxial muscles of the neck
deep circumflex iliac a.	a. circumflexa ilium profunda (NAV)	from the abdominal aorta (carnivores) or the external iliac a. (other species)	this a. arises in the caudal part of the abdomen and supplies the caudal flank and some of the thigh; in ruminants and the horse it also extends further cranially; it divides into cranial and caudal branches that run mostly between the transverse abdominis and the internal abdominal oblique muscles
deep femoral a.	a. profunda femoris (NAV)	from the external iliac a. before the femoral a. is formed	the a. passes caudally towards the adductor muscles of the thigh; it gives off the pudendoepigastric trunk; its major terminal branch is the medial circumflex femoral a.
deep lingual a.	a. profunda linguae (NAV)	the lingual a.	the mobility of the tongue demands that this a. runs a flexuous course within the depths of the tongue; it runs between the hyoglossus and genioglossus, giving off dorsal lingual branches
deep palmar arch	arcus palmaris profundus (NAV), subcarpal arch	from the deep palmar branch of the radial a. (all species) plus other aa. that vary according to species	the deep palmar arch forms an anastomotic loop on the flexor surface of the carpus which gives off the palmar metacarpal aa. that run down between the metacarpal bones; the loop encourages a reliable source of blood to the digits, even if some vessels are compressed
deep plantar arch	arcus plantaris profundus (NAV)	from the lateral and medial plantar aa. on the caudal and distal aspect of the hock	this anastomotic loop gives origin to the plantar metatarsal aa. in like manner to the deep palmar arch of the forelimb
deep temporal aa.	a. temporalis profunda caudalis/rostralis (NAV)	from the maxillary a. or, in cats, from the rete mirabile	there is only a single (caudal) vessel in the small ruminants but an additional rostral a. in others; they are mainly aa. to the temporal muscle
descending aorta	aorta descendens (NAV), dorsal aorta	from the aortic arch	this, the longest segment of the aorta, is made up of thoracic and abdominal parts; *see* thoracic aorta and abdominal aorta
descending genicular a.	a. genus descendents (NAV)	from the femoral a.	this vessel runs down the inside of the thigh to the stifle joint, supplying branches to the distal ends of the quadriceps and to the joint itself
descending palatine a.	a. palatina descendents (NAV)	a terminal branch of the maxillary a.	the a. runs a short course within the pterygopalatine fossa before dividing into sphenopalatine, and greater and lesser palatine aa.; these branches supply the nasal chambers and the hard and soft palates

Table continued over page

9 Arteries *(Continued)*

Artery	Other names	Origin	Comments
digital aa.	*see* dorsal, palmar and plantar proper digital aa., dorsal, palmar and plantar common digital aa. and, for horses, palmar and plantar digital aa.		
distal caudal femoral a.	a. caudalis femoris distalis (NAV)	from the femoral a.	the distal member of three aa. that are directed caudally into the medial muscles of the thigh
dorsal a. of the clitoris	a. dorsalis clitoridis (NAV)	from the a. of the clitoris	the homologue of the dorsal a. of the penis of the male
dorsal a. of the penis	a. dorsalis penis (NAV)	from the a. of the penis	this is the a. that runs along the dorsum of the penis that, in stallions, receives augmentation from the middle and cranial penile aa.
dorsal carpal rete	rete carpi dorsale (NAV)	from the cranial interosseous and other aa.	this is a delicate network over the dorsum of the carpus that gives rise to the dorsal metacarpal aa.
dorsal common digital aa. (forelimb)	aa. digitales dorsales communes (NAV)	from the superficial dorsal arch (if present) or various antebrachial aa.	these aa. run superficially between the metacarpal bones and unite distally with the deeper dorsal metacarpal aa.; they give origin to the dorsal proper digital aa.
dorsal common digital aa. (hindlimb)	aa. digitales dorsales communes (NAV)	from the cranial branch of the saphenous a. (carnivores only)	these aa. run specifically between the metatarsal bones and unite distally with the deeper dorsal metatarsal aa.; they give origin to the dorsal proper digital aa., as in the forelimb
dorsal costoabdominal a.	a. costoabdominalis dorsalis (NAV)	from the thoracic aorta	this a. is effectively the last of the dorsal intercostals but because it lies caudal to the last rib also supplies some of the abdominal wall
dorsal intercostal aa.	aa. intercostales dorsales (NAV)	most arise from the thoracic aorta but the first few come from the costocervical trunk, the supreme intercostal or other aa.	these paired segmental aa. mostly run subpleurally close to the caudal border of the rib between the nerve cranially and the vein caudally (= 'NAV'); collateral branches may pass to the cranial border of the rib; most give off dorsal, cutaneous and mammary branches; the vessel terminates by anastomosing with the ventral intercostal branches of the internal thoracic a.
dorsal metacarpal aa.	aa. metacarpeae dorsales (NAV)	from the dorsal carpal rete	these aa. run between the metacarpal bones and unite distally with the more superficial dorsal common digital aa; they give origin to the dorsal proper digital aa.
dorsal nasal a.	a. dorsalis nasi (NAV)	from the facial a. (horses), the infraorbital a. (dogs) or the malar a. (ruminants)	this a. runs along the nasal bone supplying the dorsal part of the muzzle and, in the horse, the nasal diverticulum
dorsal pedal a.	a. dorsalis pedis (NAV)	the continuation of the cranial tibial a.	this major a. to the foot crosses the flexor aspect of the hock; in most species it gives off lateral and medial tarsal aa. and one or more perforating tarsal aa.; in the horse it continues as the large dorsal metatarsal a.; in carnivores it turns laterally as the arcuate a. that then gives off the series of dorsal metatarsal aa.
dorsal perineal a.	a. perinealis dorsalis (NAV)	from the vaginal a. (ruminants and pigs) or the caudal gluteal a. (carnivores)	this a. contributes to the supply of the external and sphincter and adjacent parts of the perineum

dorsal proper digital aa.	aa. digitales dorsales propriae (NAV)	from the division of the dorsal common digital aa.	with the palmar (or plantar) proper digital aa. these aa. provide blood to the toes; they are named axial or abaxial according to their relation to the axis of the foot
dorsal scapular a.	a. scapularis dorsalis (NAV), transverse a. of the neck, transverse colli a.	from the costocervical trunk (dogs, ruminants and horses) or the subclavian a. (pigs)	an a. that runs dorsally supplying the cervical part of the ventral serrate muscle and ending in the muscles beneath the withers
ductus arteriosus (NAV)		the pulmonary trunk	the ductus develops from the left sixth aortic arch that unites the pulmonary trunk with the aorta; it serves as a pulmonary bypass in the fetus and usually closes a short time after birth; its remnant in the adult is the ligamentum arteriosum
episcleral aa.	aa. episclerales (NAV)	the long posterior ciliary aa., and the muscular branches of the external ophthalmic a.	these vessels supply the sclera from the external surface
external carotid a.	a. carotis externa (NAV)	the terminal branch of the common carotid a.	this large vessel supplies the jaws, face and superficial structures over the cranium and, in ruminants and cats, also contributes substantially to the blood supply to the brain; its major branches are the occipital, cranial laryngeal, ascending pharyngeal, lingual, facial (or linguofacial trunk), caudal auricular, parotid, superficial temporal and maxillary aa.
external ethmoid a.	a. ethmoidalis externa (NAV)	external ophthalmic a.	the continuation of the external ophthalmic a. that enters the cranium through the ethmoidal foramen to join the internal ethmoidal a. with which it forms a small rete; it gives off the rostral meningeal a. and some nasal branches that supply the ethmoturbinates
external iliac aa.	aa. iliaca externa (NAV)	from the abdominal aorta at the level of the last one or two lumbar vertebrae	this a. is the major parent a. for the hindlimb; it also contributes to the body wall and in some species makes some contribution to the pelvic viscera; in most species it gives off the deep circumflex iliac, the caudal abdominal and the deep femoral aa. before escaping into the thigh as the femoral a.
external maxillary a.	*See* linguofacial trunk		
external ophthalmic a.	a. ophthalmica externa (NAV)	the maxillary a.	this a. arises in the depth of the orbit and supplies both the bulb of the eye and the adnexa; its main branches are typically the supraorbital, lacrimal and long posterior ciliary aa.
external pudendal a.	a. pudenda externa (NAV)	from the pudendoepigastric trunk, or occasionally from the deep femoral a.	this a. passes through the inguinal canal, emerging at the medial border of the superficial inguinal ring where its branches supply the ventral body wall and parts of the external genitalia; its main branches are the caudal superficial epigastric a. and either the ventral scrotal or ventral labial branch, and the cranial a. of the penis or caudal mammary a.
external thoracic a.	a. thoracica externa (NAV). *See also* lateral thoracic a.	the axillary a.	this is one of the major aa. to supply the pectoral muscles; in the pig it gives rise to the lateral thoracic a.
facial a.	a. facialis (NAV)	from the external carotid a. (dogs and pigs) or the linguofacial trunk (cattle and horses)	the a. begins by coursing medial to the ventral border of the mandible, then crosses to the lateral side and runs over the cheek by the edge of the masseter muscle; it can be used for taking the pulse as it crosses the mandible; depending on the species it gives off submental, sublingual, superior and inferior labial, lateral and dorsal nasal, and angularis oculi aa.; the vessel is missing in sheep and goats and small in pigs

Table continued over page

9 Arteries *(Continued)*

Artery	Other names	Origin	Comments
femoral a.	a. femoralis (NAV)	the direct continuation of the external iliac a.	it runs through the femoral canal and down the inside of the thigh to the caudal aspect of the stifle joint where it becomes the popliteal a., it is a useful a. on which to feel the pulse where it lies between the sartorius and pectineus muscles just cranial to the femoral vein; its main branches are the lateral circumflex femoral, descending genicular and saphenous aa., and the proximal, middle and distal caudal femoral aa.
gastric aa.	*see* left and right gastric aa., left and right gastroepiploic aa., short gastric aa. and gastroduodenal a.		
gastroduodenal a.	a. gastroduodenalis (NAV)	from the hepatic a.	the a. courses to the duodenum where it divides into the right gastroepiploic and the cranial pancreaticoduodenal aa.
genital aa.	*see* ovarian, testicular, uterine, vaginal and prostatic aa.		
greater palatine a.	a. palatina major (NAV)	from the descending palatine a.	this a. runs through the palatine canal in the hard palate and continues forwards in the rostral palatine groove; it supplies both the hard palate and, via the palatine fissure, the rostral floor of the ventral nasal meatus
hemorrhoidal aa.	*see* cranial, middle and caudal rectal aa.		
hepatic a.	a. hepatica (NAV)	one of the three main branches of the celiac a.	the a. runs to the liver which it supplies and ends by dividing into the right gastric and gastroduodenal aa.
hypogastric a.	*see* internal iliac a.		
ileal aa.	aa. ilei (NAV)	from the cranial mesenteric a.	a series or bundle of ileal aa. leave the cranial mesenteric and form vascular arcades within the mesoileum; these arcades often change their pattern along the gut, providing some indication of the segment exposed at surgery; the aa. are in continuity with the jejunal and ileocolic aa.
ileocecocolic a.	*see* ileocolic a.		
ileocolic a.	a. ileocolica (NAV), ileocecocolic a.	from the cranial mesenteric a.	this a. always supplies the segments of gut around the ileocolic junction and, depending on the species, may supply other parts too; it may give off right and middle colic aa. and one or more cecal aa. in addition to the ileal and colic branches
iliacofemoral a.	a. iliacofemoralis (NAV)	from the obturator a.	this a. crosses the ventral surface of the ilium to supply the cranial muscles of the thigh and the hip joint; it is only present in the horse
iliolumbar a.	a. iliolumbalis (NAV)	from the internal iliac a. (ruminants and pigs), the cranial gluteal a. (cats and horses) or the internal iliac a. (dogs)	an a. that typically supplies the hypaxial muscles before passing beneath the shaft of the ilium to reach the tensor fasciae latae and adjacent muscles

inferior alveolar a.	a. alveolaris inferior (NAV)	from the maxillary a.	before this a. enters the mandibular foramen it gives off the mylohyoid branch; it courses along the mandibular canal supplying the jaw and teeth before emerging as the mental branches which supply the lower lip and chin
inferior labial a.	a. labialis inferior (NAV), mandibular labial a., a. of the lower lip	from the facial a. (most species), the buccal a. (pigs) or the transverse facial a. (sheep and goats)	in most species this is the first vessel to be given off the facial a. after it has emerged onto the face; it typically runs a long course parallel with the mandible to reach the lower lip
infraorbital a.	a. infraorbitalis (NAV)	a terminal branch of the maxillary a.	the a. enters the maxillary foramen to pass along the infraorbital canal; it gives off the malar a. in horses and dogs, dental branches in all, and in some species dorsal or lateral nasal branches
intercostal aa.	*see* dorsal intercostal aa.		the intercostal aa. form anastomotic loops in which the dorsal intercostal aa. unite with the ventral intercostal branches of the internal thoracic a.
interdigital a.	a. interdigitalis (NAV)	from the dorsal and palmar (or plantar) common digital aa.	these aa. communicate between the palmar (or plantar) and the dorsal common digital aa.
internal carotid a.	a. carotis interna (NAV)	one of the terminal branches of the common carotid a.	a major supplier of blood to the brain; in horses this a. lies within a mucosal fold that hangs from the roof of the guttural pouch where it is vulnerable to erosion from fungal infections; in ruminants and cats the extracranial part disappears in adults; in dogs the artery runs through the carotid canal; the a. may course through the cavernous and other dural sinuses where heat exchange may take place
internal ethmoidal a.	a. ethmoidalis interna (NAV)	from the rostral cerebral a.	this small a. runs forwards to the cribriform plate and forms a rete with the external ethmoidal a. before supplying the ethmoturbinates
internal iliac a.	a. iliaca interna (NAV), hypogastric a.	this a. forms the terminal division of aorta	this large a. arises near the penultimate lumbar vertebra and runs towards or beyond the pelvic surface of the shaft of the ilium; it is short in horses and carnivores and long in pigs and ruminants; it, or its branches, supply the pelvic viscera ('visceral branches') or the pelvic wall ('parietal branches'); its terminal divisions are the caudal gluteal and internal pudental aa. and it or its branches give rise to the lumbar, iliolumbar, cranial gluteal and umbilical aa.
internal maxillary a.	*see* maxillary a.		
internal ophthalmic a.	ophthalmica interna (NAV)	from the rostral cerebral a. or the rostral epidural rete mirabile (cattle)	a slight vessel in domestic mammals that courses with the optic nerve to the eye, receives an anastomotic branch from the external ophthalmic a. and continues as the central a. of the retina
internal pudendal a.	a. pudenda interna (NAV)	one of the terminal branches of the internal iliac a.	the a. is particularly long in carnivores and horses in which it mimics the course of the internal iliac of other species; in horses and dogs it gives off the prostatic or vaginal a. to the pelvic viscera; in most species it gives off the urethral, ventral perineal and penile or clitoral aa.; it may also supply the vestibular aa.
internal spermatic a.	*see* testicular a.		
internal thoracic a.	a. thoracica interna (NAV)	from the subclavian a.	this a. runs mostly on the dorsal surface of the sternum, ventral to the transverse thoracic muscle; it gives off thymic, mediastinal and perforating branches to the mammary glands in those with pectoral mammae, and a series of ventral intercostal branches; it terminates by dividing into the musculophrenic and cranial epigastric aa.

Table continued over page

9 Arteries *(Continued)*

Artery	Other names	Origin	Comments
jejunal aa.	aa. jejunales (NAV)	from the cranial mesenteric a.	a series or bundle of jejunal aa. leave the cranial mesenteric a. and form vascular arcades in the mesojejunum; they anastomose orally with the duodenal branch of the caudal pancreaticoduodenal a. and aborally with the ileal aa.
labyrinthine a.	a. labyrinthi (NAV)	from the basilar a. or the caudal cerebellar a.	this vessel runs into the internal acoustic meatus with the vestibulocochlear nerve to supply the inner ear.
lacrimal a.	a. lacrimalis (NAV)	from the external ophthalmic a. or the maxillary a. (cat)	a branch to the lacrimal gland and adjacent regions
lateral circumflex femoral a.	a. circumflexa femoris lateralis (NVA)	from the femoral a.	this a. supplies parts of the quadriceps, the hip joint and the cranial part of the thigh; it divides into ascending, descending and transverse branches
lateral nasal a.	a. lateralis nasi (NAV), ramus lateralis nasi rostralis (NAV-ruminants)	from the facial a. (horses) or the infraorbital a. (dogs and pigs)	an a. to the side of the muzzle
lateral plantar a.	a. plantaris lateralis (NAV)	from the caudal branch of the saphenous a.	this a. runs over the lateral side of the plantar aspect of the hock; it is a major contributor to the deep plantar arch from which the plantar metatarsal aa. arise
lateral tarsal a.	a. tarsea lateralis (NAV)	from the dorsal pedal a.	this is a small a. that supplies the dorsolateral parts of the hock in all species bar the horse
lateral thoracic a.	a. thoracica lateralis (NAV), formerly called the external thoracic a.	from the axillary a. (carnivores) or the external thoracic a. (pigs)	it is found only in the pig and carnivores and runs in the axilla between the deep pectoral and the latissimus dorsi; it also gives off lateral mammary branches
left colic a.	a. colica sinistra (NAV)	from the caudal mesenteric a.	the a. runs a straight, cranially directed course within the mesocolon in most species, supplying the descending colon; the extensive small colon of the horse means the a. is divided into several long branches in this species
left coronary a.	a. coronaria sinistra (NAV)	the left sinus of the aortic bulb	the vessel runs between the atria and the ventricles and emerges onto the surface of the heart just caudal to the pulmonary trunk; the paraconal branch runs in the interventricular groove to the apex of the heart while the circumflex runs in the coronary groove in which it ends in pigs and horses; in dogs and ruminants it continues as a subsinuosal branch
left gastric a.	a. gastrica sinistra (NAV)	one of the three main branches of the celiac a., sometimes arising from the splenic a.	the a. reaches the cardia via the gastrophrenic ligament and runs along the lesser curvature to anastomose with the right gastric a.; in ruminants it passes cranioventrally over the right side of the rumen to reach the abomasum where it becomes the left gastroepiploic a.
left gastroepiploic a.	a. gastroepiploica sinistra (NAV)	from the splenic a. (most species) or the left gastric a. (ruminants)	the a. runs along the greater curvature of the stomach (or the abomasum) and anastomoses with the right gastroepiploic a.; it gives off epiploic branches to the omentum and short gastric aa. to the stomach
left ruminal a.	a. ruminalis sinistra (NAV)	the celiac a. or one of its branches	despite its name the a. runs first on the right of the rumen, then passes along the cranial groove to gain the left longitudinal groove of the rumen

lesser palatine a.	a. palatina minor (NAV)	from the descending palatine a. (most species) or the maxillary a. (cat)	this vessel supplies the soft palate
ligamentum arteriosum (NAV)		the pulmonary trunk	this ligament is the atrophied remnant of the ductus arteriosus; the left recurrent laryngeal nerve passes around it; in aberrant cases it can contribute to the formation of congenital vascular rings around the esophagus
lingual a.	a. lingualis (NAV)	the external carotid a. (dogs, pigs, sheep and goats) or the linguofacial trunk (horses and cattle)	a large branch of the external carotid that is the principal a. to the tongue; once it reaches the root of the tongue it is called the deep lingual a.; in some species it gives off ascending palatine, perihyoid and sublingual branches
linguofacial trunk	truncus linguofacialis (NAV), external maxillary a.	the external carotid a.	an arterial pattern found in horses and cattle in which the lingual and facial aa. share a common origin
long posterior ciliary aa.	aa. ciliares posteriores longae (NAV)	from the external ophthalmic a. (ruminants) or from the union of both the internal and external ophthalmic aa. (others)	these vessels pierce the posterior part of the sclera and run forwards between the choroid and sclera to the ciliary body; they give off the short posterior ciliary aa. to the choroid and the episcleral aa. to the external surface of the sclera
lumbar aa.	aa. lumbales (NAV)	from the abdominal aorta and median sacral a.	these are paired segmental aa. that supply the local vertebrae, spinal cord, skin and back muscles and may contribute to the dorsal part of the flank
malar a.	a. malaris (NAV)	from the infraorbital a. (dogs and horses) or the maxillary a. (ruminants and pigs)	an a. that runs on the floor of the orbit forwards the medial corner of the eye, supplying the eyelids and adjacent structures
mandibular alveolar a.	*see* inferior alveolar a.		
mandibular labial a.	*see* inferior labial a.		this name for the inferior labial a. appeared in earlier editions of the NAV
maxillary a.	a. maxillaris (NAV), internal maxillary a.	from the external carotid a.	this continuation of the external carotid a. mainly supplies the orbit and upper jaw and in some species the brain; its main branches typically include the inferior alveolar, rostral tympanic, middle meningeal, deep temporal, external ophthalmic, buccal, infraorbital and descending palatine aa.
maxillary labial a.	*see* superior labial a.		this name for the superior labial a. appeared in earlier editions of the NAV
medial circumflex femoral a.	a. circumflexa femoris medialis (NAV)	the a. is a terminal branch of the deep femoral a.	this a. runs in the adductors and some parts of the hamstrings; it gives off obturator, acetabular, deep, ascending and transverse branches; the deep branch anastomoses with the lateral circumflex femoral a.
medial palmar a.	a. digitalis palmaris communis II (NAV—horse)	a continuation of the median a. beyond the carpus	this is the largest a. of the cannon region of the horse's forelimb; it runs between the tendons of the interosseous and deep digital flexor muscles; it divides in the distal quarter of the metacarpus into medial and lateral palmar (proper) digital aa.
medial plantar a.	a. plantaris medialis (NAV)	from the caudal branch of the saphenous a.	this a. runs over the medial side of the plantar aspect of the hock; it is a major contributor to the deep plantar arch from which the plantar metatarsal aa. arise
medial tarsal a.	a. tarsea medialis (NAV)	from the dorsal pedal a.	this is a small a. that supplies the dorsomedial parts of the hock in all species bar the horse
median a.	a. mediana (NAV)	the continuation of the brachial a.	this is the major a. of the forearm except in the cat; it begins just distal to the elbow where, in the horse, it can be used to take the pulse; it courses down the caudomedial aspect of the forearm and typically gives off the radial a. and in some species the deep antebrachial a. before contributing to the palmar carpal arches

Table continued over page

9 Arteries *(Continued)*

Artery	Other names	Origin	Comments
median caudal a.	a. caudalis mediana (NAV), middle tail a.	a direct continuation of the median sacral a. (most species) or the left or right caudal gluteal a. (horses)	this is usually the largest a. of the tail and runs in the midline on its ventral surface (unpaired); in some species hemal arches or chevron bones protect the a. as it passes over the intervertebral joints; the a. can be used for taking the pulse, especially in cattle
median sacral a.	a. sacralis mediana (NAV)	from the terminal trifurcation of the aorta	the a. is a direct continuation of the aorta that leads directly into the median caudal a.; it gives off sacral branches, and is often absent from the horse
meningeal aa.	*see* rostral, middle and caudal meningeal aa.		
middle a. of the penis/clitoris	a. penis/clitoridis media (NAV)	from the obturator a.	this a., only found in horses, is a major source of blood to the penis or clitoris
middle caudal femoral a.	a. caudalis femoris media (NAV)	from the femoral a.	the middle member of three aa. that are directed caudally into the medial muscles of the thigh
middle cerebral a.	a. cerebri media (NAV)	from the cerebral arterial circle near the termination of the internal carotid a.	this is the largest vessel supplying the brain; it runs over the ventral and lateral surface to supply much of the cerebral cortex; it gives off choroidal and cortical branches
middle colic a.	a. colica media (NAV)	from the cranial mesenteric a. (ruminants), the ileocolic a. (dogs) or the right colic a. (pigs and horses)	this is a relatively small a. that supplies the transverse colon; it anastomoses with the right and left colic aa.
middle meningeal a.	a. meningea media (NAV)	from the maxillary a. (dogs, pigs and horses) or the occipital a. (ruminants)	the a. enters the cranium via the foramen ovale in dogs and ruminants, and via the foramen lacerum orale in horses and pigs; it ramifies in the dura; in pigs it supplies a branch to the rostral epidural rete mirabile
middle rectal a.	a. rectalis media (NAV)	from the vaginal or prostatic a.	this is the terminal branch of the genital a. and it anastomoses in the rectal wall with the cranial and caudal rectal aa.
musculophrenic a.	a. musculophrenica (NAV)	from the internal thoracic a.	this terminal branch of the internal thoracic a. runs subperitoneally between the interdigitations of the diaphragm and transverse abdominis muscles; it gives off ventral intercostal branches
obturator a.	a. obturatoria (NAV)	from the cranial gluteal a. (most species), the iliolumbar a. (pigs) or the internal iliac a. (sheep)	the a. runs along the shaft of the ilium to the cranial border of the obturator foramen which it navigates before joining (in some species) branches of the deep femoral a.; in horses it gives off the iliacofemoral and the middle penile (or clitorine) aa; it is usually absent from dogs and cattle.
occipital a.	a. occipitalis (NAV)	from the external carotid a. (dogs and horses) or the internal carotid a. (pigs and ruminants)	this a. arises just after the terminal bifurcation of the common carotid a. and runs to the muscles of the nape and poll; it usually anastomoses with the vertebral a. and thus contributes to the basilar a.; typically it gives off condylar and caudal meningeal aa.
omocervical a.	*see* superficial cervical a.		

ovarian a.	a. ovarica (NAV)	from the abdominal aorta	like the testicular a. the terminal part of the ovarian a. is highly contorted and intimately related to the ovarian vein—a relationship that may serve for transvascular hormonal exchange; it gives off a tubal and a uterine branch (formerly called the cranial uterine a.)
palatine aa.	*see* ascending, descending, greater and lesser palatine aa. and the sphenopalatine a.		
palmar common digital aa.	aa. digitales palmares communes I–IV (NAV), medial palmar a. (horses)	from the superficial palmar arch (if present) or branches of the median, radial and other aa.	these aa. provide the principal blood supply to the toes; they run between the metacarpal bones and distally unite with the palmar metacarpal aa. to form larger vessels that divide between the digits into the palmar proper digital aa.
palmar (digital) aa. (horses)	a. digitalis lateralis/medialis (NAV), a. digitalis palmaris propria III (NAV)	from the medial palmar a.	this is a special, simpler, name applied to the palmar proper digital arteries of the horse; the medial and lateral aa. run on the palmar surface of the pastern and end by uniting in the solar canal of the distal phalanx in a terminal arch
palmar metacarpal aa.	aa. metacarpeae palmares (NAV)	from the deep palmar arch	these aa. are deep vessels that run between the metacarpal bones and distally unite with the palmar common digital aa.
palmar proper digital aa.	aa. digitales palmares propriae (NAV)	from the division of the palmar common digital aa.	with the dorsal proper digital aa. these vessels make up the blood supply to the toes; they are named axial or abaxial according to their relation to the axis of the foot (except in horses where they are termed simply lateral or medial)
pancreatic aa.	*see* cranial and caudal pancreaticoduodenal aa.		
penile aa.	*see* a. of the penis and a. of the penile bulb, and cranial, dorsal, deep and middle aa. of the penis		
perforating tarsal aa.	a. tarsea perforans distalis/proximalis (NAV)	from the dorsal pedal a.	a distal perforating tarsal a. is found in all species except carnivores (pigs have a proximal one too); the a. passes through the tarsus to contribute to the deep plantar arch
perineal aa.	*see* dorsal and ventral perineal aa.		
phrenic aa.	*see* caudal and cranial phrenic phrenicoabdominal and musculophrenic aa.		
phrenicoabdominal a.		from the abdominal aorta	this a. is found in carnivores and is a common trunk of the caudal phrenic and cranial abdominal aa. of other species
plantar common digital aa.	aa. digitales plantares communes I–IV (NAV)	from the medial plantar a. or the deep plantar arch	these are the superficial aa. on the sole of the foot; they unite with the plantar metatarsal aa. and perforating branches from the dorsum to form larger vessels that divide between the digits to form the plantar proper digital aa.
plantar digital aa. (horses)	a. digitalis lateralis/medialis (NAV), a. digitalis plantaris propria III (NAV)	from the perforating branch of the dorsal metatarsal a. plus a number of small uniting vessels	these aa. are essentially similar to the palmar digital aa. of the forelimb, differing only in their origin

Table continued over page

9 Arteries *(Continued)*

Artery	Other names	Origin	Comments
plantar metatarsal aa.	aa. metatarseae plantares (NAV)	from the deep plantar arch	these aa. are deep vessels that run between the metatarsal bones and distally unite with the plantar common digital aa.
plantar proper digital aa.	aa. digitales plantares propriae (NAV)	from the division of the plantar common digital aa.	with the dorsal proper digital aa. these vessels make up the blood supply to the toes; they are named axial or abaxial according to their relation to the axis of the foot (except in horses where they are termed simply lateral or medial)
popliteal a.	a. poplitea (NAV)	this is continuation of the femoral a.	the a. is located close to the caudal surface of the stifle joint; it runs between the heads of the gastrocnemius and gives off the caudal tibial a. and, in some species, a crural interosseous a. before continuing as the cranial tibial a.; it supplies numerous branches to the stifle joint and its articular rete
posterior ciliary aa.	*see* long and short posterior ciliary aa.		
posterior conjunctival aa.	aa. conjunctivales posteriores (NAV)	from the external ophthalmic a. or its branches	these vessels run along the sclera to reach the conjunctival fornices
proper digital aa.	*see* palmar, plantar and dorsal proper digital aa.	arise from the division of the common digital aa.	the basic scheme of the arterial supply to the digits is for each digit to be supplied with four aa., one located at each quadrant; they are derived from the division of the dorsal and palmar common digital aa.
prostatic a.	a. prostatica (NAV), urogenital a., urethrogenital a.	from the internal pudendal a. (horses and carnivores) or the internal iliac a. (pigs and ruminants)	this is the main a. of the pelvic viscera in males; it is homologous with the vaginal a.; it passes over the side of the rectum and gives off a caudal vesical a. and an a. of the deferent duct and, after supplying the prostate, ends as the middle rectal a.
proximal caudal femoral a.	a. caudalis femoris proximalis (NAV)	from the femoral a.	the proximal member of three aa. that are directed caudally into the medial muscles of the thigh
pudendoepigastric trunk	truncus pudendoepigastricus (NAV)	from the deep femoral a., or rarely, the external iliac a.	this is a short a. that runs forwards from the pubic brim to the medical part of the deep inguinal ring, where it divides into the caudal epigastric and the external pudendal aa.
pulmonary aa.	a. pulmonalis dextra/sinistra (NAV)	the pulmonary trunk	the right and left pulmonary aa. arise from the pulmonary trunk; the right a. passes ventral to the trachea to reach the hilus; each a. divides into lobar aa. that tend to run on the lateral side of the companion bronchi
pulmonary trunk	truncus pulmonalis (NAV)	the right ventricle	a short, elastic a. of similar diameter to the aorta but with somewhat thinner walls; it rapidly divides into the right and left pulmonary aa.
radial a.	a. radialis (NAV)	from the median a.	the site of origin of the a. varies between species, it arising in the proximal forearm in the dog and the distal forearm in the horse and cat; it gives off dorsal and palmar branches to the carpal rete and carpal arches
rectal aa.	*see* cranial, middle and caudal rectal aa.		
recurrent ulnar a.	a. recurrens ulnaris (NAV)	from the ulnar a.	this a. unites the ulnar and collateral ulnar aa. of carnivores

renal a.	a. renalis (NAV)	from the abdominal aorta	the renal aa. arise beneath the first to the fourth lumbar vertebrae depending on the species, the right usually cranial to the left; they transmit about one fifth of the cardiac output; each divides into dorsal and ventral branches which give off an array of interlobar aa. within the substance of the kidney; the a. also has caudal adrenal and ureteric branches
rete carpi dorsale	*see* dorsal carpal rete		
rete mirabile branches	ramus and rete mirabile epidurale rostrale (NAV)	the maxillary a. or its branches	ruminants usually have rostral and caudal branches that pierce the oval and orbitorotund foramina to supply the epidural rete
reticular a.	a. reticularis (NAV)	from the left ruminal a.	this a. runs along the left side of the rumen and before entering the ruminoreticular groove gives off esophageal branches and sometimes phrenic branches
right colic a.	a. colica dextra (NAV), aa. colicae dextrae (NAV—ruminants)	from the cranial mesenteric a. (pigs and horses) or the ileocolic a. (carnivores and ruminants)	this a. provides the principal supply to the ascending colon and is thus large in herbivores which have a well-developed ascending colon; its branches pass over and along the coils of the spiral colon of ruminants and pigs, and between the dorsal and ventral segments of the large colon of the horse; it is in continuity with branches of the middle colic and ileocolic aa.
right coronary a.	a. coronaria dextra (NAV)	the right sinus of the aortic bulb	the vessel runs between the atria and ventricles to emerge onto the cranial surface of the heart to the right of the pulmonary trunk; its circumflex branch runs in the coronary groove where it fades out in dogs and ruminants; in pigs and horses it continues as the subsinuosal branch within the subsinuosal interventricular groove
right gastric a.	a. gastrica dextra (NAV)	from the hepatic a.	the a. courses to the pyloric region in the lesser omentum and anastomoses with the left gastric a.; in ruminants the a. first joins the duodenum and runs orally to the pylorus; it gives off pancreatic and gastric branches
right gastroepiploic a.	a. gastroepiploica dextra (NAV)	one of the terminal branches of the gastroduodenal a.	the a. runs along the greater curvature of the stomach or the abomasum and anastomoses with the left gastroepiploic a.; it gives off epiploic branches to the omentum and short gastric aa. to the stomach
right ruminal a.	a. ruminalis dextra (NAV)	usually from the splenic a.	this a. is the principal supply to the rumen; it runs caudally along the right face of the organ, and then within the right accessory, caudal and left longitudinal grooves, giving off right and left, dorsal and ventral coronary aa.
rostral auricular a.	a. auricularis rostralis (NAV)	from the superficial temporal a.	this branch ascends behind the temporomandibular joint to ramify in the rostral auricular and temporal muscles
rostral cerebellar a.	a. cerebelli rostralis (NAV)	from the caudal communicating a.	the vessel runs around the brain stem between the colliculi and the cerebellar hemispheres to the vermis, supplying these structures en route
rostral cerebral a.	a. cerebri rostralis (NAV)	from the internal carotid a.	this artery runs from the internal carotid a. forwards to the longitudinal fissure of the brain where it unites with its fellow; it may give off a separate bridging rostral communicating a. that unites with its fellow; its final course is along the corpus callosum; it gives off the internal ophthalmic and internal ethmoidal aa.
rostral communicating a.	a. communicans rostralis (NAV)	from the rostral cerebral a.	the union between the two rostral cerebral aa. is often by this separate small vessel
rostral meningeal a.	a. meningea rostralis (NAV)	from the external or internal ethmoidal aa.	this a. supplies the dura of the rostral part of the cranium

Table continued over page

9 Arteries *(Continued)*

Artery	Other names	Origin	Comments
saphenous a.	a. saphena (NAV)	from the femoral a. in the proximal part of the thigh	the a. runs a superficial course over the medial aspect of the limb, often dividing near the stifle into cranial and caudal branches; the cranial branch reaches the hock and in some forms the dorsal common digital a.; the caudal branch runs to the sole where it gives off the lateral and medial plantar aa.
short gastric aa.	aa. gastricae breves (NAV)	from the splenic a.	these are short vessels that detach from the splenic a. and supply the greater curvature of the fundic region of the simple stomach
short posterior ciliary aa.	aa. ciliares posteriores breves (NAV)	the long posterior ciliary aa.	these vessels arise from the long posterior ciliary aa. and pierce the sclera near the optic nerve; they supply the choroid
sphenopalatine a.	a. sphenopalatina (NAV)	from the descending palatine a.	this vessel runs rapidly through the sphenopalatine foramen to enter the nasal chambers where it gives off the lateral and septal caudal nasal aa. that supply the richly vascular nasal mucous membrane
splenic a.	a. lienalis (NAV)	one of the three main branches of the celiac a.	it not only supplies the spleen (by splenic branches) but also continues as the left gastroepiploic a. (in simple stomached animals); it gives off the short gastric aa. to the stomach and epiploic branches to the omentum; in ruminants it gives off the right ruminal a. and pancreatic branches
stylomastoid a.	a. stylomastoidea (NAV)	the caudal auricular a. (dogs, ruminants), condylar a. (pigs) or deep auricular a. (horses)	a small a. that passes along the facial nerve through the stylomastoid foramen to supply the middle ear
subcarpal arch	*see* deep palmar arch		
subclavian a.	a. subclavia (NAV)	the right a. always arises from the brachiocephalic trunk; the left a. also arises from the brachiocephalic in horses and ruminants and from the aortic arch in pigs and dogs	this is the principal a. to the limb, continuing as the axillary a.; its main branches in the dog are the vertebral a., the costocervical trunk, and the superficial cervical and internal thoracic aa.; in pigs and ruminants the deep cervical a. also arises from it; in horses the vertebral a. comes off the costocervical trunk instead
sublingual a.	a. sublingualis (NAV)	from the lingual a. (pigs and ruminants) or the submental a. (dogs and horses)	the a. runs along the dorsal surface of the geniohyoid muscle, supplying the ventral parts of the tongue, the floor of the mouth, the frenulum linguae and the sublingual glands
subscapular a.	a. subscapularis (NAV)	from the axillary a.	a large a. that runs along the caudal border of the scapula; it gives off the caudal circumflex humeral, thoracodorsal and circumflex scapular aa. which, with the parent a., mainly supply the muscles caudal to the shoulder
superficial brachial a.	a. superficialis brachialis	from the brachial a.	this a. is only present in carnivores; it runs over the flexor aspect of the elbow and becomes the cranial superficial antebrachial a.
superficial cervial a.	a. cervicalis superficialis (NAV), omocervical a.	from the subclavian a.	this a. supplies the muscles around the base of the neck and the shoulder; it gives off deltoid, ascending and prescapular branches and the suprascapular a.
superficial circumflex iliac a.	a. circumflexa ilium superficialis (NAV)	from the femoral a. (dogs) or lateral circumflex femoral a. (cats)	this a., found only in carnivores, supplies the muscles on the cranial aspect of the thigh beneath the ilium

superficial cranial epigastric a.	a. epigastrica cranialis superficialis (NAV)	from the cranial epigastric a.	this a. of carnivores and ruminants runs caudally in the subcutis from near the xiphoid; it gives off mammary branches in carnivores
superficial dorsal arch	arcus dorsalis superficialis (NAV)	the cranial superficial antebrachial a. and the dorsal carpal branch of the cranial interosseous and sometimes other aa.	this delicate vascular network over the dorsum of the carpus is not always present; it gives off the dorsal common digital aa.
superficial palmar arch	arcus palmaris superficialis (NAV), supracarpal ach	from the superficial palmar branch of the radial a. plus a major vessel that varies according to species	the superficial palmar arch forms an anastomotic loop on the flexor surface of the metacarpus which gives off the palmar common digital aa. that run between the metacarpal bones; unlike the deep arch the superficial arch is sometimes absent
superficial temporal a.	a. temporalis superficialis (NAV)	the external carotid a.	one of the terminal branches of the external carotid that typically supplies the region between the ear and eye and usually gives off the transverse facial, rostral auricular and lateral palpebral aa.; in ruminants it also gives off the cornual a.
superior labial a.	a. labialis superior (NAV), maxillary labial a., a. of the upper lip	from the facial a. (most species), the buccal a. (pigs) or the transverse facial a. (sheep and goats)	in the horse this is the second vessel to be given off the facial a. after it has emerged onto the face; it typically runs a course parallel with the mandible to reach the upper lip
supracarpal arch	*see* superficial palmar arch		
supraorbital a.	a. supraorbitalis (NAV)	from the external ophthalmic or neighboring aa.	a small vessel that supplies the eyelids and adjacent forehead; in the horse it passes through the supraorbital foramen; it is absent in the dog
suprarenal aa.	*see* adrenal aa.		
suprascapular a.	a. suprascapularis (NAV)	from the superficial cervical a. (dogs and sheep), the caudal circumflex humeral a. (pigs) or the axillary a. (horses and cattle)	this a. supplies the stabilizing muscles of the shoulder, especially the supraspinatus and infraspinatus; it gives off an acromial branch in some species
supratrochlear a.	a. supratrochlearis (NAV)	from the external ophthalmic a.	a branch best developed in pigs that supplies the medial side of the orbit and upper eyelid
supreme intercostal a.	a. intercostalis suprema (NAV)	from the costocervical trunk	this vessel runs inside the thorax by the side of the vertebral bodies and gives origin to the first few dorsal intercostal aa.; it is absent in the dog
tail aa.	*see* median caudal a.	the median sacral and caudal gluteal aa.	there are typically nine main aa. running along the tail; paired lateral caudal, dorsolateral caudal, ventrolateral caudal and ventral caudal aa., and the unpaired median caudal a., which is the largest
testicular a.	a. testicularis (NAV), internal spermatic a.	from the abdominal aorta	the origin of this a. reflects the embryological origin of the gonad; its course is initially straight until it reaches the internal inguinal ring where it forms a major component of the spermatic cord; from here it becomes highly contorted and is embedded in the pampiniform plexus of veins that probably function for heat exchange; it reaches the testis at the head of the epididymis and gives off branches to the epididymis and deferent duct

Table continued over page

9 Arteries *(Continued)*

Artery	Other names	Origin	Comments
thoracic aorta	aorta thoracica (NAV)	in the strict sense from the termination of the aortic arch, but usually from the left ventricle	this is the intrathoracic part of the descending aorta that runs beneath the vertebral bodies to pierce the diaphragm at the aortic hiatus; its main branches are the dorsal intercostal, costoabdominal and broncho-esophageal aa., and in the horse the cranial phrenic aa.
thoracic vertebral a.	a. vertebralis thoracica (NAV)	from the costocervical trunk	this a. of the dog performs a similar role to the supreme intercostal of other species by giving off the second and third dorsal intercostal aa.
thoracodorsal a.	a. thoracodorsalis (NAV)	from the subscapular a.	this a. runs along the medial surface of the latissimus dorsi muscle, which it supplies together with the pectorals and axillary lymph centre
thyroid aa.	*see* cranial and caudal thyroid aa.		
transverse colli a.	*see* dorsal scapular a.		
transverse cubital a.	a. transversa cubiti (NAV)	from the brachial a. near the elbow	this a. crosses the flexor aspect of the elbow and supplies the carpal and digital extensors and other local muscles before passing down the forearm
transverse facial a.	a. transversa faciei (NAV)	the superficial temporal a.	the vessel runs over the masseter, to which it sends branches; in ruminants the rostral end is large and supplies aa. to the upper and lower lips
ulnar a.	a. ulnaris (NAV)	from the common interosseous a. (dogs) or the caudal interosseous a. (cats)	this vessel is only found in carnivores; it runs amidst the flexors of the carpus and paw with the ulnar nerve, giving off the recurrent ulnar a.
umbilical a.	a. umbilicalis (NAV)	from the internal iliac a. (carnivores, pigs and cattle) or the internal pudendal a. (horses)	this a. conducts blood to the placenta via the navel and umbilical cord in the fetus; it reaches the umbilicus by coursing in the lateral ligament of the bladder and accompanying the urachus; in the adult its distal remnant forms the round ligament of the bladder in the free border of the lateral ligament; depending on the species it may give off the cranial vesical and uterine aa. and the a. of the ductus deferens
urethral a.	a. urethralis (NAV)	from the internal pudendal a.	the a. supplies the pelvic urethra, especially its more caudal part; it is absent in the horse
urethrogenital a.	*see* vaginal a. and prostatic a.		
urogenital a.	*see* vaginal a. and prostatic a.		
uterine a.	a. uterina (NAV), middle uterine a., caudal uterine a.	from the umbilical a. (pigs and ruminants), the external iliac a. (horses) or the vaginal a. (carnivores)	this is the main a. to the uterus in all species; it runs in the broad ligament, dividing into several branches that anastomose with the uterine branches of the ovarian and vaginal aa.; it enlarges strikingly during pregnancy; when palpated in pregnant cows it yields a characteristic fremitus or thrill from about the third month of pregnancy
vaginal a.	a. vaginalis (NAV), urogenital a., urethrogenital a.	from the internal pudendal a. (horses and carnivores) or the internal iliac a. (pigs and ruminants)	this a., the homologue of the prostatic a. of the male, gives off a uterine a. or branch, and a dorsal perineal a. in pigs and ruminants; as in the male it gives off a caudal vesical a. and ends as the middle rectal a.

ventral perineal a.	a. perinealis ventralis (NAV)	a terminal branch of the internal pudendal a.	this a. supplies the perineum; it usually gives off the caudal rectal a. to the anus and dorsal labial or scrotal branches; in cattle it contributes a branch to the mammary gland.
vertebral a.	a. vertebralis (NAV)	from the subclavian a. (dogs), the costocervical trunk (horses), or the left subclavian a. (left a.) or the brachiocephalic trunk (right a.) (pigs and ruminants)	this a. runs mostly in the transverse canal of the cervical vertebrae, giving off spinal rami that supply the spinal cord and vertebral bodies; after anastomosing with the occipital a. it enters the vertebral canal via the lateral vertebral foramen of the atlas; it unites with its fellow to form the basilar a., which supplies the caudal part of the brain in dogs and horses; in the ox the a. mostly enters the vertebral canal between the axis and the third cervical vertebra and contributes to the blood supply to the whole brain; in the sheep it usually contributes little to the cerebral flow; its significance relates to the maintenance of consciousness during ritual slaughter
vesical aa.	*see* cranial and caudal vesical aa.		
vestibular a.	a. vestibularis (NAV)	from the internal pudendal a.	this a. is restricted to cows and supplies the wall of the vaginal vestibule

Table prepared by John Grandage.

10 Bones

Bone	Other names	Comments
accessory carpal bone	os carpi accessorium (NAV), os pisiforme (NAV), pisiform	the atypical carpal bone that projects to the palmar side of the wrist or knee; it serves as a sesamoid bone for flexors of the carpus
aitch-bone		*see* hip bone
angulare (NAA)		*see* mandible
ankle bone		*see* talus
anvil		*see* incus
apparatus hyoideus (NAV)		*see* hyoid bone
articulare (NAA)		*see* mandible
astragalus		*see* talus
atlas (NAV)	C1, first cervical vertebra	a specialized ring-like cervical vertebra that has no body, a wide vertebral canal for accommodation of the tooth-like process (dens), broad wing-like transverse processes and articular surfaces for synovial joints with the occipital condyle(s) and the axis
axis (NAV)	C2, dentata, epistropheus, second cervical vertebra	a specialized cervical vertebra that forms a pivot joint with the atlas through the tooth-like process (dens) that it bears on the cranial end of its body
baculum		*see* os penis
basihyoid bone	basihyal, basihyoideum (NAV), os basibrachiale rostrale (NAA), corpus ossis hyoidei	the unpaired, median, body of the hyoid bone, found near the root of the tongue; it usually bears horns that articulate with the skull and with the larynx
basioccipital	os basioccipitale (NAV)	the bone that forms the floor of the caudal part of the skull and which in birds bears a single condyle for articulation with the vertebral column
basisphenoid	os basisphenoidale (NAV)	a bone at the base of the skull between the basioccipital and presphenoid, from which it is separated by cartilaginous joints; its dorsal surface is dished to receive the pituitary and it bears a pair of large temporal wings, the alisphenoids
breastbone		*see* sternum
calcaneus (NAV)	calcaneum, fibular tarsal bone, heel bone, os calcis	the elongated tarsal bone beneath the point of the hock that bears a tuber on its summit for muscle insertion
cannon bone		*see* metacarpal bones 1–5, metatarsal bones 1–5
capitate		*see* carpal bone III
carpal bones	ossa carpi (NAV), wrist bones	primitively 12 bones in three rows; now from two bones (e.g. fowl) to eight bones (e.g. horse) disposed in two rows
carpal bone I	C1, first carpal, os carpale I (NAV), trapezium (NAV)	the first and most medial of the distal row of carpal bones, often missing in the horse and some other species
carpal bone II	C2, os carpale II (NAV), os trapezoideum (NAV), second carpal, trapezoid	the second bone from the medial side of the distal row of carpal bones; in ruminants it is fused to carpal bone III
carpal bone III	C3, capitate, magnum, os carpale III (NAV), os capitatum (NAV), third carpal	the third of the four bones in the distal row of carpal bones; it is large in the horse and in ruminants it is fused to carpal bone II
carpal bone IV	C4, fourth carpal, hamate, os carpale IV (NAV), os hamatum (NAV)	the most lateral of the distal row of carpal bones; in carnivores it articulates with metacarpals 4 and 5
carpometacarpus (NAA)		the largest bony element of the manus (hand) of a bird's wing, made up of several fused metacarpal, carpal and phalangeal bones

10 Bones *(Continued)*

Bone	Other names	Comments
caudal vertebrae	coccygeal vertebrae, tail bones, vertebrae caudales (NAV)	the relatively simple bones of the tail that often consist of a body only, although the proximal ones bear a neural arch and hemal processes; numbers vary widely both within and between species from three to 25
central tarsal bone	centrale, os naviculare (NAV), os tarsi centrale (NAV), scaphoid	the bone in the center of the hock sandwiched between the talus and the distal tarsals; it is fused to the fourth tarsal bone in ruminants
centrale		*see* central tarsal bone
ceratobranchial	os ceratobranchiale (NAA)	the bone forming the first (ventral) part of the horns of the avian hyoid apparatus
ceratohyoid	ceratohyoideum (NAV)	the segment of the mammalian hyoid apparatus that runs cranially from the basihyoid to the eiphyoid on each side
cervical vertebrae	vertebrae cervicales (NAV)	the vertebrae of the neck; typically seven in mammals and a variable number (14–25) in birds; characterized by the presence of a transverse foramen that conducts the vertebral vessels
cheekbone		*see* zygomatic
clavicle	clavicula (NAV) collarbone, furcula (NAA), wishbone	a bracing element of the shoulder girdle that runs from the sternum to the scapula; it is well developed in animals that grasp but is reduced or absent from most domestic mammals; in birds the two clavicles are fused to form the wishbone (furcula) which may not meet the sternum
clod bone		*see* humerus
coccyx (NAA)		*see* pygostyle
coffin bone		*see* distal phalanx
collar bone		*see* clavicle
columella (NAA)	stapes	the only auditory ossicle of birds; it extends from the tympanic membrane to the vestibular window
coracoid	coracoideum (NAA)	a large bone of the avian thoracic girdle that runs from the scapula to the sternum; it braces the shoulder against the pull of the flight muscles; in eutherian mammals it is reduced to a process born on the scapula
costae (NAV)		*see* ribs
costae fluctuantes (NAV)		*see* floating ribs
costae spuriae (NAV)		*see* false ribs
costae sternales (NAV)		*see* true ribs
costae verae (NAV)		*see* true ribs
cuboid		*see* tarsal bone IV
cuneiform		*see* ulnar carpal bone, tarsal bone I, tarsal bone II, tarsal bone III
dentary		*see* mandible
dentata		*see* axis
distal phalanx	coffin bone, os unguiculare (NAV, carnivores), os ungulare (NAV, ungulates), P3, pedal bone, phalanx distalis (NAV), terminal phalanx, os pedis	the terminal bone of the digit; it articulates with the adjacent phalanx at the distal interphalangeal joint; in ungulates it supports the hoof, while in carnivores it bears an ungual crest that supports the claw matrix and an ungual process that supports the claw itself
distal sesamoid	navicular bone (horses), os sesamoideum distale (NAV)	the sesamoid bone found on the palmar or plantar surface of the coffin joint (distal interphalangeal joint) of ungulates, over which the deep digital flexor tendon plays

Table continued over page

10 Bones *(Continued)*

Bone	Other names	Comments
dorsal sesamoids	ossa sesamoidea dorsalia (NAV)	the sesamoid bones found in the extensor tendons as they pass over the joints of the digit; found in cattle, dogs and some other species
ear ossicles	ossicula auditus (NAV)	the chain of bones that conducts auditory impulses from the eardrum to the inner ear and that serves to convert oscillations in air to oscillations in fluid. *See* malleus, incus and stapes. In birds it consists of a single bone, the columella (q.v.)
ectethmoid bone	os ectethmoidale (NAA)	the lateral part of the ethmoid complex of the avian skull
entoglossal bone	os entoglossum (NAA), paraglossal bone	the part of the avian hyoid apparatus that lies within the tongue; it is usually shaped like an arrow-head
epibranchial bone	os epibranchiale (NAA)	the bone forming the end of the horns of the avian hyoid apparatus
epihyoid bone	epihyoideum (NAV)	the paired bone that makes up the segment of the mammalian hyoid apparatus between the ceratohyoid and the stylohyoid on each side; the bone is much reduced in horses
epistropheus		*see* axis
ethmoid bone	os ethmoidale (NAV). *See also* ectethmoid, mesethmoid	the bone forming the rostral boundary of the cranium; it is made up of a cribriform plate (through which olfactory nerves enter the cranium), a perpendicular plate (a caudal continuation of the nasal septum), and paired lateral masses composed of a labyrinth of ethmoturbinates (that include the dorsal and middle nasal conchae) that occupy the nasal chambers
exoccipital	os exoccipitale (NAA), the lateral part of the occipital	the paired skull bones that flank the foramen magnum and which in mammals bear condyles for articulation with the atlas
false ribs	costae spuriae (NAV)	ribs that do not articulate directly with the sternum; there are four pairs in the dog and cat, five in ruminants, seven or eight in pigs, and ten in horses
femur (NAV)	os femoris (NAV), roundbone, thigh bone	the long bone of the thigh; its spheroidal head articulates in the acetabulum, and its distal knuckle with the tibia; the neck is stout in the horse, less so in ruminants and pigs, and narrower still in dogs and cats; the femur possesses trochanters (processes) for muscular attachment—the third is conspicuous in the horse and rabbit
fibula (NAV)	brooch bone	the smaller of the two bones of the calf or leg that articulates with the tibia and in some species forms the lateral wall of the hock (ankle) joint; it is reduced or absent in ruminants and horses
fibular tarsal bone		*see* calcaneus
floating ribs	costae fluctuantes (NAV)	false ribs, whose distal ends do not unite with adjacent ribs; there is typically one pair in dogs, cats and pigs, and none in ruminants and horses
frontal bone	os frontale (NAV)	the membrane bone of the forehead; it is paired in domestic animals, but is usually single in the human skull
furcula (NAA)		*see* clavicle
hamate		*see* carpal bone IV
hammer		*see* malleus
hip bone	aitch-bone, innominate bone, os coxae (NAV)	a compound bone, made up of the ilium, ischium and pubis, that meets and usually fuses with its fellow at the pelvic symphysis ventrally and forms a joint with the sacrum dorsally; the three components meet at the cup-shaped acetabulum

10 **Bones** *(Continued)*

Bone	Other names	Comments
hock bones		*see* tarsal bones
holy bone		*see* sacrum
humerus (NAV)	arm bone, clod bone	the long bone of the upper arm that contributes to the shoulder and elbow joints
hyoid bone	apparatus hyoideus (NAV), hyoid apparatus, os hyoideum (NAV)	the paired chain of bones that serves to suspend the larynx and tongue from the skull. *See* individual bones: basihyoid, ceratohyoid, epihyoid, thyrohyoid, stylohyoid and tympanohyoid (mammals), and basibranchial ceratobranchial, entoglossal, epibranchial and urohyal (birds)
ilium	haunch bone, hook bone, os ilium (NAV)	the cranial part of the hip bone; it forms a firm joint with the sacrum and caudally at the acetabulum a fixed joint with the pubis and ischium; in large herbivores it is flared and bears a conspicuous coxal tuber that supports the body wall; in dogs and cats its cranial margin forms a rounded iliac crest
incisive bone	os incisivum (NAV), premaxilla	the paired bone at the front of the upper jaw that bears the incisor teeth
incus (NAV)	anvil	the middle of the mammalian ear ossicles; it lies between the malleus and stapes
innominate bone		*see* hip bone
intermediate carpal bone	lunar bone, os carpi intermedium (NAV), os lunatum (NAV), semilunar bone	the middle bone in the proximal row of carpals; in dogs and cats it is fused to the radial carpal bone
intermediate phalanges	phalanges intermediae (NAA)	the bones of the avian toes that lie between the proximal and distal phalanges; in the fowl digit 1 has zero, 2 has one, 3 has two, and 4 has three bones
interparietal bone	inca bone, os interparietale (NAV)	a skull bone found in the midline between the two parietals that often ossifies from two centers and bears the sagittal crest externally and the tentorial process on its deep face
ischium	pin bone, os ischii (NAV)	the caudal bone of the hip; it usually meets its fellow in the midline and the other components of the hip bone at the acetabulum; it bears the sciatic tubers that are subcutaneous in dogs and ruminants
jugal	os jugale (NAA). *See also* zygomatic bone (mammals)	the bone of the cheek; in birds it is involved in cranial kinesis (opening of the upper jaw)
kneecap		*see* patella
knucklebone		*see* talus
lacrimal bone	os lacrimale (NAV), os prefrontale (NAA), prefrontal bone (birds)	the delicate plate of bone forming the medial and ventral wall of the orbit that contains the first part of the tear duct; in some species it contains parts of the paranasal sinuses
lumbar vertebrae	backbone, vertebrae lumbales (NAV)	the vertebrae of the loins; there are usually seven in dogs and cats, and six in horses, pigs and ruminants; they bear long transverse processes that project laterally in ungulates and cranioventrally in carnivores
lunar bone		*see* intermediate carpal bone
magnum		*see* carpal bone III
malar		*see* zygomatic
malleus (NAV)	hammer	the ear ossicle attached to the inner surface of the eardrum

Table continued over page

10 Bones *(Continued)*

Bone	Other names	Comments
mandible	dentary, mandibula (NAV), lower jawbone; composed of six separate bones in birds and reptiles—the ossa mandibulae (NAA); os dentale, supraangulare, angulare, spleniale, prearticulare, articulare	the two halves are separate in carnivores and ruminants but fused in adult horses, pigs and humans composed of six separate bones in birds and reptiles —the ossa mandibulae (NAA)
maxilla (NAV)	os maxillare (NAA), upper jawbone	the principal bone of the upper jaw that bears the canine and cheek teeth and is frequently excavated to house the maxillary paranasal sinus(es)
mesethmoid bone	os mesethmoidale (NAA)	the skull bone of birds that forms a vertical interorbital septum
metacarpal bones 1–5	cannon bone (ungulates), ossa metacarpalia I–V (NAV), pastern bones (carnivores), splint bones (horses)	the bones of the palm that extend from the wrist or knee to the digits; in horses only the third is well developed, with 2 and 4 as splint bones; in ruminants 3 and 4 are fused
metatarsal bones 1–5	cannon bone (ungulates), ossa metatarsalia I–V (NAV), pastern bones (carnivores), splint bones (horses)	the bones of the sole that extend from the hock or ankle to the digits; in horses only the third is well developed, with 2 and 4 as splint bones; in ruminants 3 and 4 are fused
middle phalanx	os coronale (NAV), phalanx media (NAV), P2, second phalanx, small pastern bone	the middle bone of those digits that have three phalanges; in horses it lies between the pastern and coffin joints
nasal bone	os nasale (NAV)	a pair of bones forming the crest of the muzzle; the distal end is pointed in horses, double in cattle
nasal conchae	os conchae nasalis ventralis (NAV), turbinals, turbinate bones	the delicate scroll-like bones that occupy the nasal chambers and support the nasal mucous membrane; the dorsal conchae belong to the ethmoturbinate part of the ethmoid bone
navicular bone		*see* distal sesamoid, central tarsal bone
notarium (NAA)	os dorsale (NAA)	a specialized bone of the back of certain birds (e.g. fowl); formed from the fusion of from two to five vertebrae of the thoracic region
occipital bone	os occipitale (NAV)	the cranial bone that surrounds the foramen magnum; made up of basal, lateral and squamous parts; in birds it is considered to be composed of the basioccipital, exoccipital and supraoccipital parts (q.v.)
orbitosphenoid	os orbitosphenoidale (NAA)	*see also* presphenoid
os basibranchiale caudale (NAA)		*see* urohyal
os basibranchiale rostrale (NAA)		*see* basihyoid
os calcis		*see* calcaneus
os compedale (NAV)		*see* proximal phalanx
os coronale (NAV)		*see* middle phalanx
os coxae (NAV)		*see* hip bone
os cuboideum (NAV)		*see* tarsal bone IV
os cuneiforme intermedium (NAV)		*see* tarsal bone II
os cuneiforme laterale (NAV)		*see* tarsal bone III
os cuneiforme mediale (NAV)		*see* tarsal bone I
os dentale (NAA)		*see* mandible
os dorsale (NAA)		*see* notarium

10 Bones *(Continued)*

Bone	Other names	Comments
os hamatum (NAV)		*see* carpal bone IV
os ilium (NAV)		*see* ilium
os incisivum (NAV)		*see* incisive bone
os ischium (NAV)		*see* ischium
os lunatum (NAV)		*see* intermediate carpal bone
os naviculare (NAV)		*see* central tarsal bone, distal sesamoid
os pelvicum (NAA)		*see* synsacrum
os penis (NAV)	baculum, penis bone	the bone present in the penis of dogs, cats, seals, bats, some primates and rodents and other groups of mammals; it serves to support the organ
os pterygopalatinum (NAA)		*see* palatine bone
ossa carpi (NAV)		*see* carpal bones
ossa cordis (NAV)	heart bones	one or two small bones found within the fibrous skeleton of the heart of cattle, horses and some other animals
ossa tarsi (NAV)		*see* tarsal bones
os scaphoideum (NAV)		*see* radial carpal bone
ossicula auditus (NAV)		*see* ear ossicles
os squamosum (NAA)		*see* temporal bone
os suffraginis		*see* proximal phalanx
os tali		*see* talus
os trapezoideum (NAV)		*see* carpal bone II
os triquetrum (NAV)		*see* ulnar carpal bone
os unguiculare (NAV)		*see* distal phalanx
os ungulare (NAV)		*see* distal phalanx
otic bones	ossa otica (NAA), ear capsule bones: epiotic, opisthotic, and pro-otic bones	these avian bones correspond to the petrous and tympanic parts of the mammalian temporal bone
palatine bone	os palatinum (NAV), os pterygopalatinum	a paired bone found at the caudal margin of the hard palate, sometimes hollowed to contain a paranasal air sinus
paraglossal bone		*see* entoglossal bone
parasphenoid	os parasphenoidale (NAA)	part of the primitive sphenoid complex of birds and lower vertebrates
parietal bone	os parietale (NAV)	one of a pair of large membrane bones of the roof of the skull between the frontals and occipital
pastern bones		*see* proximal phalanx, middle phalanx, metacarpal bones 1–5, and metatarsal bones 1–5
patella (NAV)	kneecap	the largest sesamoid bone of the body, found in the tendon of the quadriceps muscle as it passes over the stifle (knee) joint; it is triangular in animals that have three patellar ligaments, and rod-like in animals with a single ligament; it is sometimes complemented with patellar cartilages and parapatellar cartilages
pedal bone		*see* distal phalanx
phalanges		*see* proximal phalanx, middle phalanx, intermediate phalanges, distal phalanx
pin bone		*see* ischium
pisiform		*see* accessory carpal bone

Table continued over page

10 Bones *(Continued)*

Bone	Other names	Comments
ploughshare bone		*see* pygostyle, vomer
prearticulare (NAA)		*see* mandible
prefrontal bone		*see* lacrimal bone
premaxilla	os premaxillare (NAA), the incisive bone (q.v.) of mammals	the largest bone of the upper beak of birds; it is subject to wide variation associated with beak shape
presphenoid	os presphenoidale (NAV)	the more rostral of the sphenoid bones; it lies beneath the optic chiasm and bears a pair of small orbital wings (orbitosphenoids)
proximal phalanx	large pastern bone (ungulates), os compedale (NAV), os suffraginis (ungulates), phalanx proximalis (NAV), Pl, pastern bone (ungulates)	the most proximal of the bones of the digit that in ungulates contributes to the fetlock and pastern joints
proximal sesamoids	ossa sesamoidea proximalia (NAV)	the pair of bones associated with the interosseous muscle that is found on the palmar surface of the metacarpophalangeal or metatarsophalangeal joint of each digit
pterygoid bone	os pterygoideum (NAV)	one of a pair of small skull bones associated with the caudal nares and often fused to the sphenoid
pterygopalatine bone		*see* palatine bone
pubis (NAV)		the medial element of the hip bone; it meets with its fellow in the midline to form the ventral boundary of the pelvic inlet; in most birds the two pubes do not meet at the symphysis but are directed caudally
pygostyle	coccyx (NAA), ploughshare bone, pygostylus (NAV), rump post, urostyle	the tailbone of birds, made up of three to six fused caudal vertebrae
quadrate	quadratum (NAA). *See also* incus	a small avian skull bone that forms a joint with the lower jaw and with adjacent elements in the skull; the incus is its mammalian homolog
quadratojugal	os quadratojugale (NAA)	a caudal bone of the avian cheek
radial carpal bone	os carpi radiale (NAV), os scaphoideum (NAV), radiointermediate, scaphoid, scapholunare	the most medial of the proximal row of carpal bones; in some species it represents the fusion of more than one carpal element; in birds it is one of the two remaining carpal bones
radius (NAV)		one of the two bones of the forearm; it bears a head for articulation with the humerus and a distal extremity for articulation with the carpus; in ungulates it is more or less fused with the ulna
ribs	costae (NAV)	the serially arranged, paired, long, thin, curved bones that form the lateral walls of the chest; they are made up of a dorsal (vertebral) bony part and a ventral cartilaginous part (mammals) or a bony sternal part (birds). *See also* true ribs, false ribs, floating ribs
rostral bone	os rostrale (NAV)	the bone of the snout that is best developed in pigs but is also found in cattle
rump post		*see* pygostyle
sacrum	holy bone, os sacrum (NAV), vertebrae sacrales (NAV)	the series of fused vertebrae that lie between the two hip bones; usually made up of five bones in horses and cattle, four in sheep and pigs, and three in dogs and cats
scaphoid		*see* radial carpal bone, central tarsal bone
scapula (NAV)	shoulder-blade	the principal bone of the mammalian thoracic girdle; typically flat and triangular, bearing a spine on its lateral surface and an articular glenoid at its ventral or lateral extremity for the shoulder joint; usually long, thin and flat in birds

10 Bones *(Continued)*

Bone	Other names	Comments
scleral bones	ossa sclerae (NAA)	the overlapping plates of bone that occupy the sclera of the avian eye near its corneal junction
semilunar		*see* intermediate carpal bone
sesamoids		*see* distal dorsal proximal
shoulder-blade		*see* scapula
sphenoid bones		*see* basisphenoid, presphenoid
spleniale (NAA)		*see* mandible
splint bones		*see* metacarpal bones 1–5, metatarsal bones 1–5
squamous		*see* temporal
stapes (NAV)	stirrup, columella	the third and deepest of the mammalian ear ossicles; it is shaped like a stirrup and its footplate oscillates against the oval window of the inner ear; in birds only the stapes is represented—*see* columella
sternal ribs		*see* true ribs
sternum (NAV)	breastbone	the median bone of the ventral thorax that articulates with true ribs; in mammals it is composed of a manubrium, body and xiphoid made up of individual sternebrae and cartilages (six sternebrae in pigs, seven in horses and ruminants, eight in cats and dogs); in birds the bone is large and variable; in flying birds it bears a carina or keel
stirrup		*see* stapes
stylohyoid bone	stylohyal, stylohyoideum (NAV)	the paired bone that makes up the segment of the mammalian hyoid apparatus between the epihyoid and the tympanohyoid on each side
supraangulare (NAA)		*see* mandible
supraoccipital	os supraoccipitale (NAA), the squamous part of the occipital bones	the largest part of the occipital bone; it makes up the roof of the foramen magnum and is the site of insertion of the nuchal ligament in some species
sutural bones	ossa suturarum (NAV), wormian bones	inconstant and variable bones that appear along the sutures of the skull, especially around the sites of the fontanelles
synsacrum (NAA)	os pelvicum, pelvic vertebrae	a rigid part of the avian skeleton, made up of fused lumbar and sacral vertebrae with some contributions from the thoracic and caudal vertebrae and the pelvic girdle
talus (NAV)	ankle bone, astragalus, knucklebone, os tali, tibial tarsal bone	the large tarsal bone that forms a mobile joint with the tibia at the hock, that bears a pulley-like surface (trochlea) at the proximal surface, and in some species, such as ruminants, a distal trochlea too
tarsal bones	hock bones, ossa tarsi (NAV)	the bones of the ankle or hock; primitively there were about 12 bones; in modern tetrapods there are about seven or fewer; in modern birds the tarsal bones are incorporated into the tibiotarsus and tarsometatarsus
tarsal bone I	os tarsale I (NAV), os cuneiforme mediale (NAV), first tarsal, medial cuneiform, T1	the most medial of the distal row of tarsal bones; in horses it is fused with tarsal bone II
tarsal bone II	os tarsale II (NAV), os cuneiforme intermedium (NAV), middle cuneiform, second tarsal, T2	the second of the distal row of tarsal bones; in horses it is fused with tarsal bone I
tarsal bone III	os tarsale III (NAV), os cuneiforme laterale (NAV), lateral cuneiform, third tarsal, T3	the third of the distal row of tarsal bones; in horses it is large for articulation with the cannon bone
tarsal bone IV	os tarsale IV (NAV), os cuboideum (NAV), cuboid, fourth tarsal, T4	the most lateral of the distal row of tarsal bones; it articulates with both the fourth and fifth metatarsals; in ruminants it is fused with the central tarsal bone

Tables continued over page

10 Bones *(Continued)*

Bone	Other names	Comments
tarsometatarsus (NAA)	cannon bone	the avian bone formed from the fusion of metatarsal bones II, III and IV and some distal tarsals
temporal bone	os temporale (NAV), os squamosum (NAA)	the bone making up a large part of the side of the skull; composed of a petrous part (pars petrosa) that houses the inner ear, tympanic (pars tympanica) and endotympanic (pars endotympanica—cat) parts that house the middle and part of the external ear, and a squamous part (pars squamosa) that contributes to the cranial wall and jaw articulation in mammals
thoracic vertebrae	vertebrae thoracicae (NAV), dorsal vertebrae	the vertebrae of the chest; characterized by facets for articulation with ribs; typically 13 in cats, dogs, cattle and sheep, 15 in pigs and 18 in horses; in birds they are often fused—*see* notarium, synsacrum
thyrohyoid bone	thyrohyoideum (NAV)	the paired bone that makes up the segment of the mammalian hyoid apparatus between the basihyoid and the thyroid cartilage on each side
tibia (NAV)	shinbone	the larger and more medial of the two bones of the 'crus' or 'leg' proper, articulating proximally, at the stifle joint, with the femur and fibula and distally, at the hock joint, with the talus and fibula—*see* tibiotarsus
tibial tarsal bone		*see* talus
tibiotarsus (NAA)	drumstick, shankbone	the large limb bone of birds that extends from the stifle to the ankle joints and that is composed of both tibial and tarsal elements
trapezium (NAV)		*see* carpal bone I
trapezoid		*see* carpal bone II
true ribs	costae sternales (NAV), costae verae (NAV), sternal ribs	ribs that articulate with the sternum; there are typically nine in dogs and cats, eight in horses and ruminants, and seven in pigs
turbinate bones		*see* nasal conchae
tympanohyoid	tympanohyoideum (NAV), tympanohyal	the paired element that makes up the segment of the mammalian hyoid apparatus between the stylohyoid and the skull on each side; it usually remains cartilaginous
ulna (NAV)		one of the two bones of the forearm; its proximal end is elongated to form the olecranon at the elbow; the narrow distal end articulates with the carpus; in horses the distal end is incorporated into the radius
ulnar carpal bone	os carpi ulnare (NAV), os triquetrum (NAV), cuneiform	the most lateral of the proximal row of carpal bones; amongst others it articulates with the accessory carpal bone; in birds it is one of the two carpal bones
urohyal	os basibranchiale caudale (NAA), urohyoid, keel	a caudally directed median element in the avian hyoid apparatus
urostyle		*see* pygostyle
vertebrae		*see* cervical vertebrae, thoracic vertebrae, lumbar vertebrae, caudal vertebrae, notarium, sacrum, synsacrum, pygostyle
vomer (NAV)	ploughshare bone, share bone	a gutter-shaped bone that supports the floor of the cartilaginous nasal septum
wishbone		*see* clavicle
wormian bones		*see* sutural bones
zygomatic	os zygomaticum (NAV), cheekbone, jugal, malar	the principal bone of the zygomatic arch

Table prepared by John Grandage.

11 Joints

Joint	Other names	Comments
accessory carpal joint	articulatio ossis carpi accessorii (NAV)	the synovial joint between the accessory carpal and ulnar carpal bones; this, the only joint in ruminants, is supplemented in many species by a second joint between the accessory carpal and the ulna (or fused radius and ulna); it is supported by several accessory carpal ligaments
amphiarthrosis		an outmoded term for a slightly moveable cartilaginous joint such as a symphysis (q.v.)
ankle joint		an ambiguous term in veterinary science that refers either to the hock joint (see tarsal joints) or to the fetlock joint (see metacarpophalangeal joint)
antebrachiocarpal joint	articulatio antebrachiocarpea (NAV), radiocarpal joint	the composite joint between the radius and ulna and the proximal row of carpal bones. In ungulates it allows much palmar flexion but is prevented from dorsal flexion by stop facets and palmar ligaments; it permits a range of motions in carnivores
atlantoaxial joint	articulatio atlantoaxialis (NAV), 'NO' joint	the pivot joint between the dens of the axis and the fovea in the atlas that mainly allows rotation of the head on the neck; the dens is anchored by a ligament to the floor of the atlas (horses), or to the margin of the foramen magnum (dog, cat, pig); in birds it may be divided into several components
atlanto-occipital joint	articulatio atlantooccipitalis (NAV), 'YES' joint	the synovial joint between the atlas and the paired occipital condyles (mammals) or single occipital condyle (birds) that allows nodding and a limited amount of lateral motion
carpal joint	articulatio carpi (NAV), knee joints (ungulates), wrist joints	the several synovial joints of the carpus, comprising the antebrachiocarpal, middle carpal, carpometacarpal, intercarpal, intermetacarpal and accessory carpal joints (qq.v.), these joints act mainly as a hinge supported by collateral ligaments and probably serve as shock absorbers
carpometacarpal joints	articulationes carpometacarpeae (NAV)	the synovial joints between the distal row of carpal bones and the metacarpal bones; the joint cavity usually communicates with that of the middle carpal joint; movements are restricted
cartilage joints	articulationes cartilagineae (NAV)	joints in which the uniting tissue is cartilaginous and which serve to allow movement or growth; *see* synchondrosis, symphysis
coffin joint		*see* distal interphalangeal joint
composite joint	articulatio composita (NAV)	a synovial joint in which more than two bones take part, such as the carpal, tarsal or stifle joints
condylar joint	articulatio condylaris (NAV)	a synovial joint that allows motion in two planes, such as an ellipsoid or sellar joint (qq.v.)
coronal suture	sutura coronalis (NAV)	the suture between the frontal and parietal bones
costochondral joints	articulationes costochondrales (NAV)	the fibrous joints between ribs and their cartilages; cf. intrachondral joints
costovertebral joints	articulationes costovertebrales (NAV), juncturae costarum (NAA), rib joints	the joints between the ribs and the vertebral column; one part unites the head of the rib to the bodies of adjacent vertebrae, the other unites the tubercle of the rib to the transverse process of the more caudal vertebra; the more caudal joints tend to be simpler and allow greater mobility
cranial synchondroses	synchondroses cranii (NAV)	the cartilaginous joints between the bones at the base of the skull—the presphenoid, basisphenoid and basioccipital
diarthroses		*see* synovial joints

Table continued over page

11 Joints *(Continued)*

Joint	Other names	Comments
distal interphalangeal joint(s)	articulationes interphalangeae distales manus/pes (NAV), coffin joint (ungulates)	the joint(s) between the middle and distal phalanges that in some species also incorporates a distal sesamoid; motion is either restricted (ungulates), modest (dogs) or extensive (cats)
ear ossicle joints	articulationes ossiculorum auditus (NAV): articulatio incudomallearis (NAV), and articulatio incudostapedia (NAV)	the synovial joints between the three ear ossicles, noted for their minute size and elastic ligaments, they comprise the incudomallear joint between the malleus (hammer) and incus (anvil), and the incudostapedial joint between the incus and stapes (stirrup)
elbow joint	articulatio cubiti (NAV), junctura cubiti (NAA)	a composite joint between the humerus, radius and ulna. In ungulates it is a simple hinge between the condyle of the humerus and the fused radius and ulna; in others it also allows some supination, in which the head of the radius rotates upon the capitulum of the humerus and around a fixed ulna
ellipsoidal joint	articulatio ellipsoidea (NAV)	a joint between egg- and spoon-shaped articular surfaces that allows motion in only two planes
femoropatellar joint	articulatio femoropatellaris (NAV)	the synovial joint between the patella and the trochlea of the femur; the patella is united to the tibial tubercle via a single patellar ligament in small animals and three patellar ligaments in large animals; it is stabilized in the trochlear groove by paired collateral ligaments and by patellar cartilages of various forms in the different species
femorotibial joint	articulatio femorotibialis (NAV); *see* stifle joint	the synovial joint between the paired femoral and tibial condyles that is of complex form primarily to serve as a hinge-joint but also to allow some rotation, and contains paired fibrocartilaginous, semilunar menisci that make the joint congruent; it is stabilized by cruciate, collateral and meniscal ligaments
fetlock joint		the metacarpophalangeal and metatarsophalangeal joints (qq.v.) of ungulates, especially the horse
fibrous joints	articulationes fibrosae (NAV), junctura fibrosa (NAA)	joints in which the uniting tissue is fibrous and which serve to allow movement or growth; *see* gomphoses, sutures, syndesmoses
frontonasal hinge	craniofacial hinge, nasal-frontal hinge	the fibrous joint between the upper jaw and the skull of birds that is part of the mechanism of cranial kinesis, which allows both jaws to participate in opening and closing
ginglymus (NAV)		*see* hinge-joint
gomphosis (NAV)	articulatio dentoalveolaris (NAV), peg-and socket joint	the suspension of a tooth in its socket by means of a periodontal membrane; it allows very limited movement
hinge-joint	ginglymus (NAV)	a synovial joint that allows motion in only one plane, such as flexion and extension, and which is usually stabilized by a pair of collateral ligaments
hip joint	articulatio coxae (NAV), coxofemoral joint	the ball-and-socket joint between the head of the femur and the acetabulum of the hip bone; it allows three planes of motion and has a roomy joint capsule; a ligament of the femoral head limits adduction and, in horses, an accessory ligament restricts abduction. Birds possess an additional joint between the femoral trochanter and the antirochanter of the synsacrum
hock joint		*see* tarsal joints
humeral joint		*see* shoulder joint
humeroradial joint	articulatio humeroradialis (NAV)	a component of the elbow joint between the head of the radius and the capitulum of the humerus. In all species the joint acts as a hinge, but in animals that can supinate their forearms (e.g. dogs) the radius also is able to rotate against the capitulum

11 **Joints** *(Continued)*

Joint	Other names	Comments
humeroulnar joint	articulatio humeroulnaris (NAV)	the major component of the elbow joint, in which the trochlear notch of the ulna engages the trochlea of the humerus to make a simple hinge supported by collateral ligaments
incudomallear joint		*see* ear ossicle joints
incudostapedial joint		*see* ear ossicle joints
intercarpal joints	articulationes intercarpeae (NAV)	the synovial joints between the lateral and medial surfaces of the carpal bones that allow them to shuffle against one another
intermandibular joint	articulatio intermandibularis (NAV), mandibular symphysis	the joint between the two halves of the mandible that allows each half to rotate axially; it is partly fibrous and partly cartilaginous; it is mobile in ruminants and carnivores but becomes a fixed synostosis in pigs and horses
intermetacarpal joints	articulationes intermetacarpeae (NAV)	the small synovial joints between the proximal ends of the metacarpals; they communicate with the carpometacarpal joints and allow only small amounts of movement
interphalangeal joints		*see* proximal interphalangeal joints; distal interphalangeal joints
intersternal joints		*see* sternal joints
intertarsal joint	articulatio intertarsalis (NAA)	the avian homologue of the mammalian hock joint, in which the tarsal elements have either fused to the tibia or to the metatarsus
intertransverse joints	articulationes intertransversariae lumbales (NAV), articulatio intertransversaria lumbosacralis (NAV)	synovial joints between the transverse processes of adjacent lumbar vertebrae and between the sacrum and last lumbar vertebra of the horse that serve to restrict lateral bending of the spine
intervertebral joints		*see* atlantoaxial joint, intertransverse joints, zygapophyseal joints, intervertebral symphysis
intervertebral symphysis	intercentral joints, articulationes intercorporea (NAA), symphysis intervertebralis (NAV)	the moveable joint between the bodies of adjacent vertebrae that is united by a fibrocartilaginous intervertebral disc and supported by dorsal and ventral longitudinal ligaments (mammals); in birds most joints are either synostoses or saddle-shaped synovial joints
intrachondral joints	articulationes intrachondrales (NAV)	the synovial joints that occur within the costal cartilages of several ribs of ruminants, near the costochondral junctions
knee joint		an ambiguous term in veterinary science, referring to either the stifle joint or the carpal joints (qq.v)
knuckle		the metacarpophalangeal and interphalangeal joints (qq.v.) of the hand
lambdoidal suture	sutura lambdoidea (NAV)	the suture between the parietal and occipital bones
manubriosternal joint	articulatio synovialis manubriosternalis (NAV)	the first intersternebral joint, which develops as a cartilage joint but later becomes synovial in ruminants and pigs
metacarpo-/metatarso-phalangeal joints	articulationes metacarpo-/metatarsophalangeae (NAV), fetlock joints (ungulates), knuckles (primates)	the joints between the distal ends (heads) of the metacarpals and the proximal phalanges, each usually incorporating two sesamoid bones; in ungulates the joints are restricted to a simple hinge, whereas in others the rounded heads of the metacarpals permit other motions
middle carpal joint	articulatio mediocarpea (NAV), midcarpal joint	the composite joint between the proximal and distal rows of carpal bones; its cavity communicates with that of the carpometacarpal joint. In ungulates the bones bear stop facets that prevent dorsal flexion

Table continued over page

11 Joints *(Continued)*

Joint	Other names	Comments
pastern joint		the proximal interphalangeal joint (q.v.) of ungulates
pelvic symphysis	pubic symphysis (human), symphysis pelvina (NAV)	the cartilaginous joint between the two hip bones that usually involves both the pubes and ischia, in most domestic species the symphysis fuses at about the time of maturity; in some species (e.g. human) it remains a cartilaginous joint throughout life. It is absent from most birds
pivot joint		*see* trochoid joint
plane joint	arthrodial joint, articulatio plana (NAV), gliding joint	a synovial joint in which the articular surfaces are flat and allow gliding motions
proximal interphalangeal joints	articulationes interphalangeae proximales, manus/pes (NAV), knuckle (primates), pastern joint (ungulates)	the synovial joint(s) between the proximal and middle phalanges that is typically a simple hinge-joint supported by collateral ligaments. At rest the bones are at right-angles in digitigrade animals (e.g. dogs) and in a straight line in ungulates
pubic symphysis		*see* pelvic symphysis
radiocarpal joint		*see* antebrachiocarpal joint
radioulnar joints	articulatio radioulnaris proximalis/distalis (NAV)	joints between the radius and ulna found in animals that can supinate their forearms. A proximal synovial joint forms part of the elbow joint, with the margin of the radial head articulating with the notch in the ulna; the radius and ulna are united along most of the forearm by an interosseous, antebrachial membrane, while a small synovial joint at the distal end completes the articulation
sacroiliac joint	articulatio sacroiliaca (NAV), sacroiliac synchondrosis	the joint between the auricular surfaces of the wings of the ilium and sacrum; it allows only limited movement, is partly cartilaginous (craniodorsally) and partly synovial (caudoventrally), and contains numerous intra-articular ligaments
sagittal suture	sutura sagittalis (NAV)	the suture between the two parietal bones
schindylesis		a wedge-and-groove type of suture
sellar joint	articulatio sellaris (NAV), saddle joint	a synovial joint in which the articular surfaces are shaped like a saddle and permit motion in only two planes
shoulder joint	articulatio humeralis (NAA), articulatio humeri (NAV), humeral joint	the ball-and-socket joint between the glenoid of the scapula and the head of the humerus that permits motion in three planes, has an extensive joint capsule and ligaments that are weak or absent (mammals); in birds the coracoid also contributes to the glenoid
simple joint	articulatio simplex (NAV)	a synovial joint in which only two bones articulate
spheroidal joint	articulatio spheroidea (NAV), ball-and-socket joint, cotyloid joint	the most freely moveable of all synovial joints, in which a rounded head sits in a hollow cup, usually characterized by few ligaments and abundant surrounding musculature
sternal joints	intersternal joints, intersternebral joints, synchondroses sternales (NAV)	cartilaginous joints between adjacent sternebrae that tend to ossify with increasing age yet rarely ankylose to form a single bone; they allow little or no movement. In ruminants the first intersternal joint is synovial
sternocostal joints	articulationes sternocostales (NAV)	synovial joints between the costal cartilages of true ribs (mammals) or sternal ribs (birds) and the sternum
stifle joint	articulatio genus (NAV), junctura genus (NAA), knee joint (bipeds)	the composite joint between the femur, tibia and patella, made up of the femorotibial and femoropatellar joints, qq.v. In birds the joint is further complicated by a femorofibular joint

11 Joints *(Continued)*

Joint	Other names	Comments
suture	sutura (NAV), seam	a fibrous joint between membrane bones; it may be saw-toothed (sutura serrata), overlapping (sutura squamosa), interleaved (sutura foliata), abutting (sutura plana) or a wedge-and-groove (a schindylesis). Sutures mostly serve to allow growth with limited movement. Each is named according to the participating bones, e.g. internasal suture, except for the coronal, sagittal and lambdoidal sutures (qq.v.)
symphysis (NAV)	amphiarthrosis (outmoded)	a cartilaginous joint that allows limited movement, such as between the vertebral bodies
synarthrosis		a fixed joint: *see* suture, synchondrosis, synostosis
synchondrosis (NAV)		a fixed cartilaginous joint, such as that between the shaft of a bone and its epiphysis, which serves to allow growth but no movement
syndesmosis (NAV)		any fibrous joint that allows at least a modest amount of movement
synostosis (NAV)	ankylosis	a former fibrous or cartilaginous joint that has become ossified and is immovable
synovial joints	articulationes synoviales (NAV), diarthroses	freely moveable joints in which the bearing surfaces of the bones are clothed with articular cartilage, lubricated with synovial fluid and united by a joint capsule that has a synovial lining and a fibrous exterior
synsacral joints	articulationes synsacri (NAA)	the synostoses between the vertebral bodies, spines transverse processes and ilia of the avian synsacrum
tarsal joints	ankle joints (bipeds), articulatio tarsi (NAV), hock joint (quadrupeds), intertarsal joint (birds)	a composite synovial joint between the tibia and fibula, the individual tarsal bones and the metatarsals; the most mobile of these is the hinge-joint between the tibia and fibula and the talus (tarsocrural joint); the several remaining joints mostly allow only limited movement, because they are united by strong collateral, plantar and dorsal ligaments; the joints are called calcaneocuboid, centrodistal, intermetatarsal, intertarsal, talocalcaneal, talocalcaneocentral and tarsometatarsal joints
temporomandibular joint	articulatio temporomandibularis (NAV), jaw joint	the synovial joint between the condylar process of the mandible and the mandibular fossa of the temporal bone; the articular cartilage on the mandible is fibrous and the cavity is divided by an articular disk; it is modified to allow mostly hinge motion in carnivores, to-and-fro motion in rodents, and side-to-side movements in other herbivores
tibiofibular joints	articulatio tibiofibularis proximalis/distalis (NAV)	synovial joints between the proximal and distal ends of the fibula with the tibia; both joints occur in carnivores but the joint is variable, depending on the development of the fibula; in ruminants the distal end is represented as a separate bone and the proximal end is fused to the tibia
trochoid joint	articulatio trochoidea (NAV), pivot joint	a synovial joint that allows only rotation, such as between the human radius and ulna or between the dens and atlas
zygapophyseal joints	articulationes processuum articularium (NAV), articulationes zygapophysalis (NAA), facet joints, interneural joints, juncturae zygapophyseales	the synovial joints between the articular processes of adjacent vertebrae that mostly allow sliding motions

Table prepared by John Grandage.

12 Ligaments

Ligament	Other names	Origin	Insertion	Comments
accessory carpal ligg.	lig. accessorio-carpoulnare (NAV), etc.	the lateral and distal parts of the accessory carpal bone	the lateral side of the ulna, ulnar carpal, 4th carpal and 5th metacarpal bones	four strong and distinct ligg. are included under this general name
accessory lig. (of deep digital flexor)	carpal check lig., inferior check lig., lig. accessorium (NAV), subcarpal check lig.	the distal row of the carpal bones via the palmar carpal lig.	the deep digital flexor tendon, near the middle of the cannon bone	in horses: a purely fibrous head of the deep digital flexor muscle; part of stay-apparatus
accessory lig. (of hip joint)	lig. accessorium ossis femoris (NAV)	prepubic tendon	the fovea of femoral head	unique to horses; restricts abduction
accessory lig. (of superficial digital flexor)	lig. accessorium (NAV), radial check lig., superior check lig.	the distal end of the radius	the superficial digital flexor tendon, near the carpus	in horses: a strong, thin, fibrous head to the superficial digital flexor muscle
alar ligg.	ligg. alaria (NAV)	the apex of the dens of the axis	the lateral parts of the foramen magnum	in carnivores and pigs
annular lig. (of radius)	lig. anulare radii (NAV)	the edge of the medial coronoid process of the ulna	the edge of the lateral coronoid process of the ulna	it forms a loop within which the head of the radius can rotate
apical lig. of dens	lig. apicis dentis (NAV)	the apex of the dens of the axis	the ventral part of the foramen magnum	in all bar horses: *see* longitudinal lig. of dens
anterior cruciate lig.	*see* cranid cruciate lig.			
broad sacrotuberous lig.	lig. sacrotuberale latum (NAV). *See also* sacrotuberous lig.	the lateral border of the sacrum and first two tail vertebrae	the sciatic spine and sciatic tuber, leaving two gaps: sciatic foramina	in ungulates, this broad sheet forms the lateral pelvic wall
carpal check lig.	*see* accessory lig. (of deep digital flexor)			
caudal cruciate lig.	lig. cruciatum caudale (NAV), medial cruciate lig., posterior cruciate lig.	the lateral part of the popliteal notch of the tibia	the cranial part of the intercondylar fossa on the medial femoral condyle	permits flexion and rotation but limits caudal motion of the tibia
caudal lig. (of temporomandibular joint)	lig. caudale (NAV)	the retroarticular process of temporal bone	the caudal surface of the neck of the mandibular condyle	an elastic lig.
check ligg.	*see* accessory ligg. of digital flexors (deep and superficial)			
collateral ligg.	ligg. collateralia (NAV)	close to the margin of the male articular surface of a hinge-joint	near the center of curvature of the female articular surface	found on the sides of hinge-joints; they are present in all joints distal to the hip and shoulder
collateral patellar ligg.	*see* femoropatellar ligg.			
collateral sesamoidean ligg. (of fetlock, etc.)	ligg. sesamoidea collateralia (NAV)	the epicondyles of the head of the metacarpal	the abaxial borders of the proximal sesamoid bones	these ligg. make the sesamoids track in one plane
collateral sesamoidean ligg. (of coffin bone, etc.)	ligg. sesamoidea collateralia (NAV), suspensory ligg. of distal sesamoid bone, suspensory navicular ligg.	the abaxial borders of the distal end of the proximal phalanx	the ends of the distal sesamoid bone	these ligg. suspend the sesamoid; it is held in place distally by the unpaired sesamoid lig.
conjugal lig.	*see* intercapital lig.			
coracohumeral lig.	lig. coracohumerale (NAV)	the coracoid process of the scapula	the tubercles of the humerus	well-developed in primates to help suspend the arm

12 Ligaments *(Continued)*

Ligament	Other names	Origin	Insertion	Comments
costotransverse lig.	lig. colli costae, lig. costotranversarium (NAV), lig of the tubercle	the transverse process of each thoracic vertebra	the non-articular part of the tubercle of a rib	the strongest lig. binding a rib to a vertebra
costoxiphoid lig.	lig. costoxiphoidea (NAV)	the internal surface of the costal cartilages of the last true ribs	the dorsal surface of the xiphoid process	it supports the xiphoid process
cranial cruciate lig.	anterior cruciate lig., lateral cruciate lig., lig. cruciatum craniale (NAV)	the cranial part of the intercondylar area of the tibia	the caudal part of the intercondylar fossa on the lateral femoral condyle	permits flexion and rotation but limits forward motion of the tibia
cruciate ligg.	*see* cranial cruciate lig., caudal cruciate, distal interdigital, and cruciate sesamoidean ligg.			various ligg. found in different parts of the body that are disposed in a cross
cruciate sesamoidean ligg.	ligg. sesamoideum cruciata (NAV)	the bases of the proximal sesamoid bones	the diagonally opposite side of the proximal phalanx	a short and deep member of the series of sesamoidean ligg.
digital annular ligg.	proximal and distal digital annular ligg., lig. anulare digiti (NAV)	the sides of the proximal and middle phalanges and the overlying fascia	the opposite sides to those for the origin	broad (e.g., horse) or narrow (ox, dog) hoop-like bands that hold down the flexors over the pastern
distal interdigital lig.	ligg. interdigitalia distalia (NAV), cruciate ligg.	the abaxial eminences at the proximal end of the middle phalanx	the axial ends of the distal sesamoid bones	an important lig. of ruminants that prevents the toes from spreading
dorsal atlantoaxial lig.	lig. atlantoaxiale dorsale (NAV)	the cranial end of the spinous process of the axis	the caudal border of the dorsal arch of the atlas	it limits all extreme motions of the joint
dorsal carpal ligg.	lig. radiocarpeum dorsale (NAV), etc., dorsal intercarpal ligg.	eminences on the dorsal side of the radius, ulna and proximal carpals	eminences on the dorsal side of the distal carpals and metacarpals	at least four separate ligg. have been identified that are included under this general name
dorsal longitudinal lig.	lig. longitudinale dorsale (NAV)	the dorsal surface of all vertebrae caudal to the atlas . . .	. . . extending from the dens of the axis to the tail	forms the floor of the vertebral canal; narrowest in the middle of each body
dorsal sacroiliac ligg.	ligg. sacroiliaca dorsalia (NAV)	the caudal parts of the sacral wing, and in large animals the spinous processes of the sacrum	the sacral tuber and adjacent parts of the ilium	in large animals the ligg. are in two parts: a funicular part to the sacral spines and a membranous part to the sacral wing
dorsal tarsal ligg.	ligg. tarsi dorsalia	various points on the dorsal aspect of the hock, esp. the medial side of the talus	various points on the dorsal aspect of the hock, esp. the central tarsal and the distal row of the tarsal bones	these are strong to limit the amount of intratarsal motion; they complement the even stronger plantar tarsal ligg.
femoropatellar ligg.	ligg. femoropatellare laterale/mediale, (NAV), collateral patellar ligg.	the lateral and medial epicondyles of the femur	the sides of the patella	in small animals the ligg. merge with the femoral fascia
glenohumeral ligg.	ligg. glenohumeralia (NAV)	the margin of the glenoid	the margin of the humeral head, near the tubercles	weak, broad, slack varied, indistinct ligg. best developed in the human shoulder

Table continued over page

12 Ligaments *(Continued)*

Ligament	Other names	Origin	Insertion	Comments
iliofemoral lig.	lig. iliofemorale (NAV)	the iliac part of the acetabular rim	the neck of the femur	a slight thickening of the hip-joint capsule
iliolumbar lig.	lig. iliolumbale (NAV)	the margins of the transverse processes of the lumbar vertebrae	the ventral surface of wing of the ilium	conspicuous in horses and cattle; it merges with the intertransverse lig.
inferior check lig.	*see* accessory lig. (of deep digital flexor)			
inguinal lig.	lig. inguinale (NAV), arcus inguinalis, (NAV), Poupart's lig.	the tuber coxae and adjacent parts of the ilium	the lateral margin of the prepubic tendon, adjacent to the pubis	it is the caudal part of the aponeurosis of the external abdominal oblique muscle
interarcuate ligg.	*see* ligg. flava			
intercapital lig.	conjugal lig., lig. intercapitale (NAV)	the groove in the head of the rib	the corresponding groove in the opposite rib	in most species the lig. is missing from the first pair and last few pairs of ribs
intersesamoidean ligg.	*see* palmar ligg.			
interosseous lig. of forearm	lig. interosseum antebrachii (NAV)	the rough area on the proximal ulna	the rough area on the proximal radius	only in carnivora
interspinous ligg.	ligg. interspinalia (NAV)	the caudal border of the spinous processes of the vertebrae	the cranial border of the spinous processes of the next caudal vertebra	ligg. made up of fiber bundles most obvious in thoracolumbar vertebrae
intertransverse ligg.	ligg. intertransversaria (VAV)	the caudal border of the transverse processes of the vertebrae	the cranial border of the transverse processes of the next caudal vertebra	ligg. made up of bundles of fibers, only conspicuous in lumbar vertebrae
intra-articular lig.	conjugal lig., lig. capitis costae intra-articulare (NAV)	the groove in the head of a rib	the intervertebral disk, the cranial vertebra, and the opposite rib (*see* intercapital lig.)	the precise form of the lig. varies according to the particular rib involved
ischiofemoral lig.	lig. ischiofemorale (NAV)	the sciatic part of the acetabular rim	the neck of the femur	a slight thickening of the hip-joint capsule
lateral cruciate lig.	*see* cranial cruciate lig.			
lateral lig. (of atlanto-occipital joint)	lig. laterale (NAV)	the lateral part of the dorsal arch of the atlas	the jugular process of the occipital bone	appears to restrict turning the head too far to the side.
lateral lig. (of temporomandibular joint)	lig. laterale (NAV)	the lateral margin of mandibular fossa of temporal bone	the lateral pole of the condyloid process of the mandible	a strong, ill-defined thickening of the joint capsule
ligg. flava (NAV)	interarcuate ligg., yellow ligg.	the caudal border of the arch of a vertebra	the cranial border of the arch of the more caudal vertebra	a thin membranous lig. composed of elastic tissue
lig. of femoral head	lig. capitis ossis femoris (NAV), lig. teres femoris, round lig. (of femur)	the acetabular fossa	the fovea in the head of the femur	limits adduction; absent from aquatic mammals, sloths
lig. of sciatic arch	lig. arcuatum ischiadicum (NAV)	the caudal border of one ischium along the sciatic arch . . .	. . . to the caudal border of the other ischium	this lig. in concert with the pubic lig. helps stabilize the pelvic symphysis
lig. teres femoris	*see* lig. of femoral head			
longitudinal lig. of dens	lig. longitudinale dentis (NAV)	the dorsal surface of the dens of the axis	inside the ventral arch of the atlas, cranial to fovea	in horses; cf. apical lig. of dens

12 Ligaments (*Continued*)

Ligament	Other names	Origin	Insertion	Comments
medial cruciate lig.	*see* caudal cruciate lig.			
meniscal ligg.	lig. transversum genus (NAV) (= inter-meniscal lig.). *See also* meniscofemoral lig.	each horn of the menisci of the stifle joint	the adjacent intercondylar area of the tibia	these ligg. tether the menisci, while allowing them to glide on the tibia
meniscofemoral lig.	lig. meniscofemorale (NAV)	the caudal horn of the lateral meniscus of the stifle	the caudal part of the intercondylar fossa	prevents over-extension and rotation of the stifle when fully extended
nuchal lig.	back-strap, lig. nuchae (NAV), paddy-whack	a cranial continuation of the supraspinous lig. from the spines of the first few thoracic vertebrae	the dorsal spine of axis (most mammals), external occipital protuberance and 3rd to 6th cervical vertebrae (large mammals)	an elastic lig., best developed in large animals, that helps support the head; made up of a funicular part to the occiput or axis, and a laminar part (horse, ox) to other cervical vertebrae
oblique sesamoidean ligg.	ligg. sesamoidea obliqua (NAV)	the distal border of the palmar lig. and the proximal sesamoid bones	a V-shaped ridge on the palmar surface of the middle phalanx	with the straight lig., the strongest of the sesamoidean ligg.
orbital lig.	lig. orbitale (NAV)	the zygomatic process of frontal bone	the frontal process of zygomatic bone	it completes the bony orbit in species in which there is a gap (e.g. dogs); relatively larger in brachycephalics
palmar annular lig. (of fetlock)	lig. anulare palmare (NAV)	the fascia and ligg. over the sides of the fetlock . . .	. . . to the same fascia and ligg. on the opposite side	this lig. holds the digital flexors in place during flexion of the fetlock
palmar carpal ligg.	lig. radiocarpeum palmare (NAV), etc.	the eminences on the palmar side of the radius, ulna and proximal carpals	the eminences on the palmar side of the distal carpals and metacarpals	at least six separate ligg. have been identified that are included under this general name
palmar ligg. (of fetlock/metacarpo-phalangeal joint)	ligg. palmaria (NAV), intersesamoidean lig.	one of the proximal sesamoid bones . . .	. . . to the other of the proximal sesamoid bones	a fibrocartilaginous pad that extends beyond the sesamoid bones and forms a bearing surface for the deep digital flexor
palmar ligg. (of pastern joint)	ligg. palmaria (NAV)	the palmar margin of the distal articular surface of the proximal phalanx	the palmar margin of the proximal articular surface of the middle phalanx	these ligg. are well developed in large animals, when up to four per digit may be present
patellar lig./ligg.	lig. patellae (NAV), lig. patellae laterale/inter-medium/mediale (NAV—large animals), straight patellar ligg.	the apex of the patella; in large animals the lateral border and patellar cartilage too	the tibial tuberosity	in horses and cattle there are three patellar ligg., in small animals only one
plantar ligg. (of hind fetlock)	*see* palmar ligg. (of fetlock/metacarpo-phalangeal joint) of which it is the hindlimb homolog			

Table continued over page

12 Ligaments *(Continued)*

Ligament	Other names	Origin	Insertion	Comments
plantar tarsal ligg.	ligg. tarsi plantaria (NAV)	various points on the plantar aspect of the hock, but esp. the calcaneus	various points on the plantar surface of the hock, but esp. the distal tarsals and metatarsals	a very strong compound lig. that takes the strain of the Achilles tendon and keeps the hock straight
posterior cruciate lig.	*see* caudal cruciate lig.			
proximal interdigital lig.	lig. interdigitale proximale (NAV)	the axial surfaces of the middles of the proximal phalanges	the opposing phalanx of the adjacent digit a little more distally, to form a cross	an important lig. of ruminants that limits the amount the toes may spread
pubic lig.	lig. pubicum craniale (NAV)	the pubic pecten (brim) on one side . . .	. . . to the pubic pecten on the other side	with the lig. of the sciatic arch, it reinforces the pelvic symphysis
pubofemoral lig.	lig. pubofemorale (NAV)	the pubic part of the acetabular rim	the neck of the femur	a slight thickening of the hip-joint capsule
radial check lig.	*see* accessory lig. (of superficial digital flexor)			
radiate lig. (of rib)	lig. capitis costae radiatum (NAV)	the bodies of the thoracic vertebrae	the neck of the rib	a fan-shaped lig. on the ventral aspect of the joint
round lig.	*see* lig. of femoral head			
sacroiliac ligg. (interosseous part)	ligg. sacroiliaca interossea (NAV). *See also* dorsal sacroiliac ligg., ventral sacroiliac ligg.	the auricular area and adjacent parts of the sacrum	the auricular area and adjacent parts of the ilium	these complex, short intra-articular ligg. are assisted by the dorsal and ventral ligg., q.v.
sacrotuberous lig.	lig. sacrotuberale (NAV). *See also* broad sacrotuberous lig.	the caudolateral part of the sacrum and adjacent first tail vertebra	the lateral angle of the sciatic tuber	in carnivores; this thick strong lig. is readily palpable and stabilizes the sacroiliac joint
sesamoidean ligg.	*see also* straight, oblique, short, cruciate, inter- and collateral sesamoidean ligg.	the distal surface of the proximal sesamoid bones	the palmar surface of the middle and proximal phalanges	the functional insertion of the interosseous muscle
short sesamoidean ligg.	ligg. sesamoideum brevia (NAV)	the distal border of the proximal sesamoid bones	the proximal border of the proximal phalanx	the shortest, deepest and weakest of the sesamoidean ligg.
sternal lig.	lig. sterni (NAV)	the dorsal surface of the manubrium	the dorsal surface of the xiphoid	a homologue of the longitudinal ligg. of vertebral column
straight sesamoidean lig.	lig. sesamoideum rectum (NAV)	the distal border of the palmar lig. and the proximal sesamoid bones	the complementary cartilage of the middle phalanx	the only one of the sesamoidean ligg. to reach the middle phalanx
sternocostal radiate ligg.	ligg. sternocostalia radiata (NAV)	the dorsal and ventral surfaces of the sternum	the costal cartilages	the ligg. serve as reinforcements of the joint capsules
subcarpal check lig.	*see* accessory lig. (of deep digital flexor)			
superior check lig.	*see* accessory lig. (of superficial digital flexor)			
supraspinous lig.	lig. supraspinale (NAV)	the spinous processes of the thoracic vertebrae	the spinous processes of lumbar, sacral and caudal vertebrae	a ligament that limits excessive spinal flexion

12 **Ligaments** (*Continued*)

Ligament	Other names	Origin	Insertion	Comments
suspensory lig. (of proximal sesamoid bones)	interosseous muscle, mm. interossei (NAV), middle interosseous	the distal row of carpal bones and the proximal parts of the metacarpals	the proximal sesamoid bones, the common extensor tendon, and via the sesamoidean ligg., the palmar surface of the proximal and middle phalanges	one of the major passive supports for the fetlock joint in the horse; in other species it is a fleshy muscle
suspensory lig. (of distal sesamoid bone)	*see* collateral sesamoidean ligg.			
tarsal ligg.	*see* dorsal tarsal ligg., plantar tarsal ligg., collateral ligg.			over 30 separate ligg. of the hock are described
transverse acetabular lig.	lig. transversum acetabuli (NAV)	one horn of the lunate face of the acetabulum . . .	. . . to the other horn of the lunate face	the lig. bridges the acetabular notch to become part of the articular surface
transverse atlantal lig.	lig. transversum atlantis (NAV)	one side of the arch of the atlas . . .	. . . to the other side of the arch	in carnivores, pigs; it holds the dens against the ventral arch of the atlas
transverse humeral lig.	lig. transversum humerale	the greater tubercle of the humerus	the lesser tubercle of the humerus	the lig. holds the tendon of the biceps brachii in the intertubercular groove
transverse lig. of stifle	*see* meniscal ligg.			
ungual cartilage ligg.	ligg. chondro-compedalia (NAV), etc.	the borders of the ungual cartilage of the distal phalanx of the horse	all three phalanges	only in Equidae; made up of five groups of ligg. that anchor the cartilage
unpaired distal sesamoidean lig.	lig. sesamoideum distale impar (NAV)	the flexor surface of the distal phalanx	the distal surface of the distal sesamoid bone	in ungulates; this lig. binds the navicular bone to the coffin joint
ventral longitudinal lig.	lig. longitudinale ventrale (NAV)	the ventral surface of all vertebrae caudal to the axis . . .	. . . extending from neck to tail	best developed in the lumbar region
ventral sacroiliac ligg.	ligg. sacroiliaca ventralia (NAV)	an extensive area around the sacroiliac joint on the wing of the sacrum	a large area of the ventral surface of the wing of the ilium	these ligg. are complemented by dorsal and interosseous ligg.
yellow ligg.	*see* ligg. flava			

Table prepared by John Grandage.

13 Muscles

PART 13.1. MUSCLES OF THE HEAD AND NECK*

Muscle	Other names	Origin	Insertion	Innervation	Comments
		13.1A Muscles of the muzzle and lips			
buccinator	m. buccinator (NAV), the trumpeter's m.	from the lips and alveolar borders of the jaws over the cheeks	a longitudinal raphe between the two origins	the buccal branches of the facial nerve	this cheek muscle helps control food in the vestibule of the mouth; it is made up of several parts
caninus	m. caninus (NAV), lateral dilator of nostril	in the horse: the maxilla near the end of the facial crest	the lateral wing of the nostril	the buccal branch of the facial nerve	it dilates the nostril; it is well developed in the horse
cutaneous colli	*see* platysma				
cutaneous faciei	*see* platysma				
depressor of the lower lip	m. depressor labii inferioris (NAV) or mandibularis	the alveolar border of the mandible as far caudad as the masseter	the stroma of the lower lip	the ventral buccal branch of the facial nerve	absent from carnivores; may merge with buccinator
depressor of the upper lip	m. depressor labii superioris (NAV), depressor rostri	facial tubercle (ox) or end of the facial crest	the snout, below the nostril	the dorsal buccal branch of the facial nerve	especially well-developed in the pig
dilator of nostril	m. dilator naris apicalis (NAV), transverse nasal muscle	the medial border of the nostril	its fellow in the midline	the buccal branch of the facial nerve	well-developed in the horse. *See also* caninus
incisive mm.	m. incisivus superioris/ inferioris (NAV)	the alveolar borders of the incisor teeth	fibers radiate away from their origins into the lips	the buccal branches of the facial nerve	these muscles hold the lips close against the jaws and assist the orbicularis oris
levator nasolabialis	m. levator nasolabialis (NAV)	mostly from the nasal bones	the upper lip and adjacent parts of the muzzle	the branches of the facial nerve	derived from the deep part of the sphincter colli muscle
levator of the upper lip	m. levator labii superioris (NAV) or maxillaris	the side of face (species vary) beneath the levator nasolabialis	fascicles into upper lip, except in horses, in which it inserts by a common tendon with its fellow	the dorsal buccal branch of facial nerve	involved in Flehmen response
orbicularis oris	m. orbicularis oris (NAV)	within the stroma of the lips	the skin of the lips or remaining within the stroma	the buccal branches of the facial nerve	the muscle to close the mouth (rima oris)
platysma (NAV)	the NAV subdivides this m. into m. cutaneous colli and m. cutaneous faciei	the dorsal superficial fascia of the neck; fibers run between the deep and superficial layers of the sphincter colli	the commissures of the lips after running forwards over the parotid and cheek	the buccal branches of the facial nerve	a sheet of muscle that makes up the bulk of the cutaneous muscle of the neck and face

* Some muscles may belong with equal validity to other divisions or subdivisions; most avian and reptilian muscles have been omitted as have most smooth muscles and a few trivial ones.

13 Muscles *(Continued)*

PART 13.1 Head and neck *(Continued)*

Muscle	Other names	Origin	Insertion	Innervation	Comments
13.1B. Muscles of the tongue					
genioglossus	m. genioglossus (NAV)	the medial surface of the mandible caudal to the symphysis	it is fan-shaped and runs in a sagittal plane to the dorsum of the tongue	the hypoglossal nerve	acts to depress the tongue, especially along its axis
hyoglossus	m. hyoglossus (NAV)	the lateral side of the basihyoid and adjacent bones	the root and caudal two-thirds of the tongue	the hypoglossal nerve	acts to retract and depress the tongue
intrinsic m. of tongue	m. lingualis proprius (NAV), proper muscle of the tongue	various parts within the substance of the tongue	various parts within the substance of the tongue	the hypoglossal nerve	fibres run in many directions; produce complex motions such as protrusion
styloglossus	m. styloglossus (NAV)	the lateral side of the stylohyoid bone	various parts of the tongue, but especially the tip	the hypoglossal nerve	acts to retract the tongue
13.1C. Muscles of the pharynx					
caudal pharyngeal constrictors	mm. constrict-ores pharyngis caudales (NAV)	the lateral wall of the thyroid and crioid cartilages	the median raphe in the roof of the pharynx	the pharyngeal plexus	made up of the thyropharyngeal and crico-pharyngeal muscles
caudal stylopharyngeus	m. stylopharyn-geus caudalis (NAV)	the medial face of the stylohyoid bone	the dorsolateral wall of the pharynx	the pharyngeal plexus	a ditator of the pharynx
ceratopharyngeus	*see* middle pharyngeal constrictor				
chondropharyngeus	*see* middle pharyngeal constrictor				
cricopharyngeus	m. cricopharyn-geus (NAV)	the lateral wall of the arch of the cricoid cartilage	the fibers meet at the median fibrous raphe	the pharyngeal plexus	the most caudal of the pharyngeal constrictors
hyopharyngeus	*see* middle pharyngeal constrictor				
levator of the soft palate	m. levator veli palatini (NAV)	the tympanic part of the temporal bone	it spreads out from the wall of the pharynx into the soft palate	the pharyngeal plexus	it runs caudal and parallel to the tensor of the soft palate; it raises the soft palate
middle pharyngeal constrictor	m. constrictor pharyngis medius (NAV), m. hyopharyngeus (NAV)	mainly from the dorsal end of the thyrohyoid bone	the muscle fans out to meet its fellow on the median raphe in the pharyngeal roof	the pharyngeal plexus	it was formerly divided into small ceratopharyngeal and large chondropharyngeal components
palatinus	m. palatinus (NAV)	the caudal rim of the hard palate	the aponeurosis of the soft palate	the pharyngeal plexus	this small muscle runs longitudinally; it shortens the palate
palatopharyngeus	m. palato-pharyngeus (NAV)	the palatine bone and soft palate	the median fibrous raphe in the roof of the pharynx	the pharyngeal plexus	the most rostral of the pharyngeal constrictors; it mainly shortens the pharynx

Table continued over page

13 Muscles (*Continued*)

PART 13.1 Head and neck (*Continued*)

Muscle	Other names	Origin	Insertion	Innervation	Comments
pharyngeal constrictors	*see* rostral, middle and caudal pharyngeal constrictor				
pterygopharyngeus	m. pterygo-pharyngeus (NAV)	the pterygoid bone and soft palate	the median fibrous raphe in the roof of the pharynx	the pharyngeal plexus	the most dorsal pharyngeal constrictor; it shortens the pharynx
rostral pharyngeal constrictors	mm. con-strictores pharyngis rostrales (NAV), *see* palato- and pterygopharyngeus				
rostral stylopharyngeus	m. stylopharyn-geus rostralis (NAV)	the rostral border of the stylohyoid bone	the median raphe in the roof of the pharynx	the pharyngeal plexus	in ruminants it is an additional rostral pharyngeal constrictor that acts as a nasopharyn-geal sphincter
stylopharyngeus	*see* rostral stylopharyngeus and caudal stylopharyngeus				
tensor of the soft palate	m. tensor veli palatini (NAV)	various parts of the temporal bone and the auditory tube	fibers pass around the hamulus of the pterygoid to fan into the aponeurosis of the soft palate	the pharyngeal plexus	it runs parallel to the tensor of the soft palate; it tenses the soft palate
thyropharyngeus	m. thyropharyn-geus (NAV)	the lateral wall of the lamina of the thyroid cartilage	the fibers meet at the median fibrous raphe	the pharyngeal plexus	part of the caudal pharyngeal constrictor

13.1D. Muscles of the hyoid apparatus

Muscle	Other names	Origin	Insertion	Innervation	Comments
ceratohyoid	m. cerato-hyoideus (NAV)	the cranial border of the thyrohyoid bone	the caudal border of the cerato-hyoid bone	the glosso-pharyngeal nerve	a small triangular muscle that reduces the angle between the hyoid bones
cricothyroid	m. cricothy-roideus (NAV)	the arch and caudal border of the cricoid cartilage	the caudal border of the thyroid lamina	the cranial laryngeal nerve	it depresses the thyroid and so lengthens the vocal folds
geniohyoid	m. geniohyoideus (NAV)	the mandible, by the symphysis	the lingual process of the hyoid bone or the basihyoid	the hypoglossal nerve	it pulls the hyoid forwards; in concert with the sternohyoid, it expands the pharynx
mylohyoid	m. mylohyoideus (NAV)	the medial face of the alveolar border of the mandible	a midline raphe beneath the tongue and the basihyoid	the mylohyoid branch of the mandibular nerve	a thin, sheet-like muscle that acts like a sling to lift the tongue
occipitohyoid	m. occipito-hyoideus (NAV), jugulohyoid	the jugular process of the occipital bone	the proximal end of the stylohyoid bone	the facial nerve	a small muscle that retracts the hyoid apparatus

13 Muscles (*Continued*)

PART 13.1 Head and neck (*Continued*)

Muscle	Other names	Origin	Insertion	Innervation	Comments
omohyoid	*see under* Muscles of the neck				
sternohyoid	*see under* the Muscles of the neck				
stylohyoid muscle	m. stylohyoideus (NAV)	the muscular angle of the stylohyoid bone	the ends of the basihyoid bone	the facial nerve	it elevates the roof of the tongue and compresses the pharynx
thyrohyoid	m. thyrohyoideus (NAV)	an oblique line on the lamina of the thyroid cartilage	the thyrohyoid bone	the hypoglossal nerve	a small muscle that acts to draw the larynx closer to the tongue
tranverse hyoid	m. hyoideus transversus (NAV)	the medial face of the ceratohyoid bone	the homologous point on the bone of the other side	the glosso-pharyngeal nerve	to draw the two halves of the hyoid together

13.1E. Muscles of the larynx

Muscle	Other names	Origin	Insertion	Innervation	Comments
cricoarytenoid	*see* dorsal and lateral crico-arytenoid				
dorsal cricoarytenoid	m. cricoaryten-oideus dorsalis (NAV)	the median ridge and lamina of the thyroid cartilage	fibers converge to insert on the muscular process of the arytenoid cartilage	the recurrent laryngeal nerve	the only muscle to dilate the rima glottidis; it does so by rotating the arytenoid cartilage. Becomes paretic in roaring horses
hyoepiglotticus	m. hyoepi-glotticus (NAV)	the medial surface of the ceratohyoid bone	the midline with its fellow that joins the ventral surface of the epiglottis	the hypoglossal nerve	a small muscle that depresses the epiglottis onto the tongue
lateral cricoarytenoid	m. cricoaryten-oideus lateralis (NAV)	the rostral border of the arch of the cricoid cartilage	the vocal process of the arytenoid cartilage	the recurrent laryngeal nerve	serves to close the rima glottidis
sternothyroid	*see under* Muscles of the neck				
thyroarytenoid	m. thyroaryten-oideus (NAV). *See also* ventricular m., vocal m.	the medial surface of the lamina of the thyroid cartilage	the vocal process of the arytenoid cartilage	the recurrent laryngeal nerve	this muscle has distinct parts within the vocal and vestibular folds; it slackens the folds and closes the rima
transverse arytenoid	m. arytenoideus transversus (NAV)	the dorsal surface of the arytenoid cartilages	a median fibrous raphe	the recurrent laryngeal nerve	serves to close the intra-cartilaginous parts of the rima glottidis
ventricular m.	m. ventricularis (NAV), oral thyroarytenoid m., vestibular m. (of larynx)	the lamina of the thyroid cartilage; in dogs the cuneiform process of the arytenoid	the muscular process of the arytenoid	the recurrent laryngeal nerve	part of the thyroarytenoid m.; it closes the glottis and dilates the laryngeal saccule (when present)
vestibular m. (of larynx.)	*see* ventricular m.				

Table continued over page

13 Muscles *(Continued)*

PART 13.1 Head and neck *(Continued)*

Muscle	Other names	Origin	Insertion	Innervation	Comments
vocalis	m. vocalis (NAV), aboral thyroarytenoid m.	the body of the thyroid cartilage	the vocal process of the arytenoid	the recurrent laryngeal nerve	part of the thyroarytenoid m.; it closes the glottis and slackens the vocal fold
		13.1F. Muscles of the eye and eyelids			
bulbar mm.	mm. bulbi (NAV), extrinsic muscles of the eye, eye muscles, etc.	mostly from the common tendinous ring around the optic foramen	the scleral surface mostly in front of the equator	the oculomotor, trochlear and abducent nerves	the six (human) or seven (domestic mammals) muscles that move the eyeball; *see* dorsal oblique, dorsal rectus, lateral rectus, medial rectus, retractor bulbi, ventral oblique, ventral rectus
corrugator supercilii	*see* levator of the medial angle of the eye				
dorsal oblique	m. obliquus dorsalis (NAV), m. obliquus superior bulbi (NA)	in the depths of the orbit near ethmoid foramen	it inserts near the equator, between the dorsal and lateral recti	the trochlear nerve	the muscle first runs forward on the medial side of the orbit, before bending round the trochlea
dorsal rectus	m. rectus dorsalis (NAV), m. rectus superior bulbi (NA)	the common tendinous ring around the optic foramen	the upper part of the sclera in front of the equator	the oculomotor nerve	the muscle turns the eye upwards
lateral rectus	m. rectus lateralis (NAV), m. rectus lateralis bulbi (NA)	the common tendinous ring around the optic foramen	the lateral part of the sclera in front of the equator	the abducent nerve	the muscle turns the eye outwards
levator of the medial angle of the eye	m. levator anguli oculi medialis (NAV), corrugator supercilii	the frontal bone above and medial to the orbit	the upper eyelid	the auriculo-palpebral branch of the facial nerve	a small muscle in the domestic species
levator of the upper eyelid	m. levator palpebrae superioris (NAV)	the pterygoid crest	by a thin tendon in the upper eyelid	the oculomotor nerve	a muscle of the eyelids not innervated by the facial nerve
malaris	m. malaris (NAV)	the fascia in front of the eye	the lower eyelid	the facial nerve	a small and inconstant muscle
medial rectus	m. rectus medialis (NAV), m. rectus medialis bulbi (NA)	the common tendinous ring around the optic foramen	the medial part of the sclera in front of the equator	the oculomotor nerve	the muscle turns the eye medially and is used in convergence
oblique mm.	*see* dorsal oblique, ventral oblique				
orbicularis oculi	m. orbicularis oculi (NAV)	the skin and stroma of the eyelids; the palpebral ligament	the skin of the eyelids and the palpebral ligament	the auriculo-palpebral branch of the facial nerve	the muscle to close the eyes (rima palpebrarum)

13 Muscles (*Continued*)

PART 13.1 Head and neck (*Continued*)

Muscle	Other names	Origin	Insertion	Innervation	Comments
retractor bulbi	m. retractor bulbi (NAV)	the common tendinous ring around the optic foramen	the sclera at the back of the eye	the abducent nerve	not found in the human orbit; a muscle in four parts that pulls the eyeball into the orbit
retractor of the lateral angle of the eye	m. retractor anguli oculi lateralis (NAV)	the fascia near the zygomatic arch (dogs)	the lateral corner of the eye	the auriculo-palpebral nerve	a small muscle of facial expression
straight mm. of the eye	*see* dorsal, lateral, ventral and medial rectus				
ventral oblique	m. obliquus ventralis (NAV), m. obliquus inferior bulbi (NA)	in the medial wall of the orbit behind the lacrimal fossa	it inserts near the equator, between the ventral and lateral recti	the oculomotor nerve	the shortest of the bulbar mm.
ventral rectus	m. rectus ventralis (NAV), m. rectus inferior bulbi (NA)	the common tendinous ring around the optic foramen	the lower part of the sclera in front of the equator	the oculomotor nerve	the muscle turns the eye downwards
zygomatic	m. zygomaticus (NAV); the smiling m.	the fascia over the masseter muscle; in dogs the scutular cartilage	the commissures of the mouth intermingling with the orbicularis oris	the auriculopal-pebral branch of the facial nerve	a thin ribbon-like muscle
13.1G Muscles of the ear and forehead					
caudal auricular mm.	caudal ear mm., mm. auriculares caudales (NAV), m. cervico-scutularis and mm. cervico-auricularis	the fascia of the neck and occiput	the scutiform cartilage and caudal part of the conchal cartilage	the caudal auricular branch of the facial nerve	a group of about four muscles that mostly draw the ear backwards
dorsal auricular mm.	dorsal ear mm., mm. auriculares dorsales (NAV), mm. inter-scutularis, parietoscutularis, parietoauricularis	the fascia over the scutiform cartilage and the top of the head	the scutiform cartilage and dorsal surface of the conchal cartilage	the auriculopal-pebral branch of the facial nerve	a group of two or three muscles on the top of the head that help erect the ear
rostral auricular mm.	anterior ear mm., mm. auriculares rostrales (NAV)	the fascia over the scutiform cartilage and rostral part of the forehead	the rostral part of the dorsal surface of the conchal cartilage	the auriculopal-pebral branch of the facial nerve	a group of about eight muscles that draw the ear forwards, etc.
stapedius	m. stapedius (NAV)	the mastoid wall of the middle ear	the neck of the stapes	the stapedial branch of the facial nerve	one of the smallest of all muscles; it dampens ossicle oscillation
tensor tympani	m. tensor tympani (NAV)	the wall of the bony auditory tube	the upper end of the handle of the malleus	the trigeminal nerve via the otic ganglion	it tenses the eardrum and dampens the oscillations

Table continued over page

13 Muscles *(Continued)*

PART 13.1 Head and neck *(Continued)*

Muscle	Other names	Origin	Insertion	Innervation	Comments
ventral auricular mm.	ventral ear mm., mm. auriculares ventrales (NAV), mm. parotido-auricularis, styloauricularis	the fascia over the parotid gland	the fibers run dorsally to insert on the antitragus of the auricular cartilage	the cervical branch of the facial nerve	a small but distinct group of muscles that help depress and retract the ear
		13.1H Muscles of mastication			
digastric	m. digastricus (NAV), biventer	the jugular process of the occipital bone	the ventral border of the mandible	the mylohyoid branch of the trigeminal nerve and the facial nerve (to cranial and caudal bellies)	it opens the jaw; it is not always clear that it is made up of two bellies (e.g. in the dog)
lateral pterygoid	m. pterygoideus lateralis (NAV), external pterygoid	the lateral part of the sphenoid bone	the medial face of the neck and condyle of the mandible	the mandibular branch of the trigeminal	a small muscle that pulls the jaw forwards or to the side
masseter	m. masseter (NAV)	the zygomatic arch and facial crest	the lateral face of the mandible, especially its ramus	the mandibular branch of the trigeminal	relatively large in herbivores; it acts to close the jaw
medial pterygoid	m. pterygoideus medialis (NAV), internal pterygoid	the lateral part of the sphenoid, pterygoid and palatine bones	the medial face of the ramus of the mandible	the mandibular branch of the trigeminal	it closes the jaw and also helps to pull it to the side, as in chewing the cud
temporal	m. temporalis (NAV)	the surface and crest-like border to the temporal fossa	the coronoid process of the mandible	the mandibular branch of the trigeminal	it closes the jaw; relatively small in herbivores
		13.1I Muscles of the neck			
biventer	m. biventer cervicis (NAV)	the spines of the first few thoracic vertebrae	the occipital bone beneath the nuchal crest	the dorsal branches of the last six cervical nerves	the more dorsal half of the semispinalis capitis muscle
brachiocephalic	*see under* Muscles of the Forelimb				
caudal oblique m. of the head	m. obliquus capitis caudalis (NAV)	the side of the spinous process of the axis	the dorsal surface of the wing of the atlas	the dorsal branch of the second cervical nerve	a large muscle that rotates the atlas and head
cervical iliocostal	m. iliocostal cervicis (NAV), ascending cervical	the angles of the first few ribs	the transverse processes of the last few cervical vertebrae	the cervical nerves	the cranial part of the iliocostal muscle
complexus	m. complexus (NAV)	the transverse and articular processes of the thoracic and cervical vertebrae	the occipital bone beneath the nuchal crest	the dorsal branches of the last six cervical nerves	the more ventral half of the semispinalis capitis muscle
cranial oblique m. of the head	m. obliquus capitis cranialis (NAV)	the ventral surface of the wing of the atlas	the jugular and mastoid processes; the nuchal crest	the dorsal branch of the first cervical nerve	a large muscle that extends and bends the head sideways

13 **Muscles** (*Continued*)

PART 13.1 Head and neck (*Continued*)

Muscle	Other names	Origin	Insertion	Innervation	Comments
cutaneous m. of the neck	m. cutaneous colli (NAV)	the dorsal superficial fascia of the neck; fibres run between the deep and superficial layers of the sphincter colli	the commissures of the lips after running forwards over the parotid and cheek	the buccal branches of the facial nerve	part of the platysma
dorsal straight mm. of the head	m. rectus capitis dorsalis major/minor (NAV)	the spine of the axis (major); the dorsal arch of the atlas (minor)	the occipital bone, dorsal to the foramen magnum	the dorsal branch of the first cervical nerve	a group of deep muscles beneath the poll that extends the head
intertransverse	m. intertrans-versarii dorsales and ventrales cervicis (NAV)	the transverse processes of the cervical vertebrae	the transverse and articular processes of the cervical vertebrae	the cervical nerves	deep, short, muscles on the side of the neck, divided into dorsal and ventral parts
lateral straight m. of the head	m. rectus capitis lateralis (NAV)	the ventral arch of the atlas, next to the ventral straight m.	the jugular process of the occipital bone	the ventral branch of the first cervical nerve	a small muscle beneath the atlas that flexes the head
long m. of the head	m. longus capitis (NAV), rectus capitis ventralis major	the transverse processes of cervical vertebrae 3–5	the base of the skull on the basioccipital or basisphenoid	the ventral branches of the cervical nerves	a flexor of the head and part of the neck
longest m. of the atlas	m. longissimus atlantis (NAV)	the transverse processes of the first few thoracic vertebrae	the wing of the atlas	the dorsal branches of the last six cervical nerves	it runs in company with the longest muscle of the head
longest m. of the head	m. longissimus capitis (NAV)	the transverse processes of the first few thoracic vertebrae	the mastoid process of the temporal bone	the dorsal branches of the last six cervical nerves	the most cranial division of the longissimus group of muscles
long m. of the neck	m. longus colli (NAV)	the ventral surface of the bodies of thoracic vertebrae 1–6 and the transverse processes of the cervical vertebrae	the bodies and transverse processes of the cervical vertebrae	the ventral branches of the cervical nerves	a flexor of the neck that lies adjacent to the spine and is in contact with its fellow of the other side
multifidi	mm. multifidi (NAV)	the articular processes of the last four or five cervical vertebrae	the spinous and articular processes of the cervical vertebrae	the dorsal branches of the last six cervical nerves	the deepest of all the cervical muscles
oblique mm. of the head	*see* cranial oblique m. of the head, caudal oblique m. of the head				
omohyoid	m. omohyoideus (NAV)	the subscapular fascia near the shoulder joint; or the transverse processes of the last cervical vertebrae (ox)	the basihyoid bone	the ventral branch of the first cervical nerve	best developed in the horse; more weakly developed in other species; absent from the dog

Table continued over page

13 Muscles *(Continued)*

PART 13.1 Head and neck *(Continued)*

Muscle	Other names	Origin	Insertion	Innervation	Comments
omotransversarius	*see under* Muscles of the Forelimb				
rhomboids	*see under* Muscles of the Forelimb				
scalene mm.	mm. scalenus ventralis, medius and dorsalis (NAV)	the cranial border of the first rib and in some, the lateral side of the first few ribs	the transverse processes of the last four cervical vertebrae	the ventral branches of the cervical and thoracic nerves	variously subdivided in domestic species; has respiratory and neck-moving actions
semispinalis capitis	*see* biventer m., complexus m.				
sphincter colli	m. sphincter colli superficialis and profundus (NAV)	the superficial fascia of the throat and face	the skin of the throat, lips and adjacent regions	the buccal branches of the facial nerve	slender muscle strands variously disposed; some facial muscles are derived from the deep division
spinalis	*see under* Muscles of the Back				
splenius	m. splenius capitis/cervicis (NAV)	the spines of the first three or four thoracic vertebrae	the nuchal crest and transverse processes of cervical vertebrae 1–5	the dorsal branches of the last six cervical nerves	acts to elevate the head or to turn it and the neck to one side
sternocephalic	m. sterno-cephalicus	the manubrium of the sternum	the caudal border of the mandible and/or the mastoid and/or the occipital parts of the skull	the ventral branch of the accessory nerve (the eleventh cranial nerve)	in some species mandibular, mastoid or occipital parts can be identified
sternomandibularis	*see* sternocephalic				
sternothyrohyoid	m. sternohyoid-eus and m. sternothyroideus (NAV)	the manubrium of the sternum	the lamina of the thyroid cartilage and the basihyoid bone	the ventral branches of the first and second cervical nerves	may be mostly single (e.g. horse) or mostly double (e.g. dog)
straight mm. of the head	*see* dorsal, ventral and lateral straight mm. of the head				
trapezius	*see under* Muscles of the Forelimb				
ventral serrate	*see under* Muscles of the Forelimb				
ventral straight m. of the head	m. rectus capitis ventralis (NAV)	the ventral arch of the atlas	the basioccipital bone, ventral to the foramen magnum	the ventral branch of the first cervical nerve	a small muscle beneath the atlas that flexes the head

13 Muscles *(Continued)*

PART 13.2 MUSCLES OF THE TRUNK*

Muscle	Other names	Origin	Insertion	Innervation	Comments
anal sphincters	*see* external anal sphincter/ internal anal sphincter	as sphincter mm. neither have distinct origins	as sphincter mm. neither have distinct insertions	the internal m. is innervated by autonomic fibres, the external m. by somatic fibres	the two mm. are disposed concentrically; in some species anal sacs lie between them
biventer	*see under* Muscles of the Head and Neck				
brachiocephalic	*see under* Muscles of the Forelimb				
bulbocavernosus	*see* bulbospongiosus				
bulboglandularis	m. bulboglandularis (NAV)	the raphe over the dorsal part of the pelvic urethra (pig)	the m. spreads out over the surface of the bulbourethral glands	probably the perineal branch of the pudendal nerve	the m. is well-developed in pigs; striated, and may be derived from urethral, ischiourethral or bulbospongiosus mm.
bulbospongiosus	m. bulbospongiosus (NAV), bulbocavernosus	a median raphe at the sciatic arch; the wall of the corpus cavernosum	fibers unite with their fellows to encircle the urethra or form U-shaped loops ventral to it	the perineal branch of the pudendal nerve	pulsatile contraction during ejaculation and, in some species, during urination; in the female *see* vestibular and vulvar constrictors
caudal preputial m.	m. preputialis caudalis (NAV), retractor preputii	the superficial fascia near the inguinal region	the mm. from each side meet in a loop beneath the prepuce	the lateral thoracic nerve	the m. is best developed (but variably) in bulls
coccygeus	m. coccygeus (NAV)	the medial side of the sciatic spine	the transverse processes of the first few coccygeal vertebrae	the sacral nerves, often via the pudendal or caudal rectal nerve	the most lateral of the mm. that make up the pelvic diaphragm
complexus	*see under* Muscles of the Head and Neck				
cranial preputial m.	m. preputialis cranialis (NAV), protractor preputii	the superficial fascia near the xiphoid	the mm. from each side meet in a loop beneath the prepuce	the lateral thoracic nerve	it supports the prepuce and restores its position after erection
cremaster	m. cremaster (NAV)	the iliac fascia by the caudal border of the internal abdominal oblique m.	the parietal layer of the vaginal tunic of the testis	the genitofemoral nerve	the m. passes through the inguinal canal and raises the testis
cutaneous mm.	bark m., panniculus carnosus	the superficial fascia of various regions	the skin of various regions	the lateral thoracic, facial and some other nerves	many individually named mm.; well developed in echidnas, hedgehogs and armadillos

Table continued over page

* Some muscles may belong with equal validity to other divisions or subdivisions; most avian and reptilian muscles have been omitted as have most smooth muscles and a few trivial ones.

13 Muscles (*Continued*)

PART 13.2 Trunk (*Continued*)

Muscle	Other names	Origin	Insertion	Innervation	Comments
cutaneous trunci	subdivisions of this m. include: preputial, supramammary and omobrachial	the hypodermis of the gluteal region	fibres run longitudinally before terminating near the axilla	the lateral thoracic (= motor n.); sensory innervation to the overlying skin is via the segmental spinal nn.	the dual nerve supply is useful in the cutaneous trunci reflex; the preputial m. (q.v.) is derived from it
diaphragm	diaphragma (NAV), skirt	the costal cartilages of the last true ribs and the false ribs; the lumbar vertebrae and the xiphoid cartilage	a central tendon	the left and right phrenic nerves; intercostal nerves	the partition between thorax and abdomen that is the main inspiratory m.; it also regulates pressure in the thorax and abdomen
diaphragm (pelvic)	*see* levator ani and coccygeus				
dorsal serrate (cranial and caudal parts)	m. serratus dorsalis cranialis/ caudalis (NAV)	the thoraco-lumbar fascia	the cranial part to the lateral side of the middle ribs; the caudal part to the caudal ribs	the thoracic nerves	the cranial part draws the ribs forwards (during inspiration); the caudal part draws the ribs back (during expiration)
erector of penis	*see* ischio-cavernosus				
erector of spine	m. erector spinae (NAV), sacrospinal m.	the spines of the lumbar and sacral vertebrae and the iliac crest via an extensive aponeurosis	numerous complex insertions involving the ribs, vertebrae and skull	the dorsal branches of the spinal nerves	a complex of mm. that are mostly fused caudally but which subdivide into longissimus, iliocostal and spinal parts more cranially
external abdominal oblique	m. obliquus externus abdominis (NAV)	the lateral surface of the ribs and the thoracolumbar fascia	the linea alba and the prepubic tendon, fibers running obliquely caudoventrally	the intercostal, costoabdominal and lumbar nerves	the most superficial of the abdominal mm.; it has a large ventral aponeurosis
external anal sphincter	m. sphincter ani externus (NAV)	as the m. is a sphincter only a few fibers are attached to neighboring soft tissue such as the fascia below the tail	most fibers embrace the anal canal and each other; a few blend ventrally with the perineal body and the genitalia	the anal branch of the pudendal nerve	the m. is made up of subcutaneous, superficial and deep parts; it is a striated m. under voluntary control
external intercostals	mm. intercostales externi (NAV)	the caudal border of each rib	the cranial border of the next rib at a more ventral point	the intercostal nerves	inspiratory mm. that may also act during forced expiration
iliacus	*see under* Muscles of the Hindlimb				
iliocostal	m. iliocostalis (NAV)	the iliac crest, the septum between it and the longissimus m., and the caudal ribs	the ribs and the transverse process of the seventh cervical vertebra	the dorsal branches of the spinal nerves	it is the lateral division of the epaxial mm.; it has both lumbar and thoracic parts

13 Muscles (*Continued*)

PART 13.2 Trunk (*Continued*)

Muscle	Other names	Origin	Insertion	Innervation	Comments
iliopsoas	*see under* Muscles of the Hindlimb				
intercostals	*see* external and internal intercostals, and subcostals				
internal abdominal oblique	m. obliquus internus abdominis (NAV)	the thoraco-lumbar fascia, the inguinal ligament and the ilium	the linea alba, the prepubic tendon and the last few ribs; fibers run cranioventrally	the intercostal, costoabdominal and lumbar nerves	the middle of the mm. of the flank; it is thick and fleshy near the tuber coxae
internal anal sphincter	m. sphincter ani internus (NAV)	the wall of the anal canal	the wall of the anal canal	autonomic fibers from the pelvic and hypogastric nerves via the pelvic plexus	an involuntary, smooth m. that is the thickened terminal part of the circular m. of the alimentary canal
internal intercostals	mm. intercostales interni (NAV)	the caudal border of each rib	the cranial border of the next rib at a more dorsal point	the intercostal nerves	expiratory mm. that may also act during forced inspiration to brace the intercostal tissues
intertransverse mm.	mm. intertrans-versarii (NAV)	the transverse processes of the vertebrae	the transverse processes of adjacent or nearby vertebrae	the dorsal and ventral branches of adjacent spinal nerves	a complex group of small, deep mm. in all parts of the spine
ischiocavernosus	m. ischiocavernosus (NAV), erector of the penis or clitoris	the sciatic tuber behind the crus of the penis or clitoris	the sides and ventral surface of the crus of the penis or clitoris	the perineal branch of the pudendal nerve	it compresses the crus of the penis or clitoris so erecting the corpus cavernosum distally
ischiourethralis	m. ischio-urethralis (NAV)	the dorsal surface of the sciatic arch	the ventral surface of the pelvic urethra	the perineal branch of the pudendal nerve	it probably aids erection by compression of the dorsal veins of the penis
latissimus dorsi	*see under* Muscles of the Forelimb				
levator ani	m. levator ani (NAV), medial coccygeus	the medial surface of the sciatic spine	the perineal body, external anal sphincter and coccygeal vertebrae	the sacral nerves, usually via the pudendal or caudal rectal nerve	a principal part of the pelvic diaphragm very well developed in the human pelvis
levators of ribs	mm. levatores costarum (NAV)	the transverse processes of the last cervical and the thoracic vertebrae	the cranial borders of the ribs near the angles	the intercostal nerves	small inspiratory segmental mm. that draw the ribs forwards
longissimus	m. longissimus (NAV), eye m., longissimus dorsi, long dorsi	the iliac crest, and the spinous and other processes of the lumbar and thoracic vertebrae	the transverse processes of the thoracic and cervical vertebrae, and the temporal bone	the dorsal branches of the spinal nerves	the large, middle division of the epaxial mm.; has lumbar, thoracic cervical and capital parts; *see* erector of spine

Table continued over page

13 Muscles (*Continued*)

PART 13.2 Trunk (*Continued*)

Muscle	Other names	Origin	Insertion	Innervation	Comments
multifidi	mm. multifidi (NAV)	a complex set of mm. that arise mainly from the articular processes of the vertebrae	short and long varieties insert mainly into the spinous processes of the more cranial vertebrae	the medial branches of the dorsal divisions of the segmental spinal nerves	numerous, short, individual, overlapping mm. from the sacrum to the axis
omotransverse	*see under* Muscles of the Forelimb				
pectorals	*see under* Muscles of the Forelimb				
pelvic diaphragm	diaphragma pelvis (NAV). *See* levator ani and coccygeus				
preputial mm.	*see* cranial and caudal preputial mm.				
protractor preputii	*see* cranial preputial m.				
psoas mm.	*see under* Muscles of the Hindlimb				
quadratus lumborum	m. quadratus lumborum (NAV)	the lumbar transverse processes and the last ribs	the ventral surface of the wing of the sacrum	the intercostal and lumbar nerves	the psoas mm. lie ventral to it
rectus abdominis	m. rectus abdominis (NAV)	the caudal part of the sternum and the adjacent costal cartilages	the pubis by means of the prepubic tendon	the intercostal, costoabdominal, and lumbar nerves	tendinous intersections cross the m. transversely
rectus thoracis	m. rectus thoracis (NAV), transverse costarum	the lateral face of the first rib	the ventral ends of the first few ribs	the intercostal nerves	despite its name and position it is not homologous with the rectus abdominis
retractor of the clitoris	m. retractor clitoridis (NAV)	the last sacral or first few caudal vertebrae	partly around the anus; most to the clitoris	the perineal branch of the pudendal nerve	a feeble homolog of the retractor penis
retractor penis	m. retractor penis (NAV)	the last sacral or first few caudal vertebrae	partly around the anus; mostly on the ventral surface of the penis near the preputial fornix	the perineal branch of the pudendal nerve	mostly smooth m.
retractor preputii	*see* caudal preputial m.				
retractor of the ribs	m. retractor costae (NAV)	the transverse processes of the first few lumbar vertebrae	the caudal border of the last rib	the lumbar nerves	it acts as an expiratory m. by drawing the ribs backwards
rhomboids	*see under* Muscles of the Forelimb				
rotators	mm. rotatores (NAV)	the transverse processes of the vertebrae	short and long varieties insert onto the spinous processes of the two vertebrae more cranial to it	medial branches of the dorsal divisions of the segmental spinal nerves	the deepest of the transversospinalis mm.

13 Muscles *(Continued)*

PART 13.2 Trunk *(Continued)*

Muscle	Other names	Origin	Insertion	Innervation	Comments
sacrocaudal mm.	mm. sacrocaudalis ventralis/dorsalis medialis/lateralis (NAV)	various parts of the sacral and first few tail vertebrae	various parts of the more distal members of the caudal vertebrae	the sacral and caudal nerves	a series of eight mm. arranged in dorsal and ventral arrays
scalene mm.	*see under* Muscles of the Head and Neck				
semispinalis	m. semispinalis (NAV), semispinal m.	the transverse processes of the vertebrae	the spines of the more cranial vertebrae	the dorsal divisions of the segmental spinal nerves	frequently fused with the spinalis m.; present in thoracic, cervical and capital parts
spinalis	m. spinalis (NAV), spinal m.	the tips of the spines of the verterbae	the spines of the more cranial vertebrae	the dorsal divisions of the segmental spinal nerves	frequently fused with the semispinalis m.
subclavius	*see under* Muscles of the Forelimb				
subcostals	mm. subcostales (NAV)	the caudal borders of the ribs near their vertebral ends	the cranial borders of ribs more than one away from the origin	the intercostal nerves	an occasional derivative of the internal intercostal, e.g. over ribs 9–11 of dogs
supramammary	m. supra-mammarius cranialis/caudalis (NAV)	the superficial fascia near the xiphoid	passes under the mammae to reach the public region	the lateral thoracic nerve	present in the bitch; it is the homologue of the preputial mm. of the male
tail mm.	*see* sacrocaudal and inter-transverse mm.				
transverse abdominis	m. transversus abdominis (NAV)	the transverse processes of the lumbar vertebrae and the medial surfaces of the asternal ribs	the linea alba and the xiphoid cartilage	the intercostal, costoabdominal and lumbar nerves	the deepest of the abdominal mm. with long fibers
transverse thoracic	m. transversus thoracis (NAV), false skirt	the dorsal surface of the sternum or the sternal ligament	the costal cartilages of most of the true ribs	the intercostal nerves	the m. draws the two halves of the thorax together, thus assisting expiration
transversospinalis	m. transverso-spinalis (NAV)	a complex set of mm. that arise from the spinous, transverse and other processes of the vertebrae	fascicles run between vertebrae that are adjacent to, close to, or at some distance from one another	the medial branches of the dorsal divisions of the segmental spinal nerves	the most medial of the epaxial mm.; made up of the semispinalis, multifidi and rotators
trapezius	*see under* Muscles of the Forelimb				
urethralis	m. urethralis (NAV)	the m. surrounds the pelvic urethra	it is made up of longitudinal and transverse fibers	the perineal branch of the pudental nerve	it is present in both males and females
ventral serrate	*see under* Muscles of the Forelimb				

Table continued over page

13 Muscles *(Continued)*

PART 13.2 Trunk *(Continued)*

Muscle	Other names	Origin	Insertion	Innervation	Comments
vestibular constrictor (of vulva)	m. constrictor vestibuli (NAV)	the m. is a sphincter that lies cranial to the constrictor of the vulva	it is incomplete dorsally	the perineal branch of the pudendal nerve	with the vulvar constrictor it is the homologue of the male bulbo-spongiosus m.
vulvar constrictor	m. constrictor vulvae (NAV)	the m. is a sphincter that is continuous with the external anal sphincter	it lies within the labia	the perineal branch of the pudendal nerve	with the vestibular constrictor it is the homologue of the male bulbo-spongiosus m.

PART 13.3 MUSCLES OF THE FORELIMB

Muscle	Other names	Origin	Insertion	Innervation	Comments
abductor of digit 2	m. abductor digit II (NAV)	the palmar face of the second metacarpal bone of the pig	the first phalanx of digit 2	the deep branch of the ulnar nerve	one of the stronger intrinsic mm. of the pig's trotter
abductor of digit 5	m. abductor digit V (NAV), abductor digiti quinti	the accessory carpal bone	the lateral sesamoid bone in common with the flexor of digit 5	the deep branch of the ulnar nerve	one of the stronger intrinsic mm. of the paw
abductor digiti quinti	*see* abductor of digit 5				
abductor pollicis brevis	m. abductor digiti I [pollicis] brevis (NAV), short abductor of the thumb	connective tissue at the base of the dewclaw	the medial surface of the proximal phalanx of the dewclaw	the deep branch of the ulnar nerve	the most medial of the three tiny mm. that supply the dewclaw of carnivores
abductor pollicis longus	*see* oblique extensor (of carpus)				
adductor of digit 1	*see* adductor pollicis				
adductor of digit 2	m. adductor digit II (NAV), adductor of the second digit	the flexor retinaculum of the carpus	the lateral surface of the proximal phalanx of digit 2	the deep branch of the ulnar nerve	with the adductor of digit 5 this m. pulls the toes of a paw together
adductor of digit 5	m. adductor digiti V (NAV), adductor of the fifth digit, adductor digiti quinti	the flexor retinaculum of the carpus	the medial surface of metacarpal 5 and the proximal phalanx of digit 5	the deep branch of the ulnar nerve	with the adductor of digit 2 this m. pulls the toes of a paw together
adductor digiti quinti	*see* adductor of digit 5				
adductor pollicis	m. adductor digiti I [pollicis] (NAV), adductor of the thumb	connective tissue at the base of the dewclaw	the lateral side of the proximal phalanx of the dewclaw	the deep branch of the ulnar nerve	the most lateral and stoutest of three special mm. of the dewclaw of carnivores
anconeus	m. anconeus (NAV)	the epicondylar crest and adjacent caudal surface of the humerus	the lateral surface of the olecranon	the radial nerve	a small m. that occupies the space between the triceps and the olecranon fossa

13 Muscles (*Continued*)

PART 13.3 Forelimb (*Continued*)

Muscle	Other names	Origin	Insertion	Innervation	Comments
articular m. of shoulder	m. articularis humeri (NAV), capsularis	the caudal rim of the glenoid cavity	the neck of the humerus	the axillary nerve	small and of doubtful function; found in horses and occasionally pigs
biceps	m. biceps brachii (NAV)	the supraglenoid tubercle	the radial tuberosity and the tendon of the radial carpal extensor	the musculo-cutaneous nerve	a biarticular m. that flexes the elbow and extends the shoulder
brachialis	m. brachialis (NAV)	the caudal surface of the proximal half of the humerus	the medial borders of the radius and ulna	the musculo-cutaneous nerve	an exclusive flexor of the elbow
brachiocephalic	m. brachio-cephalicus (NAV)	depending on the species, various parts of the nuchal crest, mastoid process, nape and adjacent regions	the distal part of the crest of the humerus between the biceps and the brachialis	the dorsal and ventral branches of the accessory nerve and the axillary nerve	a m. that is divided into two parts by the clavicle or the clavicular tendon; *see* cleidocephalic and cleidobrachial mm.
brachioradialis	m. brachioradialis (NAV), long supinator	the lateral supracondylar ridge of the humerus	the distal end of the radius	the radial nerve	a supinator that is absent from many animals; well developed in the cat, weak in the dog, large in the human arm
capsularis	*see* articular m. of shoulder				
cleidobrachial	m. cleidobrachialis (NAV)	the clavicle or the clavicular tendon and the cleidocephalic m.	the distal part of the crest of the humerus	the accessory and axillary nerves	this m. makes up the distal segment of the brachiocephalic m.
cleidocephalic	m. cleido-cephalicus (NAV)	the nuchal crest, mastoid process, nape and adjacent regions depending on the species	the clavicle or the clavicular tendon and the cleido-brachial m.	the accessory nerve	the m. is divided into cervical, mastoid and occipital parts, which were formerly regarded as a separate mm.
cleidocervical	m. cleido-cervicalis, m. cleidocephalicus pars cervicalis (NAV)	the dorsal midline raphe over the cranial half of the neck	the clavicle or the clavicular tendon and the cleido-brachial m.	the accessory nerve	amongst the domestic animals it is only well developed in cats and dogs
cleidomastoid	m. cleido-mastoideus, m. cleidocephalicus pars mastoideus (NAV)	the mastoid process of the temporal bone	the clavicle or the clavicular tendon and the cleidobrachial m.	the accessory nerve	this part of the cleidocephalic is present in all of the domestic mammals
cleidooccipital	m. cleido-occipitalis, m. cleidocephalicus pars occipitalis (NAV)	the nuchal crest and sometimes adjacent regions of the neck	the clavicle or the clavicular tendon and the cleidobrachial m.	the accessory nerve	it is best developed in pigs and ruminants
cleidotrans-versarius	*see* omotransverse				

Table continued over page

13 Muscles (*Continued*)

PART 13.3 Forelimb (*Continued*)

Muscle	Other names	Origin	Insertion	Innervation	Comments
common digital extensor	m. extensor digitorum communis (NAV)	the lateral epicondylar crest of the humerus; in some, the radius and ulna too	the proximal ends of the distal phalanges of digits 2–5	the radial nerve	in ruminants a distinct medial belly is present that supplies digit 3
coracobrachial	m. coracobrachialis (NAV)	the coracoid process of the scapula	on either side of the tuberosity for the teres major	the musculo-cutaneous nerve	a small m. that crosses the shoulder and has, presumably, an adductor function
deep digital flexor	m. flexor digitorum profundus (NAV), flexor perforans	the medial epicondyle of the humerus and the medial surfaces of the olecranon and radius; in some species an accessory head from the palmar carpal ligament	the semilunar line on the solar surface of the distal phalanx	the median and/or the ulnar nerve	the accessory head in horses is also called the subcarpal or inferior check ligament
deep pectoral	m. pectoralis profundus (NAV), m. pectoralis ascendents (NAV alternative), ascending pectoral, caudal deep pectoral, minor pectoral (human)	all or most of the sternebrae, the fascia over the xiphoid and the costal cartilages	the greater and lesser tubercles of the humerus	the pectoral nerves	the m. is a strong retractor and adductor of the forelimb; insertions vary between species
deltoid	m. deltoideus (NAV)	the spine of the scapula, the acromion and the clavicle	the deltoid tuberosity and brachial fascia	the axillary nerve	a shoulder flexor and abductor with scapular, acromial and clavicular heads
descending pectoral	m. pectoralis descendens (NAV), cranial superficial pectoral	the manubrium and adjacent parts of the ribs and sternum	the crest of the humerus, and the brachial and antebrachial fascia	the pectoral nerves	this is the most cranial and superficial of the pectorals
digital flexors	*see* deep and superficial digital flexors				
extensor carpi radialis	*see* radial extensor of the carpus				
extensor carpi ulnaris	*see* ulnaris lateralis				
extensor of digit 2	m. extensor digiti II (NAV)	the proximal end of the ulna	it fuses with the tendon of the common digital extensor to the second digit	the radial nerve	readily identifiable in the pig
flexor carpi radialis	*see* radial flexor of the carpus				
flexor carpi ulnaris	see ulnar flexor of the carpus				

13 Muscles *(Continued)*

PART 13.3 Forelimb *(Continued)*

Muscle	Other names	Origin	Insertion	Innervation	Comments
flexor of digit 2	m. flexor digiti II (NAV)	the deep flexor tendon	the proximal phalanx and adjacent tissue of digit 2	the deep branch of the ulnar nerve	in domestic mammals the m. is only of significance in the pig
flexor of digit 5	m. flexor digiti V (NAV), flexor digiti quinti	the accessory carpal ligament	a common tendon with the abductor of digit 5	the deep branch of the ulnar nerve	one of four short mm. that act on the palmar side of digit 5
flexor digitorum brevis	*see* short digital flexor				
flexor pollicis brevis	m. flexor digiti I [pollicis] brevis (NAV), short flexor of the thumb	the connective tissue at the base of the dewclaw	the sesamoid bone at the base of the proximal phalanx	the deep branch of the ulnar nerve	the middle of the three small, short mm. that act on the dewclaw of carnivores
infraspinatus	m. infraspinarus (NAV)	the infraspinous fossa and cartilage of the scapula	the greater tubercle of the humerus	the suprascapular nerve	a stabilizing m. and abductor of the shoulder
interflexors	mm. interflexorii (NAV)	the tendon of the deep digital flexor	the tendon of the superficial digital flexor	the median nerve	a m. with several possible homologues; true function obscure
interosseous	mm. interossei (NAV), suspensory ligament (horse)	the proximal ends of the metacarpal bones	the proximal sesamoid bones and, indirectly, the proximal phalanges and the digital extensor tendons	the ulnar nerve	four mm. in each dog paw; fleshy in carnivores and the pig; mostly fibrous in ruminants and horses
lateral digital extensor	m. extensor digitorum lateralis (NAV), extensor digiti minimi (man)	the lateral collateral ligament of the elbow and adjacent parts	the proximal ends of the proximal phalanges of digits 3–5, or the tendons of the common extensor at this point	the radial nerve	the number of tendons varies from four in the cat to one in the horse and the human arm
latissimus dorsi	m. latissimus dorsi (NAV), broadest m. of the back	an aponeurosis continuous with the thoracolumbar fascia over the caudal thorax and loins	the teres tubercle or the crest of the lesser tubercle	the thoracodorsal nerve	one of the major retractors of the forelimb; it makes up most of the dorsal fold of the human axilla
lumbricales	mm. lumbricales (NAV)	the abaxial borders of the tendons of the deep digital flexor	the proximal ends of the proximal phalanges of digits 3–5 on the palmomedial side	the deep branch of the ulnar nerve	pale flimsy mm. that lie mostly between the superficial and deep digital flexors
m. of Phillips	extensor of the fourth and fifth digits; the radial head of the common digital extensor	the proximal end of the radius as a separate head of the common digital extensor (in horses)	a tendinous slip off the common digital extensor that joins the tendon of the lateral digital extensor	the radial nerve	its tendon can take on a number of different forms over the metacarpus

Table continued over page

13 Muscles (*Continued*)

PART 13.3 Forelimb (*Continued*)

Muscle	Other names	Origin	Insertion	Innervation	Comments
m. of Thiernesse	the ulnar head of the common digital extensor	the proximal end of the ulna as a separate head of the common digital extensor (in horses)	a delicate tendon descends on the medial side of the common digital extensor tendon to end on the proximal phalanx	the radial nerve	an uncommon variation of the common digital extensor that may correspond to the extensor of digit 2
oblique extensor (of carpus)	m. abductor digiti I [pollicis] longus (NAV), long abductor of the thumb	the lateral border of the middle of the radius and ulna	the proximal end of metacarpal 1, or 2 in the horse	the radial nerve	the belly is partly covered by the common digital extensor
omotransverse	m. omotrans-versarius (NAV), cleidotrans-versarius	the acromion, the spine of the scapula, or the fascia over the shoulder	the caudal border of the wing of the atlas; in horses the transverse processes of cervical vertebrae 2–4 also	the ventral branches of the cervical nerves	the m. overlies the superficial cervical lymph node, and may fuse with or course deep to the brachiocephalic
pectorals	*see* superficial pectorals, deep pectoral, subclavius				
Phillips' m.	*see* m. of Phillips				
pronator quadratus	m. pronator quadratus (NAV)	the medial interosseous border of the ulna	the medial border of the radius	the median nerve	in carnivores but not in ungulates
pronator teres	m. pronator teres (NAV)	the medial epicondyle of the humerus	the medial border and cranial surface of the proximal radius	the median nerve	in carnivores but not ungulates, in which it is reduced to a ligament
radial extensor of the carpus	m. extensor carpi radialis (NAV)	the lateral epicondylar crest of the humerus	the tuberosities on the proximal ends of the dorsal surface of meta-carpal 3 (and 2)	the radial nerve	long and short heads are recognizable in cats and in some dogs
radial flexor of the carpus	m. flexor carpi radialis (NAV)	the medial epicondyle of the humerus	the proximal end of metacarpal 2 and sometimes metacarpal 3	the median nerve	the m. has a long thin tendon of insertion
rhomboids	mm. rhomboideus thoracis/cervicis/capitis (NAV)	the occiput, the dorsal midline of the neck and the thoracic spines	the medial surface of the scapular cartilage or the dorsal border of the scapula	the ventral branches of cervical and thoracic nerves	the divisions into parts vary among species; the m. forms the hump of Indian breeds of cattle
short digital flexor	m. flexor digitorum brevis (NAV), palmaris brevis accessorius	the dorsal surface of the superficial digital flexor tendon	the palmar surface of the meta-carpophalangeal joint of digit 5 (dogs) and digits 3–5 (cats)	the deep branch of the ulnar nerve	only found in carnivores; well developed in cats
subclavius	m. subclavius (NAV), cranial deep pectoral, prescapular part of the deep pectoral	the manubrium and adjacent parts of the sternum and ribs	the cranial border of the scapula and the clavicle	the cranial pectoral nerve or the subclavian nerve	the m. is large in the pig and horse

13 Muscles *(Continued)*

PART 13.3 Forelimb *(Continued)*

Muscle	Other names	Origin	Insertion	Innervation	Comments
subscapular	m. subscapularis (NAV)	the subscapular fossa	the lesser tubercle of the humerus	the subscapular nerve	a stabilizing m. and adductor of the shoulder
superficial digital flexor	m. flexor digitorum superficialis (NAV), flexor perforatus	the medial epicondyle of the humerus; in some species there is an accessory head from the distal radius	the proximal extremity of the middle phalanx	the median and/or the ulnar nerve	the accessory head in horses is also called the radial check ligament
superficial pectorals	mm. pectorales superficiales (NAV)	the manubrium and adjacent parts of the ribs and sternum	the crest of the humerus, and the antebrachial fascia	pectoral nerves	these mm. vary between species; see the two components: transverse and descending pectoral
supinator	m. supinator (NAV)	the lateral epicondyle of the humerus	the cranial surface of the radius	the radial nerve	this m. is a synergist of the brachioradialis
supraspinatus	m. supraspinatus (NAV)	the supraspinous fossa, spine and cartilage of the scapula	the greater and lesser tubercles of the humerus	the suprascapular nerve	a stabilizing m. and extensor of the shoulder
suspensory lig.	*see* interosseous				
tensor of the antebrachial fascia	m. tensor fasciae antebrachii (NAV)	the latissimus dorsi, especially its ventral border	the olecranon and the deep fascia of the forearm	the radial nerve	a thin broad m. whose action is similar to the long head of the triceps
teres major	m. teres major (NAV)	the caudal angle of the scapula	the teres tubercle	the axillary nerve	it flexes the shoulder and rotates the limb inwards
teres minor	m. teres minor (NAV)	the middle of the caudal border of the scapula	the greater and deltoid tubercles	the axillary nerve	a small m. that flexes the shoulder and rotates the arm outwards
Thiernesses's m.	*see* m. of Thiernesse				
transverse pectoral	m. pectoralis transversus (NAV), caudal superficial pectoral	the manubrium and adjacent parts of the ribs and sternum	the crest of the humerus and the antebrachial fascia	the pectoral nerves	one of the two superficial pectorals
trapezius	m. trapezius (NAV), cucullaris	the dorsal midline raphe and supraspinous ligament from about the third cervical to the tenth thoracic vertebra	the cervical part inserts along the whole scapular spine, the thoracic part only along the proximal part of the spine	the dorsal branch of the accessory nerve	in combination the right and left mm. resemble a shawl or cowl draped over the withers, hence the name cucullaris
triceps—accessory head	m. triceps brachii, caput accessorium (NAV)	the caudal surface of the humerus	the olecranon of the ulna	the radial nerve	it is found in carnivores in which it is surrounded by other heads

Table continued over page

13 Muscles (*Continued*)

PART 13.3 Forelimb (*Continued*)

Muscle	Other names	Origin	Insertion	Innervation	Comments
triceps—lateral head	m. triceps brachii, caput laterale (NAV)	the tricipital line of the humerus	the lateral side of the summit of the olecranon	the radial nerve	it often merges with the long head
triceps—long head	m. triceps brachii, caput longum (NAV)	the caudal angle and caudal border of the scapula	the summit of the olecranon	the radial nerve	usually the largest head of the triceps; the only head to be biarticular
triceps—medial head	m. triceps brachii, caput mediale (NAV)	the medial surface of the humerus	the medial side of the summit of the olecranon	the radial nerve	often the smallest of the three heads
ulnar carpal extensor	*see* ulnaris lateralis				
ulnar flexor of the carpus	m. flexor carpi ulnaris (NAV)	the medial epicondyle of the humerus and the medial surface of the ulna	the accessory carpal bone	the ulnar nerve	the humeral head is much the larger
ulnaris lateralis	m. extensor carpi ulnaris (NAV), m. ulnaris lateralis (NAV alternative)	the lateral epicondyle of the humerus caudal to the collateral ligament of the elbow	the accessory carpal bone; the fourth or fifth metacarpal bone	the radial nerve	despite its radial innervation and name, in most species it is a flexor of the carpus
ventral serrate	m. serratus ventralis cervicis/thoracis (NAV), the cervical and thoracic ventral serrates	the transverse processes of the last five cervical vertebrae and the first eight to ten ribs	the serrated face of the medial surface of the scapula	the ventral branches of the cervical nerves and the long thoracic nerve	the right and left mm. act together to suspend the cranial part of the trunk like a sling between the forelimbs

PART 13.4 MUSCLES OF THE HINDLIMB

Muscle	Other names	Origin	Insertion	Innervation	Comments
abductor cruris caudalis	*see* caudal crural abductor				
abductor of digit 1	*see* abductor hallucis				
abductor of digit 2	m. abductor digiti II (NAV)	the plantar face of the second metatarsal bone	the first phalanx of digit 2	the tibial nerve	found in pigs
abductor of digit 5	m. abductor digiti V (NAV), abductor digiti quinti	the calcaneus	the proximal phalanx of digit 5; sometimes its superficial flexor tendon	the tibial nerve	it consists of two parts, and in the dog is partly tendinous
abductor hallucis	m. abductor digiti I [hallucis] (NAV), abductor of the big toe	connective tissue on the plantar surface of the tarsus	the base of the proximal phalanx of digit 1	the tibial nerve	absent from most domestic mammals; occurs in some primates
accessory flexor	*see* quadratus plantae				
accessory gluteal	m. gluteus accessorius (NAV). *See also* pirformis	the gluteal line on the dorsal surface of the ilium	the greater trochanter of the femur	the cranial gluteal nerve	the m. is a deep portion of the middle gluteal; not present in carnivores

13 Muscles *(Continued)*

PART 13.4 Hindlimb *(Continued)*

Muscle	Other names	Origin	Insertion	Innervation	Comments
adductor	m. adductor (NAV). *See also* short, long and great adductors	the ventral surface of the pelvis and the symphyseal tendon of the gracilis	the rough face of the femur	the obturator nerve	the m. is made up of three or four parts which are variably fused in each species
adductor brevis	*see* short adductor				
adductor of digit 1	*see* adductor hallucis				
adductor of digit 2	m. adductor digiti II (NAV), adductor of the second digit	the plantar surface of the tarsus	the lateral surface of the proximal phalanx of digit 2	the tibial nerve	with the adductor of digit 5 this m. pulls the toes of a paw together
adductor of digit 5	m. adductor digiti V (NAV), adductor of the fifth digit, adductor digiti quinti	the plantar surface of the tarsus	the medial surface of the metatarsal and proximal phalanx of digit 5	the tibial nerve	with the adductor of digit 2 this m. pulls the toes of a paw together
adductor hallucis	m. adductor digiti I [hallucis] (NAV), adductor of the big toe	connective tissue at the distal end of the tarsus	the lateral side of the proximal phalanx of digit 1	the tibial nerve	absent from most domestic species; large in the human foot
adductor longus	*see* long adductor				
adductor magnus	*see* great adductor				
articular m. of hip	m. articularis coxae (NAV), capsularis coxae	the cranial rim of the acetabulum	the proximal end of the femur after passing over the joint capsule	the cranial gluteal nerve	in horses and carnivores; it may have a receptor function
articular m. of stifle	m. articularis genus (NAV), capsularis genus	the cranial surface of the femur just proximal to the trochlea	with the quadriceps m. onto the tibial tuberosity	the femoral nerve	in carnivores; it may function to tense the pouch of the stifle joint capsule
biceps	*see* biceps femoris and gluteobiceps				
biceps femoris	m. biceps femoris (NAV)	the sacrotuberous ligament and sciatic tuber (all spp): the spinous and transverse processes of the last sacral vertebrae (horses, pigs and ruminants)	the fascia lata crural fascia, patella, patellar ligament, tibia and calcanean tuber	branches of the sciatic nerve: the caudal gluteal nerve and muscular branches of the tibial nerve	the m. is large, complex, and varied between species; it is one of the hamstrings and one of the principal extensors of the hip
caudal crural abductor	m. abductor cruris caudalis (NAV), the tenuissimus	the distal end of the sacro-tuberous ligament	the crural fascia on the lateral side	the fibular nerve	a long ribbon-like m. found in dogs and, in more rudimentary form, in cats

Table continued over page

13 Muscles *(Continued)*

PART 13.4 Hindlimb *(Continued)*

Muscle	Other names	Origin	Insertion	Innervation	Comments
caudal tibial	m. tibialis caudalis (NAV)	the caudal surface of the tibia and fibula	the plantar surface of the distal phalanges of the major digits; the medial face of tarsus (carnivores)	the tibial nerve	one of the deep digital flexors except in carnivores in which it is an independent m.
caudofemoral	*see* gluteofemoral				
cranial tibial	m. tibialis cranialis (NAV)	the proximal tibia and crural fascia	the proximal end of metatarsal 3; via the medial (cunean) tendon, tarsal bones 1 and 2 (horse)	the peroneal nerve	the m. is superficial in carnivores but is partly concealed by the long extensor and peroneus tertius in others
deep digital flexors	mm. flexores digitorum profundus (NAV)	the caudal surfaces of the tibia and fibula	the plantar aspect of the distal phalanx of the major digits	the tibial nerve	a composite m. of three parts; *see* lateral and medial digital flexors and the caudal tibial m.
deep gluteal	m. gluteus profundus (NAV)	the shaft of the ilium and the spine of the ischium	the greater trochanter	the cranial gluteal nerve	a small gluteal m. that acts more as an abductor than as a hip extensor
digital flexors	*see* deep, superficial, lateral, medial and short digital flexors, and the caudal tibial m.				
extensor digitorum longus	*see* long digital extensor				
extensor hallucis longus	*see* long extensor of the hallux				
external obturator	m. obturatorius externus (NAV), m. obturatorius externus pars intrapelvina (NAV, ruminants)	the ventral surface of the pelvis around the obturator foramen (all species); the inner surface also in ruminants and pigs	the trochanteric fossa	the obturator nerve	the m. is called external because it lies outside the pelvis despite it lying deeply; the intrapelvic part was formerly known as the internal obturator
fibular mm.	*see* peroneus brevis, longus and tertius				
flexor accessorius	*see* quadratus plantae				
flexor digitorum brevis	*see* short digital flexor				
flexor hallucis brevis	m. flexor digiti I [hallucis] brevis (NAV), short flexor of the big toe	the connective tissue at the base of the dewclaw	the base of the proximal phalanx of digit I	the tibial nerve	only present in carnivores if the hind dewclaw is complete
flexor hallucis longus	*see* lateral digital flexor				

13 Muscles (*Continued*)

PART 13.4 Hindlimb (*Continued*)

Muscle	Other names	Origin	Insertion	Innervation	Comments
gastrocnemius	m. gastrocnemius (NAV)	lateral and medial heads from the supracondyloid tuberosities of the distal femur	the calcaneal tuber	the tibial nerve	the major component of the triceps surae
gemelli	mm. gemelli (NAV)	the lateral side of the ramus of the ischium	the trochanteric fossa	the sciatic nerve	the single m. of the domestic mammals is formed from the fusion of two parts
gluteals	*see* accessory, deep, middle and superficial gluteal, gluteobiceps, gluteofemoral and piriformis	the dorsal surface of the ilium and adjacent regions	mostly to the greater and the third trochanters of the femur	the cranial and caudal gluteal nerves	a major group of extensor mm. of the hip that act synergistically with the hamstrings
gluteobiceps	m. gluteobiceps (NAV)	the broad sacrotuberous ligament and the sciatic tuber	the fascia lata, crural fascia, patella, patellar ligament, tibia and calcaneal tuber	the caudal gluteal nerve	the m. represents a fusion of the cranial part of the biceps and the superficial gluteal; in pigs and ruminants
gluteofemoral	m. gluteofemoralis (NAV), caudofemoral, cranial crucial abductor	the second to fourth tail vertebrae	the fascia lata and the patella	the caudal gluteal nerve	amongst the domestic mammals the m. is unique to the cat
gracilis	m. gracilis (NAV)	the symphyseal tendon beneath the pelvic symphysis, in common with the adductor	the fascia over the medial surface of the stifle joint and thus, indirectly, the tibia	the obturator nerve	the m. is broad in the domestic mammals despite its name
great adductor	m. adductor magnus (NAV)	the ventral surface of the pelvis and the symphyseal tendon	the rough face of the femur	the obturator nerve	the largest of the adductors; fused with the short adductor in ruminants and pigs
hamstrings	an informal grouping of mm.; *see* biceps femoris, semitendinosus and semimembranosus	various parts of the sacrum, ischium and associated ligaments	the fascia lata, crural fascia, patella, patellar ligaments, tibia and calcaneal tuber (the 'strings')	branches of the caudal gluteal and sciatic nerves	the major group of extensors of the hip that act in concert with the gluteals for forward propulsion
iliacus	m. iliacus (NAV), iliac m.	the ventral surface of the wing of the ilium	the lesser trochanter of the femur	the femoral nerve	a part of the iliopsoas m. that acts to flex the hip joint
iliopsoas	m. iliopsoas (NAV), fillet steak m.	the bodies of most of the lumbar vertebrae and the ventral surface of the wing of the ilium	the lesser trochanter of the femur	the ventral branches of the lumbar nerves	the tender m. of fillet steak; made up of the psoas major and iliacus mm.

Table continued over page

13 Muscles (*Continued*)

PART 13.4 Hindlimb (*Continued*)

Muscle	Other names	Origin	Insertion	Innervation	Comments
interflexors	mm. interflexorii (NAV)	the tendon of the deep digital flexor with the suspensory ligament of the pad	the tendons of the superficial digital flexor, more distally	the tibial nerve	only found in carnivores, in which they are paired (unpaired in the forefoot)
intermediate vastus	m. vastus intermedius (NAV)	the cranial surface of the femur	the patella and thus, indirectly, the tibial tuberosity	the femoral nerve	the least distinct of the three vasti and the smallest of the quadriceps
internal obturator	m. obturatorius internus (NAV)	the inner surface of the pelvis around the obturator foramen	the trochanteric fossa after passing over the lesser sciatic notch	the caudal gluteal nerve	present in horses and carnivores; *see also* the external obturator with which it can be confused
interosseous	mm. interossei (NAV), suspensory ligament (horse)	the proximal ends of the metatarsal bones	the proximal sesamoid bones and, indirectly, the proximal phalanges	the tibial nerve	four mm. in each dog paw; fleshy in carnivores and the pig, mostly fibrous in horses and ruminants
lateral digital extensor	m. extensor digitorum lateralis (NAV)	the lateral collateral ligament of the stifle and adjacent parts	the long digital extensor tendon (horse); middle phalanx of digit 4 (ruminants); the proximal phalanx of digit 5 (carnivores)	the peroneal nerve	the m. lies deep or caudal to the peroneus longus
lateral digital flexor	m. flexor digitorum lateralis (NAV); formerly called flexor hallucis longus	the caudal surface of the tibia and fibula	the plantar surface of the distal phalanges of the major digits	the tibial nerve	the deepest and largest of the three deep digital flexors
lateral vastus	m. vastus lateralis (NAV)	the cranial and lateral surface of the femur	the patella and thus, indirectly, the tibial tuberosity	the femoral nerve	one of the four components of the quadriceps
long adductor	m. adductor longus (NAV); confused with the short adductor in some texts	the ventral surface of the pubis	the rough face of the femur	the obturator nerve	found independently only in the cat; in others it is fused with the pectineus
long digital extensor	m. extensor digitorum longus (NAV), extensor of digit 3	the extensor fossa of the femur, with the peroneus tertius	the proximal ends of the distal phalanges of digits 2–5	the peroneal nerve	depending on species the m. has one to three bellies and one to four tendons
long digital flexor	*see* medial digital flexor				
long extensor of the hallux	m. extensor digiti I [hallucis] longus (NAV), long extensor of the first digit	the middle part of the fibula	the proximal phalanx of digit 2 (carnivores and pigs); the metatarsals (sheep); the big toe (primates)	the peroneal nerve	absent from cattle and horses

13 Muscles *(Continued)*

PART 13.4 Hindlimb *(Continued)*

Muscle	Other names	Origin	Insertion	Innervation	Comments
long peroneal	*see* peroneus longus				
lumbricales	mm. lumbricales (NAV)	the abaxial borders of the tendons of the deep digital flexor	the proximal ends of the proximal phalanges of digits 3–5	the tibial nerve	pale mm. of horses and carnivores
medial digital flexor	m. flexor digitorum medialis (NAV); formerly called long digital flexor	the caudal surface of the tibia and fibula	the plantar aspect of the distal phalanx of the major digits	the tibial nerve	the medial component of the deep digital flexors; its tendon joins that of the lateral flexor distal to the hock
medial vastus	m. vastus medialis (NAV)	the cranial and medial surface of the femur	the patella and thus, indirectly, the tibial tubercle	the femoral nerve	one of the four components of the quadriceps
middle gluteal	m. gluteus medius (NAV). *See also* accessory gluteal	the iliac crest, the gluteal surface of the ilium, and (in horses) the aponeurosis of the longissimus lumborum	the greater trochanter of the femur	the cranial gluteal nerve	a large m.; the largest m. of the horse, in which it extends unusually far forward over the loins
obturators	*see* external and internal obturator				
pectineus	m. pectineus (NAV)	the pecten of the pubis and the iliopubic eminence	the medial lip of the rough face of the femoral shaft	the obturator and/or the femoral nerves	a strong spindle-shaped m. that forms the caudal boundary of the femoral canal
peroneus brevis	m. peroneus brevis (NAV), fibularis brevis, short peroneal	the lateral surface of the distal two-thirds of the fibula	the proximal end of the fifth metatarsal	the peroneal nerve	only present in carnivores, even then as a weak m.
peroneus longus	m. peroneus longus (NAV), fibularis longus, long peroneal	the proximal end of the fibula and adjacent regions	after a lateral course it inserts on the first or second tarsals or the first metatarsal	the peroneal nerve	absent from horses; it acts to pronate the foot
peroneus tertius	m. peroneus tertius (NAV), fibularis tertius, third peroneal, femorotarsal tendon	the extensor fossa of the femur	the distal tarsal bones and the metatarsals, varying with species	the peroneal nerve	absent from carnivores, fleshy in pigs and ruminants, and fibrous in horses
piriformis	m. piriformis (NAV)	the last sacral vertebra and the sacrotuberous ligament	the greater trochanter in common with the middle gluteal m.	the caudal gluteal nerve	this is a separate m. in carnivores; in others it fuses with the middle gluteal
popliteus	m. popliteus (NAV)	the popliteal fossa on the lateral condyle of the femur	caudomedial surface of the tibia	the tibial nerve	a m. concerned with rotating (pronating) the distal limb
psoas major	m. psoas major (NAV)	the bodies of the lumbar vertebrae	the lesser trochanter of the femur	the ventral branches of the lumbar nerves	the larger part of the iliopsoas complex that acts to flex the hip

Table continued over page

13 Muscles *(Continued)*

PART 13.4 Hindlimb *(Continued)*

Muscle	Other names	Origin	Insertion	Innervation	Comments
psoas minor	m. psoas minor (NAV)	the bodies of the last few thoracic and first few lumbar vertebrae	the iliopectineal eminence of the pelvis	the ventral branches of the lumbar nerves	the m. has a shiny tendon that is conspicuous in the abdominal roof
quadratus femoris	m. quadratus femoris (NAV)	the ventral surface of the ischium beneath the sciatic tuber	the caudal surface of the femur near the lesser trochanter	the sciatic nerve	a smaller extensor and supinator of the limb
quadratus plantae	m. quadratus plantae (NAV), m. flexor accessorius (NAV alternative)	the plantar and lateral surfaces of the calcaneus	the tendon of the deep digital flexors	the tibial nerve	this small m. is effectively the tarsal head of the deep digital flexors; only in carnivors
quadriceps	m. quadriceps femoris (NAV). *See also* rectus femoris, and lateral, medial and intermediate vastus mm.	the shaft of the femur (the three vastus mm.) and the body of the ilium (the rectus femoris)	the patella and thus, indirectly, the tibial tuberosity	the femoral nerve	separation into four heads is not always easy
rectus femoris	m. rectus femoris (NAV)	the body of the ilium just in front of the acetabulum	the base of the patella and thus, indirectly, the tibial tuberosity	the femoral nerve	the only biarticular member of the quadriceps; it extends the stifle and flexes the hip
sartorius	m. sartorius (NAV), tailor's m.	the coxal tuber (carnivores) or the iliac fascia and body of the ilium (others)	the fascia over the medial aspect of the stifle	the saphenous nerve or the cranial branch of the femoral nerve	in dogs the m. is divided into cranial and caudal bellies
semimembranosus	m. semi-membranosus (NAV), the semimem	the sciatic tuber (all species); the sacrosciatic ligament (horse)	the medial aspect of the stifle joint	the caudal gluteal and tibial branches of the sciatic nerve	the vertebral head contributes to the rounded rump of the horse
semitendinosus	m. semi-tendinosus (NAV), the semiten	the sciatic tuber (all species); the spinous and transverse processes of the caudal vertebrae (pigs and horses)	the medial aspect of the stifle joint, the tibial crest and the calcaneal tendon	the caudal gluteal and tibial branches of the sciatic nerve	the vertebral head accounts for the rounded rump of the pig and horse; it is one of the hamstrings; not notably tendinous in the domestic mammals
short adductor	m. adductor brevis (NAV); confused with the long adductor in some texts	the ventral surface of the pubic tubercle	the rough face of the femur just distal to the lesser trochanter	the obturator nerve	in ruminants and pigs the m. is fused with the great adductor
short digital extensor	m. extensor digitorum brevis (NAV)	connective tissue over the dorsum of the hock	via the tendons of the long digital extensor to digits 2, 3 and 4	the peroneal nerve	best developed in carnivores and pigs, in which it is divided into three parts
short digital flexor	m. flexor digitorum brevis (NAV)	the dorsal surface of the superficial digital flexor tendons	the tendons of the deep digital flexor: digit 5 in dogs and digits 3–5 in cats	the tibial nerve	only found in carnivores; well developed in cats

13 **Muscles** *(Continued)*

PART 13.4 Hindlimb *(Continued)*

Muscle	Other names	Origin	Insertion	Innervation	Comments
short flexor of digit 1	*see* flexor hallucis brevis				
short flexor of the hallux	*see* flexor hallucis brevis				
short peroneal	*see* peroneus brevis				
soleus	m. soleus (NAV)	the proximal end of the fibula	the calcaneal tendon and tuber	the tibial nerve	absent from dogs, broad in pigs, narrow in most other species
superficial digital flexor	m. flexor digitorum superficialis (NAV)	the supra-condyloid fossa of the femur	partly on the point of the hock and mainly on the middle phalanges of weight-bearing digits	the tibial nerve	in horses the m. is mostly fibrous and synchronizes the action of the hock and stifle
superficial gluteal	m. gluteus superficialis (NAV), gluteus maximus (man). *See also* gluteobiceps	the sacrum and first caudal vertebra, the sacrotuberous ligament, the gluteal fascia and the coxal tuber	the greater trochanter (most species) or the third trochanter (horses)	the caudal gluteal nerve	a small m. in domestic mammals though big in humans, in which it forms most of the buttocks
suspensory lig.	*see* interosseous mm.				
tensor fasciae latae	m. tensor fasciae latae (NAV)	the coxal tuber	the fascia lata	the cranial gluteal nerve	in pigs, horses and ruminants it unites with the superficial gluteal
tenuissimus	*see* caudal crural abductor				
third peroneal	*see* peroneus tertius				
triceps surae	m. triceps surae (NAV), the triceps of the calf	the distal end of the femur and the proximal fibula	the calcaneal tuber on the point of the hock	the tibial nerve	more commonly known as gastrocnemius and soleus
vasti	*see* lateral, intermediate and medial vastus mm.				

Table prepared by John Grandage.

14 Nerves

Nerve	Other names	Origin	Branches	Type, distribution and comments
abducent n.	n. abducens, (NAV), sixth cranial n.	the pons, beneath the floor of the fourth ventricle		a motor n. to the lateral rectus and rectractor bulbi muscles
accessory n.	n. accessorius (NAV), eleventh cranial n., spinal accessory n., n. of Willis	it has both cranial roots from the medulla and spinal roots from the first few cervical segments of the spinal cord	internal and external, the external further dividing into dorsal and ventral branches	the internal branch contributes to the vagus and hence supplies the palate, pharynx and larynx; the external branch supplies the sleeve of superficial muscles around the neck that includes the trapezius, the brachiocephalic and sternocephalic
accessory palatine n.	n. palatinus accessorius (NAV)	the greater palatine n.		one or more small sensory nn. that traverse minor foramina in the palatine bone to supply parts of the hard and soft palates
acoustic n.	*see* vestibulocochlear n.			
ampullary nn.	n. ampullaris anterior, lateralis and posterior (NAV), n. utriculoampullaris (NAV)	the vestibular n.		the three special sensory nn. from the semicircular canals; the nn. run from the crista of the ampulla of each canal
ansa axillaris (NAV)		the union of the musculocutaneous and axillary nn.		only present in ungulates; just distal to the axillary artery
ansa cervicalis (NAV)	loop of the hypoglossal n.	the ventral division of C1 (cervical n. 1) and sometimes C2 and C3	the loop connects with the hypoglossal n.	the loop apparently contributes motor fibers to some of the strap muscles of the neck
antebrachial nn.	*see* caudal and lateral cutaneous antebrachial nn. and cranial and medial cutaneous nn. of the forearm			
auriculopalpebral n.	n. auriculopalpebralis (NAV)	the facial n.	rostral auricular, zygomatic and palpebral branches	the n. contributes to the rostral auricular plexus over the forehead and is motor to some of the ear and most of the eyelid muscles
auriculotemporal n.	n. auriculotemporalis (NAV)	the mandibular n.	the n. of the external acoustic meatus; rostral auricular nn; transverse facial branch	a sensory n. to the ear, temple, cheek and the side of the face; it supplies the guttural pouch (horse), the parotid gland, the external acoustic meatus and the tympanic membrane
axillary n.	n. axillaris (NAV)	the cervical nn. C7 and C8 (and occasionally C6)	after muscular branches it gives off a craniolateral cutaneous n. of the arm and a cranial cutaneous n. of the forearm	the n. supplies most flexors of the shoulder (the teres major and minor and the deltoid muscles) and twigs to the subscapular and brachiocephalic muscles

brachial plexus	plexus brachialis (NAV)	the ventral divisions of cervical nn. C5 to C8 and thoracic nn. T1 and T2	about a dozen large branches to the forelimb and some of its extrinsic muscles	the plexus roots unite in various ways to form trunks and then fasciculi that give rise to the dorsal scapular, subclavian, suprascapular, subscapular, musculocutaneous, axillary, pectoral, long and lateral thoracic, thoracodorsal, radial, median and ulnar nn.
buccal branches	rami buccales (NAV)	the facial n.		the main terminal branches of the facial n. that supply the muscles of expression over the cheeks, lips and muzzle; they should not be confused with the buccal *nerve*, which is sensory
buccal n.	n. buccalis (NAV)	the mandibular n.		a sensory n. to the mucous membrane and skin of the cheek that should not be confused with the motor buccal *branches* of the facial n. (above)
cardiac nn.	nn. cardiaci cervicales/thoracici (NAV)	mainly from the middle cervical and the thoracic sympathetic ganglia		these nn. provide the sympathetic innervation to the heart; the parasympathetic innervation is supplied by the depressor n. and the cardiac branches of the vagus
caroticotympanic nn.	nn. caroticotympanici (NAV)	the internal carotid plexus	the tympanic plexus	tiny nn. that convey sympathetic fibers to the tympanic plexus
carotid nn.	nn. caroti externi (NAV), n. caroticus internus	the cranial cervical sympathetic ganglion		these fine sympathetic nn. run with the carotid arteries to the carotid plexus
caudal nn.	nn. caudales (NAV), nn. coccygei (NAV alternative), tail nn.	the conus medullaris of the spinal cord	dorsal and ventral branches	there are typically about five pairs of caudal nn. in the domestic mammals; the two primary branches of each unite to form a dorsal and a ventral caudal plexus or trunk; the nn. are motor and sensory to the tail
caudal auricular n.	n. auricularis caudalis (NAV)	the facial n.		one or two nn. leave the facial n. on its emergence from the stylomastoid foramen and supply the platysma and caudal ear muscles
caudal clunial nn.	nn. clunium caudales (NAV)	the ventral branches of the sacral nn. usually via the caudal cutaneous femoral n.		sensory nn. over the sciatic tubers that stream out of the ischiorectal fossa
caudal cutaneous antebrachial n.	n. cutaneus antebrachii caudalis (NAV)	the ulnar n.		one of the four sensory nn. of the forearm
caudal cutaneous femoral n.	n. cutaneus femoris caudalis (NAV)	the ventral branches of the first few sacral nn.	the perineal nn. and caudal clunial nn.	the n. supplies the skin around the sciatic tubers and the caudal aspect of the thigh
caudal cutaneous sural n.	n. cutaneus surae caudalis (NAV), lateral plantar cutaneous sural n. (horses)	the tibial n.		a sensory n. to the plantar aspect of the hock and metapodium
caudal gluteal n.	n. gluteus caudalis (NAV)	mainly the sacral roots of the lumbosacral trunk	it supplies branches to the superficial gluteal and piriformis muscles	the n. leaves the lumbosacral trunk after escaping from the pelvis via the greater sciatic foramen

Table continued over page

14 Nerves *(Continued)*

Nerve	Other names	Origin	Branches	Type, distribution and comments
caudal iliohypogastric n.	n. iliohypogastricus caudalis (NAV)	the ventral branch of the second lumbar n, provided there are at least seven lumbar vertebrae	lateral and ventral cutaneous branches	the iliohypogastric n. is duplicated into cranial and caudal nn. in animals with more than six lumbar vertebrae; the n. supplies the muscles and skin over a segment of the flank
caudal laryngeal n.	n. laryngeus caudalis (NAV)	the recurrent laryngeal n.		motor n. to all the intrinsic muscles of the larynx except the cricothyroid
caudal lateral cutaneous n. of the arm	n. cutaneus brachii lateralis caudalis (NAV)	the radial n. as it winds around the brachial groove		this is a sensory n. to the skin just proximal to the elbow on its lateral side; the radial n. gives off several other cutaneous nn.
caudal nasal n.	n. nasalis caudalis (NAV)	the pterygopalatine n.	the nasopalatine n.	a sensory n. that passes through the sphenopalatine foramen to innervate the mucous membrane of the nasal chambers
caudal rectal nn.	nn. rectales caudales (NAV), middle haemorrhoidal n. (for one variant)	the pudendal n. or from the same sacral nn. as the pudendal n.	muscular and cutaneous branches	it may be duplicated and is subject to other variations; it is sensory to the skin of the anus and adjacent regions (with the superficial perineal n.) and is motor to the levator ani
cervical nn.	nn. cervicales (NAV), C1–C8 (mammals)	the cervical spinal cord	a segmental distribution to the neck and to plexuses that supply the ear, diaphragm and forelimb	most mammals have eight pairs of cervical nn. which lie cranially and caudally to the seven cervical vertebrae
cervical plexus	plexus cervicalis (NAV)	the ventral divisions of cervical nn. 1–4	the transverse cervical, great auricular and supraclavicular nn. and the ansa cervicalis	the plexus communicates with the cranial nn. via the ansa cervicalis
ciliary nn.	*see* short and long ciliary nn.			
clunial nn.	nn. clunium craniales/medii/caudales (NAV)	the dorsal and ventral branches of the sacral nn., and the dorsal branches of the lumbar nn.		these are mainly sensory nn. to the loins, rump, buttocks, and the outside and caudal parts of the thigh; *see* cranial, middle and caudal clunial nn.
cochlear n.	n. cochlearis (NAV)	the vestibulocochlear n.	the spiral ganglion	a special sensory n. that conducts auditory impulses from the spiral ganglion of the cochlea
common fibular n.	n. fibularis communis (NAV), n. peroneus communis (NAV alternative), common peroneal n.	the sciatic n. about half way down the thigh	the lateral cutaneous sural n., the deep and superficial fibular nn.	relatively few branches are given off this major termination of the sciatic n. before it divides into its superficial and deep branches just distal to the stifle joint
common peroneal n.	*see* common fibular n.			

cornual n.	ramus cornualis (NAV), cornual branch of the zygomaticotemporal n., horn n., rami cornuales (NAV, goats), cornual branch of the infratrochlear n.	the zygomaticotemporal branch of the zygomatic n. from the maxillary n.; the infratrochlear n. from the ophthalmic n. (goats); the first cervical n. may also contribute	the n. branches before reaching the base of the horn and supplying the corium	the sensory nn. to the horn; the principal n. is accompanied by an artery and vein; in cattle it can be blocked for local anesthesia as it emerges from the temporal fossa about midway between the base of the horn and the postorbital bar; the cornual n. of cattle was formerly thought to be a branch of the lacrimal n.
costoabdominal n.	n. costoabdominalis (NAV), subcostal n. (man)	the ventral branch of the last thoracic n.	as for the intercostal nn.	this n. closely resembles an intercostal n. but is given a different name because it lies caudal to the last rib rather than between the ribs
cranial nn.	nn. craniales (NAV)	within the cranium	*see* individual nn.	twelve pairs are recognized: *see* olfactory, optic, oculomotor, trochlear, trigeminal, abducent, facial, vestibulocochlear, glossopharyngeal, vagus, accessory and hypoglossal nn.
cranial clunial nn.	nn. clunium craniales (NAV)	the dorsal primary branches of the lumbar nn.		the cranial of three groups of sensory nn. to the rump (= clunes); these nn. supply the skin over the loins and in front of the hip
cranial cutaneous n. of the forearm	n. cutaneus antebrachii cranialis (NAV)	the cranial lateral cutaneous n. of the arm, a branch of the axillary n.		the n. is a continuation of the cranial lateral cutaneous n. of the arm; in the dog it runs with the medial branch of the superficial radial n.
cranial gluteal n.	n. gluteus cranialis (NAV)	mainly the last one or two lumbar and the first sacral nn. via the lumbosacral trunk	it gives off branches to the muscles over the cranial part of the rump	the n. leaves the lumbosacral trunk after escaping from the pelvis via the greater sciatic foramen; it supplies the gluteal and tensor fasciae latae muscles
cranial iliohypogastric n.	n. iliohypogastricus cranialis (NAV)	the ventral branch of the first lumbar n.	lateral and ventral cutaneous branches	the iliohypogastric n. is duplicated into cranial and caudal nn. in animals with more than six lumbar vertebrae; the n. supplies the muscles and skin over a segment of the flank
cranial laryngeal n.	n. laryngeus cranialis (NAV)	the vagus n.	internal and external branches; the depressor n.	the internal branch supplies the mucous membrane lining the larynx while the external supplies the cricothyroid muscle; the depressor n. runs to the heart
cranial lateral cutaneous n. of the arm	n. cutaneus brachii lateralis cranialis (NAV)	the axillary n.	the cranial cutaneous n. of the forearm	this is the sensory termination of the axillary n. that extends along the cranial aspect of the arm
cutaneous colli n.	*see* transverse cervical n.			
cutaneous nn. of the forearm	*see* caudal and lateral cutaneous antebrachial nn., and cranial and medial cutaneous nn. of the forearm			
deep branch of the radial n.	n. radialis, ramus profundus (NAV)	the parent radial n. within the brachial groove	muscular branches	a motor n. that plunges into the extensor muscles of the forearm and digit close to their origins near the elbow

Table continued over page

14 Nerves (*Continued*)

Nerve	Other names	Origin	Branches	Type, distribution and comments
deep fibular n.	n. fibularis profundus (NAV), n. peroneus profundus (NAV alternative)	the common fibular n. just distal to the stifle	muscular branches and the dorsal metatarsal nn.	it supplies the long and lateral digital extensors, the cranial tibial and the peroneus tertius muscles; it divides over the hock into lateral and medial branches that supply the short extensor muscles before becoming the dorsal metatarsal nn.
deep perineal n.	n. perinealis profundus (NAV)	the pudendal n., as one branch (ox) or as several branches (dog)		it supplies the striated muscle of the perineum and the skin of the scrotum, prepuce and, in some, the caudal part of the udder
deep peroneal n.	*see* deep fibular n.			
deep petrosal n.	n. petrosus profundus (NAV), deep vidian n.	the carotid artery plexus	the n. of the pterygoid canal	the n. carries postganglionic sympathetic fibers from the cranial cervical ganglion to the greater petrosal n.
deep temporal nn.	nn. temporales profundi (NAV)	the masticatory n.		two or three branches are motor nn. to the temporal muscles
depressor n.	n. depressor (NAV)	the cranial laryngeal n.		the n. runs with the vagus or sympathetic nerves to the myocardium; its stimulation lowers blood pressure
digital nn.	nn. digitales	various nn.		strictly, the digital nn. are any of those nn. to the fingers and toes that are not formed from the common digital nn., i.e. those nn. that are not 'proper digital nn.'
dorsal common digital nn. (forelimb)	nn. digitales dorsales communes (NAV)	the lateral and medial branches of the superficial radial n.; the dorsal branch of the ulnar n.	the proper dorsal digital nn.	these are the superficial nn. over the dorsum of the metapodium; they are called common nn. because they are common to two digits and terminate by dividing into proper digital nn.; carnivores have four, pigs three, ruminants two and horses none
dorsal common digital nn. (hindlimb)	n. digitalis dorsalis communis II/III/IV (NAV)	the superficial and deep fibular nn.	the dorsal proper digital nn.	in the hindlimb these nn. arise mainly from the superficial peroneal n.; they unite with the deeper dorsal metatarsal nn. derived from the deep fibular n.
dorsal metatarsal nn.	n. metatarseus II/III/IV (NAV)	the deep fibular n.		these nn. often unite with the dorsal common digital nn. of the paw
dorsal n. of clitoris	n. dorsalis clitoridis (NAV)	the termination of the pudendal n.		the n. is sensory to the clitoris
dorsal n. of penis	n. dorsalis penis (NAV)	the termination of the pudendal n.		the n. is sensory to the penis and prepuce
dorsal n. of scapula	n. dorsalis scapulae (NAV)	the fifth cervical n.		it supplies motor fibers to the rhomboid muscle
dorsal proper digital nn.	nn. digitales dorsales proprii (NAV)	the dorsal common digital nn.		these are the main nn. to the dorsum of the foot formed from the division of the common dorsal digital nn.; they are absent from the horse

dorsal thoracic n.	*see* thoracodorsal n.			
dorsal vagal trunk	truncus vagalis dorsalis (NAV), dorsal esophageal trunk	the right and left vagus nn.	branches to the celiac ganglion, stomach and intestines	this n. with its ventral partner enters the abdomen at the esophageal hiatus and provides the major parasympathetic supply to the alimentary tract
eighth cranial n.	*see* vestibulocochlear n.			
eleventh cranial n.	*see* accessory n.			
ethmoidal n.	n. ethmoidalis (NAV)	the nasociliary n.	lateral and medial nasal branches	the n. enters the cranium via the ethmoidal foramen, escapes again through the cribriform plate to supply sensory fibers to the dorsal part of the nasal chambers
external acoustic meatus n.	n. meatus acustici externi (NAV)	the auriculotemporal n.		it is sensory to the external acoustic meatus and to the tympanic membrane
external spermatic n.	*see* genitofemoral n.			
facial n.	n. facialis (NAV), n. intermediofacialis (NAV alternative), seventh cranial n.	the caudal border of the pons at the lateral extremity of the trapezoid body	the greater petrosal n.; the stapedial n.; the caudal auricular n.; the auriculopalpebral n.; the intermediate n.	a derivative of the second branchial arch; the n. traverses the facial canal in the temporal bone and ramifies over the cheek and temple; a mixed n. whose clinical significance relates to its motor supply to the muscles of facial expression
femoral n.	n. femoralis (NAV)	mainly the ventral branches of the fourth and fifth lumbar nn.	muscular rami and the saphenous n.	it forms within the substance of the iliopsoas and leaves the abdomen with that muscle; it innervates both the iliopsoas and all four heads of the quadriceps but probably has no cutaneous branches (except for its saphenous branch)
fibular nn.	*see* common superficial and deep fibular nn.			
fifth cranial n.	*see* trigeminal n.			
first cranial n.	*see* olfactory nn.			
fourth cranial n.	*see* trochlear n.			
frontal n.	n. frontalis (NAV)	the ophthalmic n.	the frontal sinus n.; the supraorbital n.; the supratrochlear n.	a sensory n. that arises within the orbit and often escapes through the supraorbital foramen to be part of a plexus over the forehead
frontal sinus n.	n. sinuum frontalium (NAV)	the frontal n.		a sensory n. to the frontal sinus
genitofemoral n.	n. genitofemoralis (NAV), external spermatic n.	the ventral branches of the third and fourth lumbar nn.	genital and femoral branches	it is the most cranial n. in the lumbosacral plexus; it supplies the psoas and cremaster muscles, runs through the inguinal canal and supplies the skin and genitalia around the superficial inguinal ring

Table continued over page

14 Nerves *(Continued)*

Nerve	Other names	Origin	Branches	Type, distribution and comments
glossopharyngeal n.	n. glossopharyngeus (NAV), ninth cranial n.	filaments from the side of the medulla	proximal and distal ganglia; the tympanic n.; pharyngeal plexus	a mixed n. that innervates the structures derived from the third branchial arch including the throat muscles and salivary glands; it does so mostly via the pharyngeal plexus (with the vagus)
gray rami communicantes	gray communicating branches	from the sympathetic trunk	to the ventral branches of most of the thoracic and lumbar spinal nn.	in some animals it is possible to distinguish these rami (containing postganglionic nonmyelinated sympathetic fibers) from white rami (containing preganglionic myelinated sympathetic fibers), but in many animals both types of fiber are found within the same ramus
great auricular n.	n. auricularis magnus (NAV)	the ventral division of the second cervical n.		a sensory n. to the parotid region and the convex surface of the ear
greater occipital n.	n. occipitalis major (NAV)	the dorsal division of the second cervical n.		it ramifies in the skin of the poll
greater palatine n.	n. palatinus major (NAV)	the pterygopalatine n.	the accessory palatine nn.	a large sensory n. to the hard palate, gums and the floor of the nasal chambers
greater petrosal n.	n. petrosus major (NAV), greater superficial petrosal n.	the facial n.	the n. of pterygoid canal	a mixed n. that consists mainly of taste fibers to the palate and parasympathetic fibers to the lacrimal gland and some mucous glands
greater splanchnic n.	n. splanchnicus major (NAV), the thoracic splanchnic n.	the thoracic sympathetic ganglia excluding the first five and last one or two		it passes from the thorax into the abdomen to end mainly in the celiacomesenteric plexus; it supplies filaments to the thoracic aorta and the adrenal medulla
hypogastric n.	n. hypogastricus (NAV)	the caudal mesenteric ganglion	branches to the pelvic plexus	this n. consists largely of postganglionic sympathetic fibers that are ultimately distributed to the pelvic viscera via the pelvic plexus
hypoglossal n.	n. hypoglossus (NAV), twelfth cranial n.	the caudal part of the medulla	lingual branches	the motor n. to the muscles of the tongue and to the geniohyoid
iliohypogastric n.	n. iliohypogastricus (NAV). *See also* cranial and caudal iliohypogastric nn.	the ventral branch of the first lumbar n.	lateral and ventral cutaneous branches	in animals with six lumbar vertebrae or fewer this n. is not qualified with the adjective cranial or caudal as it is in those with seven; it supplies the muscles and skin over a segment of flank
ilioinguinal n.	n. ilioinguinalis (NAV)	the ventral branch of the second or third lumbar n.	lateral and ventral cutaneous branches	this n. is from the second lumbar spinal n. in animals with six lumbar vertebrae or fewer, and from the third spinal nerve in animals with seven lumbar vertebrae or more; it supplies muscles and skin over a segment of the flank
inferior alveolar n.	n. alveolaris inferior (NAV), mandibular alveolar n.	the mandibular n.	the mylohyoid n.; the mental nn.	the terminal motor and sensory branch of the mandibular n. that ramifies in the lower jaw, its teeth and the lower lip

infraorbital n.	n. infraorbitalis (NAV)	the maxillary n.	alveolar, nasal and labial branches	the sensory n. to the muzzle; it is large in all domestic mammals, especially the pig
infratrochlear n.	n. infratrochlearis (NAV)	the ophthalmic n. or its nasociliary branch	palpebral, sinus and cornual branches	a sensory n. to the medial angle of the eye, third eyelid, lacrimal caruncle, ducts and sac, the frontal sinus and, in horned ruminants, the rostrolateral surface of the base of the horn
intercostal nn.	nn. intercostales (NAV), rami ventrales nn. thoracici (NAV)	these nn. are formed from all the ventral branches of the thoracic nn. except for the first and last	the rami communicates; lateral and ventral cutaneous branches; the intercostobrachial n.	the first intercostal n. is only a small portion of the ventral branch of the first thoracic n.; typically each intercostal n. runs adjacent to the pleura with an artery and vein near the caudal border of a rib; the last few nn. also supply part of the flank
intercostobrachial n.	n. intercostobrachialis (NAV)	the lateral cutaneous rami of some of the cranial intercostal nn plus fibers from the lateral thoracic n.	branches to the skin near the elbow and the omobrachial cutaneous muscle	the n. contains motor fibers (in ruminants and the horse) which are derived from the lateral thoracic n. and supply the omobrachial muscle
intermediate n.	n. intermedius (NAV), Wrisberg's n.	the smaller, sensory root of the facial n.	branches to the geniculate ganglion and the chorda tympani	a special sensory n. for taste from the rostral parts of the tongue (about two-thirds in humans, about four-fifths in domestic mammals) and secretomotor parasympathetic fibers to sublingual, mandibular and other salivary glands
interosseous antebrachial n.	n. interosseus antebrachii (NAV)	the median n.		a small n. that penetrates the interosseous membrane before innervating the pronator quadratus
Jacobson's n.	*see* tympanic n.			
jugular n.	n. jugularis (NAV)	the cranial cervical ganglion		this sympathetic n. sends fibers to the distal ganglion of the glossopharyngeal n. and to the proximal ganglion of the vagus
lacrimal n.	n. lacrimalis (NAV)	the ophthalmic n. joined by the zygomaticotemporal n.		a sensory n. to the upper eyelid that receives secretomotor fibers from the zygomaticotemporal n. which ramify in the lacrimal gland
lateral cutaneous antebrachial n.	n. cutaneus antebrachii lateralis (NAV)	the superficial branch of the radial nerve		this cutaneous n. supplies dorsal and lateral aspects of the forearm; the parent n. also supplies the dorsal aspect of the manus in all species except the horse
lateral cutaneous femoral n.	n. cutaneus femoris lateralis (NAV)	the ventral branch of the third or fourth lumbar n.		this caudal n. of the flank pierces the body wall beneath the coxal tuber and supplies the front and lateral parts of the thigh
lateral cutaneous sural n.	n. cutaneus surae lateralis (NAV), lateral cutaneous n. of the calf	the common fibular n.		a sensory n. to the lateral side of the calf just distal to the stifle joint
lateral palmar n.	*see* palmar nn.			

Table continued over page

14 Nerves (*Continued*)

Nerve	Other names	Origin	Branches	Type, distribution and comments
lateral plantar cutaneous sural n. (horses)	*see* caudal cutaneous sural n.			
lateral pterygoid n.	n. pterygoideus lateralis (NAV)	the mandibular n.		a motor n. to the lateral pterygoid muscle
lateral thoracic n.	n. thoracicus lateralis (NAV)	mainly from the eighth cervical n. and the first thoracic n. via the brachial plexus	branches to the pectoral muscle and to the cutaneous trunci	this is the only motor n. to the cutaneous trunci—its ability to induce twitches in the flank skin is used to assess the integrity of the spinal cord between the brachial plexus and the spinal n. receiving the sensory stimulus
least splanchnic n.	n. splanchnicus imus (NAV)	the last thoracic ganglion		an uncommon variant that conveys sympathetic fibers to the renal plexus
lesser palatine n.	n. palatinus minor (NAV)	the pterygopalatine n.		a mainly sensory n. to the soft palate and palatine tonsil; it also contains some autonomic fibers and taste fibers
lesser petrosal n.	n. petrosus minor (NAV)	the tympanic n. via the tympanic plexus		the continuation of the tympanic n. (from the ninth cranial n.) that runs to the otic ganglion and thence to the parotid gland
lesser splanchnic n.	n. splanchnicus minor (NAV)	the last one or two thoracic ganglia		it passes from the thorax into the abdomen to end mainly in the celiacomesenteric plexus with a similar distribution to the greater splanchnic n.; sometimes absent
lingual n.	n. lingualis (NAV)	the mandibular n.	the sublingual n.	the general sensory n. (excluding taste) to the tongue, the floor of the mouth and the gums of the lower jaw
long ciliary nn.	nn. ciliares longi (NAV)	the nasociliary n.		general sensory nn. to the cornea and sympathetic fibers to the dilator of the pupil; two or three pierce the sclera near the optic n.
long thoracic n.	n. thoracicus longus (NAV)	the more cranial roots of the brachial plexus	branches to the ventral serrate muscle	the n. runs along the side of the chest over the ventral serrate muscle
lumbar nn.	nn. lumbales (NAV)	the lumbar part of the spinal cord	dorsal and ventral primary divisions	these are typical segmental spinal nn. distributed to the epaxial muscles and flank; the ventral divisions often have individual names and most contribute to the lumbosacral plexus
lumbar plexus	plexus lumbalis (NAV)	the ventral branches of about the last five lumbar nn.	about five named nn. to the flank, groin, thigh, leg and genitalia, and a contribution to the sacral plexus	the lumbar plexus gives origin to the ilioinguinal, genitofemoral, lateral cutaneous femoral, femoral and obturator nn., and to the lumbosacral trunk to make up the lumbosacral plexus
lumbar splanchnic nn.	nn. splanchnici lumbales (NAV)	the lumbar sympathetic ganglia		these form a variable series of paired nn. that run from the sympathetic trunk to the prevertebral ganglia around the ventral surface of the abdominal aorta

lumbosacral plexus	plexus lumbosacralis (NAV)	the ventral branches of the last five lumbar nn. and the sacral nn.	about 15 nerves are given off to the flank, pelvis, tail, and hindlimb	the plexus roots unite in various ways to form trunks and then fasciculi that give rise to named nn.; *see* lumbar plexus and sacral plexus
lumbosacral trunk	truncus lumbosacralis (NAV)	mainly from the last two or three lumbar and the first two sacral nn.	the cranial and caudal gluteal nn., and the sciatic n.	the largest and most important part of the lumbosacral plexus that continues as the sciatic n.
major palatine n.	*see* greater palatine n.			
major petrosal n.	*see* greater petrosal n.			
mammary nn.	rami mammarii laterales/mediales (NAV)	from the lateral and ventral branches of the intercostal nn.		these branches of the intercostal nn. only apply to animals with pectoral and abdominal mammary glands
mandibular n.	n. mandibularis (NAV)	trigeminal n.	the masticatory n.; the lateral and medial pterygoid nn.; the n. to the tensor tympani; the n. to the tensor of the soft palate; the buccal n.; the auriculotemporal n.; the lingual n.; the inferior alveolar n.	one of the three divisions of the trigeminal n.; it carries both sensory and motor fibers; it carries information from the ear, the side of the face, the temple, the lower jaw, the lower lip and the mouth; it provides the motor supply to the muscles of mastication
mandibular alveolar n.	*see* inferior alveolar n.			
masseteric n.	n. massetericus (NAV)	the masticatory n.		the motor n. to the masseter muscle; it passes over the mandibular notch
masticatory n.	n. masticatorius (NAV)	the mandibular n.	the masseteric n.; the deep temporal nn.	the motor n. to the muscles of mastication made up of the fused masseteric and deep temporal nn.; these may arise separately from the mandibular n.
maxillary n.	n. maxillaris (NAV)	the trigeminal n.	the zygomatic n.; the pterygopalatine n.; the infraorbital n.; the pterygoid canal n.	a sensory division of the trigeminal n. that supplies the lips, gums and teeth of the upper jaw, the muzzle, nose and nasal chambers, and the front of the face below the eyes
medial cutaneous n. of the forearm	n. cutaneus antebrachii medialis (NAV), medial antebrachial cutaneous n.	the musculocutaneous n.	the n. ramifies in the skin of the forearm	this n. is sensory to the medial side of the forearm as far as the carpus in dogs; in horses its territory is more extensive and reaches as far distally as the fetlock
medial palmar n.	*see* palmar nn.			
medial plantar n.	*see* plantar nn.			
medial pterygoid n.	n. pterygoideus medialis (NAV)	the mandibular n.		a motor n. to the medial pterygoid muscle

Table continued over page

14 Nerves (*Continued*)

Nerve	Other names	Origin	Branches	Type, distribution and comments
median n.	n. medianus (NAV)	the more caudal roots of the brachial plexus, typically C8 and T1	the branches vary according to species but typically include an interosseous antebrachial n. and two or more common palmar digital nn.	a large n. from the brachial plexus that innervates the pronators of the forearm and most of the digital flexors (flexor carpi radialis, superficial digital flexor, radial and humeral heads of the deep digital flexor); it is also a major sensory n. to the foot
mental nn.	n. mentalis (NAV, horse, ruminants); nn. mentales (NAV, carnivores, pigs)	the inferior alveolar n.		a sensory n. to the lower lip; in some species (dogs, pigs) there is more than one mental foramen from which the nn. escape
middle clunial nn.	nn. clunium medii (NAV)	the lateral branches of the dorsal primary branches of the sacral nn.		the middle of three groups of sensory nn. to the rump (= clunes); these nn. supply the skin over the hip joint and the lateral side of the upper thigh
minor palatine n.	*see* lesser palatine n.			
minor petrosal n.	*see* lesser petrosal n.			
musculocutaneous n.	n. musculocutaneus (NAV)	cervical nn. C7 and C8 via the brachial plexus; (C5-7 in humans)	proximal and distal muscular branches, the ansa axillaris, and the medial cutaneous n. of the forearm	it supplies motor fibers to the flexor muscles of the elbow (the biceps brachii and the brachialis) and to the coracobrachialis
mylohyoid n.	n. mylohyoideus (NAV)	the inferior alveolar n.		a motor n. to the mylohyoid muscle and the rostral belly of the digastric muscle
nasociliary n.	n. nasociliaris (NAV)	the ophthalmic n.	the n. to the ciliary ganglion; the long ciliary nn.; the ethmoidal n.; the infratrochlear n.	a sensory n. that is the continuation of the parent ophthalmic n. and whose branches supply the nose and medial canthus of the eye (see individual nn.)
nasopalatine n.	n. nasopalatinus (NAV)	the caudal nasal n. (from the pterygopalatine n.)		a terminal sensory n. of the maxillary n. that pierces the palatine fissure from the floor of the nose to supply the hard palate
nn. erigentes	*see* pelvic nn.			
ninth cranial n.	*see* glossopharyngeal n.			
obturator n.	n. obturatorius (NAV)	mainly from the ventral branches of the fourth, fifth and sixth lumbar nn.	branches to the adductor muscles of the thigh: i.e. the gracilis, adductor, pectineus and external obturator	the n. is vulnerable to crush injuries as it courses adjacent to the shaft of the ilium prior to escaping through the obturator foramen to innervate the adductor muscles
oculomotor n.	n. oculomotorius (NAV), third cranial n.	the ventral surface of the cerebral crus of the midbrain	dorsal and ventral branches; the ciliary ganglion lies on the ventral branch from which short ciliary nn. are given off	the n. divides on entering the orbit: the dorsal branch supplies the dorsal rectus and levator of the upper lid, and the ventral branch supplies the ventral and medial straight and the ventral oblique muscles; it also carries parasympathetic fibers to the ciliary ganglion that are motor to the pupillary sphincter and the ciliary muscle

olfactory nn.	nn. olfactorii (NAV), first cranial n.	the olfactory bulb within the rostral cerebral fossa	about 20 bundles through the cribriform plate	special sensory nonmyelinated nn. to the olfactory mucous membrane supported mainly on the ethmoturbinates
ophthalmic n.	n. ophthalmicus (NAV)	the trigeminal n.	the lacrimal n.; the frontal n.; the nasociliary n.; the infratrochlear n.	the smallest of the three primary divisions of the trigeminal; it is a sensory n. to the eye and orbit, the forehead and parts of the nose
optic n.	n. opticus (NAV), second cranial n.	the optic chiasma		the special sensory n. that mediates vision and runs a sinuous course from the optic disk to the optic chiasma; it is regarded as an outgrowth of the brain and is clothed in meninges
palatine nn.	*see* greater and lesser palatine nn.			
palmar nn. (horses)	n. palmaris medialis/lateralis (NAV), n. digitalis palmaris communis II/III (NAV alternative)	the median and ulnar nn.	the palmar digital nn.	these are the two large sensory nn. of the metacarpal region of the horse found between the digital flexors and the interosseous muscle; they are united in the mid-cannon region by a communicating branch
palmar common digital nn.	n. digitalis palmaris communis I/II/III/IV (NAV), medial and lateral palmar nn. (horses)	the terminal divisions of the median and ulnar nn.	the proper palmar digital nn.	these are the superficial nn. over the palmar aspect of the metapodium; they are sensory nn.; the deep nn. are termed palmar metacarpal nn. and include motor fibers
palmar digital nn.	n. digitalis palmaris medialis/lateralis (NAV), proper palmar digital nn.	the medial and lateral palmar nn.	a dorsal branch	the sensory nn. to the horse's foot that begin at the fetlock joint; here they give off the dorsal branch which supplies the dorsum of the pastern and hoof
palmar metacarpal nn.	nn. metacarpei palmares (NAV)	the deep branches of the median and ulnar nn.	muscular branches	these are the deep nn. of the metapodial region
pectoral nn.	nn. pectorales caudales/craniales (NAV), ventral thoracic nn.	all the roots of the brachial plexus	branches to the pectoral muscles	the nn. are variable; a cranial group supplies the superficial pectoral muscles and a caudal group the deep pectoral muscles
pelvic nn.	nn. pelvini (NAV), pelvic splanchnic nn., nn. erigentes	the ventral branches of the sacral nn.		the nn. are predominantly parasympathetic to the pelvic plexus but also contain a few sympathetic fibers as they become distributed to the pelvic viscera
pelvic splanchnic n.	*see* pelvic nn.			
perineal nn.	*see* superficial and deep perineal nn.			
peroneal nn.	*see* common, superficial and deep fibular nn.			
phrenic n.	n. phrenicus (NAV)	typically the cervical nn. C6 and C7 (horse), C5, C6 and C7 (dog) or C3, C4 and C5 (human)	pericardial branches	the n. provides motor fibers to the diaphragm; its course from the cervical spinal cord reflects the embryological origin of the muscle

Table continued over page

14 Nerves *(Continued)*

Nerve	Other names	Origin	Branches	Type, distribution and comments
plantar nn.	n. plantaris medialis/lateralis (NAV)	the terminal branches of the tibial n.	the plantar common digital nn.	the homologue of the palmar n. of the forelimb
plantar common digital nn.	n. digitalis plantaris communis II/III/IV (NAV), medial and lateral plantar nn. (horses)	the terminal divisions of the medial plantar n. (from the tibial n.)	the proper plantar digital nn.	these are the superficial nn. over the plantar aspect of the metapodium; they are sensory nn.; the deep nn. are termed plantar metatarsal nn.
plantar metatarsal nn.	nn. metatarsei plantares (NAV)	the lateral plantar n. (from the tibial n.)	these nn. unite with the plantar common digital nn.	these are the deep nn. over the plantar aspect of the metapodium
pneumogastric n.	*see* vagus n.			
proper digital nn.	nn. digitales proprii (NAV)	the common digital nn.		the proper digital nn. are derived from the division of a common digital n.; they 'properly' belong to one digit rather than being common to more than one like their parent n.; there are typically four proper digital nn. per digit—two dorsal, two palmar
proper palmar digital nn.	n. digitalis palmaris proprius I/II/III/IV/V (NAV)	the common palmar digital nn.		there are typically two of these nn. per digit, the axial and abaxial
pterygoid nn.	*see* lateral and medial pterygoid nn.			
pterygoid canal, n. of	n. canalis pterygoidei (NAV), vidian n.	the greater and deep petrosal nn.		the n. receives parasympathetic and sensory fibers from the greater petrosal n. and sympathetic fibers from the deep petrosal n.; they course in the pterygoid canal to the pterygopalatine ganglion; the ganglion supplies the lacrimal, palatine and nasal glands
pterygopalatine n.	n. pterygopalatinus (NAV)	the maxillary n.	the major and minor palatine nn.; the caudal nasal n.	a short n. that detaches from the maxillary n. in the pterygopalatine fossa, that bears a number of small ganglia, and whose terminal branches supply the palate and the nasal chambers
pudendal n.	n. pudendus (NAV)	usually from all the sacral nn. in the dog (S1–S3), and the more caudal ones (S2–S4) in the horse and ruminants	the deep and superficial perineal nn., some cutaneous nn. and finally the dorsal n. of the penis or clitoris	this is a large n. that is sensory to the perineum, rectum and genitalia, and often motor to the striated muscles of the perineum; its precise form and course vary between species
radial n.	n. radialis (NAV)	mainly the last two cervical and the first thoracic nn. via the brachial plexus	the muscular branch, deep branch and superficial branch (of the radial n.); the caudal lateral cutaneous n. of the arm	one of the largest nn. from the brachial plexus; it provides motor fibers to the extensor muscles of the elbow, carpus and digit, and to the supinators of the paw; it also conveys sensory cutaneous fibers from some lateral and cranial parts of the limb
rami communicantes (NAV)	communicating branches	the ventral branches of most of the thoracic and lumbar spinal nn.	to and from the sympathetic trunk and the spinal nn.	these nerves unite the sympathetic trunks with the central nervous system via the thoracolumbar spinal nerves. *See also* gray and white rami communicantes

recurrent laryngeal n.	n. laryngeus recurrens (NAV)	the vagus n.	tracheal and esophageal branches; caudal laryngeal n.	the n. that embryologically supplies the sixth branchial arch including parts of the larynx, trachea and esophagus; it is sensory as far cranial as the vocal folds and motor to most of the laryngeal muscles; the right n. loops over the right subclavian artery, the left n. around the ligamentum arteriosum
rostral auricular nn.	nn. auriculares rostrales (NAV)	the auriculotemporal n.		a sensory n. to the external ear and adjacent regions of the temple
sacral nn.	nn. sacrales (NAV)	the sacral segments of the spinal cord (usually found within the lumbar part of the vertebral column)	dorsal and ventral branches that leave the sacrum by separate foramina	the ventral divisions contribute to the lumbosacral plexus with both somatic and autonomic components
sacral plexus	plexus sacralis (NAV), sciatic plexus	the ventral divisions of the sacral nn. and the lumbosacral trunk	the cranial and caudal gluteal, caudal cutaneous femoral, caudal clunial, sciatic, pudendal, pelvic and caudal rectal nn.	the plexus is rarely considered in isolation—in conjunction with the lumbar plexus it makes up the lumbosacral plexus
sacral splanchnic nn.	nn. splanchnici sacrales (NAV)	the sacral sympathetic ganglia		these form a variable series of tiny paired nn. that run from the sacral sympathetic trunk to form a plexus around the iliac vessels
saphenous n.	n. saphenus (NAV)	the femoral n.	a muscular and a cutaneous branch	the muscular branch supplies the sartorius, the cutaneous branch the craniomedial parts of the thigh, leg, hock and foot
second cranial n.	*see* optic n.			
seventh cranial n.	*see* facial n.			
sciatic n.	n. ischiadicus (NAV), ischiatic n.	mainly the last lumbar and the first sacral nn. via the lumbosacral trunk	it gives off muscular branches to the hamstrings and finally divides into the fibular and tibial nn.	this is the largest n. in the body; it begins at the greater sciatic foramen and courses over the deep gluteal muscle and down the caudal aspect of the thigh, giving twigs to muscles on the way
short ciliary nn.	nn. ciliares breves (NAV)	the ciliary ganglion		about a dozen delicate filaments convey mainly parasympathetic fibers from the ciliary ganglion to the sphincter pupillae and ciliary muscle
sixth cranial n.	*see* abducent n.			
spinal nn.	nn. spinales (NAV)	a series of dorsal and ventral rootlets from the spinal cord	after escaping from the vertebral canal through an intervertebral foramen, each n. divides into dorsal and ventral primary branches (or divisions)	paired nn. arranged serially and segmentally and named (in mammals) according to the vertebra cranial to them (except for the cervical spinal nn. in which the first emerges cranial to and the second caudal to the atlas, the third caudal to the axis, etc.); in birds all spinal nn. are best numbered sequentially from behind the cranium because of difficulties in distinguishing spinal regions

Table continued over page

14 Nerves *(Continued)*

Nerve	Other names	Origin	Branches	Type, distribution and comments
splanchnic nn.	*see* greater, lesser, least, lumbar and sacral splanchnic nn.			these nn. are all sympathetic nn.; the so-called pelvic splanchnic nn. contain mostly parasympathetic fibers and are now known as the pelvic nn.
stapedial n.	n. stapedius (NAV)	the facial n.		a tiny motor n. to the minute stapedius muscle within the middle ear
subclavian n.	n. subclavius (NAV)	the cervical nn. C5 and C6 via the brachial plexus		the motor n. to the subclavius muscle
sublingual n.	n. sublingualis (NAV)	the lingual n.		a sensory n. that supplies the ventral surface of the tongue and the floor of the mouth; it also conveys parasympathetic fibers to the sublingual glands
suboccipital n.	n. suboccipitalis (NAV)	the dorsal division of the first cervical n.	to the muscles over the nape	the motor n. supplies some ear muscles, the major and minor straight muscles of the head, and a few other muscles
subscapular n.	n. subscapularis (NAV)	the cervical nn. C6 and C7 via the brachial plexus	to the subscapular muscle	despite its short course the n. is long to allow movement of the forelimb
superficial branch of the radial n.	n. radialis, ramus superficialis (NAV)	the parent radial n. within the brachial groove	the lateral cutaneous antebrachial n.; the common dorsal digital nn.; lateral and medial branches	this sensory n. divides in some species into lateral and medial branches that run down the cranial aspect of the forearm on either side of the cephalic vein
superficial fibular n.	n. fibularis superficialis (NAV), n. peroneus superficialis (NAV alternative)	the common fibular n.	it gives off muscular and cutaneous rami before branching into the dorsal common digital nn.	the n. supplies branches to the lateral digital extensor and the peroneus brevis muscle and terminates as sensory nn. to the dorsum of the paw
superficial perineal n.	n. perinealis superficialis (NAV)	the pudendal n.		the n. is sensory to the skin of the perineal region, including the anus and vulva
superficial peroneal n.	*see* superficial fibular n.			
supraclavicular nn.	nn. supraclaviculares (NAV)	the ventral branch of the fifth or sixth cervical n.	dorsal, middle and ventral branches	these are bundles of cutaneous nn. of variable origin between species that supply the ventral aspect of the caudal neck, the shoulder and pectoral regions
supraorbital n.	n. supraorbitalis (NAV)	the frontal n.		the continuation of the frontal n. that, in the horse, passes through the supraorbital foramen to deliver sensory fibers to the forehead and upper eyelid; not present in ruminants or dogs
suprascapular n.	n. suprascapularis (NAV)	the cervical n. C6 (and C7) via the brachial plexus	to the supra- and infraspinatus muscles	this cranial member of the nn. from the brachial plexus is vulnerable to trauma as it passes over the neck of the scapula—its bruising here causes the condition of 'sweeny'

supratrochlear n.	n. supratrochlearis (NAV)	the frontal n.		a terminal branch of the frontal n. of the pig that carries sensory fibers to the medial corner of the upper eyelid
sural nn.	*see* lateral and caudal cutaneous sural nn.			
sympathetic trunk	truncus sympathicus (NAV), sympathetic chain	preganglionic sympathetic fibers by way of the (white) rami communicantes	postganglionic sympathetic fibers via the (gray) rami communicantes; many named nn.	this is the most conspicuous part of the sympathetic nervous system; paired ganglionated trunks run outside the vertebral canal; the principal nn. that issue from the ganglia are the greater, lesser, least, lumbar and sacral splanchnic nn., the cardiac nn., the vertebral n. and the jugular n.
tail nn.	*see* caudal nn.			
temporal nn.	*see* deep temporal n.			
tensor of soft palate, n. of	n. tensoris veli palatini (NAV)	the mandibular n. via the medial pterygoid n.		a motor n. to this muscle
tensor tympani, n. of	n. tensoris tympani (NAV), n. musculi tensoris tympani (NA)	the mandibular n. via the medial pterygoid n.		a motor n. to this muscle
tenth cranial n.	*see* vagus n.			
terminal n.	n. terminalis (NAV)	an olfactory n.? the lamina terminalis, or the hypothalamus depending on species		the n. is listed under the olfactory nn. yet is regarded by some as a separate entity that supplies the nasal mucosa; it may be an osmoreceptor or a rostral extension of the sympathetic nervous system
third cranial n.	*see* oculomotor n.			
thoracic nn.	nn. thoracici (NAV)	from the thoracic segments of the spinal cord	each n. typically divides into dorsal and ventral (= intercostal) branches; the first two nn. contribute to the brachial plexus	these are paired spinal nn. that are named according to the vertebra that is immediately cranial to them; there are typically 13 pairs in the dog and cat, and 18 pairs in the horse; the primary dorsal branch further divides into lateral and medial branches; *see* intercostal nn.
thoracic splanchnic n.	*see* greater splanchnic n.			
thoracodorsal n.	n. thoracodorsalis (NAV), dorsal thoracic n.	usually the middle root(s) of the brachial plexus (C8)		the n. is motor to the latissimus dorsi muscle; it runs on the medial surface of the muscle
tibial n.	n. tibialis (NAV)	the sciatic n. about half way down the thigh	muscular and cutaneous rami, the caudal cutaneous sural n. and the plantar nn.	this direct continuation of the sciatic n. supplies the caudal muscles of the calf: popliteus, gastrocnemius, soleus and the superficial and deep digital flexors; it terminates as the plantar nn.
transverse cervical n.	n. transversus colli (NAV), transverse colli n., cutaneous n. of the neck	the ventral division of the second cervical n.	cranial and caudal branches	a cutaneous n. that supplies the ventral aspect of the neck and part of the intermandibular space

Table continued over page

14 Nerves *(Continued)*

Nerve	Other names	Origin	Branches	Type, distribution and comments
transverse colli n.	*see* transverse cervical n.			
trigeminal n.	n. trigeminus (NAV), fifth cranial n.	the lateral surface of the pons	the ophthalmic n.; the maxillary n.; the mandibular n.	the largest of the cranial nn.; it is the main sensory n. to the head and has a motor root to the muscles of mastication (those of the mandibular branchial arch of the embryo)
trochlear n.	n. trochlearis (NAV), fourth cranial n., pathetic n.	the n. emerges from the brainstem just behind the caudal colliculus		the most slender of the cranial nn.; it provides the motor fibers to the dorsal oblique muscle of the eye and has the longest intracranial course of all the cranial nn.
twelfth cranial n.	*see* hypoglossal n.			
tympanic n.	n. tympanicus (NAV), Jacobson's n.	the distal (= petrosal) ganglion of the glossopharyngeal n.	the tympanic plexus; the lesser petrosal n.; the caroticotympanic nn.	thought to be a general sensory and parasympathetic n.; it courses in a canal between the petrous and tympanic parts of the temporal bone to reach the tympanic plexus; the plexus, in turn, supplies the middle ear and the parotid gland via the lesser petrosal n.
ulnar n.	n. ulnaris (NAV)	the most caudal member of the brachial plexus, receiving most fibers from T1	the caudal cutaneous antebrachial n.; the common digital nn.; a deep branch	a major n. in the brachial plexus that innervates the flexor carpi ulnaris, the ulnar head of the deep flexor and the muscles of the paw; it is sensory to the caudal aspect of the forearm and to the lateral aspect of the manus
utricular n.	n. utricularis (NAV), n. utriculoampullaris (NAV)	the vestibular n.		the n. to the macula of the utricle
vagosympathetic trunk	truncus vagosympathicus (NAV)	the vagus n. and cervical sympathetic trunk		the combined vagus and cervical sympathetic nn. in the neck located within the carotid sheath; in cats the sympathetic trunk remains separate from the vagus
vagus n.	n. vagus (NAV), tenth cranial n., pneumogastric n.	the lateral aspect of the medulla	the cranial and recurrent laryngeal nn.; the dorsal and ventral vagal trunks	a mixed n. that provides sensory fibers to the ear, pharynx and larynx, motor fibers to the pharynx, larynx and esophagus, and parasympathetic and sensory fibers to most of the thoracic and abdominal viscera; the longest of the cranial nn.
ventral vagal trunk	truncus vagalis ventralis (NAV), ventral esophageal trunk	the right and left vagus nn.	branches to the stomach and intestines	this n. with its dorsal partner enters the abdomen at the esophageal hiatus and provides the major parasympathetic supply to the alimentary tract
vertebral n.	n. vertebralis (NAV)	the cervicothoracic ganglion		this sympathetic n. follows the vertebral artery of the neck, supplying delicate branches to the spinal nn. and meninges
vestibular n.	n. vestibularis (NAV)	the vestibulocochlear n.	the utricular and ampullary nn.	the vestibular part of the eighth cranial n. that carries sensory information from the semicircular canals, utricle and saccule of the inner ear

vestibulocochlear n.	n. vestibulocochlearis (NAV); eighth cranial n.; acoustic n.	the trapezoid body just caudal to the facial n. and pons	the vestibular n.; the cochlear n.	the short n. that conveys impulses concerned with hearing and balance from the inner ear
vomeronasal n.	n. vomeronasalis (NAV)	the olfactory nn.		delicate nn. to the vomeronasal organ that are thought to mediate a unique gustatory or olfactory sense
white rami communicantes	white communicating branches	the ventral branches of most thoracic and lumbar spinal nn.	to the sympathetic trunk	in some animals it is possible to distinguish these rami (containing preganglionic myelinated sympathetic fibers) from gray rami (containing postganglionic nonmyelinated sympathetic fibers), but in many animals both types of fiber are found within the same ramus
Willis's n.	*see* accessory n.			
zygomatic n.	n. zygomaticus (NAV)	the maxillary n.	zygomaticotemporal and zygomaticofacial branches	the first branch of the maxillary n. in the pterygopalatine fossa; it conveys sensory information from around the lateral corner of the eye and the zygomatic arch
zygomaticotemporal n.	ramus zygomaticotemporalis (NAV)	the zygomatic n.	the cornual n. in ruminants	a communicating n. between the zygomatic and the lacrimal nn. that contains secretomotor fibers which ramify in the lacrimal gland

Table prepared by John Grandage.

15 Veins

For brevity, this Table lists only selected veins; in general it only includes those which have either clinical or functional significance or which do not have a similar course and distribution to the arteries of the same name (see Table 9).

Vein	Other names	Destination	Comments
accessory cephalic v.	v. cephalica accessoria (NAV)	it drains into the cephalic v.	this is the superficial v. of the dorsum of the foot that ascends over the carpus to join the cephalic v. in the distal part of the forearm
allantoic v.	*see* umbilical v.		
angular v. of the eye	v. angularis oculi (NAV)	it drains both into the facial v. and the external ophthalmic v.	the v. is of significance for intravenous injection, especially of radiographic contrast agents; the vein's deep communication with the dural venous sinuses enables them to be made radiopaque for diagnostic x-ray purposes; the v. lies subcutaneously rostral to the medial corner of the eye
auricular vv.	*see* ear veins		
axillobrachial v.	v. axillobrachialis (NAV)	it drains into the axillary v.	this v. is a dorsal continuation of the cephalic v. as it reaches the shoulder; it passes caudal to the humerus, receiving tributaries from the triceps before it reaches the axillary v.
azygos vv.	*see* right and left azygos vv., and right and left hemiazygos vv.	the coronary sinus (for the left v.) or the roof of the right atrium (for the right v.)	the azygos system of vv. drains the dorsal thoracic wall; azygos literally means unpaired even though the vv. develop from the paired embryonic cardinal vv.; usually most of one side disappears leaving a single right or left azygos; caudal segments of the other side may persist as a right or a left hemiazygos v.; both right and left azygos vv. are present in ruminants, only the right in carnivores and horses, and usually only the left in pigs
basilar sinus	sinus basilaris (NAV)	this sinus opens into the vertebral venous plexus	the sinus passes through the foramen magnum into the vertebral venous plexuses communicating variously with the more rostral sinuses; in carnivores interbasilar sinuses unite the two
bijugular trunk	truncus bijugularis (NAV)	it drains into the cranial vena cava	this is the short vessel found near the thoracic inlet where the right and left external jugular vv. unite; it is commonly found in horses and pigs; note that the name does not apply, strictly, to the union of internal and external jugulars on one side to form a common trunk, or to the union of the two internal jugulars as occurs in cattle.
bronchial vv.	vv. bronchiales (NAV)	these drain into the azygos v., in some cases via a broncho-esophageal v.	the peripheral part of the bronchial venous drainage empties directly into the pulmonary vv. (diluting its oxygen content infinitessimally); the true bronchial vv. only drain the larger parts of the bronchial tree and empty into the systemic venous system
buccal v.	v. buccalis (NAV)	it drains into the maxillary v., usually via the pterygoid plexus	this vessel is best developed in horses in which it undergoes a remarkable dilatation (sinus v. buccalis—NAV) as it passes beneath the masseter muscle
buccinator v.	*see* deep facial v.		
canal of Schlemm	*see* scleral venous sinus/plexus		

cardiac vv.	vv. cordis (NAV)	mostly these drain into the right atrium via the coronary sinus; a few open elsewhere	most cardiac vv. run much of their course beneath the epicardium, often as paired companion vv. that flank a radicle of the coronary arteries; *see* great, middle, right, and smallest cardiac vv., and the coronary sinus
caudal vv.	*see* tail vv.		
caudal mesenteric v.	v. mesenterica caudalis (NAV)	it opens into the portal v.	this is the smallest of the tributaries of the portal v., carrying venous blood from the descending colon; its tributaries include the middle and left colic vv. and the cranial rectal v.
caudal vena cava	v. cava caudalis (NAV), postcava, inferior vena cava	it leads into the sinus venarum of the right atrium	the most capacious of all the great vv.; it arises from the union of the paired common iliac vv., and runs forwards to the right of the aorta; it makes brief but intimate contact with the liver (receiving the hepatic vv.), pierces the diaphragm at the foramen venae cavae (receiving the cranial phrenic vv.) and finally runs through the caudal thorax in its own fold of pleura (plica venae cavae) to the right atrium; it is often duplicated in diving mammals; it carries the venous return from most of the hind half of the animal
cavernous sinus	sinus cavernosus (NAV)	into the ventral petrosal or basilar sinuses and out of the cranium via several emissary vv.	these are large paired sinuses that flank the pituitary and lie beneath the hypothalamus; they receive venous blood from the orbit that seems to serve as a cooling device for the internal carotid artery (or especially the rete mirabile) that runs through it; the two sinuses are converted into a ring by the intercavernous sinuses
cephalic v.	v. cephalica (NAV)	into the external jugular v. and the omobrachial v. (dogs) or the superficial cervical v. (cats)	this is the large superficial v. of the forelimb, that runs on the cranial aspect of the forearm and arm and that is used routinely for venipuncture in many species; it begins on the medial and palmar side of the paw and is augmented by the accessory cephalic v.; dorsally it passes under the brachiocephalic to reach the jugular (this part was formerly called the distal communicating branch)
cerebellar vv.	vv. cerebelli dorsales/ventrales (NAV)	these vv. drain into the transverse sigmoid or basilar sinuses	these are fine vessels that, dorsally, run on the surface of the cerebellum and flank the vermis, and, ventrally, run between the cerebellar hemispheres and the medulla
cerebral vv.	vv. cerebri (NAV), veins of the brain	these vv. drain into the dural sinuses	these vv. are unusual in their absence of valves, their lack of accompanying arteries, and their thin walls; *see* dorsal, ventral and great cerebral vv., and cerebellar vv.
coccygeal vv.	see tail vv.		
common cardinal v.	v. cardinalis communis (NE), duct of Cuvier	this embryonic v. drains into the sinus venosus of the heart	this v. is the terminal vessel that receives blood from the fetal head and trunk via the precardinal and postcardinal vv.
common iliac v.	v. iliaca communis (NAV)	the confluence of the two vv. forms the origin of the caudal vena cava	the vessel is formed from the union of the internal and external iliac vv. (they normally remain separate in the arterial system)
cornual v.	v. cornualis (NAV)	this v. empties into the maxillary v.	the v. receives blood from the horn via dorsal and ventral branches; these unite near the base of the horn and pass along the border of the temporal line
coronary sinus	sinus coronarius (NAV)	this opens into the right atrium just ventral to the entrance of the caudal vena cava	the sinus serves as the terminal vessel for most of the venous drainage of the heart; it runs in the caudal part of the coronary groove and receives the great and middle cardiac vv.; its origin is indicated by the receipt of the left azygos v. (pigs and ruminants) or the left oblique atrial v. (horses and carnivores); its atrial opening is guarded by a valvular flap, most obvious in horses

Table continued over page

15 Veins *(Continued)*

Vein	Other names	Destination	Comments
cranial mesenteric v.	v. mesenterica cranialis (NAV)	this opens into the portal v.	the largest of the tributaries of the portal v.; it typically receives drainage from the caudal pancreaticoduodenal, jejunal, ileal, ileocolic, cecal and sometimes the right and middle colic vv.
cranial phrenic vv.	vv. phrenicae craniales (NAV)	these vv. drain straight into the caudal vena cava	these vv. are conspicuous within the tendinous center of the diaphragm where they are odd because they are obliged to adopt a highly flattened form
cranial rectal v.	v. rectalis cranialis (NAV)	this drains mainly into the caudal mesenteric v.	this v. is of interest because it forms a link between the systemic vv. represented by the middle and caudal rectal vv. and the portal vv. with which it makes most connection; obstruction to portal blood flow may thus dilate the rectal vv.; moreover it indicates that drugs administered per rectum may be absorbed into the systemic circulation and can bypass the liver
cranial vena cava	v. cava cranialis (NAV), precava, superior vena cava	this v. drains directly into the sinus venarum of the right atrium	this becomes the widest vein of the body as it drains into the heart; it is valveless and is formed from the union of the two external jugular vv. (horses), from all four jugulars (cattle) or from the two brachiocephalic vv. (dogs and pigs); it may also receive costocervical, vertebral, internal thoracic and right azygos vv.
deep facial v.	v. profunda faciei (NAV), reflex v., buccinator v.	the v. drains into the facial v. rostrally and various other vessels on its course to the pterygopalatine fossa	this v. unites the superficial and deep set of facial vv.; in the horse it dilates to form a sinus (sinus v. profundae faciei—NAV), which is the middle of the three large venous sinuses of the horse's cheek; their position beneath the masseter muscle suggests they serve as a reservoir for blood that can be emptied by muscular contraction
diploic vv.	vv. diploicae (NAV)	usually these vv. drain into the sagittal sinus but there are variations	these are vv. that drain the diploe or marrow of the bones of the skull roof; three are named: the frontal, parietal and occipital diploic vv.
dorsal cerebral vv.	vv. cerebri dorsales (NAV)	they open into the dorsal group of dural sinuses, especially the dorsal sagittal sinus	these form a series of paired vessels on the dorsal surface of the cerebral cortex; they are not necessarily symmetrical
dorsal petrosal sinus	sinus petrosus dorsalis (NAV)	it opens into the transverse sinus	this paired sinus runs caudodorsally from the region of the piriform lobe into the transverse sinus, coursing in the root of the tentorium cerebelli
duct of Cuvier	*see* common cardinal v.		
ductus venosus (NE)		it opens into the caudal vena cava with the hepatic vv.	this is a fetal vessel within the substance of the liver that unites the umbilical v. with the caudal vena cava, thus allowing oxygenated placental blood to bypass the liver; it is present in all young embryos but becomes vestigial in the horse and pig; even in other species it tends to become reduced towards the end of gestation; it is obliterated shortly after birth

dural sinuses	sinus durae matris (NAV), dural venous sinuses, sinuses of the dura mater	all the sinuses ultimately open into emissary vv. that convey the blood through cranial foramina to the internal jugular, vertebral and maxillary vv. and to the vertebral venous plexuses	dural sinuses mostly occupy spaces between adjacent leaves of dura mater, especially between the periosteal and meningeal sheets; they are typically divided into dorsal and ventral sets that have limited communication with each other; they serve as vessels into which cerebral vv. empty and into which some extracranial veins from the orbit also drain; being valveless, flow can be in either direction; some are invaginated by arachnoid granulations for the drainage of cerebrospinal fluid; for individual sinuses *see the dorsal set*: sagittal, transverse, temporal, sigmoid, dorsal petrosal and straight sinuses; *the ventral set*: basilar, ventral petrosal, cavernous and intercavernous sinuses
ear vv.	auricular vv.	these typically drain into the maxillary v.	several auricular vv. run mostly over the caudal surface of the earflap; depending on the species there are lateral, intermediate, medial and rostral vv.; these and the deep auricular v. empty into the maxillary v. either via the caudal auricular or the superficial temporal vv.; in some species (e.g. rabbits, elephants) these vv. serve for cooling; the lateral and medial vv. run near the margin of the helix and are useful for venipuncture in rabbits and pigs; the lateral auricular is the v. of choice in pigs
emissary vv.	vv. emissariae (NAV)	these vv. unite the dural venous sinuses with several extracranial vv. such as the ophthalmic plexus, internal jugular v., vertebral v. and various tributaries of the maxillary v.	the emissary vv. allow venous blood within the cranium to escape through about twenty cranial foramina to enter the extracranial vv.; they include the mastoid and occipital emissary vv., the emissary vv. of the carotid and hypoglossal canals and of the jugular, oval, orbital, retroarticular, round and orbitorotund foramina, and the emissary v. of the foramen lacerum; emissary vv. are without valves and can convey blood either centrally or peripherally
esophageal vv.	vv. esophageae (NAV)	most drain into the azygos v., in some cases via a broncho-esophageal v., and into a tributary of the portal v.	the esophageal vv. serve as a watershed between drainage via the systemic and portal systems; any obstruction of the portal blood flow may cause enlargement or varicosities of the thoracic esophageal vv.
external jugular v.	v. jugularis externa (NAV)	it either drains into a brachiocephalic v. (dogs, some pigs) or a bijugular trunk (cattle, horses) before becoming the cranial vena cava	this is the principal venous pathway from the head in domestic mammals; the v. mostly runs subcutaneously in the jugular groove of the neck (which usually lies between the sternocephalic muscle ventrally and the brachiocephalic dorsally); it is the vessel of choice for venipuncture in large animals; it arises from the confluence of the linguofacial and maxillary vv.
external vertebral plexus	plexus vertebralis externus dorsalis/ventralis (NAV)	the plexus unites with the internal vertebral plexus and a variety of local extravertebral vv.	this plexus is located just outside the intervertebral foramina, and is not well developed in domestic mammals except in the cervical region; its function complements that of the more important internal vertebral plexus
great cardiac v.	v. cordis magna (NAV)	it drains into the coronary sinus	this v. takes most of the coronary venous return; it arises at the apex of the heart, ascends the paraconal ventricular groove and runs in the caudal part of the coronary groove to open into the coronary sinus and right atrium
great cerebral v.	v. cerebri magna (NAV)	it drains into the straight sinus	the unpaired v. is the channel for venous return from the deep structures of the cerebrum; its tributaries include the v. of the corpus callosum (v. corporis callosi—NAV) and various internal cerebral vv. (vv. cerebrae internae—NAV) that receive blood from the thalamus, choroid plexuses etc.
great saphenous v.	*see* medial saphenous v.		

Table continued over page

15 Veins (*Continued*)

Vein	Other names	Destination	Comments
hepatic vv.	vv. hepaticae (NAV)	drain directly into the caudal vena cava	these vessels lie totally within the liver parenchyma and open directly into the vena cava as it passes adjacent to or through the liver; it is possible to identify right, left and middle vv. from the individual lobes
hepatic portal v.	*see* portal v.		
hepatic sinus		it lies within the caudal vena cava	this is a large dilation of the caudal vena cava and the hepatic veins where they become confluent just caudal to the diaphragm in diving mammals; the sinus works as a temporary reservoir during dives when venous return is restricted by the caval sphincter located just cranial to it
hyoid arch	arcus hyoideus (NAV)	it unites right and left lingual or linguofacial vv.	this is a superficial vessel that runs transversely across the throat; it is not present in the horse
intercavernous sinuses	sinus intercavernosi (NAV)	these sinuses open laterally into the two cavernous sinuses	the intercavernous sinuses cross in front of and behind the pituitary gland, forming a vascular ring
internal jugular v.	v. jugularis interna (NAV)	it usually drains into the external jugular v. (carnivores, pigs) or into the bijugular trunk (cattle)	this is a small v. in domestic mammals; it is absent from sheep and horses; after emerging from the hypoglossal canal it runs most of its course down the neck in company with the common carotid artery in the carotid sheath
internal vertebral plexus	plexus vertebralis internus ventralis (NAV), vertebral venous sinuses, longitudinal vertebral sinuses	this plexus is united with the extravertebral vv. at every intervertebral foramen	these paired, thin-walled, valveless sinuses run the length of the vertebral canal on its floor in the epidural fat; they drain the vertebrae and spinal cord but more importantly serve as an alternative venous pathway for blood returning to the heart, especially when local pressure changes (e.g. a twisted neck or compressed abdomen) compromise the orthodox route; *see* intervertebral vv.
intervertebral vv.	vv. intervertebrales (NAV)	these vv. unite the internal and external vertebral plexuses	these paired vv. pass through the intervertebral foramina along the whole spine; they unite vv. such as the vertebral and azygos vv. and caudal vena cava with the internal vertebral plexus, thus allowing an alternative route for venous return when the extravertebral vv. are compressed
jugular vv.	*see* internal and external jugular vv.		the term jugular by itself (without the adjective internal or external) usually refers to the larger vessel, i.e. the external jugular in domestic mammals or the internal jugular in the human
lateral saphenous v.	v. saphena lateralis/parva (NAV), small saphenous v.	it empties into the distal caudal femoral v. (carnivores) or the medial circumflex femoral (pigs and ruminants)	this v. is conspicuous in dogs as it runs proximally in the subcutaneous tissue above the hock; though it is a prominent vein, its flexuous course and its loose tethering to the skin make it less than ideal for venipuncture; it anastomoses with the medial saphenous v. and usually has cranial and caudal tributaries; the v. is small in horses
left azygos v.	v. azygos sinistra (NAV)	it opens into the coronary sinus	this v. receives drainage from the intercostal vv. above and caudal to the heart and from the esophageal and bronchial vv; its extent varies and it often arises caudal to the diaphragm, which it pierces through the aortic hiatus; it is found only in ruminants and pigs
left hemiazygos v.	v. hemiazygos sinistra (NAV)	it drains into the right azygos v.	a caudal remnant of the left cardinal vv.; found only in horses and carnivores

maxillary v.	v. maxillaris (NAV)	it drains into the external jugular v.	this is one of the two principal tributaries of the jugular v.; it receives much of the drainage from the face and begins in most species as a plexus of vv., the pterygoid plexus
medial saphenous v.	v. saphena medialis/magna (NAV), great saphenous v.	it opens into the femoral v.	this is a large v. that runs on the medial side of the shank and thigh; it receives venous drainage from its cranial and caudal branches which pass over the flexor and extensor aspects of the hock respectively; the branches are fed in turn by the dorsal common digital vv. and medial and lateral plantar vv., there is communion between the great saphenous and the lateral saphenous vv. as well as with the deep vv.
median cubital v.	v. mediana cubiti (NAV)	it drains into the cephalic v.	this v. is located over the flexor surface of the elbow; it unites the median v. with the cephalic v.
middle cardiac v.	v. cordis media (NAV)	it drains into the terminal part of the coronary sinus	this v. arises near the apex of the heart and ascends the subsinuosal interventricular groove
milk v.	v. mammaria cranialis (NAV), v. epigastrica caudalis superficialis (NAV), subcutaneous abdominal v.	it drains into both the external pudendal v. and, via the milk well, into the internal thoracic v.	the name of this v. is applied particularly to that of the lactating cow in which it is grossly distended, varicose and conspicuous as it runs its tortuous subcutaneous course on the floor of the abdomen from the udder forwards; it develops from the cranial and caudal superficial epigastric vv. whose delicate anastomoses during youth become grossly distended with the first calving; valves become incompetent and venous flow is directed cranially (even along the caudal part which formerly only conducted caudally); the v. is important for venipuncture in cows
omobrachial v.	v. omobrachialis (NAV), communicating branch of the cephalic v.	it drains into the external jugular v.	this v. unites the cephalic v. of the forelimb with the external jugular v.; it runs superficially over the deltoid and brachiocephalic muscles to reach the jugular v. in its furrow; only in carnivores
omphalomesenteric v.	*see* vitelline v.		
ophthalmic plexus	plexus ophthalmicus (NAV)	this plexus drains into both the cavernous sinus and tributaries of the facial v.	this plexus is found within the periorbita, and is made up of the dorsal and ventral external ophthalmic vv. that communicate both centrally with the dural sinuses and peripherally with the facial vessels; its drainage area corresponds to that supplied by the external ophthalmic artery
ovarian v.	v. ovarica (NAV)	into the renal v., caudal vena cava, or common iliac v.	the v. tends to terminate more cranially in carnivores, especially on the left, and more caudally in ruminants; the v. is plexiform as it passes over the ovarian a., and somewhat resembles the pampiniform plexus in the male; it may serve for transvascular hormonal exchange
pampiniform plexus	plexus pampiniformis (NAV)	the plexus unites into a single testicular v.	the plexus consists of a large number of delicate venules that intimately embrace the tortuous testicular a.; the arrangement serves for heat exchange and the maintenance of a cool testicular blood supply
petrosal sinuses	*see* dorsal and ventral petrosal sinuses		

Table continued over page

15 Veins *(Continued)*

Vein	Other names	Destination	Comments
portal v.	v. portae (NAV), v. portae hepatis (NA), hepatic portal v.	into the liver at its porta, where it divides into interlobar and interlobular vv.	this v. conveys blood from the capillary bed of the abdominal digestive organs to a secondary capillary (sinusoidal) bed within the liver; it provides the so-called functional circulation (80% of the volume) to the liver; its tributaries typically include the splenic v. (corresponding to the supply from the celiac a.), and the cranial and caudal mesenteric vv.; its terminal course is within the lesser omentum ventral to the epiploic foramen
pterygoid plexus	plexus pterygoideus (NAV)	this plexus drains into the maxillary v.	this is a complex set of vessels lying lateral to the medial pterygoid muscle; it frequently unites with the ophthalmic plexus and receives drainage from many vv. including the masseteric, palatine, buccal, pharyngeal and deep temporal vv.
pulmonary vv.	v. pulmonales (NAV)	these vv. drain into the left atrium	these vessels lie mostly within the substance of the lung and convey oxygenated blood from the pulmonary alveolar capillaries to the heart; they run either with the bronchi (cattle) or, for part of the course, intersegmentally (sheep, dogs, pigs and horses); they typically run on the medial sides of the bronchi, are valveless and also carry some of the bronchial venous drainage; they open via five to eight ostia into the left atrium
reflex v.	*see* deep facial v.		
renal v.	v. renalis (NAV)	it opens directly into the caudal vena cava	the left renal v. is longer than the right because it has to cross the aorta to reach the caudal vena cava; in carnivores it often receives the ovarian or testicular v. as well as the adrenal vv.
renal portal v.	v. portalis renalis caudalis/cranialis (NAA)	this v. opens into the common iliac v., the caudal mesenteric v. and the kidney tissue itself	a renal portal system is found in vertebrates other than mammals and is derived from the embryonic postcardinal vv.; venous blood from the hind part of the body is transported to the kidneys by the renal portal v. to complement the supply from the renal arteries; in birds, cranial and caudal renal portal vv. receive blood from the external iliac v. and channel it into the kidneys by afferent renal branches; a direct connection between the portal v. and the common iliac v. is retained and guarded by a portal valve that regulates blood flow to the kidneys; some renal portal flow can also bypass the kidneys via connections with the caudal mesenteric v. and the vertebral venous sinuses
right azygos v.	v. azygos dextra (NAV)	it opens into the roof of the right atrium near the junction with the cranial vena cava	this v. drains the intercostal vv. and is formed from the embryonic postcardinal v.; it arises within the abdomen, passes through the aortic hiatus and may receive a left hemiazygos v. (horses and dogs); in ruminants it drains a more limited area; it is usually absent from pigs
right cardiac vv.	vv. cordis dextrae (NAV), vv. cordis anteriores (NA), small cardiac vv.	these vv. drain by a common vessel into the right atrium	these form a series of small vessels that drain the myocardium of the right ventricle and that open through orifices into the right atrium between the pectinate muscles
right hemiazygos v.	v. hemiazygos dextra (NAV)	it drains into the left azygos v.	the caudal remnant of the right cardinal vv., it is found only in ruminants and pigs and drains the caudal part of the dorsal thoracic wall

sagittal sinuses	sinus sagittalis dorsalis/ventralis (NAV)	the sinus terminates at the transverse sinus	this unpaired dural sinus runs in the midline within the falx cerebri; in animals with large brains there are usually dorsal and ventral sinuses; the wall is pocked by lateral lacunae for the invagination of arachnoid granulations
Schlemm's canal	*see* scleral venous sinus/plexus		
scleral venous sinus/plexus	sinus venosus sclerae (NAV), plexus venosus sclerae (NAV), Schlemm's canal	the sinus drains into the anterior ciliary vv.	this annular sinus is found within the sclera near the corneoscleral limbus; when it is predominantly a single vessel it is known as a sinus (as in some primates), and when composed of multiple vessels, as a plexus (domestic mammals); it drains the effluent aqueous humor which reaches it from the anterior chamber through the spaces of the corneoiridial angle
sigmoid sinus	sinus sigmoideus (NAV)	this sinus empties into the emissary v. of the jugular foramen	this dural sinus is one of the two main effluent passages for the transverse sinus; it runs an S-shaped course around the petrous temporal bone before entering the emissary v. of the jugular foramen
small cardiac vv.	*see* right and smallest cardiac vv.		
smallest cardiac vv.	vv. cordis minimi (NAV), thebesian vv.	these vv. drain by numerous openings into all four heart chambers	these are tiny vv. that open directly into the heart chambers from the myocardium; in the left ventricle the venous blood they discharge dilutes (by a small amount) the oxygenated blood from the lungs
small saphenous v.	*see* lateral saphenous v.		
splenic v.	v. lienalis (NAV)	this drains into the portal v.	this vessel is typically one of the three or four main tributaries of the portal v.; it receives pancreatic, left gastric, left gastroepiploic, short gastric and caudal esophaeal tributaries
spur v.	*see* superficial thoracic v.		
straight sinus	sinus rectus (NAV)	this sinus usually empties into the sagittal sinus near its junction with the transverse sinus	this dural sinus is the direct continuation within the dura of the great cerebral v.; it thus collects blood from the deeper cerebral structures
superficial thoracic v.	v. thoracica superficialis (NAV), spur v. (horses)	it drains into the axillary v. (cattle) or the thoracodorsal v. (horses)	this v. has no arterial companion; in horses its conspicuous course in the subcutaneous tissue of the ventral thorax has prompted its common name 'spur vein'
tail vv.	v. caudalis mediana/lateralis/etc. (NAV), caudal vv., coccygeal vv.	these vv. drain mostly into the median sacral and caudal gluteal vv.	there are several veins draining the tail; the main ones in carnivores are the lateral tail vv.; in cattle the large, unpaired, median tail v. is used for tail bleeding—it runs in the ventral midline adjacent to the artery (to the left or right) as far as the fourth caudal vertebra and thereafter it lies deep (dorsal to) the artery
temporal sinus	sinus temporalis (NAV)	this sinus empties into the emissary v. of the retroarticular foramen	this dural sinus is one of the two main effluent passages for the transverse sinus; it runs most of its course within the temporal canal (if present) or temporal meatus, before entering the emissary v. of the retroarticular foramen
testicular v.	v. testicularis (NAV), internal spermatic v.	it drains into the renal v. in most dogs and some others, or into the caudal vena cava or common iliac v.	the v. terminates more caudally in ruminants and more cranially in carnivores; its tributaries run over the surface of the testis before forming a dense, intricate pampiniform plexus over the testicular a. in the distal part of the spermatic cord

Table continued over page

15 Veins *(Continued)*

Vein	Other names	Destination	Comments
thebesian vv.	*see* smallest cardiac vv.		
transverse cubital v.	v. transversa cubiti (NAV), distal collateral radial v.	it drains into neighboring vv. such as the cephalic v.	a small vessel that crosses the flexor aspect of the elbow, proximal to the medial cubita v.
transverse facial v.	v. transversa faciei (NAV)	it drains into the superficial temporal v.	this v. is unusually dilated in the horse to form a sinus (sinus v. transversae faciei—NAV) just ventral to the facial crest beneath the origin of the masseter muscle
transverse sinus	sinus transversus (NAV)	this sinus opens into two others, the temporal and sigmoid sinuses	this large dural sinus runs transversely between the cerebral and cerebellar hemispheres; it is housed within the transverse canal (or groove) in the roof of the cranium; it begins in the midline at the confluence of the sinuses (where straight and sagittal sinuses meet) and more laterally is joined by the dorsal petrosal sinus
umbilical v.	v. umbilicalis (NE), allantoic v.	it opens into the ductus venosus, the left lobe of the liver, and into the right lobe of the liver with the portal v.	this fetal vessel conducts oxygenated blood from the placenta to the fetus; its placental tributaries unite into paired vessels that wind round the umbilical cord parallel to the umbilical arteries (ruminants and carnivores) or surrounded by them (pigs and horses) to join into a single vessel at the navel (the right v. degenerating in the early embryo); the left v. runs in the free margin of the falciform ligament to the umbilical fissure of the liver where, after detaching branches to the left lobe, it unites with the ductus venosus and portal v.; the v. has a thick wall resembling an artery; after birth its lumen obliterates and it gradually atrophies to become the round ligament of the liver or disappear altogether
ventral cerebral vv.	vv. cerebri ventrales (NAV)	these usually drain into the dorsal petrosal sinus	there is often only one of these; it drains the cortex of the temporal lobe
ventral petrosal sinus	sinus petrosus ventralis (NAV)	it unites the cavernous sinus with the sigmoid or basilar sinuses and communicates with several emissary vv.	this paired sinus runs caudally on the floor of the cranium from the cavernous sinus to adjacent sinuses; in the dog it contains the carotid artery
vertebral plexuses	*see* internal and external vertebral plexus		
vitelline v.	v. vitellina (NE), omphalomesenteric v.	this v. drains initially into the sinus venosus of the heart and later into the portal vein	this is an embryonic v. that carries nutrients from the yolk sac to the liver and heart; in the early embryo the paired vv. run to the sinus venosus of the heart; they course through the septum transversum and the liver anlage and, as the yolk sac declines in importance, lose parts of the left and right vessel and become modified to form part of the portal v.; they are of more sustained importance in birds and reptiles which have large heavy yolks
vorticose vv.	vv. vorticosae (NAV)	these vv. drain into the ophthalmic plexus	there are usually about four of these vv. that are the principal drainage from the choroid, leaving the eyeball near its equator

Table prepared by John Grandage.

Clinical

16 Causes of mastitis

Name of agent	Type of agent	Clinical type of mastitis
Cattle (and buffalo)		
Acholeplasma laidlawii	Bacterium	Found in mastitic milk; doubtful pathogenicity
Actinomyces bovis	Bacterium	Sub-subacute
Actinomyces pyogenes	Bacterium	Peracute
Actinomyces ulcerans	Bacterium	Subacute
Aspergillus fumigatus	Fungus	Acute, abscess formation
Aspergillus nidulans	Fungus	Acute, abscess formation
Bacillus cereus	Bacterium	Peracute gangrenous, acute
Candida spp.	Yeast	Acute
Cryptococcus neoformans	Yeast	Acute
Enterobacter aerogenes	Bacterium	Peracute
Escherichia coli	Bacterium	Peracute
Fusobacterium necrophorum	Bacterium	Subacute suppurative
Klebsiella spp.	Bacterium	Peracute
Leptospira interrogans serovar hardjo	Bacterium	Acute all quarters
Leptospira interrogans serovar pomona	Bacterium	Acute
Mycobacterium bovis	Bacterium	Chronic
Mycobacterium fortuitum	Bacterium	Acute
Mycoplasma alkalescens	Bacterium	Acute all quarters
Mycoplasma bovigenitalium	Bacterium	Acute all quarters
Mycoplasma agalactiae var. *bovis* (*M. bovis*)	Bacterium	Acute all quarters
Nocardia asteroides	Bacterium	Acute, subacute
Nocardia brasiliensis	Bacterium	Acute, subacute
Nocardia farcinica	Bacterium	Acute, subacute
Pasteurella haemolytica	Bacterium	Peracute
Pasteurella multocida	Bacterium	Peracute
Pichia spp.	Fungus	Acute
Prototheca trispora	Alga	Chronic
Prototheca zopfi	Alga	Chronic
Pseudomonas aeruginosa (pyocyanea)	Bacterium	Peracute
Saccharomyces spp.	Yeast	Peracute (summer mastitis)
Serratia marcescens	Bacterium	Mild chronic
Staphylococcus aureus	Bacterium	Peracute, acute, chronic
Staphylococcus epidermidis	Bacterium	Sub-subacute
Streptococcus agalactiae	Bacterium	Acute, subacute
Streptococcus dysgalactiae	Bacterium	Acute
Streptococcus faecalis	Bacterium	Acute
Streptococcus pneumoniae	Bacterium	Peracute
Streptococcus pyogenes	Bacterium	Acute
Streptococcus uberis	Bacterium	Acute
Streptococcus equi subsp. *zooepidemicus*	Bacterium	Subacute, chronic
Torulopsis spp.	Yeast	Acute
Trichosporon spp.	Fungus	Acute
Sheep		
Actinobacillus lignieresi	Bacterium	Not specified
Actinomyces pyogenes	Bacterium	Acute, purulent
Escherichia coli	Bacterium	Peracute
Pasteurella haemolytica	Bacterium	Peracute gangrenous
Pasteurella multocida	Bacterium	Acute
Pseudomonas aeruginosa	Bacterium	Peracute gangrenous
Staphylococcus aureus	Bacterium	Peracute gangrenous
Streptococcus agalactiae	Bacterium	Acute

16 Causes of mastitis *(Continued)*

Name of agent	Type of agent	Clinical type of mastitis
Streptococcus dysgalactiae	Bacterium	Acute
Streptococcus uberis	Bacterium	Acute
Goats		
Actinomyces pyogenes	Bacterium	Acute
Escherichia coli	Bacterium	Peracute
Mycoplasma agalactiae agalactiae	Bacterium	Acute
Staphylococcus aureus	Bacterium	Peracute gangrenous
Streptococcus agalactiae	Bacterium	Acute
Streptococcus dysgalactiae	Bacterium	Acute
Streptococcus pyogenes	Bacterium	Acute
Yersinia pseudotuberculosis	Bacterium	Acute
Pigs		
Aerobacter aerogenes	Bacterium	Mastitis-metritis-agalactia
Escherichia coli	Bacterium	Mastitis-metritis-agalactia
Klebsiella spp.	Bacterium	Mastitis-metritis-agalactia
Pseudomonas aeruginosa	Bacterium	Not specified
Staphylococcus aureus	Bacterium	Acute
Streptococcus agalactiae	Bacterium	Acute
Streptococcus dysgalactiae	Bacterium	Acute
Streptococcus uberis	Bacterium	Acute

17 Estrous cycles in animals

Species	Estral cycle (inter-estrous interval in days)	Duration of estrus (hours)	Time of ovulation	Comments
Cow	21	18	12 hours after estrus ends	
Ewe	17	36	30 hours after estrus begins	Some breeds seasonal only
Goat doe	20	40	30 hours after estrus begins	Seasonal only
Sow	21	45	36 hours after estrus begins	Tend to anestrus in winter
Mare	21	120–150	last day of estrus	Seasonal only
Bitch	210–240	7–9 days	1st or 2nd estrus day	
Queen	16	5–6 days	ovulation induced 20–74 hours after coitus	Seasonal only

18 Body temperature equivalents

Celsius (°C)		Fahrenheit (°F)
0	Freezing	32
36.0		96.8
36.5		97.7
37.0		98.6
37.5		99.5
38.0		100.4
38.5		101.3
39.0		102.2
39.5		103.1
40.0		104.0
40.5		104.9
41.0		105.8
41.5		106.7
42.0		107.6
100	Boiling	212

19 Eruption of teeth in domestic animals

Animal	Deciduous		Permanent	
Cat	$2(I\frac{3}{3}\ C\frac{1}{1}\ P\frac{3}{2})$[a]		$2(I\frac{3}{3}\ C\frac{1}{1}\ P\frac{3}{2}\ M\frac{1}{1})$[a]	
	Incisors:	3–4 weeks[b]	Incisors:	3.5–5.5 months[ab]
	Canines:	3–4 weeks	Canines:	5.5–6.5 months
	Premolars:	5–6 weeks	Premolars:	4–5 months
			Molars:	5–6 months
Dog	$2(I\frac{3}{3}\ C\frac{1}{1}\ P\frac{3}{3})$		$2(I\frac{3}{3}\ C\frac{1}{1}\ P\frac{4}{4}\ M\frac{2}{3})$	
	Incisors:	4–6 weeks	Incisors:	3–5 months
	Canines:	3–5 weeks	Canines:	5–7 months
	Premolars:	5–6 weeks	Premolars:	4–6 months
			Molars:	4–7 months
Pig	$2(I\frac{3}{3}\ C\frac{1}{1}\ P\frac{3}{3})$		$2(I\frac{3}{3}\ C\frac{1}{1}\ P\frac{4}{4}\ M\frac{3}{3})$	
	Incisors 1 and 2:	1–3 weeks	Incisors:	8–18 months
	Incisor 3:	Before birth	Canines:	8–12 months
	Canine:	Before birth	Premolar 1:	3.5–6.5 months
	Premolars:	1–10 weeks	Premolars	12–16 months
			2–4:	4–6 months
			Molar 1:	7–13 months
			Molar 2:	17–22 months
			Molar 3:	
Sheep	$2(I\frac{0}{4}\ C\frac{0}{0}\ P\frac{3}{3})$		$2(\frac{0}{4}\ C\frac{0}{0}\ P\frac{3}{3}\ M\frac{3}{3})$	
	Incisors:	Before birth—up to 8 days[c]	Incisor 1:	1–1.5 yr
		Before birth—up to 4 weeks[c]	Incisor 2:	1.5–2 yr
	Premolars:		Incisor 3:	2.5–3 yr
			Incisor 4:	3–4 yr
			Premolars:	21–24 months
			Molar 1:	3 months
			Molar 2:	9 months
			Molar 3:	18 months
Ox	$2(I\frac{0}{4}\ C\frac{0}{0}\ P\frac{3}{3})$		$2(I\frac{0}{4}\ C\frac{0}{0}\ P\frac{3}{3}\ M\frac{3}{3})$	
	Incisors:	Before birth—up to 2–14 days postnatal[c]	Incisor 1:	1.5–2 yr
			Incisor 2:	2–2.5 yr
	Premolars:	Before birth—up to 2–3 weeks[c]	Incisor 3:	3 years
			Incisor 4:	3.5–4 yr
			Premolars:	2–3 yr
			Molar 1:	5–6 months
			Molar 2:	15–18 months
			Molar 3:	24–28 months
Horse	$2(I\frac{3}{3}\ C\frac{1}{1}\ P\frac{3}{3})$		$2(I\frac{3}{3}\ C\frac{1}{1}\ P\frac{3}{3}$ or $\frac{4}{3}\ M\frac{3}{3})$	
	Incisor 1:	1 week	Incisor 1:	2.5 yr
	Incisor 2:	1 month	Incisor 2:	3.5 yr
	Incisor 3:	5–9 months	Incisor 3:	4.5 yr
	Canines:	Never erupt	Canine:	4–5 yr
	Premolars:	Before birth or 1st week postnatal	Premolar 1:	5–6 months
			Premolar 2:	2.5 yr
			Premolar 3:	3 yr
			Premolar 4:	4 yr
			Molar 1:	1 yr
			Molar 2:	2 yr
			Molar 3:	3.5–4.0 yr

Reproduced with permission from Noden D.M. and Delahunta A.D. (1985) *Embryology of Domestic Animals* (1st Edn). Williams & Wilkins, Baltimore.

[a] I, C, P, M = incisor, canine, premolar and molar teeth.

[b] All ages postnatal unless otherwise indicated.

[c] Late maturing breeds.

20 Collective nouns, gender groups

Species (adj.)	Neonate	Young male	Young female	Adult male	Adult female	Group noun
Alpaca[a]	Cria	Tui	Tui	Machos	Hembra	Punta
Camel (camelid)	Calf			Bull	Cow	Herd
Cat (feline)	Kitten			Tom	Queen	Cluster
Cattle (bovine)	Calf	Bull calf, bullock	Heifer calf	Bull	Cow	Herd
Deer Large (cervine)[b]	Calf	Pricket		Buck or Stag	Doe	Bunch (hinds), herd
Deer Small (cervine)[c]	Fawn, kid	Pricket		Buck	Doe	Herd
Dog (canine)	Pup or puppy	Dog pup	Bitch pup	Dog	Bitch	Pack
Donkey or ass (asinine)	Foal	Colt	Filly	Jack	Jenny	Herd
Elephant	Calf			Bull	Cow	Herd
Elk[d]	Calf			Bull	Cow	Herd
Ferret (musteline)	Kit			Buck or jack or hob	Bitch or jill	Cast
Fish (piscine)	Fingerling or fry					Shoal
Fox (vulpine)	Cub			Dog	Vixen	Lead
Geese, domestic (anserine)	Gosling			Gander	Goose	Skein (in flight), Gaggle (on ground)
Goat (caprine)	Kid	Buck kid	Doe kid	Buck or Billy	Doe or nanny	Flock
Hare (leprine)	Leveret			Buck	Doe	Drove
Horse (equine)	Foal	Colt	Filly	Stallion or stud	Mare	Band or herd
Kangaroo (macropine)	Joey or pouch young			Buck or boomer	Doe	Herd
Lion (leonine)	Cub			Lion	Lioness	Pride
Pheasant	Poult			Buck	Doe	Colony or banquet
Pig (porcine)	Piglet	Barrow (castrate)	Gilt	Boar	Sow	Herd
Poultry	Chick or poult			Rooster or cock	Hen	Flock
Rabbit	Nestling or kitten			Buck	Doe	Warren
Rat (murine)	Nestling			Buck	Doe	Colony
Sheep (ovine)	Lamb	Ram lamb	Ewe lamb	Ram	Ewe	Flock
Snake (ophidian)	Hatchling					Den, pit or nest
Turkey	Poult			Gobbler or tom	Hen	Flock
Whale	Calf			Bull	Cow	Pod
Swan	Cygnet			Cob	Pen	Flock
Ostrich	Chick			Male	Hen	Troupe
Bee (apian)				Drone	Queen bee	Swarm or hive
Emu	Chick	Blackhead	Blackhead	Cock	Hen	Flock or group

[a] Same nomenclature for all South American camelids, i.e. vicuna, alpaca, guanaco and llama.

[b] Large deer—Red, Japanese, Sika.

[c] Small deer – roe, fallow, muntjac, Chinese water deer.

[d] Elk and moose, wapiti and reindeer.

Note: for a more literary treatment of this subject the reader is directed to Rex Collings, *A Crash of Rhinoceroses; a Dictionary of Collective Nouns*. Moyer Bell, Wakefield, Rhode Island and London.

21 Conversion table of weight to body surface area (in square meters) for dogs*

Kg	M^2	Kg	M^2
0.5	0.06	26.0	0.88
1.0	0.10	27.0	0.90
2.0	0.15	28.0	0.92
3.0	0.20	29.0	0.94
4.0	0.25	30.0	0.96
5.0	0.29	31.0	0.99
6.0	0.33	32.0	1.01
7.0	0.36	33.0	1.03
8.0	0.40	34.0	1.05
9.0	0.43	35.0	1.07
10.0	0.46	36.0	1.09
11.0	0.49	37.0	1.11
12.0	0.52	38.0	1.13
13.0	0.55	39.0	1.15
14.0	0.58	40.0	1.17
15.0	0.60	41.0	1.19
16.0	0.63	42.0	1.21
17.0	0.66	43.0	1.23
18.0	0.69	44.0	1.25
19.0	0.71	45.0	1.26
20.0	0.74	46.0	1.28
21.0	0.76	47.0	1.30
22.0	0.78	48.0	1.32
23.0	0.81	49.0	1.34
24.0	0.83	50.0	1.36
25.0	0.85		

* Although the above chart was compiled for dogs, it can also be used for cats. A formula for more precise values follows:

$$\text{BSA in } M^2 = \frac{K \times W^{2/3}}{10^4}$$

Given that
BSA = body surface area
M^2 = sq meters
W = weight in g
K = 10.1 (dogs), 10.0 (cats)

Reproduced with permission from Kirk et al. *Current Veterinary Therapy IX. Small Animal Practice.* W.B. Saunders, Philadelphia.

22 Important venomous snakes

Family	Type of fangs	Common names	Type of venom	Distribution	Remarks
Colubridae	Rear, immovable, grooved	Colubrids	Mostly mild	Warm parts of both hemispheres	Over 1000 species, the few poisonous ones not dangerous
		Boomslang	Hemorrhagin	South Africa	Arboreal, timid
Elapidae	Front, immovable, grooved	Elapids	Predominantly neurotoxin	Mostly in Old World	Over 150 species, very poisonous
		Cobras	Mostly neurotoxin	Africa, India, Asia, Philippines, Celebes	Spitting cobra in Africa aims at eyes
		Kraits	Strong neurotoxin	India, Southeast Asia, Indonesia	Sluggish, often buried in dust
		Mambas	Neurotoxin	Tropical West Africa	Arboreal
		Blacksnake	Neurotoxin	Australia	Large snake, wet terrain
		Copperhead	Neurotoxin	Australia, Tasmania, Solomons	Damp environment
		Brown snake	Neurotoxin	Australia, New Guinea	Slender
		Tiger snake	Strong neurotoxin	Australia	Dry environment, aggressive, very dangerous
		Death adder	Neurotoxin	Australia, New Guinea	Sandy terrain
		Coral snakes	Neurotoxin	United States, tropical America	About 26 species, 2 in southern United States
Hydrophiidae	Front, immovable, hollow	Sea snakes	Some mild, others very toxic	Tropical, Indian and Pacific Oceans	Rudder-like tail, gentle, over 50 species

Viperidae	Front, movable, hollow	True vipers; viperines; viperids	Predominantly hemotoxin	Entirely in Old World	About 50 species
		European viper	Hemotoxin	Europe (rare), North Africa, Near East	Dry rocky country
		Russell's viper	Hemotoxin	Southeast Asia, Java, Sumatra	Mostly open terrain, deadly
		Sand vipers	Hemotoxin	Northern Sahara	Buried in sand
		Puff adder	Hemotoxin	Arabia, Africa	Open terrain, sluggish
		Gaboon viper	Neurotoxin and hemotoxin	Tropical West Africa	Forests, deadly
		Rhinoceros viper	Hemotoxin	Tropical Africa	Wet forests
Crotalidae	Front, movable, hollow	Pit vipers; crotalids; crotalines	Predominantly hemotoxin	Old and New Worlds; none in Africa	Over 80 species, pit between eye and nostril
		Habu viper	Neurotoxin	Warmer parts of East Asia, Ryukyu Islands	Caves and dry rocky country
		Rattlesnakes	Predominantly hemotoxin	North, Central, and South America	South American form neurotoxic
		Bushmaster	Hemotoxin	Central and South America	Wet forests, large
		Fer-de-lance	Hemotoxin	Central America, Northern South America, few West Indies	Common on plantations
		Palm vipers	Hemotoxin	Southern Mexico, Central and South America	Arboreal, small, greenish, bites face
		Copperhead	Hemotoxin	United States	Dry stony terrain
		Water moccasin	Hemotoxin	Southeast United States to Texas	Swamps
		Asiatic pit vipers	Hemotoxin	Southeast Asia, Taiwan	Most arboreal

Reproduced with permission from *Dorland's Illustrated Medical Dictionary*. 28th Edn. W.B. Saunders, Philadelphia.

23 Aquaculture: major finfish, molluscs and crustaceans used in aquaria (A), consumption (C) and sport (S) (major species shown in bold)

Scientific name	Common name	A	C	S	Location
FINFISH					
Acipenser transmontanus	White sturgeon		•		Northern hemisphere
Amphiprion chrysopterus	Anemone (clown) fish	•			Worldwide
Anguilla australis	Shortfin eel		•		Australia
Anguilla renhartii	Longfin eel		•		Australia
Anguilla anguilla	European eel		•		Europe
Anguilla japonica	Japanese eel		•		Asia
Artromotus ocellatus	Oscar	•			Worldwide
Barbus conchonius	Cherry barb	•			Worldwide
Betta splendens	Siamese fighting fish	•			Worldwide
Bidyanus bidyanus	Silver perch		•	•	Australia
Botia macracanthus	Clown perch	•			Worldwide
Brachydania rerio	Zebra danio	•			Worldwide
Carassius auratus	Goldfish				
	Crucian carp	•			Worldwide
Catla catla	Indian major carp		•		India/Pakistan
Channa striatus	Striped snakehead		•		Asia
Channa punctatus	Snakehead		•		Asia
Channos channos	Milk fish		•		Asia
Cirrhinus mrigala	Indian carp		•		India/Pakistan
Clarias batrachus	Walking catfish		•		Asia
Clarias macrocephalus	Asian catfish		•		Asia
Coregonus peled	Whitefish		•	•	Europe
Coregonus mukrun	Whitefish		•	•	Europe
Coryphaena hippurus	Mahi mahi, Dolphin fish		•		Pacific
Ctenopharyngodon idella	Grass carp		•		Northern hemisphere
Cyprinus carpio	European carp, Koi carp	•	•	•	Worldwide
Epinephelus akaara	Redspotted grouper		•		Asia
Epinephelus moara	Kelp grouper		•		Asia
Epinephelus septemfasciatus	Sevenband grouper		•		Asia
Epinephelus malabaricus	Brownspotted grouper		•		Asia
Epinephelus taurina	Greasy grouper		•		Asia
Etroplus maculatus	Chromide cichlid	•			Worldwide
Hyphessobrycon innesi	Neon tetra	•			Worldwide
Hippoglossus hippoglossus	Halibut		•		Europe
Hypophthalicthys molitrix	Bighead carp		•		Northern hemisphere
Hypophthalnicthys rabilis	Silver carp		•		Northern hemisphere
Ictalurus punctatus	Channel catfish		•		USA
Ictalurus furcatus	Blue catfish		•		USA
Lates calcarifer	Barramundi		•	•	Australia, South East Asia
Micropterus salmoides	Large-mouthed bass		•	•	USA
Micropterus dolomieui	Small-mouthed bass		•	•	USA
Morone saxatilis	Striped bass		•	•	USA
Morone chrysops	White bass		•	•	USA
Mugil cephalus	Striped mullet		•		Worldwide
Oncorhynchus mykiss	Rainbow trout		•	•	Worldwide temperate
Oncorhynchus tschawytscha	Chinook salmon		•	•	Worldwide temperate
Oncorhynchus rhodurus	Amago		•		Japan
Oncorhynchus kisutch	Coho salmon		•		USA, Japan, Chile
Oncorhynchus masou	Masu salmon		•		Japan
Oncorhynchus nerka	Sockeye salmon			•	USA

23 Aquaculture *(Continued)*

Scientific name	Common name	A	C	S	Location
Oncorhynchus gorbuscha	Pink salmon		●	●	USA
Oncorhynchus keta	Chum salmon		●	●	USA
Oplegnathus fasciatus	Japanese parrotfish		●		Japan
Oplegnathus punctatus	Rock porgy		●		Japan
Oryzias latipes	Medaka	●			Worldwide
Pagrus auratus	Snapper, red sea bream		●		Indo-pacific
Paralichythys olivaceus	Japanese flounder		●		Japan
Pelvichachromis taeneatus	Dwarf cichlid	●			Worldwide
Plecoglossus altivelis	Ayu		●		Japan
Poecilia reticulata	Guppy	●			Worldwide
Poecilia sphenops	Black molly	●			Worldwide
Pseudocaranx dentex	Silver trevally, striped jack		●		Pacific
Puntus goniocarpus	Java carp		●		South East Asia
Pterophyllum scalare	Anglefish	●			Worldwide
Salmo salar	Atlantic salmon		●	●	Worldwide temperate
Salmo trutta	Brown trout		●	●	Worldwide temperate
Salvelinus fontinalis	Brook trout			●	Worldwide temperate
Salvelinus namaykush	Lake trout			●	USA, Canada
Salvelinus alpinus	Arctic char		●	●	Northern hemisphere
Salvelinus fontinalis X Salvelinus namaycush	Splake			●	USA, Canada
Scophthalmus maximus	Turbot		●		Europe
Seriola quinqueradiata	Japanese yellowtail		●		Japan
Seriola dumerili	Purplish amberjack		●		Japan
Sparus aurata	Sea bream		●		Europe
Symphysodon discus	Discus	●			Worldwide
Takifugu rubrifes	Tiger puffer		●		Japan
Thunnus thynnus	Northern bluefin tuna		●		Japan
Thunnus albacares	Yellowfin tuna		●		Pacific
Thunnus maccoyii	Southern bluefin tuna		●		Australia
Tilapia mossambica	Tilapia		●		Worldwide
Tilapia niloticus	Nile tilapia		●	●	Worldwide
Trichogaster pectoralis	Snake skin gourami		●		Asia
Trichogaster trichopterus	Three-spot gourami	●			Asia
Xiphophorus maculatus	Platyfish	●			Worldwide
Xiphophorus helleri	Swordtail	●			Worldwide
MOLLUSCS (for consumption)					
Argopecten irradians	Bay scallop				Northern hemisphere
Crassostrea angulata	Portuguese oyster (may be identical with Pacific oyster)				Portugal, Spain, France
Crassostrea gigas	Pacific oyster				Worldwide
Crassostrea virginica	Eastern (American) oyster				USA
Haliotus rubra	Blacklip abalone				Australia
Haliotus laevigata	Greenlip abalone				Australia
Haliotus rufescens	Red abalone				USA
Mercenaria mercenaria	Hard clam				USA
Mytilus edulis	Blue mussel				Worldwide
Ostrea angasi	Flat oyster				Australia
Ostrea edulis	Edible (European) oyster				Europe
Panope abrupta	Geoduck				USA
Patinopectin yessoensis	Japanese scallop				Northern hemisphere
Pecten fumatus	Scallop				Australia
Perna canaliculus	Green mussel				New Zealand
Pinctada maxima	Pearl oyster				Pacific and Indian oceans
Saccostrea commercialis	Sydney rock oyster				Australia
Siliqua patula	Pacific razor clam				USA
Tapes philippinarum	Manila clam				Northern hemisphere
Tridacna gigas	Giant clam				Indo-pacific

23 **Aquaculture** *(Continued)*

Scientific name	Common name	Location
CRUSTACEANS (for consumption)		
Astacus astacus	European crayfish	Europe
Cherax tenuimanus	Marron	Australia
Cherax quadricarinatus	Redclaw	Australia, USA
Cherax destructor	Yabby	Australia
Homarus americans	American lobster	USA
Homarus gammarus	European lobster	Europe
Jasus edwardsii	Southern rock lobster	Australia
Macrobrachium rosenbergii	Giant freshwater prawn	Asia, Australia
Nephrops norvegicus	Norwegian lobster	Scandinavia
Pacifastacus leniusculus	American crayfish	USA, Europe
Panulirus cygnus	Western rock lobster	Australia
Penaeus monodon	Giant tiger prawn	Pacific
Penaeus japonicus	Kuruma prawn	Pacific
Penaeus esculentus	Brown tiger prawn	Australia
Penaeus vannamei	Pacific white prawn	Americas
Penaeus stylirostris	Blue prawn	Americas
Penaeus semisulcatus	Green tiger prawn	Indo-pacific
Penaeus merguiensis	Banana prawn	Indo-pacific
Penaeus chinesis	White prawn	Northern Asia
Procambarus clarkii	Red swamp crawfish	USA

Table prepared by B. Munday, University of Tasmania.